Williams
GYNECOLOGY

Williams GYNECOLOGY

THIRD EDITION

Barbara L. Hoffman, MD
John O. Schorge, MD
Karen D. Bradshaw, MD
Lisa M. Halvorson, MD
Joseph I. Schaffer, MD
Marlene M. Corton, MD

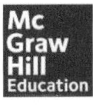
McGraw Hill Education

New York   Chicago   San Francisco   Lisbon   London   Madrid   Mexico City
Milan   New Delhi   San Juan   Seoul   Singapore   Sydney   Toronto

Williams Gynecology, Third Edition

Copyright 2016, 2012, 2008 by McGraw-Hill Education. All rights reserved. Printed in the United States of America. Except as permitted under the United States copyright Act of 1976, no part of this publication may be reproduced or distributed in any form or by any means, or stored in a data base or retrieval system, without the prior written permission of the publisher.

1 2 3 4 5 6 7 8 9 0   DOW/DOW   20 19 18 17 16

ISBN 978-0-07-184908-1
MHID 0-07-184908-4

This book was set in Adobe Garamond by Aptara, Inc.
The editors were Andrew Moyer and Regina Y. Brown.
The production supervisor was Richard Ruzycka.
Project management was provided by Indu Jawwad, Aptara, Inc.
The designer was Alan Barnett.
The cover designer was Dreamit, Inc.
The illustration manager was Armen Ovsepyan.
RR Donnelley was printer and binder.

Library of Congress Cataloging-in-Publication Data

Williams gynecology / [edited by] Barbara L. Hoffman [and 5 others]. – Third edition.
      p. ; cm.
  Gynecology
  Includes bibliographical references and index.
  ISBN 978-0-07-184908-1 (hardcover : alk. paper) –
  ISBN 0-07-184908-4 (hardcover : alk. paper)
  I. Hoffman, Barbara L., editor.   II. Title: Gynecology.
  [DNLM: 1. Genital Diseases, Female.   2. Gynecologic Surgical Procedures. 3. Gynecology. WP 140]
  RG101
  618.1—dc23   2015035428

McGraw-Hill books are available at special quantity discounts to use as premiums and sales promotions, or for use in corporate training programs. To contact a representative please e-mail us at bulksales@mcgraw-hill.com.

DEDICATION

This edition of *Williams Gynecology* is dedicated to David L. Hemsell, MD, who served as Director of the Division of Gynecology at the University of Texas Southwestern Medical Center and Parkland Memorial Hospital for more than 20 years. During this tenure, his national awards have included a Meritorious Achievement award from the Infectious Diseases Society of America and an Outstanding Service award from the American College of Obstetricians and Gynecologists.

Early in his training, Dr. Hemsell joined the Air Force and served our country as a Flight Medical Officer. In these years, he pursued specialty training in reproductive endocrinology with Dr. Paul MacDonald. He joined our faculty as the Division Director of Gynecology in 1977. In addition to his Director role, Dr. Hemsell was the Chief of Gynecology at Parkland Memorial Hospital and Medical Director of the Parkland Obstetrics and Gynecology Emergency Room. In these roles, Dr. Hemsell created an environment in which evidence-based medicine was the standard for care. Accordingly, patients, residents, and junior faculty all benefitted from this scientific health care approach. He also served as Director of the Faculty Sexual Assault Examination and Testimony Program. In that role, he coordinated the examinations of many thousands of sexual assault victims and the collection of legal evidence. As a result of his efforts, Dallas County has a system regarded as among the best in medical and legal care for these victims.

During his academic career, Dr. Hemsell added foundational knowledge regarding the etiology, pathogenesis, and treatment of female pelvic infections, especially those following gynecologic surgeries. With this expertise, he served as journal reviewer for multiple journals. He has added to academic knowledge through his nearly 50 book chapters and 100 peer-reviewed articles on multiple gynecologic topics.

For us in the Department of Obstetrics and Gynecology, Dr. Hemsell plays an important role of mentor and colleague. His experience and clinical expertise are invaluable and provide a valuable sounding board for challenging gynecology cases. On so many levels, we have benefitted greatly from his academic and clinical contributions.

CONTENTS

SECTION 1

BENIGN GENERAL GYNECOLOGY

SECTION 2

REPRODUCTIVE ENDOCRINOLOGY, INFERTILITY, AND THE MENOPAUSE

SECTION 3

FEMALE PELVIC MEDICINE AND RECONSTRUCTIVE SURGERY

SECTION 4

GYNECOLOGIC ONCOLOGY

SECTION 5

ASPECTS OF GYNECOLOGIC SURGERY

SECTION 6

ATLAS OF GYNECOLOGIC SURGERY

EDITORS

Barbara L. Hoffman, MD
Associate Professor, Department of Obstetrics and Gynecology
University of Texas Southwestern Medical Center at Dallas

John O. Schorge, MD, FACOG, FACS
Chief of Gynecology and Gynecologic Oncology
Associate Professor, Department of Obstetrics and Gynecology
Massachusetts General Hospital–Harvard Medical School

Karen D. Bradshaw, MD
Holder, Helen J. and Robert S. Strauss and Diana K.
   and Richard C. Strauss Chair in Women's Health
Director, Lowe Foundation Center for Women's Preventative
   Health Care
Professor, Department of Obstetrics and Gynecology
Professor, Department of Surgery
University of Texas Southwestern Medical Center at Dallas

Lisa M. Halvorson, MD
Bethesda, Maryland

Joseph I. Schaffer, MD
Holder, Frank C. Erwin, Jr. Professorship in Obstetrics and
   Gynecology
Director, Division of Gynecology
Director, Division of Female Pelvic Medicine
   and Reconstructive Surgery
Professor, Department of Obstetrics and Gynecology
University of Texas Southwestern Medical Center at Dallas
Chief of Gynecology, Parkland Memorial Hospital, Dallas

Marlene M. Corton, MD, MSCS
Director, Anatomical Education and Research
Professor, Department of Obstetrics and Gynecology
University of Texas Southwestern Medical Center at Dallas

Atlas Art Director

Lewis E. Calver, MS, CMI, FAMI
Associate Professor, Department of Obstetrics and Gynecology
University of Texas Southwestern Medical Center at Dallas

CONTRIBUTORS

April A. Bailey, MD
Assistant Professor, Department of Radiology
Assistant Professor, Department of Obstetrics and Gynecology
University of Texas Southwestern Medical Center at Dallas
Chapter 2: Techniques Used for Imaging in Gynecology
Co-Director of Radiologic Images for Williams Gynecology

Sunil Balgobin, MD
Assistant Professor, Department of Obstetrics and Gynecology
University of Texas Southwestern Medical Center at Dallas
Chapter 40: Intraoperative Considerations

Karen D. Bradshaw, MD
Holder, Helen J. and Robert S. Strauss and Diana K. and Richard C. Strauss Chair in Women's Health
Director, Lowe Foundation Center for Women's Preventative Health Care
Professor, Department of Obstetrics and Gynecology
Professor, Department of Surgery
University of Texas Southwestern Medical Center at Dallas
Chapter 13: Psychosocial Issues and Female Sexuality
Chapter 18: Anatomic Disorders
Chapter 21: Menopausal Transition
Chapter 22: The Mature Woman

Anna R. Brandon, PhD, MCS, ABPP
Women's Mood Disorders Center
Department of Psychiatry
University of North Carolina at Chapel Hill School of Medicine
Department of Psychiatry
University of Texas Southwestern Medical Center at Dallas
Chapter 13: Psychosocial Issues and Female Sexuality

Matthew J. Carlson, MD
Assistant Professor, Department of Obstetrics and Gynecology
University of Texas Southwestern Medical Center at Dallas
Chapter 34: Uterine Sarcoma

Kelley S. Carrick, MD
Professor, Department of Pathology
University of Texas Southwestern Medical Center at Dallas
Director of Surgical Pathology Images for Williams Gynecology

Marlene M. Corton, MD, MSCS
Director, Anatomical Education and Research
Professor, Department of Obstetrics and Gynecology
University of Texas Southwestern Medical Center at Dallas
Chapter 25: Anal Incontinence and Functional Anorectal Disorders
Chapter 38: Anatomy
Chapter 43: Surgeries for Benign Gynecologic Disorders
Chapter 45: Surgeries for Pelvic Floor Disorders

Kevin J. Doody, MD
Director, Center for Assisted Reproduction, Bedford, TX
Clinical Professor, Department of Obstetrics and Gynecology
University of Texas Southwestern Medical Center at Dallas
Chapter 20: Treatment of the Infertile Couple

David M. Euhus, MD
Professor, Department of Surgery
Johns Hopkins Hospital/University
Chapter 12: Breast Disease

Rajiv B. Gala, MD, FACOG
Vice-Chair, Department of Obstetrics and Gynecology
Residency Program Director, Department of Obstetrics and Gynecology
Ochsner Clinic Foundation
Associate Professor of Obstetrics and Gynecology
University of Queensland
Ochsner Clinical School
Chapter 7: Ectopic Pregnancy
Chapter 39: Preoperative Considerations
Chapter 42: Postoperative Considerations

William F. Griffith, MD
Medical Director, OB/GYN Emergency Services
Director, Vulvology Clinic
Co-Director, Dysplasia Services
Parkland Health and Hospital System, Dallas, Texas
Associate Professor, Department of Obstetrics and Gynecology
University of Texas Southwestern Medical Center at Dallas
Chapter 4: Benign Disorders of the Lower Genital Tract
Chapter 29: Preinvasive Lesions of the Lower Genital Tract

Lisa M. Halvorson, MD
Bethesda, Maryland
Chapter 6: First-Trimester Abortion
Chapter 15: Reproductive Endocrinology
Chapter 16: Amenorrhea
Chapter 19: Evaluation of the Infertile Couple

Cherine A. Hamid, MD
Medical Director—Gynecology
Parkland Health and Hospital Systems, Dallas, Texas
Associate Professor, Department of Obstetrics and Gynecology
University of Texas Southwestern Medical Center at Dallas
Chapter 40: Intraoperative Considerations

Barbara L. Hoffman, MD
Associate Professor, Department of Obstetrics and Gynecology
University of Texas Southwestern Medical Center at Dallas
Chapter 1: Well Woman Care
Chapter 8: Abnormal Uterine Bleeding
Chapter 9: Pelvic Mass
Chapter 10: Endometriosis
Chapter 11: Pelvic Pain
Chapter 40: Intraoperative Considerations
Chapter 43: Surgeries for Benign Gynecologic Disorders
Chapter 45: Surgeries for Pelvic Floor Disorders

Siobhan M. Kehoe, MD
Assistant Professor, Department of Obstetrics and Gynecology
University of Texas Southwestern Medical Center at Dallas
Chapter 33: Endometrial Cancer

Kimberly A. Kho, MD, MPH, MSCS, FACOG
Assistant Professor, Department of Obstetrics and Gynecology
Director of Gynecology, Southwestern Center for Minimally Invasive Surgery
University of Texas Southwestern Medical Center at Dallas
Chapter 41: Minimally Invasive Surgery Fundamentals
Chapter 44: Minimally Invasive Surgery

Jayanthi S. Lea, MD
Patricia Duniven Fletcher Distinguished Professor in Gynecologic Oncology
Director, Gynecologic Oncology Fellowship Program
Associate Professor, Department of Obstetrics and Gynecology
University of Texas Southwestern Medical Center at Dallas
Chapter 31: Vulvar Cancer
Chapter 46: Surgeries for Gynecologic Malignancies

Eddie H. McCord, MD
Associate Professor, Department of Obstetrics and Gynecology
University of Texas Southwestern Medical Center at Dallas
Chapter 3: Gynecologic Infection

David Scott Miller, MD, FACOG, FACS
Holder, Dallas Foundation Chair in Gynecologic Oncology
Medical Director of Gynecology Oncology
Parkland Health and Hospital System, Dallas, Texas
Director, Gynecologic Oncology Fellowship Program
Director of Gynecologic Oncology
Professor, Department of Obstetrics and Gynecology
University of Texas Southwestern Medical Center at Dallas
Chapter 33: Endometrial Cancer
Chapter 34: Uterine Sarcoma

Elysia Moschos, MD
Professor, Department of Obstetrics and Gynecology
University of Texas Southwestern Medical Center at Dallas
Administrative Director of Gynecologic Ultrasound
Parkland Health and Hospital System
Chapter 2: Techniques Used for Imaging in Gynecology
Co-Director of Radiologic Images for Williams Gynecology

David M. Owens, MD
Assistant Professor, Department of Obstetrics and Gynecology
University of Texas Southwestern Medical Center at Dallas
Chapter 11: Pelvic Pain

Mary Jane Pearson, MD
Director, Third-year & Fourth-Year Medical Student Programs
Professor, Department of Obstetrics and Gynecology
University of Texas Southwestern Medical Center at Dallas
Chapter 1: Well Woman Care

David D. Rahn, MD
Associate Professor, Department of Obstetrics and Gynecology
University of Texas Southwestern Medical Center at Dallas
Chapter 3: Gynecologic Infection
Chapter 23: Urinary Incontinence

Debra L. Richardson, MD, FACOG
Assistant Professor, Department of Obstetrics and Gynecology
University of Texas Southwestern Medical Center at Dallas
Chapter 30: Cervical Cancer
Chapter 32: Vaginal Cancer

David E. Rogers, MD, MBA
Associate Professor, Department of Obstetrics and Gynecology
University of Texas Southwestern Medical Center at Dallas
Chapter 11: Pelvic Pain

Anthony H. Russell
Associate Professor
Department of Radiation Oncology
Massachusetts General Hospital—Harvard Medical School
Chapter 28: Principles of Radiation Therapy

Andrea L. Russo, MD
Assistant Professor
Department of Radiation Oncology
Massachusetts General Hospital—Harvard Medical School
Chapter 28: Principles of Radiation Therapy

John O. Schorge, MD, FACOG, FACS
Chief of Gynecology and Gynecologic Oncology
Associate Professor, Department of Obstetrics and Gynecology
Massachusetts General Hospital—Harvard Medical School
Chapter 27: Principles of Chemotherapy
Chapter 33: Endometrial Cancer
Chapter 34: Uterine Sarcoma
Chapter 35: Epithelial Ovarian Cancer
Chapter 36: Ovarian Germ Cell and Sex Cord-Stromal Tumors
Chapter 37: Gestational Trophoblastic Disease
Chapter 46: Surgeries for Gynecologic Malignancies

Joseph I. Schaffer, MD
Holder, Frank C. Erwin, Jr. Professorship in Obstetrics and Gynecology
Chief of Gynecology
Parkland Health and Hospital System, Dallas, Texas
Director, Division of Gynecology
Director, Division of Female Pelvic Medicine and Reconstructive Surgery
Professor, Department of Obstetrics and Gynecology
University of Texas Southwestern Medical Center at Dallas
Chapter 24: Pelvic Organ Prolapse
Chapter 45: Surgeries for Pelvic Floor Disorders

Geetha Shivakumar, MD, MS
Mental Health Trauma Services, Dallas VA Medical Center
Assistant Professor, Department of Psychiatry
University of Texas Southwestern Medical Center at Dallas
Chapter 13: Psychosocial Issues and Female Sexuality

Gretchen S. Stuart, MD, MPHTM
Director, Family Planning Program
Director, Fellowship in Family Planning
Assistant Professor, Department of Obstetrics and Gynecology
University of North Carolina at Chapel Hill
Chapter 5: Contraception and Sterilization

Mayra J. Thompson, MD, FACOG
Professor, Department of Obstetrics and Gynecology
University of Texas Southwestern Medical Center at Dallas
Chapter 41: Minimally Invasive Surgery Fundamentals
Chapter 44: Minimally Invasive Surgery

Clifford Y. Wai, MD
Director, Fellowship Program in Female Pelvic Medicine and
    Reconstructive Surgery
Associate Professor, Department of Obstetrics and Gynecology
University of Texas Southwestern Medical Center at Dallas
Chapter 23: Urinary Incontinence
Chapter 26: Genitourinary Fistula and Urethral Diverticulum

Claudia L. Werner, MD
Medical Director of Dysplasia Services
Co-Director Vulvology Clinic
Parkland Health and Hospital System, Dallas, Texas
Professor, Department of Obstetrics and Gynecology
University of Texas Southwestern Medical Center at Dallas
Chapter 4: Benign Disorders of the Lower Genital Tract
Chapter 29: Preinvasive Lesions of the Lower Genital Tract

Ellen E. Wilson, MD
Director of Pediatric and Adolescent Gynecology Program
Children's Medical Center, Dallas, Texas
Associate Professor, Department of Obstetrics and Gynecology
University of Texas Southwestern Medical Center at Dallas
Chapter 14: Pediatric Gynecology
Chapter 17: Polycystic Ovarian Syndrome and Hyperandrogenism

ARTISTS

Atlas Art Director

Lewis E. Calver, MS, CMI, FAMI
Associate Professor, Department of Obstetrics and Gynecology
University of Texas Southwestern Medical Center at Dallas

Contributing Atlas Artists

Katherine Brown
Graduate, Biomedical Communications Graduate Program
University of Texas Southwestern Medical Center at Dallas

SangEun Cha
Graduate, Biomedical Communications Graduate Program
University of Texas Southwestern Medical Center at Dallas

T. J. Fels
Graduate, Biomedical Communications Graduate Program
University of Texas Southwestern Medical Center at Dallas

Erin Frederikson
Graduate, Biomedical Communications Graduate Program
University of Texas Southwestern Medical Center at Dallas

Alexandra Gordon
Graduate, Biomedical Communications Graduate Program
University of Texas Southwestern Medical Center at Dallas

Kimberly Hoggatt Krumwiede, MA, CMI
Associate Professor, Health Care Sciences—Education and Research
University of Texas Southwestern Medical Center at Dallas

Richard P. Howdy, Jr.
Former Instructor, Biomedical Communications Graduate Program
University of Texas Southwestern Medical Center at Dallas

Belinda Klein
Graduate, Biomedical Communications Graduate Program
University of Texas Southwestern Medical Center at Dallas

Anne Matuskowitz
Graduate, Biomedical Communications Graduate Program
University of Texas Southwestern Medical Center at Dallas

Lindsay Oksenberg
Graduate, Biomedical Communications Graduate Program
University of Texas Southwestern Medical Center at Dallas

Jordan Pietz
Graduate, Biomedical Communications Graduate Program
University of Texas Southwestern Medical Center at Dallas

Marie Sena
Graduate, Biomedical Communications Graduate Program
University of Texas Southwestern Medical Center at Dallas

Maya Shoemaker
Graduate, Biomedical Communications Graduate Program
University of Texas Southwestern Medical Center at Dallas

Jennie Swensen
Graduate, Biomedical Communications Graduate Program
University of Texas Southwestern Medical Center at Dallas

Amanda Tomasikiewicz
Graduate, Biomedical Communications Graduate Program
University of Texas Southwestern Medical Center at Dallas

Kimberly VanExel
Graduate, Biomedical Communications Graduate Program
University of Texas Southwestern Medical Center at Dallas

Kristin Yang
Graduate, Biomedical Communications Graduate Program
University of Texas Southwestern Medical Center at Dallas

PREFACE

The first edition of *Williams Obstetrics* was published over a century ago. Since then, the editors of this seminal text have presented a comprehensive and evidenced-based discussion of obstetrics. Patterned after our patriarch, *Williams Gynecology* provides a thorough presentation of gynecology's depth and breadth. In Section 1, general gynecology topics are covered. Sections 2 provides chapters covering reproductive endocrinology and infertility. The developing field of female pelvic medicine and reconstructive surgery is presented in Section 3. In Section 4, gynecologic oncology is discussed.

Traditionally, gynecologic information has been offered within the format of either a didactic text or a surgical atlas. However, because the day-to-day activities of a gynecologist blends these two, so too did we. The initial four sections of our book describe the evaluation and medical treatment of gynecologic problems. The remaining two sections focus on the surgical patient. Section 5 offers detailed anatomy and a discussion of perioperative considerations. Our final section presents an illustrated atlas for the surgical correction of conditions described in Sections 1 through 4. To interconnect this content, readers will find page references within one chapter that will direct them to complementary content in another.

Although discussions of disease evaluation and treatment are evidence based, our text strives to assist the practicing gynecologist and resident. Accordingly, chapters are extensively complemented by illustrations, photographs, diagnostic algorithms, and treatment tables.

ACKNOWLEDGMENTS

During the creation and production of our textbook, we were lucky to have the assistance and support of countless talented professionals both within and outside our department.

First, a task of this size could not be completed without the unwavering support provided by our Department Chairman, Dr. Steven Bloom, and Vice-Chairman, Dr. Barry Schwarz. Their financial and academic endorsement of our efforts has been essential. Without their academic vision, this undertaking could not have flourished.

In constructing a compilation of this breadth, the expertise of physicians from several departments was needed to add vital, contemporaneous information. We were fortunate to have Dr. April Bailey, with joint appointments in the Department of Radiology and Department of Obstetrics and Gynecology, add her insight and knowledge as a specialist in radiology. Her many stunning images contribute to the academic richness of this edition. From the Department of Pathology, Dr. Kelley Carrick also shared generously from her cadre of outstanding images. She translated her extensive knowledge of gynecologic pathology into concepts relevant for the general gynecologist. From the Department of Surgery at Johns Hopkins University, Dr. David Euhus lent his considerable knowledge of breast disease to contribute both classic and state-of-the-art information to his truly comprehensive chapter, founded on his broad research and clinical expertise. From the Department of Psychiatry here at the University of Texas Southwestern Medical Center at Dallas and from the University of North Carolina at Chapel Hill School of Medicine, we were lucky to have Drs. Geetha Shivakumar and Anna Brandon provide an extensive discussion of psychosocial issues. They expertly distilled a broad topic into a logically organized, practical, and complete presentation. In addition, Dr. Gretchen Stuart, formerly of our department and now a faculty member at the Department of Obstetrics and Gynecology of the University of North Carolina at Chapel Hill, lent her considerable talents in summarizing contraceptive methods and sterilization techniques. Many warm thanks are extended to Dr. Rajiv Gala, also formerly of our department and now of the Ochsner Clinic. Rajiv masterfully organized and summarized chapters on ectopic pregnancy and perioperative practice. His extensive review of the literature and evidence-based writing shines through these chapters. In this edition, new contributors include Drs. Anthony Russell and Andrea Russo from the Department of Radiation Oncology at Massachusetts General Hospital—Harvard Medical School. In their chapter on radiation therapy, they adeptly provided clear explanations of this therapy's fundamentals and offered extensive suggestions for clinical management of patient complications that may be encountered.

Within our own department, the list is too long and the words are too few to convey our heartfelt thanks to all of our department members for their generous contributions. From our Gynecology Division, many thanks are extended to Drs. Elysia Moschos and April Bailey, who sculpted a clear and detailed summary of traditional and new gynecologic imaging tools. In this edition, these two authors updated radiologic images as needed to present ultimate examples of normal anatomy and gynecologic pathology. We were also lucky to have experts in the field of preinvasive lesions of the lower genital tract, Drs. Claudia Werner and William Griffith. They crafted an information-packed discussion of this topic. In addition, Dr. Griffith has been a steadfast advocate of our project and has added extensive photographic content to many of our chapters. Drs. David Rahn and Eddie McCord teamed to update the chapter on gynecologic infection. Their extensive patient-care experience and rigorous literature review added greatly to the academic and clinical value of this chapter. We were also fortunate to have the expert writing talents of Drs. Mayra Thompson and Kimberly Kho, who provided a compelling and comprehensive discussion of minimally invasive surgery. Our textbook benefitted greatly from the clinical savvy and teaching-centric information that David Rogers and David Owens provided to their chapter. Also, Dr. Rogers has been a long-time supporter of our textbook. We are indebted to him for many of the classic surgical photographs in this edition. Intraoperative fundamentals were thoroughly and logically presented by Drs. Cherine Hamid and Sunil Balgobin. Their strengths in clinical practice and resident teaching are evident in their well-organized and essential chapter. Once again, blending experience and academic fundamentals, Dr. Mary Jane Pearson offered a comprehensive but concise primer on well care for the gynecologic patient.

Our Reproductive Endocrinology and Infertility Division provided other talented physicians and writers. Dr. Kevin Doody lent his considerable clinical and academic prowess in the treatment of infertility. He penned a chapter that clearly describes the state of the art in this field. Dr. Doody was also a kind benefactor with his spectacular clinical photographs on the topic and contributed these generously to numerous chapters. In addition, Dr. Ellen Wilson brought her wealth of clinical experience to chapters on pediatric gynecology and androgen excess. Drawing from her academic and clinical expertise, she crafted chapters that presented practical, prescriptive, and comprehensive discussions of these topics.

Dr. Marlene Corton is a skilled urogynecologist and has written extensively on pelvic anatomy. We were thrilled to have her create stunning chapters on anatomy and anal incontinence. Also from the Urogynecology and Female Pelvic Reconstruction Division, Drs. Clifford Wai and David Rahn added expanded content to their chapter on urinary incontinence. Dr. Wai also masterfully updated his chapter on vesicovaginal fistula and urethral diverticulum. Special thanks are extended to Dr. Ann Word and her contributions to our chapter on pelvic organ prolapse. Her expertise in extracellular matrix remodeling of the female reproductive tract added fundamental content to the discussion of prolapse physiology.

Dr. David Miller generously contributed his talents without hesitation, and we are indebted to him for his altruism toward our project. In addition, the Division of Gynecologic Oncology offered a deep bench of talented writers. The topic of vulvar cancer was thoroughly covered by Dr. Jayanthi Lea. Dr. Lea also assisted with updating our atlas and added essential steps for minimally invasive approaches. Her strengths in clinical practice and resident teaching are evident in her well-organized and evidence-based chapters. We also benefitted from Dr. Debra Richardson's comprehensive presentation and clinical discussions of cervical and vaginal cancer in her two chapters. She has been a true advocate of both the text and study guide. Dr. Siobhan Kehoe described with clarity and clinical relevance the care and treatment of women with endometrial cancer. We were appreciative of Dr. Matthew Carlson, who teamed with David Miller to present the varied pathology and treatment of uterine sarcoma.

With this edition, several of our valued authors have turned their efforts to other promising pursuits. We are grateful to Drs. F. Gary Cunningham, Bruce Carr, David Hemsell, Larry Word, and Phuc Nguyen for their prior contributions to *Williams Gynecology*. All with well-known and well-established careers, they generously contributed their academic skills without hesitation. We are indebted to them for their altruism toward our project.

Of these academicians, Dr. F. Gary Cunningham provided the academic vision that led to the creation of this text. Dr. Cunningham has been the senior author for seven editions of Williams Obstetrics, spanning over 25 years. As such, we benefited greatly from his writing genius, his meticulous organization, and his tenacity to task. His dedication to evidence-based medicine established the foundation on which our textbook was built. We feel privileged to have learned the craft of clear, concise academic summary from a consummate master.

New beautiful and detailed artwork in our atlas this edition was drawn by Mr. Lewis Calver, here at the University of Texas Southwestern Medical Center at Dallas. Again for this edition, he paired his academic talents with Dr. Marlene Corton to create updated hysterectomy and urogynecologic images. Both of these anatomists committed countless hours in the cadaver laboratory and in the library to create academically new presentations. These renderings were crafted and tailored with the gynecologic surgeon in mind to depict important techniques and anatomy for these surgeries. Dr. Jayanthi Lea joined this gifted duo to add complementary and informative illustrations to her description of minimally invasive cancer surgeries.

We also acknowledge the efforts of our atlas artists from the first two editions: Marie Sena, Erin Frederikson, Jordan Pietz, Maya Shoemaker, SangEun Cha, Alexandra Gordon, Jennie Swensen, Amanda Tomasikiewicz, and Kristin Yang. Additionally, alumni from the Biomedical Communications Program at the University of Texas Southwestern Medical Center provided seminal pieces. These alumni include Katherine Brown, Thomas "T. J." Fels, Belinda Klein, Anne Matuskowitz, Lindsay Oksenberg, Kimberly VanExel, and faculty member Richard P. Howdy, Jr. Also, Ms. Kimberly Hoggatt Krumwiede graciously provided several image series to help clarify the steps and missteps of reproductive tract development.

Within our text, images add powerful descriptive content to our words. Accordingly, many, many thanks are extended to those who donated surgical and clinical photographs. Of our contributors, many beautiful photographs within our book were taken by Mr. David Gresham, Chief Medical Photographer at the University of Texas Southwestern Medical Center. Dave's eye for detail, shading, and composition allowed even simple objects to shine and be illustrated to their full potential. He has been an advocate and valued consultant. Our pathology images were presented at their best thanks to Mr. Mark Smith, a graphics designer here at the University of Texas Southwestern Medical Center. His expertise with micrographs improved the clarity and visual aesthetic of many our microscopic images.

The providers in the Obstetrics and Gynecology Emergency Services (OGES) at Parkland Hospital were huge allies in our acquisition of images to illustrate normal and abnormal gynecologic findings. The skilled women's health care nurse practitioners have been true supporters of our efforts, and we sincerely thank them.

We are truly indebted to our administrative staff. For this project, we were lucky to have Ms. Sandra Davis serve as our primary administrative assistant. We are greatly appreciative of her tremendous efforts, professionalism, and efficiency. Ms. Ellen Watkins was a valuable assistant in obtaining needed journal articles. She truly helped to keep our project evidence-based. None of our image and text production would have been possible without the brilliant information technology team in our department. Knowledgeable and responsive, Mr. Charles Richards and Mr. Thomas Ames have supported our project since the first edition. We could not do our job without their expertise.

Williams Gynecology was sculpted into its final form by the talented and dedicated group at McGraw-Hill Education. Once again, Ms. Alyssa Fried has brought her considerable intelligence, energetic work ethic, and creativity to our project. Her attention to detail and organizational talents have kept our project on track with efficiency and style. Our words fall well short in expressing our gratitude to her. Ms. Samantha Williams served as assistant to Ms. Fried, and we extend warm thanks for her tremendous support. Her efficiency, professionalism, hard work, accuracy, and positive attitude made coordination of this project a dream. Mr. Andrew Moyer joined our project during its final sculpting. He has taken our project under his care and has adeptly shepherded it to completion with a calm and efficient style. We happily look forward to many future collaborative editions together.

Without the thoughtful, creative efforts of many, our textbook would be a barren wasteland of words. Integral to this process are Armen Ovsepyan, at McGraw-Hill Education, and Alan Barnett of Alan Barnett Design. Mr. Richard Ruzycka served as production supervisor for this edition of our textbook. He adeptly kept our project on track through an array of potential hurdles. Special thanks are extended to Mr. Joseph Varghese and Dr. Shetoli Zhimomi at Thomson Digital. They and their artistic team assisted us in revising many of our text images. Their attention to detail and accurate renderings added important academic support to our words.

Our text took its final shape under the watchful care of our compositors at Aptara, Inc. Specifically, we thank Ms. Indu Jawwad for her talents in skillfully and expediently coordinating and overseeing composition. Her dedicated attention to detail and organization were vital to completion of our project. Her pleasant professionalism was appreciated daily. Also at Aptara, Mr. Shashi Lal Das served a crucial task of quality control and assisted in creating beautiful chapter layouts to highlight our content aesthetically and informatively. Special thanks go to Ms. Kristin Landon. As copyeditor for now several editions of both *Williams Obstetrics* and *Williams Gynecology*, Kristin has added precision and clarity to our efforts. Her pleasant and patient professionalism has made our text better.

We offer a sincere "thank you" to our residents in training. Their curiosity keeps us energized to find new and effective ways to convey age-old as well as cutting-edge concepts. Their logical questions lead us to holes in our text, and thereby, always help us to improve our work. Moreover, many of the photographs in this textbook were gathered with the help of our many residents.

In addition, the contributors to this text owe a significant debt to the women who have allowed us to participate in their care. The images and clinical expertise presented in this text would not have been possible without their collaborative spirit to help us move medical knowledge forward.

Last, we offer an enthusiastic and heartfelt "thank you" to our families and friends. Without their patience, generosity, and encouragement, this task would have been impossible. For them, too many hours with "the book" left them with new responsibilities. And importantly, time away from home left precious family memories and laughs unrealized. We sincerely thank you for your love and support.

BENIGN GENERAL GYNECOLOGY

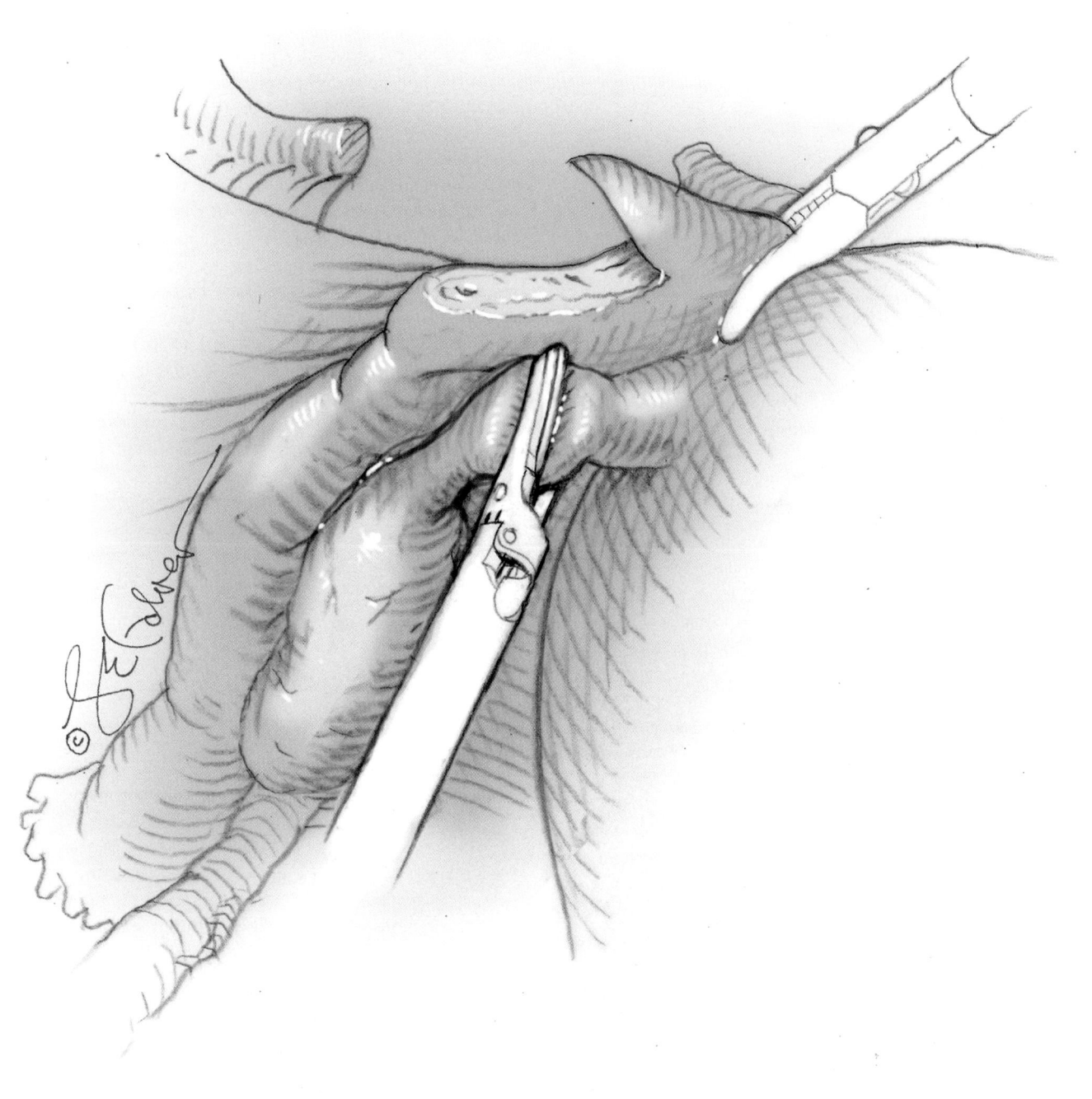

CHAPTER 1

Well Woman Care

Serving as both specialist and primary care provider, a gynecologist has an opportunity to diagnose and treat a wide variety of diseases. Once problems are identified, clinicians, in consultation with the patient, determine how best to manage chronic medical issues based on their experience, practice patterns, and professional interests. Although some conditions may require referral, gynecologists play an essential role in patient screening, in emphasizing ideal health behaviors, and in facilitating appropriate consultation for care beyond their scope of practice.

Various organizations provide preventive care recommendations and update these regularly. Commonly accessed guidelines are those from the American College of Obstetricians and Gynecologists (ACOG), Centers for Disease Control and Prevention (CDC), U.S. Preventive Services Task Force (USPSTF), and American Cancer Society.

MEDICAL HISTORY

During a comprehensive well-woman visit, patients are first queried regarding new or ongoing illness. To assist with evaluation, complete medical, social, and surgical histories are obtained and include obstetric and gynecologic events. Gynecologic topics usually cover current and prior contraceptives; results from prior sexually transmitted disease (STD) testing, cervical cancer screening, or other gynecologic tests; sexual history, described in Chapter 3 (p. 60); and menstrual history, outlined in Chapter 8 (p. 182). Obstetric questions chronicle circumstances around deliveries, losses, or complications. Current medication lists include both prescription and over-the-counter drugs and herbal agents. Also, prior surgeries, their indications, and complications are sought. A social history covers smoking and drug or alcohol abuse. Screening for intimate partner violence or depression can be completed, as outlined on page 18 and more fully in Chapter 13 (p. 298). Discussion might also assess the patient's support system and any cultural or spiritual beliefs that might affect her general health care. A family history helps identify women at risk for familial or multifactorial disease such as diabetes or heart disease. In families with prominent breast, ovarian, or colon cancer, genetic evaluation may be indicated, and criteria are outlined in Chapters 33 (p. 707) and 35 (p. 736). Moreover, a significant family clustering of thromboembolic events may warrant testing, as describe in Chapter 39 (p. 836), especially prior to surgery or hormone initiation. Last, a review of systems, whether performed by the clinician or office staff, may add clarity to new patient problems.

For adults, following historical inventory, a complete physical examination is completed. Many women present to their gynecologist with complaints specific to the breast or pelvis. Accordingly, these are often areas of increased focus, and their evaluation is described next.

PHYSICAL EXAMINATION

■ Breast Examination
Clinical Evidence

Self breast examination (SBE) is an examination performed by the patient herself to detect abnormalities. However, studies have shown that SBE increases diagnostic testing rates for ultimately benign breast disease and is ineffective in lowering breast cancer mortality rates (Kösters, 2008; Thomas, 2002). Accordingly, several organizations have removed SBE from their recommended screening practices (National Cancer Institute, 2015; Smith, 2015; U.S. Preventive Services Task Force, 2009). That said, the American College of Obstetricians and Gynecologists (2014b) and the American Cancer Society (2014) recommend breast self-awareness as another method of patient self-screening.

Self-awareness focuses on breast appearance and architecture and may include SBE. Women are encouraged to report any perceived breast changes for further evaluation.

In contrast, clinical breast examination (CBE) is completed by a clinical health-care professional and may identify a small portion of breast malignancies not detected with mammography. Additionally, CBE may identify cancer in young women, who are not typical candidates for mammography (McDonald, 2004). One method includes visual inspection combined with axillary and breast palpation, which is outlined in the following section.

The American College of Obstetricians and Gynecologists (2014b) recommends that women receive a CBE every 1 to 3 years between ages 20 and 39. At age 40, CBE is completed annually. That said, the USPSTF (2009) and the American Cancer Society report insufficient evidence to recommend routine CBE (Oeffinger, 2015).

Breast Examination

Initially during CBE, the breasts are viewed as a woman sits on the table's edge with hands placed at her hips and with pectoralis muscles flexed (Fig. 1-1). Alone, this position enhances asymmetry. Additional arm positions, such as placing arms above the head, do not add vital information. Breast skin is inspected for breast erythema; retraction; scaling, especially over the nipple; and edema, which is termed peau d'orange change. The breast and axilla are also observed for contour symmetry.

Following inspection, axillary, supraclavicular, and infraclavicular lymph nodes are palpated most easily with a woman seated and her arm supported by the examiner (Fig. 1-2). The axilla is bounded by the pectoralis major muscle ventrally and

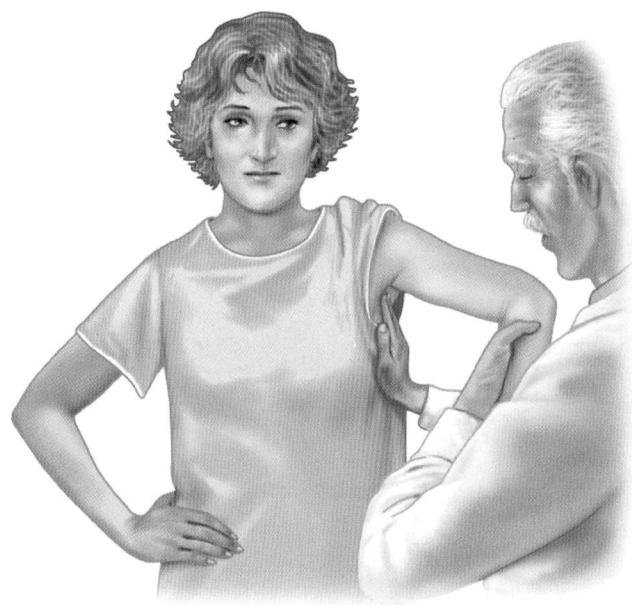

FIGURE 1-2 One method of axillary lymph node palpation. Finger tips extend to the axillary apex and compress tissue against the chest wall in the rolling fashion shown in Figure 1-4. The patient's arm is supported by the examiner.

the latissimus dorsi muscle dorsally. Lymph nodes are detected as the examiner's hand glides from high to low in the axilla and momentarily compresses nodes against the lateral chest wall. In a thin patient, one or more normal, mobile lymph nodes less than 1 cm in diameter may commonly be appreciated. The first lymph node to become involved with breast cancer metastasis (the sentinel node) is nearly always located just behind the midportion of the pectoralis major muscle belly.

After inspection, breast palpation is completed with a woman supine and with one hand above her head to stretch breast tissue across the chest wall (Fig. 1-3). Examination includes breast tissue bounded by the clavicle, sternal border, inframammary crease, and midaxillary line. Breast palpation within this pentagonal area is approached in a linear fashion. Technique uses the finger pads in a continuous rolling, gliding circular motion (Fig. 1-4). At each palpation point, tissues is assessed both superficially and deeply (Fig. 1-5). During CBE, intentional attempts at nipple discharge expression are not required unless a *spontaneous* discharge has been described by the patient.

If abnormal breast findings are noted, they are described by their location in the right or left breast, clock position, distance from the areola, and size. Evaluation and treatment of breast and nipple diseases are described more fully in Chapter 12 (p. 275).

During examination, patients are educated that new axillary or breast masses, noncyclic breast pain, spontaneous nipple discharge, new nipple inversion, and breast skin changes such as dimpling, scaling, ulceration, edema, or erythema should prompt evaluation. This constitutes breast self-awareness. Patients who desire to perform SBE are counseled on its benefits, limitations, and potential harms and instructed to complete SBE the week after menses.

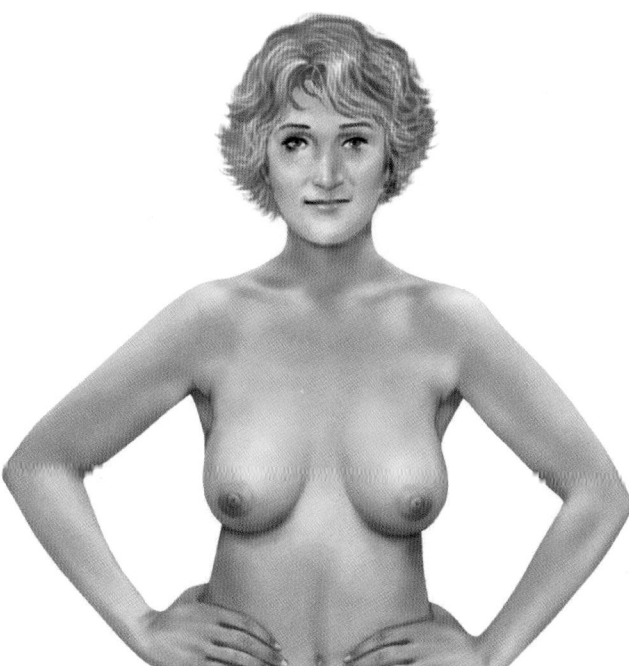

FIGURE 1-1 During visual breast inspection, hands are pressed against the waist to flex the pectoralis muscles. With the patient leaning slightly forward, breasts are visually inspected for breast contour asymmetry or skin dimpling.

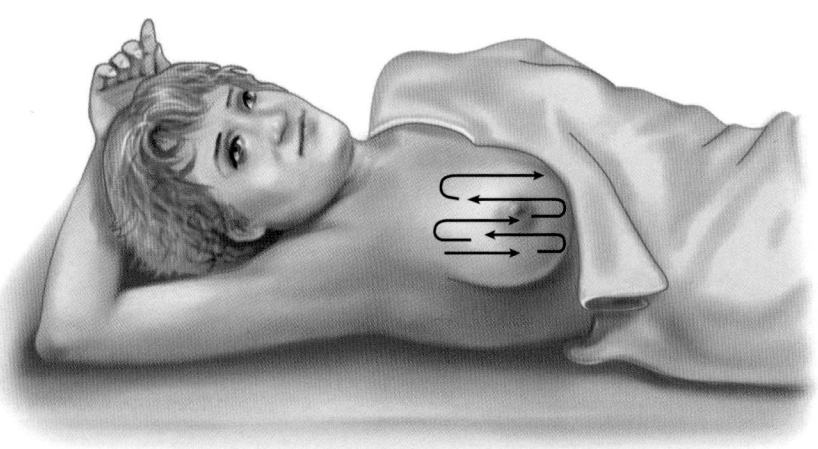

FIGURE 1-3 Recommended patient positioning and direction of palpation during clinical breast examination.

■ Pelvic Examination

This examination is typically performed with a patient supine, legs in dorsal lithotomy position, and feet resting in stirrups. The head of the bed is elevated 30 degrees to relax abdominal wall muscles for bimanual examination. A woman is assured that she may stop or pause the examination at any time. Moreover, each part of the evaluation is announced or described before its performance.

Inguinal Lymph Nodes and Perineal Inspection

Pelvic cancers and infections may drain to the inguinal lymph nodes, and these are palpated during examination. Following this, a methodical inspection of the perineum extends from the mons ventrally, to the genitocrural folds laterally, and to the anus. Notably, infections and neoplasms that involve the vulva can also involve perianal skin. Some clinicians additionally palpate for Bartholin and paraurethral gland pathology. However, in most cases, patient symptoms and asymmetry in these areas will dictate the need for this specific evaluation.

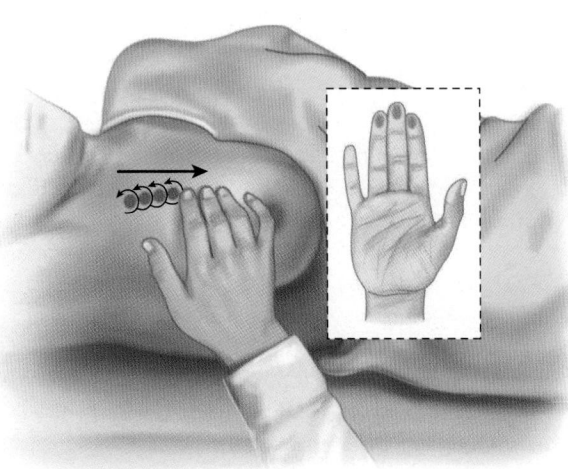

FIGURE 1-4 Recommended palpation technique. The finger pads and a circular rolling motion are used to palpate the entire breast.

Speculum Examination

Both metal and plastic specula are available for this examination, each in various sizes to accommodate vaginal length and laxity. The plastic speculum may be equipped with a small light that provides illumination, whereas metal specula require an external light source. Preference between these two types is provider dependent. The vagina and cervix are typically viewed after placement of either a Graves or Pederson speculum (Fig. 1-6). Prior to insertion, a speculum may be warmed with running water or by warming lights built into some examination tables. Additionally, lubrication may add comfort to insertion. Griffith and colleagues (2005) found that gel lubricants did not increase unsatisfactory Pap smear cytology rates or decrease *Chlamydia trachomatis* detection rates compared with water lubrication. If gel lubrication is used, a dime-sized aliquot is applied sparingly to the outer surface of the speculum blades.

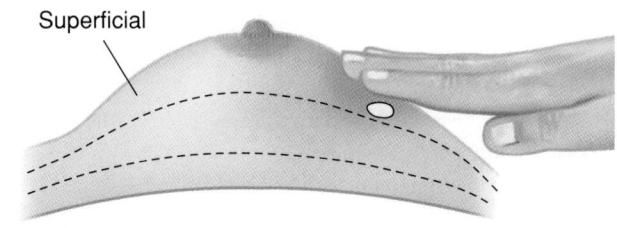

Superficial

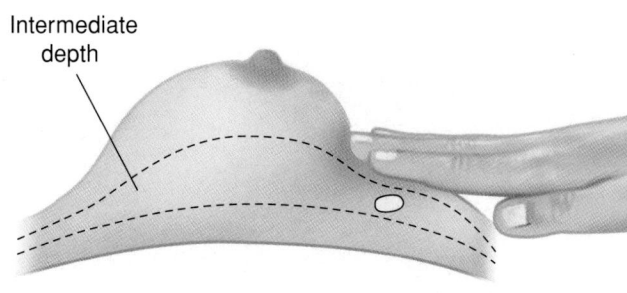

Intermediate depth

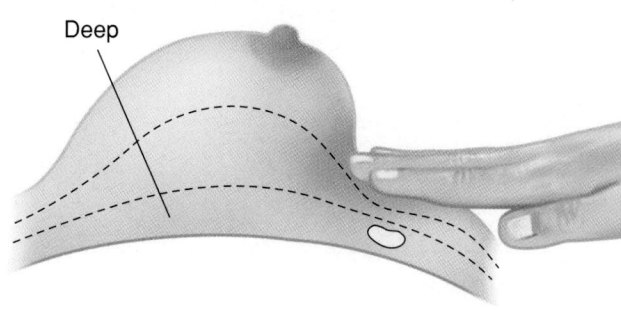

Deep

FIGURE 1-5 Palpation through several depths at each point along the linear path.

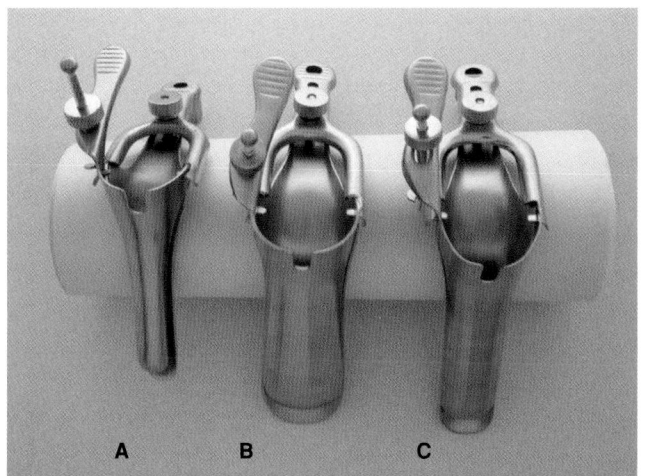

FIGURE 1-6 Vaginal specula. **A.** Pediatric Pederson speculum. This may be selected for child, adolescent, or virginal adult examination. **B.** Graves speculum. This may be selected for examination of parous women with relaxed and collapsing vaginal walls. **C.** Pederson speculum. This may be selected for sexually active women with adequate vaginal wall tone. (Used with permission from US Surgitech, Inc.)

Immediately before insertion, the labia minora are gently separated, and the urethra is identified. Because of urethral sensitivity, the speculum is inserted well below the meatus. Alternatively, prior to speculum placement, an index finger may be placed in the vagina, and pressure placed posteriorly against the bulbospongiosus muscle. A woman is then encouraged to relax this posterior wall to improve comfort with speculum insertion. This practice may prove especially helpful for women undergoing their first examination and for those with infrequent coitus, dyspareunia, or heightened anxiety.

With speculum insertion, the vagina commonly contracts, and a woman may note pressure or discomfort. A pause at this point typically is followed by vaginal muscle relaxation. As the speculum bill is completely inserted, it is angled approximately 30 degrees downward to reach the cervix. Commonly, the

uterus is anteverted, and the ectocervix lies against the posterior vaginal wall (Fig. 1-7).

As the speculum is opened, the ectocervix can be identified. Vaginal walls and cervix are inspected for masses, ulceration, or unusual discharge. As outlined in Chapter 29 (p. 632), cervical cancer screening is often completed, and additional swabs for culture or microscopic evaluation can also be collected. Screening for *Neisseria gonorrhoeae* and *Chlamydia trachomatis* and other STDs is listed in Table 1-1.

Bimanual Examination

Most often, the bimanual examination is performed after the speculum evaluation. Some clinicians prefer to complete the bimanual portion first to better identify cervical location prior to speculum insertion. Either process is appropriate. Uterine and adnexal size, mobility, and tenderness can be assessed during bimanual examination. For women with prior hysterectomy and adnexectomy, bimanual examination is still valuable and can be used to exclude other pelvic pathology.

During this examination, a gloved index and middle finger are inserted together into the vagina until the cervix is reached. For cases of latex allergy, nonlatex gloves are available. To ease insertion, a water-based lubricant can be initially applied to these gloved fingers. Once the cervix is reached, uterine orientation can be quickly assessed by sweeping the index finger inward along the ventral surface of the cervix. In those with an anteverted position, the uterine isthmus is noted to sweep upward, whereas in those with a retroverted position, a soft bladder is palpated. However, in those with a retroverted uterus, if a finger is swept along the cervix's dorsal aspect, the isthmus is felt to sweep downward. With a retroverted uterus, this same finger is continued posteriorly to the fundus and then side-to-side to assess uterine size and tenderness.

To determine the size of an anteverted uterus, fingers are placed beneath the cervix, and upward pressure tilts the fundus toward the anterior abdominal wall. A clinician's opposite

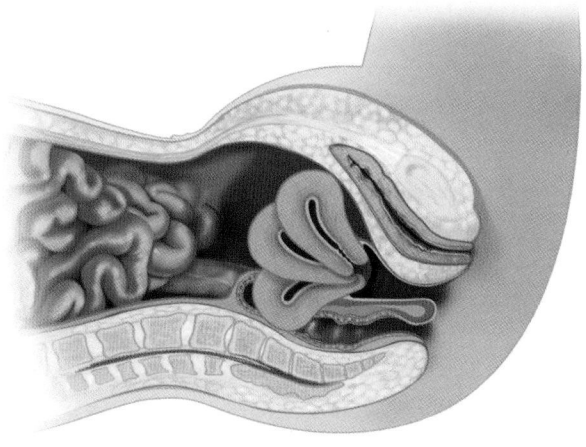

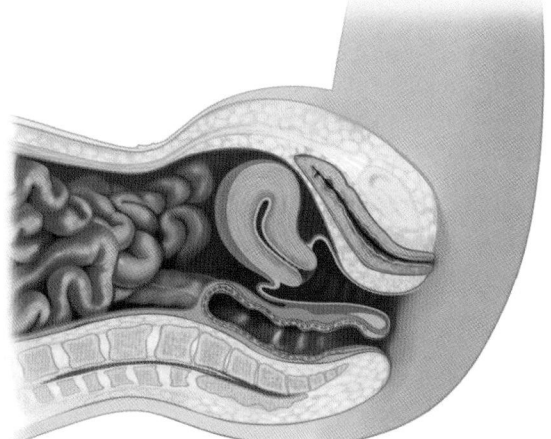

FIGURE 1-7 Uterine positions. **A.** Uterine position may be anteverted, midplane, or retroverted. **B.** As shown here, the uterine fundus can be flexed forward, and this is termed anteflexion. Similarly, the fundus may be flexed backward to create a retroverted uterus.

TABLE 1-1. Sexually Transmitted Disease Screening Guidelines for Nonpregnant, Sexually Active Asymptomatic Women

Infectious Agent	Screening Recommendations	Risk Factors
Chlamydia trachomatis + *Neisseria gonorrhoeae*	All <25 yr: annually Those older with risk factors: annually	New or multiple partners; inconsistent condom use; sex work; current or prior STD
Treponema pallidum	Those with risk factors	Sex work; confinement in adult correction facility; MSM
HIV virus	All 13–64 yr: one time[a] Those with risk factors: periodically	Multiple partners; injection drug use; sex work; concurrent STD; MSM; at-risk partners; initial TB diagnosis
Hepatitis C virus	All born from 1945 to 1965: one time Those with risk factors: periodically	Injection/intranasal drug use; dialysis; infected mother; blood products before 1992; unregulated tattoo; high-risk sexual behavior
Hepatitis B virus	Those with risk factors	HIV-positive; injection drug use; affected family or partner; MSM; multiple partners; originate from high-prevalence country
HSV	No routine screening	

[a]Centers for Disease Control and Prevention (2015) and American College of Obstetricians and Gynecologists (2014d) recommend one-time screening between ages 13 and 64 years. The U.S. Preventive Services Task Force (2014b) uses a 15–65 year age range.
HIV = human immunodeficiency virus; HSV = herpes simplex virus; MSM = men having sex with men; STD = sexually transmitted disease; TB = tuberculosis.
Data from Centers for Disease Control and Prevention (2015) and American College of Obstetricians and Gynecologists (2014d); U.S. Preventive Services Task Force (2004a, 2005, 2014a,b).

hand is placed against the abdominal wall to locate the upward fundal pressure (Fig. 1-8).

To assess adnexa, the clinician uses two vaginal fingers to lift the adnexa from the cul-de-sac or from Waldeyer fossa toward the anterior abdominal wall. The adnexa is trapped between these vaginal fingers and the clinician's other hand, which is exerting downward pressure against the lower abdomen. For those with a normal-sized uterus, this abdominal hand is typically best placed just above the inguinal ligament.

Rectovaginal Examination

The decision to perform rectovaginal evaluation varies among providers. Some prefer to complete this evaluation on all adults, whereas others elect to perform rectovaginal examination for those with specific indications. These may include pelvic pain, an identified pelvic mass, rectal symptoms, or risks for colon cancer.

Gloves are changed between bimanual and rectovaginal examinations to avoid contamination of the rectum with potential vaginal pathogens. Similarly, if fecal occult blood testing is to be done at this time, the glove is changed after bimanual examination to minimize false-positive results. Initially, an index finger is placed into the vagina and a middle finger into the rectum (Fig. 1-9). These fingers are swept against one another in

a scissoring fashion to assess the rectovaginal septum for scarring or peritoneal studding. The index finger is removed, and the middle finger completes a circular sweep of the rectal vault to exclude masses. If immediate fecal occult blood testing is indicated, it may be performed with a sample from this portion of the examination. As noted later, this single fecal occult blood testing does not constitute adequate colorectal cancer screening.

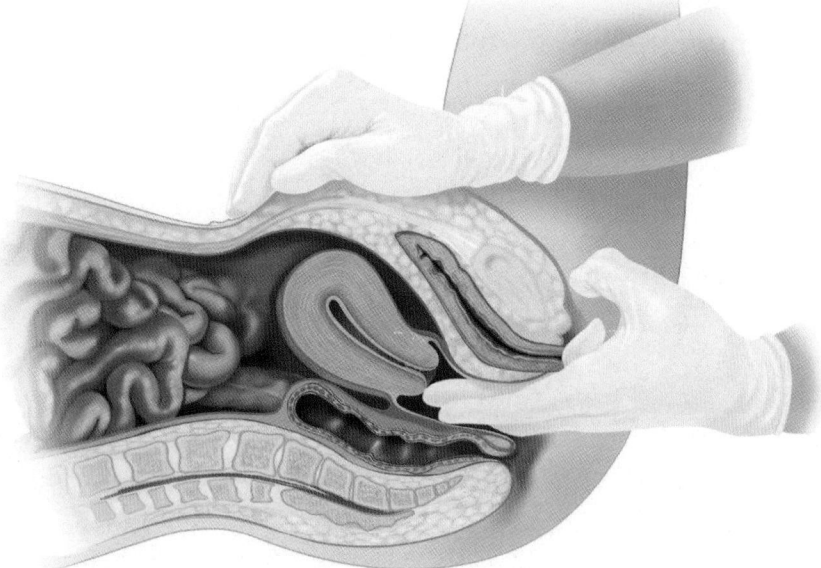

FIGURE 1-8 Bimanual examination. Fingers beneath the cervix lift the uterus toward the anterior abdominal wall. A hand placed on the abdomen detects upward pressure from the uterine fundus. Examination allows assessment of uterine size, mobility, and tenderness.

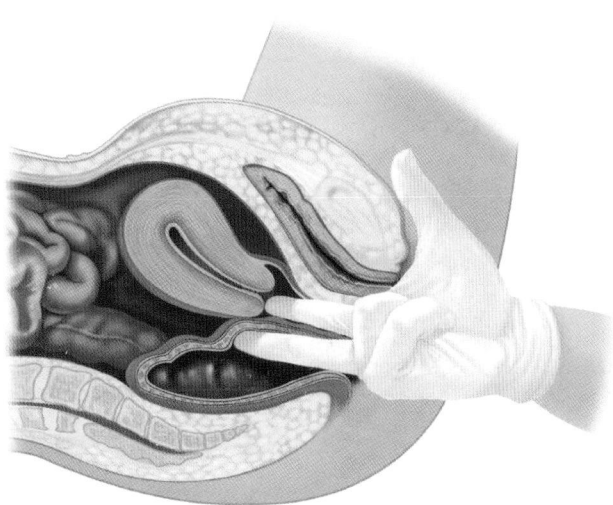

FIGURE 1-9 Rectovaginal examination.

Examination Interval

Periodic health evaluation and screening can prevent or detect numerous medical conditions. Moreover, periodic visits also foster a patient-physician partnership to help guide a woman through adolescence, reproductive years, and past menopause.

An initial reproductive health visit is recommended between ages 13 and 15 years (American College of Obstetricians and Gynecologists, 2014e). This visit initiates a discussion between an adolescent and health-care provider on issues of general reproductive health, puberty, menstruation, contraception, and STD protection. Although not mandated, a pelvic examination may be necessary if gynecologic symptoms are described. Adolescents may prefer to include parents in their gynecologic health care. However, as discussed in Chapter 14 (p. 320), adolescents may seek care for STDs, substance abuse, contraception, or pregnancy without parental permission (American College of Obstetricians and Gynecologists, 2014a).

For women older than 21 years, the American College of Obstetricians and Gynecologists (2014f) recommends annual well woman visits, during which physical and pelvic examinations are completed. Pelvic evaluation contains those components listed on page 4, namely, inspection and speculum, bimanual, and rectal examinations. However, evidence neither supports nor refutes the value of annual pelvic evaluation in asymptomatic women. Thus, exclusion of this portion is a shared decision following patient-provider discussion. Women with gynecologic complaints are encouraged to permit this examination.

One topic in this conversation is cervical cancer screening. For many women, the appropriate screening interval may not be annually, and specific screening methods and schedules are discussed in Chapter 29 (p. 634). Second, in the past, endocervical swabs for gonorrhea and chlamydia infection screening during speculum examination were preferred. Now, such screening can be completed with similar accuracy using nucleic acid amplification testing of urine, vaginal, or endocervical samples.

Other professional organizations have also published statements regarding preventive care visits. The Institute of Medicine (2011) recommends at least one annual well woman visit to obtain preventive services, including preconception and prenatal care. However, investigators from the American College of Physicians (ACP) reviewed pelvic examination benefits and harms in asymptomatic adult women (Qaseem, 2014). These authors describe scarce data to determine the ideal interval for routine pelvic examination. Accordingly, the ACP recommends against screening pelvic examination for asymptomatic, nonpregnant adult women. Thus, again, with each annual visit, a discussion of benefits and risks and an agreement to examination is prudent.

PREVENTIVE CARE

Gynecologists have an opportunity to evaluate their patients for leading causes of female morbidity and mortality and intervene accordingly. Thus, familiarity with various screening guidelines is essential. In 2014, recommendations by the American College of Obstetricians and Gynecologists (2014f) were updated. The USPSTF (2014) regularly revises its screening guidelines, which can be accessed at www.USPreventiveServicesTaskForce.org. These, along with other specialty-specific recommendations, offer valuable guidance for clinicians providing preventive care. Many of these topics are covered in other text chapters. Some remaining important subjects are present in the following sections.

Immunization

The need for new or repeat administration of vaccines should be reviewed periodically. Some vaccines are recommended for all adults, whereas others are indicated because of patient comorbidities or occupational exposure risks. For most healthy adults who have completed the indicated childhood and adolescent immunization schedules, those that warrant consideration are listed in Table 1-2. This table summarizes recommended schedules, precautions, and contraindications for these adult vaccines. As of 2015, a link is provided to the full schedules at: http://www.cdc.gov/vaccines/schedules/.

In general, any vaccine may be coadministered with another type at the same visit. Notably, the influenza vaccine is available in several formulations. Vaccines for human papillomavirus infection prevention, Gardasil and Cervarix, are discussed additionally in Chapter 29 (p. 630).

Cancer Screening
Colon Cancer

In the United States, nearly 64,000 new cases of colorectal cancer are predicted, and this malignancy is the third leading cause of cancer death in women, behind lung and breast cancer (Siegel, 2015). Incidence and mortality rates from this cancer have declined during the past two decades, largely due to improved screening tools. However, adherence to colorectal cancer screening guidelines for women is usually less than 50 percent (Meissner, 2006).

Guidelines recommend screening average-risk patients for colorectal cancer beginning at age 50 with any of the methods shown in Table 1-3 (Smith, 2015). Screening is selected from either of two method categories. The first is capable of identifying both cancer *and* precancerous lesions. The second group of methods primarily detects only cancer and includes the fecal occult blood test, fecal immunochemical test, and stool DNA tests.

Of these, colonoscopy is often the preferred test for colorectal cancer screening. For the patient with average risk and normal findings, testing is repeated in 10 years. In the United States,

TABLE 1-2. Summary of Recommendations for Adult Immunization

Vaccine and Route	Reason to Vaccinate	Vaccine Administration	Contraindications and Precautions[a,b]
Influenza	• All adults	• Yearly • October is ideal, or as long as virus is circulating • Several vaccine types and forms available[c]	**Precaution** • GBS within 6 wk of prior vaccine
Pneumococcal **PCV13** **PPSV23** *Give IM or SC*	• ≥65 yr • Smokers; long-term care residents • Chronic illness; asplenia; immunocompromise	• Age ≥65: PCV13, then PPSV23 after 6 months • Smoker aged 19–64: PPSV23 alone • Variant regimens for other indications[d]	
Hepatitis B *Give IM*	• Adult wishing immunity • Contact risks; travelers to endemic areas[e] • Chronic liver disease; ESRD; HIV; DM	• Three doses: 0, 1, and 4 months	
Hepatitis A *Give IM*	• Adult wishing immunity • Contact risks; travelers to endemic areas[e] • Chronic liver disease	• Two doses: 0 and 6 months	
Td **Tdap** *Give IM*	• Adults without prior vaccination • Pregnancy	• Primary series: Td given at 0, 1, and 7 months. If 19–64 yr, one of the three doses is Tdap • Td booster every 10 yr after primary series. If 19–64 yr, a one-time Tdap replaces one of the Td doses • At-risk wounds: booster Td dose if ≥5 yr since prior dose • Pregnancy: Tdap dose at 27–36 wk regardless of prior dosing	**Contraindication** • Tdap: encephalopathy after prior vaccine **Precaution** • GBS within 6 wk of prior vaccine • Tdap: unstable neurologic condition
Varicella *Give SC*	• Adults without immunity	• Two doses: 0 and 1 month • Nonimmune gravida: give postpartum	**Contraindications** • Pregnancy • Immunocompromise **Precaution** • Recent antibody-containing blood products • Hold "-cyclovir" antivirals[f] for 14 days after vaccine
Zoster *Give SC*	• Those ≥60 yr	• One dose	**Contraindications** • Immunocompromise • Pregnancy **Precaution** • Hold "-cyclovir" antivirals[f] for 14 days after vaccine

(Continued)

TABLE 1-2. Summary of Recommendations for Adult Immunization *(Continued)*

Vaccine and Route	Reason to Vaccinate	Vaccine Administration	Contraindications and Precautions[a,b]
Meningococcal MCV4 *Give IM* **MPSV4** *Give SC*	• Asplenia • Contact risks; travelers to endemic areas[e] • College freshmen	• One dose • Two initial doses for asplenia: 0 and 2 months • Age ≤55, use MCV4 • Age ≥56, use MPSV4 • Repeat MCV4 every 5 yr if risk persists	
MMR *Give SC*	• Adults without immunity	• One dose • Nonimmune gravida: give postpartum	**Contraindications** • Immunocompromise • Pregnancy **Precaution** • Prior thrombocytopenia • Recent antibody-containing blood products
HPV *Give IM*	• All females 11–26 yr	• Three doses: 0, 1, and 6 months	**Precaution** • Pregnancy

[a]Previous anaphylactic reaction to any of a vaccine's components serves as a contraindication for any vaccine.
[b]Moderate to severe illness is a precaution to vaccination. Mild illness is not a contraindication.
[c]Several influenza vaccines are available and listed at: http://www.cdc.gov/mmwr/preview/mmwrhtml/mm6332a3.htm#Tab.
[d]Full guidelines found at http://www.cdc.gov/vaccines/schedules/downloads/adult/adult-combined-schedule.pdf.
[e]A list is found at http://wwwnc.cdc.gov/travel/yellowbook/2010/table-of-contents.aspx.
[f]These include acyclovir, famciclovir, valacyclovir.
DM = diabetes mellitus; ESRD = end-stage renal disease; GBS = Guillain-Barré syndrome; HIV = human immunodeficiency virus; HPV = human papillomavirus; IM = intramuscular; IV = intravenous; MCV4 = meningococcal conjugate vaccine; MMR = measles, mumps, rubella; MPSV4 = meningococcal polysaccharide vaccine; PCV = pneumococcal conjugate vaccine; PPSV = pneumococcal polysaccharide vaccine; SC = subcutaneous; Td = tetanus, diphtheria; Tdap = tetanus, diphtheria, activated pertussis.
Data from Kim DK, Bridges CB, Harriman HK, et al: Advisory Committee on Immunization Practices recommended immunization schedule for adults aged 19 years or older: United States, 2015. Ann Intern Med 162:214, 2015.

flexible sigmoidoscopy is used less frequently. Its limitations include that only the distal 40 cm of colon are seen, and if lesions are found, then colonoscopy is still needed. A final suitable option—computed tomographic (CT) colonography—is not often covered by insurance plans.

Fecal occult blood testing (gFOBT) is an adequate *annual* screening method when two or three stool samples are self-collected by the patient, and the cards are returned for analysis. This method relies on a chemical oxidation reaction between the heme moiety of blood and alpha guaiaconic acid, a component of guaiac paper. Heme catalyzes the oxidation of alpha guaiaconic acid by hydrogen peroxide, the active component in the developer. This oxidation reaction yields a blue color (Sanford, 2009). Red meat, raw cauliflower, broccoli, members of the radish family, and melons have similar oxidizing ability and may yield false-positive results. Vitamin C may preemptively react with the reagents and lead to false-negative results. All of these are eliminated for 3 days before testing. Additionally, women should avoid nonsteroidal antiinflammatory drugs (NSAIDs) 7 days prior to testing to limit risks of gastric irritation and bleeding. These restrictions are cumbersome for some patients and lead to noncompliance with recommended testing.

Alternatively, the fecal immunochemical test (FIT) relies on an immune reaction to human hemoglobin. Similar to FOBT, the FIT test is performed for annual screening on two or three patient-collected stool samples and does not require pretesting dietary limitations. Advantages to FIT include greater specificity for human blood and thus fewer false-positive results from dietary meat and vegetables and fewer false-negative results due to vitamin C. As another option, screening may be completed with stool DNA (sDNA) testing. One FDA-approved test, Cologuard, screens stool for both DNA and hemoglobin biomarkers that are associated with colorectal cancer (Imperiale, 2014). Positive test results from any of these three warrant further evaluation by colonoscopy.

During patient evaluation of pelvic complaints such as pain, a gynecologist not uncommonly performs gFOBT testing on a single stool sample obtained during digital rectal examination. Although potentially helpful diagnostically, this single stool sample is not considered adequate colorectal cancer screening.

These guidelines are appropriate for those with average risk. High-risk factors include a personal history of colorectal cancer or adenomatous polyps, a first-degree relative with colon cancer or adenomas, chronic inflammatory bowel disease, known or

TABLE 1-3. Screening Guidelines for the Early Detection of Colorectal Cancer and Adenomas for Average-risk Women Aged 50 years and Older

Tests That Detect Adenomatous Polyps and Cancer[a]		
Test	**Interval**	**Key Issues for Informed Decisions**
Colonoscopy	10 years	Bowel prep required; conscious sedation provided
FSIG	5 years	Bowel prep required, sedation usually not provided. Positive findings usually merit colonoscopy
Barium enema (DCBE)	5 years	Bowel prep required; polyps ≥6 mm merit colonoscopy
Colonography (CTC)	5 years	Bowel prep required; polyps ≥6 mm merit colonoscopy
Tests That Primarily Detect Cancer[a]		
Test	**Interval**	**Key Issues for Informed Decisions**
gFOBT	Annually	Two to three stool samples collected at home are needed; a single stool sample gathered during office digital examination is not sufficient screening. Positive results merit colonoscopy
FIT	Annually	Positive results merit colonoscopy
Stool DNA (sDNA)	3 years	Positive results merit colonoscopy

[a]One method from this group is selected.
CTC = Computed tomographic colonography; DCBE = double-contrast barium enema; FIT = fecal immunochemical test; FSIG = flexible sigmoidoscopy; gFOBT = guaiac-based fecal occult blood test; sDNA = stool DNA test.
Adapted with permission from Smith RA, Manassaram-Baptiste D, Brooks D, et al: Cancer screening in the United States, 2015: a review of current American Cancer Society guidelines and current issues in cancer screening. CA Cancer J Clin 2015 Jan-Feb;65(1):30–54.

suspected hereditary syndrome such as hereditary nonpolyposis colon cancer (Lynch syndrome) or familial adenomatous polyposis (Smith, 2015).

Lung Cancer

In the United States, this cancer is estimated to account for 13 percent of all new cancers diagnosed in women in 2015 (Siegel, 2015). It is now the leading cause of cancer-related death in both men and women. All smokers should be advised of tobacco-use risks and encouraged to stop. A list of potential aids is found on page 11.

Lung cancer screening focuses on those at high risk and referral is considered for individuals with general good health, aged 55 to 74, with at least a 30-pack-year history, and who actively smoke or quit within the past 15 years. One remembers that pack-year determination is calculated by multiplying the number of packs smoked per day by the number of years the person has smoked. By convention, one pack contains 20 cigarettes. For appropriate cases, low-dose helical CT scanning is the preferred test (Smith, 2015). Although a common diagnostic test, chest radiography is not recommended as a lung cancer screening tool.

Skin Cancer

The incidence of skin cancers (melanoma and non-melanomas) has increased in the United States during the past three decades. In 2015, melanoma is expected to account for 4 percent of all cancer deaths in women (Siegel, 2015). Skin cancer risks include prolonged sun exposure, family or personal history of skin cancer, fair skin, light hair or freckling, numerous moles, immunosuppression,

and aging (American Cancer Society, 2013). The USPSTF notes insufficient evidence to recommend whole body screening by physician or patient for skin cancer in the general adult population (Wolff, 2009). It does advise clinicians to use the "ABCD" system—asymmetry, border irregularity, color, and diameter (>6 mm) to evaluate skin lesions of concern and refer appropriately.

■ Lifestyle Changes
Smoking

Cigarette smoking is the single most preventable cause of death in the United States and has been linked with certain cancers, cardiovascular disease, chronic lung diseases, and stroke. Moreover, specific to women's health, smoking is linked to diminished fertility, pregnancy complications, and postoperative complications. These are discussed in greater detail in their respective chapters.

Despite these known negative health outcomes, in 2003, only 64 percent of smokers who had routine examinations in the United States were advised by a physician to quit smoking (Torrijos, 2006). Guidelines from the U.S. Department of Health and Human Services encourage a brief behavioral patient intervention model found on page 12. Patients can also be referred to the National Cancer Institute's smoking cessation website: www.smokefree.gov. This site provides free, evidence-based information and professional assistance to help the immediate and long-term needs of those trying to quit. Unless contraindicated, pharmacologic treatments to aid smoking cessation can be offered to all interested women and

TABLE 1-4. Drugs Used for Smoking Cessation

Agent	Brand Name	Initial Dosing	Maintenance	Drug Tapering	Therapy Duration
Nicotine Replacement					
Patch[d]	Habitrol Nicoderm CQ	If >10 CPD: a 21-mg patch is reapplied daily wk 1–6 If <10 CPD: 14-mg patch daily for wk 1–6	14-mg patch is used wk 7–8 —	7-mg patch is used wk 9–10 7-mg patch is used wk 7–8	8–12 wk
Gum[d]	Nicorette 2 mg 4 mg (if ≥25 CPD)	1 piece every 1–2 hr for wk 1–6 (maximum 24 pieces/d)	1 piece every 2–4 hr for wk 7–9	1 piece every 4–8 hr for wk 10–12	12 wk
Lozenge[b]	Commit 2 mg 4 mg (if smokes <30 min after waking)	1 piece every 1–2 hr for wk 1–6 (maximum 20 pieces/d)	1 piece every 2–4 hr for wk 7–9	1 piece every 4–8 hr for wk 10–12	12 wk
Inhaler[d]	Nicotrol		6 (average use) to 16 cartridges puffed qd for 12 wk	Use is then tapered	12–24 wk
Nasal spray[d]	Nicotrol		1 dose = 1 spray to each nostril per hr (maximum 5 doses/hr & 40/d)	Use is then tapered starting wk 9	12–24 wk
Nicotine Agonists					
Varenicline[c]	Chantix	0.5 mg PO qd for 3 d, then 0.5 mg PO bid for next 4 d	Then 1 mg PO bid		12 wk
CNS Agents					
Bupropion[c]	Wellbutrin SR Zyban	1–2 wk prior to cessation: 150 mg PO qd for 3 d	Then 150 mg PO bid		7–12 wk; may use for 6 mo.
Nortriptyline[a,d]		25 mg PO qd with gradual increase	75–100 mg PO qd		12 wk; may use for 6 mo.
Clonidine[a,c]	Catapres	0.1 mg PO bid, increase by 0.10 mg/d each wk as needed	0.15–0.75 mg PO qd		3–10 wk
	Catapres-TTS	0.1-mg transdermal patch is changed weekly	0.1- to 0.2-mg transdermal patch weekly		

[a]Recommended as second-line agents by U.S. Public Health Service clinical guidelines, 2008.
[b]Has not been evaluated by the Food and Drug Administration (FDA) for pregnancy.
[c]Considered an FDA pregnancy category C drug.
[d]Considered an FDA pregnancy category D drug.
bid = twice daily; CNS = central nervous system; CPD = cigarettes per day; PO = orally; qd = daily.
Data from Fiore MC, Jaen CR, Baker TB, et al: Treating tobacco use and dependence: 2008 update. Rockville, U.S. Department of Health and Human Services, 2008.

are listed in Table 1-4. Gynecologists who are proficient in the use of these therapies may prescribe. Referral is also appropriate (American College of Obstetricians and Gynecologists, 2014c).

Exercise

Exercise has known benefits in preventing coronary artery disease, diabetes, osteoporosis, obesity, depression, insomnia, and breast and colon cancer (Brosse, 2002; Knowler, 2002; Lee, 2003; Vuori, 2001; Youngstedt, 2005). Many of these associations may result from the effects of exercise to lower blood pressure, decrease low-density lipoprotein cholesterol and triglyceride levels, increase high-density lipoprotein cholesterol levels, improve blood sugar control, and reduce weight (Braith, 2006; Pescatello, 2004; Sigal, 2004).

SECTION 1

TABLE 1-5. Definitions of Abnormal Weight for Adults and Adolescents Using Body Mass Index

Age Group	Underweight	Overweight	Obese
Adult	<18.5	25–29.9	≥30
Adolescent	<5th percentile for age	Between 85th and 95th percentile for age	>95th percentile for age

Despite these known benefits, based on U.S. government thresholds, only 45 percent of women in 2012 were considered sufficiently active (Blackwell, 2014). Recommendations from the U.S. Department of Health and Human Services (2008) include moderate-intensity activity such as walking, water aerobics, or yard work for at least 150 minutes each week *or* vigorous-intensity activities such as running, swimming laps, or aerobic dancing for 75 minutes each week. Activities can be performed in episodes of at least 10 minutes that are apportioned throughout the week. Additional health benefits are gained with physical activity beyond these amounts.

Although exercise programs have traditionally emphasized dynamic, aerobic lower-extremity exercise, research supports complementary resistance training to improve muscular strength and endurance, cardiovascular function, metabolism, coronary risk factors, weight management, and quality of life (Williams, 2007). Accordingly, government guidelines also encourage biweekly muscle-strengthening activities that involve all the major muscle groups. A fuller listing of general physical activities and their intensity description is found in the publication *2008 Physical Activity Guidelines for Americans* at the CDC website: www.health.gov/paguidelines/guidelines.

To change any type of health-related behavior, counseling can be brief yet effective. One method is the five A's system, which in this example is tailored for exercise (Fiore, 2008).

- Ask: if she is physically active now
- Advise: her about the benefits of regular physical activity
- Assess: her willingness to change and decide if she is in a (1) precontemplation, (2) contemplation phase, (3) preparation, or (4) action phase. Her stage of readiness guides further discussion
- Assist: her by recommending local exercise programs
- Arrange: for follow-up evaluation to assess progress

For those with certain comorbidities, clearance by other health care providers may be indicated. For this, the Physical Activity Readiness Questionnaire helps identify women with risk factors who merit further evaluation and is available at: www.csep.ca/cmfiles/publications/parq/par-q.pdf.

■ Obesity
Associated Risks and Diagnosis

In 2010, nearly 36 percent of women in the United States were obese, and almost twice that many were overweight (Flegal, 2012). Possible consequences of obesity include diabetes mellitus, metabolic syndrome, nonalcoholic fatty liver, cholelithiasis, hypertension, osteoarthritis, nonobstructive sleep apnea, and renal disease. Gynecologic issues related to obesity include abnormal menstruation, risks for endometrial neoplasia, and worsening polycystic ovary syndrome. Moreover, some hormonal contraceptives may have lower efficacy in obese women. Despite these considerable consequences, one study showed

that fewer than half of physicians are comfortable discussing obesity (Schuster, 2008). Even if not trained as weight management specialists, clinicians ideally screen for obesity, provide initial obesity evaluation and management, and refer as needed.

Screening is accomplished with calculation of body mass index (BMI) or less commonly, waist circumference. BMI, although not a direct measure of body fat content, is valuable in assessing the risk for weight-related complications. The following calculations can be used:

$$BMI = (Wt\ in\ lb/(Ht\ in\ inches \times Ht\ in\ inches)) \times 703$$
$$BMI = Wt\ in\ kg/(Ht\ in\ meters \times Ht\ in\ meters)$$

More simply, an online calculator can be found at: www.cdc.gov/healthyweight/assessing/bmi/adult_bmi/english_bmi_calculator/bmi_calculator.html. For adolescents (and children), BMI is adjusted for age and gender and calculated as a percentile. A BMI calculator for adolescents can be found at http://apps.nccd.cdc.gov/dnpabmi/.calculator.aspx. Table 1-5 reflects the definitions for underweight, overweight, and obesity for adolescents and adults.

Waist circumference positively correlates with abdominal fat content, which is a risk factor for poor health outcomes. Waist circumference is measured at the level of the iliac crests at the end of normal expiration. Values greater than 35 inches (88 cm) are considered elevated (National Heart, Lung, and Blood Institute, 2000).

No standard single or panel laboratory test is indicated for an obese woman. Evaluation for comorbidities is tailored to the patient, taking into consideration her family and social histories (Table 1-6). Blood pressure measurement, fasting lipid and glucose screening, and thyroid function testing can all be considered for the obese patient during initial evaluation.

TABLE 1-6. Obesity Comorbid Risk Factors

Coronary heart disease (CHD)
Other atherosclerotic disease
Diabetes mellitus
Sleep apnea
Cigarette smoking
Chronic hypertension
Abnormal lipid levels
Family history of early CHD
Gynecologic abnormalities
    Abnormal uterine bleeding
    Endometrial neoplasia
Osteoarthritis
Gallstones

Data from National Heart, Lung, and Blood Institute: The practical guide: identification, evaluation, and treatment of overweight and obesity in adults. National Institutes of Health Publication No. 98–4084, Bethesda, 2000.

For a woman with elevated BMIs, a clinician should assess her readiness for change and thereby, provide appropriate guidance, support, or referral. In addition, questions regarding previous attempts at weight loss, social hurdles that impede diet and exercise change, and detrimental eating habits are discussed in a nonjudgmental manner.

Treatment

Effective weight loss is best obtained with proper nutrition and consistent physical activity. Table 1-7 illustrates recommended guidelines to direct therapy for overweight or obese women. A detailed discussion of dietary weight loss extends beyond this chapter's scope, but several clinician and patient aids can be found in *The Practical Guide to Identification, Evaluation and Treatment of Overweight or Obesity in Adults*, available at: www.nhlbi.nih.gov/guidelines/obesity/prctgd_c.pdf.

In general, for the adult patient, a 10-percent weight loss within 6 months is realistic. According to the American Heart Association, suitable options are diets with 1200 to 1500 kcal/day or diets that incorporate a 500 or 750-kcal/d deficit (Jensen, 2014). No single diet plan is espoused as the gold standard for every patient, and the ideal regimen is one that can be adhered to.

In addition to diet and exercise, pharmacologic or surgical options may be implemented for selected obese patients. Four agents are FDA-approved for long-term obesity treatment. First, orlistat (Xenical) is a reversible inhibitor of gastric and pancreatic lipases and leads to a 30-percent blockage of dietary fat absorption (Henness, 2006). This drug is prescribed as 120-mg capsule taken orally three times daily with meals but is also available over-the-counter in 60-mg capsules (Alli), also taken three times daily. Associated malabsorption can lead to deficiencies of the fat-soluble vitamins A, D, E, and K, and all patients should receive a daily supplement enriched with these vitamins. Severe liver injury has been reported rarely, and new labeling reflects this risk (Food and Drug Administration, 2010).

Another medication, lorcaserin (Belviq) is a serotonin 2C receptor agonist used to suppress appetite (Fidler, 2011; Smith, 2010). One 10-mg tablet is taken orally twice daily. A third agent combines phentermine and topiramate (Qsymia)(Gadde, 2011). Doses begin at 3.75 mg/23 mg orally daily and are gradually titrated upward as needed to a maximum dose of 15 mg/92 mg daily. This drug has fetotoxicity potential and prescribing providers participate in a Qsymia Risk Evaluation and Mitigation Strategy program. Last, liraglutide (Saxenda) is a glucagon-like peptide-1 receptor agonist delivered by subcutaneous injection (Astrup, 2009). Dosing begins at 0.6 mg daily and is gradually escalated weekly to reach a 3-mg daily dose. Important poten-

tial risks include medullary thyroid carcinoma and pancreatitis. These last three agents are indicated for those with BMIs of 30 or greater, or 27 or greater if weight-associated comorbid risks exist.

As another adjunct, bariatric surgery may be selected for those with BMIs of 40 or greater, or with BMIs at or above 35 if other comorbid conditions are present (Jensen, 2014). Of available laparoscopic procedures, three are more commonly performed. Two are considered restrictive (limit intake), whereas bypass surgery promotes malabsorptive weight loss. First of these, gastric banding places an adjustable plastic ring around the stomach to limit food intake. Second, sleeve gastrectomy partitions off the lateral stomach by a staple line, and the remaining smaller stomach has a tubular, sleeve appearance. Last, the Roux-en-Y gastric bypass creates a small stomach pouch that is connected directly to the jejunum to bypass the duodenum. This reduces calorie and nutrient absorption. These surgeries lead to substantial weight loss in individuals with morbid obesity and have been linked with improvement in comorbid risk factors and decreased mortality rates (Hutter, 2011). With these, surgical complications are infrequent but can be serious and include gastrointestinal leaks at staple or suture lines, stomal obstruction or stenosis, thromboembolism, and bleeding (Jackson, 2012).

Following bariatric surgery, patients are advised to delay pregnancy for 12 to 24 months (American College of Obstetricians and Gynecologists, 2013). Rapid weight loss during this time poses theoretical risks for intrauterine fetal-growth restriction and nutritional deprivation. However, as weight is lost, fertility rates overall appear to be improved, and risks for pregnancy increase (Merhi, 2009). Thus, effective contraception is needed. Most contraceptive methods appear to be as effective in women with elevated BMIs compared with normal-weight controls. However, the contraceptive patch (OrthoEvra) is less effective in those weighing more than 90 kg (Zieman, 2002). Specific to those with malabsorptive bariatric surgery types, oral contraception efficacy may be lower due to poor absorption (Centers for Disease Control and Prevention, 2013). Last, due to its risk for associated weight gain, depot medroxyprogesterone acetate (Depo-Provera) may be an unpopular choice in women trying to lose weight.

■ Cardiovascular Disease

In 2010, nearly 34 percent of the female population was affected by cardiovascular disease (CVD), and more than 400,000 women died from its complications (Go, 2014). Stratification of CVD predispositions can identify vulnerable patients for management or referral (Table 1-8). Ideal goals for exercise, glucose and lipid levels, blood pressure, and smoking cessation

TABLE 1-7. Treatment Recommendations According to BMI

Treatment	BMI 25–26.9	BMI 27–29.9	BMI 30–34.9	BMI 35–39.9	BMI ≥40
Diet, activity, behavioral therapy	WCM	WCM	+	+	+
Pharmacotherapy	—	WCM	+	+	+
Surgery	—	—	—	WCM	+

+ represents the use of indicated treatment regardless of comorbidities; BMI = body mass index; WCM = with comorbidities.
Data from Jensen MD, Ryan DH, Apovian CM, et al: 2013 AHA/ACC/TOS guideline for the management of overweight and obesity in adults: a report of the American College of Cardiology/American Heart Association Task Force on Practice Guidelines and The Obesity Society. Circulation 129(25 Suppl 2):S102, 2014.

are discussed in other sections of this chapter. Specific dietary intake recommendations for women are listed in Table 1-9.

Chronic Hypertension

Nearly 41 million American women are hypertensive. The risk of hypertension increases with age and is increased for black women compared with those of other races (Go, 2014). Chronic hypertension increases the risks for myocardial infarction, stroke, congestive heart failure, renal disease, and peripheral vascular disease. Moreover, chronic hypertension and its potential therapies may limit contraception choices for some women. Thus, gynecologists should be familiar with criteria used to diagnose hypertension. Although many may choose to refer their patients for treatment of hypertension, gynecologists should be aware of target goals and long-term risks associated with this disease.

For adult screening, the American Heart Association (2014) recommends blood pressure assessment starting at age 20 and evaluation repeated every 2 years if initially normal. For patients with elevated pressures, assessment is at least annually.

TABLE 1-8. Classification of Cardiovascular Disease (CVD) in Women

≥1 assigns high-risk status	Known CHD or CVD Peripheral arterial disease Aortic aneurysm End-stage renal disease Diabetes mellitus
≥1 assigns at-risk status	Smoking SBP ≥120 or DBP ≥80 mm Hg, or treated hypertension Total cholesterol ≥200 mg/dL, HDL <50 mg/dL, or treated dyslipidemia Obesity Poor diet Physical inactivity Family history of premature CVD Metabolic syndrome Collagen-vascular disease Prior PIH or gestational DM
Ideal, if all present	Total cholesterol <200 mg/dL BP <120/<80 mm Hg Fasting blood glucose <100 mg/dL Body mass index <25 Abstinence from smoking Physically activity Healthy diet: see Table 1-9

BP = Blood pressure; CHD = coronary heart disease; CVD = cardiovascular disease; DBP = diastolic blood pressure; DM = diabetes mellitus; GDM = gestational diabetes; HDL = high-density lipoprotein; PIH = pregnancy-induced hypertension; SBP = systolic blood pressure.
Adapted with permission from Mosca L, Benjamin EJ, Berra K, et al: Effectiveness-based guidelines for prevention of cardiovascular disease in women—2011 update: a guideline from the american heart association, Circulation 2011 Mar 22;123(11):1243–1262.

TABLE 1-9. Specific Dietary Intake Recommendations for Women

Food	Serving
Fruits/vegetables	≥4.5 cups/d
Fish	2/wk
Fiber	30 g/d
Whole grains	3/d
Sugar	≤5/wk
Nuts, legumes	≥4/wk
Saturated fat	<7%/total energy intake
Cholesterol	<150 mg/d
Alcohol	≤1/d
Sodium	<1500 mg/d
trans-Fatty acids	None

Adapted with permission from Mosca L, Benjamin EJ, Berra K, et al: Effectiveness-based guidelines for prevention of cardiovascular disease in women—2011 update: a guideline from the american heart association, Circulation 2011 Mar 22;123(11):1243–1262.

With screening, blood pressures are best taken with a woman seated in a chair with the tested arm resting on a table, at the level of the heart. Ideally, the patient has been able to rest quietly for a few minutes prior to measurement and to have refrained from tobacco and caffeine use immediately prior to testing. An appropriately sized cuff is selected, and the cuff bladder should encircle at least 80 percent of the arm. Hypertension is diagnosed if readings are elevated on at least two separate office visits over one or more weeks. *Prehypertension* is diagnosed if readings fall in the range 130–139/80–89 mm Hg. Notably, women with prehypertension are at significantly increased risk of developing hypertension later (Wang, 2004). Additionally, compared with normal blood pressure readings, prehypertension is associated with greater risks for CVD (Mainous, 2004).

If hypertension is diagnosed, further examination should exclude underlying causes of hypertension and resultant end-organ disease (Table 1-10). With the diagnosis of chronic hypertension, assessment then follows for both modifiable and nonmodifiable CVD risk factors. Thus, routine laboratory tests recommended before initiating therapy include an electrocardiogram, urinalysis, blood glucose, hematocrit, lipid profile, thyroid testing, and serum potassium and creatinine measurement. A more extensive search for identifiable causes is not generally indicated unless hypertension is not controlled with initial treatment (Chobanian, 2003).

For treatment, lifestyle changes that mirror those for CVD are encouraged (see Table 1-9). However, if blood pressure is significantly elevated or resistant to lifestyle modification alone, then pharmacologic treatment may be needed to decrease long-term complications. Recommendations from the Eighth Joint National Committee (JNC 8) are shown in Table 1-11 (James, 2014).

Stroke

This is the third leading cause of death in the United States, and in 2010, approximately 425,000 American women suffered a new or recurrent stroke (Go, 2014). Gender-specific risk factors for stroke in women include hypertension, atrial fibrillation, migraines with aura, and oral contraceptive use. Aspirin is recommended

TABLE 1-10. Identifiable Causes of Hypertension

Chronic renal disease
Chronic corticosteroid therapy and Cushing syndrome
Coarctation of the aorta
Drug-induced or drug-related
    Nonsteroidal antiinflammatory drugs
    Cocaine and amphetamines
    Sympathomimetics (decongestants, anorectics)
    Combination hormonal contraception
    Adrenal steroids
    Cyclosporine and tacrolimus
    Erythropoietin
    Licorice
    Herbal medicines (ephedra, ma huang)
Pheochromocytoma
Primary aldosteronism
Renovascular disease
Sleep apnea
Thyroid or parathyroid disease

TABLE 1-12. Interpretation of Cholesterol and Triglyceride Levels

Lipoprotein (mg/dL)	Interpretation
Total cholesterol	
<200	Optimal
200–239	Borderline elevated
≥240	Elevated
LDL cholesterol	
<100	Optimal
100–129	Near optimal
130–159	Borderline elevated
160–189	Elevated
≥190	Very elevated
HDL cholesterol	
<40	Low
≥60	Elevated
Triglycerides	
<150	Optimal
150–199	Borderline elevated
200–499	Elevated
≥500	Very elevated

HDL = high-density lipoprotein; LDL = low-density-lipoprotein. Data from National Cholesterol Education Program: Detection, evaluation, and treatment of high blood cholesterol in adults (Adult Treatment Panel III). National Institutes of Health Publication No.01–3670, Bethesda, 2001.

as prevention for stroke in normotensive women aged 65 years or older for whom the lowered risks for ischemic stroke and myocardial infarction outweigh the risks for gastrointestinal bleeding and hemorrhagic stroke (Bushnell, 2014). There is no consensus as to the optimal dose or frequency of aspirin for prevention. Options are 81 mg daily or 100 mg every other day.

■ Dyslipidemia

Hypercholesterolemia

Data support that low-density lipoprotein cholesterol (LDL) is the primary atherogenic agent. Although previously believed merely to collect passively within vessel walls, LDL is now felt to be a potent proinflammatory agent and creates the chronic inflammatory response characteristic of atherosclerosis. Logically, elevated levels of total and LDL cholesterol are associated with increased rates of coronary artery disease, ischemic stroke, and other atherosclerotic vascular complications (Horenstein, 2002; Law, 1994).

Preventively, the National Cholesterol Education Program Adult Treatment Panel-III (ATP-III) (2001) recommends that all adults 20 years and older be screened with a fasting serum lipoprotein profile once every 5 years. This profile includes measurement of total, LDL, and high-density lipoprotein (HDL) cholesterol

levels and triglyceride concentrations. Table 1-12 lists interpretation of these levels. Notably, if other comorbid risks for coronary heart disease are present, then LDL goals are more stringent.

Lowering LDL levels has been associated with reduced rates of myocardial infarction and stroke (Goldstein, 2006; Sever, 2003). Initial management usually begins with lifestyle and dietary changes, discussed earlier for CVD, and outlined by the American Heart Association (Eckel, 2014). If these modifications are unsuccessful, this organization recommends lipid-lowering treatment consideration for: (1) those with known CVD, (2) those with LDL cholesterol levels at or above 190 mg/dL, (3) those aged 40 to 75 years with diabetes and LDL cholesterol levels of 70 mg/dL or more, and (4) those

TABLE 1-11. Initial Drug Therapy for Adults with Hypertension

Health Status	Goal BP	Treatment
General ≥60 yr	<150/90	Nonblack: thiazide-type diuretic, ACEI, ARB, or CCB
General <60 yr	<140/90	Black: thiazide-type diuretic or CCB
Diabetes	<140/90	
Renal disease	<140/90	ACEI or ARB

ACEI = angiotensin-converting enzyme inhibitor; ARB = angiotensin-receptor blocker; BP = blood pressure; CCB = calcium-channel blocker.
Data from James PA, Oparil S, Carter BL, et al: 2014 evidence-based guideline for the management of high blood pressure in adults: report from the panel members appointed to the Eighth Joint National Committee (JNC 8). JAMA 311(5):507, 2014.

aged 40 to 75 years with LDL cholesterol levels of 70 mg/dL or higher and an estimated 10-year risk of a cardiovascular event that is at least 7.5 percent (Stone, 2014).

Hypertriglyceridemia

Triglycerides are delivered to tissues by very-low-density lipoprotein (VLDL), which is synthesized and secreted by the liver. This triglyceride-rich lipoprotein is taken up by adipose and muscle, where triglycerides are cleaved from VLDL. Ultimately, a VLDL remnant is created that is atherogenic. For this reason, triglyceride levels can be used as one marker for atherogenic lipoproteins, and high triglyceride levels have been linked to increases in CVD (Assmann, 1996; Austin, 1998). Its clinical importance is also underscored by its inclusion as one criterion for the metabolic syndrome.

Hypertriglyceridemia is diagnosed based on criteria found in Table 1-12. For most with mild or moderate triglyceride elevation, recommendations from American Heart Association emphasize diet changes and weight loss (Miller, 2011). Alternatively, for those with triglyceride levels of 500 mg/dL or greater, treatment goals focus primarily on triglyceride level lowering to prevent pancreatitis.

■ Diabetes Mellitus

Diabetes is common, and approximately 13.4 million adult women in the United States are diabetic (Centers for Disease Control and Prevention, 2014). The long-term consequences of this endocrine disorder are serious and include coronary heart disease, stroke, peripheral vascular disease, periodontal disease, nephropathy, neuropathy, and retinopathy.

The USPSTF (2014b) recommends diabetes screening for asymptomatic adults with blood pressure of 135/80 mm Hg or greater. For normotensive adults, screening is individualized based on risks. However, the American Diabetes Association (2015) recommends that screening be considered at 3-year intervals beginning at age 45, particularly in those with BMIs of 25 or above. Moreover, testing is considered at a younger age or completed more often in those who are overweight and have one or more of the other risk factors shown in Table 1-13.

Diabetes and prediabetes may be diagnosed by various laboratory tests listed in Table 1-14. Laboratory measurement of plasma glucose concentration is performed on venous samples, and the aforementioned values are based on the use of such methods. Capillary blood glucose testing using a blood glucometer is an effective monitoring tool but is not currently recommended for diagnostic use.

For those diagnosed with diabetes, referral to a specialist is usually indicated. Delayed onset and slower progression of many diabetic complications has been shown to follow control of elevated blood glucose levels (Cleary, 2006; Fioretto, 2006; Martin, 2006). Control can be achieved with diet modification alone or combined with oral hypoglycemic agents or injectable insulin. To lower diabetic morbidity, therapy goals for otherwise normal patients include hemoglobin A₁c levels below 7 percent, preprandial glucose between 80 and 130 mg/dL, blood pressure readings below 120/80 mm Hg, low-density lipoprotein (LDL) levels below 100 mg/dL, HDL levels above 50 mg/dL, triglyceride levels below 150 mg/dL, weight loss, and smoking cessation (American Diabetes Association, 2015).

TABLE 1-13. Adult Risk Factors for Diabetes Mellitus

Age ≥45 years
Body mass index ≥25
Affected first-degree relative
Physical inactivity
Ethnicity: African-, Hispanic-, Native-, and Asian-Americans; Pacific Islanders
Prior prediabetes-range test values
Prior gestational diabetes mellitus or delivery of a baby weighing >9 lb
Hypertension: ≥140/90 mm Hg
HDL cholesterol ≤35 mg/dL and/or triglyceride level ≥250 mg/dL
Polycystic ovary syndrome
Conditions associated with insulin resistance
Existing cardiovascular disease

HDL = high-density lipoprotein.
Data from American Diabetes Association, 2015 American Diabetes Association: Standards of medical care in diabetes—2015. Diabetes Care 38:S1, 2015.

Patients with "prediabetes," that is, impaired fasting glucose or impaired glucose tolerance, have an increased risk for developing diabetes. To avert or delay diabetes, management includes increased physical activity, weight loss, drugs such as metformin, nutritional counseling, and yearly diabetes screening. Metformin is considered especially for those with BMI above 35, age younger than 60 years, and prior gestational diabetes (American Diabetes Associations, 2015).

TABLE 1-14. American Diabetes Association Criteria

Diagnostic Criteria for Diabetes Mellitus

HbA₁c ≥6.5%
or
Fasting plasma glucose ≥126 mg/dL. Fasting is no caloric intake for at least 8 hr
or
2-hr plasma glucose ≥200 mg/dL during an OGTT
or
Symptoms of diabetes plus random plasma glucose concentration ≥200 mg/dL. Classic symptoms of diabetes include polyuria, polydipsia, and unexplained weight loss

Criteria for Increased Diabetes Risk (prediabetes)

Fasting plasma glucose: 100–125 mg/dL
or
2-hr plasma glucose during 75-g OGTT: 140–199 mg/dL
or
HbA₁c: 5.7–6.4%

HbA₁c = hemoglobin A₁c; OGTT = oral glucose tolerance test.
Data from American Diabetes Association: Diagnosis and classification of diabetes mellitus, Diabetes Care. 2008 Jan;31 Suppl 1:S55–S60.

TABLE 1-15. Diagnostic Criteria for Metabolic Syndrome in Women

Criteria	Thresholds
Waist circumference	≥88 cm (≥35 in)
Triglycerides	≥150 mg/dL
HDL cholesterol	<50 mg/dL
Blood pressure	≥130/85 mm Hg
Fasting glucose	≥110 mg/dL

Drug treatment for any of these conditions is considered a positive criterion.
HDL = high-density lipoprotein.
Adapted with permission from Grundy SM, Cleeman JI, Daniels SR, et al: Diagnosis and management of the metabolic syndrome: an American Heart Association/National Heart, Lung, and Blood Institute scientific statement, Circulation 2005 Oct 25;112(17):2735–2752.

Metabolic Syndrome

This syndrome is a clustering of major cardiovascular disease risk factors (Table 1-15). At present, a single unifying cause of the metabolic syndrome has not been identified, and it may be precipitated by multiple underlying risk factors. Of these, abdominal obesity and insulin resistance appear important (Grundy, 2005).

This syndrome is common, and in 2010, 22 percent of U.S. women met diagnostic criteria. Although genders appear equally affected, Mexican Americans show the highest prevalence, and incidence appears to increase in all ethnicities with age (Beltrán-Sánchez, 2014). The sequelae associated with metabolic syndrome are significant and include an increased risk of diabetes and mortality from coronary heart disease, CVD, and all causes (Lorenzo, 2003; Malik, 2004; Sattar, 2003). Among those with metabolic syndrome, risks are further increased, by cigarette smoking and elevated LDL cholesterol levels.

Goals of clinical management include reducing risks for clinical atherosclerotic disease and for diabetes. Accordingly, primary therapy for metabolic syndrome focuses on lifestyle modification, particularly weight reduction and increased exercise. During evaluation, each metabolic syndrome component is addressed and treated in accordance with current guidelines, as discussed in earlier sections.

Thyroid Disease

The risk of thyroid disease increases with age, and dysfunction is more common in women. Accordingly, the American Thyroid Association recommends that adults, especially women, be screened for thyroid dysfunction by measurement of a serum thyroid-stimulating hormone (TSH) concentration. This begins at age 35 years and is repeated every 5 years thereafter (Garber, 2012). Moreover, individuals with clinical manifestations potentially attributable to thyroid dysfunction and those with risk factors for its development may require more frequent testing. People at higher risk for thyroid dysfunction include the elderly and those with prior neck radiation, thyroid surgery, autoimmune disease, affected first-degree relative, psychiatric disorders, or lithium use. In contrast, the U.S. Preventive Service Task Force (2004b) has found insufficient evidence to recommend for or against routine screening in asymptomatic women.

Geriatric Screening

Women are now living longer, and the current life expectancy for women in the United States is 81 years (Arias, 2014). As a woman moves past menopause, many of her health care needs may not be gynecologic. However, a family may often contact a patient's gynecologist first regarding a member's lack of independent function or memory loss.

Of these, functional status is a patient's ability to perform both basic and complex activities for independent living. Basic activities are grooming and toileting, whereas checkbook balancing, bill paying, and housekeeping tasks are more complex, instrumental activities of daily living (Katz, 1963; Lawton, 1969). Declines in functional status are linked to increased risks of hospitalization, institutionalization, and death (Walston, 2006). Identification of functional status loss may permit early intervention.

Second, loss of cognitive function may present as short- and long-term memory loss, difficulty with problem solving, or inattention to personal hygiene. Although not expert in recognition of cognitive problems, a gynecologist can perform initial screening and provide results that either reassure the patient and her family or prompt more formal evaluation by a geriatrician or neurologist.

For dementia, the Mini Mental Status Exam or, more recently, the Mini-Cog Test can screen for cognitive impairment in the primary care setting (Borson, 2000, 2006; Folstein, 1975). The Mini-Cog test requires approximately 3 minutes to administer and begins by giving the patient three items to remember early in the interview. Later in discussion, she is asked to recall those three items. For the clock-drawing test, a person is asked to draw a clock with the hands at a specific time, such as 8:30. A correct clock has numbers 1 through 12 labeled correctly in a clockwise fashion, with two arms (of any length) pointing at the correct numbers for the time requested. Any error or refusal to complete the clock is considered abnormal. An algorithm for scoring the Mini-Cog is shown in Figure 1-10. For a Mini-Cog Test result suggestive of dementia, referral to an internist, geriatrician, or neurologist, as available to the patient in that community, is indicated.

Mental Health

Depression and Intimate Partner Violence

For women of all ages, these problems are pervasive and account for significant morbidity and mortality. Each is discussed in

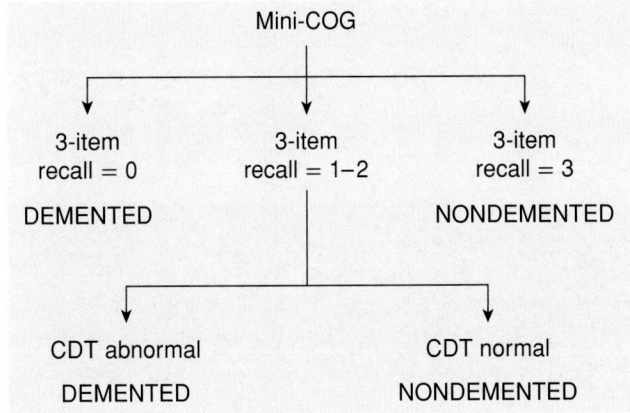

FIGURE 1-10 The Mini-Cog Test. CDT = clock-drawing test. (Modified with permission from Borson S, Scanlan J, Brush M, et al: The Mini-Cog: a cognitive "vital signs" measure for dementia screening in multi-lingual elderly. Int J Geriatr Psychiatry 2000 Nov;15(11):1021–1027.)

detail in Chapter 13 and should be routinely screened for at routine health visits. Simple questions such as "During the past 2 weeks, have you felt down, depressed, or hopeless?" and "Have you felt little interest or pleasure in doing things?" are often effective (Whooley, 1997). These two questions constitute the Personal Health Questionnaire-2 (PHQ2), a validated screening tool for depression (Kroenke, 2003). Any positive screening test should prompt further evaluation for depression as outlined in Chapter 13 (p. 298).

For intimate partner violence, American College of Obstetricians and Gynecologists (2012a) guidelines recommend that physicians routinely ask direct, specific questions regarding abuse. General introductory statements such as "Because abuse and violence are so common in women's lives, I've begun to ask about it routinely" can help a health care provider introduce this subject for discussion.

Insomnia

Insomnia is common, and its definition includes: (1) difficulty initiating sleep, (2) trouble maintaining sleep, and (3) early waking. Insomnia may be primary or may be secondary to other conditions such as depression, time-zone travel, restless leg syndrome, stimulant use, and sleep apnea (National Institutes of Health, 2005). Accordingly, historical inventory investigates and treatment addresses these and other secondary causes.

Treatment of primary insomnia is typically cognitive-behavioral or pharmacologic. Cognitive therapy is aimed at changing patients' beliefs and attitudes regarding sleep. Behavioral therapies are varied and include those that control sleep timing and duration; attempt to improve the bedroom environment; or focus on relaxation or biofeedback techniques (Morgenthaler, 2006; Silber, 2005). Medications may be used to aid sleep, and most agents are of the benzodiazepine family (Table 1-16).

TABLE 1-16. Insomnia Medications Approved by the U.S. Food and Drug Administration

Medication: Brand	Dose
Benzodiazepines	
Temazepam: Restoril	7.5–30 mg
Estazolam: ProSom	0.5–2 mg
Triazolam: Halcion	0.125–0.25 mg
Flurazepam: Dalmane	15–30 mg
Quazepam: Doral	7.5–15 mg
Benzodiazepine-Receptor Agonists	
Eszopiclone: Lunesta	1–3 mg
Zolpidem: Ambien,	5–10 mg
Ambien CR[a]	6.25–12.5 mg
Intermezzo[b]	1.75 mg
Zaleplon: Sonata	5–20 mg
Melatonin-Receptor Agonist	
Ramelteon: Rozerem	8 mg

[a]Extended release form.
[b]Indicated for middle-of-night awakening.

■ Preconceptional Counseling

Value lies in counseling women before conception so that each pregnancy is planned with the goal to achieve the best maternal and fetal outcomes. With this in mind, topics found in Table 1-17 are ideally addressed (American College of Obstetricians and Gynecologists, 2012b; Jack, 2008).

TABLE 1-17. Preconceptional Counseling Topics

Condition	Recommendations for Preconceptional Counseling
Abnormal weight	Calculate BMI yearly. *BMI ≥25 kg/m²:* Counsel on diet. Test for DM and metabolic syndrome if indicated *BMI ≤18.5 kg/m²:* Assess for eating disorder
Heart disease	Counsel on cardiac risks during pregnancy. Optimize cardiac function, offer effective BCM during this time. Discuss warfarin, ACE inhibitor, and ARB teratogenicity, and if possible, switch to less dangerous agent when conception planned. Offer genetic counseling to those with congenital cardiac anomalies. Review infective endocarditis risks (Nishimura, 2014)
Hypertension	Counsel on specific risks during pregnancy. Assess those with long-standing HTN for ventricular hypertrophy, retinopathy, and renal disease. Counsel women taking ACE inhibitors and ARBs on drug teratogenicity, on effective BCM during use, and on the need to switch agents prior to conception
Asthma	Counsel on asthma risks during pregnancy. Optimize pulmonary function and offer effective BCM during this time. Treat women with pharmacological step therapy for chronic asthma based on ACOG-ACAAI (2000) recommendations
Thrombophilia	Question for personal or family history of thrombotic events or recurrent poor pregnancy outcomes. If found, counsel and screen those contemplating pregnancy. Offer genetic counseling to those with known thrombophilia. Discuss warfarin teratogenicity, offer effective BCM during use, and switch to a less teratogenic agent, if possible, prior to conception

(Continued)

TABLE 1-17. Preconceptional Counseling Topics *(Continued)*

Condition	Recommendations for Preconceptional Counseling
Renal disease	Counsel on specific risks during pregnancy. Optimize blood pressure control and offer effective BCM during this time. Counsel women taking ACE inhibitors and ARBs on their teratogenicity, on effective BCM during use, and on the need to switch agents prior to conception
GI disease	*Inflammatory bowel disease:* Counsel affected women on subfertility risks and risks of adverse pregnancy outcomes. Discuss teratogenicity of MTX and the other immunomodulators, about which less is known, e.g., mycophenolate mofetil. Offer effective BCM during their use and switch agents, if possible, prior to conception
Liver disease	*Hepatitis B:* Vaccinate all high-risk women prior to conception (Table 1-2, p. 8). Counsel chronic carriers on transmission prevention to partners and fetus *Hepatitis C:* Screen high-risk women. Counsel affected women on risks of disease and transmission. Refer for treatment, discuss ramifications of treatment during pregnancy, and offer effective BCM
Hematologic disease	*Sickle-cell disease:* Screen all black women. Counsel those with trait or disease. Test partner if desired *Thalassemias:* Screen women of Southeast Asian or Mediterranean ancestry
Diabetes	Advocate good glucose control, especially in periconceptional period to decrease known teratogenicity of overt diabetes. Evaluate for retinopathy, nephropathy, hypertension, etc.
Thyroid disease	Screen those with thyroid disease symptoms. Ensure iodine-sufficient diet. Treat overt hyper- or hypothyroidism prior to conception. Counsel on risks to pregnancy outcome
CT disease	*RA:* Counsel on flare risk after pregnancy. Discuss MTX and leflunomide teratogenicity. Offer effective BCM during their use and switch agents prior to conception. *SLE:* Counsel on risks during pregnancy. Optimize disease. Discuss mycophenolate mofetil and cyclophosphamide teratogenicity; offer effective BCM during their use. If possible, switch agents prior to conception
Neurologic and psychiatric disorders	*Depression:* Screen for symptoms. If affected, counsel on risks of treatment and of untreated illness and high risk of peripartum exacerbation *Seizure disorder:* Optimize seizure control using monotherapy if possible
Skin disease	Discuss isotretinoin and etretinate teratogenicity, offer effective BCM during their use, switch agents prior to conception
Cancer	Counsel on fertility preservation options prior to cancer therapy and on decreased fertility following certain agents. Offer genetic counseling to those with mutation-linked cancers. Evaluate cardiac function in those given cardiotoxic agents, such as adriamycin. Obtain mammography for those given childhood chest radiotherapy. Discuss SERM teratogenicity, effective BCM during its use, and need to switch agents prior to conception. Review chemotherapy and discuss possible teratogenic effects if continued during pregnancy
Infectious disease	*Influenza:* Vaccinate all women prior to flu season *Malaria:* Avoid travel to endemic areas; offer effective BCM or chemoprophylaxis for those planning pregnancy *Rubella:* Assess immunity; vaccinate as needed and offer effective BCM during next 3 months *Tuberculosis:* Screen high-risk women and treat *Tetanus:* Update vaccination, as needed *Varicella:* Assess immunity; vaccinate as needed and offer effective BCM during next 3 months
STD	*Gonorrhea, syphilis, chlamydial infection:* Screen per Table 1-1 (p. 6) and treat as indicated *HIV:* Discuss initiation of treatment prior to conception to decrease perinatal transmission. Offer effective BCM to those not desiring conception *HPV:* Provide screening per guidelines (Chap. 29, p. 629). Vaccinate as indicated *HSV:* Provide serological screening to asymptomatic women with affected partners. Counsel affected women on risks of perinatal transmission and of preventive measures during the third trimester and labor

ACAAI = American College of Allergy, Asthma, and Immunology; ACE = angiotensin-converting enzyme; ACOG = American College of Obstetricians and Gynecologists; BCM = birth control method; ARB = angiotensin-receptor blocker; BMI = body mass index; HIV = human immunodeficiency virus; HPV = human papillomavirus; HSV = herpes simplex virus; HTN = hypertension; MTX = methotrexate; NSAID = nonsteroidal antiinflammatory drug; RA = rheumatoid arthritis; SERM = selective estrogen-receptor modulator; SLE = systemic lupus erythematosus; STD = sexually transmitted disease. Data from American College of Obstetricians and Gynecologist, 2012b; Jack, 2008; Kim, 2015.

REFERENCES

American Cancer Society: Skin cancer prevention and early detection. 2013. Available at: http://www.cancer.org/acs/groups/cid/documents/webcontent/003184-pdf.pdf. Accessed February 11, 2015

American Cancer Society: Breast cancer prevention and early detection. 2014. Available at: http://www.cancer.org/acs/groups/cid/documents/webcontent/003165-pdf.pdf. Accessed February 11, 2015

American College of Obstetricians and Gynecologists: Adolescent confidentiality and electronic health records. Committee Opinion No. 599, May 2014a

American College of Obstetricians and Gynecologists: Bariatric surgery and pregnancy. Practice Bulletin No. 105, June 2009, Reaffirmed 2013

American College of Obstetricians and Gynecologists: Breast cancer screening. Practice Bulletin No. 122, August 2011, Reaffirmed 2014b

American College of Obstetricians and Gynecologists: Guidelines for Women's Health Care, 4th ed. Washington, 2014c

American College of Obstetricians and Gynecologists: Intimate partner violence. Committee Opinion No. 518, February 2012a

American College of Obstetricians and Gynecologists: Routine human immunodeficiency virus screening. Committee Opinion No. 596, May 2014d

American College of Obstetricians and Gynecologists: The importance of preconception care in the continuum of women's health care. Committee Opinion No. 313, September 2005, Reaffirmed 2012b

American College of Obstetricians and Gynecologists: The initial reproductive health visit. Committee Opinion No. 598, May 2014e

American College of Obstetricians and Gynecologists: Well-woman visit. Committee Opinion No. 534, August 2012, Reaffirmed 2014f

American College of Obstetricians and Gynecologists (ACOG) and American College of Allergy, Asthma and Immunology (ACAAI): The use of newer asthma and allergy medications during pregnancy. Ann Allergy Asthma Immunol 84(5):475, 2000

American Diabetes Association: Standards of medical care in diabetes—2015. Diabetes Care 38:S1, 2015

American Heart Association: Understanding Blood Pressure Readings. 2014. Available at: http://www.heart.org/HEARTORG/Conditions/HighBlood Pressure/AboutHighBloodPressure/Understanding-Blood-Pressure-Readings_UCM_301764_Article.jsp. Accessed July 14, 2015

Arias E: United States life tables, 2010. Natl Vital Stat Rep 63(7):1, 2014

Assmann G, Schulte H, von Eckardstein A: Hypertriglyceridemia and elevated lipoprotein(a) are risk factors for major coronary events in middle-aged men. Am J Cardiol 77(14):1179, 1996

Astrup A, Rössner S, Van Gaal L, et al: Effects of liraglutide in the treatment of obesity: a randomised, double-blind, placebo-controlled study. Lancet 374(9701):1606, 2009

Austin MA, Hokanson JE, Edwards KL: Hypertriglyceridemia as a cardiovascular risk factor. Am J Cardiol 81(4A):7B, 1998

Beltrán-Sánchez H, Harhay MO, Harhay MM, et al: Prevalence and trends of metabolic syndrome in the adult U.S. population, 1999–2010. J Am Coll Cardiol 62(8):697, 2013

Blackwell DL, Lucas JW, Clarke TC: Summary health statistics for U.S. adults: national health interview survey, 2012. Vital Health Stat 10(260):1, 2014

Borson S, Scanlan J, Brush M, et al: The Mini-Cog: a cognitive "vital signs" measure for dementia screening in multi-lingual elderly. Int J Geriatr Psychiatry 15:1021, 2000

Borson S, Scanlan J, Watanabe J, et al: Improving identification of cognitive impairment in primary care. Int J Geriatr Psychiatry 21:349, 2006

Braith RW, Stewart KJ: Resistance exercise training: its role in the prevention of cardiovascular disease. Circulation 113(22):2642, 2006

Brosse AL, Sheets ES, Lett HS, et al: Exercise and the treatment of clinical depression in adults: recent findings and future directions. Sports Med 32:741, 2002

Bushnell C, McCullough L: Stroke prevention in women: synopsis of 2014 American Heart Association/American Stroke Association Guidelines. Ann Intern Med 160:853, 2014

Centers for Disease Control and Prevention: National diabetes statistics report: estimates of diabetes and its burden in the United States, 2014. Atlanta, U.S. Department of Health and Human Services, 2014

Centers for Disease Control and Prevention: Sexually transmitted diseases treatment guidelines, 2014. MMWR xx(xx):1, 2015

Centers for Disease Control and Prevention: U.S. Selected Practice Recommendations for Contraceptive Use, 2013. MMWR Recomm Rep 62(5):1, 2013

Chobanian AV, Bakris GL, Black HR, et al: The Seventh Report of the Joint National Committee on Prevention, Detection, Evaluation, and Treatment of High Blood Pressure: the JNC 7 report. JAMA 289(19):2560, 2003

Cleary PA, Orchard TJ, Genuth S, et al: The effect of intensive glycemic treatment on coronary artery calcification in type 1 diabetic participants of the Diabetes

Control and Complications Trial/Epidemiology of Diabetes Interventions and Complications (DCCT/EDIC) Study. Diabetes 55(12):3556, 2006

Eckel RH, Jakicic JM, Ard JD, et al: 2013 AHA/ACC guideline on lifestyle management to reduce cardiovascular risk: a report of the American College of Cardiology/American Heart Association Task Force on Practice Guidelines. Circulation 129(25 Suppl 2):S76, 2014

Fidler MC, Sanchez M, Raether B, et al: A one-year randomized trial of lorcaserin for weight loss in obese and overweight adults: the BLOSSOM trial. J Clin Endocrinol Metab 96(10):3067, 2011

Fiore MC, Jaen CR, Baker TB, et al: Treating tobacco use and dependence: 2008 update. Rockville, U.S. Department of Health and Human Services, 2008

Fioretto P, Bruseghin M, Berto I, et al: Renal protection in diabetes: role of glycemic control. J Am Soc Nephrol 17(4 Suppl 2):S86, 2006

Flegal KM, Carroll MD, Kit BK, et al: Prevalence of obesity and trends in the distribution of body mass index among US adults, 1999–2010. JAMA 307(5):491, 2012

Folstein M, Folstein S, McHugh P: "Mini-mental state". A practical method for grading the cognitive state of patients for the clinician. J Psychiatr Res 12:189, 1975

Food and Drug Administration: Completed safety review of Xenical/Alli (orlistat) and severe liver injury. 2010. http://www.fda.gov/Drugs/DrugSafety/PostmarketDrugSafetyInformationforPatientsandProviders/ucm213038.htm. Accessed February 13, 2015

Gadde KM, Allison DB, Ryan DH, et al: Effects of low-dose, controlled-release, phentermine plus topiramate combination on weight and associated comorbidities in overweight and obese adults (CONQUER): a randomised, placebo-controlled, phase 3 trial. Lancet 377(9774):1341, 2011

Garber JR, Cobin RH, Gharib H, et al: Clinical practice guidelines for hypothyroidism in adults: cosponsored by the American Association of Clinical Endocrinologists and the American Thyroid Association. Endocr Pract 18(6):988, 2012

Go AS, Mozaffarian D, Roger VL, et al: Heart disease and stroke statistics—2014 update: a report from the American Heart Association. Circulation 129(3):e28, 2014

Goldstein LB, Adams RM, Alberts MJ, et al: Primary prevention of ischemic stroke: a guideline from the American Heart Association/American Stroke Association Stroke Council. Stroke 37:1583, 2006

Griffith WF, Stuart GS, Gluck KL, et al: Vaginal speculum lubrication and its effects on cervical cytology and microbiology. Contraception 72(1):60, 2005

Grundy SM, Cleeman JI, Daniels SR, et al: Diagnosis and management of the metabolic syndrome: an American Heart Association/National Heart, Lung, and Blood Institute scientific statement. Circulation 112(17):2735, 2005

Henness S, Perry CM: Orlistat: a review of its use in the management of obesity. Drugs 66(12):1625, 2006

Horenstein RB, Smith DE, Mosca L: Cholesterol predicts stroke mortality in the Women's Pooling Project. Stroke 33(7):1863, 2002

Hutter MM, Schirmer BD, Jones DB, et al: First report from the American College of Surgeons Bariatric Surgery Center Network: laparoscopic sleeve gastrectomy has morbidity and effectiveness positioned between the band and the bypass. Ann Surg 254(3):410, 2011

Imperiale TF, Ransohoff DF, Itzkowitz SH, et al: Multitarget stool DNA testing for colorectal-cancer screening. N Engl J Med 370(14):1287, 2014

Institute of Medicine Report: Clinical preventive services for women: closing the gaps. Washington, National Academies Press, 2011

Jack BW, Atrash H, Coonrod DV, et al: The clinical content of preconception care: an overview and preparation of this supplement. Am J Obstet Gynecol 199(6 Suppl 2):S266, 2008

Jackson TD, Hutter MM: Morbidity and effectiveness of laparoscopic sleeve gastrectomy, adjustable gastric band, and gastric bypass for morbid obesity. Adv Surg 46:255, 2012

James PA, Oparil S, Carter BL, et al: 2014 evidence-based guideline for the management of high blood pressure in adults: report from the panel members appointed to the Eighth Joint National Committee (JNC 8). JAMA 311(5):507, 2014

Jensen MD, Ryan DH, Apovian CM, et al: 2013 AHA/ACC/TOS guideline for the management of overweight and obesity in adults: a report of the American College of Cardiology/American Heart Association Task Force on Practice Guidelines and The Obesity Society. Circulation 129(25 Suppl 2):S102, 2014

Katz S, Ford AB, Moskowitz RW, et al: Studies of illness in the aged. The index of ADL: a standardized measure of biological and psychosocial function. JAMA 185:914, 1963

Kim DK, Bridges CB, Harriman HK, et al: Advisory Committee on Immunization Practices recommended immunization schedule for adults aged 19 years or older: United States, 2015. Ann Intern Med 162:214, 2015

Knowler WC, Barrett-Connor E, Fowler SE, et al: Reduction in the incidence of type 2 diabetes with lifestyle intervention or metformin. N Engl J Med 346:393, 2002

Kösters JP, Gøtzsche PC: Regular self-examination or clinical examination for early detection of breast cancer. Cochrane Database Syst Rev 3:CD003373, 2008

Kroenke K, Spitzer RL, Williams JB: The Patient Health Questionnaire-2: validity of a two-item depression screener. Med Care 41(11):1284, 2003

Law MR, Wald NJ, Thompson SG: By how much and how quickly does reduction in serum cholesterol concentration lower risk of ischaemic heart disease? BMJ 308(6925):367, 1994

Lawton MP, Brody EM: Assessment of older people: self-monitoring and instrumental activities of daily living. Gerontologist 9:179, 1969

Lee IM: Physical activity and cancer prevention—data from epidemiologic studies. Med Sci Sports Exercise 35(11):1823, 2003

Levin B, Lieberman DA, McFarland B, et al: Screening and surveillance for the early detection of colorectal cancer and adenomatous polyps, 2008: a joint guideline from the American Cancer Society, the U.S. Multi-Society Task Force on Colorectal Cancer, and the American College of Radiology. CA Cancer J Clin 58(3):130, 2008

Lorenzo C, Okoloise M, Williams K, et al: The metabolic syndrome as predictor of type 2 diabetes: the San Antonio heart study. Diabetes Care 26(11):3153, 2003

Mainous AG III, Everett CJ, Liszka H, et al: Prehypertension and mortality in a nationally representative cohort. Am J Cardiol 94(12):1496, 2004

Malik S, Wong ND, Franklin SS, et al: Impact of the metabolic syndrome on mortality from coronary heart disease, cardiovascular disease, and all causes in United States adults. Circulation 110(10):1245, 2004

Martin CL, Albers J, Herman WH, et al: Neuropathy among the diabetes control and complications trial cohort 8 years after trial completion. Diabetes Care 29(2):340, 2006

McDonald S, Saslow D, Alciati MH: Performance and reporting of clinical breast examination: a review of the literature. CA Cancer J Clin 54:345, 2004

Meissner HI, Breen N, Klabunde CN, et al: Patterns of colorectal cancer screening uptake among men and women in the United States. Cancer Epidemiol Biomarkers Prev 15(2):389, 2006

Merhi ZO: Impact of bariatric surgery on female reproduction. Fertil Steril 92(5):1501, 2009

Miller M, Stone NJ, Ballantyne C, et al: Triglycerides and cardiovascular disease: a scientific statement from the American Heart Association. Circulation 123(20):2292, 2011

Morgenthaler T, Kramer M, Alessi C, et al: Practice parameters for the psychological and behavioral treatment of insomnia: an update. An American Academy of Sleep Medicine report. Sleep 29(11):1415, 2006

Mosca L, Benjamin EJ, Berra K, et al: Effectiveness-based guidelines for prevention of cardiovascular disease in women—2011 update. Circulation 123:1243, 2011

National Cancer Institute: Breast Cancer Screening (PDQ®). Available at: http://www.cancer.gov/cancertopics/pdq/screening/breast/healthprofessional/page1. Accessed February 12, 2015

National Cholesterol Education Program: Detection, evaluation, and treatment of high blood cholesterol in adults (Adult Treatment Panel III). National Institutes of Health Publication No.01–3670, Bethesda, 2001

National Heart, Lung, and Blood Institute: The practical guide: identification, evaluation, and treatment of overweight and obesity in adults. National Institutes of Health Publication No. 98–4084, Bethesda, 2000

National Institutes of Health: NIH state-of-the-science conference statement on manifestations and management of chronic insomnia in adults. NIH Consens State Sci Statements 22(2):1, 2005

Nishimura RA, Otto CM, Bonow RO, et al: 2014 AHA/ACC Guideline for the Management of Patients with Valvular Heart Disease: a report of the American College of Cardiology/American Heart Association Task Force on Practice Guidelines. Circulation 129(23):e521, 2014

Oeffinger KC, Fontham, ET, Etzioni R, et al: Breast cancer screening for women at average risk 2015 guideline update from the American Cancer Society. JAMA 314(15):1599, 2015

Pescatello LS, Franklin BA, Fagard R, et al: American College of Sports Medicine position stand. Exercise and hypertension. Med Sci Sports Exercise 36(3):533, 2004

Qaseem A, Humphrey LL, Harris R, et al: Screening pelvic examination in adult women: a clinical practice guideline from the American College of Physicians. Ann Intern Med 161:67, 2014

Sanford KW, McPherson RA: Fecal occult blood testing. Clin Lab Med 29(15):523, 2009

Saslow D, Hannan J, Osuch J, et al: Clinical breast examination: practical recommendations for optimizing performance and reporting. CA Cancer J Clin 54:327, 2004

Sattar N, Gaw A, Scherbakova O, et al: Metabolic syndrome with and without C-reactive protein as a predictor of coronary heart disease and diabetes in the West of Scotland Coronary Prevention Study. Circulation 108(4):414, 2003

Schuster RJ, Tasosa J, Tenwood NA: Translational research—implementation of NHLBI Obesity Guidelines in a primary care community setting: the Physician Obesity Awareness Project. J Nutr Health Aging 12(10):764S, 2008

Sever PS, Dahlof B, Poulter NR, et al: Prevention of coronary and stroke events with atorvastatin in hypertensive patients who have average or lower-than-average cholesterol concentrations, in the Anglo-Scandinavian Cardiac Outcomes Trial—Lipid Lowering Arm (ASCOT-LLA): a multicentre randomised controlled trial. Lancet 361:1149, 2003

Siegel RL, Miller KD, Jemal A: Cancer statistics, 2015. CA Cancer J Clin 65(1):5, 2015

Sigal RJ, Kenny GP, Wasserman DH, et al: Physical activity/exercise and type 2 diabetes. Diabetes Care 27(10):2518, 2004

Silber MH: Clinical practice. Chronic insomnia. N Engl J Med 353(8):803, 2005

Smith RA, Manassaram-Baptiste D, Brooks D, et al: Cancer screening in the United States, 2015: a review of current American Cancer Society guidelines and current issues in cancer screening. CA Cancer J Clin 65(1):30, 2015

Smith SR, Weissman NJ, Anderson CM, et al: Multicenter, placebo-controlled trial of lorcaserin for weight management. N Engl J Med 363(3):245, 2010

Stone NJ, Robinson JG, Lichtenstein AH, et al: 2013 ACC/AHA guideline on the treatment of blood cholesterol to reduce atherosclerotic cardiovascular risk in adults: a report of the American College of Cardiology/American Heart Association Task Force on Practice Guidelines. Circulation 29(25 Suppl 2):S1, 2014

Thomas DB, Gao DL, Ray RM: Randomized trial of breast self-examination in Shanghai: final results. J Natl Cancer Inst 94(19):1445, 2002

Torrijos RM, Glantz SA: The US Public Health Service "treating tobacco use and dependence clinical practice guidelines" as a legal standard of care. Tob Control 15(6):447, 2006

U.S. Department of Health and Human Services: 2008 Physical activity guidelines for Americans. Available at: http://www.health.gov/PAGuidelines/pdf/paguide.pdf. Accessed February 13, 2015

U.S. Preventive Services Task Force: Screening for breast cancer. 2009. Available at: http://www.uspreventiveservicestaskforce.org/Page/Topic/recommendation-summary/breast-cancer-screening. Accessed February 12, 2015

U.S. Preventive Services Task Force: Screening for genital herpes. 2005. Available at: http://www.uspreventiveservicestaskforce.org/uspstf05/herpes/herpesrs.htm. Accessed February 13, 2015

U.S. Preventive Services Task Force: Screening for hepatitis B virus infection. 2014a. Available at: http://www.uspreventiveservicestaskforce.org/Page/Topic/recommendation-summary/hepatitis-b-virus-infection-screening-2014. Accessed February 13, 2015

U.S. Preventive Services Task Force: Screening for syphilis infection. 2004a. Available at: http://www.uspreventiveservicestaskforce.org/3rduspstf/syphilis/syphilrs.htm. Accessed February 13, 2015

U.S. Preventive Services Task Force: Screening for thyroid disease. 2004b. Available at: http://www.uspreventiveservicestaskforce.org/Page/Topic/recommendation-summary/thyroid-disease-screening. Accessed February 13, 2015

U.S. Preventive Services Task Force: The Guide to Clinical Preventive Services, 2014b. Rockville, 2014

Vuori IM: Dose-response of physical activity and low back pain, osteoarthritis, and osteoporosis. Med Sci Sports Exerc 33(6 Suppl):S551, 2001

Walston J, Hadley EC, Ferrucci L, et al: Research agenda for frailty in older adults: toward a better understanding of physiology and etiology: summary from the American Geriatrics Society/National Institute on Aging Research Conference on Frailty in Older Adults. J Am Geriatr Soc 54(6):991, 2006

Wang Y, Wang QJ: The prevalence of prehypertension and hypertension among US adults according to the new joint national committee guidelines: new challenges of the old problem. Arch Intern Med 164(19):2126, 2004

Whooley MA, Avins AL, Miranda J, et al: Case-finding instruments for depression. Two questions are as good as many. J Gen Intern Med 12(7):439, 1997

Williams MA, Haskell WL, Ades PA, et al: Resistance exercise in individuals with and without cardiovascular disease: 2007 update: a scientific statement from the American Heart Association Council on Clinical Cardiology and Council on Nutrition, Physical Activity, and Metabolism. Circulation 116(5):572, 2007

Wolff T, Tai E, Miller T: Screening for skin cancer: an update of the evidence for the U.S. Preventive Services Task Force. Ann Intern Med 150:194, 2009

Youngstedt SD: Effects of exercise on sleep. Clin Sports Med 24:355, 2005

Zieman M, Guillebaud J, Weisberg E, et al: Contraceptive efficacy and cycle control with the Ortho Evra/Evra transdermal system: the analysis of pooled data. Fertil Steril 77:S13, 2002

CHAPTER 2

Techniques Used for Imaging in Gynecology

Several technical advances made in recent decades currently allow superb imaging of female pelvic structures. As a result, use of sonography in gynecology now equals that in obstetrics. Enhancements to traditional sonography continue to fill important clinical gaps. For example, three-dimensional (3-D) imaging refinements have expanded the gynecologic indications of sonography to rival those of computed tomography (CT) and magnetic resonance (MR) imaging for many conditions. Similarly, application of MR imaging has been extended by MR-guided high-intensity focused ultrasound therapy, used for uterine leiomyoma treatment.

SONOGRAPHY

■ Physics

In sonography, the picture displayed on a screen is produced by sound waves reflected back from an imaged structure. To begin, alternating current is applied to a transducer containing piezoelectric crystals, which convert electric energy to high-frequency sound waves. A water-soluble gel applied to the skin acts as a coupling agent. Sound waves then pass through tissue layers, encounter an interface between tissues of different densities, and are reflected back to the transducer. Converted back into electric energy, they are displayed on a screen.

Dense material, such as bone, or a synthetic material, such as an intrauterine device (IUD), produces high-velocity reflected waves, also termed *echoes*, which are displayed on a screen as white. These are described as *echogenic*. Conversely, fluid is

anechoic, generates few reflected waves, and appears black on a screen. Middle-density tissues variably reflect waves to create various shades of gray, and images are described as *hypoechoic* or *hyperechoic* relative to tissues immediately adjacent to them. Images are generated so quickly—50 to 100 frames/sec—that the picture on the screen appears to move in real time.

Sound reflection is greatest when the difference between the acoustic impedance of two structures is large. This explains why cysts are so well demonstrated with sonography. Strong echoes are produced from the cyst walls, but no echoes arise from the cyst fluid. As more sound traverses the cyst, more echoes are received from the area behind the cyst, a feature known as *through transmission* or *acoustic enhancement* (Fig. 2-1). In contrast, with a dense structure, the sound passing through it is diminished, which creates a band of reduced echoes beyond it, known as *acoustic shadowing* (Fig. 2-2).

The frequency of emitted ultrasound waves is expressed in megahertz (MHz), which means million vibrations per second. The frequency is inversely related to its wavelength, such that transducers emitting pulses of high frequency generate waves of shorter length, which result in higher spatial resolution or sharpness between interfaces but achieve less penetration. Curved transducers provide a wider field of view but often generate lower frequency waves than linear transducers. Higher frequency probes (10 to 15 MHz) are used to image superficial structures, such as breast masses or lost etonogestrel implants in the upper arm. Lower frequencies are required to image deeper structures. For example, transabdominal transducers are typically in the 3- to 5-MHz range, whereas transvaginal transducers are generally 5 to 10 MHz.

■ Examination Techniques

Guidelines for sonographic examination of the female pelvis have been established by The American Institute of Ultrasound in Medicine (2014). These serve as quality assurance standards for patient care and provide assistance to practitioners performing sonography. Guidelines describe equipment and documentation and may be accessed at: http://www.aium.org/resources/guidelines/femalepelvis.pdf.

All probes are cleaned after each examination, and vaginal probes are covered by a protective sheath prior to insertion. A female staff member should always chaperone transvaginal sonography. Guidelines describe the examination steps for each organ and anatomic region in the female pelvis. For instance, for the uterus: uterine size, shape, orientation, and description of the endometrium, myometrium, and cervix are documented. The examination and its interpretation are permanently recorded,

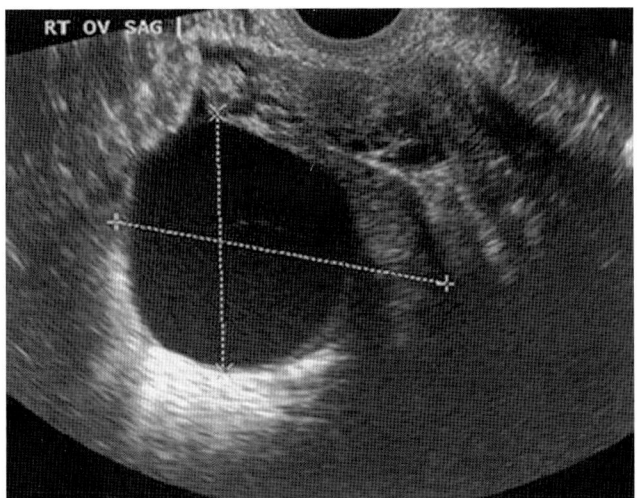

FIGURE 2-1 Transvaginal sonogram of a premenopausal ovary containing a follicular cyst. The cyst fluid appears black or anechoic. Note the white or hyperechoic area under the cyst, a sonographic feature called posterior acoustic enhancement or through transmission.

appropriately labeled, and placed in the medical record. A copy is also kept by the facility performing the study.

Gray-scale Imaging

Various examination techniques can be used for sonographic study of the female pelvis. Of these, transabdominal evaluation, using a curved-array 3- to 5-MHz transducer, is the first component of general gynecologic examinations because it provides global identification of all pelvic organs and their spatial relationships (American Institute of Ultrasound in Medicine, 2014). In a nonpregnant patient, a full bladder is preferred for adequate viewing, as it pushes the uterus upward from behind the pubic symphysis and displaces small bowel from the field of view. Moreover, the bladder acts as an *acoustic window*, to improve ultrasound wave transmission. In patients with large lesions or masses located superior to the bladder dome, transabdominal sonography provides a panoramic view for greater disease evaluation. Still, endometrial

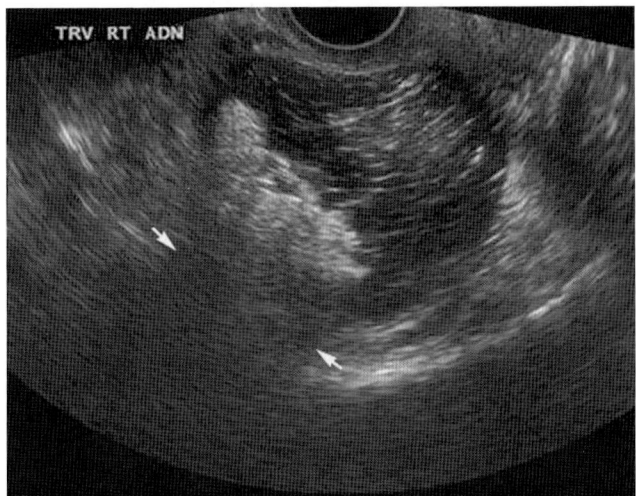

FIGURE 2-2 Transvaginal sonogram of an ovarian teratoma demonstrating posterior acoustic shadowing (*arrows*).

cavity assessment is limited with a transabdominal approach and often requires the transvaginal technique.

Transvaginal sonography (TVS) uses higher-frequency (5- to 10-MHz) transducers and is the second component of general gynecologic examinations. Because of its increased sensitivity and spatial image resolution, TVS is ideal for interrogating pelvic anatomy within the confines of the true pelvis. With larger masses, imaging may be incomplete and is complemented by transabdominal sonography.

For TVS, the probe is positioned in the vaginal fornices to place the transducer close to the region of interest and thereby lessen beam attenuation within superficial soft tissues. In contrast to transabdominal imaging, the bladder is emptied prior to a transvaginal study. TVS has few limitations. The only two absolute contraindications are imperforate hymen and patient refusal. A relative contraindication is a patient with a virginal or strictured introitus. These women, however, can usually undergo comfortable examination with proper counseling.

Transrectal and transperineal techniques employ transrectal probes and conventional transducers placed over the perineal region, respectively, for image acquisition. Much less commonly used, they are selected for indications such as pelvic floor imaging.

Harmonic Imaging

This recent modification of sonography is designed to improve tissue visualization and quality by using several frequencies at once from the transmitted ultrasound beam instead of just a single frequency. Newer probes and postprocessing features improve image resolution, particularly at surface interfaces. Visual artifacts that arise from superficial structures such as adipose are also reduced. As such, tissue harmonic imaging is routinely used in our ultrasound examinations.

Doppler Technology

This ultrasound technique can be performed with either transabdominal or transvaginal sonography to determine blood flow through pelvic organs, based on the red blood cell (RBC) velocity within vessels, especially arteries. Color Doppler captures and characterizes the spectral waveform of flow through certain vessels seen during real-time imaging. Ratios are often used to compare these different waveform components. The simplest is the systolic-diastolic ratio (S/D ratio), which compares the maximal (or peak) systolic flow with end-diastolic flow to evaluate downstream impedance to flow (Fig. 2-3). Of arterial Doppler spectral waveform parameters, the resistance index and pulsatility index are also commonly calculated. These quantitative indices estimate the impedance to RBC velocity within the artery by expressing the differences between the peak systolic and end-diastolic velocities.

A second application is *color Doppler mapping*, in which the color-coded pulsed-Doppler velocity information is superimposed on the real-time gray-scale image. The color is scaled, such that the color brightness is proportional to the flow velocity. Additionally, color Doppler also provides information regarding blood flow direction, and color is assigned to this. Flow approaching the transducer is customarily displayed in red, and flow away from it is shown in blue.

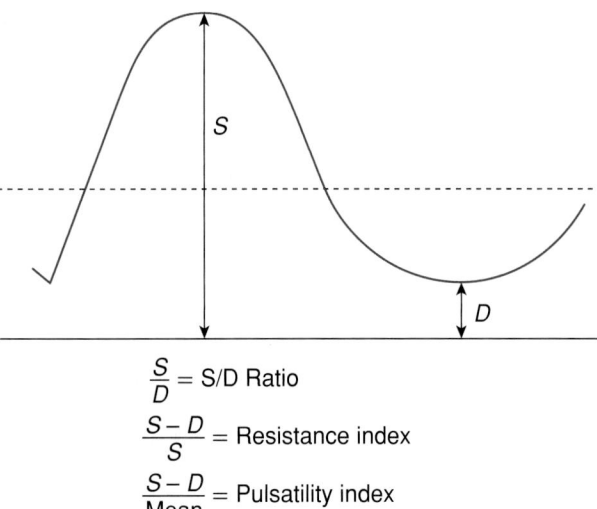

$$\frac{S}{D} = \text{S/D Ratio}$$

$$\frac{S-D}{S} = \text{Resistance index}$$

$$\frac{S-D}{\text{Mean}} = \text{Pulsatility index}$$

FIGURE 2-3 Doppler systolic–diastolic waveform indices of blood flow velocity. S represents the peak systolic flow or velocity, and D indicates the end-diastolic flow or velocity. The mean, which is the time-average mean velocity, is calculated from computer-digitized waveforms. (Reproduced with permission from Cunningham FG, Leveno KL, Bloom SL, et al: Williams Obstetrics, 24th ed. New York: McGraw-Hill Education; 2014.)

Color Doppler is not applied during every general gynecologic examination. One frequent indication is adnexal mass. Neovascularity within cancer is composed of abnormal vessels that lack smooth muscle and contain multiple arteriovenous shunts. Consequently, lower-impedance flow is expected with such masses as shown in Figure 2-4 (Kurjak, 1992; Weiner, 1992). Other indications include evaluation of ovarian masses for torsion, improved detection of extrauterine vascularity associated with ectopic pregnancy, and assessment of uterine perfusion in patients with leiomyomas and endometrial disorders (Fleischer, 2005). Due to safety concerns regarding the higher intensities generated by color and spectral Doppler, routine use of Doppler imaging in the first trimester is discouraged, unless needed for an important clinical indication.

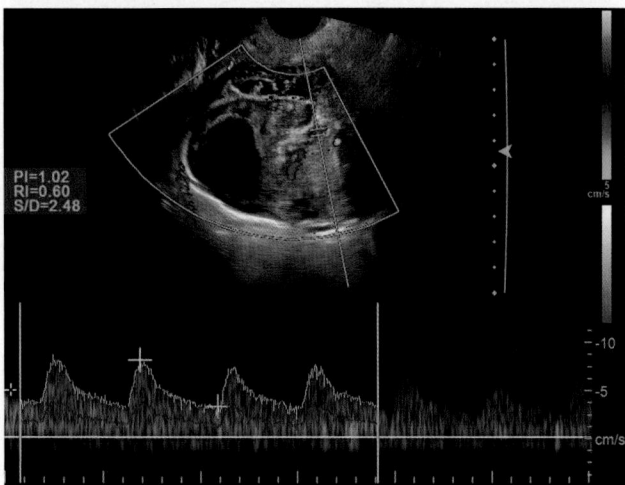

FIGURE 2-4 Complex ovarian mass with irregular cystic areas demonstrating intermediate-impedance [PI = 1.02] flow in a solid component. This mass was found to be a mucinous adenocarcinoma at surgery.

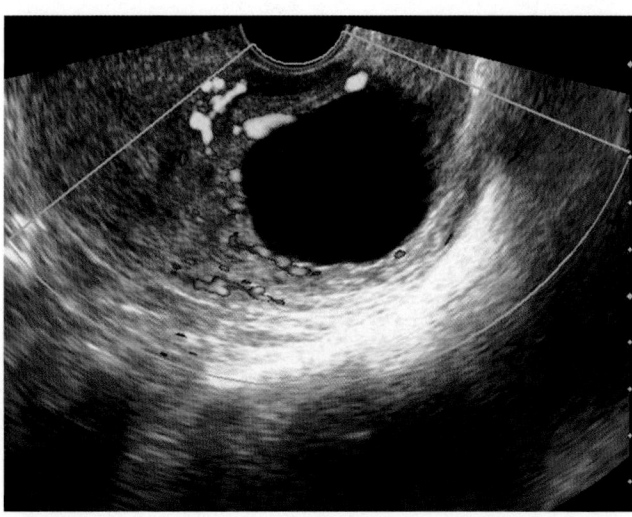

FIGURE 2-5 Power Doppler evaluation of a gestational sac in the lower uterine segment at the cesarean delivery scar. Circular flow is depicted, consistent with the peritrophoblastic flow of an implanted pregnancy.

Power Doppler imaging also maps RBC motion. It detects the energy of Doppler signals generated from moving RBCs using signal-to-noise characteristics of the vessels compared with surrounding tissues. This modality gives no information regarding blood flow direction, and thus data are displayed as a single color, usually yellow or orange. However, power Doppler is more sensitive to low-flow velocities, such as in veins and small arteries. Although employed less often than color Doppler mapping, power Doppler can gather additional information regarding endometrial and ovarian abnormalities (Fig. 2-5).

Saline Infusion Sonography

Also called sonohysterography, saline infusion sonography (SIS) displays detailed endometrial cavity anatomy by distending the cavity with sterile saline. It is commonly selected after an endometrial mass or abnormal endometrial thickness is identified during general TVS. SIS can also assist in some infertility investigations and aid viewing of the endometrial thickness if it is poorly imaged because of uterine position or pathology.

After voiding, a woman first undergoes a comprehensive TVS evaluation. A vaginal speculum is then inserted, the vagina and cervix are swabbed with an antiseptic solution, and a catheter primed with sterile saline is advanced into the cervical canal and just past the internal os. We do not routinely use a tenaculum for this. Contact with the uterine fundus is ideally avoided when advancing the catheter to avert pain or vasovagal response. It can also shear away endometrium, causing false-positive results. The speculum is carefully removed to avoid dislodging the catheter, the transvaginal probe is reinserted, and sterile saline is injected through the catheter at a rate based on the patient's tolerance. Usually not more than 20 to 40 mL is required to distend the endometrial cavity (Fig. 2-6). During this time, the cavity is observed with TVS. The sonographer scans in the longitudinal plane, imaging from one cornu to the other, and in the transverse plane, from the top of the fundus to the cervix. Endometrial surface irregularities are well delineated by the anechoic contrast of saline. At the procedure's

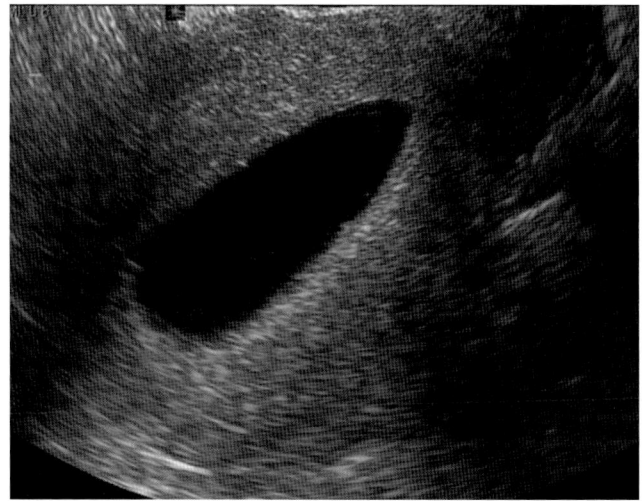

FIGURE 2-6 Saline infusion sonography of a normal endometrial cavity.

conclusion, the catheter is withdrawn under sonographic visualization. The uterine isthmus, endocervical canal, and upper vagina and vaginal fornices may also be evaluated, and this technique is referred to as *sonovaginography*. On average, the entire procedure lasts 5 to 10 minutes.

Many different catheter systems are available, including rigid systems and flexible catheters with and without attached balloons. We use a 7F SIS balloon catheter set, which tamponades the internal cervical os. This blockade prevents backflow of the distending medium and provides stable filling and adequate distention. We have found it easy to place and well tolerated (Fig. 2-7). Several distending solutions have been described, including saline, lactated Ringer solution, and 1.5-percent glycine. Sterile saline is inexpensive and provides optimal imaging. Alternatively, gel and foam substances have been developed to avoid backflow problems. However, these alternative products have not been extensively investigated and are not used widely in clinical practice.

In the premenopausal woman, SIS is best performed within the first 10 days of the menstrual cycle, and optimally on cycle days 4, 5, or 6 when the lining is thinnest. This timing is recommended to avoid misinterpreting menstrual blood clots as intrauterine pathology or missing pathology obscured by thick endometrial growth. In addition, such timing usually precludes disturbing a potential pregnancy. For the postmenopausal woman, timing of the procedure is not cycle-dependent.

Complications of SIS are minimal, and the risk of infection is less than 1 percent (Bonnamy, 2002). The American College of Obstetricians and Gynecologists (2014) recommends prophylactic antibiotics for women with prior pelvic inflammatory disease (PID) or identified hydrosalpinges. In these cases, doxycycline 100 mg orally twice daily is prescribed for 5 days. Although not strongly evidence-based, we also routinely give a single dose of doxycycline, 200 mg orally, for infection prophylaxis following SIS to immunocompromised women, such as those with diabetes, cancer, or human immunodeficiency virus infection. Prophylaxis is also given to infertile patients because of the risk for significant tubal damage associated with pelvic infection. Pain is usually minimal. In our experience, women with prior tubal ligation have greater discomfort, likely because fluid is unable to efflux through the fallopian tubes. A nonsteroidal antiinflammatory drug (NSAID) given 30 minutes prior to the procedure will typically minimize discomfort.

Contraindications to SIS include hematometra, pregnancy, active pelvic infection, or obstruction such as with an atrophic or stenotic cervix or vagina. In postmenopausal women with cervical stenosis, we have found the following techniques to be helpful: misoprostol 200 µg tablet orally the evening before and the morning of the procedure; a paracervical block with 1-percent lidocaine without epinephrine; a tenaculum on the cervix for traction; and a sonographically guided sequential cervical dilation with lacrimal duct dilators. Pisal and colleagues (2005) proposed using a 20-gauge spinal needle, inserted into the uterine cavity under sonographic guidance, to overcome severe cervical stenosis.

Hysterosalpingo-contrast Sonography

In the past, a fallopian tube could be detected with sonography only when distended by fluid, such as with obstruction. Injection

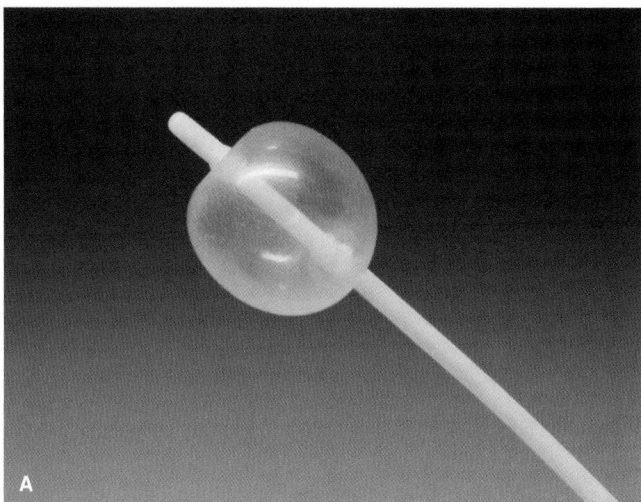

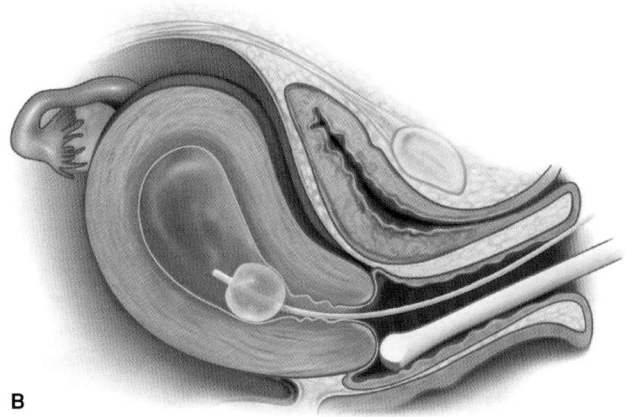

FIGURE 2-7 A. Saline infusion sonography catheter. **B.** Saline infusion sonography.

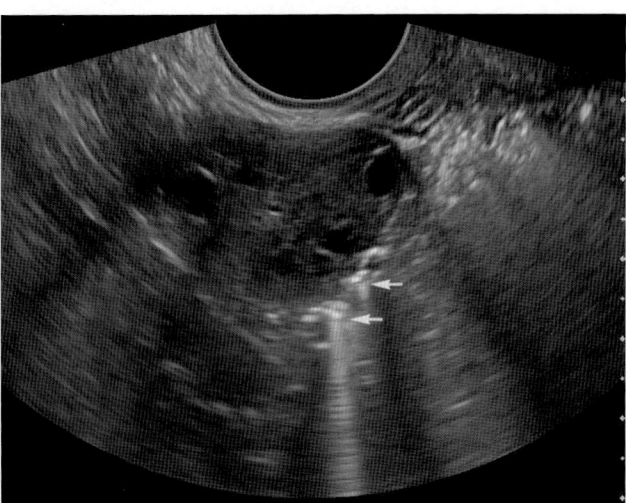

FIGURE 2-8 Transvaginal image of an ovary with echogenic bubbles adjacent to it (*arrows*) as seen during hysterosalpingo-contrast sonography (HyCoSy). The air in the saline contrast produces the bright echoes and ring-down artifacts. Visualization of these echoes adjacent to the ovary represents contrast exiting the tube, consistent with tubal patency.

of echogenic contrast during real-time sonography, called sonosalpingography, sonohysterosalpingography, or hysterosalpingo-contrast sonography (HyCoSy), is now an accurate procedure for the tubal patency assessment (Hamed, 2009).

HyCoSy is done in a manner similar to SIS. Fluid egress from the uterine cavity is blocked by a balloon catheter within the cervical canal. Using transvaginal sonography, the fallopian tubes are identified at the point where they join the uterine cornua. A hyperechoic sonographic contrast medium (Echovist, Albunex, or Infoson) is injected through the catheter to fill the cavity and then the fallopian tubes (Fig. 2-8). Alternatively, air coupled with sterile saline solution is another contrast option. With either medium choice, patent tubes appear hyperechoic as they fill with contrast. Color or pulsed Doppler techniques increase the diagnostic accuracy of HyCoSy by showing flow velocity within the tubes (Kupesic, 2007). We use the FemVue Sono Tubal Evaluation System, which simultaneously introduces air and sterile saline in a controlled fashion. The positive pressure flow of the echogenic mixture creates "scintillations" that are visually followed using real-time ultrasound. In patent tubes, flow proceeds from the uterotubal junction, through the length of the tube, and out the fimbriated end. Bubbles then surround the ovary or fill the posterior cul-de-sac. At present no large studies quantitate a risk for post-HyCoSy pelvic infection, and our periprocedural antibiotic prophylaxis mirrors our SIS protocol.

HyCoSy performed in conjunction with SIS provides a comprehensive assessment of the uterine cavity and myometrial anatomy, tubal patency, and adnexal architecture. This allows a cost-effective and time-efficient "one-stop" evaluation (Saunders, 2011). However, HyCoSy does have limitations. We have found that the entire fallopian tube often cannot be visualized due to normal tubal tortuosity. To that end, recent studies have evaluated the combination of 3-D sonography with HyCoSy to more easily view the entire tubal length

(Exacoustos, 2013; Zhou, 2012). Similar to hysterosalpingography (HSG), discussed on page 38, HyCoSy can demonstrate false occlusion from tubal spasm. In addition, a patent tube does not always correlate with normal tubal function. Last, HSG may still be needed for more accurate delineation of tubal anatomy in selected cases (Mol, 1996).

Although comparable to HSG in detecting tubal pathology, it has only recently become routinely used clinically (Heikinen, 1995; Strandell, 1999). In comparison to HSG, HyCoSy can also be performed in an outpatient setting, has lower cost, is well tolerated, avoids x-ray exposure or iodine-related allergic reaction, and provides information on uterine wall and ovarian morphology (Luciano, 2014; Savelli, 2009). The advantages of HyCoSy compared with HSG are equally valid for patient evaluation following sterilization with hysteroscopic devices. Namely, with Essure microinsert coils, tubal blockage confirmation 3 months after sterilization is mandatory (Luciano, 2011). Still, the Food and Drug Administration (FDA) and manufacturer currently recommend HSG to demonstrate tubal occlusion by Essure.

Three-dimensional Sonography

Technical Aspects. The ability to obtain certain views of pelvic organs in two dimensions is inherently limited. Transabdominally, the bony pelvis prevents scanning from the pelvic sidewall. Transvaginally, the views obtainable are restricted by the range of vaginal probe mobility. New sonography scanners now allow collection of 3-D data and representation of it on a two-dimensional (2-D) screen. This permits a more detailed assessment of the object studied, without restriction of the number and orientation of the scanning planes. With 3-D imaging, any desired plane through a pelvic organ can be obtained, regardless of the sound beam orientation during acquisition. For example, the "face-on" or coronal plane through the uterus is routinely seen in 3-D imaging but is rarely viewed during 2-D scanning. This view of the uterus is essential for assessing the external contour of the uterine fundus and the shape of the endometrial cavity for congenital uterine anomaly diagnosis.

With 3-D sonography, a volume, rather than a slice, of sonographic data is acquired and stored. The stored data can be reformatted and analyzed in numerous ways, and navigation through the saved volume can show countless planes. At any time, the volume can be retrieved, studied, reconstructed, and reinterpreted as needed. In addition, the level of energy with 3-D sonography is no higher than with 2-D, and manipulations of the obtained volumes are performed "off-line" to avoid additional ultrasound scanning time.

The three main components of 3-D sonography are volume acquisition, processing, and display. First, the preferred method to acquire volumes is automated and uses a dedicated 3-D probe that contains a mechanized drive. When these probes are activated, the transducer elements automatically sweep through the operator-selected region of interest, called a *volume box*, while the probe is held stationary.

After the appropriate volume is acquired, the user can begin to process the volume using the modes available in the ultrasound machine. The acquired volume can be displayed multiple ways. The most common is multiplanar reconstruction,

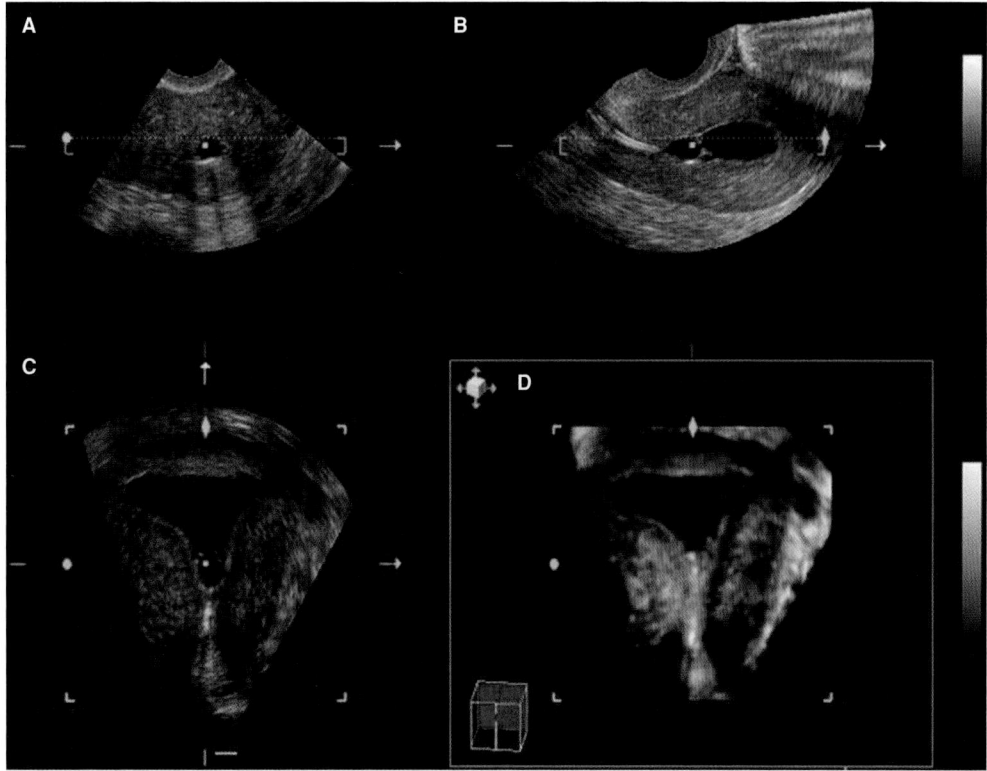

FIGURE 2-9 Multiplanar display of a 3-dimensional volume of a uterus and normal endometrial cavity during saline infusion sonography. The views were obtained from a midsagittal reference plane using the Z technique. The planes are as follows: **A.** transverse, **B.** sagittal, **C.** coronal, **D.** rendered image.

in which three perpendicular planes, sagittal (the longitudinal plane that divides the body into right and left sections), axial (the transverse plane that divides the body into cephalad and caudal sections), and coronal (the frontal plane that divides the body into ventral and dorsal sections), are displayed simultaneously. Correlation between the three planes in the multiplanar display is accomplished by placing the planar center dot at the point of interest in one plane and observing the location of the corresponding center dots in the other two planes (Fig. 2-9A-C).

Abuhamad and associates (2006) have described a straightforward postprocessing technique, called the Z technique, that aids in the manipulation of 3-D volumes of the uterus. The anatomic basis of the Z technique is such that, in aligning the midsagittal and midtransverse planes of the uterus parallel to the horizontal axis, the midcoronal plane of the uterus will easily and consistently be displayed. In addition, all or part of the saved volume can be processed into a rendered image that can be shown alone or in correlation with the multiplanar display. A rendered image is a "sum" of all the coronal planar images (Fig. 2-9D). This is the display method that has been publicized in obstetrics, when showing the image of the neonate's face in utero.

The inverse mode is a rendering technique of the entire volume in which all cystic areas within the volume become digitally opaque and all solid areas become transparent. This technique is useful when trying to see cystic areas that might be hidden in a volume, such as within an ovarian mass. Last, the volume can be displayed in parallel tomographic slices, similar to the displays used by CT and MR imaging.

3-D imaging is not without shortcomings. With 3-D sonography, the same type of acoustic artifacts that occur with 2-D imaging are encountered, such as acoustic shadowing and enhancement, refraction and reverberation, and motion artifacts from bowel peristalsis and vascular pulsation. Another potential pitfall in 3-D imaging of the pelvis involves spatial orientation within the saved volume data. Uterine flexion or version or left versus right may not be readily apparent on review of saved volumes. As such, during the preliminary real-time scanning, the operator must determine the orientation of the area of interest and notate it accordingly.

Another problem commonly encountered in 3-D transvaginal gynecologic imaging is related to the limited size of the volume box. Because of this, the entire uterus is often not acquired in a single volume. In some cases, it may be necessary to acquire two volumes, one for the cervix and a second for the uterine body. Likewise, a very large adnexal mass may not be imaged completely in any single volume of data obtained transvaginally. The size of the volume box provided by the abdominal probe is greater. Thus with 3-D sonography, a large mass may need to be imaged transabdominally instead of transvaginally.

Clinical Use. Because it can study organs in numerous scanning planes, 3-D imaging has become invaluable in gynecology to assess the uterine cavity, complex ovarian masses, ovarian fertility reserve, uterine anomalies, and interstitial pregnancies. It also can simultaneously provide anatomic and dynamic information from pelvic floor structures and from mesh implants.

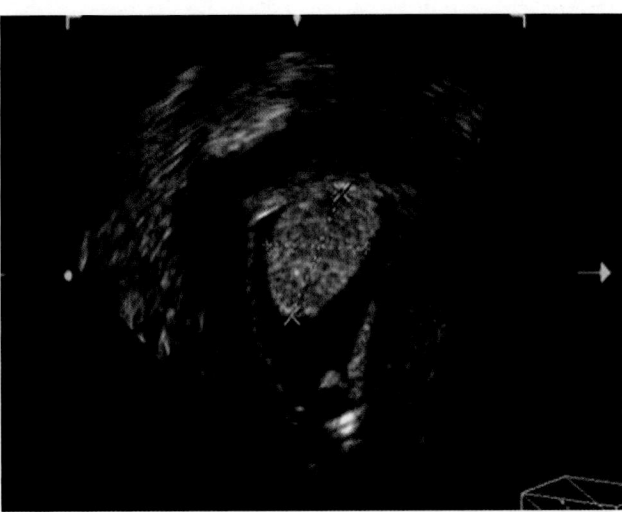

FIGURE 2-10 Three-dimensional image in the coronal plane of a polyp (*calipers*) after instillation of saline during saline infusion sonography.

Of these, mapping leiomyoma location relative to the endometrial cavity and surrounding structures is an essential step in triaging patients for treatment as discussed in Chapter 9 (p. 206). For such mapping, 3-D sonography or 3-D SIS can be used in place of conventional SIS or MR imaging. In patients receiving gonadotropin-releasing hormone (GnRH) agonists or following uterine artery embolization (UAE), 3-D sonography can also monitor leiomyoma volume reductions. However, MR imaging is more often used following UAE.

Abnormalities of the endometrium and adjacent myometrium, especially focal endometrial thickenings such as polyps, hyperplasia, and cancer, can be better defined with 3-D technology (Fig. 2-10) (Andreotti, 2006; Benacerraf, 2008). In their comparative study of 36 women with postmenopausal bleeding, Bonilla-Musoles and associates (1997) compared results from 3-D SIS with findings from TVS, 2-D SIS, transvaginal color Doppler, and hysteroscopy. Visualization of the uterine cavity and endometrial thickness with 3-D SIS was comparable to

hysteroscopy and better than the other sonographic techniques. We now routinely implement 3-D imaging for evaluation of abnormal endometria during our transvaginal studies and with all SIS procedures.

Although investigational, 3-D sonography with power Doppler angiography (3D-PDA) has been used to discriminate between benign and malignant endometrial disease in women with postmenopausal bleeding and a thickened endometrium (Alcazar, 2009). 3D-PDA can assess endometrial volume, which may more accurately represent the true tissue amount compared with a 2-D measurement of endometrial thickness. Another tool, 3-D power Doppler imaging enhanced by intravenous (IV) contrast, is also being investigated to differentiate benign endometrial polyps and endometrial cancer (Lieng, 2008; Song, 2009).

IUD positioning within the endometrial cavity can be documented adequately in most cases with traditional 2-D TVS. That said, 3-D sonography offers improved visualization, especially with the levonorgestrel-releasing IUD (Moschos, 2011). The coronal plane images, which are not possible with 2-D imaging, provide views of both the arms and shaft of the device and the relation of these to the endometrial cavity (Benacerraf, 2009). As such, patients at our institution undergoing gynecologic sonography with an IUD in situ, regardless of the study indication, have both a standard 2-D evaluation and a 3-D volume acquisition of the uterus. The coronal view of the endometrial cavity is reconstructed to establish IUD type, location, and positioning (Fig. 2-11). In addition, although the FDA still mandates a postprocedural HSG following Essure coil placement, TVS has been shown to be an acceptable method of confirmation (Fig. 2-12) (Legendre, 2010).

For adnexal mass interrogation, most agree that 3-D sonography provides detailed internal anatomy (Alcazar, 2003; Bonilla-Musoles, 1995). Moreover, the addition of power Doppler to 3-D evaluation displays the internal architecture and neovascularization also characteristic of malignant neoplasms. However, to date, 3-D power Doppler ultrasound has not shown significantly improved diagnostic accuracy compared with that

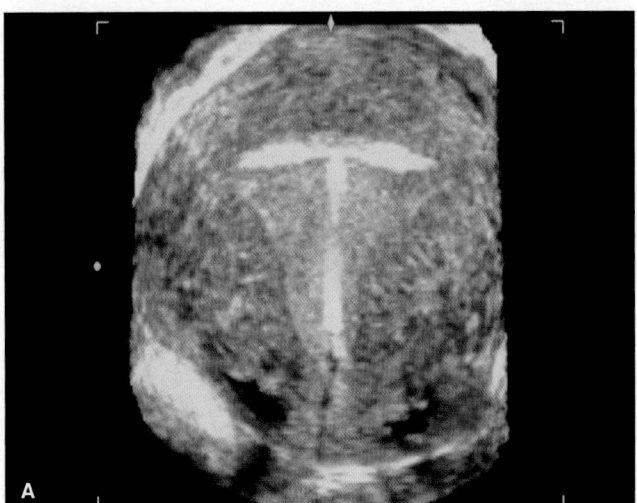
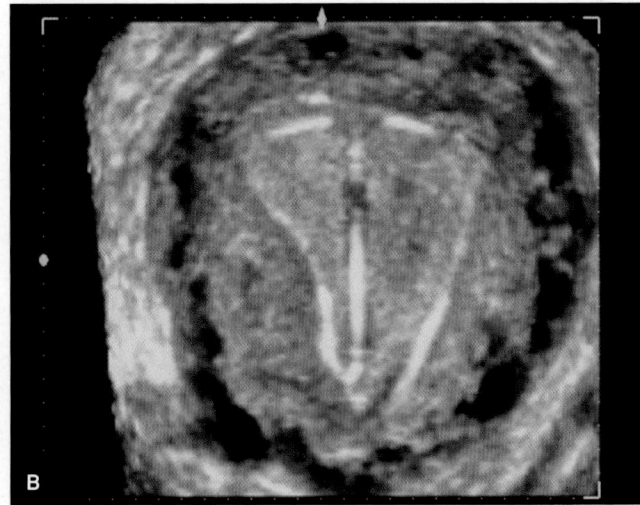

FIGURE 2-11 Intrauterine devices (IUDs). The coronal planes of 3-dimensional sonography best depict the type and positioning of the Copper T 380A IUD (ParaGard) **(A)** and levonorgestrel-releasing IUD (Mirena) **(B)** IUDs within the endometrial cavity.

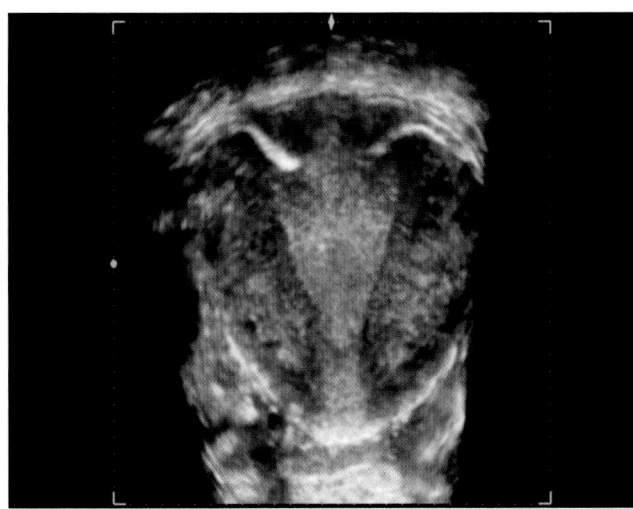

FIGURE 2-12 Essure contraception. Three-dimensional image in the coronal plane demonstrates the microinsert coils in the bilateral cornua of the uterus, corresponding to proper placement of the devices.

of gray-scale and 2-D power Doppler imaging. Further large, randomized, controlled trials are warranted (Jokubkiene, 2007).

In reproductive medicine, 3-D imaging acquires more precise ovarian volumes and follicle counts than measurements estimated from 2-D imaging. Many predict that it will become the preferred ultrasound technique for infertility ovarian evaluation (Deutch, 2009). Moreover, 3-D sonography can also examine endometrial vascularity to predict endometrial receptivity prior to ovarian stimulation (Wu, 2003).

For congenital müllerian uterine anomalies, 3-D ultrasound is now frequently used to accurately display anatomy (Ghi, 2009; Salim, 2003). It is as sensitive as hysteroscopy and as accurate as MR imaging, and it provides detailed images of both endometrial cavity shape and external fundal contour (Bermejo, 2010). Thus, because the uterine horns and fundal contour are displayed clearly in the same plane, müllerian anomalies can be differentiated (Troiano, 2004). Importantly, 3-D imaging can provide helpful details for preoperative planning.

For pelvic reconstructive surgery indications, 3-D ultrasound has been used to evaluate pelvic floor anatomy, pelvic support, and mesh implants. First, because of its composition, typical polypropylene mesh implants appear as echogenic interwoven interfaces with ultrasound. In contrast, these are poorly depicted with radiography or MR imaging. As a result, 3-D vaginal and perineal sonography is now selected for this evaluation (Dietz, 2012; Fleischer, 2012; Schuettoff, 2006). During implant interrogation, cranial aspects of mesh or retropubic mesh may be poorly imaged. For these patients, MR imaging may be helpful.

As a second indication, postprocessing reconstruction in a coronal plane improves views of the urethra and the periurethral tissue, which are inaccessible with 2-D ultrasound techniques. 3-D images are obtained with abdominal transducers using a translabial-transperineal approach or with transvaginal probes using specialized rotational transducers (Dietz, 2007, 2012; Santoro, 2011).

In women with pelvic floor dysfunction, the reconstructed tomographic ultrasound images afforded by 3-D ultrasound

are particularly useful to quantify the degree of levator ani defects (Dietz, 2010). Perhaps most importantly, 3-D imaging can provide not only anatomic but also dynamic information about pelvic floor structures, as imaging can be executed with the patient performing the Valsalva maneuver or actively contracting the pelvic floor musculature (Fleischer, 2012).

Contrast-enhanced Sonography

This newer technique couples IV contrast with traditional sonography. With contrast-enhanced sonography, the visible difference between the density (or signal intensity) of a focal lesion is compared with the surrounding normal organ tissue. Enhancement patterns within the mass itself are also assessed.

Ultrasound contrast agents used intravenously are small, stabilized microbubbles, usually 1 to 10 μm in diameter, and composed of perfluorocarbon or nitrogen gas encapsulated in albumin, phospholipid, or polymer shells. The gas-liquid interface contributes to the echogenicity of the microbubbles seen using traditional imaging. The high impedance mismatch between the microbubbles and adjacent RBCs in the blood vessels causes increased scattering and reflection of the ultrasound sound beam. This heightens the ultrasound signal and thereby increases brightness or echogenicity (Hwang, 2010). The degree of echo enhancement depends on many factors, including microbubble size, contrast agent density, compressibility of the bubbles, and the interrogating ultrasound frequency. The greater the size, density, and compressibility of the agent, the more reflection and echogenicity is elicited (Eckersley, 2002).

For ovarian cancer, contrast-enhanced sonography may highlight tumor neovascularization in developing microscopic tumors (Ferrara, 2000). In addition, because vascular channels associated with malignancy are often incompetent, the resultant extravasation of RBCs and contrast agent may be detected sonographically (Fleischer, 2008).

Other promising clinical applications of contrast-enhanced sonography currently under investigation include monitoring tumor and therapeutic angiogenesis, inflammation assessment, evaluation of ischemia and reperfusion injury, early detection of transplant rejection, and targeted drug delivery (Hwang, 2010).

Sonoelastography

Elastography is an ultrasound imaging technique that measures tissue stiffness in both physiological and pathological states. To obtain an elastographic image, a source of "stress" or "strain" promotes tissue deformation to assess this stiffness (Stoelinga, 2014).

There are three main types of ultrasound elasticity imaging: (1) elastography that tracks tissue movement during compression, typically used to interrogate veins for thrombus; (2) tracking of acoustic shear wave propagation through tissue, often used for prostate evaluation; and (3) the most common method, vibration sonoelastography (Garra, 2007). With vibration sonoelastography, low-amplitude, low-frequency shear waves propagate through the organ of interest, while real-time color Doppler techniques generate an image of tissue movement in response to the external vibrations (Taylor, 2000). For example, if a discrete, hard inhomogeneous mass, such as a tumor, lies within a region of soft tissue, the vibration amplitude is decreased at its location.

Numerous organs and diseases have been evaluated by sonoelastography, and uterine evaluation with this has gained increased attention. Potential areas of investigation include distinguishing endometrial polyps from submucous pedunculated myomas, endometrial cancer from benign endometrial thickening, cervical cancer from normal cervix, and leiomyomas from adenomyosis (Stoelinga, 2014). Moreover, identifying uterine and cervical stiffness during pregnancy may prove valuable for management of preterm or postterm complications (Molina, 2012).

Focused-ultrasound Therapy

Ultrasound energy during conventional imaging propagates harmlessly through tissue with little energy being absorbed. This energy is deposited as heat but dissipates by the cooling effects of perfusion and conduction. No harmful effects have been recorded at the intensities used for diagnostic purposes (American Institute of Ultrasound in Medicine, 2009).

If, however, the ultrasound beam carries a high level of energy and is brought into tight focus, this energy is rapidly converted into heat. When target spot temperatures rise above 55 °C, proteins are denatured, cells die, and coagulative necrosis is incited (Lele, 1977). In contrast, surrounding tissues are warmed but not to lethal temperatures. The current gynecologic use for this modality is treatment of symptomatic leiomyomas and is illustrated in Chapter 9 (p. 211).

■ Normal Sonographic Findings

Reproductive Tract Organs

In the reproductive years, a normal uterus measures approximately 7.5 × 5.0 × 2.5 cm but is smaller in prepubertal, postmenopausal, or hypoestrogenized women. Normal uterine stroma returns low-level, uniform echoes, and the position of the endometrial and endocervical canals is indicated by linear echogenic stripes, representing the interfaces between mucus and mucosa (Fig. 2-13). The cervix is best visualized transvaginally

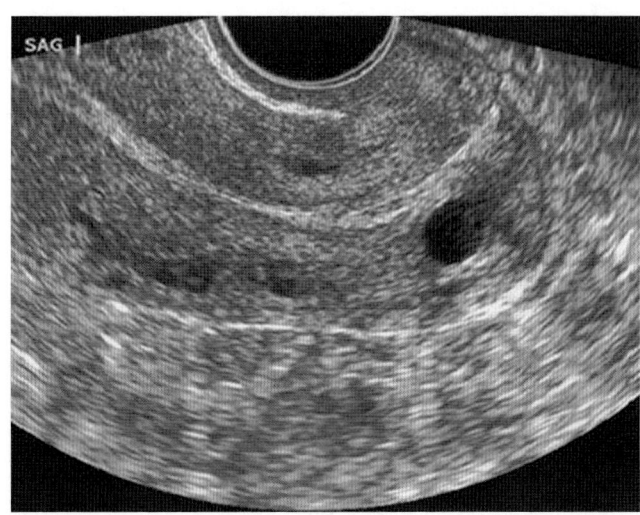

FIGURE 2-14 Transvaginal sonogram in the sagittal plane of a uterine cervix. An endocervical cyst is seen posterior to the thin, echogenic endocervical canal.

with the tip of the probe placed 2 to 3 cm from it. The endocervical canal is a continuation of the endometrial cavity and appears as a thin echogenic line (Fig. 2-14). The vagina is seen as a hypoechoic tubular structure with an echogenic lumen that curves inferiorly over the muscular perineal body at the introitus. The ovaries are ellipsoid and normally lie in the ovarian fossa with their long axes parallel to the internal iliac vessels, which lie posteriorly (Fig. 2-15). Ovarian volume ranges from 4 to 10 cubic centimeters depending on hormonal status (Cohen, 1990). This volume is calculated using the formula for the volume of an ellipse: $4/3(\pi) \times (A \times B \times C)$. In this formula, A, B, and C are the ovarian diameters in centimeters, measured in the three different planes. Ovarian follicles appear as spherical anechoic structures within the ovary and may reach a normal size of 3 cm. Normal fallopian tubes are not visible. A small amount of fluid in the posterior cul-de-sac is a normal finding and is often seen with ovulation.

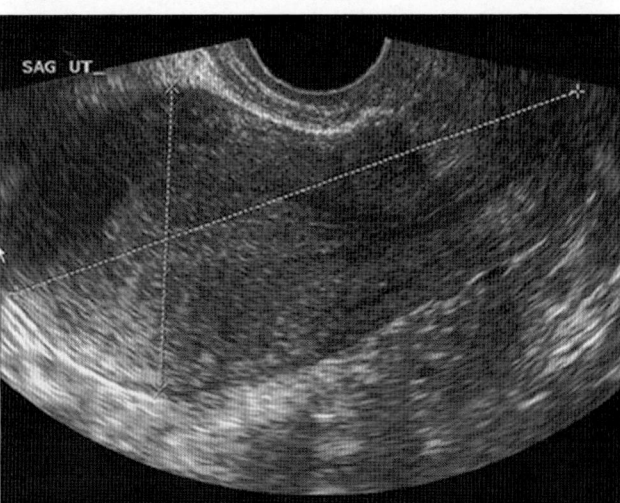

FIGURE 2-13 Transvaginal sonogram in the sagittal plane of an anteverted uterine corpus. Calipers demonstrate measurements of the uterine length (+) and the anterior-posterior dimension (×).

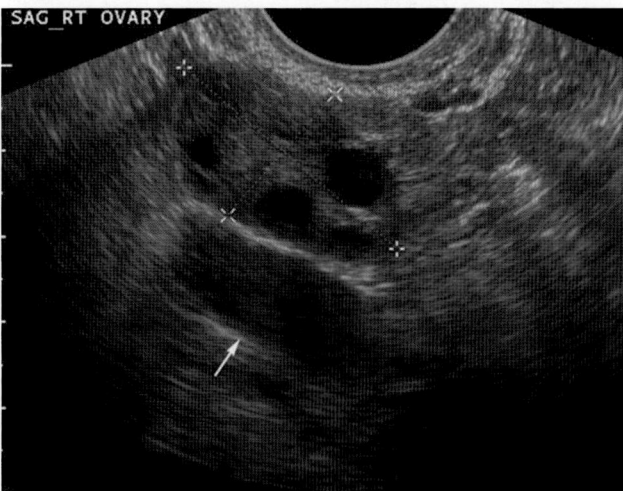

FIGURE 2-15 Transvaginal sonogram in the sagittal plane of a left ovary (calipers) in a premenopausal woman. The ovary normally lies in the ovarian fossa, anterior to the internal iliac vessel (arrow).

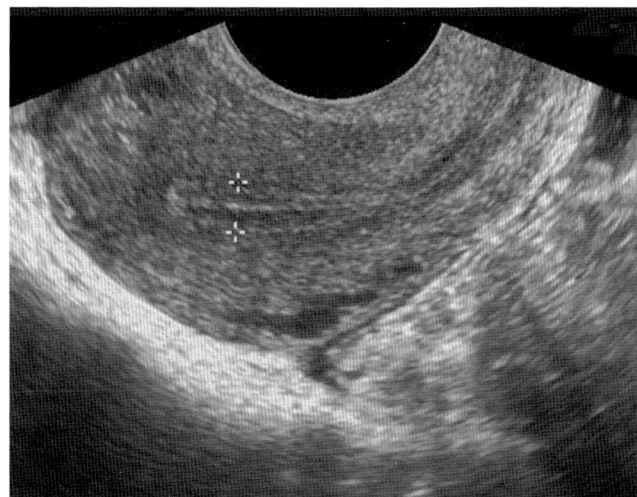

FIGURE 2-16 Transvaginal sonogram in the sagittal plane of a characteristic trilaminar proliferative endometrium. Calipers demonstrate proper measurement of the "double-layer" thickness made of the alternating hyper-hypo-hyperechogenic lines.

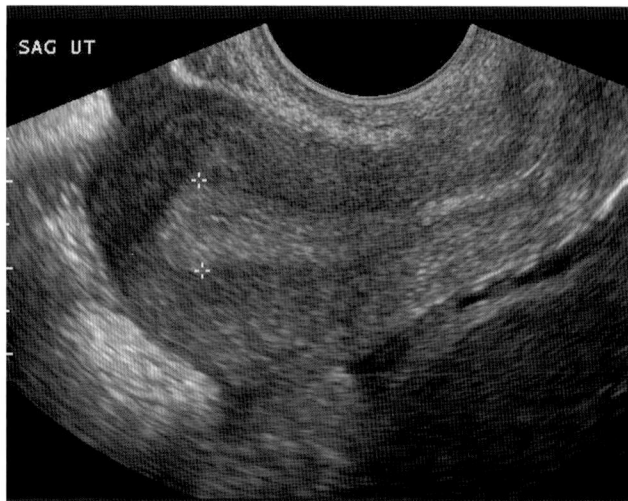

FIGURE 2-17 Transvaginal sonogram in the sagittal plane of a secretory endometrium. The endometrium, which is marked by calipers, has become uniformly echogenic.

Endometrium

Functionally, the endometrium has two main layers: the *stratum basale*, which comprises the densely cellular supporting stroma and varies little with the phase of the menstrual cycle, and the *stratum functionale*, which proliferates during each cycle and partially desquamates at menses. These layers cover the entire cavity.

Sonographically, the endometrium's appearance during the menstrual cycle correlates with the phasic changes in its histologic anatomy. During the follicular phase, when the endometrium is provided estrogen from ovarian folliculogenesis, the stratum basale appears echogenic due to spectral reflections from the mucus-laden glands. In contrast, the stratum functionale is relatively hypoechoic because of the orderly arrangement of glands that lack secretions. The central opposing surfaces of these two endometrial layers manifest as a highly reflective, thin midline stripe. Together, the three echogenic lines create the characteristic trilaminar appearance of the proliferative endometrium (Fig. 2-16).

Measurement of this endometrial thickness extends from the echogenic interface of the anterior basale layer and myometrium to the echogenic interface of the posterior basale layer and myometrium. It thus represents a "double thickness." The hypoechoic halo outside of and adjacent to the endometrium is not included in the measurement as this is actually the inner compact layer of myometrium. Sonographically, the endometrium is measured from a sagittal or long-axis image of the uterus in the plane where the central endometrial echo is seen contiguous with the endocervical canal and seen distinct from the myometrium. Endometrial thickness correlates approximately with the day of the cycle up to day 7 or 8.

With ovulation and progesterone production from the corpus luteum during the secretory phase, glandular enlargement and secretory vacuoles are seen histologically. During this phase, the endometrium achieves its maximum thickness as the

stroma becomes more vascular and edematous. Sonographically, these changes cause the endometrium to appear echogenic (Fig. 2-17).

With menstruation, the endometrium appears as a slightly irregular echogenic interface from sloughed tissue and blood. The thinnest endometrial measurements are found at conclusion of menses (Fig. 2-18).

With cessation of estrogen stimulation beginning at menopause, the endometrium atrophies, and cyclic sloughing ceases. The postmenopausal endometrium appears thin and uniform (Fig. 2-19).

Pelvic Floor

With the advent of urogynecology as a specialty, sonography is widely used to evaluate pelvic floor anatomy and function (Dietz, 2012). Various 2-D techniques, including transvaginal,

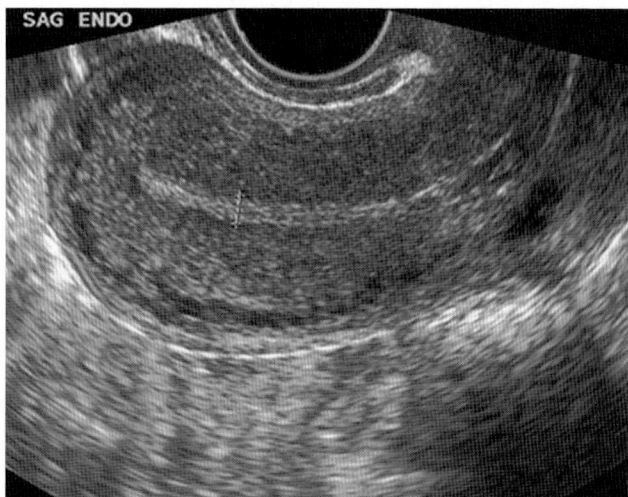

FIGURE 2-18 Transvaginal sonogram in the sagittal plane of a menstrual-phase endometrium, which is marked by calipers.

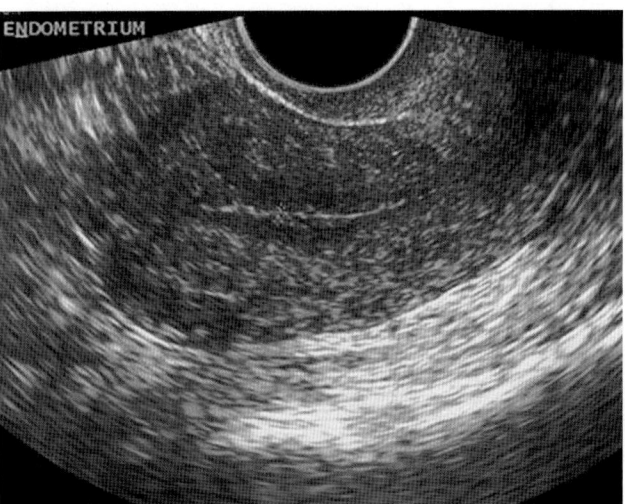

FIGURE 2-19 Transvaginal sonogram in the sagittal plane of an atrophic postmenopausal endometrium.

transrectal, transperineal, and intraurethral sonography, have been used to investigate urethral anatomy.

Transrectal sonography was the first technique used to assess anal sphincter morphology after childbirth. This method requires special equipment and distention of the anal canal. The technique has limited value in the immediate puerperium and only provides information regarding the anal sphincter. Thus, without levator ani muscle assessment, the posterior compartment is incompletely evaluated. Alternatively, anorectal morphology and the pelvic floor can both be assessed with vaginal sonography using a rotating endorectal probe or standard transvaginal probe. These methods are described further in Chapter 25 (p. 568).

Perineal sonography can also evaluate pelvic floor anatomy. The technique requires filling the bladder with approximately 300 mL of saline. With the woman either supine or erect, a

5-MHz curved-array transducer is placed in sagittal orientation to the perineum. This allows real-time imaging of the pubic symphysis, levator ani muscles, urethra, bladder neck, bladder, vagina, rectal ampulla, and anal canal simultaneously and with little transducer manipulation (Dietz, 2010). Measurements have been standardized by Schaer and coworkers (1995).

3-D ultrasound is increasingly selected to examine pelvic floor anatomy. Specifically, evaluation of pelvic anatomy, support, and mesh implants are some indications, as discussed earlier.

CLINICAL APPLICATIONS OF SONOGRAPHY

Transvaginal sonography is often preferred for early evaluation of pelvic pain, abnormal uterine bleeding, pelvic mass, early pregnancy complications, infertility practices, and early detection of ovarian and endometrial cancer. Many of these topics and their radiologic characteristics are covered in other chapters. Some remaining important subjects are presented in the following sections.

■ Intraabdominal Fluid

During general sonographic evaluation of the pelvis, a small amount of free fluid, as little as 10 mL, is commonly present in the posterior cul-de-sac (Khalife, 1998). If free fluid is seen extending to the fundus of the uterus, it is considered to be moderate in amount. Once identified, moderate free fluid should prompt further evaluation of the paracolic gutters and Morison pouch in the right upper quadrant to assess the extent of free fluid (Fig. 2-20). If fluid fills these areas, then the minimum volume of intraperitoneal fluid approximates 500 mL (Abrams, 1999; Branney, 1995). Large amounts of anechoic free peritoneal fluid generically described as ascites suggest a volume status abnormality or an infectious or inflammatory etiology. Free fluid that contains low-level echoes or echogenic

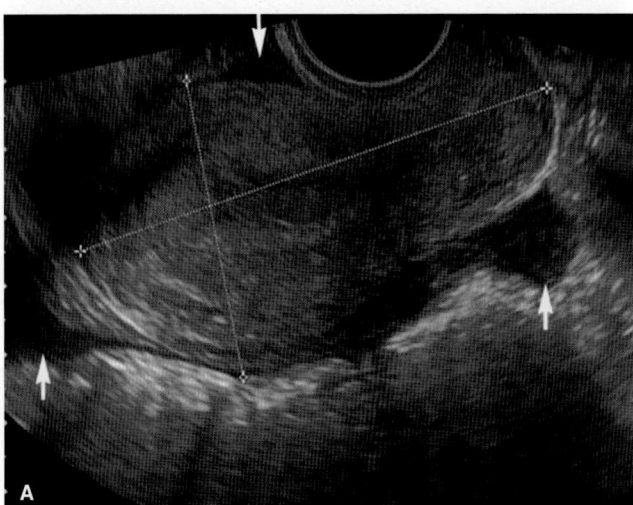

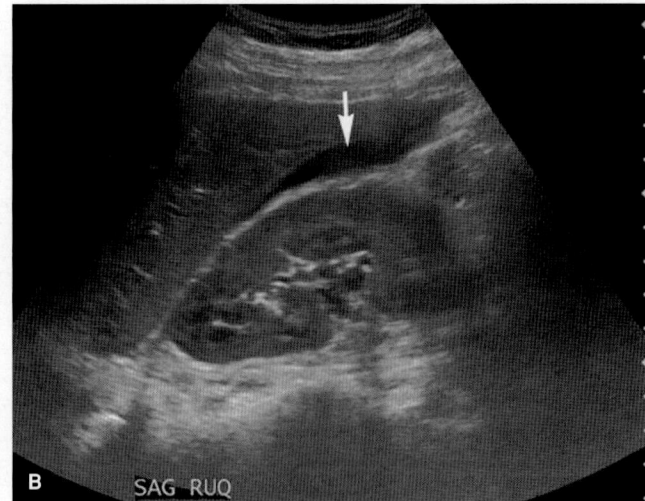

FIGURE 2-20 Hemoperitoneum. **A.** In this transvaginal image, a moderate amount of free fluid (*arrows*) is seen in the posterior cul-de-sac, above the fundus of the uterus, and in the anterior cul-de-sac. **B.** Transabdominal image of Morison pouch in the right upper quadrant. Free fluid, corresponding to the dark anechoic area (*arrow*), is visualized between the liver edge and the kidney, which suggests a large-volume hemoperitoneum.

debris is consistent with hemoperitoneum with clot, such as with a ruptured hemorrhagic cyst or ectopic pregnancy.

The sensitivity of sonography to detect free fluid has led to its increased use during emergency trauma assessments. Focused assessment with sonography for trauma (FAST) is a limited sonographic examination directed solely at identifying free fluid for the diagnosis of traumatic injury. In the context of trauma, free fluid is usually due to hemorrhage. With FAST, four specific areas are imaged: perihepatic (right upper quadrant), perisplenic (left upper quadrant), pelvis, and pericardium. FAST has significant advantages compared with diagnostic peritoneal lavage and with CT for intraperitoneal fluid identification because it is a rapid, noninvasive, bedside test. However, there is a significant false-negative rate with FAST (Scalea, 1999). This is in part due to the FAST examination being carried out early in the resuscitation phase when only a small amount of free fluid may have collected in the dependent portions of the peritoneal cavity. In addition, as its use has become more widespread, conflicts have developed regarding credentialing and whether radiologists, emergency physicians, or trauma surgeons should be performing this sonographic technique.

■ Malignant Ovarian Characteristics

Sonography is commonly the initial and often the only imaging procedure performed during pelvic and ovarian mass evaluation, as most can be correctly categorized based on gray-scale and color or power Doppler ultrasound characteristics. Found in Table 9-3 (p. 217), recommendations from a Society of Radiologists in Ultrasound consensus conference summarizes a reasonable approach to asymptomatic ovarian and other adnexal cysts imaged sonographically (Levine, 2010).

Sonography is the best preoperative diagnostic technique to determine the malignant potential of an ovarian mass (Twickler, 2010). To this end, morphologic scoring systems based on number and thickness of septa, presence and number of papillations, and proportion of solid tissue within the mass have been proposed to standardize the interpretation of findings (DePriest, 1993; Sassone, 1991). When size, morphology, and structure of adnexal masses are combined with color Doppler and spectral analysis of flow signals, the specificity and positive predictive value of sonographic diagnosis is increased (Buy, 1996; Fleischer, 1993; Jain, 1994). In a metaanalysis of 46 studies with 5159 patients, Kinkel and coworkers (2000) reported significantly higher accuracy for combined sonographic techniques compared with that of each individual technique alone. In addition, the International Ovarian Tumor Analysis (IOTA) Group has developed the most accurate mathematic model to date to calculate the malignancy risk of an adnexal mass based on sonographic features (Timmerman, 2005). We use the Ovarian Tumor Index developed by Twickler and colleagues (1999) at our institution.

Neovascularity within a malignant neoplasm produces a significant increase in color Doppler flow signals secondary to angiogenesis. These new vessels are abnormal, lack smooth muscle, and contain multiple arteriovenous shunts. Consequently, lower-impedance flow is expected with such masses as shown in Figure 2-4 (Kurjak, 1992; Weiner, 1992). Moreover, although

most benign tumors appear poorly vascularized, most malignant lesions appear well-vascularized, with flow signals in both peripheral and central regions—including within septations and solid tumor areas. Of Doppler parameters, the color content of the tumor probably reflects tumor vascularity better than any other. The overall impression of this vascularity reflects both the number and size of vessels and their functional capacity. The IOTA group scoring system uses this subjective semiquantitative assessment of flow to describe the vascular features of ovarian masses (Ameye, 2009; Timmerman, 2005). A four-point color score is used to describe tumor blood flow only within septa and solid portions of the mass (Timmerman, 2000).

These observations led many investigators to evaluate the presence, spatial distribution, and prevalence of flow signals within ovarian masses to quantify malignant characteristics. However, because of overlap of vascular parameters between malignant and benign neoplasms, a firm differential diagnosis based on spectral Doppler evaluation alone is not possible (Valentin, 1997).

■ Pelvic Inflammatory Disease

In women with acute salpingitis, pelvic sonography is commonly performed. However, large studies evaluating its sensitivity, specificity, or overall usefulness are lacking (Boardman, 1997; Cacciatore, 1992). Sonographic findings vary according to the severity of the disease. In early infection, anatomy may appear normal. With progression, early nonspecific findings include free pelvic fluid, endometrial thickening, endometrial cavity distention by fluid or gas, and indistinct borders of the uterus and ovaries. Enlarged ovaries with increased numbers of small cysts—a "polycystic ovary appearance"—has been shown to correlate with PID. With treatment, this ovarian enlargement resolves (Cacciatore, 1992).

Sonographic findings of the fallopian tubes are the most striking and specific landmarks of PID (Fig. 2-21). Although normal tubes are rarely seen unless surrounded by ascites, tubal wall inflammation allows visualization with sonography. As the

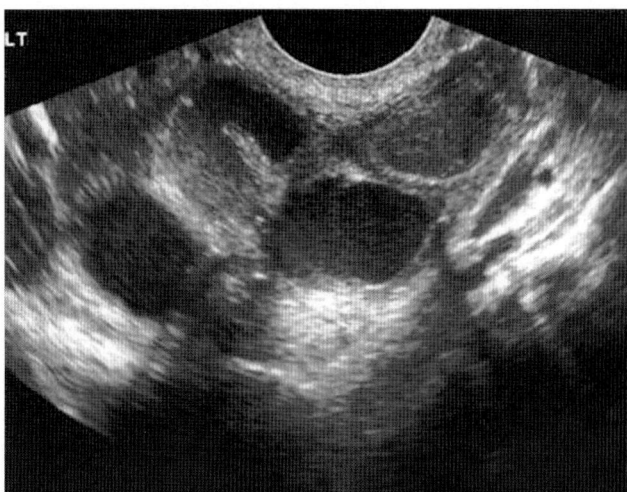

FIGURE 2-21 Transvaginal sonogram in cross-section of an inflamed, dilated tube demonstrating thickened tubal walls, incomplete septa, and echogenic fluid.

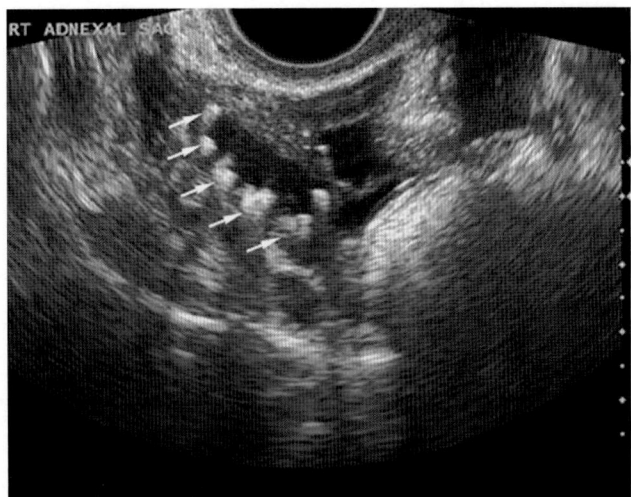

FIGURE 2-22 "Beads on a string" sign. The echogenic mural nodules shown here (*arrows*) within this tuboovarian abscess are thought to represent flattened and fibrotic endosalpingeal folds of the inflamed fallopian tube.

lumen occludes distally, the tube distends and fills with fluid. Various appearances result. The tube may become ovoid or pear shaped, filling with fluid that may be anechoic or echogenic. The tubal wall becomes thickened, measuring ≥5 mm, and incomplete septa are common as the tube folds back on itself. If the distended tube is viewed in cross section it may demonstrate the cogwheel sign, due to thickened endosalpingeal folds (Timor-Tritsch, 1998). Typically, the swollen fallopian tubes extend posteriorly into the cul-de-sac, rather than extending cephalad and anterior to the uterus as large ovarian tumors tend to do. Fluid-debris levels are often visualized in the dilated tubes, and rarely, gas-fluid levels or echogenic bubbles of gas are seen. Color and power Doppler show increased flow from hyperemia in the walls and in incomplete septa of the inflamed tubes (Tinkanen, 1993).

As the disease progresses, the ovary can become involved. When an ovary adheres to the fallopian tube, but is still visualized, it is called a tuboovarian complex. In contrast, a tuboovarian abscess results from a complete breakdown of ovarian and tubal architecture such that the separate structures are no longer identified (Fig. 2-22). If the contralateral side was not affected initially, it may become so. When both tubes are inflamed and occluded, the entire complex typically acquires a U-shape as it fills the cul-de-sac, extending from one adnexal region to the other. The lateral and posterior uterine borders become obscure, and individual tubes and ovaries cannot be distinguished. In women not responding to medical therapy, sonography or CT can be used to guide percutaneous or transvaginal drainage of these lesions.

Findings of chronic PID include hydrosalpinx. As discussed in Chapter 9, several sonographic findings such as its tubular shape, incomplete septa, and hyperechoic mural nodules can help to distinguish a hydrosalpinx from other cystic adnexal lesions (Fig. 9-23, p. 224). If color flow is detected in a hydrosalpinx, it tends to be less exuberant than flow seen in acute PID. Molander and colleagues (2002) found a higher pulsatility index in patients with a chronic hydrosalpinx (1.5 ± 0.1) than with acute PID (0.84 ± 0.04).

A small number of women with prior PID may have a peritoneal inclusion cyst. These form when ruptured ovarian cyst fluid is trapped around the ovary by adhesions. This diagnosis is suspected if the ovary is surrounded by fluid loculations created by thin septations.

■ Infertility

Sonography is employed for four main purposes in the approach to female infertility: (1) to identify abnormal pelvic anatomy; (2) to detect pathology causal or contributory to infertility; (3) to evaluate cyclic physiologic uterine and ovarian changes; and (4) to provide surveillance and visual guidance during infertility treatment.

Sonography can easily demonstrate anatomic uterine defects that may affect both gamete passage and ovum implantation. As discussed, conventional TVS can be used to visualize submucous leiomyomas and polyps, however, relationships of these lesions with the endometrial surface are better seen with SIS (see Figs. 2-6 and Fig. 8-7, p. 187). In those with a history of recurrent abortion, SIS has been used to demonstrate not only müllerian anomalies but various other uterine cavity defects in up to half of patients (Keltz, 1997). As a screening tool for cavity evaluation in this setting, it appears to be twice as accurate as HSG and TVS (Soares, 2000). Intrauterine synechiae can be seen by conventional sonography as hypoechoic lines disrupting the echogenic endometrium. These are more definitively seen during SIS as echogenic bands extending from one endometrial surface to the other (Fig. 2-23).

Transvaginal sonography is used initially to detect congenital uterine anomalies that can cause infertility or early spontaneous abortion. The addition of 3-D techniques can diagnose congenital abnormalities with a test performance similar to that of HSG, laparoscopy, and MR imaging. Thereafter, MR imaging is used to characterize and evaluate cases that are complicated or equivocal, especially preoperatively.

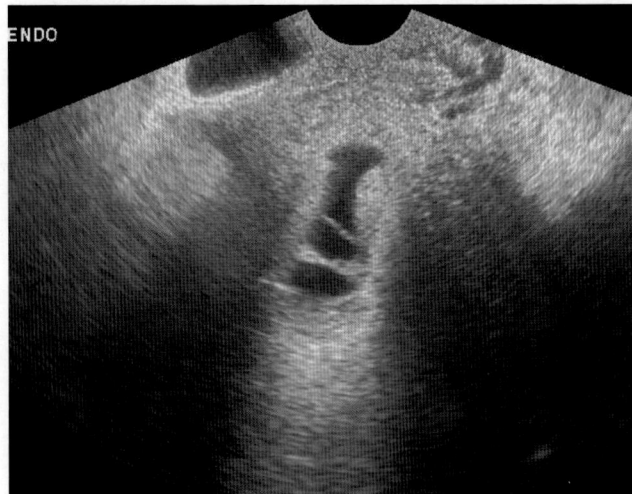

FIGURE 2-23 Asherman syndrome. Transvaginal saline infusion sonography demonstrates echogenic intrauterine synechiae.

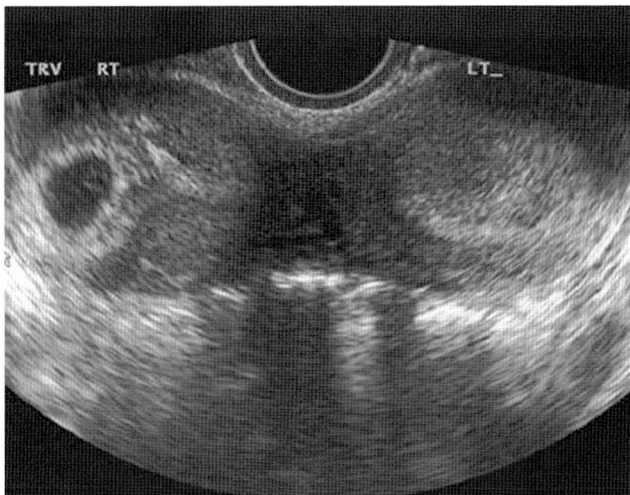

FIGURE 2-24 Uterus didelphys. Transvaginal sonogram in the transverse plane best depicts the two completely separate uterine horns. A gestational sac is evident in the right uterus.

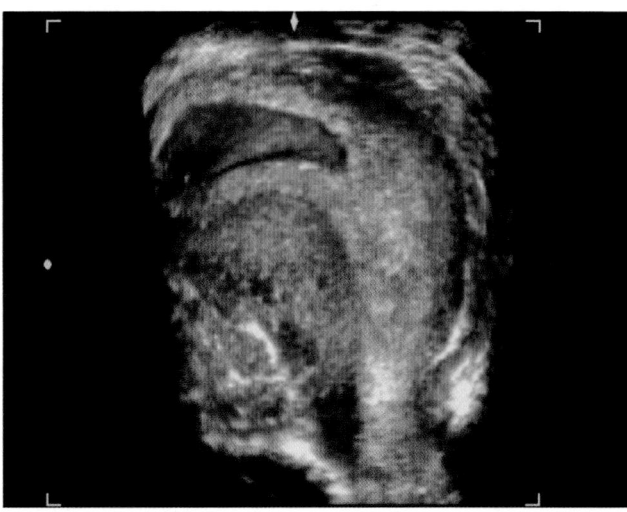

FIGURE 2-26 Unicornuate uterus. The coronal plane of 3-dimensional sonography illustrates the classic "banana" configuration. A gestational sac is seen within the endometrial cavity.

Of abnormalities, a complete fusion anomaly, such as uterus didelphys, can be accurately diagnosed by sonography. In this setting, two separate and divergent uterine horns are seen to have a deep fundal cleft between the two hemiuteri and to have a wide angle between the two endometrial cavities (Fig. 2-24). In contrast, bicornuate and septate uterine anomalies are less confidently differentiated by traditional 2-D TVS techniques. Ideally, the angle between the two endometrial cavities is ≥105° for bicornuate uterus, but ≤75° for septate uterus. The fundal contour shows a >1-cm notch for bicornuate uterus, but a <1-cm notch for septate uterus (Reuter, 1989). However, in many cases, the distinctions among complete bicornuate, partial bicornuate, and septate uteri are subtle. By measuring the relationship of the intracornual line—the line joining both horns of the uterine cavity—to the uterine fundal contour in the 3-D coronal plane, an accurate diagnosis can be made (Fig. 2-25). Similarly, arcuate versus partial septate uteri can be correctly differentiated using quantitative measurements of the depth

of fundal indentation of the endometrial cavity in the coronal plane. Combining 3-D TVS findings with SIS provides accuracy up to 90 percent to distinguish the two anomalies. Although MR imaging is frequently employed, 3-D sonography is considered by many to be the best noninvasive method for distinguishing between these uterine anomalies (Bermejo, 2010; Salim, 2003).

A unicornuate uterus without a rudimentary horn is seen as a small, well-formed elliptical uterus that deviates to one side and has a single cornu. The fundal shape is concave. With 3-D imaging, the unicornuate uterus has the classic "banana" configuration (Fig. 2-26). In 65 percent of cases, however, the unicornuate uterus is associated with a rudimentary horn, and this is difficult to recognize sonographically (Fig. 18-11, p. 419) (Jayasinghe, 2005). The dilated rudimentary horn is often misdiagnosed as a uterine or adnexal mass. Complete evaluation of these cases often requires MR imaging. With most uterine anomalies, especially if unilateral, proper positioning

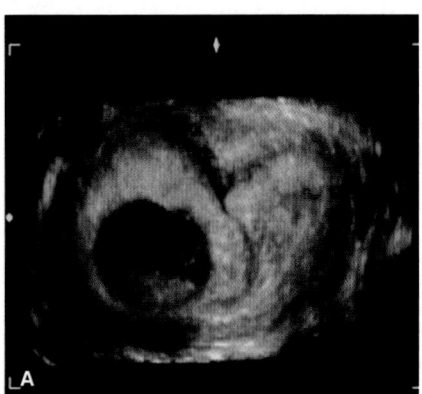
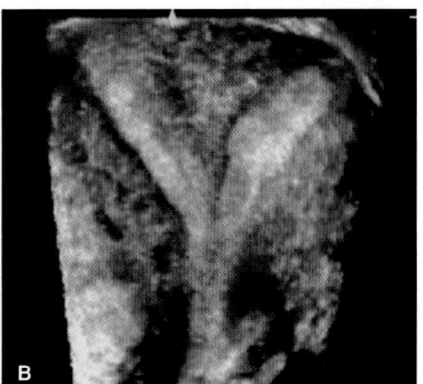
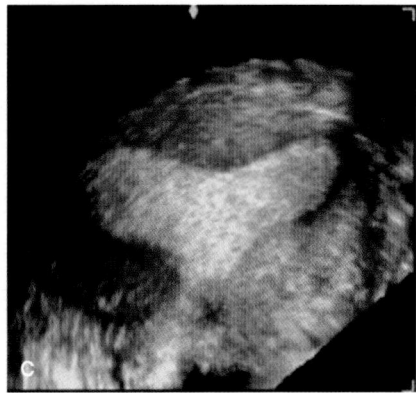

FIGURE 2-25 Three-dimensional (3-D) images of müllerian anomalies in the coronal plane. **A.** Bicornuate uterus. This 3-D rendered image demonstrates a concave external fundal contour that dips below the intercornual line consistent with a bicornuate uterus. Note the pregnancy in the right uterine horn. **B.** Septate uterus. This image depicts the normal uterine serosal contour and the narrow angle between the two small endometrial cavities characteristic of a septate uterus. As the septum ends at the uterine isthmus and does not extend into the cervix, this anomaly is properly termed *subseptate*. **C.** Arcuate uterus. This image illustrates the normal uterine serosal contour and obtuse angle of the endometrial indentation that is characteristic of an arcuate uterus.

of the kidneys should be documented with transabdominal imaging because of increased rates of associated genitourinary anomalies. Last, in women with complex anomalies associated with vaginal agenesis or imperforate hymen, hematocolpos is commonly seen, often with associated hematometra or hematosalpinx.

Pelvic endometriosis is another frequent cause of infertility. Sonography is the most common imaging procedure to evaluate suspected endometriosis, although it is mostly used to evaluate endometriotic cysts. Endometriomas exhibit a variety of sonographic appearances, the most frequent being a pelvic mass with a thick wall and diffuse low-level echoes within the cyst (Fig. 10-4, p. 236). Magnetic resonance imaging is more specific than sonography for identifying endometriomas, and thus, it is indicated in cases with unclear anatomy sonographically (Fig. 10-8). Sonography's ability to detect small implants and adhesions is limited, but it can be used to identify some cases of deep-infiltrating endometriosis.

One of the most powerful uses of sonography in the infertile patient is treatment surveillance. Sonography is used to monitor folliculogenesis both in normal and stimulated cycles. In natural cycles, observation of a developing follicle and ovulation prediction allow optimal timing for postcoital testing, human chorionic gonadotropin (hCG) administration, intercourse, insemination, and ovum collection. At ovulation, the follicle usually disappears, and fluid is observed in the cul-de-sac. At the follicular site, the corpus luteum appears as an irregular oval containing a small quantity of fluid, internal echoes, and a thick wall. In stimulated cycles, sonographic detection of too many follicles allows withholding of hCG induction to prevent ovarian hyperstimulation syndrome (Fig. 20-4, p. 456). If this develops, sonography is used to grade disease severity through measurements of ovarian size, detection of ascites, and analysis of renal flow resistances. In general, blood flow in the ovulating ovary decreases throughout the menstrual cycle. At ovulation, blood flow velocities dramatically increase in vessels surrounding the corpus luteum because of neovascularization and are seen as low-impedance waveforms. In women undergoing in vitro fertilization (IVF), low ovarian vessel impedance may correlate directly with pregnancy rates (Baber, 1988). Many infertility specialists now incorporate SIS as a first-line screening tool for uterine evaluation before embryo transfer in women undergoing IVF, ovum donation, and IVF-surrogacy (Gera, 2008; Yauger, 2008). Last, sonography can be used to guide interventional maneuvers such as oocyte retrieval and transfer of embryos into the endometrial cavity (Figs. 20-10 and 20-12, p. 464).

■ Ultrasound beyond the Pelvis

Ultrasound is used throughout the body. It is often the initial tool in radiologic evaluation, given its lack of ionizing radiation, low cost, and availability. In the abdomen, common indications for solid organ evaluation include abdominal and flank pain, jaundice, hematuria, organomegaly, or palpable mass. Abnormal blood tests, including elevated liver function tests and creatinine levels, may also be indications for an abdominal ultrasound. Typically, a limited or right upper quadrant ultrasound includes the liver, gallbladder, common bile duct, pancreas, and right kidney. A complete abdominal ultrasound adds the spleen, left kidney, and images of the aorta and inferior vena cava in the upper abdomen. Ideally, a patient has fasted prior to sonographic evaluation of the abdomen to minimize bowel gas and for adequate gallbladder distention. A renal ultrasound focuses on the kidneys, proximal collecting systems, and urinary bladder. Outside of the abdomen and pelvis, a gynecologist may select ultrasound to evaluate superficial structures, like the thyroid gland and breasts. Breast imaging is discussed in Chapter 12 (p. 278).

Compression Sonography

Compression sonography, often combined with color Doppler sonography, is the initial test currently used to detect deep-vein thrombosis (DVT) (Hanley, 2013). Sonographic evaluation of leg veins is divided into: (1) the groin and thigh examined with the patient supine; and (2) the popliteal region examined with the patient sitting or lying on her side with the thigh abducted and externally rotated. Some institutions also evaluate the calf veins. Impaired visibility, noncompressibility, and the typical echo pattern of a thrombosed vein confirm the diagnosis (Fig. 2-27).

Examination of the femoral, popliteal, and calf trifurcation veins in symptomatic patients is more than 90-percent sensitive and greater than 99-percent specific for proximal DVT (Davis, 2001). Moreover, in 220 patients with suspected DVT, Lensing and coworkers (1989) compared compression sonography with contrast venography, which is the gold standard for DVT

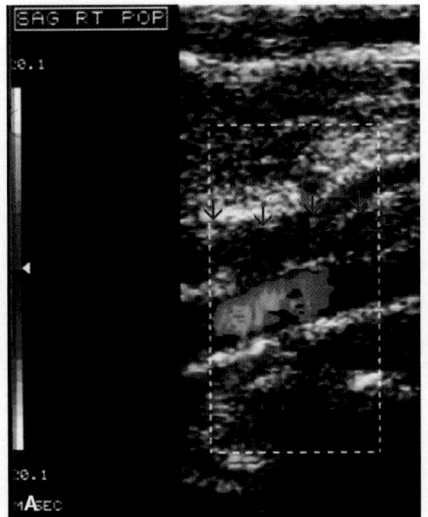
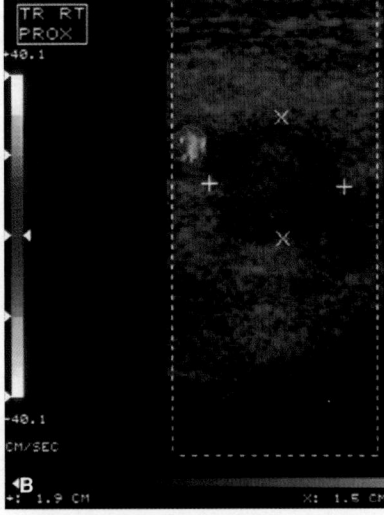

FIGURE 2-27 Sagittal (**A**) and transverse (**B**) images from a lower extremity. Color Doppler ultrasound study in a woman with popliteal vein thrombosis. **A.** Red arrows demarcate the popliteal vein with no flow suggesting clot in the lumen, which sits above the artery demonstrating normal flow as evidenced by the red color map. **B.** The transverse image shows the large size of the vein due to the thrombus (*cursors*), as well as normal flow in the artery, evidenced by the red color map.

detection. They found that both the common femoral and popliteal veins were fully compressible—no thrombosis—in 142 of 143 patients who had a normal venogram (99-percent specific). All 66 patients with proximal vein thrombosis had noncompressible femoral or popliteal veins, or both (100-percent sensitive).

For detecting calf vein thrombosis, compression sonography is significantly less reliable. Eventually, isolated calf thromboses extend into the proximal veins in up to a fourth of cases. They do so within 1 to 2 weeks of presentation and thus are usually detected by serial sonographic compression examinations (Bates, 2004). The safety of withholding anticoagulation for those symptomatic patients who have a normal compression examination has been established (Birdwell, 1998; Friera, 2002). Importantly, normal venous sonographic findings do not necessarily exclude pulmonary embolism (PE) because the thrombosis may have already embolized or because it arose from deep pelvic veins, which are inaccessible to sonographic evaluation (Goldhaber, 2004).

Ultrasound is frequently used for other vascular assessments. Sonographic screening is performed for abdominal aortic aneurysm and to evaluate solid organ vasculature. Also, vascular ultrasound incorporates spectral and color Doppler to assess the lower extremities for venous insufficiencies that may contribute to varicose veins and venous congestion.

RADIOGRAPHY

Radiographs are used in gynecologic practice in a manner similar to other medical specialties. Of frequently used studies, the *acute abdominal series* includes an upright radiograph of the chest to exclude free air under the diaphragm, an upright film of the abdomen to exclude air-fluid levels within bowel loops, and a supine image to measure bowel loop widths. It is commonly selected as an initial modality if bowel obstruction or perforation is a concern. Importantly, images from those with recent laparotomy or laparoscopy often show expected subdiaphragmatic air. In contrast, a single supine radiograph of the abdomen is called a KUB (kidneys, ureters, and bladder). It may help identify an extrauterine location of a missing IUD or a collecting-system stone.

In women with gynecologic malignancies, radiographs may also be informative. Examples are chest radiographs to screen for pulmonary metastases during cancer staging and during surveillance after initial treatment. As discussed in the next sections, several specialized radiographic procedures are especially useful or specific for gynecology.

◼ Breast Imaging

Of screening methods, mammography is the only modality clinically proven to decrease breast cancer-related mortality rates in women aged 40 to 74 years. Sensitivity of first mammography ranges from 71 to 96 percent (Humphrey, 2002). For the general population, annual screening mammography is recommended starting at age 40 for women, and a full discussion of screening criteria are found in Chapter 12 (p. 288).

During mammography, breast compression serves to immobilize the breast, to shorten exposure times, and to provide more uniform tissue thickness. These improve image quality and lower radiation doses (American College of Radiology, 2014). Digital mammography has largely replaced screen-film techniques. This lowers radiation doses, which now only approximate 1.6 mGy (Mettler, 2008). In women with breast implants, mammographic evaluation includes standard and implant-displaced mammographic views. Whether the implant is subpectoral or intramammary, to obtain these additional views, the breast implant is displaced posteriorly toward the patient's chest while the breast tissue is pulled over and in front of the implant.

Different from screening mammography, women with a palpable breast mass or clinical symptom require *diagnostic mammography*. With this, craniocaudal and mediolateral oblique views of each breast are standardly obtained, and additional views are captured as needed to evaluate specific regions of concern. At the same visit, ultrasound evaluation of the breast may add diagnostic information regarding the internal structure of a finding.

If an abnormality is identified during mammography, image-guided aspiration or biopsy is often indicated. If lesions are visible sonographically, ultrasound can guide the radiologist in real time during the biopsy. If the abnormality is not sonographically visible or if concerning calcifications are present, stereotactic and vacuum-assisted core biopsies are obtained using radiographic guidance. During stereotactic breast biopsy, the patient usually lies prone on a specialized table. The breast hangs through an opening and is compressed similar to mammography. Prior to sampling with a biopsy core needle or vacuum-assisted device, two mammographic images are obtained to precisely target the finding, and local anesthetic is administered. With vacuum-assisted biopsy, suction pulls more tissue into the needle for sampling. For abnormalities only detected with MR imaging, MR-guided biopsies are also possible, done with a technique similar to stereotactic biopsy, but performed in the MR scanner using specialized coils, localization grids, and biopsy tools.

Distinct from diagnostic breast MR imaging, *screening* breast MR imaging is reserved for specific patient groups whose lifetime breast cancer risk exceeds 20 to 25 percent as calculated by the Gail model (Chap. 12, p. 287) (Saslow, 2007). For either indication, IV gadolinium contrast is typically administered.

In women with a nipple discharge, a ductogram or galactogram may be informative. The involved duct is cannulated with a fine catheter and a small amount of contrast is injected prior to obtaining additional mammographic views (Fig. 12-7, p. 281). A full discussion of breast disease evaluation is found in Chapter 12.

◼ Intravenous Pyelography

Excretory urography, also called intravenous pyelography (IVP), is a radiographic study that provides serial imaging of the urinary tract. The initial radiograph, termed a *scout film*, helps identify radiopaque urinary calculi. Intravenous contrast is then administered, and the concentrating function of the proximal tubules renders renal parenchyma radiodense within 1–3 minutes. This *nephrogram phase* allows evaluation of renal size, contour, and axis. Next, a radiograph obtained 5 minutes after injection depicts contrast excreted into the collecting system. During this *pyelogram phase,* the calyces and proximal ureters are evaluated for symmetry and excretion promptness. Serial imaging is obtained as the more distal collecting system and bladder is opacified by contrast, and a final postvoid radiograph completes the imaging.

Up to 5 to 10 percent of women have an allergic reaction to iodide during IVP, and 1 to 2 percent of reactions are life threatening. In addition, hyperosmolar ionic contrast can be nephrotoxic because of direct tubular insult and ischemic injury. Notably, women with diabetes, renal impairment, and congestive heart failure are at high risk for this contrast nephrotoxicity. As alternatives, nonionic low and isoosmolar iodinated contrast media carry a five- to 30-fold lower incidence of allergic reactions and are less nephrotoxic (Mishell, 1997). Because of this improved safety profile, most centers no longer use intravascular hyperosmolar ionic contrast (American College of Radiology, 2013).

Preoperatively, IVP may be selected to identify urinary anomalies coexistent with reproductive tract congenital defects or confirm lower urinary tract compression by an adjacent pelvic neoplasm. However, many preoperative IVPs have been replaced with multiphasic CT urography protocols performed on multislice CT scanners (Beyersdorff, 2008). For example, although it is not a formal part of cervical cancer staging, many clinicians in the United States substitute CT imaging for IVP in cervical cancer evaluation. Of value, CT allows the cervix, parametria, uterus, adnexa, retroperitoneal lymph nodes, liver, and ureters to be imaged concurrently.

For suspected nephrolithiasis, the American College of Radiology recommends primary evaluation using noncontrast CT given its superior sensitivity for renal stones (Coursey, 2011). To evaluate hematuria, noncontrast combined with contrast-enhanced CT images (CT urography) is most appropriate due to improved sensitivity for renal and urothelial masses. Although IVP has higher in-plane spatial resolution, the current recommendations are to move immediately to initial one-step CT evaluation as CT is frequently needed regardless of IVP results to delineate abnormalities (Cowan, 2007, 2012). That said, IVP may still play a role, especially in resource-poor areas, in postoperative patients, and in those for whom radiation exposure is ideally minimized. Specifically, IVP delivers an average adult effective dose of 1 to 10 mSv, whereas CT urography carries an average adult effective dose of 10 to 30 mSv (Coursey, 2011; Ramchandani, 2008).

■ Voiding Cystourethrography and Positive Pressure Urethrography

These radiographic procedures, discussed in Chapter 26 (p. 586), are used to evaluate the female urethra. Voiding cystourethrography (VCUG) is performed by placing a small catheter into the urinary bladder to instill contrast media. For evaluation of prolapse or incontinence, the patient may be asked to Valsalva during examination. After adequate distention of the bladder, the patient is asked to urinate and images are acquired during both bladder filling and urination. If present, diverticula that open into the urethra will fill with contrast. In cases of suspected vesicovaginal or urethrovaginal fistula, the contrast trail connecting the two involved structures is seen.

In comparison, MR imaging permits superior visualization of urethral abnormalities and is more sensitive than VCUG or positive pressure urethrography (PPUG) for delineating diverticula with complex structure (Chou, 2008; Neitlich, 1998). For this reason, VCUG is currently more often used to evaluate lower urinary tract injury, such as fistulas, and patients with prolonged urinary retention, incontinence, or suspected vesicoureteral reflux.

Described in more detail in Chapter 26 (p. 586), PPUG use has declined. This stems mainly from decreasing numbers of technicians trained to complete the study, difficulty finding appropriate equipment, and the higher sensitivity of MR imaging.

■ Hysterosalpingography

This radiographic imaging technique is typically used during infertility evaluations to assess the endocervical canal, the endometrial cavity, and the fallopian tube lumina by injecting radiopaque contrast material through the cervical canal (Chap. 19, p. 438). An average HSG study is performed in 10 minutes, involves approximately 90 seconds of fluoroscopic time, and has an average radiation exposure to the ovaries of 0.01 to 0.02 Gy. As discussed previously (p. 25), hysterosalpingo-contrast sonography is used by some initially in place of HSG to assess tubal patency.

Hysterosalpingography is performed between cycle days 5 and 10. During this time, cessation of menstrual flow minimizes infection and the risk of flushing an ovum from the fallopian tube following ovulation. The test causes cramping, and an NSAID taken 30 minutes prior to the procedure may limit discomfort. To begin, a designated balloon-tipped injection catheter or acorn cannula is introduced just beyond the internal os and in the lower endometrial cavity, as this location is more comfortable for the patient. However, the catheter may also be positioned just cephalad to the external os within the endocervical canal if necessary. A paracervical block may be indicated in selected patients, such as those with cervical stenosis. Because rapid injection may cause tubal spasm, slow contrast injection of usually no more than 3 to 4 mL of contrast medium allows a clear outline of the uterine cavity. Generally, few radiographic views are needed: a preliminary view before injecting contrast, a view showing uterine cavity filling, and the third demonstrating spill of contrast from the fallopian tubes into the peritoneal cavity. An additional image with the catheter deflated and pulled back into the endocervical canal will typically be obtained at the conclusion of the examination to evaluate the lower uterine cavity and internal os.

A normal HSG may have variable appearances (Fig. 19-6, p. 439). The endometrial cavity is usually triangular or sometimes T-shaped in the anteroposterior (AP) projection. In the lateral view, it is oblong. The contour of the endometrium is usually smooth. It occasionally has polypoid filling defects that can be isolated or diffuse and can be difficult to distinguish from endometrial polyps or hyperplasia. Inadvertent injection of air bubbles introduces artifact. In these instances, SIS is often later obtained to further interrogate the endometrial cavity.

Contraindications to HSG include acute pelvic infection, active uterine bleeding, pregnancy, and iodine allergy. HSG complications are rare but can be serious. Of these, the overall risk of acute pelvic infection serious enough to require hospitalization is less than 1 percent but can reach 3 percent in women with prior pelvic infection (Stumpf, 1980). In patients with no history of pelvic infection, HSG is performed without prophylactic antibiotics. If HSG demonstrates dilated fallopian tubes, doxycycline, 100 mg orally twice daily for 5 days, is given to reduce the incidence of post-HSG PID. In patients with a history of pelvic infection, doxycycline can be administered before the procedure and continued if dilated fallopian tubes are found (American College of Obstetricians and Gynecologists, 2014). Pelvic pain, uterine perforation, and vasovagal reactions may also occur. From the contrast, allergic reaction and entry into the vascular system from high injection pressure are potential risks.

■ Selective Salpingography

In some cases, it is not possible to distinguish whether tubal blockage seen by HSG is caused by anatomic occlusion or tubal spasm. Hysteroscopic tubal cannulation can further clarify and treat many cases of proximal tubal occlusion as described in Section 44-18 (p. 1050). Alternatively, transcervical selective salpingography and tubal catheterization (SS-TC) under fluoroscopic guidance is another procedure that may be used. It is performed during the follicular phase of the cycle with the catheter forwarded through the cervix and advanced by tactile sensation to the tubal ostium. The position of the catheter is checked fluoroscopically, and if it is satisfactory, water- or oil-soluble contrast is injected. If the obstruction is overcome, the tubal contour is outlined with contrast agent. If the proximal tubal obstruction persists, a guide wire is threaded through the inner cannula of the catheter, advanced toward the obstruction, and gently manipulated to overcome the blockage. The guide wire is then withdrawn, and contrast medium is injected through the catheter to confirm patency. This fluoroscopic tool is effective at diagnosing and treating proximal tubal blockage and is discussed in Chapter 20 (p. 458) (Capitanio, 1991; Thurmond, 1991).

■ Bone Densitometry

Depending on its mineral density, bone absorbs x-rays to different degrees. Because of this, bone density can be determined, and most measurements provide site-specific information. However, these studies do not assess current or past bone remodeling rates. Thus, sequential density measurements are necessary to monitor rates of bone loss over time (Kaplan, 1995). Currently, two common methods are used. Dual-energy x-ray absorptiometry (DEXA) measures integral bone (cortical and trabecular bone) mineral density in the hip and spine. Quantitative computed tomography (QCT) evaluates bone mineral in high-turnover trabecular bone.

Of these, DEXA is the best technique for axial osteopenia determination (Fig. 21-8, p. 480). It employs two x-ray beams of differing energy levels and accurately measures bone density in the hip and spine—areas most vulnerable to osteoporotic fractures. The spine is commonly scanned between the 1st and 4th lumbar vertebrae. Measurements with DEXA are precise

and accurate; radiation dose is low—less than 5 mrem; and patient acceptability is high because the procedure time is usually only 5 to 15 minutes (Jergas, 1993). The reproducibility of DEXA bone mass measurement to identify a population at high risk for fracture is excellent. DEXA is the preferred method for bone mineral density measurement to diagnose osteoporosis (Chap. 21, p. 479). DEXA instruments that measure bone mass at peripheral sites such as the forearm are also available, but these may not predict hip fractures as accurately as direct hip measurement. Other advantages include a proven effectiveness in monitoring antifracture treatments and being the standard against which other bone imaging measures are evaluated (Blake, 2007). Disadvantageously, DEXA is a 2-D technique that cannot distinguish between cortical and trabecular bone. In addition, bone spurs, aortic calcifications, and arthritis may falsely elevate reported bone density.

Quantitative computed tomography (QCT) uses multiple x-rays to provide a cross-sectional view of the vertebral body. As the rate of turnover in trabecular bone is nearly eight times that in cortical bone, this technique can detect early metabolic changes in this highly vulnerable bone type. It provides a volumetric density, which is an advantage in situations in which DEXA may underestimate bone mineral density (Damilakis, 2007). Although its precision is excellent and it can be used to follow patients undergoing therapy, it has never been validated for World Health Organization (WHO) criteria and is not routinely used as a screening modality. Another technique is quantitative sonography (QUS). This may provide information regarding the structural organization of bone and offers the potential for greater community access to bone mass evaluation (Philipov, 2000; World Health Organization, 1994).

COMPUTED TOMOGRAPHY

This procedure involves multiple exposures of thin x-ray beams that are translated to 2-D axial images, termed a *slice*, of the particular area of interest. Multiple slices of the target body part are obtained along its length. Multiple-channel helical computed tomography, also called *spiral CT*, allows for continuous acquisition of images in a spiral and the potential for image reformatting in multiple planes. This technique is much faster and permits images to be manipulated for analysis after they have been acquired. Many variables affect radiation dose, especially slice thickness and number of cuts obtained. If a study is performed with multiple phases of contrast, each added phase or acquisition multiplies the total patient dose of radiation.

Intravenous contrast enables superior evaluation of solid organ parenchyma and vasculature. By adding IV contrast, masses become more obvious due to density differences. Dedicated thin slice evaluation of vasculature, termed CT angiography (CTA), can be done throughout the body. Although traditional (fluoroscopic) angiography is still performed, the information that cross-sectional imaging provides and its relative technical ease have increased its use. As discussed earlier, intravenous nonionic low and isoosmolar iodinated contrast media can induce nephrotoxicity and should be used with caution in patients with or at risk for renal insufficiency. Intravenous hydration before and after an examination can

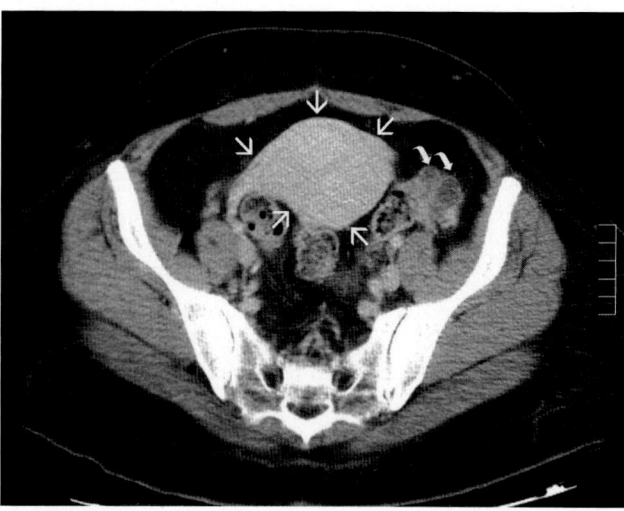

FIGURE 2-28 Computed tomography (CT) of the female pelvis in the axial plane demonstrates the normal uterus (*arrows*) as well as cysts in the left ovary (*curved arrows*).

help reduce contrast-induced nephrotoxicity. One option is 0.9-percent saline at 100 mL/hr beginning 6 to 12 hours before imaging and continuing 4 to 12 hours after the examination (American College of Radiology, 2013).

Oral contrast may enhance CT images if there is concern for gastrointestinal disease or if bowel must be differentiated from adjacent structures. Positive oral contrast is most frequently used and is dense (white) on images. Patients with documented allergies to *intravenous* contrast are rarely allergic to oral contrast. Intraluminal contrast in the rectum or urinary bladder also is dense (white) and can be used to address a specific concern, such as rectovaginal fistula or bladder injury, respectively.

■ Normal Pelvic Anatomy

The uterus is identified as a homogenous, soft tissue oval or triangle situated posterior to the bladder (Fig. 2-28). The uterine walls enhance after IV contrast. However, unlike sonography and MR imaging, the endometrium is poorly delineated by CT imaging. The cervix also may not enhance like the remainder of the uterus, and the inner stromal layer typically enhances less than the outer stromal layer (Yitta, 2011). The endocervical canal, which can be identified by MR imaging, is indistinct using CT imaging. The lateral margins of the cervix can typically be differentiated from parametrial fat because of differences in density. However, CT is not sensitive for parametrial involvement in the setting of cervical cancer (Hricak, 2005). Imaging of the vagina and vulva is very limited with CT. Typically, the ovaries are relatively hypodense, vary in appearance and position, and are usually situated lateral to the uterus.

■ Imaging Following Gynecologic Surgery

CT is well suited to diagnose potential complications of gynecologic procedures. For ureteral injuries, CT with IV contrast or CT urography is useful. To detect obstruction or injury, CT images are obtained after the kidneys have excreted the contrast and have opacified the collecting systems. High density

(white) contrast that abruptly stops within the ureter suggests obstruction. With ureteral disruption, contrast may flow freely from the injury site or may form an encapsulated collection, a urinoma (Titton, 2003).

For bladder injury, CT cystography may be informative. For this, the bladder is retrograde filled with 300 to 400 mL of dilute iodinated contrast by gravity drip. This is followed by helical CT of the bladder with multiplanar reformations (Chan, 2006). The technique is sensitive and specific for diagnosis of extraperitoneal and intraperitoneal bladder rupture and can also demonstrate vesicovaginal, ureterovaginal, or vesicoenteric fistulas (Jankowski, 2006; Yu, 2004).

CT also outperforms conventional radiography and barium studies for diagnosing bowel complications, such as small bowel obstruction (Maglinte, 1993). For characterizing an abdominal-pelvic fluid collection such as abscess or hematoma, CT with intravenous and oral contrast may be more helpful than other imaging tools (Fig. 3-8, p. 68) (Gjelsteen, 2008).

■ Gynecologic Malignancy

In most instances, sonography is the preferred initial method of evaluating the female pelvis. If additional anatomic information is needed, MR imaging is now often preferable to CT imaging because it avoids radiation exposure and iodinated IV contrast, provides excellent soft-tissue contrast, and displays pelvic structures in multiple planes. That said, CT imaging is probably the most frequently used imaging technique for evaluation and surveillance of gynecologic malignancies. Although its sensitivity for intraperitoneal metastases is limited, CT can estimate bulky metastases, such as in women with advanced ovarian cancer.

MAGNETIC RESONANCE IMAGING

With this technology, images are constructed based on the radiofrequency signal emitted by hydrogen nuclei after they have been "excited" by radiofrequency pulses in the presence of a strong magnetic field. The radiofrequency signal emitted has characteristics called *relaxation times*. These include the T1-relaxation time (longitudinal) and the T2-relaxation time (transverse). The signal intensity of one tissue compared with another, that is, the contrast, can be manipulated by adjusting parameters of the acquisition. For example, by varying the elapsed time between applications of radiofrequency pulses, which is called *repetition time,* and the time between a radiofrequency pulse and sampling the emitted signal, called the *echo delay time*, different tissue weighting can be achieved.

Sequences with a short repetition time and short echo delay time are called *T1-weighted*. Sequences with a long repetition time and long echo delay time are regarded as *T2-weighted*. As examples, the hydrogen molecules in a water-containing area, such as urine in the bladder, have longer relaxation times than those in a solid tissue such as liver. On T1-weighted images, urine in the bladder will appear dark or have low signal intensity. On T2-weighted images, the same urine will appear bright or have high signal intensity. By manipulating multiple parameters and imaging planes, MR imaging is able to achieve superior soft-tissue contrast. The strength of the magnetic field within the bore of the magnet is measured in tesla (T) (1 tesla = 10,000 gauss). For reference, the earth's magnetic field is approximately 0.5 gauss. Most clinical magnets used for MR imaging are 1.5 to 3 T or 15,000 to 30,000 gauss.

■ Technique

The standard imaging technique for the pelvis includes both T1- and T2-weighted sequences that are acquired in at least two planes, usually axial and sagittal. The T2-weighted sequence provides detailed definition of internal organ architecture, such as the zonal anatomy of the uterus and vagina, and aids identification of normal ovaries. T2-weighted images are usually superior in depicting pathologic conditions of the uterus and ovaries. The T1-weighted sequence clearly delineates organ boundaries and surrounding fat, allows optimal visualization of lymph nodes, and is necessary for tissue and fluid content characterization.

To aid accurate diagnosis, highly paramagnetic gadolinium-based contrast agents (GBCAs) are often administered prior to imaging. The most frequently used GBCA types are extracellular agents administered intravenously. Gadolinium shortens the T1 relaxation time of adjacent protons. This increases signal intensity on T1-weighted images to enhance information regarding tissue vascularity (Gandhi, 2006). Side effects are rare, and MR contrast can be used even in those with prior reactions to other contrast agents (American College of Radiology, 2004). MR contrast is given in concentrations and doses significantly lower than that used in CT imaging, undergoes renal excretion within 24 hours, and is safe for patients with mildly compromised renal function. Of note, the FDA recommends caution in administering IV GBCAs to patients with moderate to end-stage renal disease (glomerular filtration rate <30 mL/min/1.73 m^2) due to the rare but serious risk of developing nephrogenic systemic fibrosis (NSF). The risks and benefits of using GBCAs are discussed by the requesting physician and radiologist. Written informed consent from the patient is obtained if GBCA use is required for those with a severely diminished glomerular filtration rate. Providing hemodialysis immediately after administration of GBCA for patients in this category of renal compromise for the prevention of NSF has not been proven.

In addition to intravascular GBCAs, water-soluble ultrasound gel can be placed endoluminally (in the vagina and/or the rectum) to better delineate anatomy. This technique can also aid in detection of fistulas and be used to better visualize vaginal septa in the setting of müllerian anomalies (Gupta, 2014).

Additional imaging parameters include fat saturation to detect bulk fat and opposed-phase imaging to highlight microscopic fat. Diffusion-weighted imaging (DWI) with quantitative measurement of apparent diffusion coefficient (ADC) provides information regarding proton movement in tissues. Highly cellular tissues restrict random Brownian motion and yield a high DWI signal and low ADC value. This cellularity information can help identify tumors, abscesses, and lymph nodes (Moore, 2014).

■ Safety

The effects from static magnetic fields and gradient magnetic fields generated with MR imaging have been extensively studied.

TABLE 2-1. Safety of Magnetic Resonance Imaging with Some Implanted Devices

Device	Safe (S), Conditional (C), or Unsafe (U)	
	1.5 T	3 T
Intrauterine Devices		
Paragard	S	C
Mirena	S	S
Skyla	—	C
Tubal Occlusion Devices		
Essure	S	C
Adiana (Silicone)	S	S
Adiana (Radiopaque)	S	C
Filshie Clips	S	C
Hulka (Clemens) Clip	S	C
Implants		
Implanon/Nexplanon	S	S
Saline or silicone breast	S	S
Tissue expander with non-magnetic injection site	S	—
Tissue expander with magnetically localizable injection site	U	U
Biopsy Needles/Markers		
Localization wires	U	U
Biopsy needles	U	U
Coaxial needles	U	U
Breast biopsy markers (e.g., HydroMark)	S	C

To date, harmful or mutagenic effects have not been reported from MR imaging at field strengths used clinically, that is, 3 T or lower. Additionally, the American College of Radiology considers the use of MR imaging in pregnancy to be risk free, regardless of trimester. With its lack of ionizing radiation, MR imaging may be particularly useful in pregnant women for the characterization of pathology for which sonography has provided an inconclusive diagnosis. Using the ALARA (as low as reasonably achievable) principle, imaging during pregnancy is typically limited to 1.5 T. Moreover, GBCAs are not used routinely in pregnancy due to the theoretic risk of toxic gadolinium ion dissociation from its ligand into the amnionic fluid (Kanal, 2013).

Some, but not all, devices preclude MR imaging. For example, many implanted devices unique to women can be safely imaged (Table 2-1). Contraindications to entering the MR environment include mechanically, electrically, or magnetically activated implanted devices such as internal cardiac pacemakers, neurostimulators, cardiac defibrillators, electronic infusion pumps, and cochlear implants. Certain intracranial aneurysm clips and any metallic foreign body in the globe of the eye contraindicate scanning. Before the patient enters the MR environment, radiology personnel should obtain documentation of the type of patient implant (manufacturer, model, and type) and verify the MR safety rating.

Use in Gynecology

Although sonography is widely used for suspected gynecologic disease, MR imaging may add information when sonographic findings are equivocal. Specifically, its multiplanar imaging, superior soft-tissue contrast, and large field of view are distinct MR imaging advantages. Accordingly, common indications for MR imaging include distorted pelvic anatomy, large masses that are poorly delineated with sonography, indeterminate cases of adenomyosis, and endometrial disorders in poor surgical candidates. In some instances, pelvic MR imaging may help tailor clinical gynecologic and surgical management (Schwartz, 1994). Also, MR imaging is commonly selected for primary evaluation and subsequent surveillance of pelvic malignancies.

Normal Findings

The pelvic organs show generally moderate to low signal intensity on T1-weighted images. T2-weighted images of the menstrual uterus depict a high-signal-intensity endometrium; contiguous low-signal-intensity inner myometrium, which is the junctional zone; and a moderate-signal-intensity outer myometrium (Fig. 2-29) (McCarthy, 1986).

The cervix can be distinguished from the uterine body by its prominent fibrous stroma, which has an overall lower signal intensity. The internal architecture of the cervix is seen on T2-weighted images as central high signal intensity (endocervical glands and mucus) surrounded by low signal intensity (fibrous stroma) and peripheral moderate signal intensity (smooth muscle intermixed with fibrous stroma) (Lee, 1985). Similarly, T2-weighted images of the vagina display central high-signal-intensity mucosa and mucus, which is surrounded by a low-signal-intensity muscular wall (Hricak, 1988). Ovaries are normally seen on the T2-weighted sequence as moderately high-signal-intensity stroma containing very high-signal-intensity

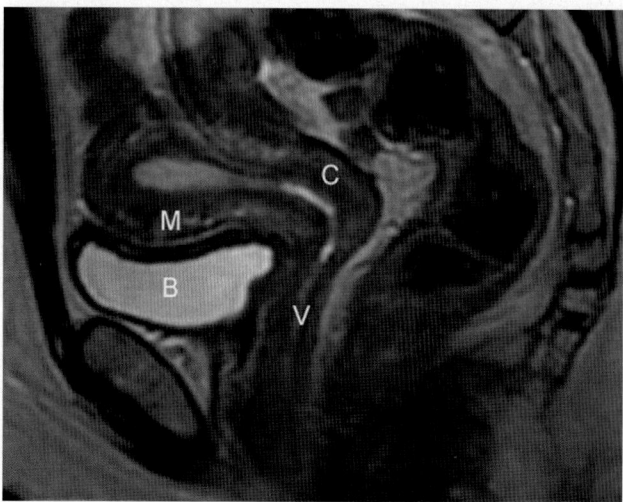

FIGURE 2-29 Sagittal T2-weighted magnetic resonance (MR) image of a normal uterus and cervix (C). B = bladder; M = myometrium; V = vagina.

follicles (Dooms, 1986). The fallopian tubes are not typically visualized. Hormonal status influences the MR appearance of all structures and reflects associated physiologic changes.

Benign Disease

Leiomyomas

Sonography remains the initial imaging technique for suspected leiomyomas, but its limited field of view, image resolution that declines with increasing patient body fat, and distorted anatomy from large or multiple myomas are potential hindrances (Wolfman, 2006). False-negative rates may reach 20 percent, and tumors <2 cm are routinely missed by TVS, even when symptomatic (Gross, 1983). Thus, MR imaging is used when TVS findings are equivocal or nondiagnostic (Ascher, 2003). For conservative myoma treatment, the effects of GnRH agonist therapy to shrink tumor volume can be quantified with MR imaging (Lubich, 1991). Moreover, MR imaging is warranted before UAE or focused-ultrasound myoma treatments and often selected prior to hysteroscopic myoma resection. In these cases, imaging verifies leiomyoma location, seeks tumor qualities that portend outcome success or failure, and excludes other causes of patient symptoms such as unsuspected malignancy or indeterminate intracavitary masses (Cura, 2006; Rajan, 2011).

As shown in Figure 2-30, leiomyomas have a variable but characteristic MR appearance and thus can be differentiated from adenomyosis or adenomyoma with 90-percent accuracy (Mark, 1987; Togashi, 1989). This is important when myomectomy is considered. Leiomyomas, even those as small as 0.5 cm, are best seen on T2-weighted images and appear as round, sharply marginated, low-signal-intensity masses relative to the myometrium. Tumors >3 cm often are heterogeneous because of varying degrees and types of degeneration (Hricak, 1986; Yamashita, 1993). With MR imaging, multiplanar views allow for accurate tumor localization as subserosal, intramural, or submucosal. Moreover, pedunculated myomas and their bridging stalk can be delineated. Of myoma types, intramural or subserosal leiomyomas are frequently circumscribed by a high-signal-intensity rim that represents edema from dilated lymphatics and veins.

Of treatment options, magnetic resonance high-intensity focused ultrasound (MR-HIFU) therapy directs a series of high-power ultrasound pulses—*sonications*—into the myoma. Without MR guidance, focused-ultrasound therapy is hampered by imprecise beam targeting. Fortunately, excellent soft-tissue resolution with MR imaging enables precise tissue targeting. Moreover, MR imaging can measure accurate, near real-time thermometry. This permits power adjustments to reach adequate treatment temperatures yet minimize thermal injury. Pulse duration lasts generally 15 seconds, and a cooling interval is inserted between pulses. The average procedure duration approximates 3½ hours (Hindley, 2004).

MR-HIFU therapy, also called MR-guided focused ultrasound (MRgFUS), is a safe and feasible minimally invasive alternative for leiomyoma treatment (Chen, 2005; Stewart, 2003). Several studies have demonstrated a relatively rapid improvement in patient symptoms, a continued decrease in the leiomyoma size over time, a quicker recovery, and few major adverse events in comparison with UAE or myomectomy

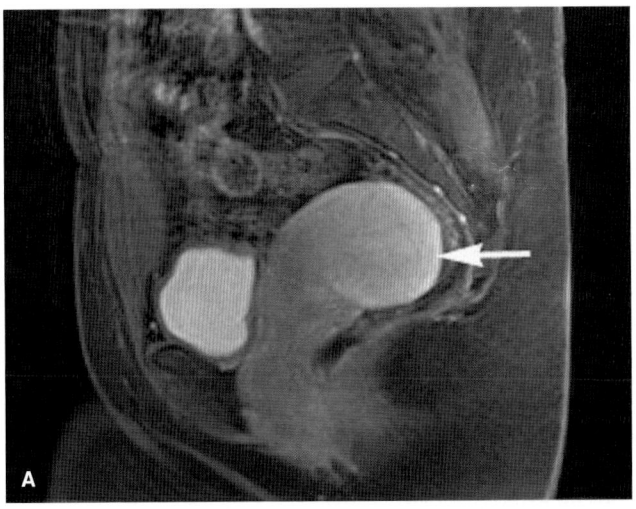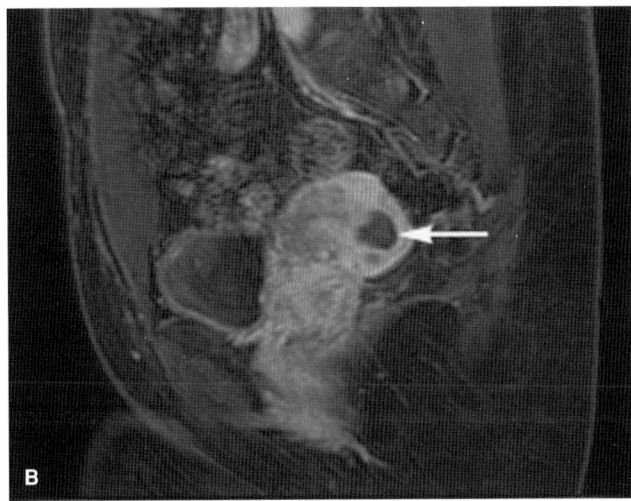

FIGURE 2-30 **A.** Sagittal T1-weighted post-contrast image demonstrates a 5.6-cm enhancing leiomyoma at the uterine fundus. **B.** Sagittal T1-weighted post-contrast image of the same patient 2 months after uterine artery embolization demonstrates lack of enhancement in the fibroid and significant interval decrease in size (now measuring 2 cm).

(Fennessy, 2007; Stewart, 2006, 2007). However, little information is available on long-term results compared with other interventional treatments. Moreover, not all patients are suitable candidates. Obstructions in the energy path such as abdominal wall scars or intraabdominal clips, total uterine size >24 weeks, a desire for future fertility, or general contraindications to MR imaging are limitations. Moreover, leiomyoma characteristics such as size, perfusion, or location near adjacent organs may limit treatment feasibility. Ongoing investigations of additional MR-HIFU indications include its use in women with symptomatic leiomyomas desiring future fertility, myomas >10 cm, and adenomyosis (Hesley, 2008; Kim, 2011a,b).

Congenital Anomalies

As discussed in Chapter 18 (p. 417), müllerian duct anomalies comprise a spectrum of developmental malformations. In the past, full evaluation required laparoscopy, laparotomy, HSG, and hysteroscopy. These invasive techniques were largely replaced by MR imaging, which has an accuracy of up to 100 percent (Carrington, 1990; Fielding, 1996). As discussed earlier, with advances in 3-D sonography techniques, sonographic evaluation with 3-D image reconstruction, with or without saline infusion, can also be used for müllerian anomaly diagnosis (p. 26).

MR imaging is particularly adept at differentiating septate and bicornuate uteri, which is imperative as these two have differing clinical implications and surgical management. Intravenous contrast is not routinely needed, but if a vaginal septum is suspected clinically, then placing ultrasound gel within the vagina prior to imaging may be helpful (Gupta, 2014). T2-weighted images and coronal planes are typically the most informative. With these, the septate uterus generally has a convex fundal contour. The bicornuate uterus typically has a significant fundal notch >1 cm, although any notch depth within 5 mm of the intercornual line qualifies for bicornuate (Behr, 2012). The endometrial cavities of a bicornuate uterus have a normal width and communicate. Although a less reliable marker, the intercornual distance with a bicornuate uterus typically measures >4 cm (Carrington, 1990; Fedele, 1989).

With a septate uterus, a fibrous septum divides the two uterine horns. Collagen has low signal intensity on both T1- and T2-weighted images, whereas the intervening myometrium of a bicornuate uterus has high signal intensity on T2-weighted images. The fundal contour of the septate uterus can be convex, flattened, or mildly concave, but if present, the fundal notch lies >5 mm above the intercornual line (Behr, 2012). Also in contrast to the bicornuate uterus, the intercornual distance of a septate uterus is not increased, and thus each uterine cavity is smaller than usual (Carrington, 1990; Forstner, 1994).

MR imaging is also used for more detailed evaluation of a unicornuate uterus, especially in evaluation for a rudimentary horn (Fig. 2-31). On MR imaging, if endometrial tissue is present within a rudimentary horn, zonal anatomy will be preserved. Moreover, communication of an endometrium-containing

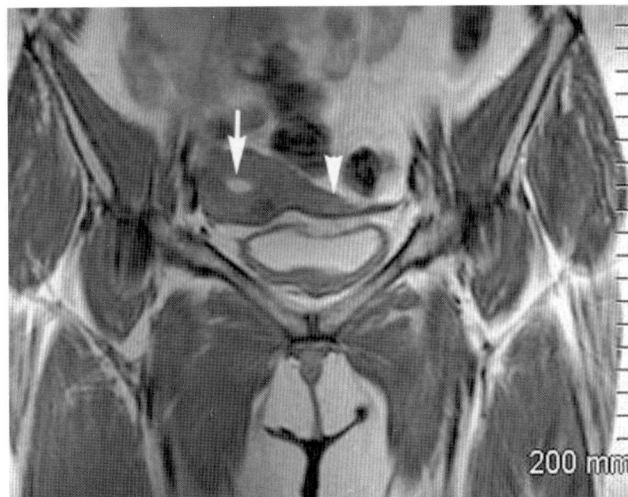

FIGURE 2-31 Unicornuate uterus. This coronal T2-weighted image demonstrates a protrusion of myometrial tissue from the left lateral uterine body (*arrowhead*). It is isointense to myometrium but does not demonstrate normal uterine zonal anatomy. Specifically, endometrium (*arrow*) is noted in the developed right uterine horn but not in the left rudimentary horn.

rudimentary horn is of considerable clinical importance (Chap. 18, p. 420). In a menstruating woman, a noncommunicating horn containing endometrium will often be evident as a hematometra when the cavity becomes distended with blood. MR imaging can also noninvasively identify uterine didelphys, agenesis, and hypoplasia.

Other Gynecologic Indications

MR imaging is equivalent or superior to sonography to diagnose adenomyosis and has a sensitivity of 88 to 93 percent and a specificity of 66 to 99 percent (Ascher, 1994; Dueholm, 2001; Reinhold, 1996). One principal advantage of MR imaging compared with sonography includes the reliability of MR imaging to diagnose adenomyosis, particularly focal adenomyomas, in the setting of concomitant pathology such as leiomyomas. Another is the reproducibility of MR imaging, which allows for accurate treatment monitoring (Reinhold, 1995).

Thickness of the-low-signal-intensity junctional zone (inner myometrium) >12 mm is diagnostic of adenomyosis on T2-weighted images (Fig. 2-32). A normal junctional zone can measure up to 8 mm, and measurements from 8 to 12 mm are considered indeterminate (Novellas, 2011). Low-signal-intensity areas of adenomyosis often contain internal ovoid and punctate foci of increased signal on both T1- and T2-weighted images. These foci are nests of ectopic endometrium with dilated endometrial glands, with or without hemorrhage (Reinhold, 1995, 1996). Contrast administration does not increase the diagnostic accuracy for adenomyosis (Outwater, 1998).

For polyps and endometrial hyperplasia, TVS and SIS are common diagnostic tools. MR imaging may be helpful if these modalities are nondiagnostic in a patient who is a poor surgical candidate for direct endometrial sampling. That said, differentiation of intracavitary myomas and endometrial polyps can be problematic with MR imaging if necrosis and inflammation are present.

For diagnosing ovarian endometriomas, MR imaging offers similar specificity to TVS (98 percent). These cysts show characteristic "shading" signal loss on T2-weighted images. The

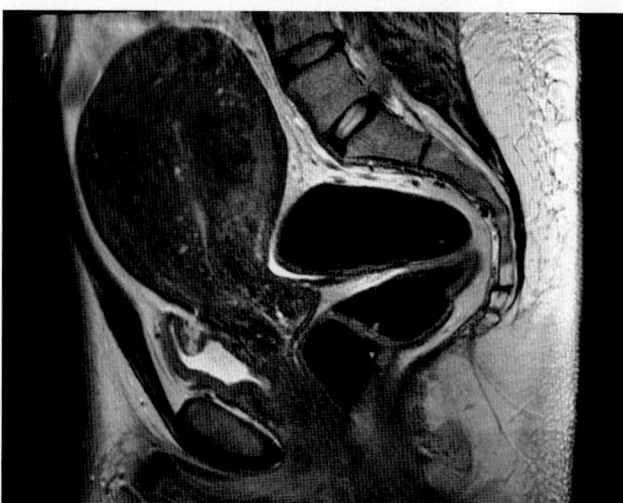

FIGURE 2-32 Sagittal T2-weighted magnetic resonance image of a uterus with diffuse adenomyosis. Adenomyosis is shown as circumferential thickening of the junctional zone.

correlating hyperintense signal on T1-weighted images originates from old blood products (Chamie, 2011). However, MR imaging differs from TVS in that it can provide evaluation for endometriosis in locations that are not easy to access sonographically or laparoscopically, especially in the setting of advanced disease. For diagnosing deep pelvic endometriosis, MR imaging has a sensitivity of 90 percent, specificity of 91 percent, and accuracy of 91 percent (Bazot, 2004). Additional features used to diagnose endometriosis include stellate margins of fibrotic plaques, tethering, and obliteration of normal pelvic spaces. On T1-weighted images, hyperintense signal foci from old hemorrhagic endometriotic disease aids diagnosis of multifocal endometriosis involving the bladder, rectum, and ureters.

For adnexal masses, MR imaging is useful to further characterize anatomy if sonography is nondiagnostic or inconclusive. MR imaging frequently provides added information regarding soft-tissue composition and the origin and extent of pelvic pathology that may be nongynecologic. Although both sonography and MR imaging are highly sensitive for the detection of adnexal malignancy, MR imaging is slightly more specific (Adusumilli, 2006; Jeong, 2000; Yamashita, 1995).

◼ Gynecologic Malignancies

For cervical cancer, imaging is not a component of strict clinical staging (Chap. 30, p. 663). That said, MR imaging is an excellent adjunct for preoperative assessment of gynecologic neoplasms. Its superior soft-tissue contrast and ability to image directly in multiple planes allow evaluation for local tumor extension and lymphadenopathy.

Although CT imaging is typically used for assessment of nodal disease and distant metastases, MR imaging consistently outperforms clinical and CT evaluation of cervical cancer in the assessment of local tumor extension (Choi, 2004; Hricak, 1996, 2007). Current recommendations for MR imaging of cervical cancer include tumors with a transverse diameter >2 cm based on physical examination, endocervical or predominately infiltrative tumors that cannot be accurately assessed clinically, and women who are pregnant or have concomitant uterine lesions that make evaluation difficult (Ascher, 2001; Hricak, 2007). When the extent of parametrial and sidewall invasion is unclear clinically, MR imaging can play an important role as it has a 95- to 98-percent negative predictive value for parametrial invasion (Hricak, 2007; Subak, 1995).

For endometrial carcinoma, surgery is currently the most accurate staging method. Preoperatively, MR imaging may assess the degree of myometrial and cervical extension, which can affect the planned hysterectomy type, extent of lymph node dissection, and decision to provide neoadjuvant intracavitary radiation (Boronow, 1984; Frei, 2000). MR imaging has a 92-percent accuracy in staging endometrial cancer, and an 82-percent accuracy in assessing myometrial invasion depth (Hricak, 1987). Thus, MR imaging is often considered if lymph node metastases are likely. Instances include a high-grade tumor; papillary or clear cell histology; cervical invasion; or need for multifactorial assessment of myometrial, cervical, and lymph node involvement (Ascher, 2001).

For ovarian neoplasms, MR imaging is reserved for evaluation when TVS or CT scanning is nondiagnostic or when high-risk surgical patients might benefit from further stratification. This stems from its increased cost, decreased availability, and longer imaging and interpretation times (Javitt, 2007). However, in a Society of Radiologists in Ultrasound consensus statement, MR imaging was recommended for simple ovarian cysts >7 cm, given sonography's limitations in detecting mural nodules in larger ovarian masses (Ekerhovd, 2001; Levine, 2010). MR imaging is also useful to determine adnexal mass origin as uterine, ovarian, or nongynecologic. For those of the ovary, MR imaging helps clarify whether the mass is neoplastic or functional and is malignant or benign. MR imaging of an adnexal mass ideally includes gadolinium-enhanced images to assess tumor vascularity and fat-saturation techniques to differentiate blood from fat (Ascher, 2001). Although histology cannot be diagnosed, findings that are suspicious for malignancy include enhancing solid components, thick septations, nodules, and/or papillary projections.

Sensitivity of MR imaging for detecting adnexal pathology ranges from 87 to 100 percent, which is comparable to sonography and CT scanning (Siegelman, 1999). The advantages of MR imaging compared with CT scanning in the evaluation of suspected ovarian cancer include its superior contrast resolution and increased sensitivity for detecting uterine invasion, extrapelvic peritoneal and lymph node metastases, and tumor extension to omentum, bowel, bone, and vessels (Low, 1995; Tempany, 2000). However, MR imaging has a lower sensitivity for implants <1 cm compared with CT (Sala, 2013).

■ Urogynecology

Pelvic floor evaluations previously performed fluoroscopically are now more often performed with MR imaging. MR imaging provides detailed soft-tissue evaluation of the female urethra, levator ani muscles, and adjacent pelvic structures in patients with incontinence or pelvic organ prolapse (Pannu, 2002). Contrast agents placed in the vagina, rectum, and/or bladder can enhance imaging.

In addition to anatomy, functional data can be obtained. For example, dynamic MR imaging is completed as the patient performs the Valsalva maneuver. With MR defecography, the patient both performs Valsalva maneuver and defecates rectal contrast (ultrasound gel) during rapid cine acquisitions. Protocols vary significantly from center to center, and upright open MR units are not universally available. At our institution, supine MR defecography is preferred to Valsalva alone (Bailey, 2014; Kumar, 2014). MR defecography can evaluate patients with pelvic organ descent, incontinence, constipation, and defecatory dysfunction. It may add information prior to complex pelvic floor reconstruction or after failed previous repairs (Macura, 2006). Grading systems of pelvic organ prolapse and pelvic floor relaxation on dynamic imaging have been developed (Barbaric, 2001; Fielding, 2000).

NUCLEAR MEDICINE

Nuclear medicine examinations are used similarly in the gynecologic patient as in other medical specialties. Small amounts of radioactive material can be ingested or injected to diagnose, and at times treat, various diseases. Thyroid studies use radioactive iodine to assess or ablate function. Bone scans may be elected to seek metastatic disease. Various renal scans can offer information regarding renal function, perfusion, and possible obstruction. Ventilation-perfusion (V/Q) scans are often used to identify pulmonary emboli. Controversy remains regarding whether pulmonary artery CTA or V/Q scan is most appropriate in pulmonary emboli evaluation. The V/Q scan does not use nephrotoxic agents and is often preferred in those with renal insufficiency. However, radiopharmaceuticals are not always readily available, and thus pulmonary artery CTA is frequently employed.

Positron emission tomography (PET) uses short-lived radiochemical compounds to serve as tracers for measuring specific metabolic processes suggestive of malignancy or infection (Juweid, 2006). This enables detection of early cancer biochemical anomalies that precede the structural changes identified by other imaging techniques. With FDG-PET, a radiolabeled analogue of glucose, 2-[^{18}F]fluoro-2-deoxy-D-glucose (FDG), is injected intravenously and is taken up by metabolically active cells such as tumor cells. PET provides a poor depiction of detailed anatomy, thus scans are frequently read side-by-side or fused with CT scans. The combination allows correlation of metabolic and anatomic data. As a result, current PET scanners are now commonly integrated with CT scanners, and the two scans can be performed during the same session.

PET/CT has become a vital clinical tool, particularly for cancer diagnosis and management. The FDG tracer highlights areas of accelerated glycolysis, which is common in neoplastic cells (Goh, 2003). Several studies have demonstrated high sensitivity and specificity of FDG-PET for the initial staging of cervical cancer, especially in patients with no evidence of extrapelvic metastatic disease by MR or CT imaging (Gjelsteen, 2008; Park, 2005). The ability of FDG-PET imaging to assess nodal status in cervical cancer has both prognostic and therapeutic implications (Fig. 2-33). Prior to lymph node radiation treatment planning, the added anatomic data obtained with PET/CT can be used to guide intensity-modulated radiotherapy (Chap. 28, p. 615). This significantly reduces the amount of radiation delivered to surrounding normal structures (Havrilesky, 2003; Wong, 2004).

INTERVENTIONAL RADIOLOGY

In gynecology, procedures often provided by interventional radiologists include image-guided biopsy or drainage. In those with advanced cervical cancer, percutaneous nephrostomy may be needed to preserve renal function or to decompress an infected collecting system. Uterine artery embolization is a vascular intervention that employs angiography to delineate the uterine arteries. Once catheterized, each artery is injected with embolic particles to occlude uterine vasculature. As discussed in Chapter 9 (p. 209), UAE can provide definitive independent treatment of uterine leiomyomas as blood flow through the uterine arteries is stopped. This leads to preferential myoma ischemia and necrosis. Although adenomyosis was initially thought to be a contraindication for UAE success, studies are now showing UAE to have durable treatment efficacy in adenomyosis (Kim, 2007). Given the frequent concomitant

SECTION 1

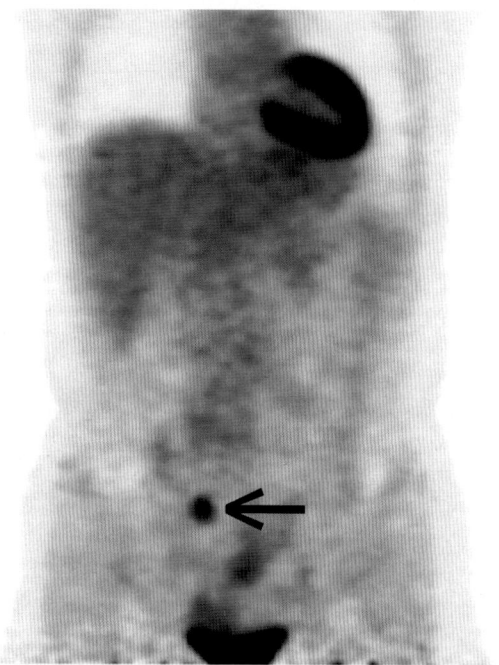 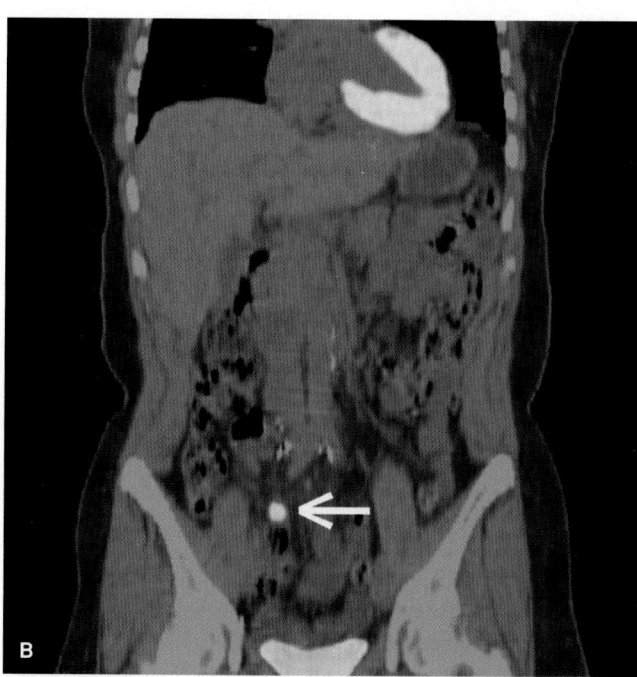

FIGURE 2-33 Positron emission tomography (PET) **(A)** and PET-computed tomography (PET-CT) fusion **(B)** images of a woman with recurrence of ovarian cancer. Arrows demarcate abnormal uptake of tracer in the pelvis that represented a 1-cm lymph node. The biopsy of this lymph node revealed recurrent ovarian cancer. (Images contributed by Dr. Dana Mathews.)

presence of adenomyosis and uterine leiomyomata, treatment success and improvement in symptoms have also been reported in populations with both diseases after UAE (Froeling, 2012). Rarely, UAE may be selected to control severe uterine bleeding in women who are not considered surgical candidates.

REFERENCES

Abrams BJ, Sukmvanich P, Seibel R, et al: Ultrasound for the detection of intraperitoneal fluid: the role of Trendelenburg position. Am J Emerg Med 17:117, 1999
Abuhamad AZ, Singleton S, Zhao Y, et al: The Z technique: an easy approach to the display of the mid-coronal plane of the uterus in volume sonography. J Ultrasound Med 25:607, 2006
Adusumilli S, Hussain HK, Caoili EM, et al: MR imaging of sonographically indeterminate adnexal masses. AJR 187:732, 2006
Alcazar JL, Galan MJ, Garcia-Manero M, et al: Three-dimensional sonographic morphologic assessment in complex adnexal masses: preliminary experience. J Ultrasound Med 22:249, 2003
Alcazar JL, Galvan R: Three-dimensional power Doppler ultrasound scanning for the prediction of endometrial cancer in women with postmenopausal bleeding and thickened endometrium. Am J Obstet Gynecol 200:44.e1, 2009
American College of Obstetricians and Gynecologists: Antibiotic prophylaxis for gynecologic procedures. Practice Bulletin No. 104, May 2009, Reaffirmed 2014
American College of Radiology: ACR Manual on Contrast Media, Version 9, 2013
American College of Radiology, American Association of Physicists in Medicine, Society for Imaging Informatics in Medicine: Practice parameter for determinants of image quality in digital mammography. Resolution No. 39, Amended 2014
American College of Radiology: Committee on Drugs and Contrast Media. Manual on Contrast Media, 5.0 ed. Reston, American College of Radiology Standards, 2004
American Institute of Ultrasound in Medicine: Guidelines for performance of the ultrasound examination of the female pelvis. 2014. Available at: http://www.aium.org/publications/guidelines/pelvis.pdf. Accessed January 25, 2015
American Institute of Ultrasound in Medicine: Official statement on heat. AIUM Bioeffects Committee, 2009

Ameye L, Valentin L, Testa AC, et al: A scoring system to differentiate malignant from benign masses in specific ultrasound-based subgroups of adnexal tumors. Ultrasound Obstet Gynecol 33:92, 2009
Andreotti RF, Fleischer AC, Mason LE Jr: Three-dimensional sonography of the endometrium and adjacent myometrium: preliminary observations. J Ultrasound Med 25:1313, 2006
Ascher SM, Arnold LL, Patt RH, et al: Adenomyosis: prospective comparison of MR imaging and transvaginal sonography. Radiology 190:803, 1994
Ascher SM, Jha RC, Reinhold C: Benign myometrial conditions: leiomyomas and adenomyosis. Top Magn Reson Imaging 14:281, 2003
Ascher SM, Takahama J, Jha RC: Staging of gynecologic malignancies. Top Magn Reson Imaging 12:105, 2001
Baber RJ, McSweeney MB, Gill RW, et al: Transvaginal pulsed Doppler ultrasound assessment of blood flow to the corpus luteum in IVF patients following embryo transfer. BJOG 95:1226, 1988
Bailey A, Khatri G, Pedrosa I, et al: Influence of rectal gel volume on study performance in women with symptomatic pelvic organ prolapse. Society of Abdominal Radiology Annual Meeting. Boca Raton, March 23–28, 2014
Barbaric ZL, Marumoto AL, Raz S: Magnetic resonance imaging of the perineum and pelvic floor. Top Magn Reson Imaging 12:83, 2001
Bates SM, Ginsberg JS: Treatment of deep-vein thrombosis. N Engl J Med 351:268, 2004
Bazot M, Darai E, Hourani R, et al: Deep pelvic endometriosis: MR imaging for diagnosis and prediction of extension of disease. Radiology 232:379, 2004
Behr S, Courtier J, Qayyum A: Imaging of müllerian duct anomalies. Radiographics 32:E233, 2012
Benacerraf BR, Shipp TD, Bromley B: Three-dimensional ultrasound detection of abnormally located intrauterine contraceptive devices which are a source of pelvic pain and abnormal bleeding. Ultrasound Obstet Gynecol 34:110, 2009
Benacerraf BR, Shipp TD, Bromley B: Which patients benefit from a 3D reconstructed coronal view of the uterus added to standard routine 2D pelvic sonography? AJR 190:626, 2008
Bermejo C, Martinez Ten P, Cantarero R, et al: Three-dimensional ultrasound in the diagnosis of Müllerian duct anomalies and concordance with magnetic resonance imaging. Ultrasound Obstet Gynecol 35:593, 2010
Beyersdorff D, Zhang J, Schoder H, et al: Bladder cancer: can imaging change patient management? Curr Opin Urol 18:98, 2008
Birdwell BG, Raskob GE, Whitsett TL, et al: The clinical validity of normal compression ultrasonography in outpatients suspected of having deep venous thrombosis. Ann Intern Med 128:1, 1998
Blake GM, Fogelman I: Role of dual-energy X-ray absorptiometry in the diagnosis and treatment of osteoporosis. J Clin Densitom 10:102, 2007

Boardman LA, Peipert JF, Brody JM, et al: Endovaginal sonography for the diagnosis of upper genital tract infection. Obstet Gynecol 90:54, 1997

Bonilla-Musoles F, Raga F, Osborne NG, et al: Three-dimensional hysterosonography for the study of endometrial tumors: comparison with conventional transvaginal sonography, hysterosalpingography, and hysteroscopy. Gynecol Oncol 65:245, 1997

Bonilla-Musoles F, Raga F, Osborne NG: Three-dimensional ultrasound evaluation of ovarian masses. Gynecol Oncol 59:129, 1995

Bonnamy L, Marret H, Perrotin F, et al: Sonohysterography: a prospective survey of results and complications in 81 patients. Eur J Obstet Gynecol Reprod Biol 102:42, 2002

Boronow RC, Morrow CP, Creasman WT, et al: Surgical staging in endometrial cancer: clinical-pathologic findings of a prospective study. Obstet Gynecol 63:825, 1984

Branney SW, Wolfe RE, Moore EE, et al: Quantitative sensitivity of ultrasound in detecting free intraperitoneal fluid. J Trauma 39:375, 1995

Buy JN, Ghossain MA, Hugol D, et al: Characterization of adnexal masses: combination of color Doppler and conventional sonography compared with spectral Doppler analysis alone and conventional sonography alone. AJR 166:385, 1996

Cacciatore B, Leminen A, Ingman-Friberg S, et al: Transvaginal sonographic findings in ambulatory patients with suspected pelvic inflammatory disease. Obstet Gynecol 80:912, 1992

Capitanio GL, Ferraiolo A, Croce S, et al: Transcervical selective salpingography: a diagnostic and therapeutic approach to cases of proximal tubal injection failure. Fertil Steril 55:1045, 1991

Carrington BM, Hricak H, Nuruddin RN, et al: Müllerian duct anomalies: MR imaging evaluation. Radiology 176:715, 1990

Chamie L, Blasalg R, Pereira R, et al: Findings of pelvic endometriosis at transvaginal US, MR imaging, and laparoscopy. Radiographics 31:E77, 2011

Chan DP, Abujudeh HH, Cushing GL Jr, et al: CT cystography with multiplanar reformation for suspected bladder rupture: experience in 234 cases. AJR 187:1296, 2006

Chen S: MRI-guided focused ultrasound treatment of uterine fibroids. Issues Emerg Health Technol 70:1, 2005

Choi SH, Kim SH, Choi HJ, et al: Preoperative magnetic resonance imaging staging of uterine cervical carcinoma: results of prospective study. J Comput Assist Tomogr 28:620, 2004

Chou CP, Levenson RB, Elsayes KM, et al: Imaging of female urethral diverticulum: an update. Radiographics 28(7):1917, 2008

Cohen HL, Tice HM, Mandel FS: Ovarian volumes measured by US: bigger than we think. Radiology 177:189, 1990

Coursey CA, Casalino DD, Remer EM, et al: ACR Appropriateness Criteria®: acute onset flank pain—suspicion of stone disease. Reston, American College of Radiology, 2011

Cowan NC: CT urography for hematuria. Nat Rev Urol 9:218, 2012

Cowan NC, Turney BW, Taylor NJ, et al: Multidetector computed tomography urography for diagnosing upper urinary tract urothelial tumour. BJU Int 99:1363, 2007

Cunningham FG, Leveno KL, Bloom SL, et al (eds): Ultrasound and Doppler. In Williams Obstetrics, 24th ed. New York, McGraw-Hill Education, 2014, p 194

Cura M, Cura A, Bugnone A: Role of magnetic resonance imaging in patient selection for uterine artery embolization. Acta Radiol 47:1105, 2006

Damilakis J, Maris T, Karantanas A: An update on the assessment of osteoporosis using radiologic techniques. Eur Radiol 17:1591, 2007

Davis JD: Prevention, diagnosis, and treatment of venous thromboembolic complications of gynecologic surgery. Am J Obstet Gynecol 184:759, 2001

DePriest PD, Shenson D, Fried A, et al: A morphology index based on sonographic findings in ovarian cancer. Gynecol Oncol 51:7, 1993

Deutch TD, Joergner I, Matson DO, et al: Automated assessment of ovarian follicles using a novel three-dimensional ultrasound software. Fertil Steril 92(5):1562, 2009

Dietz HP: Mesh in prolapse surgery: an imaging perspective. Ultrasound Obstet Gynecol 40:495, 2012

Dietz HP: Quantification of major morphological abnormalities of the levator ani. Ultrasound Obstet Gynecol 29:329, 2007

Dietz HP: The role of two- and three-dimensional dynamic ultrasonography in pelvic organ prolapse. J Minim Invasive Gynecol 17:282, 2010

Dooms GC, Hricak H, Tscholakoff D: Adnexal structures: MR imaging. Radiology 158:639, 1986

Dueholm M, Lundorf E, Hansen E, et al: Magnetic resonance imaging and transvaginal ultrasonography for the diagnosis of adenomyosis. Fertil Steril 76:588, 2001

Eckersley RJ, Sedelaar JP, Blomley MJ, et al: Quantitative microbubble enhanced transrectal ultrasound as a tool for monitoring hormonal treatment of prostate carcinoma. Prostate 51:256, 2002

Ekerhovd E, Wienerroith H, Staudach A, et al: Preoperative assessment of unilocular adnexal cysts by transvaginal ultrasonography: a comparison between ultrasonographic morphologic imaging and histopathologic diagnosis. Am J Obstet Gynecol 184:48, 2001

Exacoustos C, Di Giovanni A, Szabolcs B, et al: Automated three-dimensional coded contrast imaging hysterosalpingo-contrast sonography: feasibility in office tubal patency testing. Ultrasound Obstet Gynecol 41:328, 2013

Fedele L, Dorta M, Brioschi D, et al: Magnetic resonance evaluation of double uteri. Obstet Gynecol 74:844, 1989

Fennessy FM, Tempany CM, McDannold NJ, et al: Uterine leiomyomas: MR imaging-guided focused ultrasound surgery—results of different treatment protocols. Radiology 243:885, 2007

Ferrara KW, Merritt CR, Burns PN, et al: Evaluation of tumor angiogenesis with US: imaging, Doppler, and contrast agents. Acad Radiol 7:824, 2000

Fielding JR: MR imaging of Müllerian anomalies: impact on therapy. AJR 167:1491, 1996

Fielding JR, Dumanli H, Schreyer AG, et al: MR-based three-dimensional modeling of the normal pelvic floor in women: quantification of muscle mass. AJR 174:657, 2000

Fleischer AC: Recent advances in the sonographic assessment of vascularity and blood flow in gynecologic conditions. Am J Obstet Gynecol 193:294, 2005

Fleischer AC, Harvey SM, Kurita SC, et al: Two-/three-dimensional transperineal sonography of complicated tape and mesh implants. Ultrasound Q 28:243, 2012

Fleischer AC, Lyshchik A, Jones HW Jr, et al: Contrast-enhanced transvaginal sonography of benign versus malignant ovarian masses: preliminary findings. J Ultrasound Med 27:1011, 2008

Fleischer AC, Rodgers WH, Kepple DM, et al: Color Doppler sonography of ovarian masses: a multiparameter analysis. J Ultrasound Med 12:41, 1993

Forstner R, Hricak H: Congenital malformations of uterus and vagina. Radiology 34:397, 1994

Frei KA, Kinkel K, Bonel HM, et al: Prediction of deep myometrial invasion in patients with endometrial cancer: clinical utility of contrast-enhanced MR imaging—a meta-analysis and Bayesian analysis. Radiology 216:444, 2000

Friera A, Gimenez NR, Caballero P, et al: Deep vein thrombosis: can a second sonographic examination be avoided? AJR 178:1001, 2002

Froeling V, Scheurig-Muenkler C, Hamm B, et al: Uterine artery embolization to treat uterine adenomyosis with or without uterine leiomyomata results of symptom control and health-related quality of life 40 months after treatment. Cardiovasc Intervent Radiol 25:523, 2012

Gandhi S, Brown M, Wong J, et al: MR contrast agents for liver imaging: what, when, how. Radiographics 26:1621, 2006

Garra BS: Imaging and estimation of tissue elasticity by ultrasound. Ultrasound Q 23:255, 2007

Gera PS, Allemand MC, Tatpati LL, et al: Role of saline infusion sonography in uterine evaluation before frozen embryo transfer cycle. Fertil Steril 89:562, 2008

Ghi T, Casadio P, Kuleva M, et al: Accuracy of three-dimensional ultrasound in diagnosis and classification of congenital uterine anomalies. Fertil Steril 92:808, 2009

Gjelsteen A, Ching BH, Meyermann MW, et al: CT, MRI, PET, PET/CT, and ultrasound in the evaluation of obstetric and gynecologic patients. Surg Clin North Am 88:361, 2008

Goh AS, Ng DC: Clinical positron emission tomography imaging—current applications. Ann Acad Med Singapore 32:507, 2003

Goldhaber SZ: Pulmonary embolism. Lancet 363:1295, 2004

Gross BH, Silver TM, Jaffe MH: Sonographic features of uterine leiomyomas: analysis of 41 proven cases. J Ultrasound Med 2:401, 1983

Gupta M, Pinho D, Bailey A, et al: Endoluminal contrast for the abdominal and pelvic MRI: when, where, and how? Educational Exhibit MSE006-b, presented at the 100th Scientific Assembly and Annual Meeting of the Radiological Society of North America. November 30-December 5, 2014

Hamed HO, Shahin AY, Elsamman AM: Hysterosalpingo-contrast sonography versus radiographic hysterosalpingography in the evaluation of tubal patency. Int J Gynaecol Obstet 105:215, 2009

Hanley M, Donahue J, Rybicki FJ: ACR Appropriateness Criteria®: clinical condition: suspected lower-extremity deep vein thrombosis. Reston, American College of Radiology, 1995, Reaffirmed 2013

Havrilesky LJ, Wong TZ, Secord AA, et al: The role of PET scanning in the detection of recurrent cervical cancer. Gynecol Oncol 90:186, 2003

Heikinen H, Tekay A, Volpi E, et al: Transvaginal salpingosonography for the assessment of tubal patency in infertile women: methodological and clinical experiences. Fertil Steril 64:293, 1995

Hesley GK, Gorny KR, Henrichsen TL, et al: A clinical review of focused ultrasound ablation with magnetic resonance guidance an option for treating uterine fibroids. Ultrasound Q 24:131, 2008

Hindley J, Gedroyc WM, Regan L, et al: MRI guidance of focused ultrasound therapy of uterine fibroids: early results. AJR 183:1713, 2004

Hricak H, Chang YCF, Thurnher S: Vagina: evaluation with MR imaging. I. Normal anatomy and congenital anomalies. Radiology 169:169, 1988

Hricak H, Gatsonis C, Chi D, et al: Role of imaging in pretreatment evaluation of early invasive cervical cancer: results of the intergroup study American College of Radiology Imaging Network 6651–Gynecologic Oncology Group 183. J Clin Oncol 23(36):9329, 2005

Hricak H, Gatsonis C, Conkley F, et al: Early invasive cervical cancer: CT and MRI imaging in preoperative evaluation-ACRIN/GOG comparative study of diagnostic performance and interobserver variability. Radiology 245:491, 2007

Hricak H, Powell CB, Yu KK, et al: Invasive cervical carcinoma: Role of MR imaging in pretreatment work-up—cost minimization and diagnostic efficacy analysis. Radiology 198:403, 1996

Hricak H, Stern JL, Fisher MR, et al: Endometrial carcinoma staging by MR imaging. Radiology 162:297, 1987

Hricak H, Tscholakoff D, Heinrichs L, et al: Uterine leiomyomas: correlation of MR histopathologic findings, and symptoms. Radiology 158:385, 1986

Humphrey L, Helfand M, Chan B, et al: Breast cancer screening: a summary of the evidence for the U.S. Preventative Services Task Force. Ann Intern Med 137:347, 2002

Hwang M, Lyshchik A, Fleischer A: Molecular sonography with targeted microbubbles: current investigations and potential applications. Ultrasound Q 26:75, 2010

Jain KA: Prospective evaluation of adnexal masses with endovaginal gray-scale and duplex and color Doppler US: correlation with pathologic findings. Radiology 191:63, 1994

Jankowski JT, Spirnak JP: Current recommendations for imaging in the management of urologic traumas. Urol Clin North Am 33:365, 2006

Javitt MC, Fleischer AC, Andreotti RF, et al: Expert panel on women's imaging. Staging and follow-up of ovarian cancer. Reston (VA): American College of Radiology (ACR) 2007, p 1

Jayasinghe Y, Rane A, Stalewski H, et al: The presentation and early diagnosis of the rudimentary uterine horn. Obstet Gynecol 105:1456, 2005

Jeong Y, Outwater EK, Kang HK: Imaging evaluation of ovarian masses. Radiographics 20:144, 2000

Jergas M, Genant HK: Current methods and recent advances in the diagnosis of osteoporosis. Arthritis Rheum 36:1649, 1993

Jokubkiene L, Sladkevicius P, Valentin L: Does three-dimensional power Doppler ultrasound help in discrimination between benign and malignant ovarian masses? Ultrasound Obstet Gynecol 29:215, 2007

Juweid ME, Cheson BD: Positron-emission tomography and assessment of cancer therapy. N Engl J Med 354:496, 2006

Kanal E, Barkovich AJ, Bell C, et al: ACR guidance document for safe MR practices: 2013. J Magn Reson Imaging 37(3):501, 2013

Kaplan FS: Prevention and management of osteoporosis. Clin Symp 1995, p 47

Keltz MD, Olive DL, Kim AH, et al: Sonohysterography for screening in recurrent pregnancy loss. Fertil Steril 67:670, 1997

Khalife S, Falcone T, Hemmings R, et al: Diagnostic accuracy of transvaginal ultrasound in detecting free pelvic fluid. J Reprod Med 43:795, 1998

Kim K, Yoon S, Lee C, et al: Short-term results of magnetic resonance imaging-guided focused ultrasound surgery for patients with adenomyosis: symptomatic relief and pain reduction. Fertil Steril 95:1152, 2011a

Kim M, Kim S, Kim N, et al: Long-term results of uterine artery embolization for symptomatic adenomyosis. AJR 188:176, 2007

Kim Y, Bae D, Kim B, et al: A faster nonsurgical solution: very large fibroid tumors yielded to a new ablation strategy. Am J Obstet Gynecol 205:292, 2011b

Kinkel K, Hricak H, Lu Y, et al: US characterization of ovarian masses: a meta-analysis. Radiology 217:803, 2000

Kumar N, Khatri G, Xi Y, et al: Valsalva maneuvers versus defecation for MRI assessment of multi-compartment pelvic organ prolapse. American Roentgen Ray Society Annual Meeting, San Diego, May 4–9, 2014

Kupesic A, Plavsic BM: 2D and 3D hysterosalpingo-contrast-sonography in the assessment of uterine cavity and tubal patency. Eur J Obstet Gynecol Reprod Biol 113:64, 2007

Kurjak A, Schulman H, Sosic A, et al: Transvaginal ultrasound, color flow, and Doppler waveform of the postmenopausal adnexal mass. Obstet Gynecol 80:917, 1992

Lee JKT, Gersell DJ, Balfe DM, et al: The uterus: in vitro MR anatomic correlation of normal and abnormal specimens. Radiology 157:175, 1985

Legendre G, Gervaise A, Levaillant JM, et al: Assessment of three-dimensional ultrasound examination classification to check the position of the tubal sterilization microinsert. Fertil Steril 94:2732, 2010

Lele PP, Hazzard DG, Litz ML: Thresholds and mechanisms of ultrasonic damage to "organized" animal tissues. Symposium on Biological Effects

and Characterizations of Ultrasound Sources. US Department of Health, Education, and Welfare HEW Publication (FDA) 78–8048:224, 1977

Lensing AW, Prandoni P, Brandjes D, et al: Detection of deep-vein thrombosis by real-time B-mode ultrasonography. N Engl J Med 320:342, 1989

Levine D, Brown DL, Andreotti RF, et al: Management of asymptomatic ovarian and other adnexal cysts imaged at ultrasound: Society of Radiologists in Ultrasound consensus conference statement. Ultrasound Q 26:121, 2010

Lieng M, Qvigstad E, Dahl GF, et al: Flow differences between endometrial polyps and cancer: a prospective study using intravenous contrast-enhanced transvaginal color flow Doppler and three-dimensional power Doppler ultrasound. Ultrasound Obstet Gynecol 32:935, 2008

Low RN, Carter WD, Saleh F, et al: Ovarian cancer: comparison of findings with perfluorocarbon-exchanged MR imaging, In-111-CYT-103 immunoscintigraphy, and CT. Radiology 195:391, 1995

Lubich LM, Alderman MG, Ros PR: Magnetic resonance imaging of leiomyomata uteri: assessing therapy with the gonadotropin-releasing hormone agonist leuprolide. Magn Reson Imaging 9:331, 1991

Luciano DE, Exacoustos C, Johns DA, et al: Can hysterosalpingo-contrast sonography replace hysterosalpingography in confirming tubal blockage after hysteroscopic sterilization and in the evaluation of the uterus and tubes in infertile patients? Am J Obstet Gynecol 204:79, 2011

Luciano DE, Exacoustos C, Luciano AA: Contrast ultrasonography for tubal patency. J Minim Invasive Gynecol 21:994, 2014

Macura KJ: Magnetic resonance imaging of pelvic floor defects in women. Top Magn Reson Imaging 17:417, 2006

Maglinte DD, Gage SN, Harmon BH, et al: Obstruction of the small intestine: accuracy and role of CT in diagnosis. Radiology 188:61, 1993

Mark AS, Hricak H, Heinrichs LW: Adenomyosis and leiomyoma: differential diagnosis by means of magnetic resonance imaging. Radiology 163:527, 1987

McCarthy S, Tauber C, Gore J: Female pelvic anatomy: MR assessment of variations during the menstrual cycle and with use of oral contraceptives. Radiology 160:119, 1986

Mettler F, Huda W, Yoshizumi T, et al: Effective doses in radiology and diagnostic nuclear medicine: a catalog. Radiology 248:254, 2008

Mishell DR Jr, Stenchever MA, Droegemueller W, et al (eds): Comprehensive Gynecology, 3rd ed. St. Louis, Mosby, 1997, p 691

Mol BW, Swart P, Bossuyt PM, et al: Reproducibility of the interpretation of hysterosalpingography in the diagnosis of tubal pathology. Hum Reprod 11:1204, 1996

Molander P, Sjoberg J, Paavonen J, et al: Transvaginal power Doppler findings in laparoscopically proven acute pelvic inflammatory disease. Ultrasound Obstet Gynecol 17:233, 2002

Molina FS, Gomez LF, Florido J, et al: Quantification of cervical elastography: a reproducibility study. Ultrasound Obstet Gynecol 396:685, 2012

Moore W, Khatri G, Madhuranthakam A, et al: Added value of diffusion-weighted acquisitions in MRI of the abdomen and pelvis. AJR 202:995, 2014

Moschos E, Twickler DM: Does the type of intrauterine device affect conspicuity and position evaluation with 2D and 3D ultrasound imaging? AJR 196:1439, 2011

Neitlich JD, Foster HE, Glickman MG, et al: Detection of urethral diverticula in women: comparison of a high resolution fast spin echo technique with double balloon urethrography. J Urol 159:408, 1998

Novellas S, Chassang M, Delotte J, et al: MRI characteristics of the uterine junctional zone: from normal to the diagnosis of adenomyosis. AJR 196:1206, 2011

Outwater EK, Siegelman ES, Van Deerlin V: Adenomyosis: current concepts and imaging considerations. AJR 170:437, 1998

Pannu HK: Magnetic resonance imaging of pelvic organ prolapse. Abdom Imaging 27:660, 2002

Park W, Park YJ, Huh SJ, et al: The usefulness of MRI and PET imaging for the detection of parametrial involvement and lymph node metastasis in patients with cervical cancer. Jpn J Clin Oncol 35:260, 2005

Philipov G, Holsman M, Philips PJ: The clinical role of quantitative ultrasound in assessing fracture risk and bone status. Med J Aust 173:208, 2000

Pisal N, Sindos M, O'Riordian J, et al: The use of spinal needle for transcervical saline infusion sonohysterography in presence of cervical stenosis. Acta Obstet Gynecol Scand 84:1019, 2005

Rajan D, Margau R, Kroll R, et al: Clinical utility of ultrasound versus magnetic resonance imaging for deciding to proceed with uterine artery embolization for presumed symptomatic fibroids. Clin Radiol 66:57, 2011

Ramchandani P, Kisler T, Francis IR, et al: ACR Appropriateness Criteria®: hematuria. Reston, American College of Radiology, 2008

Reinhold C, Atri M, Mehio AR, et al: Diffuse uterine adenomyosis: morphologic criteria and diagnostic accuracy of endovaginal sonography. Radiology 197:609, 1995

Reinhold C, McCarthy S, Bret PM, et al: Diffuse adenomyosis: comparison of endovaginal US and MR imaging with histopathologic correlation. Radiology 199:151, 1996

Reuter KL, Daly DC, Cohen SM: Septate versus bicornuate uteri: errors in imaging diagnosis. Radiology 172:749, 1989

Sala E, Rockall A, Freeman S, et al: The added role of MR imaging in treatment stratification of patients with gynecologic malignancies: what the radiologist needs to know. Radiology 266:718, 2013

Salim R, Woelfer B, Backos M, et al: Reproducibility of three-dimensional ultrasound diagnosis of congenital uterine anomalies. Ultrasound Gynecol Obstet 21:578, 2003

Santoro GA, Wieczorek AP, Dietz HP, et al: State of the art: an integrated approach to pelvic floor ultrasonography. Ultrasound Obstet Gynecol 37:381, 2011

Saslow D, Boetes C, Burke W, et al: American Cancer Society guidelines for breast screening with MRI as an adjunct to mammography. CA Cancer J Clin 57:75, 2007

Sassone AM, Timor-Tritsch IE, Artner A, et al: Transvaginal sonographic characterization of ovarian disease: evaluation of a new scoring system to predict ovarian malignancy. Obstet Gynecol 78:70, 1991

Saunders RD, Shwayder JM, Nakajima ST: Current methods of tubal patency assessment. Fertil Steril 95:2171, 2011

Savelli L, Pollastri P, Guerrini M, et al: Tolerability, side effects, and complications of hysterosalpingocontrast sonography (HyCoSy). Fertil Steril 4:1481, 2009

Scalea TM, Rodriquez A, Chiu WC, et al: Focused assessment with sonography for trauma (FAST): results from an international consensus conference. J Trauma 46:466, 1999

Schaer GN, Koechli OR, Schuessler B, et al: Perineal ultrasound for evaluating the bladder neck in urinary stress incontinence. Obstet Gynecol 85:220, 1995

Schuettoff S, Beyersdorff D, Gauruder-Burmester A, et al: Visibility of the polypropylene tape after tension-free vaginal tape (TVT) procedure in women with stress urinary incontinence: comparison of introital ultrasound and magnetic resonance imaging in vitro and in vivo. Ultrasound Obstet Gynecol 27:687, 2006.

Schwartz L, Panageas E, Lange R, et al: Female pelvis: impact of MR imaging on treatment decisions and net cost analysis. Radiology 192:55, 1994

Siegelman ES, Outwater EK: Tissue characterization in the female pelvis by means of MR imaging. Radiology 212:5, 1999

Soares SR, Barbosa dos Reis MM, Camargos AF: Diagnostic accuracy of sonohysterography, transvaginal sonography, and hysterosalpingography in patients with uterine cavity diseases. Fertil Steril 73:406, 2000

Song Y, Yang J, Liu Z, et al: Preoperative evaluation of endometrial carcinoma by contrast-enhanced ultrasonography. BJOG 116:294, 2009

Stewart EA, Gedroyc WM, Tempany CMC, et al: Focused ultrasound treatment of uterine fibroid tumors: safety and feasibility of a noninvasive thermoablative technique. Am J Obstet Gynecol 189:48, 2003

Stewart EA, Gostout B, Rabinovici J, et al: Sustained relief of leiomyoma symptoms by using focused ultrasound surgery. Obstet Gynecol 110:279, 2007

Stewart EA, Rabinovici J, Tempany CMC, et al: Clinical outcomes of focused ultrasound surgery for the treatment of uterine fibroids. Fertil Steril 85:22, 2006

Stoelinga B, Hehenkamp WJK, Brolmann HAM et al: Real-time elastography for assessment of uterine disorders. Ultrasound Obstet Gynecol 43:218, 2014

Strandell A, Bourne T, Bergh C, et al: The assessment of endometrial pathology and tubal patency: a comparison between the use of ultrasonography and X-ray hysterosalpingography for the investigation of infertility patients. Ultrasound Obstet Gynecol 14:200, 1999

Stumpf PG, March CM: Febrile morbidity following hysterosalpingography: identification of risk factors and recommendations for prophylaxis. Fertil Steril 33:487, 1980

Subak LL, Hricak H, Powell CB, et al: Cervical carcinoma: computed tomography and magnetic resonance imaging for preoperative staging. Obstet Gynecol 86:43, 1995

Taylor LS, Porter BC, Rubens DJ, et al: Three-dimensional sonoelastography: principles and practices. Phys Med Biol 45:1477, 2000

Tempany C, Dou K, Silverman S, et al: Staging of advanced ovarian cancer: comparison of imaging modalities report from the Radiological Diagnostic Oncology Group. Radiology 215:761, 2000

Thurmond AS: Selective salpingography and fallopian tube recanalization. AJR 156:33, 1991

Timmerman D, Testa AC, Bourne T, et al: Logistic regression model to distinguish between the benign and malignant adnexal mass before surgery: a multicenter study by the International Ovarian Tumor Analysis Group. J Clin Oncol 23:8794, 2005

Timmerman D, Valentin L, Bourne T, et al: Terms, definitions and measurements to describe the sonographic features of adnexal tumors: a consensus opinion from the International Ovarian Tumor Analysis (IOTA) group. Ultrasound Obstet Gynecol 16:500, 2000

Timor-Tritsch IE, Lerner JP, Monteagudo A, et al: Transvaginal sonographic markers of tubal inflammatory disease. Ultrasound Obstet Gynecol 12:56, 1998

Tinkanen H, Kujansuu E: Doppler ultrasound findings in tubo-ovarian infectious complex. J Clin Ultrasound 21:175, 1993

Titton RL, Gervais DA, Hahn PF, et al: Urine leaks and urinomas: diagnosis and imaging guided intervention. Radiographics 23:1133, 2003

Togashi K, Ozasa H, Konishi I: Enlarged uterus: differentiation between adenomyosis and leiomyoma with MRI. Radiology 171:531, 1989

Troiano R, McCarthy S: Müllerian duct anomalies: imaging and clinical issues. Radiology 233:19, 2004

Twickler DM, Forte TB, Santos-Ramos R, et al: The Ovarian Tumor Index predicts risk for malignancy. Cancer 86:2280, 1999

Twickler DM, Moschos E: Ultrasound and assessment of ovarian cancer risk. AJR 194:322, 2010

Valentin L: Gray scale sonography, subjective evaluation of the color Doppler image and measurement of blood flow velocity for distinguishing benign and malignant tumor of suspected adnexal origin. Eur J Obstet Gynecol Reprod Biol 72:63, 1997

Weiner Z, Thaler I, Beck D, et al: Differentiating malignant from benign ovarian tumors with transvaginal color flow imaging. Obstet Gynecol 79:159, 1992

Wolfman DJ, Ascher SM: Magnetic resonance imaging of benign uterine pathology. Top Magn Reson Imaging 17:399, 2006

Wong TZ, Jones EL, Coleman RE: Positron emission tomography with 2-deoxy-2-[18F]fluoro-D-glucose for evaluating local and distant disease in patients with cervical cancer. Mol Imaging Biol 6:55, 2004

World Health Organization: Assessment of fracture risk and its application to screening for postmenopausal osteoporosis. WHO Reference No. WHO/TSR/843, 1994

Wu HM, Chiang CH, Huang HY, et al: Detection of the subendometrial vascularization flow index by three-dimensional ultrasound may be useful for predicting the pregnancy rate for patients undergoing in vitro fertilization-embryo transfer. Fertil Steril 79:507, 2003

Yamashita Y, Torashima M, Hatanaka Y, et al: Adnexal masses: accuracy of characterization with transvaginal US and precontrast and postcontrast MR imaging. Radiology 194:557, 1995

Yamashita Y, Torashima M, Takahashi M: Hyperintense uterine leiomyoma at T2-weighted MR imaging: differentiation with dynamic enhanced MR imaging and clinical implications. Radiology 189:721, 1993

Yauger BJ, Feinberg EC, Levens ED, et al: Pre-cycle saline infusion sonography minimizes assisted reproductive technologies cycle cancellation due to endometrial polyps. Fertil Steril 90:1324, 2008

Yitta S, Hecht E, Mausner E, et al: Normal or abnormal? Demystifying uterine and cervical contrast enhancement at multidetector CT. Radiographics 31:647, 2011

Yu NC, Raman SS, Patel M, et al: Fistulas of the genitourinary tract: a radiologic review. Radiographics 24:1331, 2004

Zhou L, Zhang X, Chen X, et al: Value of three-dimensional hysterosalpingocontrast sonography with SonoVue in the assessment of tubal patency. Ultrasound Obstet Gynecol 40:93, 2012

Gynecologic Infection

NORMAL VAGINAL FLORA

The vaginal flora of a normal, asymptomatic reproductive-aged woman includes multiple aerobic, facultative anaerobic, and obligate anaerobic species (Table 3-1). Of these, anaerobes predominate and outnumber aerobic species approximately 10 to 1 (Bartlett, 1977). These bacteria exist in a symbiotic relationship with the host and are alterable, depending on the microenvironment. They localize where their survival needs are met and have exemption from the infection-preventing destructive capacity of the human host. The function of this vaginal bacterial colonization, however, remains unknown.

Within this vaginal ecosystem, some microorganisms produce substances such as lactic acid and hydrogen peroxide that inhibit nonindigenous organisms (Marrazzo, 2006). Several other antibacterial compounds, termed *bacteriocins*, play a similar role. For protection from many of these toxic substances, a secretory leukocyte protease inhibitor is found in the vagina. This protein protects local tissues against toxic inflammatory products and infection.

Certain bacterial species normally found in vaginal flora have access to the upper reproductive tract. The female upper reproductive tract is not sterile, and the presence of these bacteria does not indicate active infection (Hemsell, 1989; Spence,

1982). Together, these findings do illustrate the potential for infection following gynecologic surgery and the need for antimicrobial prophylaxis. They also explain the potential acceleration of a local acute infection if a pathogen, such as *Neisseria gonorrhoeae,* gains access to the upper tract.

■ Vaginal pH

Typically, the vaginal pH ranges between 4 and 4.5. Although not completely understood, *Lactobacillus* species contribute by production of lactic acid, fatty acids, and other organic acids. Other bacteria can also add organic acids from protein catabolism, and anaerobic bacteria donate by amino acid fermentation.

Glycogen, which is present in healthy vaginal mucosa, provides nutrients for many vaginal ecosystem species and is metabolized to lactic acid (Boskey, 2001). Accordingly, as glycogen content within vaginal epithelial cells diminishes after menopause, this decreased substrate for acid production leads to a rise in vaginal pH. Specifically, if no pH-altering pathogens are present, a vaginal pH of 6.0 to 7.5 is strongly suggestive of menopause (Caillouette, 1997).

■ Altered Flora

Changing any element of this ecology may alter the prevalence of various species. For example, postmenopausal women not receiving estrogen replacement and young girls have a lower prevalence of *Lactobacillus* species compared with that of reproductive-aged women. However, for menopausal women, hormone replacement therapy restores vaginal lactobacilli populations, which protect against vaginal pathogens (Dahn, 2008).

Other events predictably alter lower reproductive tract flora and may lead to infection. With the menstrual cycle, transient changes in flora are observed. These are predominantly during the first days of the cycle and are presumed to be associated with hormonal changes (Keane, 1997). Menstrual fluid can also serve as a nutrient source for several bacterial species, resulting in their overgrowth. What role this plays in the development of upper reproductive tract infection following menstruation is unclear, but an association may be present. For example, women symptomatic with acute gonococcal upper reproductive tract infection characteristically are menstruating or have just completed their menses. Last, treatment with a broad-spectrum antibiotic may result in symptoms attributed to inflammation from *Candida albicans* or other *Candida* spp by eradicating other balancing species in the flora.

TABLE 3-1. Lower Reproductive Tract Bacterial Flora

Aerobes
Gram-positive
  Lactobacillus spp
  Diphtheroids
  Staphylococcus aureus
  Staphylococcus epidermidis
  Group B Streptococcus
  Enterococcus faecalis
  Staphylococcus spp
Gram-negative
  Escherichia coli
  Klebsiella spp
  Proteus spp
  Enterobacter spp
  Acinetobacter spp
  Citrobacter spp
  Pseudomonas spp

Anaerobes
Gram-positive cocci
  Peptostreptococcus spp
  Clostridium spp
Gram-positive bacilli
  Lactobacillus spp
  Propionibacterium spp
  Eubacterium spp
  Bifidobacterium spp
  Actinomyces israelii
Gram-negative
  Prevotella spp
  Bacteroides spp
  Bacteroides fragilis group
  Fusobacterium spp
  Veillonella spp
Yeast
  Candida albicans and other spp

TABLE 3-2. Bacterial Vaginosis Risk Factors

Oral sex
Douching
Black race
Cigarette smoking
Sex during menses
Intrauterine device
Early age of sexual intercourse
New or multiple sexual partners
Sexual activity with other women

an increased risk of BV is associated with sexual contact with multiple and new male and female partners, and condom use lowers the risk (Table 3-2) (Fethers, 2008). Further, rates of STD acquisition are increased in affected women, and a possible role of sexual transmission in the pathogenesis of recurrent BV has been proposed (Atashili, 2008; Bradshaw, 2006; Wiesenfeld, 2003). Successful prevention of BV is limited, but elimination or diminished use of vaginal douches may be beneficial (Brotman, 2008; Klebanoff, 2010).

Bacterial vaginosis is the most common cause of vaginal discharge among reproductive-aged women. Of symptoms, a nonirritating, malodorous vaginal discharge is characteristic, but may not always be present. The vagina is usually not erythematous, and cervical examination reveals no abnormalities.

Clinical diagnostic criteria were first proposed by Amsel and associates (1983) and include: (1) microscopic evaluation of a vaginal-secretion saline preparation, (2) release of volatile amines produced by anaerobic metabolism, and (3) determination of the vaginal pH. A saline preparation, also known as a "wet prep," contains a swab-collected sample of discharge mixed with drops of saline on a microscope slide. Clue cells are the most reliable indicators of BV and were originally described by Gardner and Dukes (1955) (Fig. 3-1). These vaginal epithelial

■ Bacterial Vaginosis

This common, complex, and poorly understood clinical syndrome reflects abnormal vaginal flora. It has been variously named, and former terms are *Haemophilus* vaginitis, *Corynebacterium* vaginitis, *Gardnerella* or anaerobic vaginitis, and nonspecific vaginitis. With bacterial vaginosis (BV), the vaginal flora's symbiotic relationship shifts for unknown reasons to one in which anaerobic species overgrow and include *Gardnerella vaginalis*, *Ureaplasma urealyticum*, *Mobiluncus* species, *Mycoplasma hominis*, and *Prevotella* species. Bacterial vaginosis (BV) is also associated with a significant reduction or absence of normal hydrogen peroxide-producing *Lactobacillus* species. Whether an altered ecosystem leads to lactobacilli disappearance or whether its disappearance results in the changes observed with BV is unclear.

In evaluating risks for BV, this condition is not considered by the Centers for Disease Control and Prevention (CDC) (2015) to be a sexually transmitted disease (STD). However,

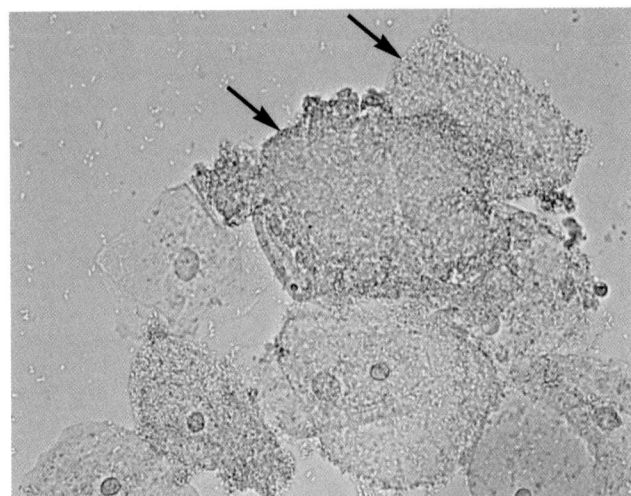

FIGURE 3-1 Photomicrograph of saline wet preparation reveals clue cells. Several of these squamous cells are heavily studded with bacteria. Clue cells are covered to the extent that cell borders are blurred and nuclei are not visible (*arrows*). (Used with permission from Dr. Lauri Campagna and Mercedes Pineda, WHNP.)

cells contain many attached bacteria, which create a poorly defined stippled cellular border. At least 20 percent of the epithelial cells should be clue cells. The positive predictive value of this test for BV is 95 percent.

Adding 10-percent potassium hydroxide (KOH) to a fresh sample of vaginal secretions releases volatile amines that have a fishy odor. This is often colloquially referred to as a "whiff test." The odor is frequently evident even without KOH. Similarly, alkalinity of seminal fluid and blood are responsible for foul-odor complaints after intercourse and with menses. The finding of both clue cells and a positive whiff test result is pathognomonic, even in asymptomatic patients.

Characteristically with BV, the vaginal pH is >4.5, and this stems from diminished acid production by bacteria. Similarly, *Trichomonas vaginalis* infection is also associated with anaerobic overgrowth and resultant elaborated amines. Thus, women diagnosed with BV should have no microscopic evidence of trichomoniasis.

Last, and used primarily in research studies rather than clinical practice, the Nugent Score is a system employed for diagnosing BV. During microscopic examination of a gram-stained vaginal discharge smear, scores are calculated by assessing bacteria staining and morphology.

Several gynecologic adverse health outcomes have been observed in women with BV. These include vaginitis, endometritis, postabortal endometritis, pelvic inflammatory disease (PID) unassociated with *N gonorrhoeae* or *Chlamydia trachomatis*, and acute pelvic infections following pelvic surgery, especially hysterectomy (Larsson, 1989, 1991, 1992; Soper, 1990). Pregnant patients with BV have an elevated risk of preterm delivery (Flynn, 1999; Leitich, 2007).

Several regimens have been proposed by the 2014 Centers for Disease Control and Prevention BV working group and are for nonpregnant women (Table 3-3). Cure rates with these regimens range from 80 to 90 percent at 1 week, but within 3 months, 30 percent of women have experienced a recurrence of altered flora. At least half have another episode of symptoms associated with this flora change, many of which are correlated with heterosexual contacts (Amsel, 1983; Gardner, 1955; Wilson, 2004). However, treatment of male sexual partners does not benefit women with this recurring condition and is not recommended. Moreover, other forms of therapy such as introduction of lactobacilli, acidifying vaginal gels, and use of probiotics have shown inconsistent effectiveness (Senok, 2009).

ANTIBIOTICS

These drugs are commonly used in gynecology to restore altered flora or treat various infections. As a group, antibiotics have been implicated in decreasing the efficacy of oral contraceptives. Fortunately, this has been proven in very few, and these are listed in Table 5-9 (p. 124).

■ Penicillins

The heart of all penicillins is a thiazolidine ring with an attached β-lactam ring and a side chain. The β-lactam ring provides antibacterial activity, which is primarily directed against gram-positive aerobic bacteria. Because of the numerous substitutions at the side chain, various antibiotics with altered antibacterial spectra and pharmacologic properties have been synthesized.

Some bacteria produce an enzyme (β-lactamase) that opens the β-lactam ring and inactivates the drug as a primary bacterial defense mechanism. Inhibitors of β-lactamase are clavulanic acid, sulbactam, and tazobactam, and these have been combined with several penicillins to enhance the activity spectrum against a broader variety of aerobic and anaerobic bacteria. Additionally, oral probenecid can be administered separately with penicillins. This drug lowers the renal-tubular secretion rate of these antibiotics and is used to increase penicillin or cephalosporin plasma levels.

Adverse reactions to penicillins may include allergic (e.g., anaphylaxis, urticaria, drug fever), neurologic (e.g., dizziness, seizure), hematologic (e.g., neutropenia, hemolytic anemia, thrombocytopenia), renal (interstitial cystitis), hepatic (elevated transaminases), or gastrointestinal (e.g., nausea, vomiting, diarrhea, pseudomembranous colitis) reactions (Mayo Clinic, 1991). Up to 10 percent of the general population may manifest an allergic reaction to penicillins. The lowest risk is associated with oral preparations, whereas the highest follows those combined with procaine and given intramuscularly. True anaphylactic

TABLE 3-3. Single-agent Bacterial Vaginosis Treatment

Recommended regimens	
Metronidazole (Flagyl)	500 mg orally twice daily for 7 days
Metronidazole gel 0.75% (Metrogel vaginal)	5 g (1 full applicator) intravaginally once daily for 5 days
Clindamycin cream[a] 2% (Cleocin, Clindesse)	5 g (1 full applicator) intravaginally at bedtime for 7 days

Alternative regimens	
Tinidazole (Tindamax)	2 g orally once daily for 2 days
Clindamycin	1 g orally once daily for 5 days
	300 mg orally twice daily for 7 days
Clindamycin ovules[a] (Cleocin)	100 mg intravaginally at bedtime for 3 days

[a]Clindamycin cream and ovules are oil-based and might weaken latex condoms and diaphragms for 5 days after use.
Reproduced with permission from Centers for Disease Control and Prevention: Sexually transmitted diseases treatment guidelines, 2015. MMWR 64(3):1, 2015.

reactions are rare, and mortality rates approximate 1 in every 50,000 treatment regimens. If penicillin allergy is noted, yet treatment is still required, desensitization can be performed relatively safely as described by Wendel and coworkers (1985) and outlined at the CDC website: http://www.cdc.gov/std/treatment/2010/penicillin-allergy.htm.

Excellent tissue penetration is achieved with these agents. Penicillin remains the primary antibiotic for treatment of syphilis, and this antibiotic family is also useful in treating skin infections, breast cellulitis, and breast abscess. The combination of amoxicillin and clavulanic acid (Augmentin) provides the best oral broad-spectrum antibiotic coverage. Moreover, the ureidopenicillins and those combined with a β-lactamase enzyme inhibitor are effective against acute community-acquired or postoperative pelvic infections. In addition, *Actinomyces israelii* infections, which are an infrequent complication of intrauterine device (IUD) use, are treated with penicillins (Westhoff, 2007).

Cephalosporins

Cephalosporins also are β-lactam antimicrobials. Substitutions at their side chains significantly alter the spectrum of activity, potency, toxicity, and half-life of these antibiotics. Organization of these qualities has resulted in their division into five generations. This classification does allow grouping based on general spectra of activity.

Rash and other hypersensitivity reactions are the most common and may develop in up to 3 percent of patients. Cephalosporins are β-lactam antibiotics and, if used in those allergic to penicillin, may create the same or accentuated response. Theoretically, this may happen in up to 16 percent of patients (Saxon, 1987). Thus, if an individual developed anaphylaxis with penicillin therapy, cephalosporin administration is contraindicated.

First-generation cephalosporins are used primarily for surgical prophylaxis and in the treatment of superficial skin cellulitis. Their activity spectrum is greatest against gram-positive aerobic cocci, with some activity against community-acquired gram-negative rods. However, there is little activity against β-lactamase producing organisms or anaerobic bacteria. Despite this inactivity against many pathogens of pelvic infection that may be acquired during surgery, there is prophylactic efficacy.

Second-generation cephalosporins have enhanced activity against gram-negative aerobic and anaerobic bacteria, with some diminution in effectiveness against aerobic gram-positive cocci. Their primary use is in surgical prophylaxis or for single-agent therapy of major community-acquired or postoperative pelvic infections, including abscess.

Third-generation cephalosporins provide gram-positive activity, even greater gram-negative coverage, and some anaerobic effects. Fourth-generation agents have a similar profile but are less susceptible to β-lactamases. Last, fifth-generation drugs, such as ceftaroline, share a similar profile but also cover methicillin-resistant *Staphylococcus aureus* (MRSA). All three groups are effective in treatment of major postoperative pelvic infections, including abscess. These agents have documented efficacy as prophylactic agents, but should be reserved for therapy.

Aminoglycosides

This family of compounds includes gentamicin, tobramycin, netilmicin, and amikacin. Gentamicin is primarily selected because of its low cost and clinical efficacy for pathogens recovered from pelvic infections. For gynecologists, it may be combined with clindamycin with or without ampicillin as a regimen for treatment of serious pelvic infections. Alternatively, gentamicin may be joined with ampicillin and metronidazole. Last, it can be used as adjuvant-agent for outpatient pyelonephritis. Aminoglycoside antibacterial activity is related to its serum/tissue concentration, and the higher the concentration, the greater the potency.

Aminoglycosides have the potential for significant patient toxicity, which can include ototoxicity, nephrotoxicity, and neuromuscular blockade. The inner ear is particularly susceptible to aminoglycosides because of selective accumulation within the hair cells and prolonged half-life within inner ear fluids. Those with vestibular toxicity complain of headaches, nausea, tinnitus, and loss of equilibrium. Cochlear toxicity leads to high-frequency hearing loss. If either of these develops, aminoglycoside administration is stopped promptly. Ototoxicity may be permanent, and risk correlates positively with therapy dose and duration.

Nephrotoxicity is reversible and may develop in up to 25 percent of patients (Bertino, 1993). Risk factors include older age, renal insufficiency, hypotension, volume depletion, frequent dosing intervals, treatment for 3 or more days, multiple antibiotic administration, or multisystem disease. Toxicity leads to a nonoliguric decrease in creatinine clearance and resultant rise in serum creatinine levels.

Neuromuscular blockade is a rare but potentially life-threatening complication and is dose-related. This family of antibiotics inhibits presynaptic acetylcholine release, blocks acetylcholine receptors, and prevents presynaptic calcium absorption. For this reason, aminoglycoside contraindications include myasthenia gravis or concurrent succinylcholine use. Blockade frequently follows rapid intravenous infusion. For this reason, aminoglycosides are ideally given intravenously over at least 30 minutes. Toxicity is usually detected before respiratory arrest, and at its first signs, intravenous calcium gluconate is administered to reverse this form of aminoglycoside toxicity.

Because of these potential adverse reactions, consideration must be given to dosing regimen. In those with normal renal function, aminoglycosides are commonly given parenterally every 8 hours. In those with reduced renal function, doses are reduced, intervals are lengthened, or both. To monitor serum concentration, provide adequate therapeutic levels, and prevent toxicity in patients given multiple daily doses, serum aminoglycoside concentrations are measured at peak (30 minutes after a 30-minute infusion or 1 hour after intramuscular [IM] injection) and at trough (immediately before a next dose). For gentamicin, tobramycin, and netilmicin, peak range ideally is 4 to 6 μg/mL, and troughs are 1 to 2 μg/mL. For amikacin, peaks and troughs are 20 to 30 μg/mL and 5 to 10 μg/mL, respectively.

Once-daily dosing has been evaluated and found to be as or less toxic than multiple daily dosing without sacrificing clinical efficacy (Bertino, 1993). Tulkens and colleagues (1988) reported that once-daily dosing of netilmicin was less toxic than administration three times daily, without jeopardizing efficacy in the treatment of women with PID. In 1992, Nicolau and associates presented pharmacokinetic data and a nomogram for administering aminoglycosides once daily, which starts with an initial dose based on creatinine clearance and subsequent dosing based on a random serum concentration drawn 8 to 12 hours later.

Carbapenems

This is a third class of β-lactam antibiotics that differ from penicillins by changes to the thiazolidine ring attached to penicillin. The three antibiotics in this family are imipenem (Primaxin), meropenem (Merrem), and ertapenem (Invanz). Adverse reactions are comparable to those of the other β-lactam antibiotics. As is true with other β-lactams, if patients have experienced a type 1 hypersensitivity reaction to either a penicillin or cephalosporin, then a carbapenem should not be administered.

These antibiotics are designed for polymicrobial bacterial infections, primarily those with resistant aerobic gram-negative bacteria not susceptible to other β-lactam agents. They should be reserved to preserve efficacy by preventing the development of resistance.

Monobactam

The marketed monobactam, aztreonam, is a synthetic β-lactam. It has a spectrum of activity similar to that of aminoglycosides, that is, gram-negative aerobic species. Like other β-lactam antibiotics, these compounds inhibit bacterial cell wall synthesis by binding to penicillin-binding proteins or causing cell lysis. Aztreonam has affinity only for the binding proteins of the gram-negative bacteria and lacks affinity for either gram-positive bacteria or anaerobic organisms. For the gynecologist, aztreonam provides coverage for gram-negative aerobic bacteria, which is usually provided by aminoglycosides, for patients with significantly impaired renal function or aminoglycoside allergy.

Clindamycin

This antibiotic is a workhorse in the treatment of serious gynecologic infections. Clindamycin is primarily active against aerobic gram-positive bacteria and most anaerobic bacteria, with little activity against aerobic gram-negative bacteria. It is also active against *C trachomatis*. *N gonorrhoeae* is moderately sensitive, and *G vaginalis,* which is typically present in BV, is very susceptible to clindamycin. It may be delivered by one of three routes: orally, intravenously, or vaginally (ovules or 2-percent cream).

The principal application of clindamycin for the gynecologist has been its combination with gentamicin and administration to women with serious community-acquired or postoperative soft-tissue infections or pelvic abscess. Its activity against MRSA has increased its use in these cases. Clindamycin is also used as monotherapy vaginally in the treatment of women with BV. Moreover, in women with early stages of hidradenitis suppurativa, some patients improve with long-term topical or oral clindamycin. Because there are parenteral and oral forms of this antibiotic, patients can transition from the more expensive parenteral therapy to oral therapy early.

Vancomycin

This is a glycopeptide antibiotic that is active only against aerobic gram-positive bacteria. It is primarily used by the gynecologist to treat patients in whom β-lactam therapy is impossible due to a type 1 allergic reaction. Additionally, an oral dose of 120 mg every 6 hours can be given to patients who have developed antibiotic-associated *Clostridium difficile* colitis and who do not respond to oral metronidazole. Last, vancomycin is often selected for MRSA infections.

Of adverse events, the most remarkable is the "red man" syndrome, which is a dermal reaction developing usually within minutes after initiation of a rapid drug infusion. The reaction, which is a response to histamine release, is an erythematous pruritic rash involving the neck, face, and upper torso. Hypotension also may develop. Intravenous administration over 1 hour or administration of an antihistamine may be protective, if given prior to infusion. Also associated with rapid administration may be painful back and chest muscle spasms.

The most significant of vancomycin's side effects is nephrotoxicity, which is enhanced with aminoglycoside therapy, as is ototoxicity. Both are associated with high serum vancomycin concentrations. For this reason, serum peak and trough concentrations are recommended and ideally range between 20 and 40 μg/mL and 5 and 10 μg/mL, respectively. The initial dose is 15 mg/kg of ideal body weight. Other side effects include reversible neutropenia that may develop after prolonged use and peripheral intravenous-catheter-related thrombophlebitis.

Metronidazole

This antibiotic is the principal therapy of trichomoniasis and commonly used for BV. Moreover, it is one of the mainstays of combination antimicrobial therapy given to women with serious postoperative or community-acquired pelvic infections, including pelvic abscess. Since it is active only against obligate anaerobes, metronidazole must be combined with agents effective against gram-positive and gram-negative aerobic bacterial species, such as ampicillin and gentamicin. It is as effective as vancomycin in the treatment of *C difficile*–associated pseudomembranous colitis.

Up to 12 percent of patients taking oral metronidazole may have nausea, and an unpleasant metallic taste has also been described. Patients should abstain from alcohol use to avoid a disulfiram-like effect and emesis. Peripheral neuropathy and convulsive seizures have been reported, are probably dose-related, and are rare.

Fluoroquinolones

Also known simply as *quinolones,* these antibiotics have become first-line agents for treating various infections because of their excellent bioavailability with oral administration, tissue penetration, broad-spectrum antibacterial activity, long half-lives, and good safety profile. As with cephalosporins, fluoroquinolones are separated into generations by their development, antibacterial activity, and pharmacokinetic properties.

Quinolones are contraindicated in children, adolescents, and pregnant and breastfeeding women because they may affect cartilage development. As a family, they are safe, and severe adverse reactions are rare. The side-effect rate ranges from 4 to 8 percent and primarily affects the gastrointestinal (GI) tract following oral administration. Central nervous system (CNS) symptoms such as headache, confusion, tremors, and seizures have been described, and these develop more frequently in patients with underlying brain disorders.

These agents are widely used by gynecologists to treat acute lower urinary tract infections and some sexually transmitted diseases. However, overuse has limited their usefulness in certain infections due to bacterial resistance (Centers for Disease Control and Prevention, 2007). If a less expensive, safer, and equally effective alternative agent is available to treat a given infection, it should be used to preserve fluoroquinolone efficacy.

■ Tetracyclines

These bacteriostatic antimicrobials are commonly used orally and inhibit bacterial protein synthesis. Doxycycline, tetracycline, and minocycline are active against many gram-positive and gram-negative bacteria, although their activity is greater against gram-positive species. Susceptible organisms also include several anaerobes, *Chlamydia* and *Mycoplasma* species, and some spirochetes. Accordingly, cervicitis, PID, syphilis, chancroid, lymphogranuloma venereum, and granuloma inguinale respond to these agents. Moreover, tetracyclines are among treatment options for community-acquired skin and soft-tissue MRSA infections. Specifically, for these infections, minocycline and doxycycline are superior to tetracycline. Tetracycline is active against *Actinomyces* species and is an alternative for treating actinomycosis. Last, these antibiotics also bind specific nonmicrobial targets, such as matrix metalloproteinases (MMPs), and are potent MMP inhibitors. As such, they provide antiinflammatory as well as antimicrobial activity for inflammatory conditions such as acne vulgaris and hidradenitis suppurativa.

With oral administration, tetracyclines can produce direct local GI irritation that manifests as abdominal discomfort, nausea, vomiting, or diarrhea. In teeth and growing bones, tetracyclines readily bind calcium, causing deformity, growth inhibition, or discoloration. Accordingly, tetracyclines are not prescribed for pregnant or nursing women or for children younger than 8 years. Sensitivity to sunlight or ultraviolet light may develop with use. Dizziness, vertigo, nausea, and vomiting may be seen with higher doses. In addition, thrombophlebitis frequently follows intravenous administration. Tetracyclines modify the normal GI flora, which can result in intestinal functional disturbances. Specifically, overgrowth of *C difficile* may lead to pseudomembranous colitis. Vaginal flora also may be altered with resultant *Candida* species overgrowth and symptomatic vulvovaginitis.

GENITAL ULCER INFECTIONS

Ulceration defines complete loss of the epidermal covering with invasion into the underlying dermis. In contrast, *erosion* describes partial loss of the epidermis without dermal penetration. These are distinguished by clinical examination. Biopsies are generally not helpful. But if taken, samples obtained from the edge of a new lesion are the most likely to be informative. Importantly, biopsy is mandatory if carcinoma is suspected, and Figure 4-2 (p. 88) illustrates technique.

Most young sexually active women in the United States who have genital ulcers will have herpes simplex infection or syphilis, but some will have chancroid, lymphogranuloma venereum, or granuloma inguinale. Essentially all are sexually transmitted and are associated with increased risk for human immunodeficiency virus (HIV) transmission. For this reason, HIV and other STD testing is offered to such patients. Sexual contacts require examination and treatment, and both require reevaluation following treatment.

■ Herpes Simplex Virus Infection

Genital herpes is the most prevalent genital ulcer disease and is a chronic viral infection. The virus enters sensory nerve endings and undergoes retrograde axonal transport to the dorsal root ganglion, where the virus develops lifelong latency. Spontaneous reactivation by various events results in anterograde transport of viral particles/protein to the surface. Here virus is shed, with or without lesion formation. It is postulated that immune mechanisms control latency and reactivation (Cunningham, 2006).

There are two types of herpes simplex virus, HSV-1 and HSV-2. Type 1 HSV is the most frequent cause of oral lesions. Type 2 HSV is found more typically with genital lesions, although both types can cause genital herpes. It is estimated that of American females aged 14 to 49 years, 21 percent have suffered a genital HSV-2 infection, and 60 percent of women are seropositive to HSV-1 (Centers for Disease Control and Prevention, 2010; Xu, 2006).

Most women who have been infected with HSV-2 lack this diagnosis because of mild or unrecognized infections. Infected patients can shed infectious virus while asymptomatic, and most infections are transmitted sexually by patients who are unaware of their infection. Most (65 percent) with active infection are women.

Symptoms

Patient symptoms at initial presentation will depend primarily on whether or not a patient during the current episode has antibody from previous exposure. If a patient has no antibody, the attack rate in an exposed person approaches 70 percent. The mean incubation period is approximately 1 week. Up to 90 percent of those who are symptomatic with their initial infection will have another episode within a year.

The virus infects viable epidermal cells, the response to which is erythema and papule formation. With cell death and cell wall lysis, blisters form (Fig. 3-2). The covering then disrupts, leaving a usually painful ulcer. These lesions develop crusting and heal, but may become secondarily infected. The three stages of lesions are: (1) vesicle with or without pustule formation, which lasts approximately a week; (2) ulceration; and (3) crusting. Virus is predictably shed during the first two phases of an infectious outbreak.

Burning and severe pain accompany initial vesicular lesions. With ulcers, urinary frequency and/or dysuria from direct

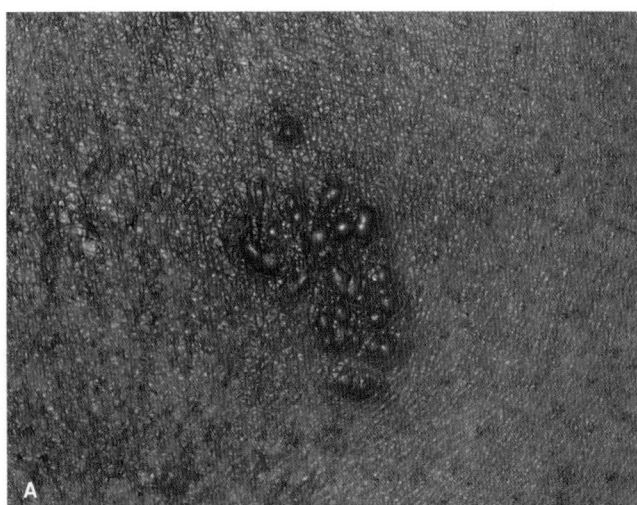
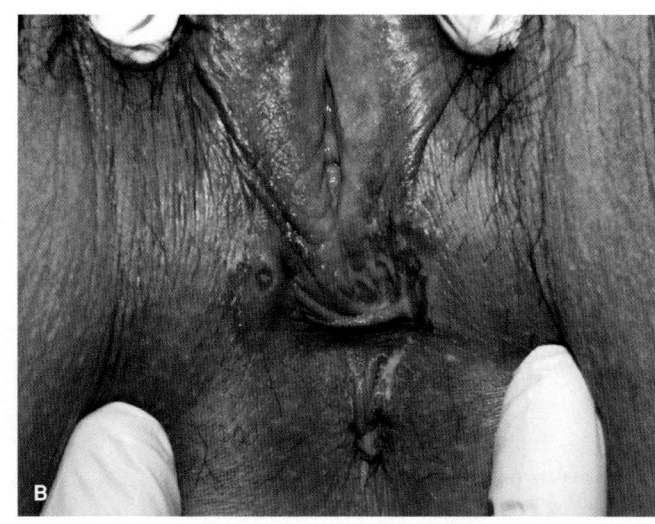

FIGURE 3-2 Genital herpetic ulcers. **A.** Vesicles prior to ulceration. **B.** Punctate (*left*) or "knife-cut" (*right*) ulcers are common lesions. (Used with permission from Dr. William Griffith.)

contact of urine with ulcers may be complaints. Local swelling can result from vulvar lesions and cause urethral obstruction. Alternatively or additionally, herpetic lesions can involve the vagina, cervix, bladder, anus, and rectum. Commonly, a woman has other signs of viremia such as a low-grade fever, headache, malaise, and myalgias.

Viral load undoubtedly contributes to the number, size, and distribution of lesions. Normal host defense mechanisms inhibit viral growth, and healing starts within 1 to 2 days. Early treatment with an antiviral medication decreases the viral load. Immune-deficient patients are at increased susceptibility but display diminished response and delayed healing.

For a previously uninfected patient, the vesicular stage is longer. The period of new lesion formation and time to healing are both longer. Pain persists for the first 7 to 10 days, and lesion healing requires 2 to 3 weeks. If a patient has had prior exposure to HSV-2, the initial episode is significantly less severe, with shorter pain and tenderness duration, and time to healing approximates 2 weeks. Virus is shed usually only during the first week.

Recurrence following HSV-2 infection is common, and almost two thirds of patients have a prodrome prior to lesion onset. Heralding paresthesias are frequently described as pruritus or tingling in the area prior to lesion formation. However, prodromal symptoms may develop without actual lesion formation. Clinical manifestations for women with recurrences are more limited, with only 1 week or less of symptoms.

Diagnosis

The gold standard for the diagnosis of genital herpes is tissue culture. Specificity is high, but sensitivity is low and declines as lesions heal. In recurrent disease, less than 50 percent of cultures are positive. Polymerase chain reaction (PCR) testing of exudate swabbed from the ulcer is many times more sensitive than culture and will probably replace it. Importantly, a negative culture result does not mean that there is no herpetic infection.

Serologic testing may also add clarity. The herpes simplex virus is surrounded by envelope glycoproteins, and of these, glycoprotein G is the antigen of interest for antibody screening.

Serologic assays can detect antibodies specific to the HSV type-specific glycoprotein G2 (HSV-2) and glycoprotein G1 (HSV-1). Assay specificity is ≥96 percent, and the sensitivity of HSV-2 antibody testing ranges from 80 to 98 percent. Importantly, with serologic screening, only IgG antibody assays are ordered. IgM testing can lead to ambiguous results as the IgM assays are not type-specific and also may be positive during a recurrent outbreak. Although these tests may be used to confirm herpes simplex infection, seroconversion following initial HSV-2 infection takes approximately 3 weeks (Ashley-Morrow, 2003). Thus, in clinically obvious cases, immediate treatment and additional STD screening can be initiated following physical examination alone. In general, STD screening for a woman found to have any STD typically includes testing directed to identify syphilis, gonorrhea, trichomoniasis, and HIV, chlamydial, and hepatitis B infections.

Serologic screening for HSV in the general population is not recommended. However, HSV serologic testing can be considered for HIV-infected individuals or for women presenting for an STD evaluation, especially for those with multiple partners and for those in demographics with high prevalence (Centers for Disease Control and Prevention, 2015). It can also add management information for couples thought but not confirmed to be discordant for infection (American College of Obstetricians and Gynecologists, 2014b).

Treatment

Clinical management is with currently available antiviral therapy. Analgesia with nonsteroidal antiinflammatory drugs or a mild narcotic such as acetaminophen with codeine may be prescribed. In addition, topical anesthetics such as lidocaine ointment may provide relief. Local care to prevent secondary bacterial infection is important.

Patient education is mandatory, and specific topics include the natural history of the disease, its sexual transmission, methods to reduce transmission, and obstetric consequences. Notably, HSV can be passed to the neonate during vaginal delivery through an infected field. A comprehensive discussion of obstetric management is found in *Williams Obstetrics*,

24th edition (Cunningham, 2014). For all women, acquisition of this infection may have significant psychological impact, and several websites provide patient information and support. The CDC website can be accessed at http://www.cdc.gov/std/Herpes/STDFact-Herpes.htm.

Women with genital herpes should refrain from sexual activity with uninfected partners when prodrome symptoms or lesions are present. Latex condom use potentially reduces the risk for herpetic transmission (Martin, 2009; Wald, 2005).

Currently available antiviral therapy includes acyclovir (Zovirax), famciclovir (Famvir), and valacyclovir (Valtrex). The CDC-recommended oral medications regimens are listed in Table 3-4. Although these agents may hasten healing and decrease symptoms, therapy does not eradicate latent virus or affect future rate of recurrent infections.

For women with established HSV-2 infection, therapy may not be necessary if their symptoms are minimal and tolerated by the patient. Episodic therapy for recurrent disease is ideally

initiated at least within 1 day of lesion outbreak or during the prodrome, if it exists. Patients may be given a prescription ahead of time so that medication is available to begin therapy with prodromal symptoms.

If episodes recur at frequent intervals, a woman may elect daily suppressive therapy, which reduces recurrences by 70 to 80 percent. Suppressive therapy may eliminate recurrences and decreases sexual transmission of virus by approximately 50 percent (Corey, 2004). Once-daily dosing may result in enhanced compliance and decreased cost.

■ Syphilis

Pathophysiology

Syphilis is an STD caused by the spirochete *Treponema pallidum*, which is a slender spiral-shaped organism with tapered ends. Women at highest risk are those from lower socioeconomic groups, adolescents, those with early onset of sexual activity, and those with a large number of lifetime sexual partners. The attack rate for this infection approximates 30 percent. In 2011, more than 49,000 cases (all stages) of syphilis were reported by state health departments in the United States (Centers for Disease Control and Prevention, 2012).

The natural history of syphilis in untreated patients can be divided into four stages. With *primary syphilis,* the hallmark lesion is the *chancre,* in which spirochetes are abundant. Classically, it is an isolated nontender ulcer with raised rounded borders and an uninfected base (Fig. 3-3). However, it may become secondarily infected and painful. Chancres are often found on the cervix, vagina, or vulva but may also form in the mouth or around the anus. This lesion can develop 10 days to 12 weeks after exposure, with a mean incubation period of 3 weeks. The incubation period is directly related to inoculum size. Without treatment, these lesions spontaneously heal in up to 6 weeks.

With *secondary syphilis,* bacteremia develops 6 weeks to 6 months after a chancre appears. Its hallmark is a maculopapular rash that may involve the entire body and includes the palms, soles, and mucous membranes (Fig. 3-4). As is true for the chancre, this rash actively sheds spirochetes. In warm, moist body areas, this rash may produce broad, pink or gray-white,

TABLE 3-4. Oral Agents for Genital Herpes Simplex Infection

First clinical episode
Acyclovir 400 mg three times daily for 7–10 days
or
Acyclovir 200 mg five times daily for 7–10 days
or
Famciclovir (Famvir) 250 mg three times daily for 7–10 days
or
Valacyclovir (Valtrex) 1 g twice daily for 7–10 days

Episodic therapy for recurrent disease
Acyclovir 400 mg three times daily for 5 days
or
Acyclovir 800 mg twice daily for 5 days
or
Acyclovir 800 mg three times daily for 2 days
or
Famciclovir 125 mg twice daily for 5 days
or
Famciclovir 1 g twice daily for 1 day
or
Famciclovir 500 mg once, then 250 mg twice daily for 2 days
or
Valacyclovir 500 mg twice daily for 3 days
or
Valacyclovir 1 g once daily for 5 days

Suppressive therapy
Acyclovir 400 mg twice daily
or
Famciclovir 250 mg twice daily
or
Valacyclovir 0.5 or 1 g once daily

Reproduced with permission from Centers for Disease Control and Prevention: Sexually transmitted diseases treatment guidelines, 2015. MMWR 64(3):1, 2015.

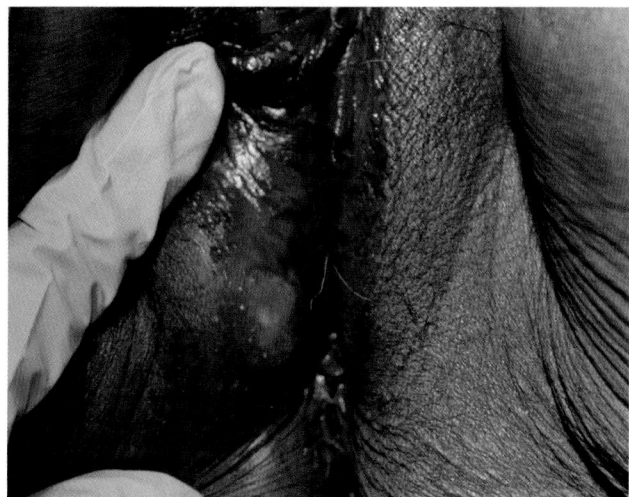

FIGURE 3-3 Vulvar syphilitic chancre.

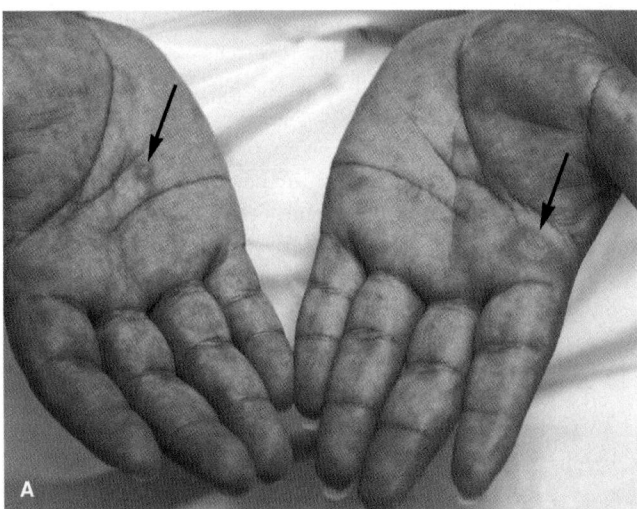
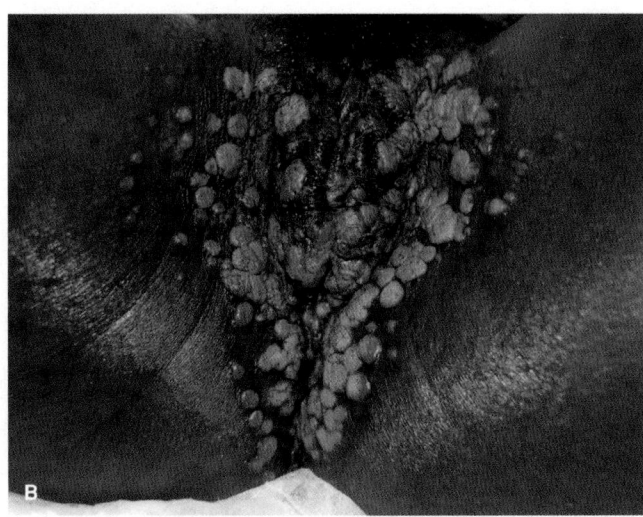

FIGURE 3-4 Secondary syphilis. **A.** Woman with multiple keratotic papules on her palms (*arrows*). With secondary syphilis, disseminated papulosquamous eruptions may be seen on the palms, soles, or trunk. (Used with permission from Dr. William Griffith.) **B.** Woman with multiple condyloma lata on her labia. Soft, flat, moist, pink-tan papules and nodules on the perineum and perianal area are typical. (Used with permission from Dr. George Wendel.)

highly infectious plaques called *condylomata lata*. Because syphilis is a systemic infection, other manifestations may include fever and malaise. Moreover, organ systems such as the kidney, liver, joints, and CNS (meningitis) can be involved.

During the first year following secondary syphilis without treatment, termed *early latent syphilis*, secondary signs and symptoms may recur. However, lesions associated with these outbreaks are not usually contagious. *Late latent syphilis* is defined as a period greater than 1 year after the initial infection.

Tertiary syphilis is the phase of untreated syphilis that may appear up to 20 years after latency. During this phase, cardiovascular, CNS, and musculoskeletal involvement become apparent. However, cardiovascular and neurosyphilis are half as common in females as in males.

Diagnosis

Spirochetes are too thin to retain Gram stain. Early syphilis is diagnosed primarily by dark-field examination or direct fluorescent antibody testing of lesion exudate. In lieu of this, presumptive diagnosis may be reached with serologic tests that are nontreponemal: (1) Venereal Disease Research Laboratory (VDRL) or (2) rapid plasma reagin (RPR) tests. Alternatively, treponemal-specific tests may be selected: (1) fluorescent treponemal antibody-absorption (FTA-ABS) or (2) *Treponema pallidum* particle agglutination (TP-PA) tests. *For population screening*, RPR or VDRL testing is appropriate. A positive test result in a woman who has not been treated previously for syphilis or a four-fold titer (two dilutions) increase in a woman previously treated for syphilis should prompt confirmation with treponemal-specific tests. Thus, *for diagnosis confirmation* in a woman with a positive nontreponemal antibody test result or with a suspected clinical diagnosis, FTA-ABS or TP-PA testing is selected. Last, *for quantitative measurement* of antibody titers to assess response to treatment, RPR or VDRL tests are typically used.

Following treatment, sequential nontreponemal tests are performed. During this surveillance, the same type of test should

be used for consistency—either RPR or VDRL. A fourfold titer decrease is required by 6 months after therapy for primary or secondary syphilis or within 12 to 24 months for those with latent syphilis or women with initially high titers (>1:32)(Larsen, 1998). These tests usually become nonreactive after treatment and with time. However, some women may have a persistent low titer, and these patients are described as *serofast*. Moreover, women with a reactive treponemal-specific test will more than likely have a positive test for the remainder of their lives, but up to 25 percent may revert to a negative result after several years.

Treatment

Penicillin is the first-line therapeutic agent for this infection, and benzathine penicillin is primarily chosen. Specific recommendations for therapy by the CDC (2015) are listed in Table 3-5.

TABLE 3-5. Treatment of Syphilis

Primary, secondary, early latent (<1 year) syphilis
Recommended regimen:
 Benzathine penicillin G, 2.4 million units IM once
 Alternative oral regimens (penicillin-allergic, nonpregnant women): Doxycycline 100 mg orally twice daily for 2 weeks

Late latent, tertiary, and cardiovascular syphilis
Recommended regimen:
 Benzathine penicillin G, 2.4 million units IM weekly times 3 doses
 Alternative oral regimen (penicillin-allergic, nonpregnant women): Doxycycline 100 mg orally twice daily for 4 weeks

Reproduced with permission from Centers for Disease Control and Prevention: Sexually transmitted diseases treatment guidelines, 2015. MMWR 64(3):1, 2015.

For patients with penicillin allergy who cannot be surveilled posttherapy or whose compliance is questioned, skin testing, desensitization, and treatment with IM benzathine penicillin is recommended (Wendel, 1985). For all patients, an acute, self-limited febrile response, termed a Jarisch-Herxheimer reaction, may develop within the first 24 hours after treatment of early disease and is associated with headache and myalgia.

As with other STDs, all patients treated for syphilis and their sexual contacts are screened for other STDs. Patients with evidence of neurologic or cardiac involvement are treated by an infectious disease specialist. After initial treatment, women are seen at 6-month intervals for clinical evaluation and serologic retesting. A fourfold dilution decrease is anticipated. If this does not occur, a patient either has failed treatment or was reinfected and should be reevaluated and retreated. Retreatment recommendations are benzathine penicillin G, 2.4 million units IM weekly for 3 weeks.

Chancroid

This is considered one of the classic STDs but is an uncommon infection in the United States. It appears as local outbreaks predominantly in black and Hispanic males. It is caused by a nonmotile, non-spore-forming, facultative, gram-negative bacillus, *Haemophilus ducreyi*. Incubation usually spans 3 to 10 days, and host access probably requires a break in the skin or mucous membrane.

Chancroid lacks a systemic reaction and prodrome. Infection presents initially with an erythematous papule that becomes pustular and ulcerates within 48 hours. Edges of these painful ulcers are usually irregular with erythematous nonindurated margins. The ulcer bases are usually red and granular and, in contrast to a syphilitic chancre, are typically soft. Lesions are frequently covered with purulent material and may become secondarily infected. The most common locations in women include the fourchette, vestibule, clitoris, and labia. Ulcers on the cervix or vagina may be nontender. Concurrently, approximately half of patients will develop unilateral or bilateral tender inguinal lymphadenopathy. If large and fluctuant, they are termed *buboes*. These may occasionally suppurate and form fistulas, the drainage from which will result in other ulcer formation.

Chancroid most commonly imitates syphilis and genital herpes. These may coexist, but uncommonly. Definitive diagnosis requires growth of *H ducreyi* on special media, but sensitivity for culture is less than 80 percent. A presumptive diagnosis can be made with identification of gram-negative, nonmotile rods on a Gram stain of lesion contents. Before obtaining either specimen, superficial pus or crusting ideally is removed with sterile, saline-soaked gauze.

For treatment, the CDC's (2015) recommended regimens for nonpregnant women include single doses of oral azithromycin (1 g) or IM ceftriaxone (250 mg). Multiple-dose options are ciprofloxacin 500 mg orally twice daily for 3 days or erythromycin base 500 mg orally three times daily for 7 days. Successful treatment leads to symptomatic improvement within 3 days, and objective evidence of improvement within 1 week. Lymphadenopathy resolves more slowly, and if fluctuant, incision and drainage may be warranted. Those with coexisting HIV infection may require longer therapy courses, and treatment failures are more common.

Accordingly, some recommend longer regimens for initial management of known HIV-infected patients.

Granuloma Inguinale

Also known as donovanosis, granuloma inguinale genital ulcerative disease is caused by the intracellular gram-negative bacterium *Calymmatobacterium* (*Klebsiella*) *granulomatis*. This bacterium is encapsulated and appears as a "closed safety pin" in stained tissue biopsy or cytology specimens. Apparently this disease is only mildly contagious, requires repeated exposures, and has a long incubation period of weeks to months.

Granuloma inguinale presents as painless inflammatory nodules that progress to highly vascular, beefy red ulcers that bleed easily on contact. If secondarily infected, they may become painful. These ulcers heal by fibrosis, which can result in scarring resembling keloids. Lymph nodes are usually uninvolved but can become enlarged, and new lesions can appear along these lymphatic drainage channels. Distant lesions have also been reported.

Diagnosis is confirmed by identification of Donovan bodies during microscopic evaluation of a specimen following Wright-Giemsa staining. Currently, there are no Food and Drug Administration (FDA)-approved PCR tests for *C granulomatis* DNA.

Treatment does stop lesion progression and may be lengthy without formation of granulation tissue in ulcer bases and reepithelialization (Table 3-6). Relapses have been reported up to 18 months after "effective" treatment. A few prospective treatment trials have been published, but these are limited. If successful, improvement will be evident within the first few treatment days.

Lymphogranuloma Venereum

This ulcerative genital disease is caused by *trachomatis* serotypes L1, L2, and L3 and is uncommon in the United States. As is true

---

TABLE 3-6. Oral Treatment for Granuloma Inguinale

Recommended regimen
Azithromycin (Zithromax) 1 g once weekly for at least 3 weeks and until lesions are completely healed

Alternative regimens
Doxycycline 100 mg twice daily as above
or
Ciprofloxacin (Cipro) 750 mg twice daily as above
or
Erythromycin base 500 mg four time daily as above
or
Trimethoprim-sulfamethoxazole DS (Bactrim DS, Septra DS) twice daily as above

DS = double strength.
Reproduced with permission from Centers for Disease Control and Prevention: Sexually transmitted diseases treatment guidelines, 2015. MMWR 64(3):1, 2015.

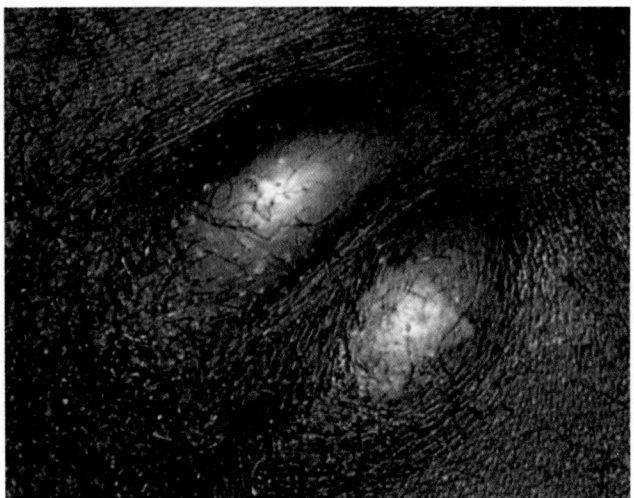

FIGURE 3-5 "Groove sign" seen with lymphogranuloma venereum. Enlarged lymph nodes matted together on either side of the inguinal ligament create this characteristic groove. (Reproduced with permission from Morse S, Ballard RC, Holmes KK, et al (eds): Atlas of Sexually Transmitted Diseases, 3rd ed. Edinburgh: Mosby; 2003.)

with other STDs, this infection is found in lower socioeconomic groups among persons with multiple sexual partners. Incubation ranges from 3 days to 2 weeks, and its clinical course is divided into three stages: (1) small vesicle or papule, (2) inguinal or femoral lymphadenopathy, and (3) anogenitorectal syndrome. Initial papules appear primarily on the fourchette and posterior vaginal wall up to and including the cervix. Repeated inoculation may result in lesions at multiple sites. These primary lesions heal quickly and without scarring.

During the second stage, sometimes referred to as the inguinal syndrome, inguinal and femoral lymph nodes progressively enlarge. Painful nodes can mat together on either side of the inguinal ligament and create a characteristic "groove sign," which appears in up to one fifth of infected women (Fig. 3-5). Moreover, enlarging nodes may rupture through the skin and lead to chronically draining sinuses. Women with lymphogranuloma venereum (LGV) commonly develop systemic infection, manifest by malaise and fever. Additionally, pneumonitis, arthritis, and hepatitis have been reported.

In the third stage of LGV, a patient develops rectal pruritus and a mucoid discharge from rectal ulcers. If these become infected, the discharge turns purulent. This presentation stems from lymphatic obstruction that follows lymphangitis and that may result in elephantiasis of external genitalia initially and fibrosis of the rectum. Stenosis of the urethra and the vagina has also been reported. Rectal bleeding is common, and a woman may complain of crampy, abdominal pain with abdominal distention, rectal pain, and fever. Peritonitis may follow bowel perforation.

LGV may be diagnosed following clinical evaluation with exclusion of other etiologies and positive chlamydial testing. Specifically, culture or immunofluorescence or nucleic acid amplification tests (NAAT) testing of samples from genital lesions, affected lymph nodes, or rectum are suitable. Moreover, a chlamydial serologic titer that is >1:64 can support the diagnosis.

For treatment, the CDC-recommended regimen (2015) is doxycycline, 100 mg orally twice daily for 21 days. Alternatively, one may use erythromycin base 500 mg orally four times daily for the same duration. Sexual contacts exposed to a patient within the prior 60 days are tested for urethral or cervical infection and treated with either standard anti-chlamydial regimen.

INFECTIOUS VAGINITIS

Symptomatic vaginal discharge most often reflects BV, candidiasis, or trichomoniasis. Bacterial vaginosis typically evokes complaints of foul discharge odor. In contrast, if abnormal discharge is associated with vulvar burning, irritation, or itching, then *vaginitis* is diagnosed. Between 7 and 70 percent of women who have vaginal discharge complaints will have no definitive diagnosis (Anderson, 2004). For those in whom identifiable infection is absent, an inflammatory diagnosis and treatment for infection should not be given. In such instances, a woman may seek reassurance, having concern about a recent sexual exposure, and STD screening may alleviate this.

Importantly, during evaluation, a clinician obtains a complete history regarding prior vaginal infections and their treatment, symptom duration, specifics of self-treatment with over-the-counter (OTC) preparations, and a complete menstrual and sexual history. The salient features of a menstrual history are outlined in Chapter 8 (p. 182). A sexual history typically includes questions regarding age at coitarche, date of most recent sexual activity, number of recent partners, gender of those partners, use of condom barrier protection, method of birth control, prior STD history, and type of sexual activity—anal, oral, or vaginal.

A thorough physical examination of the vulva, vagina, and cervix is also performed. Several etiologies may be identified in the office by microscopic examination of the discharge (Table 3-7). First, a saline preparation, described earlier, can be inspected (p. 51). In contrast, a "KOH-prep" contains a swab-collected sample of discharge mixed with several drops of 10-percent potassium hydroxide (KOH). KOH leads to osmotic swelling and then lysis of squamous cell membranes. This visually clears the microscopic view and aids identification of fungal buds or hyphae. Finally, vaginal pH analysis may add supportive information. Vaginal pH can be estimated using chemical testing paper strips. Appropriate readings are obtained by pressing a test strip directly to the upper vaginal wall and resting it there for a few seconds to absorb vaginal fluid. Once the strip is removed, its color is determined and matched to a color indicator chart on the test strip dispenser. Importantly, blood and semen are alkaline and often will artificially elevate pH. Unfortunately, inexpensive laboratory tests such as these are not as accurate as a clinician would hope (Bornstein, 2001; Landers, 2004).

■ Fungal Infection

This infection is most commonly caused by *Candida albicans*, which can be found in the vagina of asymptomatic patients and

TABLE 3-7. Characteristics of Common Vaginal Infections

Category	Complaint	Discharge	KOH "Whiff Test"	Vaginal pH	Microscopic Findings
Normal	None	White, clear	–	3.8–4.2	NA
BV	Odor, increased after intercourse and/or menses	Thin, gray or white, adherent, often increased	+	>4.5	Clue cells, bacteria clumps (saline wet prep)
Candidiasis	Itching, burning, discharge	White, curdy	–	<4.5	Hyphae and buds (10-percent KOH solution wet prep)
Trichomoniasis	Frothy discharge, odor, dysuria, pruritus, spotting	Green-yellow, frothy, adherent, increased	±	>4.5	Motile trichomonads (saline wet prep)
Bacterial[a]	Thin, watery discharge, pruritus	Purulent	–	>4.5	Many WBCs

[a]Streptococcal, staphylococcal, or *Escherichia coli.*
BV = bacterial vaginosis; KOH = potassium hydroxide; NA = not applicable; WBC = white blood cell.

is a commensal of the mouth, rectum, and vagina. Occasionally, other *Candida* species may be involved and include *C tropicalis* and *C glabrata,* among others. Candidiasis is seen more often in warmer climates and in obese patients. Additionally, immunosuppression, diabetes mellitus, pregnancy, and recent broad-spectrum antibiotic use predispose women to clinical infection. It can be sexually transmitted, and several studies have reported an association between candidiasis and orogenital sex (Bradshaw, 2005; Geiger, 1996).

With candidiasis, pruritus, pain, vulvar erythema, and edema with excoriations are frequent findings (Fig. 3-6). The typical vaginal discharge is described as curdy or cottage cheese-like. Microscopic examination of vaginal discharge with saline and

with 10-percent KOH preparations allows yeast identification. *Candida albicans* is dimorphic, with both yeast buds and hyphal forms. It may be present in the vagina as a filamentous fungus (pseudohyphae) or as germinated yeast with mycelia. Vaginal candidal culture is not routinely recommended. However, it may be warranted for those who fail empiric treatment and for women with evidence of infection yet absence of microscopic yeast.

The CDC classifies vulvovaginal candidiasis (2015) into "uncomplicated" and "complicated." Uncomplicated candidiasis cases are sporadic or infrequent, mild to moderate in symptom severity, likely caused by *Candida albicans*, and involve nonimmunocompromised women. For both uncomplicated

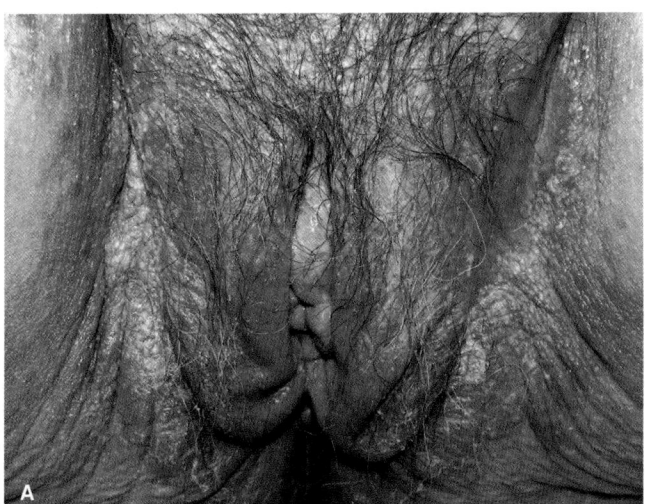
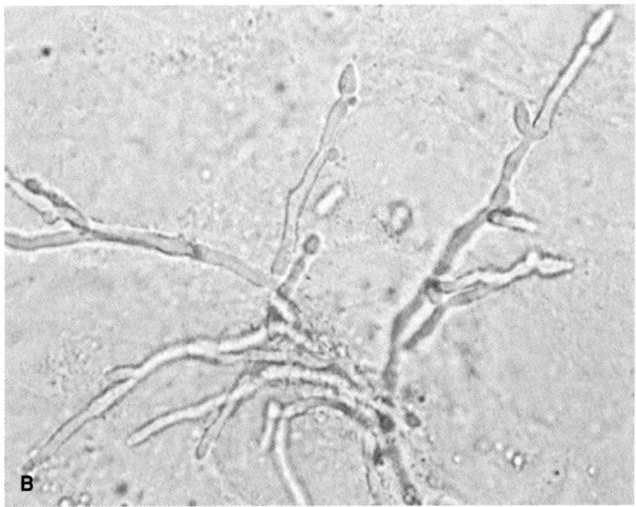

FIGURE 3-6 Candidal infection. **A.** Thick white discharge, labial erythema, and edema are seen with candidiasis. (Used with permission from Dr. William Griffith.) **B.** *Candida albicans* in a potassium hydroxide preparation. Serpentine pseudohyphae are seen. (Reproduced with permission from Hansfield HH: Vaginal infections. In Color Atlas and Synopsis of Sexually Transmitted Diseases. New York, McGraw-Hill, 2001, p 169.)

TABLE 3-8. Topical Agents (First-line Therapy) for the Treatment of Candidiasis

Drug	Brand Name	Formulation	Dosage
Butoconazole	Gynazole-1[a] Mycelex-3	2% vaginal cream 2% vaginal cream	1 app (5 g) vaginally ×1 d 1 app (5 g) vaginally ×3 d
Clotrimazole	Gyne-Lotrimin 7, Mycelex-7 Gyne-Lotrimin 3 Gyne-Lotrimin 3	1% vaginal cream 2% vaginal cream 200 mg vaginal supp	1 app vaginally for 7 d 1 app vaginally for 3 d 1 vaginal supp daily for 3 d
Clotrimazole combination pack	Gyne-Lotrimin 3 Mycelex-7	200 mg supp + 1% topical cream 100 mg supp + 1% topical cream	1 supp daily for 3 d. Use cream externally as needed 1 supp daily for 7 d. Use cream externally as needed
Clotrimazole + betamethasone	Lotrisone[a]	1% clotrimazole with 0.05% betamethasone vaginal cream	Apply cream topically twice daily[b]
Miconazole	Monistat-7 Monistat Monistat-3 Monistat-7	100 mg vaginal supp 2% topical cream 4% vaginal cream 2% topical cream	1 supp daily for 7 d Apply externally as needed 1 app vaginally for 3 d 1 app vaginally for 7 d
Miconazole combination pack	Monistat-3 Monistat-7 Monistat Dual Pack	200 mg vaginal supp + 2% topical cream 100 mg vaginal supp + 2% topical cream[b] 1200 mg vaginal supp + 2% topical cream	1 supp daily for 3 d. Use cream externally BID as needed[b] 1 supp daily for 7 d. Use cream externally BID as needed[b] 1 supp daily for 1 d. Use cream externally BID as needed
Terconazole	Terazol 3[a] Terazol 7[a] Terazol 3[a]	80 mg vaginal supp 0.4% vaginal cream 0.8% vaginal cream	1 supp daily for 3 d 1 app vaginally 7 d 1 app vaginally 3 d
Tioconazole	Monostat-1, Vagistat-1	6.5% vaginal ointment	1 app vaginally, once
Nystatin	Pyolene Nystatin/Generic	100,000 unit vaginal tablet	1 tablet daily for 14 d (best choice for 1st trimester pregnancy)
Nystatin powder	Mycostatin	100,000 units/gram	Apply to vulva twice daily for 14 d

[a]Prescription required.
[b]Maximum use recommended is 2 weeks.
app = applicatorful; supp = suppository.
Adapted with permission from Haefner H: Current evaluation and management of vulvovaginitis, Clin Obstet Gynecol 1999 Jun;42(2):184–95.

and complicated infection, effective treatment formulations are listed in Table 3-8. For uncomplicated infection, azoles are extremely effective, and women warrant specific follow-up only if therapy is unsuccessful.

However, 10 to 20 percent of women have complicated candidiasis, which implies greater symptom severity, perhaps involvement of non-*albicans* species, affected patients with relative immunosuppression, or recurrent disease. By definition, *recurrent disease* reflects four or more candidal infections during a year. For women in these complicated candidiasis categories, cultures are obtained to direct care, and longer therapy may be

needed to achieve clinical cure. Examples include local intravaginal therapy for 7 to 14 days.

For recurrent *C albicans* disease, local intravaginal therapy for 7 to 14 days or oral fluconazole (Diflucan) in 100-mg, 150-mg, or 200-mg doses once every third day for a total of three doses (day 1, 4, and 7) are options. Suppressive maintenance regimen for recurrence prevention is oral fluconazole, 100 to 200 mg weekly for 6 months. Non-*albicans* candidal species are not as responsive to topical azole therapy. For non-*albicans* recurrent infection, a 600-mg boric acid gelatin capsule intravaginally daily for 2 weeks has been successful. These capsules require a compounding pharmacy, and care is taken if children are in the household as accidental oral ingestion of boric acid capsules can be fatal.

Oral azole therapy has been associated with serum liver enzyme elevation. Thus, prolonged oral therapy may not be feasible for that reason or because of interactions with other patient medications such as calcium-channel blockers, warfarin, protease inhibitors, trimetrexate, terfenadine, cyclosporine A, phenytoin, and rifampin. In these cases, local intravaginal therapy once or twice weekly may give a similar clinical response.

■ Trichomoniasis

This protozoan infection is the most prevalent nonviral STD in the United States (Van der Pol, 2005, 2007). Unlike other STDs, its incidence appears to increase with patient age in some studies. Trichomoniasis is more often diagnosed in women because most men are asymptomatic. However, up to 70 percent of male partners of women with vaginal trichomoniasis will have trichomonads in their urinary tract.

This parasite is usually a marker of high-risk sexual behavior, and co-infection with other sexually transmitted pathogens is common, especially *N gonorrhoeae*. *Trichomonas vaginalis* has predilection for squamous epithelium, and lesions may increase accessibility to other sexually transmitted species. Vertical transmission during birth is possible and may persist for a year.

Diagnosis

Incubation with *T vaginalis* requires 3 days to 4 weeks, and the vagina, urethra, endocervix, and bladder can be infected. No symptoms are noted in up to one half of women with trichomoniasis, and such colonization can persist for months or years. However, in those with complaints, vaginal discharge is typically described as foul, thin, and yellow or green. Additionally, dysuria, dyspareunia, vulvar pruritus, vaginal spotting, and pain may be noted. At times, clinical findings are identical to those of acute PID.

With trichomoniasis, the vulva may be erythematous, edematous, and excoriated. The vagina contains the discharge just described, and subepithelial hemorrhages or "strawberry spots" dot the vagina and cervix. Trichomonads are oval anaerobic protozoa that are slightly larger than a white blood cell (WBC) and have anterior flagella (Fig. 3-7). Microscopic identification of these motile parasites in a saline preparation of the discharge is diagnostic. However, trichomonads are less motile with cooling, and slides ideally are examined within 20 minutes. Inspection of a saline preparation is highly specific, yet sensitivity is only 60 to 70 percent. In addition to microscopy, vaginal pH is often elevated.

The most sensitive diagnostic technique is culture, which is impractical because special media (Diamond media) is required and few laboratories are equipped. NAATs for trichomonal DNA are sensitive and specific but not widely available. Alternatively, the OSOM Trichomonas Rapid Test is an immunochromatographic assay, which has 88-percent sensitivity and 99-percent specificity. It is available for office use, and results are available in 10 minutes (Huppert, 2005, 2007). Trichomonads may also be noted on Pap smear screening and sensitivity approximates 60 percent (Wiese, 2000). If trichomonads are reported from a Pap smear slide, confirmation by microscopic evaluation of a saline preparation is encouraged prior to treatment (American College of Obstetricians and Gynecologists, 2013b). Women with trichomoniasis are tested for other STDs. Additionally, sexual contact(s) are evaluated or referred for evaluation.

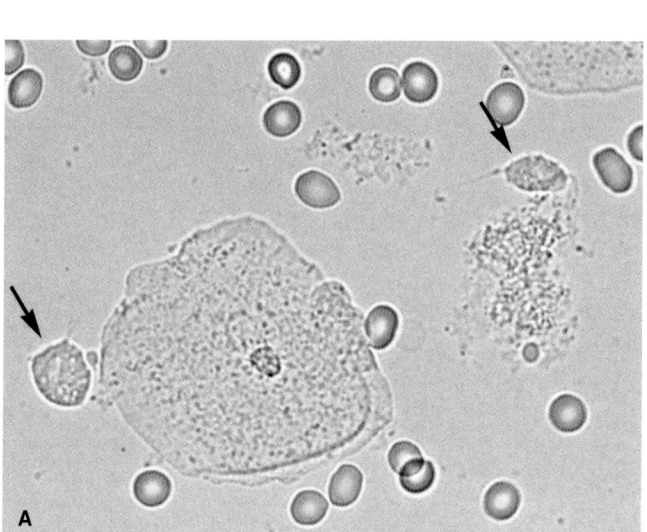
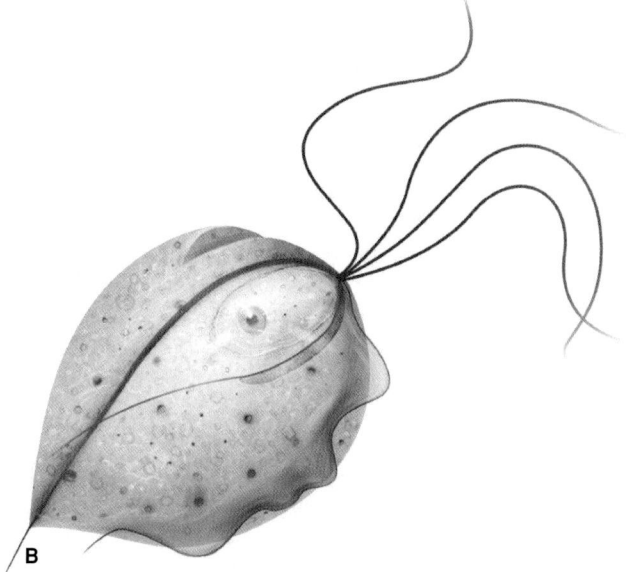

FIGURE 3-7 Trichomonads. **A.** Photomicrograph of a vaginal smear saline preparation containing trichomonads (*arrows*). One squame and many red blood cells are also present. (Used with permission from Dr. Lauri Campagna and Rebecca Winn, WHNP.) **B.** Drawing depicts anatomic features of trichomonads. Flagella allow this parasite to be motile.

Treatment

Oral regimens recommended by the CDC (2015) are either met-ronidazole 2 g once or tinidazole (Tindamax) 2 g once. Although each is effective, some report that an oral 7-day treatment regi-men with metronidazole 500 mg twice daily may be more effec-tive in compliant patients. However, compliance may be poor because of longer treatment length and metronidazole side effects (p. 54). Because of drug disulfiram-like effects, patients should abstain from alcohol during use and for 24 hours following met-ronidazole therapy and for 72 hours after tinidazole.

Affected women are retested within 3 months of treatment. Recurrence occurs in approximately 30 percent of patients. Sex partners are encouraged to seek treatment, and patients are reminded to abstain from sex until they and their partners are cured. Condom use may be protective.

Infrequently, patients may have strains that are highly resis-tant to metronidazole, but these organisms are usually sensitive to tinidazole. Culture and sensitivity are performed on speci-mens from patients with frequently recurring infections or from those who do not respond to the initial therapy and who are regimen compliant. Oral tinidazole at doses of 500 mg orally three times daily for 7 days or four times daily for 14 days have been effective in curing patients with resistant organ-isms (Sobel, 2001). Cases of allergy to these two nitroimid-azoles require desensitization by a specialist (Helms, 2008).

SUPPURATIVE CERVICITIS

■ *Neisseria gonorrhoeae*

Many women with cervical *N gonorrhoeae* are asymptomatic. For this reason, women at risk are screened periodically (Table 1-1, p. 6). Risk factors for gonococcal carriage and potential upper reproductive tract infection that merit screening are: age ≤24 years, prior or current STDs, new or multiple sexual partners, a partner with other concurrent partners, a partner with an STD, lack of barrier protection in those without a monoga-mous relationship, and commercial sex work (U.S. Preventive Services Task Force, 2014). Screening for women at low risk is not recommended.

Diagnosis

Symptomatic lower female reproductive tract gonorrhea may present as vaginitis or cervicitis. Those with cervicitis com-monly describe a profuse odorless, nonirritating, and white-to-yellow vaginal discharge. Patients may report intermenstrual or postcoital vaginal bleeding, or gentle passage of a cotton swab into the cervical os often produces endocervical bleeding. Gonococcus can also infect the Bartholin and Skene glands, the urethra, and ascend into the endometrium and fallopian tube to cause upper reproductive tract infection (p. 65).

N gonorrhoeae is a gram-negative coccobacillus that invades columnar and transitional epithelial cells, becoming intracellu-lar. For this reason, the vaginal epithelium, which is squamous cell, is not involved.

For gonococcal identification, NAATs are available and have replaced culture in most laboratories. Previously, acceptable specimens were recovered only from the endocervix or urethra.

However, newer NAAT collection kits are available for specific collection from the vagina, endocervix, or urine. For women without a cervix following hysterectomy, first-void urine sam-ples are collected. For those with a cervix, vaginal-swab speci-mens are as sensitive and specific as cervical-swab specimens. Urine samples, although acceptable, are least preferred for those with a cervix (Association of Public Health Laboratories, 2009). However, if selected, the initial urine stream, not midstream, is collected. Of note, these noncultural tests are not FDA-cleared for diagnostic identification of rectal or pharyngeal disease. Thus, cultures are obtained in those screened at these anatomic sites.

All patients with gonorrhea are tested for other STDs, and sexual contacts from the preceding 60 days are evaluated and treated or referred for this. Abstinence is practiced until therapy is completed and until they and their treated sexual partners have symptom resolution.

Expedited Partner Therapy. To prevent and control STDs, guidelines for expedited partner therapy (EPT) have been cre-ated by the CDC. EPT is the delivery of a prescription by persons infected with an STD to their sexual partners without clinical assessment of the partners or professional counseling. EPT ideally does not replace traditional strategies, such as stan-dard patient referral, when these are available. Although accept-able for treatment of heterosexual contacts with gonorrhea or chlamydial infection, data do not support EPT for trichomo-niasis or syphilis. Although sanctioned by the CDC, EPT is not legal in several states within the United States. Moreover, the risk of litigation in the event of adverse outcomes may be elevated when a practice has uncertain legal status or is outside formally accepted community practice standards (Centers for Disease Control and Prevention, 2006). The legal status of EPT in each of the 50 states can be found at: http://www.cdc.gov/std/ept/legal/default.htm.

Treatment

CDC recommendations for single-dose therapy of uncomplicated cervical, urethral, or rectal infection are outlined in Table 3-9. Importantly, widespread quinolone-resistant gonococci in the United States prompted removal of this antibiotic class from the CDC STD guidelines, and declining effectiveness of cefixime has shifted its role to an alternative agent (Centers for Disease Control and Prevention, 2015). Uncomplicated gonococcal pharyngeal infection treatment mirrors the recommended regi-men in Table 3-9. Test-of-cure cultures are not usually necessary unless an alternative to ceftriaxone is used. In cases of cephalo-sporin allergy, one potential option is single oral doses of gemi-floxacin 320 mg plus azithromycin 2 g. Another is single doses of gentamicin 240 mg IM plus oral azithromycin 2 g. For azithro-mycin allergy, ceftriaxone alone suffices. However, if the alterna-tive regimen with cefixime is used, then doxycycline, 100 mg orally twice daily for 7 days, replaces the azithromycin (Centers for Disease Control and Prevention, 2015).

■ *Chlamydia trachomatis*

This organism is among the most prevalent of the STD species recovered in the United States, and its highest prevalence is

TABLE 3-9. Single-dose Treatment of Uncomplicated Gonococcal Infection of the Cervix, Urethra, or Rectum[a]

Recommended regimen
Ceftriaxone (Rocephin) 250 mg IM[b]
PLUS
Azithromycin (Zithromax) 1 g orally once

Alternative regimen
Cefixime (Suprax) 400 mg orally once
PLUS
Azithromycin 1 g orally once

[a]Test of cure is not required. Persons with persistent symptoms of gonococcal infection or whose symptoms recur shortly after treatment are reevaluated by culture for *N gonorrhoeae*. If positive, isolates are submitted for resistance testing. Suspected treatment failures are reported to the CDC within 24 hours.
[b]Other cephalosporin options include: (1) ceftizoxime (Cefizox) 500 mg IM, (2) cefoxitin (Mefoxin) 2 g IM given with probenecid 1 g orally, or (3) cefotaxime (Claforan) 500 mg IM. Reproduced with permission from Centers for Disease Control and Prevention: Sexually transmitted diseases treatment guidelines, 2015. MMWR 64(3):1, 2015.

TABLE 3-10. Oral Treatments of Chlamydial Infection

Recommended regimen
Azithromycin 1 g once
or
Doxycycline 100 mg twice daily for 7 days

Alternative regimens
Erythromycin base 500 mg four times daily for 7 days
or
Erythromycin ethyl succinate 800 mg four times daily for 7 days
or
Levofloxacin (Levaquin) 500 mg once daily for 7 days
or
Ofloxacin (Floxin) 300 mg twice daily for 7 days

Reproduced with permission from Centers for Disease Control and Prevention: Sexually transmitted diseases treatment guidelines, 2015. MMWR 64(3):1, 2015.

found in individuals younger than 25 years. *Chlamydia* prevalence was 4.7 percent overall among sexually active females aged 14 to 24 years based on national survey estimates from 2007 to 2012 (Torrone, 2014). This increased to 13.5 percent among non-Hispanic black females. Since many with this organism are asymptomatic, women with the same risks that prompt gonococcal screening, listed on page 64, are screening candidates.

This obligate intracellular parasite is dependent on host cells for survival. It infects columnar epithelial cells, and endocervical glandular infection leads to mucopurulent discharge or endocervical secretions. If infected, the endocervical tissue is commonly edematous and hyperemic. Urethritis can also develop, and dysuria is prominent.

Microscopic inspection of secretions in a saline preparation typically reveals 20 or more leukocytes per high-power field. More specifically, culture, NAAT, and enzyme-linked immunosorbent assay (ELISA) are available for endocervical specimens. Alternatively, combined gonococcal and chlamydial tests are widely used. As with gonorrhea testing, newer NAAT collection kits permit specific collection from the vagina, the endocervix, or urine (p. 64). Vaginal-swab specimens are as sensitive and specific as cervical-swab specimens. Urine samples, although acceptable, are least preferred for women with a cervix. However, for women following hysterectomy, first-void urine samples are preferred. Again, these noncultural tests are not FDA-cleared for diagnostic identification of rectal or pharyngeal disease. If *C trachomatis* is diagnosed or suspected, then screening for other STDs is indicated.

Recommended therapy for *C trachomatis* infection is described in Table 3-10. Azithromycin has the obvious therapeutic compliance advantage of allowing clinicians to observe ingestion at the time of diagnosis. Following treatment, retesting is not recommended if symptoms resolve. To prevent further infection, abstinence is recommended until a woman and her partner(s) are treated and are asymptomatic. Sexual partner(s) are referred for evaluation, or they are examined, counseled, tested, and treated. As with gonorrhea in heterosexual partners, expedited partner therapy is sanctioned by the CDC for selected patients (p. 64).

Mycoplasma genitalium

Discovered in 1980, this bacterium's role in female lower reproductive tract pathology is poorly defined. Most women carriers are asymptomatic, but it has been linked in some but not all studies to urethritis, cervicitis, PID, and later to tubal-factor infertility (Taylor-Robinson, 2011; Weinstein, 2012). Thus, in women with persistent or recurrent urethritis, cervicitis, or PID, *M genitalium* may be considered. It has a much more established role in male urethritis (Daley, 2014). As such, gynecologists may more frequently encounter the exposed female partner of an infected male. Currently, the CDC (2015) comments that NAAT testing for exposed women and treatment of subsequently identified infections can be considered. NAATs for this organism are not widely available, but samples from voided urine, the vagina, or the endocervix are appropriate (Lillis, 2011).

For urethritis, cervicitis, or exposure coverage, azithromycin 1 g orally once is recommended. Antibiotic-resistant strains are not uncommon, and for treatment failure, moxifloxacin 400 mg once orally for 7 to 14 days may be used. This same moxifloxacin regimen for 14 days may be considered for women with PID who fail to respond after 7 to 10 days of standard regimens and in whom *M genitalium* is detected (Centers for Disease Control and Prevention, 2015; Manhart, 2011).

PELVIC INFLAMMATORY DISEASE

This is an infection of the upper female reproductive tract organs. Another diagnosis given to this disease is acute salpingitis. Although all reproductive tract organs may be involved, the organ of importance, with or without abscess formation, is the fallopian tube. Because of difficulty in accurately diagnosing this infection, its true magnitude is unknown. Many women report that they have been treated for PID when they did not have it, and vice versa. The clinical importance of diagnosing PID is emphasized by its known sequelae, which include tubal-factor infertility, ectopic pregnancy, and chronic pelvic pain. Thus, clinicians ideally carry a low threshold for diagnosing and treating PID.

■ Microbiology and Pathogenesis

The exact microbiologic pathogens in the fallopian tube cannot be known for any given patient. Studies have shown that transvaginal culture of the endocervix, endometrium, and cul-de-sac contents reveals different organisms from each site in the same patient. For that reason, treatment protocols are designed so that most potential pathogens are covered by antibiotic regimens.

Classic salpingitis is associated with and secondary to *N gonorrhoeae* infection, and *C trachomatis* is also commonly recovered (Table 3-11). Another species frequently found is *T vaginalis*. The lower reproductive tract flora in women with PID and in those with bacterial vaginosis is predominately anaerobic species. The microenvironment changes produced by BV may aid ascension of the causative organisms of PID (Soper, 2010). However, Ness and colleagues (2004) and others have shown that bacterial vaginosis is not a risk factor for PID development.

Upper tract infection is believed to be caused by bacteria that ascend from the lower reproductive tract. It is assumed that this ascension is enhanced during menstruation due to loss of endocervical barriers. The gonococcus can cause a direct inflammatory response in the human endocervix, endometrium, and fallopian tube and is one of the true pathogens of human fallopian tube epithelial cells. If normal human fallopian tube cells in cell culture are exposed to potential pathogens such as *Escherichia coli*, *Bacteroides fragilis*, or *Enterococcus faecalis*, no inflammatory response follows. If the above bacteria are introduced into a fallopian tube cell culture in which gonococci are present and have caused inflammatory damage, then an exaggerated inflammatory response results.

TABLE 3-11. Pelvic Inflammatory Disease Risk Factors

Douching
Single status
Substance abuse
Multiple sexual partners
Lower socioeconomic status
Recent new sexual partner(s)
Younger age (10 to 19 years)
Other sexually transmitted infections
Sexual partner with urethritis or gonorrhea
Previous diagnosis of pelvic inflammatory disease
Not using mechanical and/or chemical contraceptive
   barriers
Endocervical testing positive for *N gonorrhoeae* or
   C trachomatis

In contrast, intracellular *C trachomatis* does not cause an acute inflammatory response, and little *direct* permanent damage results from chlamydial tubal involvement (Patton, 1983). However, cell-mediated immune mechanisms may be responsible for subsequent tissue injury. Specifically, persistent chlamydial antigens can trigger a delayed hypersensitivity reaction with continued tubal scarring and destruction (Toth, 2000).

Last, women with pulmonary tuberculosis can develop salpingitis and endometritis. This pathogen is thought to be blood-borne, but ascension may still be a possible route. The fallopian tubes also can be infected by direct extension from inflammatory GI disease, especially ruptured abscess, for example, appendiceal or diverticular.

■ Diagnosis
Silent Pelvic Inflammatory Disease

Pelvic inflammatory disease can be segregated into "silent" PID and PID. The latter can be further subdivided into acute and chronic.

Silent PID is thought to follow multiple or continuous low-grade infection in asymptomatic women. Silent PID is not a clinical diagnosis. Rather, it is an ultimate diagnosis given to women with tubal-factor infertility who lack a history compatible with upper tract infection. Many of these patients have antibodies to *C trachomatis* and/or *N gonorrhoeae*. At laparoscopy or laparotomy, affected women may have evidence of prior tubal infection such as adhesions, but for the most part, the fallopian tubes are grossly normal. Internally, however, tubes show flattened mucosal folds, extensive deciliation of the epithelium, and secretory epithelial cell degeneration (Patton, 1989). Alternatively, hydrosalpinx may be found. Grossly, these fallopian tubes are distended along their entire length. Their distal ends are dilated and clubbed, and fimbria are replaced by or encased by smooth adhesions (Fig. 9-22, p. 224). Sonographically, a hydrosalpinx tends to be anechoic, tubular, serpentine, and often with incomplete septa (Figs. 9-23). Last, fine adhesions between the liver capsule and anterior abdominal wall may also reflect prior silent disease.

Acute Pelvic Inflammatory Disease

Symptoms and Physical Findings. The most recent diagnostic criteria presented by the CDC (2015) are for sexually active women at risk for STDs who have pelvic or lower abdominal pain and in whom other etiologies are excluded or unlikely. PID is diagnosed if uterine tenderness, adnexal tenderness, *or* cervical motion tenderness is present. One or more of the following enhances diagnostic specificity: (1) oral temperature >38.3°C (101.6°F), (2) mucopurulent cervical discharge or cervical friability, (3) abundant WBCs on saline microscopy of cervical secretions, (4) elevated erythrocyte sedimentation rate (ESR) or C-reactive protein (CRP), and (5) presence of cervical *N gonorrhoeae* or *C trachomatis*. Thus, a diagnosis of PID is one typically based on clinical findings.

With acute PID, symptoms characteristically develop during or soon following menstruation. These can include lower abdominal and/or pelvic pain, yellow vaginal discharge, heavy menstrual bleeding, fever, chills, anorexia, nausea, vomiting, diarrhea, dysmenorrhea, and dyspareunia. Patients also may have complaints suggesting urinary tract infection. Unfortunately, no single symptom is associated with a physical finding that is specific for this diagnosis. Accordingly, other possible sources of acute pelvic pain are considered and listed in Table 11-1 (p. 251).

In women with acute PID, leukorrhea or mucopurulent endocervicitis is common and is diagnosed visually and microscopically. During bimanual pelvic examination, affected women will usually have pelvic organ tenderness. Cervical motion tenderness (CMT) is typically elicited by quickly moving the cervix with examining vaginal fingers. This reflects pelvic peritonitis and can be considered a vaginal "rebound" test. If a woman has pelvic peritonitis secondary to bacteria and purulent debris that has exuded from the fimbriated end of the fallopian tube, this rapid peritoneal movement usually causes a marked pain response. Tapping the cul-de-sac with examining finger(s) will give the examiner similar information. This latter maneuver usually causes a patient significantly less pain because less inflamed peritoneum is stretched.

Abdominal peritonitis may be identified by deep probing and quick release of a hand placed on the abdomen—a test for rebound. Alternatively, an examining hand may be positioned with a palm against a woman's midabdomen and gently and quickly moved back and forth (shake). This can identify abdominal peritonitis, often with less patient discomfort.

In women with PID and peritonitis, usually only the lower abdomen is involved. However, inflammation of the liver capsule, which can accompany PID, may lead to right upper quadrant pain, a condition known as Fitz-Hugh-Curtis syndrome. Classically, symptoms of this perihepatitis include sharp, pleuritic right upper quadrant pain that accompanies pelvic pain. The upper abdominal pain may refer to the shoulder or upper arm. With auscultation, a friction rub may be heard along the right anterior costal margin. Importantly, during examination, if all abdominal quadrants are involved, suspicion for a ruptured tuboovarian abscess (TOA) is heightened.

Testing. In women with lower abdominal pain, tests directed at diagnosing PID or excluding other pain sources are selected. Pregnancy complications can be identified by serum or urine beta-human chorionic gonadotropin testing. A complete blood count (CBC) is selected as a baseline test to exclude hemoperitoneum as the cause of symptoms and identify WBC elevation. In those with significant nausea and vomiting or Fitz-Hugh-Curtis syndrome, liver enzyme values may be normal or mildly elevated. If properly collected, urinalysis findings for infection will be absent. Saline preparation of cervical or vaginal discharge will typically show sheets of leukocytes. In women with suspected acute PID, endocervical testing for both *N gonorrhoeae* and *C trachomatis* is performed as described earlier (p. 64). Screening for other STDs is also completed.

In the opinion of many, an endometrial biopsy (EMB) in women with mucopurulent secretions and suspected PID does not provide useful information to alter the diagnosis or therapy (Achilles, 2005). However, some do recommend EMB to diagnose endometritis. Polymorphonuclear leukocytes on the endometrial surface correlate with acute endometritis, whereas plasma cells in the endometrium are found with chronic endometritis. However, women with uterine leiomyomas or endometrial polyps but without PID may also often have plasma cells present in the endometrium, as do essentially all women in their lower uterine segment.

Sonography. In women with marked abdominal pain and tenderness, appreciation of upper reproductive tract organs during bimanual examination may be limited, and sonography is a primary imaging tool (Fig. 2-21, p. 33). Normal fallopian tubes are rarely imaged. However, with acute tubal inflammation, the tube swells, its lumen occludes distally, it distends, and its walls and endosalpingeal folds thicken. Characteristic findings include: (1) distended, ovoid-shaped tube filled with anechoic or echogenic fluid, (2) fallopian tube wall thickening, (3) incomplete internal septa, and (4) a "cogwheel" appearance when inflamed tubes are imaged in cross section (Timor-Tritsch, 1998). If color or power Doppler is applied, marked vascularity with low-impedance blood flow, which reflects hyperemia, is seen within thickened fallopian tube walls and if present, within septa (Molander, 2001; Romosan, 2013). Sonography may also be used to identify TOA or exclude other pathology as the pain source. If sonography does not lead to a clear diagnosis, computed-tomography (CT) scanning is often selected (Sam, 2002). Magnetic resonance (MR) imaging is a suitable alternative. In women with right upper quadrant pain suggestive of perihepatitis, chest radiography or upper abdominal sonography may be needed to exclude other pathology.

Laparoscopy. In Scandinavian countries, women suspected of having acute PID undergo laparoscopy for diagnosis. Tubal serosal hyperemia, tubal wall edema, and purulent exudate issuing from the fimbriated ends of the fallopian tubes, termed *pyosalpinx*, and pooling in the cul-de-sac confirm this diagnosis. Because of this routine practice, Hadgu and coworkers (1986) assembled criteria that preoperatively clinically predicted acute PID and assessed their validity by the absence or presence of disease at laparoscopy. Criteria included: (1) single status, (2) adnexal mass, (3) age <25 years, (4) temperature >38°C, (5) cervical *N gonorrhoeae*, (6) purulent vaginal discharge, and (7) ESR ≥15 mm/hr. The preoperative clinical diagnosis of PID was 97-percent accurate if a woman met all seven criteria, allowing avoidance of surgery. Thus, due to the risks of laparoscopy, use of clinical findings alone to diagnose PID is reasonable. In those with a less clear presentation, laparoscopy may be needed to exclude other pathology such as appendicitis or adnexal torsion.

Tuboovarian Abscess

With infection, the inflamed and suppurative fallopian tube can adhere to the ovary. Sonographically, if both tube and ovary are recognizable, the term *tuboovarian complex* is used. If inflammation proceeds, tissue planes and distinction between the two is lost, and the term *tuboovarian abscess* is applied. Tuboovarian abscesses are typically unilateral and may also involve adjacent structures that include bowel, bladder, and contralateral adnexa.

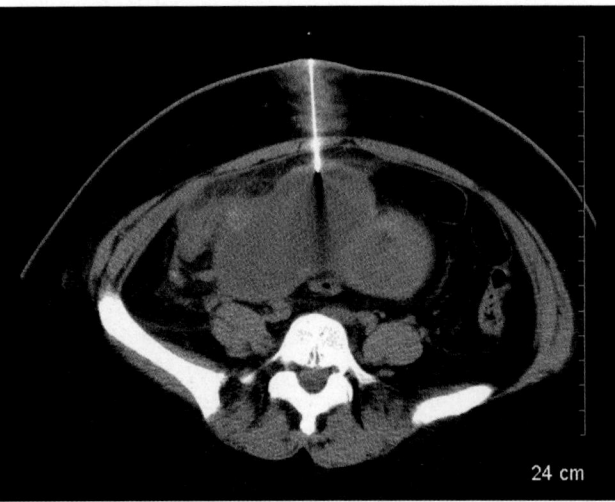

24 cm

FIGURE 3-8 Computed tomographic (CT) scan of a tuboovarian abscess undergoing percutaneous needle drainage.

With abscess progression, further structural weakening may lead to abscess rupture and potentially life-threatening peritonitis. Although PID is an important cause of TOA, these may also follow appendicitis, diverticulitis, inflammatory bowel disease, or surgery.

Classically, affected women display signs of PID and a concurrent adnexal or cul-de-sac mass. Sonographically, with TOA, a complex cystic adnexal or cul-de-sac mass with thick irregular walls, areas of mixed echogenicity, septations, and internal echoes from debris is seen (Fig. 2-22, p. 34). If the clinical picture is unclear, CT scanning may add information. A thick-walled, cystic adnexal mass with internal septations and surrounding inflammatory changes is characteristic (Fig. 3-8). Although not routinely used for TOA imaging, MR imaging usually shows a complex pelvic mass with low signal intensity on T1-weighted sequences and heterogeneously high signal intensity on T2-weighted sequences.

Microorganisms frequently cultured include *E coli*, *Bacteroides* spp, *Peptostreptococcus* spp, and aerobic *Streptococcus* spp. (Landers, 1983). Thus, broad-spectrum antibiotic coverage, including that for anaerobes, is selected for initial management of women with unruptured TOA. Most women with TOA will respond to intravenous (IV) antibiotic therapy alone and avoid the need for drainage. Combination antimicrobial regimens will predictably be more successful, and CDC (2015) recommendations for TOA complicating PID include IV regimens in Table 3-12. Parenteral antimicrobial therapy is continued until the patient has been afebrile for at least 24 hours, preferably 48 to 72 hours. In transitioning to oral therapy, doxycycline 100 mg twice daily is combined with either metronidazole 500 mg twice daily or clindamycin 450 mg four times daily to complete a 14-day course.

For those not improved within 2 to 3 days of treatment, prior to attempts at abscess drainage, antimicrobial regimen modification is indicated. Drainage plus antibiotic therapy can be considered as initial treatment for larger abscesses (≥8 cm). For this, drainage can be accomplished with or without surgery. Radiologic drainage is minimally invasive and potentially avoids the higher risks associated with general anesthesia and surgery. In general,

TABLE 3-12. Recommended Parenteral Treatment of PID

Recommended regimens

Cefotetan (Cefotan) 2 g IV every 12 hr
or
Cefoxitin (Mefoxin) 2 g IV every 6 hr
PLUS
Doxycycline 100 mg orally or IV every 12 hr

OR

Clindamycin 900 mg IV every 8 hr
PLUS
Gentamicin loading dose 2 mg/kg IV or IM followed by a maintenance dose of 1.5 mg/kg every 8 hr. Single daily dosing at 3 to 5 mg/kg per day may be substituted.

Alternative regimen

Ampicillin/sulbactam (Unasyn) 3 g IV every 6 hr
PLUS
Doxycycline 100 mg orally or IV as above

IV = intravenous; PID = pelvic inflammatory disease.
Reproduced with permission from Centers for Disease Control and Prevention: Sexually transmitted diseases treatment guidelines, 2015. MMWR 64(3):1, 2015.

pelvic collections can be emptied using transabdominal, transvaginal, transgluteal, or transrectal routes with either CT or sonographic guidance and adequate analgesia. Depending on abscess size and characteristics, contents can be removed with needle aspiration or with pigtail catheter placement and short-term drainage. In cases that are refractory or not amenable to these more conservative measures, exploratory laparoscopy or laparotomy is typically warranted. In those with TOA rupture, emergency surgery is required. Goals of surgery include abscess drainage, excision of necrotic tissues, and peritoneal cavity irrigation.

As is true in all abscesses, drainage is the key to clinical improvement. Although perhaps tempting at laparotomy, removal of the abscess is not necessary unless ovarian parenchyma is involved. This is rare. Electively opening the protective peritoneal and other tissue planes to remove tissues—especially the uterus—in the presence of acute infection does not improve patient outcome compared with percutaneous drainage. As a clinical comparison, infected Bartholin glands are not excised. Rather, they are drained and definitively treated later, when not infected, if necessary.

Infection confined within one organ, such as a pyosalpinx, responds more favorably to antimicrobial therapy because of adequate blood and lymphatic supply. This is true even if attached to an adjacent ovary. A cul-de-sac or interloop abscess is more likely to require drainage, however, because of poor blood and lymphatic supply and a less prompt response to antimicrobial therapy.

Following successful conservative treatment, bilateral adnexal abscesses cannot be equated with guaranteed infertility. In a clinical trial evaluating such patients, 25 percent of women subsequently became pregnant (Hemsell, 1993).

Chronic Pelvic Inflammatory Disease

This diagnosis is given to women who describe a history of acute PID and who have subsequent pelvic pain. Accuracy of this diagnosis clinically is orders of magnitude less than for acute PID. A hydrosalpinx might qualify as a criterion for this diagnosis. Realistically, however, it is a histologic diagnosis (chronic inflammation) made by a pathologist. Thus, the clinical utility of this diagnosis is limited.

■ Treatment of Pelvic Inflammatory Disease

The most successful patient outcomes follow early diagnosis and prompt, appropriate therapy. The primary therapy goal is to eradicate bacteria, relieve symptoms, and prevent sequelae. Tubal damage or occlusion resulting from infection may lead to infertility. Rates following one episode approximate 15 percent; two episodes, 35 percent; and three or more episodes, 75 percent (Westrom, 1975). Also, ectopic pregnancy risk is increased six- to 10-fold and may reach a 10-percent risk for those who conceive. Other sequelae include chronic pelvic pain (15 to 20 percent), recurrent infection (20 to 25 percent), and abscess formation (5 to 15 percent). Unfortunately, women with mild symptoms may remain at home for days or weeks prior to presentation for diagnosis and therapy.

Exactly where a patient is treated remains controversial. There are proposed criteria that predict better outcome for certain patients with in-hospital parenteral antimicrobial therapy (Table 3-13). However, the high cost of in-hospital treatment prevents routine hospitalization for all women given this diagnosis.

Another potential clinical decision involves management of a coexistent IUD. During the first 3 weeks after device insertion, patients have an increased IUD-associated PID risk. After this time, other PID risks are considered causative. With PID, theoretical concerns are that a coexistent IUD might worsen the infection or delay resolution. Although a provider may choose to remove the device, evidence supports leaving an IUD during treatment in those hospitalized with mild or moderate PID (Centers for Disease Control and Prevention, 2015; Tepper, 2013). Severe disease warrants IUD removal. With or without an IUD, women are treated with similar antibiotic regimens. But, if a patient fails to improve within 48 to 72 hours, the device is removed.

Oral Treatment

In women with a mild to moderate clinical presentation, outpatient treatment and inpatient therapy yield similar results. Clinical treatment with oral therapy is also appropriate for women with HIV infection and PID. These women have the same species recovered compared with non-HIV-infected patients, and their response to therapy is similar.

If women have more than moderate disease, they require hospitalization. Dunbar-Jacob and associates (2004) showed that women treated as outpatients took 70 percent of prescribed doses, and for less than 50 percent of their outpatient treatment days. If patients are treated as outpatients, an initial parenteral dose may be beneficial. Women treated as outpatients are reevaluated in approximately 72 hours by phone or in person. If women do not respond to oral therapy within 72 hours, parenteral therapy is initiated either as an inpatient or as an outpatient if home nursing care is available. This assumes that the diagnosis is confirmed at reevaluation.

Specific treatment recommendations from the CDC are found in Table 3-14. Anaerobes are believed by some to play an important role in upper tract infection and are treated. Hence, metronidazole may be added to improve anaerobic coverage. If patients have BV or trichomoniasis, then metronidazole addition is required, although perhaps not for 14 days.

Parenteral Treatment

Any woman who has criteria as outlined in Table 3-13 is hospitalized for parenteral treatment for at least 24 hours. Following this, if home parenteral treatment is available, this is a reasonable option. Alternatively, if a woman responds clinically and will be appropriately treated by one of the oral regimens in Table 3-14, then she can be discharged on those medications.

Recommendations for parenteral antibiotic treatment of PID are found in Table 3-12. Of these antibiotics, oral and parenteral routes of doxycycline have almost identical bioavailability, but parenteral doxycycline is caustic to veins. Many prospective clinical trials have shown that either of the listed cephalosporins alone, without doxycycline, will result in a clinical cure.

TABLE 3-13. Hospitalization Indications for Parenteral Treatment of PID

Pregnant
Adolescents
Drug addicts
Severe disease
Suspected abscess
Uncertain diagnosis
Generalized peritonitis
Temperature >38.3°C
Failed outpatient therapy
Recent intrauterine instrumentation
White blood cell count >15,000/mm³
Nausea/vomiting precluding oral therapy

PID = pelvic inflammatory disease.

TABLE 3-14. Outpatient Treatment of PID

Ceftriaxone (Rocephin) 250 mg IM once[a,b]
PLUS
Doxycycline 100 mg orally twice daily for 14 days
with or without
Metronidazole (Flagyl) 500 mg orally twice daily for 14 days

[a]Cefoxitin (Mefoxin) 2 g IM with 1 g oral probenecid once may replace ceftriaxone
[b]Other parenteral third-generation cephalosporins IM given in a single dose such as ceftizoxime or cefotaxime may replace ceftriaxone.
IM = intramuscular; PID = pelvic inflammatory disease.
Reproduced with permission from Centers for Disease Control and Prevention: Sexually transmitted diseases treatment guidelines, 2015. MMWR 64(3):1, 2015.

For that reason, doxycycline administration could be reserved until the patient can take oral medication. The recommendation is to continue parenteral therapy until 24 hours after the patient clinically improves, and the oral doxycycline 100 mg twice daily is continued to complete 14 days of therapy. Alternatively, if the IV gentamycin/clindamycin regimen is used, then transition to a 14-day oral agent may involve clindamycin orally four time daily or doxycycline 100 mg twice daily.

INFECTIOUS WARTS AND PAPULES

■ External Genital Warts

These lesions are created from infection with the human papillomavirus (HPV), and 86 percent of cases stem from HPV 6 or 11 (Garland, 2009). A fuller discussion of HPV pathophysiology is found in Chapter 29 (p. 627). Genital warts display differing morphologies, and appearances range from flat papules to the classic verrucous, exophytic lesions, termed condyloma acuminata (Fig. 3-9) (Beutner, 1998). Involved tissues vary, and external genital warts may develop at sites in the lower reproductive tract, urethra, anus, or mouth. They are usually asymptomatic but can be pruritic or painful depending on their size and location. Warts are typically diagnosed by clinical inspection, and biopsy is not required unless coexisting neoplasia is suspected (Wiley, 2002). Similarly, HPV serotyping is not required for routine diagnosis.

Condyloma acuminata may remain unchanged or spontaneously resolve, and the effect of treatment on future viral transmission is unclear. However, many women prefer removal, and lesions can be destroyed with sharp or electrosurgical excision, cryotherapy, or laser ablation. In addition, very large, bulky lesions may be managed with cavitational ultrasonic surgical aspiration (CUSA) (Section 43-28, p. 996).

Alternatively, topical agents can be applied to resolve lesions through various mechanisms (Table 3-15). One of these, 5-percent imiquimod cream (Aldara), is a patient-applied, immunomodulatory topical treatment for genital warts. This agent induces macrophages to secrete several cytokines, and of these, interferon-γ is probably the most important. For genital wart clearance, this cytokine stimulates a cell-mediated immune response against HPV (Scheinfeld, 2006). Another topical immune-modulating agent is a 15-percent sinecatechin ointment (Veregen) derived from green tea leaf extracts (Meltzer, 2009). Podophyllin is an antimitotic agent available in a 10- to 25-percent tincture of benzoin solution and disrupts viral activity by inducing local tissue necrosis. Podophyllin resin is no longer a first-line CDC-recommended option due to risks of systemic toxicity if used incorrectly. However, a biologically active extract of podophyllin, podofilox, also termed podophyllotoxin, is available in a 0.5-percent solution or gel (Condylox) and can be self-applied by the patient. Alternatively, trichloroacetic acid and bichloroacetic acid are proteolytic agents and are applied serially to warts by clinicians. Intralesion injection of interferon is an effective treatment for warts (Eron, 1986). However, its high cost and painful administration render it an alternative option.

Of therapy choices, no data suggest the superiority of one treatment. Thus, in general, treatment is selected based on clinical circumstances and patient and provider preferences. Importantly, no treatment option, even surgical excision, boasts 100-percent clearance rates. Indeed, clearance rates range from 30 to 80 percent. Accordingly, recurrences are common following treatment.

■ Molluscum Contagiosum

The molluscum contagiosum virus is a DNA poxvirus that is transmitted by direct human-to-human contact or by infected fomites. An incubation period of 2 to 7 weeks is typical, but can be longer. The host response to viral invasion is papular with central umbilication, giving a characteristic appearance (Fig. 3-10). It may be single or multiple and is commonly seen on the vulva, vagina, thighs, and/or buttocks. Molluscum contagiosum is contagious until lesions resolve.

These papules are typically diagnosed by visual inspection alone. However, material from a lesion can be collected on a swab, applied to a slide, and submitted to a laboratory for diagnostic staining with Giemsa, Gram, or Wright stains. Molluscum bodies, which are large intracytoplasmic structures, are diagnostic.

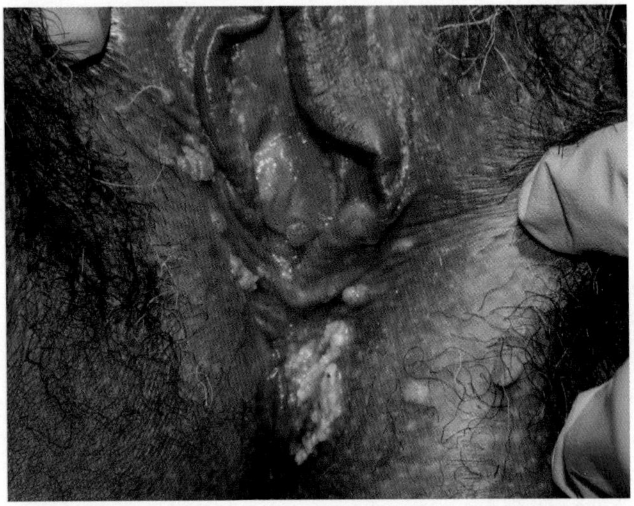

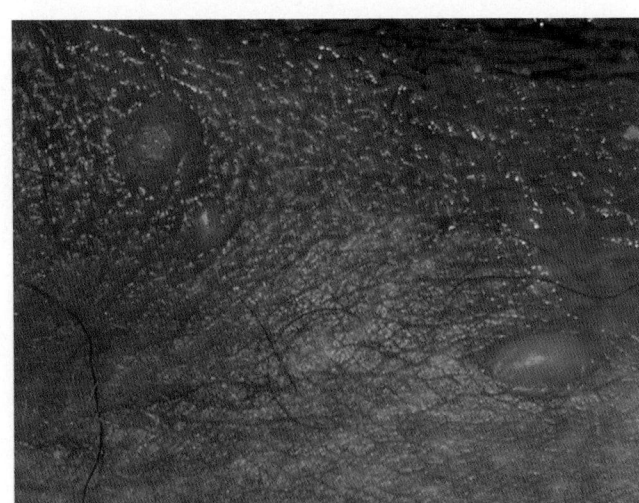

FIGURE 3-9 Condyloma acuminata. Multiple exophytic verrucous warts are seen on the labia and perineum.

FIGURE 3-10 Molluscum contagiosum. Labial lesions are flesh-colored, dome-shaped papules with central umbilication.

TABLE 3-15. Recommended Treatment of External Genital Warts

Patient-applied

Podofilox 0.5% solution or gel (Condylox). Patients should apply podofilox solution with a cotton swab, or podofilox gel with a finger, to visible genital warts twice a day for 3 days, followed by 4 days of no therapy. This cycle may be repeated, as necessary, for up to four cycles. The total wart area treated should not exceed 10 cm^2, and the total volume of podofilox should be limited to 0.5 mL per day.

or

Imiquimod 5% cream (Aldara). Patients should apply imiquimod cream once daily at bedtime, three times a week for up to 16 weeks. The treatment area should be washed with soap and water 6 to 10 hours after the application.

or

Sinecatechin 15% ointment (Veregen). This extract is applied three times daily (0.5-cm strand to each wart) using a finger to ensure wart coverage. Use is continued until warts are cleared, but not longer than 16 weeks. It is not washed off, and sexual contact is avoided when ointment is present.

Provider-administered

Cryotherapy with liquid nitrogen or cryoprobe. Repeat applications every 1 to 2 weeks.

or

Podophyllin resin 10 to 25 percent in a compound tincture of benzoin. A small amount should be applied to each wart and allowed to air dry. The treatment can be repeated weekly, if necessary. Application should be limited to <0.5 mL of podophyllin or an area of <10 cm^2 of warts per session. No open lesions or wounds should exist in the area to which treatment is administered. Some specialists suggest through washing 1 to 4 hours after application to reduce local irritation.

or

Trichloroacetic acid (TCA) or **bichloroacetic acid** (BCA) 80 to 90 percent. A small amount should be applied only to the warts and allowed to dry, at which time a white "frosting" develops. This treatment can be repeated weekly if necessary. If an excess amount of acid is applied, the treated area should be powdered with talc, sodium bicarbonate (i.e., baking soda), or liquid soap preparations to remove unreacted acid.

or

Surgical removal by tangential scissor excision, tangential shave excision, curettage, or electrosurgery.

Alternative regimens

Intralesional interferon, photodynamic therapy, topical cidofovir.

Reproduced with permission from Centers for Disease Control and Prevention: Sexually transmitted diseases treatment guidelines, 2015. MMWR 64(3):1, 2015.

Most lesions spontaneously regress within 6 to 12 months. If removal is preferred, lesions may be treated by cryotherapy, electrosurgical needle coagulation, or sharp needle-tip curettage of a lesion's umbilicated center. Alternatively, topical application of agents used in the treatment of genital warts may also be effective treatment for molluscum contagiosum (see Table 3-15).

PRURITIC INFESTATIONS

■ Scabies

Sarcoptes scabiei infect skin and result in an intensely pruritic rash. This mite is crab-shaped, and the female digs into the skin and remains there for approximately 30 days, elongating her burrow. Several eggs are laid daily and begin hatching after 3 to 4 days (Fig. 3-11). The baby mites furrow their own burrows, becoming reproductive adults in approximately 10 days. The number of adult mites present on an affected patient averages a dozen. Sexual transmission is the most likely cause of initial infection, although it can be seen in household contacts.

Burrows are thin elevated skin tracks measuring 5 to 10 mm in length. A delayed-type 4 hypersensitivity reaction to the mites,

eggs, and feces develops and results in erythematous papules, vesicles, or nodules in association with skin burrows. Secondary infection, however, may develop and hide these tracks. Most common infection sites include the hands, wrist, elbows, groin, and ankles. Itching in these areas is the predominant symptom.

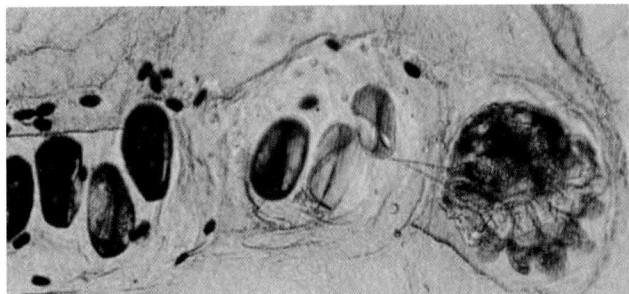

FIGURE 3-11 Burrow with *Sarcoptes scabiei*. A mite is seen at the end of a burrow (*far right*) with seven eggs and smaller fecal particles. (Reproduced with permission from Wolff K, Johnson RA, Saavedra AP: Fitzpatrick's Color Atlas and Synopsis of Clinical Dermatology, 7th ed. New York: McGraw-Hill; 2013.)

Definitive testing requires scraping across the burrow with a scalpel blade and mixing these fragments in immersion oil on a microscope slide. Identification of mites, eggs, egg fragments, or fecal pellets is diagnostic.

Once diagnosed, 5-percent permethrin cream (Elimite) is a recommended agent. A thin layer is applied from the neck downward with special attention to pruritic areas and the hands, feet, and genital regions. Ideally, all family members are treated with the exception of infants younger than 2 years. Eight to 14 hours after application, a shower or bath is taken to remove the medication. Only one application is necessary. Another option is the oral antihelminth ivermectin (Stromectol) 200 μg/kg once and then repeated 2 weeks later. Bed linens and recently worn clothing are washed to prevent reinfection. A less-preferred option is 1-percent lindane, because it is not recommended in pregnancy or in children younger than 2 years and because seizures have occurred if spread on areas with extensive dermatitis or immediately after showering. If used, a 30-g dose of cream is applied and rinsed off similar to permethrin.

An antihistamine will help reduce pruritus, which can also be treated with a hydrocortisone-containing cream in adults or with emollients or lubricating agents in infants. If these lesions become infected, antibiotic therapy may be necessary.

■ Pediculosis

Lice are small ectoparasites that measure approximately 1 mm (Fig. 3-12). Three species infest humans and include the body louse (*Pediculus humanus*), the crab louse (*Phthirus pubis*), and the head louse (*Pediculus humanus capitis*). Lice attach to the base of human hair with claws that vary in diameter between species. It is this claw's diameter that determines the infestation site. For this reason, the crab louse is found on pubic hair and other hair of similar diameter, such as axillary and facial hair, including eyelashes and eyebrows. As is true for mites, the number of lice populating a patient averages a dozen. Lice depend on frequent human blood meals, and pubic lice must travel for new attachment sites. Accordingly, pubic lice usually are sexually transmitted, whereas head and body lice may be transmitted by sharing of personal objects such as combs, brushes, and clothing.

The main symptom from louse attachment and biting is pruritus. Scratching results in erythema and inflammation, which increases blood supply to the area. Patients may develop pyoderma and fever if bites become secondarily infected. Each female adult pubic louse lays approximately four eggs a day, which are glued to the base of hairs. Incubation approximates 1 month. Their attached eggs, termed nits, can be seen attached to the hair shaft away from the skin line as hair growth progresses. These nits usually require a magnifying glass for identification. Moreover, suspicious flecks on pubic hair or in clothing can be examined microscopically to see the characteristic louse. Following diagnosis, patient screening for other STDs is encouraged. Other family members and sexual contacts require evaluation for infestation.

Pediculicides kill not only adult lice, but also the eggs. A single application is usually effective, but a second dose is recommended within 7 to 10 days to kill new hatches. Nonprescription cream rinses or shampoos contain 1-percent permethrin (Nix) or pyrethrins with piperonyl butoxide (Rid, Pronto, R&C). These remain on affected areas for 10 minutes. CDC alternative regimens include 0.5-percent malathion lotion (Ovide) applied for 8 to 12 hours. Also, ivermectin 250 μg/kg orally once can be taken and then repeated in 2 weeks.

In selected cases, 1-percent lindane shampoo can be used, but again, it is less favored due to potential toxicity. Last, eyelash and eyebrow treatment is problematic. These areas are best treated by applying petrolatum (Vaseline) with a cotton swab at night and washing it off in the morning. Bedding and infested clothing are washed and dried with a heat cycle.

In spite of treatment, pruritus may continue and can be relieved by oral antihistamines, antiinflammatory cream or ointment, or both. The patient is reevaluated after 1 week to document louse eradication.

URINARY TRACT INFECTIONS

Symptomatic acute bacterial urinary tract infections (UTIs) are among the most common bacterial infections treated by clinicians. Cystitis accounts for most of these, whereas acute pyelonephritis treatment accounts for a greater number of

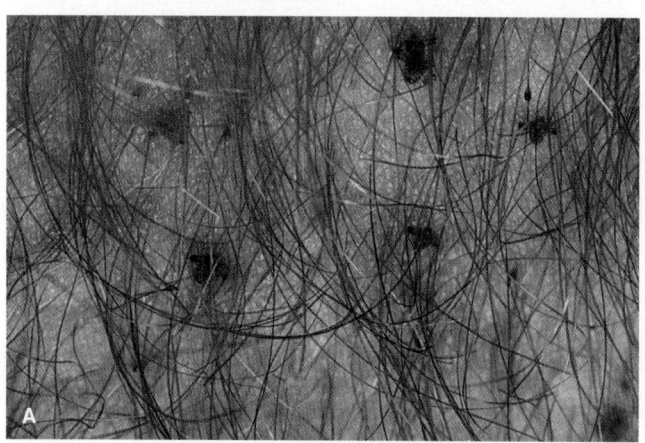

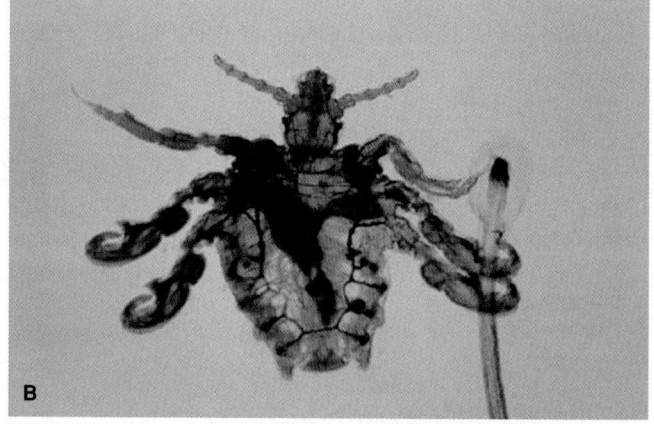

FIGURE 3-12 *Phthirus pubis.* **A.** Pubic lice are seen attached to hair. In addition, nits are seen as dark dots adhered to pubic hair. (Reproduced with permission from Morse S, Ballard RC, Holmes KK, et al (eds): Atlas of Sexually Transmitted Diseases, 3rd ed. Edinburgh: Mosby; 2003.) **B.** Photomicrograph of *Phthirus pubis.* Claw-like legs are ideally suited for clinging to hair shafts. (Used with permission from The Department of Dermaology. Naval Medical Center. Portsmouth, VA.)

hospitalizations. Because of their pelvic anatomy, women have many more UTIs than men. Bacteria ascending from the short, colonized urethra easily enter the bladder and perhaps the kidneys. Contributing to contamination, the warm moist vulva and rectum are both in close proximity. Similarly, sexual intercourse increases bladder inoculation.

Infections result from the interaction between bacteria and host. Bacterial virulence factors are important, as they enhance colonization and invasion of the lower and upper urinary tract. The principal virulence factors are increased adherence to either vaginal or uroepithelial cells and hemolysin production. The bacterial species most frequently recovered from infected urine culture is *E coli* (75–95 percent). Other identified species are *Klebsiella pneumoniae, Proteus mirabilis,* and *Staphylococcus saprophyticus* (Czaja, 2007; Echols, 1999).

Once within the bladder, bacteria may ascend within the ureters into the renal pelvis and cause upper tract infection. The renal parenchyma also can be infected by blood-borne organisms, especially during staphylococcal bacteremia. *Mycobacterium tuberculosis* gains access to the kidney through this route and also perhaps by ascension.

■ Acute Bacterial Cystitis

The most frequent presenting complaints in otherwise healthy, immunocompetent nonpregnant women are dysuria, frequency, urgency, hematuria, and incontinence. If the patient prefers, most women can be treated with a short course of antibiotics without examination, urinalysis, or urine culture for an isolated episode of acute uncomplicated bacterial cystitis. However, patients are instructed on clinical changes that merit further attention such as fever >100.4°C and persistence or recurrence of hematuria, dysuria, and frequency despite treatment. Women with these exclusions and others require evaluation to exclude other potential causes of their symptoms (Table 3-16). For example, hematuria in a postmenopausal woman may reflect cervical, uterine, or colonic bleeding evident at the time of urination. Similarly, burning with urination may indicate vulvitis.

As many as 50 percent of women who suffer an uncomplicated acute bacterial episode of cystitis will have another infection within a year. Up to 5 percent have recurring symptoms soon after treat-

TABLE 3-16. Exclusions from "Uncomplicated" Cystitis

Diabetes
Pregnancy
Immunosuppression
Symptoms >7 days
Postmenopausal hematuria
Recent UTI or urologic surgery
Documented urologic abnormalities
Recent hospital or nursing home discharge
Documented temperature above 38°C (100.4°F)
Abdominal and/or pelvic pain, nausea, vomiting
Symptoms of vaginitis (vaginal discharge/vulvar irritation)
Persisting symptoms despite >3 days of treatment of
    urinary tract infection

UTI = urinary tract infection.

ment. When symptoms develop in such women, the likelihood that a true infection is present is greater than 80 percent.

Diagnosis

Thus, for selected women with complicated or recurrent infections or with persistent or new symptoms during treatment, urinalysis and urine culture are mandatory. For a culture specimen to be informative, it must be accurately collected. A "clean catch" midstream voided urine specimen is usually sufficient. A patient is counseled on reasons for and the steps associated with urine specimen collection, which are designed to prevent contamination by other bacteria from the vulva, vagina, and rectum. More than one bacterial species identified in a urine culture usually indicates specimen collection contamination.

Initially, a patient spreads her labia and wipes the periurethral area from front to back with an antiseptic tissue. With labia spread, she begins urinating but does not collect the initial stream. A sample is then collected into a sterile specimen cup. The specimen cup is handled by the patient in such a way to avoid contamination. After collection, a urine specimen is delivered promptly to the laboratory and is plated for culture within 2 hours of collection unless it is refrigerated.

Culture. Urine culture allows accurate identification of an inciting pathogen and susceptibility testing of that pathogen to various antibiotics. Classically, significant bacteriuria is defined as $\geq 10^5$ bacteria (colony-forming units [cfu]) per milliliter of urine. If urine is collected by either suprapubic aspirate or catheterization, colony counts $\geq 10^2$ cfu/mL are diagnostic. As an exception, Hooton and colleagues (2013) demonstrated that *E coli* in midstream urine is highly predictive of bladder bacteriuria even at very low counts of 10^2 cfu/mL.

Although anaerobic bacteria are part of the vaginal, colonic, and skin flora, they rarely cause UTIs. Hence, urine culture reports do not note anaerobes except in rare instances in which the laboratory has been alerted to and specifically requested to look for an anaerobic species. Fungi can be identified on routine bacteria media and are reported but are rare causes of acute cystitis.

Culture is the gold standard, and bacterial species may be identified preliminarily, but a final urine culture report usually is not available for 48 hours. However, rapid test surrogates for culture can support a UTI diagnosis and include microscopy, nitrite testing, and leukocyte esterase testing. Empiric treatment is initially begun but modified, as needed, after culture results are available.

Culture Surrogates. *Gram staining* is a simple, rapid, and sensitive method for detecting a concentration $\geq 10^5$ cfu/mL of a bacterial species. Rapid identification allows appropriate selection of empiric antimicrobial therapy. However, realistically, such testing is typically limited to patients with complicated UTIs or acute pyelonephritis. Instead, *simple microscopic examination* of a urine specimen allows identification of both pyuria and bacteriuria. A specimen is examined expeditiously because leukocytes deteriorate quickly in urine that has not been appropriately preserved. Standards to define pyuria are inadequate, other than gross counts. Accordingly, the rapid test for leukocyte esterase has become a surrogate for the microscopic WBC count.

Leukocyte esterase testing measures esterase enzyme found in urinary leukocytes. If used alone diagnostically, this test is most beneficial for its high negative-predictive value, especially with bacterial colony counts $\geq 10^5$ cfu/mL. If one combines nitrite and leukocyte esterase testing of a clean-catch uncontaminated voided specimen, the specificity of positive test results approaches 100 percent when uropathogen colony counts are $\geq 10^5$ cfu/mL. The negative predictive value is comparable. However, if these specimens have been contaminated with vaginal or colonic bacteria or with trichomonads, the test result can be falsely positive for uropathogens. In addition, very concentrated urine or urine with significant proteinuria or glucosuria will decrease test accuracy.

Nitrites are produced from nitrates metabolized by bacteria. This is most frequently observed in the gram-negative uropathogen family typically responsible for acute UTIs in women. Unfortunately, this test does not identify *Pseudomonas* species or gram-positive pathogens such as staphylococci, streptococci, and enterococci. Moreover, first morning urine specimens are ideally tested, because more than 4 hours are required for bacteria to convert nitrates to nitrites at levels that are detectable. As a single test, the specificity of a positive nitrite test is very high when uropathogen counts are $\geq 10^5$ cfu/mL. Its negative predictive value is higher than its positive predictive value. Of note, substances that turn the urine red, such as the bladder analgesic phenazopyridine (Pyridium) or ingestion of beets, can lead to false-positive nitrite test results.

Treatment

During the past two decades, the frequency of infections caused by group B *Streptococcus* and *Klebsiella* species has increased, whereas *E coli* infection rates have diminished. Also, in many locations, sensitivity patterns in *E coli* may warrant a shift in initial empiric treatment (Table 3-17).

For significant dysuria, up to 2 days of a bladder analgesic such as phenazopyridine (Pyridium), 200 mg orally up to three times daily, may give significant relief. However, GI

TABLE 3-17. Treatment of Urinary Tract Infection	
Infection Category	**Antimicrobial Regimen**
Uncomplicated cystitis	
Recommended regimens	Nitrofurantoin macrocrystals/monohydrate (Macrobid) 100 mg twice daily for 5–7 days
	or
	Trimethoprim-sulfamethoxazole DS 160/800 mg (Bactrim DS, Septra DS) twice daily for 3 days
	or
	Trimethoprim (Bactrim, Septra) 100 mg twice daily for 3 days
	or
	Nitrofurantoin macrocrystals (Macrodantin) 100 mg four times daily for 7 days
	or
	Fosfomycin tromethamine (Monurol) single 3-g dose once
Alternative regimens	Ciprofloxacin (Cipro) 250 mg twice daily for 3 days
	or
	Norfloxacin (Noroxin) 400 mg twice daily for 3 days
	or
	Levofloxacin (Levaquin) 250 mg daily for 3 days
	or
	Specific β-lactams in 3- to 7-day regimens[a]
Outpatient pyelonephritis	
Recommended regimens	Ciprofloxacin 500 mg twice daily for 7 days[b]
	or
	Ciprofloxacin 1000 mg daily for 7 days[b]
	or
	Levofloxacin 750 mg daily for 5 days[b]
	or
	Trimethoprim-sulfamethoxazole DS 160/800 mg twice daily for 14 days[b]
Alternative regimens	Specific β-lactams in 3- to 7-day regimens for 7–14 days[a,b]

[a]Suitable agents include amoxicillin-clavulanate, cefdinir, cefaclor, cefpodomine-proxetil.
DS = double strength.
[b]If the prevalence of fluoroquinolone resistance is thought to exceed 10%, then an initial, single intravenous dose of a long-acting parenteral antimicrobial, such as 1 g of ceftriaxone or a consolidated 24-hr dose of an aminoglycoside, is recommended.
Adapted with permission from American College of Obstetricians and Gynecologists: ACOG Practice Bulletin No. 91: Treatment of urinary tract infections in nonpregnant women, Obstet Gynecol 2008 Mar;111(3):785–794.

upset, yellow-orange stained urine and clothing, and hemolysis in patients with glucose-6-phosphate dehydrogenase (G6PD) deficiency are potential side effects.

Following treatment, recurrences may develop. In those recurrently linked with intercourse, low-dose postcoital dosing with agents found in Table 3-17 is usually effective at preventing infection recurrence. A woman with two or more episodes of cystitis within 6 months or three infections within a year is considered for urologic evaluation of her urinary tract. These patients are commonly treated with daily prophylaxis for 6 months, in addition to modification of any risk factors such as diaphragm-spermicide use.

■ Asymptomatic Bacteriuria

This is defined as isolation of a specified quantitative count of bacteria in an appropriately collected urine specimen obtained from a person without symptoms or signs referable to urinary infection (Rubin, 1992). In healthy nonpregnant women, the prevalence of this condition increases with age. It is associated with sexual activity and is more common in diabetics. Moreover, one fourth to one half of elderly women in long-term care facilities have bacteriuria, which is seen primarily in those with chronic neurologic illness and functional impairment.

The Infectious Disease Society of America recommends that nonpregnant premenopausal women not be screened or treated for asymptomatic bacteriuria (Nicolle, 2005). The same is true for diabetic women and for older persons living in the community.

■ Acute Pyelonephritis

This infection may be divided into mild (no nausea or vomiting, normal to slightly elevated blood leukocyte count, and normal to low-grade fever) and severe (vomiting, dehydration, evidence of sepsis, high leukocyte count, and fever). Other symptoms include those of a lower urinary tract infection and varying degrees of back pain and tenderness to percussion over the region of the kidney(s).

Traditional therapy for this infection has included hospitalization, hydration, and intravenous antibiotic treatment for up to 2 weeks. However, studies in young healthy women with normal urinary tracts indicate that 7 to 14 days of oral therapy are sufficient for compliant women with mild infection (Gupta, 2011). In one study of more than 50 college women with acute uncomplicated pyelonephritis, resistance to trimethoprim-sulfamethoxazole was 30 percent (Hooton, 1997). Accordingly, for outpatient therapy, an oral fluoroquinolone is recommended treatment unless a pathogen is susceptible to trimethoprim-sulfamethoxazole. At initial diagnosis, clinicians may also administer a parenteral dose prior to starting oral therapy (see Table 3-17). Alternatively, if a causative organism is gram-positive, then amoxicillin-clavulanate, cefdinir, cefaclor, or cefpodomine-proxetil are recommended options (Gupta, 2011).

Hospitalization is warranted for women who display clinical indications at initial evaluation or who fail to improve with outpatient therapy. Appropriate initial IV regimens include a fluoroquinolone; an aminoglycoside with or without ampicillin; an extended-spectrum cephalosporin or extended-spectrum penicillin with or without an aminoglycoside; or a carbapenem.

TABLE 3-18. Risk Factors for Postoperative Surgical Site Infection

Smoker
Preoperative anemia
Excessive blood loss
Intraoperative hypothermia
Lower socioeconomic status
Immunocompromised patient
Recent operative site surgery
Obesity (abdominal hysterectomy)
Prolonged surgical procedure (>3.5 hr)
Foreign body placement (catheter, drain, etc.)
Perioperative HbA1c>7% or CBG >250 in diabetics

CBG = capillary blood glucose; HbA$_{1c}$ = hemoglobin A$_{1c}$.

The choice among these agents is based on local resistance data and is tailored based on culture-derived susceptibility results.

POSTOPERATIVE INFECTION

Development of a postoperative infection can create significant patient morbidity, most seriously sepsis. Risks for postoperative infection are varied and include patient and surgical factors (Table 3-18). Of these, the degree of wound contamination at the time of surgery plays an important role. Because most gynecologic surgeries are elective, a gynecologist has time to decrease microbial inoculum. Thus, BV, trichomoniasis, cervicitis, and active urinary tract or respiratory infections ideally are treated and eradicated prior to surgery.

■ Wound Classification

Since 1964, surgical wounds have been classified according to the degree of bacterial contamination of the operative site at the time of surgery. In general, as the number of operative site bacteria (inoculum) increases, so too does the postoperative infection rate.

Clean wounds are most commonly found in procedures performed for nontraumatic indications, that are without operative site inflammation, and that avoid the respiratory, alimentary, and genitourinary tracts. No breaks occur in surgical technique. Thus, most laparoscopic and adnexal surgeries are considered to be in this category. Without prophylaxis, infection rates range from 1 to 5 percent. Prophylactic antimicrobial administration does not decrease infection rates following these procedures and is not required.

Clean contaminated wounds are those in which the respiratory, gastrointestinal, genital, or urinary tract is entered under controlled conditions, without unusual bacterial contamination. Criteria further define that there is no break in surgical technique. Infection rates range from 5 to 15 percent. This group encompasses many gynecologic procedures including total hysterectomy, cervical conization, and dilatation and curettage (D & C). Of these, hysterectomy is the gynecologic procedure most frequently followed by surgical site infection. These procedures are usually elective, and only hysterectomy and obstetric

D & C require antimicrobial prophylaxis to reduce postoperative infection rates (American College of Obstetricians and Gynecologists, 2014a).

Contaminated wounds reflect operations with major breaks in sterile technique or gross GI spillage or incisions in which acute, nonpurulent inflammation is encountered (Mangram, 1999). Infection rates approximate 10 to 25 percent. For this reason, a minimum of 24 hours of perioperative antimicrobial administration is required, and delayed wound closure may be selected. Laparoscopy or laparotomy for acute salpingitis is included in this category.

Dirty wounds are typically old traumatic wounds or those that involve existing clinical infection or perforated viscera. If an abscess is present, these are considered dirty wounds. These operative sites are clinically infected at the time of surgery, and infection rates range from 30 to 100 percent. Accordingly, therapeutic antimicrobial therapy is required, and these wounds typically are allowed to close by secondary intention.

■ Surgical Site Infection Classification

The CDC provides definitions of hospital-acquired surgical site infections (SSIs). The Joint Commission currently is emphasizing this morbidity during their hospital accreditation process. Thus, hospitals are more attentive to infection rates and to the rates of individual surgeons.

In classifying SSIs, there are two categories, incisional and organ space (Fig. 3-13). Criteria for each category are detailed in Table 3-19. The incisional group is further subdivided into superficial and deep classes. Organ/space infections develop in

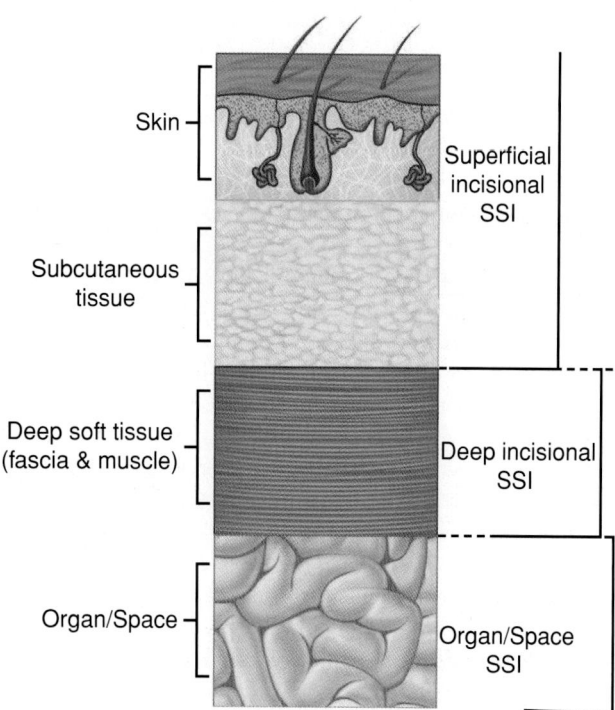

FIGURE 3-13 Anatomy and classification of surgical site infections (SSI). (Modified with permission from Mangram AJ, Horan TC, Pearson ML, et al: Guideline for prevention of surgical site infection, 1999. Hospital Infection Control Practices Advisory Committee, Infect Control Hosp Epidemiol 1999 Apr;20(4):250–278.)

spaces or organs other than that opened by the original incision or manipulated during the surgical procedure. Specific sites include the vaginal cuff, urinary tract, and intraabdominal sites. Of note, vaginal cuff infections are generally considered in the organ/space class, presuming they meet at least one of these criteria: purulent drainage from the cuff, abscess at the cuff, or pathogens cultured from fluid or tissue obtained from the cuff. Pelvic infections such as adnexal infection, pelvic abscess, or infected pelvic hematoma also fall into the category of organ/space infection.

■ Diagnosis
Physical Findings

For febrile morbidity, the most frequently used definition is an oral temperature of ≥38°C (≥100.4°F) on two or more occasions, 4 or more hours apart, and 24 or more hours following surgery. This condition is seen most often after hysterectomy, particularly abdominal hysterectomy; usually is not associated with other symptoms or signs of infection; and does not require antimicrobial therapy! It has been reported in up to 40 percent of women following abdominal and almost 30 percent of women after vaginal hysterectomy with antimicrobial prophylaxis. It resolves without antibiotic treatment in the absence of other symptoms or signs of infection.

A remote nonsurgical site may also serve as an origin of fever. These may include pulmonary complications, IV site phlebitis, and UTI. Thus, women who develop recurrent temperature elevation require a thorough history and a careful physical examination by the surgeon, seeking not only surgical but also nonsurgical causes (Fig. 42-2, p. 920).

Operative site pain (incisional, lower abdominal, pelvic, and/or lower back) following surgery is normal. However, those with an operative site infection report increasing pain at the surgery site, and increasing tenderness is present during physical examination. With superficial SSI, pain is superficial and localized to the incision. With pelvic infection, there is deep lower abdominal and/or pelvic pain, and the most common infection sites are the parametria and the vaginal surgical margin. Pelvic abscess or infected pelvic hematoma is least common, and pain is central.

Abdominal palpation is an integral part of SSI diagnosis. Avoiding an abdominal incision if present, a surgeon slowly, gently, and deeply palpates the lower abdomen over the surgical site following hysterectomy and normally elicits patient discomfort. Tenderness does not mean an acute surgical abdomen or infection. In the immediate postoperative period, this tenderness is expected and decreases quickly. Women who develop pelvic cellulitis or cuff cellulitis will have increasing tenderness at gentle depression of the lower abdominal wall over the infected area. Tenderness may be bilateral, but more commonly is more marked on one side. Peritoneal signs are not present. Cellulitis, whether it involves the parametria, adnexa, or vaginal cuff, is not associated with a mass.

In the absence of increasing lower abdominal pain and tenderness, a bimanual examination is not necessary for asymptomatic temperature elevation. However, with a combination of fever, increasing tenderness, and new-onset pain, gentle bimanual examination is required to accurately identify the infection site and to exclude or diagnose a mass. Speculum examination usually

TABLE 3-19. Criteria for Defining Surgical Site Infections (SSIs)

Superficial incisional
Involves only skin and subcutaneous tissue of the incision
Develops within 30 days of surgical procedure
Features at least one of the following:
    Purulent drainage from the superficial incision
    Bacteria in culture obtained aseptically from fluid or tissue from the superficial incision
    Incision deliberately opened by surgeon and is culture positive (or not cultured) *and* patient has at least one of the
        following incisional signs or symptoms:
        Tenderness or pain
        Heat or redness
        Localized swelling
    SSI diagnosis made by surgeon or attending physician
Stitch abscesses are not included in this category
Diagnosis of "cellulitis," by itself, does not meet criterion for SSI

Deep incisional
Involves the deep soft tissues (muscle and fascia) of the incision
Develops within 30 days of surgical procedure
Features at least one of the following:
    Purulent drainage from deep incision of surgical site (but not organ or space component)
    Deep incision that spontaneously dehisces or is deliberately opened by a surgeon and is culture-positive (or not cultured)
        and patient has at least one of the following signs or symptoms:
        Temperature ≥38°C (100.4°F)
        Localized pain or tenderness
    Abscess or other infection found by reoperation, histopathology, or radiology

Organ/space
Involves any body part that was opened or manipulated during the operative procedure, excluding the skin incision, fascia,
    or muscle layers
Develops within 30 days of the surgical procedure
Features at least one of the following:
    Purulent drainage from a drain placed through a stab wound into the organ/space
    Bacteria obtained aseptically from tissue or fluid in that organ/space
    Abscess found by reoperation, histopathology, or radiology
Vaginal cuff infection with purulence, abscess, and/or positive tissue or fluid culture is included in this category

Reproduced with pemission from Centers for Disease Control and Prevention: Procedure-associated module: surgical site infection (SSI) event, 2014.

is not required, and findings are similar with or without an existing infection. As is true for routine pelvic examination, most information at bimanual examination is obtained from the vaginal fingers. If a patient is too tender to allow adequate examination, vaginal sonography is indicated. Bowel function is usually not altered by soft-tissue cellulitis but can be by pelvic abscess or infected pelvic hematoma.

Testing

Pelvic infections following hysterectomy are polymicrobial, and for that reason, it is difficult to identify true pathogens. Research has demonstrated that bacteria recovered transvaginally from the pelves of infected and clinically uninfected women are similar. Accordingly, routine transvaginal culturing of women with cuff or pelvic cellulitis does not add useful information. Moreover, a surgeon should not wait for culture results before starting empiric broad-spectrum antibiotic therapy. However, if initial therapy

is partially effective or unsuccessful, then a culture will more predictably identify pathogen(s) since therapy will have eradicated other species. The antibiotic regimen should be changed, and culture results may direct this change. In contrast, abscess or infected hematoma fluid are cultured since those species are less likely to be vaginal contaminants. The same is true for any fluid or purulent material present in an abdominal incision.

For many postoperative SSIs, imaging is not mandatory. However, if additional anatomic information is needed, then transvaginal sonography or CT scanning are the most often used, and selection depends on clinical circumstances and suspected etiology.

■ Specific Infections

Vaginal Cuff Cellulitis

Essentially all women develop this infection at the vaginal surgical margin after hysterectomy (Fig. 3-14). Normal response

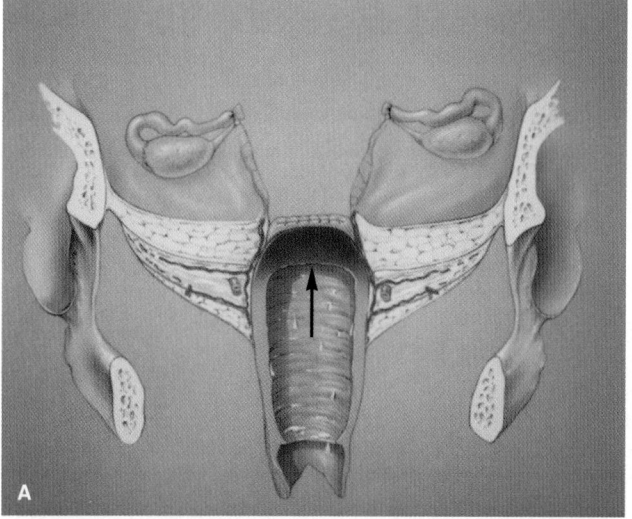

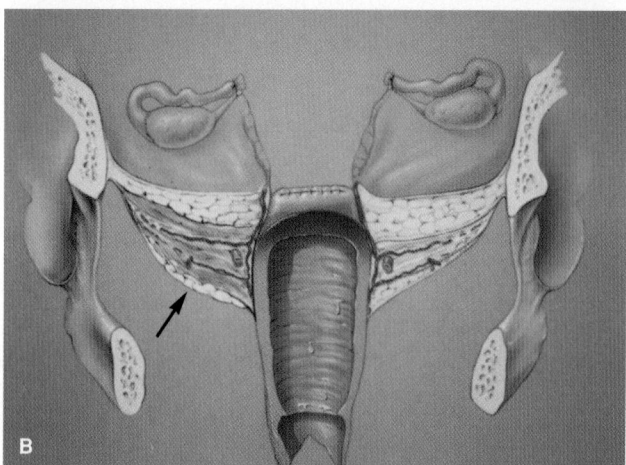

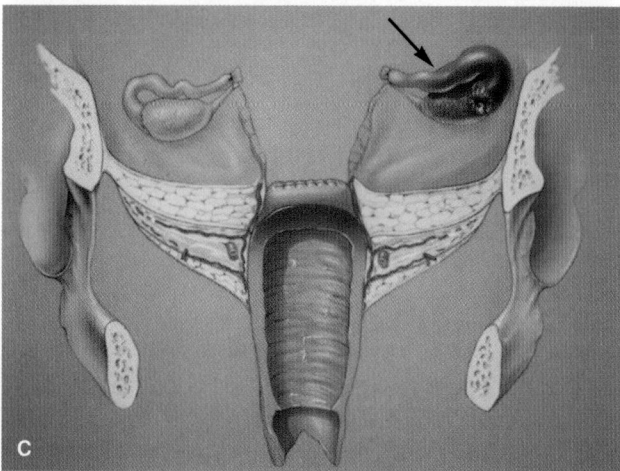

FIGURE 3-14 Organ/space infections. **A.** Vaginal cuff cellulitis. The vaginal surgical margin is edematous, hyperemic, and tender, and there are purulent secretions in the vagina. Parametria and adnexa are normal during gentle bimanual examination. **B.** Pelvic cellulitis in the right parametrium. It is indurated and tender to palpation; no mass is present. **C.** Adnexal infection after hysterectomy. The parametria are normal. Tenderness without a mass is appreciated in the adnexal area.

to healing is characterized by small-vessel engorgement, which results in erythema and heat. There is vascular stasis with endothelial leakage resulting in interstitial edema, which causes induration. This area is tender, microscopic evaluation of a wet prep reveals numerous WBCs, and purulent discharge is seen in the vagina. This process usually subsides, does not require treatment, and accordingly, does not require reporting as a SSI. The few women who do require treatment are usually those who present after hospital discharge with mild, but increasing, new-onset lower abdominal pain and have a yellow vaginal discharge. Findings are as above, but the vaginal cuff is more tender than anticipated at this interval from the initial surgical procedure. Oral antimicrobial therapy with a single broad-spectrum agent is appropriate (Table 3-20). A patient is then reevaluated in several days to assess therapeutic efficacy. This may be completed by phone or with an examination if necessary.

Pelvic Cellulitis

This is a common infection following either vaginal or abdominal hysterectomy. It develops when host humoral and cellular defense mechanisms, combined with preoperative antibiotic prophylaxis, cannot overcome the bacterial inoculum and inflammatory process at the vaginal surgical margin. The inflammatory process spreads into the parametrial region(s) resulting in lower abdominal pain, regional tenderness, and fever, usually during the late second or third postoperative day. There are no peritoneal signs and bowel and urinary function are normal, but the patient may note anorexia.

Patients are discharged on perhaps their first or second postoperative day following vaginal hysterectomy, and affected women may be at home before symptom onset. Hospitalization and treatment with an IV broad-spectrum antibiotic regimen found in Table 3-20 is indicated until a patient has been afebrile for 24 to 48 hours. She then may be redischarged home. Most patients requiring hospitalization for IV antibiotic therapy are discharged with a 5- to 7-day oral antimicrobial prescription. Single-agent therapeutic regimens have been shown in prospective randomized trials to be as effective as combination-agent regimens. These infections are polymicrobial, and the regimen selected must have coverage for gram-positive and gram-negative aerobic and anaerobic bacteria.

Adnexal Infection

This infection is uncommon and presents almost exactly like pelvic cellulitis. The difference is in the location of tenderness during bimanual pelvic examination. The cuff and parametrial areas are not usually tender, but the adnexa are. This infection also may develop after tubal ligation, surgical therapy for ectopic pregnancy, or other adnexal surgery. Empiric antibiotic regimens are identical to those for pelvic cellulitis (see Table 3-20).

Ovarian Abscess

A rare but life-threatening complication following primarily vaginal hysterectomy is ovarian abscess. Presumably with this infection, surgery is performed in the late proliferative phase of an ovulatory menstrual cycle, and ovaries are in close proximity to the vaginal surgical margin. As expected, physiologic cuff

TABLE 3-20. Empiric Antimicrobial Regiments for Postgynecologic Surgery Infections

Regimen	Dose
Single-agent intravenous	
Cephalosporin	
Cefoxitin (Mefoxin)	2 g every 6 hr
Cefotetan (Cefotan)	2 g every 12 hr
Cefotaxime (Claforan)	1–2 g every 8 hr
Penicillin ± β-lactamase inhibitor	
Piperacillin	4 g every 6 hr
Piperacillin/tazobactam (Zosyn)	3.375 g every 6 hr
Ampicillin/sulbactam (Unasyn)	3 g every 6 hr
Ticarcillin/clavulanate (Timentin)	3.1 g every 4–6 hr
Carbapenems	
Imipenem/cilastatin (Primaxin)	500 mg every 8 hr
Meropenem (Merrem)	500 mg every 8 hr
Ertapenem (Invanz)	1 g once daily
Combination agent intravenous	
Metronidazole (Flagyl) plus	Loading dose 15 mg/kg; maintenance 7.5 mg/kg every 6 hr
Ampicillin plus	2 g every 6 hr
Gentamicin	3–5 mg/kg once daily
OR	
Clindamycin plus	900 mg every 8 hr
Gentamicin	3–5 mg/kg once daily
with or without ampicillin	2 g every 6 hr
Oral agents	
Amoxicillin/clavulanate (Augmentin)	875 mg twice daily
Levofloxacin (Levoquin)	500 mg once daily
Clindamycin	300 mg every 6 hr
Metronidazole	500 mg every 6 hr

cellulitis develops normally, but when ovulation occurs, local bacteria gain access to the ovulation site and the corpus luteum. The corpus luteum often is hemorrhagic, and the blood in this functional cyst provides a perfect medium for bacterial growth.

Affected women have an essentially normal postoperative course until approximately 10 days following surgery. At this time, they experience acute unilateral lower abdominal pain, which then involves multiple quadrants. These symptoms reflect rupture of their abscess and development of generalized abdominal peritonitis. Sepsis commonly follows, and this is a true gynecologic emergency. Immediate exploratory laparotomy is necessary, with IV administration of perioperative broad-spectrum antimicrobials, abscess evacuation, and adnexectomy if easily accessible. At a minimum, necrotic tissues are debrided. After hospital discharge, oral antibiotics are typically continued for an additional 5 to 7 days, and this is variable depending on the clinical course.

Similarly, women rarely may develop a tuboovarian abscess (usually a pyosalpinx) identical to that seen as an end result of acute PID. This process can be managed medically with

IV antimicrobials, and surgery is usually not required unless rupture follows. Combination antimicrobial therapy is continued until a woman has been afebrile for 48 to 72 hours. At this point, IV antibiotics may be replaced by oral agents, which are continued outpatient to complete a 2-week course of therapy. Patients diagnosed with TOA are reevaluated approximately 3 days following hospital discharge and then again 1 and 2 weeks later to document abscess resolution.

Pelvic Abscess/Infected Pelvic Hematoma

Pelvic abscess not involving an adnexal structure may also uncommonly complicate hysterectomy (Fig. 3-15). This develops from blood, serum, and/or lymph collections following hysterectomy that provide an excellent milieu for the overgrowth of bacteria inoculated into the adjacent tissues during the surgical procedure. An alternative infection can originate within a surgical pelvic hematoma. With hematoma, a postoperative-day-1 hemoglobin classically is significantly lower than that predicted by measured intraoperative blood loss. Reoperation is not required in most instances, and fluid or blood product resuscitation suffices. Unlike women who develop tissue cellulitis following surgery and whose early symptom of infection is pain and not fever, women with an infected hematoma will have low-grade temperature elevation (>37.8°C) as their early finding. Pain is a late symptom for these women. Accordingly, women with an unexplained postoperative hemoglobin decrease are discharged with instructions to monitor their temperature twice

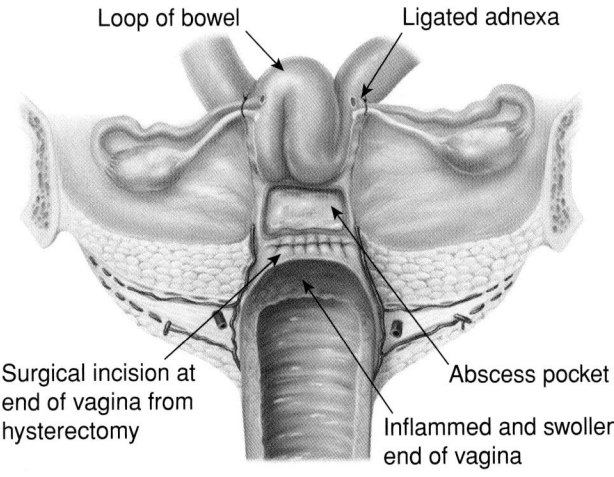

FIGURE 3-15 Pelvic abscess or infected hematoma that is extraperitoneal and cephalad to the vaginal margins.

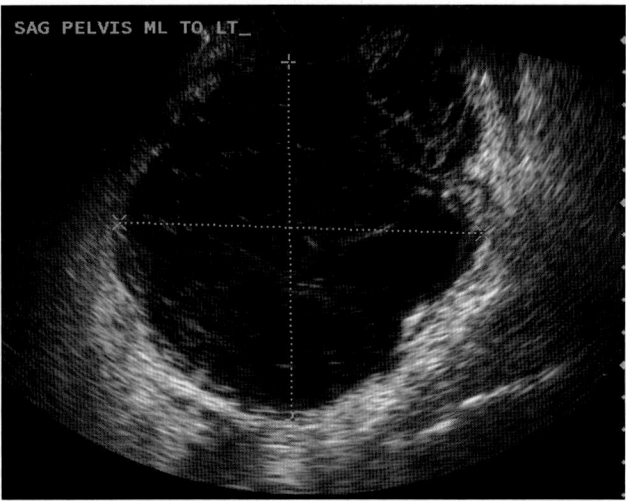

FIGURE 3-16 Transvaginal sonogram of an infected pelvic hematoma following hysterectomy. This 11 × 12 cm collection of blood and clot was drained vaginally in the operative room. (Used with permission from Dr. Elysia Moschos.)

daily for approximately 1 week. Temperatures ≥37.8°C typically warrant evaluation.

Signs and symptoms of pelvic abscess or infected hematoma are midline, and a mass is discernible centrally. Transvaginal sonography can accurately characterize the dimensions (Fig. 3-16). For both, hospital readmission for therapy is usually necessary. Combination-agent IV antimicrobial therapy is indicated, and selected regimens provide gram-positive and gram-negative aerobic and anaerobic coverage. Additionally, opening the vaginal surgical margin, if possible, to allow drainage will aid treatment and accelerate patient response. This can usually be done in a treatment room early, avoiding return to the operating room. If necessary, these can be drained with sonographic transvaginal guidance or in the operating room. These abscesses or infected hematomas usually remain confined to the extraperitoneal space, and a patient does not usually develop peritonitis. Some patients may develop diarrhea due to the proximity of the rectum, which is usually adjacent to the infected space.

Combination IV antibiotics are administered until a woman has been afebrile 48 to 72 hours. IV antibiotics may then be replaced by oral agents, which are continued outpatient to complete a 2-week course of therapy, if the abscess or hematoma is not drained. If drained, then oral agents continued for 5 to 7 days following IV agents typically is sufficient. Commonly, patients are reevaluated 3 days following hospital discharge and then again 1 and 2 weeks later to document infection resolution.

Abdominal Incision Infection

The superficial and easily accessible location of this infection aids its diagnosis. Although abdominal incision infection may develop alone or with pelvic infection following abdominal hysterectomy, it develops uncommonly after other gynecologic procedures. Unlike pelvic infection, the incidence of this infection is not altered by antimicrobial prophylaxis. Risk factors include obesity, immunosuppression, diabetes, excessive electrosurgical

coagulation use, passive drains, and coexistent skin inflammation at the time of surgical incision.

Abdominal incisions are usually the most uncomfortable following gynecologic surgery, but pain decreases daily. Erythema and heat are the first physical signs of this infection, which is usually diagnosed on the fourth or fifth postoperative day—again, after discharge from the hospital. A hematoma or seroma may develop in the abdominal wall incision without infection. If these collections are large, opening of the incision and evacuation to prevent infection in those fluids is warranted. Similarly, pus requires incision opening to ensure an intact fascia, as should be done with large seromas or hematomas.

Drainage and local care are usually the basis of successful therapy for abdominal incision infection or for large hematoma or seroma. Wet-to-dry dressings stimulate fibroblastic proliferation and development of healthy granulation tissue. Moistening the dry dressing prior to its removal will ease removal and decrease patient discomfort. At this stage, secondary closure can be considered. Importantly, wounds are irrigated with normal saline. Povidone-iodine, iodophor gauze, hydrogen peroxide, and Daiken solution are avoided as they are caustic to healing tissues. Some recommend their use early but follow with normal saline irrigation. Negative-pressure wound therapy provided by vacuum-assisted wound closure devices is available for more serious or larger wound areas that are slow to respond once the wound has a clean, granulating base (Chap. 42, p. 920).

If there is soft-tissue cellulitis adjacent to the incision, antimicrobial therapy is required. If the initial surgery was a clean procedure, then *Staphylococcus* species predominate. Following clean-contaminated or dirty procedures, isolated organisms commonly include gram-negative bacteria such as *E coli*, *Pseudomonas aeruginosa*, and *Enterobacter* species and gram-positive bacteria, namely, *Staphylococcus* and *Enterococcus* species (Kirby, 2009). Anaerobes are typically not prominent pathogens in these infections but may be present, especially following hysterectomy. Thus, these infections are usually polymicrobial. Antibiotics found in Table 3-20 are suitable regimens.

Toxic Shock Syndrome

This condition, caused by an exotoxin (TSS toxin-1) produced by *Staphylococcus aureus*, appears approximately 2 days following surgery or menstruation onset. Menstrual-associated toxic shock syndrome (TSS) rates have diminished following changes in tampon composition and use. For TSS, the vagina or wound must be colonized by a toxigenic staphylococcal strain, and the patient must lack the specific antibody that can block the superantigen.

The classic TSS symptoms include fever, malaise, and diarrhea. If postoperative, there are minimal signs of wound infection. A patient has conjunctival and pharyngeal hyperemia without purulence. The tongue is usually reddened, and the skin on the trunk is erythematous but not painful or pruritic. Temperatures are usually above 38.8°C, and orthostatic hypotension or shock may be present. This syndrome results from host cytokines released in response to superantigenic properties of the toxin. The criteria for this diagnosis are presented in Table 3-21.

TABLE 3-21. Criteria for Diagnosis of Toxic Shock Syndrome

Major criteria
Hypotension
Orthostatic syncope
Systolic BP <90 mm Hg for adults
Diffuse macular erythroderma
Temperature ≥38.8°C
Late skin desquamation, particularly on hands, palms, and soles (1–2 weeks later)

Minor criteria (organ system involvement)
Gastrointestinal: diarrhea or vomiting
Mucous membranes: oral, pharyngeal, conjunctival, and/or vaginal erythema
Muscular: myalgia or creatinine level greater than twice normal
Renal: BUN and creatinine greater than twice normal or >5 WBCs/hpf in urine, without concurrent UTI
Hematologic: platelet count <100,000 per mm³
Hepatic: SGOT, SGPT, and/or bilirubin levels greater than twice normal
Central nervous system: altered consciousness without focal localizing signs

BP = blood pressure; BUN = blood urea nitrogen; hpf = high-power field; SGOT = serum glutamic oxaloacetic transaminase; SGPT = serum glutamic pyruvic transaminase; UTI = urinary tract infection; WBC = white blood cell.

The wound, if present, is treated like any other wound. It is cultured to confirm presence of *S aureus*. However, results from other cultures (e.g., blood, throat, and cerebrospinal fluid) will be negative. To meet the strict criteria, a woman must have all major and at least three minor criteria. If this is suspected early and therapy is initiated, the complete syndrome may not develop. Serologies for Rocky Mountain spotted fever, measles, and leptospirosis must be negative. Viral infection and group A streptococci can cause a similar presentation.

While awaiting culture results for selection of specific antistaphylococcal antibiotics, empiric therapy covers both methicillin-susceptible and methicillin-resistant *S aureus*. Vancomycin (15 to 20 mg/kg/dose) can be given every 8 to 12 hours, not exceeding 2 g per dose. Some experts argue for the addition of clindamycin, but further evidence is needed. Regardless, the hallmark of therapy is entire system support with large volumes of IV fluids and electrolytes to replace massive body fluid losses from diarrhea, capillary leakage, and insensible loss. These patients may develop significant edema and are best managed in an intensive care unit. Even with appropriate management, the death rate has been reported to be as high as 5 percent because of subsequent acute respiratory distress syndrome (ARDS), disseminated intravascular coagulopathy (DIC), or hypotension unresponsive to therapy with resultant myocardial failure. This syndrome may also follow gynecologic surgical procedures such as D & C, hysterectomy, urethral suspension, and tubal ligation.

Necrotizing Fasciitis

Although described in the 1870s, it was not named until 1952, by a Parkland Hospital surgeon (Wilson, 1952). Risk factors for this postoperative incision infection are age older than 50 years, arteriosclerotic heart disease, diabetes mellitus, obesity, debilitating disease, smoking, and previous radiation therapy, all of which are associated with decreased tissue perfusion.

In our clinical service, vulvar infection in obese diabetic women is a prominent risk. Only approximately 20 percent of cases follow surgery, the majority developing after minor injuries or insect bites. Bacteria recovered from women with this infection are similar to those recovered from any postoperative gynecologic infection site, namely predominantly *E coli*, *E faecalis*, *Bacteroides* spp, *Peptostreptococcus* spp, *S aureus*, and groups A and B hemolytic streptococci.

Although this postoperative superficial incisional infection begins like any other postoperative infection with pain and erythema, its hallmark is subcutaneous and superficial fascial necrosis, manifested by excessive tissue edema in adjacent areas. There also may be associated myonecrosis. Blisters or bullae form in tissue that has become avascular and is discolored (Fig. 3-17). Crepitus or induration and edema beyond the region of visible erythema may be present. Tissue destruction is far more extensive than is evident by surface examination. The skin will slip over underlying tissue, and if incised, due to the lack of vascularity, there will be no bleeding but instead usually a thin gray transudate. Severe systemic toxicity and fever may develop. In obvious cases, no imaging is needed, and patients are prepared for surgical debridement. In less-clear cases, radiographs or CT scans, if these can be quickly obtained, may add information by revealing gas in affected tissues produced by clostridial species such as *Clostridium perfringens*.

Although broad-spectrum antibiotic administration is required, the cornerstone of treatment is prompt recognition and immediate surgical removal of necrotic tissue to a level at which viable bleeding tissue is reached. To achieve this, excision of large tissue volumes are often needed. Although this is potentially disfiguring, postponing surgery while waiting for antimicrobial activity only increases the volume of tissue death. Gynecologists may enlist assistance from a general surgeon or gynecologic oncologist if extensive debridement into the posterior perineal triangle, buttock, or inner thigh

SECTION 1

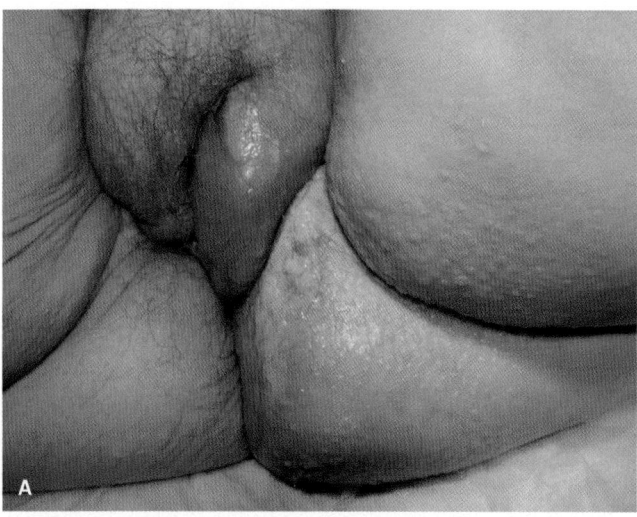
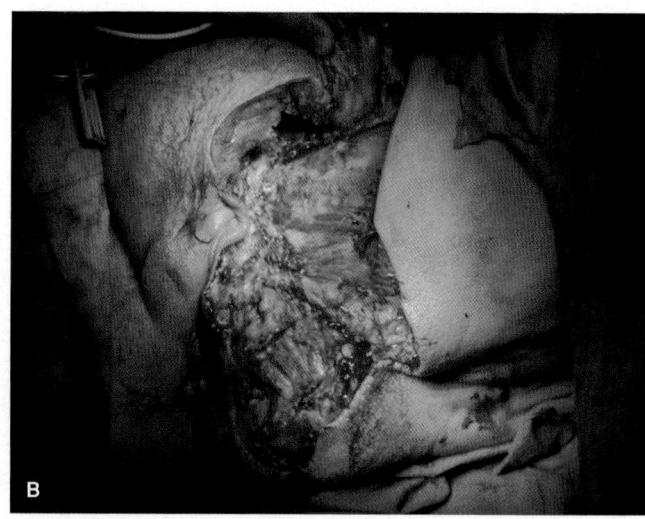

FIGURE 3-17 Vulvar necrotizing fasciitis in an obese, diabetic patient. **A.** Preoperative image of the perineum with notable edema and skin bullae. **B.** The required intraoperative resection was extensive (Used with permission from Dr. Laura Kilmer.)

is anticipated. Early fatality rates for patients with this infection approximated 20 percent in the systematic review of 1463 patients by Goh and associates (2014).

Wounds are left open and treated as wound infections as described earlier with local hydrotherapy or a wound vacuum device. Assistance from a general surgeon for potential grafting is often necessary.

Methicillin-resistant *Staphylococcus aureus*

Any of the polymicrobial infections discussed in this section may be complicated by MRSA. To cover MRSA, suitable outpatient oral antibiotics for uncomplicated infection include trimethoprim-sulfamethoxazole DS (160 mg/800 mg) twice daily, clindamycin 300 or 450 mg three times daily, doxycycline or minocycline 100 mg twice daily, or linezolid (Zyvox) 600 mg twice daily. For complicated infections, the Infectious Disease Society of America recommends MRSA coverage with IV vancomycin, IV or oral clindamycin, IV or oral linezolid 600 mg twice daily, IV daptomycin (Cubicin) 4 mg/kg once daily, or IV telavancin (Vibativ) 10 mg/kg once daily (Liu, 2011). Newer FDA-approved agents against complicated MRSA infections include ceftaroline (Teflaro), dalbavancin (Dalvance), oritavancin (Orbactive), and tedizolid (Sivextro) (Holmes, 2014). These newer drugs are expensive and may have restricted formulary use to only infectious disease specialists.

OTHER GYNECOLOGIC INFECTIONS

■ Vulvar Abscess

These infections develop similarly to other superficial abscesses but have the potential for significant expansion due to the loose areolar subcutaneous tissue in this area. Risk factors include diabetes, obesity, perineal shaving, and immunosuppression. Common isolates include *Staphylococcus*, group B *Streptococcus*, *Enterococcus* species, *E coli, and P mirabilis*. Importantly, Thurman (2008) and Kilpatrick (2010) and their coworkers found MRSA in 40 to 60 percent of cultured vulvar abscesses.

In early stages, surrounding cellulitis may be the most prominent finding and only a small or no abscess is identified. In these cases, sitz baths and oral antibiotics are reasonable treatment. When present, smaller abscesses may be treated with incision and drainage, abscess packing if indicated, and oral antibiotics to treat surrounding cellulitis. For uncomplicated infection, suitable oral agents will be broad-spectrum and will cover MRSA. Trimethoprim-sulfamethoxazole may be used alone. Two-drug therapy with clindamycin or doxycycline combined with a second-generation cephalosporin or with a fluoroquinolone is also a suitable choice, among others. However, for those with immunosuppression or diabetes, hospitalization and IV antibiotic therapy is often warranted due to increased risks for necrotizing fasciitis in these individuals. Again, coverage for MRSA is included in IV regimens (Table 3-20).

Large abscesses typically require admission for drainage under anesthesia. This provides adequate pain control for abscess drainage and for abscess cavity exploration to disrupt loculated areas of pus, as described in Section 43-21 (p. 977).

■ Bartholin Gland Duct Abscess

This infection is managed primarily by drainage (Fig. 3-18). Drainage can typically be completed in an outpatient setting and is described in Section 43-18 (p. 971). Antibiotics are commonly added to treat surrounding tissue cellulitis. The most common bacteria isolated from these abscesses include anaerobic *Bacteroides* and *Peptostreptococcus* spp and aerobic *E coli*, *S aureus*, and *E faecalis* (Bhide, 2010; Kessous, 2013). Also, *N gonorrhoeae* and *C trachomatis* may be identified (Bleker, 1990). Accordingly, polymicrobial coverage is selected, and suitable single-agent oral outpatient therapy includes, among others, trimethoprim-sulfamethoxazole, amoxicillin-clavulanate, second-generation cephalosporins, or fluoroquinolones, such as ciprofloxacin. In most cases, abscess aerobic cultures are obtained. Depending on patient risks, NAATs for *N gonorrhoeae* and *C trachomatis* and screening for other STDs may be included.

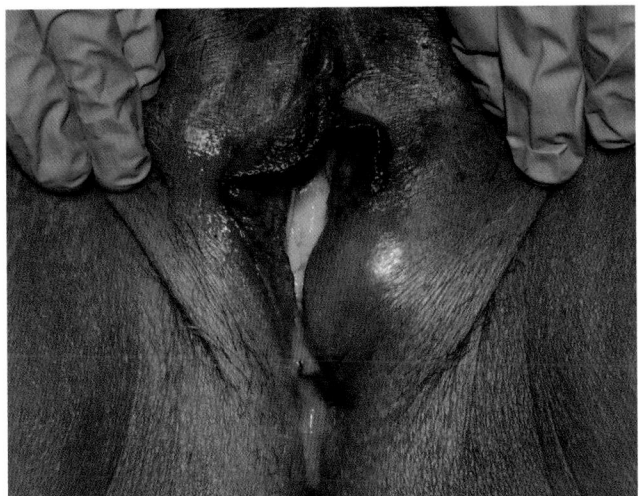

FIGURE 3-18 Bartholin gland duct abscess with some pus spontaneously draining onto the perineum.

Actinomyces Infection

Actinomyces israelii is a gram-positive, slow-growing, anaerobic bacterium found to be part of the indigenous genital flora of healthy women (Persson, 1984). Some have found it more frequently in the vaginal flora of IUD users, and rates of colonization increase with duration of IUD use (Curtis, 1981). *Actinomyces* is also identified in Pap smears, and Fiorino (1996) cited a 7-percent incidence in IUD users compared with less than 1 percent in nonusers. Pelvic infection and abscess are rare, even in those identified to harbor the bacteria. Accordingly, in the absence of symptoms, the incidental finding of *Actinomyces* on cytology may be managed by: (1) expectant management, (2) extended oral antibiotic treatment with the IUD in place, (3) IUD removal, or (4) IUD removal followed by antibiotic treatment (American College of Obstetricians and Gynecologists, 2013a). In support of conservative observation, reviews by Lippes (1999) and Westhoff (2007) suggest that asymptomatic women may retain their IUDs and do not require antibiotic treatment. With the higher rate of current IUD use, this will no doubt be an increasingly important topic. Importantly, if signs or symptoms of infection develop in women who harbor *Actinomyces*, the device is removed and antimicrobial therapy instituted. Early findings include fever, weight loss, abdominal pain, and abnormal vaginal bleeding or discharge. *Actinomyces* is sensitive to antimicrobials with gram-positive coverage, notably the penicillins.

REFERENCES

Achilles SL, Amortegui AJ, Wiesenfeld HC: Endometrial plasma cells: do they indicate subclinical pelvic inflammatory disease? Sex Transm Dis 32:185, 2005

American College of Obstetricians and Gynecologists: Antibiotic prophylaxis for gynecologic procedures. Practice Bulletin No. 104, May 2009, Reaffirmed 2014a

American College of Obstetricians and Gynecologists: Gynecologic herpes simplex virus infections. Practice Bulletin No. 57, November 2004, Reaffirmed 2014b

American College of Obstetricians and Gynecologists: Long-acting reversible contraception: implants and intrauterine devices. Practice Bulletin No. 121, July 2011, Reaffirmed 2013a

American College of Obstetricians and Gynecologists: Treatment of urinary tract infections in nonpregnant women. Practice Bulletin No. 91, March 2008, Reaffirmed 2012

American College of Obstetricians and Gynecologists: Vaginitis. Practice Bulletin No. 72. Obstet Gynecol 107:1195, May 2006, Reaffirmed 2013b

Amsel R, Totten PA, Spiegel CA, et al: Nonspecific vaginitis. Diagnostic criteria and microbial and epidemiologic associations. Am J Med 74:14, 1983

Anderson MR, Klink K, Kohrssen A: Evaluation of vaginal complaints. JAMA 291:1368, 2004

Ashley-Morrow R, Krantz E, Wald A: Time course of seroconversion by HerpeSelect ELISA after acquisition of genital herpes simplex virus type 1 (HSV-1) or HSV-2. Sex Transm Dis 30(4):310, 2003

Association of Public Health Laboratories: Laboratory diagnostic testing for *Chlamydia trachomatis* and *Neisseria gonorrhoeae*. Expert Consultation Meeting Summary Report. Atlanta, 2009

Atashili J, Poole C, Ndumbe PM, et al: Bacterial vaginosis and HIV acquisition: a meta-analysis of published studies. AIDS 22(12):1493, 2008

Bartlett JG, Onderdonk AB, Drude E, et al: Quantitative bacteriology of the vaginal flora. J Infect Dis 136(2):271, 1977

Bertino JS Jr, Booker LA, Franck PA, et al: Incidence of and significant risk factors for aminoglycoside-associated nephrotoxicity in patients dosed by using individualized pharmacokinetic monitoring. J Infect Dis 167:173, 1993

Beutner KR, Reitano MV, Richwald GA, et al: External genital warts: report of the American Medical Association Consensus Conference. AMA Expert Panel on External Genital Warts. Clin Infect Dis 27:796, 1998

Bhide A, Nama V, Patel S, et al: Microbiology of cysts/abscesses of Bartholin's gland: review of empirical antibiotic therapy against microbial culture. J Obstet Gynaecol 30(7):701, 2010

Birnbaum DM: Microscopic findings. In Knoop KJ, Stack LB, Storrow AB (eds): Atlas of Emergency Medicine, 3rd ed. New York, McGraw-Hill, 2010

Bleker OP, Smalbraak DJ, Schutte MF: Bartholin's abscess: the role of *Chlamydia trachomatis*. Genitourin Med 66:24, 1990

Bornstein J, Lakovsky Y, Lavi I, et al: The classic approach to diagnosis of vulvovaginitis: a critical analysis. Infect Dis Obstet Gynecol 9:105, 2001

Boskey ER, Cone RA, Whaley KJ, et al: Origins of vaginal acidity: high D/L lactate ratio is consistent with bacteria being the primary source. Hum Reprod 16(9):1809, 2001

Bradshaw CS, Morton AN, Garland SM, et al: Higher-risk behavioral practices associated with bacterial vaginosis compared with vaginal candidiasis. Obstet Gynecol 106:105, 2005

Bradshaw CS, Morton AN, Hocking J, et al: High recurrence rates of bacterial vaginosis over the course of 12 months after oral metronidazole therapy and factors associated with recurrence. J Infect Dis 193:1478, 2006

Brotman RM, Klebanoff MA, Nansel TR, et al: A longitudinal study of vaginal douching and bacterial vaginosis—a marginal structural modeling analysis. Am J Epidemiol 168(2):188, 2008

Caillouette JC, Sharp CF Jr, Zimmerman GJ, et al: Vaginal pH as a marker for bacterial pathogens and menopausal status. Am J Obstet Gynecol 176:1270, 1997

Centers for Disease Control and Prevention: Expedited partner therapy in the management of sexually transmitted diseases. Atlanta, U.S. Department of Health and Human Services, 2006

Centers for Disease Control and Prevention: Procedure-associated module: surgical site infection (SSI) event. 2014. Available at: http://www.cdc.gov/nhsn/PDFs/pscManual/9pscSSIcurrent.pdf. Accessed April 14, 2015

Centers for Disease Control and Prevention: Seroprevalence of herpes simplex virus type 2 among persons aged 14–49 years—United States, 2005–2008. MMWR 59(15):456, 2010

Centers for Disease Control and Prevention: Sexually transmitted disease surveillance, 2012. Atlanta, US Department of Health and Human Services, 2012

Centers for Disease Control and Prevention: Sexually transmitted diseases treatment guidelines, 2015. MMWR 64(3):1, 2015

Centers for Disease Control and Prevention: Update to CDC's sexually transmitted diseases treatment guidelines, 2006: fluoroquinolones no longer recommended for treatment of gonococcal infections. MMWR 56(14):332, 2007

Corey L, Wald A, Patel R, et al: Once-daily valacyclovir to reduce the risk of transmission of genital herpes. N Engl J Med 350:11, 2004

Cunningham AL, Diefenbach RJ, Miranda-Saksena M, et al: The cycle of human herpes simplex virus infection: virus transport and immune control. J Infect Dis 194(Suppl 1):S11, 2006

Cunningham FG, Leveno KJ, Bloom SL, (eds): Sexually transmitted infections. In Williams Obstetrics, 24th ed. New York, McGraw-Hill Education, 2014

Curtis EM, Pine L: *Actinomyces* in the vaginas of women with and without intrauterine contraceptive devices. Am J Obstet Gynecol 140:880, 1981

Czaja CA, Scholes D, Hooton TM, et al: Population-based epidemiologic analysis of acute pyelonephritis. Clin Infect Dis 45(3):273, 2007

Dahn A, Saunders S, Hammond JA, et al: Effect of bacterial vaginosis, *Lactobacillus* and Premarin estrogen replacement therapy on vaginal gene expression changes. Microbes Infect 10(6):620, 2008

Daley G, Russell D, Tabrizi S, et al: *Mycoplasma genitalium*: a review. Int J STD AIDS 25(7):475, 2014

Dunbar-Jacob J, Sereika SM, Foley SM, et al: Adherence to oral therapies in pelvic inflammatory disease. J Womens Health 13:285, 2004

Echols RM, Tosiello RL, Haverstock DC, el al: Demographic, clinical, and treatment parameters influencing the outcome of acute cystitis. Clin Infect Dis 29(1):113, 1999

Eron LJ, Judson F, Tucker S, et al: Interferon therapy for condylomata acuminata. N Engl J Med 315:1059, 1986

Fethers KA, Fairley CK, Hocking JS, et al: Sexual risk factors and bacterial vaginosis: a systematic review and meta-analysis. Clin Infect Dis 47(11):1426, 2008

Fiorino AS: Intrauterine contraceptive device-associated actinomycotic abscess and *Actinomyces* detection on cervical smear. Obstet Gynecol 87:142, 1996

Flynn CA, Helwig AL, Meurer LN: Bacterial vaginosis in pregnancy and the risk of prematurity: a meta-analysis. J Fam Pract 48:885, 1999

Gardner HL, Dukes CD: *Haemophilus vaginalis* vaginitis: a newly defined specific infection previously classified non-specific vaginitis. Am J Obstet Gynecol 69:962, 1955

Garland SM, Steben M, Sings HL, et al: Natural history of genital warts: analysis of the placebo arm of 2 randomized phase III trials of quadrivalent human papillomavirus (types 6, 11, 16, and 18) vaccine. J Infect Dis 199(6):805, 2009

Geiger AM, Foxman B: Risk factors for vulvovaginal candidiasis: a case-control study among university students. Epidemiology 7:182, 1996

Goh T, Goh LG, Ang CH, et al: Early diagnosis of necrotizing fasciitis. Br J Surg 101(1):e119, 2014

Gupta K, Hooton TM, Naber KG, et al: International clinical practice guidelines for the treatment of acute uncomplicated cystitis and pyelonephritis in women: a 2010 update by the Infectious Diseases Society of America and the European Society for Microbiology and Infectious Diseases. Clin Infect Dis 52(5):e103, 2011

Hadgu A, Westrom L, Brooks CA, et al: Predicting acute pelvic inflammatory disease: a multivariate analysis. Am J Obstet Gynecol 155:954, 1986

Haefner H: Current evaluation and management of vulvovaginitis. Clin Obstet Gynecol 42(2):184, 1999

Hansfield HH: Vaginal infections. In Color Atlas and Synopsis of Sexually Transmitted Diseases. New York, McGraw-Hill, 2001, p 169

Helms DJ, Mosure DJ, Secor WE, et al: Management of *Trichomonas vaginalis* in women with suspected metronidazole hypersensitivity. Am J Obstet Gynecol 198(4):370 e371, 2008

Hemsell DL, Hemsell PG, Wendel G Jr, et al: Medical management of severe PID avoiding operations. In Pelvic Inflammatory Disease (PID) Diagnosis and Therapy. Grafelfing, E.R. Weissenbacher, 1993, p 142

Hemsell DL, Obregon VL, Heard MC, et al: Endometrial bacteria in asymptomatic, nonpregnant women. J Reprod Med 34:872, 1989

Holmes NE, Howden BP: What's new in the treatment of serious MRSA infection? Curr Opin Infect Dis 27(6):471, 2014

Hooton TM, Roberts PL, Cox ME, et al: Voided midstream urine culture and acute cystitis in premenopausal women. N Engl J Med 369(20):1883, 2013

Hooton TM, Stamm WE: Diagnosis and treatment of uncomplicated urinary tract infection. Infect Dis Clin North Am 11:551, 1997

Huppert JS, Batteiger BE, Braslins P, et al: Use of an immunochromatographic assay for rapid detection of *Trichomonas vaginalis* in vaginal specimens. J Clin Microbiol 43:684, 2005

Huppert JS, Mortensen JE, Reed JL, et al: Rapid antigen testing compares favorably with transcription-mediated amplification assay for the detection of *Trichomonas vaginalis* in young women. Clin Infect Dis 45(2):194, 2007

Keane FE, Ison CA, Taylor-Robinson D: A longitudinal study of the vaginal flora over a menstrual cycle. Int J STD AIDS 8:489, 1997

Kessous R, Aricha-Tamir B, Sheizaf B, et al: Clinical and microbiological characteristics of Bartholin gland abscesses. Obstet Gynecol 122(4):794, 2013

Kilpatrick CC, Alagkiozidis I, Orejuela FJ, et al: Factors complicating surgical management of vulvar abscess. J Reprod Med 55(3–4):139, 2010

Kirby JP, Mazuski JE: Prevention of surgical site infection. Surg Clin North Am 89(2):365, 2009

Klebanoff MA, Nansel TR, Brotman RM, et al: Personal hygienic behaviors and bacterial vaginosis. Sex Transm Dis 37(2):94, 2010

Landers DV, Sweet RL: Tubo-ovarian abscess: contemporary approach to management. Rev Infect Dis 5(5):876, 1983

Landers DV, Wiesenfeld HC, Heine RP, et al: Predictive value of the clinical diagnosis of lower genital tract infection in women. Am J Obstet Gynecol 190:1004, 2004

Larsen SA, Johnson RE: Diagnostic tests. In Larsen SA, Pope V, Johnson RE, et al (eds): Manual of Tests for Syphilis, 9th ed., Washington D.C., Centers for Disease Control and Prevention and American Public Health Association, 1998

Larsson PG, Bergman B, Försum U, et al: Mobiluncus and clue cells as predictors of pelvic inflammatory disease after first trimester abortion. Acta Obstet Gynecol Scand 68:217, 1989

Larsson PG, Platz-Christensen JJ, Försum U, et al: Clue cells in predicting infections after abdominal hysterectomy. Obstet Gynecol 77:450, 1991

Larsson PG, Platz-Christensen JJ, Thejls H, et al: Incidence of pelvic inflammatory disease after first-trimester legal abortion in women with bacterial vaginosis after treatment with metronidazole: a double-blind, randomized study. Am J Obstet Gynecol 166:100, 1992

Leitich H, Kiss H: Asymptomatic bacterial vaginosis and intermediate flora as risk factors for adverse pregnancy outcome. Best Pract Res Clin Obstet Gynaecol 21:375, 2007

Lillis RA, Nsuami MJ, Myers L, et al: Utility of urine, vaginal, cervical, and rectal specimens for detection of *Mycoplasma genitalium* in women. J Clin Microbiol 49(5):1990, 2011

Lippes J: Pelvic actinomycosis: a review and preliminary look at prevalence. Am J Obstet Gynecol 180:265, 1999

Liu C, Bayer A, Cosgrove SE, et al: Clinical practice guidelines by the Infectious Diseases Society of America for the treatment of methicillin-resistant *Staphylococcus aureus* infections in adults and children: executive summary. Clin Infect Dis 52(3):285, 2011

Mangram AJ, Horan TC, Pearson ML, et al: Guideline for prevention of surgical site infection, 1999. Hospital Infection Control Practices Advisory Committee. Infect Control Hospital Epidemiol 20:250, 1999

Manhart LE, Broad JM, Golden MR: *Mycoplasma genitalium*: should we treat and how? Clin Infect Dis 53 Suppl 3:S129, 2011

Marrazzo JM: A persistent(ly) enigmatic ecological mystery: bacterial vaginosis. J Infect Dis 193:1475, 2006

Martin ET, Krantz E, Gottlieb SL, et al: A pooled analysis of the effect of condoms in preventing HSV-2 acquisition. Arch Intern Med 169(13):1233, 2009

Mayo Clinic: Symposium on Antimicrobial Agents. Mayo Clin Proc 66:931, 1991

Meltzer SM, Monk BJ, Tewari KS: Green tea catechins for treatment of external genital warts. Am J Obstet Gynecol 200(3):233.e1, 2009

Molander P, Sjöberg J, Paavonen J: Transvaginal power Doppler findings in laparoscopically proven acute pelvic inflammatory disease. Ultrasound Obstet Gynecol 17:233, 2001

Morse S, Long J: Infestations. In Morse S, Ballard RC, Holmes KK, et al (eds): Atlas of Sexually Transmitted Diseases. 3rd ed. Edinburgh, Mosby, 2003

Ness RB, Hillier SL, Kip KE, et al: Bacterial vaginosis and risk of pelvic inflammatory disease. Obstet Gynecol 104:761, 2004

Nicolau D, Quintiliani R, Nightingale CH: Once-daily aminoglycosides. Conn Med 56:561, 1992

Nicolle LE, Bradley S, Colgan R, et al: Infectious Diseases Society of America guidelines for the diagnosis and treatment of asymptomatic bacteriuria in adults. Clin Infect Dis 40:643, 2005

Patton DL, Halbert SA, Kuo CC, et al: Host response to primary *Chlamydia trachomatis* infection of the fallopian tube in pig-tailed monkeys. Fertil Steril 40:829, 1983

Patton DL, Moore DE, Spadoni LR, et al: A comparison of the fallopian tube's response to overt and silent salpingitis. Obstet Gynecol 73:622, 1989

Persson E, Holmberg K: A longitudinal study of *Actinomyces israelii* in the female genital tract. Acta Obstet Gynecol Scand 63:207, 1984

Romosan G, Bjartling C, Skoog L, et al: Ultrasound for diagnosing acute salpingitis: a prospective observational diagnostic study. Hum Reprod 28(6):1569, 2013

Rubin RH, Shapiro ED, Andriole VT, et al: Evaluation of new anti-infective drugs for the treatment of urinary tract infection. Infectious Diseases Society of America and the Food and Drug Administration. Clin Infect Dis 15(Suppl 1):S216, 1992

Sam JW, Jacobs JE, Birnbaum BA: Spectrum of CT findings in acute pyogenic pelvic inflammatory disease. Radiographics 22:1327, 2002

Saxon A, Beall GN, Rohr AS: Immediate hypersensitivity reactions to beta-lactam antibiotics. Ann Intern Med 107:204, 1987

Schachter J, Stephens R: Infections caused by *Chlamydia trachomatis*. In Morse S, Ballard RC, Holmes KK, et al (eds): Atlas of Sexually Transmitted Diseases, 3rd ed. Edinburgh, Mosby, 2003, p 80

Scheinfeld N, Lehman DS: An evidence-based review of medical and surgical treatments of genital warts. Dermatol Online J 12:5, 2006

Senok AC, Verstraelen H, Temmerman M, et al: Probiotics for the treatment of bacterial vaginosis. Cochrane Database Syst Rev 4:CD006289, 2009

Sobel JD, Nyirjesy P, Brown W: Tinidazole therapy for metronidazole-resistant vaginal trichomoniasis. Clin Infect Dis 33:1341, 2001

Soper DE: Pelvic inflammatory disease. Obstet Gynecol 116(2 Pt 1):419, 2010

Soper DE, Bump RC, Hurt WG: Bacterial vaginosis and trichomoniasis vaginitis are risk factors for cuff cellulitis after abdominal hysterectomy. Am J Obstet Gynecol 163:1016, 1991

Spence MR, Blanco LJ, Patel J, et al: A comparative evaluation of vaginal, cervical and peritoneal flora in normal, healthy women: a preliminary report. Sex Transm Dis 9(1):37, 1982

Taylor-Robinson D, Jensen JS: *Mycoplasma genitalium*: from Chrysalis to multicolored butterfly. Clin Microbiol Rev 24(3):498, 2011

Tepper NK, Steenland MW, Gaffield ME, et al: Retention of intrauterine devices in women who acquire pelvic inflammatory disease: a systematic review. Contraception 87(5):655, 2013

Thurman AR, Satterfield TM, Soper DE: Methicillin-resistant *Staphylococcus aureus* as a common cause of vulvar abscesses. Obstet Gynecol 112:538, 2008

Timor-Tritsch IE, Lerner JP, Monteagudo A, et al: Transvaginal sonographic markers of tubal inflammatory disease. Ultrasound Obstet Gynecol 12(1):56, 1998

Torrone E, Weinstock H: Prevalence of *Chlamydia trachomatis* genital infection among persons aged 14–39 years—United States, 2007–2012. MMWR 63(38):834, 2014

Toth M, Patton DL, Campbell LA, et al: Detection of chlamydial antigenic material in ovarian, prostatic, ectopic pregnancy and semen samples of culture-negative subjects. Am J Reprod Immunol 43(4):218, 2000

Tulkens PM, Clerckx-Braun F, Donnez J: Safety and efficacy of aminoglycosides once-a-day: experimental data and randomized, controlled evaluation in patients suffering from pelvic inflammatory disease. J Drug Dev 1:71, 1988

U.S. Preventive Services Task Force: Clinical summary. Chlamydia and gonorrhea: screening. 2014. Available at: http://www.uspreventiveservicestaskforce.org/Page/Document/ClinicalSummaryFinal/chlamydia-and-gonorrhea-screening. Accessed November 26, 2014

Van der Pol B: *Trichomonas vaginalis infection*: the most prevalent nonviral sexually transmitted infection receives the least public health attention. Clin Infect Dis 44:23, 2007

Van der Pol B, Williams JA, Orr DP, et al: Prevalence, incidence, natural history, and response to treatment of *Trichomonas vaginalis* infection among adolescent women. J Infect Dis 192:2039, 2005

Wald A, Langenberg AG, Krantz E, et al: The relationship between condom use and herpes simplex virus acquisition. Ann Intern Med 143(10):707, 2005

Weinstein SA, Stiles BG. Recent perspectives in the diagnosis and evidence-based treatment of *Mycoplasma genitalium*. Expert Rev Anti Infect Ther 10(4):487, 2012

Wendel GD Jr, Stark BJ, Jamison RB, et al: Penicillin allergy and desensitization in serious infections during pregnancy. N Engl J Med 312:1229, 1985

Westhoff C: IUDs and colonization or infection with *Actinomyces*. Contraception 75:S48, 2007

Westrom L: Effect of acute pelvic inflammatory disease on fertility. Am J Obstet Gynecol 121:707, 1975

Wiese W, Patel SR, Patel SC, et al: A meta-analysis of the Papanicolaou smear and wet mount for the diagnosis of vaginal trichomoniasis. Am J Med 108(4):301, 2000

Wiesenfeld HC, Hillier SL, Krohn MA, et al: Bacterial vaginosis is a strong predictor of *Neisseria gonorrhoeae* and *Chlamydia trachomatis* infection. Clin Infect Dis 36(5):663, 2003

Wiley DJ, Douglas J, Beutner K, et al: External genital warts: diagnosis, treatment, and prevention. Clin Infect Dis 35(Suppl 2):S210, 2002

Wilson B: Necrotizing fasciitis. Am Surg 18:416, 1952

Wilson J: Managing recurrent bacterial vaginosis. Sex Transm Infect 80:8, 2004

Wolff K, Johnson RA: Arthropod bites, stings, and cutaneous infections. In Fitzpatrick's Color Atlas and Synopsis of Clinical Dermatology, 6th ed. New York, McGraw-Hill, 2009

Xu F, Sternberg MR, Kottiri BJ, et al: Trends in herpes simplex virus type 1 and type 2 seroprevalence in the United States. JAMA 296(8):964, 2006

Benign Disorders of the Lower Genital Tract

The lower reproductive tract, comprising the vulva, vagina, and cervix, exhibits a wide spectrum of benign and neoplastic diseases. Disorder characteristics often overlap, and thus differentiating normal variants, benign disease, and potentially serious lesions can be challenging. Lower reproductive tract infection is a frequent cause and discussed in Chapter 3, whereas congenital anomalies and preinvasive neoplasia are infrequent and described in Chapters 18 (p. 404) and 29 (p. 624). The benign lesions highlighted in this chapter are common, and mastery of their identification and treatment is essential.

VULVAR ASSESSMENT

Vulvar skin is more permeable than surrounding tissues because of differences in structure, hydration, occlusion, and friction susceptibility (Farage, 2004). Accordingly, pathology can develop in this area, although frequency estimates are difficult because of patient underreporting and clinician misdiagnosis. Lesions may result from allergen or irritant exposure, infection, trauma, or neoplasia. As a result, symptoms may be acute or chronic and include pain, pruritus, dyspareunia, bleeding, and discharge. Effective therapies are available for most disorders, yet embarrassment and fear may prove significant roadblocks to care for many women.

■ General Approach to Vulvar Complaints

The initial encounter includes reassurance that the patient's complaints will be investigated thoroughly. Women often minimize and may be uncomfortable with describing their symptoms. They may relate protracted histories of assorted diagnoses and treatments by numerous providers and may voice frustration and doubt that relief is possible. Patients are not promised a cure but rather that every effort will be made to alleviate their symptoms. This can require multiple visits, tissue sampling, treatment attempts, and even a multidisciplinary plan. A patient-provider partnership approach to management enhances compliance and care satisfaction.

During counseling, the suspected diagnosis, current treatment plan, and recommended vulvar skin care are outlined. Printed materials that explain common conditions, medication use, and skin care are helpful. Patients are often relieved to learn that their complaints and conditions are not unique. Thus, referral to national websites and support groups is usually welcomed.

■ Diagnosis

History

Scheduling adequate time for the initial evaluation is a wise investment, as detailed information is essential. Symptom characterization includes descriptions of abnormal sensations, duration, precise location, and associated vaginal pruritus or discharge. Patients often refer to vulvar pruritus as vaginal, and symptom location should be clarified. A thorough medical history addresses systemic illnesses, medications, and known allergies. Obstetric, sexual, and psychosocial histories and any potentially provocative events around the time of symptom onset often suggest etiologies. Hygiene and sexual practices should be investigated in detail.

Of symptoms, vulvar pruritus is frequent with many dermatoses. Patients may have been previously diagnosed with psoriasis, eczema, or dermatitis at other body sites. Isolated vulvar pruritus may be associated with a new medication. Patients may identify foods that provoke or intensify symptoms, and in such cases, a food diary may be helpful. Most often, vulvar pruritus is due to a contact or allergic dermatitis. Common offenders include strongly scented body soaps and laundry products. Excessive washing and use of wash cloths can result in skin drying and mechanical trauma. Washing often becomes more aggressive with pruritus as patients assume their hygiene is lacking. Any of these practices can create an escalating itch-scratch cycle or exacerbate the symptoms of other preexisting dermatoses. Last, patients frequently use nonprescription remedies for relief of vulvovaginal itching or perceived odor. These products commonly contain multiple known contact allergens, and their use is discouraged (Table 4-1).

TABLE 4-1. Common Vulvar Irritants and Allergens

General Categories	Examples of Specific Agents
Antiseptics	Povidone iodine, hexachlorophene
Body fluids	Semen, feces, urine, saliva
Colored or scented toilet paper	
Condoms	Latex, lubricant, spermicide, thiuram
Contraceptive creams, jellies, foams	Nonoxynol-9, lubricants
Dyes	4-Phenylene diamine
Emollients	Lanolin, jojoba oil, glycerin
Laundry detergents, fabric softeners, dryer sheets	
Rubber products	Latex, thiuram
Sanitary baby or adult bathroom wipes	
Sanitary pads or tampons	
Soaps, bubble bath and salts, shampoos	
Topical anesthetics	Benzocaine, lidocaine
Topical antibacterials	Neomycin, bacitracin, polymyxin, framycetin, tea tree oil
Topical corticosteroids	Clobetasol propionate
Topical antifungal creams	Ethylene diamine, sodium metabisulfite

Data from American College of Obstetricians and Gynecologists, 2010; Crone, 2000; Fisher, 1973; Marren, 1992.

Physical Examination

Examination of the vulva and surrounding skin is completed using adequate lighting, optimal patient positioning, and a magnifying lens or colposcope. Both focal and generalized skin changes are carefully noted, as neoplasia may arise within a field of generalized dermatosis. Abnormal pigmentation, skin texture, nodularity, or vascularity is evaluated. Touch with a small probe such as a cotton swab defines the anatomic boundaries of generalized symptoms and precisely locates focal complaints (Fig. 4-1). A medical record diagram noting vulvar findings and symptoms aids treatment assessment over time.

Vaginal complaints or vulvar conditions without obvious etiology typically prompt vaginal examination. Careful inspection may reveal generalized inflammation or atrophy, abnormal discharge, or focal mucosal lesions such as ulcers. In these

cases, saline preparation of secretions for microscopic evaluation ("wet prep"), vaginal pH testing, and aerobic culture to detect yeast overgrowth are collected. A general skin examination, including the oral mucosa and axillae, may suggest the cause of some vulvar conditions. A focused neurologic examination to evaluate lower extremity sensation and strength as well as perineal sensation and tone may help evaluate vulvar dysesthesias.

Vulvar Biopsy

Vulvar skin changes are frequently nonspecific and typically require biopsy for accurate diagnosis. Biopsy is strongly considered if the cause of symptoms is not obvious; if initial empiric treatment fails; if the cause of symptoms is not obvious; or if focal, exophytic, or hyper-/hypopigmented lesions are present. During biopsy, ulcerative lesions are sampled at their edges, and hyper- or hypopigmented areas at their thickest region (Mirowski, 2004). Conditions with variable histologic appearance may require multiple biopsies for correct disorder classification.

The steps for vulvar biopsy are shown in Figure 4-2. First, the biopsy site is cleaned with an antimicrobial agent and infiltrated with a 1- or 2-percent lidocaine solution. Biopsy is performed most easily with a Keyes skin punch. The open, circular blade is designed to remove a shallow disc of tissue when gently pressed against the skin and rotated. Keyes punches are available in various diameters, ranging from 2 to 6 mm, and size selection is based on lesion dimensions and on whether sampling or excision is the goal. Vulvar skin and lesion thicknesses are variable, and over-rotation of or undue pressure on the Keyes punch is avoided. Too deep a biopsy will leave a depressed scar. Rotation and pressure should stop when decreased resistance is felt, signaling the dermis has been reached. The tissue disc core is then freed at its base with fine scissors. Larger punch biopsies (4 to 6 mm) may require closure with an absorbable suture.

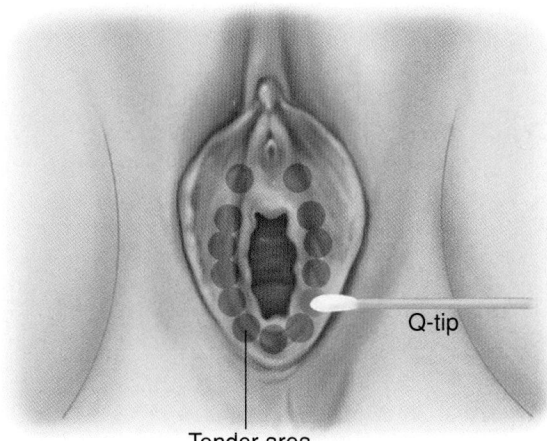

Q-tip

Tender area

FIGURE 4-1 Pain can be assessed and mapped by systematically touching a cotton-tip applicator to the vulva.

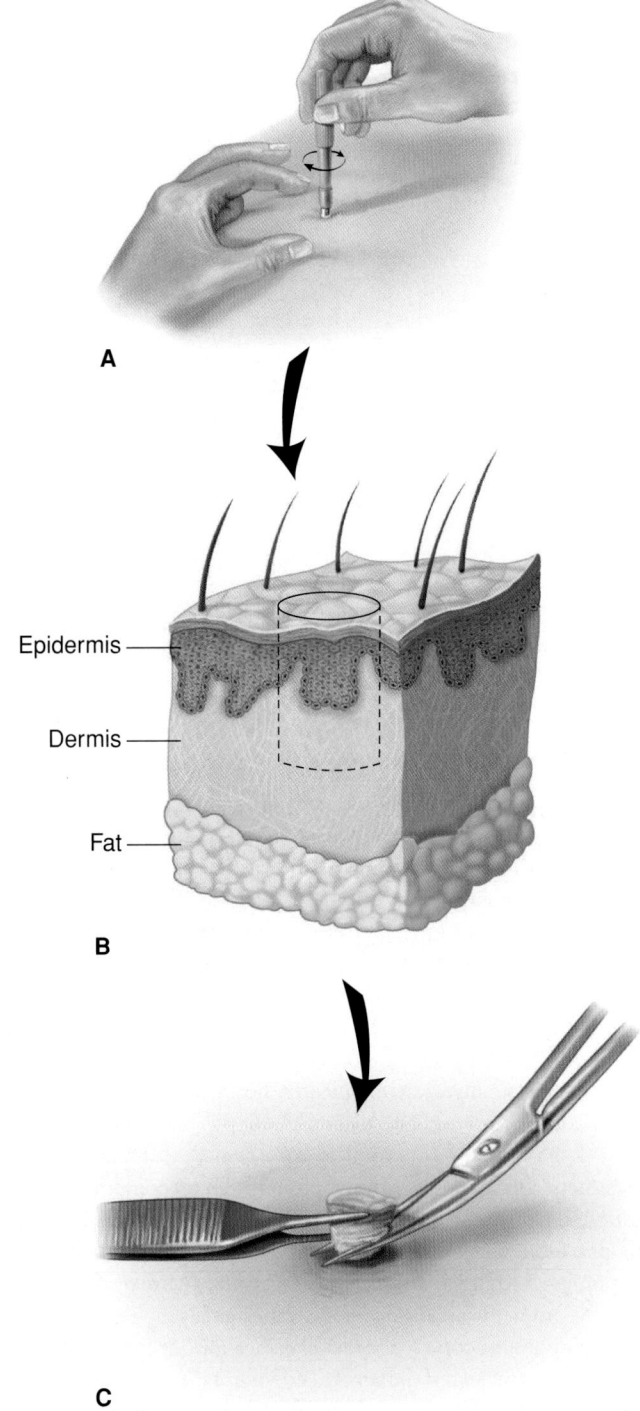

A

Epidermis

Dermis

Fat

B

C

FIGURE 4-2 Vulvar biopsy steps. **A.** A Keyes punch biopsy is placed against the biopsy site. Gentle downward pressure is exerted as the punch is rotated. **B.** A core biopsy is created that extends through the epidermis and into the dermis. **C.** The tip of a fine needle or fine forceps is used to elevate the core, while fine scissors incise its base.

For raised or pedunculated lesions, fine scissors may be used. Occasionally, a No. 15 blade scalpel is selected for larger focal lesions. Tissue is excised parallel to the natural vulvar skin folds, and the defect is sutured to aid healing and minimize scarring. Larger lesions, for which simple closure would create significant incision tension, are best excised by clinicians experienced in more advanced plastic surgery techniques.

Following biopsy, bleeding may be controlled with direct pressure, silver nitrate stick, or Monsel paste. Silver nitrate may permanently discolor the skin, which may upset the patient and confuse subsequent examinations. If needed, simple interrupted stitches using a fine, rapidly absorbable suture provide hemostasis and edge approximation. Nonnarcotic oral analgesics usually suffice to relieve postbiopsy discomfort.

VULVAR DERMATOSES

The International Society for the Study of Vulvovaginal Disease (ISSVD) provides classification systems for vulvar abnormalities. Their 2006 Classification of Vulvar Dermatoses specifically focuses on dermatoses and divides these based on biopsy-obtained histology. Their more recent terminology and organization system does not supplant the 2006 system. Instead, it classifies a broader group of dermatologic disorders that includes dermatoses, infections, and neoplasias by their similar clinical presentations to aid identification and management (Lynch, 2007, 2012). The next sections describe the more frequently encountered conditions.

■ Lichen Simplex Chronicus

An itch-scratch cycle typically leads to chronic trauma from rubbing and scratching (Lynch, 2004). Early examination reveals excoriations within a background of erythema. With chronic trauma, the skin responds by thickening, termed lichenification. Thus, in long-standing cases, vulvar skin is thick with exaggerated skin markings causing a leathery, gray appearance. Skin changes are usually bilateral and symmetric and may extend beyond the labia majora. Intense vulvar pruritus causes functional and psychologic distress, and sleep is often disrupted. Potential pruritus triggers include irritation from clothing, heat, or sweating; chemicals contained within hygiene products and topical medications; laundry products; and even food sensitivities (Virgili, 2003). A detailed history typically leads to the diagnosis.

Treatment involves halting the itch-scratch cycle. First, provocative stimuli are eliminated, and topical corticosteroid ointments help to reduce inflammation. In addition, lubricants, such as plain petrolatum or vegetable oil, and cool sitz baths help to restore the skin's barrier function. Oral antihistamine use, trimmed fingernails, and cotton gloves worn at night can help decrease scratching during sleep. If symptoms fail to resolve within 1 to 3 weeks, biopsy is indicated to exclude other pathology. Histology classically shows thickening of both the epidermis (acanthosis) and the stratum corneum (hyperkeratosis). In these refractory cases, a trial of higher-potency corticosteroid may improve symptoms.

■ Lichen Sclerosus

This classically presents in postmenopausal women, although cases are less often found in premenopausal women, children, and men (Fig. 14-8, p. 323). In a referral dermatologic clinic, lichen sclerosus was found in 1:300 to 1:1000 patients with a tendency toward whites (Wallace, 1971). Others estimate an incidence of childhood lichen sclerosus to be 1 in 900 (Powell, 2001).

The cause of lichen sclerosus remains unknown, although infectious, hormonal, genetic, and autoimmune etiologies have been suggested. Approximately 20 to 30 percent of patients with lichen sclerosus have other autoimmune disorders, such as Graves disease, types 1 and 2 diabetes mellitus, systemic lupus erythematosus, and achlorhydria, with or without pernicious anemia (Bor, 1969; Kahana, 1985; Poskitt, 1993). Accordingly, concurrent testing for these is indicated if other suggestive findings are present.

Diagnosis

Although sometimes asymptomatic, most individuals with lichen sclerosus complain of anogenital symptoms that often worsen at night. Inflammation of local terminal nerve fibers is suspected. Pruritus-induced scratching creates a vicious cycle that may lead to excoriations and vulvar skin thickening. Late symptoms can include burning and dyspareunia due to vulvar skin fragility and structural changes.

Perianal involvement is frequently seen. The typical white, atrophic papules may coalesce into porcelain-white plaques that distort normal vulvar anatomy. As a result, labia minora regression, clitoral concealment, urethral obstruction, and introital stenosis can develop. The skin generally appears thinned and crinkled. Over time, involvement may extend to the perineum and anus to form a "figure-eight" or "hourglass" shape (Fig. 4-3) (Clark, 1967). Thickened white plaques, areas of erythema, or nodularity should prompt biopsy to exclude preinvasive and malignant lesions. This characteristic clinical picture and histologic findings typically confirm the diagnosis. In long-standing cases, histologic findings may be nonspecific, and clinical suspicion will guide treatment.

Treatment and Surveillance

Curative therapies are not available for lichen sclerosus. Thus, treatment goals are symptom control and prevention of anatomic distortion. Despite its classification as a nonneoplastic dermatosis, patients with lichen sclerosus demonstrate an

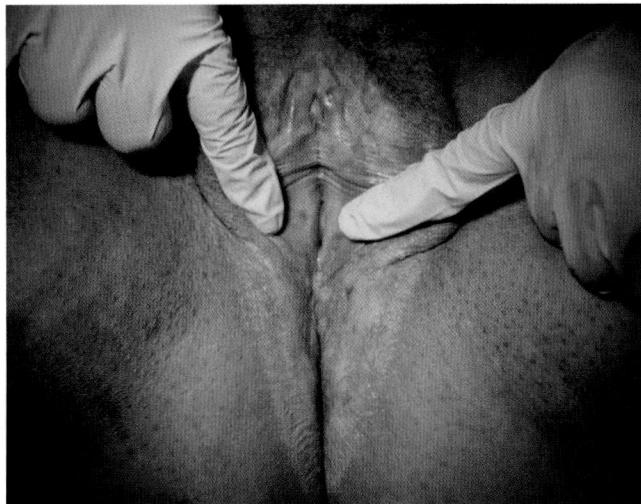

FIGURE 4-3 Vulvar lichen sclerosus. Note the thin and pale vulvar skin, loss of labia minora architecture, and labia minora fusion beneath the clitoris.

TABLE 4-2. Vulvar Care Recommendations

Avoid using gels, scented bath products, cleansing wipes, and soaps, as they may contain irritants
Use aqueous creams to clean the vulva
Avoid using a harsh washcloth to clean the vulva
Dab the vulva gently to dry
Avoid wearing tight-fitting pants
Select white cotton underwear
Avoid washing undergarments in scented washing detergents. Consider using a multirinse process with cold water to remove any remaining detergent
Consider wearing skirts and no underwear at home and at night to avoid friction and aid drying

increased risk of vulvar malignancy. Malignant transformation within lichen sclerosus develops in 5 percent of patients. Histologic cellular atypia may precede a diagnosis of invasive squamous cell carcinoma (Scurry, 1997). Accordingly, lifetime surveillance of women with lichen sclerosus every 12 months is prudent (Neill, 2010). Persistently symptomatic, new, or changing lesions should be biopsied (American College of Obstetricians and Gynecologists, 2010).

As with all vulvar disorders, hygiene recommendations focus on minimizing chemical and mechanical skin irritation (Table 4-2). The chronicity of lichen sclerosus and lack of cure elicits an array of emotions. Support groups dedicated to this condition, such as that found at www.lichensclerosus.org, offer needed psychologic support.

Corticosteroids. First-line therapy for lichen sclerosus is an ultrapotent topical corticosteroid preparation such as 0.05-percent clobetasol propionate (Temovate) or 0.05-percent halobetasol propionate (Ultravate). Ointment formulations are preferred by some providers over creams due to their protective and less irritating properties (Table 4-3). Clobetasol propionate offers effective antiinflammatory, antipruritic, and vasoconstrictive properties. Theoretic adrenocorticosuppression and iatrogenic Cushing syndrome may be risks if it is used in large doses for extended periods.

Treatment initiation within 2 years of symptom onset usually prevents significant scarring, but no treatment scheme is universally accepted for topical corticosteroid use. The currently recommended dosing schedule of the British Association of Dermatologists is 0.05-percent clobetasol propionate once nightly for 4 weeks, followed by alternating nights for 4 weeks, and finally tapering to twice weekly for 4 weeks (Neill, 2010). After this initial therapy, recommendations for maintenance therapy vary and range from tapering corticosteroids to "as needed" use to ongoing once- or twice-weekly applications. During initial treatment, some patients may also require oral antihistamines or topical 2-percent lidocaine jelly particularly at night to control itching.

Corticosteroids can also be injected into affected areas, a treatment offered by specialty clinics familiar with techniques and potential complications. One study of eight patients evaluated the efficacy of once-monthly intralesional infiltration

TABLE 4-3. Topical Medication Guide

Steroid Class Potency	Generic Name	Brand Names (available forms)
Low	Alclometasone dipropionate 0.05%	Aclovate (cream, oint.)
	Betamethasone valerate 0.01%	Valisone (cream, lotion)
	Fluocinolone acetonide 0.01%	Synalar (solution)
	Hydrocortisone 1%, 2.5%	Generic OTC versions 1% or 2.5% (cream, oint., lotion)
Intermediate	Betamethasone valerate 0.1%	Valisone (cream, lotion, oint.)
	Desonide 0.05%	DesOwen (cream, oint., lotion)
	Fluocinolone acetonide 0.025%	Synalar (cream, oint.)
	Flurandrenolide 0.025%, 0.05%	Cordran (cream, oint.)
	Fluticasone 0.005%, 0.05%	Cutivate 0.005% (oint.), 0.05% (cream)
	Hydrocortisone butyrate 0.1%	Locoid (cream, oint., solution)
	Hydrocortisone valerate 0.2%	Westcort (cream, oint.)
	Mometasone furoate 0.1%	Elocon (cream, oint., lotion)
	Prednicarbate 0.1%	Dermatop (cream, oint.)
	Triamcinolone 0.025%, 0.1%	Aristocort, Kenalog (cream, oint., lotion)
High	Amcinonide 0.1%	Cyclocort (cream, oint., lotion)
	Betamethasone dipropionate 0.05%	Diprolene, Diprosone (cream)
	Desoximetasone 0.05%, 0.25%	Topicort (cream)
	Diflorasone diacetate 0.05%	Psorcon (cream, oint.)
	Fluocinonide 0.05%	Lidex (cream, gel, oint.)
	Fluocinolone acetonide 0.2%	Synalar-HP (cream)
	Halcinonide 0.1%	Halog (cream, oint., solution)
	Triamcinolone 0.5%	Aristocort, Kenalog (cream, oint.)
Ultrapotent	Betamethasone dipropionate augmented 0.05%	Diprolene (ointment, gel)
	Clobetasol propionate 0.05%	Temovate (cream, gel, oint.)
	Diflorasone 0.05%	Psorcon (cream, oint.)
	Halobetasol propionate 0.05%	Ultravate (cream, oint.)

Oint. = ointment; OTC = over the counter.

of 25 to 30 mg of triamcinolone hexacetonide for a total of 3 months. Severity scores decreased in all categories including symptoms, gross appearance, and histopathologic findings (Mazdisnian, 1999).

Other Topical Treatments. *Estrogen cream* is not a primary therapy for lichen sclerosus. However, its addition is indicated for menopausal atrophy, labial fusion, and dyspareunia. Testosterone ointment has failed to show efficacy in trials and is no longer recommended (Bornstein, 1998; Sideri, 1994).

Retinoids are reserved for severe, nonresponsive cases of lichen sclerosus or for patients intolerant of ultrapotent corticosteroids. Topical tretinoin reduces hyperkeratosis, improves dysplastic changes, stimulates collagen and glycosaminoglycan synthesis, and induces local angiogenesis (Eichner, 1992; Kligman, 1986a,b; Varani, 1989). Virgili and colleagues (1995) evaluated the effects of topical 0.025-percent tretinoin (Retin-A, Renova) applied once daily, 5 days a week for 1 year. Complete remission of symptoms was seen in more than 75 percent of women. However, more than one quarter of patients experienced skin irritation, which is common with retinoids.

Topical calcineurin inhibitors such as tacrolimus (Protopic) and pimecrolimus (Elidel) have antiinflammatory and immuno-modulating effects. These are indicated for moderate to severe eczema and have been evaluated for lichen sclerosus (Goldstein, 2011; Hengge, 2006). Moreover, these agents, compared with topical corticosteroids, theoretically lower the risk of skin atrophy, since collagen synthesis is unaffected (Assmann, 2003; Kunstfeld, 2003). However, from a double-blind, randomized, prospective study, Funaro and associates (2014) concluded that topical clobetasol propionate was more effective in treating vulvar lichen sclerosus than topical tacrolimus. In the face of recent Food and Drug Administration (FDA) concerns regarding its link to various cancers, clinicians should exercise caution when prescribing tacrolimus for extended periods (Food and Drug Administration, 2010).

Last, *phototherapy* after pretreatment using 5-aminolevulinic acid was investigated in one small series of 12 postmenopausal women with advanced lichen sclerosus. Significant reductions in patient symptoms and short-term improvement for up to 9 months were noted (Hillemanns, 1999).

Surgery. Surgical intervention should be reserved for significant sequelae and not for primary treatment of uncomplicated lichen sclerosus. For introital stenosis, Rouzier and coworkers (2002) described marked improvements in dyspareunia and

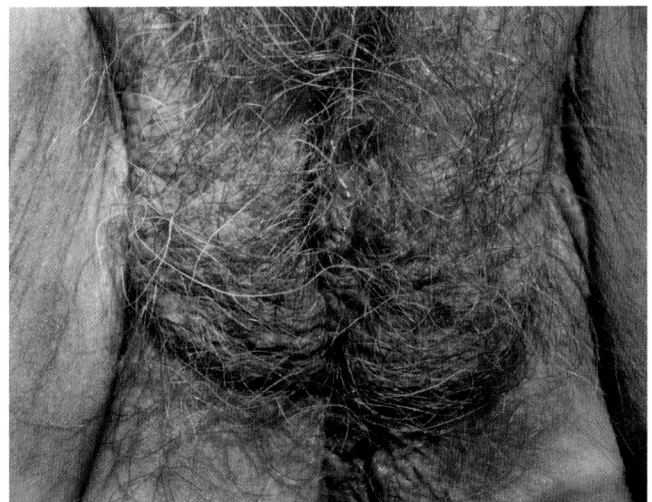

FIGURE 4-4 Vulvar contact dermatitis. Contact sites of the offending agent are seen as symmetric erythema on the vulva.

TABLE 4-4. Treatment of Vulvar Contact Dermatitis

1. Stop offending agents and/or practices
2. Correct vulvar skin barrier function
   a. Sitz bath twice daily with plain water
   b. Application of plain petrolatum
3. Treat any underlying infection
   a. Oral antifungal therapy
   b. Oral antibiotic administration
4. Reduce inflammation
   a. Topical corticosteroids twice daily for 1–3 weeks
      i. 0.05% clobetasol propionate ointment
      ii. 0.1% triamcinolone ointment
   b. Systemic corticosteroids for severe irritation
5. Break the itch-scratch cycle
   a. Cool packs (avoid ice packs, which may injure skin)
   b. Plain, cold yogurt on a sanitary napkin for 5–10 minutes
   c. Consider an SSRI (sertraline [Zoloft] 50–100 mg) or an antihistamine (hydroxyzine [Vistaril] 25–100 mg)

SSRI = selective serotonin-reuptake inhibitor.
Adapted with permission from Margesson LJ: Contact dermatitis of the vulva Dermatol Ther 2004;17(1):20–27.

---

quality of sexual intercourse if perineoplasty was performed (Section 43-22, p. 979). Vaginal dilation and corticosteroids are recommended following most surgical corrections of introital stenosis. For clitoral adhesions, surgical dissection can be used to free the hood from the glans. Reagglutination can be averted using initial nightly application of ultrapotent topical corticosteroid ointment (Goldstein, 2007).

▇ Inflammatory Dermatoses

Contact Dermatitis

A primary irritant or allergen creates vulvar skin inflammation, termed *contact dermatitis* (Fig. 4-4). This condition is common, and in unexplained cases of vulvar pruritus and inflammation, irritant contact dermatitis is diagnosed in up to 54 percent of patients (Fischer, 1996).

Irritant contact dermatitis classically presents as immediate burning and stinging upon exposure to an offending agent. In contrast, patients with *allergic contact dermatitis* experience a delayed onset and an intermittent course of pruritus and localized erythema, edema, and vesicles or bullae (Margesson, 2004). A detailed history will help distinguish between the two, and an inquiry for potential offending agents can help identify the irritant (see Table 4-1).

With allergic contact dermatitis, patch testing may aid in identifying responsible allergen(s). Alternative conditions, such as candidiasis, psoriasis, seborrheic dermatitis, and squamous cell carcinoma, can be excluded through appropriate use of cultures and biopsy.

Treatments for both entities involve elimination of the offending agent(s), restoration of the natural protective skin barrier, inflammation reduction, and scratch cessation (Table 4-4) (Farage, 2004; Margesson, 2004).

Intertrigo

Friction between moist skin surfaces produces this chronic condition. Found most often in genitocrural folds, intertrigo can also develop in the inguinal and intergluteal regions. Superimposed bacterial and fungal infections may complicate the condition.

The initial erythematous phase, if untreated, can progress to intense inflammation with erosions, exudate, fissuring, maceration, and crusting (Mistiaen, 2004). Symptoms typically include burning and itching. With long-standing intertrigo, hyperpigmentation and verrucous changes can develop.

Treatment entails the use of drying agents such as cornstarch and application of mild topical corticosteroids for inflammation. If skin changes do not respond, then seborrheic dermatitis, psoriasis, atopic dermatitis, pemphigus vegetans, or even scabies are considered. If the area is superinfected with bacteria or yeast, appropriate therapy is warranted.

To prevent recurrent outbreaks, obese patients are encouraged to lose weight. Other preventions include light-weight, loose-fitting clothing made of natural fibers, improved ventilation, and thorough drying between skin folds after bathing (Janniger, 2005).

Atopic Eczema

Classically presenting in the first 5 years of life, atopic dermatitis is a severe pruritic dermatitis that follows a chronic, relapsing course. Scaly patches with fissuring are evident. Individuals with atopic eczema may later develop allergic rhinitis and asthma (Spergel, 2003).

Topical corticosteroids and immunomodulators, such as tacrolimus, can control flares (Leung, 2004). For dry skin, moisturizing with emollients can offer relief.

Psoriasis

Approximately 1 to 2 percent of the United States' population is affected by psoriasis (Gelfand, 2005). Psoriasis is a T-cell—mediated autoimmune process in which proinflammatory

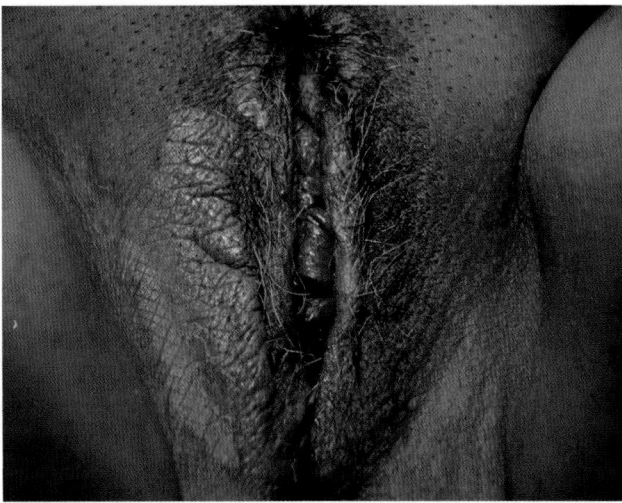

FIGURE 4-5 Psoriasis. Raised plaques are seen on the vulva. (Used with permission from Dr. Saly Thomas.)

TABLE 4-5. Differential Diagnosis of Lichen Planus

Class of Lichen Planus	Mimicking Condition
Erosive lichen planus	Lichen sclerosus
	Pemphigoid vulgaris
	Mucous membrane pemphigoid
	Behçet disease
	Plasma cell vulvitis
	Erythema multiforme major
	Stephen-Johnson syndrome
	Desquamative inflammatory vaginitis
Papulosquamous lichen planus	Molluscum contagiosum
	Genital warts
Hypertropic lichen planus	Squamous cell carcinoma

Data from Goldstein, 2005; Kaufman, 1974; Moyal-Barracco, 2004a.

cytokines induce keratinocyte and endothelial cell proliferation. Thick, red plaques covered with silvery scales are generally found on extensor limb surfaces. Occasionally, lesions involve the mons pubis or labia (Fig. 4-5). Psoriasis can be exacerbated by nervous stress and menses, with remissions experienced during summer months and pregnancy. Pruritus may be minimal or absent, and this condition is often diagnosed by skin findings alone.

Several treatments are available, and topical corticosteroids are widely used because of their rapid efficacy. High-potency corticosteroids are applied to affected areas twice daily for 2 to 4 weeks and then reduced to weekly applications. Diminishing response and skin atrophy are potential disadvantages of long-term corticosteroid use, and recalcitrant cases are best managed by a dermatologist. Vitamin D analogues, such as calcipotriene (Dovonex), although similar in efficacy to potent corticosteroids, are frequently associated with local irritation but avoid skin atrophy (Smith, 2006). Phototherapy offers short-term relief, but long-term treatment plans require a multidisciplinary team (Griffiths, 2000). For moderate to severe psoriasis, several FDA-approved immunomodulating biologic agents are available and include infliximab, adalimumab, etanercept, and ustekinumab (Smith, 2009).

Lichen Planus

This uncommon disease involves both cutaneous and mucosal surfaces and affects genders equally between ages 30 and 60 years (Mann, 1991). Although not completely understood, T-cell autoimmunity directed against basal keratinocytes is thought to underlie its pathogenesis (Goldstein, 2005). Vulvar lichen planus can present as one of three variants: (1) erosive, (2) papulosquamous, or (3) hypertrophic. Of these, erosive lichen planus is the most common vulvovaginal form and the most difficult variant to treat. Lichen planus may be drug-induced, and nonsteroidal antiinflammatory drugs, β-blocking agents, methyldopa, penicillamine, and quinine drugs have been implicated.

Diagnosis. Table 4-5 summarizes the most common imitators of lichen planus. Women typically complain of chronic vaginal discharge with intense vulvovaginal pruritus, burning pain, dyspareunia, and postcoital bleeding. On inspection, papules classically are brightly erythematous or violaceous, flat-topped, shiny polygons most commonly found on the trunk, buccal mucosa, or flexor surfaces of the extremities (Goldstein, 2005; Zellis, 1996). Lacy, white striations (Wickham striae) are frequently found in conjunction with the papules and may also be present on the buccal mucosa (Fig. 4-6). Deep, painful erosions in the posterior vestibule can extend to the labia, resulting in agglutination. With speculum insertion, vulvar skin and vaginal mucosa bleed easily. Vaginal erosions can produce adhesions and synechiae, which may lead to vaginal obliteration.

Women with suspected lichen planus require a thorough dermatologic survey looking for extragenital lesions. Nearly one quarter of women with oral lesions will have vulvovaginal

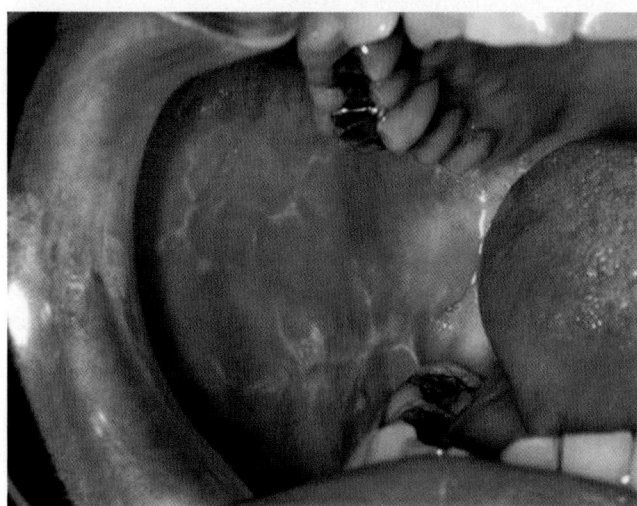

FIGURE 4-6 Oral lichen planus. Mucosal lesions manifest commonly as lacy, white striations (Wickham striae), although white papules or plaques, erosions, or blisters may also be seen. Oral lesions predominantly affect the buccal mucosa, tongue, and gingiva. (Used with permission from Dr. Edward Ellis.)

involvement, and most with erosive vulvovaginal lichen planus will have oral involvement (Pelisse, 1989). Diagnosis is confirmed by biopsy.

Vulvar Lichen Planus Treatment. Pharmacotherapy remains the first-line treatment for this condition. Additionally, vulvar care measures, discontinuing any medications associated with lichenoid changes, and psychologic support should be instituted.

Erosive vulvar lichen planus is treated initially with ultrapotent topical corticosteroid ointments, such as 0.05-percent clobetasol propionate applied daily for up to 3 months, and then slowly tapered. Refractory cases are common and may respond to a preparation containing 0.05-percent clobetasol butyrate, 3-percent oxytetracycline, and 100,000 U/g nystatin (Trimovate) (Cooper, 2006). Used in small case series, other beneficial agents include systemic corticosteroids, topical tacrolimus ointment, topical cyclosporine, and oral retinoids (Byrd, 2004; Eisen, 1990; Hersle, 1982; Morrison, 2002).

Vaginal Lichen Planus Treatment. Commonly prescribed to treat hemorrhoids, corticosteroid suppositories containing 25 mg of hydrocortisone used vaginally are helpful—specifically, if used twice daily and then tapered to maintain symptom remission (Anderson, 2002). For poorly responding patients, compounding pharmacies can provide a 100-mg hydrocortisone suppository. Potent corticosteroids are prescribed judiciously, as systemic absorption may lead to adrenocorticosuppression (Moyal-Barracco, 2004a). Combining local corticosteroid therapy with vaginal dilator use may help restore coital function in patients with moderate vaginal synechiae.

If topical medications fail, systemic treatment with prednisone 40 to 60 mg daily for up to 4 weeks may modulate symptoms (Moyal-Barracco, 2004a). Although no alternative systemic medications have been fully studied, methotrexate, hydroxychloroquine, and mycophenolate mofetil administered by providers familiar with their use are effective within a multidisciplinary approach (Eisen, 1993; Frieling, 2003; Lundqvist,

2002). Surgical adhesiolysis is a last resort. In general, vulvovaginal lichen planus is a chronic, recurrent disease for which symptomatic improvement is possible, but complete control is unlikely.

Hidradenitis Suppurativa

This chronic disease is manifested by recurrent papular lesions that may lead to abscess, fistula formation, and scarring predominantly in apocrine gland-bearing skin (Fig. 4-7). In order of frequency, affected areas include the axillae; inguinal, perianal, and perineal skin; inframammary regions; and retroauricular skin. Chronic inflammation obstructs skin follicles, with subsequent subcutaneous abscess formation, skin thickening, and deformity. Abscesses typically form sinus tracts, and the resulting disfigurement and chronic purulent drainage can be devastating physically, emotionally, and sexually.

The etiology of hidradenitis suppurativa is unknown. More than one quarter of patients will report a family history of the disease, and an autosomal dominant inheritance pattern has been hypothesized (der Werth, 2000). Although Mortimer and colleagues (1986) found higher plasma concentrations of androgens in women with hidradenitis suppurativa, others have been unable to replicate this finding (Barth, 1996).

Treatment of early cases includes local hygiene and weight reduction in patients who are obese along with topical or oral antibiotics and warm compresses. Used individually, appropriate long-term oral antibiotics and their dosages include: tetracycline, 500 mg twice daily; erythromycin, 500 mg twice daily; doxycycline, 100 mg twice daily; or minocycline, 100 mg twice daily. Topical 1-percent clindamycin solution applied twice daily may also be effective (Jemec, 1998). Additionally, a 10-week course of oral clindamycin, 300 mg twice daily, plus rifampicin, 600 mg twice daily, has shown efficacy (Gener, 2009).

As reviewed by Rhode and associates (2008), an arsenal of other treatment modalities has been reported with varying efficacies. These include cyproterone acetate (an antiandrogen available in Europe), corticosteroids, isotretinoin, cyclosporine, and infliximab. An evidence-based review of pharmacologic

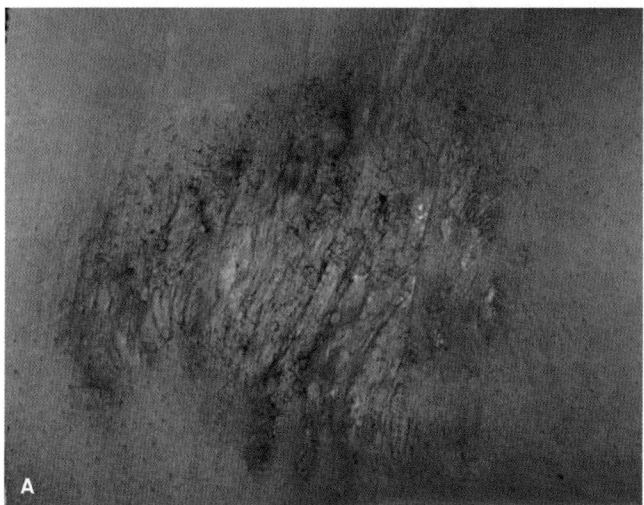
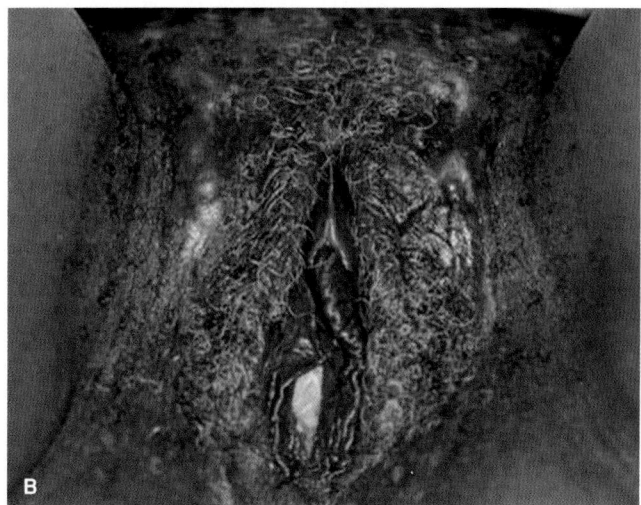

FIGURE 4-7 Hidradenitis suppurativa. **A.** Axilla shows skin puckering created by scarring from prior infection and inflammation. (Used with permission from Dr. Christine Wan.) **B.** Mons pubis with multiple draining pustules and thickened scarred skin.

interventions provided by Alhusayen (2012) suggests antibacterials and anti-tumor necrosis factor therapy are effective for hidradenitis. In late 2015, the FDA approved Humira (adalimumab) for the treatment of moderate to severe hidradenitis. Nonmedical therapies include laser and phototherapy. Severe, refractory cases may require surgical excision that often involves extensive resection of the vulva and surrounding areas. Plastic surgery techniques are often needed to close these large defects. Unfortunately, postoperative local recurrences can develop.

Aphthous Ulcers

Nearly 25 percent of women in the second and third decade of life will experience these self-limited mucosal lesions. Classically found on nonkeratinized oral mucosa, aphthous ulcers may also develop on vulvovaginal surfaces. Lesions are painful and can recur every few months. Distinguishing an aphthous ulcer from genital herpes may require appropriate cultures, serologies, and/or biopsies. Histologically, aphthous ulcers are composed of a mononuclear infiltrate with a fibrin coating. Although the etiology is unknown, some theorize the origin to be immune-mediated epithelial cell damage (Rogers, 1997). Other described triggers include stress, trauma, infection, hormonal fluctuation, and nutritional deficiencies of vitamin B_{12}, folate, iron, or zinc (Torgerson, 2006). Despite the normally self-limited nature of these ulcers, persistent lesions can lead to painful scarring (Rogers, 2003). Clinicians should consider human immunodeficiency virus testing when aphthae are large and slow to heal.

High-potency topical corticosteroids can be used at the onset of ulceration. Oral corticosteroids may be used to decrease inflammation in cases resistant to topical corticosteroids. Finally, colchicine, dapsone, and thalidomide have been shown to be effective, although they are rarely used.

VULVAR MANIFESTATIONS OF SYSTEMIC DISEASE

Systemic illnesses may initially manifest on the vulvar or vaginal mucosa as bullous, solid, or ulcerative lesions. Examples include systemic lupus erythematosus, erythema multiforme (Stevens-Johnson syndrome), pemphigus, pemphigoid, and sarcoidosis. A thorough history and physical examination usually suffice to link genital lesions with preexisting conditions. However, biopsy of vulvovaginal lesions may provide a new and unexpected diagnosis if the disorder has not yet become evident elsewhere.

■ Acanthosis Nigricans

This condition is characterized by velvety to warty, brown to black, poorly marginated plaques. These changes are typically found at skin flexures, especially on the neck, axillae, and genitocrural folds (Fig. 17-6, p. 391).

Acanthosis nigricans is commonly associated with obesity, diabetes mellitus, and polycystic ovarian syndrome. Thus, if signs or symptoms of these are present, appropriate evaluation is warranted. Common to these conditions, insulin resistance with compensatory hyperinsulinemia is thought to promote the

skin thickening of acanthosis nigricans. Insulin binds to insulin-like growth factor (IGF) receptors and leads to keratinocyte and dermal fibroblast proliferation (Hermanns-Le, 2004). Less commonly, acanthosis nigricans is caused by other insulin-resistance or fibroblast growth-factor disorders, as reviewed by Saraiya (2013).

Treatment of acanthosis nigricans has not been evaluated in randomized trials. However, weight loss can ameliorate insulin resistance, which may lead to plaque improvement. In those prescribed metformin for glucose control, improved acanthosis nigricans has been demonstrated (Romo, 2008). Topical keratinolytics and exfoliants may have benefit (Levy, 2012).

■ Crohn Disease

Up to one third of women with Crohn disease suffer from anogenital involvement, which may precede gastrointestinal (GI) symptoms and a Crohn disease diagnosis. Vulvar lesions are commonly "metastatic" in that they show typical Crohn disease granulomatous inflammation but are not contiguous with the GI involvement (Sides, 2013). However, vulvar and perianal abscesses and fistulae may extend directly from GI tract lesions. Four manifestation types are vulvar edema (usually asymmetrical), ulceration, hypertrophic lesions, and chronic abscesses (Barret, 2014). Linear "knife-cut" ulcerations and other lesions often affect inguinal, genitocrural, and interlabial folds (Fig. 4-8). All can be asymptomatic but may cause burning or pruritus.

Therapy for gastrointestinal Crohn disease generally benefits external Crohn lesions. Vulvar lesions unrelated to GI disease activity often respond to prolonged courses of oral metronidazole and corticosteroids. Anti-tumor necrosis factor alpha treatments have shown promising efficacy (Barret, 2014). Surgery often can be avoided or delayed with appropriate vulvar care, nutrition, and close collaboration with a gastroenterologist. Used as last resorts, excision of fistulous tracts or other refractory lesions and vulvectomy can be complicated by poor healing and scarring (Sides, 2013). Regardless of management, recurrence is common.

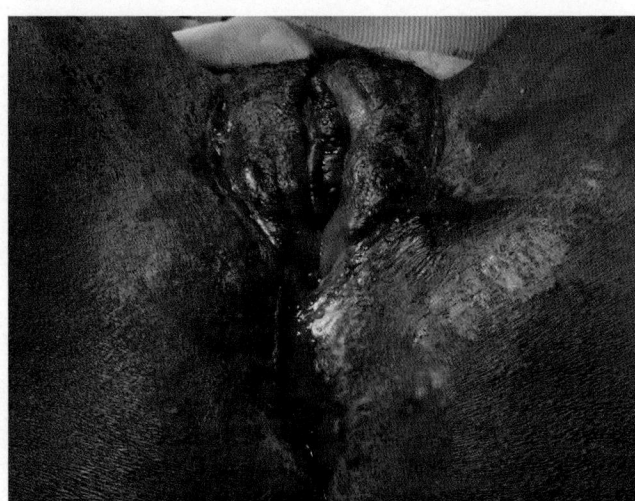

FIGURE 4-8 Vulvar Crohn disease. Knife-cut ulcers in the genitocrural folds and perineum are commonly seen with vulvar Crohn disease. (Used with permission from Dr. F. Gary Cunningham.)

■ Behçet Disease

This rare, chronic, autoinflammatory, systemic vasculitis most commonly affects patients in their twenties and thirties and those of Asian or Middle Eastern descent. Behçet disease is characterized by mucocutaneous lesions (ocular, oral, and genital) and associated systemic vasculitis. Oral and genital ulcers appear similar to aphthous ulcers and generally heal within 7 to 10 days. Nevertheless, associated pain can be debilitating. Treatment for these lesions mirrors that for aphthous ulcers.

The exact etiology of Behçet disease remains unknown, although genetic and autoimmune etiologies are suspected. Vasculitis dominates the disease process, which may involve the brain, GI tract, joints, lungs, and great vessels. Accordingly, for those suspected of Behçet disease, referral to a rheumatologist for additional testing and treatment is recommended.

DISORDERS OF PIGMENTATION

Benign variations of vulvar, perineal, and perianal skin pigmentation are commonly encountered, especially in women with darker skin. Diffuse areas of increased pigmentation are usually encountered on the labia minora and fourchette. Areas tend to be bilateral and symmetric and have an even tone and normal texture. With gentle stretching, the color attenuates evenly. This is also seen with pigment variation of chronic inflammatory dermatoses.

Various benign vulvar lesions may appear pigmented. These include benign melanosis, lentigenes, cherry hemangiomas, angiokeratomas, and seborrheic keratosis (Heller, 2013). Focal vulvar abnormalities raise concern for premalignant or malignant conditions, and prompt biopsy avoids diagnostic delay. As discussed in Chapter 29 (p. 648), high-grade intraepithelial neoplasia or invasive cancer can appear white (hyperkeratotic) or hyperpigmented and can present with or without symptoms. Melanoma is discussed in Chapter 31 (p. 688).

■ Nevus

Discrete, rounded, pigmented lesions, known as nevi or moles, are easily overlooked on the vulva. These warrant close surveillance as more than half of all melanomas arise from preexisting nevi (Kaufman, 2005). Congenital and dysplastic nevi have the most malignant potential.

Common nevi are classified into three groups: junctional, compound, and dermal, depending on whether the melanotic nevus cells are located at the epidermis-dermis junction, extend into the dermis, or evolve over time to reside entirely within the dermis. Dermal nevi may appear bluish or have normal skin coloration depending on the depth of the nevus cells and may be raised, papillary, or pedunculated.

Recommendations vary regarding biopsy of pigmented vulvar lesions. The American College of Obstetricians and Gynecologists (2008) recommends biopsy of all such lesions. Others suggest nevus-sampling criteria used elsewhere on the body in which asymmetry, uneven pigmentation, irregular borders, diameter >5 mm, and erosion or fissuring should prompt biopsy (Edwards, 2010). Burning or itching also raises concern. Histologic atypia requires full lesion excision with adequate

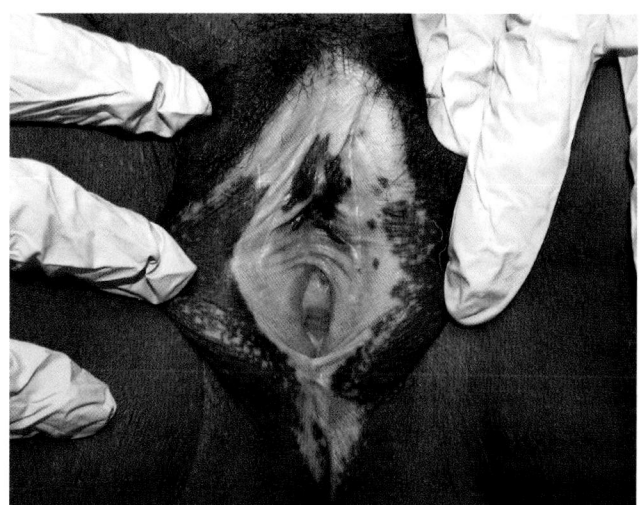

FIGURE 4-9 Vulvar vitiligo.

margins. Anatomically challenging biopsies, as with periclitoral lesions, and physical or histologic atypia may prompt referral to clinicians with specialized knowledge and experience with such lesions. Small, bland nevi that are not biopsied warrant a careful descriptive or photographic entry in the medical record and surveillance at least annually until the lesion is deemed stable. Self-examination is encouraged, and changes in lesion or symptoms are important.

■ Vitiligo

Loss of epidermal melanocytes can result in depigmented skin, termed vitiligo (Fig. 4-9). No race or ethnicity has greater risks for vitiligo, but the disease may be more disfiguring and distressing for darker-skinned individuals (Grimes, 2005).

Although etiology remains unknown, genetic factors are the most likely cause (Zhang, 2005). Approximately 20 percent of patients have at least one affected first-degree relative. Vitiligo may be mediated by an autoimmune process that destroys melanocytes. Autoimmune diseases such as Hashimoto thyroiditis, Graves disease, diabetes mellitus, rheumatoid arthritis, psoriasis, and vulvar lichen sclerosus are associated with vitiligo (Boissy, 1997; Vrijman, 2012).

Most commonly, depigmentation is symmetric and generalized, although distribution may be acral (limbs, ears) or localized. Depigmentation progression over time is variable. Sometimes confused with the epithelial changes seen with lichen sclerosus, vitiligo preserves normal skin texture and contour and is otherwise asymptomatic. There is no cure for vitiligo, and spontaneous repigmentation is rare. Several treatments for vitiligo include narrowband ultraviolet (UV) B phototherapy, excimer laser therapy, and topical immunomodulators (Baciqalupi, 2012). Most cases are self-limited and explanation of the condition alone is often sufficient.

SOLID VULVAR TUMORS

Most solid vulvar tumors are benign and arise from local tissue. Less commonly, malignant lesions arise on the vulva and are

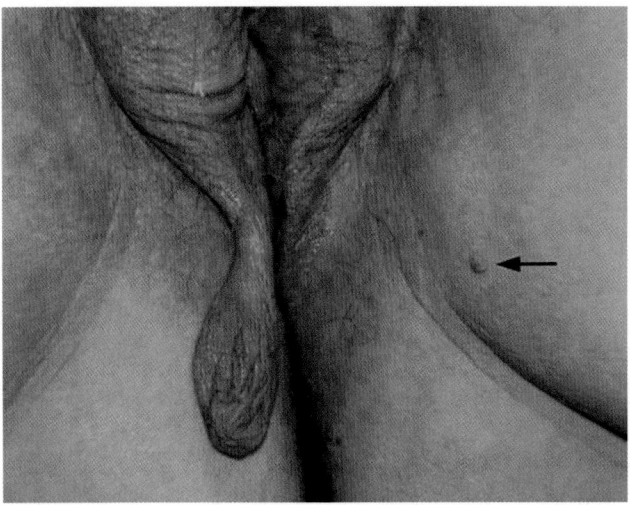

FIGURE 4-10 Vulvar acrocordons (skin tags). Lesions typically are small (*arrow*) and require no intervention. The larger vulvar acrocordon shown here was excised due to mechanical symptoms from its size.

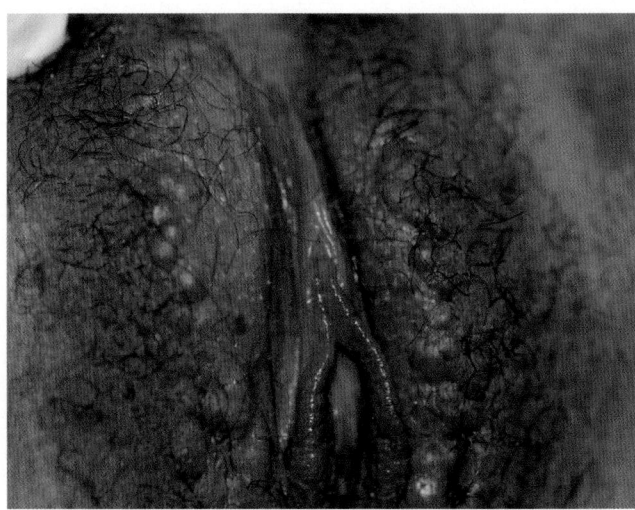

FIGURE 4-11 Vulvar syringoma. Lesions are typically arranged in clusters and may extend the length of the labia majora. Syringomas are flesh-colored or yellow and show no anatomic relationship to adjacent pubic hair follicles.

typically of squamous cell epithelial origin. Rarely, solid vulvar tumors develop as metastatic lesions. Accordingly, many growths warrant biopsy if not confidently diagnosed visually.

■ Epidermal and Dermal Lesions

Acrochordons, commonly known as skin tags, are benign, soft fibroepithelial lesions. Most often seen on the neck, axilla, or groin, these skin-colored polypoid masses are usually devoid of hair and generally measure 1 to 6 mm in diameter but can grow larger (Fig. 4-10). They are often mistaken for vulvar condylomata, and lack of therapeutic response should prompt removal for histologic analysis. Surgical removal is likewise recommended for chronic irritation or cosmetic concerns. Small lesions are easily removed under local anesthesia in an office setting. Acrochordons have been linked to diabetes mellitus, and insulin-mediated fibroblast proliferation may explain this relationship (Demir, 2002).

Seborrheic keratosis may be observed in women with concurrent lesions on the neck, face, or trunk. Sharply circumscribed, slightly raised lesions containing waxy material are typical. The malignant potential of these slow-growing lesions is minimal. Therefore, excision is offered only in cases of discomfort, disfigurement, or unclear diagnosis.

Keratoacanthoma is a rapidly growing keratinocyte proliferation originating in a pilosebaceous gland. Rarely developing on the vulva, lesions begin as firm, round papules that progress to a dome-shaped nodule with a central crater. Untreated, the lesion usually spontaneously regresses within 4 to 6 months and leaves only a slightly depressed scar. Controversy surrounds its malignant potential (Ko, 2010; Savage, 2014). Some consider keratoacanthoma benign, whereas others classify it as a well-differentiated squamous cell carcinoma. Nevertheless, its histologic resemblance to this cancer merits surgical excision in most cases with a 4- to 5-mm margin.

Syringoma is a benign eccrine (sweat gland) tumor found most frequently on the lower eyelid, neck, and face. Rarely,

the vulva may be involved bilaterally with multiple 1- to 4-mm firm papules (Fig. 4-11). The clinical appearance of vulvar syringoma is not pathognomonic. Thus, vulvar punch biopsy will establish the diagnosis and exclude malignancy. Treatment is not required. However, for those with pruritus, mild-potency topical corticosteroids and antihistamines may be helpful. In those with refractory pruritus, surgical excision or lesion ablation may be offered.

■ Subcutaneous Masses

Leiomyoma of the vulva is a rare tumor felt to arise either from smooth muscle within the vulva's erectile tissue or from transmigration through the round ligament. Surgical excision to exclude leiomyosarcoma is warranted (Nielsen, 1996).

Fibroma is a benign tumor rarely arising from deep vulvar connective tissue by fibroblast proliferation. Lesions are primarily found on the labia majora and range from 0.6 to 8 cm in diameter. Larger lesions often become pedunculated with a long stalk and may cause pain or dyspareunia. Surgical excision is indicated for symptomatic lesions or if the diagnosis is unclear.

Lipoma is a soft sessile or pedunculated mass composed of mature adipose cells. Similar to fibromas, observation is reasonable in the absence of patient complaints, although symptoms may prompt surgical excision. These lesions lack a fibrous connective tissue capsule. Thus, complete dissection may be complicated by bleeding and require a larger incision.

Ectopic breast tissue may develop along the theoretical milk lines, which extend bilaterally from the axilla through the breast and ventrally to the mons pubis. Uncommonly found in the vulva, extramammary breast tissue is hormonally sensitive and may enlarge in response to pregnancy or exogenous hormones. Uncommonly, these typically soft masses may also develop breast pathologies including fibroadenoma, Phyllodes tumor, Paget disease, and invasive adenocarcinoma.

CYSTIC VULVAR TUMORS

▇ Bartholin Gland Duct Cyst and Abscess

Mucus produced to lubricate the vulva originates in part from the Bartholin glands. Obstruction of this gland's duct is common and may follow infection, trauma, mucus changes, or congenitally narrowed ducts. However, the underlying cause is often unclear.

In some cases, cyst contents may become infected and lead to abscess formation. These tend to develop in populations with demographic profiles similar to those at high risk for sexually transmitted infections (Aghajanian, 1994). However, a wide spectrum of organisms has been cultured. *Escherichia coli* is the most common isolate, but various other gram-positive and gram-negative aerobes and anaerobes are found (Kessous, 2013; Mattila 1994; Tanaka, 2005). Infrequently, *Neisseria gonorrhoeae* or *Chlamydia trachomatis* is identified.

Diagnosis and Treatment

Most Bartholin gland cysts are small and asymptomatic except for minor discomfort during sexual contact (Fig. 4-12). With larger or infected cysts, however, patients may complain of severe vulvar pain that precludes walking, sitting, or sexual activity (Fig. 3-18, p. 318).

On physical examination, cysts typically are unilateral, round or ovoid, and fluctuant or tense. If infected, they display surrounding erythema and are tender. The mass is usually located in the inferior labia majora or lower vestibule. Whereas most cysts and abscesses lead to labial asymmetry, smaller cysts may be detected only by palpation. Bartholin abscesses on the verge of spontaneous decompression will exhibit an area of softening, where rupture will most likely occur.

Small, asymptomatic Bartholin gland duct cysts require no intervention except exclusion of neoplasia in women older than 40 years. However, a symptomatic cyst may be managed with one of several techniques. These include incision and drainage (I&D), marsupialization, and Bartholin gland excision, which are described and illustrated in Sections 43–6 through 43–8 (p. 971). Abscesses are treated with I&D or marsupialization.

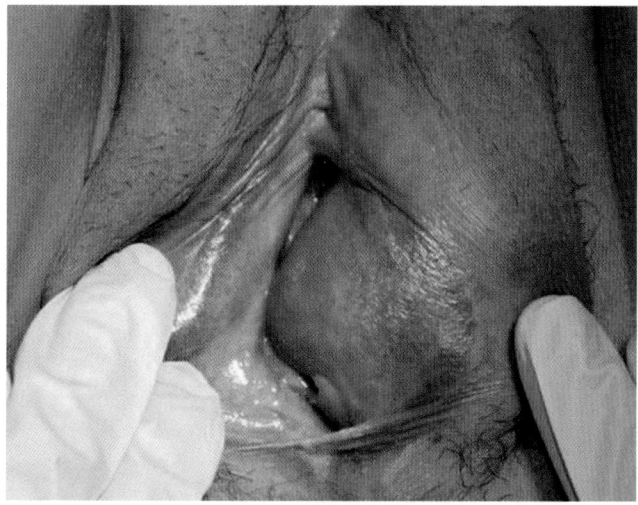

FIGURE 4-12 Bartholin gland duct cyst seen as an asymmetrical bulge in the left lower vestibule.

Malignancy

After menopause, Bartholin gland duct cysts and abscesses are uncommon and should raise concern for neoplasia. However, carcinoma of the Bartholin gland is rare, and its incidence approximates 0.1 per 100,000 women (Visco, 1996). Most are squamous carcinomas or adenocarcinomas (Heller, 2014). Given the rarity of these cancers, Bartholin gland excision is typically not indicated. Alternatively, in women older than 40 years, drainage of the cyst and biopsy of cyst wall sites adequately excludes malignancy (Visco, 1996).

▇ Urethral Diverticulum and Skene Gland

Ductal occlusion of the Skene gland or paraurethral glands may lead to paraurethral cystic enlargement and possible abscess formation. Their symptoms and treatment are described in Chapter 26 (p. 582).

▇ Epidermoid Cysts

These cysts, also known as *epidermal inclusion* or *sebaceous cysts,* are commonly found on the vulva, and less so in the vagina. Although histologically similar and lined by squamous epithelium, it is unclear if they represent separate entities. Vulvar epidermoid cysts typically form from plugged pilosebaceous units (Fig. 4-13). However, epidermoid cysts can also follow traumatic implantation of epidermal cells into deeper tissues. These cysts are variable in size, typically round or ovoid, and skin colored, yellow, or white. Generally, cysts are filled with viscous, gritty, or caseous foul-smelling material. Epidermoid cysts are generally asymptomatic and require no further evaluation. If symptomatic or secondarily infected, incision and drainage is recommended.

VULVODYNIA

In 2003, the ISSVD defined vulvodynia as "vulvar discomfort, most often described as burning pain, occurring in the absence of relevant visible findings or a specific, clinically identifiable, neurologic disorder" (Table 4-6)(Moyal-Barracco, 2004b). The term *vestibulitis* was eliminated from ISSVD terminology since inflammatory changes have not been consistently documented. Vulvar pain is described as spontaneous (unprovoked), triggered by physical pressure (provoked), or mixed. Vulvar pain described by most patients as burning, stinging, or a raw irritation is further categorized as localized or generalized.

Limited studies indicate a prevalence of vulvodynia in the general population of 3 to 11 percent (Lavy, 2007; Reed, 2004, 2014). Women from all ethnicities and a wide age range are affected. One study estimated that each year approximately 1 in 50 women will develop vulvodynia (Reed, 2008).

Vulvodynia's underlying cause is likely multifactorial and variable among individuals (Stockdale, 2014). Suspected risk factors, such as oral contraceptive pill use, genetic or immune factors, or infection (chronic yeast or human papillomavirus), remain unsupported by evidence. Whether predominantly physical or psychosocial factors trigger the pain is controversial, with strong arguments on both sides (Gunter, 2007; Lynch, 2008). Most theories propose that some local injury or noxious

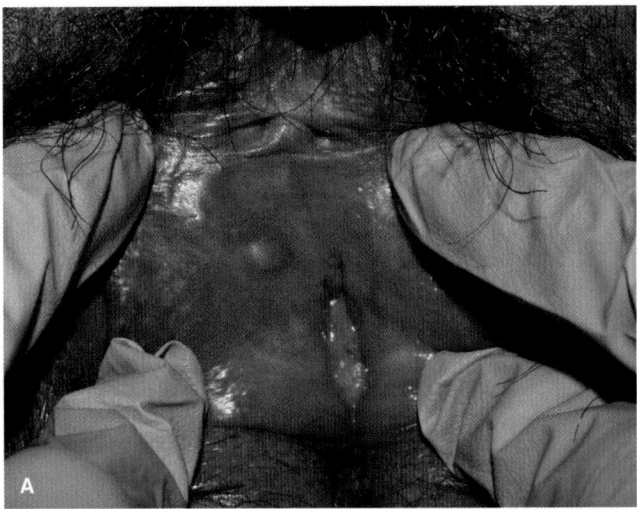 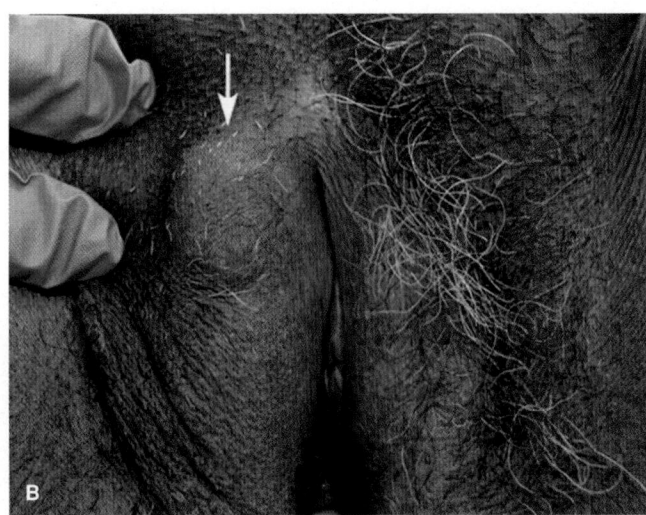

FIGURE 4-13 Epidermal inclusion cysts. **A.** This lesion on the inner labia minora required no intervention. (Used with permission from Vera bell, WHNP.) **B.** This lesion (*arrow*) on the right labia majora was excised due to patient discomfort. It was filled with tan, clay-like material. (Used with permission from Dr. Shirley Penkar.)

stimulus results in maladaptive local and/or central nervous system responses leading to a neuropathic pain syndrome (Chap. 11, p. 250). Interestingly, patients with vulvodynia have an increased prevalence of other chronic pain disorders, including interstitial cystitis, irritable bowel syndrome, fibromyalgia, and temporomandibular pain (Kennedy, 2005; Reed, 2012).

■ Diagnosis

Typically, evaluation and management attempts are delayed for years due to patient embarrassment, attempts at self-treatment, and lack of knowledge that it is a medical condition. Diagnosis

TABLE 4-6. ISSVD Terminology and Classification of Vulvar Pain

Vulvar pain related to a specific disorder
Infectious
Inflammatory
Neoplastic
Neurologic

Vulvodynia
Generalized
Provoked
Unprovoked
Mixed

Localized pain (vestibulodynia, clitorodynia, hemivulvodynia)
Provoked
Unprovoked
Mixed

Adapted with permission from the International Society for the Study of Vulvovaginal Disease (ISSVD), the International Society for the Study of Women's Sexual Health (ISSWSH), and the International Pelvic Pain Society (IPPS): 2015 Consensus terminology and classification of persistent vulvar pain.

and treatment delays, often by multiple providers, are common (Harlow, 2003, 2014).

An evidence-based algorithm for the diagnosis of vulvodynia is provided in Figure 4-14 (Haefner, 2005). Given that vulvodynia is a diagnosis of exclusion, an extensive history is critical to securing the correct diagnosis (Table 4-7) (American College of Obstetricians and Gynecologists, 2008).

Vulvodynia refers to vulvar discomfort of at least 3 to 6 months duration without an identifiable cause. Generalized or localized vulvodynia is described variably as burning, rawness, itching, or cutting pain within affected areas (Bergeron, 2001). Pain may follow a touch stimulus (allodynia) such as tight clothing, undergarments, sexual contact, or pelvic examination. Sensations may be constant, intermittent, or episodic with exacerbations noted premenstrually (Arnold, 2006).

Questioning seeks to identify frequently associated comorbid conditions or other risk factors. These may include irritable bowel syndrome, interstitial cystitis, psychologic disorders (anxiety, depression, or posttraumatic stress disorder), or a history of infectious diseases such as herpes simplex or zoster. Documentation of past surgical procedures may help identify pudendal nerve injury. A sexual history may reveal clues of past or current abuse, unfavorable coital patterns, and contraceptive modalities that could provoke vulvodynia. Additionally, clinicians inquire about recurrent candidiasis; prior genital trauma, including childbirth-related injuries; and current hygiene practices. Specifically, questions regarding use of feminine hygiene products, panty liners,

TABLE 4-7. Appropriate Vulvodynia Questions

When did the pain begin? A precipitating event?
Was the onset gradual or sudden?
Describe the pain and its intensity.
Aggravating factors? Is it provoked or unprovoked?
Relieving factors? Prior therapy?
Associated symptoms? Urinary? GI? Dermatologic?
Does pain lessen quality of life? Limit activities?

GI = gastrointestinal.

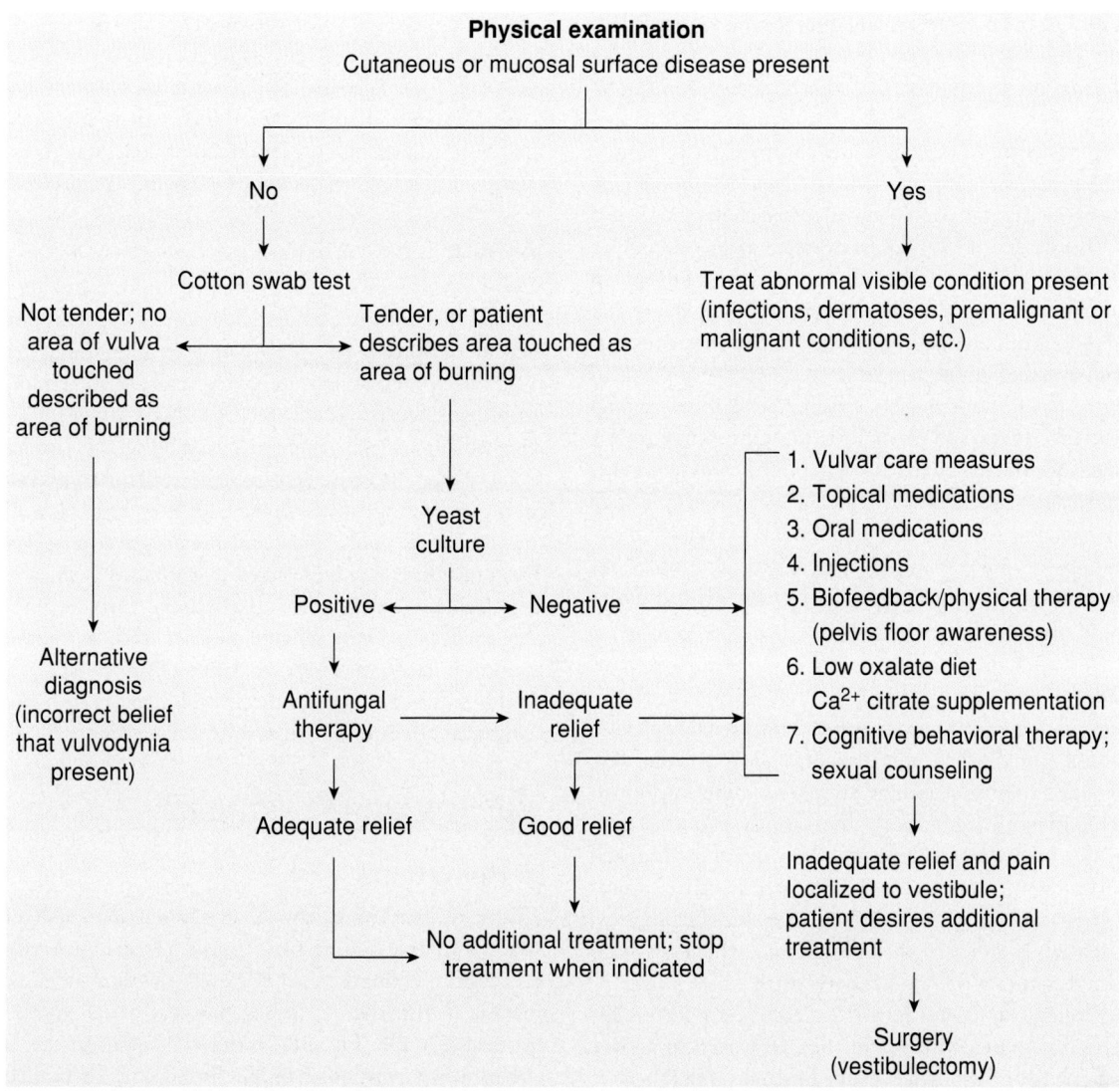

Physical examination
Cutaneous or mucosal surface disease present

No → Cotton swab test

Yes → Treat abnormal visible condition present (infections, dermatoses, premalignant or malignant conditions, etc.)

Not tender; no area of vulva touched described as area of burning

Tender, or patient describes area touched as area of burning

1. Vulvar care measures
2. Topical medications
3. Oral medications
4. Injections
5. Biofeedback/physical therapy (pelvis floor awareness)
6. Low oxalate diet Ca²⁺ citrate supplementation
7. Cognitive behavioral therapy; sexual counseling

Yeast culture

Positive ← → Negative

Alternative diagnosis (incorrect belief that vulvodynia present)

Antifungal therapy → Inadequate relief

Adequate relief   Good relief

No additional treatment; stop treatment when indicated

Inadequate relief and pain localized to vestibule; patient desires additional treatment

Surgery (vestibulectomy)

FIGURE 4-14 Algorithm for the diagnosis and treatment of vulvodynia. (Reproduced with permission from Haefner HK, Collins ME, Davis GD, et al: The vulvodynia guideline, J Low Genit Tract Dis 2005 Jan;9(1):40–51.)

laundry and body soaps, bath additives, shaving, and type of undergarment fabric worn can be helpful. Prior therapies are documented to avoid unnecessary treatment repetition.

By definition, vulvodynia lacks specific diagnostic physical signs. Therefore, a thorough examination excludes other possible pathologies. Inspection of the external vulva for lesions or irritation is followed by examination of the vestibule looking for focal, usually mild, erythema at vestibular gland openings. Use of a magnifying lens or colposcope and directed biopsies may be helpful. Of note, Bowen and colleagues (2008) found clinically relevant dermatoses in 61 percent of refractory vulvodynia patients referred to their tertiary care vulvovaginal clinic.

Systematic pain mapping of the vestibule, perineum, and inner thigh is completed, and documentation serves as a reference to assess treatment success (see Fig. 4-1). A cotton swab is used to check for allodynia and hyperesthesia. The swab end can first be unwound to form a cotton-fiber wisp. Subsequently, the wooden stick is broken to form a sharp point to retest the same areas. Pain scale scores are recorded and followed over time.

As a diagnosis of exclusion, no specific laboratory test can confirm vulvodynia, although a saline "wet prep" of vaginal secretions, vaginal pH testing, and appropriate cultures as clinically indicated for yeast and herpes virus help exclude underlying vulvovaginitis. Focal abnormalities typically prompt biopsy.

■ Treatment

Like other chronic pain conditions, vulvodynia is challenging to treat. Approximately one in 10 women with vulvodynia will experience spontaneous remission (Reed, 2008). Due to few well-designed, randomized clinical trials, no specific therapy for vulvodynia has demonstrated superiority. Often, a combination of several therapeutic approaches is required to stabilize and alleviate symptoms (Haefner, 2005; Landry, 2008). Without improvement, surgical excision is a final option. Treatment approaches to vulvodynia are described further by Haefner and associates (2005) and reviewed by Landry and colleagues (2008).

Behavioral Therapy

The first step in managing all vulvar disorders includes vulvar care as summarized in Table 4-2. Also, accurate medical information can help resolve some of the fears and questions associated with vulvodynia. The National Vulvodynia Association provides patient information and support and can be accessed online at www.nva.org.

Vulvodynia is currently seen as more complex than a simple psychosexual problem. Compared with the general population, no differences in marital contentment or psychologic distress are found (Bornstein, 1999). Nevertheless, early counseling includes a basic assessment of the intimate partner relationship and of sexual functioning. Education regarding foreplay, sexual positions, lubrication, and alternatives to vaginal intercourse is offered if potentially helpful.

Back pain, pelvic floor muscle spasm, or vaginismus may coexist with vulvodynia, and pelvic floor muscle examination is described and illustrated in Chapter 11 (p. 257). If coexistent, a physical therapist familiar with treating these concerns may provide internal and external massage, myofascial release techniques, acupressure, joint manipulation, electrical stimulation, therapeutic ultrasonography, and pelvic floor muscle retraining to improve symptoms (Bergeron, 2002).

Medications

Agents for vulvodynia treatment may be administered topically, orally, or intralesionally. Of topical agents, 5-percent lidocaine ointment applied sparingly to the vestibule 30 minutes prior to sexual intercourse can significantly decrease dyspareunia, and long-term use may promote healing by minimizing feedback pain amplification (Zolnoun, 2003). Numerous other topical anesthetic preparations are reported to have variable success. However, caution is exercised with benzocaine, which is associated with increased rates of contact dermatitis.

Eva and colleagues (2003) found decreased estrogen-receptor expression in women with vulvodynia. However, topical or intravaginal estrogen therapy has yielded mixed results.

As reported by Boardman and coworkers (2008), topical gabapentin cream is well-tolerated, effective, and avoids the potential side effects of systemic gabapentin therapy. In their study, 0.5 mL of a compounded 2-, 4-, or 6-percent gabapentin-containing cream was applied three times daily for at least 8 weeks to affected vulvar areas.

The two major classes of oral medications reported to help vulvodynia are antidepressants and anticonvulsants. However, polypharmacy is avoided by clinicians prescribing one drug at a time, and contraception use is required for reproductive-aged patients. Tricyclic antidepressants (TCAs) have become a first-line agent in the treatment of vulvodynia, and reported response rates may reach 47 percent (Munday, 2001). In our experience, amitriptyline started at doses between 5 and 25 mg orally nightly and increased as needed by 10 to 25 mg weekly yields the best results. Final daily doses do not exceed 150 to 200 mg. Importantly, compliance is encouraged during the nearly 4-week lag required to achieve significant pain relief.

Cases resistant to TCAs may be treated with the anticonvulsants gabapentin or carbamazepine (Table 11-5, p. 259) (Ben David, 1999). Oral gabapentin is initiated at a dosage of 100 mg three times daily and gradually increased over 6 to 8 weeks to a maximal daily dose of 3600 mg. Pain is reassessed every 1 to 2 weeks (Haefner, 2005).

Although topical corticosteroids generally do not help patients with vulvodynia, injections using a combination of corticosteroids and local anesthetics have been used for localized vulvodynia (Mandal, 2010; Murina, 2001). Alternatively, botulinum toxin A injections into the levator ani muscles have been reported effective for vulvodynia-related vaginismus (Bertolasi, 2009).

Surgery

Women with vulvodynia who fail to improve despite aggressive medical therapy are candidates for surgery. Options include local excision of a precise pain locus, complete resection of the vestibule (vestibulectomy), or resection of the vestibule and perineum (perineoplasty) (Section 43-22, p. 979). Traas and associates (2006) reported high success rates with vestibulectomy among women younger than 30 years. Perineoplasty is the most extensive of the three procedures. Its incision extends from just below the urethra to the perineal body, usually terminating above the anal orifice. This procedure may be selected if significant perineal scarring is suspected to contribute to dyspareunia. Overall, improvement rates for appropriately selected patients are high following vulvar excision procedures. However, surgery is reserved for those with severe, localized, long-standing vestibular pain who have failed significant attempts at conservative management.

VULVOVAGINAL TRAUMA

◼ Hematoma

This may develop in the relatively vascular vulva following straddle injury, trauma from coitus or assault, or vulvovaginal procedures. Hematomas may develop within subcutaneous tissues or within the superficial perineal pouch of the anterior perineal triangle (Fig. 38-26, p. 819). Within the latter, laceration of the vestibular bulb, clitoral crus, or branches of the internal pudendal vessels may create a sizable mass (Fig. 4-15). Given the protected anatomic location and adipose padding of the labia majora, traumatic vulvar and vaginal injuries are rare in adults. These are much more frequent in children who lack

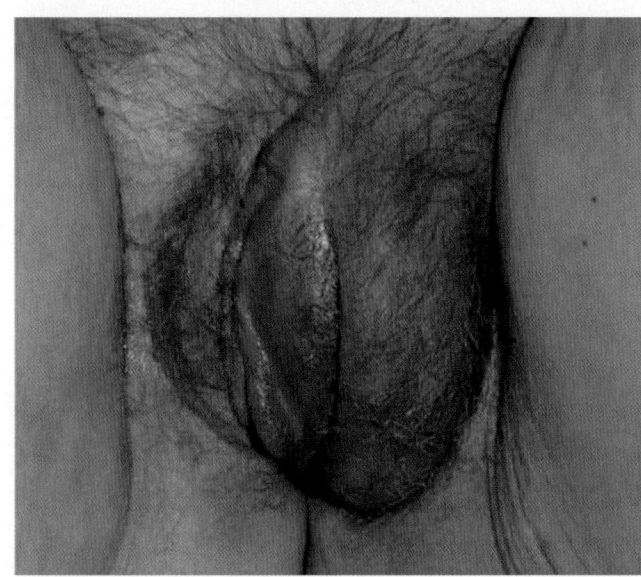

FIGURE 4-15 Vulvar hematoma.

such padding, and differentiating straddle injury and sexual abuse in children is often challenging, as injury patterns are not reliably discriminating.

Often requiring a general anesthetic, thorough examination of the vulva and vagina will estimate hematoma stability and the integrity of the surrounding bowel, bladder, urethra, and rectum. If there is no associated organ injury, the venous nature of most vulvar hematomas makes them candidates for conservative management with cool packs followed by sitz baths, pain control, and Foley catheter bladder drainage as needed. In general, vaginal hematomas measuring >4 cm or rapidly expanding are surgically explored to secure bleeding vessels. However, following incision and clot evacuation, a cavity is often seen without an identifiable bleeding vessel. To prevent reaccumulation, the cavity is closed in layers with absorbable or delayed-absorbable suture using a running or interrupted stitch closure.

Laceration

Penetrating trauma accounts for most vaginal injuries. Common causes include pelvic fracture, forced inanimate objects, coitus, and hydraulic forces such as those experienced with water skiing. Atrophic vaginal changes can predispose to injury.

With extensive laceration, examination under anesthesia is usually necessary to perform a thorough assessment and to exclude intraperitoneal damage. Moreover, if the peritoneal cavity has been breached, abdominal cavity exploration by laparotomy or laparoscopy is warranted to exclude visceral injury and supralevator or retroperitoneal hematoma.

Treatment goals include hemostasis and restoration of normal anatomy. Irrigation, debridement, and primary repair are key steps during initial management. The vaginal mucosa is typically reapproximated with running or interrupted stitches with absorbable or delayed-absorbable suture. Uncommonly, infection warrants laceration healing by secondary intention. Nonexpanding hematomas may be managed conservatively, whereas expanding masses often require evacuation and isolation of bleeding vessels. With laceration or hematoma, postoperatively, a vaginal pack can help tamponade any continued bleeding.

VAGINAL CONDITIONS

Foreign Body

Trauma or chronic irritation from a foreign body placed into the vagina can affect all ages. Objects vary by age group, and small objects may become lodged in a child's vagina during play. An adolescent may be unable to retrieve or may be unaware of a vaginal tampon or piece of a broken condom. In adults, sexual misadventure or abuse can usually explain most objects found.

Three notable items include a retained tampon or contraceptive sponge and the vaginal pessary. Women with a retained tampon or sponge typically complain of foul-smelling vaginal discharge with some associated pruritus, discomfort, or unscheduled bleeding. A history of multiple unsuccessful retrieval attempts may be elicited. In the absence of a leukocytosis, fever, or evidence of endometritis or salpingitis, simple removal

is sufficient treatment. Vaginal lavage to cleanse the vagina is not indicated and may actually increase the ascending infection risk. Toxic shock syndrome has been described with both tampons and contraceptive sponges, and its management is outlined in Chapter 3 (p. 80). Vaginal pessaries are frequently selected to conservatively treat pelvic organ prolapse or incontinence. Associated complications with these devices and their management are described fully in Chapter 24 (p. 553).

Desquamative Inflammatory Vaginitis

This uncommon, severe form of inflammatory vaginitis develops primarily in perimenopausal women, and white women appear most often affected. Although its etiology is unknown, it may represent a variant of erosive vaginal lichen planus (Edwards, 1988). Possible triggers include diarrhea or antibiotic use (Bradford, 2010). Patients typically complain of copious vaginal discharge, introital burning, and dyspareunia, all of which are refractory to common therapies. On examination, a diffuse, exudative, purulent yellow or green discharge is present on the vaginal walls and varying degrees of vestibular-vaginal erythema are noted. Microscopy reveals many polymorphonuclear and parabasal cells, but pathogens such as trichomonads or yeast forms are absent. The vaginal pH is elevated, and exclusionary test results for gonorrhea and chlamydial infection are negative. The profuse leukorrhea may lead to an erroneous diagnosis of pelvic inflammatory disease or cervicitis, but pelvic tenderness is absent. Although no randomized clinical trials are available, Sobel (2011) reports favorable outcomes with 2-percent intravaginal clindamycin cream or intravaginal hydrocortisone cream or suppositories for 4 to 6 weeks. Whether the efficacy of clindamycin is due to its antibacterial or its antiinflammatory properties is unknown (Bradford, 2010). Patients and clinicians should view this as a chronic condition with expectation of prolonged treatment courses, relapse, and need for retreatment.

Diethylstilbestrol-induced Reproductive Tract Abnormalities

In the mid-1900s, diethylstilbestrol (DES), a synthetic nonsteroidal estrogen, was prescribed to women in the United States for several pregnancy-related problems. Daughters exposed in utero to DES had congenital reproductive tract anomalies and demonstrated increased rates of vaginal clear cell adenocarcinoma (Herbst, 1971). More commonly, *vaginal adenosis,* areas of columnar epithelium within the vaginal squamous mucosa, are found in these women. Vaginal adenosis typically appears as red, granular patches. Symptoms include vaginal irritation, discharge, intermenstrual bleeding, and postcoital bleeding. A fuller discussion of DES-related defects is found in Chapter 18 (p. 423).

Gartner Duct Cyst

Most vaginal cysts are epidermoid cysts, urethral diverticula, or Gartner duct cysts. The last are uncommon vaginal cysts developing from mesonephric (wolffian) duct remnants (Chap. 18, p. 404). They are typically asymptomatic and found within the lateral vaginal wall during routine examination.

Symptoms, if present, include dyspareunia, vaginal pain, and difficulty inserting tampons. Examination reveals a tense cyst that is palpable or seen to bulge from beneath the vaginal wall. Observation is reasonable in most cases, although marsupialization or excision may be appropriate for symptomatic Gartner duct cysts.

CERVICAL CONDITIONS

■ Eversion

The squamocolumnar junction (SCJ) borders between the columnar epithelium of the endocervix and the squamous epithelium of the ectocervix. As described and illustrated in Chapter 29 (p. 625), endocervical tissue in some women may migrate outward from the endocervical canal in a process termed eversion, thought to be hormonally mediated. As a result, the SCJ lies further distally from the external cervical os. Although eversion is a normal finding, asymmetry of the columnar epithelium surrounding the cervical os can mimic an erosive lesion, and cervical biopsy can aid clarification.

■ Nabothian Cyst

Mucus-secreting columnar cells line the endocervical canal. During squamous metaplasia, squamous epithelium may cover functional glandular cells and secretions may accumulate. As this benign process continues, smooth, clear, white or yellow, rounded elevations may form and are visible during routine examination (Fig. 4-16). They also are frequently seen as well-defined anechoic sonolucency along the endocervical canal (Fig. 2-14, p. 30).

Nabothian cysts typically do not warrant therapy. However, if they grow large enough to make Pap testing or cervical examination difficult or cause symptoms, they can be opened with a biopsy forceps and drained. Moreover, if the diagnosis of a cervical mass is uncertain, biopsy for histologic confirmation is obtained.

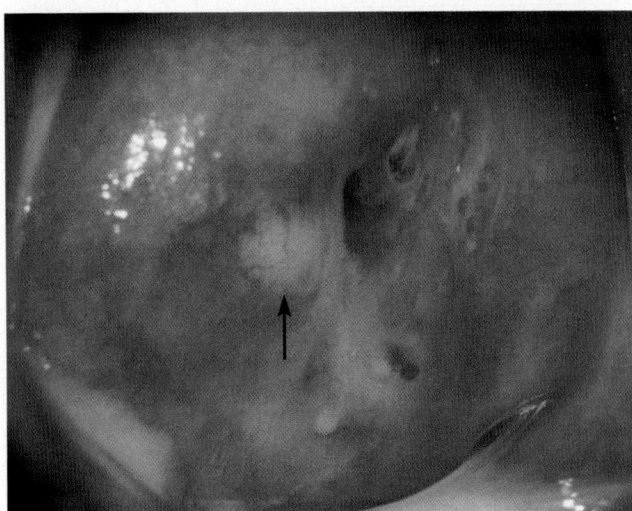

FIGURE 4-16 Cervical nabothian cyst (*arrow*) is seen as a raised, symmetric, smooth, yellow or clear lesion on the ectocervix.

■ Endocervical Polyp

One of the most common benign neoplasms of the cervix is a hyperplastic projection of endocervical tissue known as an *endocervical polyp* (Fig. 8-8, p. 188). Lesions are usually found during routine pelvic examination. They are generally asymptomatic but may be associated with leukorrhea or postcoital spotting. Additional discussion and treatment options are found in Chapter 8.

■ Cervical Stenosis

This narrowing of the cervical canal or opening may be congenital or acquired. Congenital stenosis is rare and likely due to segmental müllerian hypoplasia (Chap. 18, p. 419). In contrast, acquired stenosis is usually iatrogenic due to scarring after cervical excisional procedures such as cold-knife conization and loop electrosurgical excision. This complication is estimated to follow 1 to 2 percent of such procedures. Infection, neoplasia, severe atrophy, and radiation changes are rarer causes.

Diagnosis is based on symptoms and physical findings, as a precise and universally accepted definition is lacking. Symptoms of stenosis in menstruating women include dysmenorrhea, amenorrhea, and infertility. Postmenopausal women are usually asymptomatic until fluid, exudates, or blood accumulates behind the obstruction. The terms hydrometra (fluid), pyometra (pus), or hematometra (blood) are used to describe these conditions and are discussed additionally in Chapter 9 (p. 212). An inability to introduce a dilator into the endocervical canal is generally considered diagnostic. If obstruction is complete, a soft, enlarged uterus from trapped intracavitary fluid is sometimes palpable.

Cervical stenosis is relieved by introduction of dilators of progressively increasing diameter, which may require anesthesia. Preprocedural misoprostol may aid by softening the cervix (Chap. 41, p. 901). In postmenopausal women, pretreatment for several weeks with vaginal estrogen cream may also assist dilatation. Moreover, sonographic guidance can help avert uterine perforation, especially in postmenopausal women (Christianson, 2008). If cervical stenosis is suspected as contributory to infertility, assisted reproduction techniques may be indicated as described in Chapter 20 (p. 461).

REFERENCES

Aghajanian A, Bernstein L, Grimes DA: Bartholin's duct abscess and cyst: a case-control study. South Med J 87(1):26, 1994

Alhusayen R, Shear NH: Pharmacologic interventions for hidradenitis suppurativa: what does the evidence say? Am J Clin Dermatol 13(5):283, 2012

American College of Obstetricians and Gynecologists: Diagnosis and management of vulvar skin disorders. Practice Bulletin No. 93, May 2008, Reaffirmed 2010

American College of Obstetricians and Gynecologists: Vulvodynia. Committee Opinion No. 345, October 2006, Reaffirmed 2008

Anderson M, Kutzner S, Kaufman RH: Treatment of vulvovaginal lichen planus with vaginal hydrocortisone suppositories. Obstet Gynecol 100(2):359, 2002

Arnold LD, Bachmann GA, Rosen R, et al: Vulvodynia: characteristics and associations with comorbidities and quality of life. Obstet Gynecol 107(3):617, 2006

Assmann T, Becker-Wegerich P, Grewe M, et al: Tacrolimus ointment for the treatment of vulvar lichen sclerosus. J Am Acad Dermatol 48(6):935, 2003

Bacigalupi RM, Postolova A, Davis RS: Evidence-based, non-surgical treatments for vitiligo: a review. Am J Clin Dermatol 13(4):217, 2012

Barret M, de Parades V, Battistella M, et al: Crohn's disease of the vulva. J Crohns Colitis 8(7):563, 2014

Barth JH, Layton AM, Cunliffe WJ: Endocrine factors in pre- and postmenopausal women with hidradenitis suppurativa. Br J Dermatol 134(6):1057, 1996

Ben David B, Friedman M: Gabapentin therapy for vulvodynia. Anesth Analg 89(6):1459, 1999

Bergeron S, Binik YM, Khalife S, et al: Vulvar vestibulitis syndrome: reliability of diagnosis and evaluation of current diagnostic criteria. Obstet Gynecol 98(1):45, 2001

Bergeron S, Brown C, Lord MJ, et al: Physical therapy for vulvar vestibulitis syndrome: a retrospective study. J Sex Marital Ther 28(3):183, 2002

Bertolasi L, Frasson E, Cappelletti JY, et al: Botulinum neurotoxin type A injections for vaginismus secondary to vulvar vestibulitis syndrome. Obstet Gynecol 114(5):1008, 2009

Boardman LA, Cooper AS, Blais LR, et al: Topical gabapentin in the treatment of localized and generalized vulvodynia. Obstet Gynecol 112(3):579, 2008

Boissy RE, Nordlund JJ: Molecular basis of congenital hypopigmentary disorders in humans: a review. Pigment Cell Res 10(1–2):12, 1997

Bor S, Feiwel M, Chanarin I: Vitiligo and its aetiological relationship to organ-specific autoimmune disease. Br J Dermatol 81(2):83, 1969

Bornstein J, Heifetz S, Kellner Y, et al: Clobetasol dipropionate 0.05% versus testosterone propionate 2% topical application for severe vulvar lichen sclerosus. Am J Obstet Gynecol 178(1 Pt 1):80, 1998

Bornstein J, Zarfati D, Goldik Z, et al: Vulvar vestibulitis: physical or psychosexual problem? Obstet Gynecol 93(5 Pt 2):876, 1999

Bowen AR, Vester A, Marsden L, et al: The role of vulvar skin biopsy in the evaluation of chronic vulvar pain. Am J Obstet Gynecol 199(5):467.e1, 2008

Bradford J, Fischer G: Desquamative inflammatory vaginitis: differential diagnosis and alternate diagnostic criteria. J Low Genit Tract Dis 14(4): 306, 2010

Byrd JA, Davis MDP, Rogers RS III: Recalcitrant symptomatic vulvar lichen planus. Arch Dermatol 140(6):715, 2004

Christianson MS, Barker MA, Lindheim SR: Overcoming the challenging cervix: techniques to access the uterine cavity. J Low Genit Tract Dis 12(1):24, 2008

Clark JA, Muller SA: Lichen sclerosus et atrophicus in children. A report of 24 cases. Arch Dermatol 95(5):476, 1967

Cooper SM, Wojnarowska F: Influence of treatment of erosive lichen planus of the vulva on its prognosis. Arch Dermatol 142(3):289, 2006

Crone AM, Stewart EJ, Wojnarowska F, et al: Aetiological factors in vulvar dermatitis. J Eur Acad Dermatol Venereol 14(3):181, 2000

Demir S, Demir Y: Acrochordon and impaired carbohydrate metabolism. Acta Diabetol 39(2):57, 2002

der Werth JM, Williams HC: The natural history of hidradenitis suppurativa. J Eur Acad Dermatol Venereol 14(5):389, 2000

Edwards L: Pigmented vulvar lesions. Dermatol Ther 23(5):449, 2010

Edwards L, Friedrich EG Jr: Desquamative vaginitis: lichen planus in disguise. Obstet Gynecol 71(6 Pt 1):832, 1988

Eichner R, Kahn M, Capetola RJ: Effects of topical retinoids on cytoskeletal proteins: implications for retinoid effects on epidermal differentiation. J Invest Dermatol 98(2):154, 1992

Eisen D: The therapy of oral lichen planus. Crit Rev Oral Biol Med 4(2):141, 1993

Eisen D, Ellis CN, Duell EA, et al: Effect of topical cyclosporine rinse on oral lichen planus. A double-blind analysis. N Engl J Med 323(5):290, 1990

Eva LJ, MacLean AB, Reid WM, et al: Estrogen receptor expression in vulvar vestibulitis syndrome. Am J Obstet Gynecol 189(2):458, 2003

Farage M, Maibach HI: The vulvar epithelium differs from the skin: implications for cutaneous testing to address topical vulvar exposures. Contact Dermatitis 51(4):201, 2004

Fischer GO: The commonest causes of symptomatic vulvar disease: a dermatologist's perspective. Australas J Dermatol 37(1):12, 1996

Fisher AA: Allergic reaction to feminine hygiene sprays. Arch Dermatol 108(6):801, 1973

Food and Drug Administration: Tacrolimus (marketed as Protopic Ointment) Information, 2010. Available at: http://www.fda.gov/Drugs/DrugSafety/PostmarketDrugSafetyInformationforPatientsandProviders/ucm107845.htm. Accessed July 25, 2014

Frieling U, Bonsmann G, Schwarz T, et al: Treatment of severe lichen planus with mycophenolate mofetil. J Am Acad Dermatol 49:1063, 2003

Funaro D: A double-blind, randomized prospective study evaluating topical clobetasol propionate 0.05% versus topical tacrolimus 0.1% in patients with vulvar lichen sclerosus. J Am Acad Dermatol 71(1):84, 2014

Gelfand JMStern RS, Nijsten T: The prevalence of psoriasis in African Americans: results from a population-based study. J Am Acad Dermatol 52(1):23, 2005

Gener G, Canoui-Poitrine F, Revuz JE, et al: Combination therapy with clindamycin and rifampicin for hidradenitis suppurativa: a series of 116 consecutive patients. Dermatology 219(2):148, 2009

Goldstein AT, Burrows LJ: Surgical treatment of clitoral phimosis caused by lichen sclerosus. Am J Obstet Gynecol 196(2):126.e1, 2007

Goldstein AT, Creasey A, Pfau R, et al: A double-blind, randomized controlled trial of clobetasol versus pimecrolimus in patients with vulvar lichen sclerosus. J Am Acad Dermatol 64(6):e99, 2011

Goldstein AT, Metz A: Vulvar lichen planus. Clin Obstet Gynecol 48(4):818, 2005

Griffiths CE, Clark CM, Chalmers RJ, et al: A systematic review of treatments for severe psoriasis. Health Technol Assess 4(40):1, 2000

Grimes PE: New insights and new therapies in vitiligo. JAMA 293(6):730, 2005

Gunter J: Vulvodynia: new thoughts on a devastating condition. Obstet Gynecol Surv 62(12):812, 2007

Haefner HK, Collins ME, Davis GD, et al: The vulvodynia guideline. J Low Genit Tract Dis 9(1):40, 2005

Harlow BL, Kunitz CG, Nguyen RH, et al: Prevalence of symptoms consistent with a diagnosis of vulvodynia: population-based estimates from 2 geographic regions. Am J Obstet Gynecol 210(1):40.e1, 2014

Harlow BL, Stewart EG: A population-based assessment of chronic unexplained vulvar pain: have we underestimated the prevalence of vulvodynia? J Am Med Womens Assoc 58(2):82, 2003

Heller D: Pigmented vulvar lesions—a pathology review of lesions that are not melanoma. J Low Genit Tract Dis 17(3):320, 2013

Heller DS, Bean S: Lesions of the Bartholin gland: a review. J Low Genit Tract Dis 18(4):351, 2014

Hengge UR, Krause W, Hofmann H, et al: Multicentre, phase II trial on the safety and efficacy of topical tacrolimus ointment for the treatment of lichen sclerosus. Br J Dermatol 155(5):1021, 2006

Herbst AL, Ulfelder H, Poskanzer DC: Adenocarcinoma of the vagina. Association of maternal stilbestrol therapy with tumor appearance in young women. N Engl J Med 284(15):878, 1971

Hermanns-Le T, Scheen A, Pierard GE: Acanthosis nigricans associated with insulin resistance: pathophysiology and management. Am J Clin Dermatol 5(3):199, 2004

Hersle K, Mobacken H, Sloberg K, et al: Severe oral lichen planus: treatment with an aromatic retinoid (etretinate). Br J Dermatol 106(1):77, 1982

Hillemanns P, Untch M, Prove F, et al: Photodynamic therapy of vulvar lichen sclerosus with 5-aminolevulinic acid. Obstet Gynecol 93(1):71, 1999

International Society for the Study of Vulvovaginal Disease: 2014 Bibliography current ISSVD terminology. 2014. Available at: http://issvd.org/wordpress/wp-content/uploads/2014/02/2014-BIBLIOGRAPHY-CURRENT-ISSVD-TERMINOLOGYrev.pdf. Accessed July 26, 2014

Janniger CK, Schwartz RA, Szepietowski JC, et al: Intertrigo and common secondary skin infections. Am Fam Physician 72(5):833, 2005

Jemec GB, Wendelboe P: Topical clindamycin versus systemic tetracycline in the treatment of hidradenitis suppurativa. J Am Acad Dermatol 39(6):971, 1998

Kahana M, Levy A, Schewach-Millet M, et al: Appearance of lupus erythematosus in a patient with lichen sclerosus et atrophicus of the elbows. J Am Acad Dermatol 12(1 Pt 1):127, 1985

Kaufman RH, Faro S, Brown D: Benign Diseases of the Vulva and Vagina, 5th ed. Philadelphia, Mosby, 2005

Kaufman RH, Gardner HL, Brown D Jr, et al: Vulvar dystrophies: an evaluation. Am J Obstet Gynecol 120(3):363, 1974

Kennedy CM, Nygaard IE, Saftlas A, et al: Vulvar disease: a pelvic floor pain disorder? Am J Obstet Gynecol 192:1829, 2005

Kessous R, Aricha-Tamir B, Sheizaf B, et al: Clinical and microbiological characteristics of Bartholin gland abscesses. Obstet Gynecol 122(4):794, 2013

Kligman AM, Grove GL, Hirose R, et al: Topical tretinoin for photoaged skin. J Am Acad Dermatol 15(4 Pt 2):836, 1986a

Kligman LH: Effects of all-trans-retinoic acid on the dermis of hairless mice. J Am Acad Dermatol 15(4 Pt 2):779, 1986b

Ko CJ: Keratoacanthoma: facts and controversies. Clin Dermatol 28(3):254, 2010

Kunstfeld R, Kirnbauer R, Stingl G, et al: Successful treatment of vulvar lichen sclerosus with topical tacrolimus. Arch Dermatol 139(7):850, 2003

Landry T, Bergeron S, Dupuis MJ, et al: The treatment of provoked vestibulodynia. Clin J Pain 24:155, 2008

Lavy RJ, Hynan LS, Haley RW: Prevalence of vulvar pain in an urban, minority population. J Reprod Med 52:59, 2007

Leung KM, Margolis RU, Chan SO: Expression of phosphacan and neurocan during early development of mouse retinofugal pathway. Brain Res Dev Brain Res 152(1):1, 2004

Levy L, Zeichner JA: Dermatologic manifestation of diabetes. J Diabetes 4(1):68, 2012

Lundqvist EN, Wahlin YB, Hofer PA: Methotrexate supplemented with steroid ointments for the treatment of severe erosive lichen ruber. Acta Derm Venereol 82:63, 2002

Lynch PJ: Lichen simplex chronicus (atopic/neurodermatitis) of the anogenital region. Dermatol Ther 17(1):8, 2004

Lynch PJ: Vulvodynia as a somatoform disorder. J Reprod Med 53:390, 2008

Lynch PJ, Moyal-Barracco M, Bogliatto F, et al: 2006 ISSVD classification of vulvar dermatoses: pathological subsets and their clinical correlates. J Reprod Med 52(1):3, 2007

Lynch PJ, Moyal-Barracco M, Scurry J, et al: 2011 ISSVD terminology and classification of vulvar dermatological disorders: an approach to clinical diagnosis. J Reprod Med 16(4):339, 2012

Mandal D, Nunns D, Byrne M, et al: Guidelines for the management of vulvodynia. Br J Dermatol 162(6):1180, 2010

Mann MS, Kaufman RH: Erosive lichen planus of the vulva. Clin Obstet Gynecol 34(3):605, 1991

Margesson LJ: Contact dermatitis of the vulva. Dermatol Ther 17(1):20, 2004

Marren P, Wojnarowska F, Powell S: Allergic contact dermatitis and vulvar dermatoses. Br J Dermatol 126(1):52, 1992

Mattila A, Miettinen A, Heinonen PK: Microbiology of Bartholin's duct abscess. Infect Dis Obstet Gynecol 1(6):265, 1994

Mazdisnian F, Degregorio F, Mazdisnian F, et al: Intralesional injection of triamcinolone in the treatment of lichen sclerosus. J Reprod Med 44(4):332, 1999

Mirowski GW, Edwards L: Diagnostic and therapeutic procedures. In Edwards L (ed): Genital Dermatology Atlas. Philadelphia, Lippincott Williams & Wilkins, 2004, p 9

Mistiaen P, Poot E, Hickox S, et al: Preventing and treating intertrigo in the large skin folds of adults: a literature overview. Dermatol Nurs 16(1):43, 2004

Morrison L, Kratochvil FJ III, Gorman A: An open trial of topical tacrolimus for erosive oral lichen planus. J Am Acad Dermatol 47(4):617, 2002

Mortimer PS, Dawber RP, Gales MA, et al: Mediation of hidradenitis suppurativa by androgens. Br Med J (Clin Res Ed) 292(6515):245, 1986

Moyal-Barracco M, Edwards L: Diagnosis and therapy of anogenital lichen planus. Dermatol Ther 17(1):38, 2004a

Moyal-Barracco M, Lynch PJ: 2003 ISSVD terminology and classification of vulvodynia: a historical perspective. J Reprod Med 49(10):772, 2004b

Munday PE: Response to treatment in dysaesthetic vulvodynia. J Obstet Gynaecol 21(6):610, 2001

Murina F, Tassan P, Roberti P, et al: Treatment of vulvar vestibulitis with submucous infiltrations of methylprednisolone and lidocaine. An alternative approach. J Reprod Med 46(8):713, 2001

Neill SM, Lewis FM, Tatnall FM, et al: British Association of Dermatologists' guidelines for the management of lichen sclerosus 2010. Br J Dermatol 163(4):672, 2010

Nielsen GP, Rosenberg AE, Koerner FC, et al: Smooth-muscle tumors of the vulva. A clinicopathological study of 25 cases and review of the literature. Am J Surg Pathol 20(7):779, 1996

Pelisse M: The vulvo-vaginal-gingival syndrome. A new form of erosive lichen planus. Int J Dermatol 28(6):381, 1989

Poskitt L, Wojnarowska F: Lichen sclerosus as a cutaneous manifestation of thyroid disease. J Am Acad Dermatol 28(4):665, 1993

Powell J, Wojnarowska F: Childhood vulvar lichen sclerosus: an increasingly common problem. J Am Acad Dermatol 44(5):803, 2001

Reed BD, Crawford S, Couper M, et al: Pain at the vulvar vestibule: a web-based survey. J Low Genit Tract Dis 8:48, 2004

Reed BD, Haefner HK, Sen A, et al: Vulvodynia incidence and remission rates among adult women. Obstet Gynecol 112:231, 2008

Reed BD, Harlow SD, Sen A, et al: Relationship between vulvodynia and chronic comorbid pain conditions. Obstet Gynecol 120(1):145, 2012

Reed BD, Legocki LJ, Plegue MA, et al: Factors associated with vulvodynia incidence. Obstet Gynecol 123(2 Pt 1):225, 2014

Rhode JM, Burke WM, Cederna PS, et al: Outcomes of surgical management of stage III vulvar hidradenitis suppurativa. J Reprod Med 53:420, 2008

Rogers RS III: Complex aphthosis. Adv Exp Med Biol 528:311, 2003

Rogers RS III: Recurrent aphthous stomatitis: clinical characteristics and associated systemic disorders. Semin Cutan Med Surg 16(4):278, 1997

Romo A, Benavides S: Treatment options in insulin resistance obesity-related acanthosis nigricans. Ann Pharmacother 42(7):1090, 2008

Rouzier R, Haddad B, Deyrolle C, et al: Perineoplasty for the treatment of introital stenosis related to vulvar lichen sclerosus. Am J Obstet Gynecol 186(1):49, 2002

Saraiya A, Al-Shoha A, Brodell RT: Hyperinsulinemia associated with acanthosis nigricans, finger pebbles, acrochordons, and the sign of Leser-Trélat. Endocr Pract 19(3):522, 2013

Savage JA, Maize JC Sr: Keratoacanthoma clinical behavior: a systematic review. Am J Dermatopathol 36(5):422, 2014

Scurry JP, Vanin K: Vulvar squamous cell carcinoma and lichen sclerosus. Australas J Dermatol 38(Suppl 1): 2, 1997

Sideri M, Origoni M, Spinaci L, et al: Topical testosterone in the treatment of vulvar lichen sclerosus. Int J Gynaecol Obstet 46(1):53, 1994

Sides C, Trinidad MC, Heitlinger L, et al: Crohn disease and the gynecologic patient. Obstet Gynecol Surv 68(1):51, 2013

Smith CH, Anstey AV, Barker JN, et al: British Association of Dermatologists' guideline for biologic interventions for psoriasis 2009. Br J Dermatol 161(5):987, 2009

Smith CH, Barker JN: Psoriasis and its management. BMJ 333(7564):380, 2006

Sobel JD, Reichman O: Diagnosis and treatment of desquamative inflammatory vaginitis. Am J Obstet Gynecol 117(4):850, 2011

Spergel JM, Paller AS: Atopic dermatitis and the atopic march. J Allergy Clin Immunol 112(Suppl 6):S118, 2003

Stockdale CK, Lawson HW: 2013 Vulvodynia Guideline update. J Low Genit Tract Dis 18(2):93, 2014

Tanaka K, Mikamo H, Ninomiya M, et al: Microbiology of Bartholin's gland abscess in Japan. J Clin Microbiol 43(8):4258, 2005

Torgerson RR, Marnach ML, Bruce AJ, et al: Oral and vulvar changes in pregnancy. Clin Dermatol 24(2):122, 2006

Traas MA, Bekkers RL, Dony JM, et al: Surgical treatment for the vulvar vestibulitis syndrome. Obstet Gynecol 107(2 Pt 1):256, 2006

Varani J, Nickoloff BJ, Dixit VM, et al: All-trans retinoic acid stimulates growth of adult human keratinocytes cultured in growth factor-deficient medium, inhibits production of thrombospondin and fibronectin, and reduces adhesion. J Invest Dermatol 93(4):449, 1989

Virgili A, Bacilieri S, Corazza M: Evaluation of contact sensitization in vulvar lichen simplex chronicus. A proposal for a battery of selected allergens. J Reprod Med 48(1):33, 2003

Virgili A, Corazza M, Bianchi A, et al: Open study of topical 0.025% tretinoin in the treatment of vulvar lichen sclerosus. One year of therapy. J Reprod Med 40(9):614, 1995

Visco AG, Del Priore G: Postmenopausal Bartholin gland enlargement: a hospital-based cancer risk assessment. Obstet Gynecol 87(2):286, 1996

Vrijman C, Kroon MW, Limpens J, et al: The prevalence of thyroid disease in patients with vitiligo: a systematic review. Br J Dermatol 167(6):1224, 2012

Wallace HJ: Lichen sclerosus et atrophicus. Trans St Johns Hosp Dermatol Soc 57(1):9, 1971

Zellis S, Pincus SH: Treatment of vulvar dermatoses. Semin Dermatol 15(1):71, 1996

Zhang XJ, Chen JJ, Liu JB: The genetic concept of vitiligo. J Dermatol Sci 39(3):137, 2005

Zolnoun DA, Hartmann KE, Steege JF: Overnight 5% lidocaine ointment for treatment of vulvar vestibulitis. Obstet Gynecol 102(1):84, 2003

CHAPTER 5

Contraception and Sterilization

Today, an ever-increasing variety of effective methods is available for fertility regulation. Although none is completely without side effects or potential danger, it remains axiomatic that contraception poses fewer risks than pregnancy (Table 5-1). Contraceptive availability is paramount for the care of women, as approximately half of pregnancies in the United States are unintended (Finer, 2014). Moreover, half of these women are using contraception at the time of conception (Henshaw, 1998). These statistics have prompted a reexamination of contraceptive counseling to prevent unplanned pregnancy (American College of Obstetricians and Gynecologists, 2011; Steiner, 2006).

Methods are now grouped according to their effectiveness. *Top-tier* or *first-tier methods* are those that are most effective and are characterized by their ease of use (Fig. 5-1). These methods require only minimal user motivation or intervention and have an unintended pregnancy rate less than 2 per 100 women during the first year of use (Table 5-2). As expected, these first-tier methods provide the longest duration of contraception after initiation and require the fewest number of return visits. Top-tier methods include intrauterine contraceptive devices, contraceptive implants, and various methods of male and female sterilization. A reduction in unintended pregnancies can be better achieved by increasing top-tier method use. Thus, although counseling is provided for all contraceptive methods, common misperceptions regarding some of the top-tier methods—especially intrauterine contraception—can also be dispelled.

Second-tier methods include systemic hormonal contraceptives that are available as oral tablets, intramuscular injections, transdermal patches, or transvaginal rings. In sum, their expected failure rate is 3 to 9 percent per 100 users during the first year. This higher rate likely reflects failure to redose at the appropriate interval. Automated reminder systems for

these second-tier methods have been repeatedly shown to have limited efficacy (Halpern, 2013).

Third-tier methods include barrier methods for men and women and fertility awareness methods such as cycle beads. Their expected failure rate is 10 to 20 percent per 100 users in the first year. However, efficacy increases with consistent and correct use.

Fourth-tier methods include spermicidal preparations, which have a failure rate of 21 to 30 percent per 100 first-year users. The withdrawal method is so unpredictable that some conclude that it does not belong among other contraceptive methods (Doherty, 2009).

MEDICAL ELIGIBILITY CRITERIA

The World Health Organization (WHO) (2010) has provided evidence-based guidance for the use of all highly effective reversible contraceptive methods by women with various health factors. These guidelines were intended to be modified by individual countries to best serve their populations specific circumstances. Thus, the Centers for Disease Control and Prevention (2010, 2011) published *United States Medical Eligibility Criteria (US MEC)* for contraceptive use in the United States. These US MEC guidelines are available and updated regularly at the CDC website: http://www.cdc.gov/reproductivehealth/UnintendedPregnancy/USMEC.htm. In the US MEC, many contraceptive methods are classified into six groups by their similarity: combination oral contraceptive (COC), progestin-only

TABLE 5-1. Birth-Related or Method-Related Deaths per 100,000 Fertile Women by Age Group

Method	15–24 Years	25–34 Years	35–44 Years
Pregnancy	5.1	5.5	13.4
Abortion	2.0	1.8	13.4
Intrauterine device	0.2	0.2	0.4
Rhythm, withdrawal	1.3	1.0	1.3
Barrier method	1.0	1.3	2.0
Spermicides	1.8	1.7	2.1
Oral contraceptives	1.1	1.5	1.4
Implants/injectables	0.4	0.6	0.5
Tubal sterilization	1.2	1.1	1.2
Vasectomy	0.1	0.1	0.1

Data from Harlap S, Kost K, Forrest JD: Preventing pregnancy, protecting health: a new look at birth control choices in the US. New York, The Alan Guttmacher Institute, 1991.

SECTION 1

Description	Method examples	Pregnancy per 100 woman years

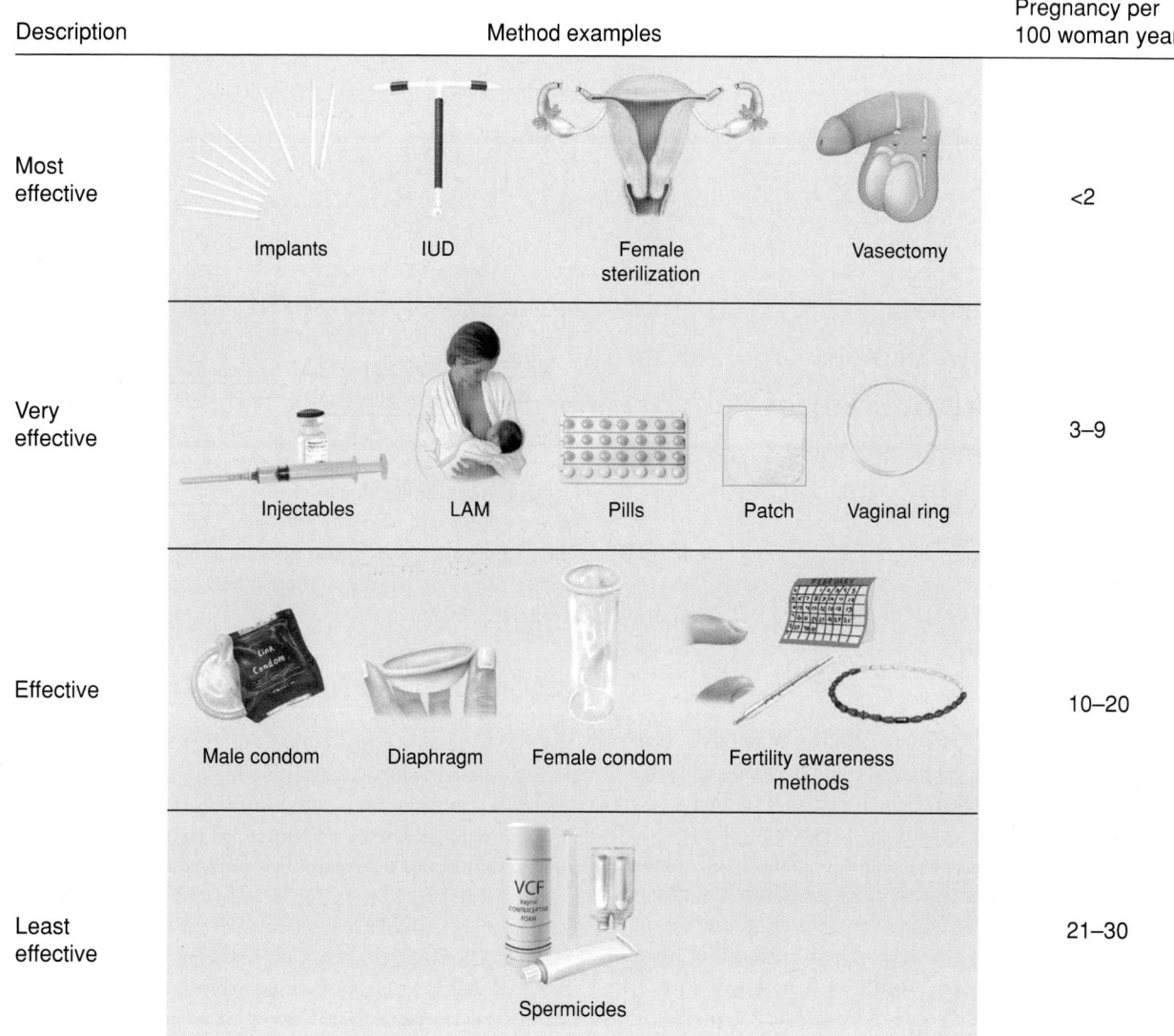

Most effective	Implants IUD Female sterilization Vasectomy	<2
Very effective	Injectables LAM Pills Patch Vaginal ring	3–9
Effective	Male condom Diaphragm Female condom Fertility awareness methods	10–20
Least effective	Spermicides	21–30

FIGURE 5-1 Contraceptive effectiveness chart. (Adapted with permission from World Health Organization, Johns Hopkins Bloomberg School of Public Health (SHSPH): Family Planning Handbook for Providers. Baltimore and Geneva, 2007.)

pill (POP), depot medroxyprogesterone acetate (DMPA), implants, levonorgestrel-releasing intrauterine system (LNG-IUS), and copper intrauterine device (Cu-IUD). For a given health condition, each method is categorized 1 through 4. The score describes a method's safety profile for a typical woman with that condition: (1) no restriction of method use, (2) method advantages outweigh risks, (3) method risks outweigh advantages, or (4) method poses an unacceptably high health risk.

■ Lactation

Among others, lactation is one factor addressed in the US MEC guidelines. Approximately 20 percent of breast-feeding women will ovulate by 3 months postpartum. Ovulation often precedes menstruation, and these women are at risk for unplanned pregnancy. For women who breast feed intermittently, effective contraception should begin as if they were not breast feeding. Moreover, contraception is essential after the first menses unless pregnancy is planned.

Of available methods, Cu-IUD in breast-feeding women has a category 1 or 2 rating (Table 5-3). Women are counseled that effects of the etonogestrel-releasing contraceptive implant (Nexplanon) or LNG-IUS and breast feeding are not known, but studies have mostly shown no adverse association (Gurtcheff, 2011). Because POPs have little effect on lactation, they are also preferred by some for use up to 6 months in women who are exclusively breast feeding. According to the American Academy of Pediatrics and the American College of Obstetricians and Gynecologists (2012), POPs and DMPA may be initiated prior to discharge regardless of breast-feeding status. For the etonogestrel implant, insertion is delayed until 4 weeks postpartum for those exclusively breast-feeding but can be inserted anytime for those not nursing. Combination hormone contraception may begin at 6 weeks following delivery, if breast feeding is well established and the infant's nutritional status is surveilled. The CDC (2011) revised the US MEC guidelines regarding the use of combined hormonal contraception during the puerperium due to the higher risk of venous thromboembolism (VTE) during these weeks.

TABLE 5-2. Contraceptive Failure Rates During the First Year of Method Use in Women in the United States

Method[a]	Perfect Use	Typical Use
Top Tier: Most Effective		
Intrauterine devices:		
Levonorgestrel system	0.2	0.2
T 380A copper	0.6	0.8
Levonorgestrel implants	0.05	0.05
Female sterilization	0.5	0.5
Male sterilization	0.1	0.15
Second Tier: Very Effective		
Combination pill	0.3	9
Vaginal ring	0.3	9
Patch	0.3	9
DMPA	0.2	6
Progestin-only pill	0.3	9
Third Tier: Effective		
Condom		
Male	2	18
Female	5	21
Diaphragm with spermicides	6	12
Fertility-awareness		24
Standard days	5	
Two day	4	
Ovulation	3	
Symptothermal	0.4	
Fourth Tier: Least Effective		
Spermicides	18	28
Sponge		
Parous women	20	24
Nulliparous women	9	12
No WHO Category		
Withdrawal	4	22
No contraception	85	85

[a]Methods organized according to tiers of efficacy.
DMPA = depot medroxyprogesterone acetate; WHO = World Health Organization.
Data from Trussell J: Contraceptive efficacy. In Hatcher RA, Trussell J, Nelson AL, et al (eds): Contraceptive Technology, 20th ed. New York, Ardent Media, 2011, p 791.

Concerns regarding contraceptive steroids and use with breast feeding are based on the theoretical and biologically plausible—but unproven—possibility that systemic progestins may interfere with initial breast milk production. Importantly, contraceptive steroids are not purported to harm the quality of breast milk. Minute quantities of the hormones are excreted in breast milk, but no adverse effects on infants have been reported. In two reviews, authors describe the lack of evidence to support a negative impact of hormonal contraception on lactation (Tepper, 2015; Truitt, 2003). The reviewers concluded that all the studies were of poor to fair quality and that randomized trials are needed.

Adolescence and Perimenopause

Females at both ends of the reproductive spectrum have unique contraceptive needs, which are discussed in Chapters 14 (p. 330) and 21 (p. 474). With adolescents, since the mid-1800s, the age of menarche has dropped. Thus, reproductive function is established many years earlier than psychosocial comprehension regarding the consequences of sexual activity. Such early sexual development may result in intermittent spontaneous sexual encounters with a naïve perception of pregnancy and sexually transmitted disease (STD) risks (Sulak, 1993). Importantly, adolescents have unintended pregnancy rates that approach 85 percent (Finer, 2014). Thus, effective contraception counseling ideally is provided *before* the onset of sexual activity. In most states, minors have explicit legal authority to consent to contraceptive services, and in many areas, publicly funded clinics provide free contraception to adolescents (Guttmacher Institute, 2014). Moreover, contraception may be provided without a pelvic examination or cervical cancer screening.

In the perimenopause, ovulation becomes irregular and fertility wanes. However, pregnancies do occur, and in women aged >40 years, nearly half of all pregnancies are unintended (Finer, 2011). Importantly, pregnancy with advanced maternal age carries an increased risk for pregnancy-related morbidity and mortality. Women in this group may also have coexistent medical problems that may preclude certain contraceptive methods. Finally, perimenopausal symptoms may be present in this group and may be improved with hormonal contraceptive methods.

TOP-TIER CONTRACEPTIVE METHODS

Intrauterine Contraception

Fears and concerns with legal liability caused this method to become almost obsolete. However, intrauterine contraception (IUC) has again gained popularity, and IUC use increased from 2 percent in 2002 to 10 percent in 2008 (Fig. 5-2) (Mosher, 2010). Still, this is much lower compared with the worldwide IUC use rate of 14 percent, and specifically with that of China

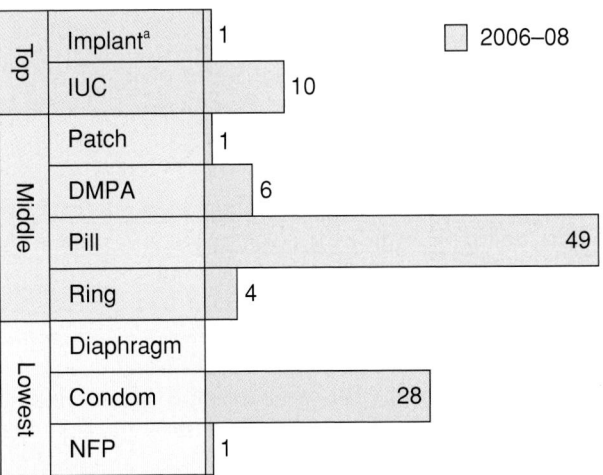

FIGURE 5-2 Rates of contraceptive use by method and by method effectiveness for years 2006–2008 in the United States. NFP = natural family planning. (Data from Mosher WD, Jones J: Use of contraception in the United States: 1982–2008, Vital Health Stat 23, 29:1, 2010.)

TABLE 5-3. U.S. Medical Eligibility Criteria for Use of Various Contraceptive Methods While Breastfeeding

Method[a]	Category	Comments
CHCs[b]		
Breastfeeding		Evidence limited. Guidelines based on theoretical concerns
<1 month	3	
>1 month	2	
Non-breastfeeding		Theoretical concerns for thrombosis risks. Blood coagulation and fibrinolysis virtually normalized by 3 weeks pp
<21 days	4	
21–42 days, with risks[c]	3	
21–42 days, with no risks	2	
>42 days	1	
DMPA, POPs, Implants		
Breastfeeding		Theoretical concerns that early use may diminish breast milk production are not supported by evidence. Limited studies
<1 month	2	
>1 month	1	
Non-breastfeeding	1	Limited evidence suggests no adverse side effects
LNG-IUS		
Breastfeeding or not		Theoretical risk of diminished breast milk production. Minimal evidence
<10 mins	2	
10 mins to ≤4 wks	2	
≥4 wks	1	
Puerperal sepsis	4	IUD insertion could worsen condition
Cu-IUD		
Breastfeeding or not		IUD placement <10 min pp is associated with lower expulsion rates compared with later IUD placement up to >72 hr pp. No comparative data for insertion >72 hr pp
<10 min	1	
10 min to ≤4 wks	2	
≥4 wks	1	At c-section, postplacental placement associated with lower expulsion rate than after vaginal delivery
		No increased risk of infection or perforation associated with pp insertion
Puerperal sepsis	4	IUD insertion could worsen condition

[a]Time reflects time from delivery.
[b]Combined hormonal contraceptive (CHC) group includes pills, vaginal ring, and patch.
[c]Associated risks that increase category score include: age ≥35, transfusion at delivery, BMI ≥30, postpartum hemorrhage, cesarean delivery, smoking, preeclampsia.
c-section = cesarean delivery; Cu-IUD = copper-bearing intrauterine device; DMPA = depot medroxyprogesterone acetate; LNG-IUS = levonorgestrel-releasing intrauterine system; POPs = progestin-only pills; pp = postpartum.
Adapted with permission from Centers for Disease Control and Prevention, 2010, 2011.

(40 percent) and northern Europe (11 percent) (United Nations, 2013).

Some barriers to IUC use in the United States include cost, politics, and provider failure to offer or encourage use of this method. To reduce the high proportion of unplanned pregnancies, the American College of Obstetricians and Gynecologists (2013b) encourages use of *long-acting reversible contraceptives (LARC)* for all appropriate candidates, including adolescents. Despite higher up-front costs, the extended span of effective IUC use results in competitive cost effectiveness compared with other contraceptive forms.

Levonorgestrel-releasing Intrauterine System

Three levonorgestrel-releasing intrauterine contraceptives are Food and Drug Administration (FDA)-approved in the United

States. Named Mirena, Skyla, and Liletta, devices are T-shaped polyethylene structures with the stem encased by a cylinder containing polydimethylsiloxane and levonorgestrel (Fig. 5-3). The cylinder has a permeable membrane that regulates continuous daily hormone release. The Mirena is currently approved for 5 years following insertion, but evidence supports use for 7 years (Thonneau, 2008). Liletta and Skyla are currently approved for 3 years. In addition to having a lower dose of progestin, Skyla is also marginally smaller in size. Mirena and Liletta have a length of 32 mm and a width of 32 mm, but with Skyla, these same dimensions measure 28 mm.

There are several progestin-mediated mechanisms by which LNG-IUS may prevent pregnancy. The progestin renders the endometrium atrophic; it stimulates thick cervical mucus that blocks sperm penetration into the uterine cavity; and it may

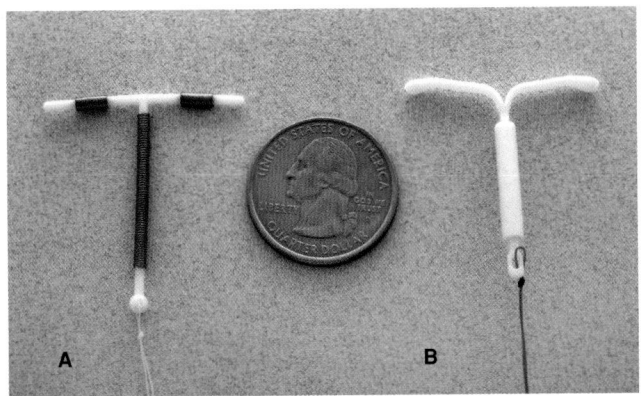

FIGURE 5-3 Intrauterine contraceptive devices: Copper-containing ParaGard T 380A (**A**) and levonorgestrel-releasing Mirena (**B**).

decrease tubal motility, thereby preventing ovum and sperm union. The progestin may also inhibit ovulation, but this is not consistent (Nilsson, 1984).

Shown in Table 5-4 are the manufacturer's contraindications to use of LNG-IUS. Women who have had a previous

---

TABLE 5-4. Manufacturer Contraindications to IUD Use

ParaGard T 380
Pregnancy or suspicion of pregnancy
Uterine abnormality with distorted uterine cavity
Acute PID, or current behavior suggesting a high risk for PID
Postpartum or postabortal endometritis in last 3 months
Known or suspected uterine or cervical malignancy
Genital bleeding of unknown etiology
Mucopurulent cervicitis
Wilson disease
Allergy to any component of ParaGard
A previously placed IUD that has not been removed

Mirena, Liletta, and Skyla
Pregnancy or suspicion of pregnancy
Uterine abnormality with distorted uterine cavity
Use for postcoital contraception
Acute PID or history of, unless there has been a subsequent intrauterine pregnancy
Postpartum endometritis or infected abortion in the past 3 months
Known or suspected uterine or cervical neoplasia
Uterine bleeding of unknown etiology
Untreated acute cervicitis or vaginitis or other lower genital tract infections
Acute liver disease or liver tumor (benign or malignant)
Increased susceptibility to pelvic infection
A previously placed IUD that has not been removed
Hypersensitivity to any component of the device
Known or suspected breast cancer or other progestin-sensitive cancer

IUD = intrauterine device; PID = pelvic inflammatory disease.
Data from Bayer HealthCare, 2014; Teva Women's Health, 2013.

---

ectopic pregnancy may be at increased risk for another because of diminished tubal motility from progestin action. In women with uterine leiomyomas, placement of the LNG-IUS may be problematic if the uterine cavity is distorted. In their metaanalysis, Zapata and associates (2010) reported the expulsion rate to be approximately 10 percent in women with coexistent leiomyomas. However, in affected women who retained the device, menstrual blood loss will be lessened in most.

Copper-T 380A Intrauterine Device

Marketed as ParaGard, this device is composed of a stem wrapped with 314 mm^2 of fine copper wire, and each arm has a 33-mm^2 copper bracelet—the sum of these is 380 mm^2 of copper. As shown in Figure 5-3, two strings extend from the base of the stem. The Cu-T 380A is approved for 10 years of continuous use, although it has been shown to prevent pregnancy with continuous use for up to 20 years (Bahamondes, 2005).

The intense local inflammatory response induced in the uterus by copper-containing devices leads to lysosomal activation and other inflammatory actions that are spermicidal (Alvarez, 1988; Ortiz, 1987). In the unlikely event that fertilization does occur, the same inflammatory actions are directed against the blastocyst. And finally, the endometrium becomes hostile for implantation.

Counseling for Intrauterine Contraception

Infection. During the modern renaissance of IUC, several improvements have resulted in safer and more effective models. That said, there are still some unwanted side effects and misconceptions surrounding their use.

First, fear of IUD-associated infections precluded use in the past by young women and those of low parity. Improved device design has mitigated these concerns appreciably. In addition, several well-designed studies have shown that sexual behavior and STDs are important risk factors.

With current devices, insertion generally does not increase the risk for pelvic infection. There is no evidence that prophylactic antibiotics are necessary with insertion for women at low risk for STDs (American College of Obstetricians and Gynecologists, 2014b; Walsh, 1998). Of the less than 1 in 100 women who develop an infection within 20 days of IUD insertion, most have a concomitant unrecognized cervical infection. Accordingly, women at higher risk for sexually transmitted lower genital tract infections are screened either before or at the time of IUD insertion (Centers for Disease Control and Prevention, 2015; Faúndes, 1998; Grimes, 2000). Alternatively, a small number of pelvic infections are presumed to be caused by intrauterine contamination with normal flora at the time of insertion. Thus, antibiotics selected for treatment of any pelvic infection within the early weeks following IUD insertion should be broad-spectrum to adequately cover all these organisms.

Long-term IUC use is not associated with an increased pelvic infection rate in women at low risk for STDs. Indeed, these long-term users have a pelvic infection rate comparable with that of COC users. Any pelvic infection after 45 to 60 days is considered sexually transmitted and appropriately treated as described in Chapter 3 (p. 69). For women who develop an infection associated with an IUD, evidence is insufficient to recommend device removal, although this is commonly done. However, close clinical reevaluation is warranted if an IUD remains (Centers for Disease Control and Prevention, 2015). In women who develop a tuboovarian abscess, the device is removed immediately after parenteral antibiotic therapy is begun.

Special concerns have arisen for women in whom *Actinomyces* species are identified in the lower genital tract, most commonly during Pap smear cytology reporting. Fiorino (1996) noted a 7-percent incidence in the Pap smears of IUD users compared with a 1-percent incidence in nonusers. Symptomatic pelvic actinomycosis is rare but tends to be indolent and severe.

Currently, in the absence of symptoms, incidental identification of *Actinomyces* species in cytologic specimens has uncertain significance. Treatment options reviewed by the American College of Obstetricians and Gynecologists (2013b) include: expectant management, an extended course of antibiotics, IUD removal, or antibiotics plus IUD removal. For women with symptomatic infection, the IUD is removed and intensive antibiotic therapy given. *Actinomyces* is susceptible to antibiotics with gram-positive coverage, notably the penicillins.

Low Parity and Adolescents. Nulliparous IUD candidates were previously precluded from IUC use because of fears of pelvic infection and induced sterility. Current studies indicate that the pelvic infection rate is not different from that discussed earlier (Lee, 1998; Society of Family Planning, 2010). Moreover, expulsion rates in nulliparas are similar to those in multiparas. A higher proportion of nulliparas will request removal of the device because of pain or bleeding, but overall, this population reports high levels of satisfaction with IUC. Specifically, after the first year, 75 to 90 percent continue use. Revised labeling now places no restrictions on IUC use based on parity. In addition, for the same reasons, *adolescent* IUD candidates may also appropriately select IUC (American College of Obstetricians and Gynecologists, 2014a). Counseling includes clear explanations of the anticipated periprocedural cramping and discomfort.

Human Immunodeficiency Virus-Infected Women. Intrauterine contraception is appropriate for affected women who are otherwise IUC candidates. Neither device type is associated with higher IUD complication rates if used in this population. Moreover, IUDs do not appear to adversely affect viral shedding or antiretroviral therapy efficacy (American College of Obstetricians and Gynecologists, 2012a).

Postabortal or Postpartum Placement. An ideal time to improve successful provision of contraception is immediately following abortion or delivery. For women with an induced or spontaneous first- or second-trimester abortion, IUC can be placed immediately after uterine evacuation.

Insertion techniques depend upon uterine size. After first-trimester evacuation, the uterine cavity length seldom exceeds 12 cm. In these instances, the IUD can be placed using the inserter provided in the package. If the uterine cavity is larger,

the IUD can be placed using ring forceps with sonographic guidance. In women for whom an IUD is placed immediately after induced abortion, the repeat induced abortion rate is only one third of the rate of women not choosing immediate IUD placement (Goodman, 2008; Heikinheimo, 2008). As perhaps expected, the risk of IUC expulsion is slightly higher when placed immediately after abortion or miscarriage, but the advantages of preventing unplanned pregnancies seem to outweigh this (Bednarek, 2011; Fox, 2011; Okusanya, 2014).

Insertion of an IUD immediately following delivery at or near term has also been studied. Placement by hand or by using an instrument has a similar expulsion rate (Grimes, 2010). As with postabortion insertion, expulsion rates by 6 months are higher than those in women whose IUD is placed after complete uterine involution. In one study, the expulsion rate in the former group was nearly 25 percent (Chen, 2010). Even in these circumstances, however, immediate placement may be beneficial because in some populations up to 40 percent of women do not return for a postpartum clinic visit (Ogburn, 2005). Finally, postpartum placement is judged to be category 1 or 2 by the US MEC, that is, its advantages consistently outweigh the risks if puerperal infection is absent (see Table 5-3).

Despite these findings, many choose to delay insertion for several weeks postpartum. Insertion at 2 weeks is quite satisfactory, and in the Parkland System Family Planning Clinics, insertion is scheduled at 6 weeks postpartum to ensure complete uterine involution.

Menstrual Changes. Commonly, IUC may be associated with changes in menstrual patterns. Women who choose the Cu-T 380A are informed that increased dysmenorrhea and bleeding with menses may develop. Objectively, no clinically significant hemoglobin changes are generally expected (Tepper, 2013). Treatment with a nonsteroidal antiinflammatory drug (NSAID) will usually diminish the amount of bleeding—even normal amounts—and also relieve dysmenorrhea (Grimes, 2006).

With the LNG-IUS, women are counseled to expect irregular spotting for up to 6 months after insertion and thereafter to expect monthly menses to be lighter or even absent. Specifically, the Mirena device is associated with progressive amenorrhea, which is reported by 30 percent of women after 2 years and by 60 percent after 12 years (Ronnerdag, 1999). As noted in Chapter 8 (p. 195), the LNG-IUS device reduces menstrual blood loss and is an effective treatment for some women with heavy menstrual bleeding (American College of Obstetricians and Gynecologists, 2014e). This is often associated with improved dysmenorrhea.

Expulsion or Perforation. Approximately 5 percent of women will spontaneously expel their IUD during the first year of use. This is most likely during the first month. Accordingly, a woman is instructed to periodically palpate the marker strings protruding from the cervical os. This can be accomplished by either sitting on the edge of a chair or squatting down and then advancing the middle finger into the vagina until the cervix is reached. Following insertion of either IUD type, women are reappointed for a visit within several weeks, usually after completion of menses. At this meeting, any side effects are addressed, and IUD placement is confirmed by visualizing the marker strings. Some recommend barrier contraception to ensure contraception during this first month. This may be especially desirable if a device has been expelled previously.

The uterus may be perforated either with a uterine sound or with an IUD. Perforations may be clinically apparent or silent. Their frequency depends on operator skill and is estimated to be approximately 1 per 1000 insertions (World Health Organization, 1987). In some cases, a partial perforation at insertion is followed by migration of the device completely through the uterine wall. Occasionally, perforation occurs spontaneously.

Marker Strings. In some cases, the IUD marker strings may not be palpated or seen during speculum examination. During the investigation, a nonpregnant patient should use alternative contraception. Possibilities include that the device was expelled silently, the device has partially or completely perforated the uterus, the woman is pregnant and the enlarging uterus has drawn the device upward, or the marker strings are temporarily hidden within the endocervical canal. An IUD should not be considered expelled unless it was seen by the patient.

Initially, an endocervical brush or similar instrument can be used to gently draw the string out of the cervical canal. If this is unsuccessful, then at least two options are available. After pregnancy has been excluded, the uterine cavity is gently probed using an instrument such as Randall stone forceps or a rod with a hooked end. The strings or device will often be found with this method. If not successful, at this juncture, or possibly as a first choice, transvaginal sonography (TVS) is performed. As described in Chapter 2 (p. 28), 3-dimensional TVS offers improved visualization (Moschos, 2011). If the device is not seen within either the uterine cavity or uterine walls, then an abdominal radiograph, with or without a uterine sound in place, may localize it. Another option includes hysteroscopy.

Management decisions depend upon where the device is located and whether there is a coexistent intrauterine pregnancy. First, a device may penetrate the uterine wall in varying degrees. It should be removed, and this approach varies by IUD location. Devices with a predominantly intrauterine location are typically managed by hysteroscopic IUD removal. In contrast, devices that have nearly completely perforated through the uterine wall are more easily removed laparoscopically.

For women with an intraabdominal IUD, an inert-material device located outside the uterus may cause harm, but not universally. Bowel perforations—both large and small—as well as bowel fistulas have been reported. Once identified laparoscopically, these inert devices can easily be retrieved via laparoscopy or less commonly by colpotomy. Conversely, an extrauterine copper-bearing device induces an intense local inflammatory reaction with adhesions. Thus, they are more firmly adhered, and laparotomy may become necessary (Balci, 2010).

In those with pregnancy and an IUD, early pregnancy identification is important. Up to approximately 14 weeks' gestation, the IUD strings may be visible within the cervix, and if

seen, they are grasped to remove the entire IUD. This action reduces subsequent complications such as late abortion, sepsis, and preterm birth (Alvior, 1973). Tatum and colleagues (1976) reported an abortion rate of 54 percent with the device left in place compared with a rate of 25 percent if it was promptly removed. More recently, a study from Israel by Ganer and coworkers (2009) reported pregnancy outcomes from 1988 to 2007 in 292 women who conceived with a Cu-IUD in place. Outcomes were compared in the two groups of women with and without IUD removal as well as with the general obstetrical population. As shown in Table 5-5, in general, the group of women with an IUD left in place had the worst outcomes. Importantly, however, the group in whom the IUD was removed still had significantly worse outcomes compared with those of the general population. Of special note, Vessey and associates (1979) had previously reported that fetal malformations were not increased in pregnancies in which the device was left in place. In the Ganer study, it is particularly worrisome that this rate was doubled compared with women in whom the device was removed. The distribution of malformations was notable in that 12 percent were skeletal malformations. In contrast, there were no chromosomal anomalies identified in fetuses born to women from the two IUD groups.

[margin note: if IUD left in place]

Because of these findings, if pregnancy continuation is desired, it is recommended that with early pregnancies the IUD be removed. However, if the strings are not visible, attempts to locate and remove the device may result in pregnancy loss. This risk must be weighed against the risk of leaving the device in place. If removal is attempted, TVS can be used. If attempts at removal are followed by evidence for infection, then antimicrobial treatment is begun and is followed by prompt uterine evacuation.

Ectopic Pregnancy. The risk of an associated ectopic pregnancy has been clarified over the past few years. IUC is effective in preventing all pregnancies. Specifically, the contraceptive effect of IUC decreases the absolute number of ectopic pregnancies by half compared with the rate in women who do not use contraception (World Health Organization, 1985, 1987). However, the IUC mechanisms of action are more effective in preventing intrauterine implantation. Thus, if IUC fails, a higher proportion of pregnancies are likely to be ectopic (Furlong, 2002).

Insertion Procedures

Before IUD insertion, the FDA requires that a woman be given a brochure detailing the side effects and apparent risks from its use. Timing of insertion influences the ease of placement as well as pregnancy and expulsion rates. When done toward the end of normal menstruation, when the cervix is usually softer and somewhat more dilated, insertion may be easier, and early pregnancy can be excluded. However, insertion is not limited to this time. For a woman who is sure she is not pregnant and does not want to be pregnant, insertion may be carried out any time during the menstrual cycle. Insertion immediately postpartum or postabortion is also feasible and discussed on page 110.

TABLE 5-5. Pregnancy Outcomes in Women Who Conceived with a Copper-Containing IUD in Place

Outcome[a]	IUD in situ (n = 98)	IUD removed (n = 194)	No IUD (n = 141,191)	p value
PROM	10.2	7.7	5.7	.021
Preterm delivery	18.4	14.4	7.3	<.001
Chorioamnionitis	7.1	4.1	0.7	<.001
Fetal growth restriction	1.0	0.5	1.7	NS
Abruption	4.1	2.1	0.7	<.001
Previa	4.1	0.5	0.5	<.001
Cesarean	32	21	13	<.001
Low birthweight				
<2500 g	11.2	13.4	6.7	<.001
<1500 g	5.1	3.6	1.1	<.001
Perinatal death	1.0	1.5	1.2	NS
Malformations	10.2	5.7	5.1	<.041

[a]Outcomes shown as percentages.
IUD = intrauterine device; NS = not significant; PROM = premature rupture of membranes.
Data from Ganer H, Levy A, Ohel I, et al: Pregnancy outcome in women with an intrauterine contraceptive device. Am J Obstet Gynecol 201:381.e1, 2009.

Prior to insertion, a pelvic examination is completed to identify uterine position and size. Abnormalities are evaluated as they may contraindicate the device. Evidence for infection such as a mucopurulent discharge or significant vaginitis is appropriately treated and resolved before insertion.

For pain management, the most effective method of analgesia has not been established, and patient and provider preference directs selection. Options include NSAIDs, topical lidocaine, or paracervical block. Misoprostol is thought to advance cervical softening to mitigate cervical dilatation pain. However, few studies have adequately evaluated these (Allen, 2009).

At the beginning of the insertion procedure, the cervical surface is cleaned with an antiseptic solution, and a tenaculum is placed on the cervical lip. The uterus is sounded to guide correct depth placement. Specific steps for IUD insertion are outlined and illustrated in Figs. 5-4 and 5-5. During insertion, if there is concern for correct IUD positioning, then placement may be checked by inspection or by sonography. If not positioned completely within the uterus, the device is removed and replaced with a new one. An expelled or partially expelled device should not be reinserted.

■ Progestin Implants

Contraception can be provided by a progestin-containing device that is implanted subdermally and releases hormone over many years. The devices are coated with a polymer to prevent fibrosis. Several systems have been developed, but only one is available in the United States. The initial implant, the Norplant System, releases levonorgestrel from six Silastic rods.

It was withdrawn from the U.S. market, and a fund has been established by the manufacturer to ensure access to patients for removal. Supposedly, the silicone-based rods caused ill-defined symptoms that were reversed with removal. A newer two-rod levonorgestrel system, Jadelle, has received FDA approval but is not marketed or distributed in the United States (Sivin, 2002). Sino-implant II is a structurally and pharmacologically similar system to Jadelle. It is manufactured in China and approved for use by several countries in Asia and Africa (Steiner, 2010).

The implant Nexplanon is currently the only subdermal contraceptive implant marketed in the United States. It is a single-rod subdermal implant containing 68 mg of a progestin—etonogestrel—and covered by an ethylene vinyl acetate copolymer. Nexplanon has replaced the earlier etonogestrel implant, Implanon.

For Nexplanon, contraception is provided by progestin released continuously to suppress ovulation, increase cervical mucus viscosity, and induce endometrial atrophy. The etonogestrel implant will provide contraception for up to 3 years. At this time, the device is removed, and another rod may be placed within the same incision site. Contraindications for this device are similar to those cited for other progestin-containing methods. Specifically, these include pregnancy, thrombosis or thromboembolic disorders, benign or malignant hepatic tumors, active liver disease, undiagnosed abnormal genital bleeding, or breast cancer (Merck, 2014). Importantly, patients are counseled that Nexplanon causes irregular bleeding that does not normalize over time. Thus, women who cannot tolerate unpredictable and irregular spotting or bleeding should select an alternative method.

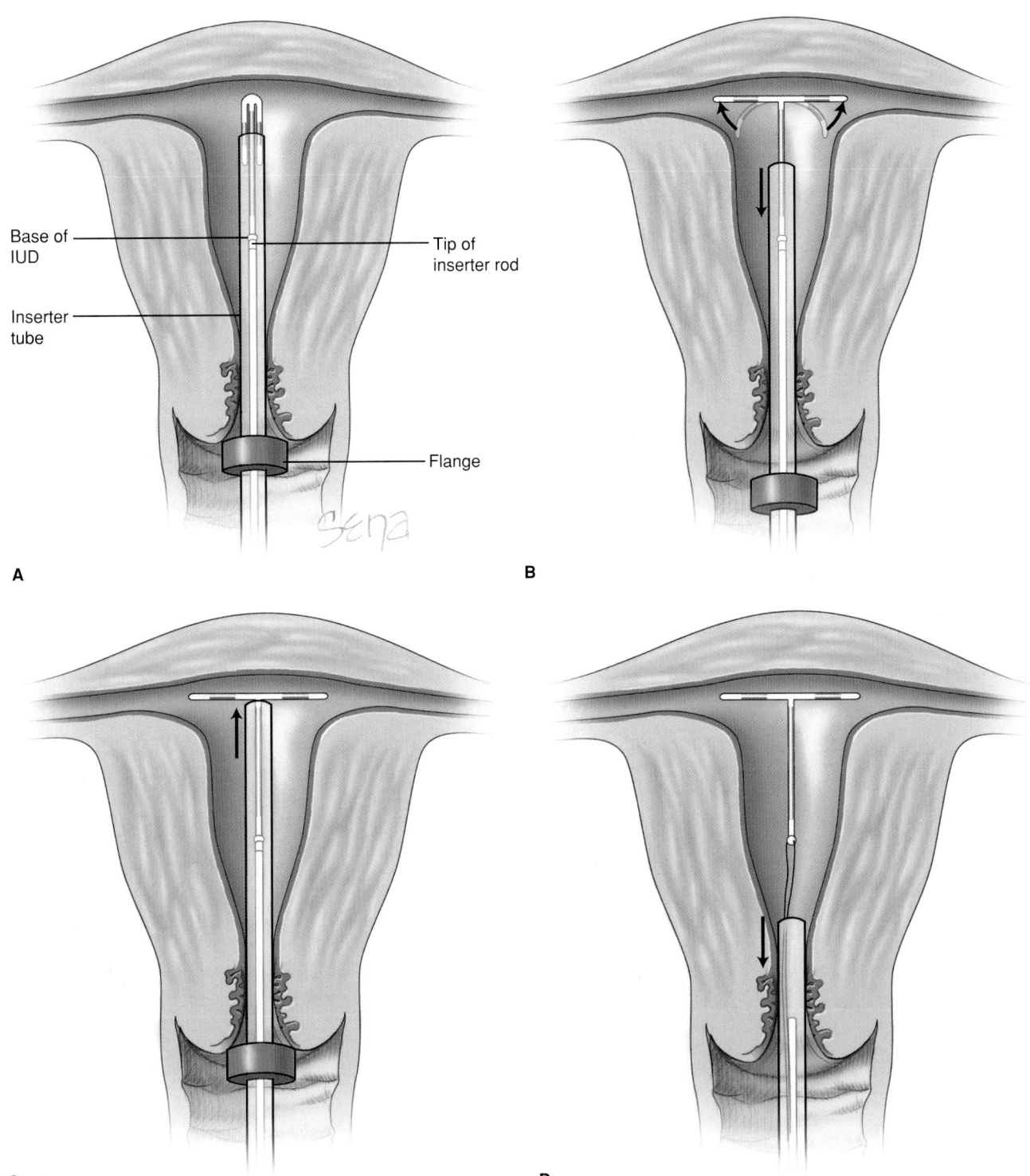

Base of IUD

Tip of inserter rod

Inserter tube

Flange

A

B

C

D

FIGURE 5-4 Insertion of ParaGard T 380A. The IUD is loaded into its inserter tube not more than 5 minutes before insertion. If longer, the malleable arms can retain "memory" of the inserter and remain bent inward. A blue plastic flange on the outside of the inserter tube is positioned from the IUD tip to reflect the uterine depth ascertained during sounding. The IUD arms should lie in the same plane as the flat portion of the blue flange. **A.** The inserter tube, with the IUD loaded, is passed into the endometrial cavity. When the blue flange abuts the cervix, insertion stops. **B.** To release the IUD arms, the solid white rod within the inserter tube is held steady while the inserter tube is withdrawn no more than 1 cm. **C.** The inserter tube is then carefully moved upward toward the top of the uterus until slight resistance is felt. **D.** First, the solid white rod and then the inserter tube are withdrawn individually. At completion, only the threads are visible protruding from the cervix. These are trimmed to allow 3 to 4 cm to extend into the vagina.

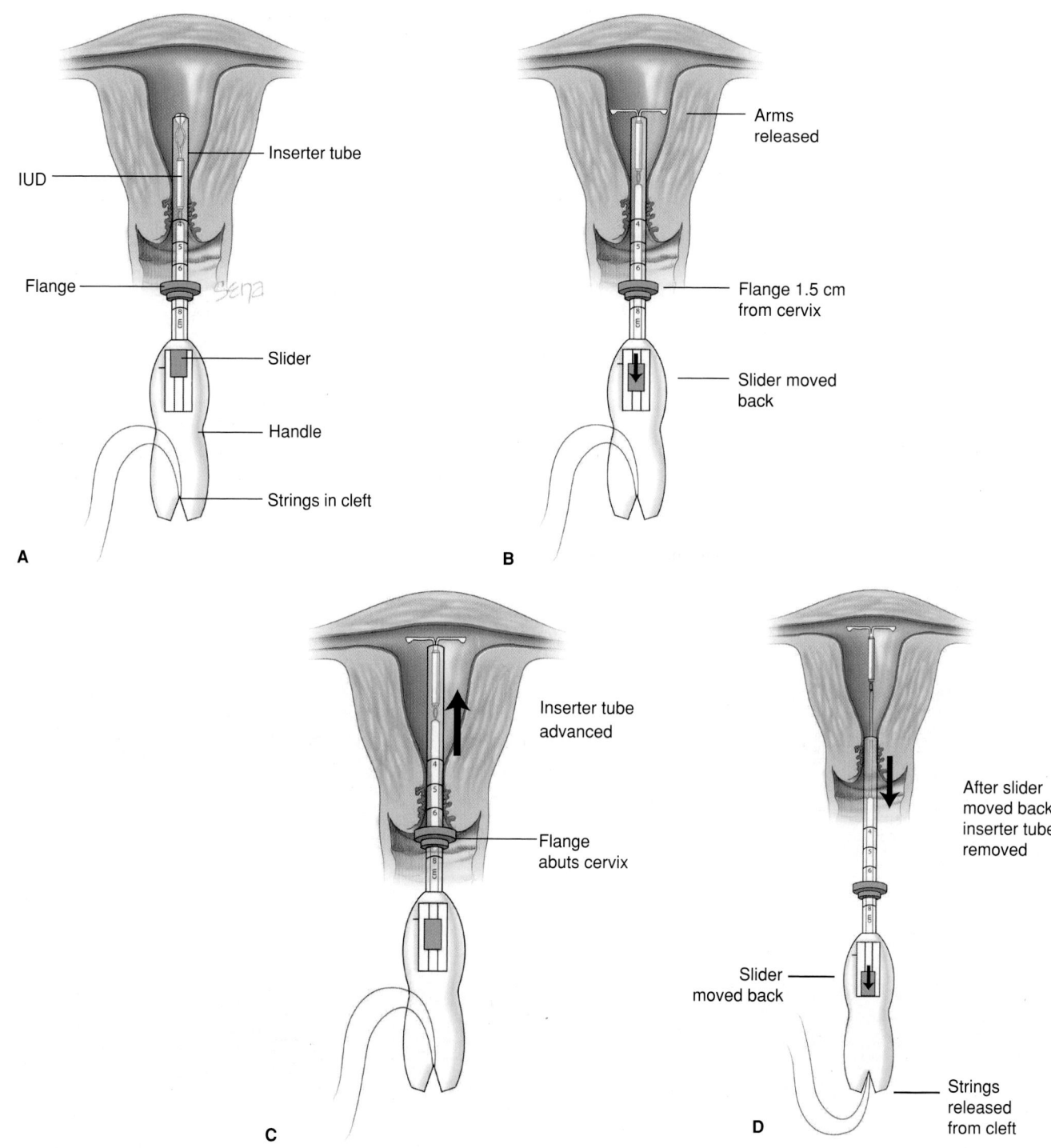

FIGURE 5-5 Insertion of Mirena intrauterine system. Threads from behind the slider are first released to hang freely. The teal-colored slider found on the handle should be positioned at the top of the handle nearest the device. The IUD arms are oriented horizontally. **A.** As both free threads are pulled outward, the Mirena IUD is drawn into the inserter tube. The threads are then moved upward from below and tightly fixed into the handle's cleft. A flange on the outside of the inserter tube is positioned from the IUD tip to reflect the depth found with uterine sounding. **B.** While inserting the Mirena device, the slider is held firmly in position at the top of the handle. Gentle traction is created by outward traction on the tenaculum to align the cervical canal with the uterine cavity. The inserter tube is gently threaded into the uterus until the flange lies 1.5 to 2 cm from the external cervical os to allow the arms to open. While holding the inserter steady, the IUD arms are released by pulling the slider back only to the raised horizontal line on the handle. This position is held for 15 to 20 seconds to allow the arms to fully open. **C.** The inserter is then gently guided into the uterine cavity until its flange touches the cervix. **D.** The device is released by holding the inserter firmly in position and pulling the slider back all the way. The threads will be released automatically. The inserter may then be removed. IUD strings are trimmed to leave approximately 3 cm visible outside the cervix.

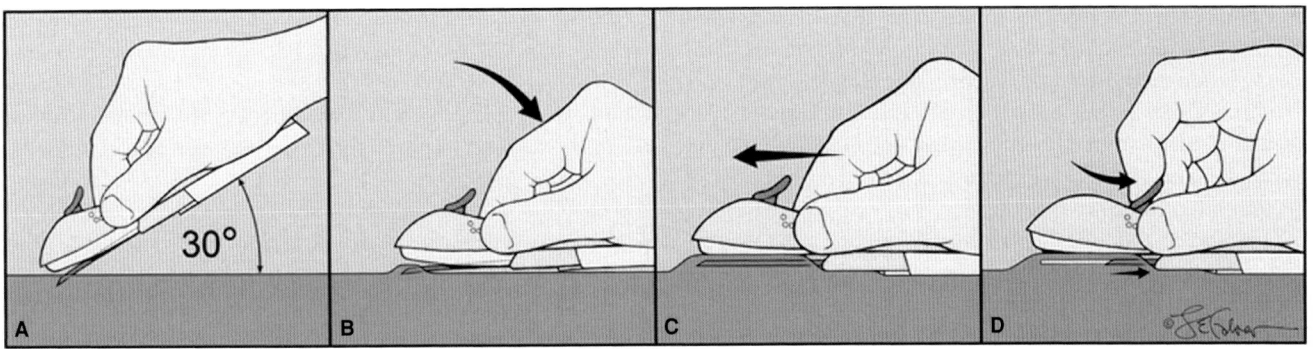

FIGURE 5-6 Nexplanon insertion. A sterile pen marks the insertion site, which is 8 to 10 cm proximal to the medial humeral condyle. A second mark is placed 4 cm proximally along the arm's long axis. The area is cleaned aseptically, and a 1-percent lidocaine anesthetic track is injected along the planned insertion path. **A.** The insertion device is grasped at its gripper bubbles found on either side, and the needle cap is removed outward. The device can be seen within the needle bore. The needle bevel then pierces the skin at a 30-degree angle. **B.** Once the complete bevel is subcutaneous, the needle is immediately angled downward to lie horizontally. **C.** Importantly, the skin is tented upward by the needle as the needle is slowly advanced horizontally and subdermally. **D.** Once the needle is completely inserted, the lever on the top of the device is pulled backward toward the operator. This retracts the needle and thereby deposits the implant. The device is then lifted away from the skin. After placement, both patient and operator should palpate the 4-cm implant.

Nexplanon is inserted subdermally along the biceps groove of the inner arm and 6 to 8 cm from the elbow (Fig. 5-6). Immediately following insertion, the provider and patient should document that the device is palpable beneath the skin. When Nexplanon is removed, this superficial location allows in-office extraction of the implant. Through a small incision large enough to admit hemostat tips, the implant is grasped and removed. If desired, a new rod can be placed through this same incision.

If Nexplanon is not palpable, it can be imaged by radiography, computed tomography (CT), sonography, or magnetic resonance (MR) imaging. Norplant and Jadelle are also radiopaque. This is an advantage compared with Implanon, which is not radiopaque and requires sonography with a 10- to 15-MHz sonographic transducer or MR imaging for identification (Shulman, 2006). In the rare event that an etonogestrel implant cannot be palpated or identified radiologically, the manufacturer can be contacted and arrangements made for etonogestrel level measurement (Merck, 2014).

■ Permanent Contraception—Sterilization

In 2011 to 2013, surgical sterilization was one of the most commonly reported forms of contraception in childbearing-aged women in the United States (Daniels, 2014). These procedures cannot be tracked accurately because most interval tubal sterilizations and vasectomies are performed in ambulatory surgical centers. However, according to the National Survey of Family Growth, approximately 643,000 female tubal sterilizations are performed annually in the United States (Chan, 2010). The two most commonly employed forms in this country are bilateral tubal ligation—frequently via laparoscopy—and hysteroscopic tubal sterilization. The latter has become popular, and in some settings, it is used in up to half of nonpuerperal female sterilizations (Shavell, 2009).

Over the past 20 years, several important multicenter studies regarding sterilization have been performed by investigators of the Collaborative Review of Sterilization (CREST) and the

Centers for Disease Control and Prevention. Data from many of these studies are subsequently described.

Female Tubal Sterilization

This is usually accomplished by occlusion or division of the fallopian tubes to prevent ovum passage and fertilization. According to the National Health Statistics Report, 27 percent of contracepting women in the United States use this method (Jones, 2012). Approximately half of tubal sterilization procedures are performed in conjunction with cesarean delivery or soon after vaginal delivery (MacKay, 2001). Accordingly, this is termed *puerperal sterilization*. The other half of tubal sterilization procedures are done at a time unrelated to recent pregnancy, that is, nonpuerperal tubal sterilization. This is also termed *interval sterilization*. In most instances, nonpuerperal tubal sterilization is accomplished via laparoscopy or hysteroscopy.

Tubal Interruption Methods. There are three methods, along with their modifications, that are used for tubal interruption. These include application of various permanent rings or clips to the fallopian tubes; electrocoagulation of a tubal segment; or ligation with suture material, with or without removal of a tubal segment. In a Cochrane review, Lawrie and colleagues (2011) concluded that all of these are effective in preventing pregnancy.

Electrocoagulation is used for destruction of a segment of tube and can be accomplished with either unipolar or bipolar current. Although unipolar coagulation has the lowest long-term failure rate, it also has the highest serious complication rate. For this reason, bipolar coagulation is favored by most (American College of Obstetricians and Gynecologists, 2013a).

Mechanical methods of tubal occlusion can be accomplished with: (1) a silicone rubber band such as the *Falope Ring* or the *Tubal Ring*, (2) the spring-loaded *Hulka-Clemens clip*—also known as the *Wolf clip*, or (3) the silicone-lined titanium *Filshie clip*. The steps to these procedures are described in Section 44-2 (p. 1006) of the surgical atlas. In a randomized trial of 2746 women, Sokal and associates (2000) compared the Tubal Ring and Filshie clip and reported similar rates of safety and 1-year pregnancy rates of 1.7 per 1000 women. All of these mechanical occlusion methods have favorable long-term success rate.

Suture ligation with tubal segment excision is more often used for puerperal sterilization. Methods include Parkland, Pomeroy, and modified Pomeroy, which are illustrated in Section 43-7 (p. 937).

The type of abdominal entry for sterilization is also variable. Laparoscopic tubal ligation is the leading method used in this country for nonpuerperal female sterilization (American College of Obstetrics and Gynecologists, 2013a). This is frequently done in an ambulatory surgical setting under general anesthesia, and the woman can be discharged several hours later. Alternatively, some choose minilaparotomy using a 3-cm suprapubic incision. This is especially popular in resource-poor countries. With either laparoscopy or minilaparotomy, major morbidity is rare. Minor morbidity, however, was twice as common with minilaparotomy in a review by Kulier and associates (2004). Finally, the peritoneal cavity can also be entered by colpotomy through the posterior vaginal fornix, although this approach is infrequently used.

Counseling. Indications for this elective procedure for sterilization include a request for sterilization with clear understanding that this is permanent and irreversible. Each woman is counseled regarding all alternative contraceptive options and their efficacy. Each woman is also informed regarding her sterilization options, which include laparoscopic or hysteroscopic tubal occlusion or bilateral total salpingectomy. The risks and benefits of each are thoroughly discussed. Many women may also have questions or misunderstanding about possible long-term outcomes after female sterilization. As with any operation, surgical risks are assessed, and occasionally the procedure may be contraindicated.

Risk-reducing Salpingectomy. The Society of Gynecologic Oncology (2013) currently recommends consideration of bilateral total salpingectomy as a preventive measure against serous ovarian and peritoneal cancers. As discussed in Chapter 35 (p. 738), this may be especially relevant for women at greatest risk for these cancers, namely, women with *BRCA1* or *BRCA2* mutation. Most pelvic serous cancers are thought to originate in the distal fallopian tube. Total salpingectomy may confer up to a 34-percent reduction in endometrioid and serous ovarian cancer rates (Erickson, 2013; Sieh, 2013). If risk-reducing salpingectomy is elected in women with BRCA mutations, the pathology requisition form should state this genetic information. This prompts more thorough tubal specimen sectioning to search for cancer and precancerous lesions, which can be found in the tubes of BRCA mutation carriers.

In low-risk women, because the ovarian cancer risk is less than 2 percent, risk-reducing salpingectomy as an isolated procedure is likely unwarranted. However, if surgery such as hysterectomy or tubal sterilization is planned, women are counseled regarding the risks and benefits of complete fallopian tube excision (Anderson, 2013). As advantages, total salpingectomy may decrease risks for subsequent tubal surgery. As disadvantages, operating time may be increased by 10 minutes, and more importantly, the degree of long-term ovarian blood supply disruption with total salpingectomy is not clearly defined (Creinin, 2014).

Regret. Invariably, some women will later express regrets about sterilization. From a CREST study, Jamieson and coworkers (2002) reported that by 5 years, 7 percent of women undergoing tubal ligation had regrets. This is not limited to female sterilization, as 6 percent of women whose husbands had undergone vasectomy had similar remorse. The cumulative probability of regret within 14 years of sterilization was 20 percent for women aged 30 or younger at sterilization compared with only 6 percent for those older than 30 years (Hillis, 1999).

No woman should undergo tubal sterilization believing that subsequent fertility is guaranteed either by surgical reanastomosis or by assisted reproductive techniques. These are technically difficult, expensive, and not always successful. Pregnancy rates vary greatly depending upon age, the amount of tube remaining, and the technology used. Pregnancy rates range from 50 to 90 percent with surgical reversal (Deffieux, 2011). Of note, pregnancies that result after tubal sterilization reanastomosis are at risk to be ectopic.

Method Failure. Reasons for interval tubal sterilization failure are not always apparent, but some have been identified. First, surgical error may occur and likely accounts for 30 to 50 percent of cases. Second, tubal fistula may complicate occlusion methods. Although usually encountered with electrocoagulation procedures, fistulas from inadequate or defective electric current delivery are now less likely because an amp meter is used routinely. In some cases, sterilization failure may follow spontaneous reanastomosis of the tubal segments. With faulty clips, occlusion can be incomplete. Last, luteal phase pregnancy may occur and describes the situation in which a woman is already pregnant when the procedure is performed. This can often be avoided by scheduling surgery during the menstrual cycle's follicular phase and by preoperative human chorionic gonadotropin (hCG) testing.

The overall failure rate reported from the CREST studies was 1.3 percent of 10,685 tubal sterilization surgeries. As shown in Figure 5-7, these rates vary for different procedures.

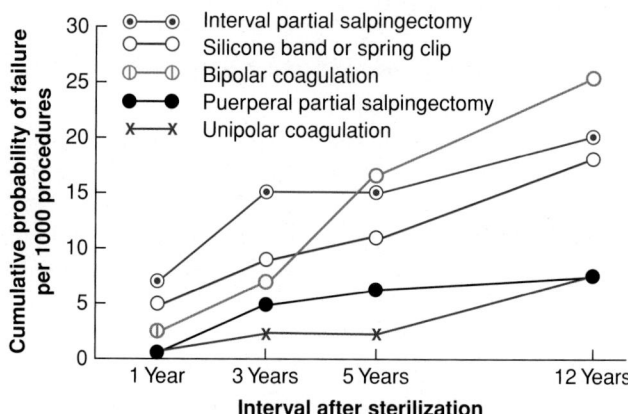

FIGURE 5-7 Data from the U.S. Collaborative Review of Sterilization (CREST) shows the cumulative probability of pregnancy per 1000 procedures by five methods of tubal sterilization. (Data from Peterson HB, Xia Z, Hughes JM, et al: The risk of pregnancy after tubal sterilization: findings from the U.S. Collaborative Review of Sterilization. Am J Obstet Gynecol 174(4):1161, 1996.)

And even with the same operation, failure rates vary. For example, with electrocoagulation, if fewer than three tubal sites are coagulated, the 5-year cumulative pregnancy rate approximates 12 per 1000 procedures. However, it is only 3 per 1000 if three or more sites are coagulated (Peterson, 1999). The lifetime increased cumulative failure rates over time are supportive that failures after 1 year are not likely due to technical errors. Indeed, Soderstrom (1985) found that most sterilization failures were not preventable.

With method failure, pregnancies following tubal sterilization have a high incidence of being ectopically implanted compared with the rate in a general gynecologic population. These rates are especially high following electrocoagulation procedures, in which up to 65 percent of pregnancies are ectopic. With failures following other methods—ring, clip, tubal resection—this percentage is only 10 percent (Peterson, 1999). Importantly, ectopic pregnancy must be excluded when any symptoms of pregnancy develop in a woman who has undergone tubal sterilization.

Other Effects. Several studies have evaluated the risk of heavy menstrual bleeding and intermenstrual bleeding following tubal sterilization, and many report no link (DeStefano, 1985; Shy, 1992). In addition, Peterson and coworkers (2000) compared long-term outcomes of 9514 women who had undergone tubal sterilization with a cohort of 573 women whose partners had undergone vasectomy. Risks for heavy menstrual bleeding, intermenstrual bleeding, and dysmenorrhea were similar in each group. Perhaps unexpectedly, women who had undergone sterilization had *decreased* duration and volume of menstrual flow, they reported *less* dysmenorrhea, but they had an *increased* incidence of cycle irregularity.

Other long-term effects have also been studied. It is controversial whether risks for subsequent hysterectomy are increased (Pati, 2000). In a CREST surveillance study, Hillis and associates (1997) reported that 17 percent of women undergoing tubal sterilization subsequently had undergone hysterectomy by 14 years. Although they did not compare this incidence with a control cohort, the indications for hysterectomy were similar to those for nonsterilized women who had undergone a hysterectomy. Women are highly unlikely to develop salpingitis following sterilization (Levgur, 2000). Tubal sterilization appears to have a protective effect against ovarian cancer, but not breast cancer (Westhoff, 2000).

Some psychological sequelae of sterilization were evaluated in a CREST study by Costello and associates (2002). These investigators reported that tubal ligation did not change sexual interest or pleasure in 80 percent of women. In the remaining 20 percent of women who reported a change, 80 percent described the changes to be positive.

Transcervical Sterilization

Mechanical Tubal Occlusion. Various methods of sterilization can be completed using a transcervical approach to reach the tubal ostia. Within each ostium, occlusion is achieved by placing either mechanical devices or chemical compounds.

Mechanical methods employ insertion of a device into the proximal fallopian tubes via hysteroscopy. One system, Essure,

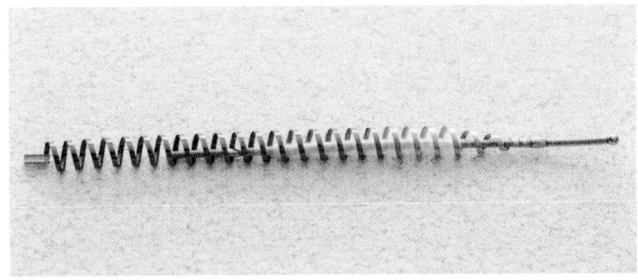

FIGURE 5-8 Microinsert used in the Essure Permanent Birth Control System.

is FDA-approved for use in the United States. A second system, Adiana Permanent Contraception, was taken off the market in 2013.

The Essure Permanent Birth Control System consists of a microinsert made of a stainless steel inner coil that is enclosed in polyester fibers. These fibers are surrounded by an expandable outer coil made of *nitinol*—a nickel and titanium alloy used in coronary artery stents (Fig. 5-8). Fibroblastic proliferation within the fibers causes tubal occlusion. The Essure technique is described in Section 44-16 (p. 1046). Analgesia provided by intravenous sedation or paracervical block will successfully alleviate pain (Cooper, 2003). In some women, general anesthesia is preferred.

By far, the overwhelming advantage of hysteroscopic sterilization is that it can be performed in the office. In addition, the procedure times average less than 20 minutes. Abnormal anatomy may preclude procedure completion. One year after placement, Essure contraceptive failure rates range from less than 1 percent to 5 percent (Gariepy, 2014; Munro, 2014).

Three months following device insertion, hysterosalpingography (HSG) is required to confirm complete occlusion (American College of Obstetricians and Gynecologists, 2012b). Prior to undergoing the procedure, patients are counseled on the importance of HSG compliance as up to half of all unplanned pregnancies after hysteroscopic sterilization may be associated with follow-up noncompliance (Cleary, 2013; Levy, 2007). Other reasons for subsequent unplanned pregnancy include incomplete occlusion (10 percent), incorrect HSG interpretation (33 percent), and an established pregnancy prior to the procedure (1 percent) (Jost, 2013; Munro, 2014). In some women, occlusion is incomplete at 3 months, and the study is then repeated at 6 months postoperatively. Until tubal occlusion is established, another method of contraception is needed. Transvaginal sonography has been investigated as an alternative confirmation tool, but currently HSG is required by the FDA (Veersema, 2011).

Pelvic pain after hysteroscopic sterilization is uncommon. If pelvic pain presents soon after the procedure, symptoms are likely to resolve by 3 months postoperatively, around the same time as the follow-up HSG (Arjona Berral, 2014; Yunker, 2015).

As with all sterilization procedures, Essure placement should be considered permanent. The success rate of subsequent spontaneous pregnancy after microsurgery tubal reversal ranges between 0 and 36 percent (Fernandez, 2014; Monteith, 2014).

Chemical Tubal Occlusion. Agents may be placed into the uterine cavity or tubal ostia to incite an inflammatory response to cause tubal occlusion. A method that has been used worldwide in more than 100,000 women consists of using an IUD-type inserter to place quinacrine pellets into the uterine fundus. It is effective, especially considering its simplicity. Pregnancy rates reported by Sokal and colleagues (2008) were 1 and 12 percent at 1 and 10 years, respectively. Although the WHO recommends against its use because of carcinogenesis concerns, it remains an important method for resource-poor countries (Castaño, 2010; Lippes, 2002).

Hysterectomy

For a woman with uterine or other pelvic disease for which hysterectomy may be indicated, this may be the ideal form of sterilization.

Male Sterilization

Vasectomy is performed each year in nearly a half million men in the United States (Magnani, 1999). The office procedure is done with local analgesia and usually takes 20 minutes or less to complete. As illustrated in Figure 5-9, a small incision is made in the scrotum, and the lumen of the vas deferens is disrupted to block sperm traveling from the testes. Compared with female tubal sterilization, vasectomy is 30 times less likely to fail and is 20 times less likely to have postoperative complications (Adams, 2009).

Sterility following vasectomy is not immediate nor is its onset reliably predictable. The time until complete expulsion of sperm stored distal to the vas deferens interruption is variable and requires approximately 3 months or 20 ejaculations (American College of Obstetricians and Gynecologists, 2013a). Thus, another form of contraception is used until azoospermia is documented. Although most recommend that semen be analyzed until two consecutive sperm counts are zero, Bradshaw and coworkers (2001) reported that a single azoospermic semen analysis is sufficient.

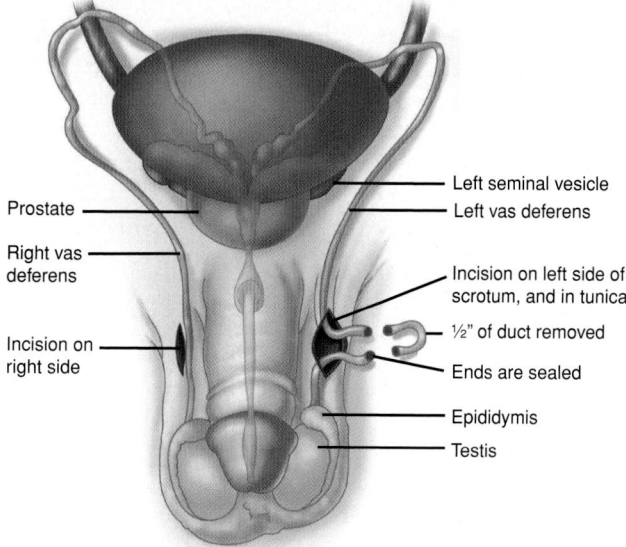

Prostate

Right vas deferens

Incision on right side

Left seminal vesicle
Left vas deferens

Incision on left side of scrotum, and in tunica

½" of duct removed

Ends are sealed

Epididymis

Testis

FIGURE 5-9 Vasectomy. On the left, the incision site is shown. On the right, a portion of the vas deferens has been excised.

Sterilization by vasectomy has a failure rate less than 1 percent (Michielsen, 2010). Causes include failure from unprotected intercourse too soon after vasectomy, incomplete vas deferens occlusion, or recanalization following suitable separation.

Fertility Restoration. After vasectomy, fertility may be restored either by surgical reanastomosis techniques or by sperm retrieval from the testis. Surgical reversal techniques and perioperative evaluation have been reviewed by the American Society for Reproductive Medicine (2008). Sperm retrieval combined with in vitro fertilization techniques avoids such reversal surgeries and is described in Chapter 20 (p. 462). From their review, Shridharani and Sandlow (2010) concluded that microsurgical reversal is cost effective, but comparative trials with sperm retrieval methods are needed.

Long-term Effects. Regret of sterilization was discussed on page 116. Other than this, long-term consequences are rare (Amundsen, 2004). However, because antibodies directed at spermatozoa frequently develop in these men, there were initial concerns that these might cause systemic disease. Putative risks were analyzed by Köhler and coworkers (2009) and include cardiovascular disease, immune-complex disorders, psychological changes, male genital cancers, and frontotemporal dementia. Their findings and those of others are not convincing for an increased risk of cardiovascular disease or accelerated atherogenesis from vasectomy (Schwingl, 2000). Moreover, rates of testicular or prostate cancers do not appear increased with this procedure (Holt, 2008; Köhler, 2009).

SECOND-TIER CONTRACEPTIVE METHODS

Contraceptives considered to be *very effective* are the hormone-containing preparations that include combination oral contraceptives, progestin-only contraceptive pills, and contraceptives with estrogens and/or progestins that are made systemically available by injection, transdermal patch, or intravaginal ring. When used as intended, these methods are highly effective, however, their efficacy is user dependent. Thus, *typical use* considers each woman's compliance with taking a daily pill, changing transdermal patches or rings, or presenting for an injection (see Table 5-2). Such "real world" use significantly diminishes their efficacy, and for women in the United States, these contraceptives have a first-year pregnancy rate of 3 to 9 per 100 users.

■ Combined Hormonal Contraceptives

These are contraceptives that contain an estrogen and a progestin. As such, several underlying conditions are considered contraindications to their use (Table 5-6). Combined hormonal contraceptives (CHCs) are available in the United States in three formats—oral contraceptive pills, the transdermal patch, and the intravaginal contraceptive ring. Because of limited data for the transdermal and transvaginal methods relative to that for COCs, their use is usually considered along with those of combined oral contraceptives.

Pharmacology

There are multiple contraceptive actions of CHCs. The most important is to inhibit ovulation by suppression of hypothalamic

Contraception and Sterilization

TABLE 5-6. Contraindications to the Use of Combination Oral Contraceptives

Pregnancy
Uncontrolled hypertension
Smokers older than 35 years
Diabetes with vascular involvement
Cerebrovascular or coronary artery disease
Migraines with associated focal neurologic deficits
Thrombophlebitis or thromboembolic disorders
History of deep-vein thrombophlebitis or thrombotic
  disorders
Thrombogenic heart arrhythmias or thrombogenic cardiac
  valvulopathies
Undiagnosed abnormal genital bleeding
Known or suspected breast carcinoma
Cholestatic jaundice of pregnancy or jaundice with pill use
Hepatic adenomas or carcinomas or active liver disease
  with abnormal liver function
Endometrial cancer or other known or suspected estrogen-
  dependent neoplasia

gonadotropin-releasing hormone, which prevents pituitary secretion of follicle-stimulating hormone (FSH) and luteinizing hormone (LH). Estrogens suppress FSH release and stabilize the endometrium to prevent intermenstrual bleeding—referred to as *breakthrough bleeding* in this setting. Progestins inhibit ovulation by suppressing LH, they thicken cervical mucus to retard sperm passage, and they render the endometrium unfavorable for implantation. Thus, CHCs have contraceptive effects from both hormones and, when taken daily for 3 out of every 4 weeks, provide virtually absolute protection against conception.

Until recently, there were only two estrogens available for use in oral contraceptives in the United States. These were *ethinyl estradiol* and its less commonly used 3-methyl ether, *mestranol*. In 2010, a third estrogen compound—*estradiol valerate*—was approved by the FDA. Most currently available progestins are *19-nortestosterone* derivatives. However, drospirenone is a spironolactone analogue, and the dose of drospirenone in COCs currently marketed has properties similar to a 25-mg dose of spironolactone (Seeger, 2007). Drospirenone displays antiandrogenic activity, and its antimineralocorticoid properties may, in theory, cause potassium retention, leading to hyperkalemia. Thus, drospirenone is not prescribed for those with renal or adrenal insufficiency or with hepatic dysfunction. Moreover, monitoring of serum potassium levels is recommended in the first month for patients chronically treated concomitantly with any drug associated with potassium retention (Bayer HealthCare Pharmaceuticals, 2012). Several studies have shown improvement in symptoms for women with premenstrual dysphoric disorder (PMDD) who use the drospirenone-containing COC, Yaz (Lopez, 2012; Yonkers, 2005). For this pill, the FDA has approved its indications to include treatment of premenstrual syndrome and moderate acne vulgaris for women requesting oral contraception.

Progestins were initially selected for their progestational potency. However, they are often compared, marketed, and prescribed based on their presumed estrogenic, antiestrogenic,

and androgenic effects. However, the doses of progestins used in combined contraceptive formulations are so low that none of these purported negative side effects are actually manifested clinically. In fact, an important effect of CHCs is increased production of sex hormone-binding globulin (SHBG) by the liver and production is promoted mostly by the estrogen component of CHCs. Elevated SHBG levels lower serum free testosterone levels and thereby limit 5α-reductase, the enzyme necessary to convert testosterone to its active form, dihydrotestosterone. For this reason, CHCs can be expected to have salutary effects on androgen-related conditions such as acne (del Marmol, 2004; Rosen, 2003; Thorneycroft, 1999).

Combined Oral Contraceptive Pills

Formulations. Hormone-containing contraceptive pills recently had a celebrated 50th anniversary in this country. These various preparations—used by approximately 16 million women in the United States in 2013—are popularly known by several names (United Nations, 2013). Among others, these include: *combination oral contraceptives (COCs), birth control pills (BCPs), oral contraceptives (OCs), oral contraceptive pills (OCPs),* and most simply, *the pill.*

Combination oral contraceptives are marketed in a bewildering variety shown in (Table 5-7 and Fig. 5-10). Currently, the daily estrogen content in most COCs varies from 20 to 50 μg of ethinyl estradiol, and most pills contain 35 μg or less. Of note, in 2011, the FDA approved the first pill containing only 10 μg of ethinyl estradiol—*Lo Loestrin Fe.* For current formulations, the lowest acceptable dose is governed by the ability to prevent unacceptable breakthrough bleeding.

With COCs, the progestin dose can be constant throughout the cycle—*monophasic pills*—but the dose frequently is varied—

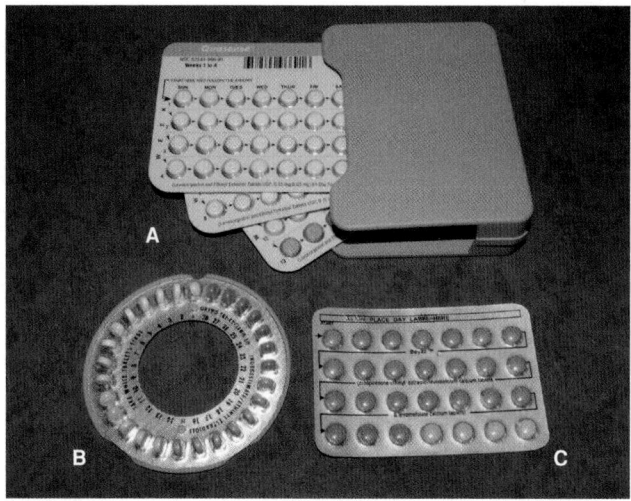

FIGURE 5-10 Various combined oral contraceptive (COC) pills. **A.** Extended-use COCs. Each of the three sequential cards of pills is taken. Placebo pills (*peach*) are found in the bottom card. **B.** 21/7 triphasic COCs. Active pills are taken for 3 weeks and are followed by seven placebo pills (*green*). With triphasic pills, the combination of estrogen and progestin varies with color changes, in this case, from white to blue to dark blue. **C.** 24/4 monophasic COCs. Monophasic pills contain a constant dose of estrogen and progestin throughout the pill pack. With 24/4 dosing regimens, the number of placebo pills is decreased to four.

TABLE 5-7. Combination Oral Contraceptive Formulations

Product Name	Estrogen	µg (days)[a]	Progestin	mg (days)
Monophasic Preparations				
20–25 µg estrogen				
Yaz, Loryna, Nikki	EE	20 (24)	Drospirenone	3.00 (24)
Beyaz[b]	EE	20 (24)	Drospirenone	3.00 (24)
Aviane, Falmina, Lessina, Orsythia	EE	20	Levonorgestrel	0.10
Loestrin 1/20, Junel 1/20, Microgestin 1/20, Gildess 1/20 Larin 1/20	EE	20	Norethindrone acetate	1.00
Loestrin Fe 1/20[c], Gildess Fe 1/20[c], Junel Fe 1/20[c], Microgestin Fe 1/20[c], Larin Fe 1/20[c]	EE	20	Norethindrone acetate	1.00
Loestrin 24 Fe[c], Minastrin 24 Fe[c] Gildess 24 Fe[c]	EE	20 (24)	Norethindrone acetate	1.00 (24)
30–35 µg estrogen				
Desogen, Ortho-Cept, Emoquette, Enskyce	EE	30	Desogestrel	0.15
Yasmin, Syeda, Yaela	EE	30	Drospirenone	3.00
Safyral[b]	EE	30	Drospirenone	3.00
Kelnor, Zovia 1/35	EE	35	Ethynodiol diacetate	1.00
Nordette, Altavera, Kurvelo, Levora, Marlissa, Portia	EE	30	Levonorgestrel	0.15
Lo/Ovral, Cryselle, Elinest	EE	30	Norgestrel	0.30
Ovcon-35, Balziva, Briellyn, Philith, Gildagia, Vyfemla	EE	35	Norethindrone	0.40
Femcon Fe[c]	EE	35	Norethindrone	0.40
Brevicon, Modicon, Nortrel 0.5/35, Wera	EE	35	Norethindrone	0.50
Ortho-Novum 1/35, Norinyl 1+35, Nortrel 1/35, Pirmella 1/35, Cyclafem w1/35, Alyacen 1/35, Dasetta 1/35	EE	35	Norethindrone	1.00
Loestrin 1.5/30, Junel 1.5/30, Microgestin 1.5/30, Gildess 1.5/30, Larin 1.5/30	EE	30	Norethindrone acetate	1.50
Loestrin Fe 1.5/30[c], Junel Fe 1.5/30[c], Microgestin Fe 1.5/30[c] Gildess Fe 1.5/30[c], Larin 1.5/30[c]	EE	30	Norethindrone acetate	1.50
Ortho-Cyclen, Sprintec, Previfem, Estarylla, Mono-Linyah	EE	35	Norgestimate	0.25
50 µg estrogen				
Ogestrel	EE	50	Norgestrel	0.50
Zovia 1/50	EE	50	Ethynodiol diacetate	1.00
Norinyl 1+50	Mes	50	Norethindrone	1.00
Multiphasic Preparations				
10 µg estrogen				
Lo Loestrin Fe[c], Lo Minastin Fe[c]	EE	10 (24) 10 (2)	Norethindrone acetate	1.00 (24)
20 µg estrogen				
Kariva, Viorele	EE	20 (21) 0 (2) 10 (5)	Desogestrel	0.15
25 µg estrogen				
Ortho Tri-Cyclen Lo	EE	25	Norgestimate	0.18 (7) 0.215 (7) 0.25 (7)
Cyclessa, Velivet	EE	25	Desogestrel	0.1 (7) 0.125 (7) 0.15 (7)

(Continued)

TABLE 5-7. Combination Oral Contraceptive Formulations *(Continued)*

Product Name	Estrogen	μg (days)[a]	Progestin	mg (days)
Multiphasic Preparations *(Continued)*				
30–35 μg estrogen				
Ortho Tri-Cyclen, Tri-Sprintec, Tri-Previfem, Tri-Linyah, Tri-Estarylla	EE	35	Norgestimate	0.18 (7) 0.215 (7) 0.25 (7)
Trivora, Enpresse, Levonest, Myzilra	EE	30 (6) 40 (5) 30 (10)	Levonorgestrel	0.05 (6) 0.075 (5) 0.125 (10)
Estrostep[c], Tri-Legest[c]	EE	20 (5) 30 (7) 35 (9)	Norethindrone acetate	1.00
Ortho-Novum 7/7/7, Alyacen 7/7/7, Cyclafem 7/7/7, Dasetta 7/7/7, Nortrel 7/7/7	EE	35	Norethindrone	0.50 (7) 0.75 (7) 1.0 (7)
Tri-Norinyl, Aranelle	EE	35	Norethindrone	0.50 (7) 1.00 (9) 0.50 (5)
Natazia	EV	3 (2) 2 (5) 2 (17) 1 (2)	Dienogest	— 2.00 (5) 3.00 (17) —
Progestin-only Preparations				
Micronor, Nor-QD, Errin, Camila, Heather, Jencycla	None		Norethindrone	0.35 (c)
Extended-cycle Preparations				
20 μg estrogen				
LoSeasonique[e]	EE	20 (84) 10 (7)	Levonorgestrel	0.10 (84)
30 μg estrogen				
Seasonale[d], Quasense[d], Introvale[d], Setlakin[d]	EE	30 (84)	Levonorgestrel	0.15 (84)
Seasonique[e], Daysee[e]	EE	30 (84) 10 (7)	Levonorgestrel	0.15 (84)
Quartette[e]	EE	20 (42) 25 (21) 30 (21) 10 (7)	Levonorgestrel	0.15 (84)

EE = ethinyl estradiol; EV = estradiol valerate; LC = levomefolate calcium; Mes = mestranol.
[a]Administered for 21 days, variations listed in parentheses.
[b]0.451 mg of levomefolate calcium, which is a form of folic acid, is found in each pill.
[c]Contains or is available in formulas that contain 75-mg doses of ferrous fumarate within the placebo pills.
[d]12 weeks of active pills, then 1 week of inert pills.
[e]12 weeks of active pills, then 1 week of ethinyl estradiol only.
Data from U.S. Food and Drug Administration: Orange book: approved drug products with therapeutic equivalence evaluations. 2014. Available at: http://www.accessdata.fda.gov/scripts/cder/ob/default.cfm. Accessed December 19, 2014.

biphasic and *triphasic pills*. In some of these, the estrogen dose is also varied during the cycle. *Multiphasic pills* were developed to reduce the amount of total progestin per cycle without sacrificing contraceptive efficacy or cycle control. The reduction is achieved by beginning with a low dose of progestin and increasing it later in the cycle. Theoretically, the lower total dose minimizes the intensity of progestin-induced metabolic changes and adverse side effects. Disadvantages of multiphasic formulations include confusion caused by the multicolored pills—in some brands there are five colors. Another side effect is breakthrough bleeding or spotting, which likely is increased compared with monophasic pills (Woods, 1992).

In a few COCs, inert placebo pills have been replaced by tablets containing iron. These have the suffix Fe added to their name. In addition, Beyaz has a form of folate—levomefolate calcium—within both its active and placebo pills.

Administration. Ideally, women would begin COCs on the first day of a menstrual cycle, in which case an additional contraceptive method is unnecessary. A more traditional schedule—the *Sunday start*—requires pill initiation on the first Sunday following the onset of menses. If menses begin on a Sunday, then pills are started that day. Last, a *quick start* method may be used in which pills are started on any day of the cycle, commonly the day prescribed. This approach improves short-term compliance (Westhoff, 2002, 2007a). Both Sunday start and quick start methods require use of an additional method for 1 week to protect against conception.

To obtain maximum efficacy and promote regular use, most manufacturers offer dispensers that provide 21 sequential color-coded tablets containing hormones, followed by seven inert tablets of another color (see Fig. 5-10B). Some newer, lower-dose pill regimens continue active hormones for 24 days, followed by 4 days of inert pills (see Fig. 5-10C). The goal of these 24/4 regimens is to improve the efficacy of very low-dose COCs. Importantly, for maximum contraceptive efficiency, each woman should adopt an effective scheme for ensuring daily—or nightly—self-administration.

During COC use, if one dose is missed, conception is unlikely with higher-dose monophasic COCs. When this is recognized, taking that day's pill plus the missed pill will minimize breakthrough bleeding. The remainder of the pill pack is then completed with one pill taken daily.

If several doses are missed, or if a dose is missed with the lower-dose pills, then two pills are taken but an effective barrier technique is added for the subsequent 7 days. The remainder of the pack is completed with one pill taken daily. Alternatively, a new pack can be started and a barrier method added as additional contraception for a week. With any scenario of missed pills, if withdrawal bleeding does not occur during the placebo pills, the pills are continued, but the woman should seek medical attention to exclude pregnancy. Fortunately, CHCs are not teratogenic if taken accidentally during early pregnancy (Lammer, 1986).

Transdermal System

There is one transdermal system available in the United States—*Ortho Evra patch*. The patch has an inner layer with an adhesive and hormone matrix and an outer water-resistant layer. The patch is applied to the buttocks, upper outer arm, lower abdomen, or upper torso but avoids the breasts. It delivers daily a dose of 150 μg of the progestin norelgestromin and 20 μg of ethinyl estradiol. A new patch is applied each week for 3 weeks, followed by a patch-free week to allow withdrawal bleeding.

In a randomized trial by Audet and associates (2001), the patch was slightly more effective than a low-dose oral contraceptive—1.2 versus 2.2 pregnancies per 100 woman years. Patch replacement was required for either complete—1.8 percent, or partial detachment—2.8 percent. In approximately 3 percent of women, a severe application-site reaction precluded further use.

Pooled data suggest that women who weigh 90 kg or more are at increased risk for pregnancy with the patch (Zieman,

2002). Other metabolic and physiologic effects mirror those seen with low-dose COCs, with the caveat that accumulated experience is limited. The patch is suitable for women who prefer weekly applications to daily dosing and who meet the other criteria for CHC administration.

Concerns have been raised that CHC delivered by the patch may be associated with an increased risk for VTE and other vascular complications. This followed reports that patch use was associated with increased hepatic synthesis of procoagulants compared with COC or vaginal ring use (Jensen, 2008; White, 2006). Although peak serum estrogen levels were lower with patch versus COC use, total exposure was greater—a relatively increased net estrogen effect (Kluft, 2008; van den Heuvel, 2005). Despite lack of a convincing clinical association, in 2008, the FDA ordered labeling for the patch to state that users *may* be at increased risk for developing VTE. Plaintiff attorneys followed with lawsuits that inevitably curtailed use of the patch method (Phelps, 2009). To date, conclusive evidence for increased morbidity with patch use compared with other CHC use is lacking (Jick, 2006, 2010a,b).

Transvaginal Ring

There is one intravaginal hormonal contraceptive available in the United States—*NuvaRing*. It is a flexible polymer ring with a 54-mm outer diameter and a 50-mm inner diameter (Fig. 5-11). Its core releases a daily dose of 15 μg ethinyl estradiol and 120 μg of the progestin etonogestrel. These doses effectively inhibit ovulation, and the failure rate is reported to be 0.65 pregnancies per 100 woman-years (Mulders, 2001; Roumen, 2001).

Prior to dispensing, the pharmacy must keep rings refrigerated. Once dispensed, their shelf life is 4 months. The ring is initially inserted within 5 days after the onset of menses. It is removed after 3 weeks for 1 week to allow withdrawal bleeding. After this, a new ring is inserted. Breakthrough bleeding is uncommon. Up to 20 percent of women and 35 percent of men reported being able to feel the ring during intercourse. If bothersome, the ring may be removed for coitus, but it should be replaced within 3 hours.

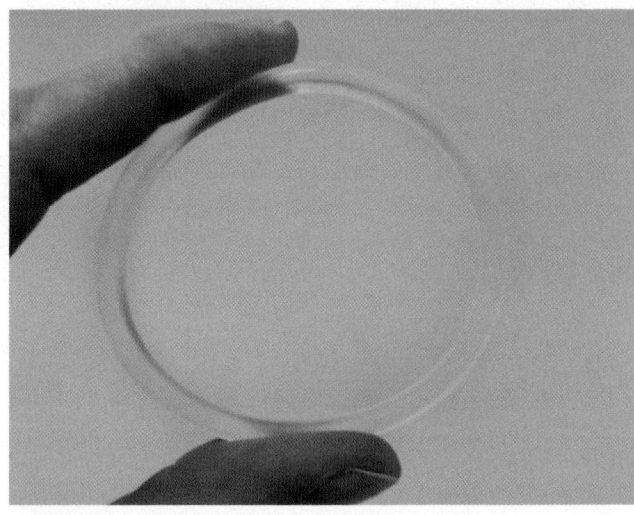

FIGURE 5-11 Estrogen- and progestin-releasing vaginal contraceptive ring.

Extended Cycle Contraception

The use of CHCs continuously for more than 28 days has become increasingly popular. Their benefits include decreased episodes of cyclic bleeding, fewer menstrual symptoms, and lower costs. Several formulations are available (see Table 5-7). Although these prepackaged cycle formulations are available, extended cycle contraception can also be achieved in other ways. The standard 21- or 28-day COC packs, with the placebo pills discarded, can be used continuously. Also, either the transdermal patch or the vaginal ring can be used without the 1-week hormone-free interval.

Several factors unique to extended-cycle CHCs are important. Some of these are shared with continuous progestin contraceptive methods such as implants or injections. The principal change is loss of menstrual normalcy that manifests as less frequent, lighter, and generally unpredictable bleeding episodes. For example, amenorrhea of 6 months or more is reported to affect 8 to 63 percent of extended cycle users. Although considered a benefit by most women, it is far from a guaranteed one. More often, women have fewer bleeding episodes per month. This allows repair of associated anemia in those who had heavy menstrual bleeding prior to extended-cycle use.

However, these characteristics also render some women reluctant to use this method, as it may be considered "unnatural" to miss monthly menses. Some are concerned that amenorrhea may be a sign of pregnancy, may diminish future fertility, or may increase endometrial neoplasia. Rather, findings support a *decreased* risk for endometrial malignancy associated with cyclic CHC use. Thus on a biological basis, it seems reasonable to conclude that this protective effect would also apply to continuous CHC use. Moreover, women who use a continuous CHC method report fewer menstrual symptoms that include headaches, fatigue, bloating, and dysmenorrhea compared with women using cyclic contraceptives (Edelman, 2014). Moreover, hypothalamic-pituitary-ovarian suppression is greater with continuous use and reduces the possibility of escape ovulation caused by delayed start of a new contraceptive cycle.

Drug Interactions

Interactions between CHCs and various other medications take two forms. First, hormonal contraceptives may interfere with the actions of some drugs shown in Table 5-8. In contrast, some drugs shown in Table 5-9 may decrease the contraceptive

TABLE 5-8. Drugs Whose Effectiveness Is Influenced by Combination Oral Contraceptives (COCs)

Interacting Drug	Documentation	Management of the Interacting Drug
Analgesics		
Acetaminophen	Adequate	Possible dose increase needed
Aspirin	Probable	Possible dose increase needed
Meperidine	Suspected	Possible dose decrease needed
Morphine	Probable	Possible dose increase needed
Anticoagulants		
Dicumarol, warfarin	Controversial	
Antidepressants		
Imipramine	Suspected	Reduce dosage about a third
Tranquilizers		
Diazepam, alprazolam	Suspected	Reduce dose
Temazepam	Possible	Possible dose increase needed
Other benzodiazepines	Suspected	Observe for increased effect
Antiinflammatories		
Corticosteroids	Adequate	Watch for increased effect, decrease dose accordingly
Bronchodilators		
Aminophylline, theophylline	Adequate	Reduce starting dose by a third
Antihypertensives		
Cyclopenthiazide	Adequate	Increase dose
Metoprolol	Suspected	Possible dose decrease needed
Other		
Troleandomycin	Suspected liver damage	Avoid
Cyclosporine	Possible	May use smaller dose
Antiretrovirals	Variable	See manufacturer or other[a]
Lamotrigine	Adequate	With monotherapy or when given with drugs that are not known to alter lamotrigine levels, then avoid COCs

[a]University of California at San Francisco (UCSF): HIV Insite, 2014.
Gaffield, 2011; Wallach, 2000.

TABLE 5-9. Drugs That May Reduce Combined Hormonal Contraceptive Efficacy

Interacting Drug	Documentation
Antituberculous	
Rifampin	Established; reduced efficacy if <50 μg EE
Antifungals	
Griseofulvin	Strongly suspected
Anticonvulsants and sedatives	
Phenytoin, phenobarbital, primidone, carbamazepine, ethosuximide	Strongly suspected; reduced efficacy if <50 μg EE; trials lacking
Antibiotics	
Tetracycline, doxycycline	Two small studies find no association
Penicillins	No association documented
Ciprofloxacin	No effect on efficacy of a 30 μg EE + desogestrel pill
Ofloxacin	No effect on efficacy of a 30 μg EE + levonorgestrel pill
Antiretrovirals	Variable effects; see manufacturer or other[a]

EE = ethinyl estradiol.
[a]University of California at San Francisco (UCSF): HIV Insite, 2014.
Data from Wallach M, Grimes DA (eds): Modern Oral Contraception. Updates from The Contraception Report. Totowa, Emron, 2000, pp 26, 90, 194.

effectiveness of CHCs. Mechanisms for these are multiple and frequently cannot be identified. In some cases, genes coding for cytochrome oxidase system enzymes are either stimulated or suppressed.

Resulting pharmacokinetic changes can decrease serum contraceptive steroid concentrations, but the ultimate effect on ovulation suppression is unknown. However, with current information, these interactions often require that the dose of contraceptive or that of the other drug be adjusted to ensure efficacy.

Combined Hormonal Contraception and Medical Disorders

A summary of health benefits associated with CHCs is found in Table 5-10. Despite this, interactions of CHCs with some chronic medical disorders may constitute relative or absolute contraindication to CHC use. These are described in the following sections.

TABLE 5-10. Some Benefits of Combination Estrogen plus Progestin Oral Contraceptives

Increased bone density
Reduced menstrual blood loss and anemia
Decreased risk of ectopic pregnancy
Improved dysmenorrhea from endometriosis
Fewer premenstrual complaints
Decreased risk of endometrial and ovarian cancer
Reduction in various benign breast diseases
Inhibition of hirsutism progression
Acne improvement
Prevention of atherogenesis
Decreased incidence and severity of acute salpingitis
Decreased activity of rheumatoid arthritis

Obese and Overweight Women. In general, CHCs are highly effective in obese women (Lopez, 2013). However, obesity may result in altered pharmacokinetics of some CHC methods. That said, data regarding overweight women are conflicting regarding increased pregnancy risk due to decreased CHC efficacy from lowered bioavailability (Brunner, 2005; Edelman, 2009; Holt, 2005; Westhoff, 2010). Importantly, in some women, obesity may be synergistic with other conditions, described next, that may render CHCs a less optimal contraceptive method.

Excessive weight gain is a concern with use of any hormonal contraceptive. Gallo and associates (2014) again concluded in their review that available evidence was insufficient to determine the influence of CHCs on weight gain, although no large effect was obvious.

Diabetes Mellitus. Higher-dose COCs were associated with insulin antagonistic properties, particularly those mediated by progestins. However, with current low-dose CHCs, these concerns have been mitigated. In healthy women, large, long-term prospective studies have found that COCs do not increase the risk for diabetes (Rimm, 1992). Moreover, these agents do not appear to increase the risk for overt diabetes in women with prior gestational diabetes (Kjos, 1998). Last, use of these contraceptives is approved for nonsmoking diabetic women who are younger than 35 years and who have no associated vascular disease (American College of Obstetricians and Gynecologists, 2013d).

Cardiovascular Disease. In general, severe cardiovascular disorders limit the use of CHCs. For less severe disorders, however, current formulations do not increase associated risks.

First, low-dose CHCs do not appreciably increase the absolute risk of clinically significant hypertension (Chasan-Taber,

1996). However, it is common practice for patients to return 8 to 12 weeks following CHC initiation for evaluation of blood pressure and other symptoms. For those with already established chronic hypertension, CHC use is permissible in those with well-controlled, otherwise uncomplicated hypertension (American College of Obstetricians and Gynecologists, 2013d). Severe forms of hypertension, especially those with end-organ involvement, usually preclude CHC use.

Women who have had a documented *myocardial infarction* should not be given CHCs. That said, these contraceptives do not increase the de novo risk for myocardial ischemia in nonsmoking women younger than 35 years (Margolis, 2007; Mishell, 2000; World Health Organization, 1997). Smoking by itself, however, is a potent risk factor for ischemic heart disease, and CHCs used after age 35 years act synergistically to increase this risk.

Cerebrovascular Disorders. Women who have had either an *ischemic* or *hemorrhagic stroke* should not use CHCs. But the incidence of strokes in nonsmoking young women is low, and use of CHCs does not increase the risk for either type of stroke (World Health Organization, 1996). This form of vascular disorder is more commonly encountered in those who smoke, have hypertension, or have migraine headaches with visual aura *and* who use CHCs (MacClellan, 2007).

Migraine headaches may be a risk factor for strokes in some young women. Curtis and coworkers (2002) reported that women using COCs who had *migraine headaches with aura* had a two- to fourfold increased risk for stroke compared with nonusers. Because of this, the WHO (2010) recommends against CHC use in this subset of migraineurs. Alternatively, the American College of Obstetricians and Gynecologists (2013d), because the absolute risk is low, has concluded that CHCs may be considered for young nonsmoking women who have migraine headaches without focal neurologic changes. For many of these women, an intrauterine contraceptive method or a progestin-only pill may be more appropriate (World Health Organization, 2010).

Venous Thromboembolism. Early in CHC history, it was apparent that *deep-vein thrombosis* and *pulmonary embolism* risks were significantly increased in women who used these contraceptives (Realini, 1985). These risks were found to be estrogen-dose related and have been appreciably lowered with evolution of low-dose formulations that contain only 10 to 35 µg of ethinyl estradiol (Westhoff, 1998). Of note, a possible increased VTE risk with drospirenone-containing COCs has been shown in two studies, and the FDA has encouraged an assessment of benefits and of VTE risks in users of these pills (Food and Drug Administration, 2012; Jick, 2011; Parkin, 2011).

Mishell and coworkers (2000) concluded that VTE risk is three- to fourfold higher in current COC users compared with nonusers. However, the risk without contraception is low—approximately 1 per 10,000 woman years—and thus the incidence with CHCs is only 3 to 4 per 10,000 woman years. Importantly, these CHC-enhanced risks appear to dissipate rapidly once contraceptive treatment is discontinued. And, of equal importance, these VTE risks are still lower than those estimated during pregnancy, which has an incidence of 5 to 6 per 10,000 woman years.

Several cofactors increase the incidence of VTE in women using estrogen-containing contraceptives or those who are pregnant or postpartum. These include one or more of the many thrombophilias, which include *protein C or S deficiency* or *factor V Leiden mutation* (Chap. 39, p. 836) (Mohllajee, 2006). Other factors that raise VTE risks are hypertension, obesity, diabetes, smoking, and a sedentary lifestyle (Pomp, 2007, 2008).

Older studies indicated a twofold increased risk for perioperative VTE in CHC users (Robinson, 1991). Data are lacking with the low-dose formulations currently used, and thus the American College of Obstetricians and Gynecologists (2013c,d) recommends balancing VTE risks against those of unintended pregnancy during the 4 to 6 weeks required preoperatively for thrombogenic effects of CHCs to dissipate.

Systemic Lupus Erythematosus. The use of CHCs in women with otherwise uncomplicated systemic lupus erythematosus (SLE) has been the "poster child" for evidence-based clinical research. In the past, and with good reason, CHCs were contraindicated in women with SLE. This was because of their underlying high risk to develop venous and arterial thrombosis along with the thrombogenic effects of older high-dose COC pills. The safety of the low-dose modern COCs in many women with SLE was shown in two randomized trials (Petri, 2005; Sánchez-Guerrero, 2005). Use of CHCs in women with SLE was reviewed by Culwell and colleagues (2009). Importantly, CHCs are not appropriate in women with SLE who have positive testing for antiphospholipid antibodies or have other known contraindications to CHC use. Affected women with these antibodies have increased clotting risks.

Seizure Disorders. Approximately 1 million women of reproductive age in the United States are diagnosed with some form of epilepsy. As shown in Tables 5-8 and 5-9, metabolism and clearance of some CHCs are appreciably altered by some, but not all, of the commonly used anticonvulsants. One mechanism with several antiepileptic drugs is potent induction of cytochrome P450 system enzymes. In turn, this increases contraceptive steroid metabolism, and serum levels of these decrease by as much as half (American College of Obstetricians and Gynecologists, 2013d; Zupanc, 2006).

These metabolic interactions usually do not result in increased seizure activity. One possible exception is combined use of CHCs and monotherapy with the anticonvulsant lamotrigine. Serum anticonvulsant levels are decreased by up to 50 percent, which may increase seizure risks (Gaffield, 2011).

Evidence-based guidelines for use of contraceptives by women with epilepsy are listed in the US MEC. Use of CHCs in epileptic women is rated as category 3, that is, theoretical or proven risks usually outweigh the method advantages. CHCs used concurrently with anticonvulsants may reduce contraceptive or anticonvulsant effectiveness. Thus, epileptic women using cytochrome P450 enhancing anticonvulsants are counseled regarding alternate contraceptive methods if feasible. If not, a COC containing at least 30 µg of ethinyl estradiol should be used. For those using lamotrigine monotherapy, CHCs are not recommended.

Although they are not CHCs, progestin-only containing preparations are also affected by use of anticonvulsants that induce the cytochrome P450 enzyme system. These result in decreased serum progestin levels and lower rates of effective ovulation suppression and pose an unacceptable risk of unplanned pregnancy.

Liver Disease. Both estrogens and progestins have known effects on hepatic function. Cholestasis and cholestatic jaundice, which develop more commonly in pregnancy, are also infrequently induced by CHC use. Because susceptibility is likely due to an inherited gene mutation of bilirubin transport, cholestasis with CHCs is more likely in women affected during a pregnancy. Discontinuing CHCs typically resolves symptoms. Whether these cholestatic effects of CHCs also raise risks for subsequent cholelithiasis and cholecystectomy is unclear. Any increased risk is likely to be small, and the known effects of increasing parity on gallbladder disease must also be considered.

Regarding women with viral hepatitis or cirrhosis, the WHO has provided recommendations (Kapp, 2009b). For women who have active hepatitis, CHCs should not be initiated, but these may be continued in women who experience a flare of their liver disease while already taking CHCs. Use of progestin-only contraception in these women is not restricted. With cirrhosis, mild compensated disease does not limit the use of CHCs or progestin-only methods. However, in those with severe decompensated disease, all hormonal types are avoided.

Neoplastic Diseases. Stimulatory effects of sex steroids on some cancers are a concern. It would appear, however, that overall these hormones do not *cause* cancer (Hannaford, 2007). A report from the Collaborative Group on Epidemiological Studies of Ovarian Cancer (2008) verified earlier studies that showed a protective effect against endometrial and ovarian cancers (Cancer and Steroid Hormone Study, 1987a,b). However, this protection wanes as duration from pill discontinuance increases (Tworoger, 2007). Reports concerning possible increased risks for premalignant and malignant changes of the liver, cervix, and breast are conflicting and are presented next.

First, *hepatic focal nodular hyperplasia* and *benign hepatic adenomas* were previously linked with older higher-dose estrogen-containing COCs. However, studies that evaluated women taking contemporary low-dose COCs reported no such association (Hannaford, 1997; Heinemann, 1998). Similarly, earlier correlations between CHCs and hepatocellular carcinoma have been refuted by the multicenter WHO Study (1989) and by Maheshwari and coworkers (2007). For women with known tumors, COCs may be used in those with focal nodular hyperplasia, but avoided in those with benign hepatic adenoma and hepatocellular carcinoma (Kapp, 2009a).

Second, *cervical dysplasia* and *cervical cancer* rates are increased in COC users. These risks increase with duration of use. But, according to the International Collaboration of Epidemiological Studies of Cervical Cancer (2007), if COC use is discontinued, by 10 years the risk becomes comparable with that of never-users. The reasons for this neoplasia risk are speculative and may be related to more frequent human papillomavirus (HPV) exposure because of decreased use of barrier

methods. It may also be related to the more frequent cytologic screening that COC users may have. Moreover, COCs may increase persistence of HPV infection and HPV oncogene expression (de Villiers, 2003). Importantly, if cervical dysplasia is treated, the recurrence rate is not increased in CHC users.

Last, *breast cancer* is stimulated by female sex steroid hormones, but it is still unclear whether CHCs have an adverse effect on tumor growth or development. The Collaborative Group on Hormonal Factors in Breast Cancer (1996) analyzed data from studies that included more than 53,000 women with breast cancer and 100,000 nonaffected women. They found a significant 1.24-fold increased risk for current COC users. This risk decreased to 1.16 for those 1 to 4 years after discontinuing COCs and 1.07 for those at 5 to 9 years. The risks were not influenced by age at first use, duration of use, family history of breast cancer, first use prior to pregnancy, or the dose or type of hormone used. This lack of correlation serves to question any causal role of COCs in breast tumorigenesis.

The Collaborative Group investigators also found that COC-associated breast tumors tended to be to be less aggressive and that cancers were detected at earlier stages. They suggested that the increased cancer diagnosis may have been because of more intensive surveillance among users. In a case-control study—4575 cases and 4682 controls—there was no relationship found with either current or past COC use and breast cancer (Marchbanks, 2002). Finally, women heterozygous for *BRCA1* or *BRCA2* gene mutations have not been shown to have an increased incidence of breast or ovarian cancer with COC use (Brohet, 2007). With regard to benign breast disease, Vessey and Yeates (2007) reported that COC use apparently *lowered* the relative risk.

HIV Infections and Antiretroviral Therapy. Women with human immunodeficiency virus (HIV) infection or acquired immunodeficiency syndrome (AIDS) require special considerations regarding contraceptive use. As outlined by the American College of Obstetricians and Gynecologists (2012a), affected women need highly effective contraception that meets several criteria. It must be compatible with highly active antiretroviral therapy (HAART), should provide a low risk for acquiring STDs, and must not increase their risk of transmitting HIV to their partners.

Although CHCs are safe for use in HIV-positive women, their metabolism may be variably altered by some HAART regimens in current use. Details of various HAART regimen interactions with CHCs are available at the University of California, San Francisco HIV InSite website: http://hivinsite.ucsf.edu/insite?page=ar-00-02.

■ Progestin-Only Contraceptives

Contraceptives that contain only a progestin were developed to obviate the unwanted side effects of estrogens. Progestins can be delivered by several routes that include tablets, injections, intrauterine devices (p. 108), and subdermal implants (p. 112).

Progestin-Only Pills

Also called *mini-pills,* POPs are taken daily. They do not reliably inhibit ovulation, but instead thicken cervical mucus and decidualize and atrophy the endometrium. Because mucus changes do not persist beyond 24 hours, to be maximally effective, a pill is ideally taken at the same time daily. Their use has not achieved widespread popularity because of a much higher incidence of irregular bleeding and a slightly higher pregnancy rate than that seen with CHCs (see Table 5-2).

POPs have minimal if any effect on carbohydrate metabolism and coagulation factors. They do not cause or exacerbate hypertension and thus may be ideal for some women at increased risk for other cardiovascular complications. Such women include those with a history of thrombosis or migraine headaches or smokers older than 35 years. Because they do not impair milk production, POPs are suitable for lactating women. When used in combination with breast feeding, POPs are virtually 100-percent effective for up to 6 months (Betrabet, 1987; Shikary, 1987).

POPs should not be taken by women with unexplained uterine bleeding, breast cancer, hepatic neoplasms, pregnancy, or active severe liver disease (Janssen-Ortho, 2014).

Compliance is essential to POP use. If a pill is taken even 4 hours late, an additional form of contraception must be used for the next 48 hours. This may contribute to another major drawback, which is a higher risk for contraceptive failure compared with CHCs. Moreover, with failure, the proportion of pregnancies that are ectopic is increased (Sivin, 1991). POP effectiveness is also decreased by some medications, and in some instances POPs should be avoided (see Tables 5-8 and 5-9).

Another disadvantage is irregular uterine bleeding. This may be characterized by amenorrhea, intermenstrual bleeding, or prolonged heavy menstrual bleeding. As with other progestin-containing contraceptive methods, functional ovarian cysts develop with a greater frequency, although they usually do not require intervention (Hidalgo, 2006; Inki, 2002).

Injectable Progestins

Formulations. There are three injectable depot progesterone preparations that are used worldwide. This method is popular in the United States and is used by approximately 6 percent of women choosing a contraceptive. Injectable progestins have mechanisms of action similar to those for oral progestins and include increased cervical mucus viscosity, creation of an endometrium unfavorable for implantation, and unpredictable ovulation suppression.

Injectable preparations include depot medroxyprogesterone acetate—marketed as *Depo-Provera*. A 150-mg dose is given by intramuscular injection every 90 days. A derivative of DMPA is marketed as *depo-subQprovera 104*, and a 104-mg dose is given subcutaneously every 90 days. Because absorption is slower with subcutaneous injections, the 104-mg dose is equivalent to the 150-mg intramuscular preparation (Jain, 2004). With either method, if the initial dose is given within the first 5 days following menses onset, no back-up contraception is necessary (Haider, 2007). A third injectable depot progestin that is not currently available in the United States is norethindrone enanthate, which is marketed as *Norgest,* and a 200-mg dose is injected intramuscularly every 2 months.

Injectable progestins have contraceptive efficacy equivalent or better than that of COCs. With perfect use, DMPA has

pregnancy rates of 0.3 percent, but typical-use failure rates are as high as 7 percent at 12 months (Kost, 2008; Said, 1986). Depot progesterone does not suppress lactation, and iron-deficiency anemia is less likely in long-term users because of less menstrual bleeding. Progestin injectables should not be taken by women with pregnancy, unexplained uterine bleeding, breast cancer, active or history of thromboembolic disease, cerebrovascular disease, or significant liver disease (Pfizer, 2014).

As with most progestin-only contraceptive methods, DMPA does not significantly affect lipid metabolism, glucose levels, hemostatic factors, liver function, thyroid function, and blood pressure (Dorflinger, 2002). Moreover, these have not been shown to increase the risk for thromboembolism, stroke, or cardiovascular disease (Mantha, 2012; World Health Organization, 1998). Despite this, manufacturer prescribing information often lists thrombosis or thromboembolic conditions as contraindications. However, for individuals with these disorders, US MEC considers progestin-containing methods category 2.

Notable Effects. Patients interested in DMPA use should be familiar with its potential effects and side effects. First, as is typical of progestin-only contraception, DMPA usually causes irregular menstrual-type bleeding. Cromer and coworkers (1994) reported that one fourth of women discontinued its use in the first year because of irregular bleeding. Amenorrhea may develop after extended use, and women are counseled about this benign effect.

Prolonged ovulation suppression may also persist after DMPA injections are stopped. In an earlier study by Gardner and Mishell (1970), one fourth of women did not resume regular menses for up to a year. Accordingly, DMPA may not be the best choice for women who plan to use contraception only briefly before attempting conception.

Bone mineral density can also be significantly diminished because of lowered estrogen levels and is most worrisome in long-term users. This loss is particularly relevant for adolescents because bone density increases most rapidly from ages 10 to 30 years (Sulak, 1999). Additionally, decreased bone mineral density may be a concern for perimenopausal women, who will shortly be entering the menopause, a time of known accelerated bone loss. These concerns prompted the FDA in 2004 to require a black-box warning that DMPA "should be used as a long-term birth control method—longer than 2 years—only if other birth-control methods are inadequate." There are some mitigating factors that balance this concern. First, although bone loss is greatest during the first 2 years, it subsequently slows appreciably. Second, most bone lost during contraceptive use is restored within 5 years after its discontinuance (Clark, 2006; Harel, 2010). In sum, the American College of Obstetricians and Gynecologists (2014c) has concluded that concerns of bone density loss should not prevent or limit use of this contraceptive method.

Of potential cancer risks, cervical carcinoma in situ rates are possibly increased with DMPA use. However, risks for cervical cancer or for hepatic neoplasms are not higher with this method (Thomas, 1995). Advantageously, ovarian and endometrial cancers are decreased (Kaunitz, 1996; World Health Organization, 1991). In addition, Skegg and colleagues (1995) pooled the results of the New Zealand and WHO case-control studies that included almost 1800 women with breast cancer. Compared with 14,000 controls, DMPA contraceptive use was associated with a twofold cancer risk in the first 5 years of use. However, the overall risk was not increased.

Of other effects, some women report breast tenderness with DMPA use. Depression has also been reported, but a causal link is unproven. Finally, although weight gain is often attributed to depot progestins, not all studies have shown this (Bahamondes, 2001; Mainwaring, 1995; Moore, 1995; Taneepanichskul, 1998). Beksinska and coworkers (2010) reported that adolescents who used intramuscular DMPA gained 2.3 kg more weight during a 4- to 5-year interval compared with weight gained by adolescents who used COCs. Subcutaneous DMPA has also been shown to cause modest weight gain in most women (Westhoff, 2007b). Because women who gain weight in the first 6 months of use are more likely to have long-term progressive weight gain, Le and colleagues (2009) suggest that these women may benefit from early counseling.

THIRD-TIER CONTRACEPTIVE METHODS

There are two types of contraceptive methods that are considered as moderately effective. One type includes barrier methods, which are designed to prevent functional sperm from reaching and fertilizing the ovum. The other category consists of fertility awareness methods. Perhaps more so than with other contraceptive methods, moderately effective methods have the highest success rates when used by couples who are dedicated to their use.

■ Barrier Methods

These methods include vaginal diaphragms and male and female condoms. As shown in Table 5-2, the reported pregnancy rate for these methods varies from 2 to 6 percent in the first year of use and is highly dependent on correct and consistent use.

Male Condom

Most condoms are made from latex rubber, and various sizes are manufactured to accommodate male anatomy. Less commonly, polyurethane or lamb cecum is used. Condoms provide effective contraception, and their failure rate when used by strongly motivated couples has been as low as 3 or 4 per 100 couple-years of exposure (Vessey, 1982). Generally, and especially in the first year of use, the failure rate is much higher.

The efficacy of condoms is enhanced appreciably with a reservoir tip. Lubricants should be water based because oil-based products destroy latex condoms and diaphragms (Waldron, 1989). Key steps to ensure maximal condom effectiveness include: (1) used with every coitus, (2) placed before penis and vagina contact, (3) withdrawn while penis still erect, (4) its base held during withdrawal, and (5) used with spermicide.

A distinct advantage of condoms is that, when used properly, they provide considerable—not absolute—protection against many STDs. Condoms also help prevent premalignant cervical changes, probably by blocking HPV transmission (Winer, 2006).

For latex-sensitive individuals, alternative condoms are available. Condoms made from lamb intestines—*natural skin*

or *lambskin condoms*—are effective, but they do not provide protection against STDs. Nonallergenic condoms are made with a synthetic thermoplastic elastomer, such as polyurethane, which is also used in some surgical gloves. These are effective against STDs but have significantly higher breakage and slippage rates compared with those of latex condoms (Gallo, 2006). In a randomized trial of 901 couples, Steiner and associates (2003) documented breakage and slippage with 8.4 percent of polyurethane condoms compared with only 3.2 percent of latex condoms. They also reported that 6-month typical pregnancy probabilities were 9.0 percent with polyurethane condoms but only 5.4 percent with latex ones.

Female Condom—Vaginal Pouch

Manufactured by many companies under different names, female condoms prevent pregnancy and STDs. One brand available in the United States is the *FC2 Female Condom*—a polyurethane cylindrical sheath with a flexible polyurethane ring at each end (Fig. 5-12). The open ring remains outside the vagina, and the closed internal ring is fitted behind the symphysis and beneath the cervix like a diaphragm (Fig. 5-13). It should not be used with a male condom because together they may slip, tear, or become displaced. In vitro tests show the female condom to be impermeable to HIV, cytomegalovirus, and hepatitis B virus. As shown in Table 5-2, the pregnancy rate is higher than with the male condom.

Diaphragm plus Spermicide

The diaphragm consists of a circular, flexible rubber dome of various diameters supported by a circumferential metal spring (Fig. 5-14). When used in combination with spermicidal jelly or cream, it can be very effective. The spermicide is applied to the cervical surface centrally in the cup and along the rim. The device is then placed in the vagina so that the cervix, vaginal fornices, and anterior vaginal wall are partitioned effectively from the remainder of the vagina and the penis. At the same time, the centrally placed spermicidal agent is held against the

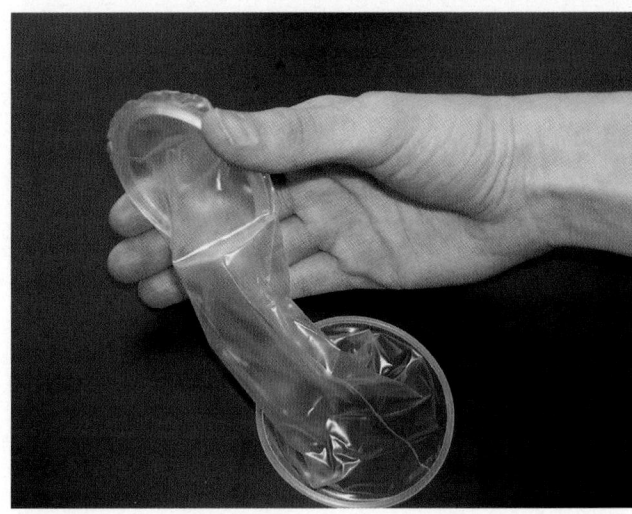

FIGURE 5-12 Female condom. (Reproduced with permission from The Cervical Barrier Advancement Society and Ibis Reproductive Health.)

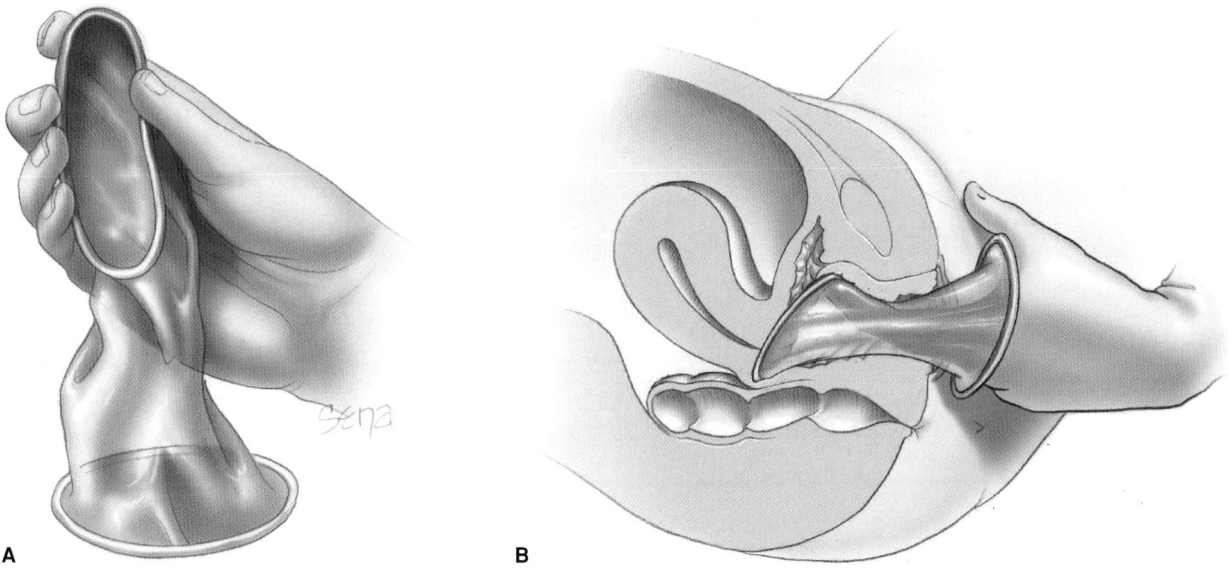

FIGURE 5-13 Female condom insertion and positioning. **A.** The inner ring is squeezed for insertion and is placed similarly to a diaphragm. **B.** The inner ring is pushed inward with an index finger.

cervix by the diaphragm. When appropriately positioned, the rim is lodged deep into the posterior vaginal fornix. Superiorly, the rim lies in close proximity to the inner surface of the symphysis immediately below the urethra (Fig. 5-15). If the diaphragm is too small, it will not remain in place. If too large, it will be uncomfortable when positioned. Because the variables of size and spring flexibility must be specified, the diaphragm is available only by prescription. Because of the requirement for proper placement, the diaphragm may not be an effective choice for women with significant pelvic organ prolapse. The malpositioned uterus can cause unstable diaphragm positioning that results in expulsion.

For use, the diaphragm and spermicidal agent can be inserted well before intercourse, but if more than 2 hours elapse, additional spermicide is placed in the upper vagina for maximum protection. Spermicide is similarly placed before

each episode of coitus. The diaphragm is not removed for at least 6 hours after intercourse. Because toxic shock syndrome has been described following its use, the diaphragm is not left in place for longer than 24 hours.

Proper diaphragm use requires a high level of motivation. Vessey and coworkers (1982) reported a pregnancy rate of only 1.9 to 2.4 per 100 woman-years for compliant users. In a small study, Bounds and colleagues (1995) reported a much higher failure rate of 12.3 per 100 woman years. The unintended pregnancy rate is lower in women older than 35 years compared with younger women.

Cervical Cap

This reusable, washable, silicone barrier device surrounds the cervix to block sperm passage and is combined with a spermicide. Marketed in the United States, FemCap is currently

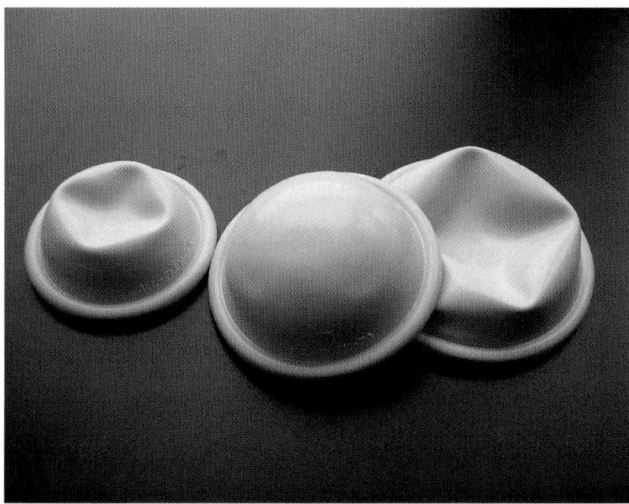

FIGURE 5-14 Group of three diaphragms. (Reproduced with permission from The Cervical Barrier Advancement Society and Ibis Reproductive Health.)

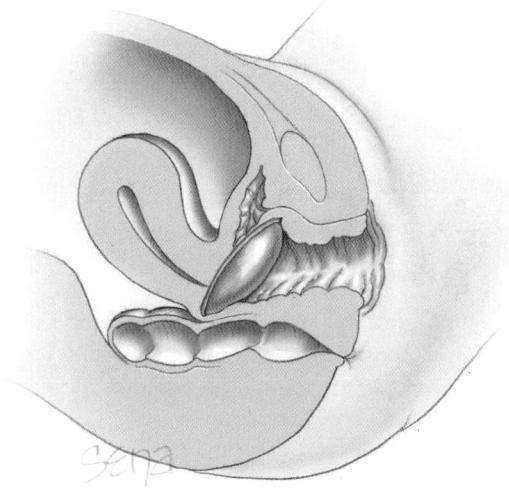

FIGURE 5-15 A diaphragm in place creates a physical barrier between the vagina and cervix.

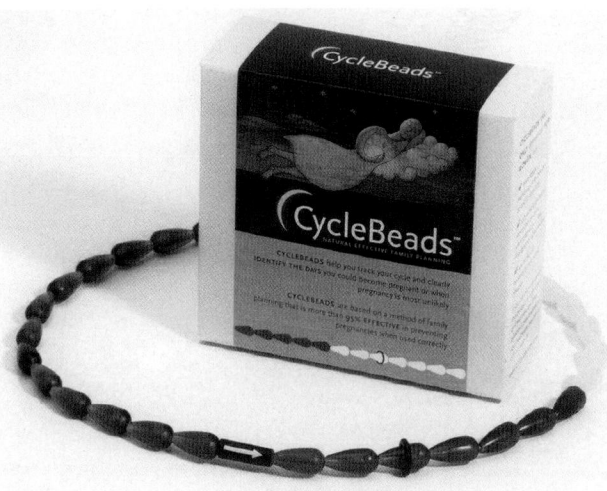

FIGURE 5-16 CycleBeads. During use, the red bead denotes menses onset, and the small black band is advanced , as directed by the arrow, for each day of the menstrual cycle. When the white beads are reached, abstinence is observed until brown beads begin again. (Reproduced with permission from Cycle Technologies.)

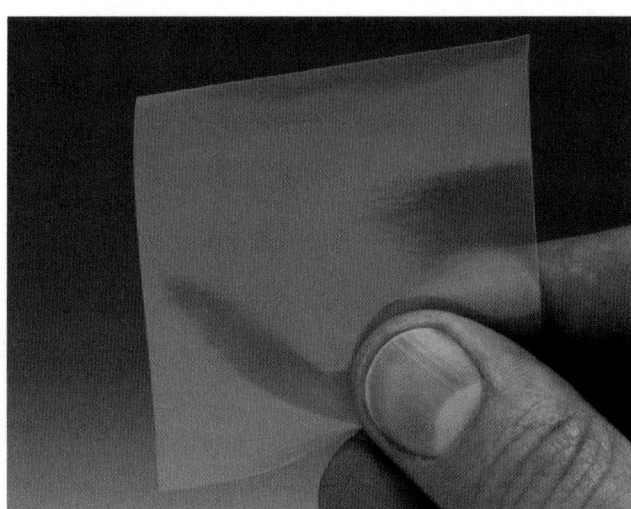

FIGURE 5-17 Vaginal contraceptive film. The film is first folded in half and then folded up and over the tip of the inserting finger. Once inserted near the cervix, the film will dissolve to provide spermicide.

available in 22-, 26-, and 30-mm diameters to accommodate differing cervical sizes. It may be inserted any time prior to intercourse and must be left in place for at least 8 hours thereafter. Spermicide dosing and redosing mirrors that with a diaphragm. Other caps formerly manufactured in the United States that might still be in use include Prentif, Vimule, Dumas, and Lea Shield.

■ Fertility Awareness-based Methods

This form of contraception is defined by the WHO (2007) as a method that involves identification of the fertile days of the menstrual cycle (Fig. 5-16). The couple may then avoid intercourse or use a barrier method during those days. The comparative efficacy of fertility-based awareness methods remains unknown (Grimes, 2004). Clearly, proper instruction is critical, and complex charting is involved. These charts, as well as detailed advice, are available from the National Fertility Awareness and Natural Family Planning Service for the United Kingdom at: http://www.fertilityuk.org and from the Natural Family Site at: http://www.bygpub.com/natural.

FOURTH-TIER CONTRACEPTIVE METHODS

■ Spermicides

These contraceptives are marketed variously as creams, jellies, suppositories, aerosol foams, and film (Fig. 5-17). They are used widely in the United States, and most are available without a prescription. Probable users include women who find other methods unacceptable. They are useful especially for women who need temporary protection, for example, during the first week after starting CHC or while nursing.

Spermicidal agents provide a physical barrier to sperm penetration and a chemical spermicidal action. The active ingredient is nonoxynol-9 or octoxynol-9. Importantly, spermicides must be deposited high in the vagina in contact with the cervix shortly before intercourse. Their duration of maximal

effectiveness is usually no more than 1 hour. Thereafter, they must be reinserted before repeat intercourse. Douching, if practiced, is avoided for at least 6 hours after intercourse.

High pregnancy rates are primarily attributable to inconsistent use rather than to method failure. Even if inserted regularly and correctly, however, foam preparations are reported to have a failure rate of 5 to 12 pregnancies per 100 woman-years of use (Trussell, 1990). If pregnancy does occur with use, spermicides are not teratogenic (Briggs, 2015).

Spermicides that primarily contain nonoxynol-9 do not provide protection against STDs. In randomized trials, Roddy and colleagues (1998) compared nonoxynol-9 with and without condom use and found no additional protective effects against chlamydial or HIV infection or gonorrhea. Long-term use of nonoxynol-9 was reported to have minimal effects on vaginal flora (Schreiber, 2006).

There is currently much interest in combined spermicide-microbicide agents. These have the advantage of protecting against STDs, including HIV (Weber, 2005). Those in the surfactant class have dual action—they destroy the sperm membrane and they also disrupt the outer envelopes or membranes of viral and bacterial pathogens. Second-generation microbicides also fortify natural defenses. Third-generation microbicides work as topical antiretroviral agents.

■ Contraceptive Sponge

The contraceptive sponge *Today* was reintroduced into the United States in 2005. Sold over the counter, it consists of a nonoxynol-9–impregnated polyurethane disc that can be inserted for up to 24 hours prior to intercourse (Fig. 5-18). The disc is moistened and placed directly against the cervix. While in place, the sponge provides contraception regardless of the number of coital episodes. For efficacy, it remains in place for 6 hours after intercourse, and to lower irritation and infection risks, it remains no longer than 30 hours (Mayer Laboratories, 2009). Although perhaps more convenient, the sponge is less effective than the diaphragm or condom.

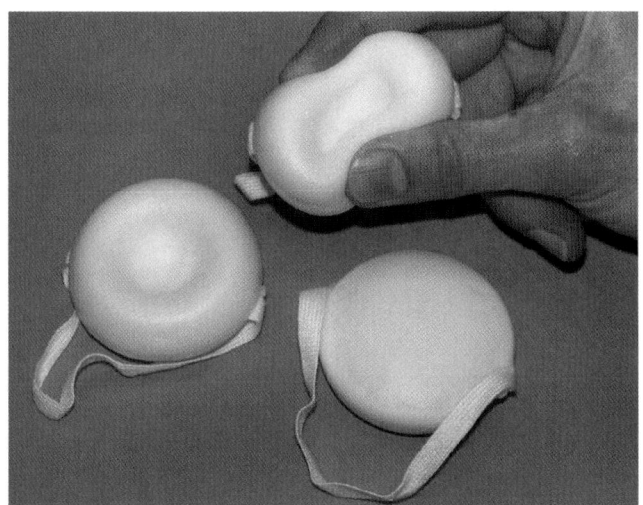

FIGURE 5-18 Vaginal sponge. When in position, the sponge dimple apposes the cervix surface, and the ribbon loop faces outward to allow easy hooking with a finger for removal.

EMERGENCY CONTRACEPTION

First popularized by the "morning-after pill" in the 1970s, emergency contraception (EC) is now widely available in other forms. These methods are appropriate for women presenting for contraceptive care following consensual but unprotected sexual intercourse or following sexual assault. There are several methods that, if used correctly, will substantially decrease the likelihood of an unwanted pregnancy in these women. According to the American College of Obstetricians and Gynecologists (2015), methods currently available include sex steroid-containing compounds, antiprogesterone compounds, and the copper-

containing IUD (Table 5-11). Importantly, because duration of use is short, women with conditions that might normally contraindicate hormonal forms may be given these for EC.

Information regarding EC is made available to health care providers or patients by several 24-hour sources:

- American Congress of Obstetricians and Gynecologists: www.acog.org
- Emergency Contraception Hotline and website: 1–888-NOT-2-LATE (888–668–2528) and www.not-2-late.com
- Reproductive Health Technologies Project: www.rhtp.org/contraception/emergency/
- Pastillas Anticonceptivas de Emergencia: www.en3dias.org.mx.

◼ Hormone-based Options
Mechanisms of Action

Hormonal contraceptives have different mechanisms of action depending on which day of the menstrual cycle intercourse occurs and which day the tablets are given (Croxatto, 2003). One major mode is inhibition or delay of ovulation (Marions, 2004). Other suggested mechanisms include endometrial changes that prevent implantation, interference with sperm transport or penetration, and impaired corpus luteum function. Despite these effects, every method used for postcoital contraception will have failures. Pregnancies that develop despite emergency hormonal contraception appear unaffected by this prophylaxis. Moreover, emergency hormonal contraception is not a form of medical abortion. Rather, this method prevents ovulation or implantation. It cannot disrupt a zygote that has implanted.

Except perhaps the copper IUD, other EC methods generally will not prevent pregnancy resulting from subsequent episodes of intercourse during the same cycle. Accordingly, use of a barrier

TABLE 5-11. Methods Available for Use as Emergency Contraception

Method	Formulation	Pills per Dose
Progestin-Only Pill		
Plan B[a]	0.75 mg levonorgestrel	1
Plan B One-Step[b]	150 mg levonorgestrel	1
SPRM Pill		
Ella[b]	30 mg ulipristal acetate	1
COC Pills[a,c]		
Ogestrel	0.05 mg ethinyl estradiol + 0.5 mg norgestrel[d]	2
Lo/Ovral, Cryselle	0.03 mg ethinyl estradiol + 0.3 mg norgestrel[d]	4
Trivora (pink), Enpress (orange)	0.03 mg ethinyl estradiol + 0.125 mg levonorgestrel	4
Aviane, Lessina	0.02 mg ethinyl estradiol + 0.1 mg levonorgestrel	5
Copper-containing IUD		
ParaGard T 380A		

[a]Treatment consists of two doses taken 12 hours apart.
[b]Treatment consists of a single dose taken once.
[c]Use of an antiemetic agent before taking the medication will lessen the risk of nausea, which is a common side effect.
[d]Norgestrel contains two isomers, and only one of these isomers is bioactive, namely levonorgestrel. Thus, the amount of norgestrel needed for efficacy is twice that of the levonorgestrel-based regimens.
COC = combination oral contraceptive; SPRM = selective progesterone-receptor modulator.

technique is recommended until the next menses. When menstruation is delayed 3 weeks past its expected onset, the likelihood of pregnancy is increased and appropriate testing is instituted.

Estrogen-Progestin Combinations

Also known as the *Yuzpe method*, these COC-containing regimens shown in Table 5-11 have been approved by the FDA for use as EC (Yuzpe, 1974). Although more effective the sooner they are taken after unprotected intercourse, pills should be taken within 72 hours of intercourse, but may be given up to 120 hours. Initial dosing is followed 12 hours later by a second dose.

Efficacy is defined by the number of pregnancies observed after treatment divided by the estimated number that would have occurred with no treatment. This *prevented fraction* ranges widely between reports and averages approximately 75 percent with COC regimens (American College of Obstetricians and Gynecologists, 2015).

Nausea and vomiting are common with COC regimens because of their high estrogen doses (Trussell, 1998a). An oral antiemetic taken at least 1 hour before each dose may reduce these bothersome symptoms. In randomized trials, a 1-hour pretreatment dose of either 50-mg meclizine or 10-mg metoclopramide was effective (Ragan, 2003; Raymond, 2000). If vomiting occurs within 2 hours of a dose, a replacement dose is given.

Progestin-only Regimens

A progestin-only method of EC is marketed as *Plan B* and *Plan B One-Step*. Plan B consists of two tablets, each containing 0.75 mg of levonorgestrel. The first dose is taken within 72 hours of unprotected coitus but may be given as late as 120 hours, and the second dose is taken 12 hours later (see Table 5-11). Ngai and associates (2005) also showed that a 24-hour interval between dosing is effective. Plan B One-Step is a single, 1.5-mg levonorgestrel dose, which is taken ideally with 72 hours or up to 120 hours following intercourse.

Most studies, including a multicenter WHO trial, indicate that the progestin-only regimens are more effective than COC regimens to prevent pregnancy (von Hertzen, 2002). The American College of Obstetricians and Gynecologists (2015) cites an approximate 50-percent decreased pregnancy rate with levonorgestrel compared with COCs. Finally, Ellertson and colleagues (2003) reported a 55-percent pregnancy prevention rate even if Plan B was taken as late as 4 to 5 days after unprotected intercourse.

Antiprogestins and Selective Progestin-receptor Modulators

These agents, described in Chapter 9 (p. 207), have contraceptive activity because they prevent progesterone-mediated endometrial preparation for implantation. There are several mechanisms by which antiprogesterone compounds achieve this. One mechanism is by progesterone-receptor modulation, and two compounds are available.

First, mifepristone (RU 486)—*Mifeprex*—is a progesterone antagonist. It either delays ovulation or impairs secretory endometrium development. Cheng and colleagues (2012) in their Cochrane review noted that mifepristone in single doses of 25 or 50 mg was superior to other hormonal EC regimens.

Mifepristone also had few side effects. In the United States, mifepristone is not used for EC because of its high cost and because it is not manufactured or marketed in an appropriate dose for EC.

A second drug, a selective progesterone-receptor modulator (SPRM), was FDA approved in 2010 for postcoital contraception. Ulipristal acetate—*Ella*—is taken as a single 30-mg tablet up to 120 hours after unprotected intercourse (Brache, 2010). Side effects include nausea and delay of subsequent menses.

■ Copper-containing Intrauterine Devices

Insertion of a copper-containing IUD is an effective postcoital contraceptive method. Fasoli and coworkers (1989) summarized nine studies that included results from 879 women who chose this as a sole method of postcoital contraception. The only pregnancy reported aborted spontaneously. Trussell and Stewart (1998b) reported that when the IUD was inserted up to 5 days after unprotected coitus, the failure rate was 1 percent. A secondary advantage is that this method also puts in place an effective 10-year method of contraception.

REFERENCES

Actavis: Liletta (levonorgestrel-releasing intrauterine system): prescribing information. Parsippany, Actavis Pharma, 2015

Adams CE, Wald M: Risks and complications of vasectomy. Urol Clin North Am 36(3):331, 2009

Allen RH, Bartz D, Grimes DA, et al: Interventions for pain with intrauterine device insertion. Cochrane Database Syst Rev 3:CD007373, 2009

Alvarez F, Brache V, Fernandez E, et al: New insights on the mode of action of intrauterine contraceptive devices in women. Fertil Steril 49(5):768, 1988

Alvior GT Jr: Pregnancy outcome with removal of intrauterine device. Obstet Gynecol 41(6):894, 1973

American Academy of Pediatrics, American College of Obstetricians and Gynecologists: Intrapartum and postpartum care of the mother. In Riley LE, Stark AR (eds): Guidelines for Perinatal Care, 7th ed. Washington, AAP/ACOG, 2012, p 204

American College of Obstetricians and Gynecologists: Adolescents and long-acting reversible contraception: implants and intrauterine devices. Committee Opinion No. 539, October 2012, Reaffirmed 2014a

American College of Obstetricians and Gynecologists: Antibiotic prophylaxis for gynecologic procedures. Practice Bulletin No. 104, May 2009, Reaffirmed 2014b

American College of Obstetricians and Gynecologists: Benefits and risks of sterilization. Practice Bulletin No. 133, February 2013a

American College of Obstetricians and Gynecologists: Depot medroxyprogesterone acetate and bone effects. Committee Opinion No. 602, June 2008, Reaffirmed 2014c

American College of Obstetricians and Gynecologists: Emergency oral contraception. Practice Bulletin No. 152, September 2015

American College of Obstetricians and Gynecologists: Gynecologic care for women with human immunodeficiency virus. Practice Bulletin No. 117, December 2010, Reaffirmed 2012a

American College of Obstetricians and Gynecologists: Hysterosalpingography after tubal sterilization. Committee Opinion No. 458, June 2010, Reaffirmed 2012b

American College of Obstetricians and Gynecologists: Increasing use of contraceptive implants and intrauterine devices to reduce unintended pregnancy. Committee Opinion No. 450, December 2009, Reaffirmed 2011

American College of Obstetricians and Gynecologists: Long-acting reversible contraception: implants and intrauterine devices. Practice Bulletin No. 121, July 2011, Reaffirmed 2013b

American College of Obstetricians and Gynecologists: Noncontraceptive uses of hormonal contraceptives. Practice Bulletin No. 110, January 2010, Reaffirmed 2014e

American College of Obstetricians and Gynecologists: Prevention of deep vein thrombosis and pulmonary embolism. Practice Bulletin No. 84, August 2007, Reaffirmed 2013c

American College of Obstetricians and Gynecologists: Use of hormonal contraception in women with coexisting medical conditions. Practice Bulletin No. 73, June 2006, Reaffirmed 2013d

American Society for Reproductive Medicine: Vasectomy reversal. Fertil Steril 90(5 Suppl):S78, 2008

Amundsen GA, Ramakrishnan K: Vasectomy: a "seminal" analysis. South Med J 97:54, 2004

Anderson CK, Wallace S, Guiahi M, et al: Risk-reducing salpingectomy as preventative strategy for pelvic serous cancer. Int J Gynecol Cancer 23(3):417, 2013

Arjona Berral JE, Rodríguez Jiménez B, Velasco Sánchez E, et al: Essure® and chronic pelvic pain: a population-based cohort. J Obstet Gynaecol 34(8):712, 2014

Audet MC, Moreau M, Koltun WD, et al: Evaluation of contraceptive efficacy and cycle control of a transdermal contraceptive patch vs an oral contraceptive: a randomized controlled trial. JAMA 285:2347, 2001

Bahamondes L, Del Castillo S, Tabares G, et al: Comparison of weight increase in users of depot medroxyprogesterone acetate and copper IUD up to 5 years. Contraception 64(4):223, 2001

Bahamondes L, Faundes A, Sobreira-Lima B, et al: TCu 380A: a reversible permanent contraceptive method in women over 35 years of age. Contraception 72(5):337, 2005

Balci O, Mahmoud AS, Capar M, et al: Diagnosis and management of intra-abdominal, mislocated intrauterine devices. Arch Gynecol Obstet 281(6):1019, 2010

Bayer HealthCare Pharmaceuticals: Mirena (levonorgestrel-releasing intrauterine system): prescribing information. Whippany, Bayer HealthCare Pharmaceuticals, 2014

Bayer HealthCare Pharmaceuticals: Skyla (levonorgestrel-releasing intrauterine system): prescribing information. Wayne, Bayer HealthCare Pharmaceuticals, 2013

Bayer HealthCare Pharmaceuticals: Yasmin, drospirenone and ethinyl estradiol tablets: prescribing information. Wayne, Bayer HealthCare Pharmaceuticals, 2012

Bednarek PH, Creinin MD, Reeves MF, et al: Immediate versus delayed IUD insertion after uterine aspiration. N Engl J Med 364(23):2208, 2011

Beksinska ME, Smit JA, Kleinschmidt I, et al: Prospective study of weight change in new adolescent users of DMPA, NET-EN, COCs, nonusers and discontinuers of hormonal contraception. Contraception 81(1):30, 2010

Betrabet SS, Shikary ZK, Toddywalla VS, et al: ICMR Task Force Study on hormonal contraception. Transfer of norethindrone (NET) and levonorgestrel (LNG) from a single tablet into the infant's circulation through the mother's milk. Contraception 35:517, 1987

Bounds W, Guillebaud J, Dominik R, et al: The diaphragm with and without spermicide. A randomized, comparative efficacy trial. J Reprod Med 40:764, 1995

Brache V, Cochon L, Jesam C, et al: Immediate pre-ovulatory administration of 30 mg ulipristal acetate significantly delays follicular rupture. Hum Reprod 25(9):2256, 2010

Bradshaw HD, Rosario DJ, James MJ, et al: Review of current practice to establish success after vasectomy. Br J Surg 88:290, 2001

Briggs GG, Freeman RK: Drugs in Pregnancy and Lactation, 10th ed. Philadelphia, Wolters Kluwer Health, 2015

Brohet RM, Goldgar DE, Easton DF, et al: Oral contraceptives and breast cancer risk in the international BRCA 1/2 carrier cohort study: a report from EMBRACE, GENEPSO, GEO-HEBON, and the IBCCS Collaborating Group. J Clin Oncol 25:5327, 2007

Brunner LR, Hogue CJ: The role of body weight in oral contraceptive failure: results from the 1995 national survey of family growth. Ann Epidemiol 15:492, 2005

Cancer and Steroid Hormone Study of the Centers for Disease Control and the National Institute of Child Health and Development: Combination oral contraceptive use and the risk of endometrial cancer. JAMA 257:796, 1987a

Cancer and Steroid Hormone Study of the Centers for Disease Control and the National Institute of Child Health and Development: The reduction in risk of ovarian cancer associated with oral-contraceptive use. N Engl J Med 316:650, 1987b

Castaño PM, Adekunle L: Transcervical sterilization. Semin Reprod Med 28(2):103, 2010

Centers for Disease Control and Prevention: Sexually transmitted diseases treatment guidelines, 2015. MMWR 64(3):1, 2015

Centers for Disease Control and Prevention: Update to CDC's U.S. Medical Eligibility Criteria for Contraceptive Use, 2010: revised recommendations for the use of contraceptive methods during the postpartum period. MMWR 60(26):878, 2011

Centers for Disease Control and Prevention: U.S. medical eligibility criteria for contraceptive use, 2010. MMWR 59(4), 2010

Chan LM, Westhoff CL: Tubal sterilization trends in the United States. Fertil Steril 94(1):1, 2010

Chasan-Taber L, Willett WC, Manson JE, et al: Prospective study of oral contraceptives and hypertension among women in the United States. Circulation 94:483, 1996

Chen BA, Reeves MF, Hayes JL, et al: Postplacental or delayed insertion of the levonorgestrel intrauterine device after vaginal delivery: a randomized controlled trial. Obstet Gynecol 116(5):1079, 2010

Cheng L, Che Y, Gülmezoglu AM: Interventions for emergency contraception. Cochrane Database Syst Rev 8:CD001324, 2012

Clark MK, Sowers M, Levy B, et al: Bone mineral density loss and recovery during 48 months in first-time users of depot medroxyprogesterone acetate. Fertil Steril 86(5):1466, 2006

Cleary TP, Tepper NK, Cwiak C, et al: Pregnancies after hysteroscopic sterilization: a systematic review. Contraception 87(5):539, 2013

Collaborative Group on Epidemiological Studies of Ovarian Cancer: Ovarian cancer and oral contraceptives: collaborative reanalysis of data of 45 epidemiological studies including 23,257 women with ovarian cancer and 87,303 controls. Lancet 371:303, 2008

Collaborative Group on Hormonal Factors in Breast Cancer: Breast cancer and hormonal contraceptives: collaborative reanalysis of individual data on 53,297 women with breast cancer and 100,239 women without breast cancer from 54 epidemiological studies. Lancet 347:1713, 1996

Cooper JM, Carignan CS, Cher D, et al: Microinsert nonincisional hysteroscopic sterilization. Obstet Gynecol 102:59, 2003

Costello C, Hillis S, Marchbanks P, et al: The effect of interval tubal sterilization on sexual interest and pleasure. Obstet Gynecol 100:3, 2002

Creinin MD, Zite N: Female tubal sterilization: the time has come to routinely consider removal. Obstet Gynecol 124(3):596, 2014

Cromer BA, Smith RD, Blair JM, et al: A prospective study of adolescents who choose among levonorgestrel implant (Norplant), medroxyprogesterone acetate (Depo-Provera), or the combined oral contraceptive pill as contraception. Pediatrics 94:687, 1994

Croxatto HB, Ortiz ME, Muller AL: Mechanisms of action of emergency contraception. Steroids 68:1095, 2003

Culwell KR, Curtis KM, del Carmen Craviotto M: Safety of contraceptive method use among women with systemic lupus erythematosus: a systematic review. Obstet Gynecol 114(2 Pt 1):341, 2009

Curtis KM, Chrisman CE, Peterson HB: Contraception for women in selected circumstances. Obstet Gynecol 99:1100, 2002

Daniels K, Daugherty J, Jones J: Current contraceptive status among women aged 15–44: United States, 2011–2013. NCHS Data Brief 173:1, 2014

Deffieux X, Morin Surroca M, et al: Tubal anastomosis after tubal sterilization: a review. Arch Gynecol Obstet 283(5):1149, 2011

del Marmol V, Teichmann A, Gertsen K: The role of combined oral contraceptives in the management of acne and seborrhea. Eur J Contracept Reprod Health Care 9(2):107, 2004

DeStefano F, Perlman JA, Peterson HB, et al: Long term risk of menstrual disturbances after tubal sterilization. Am J Obstet Gynecol 152:835, 1985

de Villiers EM: Relationship between steroid hormone contraceptives and HPV, cervical intraepithelial neoplasia and cervical carcinoma. Int J Cancer 103(6):705, 2003

Doherty IA, Stuart GS: Coitus interruptus is not contraception. Sex Transm Dis 36(12), 2009

Dorflinger LJ: Metabolic effects of implantable steroid contraceptives for women. Contraception 65(1):47, 2002

Edelman A, Micks E, Gallo MF, et al: Continuous or extended cycle vs cyclic use of combined hormonal contraceptives for contraception. Cochrane Database Syst Rev 7:CD004695, 2014

Edelman AB, Carlson NE, Cherala G, et al: Impact of obesity on oral contraceptive pharmacokinetics and hypothalamic-pituitary-ovarian activity. Contraception, 80(2):119, 2009

Ellertson C, Evans M, Ferden S, et al: Extending the time limit for starting the Yuzpe regimen of emergency contraception to 120 hours. Obstet Gynecol 101:1168, 2003

Erickson BK, Conner MG, Landen CN Jr: The role of the fallopian tube in the origin of ovarian cancer. Am J Obstet Gynecol 209(5):409, 2013

Fasoli M, Parazzini F, Cecchetti G, et al: Post-coital contraception: an overview of published studies. Contraception 39:459, 1989

Faúndes A, Telles E, Cristofoletti ML, et al: The risk of inadvertent intrauterine device insertion in women carriers of endocervical *Chlamydia trachomatis*. Contraception 58(2):105, 1998

Fernandez H, Legendre G, Blein C, et al: Tubal sterilization: pregnancy rates after hysteroscopic versus laparoscopic sterilization in France, 2006–2010. Eur J Obstet Gynecol Reprod Biol 180:133, 2014

Finer LB, Zolna MR: Shifts in intended and unintended pregnancies in the United States, 2001–2008. Am J Public Health 104(Suppl 1):S43, 2014

Finer LB, Zolna MR: Unintended pregnancy in the United States: incidence and disparities, 2006. Contraception 84(5):478, 2011

Fiorino AS: Intrauterine contraceptive device–associated actinomycotic abscess and *Actinomyces* detection on cervical smear. Obstet Gynecol 87:142, 1996

Food and Drug Administration: Drug safety communication: Updated information about the risk of blood clots in women taking birth control pills containing drospirenone. Rockville, Food and Drug Administration, 2012

Fox MC, Oat-Judge J, Severson K, et al: Immediate placement of intrauterine devices after first and second trimester pregnancy termination. Contraception 83(1):34, 2011

Furlong LA: Ectopic pregnancy risk when contraception fails. J Reprod Med 47:881, 2002

Gaffield ME, Culwell KR, Lee CR: The use of hormonal contraception among women taking anticonvulsant therapy. Contraception 83(1):16, 2011

Gallo MF, Grimes DA, Lopez LM, et al: Non-latex versus latex male condoms for contraception. Cochrane Database Syst Rev 1:CD003550, 2006

Gallo MF, Lopez LM, Grimes DA, et al: Combination contraceptives: effects on weight. Cochrane Database Syst Rev 1:CD003987, 2014

Ganer H, Levy A, Ohel I, et al: Pregnancy outcome in women with an intrauterine contraceptive device. Am J Obstet Gynecol 201:381.e1, 2009

Gardner JM, Mishell DR Jr: Analysis of bleeding patterns and resumption of fertility following discontinuation of a long-acting injectable contraceptive. Fertil Steril 21:286, 1970

Gariepy AM, Creinin MD, Smith KJ, et al: Probability of pregnancy after sterilization: a comparison of hysteroscopic versus laparoscopic sterilization. Contraception 90(2):174, 2014

Goodman S, Henlish SK, Reeves MF, et al: Impact of immediate postabortal insertion of intrauterine contraception on repeat abortion. Contraception 78:143, 2008

Grimes DA: Intrauterine device and upper-genital-tract infection. Lancet 356:1013, 2000

Grimes DA, Gallo MF, Grigorieva V, et al: Fertility awareness-based methods for contraception. Cochrane Database Syst Rev 1:CD004860, 2004

Grimes DA, Hubacher D, Lopez LM, et al: Non-steroidal anti-inflammatory drugs for heavy bleeding or pain associated with intrauterine-device use. Cochrane Database Syst Rev 4:CD006034, 2006

Grimes DA, Lopez LM, Schulz KF, et al: Immediate post-partum insertion of intrauterine devices. Cochrane Database Syst Rev 5:CD003036, 2010

Gurtcheff SE, Turok DK, Stoddard G, et al: Lactogenesis after early postpartum use of the contraceptive implant: a randomized controlled trial. Obstet Gynecol 117(5):1114, 2011

Guttmacher Institute: State policies in brief. An overview of minors' consent law. 2014. Washington, Guttmacher Institute, 2014

Haider S, Darney PD: Injectable contraception. Clin Obstet Gynecol 50(4):898, 2007

Halpern V, Grimes DA, Lopez L, et al: Strategies to improve adherence and acceptability of hormonal methods of contraception. Cochrane Database Syst Rev 10:CD004317, 2013

Hannaford PC, Kay CR, Vessey MP, et al: Combined oral contraceptives and liver disease. Contraception 55:145, 1997

Hannaford PC, Selvaraj S, Elliott AM, et al: Cancer risk among users of oral contraceptives: cohort data from the Royal College of General Practitioners' oral contraception study. BMJ 335:651, 2007

Harel Z, Johnson CC, Gold MA, et al: Recovery of bone mineral density in adolescents following the use of depot medroxyprogesterone acetate contraceptive injections. Contraception 81(4):281, 2010

Harlap S, Kost K, Forrest JD: Preventing pregnancy, protecting health: a new look at birth control choices in the US. New York, The Alan Guttmacher Institute, 1991

Heikinheimo O, Gissler M, Suhonen S: Age, parity history of abortion and contraceptive choices affect the risk of repeat abortion. Contraception 78: 149, 2008

Heinemann LA, Weimann A, Gerken G, et al: Modern oral contraceptive use and benign liver tumors: the German Benign Liver Tumor Case-Control Study. Eur J Contracept Reprod Health Care 3:194, 1998

Henshaw SK: Unintended pregnancy in the United States. Fam Plann Perspect 30:24, 1998

Hidalgo MM, Lisondo C, Juliato CT, et al: Ovarian cysts in users of Implanon and Jadelle subdermal contraceptive implants. Contraception 73(5):532, 2006

Hillis SD, Marchbanks PA, Tylor LR, et al: Poststerilization regret: findings from the United States Collaborative Review of Sterilization. Obstet Gynecol 93:889, 1999

Hillis SD, Marchbanks PA, Tylor LR, et al: Tubal sterilization and long-term risk of hysterectomy: findings from the United States Collaborative Review of Sterilization. Obstet Gynecol 89:609, 1997

Holt SK, Salinas CA, Stanford JL: Vasectomy and the risk of prostate cancer. J Urol 180(6):2565, 2008

Holt VL, Scholes D, Wicklund KG, et al: Body mass index, weight, and oral contraceptive failure risk. Obstet Gynecol 105:46, 2005

Inki P, Hurskainen R, Palo P, et al: Comparison of ovarian cyst formation in women using the levonorgestrel-releasing intrauterine system vs. hysterectomy. Ultrasound Obstet Gynecol 20(4):381, 2002

International Collaboration of Epidemiological Studies of Cervical Cancer: Cervical cancer and hormonal contraceptives: collaborative reanalysis of individual data for 16,573 women with cervical cancer and 35,509 women without cervical cancer from 24 epidemiological studies. Lancet 370:1609, 2007

Jain J, Dutton C, Nicosia A, et al: Pharmacokinetics, ovulation suppression and return to ovulation following a lower dose subcutaneous formulation of Depo-Provera. Contraception 70(1):11, 2004

Jamieson DJ, Kaufman SC, Costello C, et al: A comparison of women's regret after vasectomy versus tubal sterilization. Obstet Gynecol 99:1073, 2002

Janssen-Ortho: Micronor: prescribing information. Titusville, Janssen Ortho, 2014

Jensen JT, Burke AE, Barnhart KT, et al: Effects of switching from oral to transdermal or transvaginal contraception on markers of thrombosis. Contraception 78(6):451, 2008

Jick SS, Hagberg KW, Hernandez RK, et al: Postmarketing study of ORTHO EVRA® and levonorgestrel oral contraceptives containing hormonal contraceptives with 30 mcg of ethinyl estradiol in relation to nonfatal venous thromboembolism. Contraception 81(1):16, 2010a

Jick SS, Hagberg KW, Kaye JA: ORTHO EVRA and venous thromboembolism: an update. Contraception 81(5):452, 2010b

Jick SS, Hernandez RK: Risk of non-fatal venous thromboembolism in women using oral contraceptives containing drospirenone compared with women using oral contraceptives containing levonorgestrel: case-control study using United States claims data. BMJ 342:d2151, 2011

Jick SS, Kaye JA, Russmann S, et al: Risk of nonfatal venous thromboembolism in women using a contraceptive transdermal patch and oral contraceptives containing norgestimate and 35 µg of ethinyl estradiol. Contraception 73(3):223, 2006

Jones J, Mosher W, Daniels K: Current contraceptive use in the United States, 2006–2010, and changes in patterns of use since 1995. Natl Health Stat Report 60:1, 2012

Jost S, Huchon C, Legendre G, et al: Essure(R) permanent birth control effectiveness: a seven-year survey. Eur J Obstet Gynecol Reprod Biol 168(2):134, 2013

Kapp N, Curtis KM: Hormonal contraceptive use among women with liver tumors: a systematic review. Contraception 80(4):387, 2009a

Kapp N, Tilley IB, Curtis KM: The effects of hormonal contraceptive use among women with viral hepatitis or cirrhosis of the liver: a systematic review. Contraception 80(4):381, 2009b

Kaunitz AM: Depot medroxyprogesterone acetate contraception and the risk of breast and gynecologic cancer. J Reprod Med 45:419, 1996

Kjos SL, Peters RK, Xiang A, et al: Contraception and the risk of type 2 diabetes mellitus in Latina women with prior gestational diabetes mellitus. JAMA 280:533, 1998

Kluft C, Meijer P, LaGuardia KD, et al: Comparison of a transdermal contraceptive patch vs. oral contraceptives on hemostasis variables. Contraception 77(2):77, 2008

Köhler TS, Fazili AA, Brannigan RE: Putative health risks associated with vasectomy. Urol Clin North Am 36(3):337, 2009

Kost K, Singh S, Vaughan B, et al: Estimates of contraceptive failure from the 2002 National Survey of Family Growth. Contraception 77:10, 2008

Kulier R, Boulvain M, Walker D, et al: Minilaparotomy and endoscopic techniques for tubal sterilization. Cochrane Database Syst Rev 3:CD001328, 2004

Lammer EJ, Cordero JF: Exogenous sex hormone exposure and the risk for major malformations. JAMA 255:3128, 1986

Lawrie TA, Nardin JM, Kulier R, et al: Techniques for the interruption of tubal patency for female sterilization. Cochrane Database Syst Rev 2:CD003034, 2011

Le YC, Rahman M, Berenson AB: Early weight gain predicting later weight gain among depot medroxyprogesterone acetate users. Obstet Gynecol 114(2 Pt 1):279, 2009

Lee NC, Rubin GL, Borucki R: The intrauterine device and pelvic inflammatory disease revisited: new results from the Women's Health Study. Obstet Gynecol 72(1):1, 1988

Levgur M, Duvivier R: Pelvic inflammatory disease after tubal sterilization: a review. Obstet Gynecol Surv 55:41, 2000

Levy B, Levie MD, Childers ME: A summary of reported pregnancies after hysteroscopic sterilization. J Minim Invasive Gynecol 2007 14(3):271, 2007

Lippes J: Quinacrine sterilization: the imperative need for clinical trials. Fertil Steril 77:1106, 2002

Lopez LM, Grimes DA, Chen M, et al: Hormonal contraceptives for contraception in overweight or obese women. Cochrane Database Syst Rev 4:CD008452, 2013

Lopez LM, Kaptein AA, Helmerhorst FM: Oral contraceptives containing drospirenone for premenstrual syndrome. Cochrane Database Syst Rev 2: CD006586, 2012

MacClellan LR, Giles W, Cole J, et al: Probable migraine with visual aura and risk of ischemic stroke: the stroke prevention in young women study. Stroke 38(9):2438, 2007

MacKay AP, Kieke BA, Koonin LM, et al: Tubal sterilization in the United States, 1994–1996. Fam Plann Perspect 33:161, 2001

Magnani RJ, Haws JM, Morgan GT, et al: Vasectomy in the United States, 1991 and 1995. Am J Pub Health 89:92, 1999

Maheshwari S, Sarraj A, Kramer J, et al: Oral contraception and the risk of hepatocellular carcinoma. J Hepatol 47:506, 2007

Mainwaring R, Hales HA, Stevenson K, et al: Metabolic parameters, bleeding, and weight changes in U.S. women using progestin only contraceptives. Contraception 51:149, 1995

Mantha S, Karp R, Raghavan V, et al: Assessing the risk of venous thromboembolic events in women taking progestin-only contraception: a meta-analysis. BMJ 345:e4944, 2012

Marchbanks PA, McDonald JA, Wilson HG, et al: Oral contraceptives and the risk of breast cancer. N Engl J Med 346:2025, 2002

Margolis KL, Adami HO, Luo J, et al: A prospective study of oral contraceptive use and risk of myocardial infarction among Swedish women. Fertil Steril 88(2):310, 2007

Marions L, Cekan SZ, Bygdeman M, et al: Effect of emergency contraception with levonorgestrel or mifepristone on ovarian function. Contraception 69:373, 2004

Mayer Laboratories: Today sponge. Consumer information leaflet. Berkeley, Mayer Laboratories, 2009

Merck: Nexplanon (etonogestrel implant) prescribing information. Whitehouse Station, Merck & Co., 2014

Michielsen D, Beerthuizen R: State-of-the art of non-hormonal methods of contraception: VI. Male sterilization. Eur J Contracept Reprod Health Care 15(2):136, 2010

Mishell DR Jr: Oral contraceptives and cardiovascular events: summary and application of data. Int J Fertil 45:121, 2000

Mohllajee AP, Curtis KM, Martins SL, et al: Does use of hormonal contraceptives among women with thrombogenic mutations increase their risk of venous thromboembolism? A systemic review. Contraception 73:166, 2006

Monteith CW, Berger GS, Zerden ML: Pregnancy success after hysteroscopic sterilization reversal. Obstet Gynecol 124(6):1183, 2014

Moore LL, Valuck R, McDougall C, et al: A comparative study of one-year weight gain among users of medroxyprogesterone acetate, levonorgestrel implants, and oral contraceptives. Contraception 52:215, 1995

Moschos E, Twickler DM: Does the type of intrauterine device affect conspicuity on 2D and 3D ultrasound? AJR 196(6):1439, 2011

Mosher WD, Jones J: Use of contraception in the United States: 1982–2008. Vital Health Stat 23, 29:1, 2010

Mulders TM, Dieben T: Use of the novel combined contraceptive vaginal ring NuvaRing for ovulation inhibition. Fertil Steril 75:865, 2001

Munro MG, Nichols JE, Levy B, et al: Hysteroscopic sterilization: 10-year retrospective analysis of worldwide pregnancy reports. J Minim Invasive Gynecol 21(2):245, 2014

Ngai SW, Fan S, Li S, et al: A randomized trial to compare 24 h versus 12 h double dose regimen of levonorgestrel for emergency contraception. Hum Reprod 20:307, 2005

Nilsson CG, Lahteenmaki P, Luukkainen T: Ovarian function in amenorrheic and menstruating users of a levonorgestrel-releasing intrauterine device. Fertil Steril 41:52, 1984

Ogburn JA, Espey E, Stonehocker J: Barriers to intrauterine device insertion in postpartum women. Contraception 72(6):426, 2005

Okusanya BO, Oduwole O, Effa EE: Immediate postabortal insertion of intrauterine devices. Cochrane Database Syst Rev 6:CD001777, 2014

Ortiz ME, Croxatto HB: The mode of action of IUDs. Contraception 36:37, 1987

Parkin L, Sharples K, Hernandez RK, et al: Risk of venous thromboembolism in users of oral contraceptives containing drospirenone or levonorgestrel: nested case-control study based on UK General Practice Research Database. BMJ 342:d2139, 2011

Pati S, Cullins V: Female sterilization: evidence. Obstet Gynecol Clin North Am 27:859, 2000

Peterson HB, Jeng G, Folger SG, et al: The risk of menstrual abnormalities after tubal sterilization. N Engl J Med 343:1681, 2000

Peterson HB, Xia Z, Hughes JM, et al: The risk of pregnancy after tubal sterilization: findings from the U.S. Collaborative Review of Sterilization. Am J Obstet Gynecol 174(4):1161, 1996

Peterson HB, Xia Z, Wilcox LS, et al: Pregnancy after tubal sterilization with bipolar electrocoagulation. U.S. Collaborative Review of Sterilization Working Group. Obstet Gynecol 94:163, 1999

Petri M, Kim MY, Kalunian KC, et al: Combined oral contraceptives in women with systemic lupus erythematosus. N Engl J Med 353:2550, 2005

Pfizer: Depo-Provera: prescribing information. New York, Pfizer, 2014

Phelps JY, Kelver ME: Confronting the legal risks of prescribing the contraceptive patch with ongoing litigation. Obstet Gynecol 113(3):712, 2009

Pomp ER, le Cessie S, Rosendaal FR, et al: Risk of venous thrombosis: obesity and its joint effect with oral contraceptive use and prothrombotic mutations. Br J Haematol 139(2):289, 2007

Pomp ER, Rosendaal FR, Doggen CJ: Smoking increases the risk of venous thrombosis and acts synergistically with oral contraceptive use. Am J Hematol 83:97, 2008

Ragan RE, Rock RW, Buck HW: Metoclopramide pretreatment attenuates emergency contraceptive-associated nausea. Am J Obstet Gynecol 188:330, 2003

Raymond EG, Creinin MD, Barnhart KT, et al: Meclizine for prevention of nausea associated with use of emergency contraceptive pills: a randomized trial. Obstet Gynecol 95:271, 2000

Realini JP, Goldzieher JW: Oral contraceptives and cardiovascular disease: a critique of the epidemiologic studies. Am J Obstet Gynecol 152:729, 1985

Rimm EB, Manson JE, Stampfer MJ, et al: Oral contraceptive use and the risk of type 2 (non-insulin-dependent) diabetes mellitus in a large prospective study of women. Diabetologia 35:967, 1992

Robinson GE, Burren T, Mackie IJ, et al: Changes in haemostasis after stopping the combined contraceptive pill: implications for major surgery. BMJ 302:269, 1991

Roddy RE, Zekeng L, Ryan KA, et al: A controlled trial of nonoxynol-9 film to reduce male-to-female transmission of sexually transmitted diseases. N Engl J Med 339:504, 1998

Ronnerdag M, Odlind V: Health effects of long-term use of the intrauterine levonorgestrel-releasing system. Acta Obstet Gynecol Scand 78:716, 1999

Rosen MP, Breitkopf DM, Nagamani M: A randomized controlled trial of second- versus third-generation oral contraceptives in the treatment of acne vulgaris. Am J Obstet Gynecol 188:1158, 2003

Roumen F, Apter D, Mulders TM, et al: Efficacy, tolerability and acceptability of a novel contraceptive vaginal ring releasing etonogestrel and ethinyl estradiol. Hum Reprod 16:469, 2001

Said S, Omar K, Koetsawang S, et al: A multicentred phase III comparative clinical trial of depot-medroxyprogesterone acetate given three-monthly at doses of 100 mg or 150 mg: 1. Contraceptive efficacy and side effects. World Health Organization Task Force on Long-Acting Systemic Agents for Fertility Regulation. Special Programme of Research, Development and Research Training in Human Reproduction. Contraception 34(3):223, 1986

Sánchez-Guerrero J, Uribe AG, Jiménez-Santana L, et al: A trial of contraceptive methods in women with systemic lupus erythematosus. N Engl J Med 353:2539, 2005

Schreiber CA, Meyn LA, Creinin MD, et al: Effects of long-term use of nonoxynol-9 on vaginal flora. Obstet Gynecol 107:136, 2006

Schwingl PJ, Guess HA: Safety and effectiveness of vasectomy. Fertil Steril 73:923, 2000

Seeger JD, Loughlin J, Eng PM, et al: Risk of thromboembolism in women taking ethinylestradiol/drospirenone and other oral contraceptives. Obstet Gynecol 110:587, 2007

Shavell VI, Abdallah ME, Shade GH Jr, et al: Trends in sterilization since the introduction of Essure hysteroscopic sterilization. J Minim Invasive Gynecol 16(1):22, 2009

Shikary ZK, Betrabet SS, Patel ZM, et al: ICMR Task Force Study on hormonal contraception. Transfer of levonorgestrel (LNG) administered through different drug delivery systems from the maternal circulation via breast milk. Contraception 35:477, 1987

Shridharani A, Sandlow JL: Vasectomy reversal versus IVF with sperm retrieval: which is better? Curr Opin Urol 20(6):503, 2010

Shulman LP, Gabriel H: Management and localization strategies for the nonpalpable Implanon rod. Contraception 73(4):325, 2006

Shy KK, Stergachis A, Grothaus LG, et al: Tubal sterilization and risk of subsequent hospital admission for menstrual disorders. Am J Obstet Gynecol 166:1698, 1992

Sieh W, Salvador S, McGuire V, et al: Tubal ligation and risk of ovarian cancer subtypes: a pooled analysis of case-control studies. Int J Epidemiol 42(2):579, 2013

Sivin I: Alternative estimates of ectopic pregnancy risks during contraception. Am J Obstet Gynecol 165:1900, 1991

Sivin I, Nash H, Waldman S: Jadelle levonorgestrel rod implants: a summary of scientific data and lessons learned from programmatic experience. New York, Population Council, 2002

Skegg DC, Noonan EA, Paul C, et al: Depot medroxyprogesterone acetate and breast cancer. JAMA 273:799, 1995

Society of Family Planning: Use of the Mirena™ LNG-IUS and ParaGard™ CuT380A intrauterine devices in nulliparous women. Contraception 81:367, 2010

Society of Gynecologic Oncology: SGO Clinical Practice Statement: salpingectomy for ovarian cancer prevention. Chicago, Society of Gynecologic Oncology, 2013.

Soderstrom RM: Sterilization failures and their causes. Am J Obstet Gynecol 152:395, 1985

Sokal D, Gates D, Amatya R, et al: Two randomized controlled trials comparing the Tubal Ring and Filshie Clip for tubal sterilization. Fertil Steril 74:3, 2000

Sokal DC, Hieu do T, Loan ND, et al: Contraceptive effectiveness of two insertions of quinacrine: results from 10-year follow-up in Vietnam. Contraception 78(1):61, 2008

Steiner M, Lopez M, Grimes D, et al: Sino-implant (II)—a levonorgestrel-releasing two-rod implant: systematic review of the randomized controlled trials. Contraception 81(3):197, 2010

Steiner MJ, Dominik R, Rountree W, et al: Contraceptive effectiveness of a polyurethane condom and a latex condom: a randomized controlled trial. Obstet Gynecol 101:539, 2003

Steiner MJ, Trussell J, Mehta N, et al: Communicating contraceptive effectiveness: a randomized controlled trial to inform a World Health Organization family planning handbook. Am J Obstet Gynecol 195(1):85, 2006

Sulak PJ, Haney AF: Unwanted pregnancies: understanding contraceptive use and benefits in adolescents and older women. Am J Obstet Gynecol 168:2042, 1993

Sulak PJ, Kaunitz AM: Hormonal contraception and bone mineral density. Dialogues Contraception 6:1, 1999

Taneepanichskul S, Reinprayoon D, Khoosaad P: Comparative study of weight change between long-term DMPA and IUD acceptors. Contraception 58:149, 1998

Tatum HJ, Schmidt FH, Jain AK: Management and outcome of pregnancies associated with Copper-T intrauterine contraceptive device. Am J Obstet Gynecol 126:869, 1976

Tepper NK, Phillips SJ, Kapp N, et al: Combined hormonal contraceptive use among breastfeeding women: an updated systematic review. Contraception May 19, 2015 [Epub ahead of print]

Tepper NK, Steenland MW, Marchbanks PA, et al: Hemoglobin measurement prior to initiating copper intrauterine devices: a systematic review. Contraception 87(5):639, 2013

Teva Women's Health: ParaGard T 380A intrauterine copper contraceptive: prescribing information. Sellersville, Teva Women's Health, 2013

Thomas DB, Ye Z, Ray RM, et al: Cervical carcinoma in situ and use of depo-medroxyprogesterone acetate (DMPA). Contraception 51:25, 1995

Thonneau PF, Almont T: Contraceptive efficacy of intrauterine devices. Am J Obstet Gynecol 198(3):248, 2008

Thorneycroft IH, Stanczyk FZ, Bradshaw KD, et al: Effect of low-dose oral contraceptives on androgenic markers and acne. Contraception 60:255, 1999

Truitt ST, Fraser AB, Grimes DA, et al: Combined hormonal versus nonhormonal versus progestin-only contraception in lactation. Cochrane Database Syst Rev 2:CD003988, 2003

Trussell J: Contraceptive efficacy. In Hatcher RA, Trussell J, Nelson AL, et al (eds): Contraceptive Technology, 20th ed. New York, Ardent Media, 2011, p 791

Trussell J, Ellertson C, Stewart F: Emergency contraception. A cost-effective approach to preventing pregnancy. Womens Health Primary Care 1:52, 1998a

Trussell J, Hatcher RA, Cates W Jr, et al: Contraceptive failure in the United States: an update. Stud Fam Plann 21(1):51, 1990

Trussell J, Stewart F: An update on emergency contraception. Dialogues Contracept 5:1, 1998b

Tworoger SS, Fairfield KM, Colditz GA, et al: Association of oral contraceptive use, other contraceptive methods, and infertility with ovarian cancer risk. Am J Epidemiol 166(8):894, 2007

United Nations, Department of Economic and Social Affairs Population Division: World contraceptive patterns, 2013. New York, United Nations, 2013

University of California at San Francisco: HIV Insite: Database of antiretroviral drug interactions. 2014. Available at: http://hivinsite.ucsf.edu/insite?page=ar-00-02. Accessed December 19, 2014

U.S. Food and Drug Administration: Orange book: approved drug products with therapeutic equivalence evaluations. 2014. Available at: http://www.accessdata.fda.gov/scripts/cder/ob/default.cfm. Accessed December 19, 2014

van den Heuvel MW, van Bragt A, Alnabawy AK, et al: Comparison of ethinylestradiol pharmacokinetics in three hormonal contraceptive formulations: the vaginal ring, the transdermal patch and an oral contraceptive. Contraception 72(3):168, 2005

Veersema S, Vleugels M, Koks C, et al: Confirmation of Essure placement using transvaginal ultrasound. J Minim Invasive Gynecol 18(2):164, 2011

Vessey M, Yeates D: Oral contraceptives and benign breast disease: an update of findings in a large cohort study. Contraception 76(6):418, 2007

Vessey MP, Lawless M, Yeates D: Efficacy of different contraceptive methods. Lancet 1:841, 1982

Vessey MP, Meisler L, Flavel R, et al: Outcome of pregnancy in women using different methods of contraception. Br J Obstet Gynaecol 86:548, 1979

von Hertzen H, Piaggio G, Ding J, et al: Low dose mifepristone and two regimens of levonorgestrel for emergency contraception: a WHO multicentre randomized trial. Lancet 360:1803, 2002

Waldron T: Tests show commonly used substances harm latex condoms. Contracept Tech Update 10:20, 1989

Wallach M, Grimes DA (eds): Modern Oral Contraception. Updates from The Contraception Report. Totowa, Emron, 2000, pp 26, 90, 194

Walsh T, Grimes D, Frezieres R, et al: Randomized controlled trial of prophylactic antibiotics before insertion of intrauterine devices. Lancet 351:1005, 1998

Weber J, Desai K, Darbyshire J: The development of vaginal microbicides for the prevention of HIV transmission. PLoS Med 2(5):e142, 2005

Westhoff C, Davis A: Tubal sterilization: focus on the U.S. experience. Fertil Steril 73:913, 2000

Westhoff C, Heartwell S, Edwards S, et al: Initiation of oral contraceptive using a quick start compared with a conventional start: a randomized controlled trial. Obstet Gynecol 109:1270, 2007a

Westhoff C, Jain JK, Milsom I, et al: Changes in weight with depot medroxyprogesterone acetate subcutaneous injection 104 mg/0.65 mL. Contraception 75(4):261, 2007b

Westhoff C, Kerns J, Morroni C, et al: Quick start: novel oral contraceptive initiation method. Contraception 66:141, 2002

Westhoff CL: Oral contraceptives and thrombosis: an overview of study methods and recent results. Am J Obstet Gynecol 179:S38, 1998

Westhoff CL, Torgal AH, Mayeda ER, et al: Pharmacokinetics of a combined oral contraceptive in obese and normal-weight women. Contraception, 81(6):474, 2010

White T, Ozel B, Jain JK, et al: Effects of transdermal and oral contraceptives on estrogen-sensitive hepatic proteins. Contraception 74(4):293, 2006

Winer RL, Hughes JP, Feng Q, et al: Condom use and the risk of genital human papillomavirus infection in young women. N Engl J Med 354:2645, 2006

Woods ER, Grace E, Havens KK, et al: Contraceptive compliance with a levonorgestrel triphasic and a norethindrone monophasic oral contraceptive in adolescent patients. Am J Obstet Gynecol 166:901, 1992

World Health Organization: Acute myocardial infarction and combined oral contraceptives: results of an international multi-center case-control study. Lancet 349:1202, 1997

World Health Organization: Cardiovascular disease and use of oral and injectable progestogen-only contraceptives and combined injectable contraceptives. Results of an international, multicenter, case-control study. Contraception 57:315, 1998

World Health Organization: Combined oral contraceptives and liver cancer. Int J Cancer 43:254, 1989

World Health Organization: Depot-medroxyprogesterone acetate (DMPA) and risk of endometrial cancer. Int J Cancer 49:186, 1991

World Health Organization: Ischaemic stroke and combined oral contraceptives: results of an international, multi-center case-control study. Lancet 348:498, 1996

World Health Organization: Mechanism of action, safety and efficacy of intrauterine devices. Technical Report No. 753, Geneva, Switzerland, WHO, 1987

World Health Organization: Medical Eligibility for Contraceptive Use, 4th ed. Geneva, WHO, 2010

World Health Organization, Johns Hopkins Bloomberg School of Public Health (SHSPH): Family Planning Handbook for Providers. Baltimore and Geneva, 2007

World Health Organization Special Programme of Research, Development and Research Training in Human Reproduction, Task Force on Intrauterine Devices for Fertility Regulation: A multinational case-control study of ectopic pregnancy. Clin Reprod Fertil 3:131, 1985

Yonkers KA, Brown C, Pearlstein TB, et al: Efficacy of a new low-dose oral contraceptive with drospirenone in premenstrual dysphoric disorder. Obstet Gynecol 106:492, 2005

Yunker AC, Ritch JM, Robinson EF, et al: Incidence and risk factors for chronic pelvic pain after hysteroscopic sterilization. J Minim Invasive Gynecol 22(3):390, 2015

Yuzpe AA, Thurlow HJ, Ramzy I, et al: Post coital contraception—a pilot study. J Reprod Med 13:53, 1974

Zapata LB, Whiteman MK, Tepper NK, et al: Intrauterine device use among women with uterine fibroids: a systematic review. Contraception 82(1):41, 2010

Zieman M, Guillebaud J, Weisberg E, et al: Contraceptive efficacy and cycle control with the Ortho EvraTM/EvraTM transdermal system: the analysis of pooled data. Fertil Steril 77:S13, 2002

Zupanc M: Antiepileptic drugs and hormonal contraceptives in adolescent women with epilepsy. Neurology 66(Suppl 3):S37, 2006

CHAPTER 6

First-Trimester Abortion

The word *abortion* derives from the Latin *aboriri*–to miscarry. Abortion is defined as the spontaneous or induced termination of pregnancy before fetal viability. It is thus appropriate that miscarriage and abortion are terms used interchangeably in a medical context. But, because popular use of abortion by laypersons implies a deliberate intact pregnancy termination, many prefer miscarriage for spontaneous fetal loss. Both terms will be used throughout this chapter.

TERMINOLOGY

Defining viability has significant medical, legal, and social implications as this definition provides the line that separates abortion from preterm birth. It is usually defined by pregnancy duration and fetal birthweight for statistical and legal purposes. The National Center for Health Statistics, the Centers for Disease Control and Prevention (CDC), and the World Health Organization (WHO) all define *abortion* as any pregnancy termination—spontaneous or induced—prior to 20 weeks' gestation or with a fetus born weighing <500 g. Confusion may be introduced by state law criteria that define abortion more widely.

Technologic developments have revolutionized current abortion terminology. Transvaginal sonography (TVS) and precise measurement of serum human chorionic gonadotropin (hCG) concentrations help to identify extremely early pregnancies and to clarify intrauterine versus ectopic location. Ubiquitous application of these practices makes it possible to distinguish between a *chemical* and a *clinical* pregnancy. Another term, *pregnancy of unknown location—PUL*, aids the goal of early identification and management of ectopic pregnancy (Barnhart, 2011). Management options for ectopic gestation are described in Chapter 7 (p. 161). Of intrauterine pregnancies, those that end in a spontaneous abortion during the first trimester, that is, within the first $12^{6/7}$ weeks of gestation, are also termed *early pregnancy loss* or *early pregnancy failure*.

Approximately half of first-trimester miscarriages are *anembryonic*, that is, with no identifiable embryonic elements. The previous term *blighted ovum* for these pregnancies has fallen out of favor. The remaining pregnancies are *embryonic* miscarriages, which may be further grouped as either those with chromosomal anomalies (*aneuploid abortions*) or those with a normal chromosomal complement (*euploid abortions*).

Common terms used to describe pregnancy losses are listed here and will be discussed in this chapter. They include:

1. Spontaneous abortion—this category includes threatened, inevitable, incomplete, complete, and missed abortion. Septic abortion is used to further classify any of these that are complicated by infection.
2. Recurrent abortion—this term is variably defined, but it is meant to identify women with repetitive spontaneous abortions.
3. Induced abortion—this term is used to describe surgical or medical termination of a live fetus that has not reached viability.

SPONTANEOUS ABORTION

■ Incidence

More than 80 percent of spontaneous abortions occur during the first 12 weeks of gestation (American College of Obstetricians and Gynecologists, 2015). With first trimester losses, death of the embryo or fetus nearly always precedes spontaneous expulsion. Death of the conceptus is usually accompanied by hemorrhage into the decidua basalis. This is followed by adjacent tissue necrosis that stimulates uterine contractions and expulsion. An intact gestational sac is usually filled with fluid and may or may not contain an embryo or fetus.

The reported incidence of spontaneous abortion varies with the sensitivity of methods used to identify them. Wilcox and colleagues (1988) studied 221 healthy women through 707 menstrual cycles. They used highly specific assays sensitive to minute concentrations of maternal serum beta human chorionic gonadotropin (β-hCG) and found that 31 percent of pregnancies were lost after implantation. Importantly, two thirds of these early losses were *clinically silent*.

There are factors known to influence clinically apparent spontaneous abortion. However, it is unknown if these same factors affect clinically silent miscarriages. For example, the clinical miscarriage rate nearly doubles with maternal or paternal age greater than 40 (Gracia, 2005; Kleinhaus, 2006). Although it may seem intuitive that this difference would be similar for clinically silent miscarriages, this has not been studied.

■ Fetal Factors

As shown in Figure 6-1, approximately half of embryonic first-trimester miscarriages are aneuploid, an incidence that decreases markedly with advancing gestation at the time of pregnancy loss. In general, aneuploid fetuses abort earlier than those with a normal chromosomal complement. Kajii (1980) reported that 75 percent of aneuploid fetuses aborted before 8 weeks, while the rate of euploid abortions peaks at approximately 13 weeks. Almost 95 percent of chromosomal abnormalities in aneuploid fetuses are caused by maternal gametogenesis errors. Thus, only 5 percent are due to aberrant paternal chromosomes (Jacobs, 1980).

Aneuploid Abortion

Trisomy describes the condition in which three copies of a given chromosome are present. As shown in Table 6-1, *autosomal trisomy* is the most frequently identified chromosomal anomaly in early miscarriages. Although most trisomies result from

TABLE 6-1. Chromosomal Findings in Early Abortuses

Chromosomal Studies	Reported Incidence Range (Percent)
Normal (euploid)	
46,XY and 46,XX	45–55
Abnormal (aneuploid)	
Autosomal trisomy	22–32
Monosomy X (45,X)	5–20
Triploidy	6–8
Tetraploidy	2–4
Structural anomaly	2
Double or triple trisomy	0.7–2

Data from Eiben, 1990; Kajii, 1980; Simpson, 1980, 2007.

isolated nondisjunction, balanced structural chromosomal rearrangements are present in one partner in approximately 2 percent of couples with recurrent miscarriage (Barber, 2010). Trisomies of all chromosomes have been identified with the exception of chromosome number 1. Trisomies of number 13, 16, 18, 21, and 22 are most common. Based on a study of almost 47,000 women, the baseline risk for fetal aneuploidy was 1.4 percent. One prior miscarriage increased the risk of subsequent fetal aneuploidy to 1.67 percent. Two or three previous miscarriages increased this risk to 1.8 and 2.2 percent, respectively (Bianco, 2006).

Monosomy X (45,X) is the single most common specific chromosomal abnormality and is also known as *Turner syndrome*. Cystic hygroma, a multiloculated lymphatic malformation, is a frequent sonographic finding with this syndrome and portends a poor prognosis. Most fetuses with monosomy X spontaneously abort, but some are liveborn females (Chap. 18, p. 411). Conversely, *autosomal monosomy* is rare and incompatible with life.

Ploidy describes the number of complete chromosome sets. *Triploidy* is often associated with hydropic or molar placental degeneration (Chap. 37, p. 780). Of hydatidiform moles, partial moles are characteristically triploid. Associated triploid fetuses frequently abort early, and those born later are all grossly malformed. Advanced maternal and paternal ages do not increase the incidence of triploidy. *Tetraploid* fetuses most often abort early in gestation and are rarely liveborn.

Chromosomal structural abnormalities infrequently cause abortion. Infants with a balanced translocation who are liveborn usually appear normal but may experience recurrent pregnancy loss as discussed on page 145.

■ Euploid Abortion

The causes of euploid abortions are poorly understood, but various maternal medical disorders, genetic abnormalities, uterine defects, and environmental and lifestyle conditions have been implicated. Some of these, such as uterine anomalies or endocrinopathies, would be predicted to cause repetitive losses unless identified and treated. Others, such as genetic abnormalities, are not correctable. Paternal contribution to miscarriage is unclear and is discussed on page 145. Proposed etiologies will be discussed in the following sections, with a somewhat

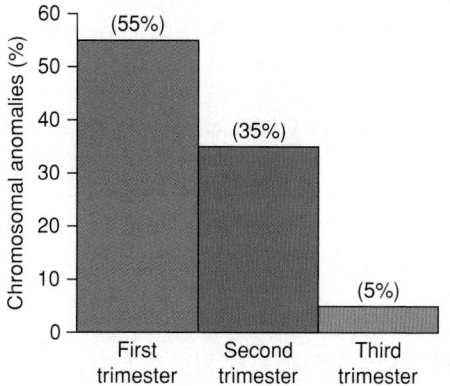

FIGURE 6-1 Frequency of chromosomal anomalies in abortuses and stillbirths during each trimester. Approximate percentages for each group are shown. (Data from Eiben, 1990; Fantel, 1980; Warburton, 1980.)

arbitrary categorization under either the isolated or recurrent pregnancy loss sections.

■ Maternal Factors
Medical Conditions

Pregnancy loss is clearly associated with diabetes mellitus and thyroid disorders (p. 149). Beyond these, few acute or chronic diseases convey early pregnancy risk. Even developing countries report that miscarriages are rarely caused by tuberculosis, malignancies, or other serious conditions.

Anorexia nervosa and *bulimia nervosa* are eating disorders reported to cause subfertility, preterm delivery, and fetal growth restriction. However, their association with miscarriages is less studied (Andersen, 2009; Sollid, 2004). *Chronic hypertension* is a common condition associated with increased rates of preeclampsia and fetal growth restriction but may not be associated with early pregnancy loss. Inflammatory bowel disease and systemic lupus erythematosus may independently increase the risk (Al Arfaj, 2010; Khashan 2012).

Women who have had multiple miscarriages are significantly more likely to have myocardial infarctions later in life. This perhaps suggests a link with underlying vascular disease (Kharazmi, 2011). Unrepaired cyanotic heart disease is likely an abortion risk, and in some, this may persist after repair (Canobbio, 1996).

Several relatively common genital tract abnormalities—especially those of the uterus—can either prevent pregnancy implantation or disrupt a pregnancy that has implanted. Of these, congenital anomalies are most often implicated, but some acquired anomalies can also cause pregnancy loss. Unless corrected, these defects typically result in repetitive pregnancy losses and thus are considered on page 147.

Infection

As an overview, only a few organisms are proven to cause abortion. In general, systemic infections likely infect the fetoplacental unit by a blood-borne route. Others may infect locally via maternal genitourinary infection or colonization.

Chlamydia trachomatis is suspected and in one study was found in 4 percent of abortuses compared with <1 percent of controls (Baud, 2011). Oakeshott and coworkers (2002) noted an association between *bacterial vaginosis* and second- but not first-trimester miscarriage. One metaanalysis showed that *Mycoplasma genitalium* infection was significantly associated with spontaneous abortion, preterm birth, and infertility (Lis, 2015).

Data concerning the abortifacient effects of some other infections are conflicting. Namely, roles for *Mycoplasma hominis, Ureaplasma urealyticum,* and human immunodeficiency virus (HIV)-1 infection in abortion are unclear (Quinn 1983a,b; Temmerman, 1992; van Benthem, 2000). Moreover in livestock, several infections cause abortion, but data remain inconclusive in humans. These include *Brucella abortus, Campylobacter fetus,* and *Toxoplasma gondii* (Feldman, 2010; Hide, 2009).

Last, infections caused by *Listeria monocytogenes,* parvovirus, cytomegalovirus, or herpes simplex virus likely have no abortifacient effects (Brown, 1997; Feldman, 2010; Yan, 2015).

Surgery

The risk of miscarriage due to a surgical procedure during pregnancy is not well studied. No currently used anesthetic agents have proven teratogenic effects when used at any gestational age. *Uncomplicated* surgical procedures—including abdominal or pelvic surgery—do not appear to increase the risk for abortion (Mazze, 1989). The American College of Obstetricians and Gynecologists (2013c) recommends that elective surgery be postponed until delivery or after. Nonurgent surgery should be performed in the second trimester, when possible, to decrease the theoretical risk for abortion or preterm contractions. Laparoscopy is also suitable, and adaptations for pregnancy are described in Chapter 41 (p. 876) (Pearl, 2011).

Ovarian tumors or cysts can be safely resected without causing pregnancy loss. An important exception involves early removal of the corpus luteum or the ovary in which it resides. If performed prior to 10 weeks' gestation, supplemental progesterone is given. Between 8 and 10 weeks, a single injection of intramuscular 17-hydroxyprogesterone caproate, 150 mg, is given at the time of surgery. If the corpus luteum is excised between 6 to 8 weeks, then two additional 150-mg injections are given 1 and 2 weeks after the first. Other suitable progesterone replacement regimens include: (1) micronized progesterone (Prometrium) 200 or 300 mg orally once daily, or (2) 8-percent progesterone vaginal gel (Crinone), one premeasured applicator vaginally daily plus micronized progesterone, 100 or 200 mg orally once daily. Supplementation is continued until 10 weeks' gestation.

Trauma seldom causes first-trimester miscarriage, and although Parkland Hospital is a busy trauma center, this is an infrequent association. Major trauma—especially abdominal—can cause fetal loss but is more likely as pregnancy advances.

Radiotherapy and Chemotherapy

In utero exposure to radiation may be abortifacient, teratogenic, or carcinogenic depending on the level of exposure and stage of fetal development. Threshold doses that cause abortion are not precisely known but definitely lie within the therapeutic doses used for maternal disease treatment (Williams, 2010). According to Brent (2009), exposure to <5 rads does not increase the miscarriage risk.

Female cancer survivors who were treated in the past with abdominopelvic radiotherapy may be at increased risk for miscarriage. Wo and Viswanathan (2009) reported an associated two- to eight-fold increased risk for miscarriages, low-birthweight and growth-restricted infants, preterm delivery, and perinatal mortality in women with prior radiotherapy. Hudson (2010) found an associated increased risk for miscarriage in those given radiotherapy and chemotherapy in the past for a childhood cancer.

Regarding chemotherapeutic agents, cases in which women with an early normal gestation are erroneously treated with methotrexate for an ectopic pregnancy are particularly worrisome. In a report of eight such cases, two viable-size fetuses had multiple malformations. An additional three patients spontaneously aborted their pregnancy (Nurmohamed, 2011). In a study of methotrexate treatment for rheumatic disease, the observed incidence of spontaneous abortion and major birth defects was statistically elevated in the patients receiving methotrexate after conception compared with disease-matched controls or women without autoimmune disease (Weber-Schoendorfer, 2014).

Medications and Vaccines

Only a few medications have been evaluated regarding the risk for early pregnancy loss. Conclusions have been difficult to derive from these studies based on multiple confounding factors including differences in doses, exposure duration, gestational age, and underlying maternal disease. Nonsteroidal antiinflammatory drugs are not linked to early pregnancy loss (Edwards, 2012). Also, oral contraceptives or spermicidal agents used in contraceptive creams and jellies are not associated with an increased miscarriage rate. When *intrauterine devices* fail to prevent pregnancy, however, the risk of abortion, and specifically septic abortion, increases substantively (Ganer, 2009; Moschos, 2011).

Most routine immunizations can be given safely during pregnancy. Fortunately, evidence to link immunization, even live-virus vaccines, with miscarriage is lacking. Two large metaanalyses clearly demonstrated no harm from the human papillomavirus (HPV) or influenza vaccine in early pregnancy (McMillan, 2015; Wacholder, 2010).

Nutritional Factors and Weight

Dietary deficiency of any one nutrient or moderate deficiency of all nutrients does not appear to be an important cause of abortion. Even in extreme cases—for example, *hyperemesis gravidarum*—abortion is rare. Dietary quality may be important as this risk may be reduced in women who consume fresh fruit and vegetables daily (Maconochie, 2007).

Data also suggest that extremes in weight can be deleterious. *Obesity* is associated with subfertility, increases the risk of miscarriage, and results in a host of other adverse pregnancy outcomes (Boots, 2014). Bellver and associates (2010a) studied 6500 women with in vitro fertilization (IVF)-conceived pregnancies and found that pregnancy and live birth rates were reduced progressively for each body mass index (BMI) unit increase. Although the risks for many adverse late-pregnancy outcomes are decreased after bariatric surgery, any salutary effects on the miscarriage rate are not clear (Guelinckx, 2009). Pregnant women who have undergone bariatric surgery are monitored for nutritional deficiencies (American College of Obstetricians and Gynecologists, 2013d).

Low BMI has also been associated with increased miscarriage risk (Helgstrand, 2005; Metwally, 2010). A cohort of more than 90,000 women demonstrated that the primary modifiable prepregnant risk factors for miscarriage are being underweight, obese, or aged 30 years or older at conception (Feodor Nilsson, 2014).

Behavior

Of these, alcohol has been well studied in pregnancy. Earlier observations were that both miscarriage and fetal anomaly rates increased with alcohol abuse rates during the first 8 weeks of gestation (Armstrong, 1992; Floyd, 1999). Such outcomes likely are dose related, although safe levels have not been identified. Maconochie (2007) observed a significantly increased

risk only with regular or heavy alcohol use. Low-level alcohol consumption did not significantly increase the abortion risk in two studies (Cavallo, 1995; Kesmodel, 2002). In contrast, Danish National Birth Cohort data suggest an adjusted hazard ratio for first-trimester fetal death of 1.66 with as few as two drinks per week (Andersen, 2012).

At least 15 percent of pregnant women admit to *cigarette smoking*. It seems intuitive that cigarettes could cause early pregnancy loss by several mechanisms that cause adverse late-pregnancy outcomes (Catov, 2008). Some studies link smoking with abortion risk and find a dose-response effect (Armstrong, 1992; Nielsen, 2006). Conversely, several others do not support this association (Rasch, 2003; Wisborg, 2003).

Excessive caffeine consumption has been associated with an increased abortion risk. Heavy intake, or approximately five cups of coffee per day—about 500 mg of caffeine—slightly increases the abortion risk (Cnattingius, 2000). Studies of "moderate" intake—less than 200 mg daily—did not demonstrate increased risk (Savitz, 2008; Weng, 2008). Currently, the American College of Obstetricians and Gynecologists (2013b) concludes that moderate consumption likely is not a major abortion risk and that any associated risk with higher intake is unsettled.

The adverse effects of illicit drugs on early pregnancy loss also are unclear. Although cocaine was linked to increased miscarriage in one study, reanalysis refuted this conclusion (Mills, 1999; Ness, 1999).

Occupation and Environment

Some environmental toxins such as benzene are implicated in fetal malformations, but data regarding miscarriage risk are less clear (Lupo, 2011). Earlier reports implicated arsenic, lead, formaldehyde, benzene, and ethylene oxide (Barlow, 1982). More recently, evidence suggests that DDT—dichlorodiphenyltrichloroethane—may raise miscarriage rates (Eskenazi, 2009). Nevertheless, DDT-containing insecticides are endorsed by the WHO (2011) for mosquito control to prevent malaria.

Few studies assess occupational exposure and abortion risks. Exposure to neither the electromagnetic fields of video display terminals nor to ultrasound increases miscarriage rates (Schnorr, 1991; Taskinen, 1990). An elevated risk has been described for dental assistants exposed to 3 or more hours of *nitrous oxide* per day in offices without gas-scavenging equipment (Rowland, 1995). In their metaanalysis, Dranitsaris and colleagues (2005) found a small incremental risk for spontaneous abortion in women who worked with *cytotoxic antineoplastic chemotherapeutic agents*.

■ Clinical Classification
Threatened Abortion

As a group, abortion can be divided clinically several ways. Commonly used categories include threatened, inevitable, incomplete, complete, and missed abortion. When the products of conception, uterus, and other pelvic organs become infected, the term septic abortion is descriptive.

Of these, *threatened abortion* is presumed when there is a bloody vaginal discharge or bleeding through a closed cervical

TABLE 6-2. Increased Incidence of Some Adverse Outcomes in Women with Threatened Abortion

Maternal	Perinatal
Placenta previa	Preterm ruptured
Placental abruption	membranes
Manual removal of placenta	Preterm birth
Cesarean delivery	Low-birthweight infant
	Fetal growth restriction
	Perinatal death

Data from Johns, 2006; Lykke, 2010; Saraswat, 2010; Wijesiriwardana, 2006.

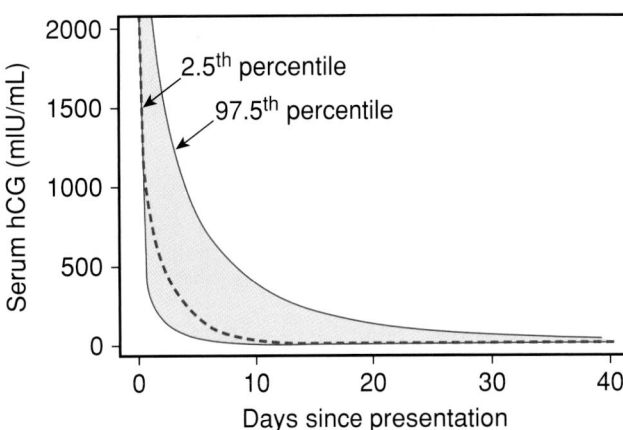

FIGURE 6-2 Composite curve describing decline in serial human chorionic gonadotropin (hCG) values starting at a level of 2000 mIU/mL following early spontaneous miscarriage. The dashed line is the predicted curve based on the summary of data from all women. The colored area within the dashed lines represent the 95-percent confidence intervals. (Data from Barnhart K, Sammel MD, Chung K, et al: Decline of serum human chorionic gonadotropin and spontaneous complete abortion: defining the normal curve. Obstet Gynecol 104:975, 2004.)

os (Hasan, 2009). In early pregnancy, bleeding is common and includes that with blastocyst implantation at the time of expected menses. Of pregnant women, approximately one quarter experience first-trimester spotting or heavier bleeding. Of these, 43 percent will subsequently miscarry. Bleeding is by far the most predictive risk factor for pregnancy loss, but this risk is substantially less if fetal cardiac activity is seen sonographically (Tongsong, 1995).

With miscarriage, bleeding usually begins first, and cramping abdominal pain follows hours to days later. There may be low-midline rhythmic cramps; persistent low backache with pelvic pressure; or dull and midline suprapubic discomfort. The combination of bleeding and pain predicts a poor prognosis for pregnancy continuation. Even if miscarriage does not follow early bleeding, the risks for later adverse pregnancy outcomes are elevated (Table 6-2). In a study of almost 1.8 million pregnancies, the risk for many of these pregnancy complications rose threefold (Lykke, 2010).

Diagnosis. A woman with an early pregnancy, vaginal bleeding, and pain should be examined. The primary goal is prompt diagnosis of an ectopic pregnancy. Serial quantitative serum β-hCG levels, progesterone levels, and transvaginal sonography, alone or in combination, can help ascertain if the fetus is alive and if it is within the uterus. Repeat evaluations are often necessary as none of these tests has 100-percent accuracy for the diagnosis of pregnancy location or fetal viability. Figure 6-2 depicts composite serum β-hCG level disappearance curves in women with bleeding who went on to have an early miscarriage (Barnhart, 2004). Several predictive models based on serum β-hCG levels done 48 hours apart have been described (Barnhart, 2010; Condous, 2007). Of these, serum β-hCG levels with a robust uterine pregnancy should increase at least 53 to 66 percent every 48 hours (Barnhart, 2004; Kadar, 1982). Seeber and associates (2006) used an even more conservative 35-percent rise after 48 hours.

With serum progesterone levels, those <5 ng/mL suggest a dying pregnancy. In contrast, values >20 ng/mL support the diagnosis of a healthy pregnancy. However, progesterone levels often lie between these thresholds, are then considered indeterminate, and thus are less informative.

Transvaginal sonography can document the location and viability of a gestation. If this cannot be done, then pregnancy of unknown location (PUL) is diagnosed. Notably, a consensus conference in 2012 concluded that prior sonographic criteria for fetal viability yielded unacceptably high rates of viable intrauterine pregnancies (IUPs) being falsely diagnosed as nonviable or as PULs (American College of Obstetricians and Gynecologists, 2015; Doubilet, 2014). Such erroneous diagnoses can lead to unnecessary surgical or medical treatment, interruption of a viable IUP, or incorrect assumption that a woman is at recurrent risk for an ectopic pregnancy. They proposed more stringent guidelines for the diagnosis of pregnancy failure (Table 6-3).

One early TVS sign of an IUP is the gestational sac. This anechoic fluid collection represents the exocoelomic cavity. It may be encircled by two echogenic external layers, the *double-decidual sign*, which represent the decidua parietalis and decidua capsularis (Fig. 6-3). The gestational sac can be seen by 4.5 weeks with maternal β-hCG levels between 1500 and 2000 mIU/mL (Barnhart, 1994; Timor-Tritsch, 1988). More recently, Connolly and colleagues (2013) reported that a threshold value of

TABLE 6-3. Society of Radiologists in Ultrasound Guidelines for Early Pregnancy Loss Diagnosis

Diagnostic Sonographic Findings
CRL ≥7 mm and no heartbeat
MSD ≥25 mm and no embryo
Absence of embryo with heartbeat ≥2 weeks after a scan showed a gestational sac without a yolk sac
Absence of embryo with heartbeat ≥11 days after a scan showed a gestational sac with a yolk sac

CRL = crown-rump length; MSD = mean sac diameter.
Data from Doubilet PM, Benson CB, Bourne T, et al: Diagnostic criteria for nonviable pregnancy early in the first trimester, N Engl J Med 2013 Oct 10;369(15):1443–1451.

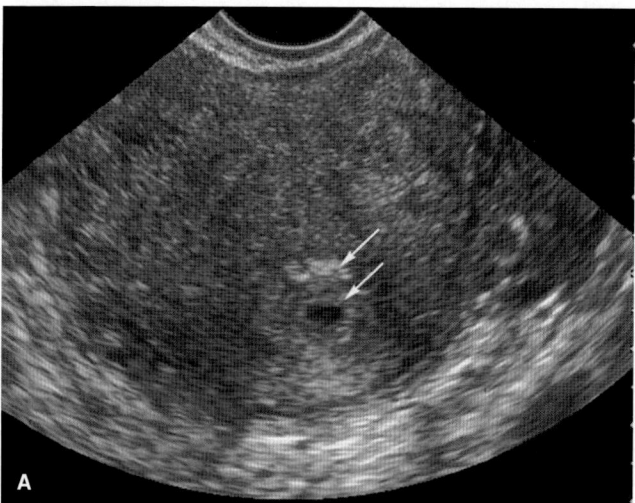

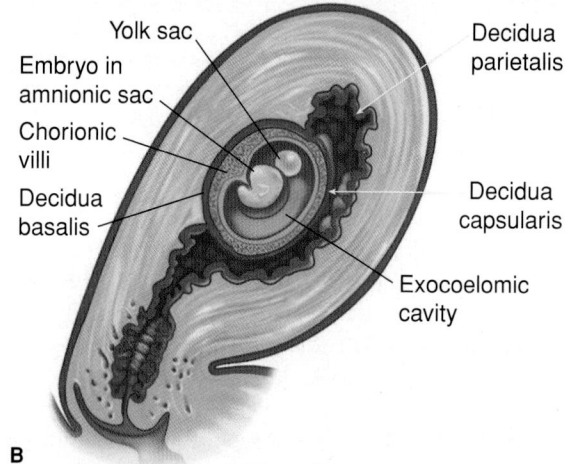

Yolk sac
Embryo in amnionic sac
Chorionic villi
Decidua basalis
Decidua parietalis
Decidua capsularis
Exocoelomic cavity

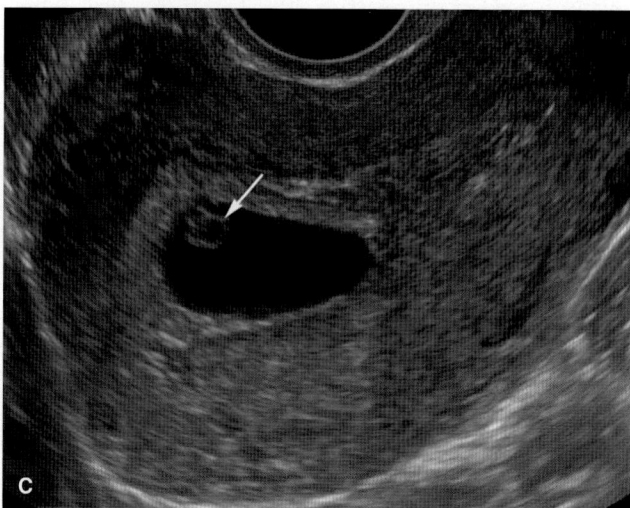

FIGURE 6-3 Early intrauterine pregnancy. **A.** Sonogram shows the anechoic gestational sac surrounded by two concentric echogenic layers, which are the inner decidua capsularis (*arrow*) and the peripheral decidua parietalis (*arrow*). **B.** The drawing shows the anatomy of an early pregnancy. **C.** The yolk sac (*arrow*) is circular and anechoic, and in this image, it lies to the right of its adjacent embryo.

3500 mIU/mL may be required to detect a gestational sac in 99 percent of cases. Importantly, a gestational sac may appear similar to other intrauterine fluid accumulations such as the *pseudogestational sac (pseudosac)* present with ectopic pregnancy (Fig. 7-4, p. 166). A pseudosac may be excluded once a definite yolk sac or embryo is seen inside the sac. The diagnosis of an IUP should be avoided if the yolk sac is not yet seen.

The yolk sac is a circular, 3- to 5-mm-diameter anechoic structure. It is typically seen within the gestational sac at approximately 5.5 weeks' gestation and with a mean sac diameter (MSD) ≥10 mm. At approximately 6 weeks' gestation, a 1- to 2-mm embryo adjacent to the yolk sac can be found (see Fig. 6-3). Absence of an embryo in a sac with a MSD of 16 to 24 mm is suspicious for pregnancy failure (Doubilet, 2014). Cardiac motion can be detected at 6 to 6.5 weeks' gestation, at an embryonic length of 1 to 5 mm. As shown in Table 6-3, absent cardiac activity at certain stages can be used to diagnose pregnancy failure.

Inevitable Abortion

Amnionic fluid leaking through a dilated cervix portends almost certain abortion. Either uterine contractions begin promptly or infection develops. Rarely is a gush of vaginal fluid during the first half of pregnancy without serious consequence.

In the rare case, fluid may have collected previously between the amnion and chorion and may not be associated with pain, fever, or bleeding. If documented, then diminished activity with observation is reasonable for some early-to-mid second-trimester gestations. After 48 hours, if no additional amnionic fluid has escaped and if there is no bleeding, cramping, or fever, then a woman may resume ambulation and pelvic rest. With bleeding, cramping, or fever, abortion is considered inevitable, and the uterus is evacuated.

Incomplete Abortion

Bleeding that follows partial or complete placental separation and that is coupled with dilation of the cervical os is termed incomplete abortion. The fetus and the placenta may remain entirely within the uterus or partially extrude through the dilated os. Before 10 weeks, they are frequently expelled together, but later, they deliver separately. Management options of incomplete abortion include curettage, medical abortion, or expectant management in clinically stable women as discussed on page 152. With surgical therapy, additional cervical dilatation may be necessary before suction curettage. In others, retained placental tissue simply lies loosely within the cervical canal and allows easy extraction with ring forceps. With miscarriage, removed products of conception are sent to pathology for standard histologic analysis. With this, products of conception are confirmed, and gestational trophoblastic disease is excluded.

Complete Abortion

In some cases, expulsion of the entire pregnancy is completed before a patient presents for care. In such cases, a history of heavy bleeding, cramping, and tissue passage at home is common. Physical examination reveals a closed cervical os. Patients are encouraged to bring in passed tissue, which may be a complete gestation, blood clots, or a decidual cast. The last is a layer of endometrium in the shape of the uterine cavity that when sloughed can appear as a collapsed sac (Fig. 7-7, p. 168).

If a gestational sac is not identified grossly in the expelled specimen, sonography is performed to differentiate a complete abortion from threatened abortion or ectopic pregnancy. Characteristic findings of a complete abortion include a thickened endometrium without a gestational sac. However, this does not guarantee a recent IUP. Condous and associates (2005) described 152 women with heavy bleeding, an empty uterus with endometrial thickness <15 mm, and a diagnosis of completed miscarriage. Six percent were subsequently proven to have an ectopic pregnancy. Thus, a diagnosis of complete abortion should not be made unless an intrauterine pregnancy was previously diagnosed sonographically or passage of a gestational sac has been confirmed. In unclear settings, serial serum β-hCG measurements aid correct diagnosis. With complete abortion, these levels drop quickly (Connolly, 2013).

Missed Abortion—Early Pregnancy Loss

The term *missed abortion* requires clarification. Historically, the term was used to describe dead products of conception that were retained for weeks or months in a uterus with a closed cervical os. Despite this, concurrent early pregnancy findings of amenorrhea, nausea and vomiting, breast changes, and uterine growth appeared normal. To elucidate these disparities, Streeter (1930) studied aborted fetuses and observed that the mean interval from death-to-abortion was approximately 6 weeks.

This historical description of missed abortion is in contrast to that defined currently based on results of serial serum β-hCG assays and TVS (Fig. 6-4). There is rapid confirmation of fetal or embryonic death—even in early pregnancies—and many women choose uterine evacuation when the diagnosis is confirmed. Many classify these as a missed abortion, although the term is used interchangeably with early pregnancy loss or pregnancy wastage (Silver, 2011).

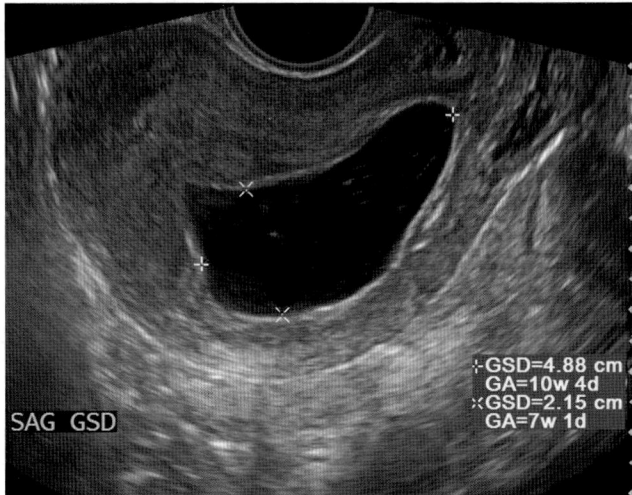

FIGURE 6-4 Transvaginal sonogram in the sagittal plane showing a gravid uterus. Calipers mark the sac borders of this anembryonic gestation.

Septic Abortion

Horrific infections and maternal deaths associated with criminal septic abortions have become rare with legalized abortion. Still, perhaps 1 to 2 percent of women with threatened or incomplete miscarriage can develop infection and sepsis syndrome. Elective abortion, either surgical or medical, is also occasionally complicated by severe and even fatal infections (Barrett, 2002; Ho, 2009). Bacteria gain uterine entry and colonize dead conception products. Organisms may invade myometrial tissues and extend to cause parametritis, peritonitis, septicemia, and rarely, endocarditis (Vartian, 1991).

Significant necrotizing infections and toxic shock syndrome have been reported due to *Clostridium perfringens*, *Clostridium sordellii*, and group A streptococcus—*S pyogenes* (Centers for Disease Control and Prevention, 2005; Daif, 2009). Clinical manifestations begin within a few days after the abortion.

Women may be afebrile when first seen with prominent endothelial injury, capillary leakage, hemoconcentration, hypotension, and a profound leukocytosis (Fischer, 2005; Ho, 2009). Maternal deaths from these clostridial species approximate 0.58 per 100,000 medical abortions (Meites, 2010).

Treatment of infected abortion or postabortal sepsis includes prompt administration of broad-spectrum antibiotics. Suitable regimens are found in Table 3-20 (p. 79). For women with septic incomplete abortion or for those with retained fragments, intravenous antimicrobial therapy is promptly followed by uterine evacuation. Most women respond to this treatment within 1 to 2 days and are discharged when afebrile. Continued oral antibiotic treatment is likely unnecessary (Savaris, 2011). Rarely, sepsis causes acute respiratory distress syndrome, acute kidney injury, or disseminated intravascular coagulopathy. In these cases, intensive supportive care is essential.

To prevent postabortal sepsis, prophylactic antibiotics are given at the time of surgical evacuation or induced abortion. The American College of Obstetricians and Gynecologists (2014b) recommends doxycycline, 100 mg orally 1 hour prior to and then 200 mg orally after the procedure.

■ Management

Unless there is serious bleeding or infection, management of spontaneous abortion can be individualized. In the case of threatened abortion, bed rest is often recommended but does not improve outcomes. Neither does treatment with a host of medications that include chorionic gonadotropin (Devaseelan, 2010). Acetaminophen-based analgesia will help relieve discomfort from cramping.

For other cases of spontaneous abortion, any of three management options is reasonable—expectant, medical, or surgical. Each has its own risks and benefits. For example, the first two are associated with unpredictable bleeding, and some women will require unscheduled curettage. Nevertheless, expectant management for suspected first-trimester miscarriage results in spontaneous resolution of pregnancy in more than 80 percent of women (Luise, 2002). Whereas surgical treatment is definitive and predictable, it is invasive and not necessary for all women (American College of Obstetricians and Gynecologists, 2015).

TABLE 6-4. Randomized Controlled Studies for Management of Early Pregnancy Loss

Study	Inclusion Criteria	No.	Treatment Arms	Outcomes
Nguyen (2005)	Incomplete SAB	149	(1) PGE$_1$, 600 μg orally (2) PGE$_1$, 600 μg orally initially and at 4 hour	60% completed at 3 d 95% at 7 d; 3% curettage
Zhang (2005)	Pregnancy failure[a]	652	(1) PGE$_1$, 800 μg vaginally (2) Vacuum aspiration	71% completed at 3 d; 16% failure 97% successful
Trinder (2006) (MIST Trial)	Incomplete SAB; missed AB	1200	(1) Expectant (2) PGE$_1$, 800 μg vaginally ±200 mg mifepristone (3) Suction curettage	50% curettage 38% curettage 5% repeat curettage
Dao (2007)	Incomplete SAB	447	(1) PGE$_1$, 600 μg orally (2) Vacuum aspiration	95% completed 100% completed
Torre (2012)	First-trimester miscarriage[b]	174	(1) Immediate—PGE$_1$, 200 μg orally Day 2—400 μg vaginally (2) Delayed—no treatment; TVS days 7 and 14	81% completed 19% curettage 57% completed 43% curettage

[a]Includes anembryonic gestation, embryonic or fetal death, without signs of incomplete SAB.
[b]Includes anembryonic gestation, embryonic or fetal death, or incomplete or inevitable SAB.
SAB = spontaneous abortion; PGE$_1$= prostaglandin E$_1$; TVS = transvaginal sonography.

With persistent or heavy bleeding, the hematocrit is determined. If there is significant anemia or hypovolemia, then pregnancy evacuation is generally indicated. In cases in which there is a live fetus, some may infrequently choose transfusion and further observation.

Several randomized studies that compared these management schemes were reviewed by Neilson (2013). A major drawback cited for between-study comparisons was varied inclusion criteria and techniques. For example, the success of medical therapy was enhanced in studies that included women with vaginal bleeding compared with those that excluded such women (Creinin, 2006). Selected studies reported since 2005 are listed in in Table 6-4. These permit some generalizations. First, success is dependent on the type of early pregnancy loss, that is, incomplete versus missed abortion. Second, expectant management of spontaneous incomplete abortion has failure rates as high as 50 percent. Medical therapy failure rates with prostaglandin E$_1$ (PGE$_1$) may be related to dose, route, and form, and rates vary from 5 to 40 percent. Last, curettage results in a quick resolution that is 95- to 100-percent successful. Importantly, subsequent pregnancy rates do not differ among these management methods (Smith, 2009).

During spontaneous miscarriage, 2 percent of D-negative women will become isoimmunized if not provided passive isoimmunization. With an induced abortion, this rate may reach 5 percent. The American College of Obstetricians and Gynecologists (2013e) recommends anti-Rh$_0$(D)immunoglobulin given as 300 μg intramuscularly (IM) for all gestational ages. Alternatively, dosing may be graduated, with 50 μg given IM for pregnancies ≤12 weeks and 300 μg given for those ≥13 weeks.

Prophylaxis with a threatened abortion is controversial, and recommendations are limited by scarce evidence-based data (Hannafin, 2006; Weiss, 2002). Up to 12 weeks' gestation, prophylaxis is optional for women with threatened abortion and a live fetus. At Parkland Hospital, we administer a 50-μg dose to all D-negative women with first-trimester bleeding.

RECURRENT MISCARRIAGE

Terms used to describe repetitive early spontaneous pregnancy losses include *recurrent miscarriage, recurrent spontaneous abortion,* and *recurrent pregnancy loss,* with the last term gaining popularity. The term *habitual abortion* was used in the past and currently is not preferred. Approximately 1 to 2 percent of fertile couples experience recurrent miscarriage, which is classically defined as three or more consecutive losses at <20 weeks' gestation or with a fetal weight <500 g. Most women with recurrent miscarriage have embryonic or early fetal loss. Recurrent anembryonic miscarriage or those with consecutive losses after 14 weeks are much less common.

Studies are difficult to compare due to a lack of standard definitions. Some investigators include women with two rather than three consecutive losses, whereas others include women with three nonconsecutive losses. Documentation of pregnancy with β-hCG levels, sonography, and/or pathological examination also varies. At minimum, recurrent miscarriage should be distinguished from sporadic pregnancy loss, which implies intervening pregnancy that reached viability.

As shown in Table 6-5, the success rate of a subsequent viable pregnancy decreases as age increases and as the number of consecutive losses increases (Brigham, 1999). Following more than 150,000 miscarriages, Bhattacharya and coworkers (2010) reported miscarriage rates as they related to the number of prior losses (Table 6-6). In both studies, the risk for subsequent miscarriage was similar following either two or three losses.

TABLE 6-5. Predicted Success Rate of Subsequent Pregnancy According to Age and Number of Previous Miscarriages

Age (yr)	No. of Previous Miscarriages			
	2	3	4	5
	Predicted Success of Subsequent Pregnancy (%)			
20	92	90	88	85
25	89	86	82	79
30	84	80	76	71
35	77	73	68	62
40+	69	64	58	52

Data from Brigham SA, Conlon C, Farquharson RG: A longitudinal study of pregnancy outcome following idiopathic recurrent miscarriage. Hum Reprod 14(11):2868, 1999.

The American Society for Reproductive Medicine (2013) has proposed that recurrent pregnancy loss (RPL) be defined by two or more failed clinical pregnancies confirmed by either sonographic or histopathologic examination. Each loss should be considered an impetus for further evaluation, and a thorough evaluation is warranted after three losses. Other considerations include maternal age and the interval between pregnancies. Evaluation and treatment are considered earlier in couples with concordant subfertility. This practice is further justified by a recent study of more than 1000 women in which those with two pregnancy losses had a prevalence of abnormal test findings similar to that of women with three or more losses (Jaslow, 2010). Remarkably, the chances for a successful pregnancy are more than 50 percent even after five losses in women younger than 45 years (Brigham, 1999).

■ Etiology

Of the many putative causes of early RPL, only three are widely accepted: parental chromosomal abnormalities, antiphospholipid antibody syndrome, and acquired or congenital uterine abnormalities. Other suspected but not proven causes are alloimmunity, endocrinopathies, and environmental toxins. As

TABLE 6-6. Predicted Miscarriage Rate with Subsequent Pregnancy Based on Number of Prior Miscarriages[a]

	Previous Pregnancy Losses			
	0	1	2	3
Pregnancies (n)	143,595	6577	700	115
Subsequent risk for miscarriage	7.0%	13.9%	26.1%	27.8%

[a] Nonconsecutive miscarriages showed the same pattern of risk as consecutive miscarriages.
Data from Bhattacharya S, Townend J, Bhattacharya S: Recurrent miscarriage: are three miscarriages one too many? Analysis of a Scottish population-based database of 151,021 pregnancies. Eur J Obstet Gynecol Reprod Biol 150:24, 2010.

discussed on page 139, very few infections are firmly associated with early pregnancy loss. It is even less likely that infections would cause recurrent miscarriage because most are sporadic or they stimulate protective maternal antibodies.

The timing of the recurrent losses may provide a clue to their etiology. For a given individual with RPL, each miscarriage tends to occur near the same gestational age (Heuser, 2010). Genetic factors most frequently result in early embryonic losses, whereas autoimmune or anatomic abnormalities more likely lead to second-trimester losses. Although many causes of RPL parallel those of sporadic miscarriage, the relative incidence differs between the two categories. For example, recurrent first-trimester losses have a significantly lower incidence of genetic abnormalities than observed in sporadic losses. In one series, the products of conception had a normal karyotype in half of recurrent miscarriages but in only a fourth of sporadic losses (Sullivan, 2004).

■ Parental Chromosomal Abnormalities

Parental Karyotype

Although these account for only 2 to 5 percent of RPL, karyotype evaluation of both parents is recommended (American Society for Reproductive Medicine, 2012). Data from 8000 couples with two or more miscarriages demonstrated structural chromosomal anomalies in 3 percent—a fivefold greater incidence than observed for the general population. In the parents, balanced reciprocal translocations accounted for 50 percent of identified abnormalities; robertsonian translocations for 24 percent; and X chromosome mosaicism such as 47, XXY—*Klinefelter syndrome*—for 12 percent. Inversions and various other anomalies made up the remainder. The women were twice as likely as the men to harbor the cytogenetic abnormality (Tharapel, 1985). The likelihood of a karyotypic abnormality does not differ between consecutive or nonconsecutive pregnancy losses (van den Boogaard, 2010).

As noted, balanced translocations are the most common structural chromosomal abnormality and result in several possible genetic outcomes in the conceptus: normal, the same balance translocation, or an unbalanced translocation (Fig. 6-5). Offspring who inherit the balanced translocation are likely to also experience recurrent miscarriage. With an unbalanced translocation, the conceptus will either spontaneously abort or produce an anomalous, frequently stillborn fetus. Thus, a history of second-trimester loss or fetal anomaly raises suspicion that one parent may have an abnormal chromosome pattern.

Sperm DNA Testing

Increasing attention has been directed to sperm aneuploidy and DNA damage as a cause of infertility and RPL. In couples with RPL, some but not all studies report higher rates of aneuploidy and DNA fragmentation in sperm from the male partner (Bellver, 2010b; Ramasamy, 2015; Robinson, 2012). Although unlikely to be as critical as maternal age, increasing paternal age was significantly associated with an increased abortion risk in one study of more than 92,000 births (Kleinhaus, 2006). This risk was lowest before age 25 years, after which it progressively increased at 5-year intervals. A detrimental effect of paternal age on pregnancy outcomes following intrauterine insemination and IVF has also

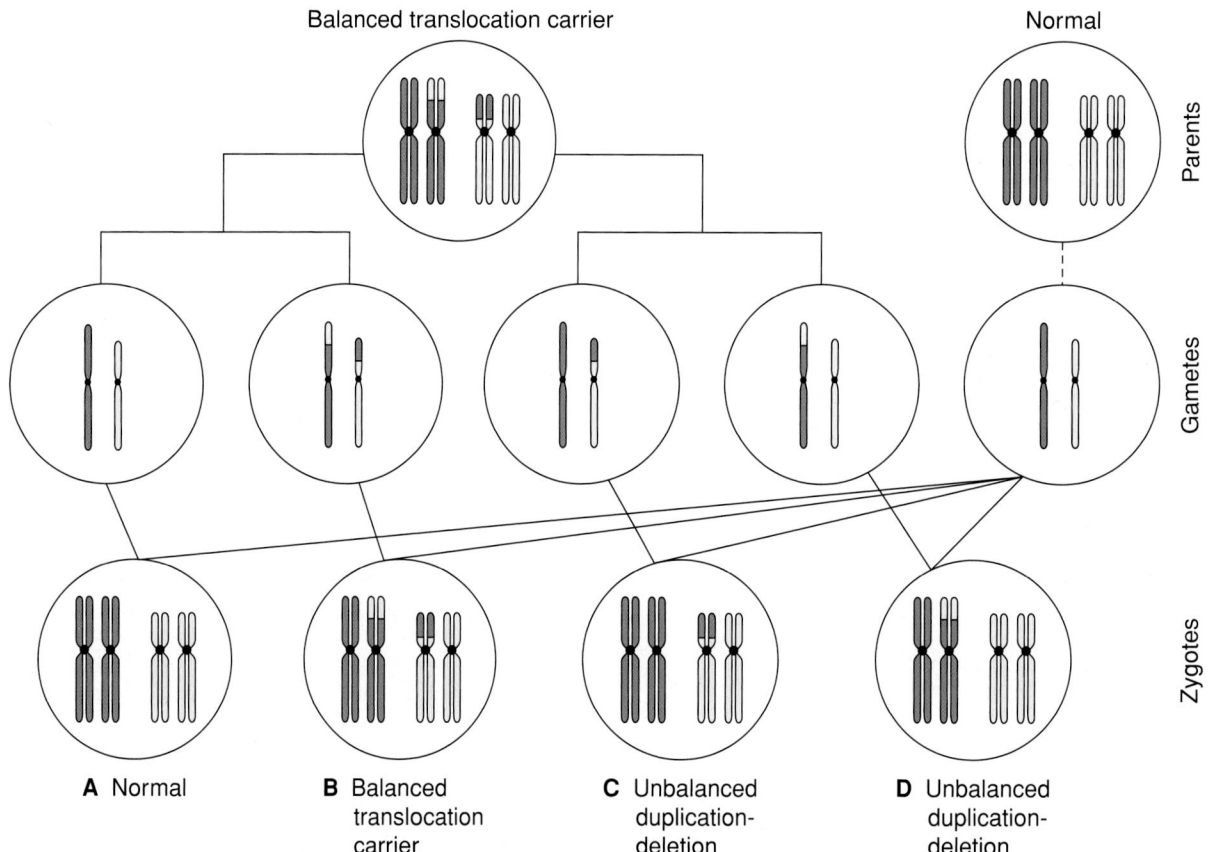

A Normal   **B** Balanced translocation carrier   **C** Unbalanced duplication-deletion   **D** Unbalanced duplication-deletion

FIGURE 6-5 Gametes produced by a balanced translocation carrier. (Reproduced with pemission from Cunningham FG, Leveno KL, Bloom SL, et al: Williams Obstetrics, 24th ed. New York: McGraw-Hill; 2014.)

been reported (Belloc, 2008; Robertshaw, 2013). However, semen analysis and assays for DNA integrity are not currently recommended as part of RPL evaluation (American Society for Reproductive Medicine, 2012).

Screening Products of Conception

Some recommend that fetal tissue be routinely analyzed for chromosomal abnormalities following a second consecutive miscarriage (Stephenson, 2006). One reason cited is that an abnormal karyotype suggests a sporadic loss and therefore does not predict an increased risk for loss with a subsequent pregnancy. Conversely, an abortus with a normal karyotype might suggest an alternative cause and imply the need for earlier evaluation.

Opponents of such routine karyotyping cite its high cost and possibility of misleading results. This applies particularly if the abnormal cells are derived from a pregnancy with placental mosaicism. Moreover, detection of a 46, XX karyotype may simply reflect contamination with maternal tissues. In sum, karyotyping of products of conception may not accurately reflect fetal karyotype. Because of the expense and limited information provided, we do not recommend this practice.

Although the cost effectiveness of karyotyping studies is not universally accepted, some are promoting the use of even more complex and expensive genetic techniques to evaluate couples with RPL (Barber, 2010). These include comparative genomic hybridization, chromosomal microarray, and copy number sequence technologies. These approaches can detect chromosomal

changes below the threshold of sensitivity for conventional cytogenetic analysis (Gao, 2012; Lui, 2015). Currently, we recommend that RPL evaluation should include a standard karyotype of both parents and that more detailed chromosomal evaluation should remain investigational.

Treatment

Individualized treatment is indicated in couples with a structural genetic abnormality. Approaches include IVF with preimplantation genetic diagnosis (PGD) or the use of donor gametes. These techniques are described in Chapter 20 (p. 466). Depending on the timing of prior losses, chorionic villus sampling or amniocentesis may also be considered. In one retrospective study of couples with known translocations, PGD was found to increase the successful pregnancy rate and decrease the length of time to conception (Fischer, 2010). Even so, the prognosis is generally good without intervention for couples with a balanced translocation. Franssen and colleagues (2006) compared couples with a balanced translocation and non-carrier couples. In both groups, 85 percent of couples had a healthy child, although the risk for miscarriage was higher in the carrier couples.

Some have recommended that PGD screening be done even in couples with normal karyotypes who have idiopathic RPL. Results from a large prospective cohort trial, however, found no support for this practice (Platteau, 2005). At this time, the American Society for Reproductive Medicine (2012) does not recommend PGD in couples who are chromosomally normal.

Anatomic Factors

Several uterine abnormalities have been implicated in RPL and other adverse pregnancy outcomes, but not infertility (Reichman, 2010). According to Devi Wold and associates (2006), 15 percent of women with three or more consecutive miscarriages will be found to have an acquired or congenital uterine anomaly. The likelihood of identifying an abnormality is similar whether a patient has experienced two, three, or four consecutive miscarriages. This suggests that cavity evaluation after two miscarriages is reasonable (Seckin, 2012).

Acquired Uterine Defects

Acquired uterine abnormalities associated with pregnancy loss include intrauterine synechiae, leiomyoma, and endometrial polyps. Of these, intrauterine synechiae—known as *Asherman syndrome*—usually result from destruction of large areas of endometrium by curettage or ablative procedures. Characteristic multiple filling defects are seen during hysterosalpingography or saline infusion sonography (Fig. 2-23, p. 34 and Fig. 19-6, p. 439). Directed hysteroscopic lysis of adhesions is preferable to curettage, as discussed and illustrated in Section 44-19 of the atlas (p. 1052). In one study, adhesiolysis decreased the miscarriage rate from 79 to 22 percent and increased successful term pregnancies from 18 to 69 percent (Katz, 1996). Other studies have reported similar outcomes with prognosis correlating with disease severity (Al-Inany, 2001; Goldenberg, 1995).

Uterine leiomyomas are found in a large proportion of adult women and can cause miscarriage, especially if located near the placental implantation site. Common sense suggests that detrimental effects should be greater for submucous compared with intramural leiomyomas, and for large versus small tumors. However, uterine cavity distortion is apparently not requisite for bad outcomes, and conclusive data are lacking (Saravelos, 2011). For example, in women undergoing IVF, pregnancy outcomes were adversely affected by submucous but not subserosal or intramural leiomyomas (Jun, 2001; Ramzy, 1998). In contrast, a metaanalysis reported increased adverse pregnancy outcomes—including miscarriage—following IVF in women with intramural myomas (Sunkara, 2010).

Currently, although based on poor-quality data, most agree that consideration be given to excision of submucosal and intracavitary leiomyomas in women with recurrent miscarriage, as discussed in Chapter 9 (p. 205). Uterine artery embolization to treat myomas may increase the risk for subsequent miscarriage and may not be advisable (Homer, 2010). Likewise, hysteroscopic removal of endometrial polyps is general recommended, although data are scant, particularly in the presence of single or small polyps.

Incompetent cervix, also known as cervical insufficiency, may develop following surgical or birth trauma and has also been associated with a molecular defect in collagen synthesis (Dukhovny, 2009). Cervical insufficiency does not cause first-trimester miscarriage but is associated with an increased risk for second-trimester loss following painless cervical dilatation after 16 to 18 weeks' gestation. Cervical incompetence is often treated surgically with cerclage placement. Interested readers are referred to Chapter 18 of *Williams Obstetrics,* 24th edition (Cunningham, 2014).

Developmental Anomalies

Congenital malformations of the müllerian ducts also may have adverse pregnancy effects. Anomalies include unicornuate, bicornuate, septate, arcuate, and didelphic uteri. Cited prevalence rates for müllerian anomalies vary widely. This is likely due to differences in the criteria set to define normalcy and in the diagnostic modality employed. Anomalies are often first detected by hysterosalpingography or routine sonography. Further characterization by 3-dimensional (3-D) sonography and magnetic resonance (MR) imaging may be helpful.

In a compilation study of more than 573,000 women, the observed incidence of anomalies was 1 in 600 in fertile women and 1 in 30 in infertile women. The overall incidence was 1 in 200 (Nahum, 1998). Much higher rates have been reported using 3-D sonography, perhaps due to greater sensitivity. Salim and associates (2003) scanned nearly 2500 women using 3-D sonography. Anomalies were identified in 24 percent of women with RPL, but in only 5 percent of controls. In a metaanalysis of publications from 1950 to 2007, Saravelos and coworkers (2008) concluded that uterine anomalies are present in approximately 17 percent of patients with RPL, 7.3 percent of infertile women, and 6.7 percent of women in the general population. The distribution of anomalies and associated loss rates are shown in Table 6-7. Unicornuate, bicornuate, and septate uteri are all associated with increased early miscarriage and second-trimester abortion, fetal malpresentation, and preterm labor (Reichman, 2010).

Demonstration of improved early pregnancy outcome following correction of a uterine anomaly has proven difficult. Nevertheless, in one observational study, pregnancy outcomes were reviewed following hysteroscopic removal of a septum in women with more than two prior miscarriages (Saygili-Yilmaz, 2003). The miscarriage rate decreased from 96 to 10 percent following surgery, and term pregnancy rates increased from zero to 70 percent. A recent metaanalysis reported that hysteroscopic metroplasty was associated with a markedly reduced

TABLE 6-7. Estimated Prevalence of Some Congenital Uterine Malformations and Their Associated Pregnancy Loss Rate

Uterine Anomaly[a]	Proportion (%)	SAB Rate (%)[b]
Bicornuate	39	40–70
Septate or unicornuate	14–24	34–88
Didelphys	11	40
Arcuate	7	—
Hypo- or aplastic	4	—

[a]Estimated overall prevalence 1:200 women (Nahum, 1998).
[b]Includes first- and second-trimester spontaneous abortions (SABs).
Data from Buttram, 1979; Nahum, 1998; Reddy, 2007; Valli, 2001.

probability of spontaneous abortion compared with untreated women (Venetis, 2014). Based on these reports and the relative safety of hysteroscopic correction, most experts recommend hysteroscopic resection of a uterine septum in women with recurrent miscarriage, as described in Section 44-17 (p. 1048) (American Society for Reproductive Medicine, 2012).

In contrast, surgical repair of a bicornuate uterus requires laparotomy and full-thickness incision of the uterine wall (Fig. 18-12, p. 422). Disadvantages to metroplasty include the requirement of cesarean delivery to prevent uterine rupture in subsequent pregnancy and the high rate of postoperative pelvic adhesion formation and subsequent infertility. Thus, surgery is generally not recommended except for women who have had a very high number of pregnancy losses. Additional discussion regarding the incidence, clinical impact, and treatment of congenital anatomic abnormalities can be found in Chapter 18 (p. 417). The use of a gestational carrier may be an option in women who are not surgical candidates.

■ Immunologic Factors

Much attention has focused on the role of the immune system in RPL. Yetman and Kutteh (1996) estimated that 15 percent of more than 1000 women with recurrent miscarriages had recognized immunologic factors. Two primary pathophysiologic models are the *autoimmune theory*—immunity against "self," and the *alloimmune theory*—immunity against antigens from another person.

Autoimmune Factors

It has been appreciated that pregnancy wastage is increased in women with systemic lupus erythematosus (Clowse, 2008). Subsequently, many women with lupus were identified to have antiphospholipid antibodies—a family of autoantibodies directed against phospholipid-binding plasma proteins (Erkan,

2011). Between 5 and 15 percent of women with RPL have clinically significant antiphospholipid antibodies compared with only 2 to 5 percent of controls (Branch, 2010).

The combination of these antiphospholipid antibodies and specific clinical findings is termed *antiphospholipid antibody syndrome—APS* (American College of Obstetrics and Gynecology, 2012). Criteria for its diagnosis are shown in Table 6-8. Positive tests are repeated at a minimum of 12 weeks with strict requirements for acceptable laboratory methods and interpretation (Miyakis, 2006). This is the only autoimmune disorder that has been clearly linked to pregnancy loss. Miscarriage due to APS most often occurs after 10 weeks. APS is more commonly associated with fetal death, preterm delivery, early-onset preeclampsia, and fetal growth restriction from placental insufficiency and placental thromboses (Clark, 2007a,b).

The mechanisms by which antiphospholipid antibodies result in miscarriage are unclear but can be divided into three general categories—thrombosis, inflammation, and abnormal placentation (Meroni, 2010). *Thrombosis* was initially thought to be due to inhibition of prostacyclin secretion by the vascular endothelium and stimulation of thromboxane A production by platelets. These actions result in vasoconstriction and increased platelet aggregation. More recently, it has been proposed that antiphospholipid antibodies act on trophoblast and endothelial surfaces to inhibit the function of annexin A5, a natural anticoagulant that prevents the activation of factor X and prothrombin (Rand, 2010). Antiphospholipid antibodies may also activate complement to intensify hypercoagulability, which leads to recurrent placental thromboses. *Acute local inflammatory responses* at the placental-maternal interface may also be induced by antiphospholipid antibodies. Finally, *placentation* may be directly affected by these antibodies through impaired decidual expression of integrins and cadherins. This can inhibit placental proliferation and syncytial development. Notably, defective decidual trophoblast invasion—not placental thrombosis—is

TABLE 6-8. Clinical and Laboratory Criteria for Diagnosis of Antiphospholipid Antibody Syndrome[a]

Clinical Criteria
Obstetric:
   One or more unexplained deaths of a morphologically normal fetus at or beyond 10 weeks
   or
   Severe preeclampsia or placental insufficiency necessitating delivery before 34 weeks
   or
   Three or more unexplained consecutive spontaneous abortions before 10 weeks
Vascular: One or more episodes of arterial, venous, or small-vessel thrombosis in any tissue or organ

Laboratory Criteria[b]
Presence of lupus anticoagulant according to guidelines of the International Society on Thrombosis and Hemostasis
or
Medium or high serum levels of IgG or IgM anticardiolipin antibodies
or
Anti-β2 glycoprotein-I IgG or IgM antibody

[a]At least one clinical and one laboratory criterion must be present for diagnosis.
[b]These tests must be positive on two or more occasions at least 12 weeks apart.
IgG = immunoglobulin G; IgM = immunoglobulin M.
Data from from Branch, 2010; Erkan, 2011; Miyakis, 2006.

the most common histologic abnormality identified in APS-related early pregnancy loss (Di Simone, 2007).

Several other *antilipid antibody idiotypes* have been described (Bick, 2006). Their measurement is expensive, frequently poorly controlled, and of uncertain relevance in the evaluation of RPL. Results are likewise inconclusive regarding testing for other antibodies including rheumatoid factor, antinuclear antibodies, and those for celiac disease. Currently, testing for these additional antibodies is not recommended during RPL evaluation.

Antiphospholipid Antibody Syndrome Treatment.
Various treatments have been proposed for women with APS and RPL (Kutteh, 2014). Several studies have compared single-agent or combination therapies using unfractionated heparin, low-molecular-weight heparin, low-dose aspirin, glucocorticoids, or intravenous immunoglobulin (IVIG). Concomitant use of glucocorticoids and heparin is generally not recommended. Compared with single treatment regimens, this combination may increase the maternal fracture risk without improving outcome. IVIG has also been discredited as described in the next section.

For women with APS, one reviewer group concluded that the combination of unfractionated heparin and low-dose aspirin significantly benefitted pregnancy outcome in those with first-trimester pregnancy losses (Ziakas, 2010). They found no improvement with low-molecular-weight heparin (LMWH) and aspirin combinations. Similar conclusions were reached in a Cochrane Database Review through 2011 (Empson, 2012). LMWH plus aspirin is appealing based on its ease of use and improved safety profile. However, until the issue is settled, unfractionated heparin is recommended.

Guidelines from the American College of Obstetricians and Gynecologists (2012) suggest that women with RPL and APS who have not had a thrombotic event receive prophylactic low-dose aspirin—81 mg orally per day—and heparin when pregnancy is diagnosed with continuation until delivery and 6 weeks postpartum. Heparin regimens vary, but unfractionated heparin—5000 to 10,000 units subcutaneously daily—is common. Some experts suggest initiating low-dose aspirin prior to conception (Kutteh, 2014). At a minimum, careful clinical surveillance to ensure early pregnancy detection seems prudent.

Alloimmune Factors
The immune tolerance of the mother to a semiallogeneic fetus remains incompletely understood (Williams, 2012). An attractive theory suggests that normal pregnancy requires the expression of blocking factors that prevent maternal rejection of paternally derived foreign fetal antigens. The pregnant woman ostensibly will not produce these blocking factors if she shares human leukocyte antigens (HLAs) with the father. Other alloimmune disorders that have been posited to cause recurrent miscarriage include altered natural killer cell activity and increased lymphocytotoxic antibodies. Berger and associates (2010) found that women with mutations of the HLA-G gene experienced recurrent miscarriages more often than women with normal haplotypes.

Various tests and treatment options have been developed to address this issue. None has withstood rigorous scrutiny. In an attempt to correct the dysregulated response to fetal antigens, proposed therapies include paternal or third-party leukocyte immunization and IVIG. Three randomized clinical trials failed to demonstrate any benefit of IVIG or placebo in patients with idiopathic miscarriage (Stephenson, 2010). Because these treatments have not been adequately tested and are potentially harmful, immunotherapy cannot currently be recommended for RPL.

Endocrinologic Factors
Luteal Phase Defect
Arredondo and Noble (2006) estimated that 8 to 12 percent of recurrent miscarriages are the result of endocrine factors. The increased incidence of miscarriage in these disorders is most frequently attributed to abnormal folliculogenesis with subsequent abnormal luteal function. This so-called *luteal phase defect (LPD)* is associated with inadequate endometrial development at implantation. Treatment for presumed LPD has included progesterone supplementation, hCG administration to enhance corpus luteum function, or ovulation induction with agents such as clomiphene citrate to generate additional corpora lutea. For this indication, none have proven beneficial. Although progesterone replacement is controversial for LPD, it is clearly indicated until 8 to 10 weeks in women who have had the supporting corpus luteum removed surgically that pregnancy (p. 139).

Thyroid Disease
Although the mechanisms by which they may adversely affect early pregnancy remain unclear, several endocrine disorders deserve discussion. These disorders include thyroid disorders, hyperprolactinemia, diabetes mellitus, and polycystic ovarian syndrome (PCOS). Of these, *thyroid disorders* have long been suspected to cause early pregnancy loss and other adverse pregnancy outcomes. Severe iodine deficiency—infrequent in developed countries—is associated with excessive miscarriage rates (Castañeda, 2002). Women suffering from hyperthyroidism have a greater risk for both spontaneous abortion and stillbirth (Andersen, 2014).

Thyroid hormone insufficiency is common, but the degree of insufficiency varies. In pregnancy, although overt hypothyroidism is rare, the incidence of subclinical hypothyroidism approximates 2 percent (Casey, 2005). Autoimmune Hashimoto thyroiditis is a usual cause, and its incidence and severity accrue with age. Despite this common prevalence, any effects of hypothyroidism on early pregnancy loss are still unclear (Krassas, 2010; Negro, 2010). That said, De Vivo (2010) reported that subclinical thyroid hormone deficiency may be associated with very early pregnancy loss.

The prevalence of abnormally high serum levels of antibodies to thyroid peroxidase or thyroglobulin is nearly 15 percent in pregnant women (Abbassi-Ghanavati, 2010; Haddow, 2011). Although most of these women are euthyroid, those with clinical hypothyroidism tend to have higher concentrations of antibodies. Even in euthyroid women, antibodies are a marker for increased miscarriage risk (Chen, 2011; Thangaratnam, 2011).

In sum, symptomatic women should undergo thyroid function testing, and overt hypo- or hyperthyroidism should be treated to prevent pregnancy complications. Screening all women with pregnancy loss is more controversial. Likewise, it is unclear whether patients with subclinical hypothyroidism or thyroid autoimmunity should receive treatment (Negro, 2006; Vissenberg, 2012).

Hyperprolactinemia

Cyclic ovulation may become dysfunctional in response to elevated serum prolactin levels such as occurs with prolactinoma. Prolactin may also have direct effects on the endometrium. Hirahara (1998) reported an increase in successful pregnancies in patients with hyperprolactinemia treated with the dopamine agonist bromocriptine. Although data are scarce, many experts still suggest measuring prolactin levels in patients with RPL.

Diabetes Mellitus

Insulin-dependent diabetes substantively increases risks for spontaneous abortion and major congenital malformations (Greene, 1999). This directly relates to the degree of periconceptional glycemic and metabolic control. Importantly, this risk is greatly mitigated with optimal metabolic control. In fact, the miscarriage rate in women with excellent control rivals that of nondiabetic women (Mills, 1988). Although diabetes itself is a recognized cause of RPL, diabetic women with recurrent loss may also have levels of insulin resistance greater than diabetic women without miscarriages (Craig, 2002). This suggests that ovarian insulin resistance may be in itself contributory, as discussed next.

Polycystic Ovarian Syndrome

Women with polycystic ovaries have generally been considered to carry an elevated miscarriage risk. However, this association has been questioned (Cocksedge, 2009). Inhibition of serum luteinizing hormone (LH) during a gonadotropin ovulation-induction cycle failed to improve pregnancy outcome in a controlled trial. This argued against a role for the elevated LH levels seen in PCOS (Clifford, 1996).

Data implicating hyperinsulinemia in pregnancy loss are somewhat stronger. Insulin modulates insulin-like growth factor actions in the ovary, thereby affecting folliculogenesis and steroid production. Retrospective and case-control studies concluded that metformin begun either before or during pregnancy decreases miscarriage rates in women with PCOS (Glueck, 2002; Nawaz, 2010). Metformin (Glucophage) lowers hepatic glucose production and increases insulin sensitivity and thereby lowers insulin levels. However, a systematic review of randomized trials found no improvement in abortion risk with metformin treatment (Palomba, 2009). At this time, routine metformin treatment for women with PCOS solely to treat pregnancy loss is not recommended.

■ Thrombophilias

Complexities of the coagulation cascade include several single-gene mutations that affect pro- or anticoagulant proteins. Mutations predisposing to thrombosis—collectively termed *thrombophilias*—are caused by mutations of the genes for factor V Leiden, prothrombin, antithrombin, and protein C and protein S. These are described further in Chapter 39 (p. 836). In the past, several of these thrombophilias were suspected to cause RPL. However, large prospective cohort studies have refuted these associations, and testing for these abnormalities for this indication is no longer recommended (American College of Obstetrics and Gynecologists, 2014d; American Society of Reproductive Medicine, 2012).

■ Evaluation and Treatment

Some considerations for evaluation and management of women with recurrent miscarriage are outlined in Table 6-9. Timing and extent of evaluation is based on maternal age, coexistent infertility, symptoms, and the level of patient anxiety. In our view, after a thorough history and clinical examination, a modicum of testing is done that is directed at likely causes. General testing may include parental karyotyping, uterine cavity evaluation, and testing for APS. There is progressively less support to screen for inherited thrombophilias, endocrine disorders, or luteal phase defect.

Unfortunately, a putative cause will be identified in only about half of couples with RPL. Empiric treatment for unexplained pregnancy loss is discouraged. Even for those with no explanatory findings, couples are cautiously assured that the chances of successfully achieving a live birth are reasonably good (Branch, 2010; Reddy, 2007). The results shown previously in Tables 6-5 and 6-6—while age dependent—forecast a reasonable prognosis for a successful subsequent pregnancy even after five recurrent losses. Although these couples are anxious to try any treatment, the lack of definitive benefits for many of these is carefully considered and appropriate counseling offered.

INDUCED ABORTION

■ Rates

The term *induced abortion* is defined as the medical or surgical termination of pregnancy before the time of fetal viability. Definitions to describe the incidence include the *abortion ratio,* which is the number of abortions per 1000 live births, and the *abortion rate,* which is the number of these per 1000 women aged 15 to 44 years.

In the United States, abortion statistics most likely are underreported. The Guttmacher Institute (2011) found that 1.2 million procedures were performed annually from 2005 through 2008. But for 2011, only about 730,322 elective abortions were reported to the CDC (Pazol, 2014). The calculated abortion ratio was 219 per 1000 live births, and the abortion rate was 13.9 per 1000 women aged 15 to 44 years. Women aged 20 to 29 years accounted for 58 percent of abortions and had the highest abortion rate. Of all abortions, 64 percent were done ≤8 weeks' gestation; 91 percent ≤13 weeks; 7 percent at 14 to 20 weeks; and only 1.4 percent were performed at ≥21 weeks.

Global statistics for abortion rates are reported by the WHO. According to its latest report, approximately 1 in 5 pregnancies were aborted worldwide in 2008 (Sedgh, 2012). Almost half of these procedures were considered unsafe.

TABLE 6-9. Tests Used for Evaluation of Couples with Recurrent Pregnancy Loss

Etiology	Diagnostic Evaluation	Possible Therapies
Genetic[a]	Karyotype partners	Genetic counseling, donor gametes
Anatomic[a]	Sonohysterography Hysterosalpingogram MR imaging	Septum transection, myomectomy, or adhesiolysis
Immunologic[a]	Lupus anticoagulant Anticardiolipin antibodies Anti-β2 glycoprotein-I antibody	Heparin + aspirin
Endocrinologic[b]	TSH Prolactin Fasting glucose, Hgb A_{1c} Day 3 FSH, estradiol Midluteal progesterone	Levothyroxine Dopamine agonist Metformin Counseling, PGD, donor oocyte IVF Progesterone
Thrombophilic[c]	Antithrombin deficiency Protein C or S deficiency Factor V Leiden mutation Prothrombin mutation Hyperhomocysteinemia	No proven treatment Folic acid
Toxic	Tobacco, alcohol use Exposure to toxins, chemicals Obesity	Eliminate consumption Behavior modification Weight loss

[a]Testing for these disorders is generally supported by the literature and expert opinion. One or a combination of these tests may be indicated.
[b]Ongoing controversy regarding testing.
[c]Current recommendations against testing. Included for historic reference.
FSH = follicle-stimulating hormone; IVF = in vitro fertilization; MR = magnetic resonance; PGD = pre-implantation diagnosis; TSH = thyroid-stimulating hormone.
Data from Brezina, 2013; Reddy, 2007; Fritz, 2011.

Classification

Abortions are performed for various indications that include social, economic, or emotional reasons. Although not formal categories, many choose to define induced abortion as: (1) indicated or therapeutic or (2) elective or voluntary.

First, medical and surgical disorders may provide a maternal-health indication for pregnancy termination. These include persistent cardiac decompensation, pulmonary arterial hypertension, advanced hypertensive vascular disease, diabetes with end-stage organ failure, and malignancy. In cases of rape or incest, most consider termination reasonable. The most common indication currently is to prevent birth of a fetus with a significant anatomic, metabolic, or mental deformity. Defining the seriousness of a fetal deformity is complicated by social, legal, and political mores.

The interruption of pregnancy before viability at the request of the woman, but not for medical reasons, is usually termed elective or voluntary abortion. Most abortions done today are elective, and thus, it is one of the most frequently performed procedures. From the Guttmacher Institute, Jones and Kavanaugh (2011) estimate that a third of American women will have at least one elective abortion by age 45.

Abortion in the United States

Legality

The legality of elective abortion was established by the United States Supreme Court in the case of *Roe v. Wade*. The Court defined the extent to which states might regulate abortion and ruled that first-trimester procedures must be left to the medical judgment of the physician. After this, the state could regulate abortion procedures in ways reasonably related to maternal health. Finally, subsequent to viability, the state could promote its interest in the potential of human life and regulate and even proscribe abortion, except for the preservation of the life or health of the mother.

Other legislation soon followed. The 1976 Hyde Amendment forbids use of federal funds to provide abortion services except in case of rape, incest, or life-threatening circumstances. The Supreme Court in 1992 reviewed *Planned Parenthood v. Casey* and upheld the fundamental right to abortion, but established that regulations before viability are constitutional as long as they do not impose an "undue burden" on the woman. Subsequently, many states passed legislation that imposes counseling requirements, waiting periods, parental consent or notification for minors, facility requirements, and funding restrictions. One major choice-limiting decision was the 2007 Supreme Court decision that reviewed *Gonzales v. Carhart* and upheld the 2003 Partial-Birth Abortion Ban Act. This was problematic because there is no medically approved definition of partial-birth abortion. According to the Guttmacher Institute, 41 states set new limits on abortion during 2011 and 2012 (Tanner, 2012). In two strongly worded Committee Opinions, the American College of Obstetricians and Gynecologists (2014a,c) calls for increased advocacy to overturn restrictions, improve access, and codify abortion as a fundamental component of women's health care. The College (2013e) supports the legal right of women to obtain an abortion prior to fetal viability and considers this a medical matter between a woman and her physician.

Training in Abortion Techniques

Because of its inherent controversial aspects, abortion training for residents and postgraduate fellows has been both championed and assailed. The Accreditation Council for Graduate Medical Education mandated in 1996 that Obstetrics and Gynecology residency education include access to experience with induced abortion. The American College of Obstetricians and Gynecologists (2014c) outlines legislative, institutional, and social barriers to abortion training and supports the use of "opt-out" programs. In these, abortion training is integrated as a standard part of the residency schedule, but residents with religious or moral objections can decline to participate. The Kenneth J. Ryan Residency Training Program was established in 1999 to improve residency training in abortion and family planning. By 2013, 59 Ryan programs had been started in the United States and in Canada. Disappointingly, a recent survey of United States residency programs determined that no abortion training was available in 16 percent of programs and that 30 percent continue to use the "opt-in" approach (Turk, 2014).

Other programs teach residents technical aspects through management of early incomplete and missed abortions and through pregnancy interruption for fetal death, severe fetal anomalies, and life-threatening medical or surgical disorders (Steinauer, 2005). Freedman and coworkers (2010) rightly emphasize that abortion training should include discussion of the social, moral, and ethical aspects of the procedure.

Formal fellowships in Family Planning are 2-year postgraduate programs. By 2010, these were located in 22 departments of obstetrics and gynecology at academic centers nationwide. Training includes experience with high-level research and with all methods of pregnancy prevention and termination.

Abortion Providers

The American College of Obstetricians and Gynecologists (2013f) respects the need and responsibility of health-care providers to determine their individual positions on induced abortion. It also emphasizes the need to provide standard-of-care counseling and timely referral if providers have individual beliefs that preclude pregnancy termination. From a mail survey of 1800 obstetrician-gynecologists, 97 percent had encountered women seeking an abortion, but only 14 percent performed them (Stulberg, 2011). Still, most practitioners help women find an abortion provider (Harris, 2011). In any event, any

physician who cares for women must be familiar with various abortion techniques so that complications can be managed or referrals made for suitable care.

■ Counseling before Elective Abortion

Three basic choices are available to a woman considering an abortion: (1) continued pregnancy with its risks and parental responsibilities; (2) continued pregnancy with arranged adoption; or (3) termination of pregnancy with its risks. Knowledgeable and compassionate counselors should objectively describe and provide information regarding these choices so that a woman or couple can make an informed decision (Baker, 2009; Templeton, 2011).

ABORTION TECHNIQUES

In the absence of serious maternal medical disorders, abortion procedures do not require hospitalization. With outpatient abortion, capabilities for cardiopulmonary resuscitation and for immediate transfer to a hospital must be available.

First-trimester abortion can be performed either medically or surgically by several methods that are listed in Table 6-10. Distinctive features of each technique were reviewed by the American College of Obstetricians and Gynecologists (2009). Results with either surgical or medical methods are comparable with those for spontaneous miscarriage as previously shown in Table 6-4. Both have a high success rate—95 percent with medical and 99 percent with surgical techniques.

With medical therapy, surgery is usually avoided as is the need for sedation (Table 6-11). Medical terminations have lower average costs and may allow for more privacy during the termination. However, medical abortion may extend for days up to a few weeks, bleeding is usually heavier and less predictable, and incomplete abortion is more common with medical versus surgical abortion (Niinimäki, 2009; Robson, 2009). Likely for these reasons, only 10 percent of abortions in the United States are managed using medical methods (Templeton, 2011).

TABLE 6-10. Techniques Used for First Trimester Abortion[a]

Approach	Technique
Surgical	Dilatation and curettage Vacuum aspiration Menstrual aspiration

Medical	Prostaglandins E_2, $F_{2\alpha}$, E_1, and analogues
	    Vaginal insertion
	    Parenteral injection
	    Oral ingestion
	Antiprogesterones—RU 486 (mifepristone)
	    and epostane
	Methotrexate—intramuscular or oral
	Various combinations of the above

[a]All procedures are aided by pretreatment using hygroscopic cervical dilators.

TABLE 6-11. Comparison of Medical versus Surgical Abortion

Factor	Medical	Surgical
Invasive	Usually no	Yes
Pain	More	Less
Vaginal bleeding	Prolonged, unpredictable	Light, predictable
Incomplete abortion	More common	Uncommon
Failure rate	2–5%	1%
Severe hemorrhage	0.1%	0.1%
Infection rate	Low	Low
Anesthesia	Usually none	Yes
Time involved	Multiple visits, follow-up exam	Usually one visit, no follow-up exam

Data from American College of Obstetricians and Gynecologists, 2015; Templeton, 2011.

◼ Surgical Abortion

Surgical pregnancy termination includes a transvaginal approach through an appropriately dilated cervix. Rarely, pregnancies are evacuated transabdominally by either hysterotomy or hysterectomy. Of transvaginal procedures, electric vacuum aspiration is the most commonly used form and is illustrated in Chapter 43 (p. 966). Alternatively, manual vacuum aspiration is done with a similar cannula that attaches to a handheld syringe for its vacuum source.

Cervical Preparation

For transvaginal evacuation, preoperative cervical ripening softens and slowly dilates the cervix to minimize trauma from mechanical dilatation. This preparation is typically associated with less pain, a technically easier procedure, and shorter operating times (Kapp, 2010). Of methods, hygroscopic dilators draw water from cervical tissues and expand to gradually dilate the cervix. One type is derived from various species of *Laminaria* algae that are harvested from the ocean floor (Chap. 43, p. 966). Another is *Dilapan-S,* which is composed of an acrylic-based gel.

Schneider and associates (1991) described 21 cases in which women who had a hygroscopic dilator placed changed their minds. Of 17 women who chose to continue their pregnancy, 14 carried to term, two delivered preterm, and one miscarried 2 weeks later. None suffered infection-related morbidity, including three untreated women with cervical cultures positive for *Chlamydia trachomatis.* In spite of this generally reassuring report, it seems prudent to presume irrevocability with regard to dilator placement and abortion.

Medications may also be used for cervical preparation. In the metaanalysis by Kapp (2010), efficacy of these medications was found to be similar to that of hygroscopic dilators. The most common is misoprostol (Cytotec), which is used off-label, and patients are counseled accordingly (Tang, 2013). The dose is 400 to 600 μg administered orally, sublingually, or placed into the posterior vaginal fornix (Meirik, 2012). Marginal benefits ascribed to misoprostol included easier cervical dilatation and a lower composite complication rate.

Another effective cervical-ripening agent is the progesterone antagonist *mifepristone* (Mifeprex). With this, 200 to 600 μg is given orally. Other options include formulations of *prostaglandins* E_2 and $F_{2\alpha}$, which have unpleasant side effects and are usually reserved as second-line drugs for cervical ripening (Kapp, 2010).

Electric Vacuum Aspiration

In this method, also known as dilatation and curettage (D & C), a rigid cannula attached to an electric-powered vacuum source empties the uterus. This may be coupled with sharp curettage. To begin, the surgeon first dilates the cervix. The pregnancy is then evacuated by suctioning out the contents—suction curettage, by mechanically scraping out the contents—sharp curettage, or both. Curettage—either sharp or suction—is recommended for gestations ≤15 weeks. According to one review, the use of suction curettage is superior if available (Tunçalp, 2010). Curettage usually requires sedation or analgesia. In addition to intravenously or orally administered sedatives, success has been reported with paracervical lidocaine blockade, with or without other analgesics (Renner, 2012). Perioperative antibiotic prophylaxis is also recommended as described on page 143.

Menstrual Aspiration

Aspiration of the endometrial cavity within 1 to 3 weeks after a missed menstrual period has been referred to as *menstrual extraction, menstrual induction, instant period, traumatic abortion,* and *mini-abortion.* The procedure is done using a flexible 5- or 6-mm Karman cannula and attached syringe. The primary drawbacks are that the small pregnancy may be missed or an ectopic pregnancy can be unrecognized. To identify placenta in the aspirate, MacIsaac and Darney (2000) recommend that the syringe contents be rinsed in a strainer to remove blood, then placed in a clear plastic container with saline and examined with back lighting. Placental tissue macroscopically appears soft, fluffy, and feathery. A magnifying lens, colposcope, or microscope also can improve visualization. Despite the possibility of missing the products, Paul and coworkers (2002) reported a 98-percent success rate with more than 1000 such procedures.

Manual Vacuum Aspiration

This procedure is similar to menstrual aspiration but is used for early pregnancy failures or elective termination up to 12 weeks. Some recommend that pregnancy terminations done in the office with this method be limited to ≤10 weeks because blood loss rises sharply between 10 and 12 weeks (Masch, 2005; Westfall, 1998). For pregnancies ≤8 weeks, preprocedure cervical ripening is usually not necessary. After this time, some recommend that osmotic dilators be placed the day prior to or misoprostol given 2 to 4 hours before the procedure. Paracervical blockade with or without sedation is used. The technique employs a hand-operated 60-mL syringe and cannula. A vacuum is created in the syringe attached to the cannula, which is inserted transcervically into the uterus. The vacuum produces up to 60 mm Hg suction. Complications are similar to other surgical methods (Goldberg, 2004).

■ Medical Abortion

Throughout history, many natural substances have been given for alleged abortifacient effects. Currently, only three medications for early medical abortion have been widely studied. These are used either alone or in combination and include: (1) the antiprogestin *mifepristone*, (2) the antimetabolite *methotrexate*, and (3) the prostaglandin *misoprostol*. Mifepristone and methotrexate increase uterine contractility by reversing progesterone-induced inhibition, whereas misoprostol directly stimulates the myometrium. Clark and associates (2006) have reported that mifepristone causes cervical collagen degradation, possibly from increased expression of matrix metalloproteinase. Methotrexate and misoprostol are both teratogens, thus there must be a commitment to completing the abortion once these drugs are given.

With these three agents, several dosing schemes are effective, and some are shown in Table 6-12. For these regimens, misoprostol is either given alone or given with methotrexate or mifepristone. As discussed on page 144 and previously shown in Table 6-4, any of several regimens used for "early pregnancy loss" are also likely to be successful for elective pregnancy interruption (American College of Obstetricians and Gynecologists, 2014e).

For elective termination at ≤63 days' gestation, randomized trials by von Hertzen (2009, 2010) and Winikoff (2008) and their colleagues showed 92- to 96-percent efficacy when one of the mifepristone/misoprostol regimens was used. Similar results were reported from 10 large urban Planned Parenthood clinics (Fjerstad, 2009). In this later study, buccal misoprostol-oral mifepristone regimens were 87- to 98-percent successful for abortion induction with pregnancies <10 weeks' gestation. This rate diminished with advancing gestations. In another study of 122 women at 9 to 12 weeks' gestation, the success rate was approximately 80 percent (Dalenda, 2010). According to the American College of Obstetricians and Gynecologists (2014e), outpatient medical abortion is an acceptable alternative to surgical pregnancy termination in appropriately selected pregnant women less than 49 days' menstrual age. After this time, available data—albeit less robust—support surgical abortion as preferable. Bleeding and cramping with medical termination can be significantly worse than menstrual cramps, thus adequate analgesia, usually including a narcotic, is provided.

Administration

With the mifepristone regimens, mifepristone treatment is followed by misoprostol given at that same time or up to 72 hours later. Some prefer that misoprostol be administered on site, after which the woman typically remains for 4 hours. Symptoms are common within 3 hours and included lower abdominal pain, vomiting, diarrhea, fever, and chills/shivering. In the first few hours after misoprostol is given, if the pregnancy appears to have been expelled, an examination is done to confirm expulsion. If the pregnancy has not been expelled, a pelvic examination is performed, and the patient is discharged and appointed to return in 1 to 2 weeks. At this time, if clinical or sonographic evaluation fails to confirm completed abortion, a suction procedure usually is recommended.

With the methotrexate regimens, misoprostol is given 3 to 7 days later, and women are seen again at least 24 hours after misoprostol administration. They are next seen approximately 7 days after methotrexate is given, and sonographic examination is performed. If an intact pregnancy is seen, then another dose of misoprostol is given. Afterward, the woman is seen again in 1 week if fetal cardiac activity is present or in 4 weeks

---

TABLE 6-12. Regimens for Medical Termination of Early Pregnancy

Mifepristone/Misoprostol
[a]Mifepristone, 100–600 mg orally followed by:
[b]Misoprostol, 200–600 μg orally or 400–800 μg vaginally, buccally, or sublingually given immediately or up to 72 hours

Methotrexate/Misoprostol
[c]Methotrexate, 50 mg/m^2 intramuscularly or orally followed by:
[d]Misoprostol, 800 μg vaginally in 3–7 days. Repeat if needed 1 week after methotrexate initially given

Misoprostol Alone
[e]800 μg vaginally or sublingually, repeated for up to three doses

[a]Doses of 200 versus 600 mg are similarly effective.
[b]Oral route may be less effective; possibly more side effects, namely, nausea and diarrhea. Sublingual route has more side effects than vaginal route. Shorter intervals (6 hours) with PGE$_1$ given after mifepristone may be less effective than when given >36 hours.
[c]Efficacy similar for routes of administration.
[d]Similar efficacy when given on day 3 versus day 5.
[e]Intervals of 3–24 hours if given vaginally; of 3–4 hours if given sublingually.
Data from Borgatta, 2001; Coyaji, 2007; Creinin, 2001, 2007; Fekih, 2010; Guest, 2007; Hamoda, 2005; Honkanen, 2004; Jain, 2002; Kulier, 2011; Pymar, 2001; Raghavan, 2009; Schaff, 2000; Shannon, 2006; von Hertzen, 2003, 2007, 2009, 2010; Winikoff, 2008.

if there is no heart motion. If abortion has not occurred by the second visit, it is usually completed by suction curettage.

With regimens using solely misoprostol, an initial 800-µg dose is repeated every 3 to 24 hr for up to three doses. Importantly, misoprostol-only regimens are associated with significantly higher continuing pregnancy rates (Grossman, 2004).

The American College of Obstetricians and Gynecologists (2014e) recommends that a woman be instructed to contact her provider during these regimens if bleeding soaks two or more pads per hour for at least 2 hours. The provider can then decide whether she needs to be seen. Similarly, patients should contact their health care provider if fever develops.

Unnecessary surgical intervention in women undergoing medical abortion can be avoided by the proper interpretation of follow-up sonographic results. Specifically, if no gestational sac is seen and there is no heavy bleeding, then intervention is unnecessary. This is true even when, as is common, the uterus contains sonographically evident debris. Another study reported that a multilayered sonographic pattern indicated a successful abortion (Tzeng, 2013). Assessment of the clinical course along with bimanual pelvic examination is generally adequate. Routine postabortal sonographic examination is unnecessary (Clark, 2010). Follow-up serum β-hCG levels have shown promise in preliminary investigations (Dayananda, 2013). Increasing evidence suggest that misoprostol is a safe and effective method to fully evacuate the uterus in the case of retained products following spontaneous or surgical abortion (American College of Obstetricians and Gynecologists, 2009).

Contraindications

In many cases, contraindications to medical abortion evolved from exclusion criteria that were used in initial clinical trials and should rightly be considered relative contraindications. These include: in situ intrauterine device; severe anemia, coagulopathy, or anticoagulant use; and significant medical conditions such as active liver disease, cardiovascular disease, or uncontrolled seizure disorders. Because misoprostol diminishes glucocorticoid activity, women with disorders requiring glucocorticoid therapy are usually excluded (American College of Obstetricians and Gynecologists, 2009). In women with renal insufficiency, the methotrexate dose is modified and given with caution, or preferably, another regimen is chosen (Kelly, 2006).

ABORTION CONSEQUENCES

Potential short-term morbidity of spontaneous and induced abortion includes retained tissue, hemorrhage, and infection in approximately equal frequency (Niinimäki, 2009; von Hertzen, 2010). In a review of more than 233,000 medical abortions, there were 1530 (0.65 percent) significant adverse events. Most of these were ongoing pregnancy (Cleland, 2013). As might be predicted, complication rates increase with progressing gestation in both spontaneous and induced abortions. For example, retained tissue occurs more frequently following second-trimester loss (40 percent) compared with earlier losses (17 percent) (van den Bosch, 2008).

Of long-term sequelae, abortion-related deaths are likely underreported (Horon, 2005). With this caveat in mind, mortality rates are exceeding low. Legally induced abortion, performed by trained gynecologists, especially when performed during the first 2 months of pregnancy, has a mortality rate of less than 1 per 100,000 procedures (Grimes, 2006; Pazol, 2014). Moreover, pregnancy-associated mortality is 14-fold greater than abortion-related mortality—8 versus 0.6 deaths per 100,000 (Raymond, 2012). Early abortions are even safer, and the relative mortality risk of abortion approximately doubles for each 2 weeks after 8 weeks' gestation. The CDC identified 10 abortion-related deaths in the United States in 2010 (Pazol, 2014).

Some data suggest that certain adverse pregnancy outcomes are more common in women who have had an induced abortion (Maconochie, 2007). Specifically, several studies note an approximate 1.5-fold increased incidence of preterm delivery at 22 to 32 weeks (Hardy, 2013; Moreau, 2005; Swingle, 2009). One systematic review of 37 studies noted a significantly increased 1.35-fold risk for subsequent low-birthweight and preterm deliveries after one pregnancy termination (Shah, 2009). These risks rose along with an increased number of procedures. Multiple sharp curettage procedures may raise the subsequent risk of placenta previa, whereas vacuum aspiration procedures likely do not (Johnson, 2003). Other studies suggest that subsequent pregnancy outcomes are similar regardless of whether a prior induced abortion was completed medically or surgically (Virk, 2007).

The rates of infertility or ectopic pregnancy do not appear to be significantly increased by prior abortion. There may be exceptions if there are postabortal infections, especially those caused by chlamydial species. It may be reasonable to compare women undergoing a pregnancy termination with those having a first-trimester miscarriage, in whom the 5-year live-birth rate was approximately 80 percent following pregnancy loss (Smith, 2009).

Data relating induced abortion to overall maternal health are limited. In one case-control study, there was no evidence for excessive mental health disorders (Munk-Olsen, 2011). A review by the American College of Obstetricians and Gynecologists (2013a) concluded that there is no causal relationship between prior induced abortion and breast cancer risk.

POSTABORTAL CONTRACEPTION

Ovulation may resume as early as 2 weeks after an early pregnancy loss, whether spontaneous or induced. Lahteenmaki and Luukkainen (1978) detected LH surges 16 to 22 days after abortion in 15 of 18 women studied. Plasma progesterone levels, which had plummeted after the abortion, increased soon after the LH surges. These hormonal events agree with histological changes observed in endometrial biopsies (Boyd, 1972).

Accordingly, effective contraception should be initiated soon after abortion unless another pregnancy is desired immediately. An intrauterine device can be inserted after the procedure is completed (Bednarek, 2011; Shimoni, 2011). Alternatively, any of the hormonal contraceptive methods discussed in Chapter 5 can be initiated at this time (Madden, 2009; Reeves, 2007).

REFERENCES

Abbassi-Ghanavati M, Casey BM, Spong CY, et al: Pregnancy outcomes in women with thyroid peroxidase antibodies. Obstet Gynecol 116:381, 2010

Al Arfaj AS, Khalil N: Pregnancy outcome in 396 pregnancies in patients with SLE in Saudi Arabia. Lupus 19:1665, 2010

Al-Inany H: Intrauterine adhesions. An update. Acta Obstet Gynecol Scand 80:986, 2001

American College of Obstetricians and Gynecologists: Abortion training and education. Committee Opinion No. 612, November 2014a

American College of Obstetricians and Gynecologists: Antibiotic prophylaxis for gynecologic procedures. Practice Bulletin No. 104, May 2009, Reaffirmed 2014b

American College of Obstetricians and Gynecologists: Antiphospholipid syndrome. Practice Bulletin No. 132, December 2012

American College of Obstetricians and Gynecologists: Early pregnancy loss. Practice Bulletin No. 150, May 2015

American College of Obstetricians and Gynecologists: Increasing access to abortion. Committee Opinion No. 613, November 2014c

American College of Obstetricians and Gynecologists: Induced abortion and breast cancer risk. Committee Opinion No. 434, June 2009, Reaffirmed 2013a

American College of Obstetricians and Gynecologists: Inherited thrombophilias in pregnancy. Practice Bulletin No. 138, September 2013, Reaffirmed 2014d

American College of Obstetricians and Gynecologists: Medical management of first-trimester abortion. Practice Bulletin No. 143, March 2014e

American College of Obstetricians and Gynecologists: Misoprostol for postabortion care. Committee Opinion No. 427, February 2009

American College of Obstetricians and Gynecologists: Moderate caffeine consumption during pregnancy. Committee Opinion No. 462, August 2010, Reaffirmed 2013b

American College of Obstetricians and Gynecologists: Nonobstetric surgery during pregnancy. Committee Opinion No. 474, February 2011, Reaffirmed 2013c

American College of Obstetricians and Gynecologists: Obesity in pregnancy. Committee Opinion No. 549, January 2013d

American College of Obstetricians and Gynecologists: Prevention of Rh D alloimmunization. Practice Bulletin No. 4, May 1999, Reaffirmed 2013e

American College of Obstetricians and Gynecologists: The limits of conscientious refusal in reproductive medicine. Committee Opinion No. 385, November 2007, Reaffirmed 2013f

American Society for Reproductive Medicine: Definitions of infertility and recurrent pregnancy loss. Fertil Steril 99(1):63, 2013

American Society for Reproductive Medicine: Evaluation and treatment of recurrent pregnancy loss: a committee opinion. Fertil Steril 98(5):1103, 2012

Andersen AE, Ryan GL: Eating disorders in the obstetric and gynecologic patient population. Obstet Gynecol 114(6):1353, 2009

Andersen AM, Andersen PK, Olsen J, et al: Moderate alcohol intake during pregnancy and risk of fetal death. Int J Epidemiol 41(2):405, 2012

Andersen SL, Olsen J, Wu CS, et al: Spontaneous abortion, stillbirth and hyperthyroidism: a Danish population-based study. Eur Thyroid J 3(3):164, 2014

Armstrong BG, McDonald AD, Sloan M: Cigarette, alcohol, and coffee consumption and spontaneous abortion. Am J Public Health 82:85, 1992

Arredondo F, Noble LS: Endocrinology of recurrent pregnancy loss. Semin Reprod Med 1:33, 2006

Baker A, Beresford T: Informed consent, patient education, and counseling. In Paul M, Lichtenberg ES, Borgatta L, et al (eds): Management of Unintended and Abnormal Pregnancy. West Sussex, Wiley-Blackwell, 2009, p 48

Barber JC, Cockwell AE, Grant E: Is karyotyping couples experiencing recurrent miscarriage worth the cost? BJOG 117:885, 2010

Barlow S, Sullivan FM: Reproductive Hazards of Industrial Chemicals: an Evaluation of Animal and Human Data. New York, Academic Press, 1982

Barnhart K, Mennuti MT, Benjamin I, et al: Prompt diagnosis of ectopic pregnancy in an emergency department setting. Obstet Gynecol 84(6):1010, 1994

Barnhart K, Sammel MD, Chung K, et al: Decline of serum human chorionic gonadotropin and spontaneous complete abortion: defining the normal curve. Obstet Gynecol 104:975, 2004

Barnhart K, van Mello NM, Bourne T, et al: Pregnancy of unknown location: a consensus statement of nomenclature, definitions, and outcome. Fertil Steril 95(3):857, 2011

Barnhart KT, Sammel MD, Appleby D, et al: Does a prediction model for pregnancy of unknown location developed in the UK validate on a US population? Hum Reprod 25(10):2434, 2010

Barrett JP, Whiteside JL, Boardman LA: Fatal clostridial sepsis after spontaneous abortion. Obstet Gynecol 99:899, 2002

Baud D, Goy G, Jaton K, et al: Role of Chlamydia trachomatis in miscarriage. Emerg Infect Dis 17(9):1630, 2011

Bednarek PH, Creinin MD, Reeves MF, et al: Immediate versus delayed IUD insertion after uterine aspiration. N Engl J Med 364(21):2208, 2011

Belloc S, Cohen-Bacrie P, Benkhalifa M, et al: Effect of maternal and paternal age on pregnancy and miscarriage rates after intrauterine insemination. Reprod Biomed Online 17(3):392, 2008

Bellver J, Ayllón Y, Ferrando M, et al: Female obesity impairs in vitro fertilization outcome without affecting embryo quality. Fertil Steril 93(2):447, 2010a

Bellver J, Meseguer M, Muriel L, et al: Y chromosome microdeletions, sperm DNA fragmentation and sperm oxidative stress as causes of recurrent spontaneous abortion of unknown etiology. Hum Reprod 25(7):1713, 2010b

Berger DS, Hogge WA, Barmada MM, et al: Comprehensive analysis of HLA-G: implications for recurrent spontaneous abortion. Reprod Sci 17(4):331, 2010

Bhattacharya S, Townend J, Bhattacharya S: Recurrent miscarriage: are three miscarriages one too many? Analysis of a Scottish population-based database of 151,021 pregnancies. Eur J Obstet Gynecol Reprod Biol 150:24, 2010

Bianco K, Caughey AB, Shaffer BL, et al: History of miscarriage and increased incidence of fetal aneuploidy in subsequent pregnancy. Obstet Gynecol 107:1098, 2006

Bick RL, Baker WF Jr: Hereditary and acquired thrombophilia in pregnancy. In Bick RL (ed): Hematological Complications in Obstetrics, Pregnancy, and Gynecology. United Kingdom, Cambridge University Press, 2006, p 122

Boots CE, Bernardi LA, Stephenson MD: Frequency of euploid miscarriage is increased in obese women with recurrent early pregnancy loss. Fertil Steril 102(2):455, 2014

Borgatta L, Burnhill MS, Tyson J, et al: Early medical abortion with methotrexate and misoprostol. Obstet Gynecol 97:11, 2001

Boyd EF Jr, Holmstrom EG: Ovulation following therapeutic abortion. Am J Obstet Gynecol 113:469, 1972

Branch DW, Gibson M, Silver RM: Recurrent miscarriage. N Engl J Med 363:18, 2010

Brent RL: Saving lives and changing family histories: appropriate counseling of pregnant women and men and women of reproductive age, concerning the risk of diagnostic radiation exposures during and before pregnancy. Am J Obstet Gynecol 200(1):4, 2009

Brezina PR, Kutteh WH: Classic and cutting-edge strategies for the management of early pregnancy loss. Obstet Gynecol Clin North Am 41(1):1, 2014

Brigham SA, Conlon C, Farquharson RG: A longitudinal study of pregnancy outcome following idiopathic recurrent miscarriage. Hum Reprod 14(11):2868, 1999

Brown ZA, Selke S, Zeh J, et al: The acquisition of herpes simplex virus during pregnancy. N Engl J Med 337:509, 1997

Buttram VC Jr, Gibbons WE: Mullerian anomalies: a proposed classification (an analysis of 144 cases). Fertil Steril 32(1):40, 1979

Canobbio MM, Mair DD, van der Velde M, et al: Pregnancy outcomes after the Fontan repair. J Am Coll Cardiol 28(3):763, 1996

Casey BM, Dashe JS, Wells CE, et al: Subclinical hypothyroidism and pregnancy outcomes. Obstet Gynecol 105(2):239, 2005

Castañeda R, Lechuga D, Ramos RI, et al: Endemic goiter in pregnant women: utility of the simplified classification of thyroid size by palpation and urinary iodine as screening tests. BJOG 109:1366, 2002

Catov JM, Nohr EA, Olsen J, et al: Chronic hypertension related to risk for preterm and term small for gestational age births. Obstet Gynecol 112(2 pt 1):290, 2008

Cavallo F, Russo R, Zotti C, et al: Moderate alcohol consumption and spontaneous abortion. Alcohol 30:195, 1995

Centers for Disease Control and Prevention: Clostridium sordellii toxic shock syndrome after medical abortion with mifepristone and intravaginal misoprostol—United States and Canada, 2001–2005. MMWR 54(29):724, 2005

Chen L, Hu R: Thyroid autoimmunity and miscarriage: a meta-analysis. Clin Endocrinol 74(4):513, 2011

Clark CA, Spitzer KA, Crowther MA, et al: Incidence of postpartum thrombosis and preterm delivery in women with antiphospholipid antibodies and recurrent pregnancy loss. J Rheumatol 34(5):992, 2007a

Clark EA, Silver RM, Branch DW: Do antiphospholipid antibodies cause preeclampsia and HELLP syndrome? Curr Rheumatol Rep 9:219, 2007b

Clark K, Ji H, Feltovich H et al: Mifepristone-induced cervical ripening: structural, biomechanical, and molecular events. Am J Obstet Gynecol 194:1391, 2006

Clark W, Bracken H, Tanenhaus J, et al: Alternatives to a routine follow-up visit for early medical abortion. Obstet Gynecol 115(2 Pt 1):264, 2010

Cleland K, Creinin M, Nucatola D, et al: Significant adverse events and outcomes after medical abortion. Obstet Gynecol 121(1):166, 2013

Clifford K, Rai R, Watson H, et al: Does suppressing luteinizing hormone secretion reduce the miscarriage rate? Results of a randomized controlled trial. BMJ 312:1508, 1996

Clowse ME, Jamison M, Myers E, et al: A national study of the complications of lupus in pregnancy. Am J Obstet Gynecol 199:127.e1, 2008

Cnattingius S, Signorello LB, Anneren G, et al: Caffeine intake and the risk of first-trimester spontaneous abortion. N Engl J Med 343:1839, 2000

Cocksedge KA, Saravelos SH, Metwally M, et al: How common is polycystic ovary syndrome in recurrent miscarriage? Reprod Biomed Online 19(4):572, 2009

Condous G, Okaro E, Khalid A, Bourne T: Do we need to follow up complete miscarriages with serum human chorionic gonadotrophin levels? BJOG 112:827, 2005

Condous G, Van Calster B, Kirk E, et al: Clinical information does not improve the performance of mathematical models in predicting the outcome of pregnancies of unknown location. Fertil Steril 88(3):572, 2007

Connolly A, Ryan DH, Stuebe AM, et al: Reevaluation of discriminatory and threshold levels for serum β-hCG in early pregnancy. Obstet Gynecol 121(1):65, 2013

Coyaji K, Krishna U, Ambardekar S, et al: Are two doses of misoprostol after mifepristone for early abortion better than one? BJOG 114(3):271, 2007

Craig TB, Ke RW, Kutteh WH: Increase prevalence of insulin resistance in women with a history of recurrent pregnancy loss. Fertil Steril 78:487, 2002

Creinin MD, Huang X, Westhoff C, et al: Factors related to successful misoprostol treatment for early pregnancy failure. Obstet Gynecol 107:901, 2006

Creinin MD, Pymar HC, Schwartz JL: Mifepristone 100 mg in abortion regimens. Obstet Gynecol 98:434, 2001

Creinin MD, Schreiber CA, Bednarek P, et al: Mifepristone and misoprostol administered simultaneously versus 24 hours apart for abortion: a randomized controlled trial. Obstet Gynecol 109(4):885, 2007

Cunningham FG, Leveno KL, Bloom SL, et al (eds): Williams Obstetrics, 24th ed. New York, McGraw-Hill, 2014, pp 267, 350

Daif JL, Levie M, Chudnoff S, et al: Group A Streptococcus causing necrotizing fasciitis and toxic shock syndrome after medical termination of pregnancy. Obstet Gynecol 113(2 Pt 2):504, 2009

Dalenda C, Ines N, Fathia B, et al: Two medical abortion regimens for late first-trimester termination of pregnancy: a prospective randomized trial. Contraception 81(4):323, 2010

Dao B, Blum J, Thieba B, et al: Is misoprostol a safe, effective and acceptable alternative to manual vacuum aspiration for postabortion care? Results from a randomized trial in Burkina Faso, West Africa. BJOG 114(11):1368, 2007

Dayananda I, Maurer R, Fortin J, et al: Medical abortion follow-up serum human chorionic gonadotropin compared with ultrasonography. Obstet Gynecol 121(3):607, 2013

Devaseelan P, Fogarty PP, Regan L: Human chorionic gonadotropin for threatened abortion. Cochrane Database Syst Rev 5:DC007422, 2010

Devi Wold AS, Pham N, Arici A: Anatomic factors in recurrent pregnancy loss. Semin Reprod Med 1:25, 2006

De Vivo A, Mancuso A, Giacobbe A, et al: Thyroid function in women found to have early pregnancy loss. Thyroid 20(6):633, 2010

Di Simone N, Meroni PL, D'Asta M, et al: Pathogenic role of anti-beta2-glycoprotein I antibodies on human placenta: functional effects related to implantation and roles of heparin. Hum Reprod Update 13(2):189, 2007

Doubilet PM, Benson CB, Bourne T, et al: Diagnostic criteria for nonviable pregnancy early in the first trimester. N Engl J Med 369(15):1443, 2014

Dranitsaris G, Johnston M, Poirier S, et al: Are health care providers who work with cancer drugs at an increased risk for toxic events? A systematic review and meta-analysis of the literature. J Oncol Pharm Pract 2:69, 2005

Dukhovny S, Zutshi P, Abbott JF: Recurrent second trimester pregnancy loss: evaluation and management. Curr Opin Endocrinol Diabetes Obes 16:451, 2009

Edwards DR, Aldridge T, Baird DD, et al: Periconceptional over-the-counter nonsteroidal anti-inflammatory drug exposure and risk for spontaneous abortion. Obstet Gynecol 120(1):113, 2012

Eiben B, Bartels I, Bahr-Prosch S, et al: Cytogenetic analysis of 750 spontaneous abortions with the direct-preparation method of chorionic villi and its implications for studying genetic causes of pregnancy wastage. Am J Hum Genet 47:656, 1990

Empson M, Lassere M, Craig J, et al: Prevention of recurrent miscarriage for women with antiphospholipid antibody or lupus anticoagulant. Cochrane Database Syst Rev (2):CD002859, 2005. Edited with no change in conclusions, Issue 2, 2012

Erkan D, Kozora E, Lockshin MD: Cognitive dysfunction and white matter abnormalities in antiphospholipid syndrome. Pathophysiology 18(1):93, 2011

Eskenazi B, Chevrier J, Rosas LG, et al: The Pine River statement: human health consequences of DDT use. Environ Health Perspect 117(9):1359, 2009

Fantel AG, Shepard TH, Vadheim-Roth C, et al: Embryonic and fetal phenotypes: prevalence and other associated factors in a large study of spontaneous abortion. In Porter IH, Hook EM (eds): Human Embryonic and Fetal Death. New York, Academic Press, 1980, p 71

Fekih M, Fathallah K, Ben Regaya L, et al: Sublingual misoprostol for first trimester termination of pregnancy. Int J Gynaecol Obstet 109(1):67, 2010

Feldman DM, Timms D, Borgida AF: Toxoplasmosis, parvovirus, and cytomegalovirus in pregnancy. Clin Lab Med 30(3):709, 2010

Feodor Nilsson S, Andersen PK, Strandberg-Larsen K, et al: Risk factors for miscarriage from a prevention perspective: a nationwide follow-up study. BJOG 121(11):1375, 2014

Fischer J, Colls P, Esudero T, et al: Preimplantation genetic diagnosis (PGD) improves pregnancy outcome for translocation carriers with a history of recurrent losses. Fertil Steril 94(1):283, 2010

Fischer M, Bhatnagar J, Guarner J, et al: Fatal toxic shock syndrome associated with Clostridium sordellii after medical abortion. N Engl J Med 353:2352, 2005

Fjerstad M, Sivin I, Lichtenberg ES, et al: Effectiveness of medical abortion with mifepristone and buccal misoprostol through 59 gestational days. Contraception 80(3):282, 2009

Floyd RL, Decoufle P, Hungerford DW: Alcohol use prior to pregnancy recognition. Am J Prev Med 17:101, 1999

Franssen MTM, Korevaar JC, van der Veen F, et al: Reproductive outcome after chromosome analysis in couples with two or more miscarriages: case-control study. BMJ 332:750, 2006

Freedman L, Landy U, Steinauer J: Obstetrician-gynecologist experiences with abortion training: physician insights from a qualitative study. Contraception 81(6):525, 2010

Fritz MA, Speroff L, (eds): Recurrent early pregnancy loss. In Clinical Gynecologic Endocrinology and Infertility, 8th ed. Philadelphia, Lippincott Williams & Wilkins, 2011, p 1220

Ganer H, Levy A, Ohel I, et al: Pregnancy outcome in women with an intrauterine contraceptive device. Am J Obstet Gynecol 201:381.e1, 2009

Gao J, Liu C, Yao F, et al: Array-based comparative genomic hybridization is more informative than conventional karyotyping and fluorescence in situ hybridization in the analysis of first-trimester spontaneous abortion. Mol Cytogenet 5(1):33, 2012

Glueck CJ, Want P, Goldenberg N, et al: Pregnancy outcomes among women with polycystic ovary syndrome treated with metformin. Hum Reprod 17:2858, 2002

Goldberg AB, Dean G, Kang MS, et al: Manual versus electric vacuum aspiration for early first-trimester abortion: a controlled study of complication rates. Obstet Gynecol 103:101, 2004

Goldenberg M, Sivan E, Sharabi Z, et al: Reproductive outcome following hysteroscopic management of intrauterine septum and adhesions. Hum Reprod 10:2663, 1995

Gracia CR, Sammel MD, Chittams J, et al: Risk factors for spontaneous abortion in early symptomatic first-trimester pregnancies. Obstet Gynecol 106:993, 2005

Greene MF: Spontaneous abortions and major malformations in women with diabetes mellitus. Semin Reprod Endocrinol 17:127, 1999

Grimes DA: Estimation of pregnancy-related mortality risk by pregnancy outcome, United States, 1991 to 1999. Am J Obstet Gynecol 194:92, 2006

Grossman D: Medical methods for first trimester abortion: Reproductive Health Library practical aspects. Geneva, World Health Organization, 2004

Guelinckx I, Devlieger R, Vansant G: Reproductive outcome after bariatric surgery: a critical review. Hum Reprod Update 15(2):189, 2009

Guest J, Chien PF, Thomson MA, et al: Randomised controlled trial comparing the efficacy of same-day administration of mifepristone and misoprostol for termination of pregnancy with the standard 36 to 48 hour protocol. BJOG 114(2):207, 2007

Guttmacher Institute: US abortion rate levels off after 30-year decline. Reuters Health Information, January 12, 2011

Haddow JE, McClain MR, Palomaki GE, et al: Thyroperoxidase and thyroglobulin antibodies in early pregnancy and placental abruption. Obstet Gynecol 117:287, 2011

Hamoda H, Ashok PW, Flett GMM, Templeton A: A randomised controlled trial of mifepristone in combination with misoprostol administered sublingually or vaginally for medical abortion up to 13 weeks of gestation. BJOG 112:1102, 2005

Hannafin B, Lovecchio F, Blackburn P: Do Rh-negative women with first trimester spontaneous abortions need Rh immune globulin? Am J Obstet Gynecol 24:487, 2006

Hardy G, Benjamin A, Abenhaim HA. Effect of induced abortions on early preterm births and adverse perinatal outcomes. J Obstet Gynaecol Can 35(2):138, 2013

Harris LH, Cooper A, Rasinski KA, et al: Obstetrician-gynecologists' objections to and willingness to help patients obtain an abortion. Obstet Gynecol 118(4):905, 2011

Hasan R, Baird DD, Herring AH, et al: Association between first-trimester vaginal bleeding and miscarriage. Obstet Gynecol 114:860, 2009

Helgstrand S, Andersen AM: Maternal underweight and the risk of spontaneous abortion. Acta Obstet Gynecol Scand 84(12):1197, 2005

Heuser C, Dalton J, Macpherson C, et al: Idiopathic recurrent pregnancy loss recurs at similar gestational ages. Am J Obstet Gynecol 203(4):343.e1, 2010

Hide G, Morley EK, Hughes JM, et al: Evidence for high levels of vertical transmission in *Toxoplasma gondii*. Parasitology 136(14):1877, 2009

Hirahara F, Andoh N, Sawai K, et al: Hyperprolactinemic recurrent miscarriage and results of randomized bromocriptine treatment trials. Fertil Steril 70(2):246, 1998

Ho CS, Bhatnagar J, Cohen AL, et al: Undiagnosed cases of fatal *Clostridium*-associated toxic shock in Californian women of childbearing age. Am J Obstet Gynecol 201:459.e1, 2009

Homer H, Saridogan E: Uterine artery embolization for fibroids is associated with an increased risk of miscarriage. Fertil Steril 94(1):324, 2010

Honkanen H, Piaggio G, Hertzen H, et al: WHO multinational study of three misoprostol regimens after mifepristone for early medical abortion. BJOG 111(7):715, 2004

Horon IL: Underreporting of maternal deaths on death certificates and the magnitude of the problem of maternal mortality. Am J Public Health 95:478, 2005

Hudson MM: Reproductive outcomes for survivors of childhood cancer. Obstet Gynecol 116:1171, 2010

Jacobs PA, Hassold TJ: The origin of chromosomal abnormalities in spontaneous abortion. In Porter IH, Hook EB (eds): Human Embryonic and Fetal Death. New York, Academic Press, 1980, p 289

Jain JK, Harwood B, Meckstroth KR, et al: A prospective randomized, double-blinded, placebo-controlled trial comparing mifepristone and vaginal misoprostol to vaginal misoprostol alone for elective termination of early pregnancy. Hum Reprod 17:1477, 2002

Jaslow CR, Carney JL, Kutteh WH: Diagnostic factors identified in 1020 women with two versus three or more recurrent pregnancy losses. Fertil Steril 93(4):1234, 2010

Johns J, Jauniaux E: Threatened miscarriage as a predictor of obstetric outcome. Obstet Gynecol 107:845, 2006

Johnson LG, Mueller BA, Daling JR: The relationship of placenta previa and history of induced abortion. Int J Gynaecol Obstet 81:191, 2003

Jones RK, Kavanaugh ML: Changes in abortion rates between 2000 and 2008 and lifetime incidence of abortion. Obstet Gynecol 117(6):1358, 2011

Jun SH, Ginsburg ES, Racowsky C, et al: Uterine leiomyomas and their effect on in vitro fertilization outcome: a retrospective study. J Assist Reprod Genet 18:139, 2001

Kadar N, DeCherney AH, Romero R: Receiver operating characteristic (ROC) curve analysis of the relative efficacy of single and serial chorionic gonadotropin determinations in the early diagnosis of ectopic pregnancy. Fertil Steril 37:542, 1982

Kajii T, Ferrier A, Niikawa N, et al: Anatomic and chromosomal anomalies in 639 spontaneous abortions. Hum Genet 55:87, 1980

Kapp N, Lohr PA, Ngo TD, et al: Cervical preparation for first trimester surgical abortion. Cochrane Database Syst Rev 2:CD007207, 2010

Katz A, Ben-Arie A, Lurie S, et al: Reproductive outcome following hysteroscopic adhesiolysis in Asherman's syndrome. Int J Fertil Menopausal Stud 41:462, 1996

Kelly H, Harvey D, Moll S: A cautionary tale. Fatal outcome of methotrexate therapy given for management of ectopic pregnancy. Obstet Gynecol 107:439, 2006

Kesmodel U, Wisborg K, Olsen SF, et al: Moderate alcohol intake in pregnancy and the risk of spontaneous abortion. Alcohol 37:87, 2002

Kharazmi E, Dossus L, Rohrmann S, et al: Pregnancy loss and risk of cardiovascular disease: a prospective population-based cohort study (EPIC-Heidelberg). Heart 97(1):49, 2011

Khashan AS, Quigley EMM, McNamee R, et al: Increased risk of miscarriage and ectopic pregnancy among women with irritable bowel syndrome. Clin Gastroenterol Hepatol 10(8):902, 2012

Kleinhaus K, Perrin M, Friedlander Y, et al: Paternal age and spontaneous abortion. Obstet Gynecol 108:369, 2006

Krassas GE, Poppe K, Glinoer D: Thyroid function and human reproductive health. Endo Rev 31:702, 2010

Kulier R, Kapp N, Gülmezoglu AM, et al: Medical methods for first trimester abortion. Cochrane Database Syst Rev 11:CD002855, 2011

Kutteh WH, Hinote CD: Antiphospholipid antibody syndrome. Obstet Gynecol Clin North Am 41(1):113, 2014

Lahteenmaki P, Luukkainen T: Return of ovarian function after abortion. Clin Endocrinol 2:123, 1978

Lis R, Rowhani-Rahbar A, Manhart LE: *Mycoplasma genitalium* infection and female reproductive tract disease: a meta-analysis. Clin Infect Dis 61(3):418, 2015

Lui S, Song L, Cram DS, et al: Traditional karyotyping versus copy number variation sequencing for detection of chromosomal abnormalities associated with spontaneous miscarriage. Ultrasound Obstet Gynecol March 13, 2015 [Epub ahead of print]

Luise C, Jermy K, May C, et al: Outcome of expectant management of spontaneous first trimester miscarriage: observational study. BMJ 324:873, 2002

Lupo PJ, Symanski E, Waller DK, et al: Maternal exposure to ambient levels of benzene and neural tube defects among offspring, Texas, 1999–2004. Environ Health Perspect 119:397, 2011

Lykke JA, Dideriksen KL, Lidegaard Ø, et al: First-trimester vaginal bleeding and complications later in pregnancy. Obstet Gynecol 115:935, 2010

MacIsaac L, Darney P: Early surgical abortion: an alternative to and backup for medical abortion. Am J Obstet Gynecol 183:S76, 2000

Maconochie N, Doyle P, Prior S, et al: Risk factors for first trimester miscarriage—results from a UK-population-based case-control study. BJOG 114:170, 2007

Madden T, Westhoff C: Rates of follow-up and repeat pregnancy in the 12 months after first-trimester induced abortion. Obstet Gynecol 113:663, 2009

Masch RJ, Roman AS: Uterine evacuation in the office. Contemp Obstet Gynecol 51:66–73, 2005

Mazze RI, Källén B: Reproductive outcome after anesthesia and operation during pregnancy: a registry study of 5405 cases. Am J Obstet Gynecol 161:1178, 1989

McMillan M, Porritt K, Kralik D, et al: Influenza vaccination during pregnancy: a systematic review of fetal death, spontaneous abortion, and congenital malformation safety outcomes. Vaccine 33(18):2108, 2015

Meirik O, My Huong NT, Piaggio G, et al: Complications of first-trimester abortion by vacuum aspiration after cervical preparation with and without misoprostol: a multicentre randomized trial. Lancet 379:1817, 2012

Meites E, Zane S, Gould C: Fatal *Clostridium sordellii* infections after medical abortions. N Engl J Med 363:1382, 2010

Meroni PL, Tedesco F, Locati M, et al: Anti-phospholipid antibody mediated fetal loss: still an open question from a pathogenic point of view. Lupus 19:453, 2010

Metwally M, Saravelos SH, Ledger WL, et al: Body mass index and risk of miscarriage in women with recurrent miscarriage. Fertil Steril 94(1):290, 2010

Miyakis S, Lockshin MD, Atsumi T, et al: International consensus statement on an update of the classification criteria for definite antiphospholipid syndrome (APS). J Thromb Haemost 4:295, 2006

Mills JL, Simpson JL, Driscoll SG, et al: Incidence of spontaneous abortion among normal women and insulin-dependent diabetic women whose pregnancies were identified within 21 days of conception. N Engl J Med 319:1618, 1988

Moreau C, Kaminski M, Ancel PY, et al: Previous induced abortions and the risk of very preterm delivery: results of the EPIPAGE study. BJOG 112:430, 2005

Moschos E, Twickler DM: Intrauterine devices in early pregnancy: findings on ultrasound and clinical outcomes. Am J Obstet Gynecol 204:427.e1–6, 2011

Munk-Olsen T, Laursen TM, Pedersen CB, et al: Induced first-trimester abortion and risk of mental disorder. N Engl J Med 364(4):332, 2011

Nahum GG: Uterine anomalies. How common are they, and what is their distribution among subtypes? J Reprod Med 43(10):877, 1998

Nawaz FH, Rizvi J: Continuation of metformin reduces early pregnancy loss in obese Pakistani women with polycystic ovarian syndrome. Gynecol Obstet Invest 69(3):184, 2010

Negro R, Formoso G, Mangieri T, et al: Levothyroxine treatment in euthyroid pregnant women with autoimmune thyroid disease: effects on obstetrical complications. J Clin Endocrinol Metab 91(7):2587, 2006

Negro R, Schwartz A, Gismondi R, et al: Universal screening versus case finding for detection and treatment of thyroid hormonal dysfunction during pregnancy. J Clin Endocrinol Metab 95(4):1699, 2010

Neilson JP, Gyte GM, Hickey M, et al: Medical treatments for incomplete miscarriage (less than 24 weeks). Cochrane Database Syst Rev 3:CD007223, 2013

Ness RB, Grisso JA, Hirschinger N, et al: Cocaine and tobacco use and the risk of spontaneous abortion. N Engl J Med 340(5):333, 1999

Nguyen NT, Blum J, Durocher J, et al: A randomized controlled study comparing 600 versus 1200 μg oral misoprostol for medical management of incomplete abortion. Contraception 72:438, 2005

Nielsen A, Hannibal CG, Lindekilde BE, et al: Maternal smoking predicts the risk of spontaneous abortion. Acta Obstet Gynecol Scand 85(9):1057, 2006

Niinimäki M, Pouta A, Bloigu A, et al: Immediate complications after medical compared with surgical termination of pregnancy. Obstet Gynecol 114:795, 2009

Nurmohamed L, Moretti ME, Schechter T, et al: Outcome following high-dose methotrexate in pregnancies misdiagnosed as ectopic. Am J Obstet Gynecol 205:533.e1, 2011

Oakeshott P, Hay P, Hay S, et al: Association between bacterial vaginosis or chlamydial infection and miscarriage before 16 weeks' gestation: prospective, community based cohort study. BMJ 325:1334, 2002

Palomba S, Falbo A, Orio F Jr, et al: Effect of preconceptional metformin on abortion risk in polycystic ovary syndrome: a systematic review and meta-analysis of randomized controlled trials. Fertil Steril 92(5):1646, 2009

Paul ME, Mitchell CM, Rogers AJ, et al: Early surgical abortion: efficacy and safety. Am J Obstet Gynecol 187:407, 2002

Pazol K, Creanga AA, Burley KD, et al: Abortion surveillance–United States, 2011. MMWR 63(11):1, 2014

Pearl J, Price R, Richardson W, et al: Guidelines for diagnosis, treatment, and use of laparoscopy for surgical problems during pregnancy. Surg Endosc 25(11):3479, 2011

Platteau P, Staessen C, Michiels A, et al: Preimplantation genetic diagnosis for aneuploidy screening in patients with unexplained recurrent miscarriages. Fertil Steril 83(2):393, 2005

Pymar HC, Creinin MD, Schwartz JL: Mifepristone followed on the same day by vaginal misoprostol for early abortion. Contraception 64:87, 2001

Quinn PA, Shewchuck AB, Shuber J, et al: Efficacy of antibiotic therapy in preventing spontaneous pregnancy loss among couples colonized with genital mycoplasmas. Am J Obstet Gynecol 145:239, 1983a

Quinn PA, Shewchuck AB, Shuber J, et al: Serologic evidence of *Ureaplasma urealyticum* infection in women with spontaneous pregnancy loss. Am J Obstet Gynecol 145:245, 1983b

Raghavan S, Comendant R, Digol I, et al: Two-pill regimens of misoprostol after mifepristone medical abortion through 63 days' gestational age: a randomized controlled trial of sublingual and oral misoprostol. Contraception 79(2):84, 2009

Ramasamy R, Scovell JM, Kovac JR, et al: Fluorescence in situ hybridization detects increased sperm aneuploidy in men with recurrent pregnancy loss. Fertil Steril 103(4):906, 2015

Ramzy AM, Sattar M, Amin Y, et al: Uterine myomata and outcome of assisted reproduction. Hum Reprod 13:198, 1998

Rand JH, Wu XX, Quinn AS, et al: The annexin A5-mediated pathogenic mechanism in the antiphospholipid syndrome: role in pregnancy losses and thrombosis. Lupus 19(4):460, 2010

Rasch V: Cigarette, alcohol, and caffeine consumption: risk factors for spontaneous abortion. Acta Obstet Gynecol Scand 82:182, 2003

Raymond E, Grimes D: The comparative safety of legal induced abortion and childbirth in the United States. Obstet Gynecol 119(2, Part 1):215, 2012

Reddy UM: Recurrent pregnancy loss: nongenetic causes. Contemp OB/GYN 52:63, 2007

Reeves MF, Smith KJ, Creinin MD: Contraceptive effectiveness of immediate compared with delayed insertion of intrauterine devices after abortion. Obstet Gynecol 109:1286, 2007

Reichman DE, Laufer MR: Congenital uterine anomalies affecting reproduction. Best Pract Res Clin Obstet Gynecol 24(2):193, 2010

Renner RM, Nichols MD, Jensen JT, et al: Paracervical block for pain control in first-trimester surgical abortion. Obstet Gynecol 119:1030, 2012

Robertshaw I, Khoury J, Abdallah ME, et al: The effect of paternal age on outcome in assisted reproductive technology using the ovum donation model. Reprod Sci 21(5):590, 2014

Robinson L, Gallos ID, Conner SJ, et al: The effect of sperm DNA fragmentation on miscarriage rates: a systematic review and meta-analysis. Hum Reprod 27(10):2908, 2012

Robson SC, Kelly T, Howel D, et al: Randomised preference trial of medical versus surgical termination of pregnancy less than 14 weeks' gestation (TOPS). Health Technol Assess 13(53):1, 2009

Rowland AS, Baird DD, Shore DL, et al: Nitrous oxide and spontaneous abortion in female dental assistants. Am J Epidemiol 141:531, 1995

Salim R, Regan L, Woelfer B, et al: A comparative study of the morphology of congenital uterine anomalies in women with and without a history of recurrent first trimester miscarriage. Hum Reprod 18:162, 2003

Saraswat L, Bhattacharya S, Maheshwari A, et al: Maternal and perinatal outcome in women with threatened miscarriage in the first trimester: a systematic review. BJOG 117:245, 2010

Saravelos SH, Cocksedge KA, Li TC: Prevalence and diagnosis of congenital uterine anomalies in women with reproductive failure: a critical appraisal. Hum Reprod Update 14(5):415, 2008

Saravelos SH, Yan J, Rehmani H, et al: The prevalence and impact of fibroids and their treatment on the outcome of pregnancy in women with recurrent miscarriage. Hum Reprod 26:3274, 2011

Savaris RF, Silva de Moraes G, Cristovam RA, et al: Are antibiotics necessary after 48 hours of improvement in infected/septic abortions? A randomized controlled trial followed by a cohort study. Am J Obstet Gynecol 204:301.e1, 2011

Savitz DA, Chan RL, Herring AH, et al: Caffeine and miscarriage risk. Epidemiology 19:55, 2008

Saygili-Yilmaz E, Yildiz S, Erman-Akar M, et al: Reproductive outcome of septate uterus after hysteroscopic metroplasty. Arch Gynecol Obstet 4:289, 2003

Schaff EA, Fielding SL, Westhoff C, et al: Vaginal misoprostol administered 1, 2, or 3 days after mifepristone for early medical abortion. A randomized trial. JAMA 284:1948, 2000

Schneider D, Golan A, Langer R, et al: Outcome of continued pregnancies after first and second trimester cervical dilatation by laminaria tents. Obstet Gynecol 78:1121, 1991

Schnorr TM, Grajewski BA, Hornung RW, et al: Video display terminals and the risk of spontaneous abortion. N Engl J Med 324:727, 1991

Seckin B, Sarikaya E, Oruc AS, et al: Office hysteroscopic findings in patients with two, three, and four or more, consecutive miscarriages. Eur J Contracept Reprod Health Care 17(5):393, 2012

Sedgh G, Singh S, Shah I, et al: Induced abortion: incidence and trends worldwide from 1995 to 2008. Lancet 379:625, 2012

Seeber BE, Sammel MD, Guo W, et al: Application of redefined human chorionic gonadotropin curves for the diagnosis of women at risk for ectopic pregnancy. Fertil Steril 86(2):454, 2006

Shah PS, Zao J, Knowledge synthesis group of determinants of preterm/LBW births: Induced termination of pregnancy and low birthweight and preterm birth: a systematic review and meta-analyses. BJOG 116(11):1425, 2009

Shannon C, Wiebe E, Jacot F: Regimens of misoprostol with mifepristone for early medical abortion: a randomized trial. BJOG 113:621, 2006

Shimoni N, Davis A, Ramos M, et al: Timing of copper intrauterine device insertion after medical abortion. Obstet Gynecol 118(3):623, 2011

Silver RM, Branch DW, Goldenberg R, et al: Nomenclature for pregnancy outcomes. Obstet Gynecol 118(6):1402, 2011

Simpson JL: Causes of fetal wastage. Clin Obstet Gynecol 50(1):10, 2007

Simpson JL: Genes, chromosomes, and reproductive failure. Fertil Steril 33(2):107, 1980

Smith LF, Ewings PD, Guinlan C: Incidence of pregnancy after expectant, medical, or surgical management of spontaneous first trimester miscarriage: long term follow-up of miscarriage treatment (MIST) randomized controlled trial. BMJ 339:b3827, 2009

Sollid CP, Wisborg K, Hjort JH, et al: Eating disorder that was diagnosed before pregnancy and pregnancy outcome. Am J Obstet Gynecol 190:206, 2004

Steinauer J, Drey EA, Lewis R, et al: Obstetrics and gynecology resident satisfaction with an integrated, comprehensive abortion rotation. Obstet Gynecol 105:1335, 2005

Stephenson MD: Management of recurrent early pregnancy loss. J Reprod Med 51:303, 2006

Stephenson MD, Kutteh WH, Purkiss S, et al: Intravenous immunoglobulin and idiopathic secondary recurrent miscarriage: a multicentered randomized placebo-controlled trial. Hum Reprod 25(9):2203, 2010

Streeter GL: Focal deficiencies in fetal tissues and their relation to intra-uterine amputation. Carnegie Institute of Washington 1930, Publication No. 414, p 5

Stulberg DB, Dude AM, Dahlquist I, et al: Abortion provision among practicing obstetrician-gynecologists. Obstet Gynecol 1189:609, 2011

Sullivan AE, Silver RM, LaCoursiere DY, et al: Recurrent fetal aneuploidy and recurrent miscarriage. Obstet Gynecol 104:784, 2004

Sunkara SK, Khairy M, El-Toukhy T, et al: The effect of intramural fibroids without uterine cavity involvement on the outcome of IVF treatment: a systematic review and meta-analysis. Hum Reprod 25(2):418, 2010

Swingle HM, Colaizy TT, Zimmerman MB, et al: Abortion and the risk of subsequent preterm birth: a systematic review with meta-analyses. J Reprod Med 54(2):95, 2009

Tang J, Kapp N, Dragoman M, et al: WHO recommendations for misoprostol use for obstetric and gynecologic indications. Int J Gynaecol Obstet 121(2):186, 2013

Tanner L: Abortion in America: restrictions on the rise. The Associated Press, October 12, 2012

Taskinen H, Kyyrönen P, Hemminki K: Effects of ultrasound, shortwaves, and physical exertion on pregnancy outcome in physiotherapists. J Epidemiol Community Health 44:196, 1990

Temmerman M, Lopita MI, Sanghvi HC, et al: The role of maternal syphilis, gonorrhoea and HIV-1 infections in spontaneous abortion. Int J STD AIDS 3:418, 1992

Templeton A, Grimes D: A request for abortion. N Engl J Med 365(23):2198, 2011

Thangaratinam S, Tan A, Knox E, et al: Association between thyroid autoantibodies and miscarriage and preterm birth: meta-analysis of evidence. BMJ 342:d2616, 2011

Tharapel AT, Tharapel SA, Bannerman RM: Recurrent pregnancy losses and parental chromosome abnormalities: a review. BJOG 92:899, 1985

Timor-Tritsch IE, Farine D, Rosen MG: A close look at early embryonic development with the high-frequency transvaginal transducer. Am J Obstet Gynecol 159(3):676, 1988

Tongsong T, Srisomboon J, Wanapirak C, et al: Pregnancy outcome of threatened abortion with demonstrable fetal cardiac activity: a cohort study. J Obstet Gynaecol 21:331, 1995

Torre A, Huchon C, Bussieres L, et al: Immediate versus delayed medical treatment for first-trimester miscarriage: a randomized trial. Am J Obstet Gynecol 206:215.e1, 2012

Trinder J, Brocklehurst P, Porter R, et al: Management of miscarriage: expectant, medical, or surgical? Results of randomized controlled trial (miscarriage treatment (MIST) trial). BMJ 332(7552):1235, 2006

Tunçalp O, Gülmezoglu AM, Souza JP: Surgical procedures for evacuating incomplete miscarriage. Cochrane Database Syst Rev 9:CD001993, 2010

Turk JK, Preskill F, Landy U, et al: Availability and characteristics of abortion training in US ob-gyn residency programs: a national survey. Contraception 89(4):271, 2014

Tzeng CR, Hwang JL, Au HK, et al: Sonographic patterns of the endometrium in assessment of medical abortion outcomes. Contraception 88(1):153, 2013

Valli E, Zupi E, Marconi D, et al: Hysteroscopic findings in 344 women with recurrent spontaneous abortion. J Am Assoc Gynecol Laparosc 8(3):398, 2001

van Benthem BH, de Vincenzi I, Delmas MD, et al: Pregnancies before and after HIV diagnosis in a European cohort of HIV-infected women. European study on the natural history of HIV infection in women. AIDS 14:2171, 2000

van den Boogaard E, Kaandorp SP, Franssen MT, et al: Consecutive or non-consecutive recurrent miscarriage: is there any difference in carrier status? Hum Reprod 25(6):1411, 2010

van den Bosch T, Daemen A, Van Schoubroeck D, et al: Occurrence and outcome of residual trophoblastic tissue: a prospective study. J Ultrasound Med 27(3):357, 2008

Vartian CV, Septimus EJ: Tricuspid valve group B streptococcal endocarditis following elective abortion. Review Infect Dis 13:997, 1991

Venetis CA, Papadopoulos SP, Campo R, et al: Clinical implications of congenital uterine anomalies: a meta-analysis of comparative studies. Reprod Biomed Online 29(6):665, 2014

Virk J, Zhang J, Olsen J: Medical abortion and the risk of subsequent adverse pregnancy outcomes. N Engl J Med 357(7):648, 2007

Vissenberg R, van den Boogaard E, van Wely M, et al: Treatment of thyroid disorders before conception and in early pregnancy: a systematic review. Hum Reprod Update 18(4):360, 2012

von Hertzen H, Honkanen H, Piaggio G, et al: WHO multinational study of three misoprostol regimens after mifepristone for early medical abortion. I: Efficacy. BJOG 110:808, 2003

von Hertzen H, Huong NTM, Piaggio G, et al: Misoprostol dose and route after mifepristone for early medical abortion: a randomized controlled non-inferiority trial. BJOG 117(10):1186, 2010

von Hertzen H, Piaggio G, Huong NT, et al: Efficacy of two intervals and two routes of administration of misoprostol for termination of early pregnancy: a randomised controlled equivalence trial. Lancet 369(9577):1938, 2007

von Hertzen H, Piaggio G, Wojdyla D, et al: Two mifepristone doses and two intervals of misoprostol administration for termination of early pregnancy: a randomized factorial controlled equivalence trial. BJOG 116(3):381, 2009

Wacholder S, Chen BE, Wilcox A, et al: Risk of miscarriage with bivalent vaccine against human papillomavirus (HPV) types 16 and 18: pooled analysis of two randomized controlled trials. BMJ 340:c712, 2010

Warburton D, Stein Z, Kline J, et al: Chromosome abnormalities in spontaneous abortion: data from the New York City study. In Porter IH, Hook EB (eds): Human Embryonic and Fetal Death. New York, Academic Press, 1980, p 261

Weber-Schoendorfer C, Chambers C, Wacker E, et al: Pregnancy outcome after methotrexate treatment for rheumatic disease prior to or during early pregnancy: a prospective multicenter cohort study. Arthritis Rheumatol 66(5):1101, 2014

Weiss J, Malone F, Vidaver J, et al: Threatened abortion: a risk factor for poor pregnancy outcome—a population based screening study (the FASTER Trial). Am J Obstet Gynecol 187:S70, 2002

Weng X, Odouki R, Li DK: Maternal caffeine consumption during pregnancy and the risk of miscarriage: a prospective cohort study. Am J Obstet Gynecol 198:279.e1, 2008

Westfall JM, Sophocles A, Burggraf H, et al: Manual vacuum aspiration for first-trimester abortion. Arch Fam Med 7:559, 1998

Wijesiriwardana A, Bhattacharya S, Shetty A, et al: Obstetric outcome in women with threatened miscarriage in the first trimester. Obstet Gynecol 107:557, 2006

Wilcox AF, Weinberg CR, O'Connor JF, et al: Incidence of early loss of pregnancy. N Engl J Med 319:189, 1988

Williams PM, Fletcher S. Health effects of prenatal radiation exposure. Am Fam Physician 82(5):488, 2010

Williams Z: Inducing tolerance to pregnancy. N Engl J Med 367(12):1159, 2012

Winikoff B, Dzuba IG, Creinin MD, et al: Two distinct oral routes of misoprostol in mifepristone medical abortion: a randomized controlled trial. Obstet Gynecol 112(6):1303, 2008

Wisborg K, Kesmodel U, Henriksen TB, et al: A prospective study of maternal smoking and spontaneous abortion. Acta Obstet Gynecol Scand 82:936, 2003

Wo JY, Viswanathan AN: Impact of radiotherapy on fertility, pregnancy, and neonatal outcomes in female cancer patients. Int J Radiat Oncol Biol Phys 73(5):1304, 2009

World Health Organization: The use of DDT in malaria vector control: WHO position statement. 2011

Yan XC, Wang JH, Wang B, et al: Study of human cytomegalovirus replication in body fluids, placental infection, and miscarriage during the first trimester of pregnancy. J Med Virol 87(6):1046, 2015

Yetman DL, Kutteh WH: Antiphospholipid antibody panels and recurrent pregnancy loss: prevalence of anticardiolipin antibodies compared with other antiphospholipid antibodies. Fertil Steril 66:540, 1996

Zhang J, Gilles JM, Barnhart K, et al: A comparison of medical management with misoprostol and surgical management for early pregnancy failure. N Engl J Med 353:761, 2005

Ziakas PD, Pavlou M, Voulgarelis M: Heparin treatment in antiphospholipid syndrome with recurrent pregnancy loss: a systematic review and meta-analysis. Obstet Gynecol 115(6):1256, 2010

CHAPTER 7

Ectopic Pregnancy

EPIDEMIOLOGY

An ectopic or extrauterine pregnancy is one in which the blastocyst implants anywhere other than the endometrial lining of the uterine cavity. Nearly 95 percent of ectopic pregnancies implant in the fallopian tube. Other sites are shown in Figure 7-1, which reflects data from 1800 surgically treated ectopic pregnancies (Bouyer, 2002). Bilateral ectopic pregnancies are rare, and their estimated prevalence is 1 of every 200,000 pregnancies (al-Awwad, 1999).

Reported incidences rates of ectopic pregnancy are less reliable than in the past as outpatient treatment protocols render national hospital discharge statistics invalid. One estimate by Kaiser Permanente of North California was 2.07 percent of total pregnancies from 1997 to 2000 (Van Den Eeden, 2005). Hoover and colleagues (2010) queried a large claims database of privately insured women between 2002 and 2007 and calculated a rate of 0.64 percent. However, this may not accurately reflect the cases in higher-risk, lower-socioeconomic, uninsured populations. Stulberg and coworkers (2014) reviewed 2004 to 2008 Medicaid claims data from 14 states. They reported a rate of 1.4 percent and noted that black women were 46 percent more likely to experience an ectopic pregnancy than whites in this government-insured group.

Among several factors that help explain the incidence of ectopic pregnancies are: (1) greater sexually transmitted disease prevalence, (2) diagnostic tools with improved sensitivity, (3) tubal factor infertility, (4) delayed childbearing and accompanied use of assisted reproductive technology, and (5) increased intrauterine device (IUD) use and tubal sterilization, which predispose to ectopic pregnancy if the method fails (Ankum, 1996; Li, 2014a; Ljubin-Sternak, 2014).

Ectopic pregnancy remains the leading cause of early pregnancy-related death. Still, current diagnostic and treatment protocols have resulted in substantial declines in fatality rates. One analysis showed a 56-percent decline in the ectopic pregnancy mortality ratio between the 1980 to 1984 epoch and the 2003 to 2007 epoch. During this later span, African-American women were approximately three times more likely to die as a result of ectopic pregnancy complications than whites (Creanga, 2011). Inadequate access to gynecologic and prenatal care may partially explain this trend.

In most of these cases, death is directly related to severe hemorrhage from tubal rupture. Risk factors that increase the likelihood of tubal rupture include ovulation induction, serum β-human chorionic gonadotropin (β-hCG) level >10,000 IU/L, and never having used contraception (Job-Spira, 1999). Appreciation of these characteristics can aid prompt surgical intervention.

RISK FACTORS

Several risks have been linked with ectopic pregnancy (Table 7-1). Among these, documented tubal pathology, surgery to restore tubal patency, or tubal sterilization can all lead to obstruction and subsequent ectopic pregnancy. A woman with two prior ectopic pregnancies has a 10- to 16-fold increased chance for another (Barnhart, 2006; Skjeldestad, 1998).

Smoking, which may be a surrogate marker for sexually transmitted infections, increases the ectopic pregnancy risk three- to fourfold in women who smoke more than one pack of cigarettes daily (Saraiya, 1998). The increased risk of ectopic pregnancy among smokers undergoing assisted reproductive technology was verified in a metaanalysis by Waylen and associates (2009). In addition, animal studies show that smoking alters oocyte cumulus complex pick-up and embryo transport through its effects on ciliary function and smooth-muscle contraction (Shaw, 2010; Talbot, 2005).

Assisted reproductive technology (ART) for sub- or infertile couples has a 0.8-percent incidence of ectopic pregnancy per

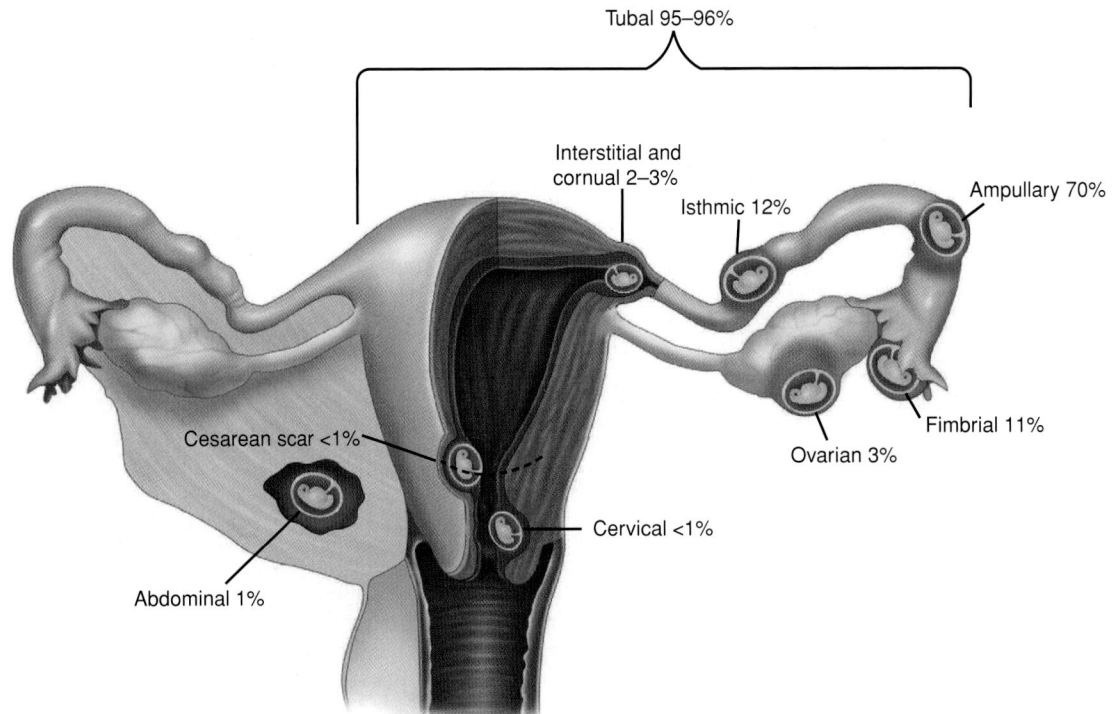

FIGURE 7-1 Various sites and frequency of ectopic pregnancies. (Reproduced with permission from Cunningham FG, Leveno KJ, Bloom SL (eds): Ectopic pregnancy. In Williams Obstetrics, 24th ed. New York, McGraw-Hill Education, 2014.)

transfer and 2.2 percent per clinical pregnancy (Coste, 2000). Interestingly, recent series note significant reductions in ectopic pregnancy rates at the time of in vitro fertilization (IVF) if frozen-thawed embryos (2.2 percent rate) are used rather than those from fresh cycles (4.6 percent) (Fang, 2015; Huang, 2014). In women undergoing IVF, the main risk factors for ectopic pregnancy are tubal factor infertility and hydrosalpinges (Strandell, 1999; Van Voorhis, 2006). Moreover, "atypical" implantation—that is, interstitial, abdominal, cervical, ovarian, or heterotopic—is more common following ART procedures. As a review, heterotopic pregnancy is

an intrauterine pregnancy coexistent with an extrauterine pregnancy.

Older reproductive-aged women, specifically women aged 35 to 44 years, carry a threefold risk of ectopic pregnancy compared with those aged 15 to 25 years (Goldner, 1993). These have been attributed to age-related hormonal changes that alter tubal function (Coste, 2000).

Contraception lowers overall pregnancy rates and thereby lowers ectopic pregnancy rates. However, if pregnancy does occur, some methods increase the relative incidence of ectopic pregnancy. Examples include the levonorgestrel-releasing intrauterine system (Mirena) and copper IUD (ParaGard). In one study of 61,448 IUD users, 118 contraceptive failures were reported, and 21 of these were ectopic (Heinemann, 2015). Progestin-only contraceptive pills also pose a slightly increased risk because of their effects to diminish tubal motility. With tubal sterilization failure, ectopic pregnancy is a concern. In one study, this risk was 3.5 times greater in women younger than 28 years at the time of sterilization. This may be in part because of age-related fecundity. Of methods, higher ectopic rates were noted with laparoscopic partial salpingectomy and electrodestruction methods (Malacova, 2014).

PATHOPHYSIOLOGY

Acute inflammation has been implicated in the tubal damage that predisposes to ectopic pregnancies. Chronic salpingitis and salpingitis isthmica nodosa also contribute (Kutluay, 1994).

Of suspected agents, recurrent chlamydial infection causes intraluminal inflammation, subsequent fibrin deposition, and tubal scarring (Hillis, 1997). Moreover, persistent chlamydial

TABLE 7-1. Risk Factors for Ectopic Pregnancy

Factor	Odds Ratio (95% CI)
Prior ectopic pregnancy	12.5 (7.5, 20.9)
Prior tubal surgery	4.0 (2.6, 6.1)
Smoking >20 cigarettes per day	3.5 (1.4, 8.6)
PID confirmed by laparoscopy or positive test for *Chlamydia trachomatis*	3.4 (2.4, 5.0)
≥3 prior spontaneous miscarriages	3.0 (1.3, 6.9)
Age ≥40 years	2.9 (1.4, 6.1)
Prior medical or surgical abortion	2.8 (1.1, 7.2)
Infertility >1 year	2.6 (1.6, 4.2)
Lifelong sexual partners >5	1.6 (1.2, 2.1)
Prior IUD use	1.3 (1.0, 1.8)

IUD = intrauterine device; PID = pelvic inflammatory disease; STD = sexually transmitted disease.
Data from Bouyer, 2003; Buster, 1999.

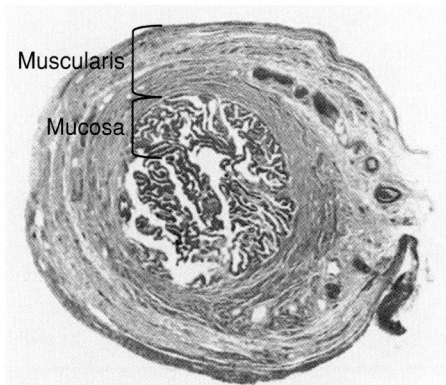

A   Normal fallopian tube

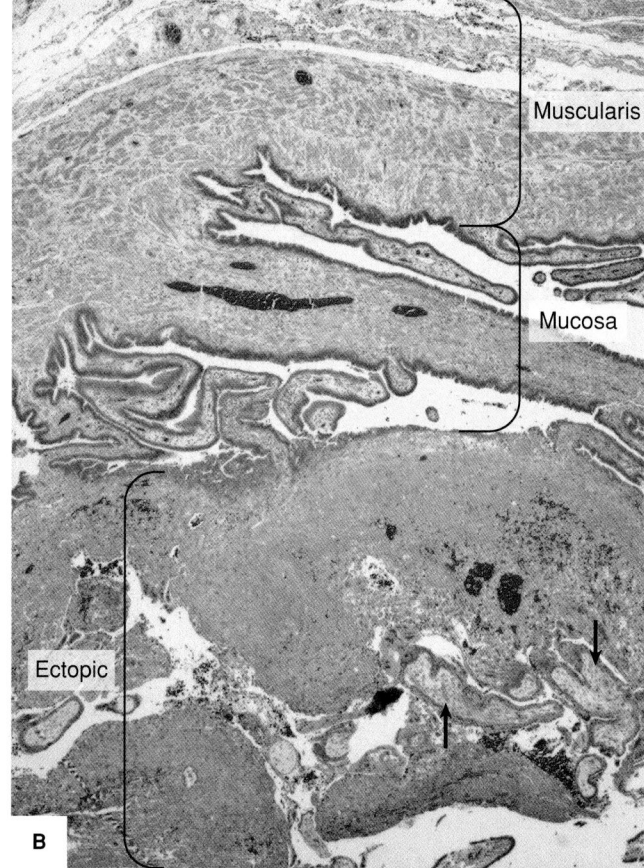

B

FIGURE 7-2 Photomicrograph of fallopian tubes. **A.** Normal ampullary portion of a fallopian tube. (Used with permission from Dr. Kelley Carrick.) **B.** Ectopic tubal pregnancy. Chorionic villi (*arrows*) can be seen within the tubal lumen. (Used with permission from Dr. Raheela Ashfaq.)

antigens can trigger a delayed hypersensitivity reaction that promotes continued scarring despite negative culture results (Toth, 2000). Whereas endotoxin-producing *Neisseria gonorrhoeae* causes virulent pelvic inflammation that has a rapid clinical onset, the chlamydial inflammatory response is chronic and peaks at 7 to 14 days.

Inflammation within the fallopian tube can also arrest embryo progress and provide a premature proimplantation signal (Shaw, 2010). Specifically, oviduct interstitial cells of Cajal are specialized pacemaker cells responsible for oviduct motility and egg transport. Infections in mice by *Chlamydia muridarum*, which is similar to human *Chlamydia trachomatis*, lead to absent spontaneous pacemaker activity and may offer another explanation of how *chlamydial infection* increases ectopic pregnancy rates in humans (Dixon, 2009).

Another factor involved with oviductal transport of embryos is the cannabinoid receptor (CB1), which is mediated by endocannabinoid signaling. Chronic exposure to nicotine can affect endocannabinoid levels and lead to fallopian tube dysfunction (Horne, 2008).

The mechanism for ectopic pregnancy in women using ART has been a conundrum because the fallopian tube is typically bypassed. Revel and colleagues (2008) sought to establish the relationship between E-cadherin, an adhesion molecule, and tubal ectopic pregnancy implantation sites. They found E-cadherin strongly localized to the tubal embryo implantation site only in women who underwent IVF. This suggests a biologic rather than mechanical factor accounting for the ectopic pregnancies associated with IVF.

Once normal tubal transport has been disrupted, fallopian tube anatomy plays an important role in tubal pregnancy genesis. Namely, the fallopian tube lacks a submucosal layer beneath its epithelium. Therefore, a fertilized ovum can easily burrow through the epithelium and implant within tube's muscularis layer (Fig. 7-2). As rapidly proliferating trophoblasts erode the muscularis layer, maternal blood pours into the spaces within the trophoblastic or the adjacent tissue.

With this process, the location of a tubal pregnancy may predict the extent of damage. Senterman and associates (1988) studied histologic samples from 84 isthmic and ampullary pregnancies. They reported that half of the ampullary pregnancies were intraluminal, and the muscularis was preserved in 85 percent of these. Conversely, isthmic gestations were found both intra- and extraluminally with greater disruption of the tubal wall. The timing of tubal rupture is also partially dependent on pregnancy location. As a rule, fallopian tubes rupture earlier if implantation is in the isthmic or ampullary portion. Later rupture is seen if the ovum implants within the interstitial portion. Rupture is usually spontaneous but can also follow trauma such as that associated with bimanual pelvic examination or coitus.

After implantation, differences in ectopic pregnancy development explain the typically divergent clinical paths between acute and chronic ectopic pregnancies. *Acute ectopic pregnancies* are those with a high serum β-hCG level at presentation. These high β-hCG levels correlate with the depth of trophoblastic invasion into the tubal wall. Greater invasion promotes concomitant severe ischemic changes and tubal wall rupture (Erol, 2015). Rapid pregnancy growth leads to an immediate diagnosis from painful tubal distention or from rupture. Indeed, these carry a higher risk of tubal rupture compared with chronic ectopic pregnancies (Barnhart, 2003c).

With *chronic ectopic pregnancy*, minor repeated ruptures or tubal abortion incites an inflammatory response that leads to formation of a pelvic mass. Its abnormal trophoblasts die early. Thus, negative or lower, static serum β-hCG levels are found. Chronic ectopic pregnancies typically rupture late, if at all, but commonly form a complex pelvic mass. In these cases, it often is the mass, rather than pain or bleeding, that prompts diagnostic surgery (Cole, 1982; Uğur, 1996).

CLINICAL MANIFESTATIONS

The classic symptom triad of ectopic pregnancy is amenorrhea followed by vaginal bleeding and ipsilateral abdominal pain. However, as women seek care earlier, the ability to diagnose ectopic pregnancy before rupture—even before the onset of symptoms—is not unusual. Of other symptoms, banal pregnancy discomforts such as breast tenderness, nausea, and urinary frequency may accompany more ominous findings. These include shoulder pain worsened by inspiration, which is caused by phrenic nerve irritation from subdiaphragmatic blood, or vasomotor disturbances such as vertigo and syncope from hemorrhagic hypovolemia.

Of physical findings, some women have orthostatic findings from hypovolemia. Birkhahn and associates (2003) employed the shock index to evaluate the severity of ruptured ectopic pregnancy. This index is the heart rate divided by systolic blood pressure and can assess trauma patients for hypovolemic or septic shock. The normal range lies between 0.5 and 0.7 for nonpregnant patients. A shock index >0.85 and a systolic blood pressure <110 mm Hg are highly suggestive of a potentially life-threatening gynecologic emergency, such as a ruptured ectopic pregnancy (Birkhahn, 2003; Polena, 2015). Despite these findings of advanced hypovolemia, normal vital signs are unreliable to exclude earlier stages of tubal rupture.

Abdominal and pelvic findings may also be notoriously scarce in many women before tubal rupture. With rupture, however, nearly three fourths will have marked tenderness on both abdominal and pelvic examination, and pain is aggravated with cervical manipulation. A pelvic mass, including fullness posterolateral to the uterus, can be palpated in approximately 20 percent of women. Initially, an ectopic pregnancy may feel soft and elastic, whereas extensive intraluminal hemorrhage produces a firmer consistency. Many times, discomfort precludes palpation of the mass, and limiting examinations may help avert iatrogenic rupture.

DIAGNOSIS

Symptoms of ectopic pregnancy can mimic multiple entities (Table 7-2). Early pregnancy complications such as threatened or missed abortion or hemorrhagic corpus luteum cyst may be difficult to differentiate. Moreover, approximately 20 percent of women with normal pregnancies have early bleeding. Several disorders not related to pregnancy can also mimic ectopic pregnancy. In general, a positive test for β-hCG usually excludes these other diagnoses. However, these conditions may exist concurrently with pregnancy—either intrauterine or ectopic. Transvaginal sonography and serial serum β-hCG measurements are the most valuable diagnostic aids to confirm clinical

TABLE 7-2. Conditions That Cause Lower Abdominal Pain

Cause	Abdominal Location	Characteristics	Associated Findings
Pregnancy			
Abortion	Midline or generalized	Crampy, episodic	(+) UCG; vaginal bleeding
Ectopic	Unilateral or generalized	Sharp or aching, continuous	(+) UCG; vaginal bleeding
Uterus and Cervix			
Endomyometritis	Lower, midline	Dull aching	Vaginal discharge, fever
Endometriosis	Lower, midline	Cyclic, aching	Possible adnexal mass
Degenerating myoma	Lower, midline	Dull aching or sharp	Irregular, enlarged uterus
Adnexal Disease			
Salpingitis	Unilateral or bilateral	Severe	Moderate to high fever
Tuboovarian abscess	Unilateral or bilateral	Dull aching or sharp	High fever; adnexal mass
Corpus luteum cyst	Lower, unilateral	Acute onset, sharp	(+/−) UCG
Adnexal torsion	Lower, unilateral	Acute onset, sharp, continuous or episodic	Adnexal mass
Other			
Appendicitis	Periumbilical or right lower	Sharp or aching, continuous	Anorexia, nausea, vomiting
Diverticulitis	Left lower	Dull aching	Fever
Cystitis	Midline, suprapubic	Acute, spasms	Dysuria, frequency
Renal calculi	Flank, radiating downward	Severe, episodic	Hematuria

UCG = urinary chorionic gonadotropin test result.

suspicions of an ectopic pregnancy. Additionally, because ectopic pregnancy can lead to significant bleeding, a hemogram is an additional fast and effective initial screen.

Laboratory Findings

Serum β-hCG Measurements

Human chorionic gonadotropin is a glycoprotein produced by syncytiotrophoblast and can be detected in serum as early as 8 days after the luteinizing hormone (LH) surge. In normal pregnancies, serum β-hCG levels rise in a log-linear fashion until 60 or 80 days after the last menses, at which time values plateau at approximately 100,000 IU/L. Given an interassay variability of 5 to 10 percent, interpretation of serial values is more reliable when performed by the same laboratory.

With a robust intrauterine pregnancy (IUP), serum β-hCG levels should increase at least 53 to 66 percent every 48 hours (Barnhart, 2004; Kadar, 1982). Seeber and associates (2006) used an even more conservative 35-percent rise after 48-hours. Past this 48 hours, allowing time for additional data may better determine the location and viability of the pregnancy. But, this is weighed against the increased chance of ectopic pregnancy rupture during these extra diagnostic days. In hemodynamically stable women, adding a third serum β-hCG level on day 4 or 7 could correct the diagnosis of a pregnancy of unknown location in an additional 7 to 13 percent of patients (Zee, 2013). Nevertheless, inadequately rising serum β-hCG levels indicate only a dying pregnancy, not its location.

Many women present with an unsure last menstrual period, and an educated guess of gestational age is made. In these cases, correlation between the serum β-hCG concentration and transvaginal sonography findings becomes especially important.

Serum Progesterone Levels

Serum progesterone concentration is used by some to aid ectopic pregnancy diagnosis when serum β-hCG levels and sonographic findings are inconclusive (Stovall, 1992). Serum progesterone concentration varies minimally between 5 and 10 weeks' gestation, thus a single value is sufficient. Mol and coworkers (1998) performed a metaanalysis of 22 studies to assess the accuracy of a single serum progesterone level to differentiate ectopic from uterine pregnancy. They found that results were most accurate when approached from the viewpoint of *healthy versus dying pregnancy*. With serum progesterone levels <5 ng/mL, a dying pregnancy was detected with *near perfect* specificity and with a sensitivity of 60 percent. Conversely, values of >20 ng/mL had a sensitivity of 95 percent with specificity approximating 40 percent to identify a healthy pregnancy. Ultimately, serum progesterone levels can be used to buttress a clinical impression, but again they *cannot* reliably differentiate between an ectopic and intrauterine pregnancy (Guha, 2014).

Sonography

High-resolution sonography has revolutionized the clinical management of women with a suspected ectopic pregnancy. With transvaginal sonography (TVS), a gestational sac is usually visible between 4½ and 5 weeks, the yolk sac appears between 5 and 6 weeks, and a fetal pole with cardiac activity is first detected at 5½ to 6 weeks. With transabdominal sonography, these structures are visualized slightly later. The sonographic diagnosis of ectopic pregnancy rests on visualization of an adnexal mass separate from the ovary (Fig. 7-3).

When the last menstrual period is unknown, serum β-hCG testing is used to define expected sonographic findings. Each institution must define a β-hCG discriminatory value for TVS, that is, the lower limit at which an examiner can reliably visualize an IUP. At most institutions, this value is a concentration between 1500 and 2000 IU/L. Accurate diagnosis by sonography is three times more likely if the initial β-hCG level is above this value. Connolly and colleagues (2013) reported evidence to suggest an even higher threshold. They noted that with live IUPs, a gestational sac was seen 99 percent of the time with a discriminatory level of 3510 IU/L. Even with β-hCG levels above the chosen discriminatory value, technical challenges such as leiomyomas, adenomyosis, multifetal gestation, or IUD can hinder the ability to accurately diagnose an intrauterine gestation (Gurel, 2007; Ko, 2014).

When β-hCG levels are above the set discriminatory value, the absence of an IUP may suggest an abnormal pregnancy. The abnormality may be an ectopic pregnancy, an incomplete abortion, or a resolving completed abortion. For example, despite total passage of products of conception with complete abortion, β-hCG testing may still be positive while original β-hCG is metabolized and cleared. Conversely, when β-hCG values lie below the discriminatory value, sonographic findings are not diagnostic in nearly two thirds of cases (Barnhart, 1999).

In an attempt to unify the language used with sonographic evaluation of early pregnancies, a consensus statement was drafted with five categories: (1) definitive ectopic pregnancy (extrauterine gestational sac with yolk sac and/or embryo), (2) probable ectopic pregnancy (inhomogeneous adnexal mass or extrauterine sac-like structure), (3) probable IUP (intrauterine echogenic sac), (4) definite IUP (intrauterine gestational sac with yolk sac and/or embryo), and (5) pregnancy of unknown location (PUL) (lacking signs of either ectopic pregnancy or IUP) (Barnhart, 2011).

Systematic sonographic evaluation is critical to establish the correct diagnosis. Most begin with the endometrial cavity. In pregnancies conceived spontaneously, identification of an IUP effectively excludes the possibility of ectopic implantation. When ART is employed, however, careful examination of the tube and ovary is performed even with an intrauterine pregnancy because heterotopic pregnancy rates may be as high as 1 per 100 (Tal, 1996). An intracavitary fluid collection caused by bleeding from the decidua can create a *pseudogestational sac*, or *pseudosac*. As shown in Figure 7-4, this one-layer collection lies typically in the midline of the uterine cavity. In contrast, a normal gestational sac is eccentrically located (Dashefsky, 1988). Another intracavitary finding is a trilaminar endometrial pattern, which represents two adjacent proliferative-phase endometrial layers (Fig. 2-16, p. 31) (Lavie, 1996). For the diagnosis of ectopic pregnancy, this finding's specificity is 94 percent but with a sensitivity of only 38 percent (Hammoud, 2005). Endometrial stripe thickness has not been well correlated with ectopic pregnancies. However, Moschos and Twickler (2008b)

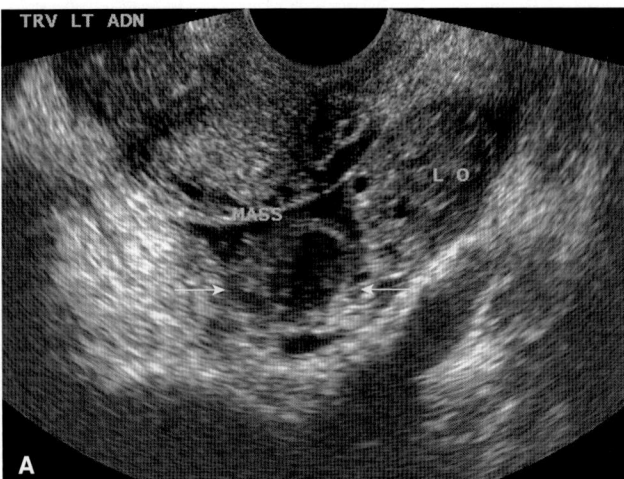

Inhomogeneous mass

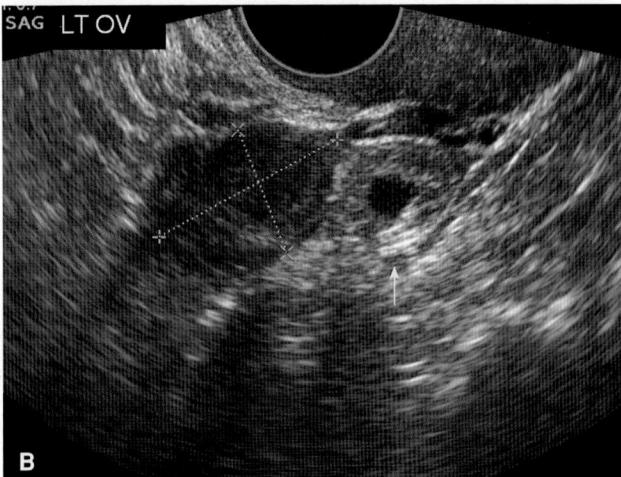

Mass with empty extrauterine sac

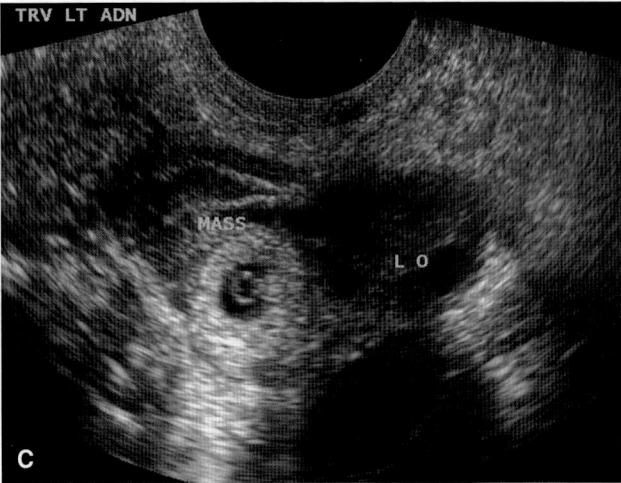

Mass with yolk sac

FIGURE 7-3 Transvaginal sonographic findings with various ectopic pregnancies. For sonographic diagnosis, an ectopic mass should be seen in the adnexa separate from the ovary and may be seen: **(A)** as an inhomogeneous adnexal mass (*yellow arrows*), **(B)** as an empty extrauterine sac with a hyperechoic ring (*arrow*), or **(C)** as a yolk sac and/or fetal pole with or without cardiac activity within an extrauterine sac. LO = left ovary. (Used with permission from Dr. Elysia Moschos.)

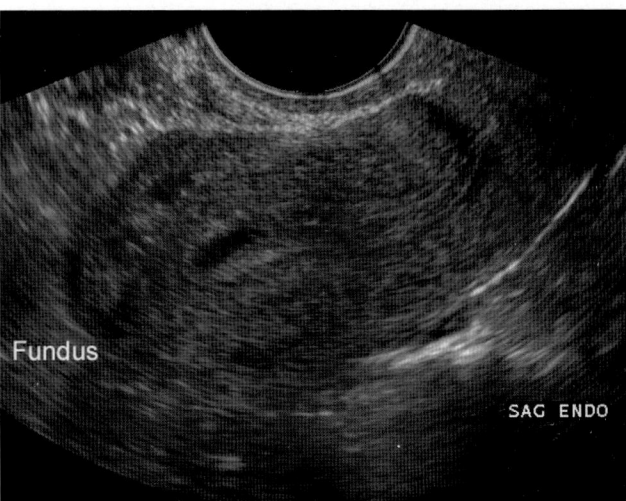

FIGURE 7-4 Transvaginal sonography of a pseudogestational sac (*arrow*) within the endometrial cavity. Note its ovoid shape and central location, which are characteristic of these fluid collections. (Used with permission from Dr. Elysia Moschos.)

determined that in PULs, none that ultimately proved to be normal IUPs had a stripe thickness <8 mm.

The fallopian tubes and ovaries are also inspected. Visualization of an extrauterine yolk sac or embryo clearly confirms an ectopic pregnancy, although such findings are less commonly seen (Paul, 2000). In some cases, a *halo* or tubal ring that surrounds an anechoic sac can be seen. According to Burry and associates (1993), this has a positive-predictive value of 92 percent and a sensitivity of 95 percent. Alternatively, an inhomogeneous complex adnexal mass is usually caused by hemorrhage within the ectopic sac or by an ectopic pregnancy that has ruptured into the tube. Overall, approximately 60 percent of ectopic pregnancies are seen as an inhomogeneous mass adjacent to the ovary; 20 percent appear as a hyperechoic ring; and 13 percent have an obvious gestational sac with a fetal pole (Condous, 2005). Brown and associates (1994) conducted a metaanalysis of 10 studies to ascertain the best transvaginal sonographic criteria to diagnose ectopic pregnancy. They reported that the finding of any adnexal mass, other than a simple ovarian cyst, was the most accurate. With this, they found a sensitivity of 84 percent, specificity of 99 percent, positive-predictive value of 96 percent, and negative-predictive value of 95 percent. However, not all adnexal masses represent an ectopic pregnancy, and integration of sonographic findings with other clinical information is necessary.

Differentiating an ectopic pregnancy from a corpus luteum cyst can be challenging. However, Swire and coworkers (2004) observed that the corpus luteum wall is less echogenic compared with both a tubal ring and the endometrium. They found that a spongelike, lacelike, or reticular pattern seen within the cyst is classic for hemorrhage (Fig. 9-16, p. 218). Moreover, a corpus luteum is found within the parenchyma of an ovary, but a markedly asymmetric appearing ovary should raise suspicion of an ectopic pregnancy (Gurel, 2007). With transvaginal color Doppler imaging, placental blood flow within the periphery of the ectopic pregnancy—the *ring of fire*—can be seen (Fig. 7-5). Although this finding can aid ectopic pregnancy diagnosis, a

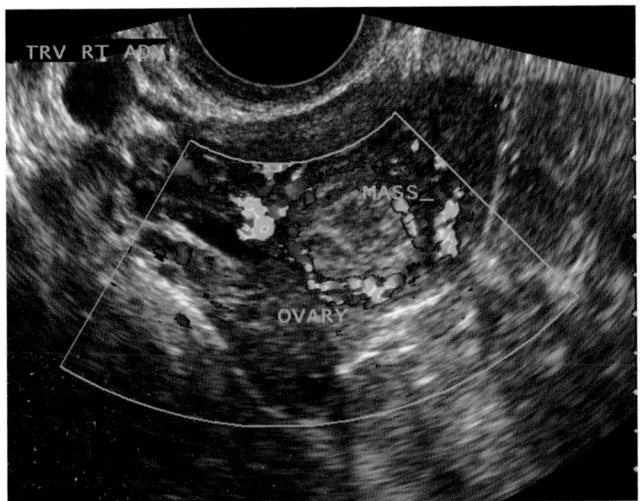

FIGURE 7-5 Color Doppler transvaginal sonography of an ectopic pregnancy. The "ring of fire" reflects placental blood flow around the periphery of the pregnancy. This finding, however, may also be seen with corpus luteum cysts.

ring of fire also can be seen with a corpus luteum of pregnancy (Pellerito, 1992). Pulsed-color Doppler sonographic measurement of resistance indices has poor sensitivity and limits its utility (Atri, 2003). Finally, to help characterize a suspicious mass, an examiner can gently palpate an adnexum that is placed between the vaginal probe and the examiner's abdominal hand during real-time scanning. A mass that moves separately from the ovary suggests a tubal pregnancy, whereas a mass that moves synchronously more likely represents a corpus luteum cyst (Levine, 2007).

During sonographic evaluation of the pelvis, TVS can detect as little as 50 mL of free peritoneal fluid in the cul-de-sac of Douglas. This may be intraabdominal bleeding or physiologic peritoneal fluid. A large volume of fluid or fluid that is echogenic is more worrisome for hemoperitoneum. In addition, transabdominal right-upper-quadrant sonographic imaging helps assess the extent of hemoperitoneum. Blood in the paracolic gutters and Morison pouch indicates significant hemorrhage. Specifically, free fluid in Morison pouch typically is not seen until a hemo-

peritoneum reaches 400 to 700 mL (Branney, 1995; Rodgerson, 2001). Detection of peritoneal fluid in conjunction with an adnexal mass is highly predictive of ectopic pregnancy (Nyberg, 1991). That said, despite technologic advances, the absence of suggestive findings does not exclude ectopic pregnancy.

■ Culdocentesis

With a 16- to 18-gauge spinal needle, the cul-de-sac of Douglas may be entered through the posterior vaginal fornix (Fig. 7-6). The aspirate characteristics, in conjunction with clinical findings, may help clarify the diagnosis. Normal-appearing peritoneal fluid is designated as a negative test. If fragments of an old clot or nonclotting blood are found in the aspirate when placed into a dry, clean test tube, then hemoperitoneum is diagnosed. If the aspirated blood clots after it is withdrawn, this may signify active intraperitoneal bleeding or puncture of an adjacent vessel. If fluid cannot be aspirated, the test can only be interpreted as unsatisfactory. Purulent fluid suggests an infection-related cause such as salpingitis or appendicitis. Feculent material may originate from a perforated colon or an inadvertent puncture of the rectosigmoid colon during culdocentesis.

Several studies have challenged the usefulness of this bedside test, and culdocentesis has been largely replaced by TVS (Glezerman, 1992; Vermesh, 1990). Sonography with findings of echogenic fluid to establish hemoperitoneum is more sensitive and specific than culdocentesis—100 and 100 percent versus 66 and 80 percent, respectively. Also, for most women, sonography is better tolerated.

■ Endometrial Evidence

Several endometrial changes are associated with ectopic pregnancy. These include decidua found in 42 percent of samples, secretory endometrium in 22 percent, and proliferative endometrium in 12 percent, all with an absence of trophoblasts (Lopez, 1994). Decidua is endometrium that is hormonally prepared for pregnancy, and the degree to which the endometrium is converted with ectopic pregnancy is variable. Thus, in addition to bleeding, women with ectopic tubal pregnancy may pass a

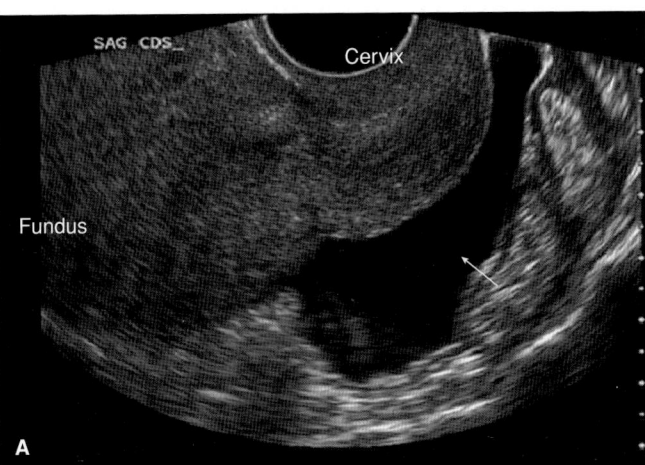 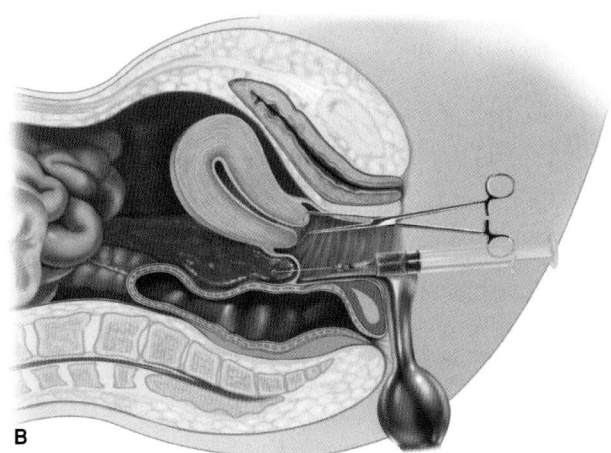

FIGURE 7-6 A. Transvaginal sonography of a fluid collection (*arrow*) in the cul-de-sac of Douglas. (Used with permission from Dr. Elysia Moschos.) **B.** Culdocentesis. With a 16- to 18-gauge spinal needle attached to a syringe, the cul-de-sac of Douglas is entered through the posterior vaginal fornix as upward traction is applied to the cervix with a tenaculum.

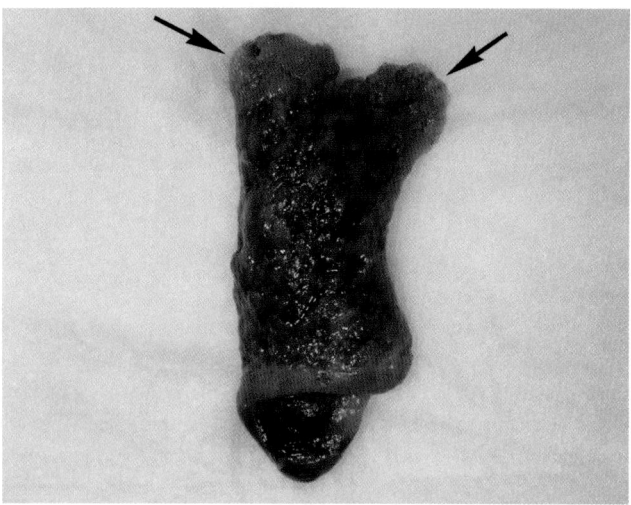

FIGURE 7-7 In this image of a decidual cast, *arrows* mark the area that conformed to the cornua. (Reproduced with permission from Cunningham FG, Leveno KJ, Bloom SL (eds): Ectopic pregnancy. In Williams Obstetrics, 24th ed. New York, McGraw-Hill Education, 2014.)

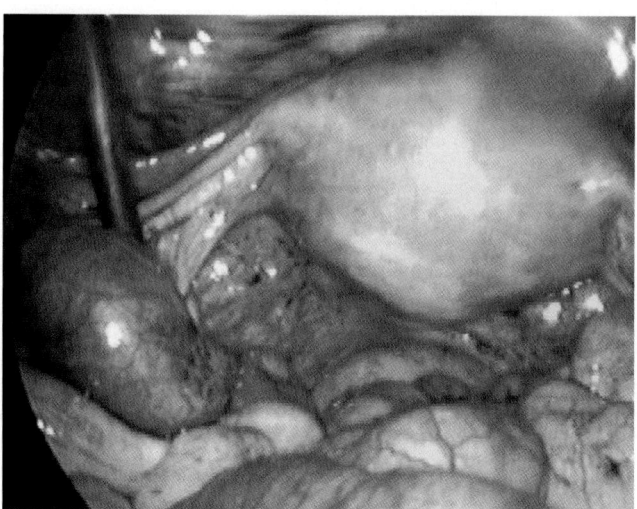

FIGURE 7-8 Laparoscopic photograph of ectopic pregnancy. A blunt probe elevates a blue, distended left tubal ampulla. (Used with permission from Dr. Kevin Doody.)

decidual cast, which is the entire sloughed endometrium that reflects the form of the endometrial cavity (Fig. 7-7). Decidual sloughing may also occur with IUP abortion. Thus, tissue is carefully evaluated visually and then histologically for evidence of a conceptus. If no clear gestational sac is visually seen or if no villi are identified histologically within the cast, then the possibility of ectopic pregnancy must still be entertained.

Before methotrexate treatment is given for ectopic pregnancy treatment, many recommend that the absence of intrauterine trophoblastic tissue be confirmed by curettage (Barnhart, 2002; Chung, 2011; Shaunik, 2011). The presumptive diagnosis of ectopic pregnancy is inaccurate in nearly 40 percent of cases without histologic exclusion of a spontaneous pregnancy loss. Nevertheless, the need, method, and risks of endometrial sampling must carefully be weighed against the limited risks of methotrexate.

Endometrial biopsy with a Pipelle catheter was studied as an alternative to curettage and found inferior. The sensitivity of obtaining chorionic villi ranged from 30 to 63 percent (Barnhart, 2003b; Ries, 2000). By comparison, frozen section of curettage fragments to identify products of conception is accurate in more than 90 percent of cases (Barak, 2005; Li, 2014b; Spandorfer, 1996).

■ Summary of Diagnostic Evaluation

Confirmation by diagnostic laparoscopy remains the gold standard for ectopic pregnancy diagnosis (Fig. 7-8). That said, with sensitive diagnostic modalities available, ectopic pregnancy can typically be diagnosed prior to surgery, and use of an evidence-based algorithm can assist. After appropriate clinical evaluation, all reproductive-aged women with any suspicion of pregnancy are tested using a sensitive urine β-hCG assay. Following positive testing, if an IUP is not confirmed by sonography, if no signs of acute intraabdominal hemorrhage are present, and if an ectopic gestation is suspected, then an evaluation such as the one depicted in Figure 7-9 may be used. Gracia and Barnhart (2001) performed a decision analysis of six diagnostic strategies

to evaluate which sequence of tests was most efficient in missing the fewest ectopic pregnancies and interrupting the fewest IUPs. They found the best strategy was to include TVS for all women with first-trimester pain or bleeding. If findings are not diagnostic, then serial serum β-hCG levels are measured. Using this strategy, only 1 percent of all potential IUPs were interrupted; no ectopic pregnancies were missed; and the average time to diagnosis was 1.46 days.

MANAGEMENT

Without intervention, an ectopic tubal pregnancy can lead to tubal abortion, tubal rupture, or spontaneous resolution. *Tubal abortion* is the expulsion of products through the fimbrial end. This tissue can then either regress or reimplant in the abdominal cavity. With reimplantation, bleeding or pain necessitating surgical intervention is a common complication. *Tubal rupture* is associated with significant intraabdominal hemorrhage. With *spontaneous resolution*, small ectopic pregnancies die and are resorbed without adverse patient effects. As with the ending of any early pregnancy, Rh status is assessed. If a woman is D negative and her partner has a blood group that is either D positive or unknown, then 300 μg anti-D immune globulin is given to prevent anti-D isoimmunization.

■ Medical Management

Medical therapy is preferred for most ectopic pregnancies, if feasible. Only methotrexate has been extensively studied as an alternative to surgical therapy. The best candidate for medical therapy is a woman who is asymptomatic and motivated and who has resources to be compliant with surveillance. Absolute contraindications for medical therapy with methotrexate include hemodynamic instability and those shown in Table 7-3 (American College of Obstetricians and Gynecologists, 2014; American Society for Reproductive Medicine, 2013). With medical therapy, some classic predictors of success are the initial serum β-hCG level, ectopic pregnancy size, and fetal cardiac activity.

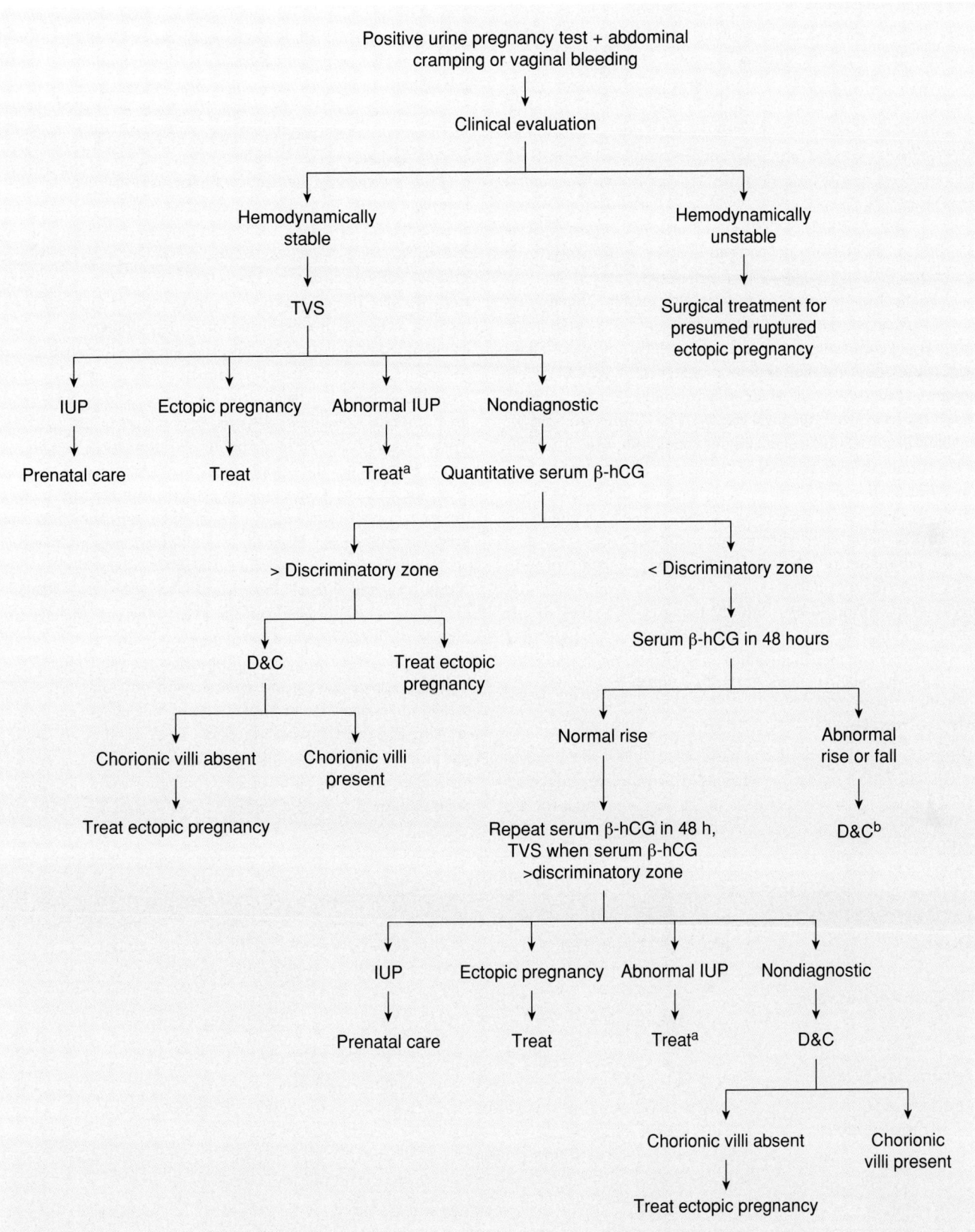

FIGURE 7-9 Algorithm of ectopic pregnancy evaluation.
[a]Abnormal IUPs may be treated by D & C, medical regimens, or expectant management as outlined in Chapter 6.
[b]Expectant management may be appropriate in a small select group of women with very low β-hCG levels that are dropping as described on page 173.
β-hCG = β-human chorionic gonadotropin; D & C = dilatation and curettage; IUP = intrauterine pregnancy; TVS = transvaginal sonography.

Of these, the β-hCG level is the single best prognostic indicator of treatment success in women given single-dose methotrexate. The prognostic value of the other two predictors may be directly related to their relationship with β-hCG concentrations. According to Lipscomb and colleagues (1999), an initial serum value <5000 IU/L was associated with a success rate of 92 percent, whereas an initial concentration >15,000 IU/L had a success rate of 68 percent. In another study, Menon and associates (2007) reported that compared with an initial serum β-hCG level of 2000 to 4999 IU/L, an initial serum β-hCG of 5000 to 9999 IU/L is nearly four times more likely to be associated with methotrexate therapy failure.

The effect of size on success rates with medical therapy has fewer supporting data, although many early trials used "large size" as an exclusion criterion. In one study, the success rate with single-dose methotrexate was 93 percent in cases with ectopic masses <3.5 cm, whereas success rates were between 87 and 90 percent when the mass was >3.5 cm (Lipscomb, 1998).

Identification of cardiac activity sonographically is a relative contraindication to medical therapy, although this is based on limited evidence. Most studies report an increased risk of failure if there is cardiac activity, however, a success rate of 87 percent has been reported (Lipscomb, 1998).

Of predictors of treatment failure, extrauterine yolk sac as a predictor of methotrexate failure has conflicting evidence (Lipscomb, 2009). Rapidly rising β-hCG levels both before (>50 percent) and during methotrexate therapy may also portend an increased failure risk (American Society for Reproductive Medicine, 2013; Dudley, 2004).

Methotrexate

This folic acid antagonist competitively inhibits the binding of dihydrofolic acid to the enzyme dihydrofolate reductase. This leads to reduced amounts of purines and thymidylate and thereby an arrest of DNA, RNA, and protein synthesis (Chap. 27, p. 596). It inhibits fast-growing tissue and is used for cancer chemotherapy and for early IUP termination. The drug can be given orally, intravenously, or intramuscularly (IM) or can be directly injected into the ectopic pregnancy sac. Currently, IM methotrexate administration is used most commonly for tubal ectopic pregnancies.

Prior to therapy, serum creatinine and β-hCG levels, a complete blood count, liver function tests, and blood type and Rh status are obtained (American Society for Reproductive Medicine, 2013). Moreover, all except blood typing are repeated prior to additional doses (Lipscomb, 2007). With administration, women are counseled to avoid the following until treatment is completed: folic acid-containing supplements, which can competitively reduce methotrexate binding to dihydrofolate reductase; nonsteroidal antiinflammatory drugs, which reduce renal blood flow and delay drug excretion; alcohol, which can predispose to concurrent hepatic enzyme elevation; sunlight, which can provoke methotrexate-related dermatitis; and coitus, which can rupture the ectopic pregnancy (American College of Obstetricians and Gynecologists, 2014). Importantly, methotrexate is a teratogen and is a Food and Drug Administration pregnancy category X. As such, it can lead to a profound embryopathy that includes intrauterine growth retardation and cardiac, craniofacial, and skeletal abnormalities (Nurmohamed, 2011).

The most common side effects of methotrexate include stomatitis, conjunctivitis, and transient liver dysfunction, although myelosuppression, mucositis, pulmonary damage, and anaphylactoid reactions have been reported with only one dose of 50 to 100 mg (Isaacs, 1996; Straka, 2004). Side effects are seen in as many as a third of women treated, however, they are usually self-limited. In some cases, leucovorin (folinic acid) is given following treatment to blunt or reverse methotrexate side effects. Such therapy is termed *leucovorin rescue* (Chap. 27, p. 597).

TABLE 7-3. Medical Treatment Protocols for Ectopic Pregnancy

	Single Dose	Multidose
Dosing	One dose; repeat if necessary	Up to four doses of both drugs until serum β-hCG level declines by 15%
Medication dosage		
Methotrexate	50 mg/m² BSA (day 1)	1 mg/kg, days 1, 3, 5, and 7
Leucovorin	NA	0.1 mg/kg days 2, 4, 6, and 8
Serum β-hCG level	Days 1, 4, and 7	Days 1, 3, 5, and 7
Indication for additional dose	• If serum β-hCG level does not decline by 15% from day 4 to day 7 • Less than 15% decline during weekly surveillance	If serum β-hCG level declines <15%, give additional dose; repeat serum β-hCG in 48 hours and compare with previous value; maximum four doses
Surveillance	Once 15% decline achieved, then weekly serum β-hCG levels until undetectable	

Methotrexate Contraindications		
Sensitivity to MTX	Intrauterine pregnancy	Peptic ulcer disease
Tubal rupture	Hepatic, renal, or hematologic dysfunction	Immunodeficiency
Breast feeding	Active pulmonary disease	

BSA = body surface area; β-hCG = β-human chorionic gonadotropin; NA = not applicable.

The single-dose and multidose methotrexate protocols shown in Table 7-3 are associated with overall resolution rates for ectopic pregnancy that approximate 90 percent. To date, Alleyassin and coworkers (2006) have completed the only randomized trial comparing single and multidose administrations. Although the study was underpowered to detect a small difference in success rates, they did observe that 89 percent in the single-dose group and 93 percent in the multidose group were successfully treated. When analyzed from the standpoint of treatment failure, single-dose therapy had a 50-percent higher failure rate compared with multidose therapy (6/54 versus 4/54). Lipscomb and colleagues (2005) reviewed their institutional experience with methotrexate therapy in 643 consecutively treated patients. They found no significant differences in treatment duration, serum β-hCG levels, or success rates between the multi- and single-dose protocols—95 and 90 percent, respectively. Barnhart and coworkers (2003a) performed a metaanalysis of 26 studies that included 1327 women treated with methotrexate for ectopic pregnancy. Single-dose therapy was more commonly used because of simplicity. It was less expensive, was easily accepted because of less intensive post-therapy monitoring, and did not require leucovorin rescue (Alexander, 1996). The major limitation was that multidose treatment had a fivefold greater chance of success than single-dose therapy. Failures included women with tubal rupture, massive intraabdominal hemorrhage, and need for urgent surgery and blood transfusions. Ultimately, most women received between one and four doses of methotrexate. Interestingly, the initial serum β-hCG value was not a valid indicator of how many doses of methotrexate a patient would need for a successful outcome (Nowak-Markwitz, 2009). In the absence of adequately powered randomized trials comparing single- with multidose therapy, we use single-dose IM methotrexate.

Single-Dose Methotrexate. This regimen is the most widely used medical treatment of ectopic pregnancy. Of various doses, the most popular is the 50 mg/m^2 body surface area (BSA) protocol (Stovall, 1993). BSA can be derived using various Internet-based BSA calculators such as: http://www.globalrph.com/bsa2.htm.

Close monitoring is imperative. A serum β-hCG level is determined prior to methotrexate administration and is repeated on days 4 and 7 following injection. Levels usually continue to rise until day 4. Comparison is then made between day 4 and 7 serum values. If there is a decline by 15 percent or more, then weekly serum β-hCG levels are drawn until they measure <2 IU/L. A decline of less than 15 percent is seen in approximately 20 percent of treated women. In such cases, a second 50 mg/m^2 dose is given, and the protocol is restarted. One review of more than 1700 cases showed that if a second dose is needed, then a day 1 serum β-hCG level <2234 IU/L could be considered a predictor of ultimate treatment success (Cohen, 2014). Approximate time to resolution for all women averages 36 days, but in some, treatment requires as long as 109 days (Lipscomb, 1998). Others have tried, without success, to develop more convenient serum β-hCG monitoring protocols (Kirk, 2007; Thurman, 2010). In the end, the original day-4-to-7 guidelines have been validated.

During the first few days following methotrexate administration, up to half of women experience abdominal pain that can be controlled with mild analgesics. This *separation pain* presumably results from tubal distention caused by tubal abortion or hematoma formation or both (Stovall, 1993). In some cases, inpatient observation with serial hematocrit determinations and gentle abdominal examinations help assess the need for surgical intervention.

Multidose Methotrexate. The most common regimen is seen in Table 7-3 and consists of up to four doses of parenteral methotrexate, followed by adjunctive doses of leucovorin 24 hours later. Serial serum β-hCG concentrations are obtained. If there is not a 15-percent decline from the previous value—for example, days 1 to 3—an additional methotrexate/leucovorin dose is given, and the serum β-hCG level is repeated 2 days later. A maximum of four doses are given, and weekly serum β-hCG level surveillance continues until values are undetectable.

A hybrid "two dose" protocol strives to balance the efficacy and convenience of the two most commonly used protocols (Barnhart, 2007). The regimen administers 50 mg/m^2 of methotrexate on days 0 and 4 without leucovorin rescue. Although the protocol is still considered experimental, no safety concerns were noted in the 101 patients treated, and the success rate approached 87 percent. A recent comparison of the single dose and "two dose" methotrexate protocols found equivalent success rates (87 and 90 percent, respectively) with a trend toward increased needs for repeated doses in the single-dose cohort (Gungorduk, 2011).

Other Medical Options

The bioavailability of oral and parenteral methotrexate is similar, but few trials have evaluated oral methotrexate for ectopic pregnancy treatment. Korhonen and coworkers (1996) randomly assigned women with candidate tubal pregnancies to be managed expectantly or to receive low-dose oral methotrexate, 2.5 mg daily for 5 days. They found no differences in primary treatment success.

Mifepristone is a progesterone antagonist and is effective for evacuation of first-trimester IUPs (Chap. 6, p. 154). Logically, the addition of mifepristone, 600 mg orally, to single-dose methotrexate might improve unruptured ectopic pregnancy resolution. However, in a randomized trial of 212 cases, success rates did not differ if mifepristone was added (Rozenberg, 2003).

Direct injection of methotrexate with sonographic or laparoscopic guidance into an ectopic pregnancy aims to minimize systemic side effects of methotrexate. Pharmacokinetic studies with 1 mg/kg of methotrexate injected either into the sac or by traditional IM injection showed similar success rates. However, fewer drug-related side effects were seen with local injection (Fernandez, 1995).

Direct injection of 50-percent glucose into the ectopic mass using laparoscopic guidance was 94-percent successful in one small prospective trial for women with serum β-hCG levels <2500 IU/L (Yeko, 1995). Gjelland and coworkers (1995) reported that the treatment success rate was significantly better in a similar population in which sonographically rather than laparoscopically guided injection was used.

Surveillance

Posttherapy monitoring assesses treatment success and screens for signs of persistent ectopic pregnancy. Most medical management protocols have well-defined surveillance schedules. In the absence of symptoms, bimanual examinations are deferred to avoid the theoretical risk of manual tubal rupture. Importantly, sonographic monitoring of ectopic mass dimensions can be misleading after serum β-hCG levels have declined to <15 IU/L. Brown and colleagues (1991) described persistent masses to be resolving hematomas rather than persistent trophoblastic tissue. For this reason, posttherapy sonography is reserved for suspected complications such as tubal rupture. Most recommend contraception for 3 to 6 months after successful medical therapy with methotrexate, as this drug may persist in human tissues for up to 8 months after a single dose (Warkany, 1978).

■ Surgical Management

Laparotomy versus Laparoscopy

At least three prospective studies have compared laparotomy with laparoscopic surgery for ectopic pregnancies (Lundorff, 1991; Murphy, 1992; Vermesh, 1989). In sum, investigators found no significant differences in overall tubal patency determined at second-look laparoscopy. This was despite higher rates of ipsilateral adhesions in the laparotomy group. Each method was followed by a similar number of subsequent intrauterine pregnancies. Fewer repeat ectopic pregnancies were noted in women treated laparoscopically, although this difference was not significant. Laparoscopy offered shorter operative times, less blood loss, fewer analgesic requirements, and shorter hospital stays. Laparoscopic surgery was significantly less successful in resolving the tubal pregnancy, but this was balanced by the just-mentioned benefits of minimally invasive surgery.

With improvements in laparoscopic equipment and with accrued experience, cases previously managed by laparotomy, such as ruptured tubal or intact interstitial pregnancies, can now be considered for laparoscopy in those with commensurate skills (Sagiv, 2001). Among experienced surgeons, shorter operating times and expedited hemorrhage control are both advantages of laparoscopic intervention for ruptured ectopic pregnancies (Cohen, 2013).

Laparotomy offers a potential advantage to laparoscopy if salpingostomy is planned. A metaanalysis using data from two trials concluded that compared with laparotomic salpingostomy, laparoscopic salpingostomy leads to one case of persistent trophoblastic disease for every 12 women undergoing the laparoscopic approach (Mol, 2008).

Laparoscopy

Two randomized trials have been completed to date to guide the choice between conservative—laparoscopic salpingostomy, and definitive—laparoscopic salpingectomy. The European Surgery in Ectopic Pregnancy (ESEP) study randomly assigned 446 women with a healthy contralateral fallopian tube to salpingectomy or salpingostomy (Mol, 2014). In the DEMETER trial

patients were also randomly selected for either of these surgeries. Similar to the ESEP study, results from the DEMETER trial showed no differences in 2-year subsequent IUP rates (64 versus 70 percent, respectively) whether salpingectomy or salpingostomy was used for ectopic pregnancy removal (Fernandez, 2013). Thus, if the contralateral fallopian tube appears normal, then salpingectomy is a reasonable treatment option that avoids the 5 to 8 percent complication rate caused by persistent or recurrent ectopic pregnancy in the same tube (Rulin, 1995).

For laparoscopic salpingectomy, many techniques have been described, and a surgical description is found in Section 44-3 (p. 1011). Lim and associates (2007) compared electrosurgical coagulation of the tube and mesosalpinx during laparoscopic salpingectomy with laparoscopic suture-loop (Endoloop) ligation. Endoloop use was associated with significantly shorter operating times (48 versus 61 minutes) and lower postoperative pain scores.

For laparoscopic salpingostomy, a woman who is hemodynamically stable and strongly desires to preserve fertility is an appropriate candidate. This applies especially if the other fallopian tube is absent or damaged. Serum β-hCG levels may be a factor in patient selection. One retrospective study found that ectopic resolution rates were lower following salpingostomy in women in whom the initial serum β-hCG level was >8000 IU/L (Milad, 1998). Supportive evidence for this comes from Natale and associates (2003), who reported that serum β-hCG levels >6000 IU/L have a high risk of implantation into the tubal muscularis.

As illustrated in Section 44-4 (p. 1013), during salpingostomy, the ectopic tissue can be flushed or grasped from the tubal incision. All free and tubal placental tissue should be meticulously removed, as retained trophoblast in the tube can lead to later invasion and bleeding. Other cases of persistent serum β-hCG levels are explained by trophoblastic tissue that is dropped during ectopic extraction and then subsequently implants intraabdominally (Bucella, 2009).

■ Medical versus Surgical Therapy

Several randomized trials have compared methotrexate treatment with laparoscopic surgery. One multicenter trial compared a multidose methotrexate protocol with laparoscopic salpingostomy and found no differences for tubal preservation and primary treatment success (Hajenius, 1997). However, in this same study group, health-related quality of life factors such as pain, posttherapy depression, and decreased perception of health were significantly impaired after systemic methotrexate compared with laparoscopic salpingostomy (Nieuwkerk, 1998).

Evidence is conflicting when single-dose methotrexate is compared with surgical intervention. In two separate studies, single-dose methotrexate was overall less successful in resolving pregnancy than laparoscopic salpingostomy, although tubal patency and subsequent uterine pregnancy rates were similar between both groups (Fernandez, 1998; Sowter, 2001). Krag Moeller and associates (2009) reported during a median surveillance period of 8.6 years that ectopic-resolution success rates were not significantly different between those managed surgically and those treated with methotrexate. Moreover, cumulative spontaneous intrauterine pregnancy rates were not different between the methotrexate group (73 percent) and the surgical group (62 percent).

Based on these studies, we conclude that women who are hemodynamically stable and in whom there is a small tubal diameter, no fetal cardiac activity, and serum β-hCG concentrations <5000 IU/L have similar outcomes with medical or surgical management. Despite lower success rates with medical therapy for women with larger tubal size, higher serum β-hCG levels, and fetal cardiac activity, medical management can be offered to the motivated woman who understands the risks of emergency surgery in the event of treatment failure.

■ Expectant Management

In select women, close observation, in anticipation that there will be spontaneous resorption of an ectopic pregnancy, is reasonable. Intuitively, it is difficult to accurately predict which woman will have an uncomplicated course with such management. Although an initial serum β-hCG concentration best predicts outcome, the range varies widely. For example, initial values <200 IU/L predict successful spontaneous resolution in 88 to 96 percent of attempts, whereas values >2000 IU/L had success rates of only 20 to 25 percent (Elson, 2004; Trio, 1995). Even with declining values, when the initial β-hCG level exceeded 2000 IU/L, the success rate was only 7 percent (Shalev, 1995). Interestingly, in this study, there was no difference in ipsilateral tubal patency or 1-year fertility rates with either success or failure of expectant management.

Close monitoring is warranted because the risk of tubal rupture persists despite low and declining serum β-hCG levels. An argument could be made that the minimal side effects of methotrexate make it preferable to a potentially prolonged surveillance and associated patient anxiety.

■ Persistent Ectopic Pregnancy

Incomplete eradication of trophoblastic tissue and its continued growth causes tubal rupture in 3 to 20 percent of women following conservative surgical or medical treatment of ectopic pregnancy (Graczykowski, 1999). Thus, abdominal pain following conservative management prompts immediate suspicion for persistent trophoblast proliferation.

Following salpingostomy, persistent ectopic pregnancy is more likely with very early pregnancies. Specifically, surgical management is more difficult because pregnancies smaller than 2 cm are harder to visualize and completely remove. To obviate this, Graczykowski and associates (1997) administered a prophylactic dose of 1 mg/m^2 methotrexate postoperatively, which reduced the incidence of persistent ectopic pregnancy and length of surveillance. Again, this is balanced against methotrexate side effects.

The optimal monitoring schedule to identify persistent ectopic pregnancy after surgical therapy has not been determined. Protocols describe serum β-hCG level monitoring from every 3 days to every 2 weeks. Spandorfer and associates (1997) estimated the risk of persistent ectopic pregnancy based on

serum β-hCG levels done on the first postoperative day after salpingostomy. They observed that if serum β-hCG levels fell by >50 percent compared with presurgical values, then there were no treatment failures within the first 9 days, and thus repeat serum β-hCG determinations 1 week after surgery were appropriate. Conversely, if serum levels fell by <50 percent, then there was a 3.5-fold increased risk of failure within the first week, thus necessitating earlier postoperative evaluation. Importantly, despite low and falling serum β-hCG concentrations, tubal rupture can still occur (Tulandi, 1991). Currently, standard therapy for persistent ectopic pregnancy is single-dose methotrexate given IM at a dose of 50 mg/m^2 BSA.

OVARIAN PREGNANCY

Ectopic implantation of the fertilized egg in the ovary is rare and is diagnosed if four clinical criteria are met. These were outlined by Spiegelberg (1878) and include: (1) the ipsilateral tube is intact and distinct from the ovary; (2) the ectopic pregnancy occupies the ovary; (3) the ectopic pregnancy is connected by the uteroovarian ligament to the uterus; and (4) ovarian tissue can be demonstrated histologically in the placental tissue. A more recent increased incidence in ovarian pregnancy likely is artifactual due to improved imaging. Risk factors are similar to those for tubal pregnancies. In one review, 24 percent of a total of 110 ovarian ectopic pregnancies were in IUD users (Ko, 2012). Nearly a third of women with an ovarian pregnancy present with hemodynamic instability because of rupture. Diagnosis is based on the classic sonographic description of a cyst with a wide echogenic outer ring on or within the ovary (Comstock, 2005). With smaller ectopic pregnancies, ovarian wedging can be considered (Ko, 2012). For larger lesions, oophorectomy is often required.

INTERSTITIAL PREGNANCY

Interstitial pregnancies implant in the proximal tubal segment that lies within the muscular uterine wall. Swelling lateral to the insertion of the round ligament is the characteristic anatomic finding (Fig. 7-10). Incorrectly, these are sometimes called cornual pregnancies, but this term describes conceptions that develop in the horns of uteri with müllerian anomalies (Lau, 1999; Moawad, 2010). In the past, interstitial pregnancies usually ruptured following 8 to 16 weeks of amenorrhea. This later gestational age at rupture is attributed to the greater distensibility of the myometrium covering the fallopian tube's interstitial segment. Risk factors are similar to others discussed, although prior ipsilateral salpingectomy is a specific risk factor for interstitial pregnancy (Lau, 1999). Because of the proximity of these pregnancies to the uterine and ovarian arteries, hemorrhage with rupture can be severe and is associated with mortality rates as high as 2.5 percent (Tulandi, 2004).

Distinct from interstitial pregnancy, the term *angular pregnancy* describes intrauterine implantation in one of the lateral angles of the uterus and medial to the uterotubal junction and round ligament. This distinction is important because angular pregnancies can sometimes be carried to term but with increased

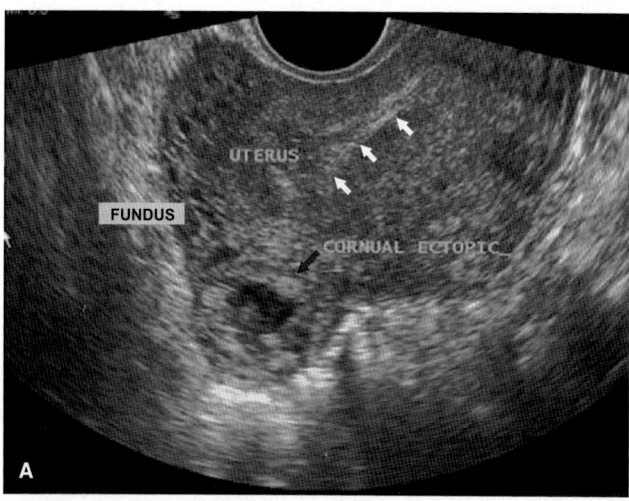
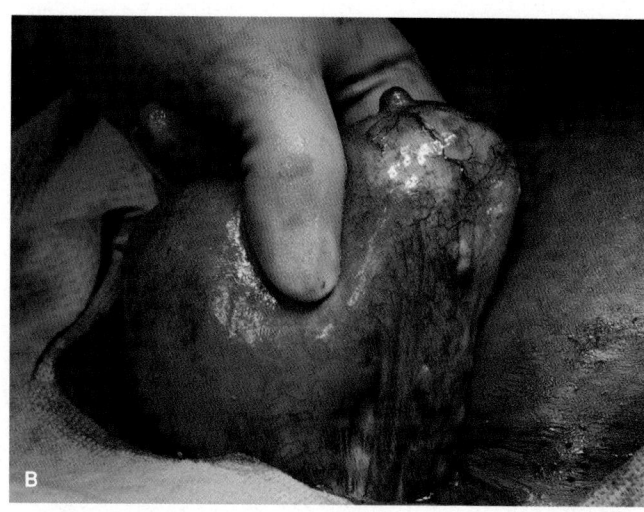

FIGURE 7-10 Interstitial pregnancy. **A.** Transvaginal sonogram, parasagittal view shows an empty uterine cavity (*white arrows*) and a mass lateral to the uterine fundus (*red arrow*). (Used with permission from Dr. Elysia Moschos.) **B.** Left-sided interstitial pregnancy prior to resection. (Used with permission from Dr. Mario Castellanos.)

risk of abnormal placentation and uterine rupture (Arleo, 2014; Jansen, 1981). Improved imaging modalities, such as 3-dimensional sonography, may help differentiate eccentrically located gestational sacs from an interstitial pregnancy (Singh, 2015; Tanaka, 2014).

For interstitial pregnancies, surgical management involves cornual resection by either laparotomy or laparoscopy (Section 43-9, p. 941). As discussed for suspected tubal pregnancy, interstitial pregnancy can now often be diagnosed early enough to consider conservative medical therapy (Bernstein, 2001). Given its low incidence, no consensus regarding prediction of success using methotrexate has been established. Jermy and colleagues (2004) reported a 94-percent success with systemic methotrexate in 17 women using a dose of 50 mg/m^2 BSA. Their series included four women in whom fetal cardiac activity was verified. Because these women have higher initial serum β-hCG levels at diagnosis, longer surveillance is usually needed. Deruelle and coworkers (2005) advocate adjuvant postmethotrexate uterine artery embolization to help avert hemorrhage and hasten ectopic pregnancy resolution. Of other therapies, uterine artery methotrexate infusion and embolization combined with systemic methotrexate has shown promising results (Hiersch, 2014; Krissi, 2014). Hysteroscopic resection or transcervical suction curettage of interstitial pregnancies has been described (Sanz, 2002; Zhang, 2004).

Following either medical or conservative surgical management, the risk of uterine rupture with subsequent pregnancies is unclear. Thus, careful observation of these women during pregnancy, along with strong consideration of elective cesarean delivery, is warranted.

CERVICAL PREGNANCY

The incidence of cervical pregnancy is reported to be between 1 in 8600 and 1 in 12,400 pregnancies (Ushakov, 1997). The incidence appears to be rising because of ART, especially IVF and embryo transfer (Ginsburg, 1994; Pattinson, 1994). A risk factor unique to cervical pregnancy is a history of dilatation and curettage in a prior pregnancy and is seen in nearly 70 percent of cases (Hung, 1996; Pisarska, 1999). Two diagnostic criteria are necessary for cervical pregnancy confirmation: (1) cervical glands are found opposite the placental attachment site, and (2) a portion of or the entire placenta is located below either the entrance of the uterine vessels or the peritoneal reflection on the anterior and posterior uterine surface (Fig. 7-11).

For most hemodynamically stable women with a first-trimester cervical pregnancy, nonsurgical management with systemic methotrexate can be offered and administered as in Table 7-3. Jeng and colleagues (2007) also described 38 cases successfully treated with methotrexate injection into the gestational sac. Resolution and uterine preservation is achieved with methotrexate regimens for gestations <12 weeks in 91 percent of cases (Kung, 1997). In selecting appropriate candidates, Hung and colleagues (1996) noted higher risks of systemic methotrexate treatment failure in those with a gestational age >9 weeks, β-hCG levels >10,000 IU/L, crown-rump length >10 mm, and fetal cardiac activity. For this reason, many induce fetal death with intracardiac or intrathoracic injection of potassium chloride (Jeng, 2007; Verma, 2009). Uterine artery embolization, either before or after methotrexate administration, may be an additional adjunct to limit bleeding complications (Cipullo, 2008; Hirakawa, 2009).

Although conservative management is feasible for many women with cervical pregnancies, surgical intervention may also be selected. Procedures include suction curettage or hysterectomy. Moreover, in those with advanced gestations or with bleeding uncontrolled by conservative methods, hysterectomy is typically required. Importantly, patients should understand the increased risk of urinary tract injury with hysterectomy due to the close proximity of the ureters to the ballooned cervix. Prior to either procedure, uterine artery embolization may be considered to limit intra- and postoperative bleeding (Nakao, 2008; Trambert, 2005). In addition, before curettage, local methotrexate injection into the amnionic sac, ligation of the descending branches of the uterine arteries, or cerclage placement at the internal os to compress feeding vessels have all been

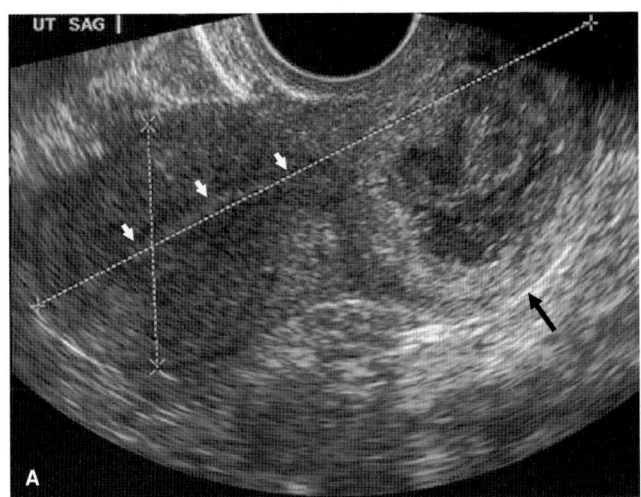

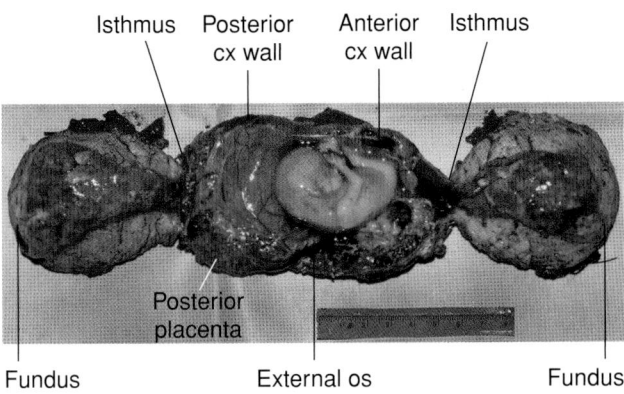

FIGURE 7-11 Cervical pregnancy. **A.** Transvaginal sonography, sagittal view of a cervical pregnancy. Sonographic findings with cervical pregnancy may include: (1) an hourglass uterine shape and ballooned cervical canal; (2) gestational tissue at the level of the cervix (*black arrow*); (3) absent intrauterine gestational tissue (*white arrows*); and (4) a portion of the endocervical canal seen interposed between the gestation and the endometrial canal. (Used with permission from Dr. Elysia Moschos.) **B.** Hysterectomy specimen containing a cervical ectopic pregnancy from a different case. (Used with permission from Dr. David Rahn.)

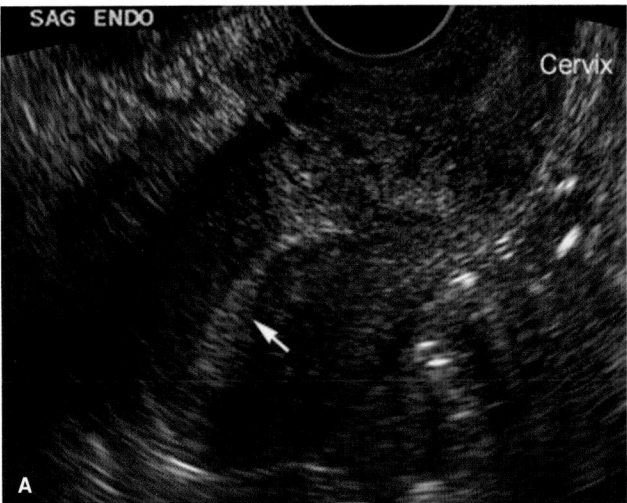

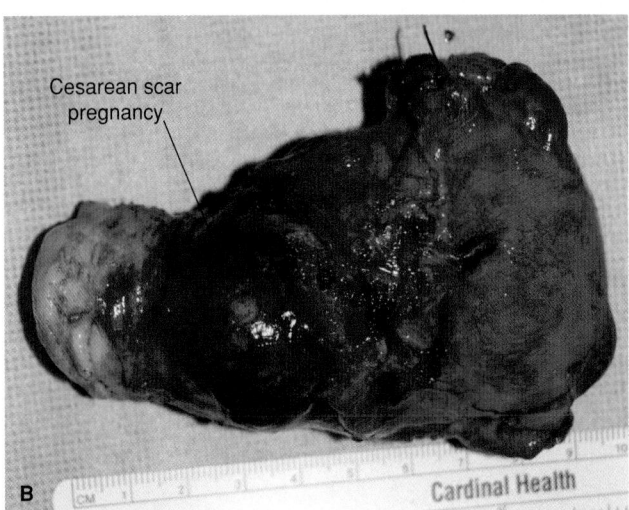

FIGURE 7-12 Cesarean scar pregnancy. **A.** Transvaginal sonogram of a uterus with a cesarean scar pregnancy (CSP) in a sagittal plane. The diagnosis is suggested by sonographic criteria indicative of CSP. First, an empty uterine cavity is identified by a bright hyperechoic endometrial stripe (*white arrow*). An empty cervical canal is similarly identified. Last, an intrauterine mass is seen in the anterior part of the uterine isthmus (*red arrows*). (Used with permission from Dr. Elysia Moschos.) **B.** Hysterectomy specimen containing a cesarean scar pregnancy. (Used with permission from Dr. Sunil Balgobin.)

described (Davis, 2008; De La Vega, 2007; Mesogitis, 2005; Trojano, 2009). Following curettage, in the event of hemorrhage, a 26F Foley catheter with a 30-mL balloon can be placed intracervically and inflated to effect hemostasis and to monitor uterine drainage (Ushakov, 1997). In addition, uterine artery embolization may be considered.

HETEROTOPIC PREGNANCY

A uterine pregnancy in conjunction with an extrauterine pregnancy is termed a *heterotopic pregnancy*. In the past, the incidence was estimated to be 1 in 30,000 pregnancies. In pregnancies resulting from ART, the heterotopic pregnancies rate approximates 0.09 percent (Perkins, 2015). For a tubal pregnancy coexistent with a uterine pregnancy, potassium chloride can be injected into the tubal pregnancy sac. Methotrexate is contraindicated due to the detrimental effects on the normal pregnancy (p. 170).

CESAREAN SCAR PREGNANCY

Implantation within the scar of a prior cesarean delivery through a microscopic tract in the myometrium is uncommon (Fig. 7-12). Similar to other ectopic pregnancies, it carries significant risks of massive hemorrhage. Reviews cite the incidence of cesarean scar pregnancy (CSP) to approximate 1 in 2000 pregnancies (Sadeghi, 2010). These microscopic tracts can also stem from other prior uterine surgery—curettage, myomectomy, operative hysteroscopy—and perhaps from manual removal of the placenta (Ash, 2007).

Differentiating between a pregnancy with low implantation and a cesarean scar pregnancy can be difficult, and several investigators have described sonographic findings (Jurkovic, 2003;

Moschos, 2008a). According to Godin (1997), four sonographic criteria should be satisfied for the diagnosis: (1) an empty uterine cavity, (2) an empty cervical canal, (3) a gestational sac in the anterior part of the uterine isthmus, and (4) absence of healthy myometrium between the bladder and gestational sac.

Treatment standards are lacking, but options include systemic or locally injected methotrexate, either alone or combined with suction curettage or hysteroscopic removal (Shen, 2012; Timor-Tritsch, 2012; Yang, 2010). Isthmic resection with a double layer closure can be performed open, laparoscopically, or robotically (Hudecek, 2014). With any of the options, uterine artery embolization may be used adjunctively to minimize hemorrhage (Zhuang, 2009). In most cases, the uterus can be preserved, although hysterectomy is also an acceptable and sometimes necessary option (Sadeghi, 2010).

OTHER ECTOPIC PREGNANCY SITES

Abdominal pregnancy is an implantation in the peritoneal cavity exclusive of tubal, ovarian, or intraligamentous implantations. These are rare and have an estimated incidence of 1 in 10,000 to 25,000 live births (Atrash, 1987; Worley, 2008). Ectopic placental implantations in less expected sites have been described in case reports and include the omentum, spleen, liver, and retroperitoneum, among others (Chin, 2010; Chopra, 2009; Gang, 2010; Martínez-Varea, 2011). Also rare, ectopic pregnancies have been reported in women with prior hysterectomy (Fylstra, 2010). Presumably, a vaginal cuff fistula, a prolapsed fallopian tube, or a cervical stump after supracervical hysterectomy allows sperm to access an ovulated ovum.

PREVENTION

Prevention is difficult because few ectopic pregnancy risk factors are modifiable (Butts, 2003). Tubal pathology carries one of the highest risks, and pelvic inflammatory disease (PID) plays a major role in tubal adhesions and obstruction. Chlamydial infections constitute nearly half of PID cases, thus efforts have been directed toward screening high-risk populations for asymptomatic infections. These include sexually active women <25 years or women with risk factors (Table 1-1, p. 6). Such screening programs in Sweden have demonstrated steady declines in both chlamydial infections and ectopic pregnancy rates, especially in women aged 20 to 24 years (Cates, 1999; Egger, 1998).

REFERENCES

al-Awwad MM, al Daham N, Eseet JS: Spontaneous unruptured bilateral ectopic pregnancy: conservative tubal surgery. Obstet Gynecol Surv 54:543, 1999

Alexander JM, Rouse DJ, Varner E, et al: Treatment of the small unruptured ectopic pregnancy: a cost analysis of methotrexate versus laparoscopy. Obstet Gynecol 88:123, 1996

Alleyassin A, Khademi A, Aghahosseini M, et al: Comparison of success rates in the medical management of ectopic pregnancy with single-dose and multiple-dose administration of methotrexate: a prospective, randomized clinical trial. Fertil Steril 85(6):1661, 2006

American College of Obstetricians and Gynecologists: Medical management of ectopic pregnancy. Practice Bulletin No. 94, 2008, Reaffirmed 2014

American Society for Reproductive Medicine: Medical treatment of ectopic pregnancy: a committee opinion. Fertil Steril 100(3):638, 2013

Ankum WM, Mol BW, Van der Veen F, et al: Risk factors for ectopic pregnancy: a meta-analysis. Fertil Steril 65:1093, 1996

Arleo EK, DeFilippis EM: Cornual, interstitial, and angular pregnancies: clarifying the terms and a review of the literature. Clin Imaging 38(6):763, 2014

Ash A, Smith A, Maxwell D: Caesarean scar pregnancy. BJOG 114(3):253, 2007

Atrash HK, Friede A, Hogue CJ: Abdominal pregnancy in the United States: frequency and maternal mortality. Obstet Gynecol 69:333, 1987

Atri M: Ectopic pregnancy versus corpus luteum cyst revisited: best Doppler predictors. J Ultrasound Med 22:1181, 2003

Barak S, Oettinger M, Perri A, et al: Frozen section examination of endometrial curettings in the diagnosis of ectopic pregnancy. Acta Obstet Gynecol Scand 84:43, 2005

Barnhart K, Hummel AC, Sammel MD, et al: Use of "2-dose" regimen of methotrexate to treat ectopic pregnancy. Fertil Steril 87(2):250, 2007

Barnhart K, Sammel MD, Chung K, et al: Decline of serum human chorionic gonadotropin and spontaneous complete abortion: defining the normal curve. Obstet Gynecol 104:975, 2004

Barnhart K, van Mello NM, Bourne T, et al: Pregnancy of unknown location: a consensus statement of nomenclature, definitions, and outcome. Fertil Steril 95(3):857, 2011

Barnhart KT, Gosman G, Ashby R, et al: The medical management of ectopic pregnancy: a meta-analysis comparing "single dose" and "multidose" regimens. Obstet Gynecol 101:778, 2003a

Barnhart KT, Gracia CR, Reindl B, et al: Usefulness of Pipelle endometrial biopsy in the diagnosis of women at risk for ectopic pregnancy. Am J Obstet Gynecol 188:906, 2003b

Barnhart KT, Katz I, Hummel A, et al: Presumed diagnosis of ectopic pregnancy. Obstet Gynecol 100:505, 2002

Barnhart KT, Rinaudo P, Hummel A, et al: Acute and chronic presentation of ectopic pregnancy may be two clinical entities. Fertil Steril 80:1345, 2003c

Barnhart KT, Sammel MD, Gracia CR, et al: Risk factors for ectopic pregnancy in women with symptomatic first-trimester pregnancies. Fertil Steril 86(1):36, 2006

Barnhart KT, Simhan H, Kamelle SA: Diagnostic accuracy of ultrasound above and below the beta-hCG discriminatory zone. Obstet Gynecol 94:583, 1999

Bernstein HB, Thrall MM, Clark WB: Expectant management of intramural ectopic pregnancy. Obstet Gynecol 97:826, 2001

Birkhahn RH, Gaeta TJ, Van Deusen SK, et al: The ability of traditional vital signs and shock index to identify ruptured ectopic pregnancy. Am J Obstet Gynecol 189:1293, 2003

Bouyer J, Coste J, Fernandez H, et al: Sites of ectopic pregnancy: a 10 year population-based study of 1800 cases. Hum Reprod 17:3224, 2002

Bouyer J, Coste J, Shojaei T, et al: Risk factors for ectopic pregnancy: a comprehensive analysis based on a large case-control, population-based study in France. Am J Epidemiol 157:185, 2003

Branney SW, Wolfe RE, Moore EE, et al: Quantitative sensitivity of ultrasound in detecting free intraperitoneal fluid. J Trauma 40(6):1052, 1995

Brown DL, Doubilet PM: Transvaginal sonography for diagnosing ectopic pregnancy: positivity criteria and performance characteristics. J Ultrasound Med 13:259, 1994

Brown DL, Felker RE, Stovall TG, et al: Serial endovaginal sonography of ectopic pregnancies treated with methotrexate. Obstet Gynecol 77:406, 1991

Bucella D, Buxant F, Anaf V, et al: Omental trophoblastic implants after surgical management of ectopic pregnancy. Arch Gynecol Obstet 280(1):115, 2009

Burry KA, Thurmond AS, Suby-Long TD, et al: Transvaginal ultrasonographic findings in surgically verified ectopic pregnancy. Am J Obstet Gynecol 168:1796, 1993

Buster JE, Pisarska MD: Medical management of ectopic pregnancy. Clin Obstet Gynecol 42:23, 1999

Butts S, Sammel M, Hummel A, et al: Risk factors and clinical features of recurrent ectopic pregnancy: a case control study. Fertil Steril 80:1340, 2003

Cates W Jr: Chlamydial infections and the risk of ectopic pregnancy. JAMA 281:117, 1999

Chin PS, Wee HY, Chern BS: Laparoscopic management of primary hepatic pregnancy. Aust N Z J Obstet Gynaecol 50(1):95, 2010

Chopra S, Keepanasseril A, Suri V, et al: Primary omental pregnancy: case report and review of literature. Arch Gynecol Obstet 279(4):441, 2009

Chung K, Chandavarkar U, Opper N, et al: Reevaluating the role of dilation and curettage in the diagnosis of pregnancy of unknown location. Fertil Steril 96(3):659, 2011

Cipullo L, Cassese S, Fasolino MC, et al: Cervical pregnancy: a case series and a review of current clinical practice. Eur J Contracept Reprod Health Care 13(3):313, 2008

Cohen A, Almog B, Satel A, et al: Laparoscopy versus laparotomy in the management of ectopic pregnancy with massive hemoperitoneum. Int J Gynaecol Obstet 123(2):139, 2013

Cohen A, Bibi G, Almog B, Tsafrir Z, et al: Second-dose methotrexate in ectopic pregnancies: the role of beta human chorionic gonadotropin. Fertil Steril 102(6):1646, 2014

Cole T, Corlett RC Jr: Chronic ectopic pregnancy. Obstet Gynecol 59(1):63, 1982

Comstock C, Huston K, Lee W: The ultrasonographic appearance of ovarian ectopic pregnancies. Obstet Gynecol 105:42, 2005

Condous G, Okaro E, Khalid A, et al: The accuracy of transvaginal ultrasonography for the diagnosis of ectopic pregnancy prior to surgery. Hum Reprod 20(5):1404, 2005

Connolly A, Ryan DH, Stuebe AM, et al: Reevaluation of discriminatory and threshold levels for serum ⊠-hCG in early pregnancy. Obstet Gynecol 121(1):65, 2013

Coste J, Fernandez H, Joye N, et al: Role of chromosome abnormalities in ectopic pregnancy. Fertil Steril 74:1259, 2000

Creanga AA, Shapiro-Mendoza CK, Bish CL, et al: Trends in ectopic pregnancy mortality in the United States: 1980–2007. Obstet Gynecol 117(4):837, 2011

Cunningham FG, Leveno KJ, Bloom SL (eds): Ectopic pregnancy. In Williams Obstetrics, 24th ed. New York, McGraw-Hill Education, 2014

Dashefsky SM, Lyons EA, Levi CS, et al: Suspected ectopic pregnancy: endovaginal and transvesical US. Radiology 169:181, 1988

Davis LB, Lathi RB, Milki AA, et al: Transvaginal ligation of the cervical branches of the uterine artery and injection of vasopressin in a cervical pregnancy as an initial step to controlling hemorrhage: a case report. J Reprod Med 53(5):365, 2008

De La Vega GA, Avery C, Nemiroff, et al: Treatment of early cervical pregnancy with cerclage, carboprost, curettage, and balloon tamponade. Obstet Gynecol 109(2 Pt 2):505, 2007

Deruelle P, Lucot JP, Lions C, et al: Management of interstitial pregnancy using selective uterine artery embolization. Obstet Gynecol 106:1165, 2005

Dixon RE, Hwang SJ, Hennig GW, et al: *Chlamydia* infection causes loss of pacemaker cells and inhibits oocyte transport in the mouse oviduct. Biol Reprod 80(4):665, 2009

Dudley PS, Heard MJ, Sangi-Haghpeykar H, et al: Characterizing ectopic pregnancies that rupture despite treatment with methotrexate. Fertil Steril 82(5):1374, 2004

Egger M, Low N, Smith GD, et al: Screening for chlamydial infections and the risk of ectopic pregnancy in a county in Sweden: ecological analysis. BMJ 316:1776, 1998

Elson J, Tailor A, Banerjee S, et al: Expectant management of tubal ectopic pregnancy: prediction of successful outcome using decision tree analysis. Ultrasound Obstet Gynecol 23:552, 2004

Erol O, Suren D, Unal B, et al: Significance of trophoblastic infiltration into the tubal wall in ampullary pregnancy. Int J Surg Pathol 23(4):271, 2015

Fang C, Huang R, Wei LN, et al: Frozen-thawed day 5 blastocyst transfer is associated with a lower risk of ectopic pregnancy than day 3 transfer and fresh transfer. Fertil Steril 103(3):655, 2015

Fernandez H, Capmas P, Lucot JP, et al: Fertility after ectopic pregnancy: the DEMETER randomized trial. Human Reprod 28(5):1247, 2013

Fernandez H, Pauthier S, Doumerc S, et al: Ultrasound-guided injection of methotrexate versus laparoscopic salpingotomy in ectopic pregnancy. Fertil Steril 63:25, 1995

Fernandez H, Yves Vincent SC, Pauthier S, et al: Randomized trial of conservative laparoscopic treatment and methotrexate administration in ectopic pregnancy and subsequent fertility. Hum Reprod 13:3239, 1998

Fylstra DL: Ectopic pregnancy after hysterectomy: a review and insight into etiology and prevention. Fertil Steril 94(2):431, 2010

Gang G, Yudong Y, Zhang G: Successful laparoscopic management of early splenic pregnancy: case report and review of literature. J Minim Invasive Gynecol 17(6):794, 2010

Ginsburg ES, Frates MC, Rein MS, et al: Early diagnosis and treatment of cervical pregnancy in an in vitro fertilization program. Fertil Steril 61:966, 1994

Gjelland K, Hordnes K, Tjugum J, et al: Treatment of ectopic pregnancy by local injection of hypertonic glucose: a randomized trial comparing administration guided by transvaginal ultrasound or laparoscopy. Acta Obstet Gynecol Scand 74:629, 1995

Glezerman M, Press F, Carpman M: Culdocentesis is an obsolete diagnostic tool in suspected ectopic pregnancy. Arch Gynecol Obstet 252:5, 1992

Godin PA, Bassil S, Donnez J: An ectopic pregnancy developing in a previous caesarian section scar. Fertil Steril 67:398, 1997

Goldner TE, Lawson HW, Xia Z, et al: Surveillance for ectopic pregnancy—United States, 1970–1989. MMWR 42:73, 1993

Gracia CR, Barnhart KT: Diagnosing ectopic pregnancy: decision analysis comparing six strategies. Obstet Gynecol 97:464, 2001

Graczykowski JW, Mishell DR Jr: Methotrexate prophylaxis for persistent ectopic pregnancy after conservative treatment by salpingostomy. Obstet Gynecol 89:118, 1997

Graczykowski JW, Seifer DB: Diagnosis of acute and persistent ectopic pregnancy. Clin Obstet Gynecol 42:9, 1999

Guha S, Ayim F, Ludlow J, et al: Triaging pregnancies of unknown location: the performance of protocols based on single serum progesterone or repeated serum hCG levels. Human Reprod 29(5):938, 2014

Gungorduk K, Asicioglu O, Yildirim G, et al: Comparison of single-dose and two-dose methotrexate protocols for the treatment of unruptured ectopic pregnancy. J Obstet Gynaecol 31(4):330, 2011

Gurel S, Sarikaya B, Gurel K, et al: Role of sonography in the diagnosis of ectopic pregnancy. J Clin Ultrasound 35(9):509, 2007

Hajenius PJ, Engelsbel S, Mol BW, et al: Randomised trial of systemic methotrexate versus laparoscopic salpingostomy in tubal pregnancy. Lancet 350:774, 1997

Hammoud AO, Hammoud I, Bujold E, et al: The role of sonographic endometrial patterns and endometrial thickness in the differential diagnosis of ectopic pregnancy. Am J Obstet Gynecol 192:1370, 2005

Heinemann K, Reed S, Moehner S, et al: Comparative contraceptive effectiveness of levonorgestrel-releasing and copper intrauterine devices: the European Active Surveillance Study for Intrauterine Devices. Contraception 91(4):280, 2015

Hiersch L, Krissi H, Ashwal E, et al: Effectiveness of medical treatment with methotrexate for interstitial pregnancy. Aust N Z J Obstet Gynaecol 54(6):576, 2014

Hillis SD, Owens LM, Marchbanks PA, et al: Recurrent chlamydial infections increase the risks of hospitalization for ectopic pregnancy and pelvic inflammatory disease. Am J Obstet Gynecol 176:103, 1997

Hirakawa M, Tajima T, Yoshimitsu K, et al: Uterine artery embolization along with the administration of methotrexate for cervical ectopic pregnancy: technical and clinical outcomes. AJR 192(6):1601, 2009

Hoover KW, Tao G, Kent CK: Trends in the diagnosis and treatment of ectopic pregnancy in the United States. Obstet Gynecol 115(3):495, 2010

Horne AW, Phillips JA III, Kane N, et al: CB1 expression is attenuated in fallopian tube and decidua of women with ectopic pregnancy. PLoS One 3(12):e3969, 2008

Huang B, Hu D, Qian K, et al: Is frozen embryo transfer cycle associated with a significantly lower incidence of ectopic pregnancy? An analysis of more than 30,000 cycles. Fertil Steril 102(5):1345, 2014

Hudecek R, Felsingerova Z, Felsinger M, et al: Laparoscopic treatment of cesarean scar ectopic pregnancy. J Gynecol Surg 30(5):309, 2014

Hung TH, Jeng CJ, Yang YC, et al: Treatment of cervical pregnancy with methotrexate. Int J Gynaecol Obstet 53:243, 1996

Isaacs JD Jr, McGehee RP, Cowan BD: Life-threatening neutropenia following methotrexate treatment of ectopic pregnancy: a report of two cases. Obstet Gynecol 88:694, 1996

Jansen RP, Elliott PM: Angular intrauterine pregnancy. Obstet Gynecol 58(2):167, 1981

Jeng CJ, Ko ML, Shen J: Transvaginal ultrasound-guided treatment of cervical pregnancy. Obstet Gynecol 109(5):1076, 2007

Jermy K, Thomas J, Doo A, et al: The conservative management of interstitial pregnancy. BJOG 111:1283, 2004

Job-Spira N, Fernandez H, Bouyer J, et al: Ruptured tubal ectopic pregnancy: risk factors and reproductive outcome: results of a population-based study in France. Am J Obstet Gynecol 180:938, 1999

Jurkovic D, Hillaby K, Woelfer B, et al: First-trimester diagnosis and management of pregnancies implanted into the lower uterine segment cesarean section scar. Ultrasound Obstet Gynecol 21(3):220, 2003

Kadar N, DeCherney AH, Romero R: Receiver operating characteristic (ROC) curve analysis of the relative efficacy of single and serial chorionic gonadotropin determinations in the early diagnosis of ectopic pregnancy. Fertil Steril 37:542, 1982

Kirk E, Condous G, Van Calster B, et al: A validation of the most commonly used protocol to predict the success of single-dose methotrexate in the treatment of ectopic pregnancy. Hum Reprod 22(3):858, 2007

Ko JK, Cheung VY: Time to revisit the human chorionic gonadotropin discriminatory level in the management of pregnancy of unknown location. J Ultrasound Med 33(3):465, 2014

Ko PC, Lo LM, Hsieh TT, et al: Twenty-one years of experience with ovarian ectopic pregnancy at one institution in Taiwan. Int J Gynaecol Obstet 119(2):154, 2012

Korhonen J, Stenman UH, Ylostalo P: Low-dose oral methotrexate with expectant management of ectopic pregnancy. Obstet Gynecol 88:775, 1996

Krag Moeller LB, Moeller C, Thomsen SG, et al: Success and spontaneous pregnancy rates following systemic methotrexate versus laparoscopic surgery for tubal pregnancies: a randomized trial. Acta Obstet Gynecol Scand 88(12):1331, 2009

Krissi H, Hiersch L, Stolovitch N, et al: Outcome, complications and future fertility in women treated with uterine artery embolization and methotrexate for non-tubal ectopic pregnancy. Eur J Obstet Gynecol Reprod Biol 182:172, 2014

Kung FT, Chang SY, Tsai YC, et al: Subsequent reproduction and obstetric outcome after methotrexate treatment of cervical pregnancy: a review of original literature and international collaborative follow-up. Hum Reprod 12:591, 1997

Kutluay L, Vicdan K, Turan C, et al: Tubal histopathology in ectopic pregnancies. Eur J Obstet Gynecol Reprod Biol 57:91, 1994

Lau S, Tulandi T: Conservative medical and surgical management of interstitial ectopic pregnancy. Fertil Steril 72:207, 1999

Lavie O, Boldes R, Neuman M, et al: Ultrasonographic "endometrial three-layer" pattern: a unique finding in ectopic pregnancy. J Clin Ultrasound 24(4):179, 1996

Levine D: Ectopic pregnancy. Radiology 245(2):385, 2007

Li C, Zhao WH, Meng CX, et al: Contraceptive use and the risk of ectopic pregnancy: a multi-center case-control study. PLoS One 9(12):e115031, 2014a

Li Y, Yang Y, He QZ, et al: Frozen section of uterine curetting in excluding the possibility of ectopic pregnancy—a clinicopathologic study of 715 cases. Clin Exp Obstet Gynecol 41(4):419, 2014b

Lim YH, Ng SP, Ng PH, et al: Laparoscopic salpingectomy in tubal pregnancy: prospective randomized trial using Endoloop versus electrocautery. J Obstet Gynaecol Res 33(6):855, 2007

Lipscomb GH: Medical therapy for ectopic pregnancy. Semin Reprod Med 25(2):93, 2007

Lipscomb GH, Bran D, McCord ML, et al: Analysis of three hundred fifteen ectopic pregnancies treated with single-dose methotrexate. Am J Obstet Gynecol 178:1354, 1998

Lipscomb GH, Givens VM, Meyer NL, et al: Comparison of multidose and single-dose methotrexate protocols for the treatment of ectopic pregnancy. Am J Obstet Gynecol 192:1844, 2005

Lipscomb GH, Gomez IG, Givens VM, et al: Yolk sac on transvaginal ultrasound as a prognostic indicator in the treatment of ectopic pregnancy with single-dose methotrexate. Am J Obstet Gynecol 200(3):338.e1, 2009

Lipscomb GH, McCord ML, Stovall TG, et al: Predictors of success of methotrexate treatment in women with tubal ectopic pregnancies. N Engl J Med 341:1974, 1999

Ljubin-Sternak S, Mestrovic T: *Chlamydia trachomatis* and genital mycoplasmas: pathogens with an impact on human reproductive health. J Pathog 2014:183167, 2014

Lopez HB, Micheelsen U, Berendtsen H, et al: Ectopic pregnancy and its associated endometrial changes. Gynecol Obstet Invest 38:104, 1994

Lundorff P, Thorburn J, Hahlin M, et al: Laparoscopic surgery in ectopic pregnancy. A randomized trial versus laparotomy. Acta Obstet Gynecol Scand 70:343, 1991

Malacova E, Kemp A, Hart R, et al: Long-term risk of ectopic pregnancy varies by method of tubal sterilization: a whole-population study. Fertil Steril 101(3):728, 2014

Martínez-Varea A, Hidalgo-Mora JJ, Payá V, et al: Retroperitoneal ectopic pregnancy after intrauterine insemination. Fertil Steril 95(7):2433.e1, 2011

Menon S, Collins J, Barnhart KT: Establishing a human chorionic gonadotropin cutoff to guide methotrexate treatment of ectopic pregnancy: a systematic review. Fertil Steril 87(3):481, 2007

Mesogitis S, Pilalis A, Daskalakis G, et al: Management of early viable cervical pregnancy. BJOG 112:409, 2005

Milad MP, Klein E, Kazer RR: Preoperative serum hCG level and intraoperative failure of laparoscopic linear salpingostomy for ectopic pregnancy. Obstet Gynecol 92:373, 1998

Moawad NS, Mahajan ST, Moniz MH, et al: Current diagnosis and treatment of interstitial pregnancy. Am J Obstet Gynecol 202(1):15, 2010

Mol BW, Lijmer JG, Ankum WM, et al: The accuracy of single serum progesterone measurement in the diagnosis of ectopic pregnancy: a meta-analysis. Hum Reprod 13:3220, 1998

Mol F, Mol BW, Ankum WM, et al: Current evidence on surgery, systemic methotrexate and expectant management in the treatment of tubal ectopic pregnancy: a systematic review and meta-analysis. Hum Reprod Update 14(4):309, 2008

Mol F, van Mello NM, Strandell A, et al: Salpingotomy versus salpingectomy in women with tubal pregnancy (ESEP study): an open-label, multicentre, randomised controlled trial. Lancet 383(9927):1483, 2014

Moschos E, Sreenarasimhaiah S, Twickler DM: First-trimester diagnosis of cesarean scar ectopic pregnancy. J Clin Ultrasound 36(8):504, 2008a

Moschos E, Twickler DM: Endometrial thickness predicts intrauterine pregnancy in patients with pregnancy of unknown location. Ultrasound Obstet Gynecol 32(7):929, 2008b

Murphy AA, Nager CW, Wujek JJ, et al: Operative laparoscopy versus laparotomy for the management of ectopic pregnancy: a prospective trial. Fertil Steril 57:1180, 1992

Nakao Y, Yokoyama M, Iwasaka T: Uterine artery embolization followed by dilation and curettage for cervical pregnancy. Obstet Gynecol 111(2 Pt 2):505, 2008

Natale A, Candiani M, Merlo D, et al: Human chorionic gonadotropin level as a predictor of trophoblastic infiltration into the tubal wall in ectopic pregnancy: a blinded study. Fertil Steril 79:981, 2003

Nieuwkerk PT, Hajenius PJ, Ankum WM, et al: Systemic methotrexate therapy versus laparoscopic salpingostomy in patients with tubal pregnancy. Part I. Impact on patients' health-related quality of life. Fertil Steril 70:511, 1998

Nowak-Markwitz E, Michalak M, Olejnik M, et al: Cutoff value of human chorionic gonadotropin in relation to the number of methotrexate cycles in the successful treatment of ectopic pregnancy. Fertil Steril 92(4):1203, 2009

Nurmohamed L, Moretti ME, Schechter T, et al: Outcome following high-dose methotrexate in pregnancies misdiagnosed as ectopic. Am J Obstet Gynecol 205(6):533.e1, 2011

Nyberg DA, Hughes MP, Mack LA, et al: Extrauterine findings of ectopic pregnancy of transvaginal US: importance of echogenic fluid. Radiology 178:823, 1991

Paul M, Schaff E, Nichols M: The roles of clinical assessment, human chorionic gonadotropin assays, and ultrasonography in medical abortion practice. Am J Obstet Gynecol 183:S34, 2000

Pattinson HA, Dunphy BC, Wood S, et al: Cervical pregnancy following in vitro fertilization: evacuation after uterine artery embolization with subsequent successful intrauterine pregnancy. Aust N Z J Obstet Gynaecol 34:492, 1994

Pellerito JS, Taylor KJ, Quedens-Case C, et al: Ectopic pregnancy: evaluation with endovaginal color flow imaging. Radiology 193(2):407, 1992

Perkins KM, Boulet SL, Kissin DM, et al: Risk of ectopic pregnancy associated with assisted reproductive technology in the United States, 2001–2011. Obstet Gynecol 125(1):70, 2015

Pisarska MD, Carson SA: Incidence and risk factors for ectopic pregnancy. Clin Obstet Gynecol 42:2, 1999

Polena V, Huchon C, Varas Ramos C, et al: Non-invasive tools for the diagnosis of potentially life-threatening gynaecological emergencies: a systematic review. PLoS One 10(2):e0114189, 2015

Revel A, Ophir I, Koler M, et al: Changing etiology of tubal pregnancy following IVP. Hum Reprod 23(6):1372, 2008

Ries A, Singson P, Bidus M, et al: Use of the endometrial pipelle in the diagnosis of early abnormal gestations. Fertil Steril 74:593, 2000

Rodgerson JD, Heegaard WG, Plummer D, et al: Emergency department right upper quadrant ultrasound is associated with a reduced time to diagnosis and treatment of ruptured ectopic pregnancies. Acad Emerg Med 8(4):331, 2001

Rozenberg P, Chevret S, Camus E, et al: Medical treatment of ectopic pregnancies: a randomized clinical trial comparing methotrexate-mifepristone and methotrexate-placebo. Hum Reprod 18:1802, 2003

Rulin MC: Is salpingostomy the surgical treatment of choice for unruptured tubal pregnancy? Obstet Gynecol 86:1010, 1995

Sadeghi H, Rutherford T, Rackow BW: Cesarean scar ectopic pregnancy: case series and review of the literature. Am J Perinatol 27(2):111, 2010

Sagiv R, Debby A, Sadan O, et al: Laparoscopic surgery for extrauterine pregnancy in hemodynamically unstable patients. J Am Assoc Gynecol Laparosc 8:529, 2001

Sanz LE, Verosko J: Hysteroscopic management of cornual ectopic pregnancy. Obstet Gynecol 99:941, 2002

Saraiya M, Berg CJ, Kendrick JS, et al: Cigarette smoking as a risk factor for ectopic pregnancy. Am J Obstet Gynecol 178:493, 1998

Seeber BE, Sammel MD, Guo W, et al: Application of redefined human chorionic gonadotropin curves for the diagnosis of women at risk for ectopic pregnancy. Fertil Steril 86(2):454, 2006

Senterman M, Jibodh R, Tulandi T: Histopathologic study of ampullary and isthmic tubal ectopic pregnancy. Am J Obstet Gynecol 159:939, 1988

Shalev E, Peleg D, Tsabari A, et al: Spontaneous resolution of ectopic tubal pregnancy: natural history. Fertil Steril 63:15, 1995

Shaunik A, Kulp J, Appleby DH, et al: Utility of dilation and curettage in the diagnosis of pregnancy of unknown location. Am J Obstet Gynecol 204(2):130.e1, 2011

Shaw JL, Dey SK, Critchley HO, et al: Current knowledge of the aetiology of human tubal ectopic pregnancy. Hum Reprod Update 16(4):432, 2010

Shen L, Tan A, Zhu H: Bilateral uterine artery chemoembolization with methotrexate for cesarean scar pregnancy. Am J Obstet Gynecol 207(5):386.e1, 2012

Singh N, Tripathi R, Mala Y, et al: Diagnostic dilemma in cornual pregnancy—3D ultrasonography may aid!! J Clin Diagn Res 9(1):QD12, 2015

Skjeldestad FE, Hadgu A, Eriksson N: Epidemiology of repeat ectopic pregnancy: a population-based prospective cohort study. Obstet Gynecol 91:129, 1998

Sowter M, Farquhar C: Changing face of ectopic pregnancy. Each centre should validate diagnostic algorithms for its own patients. BMJ 315:1312, 1997

Spandorfer SD, Menzin AW, Barnhart KT, et al: Efficacy of frozen-section evaluation of uterine curettings in the diagnosis of ectopic pregnancy. Am J Obstet Gynecol 175:603, 1996

Spandorfer SD, Sawin SW, Benjamin I, et al: Postoperative day 1 serum human chorionic gonadotropin level as a predictor of persistent ectopic pregnancy after conservative surgical management. Fertil Steril 68:430, 1997

Spiegelberg O: Zur Casuistic der Ovarialschwangerschaft. Arch Gynaekol 13:73, 1878

Stovall TG, Ling FW: Single-dose methotrexate: an expanded clinical trial. Am J Obstet Gynecol 168:1759, 1993

Stovall TG, Ling FW, Andersen RN, et al: Improved sensitivity and specificity of a single measurement of serum progesterone over serial quantitative beta-human chorionic gonadotrophin in screening for ectopic pregnancy. Hum Reprod 7:723, 1992

Straka M, Zeringue E, Goldman M: A rare drug reaction to methotrexate after treatment for ectopic pregnancy. Obstet Gynecol 103:1047, 2004

Strandell A, Thorburn J, Hamberger L: Risk factors for ectopic pregnancy in assisted reproduction. Fertil Steril 71:282, 1999

Stulberg DB, Cain LR, Dahlquist I, et al: Ectopic pregnancy rates and racial disparities in the Medicaid population, 2004–2008. Fertil Steril 102(6):1671, 2014

Swire MN, Castro-Aragon I, Levine D: Various sonographic appearances of the hemorrhagic corpus luteum cyst. Ultrasound Q 20:45, 2004

Tal J, Haddad S, Gordon N, et al: Heterotopic pregnancy after ovulation induction and assisted reproductive technologies: a literature review from 1971 to 1993. Fertil Steril 66:1, 1996

Talbot P, Riveles K: Smoking and reproduction: the oviduct as a target of cigarette smoke. Reprod Biol Endocrinol 3:52, 2005

Tanaka Y, Mimura K, Kanagawa T, et al: Three-dimensional sonography in the differential diagnosis of interstitial, angular, and intrauterine pregnancies in a septate uterus. J Ultrasound Med 33(11):2031, 2014

Thurman AR, Cornelius M, Korte JE, et al: An alternative monitoring protocol for single-dose methotrexate therapy in ectopic pregnancy. Am J Obstet Gynecol 202(2):139.e1, 2010

Timor-Tritsch IE, Monteagudo A, Santos R, et al: The diagnosis, treatment, and follow-up of cesarean scar pregnancy. Am J Obstet Gynecol 207(1):44.e1, 2012

Toth M, Patton DL, Campbell LA, et al: Detection of chlamydial antigenic material in ovarian, prostatic, ectopic pregnancy and semen samples of culture-negative subjects. Am J Reprod Immunol 43:218, 2000

Trambert JJ, Einstein MH, Banks E, et al: Uterine artery embolization in the management of vaginal bleeding from cervical pregnancy: a case series. J Reprod Med 50:844, 2005

Trio D, Strobelt N, Picciolo C, et al: Prognostic factors for successful expectant management of ectopic pregnancy. Fertil Steril 63:469, 1995

Trojano G, Colafiglio G, Saliani N, et al: Successful management of a cervical twin pregnancy: neoadjuvant systemic methotrexate and prophylactic high cervical cerclage before curettage. Fertil Steril 91(3):935.e17, 2009

Tulandi T, Al Jaroudi D: Interstitial pregnancy: results generated from the Society of Reproductive Surgeons Registry. Obstet Gynecol 103:47, 2004

Tulandi T, Hemmings R, Khalifa F: Rupture of ectopic pregnancy in women with low and declining serum beta-human chorionic gonadotropin concentrations. Fertil Steril 56:786, 1991

Uğur M, Turan C, Vicdan K, et al: Chronic ectopic pregnancy: a clinical analysis of 62 cases. Aust N Z J Obstet Gynaecol 36(2):186, 1996

Ushakov FB, Elchalal U, Aceman PJ, et al: Cervical pregnancy: past and future. Obstet Gynecol Surv 52:45, 1997

Van Den Eeden SK, Shan J, Bruce C, et al: Ectopic pregnancy rate and treatment utilization in a large managed care organization. Obstet Gynecol 105:1052, 2005

Van Voorhis BJ: Outcomes from assisted reproductive technology. Obstet Gynecol 107:183, 2006

Verma U, Goharkhay N: Conservative management of cervical ectopic pregnancy. Fertil Steril 91(3):671, 2009

Vermesh M, Graczykowski JW, Sauer MV: Reevaluation of the role of culdocentesis in the management of ectopic pregnancy. Am J Obstet Gynecol 162:411, 1990

Vermesh M, Silva PD, Rosen GF, et al: Management of unruptured ectopic gestation by linear salpingostomy: a prospective, randomized clinical trial of laparoscopy versus laparotomy. Obstet Gynecol 73:400, 1989

Warkany J: Aminopterin and methotrexate: folic acid deficiency. Teratology 17:353, 1978

Waylen AL, Metwally M, Jones GL, et al: Effects of cigarette smoking upon clinical outcomes of assisted reproduction: a meta-analysis. Human Reprod Update 15(1):31, 2009

Worley KC, Hnat MD, Cunningham FG: Advanced extrauterine pregnancy: diagnostic and therapeutic challenges. Am J Obstet Gynecol 198:297e1, 2008

Yang XY, Yu H, Li KM, et al: Uterine artery embolisation combined with local methotrexate for treatment of caesarean scar pregnancy. BJOG 117(8):990, 2010

Yeko TR, Mayer JC, Parsons AK, et al: A prospective series of unruptured ectopic pregnancies treated by tubal injection with hyperosmolar glucose. Obstet Gynecol 85:265, 1995

Zee J, Sammel MD, Chung K, et al: Ectopic pregnancy prediction in women with a pregnancy of unknown location: data beyond 48 h are necessary. Human Reprod 29(3):441, 2014

Zhang X, Liu X, Fan H: Interstitial pregnancy and transcervical curettage. Obstet Gynecol 104(2):1193, 2004

Zhuang Y, Huang L: Uterine artery embolization compared with methotrexate for the management of pregnancy implanted within a cesarean scar. Am J Obstet Gynecol 201(2):152.e1, 2009

CHAPTER 8

Abnormal Uterine Bleeding

DEFINITIONS

Abnormal uterine bleeding (AUB) may display several patterns, and descriptive terms have been updated to standardize nomenclature (Munro, 2011). For example, *heavy menstrual bleeding (HMB)* (formerly menorrhagia) defines prolonged or heavy cyclic menstruation. Objectively, menses lasting longer than 7 days or exceeding 80 mL of blood loss are determining values. The term *intermenstrual bleeding* replaces metrorrhagia. Frequently, women may complain of both patterns. The term *breakthrough bleeding* is a more informal term for intermenstrual bleeding that accompanies hormone administration. In some women, there is diminished flow or shortening of menses, *hypomenorrhea*. Women normally menstruate every 28 days ± 7 days. Cycles with intervals longer than 35 days describe a state of *oligomenorrhea*. The term *withdrawal bleeding* refers to the predictable bleeding that results from an abrupt decline in progesterone levels. Finally, *postcoital bleeding* is that prompted by vaginal intercourse.

Assessing HMB in a clinical setting has its limitations. First, patient perception of blood loss and objective measurement often fail to correlate (Chimbira, 1980b). As a result, objective methods to assess blood loss have been investigated. Hallberg and associates (1966) describe a technique to extract hemoglobin from sanitary napkins using sodium hydroxide. Hemoglobin is converted to hematin and can be measured spectrophotometrically. Although used in research, this approach in a clinical setting has obvious constraints.

Other tools used to estimate menstrual blood loss include hemoglobin and hematocrit evaluation. Hemoglobin concentrations below 12 g/dL increase the chance of identifying women with HMB. A normal level, however, does not exclude HMB, as many women with clinically significant bleeding have normal values.

Another method involves estimating the number and type of pads or tampons used by a woman during menses. Warner and colleagues (2004) found positive correlations between objective HMB and passing clots more than 1 inch in diameter and changing pads more frequently than every 3 hours. Attempts to standardize this type of evaluation have lead to development of the pictorial blood assessment chart (PBAC) (Fig. 8-1). With a scoring sheet, patients are asked to record daily the number of sanitary products that are lightly, moderately, or completely saturated. Scores are assigned as follows: 1 point for each lightly stained tampon, 5 if moderately saturated, and 10 if completely soaked. Pads are similarly given ascending scores of 1, 5, and 20, respectively. Small clots score 1 point, whereas large clots score 5. Points are then tallied for each day. Totals more than 100 points per menstrual cycle correlate with greater than 80 mL objective blood loss (Higham, 1990).

Menstrual calendars are also frequently used to evaluate abnormal bleeding and its patterns. With this, patients are asked to record dates and blood flow quality throughout the month. These calendars can be used to aid diagnosis and to document improvement during medical treatment.

INCIDENCE

Abnormal uterine bleeding is common, and etiologies include anatomic changes, hormonal dysfunction, infection, system disease, medications, and pregnancy complications (Table 8-1). As a result, AUB may affect females of all ages. Factors that influence incidence most greatly are age and reproductive status.

Prior to menarche, bleeding is investigated as an abnormal finding. In children, the vagina, rather than the uterus, is more frequently involved. Vulvovaginitis is often the cause, but dermatologic conditions, neoplasms, and trauma by accident, abuse, or foreign body are others. In addition to vaginal sources, urethra bleeding may originate from urethral prolapse or infection. True uterine bleeding usually results from increased estrogen levels, and precocious puberty, accidental exogenous ingestion, and ovarian neoplasm are considered. These are each discussed further in Chapter 14.

In adolescence, AUB results from anovulation and coagulation defects at disproportionately higher rates compared with older reproductive-aged women (Ahuja, 2010). In contrast,

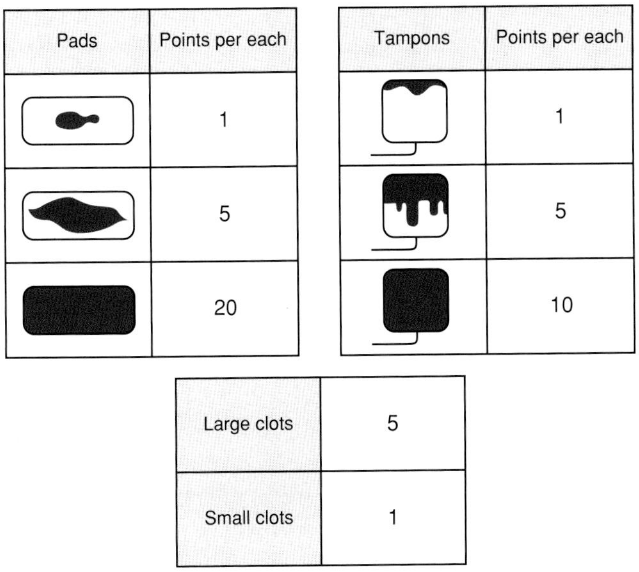

Pads	Points per each
	1
	5
	20

Tampons	Points per each
	1
	5
	10

Large clots	5
Small clots	1

FIGURE 8-1 Scoring for the pictorial bleeding assessment chart. Patients are counseled to evaluate the degree of saturation for each sanitary product used during menstruation. The total number of points are tallied for each menses. Point totals greater than 100 indicate menorrhagia.

TABLE 8-1. Differential Diagnosis of Abnormal Bleeding

Structural
Uterine—leiomyoma, adenomyosis, endometrial polyp, endometrial hyperplasia or cancer, uterine sarcoma, AVM
Cervix—endocervical polyp, dysplasia, or cancer
Vagina—cancer, postoperative granulation tissue
Fallopian tube—cancer
Ovary—sex cord-stromal tumors
Atrophic vaginal, cervical, or endometrial epithelia
Partial outflow obstruction—congenital müllerian defect, Asherman syndrome
Intrinsic endometrial

Anovulation
Immature HPO axis or aging ovarian follicles
Hypothyroidism
Hyperprolactinemia—pituitary or hypothalamic disorder
Androgen excess—PCOS, CAH, Cushing syndrome/disease
Premature ovarian failure

Pregnancy
Implantation, abortion, ectopic pregnancy, GTD

Exogenous
IUD, foreign body, trauma
Medications—sex steroids, anticoagulants, hyperprolactinemia inducing

Infection
STD, TB, chronic endometritis, postabortal or postpartum infection

Systemic abnormalities
Coagulopathies, hepatic or chronic renal failure, hyperthyroidism, obesity

AVM = arteriovenous malformation; CAH = congenital adrenal hyperplasia; GTD = gestational trophoblastic disease; HPO = hypothalamic-pituitary-ovarian axis; PCOS = polycystic ovarian syndrome; STD = sexually transmitted disease; TB = tuberculosis.

benign or malignant neoplastic growths are less frequent. Pregnancy, sexually transmitted diseases, and sexual abuse are also considered in this population.

Following adolescence, the hypothalamic-pituitary-ovarian (HPO) axis matures, and anovulatory uterine bleeding is encountered less often. With increased sexual activity, rates of bleeding related to pregnancy and sexually transmitted disease rise. The incidences of bleeding from leiomyomas and endometrial polyps also increase with age.

During the perimenopause, as with perimenarchal girls, anovulatory uterine bleeding from HPO axis dysfunction is a more frequent finding (Chap. 21, p. 472). In contrast, the incidences of bleeding related to pregnancy and sexually transmitted disease decline. With aging, risks of benign and malignant neoplastic growth increase.

After menopause, bleeding typically can be traced to a benign origin such as endometrial or vaginal atrophy or polyps. Even so, malignant neoplasms, especially endometrial carcinoma, are found more often in this age group. Less commonly, estrogen-producing ovarian carcinoma may cause endometrial hyperplasia with uterine bleeding. Similarly, ulcerative vulvar, vaginal, or cervical neoplasms can be sources. And rarely, serosanguinous discharge from a fallopian tube cancer may appear as uterine bleeding. Thus, bleeding in this demographic usually prompts evaluation to exclude these cancers.

PATHOPHYSIOLOGY

The endometrium consists of two distinct zones, the functionalis layer and the basalis layer (Fig. 8-2). The basalis layer lies in direct contact with the myometrium, is beneath the functionalis, and is less hormonally responsive. The basalis serves as a reservoir for regeneration of the functionalis layer following menses. In contrast, the functionalis layer lines the uterine cavity, undergoes dramatic change throughout the menstrual cycle, and ultimately sloughs during menstruation. Histologically, the functionalis has a surface epithelium and underlying subepithelial capillary plexus. Beneath these are organized stroma, glands, and interspersed leukocytes.

Blood reaches the uterus via the uterine and ovarian arteries. From these, the arcuate arteries arise to supply the myometrium. These in turn branch into the radial arteries, which extend toward the endometrium at right angles from the arcuate arteries (Fig. 8-3). At the endometrium-myometrium junction, the radial arteries bifurcate to create the basal and spiral arteries. The basal arteries serve the basalis layer of the endometrium and are relatively insensitive to hormonal changes. The spiral arteries stretch to supply the functionalis layer and end in a subepithelial capillary plexus.

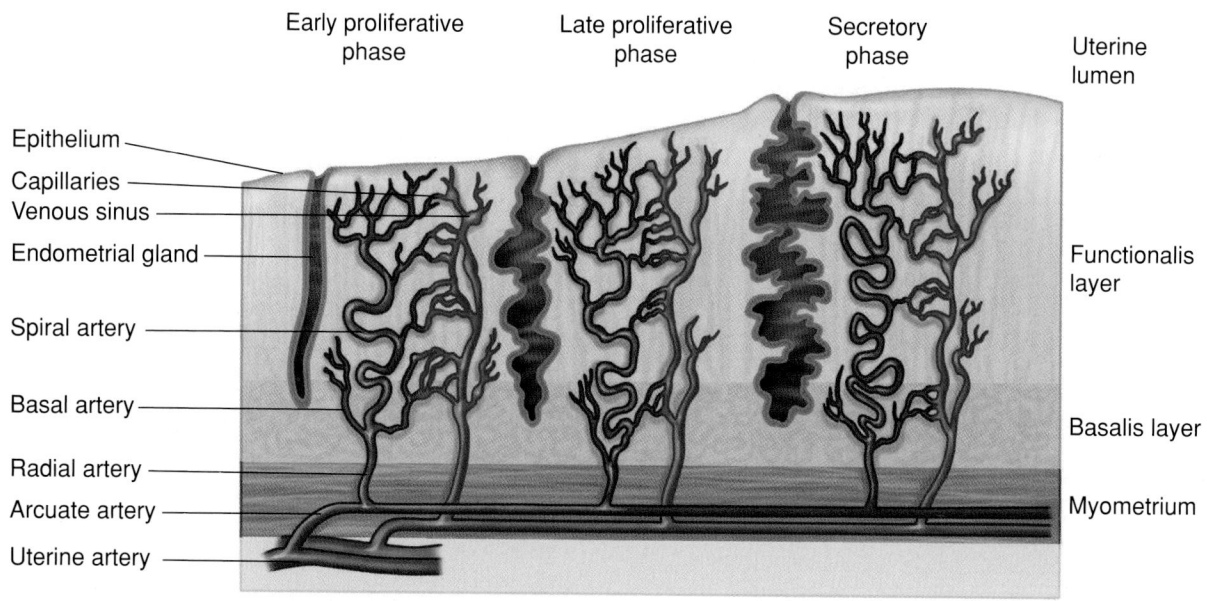

Early proliferative phase   Late proliferative phase   Secretory phase   Uterine lumen

Epithelium
Capillaries
Venous sinus
Endometrial gland

Spiral artery

Basal artery

Radial artery
Arcuate artery
Uterine artery

Functionalis layer

Basalis layer

Myometrium

FIGURE 8-2 Drawing of endometrial anatomy as it varies through the menstrual cycle.

At the end of each menstrual cycle, progesterone levels drop and lead to release of lytic matrix metalloproteinases (MMP). These enzymes break down the stroma and vascular architecture of the functionalis layer. Subsequent bleeding and sloughing of this layer constitute menstruation (Jabbour, 2006). Initially, platelet aggregation and thrombi control blood loss. In addition, the remaining endometrial arteries, under the influence of mediators, vasoconstrict to limit further bleeding (Ferenczy, 2003).

DIAGNOSIS

■ History and Physical Examination

With AUB, the diagnostic goal is exclusion of pregnancy or cancer and identification of the underlying pathology to allow

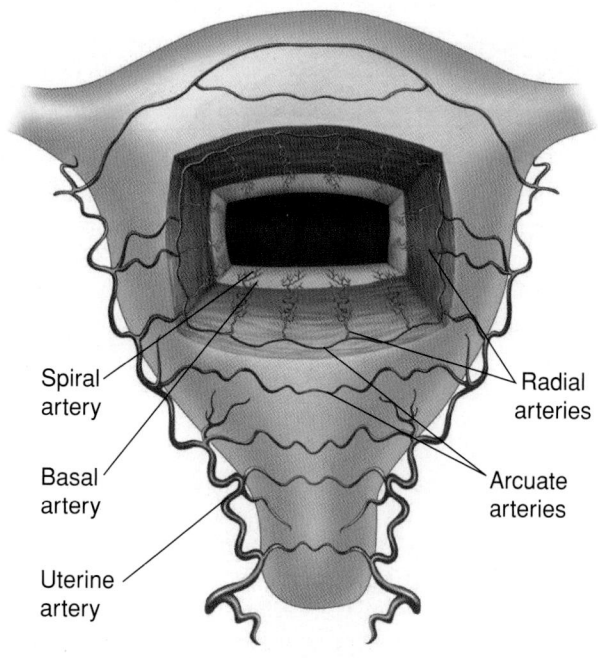

Spiral artery

Basal artery

Uterine artery

Radial arteries

Arcuate arteries

FIGURE 8-3 Drawing of uterine blood supply.

optimal treatment. During initial evaluation of abnormal bleeding, a thorough menstrual history is collected. Topics typically include age at menarche, date of last menstrual period, birth control method, and the timing and amount of bleeding. Associated symptoms such as fever, fatigue, bulk symptoms, tissue passage, or pain can also direct evaluation. Importantly, medications are reviewed, as abnormal bleeding can accompany use of nonsteroidal antiinflammatory drugs (NSAIDs), anticoagulants, and agents associated with hyperprolactinemia (Table 12-2, p. 281). Less robust evidence implicates herbal supplements such as ginseng, garlic, ginkgo, don quai, and St. John wort (Cordier, 2012).

Most gynecologic disorders do not consistently display a specific bleeding pattern, and patients may complain of HMB or intermenstrual bleeding or both. Thus, the pattern for a particular woman may be of limited value in diagnosing the underlying bleeding cause but can be used to assess improvement with treatment.

Of pain symptoms, dysmenorrhea often accompanies abnormal bleeding caused by structural abnormalities, infections, and pregnancy complications. This seems intuitive because of the role of prostaglandins in both HMB and dysmenorrhea. Painful intercourse and noncyclic pain are less frequent in women with AUB and usually suggest a structural or infectious source.

Following a historical inventory, physical examination attempts to identify findings that may suggest an etiology. Moreover, the site of uterine bleeding is confirmed, because vaginal, rectal, or urethral bleeding can present similarly. This is more difficult if there is no active bleeding, and urinalysis or stool guaiac evaluation may be helpful adjuncts.

To complement physical findings, blood tests, cervical cytology, sonography (with or without saline infusion), endometrial biopsy, and hysteroscopy are used primarily (Fig. 8-4). In many cases following history and physical examination, these tools may not be required or may be individually selected based on patient variables, suspected diagnosis, available resources, and/or provider training. Test suitability for a given patient is discussed next.

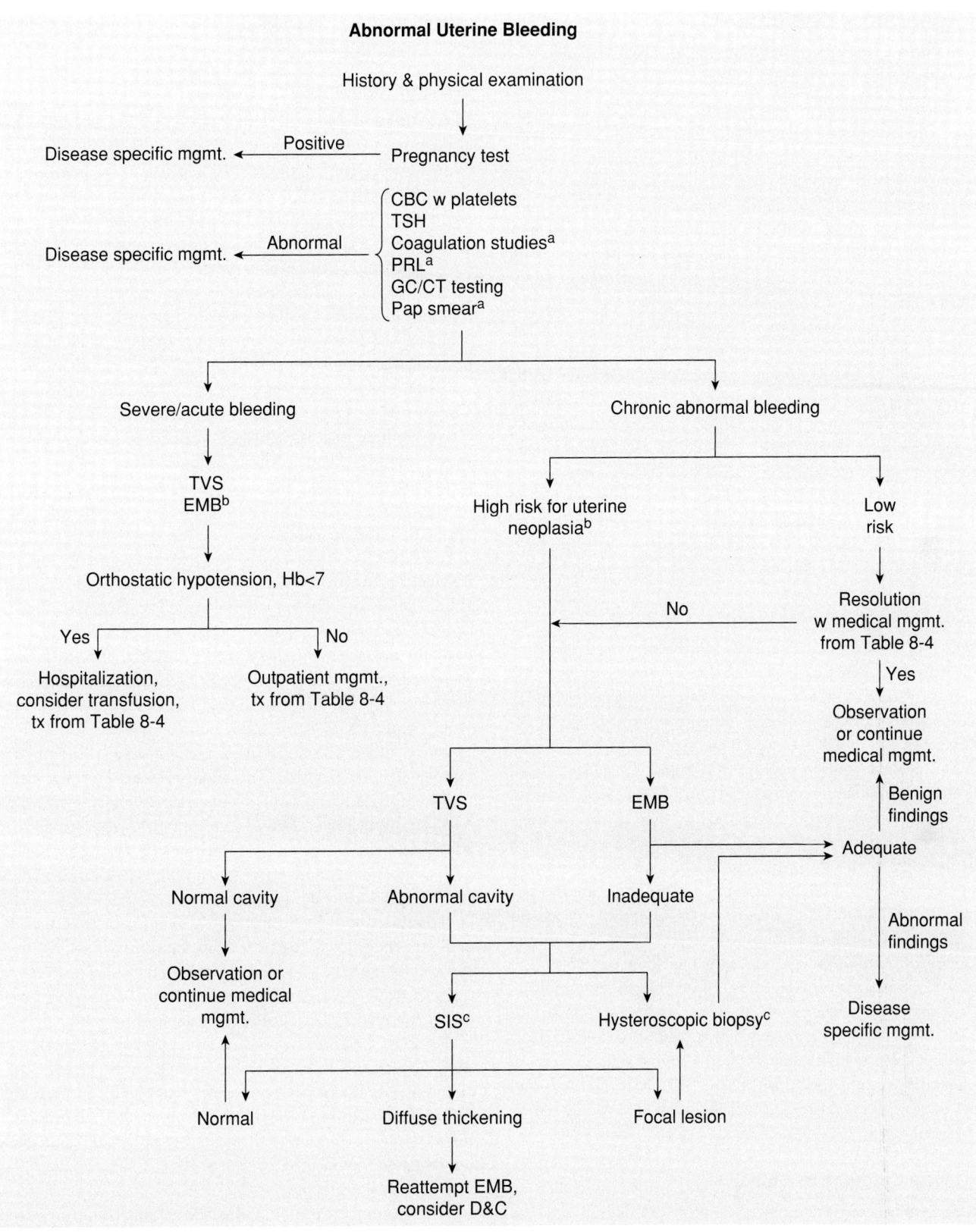

Abnormal Uterine Bleeding

FIGURE 8-4 Diagnostic algorithm to identify endometrial pathology in patients with abnormal uterine bleeding.
[a]Study obtained as indicated by patient history.
[b]Patients with chronic anovulation, obesity, ≥45 years of age, tamoxifen use, or other risks for endometrial cancer.
[c]Both comparable in sensitivity and specificity. Either or both may be selected depending on patient characteristics and physician preference (p. 186).
CBC = complete blood count; D&C = dilatation and curettage; GC/CT = *Neisseria gonorrhoeae* and *Chlamydia trachomatis*; EMB = endometrial biopsy; Hb = hemoglobin level; mgmt. = management; PRL = prolactin level; SIS = saline infusion sonography; TSH = thyroid-stimulating hormone level; TVS = transvaginal sonography; tx = treatment.

■ Laboratory Evaluation

β-Human Chorionic Gonadotropin and Hematologic Testing

Miscarriage, ectopic pregnancies, and hydatidiform moles may cause life-threatening hemorrhage. Pregnancy complications are quickly excluded with determination of urine or serum β-human chorionic gonadotropin (hCG) levels. This is typically obtained on all reproductive-aged women with a uterus.

Additionally, in women with AUB, a complete blood count (CBC) will identify anemia and the degree of blood loss. With chronic loss, erythrocyte indices will reflect a microcytic, hypochromic anemia and show decreases in mean corpuscular volume (MCV), mean corpuscular hemoglobin (MCH), and mean corpuscular hemoglobin concentration (MCHC). Moreover, in women with classic iron-deficiency anemia from chronic blood loss, an elevated platelet count may be seen. In those for whom the cause of anemia is unclear, those with profound anemia, or in those who fail to improve with oral iron therapy, iron studies are often indicated. Specifically, iron-deficiency anemia produces low serum ferritin and low serum iron levels but an elevated total iron-binding capacity. As discussed further on page 192, screening for disordered hemostasis is considered in women and adolescents with HMB and no other obvious cause.

"Wet Prep" Examination and Cervical Cultures

Cervicitis often causes intermenstrual or postcoital spotting. Accordingly, microscopic examination of a saline preparation of cervical secretions or "wet prep" can be informative. With mucopurulent discharge, sheets of neutrophils (>30 per high-power field) and red blood cells are typical. With trichomoniasis, motile trichomonads are also found. Cervicitis-related bleeding is frequently reproduced during sampling from an inflamed cervix with a friable epithelium.

The association between mucopurulent cervicitis and cervical infection with *Chlamydia trachomatis* and *Neisseria gonorrhoeae* is well established (Brunham, 1984). Thus, the Centers for Disease Control and Prevention (CDC) (2015) recommend testing for both when mucopurulent cervicitis is found. Moreover, even without frank discharge, these organisms can cause endometritis (Eckert, 2004). Thus, bleeding or spotting alone may merit screening for these two in at-risk populations listed in Table 1-1 (p. 6). Last, herpes simplex virus (HSV) may manifest as diffuse erosive and hemorrhagic ectocervical lesions (Paavonen, 1988). In patients with such findings who lack a known HSV history, directed culture or serologic testing can be obtained.

Cervical Cytology or Biopsy

Both cervical and endometrial cancers can bleed, and evidence for these tumors may be detected during diagnostic Pap smear evaluation. The most frequent abnormal cytologic results involve squamous cell pathology and may reflect cervicitis, intraepithelial neoplasia, or cancer. Less commonly, atypical glandular or endometrial cells are found. Thus, depending on the cytologic results, colposcopy, endocervical curettage, and/or endometrial biopsy may be indicated as discussed in Chapter 29 (p. 636). Moreover, at times, a visibly suspicious vaginal or cervical lesion may bleed and warrant direct biopsy with Tischler forceps.

Endometrial Biopsy

Indications. In women with AUB, sampling and histologic evaluation of the endometrium may identify infection or neoplastic lesions such as endometrial hyperplasia or cancer.

AUB is noted in 80 to 90 percent of women with endometrial cancer. The incidence and risk of this cancer increases with age, and most affected women are postmenopausal (National Cancer Institute, 2014). Thus, in postmenopausal women, the need to exclude cancer intensifies, and endometrial biopsy is typically indicated. Of premenopausal women with endometrial neoplasia, most are obese or have chronic anovulation or both. Thus, women with AUB in these two groups also warrant exclusion of endometrial cancer. Specifically, the American College of Obstetricians and Gynecologists (2012) recommends endometrial assessment in any woman older than 45 years with AUB, and in those younger than 45 years with a history of unopposed estrogen exposure such as seen in obesity or polycystic ovarian syndrome (PCOS), failed medical management, and persistent AUB.

Sampling Methods. For years, dilatation and curettage (D & C) was used for endometrial sampling. However, because of associated surgical risks, expense, postoperative pain, and need for operative anesthesia, other suitable substitutes were evaluated. In addition, investigators have demonstrated incomplete sampling and missed pathology even with D & C (Grimes, 1982; Stock, 1975).

Initial office techniques used metal curettes. Endometrial samples that are removed with these curettes show significant positive correlation with histologic results obtained from hysterectomy specimens (Stovall, 1989). Thus, they are deemed adequate sampling methods. However, disadvantages include patient discomfort and rare procedural complications such as uterine perforation and infection.

To minimize these, flexible plastic samplers have been evaluated for endometrial biopsy. Advantageously, samples from these catheters have comparable histologic findings with tissues obtained by D & C, hysterectomy, or stiff metal curette (Stovall, 1991). Moreover, they afford greater patient comfort.

Prior to performing endometrial biopsy, pregnancy is excluded in women of reproductive age. With Pipelle insertion, patients frequently note cramping, which can be allayed by a preprocedural NSAID. For some, slow transcervical intrauterine instillation of 5 mL of 2-percent lidocaine using an 18-gauge angiocatheter can lower perceived pain scores (Kosus, 2014).

After patient education and consent, a speculum is placed, and the cervix is cleansed with an antibacterial solution, such as povidone-iodine solution. In many cases, a single-tooth tenaculum is needed to stabilize the cervix and permit passage of the Pipelle through the cervical os and into the endometrial cavity. When placing the tenaculum on the anterior cervical lip, closing the clamp slowly can decrease discomfort. Some evidence also supports topical anesthetic use. Examples are 10-percent lidocaine spray immediately prior or 5-percent lidocaine/prilocaine

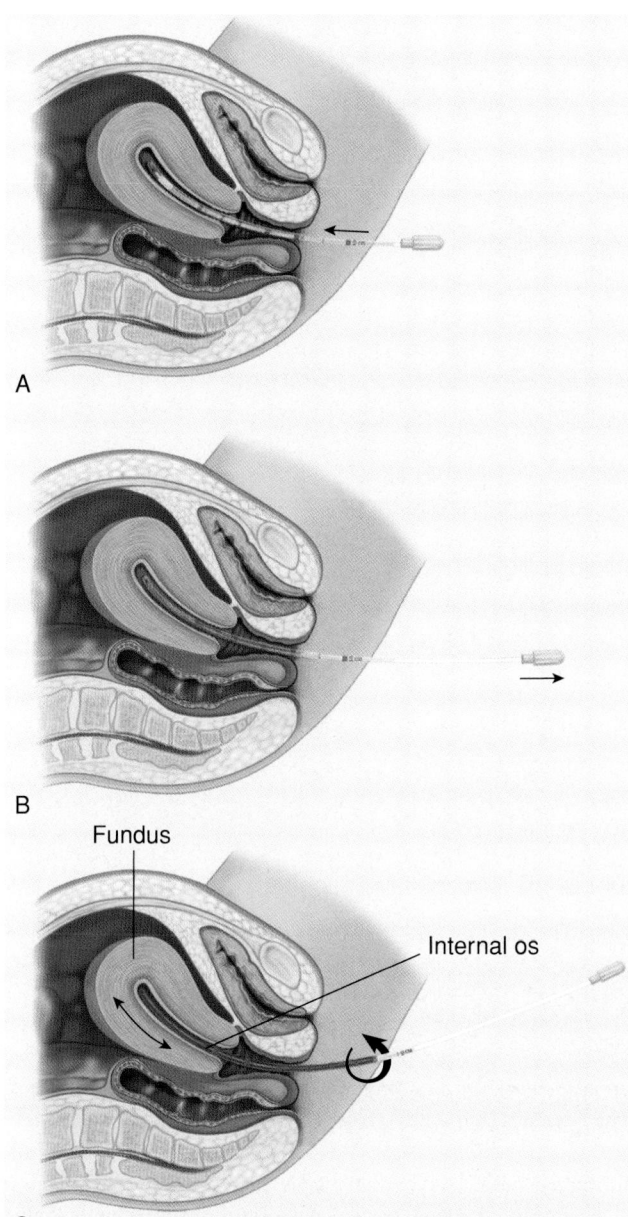

FIGURE 8-5 Steps of endometrial biopsy. **A.** During biopsy, the Pipelle is inserted through the cervical os and directed to the uterine fundus. **B.** The stilette of the Pipelle is retracted to create suction within the cylinder. **C.** Several times, the Pipelle is withdrawn to the level of the internal cervical os and advanced back to the fundus. The Pipelle is gently turned during its advance and retraction to allow thorough sampling of all endometrial surfaces.

cream (EMLA cream) 10 minutes before tenaculum placement (Davies, 1997; Zullo, 1999).

With sampling, the Pipelle is directed toward the fundus until resistance is met (Fig. 8-5). Markings on the Pipelle allow measurement of uterine depth, and this value is recorded in the procedure note. The inner Pipelle stilette is then retracted to create suction within the cylinder. Several times, the Pipelle is withdrawn to the level of the internal cervical os and advanced back to the fundus. The device is gently turned during its advance and retraction to allow thorough sampling of all endometrial surfaces. Uncommonly, a vagal response can follow Pipelle

insertion. In this instance, the procedure is terminated, and patient support is provided.

Despite its advantages, there are limitations to endometrial sampling with the Pipelle device. First, a tissue sample that is inadequate for histologic evaluation, such as from endometrial atrophy, or an inability to pass the catheter into the endometrial cavity is encountered in up to 28 percent of biopsy attempts (Smith-Bindman, 1998). Cervical stenosis and large submucous leiomyomas are classic obstructions. An incomplete evaluation often necessitates further investigation with D & C, transvaginal sonography with or without saline infusion, or diagnostic hysteroscopy (Emanuel, 1995). Second, endometrial biopsy has a cancer-detection failure rate of 0.9 percent. Thus, a positive histologic result is accurate to diagnose cancer, but a negative result does not definitively exclude it. Therefore, if an endometrial biopsy with normal tissue is obtained, but abnormal bleeding continues despite conservative treatment or if the suspicion of endometrial cancer is high, then further diagnostic efforts are warranted. Finally, endometrial sampling is associated with a greater percentage of false-negative results with focal pathology such as endometrial polyps. In a study of 639 women evaluated by diagnostic office hysteroscopy and endometrial biopsy, Svirsky and colleagues (2008) found that the sensitivity of endometrial sampling for detection of endometrial polyps and submucosal fibroids was only 8.4 and 1.4 percent, respectively. Because of these limitations with endometrial sampling, investigators have evaluated sonography, hysteroscopy, or both to replace or complement endometrial sampling.

■ Sonography
Transvaginal Sonography

With improved resolution, this technology is chosen by many instead of endometrial biopsy as a first-line tool to assess AUB. Advantageously, it allows assessment of both the myometrium and the endometrium. Thus, if AUB stems from myometrial pathology such as leiomyomas, sonography offers anatomic information that is not afforded by hysteroscopy or endometrial biopsy. In addition, transvaginal sonography (TVS) compared with these other two typically offers greater patient comfort and suitable detection of postmenopausal endometrial hyperplasia and cancer (Karlsson, 1995; Van den Bosch, 2008). That said, no tool, including TVS, is recommended for routine endometrial cancer screening in asymptomatic women (Breijer, 2012).

When the endometrium is imaged in a sagittal view, opposed endometrial surfaces appear as a hyperechoic *endometrial stripe* down the center of the uterine body (Fig. 8-6 and Fig. 2-16, p. 31). In postmenopausal women, this endometrial thickness has been correlated with endometrial cancer risk. Although endometrial thickness varies among patients, ranges have been established. Granberg and coworkers (1991) found thickness measurements of 3.4 ± 1.2 mm in postmenopausal women with atrophic endometrium, 9.7 ± 2.5 mm in those with endometrial hyperplasia, and 18.2 ± 6.2 mm in those with endometrial cancer. Subsequent investigations have similarly focused on endometrial thickness as it relates to hyperplasia and cancer risks in postmenopausal women. For endometrial cancer, negative predictive values >99 percent have been reported using a

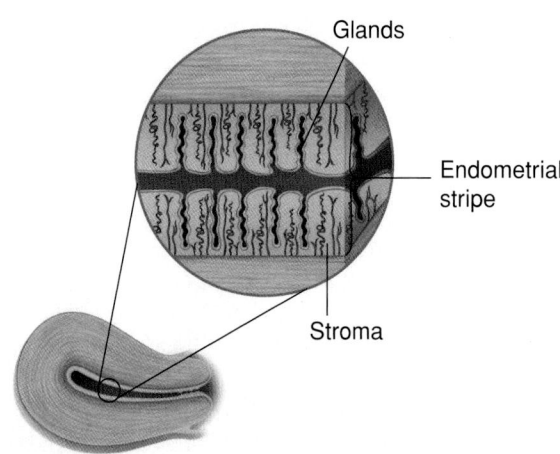

FIGURE 8-6 The sonographic endometrial stripe in a sagittal plane represents the thickness created by the apposed anterior and posterior endometrium. In premenopausal women, stripe thickness will vary during the menstrual cycle as the endometrium gradually thickens and then is sloughed.

measurement of ≤4 mm (Karlsson, 1995; Tsuda, 1997). Use of hormone replacement therapy (HRT) does not appear to affect the threshold used (Smith-Bindman, 1998). In those using cyclic HRT, completing TVS on day 4 or 5 following cycle bleeding is recommended (Goldstein, 2001). For postmenopausal women, an endometrial thickness >4 mm typically requires additional evaluation with saline infusion sonography (SIS), hysteroscopy, or endometrial biopsy.

Consensus, however, is lacking regarding the asymptomatic postmenopausal women in whom a thick endometrium is found. The American College of Obstetricians and Gynecologists (2013d) notes that this finding need not routinely prompt evaluation but that further testing is directed by coexistent patient risks. Focal lesions are common in this subgroup and thus may favor SIS or hysteroscopy if additional evaluation is indicated (Schmidt, 2009).

Researchers have also attempted to create endometrial thickness guidelines for premenopausal women. Merz and colleagues (1996) found that the normal endometrial thickness in premenopausal women did not exceed 4 mm on day 4 of the menstrual cycle, nor did it measure more than 8 mm by day 8. However, endometrial thicknesses can vary considerably among premenopausal women, and evidence-based abnormal thresholds that have been proposed range from ≥4 mm to >16 mm (Breitkopf, 2004; Goldstein, 1997; Shi, 2008). Thus, a consensus for endometrial thickness guidelines has not been established for this group. At our institution, no additional evaluation is recommended for a normal-appearing endometrium measuring ≤10 mm in a premenopausal female experiencing AUB if she has no other risk factors to prompt further testing. Risk factors for endometrial carcinoma include extended AUB, chronic anovulation, diabetes mellitus, obesity, and tamoxifen use.

Qualities other than endometrial thickness are also considered because textural changes may indicate pathology. Punctate cystic areas within the endometrium may indicate a polyp. Conversely, hypoechoic masses that distort the endometrium and originate from the inner layer of myometrium most likely are submucous

leiomyomas. Although there are no specific sonographic findings that are characteristic of endometrial cancer, some findings have been linked with greater frequency (Fig. 33-3, p. 705). For example, intermingled hypo- and hyperechoic areas within the endometrium may indicate malignancy. Endometrial cavity fluid collections and an irregular endometrial-myometrial junction have also been implicated. Thus, with these findings, even with a normal endometrial stripe width in postmenopausal patients, endometrial biopsy or hysteroscopy with biopsy is considered to exclude malignancy (Sheikh, 2000).

Although these criteria can safely reduce endometrial biopsy rates for many patients, others consider false-negative rates as too high with this strategy for evaluation of postmenopausal women (Timmermans, 2010). Some advocate hysteroscopy with direct biopsy or D & C to evaluate postmenopausal bleeding (Litta, 2005; Tabor, 2002). In other patient populations, the 4-mm guideline may also be inappropriate. For example, van Doorn and coworkers (2004) reported decreased diagnostic accuracy in diabetic or obese women, and they recommend consideration of endometrial sampling.

A major limitation of TVS is its higher false-negative rate for diagnosing focal intrauterine pathology. This results in part from the physical inability of TVS to clearly assess the endometrium when there is concurrent uterine pathology such as leiomyomas or polyps. In these cases, SIS or hysteroscopy may be informative.

Saline Infusion Sonography

This simple, minimally invasive, and effective sonographic procedure can be used to evaluate the myometrium, endometrium, and endometrial cavity (Chap. 2, p. 24). Also known as *sonohysterography* or *hysterosonography*, SIS allows identification of common masses associated with AUB such as endometrial polyps, submucous leiomyomas, and intracavitary blood clots. These masses frequently create nondescript distortion or thickening of the endometrial lining when imaged with TVS. Thus, compared with TVS, SIS typically permits superior detection of intracavitary masses and differentiation of lesions as being endometrial, submucous, or intramural (Fig. 8-7). In addition, Moschos and colleagues (2009) describe a method of endometrial biopsy during SIS using a sonography-guided Pipelle. Although not yet widely used, this technique enables directed histologic sampling of endometrial pathology and has proved superior to blind endometrial biopsy in providing a diagnosis for AUB in peri- and postmenopausal women.

SIS has also been compared with hysteroscopy to detect uterine cavitary focal lesions. De Kroon and coworkers (2003) performed a metaanalysis of 24 studies and reported SIS to equal the diagnostic accuracy of hysteroscopy. Importantly, neither hysteroscopy nor SIS can reliably discriminate between benign and malignant focal lesions. Thus, because of the malignant potential of many focal lesions, biopsy or excision of most structural lesions, when identified, is recommended for those with risk factors. For this, operative hysteroscopy is typically used.

SIS has other limitations. First, it is cycle dependent and best performed in the proliferative phase to minimize false-negative and false-positive results. For example, focal lesions may be concealed in a thick, secretory endometrium. Also, the amount of

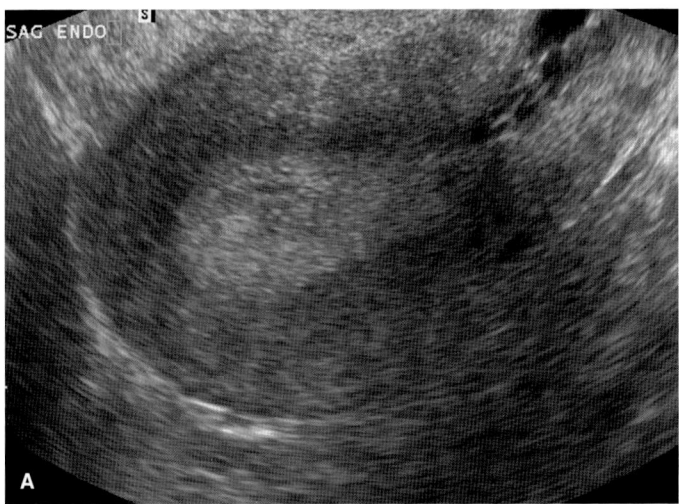 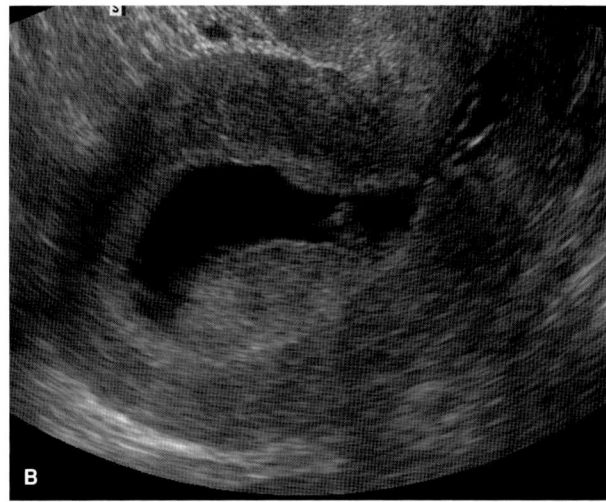

FIGURE 8-7 Transvaginal sonography of the uterus in the sagittal plane. **A.** The endometrium is thickened in this postmenopausal patient. **B.** Saline infusion sonography reveals a posterior endometrial mass and further delineates its size and qualities. (Used with permission from Dr. Elysia Moschos.)

endometrial tissue that can develop during the normal secretory phase can be mistaken for a small polyp or focal hyperplasia. Second, SIS usually has more patient discomfort than TVS, and approximately 5 percent of examinations cannot be completed because of cervical stenosis or patient discomfort. As expected, stenosis is more prevalent in postmenopausal women, and the incompletion rate mirrors that of diagnostic hysteroscopy.

Although accurate for identifying focal lesions, SIS may not add to the value of TVS for evaluation of diffuse lesions such as hyperplasia and cancer. Therefore, in postmenopausal women with AUB, and in whom the exclusion of cancer is more relevant than evaluating focal intracavitary lesions, SIS alone as an initial diagnostic tool may not have advantages over TVS.

Additional Sonographic Techniques

In selected instances, other imaging modalities can provide information beyond that obtained from TVS and SIS. Of these, color and pulsed Doppler, by demonstrating vascularity, may better highlight suspected focal abnormalities (Bennett, 2011). Similarly, 3-dimensional (3-D) sonography and 3-D SIS are most helpful to clarify focal lesions (Benacerraf, 2008; Makris, 2007). With power Doppler, finding multiple irregularly branching vessels may suggest malignancy (Opolskiene, 2007). 3-D power Doppler has been employed to differentiate malignant and benign endometrium, but its value is still undefined (Alcazar, 2009; Opolskiene, 2010). Last, although preferred to computed tomography (CT), magnetic resonance (MR) imaging is rarely needed for AUB evaluation but can display endometrium in cases in which sonographic views are obstructed.

■ Hysteroscopy

With this procedure, an endoscope, usually 3 to 5 mm in diameter, is inserted into the endometrial cavity as explained in detail in Section 44-12 (p. 1037). The uterine cavity is then distended with saline or another medium for visualization. In addition to inspection, biopsy of the endometrium allows histologic diagnosis of abnormal areas and has been shown to be

a safe and accurate means of identifying pathology. Also, focal lesions can be diagnosed and completely removed in the same session. In fact, many studies examining the accuracy of TVS or SIS for intracavitary pathology evaluation use hysteroscopy as the "gold standard" for comparison.

The main advantage of hysteroscopy is detection of intracavitary lesions such as leiomyomas and polyps that might be missed using TVS or endometrial sampling (Tahir, 1999). It also permits simultaneous removal of many lesions once identified. Thus, some advocate hysteroscopy as the primary tool for AUB diagnosis. However, the invasiveness and cost of hysteroscopy is balanced against improved diagnostic efficiency. Moreover, although accurate for identifying endometrial cancer, hysteroscopy is less accurate for endometrial hyperplasia. Accordingly, some recommend endometrial biopsy or endometrial curettage in conjunction with hysteroscopy (Ben-Yehuda, 1998; Clark, 2002).

Hysteroscopy has other limitations. Cervical stenosis will sometimes block successful introduction of the endoscope, and heavy bleeding may obscure and hinder an adequate examination. Hysteroscopy is more expensive and technically challenging than TVS or SIS. Costs can be lower with office hysteroscopy rather than that in an operative suite. However, patient discomfort may limit complete examination during some office procedures. Use of a smaller diameter or flexible hysteroscope may diminish this procedural pain (Cicinelli, 2003). In either arena, associated infection and uterine perforation have been reported, but their incidences are low (Bradley, 2002; Vercellini, 1997). Last, peritoneal seeding with malignant cells may take place during hysteroscopy via retrograde flow through the fallopian tubes in some women subsequently diagnosed with endometrial cancer (Bradley, 2004; Zerbe, 2000). Despite the risk of peritoneal contamination by cancer cells with hysteroscopy, patient prognosis overall does not appear to be worsened (Cicinelli, 2010; Polyzos, 2010). The American College of Obstetricians and Gynecologists (2011) considers hysteroscopy acceptable for AUB evaluation in those without advanced-stage uterine or cervical cancer.

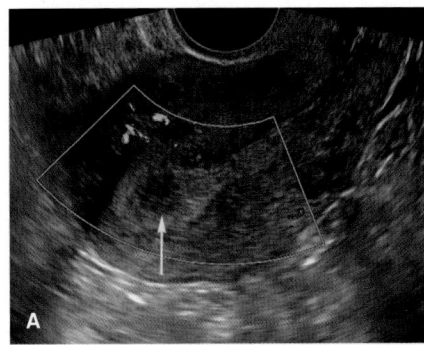 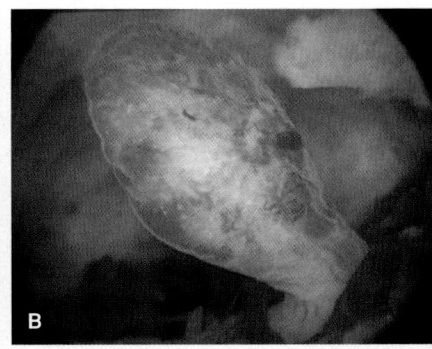 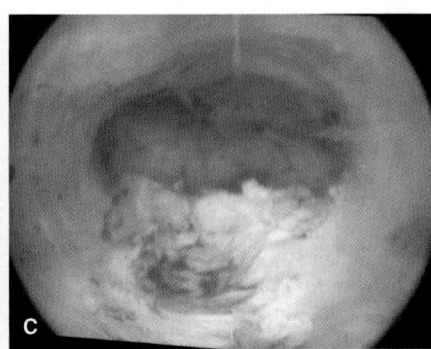

FIGURE 8-8 Endometrial polyp. **A.** Sagittal image of a uterus using transvaginal sonography with color Doppler. The yellow arrow points to the polyp, which is multicystic and hypoechoic compared with the surrounding endometrium. **B.** Hysteroscopic image of same polyp. **C.** Endometrial cavity following polyp resection. (Used with permission from Drs. David Rogers and Hilary Myears.)

■ Summary of Diagnostic Procedures

There is no one clear sequence to the use of endometrial biopsy, TVS, SIS, and hysteroscopy when evaluating AUB. None of these will distinguish all anatomic lesions with high sensitivity and specificity. That said, TVS for several reasons is a logical first step. It is well tolerated, is cost-effective, and requires relatively minimal technical skill. Additionally, it can reliably determine stripe thickness and whether a lesion is myometrial or endometrial. Once potential anatomic lesions have been identified, subsequent evaluation requires individualization. If endometrial hyperplasia or cancer is suspected, then endometrial biopsy may offer advantages. Alternatively, possible focal lesions may be best investigated with either hysteroscopy or SIS. Ultimately, the diagnostic goal is to identify and treat pathology and specifically to exclude endometrial carcinoma. Thus, selection of appropriate tests depends on their accuracy in characterizing the most likely anatomic lesions.

ETIOLOGY CLASSIFICATION

Causes of AUB are numerous and summarized by the acronym PALM-COEIN (Munro, 2011). In this International Federation of Gynecology and Obstetrics (FIGO) classification system, letters reflect Polyp, Adenomyosis, Leiomyoma, Malignancy and hyperplasia, Coagulopathy, Ovulatory disorders, Endometrial dysfunction, Iatrogenic, and those Not yet classified.

Pregnancy is not considered in this system, but AUB is encountered in 15 to 20 percent of pregnancies (Everett, 1997; Weiss, 2004). Although frequently no reason is found, bleeding may reflect early abortion, ectopic pregnancy, cervical infection, hydatidiform mole, cervical eversion, or polyp. Detailed discussions of bleeding associated with these are found in Chapters 6, 7, and 37.

STRUCTURAL ABNORMALITIES

■ Uterine Enlargement

Structural abnormalities are frequent causes of abnormal bleeding, and of these, leiomyomas are by far the most common. Myomas, adenomyosis, and isthmoceles are presented in Chapter 9. Uterine and cervical neoplasms are discussed in

Chapters 30, 33, and 34. As described in Chapter 18, partially obstructive congenital reproductive tract anomalies may at times cause chronic intermenstrual bleeding. Endometrial and endocervical structural abnormalities such as polyps and arteriovenous malformations are described here.

■ Endometrial Polyp

These soft, fleshy intrauterine growths are composed of endometrial glands, fibrous stroma, and surface epithelium. Polyps are common, and their prevalence in the general population approximates 8 percent (Dreisler, 2009a). Moreover, in those with AUB, rates range from 10 to 30 percent (Bakour, 2000; Goldstein, 1997). Intact polyps may be single or multiple, measure from a few millimeters to several centimeters, and be sessile or pedunculated (Fig. 8-8). Estrogen and progesterone have been implicated in their growth, and higher receptor levels are noted within polyps compared with adjacent normal endometrium (Leão, 2013). These hormones elongate endometrial glands, stromal tissue, and spiral arteries, leading to the characteristic polypoid appearance. Others suggest local immune disturbances contribute to polyp formation and to associated AUB and infertility (Al-Jefout, 2009; Kitaya, 2012).

Patient risk factors include increasing age, obesity, and tamoxifen use (Reslova, 1999). Although some studies suggest an association between hormone replacement therapy and polyp formation, others do not (Bakour, 2002; Dreisler, 2009a; Maia, 2004; Oguz, 2005). Use of oral contraceptive pills appear to be protective (Dreisler, 2009b). Similarly, for women taking tamoxifen, the levonorgestrel-releasing intrauterine system (LNG-IUS) was investigated and shown to lower endometrial polyp formation rates, but its ultimate effects on breast cancer recurrence are incompletely defined and a concern (Wong, 2013).

Women with polyps may have no complaints, and polyps are identified during imaging for other indications (Goldstein, 2002). More frequently, heavy cyclic or intermenstrual bleeding is an associated symptom. Bleeding may stem from surface epithelium breaks associated with chronic inflammation and vascular fragility or from apical ischemic tissue necrosis (Ferenczy, 2003). Infertility has been linked indirectly with endometrial polyps. For example, small studies have shown increased pregnancy rates and fewer early pregnancy losses in infertile women following hysteroscopic excision (Pérez-Medina, 2005; Preutthipan, 2005). The exact mechanisms related to infertility are unknown, although local inflammation may play a role as noted earlier. Also, polyps found near the tubal ostia may hinder ostium function and block sperm migration (Shokeir, 2004; Yanaihara, 2008). Accordingly, many advocate polyp removal in infertile women.

The main diagnostic tools for endometrial polyp evaluation include TVS with applied color Doppler, SIS, and hysteroscopy. Endometrial biopsy may identify polyps but has less diagnostic sensitivity. In premenopausal women, TVS is best performed prior to day 10 of the cycle to lower the risk of false-positive and false-negative findings. With TVS, an endometrial polyp may appear as a nonspecific endometrial thickening or as a round or elongated hyperechoic focal mass within the endometrial cavity. Sonolucent cystic spaces corresponding to dilated endometrial glands are seen within some polyps (Nalaboff, 2001). TVS can be augmented with color or power Doppler. Endometrial polyps typically have only one arterial feeding vessel, whereas submucous leiomyomas generally received blood flow from several vessels arising from the inner myometrium (Fig. 8-9) (Cil, 2010; Fleischer, 2003).

SIS and hysteroscopy are both accurate in identifying endometrial polyps (Soares, 2000). With SIS, polyps appear as echogenic, smooth, intracavitary masses with either broad bases or thin stalks and are outlined by fluid (see Fig. 8-9B). Hysteroscopy identifies nearly all cases of endometrial polyps (see Fig. 8-8). Another advantage of hysteroscopy is the ability to identify and remove the polyp concurrently.

The Pap smear is an ineffective tool to identify polyps. However, it occasionally incidentally leads to their identification. For example, 5 percent of postmenopausal women with benign endometrial cells identified on Pap smear are found to have endometrial polyps (Karim, 2002). Moreover, in postmenopausal women with atypical glandular cells of undetermined significance (AGUS), endometrial polyps were the most frequent underlying pathology found (Obenson, 2000).

Most polyps are benign, and premalignant or malignant transformation develops in only approximately 5 percent (Baiocchi, 2009). Thus, operative hysteroscopic polypectomy may be most effective for symptomatic women or those with risk factors for malignant transformation. These risks include postmenopausal status, larger polyp size (>1.5 cm), abnormal bleeding, and tamoxifen use (Ferrazzi, 2009; Lee, 2010). Hysteroscopically, polyps can be removed by electrosurgical resection or morcellation, as illustrated in Chapter 44 (p. 1038). During hysteroscopic polypectomy, background sampling of the endometrium is considered in those with endometrial cancer risk factors (Rahimi, 2009).

For asymptomatic women with polyps but without malignant transformation risk factors, management can be more conservative. Some advocate removal of all endometrial polyps because premalignant and malignant transformation has been identified in even asymptomatic premenopausal women (Golan, 2010). However, the transformation risk in these patients with small lesions is low, and many of these polyps spontaneously resolve or slough (Ben-Arie, 2004; DeWaay, 2002). If conservative observation is elected, the optimum surveillance for these women remains undefined.

■ Endocervical Polyp

These lesions represent overgrowths of benign endocervical stroma covered by mucinous columnar epithelium. They typically appear as single, red, smooth elongated masses extending from the endocervical canal. Polyps vary in size and range from several millimeters to 2 or 3 cm. These common growths are found more frequently in multiparas and rarely in prepubertal females. Endocervical polyps are usually asymptomatic, but they can cause intermenstrual or postcoital bleeding or symptomatic vaginal discharge. Many endocervical polyps are identified by visual inspection during pelvic examination. In other instances, they may lie higher in the endocervical canal and be found during TVS (Fig. 8-10). Last, AGUS Pap smear findings may prompt investigation and also lead to identification

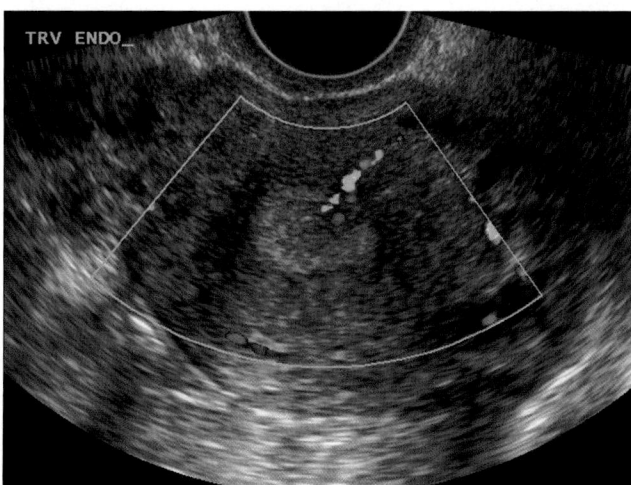

FIGURE 8-9 Transvaginal color Doppler sonography (TV-CDS) of an endometrial polyp. Color flow feature identifies a single feeder vessel, which is characteristic of a polyp. (Used with permission from Dr. Elysia Moschos.)

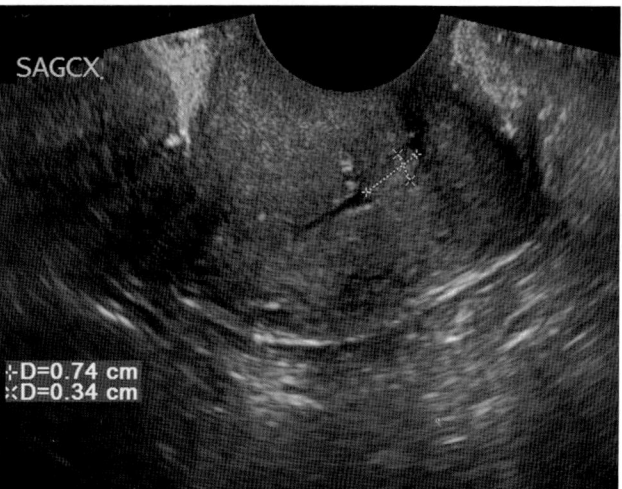

FIGURE 8-10 This transvaginal sonogram shows a sagittal view of the cervix and an endocervical polyp marked by calipers.

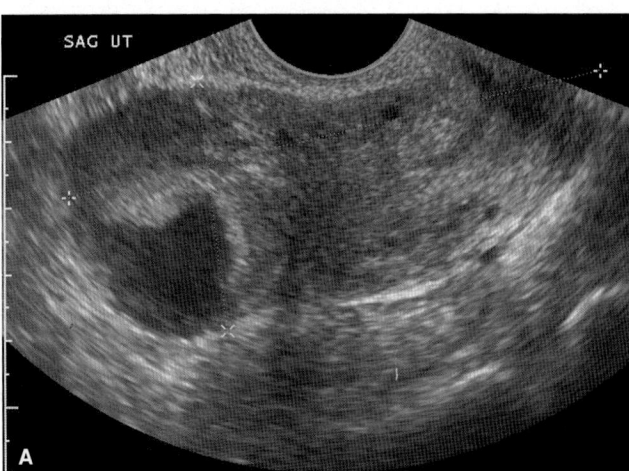
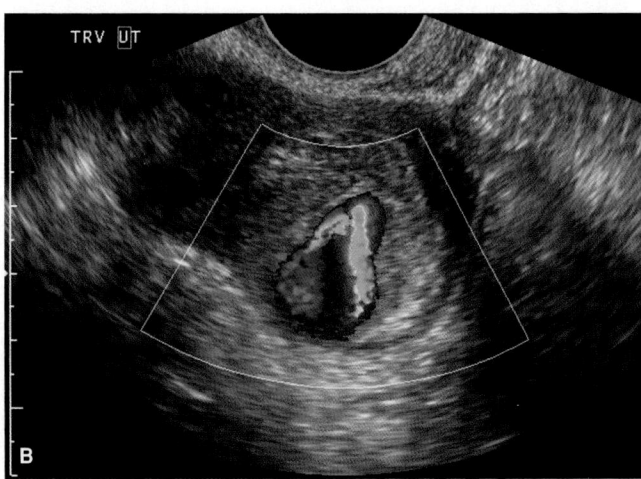

FIGURE 8-11 Transvaginal sonography of an arteriovenous malformation (AVM). **A.** Sagittal image of the uterus (*calipers*) with an irregular-shape anechoic space within the posterior fundal myometrium. **B.** Color Doppler evaluation of this area in the transverse plane demonstrates the classic mosaic color pattern of an AVM. (Used with permission from Dr. Elysia Moschos.)

of endocervical polyps higher in the endocervical canal (Burja, 1999).

Endocervical polyps are typically benign, and premalignant or malignant transformation develops in less than 1 percent (Chin, 2008; Schnatz, 2009). However, cervical cancer can present as polypoid masses and can mimic these benign lesions. Others in the differential diagnosis include condyloma acuminata, leiomyoma, decidua, granulation tissue, endometrial polyp, or fibroadenoma. Most recommend removal and histological evaluation of all polypoid lesions. However, studies have stratified affected patients by symptoms and cytology. Results showed no preinvasive disease or cancer in polyps of asymptomatic women with normal cervical cytology (Long, 2013; MacKenzie, 2009).

For removal, if the stalk is slender, endocervical polyps are grasped by ring forceps. The polyp is twisted repeatedly about the base of its stalk to strangulate its feeding vessels. With repeated twisting the base will narrow and avulse. Monsel paste (ferric subsulfate) can be applied with direct pressure to the resulting stalk stub to complete hemostasis. Rarely, a thick pedicle is found and may warrant surgical ligation and excision if heavier bleeding is anticipated. Patients are counseled that polyp recurrence rates range from 6 to 15 percent (Berzolla, 2007; Younis, 2010).

■ Arteriovenous Malformation

These consist of a mixture of arterial, venous, and small capillary-like channels with fistulous connections. Uterine arteriovenous malformation (AVM) may be congenital or acquired, and vessel sizes can vary considerably. Acquired AVMs are usually large vessels that develop with a cesarean delivery scar or form after trauma from D & C. They can also arise concurrently with cervical or endometrial cancer, with gestational trophoblastic disease, or with intrauterine device use (Ghosh, 1986). Uterine AVMs are rare and more frequently involve the corpus, but they may also be found in the cervix (Lowenstein, 2004). Affected patients often note HMB and perhaps intermenstrual bleeding that is unprovoked or that is triggered by a spontaneous miscarriage, curettage, or other intracavitary uterine surgery.

Symptoms can appear slowly or suddenly with life-threatening bleeding (Timmerman, 2003).

In some cases, AVMs are first visualized with TVS because of its ready availability and widespread use. Sonographic characteristics are nonspecific and may include anechoic tubular structures within the myometrium (Fig. 8-11). Color Doppler or power Doppler ultrasound may provide a more specific image with bright, large-caliber vessels and multidirectional flow (Tullius, 2015). Angiography aids confirmation and can be used concurrently to perform vessel embolization (Cura, 2009). CT scanning with contrast, MR imaging, SIS, and hysteroscopy have also been used to image these (Lowenstein, 2004; Timmerman, 2003).

Arteriovenous malformations are traditionally treated by hysterectomy. However, less invasive, yet effective, approaches include arterial embolization or surgical coagulation of AVM feeding vessels (Corusic, 2009; Ghosh, 1986).

EXTERNAL SOURCES

■ Intrauterine Devices

Of potential exogenous factors, intrauterine devices (IUDs), sex steroid hormone medications, and anticoagulants are typical sources. In contrast, trauma or vaginal erosion from a foreign body is infrequently encountered.

Of these, copper-containing intrauterine devices (ParaGard) can cause heavy or intermenstrual bleeding, and several explanations have been suggested. At the cellular level, prostaglandins are implicated as affecting vascular tone (Coskun, 2011). At the tissue level, endometrial vascularity, congestion, and degeneration result in interstitial hemorrhage, which may lead to intermenstrual bleeding (Shaw, 1979). At the organ level and with either IUD type, malpositioning or less commonly embedding into or perforating through the myometrium can generate AUB (Benacerraf, 2009; Kaislasuo, 2013). TVS and especially 3-D TVS can usually clarify IUD position (Moschos, 2011).

For copper IUD-related bleeding, pregnancy, infection, malpositioned device, or gross structural pathology are first excluded.

Then HMB can be treated or prevented with an empiric trial of NSAIDs taken during menses. Intermenstrual bleeding, however, is typically not improved with these agents (Godfrey, 2013). Limited evidence also supports tranexamic acid for treatment or prevention (Ylikorkala, 1983). Women with persistent or refractory bleeding may have other pathology and are managed similarly to other women with the initial complaint of AUB. However, with TVS, endometrial stripe evaluation may be limited by IUD shadowing. Importantly, endometrial biopsy with small catheters can be performed without device removal (Grimes, 2007).

With the levonorgestrel-releasing intrauterine system (LNG-IUS), marketed as Mirena, Liletta, and Skyla, unscheduled spotting or light bleeding is expected during the first several months and decreases with continued use (Centers for Disease Control and Prevention, 2013). The pathophysiology of this bleeding is not clear, but downregulation of estrogen and progesterone receptors, increased local leukocyte populations, and altered MMP levels are suggested factors (Labied, 2009). The endometrial effects of progestins are thought to predominate, and evidence is accruing that low-dose progestins increase endometrial vascular fragility (Hickey, 2002). Over time, the endometrium atrophies, and these vascular abnormalities gradually resolve at a time thought to coincide clinically with progestin-induced amenorrhea (McGavigan, 2003). Scant data guide specific treatment of problematic LNG-IUS–related bleeding, but options discussed next for other progestin-only contraception can be extrapolated.

Hormonal Therapy

Other *hormonal birth control methods* can create bleeding disturbances. Overall, menses are typically lighter with these, but intermenstrual bleeding is frequent with progestin-only methods throughout use and with combination oral contraceptive (COC) formulations during early months of use. Chronic COC-related intermenstrual bleeding is typically corrected by changing to a brand with an increased estrogen dose. In contrast, for AUB due to a progestin-only implant or depot medroxyprogesterone acetate (DMPA), bleeding can be lessened by an estrogen supplement such as daily ethinyl estradiol or conjugated equine estrogen (Premarin) or by the addition of a COC (Alvarez-Sanchez, 1996; Díaz, 1990; Said, 1996). These are provided for a few weeks. Alternatively, NSAIDs given for 5 to 7 days is reasonable, but studies show mixed results (Abdel-Aleem, 2013; Centers for Disease Control and Prevention, 2013).

With *hormone replacement therapy*, irregular spotting or bleeding is also a well-known side effect. During the first year of therapy, irregular bleeding is more likely with continuous combined therapy than sequential therapy. However, during the second year, this order is reversed (Lethaby, 2004). With continuous therapy, lower initial doses may cause less bleeding (Archer, 2007). Importantly, intrauterine pathology has been shown to be four times more frequent in patients with continued abnormal bleeding after six months of HRT use, as well as in those who have abnormal bleeding after achieving initial amenorrhea (Leung, 2003).

Of the *selective estrogen-receptor modulators (SERMs)*, raloxifene (Evista) is used to treat osteoporosis. Postmenopausal bleeding can develop with use but much less frequently and with lower rates of endometrial pathology than with HRT (Neven, 2003). Another SERM, tamoxifen, is used as an adjunct for treatment of estrogen receptor positive breast cancer. Although it diminishes estrogen action in breast tissue, tamoxifen stimulates endometrial proliferation. This SERM has been linked to hyperplasia, polyps, and carcinoma of the endometrium and to uterine sarcomas (Cohen, 2004). Thus, associated AUB warrants evaluation. However, using TVS or endometrial biopsy to screen women who use tamoxifen but who do not have abnormal bleeding has not proved effective (Barakat, 2000). Accordingly, for women without increased endometrial cancer risks but using tamoxifen, such routine surveillance is not recommended (American College of Obstetricians and Gynecologists, 2014).

Anticoagulants

Although treatment with these confers a risk of major bleeding, menstrual irregularities are also often encountered. Initially, coagulation studies including prothrombin time (PT), partial thromboplastin time (PTT), and platelet count are obtained as bleeding may be related to excess anticoagulant activity. Patients are also queried regarding recent dosage changes or antagonist medications. Physical examination is completed, and AUB evaluation components are performed as indicated.

Management of AUB can be challenging as many traditional treatment options carry thromboembolic risks. For chronic HMB, the LNG-IUS has been found to be an effective treatment in many of women using anticoagulants (Pisoni, 2006). If a surgical approach is ultimately desired, endometrial ablation or hysterectomy can be considered. Anticoagulation reversal for surgery differs depending on whether surgery is urgent or elective, and both instances are described in Chapter 39 (p. 830).

For acute severe HMB, anticoagulation is reversed, and a Foley balloon can be inserted into the intrauterine cavity and inflated to tamponade bleeding. Estrogen-containing hormonal manipulation of the endometrium and tranexamic acid are contraindicated because of their underlying risks for thromboembolism. Moreover, emergent surgery or uterine artery embolization (UAE) is associated with increased rates of intra- and postoperative bleeding or thromboembolic complications.

ENDOMETRITIS

In addition to cervicitis (p. 184), chronic endometritis has been linked to abnormal bleeding in some but not all studies (Greenwood, 1981; Pitsos, 2009). Underlying infection is often implicated, and agents of bacterial vaginosis, *Mycoplasma* species, *Neisseria gonorrhoeae*, and *Chlamydia trachomatis*, have each been identified. Thus, testing for the latter two pathogens is reasonable in sexually active patients, and positive results prompt treatment per CDC guidelines (2015). That said, vaginal cultures may not always correlate with endometrial culture (Cicinelli, 2008).

In other cases, chronic endometritis is linked to a structural cause such as endometrial polyp, IUD, or submucous leiomyoma. It may follow abortion or pregnancy.

Chronic endometritis is traditionally diagnosed histologically by plasma cell infiltration found in an endometrial sample.

In women undergoing diagnostic hysteroscopy, the diagnosis can also be suggested by endometrial hyperemia, edema, and "micropolyps" measuring <1 mm (Cicinelli, 2005).

Because infection may or may not underlie all cases of chronic endometritis, deciding whether or not to treat with antibiotics can be challenging. Moreover, few studies have evaluated the efficacy of antibiotics to resolve symptoms. At our institution, patients with documented histologic findings of endometritis are typically given a course of doxycycline, 100 mg orally twice daily for 10 days.

SYSTEMIC CAUSES

■ Kidney, Liver, and Thyroid Disease

Severe *renal dysfunction* often is accompanied by endocrine disturbances that lead to hypoestrogenism and amenorrhea or to normal estrogen levels but anovulation (Matuszkiewicz-Rowińska, 2004). In a study of 100 women with chronic renal failure undergoing dialysis, Cochrane and Regan (1997) reported that 80 percent of those menstruating complained of HMB. Of additional concern, bleeding may worsen the chronic anemia already associated with renal failure.

For AUB from anovulation, renal patients are treated with traditional methods as outlined on page 194 (Guglielmi, 2013). Of specific options, Fong and Singh (1999) report success with the LNG-IUS in renal transplant patients with HMB secondary to uterine leiomyomas. Notably, COCs may be contraindicated with severe hypertension, which commonly complicates renal disease, or with some systemic lupus erythematosus cases. Moreover, in those with renal disease, NSAIDs are avoided because they cause renal artery vasoconstriction that diminishes glomerular function.

If women with renal failure and HMB cannot take or do not respond to medical therapy, then surgical treatments are considered. Of these, Jeong and coworkers (2004) noted decreased bleeding in 87 percent of patients following endometrial ablation.

Liver dysfunction, depending on its severity, can lead to menstrual abnormalities (Stellon, 1986). With end-stage liver disease warranting transplantation, menstrual dysfunction is reported by 60 percent (de Koning, 1990). The underlying mechanism for bleeding is not clear, but as in renal failure, HPO axis dysfunction is suggested. Hemostatic dysfunction may also contribute. With the exception of von Willebrand factor, all of the coagulation proteins and most of their inhibitors are synthesized in the liver. Last, thrombocytopenia is common in women with portal hypertension and splenomegaly.

Evidenced directing the HMB treatment in women with liver disease is limited, and hormonal therapy may be inappropriate for some affected women. As outlined by the World Health Organization, in those with chronic viral hepatitis or with mild compensated cirrhosis, hormonal contraceptive use is not restricted. In those with active hepatitis or a flare of their chronic viral disease, progestin-only contraception is acceptable. Estrogen-containing products, if already in use, may be continued, whereas initiation of these is avoided. In those with severe, decompensated cirrhosis, all hormonal contraception is avoided (Kapp, 2009).

Both *hyperthyroidism* and *hypothyroidism* can cause menstrual disturbances ranging from amenorrhea to HMB. In many women, these menstrual abnormalities antedate other clinical findings of thyroid disease (Joshi, 1993). Thus, in most women with chronic AUB, measurement of serum thyroid-stimulating hormone (TSH) level is recommended. With hyperthyroidism, hypomenorrhea and oligoamenorrhea are more frequent complaints (Krassas, 2010). With severe overt hypothyroidism, women commonly present with anovulation, amenorrhea, and anovulatory AUB (p. 194). These women can also display defects in hemostasis. This may be due to decreased coagulation factor levels that have been identified in some hypothyroid patients. With either hypo- or hyperthyroidism, treatment of the underlying thyroid disorder usually corrects AUB (Krassas, 1999; Wilansky, 1989).

■ Coagulopathy

Normally, a clot forms from an aggregation of platelets, which is then stabilized by a fibrin net. Thus, many coagulation defects leading to HMB can be broadly categorized as either: (1) dysfunction of platelet adherence or (2) defects in platelet plug stabilization. First, during initial stages of hemostasis, platelets adhere to vessel wall breaks through binding of their receptors to exposed collagen. This bridging is dependent on von Willebrand factor (vWF), a plasma protein. Once bound, platelets are activated and release a potent agonist of their aggregation, thromboxane. Thus, low platelet number, defects in vWF quality or quantity, platelet receptor defects, or thromboxane inhibitors may all lead to poor platelet adherence and HMB. Second, the coagulation cascade leads to fibrin, which stabilizes aggregated platelets. Thus, defects in the clotting factors that make up these cascades may also predispose to abnormal bleeding.

In general, coagulopathies are infrequent causes of gynecologic bleeding. However, in the subset of women with HMB and normal anatomy, the incidence is significantly higher (Philipp, 2005). And in women with known inherited bleeding disorders, HMB is the most common complaint (Byams, 2011).

For diagnosis, a history of easy bruising, bleeding complications with surgery or obstetric delivery, recurrent hemorrhagic ovarian cysts, epistaxis, and gastrointestinal bleeding or a family history of bleeding disorders raises concern for coagulopathy. Laboratory screening includes a CBC with platelets, PT, PTT, and fibrinogen level (American College of Obstetricians and Gynecologists, 2013e). More frequently identified coagulopathies include von Willebrand disease, thrombocytopenia, and platelet dysfunction. Specific screening for each is discussed subsequently. Deficiencies of factor VIII and IX (hemophilia A and B) and other factor deficiencies are uncommon. Acute treatment of these disorders is by factor replacement, and long-term management is similar to that for von Willebrand disease (Mannucci, 2004).

Platelets

As described, low platelet counts may lead to AUB. *Thrombocytopenia* may be broadly categorized as resulting from disorders that: (1) increase platelet destruction, as with idiopathic thrombocytopenic purpura (ITP), (2) decrease platelet production, as with hematopoietic malignancy, or (3) increase platelet sequestration, as with splenomegaly.

Alternatively, normal platelet counts may be found, but *platelet dysfunction* leads to poor aggregation. One example is prolonged use of thromboxane inhibitors such as NSAIDs and aspirin. These drugs are often taken by women with AUB due to its close association with dysmenorrhea. Accordingly, patients are queried regarding chronic use of these drugs. Much less often, primary genetic defects in platelet receptors, such Bernard-Soulier syndrome and Glanzmann thrombasthenia, lead to platelet dysfunction and abnormal bleeding.

As a group, evidenced-based data directing the treatment of platelet-associated HMB are limited. For acute, severe HMB, platelet transfusion is considered for counts <20,000/μL or for those <50,000/μL with brisk bleeding. For those undergoing procedures, a transfusion threshold of ≤50,000/μL is used, and for major surgery, ≤100,000/μL (James, 2011). Concurrently, treatment is tailored to the underlying cause of thrombocytopenia. Long-term, with the exception of NSAIDs, treatment options include those described later for AUB secondary to endometrial dysfunction (p. 195).

Von Willebrand Disease

Von Willebrand factor (vWF) is a glycoprotein synthesized in endothelial cells and in megakaryocytes, which produce platelets. For coagulation, it is integral to platelet adherence at sites of endothelial injury and also prevents clearance of factor VIII. von Willebrand disease (vWD) has several variants, which are characterized by either diminished amount or decreased function of vWF (Table 8-2). This is an inherited bleeding disorder. In general, type 3 vWD displays autosomal recessive transmission, whereas type 1 and most subtypes of type 2 show an autosomal dominant pattern.

The disorder is more common in whites than in African-Americans, and the prevalence of vWD approximates 1 percent in the general population (Rodeghiero, 2001). However, in women with AUB and normal pelvic anatomy, vWD is found in nearly 13 percent (Shankar, 2004). Of women with vWD, nearly 75 percent complain of HMB, which typically begins with menarche (Byams, 2011).

In screening for coagulopathy as described on page 192, women with vWD may display a prolonged PTT or may have normal results. If vWD is suspected clinically, specific tests include measurement of von Willebrand-ristocetin cofactor activity, vWF antigen concentration, and factor VIII activity (James, 2009b). Of note, factor VIII and vWF levels reach a nadir during menses and are relatively increased in women using COCs. However, testing need not be rescheduled nor COCs halted to complete patient evaluation (James, 2009a). Consultation with a hematologist is often recommended because the diagnosis of vWD, especially in its mild form, can be difficult.

Treatments for women with vWD and chronic HMB mirror that listed for primary endometrial dysfunction (p. 195). Of options, COCs are often used as first-line treatment and have been noted to arrest uterine hemorrhage in 88 percent of affected women (Foster, 1995). Also, Kingman and coworkers (2004) reported that the LNG-IUS effectively decreased blood loss and induced amenorrhea in 56 percent of 16 women with an inherited bleeding disorder. DMPA (Depo-Provera), progestin-only pills, and etonogestrel implant (Nexplanon) are other options for HMB in these women. Additional treatment may also include the antifibrinolytic drug tranexamic acid (Lysteda). Importantly, agents that prevent platelet adhesion, such as aspirin or NSAIDs, are avoided (American College of Obstetricians and Gynecologists, 2013e).

For women with chronic HMB who do not respond to conventional treatment, a hematologist may be consulted for desmopressin or vWF concentrate use (Nichols, 2008). Desmopressin is a vasopressin analogue that promotes release of vWF from endothelial cells. Available in intravenous and nasal forms, its side effects include flushing, transient blood-pressure changes, nausea, or headache, but these rarely limit use. In those with chronic HMB in whom desmopressin is ineffective or contraindicated, a vWF concentrate can be chosen. Available in the United States, Humate-P or Alphanate each contains both vWF and factor VIII.

In those with vWD-related chronic HMB who no longer desire fertility, surgical intervention may be considered. Preliminary success has been found with endometrial ablation for affected women, but long-term success rates are lower than in those without a bleeding disorder (Rubin, 2004). Dilatation and curettage is ineffective long-term to control bleeding and may acutely worsen blood loss in affected women (James, 2009a). Hysterectomy is curative, although rates of bleeding complications from hysterectomy in women with vWD are higher than those of unaffected women (James, 2009c). In preparation for

TABLE 8-2. vWD Classification and Laboratory Values

Condition	Description of vWF deficiency	Bleeding propensity	vWf:RCo (IU/dL)	vWf:Ag (IU/dL)	FVIII activity
Type 1	Quantitative: partial	Mild to Moderate	<30	<30	↓ or Normal
Type 2	Qualitative	Moderate	<30	<30–200	↓ or Normal
Type 3	Quantitative: virtually complete	High	<3	<3	↓↓↓(<10 IU/dL)
Normal			50–200	50–200	Normal

FVIII = coagulation factor VIII; vWD = von Willebrand disease; vWF = von Willebrand factor; vWF:Ag = von Willebrand factor antigen; vWF:RCo = von Willebrand factor: risocetin cofactor activity.
Adapted with permission from Nichols WL, Rick ME, Ortel TL, et al: Clinical and laboratory diagnosis of von Willebrand disease: a synopsis of the 2008 NHLBI/NIH guidelines. Am J Hematol 84(6):366, 2009.

TABLE 8-3. Medical Treatment of Acute Heavy Abnormal Uterine Bleeding[a,b]

CEE[c,d]	25 mg IV every 4 hr, up to 3 doses
CEE[d,e]	2.5 mg every 6 hr
COCs[d,e] 30–50 μg	1 pill every 6 or 8 hr, up to 7 d
MPA[e]	10 mg every 4 hr
NETA[e]	5–10 mg every 4 hr
TXA[c]	10 mg/kg IV every 8 hr
TXA	1.3 g every 8 hr for 5 d

[a]Agents given orally except where noted as IV.
[b]For anemic patients, initiate oral iron supplements.
[c]If IV forms required, transition patients to oral agents once bleeding is improved.
[d]Antiemetics may aid nausea.
[e]Oral hormonal agent dosages are tapered by extending dosing from every 4–6 hr, to every 8 hr, to every 12 hr, and finally to daily. Each new dosing lasts 2 to 7 days depending on the level of concern for rebleeding.
CEE = conjugated equine estrogen (Premarin); COCs = combination oral contraceptive pills; d = day; hr = hour; IV = intravenous; MPA = medroxyprogesterone acetate; NETA = norethindrone acetate; TXA = tranexamic acid.
Data from DeVore, 1982; Munro, 2006; James, 2011.

surgical procedures, a hematologist may assist with desmopressin or vWF concentrate dosing.

For severe emergent bleeding, hormonal and antifibrinolytic options shown in Table 8-3 are implemented while clotting factor deficiencies are corrected. In addition, desmopressin can be administered (Edlund, 2002). However, desmopressin is a potent antidiuretic agent. Thus, if multiple doses or shorter dosing intervals are used, concurrent fluid restriction and monitoring for hyponatremia is advised (Rodeghiero, 2008). However, if aggressive fluid resuscitation is needed, then desmopressin may not be appropriate. In this case, vWF concentrates are used instead to quickly raise factor levels (James, 2011). Comprehensive management guidelines for vWD are also available from The National Heart, Lung, and Blood Institute at: http://www.nhlbi.nih.gov/files/docs/guidelines/vwd.pdf.

OVULATORY DISORDERS

A large percentage of women with AUB have anovulation as the underlying etiology, and the term AUB-O denotes this ovulatory dysfunction. *Dysfunctional uterine bleeding* is currently a less-preferred term for this (American College of Obstetricians and Gynecologists, 2012). With AUB-O, bleeding episodes are variable, and amenorrhea, HMB, and intermenstrual bleeding often interchange. For example, women with anovulation may be amenorrheic for weeks to months followed by irregular, prolonged, and heavy bleeding.

The underlying causes of anovulation are varied and fully described in Chapter 16 (p. 369). Regardless of the reason, if ovulation does not occur, no progesterone is produced, and a proliferative endometrium persists. At the tissue level, a chronic

proliferative endometrium is typically associated with stromal breakdown, decreased spiral arteriole density, and dilated and unstable venous capillaries (Singh, 2005). Because endometrial vessels become markedly dilated, bleeding can be severe. At the cellular level, the availability of arachidonic acid is reduced, and prostaglandin production is impaired. For these reasons, bleeding associated with anovulation is thought to result from alterations in endometrial vascular structure and prostaglandin concentration and from an increased endometrial responsiveness to vasodilating prostaglandins (Hickey, 2000, 2003).

■ Chronic Management

Ideally, AUB-O is reversed by correction of the underlying cause of anovulation. If this is not possible, chronic progestin therapy supplements the physiologic progesterone that is absent with anovulation. For women requiring contraception, COCs, progestin-only contraceptive pills, DMPA, LNG-IUS, and etonogestrel subdermal implant are options. In those not desiring contraception, cyclic monthly progesterone followed by withdrawal will typically regulate menses. Suitable oral daily doses given for 10 days each month include: (1) medroxyprogesterone acetate (MPA [Provera]), 5 or 10 mg; (2) norethindrone acetate (NETA [Aygestin]), 5 or 10 mg; or (3) micronized progesterone, 300 mg (de Lignières, 1999; Munro, 2000). As another but less frequently used choice, gonadotropin-releasing hormone (GnRH) agonists create profound hypogonadism (Chap. 9, p. 208). The induced amenorrhea can be advantageous to permit severely anemic women with HMB to rebuild their red cell volume (Vercellini, 1993). Surgery is rarely indicated for AUB-O, unless medical therapy fails, is contraindicated, or is not tolerated by the patient, or the patient has concomitant significant uterine structural lesions (American College of Obstetricians and Gynecologists, 2013b). Surgical options mirror those for abnormal bleeding associated with endometrial dysfunction, discussed on page 197.

■ Acute Hemorrhage Management

At times, women with anovulatory bleeding may have severe HMB that requires acute intervention. Fluid resuscitation is instituted as described in Chapter 40 (p. 864). Medical treatment is simultaneously administered to slow bleeding (see Table 8-3). As primary choices, equine estrogens can be given intravenously (IV) in 25-mg doses every 4 hours for up to three doses (DeVore, 1982). Once bleeding has slowed, patients can be transitioned to an oral taper using Premarin pills or more commonly COCs. These pill forms can also be selected primarily for less severe bleeding. With any of these high-dose choices, an antiemetic may be needed to control nausea. For COC administration, formulations containing at least 30 μg of ethinyl estradiol are selected, and a complete list is found in Table 5-7 (p. 120). If bleeding is significant, the regimen begins with one pill every 6 hours until the bleeding has stopped or markedly diminished. For most women, bleeding will slow within 24 to 48 hours. After bleeding has diminished, the COC dosage is decreased to one pill every 8 hours for the next 2 to 7 days and then to one pill every 12 hours for 2 to 7 days (James, 2011). A once-a-day dosage is then continued for several weeks, to be followed by withdrawal menses. This type of dose-diminishing regimen is colloquially known as a "COC taper." Effective modification of this regimen may include less frequent dosing or smaller doses. Following this taper, COCs may be stopped or continued long-term for cycle control (Munro, 2006).

As an alternative to high-dose estrogen therapy for acute HMB, high-dose MPA (10 mg) or NETA (5 to 10 mg) can be used and administered orally every 4 hours. As with oral COCs, these are then tapered once bleeding has waned. One proposed taper stretches dosing to every 6 hours for 4 days, then every 8 hours for 3 days, then every 12 hours for 2 to 14 days. The progestin is then continued daily (James, 2011). Another primary regimen uses MPA 20 mg orally three times daily combined with DMPA 150 mg intramuscularly. Here, the single depot injection serves as the taper (Ammerman, 2013).

Tranexamic acid (TXA) is also an option, and the usual IV dose is 10 mg/kg every 8 hours. As bleeding declines, transition to an oral dose of 1.3 g given three times a day can be implemented (James, 2011). Cautions for extended TXA use combined with hormonal agents are described on page 196.

With any of these medication regimens, an intrauterine Foley balloon can be inflated for brisk bleeding. This acts to tamponade the endometrial vessels while the above-listed agents exert their control.

PRIMARY ENDOMETRIAL DYSFUNCTION

This form of AUB is thought to stem predominantly from endometrial vascular dilatation alone. For example, women with ovulatory bleeding lose blood at rates three times faster than women with normal menses, but the number of spiral arterioles is not increased (Abberton, 1999). Thus, in women with ovulatory AUB, vessels supplying the endometrium are thought to have decreased vascular tone and therefore increased rates of blood loss from vasodilatation (Rogers, 2003). Several provocateurs of this change in vascular tone are suggested, especially prostaglandins. Despite these physiologic findings, AUB from endometrial dysfunction (AUB-E) has no clear diagnostic features and currently is a diagnosis of exclusion.

Acute medical treatment of severe AUB-E mirrors that for AUB due to ovulatory dysfunction as shown in Table 8-3. Chronic medical options include LNG-IUS, COCs, sustained progestins, TXA, NSAIDs, androgens, and GnRH agonists (Table 8-4).

■ Levonorgestrel-releasing Intrauterine System

In addition to providing effective contraception, this device releases sustained progestin levels within the uterine cavity. This atrophies the endometrial lining and reduces menstrual loss by 74 to 97 percent after 3 months' use (Singh, 2005; Stewart, 2001). The LNG-IUS can be used in most women, including adolescents, as a first-line treatment for HMB. It is particularly useful for reproductive-aged women with AUB-E who wish to retain fertility. Contraindications include an abnormal uterine cavity, untreated breast or reproductive tract cancer, acute liver disease or tumor, and reproductive tract infection or infection risks. Others caveats are listed in Table 5-4 (p. 109).

Of treatments for AUB-E, the LNG-IUS is one of the more extensively researched (Matteson, 2013). In randomized trials, the LNG-IUS proved more effective in decreasing menstrual blood loss than NSAIDs given during menses; than oral progesterone

TABLE 8-4. Chronic Medical Treatment of Abnormal Uterine Bleeding due to Primary Endometrial Dysfunction[a,b]

Agent	Brand	Dosage	Study
LNG-IUS	Mirena	5-yr intrauterine use	Shaaban, 2011
COCs	Table 5-7[c]	One pill daily	Fraser, 2011
DMPA	Depo-Provera	150 mg IM every 3 mo	Küçük, 2008
NETA	Aygestin	5 mg, 3 times daily, days 5–26 of cycle	Irvine, 1998
TXA[d]	Lysteda	1.3 g, 3 times daily × 5 d	Lukes, 2010
NSAID[d]			
Mefenamic acid	Ponstel	500 mg, 3 times daily × 5 d	Bonnar, 1996
Naproxen	Naprosyn	550 mg on first day, then 275 mg daily	Hall, 1987
Ibuprofen	Motrin	600 mg, daily throughout menses	Makarainen, 1986
Flurbiprofen	Ansaid	100 mg, 2 times daily × 5 d	Andersch, 1988
Danocrine	Danazol	100 mg or 200 mg, daily throughout cycle	Chimbira, 1980b
GnRH agonists	Lupron	3.75 mg, IM each month (up to 6 mo)	Thomas, 1991

[a]All agents are administered orally except GnRH agonists, DMPA, and LNG-IUS.
[b]For anemic patients, also initiate oral iron supplementation.
[c]See Table 5-7, p. 120.
[d]Begin treatment with menses onset.
COCs = combination oral contraceptive pills; DMPA = depot medroxyprogesterone acetate; GnRH = gonadotropin-releasing hormone; IM = intramuscularly; LNG-IUS = levonorgestrel-releasing intrauterine system; NETA = norethindrone acetate; NSAID = nonsteroidal antiinflammatory drug; TXA = tranexamic acid.

given 21 days each cycle; or than COCs (Irvine, 1998; Reid, 2005; Shaaban, 2011).

However, trials often evaluate HMB more generally and thus several AUB etiologies, in addition to AUB-E, are bundled. For HMB, Gupta and coworkers (2013) noted higher associated quality-of-life scores with LNG-IUS compared with several traditional oral medical options. If compared with endometrial ablation, the LNG-IUS appears to have similar therapeutic effects for HMB up to 2 years after treatment (Kaunitz, 2009). Last, one randomized trial compared LNG-IUS or hysterectomy for HMB and reported equal improvements in health status and quality of life at 1 year and again after 5 years (Hurskainen, 2001, 2004). However, by 5 years, 42 percent of those assigned to the LNG-IUS eventually underwent hysterectomy, and by 10 years, 46 percent (Heliövaara-Peippo, 2013). To summarize its efficacy, compared with most available options, the LNG-IUS provides equivalent or superior improvement in HMB for suitable candidates.

Combination Oral Contraceptive Pills

These hormonal agents effectively treat AUB-E, and when used long term, menstrual blood loss is reduced by 40 to 70 percent (Jensen, 2011; Fraser, 1991, 2011). Advantages to COC use include the additional benefits of reducing dysmenorrhea and providing contraception. Their presumed method of action is endometrial atrophy, although diminished prostaglandin synthesis and decreased endometrial fibrinolysis are other suggested actions (Irvine, 1999).

Tranexamic Acid

This antifibrinolytic drug reversibly blocks lysine binding sites on plasminogen (Fig. 8-12). In women with AUB-E, fibrinolytic activity within the endometrium is increased compared with that of women with normal menses (Gleeson, 1994). Clinically, TXA has been shown to reduce bleeding in women with AUB-E by 40 to 50 percent (Bonnar, 1996; Lukes, 2010). In addition, it requires administration only during menstruation and has few minor reported side effects that are predominantly gastrointestinal and dose-dependent. The recommended dose is two 650-mg tablets orally taken three times daily for a maximum of 5 days during menses.

Although used in other parts of the world for many years, oral TXA was approved by the U.S. Food and Drug Administration (FDA) to treat HMB in 2009. Its U.S. marketed name is Lysteda. The drug has no effect on other blood coagulation parameters such as platelet count, PTT, and PT (Wellington, 2003). Contraindications to TXA include concurrent COC use, a history of or an intrinsic risk for thromboembolic disease, disseminated intravascular coagulation, and color blindness. The last relates to animal studies showing retinal changes with TXA. Associated symptoms may not be appreciated by those with preexisting color blindness.

Nonsteroidal Antiinflammatory Drugs

These well-tolerated oral agents are commonly used to treat AUB-E, and rationale for their use stems from prostaglandin's suspected role in the pathogenesis of this endometrial dysfunction. Because women lose 90 percent of menstrual blood volume during the first 3 days of menses, NSAIDs are most effective if used with menses onset or just prior to its onset and continued throughout its duration (Haynes, 1977). Thus, one advantage is that they are taken only during menstruation. Another advantage is that frequently associated dysmenorrhea also improves with NSAIDs.

Conventional NSAIDs nonspecifically inhibit both cyclooxygenase-1 (COX-1), an enzyme critical to normal platelet function, and COX-2, which mediates inflammatory response mechanisms. Thus, conventional NSAIDs such as ibuprofen and naproxen may not be ideal considering their inhibitory effects on platelet function. However, no data show an advantage with specific COX-2 inhibitors for HMB compared with conventional NSAIDs. Among conventional NSAIDS, there are no differences in clinical efficacy, but responses to a particular agent may vary among individuals.

Although NSAIDs require only temporal dosing, are cost-effective, and are well tolerated, they often are only moderately effective for AUB-E and reduce menstrual bleeding by approximately

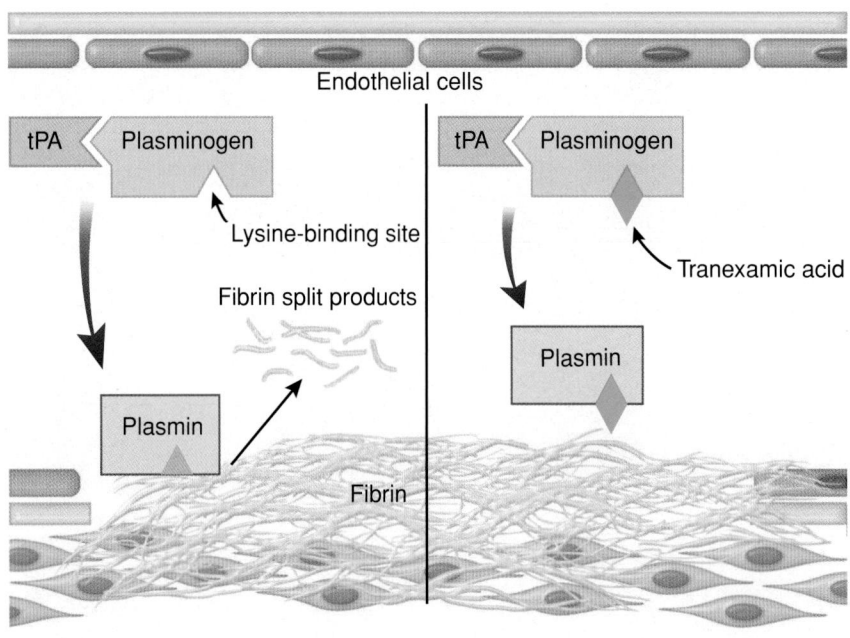

FIGURE 8-12 Tranexamic acid (TXA) mechanism of action. **A.** Normally, plasminogen binds with tissue plasminogen activator (tPA) to form plasmin. This binding degrades fibrin into fibrin degradation products and leads to clot lysis. **B.** TXA binds to the lysine-binding site on plasminogen. This new conformation blocks plasmin binding to fibrin. Fibrin strands are not broken, and a clot persists to slow bleeding.

Endothelial cells

tPA Plasminogen

Lysine-binding site

Fibrin split products

Plasmin

Fibrin

tPA Plasminogen

Tranexamic acid

Plasmin

25 percent (Lethaby, 2013a). Thus, if greater reductions in blood loss are needed, other agents in this section may prove more beneficial.

Other Hormonal Agents

In contrast to AUB-O, AUB-E is relatively unresponsive to cyclic administration of oral progestins (Kaunitz, 2010; Preston, 1995). However, women with AUB-E may respond to longer treatment schedules. NETA, 5 mg, or MPA, 10 mg, each given orally three times daily for days 5 through 26 of each menstrual cycle have proved effective (Fraser, 1990; Irvine, 1998). Unfortunately, prolonged use of high-dose progestins is often associated with side effects such as mood changes, weight gain, bloating, headaches, and atherogenic changes in the lipid profile (Lethaby, 2008). Moreover, patients may find the dosing schedule challenging.

With GnRH agonists, the profound hypoestrogenic state created induces endometrial atrophy and amenorrhea in most women. Side effects include those typical for menopause, and thus associated bone loss precludes their long-term use. This family of drugs, however, may be helpful for short-term use by inducing amenorrhea and allowing women to rebuild their red blood cell mass. Chapter 9 (p. 208) describes available agents and their dosages.

Of androgens, danazol is a derivative of the synthetic steroid 17α-ethinyl testosterone, and its net effect creates a hypoestrogenic and hyperandrogenic environment to induce endometrial atrophy. As a result, menstrual loss is reduced by approximately half, and it may even induce amenorrhea (Dockeray, 1989). For HMB, suggested dosing is 100 to 200 mg orally daily (Chimbira, 1980a). Unfortunately, this agent has significant androgenic side effects that include weight gain, oily skin, and acne. Thus, some reserve danazol as a second-line drug for short-term use prior to surgery (Bongers, 2004).

Gestrinone is derived synthetically from a 19-nortestosterone steroid nucleus. Its mechanisms of action, side effects, and indications for HMB treatment are similar to those of danazol. The recommended treatment dose is 2.5 mg orally twice weekly (Turnbull, 1990). The drug is used in the United Kingdom and other countries but is not approved for use in the United States.

Iron Therapy

Women with AUB may become anemic, and care typically is directed toward bleeding abatement and oral iron replacement. Common equivalent replacement regimens include: (1) ferrous sulfate, 325 mg tablet (contains 65 mg elemental iron) three times daily, or (2) ferrous fumarate, 200 mg tablet (contains 64 mg elemental iron) three times daily. Iron supplementation is further discussed in Chapter 39 (p. 830).

Uterine Procedures

For many women, conservative medical management may be unsuccessful or associated with significant side effects. Surgical management of HMB may include procedures to destroy the endometrium or hysterectomy.

Of these, *dilatation and curettage* is rarely used for long-term treatment of AUB because its effects are temporary.

Occasionally, D & C is performed to quickly remove a thickened endometrium and arrest severe HMB refractory to high-dose estrogen administration (American College of Obstetricians and Gynecologists, 2013c). Preprocedural TVS may be prudent as D & C may be ineffective or disadvantageous for women with an already thinned endometrial stripe.

Endometrial resection or ablation attempts to permanently remove and destroy the uterine lining. Different types use laser, radiofrequency, electrical, or thermal energies. Methods are considered first- or second-generation techniques according to when they were introduced into use and their need for concurrent hysteroscopic guidance.

Several studies that compared first- and second-generation techniques have shown them equally effective to reduce HMB (Lethaby, 2013b). Similarly equivalent efficacy is seen among the various second-generation options, which are described in Chapter 44 (p. 1043) (Daniels, 2012). After ablation, 70 to 80 percent of women experience significantly decreased flow, and 15 to 35 percent of these develop amenorrhea (Sharp, 2006). Increasing treatment failures due to endometrial regeneration accrue with time, and by 5 years following ablation, approximately 25 percent required additional surgery, in most cases hysterectomy (Cooper, 2011). However, the risk of reoperation following resection and ablation procedures is balanced by their significantly lower complication rates compared with hysterectomy.

After ablation, uterine cavity anatomy is often distorted by uterine wall agglutination and intracavitary scar bands, termed synechiae. This may pose several long-term problems. First, focal hematometra or postablation tubal sterilization syndrome (PATSS) can form from menstrual blood trapped behind synechiae. It can cause severe distention and cyclic pain (Chap. 44, p. 1043). Second, because of distorted anatomy, 33 percent of endometrial sampling attempts may be inadequate, and endometrial stripe evaluation by TVS or hysteroscopic examination may be limited (Ahonkallio, 2009). Accordingly, endometrial ablation is not routinely recommended for patients at high risk for endometrial cancer (American College of Obstetricians and Gynecologists, 2013a). Other contraindications are listed in Table 8-5.

Uterine artery embolization (UAE) is more commonly used to treat HMB secondary to uterine leiomyomas and is described in

---

TABLE 8-5. Contraindications for Endometrial Ablation

Pregnancy
Acute pelvic infection
Endometrial hyperplasia or genital tract cancer
Women at high risk for endometrial cancer[a]
Women wishing to preserve their fertility
Postmenopausal women
Expectation of amenorrhea
Large or distorted endometrial cavity[b]
Intrauterine device in place
Prior uterine surgery—classical cesarean delivery,
   transmural myomectomy

---

[a]Risks include obesity, chronic anovulation, tamoxifen use, unopposed estrogen use, and diabetes mellitus.
[b]Each device has specific cavity-size limitations.

Chapter 9 (p. 209). Rarely, this intervention may be considered emergently in women with excessive acute HMB who are not responding to conservative measures, especially those who refuse blood products or who have coagulopathic disorders. However, with the latter, coagulopathy that is severe may preclude safe femoral artery cannulation, which is requisite for UAE.

Hysterectomy, despite the above measures, ultimately is chosen by more than half of women with HMB within 5 years of their referral to a gynecologist. In at least a third of these, an anatomically normal uterus is removed (Coulter, 1991). Removal of the uterus is the most effective treatment for bleeding, and overall patient satisfaction rates are high. Disadvantages to hysterectomy include more frequent and severe intraoperative and postoperative complications compared with either conservative medical or ablative surgical procedures. Operating time, hospitalization, recovery times, and costs are also greater. The procedure and its complications are discussed in detail in Section 43-12 (p. 950).

REFERENCES

Abberton KM, Healy DL, Rogers PA: Smooth muscle alpha actin and myosin heavy chain expression in the vascular smooth muscle cells surrounding human endometrial arterioles. Hum Reprod 14:3095, 1999

Abdel-Aleem H, d'Arcangues C, Vogelsong KM, et al: Treatment of vaginal bleeding irregularities induced by progestin only contraceptives. Cochrane Database Syst Rev 10:CD003449, 2013

Ahonkallio SJ, Liakka AK, Martikainen HK, et al: Feasibility of endometrial assessment after thermal ablation. Eur J Obstet Gynecol Reprod Biol 147(1):69, 2009

Ahuja SP, Hertweck SP: Overview of bleeding disorders in adolescent females with menorrhagia. J Pediatr Adolesc Gynecol 23(6 Suppl):S15, 2010

Alcazar JL, Galvan R: Three-dimensional power Doppler ultrasound scanning for the prediction of endometrial cancer in women with postmenopausal bleeding and thickened endometrium. Am J Obstet Gynecol 200(1):44.e1, 2009

Al-Jefout M, Black K, Schulke L, et al: Novel finding of high density of activated mast cells in endometrial polyps. Fertil Steril 92(3):1104, 2009

Alvarez-Sanchez F, Brache V, Thevenin F, et al: Hormonal treatment for bleeding irregularities in Norplant implant users. Am J Obstet Gynecol 174:919, 1996

American College of Obstetricians and Gynecologists: Diagnosis of abnormal uterine bleeding in reproductive-aged women. Practice Bulletin No. 128, July 2012

American College of Obstetricians and Gynecologists: Endometrial ablation. Practice Bulletin No. 81, May 2007, Reaffirmed 2013a

American College of Obstetricians and Gynecologists: Hysteroscopy. Technology Assessment No. 7, June 2011

American College of Obstetricians and Gynecologists: Management of abnormal uterine bleeding associated with ovulatory dysfunction. Practice Bulletin No. 136, July 2013b

American College of Obstetricians and Gynecologists: Management of acute abnormal uterine bleeding in nonpregnant reproductive-aged women. Committee Opinion No. 557, April 2013c

American College of Obstetricians and Gynecologists: Tamoxifen. Committee Opinion No. 601, June 2014

American College of Obstetricians and Gynecologists: The role of transvaginal ultrasonography in the evaluation of postmenopausal bleeding. Committee Opinion No. 440, August 2009, Reaffirmed 2013d

American College of Obstetricians and Gynecologists: Von Willebrand disease in women. Committee Opinion No. 580, December 2013e

Ammerman SR, Nelson AL: A new progestogen-only medical therapy for outpatient management of acute, abnormal uterine bleeding: a pilot study. Am J Obstet Gynecol 208(6):499.e1, 2013

Andersch B, Milsom I, Rybo G: An objective evaluation of flurbiprofen and tranexamic acid in the treatment of idiopathic menorrhagia. Acta Obstet Gynecol Scand 67:645, 1988

Archer DF: Endometrial bleeding during hormone therapy: the effect of progestogens. Maturitas 57(1):71, 2007

Baiocchi G, Manci N, Pazzaglia M, et al: Malignancy in endometrial polyps: a 12-year experience. Am J Obstet Gynecol 201(5):462.e1, 2009

Bakour SH, Gupta JK, Khan KS: Risk factors associated with endometrial polyps in abnormal uterine bleeding. Int J Gynecol Obstet 76(2):165, 2002

Bakour SH, Khan KS, Gupta JK: The risk of premalignant and malignant pathology in endometrial polyps. Acta Obstet Gynecol Scand 79:317, 2000

Barakat RR, Gilewski TA, Almadrones L, et al: Effect of adjuvant tamoxifen on the endometrium in women with breast cancer: a prospective study using office endometrial biopsy. J Clin Oncol 18:3459, 2000

Benacerraf BR, Shipp TD, Bromley B: Three-dimensional ultrasound detection of abnormally located intrauterine contraceptive devices which are a source of pelvic pain and abnormal bleeding. Ultrasound Obstet Gynecol 34(1):110, 2009

Benacerraf BR, Shipp TD, Bromley B: Which patients benefit from a 3D reconstructed coronal view of the uterus added to standard routine 2D pelvic sonography? AJR 190(3):626, 2008

Ben-Arie A, Goldchmit C, Laviv Y, et al: The malignant potential of endometrial polyps. Eur J Obstet Gynecol Reprod Biol 115:206, 2004

Bennett GL, Andreotti RF, Lee SI, et al: ACR Appropriateness Criteria on abnormal vaginal bleeding. J Am Coll Radiol 8(7):460, 2011

Ben-Yehuda OM, Kim YB, Leuchter RS: Does hysteroscopy improve upon the sensitivity of dilatation and curettage in the diagnosis of endometrial hyperplasia or carcinoma? Gynecol Oncol 68:4, 1998

Berzolla CE, Schnatz PF, O'Sullivan DM, et al: Dysplasia and malignancy in endocervical polyps. J Womens Health 16(9):1317, 2007

Bongers MY, Mol BW, Brolmann HA: Current treatment of dysfunctional uterine bleeding. Maturitas 47:159, 2004

Bonnar J, Sheppard BL: Treatment of menorrhagia during menstruation: randomised controlled trial of ethamsylate, mefenamic acid, and tranexamic acid. BMJ 313:579, 1996

Bradley LD: Complications in hysteroscopy: prevention, treatment and legal risk. Curr Opin Obstet Gynecol 14(4):409, 2002

Bradley WH, Boente MP, Brooker D, et al: Hysteroscopy and cytology in endometrial cancer. Obstet Gynecol 104(5 Pt 1):1030, 2004

Breijer MC, Peeters JA, Opmeer BC, et al: Capacity of endometrial thickness measurement to diagnose endometrial carcinoma in asymptomatic postmenopausal women: a systematic review and meta-analysis. Ultrasound Obstet Gynecol 40(6):621, 2012

Breitkopf DM, Frederickson RA, Snyder RR: Detection of benign endometrial masses by endometrial stripe measurement in premenopausal women. Obstet Gynecol 104(1):2004

Brunham RC, Paavonen J, Stevens CE, et al: Mucopurulent cervicitis—the ignored counterpart in women of urethritis in men. N Engl J Med 311(1):1, 1984

Burja IT, Thompson SK, Sawyer WL Jr, et al: Atypical glandular cells of undetermined significance on cervical smears. A study with cytohistologic correlation. Acta Cytol 43:351, 1999

Byams VR, Kouides PA, Kulkarni R, et al: Surveillance of female patients with inherited bleeding disorders in United States Haemophilia Treatment Centres. Haemophilia 17 (Suppl 1):6, 2011

Centers for Disease Control and Prevention: Sexually transmitted diseases treatment guidelines, 2015. MMWR 64(3):1, 2015

Centers for Disease Control and Prevention: U.S. Selected Practice Recommendations for Contraceptive Use, 2013. MMWR 62(5):1, 2013

Chimbira TH, Anderson AB, Naish C, et al: Reduction of menstrual blood loss by danazol in unexplained menorrhagia: lack of effect of placebo. BJOG 87:1152, 1980a

Chimbira TH, Anderson AB, Turnbull A: Relation between measured menstrual blood loss and patient's subjective assessment of loss, duration of bleeding, number of sanitary towels used, uterine weight and endometrial surface area. BJOG 87:603, 1980b

Chin N, Platt AB, Nuovo GJ: Squamous intraepithelial lesions arising in benign endocervical polyps: a report of 9 cases with correlation to the Pap smears, HPV analysis, and immunoprofile. Int J Gynecol Pathol 27(4):582, 2008

Cicinelli E, De Ziegler D, Nicoletti R, et al: Chronic endometritis: correlation among hysteroscopic, histologic, and bacteriologic findings in a prospective trial with 2190 consecutive office hysteroscopies. Fertil Steril 89(3):677, 2008

Cicinelli E, Parisi C, Galantino P, et al: Reliability, feasibility, and safety of minihysteroscopy with a vaginoscopic approach: experience with 6,000 cases. Fertil Steril 80(1):199, 2003

Cicinelli E, Resta L, Nicoletti R, et al: Endometrial micropolyps at fluid hysteroscopy suggest the existence of chronic endometritis. Hum Reprod 20(5):1386, 2005

Cicinelli E, Tinelli R, Colafiglio G, et al: Risk of long-term pelvic recurrences after fluid minihysteroscopy in women with endometrial carcinoma: a controlled randomized study. Menopause 17(3):511, 2010

Cil AP, Tulunay G, Kose MF, et al: Power Doppler properties of endometrial polyps and submucosal fibroids: a preliminary observational study in women with known intracavitary lesions. Ultrasound Obstet Gynecol 35(2):233, 2010

Clark TJ, Voit D, Gupta JK, et al: Accuracy of hysteroscopy in the diagnosis of endometrial cancer and hyperplasia: a systematic quantitative review. JAMA 288:1610, 2002

Cochrane R, Regan L: Undetected gynaecological disorders in women with renal disease. Hum Reprod 12:667, 1997

Cohen I: Endometrial pathologies associated with postmenopausal tamoxifen treatment. Gynecol Oncol 94:256, 2004

Cooper K, Lee A, Chien P, et al: Outcomes following hysterectomy or endometrial ablation for heavy menstrual bleeding: retrospective analysis of hospital episode statistics in Scotland. BJOG 118(10):1171, 2011

Cordier W, Steenkamp V: Herbal remedies affecting coagulation: a review. Pharm Biol 50(4):443, 2012

Corusic A, Barisic D, Lovric H, et al: Successful laparoscopic bipolar coagulation of a large arteriovenous malformation due to invasive trophoblastic disease: a case report. J Minim Invasive Gynecol 16(3):368, 2009

Coskun E, Cakiroglu Y, Aygun BK, et al: Effect of copper intrauterine device on the cyclooxygenase and inducible nitric oxide synthase expression in the luteal phase endometrium. Contraception 84(6):637, 2011

Coulter A, Bradlow J, Agass M, et al: Outcomes of referrals to gynaecology outpatient clinics for menstrual problems: an audit of general practice records. BJOG 98:789, 1991

Cura M, Martinez N, Cura A, et al: Arteriovenous malformations of the uterus. Acta Radiol 50(7):823, 2009

Daniels JP, Middleton LJ, Champaneria R, et al: Second generation endometrial ablation techniques for heavy menstrual bleeding: network meta-analysis. BMJ 344:e2564, 2012

Davies A, Richardson RE, O'Connor H, et al: Lignocaine aerosol spray in outpatient hysteroscopy: a randomized double-blind placebo-controlled trial. Fertil Steril 67(6):1019, 1997

de Koning ND, Haagsma EB: Normalization of menstrual pattern after liver transplantation: consequences for contraception. Digestion 46:239, 1990

de Kroon CD, de Bock GH, Dieben SW, et al: Saline contrast hysterosonography in abnormal uterine bleeding: a systematic review and meta-analysis. BJOG 110:938, 2003

de Lignières B: Oral micronized progesterone. Clin Ther 21(1):41, 1999

DeVore GR, Owens O, Kase N: Use of intravenous Premarin in the treatment of dysfunctional uterine bleeding—a double-blind randomized control study. Obstet Gynecol 59:285, 1982

DeWaay DJ, Syrop CH, Nygaard IE, et al: Natural history of uterine polyps and leiomyomata. Obstet Gynecol 100:3, 2002

Díaz S, Croxatto HB, Pavez M, et al: Clinical assessment of treatments for prolonged bleeding in users of Norplant implants. Contraception 42(1):97, 1990

Dockeray CJ, Sheppard BL, Bonnar J: Comparison between mefenamic acid and danazol in the treatment of established menorrhagia. BJOG 96:840, 1989

Dreisler E, Sorensen SS, Ibsen PH, et al: Prevalence of endometrial polyps and abnormal uterine bleeding in a Danish population aged 20–74 years. Ultrasound Obstet Gynecol 33(1):102, 2009a

Dreisler E, Sorensen SS, Lose G: Endometrial polyps and associated factors in Danish women aged 36–74 years. Am J Obstet Gynecol 200(2):147.e1, 2009b

Eckert LO, Thwin SS, Hillier SL, et al: The antimicrobial treatment of subacute endometritis: a proof of concept study. Am J Obstet Gynecol 190:305, 2004

Edlund M, Blombäck M, Fried G: Desmopressin in the treatment of menorrhagia in women with no common coagulation factor deficiency but with prolonged bleeding time. Blood Coagul Fibrinolysis 13(3):225, 2002

Emanuel MH, Verdel MJ, Wamsteker K, et al: A prospective comparison of transvaginal ultrasonography and diagnostic hysteroscopy in the evaluation of patients with abnormal uterine bleeding: clinical implications. Am J Obstet Gynecol 172:547, 1995

Everett C: Incidence and outcome of bleeding before the 20th week of pregnancy: prospective study from general practice. BMJ 315:32, 1997

Ferenczy A: Pathophysiology of endometrial bleeding. Maturitas 45(1):1, 2003

Ferrazzi E, Zupi E, Leone FP, et al: How often are endometrial polyps malignant in asymptomatic postmenopausal women? A multicenter study. Am J Obstet Gynecol 200(3):235.e1, 2009

Fleischer AC, Shappell HW: Color Doppler sonohysterography of endometrial polyps and submucosal fibroids. J Ultrasound Med 22:601, 2003

Fong YF, Singh K: Effect of the levonorgesterol-releasing intrauterine system on uterine myomas in a renal transplant patient. Contraception 60(1):51, 1999

Foster PA: The reproductive health of women with von Willebrand disease unresponsive to DDAVP: results of an international survey. On behalf of the Subcommittee on von Willebrand Factor of the Scientific and Standardization Committee of the ISTH. Thromb Haemost 74(2):784, 1995

Fraser IS: Treatment of ovulatory and anovulatory dysfunctional uterine bleeding with oral progestogens. Aust N Z J Obstet Gynaecol 30(4):353, 1990

Fraser IS, McCarron G: Randomized trial of 2 hormonal and 2 prostaglandin-inhibiting agents in women with a complaint of menorrhagia. Aust N Z J Obstet Gynaecol 31:66, 1991

Fraser IS, Römer T, Parke S, et al: Effective treatment of heavy and/or prolonged menstrual bleeding with an oral contraceptive containing estradiol valerate and dienogest: a randomized, double-blind Phase III trial. Hum Reprod 26:2698, 2011

Ghosh TK: Arteriovenous malformation of the uterus and pelvis. Obstet Gynecol 68:40S, 1986

Gleeson NC: Cyclic changes in endometrial tissue plasminogen activator and plasminogen activator inhibitor type 1 in women with normal menstruation and essential menorrhagia. Am J Obstet Gynecol 171:178, 1994

Godfrey EM, Folger SG, Jeng G, et al: Treatment of bleeding irregularities in women with copper-containing IUDs: a systematic review. Contraception 87(5):549, 2013

Golan A, Cohen-Sahar B, Keidar R, et al: Endometrial polyps: symptomatology, menopausal status and malignancy. Gynecol Obstet Invest 70(2):107, 2010

Goldstein RB, Bree RL, Benson CB, et al: Evaluation of the woman with postmenopausal bleeding: Society of Radiologists in Ultrasound-Sponsored Consensus Conference statement. J Ultrasound Med 20(10):1025, 2001

Goldstein SR, Monteagudo A, Popiolek D, et al: Evaluation of endometrial polyps. Am J Obstet Gynecol 186:669, 2002

Goldstein SR, Zeltser I, Horan CK, et al: Ultrasonography-based triage for perimenopausal patients with abnormal uterine bleeding. Am J Obstet Gynecol 177(1):102, 1997

Granberg S, Wikland M, Karlsson B, et al: Endometrial thickness as measured by endovaginal ultrasonography for identifying endometrial abnormality. Am J Obstet Gynecol 164:47, 1991

Greenwood SM, Moran JJ: Chronic endometritis: morphologic and clinical observations. Obstet Gynecol 58:176, 1981

Grimes D: Intrauterine devices (IUDs). In Hatcher RA, Trussell J, Nelson AL (eds): Contraceptive Technology. New York, Ardent Media, 2007, p 123

Grimes DA: Diagnostic dilation and curettage: a reappraisal. Am J Obstet Gynecol 142:1, 1982

Guglielmi KE: Women and ESRD: modalities, survival, unique considerations. Adv Chronic Kidney Dis 20(5):411, 2013

Gupta J, Kai J, Middleton L, et al: Levonorgestrel intrauterine system versus medical therapy for menorrhagia. N Engl J Med 368(2):128, 2013

Hall P, Maclachlan N, Thorn N, et al: Control of menorrhagia by the cyclo-oxygenase inhibitors naproxen sodium and mefenamic acid. BJOG 94:554, 1987

Hallberg L, Hogdahl AM, Nilsson L, et al: Menstrual blood loss—a population study. Variation at different ages and attempts to define normality. Acta Obstet Gynecol Scand 45:320, 1966

Haynes PJ, Hodgson H, Anderson AB, et al: Measurement of menstrual blood loss in patients complaining of menorrhagia. BJOG 84:763, 1977

Heliövaara-Peippo S, Hurskainen R, Teperi J, et al: Quality of life and costs of levonorgestrel-releasing intrauterine system or hysterectomy in the treatment of menorrhagia: a 10-year randomized controlled trial. Am J Obstet Gynecol 209(6):535.e1, 2013

Hickey M, Fraser I: Human uterine vascular structures in normal and diseased states. Microsc Res Tech 60:377, 2003

Hickey M, Fraser IS: Clinical implications of disturbances of uterine vascular morphology and function. Baillieres Best Pract Res Clin Obstet Gynaecol 14:937, 2000

Hickey M, Fraser IS: Surface vascularization and endometrial appearance in women with menorrhagia or using levonorgestrel contraceptive implants. Implications for the mechanisms of breakthrough bleeding. Hum Reprod 17:2428, 2002

Higham JM, O'Brien PM, Shaw RW: Assessment of menstrual blood loss using a pictorial chart. BJOG 97:734, 1990

Hurskainen R, Teperi J, Rissanen P, et al: Clinical outcomes and costs with the levonorgestrel-releasing intrauterine system or hysterectomy for treatment of menorrhagia: randomized trial 5-year follow-up. JAMA 291:1456, 2004

Hurskainen R, Teperi J, Rissanen P, et al: Quality of life and cost-effectiveness of levonorgestrel-releasing intrauterine system versus hysterectomy for treatment of menorrhagia: a randomized trial. Lancet 357(9252):273, 2001

Irvine GA, Cameron IT: Medical management of dysfunctional uterine bleeding. Best Pract Res Clin Obstet Gynaecol 13:189, 1999

Irvine GA, Campbell-Brown MB, Lumsden MA, et al: Randomised comparative trial of the levonorgestrel intrauterine system and norethisterone for treatment of idiopathic menorrhagia. BJOG 105:592, 1998

Jabbour HN, Kelly RW, Fraser HM, et al: Endocrine regulation of menstruation. Endocr Rev 27(1):17, 2006

James AH, Kouides PA, Abdul-Kadir R, et al: Evaluation and management of acute menorrhagia in women with and without underlying bleeding disorders: consensus from an international expert panel. Eur J Obstet Gynecol Reprod Biol 158(2):124, 2011

James AH, Kouides PA, Abdul-Kadir R, et al: Von Willebrand disease and other bleeding disorders in women: consensus on diagnosis and management from an international expert panel. Am J Obstet Gynecol 201(1):12.e1, 2009a

James AH, Manco-Johnson MJ, Yawn BP, et al: Von Willebrand disease: key points from the 2008 National Heart, Lung, and Blood Institute guidelines. Obstet Gynecol 114(3):674, 2009b

James AH, Myers ER, Cook C, et al: Complications of hysterectomy in women with von Willebrand disease. Haemophilia 15(4):926, 2009c

Jensen JT, Parke S, Mellinger U, et al: Effective treatment of heavy menstrual bleeding with estradiol valerate and dienogest: a randomized controlled trial. Obstet Gynecol 117:777, 2011

Jeong KA, Park KH, Chung DJ, et al: Hysteroscopic endometrial ablation as a treatment for abnormal uterine bleeding in patients with renal transplants. J Am Assoc Gynecol Laparosc 11(2):252, 2004

Joshi JV, Bhandarkar SD, Chadha M, et al: Menstrual irregularities and lactation failure may precede thyroid dysfunction or goitre. J Postgrad Med 39:137, 1993

Kaislasuo J, Suhonen S, Gissler M, et al: Uterine perforation caused by intrauterine devices: clinical course and treatment. Hum Reprod 28(6):1546, 2013

Kapp N: WHO provider brief on hormonal contraception and liver disease. Contraception 80(4):325, 2009

Karim BO, Burroughs FH, Rosenthal DL, et al: Endometrial-type cells in cervico-vaginal smears: clinical significance and cytopathologic correlates. Diagn Cytopathol 26:123, 2002

Karlsson B, Granberg S, Wikland M, et al: Transvaginal ultrasonography of the endometrium in women with postmenopausal bleeding—a Nordic multicenter study. Am J Obstet Gynecol 172:1488, 1995

Kaunitz AM, Bissonnette F, Monteiro I, et al: Levonorgestrel-releasing intrauterine system or medroxyprogesterone for heavy menstrual bleeding: a randomized controlled trial. Obstet Gynecol 116(3):625, 2010

Kaunitz AM, Meredith S, Inki P, et al: Levonorgestrel-releasing intrauterine system and endometrial ablation in heavy menstrual bleeding: a systematic review and meta-analysis. Obstet Gynecol 113:1104, 2009

Kingman CE, Kadir RA, Lee CA, et al: The use of levonorgestrel- releasing intrauterine system for treatment of menorrhagia in women with inherited bleeding disorders. BJOG 111(12):1425, 2004

Kitaya K, Tada Y, Taguchi S, et al: Local mononuclear cell infiltrates in infertile patients with endometrial macropolyps versus micropolyps. Hum Reprod 27(12):3474, 2012

Kosus N, Kosus A, Demircioglu RI, et al: Transcervical intrauterine levobupivacaine or lidocaine infusion for pain control during endometrial biopsy. Pain Res Manag 19(2):82, 2014

Krassas GE, Pontikides N, Kaltsas T, et al: Disturbances of menstruation in hypothyroidism. Clin Endocrinol 50:655, 1999

Krassas GE, Poppe K, Glinoer D: Thyroid function and human reproductive health. Endocr Rev 31(5):702, 2010

Küçük T, Ertan K: Continuous oral or intramuscular medroxyprogesterone acetate versus the levonorgestrel releasing intrauterine system in the treatment of perimenopausal menorrhagia: a randomized, prospective, controlled clinical trial in female smokers. Clin Exp Obstet Gynecol 35(1):57, 2008

Labied S, Galant C, Nisolle M, et al: Differential elevation of matrix metalloproteinase expression in women exposed to levonorgestrel-releasing intrauterine system for a short or prolonged period of time. Hum Reprod 24(1):113, 2009

Leão RB, Andrade L, Vassalo J, et al: Differences in estrogen and progesterone receptor expression in endometrial polyps and atrophic endometrium of postmenopausal women with and without exposure to tamoxifen. Mol Clin Oncol 1(6):1055, 2013

Lee SC, Kaunitz AM, Sanchez-Ramos L, et al: The oncogenic potential of endometrial polyps: a systematic review and meta-analysis. Obstet Gynecol 116(5):1197, 2010

Lethaby A, Duckitt K, Farquhar C: Non-steroidal anti-inflammatory drugs for heavy menstrual bleeding. Cochrane Database Syst Rev 1:CD000400, 2013a

Lethaby A, Irvine G, Cameron I: Cyclical progestogens for heavy menstrual bleeding. Cochrane Database Syst Rev 1:CD001016, 2008

Lethaby A, Penninx J, Hickey M, et al: Endometrial resection and ablation techniques for heavy menstrual bleeding. Cochrane Database Syst Rev 8:CD001501, 2013b

Lethaby A, Suckling J, Barlow D, et al: Hormone replacement therapy in postmenopausal women: endometrial hyperplasia and irregular bleeding. Cochrane Database Syst Rev 3:CD000402, 2004

Leung PL, Tam WH, Kong WS, et al: Intrauterine pathology in women with abnormal uterine bleeding taking hormone replacement therapy. J Am Assoc Gynecol Laparosc 10(2):260, 2003

Litta P, Merlin F, Saccardi C, et al: Role of hysteroscopy with endometrial biopsy to rule out endometrial cancer in postmenopausal women with abnormal uterine bleeding. Maturitas 50:117, 2005

Long ME, Dwarica DS, Kastner TM, et al: Comparison of dysplastic and benign endocervical polyps. J Low Genit Tract Dis 17(2):142, 2013

Lowenstein L, Solt I, Deutsch M, et al: A life-threatening event: uterine cervical arteriovenous malformation. Obstet Gynecol 103:1073, 2004

Lukes AS, Moore KA, Muse KN, et al: Tranexamic acid treatment for heavy menstrual bleeding: a randomized controlled trial. Obstet Gynecol 116(4):865, 2010

MacKenzie IZ, Naish C, Rees CM, et al: Why remove all cervical polyps and examine them histologically? BJOG 116(8):1127, 2009

Maia H Jr, Maltez A, Studard E, et al: Effect of previous hormone replacement therapy on endometrial polyps during menopause. Gynecol Endocrinol 18:299, 2004

Makarainen L, Ylikorkala O: Ibuprofen prevents IUCD-induced increases in menstrual blood loss. BJOG 93:285, 1986

Makris N, Kalmantis K, Skartados N, et al: Three-dimensional hysterosonography versus hysteroscopy for the detection of intracavitary uterine abnormalities. Int J Gynaecol Obstet 97(1):6, 2007

Mannucci PM, Duga S, Peyvandi F: Recessively inherited coagulation disorders. Blood 104:1243, 2004

Matteson KA, Rahn DD, Wheeler TL 2nd, et al: Nonsurgical management of heavy menstrual bleeding: a systematic review. Obstet Gynecol 121(3):632, 2013

Matuszkiewicz-Rowinska J, Skorzewska K, Radowicki S, et al: Endometrial morphology and pituitary-gonadal axis dysfunction in women of reproductive age undergoing chronic haemodialysis—a multicentre study. Nephrol Dial Transplant 19:2074, 2004

McGavigan CJ, Dockery P, Metaxa-Mariatou V, et al: Hormonally mediated disturbance of angiogenesis in the human endometrium after exposure to intrauterine levonorgestrel. Hum Reprod 18:77, 2003

Merz E, Miric-Tesanic D, Bahlmann F, et al: Sonographic size of uterus and ovaries in pre- and postmenopausal women. Ultrasound Obstet Gynecol 7(1):38, 1996

Moschos E, Ashfaq R, McIntire DD, et al: Saline-infusion sonography endometrial sampling compared with endometrial biopsy in diagnosing endometrial pathology. Obstet Gynecol 113(4):881, 2009

Moschos E, Twickler DM: Does the type of intrauterine device affect conspicuity on 2D and 3D ultrasound? AJR 196(6):1439, 2011

Munro MG: Medical management of abnormal uterine bleeding. Obstet Gynecol Clin North Am 27(2):287, 2000

Munro MG, Critchley HO, Fraser IS: The FIGO classification of causes of abnormal uterine bleeding in the reproductive years. Fertil Steril 95(7):2204, 2011

Munro MG, Mainor N, Basu R, et al: Oral medroxyprogesterone acetate and combination oral contraceptives for acute uterine bleeding: a randomized controlled trial. Obstet Gynecol 108(4):924, 2006

Nalaboff KM, Pellerito JS, Ben Levi E: Imaging the endometrium: disease and normal variants. Radiographics 21:1409, 2001

National Cancer Institute: Surveillance, Epidemiology, and End Results Program: cancer of the corpus and uterus, NOS (invasive). SEER incidence and U.S. death rates, age-adjusted and age-specific rates, by race. Available at: http://seer.cancer.gov/csr/1975_2011/browse_csr.php?sectionSEL=7&pageSEL=sect_07_table.07.html. Accessed September 9, 2014

Neven P, Lunde T, Benedetti-Panici P, et al: A multicentre randomised trial to compare uterine safety of raloxifene with a continuous combined hormone replacement therapy containing oestradiol and norethisterone acetate. BJOG 110(2):157, 2003

Nichols WL, Hultin MB, James AH, et al: Von Willebrand disease (VWD): evidence-based diagnosis and management guidelines, the National Heart, Lung, and Blood Institute (NHLBI) Expert Panel report (USA). Haemophilia 14(2):171, 2008

Nichols WL, Rick ME, Ortel TL, et al: Clinical and laboratory diagnosis of von Willebrand disease: a synopsis of the 2008 NHLBI/NIH guidelines. Am J Hematol 84(6):366, 2009

Obenson K, Abreo F, Grafton WD: Cytohistologic correlation between AGUS and biopsy-detected lesions in postmenopausal women. Acta Cytolog 44:41, 2000

Oguz S, Sargin A, Kelekci S, et al: The role of hormone replacement therapy in endometrial polyp formation. Maturitas 50(3):231, 2005

Opolskiene G, Sladkevicius P, Jokubkiene L, et al: Three-dimensional ultrasound imaging for discrimination between benign and malignant endometrium in women with postmenopausal bleeding and sonographic endometrial thickness of at least 4.5 mm. Ultrasound Obstet Gynecol 35(1):94, 2010

Opolskiene G, Sladkevicius P, Valentin L: Ultrasound assessment of endometrial morphology and vascularity to predict endometrial malignancy in women with postmenopausal bleeding and sonographic endometrial thickness ≥4.5 mm. Ultrasound Obstet Gynecol 30(3):332, 2007

Paavonen J, Stevens CE, Wolner-Hanssen P, et al: Colposcopic manifestations of cervical and vaginal infections. Obstet Gynecol Surv 43:373, 1988

Pérez-Medina T, Bajo-Arenas J, Salazar F, et al: Endometrial polyps and their implication in the pregnancy rates of patients undergoing intrauterine insemination: a prospective randomised study. Hum Reprod 20:1632, 2005

Philipp CS, Faiz A, Dowling N, et al: Age and the prevalence of bleeding disorders in women with menorrhagia. Obstet Gynecol 105:61, 2005

Pisoni CN, Cuadrado MJ, Khamashta MA, et al: Treatment of menorrhagia associated with oral anticoagulation: efficacy and safety of the levonorgestrel releasing intrauterine device (Mirena coil). Lupus 15(12):877, 2006

Pitsos M, Skurnick J, Heller D: Association of pathologic diagnoses with clinical findings in chronic endometritis. J Reprod Med 54(6):373, 2009

Polyzos NP, Mauri D, Tsioras S, et al: Intraperitoneal dissemination of endometrial cancer cells after hysteroscopy: a systematic review and meta-analysis. Int J Gynecol Cancer 20(2):261, 2010

Preston JT, Cameron IT, Adams EJ, et al: Comparative study of tranexamic acid and norethisterone in the treatment of ovulatory menorrhagia. BJOG 102:401, 1995

Preutthipan S, Herabutya Y: Hysteroscopic polypectomy in 240 premenopausal and postmenopausal women. Fertil Steril 83:705, 2005

Rahimi S, Marani C, Renzi C, et al: Endometrial polyps and the risk of atypical hyperplasia on biopsies of unremarkable endometrium: a study on 694 patients with benign endometrial polyps. Int J Gynecol Pathol 28(6):522, 2009

Reid PC, Virtanen-Kari S: Randomised comparative trial of the levonorgestrel intrauterine system and mefenamic acid for the treatment of idiopathic menorrhagia: a multiple analysis using total menstrual fluid loss, menstrual blood loss and pictorial blood loss measurements. BJOG 112:1121, 2005

Reslova T, Tosner J, Resl M, et al: Endometrial polyps. A clinical study of 245 cases. Arch Gynecol Obstet 262:133, 1999

Rodeghiero F: Management of menorrhagia in women with inherited bleeding disorders: general principles and use of desmopressin. Haemophilia 14 (Suppl 1):21, 2008

Rodeghiero F, Castaman G: Congenital von Willebrand disease type I: definition, phenotypes, clinical and laboratory assessment. Best Pract Res Clin Haematol 14(2):321, 2001

Rogers PA, Abberton KM: Endometrial arteriogenesis: vascular smooth muscle cell proliferation and differentiation during the menstrual cycle and changes associated with endometrial bleeding disorders. Microsc Res Tech 60:412, 2003

Rubin G, Wortman M, Kouides PA: Endometrial ablation for von Willebrand disease-related menorrhagia—experience with seven cases. Haemophilia 10: 477, 2004

Said S, Sadek W, Rocca M, et al: Clinical evaluation of the therapeutic effectiveness of ethinyl oestradiol and oestrone sulphate on prolonged bleeding in women using depot medroxyprogesterone acetate for contraception. Hum Reprod 11:1, 1996

Schmidt T, Breidenbach M, Nawroth F, et al: Hysteroscopy for asymptomatic postmenopausal women with sonographically thickened endometrium. Maturitas 62(2):176, 2009

Schnatz PF, Ricci S, O'Sullivan DM: Cervical polyps in postmenopausal women: is there a difference in risk? Menopause 16(3):524, 2009

Shaaban MM, Zakherah MS, El-Nashar SA, et al: Levonorgestrel-releasing intrauterine system compared to low dose combined oral contraceptive pills for idiopathic menorrhagia: a randomized clinical trial. Contraception 83(1):48, 2011

Shankar M, Lee CA, Sabin CA, et al: von Willebrand disease in women with menorrhagia: a systematic review. BJOG 111:734, 2004

Shaw ST Jr, Macaulay LK, Hohman WR: Vessel density in endometrium of women with and without intrauterine contraceptive devices: a morphometric evaluation. Am J Obstet Gynecol 135:202, 1979

Sharp HT: Assessment of new technology in the treatment of idiopathic menorrhagia and uterine leiomyomata. Obstet Gynecol 108(4):990, 2006

Sheikh M, Sawhney S, Khurana A, et al: Alteration of sonographic texture of the endometrium in post-menopausal bleeding. A guide to further management. Acta Obstet Gynecol Scand 79:1006, 2000

Shi AA, Lee SI: Radiological reasoning: algorithmic workup of abnormal vaginal bleeding with endovaginal sonography and sonohysterography. AJR 191(6 Suppl):S68, 2008

Shokeir TA, Shalan HM, El Shafei MM: Significance of endometrial polyps detected hysteroscopically in eumenorrheic infertile women. J Obstet Gynecol Res 30:84, 2004

Singh RH, Blumenthal P: Hormonal management of abnormal uterine bleeding. Clin Obstet Gynecol 48:337, 2005

Smith-Bindman R, Kerlikowske K, Feldstein VA, et al: Endovaginal ultrasound to exclude endometrial cancer and other endometrial abnormalities. JAMA 280:1510, 1998

Soares SR, Barbosa dos Reis MM, Camargos AF: Diagnostic accuracy of sonohysterography, transvaginal sonography, and hysterosalpingography in patients with uterine cavity diseases. Fertil Steril 73:406, 2000

Stellon AJ, Williams R: Increased incidence of menstrual abnormalities and hysterectomy preceding primary biliary cirrhosis. Br Med J (Clin Res Ed) 293:297, 1986

Stewart A, Cummins C, Gold L, et al: The effectiveness of the levonorgestrel-releasing intrauterine system in menorrhagia: a systematic review. BJOG 108:74, 2001

Stock RJ, Kanbour A: Prehysterectomy curettage. Obstet Gynecol 45:537, 1975

Stovall TG, Ling FW, Morgan PL: A prospective, randomized comparison of the Pipelle endometrial sampling device with the Novak curette. Am J Obstet Gynecol 165:1287, 1991

Stovall TG, Solomon SK, Ling FW: Endometrial sampling prior to hysterectomy. Obstet Gynecol 73:405, 1989

Svirsky R, Smorgick N, Rozowski U, et al: Can we rely on blind endometrial biopsy for detection of focal intrauterine pathology? Am J Obstet Gynecol 199(2):115.e1, 2008

Tabor A, Watt HC, Wald NJ: Endometrial thickness as a test for endometrial cancer in women with postmenopausal vaginal bleeding. Obstet Gynecol 99:663, 2002

Tahir MM, Bigrigg MA, Browning JJ, et al: A randomised controlled trial comparing transvaginal ultrasound, outpatient hysteroscopy and endometrial biopsy with inpatient hysteroscopy and curettage. BJOG 106:1259, 1999

Thomas EJ, Okuda KJ, Thomas NM: The combination of a depot gonadotrophin releasing hormone agonist and cyclical hormone replacement therapy for dysfunctional uterine bleeding. BJOG 98(11):1155, 1991

Timmerman D, Wauters J, Van Calenbergh S, et al: Color Doppler imaging is a valuable tool for the diagnosis and management of uterine vascular malformations. Ultrasound Obstet Gynecol 21:570, 2003

Timmermans A, Opmeer BC, Khan KS, et al: Endometrial thickness measurement for detecting endometrial cancer in women with postmenopausal bleeding: a systematic review and meta-analysis. Obstet Gynecol 116(1):160, 2010

Tsuda H, Kawabata M, Kawabata K, et al: Improvement of diagnostic accuracy of transvaginal ultrasound for identification of endometrial malignancies by using cutoff level of endometrial thickness based on length of time since menopause. Gynecol Oncol 64:35, 1997

Tullius TG Jr, Ross JR, Flores M, et al: Use of three-dimensional power Doppler sonography in the diagnosis of uterine arteriovenous malformation and follow-up after uterine artery embolization: Case report and brief review of literature. J Clin Ultrasound 43(5):327, 2015

Turnbull AC, Rees MC. Gestrinone in the treatment of menorrhagia. BJOG 97(8):713, 1990

Van den Bosch T, Verguts J, Daemen A, et al: Pain experienced during transvaginal ultrasound, saline contrast sonohysterography, hysteroscopy and office sampling: a comparative study. Ultrasound Obstet Gynecol 31(3):346, 2008

Van Doorn LC, Dijkhuizen FP, Kruitwagen RF, et al: Accuracy of transvaginal ultrasonography in diabetic or obese women with postmenopausal bleeding. Obstet Gynecol 104:571, 2004

Vercellini P, Cortesi I, Oldani S, et al: The role of transvaginal ultrasonography and outpatient diagnostic hysteroscopy in the evaluation of patients with menorrhagia. Hum Reprod 12(8):1768, 1997

Vercellini P, Fedele L, Maggi R, et al: Gonadotropin releasing hormone agonist for chronic anovulatory uterine bleeding and severe anemia. J Reprod Med 38(2):127, 1993

Warner PE, Critchley HO, Lumsden MA, et al: Menorrhagia I: measured blood loss, clinical features, and outcome in women with heavy periods: a survey with follow-up data. Am J Obstet Gynecol 190:1216, 2004

Weiss JL, Malone FD, Vidaver J, et al: Threatened abortion: a risk factor for poor pregnancy outcome, a population-based screening study. Am J Obstet Gynecol 190:745, 2004

Wellington K, Wagstaff AJ: Tranexamic acid: a review of its use in the management of menorrhagia. Drugs 63:1417, 2003

Wilansky DL, Greisman B: Early hypothyroidism in patients with menorrhagia. Am J Obstet Gynecol 160:673, 1989

Wong AW, Chan SS, Yeo W, et al: Prophylactic use of levonorgestrel-releasing intrauterine system in women with breast cancer treated with tamoxifen: a randomized controlled trial. Obstet Gynecol 121(5):943, 2013

Yanaihara A, Yorimitsu T, Motoyama H: Location of endometrial polyp and pregnancy rate in infertility patients. Fertil Steril 90(1):180, 2008

Ylikorkala O, Viinikka L: Comparison between antifibrinolytic and antiprostaglandin treatment in the reduction of increased menstrual blood loss in women with intrauterine contraceptive devices. BJOG 90(1):78, 1983

Younis MTS, Iram S, Anwar B, et al: Women with asymptomatic cervical polyps may not need to see a gynaecologist or have them removed: an observational retrospective study of 1126 cases. Eur J Obstet Gynecol Reprod Biol 150(2):190, 2010

Zerbe MJ, Zhang J, Bristow RE, et al: Retrograde seeding of malignant cells during hysteroscopy in presumed early endometrial cancer. Gynecol Oncol 79(1):55, 2000

Zullo F, Pellicano M, Stigliano CM, et al: Topical anesthesia for office hysteroscopy. A prospective, randomized study comparing two modalities. J Reprod Med 44(10):865, 1999

CHAPTER 9

Pelvic Mass

Pelvic masses are common and may involve reproductive organs or nongynecologic structures. Affected women can be symptom-free or may complain of pain, pressure, dysmenorrhea, infertility, or uterine bleeding. Treatment varies with patient age and therapeutic goals. Medical management is possible for many with pelvic masses, but for others, procedural interventions offer highest success rates.

DEMOGRAPHIC FACTORS

Of associated factors, pelvic mass rates and underlying pathology change with age. In prepubertal girls, most gynecologic pelvic masses involve the ovary. Even before puberty, ovaries are active, and masses are often functional, rather than neoplastic, cysts (de Silva, 2004). Of neoplastic lesions, most are benign germ cell tumors, especially mature cystic teratomas (dermoid cysts) (Brown, 1993). Malignant ovarian tumors in children and adolescents are rare, and this age group accounts for only 1.2 percent of all ovarian cancers (National Cancer Institute, 2014). Most cancers are germ cell tumors, and among children and adolescents, rates increase with age (American Cancer Society, 2014).

In adolescents, the incidence and type of ovarian pathology in general mirrors that of prepubertal girls. However, with the onset of reproductive function, pelvic masses in adolescence may also include endometriomas and the sequelae of pelvic inflammatory disease (PID) and pregnancy.

In adult women, the differential diagnosis for a pelvic mass expands. Uterine enlargement due to pregnancy, functional ovarian cysts, and leiomyoma are among the most common. Endometrioma, mature cystic teratoma, acute or chronic tuboovarian abscess (TOA), and ectopic pregnancies are other frequent causes. Most pelvic masses in this age group are benign, but malignancy rates increase with age.

In postmenopausal women, with cessation of reproductive function, the causes of pelvic mass also change. Simple ovarian cysts and leiomyomas are still frequent. Menopause typically results in leiomyoma atrophy, but some uterine bulk may still persist. Importantly, malignancy is a more frequent cause in this demographic group. Ovarian cancer accounts for nearly 3 percent of new cancers among all women (American Cancer Society, 2014). Uterine tumors, including adenocarcinoma and sarcoma, can enlarge the uterus.

LEIOMYOMAS

Uterine enlargement most frequently reflects pregnancy or leiomyomas. Less often, enlargement is from adenomyosis, hematometra, an adhered adnexal mass, or malignancy. Of these, leiomyomas are benign smooth muscle neoplasms that typically originate from the myometrium. They are often referred to as *uterine myomas*, and they are colloquially called *fibroids*. Their incidence among women is generally cited as 20 to 25 percent, but is as high as 70 to 80 percent in studies using histologic or sonographic examination (Baird, 2003; Cramer, 1990). The health care consequences of these tumors are substantial. From 1998 to 2005, 27 percent of inpatient gynecologic admissions were for uterine leiomyoma care (Whiteman, 2010).

■ Pathophysiology
Pathology

Grossly, leiomyomas are round, rubbery tumors that when bisected display a whorled pattern. They possess a distinct autonomy from their surrounding myometrium because of a thin, outer connective tissue layer (Fig. 9-1). This clinically important cleavage plane allows leiomyomas to be easily "shelled" from the uterus during surgery. Histologically, leiomyomas contain elongated smooth-muscle cells aggregated in dense bundles. Mitotic activity, however, is rare and is a key point in differentiation from malignant leiomyosarcoma.

The typical appearance of leiomyomas may change if smooth muscle is replaced with various degenerative substances

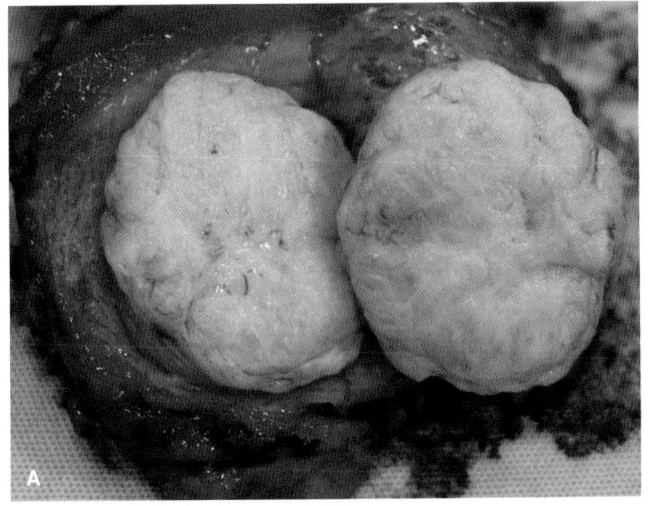

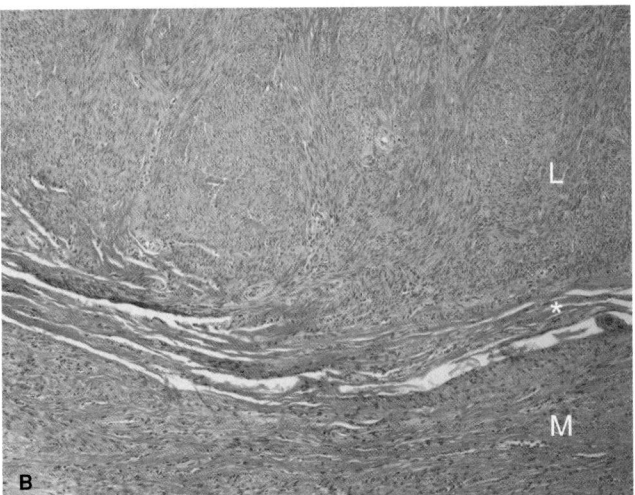

FIGURE 9-1 The appearance of leiomyomas will vary depending on the degree and type of degeneration present. **A.** In this bisected uterine fundus, a typical off-white, whorled leiomyoma lies distinct from the surrounding myometrium. **B.** Microscopically, leiomyomas (*L*) are composed of bland, spindled smooth-muscle cells characterized by elongate, blunt-ended nuclei and tapered eosinophilic cytoplasm. The cells are arranged in interlacing fascicles that intersect at right angles. Leiomyomas are usually well-circumscribed, and the interface (*asterisk*) between the myoma and adjacent myometrium can be seen grossly and microscopically. These tumors are usually more cellular than the surrounding myometrium (*M*). (Used with permission from Dr. Kelley Carrick.)

following necrosis. This process is collectively termed *degeneration*, and the replacement substances dictate the naming of these degenerative types. Forms include hyaline, calcific, cystic, myxoid, red, and fatty, and these gross changes should be recognized as normal variants. Necrosis and degeneration develop frequently in leiomyomas because of the tenuous blood supply within these tumors. Leiomyomas have a lower arterial density compared with the surrounding normal myometrium. Moreover, their lack of vascular organization leaves some tumors vulnerable to hypoperfusion and ischemia (Forssman, 1976). As discussed later, acute pain may accompany degeneration.

Pathogenesis

Each leiomyoma is derived from a single progenitor myocyte. Thus, multiple tumors within the same uterus each show independent cytogenetic origins (Townsend, 1970). Several unique defects involving chromosomes 6, 7, 12, and 14 and others correlate with rates and direction of tumor growth (Brosens, 1998). Of specific gene mutations, those involving *MED12* and *HMGA2* genes, and less commonly *COL4A5-A6* or *FH* genes, account for most leiomyomas (Mehine, 2014). Of these, fumarate hydratase (*FH*) gene mutations are rare but lead to the *hereditary leiomyomatosis and renal cell cancer (HLRCC) syndrome.* This is characterized by cutaneous and uterine leiomyomas and renal cell cancer (Mann, 2015). Future determination of each mutation's role in leiomyoma formation is anticipated to aid treatment development.

Following their genesis, uterine leiomyomas are estrogen and progesterone sensitive tumors. Consequently, they develop during the reproductive years. After menopause, leiomyomas generally shrink, and new tumor development is infrequent. These sex steroid hormones likely mediate their effect by stimulating or inhibiting transcription or cellular growth-factor production.

Leiomyomas themselves create a hyperestrogenic environment, which appears requisite for their growth and maintenance. First, compared with normal myometrium, leiomyoma cells contain a greater density of estrogen receptors, which results in greater estradiol binding. Secondly, these tumors convert less estradiol to the weaker estrone (Englund, 1998; Otubu, 1982; Yamamoto, 1993). A third mechanism involves higher levels of cytochrome P450 aromatase in leiomyomas compared with normal myocytes (Bulun, 1994). This specific enzyme catalyzes the conversion of androgens to estrogen (Chap. 15, p. 337).

Some conditions also provide sustained estrogen exposure that encourages leiomyoma formation. For example, the increased years of persistent estrogen production found with early menarche and with an increased body mass index (BMI) are each linked with a greater leiomyoma risk (Velez Edwards, 2013; Wise, 2005). Obese women produce more estrogens from increased conversion of androgens to estrogen in adipose tissue by aromatase. They also display decreased hepatic production of sex hormone binding globulin (Glass, 1989). Women with polycystic ovarian syndrome (PCOS) have a higher risk of myoma formation, which may stem from the sustained estrogen exposure that accompanies chronic anovulation (Wise, 2007).

Of other factors, estrogen and progesterone hormone treatment in premenopausal women probably has no significant inductive effect on leiomyoma formation. With few exceptions, combination oral contraceptive (COC) pills either lower or have no effect on this risk (Chiaffarino, 1999; Parazzini, 1992).

Smoking alters estrogen metabolism and lowers physiologically active serum estrogen levels (Soldin, 2011). This may explain why women who smoke generally have a lower risk for leiomyoma formation.

As with estrogen, leiomyomas carry a higher progesterone receptor density compared with their surrounding myometrium. Progesterone is considered the critical mitogen for uterine leiomyoma growth and development, and estrogen functions to upregulate and maintain progesterone receptors (Ishikawa, 2010). Thus, cell proliferation, extracellular matrix accumulation, and cell hypertrophy, which all lead to leiomyoma growth, are controlled by progesterone directly and in a permissive role by estrogen.

This relationship is supported by evidence that the antiprogestins mifepristone and ulipristal induce atrophy in most leiomyomas (Donnez, 2012a; Murphy, 1993). Moreover, in women treated with gonadotropin-releasing hormone (GnRH) agonists, leiomyomas typically decrease in size. However, if progestins are given simultaneously with GnRH agents, there is typically *increased* leiomyoma growth (Carr, 1993).

Clinically, this relationship may be important when prescribing sex steroid hormones. In postmenopausal women, hormone replacement therapy (HRT) has either a stimulatory or no effect on growth (Polatti, 2000; Reed, 2004). Palomba and associates (2002) found that higher doses of medroxyprogesterone acetate (MPA) were associated with leiomyoma growth and recommended using the lowest possible dose of MPA in these patients.

Of other factors associated with myoma development, race and age are notable risks. Myomas are rare in adolescence but increase with age during the reproductive years. In a study by Baird and coworkers (2003), the cumulative incidence by age 50 years was nearly 70 percent in whites and more than 80 percent in African-American women. Lower rates of leiomyomas are linked with pregnancy. Those who have higher parity, have had a more recent pregnancy, and have breastfed all display lower incidences of myoma formation (Terry, 2010). Leiomyomas are more common in African-American women compared with white, Asian, or Hispanic women. Thus, as noted earlier, heredity and specifically gene mutations play a seminal role in myoma development.

■ Uterine Leiomyoma Classification

These tumors are classified based on their location and direction of growth (Fig. 9-2). *Subserosal leiomyomas* originate from myocytes adjacent to the uterine serosa, and their growth is directed outward. When these are attached only by a stalk to

their progenitor myometrium, they are called *pedunculated leiomyomas*. *Parasitic leiomyomas* are subserosal variants that attach themselves to nearby pelvic structures from which they derive vascular support. These myomas then may or may not detach from the parent myometrium. *Intramural leiomyomas* are those with growth centered within the uterine walls. Finally, *submucous leiomyomas* are proximate to the endometrium and grow toward and bulge into the endometrial cavity. For endoscopic resection evaluation, submucous leiomyomas are further classified by their depth of involvement. The European Society of Hysteroscopy and the International Federation of Gynecology and Obstetrics (FIGO) defines leiomyomas as: type 0, if the mass is located entirely within the uterine cavity; type 1, if less than 50 percent is located within the myometrium; and type 2, if greater than 50 percent of the mass is surrounded by myometrium (Wamsteker, 1993). To aid abnormal uterine bleeding research, this numerical classification was expanded by FIGO to similarly assign subclassifying numbers to intramural, subserosal, and parasitic leiomyomas (Munro, 2011).

Of tumors outside the uterine corpus, only about 0.4 percent develop in the cervix (Tiltman, 1998). Leiomyomas have also been found infrequently in the ovary, fallopian tube, broad ligament, vagina, and vulva.

Leiomyomatosis

Extrauterine smooth-muscle tumors, which are benign yet infiltrative, may develop in women with concurrent or prior uterine leiomyomas, and this condition is termed leiomyomatosis. In such cases, malignant metastases from a leiomyosarcoma must be excluded.

Intravenous leiomyomatosis invades and extends serpiginously into the uterine veins, other pelvic veins, vena cava, and even cardiac chambers. As such, this rare tumor may lead to classic leiomyoma complaints or to uncharacteristic ones such as right-sided congestive cardiac symptoms. Tumors are usually amenable to resection. Although these are histologically benign, recurrence rates may reach 28 percent (Wang, 2012).

Benign metastasizing leiomyomas derive from morphologically benign uterine leiomyomas that disseminate hematogenously. Lesions have been found most often in the lungs, and less so in lymph nodes, bone, brain, and heart. Classically, these are found in women who have a recent or distant history of pelvic surgery.

Disseminated peritoneal leiomyomatosis (DPL) is benign and appears as multiple small peritoneal nodules on abdominal cavity or abdominal organs surfaces. As such, DPL intraoperatively and radiologically looks like widespread peritoneal metastatic malignancy. DPL is usually found in women of reproductive age, and 70 percent are associated with pregnancy or COC use (Bisceglia, 2014).

Last, with the increased use of electromechanical morcellation during minimally invasive myomectomy or hysterectomy, multiple small peritoneal leiomyomas may be found later after the primary surgery. Secondary implantation of myoma remnants is implicated, and these present similarly to parasitic leiomyomas or DPL (Kho, 2009). A full discussion of this topic is found in Chapter 41 (p. 896).

Treatments for all these benign conditions may involve hysterectomy with oophorectomy, tumor debulking, and agents

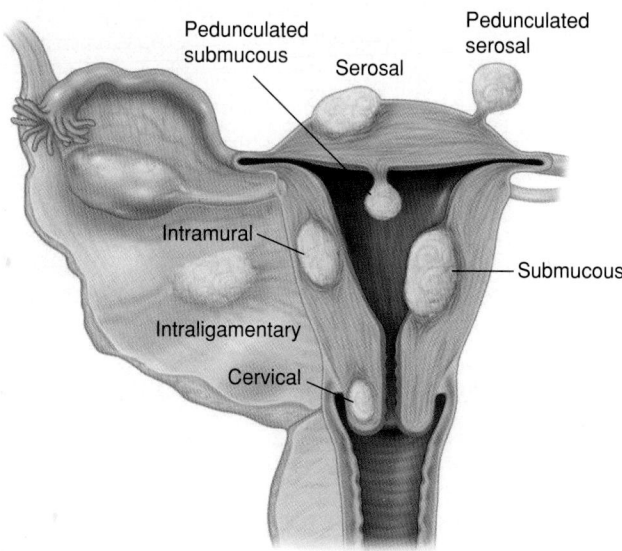

FIGURE 9-2 Leiomyomas can be categorized as shown. However, the borders of most leiomyomas overlap these distinct regions.

that lower estrogen and/or progestin levels. Pharmaceutical choices include GnRH agonists, aromatase inhibitors, selective estrogen-receptor modulators, or antiprogestins (Lewis, 2013; Taveira-DaSilva, 2014).

■ Symptoms

Bleeding

Most women with leiomyomas are asymptomatic. However, affected women may complain of bleeding, pain, pressure, or infertility. In general, symptom risk increases with myoma size and number. Bleeding is common, especially heavy menstrual bleeding (HMB), and dilated endometrial venules are implicated. Dysregulation of local vasoactive growth factors is thought to promote this vasodilatation. When engorged venules are disrupted at the time of menstrual sloughing, bleeding from these markedly dilated vessels overwhelms the usual hemostatic mechanisms (Stewart, 1996). For this reason, subserosal, intramural, and submucous tumors all have a propensity to cause HMB (Wegienka, 2003).

Pressure and Pain

A sufficiently enlarged uterus can cause chronic pressure, urinary frequency, incontinence, or constipation. Rarely, leiomyomas extend laterally to compress a ureter and lead to obstruction and hydronephrosis. Aside from pressure, patient may also note dysmenorrhea, dyspareunia, or noncyclical pelvic pain (Lippman, 2003; Moshesh, 2014).

Acute pelvic pain is a less frequent complaint but is most often seen with a degenerating or prolapsing leiomyoma. Rare tumor complications include torsion of a subserosal pedunculated leiomyoma, acute urinary retention, or deep-vein thromboembolism (Gupta, 2009). With leiomyoma degeneration, tissue necrosis classically causes acute pain, fever, and leukocytosis. This constellation mimics other acute pelvic pain sources. Thus, sonography is typically performed to help identify a cause, and usually a nondescript leiomyoma is found. Computed tomography (CT) may also be obtained, especially if clear interpretation of pelvic anatomy is obscured by multiple large leiomyomas or if appendicitis, nephrolithiasis, diverticulitis, or others are considered. Treatment of myoma degeneration is nonsurgical and includes analgesics and antipyretics as needed. However, broad-spectrum antibiotics are often administered, as differentiating between leiomyoma degeneration and acute endomyometritis can be difficult. In most cases, symptoms improve within 24 to 48 hours. Pain stemming from tumor degeneration classically follows uterine artery embolization (UAE), and treatment with analgesics usually suffices as discussed on page 209.

Women with prolapse of a tumor from the endometrial cavity will typically note cramping or acute pain as the tumor stretches the endocervical canal to pass through. Associated bleeding or serosanguinous discharge is common. Visual inspection is usually diagnostic (Fig. 9-3). However, sonography is often performed to evaluate the size and number of other uterine leiomyomas and exclude other possible sources of pain. Surgical treatment involves severing the leiomyoma from its stalk as described in detail in Section 43-11 (p. 948).

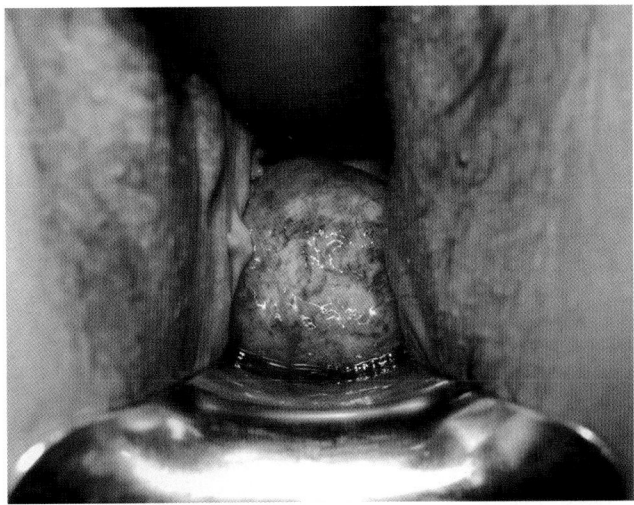

FIGURE 9-3 This round, hyperemic leiomyoma and its elongated stalk have prolapsed from the uterine cavity, through the cervix, and into the vagina. (Used with permission from Dr. David Rogers.)

Infertility and Pregnancy Wastage

Leiomyomas can diminish fertility, but only 1 to 3 percent of infertility cases are due solely to leiomyomas (Buttram, 1981; Donnez, 2002). Their putative effects include occlusion of tubal ostia and disruption of the normal uterine contractions that propel sperm or ova. Distortion of the endometrial cavity may diminish implantation and sperm transport. Importantly, leiomyomas are associated with endometrial inflammation and vascular changes that may disrupt implantation (American Society for Reproductive Medicine, 2008).

Of myomas, subfertility is more closely associated with submucous leiomyomas than with tumors located elsewhere. Improved pregnancy rates following hysteroscopic resection have provided most of the indirect evidence for this link (Casini, 2006; Surrey, 2005). In contrast, evidence does not implicate subserosal tumors. For intramural leiomyomas that do not distort the endometrial cavity, the relationship with subfertility is more tenuous. Several investigators have reported equally good in vitro fertilization (IVF) success rates in women with and without leiomyomas that did not distort the endometrial cavity (Oliveira, 2004; Yan, 2014). Others, however, have reported adverse fertility effects from such intramural leiomyomas (Eldar-Geva, 1998; Hart, 2001). Importantly, the strength of this evidence must be weighed against the morbidity associated with myomectomy. Namely, peritubal or intrauterine adhesions can threaten fertility, and myometrial defects risk uterine rupture during subsequent pregnancies.

Both uterine leiomyoma and spontaneous miscarriage are common, and an association between these has not been shown convincingly. Moreover, there is no conclusive evidence that surgical treatment reduces miscarriage rates (American Society for Reproductive Medicine, 2012b; Pritts, 2009).

Other Clinical Manifestations

Less than 0.5 percent of women with leiomyomas develop *myomatous erythrocytosis syndrome*. This may result from excessive erythropoietin production by the kidneys or by the leiomyomas themselves (Vlasveld, 2008). In either case, red cell mass returns to normal following hysterectomy.

Leiomyomas occasionally may cause *pseudo-Meigs syndrome*. Traditionally, Meigs syndrome consists of ascites and pleural effusions that accompany a benign ovarian fibroma. However, any pelvic tumor including large, cystic leiomyomas or other benign ovarian cysts can cause this. The presumed etiology stems from discordancy between the arterial supply and the venous and lymphatic drainage from the leiomyomas. If due to myomas, resolution of ascites and hydrothorax follows hysterectomy or myomectomy.

■ Diagnosis

Leiomyomas are often detected by pelvic examination with findings of uterine enlargement, irregular contour, or both. In reproductive-aged women, uterine enlargement prompts determination of a urine or serum β-human chorionic gonadotropin (hCG) level. Sonography is initially done to define pelvic anatomy. Transvaginal sonography (TVS) provides superior resolution, but some uteri are so large that transabdominal sonography is needed to image the entire corpus. The sonographic appearances of leiomyomas vary from hypo- to hyperechoic depending on the ratio of smooth muscle to connective tissue and whether there is degeneration (Fig. 9-4). Calcification and cystic degeneration create the most sonographically distinctive changes. Calcifications appear hyperechoic and commonly rim the tumor or are randomly scattered throughout the mass. Cystic or myxoid degeneration typically fills the leiomyoma with multiple, smooth-walled, round, irregularly sized but generally small hypoechoic or anechoic areas.

If HMB, dysmenorrhea, or infertility accompanies a pelvic mass, then the endometrial cavity is evaluated for submucous leiomyomas, endometrial polyps, congenital anomalies, or synechiae. With focal lesions such as submucous leiomyomas, the endometrium appears thick or irregular during TVS, and adjunct imaging tools may help clarify anatomy. Of these, saline infusion sonography (SIS) or hysteroscopy may provide additional cavity information (Figs. 9-5 and 9-6), and their

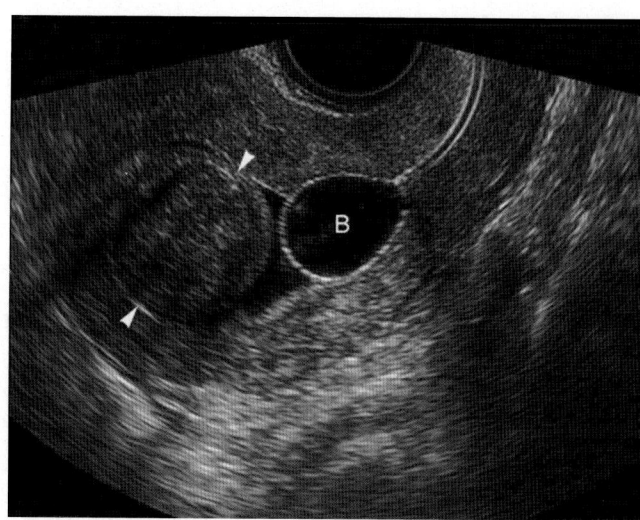

FIGURE 9-5 Submucous fibroid is clearly outlined during saline infusion sonography (SIS) (*arrowheads*). The SIS catheter balloon is seen in the lower uterine cavity (*B*). (Used with permission from Dr. Elysia Moschos.)

advantages are described in Chapters 2 and 8. Also, three-dimensional (3-D) TVS and 3-D SIS can be valuable (Fig. 9-7). Leiomyomas have characteristic vascular patterns that can be identified by color and power Doppler techniques. A peripheral circumferential rim of vascularity from which a few vessels arise to penetrate into the center of the tumor is a classic finding. As such, Doppler imaging can be used to help differentiate an extrauterine leiomyoma from another pelvic mass or a submucous leiomyoma from an endometrial polyp. For the infertile woman, the endometrial cavity can be evaluated with hysterosalpingography (HSG) or hysterosalpingo-contrast sonography HyCoSy (Chap. 2, p. 25). This offers the advantage to also define tubal patency.

When imaging is limited by body habitus or distorted anatomy, magnetic resonance (MR) imaging may be required. Although used less often for myoma evaluation, this tool allows more accurate assessment of the size, number, and location of

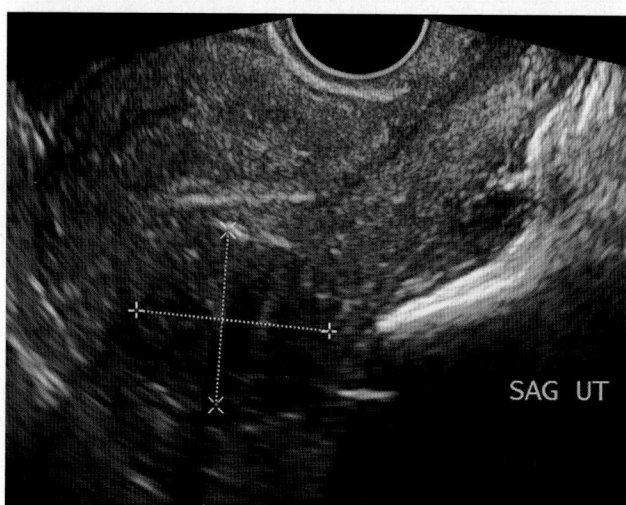

FIGURE 9-4 Transvaginal sonogram of an intramural leiomyoma. (Used with permission from Dr. Elysia Moschos.)

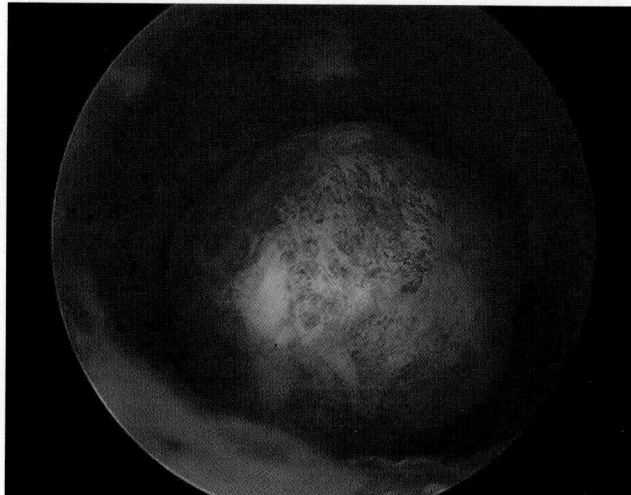

FIGURE 9-6 Hysteroscopic photograph of a submucous leiomyoma prior to resection. (Used with permission from Dr. Karen Bradshaw.)

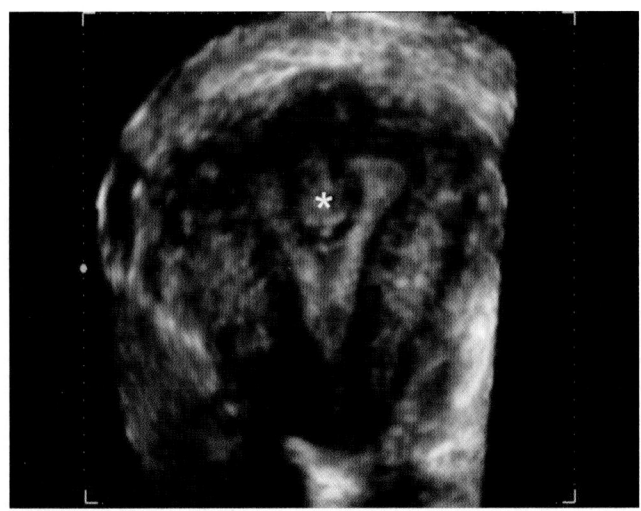

FIGURE 9-7 3-D transvaginal sonogram of a submucous leiomyoma (*asterisk*). (Used with permission from Dr. Elysia Moschos.)

leiomyomas, which may help identify appropriate candidates for hysterectomy alternatives such as myomectomy or UAE. Importantly, MR imaging can also aid differentiation of an intramural leiomyoma, which is a suitable indication for myomectomy, from a focal, compact collection of adenomyosis, which is poorly suited for enucleation.

■ Management

Observation

Regardless of their size, asymptomatic leiomyomas usually can be observed and surveilled with an annual pelvic examination. At times, adnexal assessment may be hindered by large uterine size or irregular contour, and adequate uterine and adnexal assessment can both be limited by patient obesity. In these cases, some may choose to add annual sonographic surveillance (Cantuaria, 1998).

Leiomyomas in general are slow-growing. A longitudinal sonography-based study showed the average diameter growth to be only 0.5 cm/yr, although diameter growth greater than 3 cm/yr has been observed (DeWaay, 2002). Moreover, growth rates of leiomyomas within the same patient will vary widely, and some tumors will even spontaneous regress (Peddada, 2008). Therefore, predicting myoma growth or symptom onset

is difficult, and watchful waiting may be the best option for an asymptomatic patient.

In the past, most preferred surgical removal of a large, asymptomatic leiomyomatous uterus because of concerns regarding increased later operative morbidity and cancer risks. These concerns have been disproven, and thus otherwise asymptomatic women with large leiomyomas can also be managed expectantly (Parker, 1994). In addition, most infertile women with uterine leiomyomas are initially managed expectantly. For those with symptomatic tumors, conception attempts closely follow surgery, if possible, to limit tumor recurrence before conception.

As discussed in the next section, in some women with symptomatic leiomyomas, long-term medical therapy may be preferred (Table 9-1). In others, medical therapy is used as a short-term preoperative adjunct. Also, because these tumors typically regress postmenopausally, some women choose medical treatment to relieve symptoms in anticipation of menopause.

Sex Steroid Hormones

Both COCs and progestins have been used to induce endometrial atrophy and to decrease prostaglandin production in women with leiomyomas. Friedman and Thomas (1995) studied 87 women with myomas and reported that women taking low-dose COCs had significantly shorter menses and no evidence of uterine enlargement. Few studies have evaluated DMPA specifically for leiomyoma-related bleeding, and its use is extrapolated from its effects in nonmyomatous uteri. Also, the levonorgestrel-releasing intrauterine system (LNG-IUS), marketed as Mirena, in small studies improves leiomyoma-related HMB (Sayed, 2011; Socolov, 2011). Importantly, tumors that distort the endometrial cavity preclude LNG-IUS use (Bayer, 2014). Also, compared with women without leiomyomas, those with tumors experience higher device expulsion rates (Youm, 2014).

For these reasons, sex steroid contraceptives are a reasonable treatment option for menses-related leiomyoma symptoms. However, because of the unpredictable effects of progestins on leiomyoma growth described earlier (p. 203), the American College of Obstetricians and Gynecologists (2012a) recommends close monitoring of leiomyoma and uterine size.

As noted, progesterone is considered essential for myoma growth and antiprogestins agents are another potential option. Physiologically, progesterone can bind to either progesterone receptor A (PR-A) or B (PR-B). Of these, PR-A is found in

TABLE 9-1. Indications for the Medical Treatment of Uterine Leiomyoma

Agent	NSAID	COC	DMPA	LNG-IUS	GnRH agonist	Ulipristal[a]
Symptom						
Dysmenorrhea	+	+	+	+	+	+
Menorrhagia	–	+	+	+	+	+
Pelvic pressure	–	–	–	–	+	+
Infertility	–	–	–	–	+	–

[a]Available in Europe and Canada for preoperative use for this indication.
COC = combination oral contraceptive pills; DMPA = depot medroxyprogesterone acetate; GnRH = gonadotropin-releasing hormone; LNG-IUS = levonorgestrel-releasing intrauterine system (Mirena); NSAID = nonsteroidal antiinflammatory drug.

leiomyomas in greater amounts than PR-B (Viville, 1997). Specific agents can competitively bind these receptors. Agents are classified as antiprogestins if they universally prompt antagonist effects. However, agents are termed selective progesterone-receptor modulators (SPRMs) if they exert antiprogestational effects in some tissues but progestational effects in others.

Of antiprogestins, mifepristone, also known as RU-486, diminishes leiomyoma volume by approximately half. Various doses have been used and range from 2.5 to 10 mg given orally daily for 3 to 6 months (Carbonell Esteve, 2008, 2012). Mifepristone therapy, however, has several drawbacks. First, approximately 40 percent of treated women complain of vasomotor symptoms. Second, its antiprogestational effects expose the endometrium to unopposed estrogen. The spectrum of endometrial findings range from simple endometrial hyperplasia to a newer category described as *progesterone-receptor modulator-associated endometrial changes* (Mutter, 2008). This concern for endometrial stimulation currently limits mifepristone's use to 3 to 6 months. As a final concern, mifepristone (Mifeprex) is currently Food and Drug Administration (FDA)-approved solely for early pregnancy termination. It is manufactured only as 200-mg tablets, a dose well above that needed for leiomyoma therapy.

Ulipristal acetate is a SPRM that has similar effects to mifepristone. Currently marketed outside the United States, ulipristal acetate (Esmya), given as 5- or 10-mg oral daily doses, controls leiomyoma-related bleeding in 90 percent of patients. It performs comparably with leuprolide acetate (Donnez, 2012a,b). Again, endometrial concerns currently limit its use solely to that of a preoperative adjunct. Other SPRMs are also under investigation, but none are currently commercially available for leiomyoma treatment.

Other sex steroid hormone options include the androgens, danazol and gestrinone, which shrink leiomyoma volume and improve bleeding symptoms (Coutinho, 1989; De Leo, 1999). Unfortunately, their prominent side effects, which include acne and hirsutism, preclude their use as first-line agents.

GnRH Receptor Agents

These compounds are synthetic derivatives of the GnRH decapeptide. They are inactive if taken orally, but intramuscular (IM), subcutaneous, and intranasal preparations are available. Leuprolide acetate (Lupron) is FDA-approved for leiomyoma treatment and is available in a 3.75-mg monthly dose or 11.25-mg 3-month dose, both given IM. Less frequently used GnRH agonists include goserelin (Zoladex), administered as a 3.6-mg monthly or 10.8-mg 3-month subcutaneous depot implant; triptorelin (Trelstar), given as a 3.75-mg monthly or 11.25-mg 3-month IM injection; and nafarelin (Synarel), used in a 200-μg twice-daily nasal spray regimen. These latter three are not specifically FDA-approved for leiomyoma treatment, but their off-label use has been shown effective.

GnRH agonists shrink leiomyomas by targeting the growth effects of estrogen and progesterone. Initially, these agonists stimulate receptors on pituitary gonadotropes to cause a supraphysiological release of both luteinizing hormone (LH) and follicle-stimulating hormone (FSH). Also called a *flare*, this phase typically lasts 1 week. With their long-term action, however,

agonists downregulate receptors in gonadotropes, thus creating desensitization to further GnRH stimulation. Correspondingly, decreased gonadotropin secretion leads to suppressed estrogen and progesterone levels 1 to 2 weeks after initial GnRH agonist administration (Broekmans, 1996).

Results with GnRH agonist treatment include dramatic decreases in uterine and leiomyoma volume. Most women experience a mean decrease in uterine volume of 40 to 50 percent, and most of this occurs during the first 3 months of therapy. Clinical benefits of reduced leiomyoma volumes include pain relief and diminished HMB, usually amenorrhea. During this time, anemic women are given oral iron therapy to rebuild red cell mass and increase iron stores (Filicori, 1983). GnRH agonist treatment typically is continued for 3 to 6 months. Following their discontinuance, normal menses resume in 4 to 10 weeks. Unfortunately, leiomyoma then regrow, and uterine volumes regain pretreatment sizes within 3 to 4 months (Friedman, 1990). Despite regrowth, Schlaff and coworkers (1989) reported symptom relief for approximately 1 year in half of women given GnRH agonists.

GnRH agonists have significant costs, risks, and side effects. Side effects result from the profound drop in serum estrogen levels, mirror those of menopause, and develop in up to 95 percent of women treated with these drugs (Letterie, 1989). Despite this, less than 10 percent of patients terminate treatment secondary to side effects (Parker, 2007). Importantly, 6 months of agonist therapy can result in a 6-percent loss in trabecular bone, not all of which may be recouped following discontinuation (Scharla, 1990). As a result, these agents alone are not recommended for longer than 6 months of use.

To obviate side effect severity, several medications have been added to GnRH agonist treatment. The goal of this "add-back therapy" is to counter side effects—most importantly vasomotor symptoms and bone loss—without mitigating the shrinking action on uterine and leiomyoma volume. This is made possible by the fact that the estrogen level required to improve vasomotor symptoms and minimize bone loss is below the estrogen threshold that would restimulate leiomyomas growth. Mizutani and associates (1998) found that GnRH agonists suppress leiomyoma cell proliferation and induce cell apoptosis at the fourth week of GnRH agonist therapy. They proposed that add-back therapy be withheld until after this time. Because of these and other observations, add-back therapy is typically begun 1 to 3 months following GnRH agonist initiation.

Add-back therapy traditionally includes estrogen combined with a progestin, and those studied have generally been low-dose preparations equivalent to menopausal HRT. An oral regimen of MPA, 10 mg (days 16–25), combined with equine estrogen, 0.3 to 0.625 mg (days 1–25), or a continuous daily regimen of MPA 2.5 mg and equine estrogen 0.3 mg to 0.625 mg may be used.

Add-back therapy with selective estrogen-receptor modulators (SERMs), such as tibolone and raloxifene, has also been shown to prevent bone loss. Advantages of SERMs include the ability to begin them concurrently with GnRH agonist treatment without negating the agonist effects of leiomyoma shrinkage. Unfortunately, a high percentage of women complain of vasomotor symptoms while taking SERMs (Palomba, 1998,

2004). Raloxifene is associated with greater venous thromboembolism risks (Goldstein, 2009).

Because of the limitations of GnRH agonist therapy, the American College of Obstetricians and Gynecologists (2014a) recommends that it not be used longer than 6 months without add-back therapy. Short-term, preoperative GnRH agonist use offers several advantages. Their use decreases HMB and may allow correction of anemia. Decreased uterine size as a result of treatment may allow a less complicated or extensive surgical procedure. For example, hysterectomy or myomectomy may be performed through a smaller laparotomy incision or by vaginal or minimally invasive surgery (MIS) approaches. This advantage may be less robust for GnRH agonist use prior to hysteroscopic myomectomy and is discussed in that section of the atlas (p. 1040).

In contrast to agonists, *GnRH antagonists* are available. Two agents in this class, cetrorelix and ganirelix, are currently FDA-approved for infertility use in women undergoing controlled ovarian hyperstimulation. However, a limitation of these drugs is that they are daily injectables. Also, a depot form of cetrorelix did not provide adequate or consistent suppression of estrogen production or leiomyoma growth (Felberbaum, 1998). A new agent, elagolix, is a nonpeptide oral GnRH antagonist that is currently being evaluated for both endometriosis and leiomyoma treatment (Diamond, 2014).

Nonhormonal Options

Tranexamic acid (TXA) is an antifibrinolytic agent described fully in Chapter 8 (p. 196). Studies have not evaluated TXA specifically for myoma-related HMB, but subgroup analysis does provide some support for its use for myoma-related bleeding (Eder, 2013).

The benefits of NSAIDs for leiomyoma-related bleeding are less clear, and the few studies have conflicting results (Anteby, 1985; Mäkäräinen, 1986; Ylikorkala, 1986). Thus, although NSAIDs are potentially helpful for myoma-related dysmenorrhea, available data do not support their use as sole agents for leiomyoma-related HMB.

Because aromatase levels are higher with myomas, aromatase inhibitors (AIs) for leiomyoma treatment seem logical. However, only a few small studies have evaluated short-term use of the oral nonsteroid AIs, letrozole and anastrozole (Parsanezhad, 2010; Varelas, 2007). As with GnRH agonists, the induced profound systemic hypoestrogenism leads to menopausal symptoms and potential bone loss. Moreover, their use is associated with increased FSH release, which could cause multiple follicular cyst formation. Larger prospective studies are needed to define their clinical role.

Radiologic Interventions

Uterine Artery Embolization. This is an is an angiographic interventional procedure that delivers polyvinyl alcohol microspheres or other synthetic particulate emboli into both uterine arteries. Uterine blood flow is thereby obstructed, producing ischemia and necrosis. Because vessels serving leiomyomas have a larger caliber, these microspheres are preferentially directed to the tumors, sparing the surrounding myometrium.

During UAE, an angiographic catheter is placed in one femoral artery and advanced under fluoroscopic guidance to

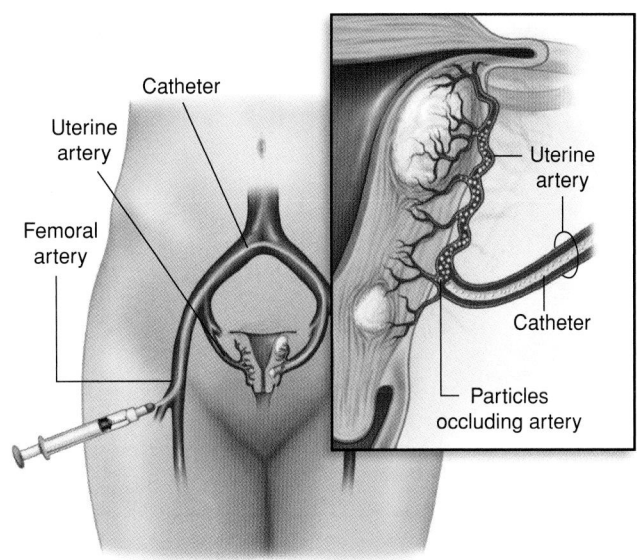

FIGURE 9-8 Diagram of uterine artery embolization (UAE).

sequentially catheterize both uterine arteries (Figs. 9-8 and 9-9). Failure to embolize both uterine arteries allows existing collateral circulation between the two uterine arteries to sustain leiomyoma blood flow and is associated with a significantly lower success rates (Bratby, 2008).

UAE is a management option for women with documented uterine leiomyomas who have significant symptoms despite medical management and who might otherwise be considered a candidate for hysterectomy or myomectomy. Based on current evidence and discussed later, women who have not completed childbearing may be better served by myomectomy (Gupta, 2012; Mara, 2008). Other patient limitations are listed in Table 9-2, and many are associated with altered vascular anatomy. This is a reason why GnRH agonists are not recommended prior to UAE. In addition, pedunculated submucous tumors are not suitable as these tumors can infarct and slough. Pedunculated subserosal tumors were previously excluded for similar reasons. But based on additional data, the Society of Interventional Radiology removed this caveat (Dariushnia, 2014).

Prior to UAE, a woman undergoes a thorough evaluation by her gynecologist. Components include current cervical cancer screening and negative testing for *Neisseria gonorrhoeae* and *Chlamydia trachomatis*. Endometrial biopsy is completed in those with endometrial cancer risk factors (Chap. 8, p. 184). Complete blood count, creatinine level, prothrombin time (PT), and partial thromboplastin time (PTT) are also obtained.

Following UAE, pain management typically requires a 24- to 48-hour hospital admission. After discharge, most patients have pain controlled with NSAIDs and have a rapid return to daily activities. However, as a result of leiomyoma necrosis, approximately 10 percent of patients develop significant postprocedural symptoms and require hospital readmission (Hehenkamp, 2005, 2006). The *postembolization syndrome,* seen in approximately 25 percent of cases, usually lasts 2 to 7 days and is classically marked by pelvic pain, nausea, low-grade fever, mild white blood cell count elevation, and malaise (Edwards, 2007). Symptom intensity varies, and management

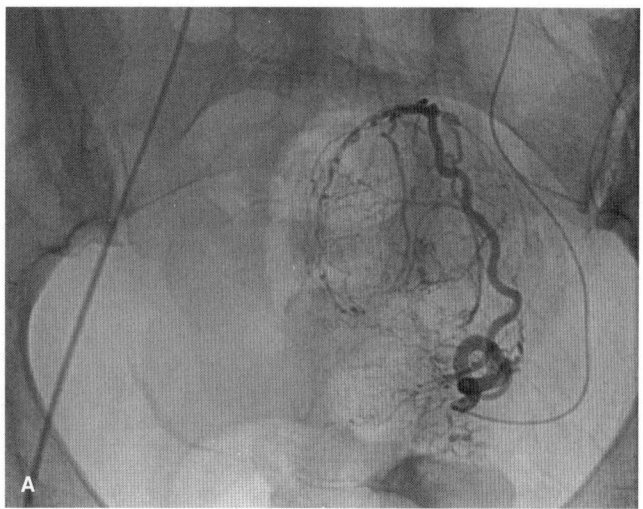
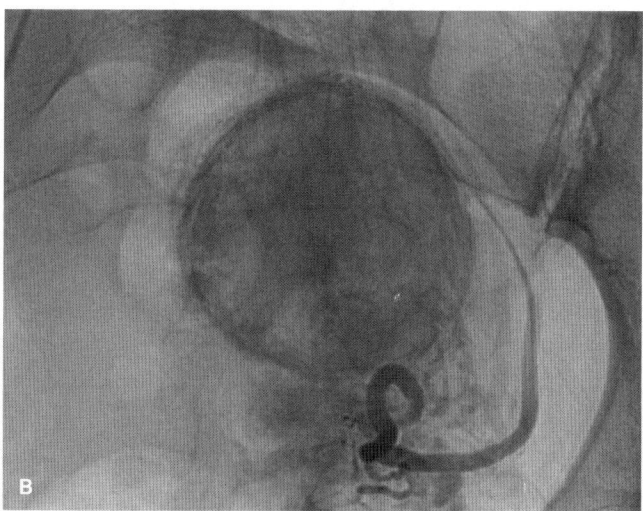

FIGURE 9-9 Fluoroscopic images obtained during uterine artery embolization (UAE). **A.** Before embolization, the leiomyoma can be identified by its numerous, hypertrophied, tortuous arteries wrapping around its periphery and extending within it. **B.** After embolization, most of the blood vessels are occluded by particles and appear truncated. Leiomyomas are again easily visualized and appear dark and smudged as the contrast/particle mixture stagnates within the tumor. (Used with permission from Dr. Samuel C. Chao.)

includes supportive care and analgesia. Because symptoms stem from myoma necrosis, antibiotics are not typically required but may be administered if infectious endomyometritis is an alternative diagnosis.

Embolization is effective for leiomyoma-related symptoms. Several randomized controlled trials have shown high rates of patient satisfaction and symptom improvement (Edwards, 2007; Hehenkamp, 2008). Compared with hysterectomy, UAE is associated with shorter hospitalization, reduced 24-hour pain scores, and earlier return to daily activities. UAE also compares favorably with myomectomy for symptom relief (Goodwin, 2006; Manyonda, 2012). However, some patients do not achieve adequate improvement. Namely, long-term surveillance reveals that approximately 26 to 37 percent of UAE-treated patients will require a subsequent procedure, which in many cases is hysterectomy (Moss, 2011; Van der Kooij, 2010).

There are several complications associated with UAE. Leiomyoma tissue passage is common and likely is seen only with leiomyomas that initially have contact with the endometrial surface. Necrotic leiomyomas that pass into the vagina usually can be removed in the office. Those that do not pass spontaneously from the uterine cavity or that remain firmly attached to the uterine wall may require dilatation and evacuation (Spies, 2002). Groin hematoma and prolonged vaginal discharge are other frequent complications. Brief amenorrhea and associated transiently elevated FSH levels may last a few menstrual cycles after UAE. Permanent amenorrhea, however, develops occasionally, and more often in older reproductive-aged patients (Hehenkamp, 2007). This complication likely results from concurrent embolization of the ovaries via anastomoses between the uterine and ovarian arteries. Rarely, embolization may incite necrosis in surrounding tissues such as the uterus, adnexa, bladder, and soft tissues.

Pregnancy subsequent to UAE can pose complications. Although the number of evaluable pregnancies is small, consistent problems include increased rates of miscarriage, postpartum hemorrhage, and cesarean delivery (Homer, 2010). Other complications, noted by some but not all studies, are higher rates of preterm delivery, fetal malpresentation, fetal growth restriction, and abnormal placentation (Goldberg, 2004; Pron, 2005; Walker, 2006).

In sum, UAE has typically low major complication rates and high symptom-relief scores. However, these are balanced against the need for ultimate reintervention in a significant number of women.

Magnetic Resonance-guided Focused Ultrasound (MRgFUS). This is also called MR-guided high intensity focused ultrasound (MR-HIFU). With this FDA-approved

TABLE 9-2. UAE Absolute and Relative Contraindications

Absolute

Pregnancy
Active uterine or adnexal infection
Suspected reproductive tract malignancy[a]

Relative	Reason
Coagulopathy	Bleeding complications
Renal impairment	Renal effects of contrast
Severe contrast allergy	Allergic reaction
Desire for future fertility	Pregnancy complications
Uterine size >20–24 weeks	Difficult to embolize
Prior salpingectomy or SO	Altered arterial anatomy
Prior pelvic radiation	Altered arterial anatomy
Large hydrosalpinx	Increased infection risk
GnRH agonist use	Narrows vascularity

[a]Unless performed as an adjunct to treatment.
GnRH = gonadotropin-releasing hormone; SO = salpingo-oophorectomy; UAE = uterine artery embolization.
Data from American College of Obstetricians and Gynecologists, 2014a; American Society for Reproductive Medicine, 2008; Dariushnia, 2014; Stokes, 2010.

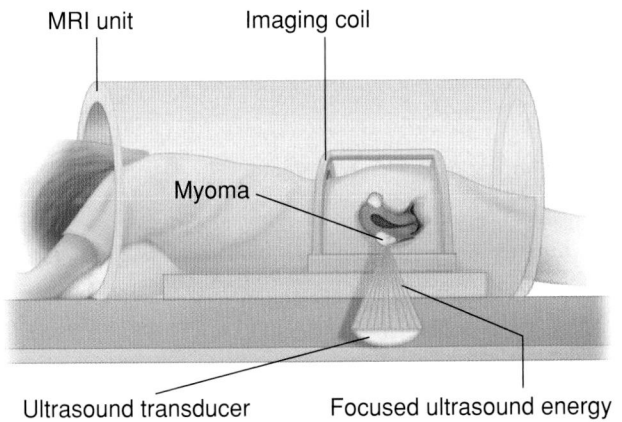

MRI unit   Imaging coil

Myoma

Ultrasound transducer   Focused ultrasound energy

FIGURE 9-10 Diagram of magnetic resonance-guided focused ultrasound.

intervention, ultrasound energy is focused to heat and incite coagulative necrosis in selected myomas (Fig. 9-10). Concurrent MR imaging enables precise targeting and provides real-time tissue temperature feedback to limit surrounding thermal injury. During sessions lasting 2 to 3 hours, a patient lies prone within the MR imaging unit, and the bladder is continuously drained. Manufacturer contraindications are general contraindications to MR imaging, pregnancy, and energy-path obstructions such as abdominal wall scars, bowel, or foreign bodies. Other study exclusions have included future fertility desires, current pelvic infection, other uterine pathology, menopause, myoma size >10 cm, and uterine size >24 weeks. Also, myomas with poor perfusion characteristics, pedunculated serosal or submucous myomas, or those near vital structures increase failure rates or injury risks. Moreover, each session has limits on total myoma volume treated and on time, which may leave some myomas untreated.

Advantageously, MRgFUS is noninvasive, requires only conscious sedation, and is associated with rapid recovery and return to daily activities. In early prospective studies, MRgFUS improves quality-of-life scores and is well tolerated (Hindley, 2004). Complications have included skin burns, adjacent tissue injury, and venous thromboembolism. Notably, similar to UAE, symptoms relief wanes with time, and ≥12 months following MRgFUS, 8 to 24 percent of women seek alternative procedures for their symptoms, including hysterectomy (Machtinger, 2012; Okada, 2009). Compared with UAE in one small nonrandomized study, MRgFUS showed superior symptom improvement at 5 years (Froeling, 2013). Results from an ongoing randomized controlled trial comparing these two are awaited.

Surgery

Hysterectomy. For women with persistent symptoms despite conservative therapy, surgery is necessary for many with myomas. Options include hysterectomy, myomectomy, endometrial ablation, and myolysis. Of these, hysterectomy is the definitive and most common surgery. In 2007, nearly 540,000 hysterectomies were performed, and 43 percent of cases had a diagnosis of leiomyoma (Wechter, 2011). Hysterectomy is effective for myoma symptoms, and a study of 418 women undergoing hysterectomy found satisfaction rates greater than 90 percent (Carlson, 1994). There were marked improvements

in pelvic pain, urinary symptoms, fatigue, psychological symptoms, and sexual dysfunction. However, benefits are balanced against the risks of major surgery.

Hysterectomy can be performed vaginally, abdominally, or laparoscopically depending on patient and uterine factors. With hysterectomy, removal of the ovaries may or may not be desired. Prophylactic salpingectomy to lower ovarian cancer risk is another consideration. The decision making for each is presented fully in Section 43-12 (p. 950).

Myomectomy. This uterus-preserving surgery excises myomas and is considered for women who desire fertility preservation or who decline hysterectomy. This can be performed hysteroscopically, laparoscopically, or via laparotomy. In general, predominantly intracavitary myomas are resected hysteroscopically, whereas subserosal or intramural myomas require laparotomy or laparoscopy for excision.

Hysteroscopic resection is an incisionless, day-surgery procedure that affords quick recovery. Resection is most effective with type 0 and type 1 tumors, and other surgical evaluation aspects are discussed in Chapter 44 (1040). For myoma-related HMB, long-term effectiveness ranges from 85 to 90 percent (Derman, 1991; Emanuel, 1999). Infertility is improved following removal, as previously described on page 205. However, despite its advantages, hysteroscopic resection is possible for only a small subset of myomas.

For women with subserosal or intramural myomas, surgeons must use a laparotomic or laparoscopic approach to enucleate tumors buried in the muscular uterine walls and then reconstruct normal anatomy. As such, surgical complexity and subsequent risks are increased. This type of myomectomy usually improves pain and bleeding. For example, HMB improves in approximately 70 to 80 percent of patients (Buttram, 1981; Olufowobi, 2004).

When selecting a surgical approach for subserosal or intramural myomas, several factors are weighed. Laparoscopic leiomyoma resection yields successful outcomes and recurrence rates comparable to those for laparotomy (Rossetti, 2001). Advantageously, shorter hospital stays and less febrile morbidity, blood loss, adhesion formation, and pain are found with laparoscopic resection compared with laparotomy (Mais, 1996; Takeuchi, 2002). However, limitations to a laparoscopic approach include myoma size, number, and location, and laparoscopic surgical skills, especially multilayer suturing of the leiomyoma beds following enucleation. In general, large intramural and multiple myomas require higher skill levels. Also, seeding the abdominal cavity with myomatous implants is a concern with intraabdominal morcellation, and tissue extraction options are described in Chapter 41 (p. 896). To overcome some of these limits, minilaparotomy techniques may be selected. However, as with larger laparotomy incisions, minilaparotomy is faster than laparoscopic myomectomy but still underperforms laparoscopy regarding patient pain scores, hospital stay, and blood loss (Alessandri, 2006; Palomba, 2007). Also, robot-assisted myomectomy has been described. In general, this offers similar MIS advantages but longer operating times. Moreover, due to poor tactile feedback from robotic instruments, myomas may be missed and lead to higher recurrence rates (Griffin, 2013).

In sum, for those considering myomectomy, hysteroscopic resection is preferred when possible. For remaining cases, abdominal approach selection varies depending on myoma characteristics and surgeon skill. That said, MIS offers decreased postoperative pain and comparable complication rates, although long-term durability data are limited.

Myomectomy versus Hysterectomy. In women not seeking pregnancy, risk and benefits aid the decision between myomectomy and hysterectomy. Again, for intracavitary lesions, hysteroscopic resection is preferred. For intramural or subserosal lesions, open myomectomy compared with open hysterectomy yields similar blood loss, intraoperative injuries, and febrile morbidity (Iverson, 1996; Sawin, 2000). However, if laparoscopic approaches are examined, one study showed laparoscopic myomectomy resulted in greater blood loss, higher rates of transfusion and conversion to laparotomy, but lower risks of bladder injury compared with laparoscopic hysterectomy (Odejinmi, 2015).

Moreover, with all myomectomy approaches, symptom relief may be incomplete and prompt additional interventions. Also, myomas can redevelop. Specifically, recurrence rates following myomectomy range from 40 to 50 percent (Acien, 1996; Fedele, 1995). Last, compared with hysterectomy, myomectomy leads to a greater risk for postoperative intraabdominal adhesions (Stricker, 1994).

Endometrial Ablation. There are several tissue-destructive modalities that cause endometrial ablation, and they are discussed in Section 44-15 (p. 1043). These techniques are effective for women with abnormal uterine bleeding from endometrial dysfunction (AUB-E). But when used as a sole technique for myoma-related bleeding, the failure rate approaches 40 percent (Goldfarb, 1999; Yin, 1998). In addition, most of these modalities have limitations regarding cavity length and degree of cavity distortion. That said, studies have shown efficacy if treating submucous myomas measuring ≤3 cm (Glasser, 2009; Sabbah, 2006; Soysal, 2001).

In other instances, ablation can be used instead as an adjunct following hysteroscopic leiomyoma resection in women with HMB. The few studies that have evaluated this have shown greater improvement in HMB following resection coupled with ablation than with resection alone (Indman, 1993; Loffer, 2005).

Myolysis and Other Approaches. Myolysis describes myoma puncture with tools to permit mono- or bipolar cautery, laser vaporization, or cryotherapy. All of these incite myoma necrosis and subsequent shrinkage. Of these, the Acessa system uses a monopolar radiofrequency needle that is inserted transabdominally into each myoma during laparoscopy, as illustrated in Figure 41-11 p. 885). With this newer approach, early evidence shows patient symptom improvement, and a reintervention rate of 11 percent at 3 years. However, data regarding long-term symptom relief, recurrence rates, and effects on fertility and pregnancy are lacking (Berman, 2014).

Another option is laparoscopic uterine artery occlusion (LUAO). This attempts to achieve myoma devascularization and necrosis by surgically sealing both uterine arteries near their origin from the internal iliac artery as well as both ovarian arteries (Ambat, 2009). The reintervention rate at 4 years is 28 percent, similar to UAE (Hald, 2009). For now, the requirement for advanced surgical skills, treatment failure rates, and scarce high-quality data limit this procedure's use.

HEMATOMETRA

In this condition, menstrual outflow obstruction traps blood and distends the uterus. Depending on the level of the genital tract blockage, blood can variably distend the vagina (hematocolpos), the uterus (hematometra), and fallopian tubes (hematosalpinx). Obstruction may be congenital, and these are described in Chapter 18. Acquired abnormalities such as scarring and neoplasms may also obstruct menstrual flow. As such, hematometra may follow radiation treatment, prolonged hypoestrogenism with atrophy, or surgeries of the endometrial cavity or endocervical canal, particularly endometrial ablation and cervical conization. Other predisposing conditions are Asherman syndrome or malignancies of the uterus or cervix.

Women with hematometra classically complain of cyclic, midline pain. Low back pain and pelvic fullness can also be noted, and with total obstruction, there is amenorrhea. If significant, a large uterus can even compress the bladder or rectum and yield urinary retention or constipation. With partial obstruction, blood may erratically drain around the blockage and can be foul. Last, blood may become infected, and pyometra creates fever and leukocytosis.

Pelvic examination findings include an enlarged, soft, or even cystic midline uterine corpus that may be tender to palpation. These findings mimic early pregnancy, leiomyoma cystic degeneration, leiomyosarcoma, and gestational trophoblastic disease. Thus, urine or serum β-hCG assay is obtained in reproductive-aged women. Importantly, in cases in which the underlying cause is unclear, endocervical and endometrial biopsy are usually indicated to exclude malignancy.

Sonography is a principal diagnostic tool, and imaging shows a smooth, symmetric hypoechoic enlargement of the uterine cavity (Fig. 9-11). Low-level internal echoes are often

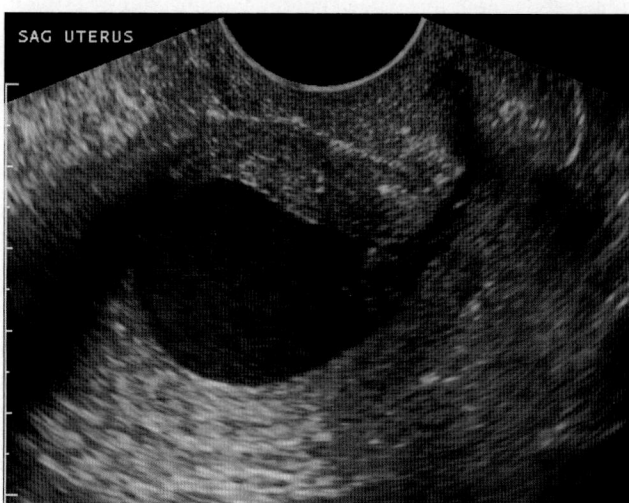

FIGURE 9-11 Sonographic transvaginal sagittal image of hematometra. The uterine walls and proximal cervix are dilated by retained blood, which appears hypoechoic. (Used with permission from Dr. Elysia Moschos.)

present. A hematosalpinx is seen less commonly and is identified as hypoechoic tubular distentions lateral to the uterus. Although typically not required for the diagnosis, MR imaging can be used in some cases to help localize the obstruction and to provide additional anatomic information.

For most cases of hematometra, relief of the obstruction and blood evacuation are the goals. Cervical dilatation in the clinic or operating suite usually relieves the accumulation. Some have described hysteroscopy following dilatation to access blood pockets and to lyse adhesions in cases complicated by uterine synechiae (Cooper, 2000). Congenital abnormalities may require more extensive procedures to correct the obstruction (Chap. 18, p. 415).

ADENOMYOSIS

■ Pathophysiology

Adenomyosis is characterized by uterine enlargement caused by ectopic rests of endometrium—both glands and stroma—located deep within the myometrium. These rests may be scattered throughout the myometrium—*diffuse adenomyosis*, or may form a localized nodular collection—*focal adenomyosis*. Although either form may be suspected clinically, the diagnosis is usually based on histologic findings in surgical specimens. Accordingly, reported incidences in hysterectomy specimens vary depending on the histologic criteria and the degree of sectioning, but range from 20 to 40 percent in large series (Vercellini, 2006). In one gynecology clinic population undergoing TVS, adenomyosis was suspected sonographically in 21 percent of women (Naftalin, 2012).

On gross examination, the uterus is often globally enlarged, but this rarely exceeds that of a 12-week pregnancy. The surface contour is usually smooth, regular, reddish, and soft. The grossly cut uterine surface typically appears spongy and trabeculated with focal areas of hemorrhage (Fig. 9-12). The ectopic foci of glands and stroma that are found in the myometrium in adenomyosis originate from the basalis layer. Because cells

from the basalis layer do not undergo the typical proliferative and secretory changes during the menstrual cycle, hemorrhage within these foci is minimal.

The most widely held theory regarding adenomyosis development describes the downward invagination of the endometrial basalis layer into the myometrium. The endometrial-myometrial interface is unique in that it lacks an intervening submucosa. Accordingly, even in normal uteri, the endometrium commonly invades the myometrium superficially (Benagiano, 2012). Mechanisms that incite deep myometrial invasion are unknown. In some cases, myometrial vulnerability stems from prior pregnancy or uterine surgery. Estrogen and progesterone likely play a role in its development and maintenance. For example, adenomyosis develops during the reproductive years and regresses after menopause. Regardless of the permissive cause, cell migration and invasion proceed.

Parity and age are significant risk factors for adenomyosis (Templeman, 2008). Specifically, nearly 90 percent of cases are in parous women, and nearly 80 percent develop in women in their 40s and 50s (Bird, 1972; Lee, 1984). Adenomyosis is also associated with aromatase expression and higher tissue estrogen levels (Yamamoto, 1993). This similar increase is also seen in leiomyomas, endometrial hyperplasia, and endometriosis, which are often coexistent with adenomyosis (Ferenczy, 1998). However, as discussed in Chapter 10, endometriosis differs epidemiologically from adenomyosis and is thought to arise from another mechanism.

Of other factors, adenomyosis is found more frequently in women taking the selective estrogen-receptor modulator tamoxifen (Parazzini, 1997). COC pill use does not appear to be a risk.

■ Diagnosis

Approximately one third of women with adenomyosis have symptoms, and HMB and dysmenorrhea are common. Perhaps 10 percent complain of dyspareunia. Symptom severity correlates with increasing number of ectopic foci and extent of

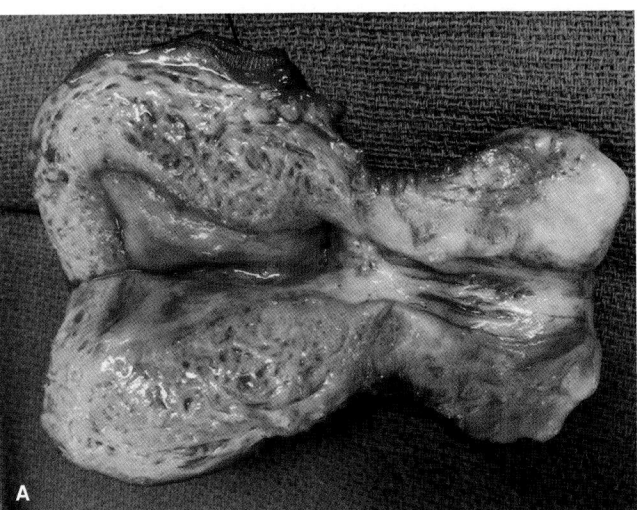
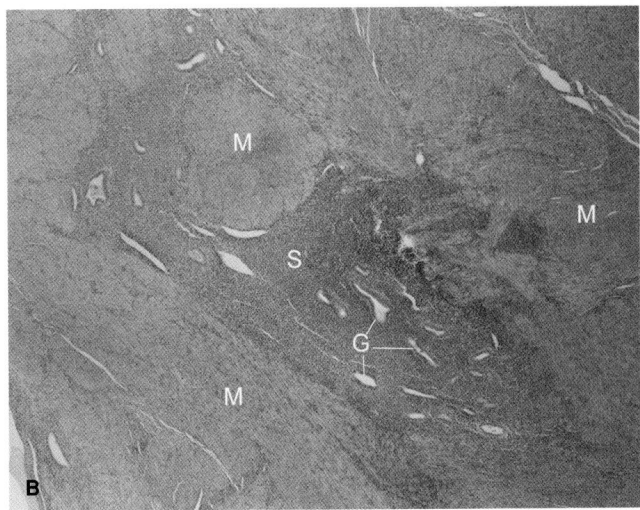

FIGURE 9-12 Adenomyosis. **A.** Gross bisected uterine specimen. Note the spongy, trabeculated myometrial texture. (Used with permission from Dr. Raheela Ashfaq.) **B.** In adenomyosis, endometrial glands (*G*) and their surrounding stroma (*S*) originate from the endometrial basalis, which dips irregularly into the myometrium (*M*). (Used with permission from Dr. Kelley Carrick.)

invasion (Levgur, 2000). The pathogenesis of these symptoms is unknown, although myometrial contractility and markers of inflammation are implicated (Guo, 2013; Liu, 2011; Mechsner, 2010). Any link with subfertility is unclear, as data are scarce and of poor quality (Maheshwari, 2012; Tomassetti, 2013).

For many years, the diagnosis of adenomyosis in most cases has been made retrospectively following hysterectomy and histologic examination. Serum measurement of cancer antigen 125 (CA125), one tumor marker, is unhelpful. Although CA125 levels are typically elevated in women with adenomyosis, they may also be elevated in those with leiomyomas, endometriosis, pelvic infection, and pelvic malignancies (Kil, 2015).

Transabdominal sonography does not consistently identify the often subtle myometrial changes of adenomyosis, thus, imaging with TVS is preferred (Bazot, 2001). In comparison, MR imaging may be equal or slightly superior to TVS (Dueholm, 2001; Reinhold, 1996). Thus, MR imaging may be most appropriate when the diagnosis is inconclusive, when further delineation would affect patient management, or when coexisting uterine myomas distort anatomy (American College of Obstetricians and Gynecologists, 2014b). With TVS, findings of diffuse adenomyosis may include: (1) anterior or posterior myometrial wall appearing thicker than its counterpart, (2) myometrial texture heterogeneity, (3) small myometrial hypoechoic cysts, which are cystic glands within ectopic endometrial foci, (4) striated projections extending from the endometrium into the myometrium, (5) ill-defined endometrial echo, and (6) a globally enlarged uterus (Fig. 9-13). With application of color or power Doppler, diffuse vascularity may be seen in affected myometrium. Because these findings are often subtle, operator experience influences diagnostic accuracy more than with other pelvic pathology.

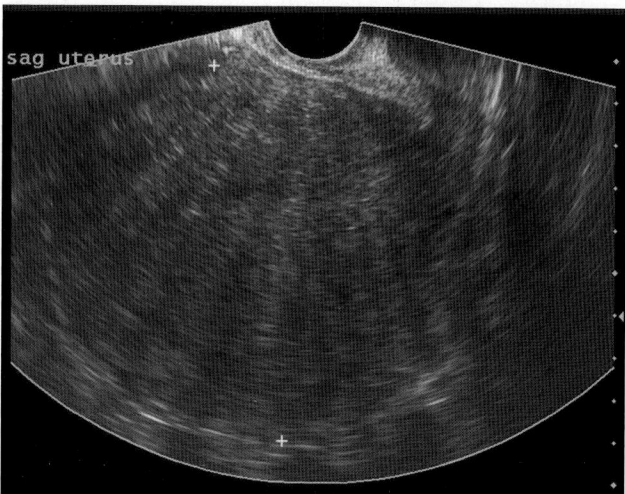

FIGURE 9-13 Transvaginal sagittal uterine image displaying globular uterine enlargement and heterogeneous myometrial texture. Uterine wall thickening can show anteroposterior asymmetry, and here the posterior wall is thicker. In this image, the endomyometrial junction is also poorly defined. Last, a "shutter blind" effect is thought to reflect endometrial gland invasion into the subendometrial tissue and appears as echogenic linear striations. (Used with permission from Dr. Elysia Moschos.)

Focal adenomyosis appears as a discrete hypoechoic nodule(s) that may sometimes be differentiated from leiomyomas by its poorly defined margins, elliptical rather than globular shape, minimal mass effect on surrounding tissues, lack of calcifications, and presence of anechoic cysts of varying diameter (Levy, 2013).

■ Management

The main objective of treatment is relief of pain and bleeding. Although supportive data specific to adenomyosis are scant, conservative therapy for symptomatic adenomyosis is similar to that for endometriosis. First, cyclic NSAIDs are often given with menses. COCs and progestin-only regimens can be used to induce endometrial atrophy and decrease endometrial prostaglandin production to improve dysmenorrhea and HMB. The LNG-IUS is also effective for treatment of adenomyosis-related bleeding (Sheng, 2009). Notably, expulsion rates may be higher in affected women (Youm, 2014). GnRH agonists are another effective choice, although their expense and hypoestrogenic side effects typically limit their long-term use. These agonists may be most helpful for women with adenomyosis-related subfertility or as relief prior to surgical treatment (Fedele, 2008). Although danazol may be considered, it is often a less desirable option due to its androgenic side effects.

Hysterectomy is definitive treatment. As with other conditions, surgical route selection is influenced by uterine size and associated uterine or abdominopelvic pathology. Alternatively, endometrial ablation or endometrial resection using hysteroscopy has successfully treated HMB caused by adenomyosis (Preutthipan, 2010). However, complete eradication of deep adenomyosis is problematic and is responsible for a significant number of treatment failures (Wishall, 2014). Because of this, McCausland and McCausland (1996) recommended sonography or MR imaging prior to ablation to identify these deep lesions and thereby allow better patient selection. Another caveat is that any injury to the endometrial lining, including ablation, may be the initiating insult that activates endometrial tissue to invade the myometrium, thus *causing* adenomyosis. Adenomyosis has been found in 45 to 65 percent of hysterectomy specimens following failed ablation (Gonzalez Rios, 2015; Shavell, 2012).

UAE has also been used to relieve symptoms for some women with adenomyosis, although study sizes are small (Chen, 2006; Kim, 2007). Investigators following women 1 to 5 years after UAE found 65 percent were still improved (Popovic, 2011). For focal adenomyosis, MRgFUS has been effective in a few small case series (Fukunishi, 2008; Yang, 2009).

OTHER UTERINE ENTITIES

Myometrial hypertrophy is global uterine enlargement without identifiable pathology, especially in those with high parity (Fraser, 1987). Also known as gravid hypertrophy, this condition results from myometrial fiber enlargement and not hyperplasia or interstitial fibrosis (Traiman, 1996). One definition includes uterine weights exceeding 130 g for nulliparas and 210 g for multiparas (Zaloudek, 2011). Symptoms are infrequent, but HMB is a common complaint.

Uterine or cervical diverticula are sacculations that communicate with and extend out from the endometrial cavity or endocervical canal. A small number are thought to be congenital anomalies developing from a localized duplication of the distal müllerian duct on one side (Engel, 1984). More often, these are acquired, develop after cesarean delivery, and are thought to arise at sites of partial uterine dehiscence. The terms *cesarean scar defect* or *isthmocele* are used for these iatrogenic niches in the myometrium. Cesarean scar defects may lead to postmenstrual spotting or intermenstrual bleeding (Bij de Vaate, 2011). Niches can serve as a passive repository for menstrual blood and release it during postmenstrual days. An alternative explanation describes fragile vessels in the niche that cause bleeding (van der Voet, 2014). Rarely, these sacs may become secondarily infected (Ou, 2011).

Although niches can be seen during TVS, defects are best imaged by SIS or HSG (Roberge, 2012). Hysteroscopy can also identify these. Treatment includes hysterectomy, hysteroscopic resection of niche edges, or laparoscopic excision of the involved myometrium followed by reapproximation of muscle edges (Api, 2015; Gubbini, 2011). Data are limited regarding superiority of one over another.

OVARIAN CYSTS AS A GROUP

Ovarian masses are a frequent finding in general gynecology, and most are cystic (Fig. 9-14). Histologically, ovarian cysts are often divided into those derived from neoplastic growth, *ovarian cystic neoplasms*, and those created by disruption of normal ovulation, *functional ovarian cysts*. Differentiation of these is not always clinically apparent using either imaging tools or tumor markers. Thus, ovarian cysts are often managed as a single composite clinical entity, and the next sections describe this general approach. Later sections discuss discrete pathologies.

The exact mechanisms leading to cyst formation are unclear. Angiogenesis is an essential component of both the follicular and luteal phases of the ovarian cycle. It also is a component of various pathologic ovarian processes, including follicular cyst

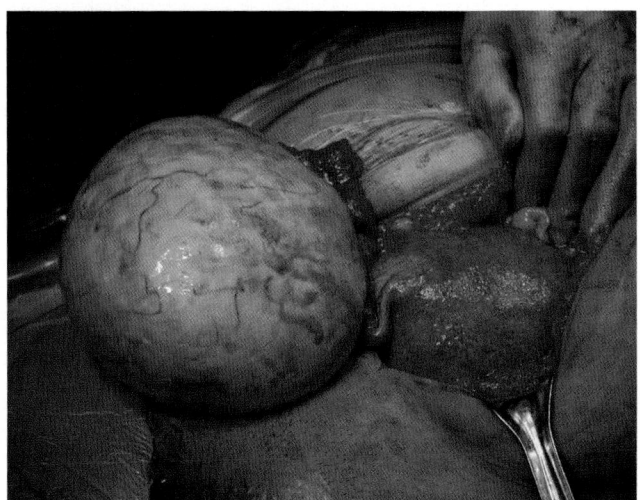

FIGURE 9-14 Intraoperative photograph of a large benign mucinous cystadenoma. The fimbriated end of the fallopian tube is seen above the ovary, and the uterus lies to the right.

formation, PCOS, ovarian hyperstimulation syndrome, and benign and malignant ovarian neoplasms.

The incidence of ovarian cysts varies only slightly with patient demographics and ranges from 5 to 15 percent (Dorum, 2005; Millar, 1993). Functional ovarian cysts make up a large portion. Neoplasms constitute most of the remainder, and these predominantly are benign. In their review of U.S. inpatient hospitalizations for 2010, Whiteman and colleagues (2010) reported that approximately 7 percent of gynecologic admissions were for benign ovarian cysts.

However, despite continuous improvement in diagnostic methods, it is often impossible to clinically differentiate between benign and malignant conditions. Thus, management must balance concerns of performing an operation for an innocent lesion with the risk of not removing an ovarian malignancy.

■ Symptoms

Most women with ovarian cysts are asymptomatic. If symptoms develop, pain is common. Dysmenorrhea may indicate endometriosis with an associated endometrioma. Intermittent or acute severe pain with vomiting often accompanies torsion. Other causes of acute pain include cyst rupture or tuboovarian abscess. In contrast, pressure or ache may be the sole symptom and can result from ovarian capsule stretching. In advanced ovarian malignancies, women may note increased abdominal girth and early satiety from ascites or from an enlarged ovary. In some women, evidence of hormonal disruption can be found. For example, excess estrogen production from granulosa cell stimulation may disrupt normal menstruation or initiate bleeding in prepubertal or postmenopausal patients. Increased androgens produced by theca cell stimulation can virilize women.

■ Diagnosis

Many ovarian cysts are asymptomatic and found incidentally on routine pelvic examination or during imaging studies for another indication. Findings vary, but typically masses are mobile, cystic, nontender, and found lateral to the uterus.

Serum β-hCG testing is invaluable in the evaluation of adnexal pathology. Detection of serum β-hCG may indicate ectopic pregnancy or a corpus luteum of pregnancy. Less commonly, β-hCG can also serve as a tumor marker in defining germ cell neoplasms.

Tumor markers are typically proteins produced by tumor cells or by the body in response to tumor cells. Of markers used, CA125 is a glycoprotein produced by mesothelial cells that line the peritoneal, pleural, and pericardial cavities. CA125 serum levels are often elevated in women with epithelial ovarian cancer. Unfortunately, CA125 is not a tumor-specific antigen, and concentrations are increased in up to 1 percent of healthy controls. Levels may also rise in women with nonmalignant disease such as leiomyomas, endometriosis, adenomyosis, and salpingitis. Despite these limitations, serum CA125 determinations may be helpful and are often obtained if ovarian cysts are large or have sonographically worrisome signs. Cysts in patients who are postmenopausal or are *BRCA* gene mutation carriers may also warrant CA125 level evaluation (Chap. 35, p. 737). Of other markers, serum alpha-fetoprotein (AFP) levels can be elevated in those rare patients with an endodermal sinus tumor or embryonal carcinoma. Increased serum levels of β-hCG may indicate an ovarian choriocarcinoma, a mixed germ cell tumor, or embryonal carcinoma. Inhibin A and B are markers for granulosa cell tumors. Last, lactate dehydrogenase (LDH) levels may be increased in those with dysgerminoma, whereas elevated carcinoembryonic antigen (CEA) and cancer antigen 19–9 (CA19–9) levels arise from secretions of mucinous epithelial ovarian carcinomas.

Sonography is a first-line tool to evaluate pelvic masses. Transabdominal scanning is performed first to avoid missing a large cyst that lies outside the pelvis. For lesions confined within the true pelvis, TVS has superior resolution. Characteristic findings for specific types of ovarian cysts have been described and have also been defined to discriminate malignant from benign lesions (Table 9-3).

Traditional gray-scale sonography can be augmented with color flow Doppler. Transvaginal color Doppler sonography (TV-CDS) may add information regarding lesion structure, malignant potential, and possible torsion. However, for assessing simple ovarian cysts and the risk of malignancy, TV-CDS typically provides no significant advantage compared with conventional TVS (Vuento, 1995). CT or MR imaging of an ovarian cyst may clarify situations in which anatomy or patient habitus complicates sonographic imaging. However, in most clinical settings, sonography alone is suitable (Outwater, 1996).

◼ Management
Observation

In prepubertal and reproductive-aged women, most ovarian cysts are functional and spontaneously regress within 6 months of identification. For postmenopausal women with a simple ovarian cyst, expectant management may also be reasonable if several criteria are met. These are: (1) sonographic evidence of a thin-walled, unilocular cyst, (2) cyst diameter less than 5 cm, (3) no cyst enlargement during surveillance, and (4) normal serum CA125 level (Nardo, 2003). The American College of Obstetricians and Gynecologists (2013) notes that simple cysts up to 10 cm in diameter by sonographic evaluation may safely be followed even in postmenopausal women.

Surgery

There is considerable morphologic similarity among cyst types and between those that are malignant and benign. For diagnosis, ovarian cyst aspiration is usually avoided because of possible intraperitoneal seeding by early-stage ovarian cancer. Moreover, nondiagnostic, false-positive and false-negative results are common (Martinez-Onsurbe, 2001; Moran, 1993). Accordingly, for many cases, excision of the cyst serves as the definitive diagnostic tool.

With suspected ovarian cancers, optimal surgical resection and proper staging by a gynecologic oncologist during the primary operation are major factors in long-term patient survival. Thus, women with pelvic masses and preoperative findings suspicious for malignancy are generally referred. The American College of Obstetricians and Gynecologists (2011) and Society of Gynecologic Oncology have jointly presented guidelines

regarding clinical criteria that should prompt preoperative referral to a gynecologic oncologist (Table 9-4).

For the generalist, cysts presumed to be benign may be excised or the whole ovary may be removed. Of these, cystectomy offers the advantage of ovarian preservation, but at the risk of cyst rupture and content spill. With ovarian cancer, such spill and subsequent malignant seeding can worsen patient prognosis. Thus, the decision for one surgical technique in preference over the other is influenced by lesion size, patient age, and intraoperative findings. For example, in premenopausal women, smaller lesions generally require only cystectomy with preservation of reproductive function. Larger lesions may necessitate oophorectomy because of increased risks of cyst rupture during enucleation, difficulty in reconstructing ovarian anatomy following large cyst removal, and the greater risk of malignancy in these bigger cysts. However, in postmenopausal women, oophorectomy is preferred because the risk for cancer is higher and comparative benefits of ovarian salvage are limited (Okugawa, 2001).

Clinical findings of an unexpected malignancy at the time of surgery will dictate further actions. Multiple small lesions studding the peritoneal surface, ascites, and exophytic growths extending from the ovarian capsule should prompt collection of peritoneal fluid for cytologic study and intraoperative frozen section analysis. If cancer is found, gynecologic oncologists are ideally consulted intraoperatively. At minimum, limited clinical staging, as discussed in Chapter 35 (p. 748), can be completed.

The surgical route is also dictated by clinical factors. Laparoscopy has many patient advantages and is safe for cystectomy and oophorectomy in appropriately selected women (Mais, 1995; Yuen, 1997). Thus, if benign disease is anticipated, this is a frequently used approach. However, large cysts may obstruct laparoscopic instrument mobility and may not fit into endoscopic sacs for contained removal.

For medium-sized cysts, laparotomy incisions can usually be minimized. As a result, most who undergo minilaparotomy can be discharged the day of surgery. Although minilaparotomy typically offers shorter operative times, lower rates of cyst rupture, and greater cost savings compared with laparoscopy, this approach can limit a surgeon's ability to lyse adhesions and inspect peritoneal surfaces for signs of ovarian malignancy.

Women with large cysts are best managed by laparotomy. With a greater potential for malignancy, a midline vertical incision provides a surgical field large enough for oophorectomy without tumor rupture and for surgical staging if malignancy is found. In those with a low risk of malignancy and a moderate-sized cyst, laparotomy through a low transverse incision may be appropriate and offer the advantages of this incision (Chap. 43, p. 929).

FUNCTIONAL OVARIAN CYSTS

These are common, originate from ovarian follicles, and are created during follicle maturation and ovulation. They are subcategorized as either *follicular cysts* or *corpus luteum cysts* based on both their pathogenesis and histologic qualities. They are not neoplasms and derive their mass from accumulation of intrafollicular fluids rather than cellular proliferation. With follicular

TABLE 9-3. Recommended Management of Asymptomatic Ovarian Masses Found with Imaging

Type of Ovarian Mass	Recommendation
Cysts with Benign Qualities	
Simple Cyst	Simple cysts, regardless of patient age, are typically benign
Premenopausal	
≤3 cm diameter	Normal anatomic finding
≤5 cm diameter	No additional treatment required
>5 but ≤7 cm diameter[a]	TVS repeated in 6–12 wks to document resolution; if persistent, then yearly TVS[b]
>7 cm diameter[a]	MRI or surgical evaluation
Postmenopausal	
≤1 cm diameter	Normal anatomic finding
≤5 cm diameter[a]	CA125 level; if normal level, then TVS repeated in 6–12 wks; if persistent cyst, then yearly TVS[b]
>7 cm diameter[a]	MRI or surgical evaluation
Hemorrhagic Cyst[c]	
Premenopausal	
≤3 cm diameter CL	Normal anatomic finding
≤5 cm diameter	No additional treatment required
>5 but ≤7 cm diameter	TVS repeated in 6–12 wks; if persistent, then consider MRI or surgical evaluation
Early postmenopausal[d] Any size	CA125 level; if normal, then TVS repeated in 6–12 wks; if persistent cyst, then consider MRI or surgical evaluation
Late postmenopausal[d] Any size	Surgical evaluation
Endometrioma	TVS repeated in 6–12 wks; if persistent, then yearly TVS[b]
Mature cystic teratoma	If not surgically removed[e], then yearly TVS[b]
Hydrosalpinx	May be observed as clinically indicated
Peritoneal inclusion cyst	May be observed as clinically indicated
Cysts with Indeterminate, but Probably Benign Qualities	
Indeterminate for: hemorrhagic cyst, mature cystic teratoma, endometrioma	
Premenopausal	TVS repeated in 6–12 wks; if persistent cyst, then consider surgical evaluation or MRI
Postmenopausal	Consider surgical evaluation
Thin-walled cyst with single thin septation or focal cyst wall calcification	Same as for simple cyst
Multiple thin septations (<3 mm)	Consider surgical evaluation
Nodule (non-hyperechoic) without flow	Consider surgical evaluation or MRI
Cysts with Qualities Suggesting Malignancy	
Thick (>3 mm) irregular septations	Consider surgical evaluation
Nodule with blood flow	Consider surgical evaluation

[a]The American College of Obstetricians and Gynecologists (ACOG) (2013) recommends a threshold up to 10 cm for simple cysts in all age groups.
[b]Shorter time interval may be selected for surveillance as clinically indicated.
[c]Color Doppler as an adjunct is recommended to exclude solid components.
[d]All postmenopausal women with an adnexal mass also undergo breast examination, digital rectal examination, and mammography, if not already performed in the last year due to the high rate of metastasis from other primary tumors to the ovary.
[e]Some studies have found that stable small dermoid cysts may be observed in premenopausal women.
CA125 = cancer antigen 125; CL = corpus luteum; MRI = magnetic resonance imaging; TVS = transvaginal sonography.
Data from American College of Obstetricians and Gynecologists, 2013; Harris, 2013; Levine, 2010.

TABLE 9-4. Referral of a Pelvic Mass Suspicious for Malignancy to a Gynecologic Oncologist

Premenopausal woman
Very elevated CA125 level
Ascites
Evidence of abdominal or distant metastasis

Postmenopausal woman
Elevated CA125 level
Ascites
Nodular or fixed pelvic mass
Evidence of abdominal or distant metastasis

CA125 = cancer antigen 125.
Data from American College of Obstetricians and Gynecologists: The role of the generalist obstetrician-gynecologist in the early detection of ovarian cancer. Committee Opinion No. 477, March 2011.

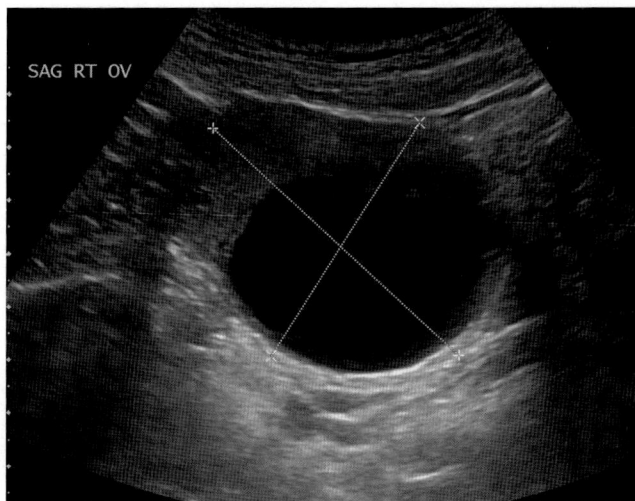

FIGURE 9-15 Sonographic transvaginal sagittal image of an ovary (*calipers*) containing a follicular cyst. Note the smooth walls and lack of internal echoes. (Used with permission from Dr. Elysia Moschos.)

cyst formation, hormonal dysfunction prior to ovulation results in expansion of the follicular antrum with serous fluid. In contrast, excessive hemorrhage from the vascular corpus luteum following ovulation may fill its center to create a corpus luteum cyst. Thus, follicular and corpus luteum cysts differ in their genesis, but symptoms and management are similar.

■ Associated Factors

Of potential factors, high-dose COCs suppress ovarian activity and protect against cyst development (Ory, 1974). However, in subsequent studies with low-dose pills, COCs provided only modest protective effects (Holt, 2003; Lanes, 1992). By contrast, the incidence of follicular cysts is increased with many progestin-only contraceptives. Recall that continuous, low-dose progestins do not completely suppress ovarian function. As a result, dominant follicles may develop in response to gonadotropin secretion, yet the normal ovulatory process is frequently disrupted, and follicular cysts develop. Clinically, follicular cysts are found with greater frequency in those using the LNG-IUS and progestin-releasing implants (Hidalgo, 2006; Nahum, 2015).

Both pre- and postmenopausal women treated with tamoxifen for breast cancer have an increased risk for benign ovarian cyst formation (Chalas, 2005). Premenopausal women and women with greater BMI are disparately affected. Most are functional cysts that resolve with time whether tamoxifen treatment is continued or discontinued (Cohen, 2003). If small simple cysts are found, sonographic surveillance is reasonable. If clinical signs of malignancy are present, then surgical exploration is indicated, and tamoxifen is discontinued. Of other SERMs, bazedoxifene, raloxifene, and ospemifene do not appear to increase ovarian cyst rates (Archer, 2015).

Several epidemiologic studies have linked smoking with functional cyst development (Holt, 2005; Wyshak, 1988). Although the exact mechanism(s) is unknown, changes in gonadotropin secretion and ovarian function are suspected (Michnovicz, 1986).

■ Diagnosis and Treatment

Functional cysts are managed similarly to other cystic ovarian lesions. Consequently, sonography is initially performed. Typical follicular cysts are completely rounded anechoic lesions with thin, regular walls (Fig. 9-15). Conversely, corpus luteum cysts are termed "great imitators" because of their varied sonographic characteristics (Fig. 9-16). Imaging with transvaginal

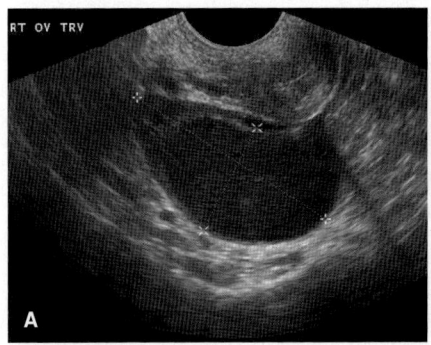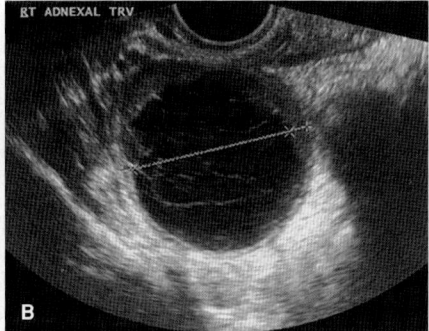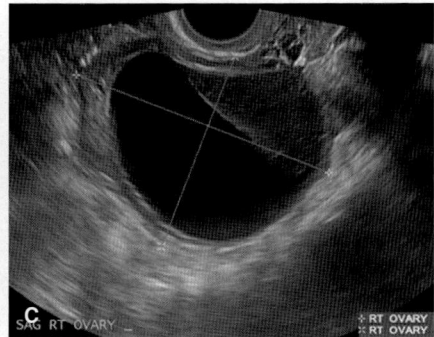

FIGURE 9-16 Sonographic transvaginal images of hemorrhagic corpus luteum cysts. **A.** Diffuse low-level echoes, which are commonly associated with hemorrhage, are seen throughout this smooth-walled cyst. **B.** With evolution of the clot, a lacy reticular pattern develops. **C.** As the clot hemolyzes, a distinct line often forms between the serum and retracting clot. With further retraction, the clot may appear as an intramural nodule. (Used with permission from Dr. Elysia Moschos.)

color Doppler typically displays a brightly colored ring because of their increased surrounding vascularity. This *ring of fire* is also common to ectopic pregnancies (Fig. 7-5 p. 167).

If asymptomatic, women with findings of a functional ovarian cyst may be observed. Evidence does not support the use of COCs to hasten resolution (Grimes, 2014). Surgical excision may be reasonable for large persistent cysts, usually those >10 cm. Progressively enlarging cysts are typically removed.

▦ Theca Lutein Cysts

These are an uncommon type of follicular cyst, characterized by luteinization and hypertrophy of their theca interna layer. Bilateral, multiple smooth-walled cysts form and range in size from 1 to 4 cm in diameter. Termed *hyperreactio lutealis*, this condition is thought to be prompted by elevated LH or β-hCG levels. Commonly associated conditions include gestational trophoblastic disease, multifetal gestation, placentomegaly, and ovarian hyperstimulation during assisted reproductive techniques (Fig. 37-4, p. 782). These cysts typically resolve spontaneously following removal of the stimulating hormone source. However, prior to this, these bulky ovaries are at risk for torsion.

BENIGN NEOPLASTIC OVARIAN CYSTS

These lesions, plus functional ovarian cysts, constitute most ovarian masses. Ovarian neoplasms can be distinguished histologically depending on their cell type of origin. These are grouped as epithelial tumors, germ cell tumors, sex cord-stromal tumors, and others shown in Table 9-5. Of benign ovarian neoplasms, serous and mucinous cystadenomas and mature cystic teratoma are the most common (Pantoja, 1975).

▦ Ovarian Teratoma

These belong to the germ cell family of ovarian neoplasms. Teratomas arise from a single germ cell, and therefore may contain any of the three germ layers—ectoderm, mesoderm, or endoderm. These layers are typically disorganized. Teratomas are classified as:

Immature teratoma—This neoplasm is malignant and described in Chapter 36 (p. 765). Immature tissues from one, two, or all three germ cell layers are found and often coexist with mature elements.

Mature teratoma—This benign tumor contains mature forms of the three germ cell layers:

1. Mature cystic teratoma develops into a cyst, is common, and is also called *benign cystic teratoma* or *dermoid cyst*.
2. Mature solid teratoma has elements formed into a solid mass.
3. Fetiform teratoma or homunculus forms a doll-shape, as the germ cell layers display considerable normal spatial differentiation.

Monodermal teratoma—This benign tumor is composed either solely or predominantly of only one highly specialized tissue type. Of the monodermal teratomas, those composed dominantly of thyroid tissue are termed *struma ovarii*.

TABLE 9-5. WHO Histologic Classification of Ovarian Tumors

Epithelial
  Serous
  Mucinous
  Endometrioid
  Clear cell
  Brenner
  Seromucinous

Mesenchymal
  Endometrioid stromal sarcoma

Mixed Epithelial/Mesenchymal
  Adenosarcoma
  Carcinosarcoma

Sex cord-stromal tumors
  Pure stromal
  Fibroma
  Thecoma
  Leydig cell
  Steroid cell
  Pure sex cord
  Juvenile granulosa cell
  Adult granulosa cell
  Sertoli cell

Mixed sex cord-stromal tumors
  Sertoli-Leydig cell

Germ cell tumors
  Dysgerminoma
  Yolk sac
  Embryonal carcinoma
  Choriocarcinoma
  Mature teratoma
  Immature teratomas

Germ cell/sex cord-stromal tumor
  Gonadoblastoma

WHO = World Health Organization.
Adapted with permission from Kurman RJ, Carcangiu ML, Herrington CS, et al (eds): WHO Classification of Tumours of Female Reproductive Organs, 4th ed. Lyon, International Agency for Research on Cancer, 2014.

Of these teratoma types, mature cystic teratoma is by far the most common. These benign tumors comprise approximately 10 to 25 percent of all ovarian neoplasms and 60 percent of all benign ovarian neoplasms (Koonings, 1989; Peterson, 1955). These cystic tumors are typically slow growing, and most measure between 5 and 10 cm (Comerci, 1994). They are bilateral in approximately 10 percent of cases (Peterson, 1955). When sectioned, most cysts appear unilocular and typically contain one area of localized growth, which protrudes into the cystic cavity. Alternatively designated as *Rokitansky protuberance, dermoid plug, dermoid process, dermoid mamilla, or embryonal rudiment,* this protuberance can be absent or multiple.

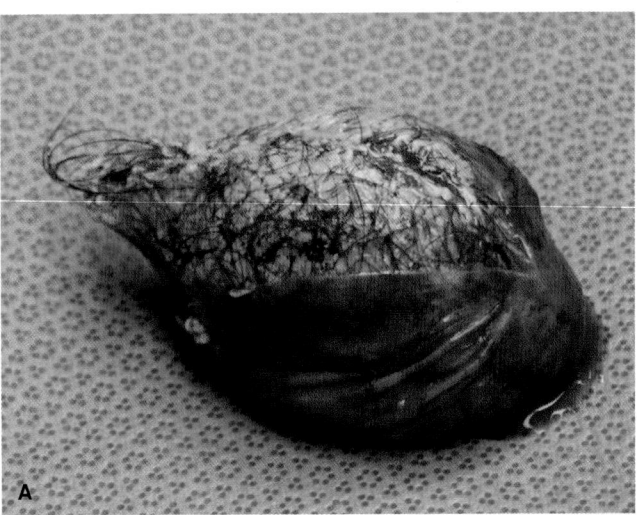
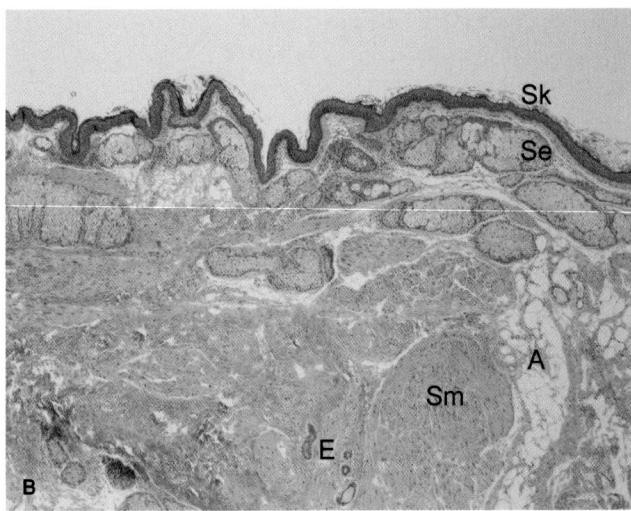

FIGURE 9-17 A. A sectioned mature cystic teratoma following cystectomy. Abundant hair and sebum, characteristic of these neoplasms, is evident. **B.** In this classic histologic example, ectodermal elements include skin (*Sk*), sebaceous (*Se*), and eccrine (*E*) glands, whereas mesodermal elements are smooth muscle (*Sm*) and adipose (*A*).

Microscopically, endodermal or mesodermal derivatives may be found, but ectodermal elements usually predominate. The cyst is typically lined with keratinized squamous epithelium and contains abundant sebaceous and sweat glands. Hair and fatty secretions are often found within (Fig. 9-17). At times, bone and teeth are also identified. The Rokitansky protuberance is usually the site where the most varied tissue types are found and is also a common location of malignant transformation. Malignant transformation develops in 0.06 to 2 percent of cases and typically in older women (Choi, 2014; Rim, 2006). Most malignant cases are squamous cell carcinoma.

The diverse tissues found within teratomas do not arise by fertilization of an ovum by sperm. Instead, they are thought to develop from genetic material contained within a single oocyte by asexual *parthenogenesis*. As a result, almost all mature cystic teratomas have a 46,XX karyotype (Linder, 1975).

Mature cystic teratomas can often undergo torsion, but cyst rupture is rare. Presumably, their thick cyst wall resists rupture compared with other ovarian neoplasms. If cysts do spill, acute peritonitis is common, and Fielder and associates (1996) attributed peritonitis to the sebum and hair contents. They showed the benefits of intraoperative lavage to prevent peritonitis and adhesion formation. Chronic leakage of teratoma contents is rare but can lead to granulomatous peritonitis.

Symptoms from these teratomas are similar to those of other ovarian cysts. However, ovarian teratomas can rarely cause immune-mediated encephalitis. Neurologic symptoms stem from antibodies to *N*-methyl-d-aspartate receptors (NMDARs), which have critical roles in synaptic transmission. The teratomas contain primitive neural tissue, which presumably provides the antigen that prompts NMDAR antibody formation. Teratoma resection is essential to resolution, which can often be dramatic. Resection may be combined with immunotherapy. In one large series of 100 patients, 75 percent recovered, but 25 percent died or survived with severe deficits (Dalmau, 2008).

Sonography is the main imaging tool, and mature cystic teratomas display several characteristic features (Fig. 9-18). First,

fat-fluid or hair-fluid levels are seen as a distinct linear demarcation where serous fluid interfaces with sebum, which is liquid at body temperature. When floating, hair forms accentuated lines and dots that represent hair in longitudinal and transverse planes. The Rokitansky protuberance is a rounded mural nodule that measures 1 to 4 cm, is predominantly hyperechoic, and creates an acute angle with the cyst wall. Last, the "tip of the iceberg" sign is created by amorphous echogenic interfaces of fat, hair, and tissues in the foreground that shadow and thus obscure structures behind it (Guttman, 1977). Notably, these findings are not exclusive to mature cystic teratomas. For example, Patel and associates (1998) reported modest positive predictive values for these findings individually. However, they described values of 100 percent when two or more were found within a given lesion.

For most women with mature cystic teratoma, surgical excision provides a definitive diagnosis, affords relief of symptoms, and prevents torsion, rupture, and malignant degeneration.

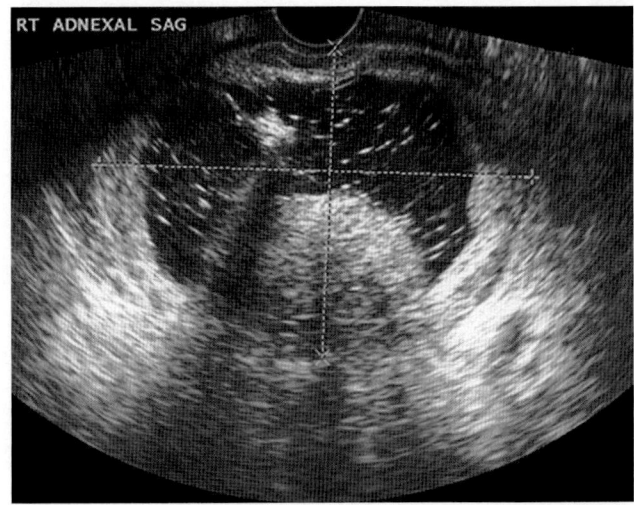

FIGURE 9-18 Sonogram revealing characteristics of mature cystic teratoma. (Used with permission from Dr. Elysia Moschos.)

Laparoscopy is appropriate, and surgical route is selected as for other ovarian masses (p. 216). To prevent granulomatous peritonitis, the cyst can be enucleated over laparotomy sponges or an endoscopic bag to capture cyst spill (Kondo, 2010). Moreover, copious pelvic irrigation is a final surgical step. In the past, most recommended that the opposite ovary be explored because of the high frequency of bilateral lesions. However, given the accuracy of current sonographic imaging, these procedures are no longer indicated with a normal-appearing contralateral ovary (Comerci, 1994).

Although most of these masses are surgically removed, a few studies have supported surveillance only for cysts measuring <6 cm in premenopausal women, especially those desiring future fertility (Alcázar, 2005; Hoo, 2010). These studies document slow tumor growth that averages less than 2 mm/yr. If not removed, sonographic surveillance is recommended every 6 to 12 months initially (Levine, 2010).

■ Benign Serous and Mucinous Tumors

These are members of the surface epithelial neoplasia group, and both are lined by cells similar to those lining the fallopian tube. *Benign serous tumors* are typically thin-walled, unilocular cysts filled with serous fluid (Fig. 9-19). They are bilateral in up to 20 percent of cases. *Benign mucinous tumors* are typically thicker-walled, mucoid-containing tumors that may be small but can often attain large diameters. They may be uni- or multilocular.

In categorizing tumors within the epithelial family, benign tumors are designated as *adenomas*; malignant tumors, as *carcinomas*; and those with exuberant cellular proliferation without invasive behavior as *low malignant potential* (Chen, 2003). The prefix cyst- describes predominantly cystic neoplasms with intracystic growth. Thus, *serous cystadenoma* describes a benign, mainly cystic tumor of the ovarian epithelial tumor group (Prat, 2009).

SOLID OVARIAN MASSES

Completely solid ovarian masses typically are benign. That said, these masses are still removed because of the inability to exclude malignancy in these tumors. Ovarian tumors that may present as a solid masses include: sex cord-stromal tumors, Krukenberg tumor, ovarian leiomyoma and leiomyosarcoma, carcinoid, primary lymphoma, and transition cell tumors, also called Brenner tumors (Fig. 9-20). The most common of these are the fibroma and fibrothecoma, both typically benign sex cord-stromal tumors and discussed in Chapter 36 (p. 771).

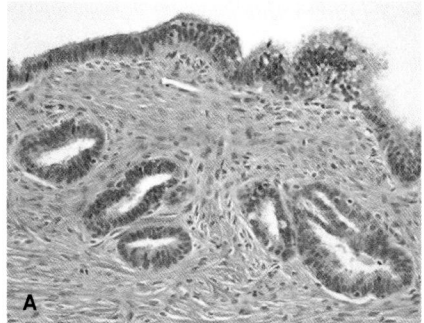
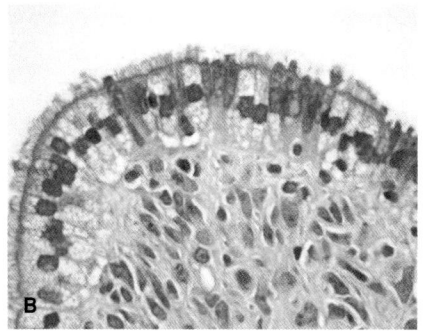

Serous cystadenoma

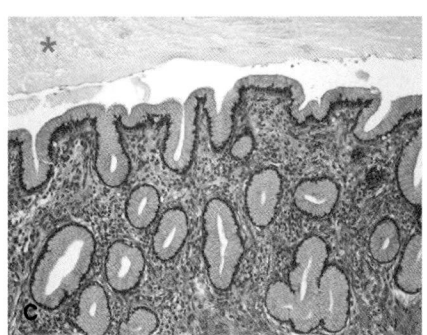
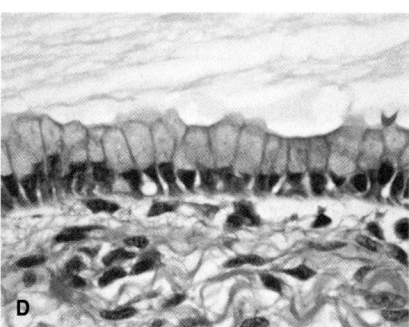

Mucinous cystadenoma

FIGURE 9-19 Serous **(A,B)** and mucinous **(C,D)** cystadenoma. **A.** This simple cyst has a fibrous wall and is lined by a single layer of benign, columnar tubal-type epithelium with cilia. Surface epithelium invaginations are cut tangentially and give the illusion of smaller subepithelial rests. **B.** High-power view of its ciliated, tubal-type lining. **C.** Mucinous cystadenomas are typically multiloculated cysts lined by a single layer of benign mucin-containing epithelium. Mucinous fluid is secreted by the epithelium and contained within the cystic mass. In this image, it is the amorphous material above the epithelium and is stained pink (*asterisk*). **D.** High-power view of simple columnar, mucin-containing epithelium. (Used with permission from Dr. Kelley Carrick.)

Solid adnexal masses may also represent nonneoplastic conditions. Ovarian remnant syndrome and ovarian retention syndrome stem from persistent functional ovarian tissue following surgery. These conditions most commonly cause pain and are discussed in detail in Chapter 11 (p. 261). Rarely,

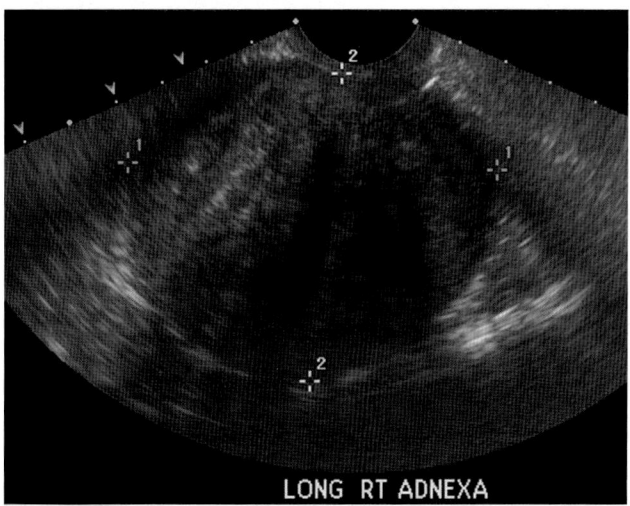

FIGURE 9-20 Transvaginal sonogram of a benign ovarian fibroma.

LONG RT ADNEXA

congenital accessory ovaries may confuse sonographic findings and are discussed in Chapter 18 (p. 423).

ADNEXAL TORSION

Torsion involves the twisting of adnexal components. Most often, the ovary and fallopian tube rotate as a single entity. Infrequently, an ovary may alone turn about its mesovarium, and rarely a fallopian tube twists alone about the mesosalpinx. Normal adnexa can twist, but in 50 to 80 percent of cases unilateral ovarian masses are identified (Nichols, 1985; Warner, 1985). Adnexal torsion accounts for 3 percent of gynecologic emergencies. Although this most commonly occurs during the reproductive years, postmenopausal women can also be affected. A disproportionate number of cases of adnexal torsion develop during pregnancy, and these compose 20 to 25 percent of all torsion cases.

Adnexal masses with increased mobility have greater torsion rates. Congenitally long uteroovarian ligaments create excessively mobile mesovaria or fallopian tubes and may increase the risk in even normal adnexa. Similarly, pathologically enlarged ovaries with a diameter >6 cm will typically rise from the true pelvis. Without these bony confines, mobility and torsion risk are increased. Accordingly, the highest rates of torsion are in adnexal masses measuring 6 to 10 cm (Houry, 2001). Torsion of the adnexa more commonly involves the right adnexa, likely because the mobility of the left ovary is limited by the sigmoid colon (Hasiakos, 2008).

Two key points assist in initially maintaining blood flow to the involved adnexal structures despite twisting of their vascular pedicles. First, adnexa are supplied from the respective adnexal branches of both the uterine and ovarian vessels. During torsion, one of these, but not the other, may be involved. Second, although low-pressure veins draining the adnexa are compressed by the twisting pedicle, high-pressure arteries initially resist compression. As a result of this continued inflow but arrested egress of blood, the adnexa become congested and edematous

but do not infarct. Because of this, cases of early torsion can often be conservatively managed at the time of surgery. With continued stromal swelling, however, arteries may become compressed, leading to infarction and necrosis that necessitate adnexectomy. Grossly, twisted adnexa are enlarged and often appear hemorrhagic (Fig. 9-21).

■ Diagnosis

Classically, the woman with adnexal torsion complains of sharp lower abdominal pain with sudden onset that worsens intermittently over several hours. The pain usually is localized to the involved side, with radiation to the flank, groin, or thigh. Low-grade fever suggests adnexal necrosis. Nausea and vomiting frequently accompany the pain.

Lack of clear physical findings can make diagnosis difficult. An adnexal mass may not be palpable, and during its early stages, significant discomfort may not be elicited during examination. Sonography plays an essential role. However, sonographic findings can vary widely depending on the degree of vascular compromise, the characteristics of any associated intraovarian or intratubal mass, and the presence or absence of adnexal hemorrhage. Sonographically, torsion may mimic ectopic pregnancy, tuboovarian abscess, hemorrhagic ovarian cyst, and endometrioma. Accordingly, rates of correct diagnosis range from 50 to 75 percent (Graif, 1984; Helvie, 1989).

Despite these limitations, specific findings have been described. First, multiple follicles rimming an enlarged ovary reflects ovarian congestion and edema described earlier. The twisted pedicle may also appear as a bull's-eye target, whirlpool, or snail shell, that is, a rounded hyperechoic structure with multiple, inner, concentric hypoechoic rings. In affected women, transvaginal color Doppler sonography may show disruption of normal adnexal blood flow. However, in some cases, incomplete or intermittent torsion may variably display both venous and arterial flow during TV-CDS. Thus, disruption of vascular flow is highly suggestive of torsion. But torsion should

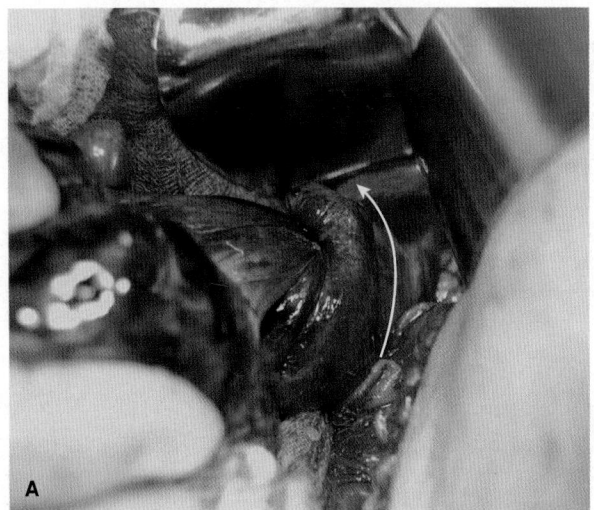
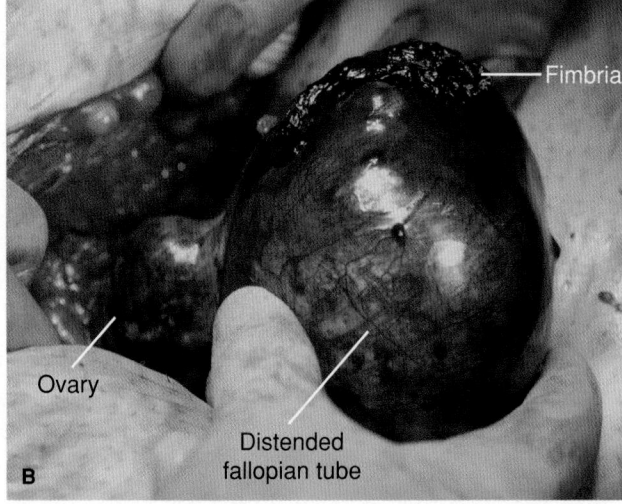

FIGURE 9-21 Intraoperative photographs of adnexal torsion. **A.** Twisting of the infundibulopelvic ligament leads to strangulation of ovarian vessels within it. **B.** A cyanotic ovary and fallopian tube result and are shown here. Hemorrhage into the tubal walls created this massively dilated fallopian tube. Dusky fimbria are seen at the end of the tube. (Used with permission from Dr. Jason Harn.)

not be excluded on the basis of a normal Doppler study alone, especially with clinically suggestive signs and symptoms.

Last, CT or MR imaging is usually not required. These may be helpful in complicated cases or in those with ambiguous clinical presentation such as seen with incomplete or chronic torsion (Rha, 2002).

■ Management

Salvage of the involved adnexa, resection of any associated cyst or tumor, and possible oophoropexy are treatment goals. Findings of adnexal necrosis or rupture with hemorrhage, however, may necessitate removal of adnexal structures.

Torsion may be evaluated by laparoscopy or laparotomy. Previously, adnexectomy was usually done to avoid possible thrombus release and subsequent embolism during untwisting. Evidence does not support this. McGovern and coworkers (1999) reviewed nearly 1000 cases of torsion and found the rare occurrence of pulmonary embolism in only 0.2 percent. These cases of embolism were associated with adnexal excision, and none were linked to untwisting of the pedicle. In a study of 94 women with adnexal torsion, Zweizig and associates (1993) reported no increased morbidity in women undergoing untwisting of the adnexa compared with those undergoing adnexectomy.

For these reasons, detorsion of the adnexa is generally recommended. Within minutes following untwisting, congestion is relieved, and ovarian volume and cyanosis typically diminish. For many, absence of these changes may prompt adnexal removal. A persistently black-bluish ovary, however, is not pathognomonic for necrosis, and the ovary may still recover. Cohen and colleagues (1999) reviewed 54 cases in which adnexa were preserved regardless of their appearance following detorsion. They reported functional integrity and successful subsequent pregnancy in almost 95 percent. Bider and coworkers (1991) observed no increased postoperative infection morbidity in cases similarly managed. Because adnexal necrosis may still occur, conservative management requires postoperative vigilance for fever, leukocytosis, and peritoneal signs.

Following detorsion, there is no consensus as to the management of the adnexa. Specific ovarian lesions should be excised. Cystectomy in a hemorrhagic, edematous ovary, however, may technically be difficult. Therefore, some recommend cystectomy if the mass persists for 6 to 8 weeks after primary intervention (Rody, 2002).

The retorsion rate among fertile women was 28 percent in one review of 38 publications (Hyttel, 2015). To minimize these rates, unilateral or bilateral oophoropexy has been described and may be considered (Djavadian, 2004). Techniques to secure the ovary vary. These include shortening of the uteroovarian ligament with a running stitch through the ligament or suturing of either the ovary or the uteroovarian ligament to the posterior aspect of the uterus, the lateral pelvic wall, or the round ligament (Fuchs, 2010; Weitzman, 2008). However, the effects of this positioning on later ovum uptake and fertility are unclear.

Management during pregnancy does not differ. However, if the corpus luteum is removed before 10 weeks' gestation, progestational support is recommended until 10 weeks' gestation

to maintain the pregnancy. Suitable regimens include: (1) micronized progesterone (Prometrium) 200 or 300 mg orally once daily; (2) 8-percent progesterone vaginal gel (Crinone) one premeasured applicator vaginally daily plus micronized progesterone 100 or 200 mg orally once daily; or (3) intramuscular 17-hydroxyprogesterone caproate (Delalutin), 150 mg. With the last option, if between 8 and 10 weeks, then only one injection is required immediately after surgery. If the corpus luteum is excised between 6 to 8 weeks, then two additional doses should be given 1 and 2 weeks after the first.

PARAOVARIAN MASSES

Most paratubal/paraovarian cysts are not neoplastic and are either distended remnants of the paramesonephric duct or mesothelial inclusion cysts. One autopsy series cited a rate of approximately 5 percent of adnexal cysts (Dorum, 2005). The most common paramesonephric cyst is the *hydatid of Morgagni*, which is pedunculated and typically dangles from one of the fimbria. Neoplastic paraovarian cysts are rare and histologically resemble tumors of ovarian origin. They are usually cystadenomas or cystadenofibromas and rarely malignant (Korbin, 1998).

These cysts are most commonly identified in asymptomatic women at the time of surgery or sonography for other gynecologic problems. If symptoms develop, they mimic those of ovarian cysts. They are infrequently associated with complications such as hemorrhage, rupture, or torsion (Genadry, 1977).

Transvaginal sonography is often used as a primary evaluation tool for symptomatic women, and most of these cysts have thin, smooth walls and anechoic centers. However, sonography and MR imaging have limitations in differentiating between paraovarian and ovarian pathology (Ghossain, 2005). Thus, many women are managed as if diagnosed with a comparable ovarian cyst. When surgically managed, cystectomy or, less frequently, drainage and fulguration of the cyst wall are performed. When small and noted as an incidental intraoperative finding, these are generally excised, although this is not an evidence-based practice.

Of solid paraovarian tumors, leiomyomas are the most common and have pathophysiology identical to those within myometrium. Infrequently, congenital anomalies such as an accessory or supernumerary ovary, rudimentary uterine horn, or pelvic kidney may present as a pelvic mass with or without symptoms. One rare solid paraovarian tumor arises as a remnant of the wolffian duct and has been termed the *female adnexal tumor of probable wolffian origin* (Devouassoux-Shisheboran, 1999). As described in Chapter 18 (p. 417), wolffian duct remnants are such that this rare tumor develops within the broad ligament or along the mesosalpinx (Kariminejad, 1973). Other rare paraovarian solid tumors include sarcomas, lymphoma, adenocarcinoma, pheochromocytoma, and choriocarcinoma.

Most paraovarian solid tumors are asymptomatic and identified on routine pelvic examination. Occasionally, there is unilateral pelvic and abdominal pain. Sonography and MR imaging are used to visualize these masses, although accurate differentiation between benign and malignant lesions is typically not possible. Thus, most solid masses are surgically removed.

FALLOPIAN TUBE PATHOLOGY

■ Hydrosalpinx

Fallopian tube neoplasms are rare, and most fallopian tube masses involve ectopic pregnancy or the sequelae of PID. Of these, hydrosalpinx is a chronic cystic swelling of the fallopian tube that forms following distal tubal obstruction. Causes include PID and endometriosis and rarely fallopian tube cancer. Grossly, the fine fimbria and tubal ostia are obliterated and replaced by a smooth, clubbed end (Fig. 9-22). The ballooned, thin walls of the elongated tube are translucent, and the tube is typically distended with a clear serous fluid. The ipsilateral ovary may be adhered to the hydrosalpinx.

Hydrosalpinx may be found in asymptomatic women during pelvic examination or sonography done for other indications. Some women note infertility or chronic pelvic pain. The differential diagnosis mimics that for other cystic pelvic lesions. In general, no laboratory test is helpful, and serum CA125 level testing for presumed ovarian malignancy is typically negative.

Sonographic interrogation shows a thin-walled, hypoechoic cystic fusiform structure with incomplete septa (Fig. 9-23). In some, multiple hyperechoic mural nodules measuring 2 to 3 mm arch around the inner circumference of the tube to create the *beads on a string* sign. These nodules represent fibrotic endosalpingeal folds.

Management varies depending on the conviction of diagnosis, desire for future fertility, and associated symptoms. In asymptomatic women who have completed childbearing, and in whom the sonographic evidence supports the diagnosis of hydrosalpinx, expectant management is typical. In those with pelvic pain or infertility, or in whom the diagnosis is uncertain, diagnostic laparoscopy is often chosen.

For women not wishing to preserve fertility, laparoscopic treatment may include lysis of adhesions and salpingectomy. Conversely, in women who desire fertility, surgical intervention

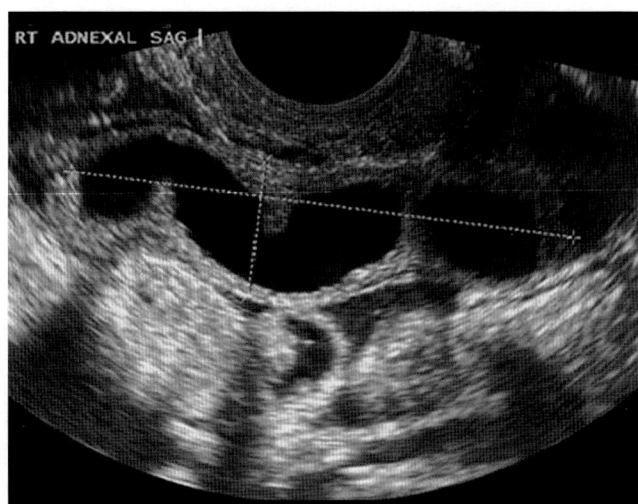

FIGURE 9-23 Transvaginal sonogram of hydrosalpinx. Incomplete septa, which are folds of the dilated tube, are seen within this fusiform, fluid-filled structure. (Used with permission from Dr. Elysia Moschos.)

depends on the degree of tubal damage. As the degree of tubal distortion increases, fertility rates decrease. In women with mild tubal disease, laparoscopic neosalpingostomy has resulted in 80-percent pregnancy rates and is a reasonable approach (Fig. 20-7, p. 459) (Schlaff, 1990). In those with severe tubal disease, IVF may offer a greater chance at conception.

Of note, women with a hydrosalpinx who undergo IVF have approximately half the pregnancy rate of other women (Camus, 1999; Zeyneloglu, 1998). The explanation is unclear, and theories include toxic hydrosalpinx fluid, lowered growth factor concentrations, and mechanical flushing of embryos by excess fluid (Loutradis, 2005; Lu, 2013; Strandell, 2002). If hydrosalpinges are resected prior to IVF, subsequent rates of pregnancy, implantation, and live births are improved (Dechaud, 1998; Johnson, 2010; Strandell, 1999). Thus, the American Society for Reproductive Medicine (2012) recommends such surgery prior to IVF. Some evidence shows that Essure inserts may sufficiently occlude the tube for this purpose (Arora, 2014).

■ Benign Neoplasms

These are rare in the fallopian tube. The most common benign tumor is mesothelioma, which is found in less than 1 percent of hysterectomy specimens (Pauerstein, 1968). Previously termed adenomatoid tumors, these 1- to 2-cm, well-circumscribed solid nodules arise in the tubal wall (Salazar, 1972). Tubal leiomyomas are uncommon and derive from the smooth muscle of the tubal muscularis, from the broad ligament, or from vessels in either location.

Microscopically, the epithelium of the fallopian tube contains an intermixing of both ciliated and secretory cells. The secretory cell population increases with age, and cellular outgrowths can be seen histologically that contain only secretory cells (Li, 2013). These benign secretory cell outgrowths (SCOUTs) and their link to serous tubal intraepithelial carcinoma (STIC) and pelvic

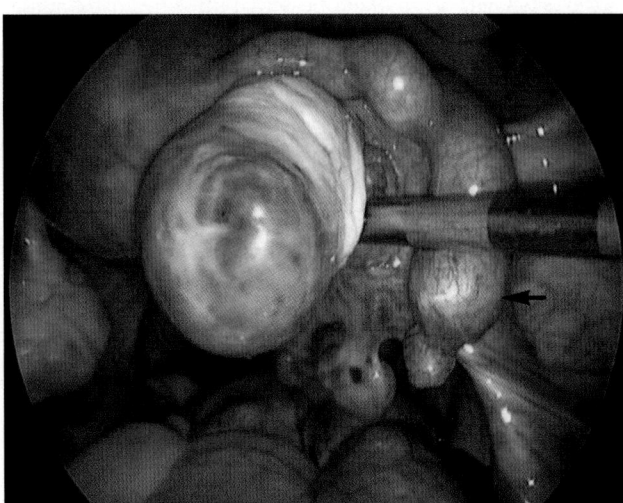

FIGURE 9-22 Laparoscopic photograph of a hydrosalpinx. Note the thin-walled ballooned fallopian tube and its clubbed end (*arrow*) stretching from the cornua and draping around the blunt probe. A typical corpus luteum cyst is seen at the distal end of the ovary. (Used with permission from Dr. Karen Bradshaw.)

serous carcinoma are current research topics (Mehrad, 2010). These are described in Chapter 35 (p. 740).

◼ Tuboovarian Abscess

This is an inflammatory mass involving the fallopian tube, ovary, and often surrounding structures. If an ovary adheres to the fallopian tube, but is still visualized, it is called a *tuboovarian complex*. In contrast, a *tuboovarian abscess* results from a complete breakdown of ovarian and tubal architecture such that the separate structures are no longer identified. Either is usually a consequence of PID, although occasionally endometritis and pelvic malignancy may be the generative source. Affected women usually have lower abdominal pain, fever, leukocytosis, and unilateral or bilateral adnexal masses. These abscesses and their management are more fully discussed in Chapter 3 (p. 68).

REFERENCES

Acien P, Quereda F: Abdominal myomectomy: results of a simple operative technique. Fertil Steril 65(1):41, 1996

Alcázar JL, Castillo G, Jurado M, et al: Is expectant management of sonographically benign adnexal cysts an option in selected asymptomatic premenopausal women? Hum Reprod 20(11):3231, 2005

Alessandri F, Lijoi D, Mistrangelo E, et al: Randomized study of laparoscopic versus minilaparotomic myomectomy for uterine myomas. J Minim Invasive Gynecol 13(2):92, 2006

Ambat S, Mittal S, Srivastava DN, et al: Uterine artery embolization versus laparoscopic occlusion of uterine vessels for management of symptomatic uterine fibroids. Int J Gynaecol Obstet 105(2):162, 2009

American Cancer Society: Cancer facts and figures 2014. Atlanta, American Cancer Society, 2014

American College of Obstetricians and Gynecologists: Alternatives to hysterectomy in the management of leiomyomas. Practice Bulletin No. 96, August 2008, Reaffirmed 2014a

American College of Obstetricians and Gynecologists: Diagnosis of abnormal uterine bleeding in reproductive-aged women. Practice Bulletin No. 128, July 2012, Reaffirmed 2014b

American College of Obstetricians and Gynecologists: Management of adnexal masses. Practice Bulletin No. 83, 2007, Reaffirmed 2013

American College of Obstetricians and Gynecologists: The role of the generalist obstetrician-gynecologist in the early detection of ovarian cancer. Committee Opinion No. 477, March 2011

American Society for Reproductive Medicine: Committee opinion: role of tubal surgery in the era of assisted reproductive technology. Fertil Steril 97(3):539, 2012a

American Society for Reproductive Medicine: Evaluation and treatment of recurrent pregnancy loss: a committee opinion. Fertil Steril 98(5):1103, 2012b

American Society for Reproductive Medicine: Myomas and reproductive function. Fertil Steril 90(Suppl 3):S125, 2008

Anteby SO, Yarkoni S, Ever Hadani P: The effect of a prostaglandin synthetase inhibitor, indomethacin, on excessive uterine bleeding. Clin Exp Obstet Gynecol 12(3–4):60, 1985

Api M, Boza A, Gorgen H, et al: Should cesarean scar defect be treated laparoscopically? A case report and review of the literature. J Minim Invasive Gynecol June 26, 2015 [Epub ahead of print]

Archer DF, Carr BR, Pinkerton JV, et al: Effects of ospemifene on the female reproductive and urinary tracts: translation from preclinical models into clinical evidence. Menopause 22(7):786, 2015

Arora P, Arora RS, Cahill D, et al: Essure® for management of hydrosalpinx prior to in vitro fertilisation—a systematic review and pooled analysis. BJOG 121(5):527, 2014

Baird DD, Dunson DB, Hill MC, et al: High cumulative incidence of uterine leiomyoma in black and white women: ultrasound evidence. Am J Obstet Gynecol 188(1):100, 2003

Bayer HealthCare Pharmaceuticals: Mirena (levonorgestrel-releasing intrauterine system). Highlights of prescribing information, 2014. Available at: http://labeling.bayerhealthcare.com/html/products/pi/Mirena_PI.pdf. Accessed May 14, 2015

Bazot M, Cortez A, Darai E, et al: Ultrasonography compared with magnetic resonance imaging for the diagnosis of adenomyosis: correlation with histopathology. Hum Reprod 16(11):2427, 2001

Benagiano G, Habiba M, Brosens I: The pathophysiology of uterine adenomyosis: an update. Fertil Steril 98(3):572, 2012

Berman JM, Guido RS, Garza Leal JG, et al: Three-year outcome of the halt trial: a prospective analysis of radiofrequency volumetric thermal ablation of myomas. J Minim Invasive Gynecol 21(5):767, 2014

Bider D, Mashiach S, Dulitzky M, et al: Clinical, surgical and pathologic findings of adnexal torsion in pregnant and nonpregnant women. Surg Gynecol Obstet 173(5):363, 1991

Bij de Vaate AJ, Brölmann HA, van der Voet LF, et al: Ultrasound evaluation of the cesarean scar: relation between a niche and postmenstrual spotting. Ultrasound Obstet Gynecol 37(1):93, 2011

Bird CC, McElin TW, Manalo-Estrella P: The elusive adenomyosis of the uterus—revisited. Am J Obstet Gynecol 112(5):583, 1972

Bisceglia M, Galliani CA, Pizzolitto S, et al: Leiomyomatosis peritonealis disseminata: report of 3 cases with extensive review of the literature. Adv Anat Pathol 21(3):201, 2014

Bratby MJ, Hussain FF, Walker WJ: Outcomes after unilateral uterine artery embolization: a retrospective review. Cardiovasc Intervent Radiol 31(2):254, 2008

Broekmans FJ: GnRH agonists and uterine leiomyomas. Human Reprod 11(Suppl 3):3, 1996

Brosens I, Deprest J, Dal Cin P, et al: Clinical significance of cytogenetic abnormalities in uterine myomas. Fertil Steril 69(2):232, 1998

Brown MF, Hebra A, McGeehin K, et al: Ovarian masses in children: a review of 91 cases of malignant and benign masses. J Pediatr Surg 28(7):930, 1993

Bulun SE, Simpson ER, Word RA: Expression of the CYP19 gene and its product aromatase cytochrome P450 in human uterine leiomyoma tissues and cells in culture. J Clin Endocrinol Metab 78(3):736, 1994

Buttram VC Jr, Reiter RC: Uterine leiomyomata: etiology, symptomatology, and management. Fertil Steril 36(4):433, 1981

Camus E, Poncelet C, Goffinet F, et al: Pregnancy rates after in-vitro fertilization in cases of tubal infertility with and without hydrosalpinx: a meta-analysis of published comparative studies. Hum Reprod 14(5):1243, 1999

Cantuaria GH, Angioli R, Frost L, et al: Comparison of bimanual examination with ultrasound examination with ultrasound examination before hysterectomy for uterine leiomyoma. Obstet Gynecol 92(1):109, 1998

Carbonell Esteve JL, Acosta R, et al: Mifepristone for the treatment of uterine leiomyomas: a randomized controlled trial. Obstet Gynecol 112(5):1029, 2008

Carbonell Esteve JL, Riverón AM, et al: Mifepristone 2.5 mg versus 5 mg daily in the treatment of leiomyoma before surgery. Int J Womens Health 4:75, 2012

Carlson KJ, Miller BA, Fowler FJ Jr: The Maine Women's Health Study: II. Outcomes of nonsurgical management of leiomyomas, abnormal bleeding, and chronic pelvic pain. Obstet Gynecol 83(4):566, 1994

Carr BR, Marshburn PB, Weatherall PT, et al: An evaluation of the effect of gonadotropin-releasing hormone analogs and medroxyprogesterone acetate on uterine leiomyomata volume by magnetic resonance imaging: a prospective, randomized, double blind, placebo-controlled, crossover trial. J Clin Endocrinol Metab 76(5):1217, 1993

Casini ML, Rossi F, Agostini R, et al: Effect of the position of fibroids on fertility. Gynecol Endocrinol 22:106, 2006

Chalas E, Costantino JP, Wickerham DL, et al: Benign gynecologic conditions among participants in the Breast Cancer Prevention Trial. Am J Obstet Gynecol 192(4):1230, 2005

Chen CL, Liu P, Zeng BL, et al: Intermediate and long term clinical effects of uterine arterial embolization in treatment of adenomyosis. Zhonghua Fu Chan Ke Za Zhi 41(10):660, 2006

Chen VW, Ruiz B, Killeen JL, et al: Pathology and classification of ovarian tumors. Cancer 97(S10):2631, 2003

Chiaffarino F, Parazzini F, La Vecchia C, et al: Use of oral contraceptives and uterine fibroids: results from a case-control study. BJOG 106(8):857, 1999

Choi EJ, Koo YJ, Jeon JH, et al: Clinical experience in ovarian squamous cell carcinoma arising from mature cystic teratoma: a rare entity. Obstet Gynecol Sci 57(4):274, 2014

Cohen I, Potlog-Nahari C, Shapira J, et al: Simple ovarian cysts in postmenopausal patients with breast carcinoma treated with tamoxifen: long-term follow-up. Radiology 227(3):844, 2003

Cohen SB, Oelsner G, Seidman DS, et al: Laparoscopic detorsion allows sparing of the twisted ischemic adnexa. J Am Assoc Gynecol Laparosc 6(2):139, 1999

Comerci JT Jr, Licciardi F, Bergh PA, et al: Mature cystic teratoma: a clinicopathologic evaluation of 517 cases and review of the literature. Obstet Gynecol 84(1):22, 1994

Cooper JM, Brady RM: Late complications of operative hysteroscopy. Obstet Gynecol Clin North Am 27(2):367, 2000

Coutinho EM, Gonçalves MT: Long-term treatment of leiomyomas with gestrinone. Fertil Steril 51(6):939, 1989

Cramer SF, Patel A: The frequency of uterine leiomyomas. Am J Clin Pathol 94(4):435, 1990

Dalmau J, Gleichman AJ, Hughes EG, et al: Anti-NMDA-receptor encephalitis: case series and analysis of the effects of antibodies. Lancet Neurol 7(12):1091, 2008

Dariushnia SR, Nikolic B, Stokes LS, et al: Quality improvement guidelines for uterine artery embolization for symptomatic leiomyomata. J Vasc Interv Radiol 25(11):1737, 2014

De Leo V, la Marca A, Morgante G: Short-term treatment of uterine fibromyomas with danazol. Gynecol Obstet Invest 47(4):258, 1999

de Silva KS, Kanumakala S, Grover SR, et al: Ovarian lesions in children and adolescents—an 11-year review. J Pediatr Endocrinol 17(7):951, 2004

DeWaay DJ, Syrop CH, Nygaard IE, et al: Natural history of uterine polyps and leiomyomata. Obstet Gynecol 100(1):3, 2002

Dechaud H, Daures JP, Arnal F, et al: Does previous salpingectomy improve implantation and pregnancy rates in patients with severe tubal factor infertility who are undergoing in vitro fertilization? A pilot prospective randomized study. Fertil Steril 69(6):1020, 1998

Derman SG, Rehnstrom J, Neuwirth RS: The long-term effectiveness of hysteroscopic treatment of menorrhagia and leiomyomas. Obstet Gynecol 77(4):591, 1991

Devouassoux-Shisheboran M, Silver SA, Tavassoli FA: Wolffian adnexal tumor, so-called female adnexal tumor of probable Wolffian origin (FATWO): immunohistochemical evidence in support of a Wolffian origin. Hum Pathol 30(7):856, 1999

Diamond MP, Carr B, Dmowski WP, et al: Elagolix treatment for endometriosis-associated pain: results from a phase 2, randomized, double-blind, placebo-controlled study. Reprod Sci 21(3):363, 2014

Djavadian D, Braendle W, Jaenicke F: Laparoscopic oophoropexy for the treatment of recurrent torsion of the adnexa in pregnancy: case report and review. Fertil Steril 82(4):933, 2004

Donnez J, Jadoul P: What are the implications of myomas on fertility? A need for a debate? Human Reprod 17(6):1424, 2002

Donnez J, Tatarchuk TF, Bouchard P, et al: Ulipristal acetate versus placebo for fibroid treatment before surgery. N Engl J Med 366(5):409, 2012a

Donnez J, Tomaszewski J, Vázquez F, et al: Ulipristal acetate versus leuprolide acetate for uterine fibroids. N Engl J Med 366(5):421, 2012b

Dorum A, Blom GP, Ekerhovd E, et al: Prevalence and histologic diagnosis of adnexal cysts in postmenopausal women: an autopsy study. Am J Obstet Gynecol 192(1):48, 2005

Dueholm M, Lundorf E, Hansen ES, et al: Magnetic resonance imaging and transvaginal ultrasonography for the diagnosis of adenomyosis. Fertil Steril 76(3):588, 2001

Eder S, Baker J, Gersten J, et al: Efficacy and safety of oral tranexamic acid in women with heavy menstrual bleeding and fibroids. Womens Health (Lond Engl) 9(4):397, 2013

Edwards RD, Moss JG, Lumsden MA, et al: Uterine-artery embolization versus surgery for symptomatic uterine fibroids. N Engl J Med 356(4):360, 2007

Eldar-Geva T, Meagher S, Healy DL, et al: Effect of intramural, subserosal, and submucosal uterine fibroids on the outcome of assisted reproductive technology treatment. Fertil Steril 70(4):687, 1998

Emanuel MH, Wamsteker K, Hart AA, et al: Long-term results of hysteroscopic myomectomy for abnormal uterine bleeding. Obstet Gynecol 93(5 Pt 1):743, 1999

Engel G, Rushovich AM: True uterine diverticulum. A partial mullerian duct duplication? Arch Pathol Lab Med 108(9):734, 1984

Englund K, Blanck A, Gustavsson I, et al: Sex steroid receptors in human myometrium and fibroids: changes during the menstrual cycle and gonadotropin-releasing hormone treatment. J Clin Endocrinol Metab 83(11):4092, 1998

Fedele L, Bianchi S, Frontino G: Hormonal treatments for adenomyosis. Best Pract Res Clin Obstet Gynaecol 22(2):333, 2008

Fedele L, Parazzini F, Luchini L, et al: Recurrence of fibroids after myomectomy: a transvaginal ultrasonographic study. Hum Reprod 10(7):1795, 1995

Felberbaum RE, Germer U, Ludwig M, et al: Treatment of uterine fibroids with a slow-release formulation of the gonadotrophin releasing hormone antagonist Cetrorelix. Hum Reprod 13(6):1660, 1998

Ferenczy A: Pathophysiology of adenomyosis. Hum Reprod Update 4(4):312, 1998

Fielder EP, Guzick DS, Guido R, et al: Adhesion formation from release of dermoid contents in the peritoneal cavity and effect of copious lavage: a prospective, randomized, blinded, controlled study in a rabbit model. Fertil Steril 65(4):852, 1996

Filicori M, Hall DA, Loughlin JS, et al: A conservative approach to the management of uterine leiomyoma: pituitary desensitization by a luteinizing hormone-releasing hormone analogue. Am J Obstet Gynecol 147(6):726, 1983

Forssman L: Distribution of blood flow in myomatous uteri as measured by locally injected 133Xenon. Acta Obstet Gynecol Scand 55(2):101, 1976

Fraser IS: Menorrhagia due to myometrial hypertrophy: treatment with tamoxifen. Obstet Gynecol 70(3 Pt 2):505, 1987

Friedman AJ, Lobel SM, Rein MS, et al: Efficacy and safety considerations in women with uterine leiomyomas treated with gonadotropin-releasing hormone agonists: the estrogen threshold hypothesis. Am J Obstet Gynecol 163(4 Pt 1):1114, 1990

Friedman AJ, Thomas PP: Does low-dose combination oral contraceptive use affect uterine size or menstrual flow in premenopausal women with leiomyomas? Obstet Gynecol 85(4):631, 1995

Froeling V, Meckelburg K, Schreiter NF, et al: Outcome of uterine artery embolization versus MR-guided high-intensity focused ultrasound treatment for uterine fibroids: long-term results. Eur J Radiol 82(12):2265, 2013

Fuchs N, Smorgick N, Tovbin Y, et al: Oophoropexy to prevent adnexal torsion: how, when, and for whom? J Minim Invasive Gynecol 17(2):205, 2010

Fukunishi H, Funaki K, Sawada K, et al. Early results of magnetic resonance-guided focused ultrasound surgery of adenomyosis: analysis of 20 cases. J Minim Invasive Gynecol 15:571, 2008

Genadry R, Parmley T, Woodruff JD: The origin and clinical behavior of the parovarian tumor. Am J Obstet Gynecol 129(8):873, 1977

Ghossain MA, Braidy CG, Kanso HN, et al: Extraovarian cystadenomas: ultrasound and MR findings in 7 cases. J Comput Assist Tomogr 29(1):74, 2005

Glass AR: Endocrine aspects of obesity. Med Clin North Am 73(1):139, 1989

Glasser MH, Heinlein PK, Hung YY: Office endometrial ablation with local anesthesia using the HydroThermAblator system: comparison of outcomes in patients with submucous myomas with those with normal cavities in 246 cases performed over 5(1/2) years. J Minim Invasive Gynecol 16(6):700, 2009

Goldberg J, Pereira L, Berghella V, et al: Pregnancy outcomes after treatment for fibromyomata: uterine artery embolization versus laparoscopic myomectomy. Am J Obstet Gynecol 191(1):18, 2004

Goldfarb HA: Combining myoma coagulation with endometrial ablation/resection reduces subsequent surgery rates. JSLS 3(4):253, 1999

Goldstein SR, Duvernoy CS, Calaf J, et al: Raloxifene use in clinical practice: efficacy and safety. Menopause 16(2):413, 2009

Gonzalez Rios AR, Fouad L, Lam MC, et al: Failed endometrial ablation: who is at risk? Obstet Gynecol 125 (Suppl 1):24S, 2015

Goodwin SC, Bradley LD, Lipman JC, et al: Uterine artery embolization versus myomectomy: a multicenter comparative study. Fertil Steril 85(1):14, 2006

Graif M, Shalev J, Strauss S, et al: Torsion of the ovary: sonographic features. AJR 143(6):1331, 1984

Griffin L, Feinglass J, Garrett A, et al: Postoperative outcomes after robotic versus abdominal myomectomy. JSLS 17(3):407, 2013

Grimes DA, Jones LB, Lopez LM, et al: Oral contraceptives for functional ovarian cysts. Cochrane Database Syst Rev 4:CD006134, 2014

Gubbini G, Centini G, Nascetti D, et al: Surgical hysteroscopic treatment of cesarean-induced isthmocele in restoring fertility: prospective study. J Minim Invasive Gynecol 18(2):234, 2011

Gupta JK, Sinha A, Lumsden MA, et al: Uterine artery embolization for symptomatic uterine fibroids. Cochrane Database Syst Rev 5:CD005073, 2012

Gupta S, Manyonda IT: Acute complications of fibroids. Best Pract Res Clin Obstet Gynaecol 23(5):609, 2009

Guo SW, Mao X, Ma Q, et al: Dysmenorrhea and its severity are associated with increased uterine contractility and overexpression of oxytocin receptor (OTR) in women with symptomatic adenomyosis. Fertil Steril 99(1):231, 2013

Guttman PH Jr: In search of the elusive benign cystic ovarian teratoma: application of the ultrasound "tip of the iceberg" sign. J Clin Ultrasound 5(6):403, 1977

Hald K, Noreng HJ, Istre O, et al: Uterine artery embolization versus laparoscopic occlusion of uterine arteries for leiomyomas: long-term results of a randomized comparative trial. J Vasc Interv Radio 20(10):1303, 2009

Harris RD, Javitt MC, Glanc P, et al: ACR Appropriateness Criteria® clinically suspected adnexal mass. Ultrasound Q 29(1):79, 2013

Hart R, Khalaf Y, Yeong CT, et al: A prospective controlled study of the effect of intramural uterine fibroids on the outcome of assisted conception. Hum Reprod 16(11):2411, 2001

Hasiakos D, Papakonstantinou K, Kontoravdis A, et al: Adnexal torsion during pregnancy: report of four cases and review of the literature. J Obstet Gynaecol Res 34(4 Pt 2):683, 2008

Hehenkamp WJ, Volkers NA, Birnie E, et al: Pain and return to daily activities after uterine artery embolization and hysterectomy in the treatment of symptomatic uterine fibroids: results from the randomized EMMY trial. Cardiovasc Intervent Radiol 29(2):179, 2006

Hehenkamp WJ, Volkers NA, Birnie E, et al: Symptomatic uterine fibroids: treatment with uterine artery embolization or hysterectomy—results from the randomized clinical Embolisation versus Hysterectomy (EMMY) trial. Radiology 246(3):823, 2008

Hehenkamp WJ, Volkers NA, Broekmans FJ, et al: Loss of ovarian reserve after uterine artery embolization: a randomized comparison with hysterectomy. Hum Reprod 22(7):1996, 2007

Hehenkamp WJ, Volkers NA, Donderwinkel PF, et al: Uterine artery embolization versus hysterectomy in the treatment of symptomatic uterine fibroids (EMMY trial): peri- and postprocedural results from a randomized controlled trial. Am J Obstet Gynecol 193(5):1618, 2005

Helvie MA, Silver TM: Ovarian torsion: sonographic evaluation. J Clin Ultrasound 17(5):327, 1989

Hidalgo MM, Lisondo C, Juliato CT, et al: Ovarian cysts in users of Implanon and Jadelle subdermal contraceptive implants. Contraception 73(5):532, 2006

Hindley J, Gedroyc WM, Regan L, et al: MRI guidance of focused ultrasound therapy of uterine fibroids: early results. AJR 183(6):1713, 2004

Holt VL, Cushing-Haugen KL, Daling JR: Oral contraceptives, tubal sterilization, and functional ovarian cyst risk. Obstet Gynecol 102(2):252, 2003

Holt VL, Cushing-Haugen KL, Daling JR: Risk of functional ovarian cyst: effects of smoking and marijuana use according to body mass index. Am J Epidemiol 161(6):520, 2005

Homer J, Saridogan E: Uterine artery embolization for fibroids is associated with an increase risk of miscarriage. Fertil Steril 94(1):324, 2010

Hoo W, Yazebek J, Holland T, et al: Expectant management of ultrasonically diagnosed ovarian dermoid cysts: is it possible to predict the outcome? Ultrasound Obstet Gynecol 36(2):235, 2010

Houry D, Abbott JT: Ovarian torsion: a fifteen-year review. Ann Emerg Med 38(2):156, 2001

Hyttel TE, Bak GS, Larsen SB, et al: Re-torsion of the ovaries. Acta Obstet Gynecol Scand 94(3):236, 2015

Indman PD: Hysteroscopic treatment of menorrhagia associated with uterine leiomyomas. Obstet Gynecol 81(5 (Pt 1)):716, 1993

Ishikawa H, Ishi K, Serna VA, et al: Progesterone is essential for maintenance and growth of uterine leiomyomata. Endocrinology 151(6):2433, 2010

Iverson RE Jr, Chelmow D, Strohbehn K, et al: Relative morbidity of abdominal hysterectomy and myomectomy for management of uterine leiomyomas. Obstet Gynecol 88(3):415, 1996

Johnson NP, van Voorst S, Sowter MC: Surgical treatment for tubal disease in women due to undergo in vitro fertilisation. Cochrane Database Syst Rev 1:CD002125, 2010

Kariminejad MH, Scully RE: Female adnexal tumor of probable Wolffian origin. A distinctive pathologic entity. Cancer 31(3):671, 1973

Kho KA, Nezhat C: Parasitic myomas. Obstet Gynecol 114(3):611, 2009

Kil K, Chung JE, Pak HJ, et al: Usefulness of CA125 in the differential diagnosis of uterine adenomyosis and myoma. Eur J Obstet Gynecol Reprod Biol 185:131, 2015

Kim MD, Kim S, Kim NK, et al: Long-term results of uterine artery embolization for symptomatic adenomyosis. AJR 188:176, 2007

Kondo W, Bourdel N, Cotte B, et al: Does prevention of intraperitoneal spillage when removing a dermoid cyst prevent granulomatous peritonitis? BJOG 117(8):1027, 2010

Koonings PP, Campbell K, Mishell DR Jr, et al: Relative frequency of primary ovarian neoplasms: a 10-year review. Obstet Gynecol 74(6):921, 1989

Korbin CD, Brown DL, Welch WR: Paraovarian cystadenomas and cystadenofibromas: sonographic characteristics in 14 cases. Radiology 208(2):459, 1998

Kurman RJ, Carcangiu ML, Herrington CS, et al (eds): WHO Classification of Tumours of Female Reproductive Organs, 4th ed. Lyon, International Agency for Research on Cancer, 2014

Lanes SF, Birmann B, Walker AM, et al: Oral contraceptive type and functional ovarian cysts. Am J Obstet Gynecol 166(3):956, 1992

Lee NC, Dicker RC, Rubin GL, et al: Confirmation of the preoperative diagnoses for hysterectomy. Am J Obstet Gynecol 150(3):283, 1984

Letterie GS, Coddington CC, Winkel CA, et al: Efficacy of a gonadotropin-releasing hormone agonist in the treatment of uterine leiomyomata: long-term follow-up. Fertil Steril 51(6):951, 1989

Levgur M, Abadi MA, Tucker A: Adenomyosis: symptoms, histology, and pregnancy terminations. Obstet Gynecol 95(5):688, 2000

Levine D, Brown DL, Andreotti RF, et al: Management of asymptomatic ovarian and other adnexal cysts imaged at US: Society of Radiologists in Ultrasound Consensus Conference Statement. Radiology 256(3):943, 2010

Levy G, Dehaene A, Laurent N, et al: An update on adenomyosis. Diagn Interv Imaging 94(1):3, 2013

Lewis EI, Chason RJ, DeCherney AH, et al: Novel hormone treatment of benign metastasizing leiomyoma: an analysis of five cases and literature review. Fertil Steril 99(7):2017, 2013

Li J, Ning Y, Abushahin N, et al: Secretory cell expansion with aging: risk for pelvic serous carcinogenesis. Gynecol Oncol 131(3):555, 2013

Linder D, McCaw BK, Hecht F: Parthenogenic origin of benign ovarian teratomas. N Engl J Med 292(2):63, 1975

Lippman SA, Warner M, Samuels S, et al: Uterine fibroids and gynecologic pain symptoms in a population-based study. Fertil Steril 80(6):1488, 2003

Liu X, Nie J, Guo SW: Elevated immunoreactivity to tissue factor and its association with dysmenorrhea severity and the amount of menses in adenomyosis. Hum Reprod 26(2):337, 2011

Loffer FD: Improving results of hysteroscopic submucosal myomectomy for menorrhagia by concomitant endometrial ablation. J Minim Invasive Gynecol 12(3):254, 2005

Loutradis D, Stefanidis K, Kousidis I, et al: Effect of human hydrosalpinx fluid on the development of mouse embryos and role of the concentration of growth factors in culture medium with and without hydrosalpinx fluid. Gynecol Endocrinol 20(1):26, 2005

Lu S, Peng H, Zhang H, et al: Excessive intrauterine fluid cause aberrant implantation and pregnancy outcome in mice. PLoS One 8(10):e7844, 2013

Machtinger R, Inbar Y, Cohen-Eylon S, et al: MR-guided focus ultrasound (MRgFUS) for symptomatic uterine fibroids: predictors of treatment success. Hum Reprod 27(12):3425, 2012

Maheshwari A, Gurunath S, Fatima F, et al: Adenomyosis and subfertility: a systematic review of prevalence, diagnosis, treatment and fertility outcomes. Hum Reprod Update 18(4):374, 2012

Mais V, Ajossa S, Guerriero S, et al: Laparoscopic versus abdominal myomectomy: a prospective, randomized trial to evaluate benefits in early outcome. Am J Obstet Gynecol 174(2):654, 1996

Mais V, Ajossa S, Piras B, et al: Treatment of nonendometriotic benign adnexal cysts: a randomized comparison of laparoscopy and laparotomy. Obstet Gynecol 86(5):770, 1995

Mäkäräinen L, Ylikorkala O: Primary and myoma-associated menorrhagia: role of prostaglandins and effects of ibuprofen. BJOG 93(9):974, 1986

Mann ML, Ezzati M, Tarnawa ED, et al: Fumarate hydratase mutation in a young woman with uterine leiomyomas and a family history of renal cell cancer. Obstet Gynecol 126(1):90, 2015

Manyonda IT, Bratby M, Horst JS, et al: Uterine artery embolization versus myomectomy: impact on quality of life—results of the FUME (Fibroids of the Uterus: Myomectomy versus Embolization) Trial. Cardiovasc Intervent Radiol 35(3):530, 2012

Mara M, Maskova J, Fucikova Z, et al: Midterm clinical and first reproductive results of a randomized controlled trial comparing uterine fibroid embolization and myomectomy. Cardiovasc Intervent Radiol 31(1):73, 2008

Martinez-Onsurbe P, Ruiz VA, Sanz Anquela JM, et al: Aspiration cytology of 147 adnexal cysts with histologic correlation. Acta Cytol 45(6):941, 2001

McCausland AM, McCausland VM: Depth of endometrial penetration in adenomyosis helps determine outcome of rollerball ablation. Am J Obstet Gynecol 174(6):1786, 1996

McGovern PG, Noah R, Koenigsberg R, et al: Adnexal torsion and pulmonary embolism: case report and review of the literature. Obstet Gynecol Surv 54(9):601, 1999

Mechsner S, Grum B, Gericke C, et al: Possible roles of oxytocin receptor and vasopressin-1α receptor in the pathomechanism of dysperistalsis and dysmenorrhea in patients with adenomyosis uteri. Fertil Steril 94(7):2541, 2010

Mehine M, Mäkinen N, Heinonen HR, et al: Genomics of uterine leiomyomas: insights from high-throughput sequencing. Fertil Steril 102(3):621, 2014

Mehrad M, Ning G, Chen EY, et al: A pathologist's road map to benign, precancerous, and malignant intraepithelial proliferations in the fallopian tube. Adv Anat Pathol 17(5):293, 2010

Michnovicz JJ, Hershcopf RJ, Naganuma H, et al: Increased 2-hydroxylation of estradiol as a possible mechanism for the anti-estrogenic effect of cigarette smoking. N Engl J Med 315(21):1305, 1986

Millar DM, Blake JM, Stringer DA, et al: Prepubertal ovarian cyst formation: 5 years' experience. Obstet Gynecol 81(3):434, 1993

Mizutani T, Sugihara A, Nakamuro K, et al: Suppression of cell proliferation and induction of apoptosis in uterine leiomyoma by gonadotropin-releasing hormone agonist (leuprolide acetate). J Clin Endocrinol Metab 83(4):1253, 1998

Moran O, Menczer J, Ben Baruch G, et al: Cytologic examination of ovarian cyst fluid for the distinction between benign and malignant tumors. Obstet Gynecol 82(3):444, 1993

Moshesh M, Olshan AF, Saldana T, et al: Examining the relationship between uterine fibroids and dyspareunia among premenopausal women in the United States. J Sex Med 11(3):800, 2014

Moss JG, Cooper KG, Khaund A, et al: Randomised comparison of uterine artery embolisation (UAE) with surgical treatment in patients with symptomatic uterine fibroids (REST trial): 5-year results. BJOG 118(8):936, 2011

Munro MG, Critchley HO, Fraser IS, et al: The FIGO classification of causes of abnormal uterine bleeding in the reproductive years. Fertil Steril 95(7):2204, 2011

Murphy AA, Kettel LM, Morales AJ, et al: Regression of uterine leiomyomata in response to the antiprogesterone RU 486. J Clin Endocrinol Metab 76(2):513, 1993

Mutter GL, Bergeron C, Deligdisch L, et al: The spectrum of endometrial pathology induced by progesterone receptor modulators. Mod Pathol 21(5):591, 2008

Naftalin J, Hoo W, Pateman K, et al: How common is adenomyosis? A prospective study of prevalence using transvaginal ultrasound in a gynaecology clinic. Hum Reprod 27(12):343, 2012

Nahum GG, Kaunitz AM, Rosen K, et al: Ovarian cysts: presence and persistence with use of a 13.5 mg levonorgestrel-releasing intrauterine system. Contraception 91(5):412, 2015

Nardo LG, Kroon ND, Reginald PW: Persistent unilocular ovarian cysts in a general population of postmenopausal women: is there a place for expectant management? Obstet Gynecol 102(3):589, 2003

National Cancer Institute: SEER stat fact sheets: ovary cancer. 2014. Available at: http://seer.cancer.gov/statfacts/html/ovary.html. Accessed October 26, 2014

Nichols DH, Julian PJ: Torsion of the adnexa. Clin Obstet Gynecol 28(2):375, 1985

Odejinmi F, Maclaran K, Agarwal N: Laparoscopic treatment of uterine fibroids: a comparison of peri-operative outcomes in laparoscopic hysterectomy and myomectomy. Arch Gynecol Obstet 291(3):579, 2015

Okada A, Morita Y, Fukunishi H, et al: Non-invasive magnetic resonance-guided focused ultrasound treatment of uterine fibroids in a large Japanese population: impact of the learning curve on patient outcome. Ultrasound Obstet Gynecol 34(5):579, 2009

Okugawa K, Hirakawa T, Fukushima K, et al: Relationship between age, histological type, and size of ovarian tumors. Int J Gynaecol Obstet 74(1):45, 2001

Oliveira FG, Abdelmassih VG, Diamond MP, et al: Impact of subserosal and intramural uterine fibroids that do not distort the endometrial cavity on the outcome of in vitro fertilization-intracytoplasmic sperm injection. Fertil Steril 81(3):582, 2004

Olufowobi O, Sharif K, Papaionnou S, et al: Are the anticipated benefits of myomectomy achieved in women of reproductive age? A 5-year review of the results at a UK tertiary hospital. J Obstet Gynaecol 24(4):434, 2004

Ory H: Functional ovarian cysts and oral contraceptives. Negative association confirmed surgically. A cooperative study. JAMA 228(1):68, 1974

Otubu JA, Buttram VC, Besch NF, et al: Unconjugated steroids in leiomyomas and tumor-bearing myometrium. Am J Obstet Gynecol 143(2):130, 1982

Ou YC, Huang KH, Lin H, et al: Sepsis secondary to cesarean scar diverticulum resembling an infected leiomyoma. Taiwan J Obstet Gynecol 50(1):100, 2011

Outwater EK, Mitchell DG: Normal ovaries and functional cysts: MR appearance. Radiology 198(2):397, 1996

Palomba S, Affinito P, Tommaselli GA, et al: A clinical trial of the effects of tibolone administered with gonadotropin-releasing hormone analogues for the treatment of uterine leiomyomata. Fertil Steril 70(1):111, 1998

Palomba S, Orio F Jr, Russo T, et al: Gonadotropin-releasing hormone agonist with or without raloxifene: effects on cognition, mood, and quality of life. Fertil Steril 82(2):480, 2004

Palomba S, Sena T, Morelli M, et al: Effect of different doses of progestin on uterine leiomyomas in postmenopausal women. Eur J Obstet Gynecol Reprod Biol 102(2):199, 2002

Palomba S, Zupi E, Russo T, et al: A multicenter randomized, controlled study comparing laparoscopic versus minilaparotomic myomectomy: short-term outcomes. Fertil Steril 88(4):942, 2007

Pantoja E, Rodriguez-Ibanez I, Axtmayer RW, et al: Complications of dermoid tumors of the ovary. Obstet Gynecol 45(1):89, 1975

Parazzini F, Negri E, La Vecchia C, et al: Oral contraceptive use and risk of uterine fibroids. Obstet Gynecol 79(3):430, 1992

Parazzini F, Vercellini P, Panazza S, et al: Risk factors for adenomyosis. Hum Reprod 12(6):1275, 1997

Parker WH: Etiology, symptomatology, and diagnosis of uterine myomas. Fertil Steril 87(4):725, 2007

Parker WH, Fu YS, Berek JS: Uterine sarcoma in patients operated on for presumed leiomyoma and rapidly growing leiomyoma. Obstet Gynecol 83(3):414, 1994

Parsanezhad ME, Azmoon M, Alborzi S, et al: A randomized, controlled clinical trial comparing the effects of aromatase inhibitor (letrozole) and gonadotropin-releasing hormone agonist (triptorelin) on uterine leiomyoma volume and hormonal status. Fertil Steril 93(1):192, 2010

Patel MD, Feldstein VA, Lipson SD, et al: Cystic teratomas of the ovary: diagnostic value of sonography. AJR 171(4):1061, 1998

Pauerstein CJ, Woodruff JD, Quinton SW: Development patterns in "adenomatoid lesions" of the fallopian tube. Am J Obstet Gynecol 100(7):1000, 1968

Peddada SD, Laughlin SK, Miner K, et al: Growth of uterine leiomyomata among premenopausal black and white women. Proc Natl Acad Sci USA 105(50):19887, 2008

Peterson WF, Prevost EC, Edmunds FT, et al: Benign cystic teratomas of the ovary: a clinico-statistical study of 1,007 cases with a review of the literature. Am J Obstet Gynecol 70(2):368, 1955

Polatti F, Viazzo F, Colleoni R, et al: Uterine myoma in postmenopause: a comparison between two therapeutic schedules of HRT. Maturitas 37(1):27, 2000

Popovic M, Puchner S, Berzaczy D, et al: Uterine artery embolization for the treatment of adenomyosis: a review. J Vasc Interv Radiol 22(7):901, 2011

Prat J: Ovarian serous and mucinous epithelial-stromal tumors. In Robboy SJ, Mutter GL, Prat J, et al (eds): Robboy's Pathology of the Female Reproductive Tract, 2nd ed. Churchill Livingstone Elsevier, 2009, p 611

Preutthipan S, Herabutya Y: Hysteroscopic rollerball endometrial ablation as an alternative treatment for adenomyosis with menorrhagia and/or dysmenorrhea. J Obstet Gynaecol Res 36(5):1031, 2010

Pritts EA, Parker WH, Olive DL: Fibroids and infertility: an updated systematic review of the evidence. Fertil Steril 91(4):1215, 2009

Pron G, Mocarski E, Bennett J, et al: Pregnancy after uterine artery embolization for leiomyomata: the Ontario multicenter trial. Obstet Gynecol 105(1):67, 2005

Reed SD, Cushing-Haugen KL, Daling JR, et al: Postmenopausal estrogen and progestogen therapy and the risk of uterine leiomyomas. Menopause 11(2):214, 2004

Reinhold C, McCarthy S, Bret PM, et al: Diffuse adenomyosis: comparison of endovaginal US and MR imaging with histopathologic correlation. Radiology 199(1):151, 1996

Rha SE, Byun JY, Jung SE, et al: CT and MR imaging features of adnexal torsion. Radiographics 22(2):283, 2002

Rim SY, Kim SM, Choi HS: Malignant transformation of ovarian mature cystic teratoma. Int J Gynecol Cancer 16(1):140, 2006

Roberge S, Boutin A, Chaillet N, et al: Systematic review of cesarean scar assessment in the nonpregnant state: imaging techniques and uterine scar defect. Am J Perinatol 29(6):465, 2012

Rody A, Jackisch C, Klockenbusch W, et al: The conservative management of adnexal torsion—a case-report and review of the literature. Eur J Obstet Gynecol Reprod Biol 101(1):83, 2002

Rossetti A, Sizzi O, Soranna L, et al: Long-term results of laparoscopic myomectomy: recurrence rate in comparison with abdominal myomectomy. Hum Reprod 16(4):770, 2001

Sabbah R, Desaulniers G: Use of the NovaSure Impedance Controlled Endometrial Ablation System in patients with intracavitary disease: 12-month follow-up results of a prospective, single-arm clinical study. J Minim Invasive Gynecol 13(5):467, 2006

Salazar H, Kanbour A, Burgess F: Ultrastructure and observations on the histogenesis of mesotheliomas, "adenomatoid tumors", of the female genital tract. Cancer 29(1):141, 1972

Sawin SW, Pilevsky ND, Berlin JA, et al: Comparability of perioperative morbidity between abdominal myomectomy and hysterectomy for women with uterine leiomyomas. Am J Obstet Gynecology 183(6):1448, 2000

Sayed GH, Zakherah MS, El-Nashar SA, et al: A randomized clinical trial of a levonorgestrel-releasing intrauterine system and a low-dose combined oral contraceptive for fibroid-related menorrhagia. Int J Gynaecol Obstet 112(2):126, 2011

Scharla SH, Minne HW, Waibel-Treber S, et al: Bone mass reduction after estrogen deprivation by long-acting gonadotropin-releasing hormone agonists and its relation to pretreatment serum concentrations of 1,25-dihydroxyvitamin D3. J Clin Endocrinol Metab 70(4):1055, 1990

Schlaff WD, Hassiakos DK, Damewood MD, et al: Neosalpingostomy for distal tubal obstruction: prognostic factors and impact of surgical technique. Fertil Steril 54(6):984, 1990

Schlaff WD, Zerhouni EA, Huth JA, et al: A placebo-controlled trial of a depot gonadotropin-releasing hormone analogue (leuprolide) in the treatment of uterine leiomyomata. Obstet Gynecol 74(6):856, 1989

Shavell VI, Diamond MP, Senter JP, et al: Hysterectomy subsequent to endometrial ablation. J Minim Invasive Gynecol 19(4):459, 2012

Sheng J, Zhang WY, Zhang JP, et al: The LNG-IUS study on adenomyosis: a 3-year follow-up study on the efficacy and side effects of the use of levonorgestrel intrauterine system for the treatment of dysmenorrhea associated with adenomyosis. Contraception 79(3):189, 2009

Socolov D, Blidaru I, Tamba B, et al: Levonorgestrel releasing-intrauterine system for the treatment of menorrhagia and/or frequent irregular uterine bleeding associated with uterine leiomyoma. Eur J Contracept Reprod Health Care 16(6):480, 2011

Soldin OP, Makambi KH, Soldin SJ, et al: Steroid hormone levels associated with passive and active smoking. Steroids 76(7):653, 2011

Soysal ME, Soysal SK, Vicdan K: Thermal balloon ablation in myoma-induced menorrhagia under local anesthesia. Gynecol Obstet Invest 51(2):128, 2001

Spies JB, Spector A, Roth AR, et al: Complications after uterine artery embolization for leiomyomas. Obstet Gynecol 100(5 Pt 1):873, 2002

Stewart EA, Nowak RA: Leiomyoma-related bleeding: a classic hypothesis updated for the molecular era. Hum Reprod Update 2(4):295, 1996

Stokes LS, Wallace MJ, Godwin RB, et al: Quality improvement guidelines for uterine artery embolization for symptomatic leiomyomas. J Vasc Interv Radiol 21:1153, 2010

Strandell A, Lindhard A: Why does hydrosalpinx reduce fertility? The importance of hydrosalpinx fluid. Hum Reprod 17(5):1141, 2002

Strandell A, Lindhard A, Waldenstrom U, et al: Hydrosalpinx and IVF outcome: a prospective, randomized multicentre trial in Scandinavia on salpingectomy prior to IVF. Hum Reprod 14(11):2762, 1999

Stricker B, Blanco J, Fox HE: The gynecologic contribution to intestinal obstruction in females. J Am Coll Surg 178(6):617, 1994

Surrey ES, Minjarez DA, Stevens JM, et al: Effect of myomectomy on the outcome of assisted reproductive technologies. Fertil Steril 83(5):1473, 2005

Takeuchi H, Kinoshita K: Evaluation of adhesion formation after laparoscopic myomectomy by systematic second-look microlaparoscopy. J Am Assoc Gynecol Laparosc 9(4):442, 2002

Taveira-DaSilva AM, Alford CE, Levens ED, et al: Favorable response to antigonadal therapy for a benign metastasizing leiomyoma. Obstet Gynecol 119(2 Pt 2):438, 2012

Templeman C, Marshall SF, Ursin G, et al: Adenomyosis and endometriosis in the California Teachers Study. Fertil Steril 90:415–424. 2008

Terry KL, De Vivo I, Hankinson SE, et al: Reproductive characteristics and risk of uterine leiomyomata. Fertil Steril 94(7):2703, 2010

Tiltman AJ: Leiomyomas of the uterine cervix: a study of frequency. Int J Gynecol Pathol 17(3):231, 1998

Tomassetti C, Meuleman C, Timmerman D, et al: Adenomyosis and subfertility: evidence of association and causation. Semin Reprod Med 31(2):101, 2013

Townsend DE, Sparkes RS, Baluda MC, et al: Unicellular histogenesis of uterine leiomyomas as determined by electrophoresis by glucose-6-phosphate dehydrogenase. Am J Obstet Gynecol 107(8):1168, 1970

Traiman P, Saldiva P, Haiashi A, et al: Criteria for the diagnosis of diffuse uterine myohypertrophy. Int J Gynaecol Obstet 54(1):31, 1996

Van der Kooij SM, Hehenkamp WJ, Wolkers NA, et al: Uterine artery embolization vs hysterectomy in the treatment of symptomatic uterine fibroids: 5-year outcome from the randomized EMMY trial. Am J Obstet Gynecol 203:105.e1, 2010

Van der Voet LF, Vervoort AJ, Veersema S, et al: Minimally invasive therapy for gynaecological symptoms related to a niche in the caesarean scar: a systematic review. BJOG 121(2):145, 2014

Velez Edwards DR, Baird DD, Hartmann KE: Association of age at menarche with increasing number of fibroids in a cohort of women who underwent standardized ultrasound assessment. Am J Epidemiol 178(3):426, 2013

Varelas FK, Papanicolaou AN, Vavatsi-Christaki N, et al: The effect of anastrazole on symptomatic uterine leiomyomata. Obstet Gynecol 110(3):643, 2007

Vercellini P, Viganò P, Somigliana E, et al: Adenomyosis: epidemiological factors. Best Pract Res Clin Obstet Gynaecol 20(4):465, 2006

Viville B, Charnock-Jones DS, Sharkey AM, et al: Distribution of the A and B forms of the progesterone receptor messenger ribonucleic acid and protein in uterine leiomyomata and adjacent myometrium. Hum Reprod 12(4):815, 1997

Vlasveld LT, de Wit CW, Vermeij RA, et al: Myomatous erythrocytosis syndrome: further proof for the pathogenic role of erythropoietin. Neth J Med 66(7):283, 2008

Vuento MH, Pirhonen JP, Makinen JI, et al: Evaluation of ovarian findings in asymptomatic postmenopausal women with color Doppler ultrasound. Cancer 76(7):1214, 1995

Walker WJ, McDowell SJ: Pregnancy after uterine artery embolization for leiomyomata: a series of 56 completed pregnancies. Am J Obstet Gynecol 195(5):1266, 2006

Wamsteker K, Emanuel MH, de Kruif JH: Transcervical hysteroscopic resection of submucous fibroids for abnormal uterine bleeding: results regarding the degree of intramural extension. Obstet Gynecol 82(5):736, 1993

Wang J, Yang J, Huang H, et al: Management of intravenous leiomyomatosis with intracaval and intracardiac extension. Obstet Gynecol 120(6):1400, 2012

Warner MA, Fleischer AC, Edell SL, et al: Uterine adnexal torsion: sonographic findings. Radiology 154(3):773, 1985.

Wechter ME, Stewart EA, Myers ER, et al: Leiomyoma-related hospitalization and surgery: prevalence and predicted growth based on population trends. Am J Obstet Gynecol 205(5):492.e1, 2011

Wegienka G, Baird DD, Hertz-Picciotto I, et al: Self-reported heavy bleeding associated with uterine leiomyomata. Obstet Gynecol 101(3):431, 2003

Weitzman VN, DiLuigi AJ, Maier DB, et al: Prevention of recurrent adnexal torsion. Fertil Steril 90(5):2018.e1, 2008

Whiteman MK, Kuklina E, Jamieson DJ, et al: Inpatient hospitalization for gynecologic disorders in the United States. Am J Obstet Gynecol 202(6):541.e1, 2010

Wise LA, Palmer JR, Spiegelman D, et al: Influence of body size and body fat distribution on risk of uterine leiomyomata in U.S. black women. Epidemiology 16(3):346, 2005

Wise LA, Palmer JR, Stewart EA, et al: Polycystic ovary syndrome and risk of uterine leiomyomata. Fertil Steril 87(5):1108, 2007

Wishall KM, Price J, Pereira N, et al: Postablation risk factors for pain and subsequent hysterectomy. Obstet Gynecol 124(5):904, 2014

Wyshak G, Frisch RE, Albright TE, et al: Smoking and cysts of the ovary. Int J Fertil 33(6):398, 1988

Yamamoto T, Noguchi T, Tamura T, et al: Evidence for estrogen synthesis in adenomyotic tissues. Am J Obstet Gynecol 169(3):734, 1993

Yan L, Ding L, Li C, et al: Effect of fibroids not distorting the endometrial cavity on the outcome of in vitro fertilization treatment: a retrospective cohort study. Fertil Steril 101(3):716, 2014

Yang Z, Cao YD, Hu LN, et al: Feasibility of laparoscopic high intensity focused ultrasound treatment for patients with uterine localized adenomyosis. Fertil Steril 91:2338, 2009

Yin CS, Wei RY, Chao TC, et al: Hysteroscopic endometrial ablation without endometrial preparation. Int J Gynaecol Obstet 62(2):167, 1998

Ylikorkala O, Pekonen F: Naproxen reduces idiopathic but not fibromyoma-induced menorrhagia. Obstet Gynecol 68(1):10, 1986

Youm J, Lee HJ, Kim SK, et al: Factors affecting the spontaneous expulsion of the levonorgestrel-releasing intrauterine system. Int J Gynaecol Obstet 126(2):165, 2014

Yuen PM, Yu KM, Yip SK, et al: A randomized prospective study of laparoscopy and laparotomy in the management of benign ovarian masses. Am J Obstet Gynecol 177(1):109, 1997

Zaloudek C, Hendrickson M, Soslow RA: Mesenchymal tumors of the uterus. In Kurman RJ, Ellenson LH, Ronnett BM (eds): Blaustein's Pathology of the Female Genital Tract, 6th ed. New York, Springer, 2011

Zeyneloglu HB, Arici A, Olive DL. Adverse effects of hydrosalpinx on pregnancy rates after in vitro fertilization-embryo transfer. Fertil Steril 70(3):492, 1998

Zweizig S, Perron J, Grubb D, et al: Conservative management of adnexal torsion. Am J Obstet Gynecol 168(6 Pt 1):1791, 1993

CHAPTER 10

Endometriosis

Endometriosis is a common benign disorder defined as the presence of endometrial glands and stroma outside of the normal location. Implants of endometriosis are most often found on the pelvic peritoneum, but other frequent sites include the ovaries and uterosacral ligaments. Endometrial tissue located within the myometrium is termed adenomyosis and discussed in Chapter 9 (p. 213). Women with endometriosis may be asymptomatic, subfertile, or suffer varying degrees of pelvic pain. This is an estrogen-dependent disease and thus lends itself to hormone-based treatment. However, in those with disease refractory to medical management, surgery may be required.

INCIDENCE

The incidence of endometriosis is difficult to quantify, as women with the disease are often asymptomatic. Moreover, imaging modalities have low sensitivities for small implants (Wall, 2015). The primary method of diagnosis is laparoscopy, with or without biopsy for histologic diagnosis (Dunselman, 2014). Using this standard, the annual incidence of surgically diagnosed endometriosis was 1.6 cases per 1000 women aged between 15 and 49 years (Houston, 1987). In asymptomatic women, the prevalence of endometriosis ranges from 6 to 11 percent, depending on the population studied and mode of diagnosis (Buck Louis, 2011; Mahmood, 1991). However, because of its link with infertility and pelvic pain, endometriosis is notably more prevalent in subpopulations of women with these complaints. From

studies, the prevalence lies between 20 to 50 percent in infertile women, and in those with pelvic pain, it ranges from 40 to 50 percent (Balasch, 1996; Eskenazi, 2001; Meuleman, 2009). In adolescents, Janssen and coworkers (2013) reported that nearly two thirds of adolescents undergoing diagnostic laparoscopy for pelvic pain had evidence of endometriosis.

Previously, white women were thought to be disproportionately affected. More recent studies have provided variable results. Some show greater rates for whites and Asians, whereas others have found no statistically significant differences in endometriosis prevalence among any racial or ethnic groups (Jacoby, 2010). Of other patient characteristics, lower body mass appears to positively correlate with endometriosis risk (Peterson, 2013; Shah, 2013).

PATHOPHYSIOLOGY

◼ Pathogenesis

The definitive cause of endometriosis remains unknown, but theories have been proposed. A more favored one describes retrograde menstruation through the fallopian tubes (Sampson, 1927). These refluxed endometrial fragments invade the peritoneal mesothelium and develop a blood supply for implant survival and growth. Supporting data include a report that surgical obliteration of the outflow tract in baboons induces endometriosis (D'Hooghe, 1997). In correlation, women with outflow tract obstruction also have a high incidence of endometriosis, which often resolves following obstruction relief (Sanfilippo, 1986; Williams, 2014). Importantly however, most women have retrograde menstruation (Halme, 1984). Thus, other factors, such as immunologic and angiogenic components, likely aid implant persistence.

Another hypothesis, the stem cell theory, implicates undifferentiated endometrial cells that initially reside in the endometrium's basalis layer. These cells differentiate into epithelial, stromal, and vascular cells as the endometrium is routinely regenerated each cycle. If displaced to an ectopic location, such as by retrograde menstruation, these stem cells may give rise to endometriosis (Valentijn, 2013).

Aberrant lymphatic or vascular spread of endometrial tissue has also been implicated (Jerman, 2015). Lymphatic spread of endometriosis to pelvic sentinel lymph nodes is noted in affected women (Mechsner, 2008; Tempfer, 2011). Findings of endometriosis in unusual locations, such as the groin, also bolster this theory (Mourra, 2015). Last, cases in which no peritoneal implants are found, but solely isolated retroperitoneal lesions are noted, implicate lymphatic spread (Moore, 1988).

Another theory concerns coelomic metaplasia and suggests that the parietal peritoneum is pluripotent and can undergo metaplastic transformation to tissue histologically identical to normal endometrium. Because the ovary and the progenitor of the endometrium, the müllerian ducts, are both derived from coelomic epithelium, such metaplasia may help explain endometriosis involving the ovary. This process may also underlie cases of endometriosis in those without menstruation, such as premenarchal girls and males treated with estrogen and orchiectomy for prostate cancer (Marsh, 2005; Taguchi, 2012). Last, a theory purports that müllerian remnants left along their embryonic path undergo abnormal differentiation (Batt, 2013; Signorile, 2012).

■ Anatomic Sites

Endometriosis may develop anywhere within the pelvis and on other extrapelvic peritoneal surfaces. Most commonly, endometriosis is found in the dependent areas of the pelvis. As such, the anterior and posterior cul-de-sacs, other pelvic peritoneum, the ovary, and uterosacral ligaments are frequently involved. Additionally, the rectovaginal septum, ureter, and bladder and rarely, pericardium, surgical scars, and pleura may be affected. One pathologic review revealed that endometriosis has been identified on all organs except the spleen (Markham, 1989). Implants may be superficial or they may be *deep infiltrating endometriosis (DIE)*, that is, infiltrative forms that involve vital structures such as bowel, bladder, and ureters (Koninckx, 2012; Vercellini, 2004). Some definitions of DIE also quantify invasion as >5 mm (Koninckx, 1994).

As just noted, ovarian endometriomas are frequent manifestations of endometriosis (Fig. 10-1). These smooth-walled, dark-brown ovarian cysts are filled with a chocolate-appearing fluid and may be unilocular or, when larger, multilocular. Their pathogenesis is unclear, yet three theories include invagination of ovarian cortex implants, coelomic metaplasia, and secondary involvement of functional ovarian cysts by endometrial implants located on the ovarian surface (Vignali, 2002).

■ Molecular Mechanisms

Endometriosis is an estrogen-dependent, chronic inflammatory disease with aberrant growth of ectopic endometrial tissue. In this discussion, *eutopic endometrium* is that which lines the uterine cavity, whereas *ectopic endometrium* describes that outside the cavity. In affected patients, ectopic endometrial implants show molecular differences from the eutopic endometrium of unaffected women. The disturbed molecular mechanisms in this disease are yet to be completely defined. However, suspected underpinnings include an environment of estrogen dominance, estrogen dependence, and progesterone resistance within implants; inflammation; escape from immune clearance; local invasion and neurovascularity development; and genetic predisposition.

Estrogen and Progesterone

Estrogen plays a causative role in endometriosis formation and is derived from multiple sources. First, most estrogen in women is produced directly by the ovaries. Second, peripheral tissues also produce estrogens through conversion of ovarian and

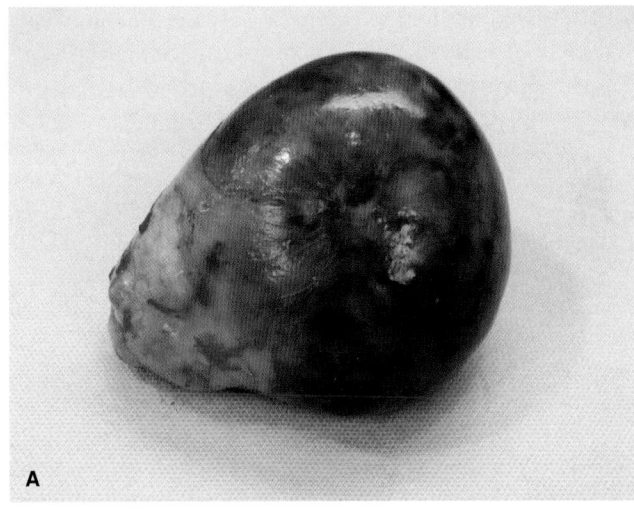

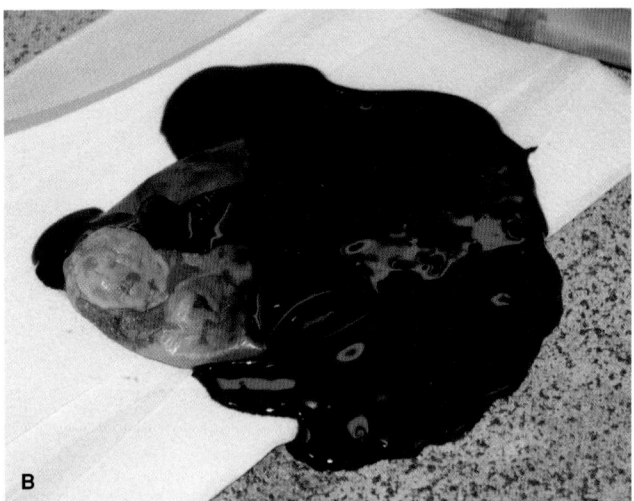

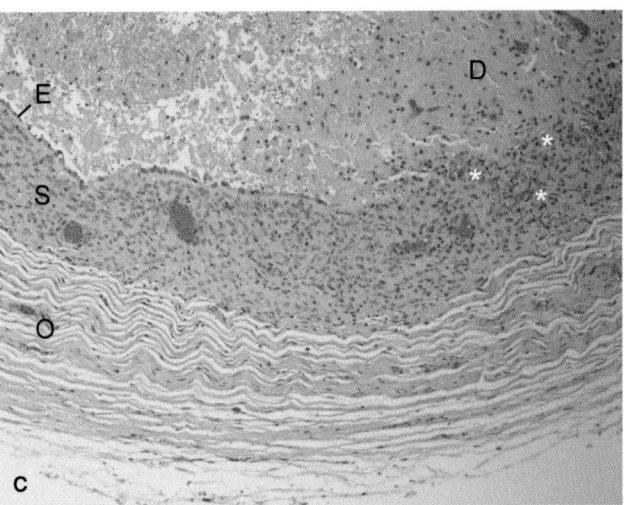

FIGURE 10-1 Endometrioma. **A.** Surgical specimen of an ovary containing an endometrioma. **B.** Dark, chocolate-like fluid had filled this cyst. (Used with permission from Dr. Roxanne Pero.) **C.** In ovarian endometriomas, endometrial-type epithelium (*E*) and subjacent stroma (*S*) line the cyst, and are bordered peripherally by ovarian stroma (*O*). The golden brown pigment in the cyst wall (*asterisks*) is hemosiderin, indicating remote hemorrhage. Debris composed of necrotic and degenerating cells and remote hemorrhage occupies the interior of the cyst (*D*). It is the remote hemorrhage that confers the chocolate-like color to cyst fluid.

adrenal androgens by the enzyme aromatase. Endometriotic implants express aromatase and 17β-hydroxysteroid dehydrogenase type 1, which are the enzymes responsible for conversion of androstenedione to estrone and of estrone to estradiol, respectively. Implants, however, are deficient in 17β-hydroxysteroid dehydrogenase type 2, which inactivates estrogen (Kitawaki, 1997; Zeitoun, 1998). This enzymatic combination ensures that implants create an estrogenic environment. Moreover, it provides the rationale for aromatase inhibitor use to diminish aromatase activity in refractory clinical cases (p. 241). Last, the endometriotic stromal cell uniquely expresses the full complement of genes in the steroidogenic cascade, which is sufficient to convert cholesterol to estradiol itself (Bulun, 2012).

In addition to an estrogenic environment, normal progesterone effects are attenuated in endometriosis. This progesterone resistance is thought to stem from an overall low concentration of progesterone receptors within implants (Attia, 2000). Specifically, pathological overexpression of estrogen receptor β in endometriosis suppresses estrogen receptor α expression. This diminishes estradiol-mediated induction of the progesterone receptor in endometriotic cells (Xue, 2007).

As one consequence of this resistance, survival of refluxed endometrium in affected women may be bolstered. Namely, normal endometrium does not express aromatase and has elevated levels of 17β-hydroxysteroid dehydrogenase type 2 in response to progesterone (Satyaswaroop, 1982). As a result, progesterone antagonizes the estrogen effects in normal endometrium during the luteal phase. Endometriosis, however, manifests a relative progesterone-resistant state, which prevents this antagonism in its implants.

Progesterone resistance may also enhance implantation of refluxed endometrium. Invasion of the mesothelium can be aided by matrix metalloproteinases (MMPs). These are a group of collagenase proteins that can digest and remodel extracellular matrix and are implicated in endometrial turnover during normal menstruation. Of the various MMPs, MMP-3 expression is significantly increased in women with endometriosis compared with healthy controls, and its expression is significantly elevated during the luteal phase (Kyama, 2006). Progesterone represses MMP activity (Itoh, 2012). Thus, in affected patients, progesterone resistance within these implants may augment the MMP activity necessary for implant invasion.

Inflammation

Prostaglandin E₂ (PGE₂) is the most potent inducer of aromatase activity in endometrial stromal cells (Noble, 1997). Estradiol produced in response to the increased aromatase activity subsequently augments PGE₂ production by stimulating the cyclooxygenase type 2 (COX-2) enzyme in uterine endothelial cells (Gurates, 2003). This creates a positive feedback loop and potentiates the estrogenic effects on endometriosis proliferation. As discussed on page 239, nonsteroidal antiinflammatory drugs (NSAIDs) are used clinically to reduce prostaglandin formation and thereby decrease endometriosis-linked pain.

Immune System

With retrograde menstruation, refluxed menstrual tissue in most women is usually cleared by macrophages, natural killer (NK) cells, and lymphocytes. For this reason, immune system dysfunction is one likely mechanism for endometriosis establishment (Seli, 2003). Of these immune cells, macrophages serve as scavengers, and increased numbers are found in the peritoneal cavity of women with endometriosis (Haney, 1981; Olive, 1985b). Although this increased population might logically act to suppress endometrial proliferation, macrophages in these affected women actually stimulate endometriotic tissue (Braun, 1994).

Of other immune system players, NK cells have cytotoxic activity against foreign cells. Although NK cell numbers are unaltered in the peritoneal fluid of affected women, the NK cell cytotoxicity against endometrium is decreased (Ho, 1995; Wilson, 1994).

Cellular immunity may also be disordered in women with endometriosis, and T lymphocytes are implicated. For example, in patients with endometriosis compared with unaffected individuals, total lymphocyte numbers or helper/suppressor subpopulation ratios do not differ in peripheral blood. However, peritoneal fluid lymphocyte numbers are increased (Steele, 1984). Also, the cytotoxic activity of T lymphocytes against autologous endometrium in affected women is impaired (Gleicher, 1984).

Humoral immunity is also altered in affected women and is thought to play a role. Endometrial antibodies of the IgG class are more frequently detected in the sera of women with endometriosis (Odukoya, 1995). One study also identified IgG and IgA autoantibodies against endometrial and ovarian tissues in the sera and in cervical and vaginal secretions of affected women (Mathur, 1982). These results suggest that endometriosis may be, in part, an autoimmune disease.

Cytokines are small, soluble immune factors involved in signaling of other immune cells. Numerous cytokines, especially interleukins, are suspected in endometriosis pathogenesis. Of specific interest, increased levels of interleukin-1β (IL-1β), IL-6, and IL-8 have been identified in relevant tissues and fluids (Arici, 1998; Mori, 1991; Tseng, 1996).

Other cytokines and growth factors are associated with endometriosis establishment. For example, both monocyte chemoattractant protein-1 (MCP-1) and RANTES (regulated on activation, normal T-cell expressed and secreted) can attract monocytes. Levels of these cytokines are increased in the peritoneal fluid of those with endometriosis and positively correlate with disease severity (Arici, 1997; Khorram, 1993). In addition, vascular endothelial growth factor (VEGF) is an angiogenic growth factor, which is upregulated by estradiol in endometrial stromal cells and peritoneal fluid macrophages. Levels of this factor are increased in the peritoneal fluid of affected women (McLaren, 1996). Although the exact role of these cytokines is unclear, perturbations in their expression and activity further support an immunologic role in endometriosis development.

Genetics

No mendelian genetic inheritance pattern has been identified for endometriosis. But, the increased incidence in first-degree relatives suggests a polygenic/multifactorial pattern. For example, in population studies, 4 to 8 percent of the female siblings or mothers of affected women had endometriosis (Dalsgaard,

2013). Other research revealed that women with endometriosis and an affected first-degree relative were more likely to have severe endometriosis (61 percent) than women without an affected first-degree relative (24 percent) (Malinak, 1980). Studies also demonstrate concordance for endometriosis in monozygotic twin pairs (Saha, 2015; Treloar, 1999).

To assist with identifying candidate genes, population-based genome-wide association studies (GWASs) have been performed. These studies are founded on the principle that common diseases, such as endometriosis, are caused by genetic variants that are common themselves. With GWAS, a set of several 100,000 common single nucleotide polymorphisms (SNPs or single DNA base-pair changes) are selected to provide the maximum coverage of the genome. Their frequencies are then compared between affected and unaffected groups. From GWASs of endometriosis, several candidate genes and chromosomes have been identified for further study (Burney, 2013).

CLASSIFICATION

The primary method of endometriosis diagnosis is visualization of endometriotic lesions by laparoscopy, with or without biopsy for histologic confirmation. The extent of endometriosis can vary widely between individuals, and thus, one classification by the American Society for Reproductive Medicine (1997) allows disease to be quantified (Fig. 10-2). With this, endometriosis on the peritoneum, ovaries, fallopian tubes, and cul-de-sac is scored at surgery. At these sites, points are assigned for disease surface area, degree of invasion, morphology, and extent of associated adhesions. Also, endometriotic lesions are morphologically categorized as white, red, or black. In this system, endometriosis is classified as stage I (minimal), stage II (mild), stage III (moderate), and stage IV (severe).

Advantages of this system are its widespread implementation, its ease of use, and its four simple-to-comprehend stages. However, the system has limitations. It correlates poorly with infertility and pain symptoms (Guzick, 1997; Vercellini, 1996). For example, women with extensive disease (stage IV) may note few complaints, whereas those with minimal disease (stage I) may have significant pain or subfertility or both. This poor predictive ability stems in part from scores that are derived from subjective visual examination. Moreover, disease involving ureter, bowel, or other extrapelvic sites is not scored (Adamson, 2013). To address these shortcomings, other systems have been developed but are yet to be widely used. These include the ENZIAN staging system to better represent DIE and the Endometrial Fertility Index (Adamson, 2010; Haas, 2011).

SYMPTOMS

Pain

As noted, women with endometriosis may be asymptomatic, but chronic pelvic pain (CPP) or subfertility is common (Ballard, 2008). Of endometriosis-associated CPP, dysmenorrhea, dyspareunia, and noncyclic pain are frequent types. Less often and described on page 234, affected women may also complain of dyschezia (pain with defecation), dysuria, or abdominal wall pain.

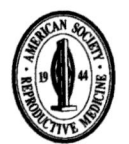

AMERICAN SOCIETY FOR REPRODUCTIVE MEDICINE REVISED CLASSIFICATION OF ENDOMETRIOSIS

Patient's Name _____   Date_____
Stage I   (Minimal) - 1-5
Stage II (Mild)   - 6-15   Laparoscopy_____ Laparotomy_____ Photography_____
Stage III (Moderate) - 16-40   Recommended Treatment_____
Stage IV (Severe)   - >40
Total_____   Prognosis_____

		<1cm	1-3cm	>3cm
PERITONEUM	**ENDOMETRIOSIS**			
	Superficial	1	2	4
	Deep	2	4	6
OVARY	R Superficial	1	2	4
	Deep	4	16	20
	L Superficial	1	2	4
	Deep	4	16	20

		Partial	Complete
	POSTERIOR CULDESAC OBLITERATION	4	40

		<1/3 Enclosure	1/3-2/3 Enclosure	>2/3 Enclosure
	ADHESIONS			
OVARY	R Filmy	1	2	4
	Dense	4	8	16
	L Filmy	1	2	4
	Dense	4	8	16
TUBE	R Filmy	1	2	4
	Dense	4*	8*	16
	L Filmy	1	2	4
	Dense	4*	8*	16

*If the fimbriated end of the fallopian tube is completely enclosed, change the point assignment to 16.

Denote appearance of superficial implant types as red [(R), red, red-pink, flamelike, vesicular blobs, clear vesicles], white [(W), opacifications, peritoneal defects, yellow-brown], or black [(B) black, hemosiderin deposits, blue]. Denote percent of total described as R____%, W____% and B____%. Total should equal 100%.

Additional Endometriosis: _____   Associated Pathology: _____

To Be Used with Normal Tubes and Ovaries

To Be Used with Abnormal Tubes and/or Ovaries

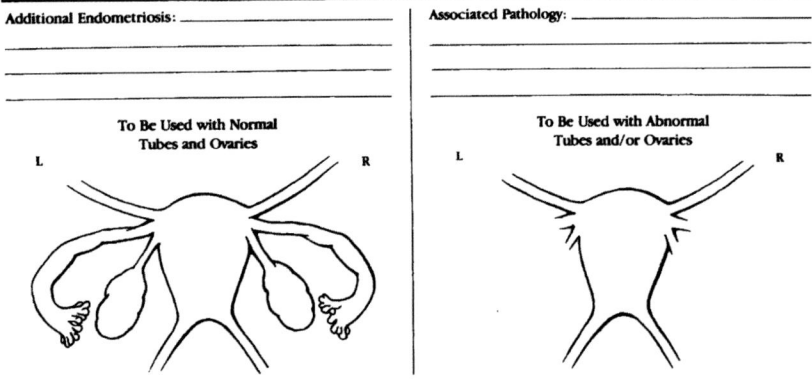

FIGURE 10-2 Reproduced with permission from American Society for Reproductive Medicine: Revised American Society for Reproductive Medicine classification of endometriosis, Fertil Steril 1997 May;67(5):817–821.

At the molecular level, the underlying cause of pain is unclear, but proinflammatory cytokines and prostaglandins released by endometriotic implants may be one source (Bulun, 2009). Other investigations implicate nerve growth into endometriotic implants (Barcena de Arellano, 2011; McKinnon, 2012). Once established, continued exposure of these sensory nerves to the inflammatory environment within the implants can lead to central sensitization and CPP, as described in Chapter 11 (p. 250) (As-Sanie, 2013; Bajaj, 2003). The variability of implant location and these chemical influences help explain the differing pain manifestations experienced by women with endometriosis. That said, typical pain scoring tools such as the visual analogue scale and the numerical rating scale are suitable for initial assessment and for evaluation of treatment efficacy (Fig. 11-3, p. 255) (Bourdel, 2015).

Of pain types, endometriosis-associated dysmenorrhea typically precedes menses by 24 to 48 hours. Compared with primary dysmenorrhea, this pain is thought to be more severe and is less responsive to NSAIDs and combination oral contraceptives (Allen, 2009; Opoku-Anane, 2012). Presence of DIE also positively correlates with dysmenorrhea severity (Lafay Pillet, 2014).

Endometriosis-associated dyspareunia is often related to rectovaginal septum, uterosacral ligament, or posterior cul-de-sac disease, although other involved sites can cause painful intercourse (Vercellini, 2007, 2012). Tension on diseased uterosacral ligaments during intercourse may trigger this pain (Fauconnier, 2002). Although some women with endometriosis describe a history of dyspareunia since coitarche, endometriosis-associated dyspareunia is suspected if pain develops after years of pain-free intercourse (Ferrero, 2005).

Noncyclic chronic pelvic pain (CPP) is another frequent symptom of endometriosis. Approximately 33 percent of women with CPP are found to have endometriosis at the time of laparoscopy (Howard, 2003). This percentage is higher in adolescents with CPP (Janssen, 2013). Some studies correlate pain severity with advanced-stage disease, whereas other studies do not (Fedele, 1992; Hsu, 2011).

The focus of chronic pain may vary. If the rectovaginal septum or uterosacral ligaments are involved with disease, pain may radiate to the rectum or lower back. Alternatively, pain radiating down the leg and causing cyclic sciatica may reflect sciatic nerve involvement (Possover, 2011). That said, pain may correlate poorly with pelvic disease location (Hsu, 2011).

■ Infertility

The incidence of endometriosis in women with subfertility is 20 to 30 percent (Waller, 1993). In addition, although wide variability is reported, patients with infertility appear to have a greater incidence of endometriosis than fertile controls (13 to 33 percent versus 4 to 8 percent) (D'Hooghe, 2003; Strathy, 1982). Furthermore, Matorras and colleagues (2001) noted an increased prevalence of more severe stages of endometriosis in women with infertility.

Adhesions are one intuitive explanation for endometriosis-related infertility. These may impair normal oocyte pick-up and transport by the fallopian tube. Beyond mechanical impairment,

numerous subtle defects also appear to be involved. Such defects include perturbations in follicle development, ovulation, sperm function, embryo quality and development, and implantation (Macer, 2012; Stilley, 2012).

A link between infertility and milder forms of endometriosis is less well supported (D'Hooghe, 1996; Schenken, 1980). An association is suggested by the differing prevalence of endometriosis between infertile and fertile women. For example, Rodriguez-Escudero and associates (1988) reported that women with minimal endometriosis had a 12-month cumulative pregnancy rate of 47 percent, which is below that of normal fertile women. Furthermore, a prospective cohort study demonstrated that women with minimal or mild endometriosis had a fecundity similar to that of those with unexplained infertility.

In moderate to severe endometriosis (stage III to IV), tubal and ovarian architecture are often distorted. As a result, impaired fertility would be expected. Few studies report fecundity rates in women with severe endometriosis. One investigation comparing mild, moderate, and severe endometriosis revealed a monthly fecundity rate of 8.7 percent in those with mild disease, 3.2 percent with moderate disease, and no pregnancies with severe disease (Olive, 1985a). In another, women with severe endometriosis undergoing in vitro fertilization (IVF) had poorer implantation and pregnancy rates compared with those with mild disease (Harb, 2013).

■ Symptoms from Specific Sites
Rectosigmoid Lesions

Defecatory pain develops much less often than other types of CPP in affected patients. Complaints may be chronic or cyclic, and they can be associated with constipation, diarrhea, or cyclic hematochezia (Roman, 2013). Thus, gastrointestinal causes of CPP are also entertained during evaluation (Chap. 11, p. 265). The origin of symptoms can be fixation of the rectum to adjacent anatomic structures or rectal wall inflammation.

Symptoms may also stem from DIE of the gastrointestinal tract, which complicates 5 to 12 percent of proven endometriosis cases. Bowel DIE predominantly involves rectosigmoid colon and much less so the small bowel, cecum, or appendix (Ruffo, 2014b). Lesions are usually confined to the subserosa and muscularis propria. Thus, colonoscopy offers poor diagnostic sensitivity (Milone, 2015). Rarely, more severe cases may involve the bowel wall transmurally and lead to intestinal obstruction or a clinical picture suggesting malignancy (Kaufman, 2011; Ruffo, 2014a).

For diagnosis, rectal DIE can be imaged by transvaginal sonography (TVS), and sensitivity approximates 80 percent. However, TVS techniques used to diagnose DIE have a learning curve, and these are predominantly performed at tertiary care centers (Tammaa, 2014). Magnetic resonance (MR) imaging can clarify anatomy and degree of invasion, especially preoperatively (Bazot, 2009; Wall, 2015). Laparoscopy typically provides the definitive diagnosis.

Without obstructing symptoms, women may be considered for conservative management with hormonal therapy. However, treatment is often surgical, and cases often warrant a surgeon skilled in bowel surgery. Variables such as anatomic site, DIE depth, lesion size, and number of foci influence surgery. Colorectal segment resection may be needed. Less invasive techniques that shave down the lesion without opening the rectum or that excise discrete nodules are also described (Alabiso, 2015).

Urinary Tract Lesions

Logically, endometriosis should be considered if urinary tract symptoms persist despite negative urine culture results. Symptoms, if present, are more common with bladder disease. These include dysuria, suprapubic pain, urinary frequency, urgency, and hematuria (Gabriel, 2011; Seracchioli, 2010). Costovertebral angle pain may reflect ureteral endometriosis with obstruction and hydronephrosis that can progress eventually to kidney function loss (Knabben, 2015).

In a large series by Antonelli and coworkers (2006), the prevalence of urinary tract DIE was 2.6 percent. In this series of 31 patients, 12 had bladder endometriosis, 15 had ureteral endometriosis, and four had both ureteral and bladder involvement. TVS has suitable accuracy for bladder DIE but is less sensitive for ureteral disease (Exacoustos, 2014a). In unclear cases, MR imaging can add additional anatomic information. In light of associated symptoms with urinary tract DIE, cystoscopy with biopsy can also help clarify the diagnosis.

Treatment is either medical or surgical. If elected, surgery for bladder invasion is typically partial cystectomy. Surgeries for ureteral involvement vary by disease severity and include: (1) freeing the tethered ureter by ureterolysis, (2) segmental resection and reanastomosis, or (3) ureter reimplantation into the bladder, that is, ureteroneocystotomy (Seracchioli, 2010).

Anterior Abdominal Wall

Some individuals with abdominal pain can have anterior abdominal wall endometriomas. Most of these lesions develop in the abdominal scar after uterine surgery or cesarean delivery, whereas others form unrelated to prior operations (Fig. 10-3) (Ding, 2013). Implants usually are found within the subcutaneous layer, are palpable, and may involve the adjacent fascia. Less often, the rectus abdominis muscle is infiltrated (Mostafa, 2013). Diagnostic tools are variably employed, and abdominal wall sonography, computed tomography (CT), MR imaging, and fine-needle aspiration are options. The decision to perform concurrent TVS is typically guided by whether CPP symptoms coexist.

In most instances, implants are surgically excised for pain relief and diagnosis. For small implants, preoperative imaging may not be needed. But with larger implants and concerns for fascial or rectus abdominis muscle involvement, CT or MR imaging can aid surgery planning (Ecker, 2014). Large fascial defects following excision may require mesh to close the defect.

Thoracic Lesions

Thoracic endometriosis defines implants inside the thoracic cavity that lead to symptoms described as menstrual or synonymously called "catemenial." These include cyclic chest or shoulder pain, hemoptysis, or pneumothorax, which predominantly occurs on

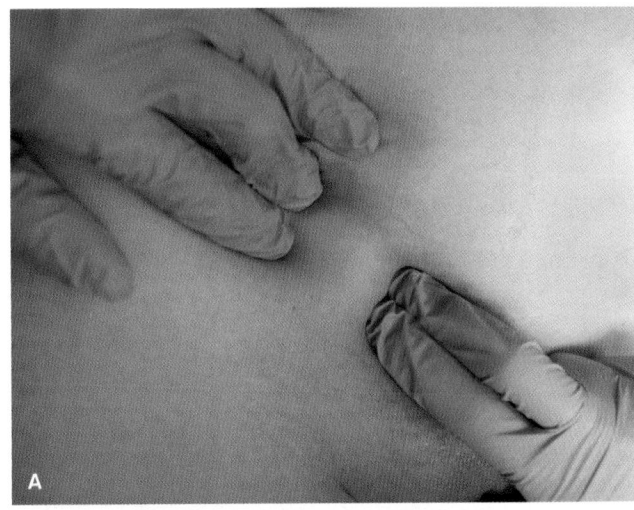

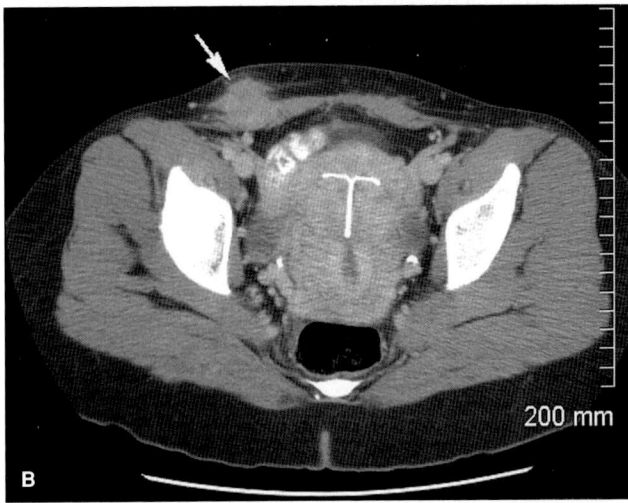

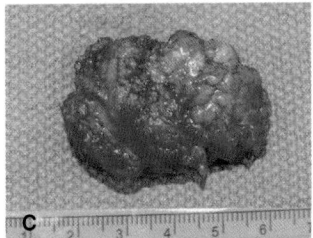
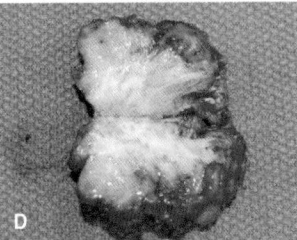

FIGURE 10-3 Endometriosis within a Pfannenstiel incision scar. **A.** Preoperative photograph delineates the borders of the mass. **B.** Computed tomography image shows a subcutaneous mass (*arrow*) extending down to the anterior abdominal wall fascia on the left. **C.** Excised mass. **D.** Bisected mass shows white fibrous scarring within yellow subcutaneous fat. Pathologic evaluation confirmed endometriosis. (Used with permission from Dr. Christi Capet.)

the right (Haga, 2014; Rousset-Jablonski, 2011). Chest CT is preferred imaging (Rousset, 2014). For pneumothorax, minimally invasive thorascopic surgery is usually indicated. This is often coupled with several months of postoperative gonadotropin-releasing hormone (GnRH) or of progestin therapy identical to that for pelvic endometriosis treatment (Alifano, 2010). Hemoptysis, depending on findings, may be treated hormonally or surgically.

DIAGNOSTIC EVALUATION

Physical Examination

For the most part, endometriosis is a disease confined to the pelvis. Accordingly, visual cues are often lacking. Some exceptions include endometriosis within an episiotomy scar or surgical scar, most often within a Pfannenstiel incision (Koger, 1993; Zhu, 2002). Rarely, endometriosis may develop spontaneously within the perineum or perianal region (Watanabe, 2003). Occasionally, blue or red powder-burn lesions are seen on the cervix or the posterior vaginal fornix. These lesions can be tender or bleed with contact. One study found that speculum examination displayed endometriosis in 14 percent of patients diagnosed with DIE (Chapron, 2002).

During bimanual examination, pelvic organ palpation often reveals suggestive anatomic abnormalities. Uterosacral ligament nodularity and tenderness may reflect active disease or scarring along the ligament. An enlarged, cystic adnexal mass may represent an ovarian endometrioma, which can be mobile or adhered to other pelvic structures. A retroverted, fixed, tender uterus and a firm, fixed posterior cul-de-sac are among other findings. Pelvic nodularities secondary to endometriosis may be more easily detected by bimanual examination during menses (Koninckx, 1996). However, examination is generally inaccurate in assessing the extent of endometriosis, especially if the lesions are extragenital. Last, rectal examination may reveal rectovaginal septum nodularity or tenderness.

Laboratory Testing

Laboratory investigations are often undertaken to exclude other causes of pelvic pain that are listed in Table 11-1 (p. 251). Initially, a complete blood count (CBC), human chorionic gonadotropin assay, urinalysis and urine cultures, vaginal cultures, and cervical swabs may be collected to exclude infections or pregnancy complications. If urinary tract endometriosis is suspected, then renal function can also be assessed by creatinine levels.

Numerous serum markers have been studied as possible diagnostic tools. Cancer antigen 125 (CA125) is a glycoprotein that is found in fallopian tube epithelium, endometrium, endocervix, pleura, and peritoneum. As discussed in Chapter 35 (p. 737), this marker is used in ovarian cancer evaluation and surveillance. Recognized by monoclonal antibody assays, elevated CA125 levels positively correlate with endometriosis severity (Hornstein, 1995a). Unfortunately, the assay has poor sensitivity in detecting mild endometriosis and appears to be a better diagnostic test for stage III or IV endometriosis (Mol, 1998; Santulli, 2015). Although the role of this assay in clinical practice is uncertain, it may be useful in the presence of a sonographically detected ovarian cyst suggestive of an endometrioma.

As for other serum markers, May and colleagues (2010) completed a systematic review of more than 100 putative biomarkers. They were unable to identify a single biomarker or biomarker panel that they felt was clinically useful.

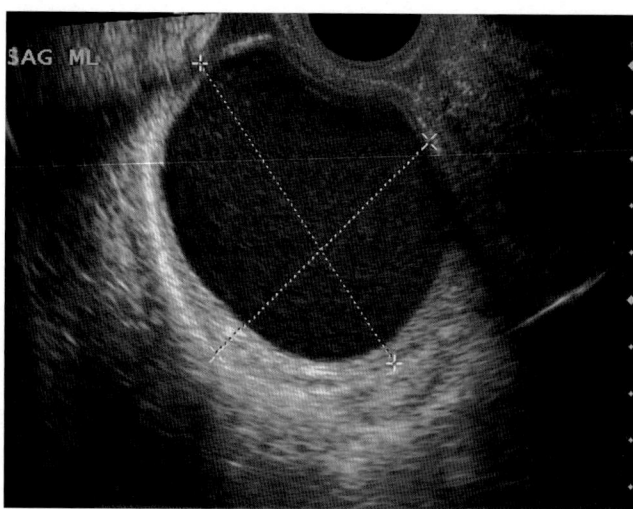

FIGURE 10-4 Transvaginal sonogram demonstrating ovarian endometrioma. A cyst with diffuse internal low-level echoes is seen.

Diagnostic Imaging

Many women with endometriosis present with CPP, and TVS is an initial imaging tool. It is accurate in detecting endometriomas and aids exclusion of other causes of pelvic pain. However, imaging of superficial endometriosis or endometriotic adhesions is inadequate. Small endometriotic plaques or nodules may occasionally be seen, but these findings are inconsistent (Wall, 2015).

Endometriomas can be diagnosed by TVS with adequate sensitivity in most settings if they are 20 mm in diameter or greater. Sensitivity and specificity of TVS to diagnose endometriomas range from 64 to 90 percent and from 22 to 100 percent, respectively (Moore, 2002). An endometrioma classically is cystic with homogeneous, low-level internal echoes, often described as "ground glass" echogenicity. There is normal surrounding ovarian tissue (Fig. 10-4). As such, these may have an identical appearance to hemorrhagic corpus luteum cysts. Although endometriomas are most often unilocular, one to four thin septations can be found (Van Holsbeke, 2010). Less typically, these cysts can display thick septations or walls. Also less often, echogenic wall foci that lack flow when color Doppler is applied can be seen and are typically depositions of blood or blood components (Bhatt, 2006). Color Doppler TVS often demonstrates pericystic, but not intracystic, flow. Although endometriomas can be found in postmenopausal women, they are less common and more often are multilocular compared with those in reproductive-aged women.

As noted previously (p. 234), TVS for DIE involving the bowel and bladder has suitable accuracy (Exacoustos, 2014a; Hudelist, 2011). That said, for the diagnosis of rectal endometriosis, TVS is highly operator dependent, and experience is often lacking (Dunselman, 2014). Thus, MR imaging may clarify anatomy for equivocal sonographic findings and offers superior resolution at soft tissue interfaces (Fig. 10-5). In some cases with DIE, MR imaging can assist preoperative planning.

CT scanning plays a limited role in the evaluation of endometriosis. This is because TVS images endometriomas well, and CT has poor sensitivity for small implants and plaques. That said, chest CT is preferred for thoracic endometriosis. CT is

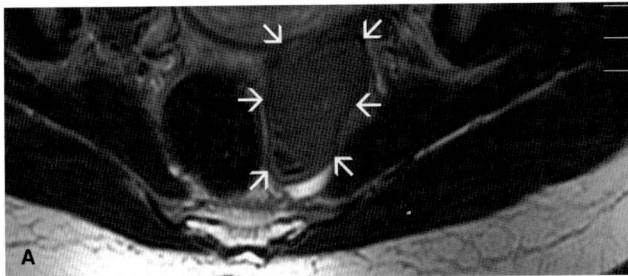

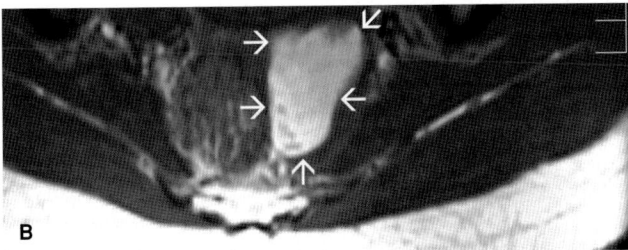

FIGURE 10-5 Magnetic resonance images of an endometrioma (*arrows*) just lateral to the rectum. **A.** Consistent with subacute blood, low-intensity signals are found on T-2 weighted sequences. **B.** High-intensity signals are seen on T-1 weighted sequences. (Used with permission from Dr. Diane Twickler.)

suitable for abdominal wall endometrioma evaluation. Also, in selected cases, CT may have a role to evaluate bowel or ureteral endometriosis (Exacoustos, 2014b).

Diagnostic Laparoscopy

Although imaging can add clinical information, laparoscopy is the primary method used for diagnosing endometriosis (American College of Obstetricians and Gynecologists, 2014b). Surgical findings vary and may include discrete endometriotic lesions, endometrioma, or adhesions. Implants are typically found on pelvic organ serosa and pelvic peritoneum. Lesions are variably colored and can be <u>red</u> (red, red-pink, or clear), <u>white</u> (white or yellow-brown), and <u>black</u> (black or black-blue) (Fig. 10-6). White and red lesions most commonly correlate with the characteristic histologic findings of endometriosis (Jansen, 1986). Dark lesions are pigmented by hemosiderin deposition from trapped menstrual debris. In addition to color differences, endometriotic lesions may differ morphologically. They can appear as <u>smooth blebs</u> on peritoneal surfaces, as <u>holes</u> or defects within the peritoneum, or as <u>flat stellate lesions</u> whose points are formed by surrounding scar tissue. Endometriotic lesions may be superficial or may deeply invade the peritoneum or pelvic organs.

Endometriomas are easily identified during laparoscopy. Laparoscopic visualization of ovarian endometriomas has a sensitivity and specificity of 97 percent and 95 percent, respectively (Vercellini, 1991). Because of this, ovarian biopsy is rarely required for diagnosis.

Pathologic Analysis

Current guidelines do not require biopsy and histologic evaluation for the diagnosis of endometriosis. However, some suggest

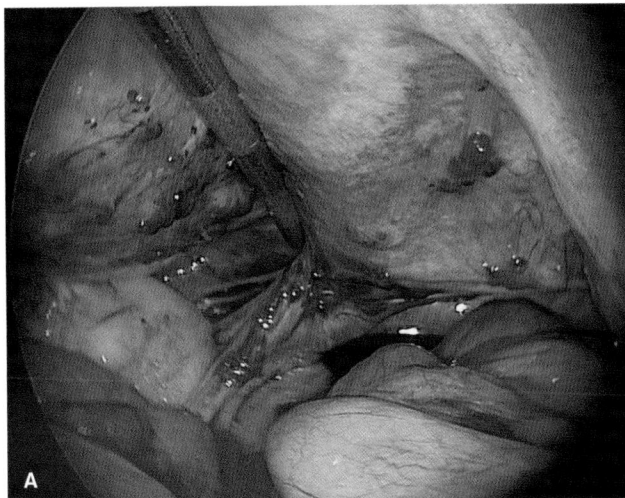

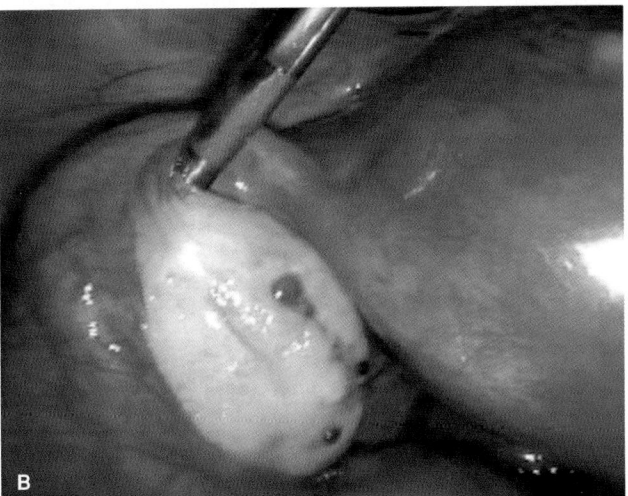

FIGURE 10-6 Endometriosis diagnosed during laparoscopy. **A.** Several red and clear endometriotic lesions seen on the pelvic peritoneum of the posterior cul-de-sac. **B.** Several brown-black lesions on the ovarian surface. (Used with permission from Dr. David Rogers.)

that relying solely on laparoscopic findings in the absence of histologic confirmation often results in overdiagnosis (Buck Louis, 2011; Wykes, 2004). Specifically, the greatest discordance between laparoscopic and histologic findings is noted in scarred lesions (Walter, 2001). Histologic diagnosis <u>requires</u> <u>both endometrial glands and stroma found outside the uterine cavity</u> (Fig. 10-7). Additionally, hemosiderin deposition is frequently seen. The gross appearance of endometriotic lesions often suggests certain microscopic findings. For example, if examined microscopically, red lesions are frequently vascularized, whereas white lesions more often display fibrosis and few vessels (Nisolle, 1997).

TREATMENT

Therapy for endometriosis depends on a woman's specific complaints, symptom severity, location of endometriotic lesions, goals for treatment, and desire to conserve future fertility. As

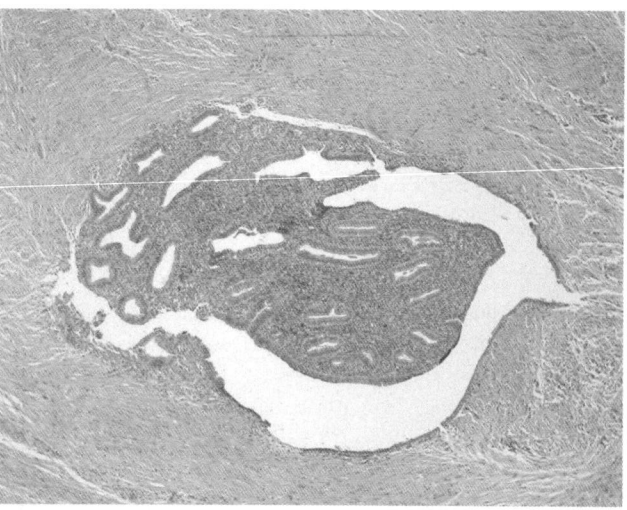

FIGURE 10-7 Endometriosis. This focus of endometrial glands and stroma was identified in the abdominal wall at the lateral aspect of a cesarean delivery scar. (Used with permission from Dr. Kelley Carrick.)

shown in Figure 10-8, determining whether a patient is seeking treatment for infertility or pain is essential, as therapy for these two is different.

If pain is prominent and conception is not currently desired, then medical therapy is typically selected. Treatment strives to atrophy ectopic endometrium and diminish disease-associated inflammation. Available agents include NSAIDs, sex steroid hormones, GnRH agents, and aromatase inhibitors. In general, suitable starting regimens are NSAIDS alone or combined with oral contraceptive pills or with a progestin. These agents may be initiated if endometriosis is suspected in a woman with CPP or may be started following diagnostic laparoscopy. If initial therapy fails to control pain following laparoscopy, then use of a different medication is reasonable. If initial empiric therapy is ineffective, then either diagnostic laparoscopy or medication change is suitable (American College of Obstetricians and Gynecologists, 2014b). Of note, although medical treatment improves pain, relapse rates are high with therapy discontinuation.

If infertility is the presenting symptom, then fertility-preserving treatment without ovulation suppression will be required, as outlined on page 243. In contrast, if the patient

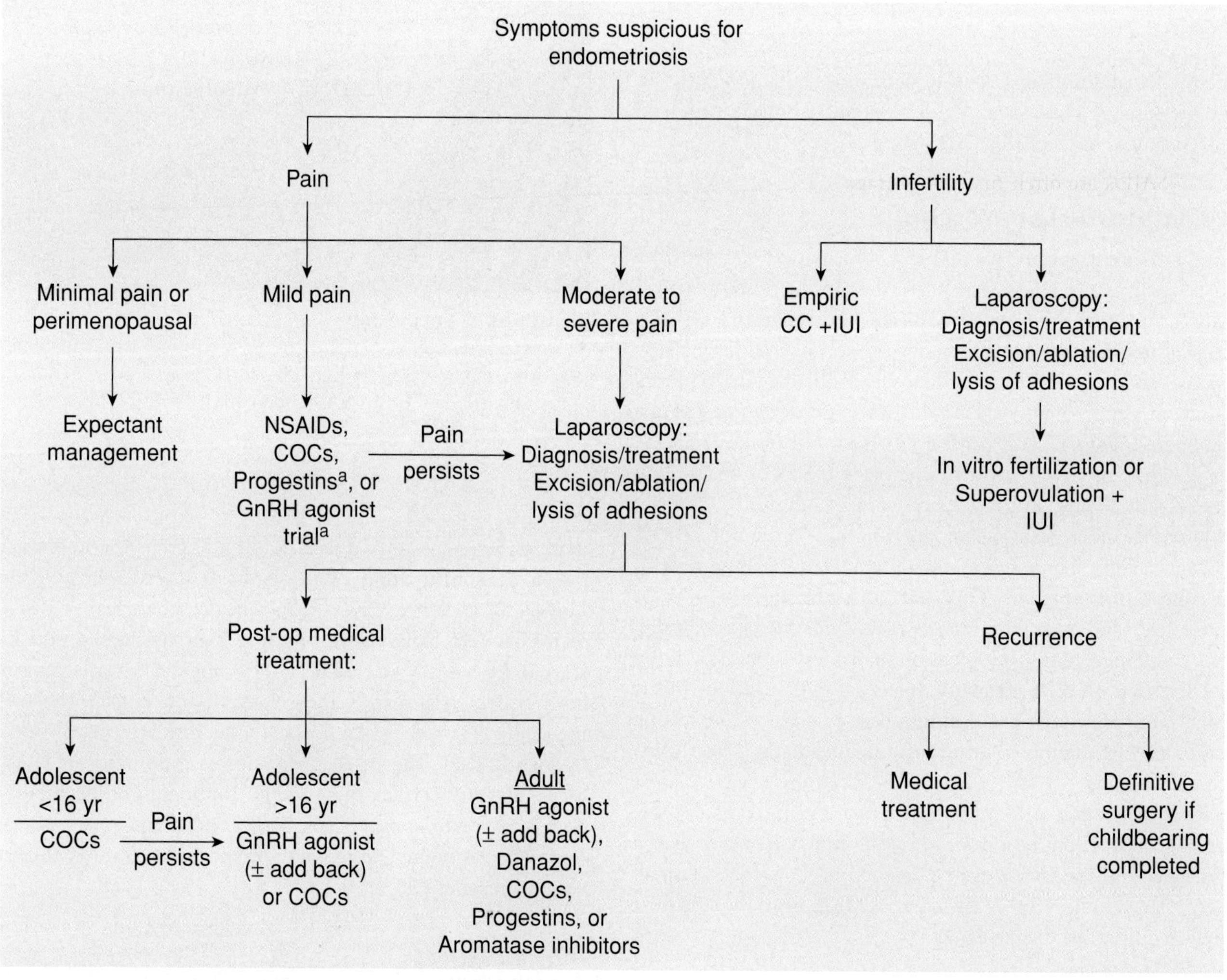

Symptoms suspicious for endometriosis

Pain

- Minimal pain or perimenopausal → Expectant management
- Mild pain → NSAIDs, COCs, Progestins[a], or GnRH agonist trial[a] → Pain persists → Laparoscopy: Diagnosis/treatment Excision/ablation/ lysis of adhesions
- Moderate to severe pain → Laparoscopy: Diagnosis/treatment Excision/ablation/ lysis of adhesions

Post-op medical treatment:

- Adolescent <16 yr — COCs → Pain persists → Adolescent >16 yr — GnRH agonist (± add back) or COCs
- Adult — GnRH agonist (± add back), Danazol, COCs, Progestins, or Aromatase inhibitors

Infertility

- Empiric CC +IUI
- Laparoscopy: Diagnosis/treatment Excision/ablation/ lysis of adhesions → In vitro fertilization or Superovulation + IUI

Recurrence

- Medical treatment
- Definitive surgery if childbearing completed

FIGURE 10-8 Diagnostic and treatment algorithm for women with presumptive or proven endometriosis. COCs = combination oral contraceptive pills; GnRH = gonadotropin-releasing hormone; IUI = intrauterine insemination; NSAIDs = nonsteroidal antiinflammatory drugs.
[a]Agents not recommended for adolescents younger than 16 years.

has severe, recalcitrant pain and has completed childbearing, definitive surgery may be warranted, as described on page 243.

Medical Treatment of Pain

Expectant Management

For many women, symptoms will preclude them from choosing expectant management. However, for those with mild symptoms or for asymptomatic women diagnosed incidentally, expectant management may be appropriate (Moen, 2002). Sutton and associates (1997) expectantly managed patients initially diagnosed by laparoscopy with minimal to moderate endometriosis. At second-look laparoscopy after 1 year, 29 percent of women had disease regression, 42 percent remained unchanged, and 29 percent had disease progression. Other investigators have shown similar rates of disease regression with expectant management (Thomas, 1987). These studies are confined to patients with minimal to moderate endometriosis. There are no well-designed trials examining the effect of expectant management on severe endometriosis.

Nonsteroidal Antiinflammatory Drugs

Both COX-1 and -2 enzymes promote synthesis of prostaglandins involved in the pain and inflammation associated with endometriosis. Specifically, endometriotic tissue expresses COX-2 at greater levels than eutopic endometrium (Cho, 2010). Accordingly, therapy aimed at lowering these prostaglandin levels plays a role in alleviating endometriosis-associated pain. As such, NSAIDs are often first-line therapy in women with primary dysmenorrhea or pelvic pain with suspected or known endometriosis. That said, study evidence supporting NSAIDs for this disease is scant and is extrapolated from efficacy data in primary dysmenorrhea (Kauppila, 1985; Marjoribanks, 2010).

The NSAIDs listed in Table 10-1 nonselectively inhibit both COX-1 and COX-2 enzymes. In contrast, selective COX-2 inhibitors specifically inhibit the COX-2 isoenzyme. Due to the cardiovascular risks with long-term use of selective COX-2 inhibitors, these medications are used at the lowest possible dose and for the shortest duration necessary (Jones, 2005). Thus, drugs in Table 10-1 are primarily selected.

Combination Hormonal Contraceptives

These agents are a mainstay for the treatment of endometriosis-related pain. They inhibit gonadotropin release, decrease menstrual flow, and decidualize implants. As such, abundant study evidence supports use of combination oral contraceptive (COC) pills or the contraceptive patch or ring to relieve endometriosis-related pain (Harada, 2008; Vercellini, 1993, 2010). These provide contraception and other noncontraceptive benefits, which are balanced against risks enumerated in Chapter 5 (p. 119).

COCs can be used conventionally in a cyclic regimen or may be used continuously, without a break for withdrawal menses. The continuous regimen decreases the frequency of painful menses and improves CPP (Guzick, 2011). For endometriosis-related pain, monophasic or multiphasic COCs are both suitable. Additionally, low-dose COCs (containing ≤20 μg ethinyl estradiol) have not proved superior to conventional-dose COCs for endometriosis treatment, but lower doses may lead to higher rates of abnormal uterine bleeding (Gallo, 2013).

Progestins

This family of hormones is often used for endometriosis therapy. Progestational agents are known to antagonize estrogenic effects on the endometrium, causing initial decidualization and subsequent endometrial atrophy. For endometriosis treatment, progestins can be administered as an oral progestin pill, depot medroxyprogesterone acetate (DMPA) (Depo-Provera), norethindrone acetate (NETA), or a levonorgestrel-releasing intrauterine system.

As supporting evidence, one randomized trial compared the effect of oral medroxyprogesterone acetate (MPA) 100 mg daily given for 6 months and placebo. At second-look laparoscopy, partial or total resolution of peritoneal implants was noted in 60 percent of progestin-treated women compared with 18 percent of the placebo group. Furthermore, pelvic pain and defecatory pain were significantly reduced (Telimaa, 1987). Side effects of high-dose MPA included acne, edema, weight gain, and irregular menstrual bleeding. In practice, MPA is prescribed in oral dosages ranging from 20 to 100 mg daily.

Alternatively, MPA may be given intramuscularly in depot form in a dosage of 150 mg every 3 months. In depot form, MPA may delay resumption of normal menses and ovulation and thus is less suitable for women contemplating imminent pregnancy. Subcutaneous formulation of MPA, marketed as Depo-SubQ Provera 104, is also effective (Schlaff, 2006).

As discussed in Chapter 5 (p. 127), the Depo-Provera package insert carries a "black box warning." This describes that

TABLE 10-1. Commonly Used Oral Nonsteroidal Antiinflammatory Drugs (NSAIDs) in the Treatment of Endometriosis-Associated Dysmenorrhea

Generic Name	Trade Name	Dosage
Ibuprofen	Motrin, Advil, Nuprin	400 mg every 4–6 hr
Naproxen	Naprosyn, Aleve	500 mg initially, then 250 mg every 6–8 hr
Naproxen sodium	Anaprox	550 mg initially, then 275 mg every 6–8 hr
Mefenamic acid	Ponstel	500 mg initially, then 250 mg every 6 hr
Ketoprofen	Orudis, Oruvail	50 mg every 6–8 hr

prolonged DMPA use may result in bone density loss, that this loss is greater with increasing duration of use, and that the loss may not be completely reversible. Labeling recommends limiting use to 2 years unless other contraceptive methods are inadequate. Thus, the risks and benefits of treatment are weighed if contemplating long-term DMPA therapy. Bone density surveillance with dual energy x-ray absorptiometry (DEXA) scanning is not recommended (American College of Obstetricians and Gynecologists, 2014a).

NETA is a 19-nortestosterone synthetic progestin that has been used to treat endometriosis. In one study, investigators administered an initial oral dosage of NETA, 5 mg daily, with increases of 2.5 mg daily until amenorrhea or a maximal dosage of 20 mg daily was reached. They found an approximately 90-percent reduction in dysmenorrhea and pelvic pain (Muneyyirci-Delale, 1998). As discussed on page in the next section, NETA is also used as adjunct therapy with GnRH agents to blunt the bone loss linked with those drugs.

Dienogest is another 19-nortestosterone synthetic progestin suitable for endometriosis. In one randomized study, it was significantly more effective than placebo for reducing endometriosis-associated pain when used orally at a dosage of 2 mg daily (Strowitzki, 2010a). Other trials show efficacy equivalent to that of GnRH agonists (Harada, 2009; Strowitzki, 2010b). Currently, this progestin as a sole agent is not available in the United States.

The levonorgestrel-releasing intrauterine system (LNG-IUS) (Mirena) delivers levonorgestrel directly to the endometrium and is effective for up to 5 years. This intrauterine device has traditionally been used for contraception, but data are accruing for endometriosis treatment. One small randomized trial that incorporated second-look laparoscopy showed improved endometriosis stage with both LNG-IUS and the comparator GnRH treatment. Other small randomized trials have shown symptom improvement when compared against expectant management, DMPA, or GnRH agonists (Petta, 2005; Tanmahasamut, 2012; Vercellini, 2003b; Wong, 2010). However, in patients with bowel endometriosis, the LNG-IUS may be ineffective for symptom control (Hinterholzer, 2007). Contraindications to LNG-IUS use are listed in Chapter 5 (p. 109).

Intuitively, the implant that chronically releases the progestin etonogestrel might be considered for endometriosis. Data regarding its efficacy for this indication are limited. One small randomized study comparing the implant and the LNG-IUS reported comparable efficacy (Walch, 2009).

GnRH Agonists

Endogenous pulsatile release of GnRH prompts secretory activity of the gonadotropes within the anterior pituitary. Gonadotropin release from the pituitary then leads to ovarian steroidogenesis and ovulation. However, continuous, nonpulsatile GnRH administration results in pituitary desensitization and subsequent loss of ovarian steroidogenesis. These features allow pharmacologic use of GnRH agonists for endometriosis treatment. With loss of ovarian estradiol production, the hypoestrogenic environment removes the stimulation normally provided to the endometriotic implants and creates a pseudomenopausal state during treatment. In addition to their direct

effect on estrogen production, GnRH agonists also reduce COX-2 levels in patients with endometriosis, providing another mechanism of treatment (Kim, 2009).

GnRH agonists are inactive if taken orally, but intramuscular, subcutaneous, and intranasal preparations are available. Leuprolide acetate (Lupron Depot) is available in a 3.75-mg monthly dose or an 11.25-mg 3-month dose, both given IM. Less frequently used GnRH agonists include goserelin (Zoladex) administered as a 3.6-mg monthly or a 10.8-mg 3-month subcutaneous depot implant; triptorelin (Trelstar) given as a 3.75-mg monthly IM injection; and nafarelin (Synarel) used in a 200-mg twice-daily nasal spray regimen. All of these except triptorelin carry specific Food and Drug Administration (FDA) approval for endometriosis treatment.

Pain Improvement. Empirically, GnRH agonists may be used *prior to laparoscopy* in women with CPP and clinical suspicion of endometriosis. In a study by Ling and associates (1999), after 3 months of GnRH agonist treatment, pain scores significantly declined compared with those after placebo. Subsequent laparoscopy revealed that 93 percent of these women had surgically diagnosed endometriosis. Similarly, in suspected cases, depot leuprolide acetate may be used empirically *in lieu of laparoscopy* for satisfactory symptom improvement. That said, an empiric GnRH trial is not routinely offered to patients younger than 16 years because GnRH agonist effects on long-term bone mineral density (BMD) have not been adequately studied in this age group.

In those with *surgically confirmed* endometriosis, numerous studies demonstrate the effectiveness of GnRH agonist therapy to improve pain symptoms (Brown, 2010). The GnRH agonists provide greater relief when administered for 6 months compared with 3 months (Hornstein, 1995b). As noted in the prior sections, GnRH agonists compares favorably with other drugs used for endometriosis treatment. Although GnRH is effective, its cost and side effects often favor trials of COCs or progestins first.

Add-back Therapy. Concerns regarding the effects of prolonged hypoestrogenism preclude extended treatment with GnRH agonists. Hypoestrogenic symptoms include hot flushes, insomnia, reduced libido, vaginal dryness, and headaches. Moreover, both spine and hip BMD decrease at 3 and 6 months of GnRH agonist therapy, with only partial recovery at 12 to 15 months after treatment (Orwoll, 1994). Because of the increased osteoporosis risk, therapy is usually limited to the shortest possible duration—usually no greater than 6 months.

Estrogen may be added to GnRH agonist therapy to counteract bone loss and is termed add-back therapy. With the addition of such hormonal add-back therapy, a GnRH agonist may occasionally be used longer than 6 months (American College of Obstetricians and Gynecologists, 2014b). The goal of add-back therapy is to supply enough estrogen to minimize GnRH agonist side effects while still maintaining a hypoestrogenic state sufficient to suppress endometriosis. Barbieri (1992) explained that tissues have varied sensitivity to estrogen, and a concentration of estrogen that will partially prevent bone loss may not stimulate endometrial growth. This "estrogen threshold" has not been established but is thought to approximate 30 to 40 pg/mL of estradiol.

Several regimens are suitable and appear equally efficacious (Wu, 2014). In one study, NETA 5 mg orally given daily, with or without conjugated equine estrogen (Premarin) 0.625 mg orally daily, for 12 months provided extended pain relief beyond the duration of treatment and preserved BMD (Hornstein, 1998). Another regimen of transdermal estradiol 25 μg plus daily 5 mg oral MPA showed that the GnRH agonist remained effective in reducing endometriosis pain (Edmonds, 1996). In addition, traditional COCs may be used effectively as add-back agents.

The extent of BMD decline has been evaluated with add-back therapy. Although bone loss was noted in all patients undergoing GnRH agonist treatment, the extent of loss was lower in the add-back group (Edmonds, 1994). Quality of life is also improved with add-back therapy (Zupi, 2004).

Such therapy can be initiated either immediately with the GnRH agonist or after 3 to 6 months of agonist therapy. However, little benefit is gained by deferring add-back therapy, and patients who receive add-back concurrently with agonist therapy have reduced bone loss (Al-Azemi, 2009; Kiesel, 1996). Supplemental calcium as a 1000-mg total daily dose is recommended along with add-back regimens (American College of Obstetricians and Gynecologists, 2014b).

GnRH Antagonists

GnRH antagonists are a newer category of GnRH analogues capable of suppressing gonadotropin production. Unlike GnRH agonists, GnRH antagonists do not produce an initial release or *flare* of gonadotropins. Thus, suppression of gonadotropins and sex steroid hormones is immediate.

GnRH antagonists are mainly used for suppression of premature ovulation during IVF cycles. They have not been well studied for endometriosis treatment. Küpker and colleagues (2002) evaluated the effect of the antagonist cetrorelix in 15 endometriosis patients. They administered subcutaneous injections of cetrorelix at a dosage of 3 mg weekly for 8 weeks. Patients were symptom free during treatment, and second-look laparoscopy revealed disease regression in 60 percent of study participants. That said, long-term depot forms are not currently available.

Of newer agents, a nonpeptide, orally bioactive GnRH antagonist, elagolix, is undergoing evaluation. One 24-week randomized trial showed similar efficacy between elagolix and DMPA for endometriosis-associated pain (Carr, 2014).

Aromatase Inhibitors

As noted earlier (p. 231), in endometriotic tissue, estrogen may be produced locally through aromatization of circulating androgens. This may clarify postmenopausal endometriosis or may explain cases in which symptoms persist despite conventional treatment. Hormonal strategies described in prior sections target ovarian estrogen production but have little effect on estrogens produced from other sources. In contrast, the aromatase inhibitors (AIs) block aromatase action and estradiol production in both the ovary and extraovarian sites. As a result, estrogen levels are dramatically suppressed, and AIs have hypoestrogenic side-effect profiles similar to those of GnRH agonists (Pavone, 2012). AIs used clinically include anastrozole (Arimidex) and letrozole (Femara).

In addition to hypoestrogenic side effects, a second concern is ovarian cyst formation. As explanation and shown in Figure 20-3 (p. 455), by blocking the conversion of androgens to estrogens in ovarian granulosa cells, AIs reduce the negative feedback at the pituitary–hypothalamus level. This leads to increased GnRH secretion. Resulting elevations in luteinizing hormone (LH) and follicle-stimulating hormone promote increased ovarian follicular development. Therefore, combining AI with a progestins or COCs helps blunt this side effect (Shippen, 2004).

Small studies that combined aromatase inhibitors with NETA or with COCs support this approach for pain relief (Amsterdam, 2005; Ferrero, 2009). However, due to side effects and limited data, such AI combinations are usually prescribed to women after other options for medical or surgical treatment have been exhausted (Dunselman, 2014).

Selective Progesterone-Receptor Modulators

Progestins produce agonist effects upon binding to progesterone receptors. In contrast, progesterone antagonists and selective progesterone-receptor modulators (SPRMs) are agents that vary in their progesterone-receptor binding. Progesterone antagonists universally bind to and inactivate these receptors. SPRMS, depending on their individual pharmacologic profile, may activate or inactive progesterone receptors variably within different tissue types (Chap. 15, p. 364). Currently, these are not used in the United States to treat endometriosis.

Of progesterone antagonists, mifepristone (RU-486; Mifeprex) is FDA-approved solely for early pregnancy termination. Studied in women with endometriosis, mifepristone reduced pelvic pain and extent of endometriosis (Kettel, 1996). However, as a side effect, its antiprogestational effects expose the endometrium to chronic unopposed estrogen. Resulting endometrial changes range from simple endometrial hyperplasia to a new category described as progesterone-receptor-modulator–associated endometrial changes (PAEC) (Mutter, 2008). The clinical significance of PAEC is still unclear.

Of SPRMs, ulipristal acetate is available in the United States for emergency contraception as Ella and in Europe for presurgical treatment of leiomyomas as Esmya. Again, long-term endometrial safety for both eutopic and ectopic endometria is unclear with this SPRM, and this limits its chronic use at this time. Most other SPRMs are still experimental.

Androgens

These drugs are now used as second-line agents for endometriosis due to their androgenic side effects. Of these, danazol is a synthetic 17α-ethinyl testosterone derivative. Its predominant action suppresses the midcycle LH surge to promote chronic anovulation (Floyd, 1980). Danazol occupies receptor sites on sex hormone-binding globulin (SHBG) and thereby increases serum free testosterone levels. It also binds directly to androgen and progesterone receptors. As a result, danazol creates a hypoestrogenic, hyperandrogenic state that induces endometrial atrophy in endometriotic implants (Fedele, 1990). Regarding efficacy, danazol given orally at dosages of 200 mg three times daily proved superior to placebo to diminish endometriotic implants and pelvic pain symptoms after 6 months of therapy (Telimaa, 1987).

The recommended dosage of danazol is 600 to 800 mg orally daily. Unfortunately, significant androgenic side effects develop and include acne, hot flushes, hirsutism, adverse serum lipid profiles, voice deepening (possibly irreversible), elevation of liver enzyme levels, and mood changes. Moreover, due to possible teratogenicity, this medication should be taken in conjunction with effective contraception. Because of its adverse side-effect profile, danazol is prescribed less frequently, and if administered, its duration is limited.

Gestrinone (ethylnorgestrienone; R2323) is an antiprogestational agent prescribed in Europe for endometriosis. It has antiprogestational, antiestrogenic, and androgenic effects. Gestrinone equals the effectiveness of danazol and of GnRH agonists for relief of endometriosis-related pain (Prentice, 2000). Furthermore, during 6 months of treatment, gestrinone was not associated with the bone density loss commonly seen with GnRH agonist use and was more effective in persistently decreasing moderate to severe pelvic pain (Gestrinone Italian Study Group, 1996). Disadvantageously, gestrinone appears to lower high-density lipoprotein (HDL) levels. Gestrinone is administered orally, 2.5 to 10 mg weekly, given daily or three times weekly.

■ Surgical Treatment of Endometriosis-Related Pain

Lesion Removal and Adhesiolysis

Because laparoscopy is the primary method for endometriosis diagnosis, surgical treatment at the time of diagnosis is an attractive option. Numerous studies have examined removal of endometriotic lesions, through either excision or ablation. In one randomized trial, diagnostic laparoscopy alone was compared with laparoscopic endometriotic lesion ablation plus uterine nerve ablation. In the ablation group, 63 percent of women attained significant symptom relief compared with 23 percent in the expectant management group (Jones, 2001).

The optimal method to address endometriotic implants for maximal symptom relief is controversial. First, laser ablation does not appear to be more effective than conventional electrosurgical ablation of endometriosis (Blackwell, 1991). Second, ablation and excision both appear to perform suitably. In one randomized trial, ablation was compared with excision of lesions in women with stage I or II endometriosis. At 6 months, similar reductions in pain scores were found (Wright, 2005). Another study showed no significant difference between ablation and excision at 12 months (Healey, 2010). However, at 5 years, the need for further hormonal or analgesic treatment was greater in the ablation group (Healey, 2014). For deeply infiltrative endometriosis, some authors have advocated radical surgical excision, although well-designed trials are lacking (Chapron, 2004).

Unfortunately, recurrence is common following surgical excision. Jones and associates (2001) demonstrated pain recurrence in 74 percent of patients at a mean time of 73 months postoperatively. The median time for recurrence was 20 months. After surgery for pain-related endometriosis, postoperative medical treatment may be elected to extend pain relief or treat residual pain. For this, the most rigorous evidence supports COCs or the LNG-IUS (Somigliana, 2014).

Adhesiolysis is postulated to effectively treat pain symptoms in women with endometriosis by restoring normal anatomy. However, most studies are poorly designed and retrospective. As a result, a definitive link between adhesions and pelvic pain is unclear (Hammoud, 2004). For example, one randomized trial demonstrated no overall pain relief from adhesiolysis compared with expectant management (Peters, 1992). However, within this study, one woman with severe, dense vascularized bowel adhesions experienced pain relief following adhesiolysis.

Adhesion prevention during endometriosis surgery emphasizes sound surgical techniques described in Chapter 40 (p. 841). Of adhesion-prevention agents available in the United States, small studies show lower adhesions reformation rates with use of the cellulose barrier Interceed in endometriosis cases (Mais, 1995a; Sekiba, 1992). But, as noted by the American Society for Reproductive Medicine (2013), although peritoneal instillates and barriers may reduce postoperative adhesions, this has not translated clinically into improved pain, fertility, or bowel obstruction rates.

Endometrioma Resection

Endometriomas are typically treated surgically to exclude malignancy or treat associated pain. To determine the best technique, total ovarian cystectomy compared against aspiration coupled with cyst wall ablation has been studied. Findings note that cystectomy lowers endometrioma recurrence rates and pain symptoms and improves subsequent spontaneous pregnancy rates (Dan, 2013; Hart, 2008). During surgery, ideally normal ovarian tissue is preserved. Toward this goal, electrosurgical coagulation of bleeding sites should be limited. As alternatives, some have described use of dilute vasopressin or suture (Pergialiotis, 2015; Qiong-Zhen, 2014). Other technical steps are described in Chapter 44 (p. 1015). Despite cystectomy, endometriomas may recur. Liu and coworkers (2007) found an approximately 15 percent recurrence rate at 2 years following initial surgery.

Importantly, women who undergo endometrioma excision may subsequently have a reduced *ovarian reserve,* that is, the capacity to provide ova capable of fertilization (Somigliana, 2012). Additionally, surgery increases risks for adhesion formation. Both effects may diminish future fertility. Accordingly, in a woman who is asymptomatic, has a small endometrioma that displays classic findings, has a known endometriosis diagnosis, and has normal or stable CA125 levels, surveillance is an option (American College of Obstetricians and Gynecologists, 2013, 2014b). This approach may benefit asymptomatic women with recurrent endometriomas, as repeat surgery can again diminish reserve (Ferrero, 2015). Following initial diagnosis of an endometrioma, repeat TVS is recommended 6 to 12 weeks later to exclude a hemorrhagic cyst. Endometriomas may then be sonographically surveilled in asymptomatic women yearly or sooner, at the clinician's discretion (Levine, 2010). The main disadvantage to observation is an inability to exclude ovarian malignancy, and thus patient counseling is essential.

Presacral Neurectomy

For some women, transection of presacral nerves lying within the presacral space may provide relief of chronic pelvic pain (Fig. 38-23, p. 816). Results from a randomized trial revealed significantly greater pain relief at 12 months postoperatively in women treated with presacral neurectomy (PSN) and endometriotic excision compared with that from endometriotic excision alone (86 percent versus 57 percent) (Zullo, 2003). However, all of these women had midline pain. One metaanalysis demonstrated a significant decrease in pelvic pain after PSN compared with that following more conservative procedures, but only in those with midline pain (Proctor, 2005). Neurectomy may be performed laparoscopically, but it is technically challenging. Due to involved nerve disruption, postoperative constipation and voiding dysfunction are common (Huber, 2015). For these reasons, PSN is used in a limited manner and not recommended routinely for management of endometriosis-related pain.

Laparoscopic Uterosacral Nerve Ablation

There is no evidence that laparoscopic uterosacral nerve ablation (LUNA) is effective in treating endometriosis-related pain (Vercellini, 2003a). In a randomized trial of 487 women with chronic pelvic pain lasting longer than 6 months, with or without minimal endometriosis, LUNA did not improve pain, dysmenorrhea, dyspareunia, or quality-of-life scores compared with laparoscopy without pelvic denervation (Daniels, 2009).

Abdominal versus Laparoscopic Approach

All of the surgical procedures listed above can be completed through open or laparoscopic approaches. First, for benign ovarian masses such as endometriomas, strong evidence supports laparoscopy (Mais, 1995b; Yuen, 1997). Laparoscopic treatment of endometrioma carries an associated 5-percent risk for conversion to laparotomy. However, because of its efficacy and low rates of postoperative morbidity, laparoscopy is a preferred route when feasible (Canis, 2003).

For excision of endometriotic implants, studies also demonstrate effectiveness and low morbidity rates with laparoscopy. Moreover, adhesiolysis is preferred via laparoscopy when safe, and laparoscopy leads to less de novo adhesion formation than laparotomy (Gutt, 2004). Laparoscopic presacral neurectomy appears to be as effective as laparotomy (Nezhat, 1992; Redwine, 1991).

Hysterectomy

This procedure is the definitive and most effective therapy for women with endometriosis who do not wish to retain fertility. It is appropriate for women with intractable pain, adnexal masses, or multiple previous conservative therapies or surgeries (American College of Obstetricians and Gynecologists, 2014b). Hysterectomy for patients with endometriosis may suitably be completed laparoscopically, abdominally, or vaginally. However, adhesions and distorted anatomy secondary to endometriosis often makes a laparoscopic or vaginal approach difficult. In addition, the need to remove ovaries may make a vaginal approach less feasible. Accordingly, the choice of procedure will depend on equipment availability, operator experience, and extent of disease.

Oophorectomy. Prior to hysterectomy for endometriosis, oophorectomy is discussed. A general discussion of risks and benefits is found in Chapter 43 (p. 950). Specific to endometriosis,

the benefits of pain relief and reoperation risks are measured against complications of hypoestrogenism. In one study, of those with hysterectomy and bilateral salpingo-oophorectomy (BSO), 10 percent had recurrent chronic pelvic pain and 4 percent required reoperation. Compared with these women, those choosing ovarian conservation had a sixfold greater risk of recurrent pain and an eightfold greater risk of requiring additional surgery (Namnoum, 1995). In a second study, among all those choosing hysterectomy, ovarian conservation doubled the reoperation rate compared with those undergoing BSO (Shakiba, 2008). Moreover, in a subanalysis of those older than 40, ovary conservation lead to a sevenfold greater reoperation rate than BSO. However, in those younger than 40, reoperation rates did not differ whether ovaries were retained or removed. The American College of Obstetricians and Gynecologists (2014b) notes that ovarian conservation can be considered in patients undergoing hysterectomy if ovaries appear normal.

In epidemiologic studies, women with prior endometriosis have slightly increased ovarian cancer rates and higher proportions of clear cell and endometrioid subtypes (Kim, 2014; Pearce, 2012; Somigliana, 2006). That said, consensus guidelines do not recommend management changes in relation to this cancer risk (Dunselman, 2014).

Postoperative Hormone Replacement. Women with surgical menopause are usually younger and would likely benefit from estrogen replacement. Options are discussed in Chapter 22. Although evidence is lacking, some suggest that treatment in these women continue until the time of expected natural menopause.

Unopposed estrogen is appropriate for hypoestrogenic women without a uterus, but disease recurrence has been reported with this therapy in women with severe endometriosis first treated with hysterectomy and BSO (Taylor, 1999). Symptoms required repeat surgery and did not recur with adjuvant combined estrogen and progestin regimens. Additionally, cases of endometrial carcinoma have been reported in women with endometriosis who were treated with unopposed estrogen after hysterectomy and BSO (Reimnitz, 1988; Soliman, 2006). This is rare and may arise from incompletely resected pelvic endometriosis. Therefore, adding a progestin to estrogen replacement therapy can be considered in women with severe endometriosis treated surgically (Moen, 2010). Again, the risks of malignancy are balanced against the adverse lipid changes and breast cancer risks associated with adding progesterone to hormone replacement therapy.

The optimal timing for hormone replacement initiation following hysterectomy with BSO is support by limited data. One small study showed no significant differences in postoperative recurrent pain rates whether hormones were initiated immediately after surgery or were delayed (Hickman, 1998).

■ Treatment of Endometriosis-Related Infertility

For an asymptomatic woman with infertility, laparoscopy solely to exclude endometriosis is unwarranted (American Society for Reproductive Medicine, 2012). For those with endometriosis-related pain undergoing medical therapy, treatment does not raise fecundity (Hughes, 2007).

For women with infertility and minimal to mild endometriosis, surgical ablation has been suggested to be beneficial, although the effect appears small (Marcoux, 1997). However, other researchers did not report a fertility benefit to surgical ablation for mild to moderate endometriosis (Parazzini, 1999). A metaanalysis of these two studies did demonstrate an advantage for laparoscopic surgery compared with diagnostic laparoscopy (Jacobson, 2010).

Moderate to severe endometriosis may be treated with surgery to restore normal anatomy and tubal function. However, well-designed trials examining the role of surgery for subfertility in women with severe endometriosis are limited (Crosignani, 1996). In infertile women with stage III/IV endometriosis, clinicians can consider operative laparoscopy, instead of expectant management, to increase spontaneous pregnancy rates (Dunselman, 2014). However, after initial unsuccessful surgery for infertility, IVF is preferable to reoperation (Pagidas, 1996).

Alternatively, patients with endometriosis and infertility are candidates for fertility treatments such as controlled ovarian hyperstimulation, intrauterine insemination, and IVF (Chap. 20, p. 449). Logically, age and disease stage factor into treatment decisions.

REFERENCES

Adamson GD: Endometriosis Fertility Index: is it better than the present staging systems? Curr Opin Obstet Gynecol 25(3):186, 2013

Adamson GD, Pasta DJ: Endometriosis fertility index: the new, validated endometriosis staging system. Fertil Steril 94(5):1609, 2010

Alabiso G, Alio L, Arena S, et al: How to manage bowel endometriosis: the ETIC approach. J Minim Invasive Gynecol 22(4):517, 2015

Al-Azemi M, Jones G, Sirkeci F, et al: Immediate and delayed add-back hormonal replacement therapy during ultra long GnRH agonist treatment of chronic cyclical pelvic pain. BJOG 116:1646, 2009

Alifano M: Catamenial pneumothorax. Curr Opin Pulm Med 16(4):381, 2010

Allen C, Hopewell S, Prentice A, et al: Nonsteroidal anti-inflammatory drugs for pain in women with endometriosis. Cochrane Database Syst Rev 2:CD004753, 2009

American College of Obstetricians and Gynecologists: Depot medroxyprogesterone acetate and bone effects. Committee Opinion No. 602, June 2014a

American College of Obstetricians and Gynecologists: Management of adnexal masses. Practice Bulletin No. 83, July 2007, Reaffirmed 2013

American College of Obstetricians and Gynecologists: Management of endometriosis. Practice Bulletin No. 114, July 2010, Reaffirmed 2014b

American Society for Reproductive Medicine: Endometriosis and infertility: a committee opinion. Fertil Steril 98(3):591, 2012

American Society for Reproductive Medicine: Revised American Society for Reproductive Medicine classification of endometriosis: 1996. Fertil Steril 67:817, 1997

American Society for Reproductive Medicine: Treatment of pelvic pain associated with endometriosis: a committee opinion. Fertil Steril 101(4):927, 2014

Amsterdam LL, Gentry W, Jobanputra S, et al: Anastrozole and oral contraceptives: a novel treatment for endometriosis. Fertil Steril 84:300, 2005

Antonelli A, Simeone C, Zani D, et al: Clinical aspects and surgical treatment of urinary tract endometriosis: our experience with 31 cases. Eur Urol 49:1093, 2006

Arici A, Oral E, Attar E, et al: Monocyte chemotactic protein-1 concentration in peritoneal fluid of women with endometriosis and its modulation of expression in mesothelial cells. Fertil Steril 67:1065, 1997

Arici A, Seli E, Zeyneloglu HB, et al: Interleukin-8 induces proliferation of endometrial stromal cells: a potential autocrine growth factor. J Clin Endocrinol Metab 83:1201, 1998

As-Sanie S, Harris RE, Harte SE, et al: Increased pressure pain sensitivity in women with chronic pelvic pain. Obstet Gynecol 122(5):1047, 2013

Attia GR, Zeitoun K, Edwards D, et al: Progesterone receptor isoform A but not B is expressed in endometriosis. J Clin Endocrinol Metab 85:2897, 2000

Bajaj P, Bajaj P, Madsen H, et al: Endometriosis is associated with central sensitization: a psychophysical controlled study. J Pain 4(7):372, 2003

Balasch J, Creus M, Fabregues F, et al: Visible and non-visible endometriosis at laparoscopy in fertile and infertile women and in patients with chronic pelvic pain: a prospective study. Hum Reprod 11:387, 1996

Ballard KD, Seaman HE, de Vries CS, et al: Can symptomatology help in the diagnosis of endometriosis? Findings from a national case–control study—part 1. BJOG 115(11):1382, 2008

Barbieri RL: Hormone treatment of endometriosis: the estrogen threshold hypothesis. Am J Obstet Gynecol 166:740, 1992

Barcena de Arellano ML, Arnold J, Vercellino F, et al: Overexpression of nerve growth factor in peritoneal fluid from women with endometriosis may promote neurite outgrowth in endometriotic lesions. Fertil Steril 95(3):1123, 2011

Batt RE, Yeh J: Müllerianosis: four developmental (embryonic) mullerian diseases. Reprod Sci 20(9):1030, 2013

Bazot M, Lafont C, Rouzier R, et al: Diagnostic accuracy of physical examination, transvaginal sonography, rectal endoscopic sonography, and magnetic resonance imaging to diagnose deep infiltrating endometriosis. Fertil Steril 92(6):1825, 2009

Bhatt S, Kocakoc E, Dogra VS: Endometriosis: sonographic spectrum. Ultrasound Q 22(4):273, 2006

Blackwell RE: Applications of laser surgery in gynecology. Hype or high tech? Surg Clin North Am 71:1005, 1991

Bourdel N, Alves J, Pickering G, et al: Systematic review of endometriosis pain assessment: how to choose a scale? Hum Reprod Update 21(1):136, 2015

Braun DP, Muriana R, Gebel H, et al: Monocyte-mediated enhancement of endometrial cell proliferation in women with endometriosis. Fertil Steril 61:78, 1994

Brown J, Pan A, Hart RJ: Gonadotrophin-releasing hormone analogues for pain associated with endometriosis. Cochrane Database Syst Rev 12:CD008475, 2010

Buck Louis GM, Hediger ML, Peterson CM, Incidence of endometriosis by study population and diagnostic method: the ENDO study. Fertil Steril 96(2):360, 2011

Bulun SE: Endometriosis. N Engl J Med 360(3):268, 2009

Bulun SE, Monsavais D, Pavone ME, et al: Role of estrogen receptor-β in endometriosis. Semin Reprod Med 30(1):39, 2012

Burney RO: The genetics and biochemistry of endometriosis. Curr Opin Obstet Gynecol 25(4):280, 2013

Canis M, Mage G, Wattiez A, et al: The ovarian endometrioma: why is it so poorly managed? Laparoscopic treatment of large ovarian endometrioma: why such a long learning curve? Hum Reprod 18:5, 2003

Carr B, Dmowski WP, O'Brien C, et al: Elagolix, an oral GnRH antagonist, versus subcutaneous depot medroxyprogesterone acetate for the treatment of endometriosis: effects on bone mineral density. Reprod Sci 21(11):1341, 2014

Chapron C, Chopin N, Borghese B, et al: Surgical management of deeply infiltrating endometriosis: an update. Ann NY Acad Sci 1034:326, 2004

Chapron C, Dubuisson JB, Pansini V, et al: Routine clinical examination is not sufficient for diagnosing and locating deeply infiltrating endometriosis. J Am Assoc Gynecol Laparosc 9:115, 2002

Cho S, Park SH, Choi YS, et al: Expression of cyclooxygenase-2 in eutopic endometrium and ovarian endometriotic tissue in women with severe endometriosis. Gynecol Obstet Invest 69:93, 2010

Crosignani PG, Vercellini P, Biffignandi F, et al: Laparoscopy versus laparotomy in conservative surgical treatment for severe endometriosis. Fertil Steril 66(5):706, 1996

Dalsgaard T, Hjordt Hansen MV, Hartwell D, et al: Reproductive prognosis in daughters of women with and without endometriosis. Hum Reprod 28(8):2284, 2013

Dan H, Limin F: Laparoscopic ovarian cystectomy versus fenestration/coagulation or laser vaporization for the treatment of endometriomas: a meta-analysis of randomized controlled trials. Gynecol Obstet Invest 76(2):75, 2013

Daniels J, Gray R, Hills RK, et al: Laparoscopic uterosacral nerve ablation for alleviating chronic pelvic pain: a randomized controlled trial. JAMA 302:955, 2009

D'Hooghe TM: Clinical relevance of the baboon as a model for the study of endometriosis. Fertil Steril 68:613, 1997

D'Hooghe TM, Bambra CS, Raeymaekers BM, et al: The cycle pregnancy rate is normal in baboons with stage I endometriosis but decreased in primates with stage II and stage III-IV disease. Fertil Steril 66:809, 1996

D'Hooghe TM, Debrock S, Hill JA, et al: Endometriosis and subfertility: is the relationship resolved? Semin Reprod Med 21:243, 2003

Ding Y, Zhu J: A retrospective review of abdominal wall endometriosis in Shanghai, China. Int J Gynaecol Obstet 121(1):41, 2013

Dunselman GA, Vermeulen N, Becker C, et al: ESHRE guideline: management of women with endometriosis. Hum Reprod 29(3):400, 2014

Ecker AM, Donnellan NM, Shepherd JP, et al: Abdominal wall endometriosis: 12 years of experience at a large academic institution. Am J Obstet Gynecol 211(4):363.e1, 2014

Edmonds DK: Add-back therapy in the treatment of endometriosis: the European experience. BJOG 103(Suppl 14):10, 1996

Edmonds DK, Howell R: Can hormone replacement therapy be used during medical therapy of endometriosis? BJOG 101 (Suppl 10):24, 1994

Eskenazi B, Warner M, Bonsignore L, et al: Validation study of nonsurgical diagnosis of endometriosis. Fertil Steril 76:929, 2001

Exacoustos C, Malzoni M, Di Giovanni A, et al: Ultrasound mapping system for the surgical management of deep infiltrating endometriosis. Fertil Steril 102(1):143, 2014a

Exacoustos C, Manganaro L, Zupi E: Imaging for the evaluation of endometriosis and adenomyosis. Best Pract Res Clin Obstet Gynaecol 28(5):655, 2014b

Fauconnier A, Chapron C, Dubuisson JB, et al: Relation between pain symptoms and the anatomic location of deep infiltrating endometriosis. Fertil Steril 78:719, 2002

Fedele L, Bianchi S, Bocciolone L, et al: Pain symptoms associated with endometriosis. Obstet Gynecol 79:767, 1992

Fedele L, Marchini M, Bianchi S, et al: Endometrial patterns during danazol and buserelin therapy for endometriosis: comparative structural and ultrastructural study. Obstet Gynecol 76:79, 1990

Ferrero S, Camerini G, Seracchioli R, et al: Letrozole combined with norethisterone acetate compared with norethisterone acetate alone in the treatment of pain symptoms caused by endometriosis. Hum Reprod 24(12):3033, 2009

Ferrero S, Esposito F, Abbamonte LH, et al: Quality of sex life in women with endometriosis and deep dyspareunia. Fertil Steril 83:573, 2005

Ferrero S, Scala C, Racca A, et al: Second surgery for recurrent unilateral endometriomas and impact on ovarian reserve: a case-control study. Fertil Steril 103(5):1236, 2015

Floyd WS: Danazol: endocrine and endometrial effects. Int J Fertil 25:75, 1980

Gabriel B, Nassif J, Trompoukis P, et al: Prevalence and management of urinary tract endometriosis: a clinical case series. Urology 78(6):1269, 2011

Gallo MF, Nanda K, Grimes DA, et al: 20 μg versus >20 μg estrogen combined oral contraceptives for contraception. Cochrane Database Syst Rev 8:CD003989, 2013

Gestrinone Italian Study Group: Gestrinone versus a gonadotropin-releasing hormone agonist for the treatment of pelvic pain associated with endometriosis: a multicenter, randomized, double-blind study. Fertil Steril 66:911, 1996

Gleicher N, Dmowski WP, Siegel I, et al: Lymphocyte subsets in endometriosis. Obstet Gynecol 63:463, 1984

Gurates B, Bulun SE: Endometriosis: the ultimate hormonal disease. Semin Reprod Med 21:125, 2003

Gutt CN, Oniu T, Schemmer P, et al: Fewer adhesions induced by laparoscopic surgery? Surg Endosc 18:898, 2004

Guzick DS, Huang LS, Broadman BA, et al: Randomized trial of leuprolide versus continuous oral contraceptives in the treatment of endometriosis-associated pelvic pain. Fertil Steril 95(5):1568, 2011

Guzick DS, Silliman NP, Adamson GD, et al: Prediction of pregnancy in infertile women based on the American Society for Reproductive Medicine's revised classification of endometriosis. Fertil Steril 67:822, 1997

Haas D, Chvatal R, Habelsberger A, et al: Comparison of revised American Fertility Society and ENZIAN staging: a critical evaluation of classifications of endometriosis on the basis of our patient population. Fertil Steril 95(5):1574, 2011

Haga T, Kataoka H, Ebana H, et al: Thoracic endometriosis-related pneumothorax distinguished from primary spontaneous pneumothorax in females. Lung 192(4):583, 2014

Halme J, Hammond MG, Hulka JF, et al: Retrograde menstruation in healthy women and in patients with endometriosis. Obstet Gynecol 64:151, 1984

Hammoud A, Gago LA, Diamond MP: Adhesions in patients with chronic pelvic pain: a role for adhesiolysis? Fertil Steril 82:1483, 2004

Harb H, Gallos I, Chu J, et al: The effect of endometriosis on in vitro fertilisation outcome: a systematic review and meta-analysis. BJOG 120, 1308, 2013

Haney AF, Muscato J, Weinberg JB: Peritoneal fluid cell populations in infertility patients. Fertil Steril 35:696, 1981

Harada T, Momoeda M, Taketani Y, et al: Dienogest is as effective as intranasal buserelin acetate for the relief of pain symptoms associated with endometriosis—a randomized, double blind, multicentre trial. Fertil Steril 91(3):675, 2009

Harada T, Momoeda M, Taketani Y, et al: Low-dose oral contraceptive pill for dysmenorrhea associated with endometriosis: a placebo-controlled, double-blind, randomized trial. Fertil Steril 90:1583, 2008

Hart RJ, Hickey M, Maouris P, Buckett W. Excisional surgery versus ablative surgery for ovarian endometriomata. Cochrane Database Syst Rev 2:CD004992, 2008

Healey M, Ang WC, Cheng C: Surgical treatment of endometriosis: a prospective randomized double-blinded trial comparing excision and ablation. Fertil Steril 94(7):2536, 2010

Healey M, Cheng C, Kaur H: To excise or ablate endometriosis? A prospective randomized double-blinded trial after 5-year follow-up. J Minim Invasive Gynecol 21(6):999, 2014

Hickman TN, Namnoum AB, Hinton EL, et al: Timing of estrogen replacement therapy following hysterectomy with oophorectomy for endometriosis. Obstet Gynecol 91(5 Pt 1):673, 1998

Hinterholzer S, Riss D, Brustmann H: Symptomatic large bowel endometriosis in a woman with a hormonal intrauterine device: a case report. J Reprod Med 52:1055, 2007

Ho HN, Chao KH, Chen HF, et al: Peritoneal natural killer cytotoxicity and CD25+ CD3+ lymphocyte subpopulation are decreased in women with stage III-IV endometriosis. Hum Reprod 10:2671, 1995

Hornstein MD, Harlow BL, Thomas PP, et al: Use of a new CA 125 assay in the diagnosis of endometriosis. Hum Reprod 10:932, 1995a

Hornstein MD, Surrey ES, Weisberg GW, et al: Leuprolide acetate depot and hormonal add-back in endometriosis: a 12-month study. Lupron Add-Back Study Group. Obstet Gynecol 91:16, 1998

Hornstein MD, Yuzpe AA, Burry KA, et al: Prospective randomized double-blind trial of 3 versus 6 months of nafarelin therapy for endometriosis associated pelvic pain. Fertil Steril 63:955, 1995b

Houston DE, Noller KL, Melton LJ III, et al: Incidence of pelvic endometriosis in Rochester, Minnesota, 1970–1979. Am J Epidemiol 125:959, 1987

Howard FM: The role of laparoscopy in the chronic pelvic pain patient. Clin Obstet Gynecol 46(4):749, 2003

Hsu AL, Sinaii N, Segars J, et al: Relating pelvic pain location to surgical findings of endometriosis. Obstet Gynecol 118(2 Pt 1):223, 2011

Huber SA, Northington GM, Karp DR: Bowel and bladder dysfunction following surgery within the presacral space: an overview of neuroanatomy, function, and dysfunction. Int Urogynecol J 26(7):941, 2015

Hudelist G, English J, Thomas AE, et al: Diagnostic accuracy of transvaginal ultrasound for non-invasive diagnosis of bowel endometriosis: systematic review and meta-analysis. Ultrasound Obstet Gynecol 37(3):257, 2011

Hughes E, Brown J, Collins JJ, et al: Ovulation suppression for endometriosis. Cochrane Database Syst Rev 3:CD000155, 2007

Itoh H, Kishore AH, Lindqvist A, et al: Transforming growth factor β1 (TGFβ1) and progesterone regulate matrix metalloproteinases (MMP) in human endometrial stromal cells. J Clin Endocrinol Metab 97:888, 2012

Jacobson TZ, Duffy JM, Barlow D, et al: Laparoscopic surgery for subfertility associated with endometriosis. Cochrane Database Syst Rev 1:CD001398, 2010

Jacoby VL, Fujimoto VY, Giudice LC, et al: Racial and ethnic disparities in benign gynecologic conditions and associated surgeries. Am J Obstet Gynecol 202(6):514, 2010

Jansen RP, Russell P: Nonpigmented endometriosis: clinical, laparoscopic, and pathologic definition. Am J Obstet Gynecol 155:1154, 1986

Janssen EB, Rijkers AC, Hoppenbrouwers K, et al: Prevalence of endometriosis diagnosed by laparoscopy in adolescents with dysmenorrhea or chronic pelvic pain: a systematic review. Hum Reprod Update 19(5):570, 2013

Jerman LF, Hey-Cunningham AJ: The role of the lymphatic system in endometriosis: a comprehensive review of the literature. Biol Reprod 92(3):64, 2015

Jones KD, Haines P, Sutton CJ: Long-term follow-up of a controlled trial of laser laparoscopy for pelvic pain. J Soc Laparoendosc Surg 5:111, 2001

Jones SC: Relative thromboembolic risks associated with COX-2 inhibitors. Ann Pharmacother 39:1249, 2005

Kaufman LC, Smyrk TC, Levy MJ, et al: Symptomatic intestinal endometriosis requiring surgical resection: clinical presentation and preoperative diagnosis. Am J Gastroenterol 106(7):1325, 2011

Kauppila A, Rönnberg L: Naproxen sodium in dysmenorrhea secondary to endometriosis. Obstet Gynecol 65(3):379, 1985

Kettel LM, Murphy AA, Morales AJ, et al: Treatment of endometriosis with the antiprogesterone mifepristone (RU486). Fertil Steril 65:23, 1996

Khorram O, Taylor RN, Ryan IP, et al: Peritoneal fluid concentrations of the cytokine RANTES correlate with the severity of endometriosis. Am J Obstet Gynecol 169:1545, 1993

Kiesel L, Schweppe KW, Sillem M, et al: Should add-back therapy for endometriosis be deferred for optimal results? BJOG 103(Suppl 14):15, 1996

Kim HS, Kim TH, Chung HH, et al: Risk and prognosis of ovarian cancer in women with endometriosis: a meta-analysis. Br J Cancer 110:1878, 2014

Kim YA, Kim MR, Lee JH, et al: Gonadotropin-releasing hormone agonist reduces aromatase cytochrome P450 and cyclooxygenase-2 in ovarian endometrioma and eutopic endometrium of patients with endometriosis. Gynecol Obstet Invest 68:73, 2009

Kitawaki J, Noguchi T, Amatsu T, et al: Expression of aromatase cytochrome P450 protein and messenger ribonucleic acid in human endometriotic and adenomyotic tissues but not in normal endometrium. Biol Reprod 57:514, 1997

Knabben L, Imboden S, Fellmann B, et al: Urinary tract endometriosis in patients with deep infiltrating endometriosis: prevalence, symptoms, management, and proposal for a new clinical classification. Fertil Steril 103(1): 147, 2015

Koger KE, Shatney CH, Hodge K, et al: Surgical scar endometrioma. Surg Gynecol Obstet 177:243, 1993

Koninckx PR, Meuleman C, Oosterlynck D, et al: Diagnosis of deep endometriosis by clinical examination during menstruation and plasma CA-125 concentration. Fertil Steril 65:280, 1996

Koninckx PR, Oosterlynck D, D'Hooghe T, et al: Deeply infiltrating endometriosis is a disease whereas mild endometriosis could be considered a nondisease. Ann NY Acad Sci 734:333, 1994

Koninckx PR, Ussia A, Adamyan L, et al: Deep endometriosis: definition, diagnosis, and treatment. Fertil Steril 98(3):564, 2012

Küpker W, Felberbaum RE, Krapp M, et al: Use of GnRH antagonists in the treatment of endometriosis. Reprod Biomed Online 5:12, 2002

Kyama CM, Overbergh L, Debrock S, et al: Increased peritoneal and endometrial gene expression of biologically relevant cytokines and growth factors during the menstrual phase in women with endometriosis. Fertil Steril 85(6):1667, 2006

Lafay Pillet MC, Huchon C, Santulli P, et al: A clinical score can predict associated deep infiltrating endometriosis before surgery for an endometrioma. Hum Reprod 29(8):1666, 2014

Levine D, Brown DL, Andreotti RF, et al: Management of asymptomatic ovarian and other adnexal cysts imaged at US: Society of Radiologists in Ultrasound Consensus Conference Statement. Ultrasound Q 26(3):121, 2010

Ling FW: Randomized controlled trial of depot leuprolide in patients with chronic pelvic pain and clinically suspected endometriosis. Obstet Gynecol 93:51, 1999

Liu X, Yuan L, Shen F, et al: Patterns of and risk factors for recurrence in women with ovarian endometriomas. Obstet Gynecol 109(6):1411, 2007

Macer ML, Taylor HS: Endometriosis and infertility: a review of the pathogenesis and treatment of endometriosis-associated infertility. Obstet Gynecol Clin North Am 39(4):535, 2012

Mahmood TA, Templeton A: Prevalence and genesis of endometriosis. Hum Reprod 6(4):544, 1991

Mais V, Ajossa S, Marongiu D, et al: Reduction of adhesion reformation after laparoscopic endometriosis surgery: a randomized trial with an oxidized regenerated cellulose absorbable barrier. Obstet Gynecol 86(4 Pt 1):512, 1995a

Mais V, Ajossa S, Piras B, et al: Treatment of nonendometriotic benign adnexal cysts: a randomized comparison of laparoscopy and laparotomy. Obstet Gynecol 86:770, 1995b

Malinak LR, Buttram VC Jr, Elias S, et al: Heritage aspects of endometriosis. II. Clinical characteristics of familial endometriosis. Am J Obstet Gynecol 137:332, 1980

Marcoux S, Maheux R, Berube S: Laparoscopic surgery in infertile women with minimal or mild endometriosis. Canadian Collaborative Group on Endometriosis. N Engl J Med 337:217, 1997

Marjoribanks J, Proctor M, Farquhar C, et al: Nonsteroidal anti-inflammatory drugs for dysmenorrhoea. Cochrane Database Syst Rev 1:CD001751, 2010

Markham SM, Carpenter SE, et al: Extrapelvic endometriosis. Obstet Gynecol Clin North Am 16:193, 1989

Marsh EE, Laufer MR: Endometriosis in premenarcheal girls who do not have an associated obstructive anomaly. Fertil Steril 83(3):758, 2005

Mathur S, Peress MR, Williamson HO, et al: Autoimmunity to endometrium and ovary in endometriosis. Clin Exp Immunol 50:259, 1982

Matorras R, Rodriguez F, Pijoan JI, et al: Women who are not exposed to spermatozoa and infertile women have similar rates of stage I endometriosis. Fertil Steril 76:923, 2001

May KE, Conduit-Hulbert SA, Villar J, et al: Peripheral biomarkers of endometriosis: a systematic review. Hum Reprod Update 16(6):651, 2010

McKinnon B, Bersinger NA, Wotzkow C, et al: Endometriosis-associated nerve fibers, peritoneal fluid cytokine concentrations, and pain in endometriotic lesions from different locations. Fertil Steril 97(2):373, 2012

McLaren J, Prentice A, Charnock-Jones DS, et al: Vascular endothelial growth factor is produced by peritoneal fluid macrophages in endometriosis and is regulated by ovarian steroids. J Clin Invest 98:482, 1996

Mechsner S, Weichbrodt M, Riedlinger WF, et al: Estrogen and progestogen receptor positive endometriotic lesions and disseminated cells in pelvic sentinel lymph nodes of patients with deep infiltrating rectovaginal endometriosis: a pilot study. Hum Reprod 23(10):2202, 2008

Meuleman C, Vandenabeele B, Fieuws S, et al: High prevalence of endometriosis in infertile women with normal ovulation and normospermic partners. Fertil Steril 92:68, 2009

Milone M, Mollo A, Musella M, et al: Role of colonoscopy in the diagnostic work up of bowel endometriosis. World J Gastroenterol 21(16):4997, 2015

Moen MH, Rees M, Brincat M, et al: EMAS position statement: managing the menopause in women with a past history of endometriosis. Maturitas 67(1):94, 2010

Moen MH, Stokstad T: A long-term follow-up study of women with asymptomatic endometriosis diagnosed incidentally at sterilization. Fertil Steril 78(4):773, 2002

Mol BW, Bayram N, Lijmer JG, et al: The performance of CA-125 measurement in the detection of endometriosis: a meta-analysis. Fertil Steril 70:1101, 1998

Moore J, Copley S, Morris J, et al: A systematic review of the accuracy of ultrasound in the diagnosis of endometriosis. Ultrasound Obstet Gynecol 20:630, 2002

Moore JG, Binstock MA, et al: The clinical implications of retroperitoneal endometriosis. Am J Obstet Gynecol 158:1291, 1988

Mori H, Sawairi M, Nakagawa M, et al: Peritoneal fluid interleukin-1 beta and tumor necrosis factor in patients with benign gynecologic disease. Am J Reprod Immunol 26:62, 1991

Mostafa HA, Saad JH, Nadeem Z, et al: Rectus abdominis endometriosis. A descriptive analysis of 10 cases concerning this rare occurrence. Saudi Med J 34(10):1035, 2013

Mourra N, Cortez A, Bennis M, et al: The groin: an unusual location of endometriosis—a multi-institutional clinicopathological study. J Clin Pathol 68(7):579, 2015

Muneyyirci-Delale O, Karacan M: Effect of norethindrone acetate in the treatment of symptomatic endometriosis. Int J Fertil Womens Med 43:24, 1998

Mutter GL, Bergeron C, Deligdisch L, et al: The spectrum of endometrial pathology induced by progesterone receptor modulators. Mod Pathol 21(5):591, 2008

Namnoum AB, Hickman TN, Goodman SB, et al: Incidence of symptom recurrence after hysterectomy for endometriosis. Fertil Steril 64:898, 1995

Nezhat C, Nezhat F: A simplified method of laparoscopic presacral neurectomy for the treatment of central pelvic pain due to endometriosis. BJOG 99:659, 1992

Nisolle M, Donnez J: Peritoneal endometriosis, ovarian endometriosis, and adenomyotic nodules of the rectovaginal septum are three different entities. Fertil Steril 68:585, 1997

Noble LS, Takayama K, Zeitoun KM, et al: Prostaglandin E2 stimulates aromatase expression in endometriosis-derived stromal cells. J Clin Endocrinol Metab 82:600, 1997

Odukoya OA, Wheatcroft N, Weetman AP, et al: The prevalence of endometrial immunoglobulin G antibodies in patients with endometriosis. Hum Reprod 10:1214, 1995

Olive DL, Stohs GF, Metzger DA, et al: Expectant management and hydrotubations in the treatment of endometriosis-associated infertility. Fertil Steril 44:35, 1985a

Olive DL, Weinberg JB, Haney AF: Peritoneal macrophages and infertility: the association between cell number and pelvic pathology. Fertil Steril 44:772, 1985b

Opoku-Anane J, Laufer MR: Prevalence of endometriosis in adolescent girls with chronic pelvic pain not responding to conventional therapy. Have we underestimated? J Pediatr Adolesc Gynecol 25(2):e50, 2012

Orwoll ES, Yuzpe AA, Burry KA, et al: Nafarelin therapy in endometriosis: long-term effects on bone mineral density. Am J Obstet Gynecol 171:1221, 1994

Pagidas K, Falcone T, Hemmings R, et al: Comparison of reoperation for moderate (stage III) and severe (stage IV) endometriosis-related infertility with in vitro fertilization-embryo transfer. Fertil Steril 65:791, 1996

Parazzini F: Ablation of lesions or no treatment in minimal-mild endometriosis in infertile women: a randomized trial. Gruppo Italiano per lo Studio dell'Endometriosi. Hum Reprod 14:1332, 1999

Pavone ME, Bulun SE: Aromatase inhibitors for the treatment of endometriosis. Fertil Steril 98(6):1370, 2012

Pearce CL, Templeman C, Rossing MA, et al: Association between endometriosis and risk of histological subtypes of ovarian cancer: a pooled analysis of case-control studies. Lancet Oncol 13(4):385, 2012

Pergialiotis V, Prodromidou A, Frountzas M, et al: The effect of bipolar electrocoagulation during ovarian cystectomy on ovarian reserve: a systematic review. Am J Obstet Gynecol April 13, 2015 [Epub ahead of print]

Peters AA, Trimbos-Kemper GC, Admiraal C, et al: A randomized clinical trial on the benefit of adhesiolysis in patients with intraperitoneal adhesions and chronic pelvic pain. BJOG 99:59, 1992

Peterson CM, Johnstone EB, Hammoud AO, et al: Risk factors associated with endometriosis: importance of study population for characterizing disease in the ENDO Study. Am J Obstet Gynecol 208(6):451.e1, 2013

Petta CA, Ferriani RA, Abrao MS, et al: Randomized clinical trial of a levonorgestrel-releasing intrauterine system and a depot GnRH analogue for the treatment of chronic pelvic pain in women with endometriosis. Hum Reprod 20:1993, 2005

Possover M, Schneider T, Henle KP: Laparoscopic therapy for endometriosis and vascular entrapment of sacral plexus. Fertil Steril 95(2):756, 2011

Prentice A, Deary AJ, Bland E: Progestagens and anti-progestagens for pain associated with endometriosis. Cochrane Database Syst Rev 2:CD002122, 2000

Proctor ML, Latthe PM, Farquhar CM, et al: Surgical interruption of pelvic nerve pathways for primary and secondary dysmenorrhoea. Cochrane Database Syst Rev 4:CD001896, 2005

Qiong-Zhen R, Ge Y, Deng Y, et al: Effect of vasopressin injection technique in laparoscopic excision of bilateral ovarian endometriomas on ovarian reserve: prospective randomized study. J Minim Invasive Gynecol 21(2):266, 2014

Redwine DB: Conservative laparoscopic excision of endometriosis by sharp dissection: life table analysis of reoperation and persistent or recurrent disease. Fertil Steril 56:628, 1991

Reimnitz C, Brand E, Nieberg RK, et al: Malignancy arising in endometriosis associated with unopposed estrogen replacement. Obstet Gynecol 71:444, 1988

Rodriguez-Escudero FJ, Neyro JL, Corcostegui B, et al: Does minimal endometriosis reduce fecundity? Fertil Steril 50:522, 1988

Roman H, Bridoux V, Tuech JJ, et al: Bowel dysfunction before and after surgery for endometriosis. Am J Obstet Gynecol 209(6):524, 2013

Rousset P, Rousset-Jablonski C, Alifano M, et al: Thoracic endometriosis syndrome: CT and MRI features. Clin Radiol 69(3):323, 2014

Rousset-Jablonski C, Alifano M, Plu-Bureau G, et al: Catamenial pneumothorax and endometriosis-related pneumothorax: clinical features and risk factors. Hum Reprod 26(9):2322, 2011

Ruffo G, Crippa S, Sartori A, et al: Management of rectosigmoid obstruction due to severe bowel endometriosis. Updates Surg 66(1):59, 2014a

Ruffo G, Scopelliti F, Manzoni A, et al: Long-term outcome after laparoscopic bowel resections for deep infiltrating endometriosis: a single-center experience after 900 cases. Biomed Res Int 2014:463058, 2014b

Saha R, Pettersson HJ, Svedberg P, et al: The heritability of endometriosis. Fertil Steril July 22, 2015 [Epub ahead of print]

Sampson JA: Peritoneal endometriosis due to menstrual dissemination of endometrial tissue into the peritoneal cavity. Am J Obstet Gynecol 14:442, 1927

Sanfilippo JS, Wakim NG, Schikler KN, et al: Endometriosis in association with uterine anomaly. Am J Obstet Gynecol 154:39, 1986

Santulli P, Streuli I, Melonio I, et al: Increased serum cancer antigen-125 is a marker for severity of deep endometriosis. J Minim Invasive Gynecol 22(2):275, 2015

Satyaswaroop PG, Wartell DJ, Mortel R: Distribution of progesterone receptor, estradiol dehydrogenase, and 20 alpha-dihydroprogesterone dehydrogenase activities in human endometrial glands and stroma: progestin induction of steroid dehydrogenase activities in vitro is restricted to the glandular epithelium. Endocrinology 111:743, 1982

Schenken RS, Asch RH: Surgical induction of endometriosis in the rabbit: effects on fertility and concentrations of peritoneal fluid prostaglandins. Fertil Steril 34:581, 1980

Schlaff WD, Carson SA, Luciano A, et al: Subcutaneous injection of depot medroxyprogesterone acetate compared with leuprolide acetate in the treatment of endometriosis-associated pain. Fertil Steril 85(2):314, 2006

Sekiba K: Use of Interceed(TC7) absorbable adhesion barrier to reduce postoperative adhesion reformation in infertility and endometriosis surgery. The Obstetrics and Gynecology Adhesion Prevention Committee. Obstet Gynecol 79(4):518, 1992

Seli E, Arici A: Endometriosis: interaction of immune and endocrine systems. Semin Reprod Med 21:135, 2003

Seracchioli R, Mabrouk M, Montanari G, et al: Conservative laparoscopic management of urinary tract endometriosis (UTE): surgical outcome and long-term follow-up. Fertil Steril 94(3):856, 2010

Shah DK, Correia KF, Vitonis AF, et al: Body size and endometriosis: results from 20 years of follow-up within the Nurses' Health Study II prospective cohort. Hum Reprod 28(7):1783, 2013

Shakiba K, Bena JF, McGill KM, et al: Surgical treatment of endometriosis: a 7-year follow-up on the requirement for further surgery. Obstet Gynecol 111(6):1285, 2008

Shippen ER, West WJ Jr: Successful treatment of severe endometriosis in two premenopausal women with an aromatase inhibitor. Fertil Steril 81(5):1395, 2004

Signorile PG, Baldi F, Bussani R, et al: Embryologic origin of endometriosis: analysis of 101 human female fetuses. J Cell Physiol 227(4):1653, 2012

Soliman NF, Hillard TC: Hormone replacement therapy in women with past history of endometriosis. Climacteric 9(5):325, 2006

Somigliana E, Berlanda N, Benaglia L, et al: Surgical excision of endometriomas and ovarian reserve: a systematic review on serum antimüllerian hormone level modifications. Fertil Steril 98(6):1531, 2012

Somigliana E, Vercellini P, Vigano P, et al: Postoperative medical therapy after surgical treatment of endometriosis: from adjuvant therapy to tertiary prevention. J Minim Invasive Gynecol 21(3):328, 2014

Somigliana E, Vigano P, Parazzini F, et al: Association between endometriosis and cancer: a comprehensive review and a critical analysis of clinical and epidemiological evidence. Gynecol Oncol 101:331, 2006

Steele RW, Dmowski WP, Marmer DJ: Immunologic aspects of human endometriosis. Am J Reprod Immunol 6:33, 1984

Stilley JA, Birt JA, Sharpe-Timms KL: Cellular and molecular basis for endometriosis-associated infertility. Cell Tissue Res 349(3):849, 2012

Strathy JH, Molgaard CA, Coulam CB, et al: Endometriosis and infertility: a laparoscopic study of endometriosis among fertile and infertile women. Fertil Steril 38:667, 1982

Strowitzki T, Faustmann T, Gerlinger C, et al: Dienogest in the treatment of endometriosis-associated pelvic pain: a 12-week, randomized, double-blind, placebo-controlled study. Eur J Obstet Gynecol Reprod Biol 151(2):193 2010a

Strowitzki T, Marr J, Gerlinger C, et al: Dienogest is as effective as leuprolide acetate in treating the painful symptoms of endometriosis: a 24-week, randomized, multicentre, open-label trial. Hum Reprod 25(3):633, 2010b

Sutton CJ, Pooley AS, Ewen SP, et al: Follow-up report on a randomized controlled trial of laser laparoscopy in the treatment of pelvic pain associated with minimal to moderate endometriosis. Fertil Steril 68:1070, 1997

Taguchi S, Enomoto Y, Homma Y: Bladder endometriosis developed after long-term estrogen therapy for prostate cancer. Int J Urol 19(10):964, 2012

Tammaa A, Fritzer N, Strunk G, et al: Learning curve for the detection of pouch of Douglas obliteration and deep infiltrating endometriosis of the rectum. Hum Reprod 29(6):1199, 2014

Tanmahasamut P, Rattanachaiyanont M, Angsuwathana S, et al: Postoperative levonorgestrel-releasing intrauterine system for pelvic endometriosis-related pain: a randomized controlled trial. Obstet Gynecol 119(3):519, 2012

Taylor M, Bowen-Simpkins P, Barrington J: Complications of unopposed oestrogen following radical surgery for endometriosis. J Obstet Gynaecol 19:647, 1999

Telimaa S, Puolakka J, Ronnberg L, et al: Placebo-controlled comparison of danazol and high-dose medroxyprogesterone acetate in the treatment of endometriosis. Gynecol Endocrinol 1:13, 1987

Tempfer CB, Wenzl R, Horvat R, et al: Lymphatic spread of endometriosis to pelvic sentinel lymph nodes: a prospective clinical study. Fertil Steril 96(3):692, 2011

Thomas EJ, Cooke ID: Successful treatment of asymptomatic endometriosis: does it benefit infertile women? Br Med J (Clin Res Ed) 294:1117, 1987

Treloar SA, O'Connor DT, O'Connor VM, et al: Genetic influences on endometriosis in an Australian twin sample. Fertil Steril 71:701, 1999

Tseng JF, Ryan IP, Milam TD, et al: Interleukin-6 secretion in vitro is upregulated in ectopic and eutopic endometrial stromal cells from women with endometriosis. J Clin Endocrinol Metab 81:1118, 1996

Valentijn AJ, Palial K, Al-Lamee H, et al: SSEA-1 isolates human endometrial basal glandular epithelial cells: phenotypic and functional characterization and implications in the pathogenesis of endometriosis. Hum Reprod 28(10):2695, 2013

Van Holsbeke C, Van Calster B, Guerriero S, et al: Endometriomas: their ultrasound characteristics. Ultrasound Obstet Gynecol 35(6):730, 2010

Vercellini P, Aimi G, Busacca M, et al: Laparoscopic uterosacral ligament resection for dysmenorrhea associated with endometriosis: results of a randomized, controlled trial. Fertil Steril 80:310, 2003a

Vercellini P, Barbara G, Somigliana E, et al: Comparison of contraceptive ring and patch for the treatment of symptomatic endometriosis. Fertil Steril 93:2150, 2010

Vercellini P, Fedele L, Aimi G, et al: Association between endometriosis stage, lesion type, patient characteristics and severity of pelvic pain symptoms: a multivariate analysis on 1000 patients. Hum Reprod 22(1):266, 2007

Vercellini P, Frontino G, De Giorgi O, et al: Comparison of a levonorgestrel-releasing intrauterine device versus expectant management after conservative surgery for symptomatic endometriosis: a pilot study. Fertil Steril 80(2):305, 2003b

Vercellini P, Frontino G, Pietropaolo G, et al: Deep endometriosis: definition, pathogenesis, and clinical management. J Am Assoc Gynecol Laparosc 11(2):153, 2004

Vercellini P, Somigliana E, Buggio L, et al: "I can't get no satisfaction": deep dyspareunia and sexual functioning in women with rectovaginal endometriosis. Fertil Steril 98(6):1503, 2012

Vercellini P, Trespidi L, Colombo A, et al: A gonadotropin-releasing hormone agonist versus a low-dose oral contraceptive for pelvic pain associated with endometriosis. Fertil Steril 60:75, 1993

Vercellini P, Trespidi L, De Giorgi O, et al: Endometriosis and pelvic pain: relation to disease stage and localization. Fertil Steril 65:299, 1996

Vercellini P, Vendola N, Bocciolone L, et al: Reliability of the visual diagnosis of ovarian endometriosis. Fertil Steril 56:1198, 1991

Vignali M, Infantino M, Matrone R, et al: Endometriosis: novel etiopathogenetic concepts and clinical perspectives. Fertil Steril 78(4):665, 2002

Walch K, Unfried G, Huber J, et al: Implanon versus medroxyprogesterone acetate: effects on pain scores in patients with symptomatic endometriosis—a pilot study. Contraception 79(1):29, 2009

Wall DJ, Javitt MC, Glanc P, et al: ACR Appropriateness Criteria® infertility. Ultrasound Q 31(1):37, 2015

Waller KG, Lindsay P, Curtis P, et al: The prevalence of endometriosis in women with infertile partners. Eur J Obstet Gynecol Reprod Biol 48:135, 1993

Walter AJ, Hentz JG, Magtibay PM, et al: Endometriosis: correlation between histologic and visual findings at laparoscopy. Am J Obstet Gynecol 184:1407, 2001

Watanabe M, Kamiyama G, Yamazaki K, et al: Anal endosonography in the diagnosis and management of perianal endometriosis: report of a case. Surg Today 33:630, 2003

Williams CE, Nakhal RS, Hall-Craggs MA, et al: Transverse vaginal septae: management and long-term outcomes. BJOG 121(13):1653, 2014

Wilson TJ, Hertzog PJ, Angus D, et al: Decreased natural killer cell activity in endometriosis patients: relationship to disease pathogenesis. Fertil Steril 62:1086, 1994

Wong AY, Tang LC, Chin RK: Levonorgestrel-releasing intrauterine system (Mirena) and Depot medroxyprogesterone acetate (Depoprovera) as long-term maintenance therapy for patients with moderate and severe endometriosis: a randomised controlled trial. Aust N Z J Obstet Gynaecol 50(3):273, 2010

Wright J, Lotfallah H, Jones K, et al: A randomized trial of excision versus ablation for mild endometriosis. Fertil Steril 83:1830, 2005

Wykes CB, Clark TJ, Khan KS: Accuracy of laparoscopy in the diagnosis of endometriosis: a systematic quantitative review. BJOG 111(11):1204, 2004

Wu D, Hu M, Hong L, et al: Clinical efficacy of add-back therapy in treatment of endometriosis: a meta-analysis. Arch Gynecol Obstet 290(3):513, 2014

Xue Q, Lin Z, Cheng YH, et al: Promoter methylation regulates estrogen receptor 2 in human endometrium and endometriosis. Biol Reprod 77(4):681, 2007

Yuen PM, Yu KM, Yip SK, et al: A randomized prospective study of laparoscopy and laparotomy in the management of benign ovarian masses. Am J Obstet Gynecol 177:109, 1997

Zeitoun K, Takayama K, Sasano H, et al: Deficient 17 beta-hydroxysteroid dehydrogenase type 2 expression in endometriosis: failure to metabolize 17 beta-estradiol. J Clin Endocrinol Metab 83:4474, 1998

Zhu L, Wong F, Lang JH: Perineal endometriosis after vaginal delivery—clinical experience with 10 patients. Aust N Z J Obstet Gynaecol 42:565, 2002

Zullo F, Palomba S, Zupi E, et al: Effectiveness of presacral neurectomy in women with severe dysmenorrhea caused by endometriosis who were treated with laparoscopic conservative surgery: a 1-year prospective randomized double-blind controlled trial. Am J Obstet Gynecol 189:5, 2003

Zupi E, Marconi D, Sbracia M, et al: Add-back therapy in the treatment of endometriosis-associated pain. Fertil Steril 82:1303, 2004

Pelvic Pain

Pain in the lower abdomen and pelvis is a common complaint. But, pain is subjective and often ambiguous, and thus, difficult to diagnose and treat. To assist, clinicians ideally understand the mechanisms underlying human pain perception, which involves complex physical, biochemical, emotional, and social interactions. Providers are obligated to search for organic sources of pain, but equally important, avoid overtreatment of a condition that is minor or short lived.

PAIN PATHOPHYSIOLOGY

Pain is a protective mechanism meant to warn of an immediate threat and to prompt withdrawal from noxious stimuli. Pain is usually followed by an emotional response and inevitable behavioral consequences. These are often as important as the pain itself. The mere threat of pain may elicit emotional responses even in the absence of actual injury.

When categorized, pain may be considered *somatic* or *visceral* depending on the type of afferent nerve fibers involved. Additionally, pain is described by the physiologic steps that produce it and can be defined as *inflammatory* or *neuropathic* (Kehlet, 2006). Both categorizations are helpful for diagnosis and treatment.

■ Somatic or Visceral Pain

Somatic pain stems from nerve afferents of the somatic nervous system, which innervates the parietal peritoneum, skin, muscles, and subcutaneous tissues. Somatic pain is typically sharp and localized. It is found on either the right or left within dermatomes that correspond to the innervation of involved tissues (Fig. 11-1).

In contrast, visceral pain stems from afferent fibers of the autonomic nervous system, which transmits information from the viscera and visceral peritoneum. Noxious stimuli typically include stretching, distention, ischemia, necrosis, or spasm of abdominal organs. The visceral afferent fibers that transfer these stimuli are sparse. Thus, the resulting diffuse sensory input leads to pain that is often described as a generalized, dull ache.

Visceral pain often localizes to the midline because visceral innervation of abdominal organs is usually bilateral (Flasar, 2006). As another attribute, visceral afferents follow a segmental distribution, and visceral pain is typically localized by the brain's sensory cortex to an approximate spinal cord level that is determined by the embryologic origin of the involved organ. For example, pathology in midgut organs, such as the small bowel, appendix, and caecum, causes perceived periumbilical pain. In contrast, disease in hindgut organs, such as the colon and intraperitoneal portions of the genitourinary tract, causes midline pain in the suprapubic or hypogastric area (Gallagher, 2004).

Visceral afferent fibers are poorly myelinated, and action potentials can easily spread from them to adjacent somatic nerves. As a result, visceral pain may at times be referred to dermatomes that correspond to these adjacent somatic nerve fibers (Giamberardino, 2003). In addition, both peripheral somatic and visceral nerves often synapse in the spinal cord at the same dorsal horn neurons. These neurons, in turn, relay sensory information to the brain. The cortex recognizes the signal as coming from the same dermatome regardless of its visceral or somatic nerve origin. This phenomenon is termed *viscerosomatic convergence* and makes it difficult for a patient to distinguish internal organ pain from abdominal wall or pelvic floor pain (Fig. 11-2) (Perry, 2003).

Viscerosomatic convergence explains the dermatomal distribution of some visceral pain. In contrast, *direct intraspinal neuronal reflexes* permit transmission of visceral nociceptive input to other pelvic viscera (viscerovisceral reflex), to muscle (visceromuscular reflex), and to skin (viscerocutaneous reflex). These intraspinal reflexes may explain why patients with endometriosis or interstitial cystitis manifest other pain syndromes such as vestibulitis, pelvic floor myalgia, or irritable bowel syndrome (IBS). Thus, unless the underlying chronic visceral pain source is identified and properly treated, referred pain and secondary pain syndromes may not be successfully eliminated (Perry, 2000).

■ Inflammatory Pain

With acute pain, noxious stimuli such as a knife cut, burn, or crush injury activate sensory pain receptors, more formally

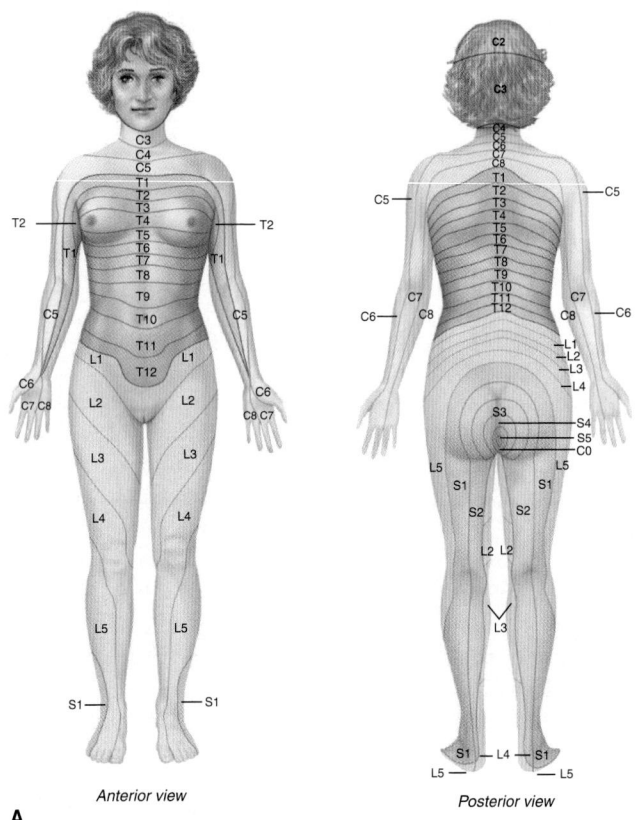

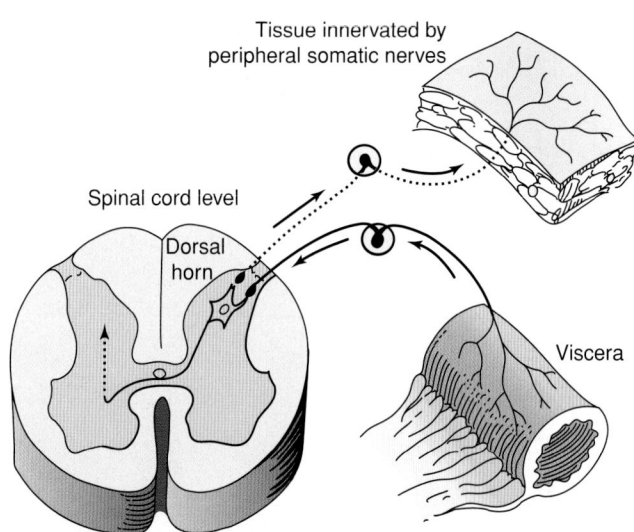

FIGURE 11-2 Viscerosomatic convergence. Pain impulses originating from an organ may affect dorsal horn neurons that are synapsing concurrently with peripheral somatic nerves. These impulses may then be perceived by the brain as coming from a peripheral somatic source such as muscle or skin rather than the diseased viscera. (Reproduced with permission from Howard FM, Perry CP, Carter JE, et al (eds): Pelvic Pain: Diagnosis and Management. Philadelphia: Lippincott Williams & Wilkins; 2000.)

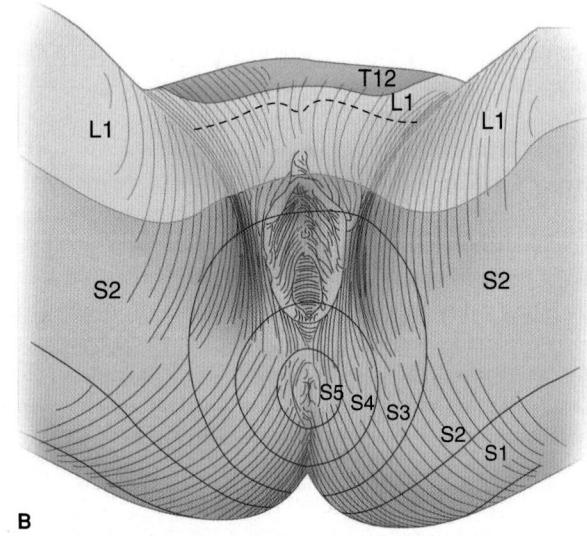

FIGURE 11-1 Dermatome maps. A dermatome is an area of skin supplied by a single spinal nerve. **A.** Body dermatomes. **B.** Perineal dermatomes. (Adapted with permission from Steege JF, Metzger DA, Levy BS (eds): Chronic Pelvic Pain: an Integrated Approach. Philadelphia: WB Saunders; 1998.)

termed *nociceptors*. Action potentials travel from the periphery to dorsal horn neurons in the spinal cord. Here, reflex arcs may lead to immediate muscle contraction, which removes and protects the body from harm. Additionally, within the spinal cord, sensory information is augmented or dampened and may then be transmitted to the brain. In the cortex, it is recognized as pain (Janicki, 2003). After an acute stimulus is eliminated, nociceptor activity quickly diminishes.

If tissues are injured, then inflammation usually follows. Body fluids, along with inflammatory proteins and cells, are

called to the injury site to limit tissue damage. Because cells and most inflammatory proteins are too large to cross normal endothelium, vasodilation and increased capillary permeability are required features of this response. Chemical mediators of this process are prostaglandins, which are released from the damaged tissue, and cytokines, which are produced in white blood cells and endothelial cells. Cytokines include interleukins, tissue necrosis factors, and interferons. These sensitizing mediators are released into affected tissues and lower the conduction threshold of nociceptors. This is termed *peripheral sensitization*. Similarly, neurons within the spinal cord and/or brain display increased excitability, termed *central sensitization*. As a result, within inflamed tissues, the perception of pain is increased relative to the strength of the external stimulus (Kehlet, 2006). Normally, as inflammation decreases and healing ensues, the increased sensitivity to stimuli and thus the perception of pain subsides.

■ Neuropathic Pain

In some individuals, sustained noxious stimuli can lead to persistent central sensitization and to a permanent loss of neuronal inhibition. As a result, a decreased threshold to painful stimuli remains despite resolution of the inciting stimuli (Butrick, 2003). This persistence characterizes *neuropathic pain*, which is felt to underlie many chronic pain syndromes. During central sensitization, neurons within spinal cord levels above or below those initially affected may eventually become involved. This phenomenon results in chronic pain that may be referred across several spinal cord levels. In addition, some evidence suggests that chronic pain states are also associated with regional brain morphology changes in regions known to regulate pain. This has been described as maladaptive central nervous system (CNS) plasticity in response to prolonged nociceptive input (As-Sanie, 2012). The concept of neuropathic pain helps explain in part why many patients with chronic pain have discomfort disproportionately greater than the amount of coexistent disease found.

Thus, in assessing patients with chronic pain, a clinician may find an ongoing inflammatory condition. In these cases, inflammatory pain dominates, and treatment is directed at resolving the underlying inflammatory condition. However, for many patients, evaluation may reveal no or minimal current pathology. In these cases, pain is neuropathic, and treatment thus focuses on management of pain symptoms themselves.

ACUTE PAIN

The definition of acute lower abdominal pain and pelvic pain varies based on duration, but in general, discomfort is present less than 7 days. The sources of acute lower abdominal and pelvic pain are extensive, and a thorough history and physical examination can aid in narrowing the list (Table 11-1). With acute pain, a timely and accurate diagnosis is the goal and ensures the best medical outcome. Thus, although history and examination are described separately here, in clinical settings they often are performed almost simultaneously for optimal results.

■ History

In addition to a thorough medical and surgical history, a verbal description of the pain and its associated factors is essential. For example, duration can be informative, and pain with abrupt

onset may be more often associated with organ torsion, rupture, or ischemia. The nature of pain may add value. Patients with acute pathology involving pelvic viscera may describe *visceral pain* that is midline, diffuse, dull, achy, or cramping. One example is the midline periumbilical pain of early appendicitis. Patients may repeatedly shift or roll to one side to find a comfortable position.

The underlying pelvic pathology may extend from the viscera to inflame the adjacent parietal peritoneum. In these cases, sharp *somatic pain* is described, which is localized, often unilateral, and focused to a specific corresponding dermatome. Again using appendicitis as an example, the classic migration of pain to the site of peritoneal irritation in the right lower quadrant illustrates acute somatic pain. In other instances, sharp, localized pain may originate, not from the parietal peritoneum, but from pathology in specific muscles or in isolated areas of skin or subcutaneous tissues. In either instance, with somatic pain, patients classically rest motionless to avoid movement of the affected peritoneum, muscle, or skin.

Colicky pain may reflect bowel obstructed by adhesion, neoplasia, stool, or hernia. It can also stem from increased bowel peristalsis in those with irritable or inflammatory bowel disease or infectious gastroenteritis. Alternatively, colic may follow forceful uterine contractions with the passage of products of conception, pedunculated submucous leiomyomas, or endometrial polyps. Last, stones in the lower urinary tract may cause spasms of pain as they are passed.

Associated symptoms may also direct diagnosis. For example, absence of dysuria, hematuria, frequency, or urgency will exclude urinary pathology in most instances. Gynecologic causes are often associated with vaginal bleeding, vaginal discharge, dyspareunia, or amenorrhea. Alternatively, exclusion of diarrhea, constipation, or gastrointestinal bleeding lowers the probability of gastrointestinal (GI) disease.

Vomiting complaints, however, are less informative, although the temporal relationship of vomiting to the pain may be helpful. In the acute surgical abdomen, if vomiting occurs, it usually follows as a response to pain and results from vagal stimulation. This vomiting is typically severe and develops without nausea. For example, vomiting has been found in approximately 75 percent of adnexal torsion cases (Descargues, 2001; Huchon, 2010). Thus, the acute onset of unilateral pain that is severe and associated with a tender adnexal mass in a patient with vomiting alerts one to the increased probability of adnexal torsion. Conversely, if vomiting is noted prior to the onset of pain, a surgical abdomen is less likely (Miller, 2006).

In general, well-localized pain or tenderness, persisting for longer than 6 hours and unrelieved by analgesics, has an increased likelihood of acute peritoneal pathology.

■ Physical Examination

Examination begins with patient observation during initial questioning. Her general appearance, including facial expression, diaphoresis, pallor, and degree of agitation, often indicates the urgency of the clinical condition.

Elevated temperature, tachycardia, and hypotension will prompt an expedited evaluation, as the risk for intraabdominal

---

TABLE 11-1. Etiologies of Acute Lower Abdominal and Pelvic Pain

Gynecologic

PID	Dysmenorrhea
Tuboovarian abscess	Mittelschmerz
Ectopic pregnancy	Ovarian mass
Incomplete abortion	Ovarian torsion
Prolapsing leiomyoma	Obstructed outflow tract

Gastrointestinal

Gastroenteritis	Inflammatory bowel disease
Colitis	Irritable bowel disease
Appendicitis	Obstructed small bowel
Diverticulitis	Mesenteric ischemia
Constipation	Malignancy

Urologic

Cystitis	Urinary tract stone
Pyelonephritis	Perinephric abscess

Musculoskeletal

Hernia	Abdominal wall trauma

Miscellaneous

Peritonitis	Sickle cell crisis
Diabetic ketoacidosis	Vasculitis
Herpes zoster	Abdominal aortic aneurysm
Opiate withdrawal	rupture

PID = pelvic inflammatory disease.

pathology increases with their presence. Constant, low-grade fever is common in inflammatory conditions such as diverticulitis and appendicitis, and higher temperatures may be seen with pelvic inflammatory disease (PID), advanced peritonitis, or pyelonephritis.

Pulse and blood pressure evaluation ideally assess orthostatic changes if intravascular hypovolemia is suspected. A pulse increase of 30 beats per minute or a systolic blood pressure drop of 20 mm Hg or both, between lying and standing after 1 minute, is often reflective of hypovolemia. If noted, establishment of intravenous access and fluid resuscitation may be required prior to examination completion. Notably, certain neurologic disorders and medications, such as tricyclic antidepressants or antihypertensives, may also produce similar orthostatic blood pressure changes.

Abdominal examination is essential. Visual inspection of the abdomen focuses on prior surgical scars, which may increase the possibility of bowel obstruction from postoperative adhesions or incisional hernia. Additionally, abdominal distention may be seen with bowel obstruction, perforation, or ascites. After inspection, auscultation may identify hyperactive or high-pitched bowel sounds characteristic of bowel obstruction. Hypoactive sounds, however, are less informative.

Palpation of the abdomen systematically explores each abdominal quadrant and begins away from the area of indicated pain. Peritoneal irritation is suggested by rebound tenderness or by abdominal rigidity due to involuntary guarding or reflex spasm of the adjacent or involved abdominal muscles.

Pelvic examination in general is performed in reproductive-aged women, as gynecologic pathology and pregnancy complications are a common pain source in this age group. The decision to pursue this pelvic examination in geriatric and pediatric patients is based on clinical information.

Of findings, purulent vaginal discharge or cervicitis may reflect PID. Vaginal bleeding can stem from pregnancy complications, benign or malignant reproductive tract neoplasia, or acute vaginal trauma. Leiomyomas, pregnancy, and adenomyosis are common causes of uterine enlargement, and the latter two may also create uterine softening. Cervical motion tenderness reflects peritoneal irritation and can be seen with PID, appendicitis, diverticulitis, and intraabdominal bleeding. A tender adnexal mass may reflect ectopic pregnancy, tuboovarian abscess, or ovarian cyst with torsion, hemorrhage, or rupture. Alternatively, a tender mass may reflect an abscess of nongynecologic origin such as one involving the appendix or colon diverticulum.

Rectal examination can add information regarding the source and size of pelvic masses and the possibility of colorectal pathologies. Stool guaiac testing for occult blood, although less sensitive when not performed serially, is still warranted in many patients (Rockey, 2005). Those with complaints of rectal bleeding, painful defecation, or significant changes in bowel habits are examples.

In emergency departments, women with acute pain may experience waits between their initial assessment and subsequent testing. For these patients, literature supports early administration of analgesia. Fears that analgesia will mask patient symptoms and hinder accurate diagnosis have not been supported (McHale, 2001; Pace, 1996). Thus, barring significant

hypotension or drug allergy, morphine sulfate may be administered judiciously in these situations.

■ Laboratory Testing

Despite benefits from a thorough history and physical examination, the sensitivity of these two in diagnosing abdominal pain is low (Gerhardt, 2005). Thus, laboratory and diagnostic testing are typically required. In women with acute abdominal pain, pregnancy complications are common. Thus, either urine or serum β-human chorionic gonadotropin (hCG) testing is recommended in those of reproductive age without prior hysterectomy. Complete blood count (CBC) can identify hemorrhage, both uterine and intraabdominal, and can assess the possibility of infection. Urinalysis can be used to evaluate possible urolithiasis or cystitis. In addition, microscopic evaluation and culture of vaginal discharge may add support to clinically suspected cases of PID.

■ Radiologic Imaging

Sonography

In women with acute pelvic pain, several imaging options are available. However, transvaginal and transabdominal pelvic sonography are preferred modalities if an obstetric or gynecologic cause is suspected (Andreotti, 2011). Sonography provides a high sensitivity for detection of structural pelvic pathology. It is widely available, can usually be obtained quickly, requires little patient preparation, is relatively noninvasive, and avoids ionizing radiation. Disadvantageously, examination quality is affected by the skill and experience of the sonographer.

In most cases, the transvaginal approach offers superior resolution of the reproductive organs. Transabdominal sonography may still be necessary if the uterus or adnexal structures are significantly large or if they lie beyond the transvaginal probe's field of view. Color Doppler imaging during sonography permits evaluation of the vascular qualities of pelvic structures. In women with acute pain, the addition of Doppler studies is particularly useful if adnexal torsion or ectopic pregnancy is suspected (Twickler, 2010). Less common causes of acute pain amenable to sonographic diagnosis are perforation of the uterine wall by an intrauterine device (IUD) or hematometra caused by menstrual outflow obstruction from müllerian agenesis anomalies. For these, 3-dimensional (3-D) transvaginal sonography has become invaluable (Bermejo, 2010; Moschos, 2011).

Computed Tomography

Computed tomography (CT) and multidetector computed tomography (MDCT) are increasingly used to evaluate acute abdominal pain in adults. CT offers a global examination that can identify numerous abdominal and pelvic conditions, often with a high level of confidence (Hsu, 2005). Compared with other imaging tools, it has superior performance in identifying GI and urinary tract causes of acute pelvic and lower abdominal pain (Andreotti, 2011). For example, noncontrasted renal colic CT has largely replaced conventional intravenous pyelography to search for ureteral obstruction. For appendicitis, one study found that the false-positive diagnosis rate among adults decreased from

24 to 3 percent from 1996 to 2006. Investigators noted that this decrease correlated with the increased rate of CT use during the same interval (Raman, 2008). Appendiceal perforation also decreased from 18 to 5 percent. Considering that the false-positive diagnosis of appendicitis in women is as high as 42 percent, this certainly represents an improvement in clinical outcomes. For evaluation of GI abnormalities such as appendicitis, the combination of both oral and intravenous contrast is preferred.

In addition to its high sensitivity, CT has several advantages for most nongynecologic disorders. It is extremely fast; is not perturbed by gas, bone, or obesity; and is not operator dependent. Disadvantages include occasional unavailability, high cost, inability to use contrast media in patients who are allergic or have renal dysfunction, and exposure to low levels of ionizing radiation (Leschka, 2007).

The debate regarding CT safety and possible overuse is ongoing (Brenner, 2007). Of major concern is the potential increased cancer risk directly attributable to ionizing radiation, which is estimated to be even higher in younger patients and women (Einstein, 2007). Radiation doses from CT are generally considered to be 100 to 500 times those from conventional radiography (Smith-Bindman, 2010). Investigators in a large multicenter analysis found the median effective radiation dose from a multiphase abdomen and pelvic CT scan was 31 mSv, and this correlates with a lifetime attributable risk of four cancers per 1000 patients (Smith-Bindman, 2009). By way of comparison, health care workers are generally limited to 100 mSv over 5 years with a maximum of 50 mSv allowed in any given year (Fazel, 2009). But, in the acute clinical setting, CT imaging benefits frequently outweigh these risks.

Other Imaging

In some instances, plain film radiography is selected. Although its sensitivity is low for most gynecologic conditions, it still may be informative if bowel obstruction or perforation is suspected (Leschka, 2007). Dilated loops of small bowel, air-fluid levels, free air under the diaphragm, or the presence or absence of colonic gas are all significant findings when attempting to differentiate between a gynecologic and GI cause of acute pain.

Magnetic resonance (MR) imaging is becoming an important tool for women with acute pelvic pain if initial sonography is nondiagnostic. Common reasons for noninformative sonographic evaluations include patient obesity and pelvic anatomy distortion secondary to large leiomyomas, müllerian anomalies, or exophytic tumor growth. As a first-line tool, MR imaging is often selected for pregnant patients, for whom ionizing radiation exposure should be limited. However, for most acute disorders, it provides little advantage over 3-D sonography or CT (Bermejo, 2010; Brown, 2005). Lack of availability can be a disadvantage after hours, on weekends, or in smaller hospitals and emergency departments.

■ Laparoscopy

Operative laparoscopy is the primary treatment for suspected appendicitis, adnexal torsion, ectopic pregnancy, and ruptured ovarian cyst associated with ongoing symptomatic hemorrhage. Moreover, diagnostic laparoscopy may be useful if no pathology

can be identified by conventional diagnostics. However, in stable patients with acute abdominal pain, noninvasive testing is typically exhausted before this approach is considered (Sauerland, 2006).

The decision to perform a surgical procedure for acute pelvic pain can be challenging. If the patient is clinically stable, the decision can be made in a timely manner, with appropriate evaluation and consultation completed preoperatively. In a less stable patient with signs of peritoneal irritation, possible hemoperitoneum, organ torsion, shock, and/or impending sepsis, the decision to operate is made decisively unless there are overwhelming clinical contraindications to immediate surgery.

CHRONIC PAIN

Persistent pain may be visceral, somatic, or mixed in origin. As a result, it may take several forms in women that include chronic pelvic pain (CPP), dysmenorrhea, dyspareunia, dysuria, musculoskeletal pain, intestinal cramping, or vulvodynia. Each of these forms is described here except for vulvodynia, discussed in Chapter 4 (p. 97). The list of pathologies that may underlie these symptoms is extensive and includes both psychological and organic disorders (Table 11-2). Moreover, pathology in one organ can commonly lead to dysfunction in adjacent systems. As a result, a woman with chronic pain may have more than one cause of pain and overlapping symptoms. A comprehensive evaluation of multiple organ systems and psychologic state is essential for complete treatment.

CHRONIC PELVIC PAIN

This common gynecologic problem has an estimated prevalence of 15 percent in reproductive-aged women (Mathias, 1996). No definition is universally accepted. However, many investigators define chronic pelvic pain as: (1) noncyclic pain that persists for 6 or more months; (2) pain that localizes to the anatomic pelvis, to the anterior abdominal wall at or below the umbilicus, or to the lumbosacral back or buttocks; and (3) pain sufficiently severe to cause functional disability or lead to medical intervention (American College of Obstetricians and Gynecologists, 2010).

Causes of CPP fall within a broad spectrum, but endometriosis, symptomatic leiomyomas, and IBS are often diagnosed. Of these, endometriosis is a frequent cause, but it typically is also associated with cyclic symptoms. It is discussed fully in Chapter 10 (p. 230). Chronic pain secondary to leiomyomas is described in Chapter 9 (p. 205).

The pathophysiology of CPP is unclear in many patients, but evidence supports a significant association with neuropathic pain, described earlier (p. 250). CPP shows increased association with IBS, interstitial cystitis, and vulvodynia, which are considered by many to be chronic visceral pain syndromes stemming from neuropathic pain (Janicki, 2003).

■ History

More than with many other gynecologic complaints, a detailed history and physical examination are integral to diagnosis. A pelvic pain questionnaire can be used initially to obtain

TABLE 11-2. Diseases That May Be Associated with Chronic Pelvic Pain in Women

Gynecologic

Endometriosis	Reproductive tract cancer	Chronic PID
Adenomyosis	Pelvic muscle trigger points	Chronic endometritis
Leiomyomas	Intrauterine contraceptive device	Vestibulitis
Abdominal adhesions	Outflow tract obstruction	Pelvic congestion syndrome
Endometrial/endocervical polyps	Ovarian retention syndrome	Broad ligament herniation
Ovarian mass	Ovarian remnant syndrome	Chronic ectopic pregnancy
Adnexal cysts	Pelvic organ prolapse	Postoperative peritoneal cysts

Urologic

Chronic UTI	Urethral syndrome	Interstitial cystitis
Detrusor dyssynergia	Urethral diverticulum	Radiation cystitis
Urinary tract stone	Urinary tract cancer	

Gastrointestinal

IBS	Colitis	Celiac disease
Constipation	Inflammatory bowel disease	Chronic intermittent bowel
Diverticular disease	Gastrointestinal cancer	obstruction

Musculoskeletal

Hernias	Degenerative joint disease	Vertebral compression
Muscular strain	Levator ani syndrome	Disc disease
Faulty posture	Fibromyositis	Coccydynia
Myofascial pain	Spondylosis	Peripartum pelvic pain

Neurologic

Neurologic dysfunction	Abdominal cutaneous nerve entrapment	Spinal cord or sacral nerve tumor
Pudendal neuralgia	Neuralgia of iliohypogastric, ilioinguinal, lateral	
Piriformis syndrome	femoral cutaneous, or genitofemoral nerves	

Miscellaneous

Psychiatric disorders
Physical or sexual abuse
Shingles

IBS = irritable bowel syndrome; PID = pelvic inflammatory disease; UTI = urinary tract disease.

information. One example is available from the International Pelvic Pain Society and may be accessed at: http://www.pelvicpain.org/docs/resources/forms/History-and-Physical-Form-English.aspx. Additionally, a body silhouette diagram can be provided to patients for them to mark specific sites of pain. The McGill Pain Questionnaire and Short Form combines a list of pain descriptors with a body map for patients to mark pain sites (Melzack, 1987). Pain scales can also quantify discomfort and include visual analogue scales (VAS) and verbal descriptor scales (VDS) (Fig. 11-3). At minimum, the series of questions found in Table 11-3 may provide valuable information. As noted, many of these questions focus on gynecologic, surgical, and psychologic risk factors.

First, of gynecologic factors, CPP is more common in women than men and is often worsened by stress and menstruation. Also, pregnancy and delivery can be traumatic to neuromuscular structures and have been linked with pelvic organ prolapse, pelvic floor muscle myofascial pain syndromes, and symphyseal or sacroiliac joint pain. In addition, injury to the ilioinguinal or iliohypogastric nerves during Pfannenstiel incision for

cesarean delivery may lead to lower abdominal wall pain even years after the initial injury (Whiteside, 2003). Following delivery, recurrent, cyclic pain and swelling in the vicinity of a cesarean incision or within an episiotomy suggests endometriosis within the scar itself (Fig. 10-3, p. 235). In contrast, in a nulliparous woman with infertility, pain may stem more often from endometriosis, pelvic adhesions, or PID.

Second, prior abdominal surgery increases a woman's risk for pelvic adhesions, especially if infection, bleeding, or large areas of denuded peritoneal surfaces were involved. Adhesions were found in 40 percent of patients who underwent laparoscopy for chronic pelvic pain suspected to be of gynecologic origin (Sharma, 2011). The incidence of adhesions increases with the number of prior surgeries (Dubuisson, 2010). Last, certain disorders persist or commonly recur, and thus information regarding prior surgeries for endometriosis, adhesive disease, or malignancy are sought.

Of psychologic risk factors, CPP and sexual abuse are significantly associated (Jamieson, 1997; Lampe, 2000). A metaanalysis by Paras and associates (2009) demonstrated that sexual

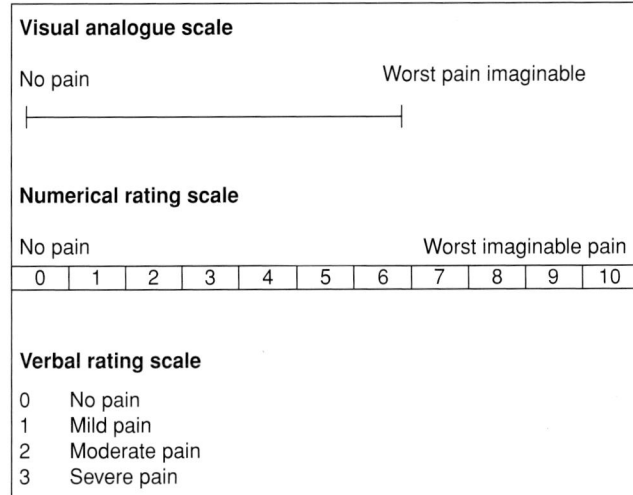

Visual analogue scale

No pain   Worst pain imaginable

├────────────────────────────────┤

Numerical rating scale

No pain   Worst imaginable pain

| 0 | 1 | 2 | 3 | 4 | 5 | 6 | 7 | 8 | 9 | 10 |

Verbal rating scale

0   No pain
1   Mild pain
2   Moderate pain
3   Severe pain

FIGURE 11-3 Rating scales for pain. The visual analogue, numeric, and verbal rating scales are shown.

abuse is linked with an increased lifetime diagnosis rate of functional bowel disorders, fibromyalgia, psychogenic seizure disorder, and CPP. Additionally, for some women, chronic pain is an acceptable means to cope with social stresses. Thus, patients are questioned regarding domestic violence and satisfaction

TABLE 11-3. Questions Relevant to Chronic Pelvic Pain

1. Describe the location, quality, severity, and timing of your pain.
2. When and how did your pain start and how has it changed?
3. What makes your pain better or worse?
4. What other symptoms or health problems do you have?
5. Do you have frequency, urgency, or bloody urine?
6. Do you have nausea or vomiting, diarrhea, constipation, or rectal bleeding?
7. Do you have pain with your periods?
8. Did your pain start initially as menstrual cramps?
9. Have you had surgery? What was the reason?
10. How many pregnancies have you had?
11. How did you deliver? Was there an episiotomy?
12. What form of birth control do you use and have you used in the past?
13. Have you ever been treated for a sexually transmitted disease or pelvic infection?
14. Do you have pain with deep penetration during intercourse?
15. Are you depressed or anxious?
16. Have you been treated for mental illness in the past?
17. Have you been or are you now being abused physically or sexually?
18. What prior evaluations or treatments have you had for your pain?
19. Have any of the previous treatments helped?
20. What medications are you taking now?
21. How has the pain affected your quality of life?
22. What do you believe or fear is causing your pain?

with family relationships. Furthermore, an inventory of depressive symptoms is essential, as depression may cause or result from CPP (Tables 13-3 and 13-4, p. 299). Other conditions bearing similarities to CPP include fibromyalgia, chronic fatigue syndrome, temporomandibular disorder, and migraine. These are referred to as functional somatic syndromes, and CPP can be comorbid with each of these (Warren, 2011).

■ Physical Examination

In a woman with chronic pain, even routine examination may be extremely painful. In those with neuropathic pain, mere light touch may elicit discomfort. Therefore, examination proceeds slowly to allow relaxation between each step. Moreover, a patient is reassured that she may ask for the examination to be halted at any time. Terms used to describe examination findings include *allodynia* and *hyperesthesia,* among others. Allodynia is a painful response to a normally innocuous stimulus, such as a cotton swab. Hyperalgesia is an extreme response to a painful stimulus.

Stance and Gait

Women with intraperitoneal pathology may compensate with changes in posture. Such adjustments can create secondary musculoskeletal sources of pain (p. 267). Alternatively, musculoskeletal structures may be the site of referred pain from these organs (Table 11-4). Thus, careful observation of a woman's posture and gait is integral.

Initially, a woman is examined while standing. Posture is evaluated anteriorly, posteriorly, and laterally. Anteriorly, symmetry of the anterior superior iliac spines (ASISs), umbilicus, and weight bearing is evaluated. If one leg bears most of the weight, the nonbearing leg is often externally rotated and slightly flexed at the knee. Next, the anterior abdominal wall and inguinal areas are inspected for abdominal wall or femoral hernias, described on page 267. Inspection of the perineum and vulva with the patient standing may identify varicosities. These are often asymptomatic or may cause superficial discomfort. Such varicosities may coexist with internal pelvic varicosities, the underlying cause of pelvic congestion syndrome (p. 261).

Posteriorly, inspection for scoliosis and of horizontal stability of the shoulders, gluteal folds, and knee creases is completed. Asymmetry may reflect musculoskeletal disorders.

Lateral visual examination searches for lordosis and concomitant kyphosis. This combination has been noted in some women with CPP and termed *typical pelvic pain posture (TPPP)* (Fig. 11-4) (Baker, 1993). Also, abnormal tilt of the pelvic bones can be assessed by simultaneously placing an open palm on each side between the posterior superior iliac spine (PSIS) and the ASIS. Normally, the ASIS lies one-quarter inch below the level of the PSIS, and greater distances may suggest abnormal tilt. Pelvic tilt may be associated with hip osteoarthritis and other orthopedic problems (Labelle, 2005; Yoshimoto, 2005).

Any observed mobility limitation can be informative. Thus, a patient is asked to bend forward at the waist. Limitation in forward flexion may reflect primary orthopedic disease or adaptive shortening of back extensor muscles. This shortening

TABLE 11-4. Musculoskeletal Origins of Chronic Pelvic Pain

Structure	Innervation	Referred Pain Site(s)
Hip	T12–S1	Lower abdomen; anterior medial thigh; knee
Lumbar ligaments, facets/disks	T12–S1	Low back; posterior thigh and calf; lower abdomen; lateral trunk; buttock
Sacroiliac joints	L4–S3	Posterior thigh; buttock; pelvic floor
Abdominal muscles	T5–L1	Abdomen; anteromedial thigh; sternum
Pelvic and back muscles		
Iliopsoas	L1–L4	Lateral trunk; lower abdomen; low back; anterior thigh
Piriformis	L5–S3	Low back, buttock; pelvic floor
Pubococcygeus	S1–L4	Pelvic floor; vagina; rectum; buttock
Obturator internal/external	L3–S2	Pelvic floor; buttock; anterior thigh
Quadratus lumborum	T12–L3	Anterior lateral trunk; anterior thigh; lower abdomen

Modified with permission from Baker PK: Musculoskeletal origins of chronic pelvic pain. Diagnosis and treatment. Obstet Gynecol Clin North Am 1993 Dec;20(4):719–742.

is seen frequently in women with chronic pain and TPPP. In such cases, patients are unable to bend over at the waist to create the normal convex curve.

Muscle weakness may also indicate orthopedic disease. A Trendelenburg test, in which a patient is asked to balance on one foot, can indicate dysfunction of hip abductor muscles or hip joint. With a positive test, when a woman elevates a leg by flexing the hip, the ipsilateral iliac crest droops.

Gait is evaluated by having the patient walk across the room. An *antalgic gait,* known as a limp, refers to a gait that minimizes weight bearing on a lower limb or joint and indicates a higher probability of musculoskeletal pain.

Sitting and Supine

A patient is next invited to sit on the examining table. Myofascial pain syndrome may involve pelvic floor muscles and often leads to a patient shifting weight to one buttock or sitting toward a chair's front edge.

With the patient supine, the anterior abdominal wall is evaluated for abdominal scars. These may be sites of hernia or nerve entrapment or may indicate a risk for intraabdominal adhesive disease. Auscultation for bowel sounds and bruits follows. Increased bowel activity may reflect irritable or inflammatory bowel diseases. Bruits prompt investigation for vascular pathology.

While supine, a woman is asked to demonstrate with one finger the point of maximal pain and then encircle the total surrounding area of involvement. Superficial palpation of the anterior abdominal wall by a clinician may reveal sites of tenderness or knotted muscle that may reflect nerve entrapment or myofascial pain syndrome (p. 268). Moreover, pain with elevation of the head and shoulders while tensing the abdominal wall muscles, *Carnett sign,* is typical of anterior abdominal wall pathology. Conversely, if the source of pain originates from inside the abdominal cavity, discomfort usually decreases with such elevation (Thomson, 1991). Moreover, Valsalva maneuver during head and shoulder elevation may display diastasis of the rectus abdominis muscle or hernias. Diastasis recti can be differentiated in most cases from a ventral hernia. Specifically, with diastasis, the borders of the rectus abdominis muscle can be palpated bilaterally along the entire length of the protrusion. Last, deep palpation of the lower abdomen may identify pathology originating from pelvic viscera. Dullness to percussion or a shifting fluid wave may indicate ascites.

Mobility is also evaluated. In most cases, a woman can elevate her leg 80 degrees from the horizontal toward her head, termed a *straight leg test.* Pain with leg elevation may be seen with lumbar disc, hip joint, or myofascial pain syndromes. Additionally, symphyseal pain with this test may indicate laxity in the symphysis pubis or pelvic girdle. Both the obturator and iliopsoas tests may indicate myofascial pain syndromes involving these muscles or disorders of the hip joint. With the obturator test, a supine patient brings one knee into 90 degrees of flexion while the same foot remains planted. The ankle is held stationary, but the knee is gently pulled laterally and then medially to assess for tenderness. With the iliopsoas test, a supine woman with

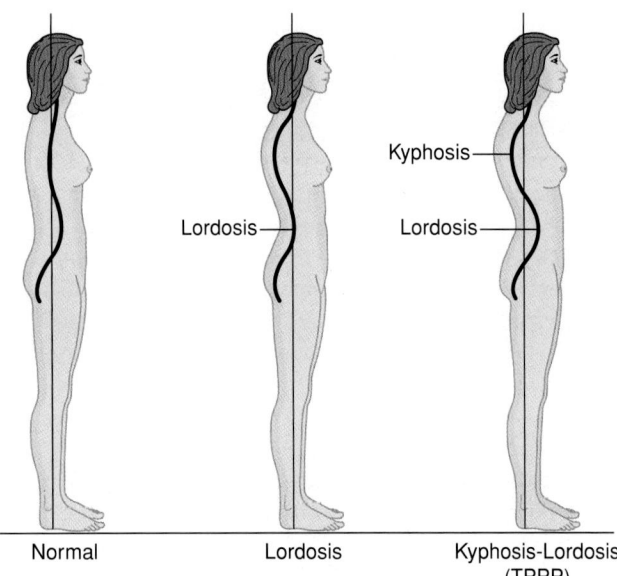

FIGURE 11-4 Concurrent lordosis and kyphosis are common postural changes associated with chronic pelvic pain. TPPP = typical pelvic pain posture.

legs extended attempts to flex each hip separately against downward resistance from the examiner's hand placed on the ipsilateral anterior thigh. If pain is described with hip flexion, the test result is positive.

Lithotomy

Pelvic examination begins with inspection of the vulva for generalized changes and localized lesions. Vulvar erythema often reflects infectious vulvitis, described in Chapter 3 (p. 60), or vulvitis stemming from dermatoses (Chap. 4, p. 88). Vulvar skin thinning may reflect lichen sclerosus or atrophic changes. The vestibular area is also examined. Erythema of the vestibule, with or without punctate lesions, may indicate vestibulitis. Following this inspection, systematic pressure point palpation of the vestibule, as shown in Figure 4-1 (p. 87), is completed

using a small cotton swab to assess for pain (allodynia). Last, the anocutaneous reflex, as described in Chapter 24 (p. 548), may also be performed to assess pudendal nerve integrity.

Prior to speculum examination, a single digit systematically evaluates the vagina. Pain elicited from pressure beneath the urethra may indicate urethral diverticulum. Pain with anterior vagina palpation under the trigone can reflect interstitial cystitis. Systematic sweeping pressure against the pelvic floor muscles along their length may identify isolated taut muscle knots from pelvic floor myofascial syndrome. Of these muscles, the pubococcygeus, iliococcygeus, and obturator internus muscles can usually be reached with a vaginal finger (Fig. 11-5). Next, insertion points of the uterosacral ligaments are palpated. Nodularity is highly suggestive of endometriosis, and palpation may reproduce dyspareunia symptoms. Cervical motion tenderness may be

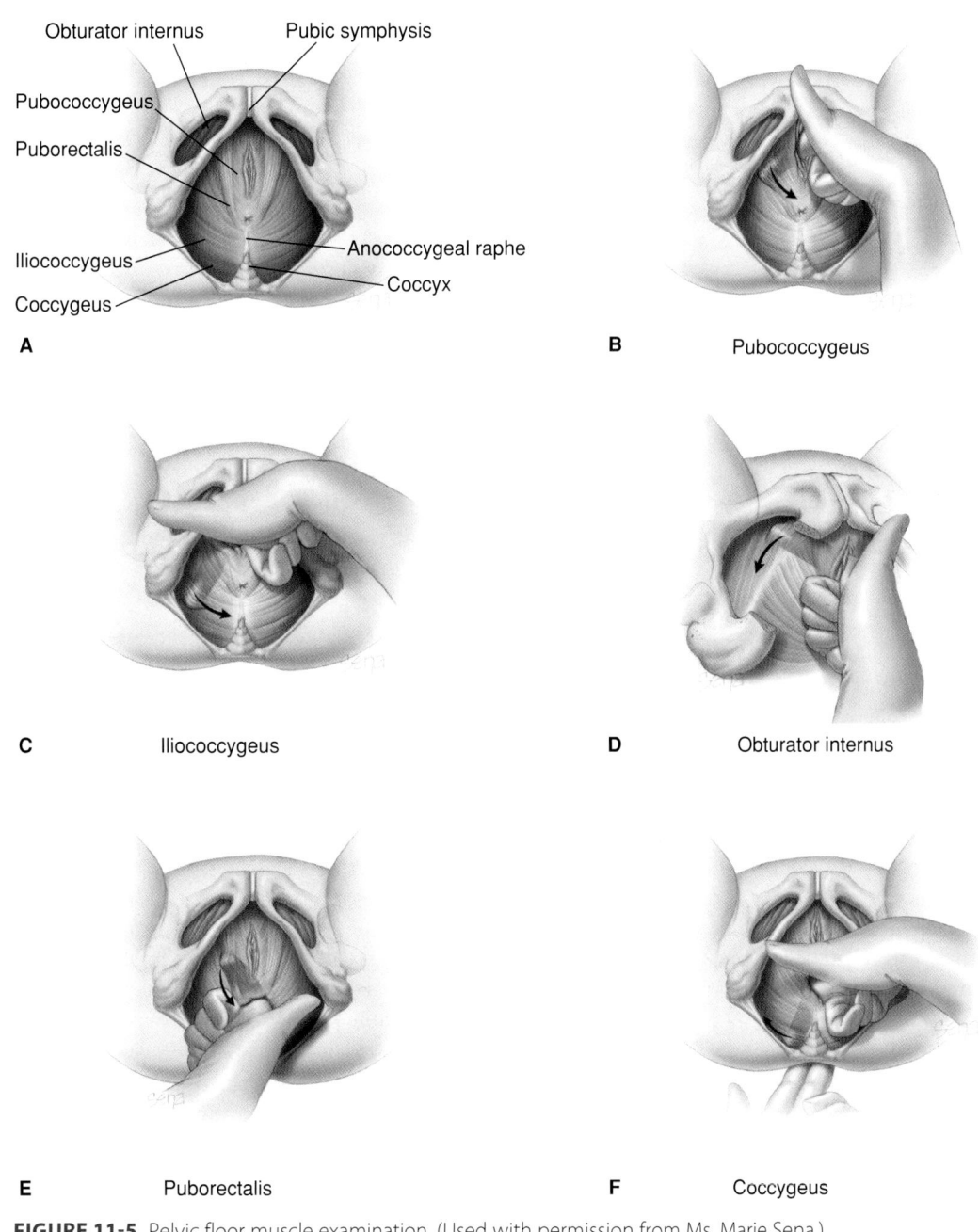

FIGURE 11-5 Pelvic floor muscle examination. (Used with permission from Ms. Marie Sena.)

noted with acute and chronic PID. If pain follows gentle movement of the coccyx, then articular disease of the coccyx, termed coccydynia, is suspected. The importance of pelvic examination sequence cannot be overstated, as information from single-digit examination may be lost if preceded by bimanual examination.

Bimanual assessment of the uterus may reveal a large uterus, often with an irregular contour, due to leiomyomas. Globular enlargement with softening is more typical of adenomyosis. Immobility of the uterus may follow scarring from endometriosis, PID, malignancy, or adhesive disease from prior surgeries. Adnexal palpation may reveal tenderness or mass. Tenderness alone may reflect endometriosis, diverticular disease, or pelvic congestion syndrome. Adnexal mass evaluation is outlined in Chapter 9 (p. 202).

Rectal examination and rectovaginal palpation of the rectovaginal septum is included. Palpation of hard stool or hemorrhoids may indicate GI disorders, whereas nodularity of the rectovaginal septum may be found with endometriosis or neoplasia. Myofascial tenderness involving the puborectalis and coccygeus muscles can be noted by sweeping the index finger with pressure across these muscles. Last, stool testing for occult blood may be performed during digital rectal examination at the initial visit. Alternatively, home test kits for occult blood are available and discussed in Chapter 1 (p. 9).

Testing

For women with CPP, diagnostic testing may add valuable information. Results from urinalysis and urine culture can indicate stones, malignancy, or recurrent infection of the urinary tract as pain sources. Thyroid disease can affect physiologic functioning and may be found in those with bowel or bladder symptoms. Thus, serum thyroid-stimulating hormone (TSH) levels are commonly assayed. Diabetes can lead to neuropathy, and glucose levels can be assessed with urinalysis or serum testing.

Radiologic imaging and endoscopy may be informative, and of these, transvaginal sonography is widely used by gynecologists to evaluate CPP. Sonography of the pelvic organs may reveal endometriomas, leiomyomas, ovarian cysts, dilated pelvic veins, and other structural lesions. In those with suspected pelvic congestion syndrome, transvaginal color Doppler ultrasound is often a primary diagnostic tool (Phillips, 2014). With sonography, patients can be imaged standing, if necessary, and while performing a Valsalva maneuver to accentuate vasculature distention. However, despite its applicability for many gynecologic disorders, sonography has poor sensitivity in identifying endometriotic implants or most adhesions. Of other modalities, CT or MR imaging often adds little additional information to that obtained with sonography. These may be selected if sonography is uninformative or if anatomy is greatly distorted.

In those with bowel symptoms, barium enema may indicate intraluminal or external obstructive lesions, malignancy, and diverticular or inflammatory bowel disease. However, flexible sigmoidoscopy and colonoscopy may offer more information because colonic mucosa can be directly inspected and biopsied if necessary.

Cystoscopy, laparoscopy, flexible sigmoidoscopy, and colonoscopy may each be employed, and patient symptoms will dictate their use. In those with symptoms of chronic pain and urinary symptoms, cystoscopy is often advised. If GI complaints predominate, then flexible sigmoidoscopy or colonoscopy may be warranted. For many women with no obvious cause of their CPP, laparoscopy is performed. Importantly, intraoperative explanations for CPP are common despite normal preoperative examinations (Cunanan, 1983; Kang, 2007). Laparoscopy allows direct identification and, in many cases, treatment of intraabdominal pathology. Therefore, laparoscopy is considered by many to be a "gold standard" for CPP evaluation (Sharma, 2011).

One laparoscopic approach to CPP is performed under local anesthesia with the patient conscious and available for questioning regarding sites of pain (Howard, 2000; Swanton, 2006). Termed *conscious pain mapping,* this technique has resulted in more targeted treatment and improved postoperative pain scores. However, its clinical use to date has been limited.

Treatment
Medical Options

In many women with CPP, an identifying source is found and treatment is dictated by the diagnosis. However, in other cases, pathology may not be identified, and treatment is directed toward dominant symptoms.

Treatment of pain typically begins with oral analgesics such as acetaminophen or nonsteroidal antiinflammatory drugs (NSAIDs) listed in Table 10-1 (p. 239). NSAIDs are particularly helpful if inflammatory states underlie the pain. Acetaminophen is a widely used and effective analgesic despite having no significant antiinflammatory properties. Of note, dosing recommendations from the Food and Drug Administration (2011) limit the maximum total daily dose of acetaminophen to 4 g.

If satisfactory relief is not achieved, then opioid analgesics such as codeine or hydrocodone may be added (Table 42-2, p. 910). Importantly, opioid maintenance therapy for CPP is considered only if all other reasonable pain control attempts have failed and if benefits outweigh harms (Chou, 2009; Howard, 2003). Opioids are most effective and least addictive if given on a scheduled basis and at doses that adequately relieve pain. If pain persists, stronger opioids such as morphine, methadone, fentanyl, oxycodone, and hydromorphone can replace milder ones. However, this is balanced against side effects. Close and regular surveillance is essential, and consultation with pain management experts may be beneficial (Baranowski, 2014; Chou, 2009). Unlike classic opioids, tramadol hydrochloride has a mild central opioid effect but also inhibits serotonin and norepinephrine reuptake.

Estrogen support is integral to endometriosis. Thus, an empiric trial of sex-steroid hormone suppression may be considered, especially in those with coexistent dysmenorrhea or dyspareunia and who lack dominant bladder or bowel symptoms. As discussed in Chapter 10 (p. 239), combination oral contraceptives, progestins, gonadotropin-releasing hormone (GnRH) agonists, and certain androgens are effective options.

For many, CPP represents neuropathic pain, and therapy with antidepressants or anticonvulsants has been extrapolated from treatment of such pain in other disorders. Tricyclic antidepressants reduce neuropathic pain independent of their antidepressant effects (Saarto, 2010). Moreover, antidepressants are a logical choice, as clinically significant depression is commonly comorbid with pain. Amitriptyline (Elavil) and its metabolite nortriptyline (Pamelor) have the best documented efficacy for neuropathic and nonneuropathic pain syndromes (Table 11-5) (Bryson, 1996). Selective serotonin-reuptake inhibitors do not have strong evidence to support their efficacy for CPP (Lunn, 2014). Of anticonvulsants, gabapentin and carbamazepine are most commonly used to reduce neuropathic pain (Moore, 2014; Wiffen, 2014).

Combining drugs with different sites or mechanisms of action may often improve pain. For example, an NSAID and an opioid may be partnered, especially in conditions in which inflammation is dominant. If muscle spasm underlies pain, then pairing a tranquilizer or a muscle relaxant with an opioid or with an NSAID may improve results (Howard, 2003).

Surgery

Nerve destruction, termed *neurolysis,* involves nerve transection or injection of a neurotoxic chemical. Nerve transection cuts a specific peripheral nerve or may be performed on an entire nerve plexus.

TABLE 11-5. Antidepressants and Antiepileptic Drugs Used in Chronic Pain Syndromes

Drug (Brand name)	Dosage	Side Effects
ANTIDEPRESSANTS		
Tricyclic antidepressants		Dry mouth, constipation, urinary retention, sedation, weight gain
Amitriptyline (Elavil)[a] Imipramine (Tofranil)[a]	For both, 10–25 mg at bedtime; increase by 10–25 mg per week up to 75–150 mg at bedtime or a therapeutic drug level	Tertiary amines have greater anticholinergic side effects
Desipramine (Norpramin)[a] Nortriptyline (Pamelor)[a]	For both, 25 mg in the morning or at bedtime; increase by 25 mg per week up to 150 mg per day or a therapeutic drug level	Secondary amines have fewer anticholinergic side effects
Selective serotonin reuptake inhibitors		
Fluoxetine (Prozac)[a] Paroxetine (Paxil)[a]	For both, 10–20 mg per day; up to 80 mg per day for fibromyalgia	Nausea, sedation, decreased libido, sexual dysfunction, headache, weight gain
Novel antidepressants		
Bupropion (Wellbutrin)[a]	100 mg per day; increase by 100 mg per week up to 200 mg twice daily (400 mg per day)	Anxiety, insomnia or sedation, weight loss, seizures (at dosages above 450 mg per day)
Venlafaxine (Effexor)[a]	37.5 mg per day; increase by 37.5 mg per week up to 300 mg per day	Headache, nausea, sweating, sedation, hypertension, seizures. Serotoninergic properties in dosages below 150 mg per day; mixed serotoninergic and noradrenergic properties in dosages above 150 mg per day
ANTIEPILEPTIC DRUGS		
First-generation agents		
Carbamazepine (Tegretol)	200 mg per day; increase by 200 mg per week up to 400 mg three times daily (1200 mg per day)	Dizziness, diplopia, nausea, aplastic anemia
Phenytoin (Dilantin)[a]	100 mg at bedtime; increase weekly up to 500 mg at bedtime	Blood dyscrasias, hepatotoxicity
Second-generation agents		
Gabapentin (Neurontin)	100–300 mg at bedtime; increase by 100 mg every 3 days up to 1800 to 3600 mg per day taken in divided doses three times daily	Drowsiness, dizziness, fatigue, nausea, sedation, weight gain
Pregabalin (Lyrica)	150 mg at bedtime for diabetic neuropathy; 300 mg twice daily for postherpetic neuralgia	Drowsiness, dizziness, fatigue, nausea, sedation, weight gain
Lamotrigine (Lamictal)[a]	50 mg per day; increase by 50 mg every 2 weeks up to 400 mg per day	Dizziness, constipation, nausea; rarely, life-threatening rashes

[a]Not approved by the Food and Drug Administration for treatment of neuropathic pain.
Reproduced with permission from Maizels M, McCarberg B: Antidepressants and antiepileptic drugs for chronic non-cancer pain, 2005 Feb 1;71(3):483–490.

Presacral neurectomy (PSN) describes interruption of somatic pain fibers from the uterus that course within the superior hypogastric plexus (Fig. 38-13, p. 806). This procedure is performed by incising the pelvic peritoneum over the sacrum and then identifying and transecting the sacral nerve plexus. In women so treated, approximately 75 percent note a greater than 50 percent decline in pain (American College of Obstetricians and Gynecologists, 2010).

However, PSN is technically challenging and requires familiarity with operating in the presacral space. Surgery has been associated with long-term constipation and urinary retention postoperatively. Infrequently, life-threatening hemorrhage may be encountered from the middle sacral vessels, which run in the presacral space.

Alternatively, *laparoscopic uterosacral nerve ablation (LUNA)* involves the destruction of nerve fibers that pass to the uterus through the uterosacral ligament. During LUNA, approximately 2 cm of uterosacral ligament near its attachment to the uterus is excised or obliterated using electrosurgery or carbon dioxide (CO_2) laser (Lifford, 2002). Based on pelvic innervation, PSN or LUNA is indicated only for treatment of centrally located pelvic pain, and both have been performed to treat refractory endometriosis-related CPP and dysmenorrhea.

Regarding efficacy, in one randomized trial, investigators performed laparoscopy with and without LUNA for 487 patients with CPP but found no difference in pain, dysmenorrhea, dyspareunia, or quality-of-life measures (Daniels, 2009). Similarly, a metaanalysis found no pain improvement difference between those who did and those who did not undergo LUNA (Daniels, 2010). Moreover, comparisons of LUNA and PSN show significantly greater long-term pain relief with PSN (Proctor, 2005). In sum, available evidence does not support frequent use of LUNA.

Hysterectomy and bilateral salpingo-oophorectomy (BSO) at times may serve as definitive management if thorough evaluation is complete and conservative therapies have failed. For many women with CPP, hysterectomy is effective in resolving pain and improving quality of life (Hartmann, 2004; Stovall, 1990). However, pain may not be resolved in a significant number of women. For example, authors of one prospective study monitored 308 women for 1 year after hysterectomy for CPP and found that 75 percent had complete discomfort resolution, 21 percent had persistent but improved pain, and 5 had unchanged or worsening pain. Pain may persist despite hysterectomy more commonly in those who are younger than 30 years, those who have mental illness, or those with no identifiable pelvic pathology (Gunter, 2003). Almost 40 percent of women with no identified pelvic pathology will have persistent pain after hysterectomy (Hillis, 1995).

Failure of hysterectomy to relieve pain may be multifactorial. First, visceral reflexes (p. 249) may produce multiple pain syndromes within the same patient. Second, hysterectomy does not address nongynecologic etiologies for pelvic pain. Last, pain from interstitial cystitis, pelvic floor myofascial syndrome, or musculoskeletal disorders may worsen following surgery due to its potentially negative effects on innervation, musculature, or vasculature.

Accordingly, before hysterectomy is considered, efforts to accurately diagnose CPP causes and to conservatively manage the pain are first exhausted. Women are given reasonable expectations for symptom relief from hysterectomy and informed of the potential for persistent or worsening pain. As with any operation, the anticipated benefits should outweigh potential risks.

If hysterectomy is planned for endometriosis, concurrent BSO is reasonable. This is more fully discussed in Chapter 10, p. 243. In one analysis of 138 women monitored for 58 months after hysterectomy with ovarian conservation for endometriosis, the relative risk for pain recurrence was 6 and relative risk for reoperation approximated 8 (Namnoum, 1995). In contrast, data regarding bilateral oophorectomy efficacy at time of hysterectomy for idiopathic CPP are lacking and are individualized.

■ Specific Causes of Chronic Pelvic Pain
Pelvic Adhesions

Adhesions are fibrous connections between opposing organ surfaces or between an organ and abdominal wall, at sites where there should be no connection. They vary in vascularity and thickness. These fibrous connections are common, and in laparoscopies performed for CPP, adhesions are found in approximately one quarter of cases (Howard, 1993). However, not all adhesive disease creates pain. For example, Thornton and associates (1997) found no relationship between pelvic pain and intraabdominal adhesions.

In those with pain, adhesions are believed to stretch the peritoneum or organ serosa as it moves. This theory is supported by studies using conscious pain mapping, in which filmy adhesions that allowed significant movement between two structures had the highest association with pain, whereas adhesions that prohibited movement had the lowest pain scores. Moreover, adhesions that had a relationship to the peritoneum had a high association with pain (Demco, 2004). Sensory nerve fibers have been identified histologically, ultrastructurally, and immunohistochemically in human peritoneal adhesions obtained at laparotomy, lending additional support to the above theories (Suleiman, 2001).

Risks for adhesions include prior surgery, prior intraabdominal infection, and endometriosis. Less commonly, inflammation from radiation, chemical irritation, or foreign-body reaction may be causes. Pain is typically aggravated by sudden movement, intercourse, or other specific activities.

Laparoscopy is the primary tool used to diagnose adhesions. In general, sonography lacks sensitivity. However, Guerriero and coworkers (1997) noted a positive correlation with ovarian adhesions if the ovarian surface borders appeared blurred or if the ovary appeared immediately adjacent to the uterus and this intimate position persisted despite transducer manipulation of both.

Surgical lysis is often used to treat pain symptoms, and several observational studies have shown pain improvement (Fayez, 1994; Steege, 1991; Sutton, 1990). However, two randomized studies comparing adhesion lysis with expectant management found no difference in pain scores after 1 year (Peters, 1992; Swank, 2003). Others who support the continued judicious use of adhesiolysis in the treatment of pelvic pain question the statistical methods used in these studies (Roman, 2009). When performed, adhesiolysis is associated with a significant risk of adhesiogenesis, especially in cases involving endometriosis (Parker, 2005). Thus, the decision to lyse adhesions is individualized.

If adhesiolysis is performed, steps are taken to minimize reformation (Hammoud, 2004). Gentle tissue handling, adequate hemostasis, and minimally invasive techniques are essential. Many studies have evaluated the efficacy of various instillates and barriers placed over organs following surgery to minimize adhesion formation. Bioresorbable sheets that are Food and Drug Administration (FDA)-approved and often used in gynecology include brands Seprafilm and Interceed. One peritoneal instillate is icodextrin solution (Adept Adhesion Reduction Solution). Of these options, the American Society for Reproductive Medicine (2013) notes that barrier sheets reduce postoperative adhesions but also state that no substantial evidence shows their use decreases pain. They also report "insufficient evidence to recommend peritoneal instillates." Similarly, two Cochrane reviews reported insufficient evidence regarding the efficacy of any of these agents (Ahmad, 2014; Hindocha, 2015).

Ovarian Remnant Syndrome and Ovarian Retention Syndrome

After oophorectomy, remnants of an excised ovary may create symptoms that are termed *ovarian remnant syndrome.* Distinction is made between this syndrome and ovarian retention syndrome, also known as residual ovary syndrome. *Ovarian retention syndrome* involves symptoms stemming from an ovary intentionally left at the time of previous gynecologic surgery (El Minawi, 1999). Although differentiated by the amount of ovarian tissue involved, both syndromes have nearly identical symptoms and are diagnosed and treated similarly.

Although an uncommon cause of CPP, women with symptomatic ovarian remnants most typically complain of chronic or cyclic pain or dyspareunia. Those with BSO performed for endometriosis may be at particular risk (Kho, 2012). The onset of symptoms is variable and may begin years following surgery (Nezhat, 2005). Women with these syndromes may have a pelvic mass palpable on bimanual examination. Sonography is often informative. In those with ovarian remnants, ovaries may be identified in some cases by a thin rim of ovarian cortex surrounding a coexistent ovarian cyst (Fleischer, 1998). Indeterminate cases may require CT or MR imaging. In cases where ureteral compression is suspected, radiographic or CT pyelography or MR imaging may be warranted. Laboratory testing, specifically follicle-stimulating hormone (FSH) levels, can aid diagnosis in reproductive-aged women with prior BSO. If these levels lie in the premenopausal range, then retained ovarian tissue is likely (Magtibay, 2005).

Although medical treatment has included hormonal manipulation to suppress functioning tissue, surgical excision is required in most symptomatic cases (Lafferty, 1996). Because the ureter is commonly intimately involved with adhesions encasing a remnant, laparotomy is prudent in some cases. However, surgeons with advanced skills in minimally invasive surgery can achieve successful outcomes (Nezhat, 2005; Zapardiel, 2012).

Pelvic Congestion Syndrome

Retrograde blood flow through incompetent valves can often create tortuous, congested ovarian or pelvic veins. Chronic pelvic ache, pressure, and heaviness may result and is termed *pelvic congestion syndrome* (Beard, 1988). Currently, it is not clear whether congestion results from mechanical dilatation, ovarian hormonal dysfunction, or both. Higher rates of ovarian varicosities and pelvic congestion syndrome are noted in parous women. A mechanical theory describes a dramatic increase in pelvic vein diameter during late pregnancy that leads to ovarian vein valve incompetence and pelvic varicosities. Estrogen is implicated in pelvic congestion syndrome in that it acts as a venous dilator. Moreover, pelvic congestion syndrome resolves following menopause, and antiestrogenic medical therapy has been shown to be effective (Farquhar, 1989; Gangar, 1993). Most likely, both factors play roles. The cause of pain with pelvic congestion remains unclear, but increased dilatation, concomitant stasis, and release of local nociceptive mediators have been suggested.

Affected women may describe pelvic ache or heaviness that may worsen premenstrually, after prolonged sitting or standing, or following intercourse. On physical examination, tenderness at the junction of the middle and lateral thirds of a line drawn between the symphysis and anterior superior iliac spine or direct ovarian tenderness may be found. In addition, varicosities in the thigh, buttocks, perineum, or vagina may be associated (Venbrux, 1999).

The left ovarian venous plexus drains into the left ovarian vein, which empties into the left renal vein. The right ovarian vein generally drains directly into the inferior vena cava. Both ovarian veins have numerous trunks, any of which may be involved. Clinical practice guidelines recommend noninvasive sonography or CT or MR venography for suspected cases. Sonographic findings with applied Doppler include a dilated tortuous ovarian vein with a diameter ≥6 mm, slow blood flow ≤3 cm/sec, and a dilated arcuate vein in the myometrium that communicates to the pelvic varicosities (Fig. 11-6) (Park, 2004). With positive findings, then retrograde ovarian and internal iliac venography is preferred if intervention is planned (Gloviczki, 2011).

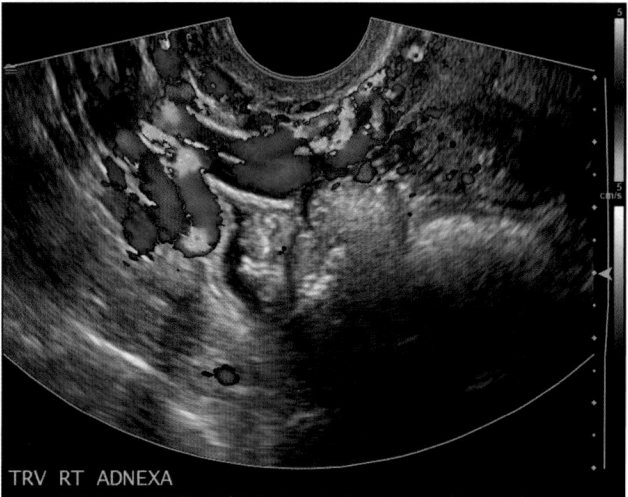

FIGURE 11-6 Color Doppler transvaginal image of tortuous and dilated pelvic vessels in the right adnexa in a patient with chronic pelvic pain. (Used with permission from Dr. Elysia Moschos.)

Diagnostic laparoscopy can also identify varicosities. However, because all these modalities are performed while a woman is supine or in Trendelenburg position, varicosities often decompress and may be missed. CO_2 insufflation pressure also contributes to the high false-negative rate of laparoscopy to diagnose pelvic varicosities.

Common treatments for pelvic congestion syndrome are hormonal suppression, ovarian vein embolization, or hysterectomy with BSO. First, medical treatment with medroxyprogesterone acetate, 30 mg orally daily, or with a GnRH agonist is effective for some women with pelvic congestion syndrome, although symptoms typically recur after medication is discontinued (Reginald, 1989; Soysal, 2001). Second, embolization appears to afford effective treatment, and pain improves in 70 to 80 percent of women (Hansrani, 2015). Third, Beard and coworkers (1991) studied 36 patients who underwent hysterectomy and BSO for pelvic congestion syndrome and intractable pelvic pain. Although 12 of 36 had residual pain at 1 year, only one patient had pain affecting daily life. They concluded that pain and quality-of-life scores were improved. Importantly, none of these options are definitive, and evidence-based studies supporting their efficacy are limited.

DYSMENORRHEA

Cyclic pain with menstruation is common and accompanies most menses (Weissman, 2004). This pain is classically described as cramping and is often accompanied by low backache, nausea and vomiting, headache, or diarrhea. The term *primary dysmenorrhea* describes cyclic menstrual pain without an identifiable associated pathology, whereas *secondary dysmenorrhea* frequently complicates endometriosis, leiomyomas, PID, adenomyosis, endometrial polyps, and menstrual outlet obstruction. For this reason, secondary dysmenorrhea may be associated with other gynecologic symptoms, such as dyspareunia, dysuria, abnormal bleeding, or infertility.

Compared with secondary dysmenorrhea, primary dysmenorrhea more commonly begins shortly after menarche. Pain characteristics, however, typically fail to permit differentiation between the two types, and primary dysmenorrhea is usually diagnosed following exclusion of known associated causes.

When other factors are removed, primary dysmenorrhea equally affects women regardless of race and socioeconomic status. However, increased pain duration or severity is positively associated with earlier age at menarche, long menstrual periods, smoking, and increased body mass index (BMI). In contrast, parity appears to improve symptoms (Harlow, 1996; Sundell, 1990).

Pathophysiologically, prostaglandins are implicated in dysmenorrhea. During endometrial sloughing, endometrial cells release prostaglandins as menstruation begins. Prostaglandins stimulate myometrial contractions and ischemia. Women with more severe dysmenorrhea have higher levels of prostaglandins in menstrual fluid, and these levels are highest during the first 2 days of menstruation. Prostaglandins are also implicated in secondary dysmenorrhea. However, anatomic mechanisms are also suspected, depending on the type of accompanying pelvic disease.

■ Diagnosis

In women with menstrual cramps and no other associated findings or symptoms, no additional evaluation may be initially required, and empiric therapy can be prescribed (Proctor, 2006). In women at risk for PID, cultures for *Chlamydia trachomatis* and *Neisseria gonorrhoeae* are prudent. Moreover, if pelvic evaluation is incomplete due to body habitus, then transvaginal sonography may be informative to exclude structural pelvic pathology.

■ Treatment

Of options, NSAIDs are often preferred. Because prostaglandins are suspected in the genesis of dysmenorrhea, NSAID administration is logical, and studies support their use (Marjoribanks, 2010). These drugs and their dosages are found in Table 10-1 (p. 239).

Steroid hormone contraception leads to endometrial atrophy and in turn lower endometrial prostaglandin levels. Of choices, combination hormone birth control methods are believed to improve dysmenorrhea by lowering prostaglandin production. Studies of combination oral contraceptives (COCs) note improved dysmenorrhea in many users (Brill, 1991; Wong, 2009). In addition, extended or continuous administration of COCs, described in Chapter 5 (p. 123), may be helpful for women with pain not controlled by the traditional cyclic pill schedule (Sulak, 1997). Progestin-only contraceptives are also used for dysmenorrhea. Namely, the levonorgestrel-releasing intrauterine system (LNG-IUS), depot medroxyprogesterone acetate injection, and progestin-releasing implanted rods all are reasonable choices (Lindh, 2013).

GnRH agonists and androgens are other options. The estrogen-lowering effects of these lead to endometrial atrophy and diminished prostaglandin production. Although GnRH agonists and androgens such as danazol lessen dysmenorrhea, their substantial side effects preclude their routine and long-term use. A fuller discussion and dosages for these agents and their side effects are found in Chapter 10 (p. 240).

Complementary and alternative medicine has been evaluated for dysmenorrhea. Oral vitamins E, fish oil, low-fat diet, and Chinese herbal medicine have all been shown to improve dysmenorrhea. However, evidence derives from small and typically nonrandomized trials (Barnard, 2000; Harel, 1996; Zhu, 2008; Ziaei, 2001). Additionally, data are limited but positive toward the use of exercise, topical heat, acupuncture, and transcutaneous electrical nerve stimulation (TENS) (Akin, 2001; Brown, 2010; Proctor, 2002; Smith, 2011).

Cases of dysmenorrhea refractory to conservative management are unusual, and in such instances, surgery may be indicated. Hysterectomy is effective in treating dysmenorrhea, but those desiring future fertility may decline it. For these women, presacral neurectomy can be considered.

DYSPAREUNIA

This is a frequent gynecologic complaint, and in reproductive-aged women in the United States, the 12-month prevalence is 15 to 20 percent (Glatt, 1990; Laumann, 1999). Painful intercourse may be associated with vulvar, visceral, musculoskeletal, neurogenic, or psychosomatic disorders. Coexistent etiologies may also lead to similar symptoms. For example, women with vulvodynia have been shown in many cases to have coexistent pelvic floor muscle spasm, both of which may cause dyspareunia (Reissing, 2005). Because of the frequent association between dyspareunia and CPP and frequent overlap of etiologies, physical examination and diagnostic testing often follow that for women with CPP (p. 253).

Dyspareunia may be subclassified as *insertional,* that is, pain with vaginal entry, or *deep,* which is associated with deep penetration. Of insertional dyspareunia cases, vulvodynia, vulvitis, and poor lubrication form the majority. Of deep dyspareunia cases, endometriosis, pelvic adhesions, and bulky leiomyomas are frequent causes. In many women, both insertional and deep dyspareunia may be present.

Additional terms include *primary dyspareunia,* which describes the onset of painful intercourse coincident with coitarche, and *secondary dyspareunia,* which is painful intercourse that follows an earlier period of pain-free sexual activity. Sexual abuse, female genital mutilation, and congenital anomalies most frequently lead to primary dyspareunia, whereas sources of secondary dyspareunia are more varied. Last, dyspareunia is clarified as *generalized,* occurring in all episodes of intercourse, or as *situational,* associated with only specific partners or sexual positions. Recent changes in the Diagnostic and Statistical Manual of Mental Disorders (DSM-5) have merged dyspareunia and vaginismus into the term *genito-pelvic pain/penetration disorder* (American Psychiatric Association, 2013).

Diagnosis

During history taking, patients are questioned regarding associated symptoms such as vaginal discharge, vulvar pain, dysmenorrhea, CPP, dysuria, or scant lubrication. Onset of symptoms and their temporal association with obstetric delivery, pelvic surgery, or sexual abuse is often informative. In addition, dyspareunia may be found in those who breast feed, presumably because of hypoestrogenism-derived vaginal atrophy seen with lactation (Buhling, 2006; Signorello, 2001). Psychosocial topics such as relationship satisfaction or depression are also covered.

Inspection of the vulva mirrors that for chronic pain. In particular, generalized erythema, episiotomy scars, or atrophy is sought. Erythema may indicate contact or allergic dermatitis or infection, particularly fungal infection. Accordingly, a historical inventory of potential skin irritants, a saline slide preparation, vaginal pH testing, and vaginal cultures are performed. Specifically, a vaginal fungal culture may be required in some cases as several noncandidal species may be poorly detected if microscopic analysis is solely used (Haefner, 2005).

Some studies, but not all, have found a positive correlation between degree of pelvic organ prolapse and dyspareunia (Burrows, 2004; Ellerkmann, 2001). If noted, its degree is assessed as described in Chapter 24 (p. 548).

Physical examination evaluates the distal, mid-, and proximal vagina. Evaluation may first begin with palpation of the Bartholin and paraurethral glands. Additionally, cotton-swab testing is used to map painful areas (Fig. 4-1, p. 87). Next, insertion of a single digit into the distal vagina may elicit

vaginismus, that is, reflex contraction of the muscles associated with distal vaginal penetration (Basson, 2010). This contraction response is normal, but prolonged spasm of the bulbospongiosus, pubococcygeus, piriformis, and obturator internus muscles may cause pain. Spasm is thought to be a conditioned response to current or former physical pain.

With deeper digital examination, midvaginal pain may be triggered. This may be seen with interstitial cystitis, in congenital anomalies, or following radiation therapy or pelvic reconstructive surgeries.

Deep dyspareunia is more commonly caused by disorders that also cause CPP. Focal points of this vaginal examination are discussed on page 257. Similarly, diagnostic testing for deep dyspareunia in large part mirrors that for CPP. Urine and vaginal cultures may indicate infection, and radiologic imaging may reveal structural visceral disease.

Treatment

Resolution of dyspareunia is highly dependent on the underlying cause. For those with vaginismus, structured desensitization is effective. Patients gradually gain control in comfortably inserting dilators of increasing size into the introitus. Concurrent psychological counseling in such cases is often warranted. Poor lubrication may be countered with education directed toward adequate arousal techniques and use of external lubricants. As discussed in Chapter 22, estrogen cream or the selective estrogen-receptor modulator ospemifene (Osphena) will usually resolve genitourinary syndrome of menopause, which is the new preferred term for vulvovaginal atrophy.

Surgery may be indicated for structural pathologies and may include ablation of endometriosis, lysis of adhesions, and restoration of normal anatomy. For those with dyspareunia confidently attributed to a retroverted uterine position, uterine suspension has been shown, albeit in small studies, to be effective (Perry, 2005).

DYSURIA

Evaluation of dysuria begins with a careful pelvic inspection to exclude vaginitis, vulvar lesions, and urethral diverticulum. A voiding diary can be informative, and for those with associated dyspareunia, a sexual history is obtained. The most common cause of dysuria is infection, and urinalysis and urine culture are therefore initial tests. Similarly, *C trachomatis* and herpes simplex virus infections are excluded. For those with chronic dysuria, urodynamic studies may help to identify those with detrusor overactivity, significantly decreased compliance, or bladder outlet obstruction (Chap. 23, p. 526). Cystoscopy is used to identify the hallmark mucosal findings of interstitial cystitis and exclude neoplastic growths or stones (Irwin, 2005). Adjunctively, sonography or laparoscopy may be indicated to exclude structural pelvic pathology or endometriosis.

Interstitial Cystitis/Painful Bladder Syndrome

This chronic inflammatory disorder of the bladder is typified by frequency, urgency, and pelvic pain. With interstitial cystitis (IC), this triad is found in combination with characteristic mucosal changes and reduced bladder capacity. In contrast to cases with classic IC findings, *painful bladder syndrome* describes chronic IC symptoms in those who lack cystoscopic findings of IC or other bladder pathology (Abrams, 2002).

The prevalence of IC in the United States is variable and cited at 0.5 to 3 percent (Berry, 2011; Jones, 1997). It is diagnosed more commonly in women, in whites, in smokers, and in those in their 40s (Kennedy, 2006; Propert, 2000). There is a strong association between IC and endometriosis. The two conditions share similar symptoms, and many patients evaluated for chronic pelvic pain have been found to have either one or both conditions (Butrick, 2007; Paulson, 2007). In addition, IC is association with IBS, generalized pain disorders, fibromyalgia, pelvic floor dysfunction, and depression (Aaron, 2000; Clauw, 1997; Novi, 2005; Peters, 2007).

The exact cause of IC is unknown, and current theories include increased mucosal permeability or mast cell activation (Sant, 2007; Warren, 2002). Glycosaminoglycans are an important component of the mucin layer that covers and protects the bladder urothelium. One theory explains that IC symptoms originate from a defect in the protective bladder glycosaminoglycan component. This leads to increased permeability of the bladder mucosa (Parsons, 2003).

Diagnosis

IC is considered in women with unexplained chronic pelvic pain and voiding symptoms. Warren and colleagues (2006) found that the key descriptor "pelvic pain" fit 100 percent of an affected population. Other relevant descriptors are "pressure" and "discomfort" (Sirinian, 2005). Of voiding complaints, frequency, urgency, nocturia, and pain with bladder filling or emptying are often reported. Dyspareunia and postcoital ache are common. As with most chronic pain syndromes, symptoms may worsen premenstrually. Given the broad spectrum of triggers (alcohol, caffeine, smoking, spicy foods, citrus fruits and juices, carbonated drinks, and potassium), patients may not relate exacerbation of their symptoms to these. Cranberry juice, frequently advised for urinary tract infection, can acutely exacerbate pain from IC.

Single-digit vaginal examination in the patient with IC may demonstrate urethral or anterior vaginal/bladder base tenderness as well as pelvic floor hypertonus, tenderness, or trigger points. The basic laboratory examination includes urinalysis and culture, and unevaluated microhematuria typically prompts cytology, especially in smokers, to exclude neoplasia. Cystoscopy and urodynamic studies may add clarity to complex presentations or exclude of other entities that mimic IC. However, consensus on cystoscopic or urodynamic criteria for IC is lacking (Hanno, 2011). Cystoscopically, *Hunner ulcers* are reddish-brown mucosal lesions with small vessels radiating toward a central scar (Fig. 11-7). These ulcers are rare but considered diagnostic for IC. The more common finding is *glomerulations,* which are small petechiae or submucosal hemorrhages. However, these may be present in patients without IC symptoms and undergoing cystoscopy for other indications (Waxman, 1998). Urodynamic testing may reveal sensory urgency at low bladder volumes, decreased compliance, and decreased capacity. The potassium sensitivity test (PST) indicates increased urothelial permeability

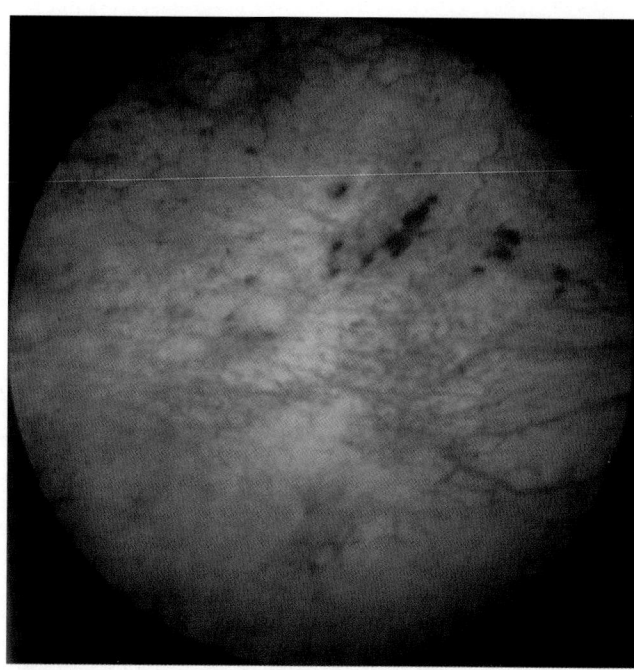

FIGURE 11-7 Cystoscopic photograph displays Hunner ulcers. (Reproduced with permission from Reuter HJ: Bladder. In Atlas of Urologic Endoscopy Diagnosis and Treatment. New York, Thieme Medical Publishers, 1987, p 85.)

but is painful and may trigger a severe symptom flare. Moreover, a negative result does not eliminate suspicion for IC. In one study, 25 percent of patients meeting strict IC criteria had a negative PST result (Parsons, 1998).

Given the broad symptom spectrum, its frequent association with other pelvic pain syndromes, and symptoms that overlap with other pain disorders, diagnosing IC can be challenging. Moreover, uniform consensus on diagnostic criteria is lacking. Thus, the diagnosis of interstitial cystitis remains clinical and is mostly one of exclusion. Not surprisingly, misdiagnosis, underdiagnosis, or delayed diagnosis of IC is common.

Treatment

The American Urological Association has provided evidence-based guidelines for IC management (Hanno, 2011, 2015). First-line treatment provides patient education and behavioral modification, especially avoidance of bladder irritants. Second-tier options are pelvic floor physical therapy to resolve trigger points or pelvic floor hypertonus or to implement pharmacological management. Suitable agents include amitriptyline, cimetidine, hydroxyzine, or pentosan polysulfate sodium (Elmiron), which is a weak anticoagulant. Also, intravesical therapy may consist of direct bladder instillation of heparin, lidocaine, or dimethyl sulfoxide (DMSO). For patients who do not respond, cystoscopy coupled with short-duration, low-pressure bladder distention and fulguration of Hunner ulcers may afford relief. FDA approval is lacking for treatment with cyclosporin A, intradetrusor botulinum toxin A, or sacral neuromodulation, which is described in Section 45-12 (p. 1085). However, their use may be considered in patients who fail to respond to other therapies. Major surgery such as cystoplasty or urinary diversion is performed rarely for carefully selected patients in whom all other therapies have failed to provide adequate symptom control.

GASTROINTESTINAL DISEASE

In numerous cases, GI disease is found as an underlying cause of chronic pelvic pain. GI causes may be organic or functional (see Table 11-1). Thus, initial screening may follow that for CPP. However, symptoms such as fever, GI bleeding, weight loss, anemia, and abdominal mass will prompt a stronger search for organic pathology. Investigations may include sigmoidoscopy or colonoscopy to exclude inflammation, diverticula, or tumors. For those with diarrhea, stool examination for leukocytes or for ova and parasites may be indicated. Moreover, serologic testing for celiac disease can be valuable. When indicated, sonography may aid in distinguishing GI from gynecologic pathology.

■ Colonic Diverticular Disease

Colon diverticula are small defects in the muscular layer of the colon through which colonic mucosa and submucosa herniate. Diverticular disease is common and typically affects the sigmoid or descending colon. Chronic symptoms include abdominal pain that localizes to the left lower quadrant, obstipation, and rectal fullness. More seriously, diverticula may cause acute or chronic GI bleeding or may become infected. Clinically, infection can be difficult to distinguish from PID or tuboovarian abscess. In these cases, CT is the preferred imaging technique and has a sensitivity for diagnosis exceeding 90 percent and a specificity approaching 100 percent (Ambrosetti, 1997).

Chronic diverticular disease is usually treated with a high-fiber diet and long-term suppressive therapy with antibiotics. With acute severe infection, hospitalization, parenteral antibiotics, surgical or percutaneous abscess drainage, or partial colectomy may be required. Suspected rupture of a diverticular abscess with peritonitis is an indication for immediate surgical exploration (Jacobs, 2007).

■ Celiac Disease

This is an inherited autoimmune intolerance to gluten, which is a component of wheat, barley, or rye. In affected individuals, gluten ingestion creates an immune-mediated reaction that damages the small intestine mucosa and leads to varying degrees of malabsorption. Thus, treatment dictates a gluten-free diet for life (Rubio-Tapia, 2013). Celiac disease is common, and its incidence in the general population approaches 1 percent (Green, 2007). Its incidence is suspected to be even higher if those with GI symptoms are screened. There is a gender bias to the disease, and two to three times as many women as men are affected (Green, 2005).

The most common presenting symptoms are abdominal pain and diarrhea. Other findings include weight loss, osteopenia, and fatigue from anemia, all of which stem from malabsorption. In addition, celiac disease has been associated with infertility, although the mechanism is not understood (Tersigni, 2014).

Celiac disease is suspected in those with characteristic findings and in those with a family history of the disorder. Diagnosis requires both duodenal biopsy and a positive response to a gluten-free diet. However, numerous patients presenting with abdominal pain and diarrhea do not have celiac disease. Thus, to avoid unnecessary biopsy, many physicians will screen with noninvasive serologic tests. Of these, serologic screening for IgA antitissue transglutaminase antibodies is preferred and is performed while patients maintain a gluten-containing diet during testing (Rubio-Tapia, 2013).

■ Functional Bowel Disorders

Also known as *functional gastrointestinal disorders (FGIDs)*, this group of functional disorders has symptoms attributable to the lower GI tract and includes those listed in Table 11-6. In defining these chronic conditions, symptoms must have begun more than 6 months previously and have occurred more than 3 days a month during the last 3 months (Longstreth, 2006). The diagnosis always presumes the absence of a structural or biochemical explanation for symptoms (Thompson, 1999).

Irritable Bowel Syndrome

This functional bowel disorder is defined as abdominal pain that improves with defecation and is associated with a change in bowel habits. Subtypes are divided by the predominant stool pattern and include constipative, diarrheal, and mixed categories. Although defining criteria are listed in Table 11-6, other symptoms that support the diagnosis include abnormal stool frequency or stool form, straining, urgency, passing mucus, and bloating (Longstreth, 2006).

IBS is common, and its general population prevalence is estimated to approximate 10 percent (Canavan, 2014; Lovell, 2012). The prevalences of diarrhea-predominant and constipation-predominant IBS are equivalent (Saito, 2002).

The pathophysiology of IBS is complex, and neural, hormonal, genetic, environmental, and psychosocial factors are variably involved (Drossman, 2002). The primary mechanism of IBS, however, is thought to stem from poorly regulated interactions between the CNS and the enteric nervous system (ENS). Such brain-gut dysfunction may eventually cause alterations of GI mucosal immune response, intestinal motility and permeability, and visceral sensitivity. In turn, these produce abdominal pain and altered bowel function (Mayer, 2008). Specifically, serotonin (5-hydroxytryptamine, 5-HT) is involved with regulating intestinal motility, visceral sensitivity, and gut secretion and is thought to play an important role in IBS (Atkinson, 2006; Gershon, 2005).

Prior to assigning a diagnosis of IBS, clinicians ideally exclude organic disease. However, for young patients who have typical IBS symptoms and no organic disease symptoms, few tests are required. Testing is individualized, and factors that typically prompt greater evaluation include older patient age, longer duration and greater severity of symptoms, absent psychosocial factors, organic disease symptoms, and family history of GI disease.

Treatment. Nonpharmacologic approaches may improve symptoms. First, no specific diet suffices for all patients,

TABLE 11-6. Functional Gastrointestinal (GI) Disorders

Functional Bowel Disorders

Irritable bowel syndrome (IBS)	Recurrent abdominal pain or discomfort at least 3 days per month in the last 3 months associated with 2 or more of the following: (1) improved with defecation; (2) onset associated with a change in stooling frequency; (3) onset associated with a change in form of stool
Functional abdominal bloating	Must include *both* of the following: (1) recurrent feeling of bloating or visible distention at least 3 days/month in 3 months; (2) insufficient criteria for a diagnosis of functional dyspepsia, IBS, or other functional GI disorder
Functional constipation	Must include *two or more* of the following: (1) straining during at least 25% of defecations; (2) lumpy or hard stools in at least 25% of defecations; (3) sensation of incomplete evacuation for at least 25% of defecations; (4) sensation of anorectal obstruction/blockage for at least 25% of defecations; (5) manual maneuvers to aid at least 25% of defecations; (6) fewer than three defecations per week Loose stools are rarely present without the use of laxatives There are insufficient criteria for IBS
Functional diarrhea	Loose or watery stools without pain, occurring in at least 75% of stools
Unspecified functional bowel disorder	Bowel symptoms not attributable to an organic etiology that do not meet criteria for the previously defined categories

Functional Abdominal Pain

Functional abdominal pain	At least 6 months of: (1) continuous or nearly continuous abdominal pain; and (2) no or only occasional relation of pain with physiologic events (e.g., eating, defecation, or menses); (3) some loss of daily functioning; (4) pain is not feigned (e.g., malingering); (5) insufficient criteria for other functional gastrointestinal disorders that would explain the abdominal pain
Unspecified functional abdominal pain	

Adapted with permission from Longstreth GF, Thompson WG, Chey WD, et al: Functional bowel disorders, Gastroenterology 2006 Apr;130(5):1480–1491.

but foods known to trigger symptoms are logically avoided. Combination probiotics in general improve global IBS symptoms, bloating, and flatulence, although current data limit recommendation of preferred species (Ford, 2014a,c).

Drug therapy is directed toward dominant symptoms. For those with constipation-dominant IBS, commercial soluble fiber analogues or psyllium husk may help if increased dietary fiber is unsuccessful (Bijkerk, 2009). Of these, psyllium husk is gradually titrated to improve tolerability to a dosage of 3 to 5 g orally twice daily. Of note, dietary fiber is effective in treating constipation but is not effective for diarrhea-dominant IBS or for IBS-associated pain (Ruepert, 2011). Another agent, linaclotide (Linzess), a guanylate cyclase agonist, stimulates increased fluid secretion and transit time (Chey, 2012b; Rao, 2012). It is taken orally as a 290-μg capsule once daily. Alternatively, lubiprostone (Amitiza) is a GI chloride-channel activator that is taken orally twice daily as an 8-μg capsule. It also enhances intestinal fluid secretion to improve intestinal motility (Chey, 2012a; Drossman, 2009). No longer available due to cardiovascular adverse events, tegaserod (Zelnorm) was a partial serotonin-receptor agonist (Food and Drug Administration, 2012b).

For those with diarrhea-dominant symptoms, treatments often strive to slow bowel motility because as substances stay longer in the gut, more water is absorbed from fecal matter to bulk stool. Indirect evidence supports loperamide (Imodium), 2 mg orally once or twice daily (Trinkley, 2014; Weinberg,

2014). For those with severe diarrhea, alosetron (Lotronex), a selective serotonin 5-HT$_3$-receptor antagonist, interacts with ENS neuron receptors to slow bowel motility. This drug decreases pain, urgency, and stool frequency (Camilleri, 2000; Chey, 2004). However, due to cases of ischemic colitis associated with its use, alosetron is now available only through a strictly regulated FDA prescribing program (Chang, 2006; Food and Drug Administration, 2012a).

For patients with pain secondary to bowel spasm, antispasmodic agents decrease intestinal smooth muscle activity and are thought to decrease abdominal discomfort. Agents available in the United States include dicyclomine (Bentyl) and hyoscyamine sulfate (Levsin). Dicyclomine is begun at 20 mg orally four times daily and increased after 1 week to 40 mg. Hyoscyamine sulfate is dosed at 0.25 to 0.5 mg orally daily and can be increased as needed up to four times daily. Although having benefits for IBS, the anticholinergic side effects of these agents often limit their long-term use (Ruepert, 2011; Schoenfeld, 2005). Peppermint oil, another effective antispasmodic, can be taken orally as over-the-counter capsules at dosages of 550 mg once daily or 187 mg three times daily (Khanna, 2014).

Tricyclic antidepressants may help patients with IBS both by an anticholinergic effect on the gut and by mood-modifying action. Tricyclic antidepressants may slow intestinal transit time and have been shown to be effective in treatment of diarrhea-dominant IBS (Hadley, 2005). Last, psychological or behavioral treatments may help some patients (Ford, 2014b).

MUSCULOSKELETAL ETIOLOGIES

Clinical syndromes involving the muscles, nerves, and skeletal system of the lower abdomen and pelvis are frequently encountered but often overlooked by gynecologists. Importantly, unrecognized musculoskeletal pain may lead to unnecessary surgery or promote development of pelvic pain syndromes.

■ Hernia

Defects in anterior abdominal wall or femoral fascia can lead to herniation of bowel or other intraabdominal contents through these rents. Such herniation can create pain locally at the defect site or cause referred pain along the distribution of a compressed sensory nerve. Moreover, if blood supply to the contents is acutely compromised, then bowel obstruction or ischemia will require surgical intervention. Hernias that involve the anterior abdominal wall and pelvic floor are most commonly associated with CPP. Much less frequently, *sciatic hernia,* which is herniation of peritoneum and peritoneal contents through the greater sciatic foramen, and *obturator hernia,* which is that through the obturator canal, are also described sources of acute or chronic pain.

Hernias may develop at sites of inherent anatomic weakness, and common types in women include ventral, umbilical, and incisional hernias. Indirect inguinal, direct inguinal, and femoral hernias are types less often found in females. Spigelian hernias are rare. As shown in Figure 11-8, ventral hernias are caused by fascial defects typically occurring in the midline. Umbilical hernias are those involving defects of the umbilical ring. Indirect inguinal hernias are those in which abdominal contents herniate through the internal inguinal ring and into the inguinal canal. As shown in Figure 11-9, contents may then exit the external inguinal ring. In contrast, contents of a direct inguinal hernia bulge through a fascial defect within Hesselbach triangle. Spigelian hernias can occur anywhere along the lateral border of the rectus abdominis muscle. However, the most frequent location is this border's intersection point with the arcuate line.

Conditions that increase intraabdominal pressure such as pregnancy, ascites, peritoneal dialysis, and chronic cough are known hernia risk factors. Congenital or acquired anatomic weakness or connective tissue disorders are also associated.

For diagnosis, patients with CPP or abdominal pain ideally are examined while standing and also during Valsalva maneuver. Because of the potential risks associated with content herniation and strangulation, hernias are typically repaired once identified. Small ventral, umbilical, or incisional hernias may be repaired

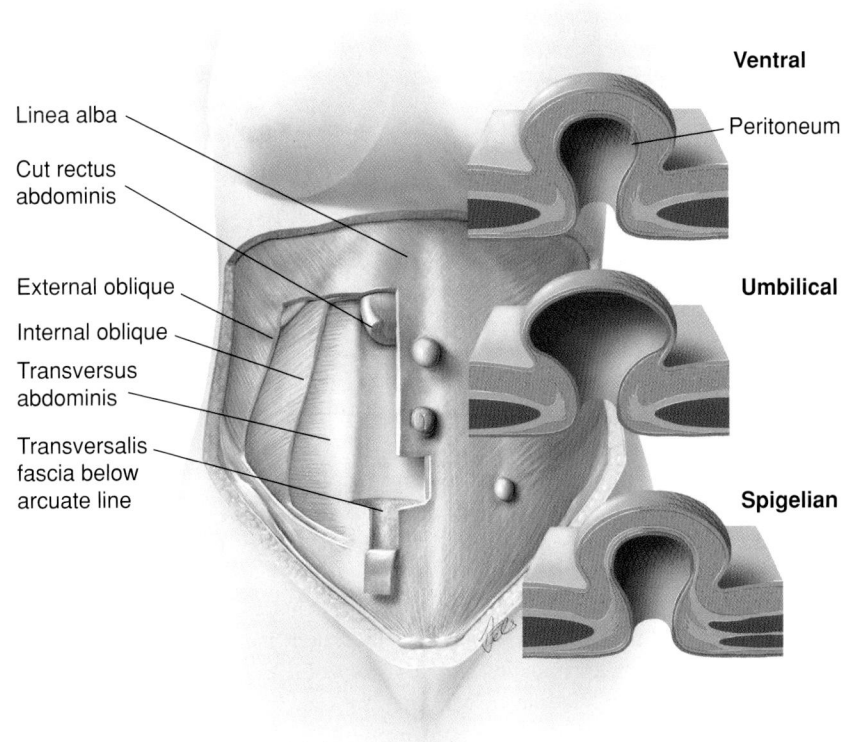

Linea alba
Cut rectus abdominis
External oblique
Internal oblique
Transversus abdominis
Transversalis fascia below arcuate line

Ventral
Peritoneum
Umbilical
Spigelian

FIGURE 11-8 Hernias that may involve the anterior abdominal wall. (Used with permission from Mr. T. J. Fels.)

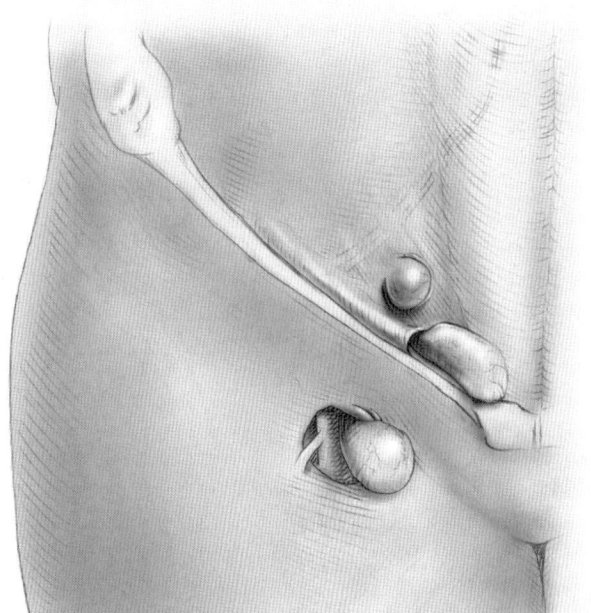

FIGURE 11-9 Indirect and direct inguinal hernias and femoral hernia. A direct hernia is cause by a fascial defect within Hesselbach triangle. The sides of this triangle are formed by the inguinal ligament, the inferior epigastric vessels, and the lateral border of the rectus abdominis muscle. An indirect hernia forms from intraabdominal contents exiting through the inguinal canal. Femoral hernias form from contents exiting through the femoral ring.

by gynecologic surgeons. In these cases, the hernia sac is excised and fascia reapproximated. Patients with larger hernias, which usually require mesh placement, or hernias in the inguinal area are typically referred to a general surgeon.

Myofascial Pain Syndrome

Primary musculoskeletal (MS) conditions may lead to CPP (see Table 11-2). In other cases, secondary myofascial pain syndromes can originate from endometriosis, interstitial cystitis, or IBS. Such chronic visceral inflammatory conditions can create pathologic changes in nearby muscles and/or nerves to cause abdominal wall or pelvic floor pain. Thus, awareness of these complex associations allows a physician to more effectively address all components leading to pain, rather than narrowly focusing on an isolated visceral disorder.

With myofascial pain, a hyperirritable area within a muscle promotes persistent fiber contraction (Simons, 1999). The primary reactive area within the muscle is termed a *trigger point (TrP)* and is identified as a palpable taut, ropy band. Trigger points are thought to form as the end of a metabolic crisis within a muscle. Dysfunction of a neuromuscular endplate can lead to sustained acetylcholine release, persistent depolarization, sarcomere shortening, and creation of a taut muscle band. Affected fibers compress capillaries and decrease local blood flow. The resulting ischemia leads to release of substances that activate peripheral nerve nociceptors and in turn cause pain (McPartland, 2004). A persistent barrage of nociceptive signals from TrPs may eventually lead to central sensitization and the potential for neuropathic pain (p. 250). Signals may spread segmentally within the spinal cord to cause localized or referred pain (Gerwin, 2005). TrPs can also initiate viscerosomatic convergence that can generate autonomic responses such as vomiting, diarrhea, and bladder spasm.

TrPs can affect any muscle, and those involving muscles of the anterior abdominal wall, pelvic floor, and pelvic girdle can be sources of CPP. The incidence of myofascial disease is unknown. However, in an evaluation of 500 patients with CPP, Carter (1998) found that 7 percent of patients primarily had TrPs as a source of their pain. Moreover, of nearly 1000 women evaluated for CPP, 22 percent were found to have significant tenderness of the levator ani muscles and 14 percent

had piriformis muscle tenderness (Gomel, 2007). Prevalence appears to be greatest at ages between 30 and 50 years. Risk factors are varied, although many trigger points can be traced to a prior specific trauma such as a sports injury or to chronic biomechanical overload of a muscle (Sharp, 2003). Accordingly, a detailed inventory of sports injuries, traumatic injuries, obstetric deliveries, surgeries, and work activities is essential.

Diagnosis

Having the patient mark painful sites on a body silhouette diagram can be an informative first step. Involvement of specific muscles will often give characteristic patterns. Patients typically describe the pain as aggravated by specific movement or activity and relieved by certain positions. Cold, damp exposure generally worsens pain. Pressure on a trigger point causes pain and produces effects on a target area or *referral zone*. This specific and reproducible area of referral rarely coincides with dermatologic or neuronal distribution and is the feature that differentiates myofascial pain syndromes from fibromyalgia (Lavelle, 2007).

Muscle examination may be completed by flat palpation, pincer palpation, or deep palpation depending on muscle location. Flat palpation uses fingertips to roll over superficial muscles, which are accessible only at the surface (Fig. 11-10). This technique is commonly used to assess the anterior abdominal wall. In muscles with greater accessibility, pincer palpation grasps the muscle belly between the thumb and fingers. With any of the palpation techniques, spot tenderness and taut muscle bands are sought. Classically, the involved muscle displays weakness and restricted stretch. TrP pressure may also elicit a local muscle twitch response, reproduce a patient's referred pain, or both.

Specific Muscle Groups

Anterior abdominal wall muscles—that is, the rectus abdominis, the obliques, and transversus abdominis muscles—may all develop TrPs, and somatovisceral pelvic symptoms from these muscles may include diarrhea or urinary frequency, urgency, or retention. Rectus abdominis muscle TrPs are frequently found along the linea semilunaris, which is the term for this muscle's lateral margin (Suleiman, 2001). Additional rectus abdominis TrPs may develop at the muscle's insertion into the pubic bone and also below the umbilicus. Within the external oblique

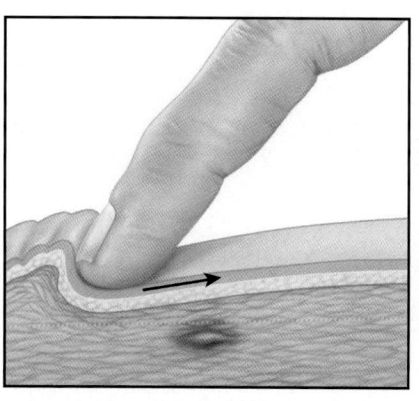
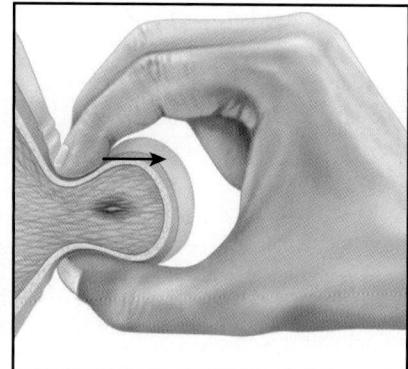
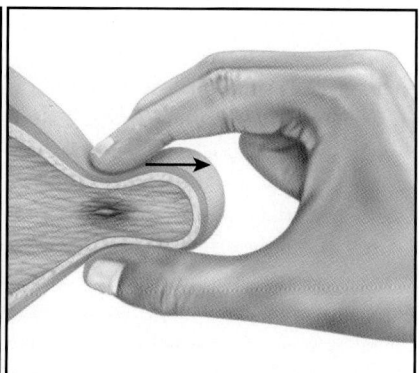

A   **B**

FIGURE 11-10 Techniques for trigger point palpation. **A.** With flat palpation, fingertips stroke across the muscle surface. **B.** With pincer palpation, the muscle is grasped and palpation for trigger points is completed as the muscle slips through the fingers.

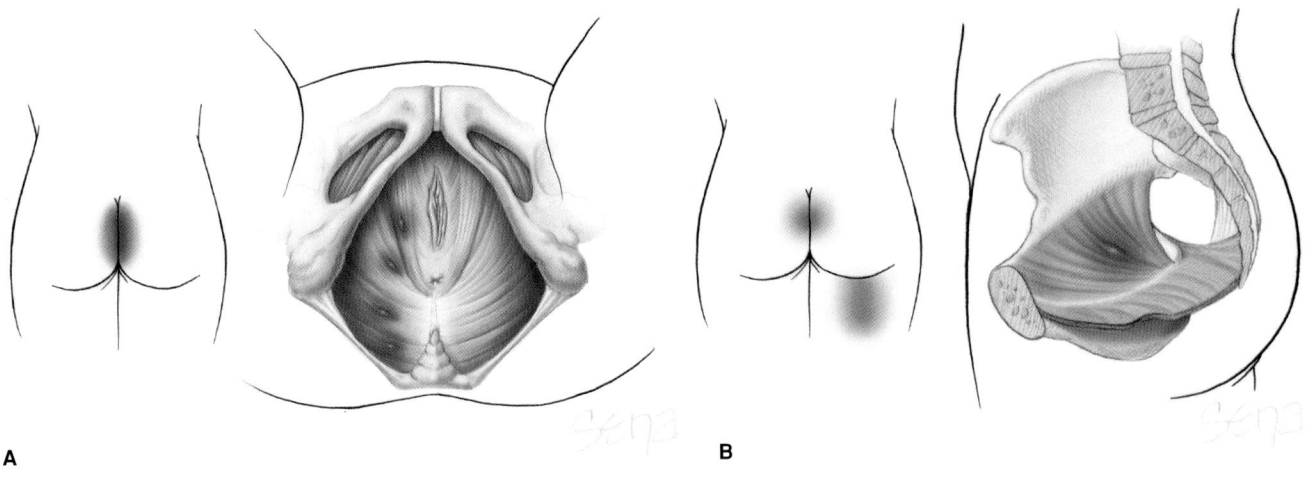

A   **B**

FIGURE 11-11 Trigger points and their extensive patterns of referred pain (*red shading*) **A.** Trigger points in the levator ani and coccygeus muscles. **B.** Trigger point in the obturator internus muscle. (Used with permission from Ms. Marie Sena.)

muscle, trigger points frequently involve its lateral attachment to the anterior iliac crest. Pain usually refers to the pubic bone.

After examination of the anterior abdominal wall, muscles of the pelvis are evaluated. Following careful inspection of the external genitalia, vaginal examination proceeds slowly with the index finger only and initially without a palpating abdominal hand. Muscles within the pelvis include the levator ani, coccygeus, obturator internus, and deep transverse perineal and piriformis muscles, and these are assessed for painful TrPs (see Fig. 11-5) (Vercellini, 2009). TrPs involving these muscles and anal sphincter muscles are frequently associated with poorly localized pain that may be described as involving the coccyx, hip, or back (Fig. 11-11). Dyspareunia is common.

Levator Ani Syndrome. Pain stemming from TrPs involving the levator ani muscles has had various names including levator ani spasm syndrome and coccydynia (see Fig. 11-11). Currently, *levator ani syndrome* is preferred. *Coccydynia* is reserved for coccygeal pain originating from skeletal trauma to the coccyx.

The levator ani muscles, including their supporting fascia, overlying parietal peritoneum, and intimately associated visceral peritoneum, are connected by common sensory nerves to the spinal cord. These provide the basis for viscerosomatic convergence (Spitznagle, 2014). Spasm of these muscles can result in lower abdominal pain, low back pain, dyspareunia, and chronic constipation.

Treatment

Regardless of TrP location, the treatment goal is TrP inactivation, which then allows stretching and release of taut muscle bands. Of methods, TrP point massage or more aggressive ischemic compression massage are effective (Hull, 2009). Biofeedback, relaxation techniques, or psychotherapy may be helpful therapy adjuncts. Analgesics, antiinflammatory drugs, muscle relaxants, or neuroleptics may also be prescribed. Finally, electrical stimulation, TrP dry needling, or TrP injection may be required. In those who are unresponsive to injection of local anesthetic agents, botulinum toxin A injection may be considered (Gyang, 2013). At our institution, as in many other

tertiary referral centers, we often consult pelvic floor physical therapy experts for many of these treatments.

■ Peripartum Pelvic Pain Syndrome

Also known as pelvic girdle pain, this condition is characterized by persistent pain that begins during pregnancy or immediately postpartum. Pain is prominent around the sacroiliac joints and symphysis and is thought to originate from injury or inflammation of the pelvic and/or lower spine ligaments. Muscle weakness, postural adjustments of pregnancy, hormonal changes, and weight of the fetus and gravid uterus are all potential contributing factors (Mens, 1996). Pelvic girdle pain is common. Significant pain is estimated to afflict approximately 20 percent of pregnant women and 7 percent of those during the 3 months following delivery (Albert, 2002; Wu, 2004). Diagnosis is usually clinical and based on findings during specific orthopedic joint manipulation tests. These are used to recreate or provoke the pain. Treatment includes physical therapy, exercise, and analgesics typically used for CPP (Vermani, 2010; Vleeming, 2008).

NEUROLOGIC ETIOLOGIES

■ Anterior Abdominal Wall Nerve Entrapment Syndromes

Nerve compression can lead to chronic pelvic pain and may involve nerves of the anterior abdominal wall or those within the pelvis. Anterior abdominal wall pain is frequently mistaken for visceral pain. Common causes include entrapment of the anterior cutaneous branches of the intercostal nerves or compression of branches of the ilioinguinal, iliohypogastric, genitofemoral nerves, and lateral femoral cutaneous nerves (Greenbaum, 1994). These peripheral nerves can be compressed either within narrow anatomic canals or rings or beneath tight ligaments, fibrous bands, or sutures. For example, each anterior cutaneous branch of an intercostal nerve traverses anteriorly through the rectus abdominis muscle. Each branch and its corresponding vessels travels through a fibrous ring found within

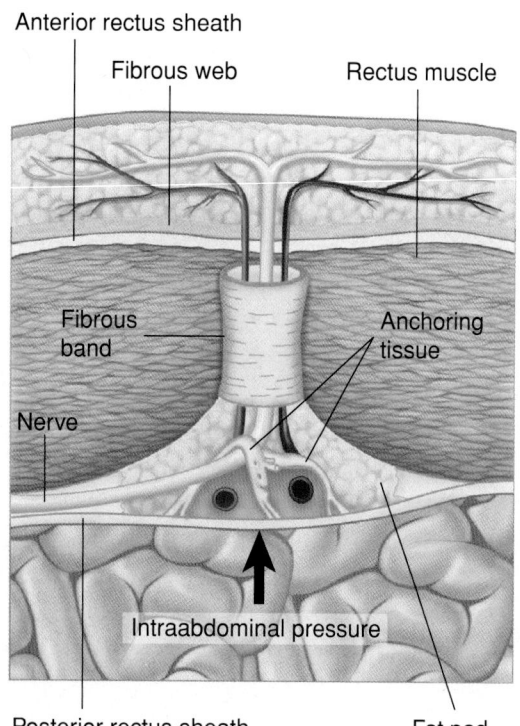

Anterior rectus sheath
Fibrous web
Rectus muscle
Fibrous band
Anchoring tissue
Nerve
Intraabdominal pressure
Posterior rectus sheath
Fat pad

FIGURE 11-12 Drawing displays nerve entrapment of the anterior cutaneous branches of one of the intercostal nerves. The nerve is compressed as it traverses the rectus abdominis muscle within a fibrous sheath. (Reproduced with permission from Greenbaum DS, Greenbaum RB, Joseph JG, et al: Chronic abdominal wall pain. Diagnostic validity and costs, Dig Dis Sci 1994 Sep;39(9):1935–1941.)

the lateral aspect of rectus abdominis muscle (Fig. 11-12). Clinically, these nerve branches are those often seen during Pfannenstiel incision creation as the anterior rectus sheath is dissected off each rectus belly (Fig. 43-2.3, p. 930). On crossing the anterior rectus sheath, each nerve branch divides and then courses within the subcutaneous layer. Within the fibrous ring, fat surrounding the neurovascular bundle appears to pad the enclosed structures (Srinivasan, 2002). However, if this bundle receives excessive intra- or extraabdominal pressure, compression of the bundle against the fibrous ring causes nerve ischemia and pain (Applegate, 1997).

Nerve entrapment, injury, or neuroma formation may also involve branches of the ilioinguinal, iliohypogastric, lateral femoral cutaneous, or genitofemoral nerves, as described in Chapter 40 (p. 845). Involvement may follow inguinal hernia repair, low transverse abdominal incisions, and lower abdominal laparoscopic trocar placement. Hypoesthesia is the more common finding with these injuries, but pain may variably develop within months of surgery or after several years.

Criteria for diagnosing nerve entrapment are clinical and include: (1) pain aggravated by patient movement or light skin pinching over the affected area and (2) pain improvement following local anesthetic injection. In general, electromyography is uninformative because it lacks adequate sensitivity (Knockaert, 1996). For local injection, 1- or 2-percent lidocaine and a 40-mg/mL concentration of triamcinolone can be combined in a 1:1 ratio. However, the corticosteroid may be omitted. Less than half a milliliter is injected at each pain site.

Injections of the mixture may be repeated if initially successful. Additional treatments can include oral analgesics, biofeedback, and gabapentin. If conservative options fail to bring sufficient relief, neurolysis with injection of 5- to 6-percent absolute alcohol or phenol, or surgical neurectomy may be required (Madura, 2005; Suleiman, 2001).

Pudendal Neuralgia

Neuralgia is sharp, severe, shooting pain that follows the distribution of the involved nerve. Pudendal nerve entrapment may create this type of pain on the perineum. The three branches of this nerve are the perineal nerve, the inferior rectal nerve, and the dorsal nerve to the clitoris (Fig. 38-28, p. 822). Thus, pain may involve, alone or in combination, the clitoris, vulva, or rectum. Pudendal neuralgia is rare, is usually unilateral, and typically develops after age 30. In affected individuals, allodynia and hyperesthesia may be extreme to the point of disability. The pain is aggravated by sitting, is relieved by sitting on a toilet seat or standing, and may progress during the day.

The diagnosis of pudendal neuralgia is clinical, and *Nantes criteria* are used by many. As inclusion criteria: pain follows the pudendal nerve innervation path, is worse with sitting, has no associated sensory loss, does not awaken patients, and is relieved by nerve blockade (Labat, 2008). Clinical suspicion may be supported by objective testing. This may include neurophysiologic testing such as pudendal nerve motor latency and electromyography (EMG), both described in Chapter 25 (p. 569). However, abnormal findings with these are not specific for pudendal neuralgia. Rarely, CT or MR imaging may be informative, although these may be performed to exclude other pathology (Khoder, 2014).

Treatment can involve physical therapy; behavioral modification; gabapentin or tricyclic antidepressants; pudendal nerve blockade, with or without corticosteroids; botulinum toxin A injection; and pudendal nerve stimulation. If these are unsuccessful, surgical nerve decompression may be elected.

Piriformis Syndrome

Compression of the sciatic nerve by the piriformis muscle may lead to buttock or low back pain in the distribution of the sciatic nerve (Broadhurst, 2004). This is termed the *piriformis syndrome*. Proposed mechanisms for compression include: contracture or spasm of the piriformis muscle from trauma, overuse and muscle hypertrophy, and congenital variations, in which the sciatic nerve or its divisions pass directly through this muscle (Hopayian, 2010).

Fishman and associates (2002) estimate the piriformis syndrome to be responsible for 6 to 8 percent of cases of low back pain and sciatica in the United States each year. Symptoms include pain and tenderness involving the buttocks, with or without radiation into the posterior thigh. Pain is worse with activity, prolonged sitting, walking, and internal rotation of the hip (Kirschner, 2009). Dyspareunia has a common but variable association and has been demonstrated in 13 to 100 percent of cases (Hopayian, 2010).

Diagnosis of the syndrome is clinical and based on findings during specific orthopedic joint manipulation tests (Michel, 2013). Nerve conduction and EMG are typically nondiagnostic.

Uncommonly, MR imaging may be helpful by identifying a swollen or enlarged piriformis muscle or anatomic muscle variants (Petchprapa, 2010). Treatment is conservative and includes physical therapy, NSAIDs, muscle relaxants, or neuropathic pain agents such as gabapentin, nortriptyline, or carbamazepine. Therapeutic injections of local anesthetics, with or without corticosteroids, or of botulinum toxin A may be used. Surgery is reserved for refractory cases.

REFERENCES

Aaron LA, Burke MM, Buchwald D: Overlapping conditions among patients with chronic fatigue syndrome, fibromyalgia, and temporomandibular disorder. Arch Intern Med 160:221, 2000

Abrams P, Cardozo L, Fall M, et al: The standardisation of terminology of lower urinary tract function: report from the Standardisation Sub-committee of the International Continence Society. Neurourol Urodyn 21:167, 2002

Ahmad G, Mackie FL, Iles DA, et al: Fluid and pharmacological agents for adhesion prevention after gynaecological surgery. Cochrane Database Syst Rev 7:CD001298, 2014

Akin MD, Weingand KW, Hengehold DA, et al: Continuous low-level topical heat in the treatment of dysmenorrhea. Obstet Gynecol 97:343, 2001

Albert HB, Godskesen M, Westergaard JG: Incidence of four syndromes of pregnancy-related pelvic joint pain. Spine 27(24):2831, 2002

Ambrosetti P, Grossholz M, Becker C, et al: Computed tomography in acute left colonic diverticulitis. Br J Surg 84:532, 1997

American College of Obstetricians and Gynecologists: Chronic pelvic pain. Practice Bulletin No. 51, March 2004, Reaffirmed May 2010

American Psychiatric Association: DSM-5: Diagnostic and Statistical Manual for Mental Disorders, 5th edition. Washington, American Psychiatric Press, 2013

American Society for Reproductive Medicine; Society of Reproductive Surgeons: Pathogenesis, consequences, and control of peritoneal adhesions in gynecologic surgery: a committee opinion. Fertil Steril 99(6):1550, 2013

Andreotti RF, Lee SI, Dejesus Allison SO, et al: ACR Appropriateness Criteria® acute pelvic pain in the reproductive age group. Ultrasound Q 27(3):205, 2011

Applegate WV, Buckwalter NR: Microanatomy of the structures contributing to abdominal cutaneous nerve entrapment syndrome. J Am Board Fam Pract 10:329, 1997

As-Sanie S, Harris RE, Napadow V, et al: Changes in regional gray matter volume in women with chronic pelvic pain: a voxel-based morphometry study. Pain 153(5):1006, 2012

Atkinson W, Lockhart S, Whorwell PJ, et al: Altered 5-hydroxytryptamine signaling in patients with constipation- and diarrhea-predominant irritable bowel syndrome. Gastroenterology 130(1):34, 2006

Baker PK: Musculoskeletal origins of chronic pelvic pain. Diagnosis and treatment. Obstet Gynecol Clin North Am 20:719, 1993

Baranowski AP, Lee J, Price C, et al: Pelvic pain: a pathway for care developed for both men and women by the British Pain Society. Br J Anaesth 112(3):452, 2014

Barnard ND, Scialli AR, Hurlock D, et al: Diet and sex-hormone binding globulin, dysmenorrhea, and premenstrual symptoms. Obstet Gynecol 95:245, 2000

Basson R, Wierman ME, van Lankveld J, et al: Summary of the recommendations on sexual dysfunctions in women. J Sex Med 7(1 Pt 2):314, 2010

Beard RW, Kennedy RG, Gangar KF, et al: Bilateral oophorectomy and hysterectomy in the treatment of intractable pelvic pain associated with pelvic congestion. BJOG 98:988, 1991

Beard RW, Reginald PW, Wadsworth J: Clinical features of women with chronic lower abdominal pain and pelvic congestion. BJOG 95:153, 1988

Bermejo C, Martínez Ten P, Cantarero R, et al: Three-dimensional ultrasound in the diagnosis of müllerian duct anomalies and concordance with magnetic resonance imaging. Ultrasound Obstet Gynecol 35(5):593, 2010

Berry SH, Elliott MN, Suttorp M et al: Prevalence of symptoms of bladder pain syndrome/interstitial cystitis among adult females in the United States. J Urol 186: 540, 2011

Bijkerk CJ, de Wit NJ, Muris JW, et al: Soluble or insoluble fibre in irritable bowel syndrome in primary care? Randomised placebo controlled trial. BMJ 339:b3154, 2009

Brenner DJ, Hall EJ: Computed tomography—an increasing source of radiation exposure. N Engl J Med 357(22):2277, 2007

Brill K, Norpoth T, Schnitker J, et al: Clinical experience with a modern low-dose oral contraceptive in almost 100,000 users. Contraception 43:101, 1991

Broadhurst NA, Simmons DN, Bond MJ: Piriformis syndrome: correlation of muscle morphology with symptoms and signs. Arch Phys Med Rehabil 85(12):2036, 2004

Brown J, Brown S: Exercise for dysmenorrhea. Cochrane Database Syst Rev 2:CD004142, 2010

Brown MA, Sirlin CB: Female pelvis. Magn Reson Imaging Clin North Am 13(2):381, 2005

Bryson HM, Wilde MI: Amitriptyline. A review of its pharmacological properties and therapeutic use in chronic pain states. Drugs Aging 8:459, 1996

Buhling KJ, Schmidt S, Robinson JN, et al: Rate of dyspareunia after delivery in primiparae according to mode of delivery. Eur J Obstet Gynecol Reprod Biol 124:42, 2006

Burrows LJ, Meyn LA, Walters MD, et al: Pelvic symptoms in women with pelvic organ prolapse. Obstet Gynaecol 104(5 Pt 1):982, 2004

Butrick CW: Interstitial cystitis and chronic pelvic pain: new insights in neuropathology, diagnosis, and treatment. Clin Obstet Gynaecol 46:811, 2003

Butrick CW: Patients with chronic pelvic pain: endometriosis or interstitial cystitis/painful bladder syndrome? JSLS 11(2):182, 2007

Camilleri M, Northcutt AR, Kong S, et al: Efficacy and safety of alosetron in women with irritable bowel syndrome: a randomised, placebo-controlled trial. Lancet 355:1035, 2000

Canavan C, West J, Card T: The epidemiology of irritable bowel syndrome. Clin Epidemiol 6:71, 2014

Carter JE: Surgical treatment for chronic pelvic pain. JSLS 2:129, 1998

Chang L, Chey WD, Harris L, et al: Incidence of ischemic colitis and serious complications of constipation among patients using alosetron: systematic review of clinical trials and post-marketing surveillance data. Am J Gastroenterol 101(5):1069, 2006

Chey WD, Chey WY, Heath AT, et al: Long-term safety and efficacy of alosetron in women with severe diarrhea-predominant irritable bowel syndrome. Am J Gastroenterol 99:2195, 2004

Chey WD, Drossman DA, Johanson JF, et al: Safety and patient outcomes with lubiprostone for up to 52 weeks in patients with irritable bowel syndrome with constipation. Aliment Pharmacol Ther 35:587, 2012a

Chey WD, Lembo AJ, Lavins BJ, et al: Linaclotide for irritable bowel syndrome with constipation: a 26-week, randomized, double-blind, placebo-controlled trial to evaluate efficacy and safety. Am J Gastroenterol 107: 1702, 2012b

Chou R, Fanciullo GJ, Fine PG, et al: Clinical guidelines for the use of chronic opioid therapy in chronic noncancer pain. J Pain 10(2):113, 2009

Clauw DJ, Schmidt M, Radulovic D, et al: The relationship between fibromyalgia and interstitial cystitis. J Psychiatr Res 31:125, 1997

Cunanan RG Jr, Courey NG, Lippes J: Laparoscopic findings in patients with pelvic pain. Am J Obstet Gynaecol 146:589, 1983

Daniels J, Gray R, Hills RK, et al: Laparoscopic uterosacral nerve ablation for alleviating chronic pelvic pain: a randomized controlled trial. JAMA 302(9):955, 2009

Daniels JP, Middleton L, Xiong T, et al: Individual patient data meta-analysis of randomized evidence to assess the effectiveness of laparoscopic uterosacral nerve ablation in chronic pelvic pain. Hum Reprod Update 16(6):568, 2010

Demco L: Pain mapping of adhesions. J Am Assoc Gynecol Laparosc 11:181, 2004

Descargues G, Tinlot-Mauger F, Gravier A, et al: Adnexal torsion: a report on forty-five cases. Eur J Obstet Gynecol Reprod Biol 98:91, 2001

Drossman DA, Camilleri M, Mayer EA, et al: AGA technical review on irritable bowel syndrome. Gastroenterology 123:2108, 2002

Drossman DA, Chey WD, Johanson JF, et al: Clinical trial: lubiprostone in patients with constipation-associated irritable bowel syndrome—results of two randomized, placebo-controlled studies. Aliment Pharmacol Ther 29:329, 2009

Dubuisson J, Botchorishvili R, Perrette S, et al: Incidence of intraabdominal adhesions in a continuous series of 1000 laparoscopic procedures. Am J Obstet Gynecol 203(2):111.e1, 2010

Einstein AJ, Henzlova MJ, Rajagopalan S: Estimating risk of cancer associated with radiation exposure from 64-slice computed tomography coronary angiography. JAMA 298(3):317, 2007

Ellerkmann RM, Cundiff GW, Melick CF, et al: Correlation of symptoms with location and severity of pelvic organ prolapse. Am J Obstet Gynecol 185:1332, 2001

El Minawi AM, Howard FM: Operative laparoscopic treatment of ovarian retention syndrome. J Am Assoc Gynecol Laparosc 6:297, 1999

Farquhar CM, Rogers V, Franks S, et al: A randomized controlled trial of medroxyprogesterone acetate and psychotherapy for the treatment of pelvic congestion. BJOG 96:1153, 1989

Fayez JA, Clark RR: Operative laparoscopy for the treatment of localized chronic pelvic-abdominal pain caused by postoperative adhesions. J Gynecol Surg 10:79, 1994

Fazel R, Krumholz HM, Wang Y, et al: Exposure to low-dose ionizing radiation from medical imaging procedures. N Engl J Med 361(9):849, 2009

Fishman LM, Dombi GW, Michaelsen C, et al: Piriformis syndrome: diagnosis, treatment and outcome—a ten-year study. Arch Phys Med Rehabil 83:295, 2002

Flasar MH, Goldberg E: Acute abdominal pain. Med Clin North Am 90:481, 2006

Fleischer AC, Tait D, Mayo J, et al: Sonographic features of ovarian remnants. J Ultrasound Med 17:551, 1998

Food and Drug Administration: FDA drug safety communication: prescription acetaminophen products to be limited to 325 mg per dosage unit; boxed warning will highlight potential for severe liver failure. Silver Springs, U.S. Food and Drug Administration, 2011

Food and Drug Administration: Lotronex (alosetron hydrochloride) information. 2012a. Available at: http://www.fda.gov/Drugs/DrugSafety/PostmarketDrugSafetyInformationforPatientsandProviders/ucm110450.htm. Accessed January 30, 2015

Food and Drug Administration: Zelnorm (tegaserod maleate) Information. 2012b. Available at: http://www.fda.gov/Drugs/DrugSafety/PostmarketDrugSafetyInformationforPatientsandProviders/ucm103223.htm. Accessed January 30, 2015

Ford AC, Moayyedi P, Lacy BE, et al: American College of Gastroenterology monograph on the management of irritable bowel syndrome and chronic idiopathic constipation. Am J Gastroenterol 109(Suppl 1):S2, 2014a

Ford AC, Quigley EM, Lacy BE, et al: Effect of antidepressants and psychological therapies, including hypnotherapy, in irritable bowel syndrome: systematic review and meta-analysis. Am J Gastroenterol 109(9):1350, 2014b

Ford AC, Quigley EM, Lacy BE, et al: Efficacy of prebiotics, probiotics, and synbiotics in irritable bowel syndrome and chronic idiopathic constipation: systematic review and meta-analysis. Am J Gastroenterol 109(10):1547, 2014c

Gallagher EJ: Acute abdominal pain. In Tintinalli JE, Kelen GD, Stapczynski JS, et al (eds): Tintinalli's Emergency Medicine: A Comprehensive Study Guide. New York, McGraw-Hill, 2004

Gangar KF, Stones RW, Saunders D, et al: An alternative to hysterectomy? GnRH analogue combined with hormone replacement therapy. BJOG 100:360, 1993

Gerhardt RT, Nelson BK, Keenan S, et al: Derivation of a clinical guideline for the assessment of nonspecific abdominal pain: the Guideline for Abdominal Pain in the ED Setting (GAPEDS) Phase 1 Study. Am J Emerg Med 23:709, 2005

Gershon MD: Nerves, reflexes, and the enteric nervous system: pathogenesis of the irritable bowel syndrome. J Clin Gastroenterol 39(4 Suppl 3):S184, 2005

Gerwin RD: A review of myofascial pain and fibromyalgia—factors that promote their persistence. Acupunct Med 23:121, 2005

Giamberardino MA: Referred muscle pain/hyperalgesia and central sensitisation. J Rehab Med (41 Suppl):85, 2003

Glatt AE, Zinner SH, McCormack WM: The prevalence of dyspareunia. Obstet Gynecol 75:433, 1990

Gloviczki P, Comerota AJ, Dalsing MC, et al: The care of patients with varicose veins and associated chronic venous diseases: clinical practice guidelines of the Society for Vascular Surgery and the American Venous Forum. J Vasc Surg 53(5 Suppl):2S, 2011

Gomel V: Chronic pelvic pain: a challenge. J Minim Invasive Gynecol 14(4):521, 2007

Green PH: The many faces of celiac disease: clinical presentation of celiac disease in the adult population. Gastroenterology 128(4 Suppl):S74, 2005

Green PH, Cellier C: Celiac disease. N Engl J Med 357(17):1731, 2007

Greenbaum DS, Greenbaum RB, Joseph JG, et al: Chronic abdominal wall pain. Diagnostic validity and costs. Dig Dis Sci 39:1935, 1994

Guerriero S, Ajossa S, Lai MP, et al: Transvaginal ultrasonography in the diagnosis of pelvic adhesions. Hum Reprod 12:2649, 1997

Gunter J: Chronic pelvic pain: an integrated approach to diagnosis and treatment. Obstet Gynecol Surv 58:615, 2003

Gyang A, Hartman M, Lamvu G: Musculoskeletal causes of chronic pelvic pain: what a gynecologist should know. Obstet Gynecol 121(3):645, 2013

Hadley SK, Gaarder SM: Treatment of irritable bowel syndrome. Am Fam Physician 72:2501, 2005

Haefner HK, Collins ME, Davis GD, et al: The vulvodynia guideline. J Lower Gen Tract Dis 9:40, 2005

Hammoud A, Gago LA, Diamond MP: Adhesions in patients with chronic pelvic pain: a role for adhesiolysis? Fertil Steril 82:1483, 2004

Hanno PM, Burks DA, Clemens JQ, et al. AUA guideline for the diagnosis and treatment of interstitial cystitis/bladder pain syndrome. J Urol 185(6):2162, 2011

Hanno PM, Erickson D, Moldwin R, et al: Diagnosis and treatment of interstitial cystitis/bladder pain syndrome: AUA guideline amendment. J Urol 193(5):1545, 2015

Hansrani V, Abbas A, Bhandari S, et al: Trans-venous occlusion of incompetent pelvic veins for chronic pelvic pain in women: a systematic review. Eur J Obstet Gynecol Reprod Biol 185C:156, 2015

Harel Z, Biro FM, Kottenhahn RK, et al: Supplementation with omega-3 polyunsaturated fatty acids in the management of dysmenorrhea in adolescents. Am J Obstet Gynecol 174:1335, 1996

Harlow SD, Park M: A longitudinal study of risk factors for the occurrence, duration and severity of menstrual cramps in a cohort of college women. BJOG 103:1134, 1996

Hartmann KE, Ma C, Lamvu GM, et al: Quality of life and sexual function after hysterectomy in women with preoperative pain and depression. Obstet Gynecol 104(4):701, 2004

Hillis SD, Marchbanks PA, Peterson HB: The effectiveness of hysterectomy for chronic pelvic pain. Obstet Gynaecol 86:941, 1995

Hindocha A, Beere L, Dias S, et al: Adhesion prevention agents for gynaecological surgery: an overview of Cochrane reviews. Cochrane Database Syst Rev 1:CD011254, 2015

Hopayian K, Song F, Riera R, et al: The clinical features of the piriformis syndrome: a systematic review. Eur Spine J 19(12):2095, 2010

Howard FM: Chronic pelvic pain. Obstet Gynecol 101:594, 2003

Howard FM: The role of laparoscopy in chronic pelvic pain: promise and pitfalls. Obstet Gynecol Surv 48:357, 1993

Howard FM, El Minawi AM, Sanchez RA: Conscious pain mapping by laparoscopy in women with chronic pelvic pain. Obstet Gynaecol 96:934, 2000

Hsu CT, Rosioreanu A, Friedman RM, et al: Computed tomography imaging of the acute female pelvis. Contemporary Diagnostic Radiology, 28(18):1, 2005

Huchon C, Fauconnier A: Adnexal torsion: a literature review. Eur J Obstet Gynecol 150(1):8, 2010

Hull M, Corton MM: Evaluation of the levator ani and pelvic wall muscles in levator ani syndrome. Urol Nurs 29(4):225, 2009

Irwin P, Samsudin A: Reinvestigation of patients with a diagnosis of interstitial cystitis: common things are sometimes common. J Urol 174:584, 2005

Jacobs D: Diverticulitis. N Engl J Med 357(20):2057, 2007

Jamieson DJ, Steege JF: The association of sexual abuse with pelvic pain complaints in a primary care population. Am J Obstet Gynecol 177:1408, 1997

Janicki TI: Chronic pelvic pain as a form of complex regional pain syndrome. Clin Obstet Gynaecol 46:797, 2003

Jones CA, Nyberg L: Epidemiology of interstitial cystitis. Urology 49(5A Suppl):2, 1997

Kang SB, Chung HH, Lee HP, et al: Impact of diagnostic laparoscopy on the management of chronic pelvic pain. Surg Endosc 21(6):916, 2007

Kehlet H, Jensen TS, Woolf CJ: Persistent postsurgical pain: risk factors and prevention. Lancet 367:1618, 2006

Kennedy CM, Bradley CS, Galask RP, et al: Risk factors for painful bladder syndrome in women seeking gynecologic care. Int Urogynecol J 17:73, 2006

Khanna R, MacDonald JK, Levesque BG: Peppermint oil for the treatment of irritable bowel syndrome: a systematic review and meta-analysis. J Clin Gastroenterol 48(6):505, 2014

Kho RM, Abrao MS: Ovarian remnant syndrome: etiology, diagnosis, treatment and impact of endometriosis. Curr Opin Obstet Gynecol 24(4):210, 2012

Khoder W, Hale D: Pudendal neuralgia. Obstet Gynecol Clin North Am 41(3):443, 2014

Kirschner JS, Foye PM, Cole JL: Piriformis syndrome, diagnosis and treatment. Muscle Nerve 40(1):10, 2009

Knockaert DC, Boonen AL, Bruyninckx FL, et al: Electromyographic findings in ilioinguinal-iliohypogastric nerve entrapment syndrome. Acta Clin Belg 51:156, 1996

Labat JJ, Riant T, Robert R, et al: Diagnostic criteria for pudendal neuralgia by pudendal nerve entrapment (Nantes criteria). Neurourol Urodyn 27(4):306, 2008

Labelle H, Roussouly P, Berthonnaud E, et al: The importance of spino-pelvic balance in L5-S1 developmental spondylolisthesis: a review of pertinent radiologic measurements. Spine 30(6 Suppl):S27, 2005

Lafferty HW, Angioli R, Rudolph J, et al: Ovarian remnant syndrome: experience at Jackson Memorial Hospital, University of Miami, 1985 through 1993. Am J Obstet Gynecol 174:641, 1996

Lampe A, Solder E, Ennemoser A, et al: Chronic pelvic pain and previous sexual abuse. Obstet Gynecol 96:929, 2000

Laumann EO, Paik A, Rosen RC: Sexual dysfunction in the United States: prevalence and predictors. JAMA 281:537, 1999

Lavelle ED, Lavelle W, Smith HS: Myofascial trigger points. Med Clin North Am 91(2):229, 2007

Leschka S, Alkadhi H, Wildermuth S, et al: Acute abdominal pain: diagnostic strategies. In Marincek B, Dondelinger RF (eds): Emergency Radiology. New York, Springer, 2007, p 411

Lifford KL, Barbieri RL: Diagnosis and management of chronic pelvic pain. Urol Clin North Am 29:637, 2002

Lindh I, Milsom I: The influence of intrauterine contraception on the prevalence and severity of dysmenorrhea: a longitudinal population study. Hum Reprod 28(7):1953, 2013

Longstreth GF, Thompson WG, Chey WD, et al: Functional bowel disorders. Gastroenterology 130:1480, 2006

Lovell RM, Ford AC: Global prevalence of, and risk factors for, irritable bowel syndrome: a meta-analysis. Clin Gastroenterol Hepatol 10:712, 2012

Lunn MP, Hughes RA, Wiffen PJ: Duloxetine for treating painful neuropathy, chronic pain or fibromyalgia. Cochrane Database Syst Rev 1:CD007115, 2014

Madura JA, Madura JA, Copper CM, et al: Inguinal neurectomy for inguinal nerve entrapment: an experience with 100 patients. Am J Surg 189:283, 2005

Magtibay PM, Nyholm JL, Hernandez JL, et al: Ovarian remnant syndrome. Am J Obstet Gynecol 193:2062, 2005

Maizels M, McCarberg B: Antidepressants and antiepileptic drugs for chronic non-cancer pain. Am Fam Physician 71:483, 2005

Marjoribanks J, Proctor M, Farquhar C, et al: Nonsteroidal anti-inflammatory drugs for dysmenorrhea. Cochrane Database Syst Rev 1:CD001751, 2010

Mathias SD, Kuppermann M, Liberman RF, et al: Chronic pelvic pain: prevalence, health-related quality of life, and economic correlates. Obstet Gynecol 87:321, 1996

Mayer E: Irritable bowel syndrome. N Engl J Med 358(16):1692, 2008

McHale PM, LoVecchio F: Narcotic analgesia in the acute abdomen—a review of prospective trials. Eur J Emerg Med 8:131, 2001

McPartland JM: Travell trigger points—molecular and osteopathic perspectives. J Am Osteopath Assoc 104:244, 2004

Melzack R: The short-form McGill Pain Questionnaire. Pain 30(2):191, 1987

Mens JM, Vleeming A, Stoeckart R, et al: Understanding peripartum pelvic pain: implications of a patient survey. Spine 21(11):1363, 1996

Michel F, Decavel P, Toussirot E, et al: The piriformis muscle syndrome: an exploration of anatomical context, pathophysiological hypotheses and diagnostic criteria. Ann Phys Rehabil Med 56(4):300, 2013

Miller SK, Alpert PT: Assessment and differential diagnosis of abdominal pain. Nurse Pract 31:38, 2006

Moore RA, Wiffen PJ, Derry S, et al: Gabapentin for chronic neuropathic pain and fibromyalgia in adults. Cochrane Database Syst Rev 4:CD007938, 2014

Moschos E, Twickler DM: Does the type of intrauterine device affect conspicuity on 2D and 3D ultrasound? AJR 196(6):1439, 2011

Namnoum AB, Hickman TN, Goodman SB, et al: Incidence of symptom recurrence after hysterectomy for endometriosis. Fertil Steril 64(5):898, 1995

Nezhat C, Kearney S, Malik S, et al: Laparoscopic management of ovarian remnant. Fertil Steril 83:973, 2005

Novi JM, Jeronis S, Srinivas S, et al: Risk of irritable bowel syndrome and depression in women with interstitial cystitis: a case-control study. J Urol 174:937, 2005

Pace S, Burke TF: Intravenous morphine for early pain relief in patients with acute abdominal pain. Acad Emerg Med 3:1086, 1996

Paras ML, Murad MH, Chen LP, et al: Sexual abuse and lifetime diagnosis of somatic disorders: a systematic review and meta-analysis. JAMA 302(5):550, 2009

Park SJ, Lim JW, Ko YT, et al: Diagnosis of pelvic congestion syndrome using transabdominal and transvaginal sonography. Am J Roentgenol 182:683, 2004

Parker JD, Sinaii N, Segars JH, et al: Adhesion formation after laparoscopic excision of endometriosis and lysis of adhesions. Fertil Steril 84:1457, 2005

Parsons CL: Prostatitis, interstitial cystitis, chronic pelvic pain, and urethral syndrome share a common pathophysiology: lower urinary dysfunctional epithelium and potassium recycling. Urology 62:976, 2003

Parsons CL, Greenberger M, Gabal L, et al: The role of urinary potassium in the pathogenesis and diagnosis of interstitial cystitis. J Urol 159(6):1862, 1998

Paulson JD, Delgado M: Relationship between interstitial cystitis and endometriosis in patients with chronic pelvic pain. JSLS 11(2):175, 2007

Perry CP: Peripheral neuropathies and pelvic pain: diagnosis and management. Clin Obstet Gynaecol 46:789, 2003

Perry CP: Somatic referral. In Howard FM, Perry CP, Carter JE, et al (eds): Pelvic Pain: Diagnosis and Management. Philadelphia, Lippincott Williams & Wilkins, 2000, p 486

Perry CP, Presthus J, Nieves A: Laparoscopic uterine suspension for pain relief: a multicenter study. J Reprod Med 50:567, 2005

Petchprapa CN, Rosenberg ZS, Sconfienza LM, et al: MR imaging of entrapment neuropathies of the lower extremity. Part 1. The pelvis and hip. Radiographics 30(4):983, 2010

Peters AA, Trimbos-Kemper GC, Admiraal C, et al: A randomized clinical trial on the benefit of adhesiolysis in patients with intraperitoneal adhesions and chronic pelvic pain. BJOG 99:59, 1992

Peters KM, Carrico DJ, Kalinowski SE, et al: Prevalence of pelvic floor dysfunction in patients with interstitial cystitis. Urology 70(1):16, 2007

Phillips D, Deipolyi AR, Hesketh RL, et al: Pelvic congestion syndrome: etiology of pain, diagnosis, and clinical management. J Vasc Interv Radiol 25(5):725, 2014

Proctor M, Farquhar C: Diagnosis and management of dysmenorrhoea. BMJ 332:1134, 2006

Proctor ML, Latthe PM, Farquhar CM, et al: Surgical interruption of pelvic nerve pathways for primary and secondary dysmenorrhoea. Cochrane Database Syst Rev 4:CD001896, 2005

Proctor ML, Smith CA, Farquhar CM, et al: Transcutaneous electrical nerve stimulation and acupuncture for primary dysmenorrhea. Cochrane Database Syst Rev 1:CD002123, 2002

Propert KJ, Schaeffer AJ, Brensinger CM, et al: A prospective study of interstitial cystitis: results of longitudinal follow-up of the interstitial cystitis data base cohort. The Interstitial Cystitis Data Base Study Group. J Urol 163:1434, 2000

Raman SS, Osuagwu FC, Kadell B, et al: Effect of CT on false positive diagnosis of appendicitis and perforation. N Engl J Med 358(9):972, 2008

Rao S, Lembo AJ, Shiff SJ, et al: A 12-week, randomized, controlled trial with a 4-week randomized withdrawal period to evaluate the efficacy and safety of linaclotide in irritable bowel syndrome with constipation. Am J Gastroenterol 107:1714, 2012

Reginald PW, Adams J, Franks S, et al: Medroxyprogesterone acetate in the treatment of pelvic pain due to venous congestion. BJOG 96:1148, 1989

Reissing ED, Brown C, Lord MJ, et al: Pelvic floor muscle functioning in women with vulvar vestibulitis syndrome. J Psychosom Obstet Gynecol 26:107, 2005

Reuter HJ: Bladder. In Atlas of Urologic Endoscopy Diagnosis and Treatment. New York, Thieme Medical Publishers, 1987, p 85

Rockey DC: Occult gastrointestinal bleeding. Gastroenterol Clin North Am 34:699, 2005

Rogers RM Jr: Basic Pelvic Neuroanatomy. In Steege JF, Metzger DA, Levy BS (eds): Chronic Pelvic Pain: an Integrated Approach. Philadelphia, WB Saunders, 1998, p 46

Roman H, Hulsey TF, Marpeau L, et al: Why laparoscopic adhesiolysis should not be the victim of a single randomized clinical trial. Am J Obstet Gynecol 200(2):136.e1, 2009

Rubio-Tapia A, Hill ID, Kelly CP, et al: ACG clinical guidelines: diagnosis and management of celiac disease. Am J Gastroenterol 108(5):656, 2013

Ruepert L, Quartero AO, de Wit NJ, et al: Bulking agents, antispasmodics and antidepressants for the treatment of irritable bowel syndrome. Cochrane Database Syst Rev 8:CD003460, 2011

Saarto T, Wiffen PJ: Antidepressants for neuropathic pain: a Cochrane review. J Neurol Neurosurg Psychiatry 81(12):1372, 2010

Saito YA, Schoenfeld P, Locke GR III: The epidemiology of irritable bowel syndrome in North America: a systematic review. Am J Gastroenterol 97: 1910, 2002

Sant GR, Kempuraj D, Marchand JE, et al: The mast cell in interstitial cystitis: role in pathophysiology and pathogenesis. Urology 69(4 Suppl):34, 2007

Sauerland S, Agresta F, Bergamaschi R, et al: Laparoscopy for abdominal emergencies: evidence-based guidelines of the European Association for Endoscopic Surgery. Surg Endosc 20:14, 2006

Schoenfeld P: Efficacy of current drug therapies in irritable bowel syndrome: what works and does not work. Gastroenterol Clin North Am 34:319, 2005

Sharma D, Dahiya K, Duhan N, et al: Diagnostic laparoscopy in chronic pelvic pain. Arch Gynecol Obstet 283(2):295, 2011

Sharp HT: Myofascial pain syndrome of the abdominal wall for the busy clinician. Clin Obstet Gynaecol 46:783, 2003

Signorello LB, Harlow BL, Chekos AK, et al: Postpartum sexual functioning and its relationship to perineal trauma: a retrospective cohort study of primiparous women. Am J Obstet Gynecol 184:881, 2001

Simons DG, Travell JG: Travell and Simons' Myofascial Pain and Dysfunction: the Trigger Point Manual, 2nd ed. Baltimore, Williams & Wilkins, 1999

Sirinian E, Azevedo K, Payne CK: Correlation between 2 interstitial cystitis symptom instruments. J Urol 173(3):835, 2005

Smith CA, Zhu X, He L, et al: Acupuncture for primary dysmenorrhoea. Cochrane Database Syst Rev 1:CD007854, 2011

Smith-Bindman R: Is computed tomography safe? N Engl J Med 363(1):1, 2010

Smith-Bindman R, Lipson J, Marcus R, et al: Radiation dose associated with common computed tomography examinations and the associated lifetime attributable risk of cancer. Arch Intern Med 169(22):2078, 2009

Soysal ME, Soysal S, Vicdan K, et al: A randomized controlled trial of goserelin and medroxyprogesterone acetate in the treatment of pelvic congestion. Hum Reprod 16:931, 2001

Spitznagle TM, Robinson CM: Myofascial pelvic pain. Obstet Gynecol Clin North Am 41(3):409, 2014

Srinivasan R, Greenbaum DS: Chronic abdominal wall pain: a frequently overlooked problem. Practical approach to diagnosis and management. Am J Gastroenterol 97:824, 2002

Steege JF, Stout AL: Resolution of chronic pelvic pain after laparoscopic lysis of adhesions. Am J Obstet Gynecol 165:278, 1991

Stovall TG, Ling FW, Crawford DA: Hysterectomy for chronic pelvic pain of presumed uterine etiology. Obstet Gynaecol 75:676, 1990

Sulak PJ, Cressman BE, Waldrop E, et al: Extending the duration of active oral contraceptive pills to manage hormone withdrawal symptoms. Obstet Gynaecol 89:179, 1997

Suleiman S, Johnston DE: The abdominal wall: an overlooked source of pain. Am Fam Physician 64:431, 2001

Sundell G, Milsom I, Andersch B: Factors influencing the prevalence and severity of dysmenorrhoea in young women. BJOG 7:588, 1990

Sutton C, MacDonald R: Laser laparoscopic adhesiolysis. J Gynecol Surg 6:155, 1990

Swank DJ, Swank-Bordewijk SCG, Hop WCJ, et al: Laparoscopic adhesiolysis in patients with chronic abdominal pain: a blinded randomised controlled multi-centre trial. Lancet 361:1247, 2003

Swanton A, Iyer L, Reginald PW: Diagnosis, treatment and follow up of women undergoing conscious pain mapping for chronic pelvic pain: a prospective cohort study. BJOG 113:792, 2006

Tersigni C, Castellani R, de Waure C, et al: Celiac disease and reproductive disorders: meta-analysis of epidemiologic associations and potential pathogenic mechanisms. Hum Reprod Update 20(4):582, 2014

Thompson WG, Longstreth GF, Drossman DA, et al: Functional bowel disorders and functional abdominal pain. Gut 45(Suppl 2):II43, 1999

Thomson WH, Dawes RF, Carter SS: Abdominal wall tenderness: a useful sign in chronic abdominal pain. Br J Surg 78:223, 1991

Thornton JG, Morley S, Lilleyman J, et al: The relationship between laparoscopic disease, pelvic pain and infertility; an unbiased assessment. Eur J Obstet Gynaecol Reprod Biol 74:57, 1997

Trinkley KE, Nahata MC: Medication management of irritable bowel syndrome. Digestion 89(4):253, 2014

Twickler DM, Moschos E: Ultrasound and assessment of ovarian cancer risk. AJR 194(2):322, 2010

Venbrux AC, Lambert DL: Embolization of the ovarian veins as a treatment for patients with chronic pelvic pain caused by pelvic venous incompetence (pelvic congestion syndrome). Curr Opin Obstet Gynecol 11:395, 1999

Vercellini P, Somigliana E, Viganò P, et al: Chronic pelvic pain in women: etiology, pathogenesis and diagnostic approach. Gynecol Endocrinol 25(3):149, 2009

Vermani E, Mittal R, Weeks A: Pelvic girdle pain and low back pain in pregnancy: a review. Pain Pract 10(1):60, 2010

Vleeming A, Albert HB, Ostgaard HC, et al: European guidelines for the diagnosis and treatment of pelvic girdle pain. Eur Spine J 17(6):794, 2008

Warren JW, Keay SK: Interstitial cystitis. Curr Opin Urol 12:69, 2002

Warren JW, Meyer WA, Greenberg P et al: Using the International Continence Society's definition of painful bladder syndrome. Urology 67:138, 2006

Warren JW, Morozov V, Howard FM: Could chronic pelvic pain be a functional somatic syndrome? Am J Obstet Gynecol 205(3):199.e1, 2011

Waxman JA, Sulak PJ, Kuehl TJ: Cystoscopic findings consistent with interstitial cystitis in normal women undergoing tubal ligation. J Urol 160:1663, 1998

Weinberg DS, Smalley W, Heidelbaugh JJ, et al: American Gastroenterological Association Institute Guideline on the pharmacological management of irritable bowel syndrome. Gastroenterology 147(5):1146, 2014

Weissman AM, Hartz AJ, Hansen MD, et al: The natural history of primary dysmenorrhoea: a longitudinal study. BJOG 111:345, 2004

Whiteside JL, Barber MD, Walters MD, et al: Anatomy of ilioinguinal and iliohypogastric nerves in relation to trocar placement and low transverse incisions. Am J Obstet Gynaecol 189:1574, 2003

Wiffen PJ, Derry S, Moore RA: Lamotrigine for chronic neuropathic pain and fibromyalgia in adults. Cochrane Database Syst Rev 12:CD006044, 2013

Wong CL, Farquhar C, Roberts H, Proctor M. Oral contraceptive pill for primary dysmenorrhoea. Cochrane Database Syst Rev 4:CD002120, 2009

Wu WH, Meijer OG, Uegaki K, et al: Pregnancy-related pelvic girdle pain (PPP), I: terminology, clinical presentation, and prevalence. Eur Spine J 13(7):575, 2004

Yoshimoto H, Sato S, Masuda T, et al: Spinopelvic alignment in patients with osteoarthrosis of the hip: a radiographic comparison to patients with low back pain. Spine 30:1650, 2005

Zapardiel I, Zanagnolo V, Kho RM, et al: Ovarian remnant syndrome: comparison of laparotomy, laparoscopy and robotic surgery. Acta Obstet Gynecol Scand 91(8):965, 2012

Zhu X, Proctor M, Bensoussan A, et al: Chinese herbal medicine for primary dysmenorrhoea. Cochrane Database Syst Rev 2:CD005288, 2008

Ziaei S, Faghihzadeh S, Sohrabvand F, et al: A randomised placebo-controlled trial to determine the effect of vitamin E in treatment of primary dysmenorrhoea. BJOG 108:1181, 2001

CHAPTER 12

Breast Disease

Breast disease in women encompasses a spectrum of benign and malignant disorders, which present most commonly as breast pain, nipple discharge, or palpable mass. The specific causes of these symptoms vary with patient age. Benign disorders predominate in young premenopausal women, whereas malignancy rates increase with advancing age. Evaluation of breast disorders usually requires the combination of a careful history, physical examination, imaging, and, when indicated, biopsy.

ANATOMY

◼ Ductal System

The glandular portion of the breast is composed of 12 to 15 independent ductal systems that each drain approximately 40 lobules (Fig. 12-1). Each lobule consists of 10 to 100 milk-producing acini that empty into small terminal ducts (Parks, 1959). Terminal ducts drain into larger collecting ducts that

merge into even larger ducts, which exhibit a saccular dilation just below the nipple called a lactiferous sinus (Fig. 12-2).

In general, only six to eight openings are visible on the nipple surface. These drain the dominant ductal systems, which account for approximately 80 percent of the breast's glandular volume (Going, 2004). Minor ducts either terminate just below the nipple surface or open on the areola near the base of the nipple. The areola itself contains numerous lubricating sebaceous glands, called Montgomery glands, which are often visible as punctate prominences.

In addition to epithelial structures, the breast is composed of varying proportions of collagenous stroma and fat. The distribution and abundance of these stromal components accounts for a breast's consistency when palpated and for its imaging characteristics.

◼ Lymphatic Drainage

Afferent lymphatic drainage of the breast is provided by dermal, subdermal, interlobar, and prepectoral systems (Fig. 12-3) (Grant, 1953). Each of these may be viewed as a lattice of valveless channels that interconnect with every other system and that ultimately drain into one or two axillary lymph nodes (the sentinel nodes). Because all of these systems are interconnected, the breast drains as a unit, and injection of colloidal dyes in any part of the breast at any level will result in accumulation of dye in the same one or two axillary sentinel lymph nodes. The axillary lymph nodes receive most of the lymphatic drainage of the breast and consequently are the nodes most frequently involved with breast cancer metastases (Hultborn, 1955). However, there are also alternate drainage pathways that do not appear to interconnect with other networks and that drain directly into internal mammary, supraclavicular, contralateral axillary, or abdominal lymph node basins.

DEVELOPMENT AND PHYSIOLOGY

During fetal development, the primordial breast arises from the basal layer of the epidermis. Before puberty, the breast is a rudimentary bud composed of a few branching ducts capped with alveolar buds, end buds, or small lobules (Osin, 1998). At puberty, usually between the ages of 10 and 13 years, ovarian estrogen and progesterone cooperate to direct organized communication between breast epithelial cells and mesenchymal cells, resulting in extensive branching of the ductal system and development of lobules (Ismail, 2003). Specific disorders of this development are discussed in Chapter 14 (p. 325). Final differentiation of the breast is mediated by progesterone and

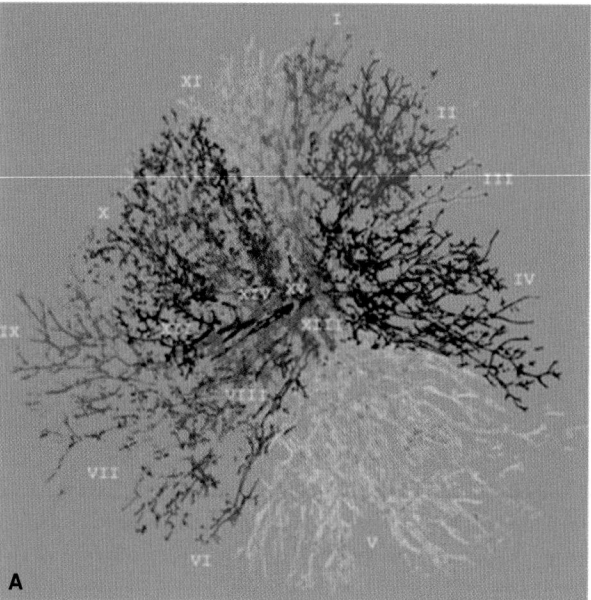

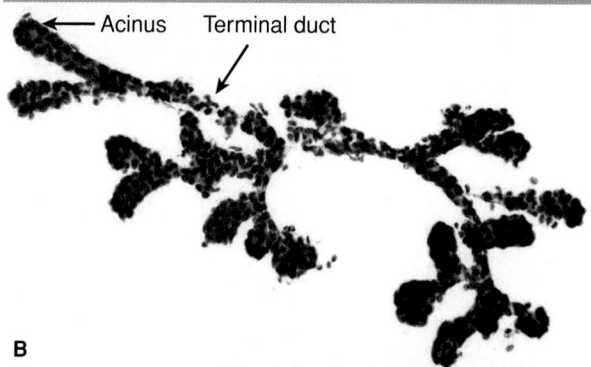

Acinus   Terminal duct

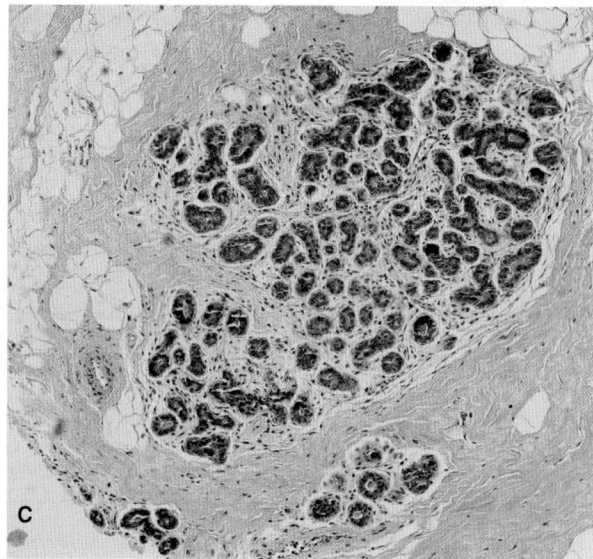

FIGURE 12-1 A. Ductal anatomy of the breast. (Reproduced with permission from Going JJ, Moffat DF: Escaping from Flatland: clinical and biological aspects of human mammary duct anatomy in three dimensions, J Pathology 2004 May;203(1):538–544.) **B.** Terminal duct—acinar structure from a fine-needle aspiration biopsy. **C.** Histology of a normal breast lobule. The terminal duct lobular units are surrounded by loosely cellular intralobular stroma, which consists of dense fibrous tissue admixed with adipocytes.

prolactin and is not completed until the first full-term pregnancy (Grimm, 2002; Ismail, 2003).

During the reproductive years, terminal ducts near the acini and the acini themselves are most sensitive to ovarian hormones and prolactin. Most forms of benign and malignant breast disease arise in these terminal duct-acinar structures. Breast epithelial cells proliferate during the luteal phase of the menstrual cycle when estrogen and progesterone levels are increased, and then undergo programmed cell death at the end of the luteal phase, when levels of these hormones decline (Anderson, 1982; Soderqvist, 1997). This effect is mediated by paracrine signaling induced by estrogen-receptor activation and is associated with an increase in the water content of the extracellular matrix (Stoeckelhuber, 2002). This is often recognized as breast fullness and tenderness in the week preceding menses.

At menopause, when ovarian estrogen production ceases, breast lobules involute, and the collagenous stroma is replaced by fat. Because estrogen receptor expression is negatively regulated by estrogen, there is an increase in estrogen receptor expression after menopause (Khan, 1997). Despite a decline in ovarian estrogen production, postmenopausal women continue to produce estrogen through the action of the enzyme aromatase, which converts adrenal androgens to estrogen (Bulun, 1994). Aromatase is found in fat, muscle, and breast tissue.

EVALUATION OF A BREAST LUMP

It is not possible to distinguish benign from malignant or cystic from solid breast masses by clinical examination. However, findings from clinical examination, interpreted in conjunction with imaging and pathology (the triple test), contribute significantly to management decisions (Hermansen, 1987).

■ Physical Examination

The breast is comma shaped, and the comma's tail corresponds to the axillary tail of Spence. This extension can be large, especially during pregnancy and lactation, and is frequently mistaken for an axillary mass.

Clinical examination of the breast begins with inspection of the breast to determine whether there is dimpling, nipple retraction, or skin changes. This examination is described in Chapter 1 (p. 2). The presence and character of expressible nipple discharge is recorded. In addition, the location of a mass is specifically documented according to its clock position and then measured along the long axis using a ruler or caliper (Fig. 12-4). The distance from the center of the nipple to the center of the mass is specified. Since numerous health care providers are typically involved in the evaluation and management of the same breast mass, the most useful entry in the clinical record will define the location and size of the mass (e.g., right breast, 2-cm mass, 3:00, 4 cm from the nipple). Although clinical examination alone can never exclude malignancy, noting that a mass has benign features such as smoothness, roundness, and mobility will factor into the ultimate decision to excise or observe a lesion. Evaluation also includes careful examination of the axillae, infraclavicular fossa, and supraclavicular fossa to identify lymphadenopathy.

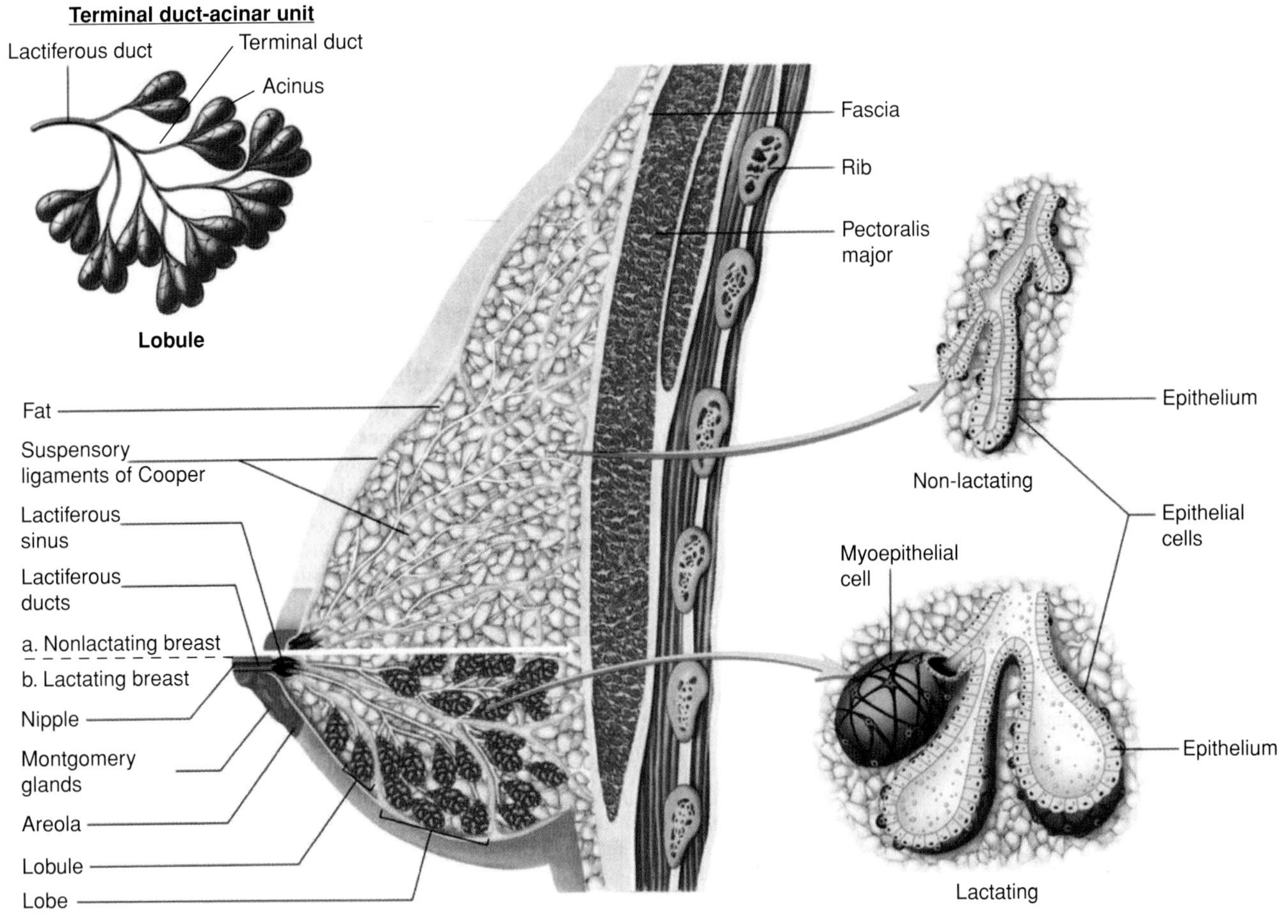

Terminal duct-acinar unit

Lactiferous duct
Terminal duct
Acinus

Lobule

Fat
Suspensory ligaments of Cooper
Lactiferous sinus
Lactiferous ducts
a. Nonlactating breast
b. Lactating breast
Nipple
Montgomery glands
Areola
Lobule
Lobe

Fascia
Rib
Pectoralis major

Epithelium

Non-lactating

Epithelial cells

Myoepithelial cell

Epithelium

Lactating

FIGURE 12-2 Breast anatomy. (Reproduced with permission from Seeley RR, Stephens TD, Tate P: Anatomy and Physiology, 7th ed. New York: McGraw-Hill; 2006.)

▇ Diagnostic Imaging

Imaging of a suspected mass may begin with mammography that includes magnification, extra compression, or extra views beyond the usual medial lateral oblique and cranial caudal views that are typically used for screening. Unlike screening mammography, diagnostic mammography may be appropriate for women of any age. In addition, sonography is invaluable for determining whether a mass is cystic or solid and is a component of most diagnostic imaging algorithms. Certain features of solid masses, such as irregular margins, internal echoes, or

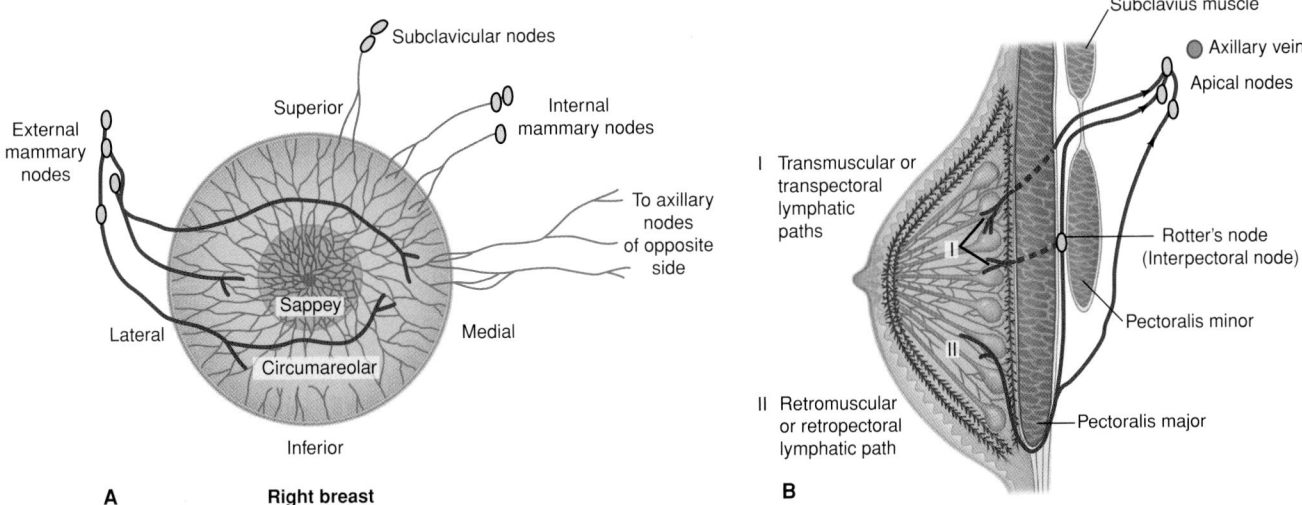

Subclavicular nodes
Superior
Internal mammary nodes
External mammary nodes
To axillary nodes of opposite side
Sappey
Lateral
Medial
Circumareolar
Inferior

A   **Right breast**

Subclavius muscle
Axillary vein
Apical nodes
I Transmuscular or transpectoral lymphatic paths
Rotter's node (Interpectoral node)
Pectoralis minor
II Retromuscular or retropectoral lymphatic path
Pectoralis major

B

FIGURE 12-3 Lymphatic drainage of the breast. **A.** Accessory drainage pathways. **B.** Classic axillary drainage pathways. (Reproduced with permission from Grant RN, Tabah EJ, Adair FE: The surgical significance of the subareolar symph plexus in cancer of the breast, Surgery 1953 Jan;33(1):71–78.)

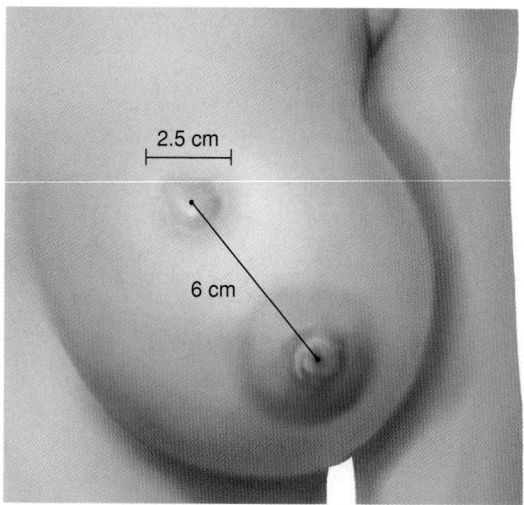

FIGURE 12-4 Recording the location of a breast mass as "Left breast, 2.5-cm mass, 10:00, 6 cm FN." FN = from the nipple.

a width-to-height ratio <1.7 may suggest malignancy (Stavros, 1995).

Diagnostic imaging results should be summarized according to the Breast Imaging Reporting and Data System (BI-RADS) classification (Table 12-1) (D'Orsi, 2013). Lesions that are graded BI-RADS 5 are highly suggestive of malignancy, and ≥95 percent of these are ultimately proven to be cancerous. Decreasing numerical grades are associated with diminishing probability of malignancy.

■ Breast Biopsy

Evaluation of a solid breast mass is completed by needle biopsy. These biopsies should be performed after an imaging test or a minimum of 2 weeks prior to an imaging test. This is because resulting tissue trauma can produce image artifacts that simulate malignancy (Sickles, 1983). Options include fine-needle aspiration (FNA) biopsy or core-needle biopsy. The trend in recent years favors core-needle biopsy (Tabbara, 2000). Although FNA takes less time to perform and is less expensive than core-needle biopsy, it is less likely to provide a specific diagnosis and has a higher insufficient sample rate (Shannon, 2001). FNA retrieves clusters of epithelial cells that may be interpreted as benign or malignant, but it cannot reliably differentiate between benign proliferative lesions and fibroepithelial neoplasms or between ductal carcinoma in situ and invasive cancer (Boerner, 1999; Ringberg, 2001).

In contrast, core-needle biopsy is performed using an automated device that takes one core at a time or is completed using a vacuum-assisted device that, once initially positioned, delivers multiple cores. Needle biopsy of solid masses should be done prior to excision, as the biopsy results contribute significantly to surgical planning (Cox, 1995).

■ Triple Test

The combination of clinical examination, imaging, and needle biopsy is called the *triple test* (Wai, 2013). When all three assessments suggest a benign lesion or all three suggest a breast cancer, the triple test is said to be concordant. A concordant benign triple test is >99-percent accurate, and breast lumps in this category can be followed by clinical examination alone at 6-month intervals. If any of the three assessments suggests malignancy, the lump should be excised regardless of results from the other two. It is always appropriate to offer excision of a fully evaluated breast lump, even after a benign concordant triple test result, as breast lumps can be a source of significant anxiety.

BENIGN LUMPS AND FIBROEPITHELIAL NEOPLASMS

■ Cysts

Most breast cysts arise from apocrine metaplasia of lobular acini. They are generally lined by a single layer of epithelium that ranges from flattened to columnar. One autopsy series that included 725 women reported microcysts in 58 percent and cysts >1 cm in 21 percent (Davies, 1964). The incidence of breast cysts peaks between 40 and 50 years, and the lifetime incidence of palpable breast cysts is estimated to be 7 percent (Haagensen, 1986).

Breast cysts are diagnosed and classified by sonography. There are three types of cysts: simple, complicated, and complex (Berg, 2003). Simple cysts are sonolucent, have a smooth margin, and show enhanced through-transmission (Fig. 12-5). These lesions do not require special management or monitoring, but they may be aspirated if painful. Recurrent cysts can be reimaged and reaspirated, but recurrent symptomatic cysts are best managed by excision.

Complicated cysts show internal echoes during sonography and can sometimes be indistinguishable from solid masses. Internal echoes are usually caused by proteinaceous debris. Consideration is given to aspirating complicated cysts. The aspirated material may be submitted for culture, if it is purulent, or for cytology, if there are worrisome clinical or imaging features. If the sonographic abnormality does not resolve completely with aspiration, a core-needle biopsy is usually performed.

Complex cysts show septa or intracystic masses during sonographic evaluation. An intracystic mass usually represents a papilloma, but medullary carcinoma, papillary carcinoma, and some infiltrating ductal carcinomas can present as complex cysts. Although some advocate core-needle biopsy for the evaluation of complex cysts, this procedure can decompress a cyst, making it difficult to localize at the time of surgery. Additionally, papillary lesions diagnosed by needle biopsy will require excision. Thus, it seems reasonable to recommend excision of all complex cysts.

■ Fibroadenoma

This represents a focal developmental abnormality of a breast lobule and as such is not a true neoplasm. Histologically, fibroadenomas are composed of glandular and cystic epithelial structures surrounded by a cellular stroma. Fibroadenomas account for 7 to 13 percent of breast clinic visits and had a prevalence of 9 percent in one autopsy series (Dent, 1988; Franyz, 1951). They often present in adolescence, are recognized most

TABLE 12-1. Breast Imaging Reporting and Data System (BI-RADS)

BI-RADS Category	Description	Examples
0	Additional views or sonography required	Focal asymmetry, microcalcifications, or a mass identified on a screening mammogram
1	No abnormalities identified	Normal fat and fibroglandular tissue
2	Not entirely normal, but definitely benign	Fat necrosis from a prior excision, stable biopsy-proven fibroadenoma, stable cyst
3	Probably benign	Circumscribed mass that has been followed for <2 years
4A	Low suspicion for malignancy, but intervention required	Probable fibroadenoma, complicated cyst
4B	Intermediate suspicion for malignancy, intervention required	Partially indistinctly marginated mass otherwise consistent with a fibroadenoma
4C	Moderate suspicion, but not classic for carcinoma	New cluster of fine pleomorphic calcifications, ill-defined irregular solid mass
5	Almost certainly malignant	Spiculated mass, fine linear and branching calcifications
6	Biopsy-proven carcinoma	Biopsy-proven carcinoma

frequently in premenopausal women, and usually spontaneously involute at menopause.

Fibroadenomas classified as benign concordant by the triple test can be safely followed without excision. Because some fibroadenomas may grow large, and because benign phyllodes tumors are often indistinguishable from fibroadenomas by imaging and needle biopsy, a fibroadenoma that is growing should be excised.

Phyllodes Tumors

These are true biphasic neoplasms characterized by epithelial-lined spaces surrounded by cellular stroma. Both the epithelial

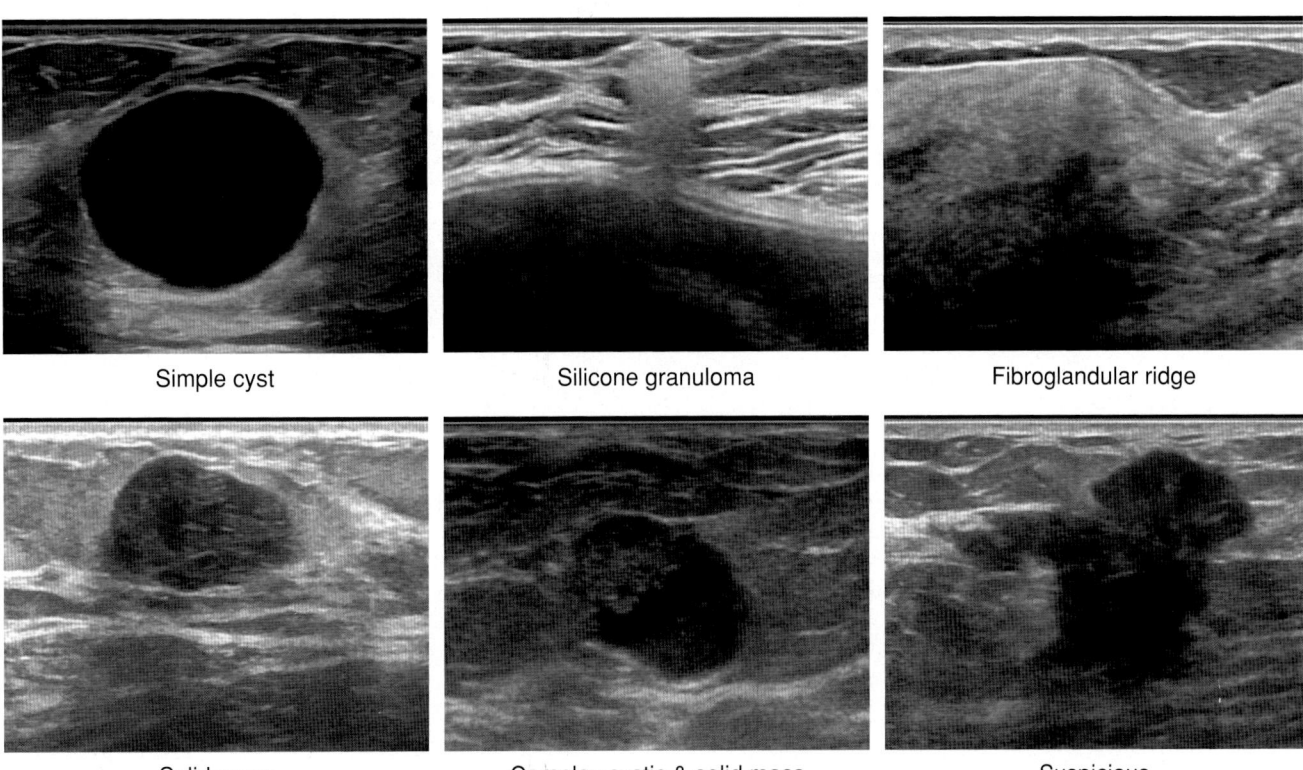

Simple cyst   Silicone granuloma   Fibroglandular ridge

Solid mass   Complex cystic & solid mass   Suspicious

FIGURE 12-5 Sonographic appearance of palpable breast masses. **A.** Simple cyst. **B.** Silicone granuloma. **C.** Fibroglandular ridge. **D.** Solid mass (benign phyllodes tumor). **E.** Complex cystic and solid mass (intracystic papillary carcinoma with low-grade ductal carcinoma in situ). **F.** Suspicious (invasive ductal carcinoma). (Used with permission from Stephen J. Seiler, MD.)

and stromal components can be monoclonal and clonally related (Karim, 2013). Phyllodes tumors are classified as benign, intermediate, or malignant, based on the degree of stromal cell atypia, number of mitoses, tumor margin characteristics, and abundance of stromal cells (Oberman, 1965). Phyllodes tumors account for less than 1 percent of breast neoplasms, and the median age at diagnosis is 40 years (Kim, 2013; Reinfuss, 1996).

Malignant phyllodes tumors can metastasize to distant organs, with lung being the primary site. Chest radiographs or chest computed-tomography (CT) scanning are appropriate staging tests for malignant cases. Phyllodes tumors rarely metastasize to lymph nodes, thus axillary staging is not required unless nodes clinically appear involved (Chaney, 2000).

Treatment consists of wide local excision with a minimum 1-cm margin. Mastectomy may be required to achieve this margin, as the median tumor size at presentation is 5 cm. Local recurrence rates for completely excised tumors range from 8 percent for benign lesions to 36 percent for malignant ones (Barth, 1999). Fibroproliferation in the surrounding breast tissue and necrosis are the strongest predictors of recurrence (Barrio, 2007). Postoperative adjuvant radiation therapy may be indicated for high-risk cases (Barth, 2009).

NIPPLE DISCHARGE

Fluid can be expressed from the nipple ducts of at least 40 percent of premenopausal women, 55 percent of parous women, and 74 percent of women who have lactated within 2 years (Wrensch, 1990). The fluid generally issues from more than one duct and may range from milky white to dark green or brown. Green coloration is related to the content of cholesterol diepoxides and does not suggest underlying infection or malignancy (Petrakis, 1988).

Multiduct discharges that are elicited only following manual expression are considered physiologic and do not require additional evaluation. However, spontaneous discharges merit evaluation (Fig. 12-6). Spontaneous milky nipple discharge, also called galactorrhea, results from various causes (Table 12-2) (Chap. 15, p. 359). Of these, pregnancy is a frequent cause of new-onset spontaneous discharge, and a bloody multiduct discharge during pregnancy is not uncommon.

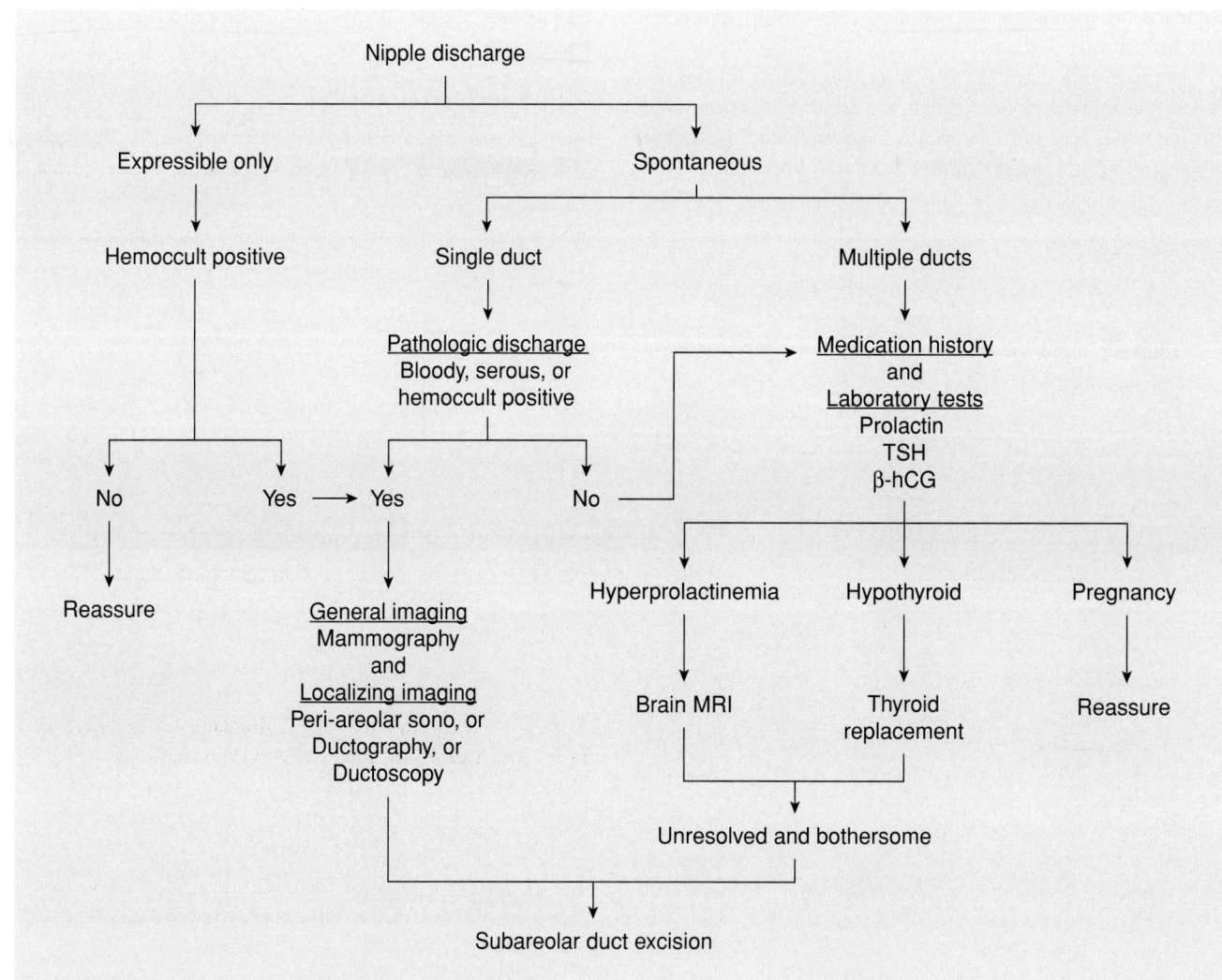

FIGURE 12-6 Diagnostic algorithm to evaluate nipple discharge. hCG = human chorionic gonadotropin; MRI = magnetic resonance imaging; TSH = thyroid-stimulating hormone.

TABLE 12-2. Causes of Galactorrhea

Idiopathic	**Systemic disorders**
	Chronic renal failure
Physiologic	Hypothyroidism
Lactation	Cirrhosis
Breast stimulation	Pseudocyesis
Stress	Seizures
	Ectopic tumor production
Hypothalamic lesions	
	Pharmacologic
Tumors	Dopamine-blocking agents:
Infiltrative disorders	Phenothiazines: chlorpromazine,
Irradiation	prochlorperazine
Trauma, surgery	Butyrophenones: haloperidol
Rathke cleft cyst	Thioxanthenes: thiothixene
	Benzamides: metoclopramide
Pituitary lesions	Risperidone
Prolactinoma	Dopamine depletors: reserpine,
Other tumors	opiates, α-methyldopa
Infiltrative disorders	H_2 antagonists: cimetidine,
Lymphocytic	ranitidine
hypophysitis	Serotonergic pathway stimulation:
Empty sella	amphetamines
	Calcium-channel blockers:
Intercostal nerve stimulation	verapamil
	Antidepressants: MAOI, TCA, SSRI
Chest wall lesions	Estrogen
Chest surgery	
Spinal cord injury	

H_2 = histamine 2; MAOI = monoamine oxidase inhibitor; TCA = tricyclic antidepressant; SSRI = selective serotonin-reuptake inhibitor.

Pathologic nipple discharge is defined as a spontaneous single-duct discharge that is serous or bloody. The rate of underlying malignancy ranges from approximately 2 percent for young women with no associated findings on imaging or physical examination to 20 percent for older women with associated findings (Cabioglu, 2003; Lau, 2005). Most pathologic nipple discharges are caused by benign intraductal papillomas, which are simple milk duct polyps (Urban, 1978). They arise in the major milk ducts, generally within 2 cm of the nipple, and contain a velvety papillary epithelium on a central fibrovascular stalk.

Evaluation of a pathologic nipple discharge begins with breast examination. Careful evaluation can frequently locate a trigger point on the areolar edge that elicits the discharge when pressed. Occult-blood testing and microscopic examination of the discharge can provide additional information. A glass slide that has been touched to the discharge and immediately fixed in 95-percent alcohol may be used for cytologic assessment. Nipple fluid samples are acellular in 25 percent of cases and thus cannot exclude an underlying malignancy (Papanicolaou, 1958). However, malignant cells, if found, are highly correlated with an underlying cancer (Gupta, 2004).

Following these examinations, diagnostic mammography and an assessment of the subareolar ducts by sonography or ductography is indicated. Diagnostic mammography is

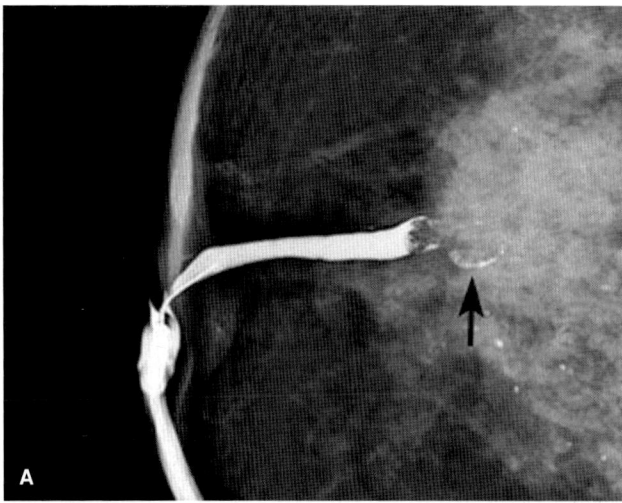

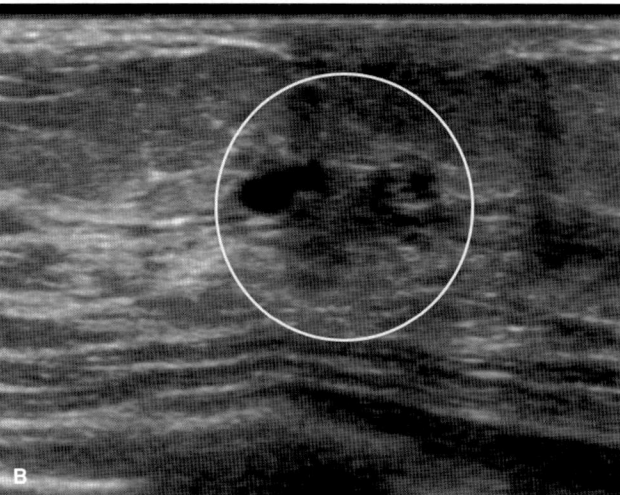

FIGURE 12-7 Imaging for a pathologic nipple discharge. **A.** Ductography shows a single dilated duct with an irregular filling defect (*arrow*). **B.** Periareolar sonogram demonstrates an irregular intraductal mass with microlobulated margins within the white circle. An excisional biopsy revealed a benign intraductal papilloma. (Used with permission from Stephen J. Seiler, MD.)

usually negative, but it may occasionally identify an underlying ductal carcinoma in situ (DCIS). Mammary ductography, also known as galactography, requires cannulating the affected duct, injecting radiocontrast, and then performing mammography (Fig. 12-7).

An evaluation of the subareolar ducts, as described above, is required to localize an intraductal lesion for subsequent excision. However, pathologic nipple discharge is *definitively* diagnosed and treated by subareolar duct excision, which is also known as microductectomy (Locker, 1988). Subareolar duct excision can also be used to treat bothersome multiduct discharges not associated with pituitary prolactinoma.

BREAST INFECTIONS

Puerperal Infections

Breast infections are generally divided into puerperal, which develop during pregnancy and lactation, and nonpuerperal.

Of these, pregnancy-related breast infection is characterized by warm, tender, diffuse breast erythema, associated with systemic signs of infection such as fever, malaise, myalgias, and leukocytosis. The most common organism is staphylococcus, and it is successfully treated with oral or intravenous antibiotics, depending on the severity. However, infection may also progress to form deep parenchymal abscesses that require surgical drainage (Branch-Elliman, 2012). Sonographic examination is highly sensitive for identifying underlying abscesses if mastitis does not improve rapidly with antibiotics or if an abscess is suggested clinically. Women with puerperal mastitis should continue to breast feed or breast pump during treatment to prevent milk stasis, which may contribute to infection progression (Thomsen, 1983). Cracked or excoriated nipples may provide entry for bacteria and are treated with lanolin-based lotions or ointments.

Appropriate antibiotics for puerperal mastitis include those covering staphylococcal species. Group A and B *Streptococcus*, *Corynebacterium*, and *Bacteroides* species and *Escherichia coli* are less frequently isolated. Commonly, cephalexin (Keflex) or dicloxacillin (Dynapen), each given at dosages of 500 mg orally four times daily, or the combination of amoxicillin and clavulanate (Augmentin), 500 mg orally three times daily, may be prescribed for 7 days. Erythromycin, 500 mg orally four times daily, will provide adequate coverage for those with a penicillin allergy. Methicillin-resistant *Staphylococcus aureus* (MRSA) is becoming a more prevalent community-acquired pathogen causing mastitis in pregnancy and the puerperium (Laibl, 2005; Stafford, 2008). If MRSA is suspected or if a patient fails to improve on an initial regimen, then trimethoprim-sulfamethoxazole double strength (Bactrim DS, Septra DS), one or two tablets orally twice daily, or clindamycin, 300 mg orally three times daily, is a suitable choice. In ill patients with extensive infection, hospitalization and intravenous (IV) antibiotics are typically required. In these complicated cases, MRSA coverage may be prudent, and clindamycin, 600 mg IV every 8 hours, or vancomycin, 1 g IV every 12 hours, can be administered. Intravenous antibiotics are typically given until the woman is afebrile for 24 to 48 hours. Oral antibiotics are then continued to complete a 7- to 10-day course.

Focal mastitis may result from an infected galactocele. A tender mass will usually be palpable at the site of skin erythema. Needle aspiration of the galactocele and antibiotics are frequently all that is required, but recurrence or progression may mandate surgical drainage.

■ Nonpuerperal Infections

Uncomplicated cellulitis in a nonirradiated breast and in a nonpuerperal setting is uncommon. Accordingly, its presence prompts imaging and biopsies to exclude inflammatory breast cancer, described on page 291.

Nonpuerperal breast abscesses are generally classified as peripheral or subareolar. Peripheral abscesses usually are skin infections such as folliculitis or infection of epidermal inclusion cysts or Montgomery glands. These abscesses are all adequately treated by drainage and antibiotics discussed in the previous section. In contrast, subareolar abscesses arise from keratin-plugged milk ducts directly behind the nipple. The abscess itself usually presents under the areola, and fistulous communications between multiple abscesses are common (Kasales, 2014). Simple drainage is associated with a recurrence rate of nearly 40 percent, thus effective treatment requires subareolar duct excision and complete removal of sinus tracts. In general, surgical drainage of nonpuerperal breast abscesses is usually always accompanied by biopsy of the abscess wall, as breast cancer occasionally presents as an abscess (Benson, 1989; Watt-Boolsen, 1987).

Idiopathic granulomatous mastitis (IGM) is not a true infection. It is included in this section because the painful masses, fluid collections, skin erythema, ulceration, and draining sinus tracts are often confused with infection. Core biopsy will show noncaseating granulomas, and fluid aspirated from apparent "abscesses" is nearly always sterile. Tissue stains can be used to exclude tuberculosis or mycotic infection. Wegener granulomatosis and sarcoidosis are considered in the initial differential diagnosis. This is a self-limiting condition that may take years to resolve. Procedures should be minimized as they will often result in painful draining sinuses. High-dose corticosteroids or methotrexate have been used for treatment, but it is not clear whether they are effective (Mohammed, 2013; Pandey, 2014).

MASTALGIA

The prevalence of breast pain is 66 percent and is higher for women nearing menopause than for younger women (Euhus, 1997; Maddox, 1989). The precise etiology of mastalgia is unknown, but it is likely related to estrogen- and progesterone-mediated changes in interstitial water content and therefore in interstitial pressure.

Mastalgia is generally classified as cyclic or noncyclic. Noncyclic mastalgia is often focal and shows no relationship to the menstrual cycle. Although focal mastalgia is frequently caused by a simple cyst, breast cancer occasionally presents as focal breast pain. Therefore, this complaint is evaluated by careful clinical examination, targeted imaging, and needle biopsy of any palpable or imaging abnormalities.

In contrast, cyclic mastalgia is usually bilateral, diffuse, and most severe during the late luteal phase of the menstrual cycle (Gateley, 1990). It remits with the onset of menstruation. Cyclic mastalgia requires no specific evaluation and is generally managed symptomatically with nonsteroidal anti-inflammatory agents (Fig. 12-8). Various other treatments have been proposed including bromocriptine, vitamin E, or oil of evening primrose. However, outcomes are no better than placebo in the best randomized clinical trials, except for bromocriptine in the subset of women with elevated prolactin levels (Kumar, 1989; Mansel, 1990). For the most severe cases, several agents are effective when administered during the last 2 weeks of the menstrual cycle. These include: (1) danazol, 200 mg orally daily; (2) the selective estrogen-receptor modifier toremifene (Fareston), 20 mg orally daily; or (3) tamoxifen (Nolvadex), 20 mg orally daily. Pregnancy must first be excluded and then avoided if these medications are used.

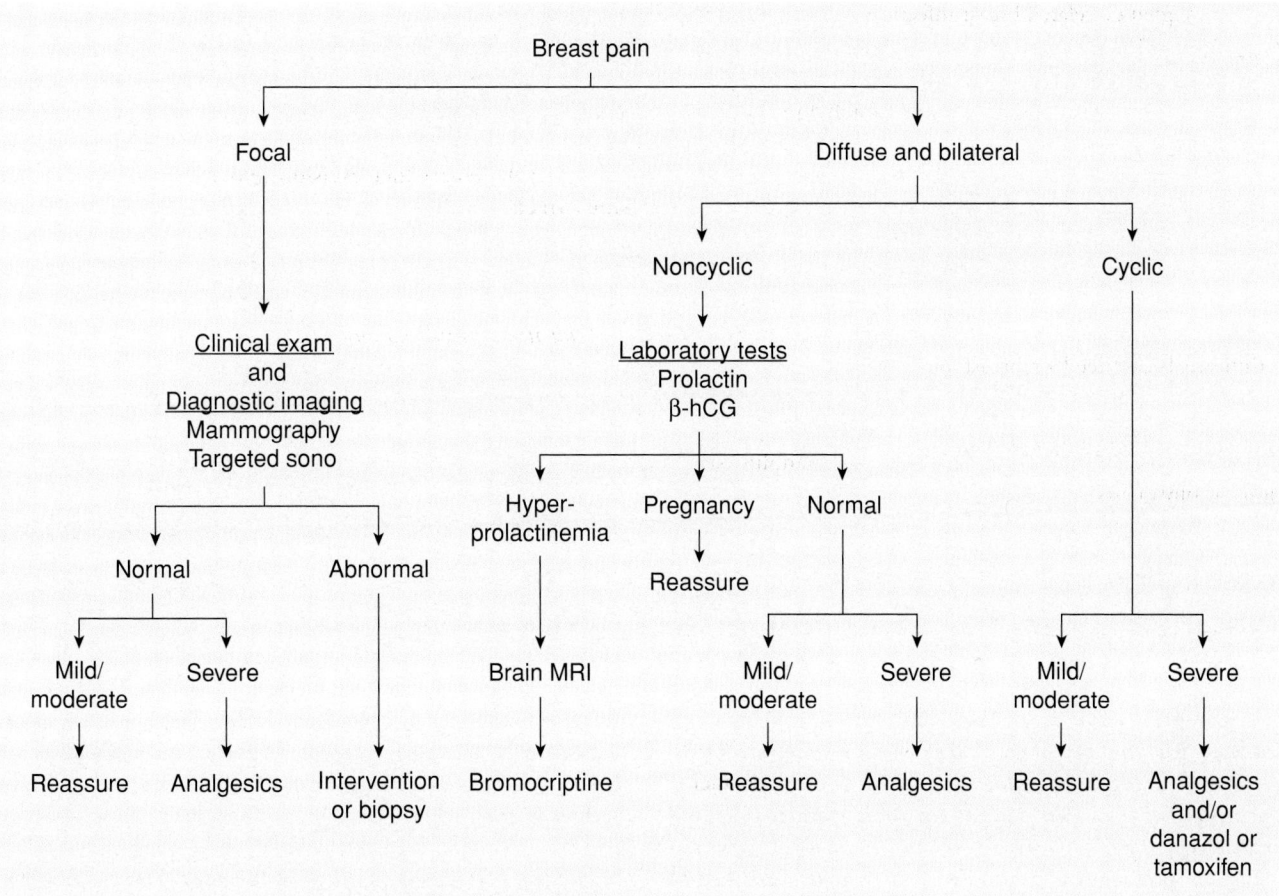

FIGURE 12-8 Diagnostic algorithm to evaluate mastalgia. Oil of evening primrose or vitamin E is frequently used for mild/moderate pain, but the effects are no better than placebo. hCG = human chorionic gonadotropin; MRI = magnetic resonance imaging.

BENIGN BREAST DISEASE

■ Benign Breast Disease without Atypia

The primary tissue components of the breast are fat, fibrous stroma, and epithelial structures. The hormonally responsive component is the epithelium, but considerable paracrine communication exists between the epithelium and stroma. The natural hormonal changes of puberty, pregnancy, lactation, and menopause drive considerable physiologic remodeling of breast tissue during a woman's lifetime, but pathologic remodeling is observed in some. This is initially characterized by acinar dilation and fibrosis, termed *nonproliferative benign breast disease.* Depending on the extent and pattern of these changes, a breast may appear mammographically dense, feel nodular to palpation, or both. The term "fibrocystic change" is often used to refer to palpably nodular breast tissue or to the histologic pattern of dilated ducts and acini invested with dense collagenous stroma. This is not a significant breast cancer risk factor and does not require any special management.

When this change is accompanied by accumulation of luminal epithelial cells (e.g., epithelial hyperplasia), it is called *benign proliferative disease* (Fig. 12-9). This change has been linked to higher levels of estrogen, insulin, and certain inflammatory cytokines, as well as reduced levels of the beneficial adipokine adiponectin (Catsburg, 2014). Benign proliferative

breast disease without atypia is a modest breast cancer risk factor with a relative risk of 1.5 to 1.9 (Dupont, 1993; Hartmann, 2005; Sneige, 2002).

■ Benign Proliferative Disease with Atypia

Atypia refers to specific alterations in the size, shape, or nuclear features of individual epithelial cells in combination with the way groups of cells are organized. Atypical proliferation of ductal cells is termed atypical ductal hyperplasia (ADH), whereas similar changes in acinar cells are termed atypical lobular hyperplasia (ALH). As more and more terminal ducts or acini become involved, the condition is recognized as ductal carcinoma in situ or lobular carcinoma in situ, respectively, which are discussed in later sections (Ringberg, 2001).

Benign proliferative disease with atypia historically accounts for 4 percent of benign breast lesions (Hartmann, 2005). However, the incidence has recently decreased coincident to reductions in hormone replacement therapy use (Menes, 2009).

It is important to recognize that the difference between ADH and low-grade ductal carcinoma in situ is based on the area occupied by the proliferative epithelial cells (Vandenbussche, 2013). Accordingly, surgical excision is usually recommended when ADH is diagnosed by core biopsy, as 4 to 38 percent of cases will be upgraded to in situ or invasive cancer.

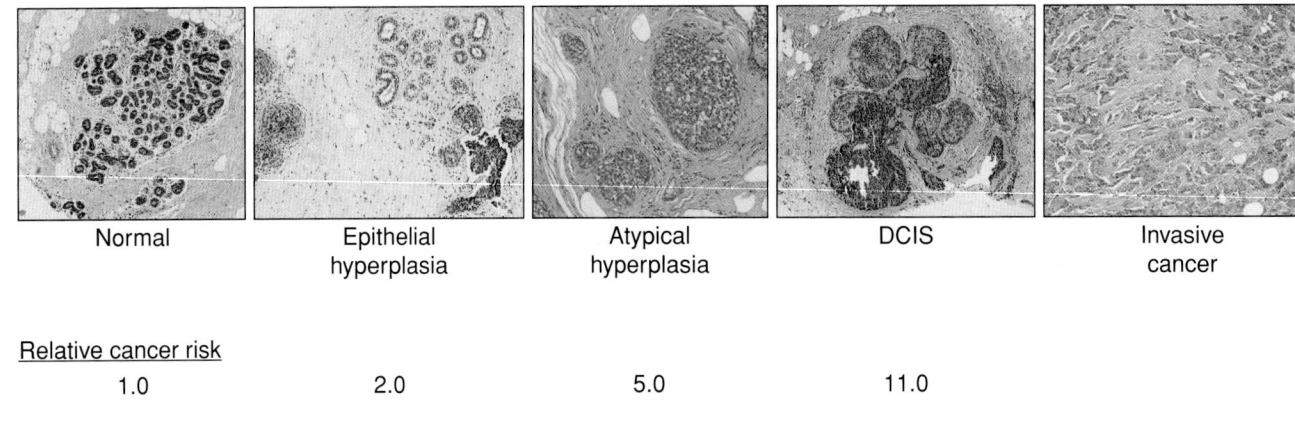

| Normal | Epithelial hyperplasia | Atypical hyperplasia | DCIS | Invasive cancer |

Relative cancer risk

1.0   2.0   5.0   11.0

Tumor suppressor gene methylation

Allelic imbalances

Oncogene amplification

FIGURE 12-9 Histologic progression from normal breast tissue to cancer. DCIS = ductal carcinoma in situ.

Chemoprevention is an excellent option for high-risk women with atypical hyperplasia. These lesions are estrogen-driven, and tamoxifen has been shown to reduce breast cancer risk by 52 to 86 percent for these women (Coopey, 2012; Fisher, 1999).

Benign proliferative disease with atypia is a marker of increased breast cancer risk. Relative risks are 4.5 to 5.0, and absolute risks approximate 1 percent per year for 20 to 30 years (Degnim, 2007; Dupont, 1993). This risk is higher for more extensive lesions. Risk does not appear to increase further with hormone replacement use.

LOBULAR CARCINOMA IN SITU

Similar to proliferative ductal lesion, lobular carcinoma in situ (LCIS) differs from ALH by the greater extent of lobular cell proliferation with LCIS and increased acini distention. LCIS is not associated with any specific mammographic or palpable features and thus is only diagnosed incidentally. Classic LCIS has not traditionally been viewed as a direct precursor of breast cancer, but this view is changing. For example, although LCIS is associated with increased risk for both breasts, women with LCIS most commonly develop carcinoma in the ipsilateral breast (Fisher, 2004b; Ottesen, 1993; Salvadori, 1991). Moreover, infiltrating lobular cancers frequently show associated LCIS, and a clonal relationship between LCIS and subsequent invasive cancer has been demonstrated (Abner, 2000; Andrade, 2012; Sasson, 2001).

As noted, LCIS is also a marker of increased breast cancer risk. The risk of subsequent breast cancer approximates 1 percent per year but is modified upward by early age at diagnosis, family history of breast cancer, and extensive disease (Bodian, 1996).

Surgical excision is recommended if LCIS is diagnosed by needle biopsy, as an associated cancer will be identified in 2 to 25 percent of cases (Buckley, 2014). Excising

to clear margins is not required (Sadek, 2013). These lesions are strongly estrogen receptor positive, and tamoxifen has been shown to reduce breast cancer risk by 56 percent in this setting (Fisher, 1999).

DUCTAL CARCINOMA IN SITU

DCIS can be understood as a condition in which cancer cells fill portions of a mammary ductal system without invading beyond the duct's basement membrane (Ringberg, 2001). Although DCIS cells have accumulated many of the DNA changes common to invasive breast cancer, they lack certain critical changes that would permit them to persist outside of the duct (Aubele, 2002). Ductal carcinoma in situ is classified as stage 0 breast cancer.

The U.S. incidence of DCIS has increased in parallel with that of invasive breast cancer during the past two decades. But, as with invasive breast cancer, the incidence has plateaued during the past several years (Virnig, 2010). DCIS currently accounts for 25 to 30 percent of all breast cancers in the United States. It is most commonly diagnosed by screening mammography as it is frequently associated with pleomorphic, linear, or branching calcifications (Fig. 12-10).

DCIS is classified by morphologic type, the presence or absence of comedonecrosis, and nuclear grade. The common morphologic types include cribriform, solid, micropapillary, and comedo (Fig. 12-11). Comedonecrosis appears as a necrotic eosinophilic core down the center of a duct packed with cancer cells. Of all of the classifying variables, nuclear grade is the most predictive for associated invasive cancer, extent of disease, and recurrence after treatment (Ringberg, 2001).

Incompletely treated DCIS may recur locally, and 50 percent of recurrences are associated with fully developed invasive breast cancer. The principal treatment of DCIS is wide excision with a negative margin. This may require mastectomy if DCIS is extensive or if there are other contraindications to breast

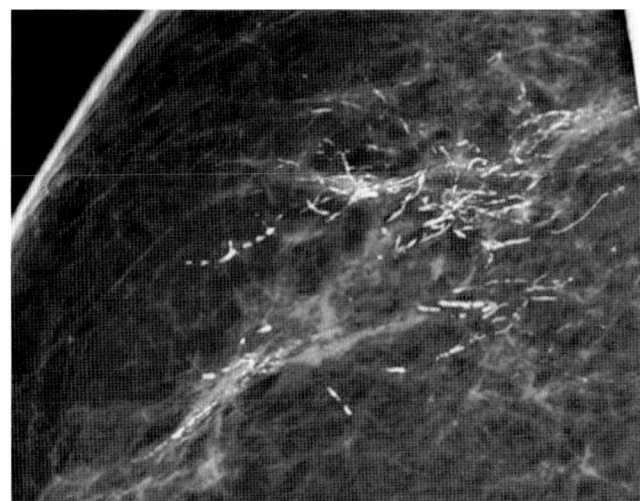

FIGURE 12-10 Fine linear-branching calcifications in a segmental distribution associated with ductal carcinoma in situ. (Used with permission from Stephen J. Seiler, MD.)

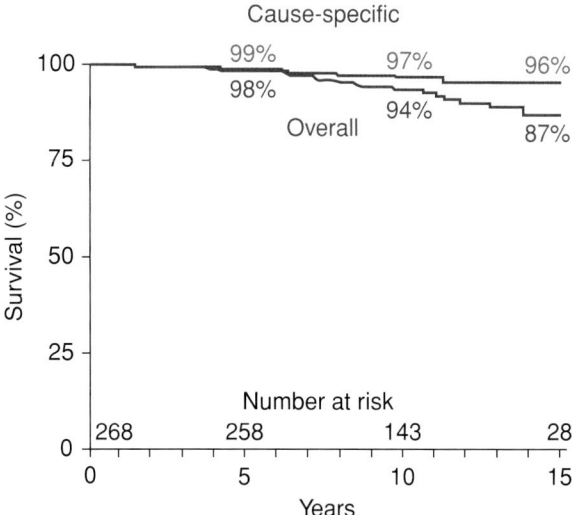

FIGURE 12-12 Cause-specific and overall survival for ductal carcinoma in situ. (Reproduced with permission from Solin LJ, Kurtz J, Fourquet A, et al: Fifteen-year results of breast-conserving surgery and breast irradiation for the treatment of ductal carcinoma in situ of the breast, J Clin Oncol 1996 Mar;14(3):754–763.)

conservation. When breast conservation is possible, postoperative breast irradiation will reduce the local recurrence rate from 18 percent to 9 percent and is considered standard adjuvant treatment (Fisher, 1993). For those treated with breast conservation and radiation, the breast cancer-specific survival rate is 96 percent (Fig. 12-12) (Solin, 1996).

Axillary staging is generally not included in the management of DCIS, although some have advocated sentinel node biopsy for large, high-grade DCIS diagnosed by needle biopsy and treated by lumpectomy, as occult invasive cancer is diagnosed in 10 percent (Wilkie, 2005). Sentinel lymph node (SLN) biopsy in conjunction with mastectomy is less contro-

versial, as it is not possible to go back and perform SLN biopsy if an occult invasive cancer is diagnosed in this setting.

Five years of tamoxifen is recommended for estrogen-receptor-positive DCIS treated by breast conservation (Fisher, 1999). Although tamoxifen is not associated with a statistically significant improvement in overall survival rates, it does significantly reduce the incidence of ipsilateral invasive cancer and also reduces the risk of contralateral breast cancer.

■ Paget Disease of the Nipple

This type of DCIS presents as a focal eczematous rash of the nipple (Fig. 12-13). Ductal carcinoma cells, responding to chemoattractants secreted by cells in the dermis, migrate to the surface of the nipple, inducing skin breakdown (Schelfhout, 2000). The condition is easily diagnosed histologically by punch biopsy or excision of the affected nipple tip after nipple-areolar blockade using local anesthetic. Evaluation also includes careful clinical examination, as an associated mass is identified in approximately 60 percent of cases (Ashikari, 1970). Among those with no palpable abnormalities, mammography will show suspicious densities or calcifications in 21 percent (Ikeda, 1993). An underlying DCIS is identified in about two thirds of cases, and an invasive cancer in approximately one third (Ashikari, 1970).

Treatment includes wide excision with negative margins. Breast conservation, which requires central breast resection including the nipple-areolar complex and all identifiable underlying disease, is followed

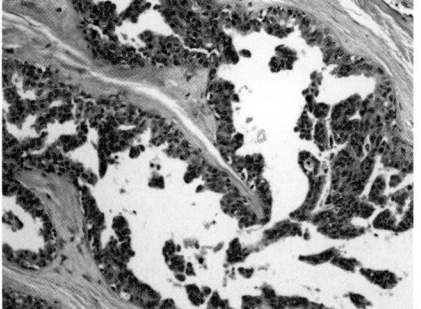

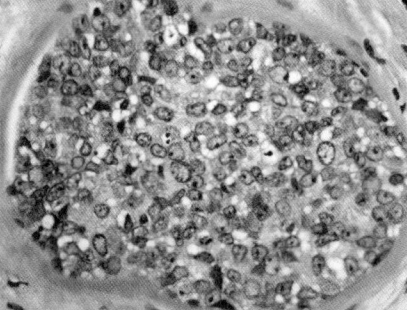

A. Cribriform DCIS, low grade

B. Micropapillary DCIS

C. Solid DCIS, high grade

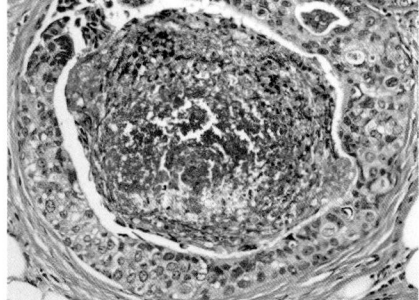

D. DCIS with comedonecrosis

FIGURE 12-11 Morphologic types of ductal carcinoma in situ (DCIS). (Used with permission from Dr. Sunati Sahoo, Pathology, UTSW Medical Center.)

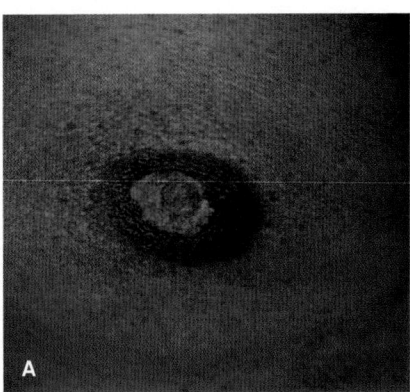
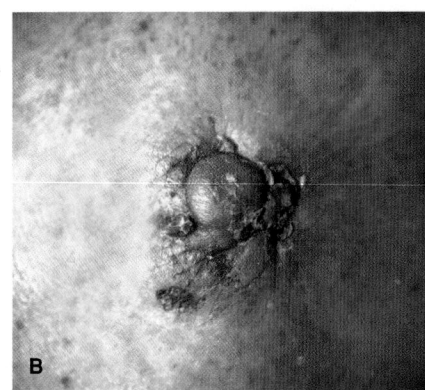
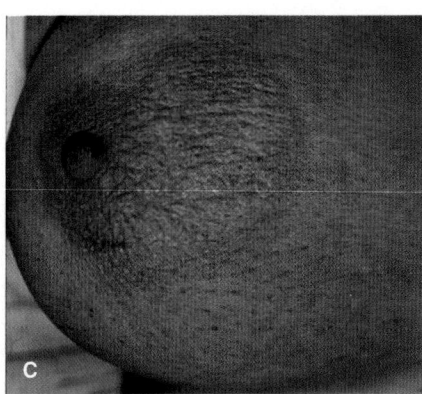

FIGURE 12-13 A. and **B.** Paget disease of the nipple. **C.** Benign reactive dermatitis. (Used with permission from Dr. Marilyn Leitch.)

by postoperative breast irradiation (Bijker, 2001). Axillary staging by sentinel node biopsy is not required unless an invasive component is identified or total mastectomy is performed.

BREAST CANCER RISK FACTORS

The most profound breast cancer risk factor is female gender. In addition, the incidence of breast cancer, as for most other cancers, increases with advancing age. Only 12 to 30 percent of breast cancer has a significant familial component, and apart from radiation exposure early in life, convincing environmental causes have not been elucidated (Baker, 2005; Locatelli, 2004). Breast cancer risk factors are listed in Table 12-3, but the strong link between ovarian function and breast tissue remodeling warrants more detailed description. In general, all of these risk factors are more prevalent in developed countries than in those that are less developed. Consequently, breast cancer is more common in industrialized cultures (Parkin, 2001).

■ Reproductive Factors
Ovulatory Cycles

Ovulatory menstrual cycles exert stress on the breast epithelium by inducing proliferation in the late luteal phase. If conception does not occur, proliferation is followed by programmed cell death (Anderson, 1982; Soderqvist, 1997). Early age at menarche is associated with earlier onset of ovulatory cycles and increased breast cancer risk (den Tonkelaar, 1996; Vihko, 1986). Conversely, early menopause, whether it is natural or surgical, is associated with a reduced breast cancer risk (Kvale, 1988). Pregnancy generates very high levels of circulating estradiol, which is associated with a transient increase in short-term risk. But pregnancy also induces terminal differentiation of breast epithelium and provides relief from ovarian cycling. Consequently, increasing parity is associated with reduced lifetime risk.

Pregnancy

The breast is unique among all human organs in that it exists as a primordium for a decade or more before entering a highly proliferative state at menarche, and then does not fully mature until the first live birth. Immature breast epithelium is more susceptible to carcinogens than postlactational epithelium (Russo, 1996). Therefore, the longer a first live birth is delayed, the greater the breast cancer risks. Relative to nulliparity, a first live birth before the age of 28 years is associated with reduced breast cancer risk, whereas one occurring later is associated with increased risk (Gail, 1989). Both early age at first live birth and greater numbers of live births are associated with reduced breast cancer risk (Layde, 1989; Pike, 1983).

■ Hormone Replacement Therapy

The postmenopausal use of combined estrogen and progestin hormone replacement therapy is a modest breast cancer risk factor, and relative risks range from 1.26 to 1.76 (Beral, 2011; Hulley, 2002; Rossouw, 2002). The risk is higher with longer durations of use and with a shorter interval between the onset of menopause and the start of the medication (Beral, 2011). Estrogen-only replacement is not convincingly associated with increased breast cancer risk, but there is a relationship with body mass index that yields a lower risk for obese women and higher risk for thin women (Anderson, 2004).

BREAST CANCER RISK STRATIFICATION AND MANAGEMENT

Approaches for managing breast cancer risk include: (1) lifestyle modification to achieve and sustain ideal body weight, (2) enhanced surveillance that includes screening magnetic resonance (MR) imaging, (3) chemoprevention with a selective estrogen-receptor modifier or an aromatase inhibitor, and (4) prophylactic surgery including oophorectomy or mastectomy for those at highest risk (Cuzick, 2014; Domchek, 2010; Goss, 2011; Heemskerk-Gerritsen, 2007; Vogel, 2010). Beyond beneficial lifestyle modification, each intervention introduces new risks, and thus breast cancer risk quantification is essential for making prevention decisions.

The American Cancer Society has endorsed screening MR imaging for women with a lifetime breast cancer risk that exceeds 20 percent (Saslow, 2010). The Food and Drug Administration (FDA) has approved tamoxifen chemoprevention for women older than 35 years with >1.7 percent breast cancer risk over 5 years. Similarly, raloxifene (Evista) is approved for increased-risk postmenopausal women. To maximize benefit and minimize harm, breast cancer risk, age, race, and prior hysterectomy all factor into chemoprevention decisions (Freedman, 2011).

TABLE 12-3. Common Risk Factors and Their Risk Ratios[a]

Genetic Risk Factors	Risk Ratio
Female gender	114
Age	4–158[b]
High-penetrance mutations: BRCA1, BRCA2, p53, STK11	26–36

Modest-penetrance mutations:
  PTEN, p16, PALB2, CDH1,
  NF1, CHEK2, ATM, BRIP1
	2.0–2.7

Family: mother, daughter, sister	1.55–1.8
Family: aunt, niece, grandmother	1.15

Genetic polymorphisms:
  FGFR2, TNRC9, MAP3K1,
  LSP1, MRPS30
	1.07–1.26

Other Factors	
Mantle radiation	5.6
Acini per lobule in benign breast tissue	
11–20	2.8
21–40	3.23
≥41	11.85
Mammographic density	
>25–50% (scattered)	2.4
>51–75% (heterogeneous)	3.4
>75% (dense)	5.3
Biopsy w LCIS	5.4
Biopsy w atypical hyperplasia	5
Increased BMD	2.0–2.5
Age at first birth >35	1.31–1.93
Obesity (BMI >30)	1.2–1.8
Any benign breast disease	1.47
Elevated circulating insulin	1.46
5 years of combined HRT	1.26–1.76
Elevated circulating estrogen	1.1–1.7
Nulliparity	1.26–1.55
Alcohol (>1 drink/day)	1.31
Age at menarche <12	1.21

[a]Risks listed by genetic or nongenetic and ordered by strength of association with breast cancer.
[b]Risk compared to women aged 20–29. The risk ratio increases approximately by 4 for every year older than 30.
BMD = bone mineral density; BMI = body mass index; HRT = hormone replacement therapy; LCIS = lobular carcinoma in situ.
Data from Beral, 2011; Bodian, 1996; Cauley, 1996; Claus, 1994; De Bruin, 2009; Easton, 2007; Freisinger, 2009; Fu, 2007; Gail, 1989; Gunter, 2009; Hankinson, 2005; Howlader, 2013; Hulley, 2002; Kotsopoulos, 2010; Lalloo, 2006; Mavaddat, 2010; McKian, 2009; Phipps, 2010; Rossouw, 2002; Santen, 2005; Welsh, 2009; Zhou, 2011.

TABLE 12-4. Genetic Syndromes Associated with Increased Breast Cancer Risk

Syndrome Name	Genetic Mutation
Hereditary breast-ovarian cancer syndrome	BRCA1, BRCA2
Li-Fraumeni	p53
Cowden	PTEN
Peutz-Jegher	STK11
Hereditary diffuse gastric cancer	CDH1
PALB2	PALB2
ATM	ATM
CHK2	CHK2
RAD51C	RAD51C

Adapted with permission from Euhus DM: Genetic testing today, Ann Surg Oncol 2014 Oct;21(10):3209–3215.

The foregoing highlights the importance of quantitative breast cancer risk stratification. Several computer models are available for this. The most thoroughly validated is the Gail model, available at http://www.cancer.gov/bcrisktool/ (Costantino, 1999; Gail, 1989; Rockhill, 2001). Although the most generally applicable model, the Gail model is insufficient when there is a strong family history of breast cancer, male breast cancer, or ovarian cancer (Euhus, 2002). Genetic models such as BRCAPRO, Tyrer-Cuzick, or BOADICEA are more appropriate in these settings (Berry, 1997; Lee, 2014; Tyrer, 2004).

■ Breast Cancer Genetics

Twin studies suggest that only 12 to 30 percent of breast cancer is primarily genetic in origin, and modeling studies implicate autosomal dominant inheritance of single genes as the most important mechanism (Lichtenstein, 2000; Locatelli, 2004; Risch, 2001). As such, genetic testing is one of the most powerful risk stratification tools available. It can identify women at very high risk for cancer who could reasonably consider risk-reducing surgery. In breast cancer patients, it can also contribute directly to decisions regarding surgery, radiation, and systemic therapies (Euhus, 2013). Mutations in *BRCA1* or *BRCA2* genes are the most frequently identified germline alterations in familial breast cancer, but the list of predisposition genes is growing (Table 12-4). Commercialized massive parallel sequencing, namely, next-generation sequencing, now allows testing for mutations in a few to dozens of genes simultaneously (Euhus, 2015).

Obtaining a reasonably detailed cancer family history is essential for identifying individuals who may benefit from genetic counseling and testing. At a minimum, the relationship and age at diagnosis is recorded for every cancer in the family. Family histories that may suggest inherited susceptibility include early-onset breast cancer (<50 years), bilateral breast cancer, male breast cancer, multiple affected relatives in one generation, breast cancer in multiple generations, development of cancers that are known to be associated with a particular syndrome, and two or more cancers in one relative, especially if they develop at an early age.

■ Hereditary Breast-Ovarian Cancer Syndrome

This syndrome accounts for 5 to 7 percent of breast cancers in the United States and is most frequently caused by *BRCA1* or *BRCA2* mutation (Malone, 2000). Hallmarks of the form linked with *BRCA1* include early age at breast cancer diagnosis (median 44 years); high-grade, estrogen- and progesterone-receptor negative breast cancers; and associated ovarian cancer (Foulkes, 2004). Other associated cancers are pancreatic cancer and melanoma.

For *BRCA1* mutation carriers, the lifetime breast cancer risk ranges from 45 to 81 percent, and ovarian cancer risk from 16 to 54 percent (Antoniou, 2008; Brohet, 2014; Ford, 1998; King, 2003; Mavaddat, 2013). Individuals who have developed both breast and ovarian cancer have an 86-percent probability of carrying a *BRCA* mutation (Cvelbar, 2005).

Among *BRCA2* carriers, lifetime risk for breast cancer ranges from 27 to 85 percent, and ovarian cancer risk from 6 to 27 percent. Women with *BRCA2* mutations develop breast cancer later in life than *BRCA1* carriers, thus age at diagnosis is not usually a good criterion for recognizing this syndrome (Panchal, 2010). Similar to sporadic breast cancer, most *BRCA2*-associated breast cancers are hormone receptor positive (Lakhani, 2002). Ovarian cancer is an associated cancer but develops less frequently than it does in *BRCA1*-affected families. Five to 13 percent of male breast cancers are associated with *BRCA2* mutations. Lifetime breast cancer risk is estimated at 1.8 percent for men with *BRCA1* mutations and 8.3 percent for *BRCA2* (Tai, 2007).

For affected women, early premenopausal bilateral oophorectomy reduces breast cancer risk by 37 to 72 percent and also lowers breast cancer-specific and all-cause mortality rates (Domchek, 2010; Finch, 2014; Kauff, 2008). This is discussed further in Chapter 35 (p. 736). Bilateral prophylactic mastectomy reduces breast cancer risk by more than 90 percent but has not yet been shown to improve survival rates (Hartmann, 2001; Heemskerk-Gerritsen, 2007; Meijers-Heijboer, 2001).

With the introduction of next-generation sequencing panel tests, clinicians are increasingly confronted with rare syndromes for which there are scarce data to guide management (see Table 12-4) (Euhus, 2015). Involvement of professional genetic counselors and careful assessment of a three-generation family cancer history is essential for estimating and managing cancer risk.

Surgical options for breast cancers that arise in the context of an inherited predisposition syndrome are the same as for sporadic breast cancers (Pierce, 2010). However, patients are counseled that the risk of an ipsilateral second primary breast cancer in a preserved breast can be as high as 3 to 4 percent annually (Haffty, 2002; Seynaevea, 2004). Moreover, lifetime contralateral breast cancer risk is 83 percent for *BRCA1* mutation carriers and 62 percent for *BRCA2* carriers, and growing evidence supports bilateral mastectomy to improve survival rates (Evans, 2013; Mavaddat, 2013; Metcalfe, 2014).

BREAST CANCER SCREENING

In the United States, digital mammography has largely replaced film-screen mammography, and 3-dimensional (3-D) tomosynthesis is gradually replacing 2-D mammography. This technique generates hundreds of images as the x-ray source arcs over the top of the breast. Digital reconstruction allows a radiologist to visually scroll through breast images and significantly attenuates overlying breast densities at each level (Kopans, 2013). Compared with 2-D mammography, tomosynthesis reduces the false-positive rate (recall rate) by 15 to 30 percent and increases the cancer detection rate by 10 to 29 percent (Greenberg, 2014; Haas, 2013; Skaane, 2013). This is achieved with slightly higher radiation doses (Feng, 2012).

■ The Screening Mammography Controversy

In 2009, the U.S. Preventive Services Task Force recommended biennial screening mammography for women aged 50 to 74 years and individualized screening decisions for women aged 40 to 49. Several influential organizations including the American College of Obstetricians and Gynecologists (2014) and the American College of Radiology suggest that yearly screening mammography begin at age 40 (Lee, 2010). The American Cancer Society recommends yearly screening beginning at age 45, but with an opportunity to begin at age 40. They promote a transition to biennial screening at age 55, although yearly screening may be elected (Oeffinger, 2015). The controversy centers on: (1) the true mortality rate benefit, (2) the harm from false-positive results, and (3) the harm from diagnosing clinically irrelevant breast cancers.

However, most data available for addressing these issues are derived from eight large, but older, randomized prospective trials. The most recent trial was completed in the 1980s. Recent technological advances have significantly improved the sensitivity of mammography, but breast cancer treatment has also advanced, reducing the mortality rate improvement from early detection. Based on 30-year-old data, it is generally agreed that screening mammography starting at age 50 reduces breast cancer mortality rates by approximately 27 percent, and one metaanalysis reported an 18-percent reduction for women aged 40 to 49 (Hendrick, 1997; Kerlikowske, 1997). However, screen-detected breast cancer is a heterogeneous disease. Some cancers will eventually develop clinical metastases no matter how small they are when first detected, and some will never become lethal no matter how long diagnosis is delayed. This latter form is the one most likely to be detected by periodic screening (length time bias).

The practice of screening mammography is based on the assumption that early intervention in some subgroup of tumors will interrupt progression and save lives. Since the introduction of screening mammography more than three decades ago, there has been a large increase in the detection of early-stage breast cancer but only a small decrease in the diagnosis of node-positive or metastatic disease (Bleyer, 2012). This suggests that many breast cancers will never progress (overdiagnosed) and that the fraction of breast cancers whose progression can be interrupted by surgery may be modest.

For now, annual mammography beginning at age 40 as recommended by several professional societies is reasonable, but women are counseled of the risks and benefits. Among 1000 U.S. women aged 50 years who are screened annually for a decade, 0.3 to 3.2 are estimated to avoid a breast cancer death, 490 to 670 will have at least 1 false alarm, and 3 to 14 will be overdiagnosed and treated needlessly (Welch, 2014). There is no arbitrary age above which screening should cease. Women should have at least 10 years of remaining life to realize a mortality benefit from screening mammography (Lee, 2013).

Breast Magnetic Resonance Imaging

Breast MR imaging is commonly used as an adjunct to screen high-risk women and to establish disease extent in certain breast cancer patients. It is more sensitive for breast cancer detection than is mammography, but it is expensive and has a high false-positive rate. In addition, some evidence links its use with increased mastectomy rates but without reducing reexcision rates or improving breast cancer outcome (Houssami, 2013, 2014; Pilewskie, 2014; Turnbull, 2010).

Annual screening breast MR imaging is frequently selected for genetically high-risk women and in women with a lifetime breast cancer risk exceeding 20 percent (Saslow, 2010). This increases the diagnosis of smaller, lymph node negative breast cancers but does not improve survival rates (Gareth, 2014; Moller, 2013).

Breast MR imaging is not routinely performed in women with newly diagnosed breast cancer. Its primary value is assessing response to neoadjuvant chemotherapy in women contemplating breast conservation and evaluating women with breast cancer metastatic to axillary lymph nodes from an unknown primary (Morrow, 2011). Additionally, it can aid establishing the extent of disease prior to breast conservation for a subset of patients in whom uncertainty persists after careful clinical examination, mammography, and sonography.

Other Breast Imaging Modalities

Adding almost any imaging modality to screening mammography will incrementally increase the cancer detection rate but at the cost of an increased false-positive rate and more biopsies. Modalities that are occasionally useful, but not recommended for routine use, include screening sonography, breast-specific gamma imaging, and breast positron emission tomography (PET) (Kalinyak, 2014; Merry, 2014; Rechtman, 2014). These latter two tests are associated with significantly higher radiation exposure. Evidence is accumulating that medical radiation exposure before age 30 can increase breast cancer risk, and thus caution is advised (Berrington de Gonzalez, 2009; Pijpe, 2012).

Screening Physical Examination

The value of a screening clinical breast examination (CBE) performed by health care providers should not be neglected (Jatoi, 2003). Four of the large, randomized mammography trials mentioned earlier collected information on CBE and found that 44 to 74 percent of the breast cancers were detected by this approach. Sensitivity and specificity were higher for CBE than mammography among young women.

In contrast, enthusiasm for patients to perform breast self-examination (BSE) has diminished after a very large randomized trial from Shanghai, China, found no improvement in mortality rates (Thomas, 2002). Although there is less interest in promoting regimented BSE, encouraging women to remain breast-aware is reasonable.

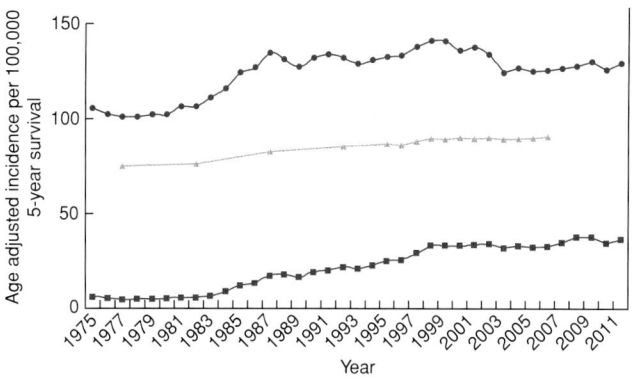

FIGURE 12-14 Trends in breast cancer incidence and survival in the United States. Curve of decreasing breast cancer rates in U.S. ● = incidence of invasive breast cancer; ▲ = incidence in situ; ■ = 5-year survival. (Data from Howlader N, Noone AM, Krapcho M, et al: SEER Cancer Statistics Review, 1975–2010, National Cancer Institute. 2013. Available at: http://seer.cancer.gov/archive/csr/1975_2010/. Accessed August 7, 2014.)

INVASIVE BREAST CANCER

In the United States, breast cancer is the most common cancer in women and the second most frequent cause of cancer-related mortality (second to lung) (Siegel, 2014). Although the incidence of breast cancer increased steadily in this country through the 1980s and 1990s, it has leveled at approximately 125 cases per year per 100,000 postmenopausal women and is declining for some ethnicities. Concurrently, survival rates steadily improve (Fig. 12-14) (Howlader, 2013).

Tumor Characteristics

Primary cancers of the breast comprise 97 percent of malignancies affecting the breast, whereas 3 percent represent metastases from other sites. The most common of these, in descending order, are the contralateral breast, sarcoma, melanoma, serous epithelial ovarian cancer, and lung cancer (DeLair, 2013). Cancers of mammary epithelial structures account for most of primary breast cancer. Infiltrating ductal carcinoma is the most common form of invasive breast cancer (~80 percent), and infiltrating lobular carcinoma is the second most frequent (~15 percent). Other malignancies such as phyllodes tumors, sarcoma, and lymphoma form the remainder.

Apart from stage, the primary tumor characteristics that most influence prognosis and treatment decisions are hormone receptor status, nuclear grade, and Her-2/neu expression (Harris, 2007). Approximately two thirds of breast cancers are estrogen- and progesterone-receptor positive. This feature is generally associated with a better prognosis and more treatment options.

Her-2/neu is a membrane tyrosine kinase that cooperates with other Her-family receptors to generate proliferation and survival signals in breast cancer cells. Approximately 25 percent of breast cancers have increased expression of Her-2/neu (Masood, 2005). The list of medications that specifically target HER2 overexpressing breast cancer is growing and includes trastuzumab (Herceptin), trastuzumab emtansine (Kadcyla), pertuzumab (Perjeta), neratinib, and lapatinib (Tykerb)(Tolaney, 2014).

Gene expression profiling has identified several "intrinsic subtypes" of breast cancer with prognostic significance (Cadoo,

SECTION 1

TABLE 12-5. Breast Cancer Surgical Staging

T Stage		Stage Grouping			
Tis	In situ	0	Tis	N0	M0
T1mi	≤1mm	IA	T1	N0	M0
T1	≤2 cm	IB	T1	N1mi	M0
T2	>2 cm but ≤5 cm	IIA	T0	N1	M0
T3	>5 cm		T1	N1	M0
T4	Involvement of skin or chest wall or		T2	N0	M0
	inflammatory cancer	IIB	T2	N1	M0
			T3	N0	M0
N Stage		IIIA	T0	N2	M0
N0	No lymph node involvement		T1	N2	M0
N0i+	≤ 0.2 mm metastasis		T2	N2	M0
N1mi	> 0.2 mm and/or > 200 cells but < 2mm		T3	N1	M0
N1	1–3 nodes		T3	N2	M0
N2	4–9 nodes	IIIB	T4	N0	M0
N3	≥ 10 nodes or any infraclavicular nodes		T4	N1	M0
			T4	N2	M0
M Stage		IIIC	Any T	N3	M0
		IV	Any T	Any N	M1
M0	No distant metastases				
M1	Distant metastases				

2013). Multigene assays are now available in the clinic for individualized prediction of prognosis and treatment response, especially for estrogen-receptor positive tumors (Rouzier, 2013).

■ Breast Cancer Staging

Careful breast cancer staging is essential for predicting outcome, planning treatment, and comparing treatment effects in clinical trials. Each patient is assigned both a clinical and a pathologic stage. The clinical stage is based on examination and radiographic findings, whereas the pathologic stage is based on actual tumor measurements and histologic assessments of lymph nodes after primary surgery. Surgical staging of breast cancer is based on the TNM system, which includes primary tumor size (T), regional lymph node involvement (N), and presence of distant metastases (M) (Table 12-5). For patients with a clinically negative axilla, sentinel lymph node biopsy has replaced complete axillary dissection for nodal staging (Lyman, 2014).

The most common distant metastatic site in breast cancer is bone, followed by lung, liver, and brain. Thus, for newly diagnosed breast cancer patients, a complete blood count and liver function tests including alkaline phosphatase are recommended. Whole body screening with CT of the chest, CT or MR imaging of the abdomen and pelvis, and bone scan or whole body PET/CT are only recommended for clinical suspicion of metastases or for patients with clinical stage III disease (National Comprehensive Cancer Network, 2014).

■ Breast Cancer Treatment

Breast cancer is best managed by a multidisciplinary team of breast surgeons, medical oncologists, and radiation oncologists.

Goals of surgery and radiation therapy are elimination of all local or regional tumor in a way that maximizes cosmesis and minimizes the risk of local or regional recurrence. There is some evidence that these local modalities reduce the risk of subsequent metastases and therefore increase survival rates (Darby, 2011). However, a significant proportion of patients with apparently localized disease have tumor cells detectable in their blood or bone marrow at diagnosis (Braun, 2005; Giuliano, 2011a). For these women, systemic treatment with chemotherapy, hormone manipulation, or targeted therapies is the primary approach for reducing metastasis risk and death (Dowsett, 2010; Peto, 2012).

Surgery

Halstead (1894) revolutionized the treatment of breast cancer by demonstrating improved outcome for patients treated with radical mastectomy. However, results from recent randomized clinical trials have appropriately fostered a trend toward less aggressive surgery. Specifically, lumpectomy with postoperative radiation therapy results in the same breast cancer-specific survival rate as total mastectomy (Fisher, 2002).

Axillary dissection, that is, near-complete axillary lymphadenectomy, was also once a standard part of breast cancer staging and treatment, but its role is diminishing (Rao, 2013). The procedure is still indicated for patients with clinically node positive disease at diagnosis. However, it is frequently omitted in selected patients with clinically negative nodes but positive sentinel nodes, because radiation therapy and systemic adjuvant therapies achieve the same low axillary recurrence rate and the same survival rate (Galimberti, 2013; Giuliano, 2010, 2011b). When required, axillary dissection results in lymphedema in

15 to 50 percent of women, depending on how it is measured (Morrell, 2005). Dissection is also associated with persistent shoulder or arm symptoms in up to 70 percent (Kuehn, 2000).

Radiation Therapy

After breast-conserving surgery, whole breast radiation reduces local recurrence from approximately 5 percent per year to 1 percent per year, although it may be omitted in elderly patients with favorable tumors (Fisher, 2002; Hughes, 2013). Shorter courses of partial breast irradiation may be appropriate in selected patients (Smith, 2009). Postmastectomy chest wall radiation improves survival in women with high-risk lymph node positive breast cancer (Overgaard, 1999; Ragaz, 2005). Recent clinical trial data are driving a marked increase use of extended-field radiation therapy (Early Breast Cancer Trialists' Collaborative Group, 2014).

Chemotherapy

In the past, adjuvant chemotherapy was reserved for patients with nodal metastases and was always given after definitive surgery. However, randomized prospective trials have shown that adjuvant chemotherapy also improves survival rates for high-risk node-negative patients (Fisher, 2004a). Increasingly, however, the decision for chemotherapy is influenced by specific measures of tumor biology including results from multigene assays (Rouzier, 2013; Sparano, 2008).

If used, adjuvant chemotherapy is usually administered after primary surgery but before radiation therapy. Neoadjuvant chemotherapy is given prior to definitive surgery and is gaining popularity. Neoadjuvant chemotherapy permits assessment of a given tumor's sensitivity to the selected agents, and tumor shrinkage permits less aggressive surgery (von Minckwitz, 2013).

Modern breast cancer chemotherapy often includes an anthracycline such as doxorubicin (Adriamycin), in conjunction with cyclophosphamide (Cytoxan) (Trudeau, 2005). The addition of a taxane has been shown to improve outcome (A'Hern, 2013). Platins such as cisplatin (Platinol) or carboplatin (Paraplatin) are increasingly used to replace doxorubicin when other cardiotoxic drugs such as trastuzumab are required and to treat certain tumor subtypes that have defects in homologous recombination. Chemotherapeutic agents are described more fully in Chapter 27 (p. 592).

Hormonal Therapy and Targeted Therapies

Adjuvant hormonal therapy is used for estrogen-receptor positive tumors. In pre- or postmenopausal women, one option is the selective estrogen-receptor modulator tamoxifen (Jaiyesimi, 1995). As discussed in Chapter 27 (p. 603), important side effects of tamoxifen include menopausal symptoms, increased risks of thromboembolic events, and higher rates of endometrial polyps and endometrial cancer. Although this cancer risk is increased, surveillance of the endometrium with routine transvaginal sonography or endometrial biopsy is not recommended. Endometrial evaluation is reserved for those with abnormal bleeding and follows that outlined in Chapter 8 (p. 184).

In postmenopausal women, aromatase inhibitors may be used. FDA-approved agents include anastrozole (Arimidex), letrozole (Femara), and exemestane (Aromasin) (Kudachadkar,

2005). In postmenopausal women, most circulating estradiol is derived from the peripheral conversion of androgens by the enzyme aromatase. Administration of aromatase inhibitors reduces circulating estradiol to nearly undetectable levels in these women. The addition of an aromatase inhibitor after tamoxifen is associated with a 23- to 39-percent improvement in the disease-free survival rate and a nearly 50-percent reduction in the contralateral breast cancer rate (Geisler, 2006). Although tamoxifen is commonly used as an initial antihormonal therapy in postmenopausal women, transition to an aromatase inhibitor and 10 years of treatment improves outcome (Johnston, 2014).

Unlike tamoxifen, aromatase inhibitors are associated with greater rates of bone loss and fractures. Accordingly, baseline bone mineral density testing and periodic monitoring is recommended. For women with mild or moderate bone loss, exercise and supplementation with vitamin D and calcium are encouraged. Various agents are available for managing severe loss, and a discussion of these drugs is found in Chapter 22 (p. 499).

Bisphosphonates such as zoledronic acid (Zometa) are often used to prevent cancer-treatment-induced bone loss (Hadji, 2011). In addition, the combination of aromatase inhibitors and zoledronic acid appears to improve outcome in hormone-receptor-positive breast cancer (Coleman, 2013).

Therapies that target specific biological pathways are becoming available. However, only HER2-targeted therapies are currently used routinely in early-stage breast cancer and only in HER2-amplified tumors. Targeting the mTOR pathway with everolimus (Afinitor) is now an FDA-approved strategy for advanced or metastatic hormone-receptor-positive breast cancer and is also being investigated for trastuzumab-resistant HER2-positive breast cancer (Andre, 2014; Dhillon, 2013). Comprehensive molecular profiling of tumors to identify targets for intervention is becoming more common (Frampton, 2013). Biologic agents for targeting cancer are described more fully in Chapter 27 (p. 603).

Surveillance

Long-term surveillance of breast cancer patients after treatment includes periodic history and physical examination. Women who elected breast conservation are counseled that the remaining breast tissue requires surveillance indefinitely. Ipsilateral, second primary breast cancers develop at a rate of approximately 1 percent per year and contralateral breast cancers at approximately 0.7 percent per year (Fatouros, 2005; Fisher, 1984; Gao, 2003). Laboratory and imaging tests are obtained to further evaluate specific signs or symptoms. Screening tests other than mammography to identify asymptomatic recurrences are not recommended (Khatcheressian, 2013).

Inflammatory Breast Cancer

Inflammatory breast cancer accounts for 1 to 5 percent of breast cancers (Chang, 1998; Dawood, 2010). This cancer presents with skin changes that can range from a faint red blush to a flaming-red rash associated with skin edema (peau d'orange change) (Fig. 12-15). It is distinguished from a neglected advanced primary breast cancer by its rapid onset and progression within just a few weeks. The cancer spreads rapidly throughout the entire

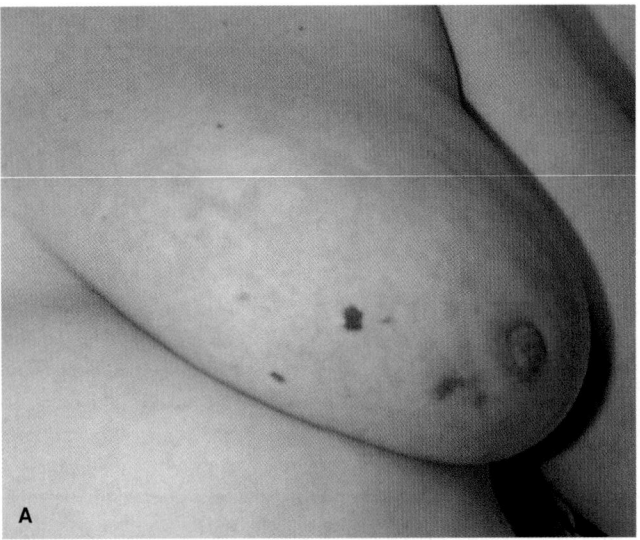
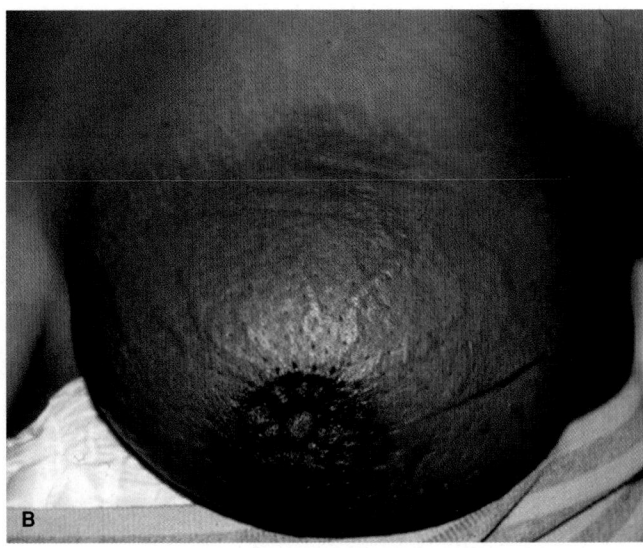

FIGURE 12-15 Photographs of inflammatory breast cancer. **A.** Subtle erythematous blush and edema in inflammatory breast cancer. **B.** Classic inflammatory breast cancer. (Used with permission from Dr. Marilyn Leitch.)

breast and creates diffuse induration. As a result, the breast may enlarge to two to three times its original volume within weeks (Taylor, 1938).

Although mastitis or even congestive heart failure can produce a similar clinical appearance, inflammatory breast cancer must be definitively excluded. This always includes diagnostic mammography and punch biopsy of the skin. However, it also may require multiple biopsies and additional imaging such as MR imaging. Treatment begins with induction chemotherapy, followed by modified radical mastectomy (total mastectomy and axillary dissection), and then postoperative chest wall irradiation with or without additional chemotherapy (Cariati, 2005). The 5-year survival rate is 30 to 55 percent, which is significantly worse than for neglected advanced primary breast cancer (Brenner, 2002; Harris, 2003).

REFERENCES

Abner AL, Connolly JL, Recht A, et al: The relation between the presence and extent of lobular carcinoma in situ and the risk of local recurrence for patients with infiltrating carcinoma of the breast treated with conservative surgery and radiation therapy. Cancer 88:1072, 2000

A'Hern RP, Jamal-Hanjani M, Szasz AM, et al: Taxane benefit in breast cancer—a role for grade and chromosomal stability. Nat Rev Clin Oncol 10(6):357, 2013

American College of Obstetricians and Gynecologists: Breast cancer screening. Practice Bulletin No. 122, August 2011, Reaffirmed 2014

Anderson GL, Limacher M, Assaf AR, et al: Effects of conjugated equine estrogen in postmenopausal women with hysterectomy: the Women's Health Initiative randomized controlled trial. JAMA 291:1701, 2004

Anderson TJ, Ferguson DP, Raab G: Cell turnover within "resting" human breast: influence of parity, contraceptive pill, age and laterality. Br J Cancer 46(3):276, 1982

Andrade VP, Ostrovnaya I, Seshan VE, et al: Clonal relatedness between lobular carcinoma in situ and synchronous malignant lesions. Breast Cancer Res 14:R103, 2012

Andre F, O'Regan R, Ozguroglu M, et al: Everolimus for women with trastuzumab-resistant, HER2-positive, advanced breast cancer (BOLERO-3): a randomised, double-blind, placebo-controlled phase 3 trial. Lancet Oncol 15:580, 2014

Antoniou AC, Cunningham AP, Peto J, et al: The BOADICEA model of genetic susceptibility to breast and ovarian cancers: updates and extensions. Br J Cancer 98:1457, 2008

Ashikari R, Park K, Huvos AG, et al: Paget's disease of the breast. Cancer 26:680, 1970

Aubele M, Werner M, Hofler H: Genetic alterations in presumptive precursor lesions of breast carcinomas. Anal Cell Pathol 24:69, 2002

Baker SG, Lichtenstein P, Kaprio J, et al: Genetic susceptibility to prostate, breast, and colorectal cancer among Nordic twins. Biometrics 61(1):55, 2005

Barrio AV, Clark BD, Goldberg JI, et al: Clinicopathologic features and long-term outcomes of 293 phyllodes tumors of the breast. Ann Surg Oncol 14:2961, 2007

Barth RJ: Histologic features predict local recurrence after breast conserving therapy of phyllodes tumors. Breast Cancer Res Treat 57:291, 1999

Barth RJ Jr, Wells WA, Mitchell SE, et al: A prospective, multi-institutional study of adjuvant radiotherapy after resection of malignant phyllodes tumors. Ann Surg Oncol 16:2288, 2009

Benson EA: Management of breast abscesses. World J Surg 13:753, 1989

Beral V, Reeves G, Bull D, et al: Breast cancer risk in relation to the interval between menopause and starting hormone therapy. J Natl Cancer Inst 103:296, 2011

Berg WA, Campassi CI, Loffe OB: Cystic Lesions of the breast: sonographic-pathologic correlation. Radiology 227:183, 2003

Berrington de Gonzalez A, Berg CD, Visvanathan K, et al: Estimated risk of radiation-induced breast cancer from mammographic screening for young BRCA mutation carriers. J Natl Cancer Inst 101:205, 2009

Berry DA, Parmigiani G, Sanchez S, et al: Probability of carrying a mutation of breast-ovarian cancer gene BRCA1 based on family history. J Natl Cancer Inst 89:227, 1997

Bijker N, Rutgers EJ, Duchateau L, et al: Breast-conserving therapy for Paget disease of the nipple: a prospective European Organization for Research and Treatment of Cancer study of 61 patients. Cancer 91:472, 2001

Bleyer A, Welch HG: Effect of three decades of screening mammography on breast-cancer incidence. N Engl J Med 367:1998, 2012

Bodian CA, Perzin KH, Lattes R: Lobular neoplasia. Long-term risk of breast cancer and relation to other factors. Cancer 78:1024, 1996

Boerner S, Fornage BD, Singletary E, et al: Ultrasound-guided fine-needle aspiration (FNA) of nonpalpable breast lesions. Cancer 87(1):19, 1999

Branch-Elliman W, Golen TH, Gold HS, et al: Risk factors for Staphylococcus aureus postpartum breast abscess. Clin Infect Dis 54(1):71, 2012

Braun S, Vogl FD, Naume B, et al: A pooled analysis of bone marrow micrometastasis in breast cancer. N Engl J Med 353:793, 2005

Brenner B, Siris N, Rakowsky E, et al: Prediction of outcome in locally advanced breast cancer by post-chemotherapy nodal status and baseline serum tumour markers. Br J Cancer 87:1404, 2002

Brohet RM, Velthuizen ME, Hogervorst FB, et al: Breast and ovarian cancer risks in a large series of clinically ascertained families with a high proportion of BRCA1 and BRCA2 Dutch founder mutations. J Med Genet 51(2):98, 2014

Buckley ES, Webster F, Hiller JE, et al: A systematic review of surgical biopsy for LCIS found at core needle biopsy—do we have the answer yet? Eur J Surg Oncol 40:168, 2014

Bulun SE, Simpson ER: Competitive RT-PCR analysis indicates levels of aromatase cytochrome P450 transcripts in adipose tissue of buttocks, thighs, and abdomen of women increase with advancing age. J Clin Endocrinol Metab 78:428, 1994

Cabioglu N, Hunt KK, Singletary S, et al: Surgical decision making and factors determining a diagnosis of breast carcinoma in women presenting with nipple discharge. J Am Coll Surg 196:354, 2003

Cadoo KA, Traina TA, King TA: Advances in molecular and clinical subtyping of breast cancer and their implications for therapy. Surg Oncol Clin North Am 22:823, 2013

Cariati M, Bennett-Britton TM, Pinder SE, et al: "Inflammatory" breast cancer. Surg Oncol 14:133, 2005

Catsburg C, Gunter MJ, Chen C, et al: Insulin, estrogen, inflammatory markers, and risk of benign proliferative breast disease. Cancer Res 74:3248, 2014

Cauley JA, Lucas FL, Kuller LH, et al: Bone mineral density and risk of breast cancer in older women: the study of osteoporotic fractures. Study of Osteoporotic Fractures Research Group. JAMA 276:1404, 1996

Chaney AW, Pollack A, Mcneese MD, et al: Primary treatment of cystosarcoma phyllodes of the breast. Cancer 89:1502, 2000

Chang S, Parker SL, Pham T, et al: Inflammatory breast carcinoma incidence and survival. The surveillance, epidemiology, and end results program of the National Cancer Institute, 1975–1992. Cancer 82:2366, 1998

Claus EB, Risch N, Thompson WD: Autosomal dominant inheritance of early-onset breast cancer. Implications for risk prediction. Cancer 73(3):643, 1994

Coleman R, de Boer R, Eidtmann H, et al: Zoledronic acid (zoledronate) for postmenopausal women with early breast cancer receiving adjuvant letrozole (ZO-FAST study): final 60-month results. Ann Oncol 24:398, 2013

Coopey SB, Mazzola E, Buckley JM, et al: The role of chemoprevention in modifying the risk of breast cancer in women with atypical breast lesions. Breast Cancer Res Treat 136:627, 2012

Costantino JP, Gail MH, Pee D, et al: Validation studies for models projecting the risk of invasive and total breast cancer incidence. J Natl Cancer Inst 91:1541, 1999

Cox CE, Reintgen DS, Nicosia SV, et al: Analysis of residual cancer after diagnostic breast biopsy: an argument for fine-needle aspiration cytology. Ann Surg Oncol 2:201, 1995

Cuzick J, Sestak I, Forbes JF, et al: Anastrozole for prevention of breast cancer in high-risk postmenopausal women (IBIS-II): an international, double-blind, randomised placebo-controlled trial. Lancet 383:1041, 2014

Cvelbar M, Ursic-Vrscaj M, Rakar S: Risk factors and prognostic factors in patients with double primary cancer: epithelial ovarian cancer and breast cancer. Eur J Gynaecol Oncol 26:59, 2005

Darby S, McGale P, Correa C, et al: Effect of radiotherapy after breast-conserving surgery on 10-year recurrence and 15-year breast cancer death: meta-analysis of individual patient data for 10,801 women in 17 randomised trials. Lancet 378:1707, 2011

Davies HH, Simons M, Davis JB: Cystic disease of the breast. Relationship to carcinoma. Cancer 17:757, 1964

Dawood S: Biology and management of inflammatory breast cancer. Expert Rev Anticancer Ther 10:209, 2010

De Bruin ML, Sparidans J, van't Veer MB, et al: Breast cancer risk in female survivors of Hodgkin's lymphoma: lower risk after smaller radiation volumes. J Clin Oncol 27:4239, 2009

Degnim AC, Visscher DW, Berman HK, et al: Stratification of breast cancer risk in women with atypia: a Mayo cohort study. J Clin Oncol 25:2671, 2007

DeLair DF, Corben AD, Catalano JP, et al: Non-mammary metastases to the breast and axilla: a study of 85 cases. Mod Pathol 26:343, 2013

den Tonkelaar I, de Waard F: Regularity and length of menstrual cycles in women aged 41–46 in relation to breast cancer risk: results from the DOM-project. Breast Cancer Res Treat 38(3):253, 1996

Dent DM, Macking EA, Wilkie W: Benign breast disease clinical classification and disease distribution. Br J Clin Pract 42 (Suppl 56):69, 1988

Dhillon S: Everolimus in combination with exemestane: a review of its use in the treatment of patients with postmenopausal hormone receptor-positive, HER2-negative advanced breast cancer. Drugs 73:475, 2013

Domchek SM, Friebel TM, Singer CF, et al: Association of risk-reducing surgery in BRCA1 or BRCA2 mutation carriers with cancer risk and mortality. JAMA 304:967, 2010

D'Orsi CJ, Sickles EA, Mendelson EB, et al (eds): ACR BI-RADS Atlas, Breast Imaging Reporting and Data System. Reston, American College of Radiology, 2013

Dowsett M, Cuzick J, Ingle J, et al: Meta-analysis of breast cancer outcomes in adjuvant trials of aromatase inhibitors versus tamoxifen. J Clin Oncol 28:509, 2010

Dupont WD, Parl FF, Hartman WH, et al: Breast cancer risk associated with proliferative breast disease and atypical hyperplasia. Cancer 71:1258, 1993

Early Breast Cancer Trialists' Collaborative Group, McGale P, Taylor C, et al: Effect of radiotherapy after mastectomy and axillary surgery on 10-year recurrence and 20-year breast cancer mortality: meta-analysis of individual patient data for 8135 women in 22 randomised trials. Lancet 383(9935):2127, 2014

Easton DF, Pooley KA, Dunning AM, et al: Genome-wide association study identifies novel breast cancer susceptibility loci. Nature 447:1087, 2007

Euhus DM: Genetic testing today. Ann Surg Oncol 21(10):3209, 2015

Euhus DM, Leitch AM, Huth JF, et al: Limitations of the Gail model in the specialized breast cancer risk assessment clinic. Breast J 8:23, 2002

Euhus DM, Robinson L: Genetic predisposition syndromes and their management. Surg Clin North Am 93(2):341, 2013

Euhus DM, Uyehara C: Influence of parenteral progesterones on the prevalence and severity of mastalgia in premenopausal women. A multi-institutional cross-sectional study. J Am Coll Surg 184:596, 1997

Evans DG, Ingham SL, Baildam A, et al: Contralateral mastectomy improves survival in women with BRCA1/2-associated breast cancer. Breast Cancer Res Treat 140:135, 2013

Fatouros M, Roukos DH, Arampatzis I, et al: Factors increasing local recurrence in breast-conserving surgery. Expert Rev Anticancer Ther 5:737, 2005

Feng SS, Sechopoulos I: Clinical digital breast tomosynthesis system: dosimetric characterization. Radiology 263:35, 2012

Finch AP, Lubinski J, Moller P, et al: Impact of oophorectomy on cancer incidence and mortality in women with a BRCA1 or BRCA2 mutation. J Clin Oncol 32:1547, 2014

Fisher B, Anderson S, Bryant J, et al: Twenty-year follow-up of a randomized trial comparing total mastectomy, lumpectomy, and lumpectomy plus irradiation for the treatment of invasive breast cancer. N Engl J Med 347:1233, 2002

Fisher B, Costantino J, Redmond C, et al: Lumpectomy compared with lumpectomy and radiation therapy for the treatment of intraductal breast cancer. New Engl J Med 328:1581, 1993

Fisher B, Dignam J, Wolmark N, et al: Tamoxifen in treatment of intraductal breast cancer: National Surgical Adjuvant Breast and Bowel Project B-24 randomised controlled trial. Lancet 353(9169):1993, 1999

Fisher B, Jeong JH, Anderson S, et al: Treatment of axillary lymph node-negative, estrogen receptor-negative breast cancer: updated findings from National Surgical Adjuvant Breast and Bowel Project clinical trials. J Natl Cancer Inst 96:1823, 2004a

Fisher ER, Fisher B, Sass R, et al: Pathologic findings from the National Surgical Adjuvant Breast Project (Protocol No. 4): XI. Bilateral Breast Cancer. Cancer 54:3002, 1984

Fisher ER, Land SR, Fisher B, et al: Pathologic findings from the National Surgical Adjuvant Breast and Bowel Project: twelve-year observations concerning lobular carcinoma in situ. Cancer 100:238, 2004b

Ford D, Easton DF, Stratton M, et al: Genetic heterogeneity and penetrance analysis of the BRCA1 and BRCA2 genes in breast cancer families. Am J Hum Genet 62:676, 1998

Foulkes WD, Metcalfe K, Sun P, et al: Estrogen receptor status in BRCA1- and BRCA2-related breast cancer: the influence of age, grade, and histological type. Clin Cancer Res 10:2029, 2004

Frampton GM, Fichtenholtz A, Otto GA, et al: Development and validation of a clinical cancer genomic profiling test based on massively parallel DNA sequencing. Nat Biotechnol 31:1023, 2013

Franyz VK, Pickern JW, Melcher GW, et al: Incidence of chronic cystic disease in so-called normal breast: a study based on 225 post-mortem examinations. Cancer 4:762, 1951

Freedman AN, Yu B, Gail MH, et al: Benefit/risk assessment for breast cancer chemoprevention with raloxifene or tamoxifen for women age 50 years or older. J Clin Oncol 29:2327, 2011

Freisinger F, Domchek SM: Clinical implications of low-penetrance breast cancer susceptibility alleles. Current oncology reports 11:8, 2009

Fu R, Harris EL, Helfand M, et al: Estimating risk of breast cancer in carriers of BRCA1 and BRCA2 mutations: a meta-analytic approach. Stat Med 26:1775, 2007

Gail MH, Brinton LA, Byar DP, et al: Projecting individualized probabilities of developing breast cancer for white females who are being examined annually. J Natl Cancer Inst 81:1879, 1989

Galimberti V, Cole BF: Axillary versus sentinel-lymph-node dissection for micrometastatic breast cancer—authors' reply. Lancet Oncol 14:e251, 2013

Gao X, Fisher SG, Emami B: Risk of second primary cancer in the contralateral breast in women treated for early-stage breast cancer: a population-based study. Int J Radiat Oncol Biol Phys 56:1038, 2003

Gareth ED, Nisha K, Yit L, et al: MRI breast screening in high-risk women: cancer detection and survival analysis. Breast Cancer Res Treat 145:663, 2014

Gateley CA, Mansel RE: Management of cyclic breast pain. Br J Hosp Med 43:330, 1990

Geisler J, Lonning PE: Aromatase inhibitors as adjuvant treatment of breast cancer. Crit Rev Oncol Hematol 57:53, 2006

Giuliano AE, Hawes D, Ballman KV, et al: Association of occult metastases in sentinel lymph nodes and bone marrow with survival among women with early-stage invasive breast cancer. JAMA 306:385, 2011a

Giuliano AE, Hunt KK, Ballman KV, et al: Axillary dissection vs no axillary dissection in women with invasive breast cancer and sentinel node metastasis: a randomized clinical trial. JAMA 305:569, 2011b

Giuliano AE, McCall L, Beitsch P, et al: Locoregional recurrence after sentinel lymph node dissection with or without axillary dissection in patients with sentinel lymph node metastases: the American College of Surgeons Oncology Group Z0011 randomized trial. Ann Surg 252:426, 2010

Going JJ, Moffat DF: Escaping from Flatland: clinical and biological aspects of human mammary duct anatomy in three dimensions. J Pathology 203(1):538, 2004

Goss PE, Ingle JN, Ales-Martinez JE, et al: Exemestane for breast-cancer prevention in postmenopausal women. N Engl J Med 364:2381, 2011

Grant RN, Tabah EJ, Adair FE: The surgical significance of the subareolar lymph plexus in cancer of the breast. Surgery 33(1):71, 1953

Greenberg JS, Javitt MC, Katzen J, et al: Clinical Performance metrics of 3D Digital breast tomosynthesis compared with 2D digital mammography for breast cancer screening in community practice. AJR 203(3):687, 2014

Grimm SL, Seagroves TN, Kabotyanski EB, et al: Disruption of steroid and prolactin receptor pattern in the mammary gland correlates with a block in lobuloalveolar development. Mol Endocrinol 16:2675, 2002

Gunter MJ, Hoover DR, Yu H, et al: Insulin, insulin-like growth factor-I, and risk of breast cancer in postmenopausal women. J Natl Cancer Inst 101:48, 2009

Gupta RK, Gaskell D, Dowle CS, et al: The role of nipple discharge cytology in the diagnosis of breast disease: a study of 1948 nipple discharge smears from 1530 patients. Cytopathology 15:326, 2004

Haagensen CD: Gross cystic disease. In Diseases of the Breast. Philadelphia, WB Saunders, 1986, p 250

Haas BM, Kalra V, Geisel J, et al: Comparison of tomosynthesis plus digital mammography and digital mammography alone for breast cancer screening. Radiology 269:694, 2013

Hadji P, Aapro MS, Body JJ, et al: Management of aromatase inhibitor-associated bone loss in postmenopausal women with breast cancer: practical guidance for prevention and treatment. Ann Oncol 22:2546, 2011

Haffty BG, Harrold E, Khan AJ, et al: Outcome of conservatively managed early-onset breast cancer by BRCA1/2 status. Lancet 359:1471, 2002

Halstead W: The results of operations for cure of cancer of the breast performed at Johns Hopkins Hospital. Johns Hopkins Hosp Bull 4:497, 1894

Hankinson SE: Endogenous hormones and risk of breast cancer in postmenopausal women. Breast Dis 24:3, 2005

Harris EE, Schultz D, Bertsch H, et al: Ten-year outcome after combined modality therapy for inflammatory breast cancer. Int J Radiat Oncol Biol Phys 55:1200, 2003

Harris L, Fritsche H, Mennel R, et al: American Society of Clinical Oncology 2007 update of recommendations for the use of tumor markers in breast cancer. J Clin Oncol 25:5287, 2007

Hartmann LC, Sellers TA, Frost MH, et al: Benign breast disease and the risk of breast cancer. N Engl J Med 353:229, 2005

Hartmann LC, Sellers TA, Schaid DJ, et al: Efficacy of bilateral prophylactic mastectomy in BRCA1 and BRCA2 gene mutation carriers. J Natl Cancer Inst 93:1633, 2001

Heemskerk-Gerritsen BA, Brekelmans CT, Menke-Pluymers MB, et al: Prophylactic mastectomy in BRCA1/2 mutation carriers and women at risk of hereditary breast cancer: long-term experiences at the Rotterdam Family Cancer Clinic. Ann Surg Oncol 14:3335, 2007

Hendrick RE, Smith RA, Rutledge JH 3rd, et al: Benefit of screening mammography in women aged 40–49: a new meta-analysis of randomized controlled trials. J Natl Cancer Inst Monogr 22:87, 1997

Hermansen C, Skovgaard Poulsen H, Jensen J, et al: Diagnostic reliability of combined physical examination, mammography, and fine-needle puncture ("triple-test") in breast tumors. A prospective study. Cancer 60:1866, 1987

Houssami N, Turner R, Macaskill P, et al: An individual person data meta-analysis of preoperative magnetic resonance imaging and breast cancer recurrence. J Clin Oncol 32:392, 2014

Houssami N, Turner R, Morrow M: Preoperative magnetic resonance imaging in breast cancer: meta-analysis of surgical outcomes. Ann Surg 257:249, 2013

Howlader N, Noone AM, Krapcho M, et al: SEER Cancer Statistics Review, 1975–2010, National Cancer Institute. 2013. Available at: http://seer.cancer.gov/archive/csr/1975_2010/. Accessed August 7, 2014

Hughes KS, Schnaper LA, Bellon JR, et al: Lumpectomy plus tamoxifen with or without irradiation in women age 70 years or older with early breast cancer: long-term follow-up of CALGB 9343. J Clin Oncol 31:2382, 2013

Hulley S, Furberg C, Barrett-Connor E, et al: Noncardiovascular disease outcomes during 6.8 years of hormone therapy: Heart and Estrogen/progestin Replacement Study follow-up (HERS II). JAMA 288:58, 2002

Hultborn KA, Larsen LG, Raghnult I: The lymph drainage from the breast to the axillary and parasternal lymph nodes, studied with the aid of colloidal Au198. Acta Radiol 45:52, 1955

Ikeda DM, Helvie MA, Frank TS, et al: Paget's disease of the nipple: radiologic-pathologic correlation. Radiology 189:89, 1993

Ismail PM, Amato P, Soyal SM, et al: Progesterone involvement in breast development and tumorigenesis—as revealed by progesterone receptor "knockout" and "knockin" mouse models. Steroids 68:779, 2003

Jaiyesimi IA, Buzdar AU, Decker DA, et al: Use of tamoxifen for breast cancer: twenty-eight years later. J Clin Oncol 13:513, 1995

Jatoi I: Screening clinical breast exam. Surg Clin North Am 83:789, 2003

Johnston SR, Yeo B: The optimal duration of adjuvant endocrine therapy for early stage breast cancer—with what drugs and for how long? Curr Oncol Rep 16:358, 2014

Kalinyak JE, Berg WA, Schilling K, et al: Breast cancer detection using high-resolution breast PET compared to whole-body PET or PET/CT. Eur J Nucl Med Mol Imaging 41:260, 2014

Karim RZ, O'Toole SA, Scolyer RA, et al: Recent insights into the molecular pathogenesis of mammary phyllodes tumours. J Clin Pathol 66:496, 2013

Kasales CJ, Han B, Smith JS Jr, et al: Nonpuerperal mastitis and subareolar abscess of the breast. AJR 202(2):W133, 2014

Kauff ND, Domchek SM, Friebel TM, et al: Risk-reducing salpingo-oophorectomy for the prevention of BRCA1- and BRCA2-associated breast and gynecologic cancer: a multicenter, prospective study. J Clin Oncol 26:1331, 2008

Kerlikowske K: Efficacy of screening mammography among women aged 40 to 49 years and 50 to 69 years: comparison of relative and absolute benefit. J Natl Cancer Inst Monogr 22:79, 1997

Khan SA, Rogers MA, Khurana KK, et al: Estrogen receptor expression in benign breast epithelium and breast cancer risk. J Natl Cancer Inst 89:37, 1997

Khatcheressian JL, Hurley P, Bantug E, et al: Breast cancer follow-up and management after primary treatment: American Society of Clinical Oncology clinical practice guideline update. J Clin Oncol 31(7):961, 2013

Kim S, Kim JY, Kim do H, et al: Analysis of phyllodes tumor recurrence according to the histologic grade. Breast Cancer Res Treat 141:353, 2013

King MC, Marks JH, Mandell JB: Breast and ovarian cancer risks due to inherited mutations in BRCA1 and BRCA2. Science 302:643, 2003

Kopans DB: Digital breast tomosynthesis: a better mammogram. Radiology 267:968, 2013

Kotsopoulos J, Chen WY, Gates MA, et al: Risk factors for ductal and lobular breast cancer: results from the Nurses' Health Study. Breast Cancer Res 12:R106, 2010

Kudachadkar R, O'Regan RM: Aromatase inhibitors as adjuvant therapy for postmenopausal patients with early stage breast cancer. CA Cancer J Clin 55:145, 2005

Kuehn T, Klauss W, Darsow M, et al: Long-term morbidity following axillary dissection in breast cancer patients—clinical assessment, significance for life quality and the impact of demographic, oncologic and therapeutic factors. Breast Cancer Res Treat 64:275, 2000

Kumar S, Mansel RE, Scanlon F: Altered responses of prolactin, luteinizing hormone and follicle stimulating hormone secretion to thyrotrophin releasing hormone/gonadotrophin releasing hormone stimulation in cyclical mastalgia. Br J Surg 71:870, 1989

Kvale G, Heuch I: Menstrual factors and breast cancer risk. Cancer 62:1625, 1988

Laibl VR, Sheffield JS, Roberts S, et al: Clinical presentation of community-acquired methicillin-resistant Staphylococcus aureus in pregnancy. Obstet Gynecol 106:461, 2005

Lakhani SR, Van De Vijver MJ, Jacquemier J, et al: The pathology of familial breast cancer: predictive value of immunohistochemical markers estrogen receptor, progesterone receptor, HER-2, and p53 in patients with mutations in BRCA1 and BRCA2. J Clin Oncol 20:2310, 2002

Lalloo F, Varley J, Moran A, et al: BRCA1, BRCA2 and TP53 mutations in very early-onset breast cancer with associated risks to relatives. Eur J Cancer 42:1143, 2006

Lau S, Küchenmeister I, Stachs A, et al: Pathological nipple discharge: surgery is imperative in postmenopausal women. Ann Surg Oncol 12:246, 2005

Layde PM, Webster LA, Baughman LA, et al: The independent associations of parity, age at first full term pregnancy, and duration of breastfeeding with the risk of breast cancer. Cancer and Steroid Hormone Study Group. J Clin Epidemiol 42:963, 1989

Lee AJ, Cunningham AP, Kuchenbaecker KB, et al: BOADICEA breast cancer risk prediction model: updates to cancer incidences, tumour pathology and web interface. Br J Cancer 110:535, 2014

Lee CH, Dershaw DD, Kopans D, et al: Breast cancer screening with imaging: recommendations from the Society of Breast Imaging and the ACR on the use of mammography, breast MRI, breast ultrasound, and other technologies for the detection of clinically occult breast cancer. J Am Coll Radiol 7:18, 2010

Lee SJ, Boscardin WJ, Stijacic-Cenzer I, et al: Time lag to benefit after screening for breast and colorectal cancer: meta-analysis of survival data from the United States, Sweden, United Kingdom, and Denmark. BMJ 346:e8441, 2013

Lichtenstein P, Holm NV, Verkasalo PK, et al: Environmental and heritable factors in the causation of cancer—analyses of cohorts of twins from Sweden, Denmark, and Finland. N Engl J Med 343:78, 2000

Locatelli I, Lichtenstein P, Yashin AI: The heritability of breast cancer: a Bayesian correlated frailty model applied to Swedish twins data. Twin Res 7(2):182, 2004

Locker AP, Galea MH, Ellis IO, et al: Microdochectomy for single-duct discharge from the nipple. Br J Surg 75:700, 1988

Lyman GH, Temin S, Edge SB, et al: Sentinel lymph node biopsy for patients with early-stage breast cancer: American Society of Clinical Oncology clinical practice guideline update. J Clin Oncol 32:1365, 2014

Maddox PR, Mansel RE: Management of breast pain and nodularity. World J Surg 13:699, 1989

Malone KE, Daling JR, Neal C, et al: Frequency of BRCA1/BRCA2 mutations in a population-based sample of young breast carcinoma cases. Cancer 88:1393, 2000

Mansel RE, Dogliotti L: European multicenter trial of bromocriptine in cyclical mastalgia. Lancet 335:190, 1990

Masood S: Prognostic/predictive factors in breast cancer. Clin Lab Med 25:809, 2005

Mavaddat N, Peock S, Frost D, et al: Cancer risks for BRCA1 and BRCA2 mutation carriers: results from prospective analysis of EMBRACE. J Natl Cancer Inst 105:812, 2013

Mavaddat N, Pharoah PD, Blows F, et al: Familial relative risks for breast cancer by pathological subtype: a population-based cohort study. Breast Cancer Res 12:R10, 2010

McKian KP, Reynolds CA, Visscher DW, et al: Novel breast tissue feature strongly associated with risk of breast cancer. J Clin Oncol 27:5893, 2009

Meijers-Heijboer H, van Geel B, van Putten WL, et al: Breast cancer after prophylactic bilateral mastectomy in women with a BRCA1 or BRCA2 mutation. N Engl J Med 345:159, 2001

Menes TS, Kerlikowske K, Jaffer S, et al: Rates of atypical ductal hyperplasia have declined with less use of postmenopausal hormone treatment: findings from the Breast Cancer Surveillance Consortium. Cancer Epidemiol Biomarkers Prev 18(11):2822, 2009

Merry GM, Mendelson EB: Update on screening breast ultrasonography. Radiol Clin North Am 52:527, 2014

Metcalfe K, Gershman S, Ghadirian P, et al: Contralateral mastectomy and survival after breast cancer in carriers of BRCA1 and BRCA2 mutations: retrospective analysis. BMJ 348:g226, 2014

Mohammed S, Statz A, Lacross JS, et al: Granulomatous mastitis: a 10 year experience from a large inner city county hospital. J Surg Res 184(1):299, 2013

Moller P, Stormorken A, Jonsrud C, et al: Survival of patients with BRCA1-associated breast cancer diagnosed in an MRI-based surveillance program. Breast Cancer Res Treat 139:155, 2013

Morrell RM, Halyard MY, Schild SE, et al: Breast cancer-related lymphedema. Mayo Clin Proc 80:1480, 2005

Morrow M, Waters J, Morris E: MRI for breast cancer screening, diagnosis, and treatment. Lancet 378:1804, 2011

National Comprehensive Cancer Network: Breast Cancer, 2014. Available at: http://www.nccn.org/professionals/physician_gls/pdf/breast.pdf. Accessed August 21, 2014

Oberman HA: Cystosarcoma phyllodes: a clinicopathologic study of hypercellular periductal neoplasms of the breast. Cancer 28:697, 1965

Oeffinger KC, Fontham, ET, Etzioni R, et al: Breast cancer screening for women at average risk 2015 guideline update from the American Cancer Society. JAMA 314:1599, 2015

Osin PP, Anbazhagan R, Bartkova J, et al: Breast development gives insights into breast disease. Histopathology 33:275, 1998

Ottesen GL, Graversen HP, Blichert-Toft M, et al: Lobular carcinoma in situ of the female breast. Short-term results of a prospective nationwide study. The Danish Breast Cancer Cooperative Group. Am J Surg Pathol 17:14, 1993

Overgaard M, Jensen MB, Overgaard J, et al: Postoperative radiotherapy in high-risk postmenopausal breast-cancer patients given adjuvant tamoxifen:

Danish Breast Cancer Cooperative Group DBCG 82c randomised trial. Lancet 353:1641, 1999

Panchal S, Bordeleau L, Poll A, et al: Does family history predict the age at onset of new breast cancers in BRCA1 and BRCA2 mutation-positive families? Clin Genet 77:273, 2010

Pandey TS, Mackinnon JC, Bressler L, et al: Idiopathic granulomatous mastitis—a prospective study of 49 women and treatment outcomes with steroid therapy. Breast J 20:258, 2014

Papanicolaou GN, Holmquist DG, Bader GM, et al: Exfoliative cytology in the human mammary gland and its value in the diagnosis of breast cancer and other diseases of the breast. Cancer 11:377, 1958

Parkin DM: Global cancer statistics in the year 2000. Lancet Oncol 2:533, 2001

Parks AG: The micro-anatomy of the breast. Ann R Coll Surg Engl 25:235, 1959

Peto R, Davies C, Godwin J, et al: Comparisons between different polychemotherapy regimens for early breast cancer: meta-analyses of long-term outcome among 100,000 women in 123 randomised trials. Lancet 379:432, 2012

Petrakis NL, Miike R, King EB, et al: Association of breast fluid coloration with age, ethnicity and cigarette smoking. Br Cancer Res Treat 11:255, 1988

Phipps AI, Li CI, Kerlikowske K, et al: Risk factors for ductal, lobular, and mixed ductal-lobular breast cancer in a screening population. Cancer Epidemiol Biomarkers Prev 19:1643, 2010

Pierce LJ, Phillips KA, Griffith KA, et al: Local therapy in BRCA1 and BRCA2 mutation carriers with operable breast cancer: comparison of breast conservation and mastectomy. Breast Cancer Res Treat 121:389, 2010

Pijpe A, Andrieu N, Easton DF, et al: Exposure to diagnostic radiation and risk of breast cancer among carriers of BRCA1/2 mutations: retrospective cohort study (GENE-RAD-RISK). BMJ 345:2012

Pike MC, Krailo MD, Henderson BE, et al: Hormonal risk factors, breast tissue age and the age-incidence of breast cancer. Nature 303:767, 1983

Pilewskie M, Olcese C, Eaton A, et al: Perioperative breast MRI is not associated with lower locoregional recurrence rates in DCIS patients treated with or without radiation. Ann Surg Oncol 21:1552, 2014

Ragaz J, Olivotto IA, Spinelli JJ, et al: Locoregional radiation therapy in patients with high-risk breast cancer receiving adjuvant chemotherapy: 20-year results of the British Columbia randomized trial. J Natl Cancer Inst 97:116, 2005

Rao R, Euhus D, Mayo HG, et al: Axillary node interventions in breast cancer: a systematic review. JAMA 310:1385, 2013

Rechtman LR, Lenihan MJ, Lieberman JH, et al: Breast-specific gamma imaging for the detection of breast cancer in dense versus nondense breasts. AJR 202:293, 2014

Reinfuss M, Mitus J, Duda K, et al: The treatment and prognosis of patients with phyllodes tumor of the breast: an analysis of 170 cases. Cancer 77:910, 1996

Ringberg A, Anagnostaki L, Anderson H, et al: Cell biological factors in ductal carcinoma in situ (DCIS) of the breast-relationship to ipsilateral local recurrence and histopathological characteristics. Eur J Cancer 37:1514, 2001

Risch N: The genetic epidemiology of cancer: interpreting family and twin studies and their implications for molecular genetic approaches. Cancer Epidemiol Biomarkers Prev 10:733, 2001

Rockhill B, Spiegelman D, Byrne C, et al: Validation of the Gail model of breast cancer risk prediction and implications for chemoprevention. J Natl Cancer Inst 93:358, 2001

Rossouw JE, Anderson GL, Prentice RL, et al: Risks and benefits of estrogen plus progestin in healthy postmenopausal women: principal results from the Women's Health Initiative randomized controlled trial. JAMA 288(3):321, 2002

Rouzier R, Pronzato P, Chereau E, et al: Multigene assays and molecular markers in breast cancer: systematic review of health economic analyses. Breast Cancer Res Treat 139:621, 2013

Russo IH, Russo J: Mammary gland neoplasia in long-term rodent studies. Environ Health Perspect 104:938, 1996

Sadek BT, Shenouda MN, Abi Raad RF, et al: Risk of local failure in breast cancer patients with lobular carcinoma in situ at the final surgical margins: is re-excision necessary? Int J Radiat Oncol Biol Phys 87:726, 2013

Salvadori B, Bartoli C, Zurrida S, et al: Risk of invasive cancer in women with lobular carcinoma in situ of the breast. Eur J Cancer 27:35, 1991

Santen RJ, Mansel R: Benign breast disorders. N Engl J Med 353:275, 2005

Saslow D, Boetes C, Burke W, et al: American Cancer Society guidelines for breast screening with MRI as an adjunct to mammography. CA Cancer J Clin 57:75, 2010

Sasson AR, Fowble B, Hanlon AL, et al: Lobular carcinoma in situ increases the risk of local recurrence in selected patients with stages I and II breast carcinoma treated with conservative surgery and radiation. Cancer 91:1862, 2001

Schelfhout VR, Coene ED, Delaey B, et al: Pathogenesis of Paget's disease: epidermal heregulin-alpha, motility factor, and the HER receptor family. J Natl Cancer Inst 92(8):622, 2000

Seeley RR, Stephens TD, Tate P: Reproductive system. In Anatomy and Physiology, 7th ed. New York, McGraw-Hill, 2006, p 1058

Seynaevea C, Verhooga LC, van de Boscha LM, et al: Ipsilateral breast tumour recurrence in hereditary breast cancer following breast-conserving therapy. Eur J Cancer 40:1150, 2004

Shannon J, Douglas-Jones AG, Dallimore NS: Conversion to core biopsy in preoperative diagnosis of breast lesions: is it justified by results? J Clin Pathol 54:762, 2001

Sickles EA, Klein DL, Goodson WH, et al: Mammography after needle aspiration of palpable breast masses. Am J Surg 145:395, 1983

Siegel R, Ma J, Zou Z, et al: Cancer statistics, 2014. CA Cancer J Clin 64:9, 2014

Skaane P, Bandos AI, Gullien R, et al: Comparison of digital mammography alone and digital mammography plus tomosynthesis in a population-based screening program. Radiology 267:47, 2013

Smith BD, Arthur DW, Buchholz TA, et al: Accelerated partial breast irradiation consensus statement from the American Society for Radiation Oncology (ASTRO). Int J Radiat Oncol Biol Phys 74:987, 2009

Sneige N, Wang J, Baker BA, et al: Clinical, histopathologic, and biologic features of pleomorphic lobular (ductal-lobular) carcinoma in situ of the breast: a report of 24 cases. Mod Pathol 15:1044, 2002

Soderqvist G, Isaksson E, von Schoultz B, et al: Proliferation of breast epithelial cells in healthy women during the menstrual cycle. Am J Obstet Gynecol 176:123, 1997

Solin LJ, Kurtz J, Fourquet A, et al: Fifteen-year results of breast-conserving surgery and breast irradiation for the treatment of ductal carcinoma in situ of the breast. J Clin Oncol 14:754, 1996

Sparano JA, Paik S: Development of the 21-gene assay and its application in clinical practice and clinical trials. J Clin Oncol 26:721, 2008

Stafford I, Hernandez J, Laibl V, et al: Community-acquired methicillin-resistant Staphylococcus aureus among patients with puerperal mastitis requiring hospitalization. Obstet Gynecol 112:533, 2008

Stavros AT, Thickman D, Rapp CL, et al: Solid breast nodules: use of sonography to distinguish between benign and malignant lesions. Radiology 196:123, 1995

Stoeckelhuber M, Stumpf P, Hoefter EA, et al: Proteoglycan-collagen associations in the non-lactating human breast connective tissue during the menstrual cycle. Histochem Cell Biol 118(3):221, 2002

Tabbara SO, Frost AR, Stoler MH, et al: Changing trends in breast fine-needle aspiration: results of the Papanicolaou Society of Cytopathology Survey. Diagn Cytopathol 22:126, 2000

Tai YC, Domchek S, Parmigiani G, et al: Breast cancer risk among male BRCA1 and BRCA2 mutation carriers. J Natl Cancer Inst 99:1811, 2007

Taylor G, Meltzer A: Inflammatory carcinoma of the breast. Am J Cancer 33:33, 1938

Thomas DB, Gao DL, Ray RM, et al: Randomized trial of breast self-examination in Shanghai: final results. J Natl Cancer Inst 94:1445, 2002

Thomsen AC, Hansen KB, Moller B: Leukocyte counts and microbiological cultivation in the diagnosis of puerperal mastitis. Am J Obstet Gynecol 146:938, 1983

Tolaney S: New HER2-positive targeting agents in clinical practice. Curr Oncol Rep 16:359, 2014

Trudeau M, Charbonneau F, Gelmon K, et al: Selection of adjuvant chemotherapy for treatment of node-positive breast cancer. Lancet Oncol 6:886, 2005

Turnbull L, Brown S, Harvey I, et al: Comparative effectiveness of MRI in breast cancer (COMICE) trial: a randomised controlled trial. Lancet 375:563, 2010

Tyrer J, Duffy SW, Cuzick J: A breast cancer prediction model incorporating familial and personal risk factors. Stat Med 23(7):1111, 2004

Urban J, Egeli R: Non-lactational nipple discharge. CA Cancer Journal Clin 28:3, 1978

U.S. Preventive Services Task Force: Screening for breast cancer: U.S. Preventive Services Task Force recommendation statement. Ann Intern Med 151(10):716, 2009

Vandenbussche CJ, Khouri N, Sbaity E, et al: Borderline atypical ductal hyperplasia/low-grade ductal carcinoma in situ on breast needle core biopsy should be managed conservatively. Am J Surg Pathol 37:913, 2013

Vihko RK, Apter DL: The epidemiology and endocrinology of the menarche in relation to breast cancer. Cancer Surv 5:561, 1986

Virnig BA, Tuttle TM, Shamliyan T, et al: Ductal carcinoma in situ of the breast: a systematic review of incidence, treatment, and outcomes. J Natl Cancer Inst 102:170, 2010

Vogel VG, Costantino JP, Wickerham DL, et al: Update of the National Surgical Adjuvant Breast and Bowel Project Study of Tamoxifen and Raloxifene (STAR) P-2 Trial: preventing breast cancer. Cancer Prev Res (Phila) 3:696, 2010

von Minckwitz G: Neoadjuvant therapy: what are the lessons so far? Hematol Oncol Clin North Am 27:767, 2013

Wai CJ, Al-Mubarak G, Homer MJ, et al: A modified triple test for palpable breast masses: the value of ultrasound and core needle biopsy. Ann Surg Oncol 20:850, 2013

Watt-Boolsen S, Rasmussen NR, Blichert-Toft M: Primary periareolar abscess in the non-lactating breast: risk of recurrence. Am J Surg 155:571, 1987

Welch HG, Passow HJ: Quantifying the benefits and harms of screening mammography. JAMA Intern Med 174:448, 2014

Welsh ML, Buist DS, Aiello Bowles EJ, et al: Population-based estimates of the relation between breast cancer risk, tumor subtype, and family history. Breast Cancer Res Treat 114:549, 2009

Wilkie C, White L, Dupont E, et al: An update of sentinel lymph node mapping in patients with ductal carcinoma in situ. Am J Surg 190:563, 2005

Wrensch WR, Petrakis NL, Gruenke LD, et al: Factors associated with obtaining nipple aspirate fluid: analysis of 1428 women and literature review. Br Cancer Res Treat 15:39, 1990

Zhou WB, Xue DQ, Liu XA, et al: The influence of family history and histological stratification on breast cancer risk in women with benign breast disease: a meta-analysis. J Cancer Res Clin Oncol 137:1053, 2011

Psychosocial Issues and Female Sexuality

Thirty years ago, psychiatrist George Engel coined the term "biopsychosocial model" to describe a developing paradigm for patient care (Engel, 1977). As shown in Figure 13-1, the model encourages treatments that consider the mind and body of a patient as two intertwining systems influenced by a third system—society. This was perhaps the first time a distinction was drawn between "disease" and "illness." Namely, disease is the pathological process, and illness is the patient's experience of that process. In keeping with this model, psychological factors have two distinct relationships with women's reproductive health. At times, they are a consequence (infertility has been linked with psychological distress). At other times, they may be an insidious cause of a health problem (increased hysterectomy rates are noted in women with a low tolerance for the physical discomfort of menstruation).

Years before Engel's work, Erik Erikson (1963) created a model that describes psychological maturation in stages across the life span. Specifically, adolescents are confronted with identity development; reproductive-aged women with intimacy concerns; peri- and early menopausal women with productivity

issues; and older women with life review. Combining Erikson's developmental model with Engel's psychosocial model provides a dimensional perspective to aid the evaluation, diagnosis, and treatment of any patient.

Not only do women use more health care services in general than men in the United States, but more women approach their physicians with psychiatric complaints, and more women have comorbid illness than men (Andrade, 2003; Kessler, 1994). Because primary care is the setting in which most patients with psychiatric illness are first seen, obstetricians and gynecologists often are the first to evaluate a woman in psychiatric distress. The clinical interview in Table 13-1 provides an example of an assessment that includes all three domains from the biopsychosocial model.

MOOD DISORDERS

Mood, anxiety, and alcohol or substance use disorders are three families of psychiatric disorders commonly seen and often comorbid with reproductive problems. These three groups are defined by specific criteria described by the *Diagnostic and Statistical Manual of Mental Disorders,* Fifth Edition (DSM-5) (American Psychiatric Association, 2013). Each family of

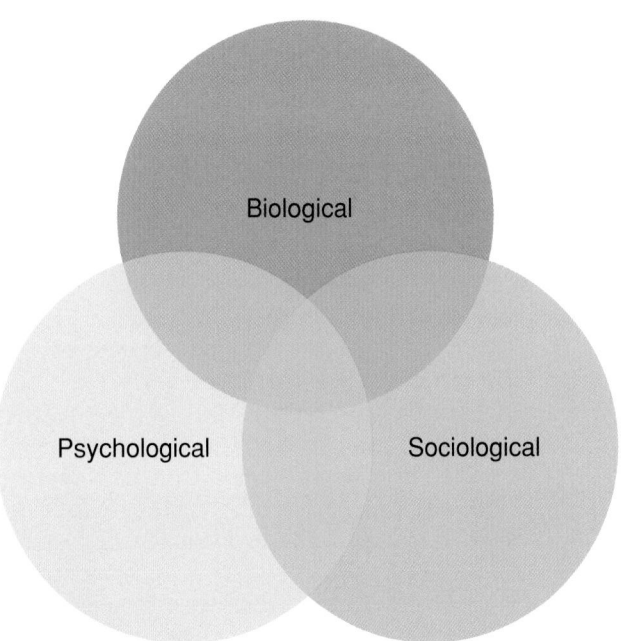

FIGURE 13-1 Biopsychosocial model. (Data from Engel GL: The need for a new medical model: a challenge for biomedicine. Science 1977 Apr 8;196(4286):129–136.)

TABLE 13-1. Psychiatric Assessment of Women

Component	Consideration
Present or past psychiatric illness	Relation to reproductive triggers: pregnancy, menses, menopause, etc.
Medications	All medications and supplements; exogenous hormones
Diet	Abnormal eating patterns; diet pills, laxatives, diuretics
Substance use	Covert use, especially of prescription drugs
Family	Including their premenstrual and postpartum mood disorders
Medical	Autoimmune disease, which can present with psychiatric symptoms
Menstrual	Premenstrual or perimenopausal symptoms
Social	Current or past sexual, physical, or emotional abuse. Note sexual preference and current relationship satisfaction
Economic	Ability to meet ongoing financial needs

Data from Burt VK, Hendrick VC: Clinical Manual of Women's Mental Health. Washington: American Psychiatric Publishing; 2005.

disorders is characterized by predominant features, and each disorder within those families is identified by specific symptoms of that feature.

Of these families, mood disorders are categorized as *depressive disorders* (major depressive disorder, persistent depressive disorder, premenstrual dysphoric disorder, other specified depressive disorder, and unspecified depressive disorder) or as *bipolar and related disorders* (bipolar I, bipolar II, cyclothymic disorder, other specified bipolar disorder, and unspecified bipolar disorder). For bipolar disorders, defining behaviors include racing thoughts, inflated grandiosity, psychomotor agitation, loquaciousness, and high-risk behavior, among others. These are severe enough to impair occupational or social relationships.

For depressive disorders, symptoms include those in Table 13-2. The lifetime prevalence in the general U.S. population approximates 20 percent (Kessler, 2005). As such, depression is a major cause of disability, and females are 1.6 times more likely than men to suffer from a major depressive episode (Substance Abuse and Mental Health Services Administration, 2013). Women also may experience one or more comorbid psychiatric disorders, most commonly an anxiety disorder and/or substance use disorder.

Self-report questionnaires are generally used to identify individuals who require further psychiatric evaluation (screening measures) and may also assess the frequency and intensity of depressive symptoms (severity measures). The Quick Inventory of Depressive Symptomatology-Self Report (QIDS-SR) is one such tool easily implemented for clinical use (Tables 13-3 and 13-4) (Rush, 2003). Further information regarding the instrument is available at www.ids-qids.org. By patient report, this questionnaire assesses symptom severity required by DSM-5 criteria to diagnosis major depressive disorder. Ultimately, diagnosing mood disorders requires assessment by a trained clinician.

ANXIETY DISORDERS

Anxiety disorders have the highest prevalence rates in the United States. Lifetime rates approximate 30 percent, and similar to depression, women are 1.6 times more likely to be diagnosed than men (Kessler, 2005). Criteria established in the DSM-5 provide guidelines to help distinguish anxiety disorders from normally expected worries (Table 13-5).

TABLE 13-2. Diagnostic Criteria for a Major Depressive Episode

A. **≥5 criteria present during the same 2-week period and represent change from previous functioning. At least one of these is:**

Depressed mood most of the day, nearly every day

Markedly diminished interest/pleasure in most activities, most of the day, most days

The balance of 5 from these:

Significant weight loss/gain, change in appetite, or failure to make expected gains

Insomnia or hypersomnia nearly every day

Psychomotor agitation or retardation nearly every day, *observable by others*

Fatigue or loss of energy nearly every day

Feelings of worthlessness or excessive or inappropriate guilt nearly every day

Diminished ability to think or concentrate or indecisiveness

Recurrent thoughts of death, recurrent suicidal ideation, plans, or attempt

B. Symptoms cause significant distress or impairment in functioning

C. Symptoms are not due to a substance or a general medical condition

D. Symptoms not accounted by other psychiatric disorder

E. No prior mania or hypomania

Data from American Psychiatric Association: Diagnostic and Statistical Manual of Mental Disorders, 5th Edition, DSM-5, Washington, American Psychiatric Association, 2013.

TABLE 13-3. The Quick Inventory of Depressive Symptomatology (16-Item) (Self-Report) (QIDS-SR$_{16}$)

CHECK THE ONE RESPONSE TO EACH ITEM THAT BEST DESCRIBES YOU FOR THE PAST SEVEN DAYS.

During the past seven days...

1. Falling Asleep:
- ☐ 0 I never take longer than 30 minutes to fall asleep.
- ☐ 1 I take at least 30 minutes to fall asleep, less than half the time.
- ☐ 2 I take at least 30 minutes to fall asleep, more than half the time.
- ☐ 3 I take more than 60 minutes to fall asleep, more than half the time.

2. Sleep During the Night:
- ☐ 0 I do not wake up at night.
- ☐ 1 I have a restless, light sleep with a few brief awakenings each night.
- ☐ 2 I wake up at least once a night, but I go back to sleep easily.
- ☐ 3 I awaken more than once a night and stay awake for 20 minutes or more, more than half the time.

3. Waking Up Too Early:
- ☐ 0 Most of the time, I awaken no more than 30 minutes before I need to get up.
- ☐ 1 More than half the time, I awaken more than 30 minutes before I need to get up.
- ☐ 2 I almost always awaken at least one hour or so before I need to, but I go back to sleep eventually.
- ☐ 3 I awaken at least one hour before I need to, and can't go back to sleep.

4. Sleeping Too Much:
- ☐ 0 I sleep no longer than 7–8 hours/night, without napping during the day.
- ☐ 1 I sleep no longer than 10 hours in a 24-hour period including naps.
- ☐ 2 I sleep no longer than 12 hours in a 24-hour period including naps.
- ☐ 3 I sleep longer than 12 hours in a 24-hour period including naps.

5. Feeling Sad:
- ☐ 0 I do not feel sad.
- ☐ 1 I feel sad less than half the time.
- ☐ 2 I feel sad more than half the time.
- ☐ 3 I feel sad nearly all of the time.

Please complete either 6 or 7 (not both)

6. Decreased Appetite:
- ☐ 0 There is no change in my usual appetite.
- ☐ 1 I eat somewhat less often or lesser amounts of food than usual.
- ☐ 2 I eat much less than usual and only with personal effort.
- ☐ 3 I rarely eat within a 24-hour period, and only with extreme personal effort or when others persuade me to eat.

-OR-

7. Increased Appetite:
- ☐ 0 There is no change from my usual appetite.
- ☐ 1 I feel a need to eat more frequently than usual.
- ☐ 2 I regularly eat more often and/or greater amounts of food than usual.
- ☐ 3 I feel driven to overeat both at mealtime and between meals.

Please complete either 8 or 9 (not both)

8. Decreased Weight (Within the Last Two Weeks):
- ☐ 0 I have not had a change in my weight.
- ☐ 1 I feel as if I have had a slight weight loss.
- ☐ 2 I have lost 2 pounds or more.
- ☐ 3 I have lost 5 pounds or more.

-OR-

9. Increased Weight (Within the Last Two Weeks):
- ☐ 0 I have not had a change in my weight.
- ☐ 1 I feel as if I have had a slight weight gain.
- ☐ 2 I have gained 2 pounds or more.
- ☐ 3 I have gained 5 pounds or more.

During the past seven days...

10. Concentration/Decision-Making:
- ☐ 0 There is no change in my usual capacity to concentrate or make decisions.
- ☐ 1 I occasionally feel indecisive or find that my attention wanders.
- ☐ 2 Most of the time, I struggle to focus my attention or to make decisions.
- ☐ 3 I cannot concentrate well enough to read or cannot make even minor decisions.

11. View of Myself:
- ☐ 0 I see myself as equally worthwhile and deserving as other people.
- ☐ 1 I am more self-blaming than usual.
- ☐ 2 I largely believe that I cause problems for others.
- ☐ 3 I think almost constantly about major and minor defects in myself.

12. Thoughts of Death or Suicide:
- ☐ 0 I do not think of suicide or death.
- ☐ 1 I feel that life is empty or wonder if it's worth living.
- ☐ 2 I think of suicide or death several times a week for several minutes.
- ☐ 3 I think of suicide or death several times a day in some detail, or I have made specific plans for suicide or have actually tried to take my life.

13. General Interest:
- ☐ 0 There is no change from usual in how interested I am in other people or activities.
- ☐ 1 I notice that I am less interested in people or activities.
- ☐ 2 I find I have interest in only one or two of my formerly pursued activities.
- ☐ 3 I have virtually no interest in formerly pursued activities.

(Continued)

TABLE 13-3. The Quick Inventory of Depressive Symptomatology (16-Item) (Self-Report) (QIDS-SR₁₆) *(Continued)*

During the past seven days...
14. Energy Level:
- ☐ 0 There is no change in my usual level of energy.
- ☐ 1 I get tired more easily than usual.
- ☐ 2 I have to make a big effort to start or finish my usual daily activities (for example, shopping, homework, cooking, or going to work).
- ☐ 3 I really cannot carry out most of my usual daily activities because I just don't have the energy.

15. Feeling Slowed Down:
- ☐ 0 I think, speak, and move at my usual rate of speed.
- ☐ 1 I find that my thinking is slowed down or my voice sounds dull or flat.
- ☐ 2 It takes me several seconds to respond to most questions, and I'm sure my thinking is slowed.
- ☐ 3 I am often unable to respond to questions without extreme effort.

During the past seven days...
16. Feeling Restless:
- ☐ 0 I do not feel restless.
- ☐ 1 I'm often fidgety, wringing my hands, or need to shift how I am sitting.
- ☐ 2 I have impulses to move about and I am quite restless.
- ☐ 3 At times, I am unable to stay seated and need to pace around.

Modified with permission from Rush AJ, Trivedi MH, Ibrahim HM, et al: The 16-item quick inventory of depressive symptomatology (QIDS), clinician rating (QIDS-C), and selfreport (QIDS-SR): a psychometric evaluation in patients with chronic major depression. Biol Psychiatry 2003 Sep 1;54(5):573–583.

TABLE 13-4. Quick Inventory of Depressive Symptomatology-Self Report (QIDS-SR₁₆) Scoring Instructions

1. Enter the highest score on any one of the four sleep items (items 1 to 4)
   Enter the highest score on any one of the four weight items (items 6 to 9)
   Enter the highest score on either of the two psychomotor items (items 15 and 16)
2. There will be one score for each of the nine Major Depressive Disorder symptom domains
3. Add the scores of the nine items (sleep, weight, psychomotor changes, depressed mood, decreased interest, fatigue, guilt, concentration, and suicidal ideation) to obtain the total score; total scores range from 0 to 27
4. 0–5: no depressive symptoms; 6–10: mild symptoms; 11–15: moderate symptoms; 16–20: severe symptoms; 21–27: very severe symptoms

Modified with permission from Rush AJ, Trivedi MH, Ibrahim HM, et al: The 16-item quick inventory of depressive symptomatology (QIDS), clinician rating (QIDS-C), and selfreport (QIDS-SR): a psychometric evaluation in patients with chronic major depression. Biol Psychiatry 2003 Sep 1;54(5):573–83.

TABLE 13-5. Diagnostic Criteria for Generalized Anxiety Disorder

A. Excessive anxiety and worry about a number of events or activities. This occurs more days than not for at least 6 months
B. The person finds it difficult to control the worry
C. The anxiety and worry are associated with ≥3 of the following six symptoms:
   Easily fatigued   Irritability
   Muscle tension   Disturbed sleep
   Difficulty concentrating Restless or keyed up
D. The anxiety, worry, or physical symptoms cause clinically significant distress or impairment in social, occupational, or other important areas of functioning
E. The disturbance is not due to physiological effects of a substance or another medical condition
F. Symptoms not better explained by another mental disorder

Data from American Psychiatric Association: Diagnostic and Statistical Manual of Mental Disorders, 5th Edition, DSM-5, Washington, American Psychiatric Association, 2013.

TABLE 13-6. Diagnostic Criteria for Substance Use Disorder

A maladaptive pattern of substance use, leading to clinically significant impairment or distress, as manifested by two or more of the following, occurring at any time in the same 12-month period:
Consumption of larger amounts or over a longer period than was intended
Desire or unsuccessful efforts to cut down
Increased time spent in activities seeking the substance
Cravings or urges
Failure to fulfill major obligations
Continued use despite recurrent problems
Giving up important social, occupational, or recreational activities
Use in physically hazardous situations
Persistent use despite knowledge of problem
Tolerance develops to the substance
Substance cessation leads to withdrawal symptoms

Data from American Psychiatric Association: Diagnostic and Statistical Manual of Mental Disorders, 5th Edition, DSM-5, Washington, American Psychiatric Association, 2013.

SUBSTANCE USE DISORDERS

In the United States, the lifetime prevalence for alcohol and substance use disorders approximates 15 percent. This diagnosis is twice as likely in males, although rates in women are increasing (Kessler, 2005). Indicators of substance misuse are found in Table 13-6. Often substance abuse disorders coexist with mood and anxiety disorders. A detailed discussion of these issues is beyond this chapter's scope, but additional information regarding alcohol and other commonly abused substances, including prescription medications, is found at: http://www.drugabuse.gov.

EATING DISORDERS

Specific feeding and eating disorders classified by the DSM-5 and relevant to women's health care are anorexia nervosa, bulimia nervosa, binge-eating disorder, and unspecified feeding or eating disorder (Tables 13-7 and 13-8). The core symptoms of both anorexia and bulimia are preoccupation with weight gain and excessive self-evaluation of weight and body shape, accompanied by either restriction of food intake (anorexia) or the use of compensatory behaviors to prevent weight gain after binge eating (bulimia). Binge-eating disorder is differentiated by consuming larger amounts of food, lacking a sense of control over the eating, but not engaging in subsequent weight-loss behaviors. These disorders are 10 to 20 times more common in females than in males, particularly in those aged 15 to 24 years (Mitchell, 2006). In young females, an estimated 4 percent suffer from anorexia, 1 to 1.5 percent from bulimia, and 1.6 percent from binge-eating disorder. While anorexia usually begins early in adolescence and peaks around age 17, bulimia nervosa typically has a later onset than anorexia and is more prevalent over the life span (Hoek, 2006). Pathological eating is also found in older women, particularly binge-eating disorder and unspecified eating disorder (Mangweth-Matzek, 2014).

The exact etiology of such abnormal consumption is unknown. However, evidence suggests a strong familial aggregation for eating disorders (Stein, 1999). In the restricting type of anorexia, the concordance rate among monozygotic twins approximates 66 percent and 10 percent for dizygotic twins (Treasure, 1989). Various biologic factors have been implicated in eating disorder development. Abnormalities in neuropeptides, neurotransmitters, and hypothalamic-pituitary-adrenal and hypothalamic-pituitary-gonadal axes are reported (Stoving, 2001). In addition, psychological and psychodynamic factors related to an absence of autonomy are thought to influence obsessive preoccupations. Although eating disorders are believed to be a Western culture phenomenon, rates are also increasing in non-Western cultures (Lai, 2013).

TABLE 13-7. Diagnostic Criteria for Anorexia Nervosa

A. Refusal to maintain body weight at or above a minimal normal weight for age and height
B. Intense fear of gaining weight or becoming fat, even though underweight
C. Disturbance in the way in which one's body weight or shape is experienced, undue influence of body weight or shape on self-evaluation, or denial of the seriousness of the current low weight

Restricting Type: No binge-eating or purging behaviors

Binge-Eating/Purging Type: Binge-eating and self-induced vomiting, or the misuse of laxatives, diuretics, or enemas

Data from American Psychiatric Association: Diagnostic and Statistical Manual of Mental Disorders, 5th Edition, DSM-5, Washington, American Psychiatric Association, 2013.

TABLE 13-8. Diagnostic Criteria for Bulimia Nervosa

A. Recurrent episodes of binge eating
Eating, in a discrete period of time, an amount of food definitely larger than most people would eat in a similar period of time under similar circumstances
A sense of lack of control over eating during the episode
B. Recurrent inappropriate compensatory behavior to prevent weight gain, such as self-induced vomiting; misuse of laxatives, diuretics, enemas, or other medications; fasting; or excessive exercise
C. Binge eating and inappropriate compensatory behaviors both occur, on average, at least once a week for 3 months
D. Self-evaluation is unduly influenced by body shape and weight
E. The disturbance does not occur exclusively during episodes of anorexia nervosa

Data from American Psychiatric Association: Diagnostic and Statistical Manual of Mental Disorders, 5th Edition, DSM-5, Washington, American Psychiatric Association, 2013.

■ Diagnosis

Anorexia nervosa is divided into two subtypes: (1) a restricting type and (2) a binge-eating/purging type, which is distinguished from bulimia by weighing less than the minimum standard for normal. Symptoms begin as unique eating habits that become more and more restrictive. Advanced symptoms may include extreme food intake restriction and excessive exercise. Up to 50 percent of anorectics also show bulimic behavior, and these types may alternate during the course of anorexic illness. Bulimic-type anorectics have been found to engage in two distinct behavior patterns, those who binge and purge and those who solely purge. The body-mass index percentile, clinical symptoms, degree of disability, and need for supervision determine clinical severity.

Diagnosis of anorexia is initially challenging as patients often defend their eating behaviors upon confrontation and rarely recognize their illness. They increasingly isolate themselves socially as their disorder progresses. Multiple somatic complaints such as gastrointestinal symptoms and cold intolerance are common. In the disorder's later stages, weight loss becomes more apparent, and medical complications may prompt patients to seek help. Findings often include dental problems, general nutritional deficiency, electrolyte abnormalities (hypokalemia and alkalosis), and decreased thyroid function. Electrocardiogram changes such as QT prolongation (bradycardia) and inversion or flattened T-waves may be noted. Rare complications include gastric dilatation, arrhythmias, seizure, and death.

Bulimia nervosa is identified by periods of uncontrolled eating of high-calorie foods (binges), followed by compensatory behaviors such as self-induced vomiting, fasting, excessive exercise, or misuse of laxatives, diuretics, or emetics. Unlike patients with anorexia, those with bulimia often recognize their maladaptive behaviors. Severity is based on the frequency of the inappropriate behaviors, clinical symptoms, and level of disability. Most bulimics have normal weights, although their weight may fluctuate. Physical changes may be subtle and include dental problems, swollen salivary glands, or knuckle calluses on the dominant hand. Termed *Russell sign,* calluses form in response to repetitive contact with stomach acid during purging (Strumia, 2005).

Binge-eating disorder is distinct from anorexia and bulimia. It is characterized by ingesting large amounts of food within a short time and is accompanied by feelings that one cannot control the amount of food eaten. Severity is assessed according to the number of gorging episodes per week. Binge-eating is associated with obesity. That said, most obese individuals do not necessarily engage in binge episodes and consume comparatively fewer calories than those with the syndrome. Prevalence in the United States approximates 1.6 percent for females and 0.8 percent for males, and in middle-aged women, binge-eating is more common than anorexia or bulimia (Mangweth-Matzek, 2014).

All these are complex disorders that affect both psychological and physical systems and are often comorbid with depression and anxiety. Rates of mood symptoms approximate 50 percent, and anxiety symptoms, 60 percent (Braun, 1994). Simple phobia and obsessive-compulsive behaviors may also coexist. In many cases, patients with anorexia have rigid, perfectionistic personalities and low sexual interest. Patients with bulimia often display sexual conflicts, problems with intimacy, and impulsive suicidal tendencies.

■ Treatment

A multidisciplinary approach benefits the treatment of eating disorders. Practice approaches include: (1) nutritional rehabilitation, (2) psychosocial treatment that includes individual and family therapies, and (3) pharmacotherapeutic treatment of concurrent psychiatric symptoms. Online resources for information and support are provided by the National Eating Disorder Association, www.edap.org and Academy for Eating Disorders, www.aedweb.org. However, health care providers should also be aware of eating disorder advocacy websites (Norris, 2006).

Data concerning the long-term physical and psychological prognosis of women with eating disorders are limited. Most may symptomatically improve with aging. However, complete recovery from anorexia nervosa is rare, and many continue to have distorted body perceptions and peculiar eating habits. Overall, the prognosis for bulimia is better than for anorexia.

MENSTRUATION-RELATED DISORDERS

Frequently, reproductive-aged women experience symptoms during the late luteal phase of their menstrual cycle. Collectively these complaints are termed *premenstrual syndrome (PMS)* or, when more severe and disabling, *premenstrual dysphoric disorder (PMDD).* Nearly 300 different symptoms have been reported and typically include both psychiatric and physical complaints. For most women, these are self-limited. However, approximately 15 percent report moderate to severe complaints that cause some impairment or require special consideration (Wittchen, 2002). Current estimates are that 3 to 8 percent of menstruating women meet the strict criteria for PMDD (Halbreich, 2003b).

■ Pathophysiology

The exact causes of these disorders are unknown, although several different biological factors have been suggested. Of these, estrogen and progesterone, as well as the neurotransmitters gamma-aminobutyric acid (GABA) and serotonin, are frequently studied.

First, estrogen and progesterone are integral to the menstrual cycle. The cyclic complaints of PMS begin following ovulation and resolve with menses. PMS is less common in women with surgical oophorectomy or drug-induced ovarian hypofunction, such as with gonadotropin-releasing hormone (GnRH) agonists (Cronje, 2004; Wyatt, 2004). Moreover, women with anovulatory cycles appear protected. One potential effect stems from estrogen and progesterone's influence on central nervous system neurotransmitters: serotonin, noradrenaline, and GABA. The predominant action of estrogen is neuronal excitability, whereas progestins are inhibitory (Halbreich, 2003a). Menstruation-related symptoms are believed to be associated with neuroactive progesterone metabolites. Of these, allopregnanolone is a potent modulator of GABA receptors, and its effects mirror those of low-dose benzodiazepines, barbiturates, and alcohol. These effects may include loss of impulse control, negative mood, and aggression or irritability (Bäckström, 2014). Wang and colleagues (1996) noted fluctuations in allopregnanolone across the various menstrual cycle phases. These changes were implicated with PMS symptom severity.

Second, evidence also supports a role for serotonergic system dysregulation in PMS pathophysiology. Decreased serotonergic activity has been noted in the luteal phase. Moreover, trials of serotonergic treatments show PMS symptom reduction (Majoribanks, 2013).

Last, sex steroids also interact with the renin-angiotensin-aldosterone system (RAAS) to alter electrolyte and fluid balance. The antimineralocorticoid properties of progesterone and possible estrogen activation of the RAAS system may explain PMS symptoms of bloating and weight gain.

■ Diagnosis

PMDD is identified in the DSM-5 by the presence of at least five symptoms accompanied by significant psychosocial or functional impairment (Table 13-9). PMS refers to the presence of numerous symptoms that are not associated with significant impairment. During evaluation, the revised criteria in DSM-5 recommend that clinicians confirm symptoms by prospective patient mood charting for at least two menstrual cycles. In certain instances, complaints may be an exacerbation of an underlying primary psychiatric condition(s). Thus, other common psychiatric conditions such as depression and anxiety disorders are excluded. Additionally, other medical conditions that have a multisystem presentation are considered. These include hypothyroidism, systemic lupus erythematosus, endometriosis,

TABLE 13-9. Diagnostic Criteria for Premenstrual Dysphoric Disorder

A. ≥5 symptoms below: occur in most cycles during the week before menses onset, improve within a few days after menses onset, and diminish in the week postmenses

B. One (or more) of the following symptoms must be present:
Marked affective lability
Marked irritability or anger or increased interpersonal conflicts
Marked depressed moods, feelings of hopelessness, or self-deprecating thoughts
Marked anxiety, tension

C. One (or more) of the following symptoms must be also present:
Decreased interest
Difficulty concentrating
Easy fatigability, low energy
Increase or decrease in sleep
Feelings of being overwhelmed
Physical symptoms such as breast tenderness, muscle or joint aches, "bloating" or weight gain
Note: Criteria A–C must be present for most menstrual cycles in the preceding year

D. Symptoms are associated with significant distress or interferences with work, school, relationships

E. The disturbance is not merely an exacerbation of another disorder such as major depression, panic disorder, persistent depressive disorder, or a personality disorder

F. Criterion A should be confirmed by prospective daily ratings in at least two symptomatic cycles

G. The symptoms are not due to physiological effects of a substance or another medical condition

Data from American Psychiatric Association: Diagnostic and Statistical Manual of Mental Disorders, 5th Edition, DSM-5, Washington, American Psychiatric Association, 2013.

anemia, fibromyalgia, chronic fatigue syndrome, fibrocystic breast disease, irritable bowel syndrome, and migraine.

■ Treatment

Therapy for PMDD and PMS include psychotropic agents, ovulation suppression, and dietary modification. Generalists may consider treatment of mild to moderate cases. However, if treatment fails or if symptoms are severe, then psychiatric referral may be indicated (Cunningham, 2009).

Selective serotonin-reuptake inhibitors (SSRIs) are considered primary therapy for psychological symptoms of PMDD and PMS, and fluoxetine, sertraline, and paroxetine are Food and Drug Administration (FDA) approved for this indication (Table 13-10). Standard dosages are administered in either continuous dosing or luteal phase (14 days prior to expected menses) dosing regimens. Several well-controlled trials of SSRIs have shown these drugs to be efficacious and well tolerated (Shah,

TABLE 13-10. List of Common Psychotropic Medications

Drug Class	Indication	Examples[a]	Brand Name	Commonly Reported Side Effects
Selective serotonin-reuptake inhibitors (SSRIs)	Depressive, anxiety, and premenstrual disorders	Fluoxetine[c] Citalopram[c] Escitalopram[c] Sertraline[c] Paroxetine[d] Fluvoxamine[c]	Prozac, Sarafem Celexa Lexapro Zoloft Paxil Luvox	Nausea, headache, insomnia, diarrhea, dry mouth, sexual dysfunction
Serotonin noradrenergic-reuptake inhibitors (SNRIs)	Depressive, anxiety, and premenstrual disorders	Venlafaxine XR[c] Duloxetine[c] Levomilnacipran[c] Desvenlafaxine[c]	Effexor Cymbalta Fetzima Pristiq	Dry mouth, anxiety, agitation, dizziness, somnolence, constipation
Tricyclic and tetracyclic antidepressants	Depressive and anxiety disorders	Desipramine[c] Nortriptyline[d] Amitriptyline[c] Doxepin[c] Maprotiline[b]	Norpramin Pamelor, Aventyl Elavil Sinequan Ludiomil	Drowsiness, dry mouth, dizziness, blurred vision, confusion, constipation, urinary retention and frequency
Benzodiazepines	Anxiety disorders	Alprazolam[d] Clonazepam[d] Diazepam[d]	Xanax Klonopin Valium	Drowsiness, ataxia, sleep changes, impaired memory, hypotension
Others	Depressive disorders	Nefazodone[c] Trazodone[c] Bupropion SR, XL[c] Mirtazipine[c] Vilazodone[c] Aripiprazole[c,e] Vertioxetine[c]	Serzone Desyrel Wellbutrin Remeron Viibryd Abilify Brintellix	Headache, dry mouth, orthostatic hypotension, somnolence Dry mouth, increased appetite, somnolence, constipation Diarrhea, nausea, dry mouth Weight gain, akathisia, extrapyramidal signs, somnolence Constipation, nausea, vomiting
	Anxiety disorders	Buspirone[b] Hydroxyzine[c]	Buspar Vistaril, Atarax	Dizziness, drowsiness, headache
	Sleep agents	Zaleplon[c] Zolpidem[c] Ramelteon[c] Eszopiclone[c]	Sonata Ambien, Intermezzo, Edluar, Zolpimist Rozerem Lunesta	Headache, somnolence, amnesia, fatigue

[a-d]Superscript reflects Food and Drug Administration pregnancy category.
[e]Adjunctive treatment in patients receiving antidepressants.
SR = sustained release; XR/XL = extended release.

2008). In addition, short-term use of anxiolytics such as alprazolam or buspirone offers added benefits to some women with prominent anxiety. However, in prescribing benzodiazepines, caution is taken in women with prior history of substance abuse (Nevatte, 2013).

Because gonadal hormonal dysregulation is implicated in the genesis of PMS symptoms, ovulation suppression is another option. There is some data to support combination oral contraceptive (COC) pills in general for premenstrual mood symptoms. Moreover, in randomized trials, *Yasmin*, a COC containing the spironolactone-like progestin drospirenone, showed therapeutic

benefits. It carries an FDA indication for PMDD treatment in women who desire contraception (Pearlstein, 2005; Yonkers, 2005). Alternatively, GnRH agonists are another means of ovulation suppression. These agents are infrequently selected due to their hypoestrogenic side effects and risks. If elected for PMDD and used longer than 6 months, add-back therapy, as discussed in Chapter 10 (p. 240), can potentially blunt these side effects. Rarely, symptoms warrant bilateral oophorectomy, and a trial of GnRH agonists prior to surgery may be prudent to determine the potential efficacy of castration. Last, the synthetic androgen danocrine (Danazol) also suppresses ovulation, but androgen-related acne and hair growth are usually poorly tolerated.

Of other possible agents, prostaglandin inhibitors such as ibuprofen and naproxen offer benefits through their antiinflammatory effects and alleviate cramping and headaches associated with PMS (Table 10-1, p. 239). Diuretics such as combined hydrochlorothiazide and triamterene (Dyazide) and spironolactone (Aldactone) may be prescribed to alleviate fluid retention and leg edema. Monitoring for potential side effects such as orthostatic hypotension and hypokalemia is critical since these can be severe.

Diet—namely, foods and beverages high in sugar and caffeine—can aggravate premenstrual symptoms in some women. Calcium, 600 mg orally twice daily, has shown benefits, theoretically by correcting deficiency-related symptoms such as muscle cramps (Thys-Jacobs, 2000). Vitamins such as pyridoxine (vitamin B_6) and vitamin E may offer some relief. Pyridoxine is a cofactor to tryptophan hydroxylase, which is the key enzyme in the serotonin synthesis (Wyatt, 1999). The recommended dose of pyridoxine is 50 to 100 mg/day, but doses exceeding 100 mg/day are avoided to prevent pyridoxine toxicity. Magnesium in combination with vitamin B_6 appears to reduce anxiety-related premenstrual symptoms (De Souza, 2000). Of nonpharmacologic alternatives to treatment, there is growing evidence assessing efficacies of acupuncture, bright-light therapy, exercise, and omega fatty acids (Brandon, 2014).

PERINATAL DISORDERS

In general, psychiatric disorders during pregnancy have a course and presentation similar to that in nonpregnant women. For this reason, there are no distinct diagnostic criteria for psychiatric disorders experienced in the context of pregnancy and the puerperium.

■ Perinatal Depression

In the revised DSM-5, a major depressive episode, with its onset during pregnancy or within 4 weeks following childbirth, is categorized by a specifier term that notes "with peripartum onset." Some women experience the first onset of depression during this time, whereas others are vulnerable for relapse (Cohen, 2006a). Etiologic studies have been inconclusive, but both hormonal changes and psychosocial stressors are implicated (Bloch, 2006; Boyce, 2005). Treatment is critical, as suicide is a leading cause of maternal death in developed countries (Centre for Maternal and Child Enquiries, 2011). Accordingly, health professionals are encouraged to thoroughly assess psychiatric and psychosocial history to enable early identification, prevention, and treatment of perinatal depression (Moses-Kolko, 2004). The American College of Obstetricians and Gynecologists (2012) currently notes insufficient evidence for *universal* peripartum depression screening but recommends that evaluation be considered for women with current depression or prior major depression. Other risks include life stress, poor social support (particularly from the partner), and maternal anxiety (Lancaster, 2010).

To screen for and assess severity of peripartum depressive symptoms, the Edinburgh Postnatal Depression Scale (EPDS) is one tool specifically developed for pregnancy (Cox, 1987). Unlike screening measures that score symptoms characteristic of pregnancy itself (appetite, weight change, sleep disturbance, and fatigue), the EPDS inquires about neurovegetative symptoms that are more specific to depression. Available in numerous languages, the EPDS is an efficient way for a clinician to identify patients at risk for perinatal depression. It is available through the American Academy of Pediatrics at: http://www2.aap.org/sections/scan/practicingsafety/toolkit_resources/module2/epds.pdf.

Antepartum

The prevalence of depression during pregnancy has been estimated to be highest (11 percent) in the first trimester, falling to 8.5 percent in the second and third trimesters. For treatment, the American Psychiatric Association and American College of Obstetricians and Gynecologists have issued pregnancy guidelines for depression management that recommend careful risk and benefit analysis of existing treatment (especially medications) (Yonkers, 2009). For major depression, psychotropic medication and psychotherapy have the largest evidence-based support (Stuart, 2014). However, data also note efficacy for several complementary interventions (Deligiannidis, 2013). The FDA (2006, 2011b) recommends careful and transparent risk assessment during pregnancy before prescribing psychotropic medications. On the other hand, women who discontinue antidepressant medication during pregnancy relapse into depression significantly more frequently than women who maintain their pharmacologic treatment (Cohen, 2006a). And as noted, suicide accounts for a significant proportion of pregnancy-associated death. Thus, a clinician must assess the risk of relapse in severely depressed women against potential risk to the newborn of antidepressant medication exposure. Additional guidance is found in *Williams Obstetrics*, 24th edition (Cunningham, 2014). Patients may benefit the most from a combination of treatment options, guided by the information available and the woman's attitudes and preferences regarding potential treatments. Nonpharmacologic and complementary approaches are also potential options for depressive symptoms during pregnancy. These include acupuncture, bright light therapy, exercise, omega fatty acid supplementation, and yoga and massage therapies (Field, 2012; Manber, 2010; Shivakumar, 2011; Su, 2008; Wirz-Justice, 2011).

Postpartum

Depression after childbirth is largely divided into three categories: "postpartum blues," postpartum depression, and postpartum psychosis. The strongest predictors of postpartum depression include prior history of depression or anxiety, family history of psychiatric illness, poor marital relationship, poor social support, and stressful life events in the previous 12 months (Boyce, 2005; Sayil, 2007).

Postpartum blues describes a transient state of heightened emotional reactivity that can develop in up to 50 percent of women. The onset is 2 to 14 days after childbirth, and its duration is less than 2 weeks (Gaynes, 2005). Blues generally require no intervention. Rest and social support contribute significantly to remission. However, postpartum blues do constitute a significant risk factor for subsequent depression during the puerperium.

Postpartum depression, as noted, includes onset during pregnancy and within 4 weeks following delivery. However, in research and most clinical settings, any depression developing within 12 months following childbirth is considered to have postpartum onset (Sharma, 2014). With this definition, the prevalence of postpartum depression approximates 15 percent of delivered women (Gaynes, 2005). Postpartum depression warrants careful assessment by a mental health professional, and treatment is initiated immediately to minimize impaired caregiving. Infants of depressed mothers exhibit cognitive, temperamental, and developmental differences compared with infants of unaffected mothers (Kaplan, 2009; Newport, 2002). SSRIs are usually first-line agents, although fluoxetine use is discouraged due to relatively high concentrations in breast milk (Sie, 2012). Several psychosocial interventions have also demonstrated efficacy in treating postpartum depression. Of these, the most significant effects have been achieved with interpersonal therapy and cognitive-behavioral therapy (Stuart, 2014). Additionally, Postpartum Support International is an excellent resource of information for both clinicians and patients. Information can be obtained at www.postpartum.net and MedEd PPD websites (http://mededppd.org/default2.asp).

Last, *postpartum psychosis* develops in less than 2 percent of new mothers, and its onset is generally within 2 weeks of childbirth (Gaynes, 2005). The risk for this severe form of depression is increased for women who have had prior mood disorders. Particularly, prior postpartum psychosis increases by 30 to 50 percent a woman's risk with subsequent deliveries (American Psychiatric Association, 2013). Evaluation and antipsychotic pharmacologic treatment is essential for these patients. Hospitalization is often indicated until the safety of mother and infant is assured.

■ Other Psychiatric Disorders

Clinicians most often focus on mood disorders during the perinatal period. However, other psychiatric illnesses such as anxiety disorders, bipolar disorder, and schizophrenia may also be present. Of these, bipolar disorders and schizophrenia are serious, recurrent psychiatric illnesses that require pharmacologic treatment. Treatment planning is critical with such patients, and decisions are made in collaboration with a psychiatric professional. The FDA (2011a) issued a safety communication alerting health care providers concerning some antipsychotic medications that are associated with neonatal extrapyramidal and withdrawal symptoms similar to the neonatal behavioral syndrome seen in those exposed to SSRIs. Thus, a careful balance must be struck between minimizing medication risk to the fetus and maternal risk from untreated or undertreated disease.

■ Perinatal Loss

With perinatal loss, many studies have focused on identifying factors that modify grieving styles, and a few have studied interventions for families after such loss. Health care providers are most helpful if they speak directly, use understandable language, and share information that would provide parents a sense of control over their situation and that would address their fears. Additional time with health professionals and a perception of being a priority are also important (DiMarco, 2001; Flenady, 2014). Since grief is individual, no generalizations can be made concerning clinical treatment in these situations. Thus, a clinician must ask a patient what she needs and wants. Couples therapy may be helpful if mother and father find it difficult to grieve congruently. Family therapy may be indicated if other children need support to process the loss and their parents' grief. Many hospitals provide support groups, and the Hygeia Foundation (http://hygeiafoundation.org) offers both useful information and online support.

MENOPAUSAL TRANSITION AND MENOPAUSE

The menopausal transition has long been investigated as a vulnerable period for emergence of mood symptoms. Anxiety, irritable mood, and sleep problems are more likely to develop in perimenopausal women than in premenopausal counterparts (Brandon, 2008; Freeman, 2006). Moreover, data suggest that rates of new-onset depression during menopausal transition are nearly twice those for premenopausal women (Cohen, 2006b). This risk persists even after adjusting for sleep disturbances and vasomotor symptoms.

Other possible risks for depression and anxiety are a prior history of depression, severe premenstrual distress, hot flushes, and disrupted sleep. Demographic predictors of increased risk during the perimenopause are lower educational status, African-American ethnicity, unemployment, and major life stressors (Bromberger, 2001; Freeman, 2006; Maartens, 2002). Moreover, psychosocial issues include a woman's recognition that her reproductive years are ending and that her children will leave to establish their own lives. Developmentally, many women are transitioning from being family focused to finding new avenues in which to invest time and energy.

Mood vulnerability during menopausal transition is believed to follow erratic physiologic fluctuations in reproductive hormones. Detailed discussion of these hormones as they relate to mood changes during this transition is found in Chapter 21 (p. 485).

■ Evaluation and Treatment

Perimenopausal women with psychological symptoms warrant a comprehensive psychosocial inventory and risk factor assessment. Since medical conditions may concurrently develop during this transition, evaluation excludes these before symptoms are considered psychosomatic. In particular, thyroid function is evaluated.

The approach to treating mood symptoms involves both pharmacotherapy and psychotherapy (Brandon, 2008). Recommended psychotropic medications are SSRIs and selective noradrenergic-reuptake inhibitors (SNRIs) such as venlafaxine (Effexor). These agents are good options for women who decline hormone therapy. Additional benefits include alleviation of vasomotor symptoms and sleep disturbance.

Studies suggest that short-term administration of estrogen is an option for perimenopausal women with depressive symptoms (Soares, 2001). However, the psychotropic role of estrogen-progesterone preparations in postmenopausal women remains unclear. Moreover, benefits are weighed against safety concerns raised by the Women's Health Initiative (WHI) Study regarding estrogen use (Chap. 22, p. 492). Of nonpharmacologic alternatives investigated to date for mood disturbance during menopause, yoga and moderate-intensity exercise have demonstrated benefit (Brandon, 2014). However, these studies are small.

LATE LIFE

According to estimates by the Census Bureau, the number of older people in the United States will significantly increase over the next decade as the "Baby Boomer" generation ages. By 2030, nearly 20 percent of the population will be older than 65 (He, 2005). Psychosocial issues addressed are significantly different for these women. Stressors may include diminished mental and physical function and loss of partner, family, or friends. Erikson identified the task of this final developmental stage of life as one of consolidation and integration. In this model, women retrospectively examine their life. They may manage their last years with integrity and with satisfaction in a life well lived, or may suffer despair, feeling that all was in vain.

According to the 2000 U.S. Census, functionally impairing mental disorders affected 11 percent of adults aged 65 to 74 and 10 percent of those older than 74 (He, 2005). Of these disorders, depression, anxiety, late-onset psychotic and paranoid disorders, and alcoholism are those most likely to be observed in clinical practice. As in the general population, anxiety is the most common psychiatric disorder in the elderly. However, the prevalence of depression is generally thought to be lower in postmenopausal women compared with reproductive-aged women. Moreover, most studies suggest that the gender gap between rates of depression closes in late life (Zarit, 1998).

■ Evaluation and Treatment

If a psychiatric disorder is suspected, careful evaluation is required to exclude underlying medical causes for these changes. For example, depression may be a comorbid disorder with or an early symptom of Alzheimer and Parkinson disease (Polidori, 2001). Alternatively, depression, anxiety, and psychosis may also result from a single medication or medication combinations.

Specific screening questionnaires for depression have been developed for the elderly, such as the Geriatric Depression Scale (Brink, 1982). This screening tool is available in various languages at: http://www.stanford.edu/~yesavage/GDS.html. In addition, neuropsychologic evaluation is helpful to discriminate between the source and nature of mood symptoms and cognitive impairment. Dementia screening is discussed in Chapter 1 (p. 17).

Recognizing the natural decline in serotonin levels with aging, many gerontologists prescribe SSRIs for their patients. However, communication among all treating physicians to coordinate medications and minimize interactions is particularly important for elderly patients.

Psychosocial treatments are often helpful for the patient and, where applicable, her caregivers. Cognitive-behavioral therapy and interpersonal therapy have both been found efficacious with the elderly. Moreover, family therapy can be of great value to those struggling with end-of-life issues, functional impairments, multiple losses, and caregiver burden. Social workers are also of tremendous value if a patient and family need to locate additional care resources.

For depression in older adults, one metaanalysis of 89 studies found that pharmacotherapy or psychotherapy achieved comparable results. In contrast, for anxiety, another analysis of 32 studies found pharmacotherapy slightly more effective than psychotherapy (Pinquart, 2006, 2007). Thus, treatment planning is individualized and assesses patient preference, contraindications, and treatment access.

SOMATIC SYMPTOM DISORDERS

Recurrent, multiple, often unexplained physical symptoms are hallmark features of *somatic symptom disorders*. These disorders are common, and their estimated prevalence in general clinical practice is 16 percent (de Waal, 2004). Their prevalence may be even higher in specialty clinics such as pain management clinics. Somatic symptom disorders are complex and poorly understood. However, symptoms cause significant distress and/or impairment in various domains of an affected individual's life. Moreover, one in four somatic symptom patients suffer from comorbid anxiety and depressive symptoms. Thus, a multidisciplinary approach is often required to effectively manage these women's symptoms.

SEXUAL ASSAULT

Sexual assault is a broad term that includes rape, unwanted genital touching, and even forced viewing of or involvement in pornography. Rape is a legal term and in the United States refers to penetration of a body orifice without consent (mouth, vagina, or anus) and with force or the threat of force or incapacity (young or old age, cognitive or physical disability, or drug or alcohol intoxication). The definition of rape includes spousal rape (Linden, 2011). Rape is often motivated by aggression and rage, with the assailant using sexual contact as a weapon for power and control.

For sexual assault, large population-based surveys indicate a lifetime prevalence of 13 to 39 percent among women and 3 percent among men (Tjaden, 2000). Certain populations are at increased risk and include the physically or mentally disabled; homeless persons; persons who are gay, lesbian, bisexual, or transgendered; alcohol and drug users; college students; and persons younger than 24 (Lawyer, 2010).

Well-known sequelae of rape include isolation, depression, anxiety, somatic symptoms, suicide attempts, and posttraumatic stress disorder (PTSD). The experience has a strong effect on the victim's subsequent health and thus is a major public health issue. Importantly, in caring for sexual assault victims, clinicians should be familiar with the complex array of reactions (emotional and physical), common injuries, and elements of proper evaluation and treatment of these patients.

■ Physical Findings

Initial evaluation of a sexual assault victim concentrates on identifying serious injuries. Although 70 percent of rape victims sustain no obvious physical injuries, 24 percent sustain minor injuries, and up to 5 percent sustain major nongenital injuries. Common nongenital injuries include bruises, cuts, scratches, and swelling (81 percent); internal injuries and unconsciousness (11 percent); and knife or gunshot wounds (2 percent) (Sommers, 2001). In the genital area, the posterior fourchette is the area most often injured. Although death is rare, the fear of death during an assault is one of the most intense reactions (Deming, 1983; Marchbanks, 1990).

Once life-threatening injuries are excluded, a patient is ideally moved to a quiet, private setting for further evaluation. A systematic, thorough, but compassionate approach to obtaining a history and collecting evidence is essential for appropriate treatment of the victim and for future prosecution of her assailant (American College of Obstetricians and Gynecologists, 2014).

■ Examination and Documentation

Although valid evidence may be collected up to 5 days after sexual assault, immediate examination increases the opportunity to obtain valuable physical evidence (Table 13-11). Consent is obtained prior to physical and genital examination and evidence collection. This step helps to reestablish a victim's sense of control and is essential for entry of evidence in a court of law (Plaut, 2004). Providers emphasize that vital information may be lost if evidence is not collected early. Moreover, evidence collection does not commit a victim to pressing criminal charges (Linden,

---

TABLE 13-11. Important Elements of Physical Examination and Evidence Collection Following Sexual Assault

Physical examination
General appearance
Affect/emotional status
Complete examination of head, body, and extremities; record injuries on body diagram
Pelvic examination, with colposcopy if available, to exclude lower reproductive tract trauma

Elements of evidence collection
Clothing collected in labeled paper bags
Swabs and smears of involved orifices and skin surfaces
Blood sample for patient blood typing to compare with assailant's type
Head hair combings; then head hairs cut or pulled from patient for comparison
Pubic hair combings; then pubic hair cut or pulled from patient for comparison
Fingernail scrapings from the patient, if the victim scratched the assailant's skin or clothing

---

1999). A patient is also counseled that she may terminate an examination if it is too emotionally or physically painful.

Most states have standardized kits for evidence collection and storage in which kits may be locked to ensure that legal evidence procedures are maintained. Documentation of all physical injuries is essential, and objective evidence of trauma (even minor) is associated with increased chances of successful prosecution. Clothing is collected as a patient undresses on a white sheet and placed in properly labeled bags (Ingemann-Hansen, 2013). Any debris, such as hair, fibers, mud, or leaves, is also collected.

Evidence gathering includes a sample of the patient's saliva and swabs of all involved orifices. A thorough pelvic examination with evidence collection is essential, even if there are no complaints of genital pain. Up to one third of victims can have traumatic genital injuries without symptoms. Common patterns of genital injury include tears of the posterior fourchette and fossa, labial abrasions, and hymenal bruising. Significant genital injuries are more common in postmenopausal or prepubertal victims. Colposcopy is used if available because this technique increases detection of more subtle injuries of the cervix and vagina. Lenahan (1998) reported that the use of colposcopy increased genital trauma recognition from 6 percent to 53 percent. In addition, a Wood's lamp may aid identification of semen on the skin, which then is collected with moistened cotton swabs. A blood sample is collected for typing, to differentiate the blood type of the victim from that of the assailant. After evidence is collected, it is signed, sealed, and locked in a secure place (Mollen, 2012; Rambow, 1992).

■ Treatment
Pregnancy Prevention

Medication prophylaxis to prevent pregnancy and common sexually transmitted diseases is provided to women following sexual assault. The risk of rape-related pregnancy approximates 5 percent per rape among reproductive-aged victims (Holmes, 1996). Most of these pregnancies, unfortunately, occur in adolescents, often the victims of incest, who never report the incident or receive medical attention. Because of variation in a woman's menstrual cycle, pregnancy prophylaxis, also termed emergency contraception, is offered to all victims with reproductive organs. Prophylaxis can be administered for up to 72 hours after rape but is most effective in the first 24 hours (Table 13-12). Some studies indicate that prophylaxis may be effective for up to 5 days following rape.

A negative pregnancy test to exclude a preexisting pregnancy is confirmed before administering emergency contraception. This is especially true for ulipristal (Ella), a progesterone antagonist, because of fetal loss risks if used in the first trimester. With estrogen/progestin combinations, side effects include nausea and vomiting, breast tenderness, and heavier menstrual period. In comparison, with levonorgestrel (Plan B), the risk of nausea and vomiting is less (Arowojolu, 2002). An antiemetic can be prescribed 30 minutes prior to hormone administration to decrease nausea (Table 42-7, p. 914).

Patients are informed that their next menses may be delayed following this prophylaxis. Although current regimens are 74 to 89 percent effective, women are counseled to return if

TABLE 13-12. Pregnancy and Sexually Transmitted Disease Prevention Following Sexual Assault

Testing
Pregnancy test (urine or serum)
Serum testing for hepatitis B surface antigen (HBsAg), HIV, and syphilis
Evaluation for *Neisseria gonorrhoeae* and *Chlamydia trachomatis* from each penetrated site
Microscopic evaluation of vaginal discharge saline preparation
If HIV PEP is planned, then CBC, serum liver function tests, and serum creatinine level

Treatment
Levonorgestrel, ulipristal, or Yuzpe method: all dosages in Table 5-11, p. 131
Ceftriaxone 125 mg intramuscularly, single dose *or* cefixime 400 mg orally, single dose
Azithromycin 1 g orally, single dose
Metronidazole 2 g orally, single dose

Optional treatment
Hepatitis B vaccination (Table 1-2, p. 8).
HIV protease-inhibitor-based PEP: lopinavir/ritonavir (Kaletra) *plus* (lamivudine or emtricitabine) *plus* zidovudine.
    One option: Kaletra 3 tablets orally twice daily with Combivir (lamivudine/zidovudine) 1 tablet twice daily for 28 days

CBC = complete blood count; HIV = human immunodeficiency virus; PEP = postexposure prophylaxis.
Data from Centers for Disease Control and Prevention: Antiretroviral postexposure prophylaxis after sexual, injection-drug use, or other nonoccupational exposure to HIV in the United States. MMWR 54(2):1, 2005; Centers for Disease Control and Prevention: Sexually transmitted diseases treatment guidelines, 2015. MMWR 64(3):1, 2015.

their next menses is more than 1 to 2 weeks late (Task Force on Postovulatory Methods of Fertility Regulation, 1998; Trussell, 1996; Yuzpe, 1982).

Sexually Transmitted Disease Prevention

The risk of acquiring sexually transmitted disease (STD) after rape has been estimated. The risk for trichomoniasis approximates 12 percent; bacterial vaginosis, 12 percent; gonorrhea, 4 percent to 12 percent; chlamydial infection, 2 to 14 percent; syphilis, 5 percent; and human immunodeficiency virus (HIV) infection, 0.1 percent (Jenny, 1990; Katz, 1997; Schwarcz, 1990). However, these risks are difficult to predict and vary by geographic location, type of assault, assailant, and presence of preexisting infections. General recommendations describe prophylaxis for hepatitis, gonorrhea, and chlamydia (see Table 13-12).

The fear of contracting HIV after sexual assault is common in survivors and is often the primary concern following rape (Baker, 1990). However, postexposure prophylaxis (PEP) against HIV remains controversial, given the low risk of transmission after a single sexual assault (Gostin, 1994). With regard to sexual exposures, the per-contact risk of HIV transmission associated with receptive penile-anal exposures is estimated to be 0.5 to 3.2 percent and with receptive penile-vaginal exposures, 0.05 to 0.15 percent (Wieczorek, 2010). Although rare, HIV transmission associated with receptive oral intercourse has been reported. Experts recommend offering PEP to candidates who are at a higher risk of being exposed to HIV and who are willing to complete the full course of medications and comply with surveillance testing (Table 13-13). The risks and side effects of these medications and need for close monitoring is discussed with patients. Nausea is a common side effect with PEP. Thus, a prescription for an antiemetic such as phenergan, to be used as needed, is commonly provided. PEP should begin within 72 hours, if indicated. For sexual assault patients presenting outside of this time frame, information is provided regarding follow-up HIV antibody testing and referral options.

Because of the emotional intensity of the experience, a woman may not recall all the information provided, and thus written instructions are helpful. Survivors are referred to local rape crisis centers and encouraged to visit within 1 to 2 days.

TABLE 13-13. HIV PEP after Sexual Assault

Assess for risk of HIV infection in the assailant and test if possible
Determine characteristics of the assault that may increase the risk of HIV transmission (i.e., mucous membrane or broken skin in contact with blood, semen, or rectal secretions)
Consider consulting an HIV specialist or the National Clinicians' Postexposure Prophylaxis Hotline: 888–448–4911
If patient is at risk for HIV from assault, discuss PEP risks and benefits
If the patient starts PEP, schedule follow-up within 7 days
If prescribing PEP, obtain CBC, serum liver function tests, and serum creatinine level
Check HIV serology at baseline, 6 weeks, and then at 3 and 6 months

CBC = complete blood count; HIV = human immunodeficiency virus; PEP = postexposure prophylaxis.

Sexual assault victims receive subsequent medical evaluation at 1 to 2 weeks, and 2 to 4 months following their rape. During these visits, examination for STDs and blood testing for HIV and syphilis is performed. Remaining hepatitis vaccinations are administered, if needed.

Psychological Response to Sexual Assault

Survivors of sexual assault may display an array of reactions that frequently include anxiety, agitation, crying, or a quiet, calm, and removed affect. In 1974, Burgess and Holmstrom first characterized the "rape trauma syndrome." They described two response phases to the trauma of sexual assault: (1) the acute disorganization phase, lasting several weeks, and (2) the reorganization phase, lasting from several weeks to years. During the acute phase, shock and disbelief, fear, shame, self-blame, humiliation, anger, isolation, grief, somatic manifestations, and loss of control are common. During the reorganization phase, feelings of vulnerability, despair, guilt, and shame may continue. Symptoms can include nonspecific anxiety, somatic complaints, or depression. Longitudinal data indicate that sexual assault survivors are at increased lifetime risk for PTSD, major depression, and suicide contemplation or attempt (Linden, 2011). Health care providers ideally enlist the input of social workers or rape crisis counselors to help evaluate the patient's immediate and future emotional and safety needs.

CHILD SEXUAL ABUSE

Sexual abuse is defined as a child engaged in sexual activities that he or she cannot comprehend, for which he or she is developmentally unprepared and cannot give consent, and/or that violate societal laws or social taboos (Kellogg, 2005). Sexual activities can include vaginal/anal intercourse, oral-genital contact, genital-genital contact, fondling, and exposure to pornography or to adults engaging in sexual activity. In the United States, the overall prevalence of child sexual abuse ranges from 11 to 32 percent for females and 4 to 14 percent for males (Sapp, 2005). Thus, indicators that prompt evaluation include: (1) statements by the child or family of abuse, (2) genital or anal

injury without concordant history of unintentional trauma, (3) semen or pregnancy identified, or (4) STD diagnosed beyond the incubation period of vertical (natal mother-to-child) transmission (Bechtel, 2010).

Determining whether genital findings in children are normal variants or indicative of assault can be difficult, and these have been categorized according to their likelihood of associated sexual abuse. An exhaustive list of normal and indeterminate signs has been compiled by Adams and colleagues (2007, 2008), and those considered diagnostic are listed in Table 13-14. A provider completing the examination should have formal training in the evaluation of suspected child sexual abuse. A list of local specialist providers can be found on the American Academy of Pediatrics Section on Child Abuse and Neglect website at http://www.aap.org/sections/childabuseneglect/. Importantly, acute injuries associated with child sexual abuse heal and resolve rapidly. Thus, examination is completed as soon as sexual assault is suspected (McCann, 2007). As signs may be subtle, a careful history and full examination are carried out with the aid of photodocumentation, preferably using a colposcope (Price, 2013).

The prevalence of STDs in child victims of sexual abuse is low (Girardet, 2009a). Thus, the decision to obtain specimens from a child is individualized. Situations that typically prompt testing include: (1) signs or complaints of genital penetration or of an STD, (2) suspected assailant with a high risk for STDs, (3) another household member with an STD, (4) abuse by a stranger, or (5) community with a high STD rate (Centers for Disease Control and Prevention, 2015).

If indicated, recommended testing includes: cultures for *Neisseria gonorrhoeae* from the pharynx, anus, and vagina; cultures for *Chlamydia trachomatis* from the anus and vagina; and culture and wet mount evaluation of a vaginal swab specimen for *Trichomonas vaginalis* infection and bacterial vaginosis. Culture rather than nucleic acid amplification tests (NAATs) are preferred. Swab specimens from vagina, rather than endocervix, are recommended for prepubertal girls (Centers for Disease Control and Prevention, 2015). Decisions regarding serologic testing for *Treponema pallidum*, HIV, and hepatitis B virus are individualized.

TABLE 13-14. Findings Diagnostic of Sexual Contact in Suspected Child Sexual Abuse

Acute genital or perianal lacerations or extensive bruising[a]
Perianal or fourchette scarring[a]
An area between 4 and 8 o'clock on the rim of the hymen where it appears to have been torn through to, or nearly to, the base
Positive genital, anal, or pharyngeal culture for *Neisseria gonorrhoeae*[b]
Confirmed diagnosis of syphilis[b]
Positive culture or saline prep for *Trichomonas vaginalis* in a child older than 1 year
Positive genital or anal culture for *Chlamydia trachomatis* in a child older than 3 years
Positive serology for HIV[b]
Pregnancy
Sperm identified in specimens taken directly from a child's body

---

[a]If other medical conditions such as Crohn disease, coagulopathy, or labial adhesion not explanatory for findings.
[b]If perinatal transmission, transmission from blood products, and needle contamination have been excluded.
HIV = human immunodeficiency virus.
Data from Adams JA: Guidelines for medical care of children evaluated for suspected sexual abuse: an update for 2008. Curr Opin Obstet Gynecol 2007 Jun;20(3):163-172; Adams JA, Kaplan RA, Starling SP, et al: Guidelines for medical care of children who may have been sexually abused. J Pediatr Adolesc Gynecol 2008 Oct;20(5):435–441.

The general concept that sexually transmissible infections found beyond the neonatal period are evidence of sexual abuse has exceptions. For example, perinatally acquired *C trachomatis* infection has, in some cases, persisted up to age 3 years in girls. Genital warts have been diagnosed in children who have no other evidence of sexual abuse. Finally, most hepatitis B virus infections in children result from household exposure to those chronically infected with the virus (Centers for Disease Control and Prevention, 2015).

Routine STD prophylaxis for children who have been sexually abused is generally not recommended due to lower rates of associated infection and a greater guarantee of scheduled follow-up. However, if the clinical setting dictates or if test results are positive for infection, antibiotics are provided. Rates of HIV transmission following sexual abuse are also very low in children (Girardet, 2009b). However, antiretroviral treatment is well tolerated by children, and PEP can be offered based on the clinical setting (Cybulska, 2012). When considered, antiretroviral PEP is initiated, similar to other prophylaxis, within the first 72 hours. The CDC (2015) recommends consulting professionals who specialize in care of HIV-infected children.

INTIMATE PARTNER VIOLENCE

The terms *domestic violence (DV), gender-based violence,* and *violence against women* encompass a multitude of abuses directed at women and girls. The United Nations Declaration on the Elimination of Violence against Women (1993) defines violence as acts that cause or have the potential to cause harm. Introduction of the term "gender-based" emphasizes that the act is rooted in inequality between women and men (Krantz, 2005). *Intimate-partner violence (IPV)* refers to harm inflicted by one intimate partner on the other, with the intention of causing pain or controlling the other's behavior. *Honor-based violence (HBV)* is most prevalent in south Asian and Middle Eastern countries, where acts are committed to maintain family honor in the community. The prevalence of HBV in the United States is increasing with increasing immigration from these areas (Dickson, 2014).

Violence against women varies and includes wife battering, sexual assault, incest, and elder abuse (Burge, 1997; Straka, 2006). Most victims know their assailant and have been assaulted more than once. The average length of victimization is 4 years for repeatedly raped women and for physically assaulted women (Tjaden, 2000).

Risks

In the United States, nearly one in four women has experienced IPV at some point in her life. Aside from youth and ethnicity, few traits characterize women who are assaulted by violent men. Peters and colleagues (2002) analyzed data from 5298 IPV reports. They found that women aged 16 to 24 years are at greatest risk for IPV, a risk that was more than twice as great as the risk for women aged 25 to 34 years. Rates of IPV decreased throughout the reproductive years and reached a nadir in women aged 65 or older. Hotaling and Sugarman (1986) in their review found only one consistent risk marker

of being an abused wife. Witnessing violence as a child was a significant risk factor in 11 of 15 studies.

Seven to 20 percent of pregnant women may be victims, and homicide is reported as the leading cause of death during pregnancy. Most cases result from partner abuse (Gazmararian, 1996; Shadigian, 2005). Therefore, screening for IPV is an important component of prenatal care.

The social and medical problem of elder abuse is escalating with an aging population. Currently, each year, approximately 1 in 10 older adults are mistreated, and 84 percent of cases are unreported (Hoover, 2014; Jayawardena, 2006). Elder abuse is divided into seven categories by The National Center on Elder Abuse: physical, emotional, and sexual abuse, financial exploitation, neglect, self-neglect, and abandonment. Of these categories, neglect is the most prevalent. It occurs most often in the home and is perpetrated most frequently by family members. Identified risk factors are caregiver stress, patient cognitive impairment, need for assistance with daily life activities, conflicted family relationships, and poor social support (Hoover, 2014).

Diagnosis

Women who have been assaulted are far more likely to seek help from their medical provider than from legal personnel, mental health professionals, or victim advocates. For years after the assault, victims have an unusually high rate of medical use and may present with psychiatric and somatic complaints (Koss, 1992). Moreover, IPV can adversely affect health, and affected women are more likely to have cardiac disease, asthma, and drink excessively compared with women without prior IPV (Bair-Merritt, 2014).

Although some clinicians may feel awkward asking patients, researchers agree that the single most important thing a physician can do for a battered woman is to ask about violence (Linden, 1999). Additionally, health care providers should ask about violence if they identify symptoms or behaviors that may be associated with victimization (Burge, 1997). These can include bruising, unexplained injuries, depression or anxiety, alcohol or drug abuse, unexplained chronic pain, isolation, inability to cope, limited access to care, noncompliance, husbands with extremely controlling behaviors or intense jealousy, or husbands with substance abuse.

Management

If a patient discloses IPV, a clinician should validate and normalize a patient's perspective. Patients are counseled that many women have assault experiences, that most are afraid to confide these, that memories of the experience can be painful, and that a fear of future assaults is a reasonable fear. Following a patient's disclosure, a clinician expresses concern for the woman's health and safety and conveys a willingness to discuss relationship issues at any time. Moreover, information describing community resources is offered. The National Domestic Violence Hotline (1–800–799–SAFE (7233)) is a nonprofit telephone referral service with access to more than 5000 women's shelters nationally.

Battery is a crime, yet few states specifically require reporting of IPV. A small number of states require mandatory arrest of batterers, and a few jurisdictions aggressively pursue cases of IPV. Accordingly, each clinician should know their state laws to properly and adequately inform their patients. In addition, providers should thoroughly document physical findings of violence. Such data may be required if criminal charges are pursued.

FEMALE SEXUALITY

Sexuality is one of the most complex and yet basic components of human behavior. Expressions of sexuality and intimacy remain important throughout life. Although basic sexual drive is biologic, its expression is determined by various psychological, social, environmental, spiritual, and learned factors. Thus, satisfaction is often less dependent on the physical components of sexuality than on the quality of the relationship and the context in which sexual behavior is undertaken.

In describing the sexual response cycle, several models have been proposed to describe normal sexual response (Kingsberg, 2013). Masters and Johnson, in 1966, were the first to offer a theoretical "human sexual response cycle" that was based on their direct observations of the anatomic and physiologic changes experienced by men and women in a laboratory setting. This was a four-stage linear cycle that they labeled as "excitement," "plateau," "orgasm," and "resolution." The cycle was independently modified by Kaplan (1979) and Leif (1977) to a triphasic model that emphasized desire—in contrast to physiologic genital arousal—as the first stage of sexual response. In 2001, Basson first published her intimacy-based circular model to help explain the multifactorial character of female sexual response (Fig. 13-2). This model includes the interplay of emotional intimacy, sexual stimuli, psychological factors, and relationship satisfaction. This model also introduces the concept of receptive/responsive desire, which is the idea that arousal often precedes desire and that women often begin a sexual encounter from a position of sexual neutrality. It encompasses

the impact of biologic and nonbiologic factors on a woman's sexual response, including motivation, interpersonal issues, cultural and religious beliefs, partner's health status, relationship quality, past sexual abuse, and distractions. Basson's model (2001, 2006) emphasizes that desire and arousal are difficult to separate, and this serves as the basis for DSM-5 classification changes. Namely, the diagnoses of hypoactive sexual desire disorder and female sexual arousal disorder are now combined and considered as female sexual interest/arousal disorder (American Psychiatric Association, 2013; Kingsberg, 2013).

■ Drive/Desire

The basis of desire and perceived arousal in women is poorly understood, but it appears to involve interactions among multiple neurotransmitters, sex hormones, and environmental factors. The biopsychosocial model of desire as outlined by Levine (1984) suggests that desire is composed of three individual but interrelated components: sexual drive, sexual beliefs, and sexual motivation. The biologic component, drive, is spontaneous and includes cravings for sexual activity, sexual dreams, unprompted sexual thoughts, and genital sensations. It is influenced by neuroendocrine mechanisms. The second component reflects a woman's beliefs and values about sex. The third component, motivation, reflects the emotional willingness to engage in sexual activity with a given partner (or alone). Motivation often carries the most weight among these components and is altered by psychological function, relationship quality, and concerns about health, occupation, or family. The interplay and input of these realms yield one's sexual interest. Thus, a clinician's differential diagnosis and assessment must be broad, and treatment incorporates a biopsychosocial/integrative approach.

■ Arousal

A woman's sexual arousal is complex and correlates positively with the sexual stimulus and its emotional context. This subconscious reflex is organized by the autonomic nervous system and processed in the limbic system in response to mental or physical stimuli that are recognized as sexual. Subjective findings of sexual arousal include vaginal and vulvar congestion, increases in vaginal lubrication, and other somatic changes such as blood pressure level, heart rate, muscle tone, respiratory rate, and temperature. However, in sexually healthy women, measurements of genital congestion and subjective arousal vary widely (Everaerd, 2000; Laan, 1995). There are also affective responses to sexual arousal. Feelings of joy and affirmation or feelings of fear, guilt, and awkwardness serve to modulate arousal.

In the basal state, clitoral corporal and vaginal smooth muscles are tonically contracted. After sexual stimulation, neurogenic and endothelial release of nitric oxide (NO) leads to clitoral cavernosal artery relaxation. The resulting arterial inflow increases intracavernosal pressure and clitoral engorgement (Cellek, 1998). The glans clitoris extrudes and sensitivity is enhanced.

In the basal state, the vaginal epithelium reabsorbs sodium from the submucosal capillary plasma transudate. However, after sexual stimulation, several neurotransmitters, including NO and vasoactive intestinal peptide, are released. These

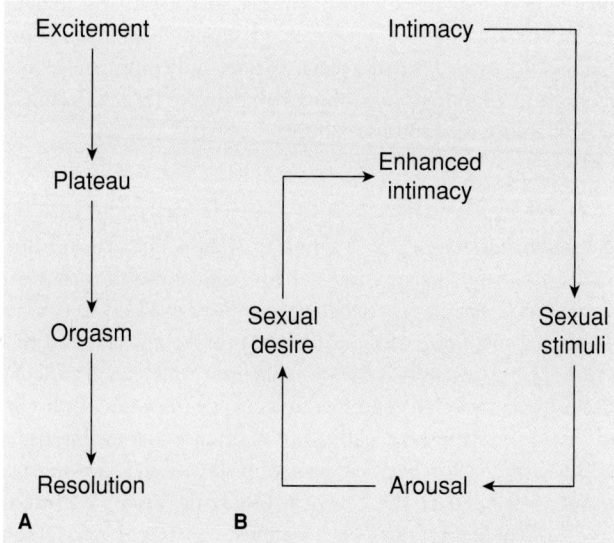

FIGURE 13-2 Models of female sexual response. (Data from Basson R: Human sex-response cycles. J Sex Marital Ther 27:33, 2001; Masters WH, Johnson VE: Human Sexual Response. Boston, Little Brown, 1966.)

modulate vaginal vascular and nonvascular smooth muscle relaxation (Palle, 1990). Submucosal capillary flow dramatically increases and overwhelms sodium reabsorption. Three to 5 mL of vaginal transudate is produced, and this enhanced lubrication aids pleasurable coitus. Smooth-muscle relaxation of the vagina increases vaginal length and luminal diameter, especially in the distal two thirds of the vagina.

■ Release and Resolution

Masters and Johnson (1966) proposed that orgasmic release is a reflex-like response that follows once a plateau of excitement has been reached or exceeded. The actual neurobiology of orgasm is unknown, although it seems to include the mesolimbic dopamine pathways and the pudendal, pelvic, and hypogastric nerves. Orgasm occurs with the release of contraction-producing agents such as serotonin and oxytocin, which lead to rhythmic contraction of the levator plate, uterus, and vagina. The physiologic and behavioral indices of orgasm involve the whole body—facial grimaces, generalized muscle myotonia, carpopedal spasms, and contractions of the gluteal and abdominal muscles. The subjective experience of orgasm includes feeling of intense pleasure with a peaking and rapid, exhilarating release. These sensations are reported to be singular, regardless of the manner in which orgasm is achieved (Newcomb, 1983). Women are unique in their ability to be multiorgasmic, that is, capable of a series of distinguishable orgasmic responses without a lowering of excitement between them.

After orgasm, the anatomic and physiologic changes of excitement reverse. In women, genital vasocongestion diminishes, and the vagina shortens and narrows. A filmy sheet of perspiration covers the body, and elevated heart and respiration rates gradually return to normal. If orgasm has occurred, there is concomitant psychologic and physical relaxation. If orgasm does not occur, a similar physiologic processes occurs, but at a slower rate.

■ Normal Variations in the Physiologic Response

Sexual function and variations in the physiologic response may be affected by many biologic and psychologic aspects of reproduction and the life cycle. First, during pregnancy, sexual function may change, and a reduction in sexual desire and coital frequency is typical (Hyde, 1996). These changes may stem from fears of causing fetal harm during intercourse or orgasm. In addition, fatigue, physical discomfort, or feeling less physically attractive are other reasons.

Women who suffer recurrent miscarriage or infertility or undergo therapeutic abortion, and even those during a normal puerperium, may have an altered physiologic and psychologic sexual response. In the puerperium, fatigue, hormonal changes, and a healing episiotomy scar may contribute to diminished frequency and enjoyment of intercourse (Srivastava, 2008). Hyde (1996) found that women who are breast feeding report less sexual activity and less satisfaction that those who were not breast feeding. The study failed to demonstrate any marked differences according to the method of delivery, although women who had cesarean delivery were more likely to resume intercourse 4 weeks postpartum than women who delivered vaginally.

For older women, baseline data from the Study of Women's Health Across the Nation (SWAN) addressed sexual behavior in 3262 women aged 42 to 52 years who were either premenopausal or in early menopausal transition. In early menopausal transition, investigators found few changes in sexual practices or function (Cain, 2003). In a group aged 40 to 69 years, Addis and associates (2006) found that 71 percent were sexually active and 65 percent reported satisfaction. Sexual dysfunction was noted in 45 percent and was associated with having a higher education level, poor health, a significant relationship, and a low mental health score.

Late in menopausal transition and with natural menopause, hormonal changes, as a consequence of the hypoestrogenic state, can interfere with physiologic response (Avis, 2000; Tan, 2012). The prevalence of sexual dysfunction is higher and ranges from 68 to 86 percent (Sarrel, 1990). Masters and Johnson (1966) described a delay in reaction time of the clitoris, delayed or absent vaginal lubrication, decreased vaginal congestion, and reduced duration of contractions with orgasm. Loss of estrogen diminishes genital blood flow, vaginal lubrication, and vaginal tissue structural integrity (Freedman, 2002; Pauls, 2005). That said, estrogen replacement in postmenopausal women improves libido and orgasm (Sarrel, 1990). Others have shown improved vaginal lubrication, blood flow, and vaginal compliance in menopausal women using systemic estrogen replacement, but these were not correlated with subjective improvements in sexual function (Berman, 1999; Semmens, 1982).

With aging, sexuality still plays an important role in physical and mental health. Klausmann (2002) and Dennerstein (2001) both suggest that even many years after menopause, an increase in desire and interest is consistently reported with a new relationship. The opportunity for sexual activity in the form of intercourse, however, is often dependent on partner issues. Both partner availability and partner health begin to shape the frequency with which this form of sexual activity occurs. In general, sexual activity declines with increasing age. Activity is reported in 30 to 78 percent of 60-year-old women, in 11 to 74 percent of those older than 70, and in 8 to 43 percent of 80-year-old women (Morley, 2003). Few data describe sexual function in those older than 80, but as the "Baby Boomer" cohort of a more sexually open group continues to age, the future holds promise for the desire to maintain this quality of life (Morley, 1992).

SEXUAL DYSFUNCTIONS

Psychiatric sexual dysfunctions are characterized by painful intercourse or disturbances in desire, arousal, orgasm, or resolution that cause marked distress and relationship difficulty (Table 13-15). Sexual dysfunction stemming from dyspareunia may also originate from gynecologic disease and is discussed more fully in Chapters 4 (p. 97) and 11 (p. 262).

Although many studies have investigated female sexual dysfunction, prevalence rates are difficult to establish due to differing criteria and measures of sexual functioning. However,

SECTION 1

TABLE 13-15. Sexual Dysfunctions

Female sexual interest/arousal disorder

Lack of or significantly reduced sexual interest/arousal for a minimum of 6 months, causing distress, and not explained by severe relationship distress (i.e., violence)

Female orgasmic disorder

Persistent or recurrent delay in, or absence of, orgasm following a normal excitement phase taking into account factors such as age, sexual experience, and the adequacy of sexual stimulation she receives, persisting for 6 months

Genitopelvic pain/penetration disorder

Recurrent or persistent genital pain in anticipation of, during, or as a result of vaginal intercourse or penetration attempts

In all the above disorders

The disturbance causes marked distress or interpersonal difficulty

Sexual dysfunction is not better accounted for by another psychiatric disorder and is not due exclusively to the direct physiologic effects of a substance or a general medical condition

Types: Lifelong versus acquired; generalized versus situational

Data from American Psychiatric Association: Diagnostic and Statistical Manual of Mental Disorders, Fifth Edition, DSM-5, Washington, American Psychiatric Association, 2013.

Hayes and colleagues (2006) estimated that 64 percent of women experience low or no sexual desire, 35 percent have difficulty achieving orgasm, and 26 percent experience sexual pain. Most difficulties last less than 6 months, but one third may persist longer.

■ Diagnosis and Treatment

Patient history is a primary diagnostic tool. Psychosocial risk factors for sexual dysfunction include comorbid psychological disorders, negative emotions, maladaptive cognitions (such as inaccurate expectations), cultural factors, lack of education regarding sexual functioning, couple distress, and absent physical attraction. Of these, psychiatric disorders such as depression and anxiety are frequently comorbid with sexual disorders. Thus, for most patients who suffer from sexual dysfunction, evaluation does not stop with an organic explanation (Bach, 2001). In accordance with the biopsychosocial approach, diagnosis of sexual disorders begins by judging if dysfunction is caused exclusively by a general medical condition, drug abuse, medication, or toxin exposure. Subsequently, evaluation for a primary psychiatric disorder follows. Assessment typically inventories a woman's ethnic, cultural, religious, and social backgrounds and includes a frank discussion about her current sexual partner(s) and sexual expectations. Clinical judgment takes into account the patient's age and sexual experience, symptom frequency and chronicity, and her perception of symptoms. Importantly, a woman is asked if the sexual difficulty is chronic or new-onset and if it persists across all situations or appears only in certain circumstances. Finally, referral to a psychiatrist or psychologist may be indicated for a thorough psychiatric interview.

Multidisciplinary treatment is ideal for patients with sexual dysfunction. A team would typically include the referring physician, gynecologist, psychologist, and a nurse-specialist. In organic disorders, it may be necessary to include specialists in urology, gastroenterology, and anesthesiology. Psychological approaches usually include some combination of sexual education, commu-nication enhancement, identification of emotional and cultural factors, cognitive-behavioral therapy, and couples therapy.

REFERENCES

Adams JA: Guidelines for medical care of children evaluated for suspected sexual abuse: an update for 2008. Curr Opin Obstet Gynecol 20:435, 2008

Adams JA, Kaplan RA, Starling SP, et al: Guidelines for medical care of children who may have been sexually abused. J Pediatr Adolesc Gynecol 20:163, 2007

Addis IB, Van Den Eeden SK, Christina L, et al: Sexual activity and function in middle-aged and older women. Obstet Gynecol 107:755, 2006

American College of Obstetricians and Gynecologists: Screening for depression during and after pregnancy. Committee Opinion No. 453, February 2010, Reaffirmed 2012

American College of Obstetricians and Gynecologists: Sexual assault. Committee Opinion No. 592, April 2014

American Psychiatric Association: Diagnostic and Statistical Manual of Mental Disorders, Fifth Edition, DSM-5, Washington, American Psychiatric Association, 2013

Andrade L, Caraveo-Anduaga JJ, Berglund P, et al: The epidemiology of major depressive episodes: results from the International Consortium of Psychiatric Epidemiology (ICPE) Surveys. Int J Methods Psychiatr Res 12(1):3, 2003

Arowojolu AO, Okewole IA, Adekunle AO: Comparative evaluation of the effectiveness and safety of two regimens of levonorgestrel for emergency contraception in Nigerians. Contraception 66(4):269, 2002

Avis NE, Stellato R, Crawford S, et al: Is there an association between menopause status and sexual functioning? Menopause 7(5):297, 2000

Bach AK, Wincze JP, Barlow DH: Sexual Dysfunction. New York, Guilford Press, 2001

Bäckström T, Bixo M, Johansson M, et al: Allopregnanolone and mood disorders. Prog Neurobiol 113:88, 2014

Bair-Merritt MH, Lewis-O'Connor A, Goel S, et al: Primary care-based interventions for intimate partner violence: a systematic review. Am J Prev Med 46(2):188, 2014

Baker TC, Burgess AW, Brickman E, et al: Rape victims' concern about possible exposure to HIV infection. J Interpers Violence 549, 1990

Basson R: Clinical practice. Sexual desire and arousal disorders in women. N Engl J Med 354(14):1497, 2006

Basson R: Human sex-response cycles. J Sex Marital Ther 27:33, 2001

Bechtel K: Sexual abuse and sexually transmitted infection in children and adolescents. Curr Opin Pediatr 22:94, 2010

Berman JR, Berman LA, Werbin TJ, et al: Clinical evaluation of female sexual function: effects of age and estrogen status on subjective and physiologic sexual responses. Int J Impot Res 11(Suppl 1):S31, 1999

Bloch M, Rotenberg N, Koren D, et al: Risk factors for early postpartum depressive symptoms. Gen Hosp Psychiatry 28(1):3, 2006

Boyce P, Hickey A: Psychosocial risk factors to major depression after childbirth. Soc Psychiatry Psychiatr Epidemiol 40(8):605, 2005

Brandon AR, Crowley SK, Gordon JL, et al: Non-pharmacologic treatments for depression related to reproductive events. Curr Psychiatr Rep 16(12):526, 2014

Brandon AR, Shivakumar G, Freeman MP: Perimenopausal depression. Curr Psychiatr 7(10):38, 2008

Braun DL, Sunday SR, Halmi KA: Psychiatric comorbidity in patients with eating disorders. Psychol Med 24(4):859, 1994

Brink TL, Yesavage JA, Lum O, et al: Screening tests for geriatric depression. Clin Gerontol 1(1):37, 1982

Bromberger JT, Meyer PM, Kravitz HM, et al: Psychologic distress and natural menopause: a multiethnic community study. Am J Public Health 91(9):1435, 2001

Burge SK: Violence against women. Prim Care 24(1):67, 1997

Burgess AW, Holmstrom LL: Rape trauma syndrome. Am J Psychiatry 131(9):981, 1974

Burt VK, Hendrick VC: Clinical Manual of Women's Mental Health. Washington, American Psychiatric Publishing, 2005, p 6

Cain VS, Johannes CB, Avis NE, et al: Sexual functioning and practices in a multi-ethnic study of midlife women: baseline results from SWAN. J Sex Res 40(3):266, 2003

Cellek S, Moncada S: Nitrergic neurotransmission mediates the non-adrenergic non-cholinergic responses in the clitoral corpus cavernosum of the rabbit. Br J Pharmacol 125(8):1627, 1998

Centers for Disease Control and Prevention: Antiretroviral postexposure prophylaxis after sexual, injection-drug use, or other nonoccupational exposure to HIV in the United States. MMWR 54(2):1, 2005

Centers for Disease Control and Prevention: Sexually transmitted diseases treatment guidelines, 2015. MMWR 64(3):1, 2015

Centre for Maternal and Child Enquiries: Saving mothers' lives: reviewing maternal deaths to make motherhood safer: 2006–08. BJOG 118(Suppl 1):1, 2011

Cohen LS, Altshuler LL, Harlow BL, et al: Relapse of major depression during pregnancy in women who maintain or discontinue antidepressant treatment. JAMA 295(5):499, 2006a

Cohen LS, Soares CN, Vitonis AF, et al: Risk for new onset of depression during the menopausal transition: the Harvard study of moods and cycles. Arch Gen Psychiatry 63(4):385, 2006b

Cox J, Holden J, Sagovsky R: Detection of postnatal depression: development of the 10-item Edinburgh postnatal depression scale. Br J Psychiatry 150:782, 1987

Cronje WH, Vashisht A, Studd JW: Hysterectomy and bilateral oophorectomy for severe premenstrual syndrome. Hum Reprod 19:2152, 2004

Cunningham FG, Leveno KL, Bloom SL, et al (eds): Psychiatric disorders. In Williams Obstetrics, 24th ed. New York, McGraw-Hill Education, 2014

Cunningham J, Yonkers KA, O'Brien S, et al: Update on research and treatment of premenstrual dysphoric disorder. Harv Rev Psychiatry 17(2):120, 2009

Cybulska B: Immediate medical care after sexual assault. Best Pract Res Clin Obstet Gynaecol 27:141, 2013

Deligiannidis KM, Freeman MP: Complementary and alternative medicine therapies for perinatal depression. Best Pract Res Clin Obstet Gynaecol 28(1):85, 2014

Deming JE, Mittleman RE, Wetli CV: Forensic science aspects of fatal sexual assaults on women. J Forensic Sci 28(3):572, 1983

Dennerstein L, Dudley E, Burger H: Are changes in sexual functioning during midlife due to aging or menopause? Fertil Steril 76(3):456, 2001

De Souza MC, Walker AF, Robinson PA, et al: A synergistic effect of a daily supplement for 1 month of 200 mg magnesium plus 50 mg vitamin B6 for the relief of anxiety-related premenstrual symptoms: a randomized, double-blind, crossover study. J Womens Health Gend Based Med 9(2):131, 2000

de Waal MW, Arnold IA, Eekhof A, et al: Somatoform disorders in general practice: prevalence, functional impairment and comorbidity with anxiety and depressive disorders. Br J Psychiatry 184:470, 2004

Dickson P: Understanding victims of honour-based violence. Community Pract 87(7):30, 2014

DiMarco MA, Menke EM, McNamara T: Evaluating a support group for perinatal loss. MCN Am J Matern Child Nurs 26(3):135, 2001

Engel GL: The need for a new medical model: a challenge for biomedicine. Science 196(4286):129, 1977

Erikson EH: Childhood and Society, 2nd ed. New York, Norton, 1963

Everaerd W, Laan E, Both S, et al: Female Sexuality. New York, John Wiley & Sons, 2000

Field T, Diego M, Hernandez-Reif M, et al: Yoga and massage therapy reduce prenatal depression and prematurity. J Body Mov Ther 16(2):204, 2012

Flenady V, Boyle F, Koopmans L, et al: Meeting the needs of parents after a stillbirth or neonatal death. BJOG 121(Suppl 4):137, 2014

Food and Drug Administration: Antipsychotic drug labels updated on use during pregnancy and risk of abnormal muscle movements and withdrawal symptoms in newborns. 2011a. Available at: http://www.fda.gov/Drugs/DrugSafety/ucm243903.htm. Accessed November 17, 2014

Food and Drug Administration: Selective serotonin reuptake inhibitors (SSRIs), selective serotonin-norepinephrine reuptake inhibitors (SNRIs), 5-hydroxytryptamine receptor agonists (triptans), 2006. Available at: http://www.fda.gov/Drugs/DrugSafety/PostmarketDrugSafetyInformationforPatientsandProviders/DrugSafetyInformationforHeathcareProfessionals/ucm085845.htm. Accessed November 17, 2014

Food and Drug Administration: Selective serotonin reuptake inhibitor (SSRI) antidepressant use during pregnancy and reports of a rare heart and lung condition in newborn babies. 2011b. Available at: http://www.fda.gov/Drugs/DrugSafety/ucm283375.htm. Accessed November 17, 2014

Freedman MA: Female sexual dysfunction. Int J Fertil Womens Med 47(1):18, 2002

Freeman EW, Sammel MD, Lin H, et al: Associations of hormones and menopausal status with depressed mood in women with no history of depression. Arch Gen Psychiatry 63(4):375, 2006

Gaynes BN, Gavin N, Meltzer-Brody S, et al: Perinatal depression: prevalence, screening accuracy, and screening outcomes. Evid Rep Technol Assess (Summ) 119:1, 2005

Gazmararian JA, Lazorick S, Spitz AM, et al: Prevalence of violence against pregnant women. JAMA 275(24):1915, 1996

Girardet RG, Lahoti S, Howard LA, et al: Epidemiology of sexually transmitted infections in suspected child victims of sexual assault. Pediatrics 124(1):79, 2009a

Girardet RG, Lemme S, Biason TA, et al: HIV post-exposure prophylaxis in children and adolescents presenting for reported sexual assault. Child Abuse Negl 33:173, 2009b

Gostin LO, Lazzarini Z, Alexander D, et al: HIV testing, counseling, and prophylaxis after sexual assault. JAMA 271(18):1436, 1994

Halbreich U: The etiology, biology, and evolving pathology of premenstrual syndromes. Psychoneuroendocrinology 28(Suppl 3):55, 2003a

Halbreich U, Borenstein J, Pearlstein T, et al: The prevalence, impairment, impact, and burden of premenstrual dysphoric disorder (PMS/PMDD). Psychoneuroendocrinology 28(Suppl 3):1, 2003b

Hayes RD, Bennett CM, Fairley CK, et al: What can prevalence studies tell us about female sexual difficulty and dysfunction? J Sex Med 3(4):589, 2006

He W, Sengupta M, Velkoff VA, et al: 65+ in the United States: 2005. Available at: http://www.census.gov/prod/2006pubs/p23–209.pdf. Accessed November 19, 2014

Hoek HW: Incidence, prevalence and mortality of anorexia nervosa and other eating disorders. Curr Opin Psychiatry 19(4):389, 2006

Holmes MM, Resnick HS, Kilpatrick DG, et al: Rape-related pregnancy: estimates and descriptive characteristics from a national sample of women. Am J Obstet Gynecol 175(2):320, 1996

Hoover RM, Polson M: Detecting elder abuse and neglect assessment and intervention. Am Fam Physician 89(6):453, 2014

Hotaling GT, Sugarman DB: An analysis of risk markers in husband to wife violence: the current state of knowledge. Violence Vict 1(2):101, 1986

Hyde JS, DeLamater JD, Plant EA, et al: Sexuality during pregnancy and the year postpartum. J Sex Res 33:143, 1996

Ingemann-Hansen O, Charles AV: Forensic medical examination of adolescent and adult victims of sexual violence. Best Pract and Res Clinic Obstet Gynaecol 27:91, 2013

Jayawardena KM, Liao S: Elder abuse at end of life. J Palliat Med 9(1):127, 2006

Jenny C, Hooton TM, Bowers A, et al: Sexually transmitted diseases in victims of rape. N Engl J Med 322(11):713, 1990

Kaplan HS: Disorders of sexual desire and other new concepts and techniques in sex therapy. In The New Sex Therapy. New York, Brunner/Mazel, 1979

Kaplan PS, Burgess AP, Sliter JK, et al: Maternal sensitivity and the learning-promoting effects of depressed and nondepressed mothers' infant-directed speech. Infancy 14(2):143, 2009

Katz MH, Gerberding JL: Postexposure treatment of people exposed to the human immunodeficiency virus through sexual contact or injection-drug use. N Engl J Med 336(15):1097, 1997

Kellogg N: The evaluation of sexual abuse in children. Pediatrics 116:506, 2005

Kessler RC, Berglund P, Demler O, et al: Lifetime prevalence and age-of-onset distributions of DSM-IV disorders in the National Comorbidity Survey Replication. Arch Gen Psychiatry 62(6):593, 2005

Kessler RC, McGonagle KA, Zhao S, et al: Lifetime and 12-month prevalence of DSM-III-R psychiatric disorders in the United States. Results from the National Comorbidity Survey. Arch Gen Psychiatry 51(1):8, 1994

Kingsberg SA, Rezaee RL: Hypoactive sexual desire in women. Menopause 20(1):1284, 2013

Klausmann D: Sexual motivation and the duration of the relationship. Arch Sex Behav 31:275, 2002

Koss MP, Heslet L: Somatic consequences of violence against women. Arch Fam Med 1(1):53, 1992

Krantz G, Garcia-Moreno C: Violence against women. J Epidemiol Community Health 59(10):818, 2005

Laan E, Everaerd W, van der Velde J, et al: Determinants of subjective experience of sexual arousal in women: feedback from genital arousal and erotic stimulus content. Psychophysiology 32(5):444, 1995

Lai CM, Mak KK, Pang JS, et al: The associations of sociocultural attitudes towards appearance with body dissatisfaction and eating behaviors in Hong Kong adolescents. Eat Behav 14(3):320, 2013

Lancaster CA, Gold KJ, Flynn HA, et al: Risk factors for depressive symptoms during pregnancy: a systematic review. Am J Obstet Gynecol 202(1):5, 2010

Lawyer S, Resnick H, Bakanic V, et al: Forcible, drug-facilitated, and incapacitated rape and sexual assault among undergraduate women. J Am Coll Health 58:453, 2010

Leif H: Inhibited sexual desire. Med Aspects Hum Sex 7:94, 1977

Lenahan LC, Ernst A, Johnson B: Colposcopy in evaluation of the adult sexual assault victim. Am J Emerg Med 16(2):183, 1998

Levine SB. An essay on the nature of sexual desire. J Sex Marital Ther 10:83–96, 1984

Linden JA: Care of the adult patient after sexual assault. N Engl J Med 365:834, 2011

Linden JA: Sexual assault. Emerg Med Clin North Am 17(3):685, 1999

Maartens LWF, Knottnerus JA, Pop VJ: Menopausal transition and increased depressive symptomatology: a community based prospective study. Maturitas 42(3):195, 2002

Manber R, Schnyer RN, Lyell D, et al: Acupuncture for depression during pregnancy: a randomized controlled trial. Obstet Gynecol 115(3):511, 2010

Mangweth-Matzek B, Hoek HW, Pope HG: Pathological eating and body dissatisfaction in middle-aged and older women. Curr Opin Psychiatry 27:431, 2014

Marchbanks PA, Lui KJ, Mercy JA: Risk of injury from resisting rape. Am J Epidemiol 132(3):540, 1990

Marjoribanks J, Brown J, O'Brien PM, et al: Selective serotonin reuptake inhibitors for premenstrual syndrome. Cochrane Database Syst Rev 6:CD001396, 2013

Masters WH, Johnson VE: Human Sexual Response. Boston, Little Brown, 1966

McCann J, Miyamoto S, Boyle C, et al: Healing of nonhymenal genital injuries in prepubertal and adolescent girls: a descriptive study. Pediatrics 120:1000, 2007

Mitchell AM, Bulik CM: Eating disorders and women's health: an update. J Midwifery Womens Health 51(3):193, 2006

Mollen CJ, Goyal MK, Frioux SM: Acute sexual assault: a review. Pediatr Emerg Care 28(6):584, 2012

Morley JE: Sexual function and the aging woman. Ann Intern Med 307, 1992

Morley JE, Kaiser FE: Female sexuality. Med Clin North Am 87(5):1077, 2003

Moses-Kolko EL, Roth EK: Antepartum and postpartum depression: healthy mom, healthy baby. J Am Med Womens Assoc 59(3):181, 2004

Nevatte T, O'Brien PM, Bäckström T, et al: ISPMD consensus on the management of premenstrual disorders. Arch Womens Ment Health 16(4):279, 2013

Newcomb MD, Bentler PM: Dimensions of subjective female orgasmic responsiveness. J Pers Soc Psychol 44(4):862, 1983

Newport DJ, Wilcox MM, Stowe ZN: Maternal depression: a child's first adverse life event. Semin Clin Neuropsychiatry 7(2):113, 2002

Norris ML, Boydell KM, Pinhas L, et al: Ana and the Internet: a review of pro-anorexia websites. Int J Eat Disord 39(6):443, 2006

Palle C, Bredkjaer HE, Ottesen B, et al: Vasoactive intestinal polypeptide and human vaginal blood flow: comparison between transvaginal and intravenous administration. Clin Exp Pharmacol Physiol 17(1):61, 1990

Pauls RN, Kleeman SD, Karram MM: Female sexual dysfunction: principles of diagnosis and therapy. Obstet Gynecol Surv 60(3):196, 2005

Pearlstein TB, Bachmann GA, Zacur HA, et al: Treatment of premenstrual dysphoric disorder with a new drospirenone-containing oral contraceptive formulation. Contraception 72:414, 2005

Peters J, Shackelford TK, Buss DM: Understanding domestic violence against women: using evolutionary psychology to extend the feminist functional analysis. Violence Vict 17 (2):255, 2002

Pinquart M, Duberstein PR: Treatment of anxiety disorders in older adults: a meta-analytic comparison of behavioral and pharmacological interventions. Am J Geriatr Psychiatry 15(8):639, 2007

Pinquart M, Duberstein PR, Lyness JM: Treatments for later-Life depressive conditions: a meta-analytic comparison of pharmacotherapy and psychotherapy. Am J Psychiatry 163(9):1493, 2006

Plaut SM, Graziottin A, Heaton PW: Sexual Dysfunction. Oxford, Health Press Limited, 2004

Polidori MC, Menculini G, Senin U, et al: Dementia, depression and parkinsonism: a frequent association in the elderly. J Alzheimer Dis 3(6):553, 2001

Price J: Injuries in prepubertal and pubertal girls. Best Pract and Res Clin Obstet Gynaecol 27:131, 2013

Rambow B, Adkinson C, Frost TH, et al: Female sexual assault: medical and legal implications. Ann Emerg Med 21:717, 1992

Rush AJ, Trivedi MH, Ibrahim HM, et al: The 16-item quick inventory of depressive symptomatology (QIDS), clinician rating (QIDS-C), and self-report (QIDS-SR): a psychometric evaluation in patients with chronic major depression. Biol Psychiatry 54(5):573, 2003

Sapp MV, Vandeven AM: Update on childhood sexual abuse. Curr Opinion Pediatr 17:258, 2005

Sarrel PM: Sexuality and menopause. Obstet Gynecol 75(4 Suppl):26S, 1990

Sayil M, Gure A, Uçanok Z: First time mothers' anxiety and depressive symptoms across the transition to motherhood: associations with maternal and environmental characteristics. Women Health 44(3):61, 2007

Schwarcz SK, Whittington WL: Sexual assault and sexually transmitted diseases: detection and management in adults and children. Rev Infect Dis 12 (S6):682, 1990

Semmens JP, Wagner G: Estrogen deprivation and vaginal function in postmenopausal women. JAMA 248(4):445, 1982

Shadigian E, Bauer ST: Pregnancy-associated death: a qualitative systematic review of homicide and suicide. Obstet Gynecol Surv 60(3):183, 2005

Shah NR, Jones JB, Aperi J, et al: Selective serotonin reuptake inhibitors for premenstrual syndrome and premenstrual dysphoric disorder: a meta-analysis. Obstet Gynecol 111:1175, 2008

Sharma V, Mazmanian D: The DSM-5 peripartum specifier: prospects and pitfalls. Arch Womens Ment Health 17(2):171, 2014

Shivakumar G, Brandon AR: Antenatal depression: a rationale for studying exercise. Depress Anxiety 28(3): 234, 2011

Sie SD, Wennink JM, van Driel JJ, et al: Maternal use of SSRIs, SNRIs and NaSSAs: practical recommendations during pregnancy and lactation. Arch Dis Child Fetal Neonatal Ed 97(6):F472, 2012

Soares CN, Almeida OP, Joffe H: Efficacy of estradiol for the treatment of depressive disorders in perimenopausal women: a double-blind, randomized, placebo-controlled trial. Arch Gen Psychiatry 58(6):529, 2001

Sommers MS, Schafer J, Zink T, et al: Injury patterns in women resulting from assault. Trauma Violence Abuse 2(3):240, 2001

Srivastava R, Thakar R, Sultan A: Female sexual dysfunction in obstetrics and gynecology. Obstet Gynecol Surv 63(8):527, 2008

Stein D, Kaye WH: Familial aggregation of eating disorders: results from a controlled family study of bulimia nervosa. Int J Eat Disord 26(2):211, 1999

Stoving RK, Hangaard J, Hagen C: Update on endocrine disturbances in anorexia nervosa. J Pediatr Endocrinol 14(5):459, 2001

Straka SM, Montminy L: Responding to the needs of older women experiencing domestic violence. Violence Against Women 12(3):251, 2006

Strumia R: Dermatologic signs in patients with eating disorders. Am J Clin Dermatol 6(3):165, 2005

Stuart S, Koleva H: Psychological treatments for perinatal depression. Best Pract Res Clin Obstet Gynaecol 28(1):61, 2014

Su KP, Huang SY, Chiu TH, et al: Omega-3 fatty acids for major depressive disorder during pregnancy: results from a randomized, double-blind, placebo-controlled trial. J Clin Psychiatry 69(4):644, 2008

Substance Abuse and Mental Health Services Administration: Results from the 2012 National Survey on Drug Use and Health: mental health findings. NSDUH Series H-47, HHS Publication No. (SMA) 13–4805, Rockville, 2013

Tan O, Bradshaw K, Carr BR: Management of vulvovaginal atrophy-related sexual dysfunction in postmenopausal women: an up-to-date review. Menopause 19(1):109, 2012

Task Force on Postovulatory Methods of Fertility Regulation: Randomized controlled trial of levonorgestrel versus the Yuzpe regimen of combined oral contraceptives for emergency contraception. Lancet 352(9126):428, 1998

Thys-Jacobs S: Micronutrients and the premenstrual syndrome: the case for calcium. J Am Coll Nutr 19(2):220, 2000

Tjaden PG, Thoennes N: Extent, nature and consequences of rape victimization: findings from the National Violence Against Women Survey. Washington, National Institute of Justice (NCJ 210346), 2000

Treasure J, Holland AJ: Genetic vulnerability to eating disorders: evidence from twin and family studies. In Remschmidt H (ed): Child and Youth Psychiatry: European Perspectives. New York, Hogrefe and Hubert, 1989, p 59

Trussell J, Ellertson C, Stewart F: The effectiveness of the Yuzpe regimen of emergency contraception. Fam Plann Perspect 28 (2):58, 1996

United Nations General Assembly (UNGA): Declaration on the elimination of violence against women. United Nations General Assembly (UNGA), 1993. Available at: http://www.un.org/documents/ga/res/48/a48r104.htm. Accessed November 19, 2014

Wang M, Seippel L, Purdy RH, et al: Relationship between symptom severity and steroid variation in women with premenstrual syndrome: study on serum pregnenolone, pregnenolone sulfate, 5 alpha-pregnane-3,20-dione and 3 alpha-hydroxy-5 alpha-pregnan-20-one. J Clin Endocrinol Metab 81(3): 1076, 1996

Wieczorek K: A forensic nursing protocol for initiating human immunodeficiency virus post-exposure prophylaxis following sexual assault. J Forensic Nurs 6(1):29, 2010

Wirz-Justice A, Bader A, Frisch U, et al: A randomized, double-blind, placebo-controlled study of light therapy for antepartum depression. J Clin Psychiatry 72(7):986, 2011

Wittchen HU, Becker E, Lieb R, et al: Prevalence, incidence and stability of premenstrual dysphoric disorder in the community. Psychol Med 32(1):119, 2002

Wyatt KM, Dimmock PW, Ismail KM, et al: The effectiveness of GnRHa with and without "add-back" therapy in treating premenstrual syndrome: a meta-analysis. BJOG 111:585, 2004

Wyatt KM, Dimmock PW, Jones PW, et al: Efficacy of vitamin B-6 in the treatment of premenstrual syndrome: systematic review. BMJ 318:1375, 1999

Yonkers KA, Brown C, Pearlstein TB, et al: Efficacy of a new low-dose oral contraceptive with drospirenone in premenstrual dysphoric disorder. Obstet Gynecol 106:492, 2005

Yonkers KA, Wisner KL, Stewart DE, et al: The management of depression during pregnancy: a report from the American Psychiatric Association and the American College of Obstetricians and Gynecologists. Gen Hosp Psychiatry 31(5):403, 2009

Yuzpe AA, Smith RP, Rademaker AW: A multicenter clinical investigation employing ethinyl estradiol combined with dl-norgestrel as postcoital contraceptive agent. Fertil Steril 37(4):508, 1982

Zarit SH, Zarit JM: Mental Disorders in Older Adults: Fundamentals of Assessment and Treatment. New York, Guilford Press, 1998

Pediatric Gynecology

Pediatric gynecology is a unique subspecialty that encompasses knowledge from various specialties including general pediatrics, gynecology, reproductive endocrinology, as well as pediatric endocrinology and pediatric urology. Treatment of a particular patient may thus require the collaboration of clinicians from one or more of these fields.

Gynecologic disorders in children can differ greatly from those encountered in the adult female. Even the simple physical examination of the genitalia differs significantly. A thorough understanding of these differences can aid in diagnosing the various gynecologic abnormalities seen in this age group.

PHYSIOLOGY AND ANATOMY

■ Hypothalamic-Pituitary-Ovarian Axis

A carefully orchestrated cascade of events unfolds in the neuroendocrine system and regulates development of the female reproductive system. In utero, gonadotropin-releasing hormone (GnRH) neurons develop in the olfactory placode. These neurons migrate through the forebrain to the arcuate nucleus of the hypothalamus by 11 weeks' gestation (Fig. 16-5, p. 376). They form axons that extend to the median eminence and to the capillary plexus of the pituitary portal system (Fig. 15-11, p. 345). Gonadotropin-releasing hormone, a decapeptide, is influenced by higher cortical centers and is released from these neurons in a pulsatile fashion into the pituitary portal plexus. As a result, by midgestation, the GnRH "pulse generator" stimulates secretion of gonadotropins, that is, follicle-stimulating hormone (FSH) and luteinizing hormone (LH), from the anterior pituitary. In turn, the pulsatile release of gonadotropins stimulates ovarian synthesis and release of gonadal steroid hormones. Concurrently, accelerated germ cell division and follicular development begins, resulting in the creation of 6 to 7 million oocytes by 5 months' gestation. By late gestation, gonadal steroids exert a negative feedback on secretion of both hypothalamic GnRH and pituitary gonadotropins. During this time, oocyte number decreases through a process of gene-related apoptosis to reach a level of 1 to 2 million by birth (Vaskivuo, 2001).

At birth, FSH and LH concentrations rise abruptly in response to the fall in placental estrogen levels and are highest in the first 3 months of life (Fig. 14-1). This transient rise in gonadotropin levels is followed by an increase in gonadal steroid concentrations, which is thought to explain instances of neonatal breast budding, minor bleeding from endometrial shedding, short-lived ovarian cysts, and transient white vaginal mucous discharge. Following these initial months, gonadotropin levels gradually decline to reach prepubertal levels by age 1 to 2 years.

The childhood years are thus characterized by low plasma levels of FSH, LH, and estradiol. Estradiol levels typically measure <10 pg/mL, and LH values are <0.3 mIU/mL. Both may be assessed if precocious development is suspected (Neely, 1995; Resende, 2007). During childhood, ovaries undergo active follicular growth and oocyte atresia. As a result of this attrition, by puberty, only 300,000 to 500,000 oocytes remain (Fritz, 2011).

■ Anatomy

Pelvic anatomy also changes during early childhood. In the neonate, sonographically, the uterus measures approximately 3.5 cm in length and 1.5 cm in width. Because the cervix is larger than the fundus, the neonatal uterus is typically spade-shaped (Fig. 14-2) (Nussbaum, 1986). An echogenic central endometrial stripe is common and reflects the transiently elevated gonadal steroid levels described earlier. Fluid is seen within the endometrial cavity in 25 percent of female newborns. Ovarian volume measures ≤1 cm^3, and small cysts are frequently found (Cohen, 1993; Garel, 2001).

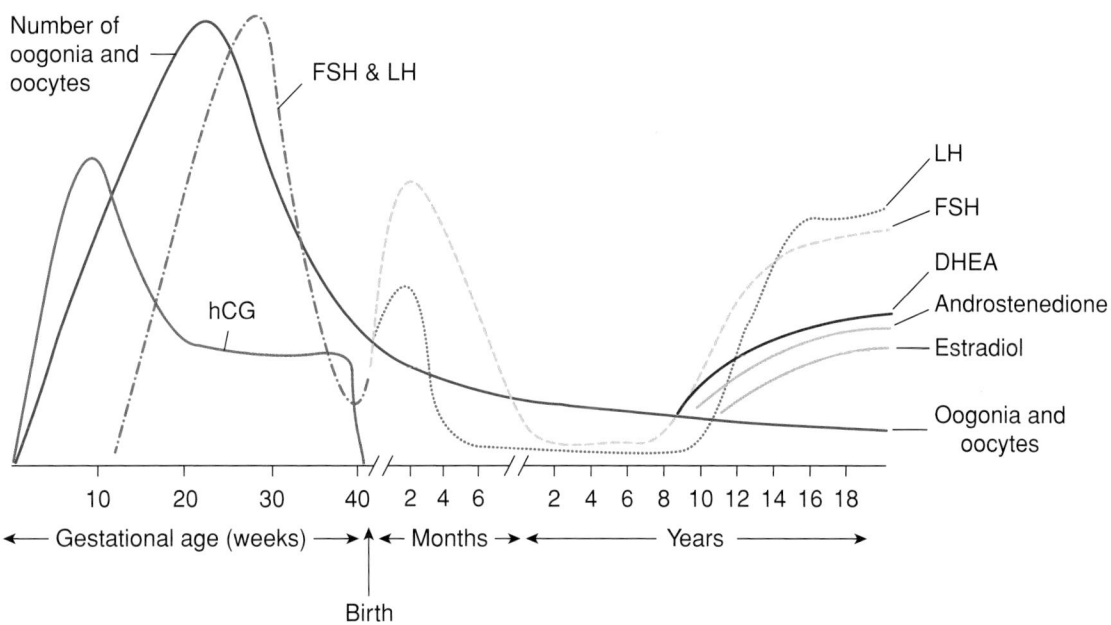

FIGURE 14-1 Variation in oocyte number and hormone levels during prenatal and postnatal periods. (DHEA = dehydroepiandrosterone; FSH = follicle-stimulating hormone; hCG = human chorionic gonadotropin; LH = luteinizing hormone.) (Reproduced with permission from Fritz M, Speroff L: Clinical Gynecologic Endocrinology and Infertility, 8th ed. Baltimore: Lippincott Williams & Wilkins; 2011.)

During childhood, the uterus measures 2.5 to 4 cm and is tubular as a result of the cervix and fundus becoming equal size. The ovaries increase in size as childhood progresses, and volumes range from 2 to 4 cm³ (Ziereisen, 2005).

■ Pubertal Changes

Puberty marks the normal physiologic transition from childhood to sexual and reproductive maturity. With puberty, primary sexual characteristics of the hypothalamus, pituitary, and ovaries initially undergo an intricate maturation process. This

maturation leads to the complex development of secondary sexual characteristics involving the breast, sexual hair, and genitalia, in addition to a limited acceleration in body growth. Each landmark of hormonal and anatomic change during this time represents a spectrum of what is considered "normal."

Marshall and Tanner (1969) recorded breast and pubic hair development in 192 English schoolgirls and created the *Tanner stages* to describe pubertal development (Fig. 14-3). Initial pubertal changes begin between ages 8 and 13 years in most North American females (Tanner, 1985). Changes before or after are categorized as either precocious puberty

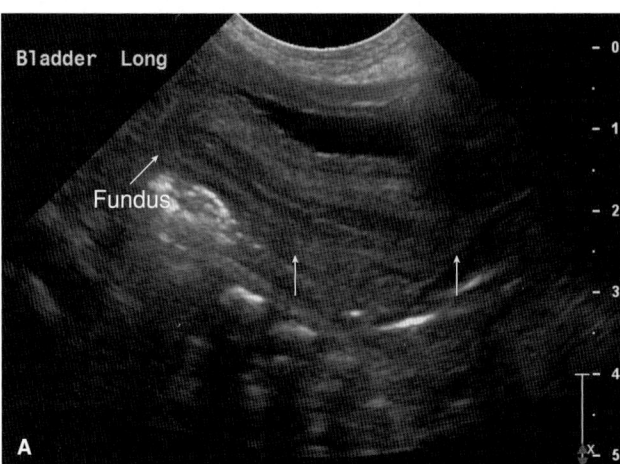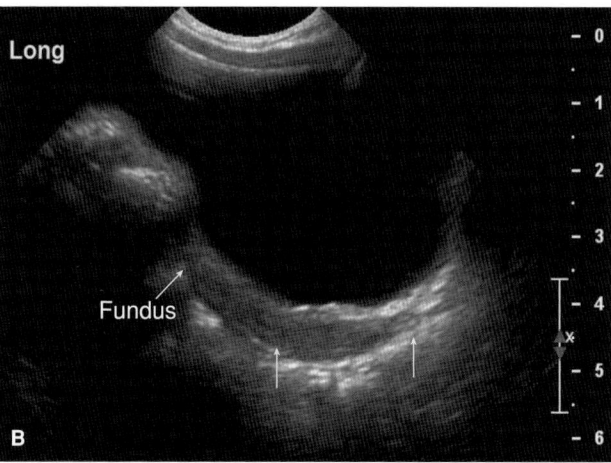

FIGURE 14-2 Transabdominal pelvic sonograms. **A.** Normal neonatal uterus. Midline longitudinal sonogram of the pelvis in this 3-day-old newborn demonstrates the uterus posterior to the bladder. Yellow arrows mark the fundus, isthmus, and cervix, respectively. The antero-posterior (AP) diameter of the cervix is greater than that of the fundus and creates a spade-shaped uterus. Due to the effect of maternal and placental hormones, a central echogenic endometrial cavity stripe is clearly visible. **B.** Normal prepubertal uterus. Midline longitudinal sonogram of the pelvis in this 3-year-old girl demonstrates the uterus posterior to the bladder. Yellow arrows mark the fundus, isthmus, and cervix, respectively. The uterus is homogeneously hypoechoic. The AP diameter of the cervix is equal to that of the fundus, and this gives the uterus a tubular shape. (Used with permission from Dr. Neil Fernandes.)

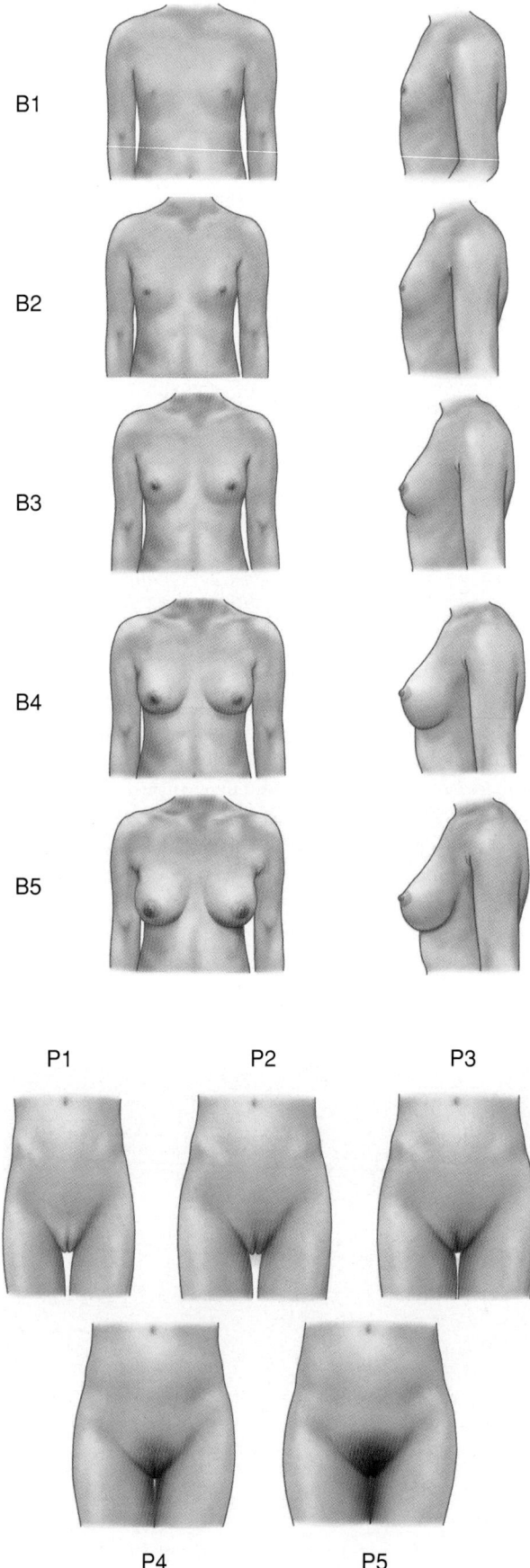

B1

B2

B3

B4

B5

P1   P2   P3

P4   P5

FIGURE 14-3 The Tanner stages of female breast and pubic hair development.

or delayed puberty and warrant evaluation. In most girls, breast budding, termed *thelarche,* is the first physical sign of puberty and begins at approximately age 10 years (Aksglaede, 2009; Biro, 2006). In a minority, pubic hair growth, known as *pubarche,* develops first. Following breast and pubic hair growth, adolescents undergo an accelerated increase in height, termed a *growth spurt,* during a 3-year span from ages 10.5 to 13.5 years.

Since these original population studies, U.S. girls have trended to start thelarche and menarche earlier. Differences in onset timing are also related to race and higher body mass index (BMI) (Biro, 2013; Rosenfield, 2009). For example, higher BMI correlates with earlier pubertal development. The mean age of menarche in white girls is 12.7 years and 6 months earlier, or 12.1, in black girls (Tanner, 1973).

GYNECOLOGIC EXAMINATION

An adolescent who has reached the age of 18 may consent to medical examination and treatment. Prior to this age, individual state laws govern whether minors can give their own consent for certain kinds of health care. Some examples include: emergency contraception, substance abuse, or sexually transmitted disease treatment. Every state has laws allowing minors to consent to care if they are emancipated, living apart from their parents, or pregnant. The Guttmacher Institute publishes an overview of Minors' Consent Law regularly at www.agi-usa.org.

A routine yearly examination of a child by her pediatrician generally includes a brief examination of the breasts and external genitalia. Congenital anomalies that are visible externally, such as imperforate hymen, may be identified. Alternatively, if parent or child has a specific complaint regarding vulvovaginal pain, rash, bleeding, discharge, or lesions, a gynecologic examination is directed toward the area of concern.

A parent or guardian should be present at the examination. This allows the child to understand that the examination is sanctioned. Moreover, clinicians can use this opportunity to inform a parent regarding findings and potential treatment. They can also emphasize the concept of inappropriate genital touching by others and parental notification if this occurs. In mid-to-late adolescence, however, a patient may prefer, for privacy reasons, not to be examined with a parent present.

"Child-friendly" objects or pictures and distracting conversation can ease fears and aid examination. Similarly, using an anatomically appropriate doll to explain the steps may decrease anxiety. The examination begins with a less-threatening approach of checking the ears, throat, heart, and lungs. Breasts are inspected. The external genital examination is best performed with the child in a frog-leg or knee-chest position to improve visualization. Occasionally, the patient may feel more comfortable sitting in a parent's lap. Sitting on a chair or examination table, the parent allows the child's legs to straddle the parent's thighs (Fig. 14-4).

Once the child is optimally positioned, each labium may be gently held with a thumb and forefinger and pulled toward the examiner and laterally. In this manner, the introitus, hymen, and lower portion of the vagina are inspected (Fig. 14-5). An

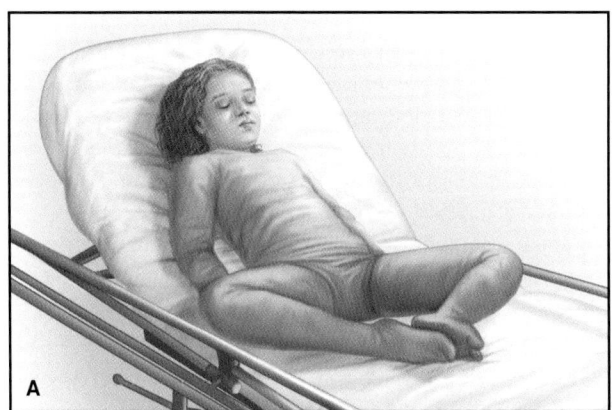

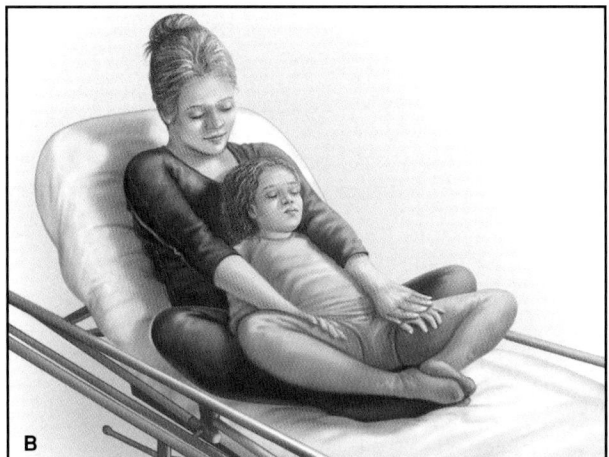

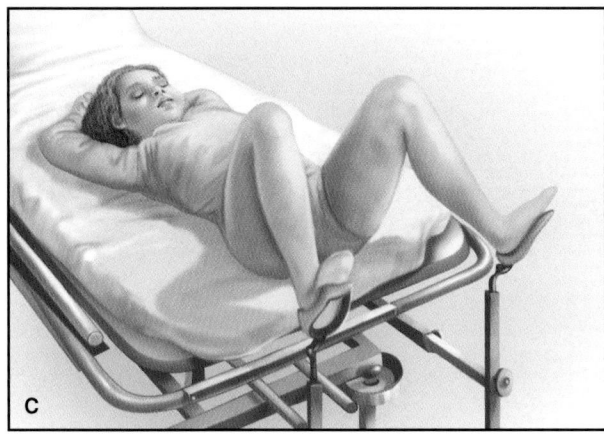

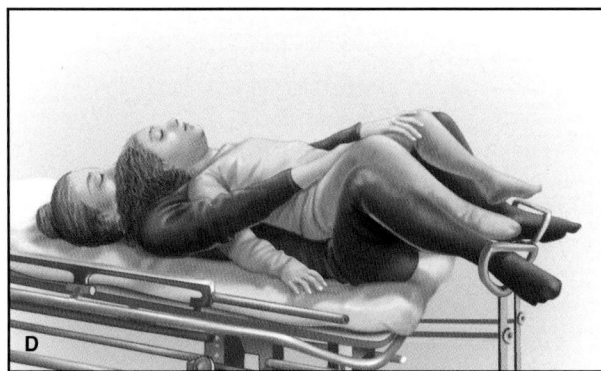

FIGURE 14-4 Various positions for examination of the pediatric patient (**A–D**).

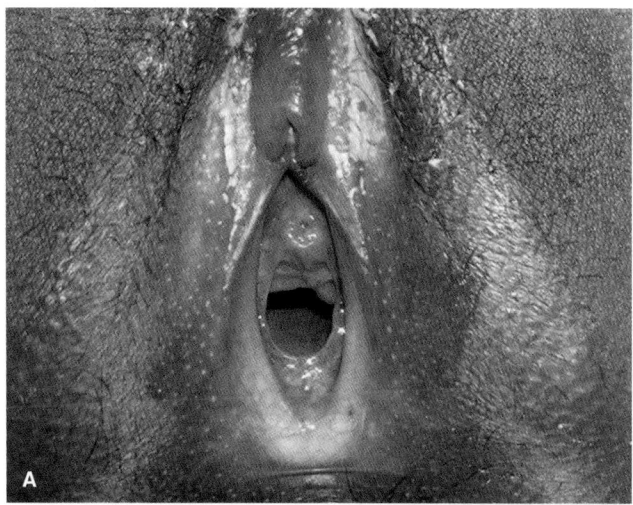

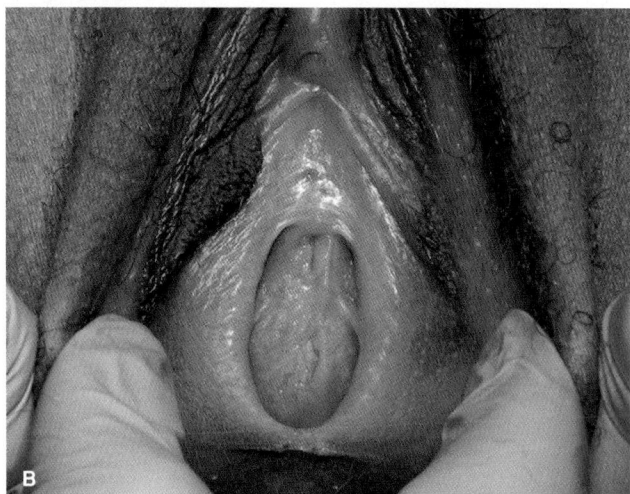

FIGURE 14-5 A. Normal prepubertal genitalia. **B.** Imperforate hymen.

internal examination is rarely necessary unless a foreign body, tumor, or vaginal bleeding is suspected. This evaluation is best accomplished under general anesthesia. Vaginoscopy may be performed using a hysteroscope or cystoscope to provide illumination as well as irrigation. During vaginoscopy, normal saline is used as the distention medium (Fig. 14-6). The labia majora are manually approximated to occlude the vagina and achieve vaginal distention.

LABIAL ADHESION

Adhesion between the labia minora begins as a small posterior midline fusion, which is usually asymptomatic. This fusion may remain an isolated minor finding or may progress toward the clitoris to completely close the vaginal orifice. Also termed *labial agglutination*, this adhesion develops in 1 to 5 percent of prepubertal girls and in approximately 10 percent of female infants within the first year of life (Berenson, 1992; Christensen, 1971).

The cause of labial adhesion is unknown, although hypoestrogenism is implicated. This fusion typically develops in a low-estrogen environment. Namely, it is seen in infants and

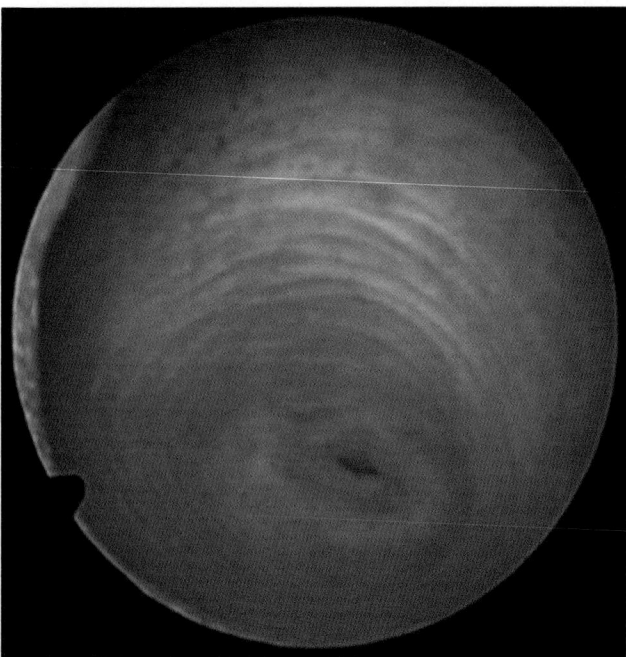

FIGURE 14-6 Photograph taken during vaginoscopy in an 8-year-old female. Typical for prepubertal girls, the cervix is almost flush with the proximal vagina.

young girls and tends to undergo spontaneous resolution at puberty (Jenkinson, 1984). Additionally, erosion of the vulvar epithelium is implicated in some cases of labial adhesion. For example, adhesion can be associated with lichen sclerosus, with herpes simplex viral infection, and with vulvar trauma following sexual abuse (Berkowitz, 1987).

The diagnosis is made visually. The labia majora appear normal, whereas the labia minora are fused with a distinct thin line of demarcation or *raphe* between them (Fig. 14-7). Extensive agglutination may leave only a ventral pinhole meatus between the labia. Located immediately beneath the clitoris, this small opening may lead to urinary dribbling as urine pools behind the adhesion. In these cases, urinary tract infection or urethritis can develop.

Treatment varies according to the degree of scarring and symptoms. In many instances, if the patient is asymptomatic, no intervention is necessary as the adhesion will typically resolve spontaneously with the rise of estrogen levels at puberty. Extensive adhesion with urinary symptoms, however, will require estrogen cream therapy. Estradiol (Estrace) cream or conjugated equine estrogen (Premarin) cream is applied to the fine, thin raphe twice daily for 2 weeks, followed by daily applications for an additional 2 weeks. A generous pea-sized amount of cream is placed with a finger or cotton-tipped applicator onto the raphe. With each application, gentle outward traction is exerted on the labia majora to help separate the adhesion. Similarly, light pressure may also be applied with the cotton applicator itself, as tolerated. After adhesion separation, a petroleum jelly (Vaseline) or vitamins A and D ointment (A&D ointment) may be applied nightly for 6 months to decrease the risk of recurrence. If the adhesion reforms during the subsequent months or years, the process may be similarly

repeated. Occasionally, with overuse of estrogen cream, local irritation, vulvar pigmentation, and minor breast budding may develop, at which time topical treatment is discontinued. These side effects are reversible once treatment is halted. Alternatively, the use of 0.05-percent betamethasone cream applied twice daily for 4 to 6 weeks is another topical option (Mayoglou, 2009; Meyers, 2006).

Manual separation of labial adhesion in an outpatient setting without analgesia is painful and thus generally not advised. In addition, recurrence is much more common. However, if the adhesion persists despite consistent use of estrogen cream, then labia minora separation may be attempted several minutes after applying 5-percent lidocaine ointment to the adhesion raphe.

If separation is not easily accomplished or tolerated, surgical separation is recommended in an operating room under general anesthesia as an outpatient procedure. Midline division of the fused labia, also termed *introitoplasty*, uses an electrosurgical fine tip and does not require suturing. To prevent repeated agglutination after surgery, an estrogen cream is applied nightly for 2 weeks. This is followed by an emollient cream nightly for at least 6 months.

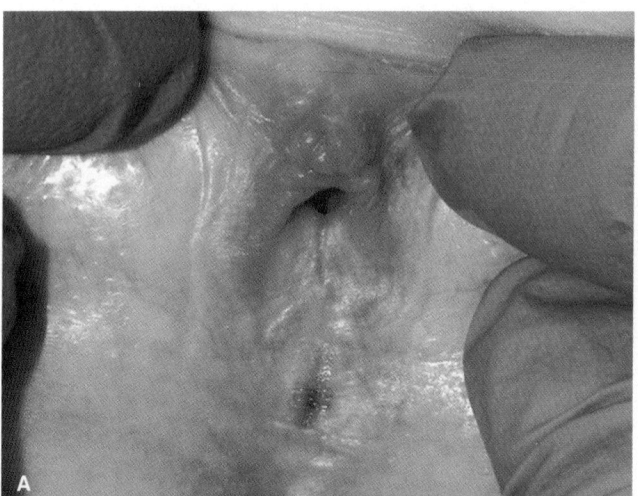

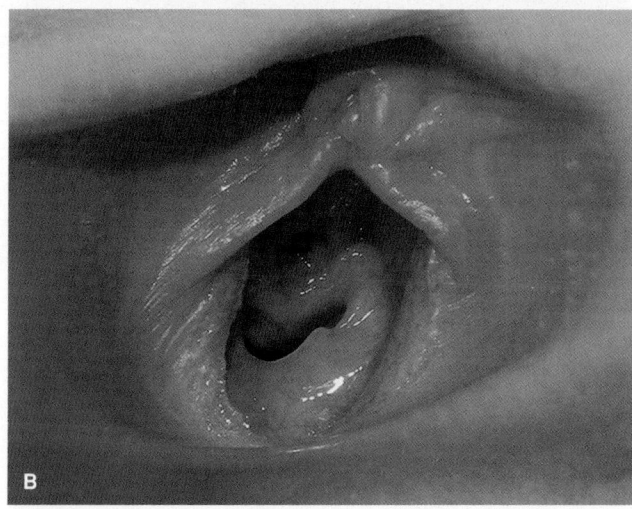

FIGURE 14-7 Labial adhesion. **A.** Labia minora are agglutinated in the midline. **B.** Resolution and restoration of normal anatomy.

CONGENITAL ANATOMIC ANOMALIES

Several anatomic and müllerian abnormalities present in early adolescence as obstructions to menstrual outflow. Described in Chapter 18, those most commonly presenting with outlet obstruction include imperforate hymen, transverse vaginal septum, cervical and vaginal agenesis with an intact uterus, obstructed (non-communicating) uterine horn, and the OHVIRA syndrome (obstructed hemivagina with ipsilateral renal agenesis) (Smith, 2007). These are often diagnosed in an adolescent with primary amenorrhea and cyclic pain. Notably, an adolescent with OHVIRA or with an obstructed uterine horn will have menses, but these often become increasingly painful over 6 to 9 months.

VULVITIS

Allergic and Contact Dermatitis

Vulvar inflammation may develop in isolation or in association with vaginitis. Allergic and contact dermatitis are common, whereas atopic dermatitis (eczema) and psoriasis are less frequent sources of itching and rash. With allergic and contact dermatitis the underlying pathophysiology varies, but the clinical appearance is usually similar. Vesicles or papules form on bright-red, edematous skin. However, in chronic cases, scaling, skin fissuring, and lichenification may be seen. In response, information regarding the degree of hygiene and continence and exposure to potential skin irritants is sought.

Typical offending agents include bubble baths and soaps, laundry detergents, fabric softeners and dryer sheets, bleach, and perfumed or colored toilet paper (Table 4-1, p. 87). Topical creams, lotions, and ointments used to soothe an area may also be an irritant to some children. For most, removing the offending agent and encouraging once- or twice-daily sitz baths is sufficient. These baths consist of placing two tablespoons of baking soda in warm water and soaking for 20 minutes. If itching is severe, an oral medication may be prescribed, such as hydroxyzine hydrochloride (Atarax) 2 mg/kg/d divided in four doses. Alternatively, a 2.5-percent topical hydrocortisone ointment can be applied twice daily for 1 week. Aside from chemical irritants, children can also develop diaper dermatitis from urine and stool exposure. Corrective measures keep the skin dry by more frequent diaper changes, or they create a moisture barrier by application of emollient creams, such as Vaseline or A&D ointment.

Lichen Sclerosus

Vulvitis may also be caused by lichen sclerosus. With this, the vulva displays hypopigmentation; atrophic, parchment-like skin; and occasional fissuring. Lesions are usually symmetrical and may form an "hourglass" appearance around the vulva and perianal areas (Fig. 14-8). Occasionally, the vulva develops dark purple vulvar ecchymoses, which may bleed. Over time, if left untreated, the periclitoral area may scar, the labia minora may become attenuated, and the posterior fourchette may fissure and bleed.

Similar to labial adhesion, lichen sclerosus can develop concurrently with hypoestrogenism or with inflammation. Lichen

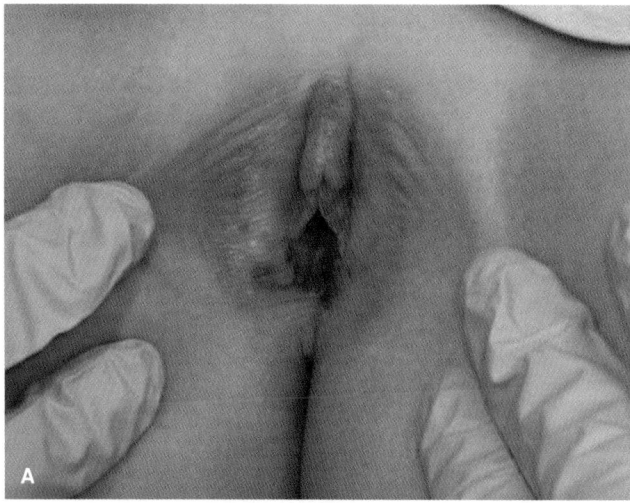

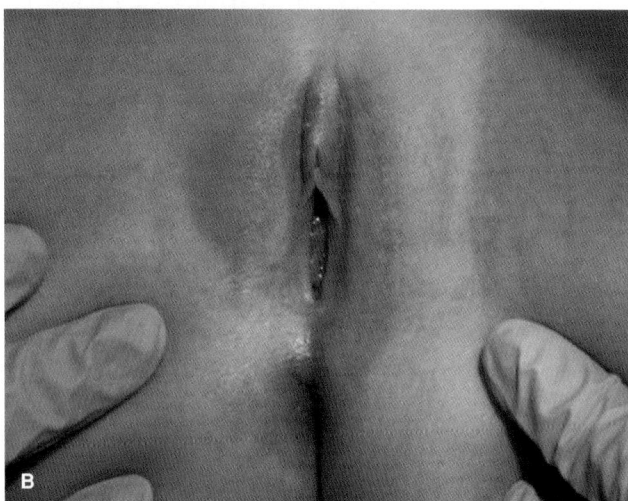

FIGURE 14-8 Lichen sclerosus before and after treatment. **A.** Findings include thin, parchment-like skin on the labia majora, ecchymoses on the labia minora and majora, and mild disease on the perianal skin. Involvement of both the vulva and perinal skin gives a figure-of-eight shape to affected areas. **B.** Skin texture and ecchymoses improved following treatment. (Used with permission from Dr. Mary Jane Pearson.)

sclerosus more commonly affects postmenopausal women and carries risks for vulvar malignancy. This association is not found in affected pediatric patients. The exact pathophysiology of lichen sclerosus is unknown, although an autoimmune process is suspected given its association with Graves thyroiditis, vitiligo, and pernicious anemia. Twin and cohort studies suggest a genetic role (Meyrick Thomas, 1986; Sherman, 2010).

Patients may complain of intense itching, discomfort, bleeding, excoriations, and dysuria. Diagnosis typically relies on visual inspection. However, rarely, a vulvar biopsy may be indicated in children if the classic skin changes are absent.

Treatment consists of topical corticosteroid cream such as 2.5-percent hydrocortisone, applied nightly to the vulva for 6 weeks. If improvement is noted, the dose may be lowered to 1-percent hydrocortisone and continued for 4 to 6 weeks. Thereafter, petroleum-based ointment use and strict attention to hygiene are recommended. Severe cases require a more potent corticosteroid such as 0.05-percent clobetasol propionate

(Temovate), applied twice daily for 2 weeks. This initial dosing is followed by an individualized regimen, which slowly tapers the dose to a once-weekly bedtime application. The long-term prognosis for childhood lichen sclerosus is unclear. Although some cases resolve at puberty, small case series suggest that as many as 75 percent of affected children have disease that persists or recurs following puberty (Berth-Jones, 1991; Powell, 2002; Smith, 2009).

◼ Infection

Some common infectious organisms that may cause prepubertal vulvitis include group A beta-hemolytic streptococcus, *Candida* species, and pinworms. With group A beta-hemolytic streptococcus, the vulva and introitus may be bright "beefy" red, and symptoms include dysuria, vulvar pain, pruritus, or bleeding. In most cases, vulvovaginal culture and clinical setting typically lead to diagnosis. Group A beta-hemolytic streptococcus is treated with an oral first-generation penicillin or cephalosporin or other appropriate antibiotic for 2 to 4 weeks.

Candidiasis is rare in prepubertal girls. It more often develops during the first year of life, after a course of antibiotics, or in females with juvenile diabetes or immunocompromise. A reddened, raised rash with well-demarcated borders and occasional satellite lesions is typical. Microscopic examination of a vaginal sample prepared with 10-percent potassium hydroxide (KOH) will help identify hyphae (Fig. 3-6, p. 61). For treatment, antifungal creams such as clotrimazole, miconazole, or butoconazole are applied to the vulva twice daily for 10 to 14 days or until the rash clears.

Enterobius vermicularis, also known as *pinworm,* can create intense vulvar itching. Nocturnal pruritus results from an intestinal infection with these 1-cm-long threadlike white worms that often exit the anus at night. Inspecting this area with a flashlight at night, parents may identify worms perianally. The "Scotch-tape test" entails pressing a piece of cellophane tape to the perianal area in the morning, affixing the tape to a slide, and visualizing parasite eggs by microscopy. Treatment is albendazole (Albenza) 200 to 400 mg in a single-dose chewable tablet.

VULVOVAGINITIS

Several months after birth, as estrogen levels wane, the vulvovaginal epithelium becomes thin and atrophic. As a result, the vulva and vagina are more susceptible to irritants and infections until puberty, and vulvovaginitis is a common prepubertal problem. Three fourths of vulvovaginitis cases in this age group are nonspecific, with culture results yielding "normal flora." Alternatively, several infectious agents, discussed subsequently, may be identified.

With nonspecific vulvovaginitis, the pathogenesis is not well defined, but known instigating factors are included in Table 14-1. Symptoms include itching, vulvar redness, discharge, dysuria, and odor. Most children and those adolescents who are not sexually active tolerate speculum examination poorly. But a vaginal swab for bacterial culture can be comfortably obtained. In cases of nonspecific vulvovaginitis, cultures typically only isolate normal vaginal flora. Culture results that reveal bowel

TABLE 14-1. Causes of Vulvovaginitis in Children

Poor vulvar hygiene
Short distance from the anus to the vagina
Inadequate front-to-back wiping after bowel movements
Lack of labial fat pads and labial hair
Nonestrogenized vulvovaginal epithelium
Vaginal foreign body
Chemical irritants such as soaps
Coexistent eczema or seborrhea
Chronic disease or altered immune status
Sexual abuse

flora suggest contamination with fecal aerobes. Treatment attempts to correct the underlying cause. Itching and inflammation may be relieved with a low-dose topical corticosteroid such as hydrocortisone, 1 or 2.5 percent. Occasionally, severe itching can lead to a secondary bacterial infection that requires oral antibiotics. Oral agents often selected are amoxicillin, an amoxicillin plus clavulanic acid combination, or a similar cephalosporin given during a 7- to 10-day course.

Infectious vulvovaginitis often presents with a malodorous, yellow or green purulent discharge, and vaginal cultures are routinely obtained in these cases. The respiratory pathogen group A beta-hemolytic streptococcus is the most common specific infectious agent found in prepubertal females and is isolated from 7 to 20 percent of girls with vulvovaginitis (Pierce, 1992; Piippo, 2000). Treatment of group A beta-hemolytic streptococcus consists of amoxicillin, 40 mg/kg, taken orally three times daily for 10 days. Less frequently, other respiratory pathogens found include: *Haemophilus influenzae, Staphylococcus aureus,* and *Streptococcus pneumoniae.* Enteric pathogens such as *Shigella* and *Yersinia* species may also be found by culture of vaginal discharge. Classically, *Shigella* species incite a mucopurulent bloody discharge, which typically follows diarrhea caused by the same organism. Treatment is with oral trimethoprim-sulfamethoxazole (TMP-SMZ), 6 to 10 mg/kg/d, divided and given every 12 hours (Bogaerts, 1992).

As discussed in Chapter 13, sexual abuse may lead to infections, including those caused by *Neisseria gonorrhoeae, Chlamydia trachomatis,* herpes simplex virus (HSV), *Trichomonas vaginalis,* and human papillomavirus (HPV). The clinical presentation of each mirrors the infectious findings in adults. Perinatal vertical transmission and latency may permit some of these to persist into infancy and childhood (Chap. 13, p. 310). Long latency and several possible modes of transmission rendered HPV especially difficult to assign origin (Fig. 14-9) (Unger, 2011). That said, child protective services are notified of any child suspected to be the victim of sexual abuse.

GENITAL TRAUMA

The prepubertal vulva is less protected from blunt injury due to the lack of labial fat pads. In addition, children are more physically active, thereby increasing the trauma risk. Fortunately, most injuries to the vulva are blunt, minor, and accidental. Sharp-object penetration, however, may cause more serious

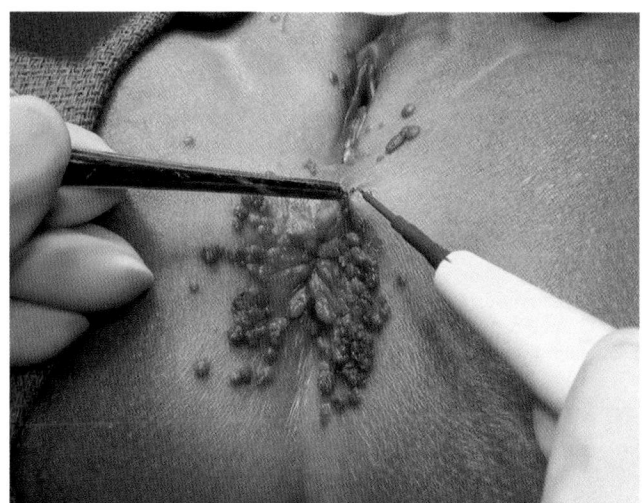

FIGURE 14-9 Surgical excision of extensive perinanal and vulvar condyloma in a prepubertal girl.

injury to the vulvovaginal area. Sexual or physical abuse is also considered. Management of vulvovaginal trauma is discussed in more detail in Chapter 4 (p. 100).

OVARIAN TUMORS

Ovarian masses, typically cysts, are common in childhood. They may be found prenatally during maternal sonographic evaluation or during prepubertal years and adolescence. Although most are benign, approximately 1 percent of all malignant tumors in this age group are ovarian (Breen, 1977, 1981).

Fetal and neonatal ovarian cysts are typically cystic and identified incidentally during maternal sonographic examination. Although the true incidence of fetal ovarian cysts is not known, some cystic development has been reported in 30 to 70 percent of female fetuses (Brandt, 1991; Lindeque, 1988). Most fetal cysts result from maternal hormonal stimulation in utero. Those during the neonatal period and infancy usually develop from the postnatal gonadotropin surge seen with the withdrawal of maternal hormones after birth. They are usually simple, unilateral, asymptomatic, and regress spontaneously by 4 months after birth, whether they are simple or complex. The risk of malignancy is low, although rupture, intracystic hemorrhage, visceral compression, and torsion followed by autoamputation of the ovary or adnexa may be uncommon complications.

For uncomplicated fetal or neonatal cysts measuring less than 5 cm in diameter, appropriate management is observation and sonographic examination every 4 to 6 weeks (Bagolan, 2002; Nussbaum, 1988; Papic, 2014). For simple cysts measuring greater than 5 cm, percutaneous cyst aspiration has been described to prevent torsion (Bryant, 2004; Noia, 2012). Large complex ovarian cysts that do not regress postnatally require surgical excision.

In children, most ovarian masses are cystic and symptoms vary. Asymptomatic cysts may be discovered incidentally during abdominal examination or during sonographic examination for some other indication. Enlarging cysts can increase abdominal girth or cause chronic pain. Hormone-secreting cysts may lead to isosexual or heterosexual precocious puberty, and thus

evaluation for signs of early pubertal development is indicated. Moreover, rupture, hemorrhage, or torsion may precipitate acute abdominal pain, similar to that seen in adults.

For imaging, a prepubertal child will not tolerate sonographic examination with a transvaginal probe. Thus, in this age group, transabdominal pelvic sonography is most frequently used. Computed tomography (CT) is helpful if a mature cystic teratoma (dermoid cyst) is suspected, as fat is better appreciated with this modality. Although magnetic resonance (MR) imaging is preferred for congenital müllerian anomaly evaluation, it is less helpful than pelvic sonography for ovarian mass determination. The most common complex cysts found in childhood and adolescence are germ cell tumors, specifically benign mature cystic teratoma (Panteli, 2009). Rarely, tumors may be malignant germ cell tumors or epithelial ovarian tumors (Schultz, 2006; Tapper, 1983).

As with those of the fetal and neonatal periods, small simple ovarian cysts without septation or internal echoes may be monitored with serial sonographic examination. Most less than 5 cm will resolve within 1 to 4 months (Thind, 1989). Persistent or enlarging cysts warrant surgical intervention, and laparoscopy is preferred. Optimal management includes fertility-sparing ovarian cystectomy with preservation of normal ovarian tissue.

Following puberty, ovarian cysts in adolescents, as in adults, are frequent. Management mirrors that of adnexal masses found in adults as described in Chapter 9 (p. 215).

BREAST DEVELOPMENT AND DISEASE

Some newborns may have minor breast budding due to transplacental passage of maternal hormones in utero. Similarly, newborn breasts may produce *witches' milk*, which is a bilateral white nipple discharge, also a result of maternal hormone stimulation. Both effects are transient and diminish over several weeks to months.

At puberty, under the influence of ovarian hormones, the breast bud grows rapidly. The epithelial sprouts of the mammary gland branch further and become separated by increasing deposition of fat. Such breast development, termed *thelarche*, begins in most girls between the ages of 8 and 13 years. Thelarche prior to age 8 or lack of breast development by age 13 is considered abnormal and investigated (p. 327).

Breast examination begins in the newborn period and extends through the prepubertal and adolescent years, as abnormalities can develop in any age group. Assessment includes inspection for accessory nipples, infection, lipoma, fibroadenoma, and premature thelarche.

■ Polythelia

Accessory nipples, also termed *polythelia*, are common and noted in 1 percent of patients. Most frequently, a small areola and nipple are found along the embryonic milk line, which extends from the axilla to the groin bilaterally. Accessory nipples are usually asymptomatic, and excision is not required. Rarely, however, they may contain glandular tissue that can lead to pain, nipple discharge, or development of fibroadenomas.

Premature Thelarche

Thelarche may begin before age 8 in some girls and if early, is most commonly seen in girls younger than 2 years. This early breast maturation is termed *premature thelarche*. It differs from precocious puberty in that it is self-limited and develops in isolation, without other signs of pubertal development. Premature thelarche is suspected when minimal breast tissue growth or nipple maturation is noted during surveillance, but the patient's height, which is measured to exclude a growth spurt, falls within established percentile curves. Monitoring body growth and breast changes alone may suffice, but in those with increased height or weight or with other pubertal changes, additional testing for precocious puberty is warranted. Thus, analysis of the patient's growth curve and Tanner stage; a radiographic bone age study; and gonadotropin measurement may be indicated (p. 328).

To explain bone age, as children develop, their bones change in size and shape. These changes can be seen radiographically and can be correlated with chronologic age. Thus, the radiographic "bone age" is the average age at which children in general reach a particular stage of bone maturation. Girls with early estrogen excess from precocious puberty show growth-rate acceleration, rapid bone age advancement, early cessation of growth, and eventual short stature because of this early cessation. Bone age can be determined at many skeletal sites, and the hand and wrist are the most commonly selected.

Premature thelarche is suggested if the bone age is synchronous and thus falls within 2 standard deviations of chronologic age. However, if the bone age is advanced by 2 or more years, puberty has begun and evaluation of precocious puberty is indicated. In those with isolated premature thelarche, serum estradiol levels may be slightly elevated, and this is seen more commonly in those who were very low-birthweight infants (Klein, 1999; Nelson, 1983). In addition, serum gonadotropin levels are in the prepubertal range. In most cases, premature breast development regresses or stabilizes, and treatment consists of reassurance with careful surveillance for other signs of precocious puberty.

Breast Shape

Growth during early breast development in girls aged 13 to 14 years may be asymmetric. The etiology is not known. However, in some cases, sports injury or surgical trauma during early breast development may lead to asymmetry (Goyal, 2003; Jansen, 2002). Examination seeks to exclude a breast mass such as a fibroadenoma or cyst. If no mass is identified, then yearly breast examinations determine the extent and persistence of asymmetry. In most cases, asymmetry will resolve by the completion of breast maturity (Templeman, 2000). Therefore, a decision toward surgical intervention is not made until full breast growth is attained. Until that time, adolescents may be fitted with padded bras or even prosthetic inserts to ensure symmetry when fully clothed.

Extremely large breasts without concurrent large breast masses can rarely develop in adolescence. Such breast hypertrophy can incite back pain, shoulder discomfort from bra-strap pressure, kyphosis, and psychologic distress. These young women will often seek reduction mammoplasty, but surgery is delayed until breast growth is completed. This is determined by serial breast measurements and is typically between the ages of 15 and 18 years.

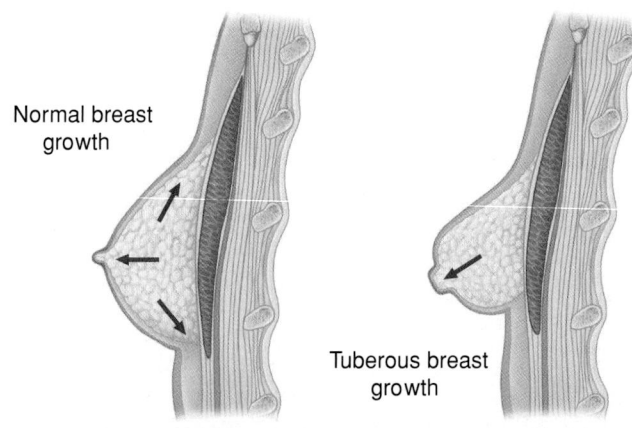

FIGURE 14-10 Comparison of normal and tuberous breast development. (Modified with permission from Grolleau JL, Lanfrey E, Lavigne B, et al: Breast base anomalies: treatment strategy for tuberous breasts, minor deformities, and asymmetry, Plast Reconstruct Surg 1999 Dec;104(7):2040–2048.)

Tuberous breasts are another growth variant (Fig. 14-10). With normal development, growth on the breast's ventral surface projects the areola forward, and circumferential peripheral growth enlarges the breast base. In some adolescents, the fascia is densely adhered to the underlying muscle and prohibits peripheral breast growth. Only forward breast growth is permitted, and *tuberous breasts* form. This appearance can also follow exogenous hormone replacement that may be prescribed to girls with a lack of breast development from genetic, metabolic, or endocrine conditions. In these conditions, to avoid tuberous development, hormone replacement is initiated at small dosages and gradually increased over time. For example, transdermal estrogen (estradiol patch), 0.025 mg, may be applied twice a week for 6 months, followed by incremental dose increases every 6 months, through doses 0.05 mg and 0.075 mg, to finally reach 0.1 mg twice a week. Medroxyprogesterone acetate (Provera), 10 mg, is given orally each day for 12 days of the month to prompt withdrawal periods. Once estrogen patch dosing has reached 0.1 mg daily, the patient may alternatively be placed on a low-dose oral contraceptive pill instead.

Absent Breast Development

Congenital absence of breast glandular tissue, termed *amastia*, is rare. More commonly, a lack of breast development results from low estrogen levels caused by constitutionally delayed puberty, chronic disease, Poland syndrome, radiation or chemotherapy, genetic disorders such as gonadal dysgenesis, or extremes of physical activity. Treatment is based on the etiology. For example, once a competitive athlete completes her career, breast development may begin spontaneously without hormonal treatment. In contrast, to prompt breast development and prevent osteoporosis, patients with gonadal dysgenesis will require some form of hormonal replacement, such as that described in the preceding section.

Breast Mass or Infection

Breast lump complaints in an adolescent often reflect fibrocystic changes. These are characterized by patchy or diffuse, bandlike thickenings. For discrete breast masses, sonography is selected to distinguish cystic from solid mass and to define cyst qualities (Garcia, 2000). In contrast, mammography has a limited role. Its limited sensitivity and specificity in young developing dense breast tissue yields high rates of false-negative results (Williams, 1986).

Actual breast cysts are found on occasion and will usually resolve spontaneously over a few weeks to months. If a cyst is large, persistent, or symptomatic, a fine-needle aspiration may be performed using local analgesia in an office setting.

Similarly, most breast masses in children and adolescents are benign and may include normal but asymmetric breast bud development, fibroadenoma, fibrocyst, lymph node, or abscess. The most common breast mass identified in adolescence is a fibroadenoma, which accounts for 68 to 94 percent of all masses (Daniel, 1968; Goldstein, 1982). Fortunately, breast cancer in pediatric populations is rare, and cancer complicated less than 1 percent of breast masses identified in this group (Gutierrez, 2008; Neinstein, 1994). Primary breast cancer may develop more frequently in pediatric patients with a history of prior radiation, especially treatment directed to the chest wall. Additionally, metastatic disease is a consideration in those with cancer.

Treatment of breast masses includes observation, needle biopsy, and surgical excision. Observation may be appropriate for small asymptomatic lesions considered to be fibroadenomas. Masses that are symptomatic, large, or enlarging are preferably excised, and techniques mirror those in the adult (Chap. 12, p. 276). For any mass not surgically excised, clinical surveillance is recommended to ensure mass stability.

Mastitis is rare in the pediatric population. Its incidence displays a bimodal distribution that peaks in the neonatal period and in children older than 10 years. The etiology in these cases is unclear, but the association with breast enlargement during these two periods has been implicated. *Staphylococcus aureus* is the most common isolate, and abscess develops more commonly than in the adult (Faden, 2005; Montague, 2013; Stricker, 2006). In adolescents, infections may be associated with lactation and pregnancy, trauma from sexual foreplay, shaving periareolar hair, and nipple piercing (Templeman, 2000; Tweeten, 1998). Infections are treated with antibiotics and occasional drainage if an abscess has formed.

VAGINAL BLEEDING

Neonates may present with vaginal bleeding during the first week of life due to the withdrawal of maternal hormones at birth. Bleeding typically resolves after a few days. Prepubertal bleeding in a child, however, merits careful evaluation (Table 14-2). Most instances of vaginal bleeding in these girls are due to local causes and can be elucidated with a simple history and physical examination. Occasionally, an examination under anesthesia with saline vaginoscopy is required for diagnosis, particularly if a foreign body is present in the upper vagina (Fig. 14-11).

PRECOCIOUS PUBERTY

Early pubertal development may be seen in both sexes, but females are much more commonly affected, with a sex ratio

TABLE 14-2. Causes of Vaginal Bleeding in Children

Foreign body
Genital tumors
Urethral prolapse
Lichen sclerosus
Vulvovaginitis
Condyloma acuminata
Trauma
Precocious puberty
Exogenous hormone usage

of 23:1 (Bridges, 1994). For girls, precocious puberty has historically been defined as breast or pubic hair development in those younger than 8 years. However, Herman-Giddens and colleagues (1997) noted that girls in the United States overall are undergoing normal pubertal development at younger ages than previously reported. In addition, racial differences exist. Puberty begins earliest in black girls, followed by Hispanic and white girls. Accordingly, to limit the proportion of girls requiring unneeded assessment for precocious puberty, some have suggested lowering the threshold age for evaluation (Herman-Giddens, 1997; Kaplowitz, 1999).

Premature pubertal development may result from various causes. These have been categorized based on pathogenesis and include central precocious puberty, peripheral precocious puberty, heterosexual precocious puberty, and temporal variation of normal puberty. Most girls evaluated are found to have normal pubertal development that has merely begun prior to standard temporal milestones and does not stem from identifiable pathology. However, because many of the underlying etiologies of precocious puberty carry significant sequelae, girls with early pubertal development are fully evaluated when identified.

■ Central Precocious Puberty (Gonadotropin Dependent)

Early activation of the hypothalamic-pituitary-ovarian axis leads to pulsatile GnRH secretion, increased gonadotropin

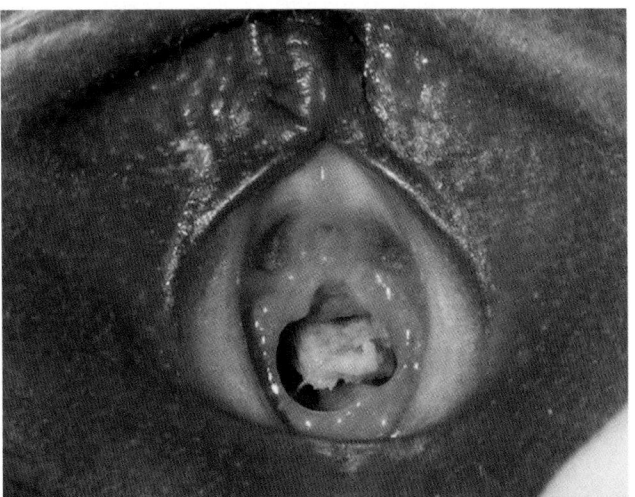

FIGURE 14-11 A clump of retained toilet paper was the foreign body found in this prepubertal girl.

formation, and in turn, increased gonadal steroid levels. Often termed *true precocious puberty*, central precocious puberty is rare and affects 1 in 5000 to 10,000 individuals in the general population (Partsch, 2002). The most common cause of central precocious puberty is idiopathic, however, central nervous system lesions must be excluded (Table 14-3).

Symptoms of central precocious puberty are similar to those of normal puberty but at an earlier age. As outlined in Table 14-4, testing includes radiographic measurement of hand and wrist bone age. In affected girls, advanced skeletal maturation is seen. In addition, serum FSH, LH, and estradiol levels are elevated for chronologic age and typically lie in the pubertal range. Early in the process, however, FSH and LH levels may be elevated only in the evenings, and a leuprolide stimulation test can be helpful. During leuprolide stimulation, baseline FSH, LH, and estradiol levels are obtained. Leuprolide (Lupron) (20 µg/kg intravenous and not to exceed 500 µg) is given, and FSH plus LH levels are measured at 1, 2, and 3 hours. An estradiol level is measured at 24 hours. Central precocious puberty is confirmed by a rise in serum LH levels following infusion. In those with elevated gonadotropin levels, MR imaging of the central nervous system may identify a cerebral abnormality associated with central precocious puberty. Pelvic sonography is performed when the estradiol level is high and gonadotropin levels are suppressed to check for ovarian cysts.

TABLE 14-3. Common Etiologies of Precocious Puberty

Central (GnRH-dependent)
Idiopathic[a]
CNS tumors
CNS anomaly
CNS infection
Head trauma
Ischemia
Iatrogenic: radiation, chemotherapy, surgical

Peripheral (GnRH-independent)
Estrogen- or testosterone-producing tumors
    (adrenal or ovarian)
Gonadotropin- or hCG-producing tumors
Congenital adrenal hyperplasia
Exogenous androgen or estrogen exposure
McCune-Albright syndrome
Ovarian follicular cysts
Primary hypothyroidism
Aromatase excess syndrome
Glucocorticoid resistance

[a]The most common cause of precocious puberty is idiopathic.
CNS = central nervous system; GnRH = gonadotropin-releasing hormone; hCG = human chorionic gonadotropin.
Data from Muir A: Precocious puberty. Pediatr Rev 2006 Oct;27(10):373–381; Nathan BM, Palmert MR: Regulation and disorders of pubertal timing. Endocrinol Metab Clin North Am 2005 Sep;34(3):617–641.

TABLE 14-4. Evaluation of Precocious Puberty[a]

Girls with signs of estrogen excess:
Radiographic bone age
FSH, LH, estradiol, TSH
Pelvic sonography
CNS magnetic resonance imaging

Girls with signs of virilization:
Radiographic bone age
FSH, LH, estradiol
DHEAS, testosterone
17α-Hydroxyprogesterone
Androstenedione
11-Deoxycortisol

Leuprolide stimulation test may help differentiate premature thelarche from true central and peripheral precocious puberty.

[a]Serum levels of the cited hormones.
CNS = central nervous system; DHEAS = dehydroepiandrosterone sulfate; FSH = follicle-stimulating hormone; GnRH = gonadotropin-releasing hormone; LH = luteinizing hormone; TSH = thyroid-stimulating hormone.

Treatment goals focus on preventing short adult height and limiting the psychologic effects of early pubertal development. Epiphyseal fusion is an estrogen-dependent process. Accordingly, girls with precocious puberty are at risk for early growth-plate closure and short stature in adulthood. Treatment consists of a GnRH agonist, which serves to downregulate pituitary gonadotropes and inhibit FSH and LH release. Estrogen levels drop, and often there is a marked regression of breast and uterine size. If therapy is instituted after menses have begun, menstrual periods will cease. Timing for the discontinuation of GnRH therapy and reinitiation of pubertal development is determined by the primary therapy goals: maximizing height, synchronizing puberty with peers, and allaying psychological distress. From a review of several studies, the mean age at treatment discontinuation was approximately 11 years (Carel, 2009).

■ Peripheral Precocious Puberty (Gonadotropin Independent)

Less commonly, elevated estrogen levels may originate from a peripheral source, such as an ovarian cyst. Termed peripheral precocious puberty, this category is characterized by lack of GnRH pulsatile release, low levels of pituitary gonadotropins, yet increased serum estrogen concentrations.

Although the originating source is variable, the most common cause is a granulosa cell tumor, accounting for more than 60 percent of cases (Emans, 2005). Other types of ovarian cysts, adrenal disorders, iatrogenic disorders, and primary hypothyroidism are additional causes (see Table 14-3). McCune-Albright syndrome is characterized by a "triad" of polyostotic fibrous dysplasia, irregular café-au-lait spots, and endocrinopathies. Precocious puberty is a frequent finding and results from estrogen production in the ovarian cysts that are common in these girls.

Testing of girls with peripheral precocious puberty finds estrogen levels that are characteristically elevated, whereas serum levels of LH and FSH are low. Bone age determination shows advanced aging, and GnRH stimulation shows no elevation in serum LH levels.

Treatment aims to eliminate estrogen. For those with exogenous exposure, halting the estrogen source, such as hormonal pills or creams, is sufficient. An estrogen-secreting ovarian or adrenal tumor will require surgical excision, and hypothyroidism is treated with thyroid hormone replacement.

■ Heterosexual Precocious Puberty

Androgen excess with signs of virilization is rare in childhood (Chap. 17, p. 389). Termed *heterosexual precocious puberty*, this condition is most commonly caused by increased androgen secretion in young females from the adrenal gland or ovary. Causes include androgen-secreting ovarian or adrenal tumors, congenital adrenal hyperplasia, Cushing syndrome, and exposure to exogenous androgens. Treatment is directed at correction of the underlying etiology.

■ Variations of Normal Puberty

Although standardized age guidelines accurately reflect the timing of pubertal development in most girls, others begin development early. Premature thelarche, premature adrenarche, and premature menarche describe the premature pubertal development of breast tissue, pubic hair, and menses, respectively. Each develops in isolation and without other evidence of pubertal development.

As described earlier (p. 327), *premature thelarche* is a diagnosis of exclusion, and evaluation for precocious puberty in these girls reveals bone ages consistent with chronologic age. Normal FSH and LH levels, normal or slightly elevated estradiol levels, normal pelvic sonographic examination, and normal growth are noted. Treatment consists of careful surveillance and reassurance that the remainder of pubertal development will progress at a normal age.

Adrenarche is the onset of dehydroepiandrosterone (DHEA) and DHEA sulfate (DHEAS) production from the adrenal zona reticularis, which can be detected around age 6 years. The phenotypic result of adrenarche is axillary and pubic hair development, termed *pubarche,* which begins in girls at approximately age 8 years (Auchus, 2004). *Premature adrenarche* is defined therefore as the growth of pubic hair prior to age 8, but other signs of estrogenization or virilization are absent. Most girls will have an increased level of DHEAS, which suggests that the adrenal gland is maturing prematurely (Korth-Schultz, 1976). Some girls with premature adrenarche are found to develop polycystic ovarian syndrome in adolescence (Ibanez, 1993; Miller, 1996). Others have a partial deficiency of 21-hydroxylase. Therefore, girls with premature adrenarche are screened for precocious puberty. When isolated, premature adrenarche treatment includes reassurance and monitoring at 3- to 6-month intervals for other signs of puberty.

Uterine bleeding that occurs once for several days or monthly, without other signs of puberty, is termed *premature menarche*. The condition is rare, and other sources of bleeding are considered and excluded first.

TABLE 14-5. Causes of Delayed Puberty

Constitutional (physiologic delay)[a]
Chronic anovulation (PCOS)
Anatomic: outlet obstruction or agenesis
Androgen insensitivity syndrome
Hypergonadotropic hypogonadism
Gonadal dysgenesis (Turner syndrome)
Pure gonadal dysgenesis (46,XX or 46,XY)
Premature ovarian failure
Hypogonadotropic hypogonadism
Central nervous system (CNS)
   CNS tumor, infection, or trauma
   Chronic disease
   GnRH deficiency (Kallman syndrome)
   Isolated gonadotropin deficiency
   Hypothyroidism
   Hyperprolactinoma
Adrenal
   Congenital adrenal hyperplasia
   Cushing syndrome
   Addison disease
Psychosocial
   Eating disorders
   Excessive exercise
   Stress, depression

[a]The most common cause of delayed puberty.
GnRH = gonadotropin-releasing hormone; PCOS = polycystic ovarian syndrome.

DELAYED PUBERTY

Puberty is considered delayed if no secondary sexual characteristics are noted by age 13, which is more than 2 standard deviations from the mean age, or if menses have not commenced by age 16. Delayed puberty affects 3 percent of adolescents. Causes include those in Table 14-5. With the exception of constitutional delay, these other abnormalities are discussed in greater detail in Chapters 16 and 18.

Constitutional delay is the most common cause, and adolescents lack both secondary sexual characteristics and pubertal growth spurt by age 13 years (Albanese, 1995; Malasanoa, 1997). The probable cause is a delay in reactivation of the GnRH pulse generator (Layman, 1994). Patients may be started on low-dose estrogen until puberty progresses, at which point estrogen may be discontinued. During low-dose estrogen treatment, it is not necessary to introduce progesterone withdrawal because in early puberty there is a similar long period of unopposed estrogen prior to ovulatory cycles.

SEXUALITY

■ Gender Identity

In most cases, phenotypic gender directs rearing practices, and girls are "raised as girls" and boys are "raised as boys."

Gender-appropriate clothes and behaviors are adopted by the child and reinforced by parental approval. Behaviors in conflict with gender are generally discouraged. However, young children will often explore various behaviors, both masculine and feminine, which make up normal experiences in the process of sex-role socialization (Mischel, 1970; Serbin, 1980).

In cases of ambiguous genitalia in the newborn, sexual assignment is more challenging. Initially, life-threatening disease such as congenital adrenal hyperplasia is excluded. As outlined in Chapter 18, gender assignment may be best delayed until test results identify genetic gender and the underlying problem.

The final gender assignment in such cases is termed the *sex of rearing* and reflects the pattern of gender behavior to be emphasized. The final determination for the sex of rearing is based not only on the individual's karyotype but also on the functional capacity of the external genitalia. For example, boys born with congenital absence of the penis, a rare disorder, are usually raised as females after bilateral orchiectomy and reconstruction of the scrotum to have the appearance of labia. If parental attitudes towards the assigned gender are consistent, most children assume the sex of rearing regardless of their genotype.

Gender dysphoria describes individuals who perceive themselves to be different from their assigned gender. In the *Diagnostic and Statistical Manual of Mental Disorders,* Fifth Edition (DSM-5), this is a recognized psychiatric diagnosis but is not considered a psychiatric disorder (American Psychiatric Association, 2013). That said, the discordance may cause depression and anxiety. One New Zealand survey of 8166 adolescents showed a prevalence of 1.2 percent for this condition (Clark, 2014). This perception can present as early as age 2 to 3 years. At our institution, the Gender Education and Care Interdisciplinary Support (GENCIS) Clinic provides a multidisciplinary approach to treating the psychological, social, and medical needs of this population of children.

Adolescent Sexuality

Adolescent sexuality develops during a period of rapid change that provides opportunities for adolescents to experience both risk-taking and health-promoting behaviors. Data from a large surveys of U.S. adolescents reveal that the percentage of those who become sexually active increases steadily after age 14 (Liu, 2015).

Adolescents view providers as an important resource for information and education regarding healthy sexual development. However, many parents and educators oppose sexuality education because of concerns that providing such information will encourage the onset of intercourse, termed *coitarche*, and will increase intercourse frequency. On the contrary, studies find that such education actually delays the onset and frequency of sexual activity, increases contraceptive use, and reduces the rate of unprotected intercourse (Kirby, 1999, 2001). One survey noted that 75 percent of adolescents attending grades 7 through 12 reported that they received classes in sexuality education (Hoff, 2000). A large percentage wanted more information on specific topics such as contraception, sexually transmitted diseases (STDs), condom use, and emotional issues.

Oral sex is now more commonplace among adolescents. The National Survey of Family Growth in 2005 reported that one in four adolescents aged 15 to 19 years who had not had vaginal intercourse reported practicing oral sex with an opposite partner. Of those adolescents who practiced sexual intercourse, 83 percent of females and 88 percent of males stated they had engaged in oral sex (Mosher, 2005). Adolescents may see oral sex as an alternative way to maintain their "virginity," prevent pregnancy, or avoid STDs, or they may perceive it as a step on the way to engaging in sexual intercourse with a dating partner.

Sexual activity and partner violence appear to have a frequent association in adolescent populations (Chap. 13, p. 311). For example, Kaestle and Halpern (2005) noted that violent victimization was more likely to occur in romantic relationships that included sexual intercourse (37 percent) compared with those that did not (19 percent). Abma and colleagues (2010) reported that among females with coitarche before age 20, 7 percent described their first intercourse as nonvoluntary.

Contraception

Despite wide availability of contraceptive options, nearly one half of pregnancies in the United States are unintended (Finer, 2014). Of adolescents, more than 20 percent do not use contraception at first intercourse, and there is a median delay of 22 months before seeking prescription methods after the sexual debut (Finer, 1998).

The most commonly used contraceptive by adolescents is the combination oral contraceptive (COC) pill. The intrauterine device and the etonogestrel implant are long-acting reversible contraceptives (LARC), and the American College of Obstetricians and Gynecologists (2014) now recommends the etonogestrel implant and the intrauterine device as first-line contraceptive options for adolescents. One study of 179 adolescents found an 85-percent continuation rate after 1 year with the levonorgestrel-releasing IUD (Paterson, 2009). Ideally, counseling begins prior to onset of sexual activity and includes discussion of emergency contraception. Many adolescents have misperceptions about contraception, including beliefs that it may cause infertility or birth defects. Such concerns may be important topics during contraceptive counseling.

Pelvic examination is not necessary when a contraceptive is prescribed if no other complaints are present. Moreover, guidelines from the American College of Obstetricians and Gynecologists (2012) note that cervical cancer screening does not usually begin until age 21 regardless of sexual activity. HIV-positive status is an exception, and full screening recommendations are described in Chapter 29 (p. 634). Sexually active adolescents are counseled and screened for gonorrhea and chlamydial infection (U.S. Preventive Services Task Force, 2014). For adolescents, the preferred method is collection of a urine sample for nucleic acid amplification testing (NAAT). Other STDs are screened as clinically indicated.

Information on HPV vaccination can also be offered. HPV vaccines, Cervarix, Gardasil 4, and Gardasil 9 are approved by the Food and Drug Administration for females aged 9 through 26 years and males ages 9 through 15. A series of three doses for girls, beginning with a first injection at age 11 or 12 years, is recommended (Kim, 2015). A second dose is administered 1 to 2 months later, and a third dose is given 6 months after the initial one. These vaccines are discussed further in Chapter 29 (p. 630).

For these types of services, the Supreme Court has ruled that minors have the right to contraceptives (*Carry v. Population Services International*). Moreover, current law dictates that all states provide consent to adolescents for treatment of "medically emancipated" conditions such as contraception, STDs, pregnancy, substance abuse, and mental health. These are legally designated medical situations for which an adolescent may receive care without the permission or knowledge of a parent or legal guardian (Akinbami, 2003).

To smooth the transition to adult care, the American College of Obstetricians and Gynecologists (2015) has published guidelines, which include ages 18 to 26 years. In addition to contraception, providers ideally discuss and screen for sexual and mental health, sleep disorders, nutrition, safety, and substance abuse.

REFERENCES

Abma JC, Martinez GM, Copen CE: Teenagers in the United States: sexual activity, contraceptive use, and childbearing, National Survey of Family Growth 2006–2008. National Center for Health Statistics. Vital Health Stat 23:30, 2010

Akinbami LJ, Gandhi H, Cheng TL: Availability of adolescent health services and confidentiality in primary care practices. Pediatrics 111:394, 2003

Aksglaede L, Sørensen K, Petersen JH, et al: Recent decline in age at breast development: the Copenhagen Puberty Study. Pediatrics 123(5):e932, 2009

Albanese A, Stanhope R: Investigation of delayed puberty. Clin Endocrinol 43:105, 1995

American College of Obstetricians and Gynecologists: Adolescents and long-acting reversible contraception: implants and intrauterine devices. Committee Opinion No. 539, October 2012, Reaffirmed 2014

American College of Obstetricians and Gynecologists: Screening for cervical cancer. Practice Bulletin No. 131, November 2012

American College of Obstetricians and Gynecologists: The transition from pediatric to adult health care: preventive care for young women aged 18–26 years. Committee Opinion No. 626, March 2015

American Psychiatric Association: Diagnostic and Statistical Manual of Mental Disorders, Fifth Edition, DSM-5, Washington, American Psychiatric Association, 2013

Auchus RJ, Rainey WE: Adrenarche—physiology, biochemistry and human disease. Clin Endocrinol 60(3):288, 2004

Bagolan P, Giorlandino C, Nahom A, et al: The management of fetal ovarian cysts. J Pediatr Surg 37:25, 2002

Berenson AB, Heger AH, Hayes JM, et al: Appearance of the hymen in prepubertal girls. Pediatrics 89:3878, 1992

Berkowitz CD, Elvik SL, Logan MK: Labial fusion in prepubescent girls: a marker for sexual abuse? Am J Obstet Gynecol 156(1):16, 1987

Berth-Jones J, Graham-Brown RA, Burns DA: Lichen sclerosus et atrophicus—a review of 15 cases in young girls. Clin Exp Dermatol 16(1):14, 1991

Biro FM, Greenspan LC, Galvez MP, et al: Onset of breast development in a longitudinal cohort. Pediatrics 132(6):1019, 2013

Biro FM, Huang B, Crawford PB, et al: Pubertal correlates in black and white girls. J Pediatr 148(2):234, 2006

Bogaerts J, Lepage P, De Clercq A, et al: Shigella and gonococcal vulvovaginitis in prepubertal central African girls. Pediatr Infect Dis J 11:890, 1992

Brandt ML, Luks FI, Filiatrault D, et al: Surgical indications in antenatally diagnosed ovarian cysts. J Pediatr Surg 26:276, 1991

Breen JL, Bonamo JF, Maxson WS: Genital tract tumors in children. Pediatr Clin North Am 28:355, 1981

Breen JL, Maxson WS: Ovarian tumors in children and adolescents. Clin Obstet Gynecol 20:607, 1977

Bridges NA, Christopher JA, Hindmarsh PC, et al: Sexual precocity: sex incidence and aetiology. Arch Dis Child 70:116, 1994

Bryant AE, Laufer MR: Fetal ovarian cysts: incidence, diagnosis and management. J Reprod Med 49:329, 2004

Carel JC, Eugster EA, Rogol A, et al: Consensus statement on the use of gonadotropin-releasing hormone analogs in children. Pediatrics 123:e752, 2009

Christensen EH, Oster J: Adhesions of labia minora (synechia vulvae) in childhood: a review and report of fourteen cases. Acta Paediatr Scand 60:709, 1971

Clark TC, Lucassen MF, Bullen P, et al: The health and well-being of transgender high school students: results from the New Zealand adolescent health survey (Youth'12). J Adolesc Health 55(1):93, 2014

Cohen HL, Shapiro M, Mandel F, et al: Normal ovaries in neonates and infants: a sonographic study of 77 patients 1 day to 24 months old. AJR 160:583, 1993

Daniel WA Jr, Mathews MD: Tumors of the breast in adolescent females. Pediatrics 41:743, 1968

Emans S, Laufer M, Goldstein D: Pediatric and Adolescent Gynecology, 5th ed. Philadelphia: Lippincott Williams & Wilkins, 2005, pp 127, 159

Faden H: Mastitis in children from birth to 17 years. Pediatr Infect Dis J 24(12):1113, 2005

Finer LB, Zabin LS: Does the timing of the first family planning visit still matter? Fam Plann Perspect 30(1):30, 1998

Finer LB, Zolna MR: Shifts in intended and unintended pregnancies in the United States, 2001–2008. Am J Public Health 104 (Suppl 1):S43, 2014

Fritz M, Speroff L: Clinical Gynecologic Endocrinology and Infertility, 8th ed. Baltimore, Lippincott Williams & Wilkins, 2011, pp 117, 393

Garcia CJ, Espinoza A, Dinamarca V, et al: Breast US in children and adolescents. Radiographics 20:1605, 2000

Garel L, Dubois J, Grignon A, et al: US of the pediatric female pelvis: a clinical perspective. Radiographics 21(6):1393, 2001

Goldstein DP, Miler V: Breast masses in adolescent females. Clin Pediatr 21:17, 1982

Goyal A, Mansel RE: Iatrogenic injury to the breast bud causing breast hypoplasia. Postgrad Med J 79(930):235, 2003

Grolleau JL, Lanfrey E, Lavigne B, et al: Breast base anomalies: treatment strategy for tuberous breasts, minor deformities, and asymmetry. Plast Reconstruct Surg 104(7):2040, 1999

Gutierrez JC, Housri N, Koniaris LG et al: Malignant breast cancer in children: a review of 75 patients. J Surg Res 147(2):182, 2008

Herman-Giddens ME, Slora EJ, Wasserman RC, et al: Secondary sexual characteristics and menses in young girls seen in office practice: a study from the Pediatric Research in Office Settings network. Pediatrics 99:505, 1997

Hoff T, Greene L, McIntosh M, et al: Sex education in America: a view from inside the nation's classrooms. Menlo Park, Henry J. Kaiser Family Foundation, 2000

Ibanez L, Potau N, Virdis R, et al: Postpubertal outcome in girls diagnosed of premature pubarche during childhood: increased frequency of functional ovarian hyperandrogenism. J Clin Endocrinol Metab 76:1599, 1993

Jansen DA, Spencer SR, Leveque JE: Premenarchal athletic injury to the breast bud as the cause for asymmetry: prevention and treatment. Breast J 8:108, 2002

Jenkinson SD, MacKinnon AE: Spontaneous separation of fused labia minora in prepubertal girls. Br Med J (Clin Res Ed) 289:160, 1984

Kaestle CE, Halpern CT: Sexual intercourse precedes partner violence in adolescent romantic relationships. J Adolesc Health 36(5):386, 2005

Kaplowitz PB, Oberfield SE: Reexamination of the age limit for defining when puberty is precocious in girls in the United States: implications for evaluation and treatment. Pediatrics 104:936, 1999

Kim DK, Bridges CB, Harriman HK, et al: Advisory Committee on Immunization Practices recommended immunization schedule for adults aged 19 years or older: United States, 2015. Ann Intern Med 162:214, 2015

Kirby D: Emerging answers: research findings on programs to reduce teenage pregnancy. The National Campaign to Prevent Teen Pregnancy, Washington, 2001

Kirby D: Reducing adolescent pregnancy: approaches that work. Contemp Pediatr 16:83, 1999

Klein KO, Mericq V, Brown-Dawson JM, et al: Estrogen levels in girls with premature thelarche compared with normal prepubertal girls as determined by an ultrasensitive recombinant cell bioassay. J Pediatr 134:190, 1999

Korth-Shcultz S, Levine LS, New M: Dehydroepiandrosterone sulfate (DS) levels, a rapid test for abnormal adrenal androgen secretion. J Clin Endocrinol Metab 42:1005, 1976

Layman LC, Reindollar RH: Diagnosis and treatment of pubertal disorders. Adolesc Med 5:37, 1994

Lindeque BG, du Toit JP, Muller LM, et al: Ultrasonographic criteria for the conservative management of antenatally diagnosed fetal ovarian cysts. J Reprod Med 33:196, 1988

Liu G, Hariri S, Bradley H, et al: Trends and patterns of sexual behaviors among adolescents and adults aged 14 to 59 years, United States. Sex Transm Dis 42(1):20, 2015

Malasanoa TH: Sexual development of the fetus and pubertal child. Clin Obstet Gynecol 40:153, 1997

Marshall WA, Tanner JM: Variations in pattern of pubertal changes in girls. Arch Dis Child 44(235):291, 1969

Mayoglou L, Dulabon L, Martin-Alguacil N, et al: Success of treatment modalities for labial fusion: a retrospective evaluation of topical and surgical treatments. J Pediatr Adolesc Gynecol 22(4):247, 2009

Meyers JB, Sorenson CM, Wisner BP, et al: Betamethasone cream for the treatment of pre-pubertal labial adhesions. J Pediatr Adolesc Gynecol 19(6):401, 2006

Meyrick Thomas RH, Kennedy CT: The development of lichen sclerosus et atrophicus in monozygotic twin girls. Br J Dermatol 114:337, 1986

Miller DP, Emans SJ, Kohane I: A follow-up study of adolescent girls with a history of premature pubarche. J Adolesc Health 18(4):301, 1996

Mischel W: Sex-typing and socialization. In Mussen PH (ed): Carmichaels Manual of Child Psychology, 3rd ed. New York, Wiley, 1970, p 3

Montague EC, Hilinski J, Andresen D, et al: Evaluation and treatment of mastitis in infants. Pediatr Infect Dis J 32(11):1295, 2013

Mosher WD, Chandra A, Jones J: Sexual behavior and selected health measures: men and women 15–44 years of age, United States, 2002. Adv Data, 362:1, 2005

Muir A: Precocious puberty. Pediatr Rev 27:373, 2006

Nathan BM, Palmert MR: Regulation and disorders of pubertal timing. Endocrinol Metab Clin North Am 34(3):617, 2005

Neely EK, Hintz RL, Wilson DM, et al: Normal ranges for immuno- chemiluminometric gonadotropin assays. J Pediatr 124(1):40, 1995

Neinstein LA: Review of breast masses in adolescents. Adolesc Pediatr Gynecol 7:119, 1994

Nelson KG: Premature thelarche in children born prematurely. J Pediatr 103:756, 1983

Noia G, Riccardi M, Visconti D, et al: Invasive fetal therapies: approach and results in treating fetal ovarian cysts. J Matern Fetal Neonatal Med 25(3):299, 2012

Nussbaum A, Sanders R, Jones M: Neonatal uterine morphology as seen on real-time US. Radiology 160:641, 1986

Nussbaum AR, Sanders RC, Hartman DS, et al: Neonatal ovarian cysts: sonographic-pathologic correlation. Radiology 168:817, 1988

Panteli C, Curry J, Kiely E, et al: Ovarian germ cell tumours: a 17-year study in a single unit. Eur J Pediatr Surg 19(2):96, 2009

Papic JC, Billmire DF, Rescorla FJ, et al: Management of neonatal ovarian cysts and its effect on ovarian preservation. J Pediatr Surg 49(6):990, 2014

Partsch CJ, Heger S, Sippell WG: Management and outcome of central precocious puberty. Clin Endocrinol 56(2):129, 2002

Paterson H, Ashton J, Harrison-Woolrych M: A nationwide cohort study of the use of the levonorgestrel intrauterine device in New Zealand adolescents. Contraception 79(6):433, 2009

Pierce AM, Hart CA: Vulvovaginitis: causes and management. Arch Dis Child 67:509, 1992

Piippo S, Lenko H, Vuento R: Vulvar symptoms in paediatric and adolescent patients. Acta Paediatrica 89:431, 2000

Powell J, Wojnarowska F: Childhood vulvar lichen sclerosus. The course after puberty. J Reprod Med 47(9):706, 2002

Resende EA, Lara BH, Reis JD, et al: Assessment of basal and gonadotropin-releasing hormone-stimulated gonadotropins by immunochemiluminometric and immunofluorometric assays in normal children. J Clin Endocrinol Metab 92(4):1424, 2007

Rosenfield RL, Lipton RB, Drum ML: Thelarche, pubarche, and menarche attainment in children with normal and elevated body mass index. Pediatrics 123:84, 2009

Schultz KA, Ness KK, Nagarajan R, et al: Adnexal masses in infancy and childhood. Clin Obstet Gynecol 49(3):464, 2006

Serbin LA: Sex-role socialization: a field in transition. In Lahey BB, Kazdin AE (eds): Advances in Clinical Child Psychology, Vol 3. New York, Plenum Publishing Corp, 1980, p 41

Sherman V, McPherson T, Baldo M, et al: The high rate of familial lichen sclerosus suggests a genetic contribution: an observational cohort study. J Eur Acad Dermatol Venereol 24(9):1031, 2010

Smith NA, Laufer MR: Obstructed hemivagina and ipsilateral renal anomaly (OHVIRA) syndrome: management and follow-up. Fertil Steril 87(4):918, 2007

Smith SD, Fischer G: Childhood onset vulvar lichen sclerosus does not resolve at puberty: a prospective case series. Pediatr Dermatol 26(6):725, 2009

Stricker T, Navratil F, Forster I, et al: Nonpuerperal mastitis in adolescents. J Pediatr 148(2):278, 2006

Tanner JM: Trend toward earlier menarche in Long, Oslo, Copenhagen, the Netherlands and Hungary. Nature 243:95, 1973

Tanner JM, Davies PWS: Clinical longitudinal standards for height and height velocity for North American children. J Pediatr 107:317, 1985

Tapper D, Lack EE: Teratomas in infancy and childhood. A 54-year experience at the Children's Hospital Medical Center. Ann Surg 198(6):398, 1983

Templeman C, Hertweck SP: Breast disorders in the pediatric and adolescent patient. Obstet Gynecol Clin North Am 27(1):19, 2000

Thind CR, Carty HM, Pilling DW: The role of ultrasound in the management of ovarian masses in children. Clin Radiol 40:180, 1989

Tweeten SS, Rickman LS: Infectious complications of body piercing. Clin Infect Dis 26(3):735, 1998

Unger ER, Fajman NN, Maloney EM, et al: Anogenital human papillomavirus in sexually abused and nonabused children: a multicenter study. Pediatrics 128(3):e658, 2011

U.S. Preventive Services Task Force: The Guide to Clinical Preventive Services, 2014. Rockville, 2014

Vaskivuo TE, Anttonen M, Herva R, et al: Survival of human ovarian follicles from fetal to adult life: apoptosis, apoptosis-related proteins, and transcription factor GATA-4. J Clin Endocrinol Metab 86:3421, 2001

Williams SM, Kaplan PA, Peterson JC, et al: Mammography in women under age 30: is there clinical benefit? Radiology 161:49, 1986

Ziereisen F, Guissard G, Damry N, et al: Sonographic imaging of the paediatric female pelvis. Eur Radiol 15:1296, 2005

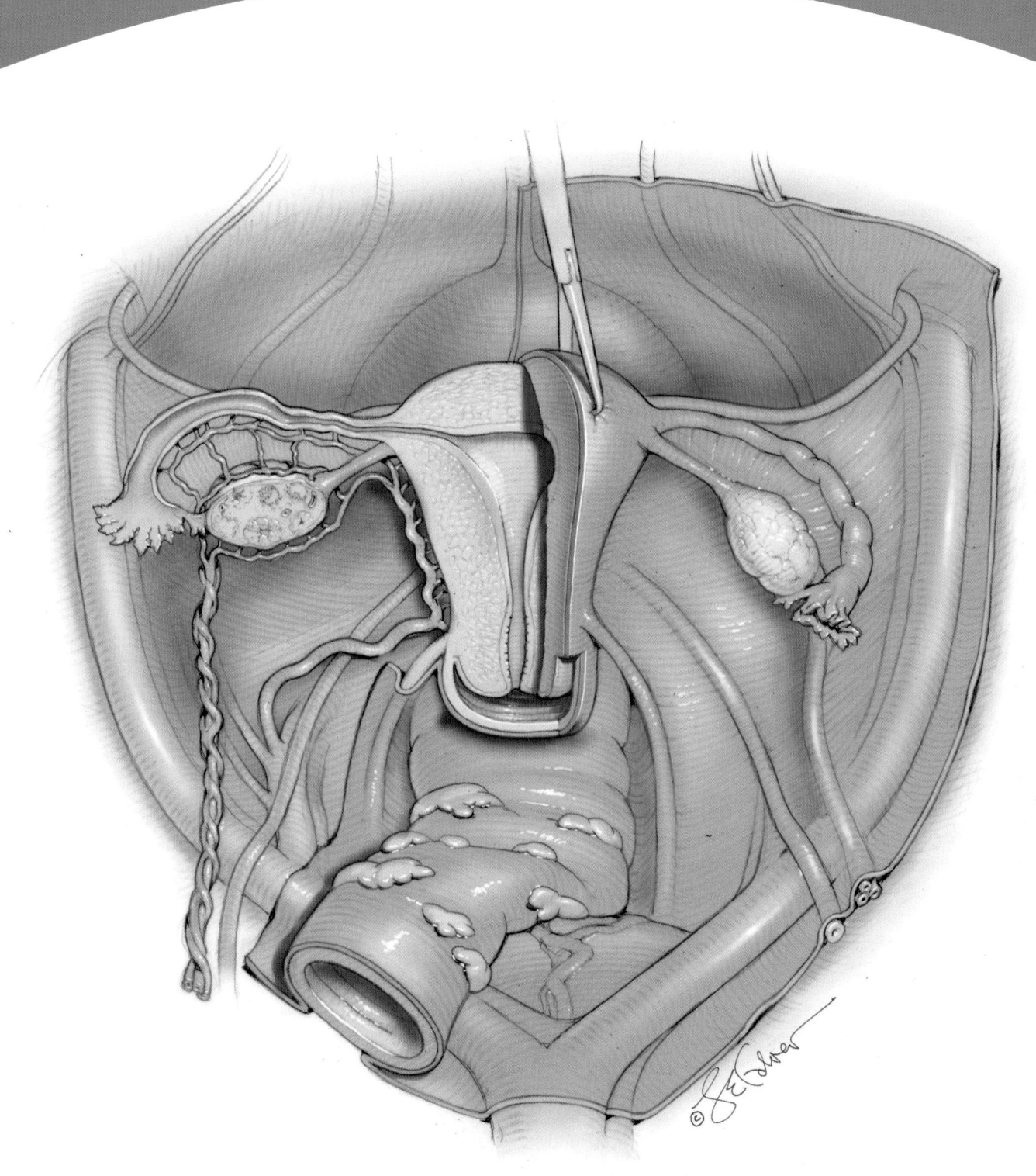

Reproductive Endocrinology

Reproductive endocrinology is the study of hormones and neuroendocrine factors that are produced by and/or affect reproductive tissues. These tissues include the hypothalamus, anterior pituitary gland, ovary, endometrium, and placenta.

A hormone is classically described as a cell product that is secreted into the peripheral circulation and that exerts its effects in distant target tissues (Fig. 15-1). This is termed *endocrine secretion*. Additional forms of cell-to-cell communication exist in reproductive physiology. *Paracrine* communication, common within the ovary, refers to chemical signaling between neighboring cells. *Autocrine* communication occurs when a cell releases substances that influence its own function. Production of a substance within a cell that affects that cell before secretion is termed an *intracrine* effect.

A neurotransmitter, in classic neural pathways, crosses a small extracellular space called a synaptic junction and binds to dendrites of a second neuron (Fig. 15-2). Alternatively, these factors are secreted into the vascular system and are transported to other tissues where they exert their effects in a process termed *neuroendocrine secretion* or *neuroendocrine signaling*. One example is gonadotropin-releasing hormone (GnRH) secretion into the portal vasculature with effects on the gonadotropes within the anterior pituitary gland.

Normal reproductive function requires precise quantitative and temporal regulation of the hypothalamic-pituitary-ovarian axis (Fig. 15-3). Within the hypothalamus, specific centers or nuclei release GnRH in pulses. This decapeptide binds to surface receptors on the gonadotrope subpopulation of the anterior pituitary gland. In response, gonadotropes secrete glycoprotein gonadotropins, luteinizing hormone (LH) and follicle-stimulating hormone (FSH), into the peripheral circulation. Within the ovary, LH and FSH bind to the theca and granulosa cells to stimulate folliculogenesis and ovarian production of steroid hormones (estrogens, progesterone, and androgens), gonadal peptides (activin, inhibin, and follistatin), and growth factors. Among other functions, these ovarian-derived factors feed back to the hypothalamus and pituitary gland to inhibit or, at the midcycle surge, to augment GnRH and gonadotropin secretion. The ovarian steroids are also critical for preparing the endometrium for placental implantation if pregnancy ensues.

HORMONE BIOSYNTHESIS AND MECHANISM OF ACTION

Hormones can be broadly classified as either steroids or peptides, each with their own mode of biosynthesis and mechanism of action. The receptors for these hormones can be divided into two groups: (1) those present on the cell surface, which in general interact with hormones that are water soluble, namely peptides, and (2) those that are primarily intracellular and interact with lipophilic hormones such as steroids. Hormones are normally present in serum and tissues in very low concentrations. Therefore, receptors must have both high affinity and high specificity for their ligand to produce the correct biologic response.

■ Peptide Hormones: LH, FSH, and hCG

The gonadotropins LH and FSH are biosynthesized and secreted by the gonadotrope subpopulation of the anterior pituitary gland. These hormones play a critical role in stimulating ovarian steroidogenesis, follicular development, and ovulation. The closely related peptide human chorionic gonadotropin (hCG) is produced by placental trophoblast and is important for maintenance of pregnancy.

LH, FSH, and hCG are heterodimers consisting of a common glycoprotein α-subunit linked to a unique β-subunit, which provides functional specificity. Although glycoprotein α- and β-subunits can be found in their unassociated form in the circulation, these "free" subunits are not known to have biologic activity. Nevertheless, their measurement may be useful in screening tests for conditions such as pituitary adenomas and pregnancy.

Endocrine action

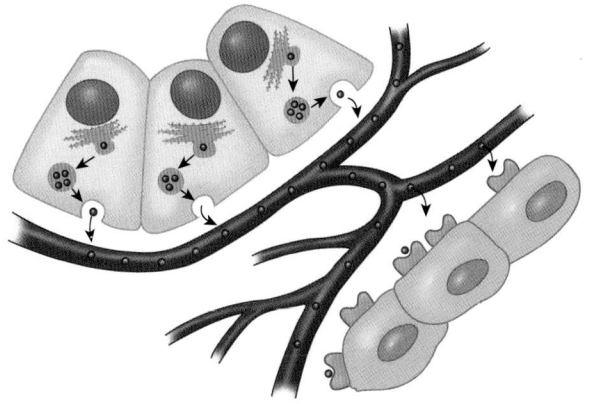

Paracrine action · · · · · Autocrine action

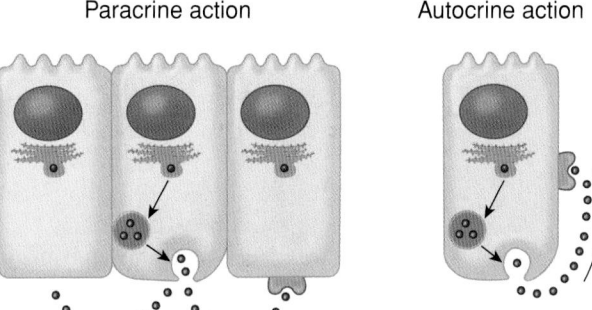

FIGURE 15-1 Different types of hormone communication. Endocrine: hormones travel through the circulation to reach their target cells. Paracrine: hormones diffuse through the extracellular space to reach their target cells, which are neighboring cells. Autocrine: hormones feed back on the cell of origin, without entering the circulation.

Neurotransmitter secretion (e.g, dopamine)

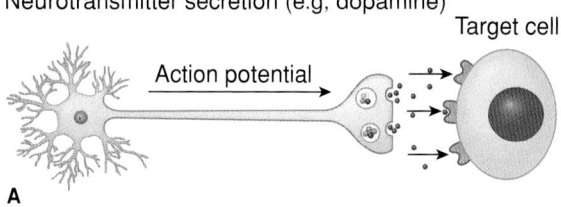

Neurohormone secretion (e.g, GnRH)

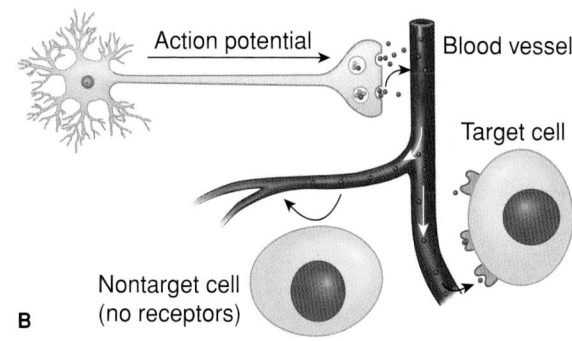

FIGURE 15-2 Types of neurotransmitter secretion. **A.** Classic neurotransmitter release and binding. Transmission of an action potential down a neural axon leads to release of neurotransmitters, which travel across a synaptic cleft to reach their target cell. **B.** Neurohormonal secretion. An action potential leads to release of neurotransmitters. In this instance, neurotransmitters enter into and travel through the circulation to reach their target organ.

The LH and hCG β-subunits are encoded by two separate genes within a gene grouping called the LH/CG cluster. The amino acid sequence of the human LH and CG β-subunits demonstrates approximately 80-percent similarity. However, the hCG β-subunit contains an additional 24-amino-acid extension on the carboxy terminus. The presence of these additional amino acids has allowed the development of highly specific assays that can distinguish LH from hCG.

In pituitary thyrotropes, the shared glycoprotein α-subunit also interacts with the thyroid-stimulating hormone β-subunit to form thyroid-stimulating hormone (TSH). This similarity between TSH and hCG can have clinical sequelae. For example, molar pregnancies frequently produce very high levels of hCG, which can bind to TSH receptors, resulting in hyperthyroidism (Walkington, 2011).

Human Chorionic Gonadotropin

This glycosylated peptide hormone is produced by the placental syncytiotrophoblast. With this molecule, the degree and type of glycosylated moieties attached to the peptide frame is variable and may indicate pregnancy stage, placental function, or pathology (Fournier, 2015). One example is the hyperglycosylated

hCG that is found more commonly in gestational trophoblastic neoplasia.

hCG can be detected in serum as early as 7 to 9 days after the LH surge. In early pregnancy, hCG levels increase rapidly, doubling approximately every 2 days. Levels of this peptide hormone peak at approximately 100,000 mIU/mL during the first trimester of pregnancy. This is followed by a relatively sharp decline in the early second-trimester concentrations and then maintenance at lower levels throughout the remainder of pregnancy.

hCG binds to LH/CG receptors on corpus luteum cells and stimulates steroidogenesis in the ovary. To maintain endometrial integrity and uterine quiescence, hCG levels are critical. Namely, hCG supports corpus luteum steroid production during early pregnancy before the placenta attains adequate steroidogenic capability. The transition in production of estrogens and progesterone from the ovary to the placenta is often called the "luteal-placental shift." In addition to effects on ovarian function, hCG exerts autocrine/paracrine effects in the placenta, promoting syncytiotrophoblast formation, trophoblast invasion, and angiogenesis.

As the placenta is the primary source for hCG production, measurement of plasma hCG levels has proved to be an effective screening tool for pregnancies with altered placental mass or function. Relatively elevated levels of hCG are observed in multifetal gestations and fetuses with Down syndrome. Lower hCG levels are observed in cases of poor placentation including ectopic pregnancy or spontaneous miscarriage. Serial hCG measurements can be very helpful to monitor these latter

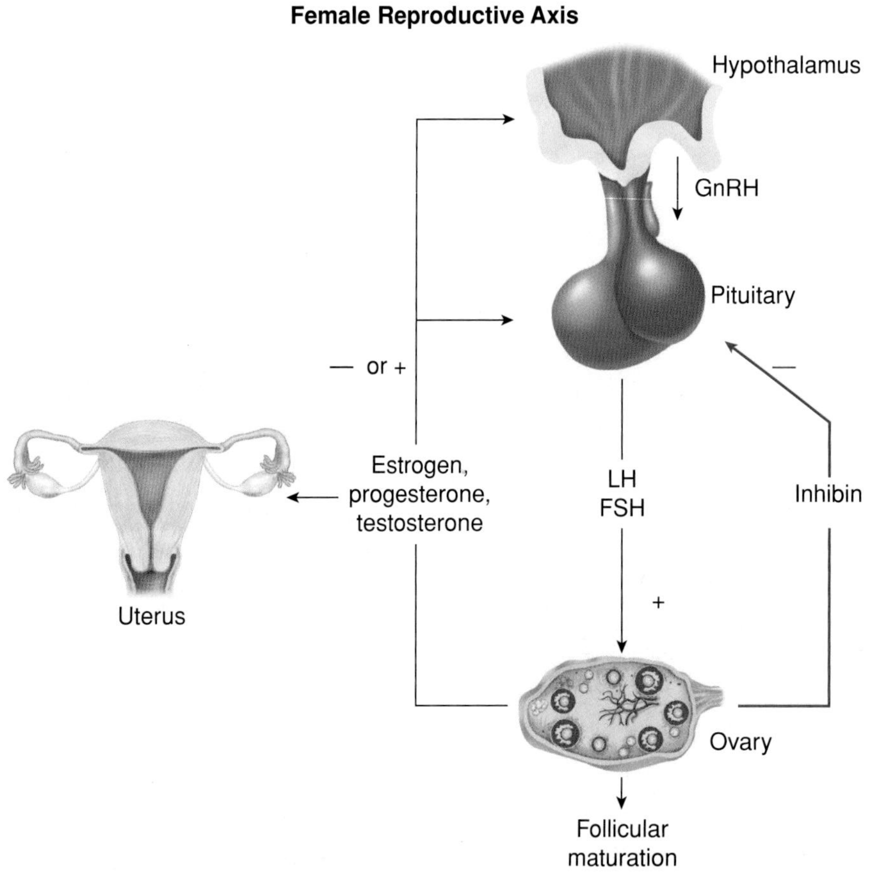

Female Reproductive Axis

Hypothalamus

GnRH

Pituitary

— or +

Estrogen,
progesterone,
testosterone

LH
FSH

Inhibin

—

Uterus

+

Ovary

Follicular
maturation

FIGURE 15-3 Positive and negative feedback loops seen with the hypothalamic-pituitary-ovarian axis. Pulsatile release of gonadotropin-releasing hormone (GnRH) leads to release of luteinizing hormone (LH) and follicle-stimulating hormone (FSH) from the anterior pituitary. Effects of LH and FSH result in follicle maturation, ovulation, and production of the sex steroid hormones (estrogen, progesterone, and testosterone). Rising serum levels of these hormones exert negative feedback inhibition on GnRH and gonadotropin release. Sex-steroid hormones vary in their effects on the endometrium and myometrium as discussed in the text. Inhibin, produced in the ovary, has a negative effect on gonadotropin release.

■ Steroid Hormones

Classification

Sex steroids are divided into three groups based on the number of carbon atoms that they contain. Each carbon in this structure is assigned a number identifier, and each ring is assigned a letter (Fig. 15-4). The 21-carbon series includes progestins, glucocorticoids, and mineralocorticoids. Androgens contain 19 carbons, whereas estrogens have 18.

Steroids are given scientific names according to a generally accepted convention in which functional groups below the plane of the molecule are preceded by the α symbol and those above the plane of the molecule are indicated by a β symbol. A Δ symbol indicates a double bond. Those steroids with a double bond between carbon atoms 5 and 6 are called Δ^5 steroids and include pregnenolone, 17-hydroxypregnenolone, and dehydroepiandrosterone. Those with a double bond between carbons 4 and 5 are termed Δ^4 steroids and include progesterone, 17-hydroxyprogesterone, androstenedione, testosterone, mineralocorticoids, and glucocorticoids.

Steroidogenesis

Sex steroid hormones are synthesized in the gonads, adrenal gland, and placenta. Cholesterol is the primary building block. All steroid-producing tissues, except the placenta, are capable of synthesizing cholesterol from the two-carbon precursor, acetate. Steroid hormone production, which involves at least 17 enzymes, primarily occurs in the mitochondria and the abundant smooth endoplasmic reticulum found in steroidogenic cells (Mason, 2002). These enzymes are members

conditions as the doubling time is relatively reliable. Markedly abnormal elevations in hCG levels are most often observed in the presence of gestational trophoblastic disease, discussed in Chapter 37 (p. 779).

Human CG is also secreted by nontrophoblastic neoplasias and can serve as a useful tumor marker. Ectopic (nonplacental) production of hCG, either the intact dimer or the β-subunit, is frequently associated with germ cell tumors and has been reported in various tumors arising from the mucosal epithelium of the cervix, bladder, lung, gastrointestinal tract, and nasopharynx. It has been postulated that hCG inhibits apoptosis in these tumors, thereby allowing rapid growth.

In addition to secretion by placental syncytiotrophoblast, hCG is produced by nonneoplastic cell types and presumably serves other functions (Cole, 2010). For example, cytotrophoblasts secrete a hyperglycosylated variant of hCG that may prove to be a sensitive marker of early pregnancy (Chuan, 2014). The pituitary gonadotropes also make small amounts of hCG. These concentrations rise in postmenopausal women and may be a rare cause of erroneously positive hCG testing in this age group (Cole, 2008).

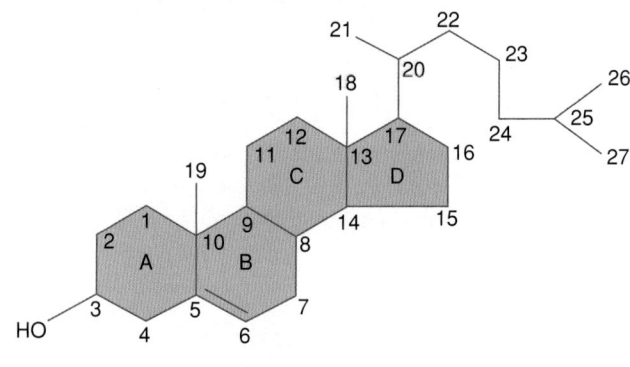

Cholesterol

FIGURE 15-4 The chemical structure of cholesterol, which is the common precursor in sex-steroid biosynthesis. All sex steroids contain the basic cyclopentanephenanthrene molecule, which consists of three 6-carbon rings and one 5-carbon ring.

TABLE 15-1. Steroidogenic Enzymes

Enzyme	Cellular Location	Reactions
P450scc	Mitochondria	Cholesterol side chain cleavage
P450c11	Mitochondria	11-Hydroxylase 18-Hydroxylase 19-Methyloxidase
P450c17	ER	17-Hydroxylase 17,20-Lyase
P450c21	ER	21-Hydroxylase
P450arom	ER	Aromatase

ER = endoplasmic reticulum.

of the cytochrome P450 superfamily. As such, genes that encode these enzymes begin with *CYP*.

Steroidogenic enzymes catalyze four basic modifications of the steroid structure: (1) side-chain cleavage (desmolase reaction), (2) conversion of hydroxyl groups to ketones (dehydrogenase reactions), (3) addition of a hydroxyl group (hydroxylation reaction), and (4) removal or addition of hydrogen to create or reduce a double bond (Table 15-1). The steroid biosynthesis pathway is shown in simplified form in Figure 15-5. This pathway is identical in all steroidogenic tissues, but the distribution of products synthesized by each tissue is determined by the presence of requisite enzymes. For example, the ovary is deficient in 21-hydroxylase and 11β-hydroxylase and thus is unable to produce corticosteroids. Of note, many steroidogenic enzymes exist as multiple isoforms, each with different precursor preferences and directional activities. As a result, specific steroids may be produced via multiple pathways in addition to the classic pathway shown in Figure 15-5 (Auchus, 2009).

Estrogens are synthesized by aromatization of C19 androgens by aromatase. The aromatase enzyme is a cytochrome P450 enzyme encoded by the gene *CYP19*. In addition to the ovary, aromatase is expressed in significant levels in adipose tissue, skin, and brain (Boon, 2010). Importantly, sufficient estrogen can be derived from peripheral aromatization to produce endometrial bleeding in postmenopausal women, especially those who are overweight or obese.

Circulating estrogens in the reproductive-aged female include estrone (E_1), estradiol (E_2), and estriol (E_3). Estradiol is the primary estrogen produced by the ovary during reproductive years. Levels are derived both from direct synthesis in the granulosa cells of developing follicles and through conversion of the less potent estrone. Estrone, the primary estrogen during menopause, is secreted primarily by the ovary. Estriol, the

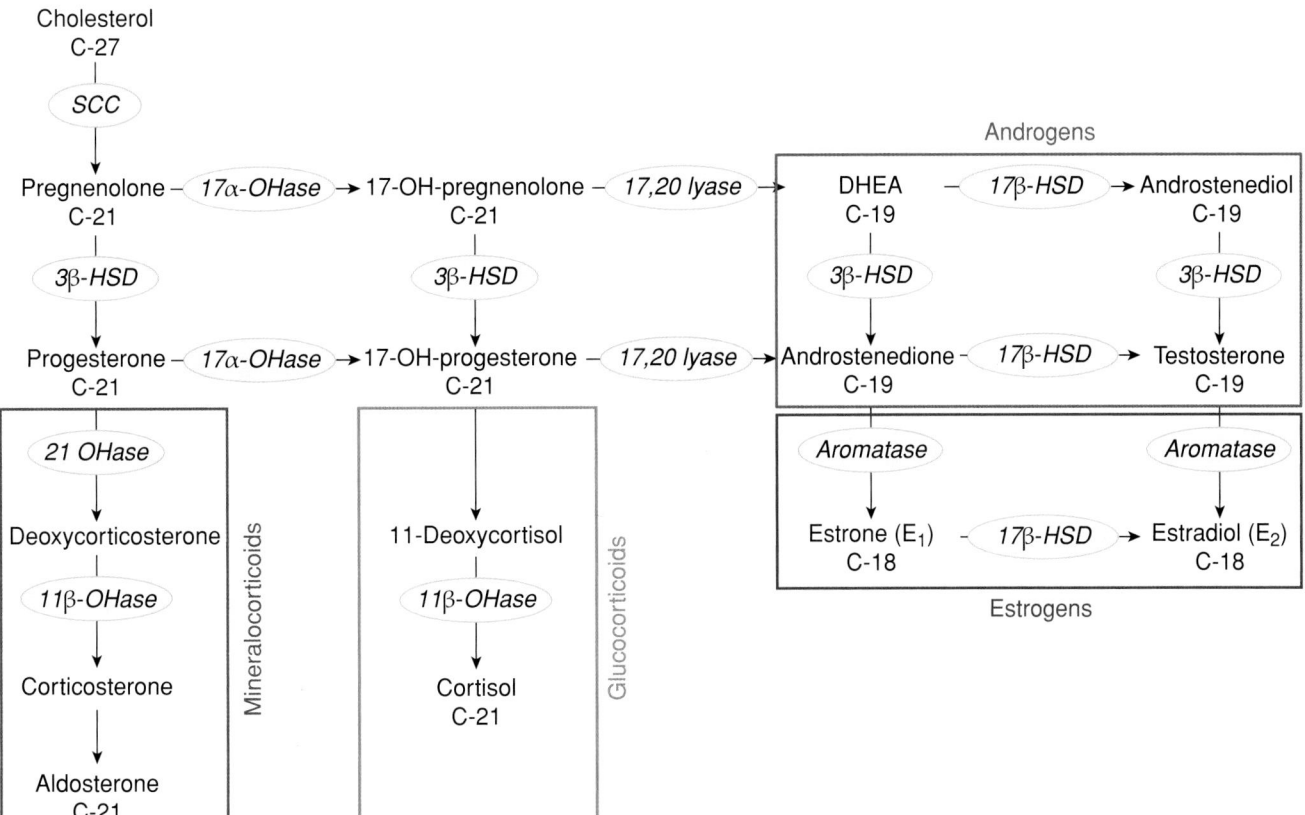

FIGURE 15-5 Steps in the steroidogenesis pathway. Enzymes are found within the blue ovals. The C-18, C-19, or C-21 designation beneath the sex steroid reflects the number of carbon atoms it contains. Colored boxing groups these pathway products. 3β-HSD = 3β-hydroxysteroid dehydrogenase; 11β-OHase = 11β-hydroxylase; 17αOHase = 17α-hydroxylase; 17β-HSD = 17β-hydroxysteroid dehydrogenase; 21OHase = 21-hydroxylase; DHEA = dehydroepiandrosterone; SCC = side-chain cleavage enzyme.

predominant estrogen during pregnancy, is primarily secreted from the placenta. However, both estrone and estriol can be converted from androstenedione in the periphery.

The ovary also produces androgens in response to LH stimulation of theca cell function. The primary products are the relatively weak androgens androstenedione and dehydroepiandrosterone (DHEA), although smaller amounts of testosterone are also secreted. Although the adrenal cortex primarily produces mineralocorticoids and glucocorticoids, it also contributes to approximately one half of the daily production of androstenedione and DHEA and essentially all of the sulfated form of DHEA (DHEAS). In women, 25 percent of circulating testosterone is secreted by the ovary, 25 percent is secreted by the adrenal gland, and the remaining 50 percent is produced by peripheral conversion of androstenedione to testosterone (Fig. 15-6) (Silva, 1987).

The adult adrenal gland is composed of three zones. Each of these zones expresses a different complement of steroidogenic enzymes and as a result synthesizes different products. The zona glomerulosa lacks 17α-hydroxylase activity but contains large amounts of aldosterone synthase (P450aldo) and therefore produces mineralocorticoids. The zona fasciculata and zona reticularis, both of which express the 17α-hydroxylase gene, synthesize glucocorticoids and androgens, respectively.

Within androgen synthesis, the 5α-reductase enzyme converts testosterone to dihydrotestosterone (DHT), a more potent androgen. DHT promotes transformation of vellus hair to terminal hair. Thus, medications that antagonize 5α-reductase are often effective in the treatment of hirsutism (Stout, 2010). This enzyme exists in two forms, each encoded by a separate gene. The type 1 enzyme is found in the skin, brain, liver, and kidneys. In contrast, the type 2 enzyme is predominantly expressed in male genitalia (Russell, 1994).

Steroid Hormone Transport in the Circulation

Most steroids in the peripheral circulation are bound to carrier proteins. These proteins may be either specific proteins, such as sex hormone-binding globulin (SHBG), thyroid-binding globulin, or corticosteroid-binding globulin, or nonspecific proteins such as albumin. Only 1 to 2 percent of androgens and estrogens are unbound or free.

Only the unbound steroid fraction is believed to be biologically active, although albumin's low affinity for sex steroids likely allows steroids bound to this protein to exert some effect. The amount of free hormone is in equilibrium with the amount of bound. In other words, the amount of free, biologically active hormone is inversely related to the amount of bound hormone, and the amount of bound hormone is a direct reflection of the levels of carrier protein. As a result, small changes in carrier protein expression can produce substantial alterations in steroid effect.

SHBG circulates as a homodimer that binds a single steroid molecule. This binding protein is primarily synthesized in the liver, although it has also been detected in the brain, placenta, endometrium, and testes. SHBG levels are increased by hyperthyroidism, pregnancy, and estrogen administration. In contrast, androgens, progestins, growth hormone (GH), insulin, and corticoids decrease SHBG levels. An increase in weight, particularly central body fat, can significantly blunt SHBG expression. In turn, this decreases bound hormone levels and increases active hormone levels (Hammond, 2012).

Clinically, unbound hormone can be technically difficult to measure, and results should be interpreted with caution. Free testosterone levels are the most commonly ordered free steroid hormone tests, but the most accurate assays are performed by only a few commercial laboratories (Rosner, 2007).

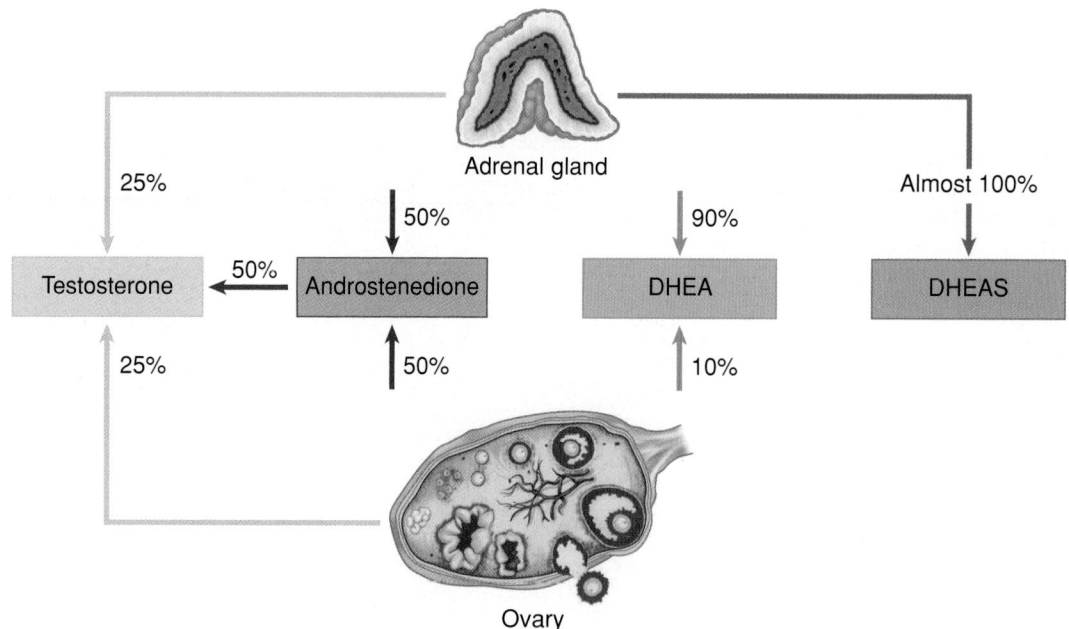

FIGURE 15-6 Contribution of the adrenal glands and ovaries to levels of androgens, dehydroepiandrosterone (DHEA), and DHEA sulfate (DHEAS).

The more available *calculated* free levels are relatively inaccurate. Moreover, free testosterone measurement is rarely necessary for clinical diagnosis in the female and is unlikely to add more information than the total testosterone level. For example, measurement of testosterone levels in patients with presumed polycystic ovarian syndrome (PCOS) is important to exclude an androgen-producing tumor, which will produce markedly elevated total testosterone levels. In contrast, normal or high-normal levels of total testosterone are consistent with the diagnosis of PCOS. Because testosterone lowers SHBG levels, patients with normal total testosterone levels, but with clinical evidence of hyperandrogenism (hirsutism and/or acne), invariably have either increased free testosterone levels or increased sensitivity of the hair follicle and sebaceous glands.

Ultimately, steroids are metabolized mainly in the liver and to a lesser extent in the kidney and intestinal mucosa. Hydroxylation of estradiol results in production of estrone or catechol estrogens. These estrogens are then conjugated to glucuronides or sulfates to form water-soluble compounds for excretion in the urine. Accordingly, administration of certain pharmacologic steroid hormones may be contraindicated in those with active liver or renal disease.

RECEPTOR STRUCTURE AND FUNCTION

Steroid hormones and peptide factors differ in their specific receptor-mediated actions, yet both eventually lead to DNA transcription and protein production in the target cell.

◼ G-Protein Coupled Receptors

These are cell-membrane-associated receptors that bind peptide factors. These receptors consist of a hydrophilic extracellular domain, an intracellular domain, and a hydrophobic transmembrane domain that spans the cell membrane seven times. When bound to hormone, these receptors undergo a conformational change, activate intracellular signaling pathways, and, through a series of phosphorylation events, ultimately modulate transcription of multiple genes within the target cell.

The gonadotropin-releasing hormone receptor (GnRH-R) is a G-protein-coupled receptor that has been identified in the ovary, testes, hypothalamus, prostate, breast, and placenta (Yu, 2011). Although data are still preliminary, GnRH and its receptor may form an autocrine/paracrine regulatory network in reproductive tissues including the ovaries and placenta in addition to the classic neuroendocrine hypothalamic-pituitary system (Kim, 2007; Lee, 2010).

Both LH and hCG bind to the same G-protein-coupled receptor known as the LH/CG receptor. Relative to LH, hCG has a slightly higher affinity for the receptor and has a longer half-life. In contrast, FSH binds to a unique G-protein-coupled receptor located on the granulosa cell membrane.

Within the ovary, the LH/CG receptor is expressed on thecal cells, interstitial cells, and luteal cells. In the granulosa cells of preantral follicles, LH/CG receptor mRNA is nearly undetectable. However, in the differentiated granulosa cells found during follicular maturation, high levels of this receptor are observed. In addition to the ovary, LH/CG and FSH receptors have also been identified in endometrium, myometrium, and placenta (Stilley, 2014; Ziecik, 2007). The function of the receptor in these extraovarian tissues is poorly understood.

◼ Steroid Hormone Receptors
Classification and Structure

The nuclear receptor superfamily consists of three receptor groups: (1) those that bind steroidal ligands, (2) those that have affinity for nonsteroidal ligands such as thyroid hormone, and (3) orphan receptors. By definition, orphan nuclear receptors do not have an identified ligand. These are believed to be constitutively active, that is, they exhibit basal or intrinsic activity. Despite their structural similarities, estrogens, progestins, androgens, mineralocorticoids, and glucocorticoids all interact with unique members of the nuclear hormone receptor family.

Free steroids diffuse into cells and combine with specific receptors (Fig. 15-7A). Members of this receptor superfamily exhibit a modular structure of distinct domains (Fig. 15-8). Each region contributes distinct activities required for full receptor function. In general, nuclear receptors have two regions that are critical for gene activation, termed activation function 1 (AF1) and activation function 2 (AF2). AF1 is located in the A/B domain and is usually ligand independent. AF2 is in the ligand-binding domain (E) and is often hormone-dependent. The highly conserved DNA-binding region (C) inserts into the DNA helix. Subsequently, steroid receptors enhance or repress gene transcription through interactions with specific DNA sequences, called hormone response elements, in the promoter region of target genes (Klinge, 2001).

Estrogen, Progesterone, and Androgen Receptors

As a a general rule, nuclear hormone receptors are localized to the cytoplasm. Following ligand binding, they then are translocated to the nucleus to exert their effects.

Two isoforms of estrogen receptors, ERα and ERβ, are encoded by separate genes (Kuiper, 1997). These receptors are differentially expressed in tissues and appear to serve distinct functions. For example, both ERα and ERβ are required for normal ovarian function. However, mice lacking ERα are anovulatory and accumulate cystic follicles, whereas ovaries missing ERβ are normal histologically despite impaired ovulation (Couse, 2000).

The progesterone receptor also exists in multiple isoforms. Encoded from a single gene, PRA and PRB are identical except for an additional 164 amino acids at the amino terminus (Conneely, 2002). Similar to estrogen receptors, the PR isoforms are not interchangeable. For example, PRA is required for normal ovarian and uterine functions but is expendable in the breast (Lydon, 1996). In contrast to the estrogen and progesterone receptor situation, only one form of the androgen receptor has been identified.

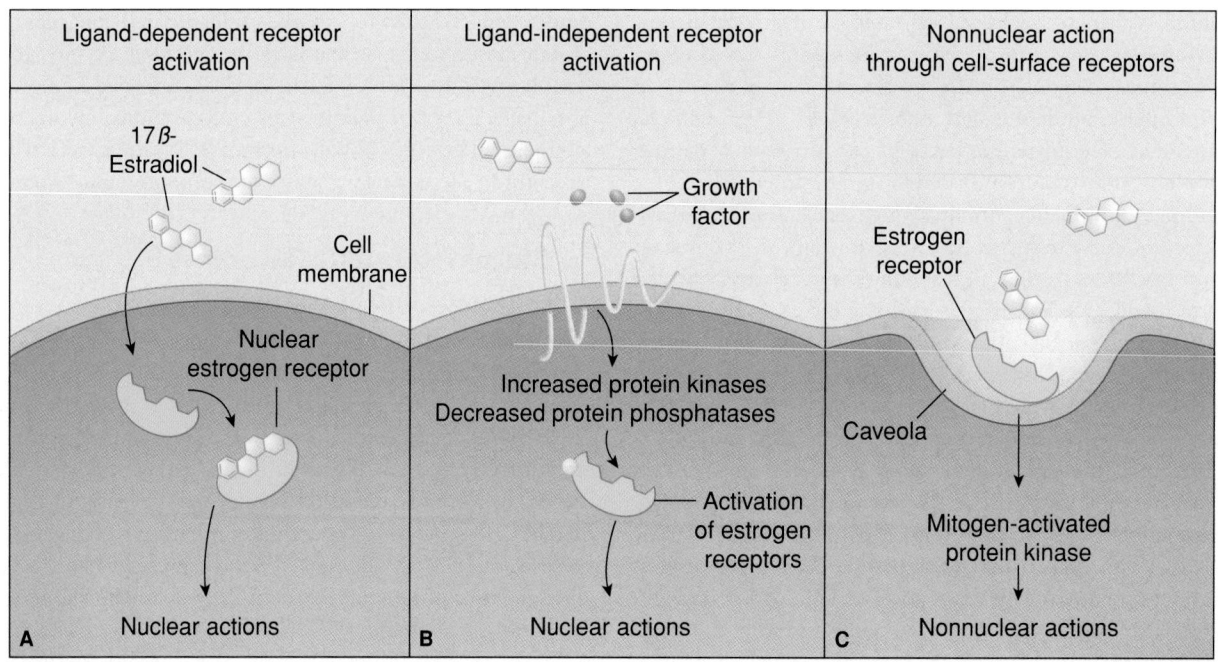

FIGURE 15-7 Estrogen-receptor ligand-dependent and ligand-independent activation. **A.** Classically, the estrogen receptor can be activated by estrogen. Unbound hormone is free to bind with empty steroid receptors found either in the cytoplasm or, more commonly, in the cell's nucleus. Hormone-bound receptors then bind to specific DNA promoter sequences. This binding typically leads to DNA transcription and eventually to specific protein synthesis. **B.** The estrogen receptor can also be activated independently of estrogen. Growth factors can increase the activity of protein kinases that phosphorylate different sites on the receptor molecule. This unbound, yet activated, receptor will then exert transcriptional effects. **C.** Nonnuclear estrogen-signaling pathways can also produce effects. Cell-membrane estrogen receptors are located in invaginations called caveolae. Estrogen binding to these estrogen receptors is linked to the mitogen-activated protein kinase pathway and results in a rapid, nonnuclear effect. (Reproduced with permission from Gruber CJ, Tschugguel W, Schneeberger C, et al: Production and actions of estrogens. N Engl J Med 2002 Jan 31;346(5):340–352.)

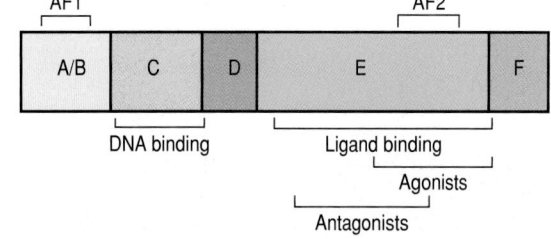

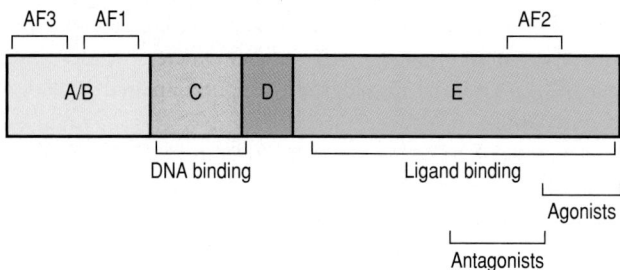

FIGURE 15-8 Drawing depicts the concept of functional domains within estrogen and progesterone receptors and notes distinct sites for ligand and DNA binding. (Reproduced with permission from Yen SS, Jaffe RB, Barbieri RL: Reproductive Endocrinology, 4th ed. Philadelphia: Saunders; 1999.)

Nongenomic Actions of Steroids

Recent studies have introduced the concept that a subset of steroids, including estrogens and progestins, may alter cell function via nongenomic effects, that is, independent of the classic nuclear hormone receptors (see Fig. 15-7C). These nongenomic effects occur rapidly and may be mediated via cell-surface receptors (Kowalik, 2013; Revelli, 1998). Pharmacologic agents under development specifically target these nongenomic effects to allow more precise therapy for steroid-sensitive disorders.

■ Receptor Expression and Desensitization

Many influences alter cellular response to sex steroids and peptide factors. The number of receptors within a cell or on the cell membrane is critical to attain maximum hormonal response. Importantly, the number of receptors on a cell can be modified through gene transcription and receptor protein degradation.

Hormonally induced negative feedback of receptors is termed *homologous downregulation* or *desensitization*. Desensitization limits the duration of a hormonal response by decreasing the cell's sensitivity to a constant, prolonged level of hormone. Within the reproductive system, desensitization is best understood for the GnRH receptor and is used clinically to produce a hypoestrogenic state. Pharmacologic agonists of GnRH, such as leuprolide acetate (Lupron), initially stimulate receptors on pituitary gonadotropes to cause a supraphysiologic release of both LH and FSH. Over a period of hours, agonists downregulate GnRH receptor sensitivity and number, thus preventing further GnRH stimulation. Correspondingly, decreased gonadotropin secretion leads to suppressed estrogen and progesterone levels 1 to 2 weeks after initial GnRH agonist administration.

IMMUNOASSAYS FOR PEPTIDE AND STEROID HORMONES

Immunoassays

These tests use antibodies to detect most polypeptide, steroid, and thyroid hormones. They are sensitive and easily automated. Hormone concentration is usually reported as international units per volume rather than mass per volume (Table 15-2). When interpreting immunoassays, several concepts must be understood. These include reference standards, the "hook effect," normal ranges, and supplementary hormone levels.

First, to minimize assay-to-assay variability, a reference material is needed to standardize assays. Reference standards serve as anchors that can provide comparability across time and methods. Such reference preparations are produced by the World Health Organization (WHO) and the National Institutes of Health (NIH). More than 20 assay standards are available to measure LH, FSH, prolactin (PRL), and hCG. Thus, knowing which reference standard is used by a specific assay is essential, as results may differ significantly. Clinically, this can become an issue in patients with possible ectopic pregnancies when serial β-hCG levels are obtained at different health care facilities.

Second, the "hook effect" can alter immunoassay result interpretation. With this effect, significantly elevated hormone levels saturate the assay's targeting antibody and create a falsely low reading. Moreover, the amount of hormone present in a sample does not necessarily correlate with the biological

TABLE 15-2. Reference Ranges for Selected Reproductive Steroids in Adult Human Serum

Steroid	Subjects	Reference Values
Androstenedione	Men	2.8–7.3 nmol/L
	Women	3.1–12.2 nmol/L
Testosterone	Men	6.9–34.7 nmol/L
	Women	0.7–2.8 nmol/L
Dihydrotestosterone	Men	1.0–3.10 nmol/L
	Women	0.07–.086 nmol/L
Dehydroepiandrosterone	Men/Women	5.5–24.3 nmol/L
Dehydroepiandrosterone sulfonate	Men/Women	2.5–10.4 μmol/L
Progesterone	Men	<0.3–1.3 nmol/L
	Women	
	Follicular	0.3–3.0 nmol/L
	Luteal	19.0–45.0 nmol/L
Estradiol	Men	<37–210 pmol/L
	Women	
	Follicular	<37–360 pmol/L
	Luteal	625–2830 pmol/L
	Midcycle	699–1250 pmol/L
	Postmenopausal	<37–140 pmol/L
Estrone	Men	37–250 pmol/L
	Women	
	Follicular	110–400 pmol/L
	Luteal	310–660 pmol/L
	Postmenopausal	22–230 pmol/L
Estrone sulfonate	Men	600–2500 pmol/L
	Women	
	Follicular	700–3600 pmol/L
	Luteal	1100–7300 pmol/L
	Postmenopausal	130–1200 pmol/L

Reproduced with permission from Yen SS, Jaffe RB, Barbieri RL: Reproductive Endocrinology, 4th ed. Philadelphia: Saunders; 1999.

activity of that hormone. For example, PRL exists in multiple isoforms, many of which are immunologically detectable but not biologically active. Similarly, varying glycosylation patterns of gonadotropins at different times during the reproductive life span are believed to alter their biologic activity.

Another caveat is a result that lies in the "normal range." For many hormones, a stated normal range is often broad. As such, the hormone level of an individual may double, but remain within the normal range even though the result is actually abnormal for that individual.

Last, the addition of other hormone levels may be necessary to define the significance of a result. In the context of the pituitary gland and its target endocrine glands, it may be adequate to measure the pituitary hormone alone. For example, high levels of circulating gonadotropins are almost invariably due to ovarian failure and loss of negative feedback. This is because pituitary overproduction of functional dimer is rare. Conversely, low gonadotropin levels can be attributed confidently to hypothalamic-pituitary dysfunction. Thus, the measurement of ovarian-derived products such as estrogen may be helpful to confirm the diagnosis but are not critical.

In other clinical scenarios, the measurement of both pituitary and target hormone levels may be indicated. For example, in many laboratories, an abnormal TSH value will lead to "reflex," that is, automatic testing for thyroid hormone levels. Low levels of both a stimulating-hormone and target hormone indicate an abnormality in either hypothalamic or pituitary function. High levels of a target-gland hormone coupled with low levels of its stimulating pituitary hormone suggest autonomous secretion by the target organ such as occurs in the hyperthyroidism of Graves disease.

Stimulation Tests

These tests may be useful when hypofunction of an endocrine organ is suspected. These tests use an endogenous stimulating hormone to assess the reserve capacity of the tissue of interest. The trophic hormone used may be a hypothalamic releasing factor such as GnRH or thyrotropin-releasing hormone (TRH). Alternatively, a substitute pituitary hormone may be used, such as hCG as a substitute for LH or leuprolide acetate for GnRH. The ability of the target gland to respond is measured by an increase in the appropriate hormone's plasma level. One example, the leuprolide stimulation test, may be used to evaluate abnormal pubertal development and is described in Chapter 14 (p. 328). Leuprolide substitutes for GnRH because clinical-grade GnRH is often unavailable (Rosenfield, 2013).

Suppression Tests

These tests may be performed when endocrine hyperfunction is suspected. For example, a dexamethasone suppression test may be given to a patient with suspected hypercortisolism (Cushing disease or syndrome). Described in full in Chapter 17 (p. 396), this test gauges the ability of dexamethasone to inhibit adrenocorticotropic hormone (ACTH) secretion and thus cortisol production by the adrenal. The failure of glucocorticoid treatment to suppress cortisol production would be consistent with primary hyperadrenalism.

THE HYPOTHALAMIC-PITUITARY AXIS

Anatomy

The hypothalamus consists of nuclei located at the base of the brain, just superior to the optic chiasm. Neurons within the hypothalamus form synaptic connections with other neurons throughout the central nervous system (CNS). A subset of the hypothalamic neurons within the arcuate, ventromedial, and paraventricular nuclei project to the median eminence. In the median eminence, a dense network of capillaries arises from the superior hypophyseal arteries. These capillaries drain into portal vessels that traverse the pituitary stalk and then form a capillary network within the anterior pituitary gland (adenohypophysis). The primary direction of this hypophyseal portal system is from hypothalamus to pituitary. However, retrograde flow also exists. This creates an ultrashort feedback loop between the pituitary gland and hypothalamic neurons. The hypothalamus is thus a critical locus for integration of information from the environment, nervous system, and other organ systems.

The anterior pituitary gland consists of endocrine cells and is derived from an invagination of Rathke pouch in the roof of the embryonic oral cavity. In contrast, the posterior pituitary gland (neurohypophysis) is neural tissue and consists of the axon terminals of magnocellular neurons arising in the supraoptic and paraventricular nuclei of the hypothalamus (Fig. 15-9).

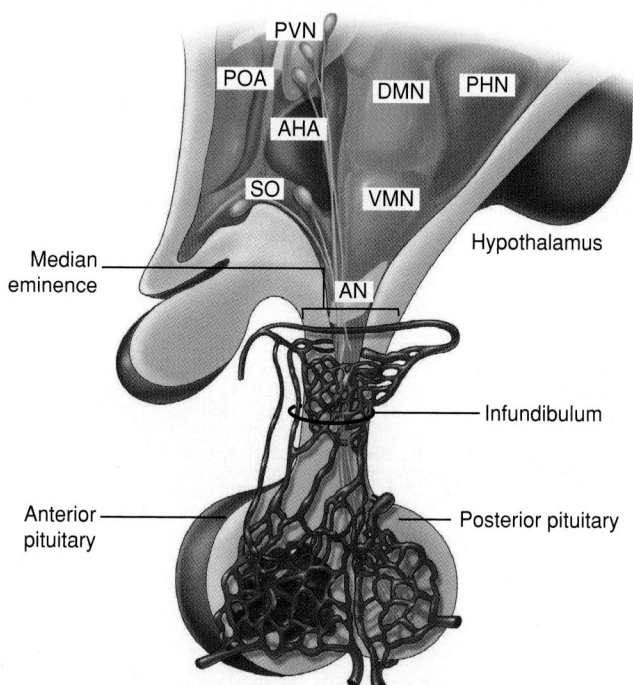

FIGURE 15-9 Sagittal section through the hypothalamus and pituitary gland with rostral structures to the left and caudal ones to the right. The hypothalamus is anatomically and functionally linked with the anterior pituitary by the portal system of blood supply. The posterior pituitary contains the axon terminals of neurons arising in the supraoptic (SO) nucleus and paraventricular nucleus (PVN) of the hypothalamus. AHA = anterior hypothalamic area; AN = arcuate nucleus; DMN = dorsomedial nucleus; PHN = posterior hypothalamic nucleus; POA = preoptic area; VMN = ventromedial nucleus. (Reproduced with permission from Cunningham FG, Leveno KJ, Bloom SL, et al: Williams Obstetrics, 23rd ed. New York: McGraw-Hill; 2010.)

Hypothalamic Neuroendocrinology

The list of known neurotransmitters continues to expand as does our understanding of their anatomic distribution, mode of regulation, and mechanism of action. Neurotransmitters can be classified as: (1) biogenic amines (dopamine, epinephrine, norepinephrine, serotonin, histamine), (2) neuropeptides, (3) acetylcholine, (4) excitatory amino neurotransmitters (glutamate, glycine, aspartic acid), (5) the inhibitory amino acid gamma-aminobutyric acid (GABA), (6) gaseous transmitters (nitric oxide, carbon monoxide), and (7) miscellaneous factors (cytokines, growth factors).

The most significant neurotransmitters in reproductive neuroendocrinology are the three monoamines: dopamine, norepinephrine, and serotonin. Clinically important neuropeptides within the reproductive axis include the endogenous opiates, kisspeptin, neuropeptide Y, galanin, and pituitary adenylate cyclase-activating peptide.

Endogenous Opiates

Central opioidergic neurons are important mediators of hypothalamic-pituitary function. Depending on the precursor peptide from which they are derived, these neuropeptides can be categorized into three classes: endorphins, enkephalins, and dynorphins. Of these, endorphins (endogenous morphines) are cleavage products of the proopiomelanocortin *POMC* gene, which also yields ACTH and α-melanocyte stimulating hormone (α-MSH) (Taylor, 1997). The endorphins serve a wide range of physiologic functions that include regulation of temperature, cardiovascular and respiratory systems, pain perception, mood, and reproduction.

Proopiomelanocortin is produced in highest concentration in the anterior pituitary gland but is also expressed in the brain, sympathetic nervous system, gonads, placenta, gastrointestinal tract, and lungs. The primary peptide synthesized from this pathway depends on the tissue source. For example, the predominant products in the brain are the opiates, whereas pituitary biosynthesis results principally in ACTH production.

Opioids in the brain play a central role in menstrual cyclicity by tonically suppressing the hypothalamic release of GnRH (Funabashi, 1994). Estrogen promotes endorphin secretion, and this is increased further with the addition of progesterone (Cetel, 1985). Thus, endorphin levels increase during the follicular phase, peak during the luteal phase, and drop markedly during menses. This pattern suggests that both opioid tone and progesterone decrease GnRH pulse frequency in the luteal phase, thus stimulating FSH secretion. For reasons that are not fully understood, opioid suppression of GnRH is relieved at the time of ovulation (King, 1984). In addition, functional hypothalamic amenorrhea due to eating disorders, intensive exercise, and stress is correlated with an increase in endogenous opiate concentrations (Chap. 16, p. 376).

Other Hypothalamic Neuropeptides

Hypothalamic kisspeptin neurons play a critical role in sexual differentiation, puberty initiation, and adult reproductive function. These neurons are part of the KNDy neuronal system, named for the coexpression of kisspeptin with neurokinin B and dynorphin. This system likely provides an important link between energy homeostasis and reproductive function. This link may stem in part from the action of the adipose-derived factor leptin, which regulates kisspeptin expression (Chehab, 2014).

Kisspeptin neurons send processes to GnRH neurons, allowing direct control of GnRH secretion. Interestingly, one group of kisspeptin neurons may mediate negative steroid feedback, whereas another is responsible for the positive feedback observed before ovulation (Lehman, 2010; Millar, 2014; Skorupskaite, 2014).

Other neurotransmitters, neuropeptide Y (NPY) and galanin, are expressed by neurons located throughout the hypothalamus and project to kisspeptin neurons, to GnRH neurons, and to other areas of the CNS that have roles in reproductive function. NPY and galanin secretion varies in response to changes in energy level as seen in anorexia and obesity. Both of these neuropeptides alter GnRH pulsatility and potentiate GnRH-induced gonadotrope secretion (Lawrence, 2011; Peters, 2009).

Pituitary adenylate cyclase-activating peptide (PACAP) is a hypothalamic peptide secreted into the pituitary portal system. It binds to receptors on anterior pituitary cells and stimulates hormone secretion including gonadotropin secretion, albeit more weakly than GnRH. Gonadotropes themselves also secrete PACAP, suggesting an autocrine/paracrine role for this hormone within the pituitary. PACAP modulates GnRH-receptor expression and, conversely, GnRH alters PACAP-receptor expression on the gonadotrope cell surface. Furthermore, pituitary PACAP gene expression is markedly increased by GnRH (Halvorson, 2014). Thus, these two important neuropeptides are functionally linked at the level of the anterior pituitary.

Anterior Pituitary Hormones

The anterior pituitary gland contains five hormone-producing cell types and their products. These include: (1) gonadotropes (which produce LH and FSH), (2) lactotropes (PRL), (3) somatotropes (GH), (4) thyrotropes (TSH), and (5) adrenocorticotropes (ACTH). Of these, gonadotropes comprise approximately 10 to 15 percent of all hormonally active cells in the anterior pituitary (Childs, 1983).

With the exception of PRL, which is under tonic inhibition, pituitary hormones are stimulated by hypothalamic neuroendocrine secretion. Both of the gonadotropins, LH and FSH, are regulated by a single releasing peptide, GnRH, which acts on the anterior pituitary's gonadotrope subpopulation. Most gonadotropes contain secretory granules that contain both LH and FSH, although a significant number of cells are monohormonal, that is, secrete only LH or only FSH.

Of the other pituitary-releasing hormones, corticotropin-releasing hormone stimulates biosynthesis and secretion of ACTH by the pituitary adrenocorticotropes. Thyrotropin-releasing hormone increases thyrotrope secretion of TSH, also known as thyrotropin. Various hypothalamic secretagogues regulate expression of somatotrope-derived growth hormone. Last, PRL expression is primarily under inhibitory regulation by dopamine. As a consequence of these regulatory mechanisms, damage to the pituitary stalk results in hypopituitarism for LH, FSH, GH, ACTH, and TSH, but an associated increase in PRL secretion.

Hypothalamic Releasing Peptides

These peptides have characteristics that are important for both their biologic function and clinical use. First, they are small peptides with short half-lives of a few minutes due to their rapid degradation. Second, hypothalamic releasing peptides are released in minute quantities and are highly diluted in the peripheral circulation. Therefore, biologically active concentrations of these factors are locally restricted to the anterior pituitary gland. Clinically, the extremely low concentrations of these hormones render them essentially undetectable in serum. Thus, levels of their corresponding pituitary factors are measured as surrogate markers.

Gonadotropin-releasing Hormone

GnRH is a decapeptide with a half-life of less than 10 minutes. Amino acid modifications generate receptor antagonists or agonists with a prolonged half-life (Fig. 15-10) (Padula, 2005). Pulsatile GnRH input is required for activation and maintenance of GnRH receptors. This characteristic is exploited clinically by administering long-acting GnRH agonists to treat steroid-dependent conditions such as endometriosis, leiomyomas, precocious puberty, breast cancer, and prostate cancer. These agonists compete with endogenous pulsatile GnRH at the receptor, depressing gonadotropin secretion and thereby decreasing serum ovarian sex steroid levels.

Humans express two forms of GnRH termed GnRH I and GnRH II (Cheng, 2005). By convention, GnRH I is the classically described hypothalamic GnRH. The GnRH II peptide has been identified in peripheral tissues and differs in receptor activation (Neill, 2002). Further research is needed to determine the overlapping and divergent functions of these two forms.

Migration of the Gonadotropin-releasing Hormone Neurons.
Many hypothalamic neurons arise within the CNS, but GnRH-containing neurons have a unique embryologic origin. Progenitor GnRH neurons originate in the medial olfactory placode and migrate along the vomeronasal nerve into the hypothalamus (Fig. 16-5, p. 376). A series of soluble factors regulate GnRH neuronal migration at specific locations along their migratory route. These factors include secreted signaling molecules such as GABA, adhesion molecules, and growth factors (Wierman, 2011). Failure of normal migration may

stem from various genetic defects in these signaling molecules and can lead to Kallmann syndrome, which is discussed in Chapter 16 (p. 375), and other forms of hypogonadotropic hypogonadism.

GnRH cell bodies are primarily located within the arcuate nucleus. From these neuronal cell bodies, GnRH is axonally transported along the tuberoinfundibular tract to the median eminence. GnRH is then secreted into the portal system that drains directly to the anterior pituitary gland and stimulates gonadotropin biosynthesis and secretion. The number of GnRH neurons in the adult is strikingly low, with only a few thousand cells dispersed within the arcuate nucleus.

The olfactory origin of GnRH neurons and nasal epithelial cells suggest a link between reproduction and olfactory signals. Compounds released by one individual that affect other members of the same species are known as *pheromones*. Pheromones obtained from the axillary secretions of women in the late follicular phase accelerate the LH surge and shorten menstrual cycles of women exposed to these chemicals. Secretions from women in the luteal phase have the opposite effects. Thus, pheromones may be one mechanism by which women who are together frequently often exhibit synchronous menstrual cycles (Stern, 1998).

A subset of GnRH neurons sends projections into other areas of the CNS, including the limbic system. These projections are not required for gonadotropin secretion, but they may play a role in modulation of reproductive behavior (Nakai, 1978; Silverman, 1987).

Pulsatile Gonadotropin-releasing Hormone Secretion.
In elegant experiments, Knobil (1974) demonstrated that pulsatile delivery of GnRH to the pituitary gonadotropes is required to achieve sustained gonadotropin secretion. As shown in Figure 15-11, continuous infusion with GnRH rapidly decreases both LH and FSH secretion, an effect that is easily reversed with a return to pulsatile stimulation.

Compared with the luteal phase, follicular phase GnRH pulsatility is characterized by increased frequency and decreased amplitude. Higher pulse frequency preferentially stimulates LH, whereas lower frequency favors FSH secretion (Thompson, 2014). Therefore, changes in GnRH pulse frequency affect the absolute levels and the ratio of LH to FSH release.

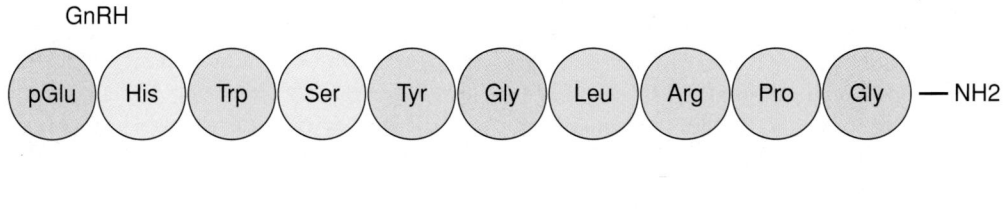

FIGURE 15-10 Schematic drawing shows the similar amino acid composition of the decapeptide gonadotropin-releasing hormone (GnRH) and of its agonist, leuprolide acetate (Lupron).

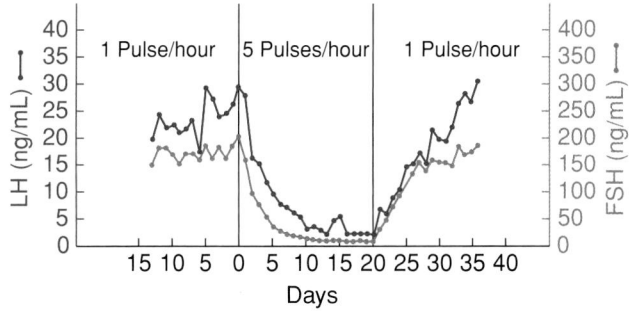

FIGURE 15-11 Graph shows changes in luteinizing hormone (LH) and follicle-stimulating hormone (FSH) levels with variation in gonadotropin-releasing hormone (GnRH) pulsatile release. (Adapted with permission from Knobil E: The neuroendocrine control of the menstrual cycle, Recent Prog Horm Res 1980;36:53–88.)

Pulsatile activity is currently believed to be an intrinsic property of GnRH neurons. Other hormones and neurotransmitters provide modulatory effects (Clayton, 1981; Yen, 1985). In animal models, estrogen increases GnRH pulse frequency and therefore leads to an increase in LH levels relative to FSH levels. In contrast, progesterone decreases GnRH pulsatility. The increase in progesterone during the luteal phase may explain the preferential stimulation of FSH observed toward the end of this phase. This rise in FSH is critical for the initiation of follicular recruitment.

■ Other Hypothalamic-Pituitary Axes

Dopamine and Prolactin

In contrast to the other anterior pituitary hormones, PRL release is primarily regulated via inhibition, specifically by dopamine. These dopamine-containing fibers arise chiefly in the hypothalamic arcuate nucleus and project to the median eminence, where dopamine enters the portal vessels (Table 15-3). Prolactin-releasing factors, although less potent, include TRH, vasopressin, vasoactive intestinal peptide (VIP), endogenous opioids, and acetylcholine.

There are five forms of the dopamine receptor divided into two groups, D_1 and D_2. Cells in the anterior pituitary gland

TABLE 15-3. Hypothalamic-Pituitary Products and Their End Organs

Hypothalamus	Pituitary	End Organ
GnRH	LH/FSH	Gonads
Dopamine	PRL	Breast
TRH	TSH	Thyroid
CRH	ACTH	Adrenal
GHRH	GH	Somatic

ACTH = adrenocorticotropin hormone; CRH = corticotropin-releasing hormone; FSH = follicle-stimulating hormone; GH = growth hormone; GHRH = growth hormone–releasing hormone; GnRH = gonadotropin-releasing hormone; LH = luteinizing hormone; PRL = prolactin; TRH = thyrotropin-releasing hormone; TSH = thyroid-stimulating hormone.

primarily express the D_2 subtypes. The medical treatment of prolactinomas has been improved in terms of both effectiveness and patient tolerance by the development of the D_2-specific ligands. For example, the dopamine agonist cabergoline is a D_2-specific ligand, whereas bromocriptine is nonspecific.

Thyrotropin-releasing Hormone

As indicated by its name, thyrotropin-releasing hormone stimulates secretion of thyroid-stimulating hormone from the anterior pituitary gland's thyrotrope subpopulation. Of note, TRH is also a potent prolactin-releasing factor and results in a clinical link between hypothyroidism and secondary hyperprolactinemia (Messini, 2010).

TSH binds to specific receptors on the plasma cell membrane of thyroid gland cells. This stimulates thyroid hormone biosynthesis. Thyroid hormone exerts negative feedback on TRH- and TSH-releasing cells.

Corticotropin-releasing Hormone

This is the primary hypothalamic factor that stimulates synthesis and secretion of ACTH. Corticotropin-releasing hormone (CRH) is distributed in multiple locations within the hypothalamus and other CNS areas. Release of CRH is stimulated by catecholaminergic input from other brain pathways and inhibited by endogenous opioids.

Corticotropin-releasing hormone binds to CRH receptors in the anterior pituitary to stimulate ACTH biosynthesis and secretion. In turn, ACTH stimulates glucocorticoid production by the adrenal's zona fasciculata and androgen production by its zona reticularis. CRH secretion is under negative-feedback regulation by circulating cortisol produced in the adrenal gland. In contrast, mineralocorticoid production by the zona glomerulosa is primarily regulated by the renin-angiotensin system. As a result, abnormalities in the CRH–ACTH pathway do not result in electrolyte disturbances.

Central CRH pathways are believed to mediate many stress responses (Kalantaridou, 2004). Clinically, in women with hypothalamic amenorrhea, CRH levels have been found to be elevated. Increased levels of CRH inhibit hypothalamic GnRH secretion by direct action and by augmenting central opioid concentrations (Fig. 16-6, p. 377). This functional pathway may explain the association between hypercortisolism and menstrual abnormalities.

Growth Hormone–releasing Hormone

Growth hormone secretion by pituitary somatotropes is stimulated by hypothalamic growth hormone-releasing hormone (GHRH) and inhibited by somatostatin. GHRH is primarily secreted by the hypothalamus, but small quantities are released by placental and immune cells. In contrast, somatostatin is widely distributed in the CNS and in the placenta, pancreas, and gastrointestinal tract.

As with GnRH, GHRH depends on pulsatile secretion to exert a physiologic effect. Exercise, stress, sleep, and hypoglycemia stimulate GH release, whereas free fatty acids and other factors related to adiposity blunt GH release. Estrogen, testosterone, and thyroid hormone also play a role in increased GH secretion.

GH stimulates skeletal and muscle growth, regulates lipolysis, and promotes the cellular uptake of amino acids. This hormone induces insulin resistance, and thus GH excess may be associated with new-onset diabetes mellitus. Most of the growth effects of GH are mediated via the insulin-like growth factors, IGF-I and IGF-II. These growth factors are produced in high quantities in the liver. Many of the target tissues in which they exert local effects also synthesize IGFs. Within the ovary, IGF-I and IGF-II stimulate granulosa cell proliferation and steroidogenesis during folliculogenesis (Silva, 2009). IGFs also suppress GH secretion through negative feedback mechanisms.

■ Posterior Pituitary Peptides

Neurons projecting to the posterior pituitary synthesize and secrete the nine-amino-acid cyclic peptides oxytocin and arginine vasopressin. Precursors for these peptides are produced in the neuronal cell body and transported down the axon in secretory granules. During transport, precursors are cleaved into mature peptides and a carrier protein—neurophysin (Verbalis, 1983). Activation of these neurons generates an axon potential that results in calcium influx and secretion of granule contents into the perivascular space. These secreted peptides then enter adjacent blood vessels for transport throughout the peripheral circulation.

Of these two peptides, oxytocin has significant roles in reproduction, specifically parturition and lactation (Kiss, 2005). The role of oxytocin in labor initiation is disputed as serum oxytocin levels are constant until the expulsive portion of labor (Blanks, 2003). Nevertheless, an increase in myometrial and decidual oxytocin-receptor expression has been noted near term, primarily due to an increase in estrogen levels.

Once labor is initiated, oxytocin is the primary mediator of myometrial contractility. Cervical and vaginal stimulation results in an acute release of oxytocin from the posterior pituitary in a process known as the *Ferguson reflex*. Clinically, oxytocin's ability to induce uterine contractions is exploited to induce or augment labor.

Vaginal distention, such as occurs with coitus, also increases oxytocin release. Based on this observation, oxytocin may be responsible for the rhythmic uterine and tubal contractions that aid sperm delivery to the oocyte. Oxytocin may also play a role in orgasm and ejaculation.

During lactation, PRL is critical for milk production in breast alveoli. The glandular cells of the alveoli are surrounded by a mesh of myoepithelial cells. Suckling triggers nerve impulses from mechanoreceptors in the nipple and areola that increase hypothalamic neuronal activity. Subsequent oxytocin release prompts the myoepithelial cells to contract and thereby express milk from the alveoli into the ducts and sinuses (Crowley, 1992). Other conditioned stimuli, such as the sight, sound, or smell of a baby or sexual arousal, will have similar effects.

Oxytocin expression has also been detected in the anterior pituitary, placenta, fallopian tubes, and gonads, with high expression in the corpus luteum (Williams, 1990). Its function in these tissues is unknown.

MENSTRUAL CYCLE

The "typical" menstrual cycle is 28 ± 7 days with menstrual flow lasting 4 ± 2 days and blood loss averaging 20 to 60 mL. By convention, the first day of vaginal bleeding is considered day 1 of the menstrual cycle. Menstrual cycle intervals vary among women and often for an individual woman at different times during her reproductive life. In a study of more than 2700 women, menstrual cycle intervals were found to be most irregular in the 2 years following menarche and the 3 years preceding menopause (Treloar, 1967). Specifically, a trend toward shorter intervals followed by interval lengthening is common during the menopausal transition. The menstrual cycle is least variable between the ages of 20 and 40 years.

When viewed from a perspective of ovarian function, the menstrual cycle can be defined as a preovulatory follicular phase and postovulatory luteal phase (Fig. 15-12). Corresponding phases in the endometrium are termed the proliferative and secretory phases (Table 15-4). For most women, the luteal phase of the menstrual cycle is stable, lasting 13 to 14 days. Thus, variations in normal cycle length generally result from variable duration of the follicular phase (Ferin, 1974).

■ The Ovary
Ovarian Morphology

The adult human ovary is oval with a length of 2 to 5 cm, a width of 1.5 to 3 cm, and a thickness of 0.5 to 1.5 cm. During the reproductive years, the ovary weighs between 5 and 10 g. It is composed of three parts: an outer cortical region, which contains both the germinal epithelium and the follicles; a medullary region, which consists of connective tissue, myoid-like contractile cells, and interstitial cells; and a hilum, which contains blood vessels, lymphatics, and nerves that enter the ovary (Fig. 15-13).

Ovaries have two interrelated functions: the generation of mature oocytes and the production of steroid and peptide hormones that create an environment in which fertilization and subsequent implantation in the endometrium can occur. Within each cycle, endocrine functions of the ovary correlate closely to the morphologic appearance and disappearance of follicles and corpus luteum.

Embryology of the Ovary

The ovary develops from three major cellular sources: (1) primordial germ cells, which arise from the endoderm of the yolk sac and differentiate into the primary oogonia; (2) coelomic epithelial cells, which develop into granulosa cells; and (3) mesenchymal cells from the gonadal ridge, which become the ovarian stroma. Additional information regarding gonadal differentiation is found in Chapter 18 (p. 404).

Primordial germ cells can be seen in the yolk sac as early as the third week of gestation (Gosden, 2013). These cells begin their migration into the gonadal ridge during the sixth week of gestation and generate primary sex cords. The ovary and testes are indistinguishable by histologic criteria until approximately 10 to 11 weeks of fetal life.

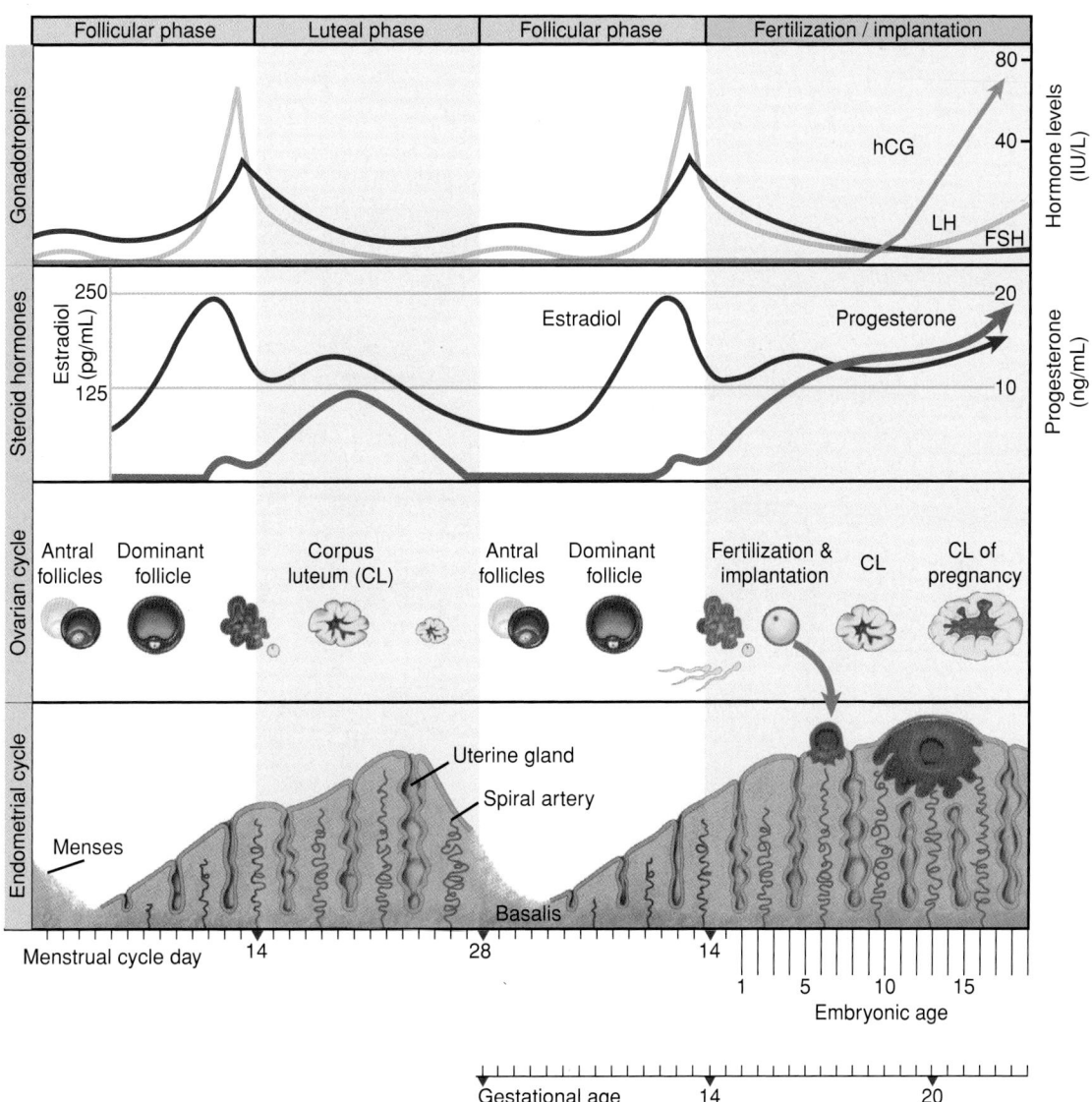

FIGURE 15-12 Gonadotropin control of the ovarian and endometrial cycles. The ovarian-endometrial cycle has been structured as a 28-day cycle. The follicular phase (days 6 to 14) is characterized by rising levels of estrogen, thickening of the endometrium, and selection of the dominant "ovulatory" follicle. During the luteal phase (days 15 to 28), the corpus luteum produces estrogen and progesterone, which prepare the endometrium for implantation. If implantation occurs, the developing blastocysts will begin to produce human chorionic gonadotropin (hCG) and rescue the corpus luteum, thus maintaining progesterone production. FSH = follicle-stimulating hormone; LH = luteinizing hormone. (Reproduced with permission from Cunningham FG, Leveno KJ, Bloom SL, et al: Williams Obstetrics, 24th ed. New York: McGraw-Hill Education; 2014.)

After the primordial cells reach the gonad, they continue to multiply through successive mitotic divisions. Starting at 12 weeks' gestation, a subset of oogonia will enter meiosis to become primary oocytes. Primary oocytes are surrounded by a single layer of flattened granulosa cells, creating a primordial follicle.

Oocyte Loss with Aging

All oogonia either develop into primary oocytes or become atretic. Classical teaching states that additional oocytes cannot be generated postnatally. This differs markedly from the male, in whom sperm are produced continuously throughout

TABLE 15-4. Menstrual Cycle Characteristics

Cycle day	1–5	6–14	15–28
Ovarian phase	Early follicular	Follicular	Luteal
Endometrial phase	Menstrual	Proliferative	Secretory
Estrogen/progesterone	Low levels	Estrogen	Progesterone

OVARY

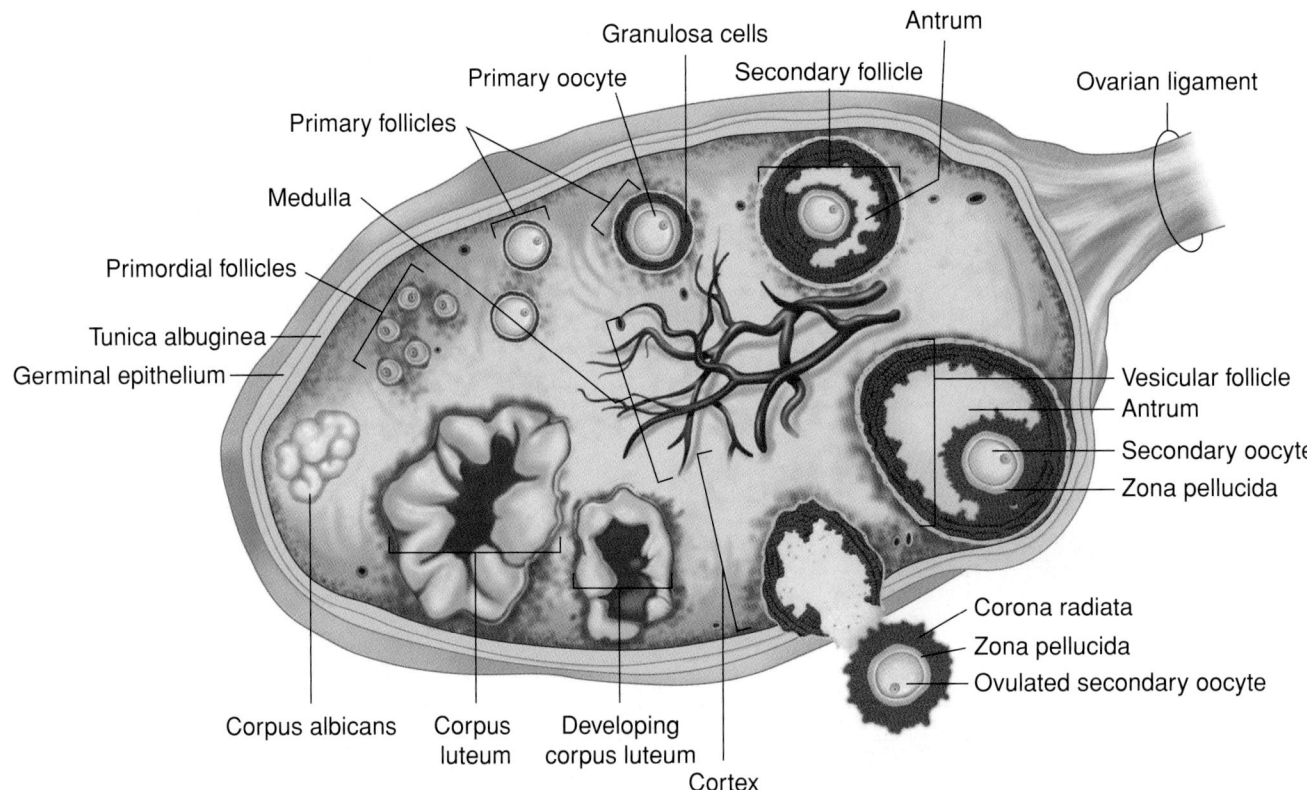

FIGURE 15-13 Ovarian anatomy and various sequential steps of follicular development.

adulthood. Exciting recent studies suggest that ovarian stem cells may be able to generate mature oocytes, providing hope for significant advances in female fertility preservation. Currently, these results remain preliminary and somewhat controversial (Notarianni, 2011; Virant-Klun, 2015).

The maximal number of oogonia is achieved at the 20th week of gestation, at which time 6 to 7 million oogonia are present in the ovary (Baker, 1963). Approximately 1 to 2 million oogonia are present at birth. Fewer than 400,000 are present at the initiation of puberty, of which fewer than 500 are destined to ovulate. Therefore, most germ cells are lost through atresia (Hsueh, 1996). Follicular atresia is thought not to be a passive, necrotic process, but rather a precisely controlled active process, namely apoptosis, which is under hormonal control. Apoptosis begins in utero and continues throughout reproductive life.

Oocyte Maturation

As previously mentioned, primary oogonia enter meiosis in utero to become primary oocytes. These oocytes are arrested in development at prophase during the first meiotic division. Meiotic progression resumes each month in a cohort of follicles. Meiosis I is completed in the oocyte destined for ovulation in response to the LH surge. Meiosis II begins, and the process is arrested, this time in the second meiotic metaphase. Meiosis II is completed only if the ovum is fertilized (Fig. 15-14).

Normal oocyte development requires cytoplasmic modifications in addition to meiotic maturation. Changes in microtubules

and actin filaments enable rearrangement of cellular organelles to allow for successful polar body extrusion and fertilization (Coticchio, 2015). The cumulus cells modulate maturation both by cell-to-cell contact via gap junctions and by secretion of paracrine factors. Our growing understanding of these factors and processes is improving in vitro maturation protocols to aid fertility preservation and infertility treatments.

Stromal Cells

Ovarian stroma contains interstitial cells, contractile cells, and connective tissue cells. These last cells provide structural support to the ovary. The group of interstitial cells that surround a developing follicle differentiates into theca cells. Under gonadotropin stimulation, these cells increase in size and develop lipid stores, characteristic of steroid-producing cells (Saxena, 1972).

Another group of interstitial cells in the ovarian hilum are known as hilus cells. These closely resemble testicular Leydig cells, and hyperplasia or neoplastic changes in hilar cells may result in excess testosterone secretion and virilization. The normal role of these cells is unknown, but their intimate association with blood vessels and neurons suggest that they may convey systemic signals to the remainder of the ovary.

■ Ovarian Hormone Production

The normal functioning ovary synthesizes and secretes estrogens, androgens, and progesterone in a precisely controlled

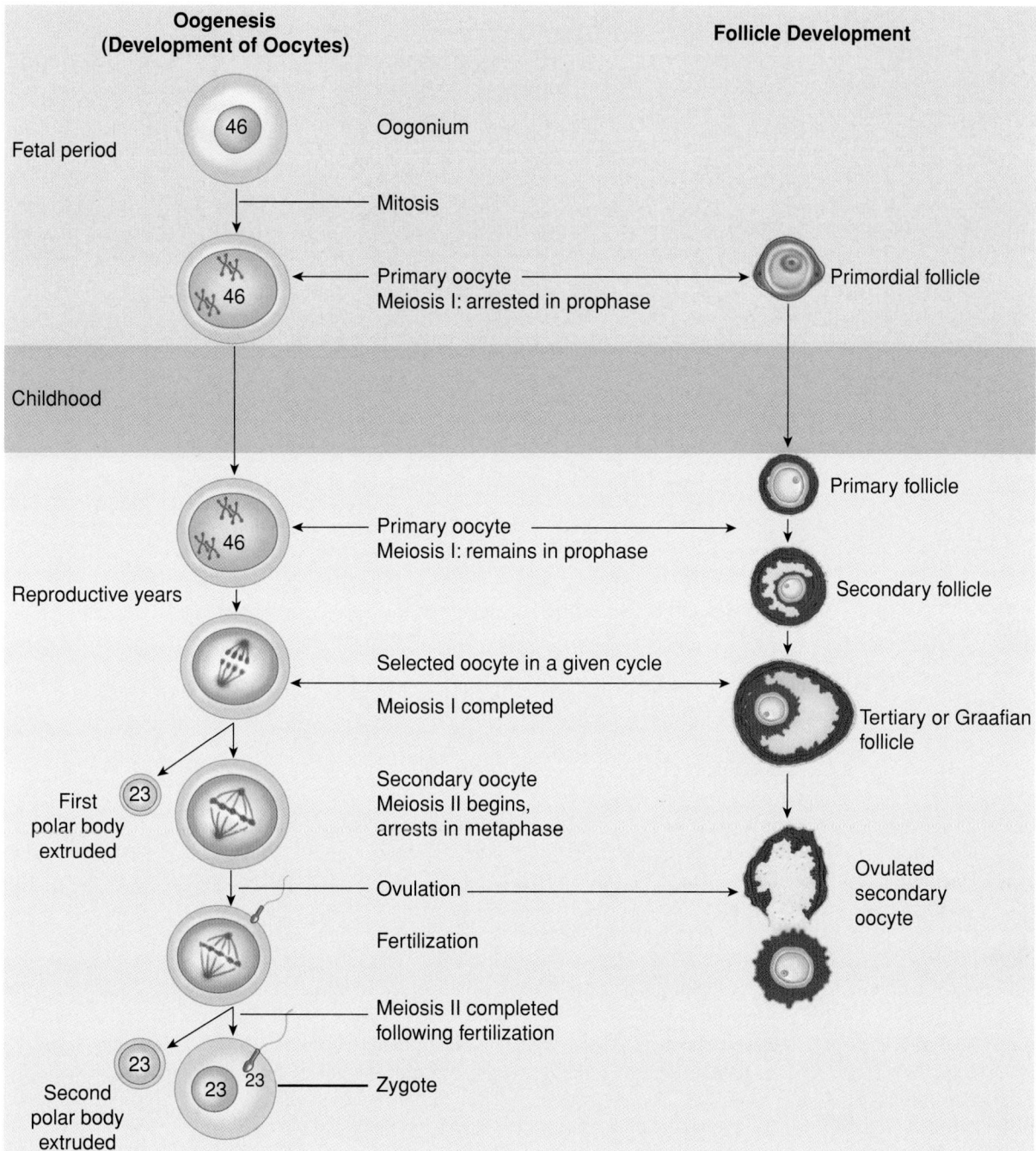

FIGURE 15-14 The steps of oocyte development and corresponding follicular maturation. In the fetal period, once the primordial germ cells arrive in the gonad, they differentiate into oogonia. Mitotic division of oogonia increases the population. Many oogonia further differentiate into primary oocytes, which begin meiosis. However, the process arrests after only prophase is completed. A primary oocyte with its surrounding epithelial cells is called a primordial follicle. In childhood, primary oocytes remain suspended in prophase. Beginning in puberty and extending through the reproductive years, several primordial follicles mature each month into primary follicles. A few of these continue development to secondary follicles. One or two secondary follicles progress to a tertiary or graafian follicle stage. At this stage, the first meiotic division completes to produce a haploid secondary oocyte and a polar body. During this process, cytoplasm is conserved by the secondary oocyte. Consequently, the polar body is disproportionately small. The secondary oocyte enters meiosis II, which then arrests in metaphase. One of the secondary oocytes is released at ovulation. If the oocyte is fertilized, completion of the second meiotic division follows. If fertilization fails to occur, then the oocyte degenerates before completion of the second meiotic division.

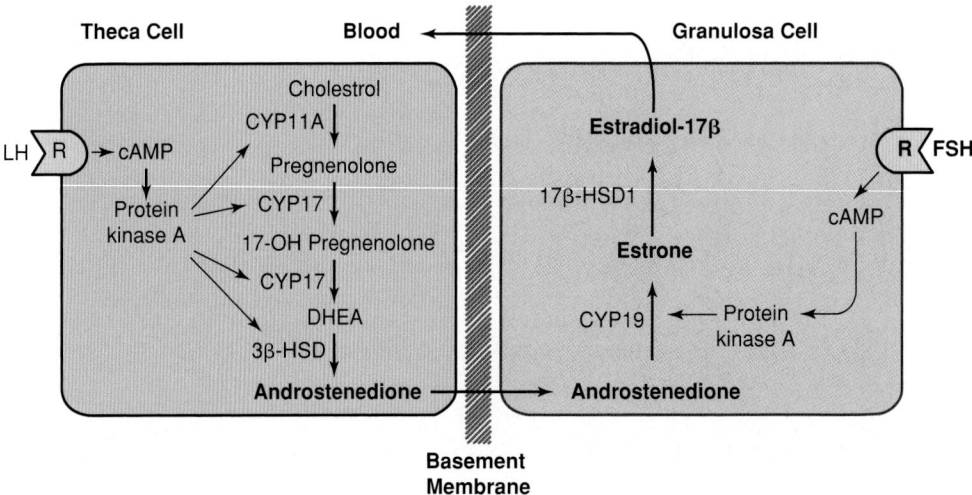

FIGURE 15-15 Diagram illustrates the two-cell theory of ovarian follicular steroidogenesis. Theca cells contain large numbers of luteinizing hormone (LH) receptors. Binding of LH to these receptors leads to cyclic AMP activation and synthesis of androstenedione from cholesterol. Androstenedione diffuses across the basement membrane of theca cells to enter granulosa cells of the ovary. Here, under the activation of follicle-stimulating hormone (FSH), androstenedione is converted by the enzyme aromatase to estrone and estradiol. cAMP = cyclic adenosine monophosphate; DHEA = dehydroepiandrosterone; 3β-HSD = 3β-hydroxysteroid dehydrogenase; 17β-HSD1 = 17β-hydroxysteroid dehydrogenase; R = receptor. (Adapted with permission from Larsen PR, Kronenberg HM, Melmed S: William's Textbook of Endocrinology, 10th edition. Philadelphia: Elsevier/Saunders; 2003.)

pattern determined, in part, by the pituitary gonadotropins, FSH and LH. The most important secretory products of ovarian steroid biosynthesis are progesterone and estradiol. However, the ovary also secretes quantities of estrone, androstenedione, testosterone, and 17α-hydroxyprogesterone. Sex steroid hormones play an important role in the menstrual cycle by preparing the uterus for implantation of a fertilized ovum. If implantation does not occur, ovarian steroidogenesis declines, the endometrium degenerates, and menstruation ensues.

Two-Cell Theory

Ovarian estrogen biosynthesis requires the combined action of two gonadotropins (LH and FSH) on two cell types (theca and granulosa cells). This concept is known as the two-cell theory of ovarian steroidogenesis (Fig. 15-15) (Peters, 1980). Until the late antral stage of follicular development, LH-receptor expression is limited to the thecal compartment, and FSH-receptor expression is limited to the granulosa cells.

Theca cells express all of the enzymes needed to produce androstenedione. This includes high levels of *CYP17* gene expression, whose enzyme product catalyzes 17-hydroxylation. This is the rate-limiting step in the conversion of progesterones to androgens (Sasano, 1989). This enzyme is absent in the granulosa cells, so they are incapable of producing the androgenic precursors needed to produce estrogens. Granulosa cells therefore rely on the theca cells. Namely, in response to LH stimulation, theca cells synthesize the androgens androstenedione and testosterone. These androgens are secreted into the extracellular fluid and diffuse across the basement membrane to the granulosa cells to provide precursors for estrogen production. In contrast to theca cells, granulosa cells have high levels of aromatase activity in response to FSH stimulation. Thus, these cells efficiently convert androgens to estrogens, primarily

the potent estrogen estradiol. In sum, ovarian steroidogenesis is dependent on the effects of LH and FSH acting independently on the theca cells and granulosa cells, respectively.

Steroidogenesis across the Life Span

Circulating levels of the gonadotropins LH and FSH vary markedly at different ages of a woman's life. In utero, the fetal human ovary has the capacity to produce estrogens by 8 weeks' gestation. However, a minimal amount of steroid is actually synthesized during fetal development (Miller, 1988). During the second trimester, the plasma levels of gonadotropins rise to levels similar to those observed in menopause (Temeli, 1985). The fetal hypothalamic-pituitary axis continues to mature during this time, becoming more sensitive to the high circulating levels of estrogen and progesterone secreted by the placenta (Kaplan, 1976). Prior to birth and in response to these high steroid levels, fetal gonadotropins fall to low levels.

After delivery, gonadotropin levels in the neonate rise abruptly due to separation from the placenta and subsequent freedom from placental steroid inhibition (Winter, 1976). The elevated gonadotropin levels persist for the first few months of life and then decline to low levels in early childhood (Schmidt, 2000). There may be multiple etiologies for the low gonadotropin levels during this period of life. The hypothalamic-pituitary axis has increased sensitivity to negative feedback, even by the low circulating levels of gonadal steroids at this stage. There may be a direct CNS role in maintaining low gonadotropin levels. In support of this mechanism, low levels of LH and FSH are found even in children with gonadal dysgenesis who lack negative feedback by gonadal steroids.

With puberty, one early sign is a sleep-associated increase in LH secretion (Fig. 15-16). Over time, increased gonadotropin secretion is noted throughout the day. An increased FSH to LH

LH secretion patterns

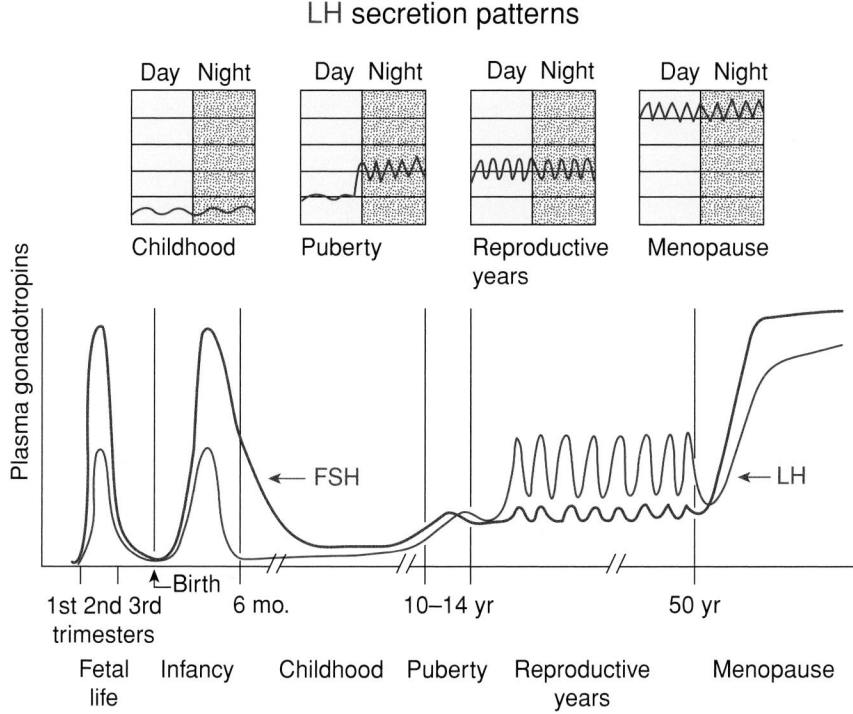

FIGURE 15-16 Variations in luteinizing hormone (LH) and follicle-stimulating hormone (FSH) during different life stages in the female. (Modified with permission from Faiman C, Winter JS, Reyes FI: Patterns of gonadotrophins and gonadal steroids throughout life, Clin Obstet Gynaecol. 1976 Dec;3(3):467–483.)

ratio is typical in the premenarchal girl and postmenopausal woman. During the reproductive years, LH exceeds FSH levels, inverting this ratio. Increased gonadotropin levels stimulate ovarian estradiol production. The rise in estrogen levels prompts the growth spurt, maturation of the female internal and external genitalia, and development of a female habitus including pubertal breast enlargement, which is termed thelarche. Activation of the pituitary-adrenal axis results in an increase in adrenal androgen production and the associated pubertal development of axillary and pubic hair, termed adrenarche or pubarche. Increased gonadotropin levels ultimately lead to ovulation and subsequent menses. The first menstrual period defines menarche. This developmental process takes approximately 3 to 4 years and is discussed further in Chapter 14 (p. 319).

Following menopause, the postmenopausal ovary contains only a few follicles. As a result, plasma estrogen and inhibin levels decrease markedly after cessation of ovulatory cycles. Through loss of this negative feedback, LH and FSH levels are strikingly elevated. Elevated LH levels can stimulate production of C-19 steroids (mainly androstenedione) in ovarian stromal cells. This ovarian-derived androstenedione and adrenal androgens can be converted by peripheral tissues to estrone, the principal serum estrogen in the postmenopausal women. The major site for the conversion of androstenedione to estrone is adipose tissue. Peripheral conversion of circulating androstenedione to estrone is directly correlated to body weight. For a given body weight, conversion is higher in postmenopausal women than in premenopausal women. These low circulating estrogen levels are usually not adequate to protect against bone loss.

■ Gonadal Peptides and the Menstrual Cycle

Of the multiple gonadal peptides, three—*inhibin, activin,* and *follistatin*—modulate gonadotrope activity in addition to effects within the ovary (de Kretser, 2002). As suggested by their names, inhibin decreases and activin stimulates gonadotrope function. Follistatin suppresses FSHβ gene expression, most likely by binding to and thereby preventing the interaction of activin with its receptor (Xia, 2009).

Inhibin and activin are closely related peptides. Inhibin consists of an α-subunit (unrelated to the LH and FSH glycoprotein α-subunit) linked by a disulfide bridge to one of two highly homologous β-subunits to form inhibin A ($\alpha\beta_A$) or inhibin B ($\alpha\beta_B$). Activin is composed of homodimers ($\beta_A\beta_A$, $\beta_B\beta_B$) or heterodimers ($\beta_A\beta_B$) of the same β-subunits as inhibin (Bilezikjian, 2012). In contrast, follistatin is structurally unrelated to either inhibin or activin.

Although originally isolated from follicular fluid, these "gonadal" peptides are expressed in the pituitary, ovary, testes, and placenta and in the brain, adrenal, liver, kidney, and bone marrow to provide diverse tissue-specific functions (Muttukrishna, 2004). Activin and follistatin most likely act as autocrine/paracrine factors in the tissues in which they are expressed, including the ovary.

In contrast, ovarian-derived inhibins circulate in significant concentrations and are believed to be critical for negative feedback of gonadotropin gene expression. Specifically, during the early follicular phase, FSH stimulates the secretion of inhibin B by the granulosa cells (Fig. 15-17) (Buckler, 1989). However, increasing levels of circulating inhibin B blunt later FSH secretion in the follicular phase. During the luteal phase, regulation of inhibin production comes under the control of LH and switches from inhibin B to inhibin A (McLachlan, 1989). Inhibin B levels peak with the LH surge, whereas inhibin A levels peak a few days later, in the midluteal phase. All inhibin levels decline with the loss of luteal function and remain low during the luteal-follicular transition and early follicular phase. The inverse relationship between circulating inhibin levels and FSH secretion is consistent with a negative-feedback role for inhibin in regulating FSH secretion.

Distinct from these three peptides, insulin-like growth factors also mediate ovarian function. Only IGF-II is involved in primordial follicle development, but both IGF-I and IGF-II stimulate growth of secondary follicles. Gonadotropins stimulate IGF-II production in theca cells, granulosa cells, and luteinized granulosa cells. Receptors for IGF are expressed on the theca and granulosa cells, supporting an autocrine/paracrine action in the follicle. FSH also mediates expression of IGF-binding proteins. This system, although complex, allows additional fine-tuning of intrafollicular activity (Silva, 2009).

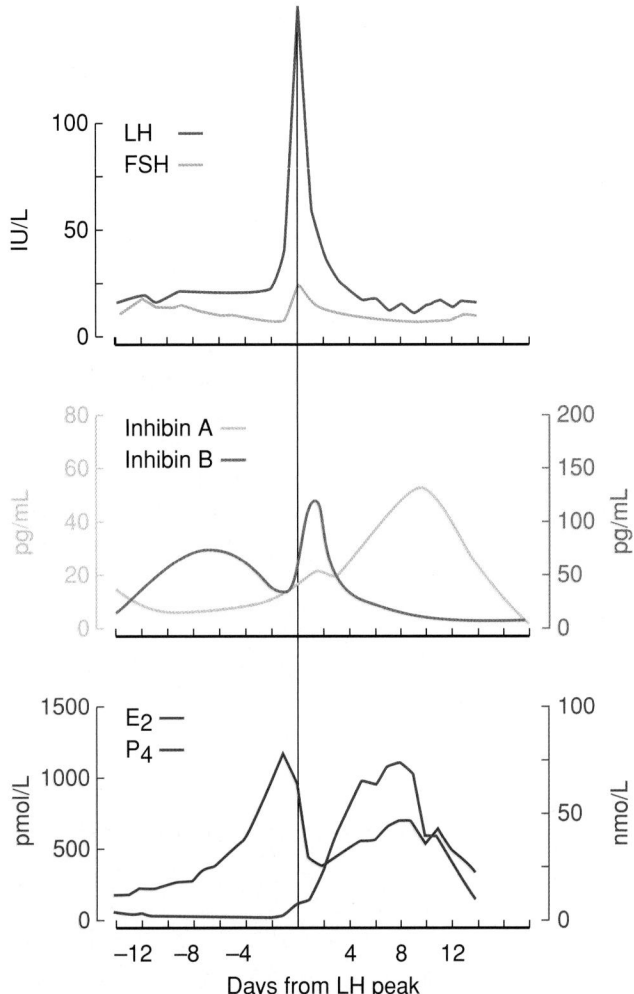

FIGURE 15-17 Graphs of gonadotropin, inhibin, and sex-steroid level changes during a normal menstrual cycle. The top graph displays peaking of luteinizing hormone (LH) (purple line) and follicle-stimulating hormone (FSH) (pink line) levels. The middle graph shows changing levels of inhibin A and inhibin B. Note that inhibin B levels (green line) peak temporally near the midcycle surge in the LH level, whereas maximal elevation of inhibin A (orange line) occurs several days following this peak. In the bottom graph, elevations in estradiol levels (red line) are noted prior to the surge in LH levels and in the midluteal phase. Progesterone levels (blue line) peak in the midluteal phase. E2 = estradiol; P4 = progesterone.

■ Follicular Development

Follicle Stages

Development begins with primordial follicles that were generated during fetal life (see Fig. 15-14). These follicles consist of an oocyte arrested in the first meiotic division surrounded by a single layer of flattened granulosa cells. The follicles are separated from the stroma by a thin basement membrane. Preovulatory follicles are avascular. As such, they are critically dependent on diffusion and on the later development of gap junctions for obtaining nutrients and clearing metabolic waste. Diffusion also allows passage of steroid precursors from the theca to the granulosa cell layer.

In the primary follicle stage, the granulosa cells of developing follicles become cuboidal and increase in number to form a pseudostratified layer. Intercellular gap junctions develop between adjacent granulosa cells and between granulosa cells and the developing oocyte (Albertini, 1974). These connections allow the passage of nutrients, ions, and regulatory factors between cells. Gap junctions also allow cells without gonadotropin receptors to receive signals from cells with receptor expression. As a result, hormone-mediated effects can be transmitted throughout the follicle.

During this stage, the oocyte begins to secrete products to form an acellular coat known as the zona pellucida. The human zona pellucida contains at least three proteins, named ZP1, ZP2, and ZP3. In current physiologic models, receptors on the acrosome head of the sperm recognize ZP3. This interaction releases acrosomal contents that permit penetration of the zona pellucida and ovum fertilization. Enzymes released from the acrosome induce alterations in ZP2 that result in hardening of the coat. This prevents fertilization of the oocyte by more than one sperm (Gupta, 2015).

Development of a secondary, or preantral, follicle includes final growth of the oocyte and a further increase in granulosa cell number. The stroma around the granulosa cell layer differentiates into the theca interna and the theca externa (Eppig, 1979).

Tertiary follicles, also called antral follicles, form from ongoing development in selected oocytes. In these, follicular fluid collects between the granulosa cells, ultimately producing a fluid-filled space known as the antrum. Granulosa cells in the antral follicle are histologically and functionally divided into two groups. The granulosa cells surrounding the oocyte form the cumulus oophorus, whereas the granulosa cells surrounding the antrum are known as mural granulosa cells. Antral fluid consists of a plasma filtrate and factors secreted by the granulosa cells. These locally produced factors, which include estrogen and growth factors, are present in substantially higher concentrations in follicular fluid than in the circulation and are likely critical for successful follicular maturation (Asimakopoulos, 2006; Silva, 2009). Further accumulation of antral fluid results in a rapid increase in follicular size and development of a preovulatory, or graafian, follicle (Hennet, 2012).

During this process, early stages of development (up to the secondary follicle) do not require gonadotropin stimulation and thus are said to be "gonadotropin-independent." Final follicular maturation requires adequate amounts of circulating LH and FSH and is therefore said to be "gonadotropin-dependent" (Butt, 1970). Of note, data suggest that progression from gonadotropin-independent to dependent stages is not as discrete as previously believed.

Concept of a Selection Window

Follicular development is a multistep process, which proceeds over at least 3 months and culminates in ovulation from a single follicle. Each month, a group of follicles known as a cohort begins a phase of semisynchronous growth. The size of this cohort appears to be proportional to the number of inactive primordial follicles within the ovaries and has been estimated at 3 to 11 follicles per ovary in young women (Hodgen, 1982; Pache, 1990). Importantly, the ovulatory follicle is recruited from a cohort that began development two to three cycles prior to the ovulatory cycle. During this time, most follicles will die as they will not be at an appropriate stage of development during the selection window.

During the luteal-follicular transition, a small increase in FSH levels is responsible for selection of the single dominant follicle that will ultimately ovulate (Schipper, 1998). As previously described, theca cells produce androgens, which are converted to estrogens by the granulosa cells. Estrogen levels increase with increased follicular size, enhance the effects of FSH on granulosa cells, and create a feed-forward action on follicles that produce estrogens.

Intrafollicular levels of the insulin-like growth factors are believed to synergize with FSH to help select the dominant follicle (Son, 2011). Additional studies have also demonstrated elevated levels of vascular endothelial growth factor (VEGF) around the follicle that will be selected. This follicle would presumably be exposed to higher levels of circulating factors such as FSH (Ravindranath, 1992).

Granulosa cells also produce inhibin B, which passes from the follicle into the plasma and specifically inhibits the release of FSH, but not of LH, by the anterior pituitary. The combined production of estradiol and inhibin B by the dominant follicle results in the decline of follicular-phase FSH levels and may be responsible at least in part for the failure of the other follicles to reach preovulatory status during any one cycle.

Estrogen-dominant Microenvironment

Ongoing follicular maturation requires the successful conversion from an "androgen-dominant" microenvironment to an "estrogen-dominant" one. At low concentrations, androgens stimulate aromatization and contribute to estrogen production. However, intrafollicular androgen levels will rise if aromatization in the granulosa cells lags behind androgen production by the thecal layer. At higher concentrations, androgens are converted to the more potent 5α-androgens, such as dihydrotestosterone. These androgens inhibit aromatase activity, cannot be aromatized to estrogens, and inhibit FSH induction of LH-receptor expression on the granulosa cells (Gervásio, 2014).

This model predicts that follicles that lack adequate FSH receptor and granulosa cell number will remain primarily androgenic and will therefore become atretic. An increased androgen-to-estrogen ratio is found in the follicular fluid of atretic follicles, and several studies have demonstrated that high estrogen levels prevent apoptosis.

IGF-I also has apoptosis-suppressing activity and is produced by granulosa cells. This action of IGF-I is suppressed by certain IGF-binding proteins that are present in the follicular fluid of atretic follicles. The action of FSH to prevent atresia may therefore result, in part, from its ability to stimulate IGF-I synthesis and suppress the synthesis of the IGF-binding proteins.

◼ Menstrual Cycle Phases

Follicular Phase

During the end of a previous cycle, estrogen, progesterone, and inhibin levels decrease abruptly with a corresponding increase in circulating FSH levels (Hodgen, 1982). As just described, this increase in FSH level is responsible for recruitment of the cohort of follicles that contains the follicle destined for ovulation. Despite general belief, sonographic studies in women have demonstrated that ovulation does not alternate sides, but occurs randomly from either ovary (Baird, 1987).

In women with waning ovarian function, the FSH level at this time of the cycle is elevated relative to that of younger women, presumably due to a loss of ovarian inhibin production in the previous luteal phase. As a result, measurement of early follicular or cycle day 3 FSH and estradiol levels is frequently performed in infertility clinics. The accelerated increase in serum FSH levels results in more robust recruitment of follicles and may explain both the shortened follicular phase observed in these older reproductive-aged women and the increased incidence of spontaneous twinning.

During the midfollicular phase, follicles produce increased amounts of estrogen and inhibin, resulting in a decline in FSH levels through negative feedback. This drop in FSH levels is believed to contribute to selection of the follicle destined to ovulate, termed the dominant follicle. Based on this theory, nondominant follicles express decreased numbers of FSH receptors and therefore are unable to respond adequately to declining FSH levels.

During most of follicular development, granulosa cell responses to FSH stimulation include an increase in granulosa cell number, an increase in aromatase expression, and, in the presence of estradiol, expression of LH receptors on the granulosa cells. With the development of LH-receptor expression during the late follicular phase, granulosa cells begin to produce small amounts of progesterone. This progesterone decreases granulosa cell proliferation, thereby slowing follicular growth (Chaffkin, 1992).

Ovulation

Toward the end of the follicular phase, estradiol levels increase dramatically. For reasons that are not completely understood but perhaps relate to changes at the kisspeptin neurons, the rapid estradiol level increase triggers a change from negative to positive feedback at both the hypothalamus and anterior pituitary gland to generate a surge in LH levels. Estradiol concentrations of 200 pg/mL for 50 hours are necessary to initiate this surge (Young, 1976). A small preovulatory increase in progesterone concentrations generates an FSH level surge, which occurs in tandem with the LH surge (McNatty, 1979). Progesterone may also augment the ability of estradiol to trigger the LH surge. These effects may explain the occasional induction of ovulation in anovulatory amenorrheic women when given progesterone to induce menses.

The LH surge acts rapidly on both the granulosa and theca cells of the preovulatory follicle to terminate the genes involved in follicular expression and turn on the genes necessary for ovulation and luteinization. In addition, the LH surge initiates the reentry of the oocyte into meiosis, expansion of the cumulus oophorus, synthesis of prostaglandins, and luteinization of granulosa cells. The mean duration of the LH surge is 48 hours, and ovulation occurs approximately 36 to 40 hours after the onset of the LH surge (Hoff, 1983; Lemarchand-Beraud, 1982). Abrupt termination of the surge is postulated to follow acutely increased steroid and inhibin secretion by the corpus luteum. Alternatively, the secretion of a gonadotropin surge-inhibiting/attenuating factor (GnSIF/AF) by either the ovary or hypothalamus is also postulated. However, the identity of this factor remains unknown (Vega, 2015).

The granulosa cells surrounding the oocyte, unlike mural granulosa cells, do not express LH receptors or synthesize progesterone. These cumulus oophorus granulosa cells develop tight gap junctions between themselves and with the oocyte. The cumulus mass that accompanies the ovulating oocyte is believed to provide a rough surface and increased size to improve oocyte "pick-up" by the tubal fimbria.

It has recently been found that amphiregulin, epiregulin, and beta-cellulin, which are epidermal growth factor-like factors, can be substituted to elicit the morphologic and biochemical events triggered by LH (Hsieh, 2009). Thus, these growth factors are part of the downstream cascade that begins with LH binding to its receptor and ends with ovulation.

Based on sonographic surveillance, extrusion of the oocyte lasts only a few minutes (Fig. 15-18) (Knobil, 1994). The exact mechanism of this expulsion is poorly defined but is not due to an increase in follicular pressure (Espey, 1974). The presence of proteolytic enzymes in the follicle, including plasmin and collagenase, suggests that these enzymes are responsible for follicular wall thinning (Beers, 1975). The preovulatory gonadotropin surge stimulates expression of tissue plasminogen activator by the granulosa and theca cells. The surge also decreases expression of plasminogen inhibitor, resulting in a marked increase in plasminogen activity (Piquette, 1993).

Prostaglandins also reach a peak concentration in follicular fluid during the preovulatory gonadotropin surge (Lumsden, 1986). Prostaglandins may stimulate smooth muscle contraction in the ovary, thereby contributing to ovulation (Yoshimura, 1987). Women undergoing infertility treatment are advised to avoid prostaglandin synthetase inhibitors in the preovulatory period to avoid luteinized unruptured follicle syndrome (LUFS) (Smith, 1996). Controversy exists as to whether LUFS should be considered pathologic or simply a sporadic event (Kerin, 1983).

Luteal Phase

Following ovulation, the remaining follicular cells differentiate into the corpus luteum, literally *yellow body* (Corner, 1956). This process, which requires LH stimulation, includes both morphologic and functional changes known as luteinization. The granulosa and theca cells proliferate and undergo hypertrophy to form granulosa-lutein cells and smaller theca-lutein cells, respectively (Patton, 1991).

During corpus luteum formation, the basement membrane that separates granulosa cells from theca cells degenerates and allows vascularization of previously avascular granulosa cells. Capillary invasion begins 2 days after ovulation and reaches the center of the corpus luteum by the fourth day. This increase in perfusion provides these luteal cells with access to circulating low-density lipoprotein (LDL), which is used to provide precursor cholesterol for steroid biosynthesis. This marked increase in blood supply can have clinical implications, as pain from a hemorrhagic corpus luteum cyst is a relatively frequent presentation to emergency rooms.

Adequate steroidogenesis in the corpus luteum depends on serum LH levels, LH receptors on luteal cells, and a sufficient number of luteal cells. Thus, it is critical that LH receptor expression on granulosa cells was appropriately induced during the prior follicular phase. Furthermore, blunted serum LH concentrations have been correlated with a shortened luteal phase. Luteal function is also influenced by gonadotropin levels from the preceding follicular phase. A reduction in LH or FSH secretion is correlated with poor luteal function. Presumably, a lack of FSH leads to a decrease in the total number of granulosa cells. Furthermore, luteal cells in these suboptimal cycles will have a decreased number of FSH-induced LH receptors and thus will be less responsive to LH stimulation.

Based on the corpus luteum's steroidogenic products, the luteal phase is considered progesterone dominant, which contrasts with the estrogen dominance of the follicular phase. Increased vascularization, cellular hypertrophy, and an increased number of intracellular organelles transform the corpus luteum into the most active steroidogenic tissue in the body. Maximal levels of progesterone production are observed in the midluteal phase and have been estimated at an impressive 40 mg of progesterone per day. Ovulation can be safely assumed to have occurred if the progesterone level exceeds 3 ng/mL on cycle day 21.

Although progesterone is the most abundant ovarian steroid during the luteal phase, estradiol is also produced in significant quantities. Estradiol levels drop transiently immediately after the LH surge. This decline may explain the midcycle spotting noticed by some women. The reason for this decrease is not known, but it may result from a direct inhibition of granulosa cell growth by increasing progesterone levels (Hoff, 1983). The decline in estradiol levels is followed by a steady increase to reach a maximum during the midluteal phase.

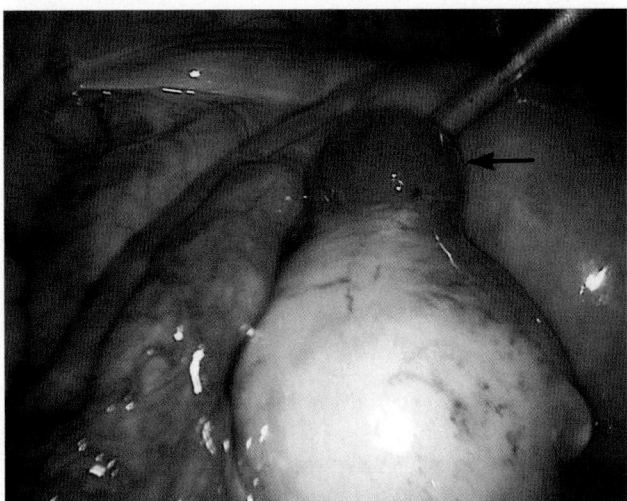

FIGURE 15-18 During laparoscopy, a stigma on the ovarian surface (*arrow*) prior to ovulation is seen. (Used with permission from Dr. David Rogers.)

The corpus luteum produces large quantities of inhibin A. This coincides with a decrease in circulating FSH levels in the luteal phase. If inhibin A levels decline at the end of the luteal phase, FSH levels rise once more to begin selection of a oocyte cohort for the next menstrual cycle.

If pregnancy does not occur, the corpus luteum regresses through a process called luteolysis. The mechanism for luteolysis is poorly understood, but luteal regression is presumed to be tightly regulated as luteal cycle length varies minimally among women. Following luteolysis, the blood supply to the corpus luteum diminishes, progesterone and estrogen secretion drop precipitously, and the luteal cells undergo apoptosis and become fibrotic. This creates the *corpus albicans* (white body).

If pregnancy occurs, hCG produced by the early gestation "rescues" the corpus luteum from atresia by binding to and activating the LH receptor on luteal cells. hCG stimulation of corpus luteum steroidogenesis maintains endometrial stability until placental steroid production is adequate to assume this function late in the first trimester. For this reason, surgical removal of the corpus luteum during pregnancy should be followed by progesterone replacement as outlined in Chapter 9 (p. 223) until approximately 10 weeks' gestation.

ENDOMETRIUM

■ Histology across the Menstrual Cycle

The endometrium consists of two layers: the *basalis layer,* which lies against the myometrium, and the *functionalis layer,* which is apposed to the uterine lumen. The basalis layer, which does not change significantly across the menstrual cycle, serves as the reserve for endometrium regeneration following menstrual sloughing. The functionalis layer is further subdivided into the more superficial *stratum compactum,* a thin layer of gland necks and dense stroma, and the underlying *stratum spongiosum* containing glands and large amounts of loosely organized stroma and interstitial tissue.

After menstruation, the endometrium is 1 to 2 mm thick. Under the influence of estrogen, the glandular and stromal cells of the functionalis layer proliferate rapidly following menses (Fig. 15-19). This period of rapid growth, the *proliferative phase,* corresponds to the ovary's follicular phase. As this phase progresses, glands become more tortuous and cells lining the glandular lumen undergo pseudostratification. The stroma remains compact. Endometrial thickness approximates 12 mm at the time of the LH surge and does not increase significantly thereafter.

Following ovulation, the endometrium transforms into a secretory tissue. The period during and after this transformation is defined as the *secretory phase* of the endometrium and correlates to the ovary's *luteal phase.* Glycogen-rich subnuclear vacuoles appear in cells lining the glands. Under further stimulation by progesterone, these vacuoles move from the glandular cells' base toward their lumen and expel their contents. This secretory process peaks on approximately postovulatory day 6, coinciding with the day of implantation. Throughout the luteal phase, glands become increasingly tortuous, and the stroma becomes more edematous. In addition, spiral arteries that feed the endometrium increase their number and coiling.

If a blastocyst does not implant and the corpus luteum is not maintained by placental hCG, progesterone levels drop and endometrial glands begin to collapse. Polymorphonuclear leukocytes and monocytes from nearby vessels infiltrate the endometrium. The spiral arteries constrict, leading to local ischemia, and lysosomes release proteolytic enzymes that accelerate tissue destruction. Prostaglandins, particularly prostaglandin $F_{2\alpha}$, are present in the endometrium and likely contribute to arteriolar vasospasm. Prostaglandin $F_{2\alpha}$ ($PGF_{2\alpha}$) also induces myometrial contractions, which may aid in expelling the endometrial tissue.

The entire endometrial functionalis layer is thought to exfoliate with menstruation, leaving only the basalis layer to provide cells for endometrial regeneration. However, in studies, the amount of tissue shed from different levels of the endometrium varies widely. Following menstruation, reepithelialization of the desquamated endometrium is initiated within 2 to 3 days after the onset of menses and completed within 48 hours.

■ Regulation of Endometrial Function
Tissue Degradation and Hemorrhage

Within the endometrium, numerous proteins maintain a delicate balance between tissue integrity and the localized destruction required for menstrual sloughing or for trophoblast invasion during implantation. Cytokines, growth factors, and steroid hormones are believed to regulate the genes encoding these tissue proteins (Critchley, 2001). Of these proteins, tissue factor, a membrane-associated protein, activates the coagulation cascade upon contact with blood. In addition, urokinase and tissue plasminogen activator (TPA) increase the conversion of plasminogen to plasmin to activate tissue breakdown. TPA activity is blocked by plasminogen activator inhibitor 1, which is present in endometrial stroma (Lockwood, 1993; Schatz, 1995). Another key mediator group, matrix metalloproteinases (MMPs), is an enzyme family with overlapping substrate specificities for collagens and other extracellular matrix components. The composition of MMPs varies within different endometrial tissues and during the menstrual cycle. Endogenous MMP inhibitors are increased premenstrually and limit MMP degradative activity.

Vasoconstriction and Myometrial Contractility

Effective menstruation depends on appropriately timed endometrial vasoconstriction and myometrial contraction. Vasoconstriction produces ischemia, endometrial damage, and subsequent menstrual sloughing. Within the endometrium, epithelial and stromal cells secrete endothelin-1, a potent vasoconstrictor. Enkephalinase, an endothelin-degrading enzyme, is expressed at its highest levels in the midsecretory endometrium (Head, 1993). However, in the late luteal phase, the drop in serum progesterone leads to a loss of enkephalinase expression. This permits increased endothelin activity promoting a physiologic environment amenable to vasoconstriction.

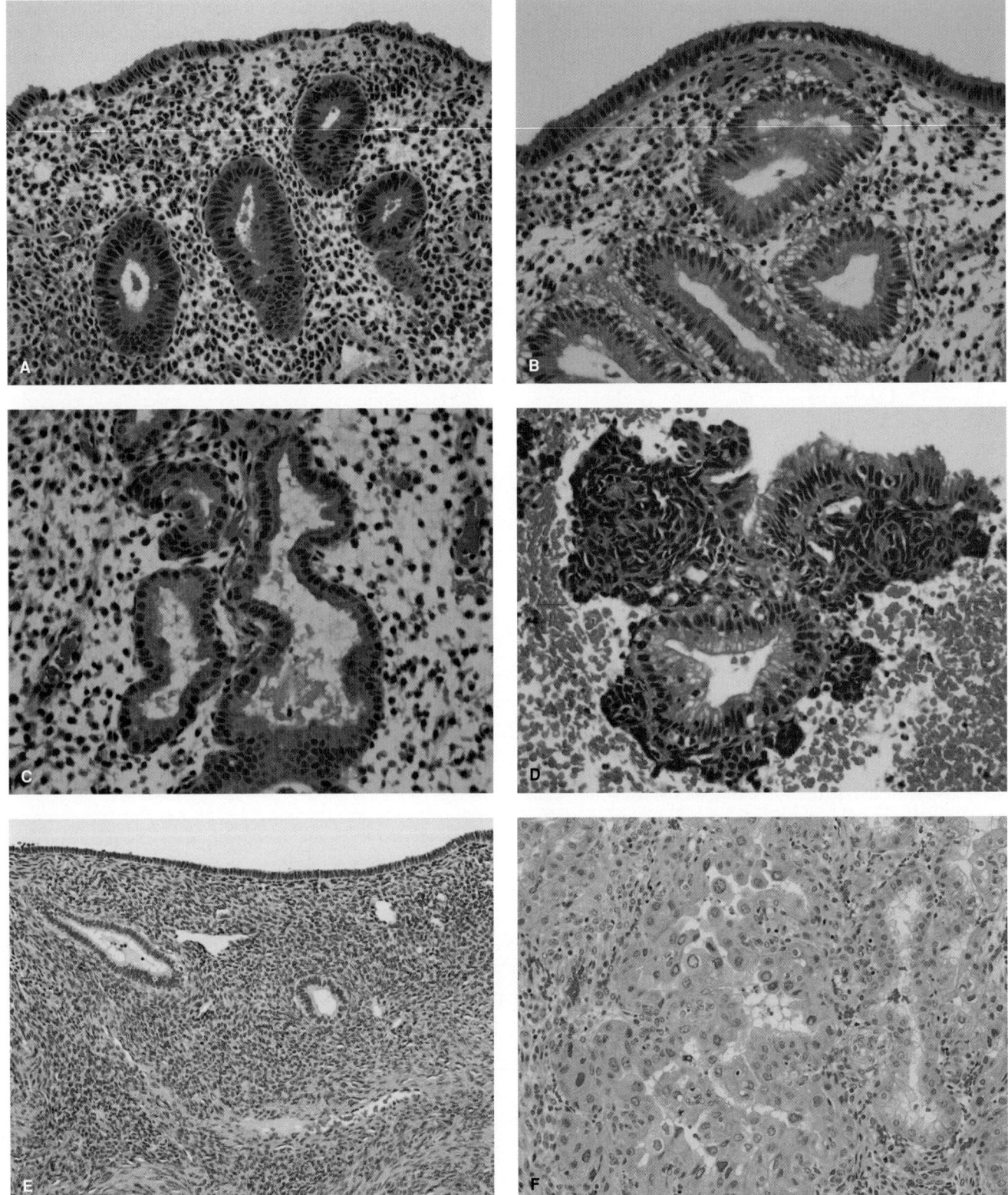

FIGURE 15-19 Endometrial changes during the menstrual cycle. **A.** Proliferative phase: straight to slightly coiled, tubular glands are lined by pseudostratified columnar epithelium with scattered mitoses. **B.** Early secretory phase: coiled glands with a slightly widened diameter are lined by simple columnar epithelium with clear subnuclear vacuoles. Stroma is variably edematous in the secretory phase. **C.** Late secretory phase: serrated, dilated glands with intraluminal secretion are lined by short columnar cells. **D.** Menstrual phase: fragmented endometrium with condensed stroma and glands with secretory vacuoles are seen in a background of blood. **E.** Atrophic endometrium: thin endometrium of the postmenopausal period has straight tubular glands lined by mitotically inactive, cuboidal epithelium. Stroma is dense and mitotically inactive. **F.** Gestational endometrium: hypersecretory glandular pattern featuring closely apposed glands with papillary infoldings and variable cytoplasmic vacuolization. The hypersecretory gland in the center shows the benign Arias-Stella reaction, with nuclear atypia characterized by variable nuclear enlargement, nuclear membrane irregularities, slight chromatin coarseness, nuclear vacuolization, and intranuclear pseudoinclusions. (Used with permission from Dr. Kelley Carrick.)

In concert with endometrial sloughing, myometrial contractions control blood loss by compressing endometrial vasculature and expelling menstrual discharge. A fall in serum progesterone decreases an enzyme that degrades prostaglandins. This increases $PGF_{2\alpha}$ activity in the myometrium and triggers myometrial contractions (Casey, 1980).

Estrogens and Progestins

The expression of estrogen and progesterone receptors in the endometrium is highly regulated across the menstrual cycle. This provides an additional mechanism for controlling steroid effects on endometrial development and function. Estrogen receptors are expressed in the nuclei of epithelial, stromal, and myometrial cells, and concentrations peak during the proliferative phase. However, during the luteal phase, rising progesterone levels decrease estrogen receptor expression. Endometrial progesterone receptors peak at midcycle in response to rising estrogen levels. By midluteal phase, progesterone receptor expression in the glandular epithelium is nearly absent, although expression remains strong in the stromal compartment (Lessey, 1988).

The proliferation and differentiation of the uterine epithelium is under the control of estradiol, progesterone, and various growth factors. The importance of estrogens for endometrial development is demonstrated by the predominance of endometrial hyperplasia seen in women receiving unopposed estrogen therapy. Estrogen interacts directly with estrogen receptors but can also indirectly induce various growth factors that include IGF-I, transforming growth factor α, and epidermal growth factor (Beato, 1989; Dickson, 1987). The effects of progesterone on endometrial growth vary among endometrial layers. Progesterone is critical for the conversion of the functionalis layer from a proliferative to a secretory pattern. Within the basalis layer, progesterone appears to promote cellular proliferation.

Growth Factors and Cell Adhesion Molecules

Numerous growth factors and associated receptors act in the endometrium. Each factor has its own pattern of expression, making it difficult to determine which factor is most critical for endometrial function (Ohlsson, 1989; Sharkey, 1995).

In addition to growth factors, cell adhesion molecules play an important role in endometrial function. These molecules fall into four classes: integrins, cadherins, selectins, and members of the immunoglobulin superfamily. Each has been implicated in endometrial regeneration and embryo implantation, discussed next.

Implantation Window

The embryo enters the uterine cavity 2 to 3 days after fertilization with implantation beginning approximately 4 days later. Studies have demonstrated that normal implantation and embryonic development require synchronous development of the endometrium and the embryo (Pope, 1988). The human blastocyst may have less stringent requirements for implantation than other species as ectopic implantation occurs relatively frequently.

Uterine receptivity can be defined as the temporal window of endometrial maturation during which trophectoderm attaches to endometrial epithelial cells with subsequent invasion into endometrial stroma. The window of implantation in the human is relatively broad, extending from day 20 through day 24 of the menstrual cycle. Precise determination of this temporal window is critical since only those factors expressed during this time act as direct functional mediators of uterine receptivity.

Endometrial receptivity is associated with loss of surface microvilli and ciliated cells and with development of cellular protrusions, called *pinopods*, on the apical surface of the endometrium. Pinopods are considered an important morphologic marker of periimplantation endometrium. Pinopod formation is known to be highly progesterone dependent (Yoshinaga, 1989).

Various factors are believed to be necessary for uterine receptivity, including cell adhesion molecules, immunoglobulins, and cytokines. Integrins have been a particularly well-studied factor in this regard (Casals, 2010). However, to date, no single integrin molecule has been determined to be the critical marker of the implantation window.

The term *luteal phase defect* describes dyssynchrony between endometrial development and menstrual cycle phase that leads to subsequent implantation failure and early pregnancy loss (Noyes, 1950; Olive, 1991). This term currently is of limited utility in clinical practice due to our inability to accurately diagnose or treat the disorder.

Following implantation, the endometrium undergoes essential remodeling by invading trophoblast. In addition, the maternal endocrine environment changes extensively because of altered maternal physiology and contributions by the placenta and fetus. A more detailed discussion of these changes can be found in *Williams Obstetrics*, 24th edition (Cunningham, 2014).

ABNORMALITIES IN THE HYPOTHALAMIC-PITUITARY AXIS

Knowledge of normal hypothalamic-pituitary axis function, described in the preceding sections, is essential to understand reproductive endocrine pathology. Classically, abnormalities in this axis result in low gonadotropin and resultant low sex steroid levels. Termed *hypogonadotropic hypogonadism*, this can be developmental or acquired. Developmental lesions due to inherited genetic defects include Kallmann syndrome and idiopathic hypogonadotropic hypogonadism. Acquired abnormalities include functional disorders (eating disorders, excessive exercise, stress) and hypothalamic-pituitary lesions due to tumor, infiltrative diseases, infarction, surgery, or radiation therapy. Information regarding hypothalamic disorders and other causes of hypogonadotropic hypogonadism can be found in Chapter 16 (p. 375). Hyperprolactinemia and pituitary adenomas are discussed here.

▪ Hyperprolactinemia
Etiology

Elevated circulating PRL levels can be caused by various physiologic activities including pregnancy, sleep, eating, and coitus.

Increased PRL levels may also be observed following chest wall stimulation such as occurs with suckling, breast examination, chest wall surgery, herpes zoster infection, or nipple piercing (Table 12-2, p. 281). PRL secretion is primarily regulated through tonic inhibition by dopamine released by the hypothalamus. PRL secretion is increased by serotonin, norepinephrine, opioids, estrogen, and TRH. Therefore, medications that block dopamine-receptor action (phenothiazines) or deplete catecholamine levels (monoamine oxidase inhibitors) may increase PRL levels (Table 12-2). Moreover, hyperprolactinemia may be caused by tumor, radiation, or infiltrative diseases such as sarcoid and tuberculosis. These can damage the pituitary stalk and thereby prevent dopamine-mediated inhibition of PRL secretion.

Primary hypothyroidism is also associated with mild elevations in serum PRL levels. Specifically, low circulating thyroid hormone levels produce a reflex increase in hypothalamic TRH levels due to loss of feedback inhibition. TRH can bind directly to anterior pituitary lactotropes and stimulate PRL production. As a rule, thyroid function tests should be performed when confirming a diagnosis of hyperprolactinemia, as a patient may require thyroid replacement rather than further evaluation for pituitary adenoma (Hekimsoy, 2010).

Prolactin-secreting adenomas, also termed prolactinomas, are the most common pituitary adenoma and the most common adenomas to be diagnosed by gynecologists. Affected women typically present with microadenomas and signs of PRL excess such as galactorrhea and amenorrhea.

Diagnosis

Hyperprolactinemia is, by definition, present in any patient with an elevated serum PRL level. Optimally, PRL levels are drawn in the morning, that is, at the time of the PRL nadir. Prior to testing, breast examination is avoided to prevent false-positive results. If a mildly elevated PRL level is found, sampling is repeated because PRL levels vary throughout the day. Moreover, many factors including the stress of venipuncture may produce false elevations.

Normal PRL levels are typically <20 ng/mL in nonpregnant women, although the upper limit of normal varies by assay.

Importantly, PRL levels rise nearly 10-fold during pregnancy and make detection of a prolactinoma difficult at this time. Occasionally, the reported PRL value will be falsely low due to a "hook effect" present in the assay (Frieze, 2002). As explained on page 341, very high levels of endogenous hormone oversaturate the test antibodies and thereby prevent required binding between a patient's PRL and the assay PRL. This problem is overcome with dilution of a patient's sample. Importantly, a mismatch between the adenoma size noted on magnetic resonance (MR) imaging and the degree of PRL level elevation should alert a clinician to either the possibility of an incorrect assay result or the likelihood that the macroadenoma is actually not primarily PRL secreting. Macroadenomas of any cell type may damage the pituitary stalk and prevent transfer of hypothalamic dopamine to the lactotropes.

Conversely, a patient may rarely have an elevated PRL level on assay despite a lack of clinical features of hyperprolactinemia. The hyperprolactinemia in these patients is thought to be secondary to alternate forms of PRL, including the so-called big or macroprolactin, which contains multimers of native PRL. Macroprolactin is not physiologically active but may be detected by PRL assays (Fahie-Wilson, 2005).

For all patients with confirmed hyperprolactinemia, MR imaging is advisable. Some advocate limiting imaging to women with a PRL level >100 ng/mL, as lower levels are most likely due to small microadenomas (Fig. 15-20). Although this is undoubtedly a safe approach in most women, mildly elevated PRL levels also may be due to pituitary stalk compression by a nonprolactin-secreting macroadenoma or a craniopharyngioma, diagnoses with severe potential consequences.

The availability of sensitive neuroimaging techniques now affords earlier diagnosis and intervention. In the past, pituitary adenomas were identified using a coned-down view of the sella turcica during standard head radiography. Although computed tomography (CT) scanning provides useful information on tumor size, bony artifacts may limit interpretation. Therefore, MR imaging, using both T1- and T2-weighted images, has become the preferred radiologic approach due to its high sensitivity and excellent spatial resolution (Ruscalleda, 2005). Frequently,

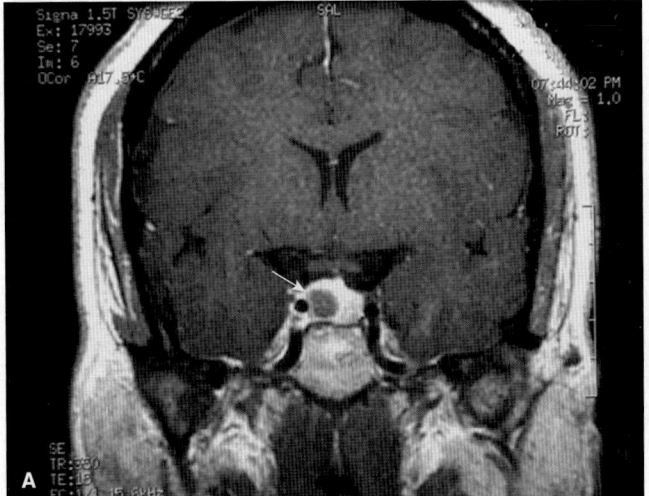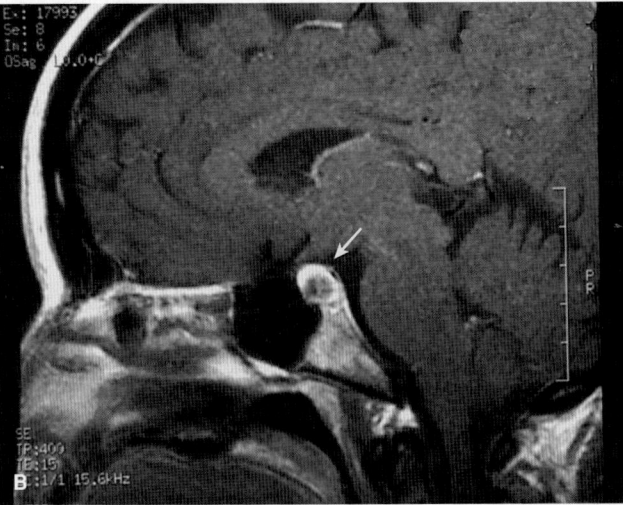

FIGURE 15-20 Magnetic resonance image of a pituitary microadenoma. **A.** Coronal image. **B.** Sagittal image.

MR imaging is performed with and without gadolinium infusion for maximum definition of tumor size and extension.

Associated Amenorrhea

The primary mechanism linking hyperprolactinemia and amenorrhea is believed to be a reflex increase in central dopamine levels. Stimulation of the dopaminergic receptors on the GnRH neurons alters GnRH pulsatility, thereby disrupting folliculogenesis. As dopamine receptors have also been identified in the ovaries, detrimental effects on folliculogenesis may also play a role. Additional mechanisms undoubtedly exist in view of the complexity of the interactions among the various hormones, peptides, and neurotransmitters that influence hypothalamic function.

■ Pituitary Adenomas

Classification

Pituitary adenomas are the most common cause of acquired pituitary dysfunction and comprise approximately 15 percent of all intracranial tumors (Melmed, 2015; Pekic, 2015). Clinically, symptoms of galactorrhea, menstrual disturbances, or infertility may lead to its diagnosis. Most tumors are benign, and only an estimated 0.1 percent of adenomas develop into frank carcinoma with metastasis (Kaltsas, 2005). Nevertheless, pituitary adenomas may cause striking abnormalities in both endocrine and nervous system function (Table 15-5).

Pituitary adenomas were historically classified as eosinophilic, basophilic, or chromophobic according to their hematoxylin and eosin staining characteristics. Tumors are now classified by their hormonal expression pattern as determined by immunohistochemistry (Fig. 15-21). Adenomas are further grouped by size into microadenomas (<10 mm in diameter) and macroadenomas (>10 mm in diameter).

The most common adenomas secrete PRL alone. However, adenomas may secrete any of the pituitary hormones either singly (monohormonal adenoma) or in combination (multihormonal adenoma). In the past, a subset of tumors was considered nonsecreting. However, with more sensitive assays, most have been determined to secrete the common α-subunit or the gonadotropin β-subunits and therefore are gonadotrope-derived. Rarely, both α- and β-subunits are secreted as functional dimeric hormone.

Symptoms

Pituitary adenomas may cause symptoms via excess hormone secretion and lead to clinical conditions such as hyperprolactinemia, acromegaly, or Cushing disease. Alternatively, adenomas may result in hormone deficiency due to damage of other pituitary cell types or the pituitary stalk by an expanding adenoma or following treatment of the primary lesion.

As might be predicted, pituitary microadenomas are typically diagnosed during evaluation of an endocrinopathy. Macroadenomas frequently present with patient symptoms from invasion of surrounding structures. The anterior pituitary gland neighbors both the optic chiasm and cavernous sinuses. Disruption of the optic chiasm by suprasellar growth of the pituitary mass may create bitemporal hemianopsia, in which the outer portion of the right and left visual fields is lost. The cavernous sinuses are a paired collection of thin-walled veins

TABLE 15-5. Clinical Features of Pituitary Adenomas

Adenoma Cell Origin (Hormone)	Clinical Syndrome	Testing[a]	Typical Results	Treatment
Lactotrope (PRL)	Galactorrhea; hypogonadism	PRL	Elevated	Dopamine agonist; surgical excision
Gonadotrope (LH, FSH, free subunits)	Silent or hypogonadism; rarely gonadotrope excess	Free α-, FSHβ-, and LHβ-subunits	Elevated	Surgical excision
Somatotrope (GH)	Acromegaly or gigantism; menstrual irregularity	IGF-I; 100-g glucose suppression test	Elevated; no GH suppression	Surgical excision; somatostatin analogues
Corticotrope (ACTH)	Cushing syndrome; menstrual irregularity	ACTH; 24-hour urinary free cortisol; dexamethasone suppression	Elevated ACTH and cortisol; no suppression	Surgical excision; ketoconazole to blunt adrenal steroidogenesis
Thyrotrope (TSH)	Thyrotoxicosis; menstrual irregularity	TSH, T_3, and T_4	All elevated	Surgical excision; PTU or methimazole; β-blockers for tachycardia

[a]All tests are serum measurements except for urinary free cortisol.

ACTH = adrenocorticotropin hormone; CRH = corticotropin-releasing hormone; FSH = follicle-stimulating hormone; GH = growth hormone; GnRH = gonadotropin-releasing hormone; IGF = insulin-like growth factor; LH = luteinizing hormone; PRL = prolactin; PTU = propylthiouracil; SHBG = sex hormone-binding globulin; TSH = thyroid-stimulating hormone; T_3 = triiodothyronine; T_4 = thyroxine.

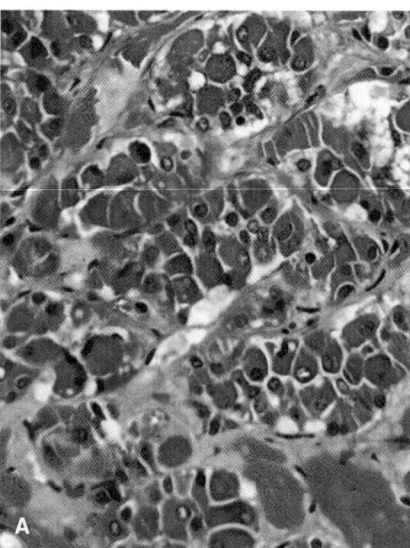 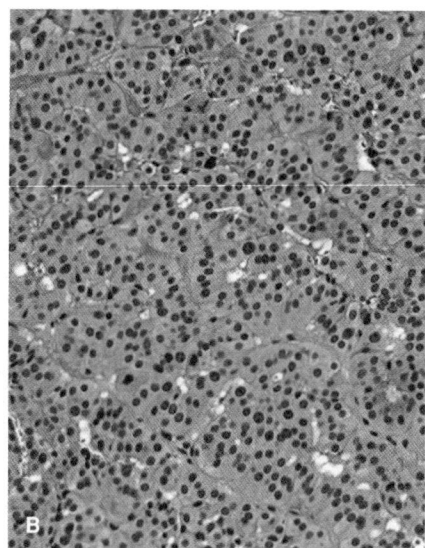 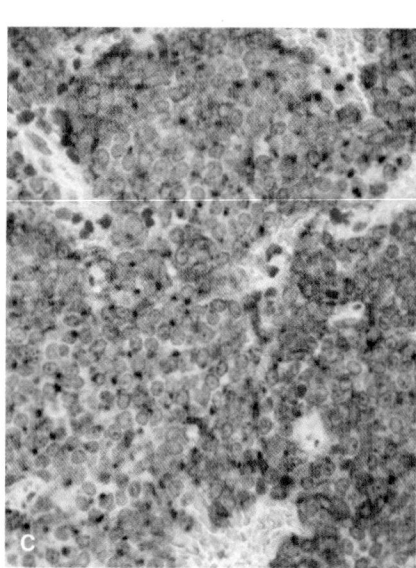

FIGURE 15-21 Photomicrographs from the anterior pituitary gland. **A.** Normal anterior pituitary gland. Secretory cells of the various types are arranged in small clusters between sinusoidal capillaries. **B.** Pituitary adenoma. In contrast to normal anterior pituitary gland, adenomas are composed of highly monomorphic cells. Note the absence of small clusters and sinusoids. **C.** Prolactin-secreting adenoma. Immunohistochemistry demonstrates expression of prolactin by many of the neoplastic cells. The dotlike pattern is characteristic of many prolactin-producing adenomas. (Used with permission from Dr. Jack Raisanen.)

located on either side of the sella turcica. Pituitary tumor compression can lead to cavernous sinus syndrome. This constellation of symptoms includes headache, visual disturbances, and cranial nerve palsies, specifically of cranial nerves III, IV, and VI.

Any pituitary mass or infiltrate can lead to reproductive dysfunction that may include delayed puberty, anovulation, oligomenorrhea, and infertility. The exact mechanisms linking adenomas to menstrual dysfunction are not well understood for many adenoma subtypes. Macroadenomas likely affect reproductive function either by compressing the pituitary stalk, which results in hyperprolactinemia, or less commonly, by directly compressing gonadotropes.

Spontaneous hemorrhage into a pituitary adenoma, termed *pituitary apoplexy*, is a rare life-threatening medical emergency. Signs and symptoms include acute visual changes, severe headache, neck stiffness, hypotension, loss of consciousness, and coma. These symptoms result from: (1) leakage of blood and necrotic material into the subarachnoid space, (2) acute hypopituitarism, and (3) a rapidly expanding hemorrhagic intrasellar mass that compresses the optic chiasm, cranial nerves, or hypothalamus and internal carotid arteries. Apoplexy may lead to severe hypoglycemia, hypotension, CNS hemorrhage, and death. Nevertheless, with rapid diagnosis and management, the outcome of patients with pituitary apoplexy is excellent (Singh, 2015). Glucocorticoid replacement is a mainstay of treatment. Surgical decompression is frequently but not invariably required.

Pregnancy and Pituitary Adenomas

The pituitary gland enlarges during pregnancy, primarily due to hypertrophy and hyperplasia of the lactotropes in response to elevated serum estrogen levels. Although the tumor can enlarge during pregnancy, the risk of clinically significant growth is small.

Tumor growth causing significant symptoms has been reported in approximately 2 percent of patients with microadenomas and 21 percent of those with macroadenomas without prior surgical or radiation treatment (Molitch, 2015). However, because significant expansion may lead to headaches or compression of the optic chiasm and blindness, visual field testing is considered in every trimester for women with macroadenomas. Although dopamine agonist therapy has been associated with an increased risk of spontaneous abortions, preterm deliveries, and congenital malformation, the data overall suggest that treatment is safe for most patients. Nevertheless, most experts advise that dopamine agonist therapy be discontinued during pregnancy when possible.

◼ Treatment of Hyperprolactinemia and Pituitary Adenomas

Most pituitary tumors grow slowly, and many cease growth after attainment of a certain size. Thus, asymptomatic patients with a microprolactinoma may be managed conservatively with serial MR imaging and serum PRL levels every 1 to 2 years as the risk of progression to a macroadenoma is <10 percent (Schlechte, 1989). These women should be followed for even mild changes in menstrual cyclicity as they are at risk for developing hypoestrogenism.

When tumors of any size are associated with amenorrhea or galactorrhea, therapy is considered (Fig. 15-22). Neurosurgical evaluation is mandatory when visual field defects or severe headaches are present. In general, first-line treatment is medical for both micro- and macroadenomas. Specifically, women should receive a dopamine agonist such as the nonspecific dopamine-receptor agonist bromocriptine (Parlodel) or the dopamine-receptor type 2 agonist cabergoline (Dostinex). Of note, the patient with hyperprolactinemia and normal imaging

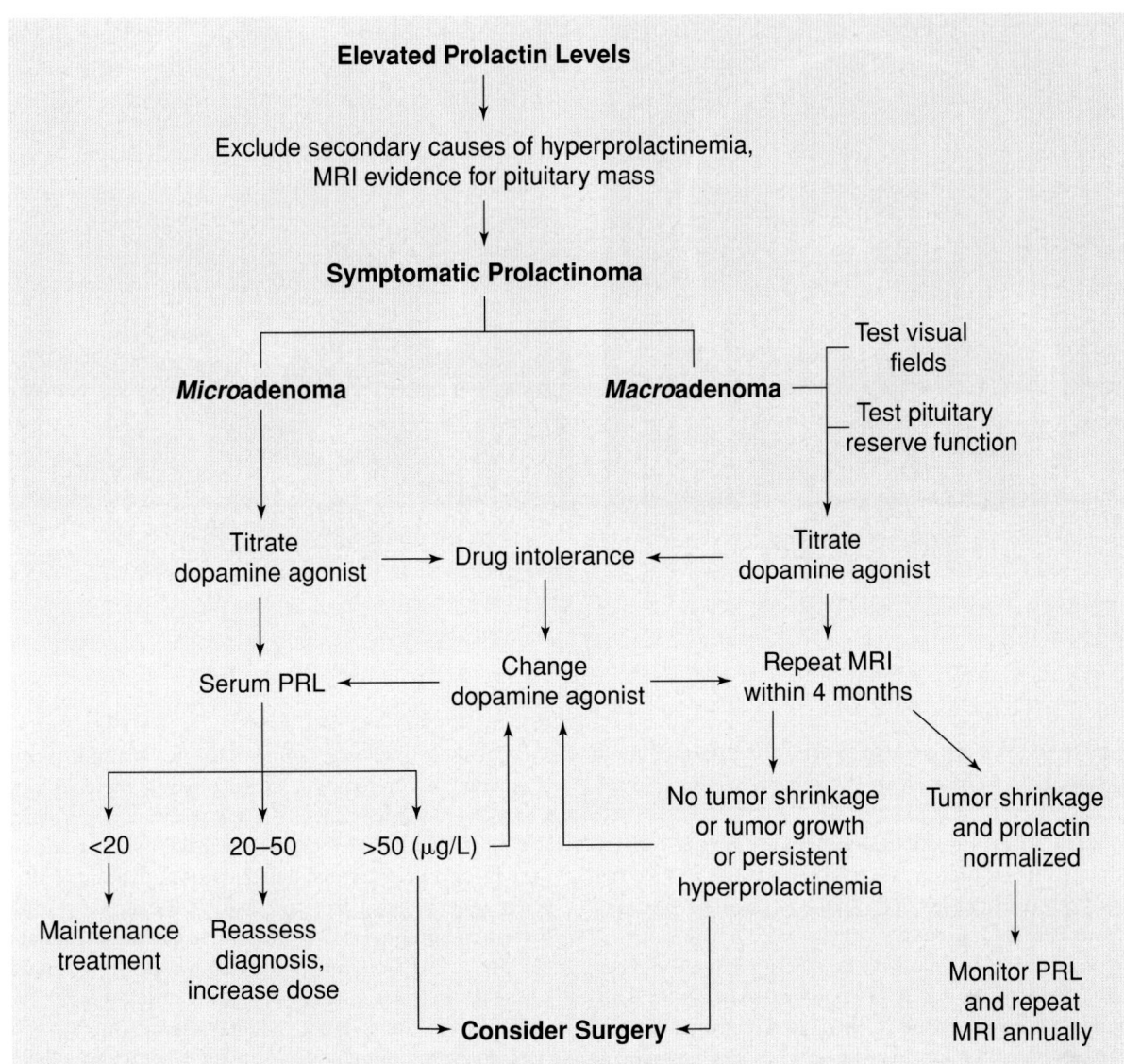

FIGURE 15-22 Algorithm describing the evaluation and treatment of pituitary adenomas. MRI = magnetic resonance imaging; PRL = prolactin. (Reproduced with permission from Kasper DL, Braunwald E, Fauci AS, et al (eds): Harrison's Principles of Internal Medicine, 17th ed. New York: McGraw-Hill; 2008.)

likely has an undetectable microadenoma and should be treated if symptomatic. The incidence of this occurring is decreasing with the advent of highly sensitive MR imaging.

Dopamine agonists decrease PRL secretion and shrink tumor size. However, bromocriptine treatment is associated with several common side effects, including headache, postural hypotension, blurry vision, drowsiness, and leg cramps. Most of these are attributable to activation of type 1 dopamine receptors. Due to its receptor specificity, cabergoline treatment is generally better tolerated than bromocriptine. Cabergoline also has a longer half-life, allowing once- or twice-weekly dosing compared with the multiple daily doses that may be required for bromocriptine. Typical initial cabergoline dosages are 0.25 mg orally twice weekly. Cabergoline has been found to be more effective than bromocriptine in normalizing PRL levels (dos Santos Nunes, 2011). Nevertheless, cabergoline can be prohibitively expensive. Most patients can tolerate bromocriptine if started at a low dose—½ tab or 0.125 mg—each night to minimize associated nausea and dizziness. This dose can be

slowly increased to three times daily as tolerated. Reliable measurement of posttreatment serum PRL levels can usually be obtained 1 month following a steady medication dose.

Neurosurgery is required for refractory tumors or those causing acutely worsening symptoms. The pituitary is approached through a transsphenoidal route whenever possible (Fig. 15-23). Complications of surgery, although rare, include intraoperative hemorrhage, a cerebrospinal fluid leak (rhinorrhea), diabetes insipidus, damage to other pituitary cell types, and meningitis (Miller, 2014).

Radiation therapy may be used for patients with surgically nonresectable, persistent, or aggressive tumors. The radiation dose necessary to stop tumor growth is lower than the dose necessary to achieve normalization of hormonal hypersecretion. More precise stereotactic radiosurgical approaches such as the gamma knife have improved radiation-beam focus, which significantly decreases local tissue damage and improves patient tolerance. Risks include optic nerve damage and delayed development of hypopituitarism (Pashtan, 2014).

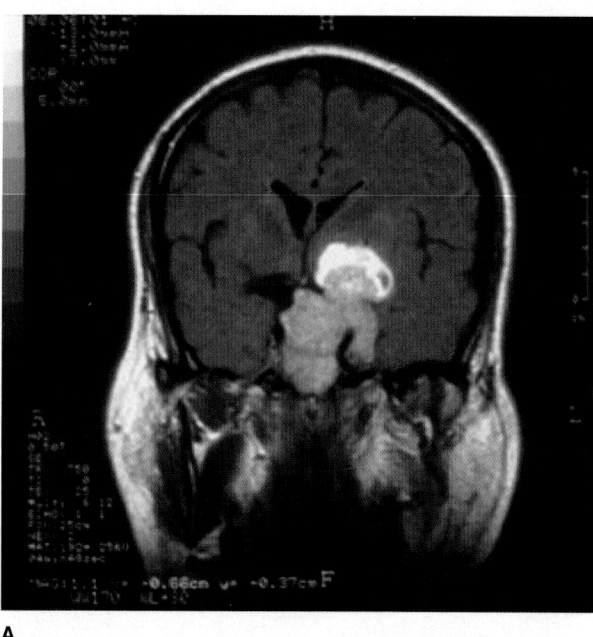
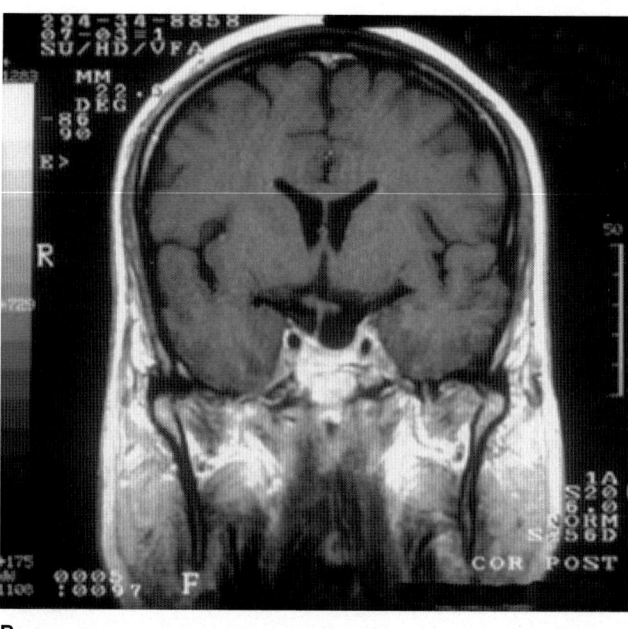

FIGURE 15-23 Magnetic resonance image of a pituitary before and after surgical resection of a macroadenoma. **A.** Preoperative coronal image reveals tumor measuring greater than 10 mm. **B.** Postoperative coronal image of the same patient following tumor excision.

DISORDERS OF PEPTIDE AND STEROID HORMONES IN REPRODUCTION

Clinical disorders may result from mutations in genes affecting hormone biosynthesis or the receptors that transduce the response. Both mechanisms have been described for pituitary peptide and steroid hormones.

First, numerous mutations have been identified in the genes that encode the LH/CG and FSH receptors. Most of the identified mutations are inactivating. These produce gonadotropin resistance of variable severity that ranges from primary amenorrhea to oligoamenorrhea and infertility (Latronico, 2013). Activating receptor mutations appear to be rare. However, a constitutively active LH/CG mutant receptor does cause a familial gonadotropin-independent precocious puberty that is limited to males (Ulloa-Aguirre, 2014). Although uncommon, mutations in the genes encoding the gonadotropin hormones themselves result in varying degrees of hypogonadism (Basciani, 2012; Kottler, 2010).

Second, gene mutation can lead to decreased function in steroid receptors. The best known of the latter is androgen insensitivity syndrome (AIS). With AIS, inactivating mutations in the androgen receptor impair the ability to respond to androgens. As a result, these 46,XY individuals have female external genitalia and scant to absent pubic and axillary hair. However, their testes do produce anti-müllerian hormone, their müllerian ducts fail to develop, and thus a blind-ending vaginal pouch without uterus or fallopian tubes results. Breasts develop in response to estrogens derived from aromatization of circulating testicular steroids (Tadokoro-Cucaro, 2014). Phenotypes of AIS are further described in Chapter 18 (p. 412).

Last, mutations in the enzymes necessary for steroidogenesis create broad clinical effects. Phenotypes depend on the location and severity of the resulting enzymatic deficiency within the steroidogenic pathway (Miller, 2011). The most common is congenital adrenal hyperplasia (CAH), typically due to a 21-hydroxylase deficiency. With severe enzymatic deficiency, affected patients have life-threatening salt wasting and female-to-male disorder of sexual differentiation (46,XX DSD). A less severe mutation may lead to "simple virilizing CAH" in which increased androgen levels are the primary hormonal abnormality (Auchus, 2015). The mildest abnormalities present as "nonclassic," "late-onset," or "adult-onset" CAH. In these patients, activation of the adrenal axis at puberty increases steroidogenesis and unmasks a mild 21-hydroxylase deficiency. Excess androgen provides negative feedback to GnRH receptors in the hypothalamus. These patients often present with hirsutism, acne, and anovulation. Thus, late-onset CAH may mimic PCOS (McCann-Crosby, 2014). Additional information regarding the CAH spectrum is found in Chapter 18 (p. 413).

ESTROGENS AND PROGESTINS IN CLINICAL PRACTICE

In gynecology, estrogen and/or progestins are used for contraception and the treatment of abnormal uterine bleeding, endometriosis, leiomyomas, PCOS, and menopausal symptoms. Specific uses are found in respective chapters on these topics. Of the various estrogen and progesterone preparations, each differs in its biologic efficacy, and clinicians should understand the reasons behind some of these differences.

■ Estrogens

Classic estrogens are C-18 steroid compounds containing a phenolic ring (Fig. 15-24). This group contains the natural estrogens—estradiol, estrone, estriol—and their derivatives

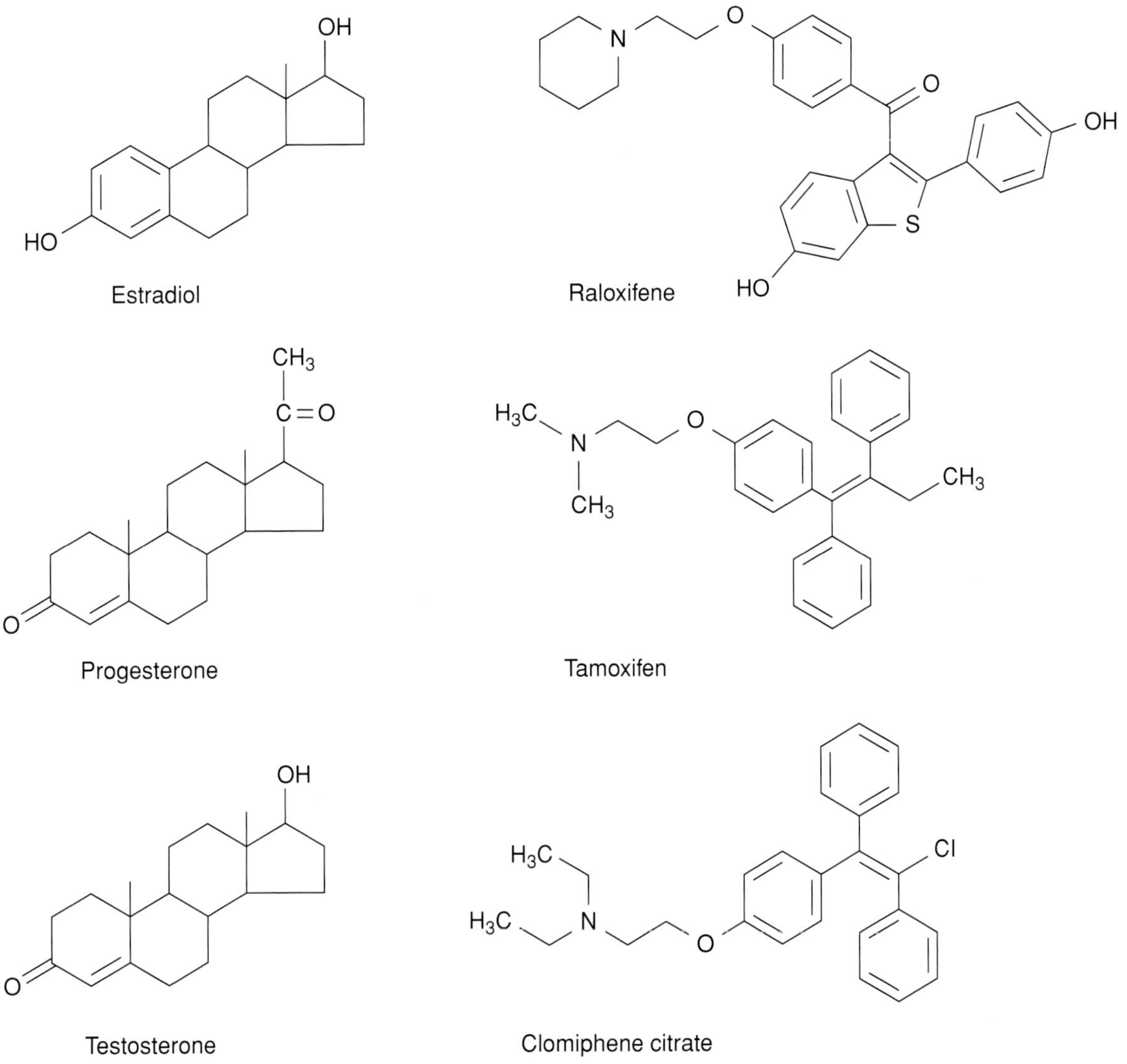

FIGURE 15-24 Chemical structures of important sex steroids and selective estrogen-receptor modulators.

as well as conjugated equine estrogens (CEE). The predominant synthetic C-18 estrogen is ethinyl estradiol, the estrogen present in combination oral contraceptives. Synthetic nonsteroidal estrogens include diethylstilbestrol (DES) and selective estrogen-receptor modulators such as tamoxifen and clomiphene citrate. Despite their variation from the classic steroid ring shape, these nonsteroidal estrogens are still able to bind to the estrogen receptor.

Of the natural estrogens, 17β-estradiol is the most potent followed by estrone and then estriol. In comparing some pharmacologically used estrogens, ethinyl estradiol, a derivative of 17β-estradiol, has been estimated to be approximately 100 to 1000 times more potent on a per weight basis than either micronized estradiol or CEE in terms of increasing SHBG levels, which is one marker of estrogen potency (Kuhl, 2005; Mashchak, 1982).

Progestogens

Although there is no formal rule, progestogens include natural progesterone and synthetic progestogens called progestins.

Only progesterone can maintain human pregnancy. Progestins can be classified as derivatives of either 19-norprogesterone or 19-nortestosterone (Kuhl, 2005). Of the 19-norprogesterones, the most commonly used are medroxyprogesterone acetate and megestrol acetate.

Most progestins used in contraceptives are derived from 19-nortestosterone. These are commonly described as first generation (norethindrone), second generation (levonorgestrel, norgestrel), or third generation (desogestrel, norgestimate). As described in Chapter 5 (p. 118), each generation has been designed to have progressively less androgenic effect. The fourth-generation progestin, drospirenone, is unique in that it is derived from spironolactone. Although it has no androgenic activity, drospirenone has an affinity for the mineralocorticoid receptor approximately five times that of aldosterone. This explains its diuretic action.

Selective Steroid-receptor Modulators

As indicated by their names, these synthetic compounds bind to their target receptors and exert tissue-specific effects,

TABLE 15-6. Agonist or Antagonist Effects of Estradiol and Selected SERMs

Drug	Breast	Bone	Lipids	Endometrium
Tamoxifen	Antagonist	Agonist	Agonist	Agonist
Raloxifene	Antagonist	Agonist	Agonist	Antagonist
Ospemifene	Neutral	Agonist	Neutral	Partial agonist
Bazedoxifene	Antagonist	Agonist	Agonist	Antagonist
Estradiol	Agonist	Agonist	Agonist	Agonist

SERM = selective estrogen-receptor modulator.
Data from Archer, 2015; Miller, 2008; Ylikorkala, 2003.

acting as agonists in some tissues and antagonists in others (Table 15-6). The best known of these are the selective estrogen-receptor modulators (SERMs) (Haskell, 2003). The variable activity among the SERMs can be attributed to differences at the molecular level. Each SERM binds to an estrogen receptor to generate a unique molecular conformation that affects the interaction of the complex with transcriptional cofactors and gene promoter regions. The response is also modified by the relative expression of ERα and ERβ receptors in the target tissue. The hormonal milieu may also be important in determining the agonist–antagonist profile of a specific SERM. For example, a SERM may act as an estrogen agonist in a low-estrogen state, such as menopause, but as a competitive antagonist in a patient with high circulating levels of the potent estrogen estradiol.

Development of new SERMs with specific agonist/antagonist profiles is an active area of current research. The SERM ospemifene (Osphena) may have favorable characteristics for long-term relief of genitourinary syndrome of menopause (Archer, 2015). Another SERM, bazedoxifene, is combined with CEE and marketed as Duavee. This coupled approach yields a drug group categorized as tissue-selective estrogen complexes (TSECs). The goal of TSECs is to craft agents with estrogen agonist/antagonist profiles that optimize clinical efficacy and safety.

More recently, selective progesterone-receptor modulators (SPRMs) have been developed to improve emergency contraception efficacy and expand treatment options for disorders includ-ing leiomyomas and endometriosis (Chwalisz, 2005). Selective androgen-receptor modulators (SARMs) are also under investigation for the treatment of osteopenia and decreased libido in women. Ideally, these will avoid the virilizing effects of testosterone treatment (Negro-Vilar, 1999).

As indicated by the preceding discussion, the agonist–antagonist effect of a steroid hormone is inextricably related to the clinical tissue of interest. Although this concept is most frequently discussed in terms of selective steroid modulators, in fact all steroid hormones within a class exert differences in their pattern of action across tissues. As a result, when a steroid is chosen for treatment, each clinical end point should be considered individually.

■ Steroid Hormone Potency

The efficacy of estrogen and progesterone treatments is altered by numerous factors such as: (1) receptor binding affinity, (2) formulation, (3) administration route, (4) metabolism, and (5) affinity for binding globulins. First, even small chemical modifications can substantially alter the biologic effects of steroid preparations. For example, the progestins in clinical use all exert progestogenic effects but may also act as weak androgens, antiandrogens, glucocorticoids, or antimineralocorticoids. These differences are likely explained by variations in binding affinity for each of these steroid receptors (Table 15-7).

Second, estrogens and progestins can be administered as oral, transdermal, vaginal, or intramuscular preparations,

TABLE 15-7. Relative Binding Affinities of Steroid Receptors and Serum Binding Globulins to Progestogens

Progestogen	PR	AR	ER	GR	MR	SHBG	CBG
Progesterone	50	0	0	10	100	0	36
Medroxyprogesterone acetate	115	5	0	29	160	0	0
Levonorgestrel	150	45	0	1	75	50	0
Etonogestrel	150	20	0	14	0	15	0
Norgestimate	15	0	0	1	0	0	0
Dienogest	5	10	0	1	0	0	0
Drospirenone	35	65	0	6	230	0	0

AR = androgen receptor; CBG = corticoid-binding globulin; ER = estrogen receptor; GR = glucocorticoid receptor; MR = mineralocorticoid receptor; PR = progesterone receptor; SHBG = sex hormone-binding globulin.
Modified with permission from Wiegratz I, Kuhl H: Progestogen therapies: differences in clinical effects? Trends Endocrinol Metab 2004 Aug;15(6):277–285.

TABLE 15-8. Relative Potency of Various Estrogens Concerning Clinical and Metabolic Parameters[a]

Estrogen	Suppression of		Increase Serum Levels of			
	Hot Flashes	FSH	HDL	SHBG	CBG	Angiotensinogen
Estradiol-17β	100	100	100	100	100	
Estriol	30	20				
CEE	120	110	150	300	150	150
Ethinyl estradiol	12,000	12,000	40,000	50,000	60,000	35,000

[a]The values are estimated on a weight basis.
CBG = corticoid-binding globulin; CEE = conjugated equine estrogens; FSH = follicle-stimulating hormone; HDL = high-density lipoprotein; SHBG = sex hormone-binding globulin.
Modified with permission from Kuhl H: Pharmacology of estrogens and progestogens: influence of different routes of administration, Climacteric 2005 Aug;8 Suppl 1:3–63.

among others. The choice of carrier molecule affects hormone bioavailability. For example, although crystalline progesterone is poorly absorbed via the intestine, dispersion of the progesterone into small particles (micronization) markedly increases surface area and uptake.

Third, oral medications pass through the intestine and the liver prior to systemic dissemination. As these tissues are sites for steroid metabolism, oral medications and their levels may be significantly altered prior to reaching their target organs. As an example, the bioavailability of orally administered micronized progesterone is less than 10 percent and compares poorly with the estimated 50- to 70-percent bioavailability for norethindrone and 100 percent for levonorgestrel. This difference is due to a high level of "first pass" metabolism of micronized progesterone but not these modified progestins (Stanczyk, 2002). As another example, the half-life of ethinyl estradiol is greatly extended relative to that of unconjugated estradiol by the presence of the ethinyl group, which impairs metabolism.

Absorption and metabolism rates may differ between individuals due to inherited or acquired differences in liver, intestinal, and renal function (Kuhl, 2005). Local metabolism will also lower steroid efficacy and can include conversion between steroids (for example, androgens to estrogens by aromatase) or within a steroid type (for example, estradiol to the weaker estrone). Diet, alcohol consumption, cigarette smoking, exercise, and stress have all been postulated to alter steroid metabolism. Thyroid disease also affects drug metabolism rates. Medications that increase hepatic enzyme activity may increase estrogen metabolism. Best understood is the ability of some antiepileptic drugs to decrease estrogen-containing contraceptive efficacy (O'Brien, 2010).

Last, steroid potency depends on affinity for the various carrier proteins produced by the liver. Only unbound hormone and to a much lesser extent, the amount bound to albumin or cortisol-binding globulin (CBG) is functionally active. Steroid bound to SHBG is considered inactive. Ethinyl estradiol is bound nearly exclusively to albumin, and this increases its bioavailability (Barnes, 2007). As shown in Table 15-7, significant differences in carrier binding are also observed for progestogens (Wiegratz, 2004).

Importantly, hormonal status affects expression of carrier proteins. Specifically, estrogens and thyroid hormone stimulate SHBG while androgens blunt serum SHBG levels. To add further complexity, it is now believed that target cells can secrete SHBG, which then acts locally as a membrane receptor to stimulate cyclic adenosine monophosphate (cAMP) intracellular signaling pathways (Rosner, 2010).

■ **Steroid Bioassays**

A limited number of studies have used bioassays to evaluate the efficacy of estrogens in women using clinical, endocrinologic, and metabolic parameters (Table 15-8) (Kuhl, 2005). As seen in animal studies, different preparations vary markedly in their potency. Of note, estrogens also demonstrate differences in terms of their tissue specificity. For example, 17β-estradiol and CEE suppress pituitary FSH to a similar extent, whereas CEE is a more potent stimulator of liver SHBG production.

REFERENCES

Albertini DF, Anderson E: The appearance and structure of intercellular connections during the ontogeny of the rabbit ovarian follicle with particular reference to gap junctions. J Cell Biol 63:234, 1974

Archer DF, Carr BR, Pinkerton JV, et al: Effects of ospemifene on the female reproductive and urinary tracts: translation from preclinical models into clinical evidence. Menopause 22(7):786, 2015

Asimakopoulos B, Koster F, Felberbaum R, et al: Cytokine and hormonal profile in blood serum and follicular fluids during ovarian stimulation with the multidose antagonist or the long agonist protocol. Hum Reprod 21:3091, 2006

Auchus RJ: Management considerations for the adult with congenital adrenal hyperplasia. Mol Cell Endocrinol 408:190, 2015

Auchus RJ: Non-traditional metabolic pathways of adrenal steroids. Rev Endocr Metab Disord 10:27, 2009

Baird DT: A model for follicular selection and ovulation: lessons from superovulation. J Steroid Biochem 27:15, 1987

Baker TG: A quantitative and cytological study of germ cells in human ovaries. Proc R Soc Lond B Biol Sci 158:417, 1963

Barnes RR, Levrant SG (eds): Pharmacology of estrogens. In Treatment of the Postmenopausal Woman. New York, Columbia University, 2007, p 767

Basciani S, Watanabe M, Mariani S, et al: Hypogonadism in a patient with two novel mutations of the luteinizing hormone β-subunit gene expressed in a compound heterozygous form. J Clin Endocrinol Metab 97(9):3031, 2012

Beato M: Gene regulation by steroid hormones. Cell 56:335, 1989

Beers WH: Follicular plasminogen and plasminogen activator and the effect of plasmin on ovarian follicle wall. Cell 6:379, 1975

Bilezikjian LM, Justice NJ, Blackler AN, et al: Cell-type specific modulation of pituitary cells by activin, inhibin and follistatin. Mol Cell Endocrinol 359(1–2):43, 2012

Blanks AM, Thornton S: The role of oxytocin in parturition. BJOG 110 (Suppl 20):46, 2003

Boon WC, Chow JD, Simpson ER: The multiple roles of estrogens and the enzyme aromatase. Prog Brain Res 181:209, 2010

Buckler HM, Healy DL, Burger HG: Purified FSH stimulates production of inhibin by the human ovary. J Endocrinol 122:279, 1989

Butt WR, Crooke AC, Ryle M, et al: Gonadotrophins and ovarian development; proceedings of the two Workshop Meetings on the Chemistry of the Human Gonadotrophins and on the Development of the Ovary in Infancy. Birmingham, 1969, Edinburgh, Livingstone, 1970

Carr BR: The ovary. In Carr BR, Blackwell RE (eds): Textbook of Reproductive Medicine, 2nd ed. Stamford, Appleton Lange, 1998, p 210

Carr BR: The ovary and the normal menstrual cycle. In Carr BR, Blackwell RE, Azziz R (eds): Essential Reproductive Medicine. New York, McGraw-Hill, 2005, p 79

Casals G, Ordi J, Creus M, et al: Osteopontin and $\alpha v \beta 3$ integrin as markers of endometrial receptivity: the effect of different hormone therapies. Reprod Biomed Online 21:349, 2010

Casey ML, Hemsell DL, MacDonald PC, et al: NAD+-dependent 15-hydroxyprostaglandin dehydrogenase activity in human endometrium. Prostaglandins 19:115, 1980

Cetel NS, Quigley ME, Yen SS: Naloxone-induced prolactin secretion in women: evidence against a direct prolactin stimulatory effect of endogenous opioids. J Clin Endocrinol Metab 60:191, 1985

Chaffkin LM, Luciano AA, Peluso JJ: Progesterone as an autocrine/paracrine regulator of human granulosa cell proliferation. J Clin Endocrinol Metab 75:1404, 1992

Chehab FF: 20 years of leptin: leptin and reproduction: past milestones, present undertakings, and future endeavors. J Endocrinol 223(1):T37, 2014

Cheng CK, Leung PC: Molecular biology of gonadotropin-releasing hormone (GnRH)-I, GnRH-II, and their receptors in humans. Endocr Rev 26:283, 2005

Childs GV, Hyde C, Naor Z, et al: Heterogeneous luteinizing hormone and follicle-stimulating hormone storage patterns in subtypes of gonadotropes separated by centrifugal elutriation. Endocrinology 113:2120, 1983

Chuan S, Homer M, Pandian R, et al: Hyperglycosylated human chorionic gonadotropin as an early predictor of pregnancy outcomes after in vitro fertilization. Fertil Steril 101(2):392, 2014

Chwalisz K, Perez MC, Demanno D, et al: Selective progesterone receptor modulator development and use in the treatment of leiomyomata and endometriosis. Endocr Rev 26:423, 2005

Clayton RN, Catt KJ: Gonadotropin-releasing hormone receptors: characterization, physiological regulation, and relationship to reproductive function. Endocr Rev 2:186, 1981

Cole LA: Biological functions of hCG and hCG-related molecules. Reprod Biol Endocrinol 8:102, 2010

Cole LA, Khanlian SA, Muller CY: Detection of perimenopause or postmenopause human chorionic gonadotropin: an unnecessary source of alarm. Am J Obstet Gynecol 198(3):275.e1, 2008

Conneely OM, Mulac-Jericevic B, DeMayo F, et al: Reproductive functions of progesterone receptors. Recent Prog Horm Res 57:339, 2002

Corner GW Jr: The histological dating of the human corpus luteum of menstruation. Am J Anat 98:377, 1956

Coticchio G, Dal Canto M, Mignini Renzini M, et al: Oocyte maturation: gamete-somatic cells interactions, meiotic resumption, cytoskeletal dynamics and cytoplasmic reorganization. Hum Reprod Update 21(4):427, 2015

Couse JF, Curtis HS, Korach KS: Receptor null mice reveal contrasting roles for estrogen receptor alpha and beta in reproductive tissues. J Steroid Biochem Mol Biol 74:287, 2000

Critchley HO, Kelly RW, Brenner RM, et al: The endocrinology of menstruation—a role for the immune system. Clin Endocrinol (Oxf) 55(6):701, 2001

Crowley WR, Armstrong WE: Neurochemical regulation of oxytocin secretion in lactation. Endocr Rev 13:33, 1992

Cunningham FG, Leveno KJ, Bloom SL, et al (eds): Implantation, embryogenesis, and placental development. In Williams Obstetrics, 24th ed. New York, McGraw-Hill Education, 2014

Cunningham FG, Leveno KJ, Bloom SL, et al (eds): Parturition. In Williams Obstetrics, 23rd ed. New York, McGraw-Hill, 2010

de Kretser DM, Hedger MP, Loveland KL, et al: Inhibins, activins, and follistatin in reproduction. Hum Reprod Update 8:529, 2002

Dickson RB, Lippman ME: Estrogenic regulation of growth and polypeptide growth factor secretion in human breast carcinoma. Endocr Rev 8:29, 1987

dos Santos Nunes V, El Dib R, Boguszewski CL, et al: Cabergoline versus bromocriptine in the treatment of hyperprolactinemia: a systematic review of randomized controlled trials and meta-analysis. Pituitary 14(3):259, 2011

Eppig JJ: A comparison between oocyte growth in coculture with granulosa cells and oocytes with granulosa cell-oocyte junctional contact maintained in vitro. J Exp Zool 209:345, 1979

Espey LL: Ovarian proteolytic enzymes and ovulation. Biol Reprod 10:216, 1974

Fahie-Wilson MN, John R, Ellis AR: Macroprolactin; high molecular mass forms of circulating prolactin. Ann Clin Biochem 42:175, 2005

Ferin M, International Institute for the Study of Human Reproduction: Biorhythms and human reproduction; a conference sponsored by the International Institute for the Study of Human Reproduction. New York, Wiley, 1974

Fournier T, Guibourdenche J, Evain-Brion D: Review: hCGs: different sources of production, different glycoforms and functions. Placenta 36 Suppl 1:S60, 2015

Frieze TW, Mong DP, Koops MK: "Hook effect" in prolactinomas: case report and review of literature. Endocr Pract 8:296, 2002

Funabashi T, Brooks PJ, Weesner GD, et al: Luteinizing hormone-releasing hormone receptor messenger ribonucleic acid expression in the rat pituitary during lactation and the estrous cycle. J Neuroendocrinol 6:261, 1994

Gervásio CG, Bernuci MP, Silva-de-Sá MF, et al: The role of androgen hormones in early follicular development. ISRN Obstet Gynecol 2014:818010, 2014

Gosden RG: Oocyte development and loss. Semin Reprod Med 31(6):393, 2013

Gruber CJ, Tschugguel W, Schneeberger C, et al: Production and actions of estrogens. N Engl J Med 346(5):340, 2002

Gupta SK: Role of zona pellucida glycoproteins during fertilization in humans. J Reprod Immunol 108:90, 2015

Halvorson LM: PACAP modulates GnRH signaling in gonadotropes. Mol Cell Endocrinol 385(1–2):45, 2014

Hammond GL, Wu TS, Simard M: Evolving utility of sex hormone-binding globulin measurements in clinical medicine. Curr Opin Endocrinol Diabetes Obes 19(3):183, 2012

Haskell SG: Selective estrogen receptor modulators. South Med J 96:469, 2003

Head JR, MacDonald PC, Casey ML: Cellular localization of membrane metalloendopeptidase (enkephalinase) in human endometrium during the ovarian cycle. J Clin Endocrinol Metab 76:769, 1993

Hekimsoy Z, Kafeşçiler S, Güçlü F, et al: The prevalence of hyperprolactinaemia in overt and subclinical hypothyroidism. Endocr J 57(12):1011, 2010

Hennet ML, Combelles CM: The antral follicle: a microenvironment for oocyte differentiation. Int J Dev Biol 56(10–12):819, 2012

Hodgen GD: The dominant ovarian follicle. Fertil Steril 38:281, 1982

Hoff JD, Quigley ME, Yen SS: Hormonal dynamics at midcycle: a reevaluation. J Clin Endocrinol Metab 57:792, 1983

Hsieh M, Zamah AM, Conti M: Epidermal growth factor-like growth factors in the follicular fluid: role in oocyte development and maturation. Semin Reprod Med 27(1):52, 2009

Hsueh AJ, Eisenhauer K, Chun SY, et al: Gonadal cell apoptosis. Recent Prog Horm Res 51:433, 1996

Kalantaridou SN, Makrigiannakis A, Zoumakis E, et al: Stress and the female reproductive system. J Reprod Immunol 62(1–2):61, 2004

Kaltsas GA, Nomikos P, Kontogeorgos G, et al: Clinical review: diagnosis and management of pituitary carcinomas. J Clin Endocrinol Metab 90:3089, 2005

Kaplan SL, Grumbach MM, Aubert ML: The ontogenesis of pituitary hormones and hypothalamic factors in the human fetus: maturation of central nervous system regulation of anterior pituitary function. Recent Prog Horm Res 32:161, 1976

Kerin JF, Kirby C, Morris D, et al: Incidence of the luteinized unruptured follicle phenomenon in cycling women. Fertil Steril 40:620, 1983

Kim HH, Mui KL, Nikrodhanond AA, et al: Regulation of gonadotropin-releasing hormone in nonhypothalamic tissues. Semin Reprod Med 25:326, 2007

King JC, Anthony EL: LHRH neurons and their projections in humans and other mammals: species comparisons. Peptides 5(Suppl 1):195, 1984

Kiss A, Mikkelsen JD: Oxytocin—anatomy and functional assignments: a minireview. Endocr Regul 39:97, 2005

Klinge CM: Estrogen receptor interaction with estrogen response elements. Nucleic Acids Res 29:2905, 2001

Knobil E: On the control of gonadotropin secretion in the rhesus monkey. Recent Prog Horm Res 30:1, 1974

Knobil E: The neuroendocrine control of the menstrual cycle. Recent Prog Horm Res 36:53, 1980

Knobil E: The Physiology of Reproduction. New York, Raven Press, 1994

Kottler ML, Chou YY, Chabre O, et al: A new FSHbeta mutation in a 29-year-old woman with primary amenorrhea and isolated FSH deficiency: functional characterization and ovarian response to human recombinant FSH. Eur J Endocrinol 162(3):633, 2010

Kowalik MK, Rekawiecki R, Kotwica J: The putative roles of nuclear and membrane-bound progesterone receptors in the female reproductive tract. Reprod Biol 13(4):279, 2013

Kuhl H: Pharmacology of estrogens and progestogens: influence of different routes of administration. Climacteric 8(Suppl 1):3, 2005

Kuiper GG, Carlsson B, Grandien K, et al: Comparison of the ligand binding specificity and transcript tissue distribution of estrogen receptors alpha and beta. Endocrinology 138:863, 1997

Latronico AC, Arnhold IJ: Gonadotropin resistance. Endocr Dev 24:25, 2013

Lawrence C, Fraley GS: Galanin-like peptide (GALP) is a hypothalamic regulator of energy homeostasis and reproduction. Front Neuroendocrinol 32:1, 2011

Lee HJ, Snegovskikh VV, Park JS, et al: Role of GnRH-GnRH receptor signaling at the maternal-fetal interface. Fertil Steril 94(7):2680, 2010

Lehman MN, Coolen LM, Goodman RL: Minireview: kisspeptin/neurokinin B/dynorphin (KNDy) cells of the arcuate nucleus: a central node in the control of gonadotropin-releasing hormone secretion. Endocrinology 151:3479, 2010

Lemarchand-Beraud T, Zufferey MM, Reymond M, et al: Maturation of the hypothalamo-pituitary-ovarian axis in adolescent girls. J Clin Endocrinol Metab 54:241, 1982

Lessey BA, Killam AP, Metzger DA, et al: Immunohistochemical analysis of human uterine estrogen and progesterone receptors throughout the menstrual cycle. J Clin Endocrinol Metab 67:334, 1988

Lockwood CJ, Nemerson Y, Krikun G, et al: Steroid-modulated stromal cell tissue factor expression: a model for the regulation of endometrial hemostasis and menstruation. J Clin Endocrinol Metab 77:1014, 1993

Lumsden MA, Kelly RW, Templeton AA, et al: Changes in the concentration of prostaglandins in preovulatory human follicles after administration of hCG. J Reprod Fertil 77:119, 1986

Lydon JP, DeMayo FJ, Conneely OM, et al: Reproductive phenotypes of the progesterone receptor null mutant mouse. J Steroid Biochem Mol Biol 56(1–6 Spec No):67, 1996

Mashchak CA, Lobo Ra, Dozono-Takano R, et al: Comparison of pharmacodynamic properties of various estrogen formulations. Am J Obstet Gynecol 144:511, 1982

Mason JI: Genetics of Steroid Biosynthesis and Function. New York, Taylor & Francis, 2002

McCann-Crosby B, Chen MJ, et al: Nonclassical congenital adrenal hyperplasia: targets of treatment and transition. Pediatr Endocrinol Rev 12(2):224, 2014

McLachlan RI, Cohen NL, Vale WW, et al: The importance of luteinizing hormone in the control of inhibin and progesterone secretion by the human corpus luteum. J Clin Endocrinol Metab 68:1078, 1989

McNatty KP, Makris A, DeGrazia C, et al: The production of progesterone, androgens, and estrogens by granulosa cells, thecal tissue, and stromal tissue from human ovaries in vitro. J Clin Endocrinol Metab 49:687, 1979

Melmed S: Pituitary tumors. Endocrinol Metab Clin North Am 44(1):1, 2015

Melmed S, Jameson JL: Disorders of the anterior pituitary and hypothalamus. In Kasper DL, Braunwald E, Fauci AS, et al (eds): Harrison's Principles of Internal Medicine, 17th ed. New York, McGraw-Hill, 2008, p 2206

Messini CI, Dafopoulos K, Chalvatzas N, et al: Effect of ghrelin and thyrotropin-releasing hormone on prolactin secretion in normal women. Horm Metab Res 42(3):204, 2010

Millar RP: New developments in kisspeptin, neurokinin B and dynorphin A regulation of gonadotropin-releasing hormone pulsatile secretion. Neuroendocrinology 99(1):5, 2014

Miller BA, Ioachimescu AG, Oyesiku NM: Contemporary indications for transsphenoidal pituitary surgery. World Neurosurg 82(6 Suppl):S147, 2014

Miller WL: Molecular biology of steroid hormone synthesis. Endocr Rev 9:295, 1988

Miller WL, Auchus RJ: The molecular biology, biochemistry, and physiology of human steroidogenesis and its disorders. Endocr Rev 32(1):81, 2011

Molitch ME: Endocrinology in pregnancy: management of the pregnant patient with a prolactinoma. Eur J Endocrinol 172(5):R205, 2015

Muttukrishna S, Tannetta D, Groome N, et al: Activin and follistatin in female reproduction. Mol Cell Endocrinol 225:45, 2004

Nakai Y, Plant TM, Hess DL, et al: On the sites of the negative and positive feedback actions of estradiol in the control of gonadotropin secretion in the rhesus monkey. Endocrinology 102:1008, 1978

Negro-Vilar A: Selective androgen receptor modulators (SARMs):a novel approach to androgen therapy for the new millennium. J Clin Endocrinol Metab 84:3459, 1999

Neill JD: GnRH and GnRH receptor genes in the human genome. Endocrinology 143:737, 2002

Notarianni E: Reinterpretation of evidence advanced for neo-oogenesis in mammals, in terms of a finite oocyte reserve. J Ovarian Res 4:1, 2011

Noyes RW, Hertig AT, Rock J: Dating the endometrial biopsy. Fertil Steril 1:3, 1950

O'Brien MD, Guillebaud J: Contraception for women taking antiepileptic drugs. J Fam Plann Reprod Health Care 36(4):239, 2010

Ohlsson R: Growth factors, protooncogenes and human placental development. Cell Differ Dev 28:1, 1989

Olive DL: The prevalence and epidemiology of luteal-phase deficiency in normal and infertile women. Clin Obstet Gynecol 34:157, 1991

O'Malley BW, Strott CA: Steroid hormones: metabolism and mechanism of action. In Yen SS, Jaffe RB, Barbieri RL (eds): Reproductive Endocrinology, 4th ed. Philadelphia, Saunders, 1999, p 128

Pache TD, Wladimiroff JW, de Jong FH, et al: Growth patterns of nondominant ovarian follicles during the normal menstrual cycle. Fertil Steril 54:638, 1990

Padula AM: GnRH analogues—agonists and antagonists. Anim Reprod Sci 88(1–2):115, 2005

Pashtan I, Oh KS, Loeffler JS: Radiation therapy in the management of pituitary adenomas. Handb Clin Neurol 124:317, 2014

Patton PE, Stouffer RL: Current understanding of the corpus luteum in women and nonhuman primates. Clin Obstet Gynecol 34:127, 1991

Pekic S, Stojanovic M, Popovic V: Contemporary issues in the evaluation and management of pituitary adenomas. Minerva Endocrinol April 22, 2015 [Epub ahead of print]

Peters EE, Towler KL, Mason DR, et al: Effects of galanin and leptin on gonadotropin-releasing hormone-stimulated luteinizing hormone release from the pituitary. Neuroendocrinology 89:18, 2009

Peters H, Joint A (eds): The Ovary: A Correlation of Structure and Function in Mammals. Berkeley, University of California Press, 1980

Piquette GN, Crabtree ME, el Danasouri I, et al: Regulation of plasminogen activator inhibitor-1 and -2 messenger ribonucleic acid levels in human cumulus and granulosa-luteal cells. J Clin Endocrinol Metab 76:518, 1993

Pope WF: Uterine asynchrony: a cause of embryonic loss. Biol Reprod 39:999, 1988

Ravindranath N, Little-Ihrig L, Phillips HS, et al: Vascular endothelial growth factor messenger ribonucleic acid expression in the primate ovary. Endocrinology 131:254, 1992

Revelli A, Massobrio M, Tesarik J: Nongenomic actions of steroid hormones in reproductive tissues. Endocr Rev 19(1):3, 1998

Rosenfield RL, Bordini B, Yu C: Comparison of detection of normal puberty in girls by a hormonal sleep test and a gonadotropin-releasing hormone agonist test. J Clin Endocrinol Metab 98(4):1591, 2013

Rosner W, Auchus RJ, Azziz R, et al: Position statement: utility, limitations, and pitfalls in measuring testosterone: an Endocrine Society position statement. J Clin Endocrinol Metab 92(2):405, 2007

Rosner W, Hryb DJ, Kahn SM, et al: Interactions of sex hormone-binding globulin with target cells. Mol Cell Endocrinol 316:79, 2010

Ruscalleda J: Imaging of parasellar lesions. Eur Radiol 15:549, 2005

Russell DW, Wilson JD: Steroid 5 alpha-reductase: two genes/two enzymes. Annu Rev Biochem 63:25, 1994

Sasano H, Okamoto M, Mason JI, et al: Immunolocalization of aromatase, 17 alpha-hydroxylase and side-chain-cleavage cytochromes P-450 in the human ovary. J Reprod Fertil 85:163, 1989

Saxena BB, Beling CG, Gandy HM, et al: Gonadotropins. New York, Wiley-Interscience, 1972

Schatz F, Aigner S, Papp C, et al: Plasminogen activator activity during decidualization of human endometrial stromal cells is regulated by plasminogen activator inhibitor 1. J Clin Endocrinol Metab 80:2504, 1995

Schipper I, Hop WC, Fauser BC: The follicle-stimulating hormone (FSH) threshold/window concept examined by different interventions with exogenous FSH during the follicular phase of the normal menstrual cycle: duration, rather than magnitude, of FSH increase affects follicle development. J Clin Endocrinol Metab 83:1292, 1998

Schlechte J, Dolan K, Sherman B, et al: The natural history of untreated hyperprolactinemia: a prospective analysis. J Clin Endocrinol Metab 68:412, 1989

Schmidt H, Schwarz HP: Serum concentrations of LH and FSH in the healthy newborn. Eur J Endocrinol 143(2):213, 2000

Sharkey AM, Dellow K, Blayney M, et al: Stage-specific expression of cytokine and receptor messenger ribonucleic acids in human preimplantation embryos. Biol Reprod 53:974, 1995

Silva JR, Figueiredo JR, van den Hurk R: Involvement of growth hormone (GH) and insulin-like growth factor (IGF) system in ovarian folliculogenesis. Theriogenology 71:1193, 2009

Silva PD, Gentzschein EE, Lobo RA: Androstenedione may be a more important precursor of tissue dihydrotestosterone than testosterone in women. Fertil Steril 48:419, 1987

Silverman AJ, Jhamandas J, Renaud LP: Localization of luteinizing hormone-releasing hormone (LHRH) neurons that project to the median eminence. J Neurosci 7:2312, 1987

Singh TD, Valizadeh N, Meyer FB, et al: Management and outcomes of pituitary apoplexy. J Neurosurg 10:1, 2015

Skorupskaite K, George JT, Anderson RA: The kisspeptin-GnRH pathway in human reproductive health and disease. Hum Reprod Update 20(4):485, 2014

Smith G, Roberts R, Hall C, et al: Reversible ovulatory failure associated with the development of luteinized unruptured follicles in women with inflammatory arthritis taking non-steroidal anti-inflammatory drugs. Br J Rheumatol 35:458, 1996

Son WY, Das M, Shalom-Paz E, et al: Mechanisms of follicle selection and development. Minerva Ginecol 63(2):89, 2011

Stanczyk FZ: Pharmacokinetics and potency of progestins used for hormone replacement therapy and contraception. Rev Endocr Metab Disord 3:211, 2002

Stern K, McClintock MK: Regulation of ovulation by human pheromones. Nature 392:177, 1998

Stilley JA, Christensen DE, Dahlem KB, et al: FSH receptor (FSHR) expression in human extragonadal reproductive tissues and the developing placenta, and the impact of its deletion on pregnancy in mice. Biol Reprod 91(3):74, 2014

Stout SM, Stumpf JL: Finasteride treatment of hair loss in women. Ann Pharmacother 44:1090, 2010

Tadokoro-Cuccaro R, Hughes IA: Androgen insensitivity syndrome. Curr Opin Endocrinol Diabetes Obes 21(6):499, 2014

Taylor HS, Vanden Heuvel GB, Igarashi P: A conserved Hox axis in the mouse and human female reproductive system: late establishment and persistent adult expression of the Hoxa cluster genes. Biol Reprod 57:1338, 1997

Temeli E, Oprescu M, Coculescu M, et al: LH and FSH levels in serum and cerebrospinal fluid (CSF) of human fetus. Endocrinologie 23(1):55, 1985

Thompson IR, Kaiser UB: GnRH pulse frequency-dependent differential regulation of LH and FSH gene expression. Mol Cell Endocrinol 385(1–2):28, 2014

Treloar AE, Boynton RE, Behn BG, et al: Variation of the human menstrual cycle through reproductive life. Int J Fertil 12(1 Pt 2):77, 1967

Ulloa-Aguirre A, Reiter E, Bousfield G, et al: Constitutive activity in gonadotropin receptors. Adv Pharmacol 70:37, 2014

Vega MG, Zarek SM, Bhagwat M, et al: Gonadotropin surge-inhibiting/attenuating factors: a review of current evidence, potential applications, and future directions for research. Mol Reprod Dev 82(1):2, 2015

Verbalis JG, Robinson AG: Characterization of neurophysin-vasopressin prohormones in human posterior pituitary tissue. J Clin Endocrinol Metab 57:115, 1983

Virant-Klun I: Postnatal oogenesis in humans: a review of recent findings. Stem Cells Cloning 8:49, 2015

Walkington L, Webster J, Hancock BW, et al: Hyperthyroidism and human chorionic gonadotrophin production in gestational trophoblastic disease. Br J Cancer 104(11):1665, 2011

Wiegratz I, Kuhl H: Progestogen therapies: differences in clinical effects? Trends Endocrinol Metab 15:277, 2004

Wierman ME, Kiseljak-Vassiliades K, Tobet S: Gonadotropin-releasing hormone (GnRH) neuron migration: initiation, maintenance and cessation as critical steps to ensure normal reproductive function. Front Neuroendocrinol 32(1):43, 2011

Williams CL, Nishihara M, Thalabard JC, et al: Duration and frequency of multiunit electrical activity associated with the hypothalamic gonadotropin releasing hormone pulse generator in the rhesus monkey: differential effects of morphine. Neuroendocrinology 52:225, 1990

Winter JS, Hughes IA, Reyes FI, et al: Pituitary-gonadal relations in infancy: 2. Patterns of serum gonadal steroid concentrations in man from birth to two years of age. J Clin Endocrinol Metab 42:679, 1976

Xia Y, Schneyer AL: The biology of activin: recent advances in structure, regulation and function. J Endocrinol 202(1):1, 2009

Yen SS, Quigley ME, Reid RL, et al: Neuroendocrinology of opioid peptides and their role in the control of gonadotropin and prolactin secretion. Am J Obstet Gynecol 152:485, 1985

Ylikorkala O, Cacciatore B, Halonen K, et al: Effects of ospemifene, a novel SERM, on vascular markers and function in healthy, postmenopausal women. Menopause 10(5):440, 2003

Yoshimura Y, Wallach EE: Studies of the mechanism(s) of mammalian ovulation. Fertil Steril 47:22, 1987

Yoshinaga K, Serono Symposia USA: Blastocyst Implantation. Boston, Adams, 1989

Young JR, Jaffe RB: Strength-duration characteristics of estrogen effects on gonadotropin response to gonadotropin-releasing hormone in women. II. Effects of varying concentrations of estradiol. J Clin Endocrinol Metab 42:432, 1976

Yu B, Ruman J, Christman G: The role of peripheral gonadotropin-releasing hormone receptors in female reproduction. Fertil Steril 95:465, 2011

Ziecik AJ, Kaczmarek MM, Blitek A, et al: Novel biological and possible applicable roles of LH/hCG receptor. Mol Cell Endocrinol 269(1–2):51, 2007

Amenorrhea

Evaluation and management of a patient with amenorrhea is common in gynecology. Specifically, the prevalence of pathologic amenorrhea ranges from 3 to 4 percent in reproductive-aged populations (Bachmann, 1982; Pettersson, 1973). Amenorrhea has classically been defined as primary (no prior menses) or secondary (cessation of menses). Although this distinction does suggest a relative likelihood of finding a particular diagnosis, the approach to diagnosis and treatment is similar for either presentation (Tables 16-1 and 16-2). Of course, amenorrhea is a normal state prior to puberty, during pregnancy and lactation, with certain hormonal medications such as continuous administration of combination oral contraceptives (COCs), and following menopause. Evaluation is considered for an adolescent: (1) who by age 13 has not menstruated or shown other evidence of pubertal development, or (2) who has reached other pubertal milestones but has not menstruated by age 15 or within 3 years of thelarche (American College of Obstetrician and Gynecologists, 2009). Secondary amenorrhea for 3 months or oligomenorrhea involving fewer than nine cycles a year is also investigated (American Society for Reproductive Medicine, 2008). In some circumstances, testing reasonably may be initiated despite the absence of these strict criteria. Examples include a patient with the stigmata of Turner syndrome, obvious virilization, or a history of uterine curettage. An evaluation for delayed puberty is also considered before the ages listed above if the patient or her parents are concerned.

NORMAL MENSTRUAL CYCLE

A differential diagnosis for amenorrhea can be constructed based on requirements for normal menses. Ovarian function in a normal menstrual cycle is divided into the follicular phase (preovulatory), ovulation, and luteal phase (postovulatory). Endometrial characteristics are partitioned into the proliferative phase (preovulatory) and secretory phase (postovulatory). Generation of a cyclic, controlled pattern of uterine bleeding requires precise temporal and quantitative regulation of several reproductive hormones (Chap. 15, p. 346).

First, the hypothalamic-pituitary-ovarian axis must be functional. The hypothalamus releases pulses of gonadotropin-releasing hormone (GnRH) into the hypophyseal portal circulation at defined frequencies and amplitude. GnRH stimulates the synthesis and secretion of the gonadotropins luteinizing hormone (LH) and follicle-stimulating hormone (FSH) by the gonadotrope cells of the anterior pituitary gland. These gonadotropins enter the peripheral circulation and act on the ovary to stimulate both follicular development and ovarian hormone production. These ovarian hormones include estrogens, progesterones, and androgens. Gonadal steroids are typically inhibitory at both the pituitary and the hypothalamus. Development of a mature follicle, however, creates a rapid rise in estrogen levels, which instead act positively to generate an LH surge. This surge is essential for ovulation.

Following ovulation, LH stimulates luteinization of the granulosa and theca cells, which had surrounded the mature oocyte, to form the corpus luteum. The corpus luteum continues to produce estrogen but also secretes high levels of progesterone. The thickened, proliferative endometrial lining produced by high circulating estrogen levels during the follicular phase is now converted to a secretory pattern by this luteal progesterone. If pregnancy occurs, the corpus luteum is "rescued" by human chorionic gonadotropin (hCG) secreted from early placental trophoblast. hCG is similar structurally to LH, shares the same receptor as LH, and assumes the role of corpus luteum support during early pregnancy. If pregnancy does not occur, then progesterone and estrogen secretion ceases, the corpus luteum regresses, and the endometrium sloughs. The pattern of this "progesterone withdrawal bleed" varies in duration and amount among women but is relatively constant across cycles for a given individual.

Amenorrhea may follow disruption of this choreographed communication. However, even with normal hormonal cycling, altered anatomy may prevent menses. The endometrium must

TABLE 16-1. Primary Amenorrhea: Frequency of Etiologies

Presentation	Frequency (%)
Hypergonadotropic hypogonadism	43
45,X and variants	27
46,XX	14
46,XY	2
Eugonadism	30
Müllerian agenesis	15
Vaginal septum	3
Imperforate hymen	1
Androgen insensitivity syndrome	1
Polycystic ovarian syndrome	7
Congenital adrenal hyperplasia	1
Cushing and thyroid disease	2
Low FSH without breast development	27
Constitutional delay	14
GnRH deficiency	5
Other CNS disease	1
Pituitary disease	5
Eating disorders, stress, excess exercise	2

CNS = central nervous system;
FSH = follicle-stimulating hormone; GnRH = gonadotropin-releasing hormone.
Data from Reindollar RH, Byrd JR, McDonough PG: Delayed sexual development: a study of 252 patients, Am J Obstet Gynecol 1981 Jun 15;140(4):371–380.

TABLE 16-2. Secondary Amenorrhea: Frequency of Etiologies[a]

Etiology	Frequency (%)
Low or normal FSH level: various	67.5
Eating disorders, stress, excess exercise	15.5
Nonspecific hypothalamic	18
Chronic anovulation (PCOS)	28
Hypothyroidism	1.5
Cushing syndrome	1
Pituitary tumor/empty sella	2
Sheehan syndrome	1.5
High FSH level: gonadal failure	10.5
46,XX	10
Abnormal karyotype	0.5
High prolactin level	13
Anatomic	7
Asherman syndrome	7
Hyperandrogenic states	2
Nonclassic CAH	0.5
Ovarian tumor	1
Undiagnosed	0.5

[a]Excluding pregnancy diagnoses.
CAH = congenital adrenal hyperplasia; FSH = follicle-stimulating hormone; PCOS = polycystic ovarian syndrome.
Adapted with permission from Reindollar RH, Novak M, Tho SP, et al: Adult-onset amenorrhea: a study of 262 patients, Am J Obstet Gynecol 1986 Sep;155(3):531–543.

be able to respond normally to hormonal stimulation, and the cervix, vagina, and introitus must be present and patent.

CLASSIFICATION SYSTEM

Numerous classification systems for the diagnosis of amenorrhea have been developed, and all have their strengths and weaknesses. One useful scheme is outlined in Table 16-3. This system divides causes of amenorrhea into anatomic versus hormonal etiologies, with further division into congenital versus acquired disorders.

As described above, normal menses require adequate ovarian production of steroid hormones. Decreased ovarian function (hypogonadism) may result either from a lack of stimulation by the gonadotropins (*hypo*gonadotropic hypogonadism) or from primary failure of the ovary (*hyper*gonadotropic hypogonadism) (Table 16-4). Several disorders are associated with relatively normal LH and FSH levels (*eu*gonadotropic), however, appropriate cyclicity is lost.

ANATOMIC DISORDERS

◼ Inherited Disorders

Anatomic abnormalities causing amenorrhea can broadly be viewed as either inherited or acquired disorders of the outflow tract (uterus, cervix, vagina, and introitus). Of these two, an inherited cause is frequent in adolescents, and pelvic anatomy is abnormal

in approximately 15 percent of women with primary amenorrhea (American Society for Reproductive Medicine, 2008). Figure 16-1 depicts the range of anatomic defects that may present with amenorrhea. These are additionally discussed in Chapter 18 (p. 404).

Lower Outflow Tract Obstruction

Amenorrhea is associated with imperforate hymen (1 in 2000 women), a complete transverse vaginal septum (1 in 70,000 women), or isolated vaginal atresia (Banerjee, 1998; Parazzini, 1990). Also, although structurally normal, labia in some girls may be severely agglutinated and can lead to obstruction. Most with agglutination are treated early with topical estrogen and/or manual separation, and outflow obstruction is thereby avoided.

Patients with outflow obstruction have a 46,XX karyotype, female secondary sexual characteristics, and normal ovarian function. Thus, the amount of uterine bleeding is normal, but its normal path for egress is obstructed or absent. Patients may note moliminal symptoms, such as breast tenderness, food cravings, and mood changes, which are attributable to elevated progesterone levels. With inherited or acquired outflow obstruction, accumulation of blood behind the blockage frequently results in cyclic abdominal pain. Intrauterine trapping of fluid (hydrometra), pus (pyometra), or blood (hematometra) creates a soft, enlarged uterus. Similarly, the terms hydrocolpos, pyocolpos, and hematocolpos describe distention of the vagina and are seen with distal obstructions. Moreover, in women

TABLE 16-3. Classification Scheme for Amenorrhea

ANATOMIC

Congenital
Müllerian agenesis (partial or complete)
Cervical atresia
Transverse vaginal septum
Imperforate hymen

Acquired
Intrauterine synechiae (Asherman syndrome)
   Dilation and curettage
   Infection (tuberculosis)
Cervical stenosis

HORMONAL/ENDOCRINOLOGIC

Hypergonadotropic hypogonadism (POF)
  Inherited/congenital
    Chromosomal (gonadal dysgenesis)
    Single gene disorders

  Acquired
    Infectious
    Autoimmune
    Iatrogenic
    Environmental
    Idiopathic

Eugonadotropic amenorrhea
  Inherited
    Polycystic ovarian syndrome
    Adult-onset congenital adrenal hyperplasia

  Acquired
    Hyperprolactinemia
    Thyroid disease
    Cushing syndrome
    Acromegaly
    Ovarian tumors (steroid producing)

Other
  End-stage kidney disease
  Liver disease
  Malignancy
  Malabsorption syndromes
  Acquired immunodeficiency syndrome

Hypogonadotropic hypogonadism
Disorders of the hypothalamus
  Inherited/congenital
    Idiopathic hypogonadotropic hypogonadism (IHH)
    Kallmann syndrome

  Acquired
    Hypothalamic amenorrhea ("functional")
      Eating disorders
      Excessive exercise
      Stress
    Destructive processes
      Tumor
      Radiation
      Trauma
      Infection
      Infiltrative disease
    Pseudocyesis

Disorders of the anterior pituitary gland
  Inherited/congenital
    Pituitary hypoplasia

  Acquired
    Macroadenoma
    Metastases
    Radiation
    Trauma
    Infarction (Sheehan syndrome)
    Infiltrative disease

with outflow blockage, an increase in retrograde menstruation may lead to endometriosis development.

Müllerian Defects

During embryonic development, the müllerian ducts give rise to the upper vagina, cervix, uterine corpus, and fallopian tubes. Agenesis during these ducts' development may be partial or complete. Accordingly, amenorrhea may result from outflow obstruction or from a lack of endometrium in cases involving uterine agenesis. In complete müllerian agenesis, often called Mayer-Rokitansky-Kuster-Hauser syndrome, patients fail to develop any müllerian structures, and examination reveals

TABLE 16-4. Categories of Amenorrhea Based on Gonadotropin and Estrogen Levels

Type of Hypogonadism	LH/FSH	Estrogen	Primary Defect
Hypergonadotropic	High	Low	Ovary
Hypogonadotropic	Low	Low	Hypothalamus/pituitary
Eugonadotropic	Normal[a]	Normal[a]	Varied

[a]Generally in normal range, but lack cyclicity.
FSH = follicle-stimulating hormone; LH = luteinizing hormone.

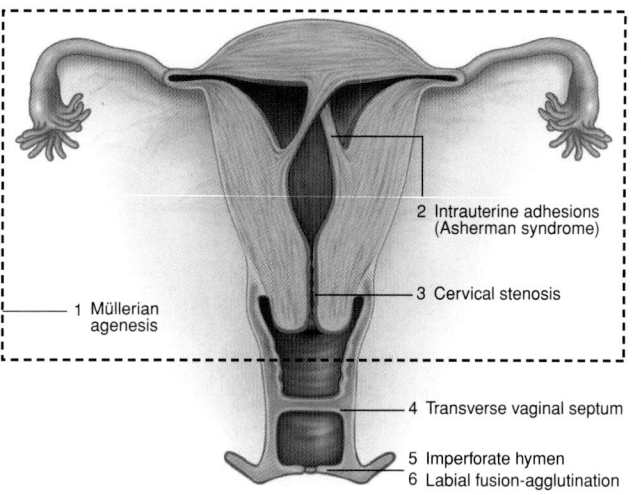

FIGURE 16-1 Anatomic defects that may lead to amenorrhea.

only a vaginal dimple (Chap. 18, p. 420). It ranks second only to gonadal dysgenesis as a cause of primary amenorrhea (Aittomaki, 2001; Reindollar, 1981).

Similar to patients with lower outflow tract obstruction, patients with müllerian anomalies have a 46,XX karyotype and normal ovarian function. Research has begun to identify candidate gene mutations that may contribute to this disorder, but details are lacking. Importantly, complete müllerian agenesis may be confused with complete androgen insensitivity syndrome. In the latter condition, the patient has a 46,XY karyotype and functioning testes. However, underlying androgen receptor mutations prevent normal testosterone binding, normal male ductal system development, and virilization. These two syndromes are compared in Table 16-5 and discussed further in Chapter 18 (p. pp. 412 and 420).

■ Acquired Disorders
Cervical Stenosis

Other abnormalities of the uterus that cause amenorrhea include cervical stenosis and extensive intrauterine adhesions. With stenosis, postoperative scarring and cervical os narrowing may follow dilatation and curettage (D & C), cervical conization, loop electrosurgical excision procedures, infection,

TABLE 16-5. Comparison of Müllerian Agenesis and Androgen Insensitivity Syndrome

Presentation	Müllerian Agenesis	Androgen Insensitivity
Inheritance pattern	Sporadic	X-linked recessive
Karyotype	46,XX	46,XY
Breast development	Yes	Yes
Axillary and pubic hair	Yes	No
Uterus	No	No
Gonad	Ovary	Testis
Testosterone	Female levels	Male levels
Associated anomalies	Yes	No

and neoplasia. Severe atrophic or radiation changes are other sources. Stenosis most commonly involves the internal os, and symptoms in menstruating women include amenorrhea or abnormal bleeding, dysmenorrhea, and infertility. Management seeks to reopen the os and is discussed in Chapter 4 (p. 102).

Intrauterine Adhesions

Also known as uterine synechiae and, when symptomatic, as Asherman syndrome, the spectrum of scarring includes filmy adhesions, dense bands, or complete obliteration of the uterine cavity (Fig. 16-2). Normally, the endometrium is divided into a functional layer, which lines the endometrial cavity, and a basal layer, which regenerates the functional layer with each menstrual cycle. Destruction of the basal endometrium prevents endometrial thickening in response to ovarian steroids. Thus, no tissue is produced or subsequently sloughed when steroid hormone levels fall at the end of the luteal phase.

Endometrial damage may follow vigorous curettage, usually in association with postpartum hemorrhage, miscarriage, or elective abortion complicated by infection. In a series of 1856 women with Asherman syndrome, 88 percent followed postabortal or postpartum uterine curettage (Schenker, 1982). Damage may also result from other uterine surgery, including metroplasty, myomectomy, or cesarean delivery, or from infection related to an intrauterine device. Although rare in the United States, tuberculous endometritis is a relatively common cause of Asherman syndrome in developing countries (Sharma, 2009). Of course, Asherman syndrome may also be an intentional outcome following uterine ablation for heavy menstrual bleeding.

Depending on the degree of scarring, patients may describe amenorrhea; in less severe cases, hypomenorrhea; or recurrent pregnancy loss due to inadequate placentation (March, 2011).

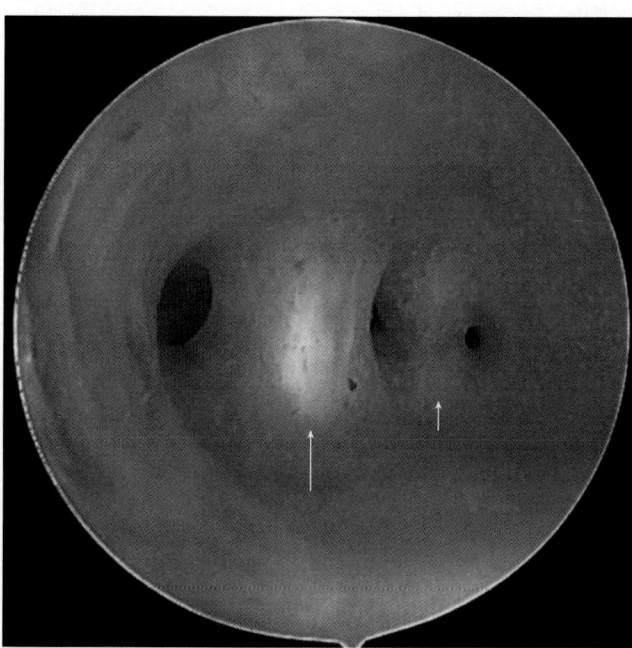

FIGURE 16-2 Hysteroscopic photograph of intrauterine adhesions (*arrows*) found with Asherman syndrome. (Used with permission from Dr. Ellen Wilson.)

In their evaluation of 292 women with intrauterine adhesions, Schenker and Margalioth (1982) noted delivery of term pregnancies in only 30 percent of 165 pregnancies. The remaining pregnancies either were spontaneously aborted (40 percent) or delivered prematurely.

If intrauterine adhesions are suspected, radiologic evaluation of the uterine cavity is performed. If information regarding tubal patency is needed, then hysterosalpingography (HSG) offers information regarding both uterine cavity and fallopian tube patency. Otherwise, saline infusion sonography (SIS) provides an excellent alternative. Intrauterine adhesions characteristically appear as irregular, angulated filling defects within the cavity (Fig. 19-6, p. 439 and Fig. 2-23, p. 34). At times, uterine polyps, leiomyomas, air bubbles, and blood clots may masquerade as adhesions. Definitive diagnosis requires hysteroscopy. To improve fertility rates or to relieve symptomatic hematometra, hysteroscopic lysis of adhesions is the preferred surgical treatment. The procedure is described in Section 44-19 (p. 1052), and fertility advantages are discussed in Chapter 20 (p. 460).

HYPERGONADOTROPIC HYPOGONADISM

The term *hypergonadotropic hypogonadism* describes any process in which: (1) ovarian function is decreased or absent (hypogonadism) and (2) due to absent negative sex-steroid feedback, the gonadotropins, LH and FSH, have increased serum levels (hypergonadotropic). This category of disorders implies primary dysfunction within the ovary rather than hypothalamic or pituitary dysfunction (Table 16-6). This process can also be termed *premature menopause* or *premature ovarian failure (POF)*, with a current trend toward the term *premature ovarian insufficiency* or *primary ovarian insufficiency (POI)*. The term ovarian insufficiency conveys the fact that ovarian function may fluctuate before complete oocyte depletion and may lead to occasional

TABLE 16-6. Differential Diagnosis of Premature Ovarian Failure

Genetic
  Chromosomal
    Normal karyotype
    Gonadal dysgenesis
  Specific gene defects
    Fragile X (FMR1 premutation)
    Galactosemia
    Other

Iatrogenic
  Ovarian surgery
  Gonadal radiation
  Systemic chemotherapy

Autoimmune disease

Toxins

Viruses

Miscellaneous

transient menses resumption or even pregnancy (Bidet, 2011). For our purposes, the term premature ovarian failure, implying permanent cessation of menses, will be used.

POF is defined as loss of oocytes and the surrounding support cells prior to age 40 years. The diagnosis is determined by two serum FSH levels that measure greater than a threshold range of 30 to 40 mIU/mL and are obtained at least 1 month apart. This definition distinguishes POF from the physiologic loss of ovarian function, which occurs with normal menopause. The incidence of POF has been estimated at 1 in 1000 women younger than 30 years and at 1 in 100 women younger than 40 (Coulam, 1986).

Careful evaluation is mandatory as the diagnosis and effective treatment may have significant implications for the patient's psychologic, cardiovascular, bone, and sexual health. The finding of a genetic disorder may also require evaluation of family members. Nevertheless, in most cases, an etiology for POF is not determined (American College of Obstetricians and Gynecologists, 2014).

■ Heritable Disorders
Gonadal Dysgenesis

Gonadal dysgenesis is the most frequent cause of POF. In this disorder, a normal complement of germ cells is present in the early fetal ovary. However, oocytes undergo accelerated atresia, and the ovary is replaced by a fibrous streak—termed a streak gonad (Figs. 16-3 and 16-4)(Simpson, 1975; Singh, 1966). Individuals with gonadal dysgenesis may present with various clinical features and can be divided into two broad groups based on whether their karyotype is normal or abnormal (Schlessinger, 2002). These are all discussed further in Chapter 18 (p. 409).

Those with normal karyotype (46,XX or 46,XY) are described as having "pure" gonadal dysgenesis. Patients with a 46,XY genotype and gonadal dysgenesis (Swyer syndrome) are phenotypically female due to absent testosterone and absent antimüllerian hormone (AMH) secretion by the dysgenetic testes. The etiology of the gonadal failure in both genetically male and female patients is poorly understood but is likely due to single gene defects or destruction of gonadal tissue in utero, perhaps by infection or toxins (Hutson, 2014).

Those with abnormal karyotype include Turner syndrome (45,X) and chromosomal mosaics such as 45,X/46,XX or 45,X/46,XY. In general, approximately 90 percent of individuals with gonadal dysgenesis from a loss of X genetic material never menstruate. The remaining 10 percent have sufficient residual follicles to experience menses and rarely may achieve pregnancy. However, the menstrual and reproductive lives of such individuals are invariably brief (Kaneko, 1990; Simpson, 1975; Tho, 1981).

As noted, in some cases of gonadal dysgenesis, a Y chromosome is present. If Y chromosomal material is found, the streak gonads are removed because nearly 25 percent of these patients will develop a malignant germ cell tumor (Chap. 36, p. 762) (Manuel, 1976). Thus, chromosomal analysis is performed in all cases of amenorrhea associated with POF, particularly before age 30. The presence of a Y chromosome cannot be determined

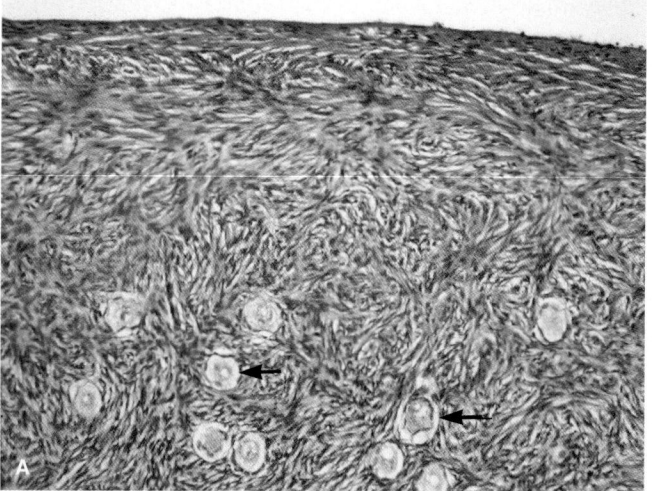
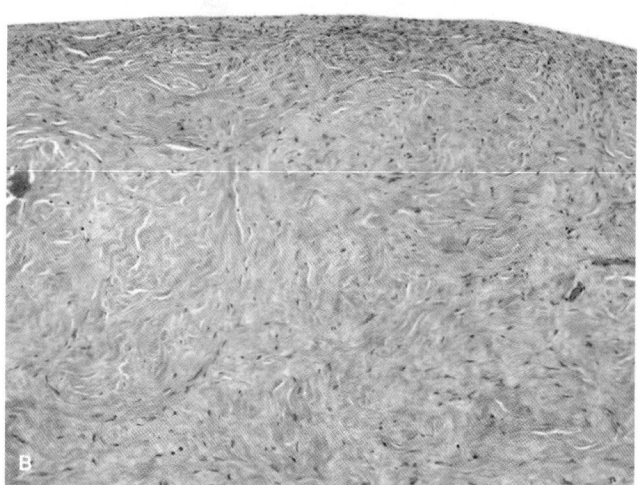

FIGURE 16-3 Photomicrographs of histologic samples. **A.** Normal premenopausal ovarian cortex with multiple primordial follicles (*arrows*). (Used with permission from Dr. Kelley Carrick.) **B.** Ovary from a woman with gonadal dysgenesis. Streak ovary showing ovarian-type stroma with no primordial follicles (Used with permission from Dr. Raheela Ashfaq.)

clinically, as only a few patients will demonstrate signs of androgen excess.

Specific Genetic Defects

In addition to chromosomal abnormalities, patients may experience POF due to single gene mutations (Cordts, 2011; Goswami, 2005). First, a significant relationship is noted between fragile X syndrome and POF (American College of Obstetricians and Gynecologists, 2010). This syndrome is caused by a triple repeat sequence mutation in the X-linked *FMR1* (fragile X mental retardation) gene. This gene is unstable, and its size can expand during parent-to-child transmission. The fully expanded mutation (>200 CGG repeats) becomes hypermethylated, resulting in silencing of gene expression. As such, this fully expanded mutation is the most common known inherited genetic cause of mental retardation and of autism. Males with the so-called premutation (50 to 200 CGG repeats) are at risk for fragile-X associated tremor/ataxia syn-

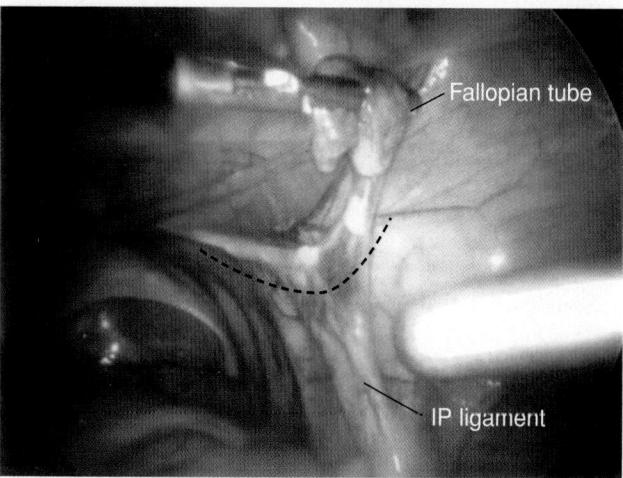

FIGURE 16-4 Photograph taken during laparoscopy of a streak gonad (*dotted line*). IP = infundibulopelvic. (Used with permission from Dr. Victor Beshay.)

drome (FXTAS). Females with the premutation have a 13- to 26-percent risk of developing POF, although the mechanism is unclear. An estimated 0.8 to 7.5 percent of sporadic POF and 13 percent of familial POF cases are due to premutations in this gene. The prevalence of premutations in women approximates 1 in 129 to 300 (Wittenberger, 2007).

Less common gene defects are *CYP17* mutations. These decrease 17α-hydroxylase and 17,20-lyase activity and thereby prevent production of cortisol, androgens, and estrogens (Fig. 15-5, p. 337). Affected patients have sexual infantilism and primary amenorrhea due to absent estrogen secretion. *Sexual infantilism* describes patients with a lack of breast development, absent pubic and axillary hair, and a small uterus. Mutations in *CYP17* also increase adrenocorticotropin hormone (ACTH) release, thereby stimulating mineralocorticoid secretion. This, in turn, leads to hypokalemia and hypertension (Goldsmith, 1967).

Mutations in genes that encode LH and FSH receptors have also been reported. These defects prevent normal responses to circulating gonadotropins, a condition termed *resistant ovary syndrome* (Aittomaki, 1995; Latronico, 2013). Identification of other single gene mutations that can cause POF is an area of active investigation. The list of implicated genes now includes those that encode both estrogen receptors (ERα and ERβ), extracellular signaling proteins (specifically, BMP15), and transcription factors FOXL2, FOX03, and SF-1 (Cordts, 2011; Goswami, 2005). The importance of these factors in maintaining ovarian function is providing further insights into normal ovarian physiology and may lead to new infertility treatments and contraceptive options.

Although frequently cited, galactosemia is a rare cause of POF. Classic galactosemia affects 1 in 30,000 to 60,000 live births. Inherited as an autosomal recessive disorder, this condition leads to abnormal galactose metabolism due to a deficiency of galactose-1-phosphate uridyl transferase, encoded by the *GALT* gene (Rubio-Gozalbo, 2010). Galactose metabolites are believed to have a direct toxic effect on many cell types, including germ cells. Potential complications include neonatal death, ataxic neurologic disease, cognitive disabilities, and cataracts. POF will develop in almost 85 percent of females if left untreated. Treatment is lifelong dietary restriction of galactose, which is present in milk-based foods. Galactosemia is frequently diagnosed during newborn screening programs or during pediatric evaluation of impaired growth and development and long before a patient would present to a gynecologist (Kaufman, 1981; Levy, 1984).

■ Acquired Abnormalities

Hypergonadotropic hypogonadism can be acquired from infection, environmental exposures, autoimmune disease, or medical treatments. Of these, infectious causes of POF are relatively rare and poorly understood, with mumps oophoritis being the most frequently reported (Morrison, 1975). Various environmental toxins have a clear detrimental effect on follicular health. These include cigarette smoking, heavy metals, solvents, pesticides, and industrial chemicals (Jick, 1977; Mlynarcikova, 2005; Sharara, 1998).

Autoimmune disorders account for an estimated 40 percent of POF cases (Hoek, 1997; LaBarbera, 1988). Ovarian failure may be one component of autoimmune pituitary polyglandular failure and accompanied by hypothyroidism and adrenal insufficiency, or it may follow other autoimmune disorders such as systemic lupus erythematosus. POF has also been associated with myasthenia gravis, idiopathic thrombocytopenic purpura, rheumatoid arthritis, vitiligo, and autoimmune hemolytic anemia (de Moraes, 1972; Jones, 1969; Kim, 1974). Although several antiovarian antibodies have been characterized, there is currently no validated serum antibody marker to assist in the diagnosis of autoimmune POF (American Society for Reproductive Medicine, 2008).

Iatrogenic ovarian failure is relatively common. This group includes patients who have undergone surgical removal of the ovaries or cystectomy due to recurrent ovarian cysts, endometriosis, or severe pelvic inflammatory disease. Alternatively, a woman may experience amenorrhea following pelvic radiation for cancer or following chemotherapy for treatment of malignancies or severe autoimmune disease.

With the latter two, the chance of developing POF is correlated with increasing radiation and chemotherapeutic dose. Patient age is also a significant factor, with younger patients less likely to develop failure and more likely to regain ovarian function over time (Gradishar, 1989). With radiotherapy, ovaries are preventively repositioned using surgery (oophoropexy), if possible, out of the anticipated radiation field prior to therapy (Terenziani, 2009). Of chemotherapeutic drugs, alkylating agents are believed to be particularly damaging to ovarian function. As discussed in Chapter 27 (p. 598), preventive adjuvant GnRH analogues may lower rates of chemotherapy-induced POF, although the efficacy of this approach remains controversial. Importantly, recent advances in oocyte and ovarian tissue cryopreservation make it likely that oocyte harvest prior to treatment will become the preferred approach when feasible. Of interest, persistent chemotherapy-induced amenorrhea appears to confer a decreased risk of breast cancer recurrence, possibly beyond that attributable to the low estrogen

levels (Swain, 2010; Zhao, 2014). Nevertheless, a substantial menopause-specific decrease in quality of life is observed in these patients (Yoo, 2013).

HYPOGONADOTROPIC HYPOGONADISM

The term *hypogonadotropic hypogonadism* implies that the primary abnormality lies in the hypothalamic-pituitary axis. As a result, poor gonadotropin stimulation of the ovaries leads to impaired follicular development. Generally in these patients, LH and FSH levels, although low, will still be in the detectable range (<5 mIU/mL). However, levels may be undetectable in patients with complete absence of hypothalamic stimulation, such as occurs in Kallmann syndrome. In addition, absent pituitary function due to abnormal development or severe pituitary damage may lead to similarly low levels. Thus, the group of hypogonadotropic hypogonadism disorders may be viewed as a continuum with perturbations leading to luteal dysfunction, oligomenorrhea, and, in the most severe presentation, amenorrhea.

■ Hypothalamic Disorders
Inherited Hypothalamic Abnormalities

Inherited hypothalamic abnormalities primarily consist of those patients with idiopathic hypogonadotropic hypogonadism (IHH). A subset has associated defects in the ability to smell (hyposmia or anosmia) and are said to have Kallmann syndrome. This syndrome can be inherited as an X-linked, autosomal dominant, or autosomal recessive disorder (Cadman, 2007; Waldstreicher, 1996). The X-linked form was the first to be characterized and follows mutation in the *KAL1* gene on the short arm of the X chromosome. Expressed during fetal development, this gene encodes an adhesion protein, named anosmin-1. As this protein is critical for normal migration of both GnRH and olfactory neurons, loss of normal anosmin-1 expression results in both reproductive and olfactory deficits (Fig. 16-5) (Franco, 1991; Soussi-Yanicostas, 1996). Kallmann patients have a normal complement of GnRH neurons, however, these neurons fail to migrate and instead remain near the nasal epithelium (Quinton, 1997). As a result, locally secreted GnRH is unable to stimulate gonadotropes in the anterior pituitary gland to release LH and FSH. In turn, marked decreases in ovarian estrogen production result in absence of breast development and menstrual cycles.

Kallmann syndrome is also associated with midline facial anomalies such as cleft palate, unilateral renal agenesis, cerebellar ataxia, epilepsy, neurosensory hearing loss, and synkinesis (mirror movements of the hands) (Winters, 1992; Zenaty, 2006). Kallmann syndrome can be distinguished from IHH by olfactory testing. This is performed easily in the office with strong odorants such as ground coffee or perfume. Interestingly, many of these patients are unaware of their deficit.

During the past 10 years, an array of autosomal genes has been identified that contribute to normal development, migration, and secretion by GnRH neurons (Caronia, 2011; Layman, 2013). Mutations in several of these genes have been described in patients with hypothalamic amenorrhea. Genes

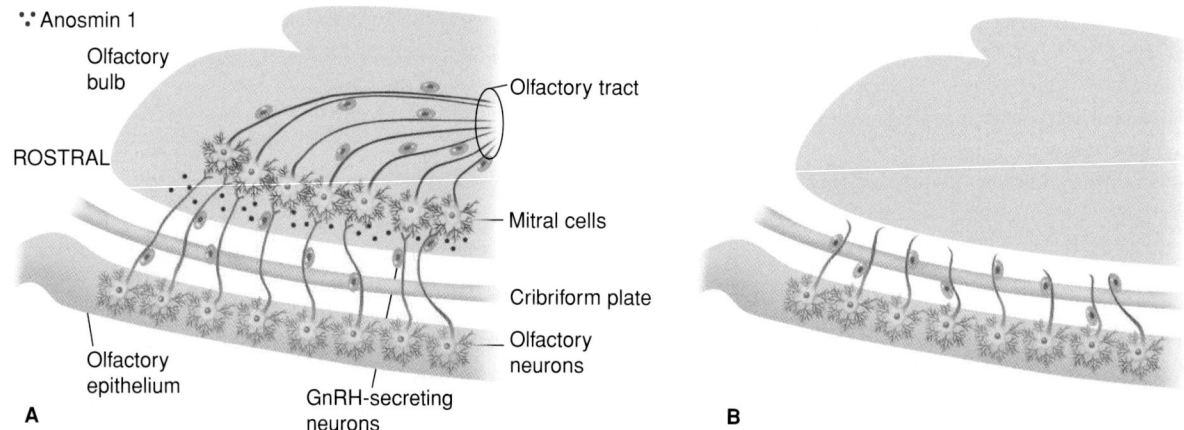

FIGURE 16-5 Normal GnRH neuron migration and the pathogenesis of Kallmann syndrome. **A.** During normal development, olfactory neurons arising in the olfactory epithelium extend their axons through the cribriform plate of the ethmoid bone to reach the olfactory bulb. Here, these axons synapse with dendrites of mitral cells, whose axons form the olfactory tract. Mitral cells secrete anosmin-1, which is the protein product of the *KAL1* gene. This protein is necessary to direct the olfactory axons to their correct location in the olfactory bulb. The GnRH-secreting neurons use this axonal path to migrate from the olfactory placode to the hypothalamus. **B.** Patients with Kallmann syndrome due to a *KAL1* mutation lack anosmin-1 expression. As a result, the axons of the olfactory neurons cannot interact properly with mitral cells, and their migration ends between the cribriform plate and olfactory bulb. As GnRH neuronal migration is dependent on this axonal trail, the GnRH secretion pathway likewise ends at this location. (Reproduced with permission from Rugarli E, Ballabio A: Kallmann syndrome. From genetics to neurobiology, JAMA 1993 Dec 8;270(22):2713–2716.)

include *FGF8, KAL1, NELF, PROK2, PROKR2,* and *CHD7.* As a result, the percentage of patients in whom this disorder need be considered idiopathic is gradually decreasing. Of note, mutation in the *CHD7* gene may cause either normosmic IHH or Kallmann syndrome, thereby blurring the distinction between these disorders.

Acquired Hypothalamic Dysfunction

Acquired hypothalamic abnormalities are much more frequent than inherited deficiencies. Most commonly, gonadotropin deficiency leading to chronic anovulation is believed to arise from functional disorders of the hypothalamus or higher brain centers. Also called "hypothalamic amenorrhea," this diagnosis encompasses three main categories: eating disorders, excessive exercise, and stress. From a teleologic perspective, amenorrhea in time of starvation or extreme stress can be seen as a mechanism to prevent pregnancy at a time in which resources are suboptimal for raising a child. Each woman appears to have her own hypothalamic "setpoint" or sensitivity to environmental factors. For example, individual women can tolerate markedly different amounts of stress without developing amenorrhea.

Eating Disorders. Anorexia nervosa and bulimia, both described in Chapter 13 (p. 301), can lead to amenorrhea. Hypothalamic dysfunction is severe in anorexia and may affect other hypothalamic-pituitary axes in addition to the reproductive axis. Amenorrhea in anorexia nervosa can precede, follow, or appear coincidentally with weight loss. In addition, even with return to normal weight, not all women with anorexia will regain normal menstrual function. Patients with premenarchal onset of anorexia are at particular risk for protracted amenorrhea (Dempfle, 2013).

Exercise-induced Amenorrhea. This is most common in women whose exercise regimen is associated with significant loss of fat, including ballet, gymnastics, and long-distance running (De Souza, 1991; Frisch, 1980). In those women who continue to menstruate, cycles are notable for their variability in cycle interval and length due to reduced hormonal function (De Souza, 1998). Puberty may be delayed in girls who begin training before menarche (Frisch, 1981).

An appreciation for the link between exercise and reproductive health has led to the concept of the *female athlete triad,* which consists of menstrual dysfunction, low energy availability with or without disordered eating, and low bone mineral density in extreme athletes. Two international symposia held in this field have begun to develop risk stratification and recommendations for this population (Duckham, 2012; Joy, 2014).

In 1970, Frisch and Revelle proposed that an adolescent girl needed to achieve a critical body weight to begin menstruating (Frisch, 1970). This mass was initially postulated to approximate 48 kilograms and was subsequently refined to a minimal body mass index (BMI) approaching normal, which is ≥19. Subsequent studies suggest that, although there is a clear correlation between body fat and reproductive function at both ends of the weight spectrum, overall energy balance better predicts the onset and maintenance of menstrual cycles (Billewicz, 1976; Johnston, 1975). For example, many elite athletes regain menstrual cyclicity following a decrease in exercise intensity prior to any gain in weight (Abraham, 1982).

Stress-induced Amenorrhea. This may be associated with clearly traumatic life events. Nevertheless, less severe life events and even positive events may be associated with stress. For example, stress-related amenorrhea is frequently associated with leaving for college, test taking, or wedding planning.

Functional Hypothalamic Amenorrhea Pathophysiology. Eating disorders, exercise, and stress may disturb menstrual

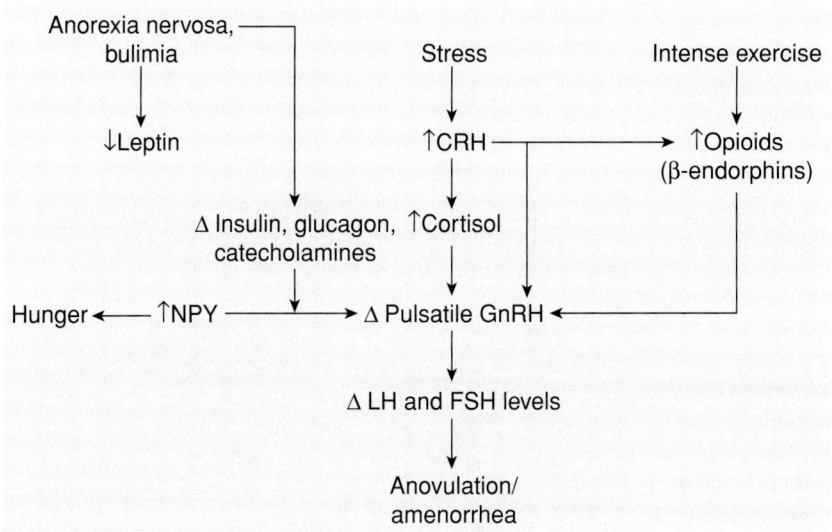

FIGURE 16-6 Diagram depicting a simplified model for the development of amenorrhea in women with eating disorders, high stress levels, or rigorous exercise. CRH = corticotropin-releasing hormone; FSH = follicle-stimulating hormone; GnRH = gonadotropin-releasing hormone; LH = luteinizing hormone; NPY = neuropeptide Y.

function through overlapping mechanisms. This observation may be in part because these problems are often concurrent. For example, women with eating disorders frequently exercise excessively and are undoubtedly under stress as they attempt to control their eating patterns. Figure 16-6 depicts a simplified model for the development of amenorrhea in these patients. It must be emphasized that each cause of functional hypothalamic amenorrhea may act via one or all of these pathways. Furthermore, in many cases, the factors known to affect reproductive function are likely acting indirectly on GnRH neurons through various neuronal subtypes that have synaptic connections to GnRH neurons.

Exercise in particular has been associated with an increase in levels of endogenous opioids (β-endorphins), producing the so-called runner's high. Opioids alter GnRH pulsatility.

As part of the stress response, each of these conditions may lead to an increase in corticotropin-releasing hormone (CRH) release by the hypothalamus, which in turn results in cortisol secretion by the adrenal gland. CRH alters the pattern of pulsatile GnRH secretion, whereas cortisol may act directly or indirectly to disrupt GnRH neuronal function.

Eating disorders are thought to disturb ovulatory function through several hormonal factors including insulin, insulin-like growth factor-1, cortisol, adiponectin, ghrelin, and leptin (Misra, 2014). First identified in 1994, leptin is a 167-amino-acid protein encoded by the *ob* gene and produced in white adipose tissue (Zhang, 1994). Leptin receptors have been identified in the central nervous system (CNS) and a wide range of peripheral tissues (Chen, 1996; Tartaglia, 1995).

Primarily produced in adipose tissue, leptin provides an important link between energy balance and reproduction, albeit one of many mechanisms (Chou, 2014; Schneider, 2004). Leptin has been termed a "satiety factor" as human leptin gene mutation results in morbid obesity, diabetes mellitus, and hypogonadism. This trio of abnormalities can be successfully reversed with recombinant human leptin treatment (Licinio, 2004).

Patients with anorexia nervosa have been found to have low circulating leptin levels (Mantzoros, 1997). It has been hypothesized that a decrease in leptin production due to weight loss could secondarily stimulate neuropeptide Y, which is known to stimulate hunger and alter GnRH pulsatility. Leptin likely acts through various additional neurotransmitters and neuropeptides including the β-endorphins and α-melanocyte-stimulating hormone (Tartaglia, 1995).

Pseudocyesis. Although rare, pseudocyesis is considered in any woman with amenorrhea and pregnancy symptoms. Pseudocyesis exemplifies the ability of the mind to control physiologic processes. More than 500 cases of pseudocyesis have been reported in the medical literature in women ranging from ages 6 to 79 years. These patients fervently believe that they are pregnant and subsequently demonstrate several pregnancy signs and symptoms, including amenorrhea.

Endocrine evaluation in a limited number of patients has suggested a pattern of hormonal derangements. These include alterations in LH pulse frequency concurrent with elevated serum androgen levels, which may explain the observed amenorrhea. Elevated serum prolactin levels and resultant galactorrhea have been noted in a subset of patients. Nocturnal growth hormone secretion also appears blunted (Tarin, 2013).

A common link in these patients is a history of severe grief, such as recent miscarriage, infant death, or longstanding infertility. Pseudocyesis may be more common in developing countries, where societal pressure to produce children may be strong (Seeman, 2014). Psychiatric treatment is generally required to treat the associated depression, which is often exacerbated when the patient is informed that she is not pregnant (Whelan, 1990).

Anatomic Destruction. Any process that destroys the hypothalamus can impair GnRH secretion and lead to hypogonadotropic hypogonadism and amenorrhea. Due to the complex neurohormonal input to the GnRH neurons, abnormalities do not need to directly interact with GnRH neurons but may operate indirectly by altering the activity of modulatory neurons.

The tumors most often associated with amenorrhea include craniopharyngiomas, germinomas, endodermal sinus tumors, eosinophilic granuloma (Hand-Schuller-Christian syndrome), gliomas, and metastatic lesions. The most common of these tumors, craniopharyngiomas, are located in the suprasellar region and frequently present with headaches and visual changes. Alternatively, impaired GnRH secretion may follow trauma, radiation, infections such as tuberculosis, or infiltrative diseases such as sarcoidosis.

■ Anterior Pituitary Gland Disorders

The anterior pituitary gland consists of gonadotropes (producing LH and FSH), lactotropes (prolactin), thyrotropes (thyroid-stimulating hormone), corticotropes (adrenocorticotropic hormone), and somatotropes (growth hormone) (Chap. 15, p. 343). Although various disorders may directly affect gonadotropes, many causes of pituitary-derived amenorrhea may also follow abnormalities in other pituitary cell types, which in turn alter gonadotrope function.

Inherited Abnormalities

In addition to mutations that underlie hypothalamic dysfunction, our understanding of genetic mechanisms that regulate normal pituitary development and function is rapidly advancing. First, patient cohorts have been described that have pituitary hormone deficiency combined with central facial and/or neurologic defects due to a failed midline fusion, a syndrome known as septo-optic dysplasia. Many of these patients carry mutations in the *PROP1* gene (Cadman, 2007). Second, mutations in genes that encode the LH or FSH β-subunits or the GnRH receptor have also been identified as rare causes of hypogonadotropic hypogonadism. Last, mutations in genes encoding the nuclear hormone receptors SF-1 and DAX1 (NR0B1) as well as genes encoding the G-protein-coupled receptor 54 (GPR54) for kisspeptin-1 are associated with hypothalamic and pituitary dysfunction (Matthews, 1993; Pallais, 2006; Seminara, 2006; Weiss, 1992).

Acquired Pituitary Dysfunction

Most pituitary dysfunction is acquired after menarche and therefore presents with normal pubertal development followed by secondary amenorrhea. Nevertheless, in rare cases, these disorders may begin prior to puberty, resulting in delayed puberty and primary amenorrhea (Howlett, 1989).

Pituitary adenomas are the most frequent cause of acquired pituitary dysfunction (Chap. 15, p. 359). These most commonly secrete prolactin, but excessive secretion of any pituitary-derived hormone can result in amenorrhea. For example, excessive ACTH secretion results in Cushing disease, which is associated with menstrual abnormalities and signs of cortisol excess. Significantly elevated serum prolactin levels (>100 ng/mL) are almost always due to a pituitary mass.

Increased serum prolactin levels are found in as many as one-tenth of amenorrheic women, and more than half of women with both galactorrhea and amenorrhea have elevated prolactin levels (the "galactorrhea-amenorrhea syndrome"). Mechanistically, dopamine is released by the hypothalamus and acts on the anterior pituitary. Dopamine is the primary regulator of prolactin biosynthesis and secretion and plays an inhibitory role. Thus, elevated prolactin levels feed back to the hypothalamus and are associated with a reflex increase in central dopamine production to lower prolactin concentrations. This rise in central dopamine levels alters GnRH neuronal function.

Pituitary tumors also may indirectly alter gonadotrope function by a mass effect. First, tumor growth may compress neighboring gonadotropes. Second, damage to the pituitary stalk can disrupt dopamine's pathway to inhibit prolactin secretion. In this latter case, resulting elevated prolactin levels lead to ele-

vated central dopamine levels that presumably interfere with menstrual function through the same mechanisms described in the previous paragraph.

As in the hypothalamus, pituitary function may also be diminished by inflammation, infiltrative disease, metastatic lesions, surgery, or radiation treatment. Although a rare condition, peripartum lymphocytic hypophysitis can be a dangerous cause of pituitary failure. Infiltrative diseases include sarcoidosis and hemochromatosis. Spontaneous hemorrhage into a pituitary adenoma, termed pituitary apoplexy, also may result in acute loss of pituitary function (Chap. 15, p. 360).

Sheehan syndrome refers to panhypopituitarism. It classically follows massive postpartum hemorrhage and associated hypotension. The abrupt, severe hypotension leads to pituitary ischemia and necrosis (Kelestimur, 2003). Patients with the most severe form develop shock due to pituitary apoplexy. Pituitary apoplexy is characterized by a sudden onset of headache, nausea, visual deficits, and hormonal dysfunction due to acute hemorrhage or infarction within the pituitary. In less severe forms, loss of gonadotrope activity in the pituitary leads to anovulation and subsequent amenorrhea. Damage to the other specific pituitary cell types lead to a failure to lactate, loss of sexual and axillary hair, and hypothyroidism or adrenal insufficiency symptoms. Pituitary cell types are differentially sensitive to damage. For this reason, prolactin secretion deficiency is the most common, followed by loss of gonadotropin and growth hormone release, loss of ACTH production, and least commonly, by decreases in thyroid-stimulating hormone (TSH) secretion (Veldhuis, 1980).

■ Other Causes of Hypogonadotropic Hypogonadism

Hypogonadotropic amenorrhea may be observed in various chronic diseases including end-stage kidney disease, liver disease, malignancies, acquired immunodeficiency syndrome, and malabsorption syndromes. The mechanisms by which these disorders result in menstrual dysfunction are poorly understood. End-stage kidney disease is associated with increased serum prolactin and altered leptin levels, both of which may disrupt normal GnRH pulsatility (Ghazizadeh, 2007). Of patients with nonalcoholic chronic liver disease, the cause of the low gonadotropin levels is unknown and is observed only in a subset of amenorrheic women (Cundy, 1991). Chronic diseases may produce amenorrhea through common mechanisms, such as stress and nutritional deficiencies. For example, patients with malabsorption due to celiac disease may have delayed menarche, secondary amenorrhea, and early menopause, which have been attributed to deficiencies in trace elements such as zinc and selenium. These are required for normal gonadotropin biosynthesis and secretion (Özgör, 2010).

EUGONADOTROPIC AMENORRHEA

Several disorders that produce amenorrhea are not associated with significantly abnormal gonadotropin levels, at least as measured at a single point in time, as is done in clinical settings. Even so, gonadotropin amplitude or pulse frequency is likely disturbed in these patients. As a result, chronic sustained sex-steroid secretion interferes with the normal feedback between the ovary and the hypothalamic-pituitary axis. Normal oocyte maturation and ovulation are impaired, and menstruation fails to occur.

Due to relatively normal gonadotropin levels, these patients will secrete estrogen and therefore can also be said to have *chronic anovulation with estrogen present*. This is in contrast to patients with ovarian failure or hypothalamic-pituitary failure, in whom estrogen levels are low or absent. This distinction may be useful during evaluation and treatment.

■ Polycystic Ovarian Syndrome

This syndrome is by far the most common cause of chronic anovulation with estrogen present and is discussed fully in Chapter 17 (p. 386). Patients with PCOS may have various menstrual presentations. First, complete amenorrhea may follow anovulation. Without ovulation, progesterone is lacking, and an absent progesterone withdrawal fails to prompt menses. In some women with PCOS, however, amenorrhea may be attributable to the ability of androgens, which are elevated in PCOS patients, to atrophy the endometrium. Alternatively, heavy menstrual or intermenstrual bleeding can result from unopposed estrogen stimulation of the endometrium. Within this unstable, thickened proliferative-phase endometrium, episodic stromal breakdown and shedding leads to irregular bleeding. Vessels may be abnormally dilated in anovulatory endometria, and bleeding may be severe. Last, women with PCOS may experience occasional ovulatory cycles, and normal withdrawal menses or pregnancy may occur.

■ Nonclassic Congenital Adrenal Hyperplasia

This condition closely mimics the presentation of PCOS with hyperandrogenism and irregular menstrual cycles. Most commonly, nonclassic congenital adrenal hyperplasia (CAH), also termed adult-onset CAH or late-onset CAH, is due to a mutation in the *CYP21A2* gene, which encodes the 21-hydroxylase enzyme. With a mild mutation, patients are asymptomatic until adrenarche, a time that requires increased adrenal steroidogenesis. Patients with CAH are unable to convert an adequate percentage of progesterone to cortisol and aldosterone, thus increasing the production of androgens (Fig. 15-5, p. 337). As in PCOS, chronically elevated androgen levels blunt follicular maturation and prevent normal cyclic feedback at the hypothalamus and pituitary gland, and thereby result in anovulation and amenorrhea.

■ Ovarian Tumor

Although uncommon, chronic anovulation with estrogen present can also be observed with ovarian tumors producing either estrogens or androgens. As discussed in Chapter 36, examples include granulosa cell tumors, theca cell tumors, and mature cystic teratomas (Aiman, 1977; Pectasides, 2008; Thomas, 2012).

■ Hyperprolactinemia and Thyroid Disorders

Although hyperprolactinemia can cause hypogonadotropic hypogonadism, as described on page 378, many hyperprolactinemic women may instead have relatively normal gonadotropin levels. As a group, however, their estrogen levels will be mildly depressed. Aside from pituitary adenomas, other circumstances significantly raise prolactin levels. First, many medications and herbs have been associated with hyperprolactinemia, galactorrhea, and disrupted menstrual cycling (Table 12-2, p. 281). The antipsychotic group of medications is a frequent cause.

Second, primary hypothyroidism may result in mildly elevated prolactin levels. One example is Hashimoto thyroiditis. In this disorder, the decrease in circulating thyroid hormone levels results in a compensatory increase in hypothalamic thyrotropin-releasing hormone (TRH) secretion. TRH prompts pituitary gland thyrotropes to produce TSH. In addition, TRH also binds to pituitary lactotropes, increasing prolactin secretion. This tight link between thyroid function and prolactin levels justifies measurement of a TSH with prolactin levels when initiating evaluation for galactorrhea or amenorrhea.

Whether due to adenoma, medications, or hypothyroidism, prolactin elevation creates a compensatory rise in central levels of dopamine, the primary inhibitor of prolactin secretion. Increased central dopamine levels alter GnRH secretion, thereby disrupting normal cyclic gonadotropin secretion and preventing ovulation. With thyroid disease, additional proposed mechanisms include direct effects of thyroid hormone and prolactin on peripheral cells as thyroid receptors are found in most cell types. Specifically, prolactin receptors have been identified in the ovary and in the endometrium. Moreover, thyroid hormone increases sex hormone-binding globulin levels, altering the levels of unbound, and thereby active, ovarian steroids.

These potentially discordant effects are reflected in the various bleeding patterns seen with thyroid disease (Krassas, 2010). Classically, hypothyroidism is stated to cause anovulation and subsequent heavy menstrual bleeding (Chap. 8, p. 192). Hyperthyroidism is implicated in amenorrhea. Nevertheless, these patterns are not strictly observed. As might be expected, the likelihood of menstrual abnormality correlates with the severity of the thyroid function disturbance (Kakuno, 2010).

EVALUATION

■ History

Figure 16-7 offers an algorithm for approaching the patient with amenorrhea. Initial questions investigate whether pubertal Tanner stages have been reached and whether menses have begun (Chap. 14, p. 319). The cycle interval, duration, and amount of menstrual flow are also characterized. Menstrual pattern changes and a description of these changes are sought. Also, the development of amenorrhea may be temporally correlated with pelvic infection, surgery, radiation therapy, chemotherapy, or other illnesses.

Surgical history focuses on prior pelvic surgery, especially intrauterine or ovarian surgery. Patients are questioned regarding postoperative infection or other surgical complications.

A review of symptoms can also be helpful. For example, new-onset headaches or visual changes may suggest a tumor of the CNS or pituitary gland. Pituitary tumors may impinge on the optic chiasm, resulting in bitemporal hemianopsia, that

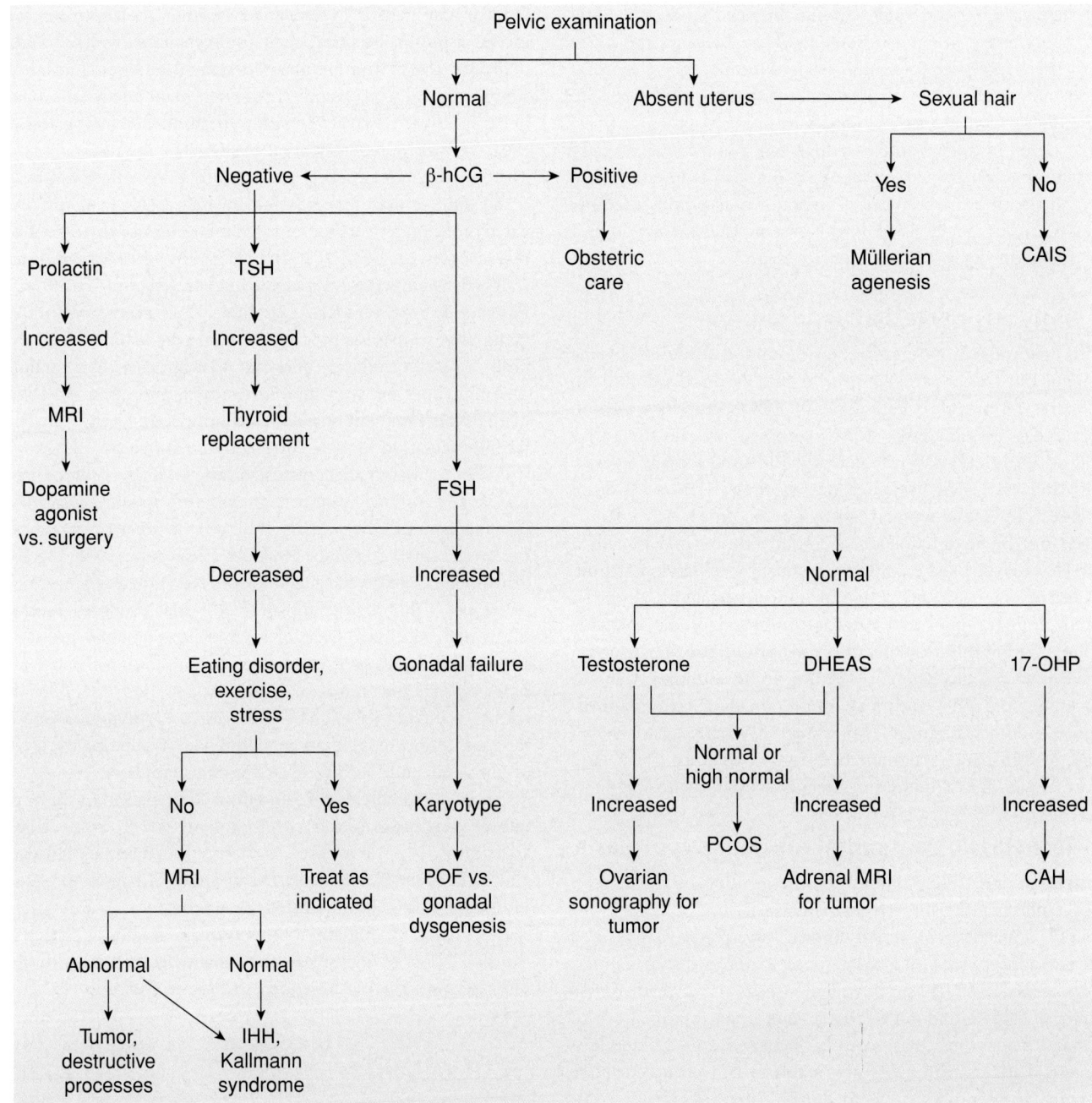

FIGURE 16-7 Diagnostic algorithm to evaluate amenorrhea. CAH = congenital adrenal hyperplasia; CAIS = complete androgen insensitivity syndrome; DHEAS = dehydroepiandrosterone sulfate; FSH = follicle-stimulating hormone; hCG = human chorionic gonadotropin; IHH = idiopathic hypogonadotropic hypogonadism; MRI = magnetic resonance imaging; 17-OHP = 17-hydroxyprogesterone; PCOS = polycystic ovarian syndrome; POF = premature ovarian failure; TSH = thyroid-stimulating hormone.

is, the loss of both right and left outer visual fields. Bilateral milky breast discharge may reflect hyperprolactinemia. Thyroid disease can be associated with heat or cold intolerance, weight changes, and sleep or bowel motility abnormalities. Hirsutism and acne are often seen with PCOS or with nonclassic CAH. Cyclic pelvic pain would suggest a reproductive tract outlet obstruction. Hot flushes and vaginal dryness point to hypergonadotropic hypogonadism, that is, POF. Of note, the range, severity, and persistence of symptoms observed in women with POF appear to exceed those experienced by women with age-appropriate menopause (Allshouse, 2015).

Important questions regarding family history include premature cessation of menses or a history of autoimmune disease, including thyroid disease, which would suggest an increased risk for POF. A history of irregular menses, infertility, or signs of excess androgen production is often noted with PCOS. Sudden neonatal death may have occurred in family members carrying mutations in the *CYP21A2* gene responsible for CAH.

The social history investigates exposure to environmental toxins, including cigarettes. Any medications are inventoried, especially those such as antipsychotics that increase prolactin levels.

■ Physical Examination

General appearance can be helpful in the evaluation of amenorrhea. A low BMI, perhaps in conjunction with tooth enamel erosion from recurrent vomiting, is highly suggestive of an eating disorder. Signs of Turner syndrome are evaluated, including short stature, webbed neck, shield-shaped chest, and others listed in Table 18-3 (p. 411) (Turner, 1972). Midline facial defects, such as cleft palate, are consistent with a developmental defect of the anterior pituitary gland. Hypertension in a prepubertal girl may reflect mutation in the *CYP17* gene and shunting of the steroidogenic pathway toward aldosterone.

Visual field defects, particularly bitemporal hemianopsia, may indicate a pituitary gland or CNS tumor. Skin is inspected for acanthosis nigricans, hirsutism, or acne, which may indicate PCOS or other hyperandrogenism causes. Supraclavicular fat, abdominal striae, and hypertension may be noted in those with Cushing syndrome. Hypothyroidism can present with an abnormally enlarged thyroid gland, delayed reflexes, and bradycardia. During breast examination, bilateral spontaneous galactorrhea implies hyperprolactinemia.

Examination of the genitalia starts by noting hair pattern. Sparse or absent axillary or pubic hair may reflect either lack of adrenarche or androgen insensitivity syndrome. Conversely, elevated androgen levels will result in a male pattern of genital hair growth. Markedly elevated levels of androgens can produce signs of virilization, most noticeably clitoromegaly (Chap. 17, p. 395). These women may also note voice deepening and male pattern balding.

Evidence of estrogen production includes a pink, moist vagina and cervical mucus. With estrogen present, vaginal smears demonstrate mostly superficial epithelial cells, whereas with atrophy, parabasal cell numbers increase (Fig. 21-9, p. 488). Low estrogen levels also manifest with a pale, thin, unrugated vagina.

Determination of reproductive tract anomalies by physical examination is described in Chapter 18 (p. 415). Rectal and digital vaginal examination may help identify a uterus above an obstruction at the level of the introitus or in the vagina. Hematocolpos suggests normal ovarian and endometrial function.

■ Testing

The differential diagnosis of amenorrhea is extensive, but evaluation of most women is relatively straightforward. For all disorders, testing may be modified by patient history and physical examination. All reproductive-aged women with amenorrhea are assumed pregnant until proven otherwise. Thus, a urinary or serum β-hCG level is almost always obtained.

Progesterone Withdrawal

Classically, patients are given exogenous progesterone and monitored for a progesterone withdrawal bleed, which follows a few days after progesterone completion (the progesterone challenge test). One regimen is medroxyprogesterone acetate (Provera) given as a 10-mg daily oral dose for 10 days. If bleeding ensues, then a woman is assumed to produce estrogen and to have a developed endometrium and patent outflow tract. If

bleeding does not follow, then a patient is given estrogen followed by progesterone treatment. A single pack of COCs works nicely for this. If a woman again fails to bleed several days after completing the 21 hormone-containing pills, then an anatomic abnormality is diagnosed.

Several factors can lead to an incorrect test interpretation. First, estrogen levels may fluctuate both in hypothalamic amenorrhea and in the early stages of ovarian failure. As a result, patients with these disorders may have at least some bleeding after progesterone withdrawal. Furthermore, women with high androgen levels, such as occurs with PCOS and CAH, may have an atrophic endometrium and fail to bleed. Specifically, up to 20 percent of women in whom estrogen is present will fail to bleed following progesterone withdrawal (Rarick, 1990). Conversely, menses may be observed after progesterone administration in up to 40 percent of women with hypothalamic amenorrhea due to stress, weight loss, or exercise and in up to 50 percent of women with POF (Nakamura, 1996; Rebar, 1990). This bleeding derives from endometrium that grew prior to amenorrhea onset.

Serum Hormone Levels

As suggested by the American Society for Reproductive Medicine (2008), it may be more reasonable to begin with hormonal evaluation in any woman found to have a normal pelvic examination (Table 16-7). First, *serum FSH levels* are typically assessed, and levels that are low suggest hypothalamic-pituitary dysfunction. An elevated FSH level is consistent with POF. FSH levels in the normal range suggest an anatomic defect or eugonadotropic hypogonadism, such as occurs in PCOS, hyperprolactinemia, or thyroid disease. Although many patients with PCOS have elevated LH to FSH level ratios >2, testing for this relationship is unnecessary as a normal ratio does not exclude this diagnosis.

If an FSH value is low, repeating this measurement and adding an LH level, which will also be low, can help confirm hypogonadotropic hypogonadism. Additional testing may include a GnRH stimulation test. Several different protocols can be employed, but one common approach provides 100 μg of GnRH as an intravenous bolus and then measures LH and FSH levels at 0, 15, 30, 45, and 60 minutes. In patients with hypogonadotropic hypogonadism or delayed puberty, although both LH and FSH levels will be blunted, FSH levels will be high relative to LH ratios during the test (Job, 1977; Yen, 1973). Although informative, use of this test has been constrained by the lack of consistently available clinical grade GnRH. More recently, providers have begun to use GnRH agonist protocols.

In contrast, an elevated FSH level strongly suggests the presence of hypergonadotropic hypogonadism, namely, POF. This diagnosis requires two FSH levels greater than a threshold range of 30 to 40 mIU/mL and obtained at least 1 month apart. At least two elevated values are required because the course of POF may fluctuate over time. This variation likely explains the occasional pregnancy that has been reported in these women. Patients keep a menstrual calendar while testing is completed because bleeding 2 weeks following an elevated serum FSH level may simply indicate that the sample was obtained during a normal midcycle gonadotropin surge.

TABLE 16-7. Tests Commonly Used in the Evaluation of Amenorrhea

Primary Laboratory Tests	Diagnosis
β-hCG	Pregnancy
FSH	Hypogonadotropic versus hypergonadotropic hypogonadism[a]
Estradiol	Hypogonadotropic versus hypergonadotropic hypogonadism
Prolactin	Hyperprolactinemia
TSH, ± fT4	Thyroid disease
Secondary Laboratory Tests	
Testosterone	PCOS and exclude ovarian tumor
DHEAS	Exclude adrenal tumor
17-OHP	Nonclassic CAH
2-hour glucose tolerance test	PCOS
Fasting lipid panel	PCOS
Autoimmune testing	POF
Adrenal antibodies (CYP21A2)	POF
Fragile X (FMR1 premutation)	POF
Karyotype	POF <35 years
Radiologic Evaluation	
Sonography	PCOS, uterine agenesis, or ovarian tumor
HSG or SIS	Müllerian anomaly or intrauterine synechiae
MR imaging	Müllerian anomaly or hypothalamic-pituitary disease

[a]Hypogonadotropic hypogonadism includes functional causes of hypothalamic amenorrhea (excessive exercise, eating disorders, and stress). Hypergonadotropic hypogonadism refers primarily to premature ovarian failure (POF).
CAH = congenital adrenal hyperplasia; DHEAS = dehydroepiandrosterone sulfate; FSH = follicle-stimulating hormone; fT4 = free thyroxine; hCG = human chorionic gonadotropin; HSG = hysterosalpingography; MR = magnetic resonance; 17-OHP = 17-hydroxyprogesterone; PCOS = polycystic ovarian syndrome; SIS = saline infusion sonography; TSH = thyroid-stimulating hormone.

As adjuncts to FSH testing, ancillary markers that will increase the sensitivity and specificity of ovarian reserve testing have been investigated. Many clinicians obtain measurements for estradiol in addition to FSH, although this has not been consistently shown to increase diagnostic accuracy. Attention has turned more recently to the use of circulating serum AMH levels (Chap. 19, p. 436) (Visser, 2012).

Prolactin and *thyroid-stimulating hormone levels* are tested in most patients with amenorrhea as prolactin-secreting adenomas and thyroid disease are relatively common and require specific treatment. Because of the relationship between hypothyroidism and prolactin levels, both hormones are measured simultaneously. If present, treatment for hypothyroidism will also normalize prolactin levels. If a TSH level is elevated, an unbound thyroxine (T_4) level is drawn to confirm clinical hypothyroidism.

Serum testosterone levels are measured in women with suspected PCOS or with clinical signs of androgen excess. Hormonal evaluation includes measurement of serum total testosterone levels. Measurement of free testosterone levels is generally unwarranted as these assays are more expensive and less reliable unless sent to a specialized laboratory. Mild elevations in testosterone levels are consistent with the diagnosis of PCOS. However, values >200 ng/dL may suggest an ovarian tumor and warrant pelvic sonography.

Serum dehydroepiandrosterone sulfate (DHEAS) production is essentially limited to the adrenal gland. Levels in high-normal range or mildly above are consistent with PCOS. Adrenal adenomas may produce circulating DHEAS levels above 700 µg/dL and merit investigation with magnetic resonance (MR) imaging or computed tomography (CT) scanning of the adrenals. Measurement of 17-hydroxyprogesterone (17-OHP) aims to identify patients with nonclassic CAH. However, confirmation of this diagnosis can be difficult due to the overlapping values among normal patients and heterozygote and homozygote carriers of mutations in the 21-hydroxylase (*CYP21A2*) gene. Accordingly, adrenal stimulation with ACTH, often colloquially termed the *cort stim test*, may be required as described in Chapter 17 (p. 395).

Other Serum Testing

At times, other serum testing may be prudent. If an eating disorder is suspected, an immediate assessment of serum electrolytes is warranted as imbalances can be life-threatening. An electrocardiogram is also considered in those patients perceived to have more severe disease. A reverse triiodothyronine (T_3) level is often elevated in patients with functional hypothalamic amenorrhea. Women with PCOS are screened for insulin resistance and lipid abnormalities as these are often found in affected patients and increase risks for diabetes and cardiovascular disease (Chap. 17, p. 391). Although no consensus exists, repeating these tests every few years is sensible.

Many patients with POF will not have a clear etiology for their disorder based on medical history or genetic testing and may reasonably be assumed to have an autoimmune cause. Recommendations for testing vary among experts, but the current recommendations focus on measurement of antiadrenal antibodies, specifically antibodies directed against 21-hydroxylase. Addition of antithyroid antibodies such as antimicrosomal/thyroid peroxidase antibodies (TPOAb) is also logical if thyroid dysfunction is suspected.

Chromosomal Analysis

Patients with gonadal dysgenesis, such as Turner syndrome, are considered for karyotyping. Classic teaching suggests that this test is unnecessary after age 30. However, consideration is given to testing patients up to age 35 because a rare individual mosaicism may retain functional oocytes and thus sustain cyclic menses longer than expected. As previously indicated, a Y-containing cell line requires bilateral oophorectomy because of the increased risk for ovarian germ cell tumors. Due to the close association between stature and abnormalities in the X-chromosome, many specialists advise karyotyping all women with POF who are shorter than 60 inches (Saenger, 2001). Chromosomal studies are also considered in any woman with a family history of POF.

Radiologic Evaluation

Any patient with hypogonadotropic hypogonadism is assumed to have an anatomic CNS or pituitary gland abnormality until proven otherwise by MR imaging or CT scanning. Thus, functional hypothalamic amenorrhea due to stress, exercise, or eating disorder is a diagnosis of exclusion. Imaging is highly sensitive for identification of destructive disorders such as tumors or infiltrative diseases of the hypothalamus or pituitary gland. Although fundamentally normal, a subset of patients with genetic causes for Kallmann syndrome or IHH will demonstrate developmental defects of the hypothalamus, olfactory bulbs, or pituitary gland during MR imaging (Klingmuller, 1987).

Reproductive tract anatomic disorders can be evaluated with several modalities depending on the suspected cause. Sonographic examination is frequently useful as a first screen for a uterus deemed grossly normal by physical examination. HSG or SIS is excellent for the detection of intrauterine synechiae or developmental anomalies. Changing trends favor SIS unless information on tubal patency is also required. Three-dimensional (3-D) sonography and 3-D SIS can also add information. MR imaging is frequently used for delineation of more complex uterine structures, such as a noncommunicating or hypoplastic uterine horn. Imaging of congenital reproductive tract anomalies is discussed further in Chapter 18 (p. 416).

TREATMENT

Treatment of amenorrhea depends on its etiology and patient goals such as a desire to treat hirsutism or seek pregnancy. Anatomic abnormalities often require surgical correction, if possible, and are discussed in Chapter 18 (p. 415). Hypothyroidism is treated with thyroid replacement, and a suggested dosage of levothyroxine is 1.6 μg/kg of body weight per day (Baskin, 2002). For most, a suitable starting dose is 50 to 100 μg of levothyroxine orally daily. TSH response is slow and levels are rechecked 6 to 8 weeks following initiation. A TSH level in the lower range of normal is the therapeutic goal. If needed, the dose may be increased by an increment of 12.5 or 25 μg (Jameson, 2012). Women with hyperprolactinemia receive a dopamine agonist, such as bromocriptine or cabergoline. Macroadenomas may require surgery if secondary deficits such as visual changes are observed. Both medical and surgical specifics of pituitary disease treatment are found in Chapter 15 (p. 360).

■ Estrogen Replacement

This therapy is instituted in essentially every patient with hypogonadism to avoid osteoporosis. Exceptions include patients with an estrogen-sensitive tumor. As in postmenopausal women, bone loss is accelerated in the first few years following estrogen deprivation. Thus, treatment is instituted quickly. Women with a uterus also require continuous or intermittent progesterone administration to protect against endometrial hyperplasia or cancer (Chap. 22, p. 494). There is no consensus, however, on an optimal regimen in these patients. Some experts recommend that women in their 20s receive higher doses of estrogen than is routinely given to postmenopausal women as this is a time of ongoing bone deposition. Frequently, it is easiest to prescribe COCs. Younger women may prefer this treatment as their friends may also use these pills, and in their minds, hormone replacement therapy may be associated with aging. Additionally, consensus is lacking on treatment duration in this patient population. For most individuals, continuation until approximately age 50, the usual age of menopause, seems reasonable.

Patients who have eating disorders or who exercise excessively will require behavior modification. In a patient with an eating disorder, psychiatric intervention is imperative due to the significant morbidity and mortality associated with this diagnosis (American Psychiatric Association, 2013; Michopoulos, 2013). Elite athletes may choose not to alter their exercise regimens and will therefore require estrogen treatment.

■ Polycystic Ovarian Syndrome

Treatment of women with PCOS may include cyclic or chronic progesterone treatment as outlined in Chapter 17 (p. 398). Insulin-sensitizing agents such as metformin (Glucophage) may be indicated in those with diabetes mellitus. In women with hyperandrogenism due to PCOS, COCs and/or spironolactone are often helpful.

Depending on its severity, nonclassic CAH in some women may be treated with low-dose corticosteroids. This partially blocks ACTH stimulation of adrenal function and thereby decreases adrenal androgen overproduction.

■ Infertility

Alternative approaches may be required in a patient who desires conception. Adequate treatment of hyperprolactinemia and thyroid disease typically results in ovulation and in normal fertility for most women. If clearly linked to infertility, anatomic abnormalities are surgically corrected whenever possible. However, depending on the type and severity of the abnormality, a surrogate to carry a gestation may be needed. POF is not reversible, and affected individuals can be offered in vitro fertilization using a donor oocyte to conceive. Assuming that behavioral modification is not successful, women with hypogonadotropic hypogonadism are referred to an infertility specialist for treatment with pulsatile GnRH or with gonadotropins. Most patients will receive gonadotropin therapy because pulsatile GnRH is more complex to administer, and GnRH is not reliably available. Women with PCOS will frequently ovulate following treatment with the selective estrogen-receptor modulator clomiphene citrate, or with an aromatase inhibitor such as letrozole. Clomiphene citrate is believed to act by transient inhibition of estrogen feedback at the hypothalamus and pituitary gland (Fig. 20-1, p. 451). This treatment, however, is not effective in those with hypogonadotropic hypogonadism as they lack significant levels of circulating estrogen.

■ Patient Education

Patients are adequately counseled regarding their diagnosis, its long-term implications, and treatment options. All women with an intact endometrium must understand the risks of unopposed estrogen action, whether the estrogen is exogenous, such as through hormone therapy, or endogenous, such as in PCOS. For hypoestrogenic women, clinicians explain the importance of estrogen replacement to protect against bone loss. As described in Chapter 22 (p. 494), estrogen may have additional benefits, which are also detailed. Last, even if not raised by the patient, the potential or lack of potential for future child-bearing is discussed.

REFERENCES

Abraham SF, Beumont PJ, Fraser IS, et al: Body weight, exercise and menstrual status among ballet dancers in training. BJOG 89(7):507, 1982

Aiman J, Nalick RH, Jacobs A, et al: The origin of androgen and estrogen in virilized postmenopausal women with bilateral benign cystic teratomas. Obstet Gynecol 49(6):695, 1977

Aittomaki K, Eroila H, Kajanoja P: A population-based study of the incidence of müllerian aplasia in Finland. Fertil Steril 76(3):624, 2001

Aittomaki K, Lucena JL, Pakarinen P, et al: Mutation in the follicle-stimulating hormone receptor gene causes hereditary hypergonadotropic ovarian failure. Cell 82(6):959, 1995

Allshouse AA, Semple AL, Santoro NF: Evidence for prolonged and unique amenorrhea-related symptoms in women with premature ovarian failure/primary ovarian insufficiency. Menopause 22(2):166, 2015

American College of Obstetricians and Gynecologists: Carrier screening for fragile X syndrome. Committee Opinion No. 469, October 2010

American College of Obstetricians and Gynecologists: Menstruation in girls and adolescents: using the menstrual cycle as a vital sign. Committee Opinion No. 349, November 2006, Reaffirmed 2009

American College of Obstetricians and Gynecologists: Primary ovarian insufficiency in adolescents and young women. Committee Opinion No. 605, July 2014

American Psychiatric Association: Diagnostic and Statistical Manual of Mental Disorders, Fifth Edition. Arlington, American Psychiatric Association, 2013

American Society for Reproductive Medicine: Current evaluation of amenorrhea. Fertil Steril 90(Supp 5):219, 2008

Bachmann GA, Kemmann E: Prevalence of oligomenorrhea and amenorrhea in a college population. Am J Obstet Gynecol 144(1):98, 1982

Banerjee R, Laufer MR: Reproductive disorders associated with pelvic pain. Semin Pediatr Surg 7(1):52, 1998

Baskin HJ, Cobin RH, Duick DS, et al: American Association of Clinical Endocrinologists medical guidelines for clinical practice for the evaluation and treatment of hyperthyroidism and hypothyroidism. Endocr Pract 8(6):457, 2002

Bidet M, Bachelot A, Bissauge E, et al: Resumption of ovarian function and pregnancies in 358 patients with premature ovarian failure. J Clin Endocrinol Metab 96(12):3864, 2011

Billewicz WZ, Fellowes HM, Hytten CA: Comments on the critical metabolic mass and the age of menarche. Ann Hum Biol 3(1):51, 1976

Cadman SM, Kim SH, Hu Y, et al: Molecular pathogenesis of Kallmann's syndrome. Horm Res 67(5):231, 2007

Caronia LM, Martin C, Welt CK, et al: A genetic basis for functional hypothalamic amenorrhea. N Engl J Med 364:215, 2011

Chen H, Charlat O, Tartaglia LA, et al: Evidence that the diabetes gene encodes the leptin receptor: identification of a mutation in the leptin receptor gene in db/db mice. Cell 84(3):491, 1996

Chou SH, Mantzoros C: 20 years of leptin: role of leptin in human reproductive disorders. J Endocrinol 223(1):T49, 2014

Cordts EB, Christofolini DM, Dos Santos AA, et al: Genetic aspects of premature ovarian failure: a literature review. Arch Gynecol Obstet 283(3):635, 2011

Coulam CB, Adamson SC, Annegers JF: Incidence of premature ovarian failure. Obstet Gynecol 67(4):604, 1986

Cundy TF, Butler J, Pope RM, et al: Amenorrhoea in women with non-alcoholic chronic liver disease. Gut 32(2):202, 1991

de Moraes RM, Blizzard RM, Garcia-Bunuel R, et al: Autoimmunity and ovarian failure. Am J Obstet Gynecol 112(5):693, 1972

Dempfle A, Herpetz-Dahlmann B, Timmesfeld N, et al: Predictors of the resumption of menses in adolescent anorexia nervosa. BMC Psychiatry 13:308, 2013

De Souza MJ, Metzger DA: Reproductive dysfunction in amenorrheic athletes and anorexic patients: a review. Med Sci Sports Exerc 23(9):995, 1991

De Souza MJ, Miller BE, Loucks AB, et al: High frequency of luteal phase deficiency and anovulation in recreational women runners: blunted elevation in follicle-stimulating hormone observed during luteal-follicular transition. J Clin Endocrinol Metab 83(12):4220, 1998

Duckham RL, Peirce N, Meyer C, et al: Risk factors for stress fracture in female endurance athletes: a cross-sectional study. BMJ Open 2(6):e001920, 2012

Franco B, Guioli S, Pragliola A, et al: A gene deleted in Kallmann's syndrome shares homology with neural cell adhesion and axonal path-finding molecules. Nature 353(6344):529, 1991

Frisch RE, Gotz-Welbergen AV, McArthur JW, et al: Delayed menarche and amenorrhea of college athletes in relation to age of onset of training. JAMA 246(14):1559, 1981

Frisch RE, Revelle R: Height and weight at menarche and a hypothesis of critical body weights and adolescent events. Science 169(943):397, 1970

Frisch RE, Wyshak G, Vincent L: Delayed menarche and amenorrhea in ballet dancers. N Engl J Med 303(1):17, 1980

Ghazizadeh S, Lessan-Pezeshkii M: Reproduction in women with end-stage renal disease and effect of kidney transplantation. Iran J Kidney Dis 1(1):12, 2007

Goldsmith O, Solomon DH, Horton R: Hypogonadism and mineralocorticoid excess. The 17-hydroxylase deficiency syndrome. N Engl J Med 277(13):673, 1967

Goswami D, Conway GS: Premature ovarian failure. Hum Reprod Update 11(4):391, 2005

Gradishar WJ, Schilsky RL: Ovarian function following radiation and chemotherapy for cancer. Semin Oncol 16(5):425, 1989

Hoek A, Schoemaker J, Drexhage HA: Premature ovarian failure and ovarian autoimmunity. Endocr Rev 18(1):107, 1997

Howlett TA, Wass JA, Grossman A, et al: Prolactinomas presenting as primary amenorrhoea and delayed or arrested puberty: response to medical therapy. Clin Endocrinol (Oxf) 30(2):131, 1989

Hutson JM, Grover SR, O'Connell M, et al: Malformation syndromes associated with disorders of sex development. Nat Rev Endocrinol 10(8):476, 2014

Jameson JL, Weetman AP: Disorders of the thyroid gland. In Longo DL, Fauci AS, Kasper DL, et al (eds): Harrison's Principles of Internal Medicine, 18th ed. New York, McGraw-Hill, 2012

Jick H, Porter J: Relation between smoking and age of natural menopause. Report from the Boston Collaborative Drug Surveillance Program, Boston University Medical Center. Lancet 1(8026):1354, 1977

Job JC, Chaussain JL, Garnier PE: The use of luteinizing hormone-releasing hormone in pediatric patients. Horm Res 8(3):171, 1977

Johnston FE, Roche AF, Schell LM, et al: Critical weight at menarche. Critique of a hypothesis. Am J Dis Child 129(1):19, 1975

Jones GS, Moraes-Ruehsen M: A new syndrome of amenorrhae in association with hypergonadotropism and apparently normal ovarian follicular apparatus. Am J Obstet Gynecol 104(4):597, 1969

Joy E, De Souza MJ, Mattiv A, et al: 2014 female athlete triad coalition consensus statement on treatment and return to play of the female athlete triad. Curr Sports Med Rep 13(4):219, 2014

Kakuno Y, Amino N, Kanoh M, et al: Menstrual disturbances in various thyroid diseases. Endocr J 57(12):1017, 2010

Kaneko N, Kawagoe S, Hiroi M: Turner's syndrome—review of the literature with reference to a successful pregnancy outcome. Gynecol Obstet Invest 29(2):81, 1990

Kaufman FR, Kogut MD, Donnell GN, et al: Hypergonadotropic hypogonadism in female patients with galactosemia. N Engl J Med 304(17):994, 1981

Kelestimur F: Sheehan's syndrome. Pituitary 6(4):181, 2003

Kim MH: "Gonadotropin-resistant ovaries" syndrome in association with secondary amenorrhea. Am J Obstet Gynecol 120(2):257, 1974

Klingmuller D, Dewes W, Krahe T, et al: Magnetic resonance imaging of the brain in patients with anosmia and hypothalamic hypogonadism (Kallmann's syndrome). J Clin Endocrinol Metab 65(3):581, 1987

Krassas GE, Poppe K, Glinoer D: Thyroid function and human reproductive health. Endocr Rev 31(5):702, 2010

LaBarbera AR, Miller MM, Ober C, et al: Autoimmune etiology in premature ovarian failure. Am J Reprod Immunol Microbiol 16(3):115, 1988

Latronico AC, Arnhold IJ: Gonadotropin resistance. Endocr Dev 24:25, 2013

Layman LC: Clinical genetic testing for Kallmann syndrome. J Clin Endocrinol Metab 98(5):1860, 2013

Levy HL, Driscoll SG, Porensky RS, et al: Ovarian failure in galactosemia. N Engl J Med 310(1):50, 1984

Licinio J, Caglayan S, Ozata M, et al: Phenotypic effects of leptin replacement on morbid obesity, diabetes mellitus, hypogonadism, and behavior in leptin-deficient adults. Proc Natl Acad Sci USA 101(13):4531, 2004

Mantzoros C, Flier JS, Lesem MD, et al: Cerebrospinal fluid leptin in anorexia nervosa: correlation with nutritional status and potential role in resistance to weight gain. J Clin Endocrinol Metab 82(6):1845, 1997

Manuel M, Katayama PK, Jones HW Jr: The age of occurrence of gonadal tumors in intersex patients with a Y chromosome. Am J Obstet Gynecol 124(3):293, 1976

March CM: Asherman's syndrome. Semin Reprod Med 29(2):83, 2011

Matthews CH, Borgato S, Beck-Peccoz P, et al: Primary amenorrhoea and infertility due to a mutation in the beta-subunit of follicle-stimulating hormone. Nat Genet 5(1):83, 1993

Michopoulos V, Mancini F, Loucks TL, et al: Neuroendocrine recovery initiated by cognitive behavioral therapy in women with functional hypothalamic amenorrhea: a randomized, controlled trial. Fertil Steril 99(7):2084, 2013

Misra M, Klibanski A: Endocrine consequences of anorexia nervosa. Lancet Diabetes Endocrinol 2(7):581, 2014

Mlynarcikova A, Fickova M, Scsukova S: Ovarian intrafollicular processes as a target for cigarette smoke components and selected environmental reproductive disruptors. Endocr Regul 39(1):21, 2005

Morrison JC, Givens JR, Wiser WL, et al: Mumps oophoritis: a cause of premature menopause. Fertil Steril 26(7):655, 1975

Nakamura S, Douchi T, Oki T, et al: Relationship between sonographic endometrial thickness and progestin-induced withdrawal bleeding. Obstet Gynecol 87(5 Pt 1):722, 1996

Özgör B, Selimoğlu MA: Coeliac disease and reproductive disorders. Scand J Gastroenterol 45(4):395, 2010

Pallais JC, Bo-Abbas Y, Pitteloud N, et al: Neuroendocrine, gonadal, placental, and obstetric phenotypes in patients with IHH and mutations in the G-protein coupled receptor, GPR54. Mol Cell Endocrinol 254–255:70, 2006

Parazzini F, Cecchetti G: The frequency of imperforate hymen in northern Italy. Int J Epidemiol 19(3):763, 1990

Pectasides D, Pectasides E, Psyrri A: Granulosa cell tumor of the ovary. Cancer Treat Rev 34(1):1, 2008

Pettersson F, Fries H, Nillius SJ: Epidemiology of secondary amenorrhea. I. Incidence and prevalence rates. Am J Obstet Gynecol 117(1):80, 1973

Quinton R, Hasan W, Grant W, et al: Gonadotropin-releasing hormone immunoreactivity in the nasal epithelia of adults with Kallmann's syndrome and isolated hypogonadotropic hypogonadism and in the early midtrimester human fetus. J Clin Endocrinol Metab 82(1):309, 1997

Rarick LD, Shangold MM, Ahmed SW: Cervical mucus and serum estradiol as predictors of response to progestin challenge. Fertil Steril 54(2):353, 1990

Rebar RW, Connolly HV: Clinical features of young women with hypergonadotropic amenorrhea. Fertil Steril 53(5):804, 1990

Reindollar RH, Byrd JR, McDonough PG: Delayed sexual development: a study of 252 patients. Am J Obstet Gynecol 140(4):371, 1981

Reindollar RH, Novak M, Tho SP, et al: Adult-onset amenorrhea: a study of 262 patients. Am J Obstet Gynecol 155(3):531, 1986

Rubio-Gozalbo ME, Gubbels CS, Bakker JA, et al: Gonadal function in male and female patients with classic galactosemia. Human Reprod Update 16(2):177, 2010

Rugarli E, Ballabio A: Kallmann syndrome. From genetics to neurobiology. JAMA 270(22):2713, 1993

Saenger P, Albertsson Wikland K, Conway GS, et al: Recommendations for the diagnosis and management of Turner syndrome. J Clin Endocrinol Metab 86(7):3061, 2001

Schenker JG, Margalioth EJ: Intrauterine adhesions: an updated appraisal. Fertil Steril 37(5):593, 1982

Schlessinger D, Herrera L, Crisponi L, et al: Genes and translocations involved in POF. Am J Med Genet 111(3):328, 2002

Schneider JE: Energy balance and reproduction. Physiol Behav 81(2):289, 2004

Seeman MV: Pseudocyesis, delusional pregnancy, and psychosis: the birth of a delusion. World J Clin Cases 2(8):338, 2014

Seminara SB: Mechanisms of disease: the first kiss—a crucial role for kisspeptin-1 and its receptor, G-protein-coupled receptor 54, in puberty and reproduction. Nat Clin Pract Endocrinol Metab 2(6):328, 2006

Sharara FI, Seifer DB, Flaws JA: Environmental toxicants and female reproduction. Fertil Steril 70(4):613, 1998

Sharma JB, Roy KK, Pushparaj M, et al: Hysteroscopic findings in women with primary and secondary infertility due to genital tuberculosis. Int J Gynaecol Obstet 104(1):49, 2009

Simpson JL: Gonadal dysgenesis and abnormalities of the human sex chromosomes: current status of phenotypic-karyotypic correlations. Birth Defects Orig Artic Ser 11(4):23, 1975

Singh | 1966 Singh RP, Carr DH: The anatomy and histology of XO human embryos and fetuses. Anat Rec 155(3):369, 1966

Soussi-Yanicostas N, Hardelin JP, Arroyo-Jimenez MM, et al: Initial characterization of anosmin-1, a putative extracellular matrix protein synthesized by definite neuronal cell populations in the central nervous system. J Cell Sci 109(Pt 7)1749, 1996

Swain SM, Jeong JH, Geyer CE, Jr: Longer therapy, iatrogenic amenorrhea, and survival in early breast cancer. N Engl J Med 362(22):2053, 2010

Tarin JJ, Hermenegildo C, Garcia-Perez MA, et al: Endocrinology and physiology of pseudocyesis. Reprod Biol Endocrinol 11:39, 2013

Tartaglia LA, Dembski M, Weng X, et al: Identification and expression cloning of a leptin receptor, OB-R. Cell 83(7):1263, 1995

2009 Terenziani M, Piva L, Meazza C, et al: Oophoropexy: a relevant role in preservation of ovarian function and pelvic irradiation. Fertil Steril 91(3):935.e15, 2009

Tho PT, McDonough PG: Gonadal dysgenesis and its variants. Pediatr Clin North Am 28(2):309, 1981

Thomas RL, Carr BR, Ziadie MS, et al: Bilateral mucinous cystadenomas and massive edema of the ovaries in a virilized adolescent girl. Obstet Gynecol 120(2 Pt 2):473, 2012

Turner H: Classic pages in obstetrics and gynecology by Henry H. Turner. A syndrome of infantilism, congenital webbed neck, and cubitus valgus. Endocrinology, vol 23, pp 566–574, 1938. Am J Obstet Gynecol 113(2):279, 1972

Veldhuis JD, Hammond JM: Endocrine function after spontaneous infarction of the human pituitary: report, review, and reappraisal. Endocr Rev 1(1):100, 1980

Visser JA, Schipper I, Laven JSE, et al: Anti-mullerian hormone: an ovarian reserve marker in primary ovarian insufficiency. Nat Rev Endocrinol 8:331, 2012

Waldstreicher J, Seminara SB, Jameson JL, et al: The genetic and clinical heterogeneity of gonadotropin-releasing hormone deficiency in the human. J Clin Endocrinol Metab 81(12):4388, 1996

Weiss J, Axelrod L, Whitcomb RW, et al: Hypogonadism caused by a single amino acid substitution in the beta subunit of luteinizing hormone. N Engl J Med 326(3):179, 1992

Whelan CI, Stewart DE: Pseudocyesis—a review and report of six cases. Int J Psychiatry Med 20(1):97, 1990

Winters SJ: Expanding the differential diagnosis of male hypogonadism. N Engl J Med 326(3):193, 1992

Wittenberger MD, Hagerman RJ, Sherman SL, et al: The FMR1 premutation and reproduction. Fertil Steril 87(3):456, 2007

Yen SS, Rebar R, VandenBerg G, et al: Hypothalamic amenorrhea and hypogonadotropinism: responses to synthetic LRF. J Clin Endocrinol Metab 36(5):811, 1973

Yoo C, Yun MR, Ahn JH, et al: Chemotherapy-induced amenorrhea, menopause-specific quality of life, and endocrine profiles in premenopausal women with breast cancer who received adjuvant anthracycline-based chemotherapy: a prospective cohort study. Cancer Chemother Pharmacol 72(3):565, 2013

Zenaty D, Bretones P, Lambe C, et al: Paediatric phenotype of Kallmann syndrome due to mutations of fibroblast growth factor receptor 1 (FGFR1). Mol Cell Endocrinol 254–255:78, 2006

Zhang Y, Proenca R, Maffei M, et al: Positional cloning of the mouse obese gene and its human homologue. Nature 372(6505):425, 1994

Zhao J, Liu J, Chen K, et al: What lies behind chemotherapy-induced amenorrhea for breast cancer patients: a meta-analysis. Breast Cancer Res Treat 145(1):113, 2014

Polycystic Ovarian Syndrome and Hyperandrogenism

Polycystic ovarian syndrome (PCOS) is a common endocrinopathy typified by oligoovulation or anovulation, signs of androgen excess, and multiple small ovarian cysts. These signs and symptoms vary widely between women and within individuals over time. Women with this endocrine disorder also have higher rates of dyslipidemia and insulin resistance, which increase long-term health risks. As a result, women with PCOS may first present to various medical specialists, including pediatricians, gynecologists, internists, endocrinologists, or dermatologists.

DEFINITION

■ Polycystic Ovarian Syndrome

In Rotterdam, The Netherlands, PCOS was redefined in a consensus meeting between the European Society of Human Reproduction and Embryology and the American Society for Reproductive Medicine (ESHRE/ASRM)—The Rotterdam ESHRE/ASRM-Sponsored PCOS Consensus Workshop Group, 2004. As shown in Table 17-1, affected individuals must meet two out of three criteria. Importantly, because other etiologies, such as congenital adrenal hyperplasia, androgen-secreting tumors, and hyperprolactinemia, may also lead to oligoovulation and/or androgen excess, these must be excluded. Thus, PCOS currently is a diagnosis of exclusion.

The Rotterdam criteria constitute a broader spectrum than that formerly put forward by the National Institutes of Health (NIH) Conference in 1990 (Zawadzki, 1990). The prominent difference is that the NIH Conference defined PCOS without regard to ovarian sonographic appearance. Last, a third organization—The Androgen Excess and PCOS Society (AE-PCOS)—has also defined criteria for PCOS (Azziz, 2006). As is shown in Table 17-1, criteria are similar among these three groups, and controversy exists as to which is most appropriate.

■ Ovarian Hyperthecosis and HAIRAN Syndrome

Ovarian hyperthecosis, often considered a more severe form of PCOS, is a rare condition characterized by nests of luteinized theca cells distributed throughout the ovarian stroma. Affected women exhibit severe hyperandrogenism and may occasionally display frank virilization signs such as clitoromegaly, temporal balding, and voice deepening (Culiner, 1949). In addition, a much greater degree of insulin resistance and acanthosis nigricans typically is found (Nagamani, 1986).

The *hyperandrogenic-insulin resistant-acanthosis nigricans (HAIRAN)* syndrome is also uncommon and consists of marked hyperandrogenism, severe insulin resistance, and acanthosis nigricans (Barbieri, 1983). The etiology of this disorder is unclear, and HAIRAN syndrome may represent either a PCOS variant or a distinct genetic syndrome. Both ovarian hyperthecosis and HAIRAN are exaggerated phenotypes of PCOS, and their treatment mirrors that for PCOS described later in this chapter.

INCIDENCE AND ETIOLOGY

PCOS is the most common endocrine disorder of reproductive-aged women and affects approximately 4 to 12 percent in general population studies (Asunción, 2000; Knochenhauer, 1998; Lauritsen, 2014). Although symptoms of androgen excess may vary among ethnicities, PCOS appears to affect all races and nationalities equally.

The underlying cause of PCOS is unknown. However, a genetic basis that is both multifactorial and polygenic is suspected, as there is a well-documented aggregation of the syndrome within families (Franks, 1997). Specifically, an increased prevalence is noted between affected individuals and their sisters (32 to 66 percent) and mothers (24 to 52 percent) (Govind, 1999; Kahsar-Miller, 2001; Yildiz, 2003). Twin studies also suggest a prominent heritable influence (Vink, 2006).

Some have suggested an autosomal dominant inheritance with expression in both females and males. For example, first-degree male relatives of women with PCOS have been shown to have significantly higher rates of elevated circulating dehydroepiandrosterone sulfate (DHEAS) levels, early balding, and insulin resistance compared with male controls (Legro, 2000, 2002).

Identification of candidate genes linked to PCOS is a major research focus, given the large potential benefit for both diagnosis and management. In general, putative genes include those involved in androgen synthesis and those associated with insulin resistance. Genome-wide association studies in Chinese women have identified variants in 11 genomic regions as potential risk factors for PCOS (Chen, 2011; Shi, 2012).

TABLE 17-1. Definition of Polycystic Ovarian Syndrome

ESHRE/ASRM (Rotterdam) 2003
Two of the three:
Clinical and/or biochemical hyperandrogenism
Oligo-/anovulation
Polycystic ovaries

NIH (1990)
To include both:
Clinical and/or biochemical hyperandrogenism
Oligo-/anovulation

AE-PCOS (2006)
To include both:
Clinical and/or biochemical hyperandrogenism
Oligo-/anovulation and/or polycystic ovaries

AE-PCOS = Androgen Excess and PCOS Society; ASRM = American Society for Reproductive Medicine; ESHRE = European Society of Human Reproduction and Embryology; NIH = National Institutes of Health. PCOS = polycystic ovarian syndrome.
Data from Azziz, 2006; The Rotterdam ESHRE/ASRM-Sponsored PCOS Consensus Workshop Group, 2004; Zawadzki, 1990.

TABLE 17-2. Consequences of Polycystic Ovarian Syndrome

Short-term consequences
Obesity
Infertility
Depression
Sleep apnea
Irregular menses
Abnormal lipid levels
Non-alcoholic fatty liver disease
Hirsutism/acne/androgenic alopecia
Insulin resistance/acanthosis nigricans

Long-term consequences
Diabetes mellitus
Endometrial cancer
Cardiovascular disease

In addition, epigenetic modification of genetic susceptibility within the maternal-fetal environment may influence adult PCOS development (Dumesic, 2014). Further investigation, however, is needed to determine the roles of these gene products in PCOS pathogenesis.

PATHOPHYSIOLOGY

Gonadotropins

Anovulation in women with PCOS is characterized by inappropriate gonadotropin secretion (Fig. 17-1). Specifically, altered gonadotropin-releasing hormone (GnRH) pulsatility leads to preferential production of luteinizing hormone (LH) compared with follicle-stimulating hormone (FSH) (Hayes, 1998; Waldstreicher, 1988). It is currently unknown whether hypothalamic dysfunction is a primary cause of PCOS or is secondary to abnormal steroid feedback. In either case, serum LH levels rise, and increased levels are observed clinically in approximately 50 percent of affected women (van Santbrink, 1997). Similarly, LH:FSH ratios are elevated and rise above 2:1 in approximately 60 percent of patients (Rebar, 1976).

Insulin Resistance

Women with PCOS also display greater degrees of insulin resistance and compensatory hyperinsulinemia than nonaffected women. Insulin resistance is defined as a reduced glucose-uptake response to a given amount of insulin. This decreased insulin sensitivity appears to stem from a postbinding abnormality in insulin receptor-mediated signal transduction (Dunaif, 1997). Both lean and obese women with PCOS are found to be more insulin resistant than nonaffected weight-matched controls (Dunaif, 1989, 1992).

Insulin resistance has been associated with an increase in several disorders including type 2 diabetes mellitus (DM), hypertension, dyslipidemia, and cardiovascular disease. Therefore, PCOS is not simply a disorder of short-term consequences such as irregular periods and hirsutism, but also one of potential long-term health consequences (Table 17-2).

Androgens

Both insulin and LH stimulate androgen production by the ovarian theca cell (Dunaif, 1992). As a result, affected ovaries secrete elevated levels of testosterone and androstenedione. Specifically, elevated free testosterone levels are noted in 70 to 80 percent of women with PCOS, and 25 to 65 percent exhibit elevated levels of DHEAS (Moran, 1994, 1999; O'Driscoll, 1994). In turn, elevated androstenedione levels contribute to an increase in estrone levels through peripheral conversion of androgens to estrogens by aromatase.

Sex Hormone-binding Globulin

Women with PCOS display decreased levels of sex hormone-binding globulin (SHBG). This glycoprotein, produced in the liver, binds most sex steroids. Only approximately 1 percent of these steroids are unbound and thus free and bioavailable. The synthesis of SHBG is suppressed by insulin as well as androgens, corticoids, progestins, and growth hormone (Bergh, 1993). Because of suppressed SHBG production, less circulating androgen is bound and thus more remains available to bind with end-organ receptors. Accordingly, some women with PCOS will have total testosterone levels in the normal range, but will be clinically hyperandrogenic due to elevated free testosterone levels.

In addition to hyperandrogenism, low SHBG levels have also been linked to impaired glucose control and a risk for developing type 2 DM (Ding, 2009). The mechanism of this association is not fully understood and may reflect a role for SHBG in glucose homeostasis. For example, Veltman-Verhulst

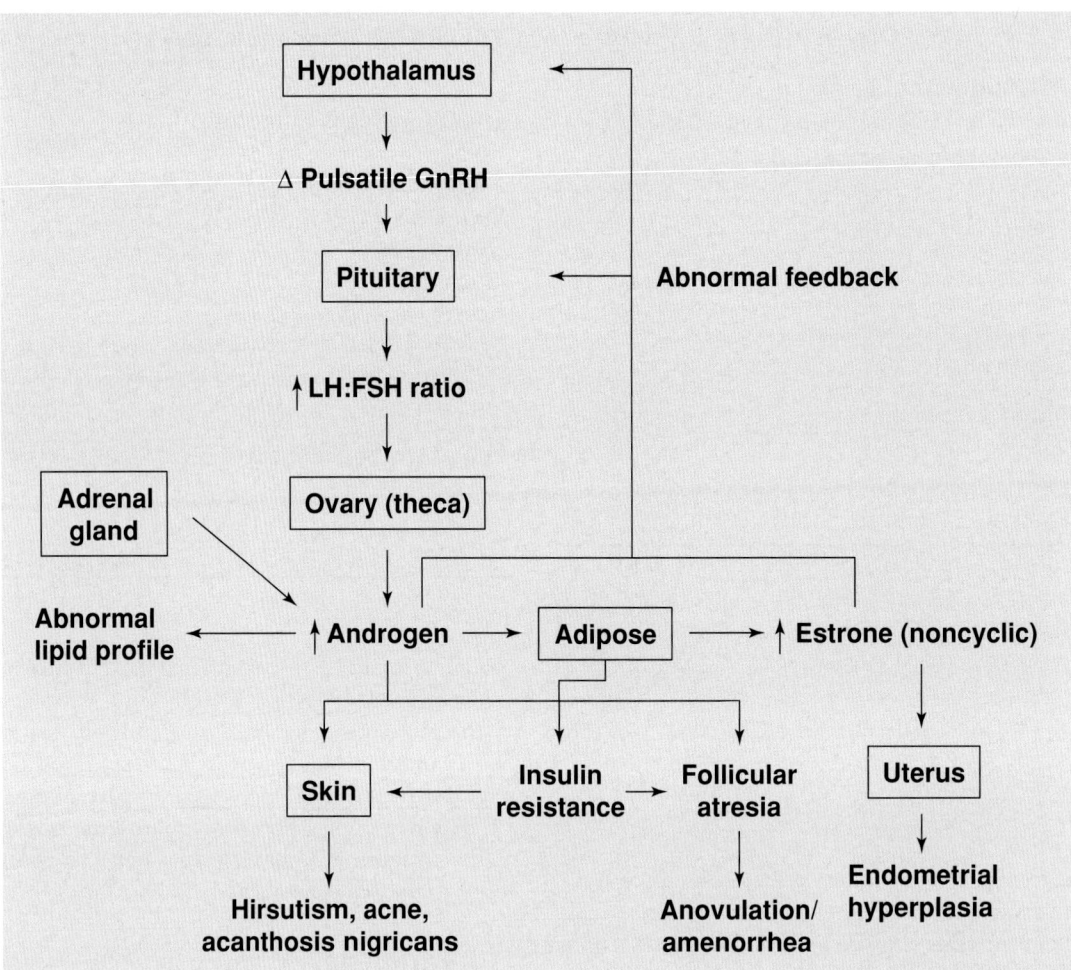

FIGURE 17-1 Model for the initiation and maintenance of polycystic ovarian syndrome (PCOS). Alterations in pulsatile gonadotropin-releasing hormone (GnRH) release may lead to a relative increase in luteinizing hormone (LH) versus follicle-stimulating hormone (FSH) biosynthesis and secretion. LH stimulates ovarian androgen production, while the relative paucity of FSH prevents adequate stimulation of aromatase activity within the granulosa cells, thereby decreasing androgen conversion to the potent estrogen estradiol.

Increased intrafollicular androgen levels result in follicular atresia. Increased circulating androgen levels contribute to abnormalities in patient lipid profiles and the development of hirsutism and acne. Increased circulating androgens can also be derived from the adrenal gland.

Elevated serum androgens (primarily androstenedione) are converted in the periphery to estrogens (primarily estrone). As conversion occurs primarily in the stromal cells of adipose tissue, estrogen production will be augmented in obese PCOS patients. This conversion results in chronic feedback at the hypothalamus and pituitary gland, in contrast to the normal fluctuations in feedback observed in the presence of a growing follicle and rapidly changing levels of estradiol. Unopposed estrogen stimulation of the endometrium may lead to endometrial hyperplasia.

Insulin resistance due to genetic abnormalities and/or increased adipose tissue contributes to follicular atresia in the ovaries as well as the development of acanthosis nigricans in the skin.

Lack of follicular development results in anovulation and subsequent oligo- or amenorrhea.

Note that this syndrome may develop from primary dysfunction of any one of a number of organ systems. For example, elevated ovarian androgen production may be due to either an intrinsic abnormality in enzymatic function and/or abnormal hypothalamic-pituitary stimulation with LH and FSH.

The common denominator is development of a self-perpetuating noncyclic hormonal pattern.

(2010) evaluated SHBG levels in women with PCOS and found an association between low SHBG levels and subsequent development of gestational diabetes mellitus.

■ Anovulation

The precise mechanism leading to anovulation is unclear, but altered GnRH pulsatility and inappropriate gonadotropin secretion have been implicated in menstrual irregularity.

Moreover, anovulation may result from insulin resistance, as a substantial number of anovulatory patients with PCOS may resume ovulatory cycles when treated with metformin, an insulin sensitizer (Nestler, 1998). It has been suggested that oligoovulatory women with PCOS exhibit a milder phenotype of ovarian dysfunction than anovulatory PCOS patients and have a more favorable response to ovulation induction agents (Burgers, 2010).

Finally, the large antral follicle cohort with increased intraovarian androgens seen in PCOS may contribute to anovulation. This is supported by the fact that some patients who have undergone ovarian wedge resection or laparoscopic ovarian drilling have improved menstrual regularity. One study demonstrated that 67 percent of PCOS patients developed regular menses following such surgery compared with only 8 percent prior to surgery (Amer, 2002).

SIGNS AND SYMPTOMS

In women with PCOS, symptoms may include menstrual irregularities, infertility, manifestations of androgen excess, or other endocrine dysfunction. Symptoms classically become apparent within a few years of puberty.

■ Menstrual Dysfunction

In women with PCOS, menstrual dysfunction may range from amenorrhea to oligomenorrhea to episodic menometrorrhagia with associated iron-deficiency anemia. In most cases, amenorrhea and oligomenorrhea result from anovulation. Namely, without ovulation and endogenous progesterone production from the corpus luteum, a normal menstrual period is not triggered. Alternatively, amenorrhea can stem from elevated androgen levels. Specifically, androgens can counteract estrogen to produce an atrophic endometrium. Thus, with markedly elevated androgen levels, amenorrhea and a thin endometrial stripe can be seen.

In contrast to amenorrhea, women with PCOS may have heavy and unpredictable bleeding. In these cases, progesterone is absent due to anovulation, and chronic estrogen exposure results. This produces constant mitogenic stimulation of the endometrium. The instability of the thickened endometrium leads to unpredictable bleeding.

Characteristically, oligomenorrhea (fewer than eight menstrual periods in 1 year) or amenorrhea (absence of menses for 3 or more consecutive months) with PCOS begins with menarche. Those with PCOS fail to establish monthly ovulatory menstrual cycles by midadolescence, and they often continue to have irregularity. However, approximately 50 percent of *all* postmenarchal girls have irregular periods for up to 2 to 4 years because of hypothalamic-pituitary-ovarian axis immaturity. Thus, due to the frequency of both irregular cycles and acne in unaffected adolescents, some advocate delaying the diagnosis of PCOS until after age 18 (Shayya, 2011).

TABLE 17-3. Medications That May Cause Hirsutism and/or Hypertrichosis

Hirsutism	Hypertrichosis
Anabolic steroids	Cyclosporine
Danazol	Diazoxide
Metoclopramide	Hydrocortisone
Methyldopa	Minoxidil
Phenothiazines	Penicillamine
Progestins	Phenytoin
Reserpine	Psoralens
Testosterone	Streptomycin

Last, some evidence suggests that PCOS patients with prior irregular cycle intervals may develop regular cycle patterns as they age. A decreasing antral follicle cohort as women enter their 30s and 40s may lead to a concurrent decrease in androgen production (Elting, 2000).

■ Hyperandrogenism

This condition is usually manifested clinically by hirsutism, acne, and/or androgenic alopecia. In contrast, signs of virilization such as increased muscle mass, voice deepening, and clitoromegaly are not typical of PCOS. Virilization reflects higher androgen levels and should prompt investigation for an androgen-producing tumor of the ovary or adrenal gland.

Hirsutism

In a female, hirsutism is defined as coarse, dark, terminal hairs distributed in a male pattern (Fig. 17-2). This is distinguished from hypertrichosis, which is a generalized increase in lanugo, that is, the soft, lightly pigmented hair associated with some medications and malignancies. PCOS accounts for 70 to 80 percent of cases of hirsutism, which typically begins in late adolescence or the early 20s. Idiopathic hirsutism is the second most frequent cause (Azziz, 2003). Additionally, various drugs may also lead to hirsutism, and their use should be investigated (Table 17-3).

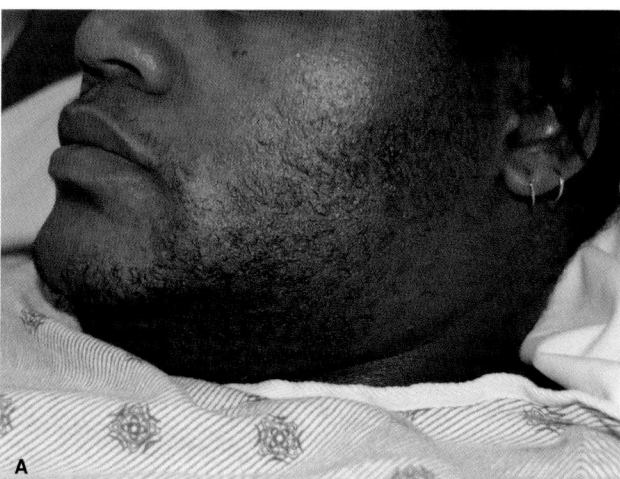

A

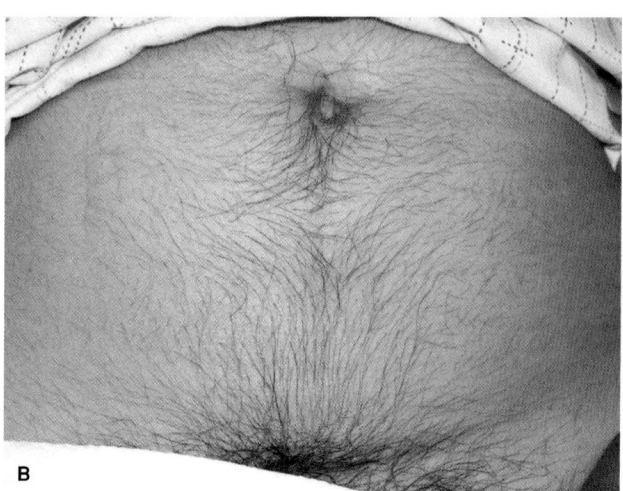

B

FIGURE 17-2 A. Facial hirsutism. (Used with permission from Dr. Tamara Chao.) **B.** Male pattern escutcheon.

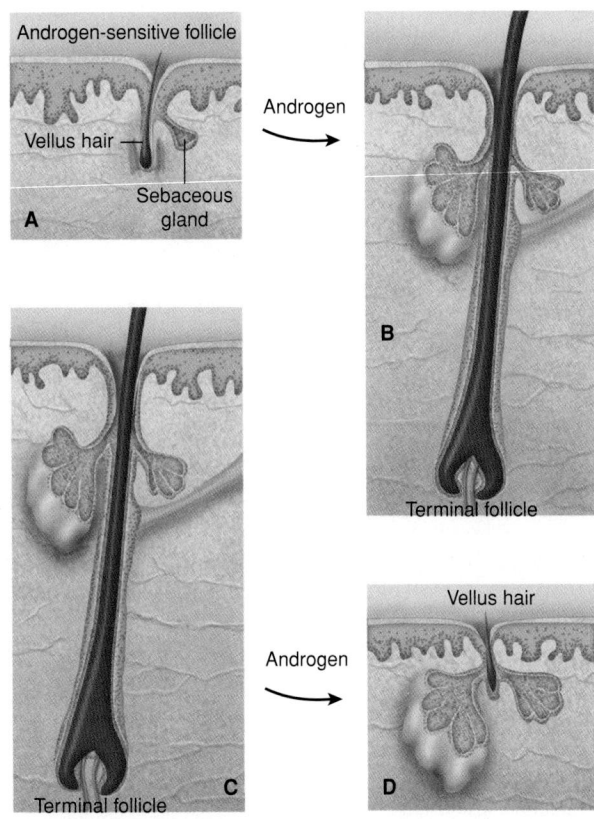

FIGURE 17-3 Androgenic effects on the pilosebaceous unit. In some hair-bearing areas, androgens stimulate sebaceous glands, and vellus follicles **(A)** are converted to terminal follicles **(B)**, leading to hirsutism. Under the influence of androgens, terminal hairs that were not previously dependent on androgens **(C)** revert to a vellus form and balding results **(D)**.

Pathophysiology of Hirsutism. Elevated androgen levels play a major role in determining the type and distribution of hair. Within a hair follicle, testosterone is converted by the enzyme 5α-reductase to dihydrotestosterone (DHT) (Fig. 17-3). Although both testosterone and DHT convert short, soft vellus hair to coarse terminal hair, DHT is markedly more effective than testosterone. Conversion is irreversible, and only hairs in androgen-sensitive areas are changed in this manner to terminal hairs. As a result the most common areas affected with excess hair growth include the upper lip, chin, sideburns, chest, and linea alba of the lower abdomen. Specifically, *escutcheon* is the term used to describe the hair pattern of the lower abdomen. In women, this pattern is triangular and overlies the mons pubis, whereas in men it extends up the linea alba to form a diamond shape.

The concentration of hair follicles per unit area does not differ between men and women, however, racial and ethnic differences do exist. Individuals of Mediterranean descent have a higher concentration of hair follicles than Northern Europeans, and a much higher concentration than Asians. For this reason, Asians with PCOS are much less likely to present with overt hirsutism than other ethnic groups. Additionally, the familial tendency for the hirsutism development is strong and stems from genetic differences in 5α-reductase activity and in target tissue sensitivity to androgens.

Ferriman-Gallwey Scoring System. To quantify the degree of hirsutism for research purposes, the Ferriman-Gallwey scoring system was developed in 1961 and later modified in 1981 (Ferriman, 1961; Hatch, 1981). Within this system, abnormal hair distribution is assessed in nine body areas and scored from 0 to 4 (Fig. 17-4). Increasing numeric scores correspond to greater hair density within a given area. Many investigators define hirsutism as a score ≥8 using the modified scoring. Because of the

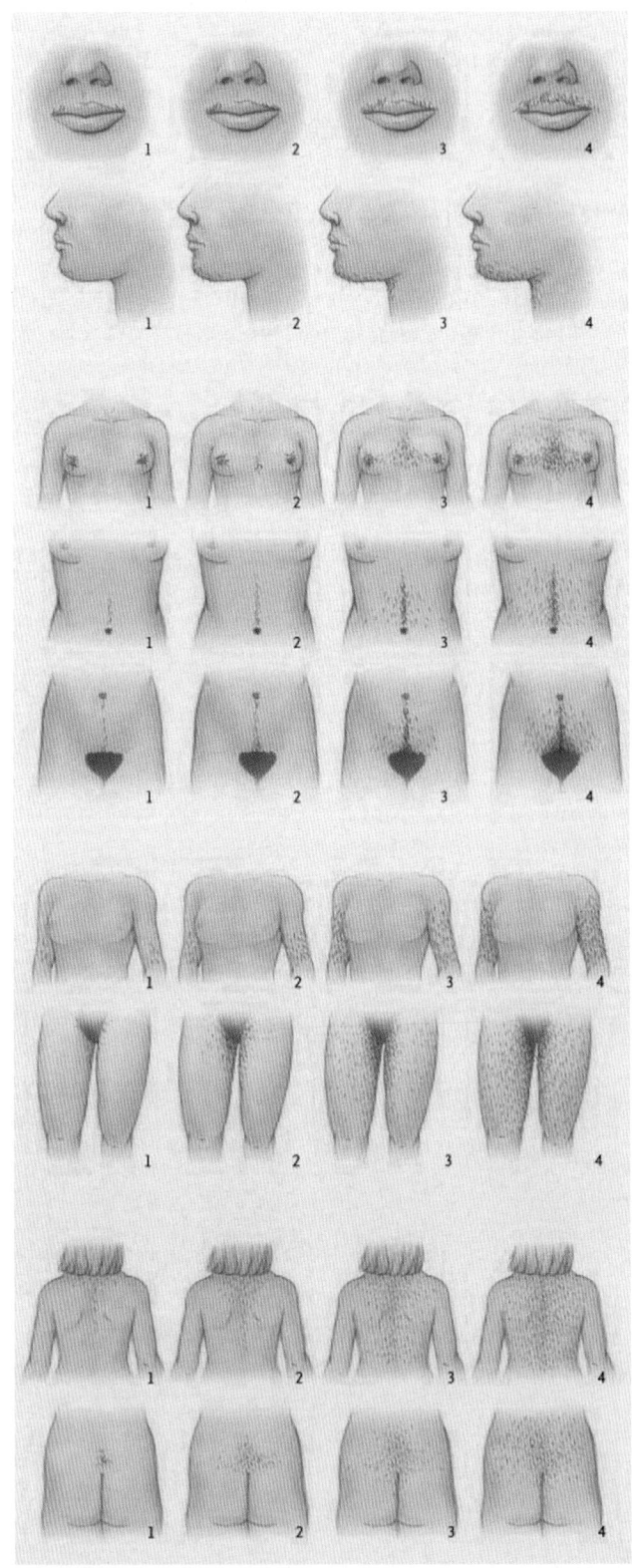

FIGURE 17-4 Depiction of the Ferriman-Gallwey system for scoring hirsutism.

lower follicle concentration in Far East Asians, the AE-PCOS Society suggests a threshold value ≥3 for this group (Escobar-Morreale, 2011).

The Ferriman-Gallwey scoring system is cumbersome and thus is not used frequently in clinical settings. Nevertheless, it may be useful for following treatment responses in individual patients. Alternatively, an abbreviated score that combines only the upper and lower abdomen and chin scores may be a suitable surrogate (Cook, 2011). Also, many specialists choose to classify hirsutism more generally as mild, moderate, or severe depending on the location and density of hair growth.

Acne

Acne vulgaris is a frequent clinical finding in adolescents. However, acne that is particularly persistent or late onset suggests PCOS (Homburg, 2004). The prevalence of acne in women with PCOS is unknown, although one study found that 50 percent of adolescents with PCOS have moderate acne (Dramusic, 1997). In addition, androgen level elevation has been reported in 80 percent of women with severe acne, 50 percent with moderate acne, and 33 percent with mild acne (Bunker, 1989). Women with moderate to severe acne have an increased prevalence (52 to 83 percent) of polycystic ovaries identified during sonographic examination (Betti, 1990; Bunker, 1989).

The pathogenesis of acne vulgaris involves four factors: blockage of the follicular opening by hyperkeratosis, sebum overproduction, proliferation of commensal *Propionibacterium acnes,* and inflammation. As in the hair follicle, testosterone is converted within sebaceous glands to its more active metabolite, DHT, by 5α-reductase. In women with androgen excess, overstimulation of androgen receptors in the pilosebaceous unit increases sebum production that eventually leads to inflammation and comedone formation (see Fig. 17-3). Inflammation leads to the main long-term side effect of acne—scarring. Accordingly, treatment is directed at minimizing inflammation, decreasing keratin production, lowering colonization of *P acnes,* and reducing androgen levels to diminish sebum production.

Alopecia

Female androgenic alopecia is a less common finding in women with PCOS. Hair loss progresses slowly and is characterized by diffuse thinning at the crown with preservation of the frontal hairline (Quinn, 2014). Its pathogenesis involves an excess of 5α-reductase activity in the hair follicle leading to a rise in DHT levels. Moreover, androgen receptor expression in these individuals is increased (Chen, 2002).

Alopecia, however, may reflect other serious disease. For this reason, affected women are also evaluated to exclude thyroid dysfunction, anemia, or other chronic illness.

■ Other Endocrine Dysfunction
Insulin Resistance

Although not well characterized, the association among insulin resistance, hyperandrogenism, and PCOS has long been recognized. The precise incidence of insulin resistance in women with PCOS has been difficult to ascertain for lack of a simple method to determine insulin sensitivity in an office setting. Although obesity is known to exacerbate insulin resistance, one

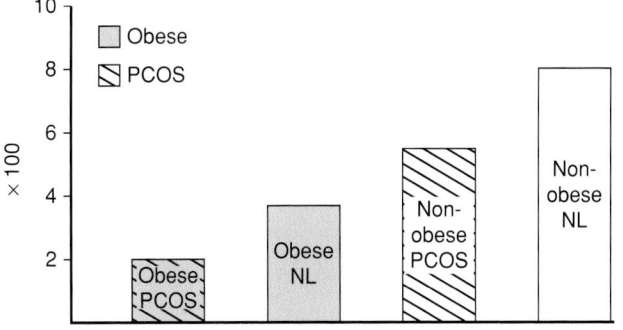

FIGURE 17-5 Insulin sensitivity is decreased in obese women with polycystic ovarian syndrome. NL = normal (those without PCOS); PCOS = polycystic ovarian syndrome. (Reproduced with permission from Dunaif A, Segal KR, Futterweit W, et al: Profound peripheral insulin resistance, independent of obesity, in polycystic ovary syndrome, Diabetes 1989 Sep;38(9):1165–1174.)

classic study demonstrated that both lean and obese women with PCOS have increased rates of insulin resistance and type 2 DM compared with weight-matched controls without PCOS (Fig. 17-5) (Dunaif, 1989, 1992).

Acanthosis Nigricans. This skin condition is characterized by thickened, gray-brown velvety plaques seen in flexure areas such as the back of the neck, axillae, inframammary creases, waist, and groin (Fig. 17-6) (Panidis, 1995). Thought to be a cutaneous marker of insulin resistance, acanthosis nigricans may be found in individuals with or without PCOS. Insulin resistance leads to hyperinsulinemia, which is believed to stimulate keratinocyte and dermal fibroblast growth, producing the characteristic skin changes (Cruz, 1992). Acanthosis nigricans develops more frequently in obese women with PCOS (50 percent incidence) than in those with PCOS and normal weight (5 to 10 percent).

As part of its differential diagnosis, acanthosis nigricans rarely can be seen with genetic syndromes or gastrointestinal tract malignancy, such as adenocarcinoma of the stomach or pancreas. To differentiate, acanthosis nigricans associated with malignancy usually has a more abrupt onset, and skin involvement is more extensive (Moore, 2008).

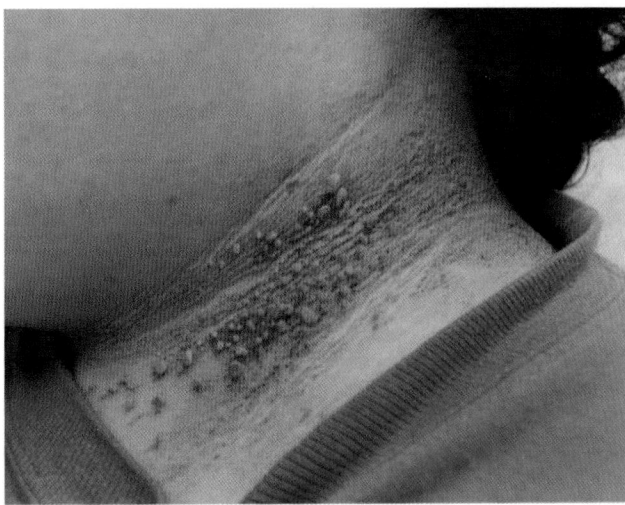

FIGURE 17-6 Acanthosis nigricans and multiple small pedunculated acrochordons (skin tags) in the neck crease. Both are dermatologic signs of insulin resistance.

Impaired Glucose Tolerance and Type 2 Diabetes Mellitus. Women with PCOS are at increased risk for impaired glucose tolerance (IGT) and type 2 DM. Based on oral glucose tolerance testing of obese women with PCOS, the prevalence of IGT and DM is approximately 30 percent and 7 percent, respectively (Legro, 1999). Even after adjusting for body mass index (BMI), women with PCOS remained more likely to have DM (Lo, 2006). Specifically, β-cell dysfunction that is independent of obesity has been reported in patients with PCOS (Dunaif, 1996a). Similar findings are reported in groups of obese and normal-weight adolescent girls with PCOS (Flannery, 2013; Palmert, 2002).

Dyslipidemia

The classic atherogenic lipoprotein profile seen in PCOS shows increased low-density lipoprotein (LDL) and triglyceride levels, elevated total cholesterol:high-density lipoprotein (HDL) ratios, but depressed HDL levels (Banaszewska, 2006). Independent of total cholesterol levels, these changes may increase the cardiovascular disease risk in women with PCOS. The prevalence of dyslipidemia in PCOS approaches 70 percent (Legro, 2001; Talbott, 1998).

Obesity

Compared with age-matched controls, women with PCOS are more likely to be obese, as reflected by elevated BMIs and waist:hip ratios (Talbott, 1995). This ratio reflects an android or central pattern of obesity, which itself is an independent risk factor for cardiovascular disease and predicts insulin resistance. As noted earlier, insulin resistance is believed to play a large role in the pathogenesis of PCOS and is often exacerbated by obesity (Dunaif, 1989). For example, obesity can worsen hyperandrogenism by lowering SHBG and therefore increasing bioavailable testosterone (Lim, 2013). Thus, obesity can have a synergistic effect on PCOS and can worsen ovulatory dysfunction, hyperandrogenism, and acanthosis nigricans.

■ Obstructive Sleep Apnea

This disorder is likely related to central obesity and insulin resistance (Fogel, 2001; Vgontzas, 2001). Women with PCOS have a 30- to 40-fold higher risk of sleep apnea compared with weight-matched controls. This suggests a link between obstructive sleep apnea and the metabolic and hormonal abnormalities associated with PCOS. Moreover, some theorize two subtypes of PCOS, that is, PCOS with or without obstructive sleep apnea. PCOS patients with this condition may be at much higher risk for DM and cardiovascular disease than women with PCOS but without obstructive sleep apnea (Nitsche, 2010).

■ Metabolic Syndrome and Cardiovascular Disease

The metabolic syndrome is characterized by insulin resistance, obesity, atherogenic dyslipidemia, and hypertension. It is associated with an increased risk of cardiovascular disease (CVD) and type 2 DM (Schneider, 2006). The prevalence of metabolic syndrome approximates 45 percent in women with PCOS compared with 4 percent in age-adjusted controls (Fig. 17-7)

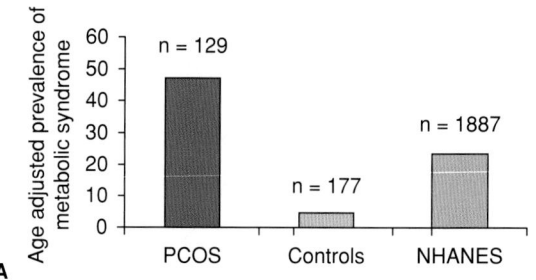

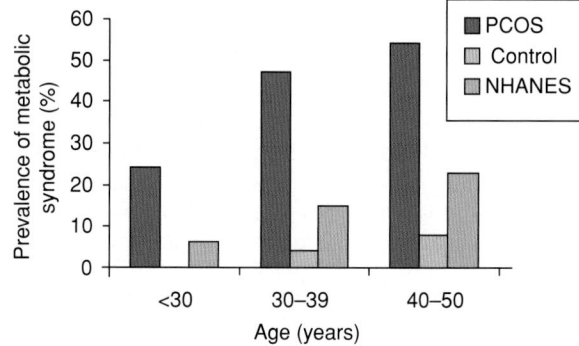

FIGURE 17-7 A. Women with polycystic ovarian syndrome (PCOS) have an increased risk of metabolic syndrome compared with age-adjusted controls and with women from the Third National Health and Nutrition Survey (NHANES III). **B.** In women with PCOS, the risk of metabolic syndrome begins earlier than in controls or those from NHANES III. NHANES III collected data from a representative sample of the noninstitutionalized civilian U.S. population from 1988 through 1994. (Reproduced with permission from Dokras A, Bochner M, Hollinrake E: Screening women with polycystic ovary syndrome for metabolic syndrome. Obstet Gynecol 2005 Jul;106(1):131–137.)

(Dokras, 2005). PCOS shares several endocrine features with the metabolic syndrome, although definitive evidence for an increased incidence of CVD in women with PCOS is lacking (Legro, 1999; Rebuffe-Scrive, 1989; Talbott, 1998). However, in a small group of women with PCOS, Dahlgren and colleagues (1992) predicted a relative risk of 7.4 for myocardial infarction. Another 10-year surveillance study showed an odds ratio of 5.91 for CVD in overweight white women with PCOS (Talbott, 1995). Thus, evidence suggests that women with PCOS should have CVD factors identified and treated (Table 1-8, p. 14) (Wild, 2010).

In addition to components of the metabolic syndrome, other markers of subclinical disease link PCOS and CVD. Women with PCOS have been found to have a greater incidence of left ventricular diastolic dysfunction and increased internal and external carotid artery stiffness (Lakhani, 2000; Tiras, 1999). Moreover, in affected women, studies have found greater endothelial dysfunction, which is described as an early event in the evolution of atherosclerosis (Orio, 2004; Tarkun, 2004).

■ Endometrial Neoplasia

In women with PCOS, the risk of endometrial cancer is increased threefold. Endometrial hyperplasia and endometrial cancer are long-term risks of chronic anovulation, and neoplastic changes in the endometrium are felt to arise from chronic unopposed estrogen (Chap. 33, p. 702) (Coulam, 1983). Moreover, the effects of hyperandrogenism, hyperinsulinemia, and obesity to lower SHBG levels and increase circulating estrogen levels may add to this risk.

Few women who develop endometrial cancer are younger than 40 years, and most of these premenopausal women are obese or have chronic anovulation or both (National Cancer Institute, 2014; Peterson, 1968). Thus, the American College of Obstetricians and Gynecologists (2012) recommends endometrial assessment in any woman older than 45 years with abnormal bleeding, and in those younger than 45 years with a history of unopposed estrogen exposure such as seen in obesity or PCOS, failed medical management, and persistent bleeding.

■ Infertility

Infertility or subfertility is a frequent complaint in women with PCOS and results from anovulatory cycles. Moreover, in women with infertility secondary to anovulation, PCOS is the most common cause (Hull, 1987). Infertility evaluation and treatment in women with PCOS is described in more detail in Chapter 20 (p. 449).

■ Pregnancy Loss

Women with PCOS who become pregnant experience an increased rate (30 to 50 percent) of early miscarriage compared with a baseline rate of approximately 15 percent in the general population (Homburg, 1998b; Regan, 1990; Sagle, 1988). The etiology of early miscarriage in women with PCOS is unclear. Initially, retrospective and observational studies showed an association between LH hypersecretion and miscarriage (Homburg, 1998a; Howles, 1987). However, one prospective study showed that lowering LH levels with GnRH agonists failed to improve outcome (Clifford, 1996).

Others have suggested that insulin resistance is related to miscarriage in these women. To lower loss rates, an insulin level lowering drug, metformin (Glucophage), has been investigated. Metformin, a biguanide, lowers serum insulin levels by reducing hepatic glucose production and increasing the sensitivity of liver, muscle, fat, and other tissues to the uptake and effects of insulin.

Some retrospective studies have indicated that women with PCOS taking metformin during pregnancy have a lower incidence of miscarriage (Glueck, 2001; Jakubowicz, 2002). In addition, a prospective study demonstrated a lower miscarriage rate for women conceiving while taking metformin compared with those using clomiphene citrate (Palomba, 2005). However, a metaanalysis of 17 studies failed to show an effect of metformin administration on miscarriage risk in women with PCOS (Palomba, 2009). Until further randomized controlled trials are performed studying the effects of metformin (a category B drug) on pregnancy outcome, the use of this medication in gestation for miscarriage prevention is not recommended.

■ Complications in Pregnancy

Several pregnancy and neonatal complications have been associated with PCOS. One large metaanalysis found that women with PCOS have a two- to threefold higher risk of gestational diabetes, pregnancy-induced hypertension, preterm birth, and perinatal mortality, unrelated to multifetal gestations (Boomsma, 2006). Metformin has been studied as a tool to mitigate these complications in those with PCOS but without DM. However, investigators in one study found that metformin treatment during pregnancy did not reduce rates of these complications (Vanky, 2010).

Many women with PCOS require the use of ovulation induction medications or in vitro fertilization to conceive. These practices substantially increase the risk of multifetal gestations, which are associated with increased rates of maternal and neonatal complications (Chap. 20, p. 466).

■ Psychologic Health

Women with PCOS may present with various psychosocial problems such as anxiety, depression, low self-esteem, reduced quality of life, and negative body image (Deeks, 2010; Dokras, 2011, 2012). If depression is suspected, screening tools such as those found in Chapter 13 (p. 298) are implemented.

DIAGNOSIS

Other potentially serious disorders may clinically appear similar to PCOS and are excluded during patient evaluation (Table 17-4). For women, who present with complaints of hirsutism, the algorithm in Figure 17-8 can be used.

■ Thyroid-stimulating Hormone and Prolactin

Thyroid disease may frequently lead to menstrual dysfunction. Thus, a serum thyroid-stimulating hormone level is typically measured during evaluation, and treatment is discussed in Chapter 16 (p. 383). Similarly, hyperprolactinemia is a well-known cause of menstrual irregularities and occasionally amenorrhea. Elevated prolactin levels lead to anovulation through inhibition of GnRH pulsatile secretion. A list of potential causes of hyperprolactinemia is found in Table 12-2 (p. 281), and treatments are described in Chapter 15 (p. 360).

■ Testosterone

Tumors of the ovary or adrenal are a rare but serious cause of androgen excess. Various ovarian neoplasms, both benign and malignant, may produce testosterone and lead to virilization. Among others, these include the stromal tumors (Chap. 36, p. 767). Importantly, an abrupt onset or sudden worsening of virilizing signs should prompt concern for a hormone-producing ovarian or adrenal tumor. Symptoms may include those in Table 17-5. Of these, hirsutism is quantified with the Ferriman-Gallwey score, whereas clitoromegaly is assessed using the clitoral index (Fig. 17-9). For the latter, clitoral length (mm) and width (mm) values are multiplied. Values greater than 35 mm^2 are abnormal (Tagatz, 1979; Verkauf, 1992).

Diagnostically, serum testosterone levels can aid ovarian tumor exclusion. Free testosterone levels are more sensitive than total testosterone levels as an indicator of hyperandrogenism. Although improving, however, current free testosterone

TABLE 17-4. Differential Diagnoses of Ovulatory Dysfunction and Hyperandrogenism

	Evaluation	Indicative Results[a]
Causes of oligo- or anovulation		
PCOS	Total T level	Mildly increased
	DHEAS level	May be mildly increased
	LH:FSH ratio	Typically >2:1
	AMH level	Increased
Hyperthyroidism	TSH level	Decreased
Hypothyroidism	TSH level	Increased
Hyperprolactinemia	PRL level	Increased
Hypogonadotropic hypogonadism	FSH, LH, E_2 levels	All decreased
POI	FSH, LH levels	Increased
	E_2 levels	Decreased
Causes of hyperandrogenism		
PCOS		
Late-onset CAH	17-OH-P level	>200 ng/dL
Androgen-secreting ovarian tumor	Total T level	>200 ng/dL
Androgen-secreting adrenal tumor	DHEAS level	>700 μg/dL
Cushing syndrome	Cortisol level	Increased
Exogenous androgen use	Toxicology screen	Increased

Summary of PCOS testing
Serum levels of FSH, LH, TSH, Total T, PRL, DHEAS, 17-OH-P
2hr-GTT, HbA1c, lipid profile
Measurement of BMI, waist circumference, BP

[a]Based on reference laboratory ranges of normal.
AMH = antimüllerian hormone; BMI = body mass index; BP = blood pressure; CAH = congenital adrenal hyperplasia; DHEAS = dehydroepiandrosterone sulfate; E_2= estradiol; FSH = follicle-stimulating hormone; GTT = glucose tolerance test; LH = luteinizing hormone; 17-OH-P = 17-hydroxyprogesterone; PCOS = polycystic ovarian syndrome; POI = premature ovarian insufficiency; PRL = prolactin; T = testosterone; TSH = thyroid-stimulating hormone.

assays lack a uniform laboratory standard (Faix, 2013). For this reason, total testosterone levels remain the best approach for identifying a possible tumor. Threshold values >200 ng/dL of total testosterone warrant evaluation for an ovarian lesion (Derksen, 1994).

Pelvic sonography is the preferred method to exclude an ovarian neoplasm in a female with very high androgen levels. Alternatively, computed tomography (CT) or magnetic resonance (MR) imaging may also be used.

■ Dehydroepiandrosterone Sulfate

This hormone is essentially produced exclusively by the adrenal gland. Therefore, serum DHEAS levels >700 μg/dL are highly suggestive of an adrenal neoplasm, and adrenal imaging with abdominal CT or MR imaging is warranted.

■ Gonadotropins

During evaluation of amenorrhea, FSH, LH, and estradiol levels are typically measured to exclude premature ovarian failure and hypogonadotropic hypogonadism (see Table 17-4). Although LH levels classically measure at least twofold higher than FSH levels, this is not found in all women with PCOS. Specifically,

one third of women with PCOS have circulating LH levels in the normal range, a finding more common in obese patients (Arroyo, 1997; Taylor, 1997). Moreover, serum LH levels are affected by sample timing within a menstrual cycle, use of oral contraceptive pills, and BMI.

■ 17-alpha Hydroxyprogesterone

The term congenital adrenal hyperplasia (CAH) describes several autosomal recessive disorders that result from complete or partial deficiency of an enzyme involved in cortisol and aldosterone synthesis, usually 21-hydroxylase or less frequently 11-hydroxylase (Fig. 15-5, p. 337). As a result of these defects, precursors are shunted into pathways leading to androgen production. Thus, depending on the enzyme affected, symptoms of CAH vary. It may present in the neonate with ambiguous genitalia and life-threatening hypotension (Chap. 18, p. 413). Alternatively, symptoms may be milder and delayed until adolescence or adulthood.

In this late-onset form of CAH, the enzyme deficiency leads to a relative cortisol deficiency. In response, adrenocorticotropic hormone (ACTH) levels are increased to normalize cortisol production. Consequent to this accommodation, adrenal gland hyperplasia and elevated androgen levels develop. Therefore,

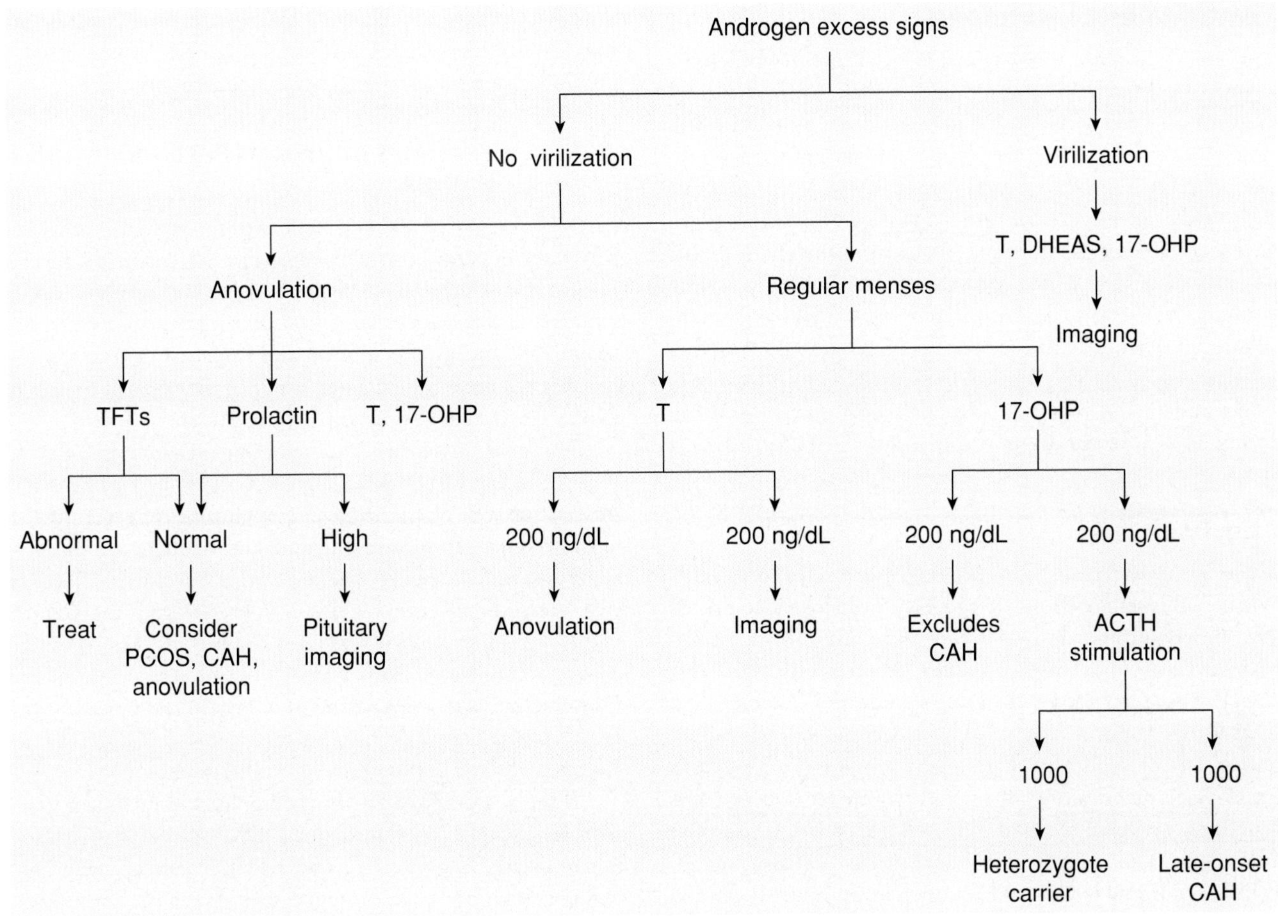

Androgen excess signs

No virilization — Virilization

Virilization branch:
Virilization → T, DHEAS, 17-OHP → Imaging

No virilization branch:
No virilization → Anovulation, Regular menses

Anovulation → TFTs, Prolactin, T, 17-OHP

TFTs → Abnormal, Normal
- Abnormal → Treat
- Normal → Consider PCOS, CAH, anovulation

Prolactin → Normal, High
- High → Pituitary imaging

Regular menses → T, 17-OHP

T → 200 ng/dL, 200 ng/dL
- 200 ng/dL → Anovulation
- 200 ng/dL → Imaging

17-OHP → 200 ng/dL, 200 ng/dL
- 200 ng/dL → Excludes CAH
- 200 ng/dL → ACTH stimulation

ACTH stimulation → 1000, 1000
- 1000 → Heterozygote carrier
- 1000 → Late-onset CAH

FIGURE 17-8 Algorithm for evaluation of androgen excess. 17-OHP = 17-hydroxyprogesterone; ACTH = adrenocorticotropin hormone; CAH = congenital adrenal hyperplasia; DHEAS = dehydroepiandrosterone sulfate; PCOS = polycystic ovarian syndrome; T = testosterone; TFTs = thyroid function tests.

symptoms of late-onset CAH reflect accumulation of precursor C19 steroid hormones. These precursors are converted to dehydroepiandrosterone, androstenedione, and testosterone. Thus, signs of hyperandrogenism predominate.

With late-onset CAH, the most commonly affected enzyme is 21-hydroxylase, and deficiency leads to accumulation of its substrate, 17-hydroxyprogesterone. Serum values are drawn in the morning from a fasting patient. Threshold values of 17-hydroxyprogesterone that measure >200 ng/dL should prompt an ACTH stimulation test. With this test, synthetic ACTH, 250 μg, is injected intravenously, and a serum 17-hydroxyprogesterone level is measured 1 hour later.

To explain this test, the ACTH given during testing stimulates uptake of cholesterol and synthesis of pregnenolone. If 21-hydroxylase activity is ineffective, steroid precursors up to and including progesterone, 17-hydroxypregnenolone, and especially 17-hydroxyprogesterone accumulate in the adrenal cortex and in circulating blood. Thus in affected individuals, serum levels of 17-hydroxyprogesterone can reach many times their normal concentrations. Levels >1000 ng/dL from blood drawn after synthetic ACTH is given are indicative of late-onset CAH.

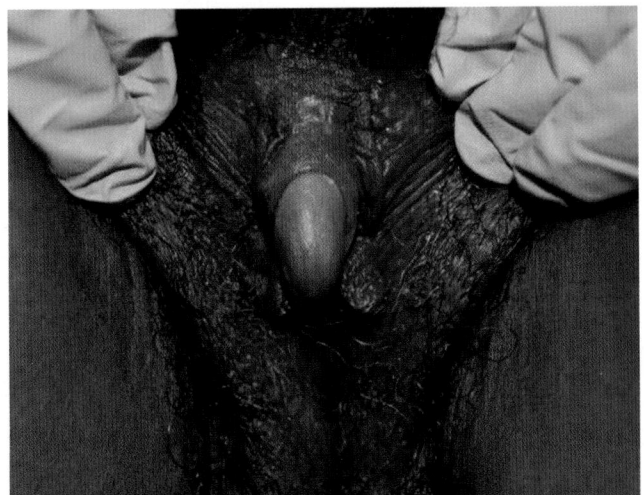

FIGURE 17-9 Photograph of woman with virilization manifest by clitoromegaly. (Reproduced with permission from Hoffman BL, Schorge JO, Schaffer JI, et al (eds): Williams Gynecology Clinical Pearls: Clitromegaly, 2nd edition. New York: McGraw-Hill; 2014.)

TABLE 17-5. Clinical Features of Virilization

Acne	Androgenic alopecia
Hirsutism	Decreased breast size
Amenorrhea	Deepening of the voice
Clitoromegaly	Increased muscle mass

■ Antimüllerian Hormone

The classic polycystic ovary contains two- to threefold more growing preantral and antral follicles than normal ovaries (Hughesdon, 1982). Within the granulosa cells of these developing follicles, the dimeric glycoprotein antimüllerian hormone (AMH) is produced, and serum AMH levels correlate closely with the number of antral follicles. Not surprisingly, AMH levels are two- to threefold higher in women with PCOS compared with nonaffected age-matched controls (Cui, 2014; Homburg, 2013). For this reason, some view AMH as a potentially useful diagnostic marker for PCOS (Pigny, 2006). That said, data regarding this marker in both PCOS and controls are incomplete and require further investigation before it can be adopted as a formal diagnostic criterion (Dewailly, 2014).

■ Cortisol

Cushing syndrome results from prolonged exposure to elevated levels of either endogenous or exogenous glucocorticoids. Of these, the syndrome is most frequently caused by administration of exogenous glucocorticoids. Alternatively, the term *Cushing disease* is reserved for cases stemming from increased adrenocorticotropin hormone (ACTH) secretion by a pituitary tumor. Cushing syndrome shares many symptoms with PCOS such as menstrual dysfunction, signs of androgen excess, truncal obesity, dyslipidemia, and glucose intolerance. Classically, moon facies and purple abdominal striae are also noted. Cushing syndrome is rare, and routine screening in all women with oligomenorrhea is not indicated. However, in those with classic Cushing findings, proximal muscle weakness, and easy bruising, screening is strongly considered (Nieman, 2008).

Initial laboratory testing investigates excessive glucocorticoid production, and three are endorsed by the Endocrine Society (Nieman, 2008). Of these, a 24-hour urine collection for urinary free cortisol excretion can be obtained. Alternatively, a dexamethasone suppression test administers 1 mg of dexamethasone orally at 11 PM, and a plasma cortisol level is measured at 8 AM the following morning. In women with a normal functioning feedback loop, administration of the corticosteroid dexamethasone lowers ACTH secretion and thus diminishes adrenal cortisol production. Normal testing values are <5 μg/dL (Crapo, 1979). However, if a woman has an exogenous or an ectopic endogenous source of cortisol, then cortisol levels during suppression testing will remain elevated. Last, using a late-night salivary cortisol level measurement, patients collect saliva samples between 11 PM and midnight on two separate evenings. Once identified, Cushing syndrome is treated based on the underlying source of excess glucocorticosteroids.

■ Measurements of Insulin Resistance and Dyslipidemia

Many women with PCOS have insulin resistance and compensatory hyperinsulinemia. Although the consensus meeting in Rotterdam suggested that tests of insulin resistance are *not* required to diagnose or treat PCOS, these tests are often used to evaluate glucose metabolism and impaired insulin secretion in these women (The Rotterdam ESHRE/ASRM-Sponsored PCOS Consensus Workshop Group, 2004).

The "gold standard" for evaluating insulin resistance has been the hyperinsulinemic euglycemic clamp. Unfortunately, this test as well as the intravenous glucose tolerance test (IV GTT) requires an intravenous line and frequent sampling, are labor and time intensive, and are not practical in a clinical setting. Accordingly, other less sensitive surrogate markers that evaluate insulin resistance are used and include: (1) 2-hour glucose tolerance test (2-hr GTT), (2) fasting serum insulin level, (3) homeostasis model assessment of insulin resistance (HOMA IR), (4) quantitative insulin sensitivity check (QUICKI), and (5) calculation of serum glucose:insulin ratios.

Of these, a 2-hr GTT is frequently used to exclude impaired glucose tolerance (IGT) and type 2 DM (Table 17-6). This test is particularly important in obese PCOS patients who are at higher risk for both. According to several organizations, women with PCOS should undergo such screening (American Diabetes Association, 2014; Conway, 2014; Fauser, 2012; Legro, 2013; Wild, 2010). Their recommendations vary as to whether all women or only specific PCOS subgroups are screened and as to the screening interval. The Amsterdam ESHRE/ASRM-Sponsored 3rd PCOS Consensus Workshop Group promotes evaluation in the following circumstances: hyperandrogenism with anovulation, acanthosis nigricans, obesity (BMI >30 kg/m² or >25 in Asian women), and a family history of DM or gestational DM. Women with PCOS may demonstrate a worsening of IGT over time, with a reported conversion rate of approximately 2 percent per year to type 2 DM. This affirms the importance of periodic assessment of glucose tolerance with a 2-hr GTT in women with PCOS (Legro, 1999, 2005). The AE-PCOS Society recommends that those with normal glucose tolerance be rescreened at least once every 2 years or more frequently if additional risks exist. Those with impaired glucose tolerance are tested annually. These

TABLE 17-6. Diagnosis of Impaired Glucose Tolerance and Diabetes Mellitus

	Normal Range	Impaired Glucose Tolerance	Diabetes Mellitus
HbA$_{1c}$	<5.7%	5.7–6.4%	≥6.5%
Fasting blood glucose level	<100 mg/dL	100–125 mg/dL	≥126 mg/dL
2-hr GTT	<140 mg/dL	140–199 mg/dL	≥200 mg/dL

2-hr GTT = 2-hour oral glucose tolerance test; HbA$_{1c}$ = hemoglobin A1c.
Data from American Diabetes Association: Standards of medical care in diabetes—2014. Diabetes Care 2014 Jan;37 Suppl 1: S14–80.

same organizations counsel against use of a fasting glucose level and note that a surrogate HbA_{1c} level can be considered.

In addition to assessment of insulin resistance, a fasting lipid profile is used to evaluate dyslipidemia. Evaluation and treatment of dyslipidemia are further described in Chapter 1 (p. 15).

■ Endometrial Biopsy

An endometrial biopsy is recommended for abnormal bleeding in any woman older than 45 years and in those younger than this with a history of unopposed estrogen exposure such as seen in obesity or PCOS, failed medical management, and persistent bleeding (American College of Obstetricians and Gynecologists, 2012). Steps of this procedure are found in Chapter 8 (p. 185).

■ Sonography

Histologically, a polycystic ovary (PCO) displays increases in the number of ripening and atretic follicles, cortical stromal thickness, and number of hilar cell nests (Hughesdon, 1982). Many of these tissue changes can be seen sonographically, and pelvic sonography is commonly used to evaluate the ovaries in women with suspected PCOS. In the NIH criteria for PCOS, sonographic evaluation is not required. However, sonography is particularly important for women with PCOS seeking fertility and in women with signs of virilization to exclude an androgen-producing ovarian cancer. A high-definition transvaginal approach is superior and has a higher detection rate of PCO than the transabdominal route. However, a transabdominal route is preferred for virginal adolescents.

Sonographic criteria for polycystic ovaries from the 2003 Rotterdam conference include ≥12 small cysts (2 to 9 mm in diameter) or an increased ovarian volume (>10 mL) or both (Fig. 17-10). Only one ovary with these findings is sufficient to define PCOS. However, criteria do not apply to women taking combination oral contraceptive pills (The Rotterdam ESHRE/ASRM-Sponsored PCOS Consensus Workshop Group, 2004).

Remarkably, studies using sonography have shown that at least 23 percent of young women have ovaries that exhibit PCO morphology, yet many of these women have no other PCOS symptoms (Clayton, 1992; Polson, 1988). In addition, a polycystic appearance of the ovaries can often be found in other conditions of androgen excess, such as congenital adrenal hyperplasia, Cushing syndrome, and exogenous use of androgenic medications. For this reason, PCO morphology found during sonographic examination is not used solely for PCOS diagnosis.

■ PCOS Diagnosis in Adolescence

Several independent *prepubertal* risk factors for PCOS have been identified. These include above-average or low birthweight for gestational age, premature adrenarche, atypical sexual precocity, and obesity with acanthosis nigricans (Rosenfield, 2007). The diagnosis of PCOS in adolescence is challenging because many symptoms of PCOS mimic the normal physiologic responses of puberty. As noted, adolescents frequently have irregular menses, and acne is common. Moreover, in adolescence, transabdominal rather than transvaginal pelvic sonography is generally performed, and image resolution is poorer. In adolescents with incomplete criteria for a firm diagnosis of PCOS, careful surveillance is warranted as they may be diagnosed at a later time (Carmina, 2010).

TREATMENT

The treatment choice for each symptom of PCOS depends on a woman's goals and the severity of endocrine dysfunction. Thus, anovulatory women desiring pregnancy will undergo significantly different treatment than adolescents with menstrual irregularity and acne. Patients often seek treatment for a singular complaint and may see various specialists such as dermatologists, nutritionists, aestheticians, and endocrinologists prior to evaluation by a gynecologist.

■ Conservative Treatment

Women with PCOS who have fairly regular cycle intervals (8 to 12 menses per year) and mild hyperandrogenism may choose not to be treated. In these women, however, periodic screening for dyslipidemia, diabetes mellitus, and metabolic syndrome is prudent.

For obese women with PCOS, important lifestyle changes focus on diet and exercise. Even modest weight loss (5 percent of body weight) can result in restoration of normal ovulatory cycles in some women. This improvement results from reductions in insulin and androgen levels, the latter mediated through increases in SHBG levels (Huber-Buchholz, 1999; Kiddy, 1992; Pasquali, 1989).

The optimal diet that best improves insulin sensitivity is not known. Diets high in carbohydrates increase insulin secretion rates, whereas diets high in protein and fat lower those rates (Bass, 1993; Nuttall, 1985). However, very-high-protein diets are concerning with respect to stresses on kidney function. Moreover, they afford only short-term weight loss initially with lesser benefits over time (Legro, 1999; Skov, 1999). Thus, it appears that a well-balanced hypocaloric diet offers the most benefit in treating obese women with PCOS.

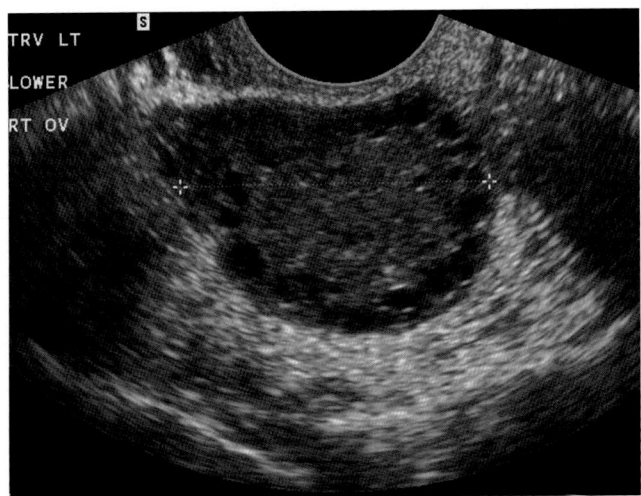

FIGURE 17-10 Transvaginal sonography displays multiple small hypoechoic cysts. (Used with permission from Dr. Elysia Moschos.)

Exercise is known to have a beneficial effect in treating patients with type 2 DM (Nestler, 1998). The most dramatic effect of lifestyle intervention was published in 2002 as the Diabetes Prevention Program. Women and men at risk for diabetes were asked to lose at least 7 percent of their weight and to exercise for 150 minutes each week. This group had a twofold greater benefit in delaying the onset of diabetes compared with a group given metformin alone. Both groups fared better than a placebo group (Knowler, 2002). Few studies, however, have looked specifically at the effect of exercise on insulin action in women with PCOS (Jaatinen, 1993). In addition to DM, women with PCOS may have comorbid risk factors for CVD. In patients with PCOS, exercise has been shown to improve cardiovascular capacity (Vigorito, 2007).

■ Treatment of Oligo- and Anovulation

Hormonal Agents

Women with oligo- or anovulation typically have fewer than eight menses per year, often skip menses for several months at a time, or simply have amenorrhea. Flow may be scanty or may be very long and heavy, resulting in iron-deficiency anemia.

A first-line treatment for menstrual irregularities is combination oral contraceptive pills (COCs), which induce regular menstrual cycles, lower androgen levels, and thin the endometrium. Specifically, COCs suppress gonadotropin release, which results in decreased ovarian androgen production. Moreover, the estrogen component increases levels of SHBG, which binds free androgen. Last, the progestin component antagonizes the endometrial proliferative effect of unopposed estrogen from PCOS, thus reducing the endometrial hyperplasia risk.

Theoretically, COCs that contain progestins with fewer androgenic properties are preferred. Such progestins include norethindrone; a third-generation progestin, such as norgestimate or desogestrel; or the newer progestin, drospirenone. However, no COC pill has shown superiority compared with another in reducing hirsutism (Sobbrio, 1990). Alternative combination hormonal contraceptive options include the contraceptive patch and vaginal ring. Before COC initiation, if a woman's last menses was more than 4 weeks prior, a pregnancy test is indicated.

In patients who are not candidates for combination hormonal contraception, progesterone withdrawal is recommended every 1 to 3 months. Examples of regimens used include: medroxyprogesterone acetate (MPA), 5 to 10 mg orally daily for 12 days, or micronized progesterone, 200 mg orally each evening for 12 days. Patients are counseled that intermittent progestins will not reduce symptoms of acne or hirsutism, nor do they provide contraception. For those requiring birth control, a continuous progestin-only contraceptive pill, depot medroxyprogesterone acetate, or a progestin-releasing implant or intrauterine device may be used and will act to thin the endometrium.

Insulin Sensitizing Agents

Although use of insulin sensitizers for PCOS has not been approved by the Food and Drug Administration (FDA), they have been found to improve both metabolic and gynecologic issues. Of these agents, metformin is the most commonly prescribed, particularly in women with impaired glucose tolerance

and insulin resistance. In clinical studies, 1500 to 2000 mg in divided doses daily with meals is typically used. More common side effects are gastrointestinal, and these can be minimized by starting at a low dose and gradually increasing the dose over several weeks to an optimal level.

Metformin decreases androgen levels in both lean and obese women with PCOS, leading to increased rates of spontaneous ovulation (Essah, 2006; Haas, 2003; Lord, 2003). Several studies demonstrate that up to 40 percent of anovulatory women with PCOS will ovulate, and many will achieve pregnancy with metformin alone (Diamanti-Kandarakis, 1998; Fleming, 2002; Neveu, 2007). Metformin is a category B drug and is safe to use as an ovulatory induction agent. As such, it may be used alone or in concert with other medications such as clomiphene citrate (Chap. 20, p. 452). Specifically, metformin has been shown to increase the ovulatory response to clomiphene citrate in patients who were previously clomiphene-resistant (Nestler, 1998). Despite these positive findings regarding metformin and ovulation induction, Legro and colleagues (2007) in a randomized prospective study of 626 women found higher live-birth rates with clomiphene citrate alone (22 percent) than with metformin alone (7 percent). Based on data, the Thessaloniki ESHRE/ASRM Sponsored PCOS Consensus Workshop Group (2008) recommends against the routine use of metformin for ovulation induction, and first-line treatment remains clomiphene citrate. They note that the addition of metformin to clomiphene citrate may be indicated for women with PCOS and glucose intolerance.

The thiazolidinediones are another class of medications also used for patients with diabetes mellitus. Similar to metformin, rosiglitazone and pioglitazone improve ovulation rates in some patients (Azziz, 2001; Dunaif, 1996b; Ehrmann, 1997). However, the glitazones are category C drugs and should be discontinued if pregnancy is achieved.

■ Hirsutism

With hirsutism treatment, a primary goal is lowering androgen levels to halt further conversion of vellus hairs to terminal ones. However, medical therapies will not eliminate hair already present. Moreover, treatments may require 6 to 12 months before clinical improvement is apparent. For this reason, clinicians should be familiar with temporary hair removal methods that may be used in the interim. Permanent cosmetic therapies can then be implemented once medications have reached maximal therapeutic effect.

Lowered Effective Androgen Levels

Several options are available to decrease androgen levels affecting hair follicles. First, as described earlier, COCs are effective in establishing regular menses and lowering ovarian androgen production.

Second, GnRH agonists lower gonadotropin levels over time, and in turn subsequently lower androgen levels. Despite their effectiveness in treating hirsutism, long-term administration of GnRH agonists is not ideal due to associated bone loss, high cost, and menopausal side effects.

Last, 5α-reductase inhibitors block conversion of testosterone to DHT. Of these, finasteride is available as a 5-mg tablet for prostate cancer (Proscar) and a 1-mg tablet for the treatment

Polycystic Ovarian Syndrome and Hyperandrogenism   **399**

CHAPTER 17

of male alopecia (Propecia). Most studies have used 5-mg daily doses for women and have found finasteride to be modestly effective for hirsutism treatment (Fruzzetti, 1994; Moghetti, 1994). Side effects are low with finasteride, although decreased libido has been noted. However, as with other antiandrogens, the risk of male fetal teratogenicity is present, and effective contraception must be used concurrently.

Eflornithine Hydrochloride

This antimetabolite topical cream is applied twice daily to affected areas and is an irreversible inhibitor of ornithine decarboxylase. This enzyme is necessary for hair follicle cell division and function, and its inhibition results in slower hair growth. It does not permanently remove hair, and thus women must continue routine methods of hair removal while using this medicine.

Eflornithine hydrochloride (Vaniqa) may require 4 to 8 weeks of use before changes are noticed. However, approximately one third of patients have marked improvement after 24 weeks of eflornithine use compared with placebo, and 58 percent showed some overall improvement in hirsutism scores (Balfour, 2001).

Androgen-receptor Antagonists

Antiandrogens are competitive inhibitors of androgen binding to the androgen receptor (Brown, 2009; Moghetti, 2000; Venturoli, 1999). Although these agents effectively treat hirsutism, they carry a risk for several side effects. Metrorrhagia may frequently develop. In addition, as antiandrogens, these drugs bear a theoretical risk of interfering with external genitalia development in male fetuses of women using such medications in early pregnancy. Accordingly, these drugs are commonly used in conjunction with oral contraceptive pills, which prompt regular menses and provide effective contraception. None of the antiandrogen agents are FDA-approved for treatment of hyperandrogenism and thus are used off-label.

Spironolactone (Aldactone), in a dosage of 50 to 100 mg orally twice daily, is the primary antiandrogen used currently in the United States. In addition to its antiandrogen effects, this drug also affects hair conversion from vellus to terminal by its direct inhibition of 5α-reductase. Spironolactone is also a potassium-sparing diuretic. As such, it is not prescribed for chronic use in combination with agents that can also raise blood potassium levels, such as potassium supplements, angiotensin-converting enzyme (ACE) inhibitors, nonsteroidal antiinflammatory drugs such as indomethacin, or other potassium-sparing diuretics.

Of less prescribed alternatives, in Europe, Canada, and Mexico, the antiandrogen cyproterone acetate is used in an oral contraceptive pill. However, this agent is not FDA-approved largely based on its potential for liver injury. Flutamide is another nonsteroidal antiandrogen marketed for the treatment of prostate cancer. It is rarely used for hirsutism, again due to its potential hepatotoxicity.

Hair Removal

Hirsutism is often treated by mechanical means, and these include both depilation and epilation techniques. In addition to hair removal, lightening hair color with bleach is a cosmetic option.

Depilation describes hair removal above the skin surface. Shaving is the most common form and does not exacerbate

hirsutism, contrary to the myth that it will increase hair follicle density. Alternatively, topical chemical depilatories are also effective. Available in gel, cream, lotion, aerosol, and roll-on forms, these agents contain calcium thioglycolate. This agent breaks disulfide bonds between hair protein chains, causing hair to break down and separate easily from the skin surface.

Epilation removes the entire hair shaft and root and includes techniques such as plucking, waxing, threading, electrolysis, and laser treatment. Threading, also known as "khite" in Arabic, is a fast method for removing entire hairs and is commonly used in the Middle East and India. Hairs are snared within an outstretched strand of twisted cotton thread and pulled out.

Although waxing and plucking allow effective temporary hair removal, permanent epilation may be achieved with thermal destruction of the hair follicle. Electrolysis, performed by a trained individual, involves placement of a fine electrode and passage of electric current to destroy individual follicles. It requires repetitive treatments over several weeks to months, can be painful, and can result in scarring.

Alternatively, laser therapy directs specific laser wavelengths to also permanently destroy follicles. During this process, termed *selective photothermolysis,* only target tissues absorb laser light and are heated. Surrounding tissues fail to absorb the selective wavelength and receive minimal thermal damage. For this reason, light-skinned women with dark hairs are better candidates for laser treatment due to the selective wavelength absorption by their hair. Advantageously, laser treatment can cover a wider surface area than electrolysis and therefore requires fewer treatments. It causes less pain, but is expensive and can result in dyspigmentation.

Prior to any epilation technique, topical anesthetics may be prescribed. Specifically, a topical cream combination of 2.5-percent lidocaine and 2.5-percent prilocaine (EMLA cream) can be applied as a thick layer that remains for 1 hour and is removed just prior to epilation. Recommended adult dosing is 1.5 g for each 2 × 2-inch area of skin treated.

■ Acne

One part of acne treatment is similar to that for hirsutism and involves lowering of androgen levels. As such, therapy may include: (1) COC pills, (2) an antiandrogen such as spironolactone, or (3) 5α-reductase inhibitors. In addition to lowering androgen levels, other therapies may be added.

In general, mild noninflammatory comedonal acne may be treated with topical retinoid monotherapy. If mild inflammatory pustules are present, topical retinoids are combined with topical antimicrobial therapy or benzoyl peroxide. Moderate to severe acne may require triple therapy with the above agents or use of oral retinoids or oral antibiotics. For this reason, women with moderate to severe acne may benefit from consultation with a dermatologist.

Topical retinoids regulate the follicular keratinocyte and normalize its desquamation. In addition, these agents also have direct antiinflammatory properties and thereby target two factors linked to acne vulgaris (Zaenglein, 2006). The most commonly used of these is tretinoin (Retin-A, Renova, others). Adapalene and tazarotene are also effective (Gold, 2006; Leyden,

2006). Initially, a pea-sized dab sufficient to cover the entire face is applied every third night and progressively increased as tolerated to nightly application (Krowchuk, 2005). Tretinoin may cause a transient worsening of acne during the first weeks of treatment. Concerning teratogenicity, tretinoin and adapalene are category C drugs and thus are not recommended for use during pregnancy or breast feeding. However, epidemiologic studies currently do not support a link between topical retinoids and birth defects (Jick, 1993; Loureiro, 2005). Tazarotene is category X and similarly is not used during these times or without highly effective contraception.

Topical benzoyl peroxide is bactericidal to *P acnes* by generating reactive oxygen species within the follicle. It also has weak comedolytic and antiinflammatory properties. Although it is the active ingredient in many over-the-counter acne products, some prescription preparations also combine benzoyl peroxide with topical clindamycin or erythromycin.

Topical antibiotics typically include erythromycin and clindamycin, whereas oral antibiotics most often used for acne include doxycycline, minocycline, and erythromycin. Oral antibiotics are more effective than topical therapies but can have various side effects such as sun sensitivity and gastrointestinal upset.

Oral isotretinoin (Accutane) successfully treats severe recalcitrant acne. Despite its efficacy, oral isotretinoin is teratogenic if taken during the first trimester of pregnancy. Malformations typically involve the cranium, face, heart, central nervous system, and thymus. Therefore, isotretinoin administration is limited to women using a highly effective method of contraception. Moreover, the iPLEDGE program is an FDA-mandated risk evaluation and mitigation strategy for isotretinoin that requires participation by involved patients, physicians, and pharmacies to eliminate embryofetal exposure.

▧ Acanthosis Nigricans

Optimal treatment for acanthosis nigricans is directed toward decreasing insulin resistance and hyperinsulinemia (Field, 1961). Specifically, a few studies have shown an improvement in acanthosis nigricans with insulin sensitizers (Walling, 2003). Other methods, including topical antibiotics, topical and systemic retinoids, keratolytics, and topical corticosteroids, have been tried with limited success (Schwartz, 1994).

▧ Surgical Therapy

Although ovarian wedge resection is now rarely performed, laparoscopic ovarian drilling restores ovulation in many women with PCOS that is resistant to clomiphene citrate (Section 44-7, p. 1021) (Farquhar, 2012). Rarely, oophorectomy is a viable option for women not seeking fertility who exhibit signs and symptoms of ovarian hyperthecosis and accompanying severe hyperandrogenism.

REFERENCES

Amer SA, Gopalan V, Li TC, et al: Long term follow-up of patients with polycystic ovarian syndrome after laparoscopic ovarian drilling: clinical outcome. Hum Reprod 17:2035, 2002

American College of Obstetricians and Gynecologists: Diagnosis of abnormal uterine bleeding in reproductive-aged women. Practice Bulletin No. 128, July 2012

American Diabetes Association: Standards of medical care in diabetes—2014. Diabetes Care 37 (Suppl 1):S14, 2014

Arroyo A, Laughlin GA, Morales AJ, et al: Inappropriate gonadotropin secretion in polycystic ovary syndrome: influence of adiposity. J Clin Endocrinol Metab 82:3728, 1997

Asunción M, Calvo RM, San Millán JL, et al: A prospective study of the polycystic ovary syndrome in unselected Caucasian women from Spain. J Clin Endocrinol Metab 85:2434, 2000

Azziz R: The evaluation and management of hirsutism. Obstet Gynecol 101: 995, 2003

Azziz R, Carmina E, Dewailly D, et al: Position statement: criteria for defining polycystic ovary syndrome as a predominantly hyperandrogenic syndrome: an Androgen Excess Society guideline. J Clin Endocrinol Metab 91:4237, 2006

Azziz R, Ehrmann D, Legro RS, et al: Troglitazone improves ovulation and hirsutism in the polycystic ovary syndrome: a multicenter, double blind, placebo-controlled trial. J Clin Endocrinol Metab 86:1626, 2001

Balfour JA, McClellan K: Topical eflornithine. Am J Clin Dermatol 2:197, 2001

Banaszewska B, Duleba A, Spaczynski R: Lipids in polycystic ovary syndrome: role of hyperinsulinemia and effects of metformin. Am J Obstet Gynecol 194: 1266, 2006

Barbieri RL, Ryan KJ: Hyperandrogenism, insulin resistance, and acanthosis nigricans syndrome: a common endocrinopathy with distinct pathophysiologic features. Am J Obstet Gynecol 147(1):90, 1983

Bass KM, Newschaffer CJ, Klag MJ, et al: Plasma lipoprotein levels as predictor of cardiovascular death in women. Arch Intern Med 153:2209, 1993

Bergh C, Carlsson B, Olsson JH, et al: Regulation of androgen production in cultured human thecal cells by insulin-like growth factor I and insulin. Fertil Steril 59:323, 1993

Betti R, Bencini PL, Lodi A, et al: Incidence of polycystic ovaries in patients with late onset or persistent acne: hormonal reports. Dermatologica 181: 109, 1990

Boomsma CM, Eijkemans MJC, Hughes EG: A meta-analysis of pregnancy outcomes in women with polycystic ovary syndrome. Hum Reprod Update 12:673, 2006

Brown J, Farquhar C, Lee O, et al: Spironolactone versus placebo or in combination with steroids for hirsutism and/or acne. Cochrane Database Syst Rev 2:CD000194, 2009

Bunker CB, Newton JA, Kilborn J, et al: Most women with acne have polycystic ovaries. Br J Dermatol 121:675, 1989

Burgers JA, Fong SL, Louwers YV, et al: Oligoovulatory and anovulatory cycles in women with polycystic ovary syndrome (PCOS): what's the difference? J Clin Endocrinol Metab 95(12):E485, 2010

Carmina E, Oberfield SE, Lobo RA: The diagnosis of polycystic ovary syndrome in adolescents. Am J Obstet Gynecol 203(3):201.e1, 2010

Chen W, Thiboutot D, Zouboulis CC: Cutaneous androgen metabolism: basic research and clinical perspectives. J Invest Dermatol 119:992, 2002

Chen ZJ, Zhao H, He L, et al: Genome-wide association study identifies susceptibility loci for polycystic ovary syndrome on chromosome 2p16.3, 2p21 and 9q33.3. Nat Genet 43(1):55, 2011

Clayton R, Ogden V, Hodgkinson J, et al: How common are polycystic ovaries in normal women and what is their significance for the fertility of the population? Clin Endocrinol 37:127, 1992

Clifford K, Rai R, Watson H, et al: Does suppressing luteinising hormone secretion reduce the miscarriage rate? Results of a randomised controlled trial. BMJ 312(7045):1508, 1996

Conway GS, Dewailly D, Diamanti-Kandarakis E, et al: The polycystic ovary syndrome: an endocrinological perspective from the European Society of Endocrinology. Eur J Endocrinol 171(4):P1, 2014

Cook H, Brennan K, Azziz R: Reanalyzing the modified Ferriman-Gallwey score: is there a simpler method for assessing the extent of hirsutism? Fertil Steril 96(5):1266, 2011

Coulam CB, Annegers JF, Kranz JS: Chronic anovulation syndrome and associated neoplasia. Obstet Gynecol 61:403, 1983

Crapo L: Cushing's syndrome: a review of diagnostic tests. Metab Clin Exp 28:955, 1979

Cruz PD Jr, Hud JA Jr: Excess insulin binding to insulin-like growth factor receptors: proposed mechanism for acanthosis nigricans. J Invest Dermatol 98(Suppl):82S, 1992

Cui Y, Shi Y, Cui L, et al: Age-specific serum antimüllerian hormone levels in women with and without polycystic ovary syndrome. Fertil Steril 102(1):230, 2014

Culiner A, Shippel S: Virilism and theca-cell hyperplasia of the ovary: a syndrome. BJOG 56:439, 1949

Dahlgren E, Janson PO, Johansson S, et al: Polycystic ovary syndrome and risk for myocardial infarction. Evaluated from a risk factor model based on a prospective population study of women. Acta Obstet Gynecol Scand 71:599, 1992

Deeks AA, Gibson-Helm ME, Teede HJ: Anxiety and depression in polycystic ovary syndrome: a comprehensive investigation. Fertil Steril 93(7):2421, 2010

Derksen J, Nagesser SK, Meinders AE, et al: Identification of virilizing adrenal tumors in hirsute women. N Engl J Med 331:968, 1994

Dewailly D, Andersen CY, Balen A, et al: The physiology and clinical utility of anti-mullerian hormone in women. Hum Reprod Update 20(3):370, 2014

Diamanti-Kandarakis E, Kouli C, Tsianateli T, et al: Therapeutic effects of metformin on insulin resistance and hyperandrogenism in polycystic ovary syndrome. Eur J Endocrinol 138:269, 1998

Ding EL, Song Y, Manson JE, et al: Sex hormone-binding globulin and risk of type 2 diabetes in women and men. N Engl J Med 361(12):1152, 2009

Dokras A, Bochner M, Hollinrake E: Screening women with polycystic ovary syndrome for metabolic syndrome. Obstet Gynecol 106:131, 2005

Dokras A, Clifton S, Futterweit W, et al: Increased prevalence of anxiety symptoms in women with polycystic ovary syndrome: systematic review and meta-analysis. Fertil Steril 97(1):225, 2012

Dokras A, Clifton S, Futterweit W, et al: Increased risk for abnormal depression scores in women with polycystic ovary syndrome: a systematic review and meta-analysis. Obstet Gynecol 117(1):145, 2011

Dramusic V, Rajan U, Wong YC, et al: Adolescent polycystic ovary syndrome. Ann NY Acad Sci 816:194, 1997

Dumesic DA, Goodarzi MO, Chazenbalk GD, Abbott DH: Intrauterine Environment and Polycystic Ovary Syndrome. Semin Reprod Med 32:159, 2014

Dunaif A: Insulin resistance and the polycystic ovary syndrome: mechanisms and implication for pathogenesis. Endocrine Rev 18:774, 1997

Dunaif A, Finegood DT: Beta-cell dysfunction independent of obesity and glucose intolerance in the polycystic ovary syndrome. J Clin Endocrinol Metab 81:942, 1996a

Dunaif A, Scott D, Finegood D, et al: The insulin-sensitizing agent troglitazone improves metabolic and reproductive abnormalities in the polycystic ovary syndrome. J Clin Endocrinol Metab 81:3299, 1996b

Dunaif A, Segal KR, Futterweit W, et al: Profound peripheral insulin resistance, independent of obesity, in polycystic ovary syndrome. Diabetes 38:1165, 1989

Dunaif A, Segal KR, Shelley DR, et al: Evidence for distinctive and intrinsic defects in insulin action in polycystic ovary syndrome. Diabetes 41:1257, 1992

Ehrmann DA, Schneider DJ, Burton E, et al: Troglitazone improves defects in insulin action, insulin secretion, ovarian steroidogenesis, and fibrinolysis in women with polycystic ovary syndrome. J Clin Endocrinol Metab 82:2108, 1997

Elting MW, Korsen TJM, Rekers-Mombarg LTM: Women with polycystic ovary syndrome gain regular menstrual cycles when aging. Hum Reprod 15:24, 2000

Escobar-Morreale HF, Carmina E, Dewailly D, et al: Epidemiology, diagnosis and management of hirsutism: a consensus statement by the Androgen Excess and Polycystic Ovary Syndrome Society. Hum Reprod Update 18(2):146, 2012

Essah PA, Apridonidze T, Iuorno MJ, et al: Effects of short-term and long-term metformin treatment on menstrual cyclicity in women with polycystic ovary syndrome. Fertil Steril 86:230, 2006

Faix JD: Principles and pitfalls of free hormone measurements. Best Pract Res Clin Endocrinol Metab 27(5):63, 2013

Farquhar C, Brown J, Marjoribanks J: Laparoscopic drilling by diathermy or laser for ovulation induction in anovulatory polycystic ovary syndrome. Cochrane Database Syst Rev 6:CD001122, 2012

Fauser BC, Tarlatzis BC, Rebar RW, et al: Consensus on women's health aspects of polycystic ovary syndrome (PCOS): the Amsterdam ESHRE/ASRM-Sponsored 3rd PCOS Consensus Workshop Group. Fertil Steril 97(1):28, 2012

Ferriman D, Gallwey JD: Clinical assessment of body hair growth in women. J Clin Endocrinol Metab 21:1440, 1961

Field JB, Johnson P, Herring B: Insulin-resistant diabetes associated with increased endogenous plasma insulin followed by complete remission. J Clin Invest 40:1672, 1961

Flannery CA, Rackow B, Cong X, et al: Polycystic ovary syndrome in adolescence: impaired glucose tolerance occurs across the spectrum of BMI. Pediatr Diabetes 14(1):42, 2013

Fleming R, Hopkinson ZE, Wallace AM, et al: Ovarian function and metabolic factors in women with oligomenorrhea treated with metformin in a randomized double blind placebo-controlled trial. J Clin Endocrinol Metab 87:569, 2002

Fogel RB, Malhotra A, Pillar G, et al: Increased prevalence of obstructive sleep apnea syndrome in obese women with polycystic ovary syndrome. J Clin Endocrinol Metab 86:1175, 2001

Franks S, Gharani N, Waterworth D, et al: The genetic basis of polycystic ovary syndrome. Hum Reprod 12:2641, 1997

Fruzzetti F, de Lorenzo D, Parrini D, et al: Effects of finasteride, a 5 alpha-reductase inhibitor, on circulating androgens and gonadotropin secretion in hirsute women. J Clin Endocrinol Metab 79(3):831, 1994

Glueck CJ, Phillips H, Cameron D, et al: Continuing metformin throughout pregnancy in women with polycystic ovary syndrome appears to safely reduce first-trimester spontaneous abortion: a pilot study. Fertil Steril 75:46, 2001

Gold LS: The MORE trial: effectiveness of adapalene gel 0.1% in real-world dermatology practices. Cutis 78(1 Suppl):12, 2006

Govind A, Obhrai MS, Clayton RN: Polycystic ovaries are inherited as an autosomal dominant trait: analysis of 29 polycystic ovary syndrome and 10 control families. J Clin Endocrinol Metab 84:38, 1999

Haas DA, Carr BR, Attia GR: Effects of metformin on body mass index, menstrual cyclicity, and ovulation induction in women with polycystic ovary syndrome. Fertil Steril 79:469, 2003

Hatch R, Rosenfield RL, Kim MH, et al: Hirsutism: implications, etiology, and management. Am J Obstet Gynecol 140:815, 1981

Hayes FJ, Taylor AE, Martin KA, et al: Use of a gonadotropin-releasing hormone antagonist as a physiologic probe in polycystic ovary syndrome: assessment of neuroendocrine and androgen dynamics. J Clin Endocrinol Metab 83:2243, 1998

Homburg R: Adverse effects of luteinizing hormone on fertility: fact or fantasy. Baillieres Clin Obstet Gynaecol 12(4):555, 1998a

Homburg R, Armar NA, Eshel A, et al: Influence of serum luteinising hormone concentrations on ovulation, conception, and early pregnancy loss in polycystic ovary syndrome. BMJ 297(6655):1024, 1998b

Homburg R, Lambalk CB: Polycystic ovary syndrome in adolescence—a therapeutic conundrum. Hum Reprod 19:1039, 2004

Homburg R, Ray A, Bhide P, et al: The relationship of serum anti-Mullerian hormone with polycystic ovarian morphology and polycystic ovary syndrome: a prospective cohort study. Hum Reprod 28(4):1077, 2013

Howles CM, Macnamee MC, Edwards RG: Follicular development and early function of conception and non-conceptional cycles after human in vitro fertilization: endocrine correlates. Hum Reprod 2:17, 1987

Huber-Buchholz MM, Carey DG, Norman RJ: Restoration of reproductive potential by lifestyle modification in obese polycystic ovary syndrome: role of insulin sensitivity and luteinizing hormone. J Clin Endocrinol Metab 84:1470, 1999

Hughesdon PE: Morphology and morphogenesis of the Stein-Leventhal ovary and of so-called "hyperthecosis". Obstet Gynecol Surv 37:59, 1982

Hull MG: Epidemiology of infertility and polycystic ovarian disease: endocrinological and demographic studies. Gynaecol Endocrinol 1:235, 1987

Jaatinen TA, Anttila L, Erkkola R, et al: Hormonal responses to physical exercise in patients with polycystic ovarian syndrome. Fertil Steril 60:262, 1993

Jakubowicz DJ, Iuorno MJ, Jakubowicz S, et al: Effects of metformin on early pregnancy loss in the polycystic ovary syndrome. J Clin Endocrinol Metab 87:524, 2002

Jick SS, Terris BZ, Jick H: First trimester topical tretinoin and congenital disorders. Lancet 341:1181, 1993

Kahsar-Miller MD, Nixon C, Boots LR, et al: Prevalence of polycystic ovary syndrome (PCOS) in first-degree relatives of patients with PCOS. Fertil Steril 75:53, 2001

Kiddy DS, Hamilton-Fairley D, Bush A, et al: Improvement in endocrine and ovarian function during dietary treatment of obese women with polycystic ovary syndrome. Clin Endocrinol (Oxf) 36:105, 1992

Kiszka AN, Wilburn-Wren KR: Clitoromegaly (update) in Hoffman BL, Schorge JO, Schaffer JI, et al (eds): Williams Gynecology, 2nd edition Online. Available at: http://accessmedicine.mhmedical.com. New York, McGraw-Hill, 2014

Knochenhauer ES, Key TJ, Kahsar-Miller M, et al: Prevalence of the polycystic ovary syndrome in unselected black and white women of the southeastern United States: a prospective study. J Clin Endocrinol Metab 83:3078, 1998

Knowler WC, Barrett-Connor E, Fowler SE, et al: Diabetes Prevention Program Research Group. Reduction in the incidence of type 2 diabetes with lifestyle intervention or metformin. N Engl J Med 346:393, 2002

Krowchuk DP: Managing adolescent acne: a guide for pediatricians. Pediatr Rev 26:250, 2005

Lakhani K, Constantinovici N, Purcell WM, et al: Internal carotid artery haemodynamics in women with polycystic ovaries. Clin Sci (Lond) 98:661, 2000

Lauritsen MP, Bentzen JG, Pinborg A, et al: The prevalence of polycystic ovary syndrome in a normal population according to the Rotterdam criteria versus revised criteria including anti-mullerian hormone. Hum Reprod 29(4):791, 2014

Legro RS: Is there a male phenotype in polycystic ovary syndrome families? J Pediatr Endocrinol Metab 13(Suppl 5):1307, 2000

Legro RS, Arslanian SA, Ehrmann DA, Hoeger KM, et al: Diagnosis and treatment of polycystic ovary syndrome: an Endocrine Society clinical practice guideline. J Clin Endocrinol Metab 98(12):4565, 2013

Legro RS, Barnhart HX, Schlaff WD, et al: Clomiphene, metformin, or both for infertility in the polycystic ovary syndrome. N Engl J Med 356(6):551, 2007

Legro RS, Gnatuk CL, Kunselman AR, et al: Changes in glucose tolerance over time in women with polycystic ovary syndrome: a controlled study. J Clin Endocrinol Metab 90:3236, 2005

Legro RS, Kunselman AR, Demers L, et al: Elevated dehydroepiandrosterone sulfate levels as the reproductive phenotype in the brothers of women with polycystic ovary syndrome. J Clin Endocrinol Metab 87:2134, 2002

Legro RS, Kunselman AR, Dodson WC, et al: Prevalence and predictors of risk for type 2 diabetes mellitus and impaired glucose tolerance in polycystic ovary syndrome: a prospective, controlled study in 254 affected women. J Clin Endocrinol Metab 84:165, 1999

Legro RS, Kunselman AR, Dunaif A: Prevalence and predictors of dyslipidemia in women with polycystic ovary syndrome. Am J Med 111:607, 2001

Leyden J, Thiboutot DM, Shalita AR, et al: Comparison of tazarotene and minocycline maintenance therapies in acne vulgaris: a multicenter, double-blind, randomized, parallel-group study. Arch Dermatol 142:605, 2006

Lim SS, Norman RJ, Davies MJ, Moran LJ, The effect of obesity on polycystic ovary syndrome: a systematic review and meta-analysis. Obes Rev 14(2):95, 2013

Lo JC, Feigenbaum SL, Yang J, et al: Epidemiology and adverse cardiovascular risk profile of diagnosed polycystic ovary syndrome. J Clin Endocrinol Metab 91(4):1357, 2006

Lord JM, Flight IH, Norman RJ: Metformin in polycystic ovary syndrome: systematic review and meta-analysis. BMJ 327:951, 2003

Loureiro KD, Kao KK, Jones KL, et al: Minor malformations characteristics of the retinoic acid embryopathy and other birth outcomes in children of women exposed to topical tretinoin during early pregnancy. Am J Med Genet A 136:117, 2005

Moghetti P, Castello R, Magnani CM, et al: Clinical and hormonal effects of the 5 alpha-reductase inhibitor finasteride in idiopathic hirsutism. J Clin Endocrinol Metab 79:1115, 1994

Moghetti P, Tosi F, Tosti A, et al: Comparison of spironolactone, flutamide, and finasteride efficacy in the treatment of hirsutism: a randomized, double blind, placebo-controlled trial. J Clin Endocrinol Metab 85:89, 2000

Moore RL, Devere TS: Epidermal manifestations of internal malignancy. Dermatol Clin 26(1):17, 2008

Moran C, Knochenhauer E, Boots LR, et al: Adrenal androgen excess in hyperandrogenism: relation to age and body mass. Fertil Steril 71:671, 1999

Moran C, Tapia MC, Hernandez E, et al: Etiological review of hirsutism in 250 patients. Arch Med Res 25:311, 1994

Nagamani M, Dinh TV, Kelver ME: Hyperinsulinemia in hyperthecosis of the ovaries. Am J Obstet Gynecol 154:384, 1986

National Cancer Institute: Surveillance, Epidemiology, and End Results Program: cancer of the corpus and uterus, NOS (invasive). SEER incidence and U.S. death rates, age-adjusted and age-specific rates, by race. Available at: http://seer.cancer.gov/csr/1975_2011/browse_csr.php?sectionSEL=7&pageSEL=sect_07_table.07.html. Accessed September 9, 2014

Nestler JE, Jakubowicz DJ, Evans WS, et al: Effects of metformin on spontaneous and clomiphene-induced ovulation in the polycystic ovary syndrome. N Engl J Med 338:1876, 1998

Neveu N, Granger L, St-Michel P, et al: Comparison of clomiphene citrate, metformin, or the combination of both for first-line ovulation induction and achievement of pregnancy in 154 women with polycystic ovary syndrome. Fertil Steril 87(1):113, 2007

Nieman LK, Biller BM, Findling JW, et al: The diagnosis of Cushing's syndrome: an Endocrine Society Clinical Practice Guideline. J Clin Endocrinol Metab 93(5):1526, 2008

Nitsche K, Ehrmann DA: Obstructive sleep apnea and metabolic dysfunction in polycystic ovary syndrome. Best Pract Res Clin Endocrinol Metab 24(5):717, 2010

Nuttall FQ, Gannon MC, Wald JL, et al: Plasma glucose and insulin profiles in normal subjects ingesting diets of varying carbohydrate, fat, and protein content. J Am Coll Nutr 4:437, 1985

O'Driscoll JB, Mamtora H, Higginson J, et al: A prospective study of the prevalence of clearcut endocrine disorders and polycystic ovaries in 350 patients presenting with hirsutism or androgenic alopecia. Clin Endocrinol 41:231, 1994

Orio F, Palomba S, Cascella T, et al: Early impairment of endothelial structure and function in young normal-weight women with polycystic ovary syndrome. J Clin Endocrinol Metab 89:4588, 2004

Palmert MR, Gordon CM, Kartashov AI, et al: Screening for abnormal glucose tolerance in adolescents with polycystic ovary syndrome. J Clin Endocrinol Metab 87(3):1017, 2002

Palomba S, Falbo A, Orio F Jr, et al: Effect of preconceptional metformin on abortion risk in polycystic ovary syndrome: a systematic review and meta-analysis of randomized controlled trials. Fertil Steril 92(5):1646, 2009

Palomba S, Orio F, Falo A, et al: Prospective parallel randomized, double-blind, double dummy controlled clinical trail comparing clomiphene citrate and metformin as the first-line treatment for ovulation induction in nonobese anovulatory women with polycystic ovary syndrome. J Clin Endocrinol Metab 90:4068, 2005

Panidis D, Skiadopoulos S, Rousso D, et al: Association of acanthosis nigricans with insulin resistance in patients with polycystic ovary syndrome. Br J Dermatol 132:936, 1995

Pasquali R, Antenucci D, Casimirri F, et al: Clinical and hormonal characteristics of obese amenorrheic hyperandrogenic women before and after weight loss. J Clin Endocrinol Metab 68:173, 1989

Peterson EP: Endometrial carcinoma in young women. A clinical profile. Obstet Gynecol 31:702, 1968

Pigny P, Jonard S, Robert Y, et al: Serum anti-Mullerian hormone as a surrogate for antral follicle count for definition of the polycystic ovary syndrome. J Clin Endocrinol Metab 91(3):941, 2006

Polson DW, Adams J, Wadsworth J, et al: Polycystic ovaries—a common finding in normal women. Lancet 1:870, 1988

Quinn M, Shinkai K, Pasch L, et al: Prevalence of androgenic alopecia in patients with polycystic ovary syndrome and characterization of associated clinical and biochemical features. Fertil Steril 101(4):1129, 2014

Rebar R, Judd HL, Yen SS, et al: Characterization of the inappropriate gonadotropin secretion in polycystic ovary syndrome. J Clin Invest 57:1320, 1976

Rebuffe-Scrive M, Cullberg G, Lundberg PA, et al: Anthropometric variables and metabolism in polycystic ovarian disease. Horm Metab Res 21:391, 1989

Regan L, Owen EJ, Jacobs HS: Hypersecretion of luteinising hormone, infertility, and miscarriage. Lancet 336:1141, 1990

Rosenfield RL: Clinical review: identifying children at risk for polycystic ovary syndrome. J Clin Endocrinol Metab 92(3):787, 2007

Sagle M, Bishop K, Ridley N, et al: Recurrent early miscarriage and polycystic ovaries. BMJ 297:1027, 1988

Schneider JG, Tompkins C, Blumenthal RS, et al: The metabolic syndrome in women. Cardiol Rev 14:286, 2006

Schwartz RA: Acanthosis nigricans. J Am Acad Dermatol 31:1, 1994

Shayya R, Chang RJ: Reproductive endocrinology of adolescent polycystic ovary syndrome. BJOG 117(2):150, 2010

Shi Y, Zhao H, Shi Y et al: Genome-wide association study identifies eight new risk loci for polycystic ovary syndrome. Nat Genet 44(9):1020, 2012

Skov AR, Toubro S, Bulow J, et al: Changes in renal function during weight loss induced by high vs. low-protein low-fat diets in overweight subjects. Int J Obes 23:1170, 1999

Sobbrio GA, Granata A, D'Arrigo F, et al: Treatment of hirsutism related to micropolycystic ovary syndrome (MPCO) with two low-dose oestrogen oral contraceptives: a comparative randomized evaluation. Acta Eur Fertil 21:139, 1990

Tagatz GE, Kopher RA, Nagel TC, et al: The clitoral index: a bioassay of androgenic stimulation. Obstet Gynecol 54(5):562, 1979

Talbott E, Clerici A, Berga SL, et al: Adverse lipid and coronary heart disease risk profiles in young women with polycystic ovary syndrome: results of a case-controlled study. J Clin Epidemiol 51:415, 1998

Talbott E, Guzick D, Clerici A, et al: Coronary heart disease risk factors in women with polycystic ovary syndrome. Arterioscler Thromb Vasc Biol 15:821, 1995

Tarkun I, Arslan BC, Canturk Z, et al: Endothelial dysfunction in young women with polycystic ovary syndrome: relationship with insulin resistance and low-grade chronic inflammation. J Clin Endocrinol Metab 89:5592, 2004

Taylor AE, McCourt B, Martin KA, et al: Determinants of abnormal gonadotropin secretion in clinically defined women with polycystic ovary syndrome. J Clin Endocrinol Metab 82:2248, 1997

The Rotterdam ESHRE/ASRM-Sponsored PCOS Consensus Workshop Group: Revised 2003 consensus on diagnostic criteria and long-term health risks related to polycystic ovary syndrome (PCOS). Hum Reprod 19:41, 2004

Thessaloniki ESHRE/ASRM-Sponsored PCOS Consensus Workshop Group: Consensus on infertility treatment related to polycystic ovary syndrome. Hum Reprod 23(3):462, 2008

Tiras MB, Yalcin R, Noyan V, et al: Alterations in cardiac flow parameters in patients with polycystic ovarian syndrome. Hum Reprod 14:1949, 1999

Vanky E, Stridsklev S, Heimstad R, et al: Metformin versus placebo from first trimester to delivery in polycystic ovary syndrome: a randomized, controlled multicenter study. J Clin Endocrinol Metab 95(12):E448, 2010 van Santbrink EJ, Hop WC, Fauser BC: Classification of normogonadotropin infertility: polycystic ovaries diagnosed by ultrasound versus endocrine characteristics of PCOS. Fertil Steril 67:452, 1997

Veltman-Verhulst SM, van Haeften TW, Eijkemans MJ, et al: Sex hormone-binding globulin concentrations before conception as a predictor for gestational diabetes in women with polycystic ovary syndrome. Hum Reprod (12):3123, 2010

Venturoli S, Marescalchi O, Colombo FM, et al: A prospective randomized trial comparing low dose flutamide, finasteride, ketoconazole, and cyproterone acetate-estrogen regimens in the treatment of hirsutism. J Clin Endocrinol Metab 84:1304, 1999

Verkauf BS, Von Thron J, O'Brien WF: Clitoral size in normal women. Obstet Gynecol 80(1):41, 1992

Vgontzas AN, Legro RS, Bixler EO, et al: Polycystic ovary syndrome is associated with obstructive sleep apnea and daytime sleepiness: role of insulin resistance. J Clin Endocrinol Metab 86:517, 2001

Vigorito C, Giallauria F, Palomba S, et al: Beneficial effects of a three-month structured exercise training program on cardiopulmonary functional capacity in young women with polycystic ovary syndrome. J Clin Endocrinol Metab 92(4):1379, 2007

Vink JM, Sadrzadeh S, Lambalk CB, et al: Heritability of polycystic ovary syndrome in a Dutch twin-family study. J Clin Endocrinol Metab 91(6):2100, 2006

Waldstreicher J, Santoro NF, Hall HJE, et al: Hyperfunction of the hypothalamic-pituitary axis in women with polycystic ovarian disease: indirect evidence of partial gonadotroph desensitization. J Clin Endocrinol Metab 66:165, 1988

Walling HW, Messingham M, Myers LM, et al: Improvement of acanthosis nigricans on isotretinoin and metformin. J Drugs Dermatol 2:677, 2003

Wild RA, Carmina E, Diamanti-Kandarakis E, et al: Assessment of cardiovascular risk and prevention of cardiovascular disease in women with the polycystic ovary syndrome: a consensus statement by the Androgen Excess and Polycystic Ovary Syndrome (AE-PCOS) Society. J Clin Endocrinol Metab 95(5):2038, 2010

Yildiz BO, Yarali H, Oguz H, et al: Glucose intolerance, insulin resistance, and hyperandrogenemia in first degree relatives of women with polycystic ovary syndrome. J Clin Endocrinol Metab 88:2031, 2003

Zaenglein AL, Thiboutot DM: Expert committee recommendations for acne management. Pediatrics 118:1188, 2006

Zawadzki JK, Dunaif A: Diagnostic criteria for polycystic ovary syndrome: towards a rational approach. In Dunaif A, Givens JR, Haseltine F, et al (eds): Polycystic Ovary Syndrome. Boston, Blackwell Scientific, 1990, p 377

CHAPTER 18

Anatomic Disorders

Early in life, embryos of male and female sex are indistinguishable from one another (Table 18-1). At critical stages of embryonic development, insults can lead to congenital anatomic disorders of the reproductive tract. Influences include genetic mutation, epigenetic factors, developmental arrest, or abnormal hormonal exposures. Disorders range from congenital absence of the vagina and uterus, to lateral or vertical fusion defects of the müllerian ducts, to external genitalia that are ambiguous. Sexual differentiation is complex and requires both hormonal pathways and morphologic development to be normal and correctly integrated. Thus, it is not surprising that neonates with genital anomalies often have multiple other malformations. Associated urinary tract defects are especially frequent and are linked to the concurrent embryonic development of both reproductive and urinary tracts (Hutson, 2014).

NORMAL EMBRYOLOGY

The urogenital tract is functionally divided into the urinary system and genital system. The urinary organs include the kidney, ureters, bladder, and urethra. The reproductive organs are the gonads, ductal system, and external genitalia. Like most organ systems, the female urogenital tract develops from multiple cell types that undergo important spatial growth and differentiation. These develop during relatively narrow time windows and are governed by time-linked patterns of gene expression (Park, 2005).

Both the urinary and genital systems develop from intermediate mesoderm, which extends along the entire embryo

TABLE 18-1. Embryonic Urogenital Structures and Their Adult Homologues

Indifferent Structure	Female	Male
Genital ridge	Ovary	Testis
Primordial germ cells	Ova	Spermatozoa
Sex cords	Granulosa cells	Seminiferous tubules, Sertoli cells
Gubernaculum	Uteroovarian and round ligaments	Gubernaculum testis
Mesonephric tubules	Epoophoron, paroophoron	Efferent ductules, paradidymis
Mesonephric ducts	Gartner duct	Epididymis, ductus deferens, ejaculatory duct
Paramesonephric ducts	Uterus, fallopian tubes, upper vagina	Prostatic utricle, appendix of testis
Urogenital sinus	Bladder, urethra Vagina Paraurethral glands Greater (Bartholin) and lesser vestibular glands	Bladder, urethra Prostatic utricle Prostate glands Bulbourethral glands
Genital tubercle	Clitoris	Glans penis
Urogenital folds	Labia minora	Floor of penile urethra
Labioscrotal swellings	Labia majora	Scrotum

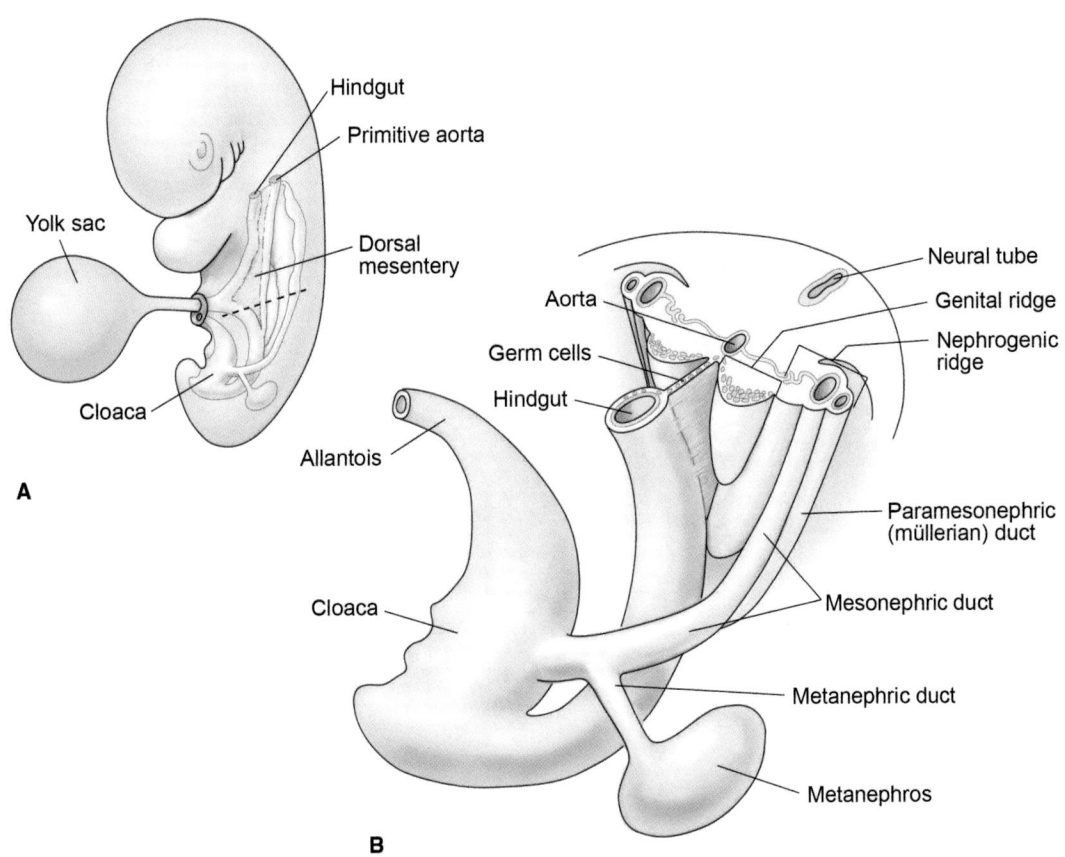

FIGURE 18-1 Early development of the embryonic genitourinary tract. **A.** In the developing embryo, the urogenital ridge forms from intermediate mesoderm lateral to the primitive aorta. The dotted line reflects the level from which part B is taken. **B.** Cross section through the embryo shows division of the urogenital ridges into the genital ridge (future gonad) and nephrogenic ridge, which contains the mesonephros and mesonephric (wolffian) ducts. The mesonephros is the primitive kidney and is connected by the mesonephric ducts to the cloaca. Primordial germ cells migrate along the dorsal mesentery of the hindgut to reach the genital ridge. Paramesonephric (müllerian) ducts develop lateral to the mesonephric ducts. (Used with permission from Kim Hoggatt-Krumwiede, MA.)

length. During initial embryo folding, a longitudinal ridge of this intermediate mesoderm develops along each side of the primitive abdominal aorta and is called the urogenital ridge. Subsequently, the urogenital ridge divides into the nephrogenic ridge and the genital ridge, also called the gonadal ridge (Fig. 18-1).

At approximately 60 days of gestation, the nephrogenic ridges develop into the mesonephric kidneys and paired mesonephric ducts, also termed wolffian ducts. These mesonephric ducts connect the mesonephric kidneys (destined for resorption) to the cloaca, which is a common opening into which the embryonic urinary, genital, and alimentary tracts join (Fig. 18-2A). Recall that evolution of the renal system passes sequentially through the pronephric and mesonephric stages to reach the permanent metanephric system. The ureteric bud arises from the mesonephric duct at approximately the fifth week of fetal life. It lengthens to become the metanephric duct (ureter) and induces differentiation of the metanephros, which will eventually become the final functional kidney.

The paired paramesonephric ducts, also termed the müllerian ducts, develop from invagination of the intermediate mesoderm at approximately the sixth week and grow alongside the mesonephric ducts (Figs. 18-1B and 18-2B). The caudal portions of the müllerian ducts approximate one another in the midline and end behind the cloaca (Fig. 18-2C). The cloaca is divided by formation of the urorectal septum by the seventh week and is separated to create the rectum and the urogenital sinus (Fig. 18-2D). The urogenital sinus is considered in three parts: (1) the cephalad or vesicle portion, which will form the urinary bladder; (2) the middle or pelvic portion, which creates the female urethra; and (3) the caudal or phallic part, which will give rise to the distal vagina and the greater vestibular (Bartholin), urethral, and paraurethral (Skene) glands. During differentiation of the urinary bladder, the caudal portion of the mesonephric ducts is incorporated into the trigone of the bladder wall. Consequently, the caudal portion of the metanephric ducts (ureters) penetrates the bladder with distinct and separate orifices (see Fig. 18-2D).

The close association between the mesonephric (wolffian) and paramesonephric (müllerian) ducts has important clinical relevance because developmental insult to either system is often associated with anomalies that involve the kidney, ureter, and reproductive tract. For example, Kenney and colleagues (1984) noted that up to 50 percent of females with uterovaginal malformations have associated urinary tract anomalies.

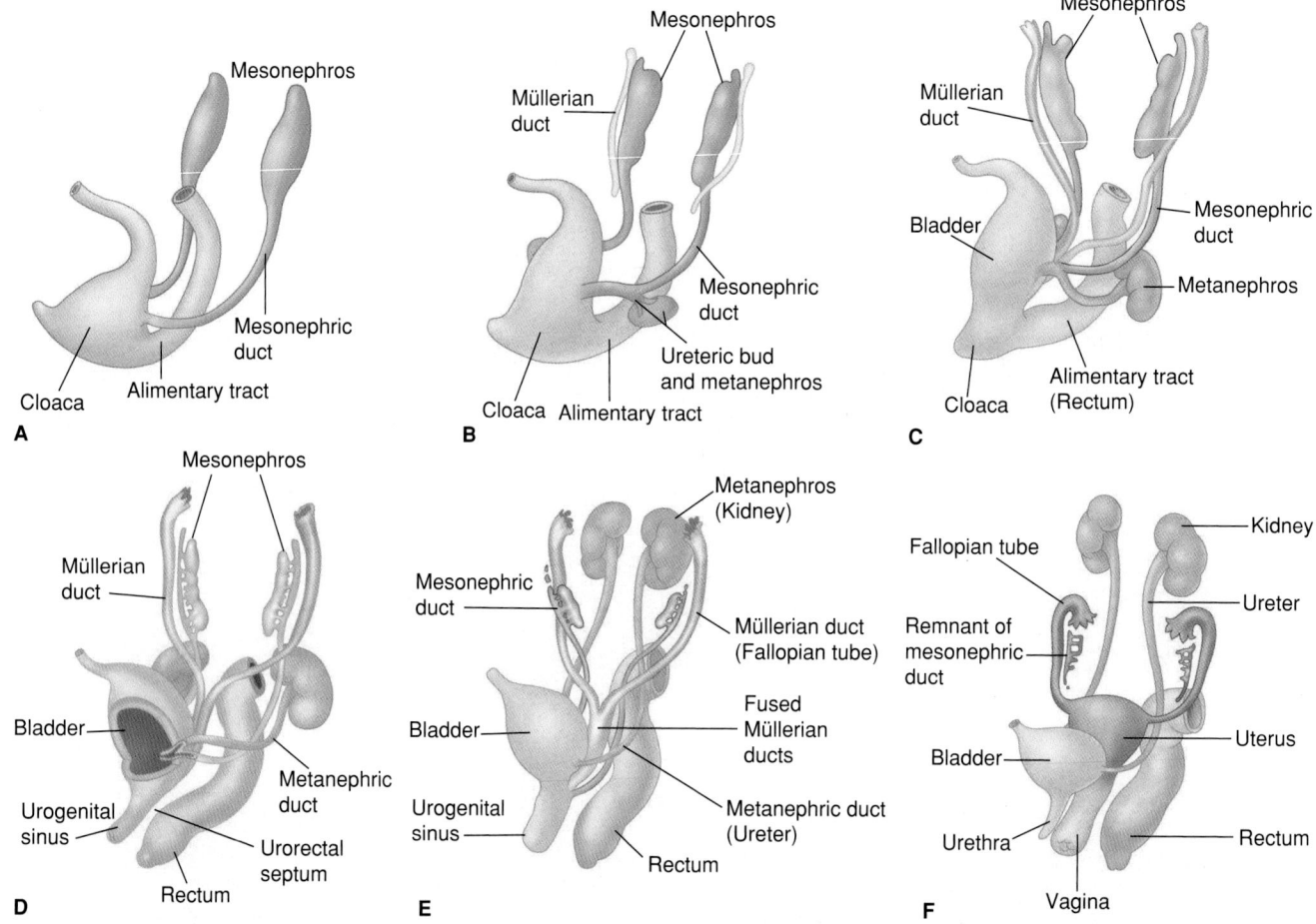

FIGURE 18-2 Embryonic development of the female genitourinary tract. (Reproduced with permission from Shatzkes DR, Haller JO, Velcek FT: Imaging of uterovaginal anomalies in the pediatric patient. Urol Radiol 1991;13(1):58–66.)

■ Gonadal Determination

Mammalian sex is determined genetically. Individuals with X and Y chromosomes normally develop as males, whereas those with two X chromosomes develop as females. Before 7 weeks of embryonic development, embryos of male and female sex are indistinguishable from one another.

During this indeterminate time, the genital ridge begins as coelomic epithelium with underlying mesenchyme. The epithelium proliferates, and cords of epithelium invaginate into the mesenchyme to create primitive sex cords. In both 46,XX and 46,XY embryos, the primordial germ cells are first identified as large polyhedral cells in the yolk sac. These germ cells migrate by amoeboid motion along the hindgut dorsal mesentery to populate the undifferentiated genital ridge (see Fig. 18-1). Thus, the major cellular components of the early genital ridge include primordial germ cells and somatic cells.

At this point, the presence or absence of gonadal determinant genes directs fetal gender development (Taylor, 2000). *Sexual determination* is the development of the genital ridge into either an ovary or testis. This depends on the genetic sex produced at fertilization, when the X-bearing oocyte is penetrated by either an X- or Y-chromosome-bearing sperm. In

humans, the gene named the *sex-determining region of the Y (SRY)* is the testis-determining factor. In the presence of *SRY*, gonads develop as testes. Other genes are important for normal gonad development and include *SOX9, SF-1, DMRT1, GATA4, WNT4, WT1, DAX1,* and *RSPO1* (Arboleda, 2014; Blaschko, 2012). Not surprisingly, mutations in any of these genes may lead to abnormal sexual determination. Moreover, gene dosage and relative expression levels play an important role (Ocal, 2011).

In males, cells in the medullary region of the primitive sex cords differentiate into Sertoli cells, and these cells organize to form the testicular cords (Fig. 18-3A). Testicular cords are identifiable at 6 weeks and consist of these Sertoli cells and tightly packed germ cells. Early in the second trimester, the cords develop a lumen and become seminiferous tubules. Development of a testis-specific vasculature is crucial for normal testicular development (Ross, 2005).

During this early development, Sertoli cells begin secreting antimüllerian hormone (AMH), also called müllerian inhibitory substance (MIS). This gonadal hormone causes regression of the ipsilateral paramesonephric (müllerian duct) system, and this involution is completed by 9 to 10 weeks' gestation (Marshall, 1978). AMH also controls the rapid gubernacular

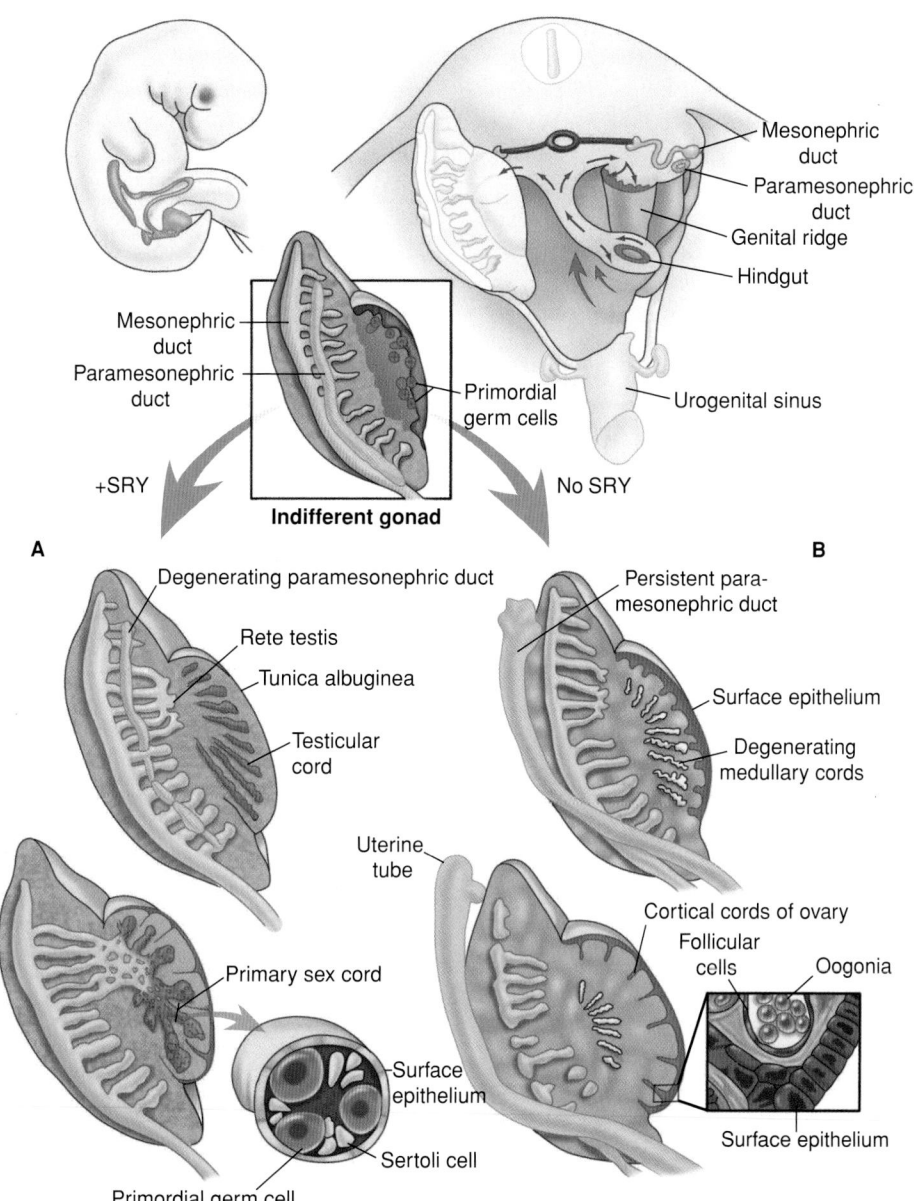

FIGURE 18-3 Development of the gonads and ductal systems in male **(A)** and female **(B)** embryos. SRY = sex-determining region of the Y.

growth necessary for the transabdominal descent of the testis. Serum AMH levels remain elevated in boys during childhood and then decline at puberty to the low levels seen in adult men. In contrast, girls have undetectable AMH levels until puberty, when serum levels become measurable. Clinically, AMH levels in mature women reflect ovarian follicle reserve and are used in fertility aspects of reproductive medicine (Chap. 19, p. 436).

In the testes, Leydig cells arise from the original mesoderm of the genital ridge and lie between the testicular cords. Their differentiation begins approximately 1 week after Sertoli cell development. The Leydig cells begin to secrete testosterone by 8 weeks' gestation due to stimulation of the testes by human chorionic gonadotropin (hCG). Testosterone acts in a paracrine manner on the ipsilateral mesonephric

(wolffian) duct to promote virilization of the duct into the epididymis, vas deferens, and seminal vesicle. In addition, the androgens testosterone and dihydrotestosterone (DHT) are essential for male phenotype development. These androgens control differentiation and growth of the internal ducts and external genitalia and also prime male differentiation of the brain.

In the female embryo, without the influence of the *SRY* gene, the bipotential gonad develops into the ovary. The pathways regulating female sex determination have remained incompletely defined, but *WNT4*, *WT1*, *FoxL2*, and *DAX1* genes are important for normal development (Arboleda, 2014; MacLaughlin, 2004). Compared with testicular development, ovarian determination is delayed by approximately 2 weeks. Development is first characterized by the absence of testicular cords in the gonad. The primitive sex cords degenerate, and the mesothelium of the genital ridge forms secondary sex cords (Fig. 18-3B). These secondary cords become the granulosa cells that band together to form the cell layer that surrounds the germ cells. Oocytes and the surrounding granulosa cells begin communication when the resting primordial follicles are stimulated to grow under the influence of follicle-stimulating hormone (FSH) at puberty. The medullary portion of the gonad regresses and forms the rete ovarii within the ovarian hilum.

Germ cells that carry two X chromosomes undergo mitosis during their initial migration to the female genital ridge. They reach a peak number of 5 to 7 million by 20 weeks' gestation. At this time, the fetal ovary demonstrates mature organization of stroma and primordial follicles containing oocytes. During the third trimester, oocytes begin meiosis but arrest during meiosis I until the oocyte undergoes ovulation after menarche. Atresia of the oocytes starts in utero, leading to a reduced number of germ cells at birth.

◼ Ductal System Development

Sexual differentiation of the mesonephric (wolffian) and paramesonephric (müllerian) ducts begins in week 7 from the influence of gonadal hormones (testosterone and AMH) and other factors. In the male, AMH forces paramesonephric regression, and testosterone prompts mesonephric duct differentiation into the epididymis, vas deferens, and seminal vesicles.

In the female, a lack of AMH allows müllerian ducts to persist. Early, these ducts grow caudally along with the mesonephric ducts. During paramesonephric duct elongation, homeobox (Hox) genes, specifically in groups 9–13, play a role in determining positional identity along the long axis of the developing duct. For example, *HoxA9* is one such gene that is expressed at high levels in areas destined to become the fallopian tube (Park, 2005). *HoxA10* and *HoxA11* are expressed in the developing uterus and in the adult uterus. These and other ovarian determinant genes play an active role in gonadal and reproductive tract morphogenesis, but mechanisms are yet to be elucidated fully (Massé, 2009; Taylor, 2000).

During their elongation, both mesonephric and paramesonephric duct systems become enclosed in peritoneal folds that later give rise to the broad ligaments of the uterus. At approximately 10 weeks' gestation and during their caudal migration, the two distal portions of the müllerian ducts approach each other in the midline and fuse even before they reach the urogenital sinus. The fused ducts form a tube called the uterovaginal canal. This tube then inserts into the urogenital sinus at Müller tubercle (Fig. 18-4).

By 12 weeks, mesonephric ducts regress from lack of testosterone. The uterine corpus and cervix differentiate, and the uterine wall thickens. Initially, the upper pole of the uterus contains a thick midline septum that undergoes dissolution to create the uterine cavity. Dissolution of the uterine septum is usually completed by 20 weeks. The unfused cephalad portions of the müllerian ducts become the fallopian tubes (Fig. 18-2F). Any failure of lateral fusion of the two müllerian ducts or failure to reabsorb the septum between them results in separate uterine horns or some degree of persistent midline uterine septum.

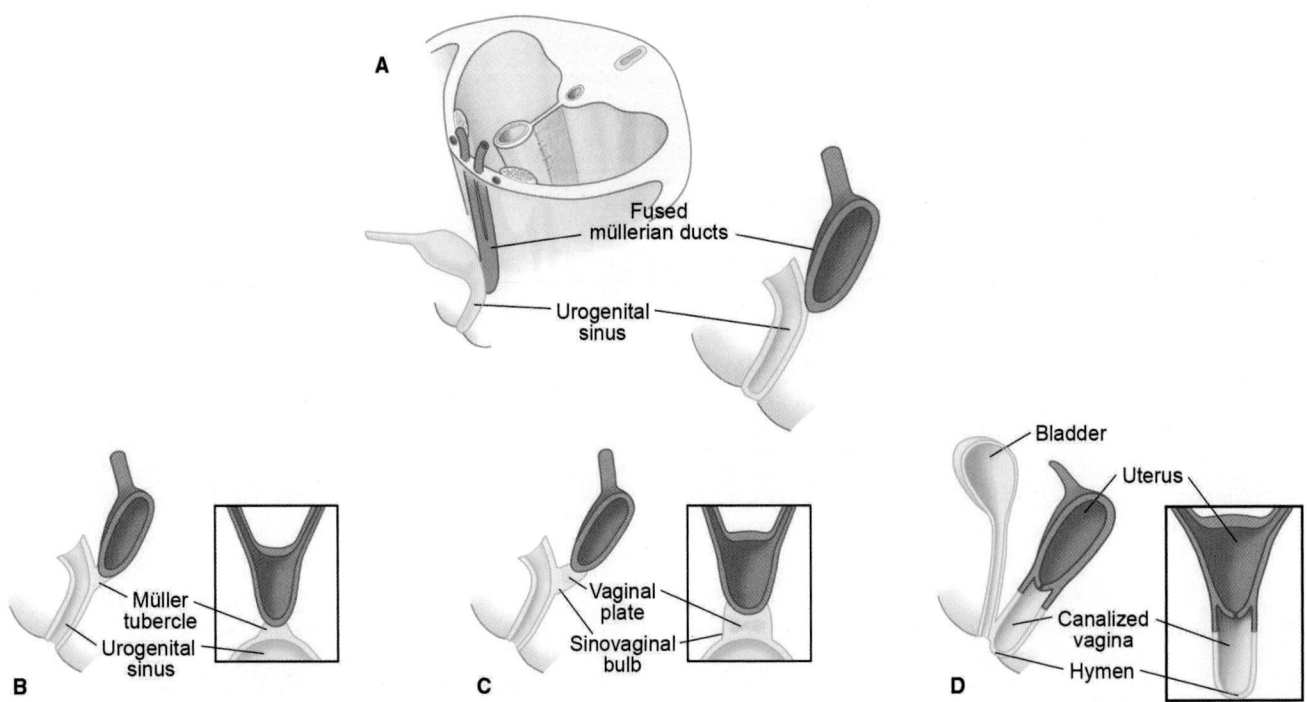

FIGURE 18-4 Development of the lower female reproductive tract. **A.** The fused müllerian ducts join the urogenital sinus at Müller tubercle (**B**). **C.** From the urogenital sinus, the sinovaginal bulbs evaginate and proliferate cranially to create the vaginal plate. **D.** Lengthening of the vaginal plate and canalization leads to development of the lower vagina. The upper vagina develops from the caudal end of the fused müllerian ducts. (Used with permission from Kim Hoggatt-Krumwiede, MA.)

Most investigators suggest that the vagina develops under influence from the müllerian ducts and estrogenic stimulation. The vagina forms partly from the müllerian ducts and partly from the urogenital sinus (Massé, 2009). Specifically, the upper two thirds of the vagina derive from the fused müllerian ducts. The distal third of the vagina develops from the bilateral sinovaginal bulbs, which are cranial evaginations of the urogenital sinus.

During vaginal development, the müllerian ducts reach the urogenital sinus at Müller tubercle (Fig. 18-4A). Here, cells in the sinovaginal bulbs proliferate cranially to lengthen the vagina and create a solid vaginal plate (Fig. 18-4B). During the second trimester, these cells desquamate, allowing full canalization of the vaginal lumen (Fig. 18-4C). The hymen is the partition that remains to a varying degree between the dilated, canalized, fused sinovaginal bulbs and the urogenital sinus. The hymen usually perforates shortly before or after birth. An imperforate hymen represents persistence of this membrane.

External Genitalia

Early development of the external genitalia is similar in both sexes. By 6 weeks' gestation, three external protuberances have developed surrounding the cloacal membrane. These are the left and right cloacal folds, which meet ventrally to form the genital tubercle (Fig. 18-5A). With division of the cloacal membrane into anal and urogenital membranes, the cloacal folds become the anal and urethral folds, respectively. Lateral to the urethral folds, genital swellings arise, and these become the labioscrotal folds. Between the urethral folds, the urogenital sinus extends onto the surface of the enlarging genital tubercle to form the urethral groove. By week 7, the urogenital membrane ruptures, exposing the cavity of the urogenital sinus to amnionic fluid.

The genital tubercle elongates to form the phallus in males and the clitoris in females. However, one is not is able to visually differentiate between male and female external genitalia until week 12. In the male fetus, dihydrotestosterone (DHT) forms locally by the 5α reduction of testosterone. DHT prompts the anogenital distance to lengthen, the phallus to enlarge, and the labioscrotal folds to fuse and form the scrotum. Sonic hedgehog (SHH) is a gene that regulates urethral tubularization in males at 14 weeks' gestation (Shehata, 2011). Specifically, DHT and SHH expression promote the urethral folds to merge and enclose the penile urethra (Fig. 18-5B). In the female fetus, without DHT, the anogenital distance does not lengthen, and the labioscrotal and urethral folds do not fuse (Fig. 18-5C). The genital tubercle bends caudally to become the clitoris, and the urogenital sinus becomes the vestibule of the vagina. The labioscrotal folds create the labia majora, whereas the urethral folds persist as the labia minora.

DISORDERS OF SEX DEVELOPMENT

Definitions

As evident from the prior discussion, abnormal sex development may involve the gonads, internal duct system, or external genitalia. Rates vary and approximate 1 in every 1000 to 4500 births (Murphy, 2011; Ocal, 2011).

Formerly, intersex disorders were subdivided as those: (1) associated with gonadal dysgenesis, (2) associated with undervirilization of 46,XY individuals, and (3) associated with prenatal virilization of 46,XX subjects. The nomenclature used to describe atypical sexual differentiation has evolved. Instead of the terms "intersex," "hermaphroditism," and "sex reversal," consensus recommends a new taxonomy based on the umbrella term, *disorder of sex development (DSD)* (Lee, 2006). Proposed classification of DSDs are: (1) sex chromosome DSDs, (2) 46,XY DSDs, and (3) 46,XX DSDs (Table 18-2) (Hughes, 2006).

Other terms describe the abnormal phenotypic findings that can be found. First, some DSDs are associated with abnormal, underdeveloped gonads, that is, *gonadal dysgenesis*. With this, if a testis is poorly formed, it is called a *dysgenetic testis*, and if an ovary is poorly formed, it is called a *streak gonad*. In affected patients, the underdeveloped gonad ultimately fails, which is indicated by elevated gonadotropin levels. Another important clinical sequela is that patients bearing a Y chromosome are at high risk of developing a germ cell tumor in the dysgenetic gonad.

A second term, *ambiguous genitalia*, describes genitalia that do not appear clearly male or female. Abnormalities may include

---

TABLE 18-2. Disorders of Sex Development (DSD) Classification

Sex Chromosome DSD
45,X Turner[a]
47,XXY Klinefelter[a]
45,X/46,XY Mixed gonadal dysgenesis
46,XX/46,XY Ovotesticular DSD

46,XY DSD
Testicular development
    Pure gonadal dysgenesis
    Partial gonadal dysgenesis
    Ovotesticular
    Testis regression
Androgen production or action
    Androgen synthesis
    Androgen receptor
    LH/HCG receptor
    Antimüllerian hormone

46,XX DSD
Ovary development
    Ovotesticular
    Testicular
    Gonadal dysgenesis
Androgen excess
    Fetal
    Maternal
    Placental

[a]And syndrome variants.
Data from Hughes IA, Houk C, Ahmed SF, et al: Consensus statement on management of intersex disorders, J Pediatr Urol 2006 Jun;2(3):148–162.

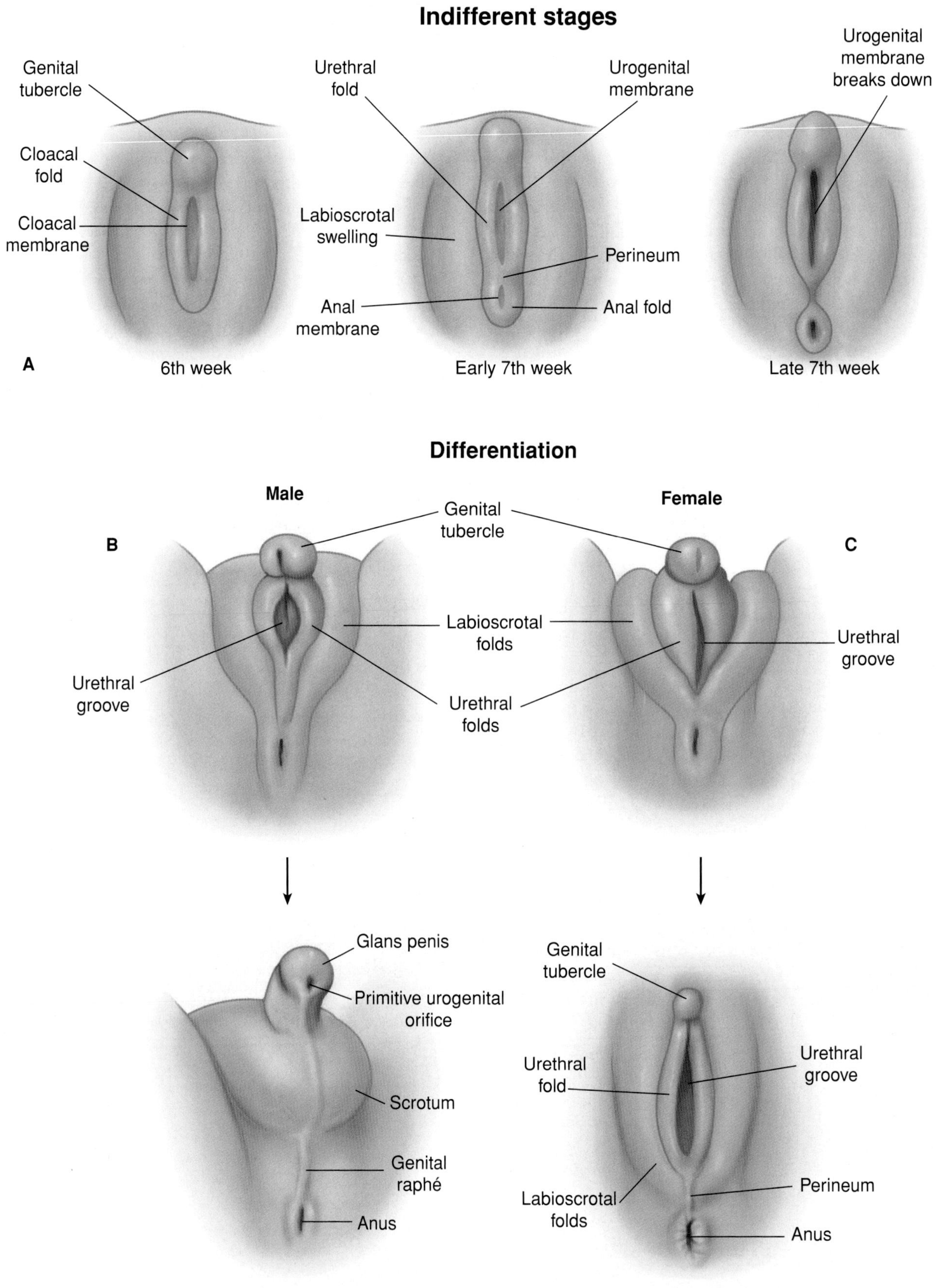

Indifferent stages

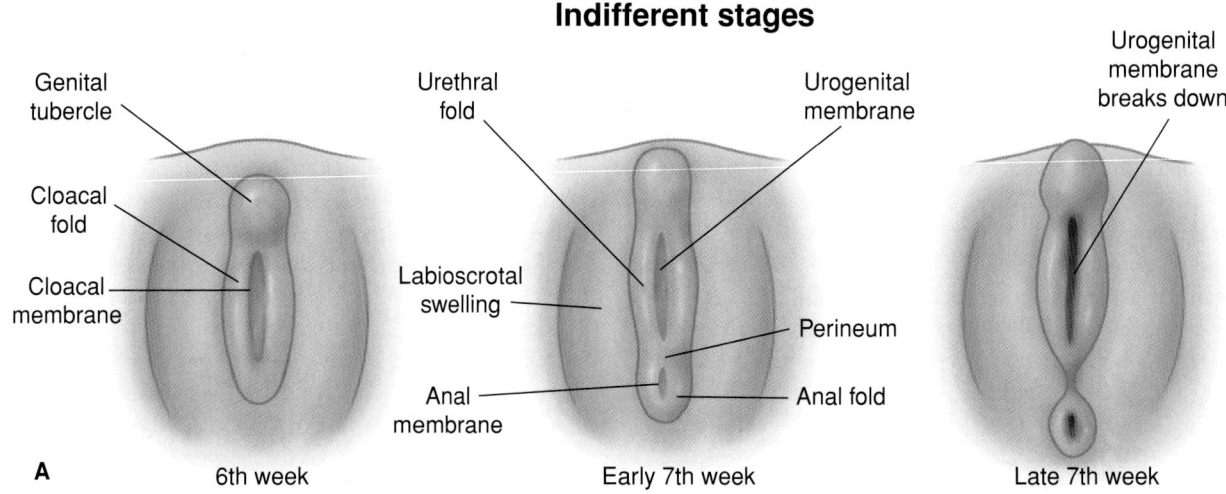

Genital tubercle

Cloacal fold

Cloacal membrane

Urethral fold

Urogenital membrane

Labioscrotal swelling

Perineum

Anal membrane

Anal fold

Urogenital membrane breaks down

A

6th week

Early 7th week

Late 7th week

Differentiation

Male

Genital tubercle

Female

B

C

Labioscrotal folds

Urethral groove

Urethral groove

Urethral folds

Glans penis

Primitive urogenital orifice

Scrotum

Genital raphé

Anus

Genital tubercle

Urethral fold

Urethral groove

Labioscrotal folds

Perineum

Anus

FIGURE 18-5 Development of the external genitalia. **A.** Indifferent stage. **B.** Virilization of external genitalia. **C.** Feminization.

hypospadias, undescended testes, micropenis or enlarged clitoris, labial fusion, and labial mass.

Last, *ovotesticular* defines conditions characterized by ovarian and testicular tissue in the same individual. It was formerly termed true hermaphroditism. In these cases, the morphology of the paired gonads can vary, and options that may be paired include a normal testis, a normal ovary, a streak gonad, a dysgenetic testis, or an ovotestis. In the last, both ovarian and testicular elements are combined within the same gonad. The gonadal location varies from abdominal to inguinal to scrotal. With ovotesticular DSDs, the internal ductal system structure depends on the ipsilateral gonad and its degree of determination. Specifically, the amount of AMH and testosterone determines the degree to which the internal ductal system is masculinized or feminized. External genitalia are usually ambiguous and undermasculinized due to inadequate testosterone.

Sex Chromosome Disorders of Sex Development

Turner and Klinefelter Syndromes

Sex chromosome DSDs typically arise from an abnormal number of sex chromosomes. Of these, Turner and Klinefelter syndromes are most frequently encountered. *Turner syndrome* is caused by de novo loss or severe structural abnormality of one X chromosome in a phenotypic female. It is the most common form of gonadal dysgenesis that leads to primary ovarian failure.

Most affected fetuses are spontaneously aborted. However, in girls with Turner syndrome who survive, phenotype varies widely, but nearly all affected patients have short stature. This results from lack of one copy of the *SHOX* gene, which resides on the short arm of the X chromosome (Hutson, 2014). The classic stigmata of Turner syndrome are listed in Table 18-3. Of these, cubitus valgus is an elbow deformity that deviates the forearm greater than 15 degrees when the arm is extended at the side. Associated problems include cardiac anomalies (especially coarctation of the aorta), renal anomalies, hearing impairment, otitis media and mastoiditis, and an increased incidence of hypertension, achlorhydria, diabetes mellitus, and Hashimoto thyroiditis. This syndrome may be recognized in childhood. However, some patients are not diagnosed until adolescence, when they present with prepubertal female genitalia and primary amenorrhea, both stemming from gonadal failure, and with short stature. The uterus and vagina are normal and capable of responding to exogenous hormones.

TABLE 18-3. Characteristic Findings of Turner Syndrome

Height 142–147 cm	High-arched palate
Micrognathia	Hearing loss
Epicanthal folds	Webbed neck
Low-set ears	Absent breast development
Shield-like chest	Widely spaced areolae
Cubitus valgus	Short fourth metacarpal
Renal abnormalities	Autoimmune disorders
Aorta coarctation	Autoimmune thyroiditis
Diabetes mellitus	

Those with a Turner variant have a structural abnormality of the second X chromosome or have a mosaic karyotype, such as 45,X/46,XX. Indeed, more than half of the girls with this syndrome have chromosomal mosaicism. Those with a Turner variant may exhibit some or all of the syndrome signs. Patients with mosaicism are more likely to have some pubertal maturation.

For patients with 45,X DSD, hormone treatment is needed to effect breast development. Our protocol uses estradiol, 0.25 mg orally daily for approximately 6 months. This begins near age 12 or at the time of delayed puberty diagnosis. The daily estradiol dose is sequentially increased each 6 months to 0.5 mg, 0.75 mg, 1 mg, and then 2 mg daily. We colloquially term this the "start low and go slow" protocol. Progesterone is begun after approximately 1 year of unopposed estrogen treatment. Each month, micronized progesterone, 200 mg orally nightly, is given for 12 nights and then stopped to permit withdrawal bleeding. This method mimics normal pubertal hormonal stimulation of breast tissue. The patient is then maintained on 2 mg of oral estradiol and monthly withdrawal to progesterone. Alternatively, a low-dose combination oral contraceptive would also be acceptable maintenance after adequate breast development has been effected.

Another sex chromosome DSD is *Klinefelter syndrome* (47,XXY), which occurs in one in 600 births or in 1 to 2 percent of all males. These individuals tend to be tall, undervirilized males with gynecomastia and small, firm testes. They have significantly reduced fertility from hypogonadism due to gradual testicular cell loss that begins shortly after testis determination (Nistal, 2014). These men are at increased risk for germ cell tumors, osteoporosis, hypothyroidism, diabetes mellitus, breast cancer, and cognitive and psychosocial problems (Aksglaede, 2013). The most common genotype of Klinefelter syndrome is XXY, although variants exist with differing numbers of X chromosomes.

Chromosomal Ovotesticular DSD

Several karyotypes can create a coexistent ovary and testis, and thus ovotesticular DSD is found in all three DSD categories (see Table 18-2). In the sex chromosome DSD group, ovotesticular DSD may arise from a 46,XX/46,XY karyotype. Here, an ovary, testis, or ovotestis may be paired. The phenotype mirrors that for ovotesticular DSDs in general described earlier on this page.

For others in the sex chromosome DSD group, ovotesticular DSD arises from a chromosomal mosaic such as 45,X/46,XY. With this karyotype, a picture of *mixed gonadal dysgenesis* shows a streak gonad on one side and a dysgenetic or normal testis on the other. The phenotypic appearance ranges from undervirilized male to ambiguous genitalia to Turner stigmata.

46,XY Disorders of Sex Development

Insufficient androgen exposure of a fetus destined to be a male leads to 46,XY DSD, formerly called male pseudohermaphroditism. The karyotype is 46,XY, and testes are frequently present. The uterus is generally absent as a result of normal embryonic AMH production by Sertoli cells. These patients are most often sterile from abnormal spermatogenesis and have a small phallus that is inadequate for sexual function. As seen in Table 18-2, etiology of 46,XY DSD may stem from abnormal testis development or from abnormal androgen production or action.

46,XY Gonadal Dysgenesis

This spectrum of abnormal gonad underdevelopment includes pure or complete, partial, or mixed 46,XY gonadal dysgenesis (see Table 18-2). These are defined by the amount of normal testicular tissue and by karyotype.

Of these, *pure gonadal dysgenesis* results from a mutation in *SRY* or in another gene with testis-determining effects (*DAX1, SF-1, CBX2*) (Hutson, 2014). This leads to underdeveloped dysgenetic gonads that fail to produce androgens or AMH. Formerly named Swyer syndrome, the condition creates a normal prepubertal female phenotype and a normal müllerian system due to absent AMH.

Partial gonadal dysgenesis defines those with gonad development intermediate between normal and dysgenetic testes. Depending on the percentage of underdeveloped testis, wolffian and müllerian structures and genital ambiguity are variably expressed.

Mixed gonadal dysgenesis is one type of ovotesticular DSD. As discussed, with mixed gonadal dysgenesis, one gonad is streak and the other is a normal or a dysgenetic testis. Of affected individuals, a 46,XY karyotype is found in 15 percent (Nistal, 2015). The phenotypic appearance is wide ranging as with partial gonadal dysgenesis.

Last, *testicular regression* can follow initial testis development. A broad phenotypic spectrum is possible and depends on the timing of testis failure.

Because of the potential for germ cell tumors in dysgenetic gonads and intraabdominal testes, affected patients are advised to undergo gonadectomy (Chap. 36, p. 762).

Abnormal Androgen Production or Action

In some cases, 46,XY DSD may stem from abnormalities in: (1) testosterone biosynthesis, (2) luteinizing hormone (LH) receptor function, (3) AMH function, or (4) androgen receptor action. First, as evident from Table 15-5, (p. 337), the sex steroid biosynthesis pathway can suffer enzymatic defects that block testosterone production. Depending on the timing and degree of blockade, undervirilized males or phenotypic females may result. Potential defective enzymes include steroid acute regulatory protein (StAR), cholesterol side-chain cleavage enzyme (P450scc), 3β-hydroxysteroid dehydrogenase type II, 17α-hydroxylase/17,20 desmolase (P450c17a), and 17β-hydroxysteroid dehydrogenase. The last two enzyme deficiencies can also cause congenital adrenal hyperplasia, and hypertension is a common feature in P450c17a deficiency. In addition to these central enzymatic defects, peripherally, abnormal 5α-reductase type 2 enzyme action leads to impaired conversion of testosterone to DHT. DHT is the active androgen in peripheral tissues, and undervirilization results.

Second, hCG/LH receptor abnormalities within the testes can lead to Leydig cell aplasia/hypoplasia and impaired testosterone production. In contrast, disorders of AMH and AMH receptors result in persistent müllerian duct syndrome (PMDS). Affected patients appear as males but have a persistent uterus and fallopian tubes due to failed AMH action.

Finally, the androgen receptor may be defective and result in androgen insensitivity syndrome (AIS). The estimated incidence of AIS ranges from 1 in 13,000 to 1 in 41,000 live births (Bangsboll, 1992; Blackless, 2000). Mutations produce a nonfunctional receptor that will not bind androgen or is unable to initiate full transcription once bound. As a result, resistance to androgens may be complete and female external genitalia are found. Alternatively, an incomplete form is associated with varying degrees of virilization and genital ambiguity. Milder forms of AIS have been described in men with severe male factor infertility and poor virilization. For those with male gender assignment, testosterone therapy via patch or injection may be needed for continued masculine response.

Patients with complete androgen-insensitivity syndrome (CAIS) appear as phenotypically normal females at birth. They often present at puberty with primary amenorrhea. External genitalia appear normal; scant or absent pubic and axillary hair is noted; the vagina is shortened or blind ending; and the uterus and fallopian tubes are absent. However, these girls develop breasts during pubertal maturation due to abundant androgen-to-estrogen conversion. Testes may be palpable in the labia or inguinal area or may be found intraabdominally.

In CAIS patients, surgical excision of the testes after puberty is recommended to decrease the associated risk of germ cell tumors, which may be as high as 20 to 30 percent (Chap. 36, p. 762) (Chavhan, 2008). Additionally, estrogen is replaced to reach physiologic levels, and a functional vagina is created either by dilation or by surgical vaginoplasty. Adequate estrogen replacement in these patients is important to maintain breast development and bone mass and to provide relief from vasomotor symptoms.

■ 46,XX Disorders of Sex Development

As seen in Table 18-2, etiology of 46,XX DSD may stem from abnormal ovarian development or from excess androgen exposure.

Abnormal Ovarian Development

Disorders of ovarian development in those with a 46,XX complement include: (1) gonadal dysgenesis, (2) testicular DSD, and (3) ovotesticular DSD.

With *46,XX gonadal dysgenesis*, similar to Turner syndrome, streak gonads develop. These lead to hypogonadism, prepubertal normal female genitalia, and normal müllerian structures, but other Turner stigmata are absent.

With *46,XX testicular DSD*, several possible genetic mutations lead to testis–like formation within the ovary (streak gonad, dysgenetic testis, or ovotestis). Defects may stem from *SRY* translocation onto one X chromosome. In individuals without *SRY* translocation, other genes with testis-determining effects are most likely present or activated. These include *WNT4, RSPO1,* or *CTNNB1* gene defects or *SOX9* gene duplication (Ocal, 2011). *SRY* guides the gonad to develop along testicular lines, and testicular hormone function is near normal.

Production of AMH prompts müllerian system regression, and androgens promote development of the wolffian system and external genitalia masculinization. Spermatogenesis, however, is absent due to a lack of certain genes on the long arm of the Y chromosome. These individuals are not usually diagnosed until puberty or during infertility evaluation.

With *46,XX ovotesticular DSD*, individuals possess a unilateral ovotestis with a contralateral ovary or testis, or bilateral ovotestes. Phenotypic findings depend on the degree of androgen exposures and mirror those for other ovotesticular DSDs (p. 411).

Androgen Excess

Discordance between gonadal sex (46,XX) and the phenotypic appearance of external genitalia (masculinized) may result from excessive fetal androgen exposure. This was previously termed female pseudohermaphroditism. In affected individuals, the ovaries and female internal ductal structures such as the uterus, cervix, and upper vagina are present. Thus, patients are potentially fertile. The external genitalia, however, are virilized to a varying degree depending on the amount and timing of androgen exposure. The three embryonic structures that are commonly affected by elevated androgen levels or ovarian development disorders are the clitoris, labioscrotal folds, and urogenital sinus. As a result, virilization may range from modest clitoromegaly to posterior labial fusion and development of a phallus with a penile urethra. Degrees of virilization can be described by the Prader score, which ranges from 0 for a normal-appearing female to 5 for a normal, virilized male.

Fetal, placental, or maternal sources may provide the excessive androgen levels. Maternally derived androgen excess may come from virilizing ovarian tumors such as luteoma and Sertoli-Leydig cell tumor or from virilizing adrenal tumors. Fortunately, these neoplasms infrequently cause fetal effects because of the tremendous ability of placental syncytiotrophoblast to convert C19 steroids (androstenedione and testosterone) to estradiol via the enzyme aromatase (Cunningham, 2014c). As another source, drugs such as testosterone, danazol, norethindrone, and other androgen derivatives may cause fetal virilization.

Of fetal sources, exposure can also arise from fetal congenital adrenal hyperplasia (CAH) due to 21-hydroxylase deficiency from *CYP21* mutation. This is a frequent cause of virilization and has an incidence approximating 1 in 14,000 live births (White, 2000). In many cases, CAH can be diagnosed antenatally, and early maternal dexamethasone therapy can ameliorate the masculine phenotype (New, 2012). In addition, androgen excess and ambiguous genitalia can also be seen with fetal 11-beta hydroxylase and 3β-hydroxysteroid dehydrogenase deficiencies, from *CYP11B1* and *HSD3B2* gene mutations, respectively (Fig. 15-5, p. 337). Mutations of *POR* gene can also disorder steroidogenesis. Cytochrome POR is a protein that transfers electrons to important cytochrome P450 enzymes and steroidogenic enzymes. Severely affected female neonates with *POR* gene mutations are virilized because of defective aromatase activity and because of the diversion of 17-hydroxyprogesterone to DHT by a "backdoor" androgen pathway (Fukami, 2013).

Of placental sources, placental aromatase deficiency from fetal *CYP19* gene mutation causes an accumulation of placental androgen and underproduction of placental estrogens. Consequently, both the mother and the 46,XX fetus are virilized (Murphy, 2011).

■ Gender Assignment

At birth, gender assignment to the normal newborn usually involves a simple assessment of the external genitalia and a straightforward joyful declaration of male or female by the obstetrician. Delivery of a newborn with DSD is a potential medical emergency and presents a serious psychosocial, diagnostic, medical, and possibly surgical challenge for a multispecialty medical team. For the unprepared obstetrician in the labor room, ambiguous external genitalia in a newborn can create possible long-lasting psychosexual and social ramifications for the individual and family. Ideally, as soon as the neonate with ambiguous genitalia is stable, parents are encouraged to hold the child. The newborn is referred to as "your baby" and not as "it" or "he/she." When discussing ambiguous development, other suggested terms used include "phallus," "gonads," "folds," and "urogenital sinus" to reference underdeveloped structures. The obstetrician explains that the genitalia are incompletely formed and emphasizes the seriousness of the situation and the need for rapid consultation and laboratory testing see (Fig. 18-6). During family education, the need for accurate determination of gender and sex of rearing is emphasized.

Because similar or identical phenotypes may have several etiologies, diagnosis of a specific DSD may require several diagnostic tools (Ocal, 2011). Relevant neonatal physical examination evaluates: (1) ability to palpate gonads in the labioscrotal or inguinal regions, (2) ability to palpate uterus during rectal examination, (3) phallus size, (3) genitalia pigmentation, and (4) presence of other syndromic features. The newborn's metabolic condition is assessed, as hyperkalemia, hyponatremia, and hypoglycemia may indicate congenital adrenal hyperplasia. The mother is examined for signs of hyperandrogenism (Thyen, 2006).

Pediatric endocrinologists and reproductive endocrinologists are consulted as soon as possible. The diagnostic evaluation of DSD includes hormone measurements, imaging, cytogenetic studies, and in some cases endoscopic, laparoscopic, and gonadal biopsy. Sonography shows the presence or absence of müllerian/wolffian structures and can locate the gonads. Sonography also can identify associated malformation such as renal abnormalities. The genetic evaluation includes karyotype, fluorescent in situ hybridization (FISH), and more recently, specific molecular studies to screen for mutations or gene dosage imbalance.

The psychologic and social implications of gender assignment and those relating to treatment are important and require a multidisciplinary approach. The current intense debate on the management of patients with DSD focuses on four major issues, namely, etiologic diagnosis, gender assignment, indications for and timing of genital surgery, and disclosure of medical information to the patient (Daaboul, 2001; de Vries, 2007). Discussions include the possible need for hormonal stimulation at puberty and potential later surgical reconstruction.

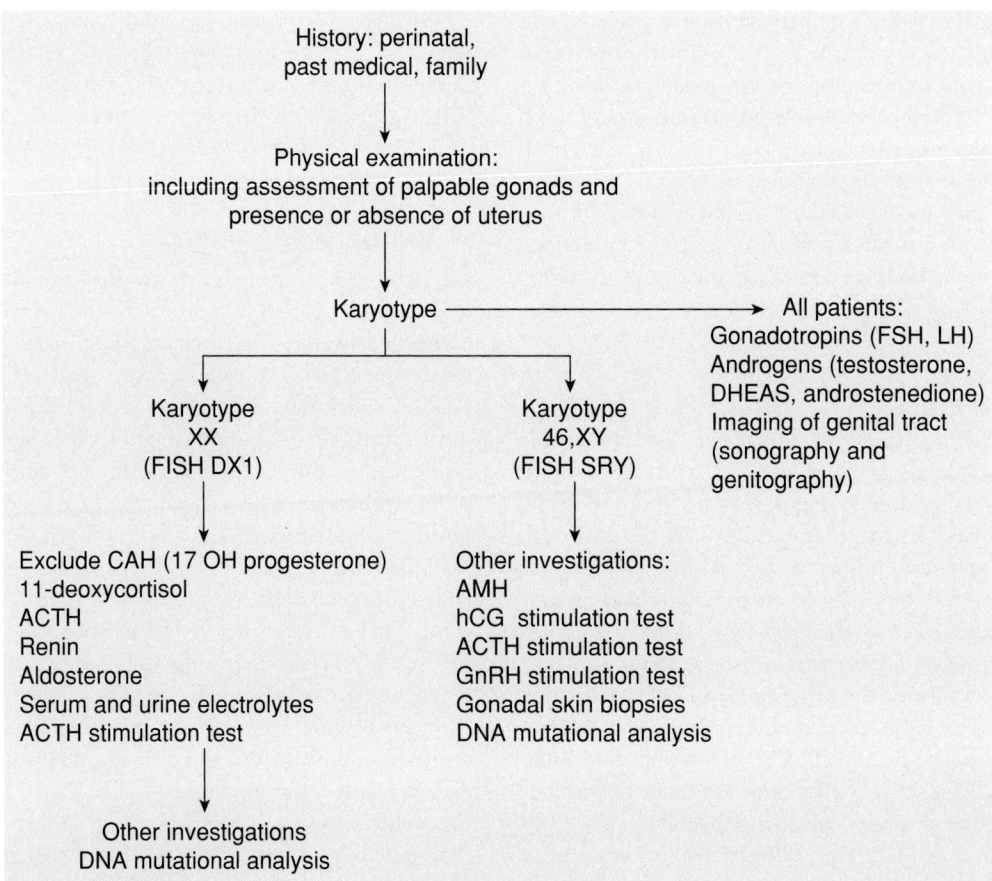

FIGURE 18-6 One algorithm for investigating disorders of sexual development. ACTH = adrenocorticotropic hormone; AMH = antimüllerian hormone; CAH = congenital adrenal hyperplasia; DHEAS = dehydroepiandrosterone sulfate; FISH = fluorescent in situ hybridization; FSH = follicle-stimulating hormone; GnRH = gonadotropin-releasing hormone; hCG = human chorionic gonadotropin; LH = luteinizing hormone; SRY = sex-determining region of the Y.

DEFECTS OF THE BLADDER AND PERINEUM

The bilaminar cloacal membrane lies at the caudal end of the germinal disc and forms the infraumbilical abdominal wall. Normally, an ingrowth of mesoderm between the ectodermal and endodermal layers of the cloacal membrane leads to formation of the lower abdominal musculature and the pelvic bones. Without reinforcement, the cloacal membrane may prematurely rupture. Bladder exstrophy is a complex and severe pelvic malformation due to premature rupture of this cloacal membrane and subsequent failure of the membrane to be reinforced by an ingrowth of mesoderm. Depending on the infraumbilical defect size and developmental stage at rupture, bladder exstrophy, cloacal exstrophy, or epispadias results.

Of these, bladder exstrophy has an estimated incidence of 1 in 50,000 newborns and is equally prevalent in males and females (Lloyd, 2013). Exstrophy is characterized by an exposed bladder lying outside the abdomen. Associated findings commonly include abnormal external genitalia and a widened symphysis pubis, caused by the outward rotation of the innominate bones. Stanton (1974) noted that 43 percent of 70 females with bladder exstrophy had associated reproductive tract anomalies. The urethra and vagina are typically short, and the vaginal

orifice is frequently stenotic and displaced anteriorly. The clitoris is duplicated or bifid, and the labia, mons pubis, and clitoris are divergent. The uterus, fallopian tubes, and ovaries are typically normal except for occasional müllerian duct fusion defects.

A complex approach is required to achieve acceptable urinary continence and external genitalia reconstruction (Laterza, 2011). Surgical closure of the exstrophy is currently performed in the first 4 years of life in stages (Massanyi, 2013). Vaginal dilatation or vaginoplasty may be required to allow satisfactory intercourse in mature females (Jones, 1973). Long term, the defective pelvic floor may predispose women to uterine prolapse (Nakhal, 2012).

DEFECTS OF THE CLITORIS

Congenital abnormalities of the clitoris are unusual but include clitoral duplication, clitoral cysts, and clitoral enlargement from excess androgen exposure. Clitoral duplication, also known as bifid clitoris, usually develops in association with bladder exstrophy or epispadias. The disorder is rare, and the incidence approximates 1 in 480,000 females (Elder, 1992).

In those with epispadias but without bladder exstrophy, visibly apparent anomalies include a widened, patulous urethra;

absent or bifid clitoris; flattened mons pubis; and labia that do not fuse anteriorly. Vertebral abnormalities and diastases of the pubic symphysis are also commonly associated. Female epispadias can be divided into three types—vestibular, subsymphyseal, and retrosymphyseal—which are differentiated by the type of urethral involvement (Schey, 1980).

Female phallic urethra is another clitoral anomaly, and the phallic urethra opens at the clitoral tip (Sotolongo, 1983). This anomaly affects 4 to 8 percent of girls with persistent cloaca and has been associated with embryonic exposure to cocaine (Karlin, 1989).

Epidermal cysts may be found on the clitoris, and inversion of epidermal cells beneath the dermis or subcutaneous tissue is the presumed pathogenesis. Cysts can reach 1 to 5 cm in diameter. Surgical removal of the cyst is the preferred treatment. Vasculature and nerve supply preservation during this procedure is important to sexual health (Johnson, 2013).

Clitoromegaly noted at birth is suggestive of fetal exposure to excessive androgens. Clitoromegaly is defined as a clitoral index greater than 10 mm^2. This index is determined by the glans length times the width. Moreover, early androgen exposure may lead to fusion of the labioscrotal folds and findings of a single perineal opening, the urogenital sinus. Labia are rugated and scrotum-like. A gonad found in the groin or labia majora, however, raises concern for 46,XY DSD.

Frequently in premature neonates, the clitoris may appear large, but it does not change size and appears to regress as the infant grows. Other causes of newborn clitoromegaly include breech presentation with vulvar swelling, chronic severe vulvovaginitis, and neurofibromatosis (Dershwitz, 1984; Greer, 1981). Clitoral reduction surgery is done typically by skilled pediatric urologists, and preservation of vasculature and nerve supply is essential.

HYMENEAL DEFECTS

The hymen is the membranous vestige of the junction between the sinovaginal bulbs and the urogenital sinus (see Fig. 18-4). It generally perforates during fetal life to establish a connection between the vaginal lumen and the perineum. Various hymeneal abnormalities include imperforate, microperforate, annular, septate, cribriform (sievelike), naviculate (boatlike), or septate types (Fig. 18-7) (Breech, 1999). Imperforate hymen follows failure of the inferior end of the vaginal plate to canalize, and its incidence approximates 1 in 1000 to 2000 females (Parazzini, 1990). Although typically sporadic, imperforate hymen in multiple family members has been reported (Stelling, 2000; Usta, 1993).

If the hymen is imperforate, blood from endometrial sloughing or mucus accumulates in the vagina. During the neonatal period, significant amounts of mucus can be secreted secondary to maternal estradiol stimulation. The newborn may have a bulging, translucent yellow-gray mass at the vaginal introitus. This condition is termed hydro/mucocolpos. Most cases are asymptomatic and resolve as the mucus is reabsorbed and estrogen levels decline. However, large hydro/mucocolpos may cause respiratory distress or may obstruct the ureters, resulting in hydronephrosis or life-threatening acute renal failure (Breech, 2009; Nagai, 2012).

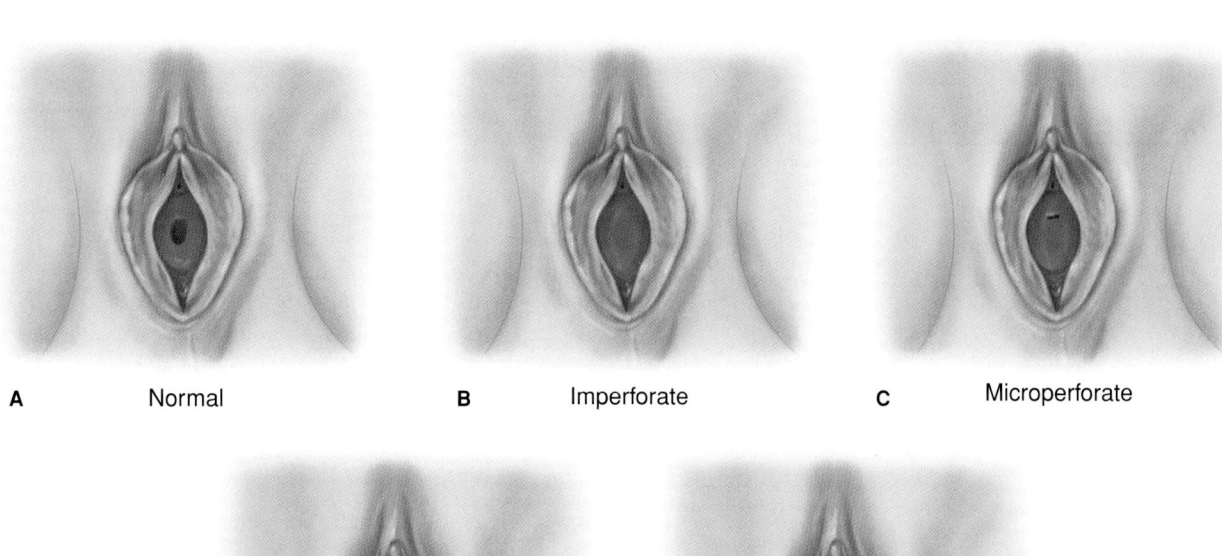

| A | Normal | B | Imperforate | C | Microperforate |

| D | Cribriform | E | Septate |

FIGURE 18-7 Types of hymens.

After menarche, adolescents with imperforate hymen present with trapped menstrual blood behind the hymen, which creates a bluish bulge at the introitus (Fig. 14-5B, p. 321). With cyclic menstruation, the vaginal canal greatly distends, and the cervix may dilate and allow formation of a hematometra and hematosalpinx. Cyclic pain, amenorrhea, abdominal pain mimicking acute abdomen, and difficulty with urination or defecation may be presenting symptoms (Bakos, 1999). Moreover, retrograde menstruation can lead to development of endometriosis. Other obstructive reproductive tract anomalies that are located more cephalad, such as transverse vaginal septum, may present similarly.

Patients with microperforate, cribriform, or septate hymen will typically complain of menstrual irregularities or difficulty with tampon placement or intercourse. Microperforate or imperforate hymen may be corrected when diagnosed and is illustrated in Section 43-17 (p. 969). Breech and Laufer (1999) advocate repair when estrogen is present to improve tissue healing, either in infancy or after thelarche, but before menarche. This timing avoids the formation of hematocolpos and possible hematometra. Laparoscopy is often performed concurrently with hymenectomy to exclude endometriosis. Importantly, clinicians should avoid needle aspiration of a hematocolpos for diagnosis or treatment. Aspiration may seed the retained blood with bacteria and increase infection risks. Moreover, recurrent hematocolpos secondary to inadequate drainage is common following needle aspiration alone.

Hymeneal cysts in the newborn must be differentiated from an imperforate hymen with hydro/mucocolpos (Nazir, 2006). These cysts typically have an opening and may regress spontaneously (Berkman, 2004). They may also be treated by incision and drainage. Simple puncture without anesthesia has also been successfully performed.

TRANSVERSE VAGINAL SEPTUM

Transverse vaginal septa are believed to arise from failed müllerian duct fusion or failed canalization of the vaginal plate (Fig. 18-8). The anomaly is uncommon, and Banerjee (1998) reported an incidence of 1 in 70,000 females. A septum may be obstructive, with mucus or menstrual blood accumulation, or nonobstructive, with mucus and blood egress.

Transverse vaginal septum can develop at any level within the vagina (Williams, 2014). Those in the upper vagina correspond to the junction between the vaginal plate and the caudal end of the fused müllerian ducts (see Fig. 18-4). Septal thickness may vary but typically is thin (1 cm). Thicker septa can measure 5 to 6 cm, and these tend to lie nearer the cervix (Rock, 1982).

In neonates and infants, obstructive transverse vaginal septum has been associated with fluid and mucus collection in the upper vagina. The resulting mass may be large enough to compress abdominal or pelvic organs. In addition, pyomucocolpos, pyometria, and pyosalpinges may develop from ascension of vaginal or perineal bacteria through small perforations within a septum (Breech, 1999). In contrast to other müllerian duct defects, transverse vaginal septum is associated with few urologic abnormalities.

Patients with transverse vaginal septum usually present with symptoms similar to those of imperforate hymen. The diagnosis

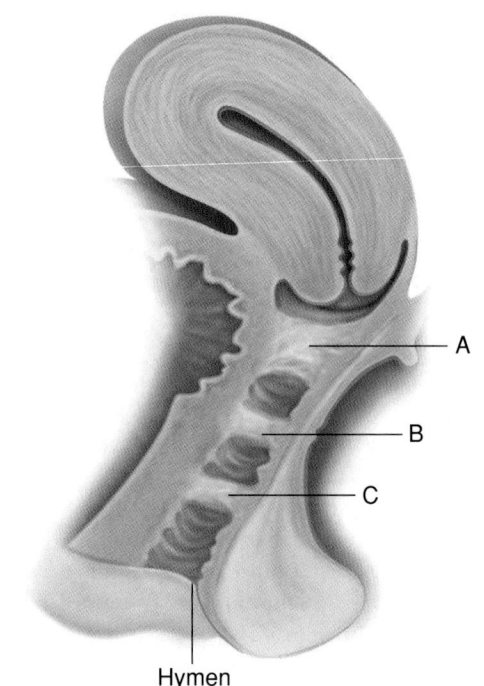

FIGURE 18-8 Potential locations of transverse vaginal septa are indicated and marked **(A–C)**. (Reproduced with permission from Rock JA, Zacur HA, Dlugi AM, et al: Pregnancy success following surgical correction of imperforate hymen and complete transverse vaginal septum, Obstet Gynecol 1982 Apr;59(4):448–451.)

is suspected when an abdominal or pelvic mass is palpated or when a foreshortened vagina and inability to identify the cervix is encountered. Diagnosis is confirmed by either sonography or magnetic resonance (MR) imaging. MR imaging is most helpful prior to surgery to determine the septal thickness and depth (Fig. 18-9). In addition, MR imaging may identify whether a cervix is present, and thereby allow differentiation of a high vaginal septum from cervical agenesis.

Surgical repair technique is dependent on septal thickness, and skin grafts or buccal mucosal grafts may occasionally be necessary to cover the defect left by excision of very thick septa. Smaller septa may be removed by excision followed by end-to-end anastomosis of the upper and lower vagina as described in Section 43-24 (p. 983). Sanfilippo (1986) recommends laparoscopy concurrently with transverse vaginal septum excision because of the high rate of endometriosis due to retrograde menstruation from outflow tract obstruction.

LONGITUDINAL VAGINAL SEPTUM

A longitudinal vaginal septum results from defective lateral fusion or incomplete reabsorption of the caudal central portion of the müllerian ducts. These septa may be partial or extend the complete vaginal length. Longitudinal septa are generally seen with partial or complete duplication of the cervix and uterus. They may also accompany anorectal malformations, and renal abnormalities are common.

Affected individuals complain of difficulty with intercourse. Vaginal bleeding may occur despite placement of a tampon, because the tampon is placed in only one of the duplicated

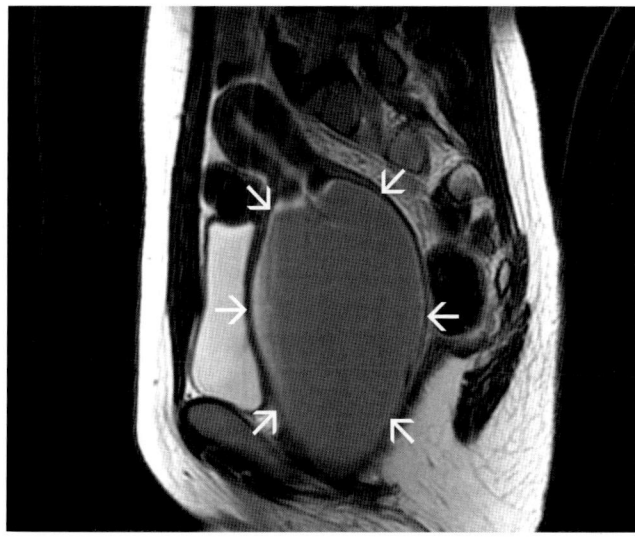

FIGURE 18-9 Magnetic resonance image of complete low transverse septum with obstruction. Marked hematocolpos is identified (*arrows*) in this 13-year-old female. The relatively low signal intensity on the T2-weighted images is consistent with subacute blood. The uterus is seen above the hematocolpos. (Used with permission from Dr. Doug Sims.)

vaginas. Nonobstructed forms can be managed conservatively unless dyspareunia develops. However, there are obstructive longitudinal vaginal septa (Fig. 18-10). Typically, the patient presents in adolescence with normal menarche, but reports worsening, monthly unilateral vaginal and pelvic pain from outflow obstruction (Carlson, 1992). During examination, a patent vagina and cervix are noted, but a unilateral vaginal and pelvic mass can be palpated. Obstructed hemivagina is almost universally associated with ipsilateral renal agenesis. The triad of uterine didelphys, obstructed hemivagina, and ipsilateral renal anomaly is the OHVIRA syndrome, also known as Herlyn-Werner-Wunderlich syndrome.

Surgical correction of a longitudinal vaginal septum consists of excision of the obstructing septum, taking precautions to avoid the urethra/bladder and rectum. With obstructive cases, sonographic guidance during excision can help in identifying the distended upper vagina (Breech, 2009). Joki-Erkkila and Heinonen (2003) followed 26 females after surgical repair of obstructive outflow tract anomalies. They found a high rate

of vaginal stricture requiring reoperation, as well as abnormal uterine bleeding, dyspareunia, and dysmenorrhea.

CONGENITAL VAGINAL CYSTS

Although in each sex the müllerian or wolffian ducts marked for degeneration normally do regress, vestigial remnants can be found and may become clinically apparent. Thus, laterally located cysts may be mesonephric (wolffian) duct remnants. The lowermost portion of the vagina derives from the urogenital sinus, which may give rise to congenital vestibular cysts (Heller, 2012).

Remnant cysts are typically located in the anterolateral wall of the vagina, although they may be found at various locations along its length. Most are asymptomatic and benign, measure 1 to 7 cm in diameter, and do not require surgical excision. Deppisch (1975) described 25 cases of symptomatic vaginal cysts and reported a wide range of symptoms. These included dyspareunia, vaginal pain, difficulty with tampon use, urinary symptoms, and palpable mass. If these cysts become infected and intervention is required during the acute phase, cyst marsupialization is preferred.

Occasionally, a remnant cyst may cause chronic symptoms and warrant excision. Pelvic MR imaging can assist prior to surgery to determine the extent of the cyst and its anatomic relationship to the ureter or bladder base (Hwang, 2009). Of note, complete vaginal cyst excision may be more difficult than anticipated, as some may extend up into the broad ligament and anatomically approximate the distal course of the ureter.

MÜLLERIAN ANOMALIES

Abnormalities of the uterus may be congenital or acquired and typically present with menstrual dysfunction, pelvic pain, infertility, or pregnancy wastage. Congenital anomalies have a heterogeneous genetic basis, and *WT1, Pax2, WNT2, PBX1,* and *HOX* genes are potentially involved (Hutson, 2014).

Various classification schemes for female reproductive tract anomalies exist, but the most commonly used system was proposed by Buttram and Gibbons (1979) and adapted by the American Society for Reproductive Medicine (former American Fertility Society, 1988). Within this system, six categories organize similar embryonic developmental defects

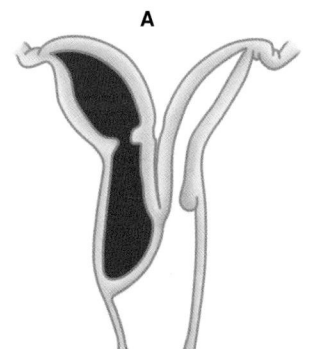 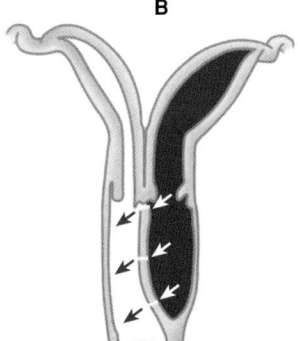 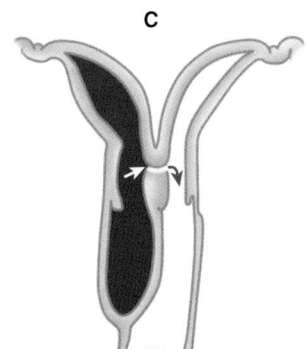

FIGURE 18-10 Uterine didelphys with obstructed hemivagina. **A.** Complete obstruction. **B.** Partial vaginal communication. **C.** Partial uterine communication. (Reproduced with permission from Rock JA, Jones HW Jr: The double uterus associated with an obstructed hemivagina and ipsilateral renal agenesis. Am J Obstet Gynecol 1980 Oct 1;138(3):339–342.)

TABLE 18-4. Classification of Müllerian Anomalies

I. Segmental müllerian hypoplasia or agenesis
   a. Vaginal
   b. Cervical
   c. Uterine
   d. Tubal
   e. Combined

II. Unicornuate uterus
   a. Rudimentary horn with cavity, communicating to unicornuate uterus
   b. Rudimentary horn with cavity, not communicating to unicornuate uterus
   c. Rudimentary horn with no cavity
   d. Unicornuate uterus without a rudimentary horn

III. Uterine didelphys

IV. Bicornuate uterus
   a. Complete bifurcation (bicollis)
   b. Partial bifurcation (unicollis)

V. Septate uterus
   a. Complete septation
   b. Partial septation

VI. Arcuate uterus

VII. Diethylstilbestrol-related anomalies

Data from American Fertility Society: The American Fertility Society classifications of adnexal adhesions, distal tubal occlusion, tubal occlusion secondary to tubal ligation, tubal pregnancies, müllerian anomalies and intrauterine adhesions, Fertil Steril 1988 Jun;49(6):944–55.

(Table 18-4). Acien (2009) and Rock (2010) have described types of uterovaginal and cervical malformations that do not adapt to the usual classification systems. Such anomalies are best described and drawn in detail in a patient's medical record for future reference.

Most cases are diagnosed during evaluation for obstetric or gynecologic problems, but in the absence of symptoms, most anomalies remain undiagnosed. Because nearly 57 percent of women with uterine defects have successful fertility and pregnancy, the true incidence of congenital müllerian defects may be significantly understated. Nahum (1998) found that the prevalence of uterine anomalies in the general population was 1 in 201 women or 0.5 percent. Dreisler and colleagues (2014) found uterine anomalies in nearly 10 percent of 622 women from the general population undergoing saline infusion sonography.

Anatomic uterine defects have long been recognized as a cause of obstetric complications. Recurrent pregnancy loss, preterm labor, abnormal fetal presentation, and prematurity constitute the major reproductive problems encountered. Cunningham and colleagues (2014a) provide a full discussion of specific müllerian abnormalities and their obstetric importance. Müllerian defects are also associated with renal anomalies in 30 to 50 percent of cases, and defects include unilateral renal agenesis, severe renal hypoplasia, horseshoe kidney, pelvic kidney, and ectopic or duplicate ureters (Sharara, 1998). Spinal anomalies have been reported in 10 to 12 percent of cases and

include wedge, supernumerary, or asymmetric and rudimentary vertebral bodies (Kimberley, 2011). The combination of müllerian and renal aplasia and cervicothoracic somite dysplasia has been described as MURCS association (Duncan, 1979). An association with Klippel-Feil syndrome has also been reported. Other anomalies associated with vaginal agenesis include ear anomalies and hearing loss, with the latter reported to be as high as 25 percent. The pattern of associated anomalies suggests an embryologic link (Kimberley, 2011).

Müllerian anomalies may be discovered during routine pelvic examinations, infertility evaluation, or surgery for other indications. Depending on clinical presentation, diagnostic tools may include hysterosalpingography (HSG), sonography, MR imaging, laparoscopy, and hysteroscopy. Each tool has limitations, but they may be used in combination to completely define anatomy. In women undergoing fertility evaluation, HSG is commonly selected for uterine cavity and tubal patency assessment. That said, HSG poorly defines the external uterine contour and can delineate only patent cavities. In other clinical settings, sonography is initially performed. Transabdominal views may help to maximize the viewing field, but transvaginal sonography (TVS) provides better image resolution. Saline infusion sonography (SIS) improves delineation of the endometrium and internal uterine morphology, but only with a patent endometrial cavity. Three-dimensional (3-D) sonography can provide uterine images from virtually any angle. Thus, coronal images can be constructed and are essential in evaluating both internal and external uterine contours. Sonography is ideally completed during the luteal phase when the secretory endometrium provides contrast from increased thickness and echogenicity (Caliskan, 2010). Several investigators have reported good concordance between 3-D TVS and MR imaging of müllerian anomalies, but MR imaging is currently preferred for imaging complex defects (Bermejo, 2010; Ghi, 2009). MR imaging provides clear delineation of both the internal and external uterine anatomy and has a reported accuracy of up to 100 percent in the evaluation of müllerian anomalies (Fedele, 1989; Pellerito, 1992). Moreover, complex anomalies and commonly associated secondary diagnoses such as renal or skeletal anomalies can be concurrently evaluated. In some women undergoing an infertility evaluation, hysteroscopy and laparoscopy may be selected to assess for müllerian anomalies; screen for endometriosis, which is often coexistent; and exclude other tubal or uterine cavity pathologies (Puscheck, 2008; Saravelos, 2008).

■ Segmental Müllerian Hypoplasia or Agenesis

Some form of müllerian aplasia, hypoplasia, or agenesis affects 1 in every 4000 to 10,000 females and is a common cause of primary amenorrhea (American College of Obstetricians and Gynecologists, 2009). Uterine agenesis follows failed development of the lower portion of the müllerian ducts during embryogenesis and usually leads to absence of the uterus, cervix, and upper part of the vagina (Oppelt, 2006). Variants may display absence of the upper vagina but presence of the uterus. Normal ovaries are found, and affected individuals otherwise develop as phenotypically normal females and present with primary amenorrhea.

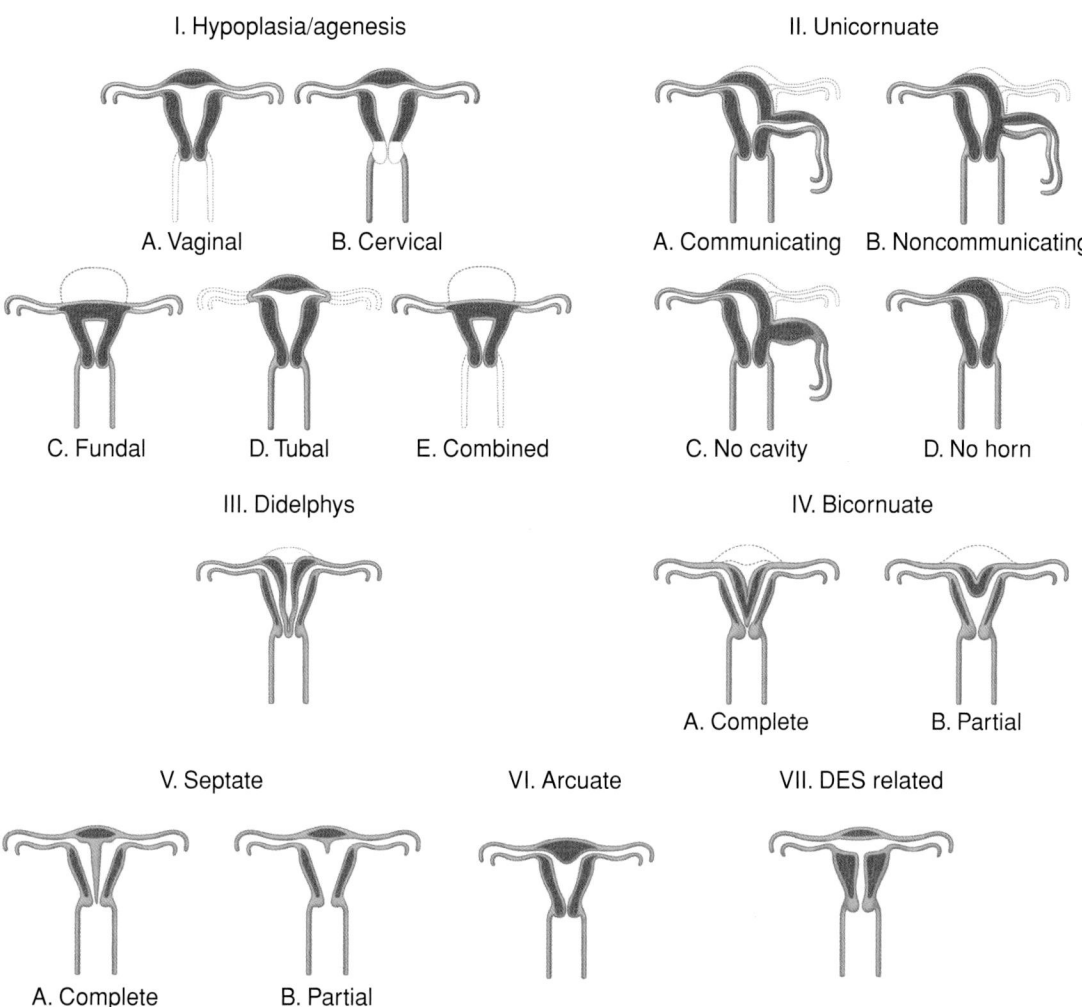

I. Hypoplasia/agenesis

A. Vaginal   B. Cervical

C. Fundal   D. Tubal   E. Combined

II. Unicornuate

A. Communicating   B. Noncommunicating

C. No cavity   D. No horn

III. Didelphys

IV. Bicornuate

A. Complete   B. Partial

V. Septate   VI. Arcuate   VII. DES related

A. Complete   B. Partial

FIGURE 18-11 Classification of müllerian anomalies. (Modified with permission from American Fertility Society: The American Fertility Society classifications of adnexal adhesions, distal tubal occlusion, tubal occlusion secondary to tubal ligation, tubal pregnancies, müllerian anomalies and intrauterine adhesions, Fertil Steril 1988 Jun;49(6):944–55.)

Vaginal Atresia

Females with vaginal atresia lack the lower portion of the vagina, but otherwise have normal pubertal maturation and external genitalia (Fig. 18-11). Embryologically, the urogenital sinus fails to contribute its expected caudal portion of the vagina (Simpson, 1999). As a result, the lower portion of the vagina, usually one-fifth to one-third of the total length, is replaced by 2 to 3 cm of fibrous tissue. In some individuals, however, vaginal atresia may extend to near the cervix.

Since most affected women have normal external genitalia and upper reproductive tract organs, vaginal atresia does not often become apparent until menarche. Adolescents generally present shortly after physiologic menarche with cyclic pelvic pain due to hematocolpos or hematometra. On physical examination, the hymeneal ring is normal. But proximal to the ring, only a vaginal dimple or small pouch is found. A rectoabdominal examination confirms midline organs. Additionally, sonographic or MR imaging will display upper reproductive tract organs. Of these, MR imaging is the most accurate diagnostic tool, as the length of the atresia, the amount of upper vaginal dilatation, and the presence of the cervix can be identified. Presence of the cervix in such cases distinguishes vaginal atresia

from müllerian agenesis. Laparoscopy, however, is often necessary when anatomy cannot be fully evaluated with radiographic studies. Treatment follows that for müllerian agenesis (p. 420).

Cervical Agenesis

Because of the common müllerian source, women with congenital absence of the cervix typically also lack the upper vagina. The uterus, however, usually develops normally (see Fig. 18-11). In addition to agenesis, Rock (2010) has described various forms of cervical dysgenesis.

Women with cervical agenesis initially present similarly to patients with other reproductive tract obstructive anomalies, that is, with primary amenorrhea and cyclic abdominal or pelvic pain. If a functional endometrium is present, a patient may have a distended uterus, and endometriosis may have developed secondary to retrograde menstrual flow. A single midline uterine fundus is the norm, although bilateral hemiuteri have also been described (Dillon, 1979).

Radiographic studies, sonography, and MR imaging aid anatomy delineation. If imaging demonstrates an obstructed uterus, hysterectomy has been recommended by some (Rock, 1984). In contrast, Niver (1980) and others report creation of an epithelialized endocervical tract and vagina. Significant morbidity, including infection, recurrent obstruction requiring hysterectomy, and death due to sepsis, however, has been reported with establishment of such a vaginal-uterine connection (Casey, 1997; Rock, 2010). Alternatively, conservative management with GnRH antagonists or agonists or with combination oral contraceptive pills may be used to suppress retrograde menses and possible endometriosis until a patient is ready for reproduction options (Doyle, 2009). Thus, the uterus may be retained for possible reproductive potential. Thijssen and associates (1990) reported a successful pregnancy using zygote intrafallopian tube transfer in a patient with cervical agenesis. Gestational surrogacy offers another viable option for these women.

Müllerian Agenesis

Congenital absence of both the uterus and vagina is termed müllerian aplasia, müllerian agenesis, or Mayer-Rokitansky-Küster-Hauser syndrome (MRKHS). In classic müllerian agenesis, patients have a shallow vaginal pouch, measuring only 1 to 2 inches deep. In addition, the uterus, cervix, and upper part of the vagina are absent. Typically, normal ovaries persist, given their separate embryonic source, and a portion of the distal fallopian tubes is present. Most patients with müllerian agenesis have only small rudimentary müllerian bulbs without endometrial activity. However, in 2 to 7 percent of women with this condition, active endometrium develops and patients typically present with cyclic abdominal pain (American College of Obstetricians and Gynecologists, 2009). Surgical excision of symptomatic rudimentary bulbs is required. With müllerian agenesis, traditional conception is impossible, but pregnancy may be achieved using oocyte retrieval, fertilization, and gestational surrogacy.

Evaluation for associated congenital renal or other skeletal anomalies is essential in individuals with müllerian hypoplasia or agenesis. As noted, approximately 15 to 36 percent of women with uterine agenesis also have defects of the urinary system, and 12 percent may have scoliosis. Skeletal malformations observed include spina bifida, sacralization (partial fusion of L5 to the sacrum), sacral bone lumbarization (nonfusion of the first and second sacral segments), and cervical vertebral anomalies. As noted earlier, MURCS syndrome displays müllerian duct aplasia, renal aplasia, and cervicothoracic somite dysplasia (Oppelt, 2006). Cardiac malformations and neurologic disturbances play a lesser role and include ventricular septal defects and unilateral hearing problems. Fifty to 60 percent of women with müllerian agenesis have secondary malformations and thus are regarded as having a complex multiorgan and multisystem syndrome.

Treatment. One treatment goal for most of these women is creation of a functional vagina. This may be accomplished conservatively or surgically. There are several conservative approaches, and each attempts to progressively invaginate the vaginal dimple to create a canal of adequate size. Graduated hard glass dilators were initially recommended by Frank (1938). Ingram (1981) modified the Frank method by affixing the dilators to a bicycle seat mounted upon a stool. This affords patients hand mobility for other activities during the 30 minutes to 2 hours spent each day for passive dilation (American College of Obstetricians and Gynecologists, 2009). Currently, firm silicon dilators are available through several medical vendors. A vagina may also be created with repeated coitus. Overall, vaginal dilatation techniques are successful in forming a functional vagina in as many as 90 percent of cases (Croak, 2003; Roberts, 2001).

Surgical procedures are seen by many as a more immediate solution to creation of a neovagina, and several methods have been reported. The method used most commonly by gynecologists is the McIndoe vaginoplasty (McIndoe, 1950). As illustrated in Section 43-25 (p. 985), a canal is created within the connective tissue between the bladder and rectum. A split-thickness skin graft obtained from the patient's buttocks or thigh is then used to line the neovagina.

Modifications of the McIndoe procedure include substitution of buccal mucosa, human amnion, or absorbable adhesion barriers as the neovaginal lining (Ashworth, 1986; Lin, 2003; Motoyama, 2003). Similarly, cutaneous or musculocutaneous flaps have been employed to line the neovagina (Williams, 1964). Also, the Davydov procedure pulls pelvic peritoneum from the pelvis into the newly created vaginal space and then to the introitus. However, bladder and ureteric injuries and vesicovaginal fistula are potential complications (Davydov, 1969).

All of these methods require a commitment to scheduled postoperative dilatation to avoid significant vaginal stricture (Breech, 1999). Accordingly, these procedures should be considered only if the patient is mature and willing to adhere to a postoperative regimen of regular intercourse or manual dilatation with dilators.

To avoid these postoperative requirements, pediatric surgeons more frequently use a segment of bowel to create the vagina. These colpoplasties most commonly use sigmoidal or ileal segments and require abdominal entry and bowel anastomosis. Many patients complain of a persistent vaginal discharge from the gastrointestinal mucosa. Kapoor (2006) reported on 14 such sigmoid vaginoplasties and noted good cosmetic results and no cases of colitis, stenosis, or excessive mucus.

Alternatively, the Vecchietti procedure uses an initial abdominal surgery to create an apparatus for passive vaginal dilatation. A synthetic sphere, attached to two wires, is placed in the vagina dimple. The wires are guided through the potential neovaginal space and into the peritoneal cavity, and then exit onto the anterior abdominal wall. The wires are placed on continuous tension, which is increased daily to stretch the blind vaginal pouch (Vecchietti, 1965).

To address uterine agenesis, uterine transplantation from a deceased donor has been described and entailed uterine harvest and revascularization. The donor uterus was supplied by its uterine and internal iliac vessels, which were anastomosed to the recipient's external iliac vessels (Ozkan, 2013). This patient with MRKH syndrome resumed menses, conceived following in vitro fertilization, but failed to sustain the gestation (Erman Akar, 2013). More work is likely to come in this area of research.

■ Unicornuate Uterus

Failure of one müllerian duct to develop and elongate results in a unicornuate uterus. This anomaly is common, and Zanetti

(1978) found an incidence of 14 percent in a series of 1160 uterine anomalies. With unicornuate uterus, a functional uterus, normal cervix, and normal round ligament and fallopian tube are found on one side. On the contralateral side, müllerian structures develop abnormally, and agenesis or more frequently a rudimentary uterine horn is identified. A rudimentary horn may communicate or more commonly not communicate with the unicornuate uterus. In addition, the endometrial cavity of the rudimentary horn may be obliterated or may contain some functioning endometrium. Active endometrium in a noncommunicating horn will eventually be symptomatic with cyclic unilateral pain and possibly with hematometra.

Women with a unicornuate uterus have an increased incidence of infertility, endometriosis, and dysmenorrhea (Fedele, 1987, 1994; Heinonen, 1983). On physical examination, the uterus is often markedly deviated, but imaging is frequently needed to further define horn anatomy (p. 418). In addition, renal sonography is performed, as 40 percent of women with a unicornuate uterus also have some degree of renal agenesis, usually ipsilateral to the anomalous side (Rackow, 2007). If anatomy is unclear, then MR imaging is selected to add information.

Women with unicornuate uterus have impaired pregnancy outcomes. A review of studies reveals a spontaneous abortion rate of 36 percent, a preterm delivery rate of 16 percent, and a live birth rate of 54 percent (Rackow, 2007). Other obstetric risks include malpresentation, fetal-growth restriction, fetal demise, and prematurely ruptured membranes (Chan, 2011; Reichman, 2009).

The pathogenesis of pregnancy loss associated with unicornuate uterus is incompletely understood, but reduced uterine capacity or anomalous distribution of the uterine artery has been suggested (Burchell, 1978). Moreover, cervical incompetence may contribute to the risk for premature delivery and second-trimester abortion. Accordingly, a unicornuate uterus is suspected in any woman with a history of pregnancy loss, premature delivery, or abnormal fetal lie.

No surgeries are currently available to enlarge the unicornuate uterus cavity. Some obstetricians recommend prophylactic cervical cerclage, but adequate trials assessing outcome are lacking. Selection of a gestational surrogate may circumvent these anatomic limitations. Other patients, however, seem to carry their pregnancies longer with each subsequent gestation and may eventually reach fetal viability prior to labor.

Pregnancy may also occur in the rudimentary horn. In noncommunicating horns, this is thought to result from the intraabdominal transit of sperm from the contralateral fallopian tube. Pregnancy in a cavitary horn regardless of communication is associated with a high rate of uterine rupture, typically prior to 20 weeks (Rolen, 1966). Because of the high maternal morbidity secondary to intraperitoneal hemorrhage, preconceptional excision of a cavitary rudimentary horn is reasonable (Heinonen, 1997; Nahum, 2002). With a rudimentary horn pregnancy, excision is indicated. Laparotomy is typical, but laparoscopy is feasible with suitable skills and well-selected cases (Kadan, 2008; Spitzer, 2009).

If the rudimentary horn is obliterated, removal is not routinely recommended. Salpingectomy or salpingo-oophorectomy on the side with the rudimentary horn, however, has been suggested to prevent ectopic pregnancy in women with a unicornuate uterus, although the ectopic pregnancy risk is low.

Uterine Didelphys

A didelphic uterus results from failed fusion of the paired müllerian ducts. This anomaly is characterized by two separated uterine horns, each with an endometrial cavity and uterine cervix. A longitudinal vaginal septum runs between the two cervices in most cases. Heinonen (1984) reported that all 26 women with uterine didelphys in his series had a longitudinal vaginal septum. Occasionally, one hemivagina is obstructed by an oblique or transverse vaginal septum (see Fig. 18-10) (Hinckley, 2003).

Uterine didelphys should be suspected if a longitudinal vaginal septum or if two separate cervices are discovered. Imaging is recommended to confirm the diagnosis as outlined on page 418.

Pregnancies develop in one of the two horns, and of the major uterine malformations, the didelphic uterus has a good reproductive prognosis. Compared with the unicornuate uterus, although the potential for uterine growth and capacity appears similar, uterine didelphys probably has an improved blood supply from collateral connections between the two horns. Alternatively, improved fetal survival may be secondary to earlier diagnosis, which favors earlier and more intensive prenatal care (Patton, 1994). Heinonen (2000) followed 36 women with uterus didelphys long term and found that 34 of 36 women (94 percent) who wanted to conceive had at least one pregnancy, and they produced 71 pregnancies. Of these pregnancies, 21 percent were spontaneously aborted, and 2 percent were ectopic. The rate for fetal survival was 75 percent; for prematurity, 24 percent; for fetal-growth restriction, 11 percent; for perinatal mortality, 5 percent; and for cesarean delivery, 84 percent. In this series, pregnancy located more often (76 percent) in the right horn than in the left. Because the spontaneous abortion rate mirrors that of women with normal uterine cavities, surgical procedures in response to pregnancy loss are rarely indicated. Thus, surgery should be reserved and only considered for highly selected patients in whom repeated late-trimester losses or premature delivery has occurred with no other apparent etiology.

Bicornuate Uterus

This anomaly is caused by incomplete fusion of the müllerian ducts. It is characterized by two separate but communicating endometrial cavities and a single uterine cervix. Failed fusion may extend to the cervix, resulting in a complete bicornuate uterus, or may be partial, causing a milder abnormality. Women with a bicornuate uterus can expect reasonable success—approximately 60 percent—in delivering a living child. As with many uterine anomalies, premature delivery is a substantial obstetric risk. Heinonen and colleagues (1982) reported a 28-percent abortion rate and a 20-percent incidence of premature labor in women with a partial bicornuate uterus. Women with a complete bicornuate uterus had a 66-percent incidence of preterm delivery and a lower fetal survival rate.

Radiologic discrimination of bicornuate uterus from the septate uterus can be challenging, however, it is important

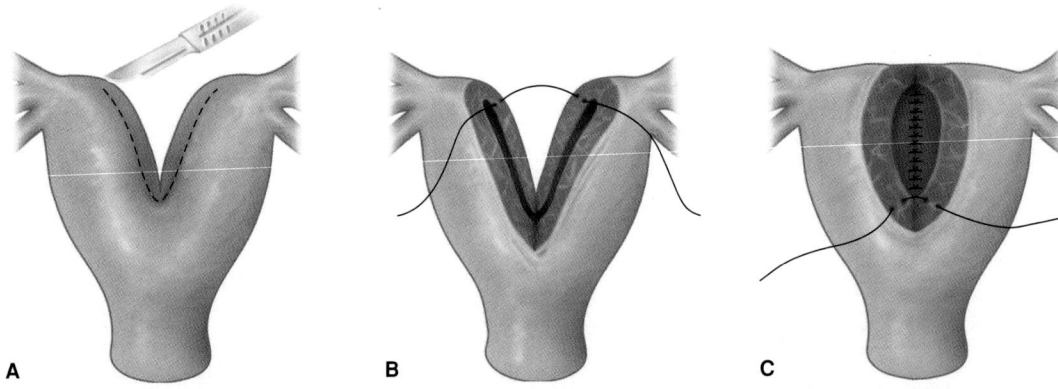

FIGURE 18-12 Strassman metroplasty is one of several techniques of bicornuate uterus repair. **A.** Excision of intervening uterine wall. **B.** Reapproximation of posterior uterine wall with a layer of myometrial sutures. **C.** Reapproximation of the anterior wall is closed similarly. Following placement of myometrial sutures, a layer of subserosal sutures is placed in the anterior and posterior walls.

because septate uterus is easily treated with hysteroscopic septal resection. Widely diverging horns seen on HSG may suggest a bicornuate uterus. An intercornual angle >105 degrees suggests bicornuate uterus, whereas one <75 degrees indicates a septate uterus. However, MR imaging is necessary to define fundal contour. With this, an intrafundal downward cleft measuring ≥1 cm is indicative of bicornuate uterus, whereas a cleft depth <1 cm indicates a septate uterus. Use of 3-D sonography also allows internal and external uterine assessment. Thus, sonography and HSG seem acceptable imaging techniques in the initial investigation. When the presumptive diagnosis is a septate uterus, laparoscopy may be performed for a definitive diagnosis and before hysteroscopic resection of the septum is initiated.

Surgical reconstruction of the bicornuate uterus is infrequently done but has been advocated in women with multiple spontaneous abortions in whom no other causative factors are identified. Strassman (1952) described the surgical technique that unified equal-sized endometrial cavities (Fig. 18-12). Reproductive outcome after unification generally has been good. In 289 women, preoperative pregnancy loss was more than 70 percent. Following surgery, more than 85 percent of pregnancies resulted in delivery of a viable infant. The actual benefit of metroplasty for a bicornuate uterus, however, has not been tested in a controlled clinical series. As in surgery for uterine didelphys, metroplasty is reserved for women in whom recurrent pregnancy loss occurs with no other identifiable cause.

■ Septate Uterus

Following fusion of the müllerian ducts, failure of their medial segments to regress can create a permanent septum within the uterine cavity. Its contours can vary widely and depend on the amount of persistent midline tissue. The septum can project minimally from the uterine fundus or can extend completely to the cervical os. Moreover, septa can develop segmentally, resulting in partial communications of the partitioned uterus (Patton, 1994). The histologic structure of septa ranges from fibrous to fibromuscular.

The true incidence of these anomalies is not known because they are usually detected only in women with obstetric complications. Although this defect does not predispose to increase rates of preterm labor or cesarean delivery, septate uterus is associated with a marked increase in spontaneous abortion rates (Heinonen, 2006). Woelfer and associates (2001) reported a first-trimester spontaneous abortion rate for septate uterus of 42 percent. Moreover, early pregnancy loss is significantly more common with a septate than with a bicornuate uterus (Proctor, 2003).

This extraordinarily high pregnancy wastage likely results from partial or complete implantation on a largely avascular septum, from distortion of the uterine cavity, and from associated cervical or endometrial abnormalities. Based on operative experience for septal defects, the blood supply to the fibromuscular septum appears markedly reduced compared with normal myometrium. In addition to spontaneous abortion, septate uterus may rarely cause fetal malformation, and Heinonen (1999) described three newborns with a limb-reduction defect born to women with septate uterus.

Diagnosis of the septate uterus follows guidelines established for the bicornuate uterus and includes HSG and/or sonography. Historically, abdominal metroplasty for septate uterus was shown to dramatically decrease fetal wastage and ultimately improve fetal survival rates (Rock, 1977; Blum, 1977). Two main disadvantages to metroplasty include the requirement of cesarean delivery to prevent uterine rupture in subsequent pregnancy and the high rate of postoperative pelvic adhesion formation and subsequent infertility.

Currently, hysteroscopic septum resection is an effective and safe alternative to treat women with septate uterus (Section 44-17, p. 1048). Typically, operative hysteroscopy is combined with concurrent laparoscopic surveillance to reduce the risk of uterine perforation. After the initial case reports by Chervenak and Neuwirth (1981), many investigators have confirmed satisfactory live birth rates with the procedure (Daly, 1983; DeCherney, 1983; Israel, 1984). In a retrospective review, Fayez (1986) evaluated reproductive outcome in women who had either an abdominal metroplasty or hysteroscopic septoplasty. They noted an 87-percent live birth rate in the hysteroscopic group compared with a 70-percent rate in the abdominal group. Similarly, Daly and associates (1989) reported impressive results after hysteroscopic surgery. Proponents of hysteroscopic resection describe reduced rates of pelvic adhesions, shortened postoperative convalescence, lowered operative morbidity, and avoidance of mandatory cesarean delivery (Patton, 1994).

Arcuate Uterus

An arcuate uterus displays only mild deviation from normal uterine development. Anatomic hallmarks include a slight midline septum within a broad fundus, sometimes with minimal fundal cavity indentation. Most clinicians report no impact on reproductive outcomes. Conversely, Woelfer and colleagues (2001) found excessive second-trimester losses and preterm labor. Surgical resection is indicated only if excessive rates of pregnancy loss are encountered and other etiologies for recurrent spontaneous abortion have been excluded.

Diethylstilbestrol-Induced Reproductive Tract Abnormalities

Diethylstilbestrol (DES), a synthetic nonsteroidal estrogen, was prescribed to an estimated 3 million pregnant women in the United States from the late 1940s through the early 1960s. Early reports claimed the drug was useful in treating abortion, preeclampsia, diabetes, hot flushes, and preterm labor (Massé, 2009). It was ineffective for these indications. Almost 20 years later, Herbst and coworkers (1971) found that DES exposure in utero was linked to the development of a "T-shaped" uterus and an increased incidence of clear cell adenocarcinomas of the vagina and cervix. The risk of this vaginal malignancy approximates 1 in 1000 exposed daughters. Daughters also have increased risks of developing vaginal and cervical intraepithelial neoplasia, suggesting that DES exposure could affect gene regulation (Herbst, 2000). DES has also been shown to suppress the *WNT4* gene and alter *Hox* gene expression in mouse müllerian ducts. This provides a plausible molecular mechanism for the uterine abnormalities, vaginal adenosis, and rarely, carcinoma observed in exposed patients (Massé, 2009).

During normal development, the vagina is originally lined by a glandular epithelium derived from the müllerian ducts. By the end of the second trimester, this layer is replaced by squamous epithelium extending up from the urogenital sinus. Failure of the squamous epithelium to completely line the vagina is termed adenosis. Although variable, it typically appears red, punctate, and granular. Common symptoms include vaginal irritation, discharge, and metrorrhagia—in particular, postcoital bleeding. Moreover, adenosis is frequently associated with vaginal clear cell adenocarcinoma.

Genitourinary malformations following DES exposure in utero have also been noted and include those of the cervix, vagina, uterine cavity, and fallopian tubes. Transverse septa, circumferential ridges involving the vagina and cervix, and cervical collars ("cockscomb cervix") have been found. Women with cervicovaginal abnormalities are more likely to have uterine anomalies, such as smaller uterine cavities, shortened upper uterine segments, and "T-shaped" and irregular cavities (Barranger, 2002). Fallopian tube abnormalities include shortened and narrowed dimensions and absent fimbria.

Males exposed to DES in utero also have structural abnormalities. Cryptorchidism, testicular hypoplasia, microphallus, and hypospadias have been reported (Hernandez-Diaz, 2002).

Women exposed to DES, in general, have impaired conception rates (Senekjian, 1988). Reduced fertility in these women is poorly understood but is associated with cervical hypoplasia

and atresia. Of those who do conceive, the incidences of spontaneous pregnancy loss, ectopic pregnancy, and preterm delivery are increased, again particularly in those with associated structural abnormalities (Goldberg, 1999). Now, more than 50 years after DES use was proscribed, most affected women are past childbearing age, but higher rates of earlier menopause and breast cancer have been reported (Hatch, 2006; Hoover, 2011).

FALLOPIAN TUBE ANOMALIES

The fallopian tubes develop from the unpaired cephalad ends of the müllerian ducts. Congenital anomalies of the fallopian tube include accessory ostia, complete or segmental absence of the fallopian tube, and several embryonic cystic remnants. The remnants of the mesonephric duct in the female include a few blind tubules, the *epoophoron*, in the mesovarium, and similar ones, collectively called the *paroophoron*, adjacent to the uterus (see Fig. 18-2F) (Moore, 2013). The epoophoron or paroophoron may develop into clinically identifiable cysts.

Remnants of the müllerian duct may be found along its embryologic course. The most common is a small, blind cystic structure attached by a pedicle to the distal end of the fallopian tube, the hydatid of Morgagni (Zheng, 2009).

Paratubal cysts are frequent incidental discoveries during gynecologic operations for other abnormalities or are found on sonographic examination (Chap. 9, p. 223). They may be of mesonephric, paramesonephric, or mesothelial origin. Most cysts are asymptomatic and slow growing and are discovered during the third and fourth decades of life.

In utero exposure to DES has been associated with various tubal abnormalities. Short, tortuous tubes or ones with shriveled fimbria and small ostia have been linked to infertility (DeCherney, 1981).

OVARIAN ANOMALIES

A *supernumerary ovary* is an ectopic ovary that has no connection with the broad, uteroovarian, or infundibulopelvic ligaments (Wharton, 1959). This rare gynecologic anomaly may be located in the pelvis, retroperitoneum, paraaortic area, colonic mesentery, or omentum. Aberrant migration of part of the genital ridge after incorporation of germ cells describes one theory (Printz, 1973).

In contrast, the term *accessory ovary* describes excess ovarian tissue nearby and connected to a normally placed ovary. Wharton (1959) estimated that both accessory ovary and supernumerary ovary were rare, finding approximately 1 case of accessory ovary in 93,000 patients and 1 case of supernumerary ovary in 29,000 autopsies. In Wharton's review, 3 of 4 patients with supernumerary ovary and 5 of 19 patients with accessory ovary had additional congenital defects, most frequently involving the genitourinary tract.

An absent ovary, with or without an associated tube, may result from congenital agenesis or from ovarian torsion with necrosis and reabsorption (Eustace, 1992; James, 1970). The incidence has been suggested to be approximately 1 in 11,240 women (Sivanesaratnam, 1986).

REFERENCES

Acien P, Acien M, Sanchez-Ferrer ML: Müllerian anomalies "without a classification": from the didelphys-unicollis uterus to the bicervical uterus with or without septate vagina. Fertil Steril 91(6):2369, 2009

Aksglaede L, Juul A: Testicular function and fertility in men and Klinefelter syndrome: a review. Eur J Endocrinol 168(4):R67, 2013

American College of Obstetricians and Gynecologists: Vaginal agenesis: diagnosis, management, and routine care. Committee Opinion No. 355, December 2006, Reaffirmed 2009

American Fertility Society: The American Fertility Society classifications of adnexal adhesions, distal tubal occlusion, tubal occlusion secondary to tubal ligation, tubal pregnancies, müllerian anomalies and intrauterine adhesions. Fertil Steril 49(6):944, 1988

Arboleda VA, Sandberg DE, Vilain E: DSDs: genetics, underlying pathologies and psychosexual differentiation. Nat Rev Endocrinol 10(10):603, 2014

Ashworth MF, Morton KE, Dewhurst J, et al: Vaginoplasty using amnion. Obstet Gynecol 67(3):443, 1986

Bakos O, Berglund L: Imperforate hymen and ruptured hematosalpinx: a case report with a review of the literature. J Adolesc Health 24(3):226, 1999

Bangsboll S, Qvist I, Lebech PE, et al: Testicular feminization syndrome and associated gonadal tumors in Denmark. Acta Obstet Gynecol Scand 71(1):63, 1992

Barranger E, Gervaise A, Doumerc S, et al: Reproductive performance after hysteroscopic metroplasty in the hypoplastic uterus: a study of 29 cases. BJOG 109(12):1331, 2002

Berkman DS, McHugh MT, Shapiro E: The other interlabial mass: hymenal cyst. J Urol 171(5):1914, 2004

Bermejo C, Martinez, Ten P, et al: Three-dimensional ultrasound in the diagnosis of Müllerian duct anomalies and concordance with magnetic resonance imaging. Ultrasound Obstet Gynecol 35:593, 2010

Blackless M, Charuvastra A, Derryck A, et al: How sexually dimorphic are we? Review and synthesis. Am J Hum Biol 12(2):151, 2000

Blaschko SD, Cunha GR, Baskin LS: Molecular mechanisms of external genitalia development. Differentiation 84(3):261, 2012

Blum M: Prevention of spontaneous abortion by cervical suture of the malformed uterus. Int Surg 62(4):213, 1977

Breech LL, Laufer MR: Müllerian anomalies. Obstet Gynecol Clin North Am 36(1):47, 2009

Breech LL, Laufer MR: Obstructive anomalies of the female reproductive tract. J Reprod Med 44(3):233, 1999

Burchell RC, Creed F, Rasoulpour M, et al: Vascular anatomy of the human uterus and pregnancy wastage. Br J Obstet Gynaecol 85(9):698, 1978

Buttram VC Jr, Gibbons WE: Müllerian anomalies: a proposed classification. (An analysis of 144 cases.) Fertil Steril 32(1):40, 1979

Caliskan E, Ozkan S, Cakiroglu Y, et al: Diagnostic accuracy of real-time 3D sonography in the diagnosis of congenital Mullerian anomalies in high-risk patients with respect to the phase of the menstrual cycle. J Clin Ultrasound 38(3):123, 2010

Carlson RL, Garmel GM: Didelphic uterus and unilaterally imperforate double vagina as an unusual presentation of right lower-quadrant abdominal pain. Ann Emerg Med 21(8):1006, 1992

Casey AC, Laufer MR: Cervical agenesis: septic death after surgery. Obstet Gynecol 90(4 Pt 2):706, 1997

Chan YY, Jayaprakasan K, Tan A, et al: Reproductive outcomes in women with congenital uterine anomalies: a systematic review. Ultrasound Obstet Gynecol 38(4):371, 2011

Chavhan GB, Parra DA, Oudjhane K, et al: Imaging of ambiguous genitalia: classification and diagnostic approach. Radiographics 28(7):1891, 2008

Chervenak FA, Neuwirth RS: Hysteroscopic resection of the uterine septum. Am J Obstet Gynecol 141(3):351, 1981

Croak AJ, Gebhart JB, Klingele CJ, et al: Therapeutic strategies for vaginal müllerian agenesis. J Reprod Med 48(6):395, 2003

Cunningham FG, Leveno KJ, Bloom SL (eds): Congenital genitourinary abnormalities. In Williams Obstetrics, 24th ed. New York, McGraw-Hill, 2014a, p 39

Cunningham FG, Leveno KJ, Bloom SL (eds): Embryogenesis and fetal morphological development. In Williams Obstetrics, 24th ed. New York, McGraw-Hill, 2014b, p 146

Cunningham FG, Leveno KJ, Bloom SL (eds): Placentation, embryogenesis, and fetal development. In Williams Obstetrics, 24th ed. New York, McGraw-Hill, 2014c, p 110

Daaboul J, Frader J: Ethics and the management of the patient with intersex: a middle way. J Pediatr Endocrinol Metab 14(9):1575, 2001

Daly DC, Maier D, Soto-Albors C: Hysteroscopic metroplasty: six years' experience. Obstet Gynecol 73(2):201, 1989

Daly DC, Walters CA, Soto-Albors CE, et al: Hysteroscopic metroplasty: surgical technique and obstetric outcome. Fertil Steril 39(5):623, 1983

Davydov SN: Colpopoeisis from the peritoneum of the uterorectal space. Akush Ginekok (Mosk) 45(12):55, 1969

DeCherney AH, Cholst I, Naftolin F: Structure and function of the fallopian tubes following exposure to diethylstilbestrol (DES) during gestation. Fertil Steril 36(6):741, 1981

DeCherney A, Polan ML: Hysteroscopic management of intrauterine lesions and intractable uterine bleeding. Obstet Gynecol 61(3):392, 1983

Deppisch LM: Cysts of the vagina: classification and clinical correlations. Obstet Gynecol 45(6):632, 1975

Dershwitz RA, Levitsky LL, Feingold M: Picture of the month. Vulvovaginitis: a cause of clitorimegaly. Am J Dis Child 138(9):887, 1984

de Vries AL, Doreleijers TA, Cohen-Kettenis PT: Disorders of sex development and gender identity outcome in adolescence and adulthood: understanding general identity development and its clinical implications. Pediatr Endocrinol Rev 4:343, 2007

Dillon WP, Mudaliar NA, Wingate MB: Congenital atresia of the cervix. Obstet Gynecol 54(1):126, 1979

Doyle JO, Laufer MR: Mayer-Rokitansky-Kuster-Hauser (MRKH) syndrome with a single septate uterus: a novel anomaly and description of treatment options. Fertil Steril 92(1):391, 2009

Dreisler E, Stampe Sørensen S: Müllerian duct anomalies diagnosed by saline contrast sonohysterography: prevalence in a general population. Fertil Steril 102(2):525, 2014

Duncan PA, Shapiro LR, Stangel JJ, et al: The MURCS association: Müllerian duct aplasia, renal aplasia, and cervicothoracic somite dysplasia. J Pediatr 95:399, 1979

Elder J: Congenital anomalies of the genitalia. In Walsh PC, Retik AB, Stamey TA, et al (eds): Campbell's Urology. Philadelphia, Saunders, 1992, p 1920

Erman Akar M, Ozkan O, Aydinuraz B, et al: Clinical pregnancy after uterine transplantation. Fertil Steril 100(5):1358, 2013

Eustace DL: Congenital absence of fallopian tube and ovary. Eur J Obstet Gynecol Reprod Biol 46(2–3):157, 1992

Fayez JA: Comparison between abdominal and hysteroscopic metroplasty. Obstet Gynecol 68(3):399, 1986

Fedele L, Dorta M, Brioschi D, et al: Magnetic resonance evaluation of double uteri. Obstet Gynecol 74:844, 1989

Fedele L, Zamberletti D, Vercellini P, et al: Reproductive performance of women with unicornuate uterus. Fertil Steril 47(3):416, 1987

Frank RT: The formation of an artificial vagina without an operation. Am J Obstet Gynecol 141:910, 1938

Fukami M, Homma K, Hasegawa T, et al: Backdoor pathway for dihydrotestosterone biosynthesis: implications for normal and abnormal human sex development. Dev Dyn 242(4):320, 2013

Ghi T, Casadio P, Kuleva M, et al: Accuracy of three-dimensional ultrasound in diagnosis and classification of congenital uterine anomalies. Fertil Steril 92(2):808, 2009

Goldberg JM, Falcone T: Effect of diethylstilbestrol on reproductive function. Fertil Steril 72(1):1, 1999

Greer DM Jr, Pederson WC: Pseudo-masculinization of the phallus. Plast Reconstr Surg 68(5):787, 1981

Hatch EE, Troisi R, Wise LA, et al: Age at natural menopause in women exposed to diethylstilbestrol in utero. Am J Epidemiol 164:682, 2006

Heinonen PK: Clinical implications of the didelphic uterus: long-term follow-up of 49 cases. Eur J Obstet Gynecol Reprod Biol 91(2):183, 2000

Heinonen PK: Clinical implications of the unicornuate uterus with rudimentary horn. Int J Gynaecol Obstet 21(2):145, 1983

Heinonen PK: Complete septate uterus with longitudinal vaginal septum. Fertil Steril 85(3):700, 2006

Heinonen PK: Limb anomalies among offspring of women with a septate uterus: a report of three cases. Early Hum Dev 56(2–3):179, 1999

Heinonen PK: Unicornuate uterus and rudimentary horn. Fertil Steril 68(2):224, 1997

Heinonen PK: Uterus didelphys: a report of 26 cases. Eur J Obstet Gynecol Reprod Biol 17(5):345, 1984

Heinonen PK, Saarikoski S, Pystynen P: Reproductive performance of women with uterine anomalies. An evaluation of 182 cases. Acta Obstet Gynecol Scand 61(2):157, 1982

Heller DS: Vaginal cysts: a pathology review. J Lower Genit Tract Dis 16(2):140, 2012

Herbst AL: Behavior of estrogen-associated female genital tract cancer and its relation to neoplasia following intrauterine exposure to diethylstilbestrol (DES). Gynecol Oncol 76(2):147, 2000

Herbst AL, Ulfelder H, Poskanzer DC: Adenocarcinoma of the vagina. Association of maternal stilbestrol therapy with tumor appearance in young women. N Engl J Med 284(15):878, 1971

Hernandez-Diaz S: Iatrogenic legacy from diethylstilbestrol exposure. Lancet 359(9312):1081, 2002

Hinckley MD, Milki AA: Management of uterus didelphys, obstructed hemivagina and ipsilateral renal agenesis. A case report. J Reprod Med 48(8):649, 2003

Hoover RN, Hyer M, Pfeiffer RM, et al: Adverse health outcomes in women exposed in utero to diethylstilbestrol. N Engl J Med 365:1304, 2011

Hughes IA, Houk C, Ahmed SF, et al: Consensus statement on management of intersex disorders. J Pediatr Urol 2(3):148, 2006

Hutson JM, Grover SR, O'Connell M, et al: Malformation syndromes associated with disorders of sex development. Nat Rev Endocrinol 10(8):476, 2014

Hwang JH, Oh MJ, Lee NW, et al: Multiple vaginal müllerian cysts: a case report and review of literature. Arch Gynecol Obstet 280(1):137, 2009

Ingram JM: The bicycle seat stool in the treatment of vaginal agenesis and stenosis: a preliminary report. Am J Obstet Gynecol 140(8):867, 1981

Israel R, March CM: Hysteroscopic incision of the septate uterus. Am J Obstet Gynecol 149(1):66, 1984

James DF, Barber HR, Graber EA: Torsion of normal uterine adnexa in children. Report of three cases. Obstet Gynecol 35(2):226, 1970

Johnson LT, Lara-Torre E, Murchison AM, et al: Large epidermal cyst of the clitoris: a novel diagnostic approach to assist in surgical removal. J Pediatr Adolesc Gynecol 26(2):e33, 2013

Joki-Erkkila MM, Heinonen PK: Presenting and long-term clinical implications and fecundity in females with obstructing vaginal malformations. J Pediatr Adolesc Gynecol 16(5):307, 2003

Jones HW Jr: An anomaly of the external genitalia in female patients with exstrophy of the bladder. Am J Obstet Gynecol 117(6):748, 1973

Kadan Y, Romano S: Rudimentary horn pregnancy diagnosed by ultrasound and treated by laparoscopy—a case report and review of the literature. J Minim Invasive Gynecol 15(5):527, 2008

Kapoor R, Sharma DK, Singh KJ, et al: Sigmoid vaginoplasty: long-term results. Urology 67(6):1212, 2006

Karlin G, Brock W, Rich M, et al: Persistent cloaca and phallic urethra. J Urol 142(4):1056, 1989

Kenney PJ, Spirt BA, Leeson MD: Genitourinary anomalies: radiologic-anatomic correlations. RadioGraphics 4:233, 1984

Kimberley N, Hutson JM, Southwell BR, et al: Vaginal agenesis, the hymen, and associated anomalies. J Pediatr Adolesc Gynecol 25:54, 2012

Laterza RM, De Gennaro M, Tubaro A, et al: Female pelvic congenital malformations. Part I: embryology, anatomy and surgical treatment. Eur J Obstet Gynecol Reprod Biol 159:26, 2011

Lee PA, Houk CP, Ahmed, et al: Consensus statement on management of intersex disorders. Pediatrics 118:488, 2006

Lin WC, Chang CY, Shen YY, et al: Use of autologous buccal mucosa for vaginoplasty: a study of eight cases. Hum Reprod 18(3):604, 2003

Lloyd JC, Wiener JS, Gargollo PC, et al: Contemporary epidemiological trends in complex congenital genitourinary anomalies. J Urol 190(4 Suppl):1590, 2013

MacLaughlin DT, Donahoe PK: Sex determination and differentiation. N Engl J Med 350(4):367, 2004

Marshall FF: Embryology of the lower genitourinary tract. Urol Clin North Am 5(1):3, 1978

Massanyi EZ, Gearhart JP, Kost-Byerly S: Perioperative management of classic bladder exstrophy. Res Rep Urol 5:67, 2013

Massé J, Watrin T, Laurent A, et al: The developing female genital tract: from genetics to epigenetics. Int J Dev Biol 53(2–3):411, 2009

McIndoe A: The treatment of congenital absence and obliterative conditions of the vagina. Br J Plast Surg 2(4):254, 1950

Moore KL, Persaud TVN, Torchia MG: The urogenital system. In The Developing Human. Philadelphia, Saunders, 2013, p 245

Motoyama S, Laoag-Fernandez JB, Mochizuki S, et al: Vaginoplasty with Interceed absorbable adhesion barrier for complete squamous epithelialization in vaginal agenesis. Am J Obstet Gynecol 188(5):1260, 2003

Murphy C, Allen L, Jamieson MA: Ambiguous genitalia in the newborn: an overview and teaching tool. J Pediatr Adolesc Gynecol 24:236, 2011

Nagai K, Murakami Y, Nagatani K, et al: Life-threatening acute renal failure due to imperforate hymen in an infant. Pediatr Int 54(2):280, 2012

Nahum GG: Rudimentary uterine horn pregnancy. The 20th-century worldwide experience of 588 cases. J Reprod Med 47(2):151, 2002

Nahum GG: Uterine anomalies. How common are they, and what is their distribution among subtypes? J Reprod Med 43(10):877, 1998

Nakhal RS, Deans R, Creighton SM, et al: Genital prolapse in adult women with classical bladder exstrophy. Int Urogynecol J 23(9):120, 2012

Nazir Z, Rizvi RM, Qureshi RN, et al: Congenital vaginal obstructions: varied presentation and outcome. Pediatr Surg Int 22(9):749, 2006

New MI, Abraham M, Yuen T, et al: An update on prenatal diagnosis and treatment of congenital adrenal hyperplasia. Semin Reprod Med 30(5):396, 2012

Nistal M, Paniagua R, Gonzalez-Peramato P, et al: Gonadal dysgenesis. Pediatr Dev Pathol 18(4):259, 2015

Nistal M, Paniagua R, Gonzalez-Peramato P, et al: Klinefelter syndrome and other anomalies in X and Y chromosomes. Clinical and pathological entities. Pediatr Dev Pathol Aug 8, 2014 [Epub ahead of print]

Niver DH, Barrette G, Jewelewicz R: Congenital atresia of the uterine cervix and vagina: three cases. Fertil Steril 33(1):25, 1980

Ocal G: Current concepts in disorders of sexual development. J Clin Res Pediatr Endocrinol 3(3):105, 2011

Oppelt P, Renner SP, Kellermann A, et al: Clinical aspects of Mayer-Rokitansky-Kuster-Hauser syndrome: recommendations for clinical diagnosis and staging. Hum Reprod 21(3):792, 2006

Ozkan O, Akar ME, Erdogan O, et al: Preliminary results of the first human uterus transplantation from a multiorgan donor. Fertil Steril 99(2):470, 2013

Parazzini F, Cecchetti G: The frequency of imperforate hymen in northern Italy. Int J Epidemiol 19(3):763, 1990

Park SY, Jameson JL: Minireview: transcriptional regulation of gonadal development and differentiation. Endocrinology 146(3):1035, 2005

Patton PE: Anatomic uterine defects. Clin Obstet Gynecol 37(3):705, 1994

Pellerito JS, McCarthy SM, Doyle MB, et al: Diagnosis of uterine anomalies: relative accuracy of MR imaging, endovaginal sonography, and hysterosalpingography. Radiology 183(3):795, 1992

Printz JL, Choate JW, Townes PL, et al: The embryology of supernumerary ovaries. Obstet Gynecol 41(2):246, 1973

Proctor JA, Haney AF: Recurrent first trimester pregnancy loss is associated with uterine septum but not with bicornuate uterus. Fertil Steril 80(5):1212, 2003

Puscheck EE, Cohen L: Congenital malformations of the uterus: the role of ultrasound. Semin Reprod Med 26(3):223, 2008

Rackow BW, Arici A: Reproductive performance of women with müllerian anomalies. Curr Opin Obstet Gynecol 19(3):229, 2007

Reichman D, Laufer MR, Robinson BK: Pregnancy outcomes in unicornuate uteri: a review. Fertil Steril 91(5):1886, 2009

Roberts CP, Haber MJ, Rock JA: Vaginal creation for müllerian agenesis. Am J Obstet Gynecol 185(6):1349, 2001

Rock JA, Jones HW Jr: The clinical management of the double uterus. Fertil Steril 28(8):798, 1977

Rock JA, Jones HW Jr: The double uterus associated with an obstructed hemivagina and ipsilateral renal agenesis. Am J Obstet Gynecol 138(3):339, 1980

Rock JA, Roberts CP, Jones HW Jr: Congenital anomalies of the uterine cervix: lessons from 30 cases managed clinically by a common protocol. Fertil Steril 94(5):1858, 2010

Rock JA, Schlaff WD, Zacur HA, et al: The clinical management of congenital absence of the uterine cervix. Int J Gynaecol Obstet 22(3):231, 1984

Rock JA, Zacur HA, Dlugi AM, et al: Pregnancy success following surgical correction of imperforate hymen and complete transverse vaginal septum. Obstet Gynecol 59(4):448, 1982

Rolen AC, Choquette AJ, Semmens JP: Rudimentary uterine horn: obstetric and gynecologic implications. Obstet Gynecol 27(6):806, 1966

Ross AJ, Capel B: Signaling at the crossroads of gonad development. Trends Endocrinol Metab 16(1):19, 2005

Sanfilippo JS, Wakim NG, Schikler KN, et al: Endometriosis in association with uterine anomaly. Am J Obstet Gynecol 154(1):39, 1986

Saravelos SH, Cocksedge KA, Li TC: Prevalence and diagnosis of congenital uterine anomalies in women with reproductive failure: a critical appraisal. Hum Reprod Update 14(5):415, 2008

Schey WL, Kandel G, Charles AG: Female epispadias: report of a case and review of the literature. Clin Pediatr (Phila) 19(3):212, 1980

Senekjian EK, Potkul RK, Frey K, et al: Infertility among daughters either exposed or not exposed to diethylstilbestrol. Am J Obstet Gynecol 158(3 Pt 1):493, 1988

Sharara FI: Complete uterine septum with cervical duplication, longitudinal vaginal septum and duplication of a renal collecting system. A case report. J Reprod Med 43(12):1055, 1998

Shatzkes DR, Haller JO, Velcek FT: Imaging of uterovaginal anomalies in the pediatric patient. Urol Radiol 13(1):58, 1991

Shehata BM, Elmore JM, Bootwala Y, et al: Immunohistochemical characterization of sonic hedgehog and its downstream signaling molecules during human penile development. Fetal Pediatr Pathol 30(4):244, 2011

Simpson JL: Genetics of the female reproductive ducts. Am J Med Genet 89(4):224, 1999

Sivanesaratnam V: Unexplained unilateral absence of ovary and fallopian tube. Eur J Obstet Gynecol Reprod Biol 22(1–2):103, 1986

Sotolongo JR Jr, Gribetz ME, Saphir RL, et al: Female phallic urethra and persistent cloaca. J Urol 130(6):1186, 1983

Spitzer RF, Kives S, Allen LM: Case series of laparoscopically resected noncommunicating functional uterine horns. J Pediatr Adolesc Gynecol 22(1):e23, 2009

Stanton SL: Gynecologic complications of epispadias and bladder exstrophy. Am J Obstet Gynecol 119(6):749, 1974

Stelling JR, Gray MR, Davis AJ, et al: Dominant transmission of imperforate hymen. Fertil Steril 74(6):1241, 2000

Strassman E: Plastic unification of double uterus. Am J Obstet Gynecol 64(1):25, 1952

Taylor HS: The role of HOX genes in the development and function of the female reproductive tract. Semin Reprod Med 18(1):81, 2000

Thijssen RF, Hollanders JM, Willemsen WN, et al: Successful pregnancy after ZIFT in a patient with congenital cervical atresia. Obstet Gynecol 76(5 Pt 2):902, 1990

Thyen U, Lanz K, Holterhus PM, et al: Epidemiology and initial management of ambiguous genitalia at birth in Germany. Horm Res 66(4):195, 2006

Usta IM, Awwad JT, Usta JA, et al: Imperforate hymen: report of an unusual familial occurrence. Obstet Gynecol 82(4 Pt 2 Suppl):655, 1993

Vecchietti G: [Creation of an artificial vagina in Rokitansky-Kuster-Hauser syndrome]. Attual Ostet Ginecol 11(2):131, 1965

Wharton LR: Two cases of supernumerary ovary and one of accessory ovary, with an analysis of previously reported cases. Am J Obstet Gynecol 78:1101, 1959

White PC, Speiser PW: Congenital adrenal hyperplasia due to 21-hydroxylase deficiency. Endocr Rev 21(3):245, 2000

Williams C, Nakhal R, Hall-Craggs M, et al: Transverse vaginal septae: management and long-term outcomes. BJOG 121(13):1653, 2014

Williams EA: Congenital absence of the vagina: a simple operation for its relief. J Obstet Gynaecol Br Commonw 71:511, 1964

Woelfer B, Salim R, Banerjee S, et al: Reproductive outcomes in women with congenital uterine anomalies detected by three-dimensional ultrasound screening. Obstet Gynecol 98(6):1099, 2001

Zanetti E, Ferrari LR, Rossi G: Classification and radiographic features of uterine malformations: hysterosalpingographic study. Br J Radiol 51(603):161, 1978

Zheng W, Robboy SJ: Fallopian tube. In Robboy SJ, Mutter GL, Prat J (eds): Robboy's Pathology of the Female Reproductive Tract. London, Churchill Livingstone, 2009, p 509

CHAPTER 19

Evaluation of the Infertile Couple

Infertility is defined as the inability to conceive after 1 year of unprotected intercourse of reasonable frequency. It can be subdivided into *primary infertility*, that is, no prior pregnancies, and *secondary infertility*, referring to infertility following at least one prior conception.

Conversely, fecundability is the ability to conceive, and data from large population studies show that the monthly probability of conceiving is 20 to 25 percent. In those attempting conception, approximately 50 percent of women will be pregnant at 3 months, 75 percent will be pregnant at 6 months, and more than 85 percent will be pregnant by 1 year (Fig. 19-1) (Guttmacher, 1956; Mosher, 1991).

Infertility is common and affects 10 to 15 percent of reproductive-aged couples. Of note, even without treatment, approximately half of women will conceive in the second year of attempting. According to the National Survey of Family Growth, the percentage of married women who reported infertility fell from 8.5 percent in 1982 to 6.0 percent in 2006 to 2010. In comparison, the percentage of women aged 15 to 44 years who had ever used infertility services increased from 9 percent in 1982 to 12 percent in 2002, with a peak of 15 percent in 1995 (Chandra, 2013, 2014). Interpretation of these data is complicated by ongoing changes in marriage rates, intentional delays in childbearing, and socioeconomic and educational status changes in a growing immigrant community. Nevertheless, well-publicized successes in infertility treatment now give patients greater hope that medical intervention will help them achieve their goal.

Most couples are more correctly considered to be *subfertile,* rather than infertile, as they will ultimately conceive if given enough time. This concept of subfertility can be reassuring to couples. However, there are obvious exceptions, such as the woman with bilaterally obstructed fallopian tubes or the azoospermic male. In general, infertility evaluation is for any couple that has failed to conceive in 1 year. But, several scenarios may prompt earlier intervention. For example, to delay assessment in an anovulatory woman or a woman with a history of severe pelvic inflammatory disease (PID) may not be appropriate. Of particular note, fecundability is highly age-related, with a significant decrease beginning at approximately 32 years of age and more rapid decline after age 37 (American Society for Reproductive Medicine, 2014a). This decline in conception rates is associated with an increase in poor pregnancy outcomes, primarily due to increased aneuploidy rates. Thus, most experts agree that evaluation is considered after only 6 months in women older than 35 years.

Prior to initiating infertility treatment, a patient's health status must be optimized for an anticipated pregnancy. Ideally, these issues are addressed prior to referral to an infertility specialist whenever possible. Topics include appropriate vaccination; screening for diabetes, infectious diseases, or genetic disorders; folic acid supplementation; weight reduction; and cessation of cigarette smoking or illicit drug use. Additional information is provided later in this chapter and in Table 1-17 (p. 18).

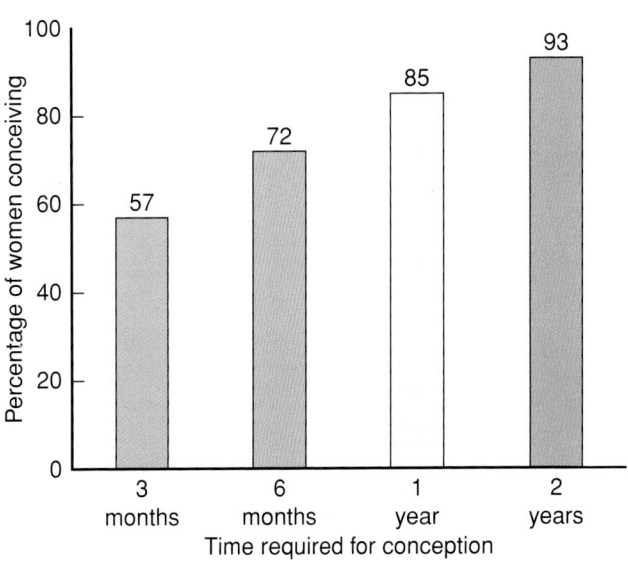

FIGURE 19-1 Time required for conception.

ETIOLOGY OF INFERTILITY

Successful pregnancy requires a complex sequence that includes ovulation, ovum pick-up by a fallopian tube, fertilization, transport of a fertilized ovum into the uterus, and implantation into a receptive uterine cavity. In the male system, sperm of adequate number and quality must be deposited at the cervix near the time of ovulation. Remembering these critical events can aid in developing an appropriate evaluation and treatment strategy.

In general, infertility can be attributed to the female partner one third of the time, the male partner one third of the time, and both partners in the remaining one third. This approximation emphasizes the value of assessing both partners before instituting therapy. Although a complete investigation may not be required before instituting therapy if a clear etiology is present, strong consideration is given to finishing testing if pregnancy is not rapidly achieved. Estimates of the incidence of various causes of infertility are shown in Table 19-1 (Abma, 1997; American Society for Reproductive Medicine, 2006).

Both partners are urged to attend the initial consultation. This time provides an excellent opportunity to educate regarding the normal conception process and methods to optimize their natural fertility. Such efforts may obviate the need for expensive and time-consuming interventions (American Society for Reproductive Medicine, 2013a). Couples are informed of the concept of a fertile window for conception. The chance of conception is increased from the 5 days preceding ovulation through the day of ovulation (Wilcox, 1995). If the male partner has normal semen characteristics, a couple ideally has daily intercourse during this period to maximize the chance of conception. Although sperm concentrations will drop with increasing coital frequency, this decrease is generally too small to significantly lower the chance of fertilization (Stanford, 2002). Couples are also reminded to avoid oil-based lubricants, which are harmful to sperm. Many myths surround the ability to conceive. Examples, such as the importance of coital position and the need to remain horizontal following ejaculation, can add undue stress to an already stressful situation and should be dispelled.

MEDICAL HISTORY

■ Female History

Gynecologic

As with any medical condition, a thorough history and physical examination is critical (American Society for Reproductive

TABLE 19-1. Etiology of Infertility

Male	25%
Ovulatory	27%
Tubal/uterine	22%
Other	9%
Unexplained	17%

Medicine, 2012a). Specifically, questions cover menstruation (frequency, duration, recent change in interval or duration, hot flushes, dysmenorrhea), prior contraceptive use, coital frequency, and infertility duration. Previous endometriosis, recurrent ovarian cysts, leiomyomas, sexually transmitted diseases, or PID is also pertinent. Because prior conception indicates ovulation and a patent fallopian tube in the patient's past, this history is sought. A prolonged time to conception may suggest borderline fertility and may increase the chance of determining an etiology. Pregnancy complications such as miscarriage, preterm delivery, retained placenta, postpartum dilatation and curettage, chorioamnionitis, or fetal anomalies are also recorded. Prior abnormal Pap testing may be relevant, particularly if a woman underwent cervical conization, which can diminish cervical mucus and cervical competence. A coital history, including frequency and timing of intercourse, is also obtained. Symptoms such as dyspareunia may point to endometriosis and a need for earlier diagnostic laparoscopy for the female partner.

Medical and Surgical

During medical history inventory, symptoms of hyperprolactinemia or thyroid disease are sought. Symptoms of androgen excess such as acne or hirsutism may point to polycystic ovarian syndrome (PCOS) or much less commonly, congenital adrenal hyperplasia. Prior chemotherapy or pelvic irradiation may suggest ovarian failure. This is also an excellent opportunity to ensure that all indicated vaccinations are current, as several are contraindicated once pregnancy is achieved (American Society for Reproductive Medicine, 2013d). Vaccine indications and schedules are found in Table 1-2 (p. 8).

Questions regarding medications include over-the-counter agents, such as nonsteroidal antiinflammatory drugs, that may adversely affect ovulation. In most instances, herbal remedies are discouraged. Women are encouraged to take a daily vitamin with at least 400 μg of folic acid to decrease the chance of neural-tube defects. In those with a previously affected child, 4 g is taken orally daily (American College of Obstetricians and Gynecologists, 2014b).

Previous pelvic and abdominal surgeries, especially if linked to endometriosis or adhesion formation, can lower fertility. As examples, operations for ruptured appendicitis or diverticulitis raise suspicion for pelvic adhesive disease or tubal obstruction or both. Prior uterine surgery can predispose to pain, bowel obstruction, or extra- or intrauterine adhesions with resultant infertility. When planning surgery, reducing adhesion formation is a priority, and meticulous surgical technique and minimally invasive surgical approaches are favored. Surgical adhesion barriers, described in Chapter 11 (p. 261), lower postoperative adhesion rates. However, no strong evidence exists that their use improves fertility, decreases pain, or lowers bowel obstruction rates (American Society for Reproductive Medicine, 2013b).

Social

A social history focuses on lifestyle factors such as eating habits. Abnormalities in gonadotropin-releasing hormone (GnRH) and gonadotropin secretion are clearly related to body mass

TABLE 19-2. Effects of Obesity and Environmental Factors on Fertility

Factor	Impact on Fertility
Obesity (BMI >35)	2-fold increase TTC
Underweight (BMI <19)	4-fold increase TTC
Smoking	1.6-fold increase RR
Alcohol (>2/day)	1.6-fold increase RR
Illicit drugs	1.7-fold increase RR
Toxins	1.4-fold increase RR
Caffeine (>250 mg/day)	45% decrease fecundability

BMI = body mass index; RR = relative risk of infertility; TTC = time to conception.
Adapted with permission from American Society for Reproductive Medicine: Optimizing natural fertility: a committee opinion, Fertil Steril 2013 Sep;100(3):631–637.

TABLE 19-3. Women's Awareness of Health Risks Associated with Smoking

Smoking Risk	Percentage Aware of Risk
Respiratory disease	99%
Heart disease	96%
Pregnancy complications	91%
Spontaneous abortion	39%
Ectopic pregnancy	27%
Infertility	22%
Early menopause	18%

Reproduced with permission from Roth LK, Taylor HS: Risks of smoking to reproductive health: assessment of women's knowledge, Am J Obstet Gynecol 2001 Apr;184(5):934–939.

indices >25 or <17 (Grodstein, 1994a). An estimated 30 to 50 percent of women, depending on race and ethnicity, are overweight or obese. Most agree that this incidence is increasing (American Society for Reproductive Medicine, 2008c; Hedley, 2004). In these women, infertility is primarily related to an increased incidence of ovulatory dysfunction, but data also suggest that fecundity is lower among ovulatory obese women. Although difficult to achieve, even modest weight reduction in overweight women is correlated with normalized menstrual cycles and subsequent pregnancies (Table 19-2).

Accumulating data also suggest that cigarette smoking lowers fertility rates (American Society for Reproductive Medicine, 2012d). At least one fifth of reproductive-aged men and women in the United States smoke cigarettes (Centers for Disease Control and Prevention, 2014). The prevalence of infertility is higher, and the time to conception is longer in women who smoke, or even those exposed passively to cigarette smoke. Moreover, smoking's negative effects on female fecundity do not appear to be overcome by assisted reproductive technologies (ART). A 5-year prospective study of 221 couples found that the risk of failing to conceive with ART was more than doubled in smokers. Each year that a woman smoked was associated with a 9-percent increase in the risk of unsuccessful ART cycles (Klonoff-Cohen, 2001).

Toxins in the smoke can accelerate follicular depletion and increase genetic mutations in gametes or early embryos (Zenzes, 2000). Smoking is associated with an increased miscarriage rate in both natural and assisted conception cycles. The mechanism for this is unclear, but the vasoconstrictive and antimetabolic properties of some cigarette smoke components such as nicotine, carbon dioxide, and cyanide may lead to placental insufficiency. Specifically, smoking has been linked to higher rates of abruption, fetal growth restriction, and preterm labor (Cunningham, 2014). In addition, smoking in pregnant women is associated with an increased risk of trisomy 21 that results from maternal meiotic nondisjunction (Yang, 1999). Admittedly, current data do not prove causation, but only correlation, between smoking and infertility or adverse pregnancy outcomes.

The effect of smoking on male fertility is more difficult to discern. Although smokers often have comparatively reduced sperm concentrations and motility, these often remain within the normal range.

Smoking is discouraged for both male and female partners planning pregnancy. The desire for pregnancy can be a powerful motivator toward cessation (Augood, 1998). Education is the most important first step (Table 19-3). If behavioral approaches fail, use of medical adjuncts such as nicotine replacement therapy, bupropion (Zyban), or varenicline (Chantix) may prove effective (Table 1-4, p. 11). Nicotine preparations are designated as category D. Bupropion and varenicline are non-nicotine Food and Drug Administration (FDA)-approved agents and carry a category C designation (Fiore, 2008). Ideally pharmacological smoking cessation therapies are best used prior to conception.

Alcohol consumption also should be limited. Heavy alcohol intake decreases fertility in women, and in men has been associated with a decrease in sperm counts and increase in sexual dysfunction (Klonoff-Cohen, 2003; Nagy, 1986). A standardized alcoholic drink is typically defined as 12 ounces of beer, 5 ounces of wine, or 1.5 ounces of hard alcohol. Based on several studies, five to eight drinks per week negatively affects female fertility (Grodstein, 1994b; Tolstrup, 2003). As alcohol is also detrimental to early pregnancy, it is prudent to advise patients to avoid excessive alcohol consumption while trying to conceive.

Caffeine is one of the most widely used pharmacologically active substances in the world. Studies evaluating a potential relationship between caffeine and impaired fertility have varied in design and resulted in conflicting findings. One large prospective trial found no association between either total caffeine intake or coffee consumption and fecundability (Hatch, 2012). Despite this, recommendations of caffeine intake moderation in infertile women seem prudent.

Illicit drugs may also affect fecundability. Marijuana suppresses the hypothalamic-pituitary-gonadal axis in both men and women, and cocaine can impair spermatogenesis (Bracken, 1990; Smith, 1987).

Environmental Factors

Increasing information suggests that some male and female infertility may result from environmental contaminants or toxins

(Giudice, 2006). Endocrine-disrupting chemicals (EDCs) have been shown to be reproductive toxicants. Examples are dioxins and polychlorinated biphenyls, as well as agricultural pesticides and herbicides, phthalates (used in making plastic materials), lead, and bisphenol A (used in the manufacture of polycarbonate plastic and resins) (Hauser, 2008; Mendola, 2008). EDC exposure is implicated to underlie a broad range of women's reproductive disorders. Lower fecundability and lower birthweight show the most solid evidence for this correlation (Caserta, 2011). Although direct links to infertility in humans are not conclusive, clinicians should counsel patients that environmental exposures to toxic substances should be avoided if possible. Currently, these cautions should be discussed carefully to avoid alarm.

Ethnicity and Family History

The ethnic background and family history of both partners influences the need for preconceptional testing. A family history of infertility, recurrent miscarriage, or fetal anomalies may point to a genetic etiology. Although the inheritance pattern is complex, data suggest that both PCOS and endometriosis occur in familial clusters. For example, a woman carries an estimated sevenfold increased risk of endometriosis over that of the general population if a single first-degree family member has the disease (Moen, 1993).

Genetic carrier screening can be offered preconceptionally or following conception. Testing before conception is often more straightforward and less stressful for the couple than delaying until pregnancy has been achieved. However, insurance carriers may decline to reimburse for this evaluation (American Academy of Pediatrics and American College of Obstetricians and Gynecologists, 2012). Preconception carrier screening also allows a couple to consider the most complete range of reproductive options. Knowing the risk of having an affected child, a couple may consider preimplantation genetic diagnosis, prenatal genetic testing, or the use of donor gametes (American College of Obstetricians and Gynecologists, 2014e). In the absence of known family history of genetic disease, it is reasonable to offer genetic carrier screening to the woman first and test the male partner only if the mother has positive results.

Specific recommendations for genetic carrier screening have been published by the American College of Obstetricians and Gynecologists (2009, 2014a,c,d), by the American College of Medical Genetics and Genomics, and by other advocacy groups and societies (Grody, 2013; Gross, 2013; Pletcher, 2006). These opinions have changed over time and continue to vary across organizations. No doubt, screening guidelines will continue to evolve as technology advances and the costs and benefits of obtaining this information become more evident. Certain disorders are more common in specific ethnic groups, although it is essential to note that there are no disorders found uniquely in a certain ethnic or racial group. Many families may be interracial and ethnic background may be unknown. For example, cystic fibrosis screening was initially recommended only for the non-Hispanic white population and those of Ashkenazi Jewish descent. However, this recommendation now extends to all individuals to account for increased numbers of

individuals with mixed ethnicity and inaccuracies based on personal reporting (Ross, 2011; Tanner, 2014).

Traditional genotyping methods detect a limited number of mutations, and these tests have been developed to be specific for the more common mutations found in the ethnic group most at risk. Expanded genotyping panels have been developed but are costly and remain limited. More recently, the cost of DNA sequencing has been greatly reduced due to the emergence of next-generation sequencing (NGS) techniques (Hallam, 2014). This allows rapid and efficient testing of many genes and thousands of mutations concurrently. Panethnic population screening by NGS for numerous genetic disorders is now technically feasible. Given that a large number of sequence variants might be identified by NGS that are not disease causing, rigorous analytic and clinical validation is required before widespread clinical application is begun (Prior, 2014).

■ Male History

Similar attention is paid to assessing the male partner's potential contribution to infertility (American Society for Reproductive Medicine, 2012b). Questions include abnormalities in pubertal development and sexual function. Erectile dysfunction, particularly in conjunction with decreased beard growth, may suggest decreased testosterone levels. Ejaculatory problems are also evaluated, including a search for developmental anomalies such as hypospadias, which could result in suboptimal semen deposition (Benson, 1997).

Sexually transmitted diseases or frequent genitourinary infections, including epididymitis or prostatitis, may lead to vas deferens inflammation and obstruction. Similarly, mumps in an adult can create testicular inflammation and damage spermatogenic stem cells (Beard, 1977). Prior cryptorchidism, testicular torsion, or testicular trauma may suggest abnormal spermatogenesis (Anderson, 1990; Cobellis, 2014). Compared with fertile males, males with unilateral or bilateral cryptorchidism have fertility rates of 80 percent and 50 percent, respectively (Lee, 1993). The reason for poor semen characteristics in these patients is unclear. The relatively warm intraabdominal temperature may cause permanent stem cell damage. Alternatively, genetic abnormalities that led to the abnormal testis location may also affect sperm production.

A history of varicocele is also obtained. A varicocele consists of dilated veins of the pampiniform plexus of the spermatic cords that drain the testes (Figs. 19-2 and 19-3). Varicoceles are believed to raise scrotal temperature, however, the negative affects of varicoceles on fertility are controversial (American Society for Reproductive Medicine, 2014b; Baazeem, 2011; Jarow, 2001). Although 30 to 40 percent of men seen in infertility clinics are diagnosed with a varicocele, nearly 20 percent of men in the general population are similarly affected. If a varicocele is suspected, it should be evaluated by a urologist, preferably one with a specific interest in infertility.

Spermatogenesis, from stem cell to mature sperm, takes nearly 90 days (Fig. 19-4). Thus, any detrimental event in the prior 3 months can adversely affect semen characteristics (Hinrichsen, 1980; Rowley, 1970). Spermatogenesis is optimal

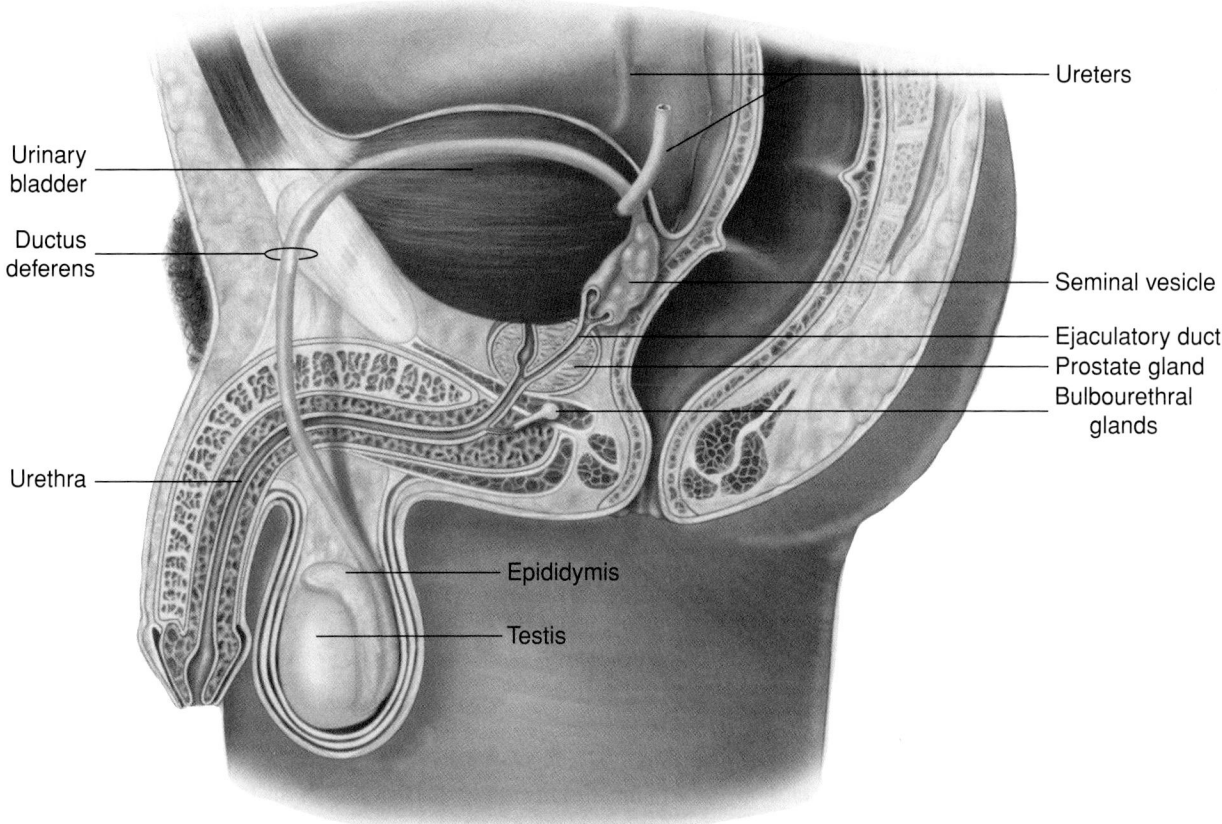

FIGURE 19-2 Male genitalia. (Reproduced with permission from McKinley M, O'Loughlin VD: Human Anatomy. New York: McGraw-Hill; 2006.)

at temperatures slightly below body temperature, hence the location of the testes outside of the pelvis. Illness with high fevers or chronic hot tub use can temporarily impair sperm quality. There is no definitive evidence that boxer underwear is advantageous.

Medical questions focus on prior chemotherapy or local radiation treatment that may damage spermatogonial stem cells. Hypertension, diabetes mellitus, and neurologic disorders can be associated with erectile dysfunction or retrograde ejaculation. Several medications are known to worsen semen characteristics,

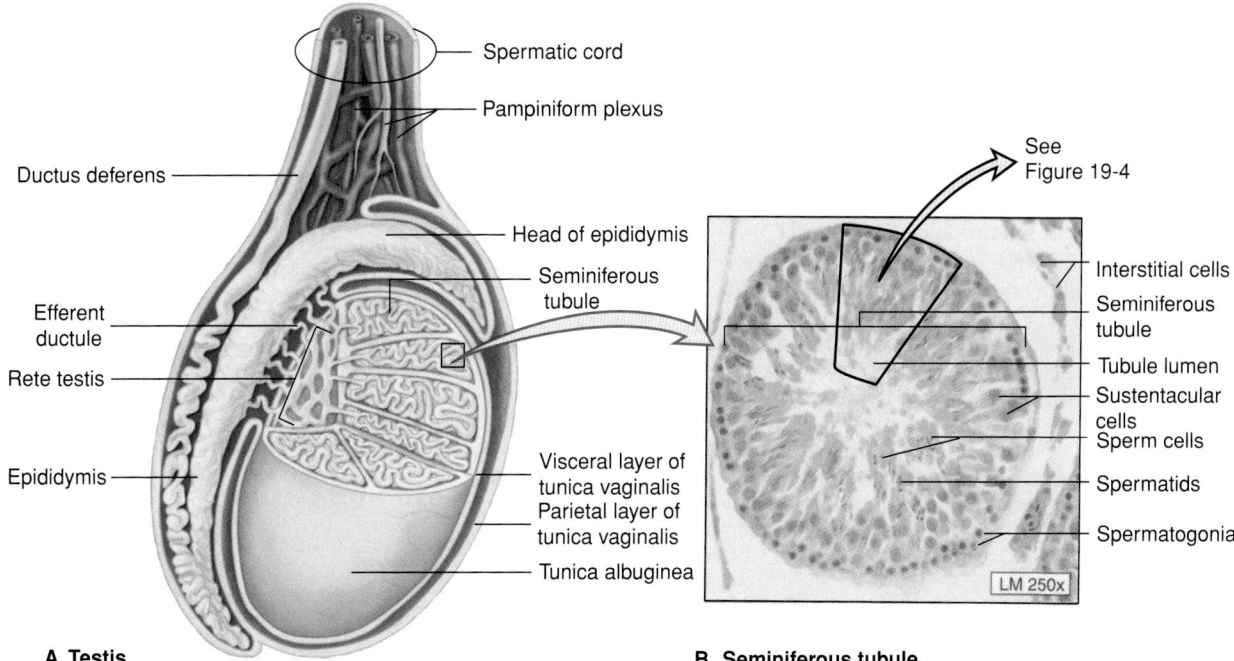

FIGURE 19-3 Male testis. **A.** Gross anatomy of a testis. **B.** Cutaway of the testis reveals the microscopic structure of a seminiferous tubule. (Reproduced with permission from McKinley M, O'Loughlin VD: Human Anatomy. New York: McGraw-Hill; 2006.)

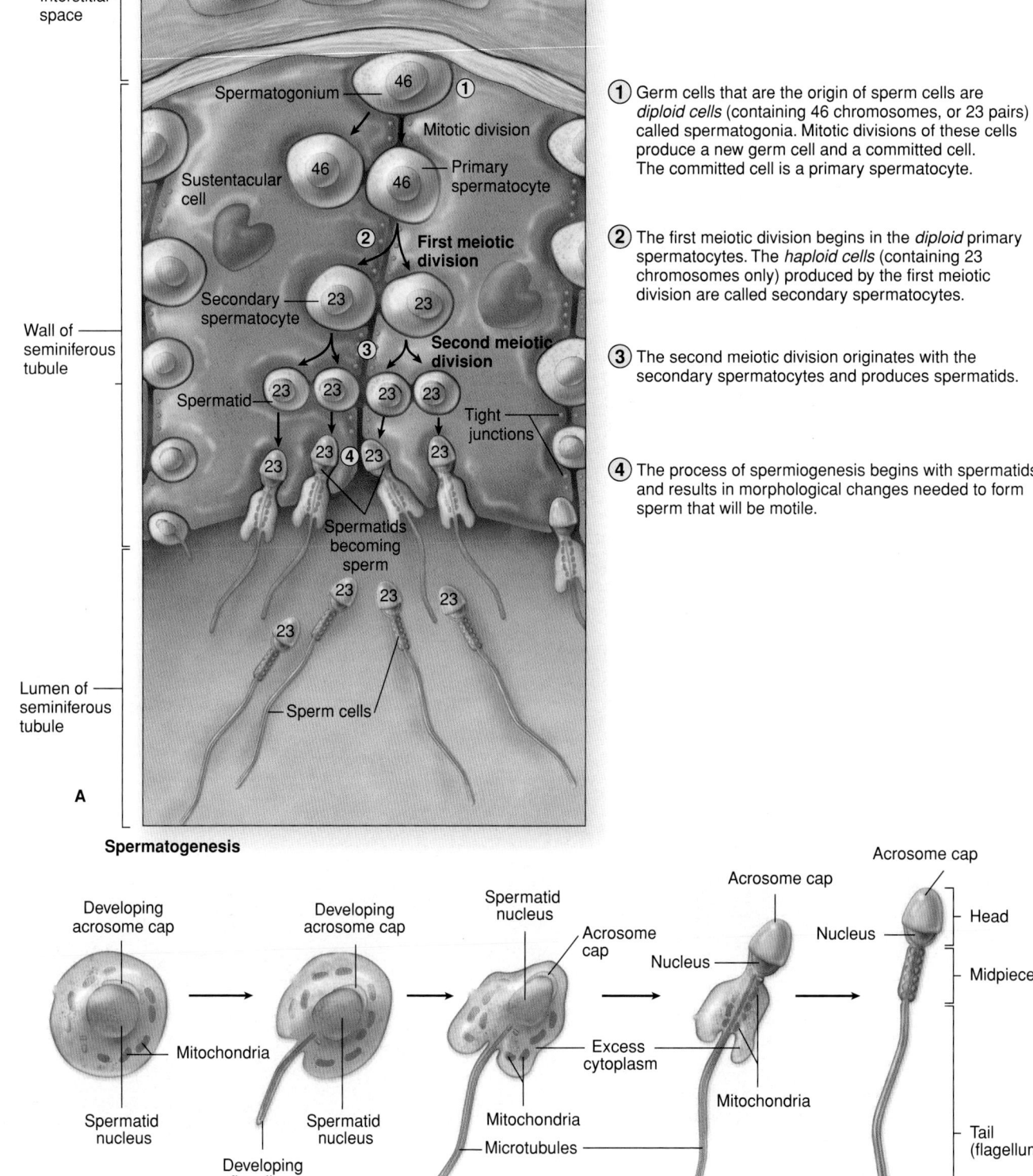

① Germ cells that are the origin of sperm cells are *diploid cells* (containing 46 chromosomes, or 23 pairs) called spermatogonia. Mitotic divisions of these cells produce a new germ cell and a committed cell. The committed cell is a primary spermatocyte.

② The first meiotic division begins in the *diploid* primary spermatocytes. The *haploid cells* (containing 23 chromosomes only) produced by the first meiotic division are called secondary spermatocytes.

③ The second meiotic division originates with the secondary spermatocytes and produces spermatids.

④ The process of spermiogenesis begins with spermatids and results in morphological changes needed to form sperm that will be motile.

FIGURE 19-4 Male testis. **A.** Cutaway of the seminiferous tubule shows the mitotic and meiotic divisions involved with spermatogenesis. **B.** Structural changes required during spermiogenesis, as sperm cells become spermatids. (Reproduced with permission from McKinley M, O'Loughlin VD: Human Anatomy. New York: McGraw-Hill; 2006.)

TABLE 19-4. Chapters with Relevant Information About Infertility

Etiology	Diagnosis	Chapter Title	Chapter Number
Ovulatory dysfunction	PCOS	PCOS and Hyperandrogenism	Chapter 17
	Hypothalamic-pituitary	Amenorrhea	Chapter 16
	Age-related	Menopausal Transition	Chapter 21
	POF	Amenorrhea	Chapter 16
Tubal disease	PID	Gynecologic Infection	Chapter 3
Uterine abnormalities	Congenital	Anatomic Disorders	Chapter 18
	Leiomyomas	Pelvic Mass	Chapter 9
	Asherman syndrome	Amenorrhea	Chapter 16
Other	Endometriosis	Endometriosis	Chapter 10

PCOS = polycystic ovarian syndrome; PID = pelvic inflammatory disease; POF = premature ovarian failure.

including cimetidine, erythromycin, gentamicin, tetracycline, and spironolactone (Sigman, 1997). Moreover, obesity, cigarettes, alcohol, illicit drugs, and environmental toxins all adversely affect semen parameters (Muthusami, 2005; Ramlau-Hansen, 2007). The increasing use of anabolic steroids also decreases sperm production by suppressing the output of intratesticular testosterone (Gazvani, 1997). Although the effects of many medications are reversible, anabolic steroid abuse may lead to lasting or even permanent damage to testicular function.

PHYSICAL EXAMINATION

▩ Examination of the Female Patient

A physical examination may provide many clues to the cause of infertility. Vital signs, height, and weight are recorded. A particularly short stature may reflect a genetic condition such as Turner syndrome. Hirsutism, alopecia, or acne indicates the need to measure androgen levels. Acanthosis nigricans is consistent with insulin resistance associated with PCOS or much less commonly, Cushing syndrome. Galactorrhea is often indicative of hyperprolactinemia. Additionally, thyroid abnormalities are sought. Many of these diagnoses and their management are discussed in greater detail in other chapters (Table 19-4).

A pelvic examination may be particularly informative. Inability to place a speculum through the introitus may raise doubts about coital frequency. The vagina should be moist and rugated, and the cervix should have a reasonable amount of mucus. Both indicate adequate estrogen production. An enlarged or irregularly shaped uterus may reflect leiomyomas, whereas a fixed uterus suggests pelvic scarring due to endometriosis or prior pelvic infection. Uterosacral nodularity or ovarian masses may additionally implicate endometriosis or less commonly, malignancy.

All women should have cervical cancer screening that is up-to-date prior to treatment. Negative cultures for *Neisseria gonorrhoeae* and *Chlamydia trachomatis* are obtained to ensure that cervical manipulation during evaluation and treatment does not cause ascending infection. The breast examination must be normal, and when indicated by age or family history, a mammogram is obtained prior to initiating hormonal treatment.

▩ Examination of the Male Patient

Most gynecologists will not feel comfortable performing a complete male physical examination. Nevertheless, parts of this evaluation are relatively easy to perform, and a gynecologist at minimum should understand the primary focus of the examination. As signs of testosterone production, normal secondary sexual characteristics such as beard growth, axillary and pubic hair, and perhaps male pattern balding should be present. Gynecomastia or eunuchoid habitus may suggest Klinefelter syndrome (47,XXY karyotype) (De Braekeleer, 1991).

The penile urethra should be at the glans tip for proper semen deposition in the vagina. Testicular length measures at least 4 cm and a minimal testicular volume is 20 mL (Charny, 1960; Hadziselimovic, 2006). Small testes are unlikely to produce normal sperm numbers. A testicular mass may indicate testicular cancer, which can present as infertility. The epididymis should be soft and nontender to exclude chronic infection. Epididymal fullness may suggest vas deferens obstruction. The prostate should be smooth, nontender, and normal size. Additionally, the pampiniform plexus of veins is palpated for varicocele (Jarow, 2001). Importantly, both vasa deferentia should be palpable. Congenital bilateral absence of the vas deferens is associated with mutation in the gene responsible for cystic fibrosis and is discussed on page 444 (Anguiano, 1992).

EVALUATION FOR ANOVULATION

The infertility evaluation can be conceptually simplified into confirmation of: (1) ovulation, (2) normal female reproductive tract anatomy, and (3) normal semen characteristics. The specifics regarding evaluation of each of these categories are detailed in the following sections and shown in Table 19-5.

Of these, ovulation may be perturbed by abnormalities within the hypothalamus, anterior pituitary, or ovaries. Hypothalamic disorders may be acquired or inherited. Acquired disorders include those due to lifestyle, for example,

TABLE 19-5.   Infertility Testing

Etiology	Evaluation
Ovulatory dysfunction	Ovulation predictor kit Early follicular FSH ± estradiol level (ovarian reserve) ± Antimüllerian hormone ± Serum measurements (TSH, prolactin, androgens) ± Ovarian sonography (antral follicle count)
Tubal/pelvic disease	Hysterosalpingography Laparoscopy + chromotubation
Uterine factors	Hysterosalpingography Transvaginal sonography/saline-infusion sonography ± Magnetic resonance imaging Hysteroscopy ± laparoscopy
Male factor	Semen analysis

FSH = follicle-stimulating hormone; TSH = thyroid-stimulating hormone.

excessive exercise, eating disorders, or stress. Alternatively, dysfunction or improper migration of the hypothalamic gonadotropin-releasing hormone neurons may be inherited, such as that which occurs in idiopathic hypogonadotropic hypogonadism (IHH) or Kallman syndrome. Thyroid disease and hyperprolactinemia may also contribute to menstrual disturbances. A full discussion of endocrine-related disorders that result in menstrual disturbances is found in Chapter 16 (p. 369).

■ Clinical Evaluation

A patient's menstrual history is an excellent predictor of regular ovulation. A woman with cyclic menses at an interval of 25 to 35 days and duration of bleeding of 3 to 7 days is most likely ovulating. Although these numbers vary widely, each woman will have her own normal pattern. Therefore, these figures typically do not vary significantly across cycles for an individual woman.

Probable ovulation is also suggested by *mittelschmerz*, which is midcycle pelvic pain associated with ovulation, or by moliminal symptoms such as breast tenderness, acne, food cravings, and mood changes. Ovulatory cycles are more likely to be associated with dysmenorrhea. Severe dysmenorrhea may suggest endometriosis.

Basal body temperature (BBT) charting has long been used to identify ovulation. This test requires that a woman's morning oral temperature be graphically charted (Fig. 19-5). Oral temperatures are usually 97.0° to 98.0°F during the follicular phase. A postovulatory rise in progesterone levels increases basal temperature by approximately 0.4° to 0.8°F. This *biphasic* temperature pattern is strongly predictive of ovulation (Bates, 1990). Nevertheless, although this test has the advantage of being inexpensive, it is insensitive in many women. Furthermore, for a couple wishing to conceive, the temperature increase follows ovulation, and therefore the window of maximal fertility has been missed (Luciano, 1990). Although this method is discussed here for completeness, most patients are better served by the use of the sensitive and readily available urinary ovulation detection kits described in the next section.

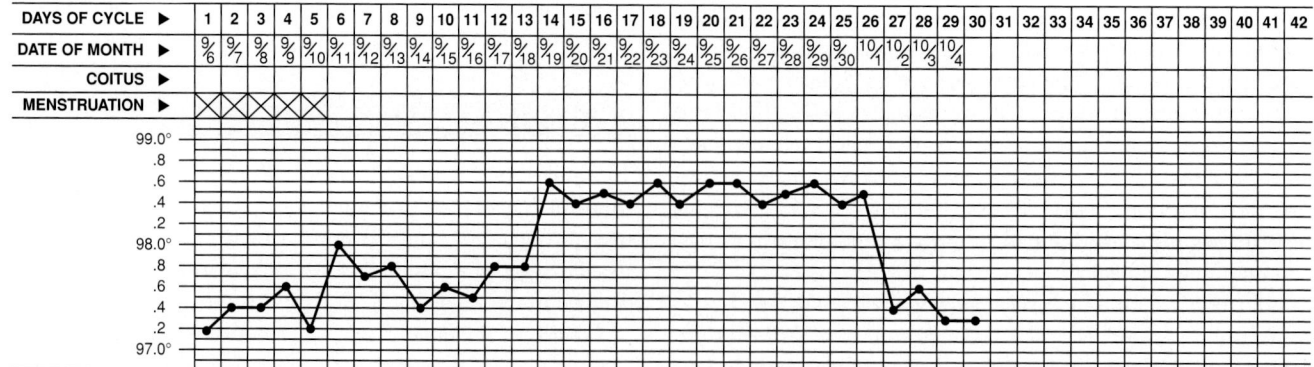

FIGURE 19-5 Biphasic pattern seen on this basal body temperature chart suggests ovulation. (Reproduced with permission from Chang WY, Agarwal SK, Azziz R: Essential Reproductive Medicine. New York: McGraw-Hill; 2005.)

Ovulation Predictor Kits

These kits measure urinary luteinizing hormone (LH) concentration by colorimetric assay. They are widely available in pharmacies, are relatively easy to use, and provide clear instructions regarding interpretation. In general, a woman begins testing 2 to 3 days prior to the predicted LH surge, and testing is continued daily. There is no clear consensus regarding the optimal time of day to test. Some specialists suggest that the concentrated first morning void is a logical time. Others are concerned that this sample may provide a false-positive result and recommend testing the second morning urine. Other clinicians reason that the serum LH peak occurs in the morning and that the greatest likelihood of detecting a urinary peak would be in the late afternoon or evening. Timing is probably not critical as long as the test is performed daily, as the LH surge spans only 48 to 50 hours. In most instances, ovulation will occur the day following the urinary LH peak (Luciano, 1990; Miller, 1996).

If equivocal results are obtained, the test can be repeated in 12 hours. In one study, urine LH surge assays were estimated to have 100-percent sensitivity and 96-percent accuracy. This is undoubtedly an overestimate of typical-use results (Grinsted, 1989; Guermandi, 2001).

Serum Progesterone

Adequate progesterone levels are required for endometrial preparation prior to implantation. This has led to the concept of *luteal phase defect (LPD)*, defined as inadequate endometrial development due to suboptimal progesterone production (American Society for Reproductive Medicine, 2012f).

Midluteal phase serum progesterone levels have long been used to document ovulation, although the sensitivity of this test has been questioned. In a classic 28-day cycle, serum is obtained on cycle day number 21 following the first day of menstrual bleeding, or 7 days following ovulation. Levels during the follicular phase are generally <2 ng/mL. Values above 4 to 6 ng/mL correlate with ovulation and progesterone production by the corpus luteum (Guermandi, 2001). Progesterone is secreted as pulses, and therefore a single measurement does not indicate overall production during the luteal phase. As a result, an absolute threshold for acceptable progesterone levels has not been clearly established. Although some clinicians empirically treat any woman with a progesterone level below approximately 10 ng/mL, the utility of this approach is unproven, and it is costly. Accordingly, the midluteal progesterone level is best regarded as an acceptable test for ovulation but not an absolute indicator of adequate luteal function.

Endometrial Biopsy

Luteal phase endometrial biopsy was hoped to reflect both corpus luteum function and endometrial response, and thereby provide more clinically relevant information than a serum progesterone level alone (Noyes, 1975). Unfortunately, the utility of this test is severely hampered by high intraobserver and interobserver variability during histologic evaluation. An out-of-phase biopsy is found nearly as frequently in fertile as in infertile women, and the overlap in incidence between the two groups is large (Balasch, 1992; Scott, 1993). In its current form, the endometrial biopsy has little predictive value and is no longer considered a routine part of infertility evaluation.

Interestingly, the timing of protein expression in the endometrial glands and stroma is being defined. Potential markers for uterine receptivity include osteopontin, cytokines (leukemia inhibitory factor, colony-stimulating factor-1, and interleukin-1), cell adhesion molecules (the integrins), ion channels, and the L-selectin ligand (Carson, 2002; Garrido-Gomez, 2014; Kao, 2003; Lessey, 1998; Petracco, 2012; Ruan, 2014). In the future, endometrial biopsies may again become part of the diagnostic evaluation if expression patterns of these proteins prove to be predictive of endometrial receptivity.

Sonography

Serial ovarian sonographic evaluations can demonstrate the development of a mature antral follicle and its subsequent collapse during ovulation. This approach is time consuming, and ovulation can be missed. However, sonography is an excellent approach for supporting the diagnosis of PCOS. Sonographic criteria for PCOS are found in Chapter 17 (p. 397).

EVALUATION FOR DIMINISHED OVARIAN RESERVE

Ovulatory status does not provide a complete picture of ovarian function. A woman may have regular, ovulatory menses but have reduced follicular response to ovarian stimulation compared with other women of similar age due to a decrease in ovarian follicles available for recruitment. In this situation, the woman is said to have decreased or diminished ovarian reserve (DOR) and in more severe presentations, primary ovarian insufficiency (POI). Although most often the result of advancing age, a decrease in ovarian reserve can occur for other reasons including smoking, genetic conditions, or prior ovarian surgery, chemotherapy, or pelvic irradiation (American College of Obstetricians and Gynecologists, 2015; American Society for Reproductive Medicine, 2012e). A more complete discussion of causes of accelerated follicular loss is found in Chapter 16 (p. 373).

Reproductive Aging

There is a clear inverse relationship between female age and fertility (Table 19-6) (American Society for Reproductive Medicine, 2014a). This loss is primarily attributable to a decrease in oocyte quality and quantity, although accumulating risk for the development of medical disorders or uterine and

TABLE 19-6. Female Aging and Infertility

Female Age (years)	Infertility
20–29	8.0%
30–34	14.6%
35–39	21.9%
40–44	28.7%

pelvic abnormalities also contributes. A classic study was performed in the Hutterites, a community that eschews contraception. After ages 34, 40, and 45, the incidence of infertility was 11 percent, 33 percent, and 87 percent, respectively. The average age at last pregnancy was 40.9 years (Menken, 1986; Tietze, 1957). Another study evaluated cumulative pregnancy rates in women using donor insemination. In women younger than 31 years, 74 percent achieved pregnancy within 1 year. These rates fell to 62 percent for women between 31 and 35 years, and further declined to 54 percent in women older than 35 (Treloar, 1998).

Ongoing atresia of nondominant follicles proceeds throughout a woman's reproductive life span (Fig. 14-1, p. 319). In addition to follicular number decline, the risks of genetic abnormalities and mitochondrial deletions in the remaining oocytes substantially increase as a woman ages (Keefe, 1995; Pellestor, 2003). These factors result in decreased pregnancy rates and increased miscarriage rates in both spontaneous and stimulated cycles. The overall miscarriage risk in women older than 40 years has been estimated to be 50 to 75 percent (Maroulis, 1991).

The follicular loss rate and age at menopause varies between women and is likely genetically determined. For example, a family history of early menopause is correlated with an increased risk of early menopause in an individual woman. In general, the age at last birth in naturally fertile populations averages 10 years prior to menopause (Nikolaou, 2003; te Velde, 2002). However, in most cases, it is impossible to predict the onset of menopause. Therefore fertility testing is ideally performed starting at age 35 in all patients desiring conception. Testing is also seriously considered in any woman with an unexplained change in menstrual cyclicity, family history of early menopause, or risk factor for POI.

An array of serum and sonographic tests has been developed to assess ovarian reserve (American Society for Reproductive Medicine, 2012e). Unfortunately, these tests lack sensitivity and positive predictive value for DOR, particularly if applied to patients at low risk for this process. In addition, these tests are more accurate as predictors of ovarian response to pharmacologic stimulation than as predictors of subsequent pregnancy. Identification of the optimal combination of tests and their appropriate interpretation continues to be refined. Currently, measurement of early follicular FSH and estradiol levels is probably the most cost-effective approach for the general practitioner. However, addition of a serum antimüllerian hormone level is moving into standard practice. Measurement of serum inhibin B levels or use of the clomiphene citrate challenge test has fallen out of favor.

Abnormal test results from any of these methods correlate with a poorer prognosis for achieving pregnancy, and referral to an infertility specialist is advisable. Conversely, a normal test does not negate the impact of a woman's age on her fertility status. This information may be useful in counseling a couple regarding prognosis. Poor results in an older woman can supply an impetus either to attempt donor oocyte in vitro fertilization (IVF) or to pursue alternatives such as adoption. Borderline results in a younger woman may suggest a need for more intensive treatment.

Follicle-stimulating Hormone and Estradiol

Measurement of serum follicle-stimulating hormone (FSH) levels in the early follicular phase is a simple and sensitive predictor of ovarian reserve (Toner, 1991). Frequently termed a "cycle day 3" FSH, this may reasonably be drawn between days 2 and 4. With declining ovarian function, the support cells (granulosa cells and luteal cells) secrete less inhibin, a peptide hormone that is responsible for inhibiting FSH secretion by the anterior pituitary gonadotropes (Chap. 15, p. 351). With loss of luteal inhibin, FSH levels rise in the early follicular phase. A value >10 mIU/mL indicates significant loss of ovarian reserve and prompts a more rapid evaluation and more intensive treatment. In a large study evaluating IVF cycles, a day-3 FSH level exceeding 15 mIU/mL predicted significantly lower pregnancy rates (Toner, 1991).

Many clinicians also measure serum estradiol levels simultaneously (Buyalos, 1997; Licciardi, 1995). Addition of an estradiol measurement may decrease the incidence of false-negative results in FSH values alone. Somewhat paradoxically, despite the overall depletion of ovarian follicles, estrogen levels in older women are elevated early in the cycle due to increased stimulation of ovarian steroidogenesis by elevated FSH levels. An early-follicular serum estradiol level >60 to 80 pg/mL is considered abnormal. Notably, reference levels for estradiol and FSH can vary between laboratories. Thus, every clinician should be familiar with their own laboratory's normal values.

Antimüllerian Hormone

This is the most recent circulating factor to be analyzed as an ovarian reserve predictor (La Marca, 2009). As suggested by its name, antimüllerian hormone (AMH) is expressed by the fetal testes during male differentiation to prevent development of the müllerian system (fallopian tubes, uterus, and upper vagina) (Chap. 18, p. 406). AMH is also expressed by the granulosa cells of small preantral follicles, with limited expression in larger follicles. This suggests that AMH plays a role in dominant follicle recruitment.

Because AMH is thought to vary minimally across the cycle, measurement of AMH levels provide an advantage compared with FSH testing. However, new studies demonstrate larger fluctuations than originally reported (Gnoth, 2015). In addition, recent or ongoing use of hormonal contraceptives may affect serum AMH levels (Johnson, 2014). At this point, it is reasonable to obtain an AMH level during the follicular phase coincident with measuring an FSH level. Notably, these recommendations may change in the near future.

Recent studies suggest that AMH levels correlate with ovarian primordial follicle number more strongly than do levels of FSH or inhibin (Hansen, 2010). Furthermore, AMH levels may drop prior to observable changes in FSH or estradiol levels, providing an earlier marker of waning ovarian function. Seifer and colleagues (2011) reported a steady decline in AMH serum levels across the reproductive life span. The median level approximated 3 ng/mL at age 25, and this dropped to 1 ng/mL at age 35 to 37. Several AMH assays are commercially available, and thus patient results are interpreted relative to normative data provided for the selected assay. Interestingly, AMH levels are increased two- to threefold in women with PCOS compared with normal cycling women (Hornburg, 2014). This observation is consistent with the multiple early follicles found in these patients.

Antral Follicle Count

Sonographic evaluation of the follicular phase antral follicle count (AFC) is commonly used as a reliable predictor for subsequent response to ovulation induction (Frattarelli, 2000; Maseelall, 2009). The number of small antral follicles reflects the size of the resting follicular pool. Antral follicles between 2 and 10 mm are counted in both ovaries. The total AFC usually ranges between 10 and 20 in a reproductive-aged woman. A count <10 predicts poor response to gonadotropin stimulation.

EVALUATION FOR FEMALE ANATOMIC ABNORMALITIES

Tubal and Pelvic Factors

Symptoms such as chronic pelvic pain or dysmenorrhea may suggest tubal obstruction, pelvic adhesions, or both. Adhesions can prevent normal tubal movement, ovum pick-up, and transport of the fertilized egg into the uterus. Etiologies include tubal disease, especially pelvic infection; endometriosis; and prior pelvic surgery.

Approximately one third to one fourth of all infertile women are diagnosed with tubal disease in developed countries (Serafini, 1989; World Health Organization, 2007). In the United States, the most common cause of tubal disease is infection with *C trachomatis* or *N gonorrhoeae*. With PID, tubal infertility has been estimated to follow in 12 percent, 23 percent, and 54 percent of women following one, two, or three cases of PID, respectively (Lalos, 1988). Nevertheless, an absent PID history is not overly reassuring, as nearly one half of patients who have tubal damage have no clinical history of antecedent disease (Rosenfeld, 1983).

In contrast, in developing countries, genital tuberculosis may account for 3 to 5 percent of infertility cases (Aliyu, 2004; Nezar, 2009). As a result, this diagnosis is considered in immigrant populations from countries with endemic infection. In these cases, tubal damage and endometrial adhesions are underlying causes. Genital tuberculosis typically follows hematogenous seeding of the reproductive tract from an extragenital primary infection. The likelihood of a return to fertility after antitubercular treatment is low, and IVF with embryo transfer remains the most reliable approach (Aliyu, 2004).

With endometriosis, chronic inflammation and intraperitoneal bleeding can lead to pelvic adhesions and subsequently impaired oocyte pick-up, compromised oocyte or embryonic uterotubal transport, or frank tubal obstruction. Endometriosis also is thought to diminish fertility via an increase in peritoneal fluid inflammatory factors, alterations in endometrial immunologic function, poor oocyte or embryonic quality, or impaired implantation (American Society for Reproductive Medicine, 2012c).

Salpingitis isthmica nodosa is an inflammatory condition of the fallopian tube, characterized by nodular thickening of its isthmic portion. Histologically, smooth muscle proliferation and diverticula of tubal epithelium contribute to this thickening. This uncommon condition typically develops bilaterally and progressively leads to ultimate tubal occlusion and infertility (Saracoglu, 1992). Treatment options include those for proximal tubal occlusion, discussed in Chapter 20 (p. 458).

Of note, a prior ectopic pregnancy, even if treated medically with methotrexate, implies the likelihood of significant tubal damage. Residual adhesions are common after even the most meticulous surgery for any pelvic pathology. This is particularly true in cases with associated pelvic inflammation due to blood or infection. Irritation caused by mature cystic teratoma (dermoid) contents may be particularly damaging.

Uterine Abnormalities

Uterine abnormalities can be either inherited (congenital) or acquired. Common congenital anomalies include uterine septum, bicornuate uterus, unicornuate uterus, and uterine didelphys. With the possible exception of a large uterine septum, the fertility effects of these anomalies have been difficult to verify, although a subset are clearly associated with pregnancy complications. As a uterine septum can now be removed relatively simply and safely with hysteroscopy, most infertility specialists will proceed with surgery if this anomaly is identified. Clinical findings and management of congenital reproductive tract anomalies are fully described in Chapter 18 (p. 417).

Acquired anomalies include intrauterine leiomyomas, polyps, and Asherman syndrome. Of these, leiomyomas may diminish fertility by proposed mechanisms including endometrial cavity distortion with associated changes in blood flow and endometrial maturation; endometrial inflammation; disordered uterine contractility that may hinder sperm or embryo transport; obstruction of the proximal fallopian tubes; or interference with ovum capture (American Society for Reproductive Medicine, 2008b; Makker, 2013; Metwally, 2012; Pritts, 2001; Samejima, 2014). Thus far, no algorithm incorporating tumor number, volume, or location accurately predicts the need to remove them, either to improve implantation rates or to decrease pregnancy complications. Of these, miscarriage, placental abruption, and preterm labor are potential problems. Nevertheless, although not supported by definitive evidence, most experts suggest removal of submucosal fibroids that significantly distort the endometrial cavity. In addition, many consider surgical excision of leiomyomas larger than 4 to 5 cm or multiple smaller tumors in this range regardless of location. Importantly, surgical benefits are weighed against postoperative complications that lower subsequent fertility. These include pelvic adhesion formation, creation of Asherman syndrome following large submucous leiomyoma removal, or the need for cesarean delivery if the full myometrial thickness is transected.

Endometrial polyps are found in an estimated 3 to 5 percent of infertile women (Farhi, 1995; Soares, 2000). The prevalence is higher in women with symptoms such as intermenstrual or postcoital bleeding. Although these complaints typically prompt hysteroscopic removal, most data have not clearly demonstrated an indication for removing polyps in otherwise asymptomatic women (Ben-Arie, 2004; DeWaay, 2002; Jayaprakasan, 2014).

TABLE 19-7.   Advantages and Disadvantages of Various Methods for Evaluating Pelvic Anatomy

	Tubal Patency	Uterine Cavity	Ovaries	Endometriosis or PAD	Developmental Defects
HSG	+	+	–	+/–	+
TVS	–	+/–	+	–	+/–
3-D TVS	–	+	+	–	+
SIS	+/–	+	+	–	+
MR imaging	–	+	+	–	+
Hysteroscopy	–	+	–	–	+ (with laparoscopy)
Laparoscopy	+	–	+	+	+ (with hysteroscopy)

HSG = hysterosalpingography; MR = magnetic resonance; PAD = pelvic adhesive disease; SIS = saline-infusion sonography; TVS = transvaginal sonography.

Of note, however, one study suggested that removal of even small polyps (<1 cm) may improve pregnancy rates following intrauterine insemination (Perez-Medina, 2005).

The presence of intrauterine adhesions, also called *synechiae*, is termed *Asherman syndrome*. This diagnosis is discussed in Chapter 16 (p. 372). Asherman syndrome develops most frequently in women with prior uterine dilation and curettage, particularly in the context of infection and pregnancy (Schenker, 1996). The clinical history will often include an acute postsurgical decrease in menstrual bleeding or even amenorrhea. A woman with an intrauterine device (IUD) complicated by infection or a woman with genital tuberculosis is also at high risk for intrauterine adhesions. Treatment of Asherman syndrome involves hysteroscopic lysis of the scar tissue as described in Chapter 20 (p. 460) and Section 44-19 (p. 1052).

■ Anatomy Evaluation

Several approaches for evaluating pelvic anatomy are: (1) hysterosalpingography (HSG), (2) transvaginal sonography (TVS) with or without saline instillation, (3) 3-dimensional (3-D) TVS, (4) hysteroscopy, (5) laparoscopy, and (6) pelvic imaging by magnetic resonance (MR) imaging. As shown in Table 19-7, each has its own advantages and disadvantages.

Hysterosalpingography

This radiographic tool can display the shape and size of the uterine cavity and define tubal status. Hysterosalpingography is generally performed on cycle days 5 through 10. At this time, few intrauterine clots should remain to block tubal outflow or give the false impression of an intrauterine abnormality. Furthermore, a woman theoretically has not ovulated or possibly conceived. For this test, iodinated contrast medium is infused through a catheter placed into the uterus. With fluoroscopy, dye is visually followed as it fills the uterine cavity, then the tubal lumen, and finally spills out of the tubal fimbria into the pelvic cavity (Fig. 19-6).

In a large metaanalysis, HSG was demonstrated to have 65-percent sensitivity and 83-percent specificity for tubal obstruction (Swart, 1995). Tubal contractions, particularly cornual spasm, can give the incorrect impression of proximal fallopian tube obstruction (a false-positive result). Much less commonly reported is a scenario in which a false-negative result is obtained when the fallopian tube is seen as patent by HSG, although subsequently it is determined to be blocked. Many causes of tubal disease affect both tubes, and thus unilateral disease is unusual. Unilateral obstruction with a normal contralateral tube is most likely due to the dye following the path of least resistance during the HSG procedure. However, laparoscopy with chromotubation is considered prior to treatment to confirm a final diagnosis.

HSG is not reliable in detecting peritubal or pelvic adhesions, although loculations of dye around the tubes may be suggestive. Thus, HSG is an excellent predictor of tubal patency but is less effective at predicting normal tubal function or the presence of pelvic adhesions. Pregnancy rates have been reported to be increased following HSG and are thought to follow flushing of intratubal debris. However, these reports described evaluation with oil-based dyes rather than water-based dyes, which are currently preferred.

HSG also provides analysis of the intrauterine cavity contour. A polyp, leiomyoma, or adhesion within the cavity will block dye diffusion and create an intrauterine "defect" in dye opacity on the radiograph (Fig. 19-7). Although false-positive results may originate from blood clots, mucus plugs, or shearing of the endometrium during placement of the intrauterine catheter, HSG accurately identifies intrauterine pathology. In one study of more than 300 women in which hysteroscopy was the gold standard, HSG was determined to be 98-percent sensitive and 35-percent specific and have a positive predictive value of 70 percent and a negative predictive value of 8 percent. Most misdiagnoses were due to an inability to distinguish polyps from submucous leiomyomas. Other studies have reported much less impressive results. For example, Soares and coworkers (2000) reported sensitivity and positive predictive values of only 50 and 30 percent, respectively, for endometrial polyp and submucous leiomyoma detection in asymptomatic patients. Nevertheless, it is clear that HSG is a helpful tool for uterine cavity evaluation.

HSG can also define developmental uterine anomalies (Fig. 19-8). A Y-shaped uterus identified during HSG may represent either a uterine septum or bicornuate uterus. In these

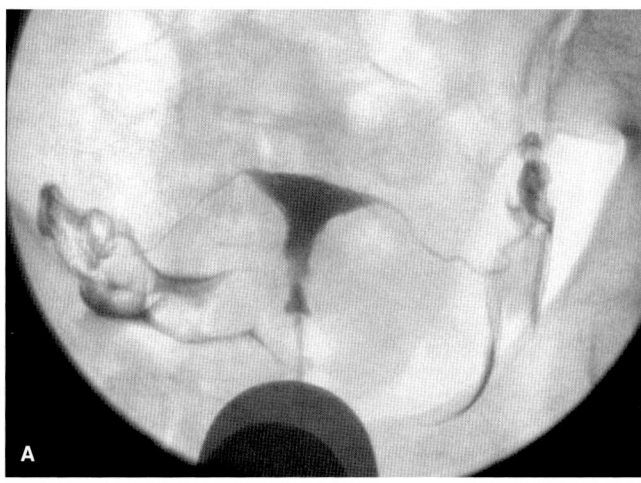

Normal

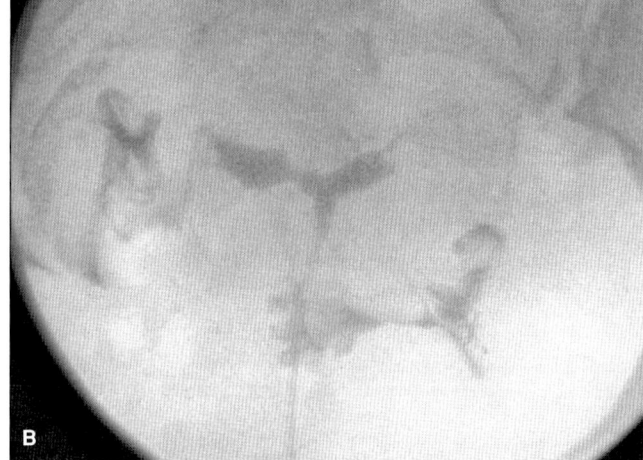

Asherman syndrome

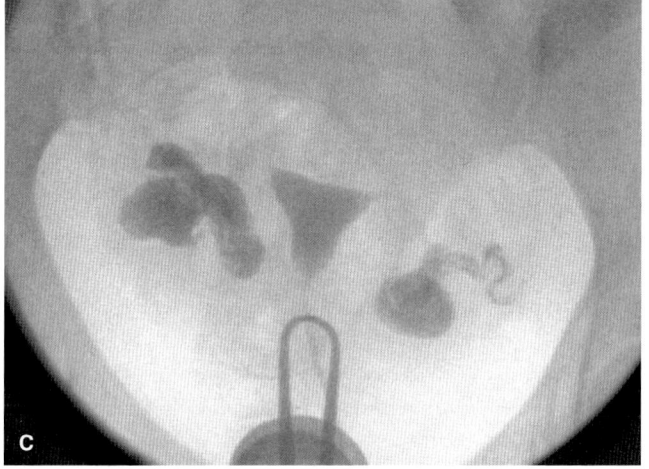

Bilateral hydrosalpinges

FIGURE 19-6 Hysterosalpingogram findings. These images are digitally reversed, causing the radiopaque contrast to appear black against a radiolucent background. **A.** Normal hysterosalpingogram. Radiopaque dye fills the uterine cavity and spills from both fallopian tubes into the peritoneal cavity. The dye catheter is seen beneath the endometrial contour. **B.** Asherman syndrome. Contrast dye fills a small and irregularly shaped endometrial cavity, often described as having a "moth-eaten" appearance. **C.** Bilateral hydrosalpinges. Note the marked tubal dilation and lack of spill of contrast medium at the fimbrial ends. (Used with permission from Dr. Kevin Doody.)

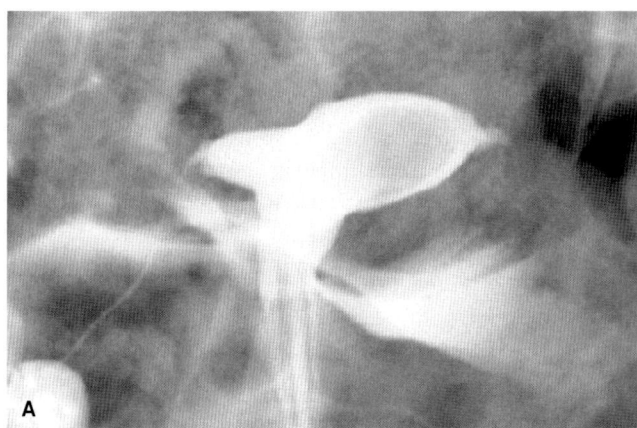
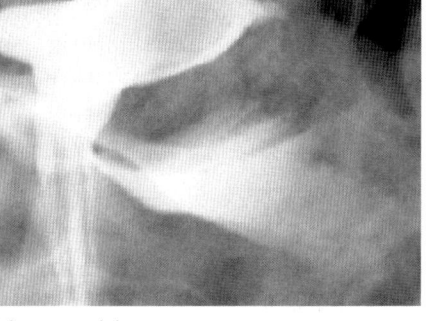

Submucous leiomyoma

Endometrial polyp

FIGURE 19-7 Appearance of leiomyoma and endometrial polyps on hysterosalpingogram (HSG). **A.** A broad-based filling defect is formed during HSG by a submucous leiomyoma. Note distortion of the left cornu by this mass. **B.** A more irregular filling defect is created by an endometrial polyp. Note that polyps generally have a less substantial attachment to the myometrium. (Used with permission from Dr. Diane Twickler.)

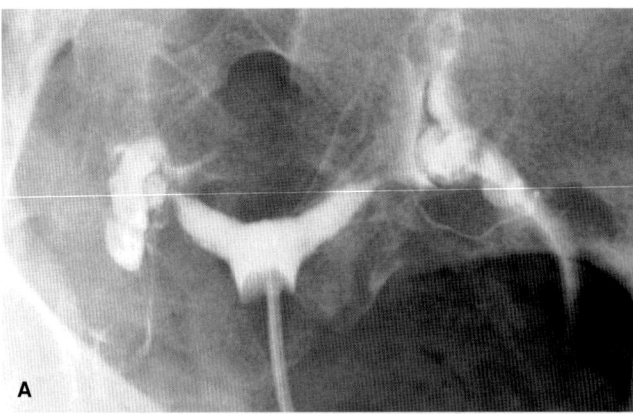

Bicornuate uterus

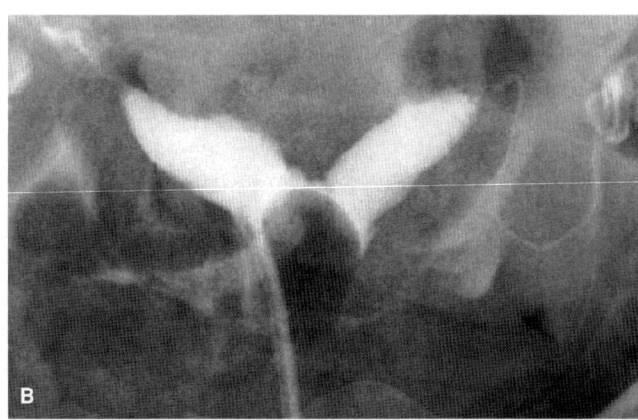

Septate uterus

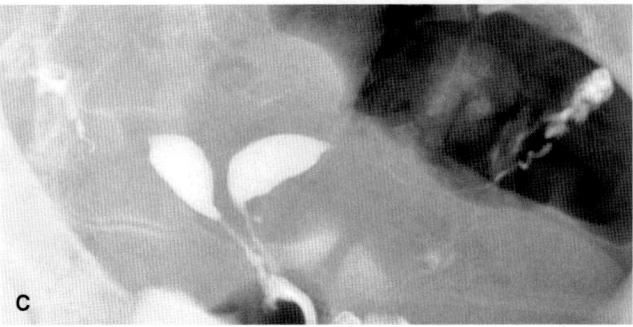

Uterine didelphys

FIGURE 19-8 Hysterosalpingogram appearance of müllerian developmental anomalies. **A.** Bicornuate uterus, due to a failure of fusion of the müllerian ducts, produces a fundal defect with wide-spaced uterine horns. **B.** Septate uterus due to a failure of resorption. This moderate septum displaces the radiopaque dye to the level of the radiolucent injector balloon. **C.** Uterine didelphys consisting of two completely separate müllerian systems including duplication of the cervix. (Used with permission from Dr. Diane Twickler.)

cases, the external contour of the uterine fundus must be evaluated using MR imaging, high-resolution sonography, 3-D TVS, or laparoscopy. With a uterine septum, a smooth fundal contour is found, whereas with a bicornuate uterus, a cleft between the two uterine horns is seen. This is an important distinction, as a septum is often resected, but a bicornuate uterus is usually not treated. In general, uterine anomalies do not cause infertility but may be associated with miscarriage or later fetal loss. Accordingly, it may be reasonable to surgically treat a uterine anomaly to improve pregnancy outcome. However, a couple must be carefully counseled that the conception rate itself is unlikely to be affected. A further discussion of the fertility effects of congenital anomalies is found in Chapter 18 (p. 417).

Sonography

Transvaginal pelvic sonography may be helpful in determining uterine anatomy, particularly during the luteal phase, when the thickened endometrium acts as contrast to the myometrium. Now more widely available, 3-D sonography is advancing discriminatory abilities (Chap. 2, p. 26).

Infusion of saline into the endometrial cavity during sonography performed in the follicular phase provides another approach to create contrast between the cavity and uterine walls. This procedure has many names including hysterosonography, sonohysterography, or saline infusion sonography (SIS). Details of this procedure are described in Chapter 2 (p. 24). SIS has a reported sensitivity of 75 percent and specificity of more than 90 percent for detecting endometrial defects. It has an acceptable positive predictive value of 50 percent and an excellent negative predictive value of 95 percent, which greatly exceeds the negative predictive value of HSG (Grimbizis, 2010; Seshadri, 2015; Soares, 2000). Moreover, SIS may be more sensitive than HSG in determining whether a cavitary defect is a pedunculated leiomyoma or a polyp (Figs. 8-7 and 9-5, pp. 187 and 206). Perhaps more importantly, SIS can help determine what portion of a submucous leiomyoma lies within the cavity. Only those with more than 50-percent of their mass within the cavity are considered for hysteroscopic resection.

The primary limitation of SIS is that it does not provide information regarding the fallopian tubes, although rapid loss of saline into the pelvis is certainly consistent with at least unilateral patency. SIS is generally less painful than HSG and does not require radiation exposure. Thus, it is preferred if information about tubal patency is not required, such as in patients who are known to require IVF for other reasons such as severe oligospermia.

Laparoscopy

Direct inspection provides the most accurate assessment of pelvic pathology, and laparoscopy is the gold standard approach. Chromotubation may be performed, and a dilute dye is injected through an acorn cannula placed against the cervix or through a balloon catheter positioned within the uterine cavity. Tubal spill is evaluated through the laparoscope (Fig. 19-9). Indigo carmine dye, if available, is preferable to methylene blue, as the methylene blue rarely may induce acute methemoglobinemia, particularly in patients with glucose-6-phosphate dehydrogenase deficiency. One 5-mL vial of indigo carmine is mixed with 50 to 100 mL of sterile saline for injection through the cervical cannula.

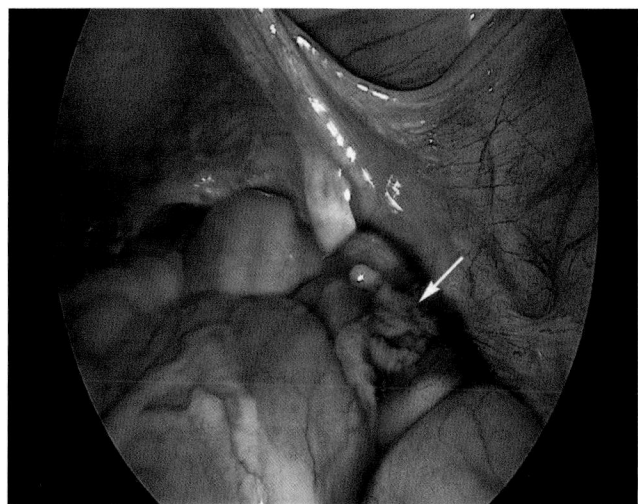

FIGURE 19-9 Chromotubation seen at laparoscopy. Note the spill of blue dye from the fimbriated end of the fallopian tube. (Used with permission from Dr. Kevin Doody.)

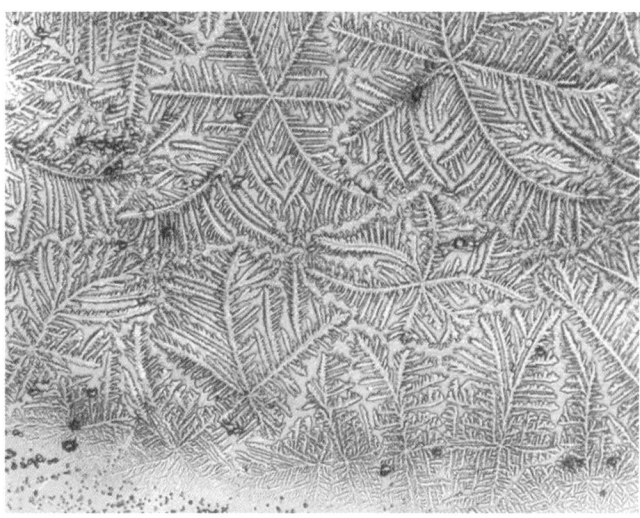

FIGURE 19-10 Ferning pattern can be seen midcycle if cervical mucus is dried on a microscope slide. A high sodium chloride concentration creates a crystalline pattern and is produced by elevated estrogen levels near ovulation.

Laparoscopy allows both diagnosis and immediate surgical treatment of abnormalities such as endometriosis or pelvic adhesions. Laparoscopic ablation of these lesions may increase subsequent pregnancy rates (Chap. 10, p. 243).

As laparoscopy is an invasive procedure, it is not advocated in place of HSG as part of the initial infertility evaluation. Exceptions include women with a history or symptoms suggestive of endometriosis or prior pelvic inflammation. However, even in these women, a preliminary HSG may be informative (De Hondt, 2005).

If laparoscopy is clearly indicated, then hysteroscopy can also be performed to evaluate the uterine cavity while the patient is under anesthesia. Moreover, in operative hysteroscopic cases, laparoscopy can help direct surgery and avoid perforation, for example, during septal incision.

Laparoscopy also may be considered in patients who fail to conceive with clomiphene or gonadotropin ovulation induction. If pelvic disease is found and treated, progression to IVF may be avoided. With improvements in IVF success rates, this latter argument is becoming less justifiable, as the cost of surgery well exceeds the cost of an IVF cycle.

Hysteroscopy

Endoscopic evaluation of the intrauterine cavity is the preferred method to define intrauterine abnormalities. Hysteroscopy can be performed in an office or operating room. With improved instrumentation, the ability to concurrently diagnose and treat abnormalities in the office is increasing. However, substantially more extensive hysteroscopic surgery is possible in the operating room. A fuller discussion of hysteroscopy and its indications is found in Chapter 41 (p. 901).

■ Cervical Factors

The cervical glands secrete mucus that is normally thick and impervious to sperm and ascending infections. High estrogen levels at midcycle change the quality of this mucus. It becomes thin and stretchy and has an increased sodium chloride concentration (Fig. 19-10). Estrogen-primed cervical mucus filters out nonsperm components of semen and forms channels that help direct sperm into the uterus. Midcycle mucus also creates a reservoir for sperm. This allows ongoing release during the next 24 to 72 hours and extends the potential time for fertilization (Katz, 1997).

Abnormalities in mucus production are most frequently observed in women who have undergone cryosurgery, cervical conization, or a loop electrosurgical excision procedure (LEEP) for treatment of cervical neoplasia. Cervical infection may also worsen mucus quality, but data are conflicting. Implicated agents include *C trachomatis*, *N gonorrhoeae*, *Ureaplasma urealyticum*, and *Mycoplasma hominis* (Cimino, 1993). Although there may be no advantage in terms of mucus quality, obtaining cultures for *C trachomatis* and *N gonorrhoeae* seems prudent to avoid causing ascending infection during HSG or intrauterine inseminations.

The postcoital test, also known as the Sims-Huhner test, was used historically to evaluate cervical mucus. For this test, a couple is requested to have intercourse on the day of ovulation. A subsequent sample of the cervical mucus is evaluated for elasticity (*Spinnbarkeit*) and the number of motile sperm per high-power field. This test has been hampered by a limited consensus on the definition of a normal test (Oei, 1995). Moreover, in a prospective, randomized trial, a normal postcoital test did not predict increased cumulative pregnancy rates (Oei, 1998).

Many infertility specialists recommend bypassing the cervix with intrauterine insemination (IUI) in any woman with prior cervical surgery, especially if she has noted a decrease in midcycle mucus production. The remaining utility of the postcoital test is for the rare couple who will not consider intrauterine insemination or do not have intrauterine insemination readily available. In regions of the world in which more specific testing cannot be obtained, a postcoital test will provide basic information regarding mucus production, appropriate intercourse practices, and presence of motile sperm.

EVALUATION OF MALE INFERTILITY

Causes of male infertility can roughly be categorized as abnormalities of sperm production or sperm function or obstruction of the ductal outflow tract.

■ Normal Spermatogenesis

During evaluation of a male infertility patient, the basics of male reproductive physiology should be understood. Analogous to the ovary, testes have two functions: the generation of mature germ cells (sperm) and the production of male hormones, primarily testosterone. The seminiferous tubules contain developing sperm and support cells called *Sertoli cells* or *sustentacular cells* (see Fig. 19-4). The Sertoli cells form tight junctions that produce a blood-testis barrier. This avascular space within the seminiferous tubules protects sperm from antibodies and toxins but also makes these cells dependent on diffusion for oxygen, nutrients, and metabolic precursors. Located between the seminiferous tubules are Leydig cells, also called *interstitial cells*, which are responsible for steroid hormone production. In simplistic terms, Leydig cells are similar to the theca cells of the ovary.

Unlike the ovary, testes contain stem cells that allow ongoing production of mature germ cells throughout a male's life. In a fertile male, approximately 100 to 200 million sperm are produced each day (Sigman, 1997). The process begins with a diploid (46,XY) spermatogonial cell, which grows and becomes a primary spermatocyte. The first meiotic division produces two secondary spermatocytes, and completion of meiosis results in four mature sperm with a haploid (23,X or 23,Y) karyotype. During this developmental process, most sperm cytoplasm is lost, mitochondria that provide energy are positioned in the sperm midpiece, and sperm flagella develop.

Production of sperm requires approximately 70 days. An additional 12 to 21 days is needed for sperm to be transported into the epididymis. Here, they further mature and gain motility (Heller, 1963; Hinrichsen, 1980; Rowley, 1970). Importantly, due to this prolonged developmental period, the results of a semen analysis reflect events during the past 3 months, not a single point in time.

To fertilize an oocyte, human sperm must undergo a process known as *capacitation*. Capacitation results in sperm hyperactivation (an extreme increase in movement) and the ability to release acrosomal contents, which allow penetration of the ovum's zona pellucida.

Normal spermatogenesis is dependent on high local levels of testosterone. LH from the anterior pituitary gland stimulates production of testosterone by the Leydig cells. FSH increases LH receptor density on the Leydig cells, thus indirectly contributing to testosterone production. In addition, FSH increases production of sex hormone-binding globulin, also called androgen-binding protein. Androgen-binding protein binds testosterone and maintains high concentrations of this hormone in the seminiferous tubules (Sigman, 1997).

In addition to hormone levels, testicular volume often reflects spermatogenesis, and a normal volume is between 15 and 25 mL. Most of this volume is provided by the seminiferous tubules. Thus, decreased testicular volume is a strong indicator of abnormal spermatogenesis.

Spermatogenesis is directed by genes on the Y chromosome. Autosomal genes also provide important contributions, which continue to be elucidated. Therefore, genetic abnormalities may adversely affect this process, as discussed later.

Male fertility likely decreases modestly with increasing age. Several studies have demonstrated that pregnancy rates decline and time to conception lengthens as male age increases. Studies of semen parameters across age suggest that sperm concentration is maintained, however, sperm motility and morphology progressively worsen (Levitas, 2007). The clinical significance of this change is unclear (Kidd, 2001). In short, although advancing male age may lower fertility, it is probably insignificant compared with aging changes in women.

■ Semen Analysis

Collection

This is a core test in male fertility evaluation. For this test, the male is asked to refrain from ejaculation for 2 to 3 days, and a specimen is collected by masturbation into a sterile cup. If masturbation is not an option, then a couple can use specially designed Silastic condoms without lubricants. Importantly, the sample should arrive in the laboratory within an hour of ejaculation to allow for optimal analysis.

The sample undergoes liquefaction, or thinning of the seminal fluid, due to enzymes from the liquid contribution of the prostate gland. This process takes 5 to 20 minutes and allows more accurate evaluation of the sperm contained in the seminal fluid. Ideally, two semen samples separated by at least a month are analyzed. In practice, frequently only a single sample is analyzed if parameters are normal.

Semen Analysis Results

The reference values for the semen analysis are shown in Table 19-8. A clinician should remember several critical aspects of this test. First, semen characteristics vary across time in a single individual. Second, semen analysis results, particularly morphologic interpretation, differ between laboratories. Thus, reference ranges for the laboratory being used should be known. Note that the concept of "reference" range is more appropriate than "normal" range. Although total motile sperm count correlates with fertility, not all males with "normal" semen parameters display normal fertility (Guzick, 2001). Conversely,

TABLE 19-8.   Semen Analysis Reference Limits

Volume	>1.5 mL[a]
Count	>15 million/mL[a]
Total Motility	>40%[a]
Morphology	>4%[a]
WBCs	<1 million/mL[b]
Round cells	<5 million/mL[b]

[a]Data from Cooper, 2010.
[b]Data from World Health Organization, 1999.
WBCs = white blood cells.

patients with semen analysis results outside the reference range may achieve pregnancy. The lack of absolute predictive value for this test is likely due to the fact that it does not provide information regarding sperm function, that is, the ultimate ability to fertilize an oocyte.

Most semen analysis reports will indicate semen volume, pH, and presence or absence of fructose. Nearly 80 percent of semen volume comes from the seminal vesicles. Seminal fluid is alkaline and is thought to protect sperm from acidity in prostatic secretions and in the vagina. Seminal fluid also provides fructose as an energy source for sperm. An acidic pH or lack of fructose is consistent with obstruction of the efferent ductal system (Daudin, 2000).

Of parameters, low semen volume often simply reflects incomplete specimen collection or short abstinence interval. However, it may indicate partial vas deferens obstruction or retrograde ejaculation. Partial or complete vas deferens obstruction may be caused by infection, tumor, prior testicular or inguinal surgery, or trauma. Retrograde ejaculation follows failed closure of the bladder neck during ejaculation and allows seminal fluid to flow backward into the bladder. Retrograde ejaculation is suspected in men with diabetes mellitus, spinal cord damage, or prior prostate or other retroperitoneal surgery that may have damaged nerves (Hershlag, 1991). Medications, particularly β-blockers, may contribute to this problem. A postejaculatory urinalysis can detect sperm in the bladder and confirm the diagnosis. If urine is properly alkalinized, these sperm are viable and can be retrieved to achieve pregnancy.

Sperm counts may be normal, or males may have low sperm counts (oligospermia), or no sperm (azoospermia) (Sharlip, 2002). Oligospermia is defined as a concentration less than 15 million sperm per milliliter, and counts below 5 million per milliliter are considered severe. The prevalence of azoospermia is approximately 1 percent of all men. Azoospermia may result from outflow tract obstruction, termed obstructive azoospermia, such as that which occurs with congenital absence of the vas deferens, severe infection, or vasectomy. Azoospermia may also follow testicular failure (nonobstructive azoospermia). In the latter case, careful centrifugation and analysis may identify a small number of motile sperm adequate for IVF use. Alternatively, this latter group may have viable sperm obtainable through either epididymal aspiration or testicular biopsy. As described later, endocrine and genetic evaluation is indicated for men with abnormal sperm counts.

Sperm movement is also assessed, and decreased sperm motility is termed *asthenospermia*. Some laboratories will distinguish between rapid (grade 3 to 4), slow (grade 2), and nonprogressive (grade 0 to 1) movement. *Total progressive motility* is the percentage of sperm exhibiting forward movement (grades 2 to 4). Asthenospermia has been attributed to prolonged abstinence, antisperm antibodies, genital tract infections, or varicocele. To differentiate between dead and nonmotile sperm, a hypoosmotic swelling test can be performed. Unlike dead sperm, living sperm can maintain an osmotic gradient. Thus, when mixed with a hypoosmotic solution, living, nonmotile sperm with normal membrane function swell and coil as fluid is absorbed (Casper, 1996). Once identified, these viable sperm may be used for intracytoplasmic sperm injection.

Abnormal sperm morphology is termed *teratospermia* or *teratozoospermia*. Kruger and colleagues (1988) developed a detailed characterization of normal sperm morphology, which showed improved correlation with fertilization rates during IVF cycles. Their criteria require careful analysis of the shape and size of the sperm head, the relative size of the acrosome in proportion to the head, and characteristics of the tail, including length, coiling, or presence of two tails. Significantly decreased fertilization rates are seen when normal morphology of the sample falls below 4 percent.

Round cells in a sperm sample may represent either leukocytes or immature sperm. White blood cells (WBCs) can be distinguished from immature sperm using various techniques, including a myeloperoxidase stain for WBCs (Wolff, 1995). True leukocytospermia is defined as greater than 1 million WBCs per milliliter and may indicate chronic epididymitis or prostatitis. In this scenario, many andrologists consider empiric antibiotic treatment prior to obtaining a repeat semen analysis. A common protocol would include doxycycline at a dosage of 100 mg orally twice daily for 2 weeks. Alternative approaches include culture of any expressible discharge or of the semen sample.

Unless a general obstetrician-gynecologist has developed a particular interest and expertise in the area of infertility, persistent abnormal semen analysis findings are an indication for referral to an infertility specialist. Although the partner may be referred directly to a urologist, it may be more reasonable to refer the couple to a reproductive endocrinologist, as the female will also require evaluation. Treatment is likely to be more complex in these couples and will typically be directed to both partners. The reproductive specialist can determine the need for further referral of the male partner to a urologist for investigation of a genetic, anatomic, hormonal, or infectious abnormality.

■ DNA Fragmentation

During the past 10 years, interest in elevated sperm DNA fragmentation as a cause of male factor infertility has increased (Sakkas, 2010; Zini, 2009). Although some degree of DNA damage is likely repaired during embryogenesis, the location and extent of damage may lower fertilization and increase miscarriage rates. Increased levels of DNA damage are associated with advanced paternal age and external factors such as cigarette smoking, chemotherapy, radiation, environmental toxins, varicocele, and genital tract infections. Studies have observed increased levels of reactive oxygen species in sperm samples with abnormal DNA fragmentation rates. In response to this observation, dietary supplementation with the antioxidants vitamin C and vitamin E has been proposed. However, data are currently lacking regarding the efficacy of this approach.

Numerous tests are currently available to analyze for DNA integrity and include the Sperm Chromatin Structure Assay (SCSA), the terminal deoxynucleotidyl transferase-mediated dUTP nick-end labeling (TUNEL) assay, the single-cell gel electrophoresis assay (COMET), and the sperm chromatin dispersion test (SCD) (American Society for Reproductive Medicine, 2013c). Each of these tests provides semiquantitative data on DNA structure. For example, the SCSA is based on the increased susceptibility of DNA with single-strand or double-strand breaks to denature in weak acid. The TUNEL assay exploits the ability of labeled nucleotides to intercalate into DNA breaks for subsequent measurement. These tests are currently hampered by a lack of consensus regarding appropriate threshold values and by conflicting data regarding their ability to predict successful pregnancy. As a result, currently evidence is insufficient to recommend the routine use of these tests in infertile couples. Nevertheless, the concept that sperm DNA integrity can be adversely affected through multiple mechanisms provides useful insight into a previously underappreciated cause of male infertility.

■ Additional Sperm Testing

Antisperm antibodies may be detected in as many as 10 percent of men. However, controversy exists regarding the negative fertility effects of antisperm antibodies found in semen. These antibodies may be particularly prevalent following vasectomy, testicular torsion, testicular biopsy, or other clinical situations in which the blood-testis barrier is breached (Turek, 1994). Treatment historically included corticosteroids, but it is unclear if this approach improves fertility. Moreover, significant side effects, including aseptic necrosis of the hip, have been reported in treated patients. Current data suggest that antisperm antibody assay does not need to be a routine component of infertility evaluation.

Numerous assays have been developed to test sperm function. These include the mannose fluorescence assay, hemizona assay, sperm penetration assay, and acrosome reaction test. The predictive significance of these assays is questionable, as they are based on highly nonphysiologic conditions and results vary widely from infertility center to infertility center. Most are no longer used and are not considered part of a basic infertility evaluation.

■ Hormonal Evaluation of the Male

Hormonal testing in the male is analogous to endocrine testing in an anovulatory female. In overview, abnormalities may be due to central defects in hypothalamic-pituitary function or due to defects within the testes. Most urologists will defer testing unless a sperm concentration is below 10 million/mL. Testing will include measurements of serum FSH and testosterone levels.

Low FSH and low testosterone levels are consistent with hypothalamic dysfunction, such as idiopathic hypogonadotropic hypogonadism or Kallman syndrome (Chap. 16, p. 375). In these patients, sperm production may be achieved with gonadotropin treatment. Although such treatment is frequently successful, at least 6 months may be required for detection of sperm production.

Elevated FSH and low testosterone levels provide evidence of testicular failure, and most men with oligospermia fall into this category. In this patient group, it is important to determine, based on testosterone levels, whether testosterone replacement is indicated. Normal spermatogenesis requires high levels of intratesticular testosterone, which cannot be achieved with exogenous testosterone. Furthermore, many of these men will lack spermatogonial stem cells. Thus, testosterone replacement will not rescue sperm production. In fact, replacement will decrease gonadotropin stimulation of remaining testicular function through negative feedback at the hypothalamus and pituitary. Unless the couple has chosen to use donor sperm, androgen supplementation is deferred during fertility treatment. However, replacement will provide other benefits, such as improved libido and sexual function, maintenance of muscle mass and bone density, and a general sense of well-being.

Additional hormonal testing may be included as part of an evaluation of the infertile male. Elevated serum prolactin levels and thyroid dysfunction affect spermatogenesis and are the most likely endocrinopathies to be detected (Sharlip, 2002; Sigman, 1997).

■ Genetic Testing of the Male

Genetic abnormalities are a relatively common cause of abnormal semen characteristics (American Society for Reproductive Medicine, 2008a). Approximately 15 percent of azoospermic men and 5 percent of severely oligospermic men will have an abnormal karyotype. Although genetic abnormalities cannot be corrected, they may have implications for the health of the patient or their offspring. Therefore, karyotyping is pursued when indicated by poor semen analysis results. The lower limit in sperm concentration for such testing varies between practitioners but lies between 3 and 10 million sperm per milliliter.

Klinefelter syndrome (47,XXY) will be a frequent finding. Klinefelter syndrome is observed in approximately 1 in 500 men in the general population and accounts for 1 to 2 percent of male infertility cases. Classically, these men are tall, undervirilized, and have gynecomastia and small, firm testes (De Braekeleer, 1991). As the phenotype varies widely, lack of these characteristics does not preclude chromosomal evaluation. Conversely, a clinician may strongly consider obtaining karyotype testing in any male with these characteristics. Autosomal abnormalities will also be found in a subset of men with severe oligospermia.

A patient with severely decreased sperm counts and a normal karyotype is offered testing for microdeletion of the Y chromosome. Up to 15 percent of men with severe oligospermia or azoospermia will have small deletions in a region of the Y chromosome termed the *azoospermia factor region (AZF)*. If the deletion is within the AZFa or AZFb subregions, then it is unlikely that viable sperm can be recovered for use in IVF. Most men with an AZFc deletion will have viable sperm at biopsy. However, these deletions should be presumed to be inherited by their offspring. The clinical significance of microdeletions in the recently identified AZFd region is unknown, as these patients have apparently normal spermatogenesis (Hopps, 2003; Kent-First, 1999; Pryor, 1997).

Obstructive azoospermia may be due to congenital bilateral absence of the vas deferens (CBAVD). Approximately 70 to 85 percent of men with CBAVD will have mutations found in the cystic fibrosis transmembrane conductance regulator gene (*CFTR* gene), although not all will have clinical cystic fibrosis

(Oates, 1994; Ratbi, 2007). Conversely, essentially all men with clinical cystic fibrosis will have CBAVD. Fortunately, testicular function in these men is usually normal, and adequate sperm may be obtained by epididymal aspiration to achieve pregnancy through IVF. Careful genetic counseling and testing of the female partner for carrier status is critical in these situations.

■ Testicular Biopsy

Evaluation of a severely oligospermic or azoospermic male may include either open or percutaneous testicular biopsy to determine whether viable sperm are present in the seminiferous tubules (Sharlip, 2002). For example, even men with testicular failure diagnosed by elevated serum FSH levels may have adequate sperm on biopsy for use in intracytoplasmic sperm injection. The biopsy specimen can be cryopreserved for future extraction of sperm during an IVF cycle. However, freshly biopsied specimens are generally felt to provide higher success rates. Thus, the biopsy may have diagnostic, prognostic, and therapeutic value.

CONCLUSION

Figure 19-11 provides an algorithm for the evaluation of an infertile couple. Details will vary between practitioners and will be affected by patient presentation. In general, the female partner has some form of testing to confirm ovulation and undergoes HSG, whereas the male partner has semen analysis performed. In older women, evaluation of an early-follicular serum FSH level is essential to ensure adequate follicular reserves. A subset of couples will decline HSG and semen analysis if the woman has a clear ovulatory defect. These couples are reminded that there is a relatively high incidence of couples having two abnormalities, one of which would be missed by this approach. These patients may be treated, but are strongly encouraged to complete the evaluation if they do not conceive within a few months. Options for treatment are discussed in Chapter 20.

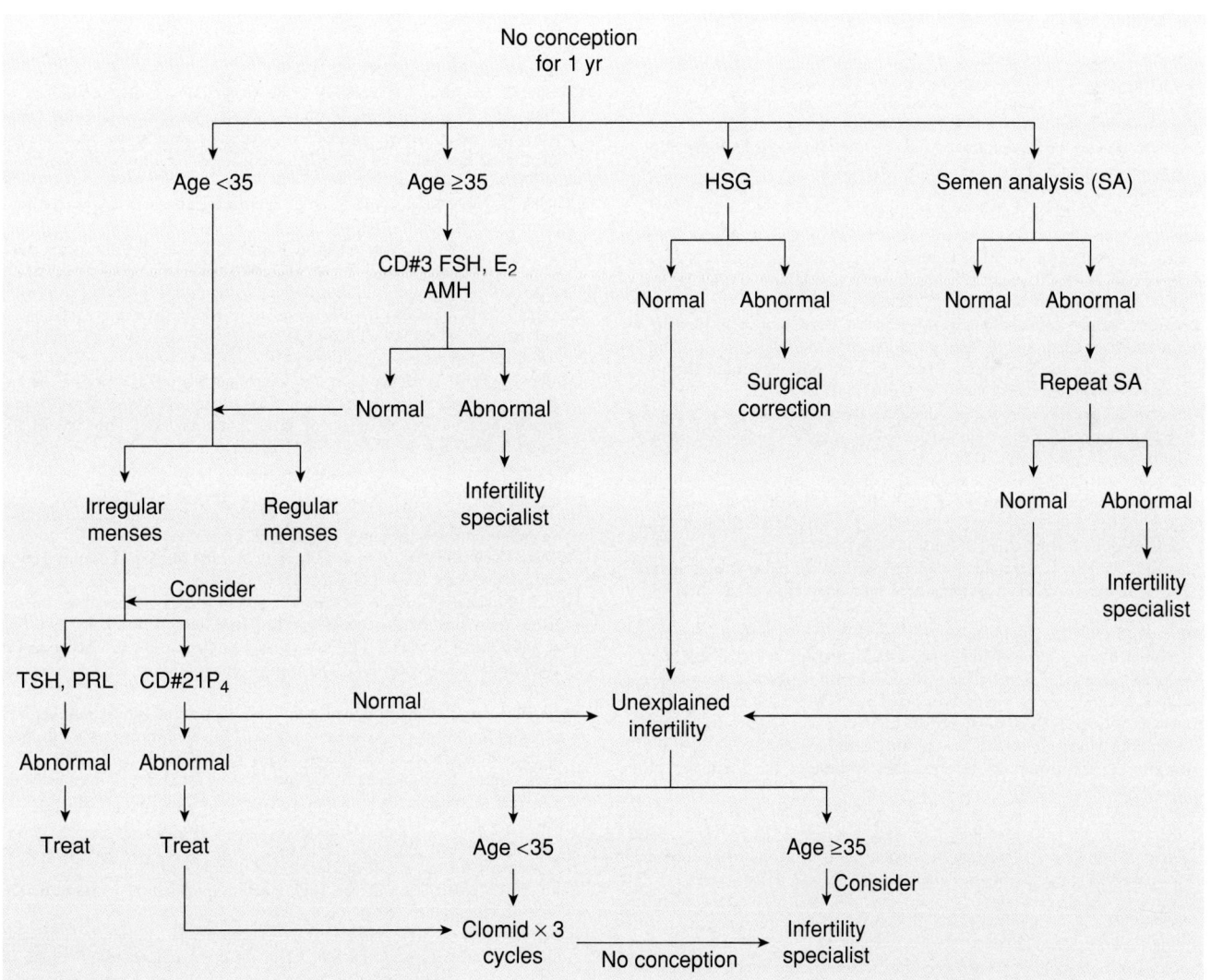

FIGURE 19-11 Diagnostic algorithm for evaluation of the infertile couple. AMH = antimüllerian hormone; CD#3 = cycle day 3; CD#21 = cycle day 21; E_2 = estradiol; FSH = follicle-stimulating hormone; HSG = hysterosalpingography; P_4 = progesterone; PRL = prolactin; SA = semen analysis; TSH = thyroid-stimulating hormone.

REFERENCES

Abma J, Chandra A, Mosher W, et al: Fertility, family planning, and women's health: new data from the 1995 National Survey of Family Growth. Vital Health Stat 23:1, 1997

Aliyu MH, Aliyu SH, Salihu HM: Female genital tuberculosis: a global review. Int J Fertil Womens Med 49:123, 2004

American Academy of Pediatrics and the American College of Obstetricians and Gynecologists: Guidelines for Perinatal Care, 7th Edition, Washington, 2012

American College of Obstetricians and Gynecologists: Carrier screening for fragile X syndrome. Committee Opinion No. 469, October 2010, Reaffirmed 2014a

American College of Obstetricians and Gynecologists: Neural tube defects. Practice Bulletin No. 44, July 2003, Reaffirmed 2014b

American College of Obstetricians and Gynecologists: Ovarian reserve testing. Practice Bulletin No. 618, January 2015

American College of Obstetricians and Gynecologists: Preconception and prenatal carrier screening for genetic diseases in individuals of Eastern European Jewish descent. Committee Opinion No. 442, October 2009

American College of Obstetricians and Gynecologists: Screening for Tay-Sachs disease. Committee Opinion No. 318, October 2005, Reaffirmed 2014c

American College of Obstetricians and Gynecologists: Spinal muscular atrophy. Committee Opinion No. 432, May 2009, Reaffirmed 2014d

American College of Obstetricians and Gynecologists: Update on carrier screening for cystic fibrosis. Committee Opinion No. 486, July 2011, Reaffirmed 2014e

American Society for Reproductive Medicine: Diagnostic evaluation of the infertile female: a committee opinion. Fertil Steril 98(2):302, 2012a

American Society for Reproductive Medicine: Diagnostic evaluation of the infertile male: a committee opinion. Fertil Steril 98(2):294, 2012b

American Society for Reproductive Medicine: Effectiveness and treatment for unexplained infertility. Fertil Steril 86(5) Suppl 1:S111, 2006

American Society for Reproductive Medicine: Endometriosis and infertility: a committee opinion. Fertil Steril 98(3):591, 2012c

American Society for Reproductive Medicine: Evaluation of the azoospermic male. Fertil Steril 90 (Suppl 3):S74, 2008a

American Society for Reproductive Medicine: Female age-related fertility decline. Fertil Steril 101(3):633, 2014a

American Society for Reproductive Medicine: Myomas and reproductive function. Fertil Steril 90(Suppl 3):S125, 2008b

American Society for Reproductive Medicine: Obesity and reproduction: an educational bulletin. Fertil Steril 90 (Suppl 3):S21, 2008c

American Society for Reproductive Medicine: Optimizing natural fertility: a committee opinion. Fertil Steril 100(3):631, 2013a

American Society for Reproductive Medicine: Pathogenesis, consequences, and control of peritoneal adhesions in gynecologic surgery: a committee opinion. Fertil Steril 99(6):1550, 2013b

American Society for Reproductive Medicine: Report on varicocele and infertility: a committee opinion. Fertil Steril 102(6):1556, 2014b

American Society for Reproductive Medicine: Smoking and infertility: a committee opinion. Fertil Steril 98(6):1400, 2012d

American Society for Reproductive Medicine: Testing and interpreting measures of ovarian reserve: a committee opinion. Fertil Steril 98(6):1407, 2012e

American Society for Reproductive Medicine: The clinical relevance of luteal phase deficiency: a committee opinion. Fertil Steril 98(5):1112, 2012f

American Society for Reproductive Medicine: The clinical utility of sperm DNA integrity testing: a guideline. Fertil Steril 99(3):673, 2013c

American Society for Reproductive Medicine: Vaccination guidelines for female infertility patients: a committee opinion. Fertil Steril 99(2):337, 2013d

Anderson J, Williamson R: Fertility after torsion of the spermatic cord. Br J Urol 65:225, 1990

Anguiano A, Oates R, Amos J, et al: Congenital bilateral absence of the vas deferens. A primarily genital form of cystic fibrosis. JAMA 267:1794, 1992

Augood C, Duckitt K, Templeton A: Smoking and female infertility: a systematic review and meta-analysis. Hum Reprod 13:1532, 1998

Baazeem A, Belzile E, Ciampi A, et al: Varicocele and male factor infertility treatment: a new meta-analysis and review of the role of varicocele repair. Eur Urol 60(4):796, 2011

Balasch J, Fabregues F, Creus M, et al: The usefulness of endometrial biopsy for luteal phase evaluation in infertility. Hum Reprod 7:973, 1992

Bates G, Garza D, Garza M: Clinical manifestations of hormonal changes in the menstrual cycle. Obstet Gynecol Clin North Am 17:299, 1990

Beard C, Benson R Jr, Kelalis P, et al: The incidence and outcome of mumps orchitis in Rochester, Minnesota, 1935 to 1974. Mayo Clin Proc 52:3, 1977

Ben-Arie A, Goldchmit C, Laviv Y, et al: The malignant potential of endometrial polyps. Eur J Obstet Gynecol Reprod Biol 115:206, 2004

Benson GS: Erection, Emission, and Ejaculation: Physiologic Mechanism, 3rd ed. St. Louis, Mosby, 1997

Bracken M, Eskenazi B, Sachse K, et al: Association of cocaine use with sperm concentration, motility, and morphology. Fertil Steril 53:315, 1990

Buyalos R, Daneshmand S, Brzechffa P: Basal estradiol and follicle-stimulating hormone predict fecundity in women of advanced reproductive age undergoing ovulation induction therapy. Fertil Steril 68:272, 1997

Carson D, Lagow E, Thathiah A, et al: Changes in gene expression during the early to mid-luteal (receptive phase) transition in human endometrium detected by high-density microarray screening. Mol Hum Reprod 8:871, 2002

Caserta D, Mantovani A, Marci R, et al: Environment and women's reproductive health. Hum Reprod Update 17(3):418, 2011

Casper R, Meriano J, Jarvi K, et al: The hypo-osmotic swelling test for selection of viable sperm for intracytoplasmic sperm injection in men with complete asthenozoospermia. Fertil Steril 65:972, 1996

Centers for Disease Control and Prevention: Current cigarette smoking among adults—United States, 2005–2013. MMWR 63(47):1108, 2014

Chandra A, Copen CE, Stephen EH: Infertility and impaired fecundity in the United States, 1982–2010: data from the National Survey of Family Growth. Natl Health Stat Report 67:1, 2013

Chandra A, Copen CE, Stephen EH: Infertility service use in the United States: data from the National Survey of Family Growth, 1982–2010. Natl Health Stat Report 73:1, 2014

Chang WY, Agarwal SK, Azziz R: Diagnostic evaluation and treatment of the infertile couple. In Carr BR, Blackwell RE, Azziz R (eds): Essential Reproductive Medicine. New York, McGraw-Hill, 2005, p 366

Charny C: The spermatogenic potential of the undescended testis before and after treatment. J Urol 38:697, 1960

Cimino C, Borruso A, Napoli P, et al: Evaluation of the importance of Chlamydia T. and/or Mycoplasma H. and/or Ureaplasma U. genital infections and of antisperm antibodies in couples affected by muco-semen incompatibility and in couples with unexplained infertility. Acta Eur Fertil 24:13, 1993

Cobellis G, Noviello C, Nino F, et al: Spermatogenesis and cryptorchidism. Front Endocrinol 5:63, 2014

Cooper TG, Noonan E, von Eckardstein S, et al: World Health Organization reference values for human semen characteristics. Hum Reprod 16(3):231, 2010

Cunningham FG, Leveno KJ, Bloom SL, et al (eds): Teratology, teratogens, and fetotoxic agents. In Williams Obstetrics, 24th ed. New York, McGraw-Hill Education, 2014

Daudin M, Bieth E, Bujan L, et al: Congenital bilateral absence of the vas deferens: clinical characteristics, biological parameters, cystic fibrosis transmembrane conductance regulator gene mutations, and implications for genetic counseling. Fertil Steril 74:1164, 2000

De Braekeleer M, Dao T: Cytogenetic studies in male infertility: a review. Hum Reprod 6:245, 1991

De Hondt A, Peeraer K, Meuleman C, et al: Endometriosis and subfertility treatment: a review. Minerva Ginecol 57:257, 2005

DeWaay DJ, Syrop CH, Nygaard IE, et al: Natural history of uterine polyps and leiomyomata. Obstet Gynecol 100:3, 2002

Farhi J, Ashkenazi J, Feldberg D, et al: Effect of uterine leiomyomata on the results of in-vitro fertilization treatment. Hum Reprod 10:2576, 1995

Fiore MC, Jaen CR, Baker TB, et al: Treating tobacco use and dependence: 2008 update. Rockville, U.S. Department of Health and Human Services, 2008

Frattarelli J, Lauria-Costab D, Miller B, et al: Basal antral follicle number and mean ovarian diameter predict cycle cancellation and ovarian responsiveness in assisted reproductive technology cycles. Fertil Steril 74:512, 2000

Garrido-Gomez T, Quinonera A, Antunez O, et al: Deciphering the proteomic signature of human endometrial receptivity. Hum Reprod 29(9):1957, 2014

Gazvani M, Buckett W, Luckas M, et al: Conservative management of azoospermia following steroid abuse. Hum Reprod 12:1706, 1997

Giudice LC: Infertility and the environment: the medical context. Semin Reprod Med 24:129, 2006

Gnoth C, Roos J, Broomhead D, et al: Antimüllerian hormone levels and numbers and sizes of antral follicles in regularly menstruating women of reproductive age referenced to true ovulation day. Fertil Steril September 15, 2015 [Epub ahead of print]

Grimbizis GF, Tsolakidis D, Mikos T, et al: A prospective comparison of transvaginal ultrasound, saline infusion sonohysterography, and diagnostic hysteroscopy in the evaluation of endometrial pathology. Fertil Steril 94(7):2720, 2010

Grinsted J, Jacobsen J, Grinsted L, et al: Prediction of ovulation. Fertil Steril 52:388, 1989

Grodstein F, Goldman M, Cramer D: Body mass index and ovulatory infertility. Epidemiology 5:247, 1994a

Grodstein F, Goldman M, Cramer D: Infertility in women and moderate alcohol use. Am J Public Health 84:1429, 1994b

Grody WW, Thompson BH, Gregg AR, et al: ACMG position statement on prenatal/preconception expanded carrier screening. Genet Med 15(6):48, 2013

Gross SJ, Pletcher BA, Monaghan KG, et al: Carrier screening in individuals of Ashkenazi Jewish descent. Genet Med 10(1):54, 2008, Reaffirmed 2013

Guermandi E, Vegetti W, Bianchi M, et al: Reliability of ovulation tests in infertile women. Obstet Gynecol 97:92, 2001

Guttmacher A: Factors affecting normal expectancy of conception. JAMA 161:855, 1956

Guzick D, Overstreet J, Factor-Litvak P, et al: Sperm morphology, motility, and concentration in fertile and infertile men. N Engl J Med 345:1388, 2001

Hadziselimovic F: Early successful orchidopexy does not prevent from developing azoospermia. Int Braz J Urol 32(5):570, 2006

Hallam S, Nelson H, Greger V, et al: Validation for clinical use of, and initial clinical experience with, a novel approach to population-based carrier screening using high-throughput, next-generation DNA sequencing. J Mol Diagn 16(2):180, 2014

Hansen KR, Hodnett GM, Knowlton N, et al: Correlation of ovarian reserve tests with histologically determined primordial follicle number. Fertil Steril 95(1):170, 2011

Hatch EE, Wise LA, Mikkelsen EM, et al: Caffeinated beverage and soda consumption and time to pregnancy. Epidemiology 23(3):393, 2012

Hauser R, Sokol R: Science linking environmental contaminant exposures with fertility and reproductive health impacts in the adult male. Fertil Steril 89(2 Suppl):e59, 2008

Hedley AA, Ogden Cl, Johnson CL, et al: Prevalence of overweight and obesity among U.S. children, adolescents, and adults, 1999–2002. JAMA 291(23):2847, 2004

Heller C, Clermont Y: Spermatogenesis in man: an estimate of its duration. Science 140:184, 1963

Hershlag A, Schiff S, DeCherney A: Retrograde ejaculation. Hum Reprod 6:255, 1991

Hinrichsen M, Blaquier J: Evidence supporting the existence of sperm maturation in the human epididymis. J Reprod Fertil 60:291, 1980

Hopps CV, Mielnik A, Goldstein M, et al: Detection of sperm in men with Y chromosome microdeletions of the AZFa, AZFb, and AZFc regions. Hum Reprod 18(8):1660, 2003

Hornburg R, Crawford G: The role of AMH in anovulation associated with PCOS: a hypothesis. Hum Reprod 29(6):1117, 2014

Jarow J: Effects of varicocele on male fertility. Hum Reprod Update 7:59, 2001

Jayaprakasan K, Polanski L, Sahu B, et al: Removal of endometrial polyps prior to infertility treatment. Cochrane Database Syst Rev 8:CD009592, 2014

Johnson LN, Sammel MD, Dillon KE, et al: Antimüllerian hormone and antral follicle count are lower in female cancer survivors and healthy women taking hormonal contraception. Fertil Steril 102(3):774, 2014

Kao L, Germeyer A, Tulac S, et al: Expression profiling of endometrium from women with endometriosis reveals candidate genes for disease-based implantation failure and infertility. Endocrinology 144:2870, 2003

Katz D, Slade D, Nakajima S: Analysis of pre-ovulatory changes in cervical mucus hydration and sperm penetrability. Adv Contracept 13:143, 1997

Keefe D, Niven-Fairchild T, Powell S, et al: Mitochondrial deoxyribonucleic acid deletions in oocytes and reproductive aging in women. Fertil Steril 64:577, 1995

Kent-First M, Muallem A, Shultz J, et al: Defining regions of the Y-chromosome responsible for male infertility and identification of a fourth AZF region (AZFd) by Y-chromosome microdeletion detection. Mol Reprod Dev 53:27, 1999

Kidd S, Eskenazi B, Wyrobek A: Effects of male age on semen quality and fertility: a review of the literature. Fertil Steril 75:237, 2001

Klonoff-Cohen H, Lam-Kruglick P, Gonzalez C: Effects of maternal and paternal alcohol consumption on the success rates of in vitro fertilization and gamete intrafallopian transfer. Fertil Steril 79:330, 2003

Kruger T, Acosta A, Simmons K, et al: Predictive value of abnormal sperm morphology in in vitro fertilization. Fertil Steril 49:112, 1988

Lalos O: Risk factors for tubal infertility among infertile and fertile women. Eur J Obstet Gynecol Reprod Biol 29:129, 1988

La Marca A, Broekmans FJ, Volpe A, et al: Anti-Mullerian hormone (AMH): what do we still need to know? Hum Reprod 24(9):2264, 2009

Lee P: Fertility in cryptorchidism: Does treatment make a difference? Endocrinol Metab Clin North Texas 22:479 1993

Lessey B: Endometrial integrins and the establishment of uterine receptivity. Hum Reprod 13(Suppl 3):247, 1998

Levitas E, Lunenfeld E, Weisz N, et al: Relationship between age and semen parameters in men with normal sperm concentration: analysis of 6022 semen samples. Andrologia 39(2):45, 2007

Licciardi F, Liu H, Rosenwaks Z: Day 3 estradiol serum concentrations as prognosticators of ovarian stimulation response and pregnancy outcome in patients undergoing in vitro fertilization. Fertil Steril 64:991, 1995

Luciano A, Peluso J, Koch E, et al: Temporal relationship and reliability of the clinical, hormonal, and ultrasonographic indices of ovulation in infertile women. Obstet Gynecol 75(3 Pt 1):412, 1990

Makker A, Goel MM: Uterine leiomyomas: effects on architectural, cellular, and molecular determinants of endometrial receptivity. Reprod Sci 20(6):631, 2013

Maroulis G: Effect of aging on fertility and pregnancy. Semin Reprod Endocrinol 9:165, 1991

Maseelall PB, Hernandez-Rey AE, Oh C, et al: Antral follicle count is a significant predictor of livebirth in in vitro fertilization cycles. Fertil Steril 91 (4 Suppl):1595, 2009

McKinley M, O'Loughlin VD: Reproductive System in Human Anatomy. New York, McGraw-Hill, 2006, p 873

Mendola P, Messer LC, Rappazzo K: Science linking environmental contaminant exposures with fertility and reproductive health impacts in the adult female. Fertil Steril 89(2 Suppl):e81, 2008

Menken J, Trussell J, Larsen U: Age and infertility. Science 233(4771):1389, 1986

Metwally M, Cheong YC, Horne AW: Surgical removal of fibroids does not improve fertility outcomes. Cochrane Database Syst Rev 11:CD003857, 2012

Miller P, Soules M: The usefulness of a urinary LH kit for ovulation prediction during menstrual cycles of normal women. Obstet Gynecol 87:13, 1996

Moen M, Magnus P: The familial risk of endometriosis. Acta Obstet Gynecol Scand 72:560, 1993

Mosher W, Pratt W: Fecundity and infertility in the United States: incidence and trends. Fertil Steril 56:192, 1991

Muthusami KR, Chinnaswamy P: Effect of chronic alcoholism on male fertility hormones and semen quality. Fertil Steril 84(4):919, 2005

Nagy F, Pendergrass P, Bowen D, et al: A comparative study of cytological and physiological parameters of semen obtained from alcoholics and non-alcoholics. Alcohol Alcohol 21:17, 1986

Nezar M, Goda H, El-Negery M, et al: Genital tract tuberculosis among fertile women: an old problem revisited. Arch Gynecol Obstet 280(5):787, 2009

Nikolaou D, Templeton A: Early ovarian ageing: a hypothesis. Detection and clinical relevance. Hum Reprod 18:1137, 2003

Noyes R, Hertig A, Rock J: Dating the endometrial biopsy. Am J Obstet Gynecol 122:262, 1975

Oates R, Amos J: The genetic basis of congenital bilateral absence of the vas deferens and cystic fibrosis. J Androl 15:1, 1994

Oei SG, Helmerhorst FM, Bloemenkamp KW: Effectiveness of the postcoital test: randomised controlled trial. BMJ 317(7157):502, 1998

Oei S, Keirse M, Bloemenkamp K, et al: European postcoital tests: opinions and practice. BJOG 102:621, 1995

Pellestor F, Andreo B, Arnal F, et al: Maternal aging and chromosomal abnormalities: new data drawn from in vitro unfertilized human oocytes. Hum Genet 112:195, 2003

Perez-Medina T, Bajo-Arenas J, Salazar F, et al: Endometrial polyps and their implication in the pregnancy rates of patients undergoing intrauterine insemination: a prospective, randomized study. Hum Reprod 20:1632, 2005

Petracco RG, Kong A, Grechukhina O, et al: Global gene expression profiling of proliferative phase endometrium reveals distinct functional subdivisions. Reprod Sci 19(10):1138, 2012

Pletcher BA, Bocian M, American College of Medical Genetics: Preconception and prenatal testing of biologic fathers for carrier status. Genet Med 8(2):13, 2006

Prior TW: Next-generation carrier screening: are we ready? Genome Med 6(8):62, 2014

Pritts E: Fibroids and infertility: a systematic review of the evidence. Obstet Gynecol Surv 56:483, 2001

Pryor J, Kent-First M, Muallem A, et al: Microdeletions in the Y chromosome of infertile men. N Engl J Med 336:534, 1997

Ramlau-Hansen CH, Thulstrup AM, Aggerholm AS, et al: Is smoking a risk factor for decreased semen quality? A cross-sectional analysis. Human Reproduction 22(1):188, 2007

Ratbi I, Legendre M, Niel F, et al: Detection of cystic fibrosis transmembrane conductance regulator (CFTR) gene rearrangements enriches the mutation spectrum in congenital bilateral absence of the vas deferens and impacts on genetic counseling. Hum Reprod 22(5):1285, 2007

Rosenfeld DL, Scholl G, Bronson R, et al: Unsuspected chronic pelvic inflammatory disease in the infertile female. Fertil Steril 39:44, 1983

Ross LF: A re-examination of the use of ethnicity in prenatal carrier testing. Am J Med Genet 158(A1):19, 2012

Roth LK, Taylor HS: Risks of smoking to reproductive health: assessment of women's knowledge. Am J Obstet Gynecol 184(5):934, 2001

Rowley M, Teshima F, Heller C: Duration of transit of spermatozoa through the human male ductular system. Fertil Steril 21:390, 1970

Ruan YC, Chen H, Chan HC: Ion channels in the endometrium: regulation of endometrial receptivity and embryo implantation. Hum Reprod Update 20(4):517, 2014

Sakkas D, Alvarez JG: Sperm DNA fragmentation: mechanisms of origin, impact on reproductive outcome, and analysis. Fertil Steril 93(4):1027, 2010

Samejima T, Koba K, Nakae H, et al: Identifying patients who can improve fertility with myomectomy. Eur J Obstet Gynecol Reprod Biol 185C:28, 2014

Saracoglu OF, Mungan T, Tanzer F: Pelvic tuberculosis. Int J Gynaecol Obstet 37:115, 1992

Schenker J: Etiology of and therapeutic approach to synechia uteri. Eur J Obstet Gynecol Reprod Biol 65:109, 1996

Scott R, Snyder R, Bagnall J, et al: Evaluation of the impact of intraobserver variability on endometrial dating and the diagnosis of luteal phase defects. Fertil Steril 60:652, 1993

Seifer DB, Baker VL, Leader B: Age-specific serum anti-Mullerian hormone values for 17,120 women presenting to fertility centers within the United States. Fertil Steril 95(2074), 2011

Serafini P, Batzofin J: Diagnosis of female infertility. A comprehensive approach. J Reprod Med 34(1):29, 1989

Seshadri S, El-Touckhy T, Douiri A, et al: Diagnostic accuracy of saline infusion sonography in the evaluation of uterine cavity abnormalities prior to assisted reproductive techniques: a systematic review and meta-analysis. Hum Reprod Update 21(2):262, 2015

Sharlip I, Jarow J, Belker A, et al: Best practice policies for male infertility. Fertil Steril 77:873, 2002

Sigman M, Jarow JP: Endocrine evaluation of infertile men. Urology 50(5):659, 1997

Smith C, Asch R: Drug abuse and reproduction. Fertil Steril 48:355, 1987

Soares S, Barbosa dos Reis M, Camargos A: Diagnostic accuracy of sonohysterography, transvaginal sonography, and hysterosalpingography in patients with uterine cavity diseases. Fertil Steril 73:406, 2000

Stanford J, White G, Hatasaka H: Timing intercourse to achieve pregnancy: current evidence. Obstet Gynecol 100:1333, 2002

Swart P, Mol B, van der Veen F, et al: The accuracy of hysterosalpingography in the diagnosis of tubal pathology: a meta-analysis. Fertil Steril 64:486, 1995

Tanner AK, Valencia CA, Rhodenizer D, et al: Development and performance of a comprehensive targeted sequencing assay for pan-ethnic screening of carrier status. J Mol Diagn 16(3):350, 2014

te Velde E, Pearson P: The variability of female reproductive ageing. Hum Reprod Update 8:141, 2002

Tietze C: Reproductive span and rate of reproduction among Hutterite women. Fertil Steril 8:89, 1957

Tolstrup J, Kjaer S, Holst C, et al: Alcohol use as predictor for infertility in a representative population of Danish women. Acta Obstet Gynecol Scand 82:744, 2003

Toner J, Philput C, Jones G, et al: Basal follicle-stimulating hormone level is a better predictor of in vitro fertilization performance than age. Fertil Steril 55:784, 1991

Treloar S, Do K, Martin N: Genetic influences on the age at menopause. Lancet 352:1084, 1998

Turek PJ, Lipshultz LI: Immunologic infertility. Urol Clin North Am 21(3):447, 1994

Wilcox A, Weinberg C, Baird D: Timing of sexual intercourse in relation to ovulation. Effects on the probability of conception, survival of the pregnancy, and sex of the baby. N Engl J Med 333:1517, 1995

Wolff H: The biologic significance of white blood cells in semen. Fertil Steril 63:1143, 1995

World Health Organization: Laboratory Manual for the Examination of Human Semen and Sperm-Cervical Mucus Interaction. Cambridge University Press, 1999

World Health Organization: Women and sexually transmitted infections. 2007. Available at: http://www.who.int/mediacentre/factsheets/fs110/en./ Accessed August 21, 2010

Yang Q, Sherman SL, Hassold TJ, et al: Risk factors for trisomy 21: maternal cigarette smoking and oral contraceptive use in a population-based case-control study. Genet Med 1(3):8, 1999

Zenzes MT. Smoking and reproduction: gene damage to human gametes and embryos. Hum Reprod Update 6(2):122, 2000

Zini A, Sigman M: Are tests of sperm DNA damage clinically useful? Pros and cons. J Androl 30:219, 2009

CHAPTER 20

Treatment of the Infertile Couple

Infertility results from diseases of the reproductive system that impair the body's ability to perform basic reproductive function. It is defined as the failure to achieve a successful pregnancy after 12 months or more of regular unprotected intercourse. Earlier evaluation and treatment may be justified based on medical history and physical findings and is warranted after 6 months for women older than 35 (American Society for Reproductive Medicine, 2012b). Ten to 15 percent of the reproductive-aged population is infertile, and men and women are equally affected.

Infertility treatment is a complex process influenced by numerous factors. Important considerations include duration of infertility, a couple's age (especially the female's), and diagnosed cause. Additionally, the level of distress experienced by a couple should be taken into account.

In general, a first step involves identification of a primary cause and contributing factors, and treatment is aimed at their direct correction. Most are treated with conventional therapies such as medication or surgery. In many cases, therapy can begin without a complete evaluation, especially if a cause is obvious. However, if pregnancy does not quickly follow, then more thorough testing is prudent.

In contrast, evaluation commonly may not yield a satisfactory explanation or may identify causes that are not amenable to direct correction. For such cases, recent advances in assisted reproduction have provided effective treatments. These approaches, however, are not without disadvantage. For example, in vitro fertilization (IVF) has been linked with higher rates of some fetal and maternal complications. Appropriate treatments may also pose ethical dilemmas for couples or their physician. For example, selective reduction of a multifetal pregnancy may improve survival chances for some fetuses but at the cost of others. Last, infertility treatment can be a financial burden, a significant source of emotional stress, or both. During consultation, an infertility specialist does not dictate treatment but offers and explains therapy options, which may include expectant management or even adoption.

LIFESTYLE THERAPIES

Weight Optimization

Ovarian function is dependent on weight. Low body-fat content is associated with hypothalamic hypogonadism. In contrast, central body fat is associated with insulin resistance and contributes to ovarian dysfunction in many women with polycystic ovarian syndrome (PCOS). Lifestyle modification in overweight infertile women with PCOS leads to a reduction of central fat and improved insulin sensitivity, decreased hyperandrogenemia, lowered luteinizing hormone (LH) concentrations, and restoration of normal fertility in many cases (Hoeger, 2001; Kiddy, 1992). Even a 5 to 10 percent reduction in body weight has been shown to be successful in these women (Crosignani, 2003; Kiddy, 1992; Pasquali, 1989). Apart from diet, exercise can also improve insulin sensitivity. Weight loss and exercise are inexpensive and should be recommended as first-line management of obese women with PCOS.

Although pharmacologic options can effectively treat anovulation if weight cannot be lost, it should be noted that obesity is a significant risk factor for obstetric and perinatal complications. Some maternal risks include higher rates of gestational diabetes, cesarean delivery, preeclampsia, unexplained stillbirth, and surgical wound infection (Cunningham, 2014). Obesity also has been associated with an increased risk of birth defects (American Society for Reproductive Medicine, 2008). Therefore, strong consideration is given to delaying treatments in morbidly obese women until their body mass index (BMI) can be reduced below 40. This is especially true if treatments involve surgical risks or risk of multifetal gestation.

Weight-loss options are discussed in Chapter 1 (p. 13). If bariatric surgery is selected, conception is ideally delayed for 12 to 18 months (American College of Obstetricians and Gynecologists, 2013). This is because rapid weight loss during this time poses theoretical risks for intrauterine fetal-growth restriction and nutritional deprivation.

Undernutrition can also be a problem. The reproductive axis is closely linked to nutritional status, and inhibitory pathways suppress ovulation in subjects with significant weight loss.

Anorexia nervosa and bulimia nervosa affect up to 5 percent of reproductive-aged women and may cause amenorrhea, infertility, and in those who do conceive, an increased likelihood of miscarriage. Fortunately, recovery may follow minimal acquisition of weight because energy balance has a more important effect than body fat mass.

■ Exercise

Physical activity has numerous health benefits. The relationship between exercise and fertility, however, is not straightforward. Competitive female athletes often experience amenorrhea, irregular cycles or luteal dysfunction, and infertility. This may be related not specifically to physical activity itself but rather to low body-fat content or physical stress associated with competition. At this time, insufficient data exist to support or discourage physical activity in infertile women without documented ovarian dysfunction associated with obesity or low body weight.

■ Nutrition

In the absence of obesity or significant undernutrition, the role of diet in infertility is unclear. High-protein diets and gluten intolerance (celiac disease) have been investigated as underlying causes in women. However, studies sizes have been small, and conflicting results found (Collin, 1996; Jackson, 2008; Meloni, 1999). In men, dietary antioxidants have been proposed as a potential way to improve male reproductive outcomes by reducing oxidative damage in sperm DNA (Ross, 2010). Although the approach is promising, large well-designed studies to guide its clinical use are needed (Patel, 2008). Additionally, the nutritional supplement carnitine had been often touted as a potential benefit for male infertility. This finding, however, has not been confirmed by a randomized, prospective trial (Sigman, 2006).

Despite a lack of conclusive benefits to nutritional supplements or diet modification in infertile couples, it does seem reasonable to recommend daily multivitamin supplementation to both. Folic acid is contained in most multivitamins, and daily doses of 400 µg orally are recommended for women attempting pregnancy to reduce the incidence of neural-tube defects in their fetuses (American College of Obstetricians and Gynecologist, 2014b).

Herbal therapies including traditional Chinese medicine and acupuncture have been proposed to enhance fertility either alone or in conjunction with standard therapies including assisted reproductive technology (ART). Smith and associates (2010) found that 29 percent of infertile couples seeking pregnancy in the United States had used complementary and alternative medicine. At this time, however, current evidence does not support a benefit of herbal/botanical therapies or acupuncture for fertility as either a primary treatment modality or an adjunct to established therapies (Cheong, 2013).

■ Stress Management

Stress has been implicated in reproductive failure. Although severe stress can result in anovulation, less significant stress may also play a role, but a mechanism has yet to be defined. Patients with higher stress levels have been found to have lower pregnancy rates when undergoing IVF treatments (Thiering, 1993). Accordingly, screening all infertile couples for evidence of anxiety or depression is a consideration. Although pharmacologic management of stress is not typically recommended during infertility treatments, a "mind/body" approach that combines psychological counseling and meditation may be reasonable for those patients manifesting high levels of anxiety (Domar, 1990).

CORRECTION OF OVARIAN DYSFUNCTION

■ Hyperprolactinemia

Prolactin is a pituitary hormone that plays an important role in various reproductive functions, and elevated levels are commonly encountered in clinical endocrinology practice. If hyperprolactinemia is found, then physiologic, pharmacologic, or other secondary causes of hormone hypersecretion are sought (Table 12-2, p. 281).

Dopamine agonists are the primary treatment of hyperprolactinemia (Chap. 15, p. 360). Surgical therapies are only considered with prolactin-secreting adenomas resistant to medical therapy. During pregnancy, if hyperprolactinemia is not associated with a pituitary lesion or a lesion is less than 10 mm (microadenoma), then dopamine-agonist therapy is stopped because the tumor expansion risk is low (Molitch, 1999). If the tumor size is 10 mm or larger (macroadenoma), bromocriptine (Parlodel) use is advised during pregnancy to avoid significant tumor growth.

■ Hypothyroidism

Thyroid disorders are prevalent in reproductive-aged individuals and affect women four to five times more often than men. In women, oligomenorrhea and amenorrhea are frequent findings. Although ovulation and conception can still occur in those with mild hypothyroidism, treatment with thyroxine usually restores a normal menstrual pattern and enhances fertility.

Subclinical hypothyroidism may also be associated with ovarian dysfunction (Strickland, 1990). Lincoln and associates (1999) found a 2-percent incidence of elevated thyroid-stimulating hormone (TSH) levels in 704 asymptomatic women seeking evaluation for infertility. Correction of hypothyroidism in those with ovarian dysfunction and elevated TSH levels led to pregnancy in 64 percent of patients. In addition, subclinical hypothyroidism may also adversely affect pregnancy outcomes, but current evidence does not support that treatment of subclinical hypothyroidism during pregnancy improves these outcomes (Casey, 2014). That said, in women seeking treatment for infertility, early detection and treatment of hypothyroidism of any degree is advised.

■ Ovulation Induction

Ovarian dysfunction is the most common indication for the use of medications to induce ovulation. These agents can also be selected for ovulatory women to increase the likelihood of pregnancy in couples with other causes of infertility or unexplained infertility. Use of these medications to promote follicular development and prompt ovulation is called *superovulation* or *ovulation enhancement*. If these agents are administered solely to stimulate follicles and egg harvesting is completed by ART, then the termed *controlled ovarian hyperstimulation* is used. In contrast, we prefer the term *ovulation induction* to describe treatment with medications to stimulate normal ovulation in women with ovarian dysfunction.

Frequent causes of ovarian dysfunction include PCOS and diminished ovarian reserve. Less often, central (hypothalamic or pituitary) disorders or thyroid dysfunction can result in infertility (Table 16-3, p. 371). Rarely, ovarian tumors or adrenal abnormalities lead to abnormal ovarian function. Treatment of ovarian dysfunction is based on the identified cause and the results of any prior attempted therapy.

Clomiphene Citrate

Clomiphene citrate (CC) is the initial treatment for most anovulatory infertile women. Chemically similar to tamoxifen, CC is a nonsteroidal triphenylethylene derivative that demonstrates both estrogen agonist and antagonist properties. Antagonist properties predominate except at very low estrogen levels. As a result, negative feedback that is normally produced by estrogen in the hypothalamus is reduced (Fig. 20-1). Gonadotropin-releasing hormone (GnRH) secretion is altered and stimulates pituitary gonadotropin release. The resulting increase in follicle-stimulating hormone (FSH) levels, in turn, drives ovarian follicular activity.

Tamoxifen has also been used successfully for ovulation induction. However, it is not approved by the Food and Drug Administration (FDA) for this indication and has not been demonstrated to have significant advantage compared with CC.

Clomiphene citrate is administered orally, typically starting on the third to fifth day after the onset of spontaneous or progestin-induced menses. Ovulation rates, conception rates, and pregnancy outcome are similar regardless whether treatment begins on cycle day 2, 3, 4, or 5. Prior to therapy, sonography is advisable to exclude signs of significant spontaneous follicular maturation or residual follicular cysts. In general at our institution, clomiphene can be administered if no follicle is >20 mm and the endometrium is less than 5 mm. A pregnancy test is also indicated after spontaneous menses. Although not a proven teratogen, CC is classified as category X by the FDA and thus is contraindicated in suspected or documented pregnancy.

The dose required to achieve ovulation correlates with body weight. However, there is no reliable way to accurately predict which dose will be required in an individual woman (Lobo, 1982). Consequently, CC is titrated empirically to establish the lowest effective dose for each patient. Treatment typically begins with a single 50-mg tablet taken daily for 5 consecutive days. Doses are increased by a 50-mg increment in each subsequent cycle until ovulation is induced. The dose of CC should not be increased if normal ovulation is confirmed. Thus, lack of pregnancy alone does not justify a dose increase. The effective dose of CC ranges from 50 mg/d to 250 mg/d, although doses in excess of 100 mg/d are not approved by the FDA. Some studies have suggested that adjunctive therapy with glucocorticoids

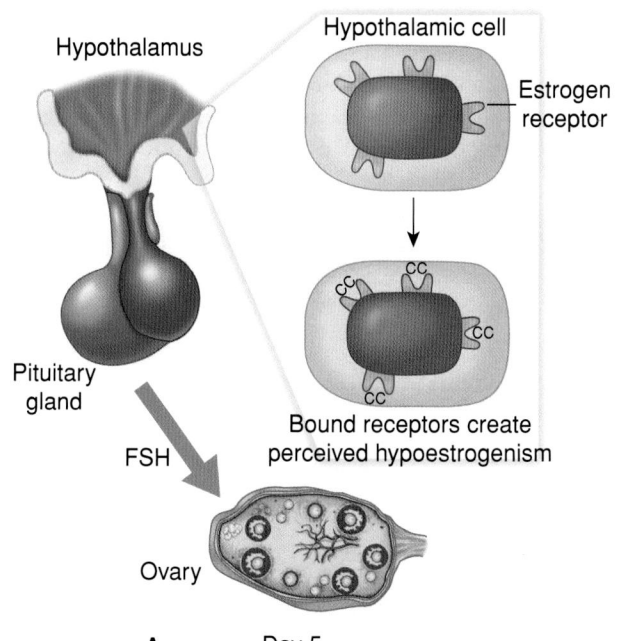
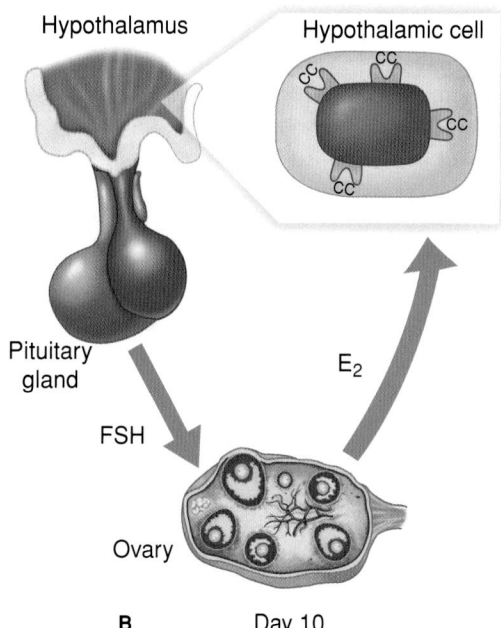

FIGURE 20-1 Effect of clomiphene citrate (CC) administration. **A.** Clomiphene binds to the estrogen receptor in the pituitary and hypothalamus. This causes an effective reduction in hypothalamic estrogen receptor number. Because of this reduced receptor number, the hypothalamus and pituitary are effectively blinded to true circulating estrogen levels and perceived hypoestrogenism results. From this, estrogen's negative feedback is interrupted centrally, and follicle-stimulating hormone (FSH) secretion increases from the anterior pituitary. This leads to maturation of multiple follicles. **B.** By the late follicular phase, because of clomiphene citrate's long retention within tissues, estrogen receptor depletion continues centrally. As a result, increased estradiol (E_2) secretion from the ovary is not capable of exerting normal negative feedback on FSH release. This leads to a growth of multiple dominant follicles and multiple ovulations.

may benefit some patients not responsive to CC alone (Elnashar, 2006; Parsanezhad, 2002). The precise mechanism is unclear, although several direct and indirect actions of dexamethasone have been suggested. This therapy may be empiric or individualized based on elevated dehydroepiandrosterone sulfate (DHEAS) levels.

In general, women failing to ovulate with 100 mg/d dosing or failing to conceive following 3 to 6 months of ovulatory response to CC should be considered candidates for alternative treatments. In a retrospective study including 428 women who received CC for ovulation induction, 84.5 percent of pregnancies achieved with treatment occurred during the first three ovulatory cycles (Gysler, 1982).

Insulin-sensitizing Agents

Although PCOS appears to be a heterogeneous disorder, many women with this condition exhibit insulin resistance (Chap. 17, p. 387). Insulin resistance leads to compensatory hyperinsulinemia and dyslipidemia. Given the strong evidence that hyperinsulinemia plays a pivotal pathogenic role in development of PCOS, it is reasonable to assume that interventions that reduce circulating insulin levels in women with PCOS may restore normal reproductive endocrine function. As discussed, weight loss, nutrition, and exercise have clearly led to reduced hyperinsulinemia, resolution of hyperandrogenism, and in some cases, resumption of ovulatory function in overweight women with PCOS. However, women may be poorly compliant, and weight loss is rarely maintained over time.

Insulin-sensitizing agents show promise in the treatment of PCOS. When administered to insulin-resistant patients, these compounds act to increase target tissue responsiveness to insulin, thereby reducing the need for compensatory hyperinsulinemia (Antonucci, 1998). Current insulin-sensitizing agents include the biguanides and thiazolidinediones (Chap. 17, p. 398).

Of these, studies suggest that metformin (Glucophage), given 500 mg orally three times daily or 850 mg twice daily with meals and administered to women with PCOS, increased the frequency of spontaneous ovulation, menstrual cyclicity, and ovulatory response to CC (Nestler, 1998; Palomba, 2005; Vandermolen, 2001). In contrast, a large, prospective, randomized, multicenter trial does not support the hypothesis that metformin, either alone or in combination with CC, improves the live-birth rate in women with PCOS (Legro, 2007).

Gonadotropins

Clomiphene citrate is easy to use and leads to ovulation in most patients (Hammond, 1983). However, pregnancy rates are disappointing and approximate ≤50 percent (Raj, 1977; Zarate, 1971). Lower than expected pregnancy rates with CC have been attributed to its long half-life and peripheral antiestrogenic effects, mainly on the endometrium and cervical mucus. For such individuals, who are often classified as "clomiphene resistant," the next step is traditionally the administration of exogenous gonadotropin preparations via injections.

As with CC, the goal of ovulation induction with gonadotropins is simply to normalize ovarian function. Ideally, the dose used is the minimum required to cause normal development of a single dominant follicle. Because the response to gonadotropins can vary greatly from individual to individual and even from cycle to cycle, intensive monitoring is required to adjust dosage and timing of ovulation.

Gonadotropin preparations vary in terms of their source (urinary or recombinant) and by the presence or absence of LH activity (Table 20-1). Traditional urinary-derived human menopausal gonadotropin (hMG) preparations contain both FSH and LH. These are extracted and purified from the urine of postmenopausal women, in whom FSH and LH levels are normally high. These preparations also contain human chorionic gonadotropin (hCG), which is mainly derived from normal pituitary secretion in postmenopausal women. LH and hCG both bind to the same receptor (luteinizing hormone/chorionic gonadotropin receptor [LHCGR]).

In contrast, in purified hMG, hCG serves as the primary source of the LH activity, although significant LH is also present in the older, nonhighly purified hMG products (Filicori, 2002). Highly purified urinary preparations allow for administration via subcutaneous route with minimal or no reaction at the injection site. Alternatives to hMG include highly purified urinary gonadotropin preparations and purified recombinant FSH.

Both LH and FSH activity are required for normal ovarian steroidogenesis and follicular development. In many cases, pure FSH preparations can be used because of adequate endogenous

TABLE 20-1. Injectable Gonadotropin Preparations Used for Ovulation Induction

Name	Product Type	FSH Activity	LH Activity	hCG Activity
Bravelle Fertinex[a]	Vial	Highly purified urinary	Minimal	Minimal
Follistim Gonal-f	Pen or vial	Highly purified recombinant	None	None
Menopur	Vial	Highly purified urinary	Minimal	Highly purified urinary
Repronex Pergonal[a] Humagon[a]	Vial	Urinary	Urinary	Urinary

[a]No longer available.
FSH = follicle-stimulating hormone; hCG = human chorionic gonadotropin; LH = luteinizing hormone.

LH production. However, for ovulation induction in patients with hypogonadotropic amenorrhea, LH activity must be provided from an exogenous source. Thus, options include hMG, recombinant LH, low-dose (diluted) urinary or recombinant hCG. Ovulation induction in women with PCOS can be performed either with FSH-only containing products or those containing both LH and FSH activity. At present, data do not support the superiority of one preparation over another.

Gonadotropin development will likely continue. A long-acting FSH is commercially available outside the United States. This recombinant molecule was created by adding a DNA sequence to the human FSH gene. This extra sequence allows for more glycosylation and hence a prolonged clearance. Low-molecular-weight molecules (nonproteins) have been identified that activate the FSH and LH receptors. However, these compounds are still in early stages of clinical development. Advantages of these nontraditional gonadotropins include oral delivery.

Most clinicians begin ovulation induction attempts at a low gonadotropin dosage of 50 to 75 IU injected daily. This is gradually increased if no ovarian response (as assessed by serum estradiol measurements) is noted after several days (Fig. 20-2). This is referred to as a "step-up" protocol. A "step-down" protocol can also be used with the advantage of a decreased duration of stimulation. However, the risk of excessive ovarian response, such as multiple follicle development or ovarian hyperstimulation syndrome, may be increased with this method. With either approach, if a patient fails to conceive, subsequent cycles may be started at higher doses based on prior response.

In general, gonadotropin stimulation in women with PCOS is less successful than in patients with hypogonadotropic amenorrhea (Balen, 1994). Women with PCOS have ovaries highly sensitive to gonadotropin stimulation. They have a higher risk of excessive ovarian response and of multifetal pregnancy than those with normal ovaries (Farhi, 1996).

Aromatase Inhibitors

Gonadotropins are associated with more effective ovulation induction and higher pregnancy rates than CC. However, gonadotropins are expensive and carry higher risks for ovarian hyperstimulation syndrome and multifetal gestation. Accordingly, aromatase inhibitors have been investigated as ovulation-inducing agents (Fig. 20-3). These drugs were originally developed for breast cancer treatment and effectively inhibit *aromatase*, a cytochrome P450 hemoprotein that catalyzes the rate-limiting step in estrogen production. Aromatase inhibitors are orally administered, easy to use, relatively inexpensive, and associated with typically minor side effects (Chap. 10, p. 241).

The most widely used aromatase inhibitor to induce ovulation in anovulatory and ovulatory infertile women is letrozole (Femara). Compared with CC, its use is associated with higher pregnancy rates following ovulation induction (Legro, 2014). When used in combination with gonadotropins, letrozole leads to lower gonadotropin requirements and may achieve pregnancy rates comparable to gonadotropin treatment alone (Casper, 2003; Mitwally, 2004). The typical dosage used is 2.5 mg to 5 mg orally daily for 5 days.

Data suggesting that letrozole use for infertility treatment might be associated with a higher risk of congenital cardiac and bone malformations in the newborn are contradictory (Biljan, 2005; Tulandi, 2006). However, in 2005, the manufacturer issued a statement to physicians worldwide advising that letrozole use in premenopausal women, specifically its use for ovulation induction, is contraindicated (Fontana, 2005). As a result, it is not likely that letrozole will gain FDA approval or widespread acceptance for ovulation induction in the near future. Larger, well-designed randomized prospective trials that confirm their safety are still needed (Franik, 2014).

A second aromatase inhibitor, anastrozole, is of the same compound class as letrozole and has also been approved for treatment of women with breast cancer. At this time, no concerns have been raised regarding its teratogenicity. However, experience with anastrozole (Arimidex) in ovulation induction at this time is limited, and ideal dosages are currently unknown. Two trials comparing anastrozole to clomiphene have not found it to be more effective than clomiphene (Tredway, 2011a,b).

Complications of Fertility Drugs

Ovarian Hyperstimulation Syndrome. This is a clinical symptom complex associated with ovarian enlargement resulting from exogenous gonadotropin therapy. Symptoms may include abdominal pain and distention, ascites, gastrointestinal problems, respiratory compromise, oliguria, hemoconcentration, and thromboembolism. These symptoms may develop during ovulation induction or in early pregnancies that were conceived through exogenous ovarian stimulation.

The etiology of ovarian hyperstimulation syndrome (OHSS) is complex, but hCG, either exogenous or endogenous (derived from a resulting pregnancy), is believed to be an early contributing factor. Development of OHSS involves increased vascular permeability and loss of fluid, protein, and electrolytes into the peritoneal cavity, which leads to hemoconcentration. Increased capillary permeability is felt to result from vasoactive substances produced by the corpus luteum. Vascular endothelial growth factor (VEGF) is thought to play a major role, and angiotensin II may also be involved. Hypercoagulability may be related to hyperviscosity following hemoconcentration. Alternatively, it may be secondary to the high estrogen levels present, and these high levels can increase coagulation factor production. Predisposing factors for OHSS include multifollicular ovaries such as with PCOS, young age, high estradiol levels during ovulation induction, and pregnancy.

Abdominal pain is prominent and caused by ovarian enlargement and accumulation of peritoneal fluid. Although sonographic examination of women with OHSS usually reveals enlarged ovaries with numerous follicular cysts and ascites, OHSS is a clinical diagnosis (Fig. 20-4). Several different classification schemes have been proposed to categorize the severity of this syndrome, and Table 20-2 lists one.

Treatment of OHSS is generally supportive. Paracentesis is typically performed transvaginally as an outpatient and can ameliorate abdominal discomfort and relieve respiratory distress. Reaccumulation of ascites may prompt additional paracenteses or rarely placement of a percutaneous "pigtail" catheter for continuous drainage. Untreated hypovolemia can lead to renal, hepatic, or pulmonary end-organ failure. Thus, fluid balance must be maintained by replacement with an isotonic fluid

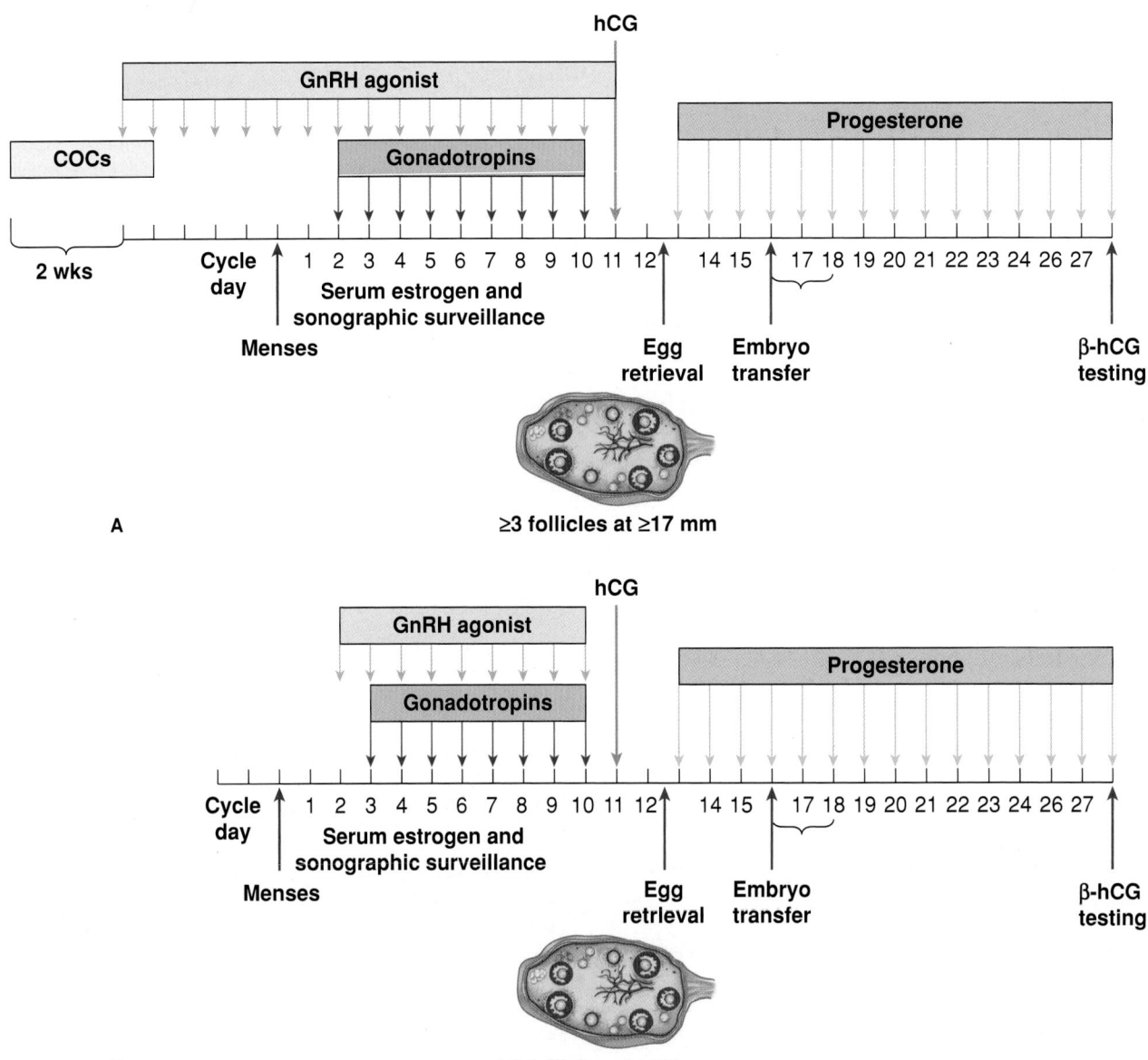

FIGURE 20-2 Drug protocols for ovulation induction. **A.** Downregulation of gonadotropin-releasing hormone (GnRH) agonist protocol. This is also known as the *long protocol*. In this diagram, the long protocol is combined with combination oral contraceptive (COC) pill pretreatment. With the long protocol, GnRH agonists are begun typically 7 days prior to gonadotropins. GnRH agonists suppress endogenous pituitary release of gonadotropins. This minimizes the risk of a premature luteinizing hormone (LH) surge and thus premature ovulation. During all protocols, serial serum estrogen levels and sonographic surveillance of follicular development accompany gonadotropin administration. Human chorionic gonadotropin (hCG) is administered to trigger ovulation when sonography shows three or more follicles measuring at least 17 mm. Eggs are retrieved 36 hours later. Embryos are transfer back to the uterus 3–5 days following retrieval. Progesterone supplementation, with either vaginal preparations or intramuscular injection, follows during the luteal phase to support the endometrium. The goal of COC pretreatment is to prevent ovarian cyst formation. One of the major drawbacks of GnRH agonist therapy is the induction of initial transient gonadotropin release or *flare*, which may lead to ovarian cyst formation. Functional ovarian cysts can prolong the duration of pituitary suppression required prior to gonadotropin initiation and may also exert a detrimental effect on follicular development because of their steroid production. Moreover, COC pretreatment may improve induction results by providing an entire cohort of follicles synchronized at the same developmental stage that will reach maturity at the same time once stimulated by gonadotropins. **B.** GnRH flare protocol. This is also known as the *short protocol*. GnRH agonists initially bind gonadotropes and stimulate follicle-stimulating hormone (FSH) and LH release. This initial flare of gonadotropes stimulates follicular development. Following this initial surge of gonadotropins, the GnRH agonist causes receptor downregulation and an ultimately hypogonadotropic state. Gonadotropin injections begin 2 days later to continue follicular growth. As with the long protocol, continued GnRH agonist therapy prevents premature ovulation. *(Continued)*

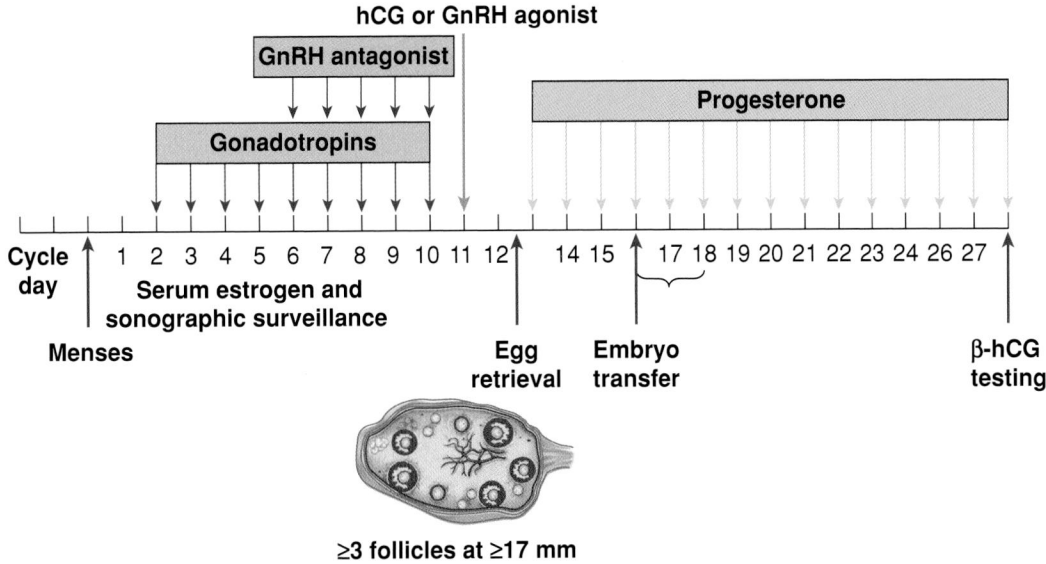

C   ≥3 follicles at ≥17 mm

FIGURE 20-2 *(Continued)* **C.** GnRH antagonist protocol. As with GnRH agonists, these agents are combined with gonadotropins to prevent premature LH surge and ovulation. This protocol attempts to minimize risk of ovarian hyperstimulation syndrome (OHSS) and GnRH side effects, such as hot flashes, headaches, bleeding, and mood changes.

such as normal saline. Monitoring of electrolytes is critical. Because of hypercoagulability in these women, prophylaxis for thromboembolism is strongly considered with severe OHSS.

During exogenous ovulation, strategies to avoid OHSS induction include decreasing follicular stimulation (a decreased FSH dose), "coasting" (withholding FSH administration for one or more days prior to the hCG trigger injection), prophylactic

treatment with volume expanders, and substitution of hCG for FSH during the final days of ovarian stimulation. With this last strategy, low-dose hCG administration can support maturation of larger ovarian follicles but is postulated to directly or indirectly increase atresia rates of small antral follicles and thereby lower OHSS rates. However, during ovulation induction, if concern for OHSS develops, then the hCG trigger can

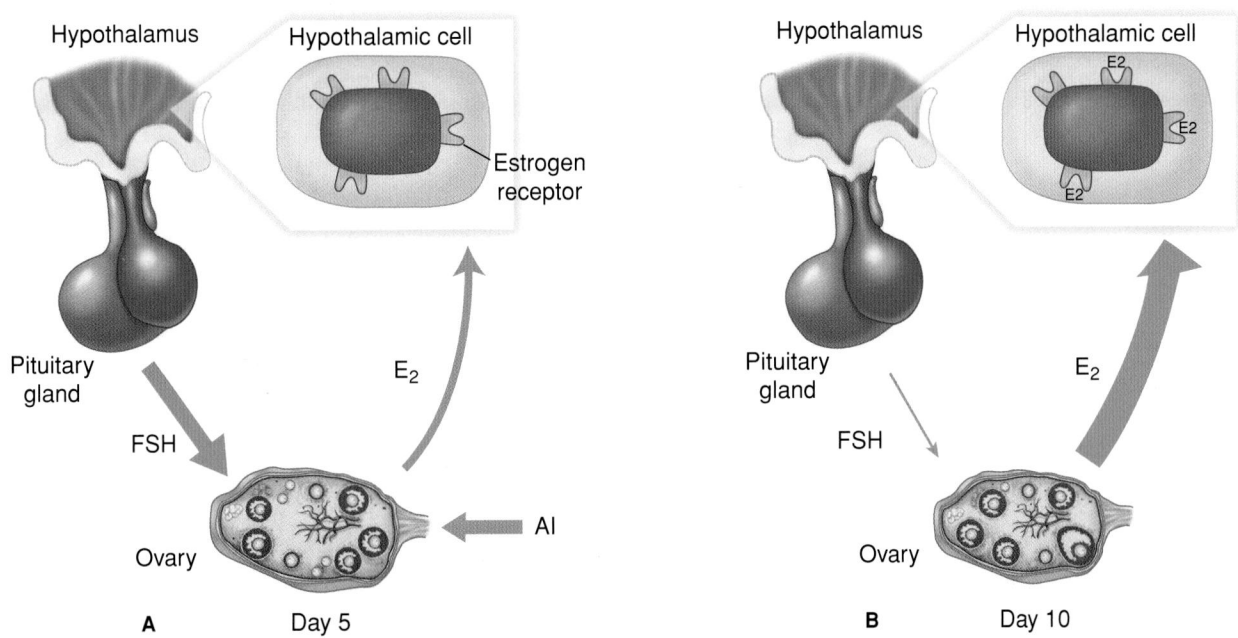

FIGURE 20-3 Effect of aromatase inhibitor (AI) administration. **A.** Administration suppresses ovarian estradiol (E_2) secretion and reduces estrogen negative feedback at the pituitary and hypothalamus. As a result, increased follicle-stimulating hormone (FSH) secretion from the anterior pituitary stimulates growth of multiple ovarian follicles. **B.** Later in the follicular phase, the effect of the aromatase inhibitor is reduced, and E_2 levels increase as a result of follicular growth. Because aromatase inhibitors do not affect estrogen receptors centrally, the increased E_2 levels result in normal central negative feedback on FSH secretion. Follicles smaller than the dominant follicle undergo atresia, with resultant monofollicular ovulation in most cases.

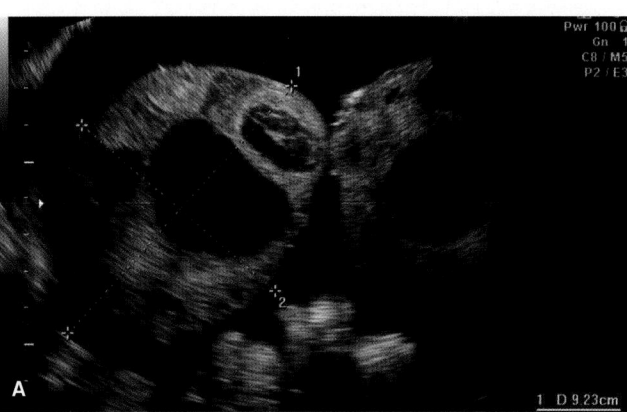 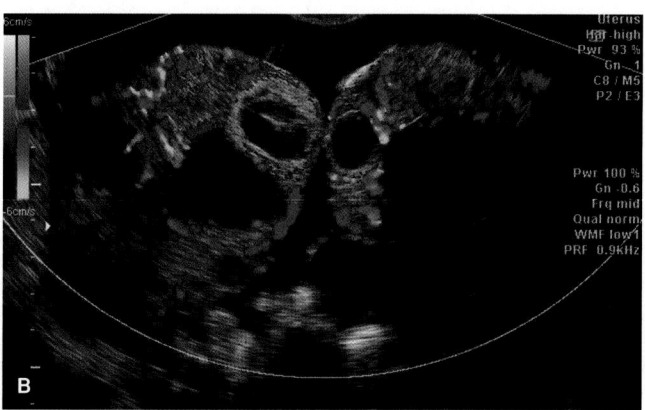

FIGURE 20-4 A. Sonogram of ovaries with multiple large cysts secondary to ovarian hyperstimulation syndrome. Ovaries are enlarged and meet in the midline. Ascites surrounds these enlarged ovaries. **B.** Color Doppler transvaginal sonography is often performed to exclude ovarian torsion in these patients.

be withheld, resulting in cycle cancellation. For these patients, IVF should often be considered rather than further attempts at ovulation induction.

OHSS can also develop with ART therapy, and the risk can be substantially reduced with appropriate precautions. Predicted high responders (e.g., high numbers of antral follicles, high AMH level, or prior high response to ovulation induction) should be stimulated with a GnRH antagonist protocol. This allows a single GnRH agonist dose to be used for the "trigger" in place of hCG. The resulting endogenous LH surge can bring about the final stages of follicle and oocyte maturation without significant OHSS risk. Moreover, prevention of pregnancy does not completely eliminate the risk of OHSS but certainly serves to limit symptom duration. Thus, an additional option in ART cycles is to freeze all embryos and forgo embryo transfer that cycle.

Multifetal Gestation. From 1980 through 1997, the number of twin births rose by more than 50 percent, and the number of higher-order multifetal births increased by more than 400 percent (Fig. 20-5) (Martin, 1999). Using data from these years, the Centers for Disease Control and Prevention (CDC) (2000) estimated that approximately 20 percent of triplets and higher-order multifetal births were attributable to spontaneous events;

40 percent were related to ovulation-inducing drugs without ART; and 40 percent resulted from ART. However, further analysis of the same data indicates that the overwhelming majority of all multifetal births result from spontaneously conceived twin gestations and that only approximately 10 percent result from IVF and related procedures.

Higher-order multifetal pregnancy is an adverse outcome of infertility treatment. In general, increased fetal number leads to greater risk of perinatal and maternal morbidity and mortality. Prematurity leads to most adverse events in these cases, but fetal-growth restriction and discordance are other potential factors.

Monozygotic gestation is also increased in ovulation induction and ART and is associated with greater fetal risks. These include a three- to fivefold higher perinatal mortality rate compared with that of dizygotic twins. Abnormal placentation also develops at higher rates. Additionally, congenital anomalies are increased two- to threefold in monozygotic twins versus singleton neonates, with an estimated incidence of 10 percent. Initially, extended embryo culture and zona manipulation were postulated to increase the risk of monozygosity. More recent, well-designed trials have refuted this contention (Franasiak, 2015; Papanikolaou, 2010).

Patients with higher-order multifetal gestations are faced with options of continuing their pregnancy with all the risks previously described, terminating the entire pregnancy, or selecting multifetal pregnancy reduction (MFPR). MFPR reduces the number of fetuses to decrease the risk of maternal and perinatal morbidity and mortality. Although MFPR lowers the risks associated with preterm delivery, it often creates profound ethical dilemmas. Moreover, multifetal reduction lowers, but does not eliminate, the risk of fetal-growth restriction in remaining fetuses. With MFPR, pregnancy loss and prematurity are primary risks. However, current data suggest that such complications have decreased as experience with the procedure has grown (Evans, 2008).

Several issues in infertility care contribute to the increased incidence of higher-order multifetal pregnancies. An infertile couple's sense of urgency may lead to a preference for more aggressive strategies involving gonadotropin treatment or for more embryos to be transferred in IVF cycles. Clinicians may feel competitive pressures to achieve higher pregnancy rates and may be inclined to turn to superovulation or IVF earlier in treatment or to transfer a greater number of embryos.

TABLE 20-2. Classification and Staging of Ovarian Hyperstimulation Syndrome	
Grade 1:	Abdominal distention/discomfort
Grade 2:	Grade 1 plus nausea and vomiting or diarrhea Ovaries enlarged 5–12 cm
Grade 3:	Sonographic evidence of ascites
Grade 4:	Clinical evidence of ascites or hydrothorax or difficulty breathing
Grade 5:	All of the above plus decreased blood volume, hemoconcentration, diminished renal perfusion and function, and coagulation abnormalities

Reproduced with permission from Whelan JG III, Vlahos NF: The ovarian hyperstimulation syndrome, Fertil Steril 2000 May;73(5):883–896.

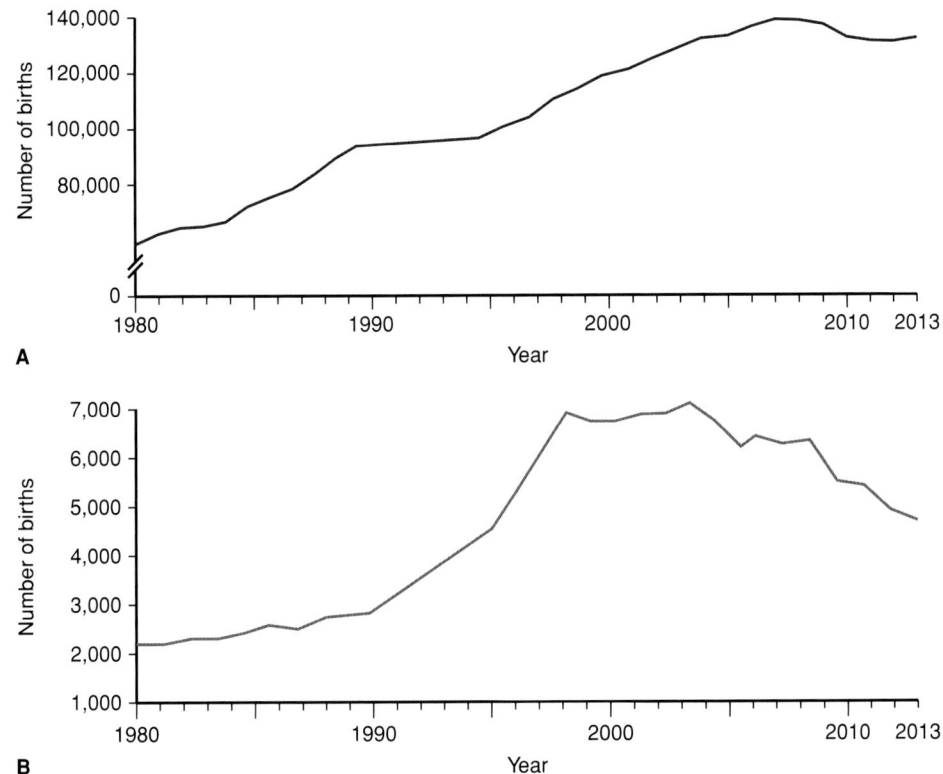

FIGURE 20-5 Trends in frequency of multifetal gestations. **A.** Number of twin births in the United States from 1980 to 2006. **B.** Number of triplet and higher-order multifetal births in the United States for the same time period. (Data from Martin JA, Hamilton BE, Osternman MH, et al: Births: final data for 2013. Natl Vital Stat Rep 64:1, 2015.)

There have been efforts to lower the rates of multifetal gestation in patients undergoing ovulation induction or superovulation by using serum estradiol limits and arbitrary sonographic criteria of follicular size. These, however, have been ineffective. In a multicenter randomized clinical trial involving 1255 ovulation induction cycles, hCG was withheld if the estradiol concentration rose above 3000 pg/mL or if more than six follicles greater than 18 millimeters in diameter were present (Guzick, 1999). Despite these limits on hCG administration, the multifetal gestation rate was still 30 percent. Although sonography and serum estradiol monitoring have not reduced the incidence of multifetal gestation or OHSS, the risk of multifetal pregnancy does correlate with the magnitude of follicular response as indicated by follicle number and serum estradiol levels. However, there is no consensus among centers regarding specific sonographic criteria or estradiol levels beyond which hCG should not be administered.

When the likelihood of multifetal gestation is felt to be excessive, IVF can be undertaken to reduce the risk. Because the number of embryos transferred can be strictly controlled, this strategy can minimize the risk of higher-order multifetal gestations. Guidelines set forth by the American Society for Reproductive Medicine and the Society for Assisted Reproductive Technology (2013a) have led to a significant reduction in triplet (and higher-order) gestations (Table 20-3). Efforts to reduce twin pregnancies through the increased use of elective single embryo transfer (eSET) are currently ongoing (American Society for Reproductive Medicine, 2012c).

Ovarian Drilling

Surgical ovarian wedge resection was the first established treatment for anovulatory PCOS patients. It was largely abandoned because of postsurgical adhesion formation, which converted endocrinologic subfertility to mechanical subfertility (Adashi, 1981; Buttram, 1975; Stein, 1939). As a result, it was replaced by medical ovulation induction with CC and gonadotropins (Franks, 1985). However, medical ovulation induction, as discussed earlier, has limitations. Accordingly, surgical therapy using laparoscopic techniques and termed *laparoscopic ovarian drilling* is an alternative in women resistant to medical therapies.

During laparoscopic ovarian drilling, electrosurgical coagulation, laser vaporization, or Harmonic scalpel may be used to create multiple perforations into the ovarian surface and stroma (Section 44-7, p. 1021). In many uncontrolled observational studies, drilling has led to temporary, higher rates of spontaneous postoperative ovulation and conception or to improved medical ovulation induction (Armar, 1990, 1993; Farhi, 1995; Greenblatt, 1987; Kovacs, 1991).

The mechanism of action with laparoscopic ovarian drilling is thought to be similar to that of ovarian wedge resection. Both procedures destroy ovarian androgen-producing tissue

TABLE 20-3. Recommended Limits on the Numbers of Embryos to Transfer

Prognosis	<35 yr	35–37 yr	38–40 yr	41–42 yr
Cleavage-stage embryos[a]				
Favorable[b]	1–2	2	3	5
All others	2	3	4	5
Blastocysts[a]				
Favorable[b]	1	2	2	3
All others	2	2	3	3

[a]Justification for transferring one additional embryo more than the recommended limit should be clearly documented in the patient's medical record.
[b]Favorable = first cycle of in vitro fertilization (IVF), good embryo quality, excess embryos available for cryopreservation, or previous successful IVF cycle.
Reproduced with permission from American Society for Reproductive Medicine, Society for Assisted Reproductive Technology: Criteria for number of embryos to transfer: a committee opinion, Fertil Steril 2013 Jan;99(1):44–6.

and reduce peripheral conversion of androgens to estrogens. Specifically, a fall in serum levels of androgens and LH and an increase in FSH levels have been demonstrated after ovarian drilling (Armar, 1990; Greenblatt, 1987). The endocrine changes following surgery are thought to convert the adverse androgen-dominant intrafollicular environment to an estrogenic one and to restore the hormonal environment to normal by correcting ovarian-pituitary feedback disturbances (Aakvaag, 1985; Balen, 1993). Thus, both local and systemic effects are thought to promote follicular recruitment and maturation and subsequent ovulation.

Risks of ovarian drilling include postoperative adhesion formation and the other risks of laparoscopic surgery (Chap. 41, p. 877). Additionally, theoretical risks of diminished ovarian reserve and premature ovarian failure remain to be well investigated. As surgery is more invasive, ovarian drilling is generally not offered prior to consideration of medical therapies.

CORRECTION OF DIMINISHED OVARIAN RESERVE

Ovarian dysfunction may result from ovarian failure or from a diminished ovarian reserve, either of which may follow normal aging, disease, cancer treatment, or ovarian surgery. Even if a woman is spontaneously menstruating, a basal (cycle day 2 or 3) FSH level above 15 IU/L predicts that medical therapies including exogenous gonadotropins will be of little benefit. For these women, the option of using donor eggs should be considered (p. 465). Expectant management may also be considered, although the likelihood of pregnancy is low. AMH can identify patients with diminished ovarian reserve prior to the elevation of basal FSH. Although patients with low AMH (<1 ng/mL) generally respond poorly to gonadotropins, some may benefit from ART.

CORRECTION OF ANATOMIC ABNORMALITIES

Anatomic distortions of the female reproductive tract are a major cause of infertility and may prevent ovum entry into the fallopian tube; impair transport of ova, sperm, or embryos; or interfere with implantation. The three primary types of anatomic abnormalities include tubal factors, peritoneal factors, and uterine factors. Each has differing effects and therefore may require different therapies.

■ Tubal Factors

Tubal occlusion can arise from congenital abnormality, infection, or iatrogenic causes. Additionally, a small subset of tubal infertility is idiopathic. Not only the cause of tubal damage but also the anatomic abnormality is important. For example, proximal tubal occlusion, distal tubal occlusion, and tubal absence differ markedly in their treatment.

Proximal tubal occlusion describes obstruction proximal to the fimbria and may develop at the tubal ostium, isthmus, or ampulla. *Midtubal occlusion* is considered a subset of proximal occlusion. Proximal tubal occlusion may be secondary to tubal resection, luminal obliteration, or simple plugging with mucus or debris. In contrast, *distal tubal occlusion* describes obstruction at the tube's fimbria. It typically results from prior pelvic infection and may be associated with concomitant adnexal adhesions.

Tubal Cannulation

Proximal tubal occlusion is often amenable to direct techniques. If diagnosed at the time of hysterosalpingography (HSG), consideration is given to performing concurrent selective salpingography. A catheter is placed such that it wedges within the tubal ostium. This allows significant hydrostatic pressure to be applied to the tube. Such pressure will likely overcome most instances of tubal spasm or plugging by mucus or debris. If tubal patency cannot be reestablished, an inner catheter with guide wire is used to cannulate the tube. This creates patency of isolated short segmental scarring in most instances. Scarring of a longer segment or luminal obliteration, however, is not amenable to correction with tubal cannulation. In these women, surgical segmental resection with reanastomosis or IVF may be considered.

Tubal Reconstruction

Proximal Tubal Obstruction. Tubal obstruction not amenable to treatment with selective salpingography has traditionally been treated surgically, and options include hysteroscopic cannulation, surgical reanastomosis, and neosalpingostomy. Although success rates of ART have risen considerably, reproductive surgery remains an important option or complement to ART for many couples.

Some types of tubal blockage have a much better prognosis with surgical therapy than others. For example, hysteroscopic cannulation of fallopian tubes can treat some types of proximal obstruction in a fashion similar to selective salpingography (Section 44-18, p. 1050). Hysteroscopic cannulation is best performed with concurrent laparoscopy to verify distal tubal patency.

Proximal obstruction not amenable to cannulation techniques can be treated with segmental resection and reanastomosis (Fig. 20-6). In most cases, this can be done as an outpatient procedure through a minilaparotomy incision. However, obstruction extending into the interstitial portion of the tube is more technically challenging to repair and more prone to repeated obstruction postoperatively. Therefore, proximal occlusion extending to the interstitial segment that cannot be treated with cannulation is best treated in most instances with IVF.

Options for proximal and midtubal occlusion resulting from prior sterilization are either tubal reanastomosis or IVF. From a patient perspective, outpatient tubal reanastomosis avoids ovarian stimulation and increased risk for multifetal gestation and provides an ability to conceive normally. In general, although the monthly probability of pregnancy following tubal reversal is likely lower than that for age-matched controls without prior sterilization, the cumulative chance of pregnancy is high. However, IVF is strongly considered if other fertility factors are present or the type of sterilization performed does not permit reconstruction. For example, in cases of sterilization completed by fimbriectomy, neosalpingostomy can be corrective.

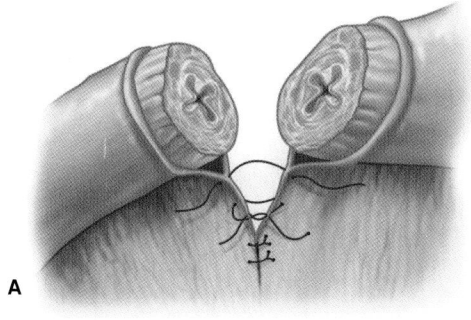

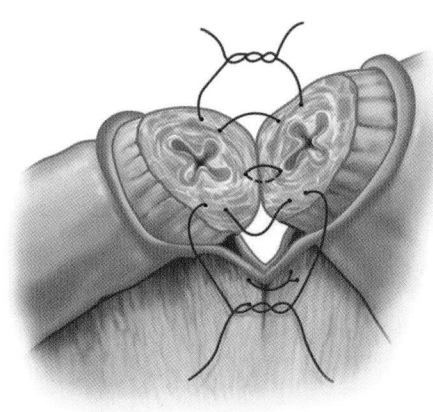

FIGURE 20-6 Surgical reanastomosis of fallopian tube segments. The scarred portion of the tube is sharply excised until nonfibrotic tubal tissues are reached. **A.** The mesosalpinx is reapproximated with interrupted stitches using 6–0 delayed-absorbable suture. **B.** The tubal muscularis is reapproximated with single stitches in each quadrant using 7–0 delayed absorbable suture. Tubal serosa is closed with interrupted or running 6–0 delayed-absorbable suture.

However, the probability of pregnancy is lower, and IVF is considered. Importantly, the risk of subsequent ectopic pregnancy following reanastomosis for midtubal occlusion is 3 to 5 percent (Gordts, 2009).

The "reversibility" of sterilization can generally be determined by review of the operative report and also the pathology report if the procedure involved segmental resection. If operative records are unavailable or suggest that reanastomosis may not be feasible, laparoscopy is performed prior to laparotomy to assess chances of surgical success.

Outpatient reversal of sterilization is most commonly done by minilaparotomy. Incision size typically varies from 3 to 6 cm depending on a patient's weight and anatomy. Some surgeons are able to complete some of these procedures by laparoscopy. Robotic control may be helpful for this but may increase operating time and expense.

Distal Tubal Obstruction. Following pelvic inflammatory disorders, normal fimbrial anatomy may be destroyed, or fimbria may be encased by adnexal adhesions. In these cases, neosalpingostomy can be performed at minilaparotomy or laparoscopy (Fig. 20-7). However, women desiring neosalpingostomy for treatment of distal occlusion are counseled that the risk of ectopic pregnancy is high, the likelihood of pregnancy is 50 percent or lower, and postoperative reocclusion

is common (Bayrak, 2006). Moreover, hydrosalpinges that are dilated more than 3 cm in diameter, that are associated with significant adnexal adhesions, or that display an obviously attenuated endosalpinx yield a poor prognosis. These tubes are best treated by salpingectomy. If both tubes are affected, bilateral salpingectomy is recommended prior to proceeding with IVF. This stems from data showing women with hydrosalpinges undergoing IVF have approximately half the pregnancy rate of other women with unaffected tubes (American Society for Reproductive Medicine, 2012a).

Uterine Factors

Three types of uterine factors have been implicated in infertility and include leiomyomas, endometrial polyps, and intrauterine adhesions. Müllerian anomalies, especially intrauterine septum or segmental agenesis, can increase infertility or pregnancy complication rates. These congenital abnormalities are described fully in Chapter 18 (p. 417). Mechanisms of infertility with these factors have not been clearly elucidated. However, the end result is decreased endometrial receptivity and reduced likelihood of embryo implantation.

Leiomyomas

Leiomyomas are common benign tumors of the uterus and have been associated with infertility in some women (Chap. 9, p. 205). Retrospective studies have suggested a benefit from surgically removing certain tumors to increase efficacy of both natural and assisted conception (Griffiths, 2006).

There are no randomized controlled trials to clearly demonstrate that myomectomy improves fertility. However, in view of the many retrospective observational studies that suggest this, it is reasonable to offer myomectomy to well-selected infertile women, especially if tumors are large or impinge on the endometrial cavity. Myomectomy can be performed using hysteroscopy, laparoscopy, or laparotomy, and selection of the approach is discussed in Chapter 9 (p. 211. Currently, no studies validate one method compared with another in terms of efficacy. Therefore, clinical judgment should determine the most appropriate technique from the standpoint of safety, restoration of normal uterine anatomy, and speed of recovery.

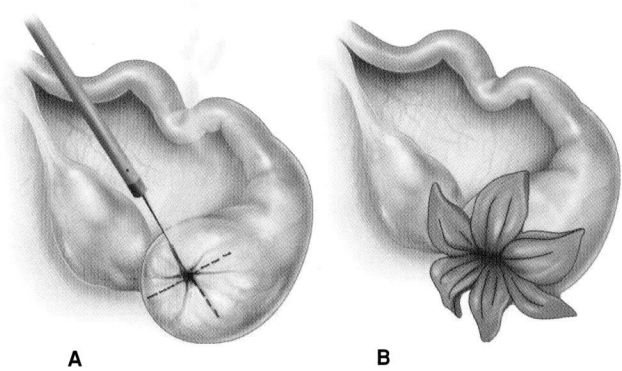

FIGURE 20-7 Neosalpingostomy. **A.** The distal end of the clubbed fallopian tube is opened sharply or with electric or laser energy. **B.** The endosalpinx is everted using Cuff or Bruhat technique.

TABLE 20-4. Number and Percentage of Pregnancies after Hysteroscopic Polypectomy (n = 204)

	Polypectomy n = 101 (%)	Control n = 103 (%)	p-value
Subsequent pregnancy	64 (63.4)	29 (28.2)	<0.001

RR 2.1 (95% CI 1.5–2.9).
Reproduced with permission from Pérez-Medina T, Bajo-Arenas J, Salazar F, et al: Endometrial polyps and their implication in the pregnancy rates of patients undergoing intrauterine insemination: a prospective, randomized study. Hum Reprod 2005 Jun;20(6):1632–1635.

Endometrial Polyps

These soft, fleshy endometrial growths are commonly diagnosed during infertility evaluation. Several studies suggest good pregnancy rates following polypectomy, although the mechanism by which polyps impair fertility has not been established. The requirement to remove even small polyps in infertile women has been previously debated. However, one prospective trial of 204 women with polyps and with an additionally diagnosed cervical factor, male factor, or unexplained infertility appears to give some clear guidance.

In this trial, women were randomized to one of two groups prior to treatment with intrauterine insemination (IUI) (Pérez-Medina, 2005). The first group underwent polypectomy. The second underwent only hysteroscopic biopsy of the polyp to obtain histologic confirmation. All patients were managed expectantly for three cycles prior to proceeding with up to four cycles of IUI. The pregnancy rate in the polypectomy group was more than twice as high regardless of initial polyp size (Table 20-4). These data suggest that endometrial polyps can significantly impair infertility treatment outcome. Thus, it would seem prudent to

perform hysteroscopic polypectomy in all infertile patients if a polyp is identified (Section 44-13, p. 1038).

Intrauterine Adhesions

Adhesions within the endometrial cavity, also called *synechiae*, can range from asymptomatic small bands to complete or near complete obliteration of the endometrial cavity. If amenorrhea or hypomenorrhea result, the condition is termed *Asherman syndrome* (Chap. 16, p. 372).

Treatment involves surgical adhesiolysis to restore normal uterine cavity size and configuration. Dilatation and curettage (D & C) and abdominal approaches have previously been used. However, with the advantages of hysteroscopy, the role of these other techniques has been minimized.

Hysteroscopic adhesion resection may range from simple lysis of a small band to extensive adhesiolysis of dense intrauterine adhesions using scissors, electrosurgical cutting, or laser energy (Section 44-19, p. 1052). However, women whose uterine fundus is completely obscured and those with a markedly narrowed, fibrotic cavity present the greatest therapeutic challenge. Several techniques have been described for these difficult cases, but outcome is far worse than in patients with small band adhesions. In those women with severe Asherman syndrome that is not amenable to reconstructive surgery, gestational carrier surrogacy is a valuable option (p. 465).

■ Peritoneal Disease

Endometriosis

This condition and its effects on infertility are extensively discussed in Chapter 10 (p. 234). In women with minimal or mild disease, evidence supporting lesion ablation is limited and use of empiric general fertility boosting procedures such as ART or superovulation combined with IUI is reasonable. These treatments have been validated to increase fecundity in women with stage I and II disease (Table 20-5) (Guzick, 1999).

TABLE 20-5. Cycle Fecundity with Stage I or II Endometriosis compared with Unexplained Infertility

	Unexplained Infertility		Endometriosis-associated Infertility		
Treatment	Guzick[a]	Deaton[a]	Chaffin[a]	Fedele[a]	Kemmann[a]
No treatment or intracervical insemination	0.02	0.033	—	0.045	0.028
IUI	0.05[b]	—	—	—	—
Clomiphene	—	—	—	—	0.066
Clomiphene/IUI	—	0.095[b]	—	—	—
Gonadotropins	0.04[b]	—	0.066	—	0.073[b]
Gonadotropins/IUI	0.09[b]	—	0.129[b]	0.15[b]	—
IVF	—	—	—	—	0.222[b]

[a]And their colleagues.
[b]p<.05 for treatment vs. no treatment.
IUI = intrauterine insemination; IVF = in vitro fertilization.
Reproduced with permission from American Society for Reproductive Medicine: Endometriosis and infertility. Fertil Steril 2006 Nov;86(5 Suppl 1):S156–S160.

Moderate and severe endometriosis results in distortion of anatomic relationships of reproductive organs. In many cases, surgical treatment may improve anatomy, and pregnancy can result (American Society for Reproductive Medicine, 2006). Unfortunately, advanced disease may prevent adequate restoration of pelvic anatomy. Therefore, a surgeon's operative findings and anticipated surgical results guide postoperative strategy. If satisfactory surgical outcome is achieved, it is reasonable to attempt pregnancy for 6 to 12 months prior to considering other options such as IVF. It should be remembered that endometriosis in some cases may recur quickly, and unnecessary delay in attempting pregnancy postoperatively is not advised.

In women with advanced endometriosis, several studies suggest that long-term treatment with GnRH agonists before initiation of a cycle may improve fecundity (Dicker, 1992; Surrey, 2002). Currently, however, this treatment strategy is not universally accepted.

If endometriomas are noted, surgical options include cyst drainage, drainage followed by cyst wall ablation, or cyst excision. These three procedures can be performed laparoscopically in nearly all circumstances given adequate surgeon experience. Simple drainage minimizes ovarian destruction but commonly results in rapid cyst recurrence. One histologic study demonstrated that a mean of 60 percent of the cyst wall (range of 10 to 98 percent) was lined by endometrium to a depth of 0.6 mm (Muzii, 2007). Thus, drainage and ablation may not destroy all endometrium to this depth. Moreover, this approach is associated with significant risk of cyst recurrence and thermal damage to the ovary. For these reasons, laparoscopic excision of the cyst wall by a stripping technique should be considered optimal treatment for most endometriomas (Section 44-5, p. 1015). Hart and coworkers (2008) compared ablative surgery and cyst excision. With excision, they noted more favorable rates of diminished pain, cyst recurrence, and spontaneous pregnancy. However, excision is inevitably accompanied by removal of normal ovarian tissue and often leads to decreased ovarian volume and diminished ovarian reserve (Almog, 2010; Exacoustos, 2004; Ragni, 2005).

Endometrioma recurrence is common. But, surgery for a recurrent endometrioma appears to be even more harmful to the ovarian reserve than primary surgery (Muzii, 2015). Thus, further ovarian surgery is individualized (American College of Obstetricians and Gynecologists, 2014a). If there is confidence in the diagnosis, it may be prudent in some cases to avoid surgery entirely when future fertility is desired.

Pelvic Adhesions

Pelvic adhesions may result from endometriosis, prior surgery, or pelvic infection and often vary in their density and vascularity. Adhesions may impair fertility by distorting adnexal anatomy and by interfering with gamete and embryo transport, even in the absence of tubal disease.

Surgical lysis may restore pelvic anatomy in some cases, but adhesions may recur, especially if they are dense and vascular. Adherence to microsurgical principles and minimally invasive surgery may help decrease adhesion formation. Although numerous adjuvants, such as adhesion barriers, have been used to reduce the risk of postoperative adhesion formation, currently none have been validated to improve fecundity (American Society for Reproductive Medicine, 2013c).

Among infertile women with adnexal adhesions, pregnancy rates after adhesiolysis are 32 percent at 12 months and 45 percent at 24 months of surveillance. These rates can be compared with 11 percent at 12 months and 16 percent at 24 months in those left untreated (Tulandi, 1990). As with severe endometriosis, clinical judgment regarding operative findings and results of surgery should guide the strategy postoperatively. IVF is the best option for those with a poor prognosis for normal anatomy restoration.

CORRECTION OF CERVICAL ABNORMALITIES

In response to follicular estradiol production, the cervix should produce abundant thin mucus. If present, this mucus acts as a conduit and functional reservoir for sperm. Accordingly, inadequate cervical mucus impairs sperm transport to the upper female reproductive tract.

Causes of abnormal or deficient mucus include infection, prior cervical surgery, use of antiestrogens (e.g., clomiphene citrate) for ovulation induction, and sperm antibodies. However, many women with decreased or hostile mucus have no history of predisposing factors.

Examination of cervical mucus may reveal gross evidence of chronic cervicitis that deserves treatment. Doxycycline, 100 mg orally twice daily for 10 days, is an appropriate therapy. In those with decreased mucus volume, treatments include short-term supplementation with exogenous estrogen, such as ethinyl estradiol, and the use of the mucolytic expectorant guaifenesin. However, the value of estrogen and guaifenesin has not been confirmed. Moreover, exogenous estrogens could have a negative effect on follicular development and ovarian function.

For these reason, most clinicians treat noninfectious, suspected cervical mucus abnormalities with IUI (Fig. 20-8). Although this approach also has not been validated with randomized prospective trials, the theoretical basis for this approach seems sound (Helmerhorst, 2005). Additionally, IUI has been

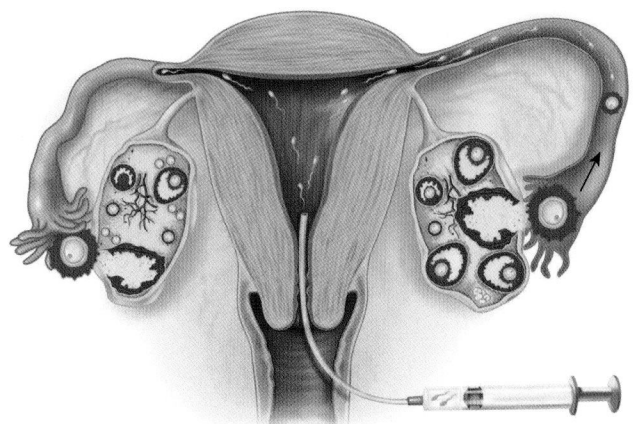

FIGURE 20-8 Intrauterine insemination (IUI). Prior to IUI, partner or donor sperm is washed and concentrated. IUI is usually combined with superovulation, and signs of impending ovulation are monitored with transvaginal sonography. At the time of suspected ovulation, a long, thin catheter is threaded through the cervical os and into the endometrial cavity. A syringe containing the sperm concentrate is attached to the catheter's distal end, and the sperm sample is injected into the endometrial cavity.

demonstrated to be effective for treatment of unexplained infertility. As a result, many clinicians forgo cervical mucus testing and proceed directly with IUI treatments in the absence of tubal disease.

CORRECTION OF MALE INFERTILITY

Male infertility has numerous causes and may include various sperm or semen volume abnormalities that are described subsequently. Accordingly, therapy should be planned only after thorough evaluation (Chap. 19, p. 442). In the absence of identifiable correctable cause, it is appropriate to offer IUI or ART as treatment options. The choice of whether to proceed initially with IUI therapies as opposed to the more intensive and expensive ART treatments is dependent on several factors. These include duration of infertility, age of the female, and history of prior treatments. If ART is considered for male factor, intracytoplasmic sperm injection (ICSI) is typically selected rather than traditional IVF (Fig. 20-9).

Abnormal Semen Volume

Aspermia is characterized by a complete lack of semen and results from failure to ejaculate. The physiology of normal ejaculation includes emission of sperm with accessory gland fluid into the urethra, simultaneous closure of the urethral sphincters, and forceful ejaculation of semen through the urethra. Emission and closure of the bladder neck are primarily alpha-adrenergically mediated thoracolumbar sympathetic reflex events with supraspinal modulation. Ejaculation is a sacral spinal reflex mediated by the pudendal nerve.

Anejaculation or anorgasmia is not rare and may stem from psychogenic factors, organic erectile dysfunction, or impaired parasympathetic sacral spinal reflex. Appropriate treatments depend on the cause and can include psychologic counseling or erectile dysfunction treatment with sildenafil citrate (Viagra) or other similar medication. Vibratory stimulation may also be effective in some instances. Electroejaculation is an invasive procedure and is generally used for men with spinal cord injuries who are unresponsive to the therapies above.

Men who always achieve orgasm but never experience prograde ejaculation or have a greatly reduced prograde volume typically have retrograde ejaculation. Therefore, administration of oral pseudoephedrine or another alpha-adrenergic agent to aid bladder neck closure is warranted. However, for many, pharmacologic methods are ineffective, and IUI may be performed using sperm processed from a voided urine specimen collected after ejaculation.

A minority of men who achieve orgasm, but not prograde ejaculation, have failure of emission. A trial of sympathomimetic agents is reasonable in these individuals as well, although pharmacologic therapies have generally provided limited success. Alternatively, testicular or epididymal extraction of sperm via aspiration or biopsy may be used in cases refractory to medication. As with electroejaculation, this technique recovers a limited number of viable sperm and is best suited for use with ICSI.

Hypospermia, that is, low semen volume (<2 mL), impairs sperm transport into cervical mucus and can be associated with decreased sperm density or motility. Retrograde ejaculation may underlie this condition, and treatment follows that just described for aspermia.

Alternatively, hypospermia may follow partial or complete ejaculatory duct obstruction. In these cases, transurethral excision of the obstruction and reanastomosis of the ejaculatory ducts has resulted in marked semen parameter improvement, and pregnancies have been achieved. However, couples are counseled that postoperative complete obstruction of the ejaculatory ducts is not rare. Thus, consideration is given to cryopreservation of sperm prior to surgical attempts in those individuals with partial obstruction.

Abnormal Sperm Count

Azoospermia is characterized by the total absence of sperm in semen. This may result from male reproductive tract obstruction or from nonobstructive causes.

Obstructive azoospermia, especially resulting from prior vasectomy or ejaculatory duct obstruction, may be amenable to surgical treatment. However, congenital bilateral absence of the vas deferens (CBAVD) is a common cause of azoospermia and

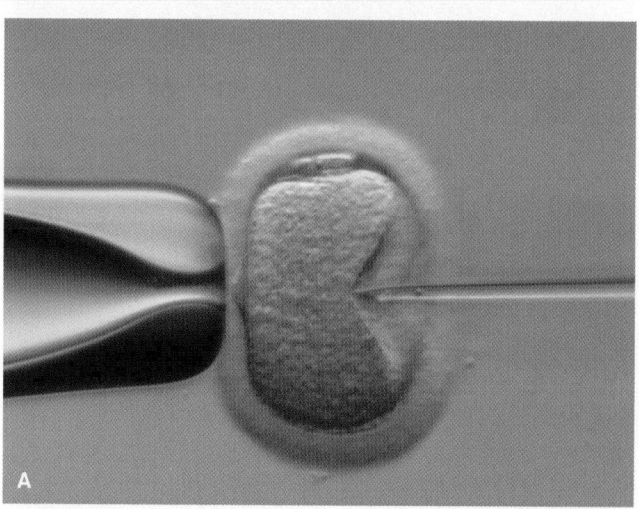
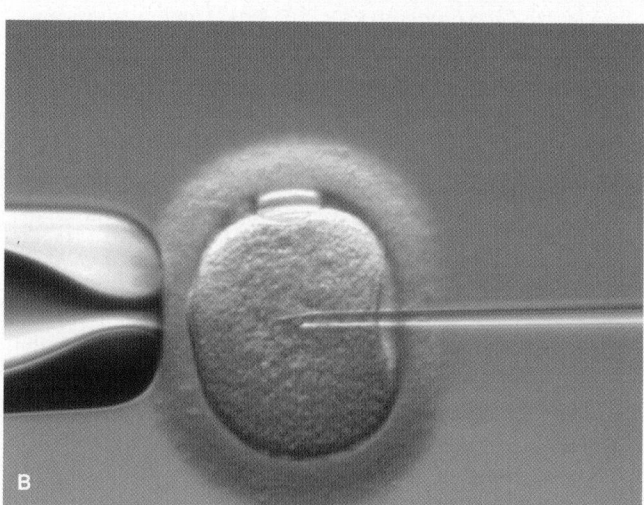

FIGURE 20-9 Photomicrographs of intracytoplasmic sperm injection.

unfortunately is not treatable surgically. In such candidates, testicular sperm extraction (TESE) may be performed in conjunction with ICSI.

Nonobstructive azoospermia may be caused by a karyotypic abnormality such as Klinefelter syndrome (47,XXY) or balanced translocation; deletion of a small portion of the Y chromosome; testicular failure; or by unexplained causes. In many cases, TESE may be combined effectively with ICSI in those with Klinefelter syndrome and Y microdeletion of the AZFc region. However, in men with Y microdeletion in the AZFa or AZFb region, this ART combination has been ineffective (Choi, 2004).

Oligospermia is diagnosed if fewer than 15 million sperm are present per milliliter of semen. Causes are varied and include hormonal, genetic, environmental (including medications), and unexplained causes. Additionally, an obstructive cause, especially ejaculatory duct obstruction, should be considered if oligospermia is seen in conjunction with low semen volume. If severe oligospermia (<5 to 10 million sperm per mL) is noted, then an evaluation similar to that for azoospermia is warranted.

Oligospermia in the absence of decreased sperm motility not uncommonly reflects hypogonadotropic hypogonadism. In general, hypogonadotropic hypogonadism is best treated with FSH and hCG administered to the male. Alternatively, clomiphene citrate and aromatase inhibitors, although not FDA-approved treatment for this indication, may be considered for some males, especially if obesity and elevated serum estradiol levels are present. Spermatogenesis is a long process lasting approximately 100 days. Thus, several months may be required to identify significant improvements in sperm density with either treatment.

Environmental factors such as excessive exposure to high temperatures should be investigated. Drug and medication history is also obtained. If an environmental factor is identified, correction may improve sperm numbers.

■ Abnormal Sperm Motility or Morphology

Asthenospermia, that is, decreased sperm motility, may be seen alone or in combination with oligospermia or other abnormal semen parameters. In general, asthenospermia does not respond to directed treatments. Expectant management may be considered especially if the duration of infertility is short and maternal age is less than 35 years. For treatment, IUI and ICSI are preferred, although IUI is generally not successful in severe cases (Centola, 1997). If fewer than 1 million motile sperm are available for insemination following semen processing or the couple has experienced more than 5 years of infertility, then ICSI is considered as initial therapy (Ludwig, 2005).

Teratozoospermia or abnormal sperm morphology is most often seen in conjunction with oligospermia, asthenospermia, and oligoasthenospermia. Directed treatments for teratozoospermia are not available, and therapy options include IUI and ART. Because teratozoospermia may commonly be accompanied by sperm function defects that may impair fertilization, ICSI is considered if ART is selected.

■ Varicocele

This results from dilatation of the pampiniform plexus of the spermatic vein and is usually left-sided (Fig. 19-3, p. 431).

Traditional treatment is surgical ligation of the internal spermatic vein. With ligation, several surgical techniques have been employed, but retroperitoneal high ligation and transinguinal ligation are the most frequently performed. More recently, interventional radiographic techniques that selectively catheterize and embolize the internal spermatic vein with sclerosing solutions, tissue adhesives, or detachable balloons or coils have been used as alternatives. Despite the widespread application of varicocele treatments, there is insufficient evidence to conclude that treatment of a clinical varicocele in couples with male subfertility improves the likelihood of conception (Evers, 2003).

UNEXPLAINED INFERTILITY

This may represent one of the most common infertility diagnoses, and its reported prevalence has reached as high as 30 percent (Dodson, 1987). The diagnosis of unexplained infertility is highly subjective and depends on the diagnostic tests performed or omitted and on their quality. Paradoxically, a diagnosis of unexplained infertility, therefore, will more often be reached if the evaluation is incomplete or poor quality (Gleicher, 2006). Nevertheless, an unexplained infertility diagnosis can, by definition, not be directly treated. Expectant management may be considered especially with infertility of short duration and with relatively young maternal age. However, if treatment is desired, then IUI, superovulation, and ART are empiric appropriate interventions to consider.

INTRAUTERINE INSEMINATION

This technique uses a thin flexible catheter to place a prepared semen sample into the uterine cavity. First, motile, morphologically normal spermatozoa are separated from dead sperm, leukocytes, and seminal plasma. This highly motile fraction is then inserted transcervically near the anticipated time of ovulation. Intrauterine insemination can be performed with or without superovulation and is appropriate therapy for treatment of cervical factors, mild and moderate male factors, and unexplained infertility.

If performed for cervical factors, IUI timed by urine LH surge is an initial strategy that achieves reasonable pregnancy rates of up to 11 percent per cycle (Steures, 2004). Although this rate is lower than that seen with superovulation combined with IUI, the side effects and costs of superovulation are avoided.

In contrast, for unexplained infertility and for male factors, IUI is most commonly performed in conjunction with superovulation. A combination of clomiphene citrate and IUI was evaluated by Deaton and colleagues (1990) in one randomized trial. The treatment group had a significantly higher pregnancy rate (9.5 percent) compared with controls (3.3 percent). Gonadotropin treatment (FSH or hMG) alone has been shown to increase the likelihood of pregnancy, but the benefit is markedly improved with the addition of IUI.

ASSISTED REPRODUCTIVE TECHNOLOGY

Assisted reproductive technology describes clinical and laboratory techniques used to achieve pregnancy in infertile couples for whom direct corrections of underlying causes are not feasible. In principle, IUI meets this definition. By convention, however, ART procedures are those that at some point require extraction and isolation of an oocyte as described in the following paragraphs.

■ In Vitro Fertilization

During IVF, mature oocytes from stimulated ovaries are retrieved transvaginally with sonographic guidance (Fig. 20-10). Sperm and ova are then combined in vitro to prompt fertilization (Fig. 20-11). If successful, viable embryos are transferred transcervically into the endometrial cavity using sonographic guidance (Fig. 20-12). As discussed earlier, prior to proceeding with IVF, hydrosalpinges are removed or tubal interruption performed to increase implantation rates and decrease the risk of miscarriage.

Similar to IUI, substantial benefit is achieved using controlled ovarian hyperstimulation prior to egg retrieval. Many ova are genetically or functionally abnormal. Thus, exposure of

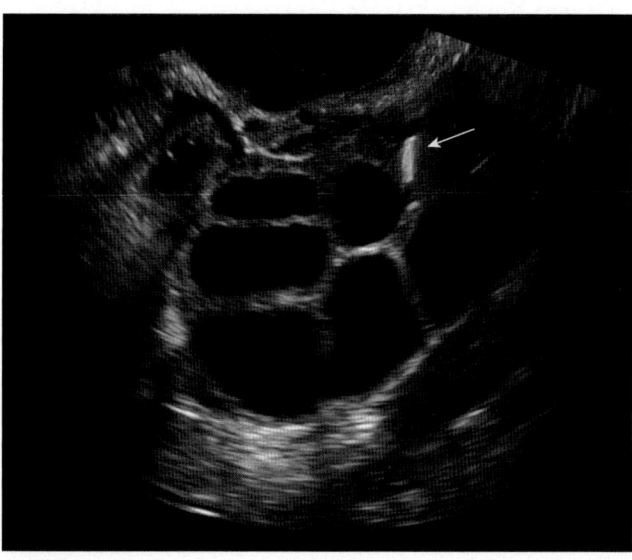

FIGURE 20-10 Sonogram demonstrates transvaginal oocyte retrieval. The needle is seen in the upper right portion of the image as a hyperechoic line (*arrow*) entering a mature follicle.

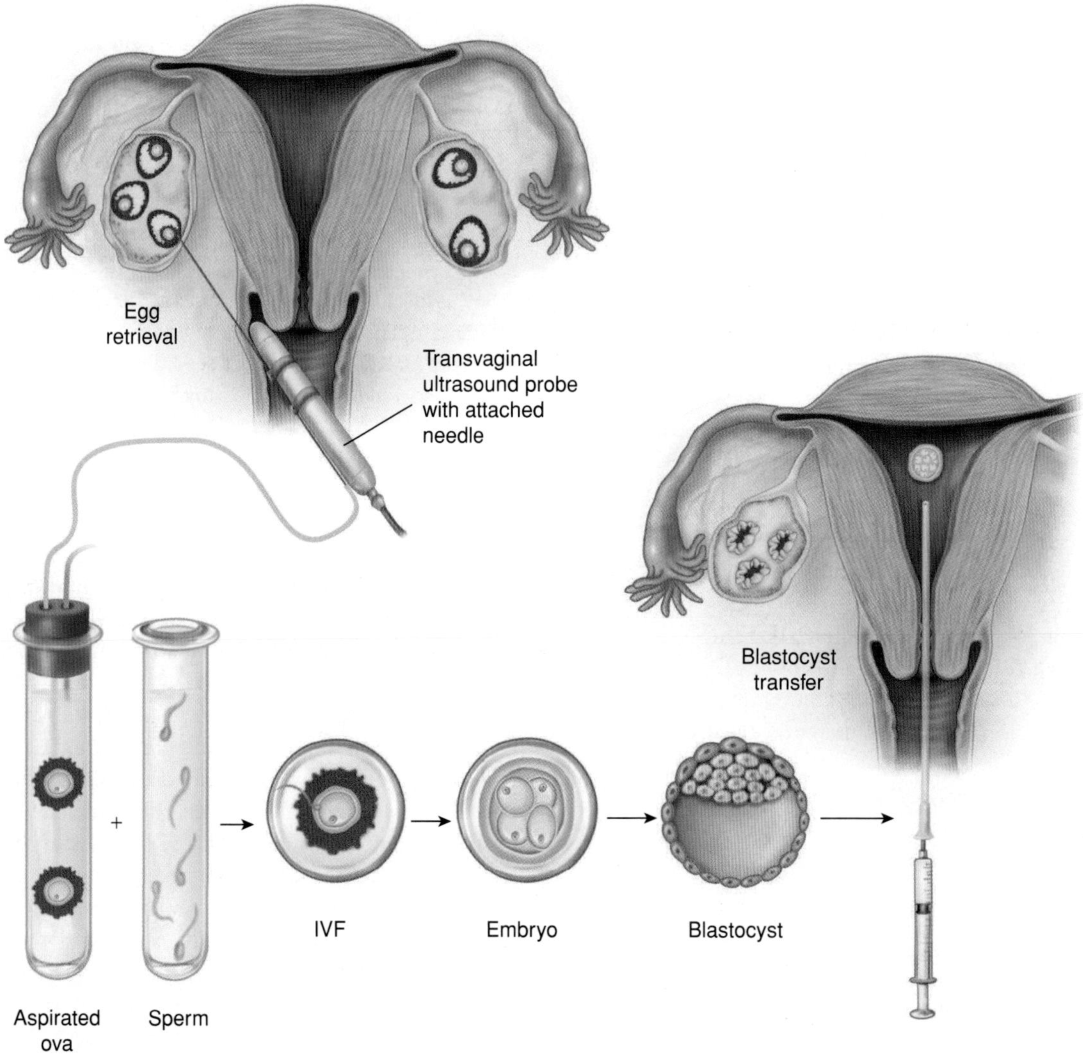

Egg
retrieval

Transvaginal
ultrasound probe
with attached
needle

Blastocyst
transfer

+

IVF

Embryo

Blastocyst

Aspirated
ova

Sperm

FIGURE 20-11 In vitro fertilization (IVF). Controlled ovarian hyperstimulation is achieved with one of the protocols displayed in Figure 20-2, and follicle maturation is monitored over several days sonographically. Near ovulation, a transvaginal approach is used to harvest eggs from the ovaries. These oocytes are fertilized in vitro, and fertilized eggs develop to the blastocyst stage. Blastocysts are then drawn up into a syringe and delivered into the endometrial cavity under sonographic guidance.

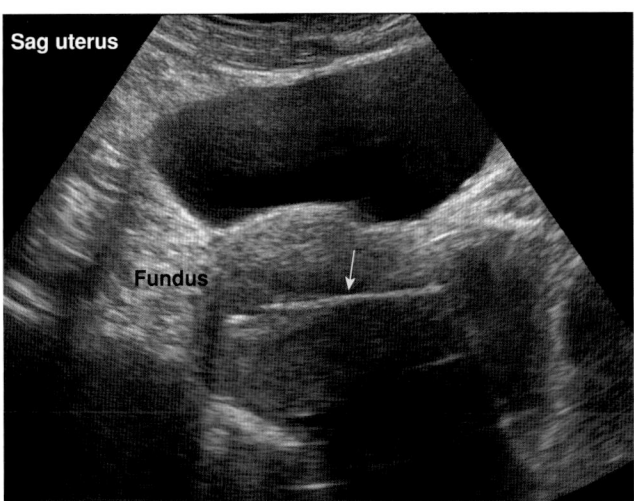

Sag uterus

Fundus

FIGURE 20-12 Embryo transfer performed using abdominal sonographic guidance for proper placement. Catheter (*arrow*) is seen within the endometrial cavity.

several ova to sperm results in an increased chance of a healthy embryo. Most often, a GnRH agonist is used in conjunction with gonadotropins (FSH or hMG). These agonists prevent the possibility of spontaneous LH surge and ovulation prior to egg retrieval. Optimally, 10 to 20 ova are harvested, and from these, one healthy embryo is ideally transferred back to the uterus.

Unfortunately, methods to determine embryo health are imperfect. Therefore, to maximize the probability of pregnancy, more than one embryo is typically transferred, thus resulting in increased risk of multifetal gestation. However, advances in culture conditions now permit embryos to be cultured to the blastocyst stage. This allows transfer of fewer embryos yet maintains high pregnancy rates (Langley, 2001).

Intracytoplasmic Sperm Injection

This variation of IVF is most applicable to male factor infertility. During the micromanipulation technique of ICSI, cumulus cells surrounding an ovum are enzymatically digested, and a single sperm is directly injected through the zona pellucida and oocyte cell membrane. Pregnancy rates with ICSI are comparable with those achieved with IVF for other causes of infertility. For azoospermic men, ICSI has made pregnancy in their partners possible. In these cases, sperm are mechanically extracted from the testicle or epididymis.

Gestational Carrier Surrogacy

This variation of IVF places a fertilized egg into the uterus of a surrogate rather than into the "intended mother." Indications are varied, and this approach may be appropriate for women with uncorrectable uterine factors, for those in whom pregnancy would pose significant health risks, and for those with repetitive unexplained miscarriage.

Gestational carrier surrogacy has legal and psychosocial issues. In most states, a surrogate is the legal parent and therefore, adoption must be completed after birth to give the intended mother her parental rights. However, a few states have adopted specific laws that extend protection to the intended parents.

Egg Donation

This may be employed in cases of infertility associated with ovarian failure or diminished ovarian reserve. Additionally, the technique may also be used to achieve pregnancy in fertile women when offspring would be at risk for maternally transmitted genetic disease. Egg donors may be known to the recipient couple or more commonly are anonymous young women recruited by an agency or IVF center.

Egg donation can be performed using "fresh" oocytes or cryopreserved eggs. Fresh egg donation cycles require synchronization of the recipient's endometrium with egg development in the donor.

To accomplish this, the egg donor completes one of the superovulation protocols outlined in Figure 20-2. Concurrently, if a recipient is not menopausal, GnRH agonists are used to suppress gonadotropin production in the receiving woman. This allows a scheduled priming of her endometrium with estrogen and progesterone. Following gonadotropin suppression, exogenous estrogen is given to the recipient. This estrogen administration begins just prior to the start of gonadotropin administration to the egg donor. After a donor receives hCG to allow the final stages of follicle and egg maturation, the recipient begins progesterone to prepare her endometrium. In the recipient, estrogen and progesterone are typically continued until late in the first trimester when placental production of these hormones is deemed to be adequate.

Gamete or Zygote Intrafallopian Transfer

Gamete intrafallopian transfer (GIFT) is similar to IVF in that egg retrieval is performed after controlled ovarian hyperstimulation. Unlike IVF, however, fertilization and early embryo development do not take place in the laboratory. Eggs and sperm are placed via catheter through the fimbria and deposited directly into the oviduct. This transfer of gametes is most commonly performed at laparoscopy. Like IUI, GIFT is most applicable for unexplained infertility and should not be considered for tubal factor causes.

This technique was most popular in the late 1980s and early 1990s. However, as laboratory techniques have improved, IVF has largely replaced GIFT. In general, GIFT is more invasive, provides less diagnostic information, and requires transfer of more than two eggs for optimal pregnancy chances, which increases the risk of higher-order multifetal gestation. Thus, the major indication for GIFT at present is to avoid the religious or ethical concerns that some patients may have with fertilization taking place outside the body.

Zygote intrafallopian transfer (ZIFT) is a variant of IVF with similarities to GIFT. Zygote transfer is not performed directly into the uterine cavity but rather into the fallopian tube at laparoscopy. If the transfer is completed after a zygote has begun to divide, the procedure is more accurately termed tubal embryo transfer (TET). Although a normal fallopian tube may provide a superior environment for the early-stage embryo, this advantage has been lessened with improvements in laboratory culture methods. Accordingly, ZIFT currently is considered most appropriately in the rare case in which transcervical transfer during IVF is technically not feasible.

■ Embryo, Oocyte, or Ovarian Tissue Cryopreservation

With IVF, many eggs are retrieved to ultimately produce one to three healthy embryos for transfer. This frequently leads to extra embryos. Successful freezing and thawing of embryos has been possible for two decades. Moreover, advances in cryoprotectants and techniques have allowed improved survival rates of embryos frozen at various developmental stages. With cryopreservation, these supernumerary embryos can yield pregnancies later, obviating the need for ovarian stimulation and egg retrieval. For some patients, avoidance of fresh transfer and cryopreservation of all embryos may improve the chance of pregnancy. This may be due to improve synchrony between the embryo and the endometrium (Doody, 2014).

Cryopreservation of unfertilized eggs had previously posed significant technical hurdles. These challenges have been largely overcome by the development of ultrarapid freezing techniques (vitrification). Because of this advancement and preliminary data confirming its safety, oocyte cryopreservation is no longer considered experimental. Egg freezing is useful in preserving the fertility potential of women facing gonadotoxic chemotherapy. This technique also provides greater timing flexibility to circumvent cycle synchronization during egg donation. As success improves, oocyte cryopreservation may assist women desiring to delay childbearing, although data are lacking regarding its efficacy in this patient population. Careful counseling is needed with regard to age and clinic-specific success rates (American Society for Reproductive Medicine, 2013a).

Distinct from oocyte freezing, ovarian tissue cryopreservation is an option to preserve reproductive potential. Candidates are patients who must urgently undergo aggressive chemotherapy and/or radiotherapy or who have other medical conditions requiring treatment that may threaten ovarian function and subsequent fertility. This fertility preservation strategy may be well suited for prepubertal girls or women with hormone-sensitive malignancies. One or both ovaries or ovarian cortex tissue is removed during laparoscopy or minilaparotomy. Postoperatively, the ovarian cortex is cut into small tissue slivers measuring 0.3- to 2-mm thick and cryopreserved. Successful pregnancies have been achieved following autologous transplantation of thawed cortical tissue into a pelvic site such as a contralateral ovary or pelvic sidewall. Some pregnancies have been achieved without further intervention, while others have required ART. Safety concerns include the risk for reintroducing a malignancy following transplantation. This risk may be greatest with blood-borne cancers such as leukemia. Although promising, this procedure is currently considered experimental (American Society for Reproductive Medicine, 2014).

■ In Vitro Maturation

This technique has been used to achieve pregnancy by aspirating antral follicles from unstimulated ovaries and culturing these immature oocytes to allow resumption and completion of meiosis in vitro. In vitro maturation (IVM) may be useful in patients with PCOS in whom stimulation poses a significant risk of OHSS. Recent data suggest that success rates with standard IVF remain superior to those with IVM (Walls, 2015).

Additionally, long-term outcomes are unknown, thus IVM is deemed experimental (American Society for Reproductive Medicine, 2013b). In the future, refinement of this technique may make possible maturation of ova from preantral follicles. This could potentially allow preservation of fertility potential but without the need for subsequent autologous transplantation for women in whom gonadotoxic chemotherapy is required.

■ Preimplantation Genetic Diagnosis or Screening

These laboratory techniques identify genetic abnormalities in eggs or embryos prior to their transfer. Thus, risk for transmission of hereditable disease is a well-established indication for *preimplantation genetic diagnosis (PGD)*. In contrast, *preimplantation genetic screening (PGS)* aims to identify embryonic aneuploidy resulting from gamete meiotic errors. Its proposed indications include recurrent miscarriage, advanced maternal age, and multiple failed IVF cycles.

PGD is no longer considered experimental, and implementation of newly developed methods for genetic analysis will likely continue to broaden its application (Society for Assisted Reproductive Technology, 2008). During this technique, cells are removed from a developing embryo. Multiple options exist regarding biopsy timing and genetic material source. Biopsy of the first and second polar body has the advantage of avoiding cell removal from the developing embryo. However, two separate micromanipulation procedures are required, and genetic abnormalities of paternal origin are not detected. Biopsy of cleavage-stage embryos (6- to 8-cell stage) allows evaluation of both maternal and paternal contribution to the genome (Fig. 20-13). However, biopsy at this stage may only partially reflect the embryo's genetic makeup if mitotic nondisjunction has occurred and embryonic mosaicism has been created. In addition, biopsied normal embryos may have a slightly decreased implantation rate. Most recently, biopsy of the trophectoderm at the blastocyst stage has been suggested to hold several advantages (Fig. 20-14). The trophectoderm is the layer from which trophoblasts and thus the placenta develop. Biopsy from this layer allows evaluation of several cells but avoids removal of fetal cells. However, biopsy of embryos at this late stage may require embryo cryopreservation following biopsy if genetic analysis cannot be performed rapidly.

Once cells are extracted, they are tested for structural aberrations and/or aneuploidy. Common testing options include single-nucleotide polymorphism (SNP) plus comparative genomic hybridization (CGH) microarrays or quantitative polymerase chain reaction. To analyze single cells for disease-specific DNA mutations, linkage analysis and DNA sequencing are generally used. Most recently, next-generation sequencing (NGS) has been used for both PGS and PGD. NGS has the potential to improve genetic diagnosis in embryos, especially in terms of high-throughput automation (Fiorentino, 2014).

■ Complications of Assisted Reproductive Technology

In most cases, ART leads to successful delivery of healthy singleton pregnancies. However, some pregnancy complications

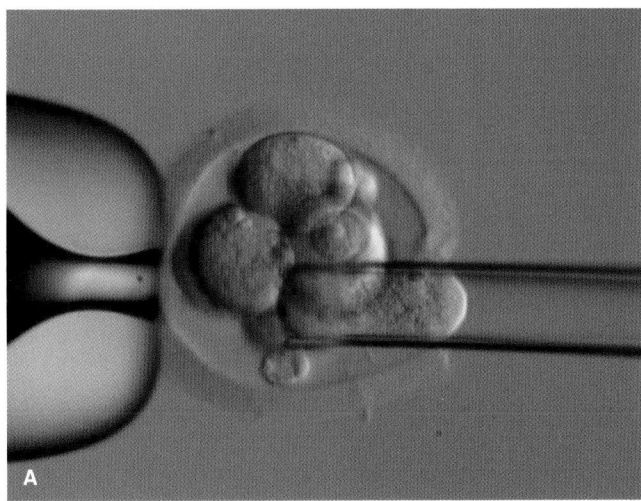

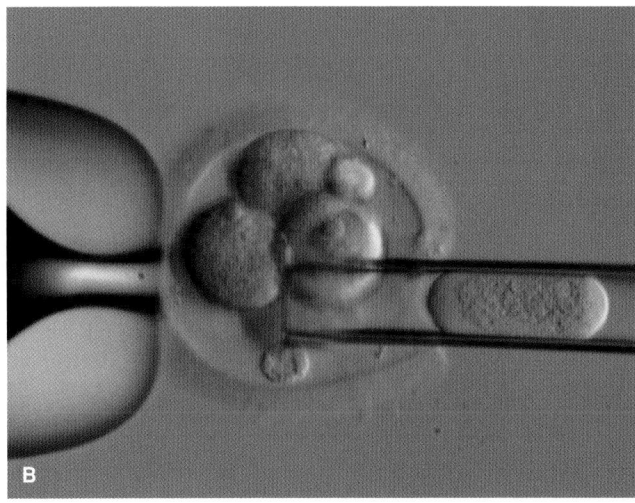

FIGURE 20-13 Photomicrographs of embryo biopsy.

may develop more frequently in those conceived using ART. Of maternal risks, preeclampsia, placenta previa, and placental abruption are more common in IVF-conceived pregnancies (Table 20-6). Of fetal risks, multifetal gestation, discussed earlier, is the most common. In addition, perinatal mortality, preterm delivery, low birthweight, and fetal-growth restriction have been implicated in IVF singleton gestations. These trends persist even following adjustment for age and parity (Reddy, 2007). Other studies, however, have not confirmed this increased risk (Fujii, 2010). Additionally, congenital anomalies and epigenetic issues are concerns (Table 20-7).

Discussions regarding the risks for congenital anomalies began shortly after the initial success of IVF and intensified following the use of ICSI. Specifically, studies do suggest a higher incidence of congenital anomalies in infants conceived with ovulation induction, IUI, or IVF compared with those from the general population (El-Chaar, 2009; Reddy, 2007). Interpretation of most published studies, however, is complex. For example, the patient population undergoing IVF is very different from the general obstetric population with respect to age and other factors. If data are adjusted for maternal age or

duration of subfertility, the risk of congenital anomalies does not appear to be increased with ART (Shevell, 2005; Zhu, 2006). This implies that much of the risk is intrinsic to the infertile couple and not related to the procedure itself.

An increase in the risk of epigenetic issues has also been reported. Although these conditions appear to be rare, their importance cannot be overstated. For review, each autosomal gene is represented by two copies, or alleles, and one copy is inherited from each parent. For most genes, both alleles are expressed simultaneously. However, approximately 150 human genes are *imprinted*, and with these genes, only one of the alleles is expressed. Imprinted genes are under control of an imprinting center that directs embryogenesis and viability. Alteration of the cellular environment can interfere with this regulation and may follow gamete manipulation or inadequate in vitro culture conditions. As a result, accelerated embryo growth, birth complications, placental abnormalities, and polyhydramnios have been observed in nonhuman mammalian ART pregnancies.

TABLE 20-6. Potential Risks in Singleton IVF-conceived Pregnancies

	Absolute Risk (%) in IVF-conceived Pregnancies	Relative Risk (vs. non IVF-conceived Pregnancies)
Preeclampsia	10.3%	1.6 (1.2–2.0)
Placenta previa	2.4%	2.9 (1.5–5.4)
Placental abruption	2.2%	2.4 (1.1–5.2)
Gestational diabetes	6.8%	2.0 (1.4–3.0)
Cesarean delivery[a]	26.7%	2.1 (1.7–2.6)

[a]Please note that most experts believe the rate of cesarean delivery to be well above the 26.7% rate quoted here.
IVF = in vitro fertilization.
Reproduced with permission from Society for Assisted Reproductive Technology: Informed consent for assisted reproduction: in vitro fertilization, intracytoplasmic sperm injection, assisted hatching, embryo cryopreservation. 2009. pp 20, 22.

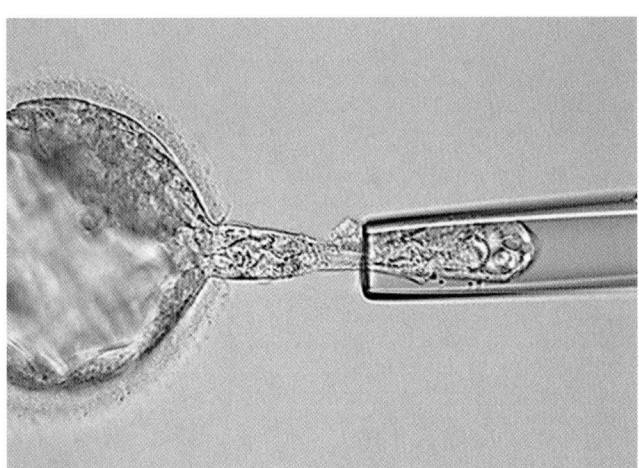

FIGURE 20-14 Photomicrograph of trophectoderm biopsy. The trophectoderm is distinct from the embryonic inner cell mass and gives rise to trophoblastic cells of the future placenta.

TABLE 20-7. Potential Risks in Singleton IVF Pregnancies

	Absolute Risk (%) in IVF Pregnancies	Relative Risk (vs. non-IVF Pregnancies)
Preterm birth	11.5	2.0 (1.7–2.2)
Low birthweight (<2500 g)	9.5	1.8 (1.4–2.2)
Very low birthweight (<1500 g)	2.5	2.7 (2.3–3.1)
Small for gestational age	14.6	1.6 (1.3–2.0)
NICU admission	17.8	1.6 (1.3–2.0)
Stillbirth	1.2	2.6 (1.8–3.6)
Neonatal mortality	0.6	2.0 (1.2–3.4)
Cerebral palsy	0.4	2.8 (1.3–5.8)
Genetic risks		
imprinting disorder	0.03	17.8 (1.8–432.9)
major birth defect	4.3	1.5 (1.3–1.8)
chromosomal abnormalities (after ICSI):		
of a sex chromosome	0.6	3.0
of another chromosome	0.4	5.7

IVF = in vitro fertilization; NICU = neonatal intensive care unit.
Reproduced with permission from Society for Assisted Reproductive Technology: Informed consent for assisted reproduction: in vitro fertilization, intracytoplasmic sperm injection, assisted hatching, embryo cryopreservation. 2009. pp 20, 22.

In humans, imprinted genes may contribute to behavior and language development, alcohol dependency, schizophrenia, and bipolar affective disorders. Imprinting may also increase risks for obesity, cardiovascular disease, and for childhood and adult cancers. Of imprinting disorders, only rates of the rare Beckwith-Wiedemann syndrome are currently suggested to be increased in human ART. Additionally, causation has not been conclusively proven. However, in view of the above increased risks, it is reasonable to consider more intensive prenatal assessment in pregnancies conceived by IVF.

Studies assessing cognitive development after ART have for the most part been reassuring, although conflicting studies do exist. Many studies are suboptimal due to small sample size, choice of comparison group, and confounding and mediating factors (Carson, 2010). Fortunately, currently available data suggest that the psychomotor development of preschool children conceived by IVF does not differ from that of naturally conceived children. Similarly, the socioemotional development of children conceived by IVF appears comparable with that of naturally conceived children (Ludwig, 2006).

CONCLUSION

The treatment of infertility is typically initiated only after a thorough investigation as outlined in the previous chapter. The initial focus is to identify lifestyle or environmental issues that may contribute to or cause the reproductive impairment. Obesity, adequate nutrition, and associated stress should not be overlooked. In general, it is desirable to correct any identifiable contributors to subfertility. In many cases, no obvious cause can be detected. In other couples, the cause(s) may be identifiable but not amenable to directed corrective therapies. In these circumstances,

generalized fertility boosting strategies may be recommended. These treatments include IUI (with or without superovulation) and ART. Importantly, superovulation and ART are not without risks, and couples should be appropriately counseled. Additionally, these techniques may involve third parties (egg, sperm, or embryo donors or gestational carriers). These procedures are associated with unique psychosocial, legal, and ethical considerations. Emerging technologies such as preimplantation genetic testing bring additional ethical issues that must be confronted and resolved by both patient and practitioner.

REFERENCES

Aakvaag A: Hormonal response to electrocautery of the ovary in patients with polycystic ovarian disease. BJOG 92:1258, 1985

Adashi EY, Rock JA, Guzick D, et al: Fertility following bilateral ovarian wedge resection: a critical analysis of 90 consecutive cases of the polycystic ovary syndrome. Fertil Steril 36:30, 1981

Almog B, Sheizaf B, Shalom-Paz E, et al: Effects of excision of ovarian endometrioma on the antral follicle count and collected oocytes for in vitro fertilization. Fertil Steril 94(6):2340, 2010

American College of Obstetricians and Gynecologists: Management of endometriosis. Practice Bulletin No. 114, July 2010, Reaffirmed 2014a

American College of Obstetricians and Gynecologists: Neural tube defects. Practice Bulletin No. 44, July 2003, Reaffirmed 2014b

American College of Obstetricians and Gynecologists: Obesity in pregnancy. Committee Opinion No. 549, January 2013

American Society for Reproductive Medicine: Committee opinion: role of tubal surgery in the era of assisted reproductive technology. Fertil Steril 97(3):539, 2012a

American Society for Reproductive Medicine: Diagnostic evaluation of the infertile female: a committee opinion. Fertil Steril 98(2):302, 2012b

American Society for Reproductive Medicine: Endometriosis and infertility. Fertil Steril 86(5 Suppl 1):S156, 2006

American Society for Reproductive Medicine: Obesity and reproduction: an educational bulletin. Fertil Steril 90(5 Suppl):S21, 2008

American Society for Reproductive Medicine: Ovarian tissue cryopreservation: a committee opinion. Fertil Steril 101(5):1237, 2014

American Society for Reproductive Medicine, Society for Assisted Reproductive Technology: Criteria for number of embryos to transfer: a committee opinion. Fertil Steril 99(1):44, 2013a

American Society for Reproductive Medicine, Society for Assisted Reproductive Technology: Elective single-embryo transfer. Fertil Steril 97(4):835, 2012c

American Society for Reproductive Medicine, Society for Assisted Reproductive Technology: In vitro maturation: a committee opinion. Fertil Steril 99(3):663, 2013b

American Society for Reproductive Medicine, Society of Reproductive Surgeons: Pathogenesis, consequences, and control of peritoneal adhesions in gynecologic surgery: a committee opinion. Fertil Steril 99(6):1550, 2013c

Antonucci T, Whitcomb R, McLain R, et al: Impaired glucose tolerance is normalized by treatment with the thiazolidinedione troglitazone. Diabetes Care 20:188, 1998

Armar N, McGarrigle H, Honour J, et al: Laparoscopic ovarian diathermy in the management of anovulatory infertility in women with polycystic ovaries: endocrine changes and clinical outcomes. Fertil Steril 53:45, 1990

Armar NA, Lachelin GC: Laparoscopic ovarian diathermy: an effective treatment for anti-oestrogen resistant anovulatory infertility in women with the polycystic ovary syndrome. BJOG 100(2):P161, 1993

Balen A, Braat D, West C, et al: Cumulative conception and livebirth rates after the treatment of anovulatory infertility: safety and efficacy of ovulation induction. Hum Reprod 9:1563, 1994

Balen A, Tan SL, Jacobs H, et al: Hypersecretion of luteinising hormone. A significant cause of infertility and miscarriage. BJOG 100:1082, 1993

Bayrak A, Harp D, Saadat P, et al: Recurrence of hydrosalpinges after cuff neosalpingostomy in a poor prognosis population. J Assist Reprod Genet 23:285, 2006

Biljan MM, Hemmings R, Brassard N, et al: The outcome of 150 babies following the treatment with letrozole or letrozole and gonadotrophins. Fertil Steril 84(Suppl 1):S95, 2005

Buttram VC, Vaquero C: Post-ovarian wedge resection adhesive disease. Fertil Steril 26:874, 1975

Carson C, Kurinczuk JJ, Sacker A, et al: Cognitive development following ART: effect of choice of comparison group, confounding and mediating factors. Hum Reprod 25(1):244, 2010

Casey BM, Cunningham FG: Endocrinologic disorders. In Cunningham FG, Leveno KL, Bloom SL, et al (eds): Williams Obstetrics, 24th ed, New York, McGraw-Hill, 2014

Casper RF: Letrozole: ovulation or superovulation? Fertil Steril 80:1335, 2003

Centers for Disease Control and Prevention: Contribution of assisted reproductive technology and ovulation-inducing drugs to triplet and higher-order multiple births—United States, 1980–1997. MMWR 49:535, 2000

Centola GM: Successful treatment of severe oligozoospermia with sperm washing and intrauterine insemination. J Androl 18:448, 1997

Cheong YC, Dix S, Hung Y, et al: Acupuncture and assisted reproductive technology. Cochrane Database Syst Rev 7:CD006920, 2013

Choi JM, Chung P, Veeck L, et al: AZF microdeletions of the Y chromosome and in vitro fertilization outcome. Fertil Steril 81:337, 2004

Collin P, Vilska S, Heinonen PK, et al: Infertility and coeliac disease. Gut 39(3):382, 1996

Crosignani PG, Colombo M, Vegetti W, et al: Overweight and obese anovulatory patients with polycystic ovaries: parallel improvements in anthropometric indices, ovarian physiology and fertility rate induced by diet. Hum Reprod 18(9):1928, 2003

Cunningham FG, Leveno KL, Bloom SL, et al (eds): Obesity. In Williams Obstetrics, 24th ed. New York, McGraw-Hill, 2014

Deaton J, Gibson M, Blackmer K, et al: A randomized, controlled trial of clomiphene citrate and intrauterine insemination in couples with unexplained infertility or surgically corrected endometriosis. Fertil Steril 54:1083, 1990

Dicker D, Goldman JA, Levy T, et al: The impact of long-term gonadotropin-releasing hormone analogue treatment on preclinical abortions in patients with severe endometriosis undergoing in vitro fertilization-embryo transfer. Fertil Steril 57:597, 1992

Dodson WC, Whitesides DB, Hughes CL, et al: Superovulation with intrauterine insemination in the treatment of infertility: a possible alternative to gamete intrafallopian transfer and in vitro fertilization. Fertil Steril 48:441, 1987

Domar AD, Seibel MM, Benson H, et al: The mind/body program for infertility: a new behavioral treatment approach for women with infertility. Fertil Steril 54: 1183, 1990

Doody KJ: Cryopreservation and delayed embryo transfer—assisted reproductive technology registry and reporting implication. Fertil Steril 102(1):27, 2014

El-Chaar D, Yang Q, Gao J, et al: Risk of birth defects increased in pregnancies conceived by assisted human reproduction. Fertil Steril 92(5):1557, 2009

Elnashar A, Abdelmageed E, Fayed M, et al: Clomiphene citrate and dexamethazone in treatment of clomiphene citrate-resistant polycystic ovary syndrome: a prospective placebo-controlled study. Hum Reprod 21(7):1805, 2006

Evans MI, Britt DW: Fetal reduction 2008. Curr Opin Obstet Gynecol 20(4):386, 2008

Evers JL, Collins JA: Assessment of efficacy of varicocele repair for male subfertility: a systematic review. Lancet 361(9372):1849, 2003

Exacoustos C, Zupi E, Amadio A, et al: Laparoscopic removal of endometriomas: sonographic evaluation of residual functioning ovarian tissue. Am J Obstet Gynecol 191(1):68, 2004

Farhi J, Soule S, Jacobs HS, et al: Effect of laparoscopic ovarian electrocautery on ovarian response and outcome of treatment with gonadotropins in clomiphene citrate-resistant patients with polycystic syndrome. Fertil Steril 64:930, 1995

Farhi J, West C, Patel A, et al: Treatment of anovulatory infertility: the problem of multiple pregnancy. Hum Reprod 11:429, 1996

Filicori M, Cognigni GE, Taraborrelli S, et al: Modulation of folliculogenesis and steroidogenesis in women by graded menotropin administration. Hum Reprod 17:2009, 2002

Fiorentino F, Bono S, Biricik A, et al: Application of next-generation sequencing technology for comprehensive aneuploidy screening of blastocysts in clinical preimplantation genetic screening cycles. Hum Reprod 29(12):2802, 2014

Fontana PG, Leclerc JM: Contraindication of Femara (letrozole) in premenopausal women. 2005. Available at: http://www.google.com/url?sa=t&rct=j&q=&esrc=s&source=web&cd=1&ved=0CCMQFjAA&url=http%3A%2F%2Fwww.novartis.ca%2Fasknovartispharma%2Fdownload.htm%3Fres%3DFemara_DHCP_E_2005_Nov.pdf%26resTitleId%3D266&ei=KPzkVP60NMyZgwT8qoK4DQ&usg=AFQjCNH2Z9u7iXhv06G82y-4xEMgWBOmxg. Accessed February 18, 2015

Franasiak JM, Dondik Y, Molinaro TA, et al: Blastocyst transfer is not associated with increased rates of monozygotic twins when controlling for embryo cohort quality. Fertil Steril 103(1):95, 2015

Franik S, Kremer JA, Nelen WL, et al: Aromatase inhibitors for subfertile women with polycystic ovary syndrome. Cochrane Database Syst Rev 2:CD010287, 2014

Franks S, Adams J, Mason H, et al: Ovulation disorders in women with polycystic ovary syndrome. Clin Obstet Gynecol 12:605, 1985

Fujii M, Matsuoka R, Bergel E, et al: Perinatal risk in singleton pregnancies after in vitro fertilization. Fertil Steril 94(6):2113, 2010

Gleicher N, Barad D: Unexplained infertility: does it really exist? Hum Reprod 21:1951, 2006

Gordts S, Campo R, Puttemans P, et al: Clinical factors determining pregnancy outcome after microsurgical tubal reanastomosis. Fertil Steril 92(4):1198, 2009

Greenblatt E, Casper RF: Endocrine changes after laparoscopic ovarian cautery in polycystic ovarian syndrome. Am J Obstet Gynecol 156:279, 1987

Griffiths A, D'Angelo A, Amso N, et al: Surgical treatment of fibroids for subfertility. Cochrane Database Syst Rev 3:CD003857, 2006

Guzick DS, Carson SA, Coutifaris C, et al: Efficacy of superovulation and intrauterine insemination in the treatment of infertility. N Engl J Med 340:177, 1999

Gysler M, March CM, Mishell DR Jr, et al: A decade's experience with an individualized clomiphene treatment regime including its effect on the postcoital test. Fertil Steril 37:161, 1982

Hammond M, Halme J, Talbert L, et al: Factors affecting the pregnancy rate in clomiphene citrate induction of ovulation. Obstet Gynecol 62:196, 1983

Hart RJ, Hickey M, Maouris P, et al: Excisional surgery versus ablative surgery for ovarian endometriomata. Cochrane Database Syst Rev 2:CD004992, 2008

Helmerhorst FM, Van Vliet HA, Gornas T, et al: Intra-uterine insemination versus timed intercourse for cervical hostility in subfertile couples. Cochrane Database Syst Rev 4:CD002809, 2005

Hoeger K: Obesity and weight loss in polycystic ovary syndrome. Obstet Gynecol Clin North Am 28:85, 2001

Jackson JE, Rosen M, McLean T, et al: Prevalence of celiac disease in a cohort of women with unexplained infertility. Fertil Steril 89(4):1002, 2008

Kiddy DS, Hamilton-Fairly D, Bush A, et al: Improvement in endocrine and ovarian function during dietary treatment of obese women with polycystic ovary syndrome. Clin Endocrinol (Oxf) 36:105, 1992

Kovacs G, Buckler H, Bangah M, et al: Treatment of anovulation due to polycystic ovarian syndrome by laparoscopic ovarian electrocautery. BJOG 98:30, 1991

Langley MT, Marek DM, Gardner DK, et al: Extended embryo culture in human assisted reproduction treatments. Hum Reprod 16:902, 2001

Legro RS, Barnhart HX, Schlaff WD, et al: Clomiphene, metformin or both for infertility in polycystic ovary syndrome. N Engl J Med 356(6):551, 2007

Legro RS, Brzyski RG, Diamond MP, et al: Letrozole versus clomiphene for infertility in the polycystic ovary syndrome. N Engl J Med 371(2):119, 2014

Lincoln SR, Ke RW, Kutteh WH: Screening for hypothyroidism in infertile women. J Reprod Med 44:455, 1999

Lobo RA, Gysler M, March CM, et al: Clinical and laboratory predictors of clomiphene response. Fertil Steril 37:168, 1982

Ludwig AK, Diedrich K, Ludwig M, et al: The process of decision making in reproductive medicine. Semin Reprod Med 23(4):348, 2005

Ludwig AK, Sutcliffe AG, Diedrich K, et al: Post-neonatal health and development of children born after assisted reproduction: a systematic review of controlled studies. Eur J Obstet Gynecol Reprod Biol 127(1):3, 2006

Martin JA, Hamilton BE, Osternman MH, et al: Births: final data for 2013. Natl Vital Stat Rep 64:1, 2015

Martin JA, Park MM: Trends in twin and triplet births: 1980–97. Natl Vital Stat Rep 47:1, 1999

Meloni GF, Desole S, Vargiu N, et al: The prevalence of celiac disease in infertility. Hum Reprod 14:2759, 1999

Mitwally MF, Casper RF: Aromatase inhibition reduces the dose of gonadotropin required for controlled ovarian hyperstimulation. J Soc Gynecol Investig 11:406, 2004

Molitch ME: Management of prolactinomas during pregnancy. J Reprod Med 44:1121, 1999

Muzii L, Achilli C, Lecce F, et al: Second surgery for recurrent endometriomas is more harmful to healthy ovarian tissue and ovarian reserve than first surgery. Fertil Steril 103(3):738, 2015

Muzii L, Bianchi A, Bellati F, et al: Histologic analysis of endometriomas: what the surgeon needs to know. Fertil Steril 87(2):362, 2007

Nestler JE, Jakubowicz DJ, Evans WS, et al: Effects of metformin on spontaneous and clomiphene-induced ovulation in the polycystic ovary syndrome. N Engl J Med 338:1876, 1998

Palomba S, Orio F, Falbo A, et al: Prospective parallel randomized, double blind, double-dummy controlled clinical trial comparing clomiphene citrate and metformin as the first-line treatment for ovulation induction in nonobese anovulatory women with polycystic ovary syndrome. J Clin Endocrinol Metab 90:4068, 2005

Papanikolaou EG, Fatemi H, Venetis C, et al: Monozygotic twinning is not increased after single blastocyst transfer compared with single cleavage-stage embryo transfer. Fertil Steril 93(2):592, 2010

Parsanezhad ME, Alborzi S, Motazedian S, et al: Use of dexamethasone and clomiphene citrate in the treatment of clomiphene citrate-resistant patients with polycystic ovary syndrome and normal dehydroepiandrosterone sulfate levels: a prospective, double-blind, placebo-controlled trial. Fertil Steril 78(5):1001, 2002

Pasquali R, Antenucci D, Casmirri F, et al: Clinical and hormonal characteristics of obese amenorrheic hyperandrogenic women before and after weight loss. J Clin Endocrinol Metab 68:173, 1989

Patel SR, Sigman M: Antioxidant therapy in male infertility. Urol Clin North Am 35(2):319, 2008

Pérez-Medina T, Bajo-Arenas J, Salazar F, et al: Endometrial polyps and their implication in the pregnancy rates of patients undergoing intrauterine insemination: a prospective, randomized study. Hum Reprod 20:1632, 2005

Ragni G, Somigliana E, Benedetti F, et al: Damage to ovarian reserve associated with laparoscopic excision of endometriomas: a quantitative rather than a qualitative injury. Am J Obstet Gynecol 193(6):1908, 2005

Raj S, Thompson I, Berger M, et al: Clinical aspects of polycystic ovary syndrome. Obstet Gynecol 49(5):552, 1977

Reddy UM, Wapner RJ, Rebar RW, et al: Infertility, assisted reproductive technology, and adverse pregnancy outcomes: executive summary of a National Institute of Child Health and Human Development workshop. Obstet Gynecol 109(4):967, 2007

Ross C, Morriss A, Khairy M, et al: A systematic review of the effect of oral antioxidants on male infertility. Reprod Biomed Online 20(6):711, 2010

Shevell T, Malone FD, Vidaver J, et al: Assisted reproductive technology and pregnancy outcome. Obstet Gynecol 106(5 Pt 1):1039, 2005

Sigman M, Glass S, Campagnone J, et al: Carnitine for the treatment of idiopathic asthenospermia: a randomized, double-blind, placebo-controlled trial. Fertil Steril 85(5):1409, 2006

Smith JF, Eisenberg ML, Millstein SG, et al: The use of complementary and alternative fertility treatment in couples seeking fertility care: data from a prospective cohort in the United States. Fertil Steril 93(7):2169, 2010

Society for Assisted Reproductive Technology: Informed consent for assisted reproduction: in vitro fertilization, intracytoplasmic sperm injection, assisted hatching, embryo cryopreservation. 2009. pp 20, 22

Society for Assisted Reproductive Technology, American Society for Reproductive Medicine: Preimplantation genetic testing: a Practice Committee opinion. Fertil Steril 90(5 Suppl):S136, 2008

Stein IF, Cohen MR: Surgical treatment of bilateral polycystic ovaries. Am J Obstet Gynecol 38:465, 1939

Steures P, van der Steeg JW, Verhoeve HR, et al: Does ovarian hyperstimulation in intrauterine insemination for cervical factor subfertility improve pregnancy rates? Hum Reprod 19:2263, 2004

Strickland DM, Whitted WA, Wians FH Jr: Screening infertile women for subclinical hypothyroidism. Am J Obstet Gynecol 163:262, 1990

Surrey ES, Silverberg KM, Surrey MW: Effect of prolonged gonadotropin-releasing hormone agonist therapy on the outcome of in vitro fertilization-embryo transfer in patients with endometriosis. Fertil Steril 78:699, 2002

Thiering P, Beaurepaire J, Jones M, et al: Mood state as a predictor of treatment outcome after in vitro fertilization/embryo transfer technology (IVF/ET). J Psychosom Res 37:481, 1993

Tredway D, Schertz JC, Beck D, et al: A phase II, prospective, randomized dose-finding comparative study evaluating anastrozole versus clomiphene citrate in infertile women with ovulatory dysfunction. Fertil Steril 95:1719, 2011a

Tredway D, Schertz JC, Beck D, et al: Anastrozole single-dose protocol in women with oligo- or anovulatory infertility: results of a randomized phase II dose-response study. Fertil Steril 95:1724, 2011b

Tulandi T, Collins JA, Burrows E, et al: Treatment-dependent and treatment-independent pregnancy among women with periadnexal adhesions. Am J Obstet Gynecol 162:354, 1990

Tulandi T, Martin J, Al-Fadhli R, et al: Congenital malformations among 911 newborns conceived after infertility treatment with letrozole or clomiphene citrate. Fertil Steril 85:1761, 2006

Vandermolen DT, Ratts VS, Evans WS, et al: Metformin increases the ovulatory rate and pregnancy rate from clomiphene citrate in patients with polycystic ovary syndrome who are resistant to clomiphene citrate alone. Fertil Steril 75:310, 2001

Walls ML, Hunter T, Keelan JA, et al: In vitro maturation as an alternative to standard in vitro fertilization for patients diagnosed with polycystic ovaries: a comparative analysis of fresh, frozen and cumulative cycle outcomes. Hum Reprod 30(1):88, 2015

Whelan JG III, Vlahos NF: The ovarian hyperstimulation syndrome. Fertil Steril 73:883, 2000

Zarate A, Herdmandez-Ayup S, Rios-Montiel A: Treatment of anovulation in the Stein-Leventhal syndrome. Analysis of ninety cases. Fertil Steril 22:188, 1971

Zhu JL, Basso O, Obel C, et al: Infertility, infertility treatment, and congenital malformations: Danish national birth cohort. BMJ 333(7570):679, 2006

Menopausal Transition

The menopausal transition is a progressive endocrinologic continuum that takes reproductive-aged women from regular, cyclic menses to a final menstrual period and ovarian senescence. With medical advancements, average life expectancy has increased, and most women can now expect to live at least one third of their lives in the menopause. Specifically, by 2020, approximately 43 million women will be aged 45 to 64 years (U.S. Census Bureau, 2014). Importantly, menopausal transition and the years of life spent in the postmenopausal state bring with them issues related to both quality of life and disease prevention and management (Lund, 2008).

DEFINITIONS

Menopause refers to a point in time that follows 1 year after the complete cessation of menstruation, and the *postmenopause* describes years following that point. The average age of women experiencing their final menstrual period (FMP) is 51.5 years, but a halt to menses from ovarian failure may occur at any age. Cessation before age 40, termed *premature ovarian failure*, is associated with an elevated follicle-stimulating hormone (FSH) level and variable causes described in Chapter 16 (p. 373). Of other definitions, the older words *perimenopause* and *climacteric* generally refer to the late reproductive years, usually late 40s to early 50s. These can be used with patients but less so in scientific settings. Here, the term *menopausal transition (MT)* is preferred (Harlow, 2012; Soules, 2001). Characteristically, MT begins with menstrual cycle irregularity and extends to 1 year after permanent cessation of menses. This reproductive aging with loss of follicular activity progresses within a wide age range (42 to 58 years). The average age at its onset is 47, and MT typically spans 4 to 7 years (Burger, 2008; McKinlay, 1992).

As chronological age is an unreliable indicator, guidelines for classifying reproductive aging have been proposed. The first classification of stages and nomenclature for female reproductive aging were developed in 2001 and updated in 2012 at the Stages of Reproductive Aging workshop (STRAW)

(Harlow, 2012). These staging criteria are guides rather than strictly applied diagnoses. Every stage may not manifest in all women, or a stage may occur out of the expected sequence. Also, the age range and duration of each stage varies for given individuals.

In the STRAW system, the anchor stage is the FMP (Fig. 21-1). Five stages precede and two stages follow the FMP. Stage –5 refers to the early reproductive period, stage –4 to the reproductive peak, and stage –3 to the late reproductive period. Stage –2 is the early MT, and stage –1 is the late MT. Stage +1a is the first year after FMP, stage +1b reflects years 2 to 5 postmenopause, and stage +2 refers to the ensuing later postmenopausal years.

INFLUENTIAL FACTORS

Several environmental, genetic, and surgical influences may alter ovarian aging. For example, smoking hastens the age of menopause by approximately 2 years (Gold, 2001; Wallace, 1979). Chemotherapy, pelvic radiation, and ovarian surgery may also lead to earlier menopause. During MT, more erratic fluctuations in female reproductive hormones lead to an array of physical and psychological symptoms as outlined in Table 21-1 (Bachmann, 2001; Dennerstein, 1993). Diet, exercise, reproductive history, socioeconomic status, body mass index (BMI), mood, climate, and individual or cultural attitudes toward

TABLE 21-1. Symptoms Associated with Menopausal Transition

Menstrual pattern	Sexual dysfunction
Shorter cycles (typical)	Vaginal dryness
Longer cycles (possible)	Decreased libido
Irregular bleeding	Dyspareunia
Vasomotor	**Somatic**
Hot flushes	Headache
Night sweats	Dizziness
Sleep disturbances	Palpitations
Psychological/cognitive	Breast pain/enlargement
Worsening PMS	Joint aches and back pain
Depression	**Others**
Irritability	Urinary incontinence
Mood swings	Dry, itchy skin
Poor concentration	Weight gain
Poor memory	

PMS = premenstrual syndrome.

					Final Menstrual Period (FMP)		
Stages:	−5	−4	−3	−2	−1	0 +1	+2
Terminology:	Reproductive			Menopausal Transition		Postmenopause	
	Early	Peak	Late	Early	Late*	Early*	Late
				Perimenopause			
Duration of Stage:	Variable			Variable		ⓐ 1 yr ⓑ 4 yrs	Until demise
Menstrual Cycles:	Variable to regular	Regular		Variable cycle length (>7 days different from normal)	≥2 Skipped cycles and an interval of amenorrhea (≥60 days)	Amen x 12 mos None	
Endocrine:	Normal FSH		↑ FSH	↑ FSH		↑ FSH	

*Stages most likely to be characterized by vasomotor symptoms   ↑ = elevated

FIGURE 21-1 The stages of reproductive aging. (Reproduced with permission from Soules MR, Sherman S, Parrott E, et al: Executive summary: stages of reproductive aging workshop (STRAW). Fertil Steril 2001 Nov;76(5):874–878.)

menopause may explain variations in reports of menopausal symptoms (O'Neil, 2011).

PHYSIOLOGIC CHANGES

In the early MT (stage −2), a woman's menstrual cycles remain regular, but the interval between cycles may be altered by 7 or more days. Typically, cycle lengths become shorter. Compared with younger women, FSH levels are elevated, and serum estrogen levels may be increased in the early follicular phase. Normal ovulatory cycles may be interspersed with anovulatory cycles during this transition, and conception can occur unexpectedly. The late MT (stage −1) is characterized by two or more skipped menses and at least one intermenstrual interval of 60 days or more due to longer and longer periods of anovulation (Soules, 2001). This overview of altered menstruation results from changes in several endocrine axes described next.

■ Hypothalamus-Pituitary-Ovarian Axis

During the reproductive years, gonadotropin-releasing hormone (GnRH) is released in a pulsatile fashion by the arcuate nucleus of the medial basal hypothalamus. It binds to GnRH receptors on the pituitary gonadotropes to stimulate cyclic luteinizing hormone (LH) and FSH release. These gonadotropins, in turn, stimulate the production of the ovarian steroids: estrogen, progesterone, and also inhibin. Estrogen and progesterone exert positive and negative feedback on pituitary gonadotropin production and on the amplitude and frequency of GnRH release. Produced by granulosa cells, inhibin also exerts an important negative influence on FSH secretion from the pituitary. This tightly regulated endocrine system leads to regular, ovulatory menstrual cycles.

Beginning in the late 40s and in early MT (stage −2), FSH levels rise slightly and bring about an increased ovarian follicular response, which raises overall estrogen levels (Jain, 2005; Klein, 1996). The monotropic FSH rise is attributed to decreased ovarian inhibin secretion rather than diminished estradiol feedback. In perimenopausal women, estradiol production fluctuates with FSH levels and can reach higher concentrations than those observed in women younger than 35. Estradiol levels generally do not drop significantly until late in MT. Despite continuing regular cyclic menstruation, progesterone levels during the early MT are lower than in mid-reproductive aged women (Santoro, 2004). Testosterone levels do not vary appreciably during the MT. That said, sex hormone-binding globulin (SHBG) production declines after the menopause and may lead to relative increased levels of free or unbound estrogen and testosterone.

Women in late MT exhibit impaired folliculogenesis and an increasing incidence of anovulation compared with women in their mid-reproductive years. Also, during this time, ovarian follicles undergo an accelerated rate of loss until eventually, in late MT, the supply of follicles is depleted. These changes, including the earlier-described FSH level increase, reflect the reduced capability of aging follicles to secrete inhibin (Reyes, 1977; Santoro, 1996). As another indicator, antimüllerian hormone (AMH) is a glycoprotein secreted by the granulosa cells of secondary and preantral follicles and indirectly reflects the primordial follicle pool (Grynnerup, 2014). Circulating AMH concentrations remain relatively stable across the menstrual cycle in reproductive-aged women and correlate with the number of early antral follicles. AMH levels decrease markedly and progressively across MT (Hale, 2007). With ovarian failure in the menopause (stage +1b), ovarian steroid hormone release ceases, and the negative-feedback loop is opened. As a result, GnRH is released at maximal frequency and amplitude. In turn, circulating FSH and LH levels rise up to fourfold higher than those in the reproductive years (Klein, 1996).

Ovary

Ovarian senescence is a process that has been shown to actually begin in utero within the embryonic ovary due to programmed oocyte atresia. From birth onward, primordial follicles continuously are activated, mature partially, and then regress. This follicular activation continues in a constant pattern that is independent of pituitary stimulation.

A more rapid depletion of ovarian follicles starts in the late 30s and early 40s and continues until a point at which the menopausal ovary is virtually devoid of follicles (Figs. 21-2 and 21-3). An average woman may experience about 400 ovulatory events during her reproductive lifetime. This represents a very small percentage of the 6 to 7 million oocytes present at the 20th week of gestation, or even the 1 to 2 million oocytes present at birth. The process of atresia of the nondominant cohort of follicles, largely independent of menstrual cyclicity, is the prime event that leads to the eventual loss of ovarian activity and menopause.

As evidence, Richardson and colleagues (1987) performed a quantitative histologic study of the endometrium and ovaries of women in MT undergoing hysterectomy for benign indications. These were coupled with a single hormonal measurement and a reproductive history from the study women aged 44 to 55 years. The women who reported regular cycles had an average of 1700 follicles in a selected ovary compared with an average of 180 follicles in the ovaries of those who reported irregular cycles.

Adrenal Steroid Levels

With advancing age, adrenal production of dehydroepiandrosterone sulfate (DHEAS) declines. In women aged 20 to

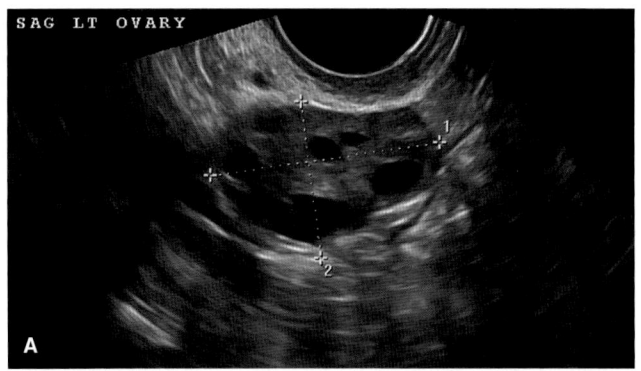

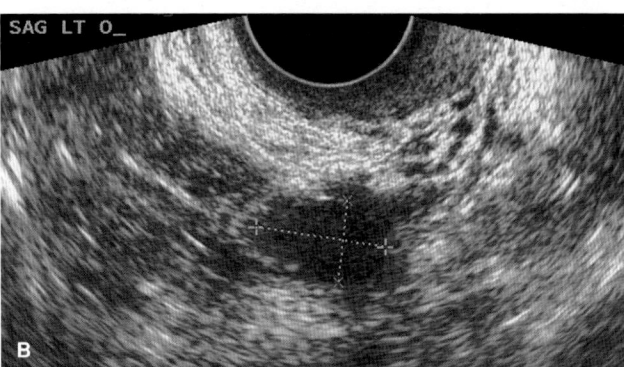

FIGURE 21-2 Transvaginal sonographic images of a pre- and postmenopausal ovary. **A.** In general, premenopausal ovaries have greater volume and contain follicles, which are seen as multiple, small, anechoic smooth-walled cysts. **B.** In comparison, postmenopausal ovaries have smaller volume and are characteristically devoid of follicular structures. (Used with permission from Dr. Elysia Moschos.)

Reproductive age ovary

Menopausal ovary

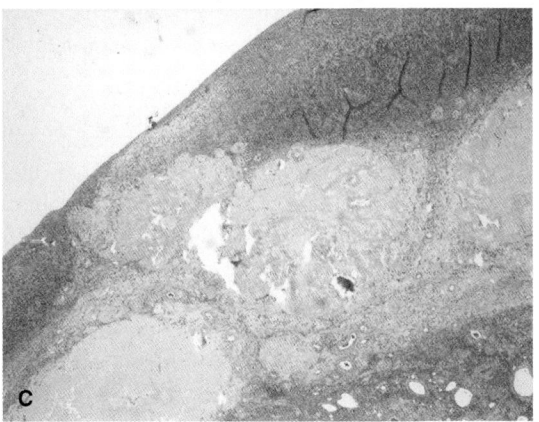

Primordial follicles

FIGURE 21-3 Microscopic differences between a reproductive-age and menopausal ovary. **A.** Reproductive-age ovary. Note preponderance of primordial follicles. **B.** High-power image of primordial follicles. **C.** The menopausal ovary shows abundance of atretic follicles and persistent corpora albicans. (Used with permission from Dr. Raheela Ashfaq.)

30 years, DHEAS concentrations peak, with an average of 6.2 μmol/L, and then decrease steadily. In women 70 to 80 years of age, DHEAS levels are diminished by 74 percent to 1.6 μmol/L. Other adrenal hormone levels fall with aging as well (Burger, 2000; Labrie, 1997). Androstenedione levels peak at ages 20 to 30 years and then decline to 62 percent of this peak level in women aged 50 to 60 years. Pregnenolone levels diminish by 45 percent from reproductive life to menopause. The ovary contributes to the production of these hormones during the reproductive years, but after menopause, only the adrenal gland continues this hormone synthesis.

Burger and associates (2000) prospectively studied 172 women during MT as a part of the Melbourne Women's Midlife Health Project. By analyzing hormone levels longitudinally in these patients, no relationship between a woman's final menstrual period and the decline in DHEAS levels was noted. Advancing age, regardless of menopausal status, determined DHEAS level decline.

Endometrium

Microscopic changes in the endometrium directly reflect systemic estrogen and progesterone levels and thus may change dramatically depending on the stage of MT. During early MT, the endometrium may reflect ovulatory cycles, which are prevalent during this time. During later MT stages, anovulation is common, and the endometrium will display an estrogenic effect that is unopposed by progesterone. Accordingly, proliferative changes or disordered proliferative changes are frequent findings on pathologic examination of endometrial biopsy samples. After menopause, the endometrium becomes atrophic due to lack of estrogen stimulation (Fig. 15-19, p. 356).

Menstrual Disturbances

During MT, abnormal uterine bleeding (AUB) is common, and Treloar (1981) found that menses were irregular in more than one half of all women in this transition. Paramsothy (2014) reported that AUB accounted for 14 percent of all hospitalizations from 1998 to 2005 among women aged 45 to 54. Anovulation is the most common cause of erratic bleeding during MT. However, because the time interval surrounding menopause is characterized by relatively high, acyclic estrogen levels and relatively low progesterone production, women in MT are at increased risk for developing endometrial hyperplasia or carcinoma. Estrogen-sensitive neoplasms, such as endometrial polyps and uterine leiomyomas, and pregnancy-related events are also considered. Many women in their late 40s do not consider themselves fertile and will cease contraception but will still have occasional ovulatory cycles. Contraception can be discontinued by all women at age 55. No spontaneous pregnancies above that age have been reported. Some women may still have menstrual bleeding above age 55, but ovulation is rare and any oocytes are likely poor quality and not viable (Gebbie, 2010).

In all women, regardless of menopausal status, the etiology of AUB should be determined as outlined in Chapter 8 (p. 180). As noted, endometrial cancer is suspected in any woman in MT with AUB. The overall incidence of endometrial cancer is approximately 0.1 percent of women in this group per year, but in women with AUB in MT, the risk increases to 10 percent (Lidor, 1986). Thus, endometrial biopsy is done to exclude malignancy.

Although endometrial neoplasia is the greatest concern during this time, endometrial biopsy frequently reveals a non-neoplastic endometrium displaying estrogen effects unopposed by progesterone. In premenopausal women, this results from anovulation. In postmenopausal women, unopposed estrogen may be derived from extragonadal endogenous estrogen production, which may result from increased aromatization of androgen to estrogen due to obesity. In addition, decreased SHBG levels lead to increased levels of free and therefore bioavailable estrogen (Moen, 2004). Less often, unopposed exogenous estrogen administration or an estrogen-producing ovarian tumor can also account for these effects in postmenopausal women.

Central Thermoregulation

Of the many menopausal symptoms that may affect quality of life, the most frequent are those related to thermoregulation dysfunction. Kronenberg (1990) tabulated all of the published epidemiologic studies and determined that vasomotor symptoms, also variably termed hot flashes, hot flushes, and night sweats, developed in 11 to 60 percent of menstruating women during MT. In the Massachusetts Women's Health Study, the incidence of hot flushes increased from 10 percent during the premenopausal period to approximately 50 percent after menses cessation (McKinlay, 1992). Hot flushes begin an average of 2 years before the FMP, and 85 percent of women who experience them will continue to experience them for more than 1 year. Of these women, 25 to 50 percent will have hot flushes for 5 years, and >15 percent may experience them for >15 years (Kronenberg, 1990). More recent studies of duration indicate that women can expect hot flushes to continue, on average, for nearly 5 years after the FMP, while more than one third of women who experience moderate/severe hot flushes will continue to have them for more than 10 years after the FMP (Freeman, 2014). Longitudinal studies show that hot flushes are associated with low exercise levels, smoking, high FSH and low estradiol levels, increasing BMI, ethnicity, lower socioeconomic status, and prior premenstrual dysphoric disorder (PMDD) or depression (Gold, 2006; Guthrie, 2005).

Vasomotor Symptoms

Thermoregulatory and cardiovascular changes that accompany a hot flush are well documented. An individual hot flush generally lasts 1 to 5 minutes, and skin temperatures rise because of peripheral vasodilation (Kronenberg, 1990). This change is particularly marked in the fingers and toes, where skin temperature can increase 10 to 15°C. Most women sense a sudden wave of heat that spreads over the body, particularly the upper body and face. Sweating begins primarily on the upper body, and it corresponds closely in time with an increase in skin conductance (Fig. 21-4). Sweating has been observed in women during 90 percent of hot flushes (Freedman, 2001).

Increases in both awake and sleep systolic blood pressure are noted with hot flushes (Gerber, 2007). In addition, heart rate rises 7 to 15 beats per minute at approximately the same

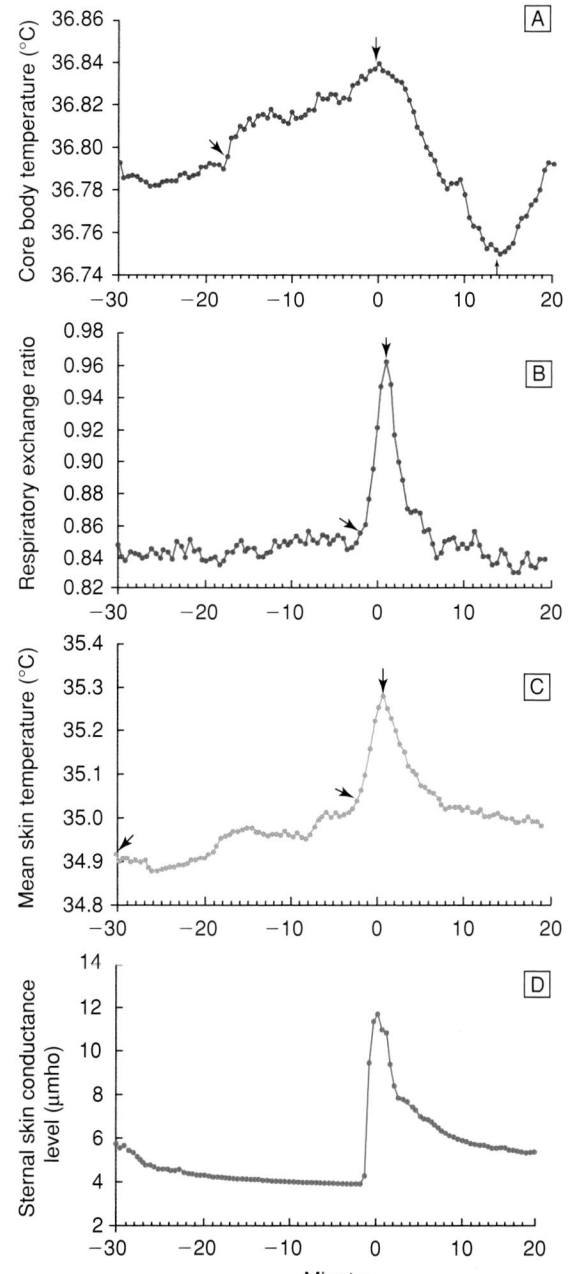

FIGURE 21-4 Physiologic changes (means) during a hot flush. **A.** Core body temperature. **B.** Respiratory exchange ratio. **C.** Skin temperature. **D.** Sternal skin conductance. Time 0 is the beginning of the sternal skin conductance response. (Reproduced with permission from Freedman RR: Biochemical, metabolic, and vascular mechanisms in menopausal hot flashes. Fertil Steril 1998 Aug;70(2):332–337.)

time as peripheral vasodilatation and sweating. Heart rate and skin blood flow usually peak within 3 minutes of the hot flush onset. Simultaneously with sweating and peripheral vasodilation, the metabolic rate also significantly rises. Hot flushes can also be accompanied by palpitations, anxiety, irritability, and panic.

Five to 9 minutes after a hot flush begins, the core temperature declines 0.1 to 0.9°C due to heat loss from perspiration and increased peripheral vasodilation (Molnar, 1981). If heat loss and sweating are significant, a woman may experience chills. Skin temperature gradually returns to normal, sometimes taking 30 minutes or longer.

Pathophysiology of Vasomotor Symptoms

The underlying physiologic steps leading to hot flushes remain an enigma, and some dysfunction of the thermoregulatory nucleus of the hypothalamus is likely. This nucleus regulates perspiration and vasodilatation, which is the primary mechanism of heat loss in humans. If exposed to higher temperatures, the nucleus activates these heat dissipation mechanisms. This maintains core body temperature in a regulated normal range, called the *thermoregulatory zone*. It is hypothesized that women who experience more severe vasomotor symptoms have a narrower thermoregulatory zone than those without symptoms. In these women, minimal changes in core body temperature induce shivering or hot flush.

Various hormones and neurotransmitters modulate hot flush frequency. Of these, estrogens play a vital role. Although there is no clear correlation between the two, estrogen withdrawal or rapid fluctuation in levels, rather than a chronically low estrogen concentration, is suspected (Erlik, 1982; Overlie, 2002). This hypothesis is supported by the fact that women with gonadal dysgenesis (Turner syndrome), who lack normal estrogen levels, do not experience hot flushes unless first exposed to estrogen and then withdrawn from treatment.

In addition to estrogen, Freedman and colleagues (1998, 2014) hypothesized that altered neurotransmitter concentrations may create a narrow thermoregulatory zone and a lowered sweating threshold. Norepinephrine is thought to be the primary neurotransmitter responsible for lowering the thermoregulatory setpoint and triggering the heat loss mechanisms associated with hot flushes (Rapkin, 2007). Plasma levels of norepinephrine metabolites are increased before and during hot flushes. Moreover, research shows that norepinephrine injections can increase core body temperature and induce a heat loss response (Freedman, 1990). Conversely, medications that decrease norepinephrine levels, such as clonidine, may reduce vasomotor symptoms (Laufer, 1982).

Estrogens are known to modulate adrenergic receptors in many tissues. Freedman and colleagues (2001) suggested that menopause-related declines in estrogen levels lower hypothalamic α_2-adrenergic receptor concentrations. In turn, a decline in presynaptic α_2-adrenergic receptor levels leads to increased norepinephrine levels, thereby causing vasomotor symptoms.

Serotonin is likely another involved neurotransmitter (Slopien, 2003). Estrogen withdrawal is associated with a decreased blood serotonin level, which is followed by upregulation of serotonin receptors in the hypothalamus. Activation of specific serotonin receptors has been shown to mediate heat loss (Gonzales, 1993). However, the role of serotonin in central regulatory pathways is complex because binding at some serotonin receptors can exert negative feedback on other serotonin receptor types (Bachmann, 2005). Therefore, the effect of a change in serotonin activity depends on the type of receptor activated. Of other potential candidates, β-endorphins and other neurotransmitters affect the thermoregulatory center and make some women more prone to hot flashes (Pinkerton, 2009).

Genetic polymorphisms and vasomotor symptom prevalence and severity may also be linked. Some polymorphisms are variants of genes encoding estrogen receptor alpha (Crandall, 2006; Malacara, 2004). Others are single nucleotide polymorphisms involved in the synthesis or metabolism of estradiol or in its conversion to more- or less-potent estrogens. Currently, it is unknown whether these genetic determinants exert their effects centrally or peripherally (Al-Safi, 2014).

In sum, studies suggest that reductions and significant fluctuations in estradiol levels lead to a decline in inhibitory presynaptic α_2-adrenergic receptor concentrations and an increase in hypothalamic norepinephrine and serotonin release. Norepinephrine and serotonin lower the setpoint in the thermoregulatory nucleus and allows heat loss mechanisms to be triggered by subtle changes in core body temperature. This current theory of hot flush pathogenesis underlies many of the treatment options discussed in Chapter 22 (p. 495).

Risk Factors for Vasomotor Symptoms

Several risk factors have been associated with an increased probability of hot flushes, including early menopause, surgical menopause, race/ethnicity, BMI, a sedentary lifestyle, smoking, and use of selective estrogen-receptor modulators (SERMs). Moreover, women exposed to high ambient temperatures may experience more frequent and severe hot flushes (Randolph, 2005). Of risks, surgical menopause is associated with a 90-percent probability of hot flushes during the first year after oophorectomy, and symptoms can be more abrupt and severe than those associated with natural menopause. Among racial and ethnic groups, hot flushes appear to be more common and more bothersome in African-American than in white women and are more common among white than among Asian women (Gold, 2001; Kuh, 1997; Thurston, 2008). These racial/ethnic differences in vasomotor symptoms persisted even after controlling for key factors such as BMI, estradiol level, hormone use, smoking, education level, and economic hardship (Al-Safi, 2014). The effect of BMI on hot flush frequency is not clear (Da Fonseca, 2013; Hunter, 2012; Wilbur, 1998).

■ Bone Structure and Metabolism

The skeleton consists of two bone types (Fig. 21-5). Cortical bone is the bone of the peripheral skeleton (arms and legs), and trabecular bone is the bone of the axial skeleton, which includes the vertebrae, pelvis, and proximal femur. Peak bone mass is influenced by genetic and endocrine factors, and opportunity in the younger years for acquiring bone mass is brief (American College of Obstetricians and Gynecologists, 2012). Almost all bone mass in the axial skeleton will be accumulated in young women by late adolescence, so the years immediately following menarche are especially important (Sabatier, 1996; Theintz, 1992). Calcium supplementation in prepubertal and pubertal girls improves bone accrual (Bonjour, 2001; Stear, 2003). Accordingly, osteoporosis prevention with weight-bearing exercise and vitamin D and calcium intake ideally begins in adolescence (Recker, 1992). Following adolescence, bone resorption is normally coupled to bone formation such that positive bone balance is achieved when skeletal maturity is attained, typically at age 25 to 35 years. Thereafter, bone mass declines at a slow, steady rate of approximately 0.4 percent each year. During menopause, the rate increases to 2 to 5 percent per year for the first 5 to 10 years and then slows to 1 percent per year. The

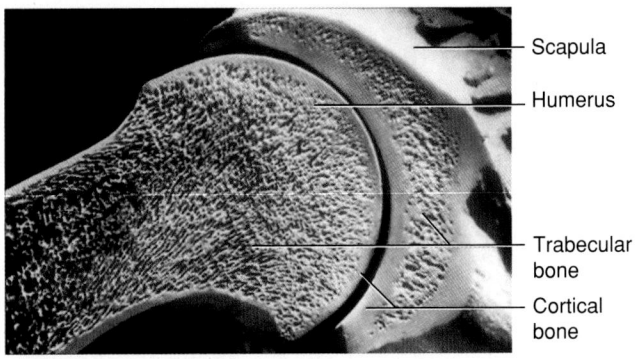

FIGURE 21-5 Photograph of bone with trabecular and cortical bone labeled. (Reproduced with permission from Saladin KS: Anatomy & Physiology, 3rd edition. New York: McGraw-Hill; 2005.)

subsequent risk of fracture from osteoporosis will depend on bone mass at the time of menopause and the rate of bone loss following menopause (Riis, 1996).

Normal bone is a dynamic, living tissue that is in a continuous process of destruction and rebuilding. This bone remodeling, also described as bone turnover, allows adaptation to mechanical changes in weight bearing and other physical activities. The process of bone remodeling involves a constant resorption of bone, carried out by multinucleated giant cells known as *osteoclasts*, and a concurrent process of bone formation, completed by *osteoblasts* (Fig. 21-6).

Activated osteoclasts secrete hydrochloric acid and collagen-degrading enzymes onto the bone surface, resulting in bone mineral dissolution and degradation of the organic matrix. After detaching from the organic matrix, the osteoclasts can relocate and begin resorption at another site on the bone surface or undergo apoptosis. Increased osteoclast activity in postmenopausal osteoporosis is mediated by the receptor activator of nuclear factor (RANK) ligand pathway. In this pathway, RANK, RANK ligand, and osteoprotegerin (OPG) are three major components (Table 21-2).

Of these, RANK ligand is expressed by osteoblasts (Bar-Shavit, 2007). This ligand binds to the RANK receptor on osteoclasts and osteoclast precursors. Binding promotes osteoclast formation, function, and survival. RANK ligand is the common

TABLE 21-2. Key Components of the RANKL/RANK/OPG Pathway

RANK ligand (RANKL)
Protein expressed by osteoblasts/bone lining cells
Binds to RANK on osteoclasts
Activation of RANK promotes osteoclast formation, function, survival

RANK
Expressed by osteoclasts and their precursor
Activated by RANKL binding

Osteoprotegerin (OPG)
Protein secreted by osteoblasts/bone lining cells
Natural inhibitor of RANKL
Blocks RANKL-mediated activation of RANK to balance bone remodeling

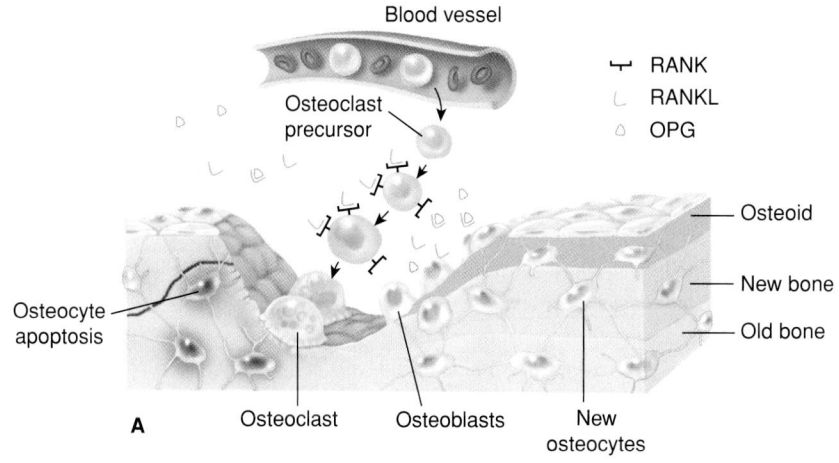

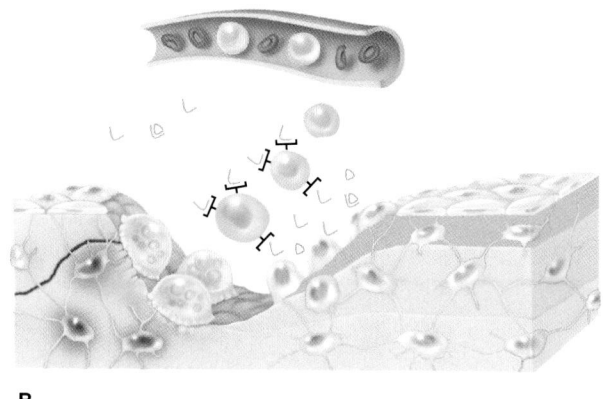

FIGURE 21-6 Bone remodeling. **A.** Osteoclasts resorb matrix, whereas osteoblasts deposit new lamellar bone. Osteoblasts that are trapped in the matrix become osteocytes. Others undergo apoptosis or form new, flattened osteoblast lining cells. Osteoblasts produce the proteins RANKL and OPG. When RANKL binds to RANK, the receptor on the surface of osteoclast progenitor cells, this promotes those cells' development, activity, and survival as osteoclasts. This leads to bone resorption. OPG serves as a counterbalance. OPG binds to RANKL and thereby, RANKL is incapable of binding with RANK to promote osteoclast development. Through this mechanism, bone resorption is limited. **B.** With hypoestrogenism, RANKL production is increased. Excessive levels of RANKL outnumber those of OPG and osteoclast development and bone resorption is favored.

is followed by the appearance of osteoblasts resulting in bone formation. In sum, resorption and formation are balanced in premenopausal women.

In postmenopausal women, decreased estrogen levels lead to increased RANK ligand expression, which may overwhelm the natural activity of OPG. Studies show that estrogen may indirectly inhibit RANK ligand expression and stimulate OPG expression. Thus, the reduction in estrogen levels associated with menopause may lead to increased RANK ligand and decreased OPG. Bone resorption follows, but osteoblasts can only partially fill resorption cavities. This results in a chronic imbalance of formation and resorption, which leads to ongoing bone loss over time. Thus, increased RANK ligand after menopause leads to excessive bone resorption and potentially postmenopausal osteoporosis (Sambrook, 2006).

■ Osteopenia and Osteoporosis
Clinical Importance

Osteoporosis is a skeletal disorder that progressively reduces bone mass and strength (typically in trabecular bone) and leads to increased fracture risks. Changes to the microstructure of bone in women with postmenopausal osteoporosis include increased cortical porosity, decreased bone mass, disrupted trabecular architecture, reduced cortical thickness, and lower mineral content of bone. Osteopenia is a precursor to osteoporosis, and the National Osteoporosis Foundation (2014) estimates that more than 10 million Americans currently have osteoporosis and another 33.6 million have osteopenia of the femoral neck.

Fracture is a frequent consequence of osteoporosis. The vertebrae, femoral neck, and wrists are most commonly fractured, and epidemiologic studies estimate that the remaining lifetime risk of common fragility fractures in white women after age 50 approximates 15 percent at each of these sites (Holroyd, 2008; Kanis, 1994). Nearly 1.5 million Americans experience osteoporotic fractures each year. Worldwide, 9 million osteoporotic fractures are estimated per year (Johnell, 2006; Lund, 2008). Fractures are associated with significant morbidity and mortality, and the risk of dying following a clinical fracture is reportedly twofold higher than for persons without fractures. The overall mortality rate from femoral neck fracture alone approximates 30 percent. In addition, only 40 percent of those who sustain a femoral neck fracture are capable of returning to their prefracture level of independence. As such, clinicians ideally educate patients regarding bone loss prevention, screen to identify bone loss early, and work with patients to implement effective management plans for osteoporosis or osteopenia.

regulator of osteoclast activity and ultimately of bone resorption. OPG is also secreted by osteoblasts and is a natural inhibitor of RANK ligand. OPG blocks RANK ligand-mediated activation of RANK and thereby limits osteoclast resorption activity. This balances bone remodeling (Kostenuik, 2005). Many different factors can affect osteoclast activity, but RANK ligand is required to mediate their effects on bone resorption. Cytokines and certain hormones stimulate the expression of RANK ligand by osteoblasts and other cells. One negative regulator of this process is estrogen, which limits the expression of RANK ligand from osteoblasts. Another regulator is OPG, a natural inhibitor of RANK ligand that sequesters and neutralizes the effects of RANK ligand.

In healthy premenopausal women, estrogen limits osteoblast expression of RANK ligand. The OPG binds to RANK ligand to further limit its availability to stimulate osteoclasts. The remaining RANK ligand binds to osteoclast precursors, which fuse and form differentiated osteoclasts for bone resorption. This

Pathophysiology

A major proportion of bone strength is determined by bone mineral density (BMD), which is grams of mineral per area and volume of bone. However, bone quality, bone strength, and fracture risk are also affected by bone remodeling rates, bone size and geometry, microarchitecture, mineralization, damage accumulation, and matrix quality. Unfortunately, all of these are more difficult to accurately assess (Kiebzak, 2003).

Primary osteoporosis refers to bone loss associated with aging and menopausal estrogen deficiency. As estrogen levels fall after menopause, its regulatory effect on bone resorption is lost. As a result, bone resorption is accelerated and is usually not balanced by compensatory bone formation. This accelerated bone loss is most rapid in the early postmenopausal years (Gallagher, 2002). If osteoporosis is caused by other diseases or medications, the term *secondary osteoporosis* is used (Stein, 2003).

The amount of bone at any point in time reflects the balance of the osteoblastic (building) and osteoclastic (resorbing) activities, which are influenced by numerous stimulating and inhibiting agents (Canalis, 2007). As noted earlier, both aging and a loss of estrogen lead to a significant increase in osteoclastic activity. Also, decreased dietary calcium intake or impaired calcium absorption from the gut lowers the serum level of ionized calcium. This stimulates parathyroid hormone (PTH) secretion to mobilize calcium from bone by stimulation of osteoclastic activity (Fig. 21-7). Increased PTH levels stimulate vitamin D production. In turn, elevated vitamin D concentrations raise serum calcium levels by several effects: (1) stimulates osteoclasts to remove calcium from bone, (2) increases intestinal calcium absorption, (3) stimulates renal calcium reabsorption, and lowers PTH production by the parathyroid glands (Molina, 2013).

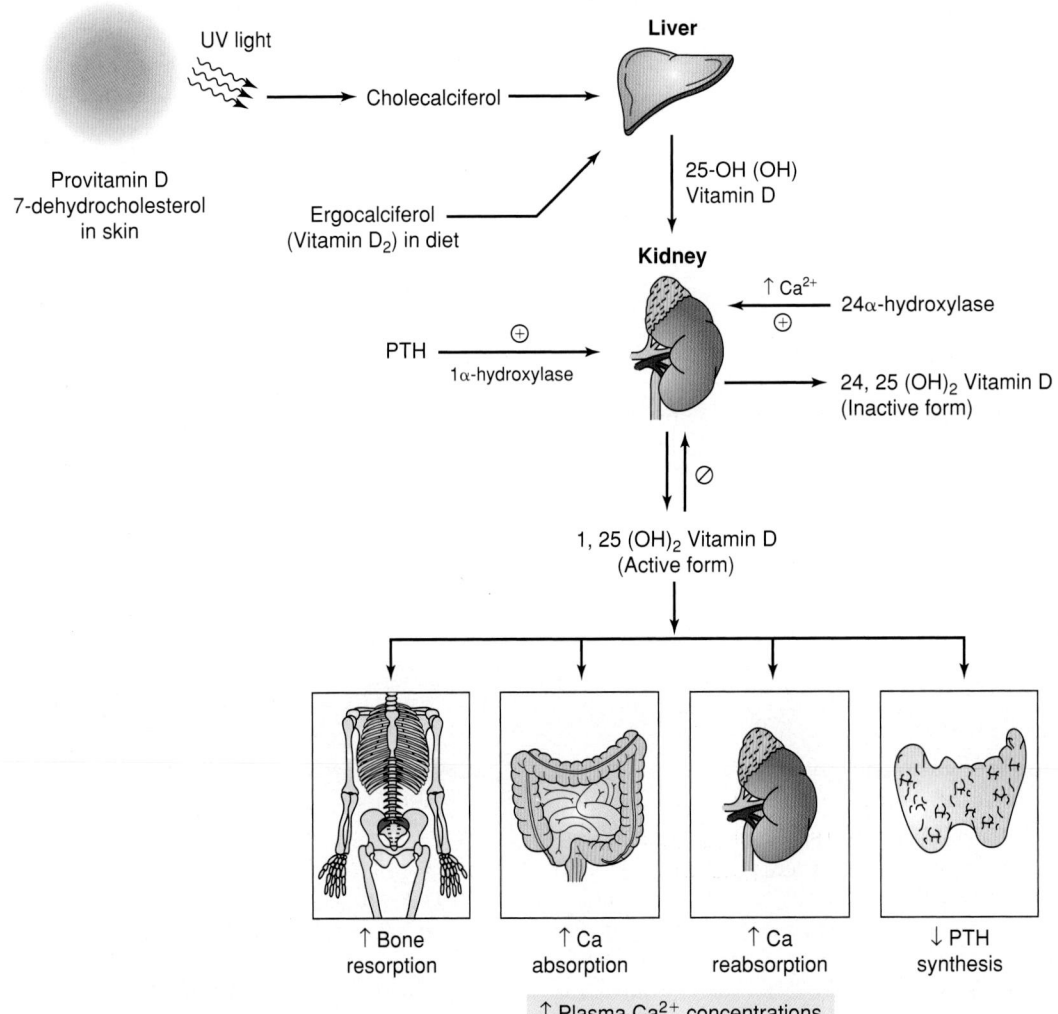

FIGURE 21-7 Vitamin D metabolism. Provitamin D (7-dehydrocholesterol) in the skin is converted to cholecalciferol by ultraviolet (UV) light. Cholecalciferol and ergocalciferol (from plants) are transported to the liver, where they undergo hydroxylation to form the major circulating form of vitamin D. A second hydroxylation step occurs in the kidney and results in the hormonally active vitamin D [1,25(OH)$_2$D$_3$], also known as calcitriol. This activation step is mediated by 1α-hydroxylase and is regulated by parathyroid hormone (PTH), Ca^{2+} levels, and vitamin D [1,25(OH)$_2$D$_3$]. The activity of 1α-hydroxylase is stimulated by PTH and inhibited by sufficient levels of Ca^{2+} and 1,25(OH)$_2$D$_3$. Vitamin D increases bone resorption, Ca^{2+} absorption from the intestine, and renal Ca^{2+} reabsorption, but it decreases PTH production by the parathyroid glands. The overall effect of vitamin D is to increase plasma Ca^{2+} concentrations. This rise in plasma Ca^{2+} levels inhibits 1α-hydroxylase and favors hydroxylation at C-24. This leads to synthesis of an inactive vitamin D metabolite—24,25(OH)$_2$D$_3$. (Reproduced with permission from Molina PE: Endocrine Physiology, 4th ed. New York: McGraw-Hill; 2013.)

In normal premenopausal women, this series of events leads to increased serum calcium levels, and PTH levels return to normal. In menopausal women, estrogen deficiency creates a greater responsiveness of bone to PTH. Thus, for any given PTH level, relatively more calcium is removed from bone.

Diagnosis

BMD is the standard used for bone mass determination and is assessed with dual-energy x-ray absorptiometry (DEXA) of the lumbar vertebrae, radius, and femoral neck (Fig. 21-8) (Marshall, 1996). The lumbar vertebrae contain primarily trabecular bone, and this bone type forms 20 percent of the skeleton. Trabecular bone is less dense than cortical bone and has a faster bone remodeling rate. Therefore, early rapid bone loss can be determined by evaluation of this site. Cortical bone is denser and more compact bone and makes up 80 percent of the skeleton. It is most abundant in the long-bone shafts of the appendicular skeleton. The greater trochanter and femoral neck contain both cortical and trabecular bone, and these sites are ideal for the prediction of femoral neck fracture risk in older women (Miller, 2002).

Normative bone mineral density values for sex, age, and ethnicity have been determined. For diagnostic purposes, results of BMD testing are reported as *T-scores.* These measure in standard deviations (SDs) the variance of an individual's BMD from that expected for a person of the same sex at peak bone mass (25 to 30 years). A T-score of –2.0 in a woman, for example, means that her BMD is two SDs below the average peak bone mass for a young woman. Definitions include those found in Table 21-3. The fourth category, "severe osteoporosis," describes patients who have a T-score below –2.5 and who have also suffered a fragility fracture. These are fractures caused by a fall from standing height or lower.

Patients are also assigned a *Z-score,* which is the standard deviation between the patient's measurement and average bone mass for a patient with the same age and weight. Z-scores lower than –2.0 (2.5 percent of the normal population of the same age) require diagnostic evaluation for *secondary osteoporosis* (Faulkner, 1999). Similarly, any patient with osteoporosis is screened for other conditions that lead to osteoporosis (Table 21-4).

The relation between BMD and fracture risk has been calculated in numerous studies. A metaanalysis by Marshall and coworkers (1996) showed that BMD is still the most readily quantifiable predictor of fracture risk for those who have not yet suffered a fragility fracture. For each standard deviation of BMD below a baseline level (either mean peak bone mass or mean for the reference population of the person's age and sex), the fracture risk approximately doubles (National Osteoporosis Foundation, 2002).

Recognizing the difficulty in measuring bone mass and bone quality accurately, the World Health Organization (WHO) developed the Fracture Risk Assessment Tool (FRAX) to assess an individual's 10-year fracture risk. The algorithm, however, is applicable only for patients who have not received pharmacotherapy. The FRAX tool is accessible online and is available for multiple countries and in different languages (http://www.shef.ac.uk/FRAX/). The online tool incorporates 11 risk factors and the femoral neck raw BMD value in g/cm^2 to calculate the 10-year fracture risk. The site also offers downloadable charts for calculating fracture risks using BMI or BMD. The FRAX algorithm identifies patients who might benefit from pharmacotherapy and is most useful for recognizing those with BMD in the osteopenic category.

Prevention

As predictors of osteoporotic fracture, the most important factors are BMD in combination with age, fracture history, ethnicity, various drug treatments, weight loss, and physical fitness. The presence of a key risk factor alerts a clinician to the need for further assessment and possibly active intervention, such as calcium and vitamin D therapy coupled with weight-bearing exercise or pharmacologic therapy (Tables 21-5 and 21-6). Treatment options for osteoporosis are discussed in Chapter 22 (p. 499).

TABLE 21-3. WHO Criteria for Bone Disease Based on Bone Mineral Density (BMD)

Normal BMD : T-score between +2.5 and −1.0
Osteopenia: T-score between −1.0 and −2.5
Osteoporosis : T-score at or below −2.5
Severe or established osteoporosis: T-score at or below −2.5 with one or more fractures

Data from National Osteoporosis Foundation: Clinician's guide to prevention and treatment of osteoporosis. Washington, National Osteoporosis Foundation, 2014.

TABLE 21-4. Secondary Causes of Osteoporosis and Recommended Testing

Primary hyperparathyroidism	Serum levels of: parathyroid hormone calcium phosphorus alkaline phosphatase
Secondary hyperparathyroidism from chronic renal failure	Renal function tests
Hyperthyroidism or excess thyroid hormone treatment	Thyroid function tests
Increased calcium excretion	24-hour urine collection for calcium and creatinine concentrations
Hypercortisolism, alcohol abuse, and metastatic cancer	Careful history and when indicated appropriate laboratory studies
Osteomalacia	Serum levels of: calcium phosphorus alkaline phosphatase 1,25-dihydroxyvitamin D

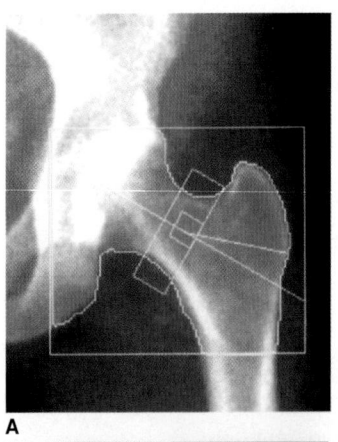

A

DXA Results Summary:

Region	Area (cm²)	BMC (g)	BMD (g/cm²)	T - Score	Z - Score
Neck	4.59	3.79	0.827	−0.2	1.0
Troch	8.57	6.65	0.775	0.7	1.5
Inter	14.62	17.48	1.196	0.6	1.2
Total	**27.79**	**27.92**	**1.005**	**0.5**	**1.3**
Ward's	1.12	0.71	0.639	−0.8	1.0

Total BMD CV 1.0%, ACF = 1.028, BCF = 0.998, TH = 6.508
WHO Classification: Normal
Fracture Risk: Not Increased

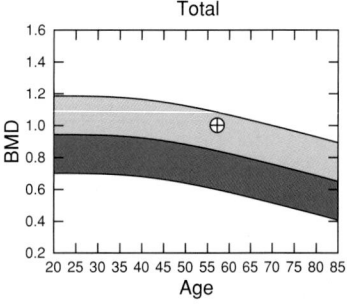

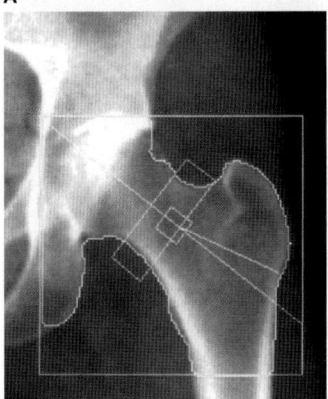

B

DXA Results Summary:

Region	Area (cm²)	BMC (g)	BMD (g/cm²)	T - Score	Z - Score
Neck	4.97	2.74	0.552	−2.7	−1.4
Troch	11.53	5.62	0.487	−2.1	−1.3
Inter	18.92	14.78	0.781	−2.1	−1.4
Total	**35.43**	**23.14**	**0.653**	**−2.4**	**−1.4**
Ward's	1.16	0.38	0.331	−3.4	−1.5

Total BMD CV 1.0%
WHO Classification: Osteopenia
Fracture Risk: Increased

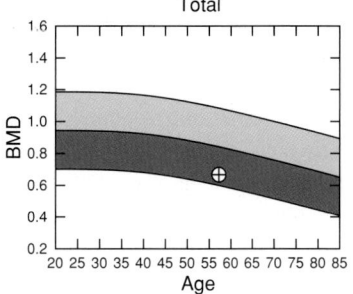

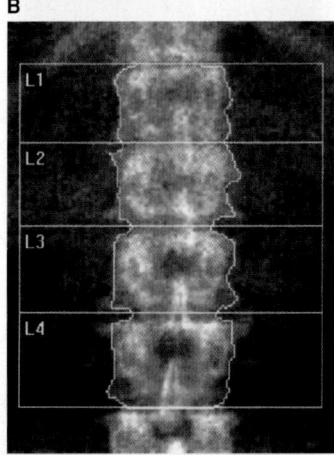

C

DXA Results Summary:

Region	Area (cm²)	BMC (g)	BMD (g/cm²)	T - Score	Z - Score
L1	12.00	12.73	1.061	1.2	2.3
L2	13.37	14.93	1.116	0.8	2.0
L3	14.03	16.56	1.181	0.9	2.1
L4	15.80	20.23	1.280	1.5	2.8
Total	**55.20**	**64.45**	**1.168**	**1.1**	**2.3**

Total BMD CV 1.0%
WHO Classification: Normal
Fracture Risk: Not Increased

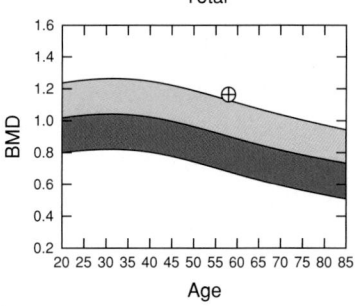

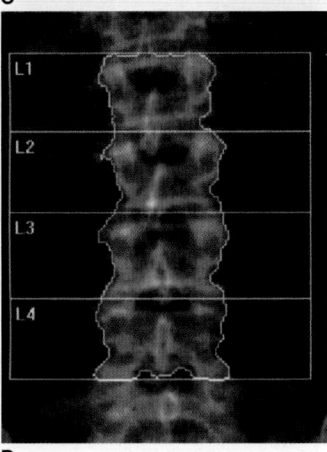

D

DXA Results Summary:

Region	Area (cm²)	BMC (g)	BMD (g/cm²)	T - Score	Z - Score
L1	11.73	8.03	0.684	−2.2	−1.0
L2	12.60	9.70	0.770	−2.3	−1.0
L3	14.59	11.70	0.802	−2.6	−1.1
L4	14.44	11.01	0.763	−3.2	−1.7
Total	**53.36**	**40.44**	**0.758**	**−2.6**	**−1.2**

Total BMD CV 1.0%, ACF = 1.028, BCF = 0.998, TH = 5.974
WHO Classification: Osteoporosis
Fracture Risk: High

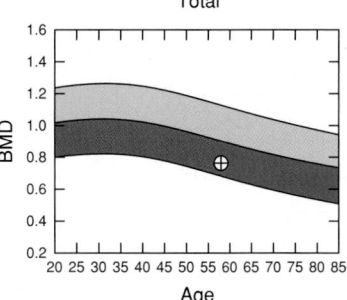

FIGURE 21-8 Dual-energy x-ray absorptiometry (DEXA) scans. **A.** DEXA report describing normal hip density. **B.** DEXA report describing osteopenia of the hip. **C.** DEXA report describing normal vertebral body density. **D.** DEXA report describing vertebral body osteoporosis. BMC = bone mineral content; BMD = bone mineral density.

TABLE 21-5. Osteoporosis Risk Factors

Major Risk Factors	Minor Risk Factors
Age >65 years	Rheumatoid arthritis
Vertebral compression fracture	History of clinical hyperthyroidism
Fragility fracture after age 40	Chronic anticonvulsant therapy
Family history of osteoporotic fracture	Low dietary calcium intake
Systemic glucocorticoid therapy for >3 months	Smoker
Malabsorption syndrome	Excessive alcohol intake
Primary hyperparathyroidism	Excessive caffeine intake
Propensity to fall	Weight <57 kg
Osteopenia apparent on radiography	>10 percent weight loss at age 25
Hypogonadism	Chronic heparin therapy
Early menopause (before age 45)	

Risk factors for osteoporotic fracture are not independent of one another. They are additive and are considered in the context of baseline age and sex-related fracture risk. For example, a 55-year-old woman with low BMD is at significantly less risk than a 75-year-old woman with the same low BMD. Similarly, a woman with low BMD and a prior fragility fracture is at considerably greater risk than another person with the same low BMD and no prior fracture.

Nonmodifiable Factors. Age is one major contributor to fracture risk. As summarized by Kanis and associates (2001), the 10-year probability of experiencing a fracture of forearm, humerus, vertebra, or femoral neck increases as much as eightfold between ages 45 and 85 years for women. Osteoporotic fractures occur most commonly in men and women older than 65 years. Medical interventions have been demonstrated to be effective only in preventing fractures in populations with an average age older than 65 years. However, most currently approved osteoporosis therapies prevent or reverse bone loss if initiated at, or soon after, age 50. Therefore, it seems prudent to begin the identification of people at high risk for osteoporosis in their 50s. As noted, BMD is currently the best quantifiable predictor of osteoporotic fracture, and screening guidelines are discussed on page 482.

As noted, a prior fragility fracture places a person at increased risk for another fracture. The increased risk is 1.5- to 9.5-fold depending on age at assessment, number of prior fractures, and site of prior fracture (Melton, 1999). Vertebral fractures are the best studied, and a vertebral fracture increases the risk of a second such fracture at least fourfold. The placebo group of a major clinical trial showed that 20 percent of those who experienced a vertebral fracture during the study period had a second vertebral fracture within 1 year (Lindsay, 2001). Vertebral fractures also indicate vulnerability at other sites, such as the femoral neck. Similarly, wrist fractures predict vertebral and femoral neck fractures.

Another nonmodifiable risk factor is race, and osteoporosis is most common in menopausal white women. In 2002, the National Osteoporosis Foundation found that 20 percent of these women have osteoporosis, and 52 percent have low BMD. Although persons of any ethnicity can develop osteoporosis, data from the Third National Health and Nutrition Examination Survey (NHANES III) show that the risk is highest among non-Hispanic white and Asian women and lowest among non-Hispanic black women. Racial and ethnic differences are important in counseling and management because fracture rates do not always correlate with BMD across ethnic groups. For example, Chinese American women typically have lower BMD than white American women, but lower rates of femoral neck and forearm fracture (Walker, 2011). It is postulated that greater cortical density and thicker trabeculae compensate for fewer trabeculae in smaller bones. Thus, both BMD and microarchitecture appear to play distinct roles in fracture vulnerability (American College of Obstetricians and Gynecologists, 2012).

TABLE 21-6. General Guidelines for Prevention of Osteoporosis in Postmenopausal Women

Counsel on osteoporosis risks
Check for secondary causes (see Table 21-4)
For women 51 and older, encourage diet containing calcium 1200 mg daily and vitamin D 800–1000 IU daily. Add supplement if diet is incomplete
Recommend regular weight-bearing and muscle-strengthening exercise
Advise against tobacco smoking and excess alcohol intake
Assess for fall risks (see Table 21-7) and modify as possible
Measure height annually
In women ≥65 years, recommend BMD testing
In postmenopausal women aged 50–65 years, recommend BMD testing based on the risk factor profile (see Table 21-5)
In those >50 with a new fracture, recommend BMD testing to determine degree of disease severity
For patients on pharmacotherapy, perform BMD testing 2 years after initiating therapy and every 2 years thereafter. However, testing frequency may be tailored to clinical situations

BMD = bone mineral density.
Data from National Osteoporosis Foundation: Clinician's guide to prevention and treatment of osteoporosis. Washington, National Osteoporosis Foundation, 2014.

Genetic influence on osteoporosis and BMD is important, and heredity is estimated to account for 50 to 80 percent of BMD variability (Ralston, 2002). The Study of Osteoporotic Fractures, for example, identified that maternal femoral neck fracture was a predictor for femoral neck fracture in a population of elderly women (Cummings, 1995). An affected maternal grandmother also raises a woman's fracture risk. Several genes have been associated with osteoporosis, but these discoveries have yet to translate into clinical application.

Modifiable Factors. Of these, exercise, in the form of progressive resistance training, may result in clinically relevant benefits to femoral neck BMD and lumbar vertebral BMD in postmenopausal women (Kelly, 2012). Greater improvements in bone mass were also associated with increases in static balance. These associations may be particularly important for reducing fall risks. Exercise results in other general health benefits that are not totally realized with pharmacological and nutritional interventions. For example, investigators note that greater increases in femoral neck BMD and lumbar vertebral BMD are also associated with declines in BMI and percent body fat (Bouchard, 2013).

Fractures are frequently associated with falls. Thus, a history of falls or factors that increase fall rates are included in a risk assessment (Table 21-7). Factors include those associated with general frailty, such as reduced muscle strength, impaired balance, low body mass, and diminished visual acuity (Delaney, 2006). Alcohol and sedative drug use are other important risks.

Therapy with glucocorticoids lasting more than 2 to 3 months is a major risk factor for bone loss and fracture, particularly among postmenopausal women. The National Osteoporosis Foundation guidelines (2014) describe a chronic daily dose of prednisone that is ≥5 mg as the threshold for assessment and clinical intervention to prevent or treat glucocorticoid-induced osteoporosis.

Osteoporosis Screening. After assessment of all potential risk factors, BMD measurement is a prominent component of strategies to confirm osteoporosis and determine disease sever-

ity. BMD testing is recommended for all menopausal women who: (1) are aged 65 years or older, (2) have one or more risk factors for osteoporosis, or (3) sustain fractures (see Table 21-5). Additionally, screening is considered for perimenopausal women if they have a specific risk factor such as prior low-trauma fracture, have a low BMI, or are taking a medication known to accelerate bone loss. Many vertebral fractures are asymptomatic, and vertebral imaging is recommended for women aged ≥70 years with a T-score ≤ −1.0 or those 65 to 69 years with a score ≤ −1.5 (National Osteoporosis Foundation, 2014). Unfortunately, Schnatz and associates (2011) found that many women are not properly screened or treated for osteoporosis and that inappropriate screening may also lead to improper management of osteoporosis and its associated complications. If therapy to increase BMD is instituted, BMD should be monitored.

Less commonly, bone markers of resorption and formation are used as an adjunct to BMD. These can be used to assess osteoporosis risk or to monitor treatment. During remodeling, osteoblasts synthesize several cytokines, peptides, and growth factors that are released into the circulation. Their concentrations thus reflect the rate of bone formation. Serum bone formation markers include osteocalcin, bone-specific alkaline phosphatase, and procollagen I carboxy-terminal propeptide (PICP). Osteoclasts produce bone degradation products that are also released into the circulation and are eventually cleared via the kidney. Main bone resorption markers include urinary deoxypyridinoline (u-DPD), urinary collagen type I cross-linked N telopeptide (u-NTX) and serum collagen type I cross-linked C telopeptide (s-CTX).

These markers of bone formation and resorption can estimate bone-remodeling rates and may help identify fast bone losers. As evaluated by these markers, bone remodeling rates increase at menopause and remain elevated and correlate negatively with BMD.

That said, most prospective studies analyzing the relationship between bone remodeling and rates of bone loss have been short-term and have been limited by the precision error of densitometry. Garnero and colleagues (1994) prospectively evaluated over 4 years the utility of bone markers to identify fast bone losers in a large cohort of healthy menopausal women. They found that higher levels of bone formation and resorption markers were significantly associated with faster and possibly greater BMD loss.

Markers of bone resorption may also be useful predictors of fracture risk and bone loss. Elevation of these markers may be associated with an increased fracture risk in elderly women, although data are not uniform. The association of markers of bone resorption with femoral neck fracture risk is independent of BMD, but a low BMD combined with high bone resorption biomarker doubles the risk associated with either of these factors alone. However, biomarker measurements are currently limited by their high variability within individuals. Additional studies with fracture endpoints are needed to confirm the usefulness of these markers in individual patients.

Biomarkers may also have value in predicting and monitoring response to potent antiresorptive therapy in clinical trials. Normalization of bone formation and resorption marker levels following therapy has been observed in prospective trials.

TABLE 21-7. Fall Risk Factors

Physiologic changes	Environmental
Prior falls	Poor lighting
Diminished balance	Unsafe footwear
Reduced muscle mass	Telephone cords
Comorbid conditions	Cluttered hallways
Arthritis	Loose rugs
Arrhythmia	Slippery/damaged flooring
Alcohol abuse	No bathroom support bars
Gait disorders	**Medications**
Balance disorders	Narcotics
Visual impairment	Anticonvulsants
Cognitive impairment	Antiarrhythmic agents
Orthostatic hypotension	Psychiatric medications
	Antihypertensive agents

Reduction in biochemical marker levels appears in some studies to be correlated with a decrease in vertebral fracture incidence but is not necessarily always predictive of response to therapies. Bone remodeling markers are not yet used for routine clinical management. Additional studies are needed to confirm their use in individual patients. However, with refinement of assay technology and better understanding of biological variability, it is likely that they will become a useful adjunct in the future for risk assessment and management.

Cardiovascular Changes

In women older than 50 years, atherosclerotic cardiovascular disease (CVD) remains the leading cause of death. CVD accounts for approximately 40 percent of deaths in women compared with about 5 percent due to breast cancer. Before menopause, women have a much lower risk for cardiovascular events compared with men their same age. Reasons for protection from CVD in premenopausal women are complex, but a significant contribution is assigned to greater high-density lipoprotein (HDL) levels in younger women, which is an effect of estrogen. However, after menopause, this benefit disappears over time such that a 70-year-old woman begins to have a CVD risk identical to that of a male of comparable age (Matthews, 1989). The risk of CVD increases exponentially for women as they enter menopause and as estrogen levels decline (Matthews, 1994; van Beresteijn, 1993). This becomes vitally important for women in MT, when preventive measures can significantly improve both life quality and quantity.

The relationship between menopause and CVD incidence was first examined in the Framingham cohort of 2873 women (Kannel, 1987). A trend showed a two- to sixfold higher incidence of CVD in postmenopausal women compared with premenopausal women in the same age range. Moreover, the increases in CVD associated with the MT are observed regardless of the age at menopause. These and other data indicate that withdrawal of estrogen may be associated with an increased CVD risk. Nonetheless, questions of whether estrogen deficiency accelerates development of CVD and whether menopausal hormone treatment can ameliorate CVD risk remain unanswered (Harman, 2014).

Cardiovascular Disease Prevention

CVD risk factors are the same for men and women and include nonmodifiable risk factors such as age and family history of CVD. Modifiable elements are hypertension, dyslipidemia, obesity, diabetes/glucose intolerance, smoking, poor diet, and lack of physical activity. Because most CVD risk factors are modifiable, significant reductions in cardiovascular morbidity and mortality rates are feasible. Since data question the widespread use of hormone treatment to avert this common problem, other strategies must be considered (Chap. 22, p. 492). Modifying strategies are discussed fully in Chapter 1 (p. 14), and some are briefly summarized here.

Of these, physical activity and its cardiovascular benefits were studied in the Women's Health Initiative (WHI). Manson and colleagues (2002) determined that walking or vigorous exercise reduced the risk of cardiovascular events in postmenopausal women regardless of their age, BMI, or ethnic background. As expected, a sedentary lifestyle correlated directly with an elevated risk for coronary events (McKechnie, 2001).

As another CVD risk factor, central fat distribution, also termed truncal obesity, in women correlates positively with increases in total cholesterol, triglyceride, and low-density lipoprotein (LDL) cholesterol levels, and negatively correlates with HDL levels (Haarbo, 1989). This atherogenic lipid profile associated with abdominal adiposity is at least partly mediated through interplay with insulin and estrogen. A strong correlation exists between the magnitude of the worsening in cardiovascular risk factors (lipid and lipoprotein changes, blood pressure, and insulin levels) and the amount of weight gained during MT (Wing, 1991).

Favorable lipoprotein profiles in young women are maintained in part by physiologic estrogen levels. Specifically, throughout adulthood HDL levels are approximately 10 mg/dL higher in women. Moreover, total cholesterol and LDL levels are lower in premenopausal women than in men (Jensen, 1990; Matthews, 1989). After menopause and with the subsequent declines in estrogen levels, this favorable effect on lipids is lost. HDL levels decrease and total cholesterol levels increase. After menopause, the risk of coronary heart disease doubles for women, and at approximately age 60, the atherogenic lipids reach levels higher than those in men. Despite these changes in atherogenic lipids following menopause, total cholesterol and LDL levels can be favorably reduced by dietary modifications, estrogen treatment, and lipid-lowering medications (Matthews, 1994).

Last, clotting parameters are known to changes with aging. Fibrinogen, plasminogen activator inhibitor-1, and factor VII levels increase and cause a relatively hypercoagulable state. This is thought to contribute to increases in CVD and cerebrovascular disease rates in older women. Aspirin is effective in the *secondary prevention* of CVD in both men and women (Antithrombotic Trialists' Collaboration, 2002). However, as discussed in Chapter 1 (p. 15), aspirin is not recommended for *primary prevention* of heart disease in women younger than 65 unless individual health benefits are judged to outweigh risks. These counterbalancing risks primarily involve aspirin-related bleeding episodes such as hemorrhagic stroke and gastrointestinal bleeding (Lund, 2008).

Weight Gain and Fat Distribution

Weight gain is a common complaint among women during MT. With aging, a woman's metabolism slows, reducing her caloric requirements. If eating and exercise habits are not altered, weight is gained (Matthews, 2001). Specifically, Espeland and associates (1997) characterized the weight and fat distribution of 875 women in the Postmenopausal Estrogen/Progestin Interventions (PEPI) trial and correlated the effects of lifestyle, clinical, and demographic factors. Women aged 45 to 54 years had significantly greater increases in weight and in hip circumference than those aged 55 to 65 years. These investigators reported that overall baseline physical activity and baseline leisure and work activities were strongly related to weight gain in the PEPI cohort. Women who reported more activity gained less weight than less active women.

Weight gain during this period is associated with fat deposition in the abdomen, increased amounts of visceral fat, and body fat redistribution (Kim, 2014). These raise the likelihood of developing insulin resistance and subsequent diabetes mellitus and heart disease (Dallman, 2004; Wing, 1991). This stems from associated alterations in cardiometabolic risks due to hormone-related declines in energy expenditure and fat oxidation (Jull, 2014). In addition, data from the Rosetta Study and the New Mexico Aging Process Study show that older adults have higher percentages of body fat than younger adults at any age due to muscle mass loss with aging (Baumgartner, 1995).

Numerous other factors underlie weight gain and include genetic factors, neuropeptides, and adrenergic nervous system activity (Milewicz, 1996). Although many women believe that noncontraceptive estrogen therapy causes weight gain, results from clinical trials and epidemiologic studies indicate that the effect of menopausal hormone therapy on body weight and girth, if any, is to blunt slightly the rate of age-related increases.

Lifestyle interventions to minimize gains in fat mass and changes in body composition and body fat distribution during MT predominantly include exercise and healthy nutrition. As discussed in Chapter 1 (p. 13), specific interventions include encouraging individuals to set realistic lifestyle goals, referral to weight loss programs, pharmacotherapy, or surgical interventions (Jull, 2014). Women exposed to a program of combined exercise and calorie-restricting dietary interventions for 54 weeks had improved body weight and reduced abdominal adiposity compared with usual activities in the control group (Simkin-Silverman, 2007). As well, significant reductions in waist circumference and body fat were maintained beyond 4 years. Hagner and coworkers (2009) found that a Nordic walking program reduced weight gain during MT.

■ Dermatologic Changes

Skin changes that may develop during MT include hyperpigmentation (age spots), wrinkles, and itching. These are caused in part by skin aging, which results from the synergistic effects of intrinsic aging and photo-aging (Guinot, 2005). Hormonal aging of the skin is also thought to be responsible for many dermal changes. These include a reduced thickness due to lower collagen content, diminished sebaceous gland secretion, loss of elasticity, and decreased blood supply (Wines, 2001). Although the effect of hormone deficiency on skin aging has been widely studied, distinguishing its contribution from those of intrinsic aging, photo-aging, and other environmental insults is difficult.

■ Dental Changes

Dental problems may also develop as estrogen levels wane in late MT. The buccal epithelium atrophies due to estrogen deprivation, resulting in decreased saliva and sensation. A bad taste in the mouth, increased incidence of cavities, and tooth loss also may occur (Krall, 1994). Oral alveolar bone loss is strongly positively correlated with osteoporosis and can lead to tooth loss. Even in women without osteoporosis, vertebral BMD correlates positively with the number of teeth. In turn,

the beneficial effect of estrogen on skeletal bone mass is also manifested in oral bone.

■ Breast Changes

The breast undergoes change during MT mainly because of hormonal withdrawal. In premenopausal women, estrogen and progesterone exert proliferative effects on ductal and glandular structures, respectively. At menopause, withdrawal of estrogen and progesterone leads to a relative reduction in breast proliferation. A significant reduction in the volume and tissue density is seen during mammography as these areas become replaced with adipose tissue. Mammography is advisable for women older than age 40, and breast imaging is fully discussed in Chapter 12 (p. 288).

■ Central Nervous System
Sleep Dysfunction and Fatigue

Sleep quality declines with age, but the menopausal transition appears to contribute to this decline in women. Women may wake several times during the night and may be drenched in sweat. The relationship between hot flushes and impaired sleep has been studied. Hollander and associates (2001) studied late reproductive-aged women and found that women with a greater incidence of hot flushes were more likely to report poor sleep than were women with fewer vasomotor symptoms. Self-reported poor sleep rates increase as women traverse MT, and it was reported in 38 percent of the 12,603 women who participated in the cross-sectional survey of the SWAN Study (Hall, 2009). As with most menopausal symptoms, severity and prevalence seem to peak during late MT, when women have prolonged amenorrhea.

Even women with few vasomotor symptoms may experience insomnia and associated menopause-related mood symptoms (Erlik, 1982; Woodward, 1994). As women age, they are more likely to experience lighter sleep and are awakened more easily by pain, sound, or bodily urges. Health issues and other chronic conditions experienced by women or by their spouse or bedmate are likely to further disrupt sleep. Arthritis, carpal tunnel syndrome, chronic lung disease, heartburn, and certain medications that are known to disrupt sleep may dramatically lower the quality and quantity of restful sleep. Nocturia, urinary frequency, and urgency, all of which are more common in menopausal women, are other notable factors.

Sleep disordered breathing (SDB), which includes various degrees of pharyngeal obstruction, is much more common in menopausal women and their mates. In women, SDB is often associated with increased BMI and declining estrogen and progesterone levels. Loud snoring can follow partial upper airway obstruction that ranges in severity from upper airway resistance to obstructive sleep apnea (Gislason, 1993).

Disturbed sleep can lead to fatigue, irritability, depressive symptoms, cognitive dysfunction, and impaired daily functioning. Commonsense education for patients during MT may prove valuable (Table 21-8). Importantly, although fatigue may stem from night sweats and poor sleep, other common potential etiologies, such as anemia or thyroid disease, among

TABLE 21-8. Fatigue Prevention Instructions

Obtain adequate sleep every night

Exercise regularly to reduce stress

Avoid long work hours and maintain your personal schedule

If stress is environmental, take vacations, switch jobs, or approach your company or family to help resolve sources of stress

Limit intake of alcohol, drugs, and nicotine

Eat a healthy, well-balanced diet

Drink adequate amounts water (8 to 10 glasses) during the early part of the day

Consider seeing a specialist in menopausal medicine

others, are also considered. In all these examples, treatment of underlying health conditions is the main focus to improve patient sleep. At times, short-term use of pharmacologic sleep aids is indicated, and these are listed in Table 1-16 (p. 18).

Cognitive Dysfunction

Memory declines with advancing age. Although no direct effect of lowered estrogen levels on memory and cognition has been determined, many investigators suspect a relationship between the two. Cognitive functioning was assessed in a cohort study of reproductive-aged and postmenopausal women not using hormone replacement therapy. In postmenopausal patients, cognitive performance declined with advancing age. This was not the case for reproductive-aged women. Premenopausal women in their 40s were less likely to exhibit cognitive decline compared with postmenopausal patients in the same decade of life. These researchers concluded that deterioration of some forms of cognitive function is accelerated after menopause (Halbreich, 1995).

In another study, Henderson and coworkers (2013) studied 643 healthy postmenopausal women not using hormone therapy who were recruited as early (<6 years after menopause) and late (>10 years after menopause) groups. Women were administered a comprehensive neuropsychological battery. Concurrently, serum free estradiol, estrone, progesterone, free testosterone, and SHBG levels were measured. Cognitive outcomes were standardized composite measures of verbal memory, executive functions, and global cognition. Endogenous sex steroid levels were unassociated with cognitive composites, but SHBG levels were positively associated with verbal memory. Results for early and late groups did not differ significantly, although progesterone concentrations were significantly positively associated with verbal memory and global cognition in early group women. Hormone levels were not significantly related to mood.

Factors accelerating cerebral degenerative changes represent potentially modifiable risks for cognitive decline (Kuller, 2003; Meyer, 1999). Investigators have studied putative risk factors and have correlated them with measures of cerebral atrophy, computed tomography (CT) densitometry, and cognitive testing among neurologically and cognitively normal, aging volunteers. Risk factors for decreased cerebral perfusion and thinning of gray and white matter densities include prior transient ischemic attacks (TIAs), hyperlipidemia, hypertension, smoking, excess alcohol consumption, and male gender, which would imply lack of estrogen. The authors encourage interventions to modify many of these risks.

Psychosocial Changes

Women have long been recognized as carrying a higher lifetime risk of developing depression than men. The World Health Organization has consistently ranked depression as a leading cause of disability in women. The risk of developing a major depressive disorder is 1.5 to 1.7 times higher in women than in men, particularly during reproductive years. A prior depressive episode (particularly if related to reproductive events) remains the strongest predictor of mood symptoms or depression during midlife. Vasomotor symptoms, anxiety, and other health-related issues also modulate depression risks (Soares, 2014).

Contemporary findings have dispelled myths that natural menopause itself is associated with depressed mood (Ballinger, 1990; Busch, 1994). However, an increased risk of depressive symptoms during MT has been repeatedly observed in population-based studies. In the Penn Ovarian Aging Study, the risk was nearly three times higher in women in MT compared with premenopausal women. Moreover, women with no history of depression were two and a half times more likely to report depressed mood during MT than during the premenopausal period (Freeman, 2004). Other cohort studies report similar findings (Bromberger, 2011; Cohen, 2006; Dennerstein, 2004; Woods, 2008). Moreover, there are a high percentage of subjects with recurrent depression during MT (Freeman, 2007). Thus, a screen for depression is prudent for women in this transition, and tools are described in Chapter 13 (p. 298).

It has been suggested that the hormonal fluctuations during early MT are responsible, in part, for this affective instability. Similarly, surgical menopause induces mood changes because of the rapid hormonal loss at this time. Soares (2005) hypothesizes that a major component of the reported emotional distress during MT may be causally related to high and erratic estradiol levels. For example, Ballinger and colleagues (1990) showed that increases in stress hormones (and probably symptoms that are stress related) are physiologically linked with high estrogen levels. They also reported that women with abnormal psychometric test scores early after menopause had higher estradiol levels than women with lower scores. Spinelli and associates (2005) showed that estrogen levels are correlated with the intensity of menopausal symptoms. A randomized, placebo-controlled menopause treatment study evaluated administered standard doses of conjugated equine estrogen (0.625 mg/d), which significantly improved sleep, but also showed an estrogen-related increase of inward-directed hostility (Schiff, 1980).

Importantly, the MT is a complex sociocultural as well as a hormonal event, and psychosocial factors may contribute to mood and cognitive symptoms. For example, women entering MT may face emotional stress from onset of a major illness, caring for an adolescent or aging parent, divorce or widowhood, and career change or retirement (LeBoeuf, 1996). Lock (1991) suggests that part of the stress reported by Western women is clearly culture-specific. Western culture emphasizes beauty and youth, and as women grow older, some suffer from a perceived loss of status, function, and control (LeBoeuf, 1996). However, the end of predictable menstruation and the end of fertility may be significant to a woman simply because it is a change, no matter how aging and the end of reproductive life are viewed by that woman and by her culture (Frackiewicz, 2000). For some women, the approach of menopause may also be perceived as a significant loss, both to women who have accepted childbearing and rearing as their major life roles and those who are childless, perhaps not by choice. For these reasons, impending menopause may be perceived as a time of loss, when depression and other psychological disorders may develop (Avis, 2000).

■ Libido Changes

Although the relationship between circulating hormones and libido has been extensively investigated, definitive data are lacking. Many studies demonstrate that other factors besides menopause may account for libido changes (Gracia, 2007). Avis and associates (2000) studied sexual function in a subgroup of 200 women in the Massachusetts Women's Health Study II who underwent natural menopause. None took hormone treatment, and all these women had sexual partners. Menopausal status was observed to be significantly related to decreased sexual interest. However, after adjustment for physical and mental health, smoking, and marital satisfaction, menopausal status no longer had a significant relationship to libido. Dennerstein (2005) prospectively evaluated 438 Australian women during 6 years of their menopausal transition. Menopause was significantly associated with dyspareunia and indirectly with sexual response. Feelings for one's partner, stress, and other social factors also indirectly affected sexual functioning.

Other investigators have demonstrated that sexual problems are more prevalent after menopause. A longitudinal study of women during MT until at least 1 year after the final menstrual period demonstrated a significant decrease in the rate of weekly coitus. Patients reported a significant decline in the number of sexual thoughts, sexual satisfactions, and vaginal lubrication after becoming menopausal (McCoy, 1985). In a study of 100 naturally menopausal women, both sexual desire and activity decreased compared with that during the premenopausal period. Women reported loss of libido, dyspareunia, and orgasmic dysfunction, with 86 percent reporting no orgasms after menopause (Tungphaisal, 1991).

■ Lower Reproductive Tract Changes

Estrogen receptors have been identified in the vulva, vagina, bladder, urethra, pelvic floor musculature, and endopelvic tissues. These structures thus share a similar hormonal responsiveness and are susceptible to estrogen deprivation. To reflect this common link, the International Society for the Study of Women's Sexual Health (ISSWSH) and The North American Menopause Society adopted the term *genitourinary syndrome of menopause (GSM)* to encompass the constellation of signs and symptoms that affect the genitourinary system after menopause (Table 21-9). As such, GSM is a syndrome that may include genital symptoms of dryness, burning, and irritation; sexual symptoms of absent lubrication, dyspareunia, and dysfunction;

TABLE 21-9. Genitourinary Syndrome of Menopause Characteristics

Symptoms	Signs
Genital dryness	Labia minora resorption
Poor lubrication	Narrowed introitus
Dyspareunia	Absent hymenal tags
Postcoital bleeding	Tissue pallor or erythema
Poor arousal, orgasm, desire	Urethral eversion
Vulvovaginal:	Urethral prolapse
irritation, burning, itching	Prominent urethral meatus
Dysuria	Recurrent UTI
Urinary frequency	Absent rugae
Urinary urgency	Fragile or fissured tissue
	Petechial hemorrhages
	Scant vaginal secretions
	Poor elasticity

UTI = urinary tract infection.
Adapted with permission from Portman DJ, Gass ML; Vulvovaginal Atrophy Terminology Consensus Conference Panel: Genitourinary syndrome of menopause: new terminology for vulvovaginal atrophy from the International Society for the Study of Women's Sexual Health and the North American Menopause Society, Menopause 2014 Oct;21(10):1063–1068.

and urinary symptoms of urgency, dysuria, and recurrent urinary tract infections (UTIs) (Portman, 2014).

Vulvovaginal Changes

Without estrogen's trophic influence, the vagina loses collagen, adipose tissue, and ability to retain water (Sarrel, 2000). As vaginal walls shrink, rugae flatten, and the vagina attains a smooth-walled, pale-pink appearance. The surface epithelium thins to only a few cell layers. This markedly reduces the ratio of superficial to basal cells, described on page 489. Moreover, the thin vaginal surface is friable and prone to submucosal petechial hemorrhages or bleeding with minimal trauma. The blood vessels in the vaginal walls narrow, and over time the vagina itself contracts and loses flexibility.

In addition, vaginal pH becomes more alkaline and a pH greater than 4.5 is typically observed with estrogen deficiency (Caillouette, 1997; Roy, 2004). An alkaline pH creates a vaginal environment less hospitable to lactobacilli and more susceptible to infection by urogenital and fecal pathogens. Hoffmann and colleagues (2014) found that the prevalence of bacterial vaginosis ranged from 23 to 38 percent in postmenopausal women, and rates increased with age. In contrast, *Candida* species were noted in 5 to 6 percent of these same women, and rates declined with aging.

In addition to vaginal changes, the vulvar epithelium gradually atrophies and secretions from sebaceous glands diminish. Subcutaneous fat in the labia majora is lost, which leads to shrinkage and retraction of clitoral prepuce and the urethra, fusion of the labia minora, and introital narrowing and then stenosis (Mehta, 2008).

Symptoms of vulvovaginal atrophy include vaginal dryness, itching, irritation, and dyspareunia. These are common complaints during MT, and prevalence estimates range from 10 to 50 percent (Levine, 2008). Treatment options include topical or systemic estrogen, SERMs, and vaginal moisturizers, which are all discussed in Chapter 22 (p. 505).

Dyspareunia and Sexual Dysfunction

Menopausal patients often note dyspareunia and other forms of sexual dysfunction. In one study, 25 percent of postmenopausal women noted some degree of dyspareunia (Laumann, 1999). These same investigators found that painful intercourse correlated with sexual problems, including lack of libido, arousal disorder, and anorgasmia. Although dyspareunia in this population is generally attributed to vaginal dryness and mucosal atrophy secondary estrogen deficiency, prevalence studies suggest that a decrement in all aspects of female sexual function is associated with midlife (Dennerstein, 2005).

Levine and associates (2008) studied 1480 sexually active postmenopausal women and found that the prevalence of vulvovaginal atrophy and of female sexual dysfunction each approximated 55 percent. They found that women with female sexual dysfunction were 3.84 times more likely to have vulvovaginal atrophy than women without such dysfunction. Estrogen deficiency diminishes vaginal lubrication, blood flow, and vasocongestion with sexual activity. These changes are coupled with the structural atrophy described in that last section. Reduced testosterone levels have been implicated in genital atrophy as well, but the relationship between testosterone and sexuality during MT remains obscure. Circulating testosterone levels decline gradually with age from the mid-reproductive years and have dropped by 50 percent by age 45. Paradoxically, studies have been unable to demonstrate that sexual dysfunction is related to decreased androgen levels in MT (O'Neil, 2011).

Urogenital conditions such as prolapse or incontinence correlate strongly with sexual dysfunction (Barber, 2002; Salonia, 2004). Patients with urinary incontinence are likely to have pelvic-floor hypotonus dysfunction, which may cause pain on deep penetration due to pelvic support instability. Hypertonic or dyssynergic pelvic-floor muscles, which are commonly seen in patients with urinary frequency, constipation, and vaginismus, are often associated with superficial pain and friction during intercourse (Handa, 2004). The presence of organ prolapse contributes to dyspareunia, as does a history of a gynecologic surgical procedure that may cause dyspareunia by shortening the vagina (Goldberg, 2001).

Menopause is also a time of life when significant psychosocial and physiological changes occur simultaneously, and concomitant illnesses arise. It is understandable that such major life changes influence sexual functioning. In the longitudinal Melbourne Midlife Study, Dennerstein and associates (1993) confirmed a significant decline in sexual functioning during MT. Sexual responsivity, libido, sexual frequency, positive feelings for a partner, and a partners' sexual performance all typically decreased, and vaginal dyspareunia rates typically increased. Other medical conditions such as arthritis, hip or lumbar joint pain, or fibromyalgia may contribute to vaginal or pelvic pain with intercourse. Pain may be due to radiation

of pain from trigger points in the trunk, buttocks, or pelvic-floor muscles, or from possible pudendal nerve entrapment. Chronic pelvic pain may also contribute to sexual dysfunction as discussed in Chapter 11 (p. 262).

Urogenital Changes

As part of GSM, urinary symptoms can include dysuria, urgency, urethral eversion or prolapse, and recurrent UTIs (Portman, 2014: Trutnovsky, 2014). Specifically, thinning of urethral and bladder mucosa underlie these. For these complaints, vaginal estrogen, discussed in Chapter 22 (p. 505), is a reasonable first option (Rahn, 2014).

The association between declining estrogen levels and incontinence is more controversial. In support of a causal link, urethral shortening associated with menopausal atrophic changes may result in genuine stress urinary incontinence. For example, Bhatia and colleagues (1989) showed that estrogen therapy may improve or cure stress urinary incontinence in more than 50 percent of treated women, presumably by exerting a direct effect on urethral mucosa coaptation (Chap. 23, p. 530). Accordingly, a trial of hormone therapy may be considered in select patients prior to surgical correction of incontinence in women with vaginal atrophy.

That said, Waetjen and coworkers (2009) evaluated women in MT and found a slight increase in stress and urge incontinence. They did find, however, a more robust association with worsening anxiety symptoms, a high baseline BMI, weight gain, and new-onset diabetes. Their conclusion was that from a public health stand point, clinicians and women should focus first on these modifiable risk factors. Other studies have also failed to find links between incontinence and menopausal status. Sherburn and colleagues (2001) performed a cross-sectional study of Australian women aged 45 to 55 years. In this population, they identified a 15-percent prevalence of incontinence. Associated risk factors included gynecologic surgery, higher BMI, UTIs, constipation, and multiparity. Subsequently, these investigators studied a subset of 373 premenopausal females to determine if MT itself was associated with an increased incidence of incontinence. In this group of women, the overall incidence was 35 percent, with no increase associated with menopause. Incontinence was most closely related to hysterectomy. More recently, Trutnovsky and associates (2014) explored the effects of menopause and hormone therapy both on stress and urge urinary incontinence. In the 382 women evaluated, the length of menopause showed no significant relationship with urinary incontinence.

In addition to incontinence, pelvic organ prolapse rates increase with advancing age. Importantly, vaginal relaxation with anterior wall, posterior wall, or apical prolapse is not a direct consequence of estrogen deprivation, as many factors play a role in pelvic floor relaxation (Chap. 24, p. 538).

PATIENT EVALUATION

Clinical goals during MT are to optimize a woman's health and well-being during and after this transition. This is an excellent time for a comprehensive health evaluation that includes a complete medical history, physical examination, and laboratory studies. Risk factors for common health problems such as obesity,

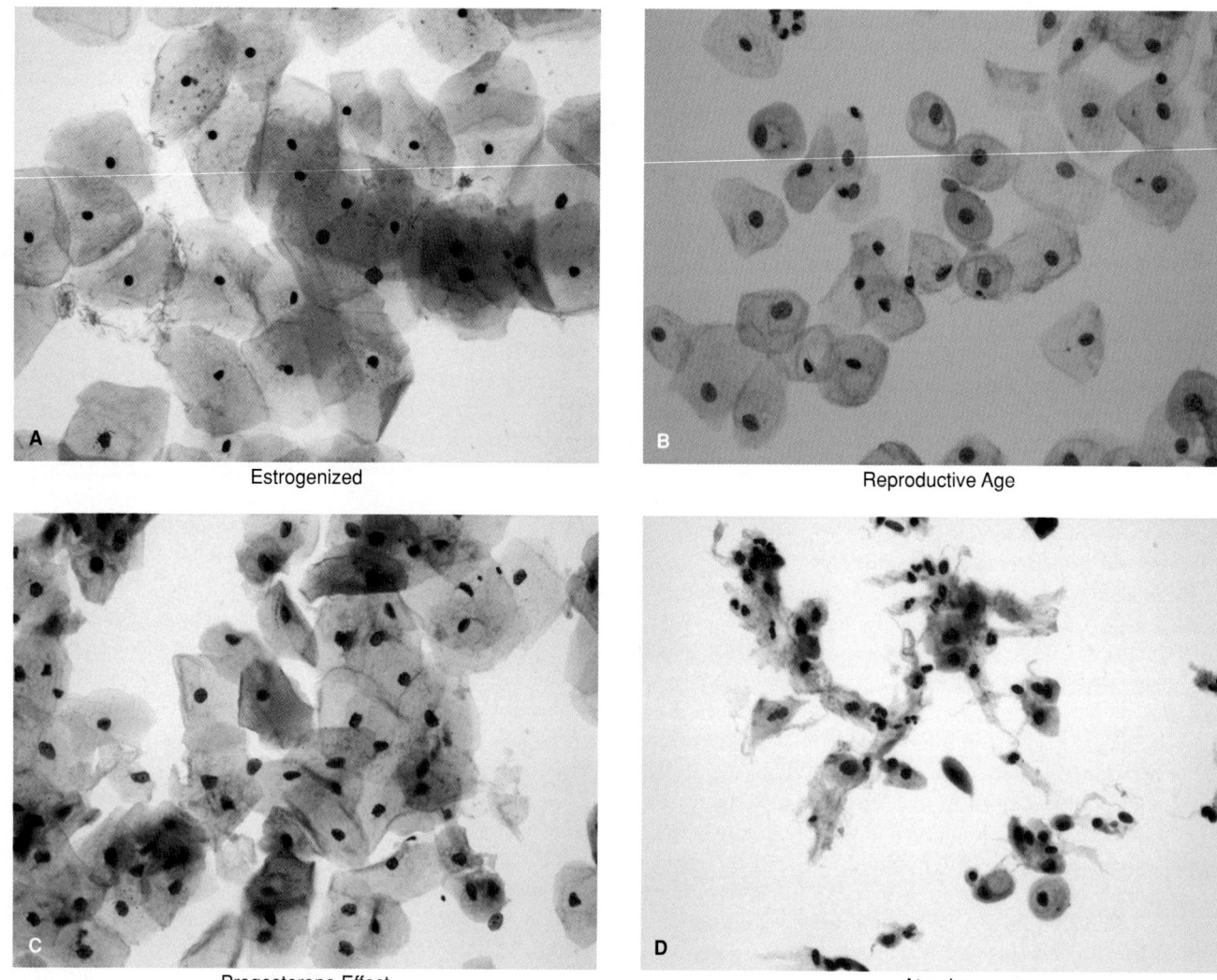

A Estrogenized

B Reproductive Age

C Progesterone Effect

D Atrophy

FIGURE 21-9 Photomicrographs of cytologic specimens illustrate key points of the maturation index. This index provides insight into the cytohormonal status of the patient and is based on a count of parabasal, intermediate, and superficial (P:I:S) cells. Generally, a predominance of superficial or superficial and intermediate cells (**A** and **B**) is seen in reproductive-aged women. **C.** A predominance of intermediate cells is seen in the luteal phase, in pregnancy, with amenorrhea, and in newborns, premenarchal girls, and women in early menopausal transition. **D.** A predominance of parabasal cells is seen in menopausal patients with atrophy. (Used with permission from Dr. Raheela Ashfaq.)

osteoporosis, heart disease, diabetes mellitus, and certain cancers are assessed and then managed. Counseling regarding diet, exercise, alcohol moderation, and smoking cessation is imperative, if applicable. Psychosocial well-being is also assessed. Clinicians may inquire directly about depression, anxiety, and sexual functioning or may choose to administer a simple questionnaire to assess for psychosocial issues (Chap. 13, p. 299).

A thorough general physical examination is performed during patient visits to document changes associated with aging and MT. Of elements, height, weight, waist circumference, and BMI are recorded and can be used to counsel women about physical exercise and weight loss or weight gain. Height loss may be associated with osteoporosis and vertebral compression fractures and thus is recorded yearly. Blood pressure monitoring effectively screens for hypertension, which is common in this population. The remaining examination notes expected physiologic changes of MT and seeks potential pathology described in earlier sections.

The diagnosis of MT can usually be made with documentation of age-appropriate symptoms and careful physical examination. Clearly, a 50-year-old woman with menstrual irregularity, hot flushes, and vaginal dryness is considered to be in MT. Other testing such as FSH or estradiol levels, described next, can be performed to document ovarian failure. However, for those in MT, FSH levels may be normal. Even when much younger women present with similar symptoms, evaluation should also include FSH measurement. If ovarian failure develops before age 40, it is usually pathologic. Thus, chromosomal abnormalities, infections, autoimmune disorders, galactosemia, cigarette smoking, or iatrogenic causes such as radiation or chemotherapy are considered (Table 16-6, p. 373).

■ Gonadotropin and Estrogen Levels

Biochemical changes, of which a woman may be unaware, may be identified prior to cycle irregularity. For example, in the early follicular phase of the menstrual cycle in many women older than 35 years, FSH levels may rise without a concurrent luteinizing hormone (LH) elevation. This finding is associated with a poor prognosis for future fertility. Specifically, a cycle day 3 FSH level greater than 10 mIU/mL is used in some in vitro fertilization (IVF) programs to route patients into donor egg programs (Chap. 20, p. 465). An FSH level greater than 40 mIU/mL has been used to document ovarian failure associated with menopause.

Estrogen levels may be normal, elevated, or low depending on the stage of MT. Only at menopause are estrogen levels extremely low or undetectable. Additionally, estrogen levels may be used to assess women's response to hormone treatment. Most clinicians prefer to reach a physiologic serum estradiol range of 50 to 100 pg/mL when selecting and adjusting replacement therapy. Women who receive estradiol pellets as replacement therapy may have elevated serum estradiol values from 300 to 500 pg/mL. These high levels are not uncommon with this replacement method but are discouraged.

■ Estrogen Maturation Index

The maturation index (MI) is an inexpensive, but less often used, means to evaluate hormonal influences in women. A specimen to measure the MI may be collected during a vaginal speculum examination at the same time cervical cancer screening is performed. The index report is read from left to right and refers to the percentage of parabasal, intermediate, and superficial squamous cells appearing on a smear, with the total sum of all three values equaling 100 percent (Fig. 21-9) (Randolph, 2005). For example, an MI of 0:40:60 represents 0 percent parabasal cells, 40 percent intermediate cells, and 60 percent superficial cells. This MI reflects adequate vaginal estrogen effects. A shift to the left indicates an increase in parabasal or intermediate cells, which denotes low estrogen effects. Conversely, a shift to the right reflects an increase in the superficial or intermediate cells, which is associated with higher estrogen levels.

An ideal MI vaginal specimen consists of freely exfoliating squamous cells from the upper third of the vaginal wall. Avoiding the cervix, the vaginal wall secretions are gently scraped with a spatula or saline-moistened swab. Immediately after collection, the specimen is transferred to a microscope slide. Cells are either suspended in a small amount of saline (as in a wet prep) or smeared to the slide and fixed with 95-percent ethanol spray fixative.

REFERENCES

Al-Safi ZA, Santoro N: Menopausal hormone therapy and menopausal symptoms. Fertil Steril 101(4):905, 2014
American College of Obstetricians and Gynecologists: Osteoporosis. Practice Bulletin No. 129, September 2012
Antithrombotic Trialists' Collaboration: Collaborative meta-analysis of randomised trials of antiplatelet therapy for prevention of death, myocardial infarction, and stroke in high risk patients. BMJ 324(7329):71, 2002
Avis NE, Stellato R, Crawford S, et al: Is there an association between menopause status and sexual functioning? Menopause 7:297, 2000
Bachmann G: Physiologic aspects of natural and surgical menopause. J Reprod Med 46(3 Suppl):307, 2001
Bachmann GA: Menopausal vasomotor symptoms: a review of causes, effects and evidence-based treatment options. J Reprod Med 50:155, 2005

Ballinger CB: Psychiatric aspects of the menopause. Br J Psychiatry 156:773, 1990
Bar-Shavit Z: The osteoclast: a multinucleated, hematopoietic-origin, bone-resorbing osteoimmune cell. J Cell Biochem 102(5):1130, 2007
Barber MD, Visco AG, Wyman JF, et al: Sexual function in women with urinary incontinence and pelvic organ prolapse. Obstet Gynecol 99:281, 2002
Baumgartner RN, Heymsfield SB, Roche AF: Human body composition and the epidemiology of chronic disease. Obes Res 3:73, 1995
Bhatia NN, Bergman A, Karram MM: Effects of estrogen on urethral function in women with urinary incontinence. Am J Obstet Gynecol 160:176, 1989
Bonjour JP, Chevalley T, Ammann P, et al: Gain in bone mineral mass in prepubertal girls 3.5 years after discontinuation of calcium supplementation: a follow-up study. Lancet 358:1208, 2001
Bouchard C: Prevention of falls, prevention of osteoporosis, or both: what is the best strategy for preventing fractures in older women? Menopause 20(10):995, 2013
Bromberger JT, Kravitz HM, Chang YF, et al: Major depression during and after the menopausal transition: Study of Women's Health Across the Nation (SWAN). Psychol Med 41(9):1879, 2011
Burger HG, Dudley EC, Cui J, et al: A prospective longitudinal study of serum testosterone, dehydroepiandrosterone sulfate, and sex hormone-binding globulin levels through the menopause transition. J Clin Endocrinol Metab 85:2832, 2000
Burger HG, Hale GE, Dennerstein L, et al: Cycle and hormone changes during perimenopause: the key role of ovarian function. Menopause 15(4 Pt 1):603, 2008
Busch CM, Zonderman AB, Costa PT Jr: Menopausal transition and psychological distress in a nationally representative sample: is menopause associated with psychological distress? J Aging Health 6:206, 1994
Caillouette JC, Sharp CF Jr, Zimmerman GJ, et al: Vaginal pH as a marker for bacterial pathogens and menopausal status. Am J Obstet Gynecol 176:1270, 1997
Canalis E, Giustina A, Bilezikian JP: Mechanisms of anabolic therapies for osteoporosis. N Engl J Med 357(9):905, 2007
Cohen LS, Soares CN, Vitonis AF, et al: Risk of new onset of depression during the menopausal transition: the Harvard Study of Moods and Cycles. Arch Gen Psychiatry 63(4):385, 2006
Crandall CJ, Crawford SL, Gold EB: Vasomotor symptom prevalence is associated with polymorphisms in sex steroid-metabolizing enzymes and receptors. Am J Med 119:552, 2006
Cummings SR, Nevitt MC, Browner WS, et al: Risk factors for hip fracture in white women. Study of Osteoporotic Fractures Research Group. N Engl J Med 332:767, 1995
Da Fonseca AM, Bagnoli VR, Souza MA, et al: Impact of age and body mass on the intensity of menopausal symptoms in 5968 Brazilian women. Gynecol Endocrinol 29(2):116, 2013
Dallman MF, la Fleur SE, Pecoraro NC, et al: Minireview: glucocorticoids—food intake, abdominal obesity, and wealthy nations in 2004. Endocrinology 145:2633, 2004
Delaney MF: Strategies for the prevention and treatment of osteoporosis during early postmenopause. Am J Obstet Gynecol 194(2 Suppl):S12, 2006
Dennerstein L, Guthrie JR, Clark M, et al: A population-based study of depressed mood in middle-aged, Australian-born women. Menopause 11(5):563, 2004
Dennerstein L, Hayes RD: Confronting the challenges: epidemiological study of female sexual dysfunction and the menopause. J Sex Med 2(Suppl 3):118, 2005
Dennerstein L, Smith AM, Morse C, et al: Menopausal symptoms in Australian women. Med J Aust 159:232, 1993
Erlik Y, Meldrum DR, Judd HL: Estrogen levels in postmenopausal women with hot flashes. Obstet Gynecol 59:403, 1982
Espeland MA, Stefanick ML, Kritz-Silverstein D, et al: Effect of postmenopausal hormone therapy on body weight and waist and hip girths. Postmenopausal Estrogen-Progestin Interventions Study Investigators. J Clin Endocrinol Metab 82:1549, 1997
Faulkner KG, von Stetten E, Miller P: Discordance in patient classification using T-scores. J Clin Densitom 2:343, 1999
Frackiewicz EJ, Cutler NR: Women's health care during the perimenopause. J Am Pharm Assoc (Wash) 40:800, 2000
Freedman RR: Biochemical, metabolic, and vascular mechanisms in menopausal hot flashes. Fertil Steril 70:332, 1998
Freedman RR: Menopausal hot flashes: mechanisms, endocrinology, treatment. J Steroid Biochem Mol Biol 142:115, 2014
Freedman RR: Physiology of hot flashes. Am J Hum Biol 13:453, 2001
Freedman RR, Woodward S, Sabharwal SC: Alpha 2-adrenergic mechanism in menopausal hot flushes. Obstet Gynecol 76:573, 1990
Freeman EW, Sammel MD, Lin H, et al: Hormones and menopausal status as predictors of depression in women in transition to menopause. Arch Gen Psychiatry 61(1):62, 2004

Freeman EW, Sammel MD, Lin H, et al: Symptoms associated with menopausal transition and reproductive hormones in midlife women. Obstet Gynecol 110(2 Pt 1):230, 2007

Freeman EW, Sammel MD, Sanders RJ: Risk of long-term hot flashes after natural menopause: evidence from the Penn Ovarian Aging Study cohort. Menopause 21(9):924, 2014

Gallagher JC, Rapuri PB, Haynatzki G, et al: Effect of discontinuation of estrogen, calcitriol, and the combination of both on bone density and bone markers. J Clin Endocrinol Metab 87:4914, 2002

Garnero P, Gineyts E, Riou JP, et al: Assessment of bone resorption with a new marker of collagen degradation in patients with metabolic bone disease. J Clin Endocrinol Metab 79:780, 1994

Gebbie AE, Hardman SM: Contraception in the perimenopause—old and new. Menopause Int 16(1):33, 2010

Gerber LM, Sievert LL, Warren K, et al: Hot flashes are associated with increased ambulatory systolic blood pressure. Menopause 14(2):308, 2007

Gislason T, Benediktsdottir B, Bjornsson JK, et al: Snoring, hypertension, and the sleep apnea syndrome. An epidemiologic survey of middle-aged women. Chest 103:1147, 1993

Gold EB, Bromberger J, Crawford S, et al: Factors associated with age at natural menopause in a multiethnic sample of midlife women. Am J Epidemiol 153:865, 2001

Gold EB, Colvin A, Avis N, et al: Longitudinal analysis of the association between vasomotor symptoms and race/ethnicity across the menopausal transition: study of women's health across the nation. Am J Public Health 96(7):1226, 2006

Goldberg RP, Tomezsko JE, Winkler HA, et al: Anterior or posterior sacrospinous vaginal vault suspension: long-term anatomic and functional evaluation. Obstet Gynecol 98:199, 2001

Gonzales GF, Carrillo C: Blood serotonin levels in postmenopausal women: effects of age and serum oestradiol levels. Maturitas 17:23, 1993

Gracia CR, Freeman EW, Sammel MD, et al: Hormones and sexuality during transition to menopause. Obstet Gynecol 109(4):831, 2007

Grynnerup AG, Lindhard A, Sorensen S: Recent progress in the utility of anti-Mullerian hormone in female infertility. Curr Opin Obstet Gynecol 26:162, 2014

Guinot C, Malvy D, Ambroisine L, et al: Effect of hormonal replacement therapy on skin biophysical properties of menopausal women. Skin Res Technol 11:201, 2005

Guthrie JR, Dennerstein L, Taffe JR, et al: Hot flushes during the menopause transition: a longitudinal study in Australian-born women. Menopause 12(4):460, 2005

Haarbo J, Hassager C, Riis BJ, et al: Relation of body fat distribution to serum lipids and lipoproteins in elderly women. Atherosclerosis 80:57, 1989

Hagner W, Hagner-Derengowska M, Wiacek M, et al: Changes in level of VO2max, blood lipids, and waist circumference in the response to moderate endurance training as a function of ovarian aging. Menopause 16(5):1009, 2009

Halbreich U, Lumley LA, Palter S, et al: Possible acceleration of age effects on cognition following menopause. J Psychiatr Res 29:153, 1995

Hale GE, Zhao X, Hughes CL, et al: Endocrine features of menstrual cycles in middle and late reproductive age and the menopausal transition classified according to the Staging of Reproductive Aging Workshop (STRAW) staging system. J Clin Endocrinol Metab 92(8):3060, 2007

Hall MH, Matthews KA, Kravitz HM, et al: Race and financial strain are independent correlates of sleep in midlife women: the SWAN sleep study. Sleep 32:73, 2009

Handa VL, Harvey L, Cundiff GW, et al: Sexual function among women with urinary incontinence and pelvic organ prolapse. Am J Obstet Gynecol 191:751, 2004

Harlow SD, Gass M, Hall JE, et al: Executive summary of the Stages of Reproductive Again Workshop + 10: addressing the unfinished agenda of staging reproductive aging. Fertil Steril 97:843, 2012

Harman SM: Menopausal hormone treatment cardiovascular disease: another look at an unresolved conundrum. Fertil Steril 101(4):887, 2014

Henderson VW, St John JA, Hodis HN, et al: Cognition, mood, and physiological concentrations of sex hormones in the early and late postmenopause. Proc Natl Acad Sci USA 110(50):20290, 2013

Hoffman JN, You HM, Hedberg EC, et al: Prevalence of bacterial vaginosis and Candida among postmenopausal women in the United States. J Gerontol B Psychol Sci Soc Sci 69 Suppl 2:S205, 2014

Hollander LE, Freeman EW, Sammel MD, et al: Sleep quality, estradiol levels, and behavioral factors in late reproductive age women. Obstet Gynecol 98:391, 2001

Holroyd C, Cooper C, Dennison E: Epidemiology of osteoporosis. Best Pract Res Clin Endocrinol Metab 22(5):671, 2008

Hunter MS, Gentry-Maharaj A, Ryan A, et al: Prevalence, frequency and problem rating of hot flushes persist in older postmenopausal women: impact of age, body mass index, hysterectomy, hormone therapy use, lifestyle and mood in a cross-sectional cohort study of 10,418 British women aged 54–65. BJOG 119(1):40, 2012

Jain A, Santoro N: Endocrine mechanisms and management for abnormal bleeding due to perimenopausal changes. Clin Obstet Gynecol 48:295, 2005

Jensen J, Nilas L, Christiansen C: Influence of menopause on serum lipids and lipoproteins. Maturitas 12(4):321, 1990

Johnell O, Kanis JA: An estimate of the worldwide prevalence and disability associated with osteoporotic fractures. Osteoporos Int 17(12):1726, 2006

Jull J, Stacey D, Beach S, et al: Lifestyle interventions targeting body weight changes during the menopause transition: a systematic review. J Obes 2014:824310, 2014

Kanis JA: Assessment of fracture risk and its application to screening for postmenopausal osteoporosis: synopsis of a WHO report. WHO Study Group. Osteoporos Int 4:368, 1994

Kanis JA, Johnell O, Oden A, et al: Ten year probabilities of osteoporotic fractures according to BMD and diagnostic thresholds. Osteoporos Int 12:989, 2001

Kannel WB: Metabolic risk factors for coronary heart disease in women: perspective from the Framingham Study. Am Heart J 114:413, 1987

Kelly GA, Kelly KS, Kohrt WM: Effect of ground and joint reaction force exercise on lumbar spine and femoral neck bone mineral density in postmenopausal women: a meta-analysis of randomized controlled trials. BMC Musculoskelet Disord 13:177, 2012

Kiebzak GM, Miller PD: Determinants of bone strength. J Bone Miner Res 18:383, 2003

Kim JH, Cho HT, Kim YJ: The role of estrogen in adipose tissue metabolism: insights into glucose homeostasis regulation. Endocr J 61(11):1055, 2014

Klein NA, Illingworth PJ, Groome NP, et al: Decreased inhibin B secretion is associated with the monotropic FSH rise in older, ovulatory women: a study of serum and follicular fluid levels of dimeric inhibin A and B in spontaneous menstrual cycles. J Clin Endocrinol Metab 81:2742, 1996

Kostenuik PJ: Osteoprotegerin and RANKL regulate bone resorption, density, geometry and strength. Curr Opin Pharmacol 5(6):618, 2005

Krall EA, Dawson-Hughes B, Papas A, et al: Tooth loss and skeletal bone density in healthy postmenopausal women. Osteoporos Int 4:104, 1994

Kronenberg F: Hot flashes: epidemiology and physiology. Ann NY Acad Sci 592:52, 1990

Kuh DL, Wadsworth M, Hardy R: Women's health in midlife: the influence of the menopause, social factors and health in earlier life. BJOG 104:923, 1997

Kuller LH, Lopez OL, Newman A, et al: Risk factors for dementia in the cardiovascular health cognition study. Neuroepidemiology 22:13, 2003

Labrie F, Belanger A, Cusan L, et al: Marked decline in serum concentrations of adrenal C19 sex steroid precursors and conjugated androgen metabolites during aging. J Clin Endocrinol Metab 82:2396, 1997

Laufer LR, Erlik Y, Meldrum DR, et al: Effect of clonidine on hot flashes in postmenopausal women. Obstet Gynecol 60:583, 1982

Laumann EO, Paik A, Rosen RC: Sexual dysfunction in the United States: prevalence and predictors. JAMA 281:537, 1999

LeBoeuf FJ, Carter SG: Discomforts of the perimenopause. J Obstet Gynecol Neonatal Nurs 25:173, 1996

Levine KB, Williams RE, Hartmann KE: Vulvovaginal atrophy is strongly associated with female sexual dysfunction among sexually active postmenopausal women. Menopause 15(4 Pt 1):661, 2008

Lidor A, Ismajovich B, Confino E, et al: Histopathological findings in 226 women with post-menopausal uterine bleeding. Acta Obstet Gynecol Scand 65:41, 1986

Lindsay R, Silverman SL, Cooper C, et al: Risk of new vertebral fracture in the year following a fracture. JAMA 285:320, 2001

Lock M: Medicine and culture: Contested meanings of the menopause. Lancet 337:1270, 1991

Lund KJ: Menopause and the menopausal transition. Med Clin North Am 92(5):1253, 2008

Malacara JM, Perez-Luque EL, Martinez-Garza S, et al: The relationship of estrogen receptor-alpha polymorphism with symptoms and other characteristics in post-menopausal women. Maturitas 49:163, 2004

Manson JE, Greenland P, LaCroix AZ, et al: Walking compared with vigorous exercise for the prevention of cardiovascular events in women. N Engl J Med 347:716, 2002

Marshall D, Johnell O, Wedel H: Meta-analysis of how well measures of bone mineral density predict occurrence of osteoporotic fractures. BMJ 312:1254, 1996

Matthews KA, Abrams B, Crawford S, et al: Body mass index in mid-life women: relative influence of menopause, hormone use, and ethnicity. Int J Obes Relat Metab Disord 25:863, 2001

Matthews KA, Meilahn E, Kuller LH, et al: Menopause and risk factors for coronary heart disease. N Engl J Med 321:641, 1989

Matthews KA, Wing RR, Kuller LH, et al: Influence of the perimenopause on cardiovascular risk factors and symptoms of middle-aged healthy women. Arch Intern Med 154:2349, 1994

McCoy NL, Davidson JM: A longitudinal study of the effects of menopause on sexuality. Maturitas 7:203, 1985

McKechnie R, Rubenfire M, Mosca L: Association between self-reported physical activity and vascular reactivity in postmenopausal women. Atherosclerosis 159:483, 2001

McKinlay SM, Brambilla DJ, Posner JG: The normal menopause transition. Maturitas 14:103, 1992

Mehta A, Bachmann G: Vulvovaginal complaints. Clin Obstet Gynecol 51 (3):549, 2008

Melton LJ III, Atkinson EJ, Cooper C, et al: Vertebral fractures predict subsequent fractures. Osteoporos Int 10:214, 1999

Meyer JS, Rauch GM, Crawford K, et al: Risk factors accelerating cerebral degenerative changes, cognitive decline and dementia. Int J Geriatr Psychiatry 14:1050, 1999

Milewicz A, Bidzinska B, Sidorowicz A: Perimenopausal obesity. Gynecol Endocrinol 10:285, 1996

Miller PD, Njeh CF, Jankowski LG, et al: What are the standards by which bone mass measurement at peripheral skeletal sites should be used in the diagnosis of osteoporosis? J Clin Densitom 5(Suppl):S39, 2002

Moen MH, Kahn H, Bjerve KS, et al: Menometrorrhagia in the perimenopause is associated with increased serum estradiol. Maturitas 47:151, 2004

Molina P: Parathyroid gland and Ca^{2+} and PO^{4-} regulation. In Endocrine Physiology, 4th ed. New York, McGraw-Hill, 2013

Molnar WR: Menopausal hot flashes: their cycles and relation to air temperature. Obstet Gynecol 57:52S, 1981

National Osteoporosis Foundation: America's bone health: the state of osteoporosis and low bone mass in our nation. Washington, The Foundation, 2002

National Osteoporosis Foundation: Clinician's guide to prevention and treatment of osteoporosis. Washington, National Osteoporosis Foundation, 2014

O'Neill S, Eden J: The pathophysiology of menopausal symptoms. Obstet Gynaecol Reprod Med 22(3):63, 2011

Overlie I, Finset A, Holte A: Gendered personality dispositions, hormone values, and hot flushes during and after menopause. J Psychosom Obstet Gynaecol 23(4):219, 2002

Paramsothy P, Harlow SD, Greendale GA, et al: Bleeding patterns during the menopausal transition in the multi-ethnic Study of Women's Health Across the Nation (SWAN): a prospective cohort study. BJOG 121:1564, 2014

Pinkerton JV, Stovall DW, Kightlinger RS: Advances in the treatment of menopausal symptoms. Womens Health (England) 5(4):361, 2009

Portman DJ, Gass ML; Vulvovaginal Atrophy Terminology Consensus Conference Panel: Genitourinary syndrome of menopause: new terminology for vulvovaginal atrophy from the International Society for the Study of Women's Sexual Health and the North American Menopause Society. Menopause 21(10):1063, 2014

Rahn DD, Carberry C, Sanses TV, et al: Vaginal estrogen for genitourinary syndrome of menopause: a systematic review. Obstet Gynecol 124(6):1147, 2014

Ralston SH: Genetic control of susceptibility to osteoporosis. J Clin Endocrinol Metab 87:2460, 2002

Randolph JF Jr, Sowers M, Bondarenko I, et al: The relationship of longitudinal change in reproductive hormones and vasomotor symptoms during the menopausal transition. J Clin Endocrinol Metab 90:6106, 2005

Rapkin AJ: Vasomotor symptoms in menopause: physiologic condition and central nervous system approaches to treatment. Am J Obstet Gynecol, 196(2):97, 2007

Recker RR, Davies KM, Hinders SM, et al: Bone gain in young adult women. JAMA 268:2403, 1992

Reyes FI, Winter JS, Faiman C: Pituitary-ovarian relationships preceding the menopause. I. A cross-sectional study of serum follicle-stimulating hormone, luteinizing hormone, prolactin, estradiol, and progesterone levels. Am J Obstet Gynecol 129:557, 1977

Richardson SJ, Senikas V, Nelson JF: Follicular depletion during the menopausal transition: evidence for accelerated loss and ultimate exhaustion. J Clin Endocrinol Metab 65:1231, 1987

Riis BJ, Hansen MA, Jensen AM, et al: Low bone mass and fast rate of bone loss at menopause: equal risk factors for future fracture: a 15-year follow-up study. Bone 19:9, 1996

Roy S, Caillouette JC, Roy T, et al: Vaginal pH is similar to follicle-stimulating hormone for menopause diagnosis. Am J Obstet Gynecol 190:1272, 2004

Sabatier JP, Guaydier-Souquieres G, Laroche D, et al: Bone mineral acquisition during adolescence and early adulthood: a study in 574 healthy females 10–24 years of age. Osteoporos Int 6:141, 1996

Saladin KS: Bone Tissue in Human Anatomy. New York, McGraw-Hill, 2005, p 158

Salonia A, Zanni G, Nappi RE, et al: Sexual dysfunction is common in women with lower urinary tract symptoms and urinary incontinence: results of a cross-sectional study. Eur Urol 45:642, 2004

Sambrook P, Cooper C: Osteoporosis. Lancet 367(9527):2010, 2006

Santoro N, Brown JR, Adel T, et al: Characterization of reproductive hormonal dynamics in the perimenopause. J Clin Endocrinol Metab 81:1495, 1996

Santoro N, Lasley B, McConnell D, et al: Body size and ethnicity are associated with menstrual cycle alterations in women in the early menopausal transition: the Study of Women's Health across the Nation (SWAN) Daily Hormone Study. J Clin Endocrinol Metab 89(6):2622, 2004

Sarrel PM: Effects of hormone replacement therapy on sexual psychophysiology and behavior in postmenopause. J Womens Health Gend Based Med 9(Suppl 1):S25, 2000

Schiff I, Tulchinsky D, Cramer D, et al: Oral medroxyprogesterone in the treatment of postmenopausal symptoms. JAMA 244:1443, 1980

Schnatz PF, Marakovits KA, Dubois M, et al: Osteoporosis screening and treatment guidelines: are they being followed? Menopause 18(10):1072, 2011

Sherburn M, Guthrie JR, Dudley EC, et al: Is incontinence associated with menopause? Obstet Gynecol 98:628, 2001

Simkin-Silverman LR, Wing RR, Boraz MA, et al: Lifestyle intervention can prevent weight gain during menopause: results from a 5-year randomized clinical trial. Ann Behav Med 26(3):212, 2003

Slopien R, Meczekalski B, Warenik-Szymankiewicz A: Relationship between climacteric symptoms and serum serotonin levels in postmenopausal women. Climacteric 6:53, 2003

Soares CN: Menopause and mood disturbance. Psychiatric Times 12:2005

Soares CN: Mood disorders in midlife women: understanding the critical window and its clinical implications. Menopause 21(2)198, 2014

Soules MR, Sherman S, Parrott E, et al: Executive summary: stages of reproductive aging workshop (STRAW). Fertil Steril 76:874, 2001

Spinelli MG: Neuroendocrine effects on mood. Rev Endocr Metab Disord 6:109, 2005

Stear SJ, Prentice A, Jones SC, et al: Effect of a calcium and exercise intervention on the bone mineral status of 16- to 18-year-old adolescent girls. Am J Clin Nutr 77:985, 2003

Stein E, Shane E: Secondary osteoporosis. Endocrinol Metab Clin North Am 32:115, 2003

Theintz G, Buchs B, Rizzoli R, et al: Longitudinal monitoring of bone mass accumulation in healthy adolescents: evidence for a marked reduction after 16 years of age at the levels of lumbar spine and femoral neck in female subjects. J Clin Endocrinol Metab 75:1060, 1992

Thurston RC, Bromberger JT, Joffe H, et al: Beyond frequency: who is most bothered by vasomotor symptoms? Menopause 5:841, 2008

Treloar AE: Menstrual cyclicity and the pre-menopause. Maturitas 3(3–4):249, 1981

Trutnovsky G, Rojas RG, Mann KP, et al: Urinary incontinence: the role of menopause. Menopause 21(4):399, 2014

Tungphaisal S, Chandeying V, Sutthijumroon S, et al: Postmenopausal sexuality in Thai women. Asia Oceania J Obstet Gynaecol 17:143, 1991

U.S. Census Bureau: 2014 National population projections. Projections of population by sex and selected age groups for the United States: 2015 to 2060. Available at: http://www.census.gov/population/projections/data/national/2014/summarytables.html. Accessed February 28, 2015

van Beresteijn EC, Korevaar JC, Huijbregts PC, et al: Perimenopausal increase in serum cholesterol: a 10-year longitudinal study. Am J Epidemiol 137:383, 1993

Waetjen LE, Ye J, Feng WY, et al: Association between menopausal transition stages and developing urinary incontinence. Obstet Gynecol 114(5):989, 2009

Walker MD, Liu XS, Stein E, et al: Differences in bone microarchitecture between postmenopausal Chinese-American and white women. J Bone Miner Res 26:1392, 2011

Wallace RB, Sherman BM, Bean JA, et al: Probability of menopause with increasing duration of amenorrhea in middle-aged women. Am J Obstet Gynecol 135:1021, 1979

Wilbur J, Miller AM, Montgomery A, et al: Sociodemographic characteristics, biological factors, and symptom reporting in midlife women. Menopause 5:43, 1998

Wines N, Willsteed E: Menopause and the skin. Australas J Dermatol 42:149, 2001

Wing RR, Matthews KA, Kuller LH, et al: Weight gain at the time of menopause. Arch Intern Med 151:97, 1991

Woods NF, Smith-DiJulio K, Percival DB, et al: Depressed mood during the menopausal transition and early postmenopause: observations from the Seattle Midlife Women's Health Study. Menopause 15(2):223, 2008

Woodward S, Freedman RR: The thermoregulatory effects of menopausal hot flashes on sleep. Sleep 17:497, 1994

The Mature Woman

The typical "mature woman" is aged 40 years or older and has completed childbearing. During their late 40s, most women enter menopausal transition. Detailed in Chapter 21, this period of physiologic change due to ovarian senescence and estrogen decline is usually completed between ages 51 and 56. Menopause marks a defining point in this transition and is defined as the point in time of permanent menstruation cessation due to loss of ovarian function. Clinically, the menopause refers to a point in time that follows 1 year after cessation of menstruation.

With ovarian senescence, declining hormone estrogen levels have specific effects. Some lead to physical symptoms, such as vasomotor symptoms and vaginal dryness, whereas others are metabolic and structural changes. These include bone loss, skin thinning, fatty replacement of the breast, lipoprotein changes, and genitourinary atrophy. As a result, postmenopausal women have unique issues associated with aging and estrogen loss that may negatively affect their individual health.

For many years, menopause was seen as a "deficiency disease" of estrogen, progesterone, and testosterone. For this reason, hormone replacement therapy has been used in one form or another for more than 100 years. The history surrounding this treatment is discussed here, as are current recommendations for the treatment of menopausal symptoms.

HORMONE TREATMENT: HISTORY AND CONTROVERSIES

Clinicians ideally provide evidence-based medicine, and seldom is a single study relied on solely to guide practice (Lobo, 2008). Thus, providers should understand the weaknesses and strengths of clinical trials to accurately counsel their patients. As one example, hormone treatment (HT) was widely prescribed to menopausal women, in good faith, based on initial observational studies. The general medical consensus was that HT, in addition to its prevention and treatment of osteoporosis, could protect against cardiovascular disease, stroke, and dementia. Subsequently, prospective, randomized controlled trials (RCTs) challenged the validity of these earlier observational studies. However, in this evaluation, clinicians must appreciate the type of population studied, the ages and risk factors of participating women, and the hormone regimens tested.

■ Early Estrogen Administration Trends

Estrogen treatment (ET) for menopausal symptom relief gained popularity in the 1960s and 1970s. Proponents promoted ET for its "preservation of youth" and prevention of chronic disease. By the mid-1970s, more than 30 million prescriptions were written for estrogen each year, and half of all menopausal women were using ET for a median of 5 years. Premarin (conjugated equine estrogen) was the fifth most prescribed drug in the marketplace.

In 1975, a study revealed a connection between endometrial cancer and ET. Investigators found a 4.5 times greater risk of this cancer in those using estrogen (Smith, 1975). As a result, the Food and Drug Administration (FDA) ordered labeling changes to state this higher risk. Progestins were then added in the 1980s to therapy regimens to significantly reduce endometrial cancer risks.

During that same time, estrogens were documented by several studies to prevent bone loss (Gambrell, 1983). Additionally, an expanding literature provided a robust affirmation of the effectiveness of menopausal HT in reducing vasomotor symptoms, maintaining bone mineral density (BMD), and preventing and treating vulvovaginal atrophy (Shulman, 2010). Several observational studies also suggested that estrogens prevented development of coronary heart disease (CHD) and other conditions, such as Alzheimer disease. However, in 1985, conflicting reports from two studies were published.

First, the Framingham Heart Study, an observational study of 1234 women, showed that those who took hormones had a 50-percent elevated risk of cardiac morbidity and more than a twofold risk for cerebrovascular disease (Wilson, 1985). In the same edition of the *New England Journal of Medicine*, a much larger observational trial, The Nurses' Health Study, with 121,964 women, found significantly lower rates of heart disease in postmenopausal women taking estrogen compared with a similar cohort not taking estrogen (Stampfer, 1985). Numerous subsequent articles reported the protective effects that combination HT provided menopausal women against cardiovascular disease and osteoporosis.

Current thinking is that that these early nonrandomized, unblinded, observational studies included samples of women who were not necessarily representative of the entire postmenopausal population. These hormone users tended to have superior access to care and to be thinner, wealthier, and healthier (Grodstein, 2003; Prentice, 2006). An additional source of confounding and possible selection bias is suggested to be the timing of HT initiation relative to the underlying state of the vasculature. Some investigators suggest that estrogen may delay the onset of the earliest stages of atherosclerosis, which are more likely to be present in younger women. However, estrogen may be ineffective or even trigger events in advanced lesions that are found in older women (Mendelsohn, 2005). This potential "window of opportunity" is supported by animal and laboratory studies (Grodstein, 2003). In sum, these study biases may have contributed to favorable outcomes attributed to estrogen in observational trials. When these biases are eliminated and the data reanalyzed, the results of earlier observational trials and later RCTs are remarkably similar.

Postmenopausal Estrogen/Progestin Interventions Trial

Because of data available in the late 1980s, estrogens were prescribed, not only for vasomotor symptom relief, but also for prevention of other conditions. In 1995, The Writing Group for the Postmenopausal Estrogen/Progestin Interventions (PEPI) Trial published results that suggested benefit for CHD risk. In this study, menopausal women with a mean age of 56 years were randomly allocated to one of five treatments: (1) placebo, (2) estrogen alone, (3) estrogen plus cyclic medroxyprogesterone acetate (MPA), (4) estrogen plus cyclic micronized progesterone, or (5) estrogen plus continuous MPA. Primary outcomes studied in the 875 women evaluated during 3 years included measurement of systolic blood pressure and of serum lipid, insulin, and fibrinogen levels. The PEPI trial documented that low-density lipoprotein (LDL) cholesterol levels declined and high-density lipoprotein (HDL) levels were increased in the four treatment groups receiving estrogens. Levels were most substantially improved in women solely given estrogen. An intermediate effect was noted in those prescribed conjugated equine estrogen (CEE) and micronized progesterone, whereas the smallest change followed CEE and MPA administration. Fibrinogen levels were increased in the placebo group compared with groups given hormones. However, no differences were identified in systolic blood pressure or glucose-challenged insulin levels. Clinical outcomes were also reported, and complications were few. Of these, all occurred in the HT-treated groups and included one cardiac arrest, two myocardial infarctions (MIs), and two cerebrovascular events.

Heart and Estrogen/Progestin Replacement Study

With results published in 1998, the Heart and Estrogen/Progestin Replacement Study (HERS) described cardiac morbidity in 2763 women with preexisting heart disease (Hulley, 1998). These women received estrogen as secondary prevention for further cardiac disease progression. First-year findings showed an increase in MIs in women who received CEE with continuous MPA. However, after average treatment duration of 4 years, rates of cardiovascular death or nonfatal MI did not differ between treatment groups.

This trial represented the first RCT at variance with prior data and created confusion for both clinicians and their patients. Beliefs that hormones prevented heart disease persisted, but the HERS data caused many investigators to question the cardioprotective effects of hormones. Subsequent HERS II results also showed that HT was not beneficial in the secondary prevention of heart disease even after 6.8 years (Grady, 2002). One reanalysis of the Nurses' Health Study focused on early hazard among women initiating HT during the monitoring period and showed a similar time trend, with early harm (Grodstein, 2001).

Women's Health Initiative

After an unsuccessful effort in 1990 to obtain FDA approval for HT as prevention for CHD, the need for RCTs to demonstrate conclusive benefit was widely acknowledged. As a result, before the results from the PEPI trial and HERS trials were available, the National Institutes of Health (NIH) launched the Women's Health Initiative (WHI) in 1993. This major study was to evaluate the putative protective effects of HT on common chronic diseases of aging. The WHI examined the effect of a single combined CEE and MPA drug compared with placebo in 16,608 healthy postmenopausal women aged 50 to 79 years (mean of 63.3 years) who had not undergone hysterectomy (Rossouw, 2002). Specific end points were evaluated: CHD, venous thromboembolism (VTE), breast cancer, colon cancer, and bone fractures. Concurrently, the study also compared CEE with placebo in postmenopausal women without a uterus (the estrogen-only arm).

As part of the original WHI study design, investigators predetermined targets for CHD (anticipated benefit) and breast cancer (anticipated risk) as primary disease end points. This design dictated that if the incidence of an end point was exceeded within a given period, the study would be terminated. Moreover, combined end points were weighted into a "global index," which if exceeded, would result in study termination. After a mean 5.2 years of monitoring, the estrogen and progestin arm of WHI was halted early upon recommendation of its Data and Safety Monitoring Board because overall risks exceeded the benefits. In July 2002, results were released to the media. This preceded journal publication of the data and timely education of health care providers. Chaos ensued while physicians and patients evaluated research facts and before recommendations could be made.

In a subsequent detailed analysis of cardiovascular end points, the hazard for cardiovascular death or nonfatal MI was 1.24. This translated into 188 actual cases in the hormone group and 147 in the placebo group (Anderson, 2004). However, there were no significant differences in coronary revascularization, hospitalization for angina, confirmed angina, acute coronary syndrome, or congestive heart failure.

To explore the timing of HT initiation, Rossouw and colleagues (2007) performed a secondary analysis of the WHI data. They looked specifically at the effect of HT on stroke and CHD rates across categories of age and years since menopause in the combined trial. Women who initiated HT closer to menopause tended to have reduced CHD risk compared with the increase in CHD risk among women more distant from menopause. In women with less than 10 years since their menopause began, the hazard ratio for CHD was 0.76. In those with 10 to 20 years since menopause, the ratio was 1.10; and with 20 or more years, 1.28.

In evaluating data by age, lower risk was found for young women and higher risk for older patients. Specifically, for the age group of 50 to 59 years, the hazard ratio for CHD was 0.93, or two fewer events per 10,000 person years; for the age group 60 to 69 years, 0.98 or 1 fewer event per 10,000 person years; and for those 70 to 79 years, 1.26 or 19 extra events per 10,000 person years. HT increased the stroke risk—the hazard ratio was 1.32—and this risk did not vary significantly by age or time since menopause. Rossouw and colleagues concluded that women who initiated HT closer to menopause tended to have reduced CHD risk compared with the increase in CHD risk among women more distant from menopause. Whether CEE or combined CEE and MPA administration improves the cardiovascular health of women who recently experienced menopause remains to be determined. Presently, evidence is insufficient to suggest that either of these regimens should be initiated or continued for primary or secondary CHD prevention (American College of Obstetricians and Gynecologists, 2013). Although this was the principal analysis conclusion, the results led providers and patients to limited HT use, even for healthy women with bothersome vasomotor symptoms during menopausal transition.

Concurrent with the WHI, a similarly constructed study, the Women's International Study of Long Duration Oestrogen after Menopause (WISDOM), began enrollment in 1999. This trial was stopped following halting of the WHI. Analyzing data collected from this study, Vickers and coworkers (2007) found that HT increases cardiovascular and thromboembolic risk when started many years after the menopause.

With this background in mind, data from no single trial can be extrapolated to all women. In the North American Menopause Society's (2012) hormone therapy position statement, they note that while the WHI is, for some outcomes, the only large long-term RCT of postmenopausal women using HT, the trial has several characteristics that limit generalization to all postmenopausal women. These include the use of only one formulation of estrogen and only one progestin. Unlike most HT studies that focused on symptomatic, recently postmenopausal women, the WHI enrolled generally healthy but older postmenopausal women. These parameters should be accounted for when applying the WHI findings to clinical practice.

CURRENT HORMONE REPLACEMENT ADMINISTRATION

■ Risks and Benefits

As a result of these and other studies, most clinicians agree that HT is associated with an increased risk of CHD in older menopausal women, and an increased risk of breast cancer, stroke,

VTE, and cholecystitis. Breast cancer appears only to be a risk factor with long-term use (>5 years). Two studies have shown an increase in ovarian cancer risk with long-term use (>10 years) but not with short-term use (<5 years) (Danforth, 2007; Lacey, 2006). However, other studies have not confirmed this risk (Noller, 2002).

In contrast, several long-term benefits are noted with HT. These include increased BMD and decreased rates of fracture and colorectal cancer. HT's effects on mortality rates have also been examined. A metaanalysis by Salpeter and associates (2004) pooled data from 26,708 participants to reveal that the mortality rate associated with HT was 0.98. Of note, HT reduced mortality rates in women younger than 60 years but not in women older than 60. These investigators suggest that once CHD is established, HT has no effect in reversing disease progression. Moreover, the incidence of cardiovascular events can potentially increase in older groups due to an increased risk for blood clots. Similarly, Rossouw and colleagues (2007) showed a nonsignificant tendency for the effects of HT on mortality rates to be more favorable in younger than older women.

■ Indications and Contraindications

Based on current literature, HT is indicated only for treatment of vasomotor symptoms and vaginal atrophy and for osteoporosis prevention or treatment. Current guidelines recommend reevaluation of the need for HT at 6- to 12-month intervals. HT is prescribed in the lowest effective dose for the shortest period of time. Accordingly, bone-specific agents would likely be more appropriate in women requiring long-term osteoporosis prevention or treatment.

For women with a uterus, a progestin is combined with an estrogen to lower risks of endometrial cancer. Progestins may be prescribed daily with estrogen, and this dosing is termed continuous therapy. Another suitable continuous oral agent is the combination of CEE plus the selective estrogen-receptor modulator (SERM) bazedoxifene. This is marketed as the drug Duavee.

Instead, HT may be provided in a cyclic regimen. For this, estrogen is administered for 25 days each month and a progestin added for the final 10 days. Drugs are withdrawn for 5 days and endometrial sloughing and bleeding follows. Another common regimen includes treatment with estrogen continuously with a progestin administered for the first 10 days of each month. Such cyclic therapy is most often used in those during menopausal transition, whereas continuous therapy is usually selected for women following menopause.

Oral progestins are most commonly prescribed, although a progestin-releasing intrauterine device (Mirena) provides another promising option for localized rather than systemic progesterone administration in postmenopausal women (Peled, 2007). In addition, combined estrogen and progestin products are available for either oral or transdermal use. Low-dose combination oral contraceptives are effective in the young perimenopausal woman and have the additional benefit of pregnancy prevention.

Importantly, estrogen is contraindicated or evaluated in women who exhibit conditions found in Table 22-1.

TABLE 22-1. Warnings and Precautions with Estrogen Administration

Estrogen should not be used in women with any of the following conditions:

Undiagnosed abnormal genital bleeding
Known, suspected, or history of breast cancer
Known or suspected estrogen-dependent neoplasia
Active or prior venous thromboembolism
Active or recent (e.g., within the past year) arterial thromboembolic disease (e.g., stroke or myocardial infarction)
Liver dysfunction or disease
Known hypersensitivity to the ingredients of the estrogen preparation
Known or suspected pregnancy

Estrogen should be used with caution in women with the following conditions:

Dementia
Gallbladder disease
Hypertriglyceridemia
Prior cholestatic jaundice
Hypothyroidism
Fluid retention plus cardiac or renal dysfunction
Severe hypocalcemia
Prior endometriosis
Hepatic hemangiomas

Data from Food and Drug Administration: Noncontraceptive estrogen drug products for the treatment of vasomotor symptoms and vulvar and vaginal atrophy symptoms—recommended prescribing information for health care providers and patient labeling, 2005.

Ultimately, the decision regarding whether or not to begin HT is a personal one, to be decided by the patient with guidance from her health care provider.

TREATMENT OF VASOMOTOR SYMPTOMS

Common early symptoms of menopause include hot flushes, insomnia, irritability, and mood disorders, which can be caused by vasomotor instability. Physical changes include vaginal atrophy, stress urinary incontinence, and skin atrophy. Long-term health risks that have been attributed to the hormonal changes from menopause include osteoporosis, cardiovascular disease, and, in some studies, Alzheimer disease, macular degeneration, and stroke.

Of these, the most frequent complaint of the menopausal transition is vasomotor symptoms. Also known as hot flushes or hot flashes, their physiology is discussed in Chapter 21 (p. 474). Following menopause, hot flushes are still pervasive and are experienced by 50 to 85 percent of postmenopausal women. Significant distress results for approximately 25 percent of women. Sleep disturbances can lead to lethargy and depressed mood.

The frequency of hot flushes does decrease with time. In the PEPI trial, the percentage of women taking placebo who experienced vasomotor symptoms declined from 56 percent at their entry into the study to 30 percent by their third year in the trial

(Greendale, 1998). Freeman and coworkers (2014) found that moderate to severe hot flushes continue on average for nearly 5 years after menopause, and more than one third of women observed for 10 years or more after menopause have these. Fifteen years after menopause, approximately 3 percent of women report frequent hot flushes, and 12 percent report moderate to severe vasomotor symptoms (Barnabei, 2002; Hays, 2003).

Several treatment options are discussed subsequently, and three have FDA approval for this indication. These are systemic estrogen, one selective serotonin-reuptake inhibitor (SSRI), and the combined CEE plus bazedoxifene agent. When deciding among the available interventions for vasomotor symptoms, the safest options are encouraged first, such as lifestyle changes, but may proceed to prescription treatments, as needed. Patient preference, symptom severity, side effects, and the presence of other comorbid conditions will influence treatment options.

■ Hormonal Therapy

Estrogen

Systemic ET is the most effective treatment for vasomotor symptoms, and the value of such treatment has been demonstrated in numerous RCTs (Nelson, 2004). MacLennan and associates (2004) performed a systematic review of 24 RCTs involving 3329 women who had moderate to severe hot flushes. These investigators found that HT reduced the frequency of hot flushes by approximately 18 events per week, that is, approximately 75 percent compared with placebo. The severity of vasomotor symptoms also was reduced significantly. Moreover, in the PEPI trial, all treatment arms were more effective than placebo in reducing vasomotor symptoms. There were no significant differences between specific hormone regimens (Greendale, 1998).

Estrogen can be administered by oral, parenteral, topical, or transdermal routes with similar effects (Table 22-2). Within these groups, several different formulation choices are available. Continuous estrogen therapy is recommended, although doses and route of administration can be changed relative to patient preference. In the United States, oral estrogens are the most popular. Transdermal estrogen patches avoid the liver's first-pass effect and offer the convenience of less frequent administration (once or twice weekly). The lowest effective dose and duration of therapy are unknown, but this "mantra" is cited by most major menopause organizations for ensuring safety. For treatment of vasomotor symptoms, the FDA has approved all oral estrogen formulations, most transdermal patch formulations, a topical gel, and one intravaginal estrogen product. All systemic HT products except for the ultra-low-dose estradiol transdermal patch (Menostar) have FDA approval for this indication (North American Menopause Society, 2012).

Progestins

These alone are somewhat effective for daily treatment of hot flushes in women for whom estrogen is contraindicated. However, adverse effects that include vaginal bleeding and weight gain may limit their use. Beyond mild reduction in number of hot flushes, progestins used as agents in combined HT offer only one additional benefit. Namely, they provide essential protection against estrogen-induced endometrial hyperplasia and endometrial cancer

TABLE 22-2.   Selected Hormonal Preparations for the Treatment of Menopausal Vasomotor Symptoms

Preparation	Generic Name	Brand Name	Available Strengths
Estrogen			
Oral[a]	CEE	Premarin	0.3, 0.45, 0.625, 0.9, or 1.25 mg
	17β-Estradiol	Estrace[b]	0.5, 1.0, or 2.0 mg
	Estradiol acetate	Femtrace	0.45, 0.9, or 1.8 mg
	10 synthetic estrogens	Enjuvia	0.3, 0.45, 0.625, 0.9, or 1.25 mg
Transdermal Patch	17β-Estradiol	Alora[b]	0.025, 0.05, 0.075, or 0.1 mg/d (patch applied twice weekly to abdomen or buttock; 8 patches/box)
	17β-Estradiol	Climara[b]	0.025, 0.0375, 0.05, 0.06 0.075, or 0.1 mg/d (patch applied to abdomen or buttock weekly; 4 patches/box)
	17β-Estradiol	Menostar[b]	14 μg/d (patch applied to abdomen weekly; 4 patches/box)
	17β-Estradiol	Vivelle-dot[b]	0.025, 0.0375, 0.05, or 0.075, 0.1 mg/d (patch applied twice weekly to abdomen; 8 patches/box)
Transdermal Gel	17β-Estradiol	Estrogel[b]	1 metered dose of gel applied daily to arm (64 doses per 93-g can)
	17β-Estradiol	Estrasorb[b]	Gel from 2 packets applied to legs daily (56 packets/carton)
	17β-Estradiol	Divigel[b]	0.25, 0.5, or 1 mg packets; Gel from 1 packet applied to thigh daily (30 packets/carton)
	17β-Estradiol	Elestrin[b]	1 metered-dose of gel applied to arm daily (30 doses per 35-g container)
	17β-Estradiol	Evamist[b]	1 to 3 metered-dose sprays to forearm daily (56 doses per pump)
Vaginal	Estradiol acetate	Femring	0.05 or 0.1 mg/d (inserted for 90 days)
Progestin			
Oral[a]	MPA	Provera	2.5, 5.0, or 10.0 mg
	Micronized progesterone	Prometrium[b]	200 mg (in peanut oil) (1 daily for 12 days each 28-d cycle)
Vaginal	Progesterone	Prochieve 4%[b]	45 mg
Combination preparations			
Oral sequential[a]	CEE + MPA	Premphase	0.625 mg CEE (red) plus 0.625 mg CEE/5.0 mg MPA (blue) (28 pills per pack; 14 red & 14 blue)[c]
Oral continuous[a]	CEE+ MPA	Prempro	0.3 mg CEE/1.5 mg MPA, or 0.45 mg CEE/1.5 mg MPA, or 0.625 mg CEE/2.5 mg MPA, or 0.625 mg CEE/5 mg MPA (28 pills per pack)
	17β-Estradiol + drospirenone	Angeliq	1 mg E$_2$/0.5 mg drospirenone (28 pills per pack)
	17β-Estradiol + NETA	Activella	1 mg E$_2$/0.5 mg NETA, or 0.5 mg E$_2$/0.1 mg NETA (28 pills per dial pack)
	Ethinyl estradiol + NETA	femhrt	2.5 μg EE/0.5 mg NETA, or 5 μg EE/1 mg NETA
Transdermal continuous	17β-Estradiol + LNG	Climara Pro	0.045 mg/d E$_2$+ 0.015 mg/d LNG (patch applied weekly)
	17β-Estradiol + NETA	CombiPatch	0.05 mg/d E$_2$+ 0.14 mg/d NETA, or 0.05 mg/d E$_2$/0.25 mg/d NETA (patch applied twice weekly to abdomen)
TSEC[a]	CEE + BZA	Duavee	0.45 mg/d CEE + 20 mg BZA

[a]One pill daily.
[b]Considered a bioidentical preparation.
[c]The first 14 pills contain estrogen and the subsequent pills (15 through 28) contain estrogen with progestin.
BZA = bazedoxifene; CEE = conjugated equine estrogen; LNG = levonorgestrel; MPA = medroxyprogesterone acetate; NETA = norethindrone acetate; TSEC = tissue selective estrogen complex.

in women with a uterus. Clinical trials have shown that progestins provide no meaningful increase in estrogen's benefits to bone. Moreover, progestins may attenuate estrogen's beneficial effects on lipids and blood flow and increase the risk for breast cancer.

Bazedoxifene

This SERM combined with CEE was FDA-approved in 2014 for the management of menopausal vasomotor symptoms in women with an intact uterus (Lobo, 2009). As with other SERMs, bazedoxifene (BZA) acts as an estrogen agonist or antagonist, depending on the tissue affected. This combination is called a *tissue-selective estrogen complex (TSEC),* and its advantage is to combine the benefits of CEE with the SERM's ability to offset estrogen stimulation of the endometrium and breast. Thus, a progestin is not required. By itself, BZA reduces BMD loss, increases the number of hot flushes, and raises VTE risks. The combination of BZA 20 mg plus CEE 0.45 mg reduces BMD loss and incidence of hot flushes but does not increase VTE rates compared with CEE and MPA. Notably, BZA acts as an antagonist in uterine tissue to prevent the endometrial hyperplasia commonly associated with unopposed estrogen (Pinkerton, 2014).

In the randomized Selective estrogens, Menopause, and Response to Therapy (SMART-2) trial, BZA plus CEE reduced hot flush frequency by 74 percent at week 12 compared with a 51-percent reduction from placebo (Pinkerton, 2009). A secondary efficacy analysis of SMART-2 data assessed sleep parameters and health-related quality of life in 318 women experiencing >7 moderate to severe hot flushes daily. Time to fall asleep, sleep disturbance, and sleep adequacy were improved with BZA plus CEE compared with placebo. This dose also significantly improved the vasomotor function score and the Menopause-Specific Quality of Life (MENQOL) questionnaire score compared with placebo (Utian, 2009). Overall the BZA plus CEE combined agent is well tolerated and effective in treated hot flushes, but its effectiveness relative to HT remains uncertain.

Bioidentical Hormones

Some women believe that conventional FDA-regulated pharmaceutical estrogens and progestins hold a clear and present danger. Ironically, more is known about the absolute risks and benefits of HT than almost any other class of drugs. Although prescriptions for estrogen and progesterone have declined significantly since publication of the WHI results, the use of "bioidentical hormones" has increased. This term invented by marketers is often used to describe custom-compounded HT products but has no clear scientific meaning (Shifren, 2014). The term now usually refers to compounds that have the same chemical and molecular structure as hormones that are produced in the body.

Custom compounding of HT may combine several hormones (e.g., estradiol, estrone, and estriol) and use nonstandard routes of administration (e.g., subdermal implants). Some of the hormones are not FDA approved (estriol) or monitored, and some compounded therapies contain nonhormonal ingredients (e.g., dyes, preservatives) that some women cannot tolerate. Moreover, custom-compounded formulations have not been tested for efficacy or safety; product information is not

consistently provided to women along with their prescription, as is required with commercially available HT; and batch standardization and purity may be uncertain. Thus, these hormones cannot be assumed to be safer than conventional pharmaceutical estrogen or progestins. Several organizations note that conventional FDA-approved HT products are preferred to custom-compounded formulations (American College of Obstetricians and Gynecologists, 2014a; North American Menopause Society, 2012). In conjunction with bioidentical hormones, salivary hormone testing to assist with hormone level adjustment is inaccurate and unreliable (Lewis, 2002; Zava, 1998).

■ Central Nervous System Agents

Several nonhormonal therapies are available to treat vasomotor symptoms (Table 22-3). Alternatively, women who are principally bothered by night sweats and sleep disruption may benefit from a trial of sleep medication, and options are listed in Table 1-16 (p. 18). Of vasomotor symptom therapies, SSRIs, selective norepinephrine-reuptake inhibitors (SNRIs), clonidine, and gabapentin have demonstrated benefits compared with placebo (American College of Obstetricians and Gynecologists, 2014b). Of these, only the SSRI paroxetine mesylate (Brisdelle) is FDA-approved for vasomotor symptom treatment.

For many, the side effects or relative ineffectiveness of these agents compared with estrogen therapy can limit their routine use for this indication. Moreover, long-term studies with any of these agents for vasomotor symptom treatment are not available.

Serotonin and Norepinephrine

As noted in Chapter 21 (p. 474), both serotonin and norepinephrine are implicated in modulation of the thermoregulatory setpoint, which is integral to hot flushes. Accordingly, SSRIs have been studied, and in two RCTs, the low-dose mesylate salt of paroxetine (LDMP) was given to postmenopausal women experiencing daily, moderate to severe hot flushes. One study lasted 12 weeks, and the other 24 weeks (Simon, 2013). In

TABLE 22-3. Nonhormonal Agents Used for Vasomotor Symptoms

Prescription (brand name)	Dose[a]
SSRI	
Paroxetine mesylate (Brisdelle)	7.5 mg
Paroxetine (Paxil)	20 mg
Venlafaxine (Effexor XR)	75 mg
Citalopram (Celexa)	20 mg
Escitalopram (Lexapro)	10–20 mg
Sertraline (Zoloft)	50 mg
Fluoxetine (Prozac, Sarafem)	20 mg
SNRI: Desvenlafaxine (Pristiq)	100 mg
Clonidine (Catapres)	0.1 mg
Gabapentin (Neurontin)	600–900 mg

[a]Oral daily dosing.
SNRI = selective norepinephrine- reuptake inhibitor;
SSRI = selective serotonin-reuptake inhibitor.

both trials, LDMP reduced the weekly *frequency* of hot flushes compared with placebo, but persistent declines in hot flush *severity* were less consistent (Carris, 2014). Following initiation, frequency reduction begins as early as 1 week after therapy, and for severity reduction, as early as 2 weeks.

Other SSRIs have also been studied. With venlafaxine extended release (Effexor XR), Evans and coworkers (2005) noted 51-percent fewer hot flushes compared with placebo. Several other trials have compared this same SSRI with gabapentin or with clonidine in breast cancer survivors with hot flushes and also showed symptom benefit from the SSRI (Boekhout, 2011; Bordeleau, 2010; Loprinzi, 2000). Joffe and associates (2014) compared venlafaxine and low-dose estrogen and noted that estradiol reduced hot flushes by 2.3 events daily compared with 1.8 for the SSRI. Both outperformed placebo.

With paroxetine (Paxil) modest improvement in hot flushes are seen compared with placebo. In one RCT, a 20-mg dose lowered hot flush frequency by 51 percent. Stearns and coworkers (2003) evaluated paroxetine CR, 12.5 mg/d and 25 mg/d dosages, compared with placebo. At both dosages, paroxetine led to approximately three fewer hot flushes per day compared with 1.8 fewer per day with placebo.

With citalopram (Celexa), mean hot flush scores were lowered by 37 to 50 percent (Barton, 2010; Kalay, 2007). With escitalopram (Lexapro), two RCTs noted significant improvement compared with placebo (Carpenter, 2012; Freeman, 2011). Of the SSRIs, fluoxetine (Prozac, Sarafem) and sertraline (Zoloft) appear to be less effective (Gordon, 2006; Grady, 2007; Loprinzi, 2002; Suvanto-Luukkonen, 2005).

Of the SNRIs, desvenlafaxine (Pristiq) significantly reduces the number of hot flushes by approximately 60 percent and their severity by 25 percent compared with placebo (Archer, 2009a,b; Speroff, 2008). A 1-year study noted that these improvements persisted (Pinkerton, 2013).

Importantly, benefits of SSRIs are balanced against drug side effects, which can include nausea, headache, diarrhea, insomnia, jitteriness, fatigue, and sexual dysfunction. With the SNRIs, hypertension may also be aggravated (Handley, 2015).

Clonidine

The centrally active α_2-adrenergic receptor agonist clonidine (Catapres) has been effective in some clinical trials (Nagamani, 1987). Many of these RCTs specifically evaluated benefits for breast cancer survivors and showed improvement in vasomotor symptoms (Boekhout, 2011; Buijs, 2009; Loibl, 2007). Notably, hypotension, dry mouth, dizziness, constipation, and sedation may limit its use. For many women, low-dose clonidine is ineffective, and thus adequate therapy may require substantially higher doses that may magnify side effects.

Gabapentin

Gabapentin (Neurontin) is structurally related to the neurotransmitter γ-aminobutyric acid (GABA), but its exact mechanism of action is unknown. Currently, gabapentin is FDA-approved to treat seizures and neuropathic pain. However, it has extensive off-label use for various other neurologic conditions.

In 2003, Guttuso and colleagues evaluated the use of gabapentin, 900 mg daily, for treatment of vasomotor symptoms.

They found a 45-percent reduction in hot flush frequency compared with a 29-percent reduction with placebo. Moreover, Reddy and coworkers (2006) conducted an RCT in which 60 postmenopausal women received gabapentin, 2400 mg/d; oral CEE, 0.625 mg/d; or placebo for 12 weeks. The reductions in the hot flush composite scores for both estrogen (72 percent) and gabapentin (71 percent) were greater than that associated with placebo (54 percent). However, headache, dizziness, and disorientation occurred in almost 25 percent of the women treated with gabapentin.

■ Complementary and Alternative Medicine

Phytoestrogens

Phytoestrogens (isoflavones) are plant-derived compounds that bind to estrogen receptors and have both estrogen agonist and antagonist properties. They are found in soy products and red clover. In sum and outlined subsequently, data supporting their effectiveness for vasomotor symptom treatment show no conclusive efficacy (Lethaby, 2013).

With soy products, although the mechanisms of action are not fully understood, they appear to bind to the estrogen receptor. For this reason, one should not assume these dietary supplements are safe for women with estrogen-dependent cancers. That said, sonographic surveillance has not shown increased endometrial thickness or altered lipid profiles in women taking isoflavones (Palacios, 2010; Quaas, 2013; Ye, 2012). For treatment of hot flushes, data supporting isoflavone efficacy are mixed (Albertazzi, 1998; Cheng, 2007; Liu, 2014; Quella, 2000). Moreover, the effects of soy protein found in various food preparations are not bioequivalent. Even soy foods are not necessarily reliable sources of biologically active isoflavones.

Flaxseed or flaxseed oil (*Linum usitatissimum*) is rich in α-linolenic acid, a form of omega-3 fatty acid. Also known as linseed, flaxseed is touted to reduce vasomotor symptoms. However, data regarding its efficacy for this indication are contradictory (Lemay, 2002; Lewis, 2006; Pruthi, 2012).

Red clover (*Trifolium pretense*) is a member of the legume family. It contains at least four estrogenic isoflavones and is therefore marketed as a phytoestrogen source. Several studies and analyses, however, have failed to demonstrate an effect over placebo in the treatment of menopausal symptoms (Geller, 2009; Nelson, 2006; Tice, 2003).

Dong quai, also translated as don kwai, dang gui, and tang kuei, is a Chinese herbal medicine derived from the root of *Angelica sinensis* and is the most commonly prescribed Chinese herbal medicine for "female problems." Within traditional Chinese medicine practice, dong quai is suggested to exert estrogenic activity. In most studies, however, its benefit cannot be substantiated (Haines, 2008; Hirata, 1997). Notably, dong quai contains numerous coumarin-like derivatives and may cause excessive bleeding or interactions with other anticoagulants. This herbal agent also contains psoralens and is potentially photosensitizing.

Black cohosh (*Cimifuga racemosa*) is also thought to have estrogenic properties, although its mechanism of action is unknown. In their Cochrane Review, Leach and Moore (2012) found insufficient evidence to support its use for vasomotor symptom relief. Although few adverse effects have been reported, the long-term safety of this product is unknown.

Phytoprogestins

Extracts, tablets, and creams derived from yams are claimed to be progesterone substitutes. Specifically, claims are made that the plant sterol dioscorea is converted into progesterone in the body and alleviates "estrogen dominance." However, there is no human biochemical pathway for bioconversion of dioscorea to progesterone in vivo.

In contrast, Mexican yam extract contains considerable diosgenin, an estrogen-like substance found in plants. Some estrogen effects might be expected from eating these yam species, but only if large quantities of raw yams are consumed. Yams from the grocery store generally are not the varieties known to contain significant amounts of dioscorea or diosgenin.

Based on the lack of bioavailability, the hormones in wild and Mexican yam would not be expected to have efficacy. Wild yam extracts are neither estrogenic nor progestational, and although many yam extract products contain no yam, some are laced with progestins. There are no published reports demonstrating the effectiveness of wild yam cream for postmenopausal symptoms. Moreover, oral ingestion does not produce serum levels.

Vitamin E

In a few studies in breast cancer survivors, vitamin E provided minimal or no vasomotor symptom improvement (Biglia, 2009; Rada, 2010).

Lifestyle Changes

Practices that lower core body temperature such as cooling the room, dressing in layers, and consuming cool drinks may temporarily help with night sweats and flushing (American College of Obstetricians and Gynecologists, 2014b). However, behavioral efforts to curb the frequency of hot flushes have no firm support in RCTs. For example, little evidence demonstrates

the efficacy of relaxation techniques, acupuncture, exercise, and yoga to control vasomotor complaints (Daley, 2014; Dodin, 2013; Newton, 2014; Saensak, 2014).

TREATMENT OF OSTEOPOROSIS

Indications

The primary goal of osteoporosis treatment is fracture prevention in women who have low BMD or additional risk factors for fracture (Fig. 22-1). Toward this end, therapy aims to stabilize or increase BMD. Treatment includes lifestyle changes and often pharmacologic therapy. The key lifestyle modifications that can decrease fracture risks of in postmenopausal women include regular weight-bearing exercise and a balanced diet with adequate calcium and vitamin D. Factors for patients to avoid include smoking, an excessively low body weight, excessive alcohol intake, and fall risks at home (Christiansen, 2013).

With pharmacologic therapy, several organizations offer guidelines. The National Osteoporosis Foundation (NOF) (2014), American Association of Clinical Endocrinologists (AACE) (Watts, 2010), and North American Menopause Society (NAMS) (2010) recommend starting therapy for: (1) all postmenopausal women with total hip, femoral neck, or spine T-scores at or below −2.5; (2) for those with an osteoporotic vertebral or hip fracture; and (3) all postmenopausal women with total hip or spine T-scores from −1.0 to −2.5 who have one or more additional risk factors for fracture, such as those in Table 21-8 (p. 480).

Drugs prescribed for fracture prevention attempt to restore and balance bone remodeling by: (1) reducing bone resorption, termed *antiresorptive agents*, or (2) stimulating bone formation, termed *anabolic agents*. Most of the bone-active agents currently available in the United States inhibit bone resorption. Estrogen, SERMs, bisphosphonates, denosumab, calcitonin, and vitamin D each have antiresorptive properties

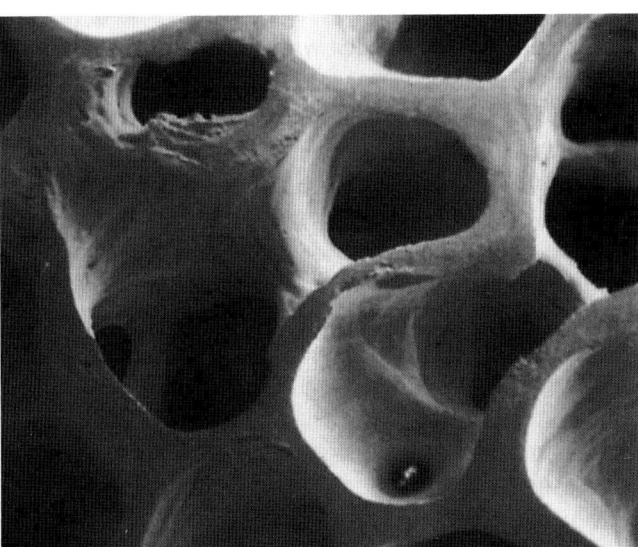 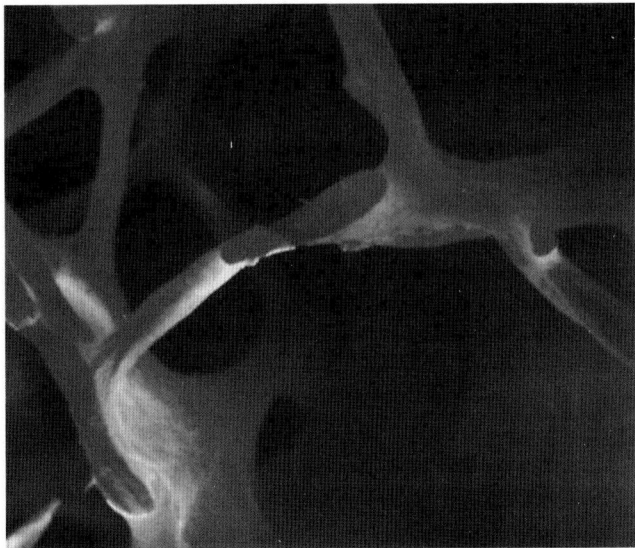

FIGURE 22-1 Electron micrographs of tissue obtained from iliac crest biopsy. Normal bone architecture in an individual with normal bone mineral density (*left*). Diminished bone architecture is seen in the biopsy from an individual with osteoporosis (*right*) (Reproduced with permission from Dempster DW, Shane E, Horbert W, et al: A simple method for correlative light and scanning electron microscopy of human iliac crest bone biopsies: qualitative observations in normal and osteoporotic subjects, J Bone Miner Res 1986 Feb;1(1):15–21.)

TABLE 22-4. Agents Approved in the United States for the Management of Osteoporosis[a]

Agent	Brand Name	Clinical Indication	
		Prevention	**Treatment**
Bisphosphonates			
Alendronate	Fosamax	5 mg pill once daily 35 mg pill once wkly	10 mg pill once daily 70 mg pill or solution once weekly
	Binosto	–	70 mg solution once weekly
Ibandronate	Boniva	2.5 mg pill once daily 150 mg pill once monthly	2.5 mg pill once daily 150 mg pill once monthly
Risedronate	Actonel	5 mg pill once daily 35 mg pill once wkly	5 mg pill once daily 35 mg pill once weekly 150 mg pill once monthly 75 mg pill on two consecutive days as a monthly dose
Risedronate (enteric coated)	Atelvia	–	35 mg pill once weekly
Zoledronate	Reclast	5 mg IV every 2 years	5 mg IV yearly
Hormones			
CEE	Premarin	0.3 mg pill daily	
Other estrogens	See Table 22-2		
Monoclonal antibody			
Denosumab	Prolia	–	60 mg SC once every 6 months
Recombinant human parathyroid hormone			
Teriparatide	Forteo	–	20 μg SC daily. 1 injection pen contains 28 doses
Salmon calcitonin			
Nasal spray	Fortical	–	1 spray = 200 IU intranasally daily (alternating nostrils daily). 1 bottle contains a 30-day supply
	Miacalcin	–	1 spray = 200 IU intranasally daily (alternating nostrils daily). 1 bottle contains a 30-day supply
Injectable	Miacalcin	–	100 units SC or IM every other day. 1 vial contains 4 doses
SERM			
Raloxifene	Evista	60 mg once daily	60 mg once daily
TSEC			
CEE/BZA	Duavee	0.45 mg/20 mg pill once daily	

[a]Oral agent unless route indicated.
BZA = bazedoxifene; CEE = conjugated equine estrogen; IM = intramuscular injection; IU = international units; IV = intravenous; SC = subcutaneous injection; SERM = selective estrogen-receptor modulator; TSEC = tissue-selective estrogen complex.

(Table 22-4). All have been shown to halt bone loss, and most also increase BMD. Improvement in BMD with therapeutic intervention varies according to bone composition. Therapies that prevent bone resorption will act most quickly on bone that has high trabecular content and rapid turnover, such as the vertebrae. Alternatively, the impact of drug therapies on the hip may be delayed because the hip is composed of approximately 50 percent trabecular and 50 percent cortical bone (Fig. 21-5, p. 476). In contrast to these antiresorptive agents, recombinant parathyroid hormone (PTH 1–34), known as teriparatide, is anabolic and leads to BMD increases.

For osteoporosis, each agent differs in its indication for prevention, for treatment, or both. HT is indicated for the prevention of osteoporosis. Bisphosphonates and SERMs can be used for prevention and for treatment. Calcitonin and teriparatide are approved for treatment. Denosumab is a monoclonal antibody to the receptor activator of nuclear factor (RANK) ligand and is approved for osteoporosis treatment.

Hormonal Therapy
Estrogen and Progesterone Replacement

As estrogen levels decline, bone-remodeling rates increase and favor bone resorption over bone formation. In observational studies, HT reduces osteoporosis-related fractures by approximately 50 percent when started soon after menopause. Continued long term, HT significantly decreases fracture rates in women with established disease (Tosteson, 2008). Results from 57 randomized, placebo-controlled trials show that HT reduces the rate of bone resorption and results in an increase in BMD (Wells, 2002). The WHI controlled trials confirmed a significant 33-percent reduction in hip fractures in healthy postmenopausal women receiving HT after an average follow-up of 5.6 years. Notably, hip fracture reduction was not limited to women with osteoporosis, as in trials of other pharmacologic agents (The Women's Health Initiative Steering Committee, 2004). Even very low estrogen doses combined with calcium and vitamin D produce significant increases in BMD compared with placebo (Ettinger, 2004; Prestwood, 2003). Specifically, oral daily 0.2-mg doses of estradiol; 0.3-mg doses of CEE; or transdermal estradiol patch delivering 0.014 mg/d are suitable.

Unfortunately, this preventive effect is lost rapidly following HT discontinuation (Barrett-Connor, 2003). Women participating in the National Osteoporosis Risk Assessment (NORA) trial who had discontinued estrogen therapy within the 5 years preceding the study demonstrated a significantly higher hip fracture risk than did women who had never received estrogen therapy. In addition, current HT users in the NORA trial had a 40-percent reduction in hip fractures, which was lost by past users. Thus, fracture risk and the potential need for an alternative therapy is ideally assessed when women discontinue HT.

Bazedoxifene

The drug that combines CEE with the SERM bazedoxifene is indicated to alleviate vasomotor symptoms and prevent postmenopausal bone loss. In the randomized SMART trials noted earlier (p. 497), investigators found a significantly increased adjusted mean percentage BMD change in the lumbar spine from baseline to 24 months in those taking BZA plus CEE compared with women using placebo (Lindsay, 2009). Findings were similar for total hip BMD. Moreover, the FDA-approved dose of CEE (0.45 mg) plus BZA (20 mg) does not cause a change in breast density or endometrial thickness compared with placebo (Pinkerton, 2014).

Raloxifene

This SERM is approved for the prevention and treatment of osteoporosis and to reduce the risk of invasive breast cancer. It activates estrogen receptors in the bone but does not appear to activate those in the breast or uterus.

Of bone loss sites, raloxifene may be most appropriate for prevention and treatment of vertebral disease. For example,

raloxifene prevented vertebral fractures in the Multiple Outcomes of Raloxifene Evaluation (MORE) trial, which enrolled 7705 postmenopausal women with osteoporosis. The beneficial effects of oral raloxifene, 60 mg/d, appeared rapidly, and clinical vertebral fracture risk was reduced by 68 percent following the first year of therapy. In addition, this effect was sustained over time. At 4 years of treatment, dosages of 60 mg daily led to a 36-percent reduction in fractures, and 120 mg each day produced a 43-percent decline (Delmas, 2002; Ettinger, 1999). However, in the MORE trial, Ettinger and associates (1999) reported that raloxifene therapy compared with placebo was not associated with significant reductions in nonvertebral fracture risks at 3 and 4 years. A more recent retrospective cohort study showed that patients treated with alendronate and raloxifene had similar adjusted fracture rates in up to 8 years of compliant treatment (Foster, 2013).

In 2012, Chung and colleagues showed that raloxifene, but not bisphosphonates, significantly suppressed circulating concentration of sclerostin, an inhibitor of bone formation, suggesting that sclerostin may in part mediate the action of estrogen on bone metabolism.

In addition to its bone effects, raloxifene may protect against breast cancer, as suggested by observational studies of various clinical trials (Barrett-Connor, 2006). The incidence of breast cancer was evaluated as a secondary end point in the MORE trial. Investigators found that raloxifene was associated with a 65-percent relative risk reduction in all breast cancers. Of specific breast cancer subtypes, they noted a 90-percent reduction in estrogen receptor–positive cancers, a 12-percent reduction in estrogen receptor–negative breast cancers, and a 76-percent relative risk reduction in invasive breast cancer.

Raloxifene may not have the same increased cardiovascular risk profile as estrogen. In a MORE post hoc analysis, 4 years of raloxifene therapy had no adverse effect on cardiovascular events in the overall cohort. Advantageously, it did result in a significant 40-percent reduction in the incidence of cardiovascular events among a subgroup of women with increased cardiovascular risk (Barrett-Connor, 2002).

Of side effects, hot flushes are associated with raloxifene therapy, although the incidence is low (Cohen, 2000). In addition, raloxifene, 60 mg daily for 4 years, has been associated with an increased risk of thromboembolic events. In one study, the relative risk associated with any dosage of raloxifene was 2.76 for deep-vein thrombosis, 2.76 for pulmonary embolism, and 0.50 for retinal vein thrombosis (Delmas, 2002). It is therefore contraindicated in patients with a history of VTE and is used with caution in women with hepatic or moderate to severe renal impairment.

Nonhormonal Antiresorptive Agents
Bisphosphonates

Four bisphosphonates are currently available and include alendronate (Fosamax, Binosto), risedronate (Actonel, Atelvia), ibandronate (Boniva), and zoledronate (Reclast). The first three are taken orally, but zoledronate is an intravenous infusion. These agents chemically bind to calcium hydroxyapatite in bone (Figs. 22-2 and 22-3). They decrease bone resorption

Bisphosphonates   **Pyrophosphates**

$$OH-\overset{\overset{O}{\|}}{P}-\overset{\overset{R_1}{|}}{\underset{\underset{R_2}{|}}{C}}-\overset{\overset{O}{\|}}{P}-OH \qquad OH-\overset{\overset{O}{\|}}{P}-O-\overset{\overset{O}{\|}}{P}-OH$$

FIGURE 22-2 The molecular structure of bisphosphonates, with two short side chains (R₁ and R₂) attached to the C core, is similar to that of the naturally occurring pyrophosphates. Variations in side-chain structure determine the strength with which the bisphosphonate binds to bone, the distribution throughout bone, and the amount of time it remains in the bone after treatment is discontinued.

by blocking the function and survival but not the formation of osteoclasts (Diab, 2012; Russell, 2008).

The oral bisphosphonates display poor bioavailability and therefore are taken on an empty stomach with adequate water for proper dissolution and absorption. In general, these agents have a favorable overall safety profile, and adverse event rates are comparable with placebo (Black, 1996; Harris, 1999). However, bisphosphonates may cause upper gastrointestinal inflammation, ulceration, and bleeding (Lanza, 2000). Thus, to aid delivery to the stomach and reduce the risk of esophageal irritation, dosing instructions are reinforced with each patient.

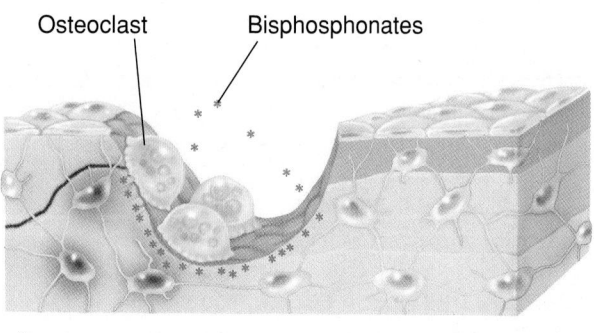

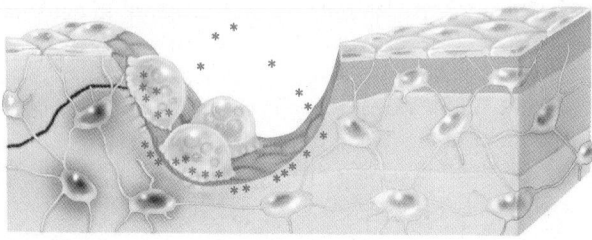

FIGURE 22-3 Bisphosphonates reduce fractures by suppressing bone resorption by osteoclasts. The molecular structure of the bisphosphonates is analogous to that of the naturally occurring pyrophosphates. **A.** Bisphosphonate concentration is increased eightfold at sites of active bone resorption. **B.** The bisphosphonates enter osteoclasts and reduce resorption through inhibition of farnesyl pyrophosphate synthase. Inhibition of this enzyme leads to disruption of osteoclast attachment to the bone surface. This halts resorption and promotes early osteoclast cell death.

First, bisphosphonates are taken in the morning with a full glass of water. During the 30 minutes following administration, no other food or beverages are consumed. Finally, women must remain upright (sitting or standing) for at least 30 minutes after ingesting the drug.

In terms of long-term safety, concerns about two uncommon adverse events have emerged: osteonecrosis of the jaw (ONJ) and atypical femur fractures (AFFs) (Diab, 2013). ONJ is defined as exposed necrotic bone in the maxillofacial region that fails to heal after 8 weeks. It can be associated with pain, paresthesia, soft tissue ulceration and swelling, and loosening of teeth. This can develop spontaneously but is generally associated with invasive dental procedures. ONJ has been described in patients receiving chronic bisphosphonate therapy for osteoporosis treatment but appears to be much more common in cancer patients receiving higher-dose bisphosphonates (Khosia, 2007).

AFFs are stress fractures that are frequently bilateral, are typically associated with minimal or no trauma, and are heralded by prodromal pain in the fracture region (Dell, 2012). One case-controlled study found that longer bisphosphonate use (5 to 9 years) was associated with a greater risk of AFFs compared with shorter use (<2 years) (Meier, 2012). One review showed that bisphosphonate exposure was associated with an increased risk of AFF and an adjusted risk ration of 1.70 (Gedmintas, 2013). However, in this analysis, the large variation in relative risks reported in the different studies suggests significant heterogeneity in the patient populations.

No causal relationship has been established between prolonged bisphosphonate exposure and either of these outcomes. Even though the risks of ONJ and AFF may increase after 5 years of bisphosphonate therapy, the likelihood remains low. The FDA suggests reevaluating individually the need for continuing bisphosphonate therapy beyond 3 to 5 years (Whitaker, 2012). A "drug holiday" may be considered because of the unique pharmacokinetics of bisphosphonate. These agents accumulate in the skeleton to create a reservoir that continues to be released for months or years after treatment. Although this provides some residual benefit in terms of fracture reduction after an initial 3- to 5-year course of therapy, continuing treatment for 10 years seems to be a better choice for high-risk patients. If a drug holiday is advised, risk is reevaluated sooner for drugs with lower skeletal affinity. Thus, reassessment may be prudent after 1 year for risedronate, 1 to 2 years for alendronate, and 2 to 3 years for zoledronate (Diab, 2014).

Alendronate. This bisphosphonate is approved for the treatment and prevention of osteoporosis. Alendronate has been shown to reduce the risk of vertebral fractures in postmenopausal women with low BMD or osteoporosis, either with or without existing vertebral fractures (Black, 1996). Alendronate also reduces nonvertebral fracture risk in women with osteoporosis. Among women with osteoporosis who participated in the Fracture Intervention Trial (FIT), the risk of nonvertebral fractures was reduced by month 24. In addition, the effects of alendronate are sustained. For example, women who used alendronate for 5 years and then discontinued use for a subsequent 5 years had nonvertebral fracture rates comparable to those of women using the drug for 10 years (Black, 2006; Bone, 2004).

Risedronate. This bisphosphonate is an effective agent in the prevention and treatment of postmenopausal osteoporosis. The strongest data supporting its efficacy stem from the Vertebral Efficacy with Risedronate Therapy (VERT) trials, conducted multinationally and also in North America. In the VERT multinational trial, Reginster and coworkers (2000) showed that risedronate reduced the risk of new vertebral fractures by 61 percent at 1 year and by 49 percent at 3 years of use. Moreover, both VERT trials found significant reductions in vertebral fractures as early as 6 months after initiation of risedronate therapy (Roux, 2004). Two extensions of these trials have provided evidence of sustained efficacy. The continuation of risedronate therapy for 2 additional years (5 years total) in the multinational VERT study was associated with a 59-percent reduction in new vertebral fractures compared with placebo.

Ibandronate. This bisphosphonate is approved for the prevention and treatment of postmenopausal osteoporosis. Ibandronate is an effective agent, and data from the Oral Ibandronate Osteoporosis Vertebral Fracture Trial in North America and Europe (BONE) trial showed that daily ibandronate lowered incident vertebral fracture risk by 62 percent (Chesnut, 2004). To improve compliance, this drug was evaluated as a once-monthly therapy. Once-monthly oral ibandronate is at least as effective and well tolerated as daily treatment (Miller, 2005; Reginster, 2006). Moreover, once-monthly administration may be more convenient and thereby improve compliance rates.

Zoledronate. This bisphosphonate is approved for the prevention and treatment of postmenopausal osteoporosis. Zoledronate is effective, and data from the Health Outcomes and Reduced Incidence with Zoledronic Acid Once Yearly (HORIZON) Pivotal Fracture Trial showed that yearly zoledronate infusion lowered incident vertebral fracture risk by 70 percent compared with placebo (Black, 2007).

Denosumab

This is a fully human monoclonal antibody to RANK ligand, which is described and illustrated in Chapter 21 (p. 476). To summarize, denosumab's binding to RANK ligand inhibits osteoclast development and activity. This in turn decreases bone resorption and increases BMD. In a manufacturer-sponsored trial, 7868 women randomly received either denosumab or placebo subcutaneously every 6 months for 3 years (Cummings, 2009). Relative risk for new radiographically diagnosed vertebral fractures was 68-percent lower in the denosumab group. The risk for hip fractures was 40-percent lower in the denosumab group. Overall incidence of significant adverse events was similar between groups.

Calcitonin

The polypeptide hormone calcitonin decreases the rate of bone absorption by inhibiting resorptive activity in osteoclasts. Calcitonin is a protein, and as such, oral administration leads to its digestion. For this reason, it is delivered as an injection or nasal spray (Fortical, Miacalcin). Salmon calcitonin nasal spray has been associated with a reduction in vertebral fracture risk among postmenopausal women with osteoporosis. In the Prevent Recurrence of Osteoporotic Fractures (PROOF) study, calcitonin nasal spray, 200 IU administered daily for up to 5 years reduced the risk of vertebral fractures by 33 percent compared with placebo. However, vertebral fracture reduction was not seen at lower (100 IU/d) or higher (400 IU/d) dosages (Chesnut, 2000). Moreover, in this study, calcitonin failed to produce significant reductions in nonvertebral fracture.

Some observational data suggest that calcitonin has an analgesic effect independent of its effect on bone (Häuselmann, 2003; Ofluoglu, 2007). This analgesic effect may make this agent particularly useful as an adjunct to other therapies for osteoporosis in women with painful, symptomatic fracture (Blau, 2003). Injectable or intranasal calcitonin is associated with an 8- to 10-percent incidence of nausea or gastric discomfort and a 10-percent incidence of local site reactions. These symptoms tend to decrease in severity with continued use. Nasal symptoms such as rhinitis occur in 3 percent of patients treated with intranasal calcitonin (Cranney, 2002).

■ Parathyroid Hormone

Recombinant parathyroid hormone (PTH 1–34), known as teriparatide, is given by daily subcutaneous injection and is approved by the FDA for the treatment of postmenopausal women with established osteoporosis, who are at high risk for fracture. Teriparatide (Forteo) increases osteoblast numbers and activity by recruiting new cells and reducing apoptosis of differentiated osteoblasts. At low daily doses of teriparatide, the anabolic effects of PTH predominate. This is in contrast to the catabolic effects generally associated with long-term, higher-dose, and chronic exposure to PTH.

Clinical studies indicate that teriparatide increases bone quality by increasing bone density, turnover, and size (Rubin, 2002). Moreover, improvements in microarchitectural elements are evident in both cancellous and cortical regions. In women with postmenopausal osteoporosis, teriparatide, 20 or 40 μg/d, administered for approximately 21 months, was associated with 65-percent and 69-percent reductions in vertebral fractures, and 35-percent and 40-percent reductions in nonvertebral fractures, respectively (Neer, 2001).

Similar findings were reported in a study of 52 women treated with concomitant teriparatide and HT compared with HT alone (Lindsay, 1997). In this study, at the end of 3 years, increases in vertebral, total hip, and total body BMD were 13.4 percent, 4.4 percent, and 3.7 percent, respectively, in the combined treatment group. The addition of alendronate to teriparatide, however, does not appear to enhance effects on BMD (Gasser, 2000). The effects of combination use of PTH with other bisphosphonates are not known.

In general, PTH is safe and well tolerated, although additional data from long-term studies are needed. The most frequent treatment-related adverse events in clinical trials of teriparatide were dizziness, leg cramps, nausea, and headache. Toxicity studies with rats have shown an increased risk of osteosarcoma. However, there are significant differences in bone metabolism between rats and humans, and the applicability of rat data to humans is unclear. That said, a black box warning has been included on the product labeling in the United States, and teriparatide use is avoided by patients at increased risk for skeletal malignancy. Use for more than 2 years is not recommended due to the potential for side effects (Tashjian, 2002).

In sum, denosumab seems to be as effective as teriparatide and zoledronate. Osteonecrosis of the jaw and fragility fractures associated with long-term bisphosphonate use are unlikely to be linked to short-acting agents such as denosumab. Because denosumab is an antibody, its potential to affect the immune system requires scrutiny. Long-term adherence to oral bisphosphonate therapy is often poor, making the relative ease of biannual injections attractive. Although teriparatide and intravenous bisphosphonates are expensive, weekly oral alendronate is available at low cost as a generic. Clinically, cost will likely play a central role in determining how these agents are selected.

■ Nonpharmacologic Therapy

Calcium

Nonpharmacologic interventions are cornerstones of osteoporosis prevention and include dietary modifications, exercise programs, fall prevention strategies, and education. Of these, adequate daily calcium intake is essential for bone maintenance. For women aged 31 to 50 years, the recommended dietary reference intake (DRI) is 1000 mg daily, and for those 51 years and older, 1200 mg is recommend daily. Ideally, these DRIs are obtained through diet alone, but supplementation is used to attain these levels if needed (Institute of Medicine, 2010; Prentice, 2013). Few women meet these goals, and calcium deficiency is widespread. For example, more than 90 percent of women fail to take in enough dietary calcium to meet DRIs put forth by the Institute of Medicine. Although poor calcium intake is observed at all ages, it appears to be most common among older individuals. Specifically, fewer than 1 percent of women 71 years or older actually meet recommended goals.

Calcium supplementation combined with vitamin D administration has been associated with reduced bone loss and decreased risk for fractures in several prospective studies (Chapuy, 1992; Dawson-Hughes, 1997; Larsen, 2004). Prentice and associates (2013) examined the health benefits and risk of calcium and vitamin D supplementation using data from the WHI. This showed a substantial reduction in hip fracture risk. Notably, supplementation must be continued long term for efficacy to be sustained.

Vitamin D

The DRI of vitamin D is 600 IU daily for a postmenopausal woman who is not at high risk for fractures or falls. For persons who have a high risk of osteoporosis or who are older than 70, 800 IU daily is recommended (Institute of Medicine, 2010). As with calcium, the prevalence of vitamin D deficiency is high, especially in the elderly. Deficiency leads to poor calcium absorption, secondary hyperparathyroidism, increased bone turnover, increased rates of bone loss, and, if severe, impaired bone mineralization. In addition, vitamin D deficiency causes muscle weakness and is associated with an increase in rates of falls. Vitamin D supplementation can reverse many of these effects and significantly reduce falls and hip fractures (Dawson-Hughes, 1997).

The metabolite 25-hydroxyvitamin D is considered to be the best clinical measure of vitamin D stores (Rosen, 2011). Vitamin D *deficiency* is defined as a 25-hydroxyvitamin D serum level below 10 ng/mL. Vitamin D *insufficiency* is a serum level of 25-hydroxyvitamin D between 10 and 30 ng/mL.

Diet

A relationship between protein intake and BMD has been reported, but a relationship with fractures has not been described. Using data from the Third National Health and Nutrition Examination Survey (NHANES III), Kerstetter and colleagues (2000) demonstrated a significant association between protein intake and total femur BMD among non-Hispanic white women aged 50 years and older. Moreover, protein supplementation (20 g/d) five times weekly for 6 months following hip fracture was associated with a 50-percent reduction in femoral bone loss at 1 year compared with placebo.

Although no specific recommendations regarding protein intake can be made based on the limited data available, it seems prudent for clinicians to ensure that their patients eat healthy diets that provide the daily DRI of protein. As put forth by the Institute of Medicine, diets ideally contain at least 46 g/d for women (Dawson-Hughes, 2002). There may be upper limits for desirable protein intake as well. Excess urinary calcium excretion has been observed in association with the large acid loads delivered by very-high-protein diets (Barzel, 1998).

Caffeine consumption does not appear to influence bone health in postmenopausal women who maintain an adequate daily intake of calcium and vitamin D. However, one longitudinal study showed that even moderate amounts of caffeine (two to three servings of coffee daily) may lead to bone loss in women with low calcium intake (<800 mg/d) (Harris, 1994).

Calcium reabsorption is directly proportional to sodium reabsorption in the renal tubule. Accordingly, increases in dietary sodium have been observed to cause increases in urinary calcium excretion and corresponding increases in biochemical markers of bone turnover. Specifically, a relationship between high sodium intake (>1768 mg/d) and lower BMD has been described (Sellmeyer, 2002). This sodium effect appears to be independent of calcium intake and activity levels. As with caffeine, sodium intake moderation is a reasonable precautionary measure until this relationship is fully understood.

Physical Preventions

Small but statistically significant increases in BMD have been observed in postmenopausal women participating in exercise programs, including aerobic exercise and resistance training (heavy weight with few repetitions). One metaanalysis of 43 RCTs concluded that lower limb resistance exercise was most effective for femur neck BMD, and combination exercise programs were most effective for vertebral BMD (Howe, 2011). Another analysis that focused on walking as exercise showed a benefit for femur neck BMD (Ma, 2013).

Although an increase in bone density may occur, especially at the sites at which the exercise is directed, benefits of exercise may likely also be due to factors other than greater BMD (Carter, 2002). For example, an association between exercise and reduced falls has been reported. Improvements in balance,

TABLE 22-5. Selected Preparations for Genitourinary Symptoms of Menopause[a]

Preparation	Generic Name	Brand Name	Dose
Vaginal cream	Conjugated estrogens	Premarin	0.625 mg per 1 g cream (0.5 g twice weekly or 0.5 g/d for 3 wks, with 1 wk off therapy. May titrate up to 2 g per application as needed) (available as 42.5 g tube)
	17β-Estradiol	Estrace	0.1 mg per 1 g cream (2–4 g/d for 1–2 wks, then 1–2 g/d for 1–2 wks, then 1–2 g 1 to 3 times weekly) (42.5 g tube)
Vaginal tablet	Estradiol	Vagifem	0.010 mg tablet (1 tablet/d for 2 wks, then 1 tablet twice weekly)
Vaginal ring	17β-Estradiol	Estring	2 mg, remains for 90 days
	Estradiol acetate	Femring	12.4-mg or 24.8-mg ring, remains for 90 days
Oral tablet	Ospemifene	Osphena	60 mg daily

[a]Most estrogen-containing products listed in Table 22-2 for the treatment of menopausal hot flushes are also approved for the treatment of vaginal dryness.

stronger muscles, better muscle tone, and stronger, more flexible bone all undoubtedly contribute to fracture reduction.

Falls are responsible for more than 90 percent of hip fractures (Carter, 2002). Sideways falls appear to be the most detrimental and were independently associated with hip fracture in a study by Greenspan and associates (1998). Therefore, fall prevention is essential for women with osteopenia or osteoporosis. Living conditions are modified to minimize falls by reducing clutter and implementing nonslip tiles, rugs with nonskid backing, and night lights.

Hip protector padding was also initially thought to reduce hip fractures in elderly adults. However, one Cochrane database analysis indicates that the effect of hip protectors to lower hip fracture risk is small, and compliance is low (Santesso, 2014). Falls and fractures often occur at night, when women are likely to have taken off their hip protectors. This may result from the bulkiness of hip protectors, which are uncomfortable to wear while sleeping (van Schoor, 2003).

TREATMENT OF SEX-RELATED ISSUES

■ Dyspareunia

Estrogen Replacement

Low estradiol levels commonly lead to the *genitourinary syndrome of menopause*. This syndrome may include but is not limited to: (1) genital symptoms of dryness, burning, and irritation; (2) sexual symptoms of lack of lubrication, discomfort or pain, and impaired function; and (3) urinary symptoms of urgency, dysuria and recurrent urinary tract infections (Portman, 2014). Data from the Yale Midlife Study showed a close relationship between serum estradiol levels and sexual problems. In this study, significantly more women with estradiol levels less than 50 pg/mL reported vaginal dryness, dyspareunia, and pain compared with women whose estradiol levels were greater than 50 pg/mL (Sarrel, 1998). Prospective records of coital behavior and concomitant steroid analysis revealed that women with estradiol levels less than 35 pg/mL reported significant reductions in coital activity.

Estrogen replacement effectively reverses atrophic changes. Vaginal atrophy and diminished vaginal mucosal elasticity, vaginal fluid secretion levels, blood flow, and sensorimotor responses are improved by either topical or systemic estrogen (Dennerstein, 2002). In one metaanalysis evaluating RCTs from 1969 to 1995, investigators found that compared with placebo, oral or vaginal estrogens significantly improved vaginal atrophy symptoms, dyspareunia, and vaginal pH (Cardozo, 1998). If oral and vaginal estrogens were compared, vaginal products had greater patient acceptance, lower systemic estradiol concentrations, yet significant improvement of dyspareunia and pH changes.

Of vaginal topical agents, available forms include creams, continuous-release rings, and tablets (Table 22-5). In comparing types during a 12-week study period, Ayton and colleagues (1996) found that a continuous low-dose estradiol-releasing vaginal ring (Estring) provided comparable relief to CEE vaginal cream used for 12 weeks. In addition, study patients found the vaginal ring significantly more acceptable than the cream. The ring is prescribed as a single unit. Each unit contains 2 mg of estradiol and is worn vaginally for 90 days and then replaced.

Alternatively, a 10-μg 17β-estradiol tablet (Vagifem) is available for vaginal application. One tablet is inserted daily for an initial 2 weeks of treatment and is followed by twice-weekly application. These tablets and CEE vaginal cream have been found to be equivalent in relieving symptoms of atrophic vaginitis (Rioux, 2000). Advantageously, women using vaginal tablets had less endometrial proliferation or hyperplasia than those using cream. Additionally, tablets were rated significantly more favorably than the cream, and their use was associated with fewer patient withdrawals from the study.

Studies of the vaginal tablets and ring have confirmed endometrial safety at 1 year, but studies of the long-term effects of low-dose vaginal ET on the endometrium are lacking. Women using vaginal ET should report any vaginal bleeding, and this bleeding should be evaluated thoroughly. Progestins typically are not prescribed to women using only low-dose vaginal estrogen products. If a woman is at high risk of endometrial cancer or is using a higher dose of vaginal ET, transvaginal ultrasound or intermittent progestogen therapy may be considered (North American Menopause Society, 2013).

Ospemifene

Marketed as Osphena, this SERM is taken orally daily in a 60-mg dose to treat moderate to severe dyspareunia from menopause-associated vulvar and vaginal atrophy. In one RCT with 826 women, ospemifene was significantly superior to placebo in improving the vaginal pH, the self-assessed severity of most bothersome symptoms, and the percentage of superficial vaginal epithelial cells (Bachmann, 2010). As noted in Chapter 21 (p. 489), superficial cells are increased relative to parabasal cells in estrogen-sufficient vaginal epithelia. Ospemifene was shown to be safe and well tolerated.

Hot flushes, a common adverse event associated with SERM use, were more frequently reported in the ospemifene groups. These did not raise discontinuation rates and were generally mild. Urinary tract infections were slightly more prevalent. The endometrial effects of ospemifene were negligible. There were no cases of endometrial hyperplasia or carcinoma and no reports of vaginal bleeding/spotting in this 3-month trial.

Vaginal Lubricants and Moisturizers

Various water-soluble vaginal lubricants are available over the counter for treatment of vaginal dryness with coitus. Most commonly used water-based lubricants include K-Y Jelly, Astroglide, and Slippery Stuff. They can be applied before intercourse to the vaginal introitus. Alternatively, a polycarbophil-based gel (Replens) offers a more sustained correction of vaginal dryness. This gel is an acidic hydrophilic insoluble polymer, which can hold water to act as a vaginal moisturizer. The polymer binds to the vaginal epithelium and is sloughed with epithelial layer turnover. In addition, the acidity of the gel helps to lower the vaginal pH to that found in premenopausal women. This vaginal moisturizer is used three times weekly, but the schedule can be individualized.

As a group, these agents are an effective first-line tool for vaginal atrophy symptoms. From their review of 44 RCTs and prospective comparative trials, Rahn and associates (2014) suggest vaginal moisturizers/lubricants or vaginal estrogen for relief in women with a sole complaint of vaginal dryness, dyspareunia, itching or burning, dysuria, or urinary urgency. For those with multiples of these, they favored vaginal estrogen therapy.

■ Libido

A decline in libido is common during menopause (Sarrel, 1990). As described in Chapter 21 (p. 486), the cause is no doubt multifactorial. Estrogen therapy can be helpful for GSM symptoms, as described in the last section. However, HT is not recommended as the sole treatment of other problems of sexual function, including diminished libido (North American Menopause Society, 2012).

Flibanserin (Addyi) is an agent that has both serotonin-receptor agonist and antagonist activity. In 2015, this agent was approved by the FDA to treat female hypoactive sexual desire disorder (HSDD). For postmenopausal women, data derive mainly from the SNOWDROP trial (Simon, 2014). In this study, flibanserin, compared with placebo, provided a significant increase in the number of satisfying sexual events (1.0 versus 0.6) and in the Female Sexual Function Index (FSFI) desire domain score (0.7 versus 0.4). Notably, these gains are measured against drug side effects that can include hypotension and syncope, especially with alcohol use. To emphasize this interaction, as part of the FDA-approval, prescribing clinicians must participate in a risk evaluation and mitigation strategy (REMS) program. An additional black box warning describes hypotension and syncope when flibanserin is administered with moderate or strong CYP3A4 inhibitors or in patients with hepatic impairment (Sprout Pharmaceuticals, 2015).

Androgen replacement in women with HSDD is a controversial topic. Although some studies have documented an association between androgen replacement and improved sexual desire, large quality trials with long-term follow-up are needed (Lobo, 2003; Pauls, 2005; Shifren, 2000). Dehydroepiandrosterone (DHEA) is an androgen precursor, and reviews of RCTs show no or only slightly improved sexual functioning in supplemented postmenopausal women (Elraiyah, 2014; Scheffers, 2015).

Symptoms of androgen insufficiency include diminished sense of well-being, persistent fatigue, sexual function changes, and low levels of serum free testosterone. Women with these findings may be offered replacement. Importantly, candidates are counseled that androgen replacement therapy is off-label and not FDA-approved. Therapy should be performed under close clinician supervision. Early effects of androgen therapy include acne and hirsutism, with one study reporting a 3-percent increased rate of acne in testosterone-therapy groups (Lobo, 2003). Long-term side effects such as male pattern baldness, voice deepening, and clitoral hypertrophy are infrequent within normal androgen levels. Androgen therapy may adversely affect the lipid profile, and long-term effects on cardiovascular and breast cancer risks are unknown (Braunstein, 2007; Davis, 2012, 2013).

TREATMENT OF DEPRESSION

Depression in women is common, with a lifetime prevalence of approximately 18 percent (Chaps. 13, p. 298). Antidepressant medications together with psychotherapy and counseling are the principal therapeutic interventions for women with depression.

HT is not considered treatment for depression, but lesser mood symptoms may be improved concurrent with resolution of hot flushes and disrupted sleep. For example, in the prospective Massachusetts Women's Health Study, hot flushes and trouble sleeping were highly related to depression and provide support for the "domino" hypothesis that menopausal symptoms are a cause of increased depressed mood at this life stage (Avis, 2001). Several controlled studies have demonstrated that HT can improve depression in *perimenopausal* women. Notably, most studies involved women with vasomotor symptoms, so it is likely that the depressed mood improvement was predominantly linked to resolution of bothersome hot flushes and sleep disruption and improved quality of life (Soares, 2001; Zweifel, 1997). Women who present with bothersome vasomotor symptoms and associated disordered mood at the time of the menopausal transition may elect a trial of HT for symptom relief. Namely, consideration may be given to those who fail to respond to a conventional first-line intervention, those who refuse to take psychotropic agents, or those who will begin HT for other acute menopausal symptoms and who could delay antidepressant therapy until determining whether estrogen treatment is sufficient.

TREATMENT OF SKIN AGING

As people age, their skin loses elasticity, collagen fibers, vascularity, and moisture. As a result, the skin lies more loosely, and lines appear where the facial muscles attach to the skin's undersurface. Many factors play a role in the rate and degree of aging. First and foremost is genetics. People with thin, dry, fair skin realize signs earlier. In addition, overexposure to sunlight and excessive use of tobacco and alcohol accelerate skin aging. Thus, prevention of skin aging includes protection from ultraviolet light, avoidance of tobacco, and limited alcohol intake.

Skin is a hormonally sensitive structure, and both estrogen and androgen receptors have been localized to skin (Hasselquist, 1980). However, it is difficult to separate hormonal deficiency from chronological skin aging and age-related environmental insults such a smoking or photo-aging from sun exposure.

The predominant evidence for an estrogen effect on skin has been derived from observational studies using various estrogen preparations with or without cyclic progestin. Thus, it is difficult to clearly separate the effects of estrogen from estrogen and progestin in many of the studies. Results of RCTs show improvement in certain skin parameters, but these were inconsistent among the trials (Maheux, 1994; Sator, 2007; Sauerbronn, 2000). In the largest RCT, Phillips and associates (2008) noted that low-dose HT did not significantly alter age-related facial skin changes in 320 women compared with placebo. Thus in balancing the risk and benefits, there is currently insufficient evidence to recommend HT to improve age-related skin characteristics.

PREVENTIVE HEALTH CARE

Leading causes of mortality for two age groups of women are found in Table 22-6. Testing and prevention strategies are aimed at reducing the incidence and effects of these causes. In addition to testing, illness prevention requires patient education to enable women to play an active role in maintaining their own health. Through dialogue and counseling, clinicians and their actively participating patients can reap the benefits of preventive care. Prevention recommendations for many of these causes of morbidity are reviewed in Chapter 1, but a select few found commonly in older populations are discussed below.

■ Alzheimer Senile Dementia

Dementia is defined as a progressive decline in intellectual and cognitive function. Its causes can be categorized into three broad groups: (1) cases in which the brain is the target of a systemic illness; (2) primary structural causes such as tumor; and (3) primary

TABLE 22-6. Leading Causes of Mortality in Women of Differing Age[a]

In those between 45 and 54 years:
Cancer
Heart disease
Accidents
Chronic liver disease
Cerebrovascular disease
Chronic lower respiratory disease
Diabetes mellitus
Suicide

In those older than 65 years:
Heart disease
Cancer
Cerebrovascular disease
Chronic lower respiratory disease
Alzheimer disease
Diabetes mellitus
Influenza and pneumonia
Chronic renal disease

[a]For each age group, causes are listed by their descending frequency.
Data from Heron M: Deaths: leading causes for 2010. Natl Vital Stat Rep 62(6):1, 2013.

degenerative diseases of the nervous system, such as senile dementia of the Alzheimer type (SDAT). It is estimated that up to 50 percent of women aged 85 years or older may suffer from senile dementia or SDAT. Early signs of dementia may be subtle, and testing strategies are found in Chapter 1 (p. 17).

The role of estrogen in the prevention of dementia is controversial. Several epidemiologic studies have suggested that HT prevents development of SDAT. Moreover, metaanalyses of observational studies found that HT was associated with a decreased risk of dementia, but it does not seem to improve established disease (Yaffe, 1998; Zandi, 2002). However, data from a large RCT found negative findings for a preventive role. Women enrolled in the Women's Health Initiative Memory Study (WHIMS), an ancillary study of the WHI, were noted to have increased rates of dementia compared with those given placebo (Shumaker, 2003, 2004). Although this increased risk was statistically significant only in the group of women >75 years, the observation nonetheless is a cause for concern in terms of its long-term implications for HT in older postmenopausal women who are well advanced in menopause. It is unclear whether, similar to CHD, concepts of critical window and timing hypotheses or if the duration of HT have an effect in the prevention of SDAT. Unfortunately, these mixed findings leave unanswered questions regarding HT's efficacy in preventing dementia in postmenopausal women. Currently, HT is not recommended for this indication.

■ Urogynecologic Disease

The development of pelvic organ prolapse and urinary incontinence is multifactorial. Thus, the effectiveness of preventive measures such as cesarean delivery, pelvic floor muscle training (Kegel exercises), and estrogen therapy is unclear. Estrogen receptors are found throughout the lower urinary and reproductive tracts. In these areas, hypoestrogenism is associated with collagen changes and diminished vascularity of the urethral subepithelial plexus. However, separating the effects of hypoestrogenism from aging in the genesis of pelvic organ prolapse and urinary incontinence is problematic and discussed in Chapters 23 (p. 515) and 24 (p. 539).

For a woman with obvious lower reproductive tract atrophic changes, a trial of vaginal estrogen treatment for urinary incontinence is reasonable. Vaginal ET reduces irritative urinary symptoms, such as frequency and urgency, and has been demonstrated to reduce the likelihood of recurrent urinary tract infections in postmenopausal women (Eriksen, 1999). However, several other studies evaluating effects of estrogen have noted either de novo development or worsening of incontinence in women using HT (Hendrix, 2005; Jackson, 2006). Accordingly, there is no current indication for the use of HT for the prevention of pelvic organ prolapse or incontinence.

In sum, the body of current evidence shows that HT prescribing is complex and should be tailored to the individual woman's risk/benefit profile. Thus dose, type, and route of administration are carefully evaluated. While clinicians spout the mantra of "lower doses for shorter periods of time," there actually are no arbitrary time limits regarding the duration of HT use in the symptomatic woman. It can be used for as long as the woman feels the benefits outweigh the risks for her. Annual or semiannual visits to reevaluate symptoms, side effects, risks, and benefits are tailored to the individual patient.

REFERENCES

Albertazzi P, Pansini F, Bonaccorsi G, et al: The effect of dietary soy supplementation on hot flushes. Obstet Gynecol 91(1):6, 1998

American College of Obstetricians and Gynecologists: Compounded bioidentical menopausal hormone therapy. Committee Opinion No. 532, August 2012, Reaffirmed 2014a

American College of Obstetricians and Gynecologists: Hormone therapy and heart disease. Committee Opinion No. 565, June 2013

American College of Obstetricians and Gynecologists: Management of menopausal symptoms. Practice Bulletin No. 141, January 2014b

Anderson GL, Limacher M, Assaf AR, et al: Effects of conjugated equine estrogen in postmenopausal women with hysterectomy: the Women's Health Initiative randomized controlled trial. JAMA 291(14):1701, 2004

Archer DF, Dupont CM, Constantine GD, et al: Desvenlafaxine for the treatment of vasomotor symptoms associated with menopause: a double-blind, randomized, placebo-controlled trial of efficacy and safety. Am J Obstet Gynecol 200(3):238.e1, 2009a

Archer DF, Seidman L, Constantine GD, et al: A double-blind, randomly assigned, placebo-controlled study of desvenlafaxine efficacy and safety for the treatment of vasomotor symptoms associated with menopause. Am J Obstet Gynecol 200(2):172.e1, 2009b

Avis NE, Crawford S, Stellato R, et al: Longitudinal study of hormone levels and depression among women transitioning through menopause. Climacteric 4(3):243, 2001

Ayton RA, Darling GM, Murkies AL, et al: A comparative study of safety and efficacy of continuous low dose oestradiol released from a vaginal ring compared with conjugated equine oestrogen vaginal cream in the treatment of postmenopausal urogenital atrophy. BJOG 103(4):351, 1996

Bachmann GA, Komi JO, Ospemifene Study Group: Ospemifene effectively treats vulvovaginal atrophy in postmenopausal women: results from a pivotal phase 3 study. Menopause 17(3):480, 2010

Barnabei VM, Grady D, Stovall DW, et al: Menopausal symptoms in older women and the effects of treatment with hormone therapy. Obstet Gynecol 100(6):1209, 2002

Barrett-Connor E, Grady D, Sashegyi A, et al: Raloxifene and cardiovascular events in osteoporotic postmenopausal women: four-year results from the MORE (Multiple Outcomes of Raloxifene Evaluation) randomized trial. JAMA 287(7):847, 2002

Barrett-Connor E, Mosca L, Collins P, et al: Effects of raloxifene on cardiovascular events and breast cancer in postmenopausal women. N Engl J Med 355(2):125, 2006

Barrett-Connor E, Wehren LE, Siris ES, et al: Recency and duration of postmenopausal hormone therapy: effects on bone mineral density and fracture risk in the National Osteoporosis Risk Assessment (NORA) study. Menopause 10(5):412, 2003

Barton DL, LaVasseur BI, Sloan JA, et al: Phase III, placebo-controlled trial of three doses of citalopram for the treatment of hot flashes: NCCTG trial N05C9. J Clin Oncol 28(20):3278, 2010

Barzel US, Massey LK: Excess dietary protein can adversely affect bone. J Nutr 128(6):1051, 1998

Biglia N, Sgandurra P, Peano E, et al: Non-hormonal treatment of hot flushes in breast cancer survivors: gabapentin vs. vitamin E. Climacteric 12(4):310, 2009

Black DM, Cummings SR, Karpf DB, et al: Randomised trial of effect of alendronate on risk of fracture in women with existing vertebral fractures. Fracture Intervention Trial Research Group. Lancet 348(9041):1535, 1996

Black DM, Delmas PD, Eastell R, et al: Once-yearly zoledronic acid for treatment of postmenopausal osteoporosis. N Engl J Med 356(18):1809, 2007

Black DM, Schwartz AV, Ensrud KE, et al: Effects of continuing or stopping alendronate after 5 years of treatment: the Fracture Intervention Trial Longterm Extension (FLEX): a randomized trial. JAMA 296(24):2927, 2006

Blau LA, Hoehns JD: Analgesic efficacy of calcitonin for vertebral fracture pain. Ann Pharmacother 37(4):564, 2003

Boekhout AH, Vincent AD, Dalesio OB, et al: Management of hot flashes in patients who have breast cancer with venlafaxine and clonidine: a randomized, double-blind, placebo-controlled trial. J Clin Oncol 29(29):3862, 2011

Bone HG, Hosking D, Devogelaer JP, et al: Ten years' experience with alendronate for osteoporosis in postmenopausal women. N Engl J Med 350(12):1189, 2004

Bordeleau L, Pritchard KI, Loprinzi CL, et al: Multicenter, randomized, cross-over clinical trial of venlafaxine versus gabapentin for the management of hot flashes in breast cancer survivors. J Clin Oncol 28(35):514, 2010

Braunstein GD: Safety of testosterone treatment in postmenopausal women. Fertil Steril 88(1):1, 2007

Buijs C, Mom CH, Willemse PH, et al: Venlafaxine versus clonidine for the treatment of hot flashes in breast cancer patients: a double-blind, randomized cross-over study. Breast Cancer Res Treat 115(3):573, 2009

Cardozo L, Bachmann G, McClish D, et al: Meta-analysis of estrogen therapy in the management of urogenital atrophy in postmenopausal women: second report of the Hormones and Urogenital Therapy Committee. Obstet Gynecol 92(4 Pt 2):722, 1998

Carpenter JS, Guthrie KA, Larson JC, et al: Effect of escitalopram on hot flash interference: a randomized, controlled trial. Fertil Steril 97(6):1399, 2012

Carris N, Kutner S, Reilly-Rogers S: New pharmacological therapies for vasomotor symptom management: focus of bazedoxifene/conjugated estrogens and paroxetine mesylate. Ann Pharmacother 48(10):1343, 2014

Carter ND, Khan KM, McKay HA, et al: Community-based exercise program reduces risk factors for falls in 65- to 75-year-old women with osteoporosis: randomized controlled trial. CMAJ 167(9):997, 2002

Chapuy MC, Arlot ME, Duboeuf F, et al: Vitamin D_3 and calcium to prevent hip fractures in the elderly women. N Engl J Med 327(23):1637, 1992

Cheng G, Wilczek B, Warner M, et al: Isoflavone treatment for acute menopausal symptoms. Menopause 14(3 Pt 1):468, 2007

Chesnut CH 3rd, Silverman S, Andriano K, et al: A randomized trial of nasal spray salmon calcitonin in postmenopausal women with established osteoporosis: the Prevent Recurrence of Osteoporotic Fractures Study. PROOF Study Group. Am J Med 109(4):267, 2000

Chesnut CH 3rd, Skag A, Christiansen C, et al: Effects of oral ibandronate administered daily or intermittently on fracture risk in postmenopausal osteoporosis. J Bone Miner Res 19:1241, 2004

Christiansen C, Chesnut CH 3rd, Adachi JD, et al: Safety of bazedoxifene in a randomized, double-blind, placebo- and active-controlled Phase 3 study of postmenopausal women with osteoporosis. BMC Musculoskelet Disord 11:130, 2010

Chung YE, Lee SH, Lee SY, et al: Long-term treatment with raloxifene, but not bisphosphonates, reduces circulating sclerostin levels in postmenopausal women. Osteoporos Int 23:1235, 2012

Cohen FJ, Lu Y: Characterization of hot flashes reported by healthy postmenopausal women receiving raloxifene or placebo during osteoporosis prevention trials. Maturitas 34(1):65, 2000

Cranney A, Tugwell P, Zytaruk N, et al: Meta-analyses of therapies for postmenopausal osteoporosis. VI. Meta-analysis of calcitonin for the treatment of postmenopausal osteoporosis. Endocr Rev 23(4):540, 2002

Cummings SR, San Martin J, McClung MR, et al: Denosumab for prevention of fractures in postmenopausal women with osteoporosis. N Engl J Med 361(8):756, 2009

Danforth KN, Tworoger SS, Hecht JL, et al: A prospective study of postmenopausal hormone use and ovarian cancer risk. Br J Cancer 96(1):151, 2007

Daley A, Stokes-Lampard H, Thomas A, et al: Exercise for vasomotor menopausal symptoms. Cochrane Database Syst Rev 11:CD006108, 2014

Davis SR: Androgen use for low sexual desire in midlife women. Menopause 20(7):795, 2013

Davis SR, Braunstein GD: Efficacy and safety of testosterone in the management of hypoactive sexual desire disorder in postmenopausal women. J Sex Med 9(4):1134, 2012

Dawson-Hughes B, Harris SS: Calcium intake influences the association of protein intake with rates of bone loss in elderly men and women. Am J Clin Nutr 75(4):773, 2002

Dawson-Hughes B, Harris SS, Krall EA, et al: Effect of calcium and vitamin D supplementation on bone density in men and women 65 years of age or older. N Engl J Med 337(10):670, 1997

Dell RM, Adams AL, Greene DF, et al: Incidence of atypical nontraumatic diaphyseal fractures of the femur. J Bone Miner Res 27:2544, 2012

Delmas PD, Ensrud KE, Adachi JD, et al: Efficacy of raloxifene on vertebral fracture risk reduction in postmenopausal women with osteoporosis: four-year results from a randomized clinical trial. J Clin Endocrinol Metab 87(8):3609, 2002

Dempster DW, Shane E, Horbert W, et al: A simple method for correlative light and scanning electron microscopy of human iliac crest bone biopsies: qualitative observations in normal and osteoporotic subjects. J Bone Miner Res 1(1):15, 1986

Dennerstein L, Randolph J, Taffe J, et al: Hormones, mood, sexuality, and the menopausal transition. Fertil Steril 77(Suppl 4):S42, 2002

Diab DL, Watts NB: Bisphosphonates in the treatment of osteoporosis. Endocrinol Metab Clinic North Am 41:487, 2012

Diab DL, Watts NB: Postmenopausal osteoporosis. Curr Opin Endocrinol Diabetes Obes 20:501, 2013

Diab DL, Watts NB: Use of drug holidays in women taking bisphosphonates. Menopause 21(2):195, 2014

Dodin S, Blanchet C, Marc I, et al: Acupuncture for menopausal hot flushes. Cochrane Database Syst Rev 7:CD00741, 2013

Elraiyah T, Sonbol MB, Wang Z, et al: Clinical review: the benefits and harms of systemic dehydroepiandrosterone (DHEA) in postmenopausal women with normal adrenal function: a systematic review and meta-analysis. J Clin Endocrinol Metab 99(10):353, 2014

Eriksen B: A randomized, open, parallel-group study on the preventive effect of an estradiol-releasing vaginal ring (Estring) on recurrent urinary tract infections in postmenopausal women. Am J Obstet Gynecol 180(5):1072, 1999

Ettinger B, Black DM, Mitlak BH, et al: Reduction of vertebral fracture risk in postmenopausal women with osteoporosis treated with raloxifene: results from a 3-year randomized clinical trial. Multiple Outcomes of Raloxifene Evaluation (MORE) Investigators. JAMA 282(7):637, 1999

Ettinger B, Ensrud KE, Wallace R, et al: Effects of ultralow-dose transdermal estradiol on bone mineral density: a randomized clinical trial. Obstet Gynecol 104(3):443, 2004

Evans ML, Pritts E, Vittinghoff E, et al: Management of postmenopausal hot flushes with venlafaxine hydrochloride: a randomized, controlled trial. Obstet Gynecol 105(1):161, 2005

Food and Drug Administration: Noncontraceptive estrogen drug products for the treatment of vasomotor symptoms and vulvar and vaginal atrophy symptoms—recommended prescribing information for health care providers and patient labeling, 2005. Available at: http://www.fda.gov/downloads/drugs/guidancecomplianceregulatoryinformation/guidances/ucm075090.pdf. Accessed April 24, 2015

Foster SA, Shi N, Curkendall S, et al: Fractures in women treated with raloxifene or alendronate: a retrospective database analysis. BMC Womens Health 13:15, 2013

Freeman EW, Guthrie KA, Caan B, et al: Efficacy of escitalopram for hot flashes in healthy menopausal women: a randomized controlled trial. JAMA 305(3):267, 2011

Freeman EW, Sammel MD, Sanders RJ: Risk of long-term hot flashes after natural menopause: evidence from the Penn Ovarian Aging Study cohort. Menopause 21(9):924, 2014

Gambrell RD Jr, Bagnell CA, Greenblatt RB: Role of estrogens and progesterone in the etiology and prevention of endometrial cancer: review. Am J Obstet Gynecol 146(6):696, 1983

Gasser JA, Kneissel M, Thomsen JS, et al: PTH and interactions with bisphosphonates. J Musculoskelet Neuronal Interact 1(1):53, 2000

Gedmintas L, Solomon DH, Kim SC: Bisphosphonates and risk of subtrochanteric, femoral shafts, and atypical femur fracture: a systemic review and meta-analysis. J Bone Miner Res 28:1729, 2013

Geller SE, Shulman LP, van Breemen RB, et al: Safety and efficacy of black cohosh and red clover for the management of vasomotor symptoms: a randomized controlled trial. Menopause 16(6):1156, 2009

Gordon PR, Kerwin JP, Boesen KG, et al: Sertraline to treat hot flashes: a randomized controlled, double-blind, crossover trial in a general population. Menopause 13(4):568, 2006

Grady D, Cohen B, Tice J, et al: Ineffectiveness of sertraline for treatment of menopausal hot flushes: a randomized controlled trial. Obstet Gynecol 109(4):823, 2007

Grady D, Herrington D, Bittner V, et al: Cardiovascular disease outcomes during 6.8 years of hormone therapy: Heart and Estrogen/progestin Replacement Study follow-up (HERS II). JAMA 288(1):49, 2002

Greendale GA, Reboussin BA, Hogan P, et al: Symptom relief and side effects of postmenopausal hormones: results from the Postmenopausal Estrogen/Progestin Interventions Trial. Obstet Gynecol 92(6):982, 1998

Greenspan SL, Myers ER, Kiel DP, et al: Fall direction, bone mineral density, and function: risk factors for hip fracture in frail nursing home elderly. Am J Med 104(6):539, 1998

Grodstein F, Clarkson TB, Manson JE: Understanding the divergent data on postmenopausal hormone therapy. N Engl J Med 348(7):645, 2003

Grodstein F, Manson JE, Stampfer MJ: Postmenopausal hormone use and secondary prevention of coronary events in the Nurses' Health Study. A prospective, observational study. Ann Intern Med 135(1):1, 2001

Guttuso T Jr, Kurlan R, McDermott MP, et al: Gabapentin's effects on hot flashes in postmenopausal women: a randomized controlled trial. Obstet Gynecol 101(2):337, 2003

Haines CJ, Lam PM, Chung TK, et al: A randomized, double-blind, placebo-controlled study of the effect of a Chinese herbal medicine preparation (Dang Gui Buxue Tang) on menopausal symptoms in Hong Kong Chinese women. Climacteric 11(3):244, 2008

Handley AP, Williams M: The efficacy and tolerability of SSRI/SNRIs in the treatment of vasomotor symptoms in menopausal women: a systematic review. J Am Assoc Nurse Pract 27(1):54, 2015

Harris SS, Dawson-Hughes B: Caffeine and bone loss in healthy postmenopausal women. Am J Clin Nutr 60(4):573, 1994

Harris ST, Watts NB, Genant HK, et al: Effects of risedronate treatment on vertebral and nonvertebral fractures in women with postmenopausal osteoporosis: a randomized controlled trial. Vertebral Efficacy With Risedronate Therapy (VERT) Study Group. JAMA 282(14):1344, 1999

Hasselquist MB, Goldberg N, Schroeter A, et al: Isolation and characterization of the estrogen receptor in human skin. J Clin Endocrinol Metab 50(1):76, 1980

Häuselmann HJ, Rizzoli R: A comprehensive review of treatments for postmenopausal osteoporosis. Osteoporos Int 14(1):2, 2003

Hays J, Ockene JK, Brunner RL, et al: Effects of estrogen plus progestin on health-related quality of life. N Engl J Med 348(19):1839, 2003

Hendrix SL, Cochrane BB, Nygaard IE, et al: Effects of estrogen with and without progestin on urinary incontinence. JAMA 293(8):935, 2005

Heron M: Deaths: leading causes for 2010. Natl Vital Stat Rep 62(6):1, 2013

Hirata JD, Swiersz LM, Zell B, et al: Does dong quai have estrogenic effects in postmenopausal women? A double-blind, placebo-controlled trial. Fertil Steril 68(6):981, 1997

Howe TE, Shea B, Dawson LJ, et al: Exercise for preventing and treating osteoporosis in postmenopausal women. Cochrane Database Syst Rev 7:CD000333, 2011

Hulley S, Grady D, Bush T, et al: Randomized trial of estrogen plus progestin for secondary prevention of coronary heart disease in postmenopausal women. Heart and Estrogen/progestin Replacement Study (HERS) Research Group. JAMA 280(7):605, 1998

Institute of Medicine: DRIs for calcium and vitamin D. 2010. Available at: http://www.iom.edu/Reports/2010/Dietary-Reference-Intakes-for-Calcium-and-Vitamin-D/DRI-Values.aspx. Accessed April 24, 2015

Jackson SL, Scholes D, Boyko EJ, et al: Predictors of urinary incontinence in a prospective cohort of postmenopausal women. Obstet Gynecol 108(4):855, 2006

Joffe H, Guthrie KA, LaCroix AZ, et al: Low-dose estradiol and the serotonin-norepinephrine reuptake inhibitor venlafaxine for vasomotor symptoms: a randomized clinical trial. JAMA Intern Med 174(7):1058, 2014

Kalay AE, Demir B, Haberal A, et al: Efficacy of citalopram on climacteric symptoms. Menopause 14(2):223, 2007

Kerstetter JE, Looker AC, Insogna KL: Low dietary protein and low bone density. Calcif Tissue Int 66(4):313, 2000

Khosia S, Burr D, Cauley J, et al: Bisphosphonate-associated osteonecrosis of the jaw: report of a task force of the American Society for Bone and Mineral Research. J Bone Miner Res 22:1479, 2007

Lacey JV Jr, Brinton LA, Leitzmann MF, et al: Menopausal hormone therapy and ovarian cancer risk in the National Institutes of Health-AARP Diet and Health Study Cohort. J Natl Cancer Inst 98(19):1397, 2006

Lanza FL, Hunt RH, Thomson AB, et al: Endoscopic comparison of esophageal and gastroduodenal effects of risedronate and alendronate in postmenopausal women. Gastroenterology 119(3):631, 2000

Larsen ER, Mosekilde L, Foldspang A: Vitamin D and calcium supplementation prevents osteoporotic fractures in elderly community dwelling residents: a pragmatic population-based 3-year intervention study. J Bone Miner Res 19(3):370, 2004

Leach MJ, Moore V: Black cohosh (Cimicifuga spp.) for menopausal symptoms. Cochrane Database Syst Rev 9:CD007244, 2012

Lemay A, Dodin S, Kadri N, et al: Flaxseed dietary supplement versus hormone replacement therapy in hypercholesterolemic menopausal women. Obstet Gynecol 100(3):495, 2002

Lethaby A, Marjoribanks J, Kronenberg F, et al: Phytoestrogens for menopausal vasomotor symptoms. Cochrane Database Syst Rev 12:CD001395, 2013

Lewis JG, McGill H, Patton VM, et al: Caution on the use of saliva measurements to monitor absorption of progesterone from transdermal creams in postmenopausal women. Maturitas 41(1):1, 2002

Lewis JE, Nickell LA, Thompson LU, et al: A randomized controlled trial of the effect of dietary soy and flaxseed muffins on quality of life and hot flashes during menopause. Menopause 13:631, 2006

Lindsay R, Gallagher JC, Kagan R, et al: Efficacy of tissue-selective estrogen complex of bazedoxifene/conjugated estrogens for osteoporosis prevention in at-risk postmenopausal women. Fertil Steril 92(3):1045, 2009

Lindsay R, Nieves J, Formica C, et al: Randomised controlled study of effect of parathyroid hormone on vertebral-bone mass and fracture incidence among postmenopausal women on oestrogen with osteoporosis. Lancet 350(9077):550, 1997

Liu ZM, Ho SC, Woo J, et al: Randomized controlled trial of whole soy and isoflavone daidzein on menopausal symptoms in equol-producing Chinese postmenopausal women. Menopause 21(6):653, 2014

Lobo R: Evidence-based medicine and the management of menopause. Clin Obstet Gynecol 51(3):534, 2008

Lobo RA, Pinkerton JV, Gass ML, et al: Evaluation of bazedoxifene/conjugated estrogens for the treatment of menopausal symptoms and effects on metabolic parameters and overall safety profile. Fertil Steril 92(3):1025, 2009

Lobo RA, Rosen RC, Yang HM, et al: Comparative effects of oral esterified estrogens with and without methyltestosterone on endocrine profiles and dimensions of sexual function in postmenopausal women with hypoactive sexual desire. Fertil Steril 79(6):1341, 2003

Loibl S, Schwedler K, von Minckwitz G, et al: Venlafaxine is superior to clonidine as treatment of hot flashes in breast cancer patients—a double-blind, randomized study. Ann Oncol 18(4):689, 2007

Loprinzi CL, Kugler JW, Sloan JA, et al: Venlafaxine in management of hot flashes in survivors of breast cancer: a randomised controlled trial. Lancet 356(9247):2059, 2000

Loprinzi CL, Sloan JA, Perez EA, et al: Phase III evaluation of fluoxetine for treatment of hot flashes. J Clin Oncol 20(6):1578, 2002

Ma D, Wu L, He Z: Effects of walking on the preservation of bone mineral density in perimenopausal and postmenopausal women: a systematic review and meta-analysis. Menopause 20(11):1216, 2013

MacLennan AH, Broadbent JL, Lester S, et al: Oral oestrogen and combined oestrogen/progestogen therapy versus placebo for hot flashes. Cochrane Database Syst Rev 4:CD002978, 2004

Maheux R, Naud F, Rioux M, et al: A randomized, double-blind, placebo-controlled study on the effect of conjugated estrogens on skin thickness. Am J Obstet Gynecol 170(2):642, 1994

Meier RP, Perneger TV, Stern R, et al: Increasing occurrence of atypical femoral fractures associated with bisphosphonate use. Arch Intern Med 172:930, 2012

Mendelsohn ME, Karas RH: Molecular and cellular basis of cardiovascular gender differences. Science 308(5728):1583, 2005

Miller PD, McClung MR, Macovei L, et al: Monthly oral ibandronate therapy in postmenopausal osteoporosis: 1-year results from the MOBILE Study. J Bone Miner Res 20(8):1315, 2005

Nagamani M, Kelver ME, Smith ER: Treatment of menopausal hot flashes with transdermal administration of clonidine. Am J Obstet Gynecol 156(3):561, 1987

National Osteoporosis Foundation: Clinician's Guide to Prevention and Treatment of Osteoporosis. Washington, National Osteoporosis Foundation, 2014

Neer RM, Arnaud CD, Zanchetta JR, et al: Effect of parathyroid hormone (1–34) on fractures and bone mineral density in postmenopausal women with osteoporosis. N Engl J Med 344(19):1434, 2001

Nelson HD: Commonly used types of postmenopausal estrogen for treatment of hot flashes: scientific review. JAMA 291(13):1610, 2004

Nelson HD, Vesco KK, Haney E, et al: Nonhormonal therapies for menopausal hot flashes: systematic review and meta-analysis. JAMA 295(17):2057, 2006

Newton KM, Reed SD, Guthrie KA, et al: Efficacy of yoga for vasomotor symptoms: a randomized controlled trial. Menopause 21(4):339, 2014

Noller KL: Estrogen replacement therapy and risk of ovarian cancer. JAMA 288(3):368, 2002

North American Menopause Society: Management of osteoporosis in postmenopausal women: 2010 position statement of the North American Menopause Society. Menopause 17(1):25, 2010

North American Menopause Society: Management of symptomatic vulvovaginal atrophy: 2013 position statement of the North American Menopause Society. Menopause 20(9):888, 2013

North American Menopause Society: The 2012 hormone therapy position statement of the North American Menopause Society. Menopause 19(3):257, 2012

Ofluoglu D, Akyuz G, Unay O, et al: The effect of calcitonin on beta-endorphin levels in postmenopausal osteoporotic patients with back pain. Clin Rheumatol 26(1):44, 2007

Palacios S, Pornel B, Vázquez F, et al: Long-term endometrial and breast safety of a specific, standardized soy extract. Climacteric 13(4):368, 2010

Pauls RN, Kleeman SD, Karram MM: Female sexual dysfunction: principles of diagnosis and therapy. Obstet Gynecol Surv 60(3):196, 2005

Peled Y, Perri T, Pardo Y, et al: Levonorgestrel-releasing intrauterine system as an adjunct to estrogen for the treatment of menopausal symptoms—a review. Menopause 14(3 Pt 1):550, 2007

Phillips TJ, Symons J, Menon S, et al: Does hormone therapy improve age-related skin changes in postmenopausal women? A randomized, double-blind, double-dummy, placebo-controlled multicenter study assessing the effects of norethindrone acetate and ethinyl estradiol in the improvement of mild to moderate age-related skin changes in postmenopausal women. J Am Acad Dermatol 59(3):397, 2008

Pinkerton JV, Archer DF, Guico-Pabia CJ, et al: Maintenance of the efficacy of desvenlafaxine in menopausal vasomotor symptoms: a 1-year randomized controlled trial. Menopause 20(1):38, 2013

Pinkerton JV, Harvey JA, Lindsay R, et al: Effects of bazedoxifene/conjugated estrogens on the endometrium and bone: a randomized trial. J Clin Endocrinol Metab 99:E189, 2014

Pinkerton JV, Utian WH, Constantine GD, et al: Relief of vasomotor symptoms with the tissue-selective estrogen complex containing bazedoxifene/conjugated estrogens: a randomized, controlled trial. Menopause 16:1116, 2009

Portman DJ, Gass ML, Vulvovaginal Atrophy Terminology Consensus Conference Panel: Genitourinary syndrome of menopause: new terminology for vulvovaginal atrophy from the International Society for the Study of Women's Sexual Health and the North American Menopause Society. Maturitas 79(3):349, 2014

Prentice RL, Langer RD, Stefanick ML, et al: Combined analysis of Women's Health Initiative observational and clinical trial data on postmenopausal hormone treatment and cardiovascular disease. Am J Epidemiol 163(7):589, 2006

Prentice RL, Pettinger MB, Jackson RD, et al: Health risks and benefits from calcium and vitamin D supplementation: Women's Health Initiative clinical trial and cohort study. Osteoporos Int 24:567, 2013

Prestwood KM, Kenny AM, Kleppinger A, et al: Ultralow-dose micronized 17beta-estradiol and bone density and bone metabolism in older women: a randomized controlled trial. JAMA 290(8):1042, 2003

Pruthi S, Qin R, Terstreip SA, et al: A phase III, randomized, placebo-controlled, double-blind trial of flaxseed for the treatment of hot flashes: North Central Cancer Treatment Group N08C7. Menopause 19(1):48, 2012

Quaas AM, Kono N, Mack WJ, et al: Effect of isoflavone soy protein supplementation on endometrial thickness, hyperplasia, and endometrial cancer risk in postmenopausal women: a randomized controlled trial. Menopause 20(8):840, 2013

Quella SK, Loprinzi CL, Barton DL, et al: Evaluation of soy phytoestrogens for the treatment of hot flashes in breast cancer survivors: a North Central Cancer Treatment Group Trial. J Clin Oncol 18(5):1068, 2000

Rada G, Capurro D, Pantoja T, et al: Non-hormonal interventions for hot flushes in women with a history of breast cancer. Cochrane Database Syst Rev 9:CD004923, 2010

Rahn DD, Carberry C, Sanses TV, et al: Vaginal estrogen for genitourinary syndrome of menopause: a systematic review. Obstet Gynecol 124(6):114, 2014

Reddy SY, Warner H, Guttuso T Jr, et al: Gabapentin, estrogen, and placebo for treating hot flashes: a randomized controlled trial. Obstet Gynecol 108(1):41, 2006

Reginster J, Minne HW, Sorensen OH, et al: Randomized trial of the effects of risedronate on vertebral fractures in women with established postmenopausal osteoporosis. Vertebral Efficacy with Risedronate Therapy (VERT) Study Group. Osteoporos Int 11(1):83, 2000

Reginster JY, Adami S, Lakatos P, et al: Efficacy and tolerability of once-monthly oral ibandronate in postmenopausal osteoporosis: 2 year results from the MOBILE study. Ann Rheum Dis 65(5):654, 2006

Rioux JE, Devlin C, Gelfand MM, et al: 17beta-estradiol vaginal tablet versus conjugated equine estrogen vaginal cream to relieve menopausal atrophic vaginitis. Menopause 7(3):156, 2000

Rosen CJ: Clinical practice. Vitamin D insufficiency. N Engl J Med 364(3):248, 2011

Rossouw JE, Anderson GL, Prentice RL, et al: Risks and benefits of estrogen plus progestin in healthy postmenopausal women: principal results from the Women's Health Initiative randomized controlled trial. JAMA 288(3):321, 2002

Rossouw JE, Prentice RL, Manson JE, et al: Postmenopausal hormone therapy and risk of cardiovascular disease by age and years since menopause. JAMA 297(13):1465, 2007

Roux C, Seeman E, Eastell R, et al: Efficacy of risedronate on clinical vertebral fractures within six months. Curr Med Res Opin 20:433, 2004

Rubin MR, Cosman F, Lindsay R, et al: The anabolic effects of parathyroid hormone. Osteoporos Int 13(4):267, 2002

Russell RG, Watts NB, Ebetino FH, et al: Mechanisms of action of bisphosphonates: similarities and differences and their potential influence on clinical efficacy. Osteoporos Int 19(6):733, 2008

Saensak S, Vutyavanich T, Somboonporn W, et al: Relaxation for perimenopausal and postmenopausal symptoms. Cochrane Database Syst Rev 7:CD008582, 2014

Salpeter SR, Walsh JM, Greyber E, et al: Mortality associated with hormone replacement therapy in younger and older women: a meta-analysis. J Gen Intern Med 19(7):791, 2004

Santesso N, Carrasco-Labra A, Brignardello-Petersen R: Hip protectors for preventing hip fractures in older people. Cochrane Database Syst Rev 3:CD001255, 2014

Sarrel P, Dobay B, Wiita B: Estrogen and estrogen-androgen replacement in postmenopausal women dissatisfied with estrogen-only therapy. Sexual behavior and neuroendocrine responses. J Reprod Med 43(10):847, 1998

Sarrel PM: Sexuality and menopause. Obstet Gynecol 75(4 Suppl):26S, 1990

Sator PG, Sator MO, Schmidt JB, et al: A prospective, randomized, double-blind, placebo-controlled study on the influence of a hormone replacement therapy on skin aging in postmenopausal women. Climacteric 10(4):320, 2007

Sauerbronn AV, Fonseca AM, Bagnoli VR, et al: The effects of systemic hormonal replacement therapy on the skin of postmenopausal women. Int J Gynaecol Obstet 68(1):35, 2000

Scheffers CS, Armstrong S, Cantineau AE, et al: Dehydroepiandrosterone for women in the peri- or postmenopausal phase. Cochrane Database Syst Rev 1:CD011066, 2015

Sellmeyer DE, Schloetter M, Sebastian A: Potassium citrate prevents increased urine calcium excretion and bone resorption induced by a high sodium chloride diet. J Clin Endocrinol Metab 87(5):2008, 2002

Shifren JL, Braunstein GD, Simon JA, et al: Transdermal testosterone treatment in women with impaired sexual function after oophorectomy. N Engl J Med 343(10):682, 2000

Shifren JL, Gass ML, NAMS Recommendations for Clinical Care of Midlife Women Working Group: The North American Menopause Society recommendations for clinical care of midlife women. Menopause 21(10):1038, 2014

Shulman LP: In search of a middle ground: hormone therapy and its role in modern menopause management. Menopause 17(5):898, 2010

Shumaker SA, Legault C, Kuller L, et al: Conjugated equine estrogens and incidence of probable dementia and mild cognitive impairment in postmenopausal women: Women's Health Initiative Memory Study. JAMA 291(24):2947, 2004

Shumaker SA, Legault C, Rapp SR, et al: Estrogen plus progestin and the incidence of dementia and mild cognitive impairment in postmenopausal women: the Women's Health Initiative Memory Study: a randomized controlled trial. JAMA 289(20):2651, 2003

Simon JA, Kingsberg SA, Shumel B, et al: Efficacy and safety of flibanserin in postmenopausal women with hypoactive sexual desire disorder: results of the SNOWDROP trial. Menopause 21(6):633, 2014

Simon JA, Portman DJ, Kaunitz AM, et al: Low-dose paroxetine 7.5 mg for menopausal vasomotor symptoms: two randomized controlled trials. Menopause 20:1027, 2013

Smith DC, Prentice R, Thompson DJ, et al: Association of exogenous estrogen and endometrial carcinoma. N Engl J Med 293(23):1164, 1975

Soares CN, Almeida OP, Joffe H, et al: Efficacy of estradiol for the treatment of depressive disorders in perimenopausal women: a double-blind, randomized, placebo-controlled trial. Arch Gen Psychiatry 58(6):529, 2001

Speroff L, Gass M, Constantine G, et al: Efficacy and tolerability of desvenlafaxine succinate treatment for menopausal vasomotor symptoms: a randomized controlled trial. Obstet Gynecol 111:77, 2008

Sprout Pharmaceuticals: Addyi: prescribing information. Raleigh, Sprout Pharmaceuticals, 2015

Stampfer MJ, Willett WC, Colditz GA, et al: A prospective study of postmenopausal estrogen therapy and coronary heart disease. N Engl J Med 313(17):1044, 1985

Stearns V, Beebe KL, Iyengar M, et al: Paroxetine controlled release in the treatment of menopausal hot flashes: a randomized controlled trial. JAMA 289(21):2827, 2003

Suvanto-Luukkonen E, Koivunen R, Sundström H, et al: Citalopram and fluoxetine in the treatment of postmenopausal symptoms: a prospective, randomized, 9-month, placebo-controlled, double-blind study. Menopause 12(1):18, 2005

Tashjian AH Jr, Chabner BA: Commentary on clinical safety of recombinant human parathyroid hormone 1–34 in the treatment of osteoporosis in men and postmenopausal women. J Bone Miner Res 17(7):1151, 2002

The Women's Health Initiative Steering Committee: Effects of conjugated equine estrogen in postmenopausal women with hysterectomy: The Women's Health Initiative Randomized Controlled Trial. JAMA 291:1701, 2004

The Writing Group for the PEPI Trial. Effects of estrogen or estrogen/progestin regimens on heart disease risk factors in postmenopausal women. Postmenopausal Estrogen/Progestin Interventions (PEPI) Trial. JAMA 273:199, 1995

Tice JA, Ettinger B, Ensrud K, et al: Phytoestrogen supplements for the treatment of hot flashes: the Isoflavone Clover Extract (ICE) Study: a randomized controlled trial. JAMA 290(2):207, 2003

Tosteson AN, Melton LJ III, Dawson-Hughes B, et al: Cost-effective osteoporosis treatment thresholds: the United States perspective. Osteoporos Int 19(4):437, 2008

Utian W, Yu H, Bobula J, et al: Bazedoxifene/conjugated estrogens and quality of life in post-menopausal women. Maturitas 63:329, 2009

van Schoor NM, Smit JH, Twisk JW, et al: Prevention of hip fractures by external hip protectors: a randomized controlled trial. JAMA 289(15):1957, 2003

Vickers MR, MacLennan AH, Lawton B, et al: Main morbidities recorded in the women's international study of long duration oestrogen after menopause (WISDOM): a randomised controlled trial of hormone replacement therapy in postmenopausal women. BMJ 335(7613):239, 2007

Watts NB, Bilezikian JP, Camacho PM, et al: American Association of Clinical Endocrinologists Medical Guidelines for Clinical Practice for the diagnosis and treatment of postmenopausal osteoporosis: executive summary of recommendations. Endocr Pract 16(6):1016, 2010

Wells G, Tugwell P, Shea B, et al: Metaanalyses of therapies for postmenopausal osteoporosis. V. Metaanalysis of the efficacy of hormone replacement therapy in treating and preventing osteoporosis in postmenopausal women. Endocr Rev 23:529, 2002

Whitaker M, Guo J, Kehoe T, Benson G. Bisphosphonates for osteoporosis—where do we go from here? N Engl J Med 366:2048, 2012

Wilson PW, Garrison RJ, Castelli WP: Postmenopausal estrogen use, cigarette smoking, and cardiovascular morbidity in women over 50. The Framingham Study. N Engl J Med 313(17):1038, 1985

Yaffe K, Sawaya G, Lieberburg I, et al: Estrogen therapy in postmenopausal women: effects on cognitive function and dementia. JAMA 279(9):688, 1998

Ye YB, Wang ZL, Zhuo SY, et al: Soy germ isoflavones improve menopausal symptoms but have no effect on blood lipids in early postmenopausal Chinese women: a randomized placebo-controlled trial. Menopause 19(7):791, 2012

Zandi PP, Carlson MC, Plassman BL, et al: Hormone replacement therapy and incidence of Alzheimer disease in older women: the Cache County Study. JAMA 288(17):2123, 2002

Zava DT, Dollbaum CM, Blen M: Estrogen and progestin bioactivity of foods, herbs, and spices. Proc Soc Exp Biol Med 217(3):369, 1998

Zweifel JE, O'Brien WH: A metaanalysis of the effect of hormone replacement therapy upon depressed mood. Psychoneuroendocrinology 22(3):189, 1997

SECTION 3

FEMALE PELVIC MEDICINE AND RECONSTRUCTIVE SURGERY

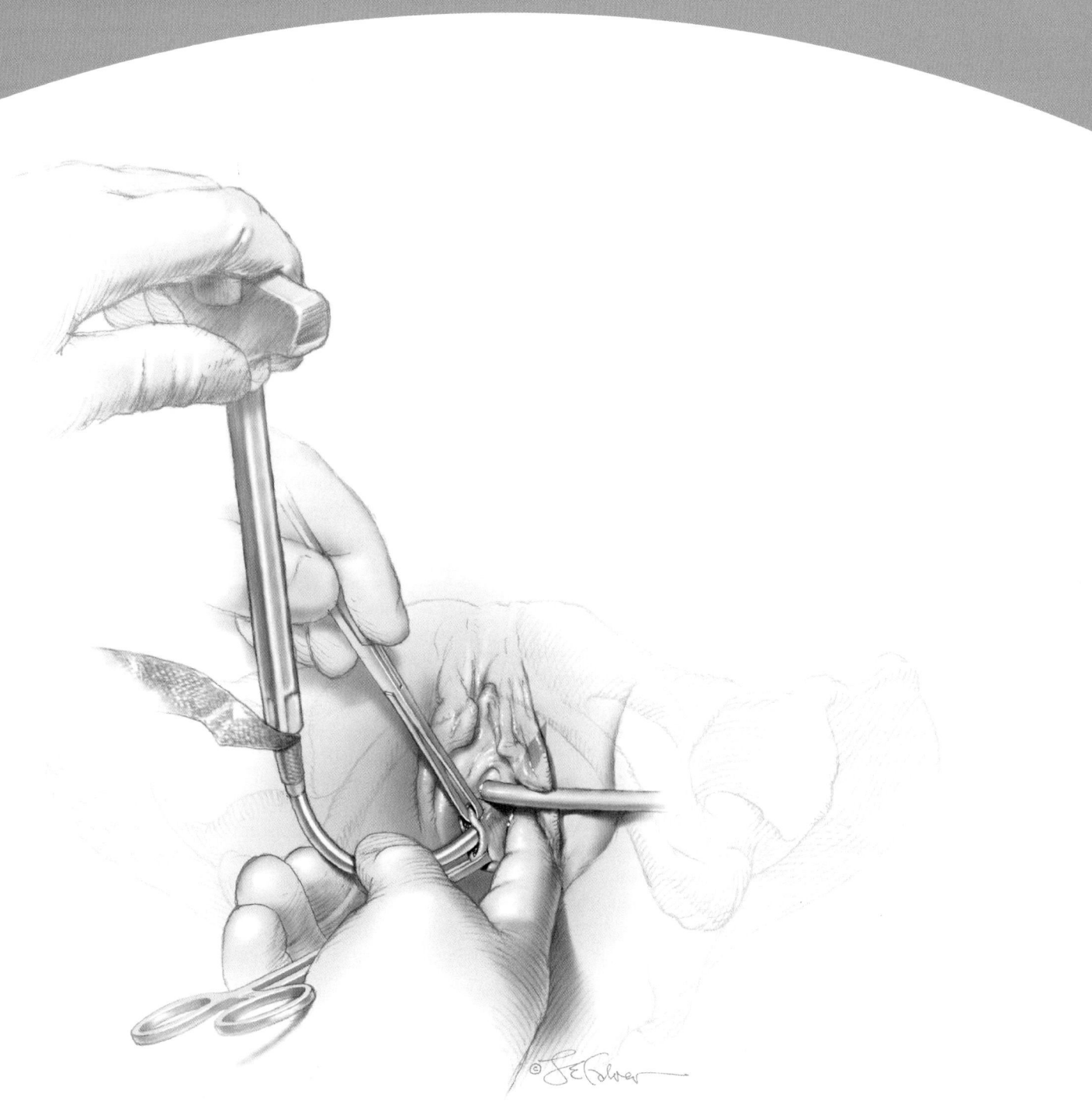

CHAPTER 23

Urinary Incontinence

DEFINITIONS

Urinary incontinence is defined as involuntary leakage of urine. This is in contrast to urine that leaks from extraurethral sources, such as with fistulas or congenital malformations of the lower urinary tract. Although incontinence is categorized into several forms, this chapter focuses on the evaluation and management of stress and urgency urinary incontinence. *Stress urinary incontinence (SUI)* is the involuntary leakage of urine with increases in intraabdominal pressure. *Urgency urinary incontinence* (previously "urge" urinary incontinence) is the involuntary leakage accompanied or immediately preceded by a perceived strong imminent need to void. A related condition, *overactive bladder*, describes urinary urgency with or without incontinence and usually with increased daytime urinary frequency and nocturia (Abrams, 2009).

According to International Continence Society guidelines, urinary incontinence is a symptom, a sign, and a condition (Abrams, 2002). For example, with SUI, a patient may complain of involuntary urine leakage with exercise or laughing. Concurrent with these symptoms, involuntary leakage from the urethra synchronous with cough or Valsalva may be observed during examination by a provider. And as a condition, SUI is objectively demonstrated during urodynamic testing if involuntary leakage of urine is seen with increased abdominal pressure and absence of detrusor muscle contraction. Under these circumstances, when the symptom or sign of SUI is confirmed with objective testing, the term *urodynamic stress incontinence* is preferred.

With urgency urinary incontinence, women have difficulty postponing urination urges and generally must promptly empty their bladder on cue and without delay. Common triggers are hand washing, running water, or exposure to cold. Urgency urinary incontinence is sometimes objectively demonstrated during urodynamic testing to correspond temporally with spontaneous detrusor muscle contractions—a condition termed *detrusor overactivity*. When both stress and urgency symptoms are present, it is called *mixed urinary incontinence*.

EPIDEMIOLOGY

In Western societies, epidemiologic studies indicate a prevalence of urinary incontinence of 25 to 51 percent and even higher among nursing home patients (Buckley, 2010; Markland, 2011). This wide range is attributed to variations in research methodologies, population characteristics, and definitions of incontinence. As part of the 2005 to 2006 National Health and Nutrition Examination Survey (NHANES), a cross-sectional group of 1961 nonpregnant, noninstitutionalized women in the United States were questioned regarding pelvic floor disorders. Urinary incontinence characterized by participants as moderate to severe leakage was identified in 15.7 percent (Nygaard, 2008). However, current available data are limited by the fact that most women do not seek medical attention for this condition (Hunskaar, 2000). It is estimated that only one in four women will seek medical advice for incontinence, due to embarrassment, limited health care access, or poor screening by health care providers (Hagstad, 1985).

Among ambulatory women with urinary incontinence, the most common type is SUI, which represents 29 to 75 percent of cases. Urgency urinary incontinence accounts for up to 33 percent of incontinence cases, whereas the remainder is attributable to mixed forms (Hunskaar, 2000). In one review, 15 percent of 64,528 women met criteria for overactive bladder with or without incontinence, and 11 percent had urgency urinary incontinence (Hartmann, 2009).

Urinary incontinence can significantly impair quality of life and lead to disrupted social relationships, embarrassment and frustration, hospitalizations due to skin breakdown and urinary tract infection (UTI), and nursing home admission. An incontinent elderly woman is 2.5 times more likely to be admitted to a nursing home than a continent one (Langa, 2002). Moreover, population projections from the U.S. Census Bureau forecast that the number of American women with urinary incontinence will increase 55 percent from 18.3 million to 28.4 million between 2010 and 2050 (Wu, 2009).

RISKS

◼ Age

The prevalence of incontinence appears to increase gradually during young adult life. For example, data from the 2005 to 2006 NHANES demonstrate a steady increase in incontinence prevalence with age: 7 percent in those aged 20 to 40 years, 17 percent for ages 40 to 60, 23 percent for ages 60 to 80, and 32 percent for those older than 80 (Nygaard, 2008).

Incontinence should not be viewed as a normal consequence of aging. However, several physiologic age-related changes in the lower urinary tract may predispose to incontinence, overactive bladder, or other voiding difficulties. First, the prevalence of involuntary detrusor contractions increases with age, and detrusor overactivity is found in 21 percent of healthy, continent community-dwelling elderly (Resnick, 1995). Both total bladder capacity and the ability to postpone voiding decreases, and these declines may lead to urinary frequency. In addition, urinary flow rates are reduced in older women and are likely due to an age-associated decrease in detrusor contractility (Resnick, 1984). In women, postmenopausal decreases in estrogen levels result in atrophy of the urethral mucosal seal, loss of compliance, and bladder irritation, which may predispose to both stress and urgency urinary incontinence. Finally, renal filtration rate and diurnal levels of antidiuretic hormone and atrial natriuretic factor change with age. These alterations shift the diurnal-predominant pattern of fluid excretion toward one with greater urine excretion later in the day (Kirkland, 1983).

◼ Other Factors

Race may influence incontinence rates, and white women are believed to have higher SUI rates than women of other races. In contrast, urgency urinary incontinence is believed to be more prevalent among African-American women. Most reports are not population-based and thus are not the best estimate of true racial differences. However, data from the Nurses' Health Study cohorts, which included more than 76,000 women, did support these racial differences (Townsend, 2010). It is not yet clear whether these differences are biologic, related to healthcare access, or affected by cultural expectations and symptom tolerance thresholds.

Body mass index (BMI) is a significant and independent risk factor for urinary incontinence of all types (Table 23-1). Specifically, the prevalence of both urgency urinary and stress incontinence increases proportionally with BMI (Hannestad, 2003). Theoretically, the increase in intraabdominal pressure

TABLE 23-1. Risk Factors for Urinary Incontinence

Age
Obesity
Smoking
Pregnancy
Childbirth
Menopause
Urinary symptoms
Cognitive impairment
Functional impairment
Chronically increased abdominal pressure
    Chronic cough
    Constipation
    Occupational lifting

that coincides with an increased BMI results in a higher intravesical pressure. This higher pressure overcomes urethral closing pressure and leads to incontinence (Bai, 2002). Encouragingly, weight loss for many can be an effective treatment and is considered a first-line option to reduce urinary incontinence rates (Dumoulin, 2014b). The prevalence of urinary incontinence significantly declines following weight loss achieved by behavior modification or with bariatric surgery (Burgio, 2007; Deitel, 1988; Subak, 2009). Even losses of 5 to 10 percent of body weight are sufficient for significant improvement in urinary incontinence (Wing, 2010).

Menopause may have a relationship with incontinence, but studies have inconsistently demonstrated an increase in urinary dysfunction rates (Bump, 1998). In those with symptoms, separating aging changes from hypoestrogenism effects is difficult. First, high-affinity estrogen receptors are found in the urethra, pubococcygeal muscle, and bladder trigone but are infrequently found elsewhere in the bladder (Iosif, 1981). Hypoestrogenic-related collagen changes and reductions in urethral vascularity and skeletal muscle volume are factors. They are thought collectively to contribute to impaired urethral function via a decreased resting urethral pressure (Carlile, 1988). Moreover, estrogen deficiency with resulting urogenital atrophy is believed to be responsible in part for urinary sensory symptoms following menopause (Raz, 1993). Despite this current evidence, it is less clear whether estrogen therapy is useful in the treatment or prevention of incontinence. Namely, systemic estrogen replacement, compared with placebo, appears to worsen incontinence, whereas topical vaginal estrogen application *may improve* incontinence (Cody, 2012; Fantl, 1994, 1996; Rahn, 2014, 2015).

Childbirth and pregnancy also play a role, and urinary incontinence prevalence is higher in parous women compared with nulliparas. The effects of childbirth may result from direct injury to pelvic muscles and connective tissue attachments. In addition, nerve damage from trauma or stretch injury can lead to pelvic muscle dysfunction. Specifically, rates of prolonged pudendal nerve latency after delivery are higher in women with incontinence compared with asymptomatic puerperal women (Snooks, 1986).

Of potential obstetric factors, one large study identified that fetal birthweight >4000 g increased the risk of all urinary incontinence types (Rortveit, 2003b). These authors also noted that cesarean delivery may offer a short-term protective effect from urinary incontinence. The adjusted odds ratio for any incontinence associated with vaginal delivery compared with that with cesarean delivery was 1.7 (Rortveit, 2003a). However, the protective effect of cesarean delivery on incontinence may dissipate after additional deliveries, decreases with age, and is not present in older women (Nygaard, 2006).

Family history may alter incontinence risks, and the urinary incontinence rates may be increased in the daughters and sisters of incontinent women. In one large survey, daughters of incontinent women had an increased relative risk of 1.3 and an absolute risk of 23 percent of having urinary incontinence. Younger sisters of incontinent women also had a greater likelihood of having any urinary incontinence (Hannestad, 2004).

Chronic obstructive pulmonary disease in women older than 60 years significantly increases urinary incontinence risks

(Brown, 1996; Diokno, 1990). Similarly, cigarette smoking is identified as an independent risk factor for urinary incontinence. Both current and former smokers have a two- to three-fold risk of incontinence compared with nonsmokers (Brown, 1996; Bump, 1992; Diokno, 1990). In one study, investigators found an association between current and former smoking and incontinence, but only for those who smoked more than 20 cigarettes daily. Severe incontinence was weakly associated with smoking regardless of cigarette number (Hannestad, 2003). Theoretically, persistently increased intraabdominal pressures are generated from a smoker's chronic cough, and collagen synthesis is diminished by smoking's antiestrogenic effects.

Hysterectomy does not appear to increase urinary incontinence rates. Studies that include pre- and postoperative urodynamic testing reveal clinically insignificant changes in bladder function. Moreover, evidence does not support avoidance of clinically indicated hysterectomy or the selection of supracervical hysterectomy as measures to prevent urinary incontinence (Vervest, 1989; Wake, 1980).

PATHOPHYSIOLOGY

■ Continence

The bladder has the capacity to accommodate large increases in volume with minimal or no increases in intravesical pressure. The ability to store urine coupled with convenient and socially acceptable voluntary emptying is *continence*. Continence requires the complex coordination of multiple components that include: muscle contraction and relaxation, appropriate connective tissue support, and integrated innervation and communication between these structures. Simplistically, during filling, urethral contraction is coordinated with bladder relaxation and urine is stored. During voiding, the urethra relaxes and the bladder contracts. These mechanisms can be challenged by uninhibited detrusor contractions, marked increases in intraabdominal pressure, and degradation or dysfunction of the various anatomic components of the continence mechanism.

■ Bladder Filling

Bladder Anatomy

The bladder wall is multilayered and contains mucosal, submucosal, muscular, and adventitial layers (Fig. 23-1). The bladder mucosa is composed of a transitional cell epithelium, supported by a lamina propria. With small bladder volumes, the mucosa appears as convoluted folds. However, with bladder filling, it is stretched and thinned. The bladder epithelium, termed *uroepithelium*, is made up of distinct cell layers. The most superficial is the umbrella cell layer, and its impermeability is thought to provide the primary urine-plasma barrier. Covering the uroepithelium is a glycosaminoglycan (GAG) layer. This GAG layer may prohibit bacterial adherence and prevents urothelial damage by acting as a protective barrier. Specifically, theories suggest that this carbohydrate polymer layer may be defective in patients with interstitial cystitis (Chap. 11, p. 263).

The muscular layer, termed the detrusor muscle, is composed of three smooth-muscle layers arranged in a plexiform fashion. This unique arrangement allows for rapid multidimensional expansion during bladder filling and is a key component to the bladder's ability to accommodate large volumes.

Innervation

Normal function of the lower urinary tract requires integration of peripheral and central nervous systems. The peripheral nervous system contains somatic and autonomic divisions (Fig. 23-2). Of these, the somatic component innervates striated muscle, whereas the autonomic division innervates smooth muscle.

The autonomic nervous system controls involuntary action and is categorized into sympathetic and parasympathetic divisions. The sympathetic system mediates its end-organ effects through epinephrine or norepinephrine acting on α- or β-adrenergic receptors (Fig. 23-3). The parasympathetic division acts through acetylcholine binding to muscarinic or nicotinic receptors. In the pelvis, autonomic fibers that supply the pelvic viscera course in the superior and inferior hypogastric plexi (Fig. 23-4).

The somatic nervous system controls voluntary movement, and the portion of this system that is most relevant to lower urinary tract function originates from Onuf somatic nucleus. This nucleus is located in the ventral horn gray matter of spinal levels S2–S4 and contains the neurons that innervate the striated urogenital sphincter complex, described next. Nerves involved with that connection include branches of the pudendal and pelvic nerves.

Urogenital Sphincter

As the bladder fills, synchronized contraction of the urogenital sphincter is integral to continence. Composed of striated muscle, this sphincter complex includes: (1) the *sphincter urethrae*, (2) the *urethrovaginal sphincter*, and (3) the *compressor urethrae*. The sphincter urethrae wraps circumferentially around the urethra. In comparison, the urethrovaginal sphincter and the compressor urethrae arch ventrally over the urethra and insert into the fibromuscular tissue of the anterior vaginal wall (Fig. 23-5).

These three muscles function as a single unit and contract to close the urethra. Contraction of these muscles circumferentially constricts the cephalad two thirds of the urethra and laterally compresses the distal one third. The sphincter urethrae is predominantly composed of slow-twitch fibers and remains tonically contracted, contributing substantially to continence at rest. In contrast, the urethrovaginal sphincter and the compressor urethrae are comprised of fast-twitch muscle fibers, which allow brisk contraction and urethra lumen closure when continence is challenged by sudden increases in intraabdominal pressure.

Innervation Important to Storage

The urogenital sphincter receives somatic motor innervation through the pudendal and pelvic nerves (Fig. 23-6). Thus, pudendal neuropathy, which may follow obstetric injury, can affect normal sphincter functioning. Additionally, prior pelvic surgery or pelvic radiation therapy may damage nerves, vasculature, and soft tissue. Such injury can lead to ineffective urogenital sphincter action and contribute to incontinence.

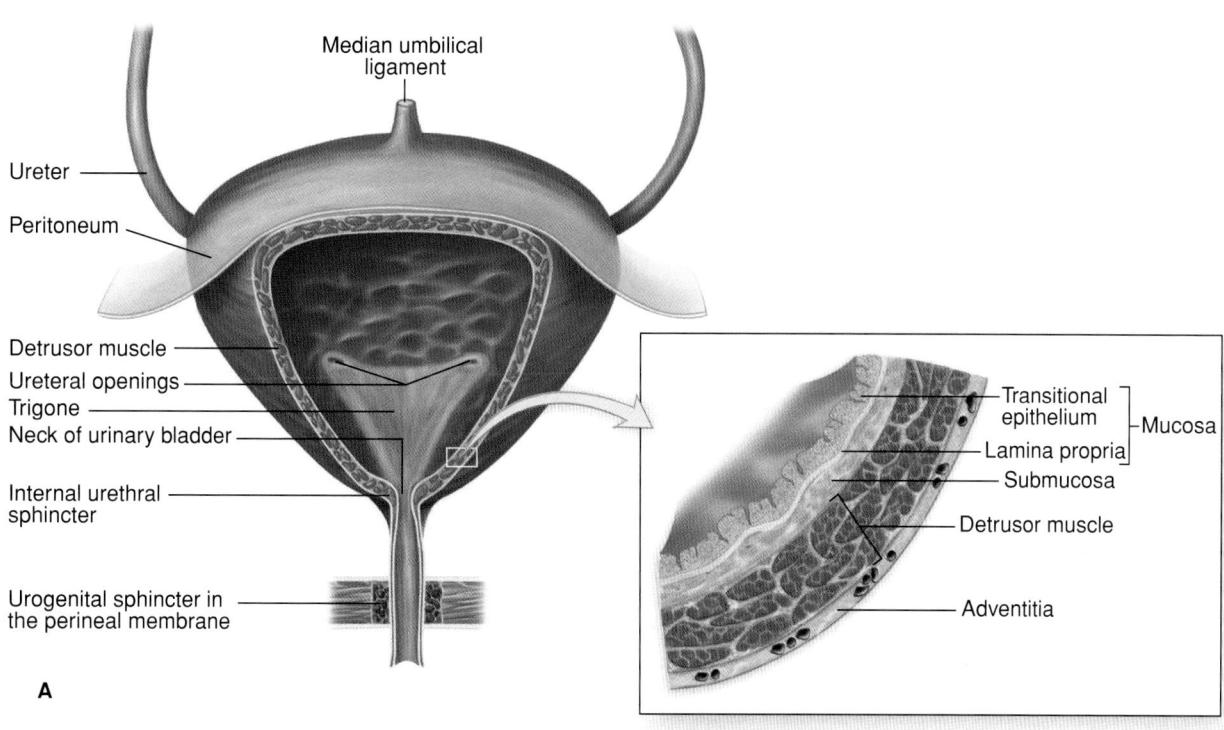

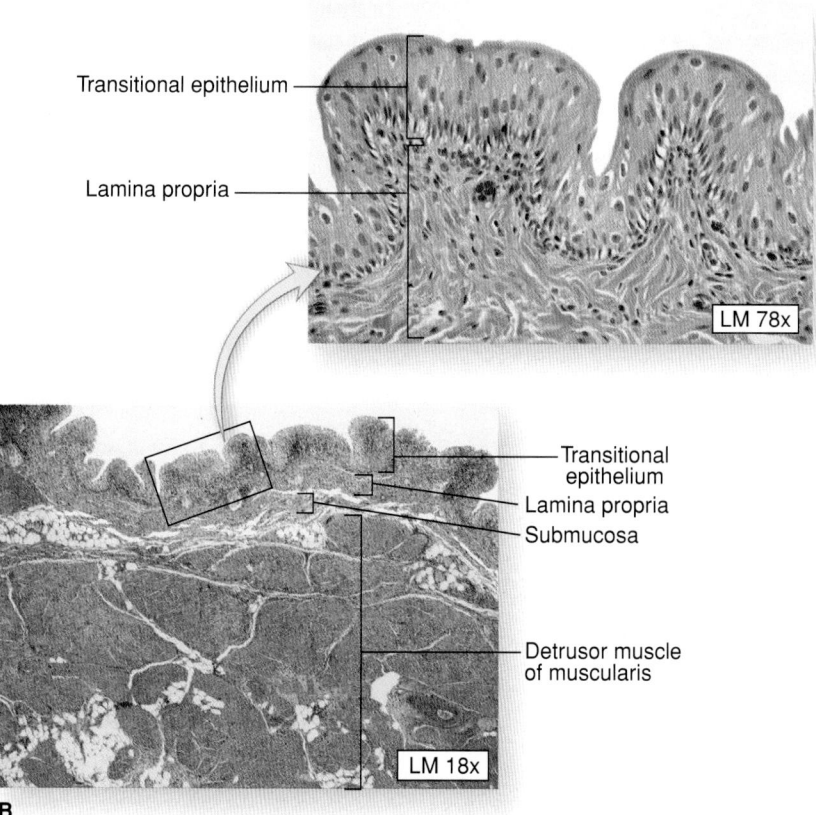

FIGURE 23-1 Bladder anatomy. **A.** Anteroposterior view of bladder anatomy. Inset: The bladder wall contains mucosal, submucosal, muscular, and adventitial layers. **B.** Photomicrograph of the bladder wall. The mucosa of an empty bladder is thrown into convoluted folds or rugae. The plexiform arrangement of muscle fibers of the detrusor muscle cause difficulty in defining its three distinct layers. (Reproduced with permission from McKinley M, O'Loughlin VD: Human Anatomy. New York: McGraw-Hill; 2006.)

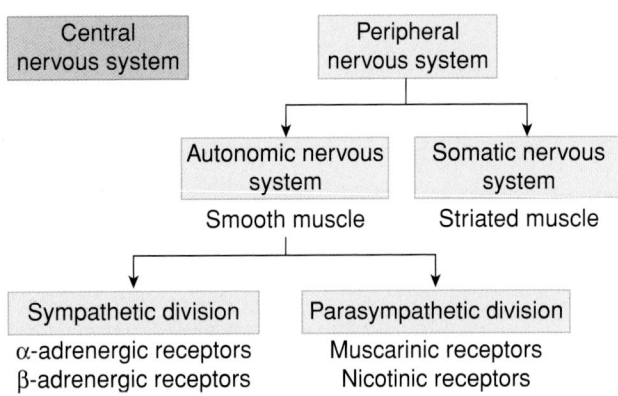

FIGURE 23-2 Divisions of the human nervous system. The peripheral nervous system includes: (1) the somatic nervous system, which mediates voluntary movements through its actions on striated muscle and (2) the autonomic nervous system, which controls involuntary motion through its actions on smooth muscle. The autonomic nervous system is further divided into the sympathetic division, which acts through epinephrine and norepinephrine binding to adrenergic receptors and (2) the parasympathetic division, which acts through acetylcholine binding to muscarinic or nicotinic receptors.

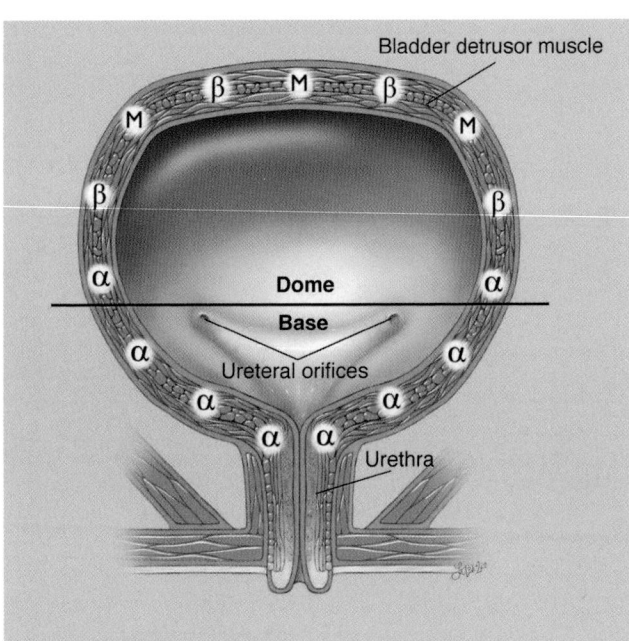

FIGURE 23-3 The bladder dome is rich in parasympathetic muscarinic receptors (M) and sympathetic β-adrenergic receptors (β). The bladder neck contains a greater density of sympathetic α-adrenergic receptors (α). (Used with permission from Lindsay Oksenberg.)

Sympathetic fibers are carried through the superior hypogastric nerve plexus and communicate with α- and β-adrenergic receptors within the bladder and urethra. β-Adrenergic receptor stimulation in the bladder dome results in smooth-muscle relaxation and assists with urine storage (Fig. 23-7). β-Agonist medication may improve overactive bladder symptoms through this mechanism of smooth muscle relaxation. In contrast, α-adrenergic receptors predominate in the bladder base and urethra. These receptors are stimulated by norepinephrine, which initiates a cascade of events that preferentially leads to urethral contraction and aids urine storage and continence. These effects of α-stimulation underlie the treatment of SUI with imipramine, a tricyclic antidepressant with adrenergic agonist properties.

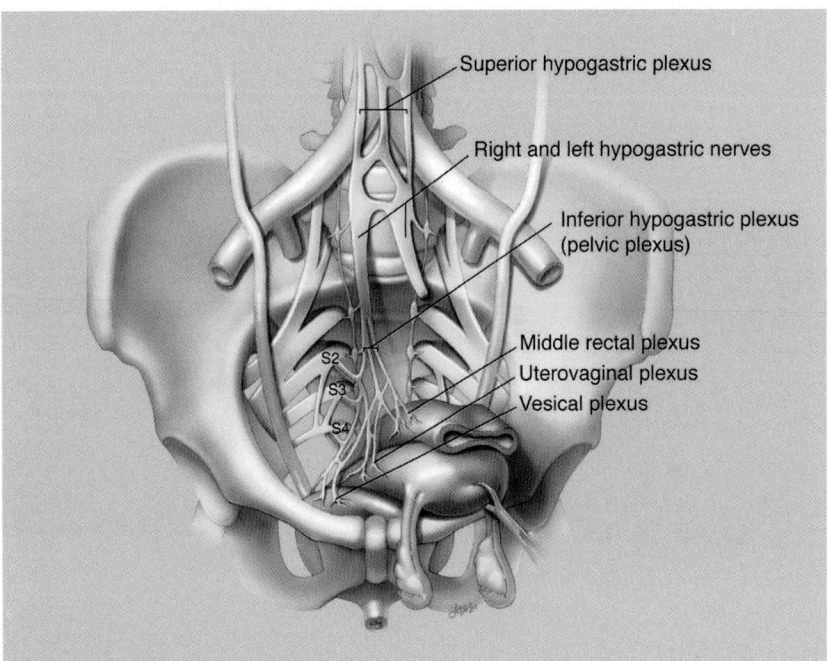

FIGURE 23-4 The inferior hypogastric plexus, also known as the pelvic plexus, is formed by visceral efferents from S2 to S4, which provide the parasympathetic component by way of the pelvic nerves. The superior hypogastric plexus primarily contains sympathetic fibers from the T10 to L2 cord segments and terminates by dividing into right and left hypogastric nerves. The hypogastric nerves and rami from the sacral portion of the sympathetic chain contribute the sympathetic component to the pelvic plexus. The pelvic plexus divides into three portions according to the course and distribution of its fibers: the middle rectal plexus, uterovaginal plexus, and vesical plexus. (Used with permission from Lindsay Oksenberg.)

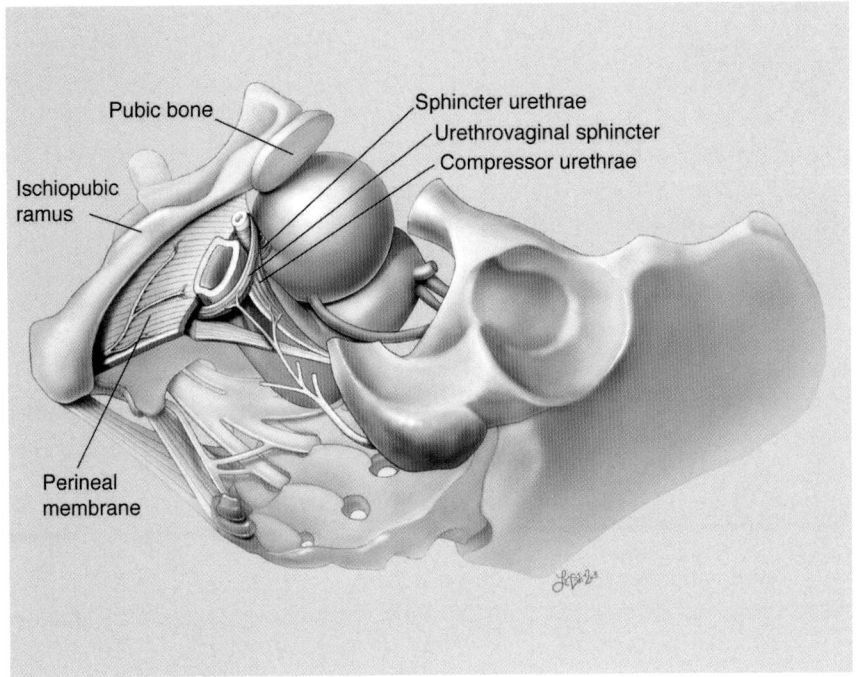

FIGURE 23-5 Striated urogenital sphincter anatomy. The perineal membrane is removed to show the three component muscles of the striated urogenital sphincter. This sphincter receives most of its somatic innervation through the pudendal nerve. (Used with permission from Lindsay Oksenberg.)

Urethral Coaptation

One key to maintaining continence is adequate urethral mucosal coaptation. The uroepithelium is supported by a connective tissue layer, which is thrown into deep folds, also known as plications. A rich capillary network runs within its subepithelial layer. This vascular network aids in urethral mucosal approximation, also termed *coaptation*, by acting like an "inflatable cushion" (Fig. 23-8). In women who are hypoestrogenic, this submucosal vasculature plexus is less prominent. In part, hormone replacement targets this diminished vascularity and and in theory, enhances coaptation to improve continence.

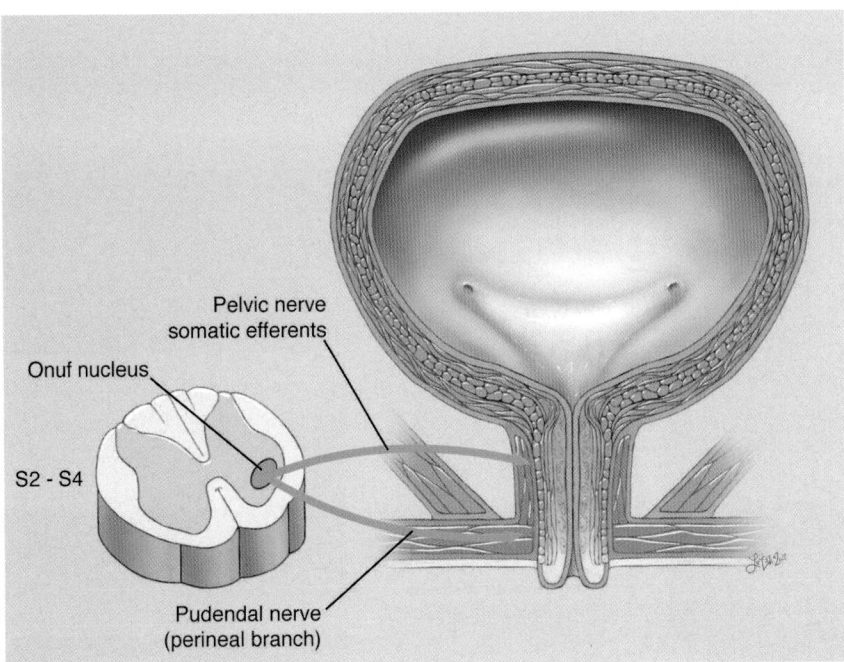

FIGURE 23-6 Onuf nucleus is found in the ventral horn gray matter of S2 through S4. This nucleus contains the neurons whose fibers supply the striated urogenital sphincter. The urethrovaginal sphincter and compressor urethrae are innervated by the perineal branch of the pudendal nerve. The sphincter urethrae is variably innervated by somatic efferents that travel in the pelvic nerves. (Used with permission from Lindsay Oksenberg.)

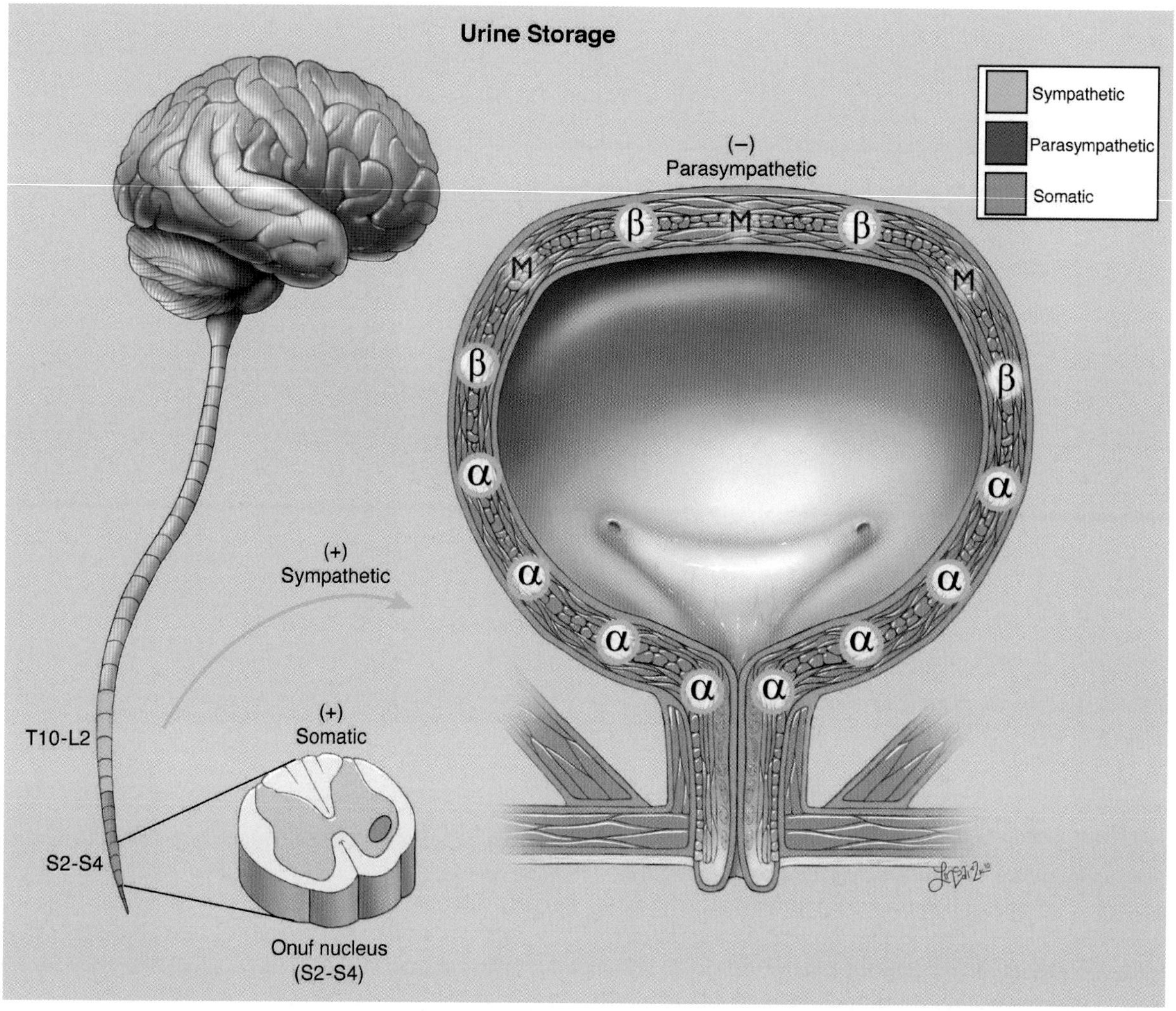

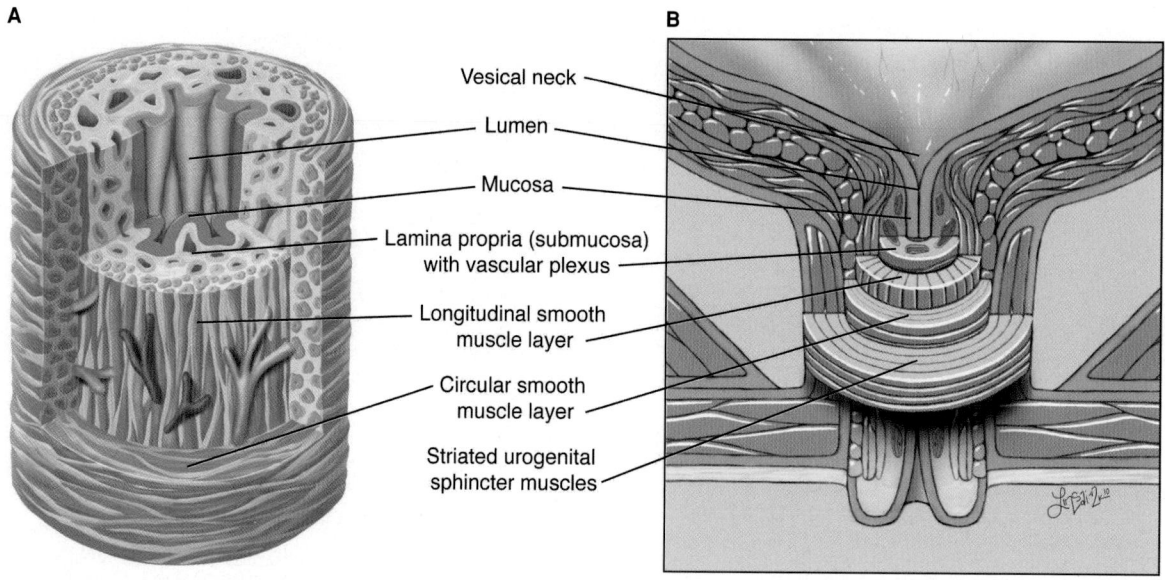

Urine Storage

FIGURE 23-7 Physiology of urine storage. Bladder distention from filling leads to: (1) α-adrenergic contraction of the urethral smooth muscle and increased tone at the vesical neck (via the T11-L2 spinal sympathetic reflex); (2) activation of urethral motor neurons in Onuf nucleus with contraction of striated urogenital sphincter muscles (via the pudendal nerve); and (3) inhibited parasympathetic transmission with decreased detrusor pressure. α = alpha adrenergic receptors; β = beta adrenergic; M = muscarinic (cholinergic). (Used with permission from Lindsay Oksenberg.)

A

B

Vesical neck

Lumen

Mucosa

Lamina propria (submucosa) with vascular plexus

Longitudinal smooth muscle layer

Circular smooth muscle layer

Striated urogenital sphincter muscles

FIGURE 23-8 Drawing of urethral anatomy. **A.** Urethral anatomy in cross section. Urethral coaptation results in part from filling of the rich subepithelial vascular plexus. The urethra contains circular and longitudinal smooth muscle layers. **B.** Vesical neck and urethral anatomy. The striated urogenital sphincter lies external to the urethral smooth muscle layers. (Used with permission from Lindsay Oksenberg.)

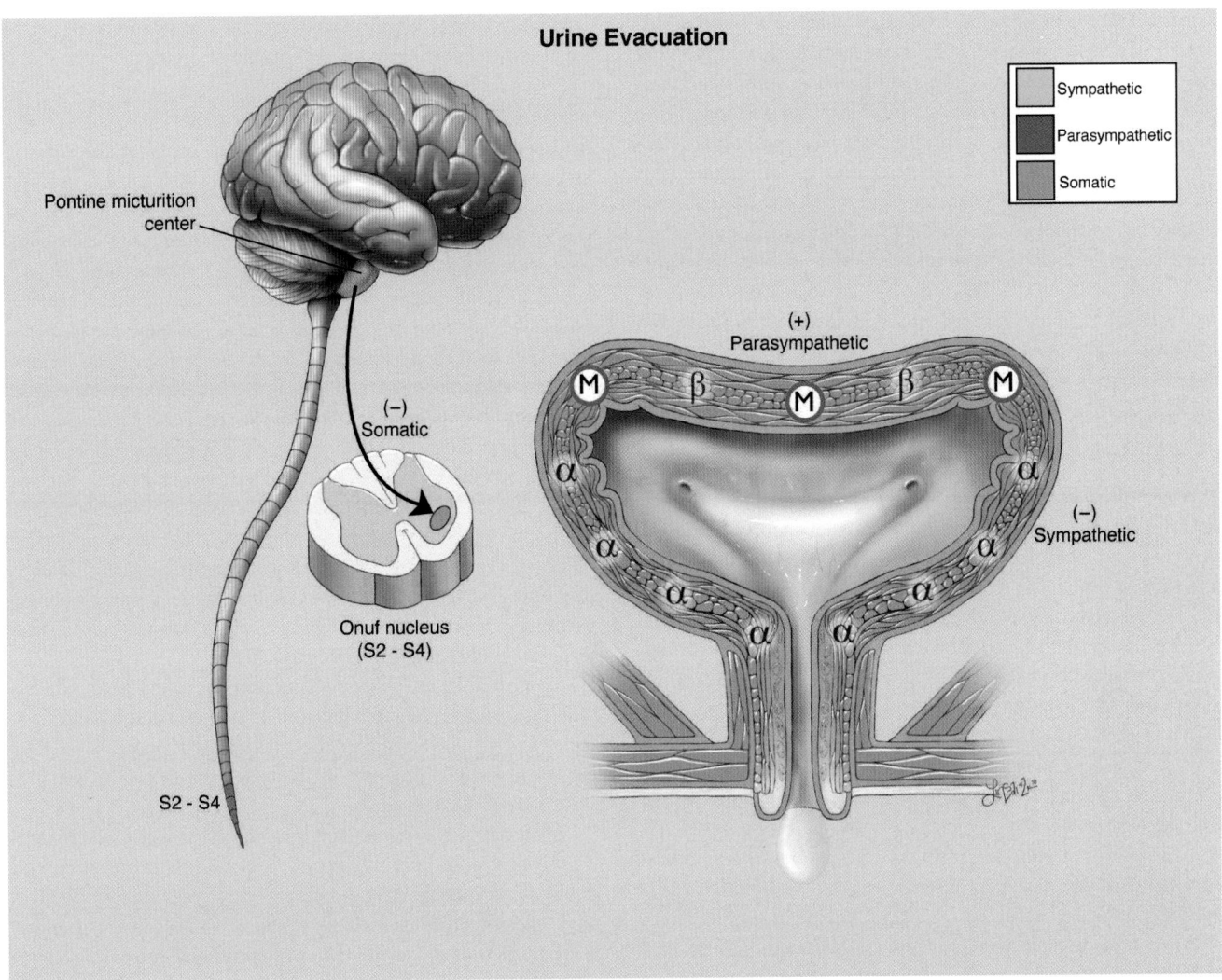

Urine Evacuation

Sympathetic
Parasympathetic
Somatic

Pontine micturition center

(+) Parasympathetic

(−) Somatic

Onuf nucleus (S2 - S4)

S2 - S4

(−) Sympathetic

FIGURE 23-9 Physiology of urine evacuation. Efferent impulses from the pontine micturition center results in inhibition of somatic fibers in Onuf nucleus and voluntary relaxation of the striated urogenital sphincter muscles. These efferent impulses also result in preganglionic sympathetic inhibition with opening of the vesical neck and parasympathetic stimulation, which results in detrusor muscarinic contraction. The net result is relaxation of the striated urogenital sphincter complex causing decreased urethral pressure, followed almost immediately by detrusor contraction and voiding. α = alpha adrenergic receptors; β = beta adrenergic; M = muscarinic (cholinergic). (Used with permission from Lindsay Oksenberg.)

■ Bladder Emptying

Innervation Related to Voiding

When an appropriate time for bladder emptying arises, sympathetic stimulation is reduced and parasympathetic stimulation is triggered. Specifically, neural impulses carried in the pelvic nerves stimulate acetylcholine release and lead to detrusor muscle contraction (Fig. 23-9). Concurrent with detrusor stimulation, acetylcholine also stimulates muscarinic receptors in the urethra and leads to outlet relaxation for voiding.

Within the parasympathetic division, acetylcholine receptors are broadly defined as muscarinic and nicotinic. The bladder is densely supplied with muscarinic receptors, which when stimulated lead to detrusor contraction. Of the muscarinic receptors, five glycoproteins designated M_1–M_5 have been identified. M_2 and M_3 receptor subtypes are predominantly responsible for detrusor smooth muscle contraction. Thus, treatment with muscarinic antagonist medication blunts detrusor contraction

to improve continence. Continence drugs that target only the M_3 receptor maximize drug efficacy yet minimize activation of other muscarinic receptors and drug side effects.

Muscular Activity with Voiding

Smooth muscle cells within the detrusor fuse with one another so that a network of low-resistance electrical pathways extends from one muscle cell to the next. Thus, action potentials can spread quickly throughout the detrusor muscle to cause rapid contraction of the entire bladder. In addition, the plexiform arrangement of bladder detrusor fibers allows multidirectional contraction and is ideally suited for rapid concentric contraction during bladder emptying.

During voiding, all components of the striated urogenital sphincter relax. Importantly, bladder contraction and sphincter relaxation must be coordinated for effective voiding. Occasionally, the urethral sphincter fails to relax during contraction of the detrusor and retention ensues. Classically, this is a possible urinary complication of spinal cord injury termed *detrusor sphincter dyssynergia* and may lead to elevated bladder pressures and vesicoureteral reflux. Women with this condition are sometimes treated with α-blocking agents to help with sphincter relaxation and to lower bladder pressures during contraction, but these may aggravate hypotension. In women without known neurologic pathology but still with inappropriately contracted pelvic floor musculature, treatment with muscle relaxants may be appropriate. These drugs purportedly relax the urethral sphincter and levator ani muscles to improve coordinated voiding.

■ Continence Theories

Anatomic Stress Incontinence

Theories on continence vary in their supportive evidence but can simplistically be distilled into those that involve anatomic stress incontinence or those that describe decreased urethral integrity (sphincteric deficiency). These theories are not mutually exclusive and in many women, both may be contributory.

First, urethral and bladder neck support is integral to continence. This anatomic support derives from: (1) ligaments along the urethra's lateral aspects, termed the pubourethral ligaments; (2) the vagina and its lateral fascial condensation; (3) the arcus tendineus fascia pelvis; and (4) levator ani muscles. A full anatomic description of these ligaments and muscles is found in Chapter 38 (p. 802).

In an ideally supported urogenital tract, increases in intraabdominal pressure are equally transmitted to the bladder, bladder base, and urethra. In women who are continent, increases in downward-directed pressure from cough, laugh, sneeze, and Valsalva maneuver are countered by supportive tissue tone provided by the levator ani muscles and vaginal connective tissue (Fig. 23-10). With loss of support, the ability of the urethra and bladder neck to close against a firm supportive "backboard" is diminished. This results in reduced urethral closing pressures, an inability to resist increases in bladder pressure, and in turn, incontinence. This mechanistic theory is the basis for surgical reestablishment of this support. Traditional procedures such as Burch and Marshall-Marchetti-Kranz (MMK)

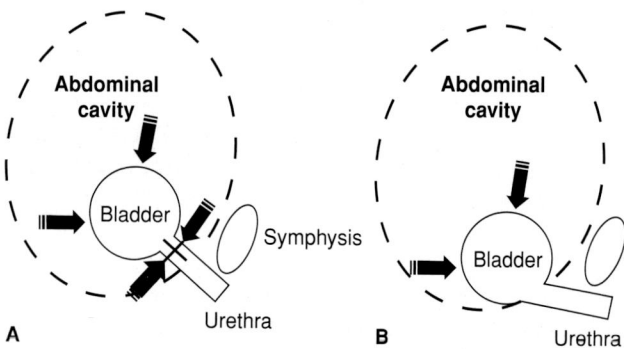

FIGURE 23-10 Drawing describes the pressure transmission theory. **A.** In women with normal support, increases in intraabdominal pressure are equally distributed to contralateral sides of the bladder and urethra. **B.** In those with poor urethral support, increases in intraabdominal pressure alter the urethrovesical angle and continence is lost.

colposuspensions attempt to return this anatomic support to the urethrovesical junction and proximal urethra.

Sphincteric Deficiency

Another way to conceptualize SUI is to consider the urethra as providing continence through the combination of: urethral mucosal coaptation, the underlying urethral vascular plexus, the combined viscous and elastic properties of the urethral epithelium, and contraction of appropriate surrounding musculature. Taken together, these components contribute to *urethral integrity*. Defects in any or a combination of these components may lead to urine leakage and have traditionally been termed *intrinsic sphincteric defect (ISD)*. For example, prior surgery in the retropubic space may cause denervation and scarring of the urethra and its supporting tissue. These effects subsequently prevent urethral closure and lead to incontinence. Specific causes are varied and include prior pelvic reconstructive surgeries, prior pelvic radiation therapy, diabetic neuropathy, neuronal degenerative diseases, and hypoestrogenism. Namely, in women with atrophic lower genital tracts, vascular changes within the plexus surrounding the urethra lead to poor coaptation and greater incontinence risks.

As noted earlier, nerve dysfunction following birth trauma may lead to defective urethral sphincter function. In addition, childbirth also often injures urethral fascial support. This clinical example highlights the intimate relationship between urethral support and integrity.

Treatments to restore urethral integrity include transurethral injection of bulking agents, surgical sling procedures, and pelvic floor muscle strengthening, which are all described in later sections. In brief, bulking agents are placed at the urethrovesical junction to elevate the epithelium and promote coaptation. Alternatively, sling procedures restore periurethral support anatomy or create partial urethral obstruction to enhance urethral integrity. Last, because the urethra exits through urogenital hiatus, levator ani muscle conditioning with Kegel exercises can bolster urethral integrity. These muscles can be contracted around the urethra when continence is challenged during sudden increases in intraabdominal pressures.

A consideration for surgical management of patients with ISD, particularly those younger than 50 years, is that a retropubic colposuspension procedure merely elevates and stabilizes the urethra and does not promote coaptation. This may be less likely to achieve satisfactory continence than a procedure directed at both anatomic stress incontinence and deficient urethral sphincter function and support (Sand, 1987). That said, a small trial randomizing incontinent women with ISD to Burch or sling procedures did not show differences in postoperative voiding function or in SUI cure rates (Culligan, 2003).

DIAGNOSIS

■ History

Symptom Clustering

Assessment of incontinence begins with a patient describing her urinary symptoms. These complaints may be collected through direct conversation but can be augmented with patient

TABLE 23-2. The Three Incontinence Questions (3IQ)

1. During the last 3 months, have you leaked urine (even a small amount)?
   a. Yes (continue questions)
   b. No (questionnaire completed)
2. During the last 3 months, did you leak urine: (mark all that apply)
   a. When you were performing some physical activity, such as coughing, sneezing, lifting, or exercise?
   b. When you had the urge or feeling that you needed to empty your bladder, but you could not get to the toilet fast enough?
   c. Without physical activity and without a sense of urgency?
3. During the last 3 months, did you leak urine *most often*: (mark only one)
   a. When you were performing some physical activity, such as coughing, sneezing, lifting, or exercise?
   b. When you had the urge or feeling that you needed to empty your bladder, but you could not get to the toilet fast enough?
   c. Without physical activity and without a sense of urgency?
   d. About equally as often with physical activity as with a sense of urgency?

The response to question 3 with (a) or (b) indicates stress-predominant or urgency-predominant incontinence, respectively, whereas (d) indicates mixed and (c) suggests another cause of incontinence.

Bladder Diary Please record the time and amount of your oral intake, urine output, urine leakage, and pad changes FOR 3 DAYS			
Time	Oral Intake	Voided Urine	Urine Leakage or Pad Change

FIGURE 23-11 Example of a urinary diary.

questionnaires. Two common forms are the Pelvic Floor Distress Inventory and the Pelvic Floor Impact Questionnaire. Both are available in long and short forms and evaluate urinary, bowel, and prolapse symptoms (Barber, 2001). Such lengthy research questionnaires may be impractical for general clinical practice. Instead, shorter validated questionnaires may easily be incorporated into the clinic setting. As shown in Table 23-2, the 3IQ has only three questions that screen for incontinence and then helps clarify the incontinence type (Brown, 2006).

During inquiry, the number of voids and pads used per day, type of pad, frequency of pad changing, and the degree of pad saturation are important. Although these specifics alone may not establish the exact type of incontinence, they do provide information regarding symptom severity and its effects on patient activities. If a woman's symptoms do not diminish her quality of life, then simple observation is reasonable. Conversely, those with bothersome symptoms warrant further evaluation.

Specific to incontinence, information that describes the circumstances in which urine leaks and specific maneuvers that incite or provoke leakage are sought. With SUI, triggers may include increases in intraabdominal pressure such as coughing, sneezing, Valsalva maneuver, or deep penetration during intercourse. Alternatively, women with urgency urinary incontinence may describe urine loss after urge sensations that typically cannot be suppressed. *Overflow incontinence* was a term used in the past to refer to women who were unable to empty their bladder well but who also had involuntary, continuous urinary leakage or dribbling and often episodes of incontinence associated with urgency. Currently, however, this is considered by many to reflect another presentation of urgency urinary incontinence.

During questioning, symptoms typically cluster into those most frequently seen with SUI or with urgency urinary incontinence (see Table 23-2). Alternatively, a significant overlap of complaints may reflect coexistent SUI and urgency urinary incontinence, that is, mixed urinary incontinence. For these reasons, pattern identification is helpful as it may direct diagnostic testing and guide initial empiric therapy.

Voiding Diary

Typically, patients may not have an entirely accurate recollection of their own voiding habits. Accordingly, to obtain a thorough record, a woman ideally completes a urinary diary (Fig. 23-11). With this, the volumes and type of each oral fluid intake, volumes of urine with each void, episodes of urinary leakage, and triggers of incontinence episodes are recorded for 3 to 7 days. During each 24-hour period, women also record times of sleep and awakening to document voluntary nocturnal voiding patterns or enuresis. Three days usually suffices to determine the general trend of incontinence.

The information gained from a voiding/urinary diary is a valuable diagnostic and sometimes therapeutic tool. The first morning void is usually the largest of the day and is a good estimate of bladder capacity. Patients often can identify patterns in intake and voiding and modify behavior. For example, a patient may recognize increased urinary frequency or urgency urinary incontinence episodes after caffeine intake. Moreover, this diary information can serve as a baseline against which treatment effectiveness can be assessed.

Urinary Symptoms

Specific patient symptoms may help differentiate incontinence types. For example, most women void eight or fewer times per day. Without a history that reflects increased fluid intake, increased voiding may indicate overactive bladder, UTI, calculi, or urethral pathology and often prompts additional evaluation. In addition, urinary frequency is commonly associated with interstitial cystitis (IC). In women with IC, the numbers of voids may commonly exceed 20 per day. Nocturia may be noted in women with urgency urinary incontinence or in those with systemic fluid management disorders such as congestive heart failure. In the latter case, treatment of the underlying condition frequently leads to symptom improvement or cure of nighttime frequency.

Urinary retention may provide clues. Often incomplete emptying can result in incontinence associated with either stress or urgency. Urethral obstruction, often manifested as an inability to void or an impeded urinary stream, is uncommon in women. Its description prompts careful evaluation for pelvic organ prolapse and underscores the importance of asking about prior pelvic/vaginal surgery or trauma that could scar or obstruct the urethra.

Of other urinary symptoms, the volume of urine lost with each episode may aid diagnosis. Large volumes are typically lost following a spontaneous detrusor contraction associated with urgency urinary incontinence and may often involve loss of the entire bladder volume. In contrast, woman with SUI usually describe smaller volumes lost. Moreover, these women often are able to contract the levator ani muscles to temporarily stop their urine stream. Another symptom, postvoid dribbling, is classically associated with urethral diverticulum, which may often be mistaken for urinary incontinence (Chap. 26, p. 582). Hematuria, although a common sign of UTI, may also indicate underlying malignancy and can cause irritative voiding symptoms.

Symptom onset may also prove informative. For example, problems beginning at menopause may suggest hypoestrogenism as an etiology. These patients may benefit from topical vaginal estrogen. In contrast, symptoms after hysterectomy or childbirth may reflect changes in tissue support or innervation.

Past Medical History

Obstetric trauma may be associated with damage to pelvic floor support, which may lead to SUI. Accordingly, information is sought regarding a prolonged labor, operative vaginal delivery, macrosomia, or postpartum catheterization for urinary retention. As alluded to earlier, urinary incontinence can be linked with several medical conditions or their treatments, which could be modified to improve incontinence. To help remember these potential contributors, a useful mnemonic is "DIAPPERS": dementia/delirium, infection, atrophic vaginitis, psychological, pharmacologic, endocrine, restricted mobility, and stool impaction (Swift, 2008).

First, continence requires the cognitive ability to recognize and react appropriately to the sensation of a full bladder, motivation to maintain dryness, sufficient mobility and manual dexterity, and ready access to a toilet. Patients with dementia or significant psychological impairments often do not have the necessary cognitive ability for continence. Women with severe physical handicaps or restricted mobility may simply not have time to reach the toilet, especially in the setting of urinary urgency/overactive bladder. Thus, this so-called functional incontinence occurs in situations in which a woman cannot reach a toilet in time because of physical, psychological, or mentation limitations. Often, this group would be continent if

these issues were absent. Simple interventions such as a bedside commode may be helpful in such cases.

Urinary tract infections cause bladder mucosal inflammation. This inflammation is thought to increase sensory afferent activity, which contributes to an overactive bladder. Similarly, estrogen deficiency can lead to atrophic epithelium of the vagina and urethra. These are associated with increased local irritation and greater risks of UTI and overactive bladder.

A detailed medication inventory is collected. Pertinent drugs include estrogen, α-adrenergic agonists, and diuretics, to name a few (Table 23-3).

Of endocrinopathies, diabetes mellitus can promote osmotic diuresis and polyuria if glucose control is poor. Polydipsia from diabetes insipidus or excessive caffeine or alcohol intake can also lead to polyuria or urinary frequency. Similarly, other disorders of impaired arginine vasopressin secretion or action may cause polyuria and nocturia (Ouslander, 2004). Conditions such as congestive heart failure, hypothyroidism, venous insufficiency, and the effects of certain medications all contribute to peripheral edema, leading to urinary frequency and nocturia when a patient is supine.

Last, stool impaction resulting from poor bowel habits and constipation can contribute to overactive bladder symptoms. This is perhaps from local irritation or direct compression against the bladder wall.

■ Physical Examination

General Inspection and Neurologic Evaluation

Initially, the perineum is inspected for evidence of atrophy, which may be noted throughout the lower genital tract. In addition, a suburethral cystic mass or dilation with transurethral expression of fluid during compression suggests a urethral diverticulum (Fig. 26-6, p. 585).

Examination of an incontinent woman also includes a detailed neurologic evaluation of the perineum. Because neurologic responses may be altered in an anxious patient who is in a vulnerable setting, signs elicited during evaluation may not signify true pathology and are interpreted with caution. Neurologic testing begins with an attempt to elicit a *bulbocavernosus reflex*. During this test, one labium majus is stroked with a cotton swab. Normally, both labia generally contract at the same time. The afferent limb of this reflex is the clitoral branch of the pudendal nerve, whereas its efferent limb is conducted through the inferior hemorrhoidal branch of the pudendal nerve. This reflex is integrated at the S2-S4 spinal cord level (Wester, 2003). Thus, reflex absence may reflect central or peripheral neurologic deficits. Second, a normal circumferential anal sphincter contraction, colloquially called an "anal wink," should follow cotton swab brushing of the perianal skin. External urethral sphincter activity requires at least some degree of intact S2-S4 innervation, and this *anocutaneous reflex* is mediated by the same spinal neurologic level. Thus, an absent wink may indicate deficits in this neurologic distribution.

Pelvic Support Assessment

Poor urethral support commonly accompanies pelvic organ prolapse. For example, women with significant prolapse are often

TABLE 23-3. Medications That May Contribute to Incontinence

Medication	Examples	Mechanism	Effect
Alcohol	Beer, wine, liquor	Diuretic effect, sedation, immobility	Polyuria, frequency
α-Adrenergic agonists	Decongestants, diet pills	IUS contraction	Urinary retention
α-Adrenergic blockers	Prazosin, terazosin, doxazosin	IUS relaxation	Urinary leakage
Anticholinergic agents		Inhibit bladder contraction, sedation, fecal impaction	Urinary retention and/or functional incontinence
Antihistamines	Diphenhydramine, scopolamine, dimenhydrinate		
Antipsychotics	Thioridazine, chlorpromazine, haloperidol		
Antiparkinsonians	Trihexyphenidyl, benztropine mesylate		
Miscellaneous	Dicyclomine, disopyramide		
Skeletal muscle relaxants	Orphenadrine, cyclobenzaprine		
Tricyclic antidepressants	Amitriptyline, imipramine, nortriptyline, doxepin		
ACE inhibitors	Enalapril, captopril, lisinopril, losartan	Chronic cough	Urinary leakage
Calcium-channel blockers	Nifedipine, nicardipine, isradipine, felodipine	Relaxes bladder, fluid retention	Urinary retention, nocturnal diuresis
COX-2 inhibitors	Celecoxib	Fluid retention	Nocturnal diuresis
Diuretics	Caffeine, HCTZ, furosemide, bumetanide, acetazolamide, spironolactone	Increases urinary frequency, urgency	Polyuria
Narcotic analgesics	Opiates	Relaxes bladder, fecal impaction, sedation	Urinary retention, and/or functional incontinence
Thiazolidinediones	Rosiglitazone, pioglitazone, troglitazone	Fluid retention	Nocturnal diuresis

ACE = angiotensin-converting enzyme; COX-2 = cyclooxygenase-2; HCTZ = hydrochlorothiazide; IUS = internal urethral sphincter; NSAID = nonsteroidal antiinflammatory drug.

unable to completely empty their bladder due to urethral kinking and obstruction. These women frequently must digitally elevate or reduce their prolapse to allow emptying. Thus, an external evaluation for prolapse, as described in Chapter 24 (p. 548), is indicated for all women with urinary incontinence. Following this evaluation for vaginal compartment defects, pelvic muscle strength is also assessed. Women with mild to moderate urinary incontinence often respond well to pelvic floor therapy, and under these circumstances, a trial of this therapy is warranted and often curative (p. 528).

Lack of distal anterior vaginal wall support and resultant urethral hypermobility during increased intraabdominal pressure may help influence choice of surgical intervention in the patient reporting SUI. These patients commonly demonstrate relaxation and descent of the distal anterior vagina with resultant urethral hypermobility during increases in intraabdominal

pressures. In patients with descent to the level of the hymen or beyond with Valsalva, urethral hypermobility is universal (Noblett, 2005). In those with SUI and lesser anterior vaginal wall prolapse, a Q-tip test may provide a more objective assessment of urethral hypermobility. However, it has become a less essential part of pelvic floor assessment due to its poor predictive value for antiincontinence surgery success.

When performed, the soft end of a cotton swab is placed into the urethra to the urethrovesical junction. Failure to insert the swab to this depth can lead to assessment errors. An application of intraurethral analgesia may prove helpful, and 1-percent lidocaine jelly is placed on the cotton swab prior to insertion. Following placement, a Valsalva maneuver is prompted, and the swab-excursion angle at rest and with Valsalva maneuver is measured. An angle change or a resting angle >30 degrees to the horizon suggests urethral hypermobility.

Bimanual and Rectovaginal Examination

In general, these portions of the pelvic examination provide fewer diagnostic clues to underlying incontinence causes. However, bimanual examination may reveal a pelvic mass or a uterus enlarged by leiomyomas or adenomyosis. These can create incontinence through increased external pressure transmitted to the bladder. In addition, stool impaction is easily identified with rectal examination.

■ Diagnostic Testing

Urinalysis and Culture

In all women with urinary incontinence, infection or urinary tract pathology must be excluded. Urinalysis and urine culture are sent at an initial visit, and infection is treated as described in Table 3-17 (p. 74). Persistent irritative voiding symptoms, despite appropriate antibiotic treatment, warrant additional evaluation for other conditions such as interstitial cystitis.

Postvoid Residual Volume

This volume is routinely measured during incontinence evaluation. After a woman voids, the postvoid residual (PVR) volume may be measured by transurethral catheterization or with a handheld sonographic bladder scanner. The latter is a portable 3-dimensional ultrasound device that scans the bladder and provides numeric results (Fig. 23-12). In general, they are quick, easy to use, and more comfortable for the patient. However, if using a handheld scanner, care must be taken in women with a leiomyomatous uterus or other pelvic mass as these may lead to a false report of a large PVR. In these instances, or if a scanner is not available, transurethral catheterization may be used to confirm residual bladder volume.

A large PVR volume may often reflect one of several problems including recurrent infection, urethral obstruction from a

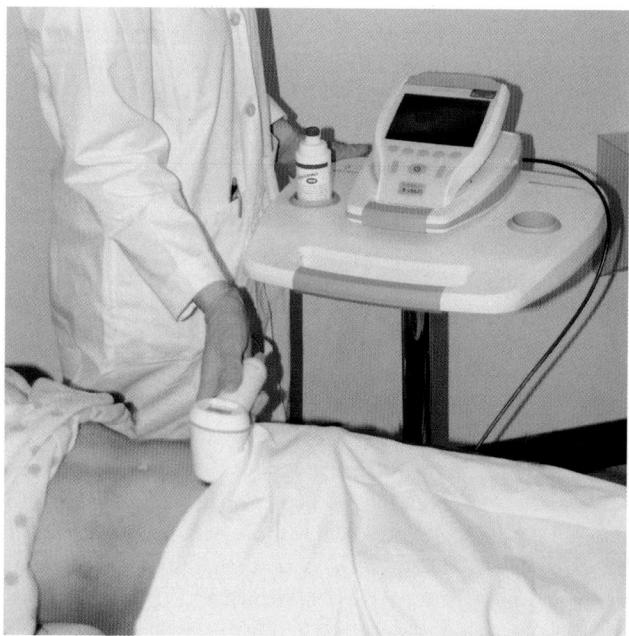

FIGURE 23-12 Handheld bladder scanner aids estimation of bladder volume.

pelvic mass, or neurologic deficits. In contrast, a normally small PVR volume is often found in those with SUI. After continence surgery, PVR measurement is a helpful indicator of a patient's ability to completely empty her bladder. Postoperative PVR determination and voiding trials are described in Chapter 42 (p. 917).

Urodynamic Studies

Surgical correction of incontinence is invasive and not without risk. However, the "bladder is an unreliable witness," and historical information may not always accurately indicate the true underlying type of incontinence (Blaivas, 1996). Thus, if initial conservative management is unsuccessful or surgical treatment is anticipated, then objective assessment is pursued. In addition, if symptoms and physical findings are incongruous, then objective *urodynamic studies (UDS)*, using simple or multichannel cystometrics, may also be indicated. For example, in a woman with mixed urinary incontinence, who has symptoms of both stress and urgency urinary incontinence, UDS may reveal that only the urgency component is responsible for her incontinence. These cases are treated with behavioral, physical, and/or pharmacologic therapy initially. Thus, if identified by UDS, these individuals can avoid unnecessary surgery. Additionally, surgical therapy may be modified if UDS reveals parameters consistent with ISD.

Despite these indications, UDS remains controversial. Leakage noted during testing is not always clinically relevant. In addition, testing may be uninformative if the original offending maneuver or situation that led to incontinence cannot be reproduced during testing. Moreover, objective confirmation of the diagnosis is not always necessary, since empiric nonsurgical therapy in women with urgency-predominant symptoms is reasonable. Also, for women with stress-predominant urinary incontinence undergoing surgical treatment, outcomes were no different 1 year later in those screened by UDS compared with those evaluated by a simple office evaluation. The office testing included demonstrable leakage during examination, urine analysis without infection, and PVR <150 mL (Nager, 2012).

Simple Cystometrics. Objective measurement of bladder function, that is, UDS, combines a battery of tests termed *cystometrics*, which may be *simple* or *multichannel*. Simple cystometrics allows determination of SUI and detrusor overactivity and measurement of first sensation, desire to void, and bladder capacity. This procedure is easily performed with room-temperature sterile normal saline, a 60-mL catheter-tipped syringe, and a urinary catheter, either Foley or Robnell. The urethra is sterilely prepared, the catheter is inserted, and the bladder is drained. A 60-mL syringe with its plunger removed is attached to the catheter and is filled upright with sterile water. Water is added in increments until a woman feels a sensation of bladder filling, urge to void, and bladder maximum capacity. A normal bladder capacity for most women ranges from 300 to 700 mL. Changes in the fluid meniscus within the syringe are monitored. In the absence of a cough or Valsalva maneuver that would raise intraabdominal pressure, an abrupt meniscus elevation indicates bladder contraction and suggests detrusor overactivity. Once bladder capacity is reached, the catheter is removed, and the woman is asked to perform a Valsalva maneuver or cough while standing. Leakage directly linked to these increases in intraabdominal pressure indicates SUI.

Simple cystometrics require inexpensive equipment and can typically be completed by most gynecologists. One limitation, however, is its inability to assess for ISD, which may preclude certain surgical options. Multichannel cystometrics can evaluate for ISD and thus may offer advantages. An interesting potential application of simple cystometrics is in the evaluation of the *continent* patient planning surgery for prolapse. With 300 mL of saline instilled in the bladder and vaginal prolapse reduced with large cotton swabs, some patients will demonstrate leakage with cough or Valsalva—perhaps when standing if not seen supine. In these women with "potential" or "occult" SUI, some may consider a prophylactic continence procedure. Currently available decision-aid tools attempt to quantify the risk of this unmasked incontinence to help patients balance concomitant continence surgery benefits and risks (Jelovsek, 2014; Wei, 2012).

Multichannel Cystometrics. This UDS type provides more information on other physiologic bladder parameters than simple cystometrics. Multichannel cystometrics more commonly is performed by urogynecologists or urologists due to the expense and limited availability of needed equipment. Testing can be performed with a woman standing or seated upright in a specialized testing chair. During evaluation, two catheters are used. One is placed into the bladder and the other into either the vagina or rectum. The vagina is preferred unless advanced prolapse is evident, as stool in the rectal vault may obstruct catheter sensors and lead to inaccurate readings. Additionally, vaginal placement for most women is more comfortable. From each of these two catheters, distinct pressure readings are obtained or calculated. These include: (1) intraabdominal pressure, (2) vesicular pressure, (3) calculated detrusor pressure, (4) bladder volume, and (5) saline-infusion flow rate. As shown in Figures 23-13 and 23-14, the various incontinence forms can be differentiated.

Uroflowmetry. Initially, women are asked to empty their bladder into a commode connected to a flowmeter (uroflowmetry). After a maximal flow rate is recorded, the patient is catheterized to measure postvoid residual volume and to ensure an empty bladder prior to further testing. This test provides information on a woman's ability to empty her bladder and can identify women with urinary retention and other types of voiding dysfunction. Presuming that a patient begins with a comfortably full bladder of 200 mL or greater, most patients can empty their bladder over 15 to 20 seconds with flow rates >20 mL/sec. Maximum flow rates <15 mL/sec, with a voided volume >200 mL, are generally considered abnormally slow. In this setting—especially if accompanied by urinary retention—voiding dysfunction is identified. This may result from obstruction from a kinked urethra in the setting of anterior vaginal wall prolapse or postoperatively after creation of antiincontinence support that is too tight. As another example, voiding dysfunction may reflect neurologic dysfunction and poor detrusor contractility, as in those with longstanding poorly controlled diabetes.

Cystometrography. Following uroflowmetry, cystometrography is performed to determine whether a woman has urodynamic stress incontinence (USI) or detrusor overactivity (DO). Additionally, this test provides information on bladder threshold volumes at which a woman senses bladder capacity. Delayed sensation or sensation of bladder fullness only with large capacities may indicate neuropathy. Conversely, extreme bladder sensitivity may suggest sensory disorders such as interstitial cystitis.

For the cystometrogram, a catheter is inserted transurethrally into the bladder and a second catheter is inserted into the vagina or rectum (see Fig. 23-14). While the patient is seated, the bladder is filled with room-temperature sterile normal saline, and the patient is asked to cough at regular intervals. Additionally, during filling, the volumes at which a first desire to void and maximal bladder capacity is reached are noted. From pressure readings, DO and/or USI may be identified.

After cystometrography, once approximately 200 mL of saline has been instilled, an abdominal *leak point pressure* is measured. The patient is asked to perform a Valsalva maneuver, and the pressure generated by the effort is measured and evidence of urine leakage is sought. If leakage is seen when a pressure of <60 cm H_2O is generated, then criteria have been met for a diagnosis of ISD. At our institution, abdominal leak point pressures are measured at a bladder volume of 200 mL, using the true zero of intravesical pressure as the baseline. However, the volume at which this test is performed varies among institutions, with some choosing to use bladder capacity and others choosing to use 150 mL as the testing volume.

Pressure Flowmetry. This evaluation usually follows cystometrography and is similar to the uroflowmetry conducted at the beginning of urodynamic testing. A woman is asked to void into a large beaker that rests on a calibrated weighted sensor. Maximum flow rate and postvoid residual volume are once again recorded. Similar to uroflowmetry, the output from the urodynamics instrumentation provides a graphical representation of the void. However, during voiding, a woman now has a microtip transducer catheter in her bladder, which provides an additional display of detrusor pressure during the void, including pressures at the point of maximum flow rate. This is particularly useful in women who may have incomplete bladder emptying, as the pressure flowmetry may suggest either an obstructive scenario (elevated maximal detrusor pressure with slow flow rate) or poor detrusor contractility (low detrusor pressure and slow flow rate).

Urethral Pressure Profile. The final part of cystometric testing is the urethral pressure profile. At our institution, we usually perform this test in the seated patient with a volume of 200 mL instilled in the bladder. However, again, this volume is often institution dependent. A catheter transducer is positioned within the bladder, and the microtip dual-sensor catheter is pulled through the urethra with the aid of an automated puller arm at a speed of 1 mm/sec. Maximum urethral closure pressure (MUCP) is determined by averaging the pressure from three pull-throughs of the thin 7F catheter. As such, the MUCP values provide important information on the intrinsic properties of the urethra and aid in diagnosis of ISD. A diagnosis of ISD is made

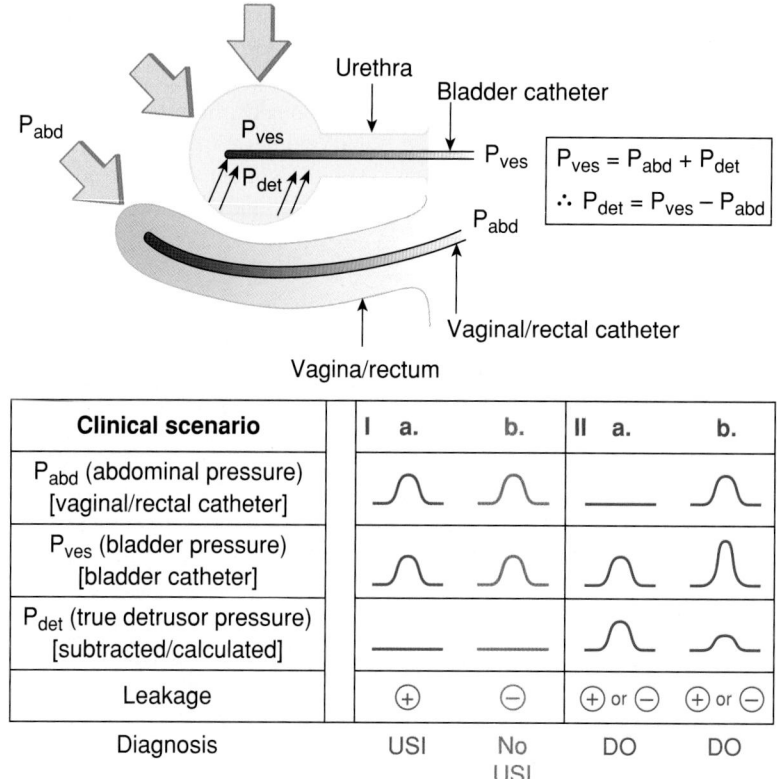

Clinical scenario	I a.	b.	II a.	b.
P_{abd} (abdominal pressure) [vaginal/rectal catheter]	⌒	⌒	—	⌒
P_{ves} (bladder pressure) [bladder catheter]	⌒	⌒	⌒	⌒
P_{det} (true detrusor pressure) [subtracted/calculated]	—	—	⌒	⌒
Leakage	⊕	⊖	⊕ or ⊖	⊕ or ⊖
Diagnosis	USI	No USI	DO	DO

FIGURE 23-13 Interpretation of multichannel urodynamic evaluation: cystometrogram. A catheter is placed in the bladder to determine the pressure generated within it (P_{ves}). The pressure in the bladder is produced from a combination of the pressure from the abdominal cavity and the pressure generated by the detrusor muscle of the bladder. Bladder pressure (P_{ves}) = Pressure in abdominal cavity (P_{abd}) + Detrusor pressure (P_{det}). A second catheter is placed in the vagina (or rectum if advanced-stage prolapse is present) to determine the pressure in the abdominal cavity (P_{abd}). As room temperature water is instilled into the bladder, the patient is asked to cough every 50 mL and the external urethral meatus is observed for leakage of urine around the catheter. The volume at first desire to void and the bladder capacity is recorded. Additionally, the detrusor pressure (P_{det}) channel is observed for positive deflections to determine if there is detrusor activity during testing. The detrusor pressure (P_{det}) cannot be measured directly by any of the catheters. However, from the first equation, we can calculate the detrusor pressure (P_{det}) by subtracting the abdominal pressure (P_{abd}) from the bladder pressure (P_{ves}):
Detrusor pressure (P_{det}) = Bladder pressure (P_{ves}) – Pressure in abdominal cavity (P_{abd})

I. Urodynamic Stress Incontinence (USI)
Urodynamic stress incontinence is diagnosed when urethral leakage is seen with increased abdominal pressure, in the *absence* of detrusor pressure.
a. +USI (Column 1): Abdominal pressure is generated with Valsalva maneuver or cough. This pressure is transmitted to the bladder and a bladder pressure (P_{ves}) is noted. The calculated detrusor pressure is zero. Leakage is observed and diagnosis of USI is assigned.
b. No USI (Column 2): Abdominal pressure is generated with Valsalva maneuver or cough. This pressure is transmitted to the bladder and a bladder pressure (P_{ves}) is noted. The calculated detrusor pressure is zero. Leakage is *not* observed. The patient is *not* diagnosed as having USI.
II. Detrusor Overactivity (DO)
Detrusor overactivity is diagnosed when the patient has involuntary detrusor contractions during testing with or without leakage.
a. +DO (Column 3): Although no abdominal pressure is observed, a vesicular pressure is noted. A calculated detrusor pressure is recorded and noted to be present. A diagnosis of DO is made regardless of whether leakage is seen or not.
b. +DO (Column 4): In this example, an abdominal pressure as well as a vesicular pressure is observed. Using only the P_{abd} and the P_{ves} channels, it is difficult to tell whether or not the detrusor muscle contributed to the pressure generated in the bladder. On subtraction, a calculated detrusor pressure is recorded. Thus, a diagnosis of DO is made, again regardless of whether leakage is seen or not.
In addition to these channels, occasionally a channel to detect electromyographic activity is used.
Flow rate = rate of fluid infusion (usually 100 mL/min); P_{abd} = pressure in abdominal cavity; P_{det} = detrusor pressure (calculated); P_{ves} = bladder pressure; Vol = volume of fluid instilled in the bladder.

if the MUCP is <20 cm H_2O or, as described in the last section, if the leak point pressure is <60 cm H_2O (McGuire, 1981). These terms and concepts provide the rationale for procedures aimed at correcting stress incontinence. Importantly, however, the values used to define ISD are not well standardized and have not been consistently found to influence surgical outcomes (Monga, 1997; Weber, 2001).

TREATMENT

■ Conservative/Nonsurgical
Pelvic Floor Strengthening

Conservative management is a reasonable initial approach to most patients with urinary incontinence. The rationale behind

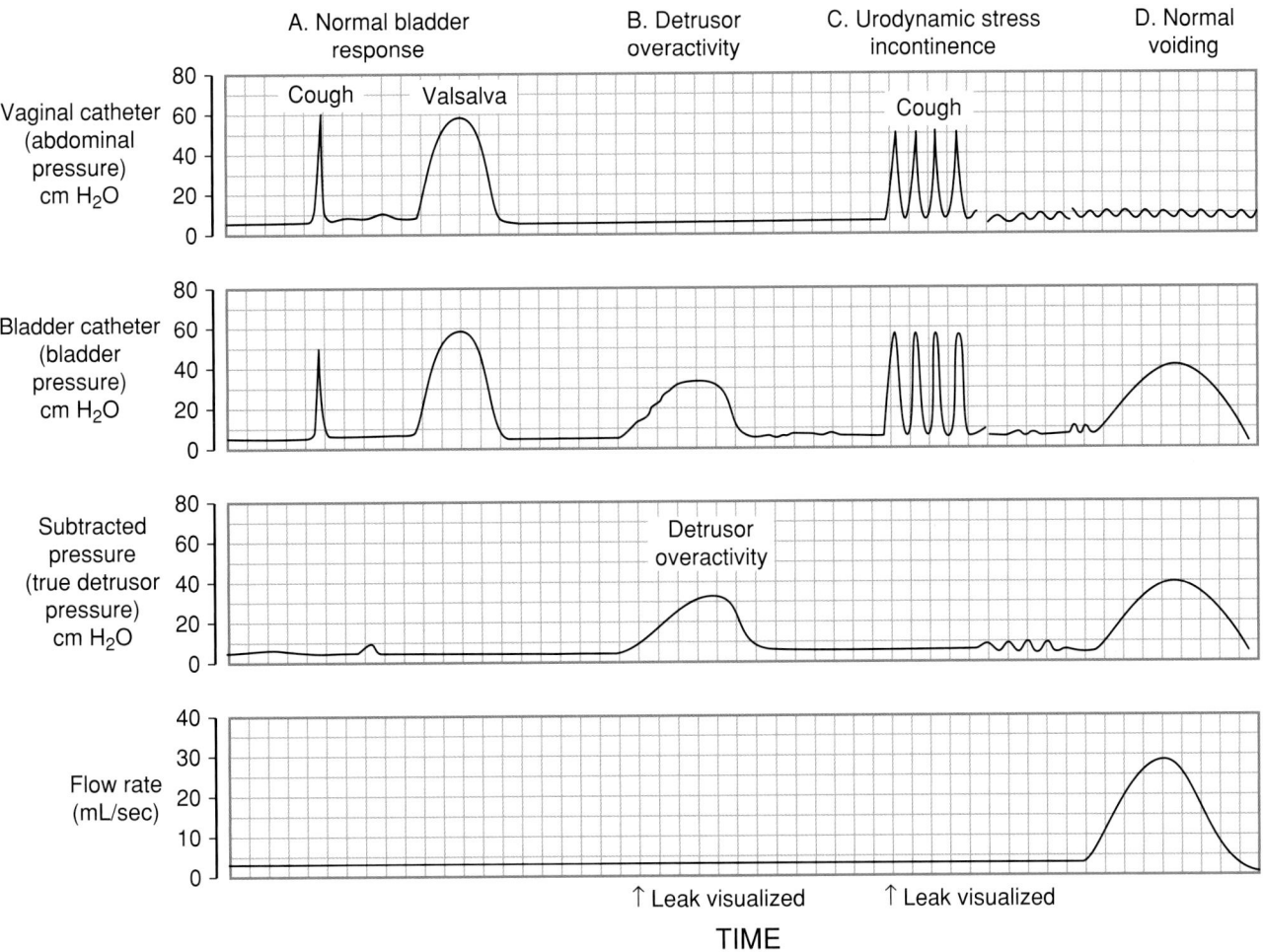

FIGURE 23-14 Multichannel cystometrics. **A.** A patient with normal function. Note that provocation by coughing or Valsalva maneuver does not provoke an abnormal rise in detrusor pressure. **B.** A patient with combined detrusor overactivity and urodynamic stress incontinence. First, spontaneous detrusor activity leads to increased bladder pressure reading in the absence of cough or Valsalva maneuver. **C.** Second, a cough alone leads to urine leakage, independent of detrusor muscle activity. **D.** At maximum capacity and on command, a detrusor contraction is generated and voiding is initiated.

conservative management is to strengthen the pelvic floor and provide a supportive "backboard" against which the urethra may close. For both SUI and urgency urinary incontinence, these fundamentals prove valuable. With SUI, pelvic floor strengthening attempts to compensate for anatomic defects. For urgency urinary incontinence, it intensifies pelvic floor muscle contractions to provide temporary continence during waves of bladder detrusor contraction. For strengthening, options include active pelvic floor exercises and passive electrical pelvic floor muscle stimulation.

Active pelvic floor muscle training (PFMT) may lessen, if not cure, urinary incontinence in women who have mild to moderate symptoms. Also known as *Kegel exercises,* PFMT entails voluntary contraction of the levator ani muscles. As with any muscle building, isometric or isotonic forms of exercise may be selected. Exercise sets are performed numerous times during the day, with some reporting up to 50 or 60 times each day. However, specific details in performance of these exercises are subject to provider preference and clinical setting.

If isotonic contractions are used for PFMT, a woman is asked to squeeze and hold contracted levator ani muscles.

Women, however, often have difficulty isolating these muscles. Frequently, patients will erroneously contract their abdominal wall muscles rather than the levators. To help localize the correct group, an individual may be instructed to identify the muscles that are tightened when snug pants are pulled up and over her hips. Moreover, in an office setting, a provider can determine if the levator ani group is contracted by placing two fingers in the vagina while Kegel exercises are performed.

At our institution, we aim to help patients achieve a sustained pelvic floor contraction of 10 seconds. We begin with the contraction duration a patient can sustain (e.g., 3 seconds) and ask them to hold for this long and then relax for one to two times this duration (e.g., 6 seconds). This squeeze and release is repeated 10 to 15 times. Three sets are performed throughout the day for a total of approximately 45 contractions. Over a series of weeks with frequent follow-up visits, the contraction duration is steadily increased. Patients thus improve the tone of their pelvic floor muscles and are usually able to more forcefully squeeze their muscles in anticipation of sudden increases of intraadominal pressure for SUI.

Alternatively, if isometric contractions are used for PFMT, a woman is asked to rapidly contract and relax the levator ani muscles. These "quick flicks" may prove advantageous if waves of urinary urgency strike. Of note, there is no value to stopping urination midstream, and women are counseled that this practice often worsens voiding dysfunction.

To augment exercise efficacy, weighted vaginal cones or obturators may be placed into the vagina during Kegel exercises. These provide resistance against which pelvic floor muscles can work.

PFMT for women with urinary incontinence compared with no treatment, placebo or sham treatment, or other inactive control treatment has been reviewed (Dumoulin, 2014a). Although interventions vary considerably, women who performed PFMT are more likely to report cure or improved incontinence and improved continence-specific quality of life than women who did not use PFMT. The exercising women also objectively demonstrated less leakage during office-based pad testing. Prognostic indicators that may predict a poor response to PFMT for SUI treatment include severe baseline incontinence, prolapse beyond the hymenal ring, prior failed physiotherapy, a history of prolonged second-stage labor, BMI >30 kg/m^2, high psychological distress, and poor overall physical health (Hendriks, 2010).

As an alternative to active pelvic floor contraction, a vaginal probe may be used to deliver low-frequency electrical stimulation to the levator ani muscles. Although the mechanism is unclear, this passive electrical stimulation may be used to improve either SUI or urgency urinary incontinence (Indrekvam, 2001; Wang, 2004). With urgency urinary incontinence, traditionally a low frequency is applied, whereas for SUI, higher frequencies are used. Electrical stimulation may be implemented alone or more commonly in combination with active PFMT.

Many behavioral techniques, often considered together as *biofeedback therapy,* measure physiologic signals such as muscle tension and then display them to a patient in real time. In general, visual, auditory, and/or verbal feedback cues are directed to the patient during these therapy sessions. Specifically, during biofeedback for active PFMT, a sterile vaginal probe that measures pressure changes within the vagina during levator ani muscle contraction is typically used. Visual readings reflect an estimate of muscle contraction strength. Treatment sessions are individualized, dictated by the underlying dysfunction, and modified based on response to therapy. In many cases, reinforcing sessions at various subsequent intervals may also prove advantageous.

Dietary

Various food groups that may have high acidity or caffeine content can lead to greater urinary frequency and urgency. Dallosso and colleagues (2003) found consumption of carbonated drinks to be associated with development of urgency urinary incontinence symptoms. Accordingly, elimination of these dietary irritants may benefit these women. In addition, certain dietary supplements such as calcium glycerophosphate (Prelief) have been shown to decrease urgency and frequency symptoms (Bologna, 2001). This is a phosphate-based product and is thought to buffer urine acidity.

Scheduled Voiding

Women with urgency urinary incontinence may feel voiding urges as frequently as every 10 to 15 minutes. Initial goals extend voidings to half-hour intervals. Tools used to achieve this include Kegel exercises during waves of urgency or mental distraction techniques during these times. Scheduled voiding, although used primarily for urgency urinary incontinence, may also be helpful for those with SUI. For these patients, regularly scheduled urination leads to an empty bladder during a greater percentage of the day. Because some women will leak urine only if bladder volumes surpass a specific threshold, frequent emptying can significantly decrease incontinence episodes.

Estrogen Replacement

Estrogen has been shown to increase urethral blood flow and increase α-adrenergic receptor sensitivity, thereby increasing urethral coaptation and urethral closure pressure. Hypothetically, estrogen may also increase collagen deposition and increase vascularity of the periurethral capillary plexus. These are purported to improve urethral coaptation. Thus, for incontinent women who are atrophic, administration of exogenous estrogen is reasonable.

Estrogen is commonly administered topically, and many different regimens are appropriate. At our institution, we use conjugated equine estrogen cream (Premarin cream) administered daily for 2 weeks, then twice weekly thereafter. Although no data are available to address the duration of treatment, women may be treated chronically with topical estrogen cream. Alternatively, oral estrogen may be prescribed if other menopausal symptoms for which estrogen would be beneficial coexist (Chap. 22, p. 494). However, despite these suggested benefits, a consensus regarding estrogen's beneficial effects on the lower urinary tract has not been reached. Specifically, some studies have shown worsening or development of urinary incontinence with systemic estrogen administration (Grady, 2001; Grodstein, 2004; Hendrix, 2005; Jackson, 2006).

■ Treatment of Stress Urinary Incontinence
Medications

Pharmaceutical treatment plays a minor role in the treatment of women with SUI. However, for women with mixed urinary incontinence, a trial of imipramine is reasonable to aid urethral contraction and closure. As discussed earlier, this tricyclic antidepressant has α-adrenergic effects, and the urethra contains a high content of these receptors.

Pessary and Urethral Inserts

Certain pessaries have been designed to treat incontinence as well as pelvic organ prolapse. These "incontinence pessaries" are designed to reduce downward excursion or funneling of the urethrovesical junction (Fig. 24-16, p. 551). This provides bladder neck support and thereby helps to reduce incontinence episodes. The success of pessary use in the treatment of urinary incontinence is variable, dependent on the amount of prolapse and other factors. Not all women are appropriate candidates for devices, nor will all desire long-term management of incontinence or prolapse with these.

TABLE 23-4. Summary of Incontinence Procedures

Procedure	Description	Indication	Comments
Midurethral slings: TVT TOT	Midurethra supported by mesh placed: by retropubic approach by transobturator approach	 SUI; ISD SUI	Effective short-term treatment, rapid post-operative recovery; TVT with long-term efficacy data; further study required to determine effectiveness of TOT in patients with ISD
Retropubic urethropexy	Pubocervical fascia attached to: Cooper ligament (Burch) or symphysis pubis (MMK)	SUI	Effective long-term treatment; requires surgeon experience; less reproducible benefits than midurethral sling procedure
Pubovaginal slings	Bladder neck supported by fascial strip attached to anterior abdominal wall	ISD; failed SUI procedure	Effective long-term treatment; may be useful when synthetic material is not desirable; requires graft isolation
Urethral injection	Bulking agent into urethral submucosa	ISD	Also for SUI in poor surgical candidates; may require several repeated injections
Needle suspension	Proximal urethra suspended by anterior abdominal wall	SUI	Low long-term success rates; no longer recommended for SUI
Paravaginal defect repair	Lateral vaginal wall attached to ATFP	Vaginal prolapse	No longer recommended for SUI

ATFP = arcus tendineus fascia pelvis; ISD = intrinsic sphincteric deficiency; MMK = Marshall-Marchetti-Krantz procedure; SUI = stress urinary incontinence; TOT = transobturator tape; TVT = tension-free vaginal tape.

A large prospective trial comparing incontinence pessaries and behavioral therapy for women with SUI demonstrated that 40 and 49 percent of patients were either much or very much improved at 3 months, respectively. The women randomized to behavioral therapy reported greater treatment satisfaction, and a greater percentage reported no bothersome incontinence symptoms (Richter, 2010b).

As an alternative to pessaries, urethral occlusive devices include *urethral inserts* (FemSoft and Reliance Urinary Control Insert) and *urethral patches* (CapSure and Re/Stor). Urethral inserts conform to the urethra and create a seal at the bladder neck to prevent accidental leakage. During routine bathroom visits, the insert is removed, discarded, and replaced with a fresh insert. Although data are limited on the effectiveness of inserts, adverse effects of mucosal irritation or superficial bacterial infection are generally minor. In an observational study of 150 women, Sirls and associates (2002) found significantly reduced rates of incontinence episodes with the FemSoft device. With urethral patches, a water-tight seal is created over the urethra after the patch adheres to surrounding periurethral skin using adhesive gel. Similarly, although success rates vary between 44 and 97 percent, these devices are associated with minimal adverse effects (Bellin, 1998; Versi, 1998).

Surgery

For those who are unsatisfied with or do not desire conservative management, surgery may be an appropriate next step for SUI. As noted earlier, urethral support is integral to continence. Thus, surgical procedures that recreate this support often diminish or cure incontinence. In general, these surgical procedures are believed to prevent bladder neck and proximal urethra descent during increases in intraabdominal pressure

and are grouped as shown in Table 23-4. General postoperative risks for continence surgeries include lower urinary tract injury, failure to correct or recurrence of SUI, and creation of de novo voiding dysfunction such as urgency or retention.

Midurethral Slings. The therapeutic mechanism of these slings is based on the integral theory hypothesized by Petros and Ulmsten (1993). In brief, control of urethral closure involves the interplay of three structures: the pubourethral ligaments, the suburethral vaginal hammock, and the pubococcygeus muscle. Loss of these supports lead to urinary incontinence and pelvic floor dysfunction. Midurethral slings are believed to recreate this structural support.

There are different variations of these procedures, but all use a vaginal approach to place synthetic mesh beneath the midurethra. Recovery from midurethral sling placement is rapid, and many gynecologists provide this surgery on an outpatient basis. As such, these are often a popular surgical treatment for SUI. Simplistically, they are classified according to the route of placement and are subdivided into those using a retropubic or a transobturator approach.

For the retropubic approach, several commercial kits are available, and one commonly used is the tension-free vaginal tape (TVT). With this, the sling (tape) is placed through a vaginal incision to create a hammock beneath the urethra. On each side of the urethra, the sling's arms are brought out to the lower anterior abdominal wall and affixed. For this procedure, sharp trocars traverse the retropubic space as illustrated in Section 45-3 of the atlas (p. 1063). Thus, bladder puncture and retropubic space vessel laceration are specific risks. Many studies attest to this procedure's efficacy (Holmgren, 2005; Song, 2009). One prospective observational study confirmed the long-term safety and efficacy of the TVT device. At 17 years, 87 percent were subjectively cured or significantly improved (Nilsson, 2013).

For the transobturator tape (TOT) approach, various kits are also available, and sling material is directed bilaterally through the obturator foramen and underneath the midurethra. The entry point overlies the proximal tendon of the adductor longus muscle of the inner thigh as shown in Section 45-4 (p. 1066). This approach was introduced with the intent to reduce the vascular and lower urinary tract injury risks that can be associated with traversing the retropubic space.

The TOT is indicated for primary SUI secondary to urethral hypermobility (p. 525). For this, subjective success rates range from 73 to 92 percent up to 5 years after surgery (Abdel-Fattah, 2012; Laurikainen, 2014; Wai, 2013). However, abundant longer-term data regarding the efficacy of transobturator approaches are lacking. Moreover, in patients with SUI secondary to ISD, the value of TOT is unclear as results are conflicting and data are limited (Miller, 2006; O'Connor, 2006; Richter, 2010a).

In comparing these two, one multicenter randomized study of 597 found no significant differences in objective and subjective success rates at 12 months between the retropubic (80.8 and 62.2 percent) and the transobturator (77.7 and 55.8 percent) routes, respectively (Richter, 2010a). The retropubic route had a significantly higher rate of postoperative voiding dysfunction requiring reoperation, whereas the transobturator route resulted in more neurologic symptoms. Overall quality of life and satisfaction scores with the two procedures were similar. Others have found similar findings with respect to procedure–related complications. Namely, the retropubic route has a higher rate of bladder injury but required a decreased use of anticholinergic medication postoperatively (Barber, 2006; Brubaker, 2011).

Modification of the TVT and TOT procedure is seen with the minimally invasive slings, sometimes called "microslings" or "minislings." With this technique, an 8-cm-long strip of polypropylene synthetic mesh is placed across and beneath the midurethra through a small vaginal incision. Mesh is not threaded through the retropubic space as with TVT, nor does it perforate the obturator membrane as with TOT. That said, lower urinary tract injury is not completely averted with this method. Initial results for the minislings suggested high objective and subjective cure rates (Neuman, 2008). However, in one study, the minisling group had a higher proportion of patients with more severe incontinence 1 year after surgery than those in the retropubic sling group (Barber, 2012).

In March 2013, the FDA issued an update regarding considerations about surgical mesh for SUI. In that statement, the established safety and efficacy of mesh sling procedures for the treatment of SUI were upheld for full-length multiincision operations. They further noted that the safety and effectiveness of minislings had not yet been adequately demonstrated.

Retropubic Urethropexy. This group includes the Burch and Marshall-Marchetti-Krantz (MMK) colposuspension procedures. Traditionally performed via laparotomy, these suspend and anchor the pubocervical fascia to the musculoskeletal framework of the pelvis (Section 45-2, p. 1061). With the advent of

less invasive procedures for SUI, such as the midurethral sling, these techniques are less commonly performed. The Burch technique uses the strength of the iliopectineal ligament (Cooper ligament) to lift the anterior vaginal wall and the periurethral and perivesicular fibromuscular tissue. In contrast, during MMK surgery, the periosteum of the symphysis pubis is used to suspend these tissues. Thus, an added risk for MMK is osteitis pubis.

Retropubic urethropexy effectively treats SUI. One-year overall continence rates range between 85 and 90 percent, and the 5-year continence rate approximates 70 percent (Lapitan, 2009). As another indication, data suggest that Burch retropubic urethropexy performed concurrently with abdominal sacrocolpopexy (ASC) may significantly reduce rates of later, postoperative de novo SUI (Chap. 24, p. 557) (Brubaker, 2008a). In support of this practice, a 7-year follow-up study showed that patients undergoing ASC and prophylactic Burch urethropexy still demonstrated lower de novo SUI rates than women receiving ASC alone (Nygaard, 2013).

Pubovaginal Slings. With this surgery, a strip of either rectus fascia or fascia lata is placed under the bladder neck and through the retropubic space. The ends are secured at the level of the rectus abdominis fascia (Section 45-5, p. 1068). This surgery has traditionally been used for SUI stemming from ISD. In addition, this procedure may also be indicated for patients with prior failed continence operations.

Urethral Bulking Agent Injection. Using cystoscopic guidance, agents can be injected into the urethral submucosa to "bulk up" the mucosa and improve coaptation. Surgical steps and agent types are illustrated in Section 45-6 (p. 1070). This option has traditionally been indicated for women who have stress incontinence associated with ISD. However, the Food and Drug Administration (FDA) has broadened criteria for their use to include patients with less severe leak point pressures. Thus, those with leak point pressures <100 cm H_2O may also be candidates (McGuire, 2006). Additionally, this office procedure is a useful alternative for women with SUI who have multiple medical problems and are thus poor surgical candidates.

Transvaginal Needle Procedures and Paravaginal Defect Repair. In the 1960s through 1980s, needle suspension procedures such as the Raz, Pereyra, and Stamey techniques were popular operations for SUI but have now largely been replaced by other methods. In brief, these surgeries use specially designed ligature carriers to place sutures through the anterior vaginal wall and/or periurethral tissues and suspend them to various levels of the anterior abdominal wall. These rely on the strength and integrity of the periurethral tissue and abdominal wall strength to correct urethral hypermobility and prevent bladder neck and proximal urethra descent. Although initial cure rates are satisfactory, the durability of these procedures decreases with time. Success rates range from 50 to 60 percent, well below rates found with other current continence procedures (Moser, 2006). Failure stemmed largely from "pull-through" of sutures at the level of the anterior vaginal wall.

In addition, abdominal paravaginal defect repair (PVDR) is a surgical procedure that corrects lateral support defects of the

TABLE 23-5. Pharmacologic Treatment of Overactive Bladder

Drug Name	Brand Name	Drug Type	Dosage[a]	Available Doses
Oxybutynin (short-acting)	Ditropan	Antimuscarinic	2.5–5 mg three times daily	5-mg tablet, 5 mg/mL syrup
Oxybutynin (long-acting)	Ditropan XL	See above	5–30 mg daily	5-, 10-, 15-mg tablet
Oxybutynin (transdermal)	Oxytrol	See above	3.9 mg/d; change patch twice weekly	36-mg patch, 8 per carton
Oxybutynin (transdermal) 10% gel 3% gel	Gelnique	See above	Apply 1 g daily Apply 3 pumps daily	1-g packet, 30 per carton 30 doses per bottle
Tolterodine (short-acting)	Detrol	See above	1–2 mg twice daily	1-, 2-mg tablet
Tolterodine (long-acting)	Detrol LA	See above	2–4 mg daily	2-, 4-mg capsule
Fesoterodine fumarate	Toviaz	See above	4–8 mg daily	4-, 8-mg tablets
Trospium chloride	Sanctura	Antimuscarinic quaternary amine	20 mg twice daily	20-mg tablet
Trospium chloride	Sanctura XR	See above	60 mg daily	60-mg tablet
Darifenacin	Enablex	M_3-selective antimuscarinic	7.5–15 mg daily	7.5-, 15-mg tablet
Solifenacin	Vesicare	M_3-selective antimuscarinic	5–10 mg daily	5-, 10-mg tablets
Imipramine hydrochloride	Tofranil	Tricyclic antidepressant, anticholinergic, α-adrenergic, antihistamine	10–25 mg one to four times daily. Begin with 10–25 mg nightly.	10-, 25-, 50-mg tablets
Mirabegron	Myrbetriq	β_3 adrenergic agonist	25–50 mg daily	25-, 50-mg tablets

[a]Oral dosing except for transdermal forms.

anterior vaginal wall. The technique involves suture attachment of the lateral vaginal wall to the arcus tendineus fascia pelvis. Currently, PVDR is primarily a prolapse-correcting operation. Although previously used to correct SUI, long-term data show this to no longer be a superior method for primary treatment of SUI (Colombo, 1996; Mallipeddi, 2001).

Treatment of Urgency Urinary Incontinence

Anticholinergic Medications

These medications appear to work at the level of the detrusor muscle by competitively inhibiting acetylcholine at muscarinic receptors (M_2 and M_3) (Miller, 2005). These agents thereby blunt detrusor contractions to reduce the number of incontinence episodes and volume lost with each. These medications are significantly better than placebo at improving symptoms of urgency urinary incontinence and overactive bladder. However, in a Cochrane database review, Nabi and colleagues (2006) reported that the reduction in baseline urgency incontinence episodes per day reflects only a modest benefit.

Oxybutynin, Tolterodine, and Fesoterodine. These frequently used drugs competitively bind to cholinergic receptors (Table 23-5). As noted, muscarinic receptors are not limited

to the bladder. Thus, drug side effects may be significant. Of these, dry mouth, constipation, and blurry vision are common, and dry mouth is a primary reason for drug discontinuation (Table 23-6). Importantly, anticholinergics are contraindicated in those with narrow-angle glaucoma.

Because of these side effects, the therapeutic goal of bladder M_3 blockade with these antimuscarinic agents is often

TABLE 23-6. Potential Anticholinergic Side Effects

Side Effect	Potential Clinical Consequence
Increased pupil size	Photophobia
Decreased visual accommodation	Blurred vision
Decreased salivation	Gingival and buccal ulceration
Decreased bronchial secretions	Small-airway mucus plugging
Decreased sweating	Hyperthermia
Increased heart rate	Angina, myocardial infarction
Decreased detrusor function	Bladder distention and urinary retention
Decreased gastrointestinal mobility	Constipation

limited. Accordingly, drug selection is tailored, and efficacy is balanced against tolerability. For example, Diokno and associates (2003) found oxybutynin to be more effective than tolterodine. However, tolterodine was associated with lower side effect rates. Tolterodine and fesoterodine have also been compared in a randomized study of 1135 patients. Fesoterodine was found to perform better than tolterodine, although once again, side effects were lowest in the tolterodine group (Chapple, 2008). A population-based study reported that only 56 percent of women felt their overactive bladder medication was effective, and half stopped taking the medication (Diokno, 2006).

Most side effects attributed to oxybutynin stem from its secondary metabolite that follows liver metabolism. Therefore, to minimize oral oxybutynin side effects, a transdermal patch was designed to decrease the "first-pass" effect of this drug. This leads to decreased liver metabolism and fewer systemic cholinergic side effects. Dmochowski and coworkers (2003) found fewer anticholinergic side effects with transdermal oxybutynin compared with long-acting oral tolterodine.

Transdermal oxybutynin (Oxytrol) is supplied as a 7.6 × 5.7 cm patch that is applied to the abdomen, hip, or buttock; worn continuously; and changed twice weekly. Each patch contains 36 mg of oxybutynin and delivers approximately 3.9 mg daily. Application-site pruritus is the most frequent side effect, and varying the application site may minimize skin reactions (Sand, 2007). A transdermal oxybutynin gel (Gelnique), available in 3- and 10-percent strengths, is applied daily to skin of the abdomen, upper arms/shoulders, or thigh, and application sites are rotated.

Imipramine. This agent is less effective than tolterodine and oxybutynin but displays α-adrenergic and anticholinergic characteristics. Therefore, it is occasionally prescribed for those with mixed urinary incontinence. Importantly, doses of imipramine used to treat incontinence are significantly lower than those used to treat depression or chronic pain. In our experience, this minimizes the theoretical risk of drug-related side effects.

Selective Muscarinic-receptor Antagonists. These drugs were introduced with the aim of reducing anticholinergic side effects. The agents are all M$_3$-receptor selective antagonists and include solifenacin (Vesicare), trospium chloride (Santura), and darifenacin (Enablex). Advantages of increased urgency warning time and decreased muscarinic side effects have been shown in randomized controlled studies (Cardozo, 2004; Chapple, 2005; Haab, 2006; Zinner, 2004). However, although the side-effect profiles of these drugs are potentially more attractive, they have not been proved superior in efficacy to nonselective muscarinic agents (Hartmann, 2009).

Mirabegron

More recently, a β$_3$-adrenergic receptor agonist, mirabegron (Myrbetriq), has been introduced into the U.S. pharmaceutical market for the treatment of urgency urinary incontinence, urgency, and frequency. Activation of these receptors results in relaxation of the detrusor smooth muscle and increased bladder capacity. Most commonly reported adverse reactions include

hypertension, nasopharyngitis, UTIs, dry mouth, and headache (Herschorn, 2013).

Sacral Neuromodulation

Urine storage and bladder emptying require a complex coordinated interaction of spinal cord and higher brain centers, peripheral nerves, urethral and pelvic floor muscles, and the detrusor muscle. If any of these levels are altered, normal micturition is lost. To overcome these problems, electrical nerve stimulation, also called neuromodulation, has been used. InterStim is the only implantable neuromodulation system approved by the FDA for treatment of refractory urgency urinary incontinence and for treatment of anal incontinence. It may be also considered for those with pelvic pain, interstitial cystitis, and defecatory dysfunction, although it is not FDA-approved for these indications. Sacral neuromodulation is not considered primary therapy and is typically offered mainly to women who have exhausted pharmacologic and conservative options.

This outpatient surgically implanted device contains a pulse generator and electrical leads that are placed into the sacral foramina to modulate bladder and pelvic floor innervation. Its mode of action is incompletely understood but may be related to somatic afferent inhibition that interrupts abnormal reflex arcs in the sacral spinal cord involved in the filling and evacuation phases of micturition.

Implantation is typically a two-stage process. Initially, leads are placed and attached to an externally worn generator (Section 45-12, p. 1085). After placement, frequency and amplitude of electrical impulses can be adjusted and tailored to maximize effectiveness. If a 50-percent or greater improvement in symptoms is noted, then internal implantation of a permanent pulse generator is planned. This procedure is minimally invasive and is typically completed in a day-surgery setting. Surgical complications are rare but may include pain or infection at the generator insertion site.

Although its use is often reserved for those who have been unsuccessfully treated with behavioral or pharmacologic therapy, this modality is effective for urinary symptom treatment. Studies have found improvement rates ranging from 60 to 75 percent, and cure rates approximating 45 percent (Janknegt, 2001; Schmidt, 1999; Siegel, 2000). Sustained improvement from baseline incontinence parameters has been shown at long-term follow-up. One 3-year study reported a 57-percent reduction in incontinence episodes per day, and similar findings were found in a separate 5-year study (Kerrebroeck, 2007; Siegel, 2000). A systematic review of 17 case series at follow-up periods of 3 to 5 years similarly reported 39 percent of patients cured and 67 percent with greater than 50-percent improvement in incontinence symptoms (Brazzelli, 2006).

Percutaneous Tibial Nerve Stimulation

Sometimes referred to as posterior tibial nerve stimulation, percutaneous tibial nerve stimulation (PTNS) is becoming a more common therapy for refractory urgency urinary incontinence. It involves percutaneous needle electrode placement into an area cephalic to the medial malleolus of the lower extremity. Electrical pulses are sent via a generator to the tibial nerve. This nerve originates from spinal roots L4-S3, and its stimulation leads to retrograde neuromodulation. Multicenter studies have demonstrated its efficacy compared with sham or with primary treatment with anticholinergic medication (Peters, 2009, 2010; MacDiarmid, 2010).

Botulinum Toxin A

Injection of botulinum toxin A (onabotulinumtoxinA) into the bladder wall is approved for the treatment of idiopathic detrusor overactivity. Three placebo-controlled studies showed the effectiveness of this treatment (Anger, 2010). All three used cystoscopic injection of 200 units of botulinum toxin A versus placebo, and each demonstrated significantly improved continence rates. Improvement occurred as early as 4 weeks after injection (Brubaker, 2008b; Flynn, 2009; Khan, 2010; Sahai, 2007). Urinary retention—defined a postvoid residual volume measuring > 200 mL—is a common side effect and developed in 27 to 43 percent of patients in these randomized trials. Most patients are asymptomatic, but patients receiving botulinum toxin A for overactive bladder or urgency urinary incontinence are counseled that temporary self-catheterization may be required after injection.

More recently, one double-blind, randomized trial compared oral anticholinergic therapy against injections of 100 units of botulinum toxin A in women with idiopathic urgency urinary incontinence. Investigators found comparable reductions in incontinence episodes. The botulinum toxin A group was less likely to complain of dry mouth and more likely to have complete resolution of urgency urinary incontinence (Visco, 2012). In the injection group, the rate of catheter use for urinary retention was only 5 percent. At our institution, we use 100 units for women with idiopathic overactive bladder.

A patient can expect the effects of the toxin to wane over time. In a small study describing the need for repeat injections, 20 patients from a cohort of 34 received a second injection, and nine patients received up to four injections. These repeat injections appear to be equally effective as the primary injection. Median time between injections is approximately 377 days (Sahai, 2010).

REFERENCES

Abdel-Fattah M, Mostafa A, Familusi A, et al: Prospective randomised controlled trial of transobturator tapes in management of urodynamic stress incontinence in women: 3-year outcomes from the evaluation of transobturator tapes study. Eur Urol 62(5):843, 2012

Abrams P, Artibani W, Cardozo L, et al: Reviewing the ICS 2002 terminology report: the ongoing debate. Neurourol Urodyn 28(4):287, 2009

Abrams P, Cardozo L, Fall M, et al: The standardisation of terminology of lower urinary tract function: report from the Standardisation Sub-committee of the International Continence Society. Am J Obstet Gynecol 187:116, 2002

Anger JT, Weinberg A, Suttorp MJ, et al: Outcomes of intravesical botulinum toxin for idiopathic overactive bladder symptoms: a systematic review of the literature. J Urol 183:2258, 2010

Bai SW, Kang JY, Rha KH, et al: Relationship of urodynamic parameters and obesity in women with stress urinary incontinence. J Reprod Med 47:559, 2002

Barber MD, Gustilo-Ashby AM, Chen CC, et al: Perioperative complications and adverse events of the MONARC transobturator tape, compared with the tension-free vaginal tape. Am J Obstet Gynecol 195:1820, 2006

Barber MD, Kuchibhatla MN, Pieper CF, et al: Psychometric evaluation of 2 comprehensive condition-specific quality of life instruments for women with pelvic floor disorders. Am J Obstet Gynecol 185(6):1388, 2001

Barber MD, Weidner AC, Sokol AI, et al: Single-incision mini-sling compared with tension-free vaginal tape for the treatment of stress urinary incontinence: a randomized controlled trial. Obstet Gynecol 119:328, 2012

Bellin P, Smith J, Poll W, et al: Results of a multicenter trial of the CapSure (Re/Stor) Continence shield on women with stress urinary incontinence. Urology 51:697, 1998

Blaivas JG: The bladder is an unreliable witness. Neurourol Urodyn 15:443, 1996

Bologna RA, Gomelsky A, Lukban JC, et al: The efficacy of calcium glycerophosphate in the prevention of food-related flares in interstitial cystitis. Urology 57(6, Suppl 1):119, 2001

Brazzelli M, Murray A, Frasier C: Efficacy and safety of sacral nerve stimulation for urinary urge incontinence. A systematic review. J Urol 175:835, 2006

Brown JS, Bradley CS, Subak KK, et al: The sensitivity and specificity of a simple test to distinguish between urge and stress urinary incontinence. Ann Int Med 144(10):715, 2006

Brown JS, Seeley DG, Fong J, et al: Urinary incontinence in older women: who is at risk? Study of Osteoporotic Fractures Research Group. Obstet Gynecol 87(5 Pt 1):715, 1996

Brubaker L, Norton PA, Albo ME, et al: Adverse events over two years after retropubic or transobturator midurethral sling surgery: findings from the Trial of Midurethral Slings (TOMUS) study. Am J Obstet Gynecol 205:498.e1, 2011

Brubaker L, Nygaard I, Richter HE, et al: Two-year outcomes after sacrocolpopexy with and without Burch to prevent stress urinary incontinence. Obstet Gynecol 112:49, 2008a

Brubaker L, Richter HE, Visco AG, et al: Refractory idiopathic urge incontinence and botulinum A injection. J Urol 180:217, 2008b

Buckley BS, Lapitan MC, Epidemiology Committee of the Fourth International Consultation on Incontinence, Paris, 2008: Prevalence of urinary incontinence in men, women, and children—current evidence: findings of the Fourth International Consultation on Incontinence. Urology 76(2):265, 2010

Bump RC, McClish DK: Cigarette smoking and urinary incontinence in women. Am J Obstet Gynecol 167:1213, 1992

Bump RC, Norton PA: Epidemiology and natural history of pelvic floor dysfunction. Obstet Gynecol Clin North Am 25:723, 1998

Burgio KL, Richter HE, Clements RH, et al: Changes in urinary and fecal incontinence symptoms with weight loss surgery in morbidly obese women. Obstet Gynecol 110(5):1034, 2007

Cardozo L, Lisec M, Millard R, et al: Randomized, double-blind placebo controlled trial of the once daily antimuscarinic agent solifenacin succinate in patients with overactive bladder. J Urol 172(5, Part 1):1919, 2004

Carlile A, Davies I, Rigby A, et al: Age changes in the human female urethra: a morphometric study. J Urol 139:532, 1988

Chapple CR, Martinez-Garcia R, Selvaggi L, et al: A comparison of the efficacy and tolerability of solifenacin succinate and extended release tolterodine at treating overactive bladder syndrome: results of the STAR Trial. Eur Urol 48:464, 2005

Chapple CR, Van Kerrebroeck PE, Jünemann KP, et al: Comparison of fesoterodine and tolterodine in patients with overactive bladder. BJU Int 102(9):1128, 2008

Cody JD, Jacobs ML, Richardson K, et al: Oestrogen therapy for urinary incontinence in post-menopausal women. Cochrane Database Syst Rev 4:CD001405, 2012

Colombo M, Milani R, Vitobello D, et al: A randomized comparison of Burch colposuspension and abdominal paravaginal defect repair for female stress urinary incontinence. Am J Obstet Gynecol 175:78, 1996

Culligan PG, Goldberg RP, Sand PK: A randomized controlled trial comparing a modified Burch procedure and a suburethral sling: long-term follow-up. Int Urogynecol J Pelvic Floor Dysfunct 14(4):229, 2003

Dallosso HM, McGrother CW, Matthews RJ, et al: The association of diet and other lifestyle factors with overactive bladder and stress incontinence: a longitudinal study in women. BJU Int 92:69, 2003

Deitel M, Stone E, Kassam HA, et al: Gynecologic-obstetric changes after loss of massive excess weight following bariatric surgery. J Am Coll Nutr 7:147, 1988

Diokno AC, Appell RA, Sand PK, et al: Prospective, randomized, double-blind study of the efficacy and tolerability of the extended-release formulations of oxybutynin and tolterodine for overactive bladder: results of the OPERA trial. Mayo Clin Proc 78:687, 2003

Diokno AC, Brock BM, Herzog AR, et al: Medical correlates of urinary incontinence in the elderly. Urology 36:129, 1990

Diokno AC, Sand PK, Macdiarmid S, et al: Perceptions and behaviors of women with bladder control problems. Fam Pract 23(5):568, 2006

Dmochowski RR, Sand PK, Zinner NR, et al: Comparative efficacy and safety of transdermal oxybutynin and oral tolterodine versus placebo in previously treated patients with urge and mixed urinary incontinence. Urology 62:237, 2003

Dumoulin C, Hay-Smith J: Pelvic floor muscle training versus no treatment, or inactive control treatments, for urinary incontinence in women. Cochrane Database Syst Rev 1:CD005654, 2014a

Dumoulin C, Hunter KF, Moore K, et al: Conservative management for female urinary incontinence and pelvic organ prolapse review 2013: summary of the 5th International Consultation on Incontinence. Neurourol Urodyn November 18, 2014b [Epub ahead of print]

Fantl JA, Cardozo L, McClish DK: Estrogen therapy in the management of urinary incontinence in postmenopausal women: a meta-analysis. First report of the Hormones and Urogenital Therapy Committee. Obstet Gynecol 83:12, 1994

Flynn M, Amundsen CL, Perevich M, et al: Short term outcomes of a randomized, double blind placebo controlled trial of botulinum A toxin for the management of idiopathic detrusor overactivity incontinence. J Urol 181(6):2608, 2009

Food and Drug Administration: Considerations about surgical mesh for SUI. 2013. Available at: http://www.fda.gov/MedicalDevices/Productsand MedicalProcedures/ImplantsandProsthetics/UroGynSurgicalMesh/ucm 345219.htm. Accessed March 14, 2015

Grady D, Brown JS, Vittinghoff E, et al: Postmenopausal hormones and incontinence: the heart and estrogen/progestin replacement study. Obstet Gynecol 97:116, 2001

Grodstein F, Lifford K, Resnick, NM, et al: Postmenopausal hormone therapy and risk of developing urinary incontinence. Obstet Gynecol 103:254, 2004

Haab F, Corcos J, Siami P, et al: Long-term treatment with darifenacin for overactive bladder: results of a 2-year, open-label extension study. BJU Int 98:1025, 2006

Hagstad A, Janson PO, Lindstedt G: Gynaecological history, complaints and examinations in a middle-aged population. Maturitas 7:115, 1985

Hannestad YS, Lie RT, Rortveit G, et al: Familial risk of urinary incontinence in women: population based cross sectional study. BMJ 329(7471):889, 2004

Hannestad YS, Rortveit G, Daltveit AK, et al: Are smoking and other lifestyle factors associated with female urinary incontinence? The Norwegian EPINCONT Study. BJOG 110:247, 2003

Hartmann KE, McPheeters ML, Biller DH, et al: Treatment of overactive bladder in women. Evidence report/technology assessment No. 187, Rockville, Agency for Healthcare Research and Quality, 2009

Hendriks EJM, Kessels AGH, de Vet HCW, et al: Prognostic indicators of poor short-term outcome of physiotherapy intervention in women with stress urinary incontinence. Neurourol Urodyn 29:336, 2010

Hendrix SL, Cochrane BB, Nygaard IE, et al: Effects of estrogen with and without progestin on urinary incontinence. JAMA 293:935, 2005

Herschorn S, Barkin J, Castro-Diaz D, et al: A phase III, randomized, double-blind, parallel-group, placebo-controlled, multicentre study to assess the efficacy and safety of the β_3 adrenoceptor agonist, mirabegron, in patients with symptoms of overactive bladder. Urology 82(2):313, 2013

Holmgren C, Nilsson S, Lanner L, et al: Long-term results with tension-free vaginal tape on mixed and stress urinary incontinence. Obstet Gynecol 106(1):38, 2005

Hunskaar S, Arnold EP, Burgio K, et al: Epidemiology and natural history of urinary incontinence. Int Urogynecol J Pelvic Floor Dysfunct 11:301, 2000

Indrekvam S, Sandvik H, Hunskaar S: A Norwegian national cohort of 3198 women treated with home-managed electrical stimulation for urinary incontinence—effectiveness and treatment results. Scand J Urol Nephrol 35:32, 2001

Iosif CS, Batra S, Ek A, et al: Estrogen receptors in the human female lower urinary tract. Am J Obstet Gynecol 141:817, 1981

Jackson SL, Scholes D, Boyko EJ, et al: Predictors of urinary incontinence in a prospective cohort of postmenopausal women. Obstet Gynecol 108:855, 2006

Janknegt RA, Hassouna MM, Siegel SW, et al: Long-term effectiveness of sacral nerve stimulation for refractory urge incontinence. Eur Urol 39:101, 2001

Jelovsek JE, Chagin K, Brubaker L, et al. A model for predicting the risk of de novo stress urinary incontinence in women undergoing pelvic organ prolapse surgery. Obstet Gynecol 123:279, 2014

Kerrebroeck PE, Voskuilen A, Heesakkers J, et al: Results of sacral neuromodulation therapy for urinary voiding dysfunction: outcomes of a prospective, worldwide clinical study. J Urol 178:2029, 2007

Khan S, Panicker J, Roosen A, et al: Complete continence after botulinum neurotoxin type A injections for refractory idiopathic detrusor overactivity incontinence: patient-reported outcome at 4 weeks. Eur Urol 57(5):891, 2010

Kirkland JL, Lye M, Levy DW, et al: Patterns of urine flow and excretion in healthy elderly people. BMJ 287:1665, 1983

Langa KM, Fultz NH, Saint S, et al: Informal caregiving time and costs for urinary incontinence in older individuals in the United States. J Am Geriatr Soc 50:733, 2002

Lapitan MC, Cody DJ, Grant AM: Open retropubic colposuspension for urinary incontinence in women. Cochrane Database Syst Rev 4:CD002912, 2009

Laurikainen E, Valpas A, Aukee P, et al: Five-year results of a randomized trial comparing retropubic and transobturator midurethral slings for stress incontinence. Eur Urol 65(6):1109, 2014

MacDiarmid SA, Peters KM, Shobeiri SA, et al: Long-term durability of percutaneous tibial nerve stimulation for the treatment of overactive bladder. J Urol 183:234, 2010

Mallipeddi PK, Steele AC, Kohli N, et al: Anatomic and functional outcome of vaginal paravaginal repair in the correction of anterior vaginal wall prolapse. Int Urogynecol J Pelvic Floor Dysfunct 12:83, 2001

Markland AD, Richter HE, Fwu CW et al: Prevalence and trends of urinary incontinence in adults in the United States, 2001 to 2008. J Urol 186(2):589, 2011

McGuire EJ: Urethral bulking agents. Nat Clin Pract Urol 3(5):234, 2006

McGuire EJ: Urodynamic findings in patients after failure of stress incontinence operations. Prog Clin Biol Res 78: 351, 1981

McKinley M, O'Loughlin VD: Urinary system. In Human Anatomy. New York, McGraw-Hill, 2006, p 843

Miller JJ, Botros SM, Akl MN, et al: Is transobturator tape as effective as tension-free vaginal tape in patients with borderline maximum urethral closure pressure? Am J Obstet Gynecol 195:1799, 2006

Miller JJ, Sand PK: Diagnosis and treatment of overactive bladder. Minerva Ginecol 57:501, 2005

Monga AK, Stanton SL: Urodynamics: prediction, outcome and analysis of mechanism for cure of stress incontinence by periurethral collagen. BJOG 104:158, 1997

Moser F, Bjelic-Radisic V, Tamussino K: Needle suspension of the bladder neck for stress urinary incontinence: objective results at 11 to 16 years. Int Urogynecol J 17:611, 2006

Nabi G, Cody JD, Ellis G, et al: Anticholinergic drugs versus placebo for overactive bladder syndrome in adults. Cochrane Database Syst Rev 4:CD0003781, 2006

Nager CW, Brubaker L, Litman HJ, et al. A randomized trial of urodynamic testing before stress-incontinence surgery. N Engl J Med 366(21):1987, 2012

Neuman M: Perioperative complications and early follow-up with 100 TVT-SECUR procedures. J Minim Invasive Gynecol 15(4):480, 2008

Nilsson CG, Palva K, Aarnio R, et al: Seventeen years' follow-up of the tension-free vaginal tape procedure for female stress urinary incontinence. Int Urogynecol J 24(8):1265, 2013

Noblett K, Lane FL, Driskill CS: Does pelvic organ prolapse quantification exam predict urethral mobility in stages 0 and I prolapse? Int Urogynecol J Pelvic Floor Dysfunct 15:268, 2005

Nygaard I: Is cesarean delivery protective? Semin Perinatol 30:267, 2006

Nygaard I, Barber MD, Burgio KL, et al. Prevalence of symptomatic pelvic floor disorders in U.S. women. JAMA 300(11):1311, 2008

Nygaard I, Brubaker L, Zyczynski HM, et al: Long-term outcomes following abdominal sacrocolpopexy for pelvic organ prolapse. JAMA 309:2016, 2013

O'Connor RC, Nanigian DK, Lyon MB, et al: Early outcomes of mid-urethral slings for female stress urinary incontinence stratified by Valsalva leak point pressure. Neurourol Urodyn 25:685, 2006

Ouslander JG: Management of overactive bladder. N Engl J Med 350(8):786, 2004

Peters KM, Macdiarmid SA, Wooldridge LS, et al: Randomized trial of percutaneous tibial nerve stimulation versus extended-release tolterodine: results from the overactive bladder innovative therapy trial. J Urol 182:1055, 2009

Peters KM, Carrico DJ, Perez-Marrero RA, et al: Randomized trial of percutaneous tibial nerve stimulation versus Sham efficacy in the treatment of overactive bladder syndrome: results from the SUmiT trial. J Urol 183:1438, 2010

Petros PE, Ulmsten UI: An integral theory of female urinary incontinence. Experimental and clinical considerations. Scand J Urol Nephrol 153(Suppl):1, 1993

Rahn DD, Carberry C, Sanses TV, et al: Vaginal estrogen for genitourinary syndrome of menopause: a systematic review. Obstet Gynecol 124(6):1147, 2014

Rahn DD, Ward RM, Sanses TV, et al: Vaginal estrogen use in postmenopausal women with pelvic floor disorders: systematic review and practice guidelines. Int Urogynecol J 26(1):3, 2015

Raz R, Stamm WE: A controlled trial of intravaginal estriol in postmenopausal women with recurrent urinary tract infections. N Engl J Med 329:753, 1993

Resnick NM: Voiding dysfunction in the elderly. In Yalla SV, McGuire EJ, Elbadawi A, et al (eds): Neurourology and Urodynamics: Principles and Practice. New York, Macmillan, 1984, p 303

Resnick NM, Elbadawi A, Yalla SV: Age and the lower urinary tract: what is normal? Neurourol Urodyn 14:577, 1995

Richter HE, Albo ME, Zyczynski HM, et al: Retropubic versus transobturator midurethral slings for stress incontinence. N Engl J Med 362(22):2066, 2010a

Richter HE, Burgio KL, Brubaker L, et al: Continence pessary compared with behavioral therapy or combined therapy for stress incontinence. A randomized controlled trial. Obstet Gynecol 115(3):609, 2010b

Rortveit G, Daltveit AK, Hannestad YS, et al: Urinary incontinence after vaginal delivery or cesarean section. N Engl J Med 348(10):900, 2003a

Rortveit G, Daltveit AK, Hannestad YS, et al: Vaginal delivery parameters and urinary incontinence: the Norwegian EPINCONT study. Am J Obstet Gynecol 189(5):1268, 2003b

Sahai A, Dowson C, Khan MS, et al: Repeated injections of botulinum toxin-A for idiopathic detrusor overactivity. Urology 75(3):552, 2010

Sahai A, Khan MS, Dasgupta P: Efficacy of botulinum toxin-A for treating idiopathic detrusor overactivity: results from a single center, randomized, double-blind, placebo controlled trial. J Urol 177(6):2231, 2007

Sand P, Zinner N, Newman D, et al: Oxybutynin transdermal system improves the quality of life in adults with overactive bladder: a multicentre, community-based, randomized study. BJU Int 99(4):836, 2007

Sand PK, Bown LW, Panganiban R, et al: The low pressure urethra as a factor in failed retropubic urethropexy. Obstet Gynecol 62:399, 1987

Schmidt RA, Jonas UD, Oleson KA, et al: Sacral nerve stimulation for treatment of refractory urinary urge incontinence. J Urol 162:352, 1999

Siegel SW, Catanzaro F, Dijkema HE, et al: Long-term results of a multicenter study on sacral nerve stimulation for treatment of urinary urge incontinence, urgency-frequency, and retention. Urology 56(6 Suppl 1):87, 2000

Sirls LT, Foote JE, Kaufman JM, et al: Long-term results of the FemSoft1 Urethral Insert for the management of female stress urinary incontinence. Int Urogynecol J 13:88, 2002

Song PH, Kim YD, Kim HT, et al: The 7-year outcome of the tension-free vaginal tape procedure for treating female stress urinary incontinence. BJU Int 104(8):1113, 2009

Snooks SJ, Swash M, Henry MM, et al: Risk factors in childbirth causing damage to the pelvic floor innervation. Int J Colorectal Dis 1:20, 1986

Subak LL, Wing R, West DS, et al: Weight loss to treat urinary incontinence in overweight and obese women. N Engl J Med 360(5):481, 2009

Swift SE, Bent AE: Basic evaluation of the incontinent female patient. In Bent AE, Cundiff GW, Swift SE (eds): Ostergard's Urogynecology and Pelvic Floor Dysfunction, 6th ed. Philadelphia, Lippincott Williams & Wilkins, 2008, p 67

Townsend MK, Curhan GC, Resnick, et al: The incidence of urinary incontinence across Asian, black, and white women in the United States. Am J Obstet Gynecol 202:378.e1, 2010

Versi E1, Griffiths DJ, Harvey MA: A new external urethral occlusive device for female urinary incontinence. Obstet Gynecol 92:286, 1998

Vervest HA, van Venrooij GE, Barents JW, et al: Non-radical hysterectomy and the function of the lower urinary tract. II: Urodynamic quantification of changes in evacuation function. Acta Obstet Gynecol Scand 68:231, 1989

Visco AG, Brubaker L, Richter HE, et al: Anticholinergic therapy vs. onabotulinumtoxinA for urgency urinary incontinence. N Engl J Med 367:1803, 2012

Wai CY, Curto TM, Zyczynski HM, et al: Patient satisfaction after midurethral sling surgery for stress urinary incontinence. Obstet Gynecol 121(5):1009, 2013

Wake CR: The immediate effect of abdominal hysterectomy on intravesical pressure and detrusor activity. BJOG 87:901, 1980

Wang AC, Wang YY, Chen MC: Single-blind, randomized trial of pelvic floor muscle training, biofeedback-assisted pelvic floor muscle training, and electrical stimulation in the management of overactive bladder. Urology 63:61, 2004

Weber AM: Leak point pressure measurement and stress urinary incontinence. Curr Womens Health Rep 1:45, 2001

Wei JT, Nygaard I, Richter HE, et al. A midurethral sling to reduce incontinence after vaginal prolapse repair. N Engl J Med 366(25):2358, 2012

Wester C, Fitzgerald MP, Brubaker L, et al: Validation of the clinical bulbocavernosus reflex. Neurourol Urodyn 22:589, 2003

Wing RR, Creasman JM, West DS, et al: Improving urinary incontinence in overweight and obese women through modest weight loss. Obstet Gynecol 116:284, 2010

Wu JM, Hundley AF, Fulton RG, et al: Forecasting the prevalence of pelvic floor disorders in U.S. women 2010 to 2050. Obstet Gynecol 114(6):1278, 2009

Zinner N, Gittelman M, Harris R, et al: Trospium chloride improves overactive bladder symptoms: a multicenter phase III trial. J Urol 171(6 Pt 1): 2311, 2004

CHAPTER 24

Pelvic Organ Prolapse

Pelvic organ prolapse is a common condition that can lead to genital tract dysfunction and diminished quality of life. *Signs* include descent of one or more of the following: the anterior vaginal wall, posterior vaginal wall, uterus and cervix, vaginal apex, or the perineum (Haylen, 2010). *Symptoms* include vaginal bulging, pelvic pressure, and splinting or digitation. Splinting is manual bolstering of the prolapse to improve symptoms, whereas digitation aids stool evacuation. For pelvic organ prolapse to be considered a disease state in a given individual, symptoms should be attributable to pelvic organ descent such that surgical or nonsurgical reduction relieves the symptoms, restores function, and improves quality of life.

EPIDEMIOLOGY

Pelvic organ prolapse (POP) affects millions of women worldwide. In the United States, it is the third most common indication for hysterectomy. Moreover, a woman has an estimated cumulative lifetime risk of 12 percent to undergo surgery for POP (Wu, 2014). Estimates of disease prevalence are hampered by lack of consistent definitions. If the validated Pelvic Organ Prolapse Quantification examination alone is used to describe pelvic organ support, 30 to 65 percent of women presenting for routine gynecologic care have stage 2 prolapse (Bland, 1999; Swift, 2000, 2005; Trowbridge, 2008). In contrast, studies that define prolapse solely based on patient symptoms show a prevalence ranging from 3 to 6 percent in the United States (Bradley, 2005; Nygaard, 2008; Rortveit, 2007).

RISK FACTORS

Obstetric-related Risks

Table 24-1 summarizes predisposing factors for POP. It develops gradually over a span of years, and its etiology is multifactorial. The relative importance, however, of each factor is not known.

Of these, vaginal childbirth is the most frequently cited risk factor. Some evidence suggests that pregnancy itself predisposes to POP. But numerous studies have clearly shown that vaginal delivery increases a woman's propensity for developing POP. In the Pelvic Organ Support Study (POSST), increasing parity was associated with prolapse risk (Swift, 2005). Specifically, the risk of POP increased 1.2 times with each vaginal delivery. In the Reproductive Risks for Incontinence Study at Kaiser (RRISK) study, Rortveit and colleagues (2007) found that the prolapse risk increased significantly in woman with one vaginal delivery (odds ratio [OR] 2.8), two (OR 4.1), or three or more (OR 5.3) deliveries compared with nulliparas. In a longitudinal study of 1011 women, vaginal delivery was associated with a significantly greater risk of prolapse to the hymen or beyond compared with cesarean delivery without labor (OR 5.6) (Handa, 2011).

Although vaginal delivery is implicated in a woman's lifetime risk for POP, specific obstetric risk factors remain controversial. These include macrosomia, prolonged second-stage labor, episiotomy, anal sphincter laceration, epidural analgesia, forceps use, and oxytocin stimulation of labor. Each is a proposed risk factor. As we await further studies, we can anticipate that although each may have an important effect, it is the cumulative sum of all events occurring as the fetus traverses the birth canal that predisposes to POP.

Currently, two obstetric interventions—elective forceps delivery to shorten second-stage labor and elective episiotomy—are not advocated. Both lack evidence of benefit and carry risks for maternal and fetal harm. First, forceps delivery is directly implicated in pelvic floor injury through its association with anal sphincter laceration. Additionally, recent evidence shows that operative vaginal birth significantly increases the odds for all pelvic floor disorders, especially prolapse (OR 7.5) (Handa, 2011). For these reasons, elective forceps delivery is not recommended to prevent pelvic floor disorders and may be a contributing factor. Likewise, at least six randomized controlled trials (RCTs) comparing elective and selective episiotomy have shown no proven benefit. These studies have shown an association with anal sphincter laceration, postpartum anal incontinence, and postpartum pain (Carroli, 2009).

Elective cesarean delivery to prevent pelvic floor disorders such as POP and urinary incontinence is controversial.

TABLE 24-1. Risk Factors Associated with Pelvic Organ Prolapse

Pregnancy
Vaginal childbirth
Menopause
   Aging
   Hypoestrogenism
Chronically increased intraabdominal pressure
   Chronic obstructive pulmonary disease
   Constipation
   Obesity
Pelvic floor trauma
Genetic factors
   Race
   Connective tissue disorders
Spina bifida

Theoretically, if all women underwent cesarean delivery, fewer women would have pelvic floor disorders. Keeping in mind that most women do *not* have these disorders, cesarean delivery on maternal request (CDMR) would subject many women to a potentially dangerous intervention who would otherwise not develop the problem. Specifically, given the 12-percent lifetime risk of undergoing surgery for prolapse, for every one woman who would avoid pelvic floor surgery later in life by undergoing primary elective cesarean delivery, approximately nine women would gain no benefit yet would nevertheless assume the potential risks of cesarean delivery. Definitive recommendations will require further studies to define the potential risks and benefits of CDMR for primary prevention of pelvic floor dysfunction (American College of Obstetricians and Gynecologists, 2013b; Patel, 2006). Currently, decisions regarding CDMR to prevent pelvic floor disorders must be individualized. That said, the American College of Obstetricians and Gynecologists (2013a) recommends against CMDR for women desiring several children given the risk of abnormal placentation with accruing cesarean deliveries.

■ Age

Data from several studies show that POP prevalence increases steadily with age (Nygaard, 2008; Olsen, 1997; Swift, 2005). In the POSST study, in women aged 20 to 59 years, the incidence of POP roughly doubled with each decade. As with other risks for POP, aging is a complex process. The increased incidence may result from physiologic aging and degenerative processes and from hypoestrogenism. Research clearly demonstrates an important role for reproductive hormones in the maintenance of connective tissues and the extracellular matrix necessary for pelvic organ support. Estrogen and progesterone receptors have been identified in the nuclei of connective tissue and smooth muscle cells of both the levator ani stroma and uterosacral ligaments (Smith, 1990, 1993). Separating the effects of estrogen deprivation from the effects of the aging process is problematic.

■ Connective Tissue Disease

Women with connective tissue disorders may be more likely to develop POP. Histologic studies have shown that in women with POP, the ratio of collagen I to collagen III and IV is decreased (Moalli, 2004). This relative decline in well-organized dense collagen is believed to contribute to weakening of vaginal wall tensile strength and an increased susceptibility to vaginal wall prolapse. In a small case series study, one third of women with Marfan syndrome and three fourths of women with Ehlers-Danlos syndrome reported a history of POP (Carley, 2000).

■ Race

Racial differences in POP prevalence have been demonstrated in several studies (Schaffer, 2005). Black and Asian women show the lowest risk, whereas Hispanic and white women appear to have the highest risk (Hendrix, 2002; Kim, 2005; Whitcomb, 2009). Although differences in collagen content have been demonstrated between races, racial differences in the bony pelvis may also play a role. For instance, black women more commonly have a narrow pubic arch and an android or anthropoid pelvis. These shapes are protective against POP compared with the gynecoid pelvis typical of most white women.

In addition, emerging evidence suggests that POP may have a genetic component. Recent genome-wide linkage studies have identified specific predisposition genes that may contribute to POP (Allen-Brady, 2015).

■ Increased Abdominal Pressure

Chronically elevated intraabdominal pressure is believed to play a role in POP pathogenesis. Elevated pressures are present with obesity, chronic constipation, chronic coughing, and repetitive heavy lifting. Higher body mass index (BMI) correlates with POP risk. In the Women's Health Initiative (WHI) trial, being overweight (BMI 25 to 30 kg/m^2) increased the POP rate by 31 to 39 percent, and obesity (BMI >30 kg/m^2) raised the POP rate 40 to 75 percent (Hendrix, 2002). With regard to lifting, a Danish study demonstrated that nursing assistants who were involved with repetitive heavy lifting were at increased risk to undergo surgical intervention for prolapse (OR 1.6) (Jorgensen, 1994). In addition, cigarette smoking and chronic obstructive pulmonary disease (COPD) have also been implicated in POP development (Gilpin, 1989; Olsen, 1997). In a matched case-control study, COPD was associated with an increased risk of future pelvic floor repair after hysterectomy (Blandon, 2009). The repetitive increases in intraabdominal pressure resulting from chronic coughing may predispose to POP. Instead, some believe that the inhaled chemical compounds in tobacco may cause tissue changes that lead to POP rather than the chronic cough itself (Wieslander, 2005).

DESCRIPTION AND CLASSIFICATION

■ Visual Descriptors

Pelvic organ prolapse is descent of the anterior vaginal wall, posterior vaginal wall, uterus (cervix), the vaginal apex after hysterectomy, rectum, or the perineum, alone or in combination. The terms *cystocele, cystourethrocele, uterine prolapse, uterine procidentia, rectocele,* and *enterocele* have traditionally been used to describe the structures behind the vaginal wall thought to be prolapsed (Fig. 24-1). However, these terms are imprecise and misleading, as they focus on what is presumed to be prolapsed rather than what is objectively noted to be prolapsed.

Although these terms are deeply entrenched in the literature, it is more clinically useful to describe prolapse in terms of what one actually sees: anterior vaginal wall prolapse, apical prolapse, cervical prolapse, posterior vaginal wall prolapse, rectal prolapse, or perineal descent.

▪ Pelvic Organ Prolapse Quantification (POP-Q)

In 1996, the International Continence Society defined a system of Pelvic Organ Prolapse Quantification (POP-Q) (Bump, 1996). Demonstrating high intra- and interexaminer reliability, the POP-Q system allows clinicians and researchers to report findings in a standardized, easily reproducible fashion. This system contains a series of site-specific measurements of a woman's pelvic organ support. Prolapse in each segment is measured relative to the hymen, which is an anatomic landmark that can be identified consistently. Six points are located with reference to the plane of the hymen: two on the anterior vaginal wall (points Aa and Ba), two at the apical vagina (points C and D), and two on the posterior vaginal wall (points Ap and Bp) (Fig. 24-2). The genital hiatus (Gh), perineal body (Pb), and total vaginal length (TVL) are also measured. All POP-Q points, except TVL, are measured during patient Valsalva and should reflect maximum protrusion.

Anterior Vaginal Wall Points

Point Aa defines a point that lies in the midline of the anterior vaginal wall and is 3 cm proximal to the external urethral meatus. This corresponds to the proximal location of the urethrovesical crease. In relation to the hymen, this point's position ranges from −3 (normal support) to +3 cm (maximum prolapse of point Aa).

Point Ba represents the most distal position of any part of the upper anterior vaginal wall, that is, the segment of vagina that normally would extend cephalad from point Aa. It is −3 cm in the absence of prolapse. In a woman with total vaginal eversion posthysterectomy, Ba would have a positive value equal to the position of the cuff from the hymen.

Apical Vaginal Points

The two apical points, C and D, which are located in the proximal vagina, represent the most cephalad locations of a normally positioned lower reproductive tract. *Point C* defines a point that is at either the most distal edge of the cervix or the leading edge of the vaginal cuff after total hysterectomy.

Point D defines a point that represents the location of the posterior fornix in a woman who still has a cervix. It is omitted in the absence of a cervix. This point represents the level of uterosacral ligament attachment to the proximal posterior cervix and thus differentiates uterosacral-cardinal ligament

Normal female pelvic anatomy

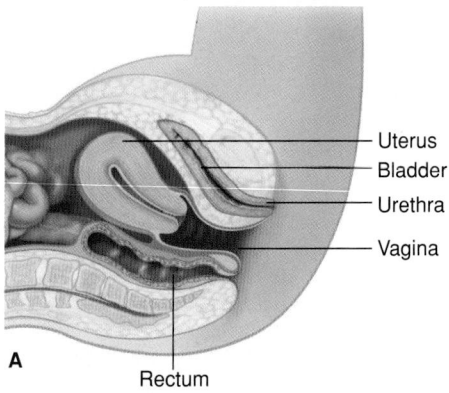

— Uterus
— Bladder
— Urethra
— Vagina

A

Rectum

Anterior vaginal wall prolapse

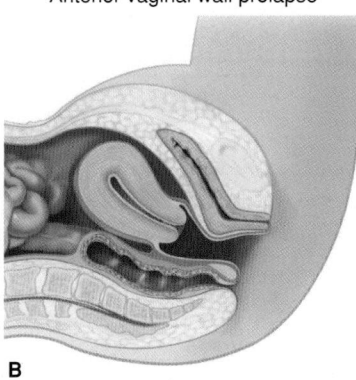

B

Distal posterior wall prolapse

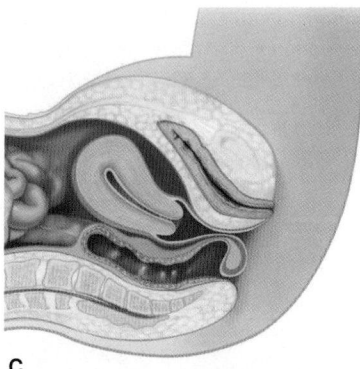

C

Apical posterior wall prolapse

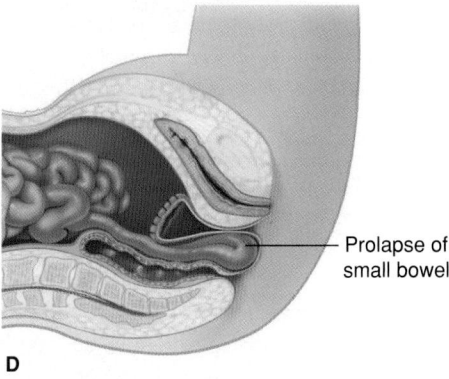

Prolapse of small bowel

D

FIGURE 24-1 Sagittal view of pelvic anatomy. **A.** Normal pelvic anatomy. **B.** Anterior vaginal wall prolapse or cystocele. **C.** Distal posterior wall prolapse or rectocele. **D.** Apical posterior wall prolapse or enterocele.

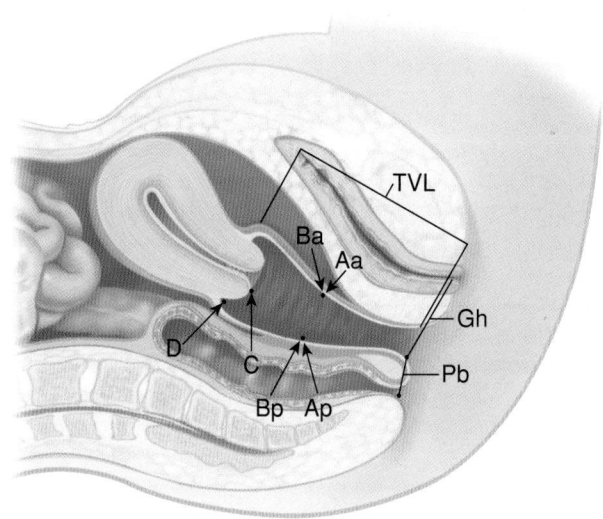

FIGURE 24-2 Anatomic landmarks used during pelvic organ prolapse quantification (POP-Q).

(see Fig. 24-2). The genital hiatus is measured from the middle of the external urethral meatus to the midline of the posterior hymenal ring. The perineal body is measured from the posterior margin of the genital hiatus to the midanal opening.

Assessment with POP-Q

With the hymenal plane defined as zero, the anatomic position of these points from the hymen is measured in centimeters. Points above or proximal to the hymen are described with a negative number. Positions below or distal to the hymen are noted using a positive number. The point measurements can be organized using a three-by-three grid as shown in Figure 24-3. Figures 24-4 and 24-5 illustrate the use of POP-Q in evaluating different examples of POP.

The degree of prolapse can also be quantified using a five-stage ordinal system as summarized in Table 24-2 (Bump, 1996). Stages are assigned according to the most severe portion of the prolapse.

support failure from cervical elongation. The *total vaginal length* (TVL) is the greatest depth of the vagina in centimeters when point C or D is reduced to its fullest position.

Posterior Vaginal Wall Points

Point Ap defines a point in the midline of the posterior vaginal wall that lies 3 cm proximal to the hymen. Relative to the hymen, this point's range of position is by definition –3 (normal support) to +3 cm (maximum prolapse of point Ap).

Point Bp represents the most distal position of any part of the upper posterior vaginal wall. By definition, this point is at –3 cm in the absence of prolapse. In a woman with total vaginal eversion posthysterectomy, Bp would have a positive value equal to the position of the cuff from the hymen.

Genital Hiatus and Perineal Body

In addition to the hymen, remaining measurements include those of the genital hiatus (Gh) and the perineal body (Pb)

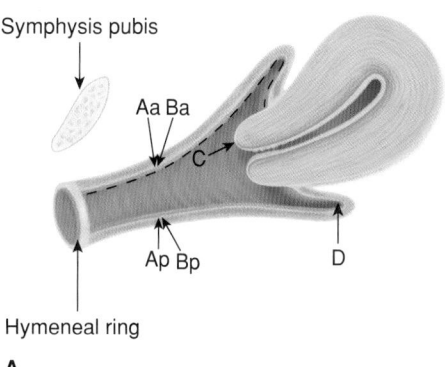

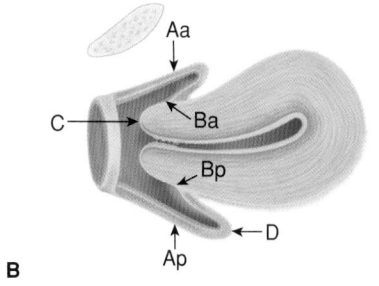

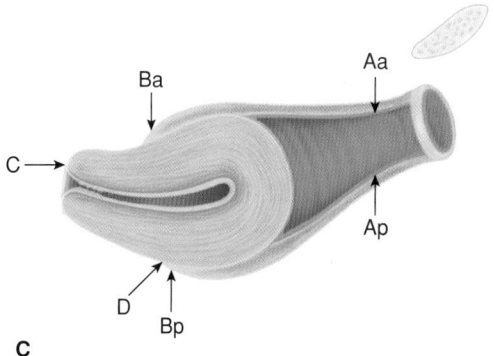

FIGURE 24-4 POP-Q depiction of varying degrees of uterine prolapse **(A–C)**.

anterior wall	anterior wall	cervix or cuff
Aa	**Ba**	**C**
genital hiatus	perineal body	total vaginal length
gh	**pb**	**tvl**
posterior wall	posterior wall	posterior fornix
Ap	**Bp**	**D**

FIGURE 24-3 Grid system used for charting in pelvic organ prolapse quantification (POP-Q).

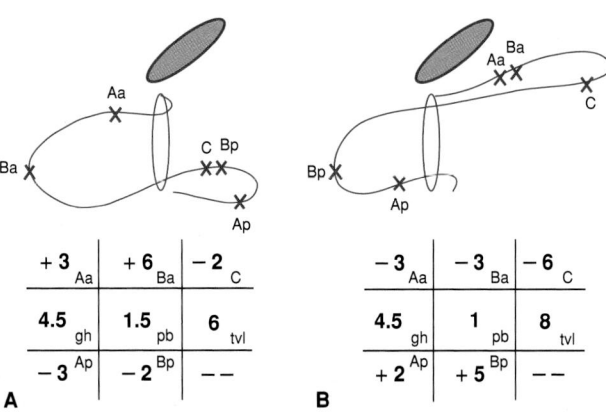

FIGURE 24-5 Grid and drawing of an anterior support defect (**A**) and posterior support defect (**B**). (Reproduced with permission from Bump RC, Mattiasson A, Bø K, et al: The standardization of terminology of female pelvic organ prolapse and pelvic floor dysfunction, Am J Obstet Gynecol 1996 Jul;175(1):10–17.)

Baden-Walker Halfway System

This descriptive tool is also used to classify prolapse during physical examination and is widely used. Although not as informative as the POP-Q, it is adequate for clinical use if each compartment (anterior, apical, and posterior) is evaluated (Table 24-3) (Baden, 1972).

PATHOPHYSIOLOGY

Pelvic organ support is maintained by complex interactions among the pelvic floor muscles, pelvic floor connective tissue, and vaginal wall. These work in concert to provide support and also maintain normal physiologic function of the vagina, urethra, bladder, and rectum. Several factors are implicated in failure of this support, but none fully explain its pathogenesis. These include genetic predisposition, loss of pelvic floor striated muscle support, vaginal wall weakness, and loss of connective attachments between the vaginal wall and the pelvic floor muscles and pelvic viscera. As noted earlier, vaginal birth and aging are two

TABLE 24-3. Baden-Walker Halfway System for the Evaluation of Pelvic Organ Prolapse on Physical Examination[a]

Grade	
Grade 0	Normal position for each respective site
Grade 1	Descent halfway to the hymen
Grade 2	Descent to the hymen
Grade 3	Descent halfway past the hymen
Grade 4	Maximum possible descent for each site

[a]Descent of the anterior vaginal wall, posterior vaginal wall, or apical prolapse can be graded with this system. Reproduced with permission from Baden WF, Walker T: Surgical Repair of Vaginal Defect. Philadelphia: JB Lippincott; 1992.

major risk factors for POP (Mant, 1997). The loss of support that evolves decades after vaginal delivery may stem from an initial insult compounded by aging and other contributors.

Levator Ani Muscle

The levator ani muscle is a pair of striated muscles composed of three regions. The *iliococcygeus muscle* forms a flat horizontal shelf spanning from one pelvic sidewall to the other (Figs. 38-7 and 38-8, p. 802). The *pubococcygeus muscle* arises from the pubic bone on either side; is attached to the walls of the vagina, urethra, anus, and perineal body; and inserts on the coccyx. The pubococcygeus muscle thereby helps suspend the vaginal wall to the pelvis. The *puborectalis muscle* forms a sling that originates from the pubic bone. This wraps around and behind the rectum. Connective tissue covers the superior and inferior fascia of the levator ani muscle. In the healthy state, baseline resting contractile activity of the levator ani muscle elevates the pelvic floor and compresses the vagina, urethra, and rectum toward the pubic bone (Fig. 38-10, p. 803). This narrows the genital hiatus and prevents prolapse of the pelvic organs.

TABLE 24-2. The Pelvic Organ Prolapse Quantification (POP-Q) Staging System of Pelvic Organ Support

Stage 0:	No prolapse is demonstrated. Points Aa, Ap, Ba, and Bp are all at −3 cm and either point C or D is between −TVL (total vaginal length) cm and −(TVL −2) cm (i.e., the quantitation value for point C or D is ≤−[TVL −2] cm). Figure 24-2 represents stage 0
Stage I:	The criteria for stage 0 are not met, but the most distal portion of the prolapse is >1 cm above the level of the hymen (i.e., its quantitation value is <−1 cm)
Stage II:	The most distal portion of the prolapse is ≤1 cm proximal to or distal to the plane of the hymen (i.e., its quantitation value is ≥−1 cm but ≤+1 cm)
Stage III:	The most distal portion of the prolapse is >1 cm below the plane of the hymen but protrudes no further than 2 cm less than the total vaginal length in centimeters (i.e., its quantitation value is >+1 cm but <+[TVL −2] cm). Figure 24-5B represents stage III Bp prolapse
Stage IV:	Essentially, complete eversion of the total length of the lower genital tract is demonstrated. The distal portion of the prolapse protrudes to at least (TVL − 2) cm (i.e., its quantitation value is ≥+[TVL − 2] cm). In most instances, the leading edge of stage IV prolapse will be the cervix or vaginal cuff scar. Figure 24-4C represents stage IVC prolapse

Data from Bump RC, Mattiasson A, Bø K, et al: The standardization of terminology of female pelvic organ prolapse and pelvic floor dysfunction, Am J Obstet Gynecol 1996 Jul;175(1):10-17.

When the levator ani muscle has normal tone and the vagina has adequate depth, the upper vagina lies nearly horizontal in the standing female. Thus, during periods of increased intraabdominal pressure, the upper vagina is compressed against the levator plate. It is theorized that when the levator ani muscle loses tone, the vagina drops from a horizontal to a semivertical position (Fig. 38-11, p. 804). This widens or opens the genital hiatus and predisposes pelvic viscera to prolapse. Without adequate levator ani muscle support, the visceral fascial attachments of the pelvic contents are placed on tension and are thought to stretch and eventually fail.

Theoretically, the levator ani muscle may sustain either direct muscle or denervation injury during childbirth, and these injuries are involved in POP pathogenesis. During second-stage labor, nerve injury from stretch or compression or both is believed to partially denervate the levator ani muscle. Denervated muscle loses tone, the genital hiatus opens, and pelvic viscera prolapse (DeLancey, 1993; Peschers, 1997; Shafik, 2000).

The experimental evidence for this theory of denervation-induced injury leading to POP has been difficult to obtain and is contradictory. Some studies demonstrate histomorphologic abnormalities in the levator ani muscle from women with prolapse and stress incontinence, whereas other studies fail to find histologic evidence of levator ani muscle denervation (Gilpin, 1989; Hanzal, 1993; Heit, 1996; Koelbl, 1989). In addition, levator ani muscle biopsies obtained from parous and nulliparous cadavers failed to find evidence of atrophy or other important muscle changes (Boreham, 2009). This suggests that pregnancy and parturition have little or no effect on levator ani muscle histomorphology. Additionally, experimental denervation of the levator ani muscle in the squirrel monkey led to significant muscular atrophy but did not affect pelvic organ support. Taken together, experimental evidence does not support a role for denervation-induced injury in POP pathophysiology.

Importantly, however, loss of skeletal muscle volume and function occurs in virtually all striated muscles during aging. Results obtained from young and older women with POP indicate that the levator ani muscle undergoes substantial morphologic and biochemical changes during aging. Thus, loss of levator tone with age may contribute to pelvic organ support failure in older women, possibly those with preexisting defects in connective tissue support. As striated muscles lose tone, ligamentous and connective tissue support of the pelvic organs must sustain more forces conferred by abdominal pressure. As connective tissues bear these loads for long periods, they stretch and may eventually fail, resulting in prolapse.

■ Connective Tissue

A continuous interdependent system of connective tissues and ligaments surrounds the pelvic organs and attaches them to the levator ani muscle and bony pelvis. The connective tissue of the pelvis is comprised of collagen, elastin, smooth muscle, and microfibers, which are anchored in an extracellular matrix of polysaccharides. The connective tissue that invests the pelvic viscera provides substantial pelvic organ support.

Of these, the *arcus tendineus fascia pelvis* is a condensation of parietal fascia covering the medial aspects of the obturator internus and levator ani muscle (Fig. 38-7, p. 801). It provides

the lateral and apical anchor sites for the anterior and posterior vagina. The arcus tendineus fascia pelvis is therefore poised to withstand descent of the anterior vaginal wall, vaginal apex, and proximal urethra. Experts now believe that a major inciting factor for prolapse is loss of connective tissue support at the vaginal apex leading to stretching or tearing of the arcus tendineus fascia pelvis. The result is apical and anterior vaginal wall prolapse.

The *uterosacral ligaments* contribute to apical support by suspending and stabilizing the uterus, cervix, and upper vagina. The ligament contains approximately 20 percent smooth muscle. Several studies have shown a decrease in the fractional area and distribution of smooth muscle in the uterosacral ligaments of women with prolapse (Reisenauer, 2008; Takacs, 2009). These studies suggest that abnormalities in uterosacral ligament support of the pelvic organs contribute to prolapse development.

Abnormalities of connective tissue and connective tissue repair may predispose women to prolapse (Norton, 1995; Smith, 1989). As noted, women with connective tissue disorders such as Ehlers-Danlos or Marfan syndrome are more likely to develop POP and urinary incontinence (Carley, 2000; Norton, 1995).

The pelvic floor fascia and connective tissues may also lose strength consequent to aging and loss of neuroendocrine signaling in pelvic tissues (Smith, 1989). Estrogen deficiency can affect the biomedical composition, quality, and quantity of collagen. Estrogen influences collagen content by increasing synthesis or decreasing degradation. Exogenous estrogen supplementation has been found to increase the skin collagen content in postmenopausal women who are estrogen deficient (Brincat, 1983). Moreover, estrogen supplementation prior to prolapse surgery and/or postoperatively is considered essential by many pelvic reconstruction surgeons. In a systematic review, Rahn and coworkers (2015) found that vaginal estrogen application before POP surgery improved the vaginal maturation index and increased vaginal epithelial thickness. This suggests a possible role in healing and future support. Although this practice may seem logical and empirically sound, evidence does not yet show improved surgical outcomes with this use of adjuvant estrogen.

■ Vaginal Wall

Abnormalities in the vaginal wall and its attachments to the pelvic floor muscles may be involved in POP pathogenesis. The vaginal wall is composed of mucosa (epithelium and lamina propria), a fibroelastic muscularis layer, and an adventitial layer that is made up of loose areolar tissue, abundant elastic fibers, and neurovascular bundles (Fig. 24-6). The muscularis and adventitial layers together form the *fibromuscular layer*, which was previously referred to as "endopelvic fascia." The fibromuscular layer coalesces laterally and attaches to the arcus tendineus fascia pelvis and superior fascia of the levator ani muscle. In the lower third of the vagina, the vaginal wall is attached directly to the perineal membrane and the perineal body. This suspensory system, together with the uterosacral ligaments, prevents the vagina and uterus from descent when the genital hiatus is open.

Abnormalities in the anatomy, physiology, and cellular biology of vaginal wall smooth muscle may contribute to POP. Specifically, in fibromuscular tissue taken at the vaginal apex from both the anterior and posterior vaginal walls, vaginal prolapse is associated with loss of smooth muscle, myofibroblast

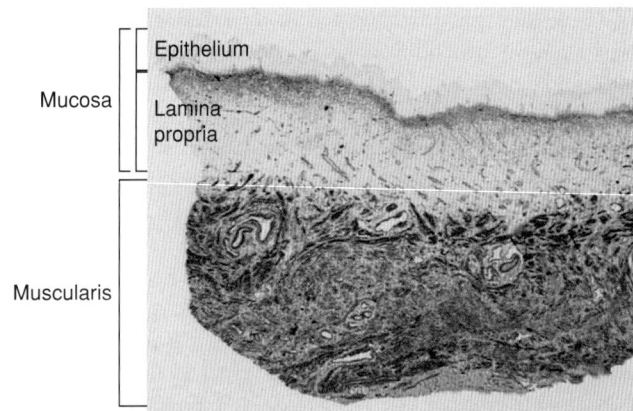

FIGURE 24-6 Photomicrograph shows a cross section of the vaginal wall. Mucosal and muscularis layers are shown here. The adventitia, which is typically seen deep to muscularis, is not shown in this section. The fibromuscular layer is comprised of muscularis and adventitial layers. (Used with permission from Dr. Ann Word.)

activation, abnormal smooth muscle phenotype, and increased protease activity (Boreham, 2001, 2002a,b; Moalli, 2005; Phillips, 2006). Additionally, abnormal synthesis or degradation of vaginal wall collagen and elastin fibers appears to contribute to prolapse.

■ The Defect Theory of Pelvic Organ Prolapse

This theory states that tears in different sites of the "endopelvic fascia" surrounding the vaginal wall allow herniation of the pelvic organs. Specifically, attenuation of the vaginal wall without loss of fascial attachments is called a *distention* cystocele or rectocele (Fig. 24-7). With distention-type prolapse, the vaginal wall appears smooth and without rugae, due to abdominal contents pressed against the vagina from within. In contrast, anterior and posterior wall defects due to loss of the connective tissue

attachment of the lateral vaginal wall to the pelvic sidewall are described as *displacement* (paravaginal) cystocele or rectocele (Fig. 24-8). With displacement-type prolapse, vaginal rugae are visible. Both defect types could result from the stretching or tearing of support tissues during second-stage labor.

Many experts now believe the primary defect leading to prolapse is loss of support at the vaginal apex. This allows the apical portions of the anterior and posterior vaginal walls to descend. As such, resuspension of the vaginal apex will restore support to both the anterior and posterior walls.

■ Levels of Vaginal Support

The vagina is a fibromuscular, flattened, cylindrical tube with three levels of support, as described by DeLancey (1992). Level I support suspends the upper or proximal vagina. Level II support attaches the midvagina along its length to the arcus tendineus fascia pelvis. Level III support results from fusion of the distal vagina to adjacent structures. Defects in each level of support result in identifiable vaginal wall prolapse: apical, anterior, and posterior.

Level I support consists of the cardinal and uterosacral ligaments attachment to the cervix and upper vagina (Fig. 38-15, p. 808). The cardinal ligaments fan out laterally and attach to the parietal fascia of the obturator internus and piriformis muscles, the anterior border of the greater sciatic foramen, and the ischial spines. The uterosacral ligaments are posterior fibers that attach to the presacral region at the level of S2 through S4. Together, this dense visceral connective tissue complex maintains vaginal length and horizontal axis. It allows the vagina to be supported by the levator plate and positions the cervix just superior to the level of the ischial spines. Defects in this support complex may lead to apical prolapse. This is frequently associated with small bowel herniation into the vaginal wall, that is, enterocele.

Level II support consists of the paravaginal attachments that are contiguous with the cardinal/uterosacral complex at the ischial spine. These are the connective tissue attachments of the

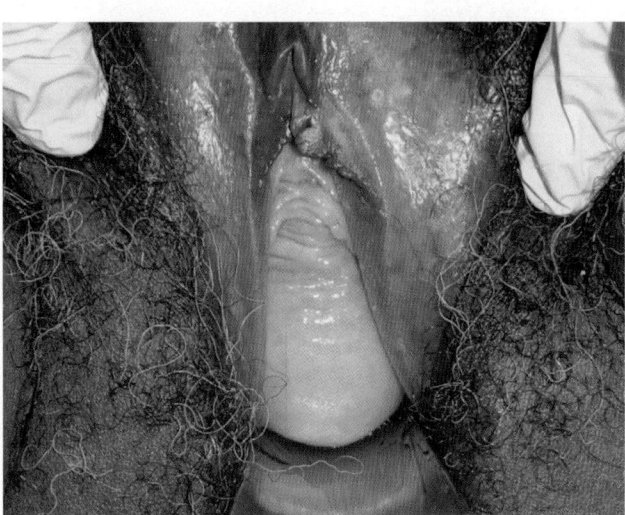

FIGURE 24-7 Photograph shows midline or distention cystocele. Note the characteristic loss of vaginal wall rugae. This contrasts with the findings in Figure 24-8.

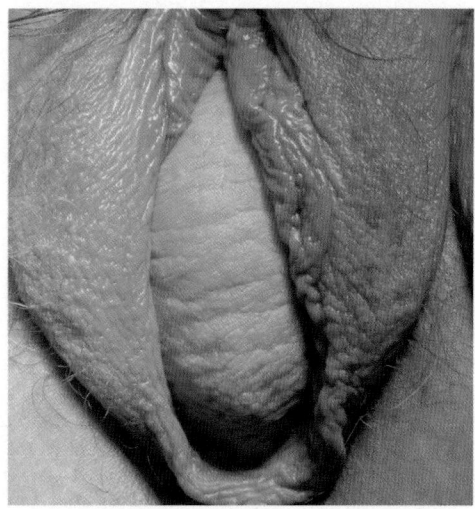

FIGURE 24-8 Photograph shows a lateral cystocele, also termed paravaginal or displacement cystocele. Rugae are present, which indicates that loss of support is lateral rather than central.

lateral vagina anteriorly to the arcus tendineus fascia pelvis and posteriorly to the arcus tendineus rectovaginalis. Detachment of this connective tissue from the arcus tendineus fascia pelvis leads to lateral or paravaginal anterior vaginal wall prolapse.

Level III support is composed of the perineal body, superficial and deep perineal muscles, and fibromuscular connective tissue. Collectively, these support the distal one third of the vagina and introitus. The perineal body is essential for distal vaginal support and proper function of the anal canal. Damage to level III support contributes to anterior and posterior vaginal wall prolapse, gaping introitus, and perineal descent.

PATIENT EVALUATION

▨ Symptoms

Pelvic organ prolapse involves multiple anatomic and functional systems and is commonly associated with genitourinary, gastrointestinal, and musculoskeletal symptoms (Table 24-4). Prolapse rarely creates severe morbidity or mortality, however, it can greatly diminish quality of life. In contrast, many women with mild to advanced prolapse lack bothersome symptoms. Thus, initial evaluation must include a careful assessment of prolapse-related symptoms and their effect on activities of daily living.

TABLE 24-4. Symptoms Associated with Pelvic Organ Prolapse

Symptoms	Other Possible Causes
Bulge symptoms	
Sensation of vaginal bulging or protrusion	Rectal prolapse
Seeing or feeling a vaginal or perineal bulge	Vulvar or vaginal cyst/mass
Pelvic or vaginal pressure	Pelvic mass
Heaviness in pelvis or vagina	Hernia (inguinal or femoral)
Urinary symptoms	
Urinary incontinence	Urethral sphincter incompetence
Urinary frequency	Detrusor overactivity
Urinary urgency	Hypoactive detrusor function
Weak or prolonged urinary stream	Bladder outlet obstruction (i.e., postsurgical)
Hesitancy	Excessive fluid intake
Feeling of incomplete emptying	Interstitial cystitis
Manual reduction of prolapse to start or complete voiding	Urinary tract infection
Position change to start or complete voiding	
Bowel symptoms	
Incontinence of flatus or liquid/solid stool	Anal sphincter disruption or neuropathy
Feeling of incomplete emptying	Diarrheal disorder
Hard straining to defecate	Rectal prolapse
Urgency to defecate	Irritable bowel syndrome
Digital evacuation to complete defecation	Rectal inertia
Splinting vagina or perineum to start or complete defecation	Pelvic floor dyssynergia
Feeling of blockage or obstruction during defecation	Hemorrhoids
	Anorectal neoplasm
Sexual symptoms	
Dyspareunia	Vaginal atrophy
Decreased lubrication	Levator ani syndrome
Decreased sensation	Vulvodynia
Decreased arousal or orgasm	Other female sexual disorder
Pain	
Pain in vagina, bladder, or rectum	Interstitial cystitis
Pelvic pain	Levator ani syndrome
Low back pain	Vulvodynia
	Lumbar disc disease
	Musculoskeletal pain
	Other causes of chronic pelvic pain

Reproduced with permission from Barber MD: Symptoms and outcome measures of pelvic organ prolapse. Clin Obstet Gynecol 2005 Sep;48(3):648–661.

TABLE 24-5. Short Form: Pelvic Floor Impact Questionnaire 7-Item (PFIQ-7)

Please select the best answer to each question below.

Name _____

Has your prolapse affected your:

1. Ability to do household chores (cooking, house cleaning, laundry)?

| _ Not at all | _ Mildly | _ Moderately | _ Severely |

2. Physical recreation such as walking, swimming, or other exercises?

| _ Not at all | _ Mildly | _ Moderately | _ Severely |

3. Entertainment activities (movies, church)?

| _ Not at all | _ Mildly | _ Moderately | _ Severely |

4. Ability to travel by car or bus more than 30 minutes from home?

| _ Not at all | _ Mildly | _ Moderately | _ Severely |

5. Participation in social activities outside your home?

| _ Not at all | _ Mildly | _ Moderately | _ Severely |

6. Emotional health (nervousness, depression)?

| _ Not at all | _ Mildly | _ Moderately | _ Severely |

7. Feeling frustrated?

| _ Not at all | _ Mildly | _ Moderately | _ Severely |

Reproduced with permission from Chapple CR, Zimmern PE, Brubaker L, et al (eds): Multidisciplinary Management of Female Pelvic Floor Disorders. Philadelphia: Elsevier; 2006.

Symptoms are carefully reviewed to determine if they are caused by the prolapse or by other etiologies. "Bulge" symptoms, which are pelvic pressure, the feeling of sitting on a ball, or heaviness in the vagina, are most likely to correlate with prolapse. Other symptoms, such as back pain, constipation, and abdominal discomfort, may coexist with prolapse but not result from it. A thorough history and physical examination will often help delineate the relationship between POP and symptoms.

During symptom inventory, several tools may be useful in assessing severity. Two commonly used questionnaires are the Pelvic Floor Distress Inventory (PFDI) and the Pelvic Floor Impact Questionnaire (PFIQ) (Barber, 2005b). The PFDI assesses urinary, colorectal, and prolapse symptoms, whereas the PFIQ seeks a diminished quality of life due to prolapse (Tables 24-5 and 24-6).

Bulge symptoms most strongly correlate with POP. These are typified by feeling or seeing a vaginal or perineal protrusion, and the sensation of pelvic pressure. Women may comment on feeling a ball in the vagina, sitting on a weight, or noting a bulge rubbing against their clothes. These symptoms worsen with prolapse progression (Ellerkmann, 2001). Specifically, women with prolapse beyond the hymen are more likely to report a vaginal bulge and have more symptoms than those with prolapse that stops above the hymen (Bradley, 2005; Tan, 2005; Weber, 2001a). If bulge symptoms are the primary complaint, successful replacement of the prolapse with nonsurgical or surgical therapy will usually provide adequate symptom relief.

Urinary symptoms often accompany POP and may include stress urinary incontinence (SUI), urgency urinary incontinence, frequency, urgency, urinary retention, recurrent urinary tract infection, or voiding dysfunction. Although these symptoms may be caused or exacerbated by POP, it should not be assumed that surgical or nonsurgical correction of prolapse will be curative. For example, irritative bladder symptoms (frequency, urgency, and urgency urinary incontinence) may not improve with prolapse replacement. Moreover, they may be unrelated to the prolapse and require alternative therapy. In contrast, urinary retention has been found to improve with prolapse treatment if the symptom is due to an obstructed urethra (FitzGerald, 2000).

For these reasons, urodynamic testing is a valuable adjunct in women with urinary symptoms who are undergoing treatment of prolapse (Chap. 23, p. 526). This testing attempts to determine the relationship between urinary symptoms and POP and will help guide therapy. Additionally, consideration may also be given to temporarily placing a pessary prior to surgery to determine if urinary symptoms improve. This may predict whether surgical reduction of prolapse will be beneficial.

Constipation is often present in women with POP, although it is generally not caused by POP. Thus, surgical repair or treatment with a pessary will not usually cure constipation and may actually worsen it. In one study of defect-directed posterior repair, constipation resolved postoperatively in only 43 percent of patients (Kenton, 1999). Therefore, if a patient's primary symptom is constipation, treatment of prolapse may not be indicated. Constipation should be viewed as a problem distinct from prolapse and evaluated separately.

Digital decompression of the posterior vaginal wall, the perineal body, or the distal rectum to evacuate the rectum is the most common defecatory symptom associated with posterior vaginal wall prolapse (Burrows, 2004; Ellerkmann, 2001). Surgical approaches to this problem provide variable success, and symptom resolution rates range from 36 to 70 percent (Cundiff, 2004; Kenton, 1999).

Anal incontinence of flatus, liquid, or solid stool may also associate with POP. On occasion, prolapse may lead to stool trapping in the distal rectum with subsequent leakage of liquid stool around retained feces. If symptoms are present, a full anorectal

TABLE 24-6. Short Form: Pelvic Floor Distress Inventory 22-Item (PFDI-22)[a]

POPDI-6

Do you usually_____, and if so how much are you bothered by:
1. experience pressure in the lower abdomen
2. experience heaviness or dullness in the abdomen or genital area
3. have a bulge or something falling out that you can see or feel in the vaginal area
4. have to push on the vagina or around the rectum to have or complete a bowel movement
5. experience a feeling of incomplete bladder emptying
6. have to push up on a bulge in the vaginal area with your fingers to start or complete urination

CRADI-8

_____, and if so how much are you bothered by it
1. Do you usually feel you need to strain too hard to have a bowel movement
2. Do you usually feel you have not completely emptied your bowels at the end of bowel movement
3. Do you usually lose stool beyond your control if your stool is well formed
4. Do you usually lose stool beyond your control if your stool is loose or liquid
5. Do you usually lose gas from the rectum beyond your control
6. Do you usually have pain when you pass your stool
7. Do you usually experience a strong sense of urgency and have to rush to the bathroom to have a bowel movement
8. Does part of your bowel ever pass through the rectum and bulge outside during or after a bowel movement

UDI-8

Do you usually have _____, and if so, how much are you bothered by:
1. frequent urination
2. leakage related to feeling of urgency
3. leaking related to activity, coughing, or sneezing
4. leakage when you go from sitting to standing
5. small amounts of urine leakage (i.e., drops)
6. difficulty emptying the bladder
7. pain or discomfort in the lower abdomen or genital area
8. pain in the middle of your abdomen as your bladder fills

[a]For each question, patients fill in the blank with each phrase underneath the question. The same multiple choice responses (not at all, mildly, moderately, and severely) used for the PFIQ-7 are used for the PFDI-22.
Reproduced with permission from Chapple CR, Zimmern PE, Brubaker L, et al (eds): Multidisciplinary Management of Female Pelvic Floor Disorders. Philadelphia: Elsevier; 2006.

evaluation is performed (Chap. 25, p. 564). Most types of anal incontinence would not be expected to improve with surgical repair of prolapse. However, if evaluation reveals an anal sphincter defect as the cause of anal incontinence, anal sphincteroplasty may be performed concurrently with prolapse repair.

Female sexual dysfunction is present in women with dyspareunia, low libido, problems with arousal, and inability to achieve orgasm. The etiology is frequently multifactorial and includes psychosocial factors, urogenital atrophy, aging, and male sexual dysfunction. Sexual dysfunction is often also seen in women with POP. However, findings from studies evaluating sexual function in women with prolapse are inconsistent. In one study, a validated sexual function questionnaire was used to compare frequency of intercourse, libido, dyspareunia, orgasmic function, and vaginal dryness in women with and without prolapse (Weber, 1995). No differences were seen between the two groups. In another cross-sectional study of 301 women, pelvic floor symptoms were associated with dyspareunia, reduced arousal, and infrequent orgasm (Handa, 2008). In addition, sexual dysfunction was worse in women with symptomatic prolapse versus those with asymptomatic prolapse. In another study of sexual function in women with prolapse, decreased activity was associated with decreased vaginal length, and one quarter of women avoided sexual activity due to pelvic floor symptoms (Edenfield, 2015). Accordingly, women with an obstructing bulge as a cause of sexual dysfunction may benefit from therapy to reduce the prolapse. Unfortunately, some prolapse procedures such as posterior repair with levator plication and vaginal placement of mesh may contribute to postoperative dyspareunia. Therefore, care is taken in planning appropriate surgical procedures for women with concomitant sexual dysfunction (Ulrich, 2015).

Pelvic and back pain is another complaint in women with POP, but little evidence supports a direct association. A cross-sectional study of 152 consecutive patients with POP did not find an association between pelvic or low back pain and prolapse after controlling for age and prior surgery (Heit, 2002). Swift and colleagues (2003) found that back and pelvic pain were common among 477 women presenting for routine annual gynecologic examination and had no relationship to POP. Some suggest that low back pain in a patient with prolapse may be caused by altered body mechanics. However, if pain is a primary symptom, other sources should be sought (Chap. 11,

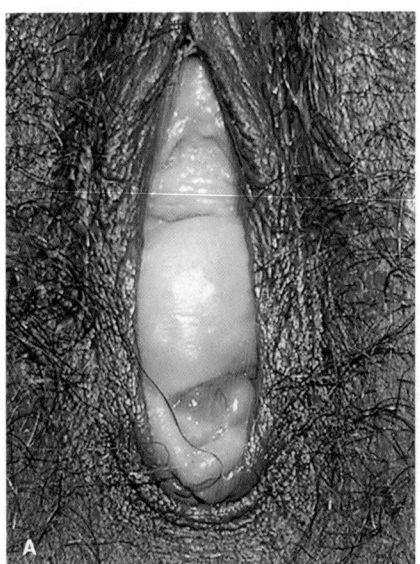 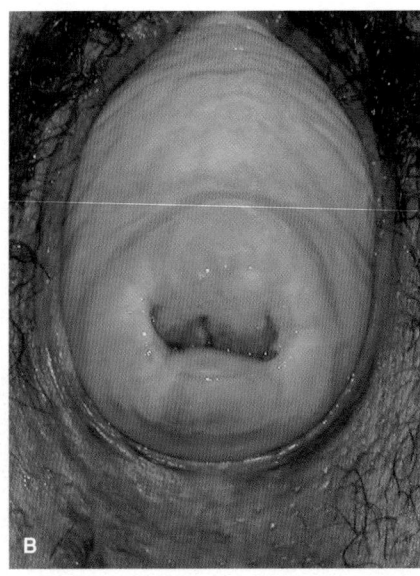 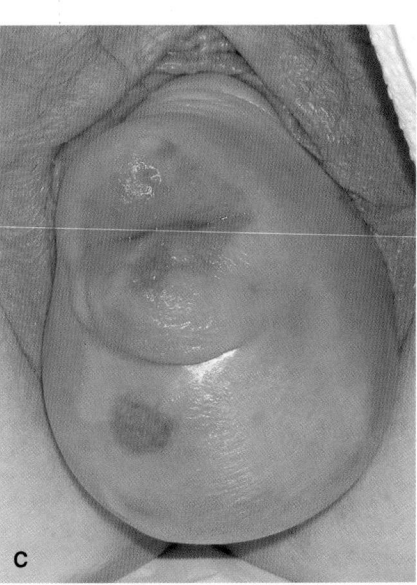

FIGURE 24-9 Degrees of pelvic organ prolapse. **A.** Stage 2. This stage is defined by the most distal edge of the prolapse lying within 1 cm of the hymenal ring. **B.** Stage 3. This stage is defined by the most distal portion of the prolapse being >1 cm below the plane of the hymen, but protruding no farther than 2 cm less than the total vaginal length in centimeters. **C.** Stage 4. This stage is defined as complete or near complete eversion.

p. 267). In the absence of an identifiable etiology, temporary pessary placement is considered to determine whether prolapse reduction will improve pain symptoms. Referral to a physical therapist may also shed light on a connection among prolapse, altered body mechanics, and pain.

Importantly, although POP is associated with varied complaints, symptoms and their severity do not always correlate well with advancing stages of prolapse. In addition, many common symptoms do not differentiate between compartments (Jelovsek, 2005; Kahn, 2005; Weber, 1998). Thus, when planning surgical or nonsurgical therapy, realistic expectations should be set with regard to symptom relief. A patient is informed that symptoms directly related to prolapse such as vaginal bulge and pelvic pressure are likely to improve with a successful anatomic repair. However, other associated symptoms such as constipation, back pain, and urinary urgency and frequency may or may not improve.

■ Physical Examination

Perineal Examination

Physical examination begins with a full body systems evaluation to identify pathology outside the pelvis. Systemic conditions such as cardiovascular, pulmonary, renal, or endocrinologic disease may affect treatment choices and should be identified early.

The initial pelvic examination is performed with a woman in lithotomy position. The vulva and perineum are examined for signs of vulvar or vaginal atrophy or other abnormalities. A neurologic examination of sacral reflexes is performed using a cotton swab. First, the *bulbocavernosus reflex* is elicited by tapping or stroking lateral to the clitoris and observing contraction of the bulbocavernosus muscle bilaterally. Second, evaluation of anal sphincter innervation is completed by stroking lateral to the anus and observing a reflexive contraction of the anus, known as the *anal wink reflex*. Intact reflexes suggest normal

sacral pathways. However, they can be absent in women who are neurologically intact.

POP examination begins by asking a woman to attempt Valsalva maneuver prior to placing a speculum in the vagina (Fig. 24-9). Patients who are unable to adequately complete a Valsalva maneuver are asked to cough. This "hands-off" approach more accurately displays true anatomy. Namely, with speculum examination, structures are artificially lifted, supported, or displaced. Importantly, this assessment helps answer three questions: (1) Does the protrusion come beyond the hymen? (2) What is the presenting part of the prolapse (anterior, posterior, or apical)? (3) Does the genital hiatus significantly widen with increased intraabdominal pressure?

During examination, a clinician verifies that the full extent of the prolapse is being seen. Specifically, a woman is asked to describe the extent of prolapse beyond the hymen during real-life activities. This degree may be conveyed in terms of inches. Alternatively, a mirror may be placed at the perineum and visual confirmation can be obtained from the patient.

Prolapse is a dynamic condition that responds to the effects of gravity and intraabdominal pressure. It frequently worsens over the course of a day or during physical activity. Thus, prolapse might not be evident during office examination early in the morning. If the full extent of prolapse cannot be demonstrated, a woman should be examined in a standing position and during Valsalva maneuver.

Vaginal Examination

If the POP-Q examination is performed, the genital hiatus (Gh) and perineal body (Pb) are measured during Valsalva maneuver (Fig. 24-10). The total vaginal length (TVL) is then measured by placing a marked ring forceps, or a ruler, at the vaginal apex and noting the distance to the hymen. A bivalve speculum is then inserted to the vaginal apex. It displaces the anterior and posterior vaginal walls, and points C and D are then measured

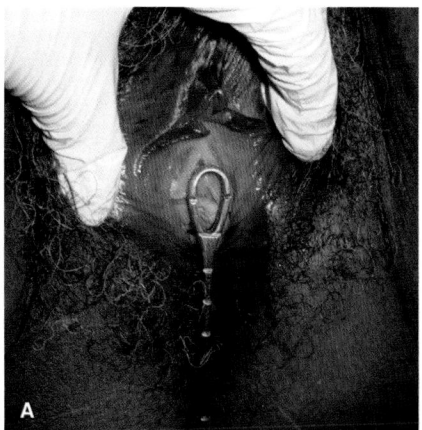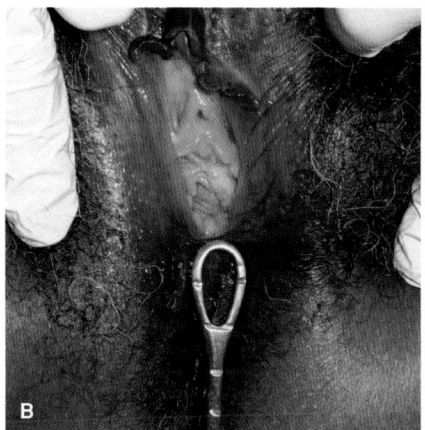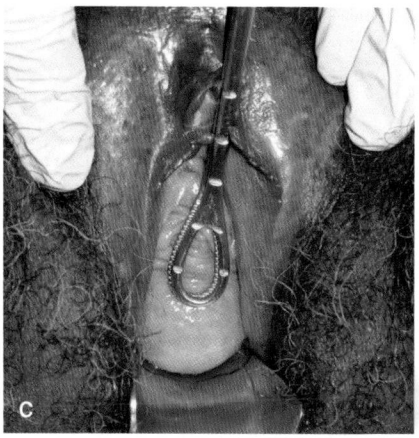

FIGURE 24-10 A. Measurement of the genital hiatus (Gh). For POP-Q evaluation, a sponge stick is used that is marked at 1-, 2-, 3-, 4-, 5-, 7.5-, and 10-cm increments. Measurement is obtained with a woman performing maximum Valsalva maneuver. **B.** Measurement of the perineal body. **C.** Measurement of points Aa and Ba. Aa is a discrete point lying 3 cm proximal to the urethral meatus and is measured in relation to the hymen. During measurement, a split speculum displaces the posterior vaginal wall, but downward traction is avoided, as this causes artificial descent of the anterior vaginal wall.

with Valsalva. The speculum is slowly withdrawn to assess descent of the apex.

A split speculum is then used to displace the posterior vaginal wall and allow for viewing of the anterior wall and measurement of points Aa and Ba. Attempts are made to characterize the anterior vaginal wall defect. Sagging lateral vaginal sulci with vaginal rugae still present suggest a *paravaginal defect*, that is, a lateral loss of support (Fig. 24-11). A central bulge and loss of vaginal rugae is called a *midline* or *central defect* (see Fig. 24-7). If loss of support appears to arise from detachment of the anterior vaginal wall's apical segment, it is termed a *transverse* or *anterior apical defect* (Fig. 24-12). Transverse defects are assessed by replacing the anterior apical segment and observing whether the prolapse descends during Valsalva maneuver. The urethra is also evaluated during anterior vaginal wall assessment, and Q-tip testing can be performed to determine urethral hypermobility (Chap. 23, p. 524).

The split speculum is then rotated 180 degrees to displace the anterior wall and allow examination of the posterior wall.

Points Ap and Bp are measured (Fig. 24-13). If the posterior vaginal wall descends, attempts are made to determine if rectocele or enterocele is present. Enterocele can only definitively be diagnosed by observing small bowel peristalsis behind the vaginal wall (Fig. 24-14). In general, bulges at the apical segment of the posterior vaginal wall should implicate enteroceles, whereas bulges in the distal posterior wall are presumed to be rectoceles. Further distinction may be found during standing rectovaginal examination. With this, a clinician's index finger is placed in the rectum and thumb on the posterior vaginal wall. Small bowel may be palpated between the rectum and vagina, confirming enterocele.

Differentiation of midline, lateral, apical, and distal defects of the anterior and posterior vaginal walls has not been shown to have good inter- or intraexaminer reliability. However, individual evaluation may help assess prolapse severity and clarify anatomy if surgical correction is planned (Barber, 1999; Whiteside, 2004).

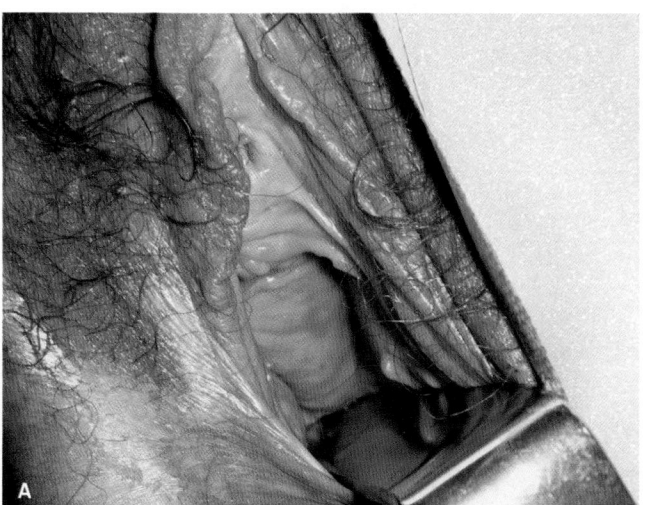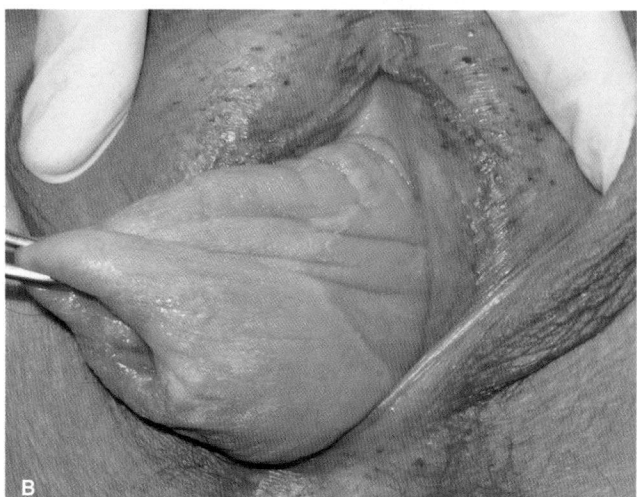

FIGURE 24-11 A. Normal lateral support as shown by normal positioning of the vaginal sulci. **B.** Complete loss of lateral support, shown as absent lateral sulci.

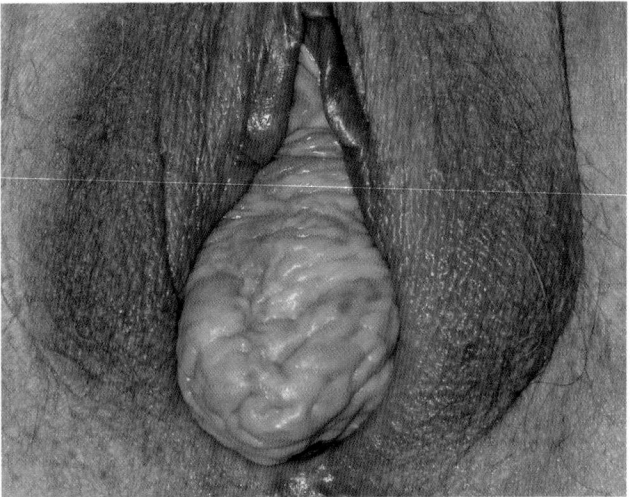

FIGURE 24-12 A transverse vaginal wall defect. Note detachment of the anterior vaginal wall from the apex and the presence of rugae, which suggests that this is not a midline or central defect.

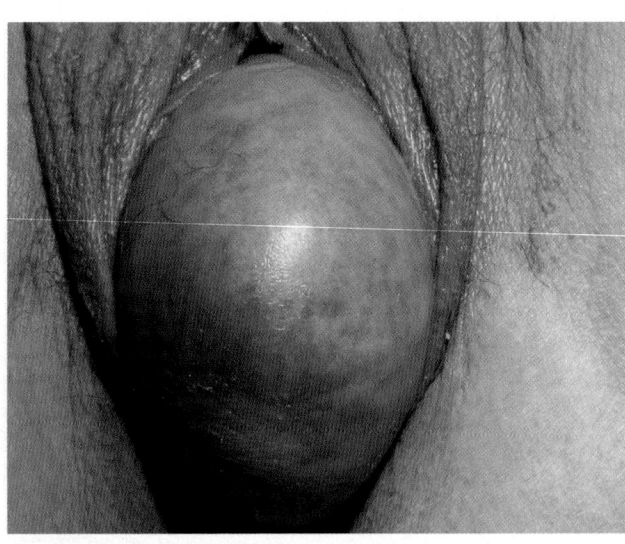

FIGURE 24-14 Enterocele. During evaluation, small bowel peristalsis may be noted behind the vaginal wall. Enterocele is most commonly noted at the vaginal apex, although anterior and posterior vaginal wall enteroceles may occur.

As mentioned, apical prolapse is believed to be the cause of most anterior and posterior wall descent. Therefore, careful attention is paid to the relationship of the apex to these structures. The apex should be replaced to its normal position. If this maneuver restores anterior and posterior support, it can be determined that the primary defect is at the apex.

Bimanual examination is performed to identify other pelvic pathology. In addition, we strongly recommend assessment of pelvic floor musculature (Fig. 11-5, p. 257). This examination is essential if pelvic floor rehabilitation is being considered as treatment. During part of the evaluation, an index finger is placed 1 to 3 cm inside the hymen, at 4 and then 8 o'clock (Fig. 24-15). Muscle resting tone and strength is assessed using the 0 through 5 Oxford grading scale, in which 5 represents normal tone and strength (Laycock, 2002). Muscle symmetry

is also evaluated. Asymmetric muscles, with palpable defects or scarring, may be associated with a prior obstetric forceps delivery, episiotomy, or laceration.

APPROACH TO TREATMENT

For women who are asymptomatic or mildly symptomatic, expectant management is appropriate. It is difficult to predict if prolapse will worsen or if symptoms will develop. In this situation, benefits of treatment are balanced against risks. Therefore, in the absence of other factors, invasive therapy is typically not selected for asymptomatic women. Pelvic floor muscle rehabilitation may be offered to a patient seeking to prevent prolapse progression. However, no data support the effectiveness of this practice (Hagen, 2011).

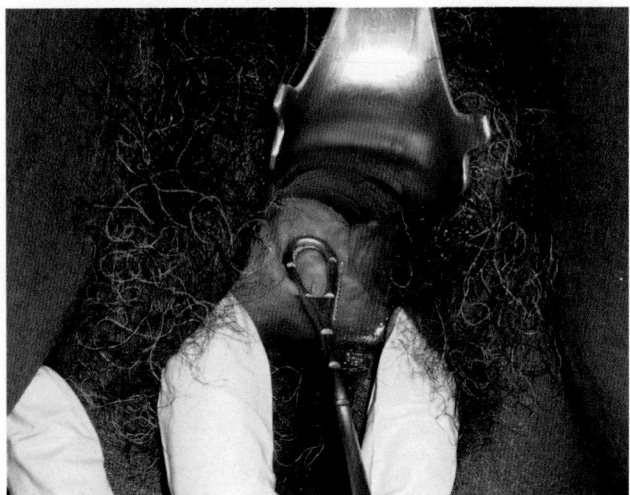

FIGURE 24-13 Split speculum displacing the anterior vaginal wall. This allows for measurement of points Ap and Bp. Ap is always defined as a discrete point lying 3 cm proximal to the hymen.

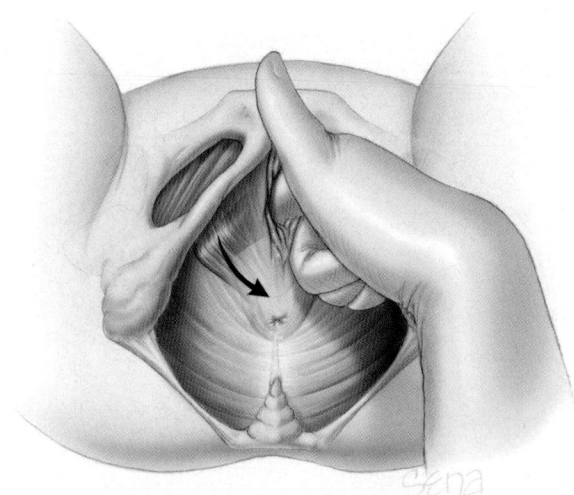

FIGURE 24-15 Pelvic floor muscle assessment. The index finger is placed 2 to 3 cm inside the hymen at 4 and 8 o'clock. Both resting and contraction tone and strength are evaluated.

For women with significant prolapse or for those with bothersome symptoms, nonsurgical or surgical therapy may be selected. Treatment choice depends on the type and severity of symptoms, age and medical comorbidities, desire for future sexual function and/or fertility, and risk factors for recurrence. Treatment goals strive to provide symptom relief, but therapy benefits should always outweigh risks.

Often a combination of nonsurgical and surgical approaches may be selected. Symptoms are ranked by severity, and options for each are discussed. An evidence-based appraisal of each option's success rate is included. In the simplest case, a patient with prolapse of the vaginal apex beyond the hymen, whose only symptom is bulge or pelvic pressure, could be offered pessary or surgical treatment. In a more complicated case, a woman with prolapse beyond the hymenal ring may note a bulge, constipation, urgency urinary incontinence, and pelvic pain. Symptoms would be ranked by severity and importance of resolution. To address all complaints, therapy might involve pessary or surgery for bulge symptoms, and nonsurgical treatment of constipation, incontinence, and pelvic pain.

NONSURGICAL TREATMENT

■ Pessary

Pessary Indications

Throughout history, various vaginal devices and materials have been used to physically support vaginal prolapse. Today's pessaries are usually made of silicone or inert plastic, and they are safe and simple to manage. Despite a long history of use, literature describing their indications, selection, and management is often anecdotal or contradictory.

The most common indication for vaginal pessary is POP. Traditionally, pessaries have been reserved for women either unfit or unwilling to undergo surgery. A survey of the American Urogynecologic Society (AUGS) membership confirmed this sentiment among gynecologists with more than 20 years in practice (Cundiff, 2000). However, the same survey showed that younger gynecologists, particularly those who described themselves as urogynecologists, used pessaries as a first-line therapy before recommending surgery.

Of other indications, pessaries may also help some women with prolapse and associated urinary incontinence. One RCT compared two pessary types for relief of prolapse symptoms and urinary complaints. This study demonstrated that pessaries provide a modest improvement in urinary obstructive, irritative, and stress symptoms (Chap. 23, p. 530) (Schaffer, 2006).

Pessaries may also be used diagnostically. As previously discussed, symptoms may not correlate with the type or severity of prolapse. Short-term pessary use may help clarify this relationship. Even if a patient declines long-term pessary use, she may agree to a short trial to determine if her chief complaint is improved or resolved. A pessary may also be placed diagnostically to identify which women are at risk for urinary incontinence after prolapse-correcting surgery (Chaikin, 2000; Liang, 2004).

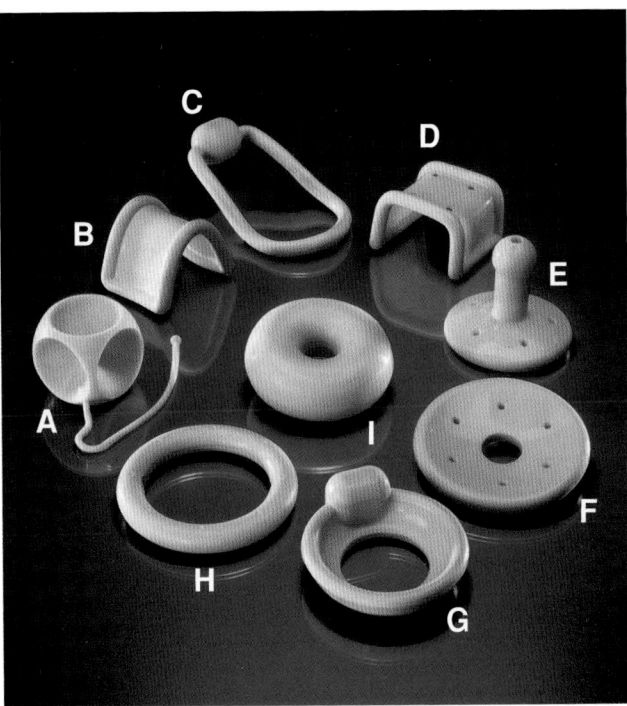

FIGURE 24-16 Types of Milex pessaries. **A.** Cube pessary. **B.** Gehrung pessary. **C.** Hodge with knob pessary. **D.** Regula pessary. **E.** Gellhorn pessary. **F.** Shaatz pessary. **G.** Incontinence dish pessary. **H.** Ring pessary. **I.** Donut pessary. (Reproduced with permission from CooperSurgical, Inc.)

Pessary Selection

Pessaries are divided into two broad categories: support and space-filling (Fig. 24-16). Support pessaries, such as the ring pessary, use a spring mechanism that rests in the posterior fornix and against the posterior aspect of the symphysis pubis. Vaginal support results from elevation of the superior vagina by the spring, which is supported by the symphysis pubis. Ring pessaries may be constructed as a simple circular ring or as a ring with support that looks like a large contraceptive diaphragm (Fig. 24-17). These are effective in women with first- and second-degree

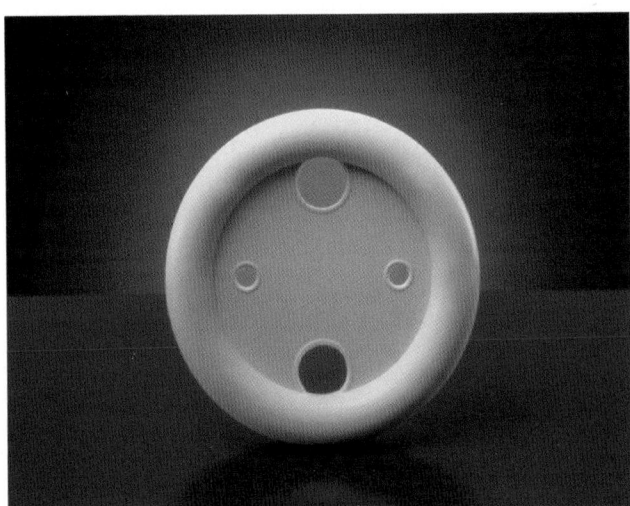

FIGURE 24-17 Milex ring pessary with support. (Reproduced with permission from CooperSurgical, Inc.)

prolapse. Also, the diaphragm portion of a support ring is especially useful in women with accompanying anterior vaginal wall prolapse. When properly fitted, the device should lie behind the pubic symphysis anteriorly and behind the cervix posteriorly.

In contrast, space-filling pessaries maintain their position by creating suction between the pessary and vaginal walls (cube), by creating a diameter larger than the genital hiatus (donut), or by both mechanisms (Gellhorn). The Gellhorn is often used for moderate to severe prolapse and for complete procidentia. It contains a concave disc that fits against the cervix or vaginal cuff and has a stem that is positioned just cephalad to the introitus. The concave disc supports the vaginal apex by creating suction, and the stem is useful for device removal. Of all pessaries, the two most commonly used and studied devices are the ring and the Gellhorn pessaries.

Patient Evaluation and Pessary Placement

A patient must be an active participant in the treatment decision to use a pessary. Its success will depend upon her ability to care for the pessary—either alone or with the assistance of a caregiver—and her willingness and availability to come for subsequent evaluations. Vaginal atrophy should be treated

before or concomitantly with pessary initiation. In women who are suitable candidates for estrogen therapy, vaginal estrogen cream is recommended (Table 22-5, p. 505). In one regimen, 1 g of conjugated equine estrogen cream (Premarin cream) is inserted nightly for 2 weeks, then two times per week thereafter.

Device selection integrates patient factors such as hormonal status, sexual activity, prior hysterectomy, and stage and site of POP. After a pessary is chosen, a woman is fitted with the largest size that can be comfortably worn. If a pessary is ideally fitted, a patient is not aware of its presence. As a woman ages and gains or loses weight, alternate sizes may be required.

Generally, a patient is fitted with a pessary while in the lithotomy position after she has emptied both her bladder and rectum. A digital examination is performed to assess vaginal length and width, and an initial estimation of pessary size is made. Figure 24-18 shows Gellhorn pessary placement. For ring pessary placement, the device is held in the clinician's dominant hand in a folded position. Lubricant is placed on either the vaginal introitus or the pessary's leading edge. While holding the labia apart, the pessary is inserted by pushing in a cephalad direction and against the posterior vaginal wall. Next,

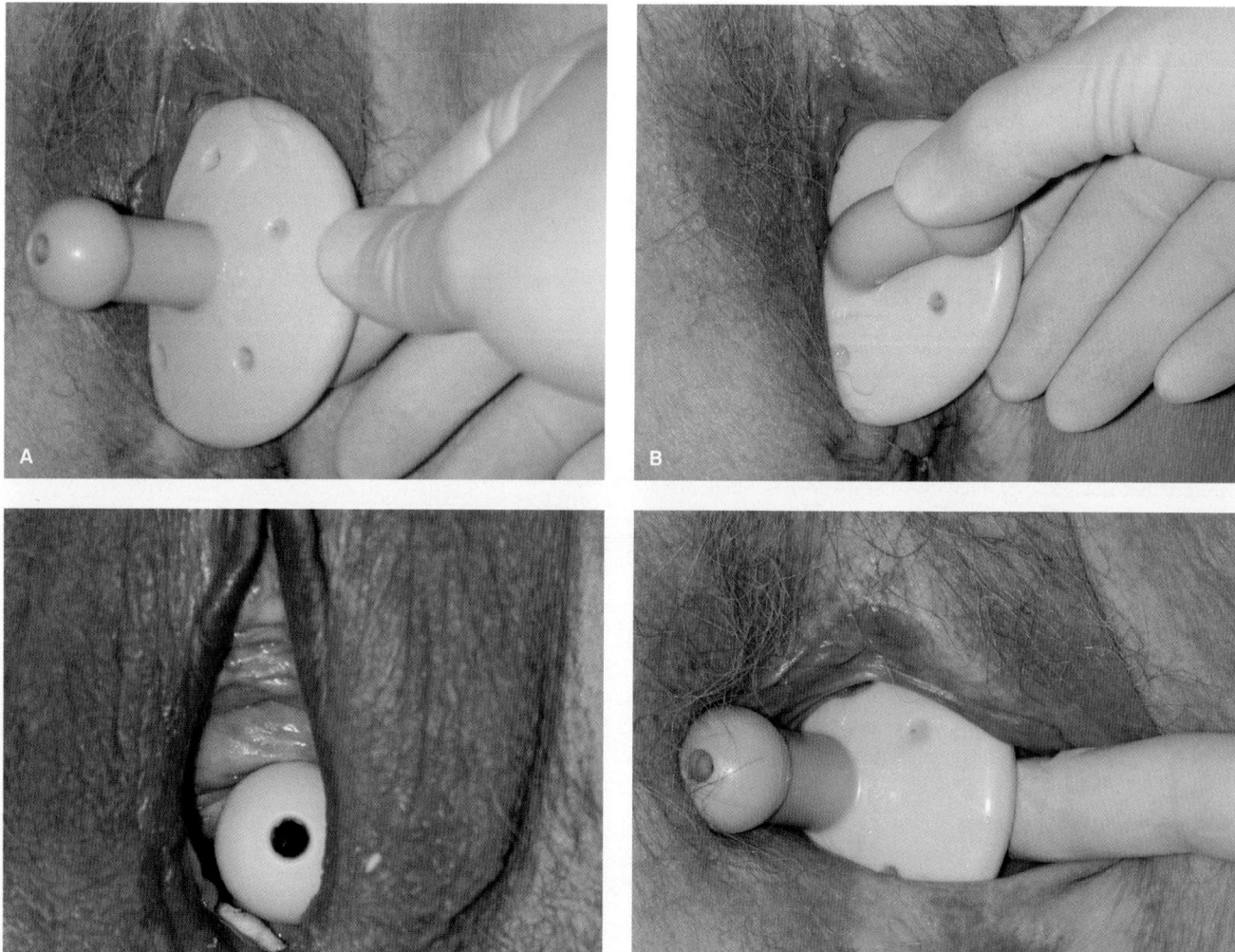

FIGURE 24-18 Technique for placement and removal of a Gellhorn pessary. Figures **A**, **B**, and **C** show placement. **D.** To remove a Gellhorn pessary, an index finger is placed behind the disk and suction is broken prior to removal.

an index finger is directed into the posterior vaginal fornix to ensure that the cervix is resting above the pessary. The clinician's finger should barely slide between the lateral edges of the ring pessary and the vaginal sidewall. The pessary should fit snugly but not tightly against the symphysis pubis and the posterior and lateral vaginal walls. Too much pressure may increase the risk for pain.

Following pessary placement, a woman is prompted to perform a Valsalva maneuver, which might dislodge an improperly fitted pessary. She should be able to stand, walk, cough, and urinate without difficulty or discomfort. Instruction on removal and placement then follows. For removal of a ring pessary, an index finger is inserted into the vagina to hook the ring's leading edge. Traction is applied along the vaginal axis to bring the ring toward the introitus. Here, it may be grasped by the thumb and index finger and removed.

Ideally, a pessary is removed nightly to weekly, washed in soap and water, and replaced the next morning. Women also receive instructions describing the management of commonly encountered problems (Table 24-7). After initial placement, a return visit may follow in 1 to 2 weeks. For patients comfortable with their pessary management, return visits may be semiannual. If the patient and the provider are motivated, most women can be taught to self-manage a pessary. For those unable or unwilling to remove and replace a device themselves, a pessary may be removed and the patient's vagina inspected at the provider's office every 2 or 3 months. Delaying visits longer than this may lead to problematic discharge and odor.

Pessary Complications

Serious complications such as erosion into adjacent organs are rare with proper use and usually result only after years of neglect. At each return visit, the pessary is removed, and the vagina is inspected for erosions, abrasions, ulcerations, or granulation tissue (Fig. 24-19). Vaginal bleeding is usually an early sign and should not be ignored. *Pessary ulcers* or abrasions are treated by changing the pessary type or size to alleviate pressure points or by removing the pessary completely until healed. Treatment of vaginal atrophy with local estrogen is commonly required. Alternatively, water-based lubricants applied to the pessary may help prevent these complications. *Prolapse ulcers* have the same appearance as pessary ulcers, however, the former result from the prolapsed bulge rubbing against patient clothing. These are treated by replacing the prolapse either with a pessary or by surgery.

Pelvic pain with pessary use is not normal. This usually indicates that the size is too large, and a smaller pessary would be more suitable. All pessaries tend to trap vaginal secretions and obstruct normal drainage to some degree. The resultant odor may be managed by encouraging more frequent nighttime device removal, washing, and reinsertion the next day.

TABLE 24-7. Guidelines for Pessary Care

Pessary type_____
     Size_____

1. After your initial pessary fitting is successful, you will be asked to return for a follow-up appointment in about 2 weeks. The purpose of this visit is to check the pessary and examine the vagina to ensure that it is healthy. Follow-up appointments will follow this schedule:
       1st year: every 3–6 months
       2nd year and beyond: every 6 months
   You may learn to care for the pessary yourself. For those patients who can remove and insert the pessary themselves, we recommend weekly overnight removal and cleansing of the pessary with soap and warm water. These patients should see the doctor at least once per year.
2. The following is a list of problems you may encounter with the pessary and our recommendations for their management.

Problem	Management
A. The pessary falls out.	Keep the pessary and notify your doctor's office. An appointment will be made. It may be possible that a change in the size or the type of pessary is needed.
B. You experience pelvic pain.	Notify your doctor's office. If the pessary has slipped and you can remove it, do so. Otherwise, have your doctor remove the pessary. A change in pessary size or type may be needed.
C. Vaginal discharge and odor.	You can douche with warm water and you may want to try using Trimo-San vaginal gel 1–3 times a week.
D. Vaginal bleeding.	Vaginal bleeding may be a sign that the pessary is irritating the lining of the vagina. Call your doctor's office and arrange an appointment.
E. Leaking from the bladder.	Sometimes, the support provided by the pessary will cause leaking from the bladder. Notify your doctor and discuss this problem.

Trimo-San gel (oxyquinolone sulfate) helps restore and maintain the normal vaginal acidity that helps reduce odor-causing bacteria.
Reproduced with permission from Farrell SA: Practical advice for ring pessary fitting and management, J SOGC 19:625, 1997.

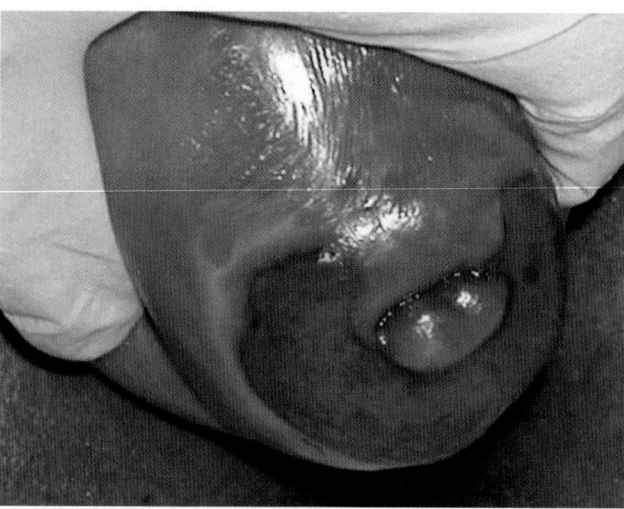

FIGURE 24-19 Granulation tissue resulting from pessary trauma.

Alternatively, a woman may use a pH-based deodorant gel such as oxyquinoline sulfate gel (Trimo-San) once or twice weekly or may douche with warm water. Trimo-San gel helps restore and maintain normal vaginal acidity that aids in reducing odor-causing bacteria.

Pelvic Floor Muscle Exercises

These exercises have been suggested as a therapy that might limit progression and alleviate prolapse symptoms. Also known as Kegel exercises, these muscle-strengthening techniques are described in Chapter 23 (p. 528). Two hypotheses describe the benefits of pelvic floor muscle exercises for prolapse prevention and treatment (Bø, 2004). First, from these exercises, women learn to consciously contract muscles before and during increases in abdominal pressure. This prevents organ descent. Alternatively, regular muscle strength training builds permanent muscle volume and structural support.

Unfortunately, high-quality scientific evidence supporting pelvic exercise for prevention and treatment of prolapse is lacking (Hagen, 2011). However, pelvic floor exercise has minimal risk and low cost. For this reason, it may be offered to asymptomatic or mildly symptomatic women who are interested in preventing prolapse progression or who decline other treatments.

SURGICAL TREATMENT

In preparing for prolapse surgery, the patient should have an understanding of the expected results, and the surgeon should have an understanding of the patient's expectations. Treatment success varies widely based on the definition of success. Thus, the surgeon and the patient must agree on the desired results. Generally, patients seek relief of symptoms, whereas surgeons may view surgical success as restoration of anatomy. In the CARE trial, absence of vaginal bulge symptoms had the strongest relationship to a patient's assessment of overall improvement and surgical success, whereas anatomic success alone did not (Barber, 2009). It is therefore recommended that surgical success be defined as absence of bulge symptoms in addition to anatomic criteria.

Obliterative Procedures

The two categories of prolapse surgery are obliterative and reconstructive. Obliterative approaches include Lefort colpocleisis and complete colpocleisis (Chap. 45, p. 1120). These can be performed for women with posthysterectomy prolapse or those retaining a uterus. These procedures involve removing vaginal epithelium, suturing anterior and posterior vaginal walls together, obliterating the vaginal vault, and effectively closing the vagina. Obliterative procedures are only appropriate for elderly or medically compromised patients who have no desire for future coital activity.

Obliterative procedures are technically easier, require less operative time, and offer superior success rates compared with reconstructive procedures. Success rates for colpocleisis range from 91 to 100 percent, although the quality of evidence-based studies supporting these rates is poor (FitzGerald, 2006). After colpocleisis, fewer than 10 percent of patients express regret, often due to loss of coital activity (FitzGerald, 2006; Wheeler, 2005). Thus, the consenting process must include an honest and thoughtful discussion with the patient and her partner regarding future sexual intercourse. Latent SUI can be unmasked with colpocleisis due to resulting downward traction on the urethra. However, the morbidity of a concurrent antiincontinence procedure may outweigh the potential incontinence risk and is considered before adding surgeries in women who may already be medically compromised.

In patients who still have a uterus, vaginal hysterectomy may be performed prior to colpocleisis. However, concurrent hysterectomy increases blood loss and operative time. Again, in compromised patients, this can counteract some of the major benefits of colpocleisis. If retention of the uterus at time of colpocleisis is planned, neoplasia is excluded preoperatively. For this, Pap testing for cervical neoplasia should be current. For endometrial neoplasia, endometrial sampling and/or sonographic interrogation of endometrial stripe thickness is performed.

Reconstructive Procedures

These surgeries attempt to restore normal pelvic anatomy and are more commonly performed for POP than obliterative procedures. Vaginal, abdominal, laparoscopic, and robotic routes may be used, and in the United States, a vaginal approach is preferred by most for prolapse repairs (Boyles, 2003; Brown, 2002).

Approach selection is individualized and factors the patient's unique characteristics and surgeon's expertise. An abdominal approach may be advantageous for women with prolapse recurrence following a vaginal approach, those with a shortened vagina, or those believed to be at higher risk for recurrence, such as young women with severe prolapse (Benson, 1996; Maher, 2004). In contrast, a vaginal approach typically offers shorter operative time and a quicker return to daily activities. Laparoscopic and robotic approaches may offer smaller incisions, decreased hospital stay, and quicker short-term recovery compared with abdominal approaches.

Of these, laparoscopic and robotic approaches to prolapse repair are becoming more common. Procedures include sacrocolpopexy, paravaginal repair, and vaginal vault suspension to the uterosacral ligaments. One randomized trial in the United Kingdom compared open and laparoscopic sacrocolpopexy and found similar anatomic and subjective outcomes after 1 year (Freeman, 2013). Perceived advantages to the laparoscopic approach such as earlier return to usual activities were not seen. Several small RCTs have compared laparoscopic and robotic sacrocolpopexy (Anger, 2014; Paraiso, 2011). In general, these studies have found similar short-term outcomes but increased cost with the robotic approach.

The prolapse surgeon should be versatile. Procedure route selection is individualized, and compelling evidence does not support one approach as superior to another. Adoption of new surgical techniques should be driven by patient motives, as determined by evidence-based medicine (American College of Obstetricians and Gynecologists, 2015).

Surgical Plan

Reconstructive prolapse repair will often involve a combination of procedures in several vaginal compartments. However, the decision regarding which compartments to repair is not always straightforward. In the past, a defect-directed approach to prolapse repair was preferred. With this strategy, all current, latent, or potential defects are evaluated and repaired. However, current expert opinion suggests that asymptomatic areas of prolapse do not always warrant repair, and correction can lead to de novo symptoms in some cases. For instance, repair of an asymptomatic posterior wall prolapse may lead to dyspareunia. Thus, surgery in general is planned to relieve *current* prolapse symptoms.

Anterior Compartment

Many procedures for anterior vaginal wall prolapse repair have been described. Historically, anterior colporrhaphy has been the most common operation, yet long-term anatomic success rates are poor. In a randomized trial of three anterior colporrhaphy techniques, Weber and associates (2001b) found a low rate of anatomic success. Specifically, satisfactory anatomic results were obtained in only 30 percent of their traditional midline plication group, 46 percent of the ultralateral repair group, and 42 percent of the group undergoing traditional plication plus lateral reinforcement with synthetic mesh. These differences were not statistically significant. Despite anatomic results that may appear suboptimal, symptom relief from anterior colporrhaphy may be acceptable. One reanalysis of data from this trial instead used clinically relevant definitions of surgical success that included no prolapse beyond the hymen, lack of prolapse symptoms, and no retreatment requested. With these, 88 percent of subjects met the definition of success (Chmielewski, 2011). Thus, if a central or midline defect is suspected, anterior colporrhaphy may be performed (Chap. 45, p. 1088).

Mesh or biomaterial may also be used in conjunction with anterior colporrhaphy or by itself. Mesh is used to reinforce the vaginal wall and is sutured in place laterally. However, the use of mesh and mesh kits for anterior vaginal wall prolapse remains controversial (American College of Obstetricians and Gynecologists, 2013b). Although recent studies show improved anatomic success when mesh is used for anterior wall repair, there are significant risks. These include mesh erosion, pain, and dyspareunia and are discussed on page 556 (Sung, 2008).

In many cases, anterior vaginal wall prolapse results from fibromuscular defects at the anterior apical segment or transverse detachment of the anterior apical segment from the vaginal apex. In these situations, an apical suspension procedure such as an abdominal sacrocolpopexy or uterosacral ligament vaginal vault suspension will resuspend the anterior vaginal wall to the apex and reduce anterior wall prolapse. With these procedures, continuity is also reestablished between the anterior and posterior vaginal fibromuscular layers to prevent enterocele formation.

Alternatively, if a lateral defect is suspected, paravaginal repair can be performed through a vaginal, abdominal, or laparoscopic route (Chap. 45, p. 1090). Paravaginal repair is performed by reattaching the fibromuscular layer of the vaginal wall to the arcus tendineus fascia pelvis.

Vaginal Apex

Support of the vaginal apex is thought by many to be an essential cornerstone of a successful prolapse repair (Brubaker, 2005a). The vaginal apex can be resuspended with several procedures that include abdominal sacrocolpopexy, sacrospinous ligament fixation, or uterosacral ligament vaginal vault suspension. These are all illustrated in Chapter 45 (p. 1098).

Of these, abdominal sacrocolpopexy suspends the vaginal vault to the sacrum using synthetic mesh. Advantages include the procedure's durability over time and conservation of normal vaginal anatomy. For example, compared with other vault suspension procedures, sacrocolpopexy offers greater vaginal apex mobility and avoids vaginal shortening. In addition, sacrocolpopexy provides enduring correction of apical prolapse, and long-term success rates approximate 90 percent. This procedure may be used primarily or as a second surgery for women with recurrences after failure of other prolapse repairs. Sacrocolpopexy may be performed as selected an abdominal, laparoscopic, or robotic procedure. When hysterectomy is performed in conjunction with sacrocolpopexy, consideration is given to performing a supracervical rather than a total abdominal hysterectomy. With the cervix left in situ, the risk of postoperative mesh erosion at the vaginal apex is believed to be diminished (McDermott, 2009). In this case, the mesh is not exposed to vaginal bacteria, which occurs when the vagina is opened with total hysterectomy (Griffis, 2006). In addition, the strong connective tissue of the cervix allows for an additional anchoring point for the permanent mesh.

Another option, sacrospinous ligament fixation (SSLF), is one of the most popular procedures for apical suspension. The vaginal apex is suspended to the sacrospinous ligament unilaterally or bilaterally using a vaginal extraperitoneal approach. After SSLF, recurrent apical prolapse is uncommon. However, anterior vaginal wall prolapse develops postoperatively in 6 to 28 percent of patients and is thought to develop from redirection of abdominal forces anteriorly (Benson, 1996; Morley, 1988; Paraiso, 1996). Complications associated with SSLF include buttock pain from nerve involvement with supporting ligatures in 3 percent of patients and vascular injury in 1 percent (Sze, 1997a,b). Although infrequent, significant and life-threatening hemorrhage can follow injury to blood vessels located near the sacrospinous ligament.

Uterosacral ligament vaginal vault suspension is another apical surgery. With this procedure, the vaginal apex is attached to remnants of the uterosacral ligament at the level of the ischial spines or higher. Performed vaginally or abdominally, the uterosacral ligament vaginal vault suspension is believed to replace the vaginal apex to a more anatomic position than SSLF, which deflects the vagina posteriorly (Barber, 2000; Maher, 2004; Shull, 2000). This procedure has been adopted by many surgeons in the United States in attempts to reduce the rates of anterior vaginal prolapse recurrence following SSLF (Shull, 2000). Although uterosacral ligament vaginal vault suspension has gained popularity, studies supporting its use are limited to retrospective case series (Amundsen, 2003; Karram, 2001; Silva, 2006). In these studies and others, anterior vaginal prolapse recurrence rates range from 1 to 7 percent, and overall recurrence rates from 4 to 18 percent. One landmark RCT compared SSLF and uterosacral ligament vaginal vault suspension and did not find significant differences in anatomic or functional outcomes between the two procedures at 2 years (Barber, 2014).

Hysterectomy at the Time of Prolapse Repair

In the United States, hysterectomy is often performed concurrently with prolapse surgery. Conversely, in many European countries, it is rarely performed during pelvic floor reconstruction. Although this has not been compared in RCTs, arguments exist for both. If apical or uterine prolapse is present, hysterectomy will more readily allow the vaginal apex to be resuspended with the previously described apical suspension procedures. If hysterectomy is not performed in the context of apical prolapse, these procedures must be modified or specific uterine suspension procedures performed (not described in this text). Alternatively, if apical or cervical prolapse is not present, hysterectomy need not be incorporated into prolapse repair.

Posterior Compartment

Posterior vaginal wall prolapse may be due to enterocele or rectocele. Enterocele is defined as herniation of the small bowel through the vaginal fibromuscular layer, usually at the vaginal apex. Discontinuity of the anterior and posterior vaginal wall fibromuscular layers allows for this herniation. Accordingly, enterocele repairs have as their goal reattachment of these fibromuscular layers. If posterior wall prolapse is due to enterocele, repair of this defect should reduce the posterior wall prolapse.

If due to rectocele, posterior vaginal wall prolapse is repaired with one of several techniques, which are illustrated in Chapter 45 (p. 1093). Of these, traditional posterior colporrhaphy aims to rebuild the fibromuscular layer between the rectum and vagina by performing a midline fibromuscular plication. The anatomic cure rate is 76 to 96 percent, and most studies report a greater than 75-percent improvement rate of bulge symptoms (Cundiff, 2004). To narrow the genital hiatus and prevent recurrence, some surgeons plicate the levator ani muscle concurrently with posterior repair. However, this practice may contribute to dyspareunia rates of 12 to 27 percent (Kahn, 1997; Mellegren, 1995; Weber, 2000). Thus, it is best avoided in women who are sexually active.

Site-specific posterior repair is an approach based on the assumption that specific tears in the fibromuscular layer can be repaired in a discrete fashion. Defects may be midline, lateral, distal, or superior. This approach is conceptually analogous to a fascial hernia, in which the fascial tear is identified and repaired. Thus, its theoretical advantage lies in its restoration of normal anatomy rather than plication of tissue in the midline. Although site-specific repair has gained wide acceptance, anatomic cure rates range from 56 to 100 percent, similar to that with traditional posterior colporrhaphy (Muir, 2007). Moreover, anatomic and functional long-term outcomes are unknown.

Mesh reinforcement with allograft, xenograft, or synthetic mesh has been used in conjunction with posterior colporrhaphy and site-specific repair to help reduce prolapse recurrence. However, the efficacy and safety of graft augmentation in the posterior vaginal wall has not been established. Paraiso and coworkers (2006) randomly assigned 105 women to posterior colporrhaphy, site-specific repair, or site-specific repair plus a graft using porcine small intestine submucosa. After 1 year, those with graft augmentation had a significantly higher anatomic failure rate (46 percent) than those who received site-specific repair alone (22 percent) or posterior colporrhaphy (14 percent). More research is needed to determine the safety, efficacy, and optimal material for posterior wall graft augmentation. Until then, the use of mesh in the posterior vaginal wall should generally be avoided.

Last, sacrocolpoperineopexy is a modification of sacrocolpopexy. It may be selected for correction of posterior vaginal wall descent when an abdominal approach is employed for other prolapse procedures or if treatment of perineal descent is necessary (Cundiff, 1997; Lyons, 1997; Sullivan, 2001). With this procedure, the posterior sacrocolpopexy mesh is extended down the posterior vaginal wall to the perineal body. In several case series, anatomic cure rates were greater than 75 percent.

Perineum

The perineal body provides distal support to the posterior vaginal wall and anterior rectal wall and anchors these structures to the pelvic floor. A disrupted perineal body will allow descent of the distal vagina and rectum and will contribute to a widened levator hiatus.

To recreate normal anatomy, perineorrhaphy is often done in conjunction with posterior colporrhaphy (Chap. 45, p. 1096). During surgery, the perineum is rebuilt through midline plication of the perineal muscles and connective tissue. Importantly, overly aggressive plication can narrow the introitus, create a posterior vaginal wall ridge, and lead to entry dyspareunia. However, in a woman who is not sexually active, high perineorrhaphy with intentional introital narrowing is believed to decrease the risk of posterior wall prolapse recurrence.

■ Mesh in Reconstructive Pelvic Surgery
Mesh Indications

Approximately 30 percent of women undergoing surgery for prolapse will require a repeat operation for recurrence (Olsen, 1997). As such, continuous efforts strive to improve surgical procedures and outcomes.

Synthetic mesh for sacrocolpopexy and midurethral slings has been widely studied and is safe and effective. Mesh erosion

TABLE 24-8. Types of Surgical Mesh

Type I:	Macroporous. Pore size >75 µm (size required for infiltration by macrophages, fibroblasts, blood vessels in angiogenesis, and collagen fibers) *GyneMesh, Atrium, Marlex, Prolene*
Type II:	Microporous. Pore size <10 µm in at least 1 dimension *Gore-Tex*
Type III:	Macroporous patch w/multifilaments or a microporous component *Teflon, Mersilene, Surgipro, Mycro Mesh*
Type IV:	Submicronic. Pore size <1 µm. Often used in association with type I mesh for intraperitoneal adhesion prevention *Silastic, Cellgard, Preclude*

Data from Amid PK: Classification of biomaterials and their related complications in abdominal wall hernia surgery. Hernia 1:15, 1997.

develops in a small percentage of cases but can be managed with local estrogen therapy and limited vaginal wall mesh excision. Rarely is excision of the entire mesh warranted. In an attempt to limit erosion rates, surgeons have used biologic material grafts, including cadaveric fascia. However, high rates of prolapse recurrence are associated with this material (FitzGerald, 1999, 2004; Gregory, 2005). Therefore, synthetic mesh is recommended for sacrocolpopexy and midurethral slings.

The use of biologic grafts or synthetic mesh for other transvaginal reconstructive pelvic surgery has expanded rapidly and in the absence of supporting long-term safety and efficacy data. Some surgeons routinely use graft or mesh augmentation, others never use it, and some use it only for limited indications. Selective use may include: (1) the need to bridge space, (2) weak or absent connective tissue, (3) connective tissue disease, (4) high risk for recurrence (obesity, chronically increased intraabdominal pressure, and young age), and (5) shortened vagina.

Despite the common use of mesh or grafts, one systematic review on their use in transvaginal prolapse repair found a lack of high-quality scientific data to support this practice (Sung, 2008). Since this review, several RCTs have found that mesh use compared with no mesh for anterior colporrhaphy yields higher short-term rates of successful prolapse treatment. However, more surgical complications and postoperative adverse events are associated with mesh use in these studies (Altman, 2011). In 2011, the Food and Drug administration (FDA) reported the potentially serious complications associated with surgical mesh for transvaginal repair of POP. Noted complications include mesh erosion, scarring, pain, and dyspareunia. Additionally, synthetic mesh may become ingrown and difficult to remove. Complications may therefore be irreversible. Thus, the FDA urges clinicians to weigh the risks versus theoretical benefit of this practice. The American College of Obstetricians and Gynecologists (2011) and AUGS (2012) echo these concerns and recommend that vaginal synthetic mesh for the treatment of POP should be reserved for high-risk women in whom the benefits outweigh the risks.

Mesh Material

Surgeons using mesh or grafts should be familiar with the different types and their characteristics. Biologic grafts may be autologous, allograft, or xenograft. *Autologous* grafts are harvested from another part of the patient's body such as rectus abdominis

fascia or thigh fascia lata. Morbidity is low but may include increased operative time, pain, hematoma, or weakened fascia at the harvest site. *Allografts* come from a human source other than the patient and include cadaveric fascia or cadaveric dermis. *Xenografts* are biologic tissue obtained from a source or species foreign to the patient such as porcine dermis, porcine small intestinal submucosa, or bovine pericardium. Biologic materials have varying biomechanical properties and, as noted earlier, are associated with high rates of prolapse recurrence. Thus, recommendations on the appropriate clinical situations for biologic material are limited.

Synthetic mesh is classified as types I through IV, based on pore size (Table 24-8) (Amid, 1997). Pore size is the most important property of synthetic mesh. Bacteria generally measure less than 1 µm, whereas granulocytes and macrophages are typically larger than 10 µm. Thus, a mesh with pore size <10 µm may allow bacterial but not macrophage infiltration and thereby predispose to infection. Accordingly, type I mesh has the lowest rate of infection compared with types II and III. Pore size is also the basis of tissue ingrowth, angiogenesis, flexibility, and strength. Pore sizes of 50 to 200 µm allow for superior tissue ingrowth and collagen infiltration. This again favors type I. Meshes are either monofilament or multifilament. Multifilament mesh has small intrafiber pores that can harbor bacteria, therefore, monofilament mesh is recommended. From these findings, consensus suggests that if synthetic mesh is used, type I monofilament is the best choice for reconstructive pelvic surgery.

Mesh or graft augmentation will undoubtedly persist due to the current poor cure rates with traditional transvaginal repairs. However, evidence to guide the surgeon and provide a patient with accurate safety and efficacy information is scant. Moreover, industry-driven, premature adoption of untested materials and procedures has historically led to unacceptable complications. For these reasons, randomized, prospective trials comparing traditional repairs with graft or mesh augmentation are needed.

■ Concomitant Prolapse and Incontinence Surgery

Prior to prolapse repairs, women should be evaluated for SUI (Chap. 23, p. 526). Those with bothersome SUI symptoms are considered for concurrent antiincontinence surgery. However, in women without SUI symptoms, latent stress incontinence may be unmasked or SUI may develop de novo following prolapse repair. Therefore, preoperative urodynamic testing with the prolapse replaced is recommended. If SUI is demonstrated, these patients also are considered for a concurrent antiincontinence operation. This has been a difficult decision for patients and surgeons because a procedure with known risks is being performed for a problem that does not currently exist and may never develop.

The CARE (Colpopexy and Urinary Reduction Efforts) trial has helped clarify this problem (Brubaker, 2006). In this trial, women undergoing abdominal sacrocolpopexy for prolapse who did not exhibit symptoms of SUI were randomized to undergo concurrent Burch colposuspension or not. Preoperative urodynamic testing was performed, but surgeons were blinded to the results. Three months after surgery, 24 percent of women in the Burch group and 44 percent of women in the control group met one or more criteria for SUI. The incontinence was bothersome in 6 percent of the Burch group and 24 percent of the control group.

These data can be interpreted in several ways. It can be argued that all women undergoing sacrocolpopexy for stage 2 or greater anterior vaginal wall prolapse should undergo Burch colposuspension, as 44 percent will develop SUI symptoms. However, the opposing argument is that only 24 percent will develop bothersome incontinence symptoms, thus three quarters of women would be subjected to an unnecessary operation.

In a similar trial, the Outcomes Following Vaginal Prolapse Repair and Mid Urethral Sling (OPUS) trial, women undergoing vaginal surgery for POP who did not have SUI symptoms were randomly assigned to receive a midurethral sling or sham incision. Twelve months after surgery, 27 percent of women in the sling group and 43 percent of women in the sham group had incontinence (Wei, 2012).

Importantly, these studies provide high-quality evidence for a surgeon to share during patient counseling. The decision to perform a concurrent antiincontinence operation in women without SUI should be individualized and based on risks, benefits, and patient goals and expectations.

REFERENCES

Allen-Brady K, Cannon-Albright LA, Farnham JM, et al: Evidence for pelvic organ prolapse predisposition genes on chromosomes 10 and 17. Am J Obstet Gynecol 212(6):771.e1, 2015

Altman D, Väyrynen T, Engh ME, et al: Anterior colporrhaphy versus transvaginal mesh for pelvic-organ prolapse. N Engl J Med 364(19):1826, 2011

American College of Obstetricians and Gynecologists: Cesarean delivery on maternal request. Committee Opinion No. 559, April 2013a

American College of Obstetricians and Gynecologists: Pelvic organ prolapse. Practice Bulletin No. 79, February 2007, Reaffirmed 2013b

American College of Obstetricians and Gynecologists: Robotic Surgery in Gynecology. Committee Opinion No. 628, March 2015

American Urogynecologic Society: Guidelines for providing privileges and credentials to physicians for transvaginal placement of surgical mesh for pelvic organ prolapse. Female Pelvic Med Reconstr Surg 18(4):194, 2012

Amid PK: Classification of biomaterials and their related complications in abdominal wall hernia surgery. Hernia 1:15, 1997

Amundsen CL, Flynn BJ, Webster GD: Anatomical correction of vaginal vault prolapse by uterosacral ligament fixation in women who also require a pubovaginal sling. J Urol 169:1770, 2003

Anger JT, Mueller ER, Tarnay C, et al: Robotic compared with laparoscopic sacrocolpopexy: a randomized controlled trial. Obstet Gynecol 123(1):5, 2014

Baden WF, Walker T: Fundamentals, symptoms and classification. In Surgical Repair of Vaginal Defect. Philadelphia, JB Lippincott, 1992, p 14

Baden WF, Walker TA: Genesis of the vaginal profile: a correlated classification of vaginal relaxation. Clin Obstet Gynecol 15:1048, 1972

Barber MD: Symptoms and outcome measures of pelvic organ prolapse. Clin Obstet Gynecol 48:648, 2005a

Barber MD, Brubaker L, Burgio KL, et al: Comparison of 2 transvaginal surgical approaches and perioperative behavioral therapy for apical vaginal prolapse: the OPTIMAL randomized trial. JAMA 311(10):1023, 2014

Barber MD, Brubaker L, Nygaard I, et al: Defining success after surgery for pelvic organ prolapse. Obstet Gynecol 114:600, 2009

Barber MD, Cundiff GW, Weidner AC, et al: Accuracy of clinical assessment of paravaginal defects in women with anterior wall prolapse. Am J Obstet Gynecol 181:87, 1999

Barber MD, Visco AG, Weidner AC, et al: Bilateral uterosacral ligament vaginal vault suspension with site-specific endopelvic fascia defect repair for treatment of pelvic organ prolapse. Am J Obstet Gynecol 183:1402, 2000

Barber MD, Walters MD, Bump RC: Short forms of two condition-specific quality-of-life questionnaires for women with pelvic floor disorders (PFDI-20 and PFIQ-7). Am J Obstet Gynecol 193:103, 2005b

Benson JT, Lucente V, McClellan E: Vaginal versus abdominal reconstructive surgery for the treatment of pelvic support defects: a prospective randomized study with long-term outcome evaluation. Am J Obstet Gynecol 175:1418, 1996

Bland DR, Earle BB, Vitolins MZ, et al: Use of the Pelvic Organ Prolapse staging system of the International Continence Society, American Urogynecologic Society, and the Society of Gynecologic Surgeons in perimenopausal women. Am J Obstet Gynecol 181:1324, 1999

Blandon RE, Bharucha AE, Melton LJ 3rd, et al: Risk factors for pelvic floor repair after hysterectomy. Obstet Gynecol 113(3):601, 2009

Bø K: Pelvic floor muscle training is effective in treatment of stress urinary incontinence, but how does it work? Int Urogynecol J 15:76, 2004

Boreham M, Marinis S, Keller P, et al: Gene expression profiling of the pubococcygeus in premenopausal women with pelvic organ prolapse. J Pelv Med Surg 4:253, 2009

Boreham MK, Miller RT, Schaffer JI, et al: Smooth muscle myosin heavy chain and caldesmon expression in the anterior vaginal wall of women with and without pelvic organ prolapse. Am J Obstet Gynecol 185:944, 2001

Boreham MK, Wai CY, Miller RT, et al: Morphometric analysis of smooth muscle in the anterior vaginal wall of women with pelvic organ prolapse. Am J Obstet Gynecol 187:56, 2002a

Boreham MK, Wai CY, Miller RT, et al: Morphometric properties of the posterior vaginal wall in women with pelvic organ prolapse. Am J Obstet Gynecol 187:1501, 2002b

Boyles SH, Weber AM, Meyn L: Procedures for pelvic organ prolapse in the United States, 1979–1997. Am J Obstet Gynecol 188:108, 2003

Bradley CS, Nygaard IE: Vaginal wall descensus and pelvic floor symptoms in older women. Obstet Gynecol 106:759, 2005

Brincat M, Moniz CF, Studd JWW, et al: Sex hormone and skin collagen content in postmenopausal women. BMJ 287:1337, 1983

Brown JS, Waetjien LE, Subak LL, et al: Pelvic organ prolapse surgery in the United States, 1997. Am J Obstet Gynecol 186:712, 2002

Brubaker L: Burch colposuspension at the time of sacrocolpopexy in stress continent women reduces bothersome stress urinary symptoms: the CARE randomized trial. J Pelvic Surg 11(Suppl 1):S5, 2005a

Brubaker L, Cundiff GW, Fine P, et al: Pelvic Floor Disorders Network. Abdominal sacrocolpopexy with Burch colposuspension to reduce urinary stress incontinence. N Engl J Med 354:1557, 2006

Bump RC, Mattiasson A, Bø K, et al: The standardization of terminology of female pelvic organ prolapse and pelvic floor dysfunction. Am J Obstet Gynecol 175:10, 1996

Burrows LJ, Meyn LA, Walters MD, et al: Pelvic symptoms in women with pelvic organ prolapse. Obstet Gynecol 104:982, 2004

Carley ME, Schaffer J: Urinary incontinence and pelvic organ prolapse in women with Marfan or Ehlers Danlos syndrome. Am J Obstet Gynecol 182:1021, 2000

Carroli G, Mignini L: Episiotomy for vaginal birth. Cochrane Database Syst Rev 1:CD000081, 2009

Chaikin DC, Groutz A, Blaivas JG: Predicting the need for anti-incontinence surgery in continent women undergoing repair of severe urogenital prolapse. J Urol 163:531, 2000

Chmielewski L, Walters MD, Weber AM, et al. Reanalysis of a randomized trial of 3 techniques of anterior colporrhaphy using clinically relevant definitions of success. Am J Obstet Gynecol 205:69.e1, 2011

Cundiff GW, Fenner D: Evaluation and treatment of women with rectocele: focus on associated defecatory and sexual dysfunction. Obstet Gynecol 104:1403, 2004

Cundiff GW, Harris RL, Coates K, et al: Abdominal sacral colpoperineopexy: a new approach for correction of posterior compartment defects and perineal descent associated with vaginal vault prolapse. Am J Obstet Gynecol 177:1345, 1997

Cundiff GW, Weidner AC, Visco AG, et al: A survey of pessary use by the membership of the American Urogynecologic Society. Obstet Gynecol 95:931, 2000

DeLancey JO: Anatomic aspects of vaginal eversion after hysterectomy. Am J Obstet Gynecol 166:1717, 1992

DeLancey JO: Anatomy and biomechanics of genital prolapse. Clin Obstet Gynecol 36:897, 1993

Edenfield AL, Levin PJ, Dieter AA, et al: Sexual activity and vaginal topography in women with symptomatic pelvic floor disorders. J Sex Med 12(2):416, 2015

Ellerkmann RM, Cundiff GW, Melick CF, et al: Correlation of symptoms with location and severity of pelvic organ prolapse. Am J Obstet Gynecol 185:1332, 2001

Farrell SA: Practical advice for ring pessary fitting and management. J SOGC 19:625, 1997

FitzGerald MP, Edwards SR, Fenner D: Medium-term follow-up on use of freeze-dried, irradiated donor fascia for sacrocolpopexy and sling procedures. Int Urogynecol J Pelvic Floor Dysfunct 15(4):238, 2004

FitzGerald MP, Kulkarni N, Fenner D: Postoperative resolution of urinary retention in patients with advanced pelvic organ prolapse. Am J Obstet Gynecol 183:1361, 2000

FitzGerald MP, Mollenhauer J, Bitterman P, et al: Functional failure of fascia lata allografts. Am J Obstet Gynecol 181:1339, 1999

FitzGerald MP, Richter HE, Sohail S, et al: Colpocleisis: a review. Int Urogynecol J 17:261, 2006

Flynn MK, Amundsen CL: Diagnosis of pelvic organ prolapse. In Chapple CR, Zimmern PE, Brubaker L, et al (eds): Multidisciplinary Management of Female Pelvic Floor Disorders. Philadelphia, 2006, p 118

Food and Drug Administration: UPDATE on serious complications associated with transvaginal placement of surgical mesh for pelvic organ prolapse: FDA safety communication. 2011. Available at: http://www.fda.gov/MedicalDevices/Safety/AlertsandNotices/ucm262435.htm. Accessed October 18, 2014

Freeman RM, Pantazis K, Thomson A, et al: A randomised controlled trial of abdominal versus laparoscopic sacrocolpopexy for the treatment of post-hysterectomy vaginal vault prolapse: LAS study. Int Urogynecol J 24(3):377, 2013

Gilpin SA, Gosling JA, Smith AR, et al: The pathogenesis of genitourinary prolapse and stress incontinence of urine. A histological and histochemical study. BJOG 96:15, 1989

Gregory WT, Otto LN, Bergstrom JO, et al: Surgical outcome of abdominal sacrocolpopexy with synthetic mesh versus abdominal sacrocolpopexy with cadaveric fascia lata. Int Urogynecol J Pelvic Floor Dysfunct 16:369, 2005

Griffis K, Evers MD, Terry CL, et al: Mesh erosion and abdominal sacrocolpopexy: a comparison of prior, total, and supracervical hysterectomy. J Pelvic Med Surg 12(1): 25, 2006

Hagen S, Stark D: Conservative management of pelvic organ prolapse in women. Cochrane Database Syst Rev 12:CD003882, 2011

Handa VL, Blomquist JL, Knoepp LR, et al: Pelvic floor disorders 5–10 years after vaginal or cesarean childbirth. Obstet Gynecol 118(4):777, 2011

Handa VL, Cundiff G, Chang HH, et al: Female sexual function and pelvic floor disorders. Obstet Gynecol 111(5):1045, 2008

Hanzal E, Berger E, Koelbl H: Levator ani muscle morphology and recurrent genuine stress incontinence. Obstet Gynecol 81:426, 1993

Haylen BT, de Ridder D, Freeman RM, et al: An International Urogynecologic Association (IUGA)/International Continence Society (ICS) joint report on the terminology for female pelvic floor dysfunction. Int Urogynecol J Pelvic Floor Dysfunct 21:5, 2010

Heit M, Benson JT, Russell B, et al: Levator ani muscle in women with genitourinary prolapse: indirect assessment by muscle histopathology. Neurourol Urodyn 15:17, 1996

Heit M, Culligan P, Rosenquist C, et al: Is pelvic organ prolapse a cause of pelvic or low back pain? Obstet Gynecol 99:23, 2002

Hendrix SL, Clark A, Nygaard I, et al: Pelvic organ prolapse in the Women's Health Initiative: gravity and gravidity. Am J Obstet Gynecol 186:1160, 2002

Jelovsek JE, Barber MD, Paraiso MFR, et al: Functional bowel and anorectal disorders in patients with pelvic organ prolapse and incontinence. Am J Obstet Gynecol 193:2105, 2005

Jorgensen S, Hein HO, Gyntelberg F: Heavy lifting at work and risk of genital prolapse and herniated lumbar disc in assistant nurses. Occup Med (Lond) 44:47, 1994

Kahn MA, Breitkopf CR, Valley MT, et al: Pelvic Organ Support Study (POSST) and bowel symptoms: straining at stool is associated with perineal

and anterior vaginal descent in a general gynecologic population. Am J Obstet Gynecol 192:1516, 2005

Kahn MA, Stanton SL: Posterior colporrhaphy: its effects on bowel and sexual function. BJOG 104:82, 1997

Karram M, Goldwassar S, Kleeman S, et al: High uterosacral vaginal vault suspension with fascial reconstruction for vaginal repair of enterocele and vaginal vault prolapse. Am J Obstet Gynecol 185:1339, 2001

Kenton K, Shott S, Brubaker L: Outcomes after rectovaginal fascia reattachment for rectocele repair. Am J Obstet Gynecol 181:1360, 1999

Kim S, Harvey MA, Johnston S: A review of the epidemiology and pathophysiology of pelvic floor dysfunction: do racial differences matter? J Obstet Gynaecol Cancer 27:251, 2005

Koelbl H, Strassegger H, Riss PA, et al: Morphologic and functional aspects of pelvic floor muscles in patients with pelvic relaxation and genuine stress incontinence. Obstet Gynecol 74:789, 1989

Laycock J: Patient assessment. In Laycock J, Haslam J (eds): Therapeutic Management of Incontinence and Pelvic Pain. Pelvic Organ Disorders. London, Springer, 2002, p 52

Liang CC, Chang YL, Chang SD, et al: Pessary test to predict postoperative urinary incontinence in women undergoing hysterectomy for prolapse. Obstet Gynecol 104:795, 2004

Lyons TL, Winer WK: Laparoscopic rectocele repair using polyglactin mesh. J Am Assoc Gynecol Laparosc 4:381, 1997

Maher CF, Qatawneh AM, Dwyer PL, et al: Abdominal sacral colpopexy or vaginal sacrospinous colpopexy for vaginal vault prolapse: a prospective randomized study. Am J Obstet Gynecol 190:20, 2004

Mant J, Painter R, Vessey M: Epidemiology of genital prolapse: observations from the Oxford Family Planning Association Study. BJOG 104:579, 1997

McDermott CD, Hale DS: Abdominal, laparoscopic, and robotic surgery for pelvic organ prolapse. Obstet Gynecol Clin North Am 36: 585, 2009

Mellegren A, Anzen B, Nilsson BY, et al: Results of rectocele repair: a prospective study. Dis Colon Rectum 38:7, 1995

Moalli PA, Shand SH, Zyczynski HM, et al: Remodeling of vaginal connective tissue in patients with prolapse. Obstet Gynecol 106:953, 2005

Moalli PA, Talarico LC, Sung VW, et al: Impact of menopause on collagen subtypes in the arcus tendineous fasciae pelvis. Am J Obstet Gynecol 190(3):620, 2004

Morley GW, DeLancey JO: Sacrospinous ligament fixation for eversion of the vagina. Am J Obstet Gynecol 158:872, 1988

Muir TW: Surgical treatment of rectocele and perineal defects. In Walters MD, Karram MM (eds): Urogynecology and Reconstructive Pelvic Surgery, 3rd ed. Philadelphia, Mosby-Elsevier, 2007, p 254

Norton PA, Baker JE, Sharp HC, et al: Genitourinary prolapse and joint hypermobility in women. Obstet Gynecol 85:225, 1995

Nygaard I, Barber MD, Burgio Kl, et al: Prevalence of symptomatic pelvic floor disorders in US women. JAMA 300(11):131, 2008

Olsen AL, Smith VJ, Bergstrom JO, et al: Epidemiology of surgically managed pelvic organ prolapse and urinary incontinence. Obstet Gynecol 89:501, 1997

Paraiso MF, Ballard LA, Walters MD, et al: Pelvic support defects and visceral and sexual function in women treated with sacrospinous ligament suspension and pelvic reconstruction. Am J Obstet Gynecol 175:1423, 1996

Paraiso MF, Barber MD, Muir TW, et al: Rectocele repair: a randomized trial of three surgical techniques including graft augmentation. Am J Obstet Gynecol 195:1762, 2006

Paraiso MF, Jelovsek JE, Frick A, et al: Laparoscopic compared with robotic sacrocolpopexy for vaginal prolapse: a randomized controlled trial. Obstet Gynecol 118(5):1005, 2011

Patel DA, Xu X, Thomason AD, et al: Childbirth and pelvic floor dysfunction: an epidemiologic approach to the assessment of prevention opportunities at delivery. Am J Obstet Gynecol 195:23, 2006

Peschers UM, Schaer GN, DeLancey JO, et al: Levator ani function before and after childbirth. BJOG 104:1004, 1997

Phillips CH, Anthony F, Benyon C, et al: Collagen metabolism in the uterosacral ligaments and vaginal skin of women with uterine prolapse. BJOG 113:39, 2006

Rahn DD, Ward RM, Sanses TV, et al: Vaginal estrogen use in postmenopausal women with pelvic floor disorders: systematic review and practice guidelines. Int Urogynecol J 26(1):3, 2015

Reisenauer C, Shiozawa T, Oppitz M, et al: The role of smooth muscle in the pathogenesis of pelvic organ prolapse—an immunohistochemical and morphometric analysis of the cervical third of the uterosacral ligament. Int Urogynecol J Pelvic Floor Dysfunct 19:383, 2008

Rortveit G, Brown JS, Thom DH, et al: Symptomatic pelvic organ prolapse: prevalence and risk factors in a population-based, racially diverse cohort. Obstet Gynecol 109(6):1396, 2007

Schaffer JI, Cundiff GW, Amundsen CL, et al: Do pessaries improve lower urinary tract symptoms? J Pelvic Med Surg 12:72, 2006

Schaffer JI, Wai CY, Boreham MK: Etiology of pelvic organ prolapse. Clin Obstet Gynecol 48:639, 2005

Shafik A, El-Sibai O: Levator ani muscle activity in pregnancy and the postpartum period: a myoelectric study. Clin Exp Obstet Gynecol 27:129, 2000

Shull BL, Bachofen C, Coates KW, et al: A transvaginal approach to repair of apical and other associated sites of pelvic organ prolapse with uterosacral ligaments. Am J Obstet Gynecol 183:1365, 2000

Silva WA, Paulks RN, Segal JL, et al: Uterosacral ligament vault suspension: five-year outcomes. Obstet Gynecol 108:255, 2006

Smith AR, Hosker GL, Warrell DW: The role of partial denervation of the pelvic floor in the aetiology of genitourinary prolapse and stress incontinence of urine. A neurophysiological study. BJOG 96:24, 1989

Smith P, Heimer G, Norgren A, et al: Localization of steroid hormone receptors in the pelvic muscles. Eur J Obstet Gynecol Reprod Biol 50:83, 1993

Smith P, Heimer G, Norgren A, et al: Steroid hormone receptors in pelvis muscles and ligaments in women. Gynecol Obstet Invest 30:27, 1990

Sullivan ES, Longaker CJ, Lee PY: Total pelvic mesh repair: a ten-year experience. Dis Colon Rectum 44:857, 2001

Sung VW, Rogers RG, Schaffer JI, et al: Graft use in transvaginal pelvic organ prolapse repair: a systematic review. Obstet Gynecol 112:1131, 2008

Swift S, Woodman P, O'Boyle A, et al: Pelvic Organ Support Study (POSST): the distribution, clinical definition, and epidemiologic condition of pelvic organ support defects. Am J Obstet Gynecol 192:795, 2005

Swift SE: The distribution of pelvic organ support in a population of female subjects seen for routine gynecologic health care. AM J Obstet Gynecol 183:277, 2000

Swift SE, Tate SB, Nicholas J: Correlation of symptoms with degree of pelvic organ support in a general population of women: what is pelvic organ prolapse? Am J Obstet Gynecol 189:372, 2003

Sze EH, Miklos JR, Partoll L, et al: Sacrospinous ligament fixation with transvaginal needle suspension for advanced pelvic organ prolapse and stress incontinence. Obstet Gynecol 89:94, 1997a

Sze HM, Karram MM: Transvaginal repair of vault prolapse: a review. Obstet Gynecol 89:466, 1997b

Takacs P, Nassiri M, Gualtieri M, et al: Uterosacral ligament smooth muscle cell apoptosis is increased in women with uterine prolapse. Reprod Sci 16:447, 2009

Tan JS, Lukaz ES, Menefee SA, et al: Predictive value of prolapse symptoms: a large database study. Int Urogynecol J Pelvic Floor Dysfunct 16:203, 2005

Trowbridge ER, Fultz NH, Patel DA, et al: Distribution of pelvis organ support in a population-based sample of middle-aged community-dwelling African American and white women in southeastern Michigan. Am J Obstet Gynecol 198:548, 2008

Ulrich D, Dwyer P, Rosamilia A, et al: The effect of vaginal pelvic organ prolapse surgery on sexual function. Neurourol Urodyn 34(4):316, 2015

Weber AM, Abrams P, Brubaker L, et al: The standardization of terminology for researchers in female pelvic floor disorders. Int Urogynecol J Pelvic Floor Dysfunct 12:178, 2001a

Weber AM, Walters MD, Ballard LA, et al: Posterior vaginal wall prolapse and bowel function. Obstet Gynecol 179:1446, 1998

Weber AM, Walters MD, Piedmonte MR, et al: Anterior colporrhaphy: a randomized trial of three surgical techniques. Am J Obstet Gynecol 185:1299, 2001b

Weber AM, Walters MD, Piedmonte MR: Sexual function and vaginal anatomy in women before and after surgery for pelvic organ prolapse and urinary incontinence. Am J Obstet Gynecol 182:1610, 2000

Weber AM, Walters MD, Schover LR: Sexual function in women with uterovaginal prolapse and urinary incontinence. Obstet Gynecol 85:483, 1995

Wei JT, Nygaard I, Richter HE, et al: A midurethral sling to reduce incontinence after vaginal prolapse repair. N Engl J Med 366:2358, 2012

Wheeler TL Jr, Richter HE, Burgio KL, et al: Regret, satisfaction, and symptoms improvement: analysis of the impact of partial colpocleisis for the management of severe pelvic organ prolapse. Am J Obstet Gynecol 193:2067, 2005

Whitcomb EL, Rortveit G, Brown JS, et al: Racial differences in pelvic organ prolapse. Obstet Gynecol 114(6):1271, 2009

Whiteside JL, Weber AM, Meyn LA, et al: Risk factors for prolapse recurrence after vaginal repair. Am J Obstet Gynecol 191:1533, 2004

Wieslander CK, Word RA, Schaffer JI, et al: Smoking is a risk factor for pelvic organ prolapse. J Pelvic Medicine & Surgery 26th Annual Scientific Meeting of the American Urogynecologic Society (AUGS), Atlanta, Georgia, p S16, 2005

Wu JM, Matthews CA, Conover MM, et al: Lifetime risk of stress urinary incontinence or pelvic organ prolapse surgery. Obstet Gynecol 123(6):1201, 2014

CHAPTER 25

Anal Incontinence and Functional Anorectal Disorders

ANAL INCONTINENCE

Although definitions are inconsistent, anal incontinence (AI) is most commonly defined as an involuntary loss of flatus, liquid, or solid stool that causes a social or hygienic problem (Abrams, 2005; Haylen, 2010). The definition of AI includes incontinence of flatus, whereas that of fecal incontinence (FI) does not.

Despite acceptance of these by healthcare professionals, one survey observed that only 30 percent of nearly 1100 community-dwelling women with FI had heard the term "fecal incontinence," and 71 percent preferred the term "accidental bowel leakage" (Brown, 2012). Thus, at a recent consensus workshop, this latter more patient-centered term was suggested for use with patients (Bharucha, 2015).

AI can lead to poor self-image and isolation, and the social and quality-of-life effects of AI are significant (Johanson, 1996). Additionally, AI increases the likelihood that an older patient will be admitted to a nursing home rather than cared for at home (Grover, 2010).

■ Epidemiology

Anal incontinence is common, and rates among men and women are similar (Madoff, 2004b; Nelson, 2004). In one National Health and Nutrition Examination Survey (NHANES), FI was also not significantly associated with race or ethnicity, education level, income, or marital status (Whitehead, 2009). Although all age groups may be affected, the AI prevalence increases with age and may reach 46 percent in older, institutionalized women (Nelson, 1998). Using data from NHANES that incorporated years 2005 through 2010, investigators noted that the prevalence of FI in women approximated 9 percent (Nygaard, 2008; Wu, 2014). Similarly, the estimated prevalence of FI in noninstitutionalized U.S. adults was 8.3 percent (18 million). Of these individuals, liquid stool incontinence was noted in 6.2 percent, mucus in 3.1 percent, and solid stool in 1.6 percent (Whitehead, 2009). The prevalence of FI increased from 2.6 percent in those aged 20 to 30 years and rose to 15.3 percent in subjects aged 70 years or older.

■ Physiology

Normal defecation and anal continence are complex processes that require: (1) a competent anal sphincter complex, (2) normal anorectal sensation, (3) adequate rectal capacity and compliance, and (4) conscious control. Logically, mechanisms responsible for FI include anal sphincter and pelvic floor weakness, reduced or increased rectal sensation, reduced rectal capacity and compliance, and diarrhea (Bharucha, 2015). In many patients these factors may be additive, and thus no single physiologic measure is consistently associated with FI.

Muscular Contributions

Essential contributors to fecal continence include the internal and external anal sphincters and the puborectalis muscle (Figs. 38-9 and 38-21, p. 803). Of these, the internal anal sphincter (IAS) is the thickened distal 3- to 4-cm longitudinal extension of the colon's circular smooth-muscle layer. It is innervated by the autonomic nervous system and provides 70 to 85 percent of the anal canal's resting pressure (Frenckner, 1975). As a result, the IAS contributes substantially to the maintenance of fecal continence at rest.

The external anal sphincter (EAS) consists of striated muscle and is primarily innervated by somatic motor fibers that course in the inferior rectal branch of the pudendal nerve (Fig. 25-1A). The EAS provides the anal canal's squeeze pressure and is mainly responsible for maintaining fecal continence when continence is threatened. At times, squeeze pressure may be voluntary or may be induced by increased intraabdominal pressure. In addition, although resting sphincter tone is generally attributed to the IAS, the EAS maintains a constant state of resting contraction and may be responsible for approximately 25 percent of anal resting pressure. During defecation, however, the EAS relaxes to allow stool passage.

The puborectalis muscle is part of the levator ani muscle group and is innervated from its pelvic surface by direct efferents from the third, fourth, and fifth sacral nerve roots (Fig. 25-1B) (Barber, 2002). Although the suggestion is controversial, it may also be innervated from its perineal surface by the inferior rectal

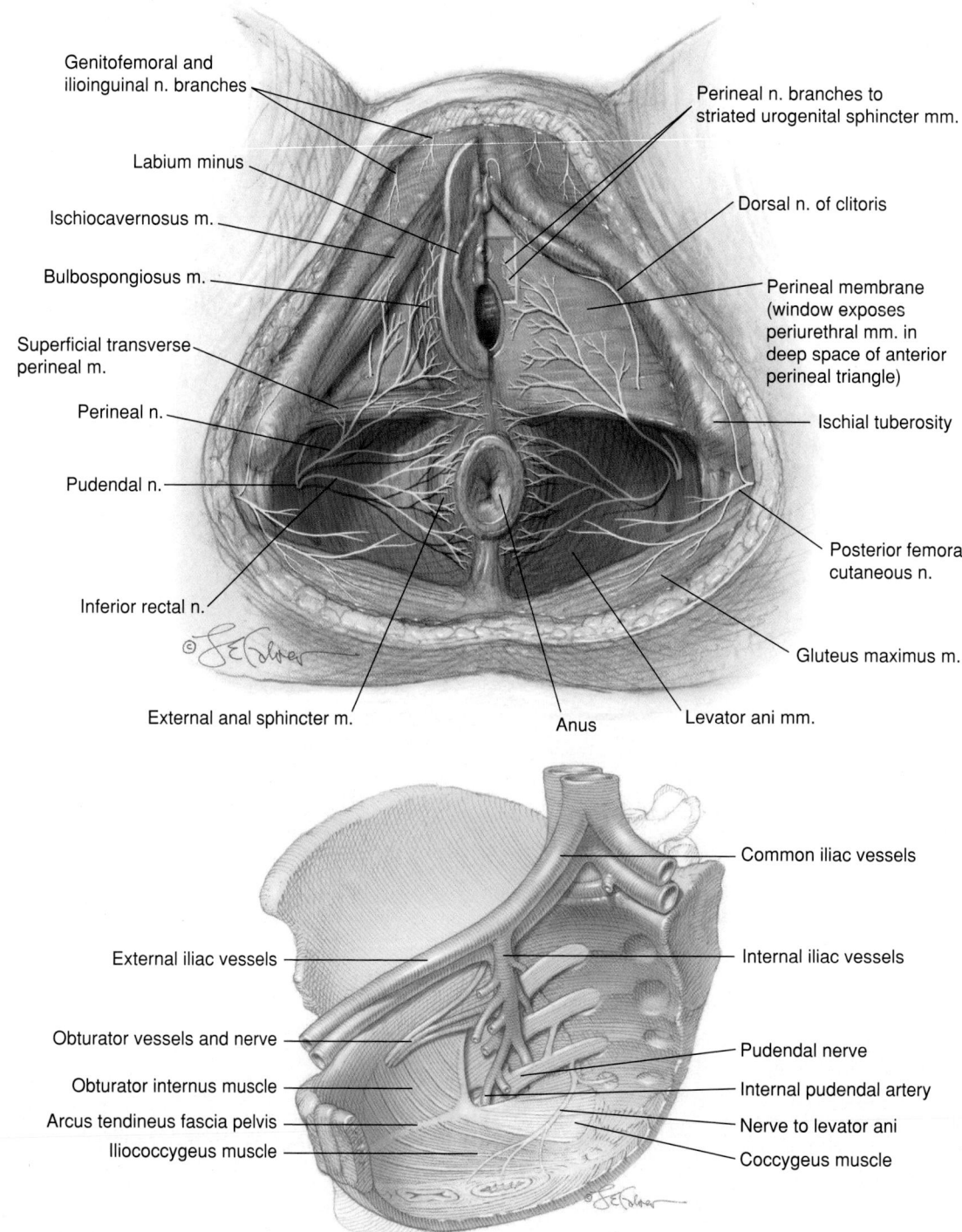

FIGURE 25-1 Innervation of the anal sphincter complex. **A.** The external anal sphincter is innervated by the pudendal nerve. **B.** Innervation of the female pelvic floor muscles from direct branches of S3-S5.

branch of the pudendal nerve. Its constant tone contributes to the anorectal angle, which aids in preventing rectal contents from entering the anus (Fig. 38-10, p. 803). Similar to the EAS, this muscle can be contracted voluntarily or in response to sudden increases in abdominal pressure.

The role of the puborectalis in maintaining stool continence remains unclear. However, it is best appreciated in women who remain continent of solid stool despite absence of the anterior arch of the external and internal sphincters, as can be seen in those with chronic fourth-degree lacerations (Fig. 25-2). With normal

puborectalis relaxation, evacuation is generally aided by the better longitudinal alignment of the rectoanal lumen. Conversely, paradoxical contraction of the puborectalis muscle during defecation may lead to impaired evacuation. Moreover, atrophy of this muscle has been associated with FI (Bharucha, 2004).

Anorectal Sensation

Innervation to the rectum and anal canal is derived from the inferior hypogastric nerve plexus that contain sympathetic and parasympathetic components and by intrinsic nerves present in

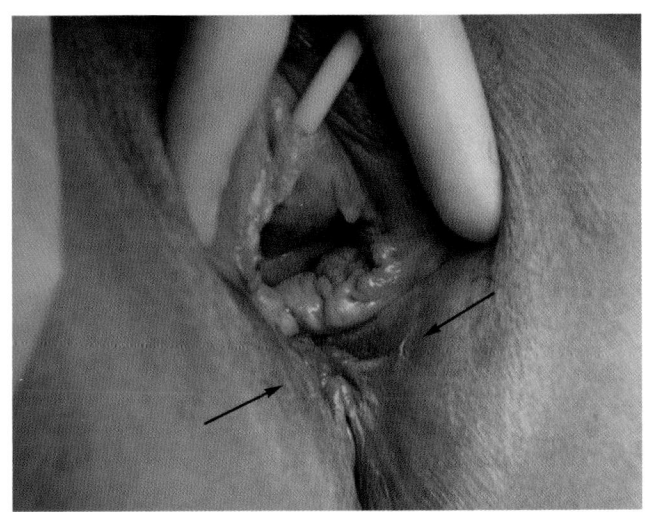

FIGURE 25-2 Chronic fourth-degree laceration with complete absence of the perineal body and the anterior portion of external anal sphincter (cloacal-like deformity). Skin dimples at 3 and 9 o'clock (*arrows*) indicate sites of retracted ends of the external anal sphincter.

the rectoanal wall (Fig. 38-13, p. 806). In addition, the inferior rectal branch of the pudendal nerve conveys sensory input from the lower anal canal and the skin around the anus. Sensory receptors within the anal canal and pelvic floor muscles can detect the presence of stool in the rectum and the degree of distention. Through these neural pathways, information regarding rectal distention and rectal contents can be transmitted and processed and the action of the sphincteric musculature coordinated.

The rectoanal inhibitory reflex (RAIR) refers to the transient relaxation of the IAS and contraction of EAS induced by rectal distention when stool first arrives in the rectum. This reflex is mediated by the intrinsic nerves in the anorectal wall and allows the sensory-rich upper anal canal to come in contact with or "sample" the rectal contents (Whitehead, 1987). Specifically, sampling refers to the process whereby the IAS relaxes, often independently of rectal distention, allowing the anal epithelium to ascertain whether rectal contents are gas, liquid, or solid stools (Miller, 1988).

Following integration of this neural information, defecation can ensue in the appropriate social setting. Alternatively, if required, defecation can generally be postponed, as the rectum can accommodate its contents and the EAS or puborectalis muscle or both can be voluntarily contracted. However, if rectal sensation is impaired, contents may enter the anal canal and may leak before the EAS can contract (Buser, 1986).

Evaluation of the RAIR may clarify the underlying etiology of AI. This reflex is absent in those with congenital aganglionosis (Hirschsprung disease) but preserved in patients with cauda equina lesions or after spinal cord transection (Bharucha, 2006).

Rectal Accommodation and Compliance

Following anal sampling, the rectum can relax to admit the increased rectal volume in a process known as accommodation. The rectum is a highly compliant reservoir that permits stool storage. As rectal volume increases, an urge to defecate is perceived. If this urge is voluntarily suppressed, the rectum relaxes to continue stool accommodation. A loss of compliance may decrease the ability of the rectal wall to stretch or accommodate, and as a result, rectal pressure may remain high. This may

place increased demands on the other components of the continence mechanism such as the anal sphincter complex.

Rectal compliance can be calculated by measuring the sensitivity to and maximal volume tolerated from a fluid-filled balloon during anorectal manometry (p. 567). Rectal compliance may be decreased in those with ulcerative and radiation proctitis. In contrast, increased compliance may be noted in certain patients with constipation, potentially signaling a megarectum.

■ Incontinence Risks

Obstetric

Abnormal defecation develops if any of the just-described components of anal continence are altered. Logically, causes of AI and defecatory disorders are diverse and are likely multifactorial (Table 25-1).

In younger, reproductive-aged women, the most common association with AI is vaginal delivery and damage to the anal sphincter muscles (Snooks, 1985; Sultan, 1993; Zetterstrom, 1999). This damage may be mechanical or neuropathic and can result in fecal and flatal incontinence at an early age. Interestingly, the incidence of FI following vaginal delivery has declined from 13 percent of primiparous women two decades ago to 8 percent in more recent series (Bharucha, 2015). This may reflect changes in obstetric practices that include decreased use of instrumented vaginal delivery and more restricted episiotomy use.

TABLE 25-1. Risk Factors for Fecal Incontinence

Obstetric	
Increasing parity	Anal sphincter damage
Medical conditions	
Obesity	Diabetes mellitus
Aging	COPD
Smoking	Chronic hypertension
Postmenopausal	Stroke
Medications	Scleroderma
Decreased activity	Pelvic radiation
Urogynecologic	
Urinary incontinence	Pelvic organ prolapse
Gastrointestinal	
Constipation	Anal abscess
Diarrhea	Anal fistula
Fecal urgency	Anal surgery
Food intolerance	Cholecystectomy
IBS	Rectal prolapse
Neuropsychiatric	
Spinal cord lesion	Myopathies
Parkinson disease	Psychosis
Spinal surgery	Nerve stretch injury
Multiple sclerosis	Cognitive dysfunction
Brain tumor	

COPD = chronic obstructive pulmonary disease;
IBS = irritable bowel syndrome.

Rates of sphincter tear during vaginal births in the United States range from 6 to 18 percent (Fenner, 2003; Handa, 2001). In one study of primiparas delivered at term, at both 6 weeks and 6 months postpartum, women who sustained anal sphincter tears during vaginal delivery had twice the risk of FI and reported more severe FI compared with women who delivered vaginally without evidence of sphincter disruption (Borello-France, 2006). In contrast, a retrospective study of 151 women with diverse obstetric histories who delivered 30 years previously reported that women with a prior sphincter disruption were more likely to have "bothersome" flatal incontinence but were not at increased risk for FI compared with women who had an isolated episiotomy or those who underwent cesarean delivery (Nygaard, 1997). Thus, other mechanisms associated with pregnancy and with aging may contribute to AI regardless of delivery mode or anal sphincter disruption. Importantly, cesarean delivery minimizes the risk of anatomic anal sphincter injury, but it does not universally protect against later AI. The National Institutes of Health (NIH) (2006) consensus conference on cesarean delivery on maternal request concluded that evidence was insufficient to support a practice of elective cesarean delivery for the prevention of pelvic floor disorders, including FI.

Other Factors

Few epidemiological studies have evaluated the risk factors for FI in the community. That said, underlying bowel disturbances, particularly diarrhea; the symptom of rectal urgency; and burden of chronic illness, are the strongest independent risk factors for FI (Bharucha, 2015). Inflammatory bowel conditions, especially with chronic diarrhea, are another common risk. Liquid stool is more difficult to control than solid, and thus FI may develop even if all components of the continence mechanism are grossly intact. Alternatively, chronic constipation with straining to defecate may damage the muscular and/or neural components of the sphincter mechanism. Similarly, other neuromuscular injury to the puborectalis and/or anal sphincter muscles, such as that associated with pelvic organ prolapse, may lead to AI.

Radiation therapy involving the rectum can result in poor compliance and loss of accommodation. Also, nervous system dysfunction in those with spinal cord injury, back surgery, multiple sclerosis, diabetes, or cerebrovascular accident may lead to poor accommodation, loss of sensation, impaired reflexes, and myopathy. Finally, loss of rectal sensation and decreased squeeze sphincter pressures can be seen with normal aging. One study suggests that even asymptomatic older nulliparous

women have anal sphincter neurogenic injury, which partly explained weak anal squeeze pressures (Bharucha, 2012).

■ Diagnosis

There is no current consensus on how best to screen for FI. Proposed barriers include poor patient understanding of the term FI, embarrassment, a belief that FI is a normal part of aging, confusion as to whom they might discuss the problem with, priority of other medical conditions, and unfamiliarity or pessimism regarding treatment options (Bharucha, 2015). In one study, less than one third of patients with FI had disclosed this to a provider (Johanson, 1996). In another that evaluated women presenting for benign gynecologic care, only 17 percent with FI were asked about the symptom by their health care provider (Boreham, 2005).

In contrast to urinary incontinence, no FI classification approach is widely accepted. However, the type (urge, passive, or mixed), etiology, and severity of FI provide some basis to categorize FI. A complete history and physical examination evaluates these prior to treatment planning and often identifies correctable problems.

History

To the patient, relevant questions are posed regarding incontinence duration and frequency, stool consistency, timing of incontinent episodes, use of sanitary protection, and incontinence-related social impairment. Additionally, risk factors noted in Table 25-1 are sought. Importantly, urge-related AI is differentiated from incontinence without awareness, as these may be associated with different underlying pathologies. For example, urgency without incontinence may reflect inability of the rectal reservoir to store stool rather than a sphincteric disorder.

To gather historical data, validated questionnaires, stooling diaries, and the Bristol Stool Scale are objective options. Of these, a patient diary of stool habits is commonly used in research, but its utility is often limited by poor patient adherence. Alternatively, questionnaires reduce patient recall bias and help standardize AI scores. Several incontinence-scoring systems provide objective measure of a patient's degree of incontinence. Four commonly used symptom severity scores are the Pescatori Incontinence Score; Wexner (Cleveland Clinic) Score; St. Marks (Vaizey) Score; and the Fecal Incontinence Severity Index (FISI) (Tables 25-2 and 25-3) (Jorge, 1993; Pescatori, 1992; Rockwood, 1999; Vaizey, 1999). All of these incorporate the type and frequency of leakage. Of these, the Vaizey Score and the FISI include symptom weighting. The inclusion of patient-assigned severity scores increases the utility of the FISI compared with other scales. The ability of the

TABLE 25-2. Fecal Incontinence Severity Index

	Two or More Times Daily	Once Daily	Two or More Times Weekly	Once Weekly	1–3 Times Monthly	Never
Gas	☐	☐	☐	☐	☐	☐
Mucus	☐	☐	☐	☐	☐	☐
Liquid stool	☐	☐	☐	☐	☐	☐
Solid stool	☐	☐	☐	☐	☐	☐

Reproduced with permission from Rockwood TH, Church JM, Fleshman JW, et al: Patient and surgeon ranking of the severity of symptoms associated with fecal incontinence: the fecal incontinence severity index, Dis Colon Rectum 1999 Dec;42(12):1525–1532.

TABLE 25-3. St. Marks (Vaizey) Incontinence Score

	Never[a]	Rarely[b]	Sometimes[c]	Weekly[d]	Daily[e]
Incontinence for solid stool	0	1	2	3	4
Incontinence for liquid stool	0	1	2	3	4
Incontinence for gas	0	1	2	3	4
Alteration in lifestyle	0	1	2	3	4
		No	Yes		
Need to wear a pad or plug		0	2		
Taking constipating medicines		0	2		
Lack of ability to defer defecation for 15 minutes		0	4		

[a]Never = no episodes in the past 4 wks.
[b]Rarely = 1 episode in the past 4 wks.
[c]Sometimes = more than 1 episode in the past 4 wks but <1 a wk.
[d]Weekly = 1 or more episodes a week but <1 daily.
[e]Daily = 1 or more episodes daily.
Add one score from each row: Minimum score = 0 = perfect continence . Maximum score = 24 = totally incontinent.
Reproduced with permission from Vaizey CJ, Carapeti E, Cahill JA, et al: Prospective comparison of faecal incontinence grading systems, 1999 Jan;44(1):77–80.

Vaizey Score to incorporate a component of fecal urgency makes this scale desirable in certain clinical trials.

In addition to symptom severity, the patient's quality-of-life decline from AI is also characterized. The validated fecal incontinence quality-of-life (FI-QOL) questionnaire is a 29-item tool designed to estimate associated worsening lifestyle, coping behavior, depression/self-perception, and embarrassment (Table 25-4) (Rockwood, 2000). Other quality-of-life scales available

TABLE 25-4. Fecal Incontinence Quality of Life Scale Composition

Scale 1: Lifestyle

I am afraid to go out
I avoid visiting friends
I avoid many things I want to do
I plan my schedule around my bowel pattern
It is difficult for me to get out and do things

I avoid traveling
I avoid traveling by plane or train
I avoid staying overnight away from home
I avoid going out to eat
I limit how much I eat before I go out

Scale 2: Coping/Behavior

I feel I have no control over my bowels
I worry about bowel accidents
The possibility of bowel accidents is always on my mind
Whenever I go someplace new, I specifically locate where the bathrooms are
I try to prevent bowel accidents by staying very near a bathroom
I can't hold my bowel movement long enough to get to the bathroom
Whenever I am away from home, I try to stay near a restroom as much as possible

I have sex less often than I would like to
I worry about not reaching the toilet in time

Scale 3: Depression/Self-perception

In general, how would you say your health is?
I am afraid to have sex
I feel depressed
During the past month, have you felt so sad, discouraged, hopeless, or had so many problems that you wondered if anything was worthwhile?

I feel different from other people
I enjoy life less
I feel like I am not a healthy person

Scale 4: Embarrassment

I leak stool without even knowing it
I worry about others smelling stool on me
I feel ashamed

Reproduced with permission from Rockwood TH, Church JM, Fleshman JW, et al: Fecal incontinence quality of life scale: quality of life instrument for patients with fecal incontinence, Dis Colon Rectum 1999 Dec;42(12):1525–1532.

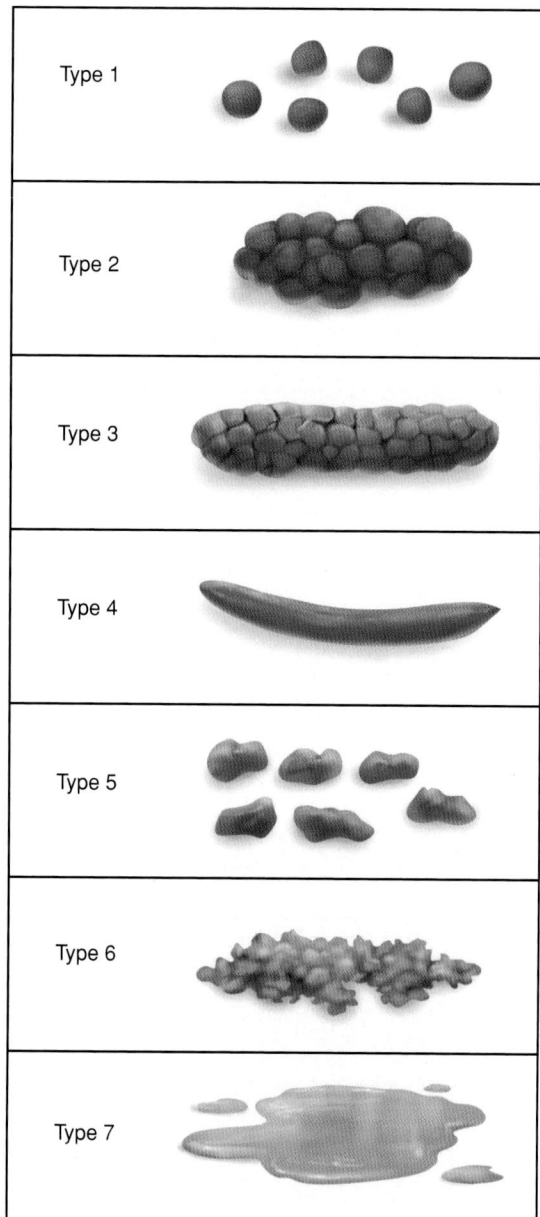

FIGURE 25-3 Bristol Stool Scale. Stools are categorized by their shape and texture. (Reproduced with permission from Lewis SJ, Heaton KW: Stool form scale as a useful guide to intestinal transit time. Scand J Gastroenterol 1997 Sep;32(9):920–924.)

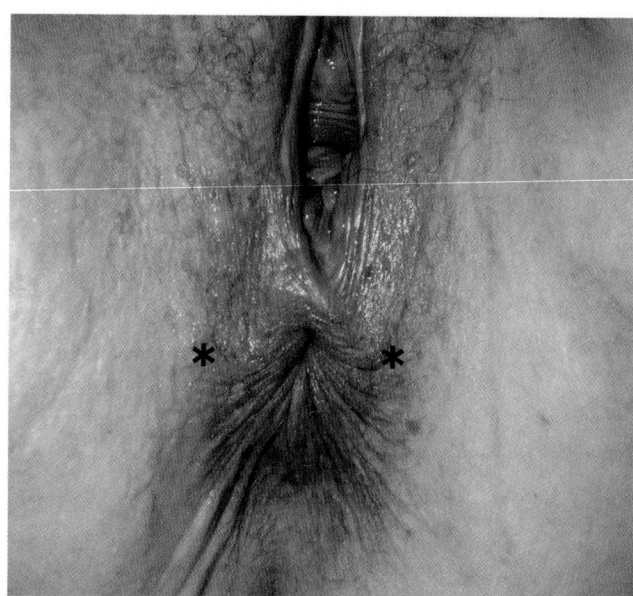

FIGURE 25-4 Photograph showing the "dovetail" sign, which is created by disruption of the anterior portion of external anal sphincter (EAS). Radial skin spikes are typically formed by attachment of skin to the EAS but are commonly absent from 10 to 2 o'clock (*asterisks*) in those with this disruption.

include the Modified Manchester Health Questionnaire and the Gastrointestinal Quality of Life Index (Kwon, 2005; Sailer, 1998). These validated tools may be used diagnostically and also following treatment to determine response.

Last, the validated Bristol Stool Scale is often selected to determine a patient's usual stool consistency (Lewis, 1997). This scale contains seven descriptions of stool characteristics and pictures of each stool type (Fig. 25-3) (Degen, 1996). Such stool consistency categorization correlates with objective measures of whole-gut transit time (Heaton, 1994).

Physical Examination

This begins with careful inspection of the anus and perineum to identify stool soiling, scars, perineal body length, hemorrhoids, anal warts, rectal prolapse, dovetail sign, or other anatomic abnormalities (Fig. 25-4). The perianal skin is gently stroked with a cotton-tipped swab to obtain the cutaneous anal reflex. Colloquially termed anal wink, circumferential contraction of the anal skin and underlying EAS is normally seen. This finding provides gross assessment of pudendal nerve integrity.

With digital rectal examination, one can assess anal resting tone, sample for gross or occult blood, and palpate masses or fecal impaction. In addition, squeeze pressure can subjectively be judged during voluntary patient contraction of the EAS around a gloved finger inserted into the anorectum. Last, during patient Valsalva maneuver, one observes for excessive perineal body descent, vaginal wall prolapse, rectal prolapse, or muscle incoordination (Fig. 25-5). With the latter, a paradoxic

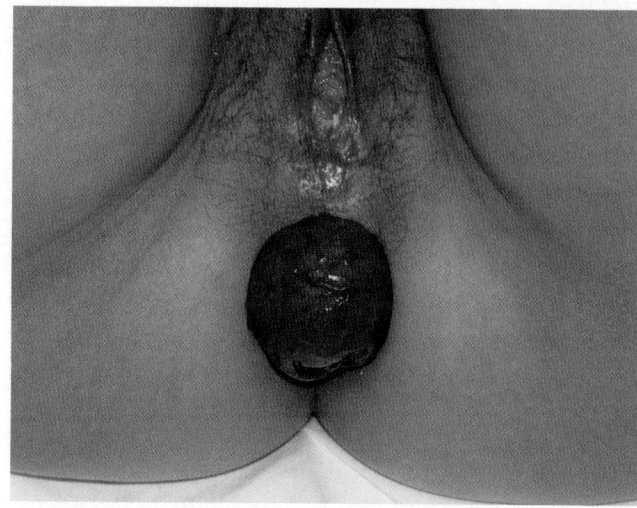

FIGURE 25-5 During patient Valsalva, a full-thickness rectal prolapse protrudes through the anal opening.

TABLE 25-5. Functional Testing for Patients with Fecal Incontinence[a]

Factors	Manometry				DG	EAUS	MRI	EMG
	Resting	Squeeze	RP	RC				
Muscle								
IAS	+					+	+	
EAS		+				+	+	+
Puborectalis					+		+	+
Rectum								
Perception			+					
Compliance				+				
Reservoir			+	+	+			
Megarectum			+		+		+	
Pelvic floor								
Perineal descent					+		+	
Anorectal angle					+		+	
Neural								
Pudendal nerve		+						+

[a]Plus sign indicates an appropriate test for a particular component of continence.
DG = defecography; EAS = external anal sphincter; EAUS = endoanal ultrasonography; EMG = electromyography; FI = fecal incontinence; IAS = internal anal sphincter; RC = rectal compliance; RP = rectal perception.
Adapted with permission from Hinninghofen H, Enck P: Fecal incontinence: evaluation and treatment. Gastroenterol Clin North Am 2003 Jun;32(2):685–706.

contraction—that is, abnormal sphincter contraction around the finger—may be elicited during patient Valsalva when an examining finger is inserted into the anorectum. Digital rectal examination is reasonably accurate relative to manometry for assessing anal resting tone and squeeze function and for identifying dyssynergia (Orkin, 2010; Tantiphlachiva, 2010).

Diagnostic Testing

Anorectal Manometry. Physical and historical findings typically guide the remainder of testing, which may include imaging and functional studies. Of these, anorectal manometry is performed mainly in academic institutions with an anophysiology laboratory prior to surgical intervention. It is a functional test that allows objective assessment of: (1) rectal compliance and rectal sensation, (2) reflexes, and (3) anal sphincter function (Table 25-5). During this test, a small flexible tube containing an inflatable balloon tip and pressure transducer is inserted into the rectum (Fig. 25-6). First, rectal compliance and sensation may be determined by sequentially inflating a rectal balloon to various volumes. Decreased rectal compliance may be noted by an inability to inflate a balloon to typical volumes without patient discomfort. This may indicate a rectal reservoir that is unable to appropriately store stool. In contrast, decreased perception of balloon insufflation may indicate neuropathy.

Second, sphincter reflexes are also assessed during pressure measurements. During balloon insufflation, relaxation of the IAS should accompany rectal distention via the rectoanal inhibitory reflex (p. 563).

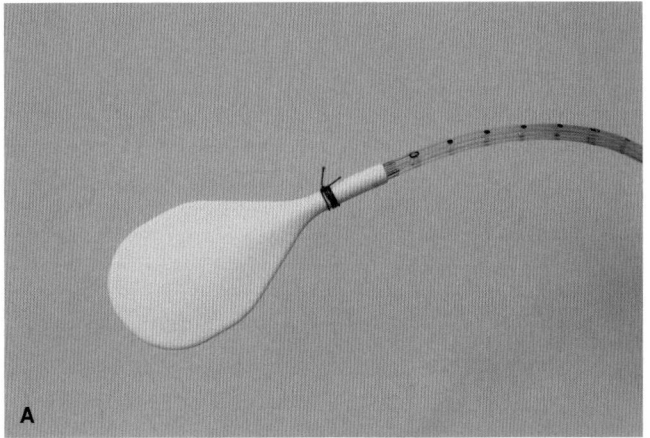
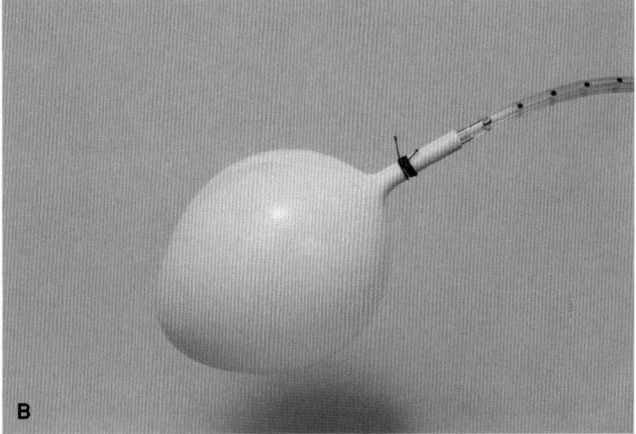

FIGURE 25-6 Manometry tube and balloon, empty **(A)** and after filling **(B)**.

Third, IAS resting pressure and EAS squeeze pressure are then measured at incremental points as the balloon is slowly withdrawn from the rectum. In general, decreased pressure readings may indicate structural disruption, myopathy, or neuropathy. As an additional test, the rectal balloon expulsion test may be performed as a patient simulates defecation and expels the balloon. The balloon expulsion test is mainly used in patients with constipation and attempts to differentiate between obstructed constipation and functional constipation (Minguez, 2004).

The main limitation with manometry is that normal values may be seen in incontinent patients and vice versa. Despite this disadvantage, anal manometry plays an important role in AI evaluation.

Endoanal Ultrasonography. Also known as transanal sonography, this technique is now the primary diagnostic imaging technique to evaluate the integrity, thickness, and length of the IAS and EAS (Fig. 25-7). It is performed for many patients during FI testing, especially if sphincter integrity is in question. The technique uses a rotating endoprobe with a ≥10-MHz transducer, which provides a 360-degree evaluation of the anal canal. Sonography gel is placed on the probe tip, which is sheathed with a condom prior to insertion into the anus. This tool allows diagnosis of anterior anal sphincter defects in women with a known history of clinically diagnosed anal sphincter disruption and also in those with unrecognized or misdiagnosed defects at the time of delivery. Prior to the common use of endoanal sonography (EAUS), women with these "occult"—that is, solely sonographically diagnosed—anal sphincter defects were labeled as having "idiopathic" FI and were not considered good candidates for surgical correction.

In addition to the anal sphincters, this modality can image the puborectalis muscle and perineal body. Oberwalder and colleagues (2004) showed that in a group of incontinent women, perineal body thickness <10 mm was associated with anal sphincter defects in 97 percent of cases, whereas perineal body thicknesses of 10 to 12 mm were associated with sphincter defect in only one third of patients with FI. Perineal body thickness >12 mm was infrequently associated with these defects.

Newer techniques may also be informative. For example, dynamic endoanal or transperineal ultrasound can permit functional assessment of the anorectum, similar to defecography, described next (Vitton, 2011).

Evacuation Proctography. During this radiographic test, also known as defecography, the rectum is opacified with a thick barium paste, and the small bowel fills with a barium suspension given orally. Radiographic or fluoroscopic imaging is then obtained while a patient is resting, contracting her sphincter, coughing, and straining to expel the barium.

This test of dynamic rectal emptying and anorectal anatomy is not widely used to assess evacuation disorders unless obstructive causes for AI are suspected. Accordingly, it may be obtained if intussusception, internal rectal prolapse, enterocele, or failed relaxation of the puborectalis muscle during defecation is a concern.

Magnetic Resonance Imaging. Magnetic resonance (MR) imaging of the anal sphincter complex can be done either with an endoanal coil placed in the anorectum or with external phased-array coils. This latter external coil technique is preferred because physical anatomy is less distorted and the lack of an intraluminal coil increases patient comfort (Van Koughnett, 2013a). MR imaging is more expensive than EAUS, and its value for anal sphincter evaluation is controversial on several points. First, EAUS is more sensitive in detecting IAS

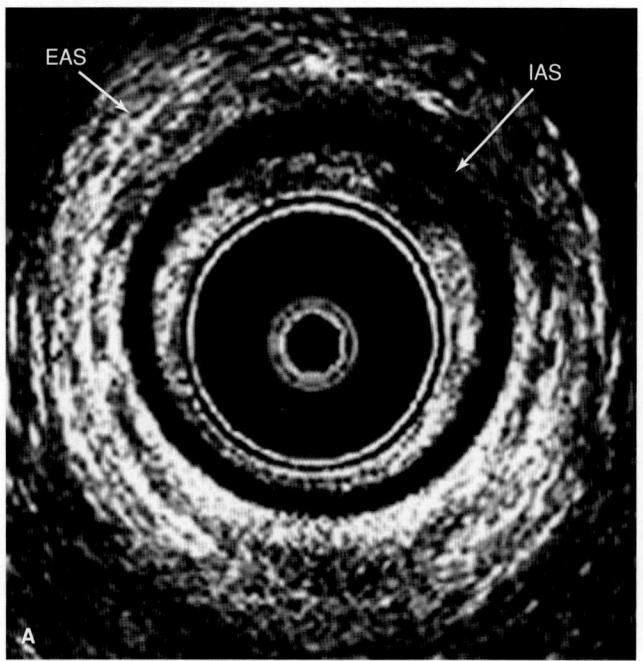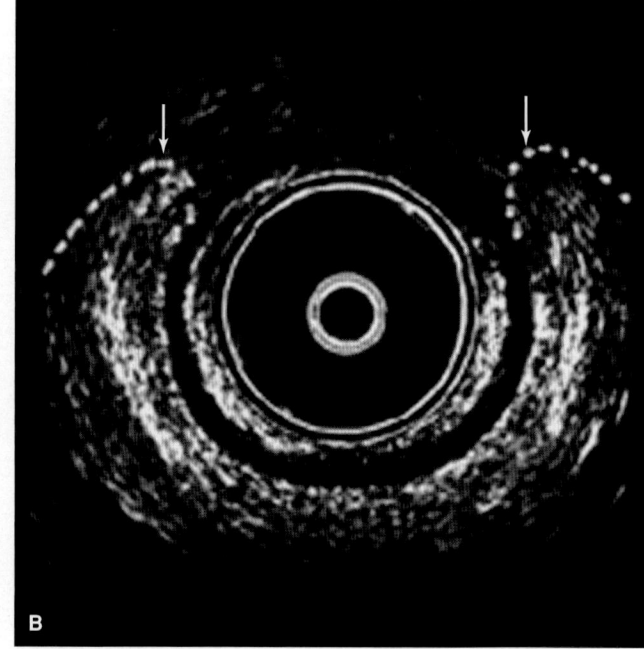

FIGURE 25-7 Cross-sectional anal endosonography images at level of mid anal canal. **A.** A woman with normal anal sphincters. **B.** Anterior defects of the external and internal anal sphincter muscles. EAS = external anal sphincter; IAS = internal anal sphincter. Dashed lines and (*arrows*) in B illustrate the ends of the torn EAS.

abnormalities, whereas MR imaging is more sensitive in visualizing EAS morphology, including atrophy (Beets-Tan, 2001; Rociu, 1999). This may have value preoperatively, as patients with EAS atrophy may have poorer results following anal sphincteroplasty compared with those without atrophy (Briel, 1999). Second, MR imaging results vary considerably among interpreters and depend on their experience level. Thus, either EAUS or MR imaging can only be recommended in FI evaluation if sufficient experience is available (Terra, 2006).

Another MR imaging modality, termed dynamic MR imaging, allows dynamic examination of rectal emptying and evaluation of pelvic floor muscles during rest, squeeze, and defecation (Gearhart, 2004; Kaufman, 2001). Thus, it simultaneously permits a survey of pelvic anatomy, organ prolapse, and defecatory function. This may be particularly appealing to patients requiring multiple anorectal tests (Khatri, 2014; Van Koughnett, 2013a). However, it is technically difficult, more expensive, and again requires an experienced radiologist. Moreover, other than avoiding the ionizing radiation of evacuation proctography, this technique offers no advantage for studying rectal function. In addition, the variability of pelvic MR imaging measurements among readers is high (Lockhart, 2008). Despite these limitations, this test has been increasingly adopted in many academic settings, including our institution.

Electromyography. This test uses a needle or surface electrode to record electrical activity of muscles at rest and during contraction. During needle electromyography (EMG), needle electrodes are inserted through the skin into a muscle, and electrical activity detected by these electrodes is displayed graphically. In evaluation of AI, EMG may be used to assess the neuromuscular integrity of the EAS and puborectalis muscle. Specifically, by measuring action potentials from muscle motor units, EMG can help clarify which portions of these muscles are contracting and relaxing appropriately. Additionally, following injury, muscle may be partially or completely denervated, and compensatory reinnervation may then follow. Patterns characteristic of such denervation and reinnervation may be identified with EMG.

Unlike needle electrodes, surface patch electrodes are placed on the darker-skinned area of the anus, cause little discomfort to the patient, and carry no risk of infection. However, this technique is prone to artifacts. In comparing the two, needle EMG is painful but provides useful information regarding sphincter innervation. Surface EMG may be best used during repetitive biofeedback sessions. In general, its use is limited to research centers.

Pudendal Nerve Terminal Motor Latency Test. This stimulation test of the pudendal nerve measures the time delay between electrical nerve stimulation and EAS motor response. This delay, also termed latency, if prolonged, may indicate pudendal nerve pathology, which may be a cause of AI.

During pudendal nerve terminal motor latency (PNTML) testing, a stimulating electrode positioned on an examiner's gloved fingertip is connected to a pulsed-stimulus generator. The pudendal nerves are transanally stimulated through the lateral walls of the rectum at the level of the ischial spines by this electrode. The action potential response of the EAS is received by recording electrodes at the base of the examining finger and registered on an oscilloscope.

Although PNTML prolongation has long been considered a marker of idiopathic FI, this test provides little information regarding FI etiology. PNTML results have been contradictory and this test is not endorsed by many experts, including the American Gastroenterological Association (Diamant, 1999). Moreover, the relationship of pudendal nerve function, typically assessed by PNTML, to sphincteroplasty outcome remains unclear (Madoff, 2004a). One study found no association between pudendal nerve status and long-term postoperative anal continence (Malouf, 2000). Accordingly, it has been replaced by more specific and sensitive tests for sphincter muscle innervation such as EMG (Barnett, 1999). Currently, needle electromyography is the only available technique for documenting neurogenic injury but is performed only in select academic centers and mostly in the context of research clinical trials.

Unfortunately, EMG and PNTML do not provide an assessment of all the peripheral nerves that innervate the anorectum. In addition, both tests are associated with patient discomfort. These significant limitations have prevented widespread acceptance or use of needle EMG and PNTML testing. Currently, anorectal neurologic injury is assessed by performing anal EMG or PNTML but only in specialized centers. Newer and less invasive approaches for documenting neurogenic injury have been described and are under investigation (Meyer, 2014; Rao, 2014).

Colonoscopy and Barium Enema. Based on the history and physical examination, these tests may be indicated to exclude inflammatory bowel conditions or malignancy.

■ Treatment

Nonsurgical Treatment

Treatment of FI is highly individualized and dependent on etiology, severity, available treatment options, and patient health. Because FI etiology is often multifactorial, treatments that target only one mechanism (such as sphincter weakness) are unlikely to benefit all patients with FI. Moreover, because current surgical outcomes are less than optimal, most patients, even those with anatomic defects, are initially treated conservatively. Of conservative options, management may include patient education, normalization of stool consistency, behavioral techniques, and daily pelvic floor muscle strengthening exercises (Whitehead, 2015).

Medical Management. For patients with minor incontinence, the use of bulking agents can thicken stool consistency and create feces that are firmer and easier to control (Table 25-6). Common side effects such as abdominal distention and bloating can be improved by starting with smaller doses or switching to a different agent. In support of this practice, a small randomized trial showed that fiber supplementation decreased diarrhea-associated FI (Bliss, 2001). However, evidence that fiber supplements benefit patients with constipation-associated FI is lacking.

Also to bulk stool, agents that slow fecal intestinal transit time can reduce overall stool volume by increasing the time available for the colon to reabsorb fluid from stool. One such agent, loperamide hydrochloride (Imodium), also increases anal resting tone and thus may even benefit patients with FI

TABLE 25-6. Medical Management of Fecal Incontinence

Treatment	Brand Name	Oral Dosage
Bulking agents		
Psyllium	Metamucil	1 tbsp. mixed into 8 oz. of water 1–3 times daily
Psyllium	Konsyl	1 tsp. mixed into 8 oz. of water 1–3 times daily
Methylcellulose	Citrucel	1 tbsp. mixed into 8 oz. of water 1–3 times daily
Loperamide hydrochloride	Imodium	2–4 mg, 1–4 times daily to a maximum daily dose of 16 mg
Diphenoxylate hydrochloride	Lomotil	5 mg, 1–4 times daily to a maximum daily dose of 20 mg
Amitriptyline	Generic	10–25 mg at bedtime; increase by 10–25 mg weekly up to 75–150 mg at bedtime or a therapeutic drug level

and no diarrhea (Read, 1982). Side effects are uncommon and include dry mouth. One ongoing trial is comparing loperamide and oral placebo for FI treatment (National Institute of Child Health and Human Development, 2014).

Diphenoxylate hydrochloride (Lomotil) is used in the same capacity as loperamide, and dosing is similar. Although diphenoxylate is a Schedule V substance, potential for physical dependence is minimal. Of other possible medications, amitriptyline is a tricyclic antidepressant that can be used to treat idiopathic FI. Although the mechanism of action is poorly understood, some of its beneficial effects may be related to its anticholinergic properties. Other agents such as cholestyramine and clonidine, an α-adrenergic agonist, have been studied, but current data are limited (Whitehead, 2015). The laxative lactulose aids some nursing home residents with FI associated with fecal impaction (Omar, 2013).

To guide drug selection, one systematic review analyzed pharmacologic agent use for FI treatment in adults (Omar, 2013). These reviewers noted that antidiarrheal drugs improve diarrhea-associated FI more than placebo, and loperamide is more effective than diphenoxylate. However, overall, they commented on the poor quality of evidence.

Bowel Management. Daily, timed, tap-water enemas or glycerin or bisacodyl suppositories (Dulcolax) may be used to empty the rectum after eating. These provide acceptable and helpful options for some patients with constipation symptoms associated with AI. These may include women with normal stool consistency but difficulty evacuating due to anatomic reasons such as rectocele with stool trapping or those with denervation and impaired rectal sensation. All these may lead to accumulation of a large mass of solid stool in the rectum and leaking of loose stool around it. Bulking agents can be used concurrently with these evacuation methods to diminish stooling between desired defecations.

Biofeedback and Pelvic Floor Therapy. Biofeedback is usually selected to increase neuromuscular conditioning. Specifically, for FI, therapy goals aim to improve anal sphincter strength, sensory awareness of stool presence, and coordination between the rectum and the anal sphincter (Rao, 1998). Treatment protocols are individualized and dictated by the underlying dysfunction. Accordingly, the number and frequency of sessions required for improvement varies, but

commonly three to six 1-hour, weekly or biweekly appointments are needed. In many cases, reinforcing sessions at various subsequent intervals are also recommended.

Biofeedback has been noted to be an effective treatment for FI, and up to 80 percent of treated patients show symptom improvement (Engel, 1974; Jensen, 1997; Norton, 2001). Despite this, one Cochrane review found insufficient evidence of biofeedback's benefits for FI (Norton, 2012). However, a randomized controlled trial by Heymen and coworkers (2009) offers support. These investigators initially provided education materials and instruction regarding fiber supplements and/or antidiarrheal medication. Patients who were adequately treated by these strategies (21 percent) were excluded from further study. The remaining 107 patients, who remained incontinent and dissatisfied, then progressed to treatment, either biofeedback or pelvic floor exercises. Biofeedback training more effectively reduced FI severity and number of days with FI. Moreover, 3 months after training, 76 percent of biofeedback patients reported adequate relief of FI symptoms compared with only 41 percent of patients treated with pelvic floor exercises. Twelve months later, biofeedback improvement persisted.

The results of this and other trials suggest that biofeedback may not be necessary for patients with milder FI symptoms. However, for those with more severe FI symptoms, instrument-assisted biofeedback is effective (Whitehead, 2015).

Pelvic Floor Muscle Strengthening. Also known as Kegel exercises, active pelvic floor muscle training (PFMT) exercises voluntary contract the levator ani muscles. Performance of these exercises is fully described in Chapter 23 (p. 528). As noted, these alone are less effective than biofeedback for patients with more severe FI symptoms (Heymen, 2009). However, exercises are safe and inexpensive and may benefit patients with mild symptoms, especially if performed in conjunction with other interventions, such as patient education, diet modification, and medical management.

In contrast to active PFMT, anal musculature can be passively stimulated electrically by electrodes. However, when used as sole therapy, electrical stimulation of the anus appears to be ineffective (Whitehead, 2015).

Surgical Treatment

Currently available FI surgical procedures are often associated with less than optimal results and with postoperative morbidity.

Accordingly, surgery is reserved for those patients with major structural abnormalities of the anal sphincter(s), those with severe symptoms, and those who fail to respond to conservative management.

Anal Sphincteroplasty. This is the most commonly performed FI corrective operation. Repair of the EAS and/or IAS is indicated for women with acquired AI and an anterior sphincter defect following an obstetric or iatrogenic injury. Two methods may be used for sphincter repair and include an end-to-end technique and an overlapping method, both described in Section 45-25 (p. 1125). The end-to-end technique is most frequently used by obstetricians to reapproximate torn ends of an anal sphincter at delivery. However, in patients remote from delivery with a sphincter defect and FI, the overlapping technique is preferred by most colorectal surgeons and urogynecologists.

With the overlapping method performed remote from delivery, short-term continence improvements of 67 percent were previously reported (Madoff, 2004a). However, recent reports show significant deterioration of continence during long-term postoperative surveillance (Bravo Gutierrez, 2004; Glasgow, 2012). In a single, retrospective study, no patients remained completely continent to liquid and solid stool at 10 years (Zutshi, 2009). Hypotheses regarding this deterioration include aging, scarring, and progressive pudendal neuropathy related either to initial injury or to repair. Patients who fail to improve after anal sphincteroplasty and who are found to have a persistent sphincter defect may be candidates for a second sphincteroplasty. However, those with an intact sphincter following repair and persistent symptoms are only considered candidates for conservative management or one of the salvage or minimally invasive surgical procedures described later.

Currently, no conclusive evidence supports that the overlapping method, if used at delivery, leads to results superior to those obtained with the traditional end-to-end method of anal sphincter repair (Farrell, 2012; Fitzpatrick, 2000; Garcia, 2005). Moreover, overlapping repair requires increased technical skills and carries the potential for increased blood loss, operating time, and pudendal neuropathy. For these reasons, the end-to-end technique is likely to remain the standard method for sphincter reapproximation at delivery until further data from randomized trials are available. Importantly, primary prevention of these lacerations should continue to be emphasized.

Diversion (Colostomy or Ileostomy). Diversion is reserved for patients with incapacitating FI who have failed other treatments (Sections 46-17 and 46-19, p. 1192). For these selected patients, such procedures can significantly improve their quality of life.

Other Major Surgeries. Of these, gracilis muscle transposition is advocated for patients who have failed sphincter repair or those with a sphincter defect too large to allow muscle reapproximation (Baeten, 1991). Dynamic gracilloplasty separates the gracilis tendon from its point of insertion at the knee, wraps the muscle around the anus, and attaches the tendon to the contralateral ischial tuberosity. To squeeze the anus closed, the gracilis muscle is then stimulated with an electrical pulse generator that is implanted in the abdominal wall. This procedure is not currently performed in the United States, as the pulse generator is not approved by the Food and Drug Administration (FDA) (Cera, 2005).

Implanting an artificial anal sphincter is another option to mimic sphincter function, but again, it is infrequently performed in the United States. With this, a fluid-inflated cuff is implanted around the anus, a reservoir balloon is placed within the abdominal wall, and a control pump is inserted into one labium majus. When fully inflated, the cuff occludes the anal canal. When defecation is desired, the control pump in the labia is squeezed to move fluid from the anal cuff into the reservoir balloon. The cuff, when fluid-empty, relaxes pressure around the anus and permits defecation. The fluid within the reservoir then returns to the anal cuff to restore circumferential pressure and continence (Christiansen, 1987).

A third procedure, postanal pelvic floor repair, has largely been abandoned. The procedure is designed to reestablish the anorectal angle and to lengthen and tighten the anal canal. Through an intersphincteric approach, sutures are placed between the ends of the iliococcygeus, pubococcygeus, puborectalis, and external anal sphincter muscles. Although originally reported to improved incontinence in up to 80 percent of patients, similar results have not been replicated (Browning, 1983; Deen, 1993; Parks, 1975).

Minimally Invasive Procedures

Sacral Nerve Stimulation. In 2011, the FDA approved sacral nerve stimulation (SNS) for FI treatment. Also known as sacral neuromodulation, this surgery is typically offered to women who have failed to adequately improve with multiple other conservative therapies, and a full description of the InterStim System procedure appears in Section 45-12 (p. 1085). To summarize, an electrode is placed near the S3 nerve root and connected to a temporary pulse generator. Electrical charges to this nerve root may modulate abnormal afferent impulses, although the exact mechanism of SNS action for FI remains unknown (Gourcerol, 2011). Patients who show ≥50 percent improvement during the temporary test phase are eligible for a permanent pulse generator.

In one prospective trial, 90 percent of 133 patients proceeded from temporary to permanent stimulation (Wexner, 2010). For this study, therapeutic success was defined as a 50-percent or greater reduction of incontinent episodes per week compared with baseline. At 12 months, 83 percent of subjects achieved therapeutic success, and 41 percent achieved 100 percent fecal continence. At 24 months, therapeutic success was found in 85 percent. At 5 years, 89 percent were deemed a therapeutic success, and 36 percent reported complete continence (Hull, 2013). Limited data are available from patients with an underlying EAS defect, but these suggest that SNS is also effective for this group (Chan, 2008; Matzel, 2011).

Percutaneous Tibial Nerve Stimulation. The posterior tibial nerve contains fibers from the sacral nerves. Stimulation of its peripheral fibers transmits impulses to the sacral nerves and reflexively neuromodulates the rectum and anal sphincters (Shafik, 2003). Percutaneous tibial nerve stimulation (PTNS) is carried out with a needle inserted through the ankle skin in a position posterior and superior to the medial malleolus. This needle is then coupled with an electronic pulse generator. Outpatient stimulation sessions usually last 30 minutes and are provided one to three times weekly. Suitable candidates have criteria similar to those for SNS.

One review of 13 studies showed that 62 to 82 percent of patients reported at least a 50-percent reduction in the frequency of FI episodes (Thomas, 2013). Compared with the InterStim System, PTNS requires repetitive treatments to maintain effectiveness. However, PTNS is a minimally invasive outpatient technique with almost no associated morbidity (Thin, 2013). A randomized controlled trial comparing SNS and PTNS in the treatment for FI is currently in progress (Marti, 2015).

Bulking Agent Injection. Injecting inert substances around the anal canal in patients with FI aims to increase resting anal canal pressure (Shafik, 1993). Although many patients with FI may be candidates for injectables, the ideal candidate is one who has seepage or mild to moderate FI, who has failed medical management, but who is not yet ready to undergo surgery (Van Koughnett, 2013b).

The results of a large multicenter randomized controlled trial support the efficacy of dextranomer injections compared with sham injections (Graf, 2011). At 3 months, 52 percent of the dextranomer-injected patients had at least a 50-percent decline in FI frequency, whereas only 31 percent of sham-treated patients achieved this reduction. A surveillance study showed that benefits persisted for 36 months (Mellgren, 2014).

Secca Procedure. This outpatient procedure is currently used in the United States to treat FI in patients with no evidence of sphincter defects or pudendal neuropathy. It delivers temperature-controlled radiofrequency energy to the IAS by means of a specifically designed anoscope. Resulting tissue heating is believed to cause collagen contraction followed by focal wound healing, remodeling, and tightening. Studies to date have involved only small cohorts. Efron and colleagues (2003) showed a median 70-percent resolution of symptoms in 50 patients. However, one retrospective series showed long-term benefit in only 22 percent, and most patients underwent additional treatments (Abbas, 2012).

Other Therapies. Several other treatment options are currently under investigation. First, a mesh sling can be inserted surgically through small incisions lateral to the anus. By a transobturator approach, the mesh is then tunneled beneath the puborectalis muscle to add support. A trial evaluating this technique has been completed, but long-term results are not yet available.

Second, a vaginally placed bowel-control device offers a nonsurgical option. The vaginal insert contains a silicone-coated stainless steel base and posteriorly directed balloon. Using a pump, the vaginal insert is inflated to collaterally occlude the rectum. Thus, its primary limitation mirrors that for vaginal pessaries, namely, that not all women are successfully fitted. In one study, this device significantly improved objective and subjective measures of FI (Richter, 2015). Approximately 86

percent of patients considered bowel symptoms "very much better" or "much better." Moreover, no serious adverse events were reported. However, longer-term outcome data are needed.

Anal plugs present another therapy option, but most current devices are uncomfortable and poorly tolerated. However, newer models made of softer material are under investigation (Meyer, 2014).

Last, magnetic beads strung on an elastic band can be inserted surgically around the anal canal to increase the resting pressure. Small studies have shown continence results comparable to the artificial anal sphincter and to SNS but with fewer complications (Whitehead, 2015). However, this device is not yet approved in the United States.

FUNCTIONAL ANORECTAL DISORDERS

In the current classification of functional gastrointestinal disorders, three functional anorectal disorders are recognized: (1) functional FI, (2) functional anorectal pain, and (3) functional defecation disorders (Table 11-6, p. 266) (Drossman, 2006). Criteria for these and other functional GI disorders have been defined by the Rome III Foundation expert consensus organization and are primarily diagnosed based on patients' reported symptoms. As with other functional disorders, organic disease is excluded prior to assignment of these diagnoses.

■ Functional Fecal Incontinence

Functional FI is defined by Rome III criteria as recurrent uncontrolled passage of fecal material for more than 3 months in an individual with anatomically normal defecatory muscles that function abnormally. As a result, fecal retention or diarrhea is common, and psychologic disorders may be associated. The etiology is varied, and causes may include disturbed intestinal motility, poor rectal compliance, impaired rectal sensation, and weakened pelvic floor muscles (Whitehead, 2001). Once diagnosed, functional FI is primarily treated with medical management or biofeedback, as described earlier.

■ Functional Anorectal Pain

Categories within this group are differentiated from one another by the duration of pain and by the presence or lack of associated puborectalis muscle tenderness. Levator ani syndrome, also known as levator ani spasm, usually presents as a pressure or ache in the upper rectum (Chap. 11, p. 269). Rome III criteria require that symptoms be present for more than 3 months; that episodes last at least 20 minutes; and that symptoms be associated with puborectalis muscle tenderness when palpated. In contrast, proctalgia fugax presents as sudden, severe anal or lower rectal pain that lasts for a few seconds to a few minutes. Pain may disrupt normal activities, but episodes rarely occur more than five times a year.

Treatments for levator ani syndrome are varied and may include, among others, trigger-point release maneuvers, biofeedback, local heat, and pharmacologic agents such as nonsteroidal antiinflammatory drugs, other analgesics, muscle relaxants, and tranquilizers. In contrast, proctalgia fugax is typically managed with reassurance.

Functional Defecation Disorders

This group of disorders includes dyssynergic defecation and inadequate defecatory propulsion disorders. Dyssynergic defecation is also called pelvic floor dyssynergia, anismus, outlet obstruction constipation, or spastic pelvic floor syndrome. It is characterized by failed relaxation of the puborectalis muscle and EAS, which is needed for normal defecation. This condition is common and is thought to account for 25 to 50 percent of chronic constipation cases (Bharucha, 2014; Wald, 1990). Symptoms include chronic straining and impaired or incomplete evacuation. Diagnosis requires confirmation by EMG, manometry, or radiologic testing that shows persistent contraction of these muscles during attempted defecation. Other causes of constipation should also be excluded.

The treatment of constipation is challenging and often ineffective. Schiller and associates (1984) showed that only 53 percent of patients were satisfied with traditional medical therapies. Biofeedback interventions for dyssynergic defecation teach patients to relax their pelvic floor and anal sphincter muscles while simultaneously increasing intraabdominal and intrarectal pressures (Valsalva maneuver). The efficacy of biofeedback compared with laxatives in treating dyssynergic defecation was demonstrated in a controlled trial by Chiarioni and coworkers (2006). Moreover, biofeedback benefits were sustained at 1-year follow-up. In a prospective randomized trial by Rao and associates (2007), biofeedback efficacy was compared with sham feedback therapy and with standard therapy (diet, exercise, laxatives) in 77 subjects with chronic constipation and dyssynergic defecation. Subjects in the biofeedback group had a greater number of complete spontaneous bowel movements and greater satisfaction with bowel function and were more likely to discontinue the use of digital maneuvers than subjects receiving standard or sham therapy. In addition, colonic transit time significantly improved in biofeedback and standard therapy subjects but not in subjects who received sham feedback, suggesting that colonic transit slowing is due to dyssynergia. These findings emphasize the importance of performing neuromuscular conditioning and modifying the underlying physiologic behavior to correct dyssynergia and improve bowel function. Based on current data, biofeedback therapy is the preferred treatment for patients with dyssynergic defecation and chronic constipation, especially for those who have failed diet, exercise, and/or laxative therapy.

Sacral nerve stimulation, described on page 571, is a promising therapeutic option for patients with intractable constipation. Although not yet approved in the United States for this indication, a prospective study showed that SNS effectively treated idiopathic slow- and normal-transit constipation refractory to conservative measures (Kamm, 2010). In this study, primary end points were increased defecation frequency, decreased straining, and decreased sensation of incomplete evacuation. Of 62 patients who underwent a temporary-generator trial, 73 percent proceeded to permanent generator implantation. Treatment success was achieved in 87 percent of these patients.

RECTOVAGINAL FISTULA

Definition and Classification

Rectovaginal fistulas (RVFs) are congenital or acquired epithelial lined tracts between the vagina and rectum. They are classified according to their location, size, and etiology. All of these features assist selection of the appropriate management and prediction of surgical repair outcome. Of factors, the underlying cause of a fistula is the most important predictor of outcome success, as it takes into account tissue and overall patient health (Table 25-7).

Most RVFs are related to obstetric events and occur in the distal third of the vagina just above the hymen (Fig. 25-8) (Greenwald, 1978; Lowry, 1988; Tsang, 1998). Defect diameters range from less than 1 mm to several centimeters, and most communicate with the rectum at or above the pectinate (dentate) line (Fig. 38-21, p. 815). In contrast, fistulas with an opening below the dentate line are also appropriately called anovaginal fistulas. Surgical management of these "low" RVFs depends on the condition of the EAS but is usually achieved by a perineal (transvaginal or transanal) approach. Midlevel RVFs are found in the middle third of the vagina, whereas

---

TABLE 25-7. Rectovaginal Fistula Risk Factors

Obstetric complications
Third- or fourth-degree laceration repair dehiscence
Unrecognized vaginal laceration during operative vaginal or precipitous delivery

Inflammatory bowel disease
Most commonly Crohn disease
Ulcerative colitis less common, as it is not a transmural disease

Infection
Most commonly cryptoglandular abscess located in the anterior aspect of the anal canal
Lymphogranuloma venereum
Tuberculosis
Bartholin abscess
Human immunodeficiency virus infection
Diverticular disease

Previous surgery in the anorectal area
Hemorrhoidectomy
Low anterior resection
Excision of rectal tumors
Hysterectomy
Posterior vaginal wall repairs

Pelvic radiation therapy

Neoplasm
Invasive cervical or vaginal cancer
Anal or rectal cancer

Trauma
Intraoperative
Coital

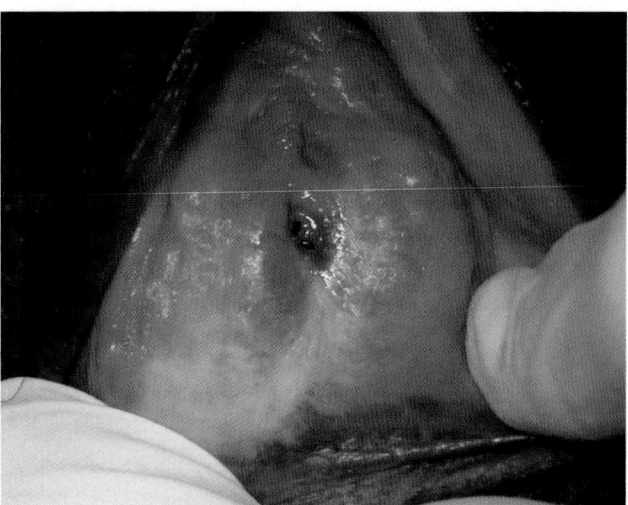

FIGURE 25-8 Rectovaginal fistula in the distal wall of the posterior vagina in a woman who sustained a fourth-degree perineal laceration.

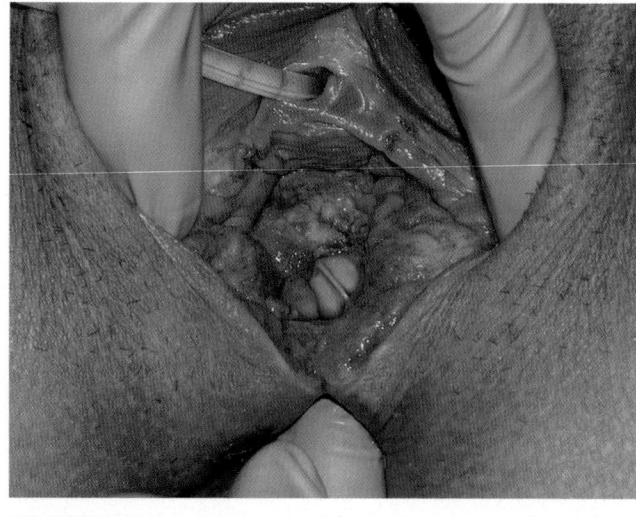

FIGURE 25-9 Large rectovaginal fistula in a woman who underwent midline episiotomy. Note that the fistula is above an intact external anal sphincter.

high rectovaginal fistulas have their vaginal communication close to the cervix or the vaginal cuff. In cases with high RVFs, fistulas may open into the sigmoid colon. These fistulas may not be readily seen during examination. They often require contrast or endoscopic studies for diagnosis and an abdominal approach for repair.

■ Diagnosis

Patients with RVF usually complain of flatus or stool leakage per vagina. They may also present with recurrent bladder or vaginal infection, rectal or vaginal bleeding, and pain. Symptoms often suggest the underlying etiology. For example, patients with obstetric injury and large defects of the anterior portion of the anal sphincters may have gross fecal incontinence. In contrast, those with an infectious or inflammatory process may complain of diarrhea, abdominal cramping, and fevers in addition to passage of stool per vagina.

During physical examination, most low RVFs can be visualized during inspection of the perineum and distal portion of the posterior vaginal wall. Rectovaginal examination allows assessment of the thickness of the perineal body and anovaginal wall and may allow palpation and visualization of the actual defect. Some RVFs that are not readily seen on initial examination can be identified by noting air bubbles at the fistula's vaginal opening after filling the vagina with water. Alternatively, methylene blue can be instilled in the rectum after a tampon is placed in the vagina. The fistula and a gross assessment of its location can be identified by inspecting the level of blue staining on the tampon following its removal.

If the fistula site is not determined by the preceding maneuvers, a contrast study is indicated. These include barium enema or computed tomography (CT) scanning.

Unless RVFs are obviously due to a prior obstetric event, a biopsy of the fistulous tract is indicated to investigate possible malignancy or inflammatory conditions. In addition, proctoscopy or colonoscopy is often warranted if inflammatory bowel disease, malignancy, or gastrointestinal infection is suspected.

■ Treatment

Treatment of RVF depends on the underlying etiology and the defect's size and location. Some women with small RVFs following obstetric trauma may be followed conservatively in anticipation of spontaneous healing of the fistulous tract (Goldaber, 1993; Rahman, 2003). If surgical repair is required, it is delayed until surrounding tissues are free of edema, induration, and infection (Wiskind, 1992).

Larger obstetric-related defects and other low fistulas are most often corrected surgically (Fig. 25-9). Surgical techniques include: (1) a transvaginal or transanal approach through episioproctotomy (conversion of the defect into a complete perineal tear, that is, a fourth-degree laceration), (2) a fistulotomy with transvaginal purse-string method of repair without episioproctotomy, or (3) a fistulotomy with a tension-free layered closure without episioproctotomy. A further description of this last operation is found in Section 45-26 of the atlas (p. 1128). Additionally, endorectal flap advancement is used by colorectal surgeons primarily for the treatment of complex perianal fistulas such as those with tract diameters >2.5 cm or those related to trauma or infection (MacRae, 1995). With flap advancement, the fistulous tract is excised, a broad-based flap of rectal wall is employed to obliterate the fistula's origin, and sphincter muscle division is avoided. Of these methods, better outcomes have been shown following RVF repair using anal sphincteroplasties compared with endorectal advancement flap (Tsang, 1998). In patients with low RVFs, preoperative endoanal ultrasonography of the EAS is important. For example, an episioproctotomy is avoided if the sphincter is intact (Hull, 2007).

Midlevel vaginal fistulas are also often due to obstetric trauma and are repaired transvaginally or transanally by a tension-free layered closure or an endorectal advancement flap. High fistulas are most commonly repaired by a transabdominal approach using bowel resection of the involved segment followed by primary bowel reanastomosis.

Success rates vary depending on the underlying cause and method of repair. Successful repairs following obstetric injury vary from 78 to 100 percent (Khanduja, 1999; Tsang, 1998). Success rates of 40 to 50 percent are reported with the rectal advancement flaps and of 74 percent with episioproctotomy (Mizrahi, 2002; Sonoda, 2002). Fistulas due to other etiologies such as radiation, cancer, or active inflammatory bowel disease are more difficult to treat successfully. In general, success rates are highest with the first surgical attempt at repair (Lowry, 1988).

REFERENCES

Abbas MA, Tam MS, Chun LJ: Radiofrequency treatment for fecal incontinence: is it effective long-term? Dis Colon Rectum 55:605, 2012

Abrams P, Cardozo L, Khoury S, et al: Incontinence. Third International Consultation on Incontinence, Monaco, 2004. Public Health Publications, 2005, p 286

Baeten CG, Konsten J, Spaans F, et al: Dynamic graciloplasty for treatment of faecal incontinence. Lancet 338(8776):1163, 1991

Barber MD, Bremer RE, Thor KB, et al: Innervation of the female levator ani muscles. Am J Obstet Gynecol 187(1):64, 2002

Barnett JL, Hasler WL, Camilleri M: American Gastroenterological Association medical position statement on anorectal testing techniques. Gastroenterology 116(3):732, 1999

Beets-Tan RG, Morren GL, Beets GL, et al: Measurement of anal sphincter muscles: endoanal US, endoanal MR imaging, or phased-array MR imaging? A study with healthy volunteers. Radiology 220(1):81, 2001

Bharucha AE: Outcome measures for fecal incontinence: anorectal structure and function. Gastroenterology 126(1 Suppl 1):S90, 2004

Bharucha AE: Pelvic floor: anatomy and function. Neurogastroenterol Motil 18(7):507, 2006

Bharucha AE, Daube J, Litchy W, et al: Anal sphincteric neurogenic injury in asymptomatic nulliparous women and fecal incontinence. Am J Physiol Gastrointest Liver Physiol 303:G256, 2012

Bharucha AE, Dunivan G, Goode PS, et al: Epidemiology, pathophysiology, and classification of fecal incontinence: state of the science summary for the National Institute of Diabetes and Digestive and Kidney Diseases (NIDDK) workshop. Am J Gastroenterol 110(1):127, 2015

Bharucha AE, Rao SC: An update on anorectal disorders for gastroenterologists. Gastroenterology 146:37, 2014

Bliss DZ, Jung HJ, Savik K, et al: Supplementation with dietary fiber improves fecal incontinence. Nurs Res 50:203, 2001

Boreham MK, Richter HE, Kenton KS, et al: Anal incontinence in women presenting for gynecologic care: prevalence, risk factors, and impact upon quality of life. Am J Obstet Gynecol 192(5):1637, 2005

Borello-France D, Burgio KL, Richter HE, et al: Fecal and urinary incontinence in primiparous women. Obstet Gynecol 108(4):863, 2006

Bravo Gutierrez A, Madoff RD, Lowry AC, et al: Long-term results of anterior sphincteroplasty. Dis Colon Rectum 47(5):727, 2004

Briel JW, Stoker J, Rociu E, et al: External anal sphincter atrophy on endoanal magnetic resonance imaging adversely affects continence after sphincteroplasty. Br J Surg 86(10):1322, 1999

Brown HW, Wexner SD, Segall MM, et al: Accidental bowel leakage in the mature women's health study: prevalence and predictors. Int J Clin Pract 66:1101, 2012

Browning GG, Parks AG: Post-anal repair for neuropathic fecal incontinence—correlation of clinical-result and anal-canal pressures. Br J Surg 70(2):101, 1983

Buser WD, Miner PB: Delayed rectal sensation with fecal incontinence. Gastroenterology 91:1186, 1986

Cera SM, Wexner SD: Muscle transposition: does it still have a role? Clin Colon Rectal Surg 18(1):46, 2005

Chan MK, Tjandra JJ: Sacral nerve stimulation for fecal incontinence: external anal sphincter defect vs. intact anal sphincter. Dis Colon Rectum 51:1015, 2008

Chiarioni G, Whitehead WE, Pezza V, et al: Biofeedback is superior to laxatives for normal transit constipation due to pelvic floor dyssynergia. Gastroenterology 130(3):657, 2006

Christiansen J, Lorentzen M: Implantation of artificial sphincter for anal incontinence. Lancet 2(8553):244, 1987

Deen KI, Oya M, Ortiz J, et al: Randomized trial comparing three forms of pelvic floor repair for neuropathic faecal incontinence. Br J Surg 80:794, 1993

Degen LP, Phillips SF: How well does stool form reflect colonic transit? Gut 39(1):109, 1996

Diamant NE, Kamm MA, Wald A, et al: AGA technical review on anorectal testing techniques. Gastroenterology 116:735, 1999

Drossman DA: The functional gastrointestinal disorders and the Rome III process. Gastroenterology 130(5):1377, 2006

Efron JE, Corman ML, Fleshman J, et al: Safety and effectiveness of temperature-controlled radio-frequency energy delivery to the anal canal (Secca procedure) for the treatment of fecal incontinence. Dis Colon Rectum 46(12):1606, 2003

Engel BT, Nikoomanesh P, Schuster MM: Operant conditioning of rectosphincteric responses in the treatment of fecal incontinence. N Engl J Med 290:646, 1974

Farrell SA, Flowerdew G, Gilmour D, et al: Overlapping compared with end-to-end repair of complete third-degree or fourth-degree obstetric tears. Three-year follow-up of a randomized controlled trial. Obstet Gynecol 120(4):803, 2012

Fenner DE, Genberg B, Brahma P, et al: Fecal and urinary incontinence after vaginal delivery with anal sphincter disruption in an obstetrics unit in the United States. Am J Obstet Gynecol 189(6):1543, 2003

Fitzpatrick M, Behan M, O'Connell PR, et al: A randomized clinical trial comparing primary overlap with approximation repair of third-degree obstetric tears. Am J Obstet Gynecol 183(5):1220, 2000

Frenckner B, Euler CV: Influence of pudendal block on the function of the anal sphincters. Gut 16(6):482, 1975

Garcia V, Rogers RG, Kim SS, et al: Primary repair of obstetric anal sphincter laceration: a randomized trial of two surgical techniques. Am J Obstet Gynecol 192(5):1697, 2005

Gearhart SL, Pannu HK, Cundiff GW, et al: Perineal descent and levator ani hernia: a dynamic magnetic resonance imaging study. Dis Colon Rectum 47:1298, 2004

Glasgow SC, Lowry AC: Long-term outcomes of anal sphincter repair for fecal incontinence: a systematic review. Dis Colon Rectum 55:482, 2012

Goldaber KG, Wendel PJ, McIntire DD, et al: Postpartum perineal morbidity after fourth-degree perineal repair. Am J Obstet Gynecol 168(2):489, 1993

Gourcerol G, Vitton V, Leroi AM, et al: How sacral nerve stimulation works in patients with faecal incontinence. Colorectal Dis 13:e203, 2011

Graf W, Mellgren A, Matzel KE, et al: Efficacy of dextranomer in stabilized hyaluronic acid for treatment of faecal incontinence: a randomised, sham-controlled trial. Lancet 377:997, 2011

Greenwald JC, Hoexter B: Repair of rectovaginal fistulas. Surg Gynecol Obstet 146(3):443, 1978

Grover M, Busby-Whitehead J, Palmer MH, et al: Survey of geriatricians on the effect of fecal incontinence on nursing home referral. J Am Geriatr Soc 58:1058, 2010

Handa VL, Danielsen BH, Gilbert WM: Obstetric anal sphincter lacerations. Obstet Gynecol 98(2):225, 2001

Haylen BT, de Ridder D, Freeman RM, et al. An International Urogynecological Association (IUGA)/International Continence Society (ICS) joint report on the terminology for female pelvic floor dysfunction. Neurourol Urodyn 29:4, 2010

Heaton KW, O'Donnell LJ: An office guide to whole-gut transit time. Patients' recollection of their stool form. J Clin Gastroenterol 19(1):28, 1994

Heymen S, Scarlett Y, Jones K, et al: Randomized controlled trial shows biofeedback to be superior to pelvic floor exercises for fecal incontinence. Dis Colon Rectum 52(10):1730, 2009

Hinninghofen H, Enck P: Fecal incontinence: evaluation and treatment. Gastroenterol Clin North Am 32:685, 2003

Hull T, Giese C, Wexner SD, et al: Long-term durability of sacral nerve stimulation therapy for chronic fecal incontinence. Dis Colon Rectum 56:234, 2013

Hull TL, Bartus C, Bast J, et al: Success of episioproctotomy for cloaca and rectovaginal fistula. Dis Colon Rectum 50(1):97, 2007

Jensen LL, Lowry AC: Biofeedback improves functional outcome after sphincteroplasty. Dis Colon Rectum 40(2):197, 1997

Johanson JF, Lafferty J: Epidemiology of fecal incontinence: the silent affliction. Am J Gastroenterol 91(1):33, 1996

Jorge JMN, Wexner SD: Etiology and management of fecal incontinence. Dis Colon Rectum 36:77, 1993

Kamm MA, Dudding TC, Melenhorst J, et al: Sacral nerve stimulation for intractable constipation. Gut 59(3):333, 2010

Kaufman HS, Buller JL, Thompson JR, et al. Dynamic pelvic magnetic resonance imaging and cystocolpoproctography alter surgical management of pelvic floor disorders. Dis Colon Rectum 44:1575, 2001

Khanduja KS, Padmanabhan A, Kerner BA, et al: Reconstruction of rectovaginal fistula with sphincter disruption by combining rectal mucosal advancement flap and anal sphincteroplasty. Dis Colon Rectum 42(11):1432, 1999

Khatri G: Magnetic resonance imaging of pelvic floor disorders. Top Magn Reson Imaging 23:259, 2014

Kwon S, Visco AG, Fitzgerald MP, et al: Validity and reliability of the modified Manchester health questionnaire in assessing patients with fecal incontinence. Dis Colon Rectum 48(2):323, 2005

Lewis SJ, Heaton KW: Stool form scale as a useful guide to intestinal transit time. Scand J Gastroenterol 32(9):920, 1997

Lockhart ME, Fielding JR, Richter HE: Reproducibility of dynamic MR imaging pelvic measurements: a multi-institutional study. Radiology 249(2):534, 2008

Lowry AC, Thorson AG, Rothenberger DA, et al: Repair of simple rectovaginal fistulas. Influence of previous repairs. Dis Colon Rectum 31(9):676, 1988

MacRae HM, McLeod RS, Cohen Z, et al: Treatment of rectovaginal fistulas that has failed previous repair attempts. Dis Colon Rectum 38(9):921, 1995

Madoff RD: Surgical treatment options for fecal incontinence. Gastroenterology 126:S48, 2004a

Madoff RD, Parker SC, Varma MG, et al: Faecal incontinence in adults. Lancet 364(9434):621, 2004b

Malouf AJ, Norton CS, Engel AF, et al: Long-term results of overlapping anterior anal-sphincter repair for obstetric trauma. Lancet 355(9200):260, 2000

Marti L: Comparison of sacral nerve modulation and pudendal nerve stimulation in treatment of fecal incontinence. Trial No. NCT 01069016. Available at: https://clinicaltrials.gov. Accessed March 16, 2015

Matzel KE: Sacral nerve stimulation for faecal incontinence: its role in the treatment algorithm. Colorectal Dis 13(Suppl. 2):10, 2011

Mellgren AM, Matzel KE, Pollack J, et al: Long-term efficacy of NASHA Dx injection therapy for treatment of fecal incontinence. Neurogastroenterol Motil 26:1087, 2014

Meyer I, Richter HE: An evidence-based approach to the evaluation, diagnostic assessment and treatment of fecal incontinence in women. Curr Obstet Gynecol Rep 3(3):155, 2014

Miller R, Lewis GT, Bartolo DC, et al: Sensory discrimination and dynamic activity in the anorectum: evidence using a new ambulatory technique. Br J Surg 75(10):1003, 1988

Minguez M, Herreros B, Sanchiz V, et al: Predictive value of the balloon expulsion test for excluding the diagnosis of pelvic floor dyssynergia in constipation. Gastroenterology 126:57, 2004

Mizrahi N, Wexner SD, Zmora O, et al: Endorectal advancement flap: are there predictors of failure? Dis Colon Rectum 45(12):1616, 2002

National Institute of Child Health and Human Development (NICHD): Pelvic Floor Disorders Network: controlling anal incontinence by performing anal exercises with biofeedback or loperamide (CAPABLe). Trial No. NCT02008565. Available at: https://clinicaltrials.gov. Accessed March 16, 2015

National Institutes of Health: NIH state-of-the-science conference: cesarean delivery on maternal request. 2006. Available at: http://consensus.nih.gov/2006/cesareanstatement.htm. Accessed March 16, 2015

Nelson R, Furner S, Jesudason V: Fecal incontinence in Wisconsin nursing homes: prevalence and associations. Dis Colon Rectum 41(10):1226, 1998

Nelson RL: Epidemiology of fecal incontinence. Gastroenterology 126(1 Suppl 1): S3, 2004

Norton C, Cody JD: Biofeedback and/or sphincter exercises for the treatment of faecal incontinence in adults. Cochrane Database Syst Rev 7:CD002111, 2012

Norton C, Kamm MA: Anal sphincter biofeedback and pelvic floor exercises for faecal incontinence in adults—a systematic review. Aliment Pharmacol Ther 15(8):1147, 2001

Nygaard I, Barber MD, Burgio KL, et al: Prevalence of symptomatic pelvic floor disorders in US women. JAMA 300:1311, 2008

Nygaard IE, Rao SS, Dawson JD: Anal incontinence after anal sphincter disruption: a 30-year retrospective cohort study. Obstet Gynecol 89(6):896, 1997

Oberwalder M, Thaler K, Baig MK, et al: Anal ultrasound and endosonographic measurement of perineal body thickness: a new evaluation for fecal incontinence in females. Surg Endosc 18(4):650, 2004

Omar MI, Alexander CE: Drug treatment for faecal incontinence in adults. Cochrane Database Syst Rev 6:CD002116, 2013

Orkin BA, Sinykin SB, Lloyd PC: The digital rectal examination scoring system (DRESS). Dis Colon Rectum 53:1656, 2010

Parks AG: Anorectal incontinence. Proc R Soc Med 68(11):681, 1975

Pescatori M, Anastasio G, Bottini C, et al: New grading and scoring for anal incontinence. Evaluation of 335 patients. Dis Colon Rectum 35(5):482, 1992

Rahman MS, Al-Suleiman SA, El-Yahia AR, et al: Surgical treatment of rectovaginal fistula of obstetric origin: a review of 15 years' experience in a teaching hospital. J Obstet Gynaecol 23(6):607, 2003

Rao SS: The technical aspects of biofeedback therapy for defecation disorders. Gastroenterologist 6(2):96, 1998

Rao SS, Coss-Adame E, Tantiphlachiva K, et al: Translumbar and transsacral magnetic neurostimulation for the assessment of neuropathy in fecal incontinence. Dis Colon Rectum 57:645, 2014

Rao SS, Seaton K, Miller M, et al: Randomized controlled trial of biofeedback, sham feedback, and standard therapy for dyssynergic defecation. Clin Gastroenterol Hepatol 5(3):331, 2007

Read M, Read NW, Barber DC, et al: Effects of loperamide on anal sphincter function in patients complaining of chronic diarrhea with fecal incontinence and urgency. Dig Dis Sci 27(9):807, 1982

Richter HE, Matthews CA, Muir T, et al: A vaginal bowel-control system for the treatment of fecal incontinence. Obstet Gynecol 125:540, 2015

Rociu E, Stoker J, Eijkemans MJ, et al: Fecal incontinence: endoanal US versus endoanal MR imaging. Radiology 212(2):453, 1999

Rockwood TH, Church JM, Fleshman JW, et al: Fecal incontinence quality of life scale: quality of life instrument for patients with fecal incontinence. Dis Colon Rectum 43(1):9, 2000

Rockwood TH, Church JM, Fleshman JW, et al: Patient and surgeon ranking of the severity of symptoms associated with fecal incontinence: the fecal incontinence severity index. Dis Colon Rectum 42(12):1525, 1999

Sailer M, Bussen D, Debus ES, et al: Quality of life in patients with benign anorectal disorders. Br J Surg 85(12):1716, 1998

Schiller LR, Santa Ana CA, Morawski SG, et al: Mechanism of the antidiarrheal effect of loperamide. Gastroenterology 86(6):1475, 1984

Shafik A: Polytetrafluoroethylene injection for the treatment of partial fecal incontinence. Int Surg 78:159, 1993

Shafik A, Ahmed I, El-Sibai O, et al: Percutaneous peripheral neuromodulation in the treatment of fecal incontinence. Eur Surg Res 35(2):103, 2003

Snooks SJ, Henry MM, Swash M: Faecal incontinence due to external anal sphincter division in childbirth is associated with damage to the innervation of the pelvic floor musculature: a double pathology. BJOG 92(8):824, 1985

Sonoda T, Hull T, Piedmonte MR, et al: Outcomes of primary repair of anorectal and rectovaginal fistulas using the endorectal advancement flap. Dis Colon Rectum 45(12):1622, 2002

Sultan AH, Kamm MA, Hudson CN, et al: Anal-sphincter disruption during vaginal delivery. N Engl J Med 329(26):1905, 1993

Tantiphlachiva K, Rao P, Attaluri A, et al: Digital rectal examination is a useful tool for identifying patients with dyssynergia. Clin Gastroenterol Hepatol 8:955, 2010

Terra MP, Beets-Tan RG, van der Hulst VP, et al: MRI in evaluating atrophy of the external anal sphincter in patients with fecal incontinence. AJR 187(4):991, 2006

Thin NN, Horrocks EJ, Hotouras A, et al: Systematic review of the clinical effectiveness of neuromodulation in the treatment of faecal incontinence. Br J Surg 100:1430, 2013

Thomas GP, Dudding TC, Rahbour G, et al: A review of posterior tibial nerve stimulation for faecal incontinence. Colorectal Dis 15:519, 2013

Tsang CB, Madoff RD, Wong WD, et al: Anal sphincter integrity and function influences outcome in rectovaginal fistula repair. Dis Colon Rectum 41(9):1141, 1998

Vaizey CJ, Carapeti E, Cahill JA, et al: Prospective comparison of faecal incontinence grading systems. Gut 44(1):77, 1999

Van Koughnett JA, da Silva G: Anorectal physiology and testing. Gastroenterol Clin North Am 42(4):713, 2013a

Van Koughnett JA, Wexner SD: Current management of fecal incontinence: choosing amongst treatment options to optimize outcomes. World J Gastroenterol 19(48): 9216, 2013b

Vitton V, Vignally P, Barthet M, et al: Dynamic anal endosonography and MRI defecography in diagnosis of pelvic floor disorders: comparison with conventional defecography. Dis Colon Rectum 54:1398, 2011

Wald A: Surgical treatment for refractory constipation—more hard data about hard stools? Am J Gastroenterol 85(6):759, 1990

Wexner SD, Coller JA, Devroede G, et al: Sacral nerve stimulation for fecal incontinence: results of a 120-patient prospective multicenter study. Ann Surg 251(3):441, 2010

Whitehead WE, Borrud L, Goode PS, et al: Fecal incontinence in U.S. adults: epidemiology and risk factors. Gastroenterology 137(2):512.e1, 2009

Whitehead WE, Rao SC, Lowry A, et al: Treatment of Fecal Incontinence: proceedings of an NIH Conference. Am J Gastroenterol 110:138, 2015

Whitehead WE, Schuster MM: Anorectal physiology and pathophysiology. Am J Gastroenterol 82(6):487, 1987

Whitehead WE, Wald A, Norton NJ: Treatment options for fecal incontinence. Dis Colon Rectum 44(1):131, 2001

Wiskind AK, Thompson JD: Transverse transperineal repair of rectovaginal fistulas in the lower vagina. Am J Obstet Gynecol 167(3):694, 1992

Wu JM, Vaughan CP, Goode PS, et al: Prevalence and trends of symptomatic pelvic floor disorders in U.S. women. Obstet Gynecol 123:141, 2014

Zetterstrom JP, Lopez A, Anzen B, et al: Anal incontinence after vaginal delivery: a prospective study in primiparous women. BJOG 106(4):324, 1999

Zutshi M, Tracey TH, Bast J, et al: Ten-year outcome after anal sphincter repair for fecal incontinence. Dis Colon Rectum 52:1089, 2009

CHAPTER 26

Genitourinary Fistula and Urethral Diverticulum

GENITOURINARY FISTULA

A genitourinary fistula is defined as an abnormal communication between the urinary (ureters, bladder, urethra) and the genital (uterus, cervix, vagina) systems. The true incidence of genitourinary fistula is unknown and varies according to whether the etiology is obstetric or gynecologic. In Asia and Africa, up to 100,000 new cases of obstetric genitourinary fistula are added each year to the estimated pool of 2 million women with unrepaired fistulas (World Health Organization, 2014). For industrialized countries, most fistulas occur iatrogenically from pelvic surgery, and the generally accepted incidence derives from data on surgeries to correct these fistulas. For example, numbers from the National Hospital Discharge Survey of inpatient women show that approximately 4.8 per 100,000 women underwent lower reproductive tract fistula repair (Brown, 2012). This likely is underestimated as many cases are unreported, unrecognized, or treated conservatively. Of genitourinary fistulas, the vesicovaginal fistula is most common and develops significantly more frequently than ureterovaginal fistulas (Goodwin, 1980; Shaw, 2014).

PATHOPHYSIOLOGY

The principles and phases of wound healing aid the understanding of genitourinary fistula pathogenesis. After injury, tissue damage and necrosis stimulate inflammation, and the process of cell regeneration begins (Kumar, 2015). Initially at the injury site, new blood vessels form, that is, *angiogenesis*. Three to 5 days after injury, fibroblasts proliferate and subsequently synthesize and deposit extracellular matrix, in particular collagen. This *fibrosis phase* determines the final strength of the healed wound. Collagen deposition peaks approximately 7 days after injury and continues for several weeks. Subsequent scar maturation and organization, termed *remodeling*, augments wound strength. These phases are interdependent and any disruption of this sequence eventually may create a fistula. Most defects tend to present 1 to 3 weeks after tissue injury. This is a time during which tissues are most vulnerable to alterations in the healing environment, such as hypoxia, ischemia, malnutrition, radiation, and chemotherapy. Edges of the wound eventually epithelialize, and a chronic fistulous tract is thus formed.

CLASSIFICATION

Although many classification systems exist for genitourinary fistula, no single system is considered the accepted standard nor is any one scheme superior in predicting surgical success. Fistulas can develop at any point between the genital and urinary systems, and one classification method reflects the anatomic communication (Table 26-1).

Vesicovaginal fistulas can also be characterized by their size and location in the vagina. They are termed *high vaginal,* when found proximally in the vagina; *low vaginal,* when noted distally; or *midvaginal,* when identified centrally. For instance, posthysterectomy vesicovaginal fistulas are often proximal, or "high" in the vagina, and located at the level of the vaginal cuff.

Others classify vesicovaginal fistula based on the complexity and extent of involvement (Table 26-2) (Elkins, 1999). In this scheme, complicated vesicovaginal fistulas are those that involve pelvic malignancy, prior radiation therapy, a shortened vaginal length, or bladder trigone; those that are distant from the vaginal cuff; or those that measure >3 cm in diameter.

In one obstetric classification system, high-risk vesicovaginal fistulas are described by their size (>4 to 5 cm in diameter); involvement of urethra, ureter(s), or rectum; juxtacervical location with an inability to visualize the superior edge; and reformation following a failed repair (Elkins, 1999).

TABLE 26-1. Classification of Genitourinary Fistula Based on Anatomic Communication

	Urinary Tract		
	Ureter	**Bladder**	**Urethra**
Vagina	Ureterovaginal	Vesicovaginal	Urethrovaginal
	Vesicoureterovaginal		
Cervix	Ureterocervical	Vesicocervical	Urethrocervical
Uterus	Ureterouterine	Vesicouterine	Not reported

A surgical classification to objectively evaluate obstetric urinary fistula repair has also been introduced (Waaldijk, 1995). In this system, type I fistulas are those that do not involve the urethral closure mechanism, type II fistulas do, and type III fistulas involve the ureter and include other exceptional fistulas. Type II fistulas are divided into: (A) without or (B) with subtotal or total urethra involvement. Type IIB fistulas are further subdivided as: (a) without or (b) with a circumferential configuration around the urethra.

To aid objective comparison of surgical outcomes, a more comprehensive and standardized classification system has been developed (Table 26-3). It integrates fistula distance from the external urethral meatus, fistula size, degree of surrounding tissue fibrosis, and extent of vaginal length reduction (Goh, 2004). This system has good inter- and intraobserver reproducibility and has demonstrated efficacy in predicting which patients are at risk of postfistula urinary incontinence and failure of closure (Goh, 2008, 2009). Despite the availability of these numerous classification systems, most clinicians will, from a practical standpoint, often use the anatomic communication and the relative position in the vagina (high, mid, low) in their initial description of the fistula.

ETIOLOGY

Congenital genitourinary fistulas are rare, but if found, are commonly associated with other renal or urogenital abnormalities. Thus, most vesicovaginal fistulas are acquired and typically result from either obstetric trauma or pelvic surgery.

TABLE 26-2. Classification of Vesicovaginal Fistulas

Simple
Size ≤3 cm
Located near the cuff (supratrigonal)
No prior radiation or malignancy
Normal vaginal length

Complicated
Prior radiation therapy
Pelvic malignancy present
Vaginal length shortened
Size >3 cm
Located distant from cuff or has trigonal involvement

■ Obstetric Trauma

In developing countries, more than 70 percent of genitourinary fistulas arise from obstetric trauma, specifically from prolonged or obstructed labor or complicated cesarean delivery (Arrowsmith, 1996; Kumar, 2009; Raassen, 2014). Their development in this setting often reflects social practices or obstetric management common to a particular community or geographic region. For example, both childbearing at a young age, before the pelvis has completely developed or fully grown, and female circumcision, more correctly termed *female genital mutilation*, may significantly narrow the vaginal introitus and obstruct labor. Prolonged obstructed labor or anatomic malpresentation of the presenting fetal part can cause pressure and ischemic necrosis of the anterior vaginal wall and bladder, subsequently resulting in fistula formation. Alternatively, the vagina may be damaged by instruments used to deliver stillborn

TABLE 26-3. Classification of Genitourinary Fistulas

This new classification divides genitourinary fistulas into four main types, depending on the distance of the fistula's distal edge from the external urinary meatus. These four types are further subclassified by the size of the fistula, extent of associated scarring, vaginal length, or special considerations.

Type 1: Distal edge of fistula >3.5 cm from external urinary meatus

Type 2: Distal edge of fistula 2.5–3.5 cm from external urinary meatus

Type 3: Distal edge of fistula 1.5 to <2.5 cm from external urinary meatus

Type 4: Distal edge of fistula <1.5 cm from external urinary meatus

(a) Size <1.5 cm, in the largest diameter
(b) Size 1.5–3 cm, in the largest diameter
(c) Size >3 cm, in the largest diameter

  i. None or only mild fibrosis (around fistula and/or vagina) and/or vaginal length >6 cm, normal capacity
  ii. Moderate or severe fibrosis (around fistula and/or vagina) and/or reduced vaginal length and/or capacity
  iii. Special consideration, e.g., postradiation, ureteric involvement, circumferential fistula, or previous repair

Data from Goh JT: A new classification for female genital tract fistula. Aust N Z J Obstet Gynaecol 2004 Dec;44(6):502–504.

infants or perform abortion. Malnutrition and limited health care in many of these countries can further diminish wound healing.

In contrast, in most developed countries, fistulas uncommonly follow obstetric procedures or deliveries. Rarely, cesarean deliveries, usually those accompanied by obstetric complications, have led to complex urinary fistula (Billmeyer, 2001). Similarly, rare cases following cervical cerclage have been reported (Massengill, 2012).

■ Pelvic Surgery

In developed countries, iatrogenic injury during pelvic surgery is responsible for 90 percent of vesicovaginal fistulas, and the accepted incidence of fistula formation after pelvic surgery is 0.1 to 2 percent (Harris, 1995; Hilton, 2012a,b; Tancer, 1992). The remaining fistulas result from procedures performed by urologists and by colorectal, vascular, and general surgeons. In industrialized countries, hysterectomy is the most common surgical precursor to vesicovaginal fistula, accounting for approximately 75 percent of fistula cases (Symmonds, 1984). When all hysterectomy types are considered, vesicovaginal fistula is estimated to complicate 0.8 per 1000 procedures (Harkki-Siren, 1998). In their review of more than 62,000 hysterectomy cases, laparoscopic hysterectomies were associated with the greatest incidence (2 per 1000), followed by abdominal (1 per 1000), vaginal (0.2 per 1000), and supracervical (0 per 1000) hysterectomies. With hysterectomy for benign disease, Duong and colleagues (2009) noted that bladder wall laceration extending into the bladder neck or a ureteral orifice (trigone) significantly increased the risk of subsequent vesicovaginal fistula.

Because most genitourinary fistulas follow pelvic surgery, prevention and intraoperative recognition of lower urinary tract injury is imperative. As discussed extensively in Chapter 40 (p. 869), intraoperative cystoscopy has been shown to improve the detection rate of lower urinary tract injuries. This in turn may ultimately translate into a lower incidence of genitourinary fistula. Thus, intraoperative cystoscopy can be a useful adjunct, particularly in cases in which the ureters or bladder are suspected to have been at increased injury risk.

■ Other Causes

Other etiologies for urinary tract fistulas include radiation therapy, malignancy, trauma, foreign bodies, infections, pelvic inflammation, and inflammatory bowel disease. Of these, *radiation therapy* induces an endarteritis that can lead to tissue necrosis and subsequent potential fistula formation. This modality is a frequent cause, and some series have reported that up to 6 percent of genitourinary fistulas can result from radiation (Lee, 1988). Although most damage following this therapy develops within weeks and months, associated fistulas have been reported to present up to 20 years after the original insult (Graham, 1967; Zoubek, 1989).

Malignancy is commonly linked with tissue necrosis and may lead to urinary fistula formation. Emmert and Kohler (1996) found a 1.8-percent incidence of rectovaginal and vesicovaginal fistula in their analysis of nearly 2100 women with cervical cancer. Thus, tissue biopsy is routinely considered

during diagnostic evaluation of women with a fistula and history of malignancy.

Trauma sustained during sexual activity or sexual assault can result in genitourinary fistula formation and has been estimated to precede 4 percent of these defects (Kallol, 2002; Lee, 1988). Foreign bodies such as a neglected pessary or vesical calculi are also documented causes (Arias, 2008; Dalela, 2003). Given that transurethral catheter placement has been linked to urethrovaginal fistula, this commonly used device should be placed, maintained, and removed with care (Dakhil, 2014). Foreign material introduced during surgery such as collagen injected transurethrally and complications resulting from synthetic mesh placement for urinary incontinence or pelvic organ prolapse are other inciting agents (Blaivas, 2014; Firoozi, 2012; Pruthi, 2000). Also, during sling surgeries, excess sling tension may increase tissue stress and necrosis. Thus, initial material selection and patient evaluation for poor wound healing risk factors are important prevention steps (Giles, 2005). Ideally, the material selected minimizes the normal foreign-body reaction, is nontoxic and nonantigenic, and is porous enough to admit immune and phagocytic cells and promote native tissue ingrowth (Birch, 2002). Mesh selection is further discussed in Chapter 24 (p. 556).

Other rare causes of fistula formation include infections such as lymphogranuloma venereum, urinary tuberculosis, pelvic inflammation, and syphilis; inflammatory bowel disease; and autoimmune disease (Ba-Thike, 1992; Monteiro, 1995). Additionally, conditions that interfere with healing such as poorly controlled diabetes mellitus, smoking, local infection, peripheral vascular disease, and chronic corticosteroid use are potential risks.

SYMPTOMS

Vesicovaginal fistula classically presents with unexplained continuous urinary leakage from the vagina after a recent operation. Depending on the size and location of the fistula, the urine amount will vary. Occasionally small-volume, intermittent leakage is mistaken for postoperative stress incontinence. For this reason, patients with new-onset urinary leakage, particularly in the setting of recent pelvic surgery, are examined thoroughly to exclude fistula formation. Other less specific symptoms of genitourinary fistula include fever, pain, ileus, and bladder irritability.

Vesicovaginal fistula may present days to weeks after the initial inciting surgery, and those following hysterectomy typically present at 1 to 3 weeks. Some fistulas, however, have longer latency, and symptoms may develop several years later.

DIAGNOSIS

A thorough history and physical examination identifies most cases of vesicovaginal fistula. Accordingly, information is documented regarding obstetric deliveries, prior surgeries, previous fistula management, and malignancy treatment, especially pelvic surgery and radiation therapy.

Physical examination is equally informative, and vaginal inspection often will identify the defect. A meticulous assessment for other fistulous tracts is performed, and their location and size noted. Visual assistance with an endoscopic lens and translucent

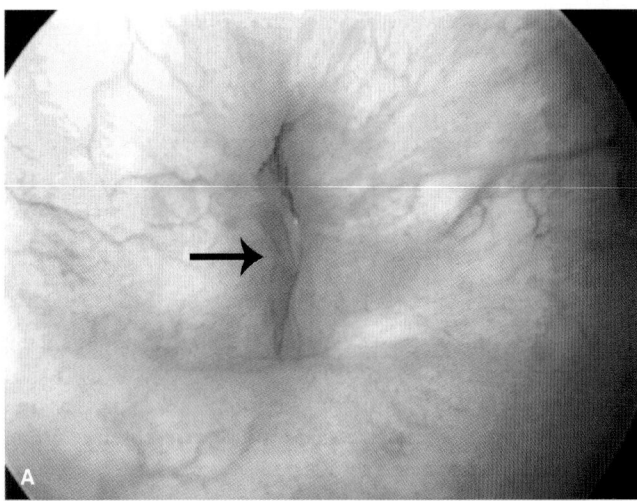
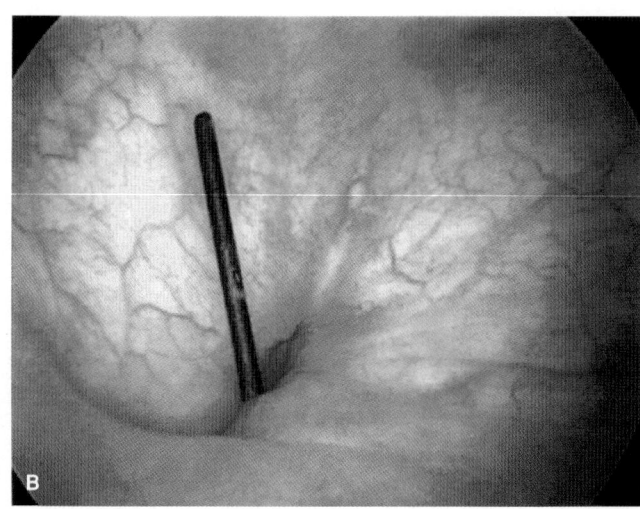

FIGURE 26-1 A. Cystoscopic view of vesicovaginal fistula (*arrow*). **B.** Probe placed through fistulous tract to aid cystoscopic visualization.

vaginal speculum can sometimes help identify a vaginal-apex fistula, which can be more difficult to detect.

It is essential to differentiate between "extraurethral" urinary leakage, as with a fistula, and "transurethral" leakage, that is, through the urethra, as with stress urinary incontinence. Occasionally, the vaginal fluid source is unclear, and a small amount of urine can easily be mistaken for vaginal discharge. Measurement of the vaginal fluid's creatinine content can sometimes be used to confirm its origin. Although creatinine levels in urine vary, with mean levels reaching 113.5 mg/dL, a value >17 mg/dL is consistent with urine (Barr, 2005). In contrast, fluid with a concentration <5 mg/dL is highly unlikely to be human urine.

Although a genitourinary fistula ideally is visualized directly, inspection at times is unrevealing. In these circumstances, retrograde bladder instillation of visually distinct solutions such as sterile milk or dilute methylene blue or indigo carmine can often indicate a fistula and aid in its localization.

If the presence of a urinary fistula is uncertain or its vaginal location is not identified, a *three-swab test*, commonly known as the "*tampon test,*" is recommended (Moir, 1973). This test is commonly performed with a tampon. However, we recommend using two to four pieces of gauze sequentially packed into the vaginal canal. A diluted solution of methylene blue or indigo carmine is instilled into the bladder using a transurethral catheter. Notably, use of the former may increase given current indigo carmine shortages. After 15 to 30 minutes of routine activity, the gauze is removed serially from the vagina, and each is inspected for dye. The specific gauze colored with dye suggests the fistula location—a proximal or high location in the vagina for the innermost gauze and a low or distal fistula for the outermost. If the distally placed sponge is stained with dye, however, confirmation that it was not contaminated by urine leaking out through the urethra, as in the case of stress urinary incontinence, is essential.

Cystourethroscopy is another valuable diagnostic tool (Fig. 26-1). It permits fistula localization, determination of its proximity to the ureteral orifices, inspection for multiple fistula sites, and assessment of surrounding bladder mucosa viability. In addition, the use of cystourethroscopy and vaginoscopy

concurrently to identify vesicovaginal fistula has been described (Andreoni, 2003).

Concomitant ureteral involvement is estimated to complicate 10 to 15 percent of vesicovaginal fistula cases and is sought during diagnostic evaluation (Goodwin, 1980). At our institution, intravenous contrast-enhanced computed tomography (CT) scanning in the excretory phase has become the preferred diagnostic test after initial cystourethroscopic survey is completed (Fig. 26-2). Selection of modalities other than CT for fistulous tract identification may be considered based on cost or availability. First, intravenous pyelography (IVP) can adequately confirm integrity of the upper collecting system and exclude ureteral involvement in a fistula. Second, retrograde pyelography may be used. Often carried out in conjunction with cystoscopy, it is performed by placing a small catheter into the distal ureter. Contrast material is injected through the catheter into one or both ureters. Fluoroscopic or conventional radiographs are then obtained. Retrograde pyelography

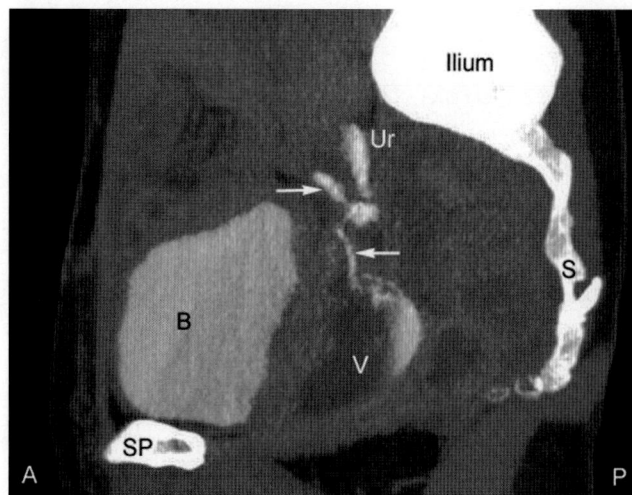

FIGURE 26-2 Ureterovaginal fistula. Both *arrows* show anomalous tracking of contrast. The lower *arrow* denotes a fistulous tract to the upper vagina. B = bladder; S = sacrum; SP = symphysis pubis; Ur = ureter; V = vagina. (Used with permission from Dr. April Bailey.)

generally has been reported to have the same diagnostic value as IVP.

In some instances resources are scarce, cost may be a limitation, and access to specialized diagnostic imaging is a challenge. With some advance planning, phenazopyridine hydrochloride (Pyridium) can be used in conjunction with the three-swab test to determine ureteral involvement, as a very rudimentary alternative to the aforementioned more sophisticated imaging. This tablet is administered orally, is excreted renally, acts as a topical bladder analgesic, and stains urine orange as a side effect. Women with suspected ureteral involvement are instructed to take a 200-mg dose a few hours before their clinic appointment. The steps of the three-swab test are then performed, as described earlier. In this case, if the most proximal (innermost) gauze is colored with orange dye, ureteral involvement is suspected. If both orange and blue dyes are seen, then involvement of both the bladder and ureter(s) is suspected.

Voiding cystourethrography (VCUG) can help confirm the presence, location, and number of fistulous tracts. In this, the bladder is filled via catheter with contrast dye, and fluoroscopic images of the lower urinary tract are obtained during patient micturition. However, CT has largely replaced this modality. Transabdominal sonography with applied color Doppler to identify flow through the fistula has been suggested as another diagnostic option (Volkmer, 2000). However, without color Doppler, sonography failed to identify 29 percent of vesicovaginal fistula cases in one study (Adetiloye, 2000).

TREATMENT

Conservative Treatment

Occasionally, genitourinary fistulas may spontaneously close during continuous bladder drainage using an indwelling urinary catheter. Approximately 12 percent of women treated by sustained catheterization alone had fistulas that healed spontaneously (Oakley, 2014; Waaldijk, 1994). Romics and colleagues (2002) found that in 10 percent of cases, urinary fistulas close spontaneously after 2 to 8 weeks of transurethral catheterization, especially if the fistula is small (2- to 3-mm diameter). Another series reported fistulas up to 2 cm in diameter spontaneously healed in 50 to 60 percent of patients treated with an indwelling catheter (Waaldijk, 1989).

Despite these series, data that correlate fistula size and success of conservative management are limited. Many reports of successful spontaneous closure with catheter drainage have been limited to fistulas that were 1 cm in size or smaller (Lentz, 2005; Ou, 2004). Many studies are vague regarding how fistula size is measured, and each series has potential for considerable bias in its selection criteria. However, in general, the larger a fistula, the less likely it is to heal without surgery.

Evidence regarding the duration of catheter drainage also varies. Regardless, many agree that if a fistula has not closed within 4 weeks, it is unlikely to do so. This may be secondary to epithelialization of the fistulous tract (Davits, 1991; Tancer, 1992). Moreover, continued urinary drainage may lead to further bladder inflammation and irritation (Zimmern, 1991). Importantly,

if attempting conservative treatment of a vesicovaginal fistula with catheter insertion and chronic drainage, urinary drainage ideally begins shortly after the inciting event.

Fibrin sealant (Tisseal, Evicel), also colloquially called fibrin glue, is formed from concentrated fibrinogen combined with thrombin to simulate the final clotting cascade stages. In gynecologic surgery, it is mainly used to control low-pressure bleeding. Although fibrin sealant has been described for the treatment of vesicovaginal fistula, it is often selected as a surgical adjunct rather than primary surgical treatment (Evans, 2003). Data regarding fibrin sealant effectiveness are sparse, and well-designed trials are lacking. Thus, fibrin sealant monotherapy may not be the initial recommended treatment in most vesicovaginal fistula cases due to potential lack of durability and thus a risk for recurrence. However, it may provide a viable alternative in patients with multiple comorbidities that contraindicate a prolonged fistula repair surgery.

In sum, a trial of conservative therapy is usually warranted and reasonable, especially if instituted shortly after the inciting event and if the fistula is small. However, gains from a conservative approach are balanced against a patient's desire for an expedited repair to resolve the leak. Thus, the timing of intervention ideally achieves a compromise between reasonable conservative efforts and addressing the patient's immediate distress and quality of life. As noted, most urinary fistulas ultimately require surgical intervention.

Surgical Treatment

Incorporating the fundamentals of genitourinary fistula repair is essential to successful resolution. These include accurate fistula delineation; adequate assessment of surrounding tissue vascularity; timely repair; multilayer, tension-free, and watertight defect closure; and postoperative bladder drainage.

Primary surgical repair of genitourinary fistula is associated with high cure rates (75 to 100 percent) (Rovner, 2012b). Factors that support this rate include adequate vascularity of the surrounding tissue, brief fistulous tract duration, no prior radiation therapy, meticulous surgical technique, and surgeon experience. The first attempt at surgical repair is usually associated with the best chance of successful healing. Surgical repair success rates specifically for obstetric fistulas are also high. Of these, 81 percent are corrected with the first attempt, and 65 percent with the second (Elkins, 1994; Hilton, 1998).

Timing of Repair

One principle of fistula repair dictates that a repair be performed in noninfected and noninflamed tissues. Early surgical intervention of uncomplicated fistulas within the first 24 to 48 hours following the inciting surgery is possible as it avoids the brisk postoperative inflammatory response. Such early closure does not affect success rates, yet it appears to reduce social and psychologic patient distress (Blaivas, 1995; Persky, 1979).

In instances of extensive and severe inflammation, we recommend delaying operative repair for 6 weeks until the inflammation subsides. During this time, a trial of catheter drainage, while the surrounding tissue has an opportunity to heal, is reasonable.

Route of Surgical Repair

Many different surgical repair options are available for vesicovaginal fistula. However, data that support an optimal route are limited, and the lack of consensus may reflect variances in surgeon experience and preference. Among important surgical considerations, ability to gain access to the fistula is essential and commonly dictates the surgical approach. Fortunately, success rates are high whether the route of repair is transvaginal or transabdominal.

Vaginal. The transvaginal approach to genitourinary fistula repair is straightforward and direct. Compared with abdominal approaches, it is associated with shorter operative times, decreased blood loss, less morbidity, and shorter hospital stays (Wang, 1990). The transvaginal route also allows easy access for the use of ancillary equipment, such as ureteral stents. This is particularly useful if the fistula is located near ureteral orifices.

One transvaginal approach used most commonly by gynecologists, the *Latzko technique*, is illustrated in Section 45-10 (p. 1078). In this technique, likened to a partial colpocleisis, the most proximal portions of the anterior and posterior vaginal walls are surgically apposed to close the defect, without completely removing the fistulous tract. This partially obliterates the upper vagina, similar to that achieved by colpocleisis. Because of the potential for vaginal shortening, this technique may not be appropriate if vaginal depth has already been compromised or if there is preexisting sexual dysfunction. If use of the Latzko technique is anticipated, patient counseling specifically addresses these issues and potential sequelae. That said, recent studies evaluating sexual function show similar or higher functioning scores following vaginal repair routes compared with abdominal routes (Lee, 2014; Mohr, 2014).

The *classical technique*, in contrast to the Latzko method, involves total excision of the fistulous tract and mobilization of the surrounding anterior vaginal wall epithelium. After tract resection, the bladder mucosa is first closed, and a watertight repair is confirmed. This is followed by closure of one or two layers of fibromuscular tissue. Vaginal epithelium is then reapproximated.

Of the two approaches, some favor incomplete fistulous tract excision (Latzko repair) to avoid weakening the surrounding tissue, enlarging the defect, and thereby potentially compromising the repair. By preserving the presumptively stronger scar tissue surrounding the fistula, it theoretically permits a more secure reapproximation of surrounding tissue.

Abdominal (Transperitoneal). With this route, the fistula is accessed and excised through an intentional cystotomy on the preperitoneal side of the bladder as shown in Section 45-10 (p. 1081). This approach is used for situations in which the fistula: (1) is located proximally in a narrow vagina, (2) lies close to the ureteral orifices, (3) is complicated by a concomitant ureteric fistula, (4) persists after prior repair attempts, (5) is large or complex in configuration, or (6) requires an abdominal interposition graft, described in the next section.

Evidence-based support for laparoscopic genitourinary fistula repair has been limited to case reports and expert opinion (Miklos, 2015; Nezhat, 1994). The technique requires advanced laparoscopic surgical skills. Accordingly, success with this approach appears to be highly dependent on surgeon experience.

Interpositional Flaps. Surrounding tissue vascularity is essential for successful genitourinary fistula healing after repair. When intervening tissues for fistula closure are thin and poorly vascularized, various tissue flaps may be placed vaginally or abdominally between the bladder and the vagina in an attempt to enhance the repair and to lend support and blood supply (Eisen, 1974; Martius, 1928). Sections 45-10 and 45-11 (p. 1081) illustrate the omental J-flap, which is an abdominal option, whereas the Martius bulbocavernosus fat pad flap is used during vaginal procedures. Although interposition flaps are useful in situations where tissue viability is in question, their utility in uncomplicated cases of vesicovaginal fistula is unclear.

■ Other Genitourinary Fistulas

Although vesicovaginal fistulas are the most common type of genitourinary fistula, other fistulas can develop and may be described based on their communication between anatomic structures. Urethrovaginal fistulas can result from surgery involving the anterior vaginal wall, in particular anterior colporrhaphy and urethral diverticulectomy (Blaivas, 1989; Ganabathi, 1994a). In developing countries, as with vesicovaginal fistula, obstetric trauma remains the most common cause of urethrovaginal fistulas. Frequently, patients present with continuous urinary drainage into the vagina or with stress urinary incontinence. The principles of repair are similar, namely, layered closure, tension-free repair, and postoperative bladder drainage. Other types of genitourinary fistula can also develop (see Table 26-1).

URETHRAL DIVERTICULUM

Paraurethral glands are found along the anterior vaginal wall and communicate directly with the urethra. A urethral diverticulum commonly forms from a cystic enlargement of one of these glands. This isolated outpouching is commonly asymptomatic and is frequently diagnosed incidentally during routine examination. However, many present with symptoms and often require surgical excision.

Urethral diverticulum is reported to develop in 1 to 6 percent of the general female population. With greater awareness and radiologic advances, rates of diagnosis are increasing (Rovner, 2012a). However, the true incidence may be underestimated because diverticula are frequently asymptomatic and thus underreported. In women with lower urinary tract symptoms, the incidence dramatically increases and may reach 40 percent (Stewart, 1981).

Urethral diverticulum is diagnosed most often in the third to sixth decades of life and more commonly in females than in males (Aldridge, 1978). A 6:1 predominance of urethral diverticula in African-Americans compared with whites has been reported, although others have found no racial predisposition (Davis, 1970; Leach, 1987).

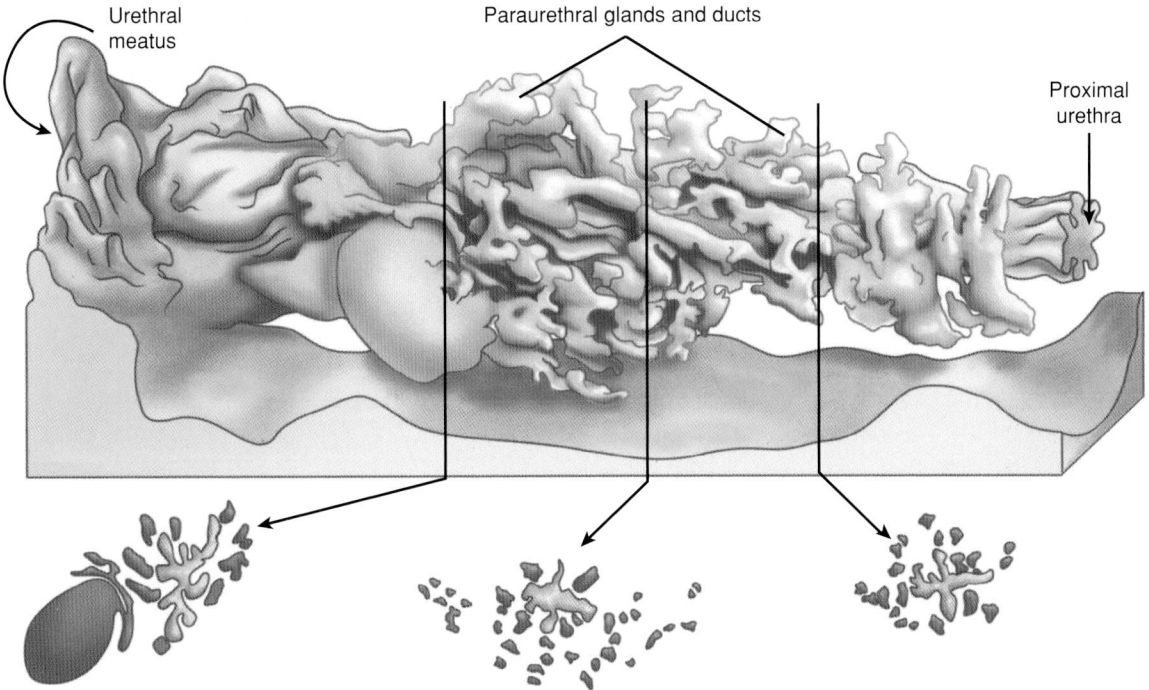

FIGURE 26-3 Complex configuration of paraurethral glands. The three smaller bottom images are cross-sectional views of the urethra and surrounding paraurethral glands. (Adapted with pemission from Huffman JW: The detailed anatomy of the paraurethral ducts in the adult human female. Am J Obstet Gynecol 1948 Jan;55(1):86–101.)

ETIOLOGY

The etiology of urethral diverticula is unclear. Although most are thought to be acquired, rare congenital diverticula have been reported. Congenital causes include persistence of embryologic remnants, defective closure of the ventral portion of the urethra, and congenital cystic dilatation of paraurethral glands (Ratner, 1949). Embryology of the female genital tract, described in Chapter 18 (p. 404), contributes to our understanding of congenital urethral diverticulum. During female development, the müllerian ducts form the upper vagina, whereas the urogenital sinus gives rise to the distal vagina, vestibule, and female urethra (Fig. 18-4, p. 408). In the vagina, müllerian mucinous columnar epithelium is replaced by squamous epithelium of the urogenital sinus. When the process of epithelial replacement is arrested, small foci of müllerian epithelium may persist and form cysts or diverticula.

More commonly, diverticula are acquired and can result from infection, birth trauma, or traumatic instrumentation. The most widely held theory regarding urethral diverticular development dates back to Routh (1890) and involves the paraurethral glands and their ducts. The paraurethral glands surround and cluster most densely along the urethra's inferolateral border (Fig. 26-3). Of these glands, the bilateral Skene glands are the most distal and typically the largest. Paraurethral glands connect to the urethral canal via a network of branching ducts. The arborizing pattern in portions of this network helps to explain the complexity of some urethral diverticula (Vakili, 2003).

Routh theorized that infection and inflammation obstruct individual ducts and lead to cystic dilatation. If these do not spontaneously resolve or if infection is not treated promptly, an abscess can form. Subsequent abscess expansion and continued inflammation may rupture the gland into the urethral lumen to create a fistulous communication between the two (Fig. 26-4). As infection clears,

the dilated diverticular sac and new communicating ostium into the urethra persist. Of infectious agents, *Neisseria gonorrhoeae* and *Chlamydia trachomatis* are organisms that were once commonly associated with urethritis and severe inflammation of the paraurethral glands. However, positive identification of these organisms is not mandatory for diagnosis, and more often than not, urethral cultures from women who have diverticula yield a polymicrobial result, which typically does not require treatment.

In addition to infection, injured urethral tissue can swell and obstruct paraurethral ducts. Logically, urethral trauma sustained during childbirth or during urethral instrumentation are suggested etiologies (McNally, 1935). Moreover, as described

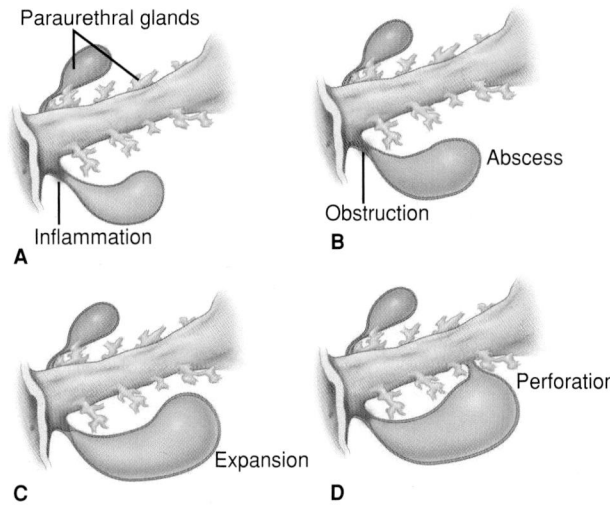

FIGURE 26-4 Mechanism of urethral diverticulum development. (Reproduced with permission from Walters MD, Karram MM (eds): Urogynecology and Reconstructive Pelvic Surgery. St. Louis: Mosby; 1999.)

earlier, different social customs and obstetric practices in the developing world can potentially contribute to urethral trauma (p. 578). In addition, female genital mutilation or repeated urethral dilatations can traumatize the urethra.

CLASSIFICATION

Early classification systems organized urethral diverticula according to their radiographic complexity and described them as: (1) simple saccular, (2) multiple, or (3) compound or complex with branching sinuses (Lang, 1959). To help standardize surgical treatment, Ginsburg and Genadry (1983) created a preoperative classification system based on urethral location. This system organized diverticula based on their urethral location and described lesions as type 1 (proximal third), type 2 (middle third), and type 3 (distal third).

In an attempt to fully incorporate all characteristics necessary to adequately assign treatment, Leach and coworkers (1993) constructed the L/N/S/C3 classification system. In this system, the diverticulum characteristics are described according to its location (L), number (N), size (S), and configuration, communication, and continence status of the patient (C3). Of these, location is described in relation to the urethra and defined as distal, mid-, or proximal urethral and as with or without extension beneath the bladder neck. In Leach's series of 61 patients, investigators found that most diverticula were in the midurethra. Logically, this distribution reflects the predominance of paraurethral glands along the middle third of the urethra. Ascertainment of the number of diverticula is important to prevent incomplete excision of multiple lesions and thus symptom persistence. Diverticulum size similarly can influence treatment. For example, some recommend concomitant interpositional tissue flaps for large diverticula. Moreover, urinary incontinence may develop de novo or persist if the diverticulum is extremely large and involves sphincter continence mechanisms.

Of the three "C"s, diverticula configuration may be described as solitary or multiloculated and as simple, saddle-shaped, or circumferential (Fig. 26-5). Preoperative delineation

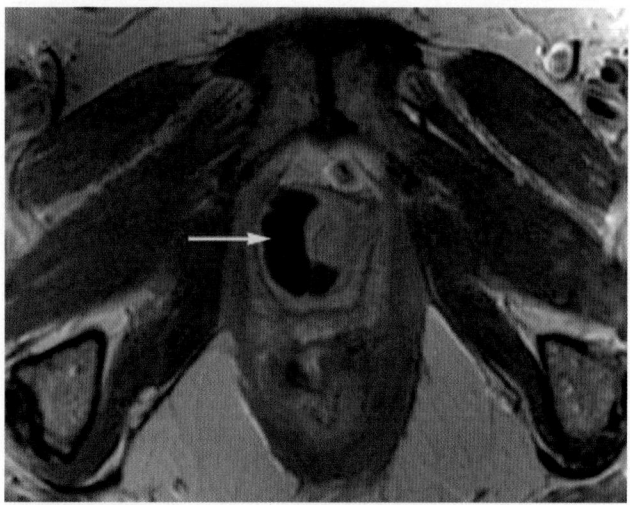

FIGURE 26-5 Magnetic resonance image of a circumferential urethral diverticulum (*arrow*) that extends around the urethra.

assists in complete surgical excision and aids preparation for an interpositional flap in those cases requiring extensive urethral resection (Rovner, 2003).

Obviously, successful repair of the urethral wall defect depends in great part on identifying the diverticular opening into the urethral canal. Thus, the communication site is sought preoperatively and classified as proximal, mid-, or distal urethral. In the previously cited study, midurethral communication sites were the most common (60 percent), followed by proximal (25 percent) and distal (15 percent) sites.

Finally, in this classification system, the continence status and urethral hypermobility of the patient are documented. Almost half of the patients in Leach's series had stress urinary incontinence, and these authors suggest that urethral hypermobility is an indication for concomitant incontinence surgery. Although several studies have documented the safety of performing concurrent bladder-neck suspension, some still consider this approach controversial due to concerns of urethral erosion (Bass, 1991; Ganabathi, 1994b; Leng, 1998; Swierzewski, 1993). Although consensus is lacking on this issue, repairing the diverticulum first and then considering antiincontinence surgery if urinary incontinence persists is reasonable. This staged fashion is a particularly realistic option because of the current array of effective minimally invasive surgical procedures, such as midurethral slings. For postoperative comparison, we typically perform baseline preoperative urodynamic testing, although this step may not be adopted by all. Importantly, these data and postoperative expectations are discussed with the patient during preoperative counseling.

SYMPTOMS

Urethral diverticula are frequently asymptomatic and discovered incidentally during gynecologic or urologic examination. However, symptoms may vary and reflect diverticulum characteristics, especially size, location, and extension. Although postvoid dribbling, dysuria, and egress of discharge through the urethra with finger compression of a suburethral mass are pathognomonic, not all women present so classically (Fig. 26-6). For most patients, symptoms are nonspecific and include pain, dyspareunia, and several urinary symptoms. Romanzi and colleagues (2000) found pain in 48 percent of affected women. Pain most likely stems from cystic dilatation and also possibly from concurrent inflammation. Those with dyspareunia may note either entry or deep dyspareunia, depending on whether diverticula are distal or proximal, respectively.

A large diverticulum can sometimes be mistaken for early-stage pelvic organ prolapse, especially when the presenting complaint is vaginal fullness, bulge, or pressure. In these cases, the palpable diverticular vaginal mass may mimic a cystocele or rectocele. In most, careful systematic palpation of the vaginal wall will distinguish prolapse from a discrete vaginal wall cyst or diverticulum.

Various lower urinary tract symptoms are frequently associated with urethral diverticulum. Specifically, urinary incontinence is noted by 35 to 60 percent of affected women (Gabanathi, 1994b; Romanzi, 2000). In addition, during micturition, urine may enter the diverticular sac, only to later spill from the sac and present as postvoid dribble or as urinary

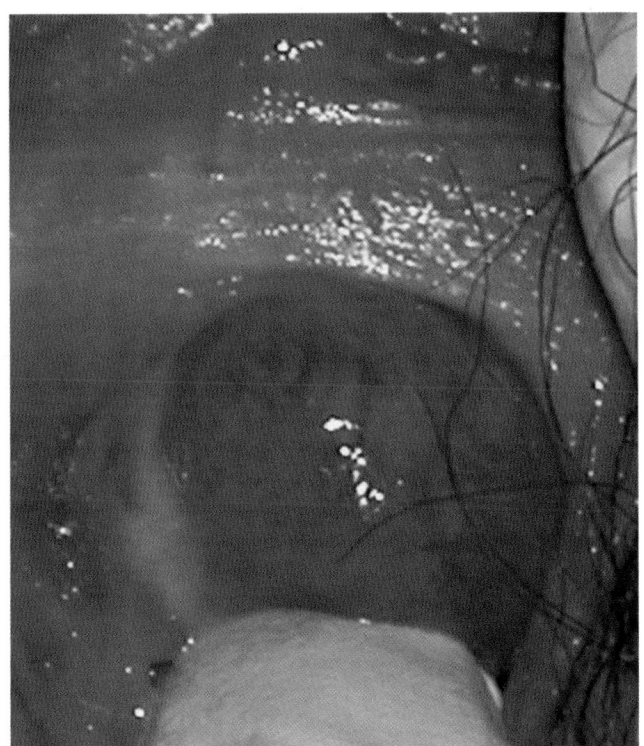

FIGURE 26-6 Transurethral expression of discharge with compression of a urethral diverticulum seen in the anterior vaginal wall.

incontinence. In contrast to urine loss, urinary retention has also been reported (Nitti, 1999). Retention frequently accompanies periurethral or diverticular sac cancers, discussed later in this section. Urinary tract infection often complicates urethral diverticulum. In their review of 60 women with diverticula, Pathi and associates (2013) found that recurrent urinary tract infection was highly specific for urethral diverticula.

Less frequently, stones may form from urine stagnation and salt precipitation within the diverticular sac. As such, stones may be singular or multiple and are usually composed of calcium oxalate or calcium phosphate. The reported frequency approximates 10 percent (Perlmutter, 1993).

Malignant transformation within a urethral diverticulum is rare and accounts for only 5 percent of urethral cancers. Most of these tumors are adenocarcinomas, although transitional cell and squamous cell carcinomas have also been identified (Clayton, 1992). Tumors typically present in the sixth or seventh decade of life, and hematuria, irritative voiding complaints, and urinary retention are common. Thus, palpation of an indurated or fixed periurethral mass, coupled with urinary obstructive symptoms, typically prompts further diagnostic evaluation and tissue biopsy (von Pechmann, 2003). Given the rarity of cancers within these diverticula, codified treatment strategies are lacking. Currently, these malignancies are treated by anterior exenteration or by diverticulectomy, alone or with adjuvant radiation therapy (Shalev, 2002).

DIAGNOSIS

For many women, urethral diverticula may be diagnosed using simply a detailed history, physical examination, and high

index of suspicion. Patient evaluation focuses on the common characteristics and symptoms noted earlier. However, despite available clinical tools, the diagnosis for many women is delayed as they may initially be treated for stress or urgency incontinence, chronic cystitis, trigonitis, urethral syndrome, vulvovestibulitis, pelvic organ prolapse, and idiopathic chronic pelvic pain. Moreover, the diverticulum itself may mimic a Gartner duct cyst, müllerian remnant vaginal cyst, vaginal epidermoid inclusion cyst, ectopic ureterocele, or endometrioma.

■ Physical Examination

The most frequent physical finding, an anterior vaginal mass beneath the urethra, is detected in 50 to 90 percent of symptomatic patients (Ganabathi, 1994b; Gerrard, 2003; Romanzi, 2000). Although urethral expression of purulent material during compression of the mass with a finger is common, failure to demonstrate transurethral expression of discharge does not exclude the diagnosis. Stenosis of the diverticular duct may obstruct sac emptying in these cases. Thus, meticulous examination and palpation is performed along the entire length of the urethra. Once diverticula are identified, their number, size, consistency, and configuration are determined.

However, physical examination alone is typically insufficient to completely characterize a mass. Of available ancillary tests, each has its advantages and disadvantages, and investigators may differ as to which is chosen primarily. Accordingly, familiarity with each modality's strengths aids selection of the most appropriate test for a given clinical setting.

■ Cystourethroscopy

Of the diagnostic procedures used to detect urethral diverticula, cystourethroscopy is the only tool that allows direct inspection of the urethra and bladder. During endoscopy, fingers pressed upward against the proximal anterior vaginal wall help occlude the bladder neck and allow the distending medium to create positive pressure and open diverticular ostia (Fig. 26-7). A zero-degree cystoscope lens allows complete radial assessment of the urethra to aid identification of diverticular ostia and at times, purulent discharge extruding from them.

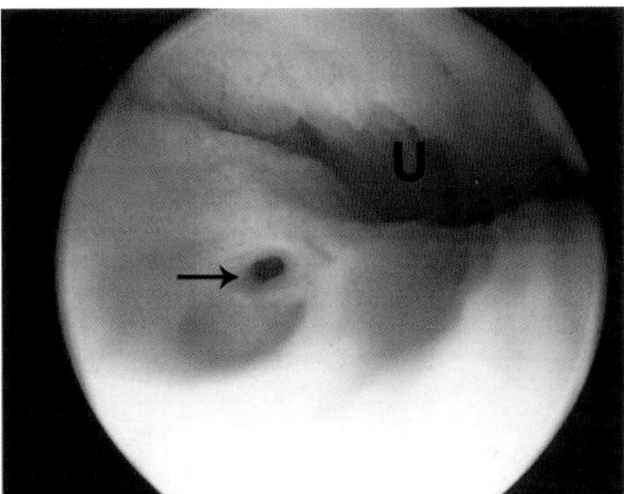

FIGURE 26-7 Diverticular opening visualized during cystourethroscopic examination (*arrow*). U = urethra.

A primary advantage to cystourethroscopy includes its accuracy for diverticulum detection (Summitt, 1992). Moreover, in those with nonspecific lower urinary tract symptoms, other causes such as urethritis, cystitis, stones, or stenosis can be excluded. Despite these advantages and its common use by urogynecologists, gynecologic generalists employ cystourethroscopy less frequently due to obstacles such as inexperience evaluating bladder and urethral mucosal anatomy, cystoscopic expertise, instrumentation costs, and credentialing challenges. Even for clinicians who are experienced with this tool, it may still fail to display all diverticula. For example, a poor seal between the cystoscope and distal urethral mucosa may lead to inadequate sac distention and failure to identify distally located diverticula. Also, diverticula whose ostia are stenotic, and thus do not communicate with the urethral lumen, can be missed. Although this endoscopy is minimally invasive, patient pain and risk of postprocedural infection are additional legitimate concerns. Last, important information regarding diverticular size and configuration may not be obtained with this tool.

Magnetic Resonance Imaging

This imaging modality has slowly become the diagnostic standard to characterize periurethral masses because of its superior resolution at soft tissue interfaces. Specifically, for detecting urethral diverticula, magnetic resonance (MR) imaging has comparable or superior sensitivity compared with other radiologic techniques (Lorenzo, 2003; Neitlich, 1998). To improve image resolution with MR imaging, an imaging coil may be placed into the rectum or vagina. The coil, which is housed inside a probe, improves the image quality of structures surrounding the rectum or vagina. Alternatively, an external plate or coil for image resolution enhancement can be used to minimize patient discomfort. Many institutions have opted for this method largely due to patient comfort, without significant loss of diagnostic accuracy. Despite MR imaging's advantages, procedure costs are balanced against the need for additional anatomic information. For a solitary diverticulum with clearly demarcated boundaries and no evidence of extension, costly and extensive imaging may not be necessary.

Other Imaging Tools

Although we use the two previously mentioned techniques most commonly, other techniques may be performed at other institutions. Of these, *voiding cystourethrogram (VCUG)* is used by some as an initial tool in urethral diverticulum evaluation. Radiographic contrast instilled into the bladder fills a diverticular sac during voiding, and postvoid radiographs then highlight sac volume. This painless, simple test has an overall reported accuracy that approximates 85 percent. However, some prefer positive-pressure urethrography as a primary diagnostic tool, since VCUG requires a diverticular communication to be patent during testing (Blander, 2001). Additionally, VCUG involves ionizing radiation exposure for the patient, although this is minimal.

Positive pressure urethrography (PPUG) also uses radiographic contrast and x-ray. With PPUG, a double-balloon, triple-lumen catheter (Trattner catheter) is inserted through the urethra, and its tip enters the bladder (Fig. 26-8). Inflating the proximal

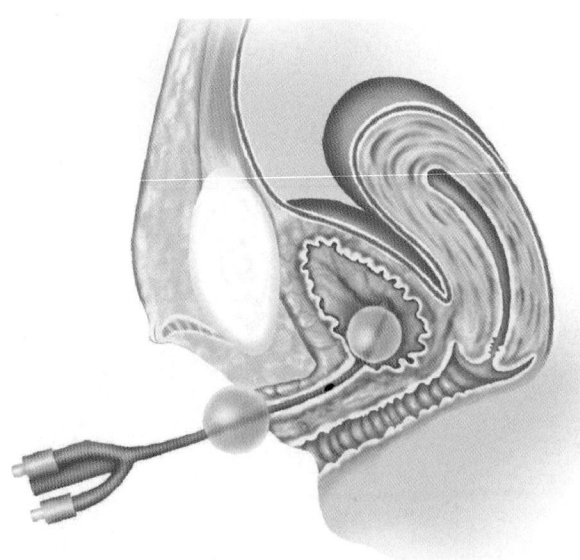

FIGURE 26-8 Trattner double-balloon catheter used to diagnose urethral diverticula. (Reproduced with permission from Greenberg M, Stone D, Cochran ST, et al: Female urethral diverticula: doubleballoon catheter study, 1981 Feb;136(2):259–264.)

balloon allows it to be pulled snug against and occlude the urethra at the urethrovesical junction. A distal balloon obstructs the distal urethra. A single catheter port between the two balloons allows instillation of radiopaque contrast, subsequent urethral distention, and expansion of the diverticulum under positive pressure. For accurately identifying diverticula, PPUG has a sensitivity surpassing that of VCUG (Golomb, 2003). Disadvantageously, PPUG can be time-consuming, technically difficult, and associated with patient discomfort and postprocedural infection risk. Additionally, similar to VCUG, diverticula may be missed if thick pus or debris prevents adequate filling with contrast medium or if the diverticular ostium is stenotic. Accordingly, although PPUG has been a primary tool for many for diagnosing urethral diverticula, fewer radiologists are proficient with the technique, and it has gradually been replaced by other modalities.

Sonography is a relatively new tool for urethral diverticulum assessment and appears to have some efficacy (Gerrard, 2003). Suggested technical advantages include visualization of diverticula that do not fill during radiographic contrast studies and characterization of diverticular wall thickness, size, and internal architecture (Yang, 2005). Transabdominal, -vaginal, -rectal, -perineal and -urethral sonographic techniques have all been described (Keefe, 1991; Vargas-Serrano, 1997). Although the endourethral technique has been reported to have excellent specificity, it is expensive and may be more invasive that the other sonographic routes (Chancellor, 1995). Advantages of sonography include patient comfort, avoidance of ionizing radiation and contrast exposure, relative low cost, and reduced invasiveness. However, in addition to its learning curve, sonography's role in urethral diverticulum diagnosis has not been clearly established. Currently, it remains an academic or adjunctive technique.

Because there is still no consensus on which modality is best used primarily, it is reasonable to begin with cystourethroscopic evaluation followed by VCUG. At our institution, if the initial evaluation is unrevealing but the diagnostic suspicion remains high or if the lesion appears more complex, then MR imaging combined with an endorectal coil or external plate may improve the resolution of images and add to the information gained.

TREATMENT

■ Acute Treatment

Women with a urethral diverticulum may present acutely with pain, urinary symptoms, or focal tenderness during examination. Conservative management is recommended in the acute phase and includes sitz baths, administration of a broad-spectrum oral antibiotic such as a cephalosporin or fluoroquinolone, and oral analgesics.

■ Chronic Diverticula

For a chronic diverticulum, a conservative approach may be elected by women who have few or no symptoms and decline surgery due to its associated risks of urethrovaginal fistula and sphincter defect incontinence. However, in women electing observation, long-term data are lacking regarding rates of subsequent symptom development, diverticulum enlargement, and eventual need for surgical excision.

Many practitioners may deliberate as to whether an enlarged inflamed cystic connection with the urethra is termed a "Skene gland cyst" or a "urethral diverticulum." Pragmatically, for those with persistent bothersome symptoms the treatment is the same with surgical intervention often indicated. Procedures include diverticulectomy, transvaginal partial ablation, and marsupialization, which are all described in Section 45-9 (p. 1075) of the atlas.

Of these, *diverticulectomy* is the most frequently chosen to treat diverticula at any site along the urethra. Excision of the entire diverticulum provides long-term correction of the urethral defect, normal urine stream, and high rates of postoperative continence. However, disadvantages include risks for postsurgical urethral stenosis, urethrovaginal fistula, potential injury to the urinary sphincter continence mechanism with subsequent incontinence, and the possibility of recurrence. For patients who also have stress urinary incontinence, some practitioners recommend concomitant placement of either a midurethral or pubovaginal sling. As noted earlier, although this practice is supported by some studies, our preference is to approach it as a staged procedure. We perform the defect repair first and later reassess the need for an antiincontinence procedure.

Another surgery, *partial diverticular sac ablation,* may be preferred for proximal diverticula to avoid bladder entry or bladder neck injury risks. Tancer and associates (1983) described this procedure, during which excess diverticular wall is excised, the diverticular neck is not removed, but remaining diverticular wall tissue is reapproximated to close the defect.

Last and less frequently, diverticulum marsupialization, also known as the Spence procedure, has been used for distal diverticula (Spence, 1970). The procedure is a meatotomy that when healed forms a new wider urethral meatus. Although simple to perform, this procedure alters the shape and function of the urethral meatus, with patients often noting spraying of their urine stream.

Other procedures described in case reports include urethroscopic transurethral electrosurgical fulguration of the diverticular sac and transurethral incision to widen the diverticular ostia (Miskowiak, 1989; Saito, 2000; Vergunst, 1996). Data are lacking, however, regarding long-term efficacy and complication rates with these techniques.

REFERENCES

Adetiloye VA, Dare FO: Obstetric fistula: evaluation with ultrasonography. J Ultrasound Med 19:243, 2000

Aldridge CW Jr, Beaton JH, Nanzig RP: A review of office urethroscopy and cystometry. Am J Obstet Gynecol 131:432, 1978

Andreoni C, Bruschini H, Truzzi JC, et al: Combined vaginoscopy-cystoscopy: a novel simultaneous approach improving vesicovaginal fistula evaluation. J Urol 170:2330, 2003

Arias BE, Ridgeway B, Barber MD. Complications of neglected vaginal pessaries: case presentation and literature review. Int Urogynecol J 19:1173, 2008

Arrowsmith S, Hamlin EC, Wall LL: Obstructed labor injury complex: obstetric fistula formation and the multifaceted morbidity of maternal birth trauma in the developing world. Obstet Gynecol Surv 51:568, 1996

Barr DB, Wilder LC, Caudill SP, et al: Urinary creatinine concentrations in the U.S. population: implications for urinary biologic monitoring measurements. Environ Health Perspect 113:192, 2005

Bass JS, Leach GE: Surgical treatment of concomitant urethral diverticulum and stress incontinence. Urol Clin North Am 18:365, 1991

Ba-Thike K, Than A, Nan O: Tuberculous vesico-vaginal fistula. Int J Gynaecol Obstet 37:127, 1992

Billmeyer BR, Nygaard IE, Kreder KJ: Ureterouterine and vesicoureterovaginal fistulas as a complication of cesarean section. J Urol 165:1212, 2001

Birch C, Fynes MM: The role of synthetic and biological prostheses in reconstructive pelvic floor surgery. Curr Opin Obstet Gynecol 14:527, 2002

Blaivas JG: Vaginal flap urethral reconstruction: an alternative to the bladder flap neourethra. J Urol 141:542, 1989

Blaivas JG, Heritz DM, Romanzi LJ: Early versus late repair of vesicovaginal fistulas: vaginal and abdominal approaches. J Urol 153:1110, 1995

Blaivas JG, Mekel G: Management of urinary fistulas due to midurethral sling surgery. J Urol 192(4):1137, 2014

Blander DS, Rovner ES, Schnall MD, et al: Endoluminal magnetic resonance imaging in the evaluation of urethral diverticula in women. Urology 57:660, 2001

Brown HW, Wang L, Bunker CH, et al: Lower reproductive tract fistula repairs in inpatient US women, 1979-2006. Int Urogynecol J 23(4):403, 2012

Chancellor MB, Liu JB, Rivas DA, et al: Intraoperative endo-luminal ultrasound evaluation of urethral diverticula. J Urol 153(1):72, 1995

Clayton M, Siami P, Guinan P: Urethral diverticular carcinoma. Cancer 70:665, 1992

Dakhil L: Urethrovaginal fistula: a rare complication of transurethral catheterization. Female Pelv Med Reconstr Surg 20:293, 2014

Dalela D, Goel A, Shakhwar SN, et al: Vesical calculi with unrepaired vesicovaginal fistula: a clinical appraisal of an uncommon association. J Urol 170:2206, 2003

Davis BL, Robinson DG: Diverticula of the female urethra: assay of 120 cases. J Urol 104:850, 1970

Davits RJ, Miranda SI: Conservative treatment of vesicovaginal fistulas by bladder drainage alone. Br J Urol 68:155, 1991

Duong TH, Gellasch TL, Adam RA: Risk factors for the development of vesicovaginal fistula after incidental cystotomy at the time of a benign hysterectomy. Am J Obstet Gynecol 201(5):512.e1, 2009

Eisen M, Jurkovic K, Altwein JE, et al: Management of vesicovaginal fistulas with peritoneal flap interposition. J Urol 112:195, 1974

Elkins TE: Surgery for the obstetric vesicovaginal fistula: a review of 100 operations in 82 patients. Am J Obstet Gynecol 170:1108, 1994

Elkins TE, Thompson JR: Lower urinary tract fistulas. In Walters MD, Karram MM (eds): Urogynecology and Reconstructive Pelvic Surgery. St. Louis, Mosby, 1999, p 355

Emmert C, Kohler U: Management of genital fistulas in patients with cervical cancer. Arch Gynecol Obstet 259:19, 1996

Evans LA, Ferguson KH, Foley JP, et al: Fibrin sealant for the management of genitourinary injuries, fistulas and surgical complications. J Urol 169:1360, 2003

Firoozi F, Ingber MS, Moore CK, et al: Purely transvaginal/perineal management of complications from commercial prolapse kits using a new prostheses/grafts complication classification system. J Urol 187(5):1674, 2012

Ganabathi K, Dmochowski R, Zimmern PE, et al: Prevention and management of urovaginal fistula. Urologia Panamericana 6:91, 1994a

Ganabathi K, Leach GE, Zimmern PE, et al: Experience with the management of urethral diverticulum in 63 women. J Urol 152:1445, 1994b

Gerrard ER Jr, Lloyd LK, Kubricht WS, et al: Transvaginal ultrasound for the diagnosis of urethral diverticulum. J Urol 169:1395, 2003

Giles DL, Davila GW: Suprapubic-vaginocutaneous fistula 18 years after a bladder-neck suspension. Obstet Gynecol 105:1193, 2005

Ginsburg D, Genadry R: Suburethral diverticulum: classification and therapeutic considerations. Obstet Gynecol 61:685, 1983

Goh JT: A new classification for female genital tract fistula. Aust N Z J Obstet Gynaecol 44:502, 2004

Goh JT, Browning A, Berhan B, et al: Predicting the risk of failure of closure of obstetric fistula and residual urinary incontinence using a classification system. Int Urogynecol J Pelvic Floor Dysfunct 19(12):1659, 2008

Goh JT, Krause HG, Browning A, et al: Classification of female genito-urinary tract fistula: inter- and intra-observer correlations. J Obstet Gynaecol Res 35(1):160, 2009

Golomb J, Leibovitch I, Mor Y, et al: Comparison of voiding cystourethrography and double-balloon urethrography in the diagnosis of complex female urethral diverticula. Eur Radiol 13:536, 2003

Goodwin WE, Scardino PT: Vesicovaginal and ureterovaginal fistulas: a summary of 25 years of experience. J Urol 123:370, 1980

Graham JB: Painful syndrome of postradiation urinary-vaginal fistula. Surg Gynecol Obstet 124:1260, 1967

Greenberg M, Stone D, Cochran ST, et al: Female urethral diverticula: double-balloon catheter study. AJR 136:259, 1981

Harkki-Siren P, Sjoberg J, Tiitinen A: Urinary tract injuries after hysterectomy. Obstet Gynecol 92:113, 1998

Harris WJ: Early complications of abdominal and vaginal hysterectomy. Obstet Gynecol Surv 50:795, 1995

Hilton P: Urogenital fistula in the UK: a personal case series managed over 25 years. BJU Int 110:102, 2012a

Hilton P, Cromwell DA: The risk of vesicovaginal and urethrovaginal fistula after hysterectomy performed in the English National Health Service—a retrospective cohort study examining patterns of care between 2000 and 2008. BJOG 119:1447, 2012b

Hilton P, Ward A: Epidemiological and surgical aspects of urogenital fistulae: a review of 25 years' experience in southeast Nigeria. Int Urogynecol J Pelvic Floor Dysfunct 9:189, 1998

Huffman JW: The detailed anatomy of the paraurethral ducts in the adult human female. Am J Obstet Gynecol 55:86, 1948

Kallol RK, Vaijyanath AM, Sinha A, et al: Sexual trauma—an unusual case of a vesicovaginal fistula. Eur J Obstet Gynecol 101:89, 2002

Keefe B, Warshauer DM, Tucker MS, et al: Diverticula of the female urethra: diagnosis by endovaginal and transperineal sonography. AJR 156:1195, 1991

Kumar V, Abbas AK, Aster JC: Inflammation and repair. In Kumar V, Abbas AK, Fausto N (eds): Robbins and Cotran Pathologic Basis of Disease. St. Louis, Saunders, 2015

Kumar A, Goyal NK, Das SK, et al: Our experience with genitourinary fistulae. Urol Int 82(4):404, 2009

Lang EK, Davis HJ: Positive pressure urethrography: a roentgenographic diagnostic method for urethral diverticulum in the female. Radiology 72:401, 1959

Leach GE, Bavendam TG: Female urethral diverticula. Urology 30:407, 1987

Leach GE, Sirls LT, Ganabathi K, et al: L N S C3: a proposed classification system for female urethral diverticula. Neurourol Urodyn 12:523, 1993

Lee D, Dillon BE, Lemack GE, et al: Long-term functional outcomes following nonradiated vesicovaginal repair. J Urol 191(1):120, 2014

Lee RA, Symmonds RE, Williams TJ: Current status of genitourinary fistula. Obstet Gynecol 72:313, 1988

Leng WW, McGuire EJ: Management of female urethral diverticula: a new classification. J Urol 160:1297, 1998

Lentz SS: Transvaginal repair of the posthysterectomy vesicovaginal fistula using a peritoneal flap: the gold standard. J Reprod Med 50:41, 2005

Lorenzo AJ, Zimmern P, Lemack GE, et al: Endorectal coil magnetic resonance imaging for diagnosis of urethral and periurethral pathologic findings in women. Urology 61:1129, 2003

Martius H: Die operative Wiederhertellung der vollkommen fehlenden Harnrohre und des Schiessmuskels derselben. Zentralbl Gynak 52:480, 1928

Massengill JC, Baker TM, Von Pechmann WS, et al: Commonalities of cerclage-related genitourinary fistulas. Female Pelvic Med Reconstr Surg 18(6):362, 2012

McNally A: A diverticulum of the female urethra. Am J Surg 28:177, 1935

Miklos JR, Moore RD: Laparoscopic extravesical vesicovaginal fistula repair: our technique and 15-year experience. Int Urogynecol J 26(3):441, 2015

Miskowiak J, Honnens dL: Transurethral incision of urethral diverticulum in the female. Scand J Urol Nephrol 23:235, 1989

Mohr S, Brandner S, Mueller MD, et al: Sexual function after vaginal and abdominal fistula repair. Am J Obstet Gynecol 211(1):74.e1, 2014

Moir JC: Vesico-vaginal fistulae as seen in Britain. J Obstet Gynaecol Br Commonw 80:598, 1973

Monteiro H, Nogueira R, de Carvalho H: Behçet's syndrome and vesicovaginal fistula: an unusual complication. J Urol 153:407, 1995

Neitlich JD, Foster HE Jr, Glickman MG, et al: Detection of urethral diverticula in women: comparison of a high resolution fast spin echo technique with double balloon urethrography. J Urol 159:408, 1998

Nezhat CH, Nezhat F, Nezhat C, et al: Laparoscopic repair of a vesicovaginal fistula: a case report. Obstet Gynecol 83:899, 1994

Nitti VW, Tu LM, Gitlin J: Diagnosing bladder outlet obstruction in women. J Urol 161:1535, 1999

Oakley SH, Brown HW, Greer JA, et al: Management of vesicovaginal fistulae: a multicenter analysis from the Fellows' Pelvic Research Network. Female Pelvic Med Reconstr Surg 20(1):7, 2014

Ou CS, Huang UC, Tsuang M, et al: Laparoscopic repair of vesicovaginal fistula. J Laparoendosc Adv Surg Tech A 14:17, 2004

Pathi SD, Rahn DD, Sailors JL, et al: Utility of clinical parameters, cystourethroscopy, and magnetic resonance imaging in the preoperative diagnosis of urethral diverticula. Int Urogynecol J 24(2):319, 2013

Perlmutter S, Huang AB, Hon M, et al: Sonographic demonstration of calculi within a urethral diverticulum. Urology 42:735, 1993

Persky L, Herman G, Guerrier K: Nondelay in vesicovaginal fistula repair. Urology 13:273, 1979

Pruthi RS, Petrus CD, Bundrick WS Jr: New onset vesicovaginal fistula after transurethral collagen injection in women who underwent cystectomy and orthotopic neobladder creation: presentation and definitive treatment. J Urol 164:1638, 2000

Raassen TJ, Ngongo CJ, Mahendeka MM: Iatrogenic genitourinary fistula: an 18-year retrospective review of 805 injuries. Int Urogynecol J 25(12):1699, 2014

Ratner M, Siminovitch M, Ritz I: Diverticulum of the female urethra with multiple calculi. Can Med Assoc J 60:510, 1949

Romanzi LJ, Groutz A, Blaivas JG: Urethral diverticulum in women: diverse presentations resulting in diagnostic delay and mismanagement. J Urol 164:428, 2000

Romics I, Kelemen Z, Fazakas Z: The diagnosis and management of vesicovaginal fistulae. BJU Int 89:764, 2002

Routh A: Urethral diverticulum. BMJ 1:361, 1890

Rovner ES: Bladder and female urethral diverticula. In Wein AJ, Kavoussi LR, Novick AC, et al (eds): Campbell-Walsh Urology, 10th ed. Philadelphia, Saunders, 2012a

Rovner ES: Urinary tract fistulae. In Wein AJ, Kavoussi LR, Novick AC, et al (eds): Campbell-Walsh Urology, 10th ed. Philadelphia, Saunders, 2012b

Rovner ES, Wein AJ: Diagnosis and reconstruction of the dorsal or circumferential urethral diverticulum. J Urol 170:82, 2003

Saito S: Usefulness of diagnosis by the urethroscopy under anesthesia and effect of transurethral electrocoagulation in symptomatic female urethral diverticula. J Endourol 14:455, 2000

Shalev M, Mistry S, Kernen K, et al: Squamous cell carcinoma in a female urethral diverticulum. Urology 59:773, 2002

Shaw J, Tunitsky-Bitton E, Barber MD, et al: Ureterovaginal fistula: a case series. Int Urogynecol J 25(5):615, 2014

Spence HM, Duckett JW Jr: Diverticulum of the female urethra: clinical aspects and presentation of a simple operative technique for cure. J Urol 104:432, 1970

Stewart M, Bretland PM, Stidolph NE: Urethral diverticula in the adult female. Br J Urol 53:353, 1981

Summitt RL Jr, Stovall TG: Urethral diverticula: evaluation by urethral pressure profilometry, cystourethroscopy, and the voiding cystourethrogram. Obstet Gynecol 80:695, 1992

Swierzewski SJ 3rd, McGuire EJ: Pubovaginal sling for treatment of female stress urinary incontinence complicated by urethral diverticulum. J Urol 149:1012, 1993

Symmonds RE: Incontinence: vesical and urethral fistulas. Clin Obstet Gynecol 27:499, 1984

Tancer ML: Observations on prevention and management of vesicovaginal fistula after total hysterectomy. Surg Gynecol Obstet 175:501, 1992

Tancer ML, Mooppan MM, Pierre-Louis C, et al: Suburethral diverticulum treatment by partial ablation. Obstet Gynecol 62:511, 1983

Vakili B, Wai C, Nihira M: Anterior urethral diverticulum in the female: diagnosis and surgical approach. Obstet Gynecol 102:1179, 2003

Vargas-Serrano B, Cortina-Moreno B, Rodriguez-Romero R, et al: Transrectal ultrasonography in the diagnosis of urethral diverticula in women. J Clin Ultrasound 25:21, 1997

Vergunst H, Blom JH, De Spiegeleer AH, et al: Management of female urethral diverticula by transurethral incision. Br J Urol 77:745, 1996

Volkmer BG, Kuefer R, Nesslauer T, et al: Colour Doppler ultrasound in vesicovaginal fistulas. Ultrasound Med Biol 26:771, 2000

von Pechmann WS, Mastropietro MA, Roth TJ, et al: Urethral adenocarcinoma associated with urethral diverticulum in a patient with progressive voiding dysfunction. Am J Obstet Gynecol 188:1111, 2003

Waaldijk K: Surgical classification of obstetric fistulas. Int J Gynaecol Obstet 49:161, 1995

Waaldijk K: The immediate surgical management of fresh obstetric fistulas with catheter and/or early closure. Int J Gynaecol Obstet 45:11, 1994

Waaldijk K: The (surgical) management of bladder fistula in 775 women in northern Nigeria. Doctoral thesis, University of Utrecht, 1989, p 85

Wang Y, Hadley HR: Nondelayed transvaginal repair of high lying vesicovaginal fistula. J Urol 144:34, 1990

World Health Organization: 10 facts on obstetric fistula. 2014. Available at: http://www.who.int/features/factfiles/obstetric_fistula/en. Accessed December 5, 2014

Yang JM, Huang WC, Yang SH: Transvaginal sonography in the diagnosis, management and follow-up of complex paraurethral abnormalities. Ultrasound Obstet Gynecol 25:302, 2005

Zimmern PE, Leach GE: Vesicovaginal fistula repair. Prob Urol 5:171, 1991

Zoubek J, McGuire EJ, Noll F, et al: The late occurrence of urinary tract damage in patients successfully treated by radiotherapy for cervical carcinoma. J Urol 141:1347, 1989

CHAPTER 26

SECTION 4
GYNECOLOGIC ONCOLOGY

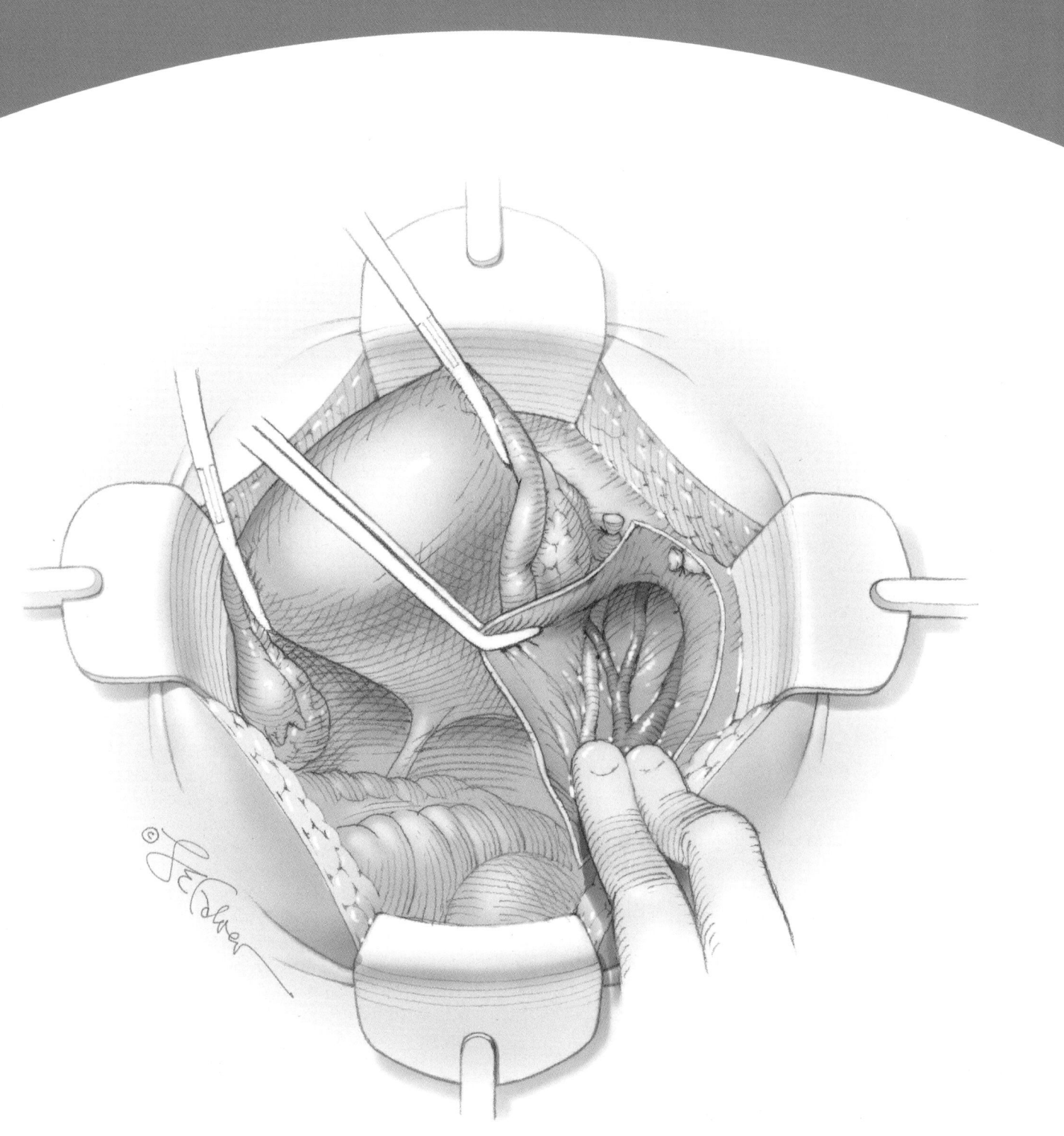

CHAPTER 27

Principles of Chemotherapy

BIOLOGY OF CANCER GROWTH

In principle, chemotherapeutic drugs are able to treat cancer and spare normal cells by exploiting inherent differences in their individual growth patterns. Each tumor type has its own characteristics, which explain why the same chemotherapy regimen is not equally effective for the whole spectrum of gynecologic cancers. Selecting appropriate drugs and limiting toxicity demands an understanding of cellular kinetics and biochemistry.

■ The Cell Cycle

All dividing cells follow the same basic sequence for replication. The *cell generation time* is the time required to complete the five phases of the cell cycle (Fig. 27-1). The G_1 phase (G = gap) involves various cellular activities, such as protein synthesis, RNA synthesis, and DNA repair. When prolonged, the cell is considered to be in the G_0 phase, that is, the resting phase. G_1 cells may either terminally differentiate into the G_0 phase or reenter the cell cycle after a period of quiescence. During the S phase, new DNA is synthesized. The G_2 (premitotic) phase is characterized by cells having twice the DNA content as they prepare for division. Finally, actual mitosis and chromosomal division takes place during the M phase.

Tumors do not typically have faster generation times. They instead have many more cells in the active phases of replication and have dysfunctional apoptosis (programmed cell death), hence proliferation. In contrast, normal tissues have a much larger number of cells in the G_0 phase. As a result, cancer cells proceeding through the cell cycle may be more sensitive to chemotherapeutic agents, whereas normal cells in G_0 are protected. This growth pattern disparity underlies the effectiveness of chemotherapeutic agents.

■ Cancer Cell Growth

Tumors are characterized by a *gompertzian growth* pattern (Fig. 27-2). Fundamentally, a tumor mass requires progressively longer times to double in size as it enlarges. When a cancer is microscopic and nonpalpable, growth is exponential. However, as a tumor enlarges, the number of its cells undergoing replication decreases due to limitations in blood supply and increasing interstitial pressure.

When tumors are in the exponential phase of gompertzian growth, they should be more sensitive to chemotherapy because a larger percentage of cells are in the active phase of the cell cycle. For this reason, metastases should be more sensitive to chemotherapy than the primary tumor. To capitalize on this potential benefit, advanced ovarian cancer is usually first treated with surgery to remove the primary tumor, debulk large masses, and leave only microscopic residual disease for the adjuvant chemotherapy to act on. In addition, when a tumor mass shrinks in response to treatment, the presumption is that a greater number of cells will enter the active phase of the cell cycle to accelerate growth. This larger percentage of replicating cells should also increase the sensitivity of a tumor to chemotherapy.

■ Doubling Time

The time needed for a tumor to double in size is commonly referred to as its *doubling time*. Whereas the cell cycle generally refers to the activity of individual tumor cells, doubling time refers to the growth of an entire heterogeneous tumor mass. In humans, the doubling times of specific tumors vary greatly. The speed with which tumors grow and double in size is largely regulated by the number of cells that are actively dividing—known as the *growth fraction*. Typically, only a small percentage of the tumor will have cells that are rapidly proliferating. The remaining cells are in the G_0 resting phase. In general, tumors that are cured by chemotherapy are those with a high growth fraction, such as gestational trophoblastic neoplasia. When tumor volume is reduced by surgery or chemotherapy, the remaining tumor cells are theoretically propelled from the G_0 phase into the more vulnerable phases of the cell cycle, rendering them susceptible to chemotherapy.

■ Cell Kinetics

Chemotherapeutic agents typically work by first-order kinetics to kill a constant *fraction* of cells rather than a constant

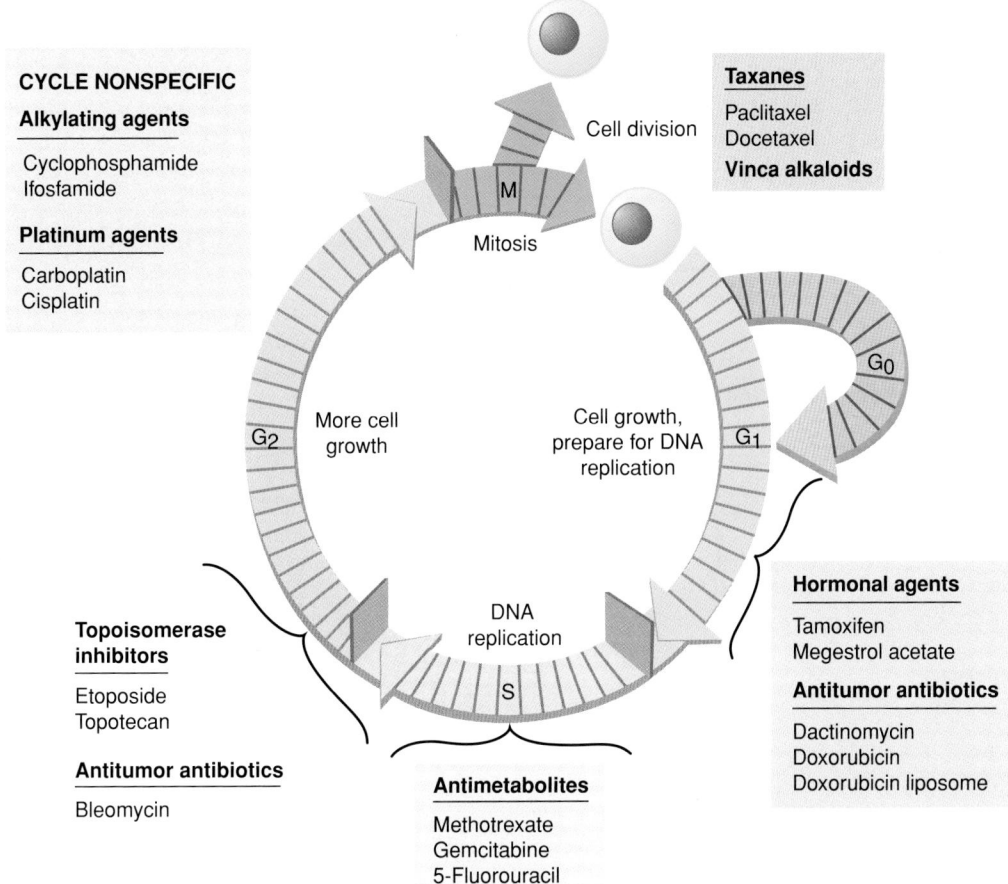

CYCLE NONSPECIFIC

Alkylating agents

Cyclophosphamide
Ifosfamide

Platinum agents

Carboplatin
Cisplatin

Taxanes

Paclitaxel
Docetaxel

Vinca alkaloids

Cell division

M

Mitosis

G_2

More cell
growth

Cell growth,
prepare for DNA
replication

G_0

G_1

Topoisomerase inhibitors

Etoposide
Topotecan

Antitumor antibiotics

Bleomycin

DNA
replication

S

Antimetabolites

Methotrexate
Gemcitabine
5-Fluorouracil

Hormonal agents

Tamoxifen
Megestrol acetate

Antitumor antibiotics

Dactinomycin
Doxorubicin
Doxorubicin liposome

FIGURE 27-1 Diagram of the cell cycle. Agents are organized according to the cell cycle stage in which they are most effective for tumor control.

number. For example, one dose of a cytotoxic drug may result in a few logs (10^2 to 10^4) of cell kill. This, however, is not curative since tumor burden may be 10^{12} cells or more. Thus, the magnitude of cell kill necessary to eradicate a tumor typically requires intermittent courses of chemotherapy. In general,

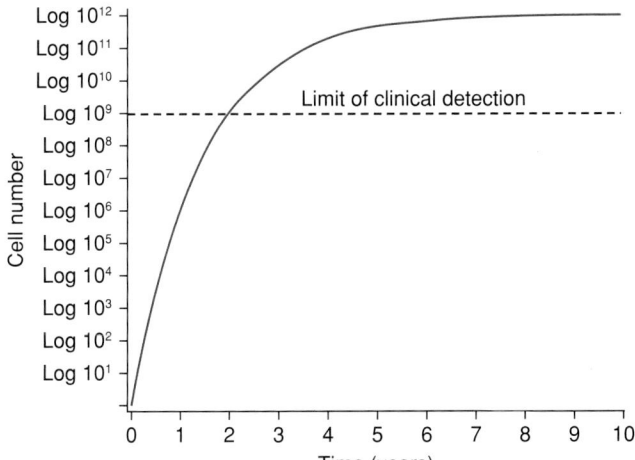

FIGURE 27-2 The gompertzian growth curve. During early stages of tumor expansion, growth is exponential, but with enlargement, tumor growth slows. Consequently, most tumors have completed their exponential growth phase at the time of clinical detection.

a cancer's curability is inversely proportional to the number of viable tumor cells at the beginning of chemotherapy.

Some drugs achieve cell kill at several phases of the cell cycle. These *cell cycle-nonspecific* agents act in all phases of replication from G_0 to the M phase. *Cell cycle-specific* agents act only on cells that are in a specific phase. By combining drugs that act in different phases of the cell cycle, the overall cell kill should be enhanced.

CLINICAL USE OF CHEMOTHERAPY

■ Clinical Setting

Chemotherapy may be used in at least five different ways. The term *induction chemotherapy* is defined as primary treatment for patients with an advanced malignancy when no feasible alternative treatment exists. *Adjuvant chemotherapy* is given to destroy remaining microscopic cells that may be present after the primary tumor is removed by surgery. *Neoadjuvant chemotherapy* refers to drug treatment directed at an advanced cancer to decrease preoperatively the extent or morbidity of a subsequent surgical resection. *Consolidation* (or *maintenance*) *chemotherapy* is given after cancer has disappeared following the initial therapy to prolong the duration of clinical remission or to prevent ultimate relapse. Therapy applied to recurrent disease or to a tumor that is refractory to initial treatment is termed *salvage* (or *palliative*) *chemotherapy*. In these incurable patients, the intent is to achieve tumor shrinkage or stability but maintain quality of life.

In general, chemotherapy is used with either curative or palliative intent. When implementing chemotherapy with curative intent, the number of courses is typically predefined. Emphasis is placed on maintaining curative dosages and adhering closely to the treatment schedule. This may lead to significant toxicity and require growth-factor support. However, for the possibility of achieving cure, these side effects are typically deemed acceptable.

Chemotherapy is often not used with curative intent, and the treating clinician must balance several factors to provide effective, compassionate palliation. Thus, in this setting, greater importance is attached to avoiding excessive toxicity. In many ways, the use of chemotherapy for palliation exemplifies the "art" of medicine. Instead of a defined number of treatment courses, a clinician must frequently revisit the treatment effectiveness and alter the dosage and timing of chemotherapy administration accordingly.

Drug Regimens

With few exceptions, single drugs administered at clinically tolerable doses do not cure cancer. However, using two or more drugs simultaneously may greatly exacerbate toxicity. Thus, in principle, the goal of combination chemotherapy is to provide maximum cell kill with minimal or tolerable adverse patient side effects. Drugs are selected based on their proven efficacy as single agents, different mechanisms of action, and toxicities that overlap minimally or not at all.

Combination chemotherapy is more effective in attacking heterogeneous populations of cells. Moreover, the use of multiple drugs with differing mechanisms of action tends to minimize the emergence of drug resistance. Typically, drugs used in combination should have clinical data indicating that their effects will be synergistic or at least additive. Drugs in combination are used at their optimal doses and schedules. Dose reductions initiated solely to allow the addition of other agents are counterproductive because most drugs must be used near their maximum tolerated dose to ensure efficacy.

Frequently, chemotherapy is combined with radiation therapy or sequenced with surgery. With chemoradiation, the goal is to achieve local control by chemically rendering the tumor more sensitive to radiation. For example, care of locally advanced cervical cancer was transformed by adding weekly cisplatin to standard radiotherapy. In addition, concurrent chemotherapy is intended to treat micrometastases outside the radiation field.

However, treatment-related toxicity is also increased. Patients previously treated with radiation therapy may have bone marrow, skin, or other body systems that are more susceptible to chemotherapy toxicity. As a result, dose reductions or delays are commonplace. Furthermore, chemotherapy is generally less effective in tumors that lie within a previously irradiated field due to increased fibrosis and capillary destruction.

Combining chemotherapy with surgery has many different applications. A woman with endometrial cancer may have nodal metastases detected during surgery, and receive pelvic radiation preceded or followed by combination chemotherapy.

Alternatively, a woman with recurrent ovarian cancer may be treated by combination chemotherapy with or without preceding secondary cytoreductive surgery. The purpose of sequencing treatment in this way is to reduce tumor bulk and thereby augment chemotherapy effectiveness. In general, adjunctive therapy is begun within a few weeks after surgery.

Directing Care of the Patient

To effectively counsel a gynecologic cancer patient and then guide her chemotherapeutic treatment course requires a comprehensive understanding of the diagnosis, alternatives, and goals of care. Coexisting conditions or tumor-related complications (e.g., deep-vein thrombosis) may need to be addressed. As the intended therapy is finalized, extensive information regarding anticipated side effects is provided to allay concerns and reduce anxiety. A consent form must be reviewed and signed by the patient, in addition to clarification of all potential logistical challenges (e.g., intravenous access).

Prior to drug infusion, a complete medical history and comprehensive physical examination are mandatory. Blood work, including a complete blood count, comprehensive metabolic panel, and tumor markers (e.g., CA125) as indicated, are drawn and reviewed before orders to begin infusion are signed. Drug administration must take place in a setting where staff are immediately available to intervene should the need arise. Afterward, the patient is provided contact numbers in case of questions, problems, or other concerns that can often develop prior to the next visit.

Typically, regular office visits shortly before or on the day of treatment allow assessment of toxicity and general health. Patient examination and review of blood work results, in the context of the tumor response and overall treatment goal, will help determine whether drugs are changed or their dosages revised. Over time, the treatment strategy is continually reassessed as circumstances change.

PHARMACOLOGIC PRINCIPLES

Dosing and Dose Intensity

Overall, treatment effectiveness depends on drug concentration and duration of exposure to critical tumor sites. Chemotherapeutic agents typically have a narrow therapeutic range or "window." Thus, doses must be calculated accurately to achieve an optimal effect above a critical threshold while avoiding undue toxicity.

Most commonly, chemotherapy doses are calculated based on the patient's body surface area (BSA) and are expressed in milligrams per meter squared (mg/m^2). BSA is a better indicator of metabolic mass than body weight because it is less affected by abnormal adipose mass. This calculation ensures that each patient receives proportionally similar drug amounts. Although height is a fixed variable, patient weights are obtained prior to every therapy course, as they may fluctuate significantly. Rarely, tissue edema or ascites must be factored, since doses should be based on weight without this coexisting fluid. The BSA is most often calculated by using a nomogram (standard reference graph table). Consistent derivation of the BSA at each visit is important, and various calculators are routinely available via software or online (http://www.globalrph.com/bsa2.htm). "Normal" adult BSA for women approximates 1.7 m^2.

Alternatively, the dosing of some drugs is more specific. For example, bevacizumab is a monoclonal antibody metabolized and eliminated via the reticuloendothelial system. It is dosed only by patient weight (mg/kg). For renally excreted drugs, such as carboplatin, dosing may be based on an estimate of the glomerular filtration rate (Calvert formula).

The amount of drug administered over time is known as the *dose intensity* (or *density*). Its primary importance is in highly responsive tumors, in which cure can be achieved with chemotherapy. However, in other less sensitive tumors, it may not be possible to increase the dose to a level sufficient to produce demonstrable benefit without producing dose-limiting toxicity. On the other hand, reducing dose intensity to decrease toxicity can produce inferior therapeutic results.

■ Administration Route and Excretion

Chemotherapy may be administered systemically or regionally. Oral, intravenous (IV), subcutaneous (SC), or intramuscular (IM) routes comprise systemic treatment options. Regional chemotherapy is aimed at delivering drugs directly into the cavity in which the tumor is located. Clearance for many agents from a body cavity is slower than from systemic circulation. As a result, cancer cells are exposed longer to higher concentrations of active agents. This technique has been most extensively studied in ovarian cancer, in which tumors are usually confined to the intraperitoneal (IP) space. Clinical studies have uniformly demonstrated a pharmacologic advantage favoring administration into the IP compartment. However, penetration into peritoneal tumor nodules by passive diffusion is often limited by the presence of intraabdominal adhesions, poor fluid circulation, fibrotic tumor encapsulation, and coexisting ascites. Because of these limitations in drug penetration, IP chemotherapy is typically administered to women with minimal residual disease.

During IV administration, several drugs known as vesicants require special care (Table 27-1). Extravasation of these into the subcutaneous tissue can result in severe pain and necrosis. These drugs require slow infusion either through a rapidly flowing peripheral IV catheter or preferably via a central venous catheter. If extravasation is suspected, the infusion is immediately stopped, the affected arm elevated, and ice packs applied. In severe cases, a plastic surgeon should be consulted.

Agent activity and toxicity is influenced dramatically by drug inactivation, elimination, or excretion. For the most part, this takes place primarily via the liver or kidneys. As a result, drug activity may be diminished and toxicity exacerbated when normal hepatic or renal function is impaired. In addition, drug toxicity is often more pronounced in the elderly or malnourished. For example, a low serum creatinine level in cachectic women may not accurately reflect underlying renal function. If a carboplatin dose is calculated using this falsely low value, the amount may be excessive and result in considerable morbidity. Instead, a preset creatinine level may need to be selected (0.8 or 1.0 mg/dL) to aid safer dosing in some patients.

■ Drug Interactions and Allergic Reaction

Most women who receive chemotherapy are prescribed medication for other noncancerous conditions, such as hypertension. Moreover, women also often receive analgesics, antiemetics, and antibiotics during chemotherapy. Most drug interactions are of little consequence, but some may lead to substantially altered drug toxicity. Drugs that are metabolized in the liver are particularly at risk for such interactions. For example, using methotrexate in a woman taking warfarin (Coumadin) will usually enhance the anticoagulant effect and thus will require a warfarin dose reduction.

An anaphylactic, allergic, or hypersensitivity reaction during or after administration of chemotherapy may develop, despite patient history review and administration of prophylactic medications. Accordingly, a treatment facility must have trained nursing staff and resources to manage these sudden, but common, issues. Prior to drug administration, a woman is instructed to report symptoms that may herald an anaphylactic reaction such as flushing, pruritus, dyspnea, tachycardia, hoarseness, or lightheadedness. Emergency equipment, such as supplemental oxygen, ventilatory face mask and bag, or intubation equipment, must be immediately available. For a localized hypersensitivity response, administration of intravenous diphenhydramine (Benadryl) and/or corticosteroids may be sufficient. However, for a generalized hypersensitivity or anaphylactic response, chemotherapy should be stopped immediately, the emergency team notified, and emergency drugs administered, such as epinephrine (0.1–0.5 mg of a 1:10,000 solution) (Table 27-2).

TABLE 27-1. Chemotherapeutic Agents and Their Association with Extravasation Injury

Vesicants	Exfoliants	Irritants	Inflammants	Neutral
Dactinomycin	Cisplatin	Carboplatin	Methotrexate	Bleomycin
Doxorubicin	Docetaxel	Etoposide		Cyclophosphamide
Paclitaxel	Liposomal doxorubicin			Gemcitabine
	Topotecan			Ifosfamide

Vesicant, agent capable of causing skin ulceration and tissue necrosis on extravasation; *exfoliant*, agent capable of causing skin exfoliation on extravasation; *irritant*, agent capable of causing skin irritation on extravasation; *inflammant*, agent capable of causing skin inflammation on extravasation.

Adapted with permission from Gershenson DM, McGuire WP, Gore M, et al (eds): Gynecologic Cancer Controversies in Management. Philadelphia: Elsevier; 2004.

TABLE 27-2. Management of Hypersensitivity Reactions

1. Stop the chemotherapy infusion
2. Assess the patient's airway, breathing, and circulation
3. Administer intravenous normal saline if hypotensive
4. Administer oxygen if dyspneic or hypoxic
5. Administer intravenous antihistamine (e.g., 50 mg intravenous diphenhydramine or 25–50 mg intravenous promethazine)
6. Administer 5 mg of nebulized salbutamol if the patient has bronchospasm
7. Administer intravenous corticosteroids (e.g., 100 mg of hydrocortisone); this may have no effect on the initial reaction, but may prevent rebound or prolonged allergic manifestations
8. If the patient does not promptly improve or has symptoms of persistent or severe hypotension or persistent bronchospasm or laryngeal edema, administer adrenaline or epinephrine (0.1–0.25 mg intravenous); further acute resuscitation measures may be required
9. Reassure the patient that the problem is a recognized and treatable one

Adapted with permission from Gershenson DM, McGuire WP, Gore M, et al (eds): Gynecologic Cancer Controversies in Management. Philadelphia: Elsevier; 2004.

Drug Resistance

In principle, larger tumor masses have a greater proportion of cells that have already developed resistance. Resistance may be intrinsic or acquired, and it may develop to one drug or to multiple agents. Intrinsic drug resistance is seen if tumors are first exposed to an agent and fail to respond. In contrast, with acquired drug resistance, tumors no longer respond to drugs to which they were initially sensitive. Sometimes, this develops with a specific drug. More often, however, acquired resistance is "pleiotropic," meaning that a cancer is resistant to multiple chemotherapy agents. This is often mediated by the P-glycoprotein or multidrug resistance pump. Advanced ovarian cancer is a good example. Most patients will initially achieve remission with platinum-based chemotherapy, but 80 percent will ultimately relapse and die from tumors that have become resistant to all cytotoxic therapy.

Evaluating Response to Chemotherapy

The effective use of chemotherapy is a dynamic process whereby a treating clinician is constantly weighing toxicity to the patient against tumor response. Numerous factors influence toxicity and include the patient's baseline nutrition, overall health, extent of disease, and prior therapy. In counseling women to continue treatment or switch to a different regimen, a clinician must have objective criteria for response (Table 27-3). The most important indicator is the *complete response rate*. For

ovarian cancer, this would include normal CA125 levels (usually <35 U/mL), physical examination findings, and imaging test results. Ultimately, women who have any possibility of cure are those who first achieve a complete response. However, if chemotherapy results in a partial response, many women still view this as advantageous compared with supportive care, even if a survival benefit is unproven.

CHEMOTHERAPEUTIC DRUGS

Antimetabolites

The antimetabolites are analogues of naturally occurring components of the metabolic pathways that lead to the synthesis of purines, pyrimidines, and nucleic acids. In most cases, they are S phase-specific agents that are most effective in rapidly growing tumors associated with short doubling times and large growth fractions (Table 27-4).

Methotrexate

This antimetabolite is U.S. Food and Drug Administration (FDA)-approved to be used solely for treatment of women with gestational trophoblastic neoplasia (GTN). It is also commonly used for the medical management of ectopic pregnancy. Methotrexate (MTX) tightly binds to dihydrofolate reductase, blocking the reduction of dihydrofolate to tetrahydrofolate (the active form of folic acid) (Fig. 27-3). As a result, thymidylate

TABLE 27-3. Clinical End Points in Evaluating Response to Chemotherapy

End Point	Definition
Complete response (CR)	Disappearance of all measurable "target" lesions
Partial response (PR)	A decrease of ≥30% in the sum of diameters of all target lesions
Progressive disease (PD)	An increase of ≥20% in the sum of diameters of target lesions or the identification of one or more new lesions
Stable disease (SD)	Neither sufficient shrinkage to qualify for PR, nor sufficient increase to qualify for PD

Data from Eisenhauer EA, Therasse P, Bogaerts J, et al: New response evaluation criteria in solid tumours: revised RECIST guideline (version 1.1). Eur J Cancer 2009 Jan;45(2):228–47.

TABLE 27-4. Chemotherapy Antimetabolites Used for Gynecologic Cancer

Generic Name	Brand Name	Indications	Routes	Common Dosages	Common Toxicity
Methotrexate	Trexall, Rheumatrex	GTN	PO, IM, IV, intrathecal	IM: 1 mg/kg on days 1, 3, 5, 7 of 8-day cycle or 30–50 mg/m^2/wk IV: 100 mg/m^2 during 30 min, then 200 mg/m^2 during 12 hr	BMD, mucositis, renal toxicity, CNS dysfunction
Gemcitabine	Gemzar	Recurrent ovarian CA, uterine sarcoma	IV	600–1250 mg/m^2/wk over 30 min × 2–3 wk	BMD, N/V/D, malaise and fever
5-Fluorouracil	Adrucil	Cervical CA, vulvar CA	IV	800–1000 mg/m^2/d during 96 hr	Mucositis, PPE
	Efudex	VAIN	Vaginal cream	3 mL QOD × 1 wk, then weekly up to 10 wk	Vulvovaginal irritation

BMD = bone marrow depression; CA = cancer; CNS = central nervous system; GTN = gestational trophoblastic neoplasia; IM = intramuscular; IV = intravenous; N/V/D = nausea, vomiting, and diarrhea; PPE = palmar-plantar erythrodysesthesia; PO = orally; QOD = every other day; VAIN = vaginal intraepithelial neoplasia.

synthetase and various steps in de novo purine synthesis are halted. This leads to arrest of DNA, RNA, and protein synthesis.

Methotrexate may be administered orally, IM, IV, or intrathecally. Most commonly, single-agent treatment of GTN involves MTX given IM as an 8-day regimen of 1 mg/kg on treatment days 1, 3, 5, and 7, or at dosages of 30 to 50 mg/m^2 once each week. Combination therapy for high-risk disease includes 100 mg/m^2 MTX given IV over 30 minutes, followed by a 200 mg/m^2 IV dose over 12 hours. With MTX, patients are counseled to avoid folate-containing supplements unless specifically directed.

MTX causes few side effects at typical doses. However, at high doses, although used infrequently, this agent can lead to fatal bone marrow toxicity. This toxicity can be prevented by "rescue" doses of leucovorin. Leucovorin is folinic acid, has activity that is equivalent to folic acid, and thus is readily converted to tetrahydrofolate. Leucovorin, however, does not require dihydrofolate reductase for its conversion. Therefore, its function is unaffected by inhibition of this enzyme by MTX. Leucovorin administration, therefore, allows for some purine and pyrimidine synthesis. Leucovorin rescue is incorporated into the 8-day alternating MTX schedule, and a 0.1 mg/kg leucovorin dose is provided orally on treatment days 2, 4, 6, and 8.

In addition to myelosuppression, renal toxicity and acute cerebral dysfunction are typically only seen at high MTX doses. Methotrexate is predominantly excreted through the kidneys, and thus women with renal insufficiency have doses reduced. Serum MTX levels are carefully monitored in these patients, as they may require prolonged leucovorin rescue.

Gemcitabine

This antimetabolite is FDA approved to be used with other agents for treatment of recurrent ovarian cancer but is also commonly used for uterine sarcoma. Gemcitabine (Gemzar) is a synthetic nucleoside analogue that undergoes multiple phosphorylations to form the active metabolite. The resulting triphosphate is subsequently incorporated into DNA as a fraudulent base pair. Following the insertion of gemcitabine, one additional deoxynucleotide is added to the end of the DNA chain before replication is terminated, and thereby, DNA synthesis is halted.

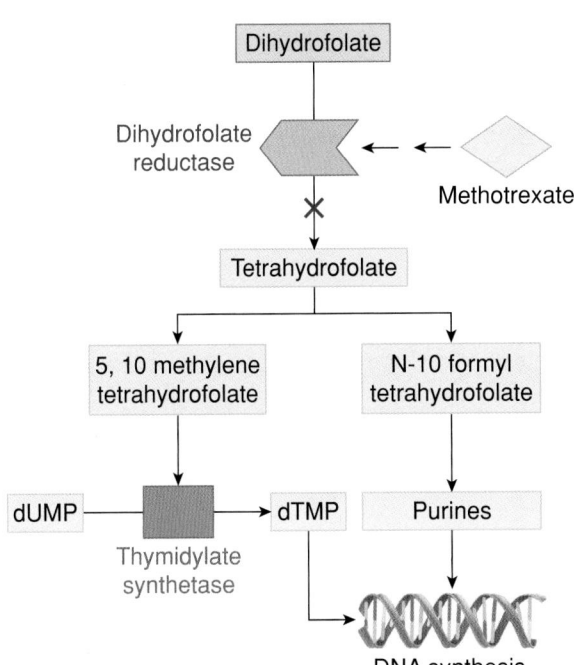

FIGURE 27-3 Methotrexate's primary target is the enzyme dihydrofolate reductase (DHFR). Inhibition of DHFR leads to partial depletion of 5,10 methylene tetrahydrofolic acid and N-10 formyl tetrahydrofolic acid, which are cofactors required for the respective synthesis of thymidylate and purines. As a result, methotrexate leads to arrested DNA, RNA, and protein synthesis. dTMP = deoxythymidine monophosphate; dUMP = deoxyuridine monophosphate.

The usual administration of gemcitabine is by 30-minute infusion. Longer durations, such as those greater than 60 min, are associated with increased toxicity due to intracellular accumulation of the triphosphate. Depending on whether it is used as a single agent or in combination, gemcitabine is typically given at doses between 600 and 1250 mg/m² once weekly for 2 to 3 weeks, followed by a week off therapy.

Myelosuppression, especially neutropenia, is the main dose-limiting side effect. Gastrointestinal (GI) toxicity, such as nausea, vomiting, diarrhea, or mucositis, is also common. Approximately 20 percent of patients will develop a flulike syndrome, including fever, malaise, headache, and chills. Pulmonary toxicity is infrequent, but reported.

5-Fluorouracil

5-Fluorouracil (5-FU) is not FDA approved for gynecologic cancer but is occasionally paired with cisplatin during chemoradiation for cervical cancer. A topical form (Efudex) can be used for vaginal intraepithelial neoplasia (VAIN) treatment as discussed in Chapter 29 (p. 646). This "false" pyrimidine antimetabolite acts principally as a thymidine synthetase inhibitor to block DNA replication.

Systemic 5-FU (Adrucil) is usually given as a 96-hour continuous IV infusion of 800 to 1000 mg/m²/d. Mucositis and/or diarrhea may be severe and dose-limiting. Hand-foot syndrome (palmar-plantar erythrodysesthesia), described on page 600, is less common but can also be dose-limiting. Myelosuppression, mainly neutropenia and thrombocytopenia, are less frequent. Nausea and vomiting are usually mild.

■ Alkylating Agents

Cyclophosphamide

The class of alkylating agents is characterized by positively charged alkyl groups that bind to negatively charged DNA to form adducts (Table 27-5). Binding leads to DNA breaks or cross-links and a halt to DNA synthesis. In general, these drugs are cell cycle-nonspecific agents.

Of alkylating agents, cyclophosphamide (Cytoxan) is FDA approved by itself or in combination for epithelial ovarian cancer treatment. Cyclophosphamide is the "C" of the EMA-CO (etoposide, methotrexate, actinomycin D, cyclophosphamide, Oncovin [vincristine]), which is a regimen prescribed for high-risk GTN. It is also used, albeit infrequently, as salvage

therapy for recurrent epithelial ovarian cancer (Bower, 1997; Cantu, 2002). Cyclophosphamide is a derivative of nitrogen mustard and is activated through a multistep process by microsomal enzymes in the liver. It promotes DNA cross-linking and DNA synthesis inhibition.

This agent may be administered IV or orally. It is typically given IV at doses of 500 to 750 mg/m² over 30 minutes every 3 weeks. Orally, a metronomic (repetitive low-dose) regimen of 50 mg daily is often used to minimize toxicity and target the tumor endothelium or stroma in combination with a biologic agent, such as bevacizumab (Chura, 2007).

Myelosuppression, mainly neutropenia, is the usual dose-limiting side effect. Cyclophosphamide is exclusively excreted by the kidneys. One of its metabolites, acrolein, can alkylate and inflame the bladder mucosa. As a result, hemorrhagic cystitis is a classic complication that may follow from 24 hours to several weeks after administration. To prevent this effect, adequate hydration is imperative to aid acrolein excretion. In addition, GI toxicity, such as nausea, vomiting, or anorexia, is common. Alopecia is typically severe. Moreover, later secondary malignancy rates are increased, particularly acute myelogenous leukemia and bladder cancer.

Of chemotherapeutic drugs, alkylating agents are believed to be particularly damaging to ovarian function. Preventatively, adjuvant GnRH agonists may lower rates of chemotherapy-induced ovarian failure, although the efficacy of this approach remains controversial (Chen, 2011; Elgindy, 2013). Through its hypoestrogenic effects, a GnRH agonist may decrease ovarian blood flow, and thereby decrease chemotherapeutic exposure of the ovaries (Blumenfeld, 2003). Alternatively, pituitary-gonadal axis inhibition may protect the germinal epithelium by inhibiting oogenesis. Last, as GnRH receptors have been identified in the ovary, GnRH agonist may act directly in the ovary to decrease granulosa cell metabolism (Peng, 1994). Importantly, advances in oocyte and ovarian tissue cryopreservation make it likely that the removal of oocytes prior to treatment will become the preferred approach when feasible.

Ifosfamide

This alkylating agent is not FDA approved for gynecologic cancers but is sometimes administered for salvage treatment of recurrent epithelial ovarian cancer, cervical cancer, and uterine sarcoma. Ifosfamide (Ifex) is a structural analogue of cyclophosphamide, differing only slightly. However, its metabolic

TABLE 27-5. Chemotherapy Alkylating Agents Used for Gynecologic Cancer

Generic Name	Brand Name	Indication	Routes	Dosages	Toxicity
Cyclophosphamide	Cytoxan	GTN, recurrent ovarian CA	PO, IV	IV: 500–750 mg/m² over 30 min, every 3 wk PO: 50 mg/d	BMD, cystitis, N/V, alopecia
Ifosfamide	Ifex	Recurrent ovarian CA, cervical CA, uterine sarcoma	IV	1.2–1.6 g/m²/d, days 1–3 of 3-wk cycle	BMD, cystitis, N/V, alopecia, CNS and renal toxicity

BMD = bone marrow depression; CA = cancer; CNS = central nervous system; GTN = gestational trophoblastic neoplasia; IV = intravenous; N/V = nausea and vomiting; PO = orally.

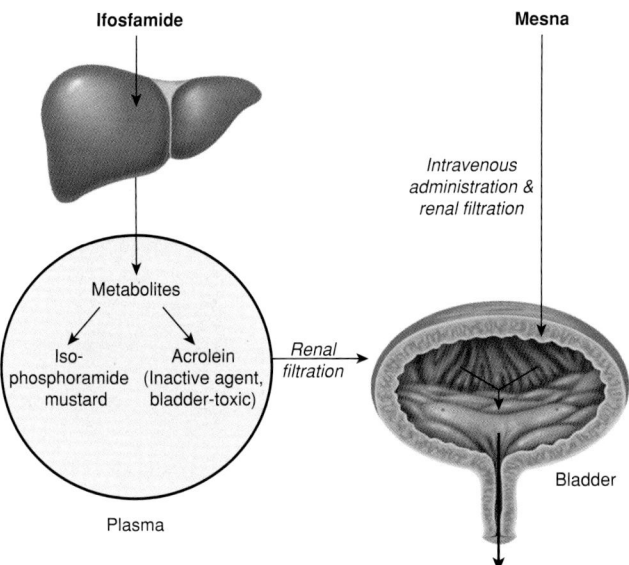

FIGURE 27-4 Ifosfamide is a prodrug, which is ultimately metabolized into active and inactive metabolites. Isophosphoramide mustard is the main active alkylating metabolite. The inactive metabolite, acrolein, is concentrated in the bladder and is bladder toxic. The drug mesna and acrolein join in the bladder to create an inactive compound, which is then excreted by the bladder. This conversion of acrolein to an inactive compound minimizes ifosfamide's bladder toxicity.

activation occurs more slowly and leads to a greater production of chloracetaldehyde, a possible neurotoxin.

Ifosfamide is administered IV, usually as a short infusion. Common doses of 1.2 to 1.6 g/m^2 are given on days 1 through 3 of a 3-week cycle. As with cyclophosphamide, adequate hydration is recommended to reduce the incidence of drug-induced hemorrhagic cystitis. In addition, concurrent mesna (Mesnex) is used to prevent severe hematuria. A mesna metabolite chemically binds with acrolein, an ifosfamide metabolite, and detoxifies acrolein in the bladder (Fig. 27-4). Other side

effects are similar to those of cyclophosphamide. However, neurotoxicity, manifested as lethargy, confusion, seizure, ataxia, hallucinations, and occasionally coma, is more likely. These symptoms are caused by the chloracetaldehyde metabolite and are reversible with removal of the drug and supportive care. The incidence of neurotoxicity is higher in the rare patient receiving high-dose therapy and also in those with impaired renal function, where a preventive dose reduction is typically necessary.

◼ Antitumor Antibiotics

Dactinomycin

The antitumor antibiotics are generally derived from microorganisms. Most antitumor antibiotics exert their cytotoxic effects by DNA intercalation during multiple phases of the cell cycle. They are considered cell-cycle specific.

In this group, dactinomycin is FDA approved to treat GTN as a single agent or as part of combination chemotherapy (Table 27-6). Dactinomycin (Cosmegen), also known as actinomycin D, is the "A" of the EMA-CO chemotherapy combination. Dactinomycin is a product of a *Streptomyces* species and becomes anchored into purine-pyrimidine DNA base pairs, resulting in DNA synthesis inhibition. It also produces toxic oxygen free radicals that cause DNA breaks. Dactinomycin is mainly excreted through the biliary system.

The usual "pulse" dosage of dactinomycin is 1.25 mg IV push every other week, but is sometimes administered as a 0.5 mg dose on days 1 through 5 every 2 to 3 weeks. Myelosuppression is the main dose-limiting side effect and may be severe. Moreover, GI toxicity, including nausea, vomiting, mucositis, and diarrhea, is often significant. Alopecia is common. As with others in the antibiotic group, dactinomycin is a potent vesicant (see Table 27-1).

Bleomycin

This antitumor antibiotic is FDA approved for malignant pleural effusion treatment or for palliative therapy of recurrent

TABLE 27-6. Chemotherapeutic Antibiotics Used for Gynecologic Cancer

Generic Name	Brand Name	Indication	Route	Dosage	Toxicity
Actinomycin D (dactinomycin)	Cosmegen	GTN	IV	1.25 mg IV push every other wk or 0.5 mg on days 1–5, every 2–3 wk	BMD, N/V/D, alopecia, vesicant
Bleomycin	Blenoxane	Germ cell or SCST ovarian CA, GTN	IV, IM, SC, intrapleural	IV: 20 U/m^2 (maximum dose of 30 U), every 3 wk	Pulmonary toxicity, fever, skin reaction
Doxorubicin	Adriamycin	Uterine sarcoma, recurrent epithelial ovarian CA	IV	45–60 mg/m^2 every 3 wk	BMD, cardiac toxicity, alopecia, vesicant
Liposomal doxorubicin	Doxil	Recurrent epithelial ovarian CA	IV	40–50 mg/m^2 over 30 min, every 4 wk	PPE, stomatitis, infusion reaction

BMD = bone marrow depression; CA = cancer; GTN = gestational trophoblastic neoplasia; IM = intramuscular; IV = intravenous; N/V/D = nausea, vomiting, and diarrhea; PPE = palmar-plantar erythrodysesthesia; SC = subcutaneous; SCST = sex cord-stromal tumor.

squamous cervical or vulvar cancer. An off-label use includes bleomycin as the "B" in BEP (bleomycin, etoposide, cisplatin) regimens, which are used as adjuvant treatment of malignant ovarian germ cell or sex cord-stromal tumors (Park, 2011; Weinberg, 2011). Additionally, it is used in GTN salvage treatment (Alazzam, 2012). Bleomycin (Blenoxane), when complexed with iron, creates activated oxygen free radicals, which cause DNA-strand breaks and cell death. It is maximally effective during the G_2 phase.

The usual dosage of bleomycin is 20 units/m² IV (maximum dose of 30 units), given every 3 weeks. Bleomycin can also be administered IM, SC, or intrapleurally. The dose is quantified by international units of "cytotoxic activity."

Pulmonary toxicity is the main dose-limiting side effect, developing in 10 percent of patients and causing death in 1 percent. Accordingly, for women prescribed bleomycin, chest radiographs and pulmonary function tests (PFTs) are performed at baseline and obtained regularly before every one or two treatment cycles. The most important PFT measurement is the diffusing capacity of the lung for carbon monoxide (DLCO). The DLCO measures the ability to transfer oxygen from the lungs to the blood stream. If the DLCO declines by 15 to 30 percent, it indicates development of restrictive lung disease. In patients receiving bleomycin, therapy may then be stopped before the onset of symptomatic pulmonary fibrosis. Fibrosis often presents clinically as pneumonitis with cough, dyspnea, dry inspiratory crackles, and infiltrates on chest radiograph. This complication is more common in patients older than 70 and with cumulative doses of greater than 400 units. Bleomycin is not myelosuppressive. However, skin reactions are common and include hyperpigmentation or erythema.

Doxorubicin

This antitumor antibiotic is FDA approved to treat epithelial ovarian cancer. Doxorubicin (Adriamycin) is also used on occasion for uterine sarcoma (Hyman, 2014; Mancari, 2014). This agent intercalates into DNA to inhibit DNA synthesis, inhibits topoisomerase II, and forms cytotoxic oxygen free radicals. The drug is metabolized extensively in the liver and eliminated through biliary excretion.

The usual dose of doxorubicin is 45 to 60 mg/m² IV, repeated every 3 weeks. Myelosuppression, particularly neutropenia, is the main dose-limiting side effect. However, cardiotoxicity is a classic complication. Patients are monitored with a multiple-gated acquisition (MUGA) radionuclide scan at baseline and periodically during therapy. The risk of cardiotoxicity is higher in women older than 70 and those with cumulative doses exceeding 550 mg/m². Ultimately, women may develop an irreversible dilated cardiomyopathy associated with congestive heart failure. Gastrointestinal toxicities are generally mild, but alopecia is universal.

Doxorubicin Hydrochloride Liposome

This antitumor antibiotic is FDA approved for the salvage treatment of recurrent epithelial ovarian cancer (Gordon, 2004). The liposomal encapsulation of doxorubicin (Doxil) dramatically alters the pharmacokinetic and toxicity profiles of the drug. Researchers developed liposomal doxorubicin to reduce cardiotoxicity and to selectively target tumor tissues.

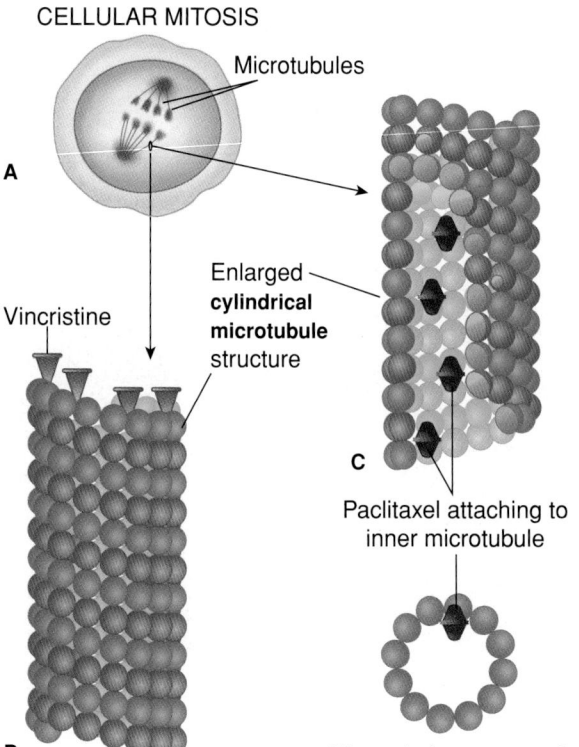

FIGURE 27-5 Diagram of taxane's and vinca alkaloid's mechanism of action. Parts B and C show magnified microtubule structure. **A.** During cellular mitosis, microtubules are essential for chromosome alignment and separation. **B.** Vincristine, one of the vinca alkaloids, attaches consistently to one end of the microtubule to inhibit microtubule assembly. **C.** Paclitaxel, one of the taxanes, binds to the inner ring of the microtubule and prohibits microtubule disassembly. In both B and C, microtubule function is impaired.

Liposomal doxorubicin may be administered as an IV infusion over 30 to 60 minutes and is dosed at 40 to 50 mg/m² every 4 weeks. In contrast to doxorubicin, administration of the encapsulated liposome is associated with minimal nausea, vomiting, alopecia, and cardiotoxicity. Infusion-related reactions develop in less than 10 percent of patients and are most common during the first treatment course. However, an increased rate of stomatitis and palmar-plantar erythrodysesthesia (PPE) is noted.

PPE is characterized by a cutaneous reaction of varying intensity. Patients may initially complain of tingling sensations on their soles and palms that generally progresses to swelling and tenderness to touch. Erythematous plaques typically develop that can become extremely painful and often lead to desquamation and skin cracking. Symptoms result from the prolonged blood levels of this time-released cytotoxic agent and may last several weeks.

■ Plant-derived Agents
Taxanes

The cytotoxic activity of all the plant-derived agents stems from the disturbance of normal assembly, disassembly, and stabilization of intracellular microtubules to halt cell division during mitosis (Fig. 27-5). The group includes the taxanes, vinca alkaloids, and topoisomerase inhibitors.

TABLE 27-7. Chemotherapeutic Plant Alkaloids Used for Gynecologic Cancer

Generic Name	Brand Name	Indications	Routes	Dosages	Toxicity
Paclitaxel	Taxol	Recurrent epithelial ovarian CA, endometrial CA, cervical CA, GTN	IV, IP	IV: 135–175 mg/m^2 every 3 wk, or 80 mg/m^2/wk for 3 weeks IP: 60 mg/m^2 on day 8 following a day-1 IV dose	HSR, peripheral neurotoxicity, BMD, alopecia, bradycardia and arrhythmia
Docetaxel	Taxotere	Recurrent epithelial ovarian CA, uterine sarcoma	IV	75–100 mg/m^2 every 3 weeks, or 35 mg/m^2/week for 3 weeks	BMD, peripheral edema, HSR, alopecia
Vincristine	Oncovin	GTN	IV	0.8–1.0 mg/m^2 every other week	Neurotoxicity, abdominal pain, alopecia
Etoposide	VP-16	Germ cell or SCST ovarian CA; recurrent epithelial ovarian CA	IV, PO	IV: 100 mg/m^2 days 1 & 2, every 2 wk, or 75–100 mg/m^2, days 1–5, every 3 wk PO: 50 mg/m^2/day for 3 wk	BMD, alopecia, secondary cancers
Topotecan	Hycamtin	Recurrent epithelial ovarian CA, cervical CA	IV	1.5 mg/m^2/d, days 1–5, every 3 wk, or 4 mg/m^2/wk for 3 wk, or 0.75 mg/m^2/d, days 1–3, every 3 wk	BMD, N/V, alopecia, fever, malaise

BMD = bone marrow depression; CA = cancer; GTN = gestational trophoblastic neoplasia; HSR = hypersensitivity reaction; HTN = hypertension; IV = intravenous; N/V = nausea and vomiting; PO = orally; SCST = sex cord-stromal tumor.

Of the taxanes, paclitaxel and docetaxel are both cell cycle-specific agents that have maximal activity during the M phase (Table 27-7). Derived from yew tree species, they act to "poison" the mitotic spindle by preventing depolymerization of the microtubules and inhibiting cellular replication.

Paclitaxel. The best-selling cancer drug ever manufactured, paclitaxel (Taxol) is FDA approved for the treatment of primary or recurrent epithelial ovarian cancer. It is also extensively used for endometrial cancers, cervical cancers, and GTN.

Paclitaxel is typically administered IV as a 3-hour infusion, but may also be given as an intraperitoneal (IP) dose. The usual IV dosage is 135 to 175 mg/m^2 every 3 weeks. Weekly paclitaxel is also effective in a regimen of 80 mg/m^2 IV for 3 consecutive weeks on a 21-day schedule ("dose-dense" regimen) for primary disease or on a 28-day schedule for recurrent disease (Katsumata, 2009; Markman, 2006). For initial therapy of optimally debulked ovarian cancer following a day-1 IV dose, paclitaxel is usually given IP on day 8 at a dose of 60 mg/m^2 (Armstrong, 2006).

Myelosuppression is the usual dose-limiting side effect. Additionally, a hypersensitivity reaction occurs in approximately one third of patients due to its formulation in Cremophor-EL, an emulsifying agent. Typically, the reaction develops within minutes of starting an initial infusion. Fortunately, the incidence can be decreased 10-fold by premedication with corticosteroids, usually dexamethasone, 20 mg orally 12 and 6 hours before paclitaxel infusion. Neurotoxicity is the principal nonhematologic dose-limiting side effect. Common symptoms include numbness, tingling, and/or burning pain in a stocking-glove distribution. Peripheral neuropathy progresses with increased paclitaxel exposure and may become debilitating. Alopecia affects almost all patients and results in total body hair loss.

Docetaxel. This taxane is not FDA approved for gynecologic cancers but is often used to treat recurrent epithelial ovarian cancer and uterine sarcoma (Gockley, 2014; Herzog, 2014b). In addition, patients with worsening peripheral neuropathy with paclitaxel are often switched to docetaxel. Clinical efficacy is similar, but docetaxel is associated with less neurotoxicity.

The usual dosage of docetaxel (Taxotere) is 75 to 100 mg/m^2 IV, repeated every 3 weeks. For recurrent ovarian cancer, weekly docetaxel is also effective at a dosage of 35 mg/m^2 IV for 3 consecutive weeks on a 28-day schedule (Tinker, 2007).

Unlike paclitaxel, myelosuppression is the main dose-limiting side effect. Fluid retention syndrome develops in approximately half of patients and manifests as weight gain, peripheral edema, pleural effusion, and ascites. Corticosteroid prophylaxis prevents most of this toxicity, as well as dermatologic side effects and hypersensitivity reactions.

Vinca Alkaloids

Vincristine, vinblastine, and vinorelbine are cell cycle-specific drugs derived from the periwinkle plant with maximal activity in the M phase. These compounds inhibit normal microtubular polymerization by binding to the tubulin subunit at a site distinct from the taxane-binding site (see Fig. 27-5). These drugs are infrequently used in gynecologic oncology. That said, vincristine is the "O" of EMA-CO combination chemotherapy for GTN treatment. The usual dosage of vincristine (Oncovin) is 0.8 to 1.0 mg/m² given IV every other week. The total individual dose is capped at 2 mg to prevent or delay neurotoxicity. This is the most common dose-limiting toxicity and may include peripheral neuropathy, autonomic nervous system dysfunction, cranial nerve palsies, ataxia, or seizures. Moreover, concurrent administration with other neurotoxic agents such as cisplatin and paclitaxel may increase severity. GI toxicity is also common, including constipation, abdominal pain, and paralytic ileus. However, myelosuppression is typically mild.

Topoisomerase Inhibitors

Topoisomerase (TOPO) enzymes unwind and rewind DNA to aid DNA replication. Topoisomerase inhibitors interfere with this function and halt DNA synthesis. This group is further divided into categories based on the specific topoisomerase enzyme they inhibit. The camptothecins inhibit TOPO I and include topotecan. The podophyllotoxins inhibit TOPO II and include etoposide.

Topotecan. This TOPO I inhibitor is a semisynthetic analogue of the alkaloid extract camptothecin. It binds to and stabilizes a transient TOPO I-DNA complex, resulting in double-strand breakage and lethal DNA damage. Topotecan (Hycamtin) is FDA approved as salvage therapy of recurrent epithelial ovarian cancer and recurrent cervical cancer (Long, 2005).

Topotecan is usually administered IV in two different schedules. Standard dosage for recurrent ovarian cancer is 1.5 mg/m² for days 1 through 5, given every 3 weeks (Gordon, 2004). However, this schedule is associated with a greater than 80-percent incidence of severe neutropenia. A less toxic regimen is 4 mg/m² weekly for 3 weeks during a 28-day schedule (Spannuth, 2007). The usual dosage when combined with cisplatin for recurrent cervical cancer is 0.75 mg/m² on days 1 through 3, given every 3 weeks (Long, 2005).

Myelosuppression, most commonly neutropenia, is the main dose-limiting side effect. GI toxicity is also frequent and includes nausea, vomiting, diarrhea, and abdominal pain. Systemic symptoms such as headache, fever, malaise, arthralgias, and myalgias are typical. Alopecia is often as complete as that seen with paclitaxel therapy.

Etoposide. This cell-cycle specific agent has maximal activity in the late S and G₂ phase. Etoposide "poisons" the TOPO II enzyme by stabilizing an otherwise transient form of the TOPO II-DNA complex. As a result, DNA cannot unwind, and double-strand DNA breaks form. This agent is not FDA approved for gynecologic cancers. However, it is often used IV as part of combination chemotherapy. Etoposide (VP-16) represents the "E" of the EMA-CO regimen, which is used for GTN. In addition, it is a component of the BEP regimen, used for ovarian germ cell or sex cord-stromal tumors. Oral etoposide may be efficacious as a single agent for salvage treatment of recurrent epithelial ovarian cancer.

The dosage of etoposide varies. In the EMA-CO regimen, 100 mg/m² is administered IV on days 1 and 2, every 2 weeks. In the BEP regimen, it is usually prescribed in dosages of 75 to 100 mg/m² IV on days 1 through 5, given every 3 weeks. The oral dosage is 50 mg/m²/d for 3 weeks, followed by a week off during a 28-day schedule.

Up to 95 percent of etoposide is protein-bound, mainly to albumin. Thus, decreased albumin levels result in a higher fraction of free drug and potentially a higher incidence of toxicity. Myelosuppression, most commonly neutropenia, is the main dose-limiting side effect. GI symptoms of nausea, vomiting, and anorexia are usually minor, except with oral administration. Most patients will develop alopecia. With etoposide, particularly if the total dose exceeds 2000 mg/m², there is a small but significant risk (approximately 1 in 1000) of later secondary malignancies. Of these, acute myelogenous leukemia is the most common.

■ Miscellaneous

Carboplatin

Several antineoplastic compounds do not clearly fit into any of the preceding categories but have similarities with alkylating agents. Among these cell-cycle nonspecific drugs are carboplatin and cisplatin.

Carboplatin (Paraplatin) produces DNA adducts that inhibit DNA synthesis. This agent is one of the most widely used, particularly in adjuvant or salvage treatment of epithelial ovarian cancer, and is FDA approved for this indication. It is also frequently used off-label for endometrial cancer.

The usual IV dose of carboplatin is calculated to a target "area under the curve" (AUC) of 6, based on the glomerular filtration rate (GFR). The Calvert equation is the most often used (carboplatin total dose [mg] = AUC × [GFR + 25]) for dose calculation. In clinical practice, the estimated creatinine clearance (CrCl) is usually substituted for the GFR and may be calculated by the Cockcroft-Gault equation (CrCl = [140 − age] × weight [kg]/0.72 × serum creatinine level [mg/100 mL]). The infusion takes 30 to 60 minutes, and dosing is repeated every 3 to 4 weeks.

Myelosuppression, most commonly thrombocytopenia, is the main dose-limiting side effect. GI toxicity and peripheral neuropathy are notably less severe than with cisplatin. Hypersensitivity reactions will eventually develop in up to 25 percent of women receiving more than six cycles.

Cisplatin

Similar to carboplatin, this agent produces DNA adducts that inhibit DNA synthesis. Cisplatin is one of the oldest and most widely used agents and is FDA approved for ovarian, cervical, and germ cell cancer. It may be given concomitantly with radiation as a radiosensitizing agent for primary treatment of cervical cancer or either as a single agent or in combination for recurrent cervical cancer. Alternatively, cisplatin is part of combination chemotherapy as the "P" of BEP, given for ovarian germ cell or sex cord-stromal tumors. However, for use in epithelial ovarian cancer, cisplatin has largely been replaced by carboplatin, except for IP therapy, due to possibly superior tissue penetration and potentially better outcomes.

TABLE 27-8. Dose and Schedule of Antiemetics to Prevent Emesis Induced by Antineoplastic Therapy of High Emetic Risk

Antiemetics	Brand Name	Single Dose Administered before Chemotherapy	Single Dose Administered Daily
5-HT₃ serotonin-receptor antagonists			
Granisetron	Kytril	Oral: 2 mg IV: 1 mg or 0.01 mg/kg	
Ondansetron	Zofran	Oral: 24 mg IV: 8 mg or 0.15 mg/kg	
Palonosetron	Aloxi	IV: 0.25 mg	
Dexamethasone	Decadron	Oral: 12 mg	Oral: 8 mg, days 2–4
Aprepitant	Emend	Oral: 125 mg	Oral: 80 mg, days 2 and 3

5-HT_3 = 5-Hydroxytryptamine-3; IV = intravenous.
Data from Kris MG, Hesketh PJ, Somerfield MR, et al: American Society of Clinical Oncology guideline for antiemetics in oncology: update 2006. J Clin Oncol 2006 Jun 20;24(18):2932–2947.

The dosage of cisplatin varies depending on the indication. In cervical cancer, dosages of 40 mg/m² IV weekly or 75 mg/m² are given every 3 weeks during radiation therapy, or 50 mg/m² IV is provided every 3 weeks for patients with recurrent disease (Long, 2005). As part of the BEP protocol, cisplatin is administered 20 mg/m² IV on days 1 through 5 every 3 weeks. Alternatively, for ovarian cancer IP chemotherapy, cisplatin is given on day 1 or 2 of a 21-day cycle at a dose of 75 to 100 mg/m² (Armstrong, 2006; Dizon, 2011).

Cisplatin has several significant toxicities. Of these, nephrotoxicity is the main dose-limiting side effect. Accordingly, patients must be aggressively hydrated before, during, and after drug administration. Mannitol (10 g) or furosemide (20 to 40 mg) may be necessary to maintain a urine output of at least 100 to 150 mL/hour. With cisplatin, electrolyte abnormalities, such as hypomagnesemia and hypokalemia, are common. In addition, severe, prolonged nausea and vomiting can be dramatic without adequate premedication (Table 27-8). Patients often describe a metallic taste and loss of appetite following treatment. Neurotoxicity, usually in the form of peripheral neuropathy, can also be dose limiting and irreversible. Ototoxicity typically manifests as high-frequency hearing loss and tinnitus. Similar to carboplatin, hypersensitivity reactions may develop with prolonged use. Overall, cisplatin is significantly more toxic than carboplatin, except for its reduced hematologic toxicity.

■ Hormonal Agents

Tamoxifen

Due to their minimal toxicity and reasonable activity, hormonal agents are often used for palliative treatment of endometrial and ovarian cancers despite lacking formal FDA approval for these indications. Of these, tamoxifen is a selective estrogen-receptor modulator. It is a nonsteroidal prodrug and is metabolized into a high-affinity estrogen-receptor antagonist in breast tissue. It does not activate the estrogen receptor and thereby blocks breast cancer cell growth. The complex is then transported into the tumor cell nucleus, where it binds to DNA and halts cellular growth and proliferation in the G_0 or G_1 phase. Antiangiogenic

effects have also been suggested. In addition to breast cancer, tamoxifen (Nolvadex) is occasionally used to treat endometrial and ovarian cancer (Fiorica, 2004; Hurteau, 2010).

Tamoxifen is orally administered, usually prescribed in doses of 20 to 40 mg for continuous daily use. Toxicity associated with tamoxifen is minimal, mainly consisting of menopausal symptoms such as hot flushes, nausea, and vaginal dryness or discharge. Moreover, some degree of fluid retention and peripheral edema develops in one third of patients. Reduced cognition and libido may also be noted during therapy.

In the endometrium, tamoxifen acts as a partial estrogen-receptor agonist. Sustained use increases the risk for endometrial polyp formation, and endometrial cancer risks triple. Moreover, thromboembolic event rates are raised, especially during and immediately after major surgery or periods of immobility. In contrast, tamoxifen prevents osteoporosis due to its partial agonist properties in bone and has beneficial effects on the serum lipid profile.

Megestrol Acetate

This agent is a synthetic derivative of progesterone that has activity on tumors through its antiestrogenic effects. As such, megestrol acetate (Megace) is most often used to treat endometrial hyperplasia, nonoperable endometrial cancer, and recurrent endometrial cancer, especially in those patients with grade 1 disease (Chap. 33, p. 706).

The usual oral dosage is 80 mg twice daily. Megestrol acetate has minimal toxicity, but patients often gain weight from a combination of fluid retention and increased appetite. Thromboembolic events are rare. Patients with diabetes mellitus are carefully monitored because of the possibility of exacerbating hyperglycemia due to its concurrent glucocorticoid activity.

BIOLOGICAL AND TARGETED THERAPY

Differing molecular pathways within normal and malignant cells have led to targeted agents that exploit these differences. Targeted therapies offer the potential for improved long-term disease control with less toxicity. Many of these novel agents are currently being evaluated in clinical trials. Thus, an overview of noncytotoxic drug development is critical for understanding future medical treatment of gynecologic cancer.

■ Antiangiogenesis Agents

Angiogenesis is a normal physiologic process that forms new blood vessels and remodels vasculature for oxygen and nutrient transport to tissues. This process is usually transient and tightly regulated by various pro- and antiangiogenic factors. However, the homeostatic balance is dysregulated in malignancy. In cancers, sustained angiogenesis leads to tumor growth and metastasis and provides access to systemic lymphatic and circulatory systems. Thus, targeted inhibition of angiogenesis is an appealing therapeutic approach.

The binding of vascular endothelial growth factor (VEGF) to the VEGF receptor is a vital first step in stimulating normal angiogenesis. Many malignancies, such as ovarian cancer, are characterized by increased levels of VEGF or other proangiogenic factors. Several novel agents interfere with this process to halt tumor growth.

Bevacizumab

This agent is a monoclonal antibody that binds to VEGF to prevent VEGF interaction with its receptor (Fig. 27-6A). Currently, bevacizumab (Avastin) is FDA-approved for persistent, recurrent, or metastatic cervical cancer, as well as relapsed platinum-resistant epithelial ovarian cancer (Pujade-Lauraine, 2014; Tewari, 2014). Its usual dosage is 15 mg/kg given IV every 3 weeks with or without cytotoxic chemotherapy. In most cases, toxicity with bevacizumab is minimal. However, GI perforation may occur in up to 10 percent of patients (Cannistra, 2007). This complication is more likely in women with preexisting inflammatory bowel disease or in those with bowel resection at their primary surgery for advanced ovarian cancer (Burger, 2014). Elevated blood pressure is common and may lead to hypertensive crisis. Other possible toxicities include incomplete wound healing, weakness, pain, nosebleed, and proteinuria.

VEGF Trap

VEGF-A is the main isoform of VEGF. It can be bound by bevacizumab, as just described, or by a recombinant "fusion protein" named VEGF Trap (aflibercept). VEGF Trap is constructed by fusing two specific portions of the VEGF receptor and the "Fc" constant region of the IgG molecule. The receptor portions provide high-affinity binding of VEGF (Fig. 27-6B). Clinical experience in gynecologic cancers is preliminary. Early reports suggest a risk of GI perforation similar to that for bevacizumab (Coleman, 2012; Gotlieb, 2012; Mackay, 2012; Tew, 2014).

Sunitinib

Receptor tyrosine kinases (RTKs) are proteins that span the plasma membrane of cells and act as receptors (Fig. 27-7C). If

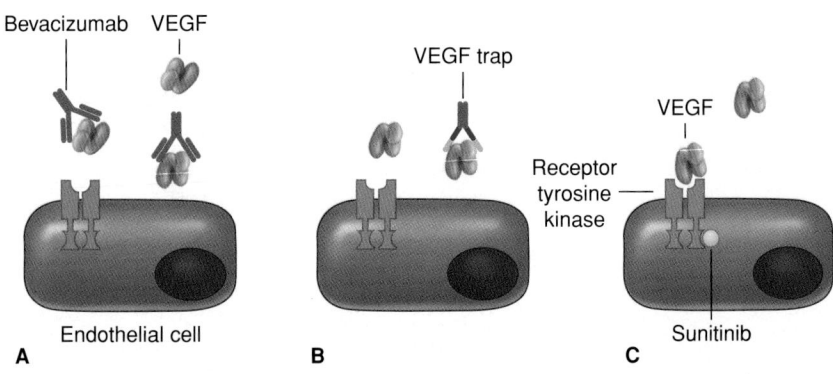

FIGURE 27-6 Mechanisms of action for three antiangiogenesis agents. **A.** Bevacizumab is a monoclonal antibody that binds vascular endothelial growth factor (VEGF). Binding prevents VEGF from combining with its endothelial-bound receptor, which is a receptor tyrosine kinase. **B.** VEGF Trap similarly binds VEGF and prevents receptor binding. **C.** Sunitinib binds with the intracellular ATP-binding sites of receptor tyrosine kinase to inhibit receptor action even though VEGF may be bound. In all three cases, angiogenesis is inhibited, and tumor growth is halted.

two side-by-side receptors bind a ligand, then an active dimer is formed. Ligands for RTKs include cytokines, hormones, and growth factors. The activated dimer then phosphorylates tyrosine residues. Phosphorylation first of the tyrosine kinase itself, and then of other proteins, activates them. By this means, RTKs regulate normal cellular processes but also play a critical role in cancer development and progression.

Sunitinib (Sutent) is an oral agent that inhibits several RTKs, including those that bind proangiogenic growth factors, such as VEGF and platelet-derived growth factor. For gynecologic cancers, the clinical efficacy of a 50 mg daily dose is currently under investigation (Baumann, 2012; Hensley, 2009).

Cediranib

Another RTK inhibitor of VEGF, cediranib (Recentin), has demonstrated significant clinical activity in relapsed ovarian cancer. With an oral daily dose of 30 mg, a 17-percent response

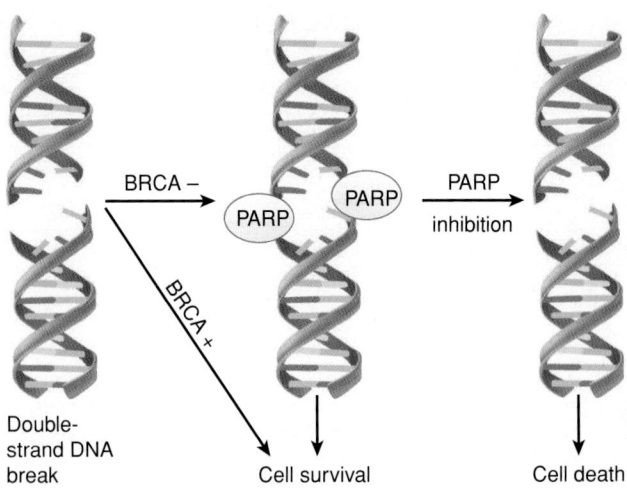

FIGURE 27-7 For DNA breaks, BRCA repairs both strands and the cell survives. With BRCA mutations and absent BRCA function, only PARP is available for DNA repair to permit cell survival. If a PARP inhibitor is administered, then DNA breaks are not repaired, and the tumor cell dies.

rate was reported when used as a single agent (Matulonis, 2009). Even more promising results have been recently observed when combined with olaparib, a poly(ADP) ribose polymerase inhibitor (Liu, 2014).

■ Mammalian Target of Rapamycin Inhibitors

The *mammalian target of rapamycin (mTOR)* is a protein kinase that regulates membrane trafficking, transcription, translation, and cell cytoskeleton maintenance. mTOR has downstream effects that include increased VEGF production. Thus, efforts to inhibit mTOR signaling also can lead to angiogenesis inhibition. Rapamycin inhibits mTOR, and analogues of this drug, such as temsirolimus (CCI-779) and everolimus (RAD001), are currently being studied for gynecologic cancer treatment (Alvarez, 2013; Fleming, 2014; Slomovitz, 2010).

■ Poly(ADP) Ribose Polymerase Inhibitors

Another promising group of targeted therapies, poly(ADP) ribose polymerase (PARP) inhibitors, exploit the differences in DNA damage repair between normal and malignant cells. During the cell cycle, DNA is routinely damaged thousands of times. The BRCA protein repairs double-strand breaks, and PARP repairs single-strand breaks. In the functioning cell, if BRCA does not repair the break, PARP will (Fig. 27-7).

Five to 10 percent of ovarian cancer patients have a germline *BRCA1* or *BRCA2* gene mutation, which predisposes them to loss of homologous DNA repair. Normal cells do not replicate their DNA as often as cancer cells, and without mutated BRCA1 or BRCA2, still have functional homologous repair. This allows them to survive PARP inhibition. Thus, only tumor cells with BRCA defects are almost entirely dependent on PARP repair. If PARP repair is prevented, damaged cancer cell DNA cannot be repaired and cells die. In contrast, normal cells are unaffected. Several PARP inhibitors are currently in development to take advantage of this unique tumor cell vulnerability.

Olaparib (AZD2281)

This PARP inhibitor is now FDA-approved for *BRCA1* and *BRCA2* mutation carriers with relapsed ovarian cancer that has demonstrated resistance to platinum drugs (Kaufman, 2015). It also has clinical activity in patients without mutations (Ledermann, 2014). As a single agent, the usual oral dose is 400 mg twice daily. The most frequent side effects are fatigue, nausea, and vomiting (Kaufman, 2015). Further encouraging studies are evaluating standard cytotoxic drugs compared against olaparib plus other targeted agents as maintenance therapy (Liu, 2014).

SIDE EFFECTS

Chemotherapy regimens, especially those including cytotoxic drugs, are universally toxic and display a narrow margin of safety. The Cancer Therapy Evaluation Program (CTEP) of the National Cancer Institute (NCI) has developed a detailed and comprehensive set of guidelines for the description and grading of toxicity.

Termed the Common Terminology Criteria for Adverse Events (CTCAE), the most recent revision is version 4.0 and is available at: http://evs.nci.nih.gov/ftp1/CTCAE/About.html.

In general, treatment modifications depend on the degree (grade) and duration of toxicity experienced during the preceding therapy course. Doses are reduced if a woman experiences a severe reaction but then may be subsequently increased if tolerance improves. However, treatment is not resumed until toxicity has resolved to baseline or "Grade 1" levels and may be delayed on a week-to-week basis to permit recovery. Dose modification and supportive care are implemented to prevent delays of greater than 2 weeks, which would otherwise compromise therapeutic efficacy. Serious myelosuppression can be partially corrected with the use of hematopoietic growth factors (p. 606). Many of the common toxicities can be prevented with proper use of premedications or alleviated with supportive measures.

■ Bone Marrow Toxicity

Myelosuppression, especially neutropenia, is the most common dose-limiting side effect of cytotoxic drugs. The absolute neutrophil count (ANC) is the critical measure when determining patient infection risk and may reflect mild ($1000–1500/mm^3$), moderate ($500–1000/mm^3$), or severe ($<500/mm^3$) neutropenia. Frequently, patients receiving therapy will have a nadir (lowest measurement) into the neutropenic range that will recover before the next scheduled course of treatment. However, if they are admitted to the hospital for fever or other condition, neutropenic precautions should be observed. Although guidelines vary, precautions include assiduous provider hand washing; provider outer gowns, gloves, and masks; and patient isolation from potential infection carriers.

Moderate degrees of anemia often develop in cancer patients receiving chemotherapy and may contribute to chronic fatigue. Frequent transfusions are not practical or recommended, and many patients will adapt to chronic anemia with minimal symptoms. Synthetic erythropoietin is infrequently indicated (p. 606).

Thrombocytopenia is less common but may predispose the patient to serious bleeding if the platelet count drops below $10,000/mm^3$. No predetermined platelet value should prompt routine transfusion, but ongoing bleeding in affected patients is a warranted indication.

■ Gastrointestinal Toxicity

Most anticancer agents are associated with some degree of nausea, vomiting, and anorexia. Typically, the emetogenic potential of a particular drug or regimen will dictate the antiemetic regimen used (Tables 27-9 and 27-10). Mild nausea and vomiting can often be managed effectively by prochlorperazine (Compazine) with or without dexamethasone (Table 42-7, p. 914). If drugs with more severe emetogenic effects such as cisplatin are administered, then ondansetron, granisetron, or palonosetron, which are 5-hydroxytryptamine antagonists, can be given IV before chemotherapy. Ondansetron (Zofran) and granisetron (Kytril) can also be provided orally to manage delayed and/or chronic nausea after chemotherapy. However, these drugs can induce significant constipation as a side effect.

TABLE 27-9. Emetic Risk of Intravenously Administered Antineoplastic Agents Used in Gynecologic Oncology

Emetic Risk	Incidence of Emesis (without antiemetics)	Agent
High	>90%	Cisplatin Cyclophosphamide ≥1500 mg/m^2 Dactinomycin
Moderate	30–90%	Carboplatin Ifosfamide Cyclophosphamide <1500 mg/m^2 Doxorubicin
Low	10–30%	Paclitaxel Docetaxel Topotecan Etoposide Methotrexate Gemcitabine
Minimal	<10%	Bevacizumab Bleomycin Vinblastine Vincristine Vinorelbine

Data from Hesketh, 2008; Kris, 2006; Roila, 2006.

Chemotherapy-related diarrhea, oral mucositis, esophagitis, and gastroenteritis are treated with supportive care.

Dermatologic Toxicity

Most drugs can cause a toxicity spectrum to the skin or subcutaneous tissues that includes hyperpigmentation, photosensitivity, nail abnormalities, rashes, urticaria, erythema, and alopecia. Many of these are drug specific and self-limited, but occasionally, they may be dose limiting. As discussed earlier, palmar-plantar erythrodysesthesia is a known toxicity of liposomal doxorubicin (p. 600). In addition, changes in skin pigmentation are seen with bleomycin, whereas nail discoloration and onycholysis have been associated with docetaxel therapy. Mild urticarial reactions are prevented or alleviated by premedication with diphenhydramine hydrochloride, 50 mg IV or orally.

One of the most emotionally distressing side effects of many chemotherapeutic agents is scalp alopecia. Fortunately, this is usually reversible. With some drugs such as paclitaxel, women will also experience loss of eyelashes, eyebrows, and other body hair. In general, techniques to minimize alopecia are unsuccessful. Instead, women are counseled regarding cosmetic options such as false eyelashes and wigs.

Neurotoxicity

Peripheral neuropathy develops commonly with cisplatin, paclitaxel, and the vinca alkaloids. Cisplatin-induced neurotoxicity usually resolves slowly, due to axonal demyelination and loss. This toxicity is related to cumulative dose and intensity. To counter this toxicity, amifostine (Ethyol) may be administered, but substitution of carboplatin will avoid much of the toxicity. Gabapentin (Neurontin) is the usual treatment for neuropathic pain, starting at a dosage of 300 mg daily. Other options to treat symptomatic peripheral neuropathy that have shown some efficacy include oral glutamine (up to 15 g twice daily) or oral vitamin B$_6$ (up to 50 mg three times daily).

With chemotherapeutic agents in general, drug dosing may need to be adjusted if peripheral neuropathy becomes problematic—for example, if a patient can no longer hold a cup of coffee. More dramatic instances of acute cerebellar syndromes, cranial nerve palsies or paralysis, and occasionally acute and chronic encephalopathies are managed with supportive care and usually with discontinuation of the offending agent.

GROWTH FACTORS

Synthetic Erythropoietins

In some clinical situations, incorporation of hematopoietic drug factors to prompt red blood cell (RBC) or granulocyte

TABLE 27-10. Drug Regimens for the Prevention of Chemotherapy-Induced Emesis by Emetic Risk Category

Emetic Risk Category (Incidence of Emesis without Antiemetics)	Antiemetic Regimens and Schedules
High (>90%)	5-HT$_3$ serotonin receptor antagonist: day 1 Dexamethasone: days 1–3 Granisetron: days 1–3
Moderate (30% to 90%)	5-HT$_3$ serotonin receptor antagonist: day 1 Dexamethasone: days 1–3
Low (10% to 30%)	5-HT$_3$ serotonin receptor antagonist: day 1 Dexamethasone: days 1–3
Minimal (<10%)	Prescribe as needed

5-HT$_3$ = 5-Hydroxytryptamine-3; see table 27-8.
Data from Kris MG, Hesketh PJ, Somerfield MR, et al: American Society of Clinical Oncology guideline for antiemetics in oncology: update 2006. J Clin Oncol 2006 Jun 20;24(18):2932–2947.

production may have merit. Of these, epoetin alfa and darbepoetin alfa are synthetic erythropoietins that have the same biologic effects as endogenous erythropoietin to stimulate RBC production. These agents are recommended for patients with chemotherapy-associated anemia who have a hemoglobin concentration that is approaching, or has fallen below, 10 g/dL. However, when used at higher hemoglobin levels, they may actually be associated with tumor progression and shorten survival (Rizzo, 2008). Moreover, several large studies have shown that despite reducing the need for RBC transfusions, erythropoiesis stimulating agents (ESAs) increase the risk for thromboembolic events and death in cancer patients treated with epoetin alfa (Aapro, 2012; Tonia, 2012). As a result, the FDA has issued a "black-box" warning to state that a higher mortality rate and/or shortened time to tumor progression were found when ESAs were dosed with the intent to achieve hemoglobin values ≥ 12 g/dL compared with placebo or observational controls. Once routinely used, these agents are now infrequently administered to gynecologic cancer patients due to safety concerns.

When used, epoetin alfa (Procrit, Eprex, and Epogen) is usually prescribed as 40,000 units SC, given weekly (Case, 2006). Beyond local pain at the injection site, this agent has minimal side effects. Possible toxicity may include diarrhea, nausea, or hypertension (Bohlius, 2006; Khuri, 2007). For darbepoetin alfa (Aranesp), the usual SC dose is 200 μg every other week or 500 μg given every 3 weeks. Darbepoetin alfa has minimal side effects beyond local pain at the injection site.

■ Granulocyte Colony-Stimulating Factors

Filgrastim and pegfilgrastim are human granulocyte colony-stimulating factors (G-CSF) produced by recombinant DNA technology. As such, these cytokines bind to hematopoietic cells and activate proliferation, differentiation, and activation of granulocyte progenitor cells. These growth factors are mainly used to prevent episodes of febrile neutropenia (ANC <1500), particularly in patients with a greater than 20-percent risk for such an event. Fortunately, none of the common regimens used in the treatment of gynecologic cancer have a risk that exceeds 20-percent, and thus growth factors are typically not required for initial prophylaxis. Instead, growth factors are usually indicated to permit a patient to maintain her treatment schedule.

Filgrastim (Neupogen) is given SC, and the usual SC dose is 5 μg/kg/d. However, patients typically are given either 300 μg or 480 μg, which is the content of manufactured vials. It should be administered at least 24 hours after chemotherapy completion. Therapy is terminated when the white blood count (WBC) exceeds 10,000/mm³ or when the absolute neutrophil count exceeds 1000/mm³ for 3 consecutive days. Toxicity with filgrastim is limited, and transient bone pain is usually mild to moderate.

Pegfilgrastim (Neulasta) acts similarly to filgrastim to stimulate production of granulocyte progenitor cells within the bone marrow. The "peg" in pegfilgrastim refers to a polyethylene glycol unit that prolongs the time it remains in the body. Pegfilgrastim is given as a single 6-mg SC injection once per chemotherapy cycle. This is usually far more convenient than daily filgrastim doses. It should not be administered during the 14 days before and within 24 hours after administration of cytotoxic chemotherapy. Transient bone pain is usually mild to moderate, but often more pronounced than with filgrastim.

CHEMOSENSITIVITY AND RESISTANCE ASSAYS

Routinely, the selection of specific chemotherapeutic agents is based on clinical literature describing outcomes for a specific gynecologic cancer. In contrast to this empiric approach, chemotherapy sensitivity and resistance assays are theoretically appealing due to the possibility of tailoring treatment. Using this strategy, viable tumor tissue is collected from the patient during surgery or other intervention (e.g., paracentesis). The sample is shipped to a specialized laboratory. Here, in vitro analysis determines whether tumor growth is inhibited by a drug or panel of drugs.

The potential of selecting effective cancer treatments while sparing unnecessary ones is intriguing, and patients may even request testing. However, no current assay has demonstrated sufficient efficacy to support its use. Thus, these assays are not recommended for individual patients outside of a clinical trial (Burstein, 2011).

CANCER DRUG DEVELOPMENT

The only proven way to improve cancer treatment success rates is to test new agents, higher doses, novel combinations of drugs, or unique ways of administering treatment. Since gynecologic cancers are relatively uncommon, most landmark Phase III studies are conducted within large collaborative groups such as the NRG Oncology Group. Promising drugs are first identified by demonstrating success in cancer cell lines or in animals inoculated with tumor. After preclinical steps are completed, novel agents proceed through four phases of clinical testing.

Phase I trials use a dose-escalating design to determine the dose-limiting toxicity, maximum tolerated dose (MTD), and pharmacokinetic parameters of the drug. Groups of three to six patients with varied tumor types are enrolled and receive escalating dose levels. The MTD is determined as the dose below which two patients experience dose-limiting toxicity. In a Phase I trial, detecting a tumor response is not critical, since enrolled patients have typically completed extensive prior therapy. However, observed responses would encourage further disease-specific Phase II trials.

After the recommended dose and treatment schedule have been defined in a Phase I trial, the regimen can proceed to Phase II. The primary goal of this trial type is to define the actual response rate in patients with a specific cancer type. Usually a measure of disease (MOD) is required to allow accurate determination of a complete response, partial response, stable disease, or progression. Typically, patients enrolled in Phase II trials have received only one prior chemotherapy regimen. This allows for a reasonable chance of response compared with subjects in Phase I studies. Secondary end points of Phase II trials include determination of the "progression-free interval," cumulative incidence of dose-limiting toxicity over multiple cycles, and overall survival rates.

Phase III randomized trials are designed to directly compare the drug with existing standard regimens in a particular stage and type of cancer. Phase III trials generally require a minimum of 150 patients per "arm" to provide adequate statistical precision. Finally, Phase IV clinical trials evaluate drugs that are already FDA approved. The goal of Phase IV trials is to study long-term drug safety and efficacy.

The emergence of biologic and targeted therapies has necessitated a reanalysis of this traditional paradigm of cancer drug development. For example, antiangiogenic agents and PARP inhibitors do not have dose-dependent toxicities to establish a MTD. Additionally, instead of measuring tumor shrinkage as an indicator of response for these cytostatic agents, new end points are being developed and validated (e.g., 6-month progression-free survival). Novel clinical trial designs will be a vital part of future drug development (Herzog, 2014a).

In general, patients are strongly encouraged to participate in appropriate Phase I, II, and III clinical trials. Doing so expands their options for treatment. In addition, the results of such studies are the primary method to improve the outcomes of women diagnosed with gynecologic cancer in the future. However, fewer than 5 percent of cancer patients currently enroll in a clinical trial.

REFERENCES

Aapro M, Jelkmann W, Constantinescu SN, et al: Effects of erythropoietin receptors and erythropoiesis-stimulating agents on disease progression in cancer. Br J Cancer 106(7):1249, 2012

Alazzam M, Tidy J, Osborne R, et al: Chemotherapy for resistant or recurrent gestational trophoblastic neoplasia. Cochrane Database Syst Rev 12:CD008891, 2012

Alvarez EA, Brady WE, Walker JL, et al: Phase II trial of combination bevacizumab and temsirolimus in the treatment of recurrent or persistent endometrial carcinoma: a Gynecologic Oncology Group study. Gynecol Oncol 129(1):22, 2013

Armstrong DK, Bundy B, Wenzel L, et al: Intraperitoneal cisplatin and paclitaxel in ovarian cancer. N Engl J Med 354(1):34, 2006

Baumann KH, du Bois A, Meier W, et al: A phase II trial (AGO 2.11) in platinum-resistant ovarian cancer: a randomized multicenter trial with sunitinib (SU11248) to evaluate dosage, schedule, tolerability, toxicity and effectiveness of a multitargeted receptor tyrosine kinase inhibitor monotherapy. Ann Oncol 23(9):2265, 2012

Blumenfeld Z: Gynaecologic concerns for young women exposed to gonadotoxic chemotherapy. Curr Opin Obstet Gynecol 15(5):359, 2003

Bohlius J, Wilson J, Seidenfeld J, et al: Recombinant human erythropoietins and cancer patients: updated meta-analysis of 57 studies including 9353 patients. J Natl Cancer Inst 98(10):708, 2006

Bower M, Newlands ES, Holden L, et al: EMA/CO for high-risk gestational trophoblastic tumors: results from a cohort of 272 patients. J Clin Oncol 15(7):2636, 1997

Burger RA, Brady MF, Bookman MA, et al: Risk factors for GI adverse events in a phase III randomized trial of bevacizumab in first-line therapy of advanced ovarian cancer: a Gynecologic Oncology Group Study. J Clin Oncol 32(12):1210, 2014

Burstein HJ, Mangu PB, Somerfield MR, et al: American Society of Clinical Oncology clinical practice guideline update on the use of chemotherapy sensitivity and resistance assays. J Clin Oncol 29(24):3328, 2011

Cannistra SA, Matulonis UA, Penson RT, et al: Phase III study of bevacizumab in patients with platinum-resistant ovarian cancer or peritoneal serous cancer. J Clin Oncol 25(33):5180, 2007

Cantu MG, Buda A, Parma G, et al: Randomized controlled trial of single-agent paclitaxel versus cyclophosphamide, doxorubicin, and cisplatin in patients with recurrent ovarian cancer who responded to first-line platinum-based regimens. J Clin Oncol 20(5):1232, 2002

Case AS, Rocconi RP, Kilgore LC, et al: Effectiveness of darbepoetin alfa versus epoetin alfa for the treatment of chemotherapy induced anemia in patients with gynecologic malignancies. Gynecol Oncol 101(3):499, 2006

Chen H, Li J, Cui T, et al: Adjuvant gonadotropin-releasing hormone analogues for the prevention of chemotherapy induced premature ovarian failure in premenopausal women. Cochrane Database Syst Rev 11:CD008018, 2011

Chura JC, Van Iseghem K, Downs LS Jr, et al: Bevacizumab plus cyclophosphamide in heavily pretreated patients with recurrent ovarian cancer. Gynecol Oncol 107(2):326, 2007

Coleman RL, Sill MW, Lankes HA, et al: A phase II evaluation of aflibercept in the treatment of recurrent or persistent endometrial cancer: a Gynecologic Oncology Group study. Gynecol Oncol 127(3):538, 2012

Dizon DS, Sill MW, Gould N, et al: Phase I feasibility study of intraperitoneal cisplatin and intravenous paclitaxel followed by intraperitoneal paclitaxel in untreated ovarian, fallopian tube, and primary peritoneal carcinoma: a gynecologic oncology group study. Gynecol Oncol 123(2):182, 2011

Eisenhauer EA, Therasse P, Bogaerts J, et al: New response evaluation criteria in solid tumours: revised RECIST guideline (version 1.1). Eur J Cancer 45:228, 2009

Elgindy EA, El-Haieg DO, Khorshid OM, et al: Gonadatrophin suppression to prevent chemotherapy-induced ovarian damage: a randomized controlled trial. Obstet Gynecol 121(1):78, 2013

Fiorica JV, Brunetto VL, Hanjani P, et al: Phase II trial of alternating courses of megestrol acetate and tamoxifen in advanced endometrial carcinoma: a Gynecologic Oncology Group study. Gynecol Oncol 92(1):10, 2004

Fleming GF, Filiaci VL, Marzullo B, et al: Temsirolimus with or without megestrol acetate and tamoxifen for endometrial cancer: a Gynecologic Oncology Group study. Gynecol Oncol 132(3):585, 2014

Gockley AA, Rauh-Hain JA, Del Carmen MG: Uterine leiomyosarcoma: a review article. Int J Gynecol Cancer 24(9):1538, 2014

Gordon AN, Tonda M, Sun S, et al: Long-term survival advantage for women treated with pegylated liposomal doxorubicin compared with topotecan in a phase 3 randomized study of recurrent and refractory epithelial ovarian cancer. Gynecol Oncol 95(1):1, 2004

Gotlieb WH, Amant F, Advani S, et al: Intravenous aflibercept for treatment of recurrent symptomatic malignant ascites in patients with advanced ovarian cancer: a phase 2, randomised, double-blind, placebo-controlled study. Lancet Oncol 13(2):154, 2012

Hensley ML, Sill MW, Scribner DR Jr, et al: Sunitinib malate in the treatment of recurrent or persistent uterine leiomyosarcoma: a Gynecologic Oncology Group phase II study. Gynecol Oncol 115(3):460, 2009

Herzog TJ, Alvarez RD, Secord A, et al: SGO guidance document for clinical trial designs in ovarian cancer: a changing paradigm. Gynecol Oncol 135(1):3, 2014a

Herzog TJ, Monk BJ, Rose PG, et al: A phase II trial of oxaliplatin, docetaxel, and bevacizumab as first-line therapy of advanced cancer of the ovary, peritoneum, and fallopian tube. Gynecol Oncol 132(3):517, 2014b

Hesketh PJ: Chemotherapy-induced nausea and vomiting. N Engl J Med 358(23):2482, 2008

Hurteau JA, Brady MF, Darcy KM, et al: Randomized phase III trial of tamoxifen versus thalidomide in women with biochemical-recurrent-only epithelial ovarian, fallopian tube or primary peritoneal carcinoma after a complete response to first-line platinum/taxane chemotherapy with an evaluation of serum vascular endothelial growth factor (VEGF): a Gynecologic Oncology Group Study. Gynecol Oncol 119(3):444, 2010

Hyman DM, Grisham RN, Hensley ML: Management of advanced uterine leiomyosarcoma. Curr Opin Oncol 26(4):422, 2014

Katsumata N, Yasuda M, Takahashi F, et al: Dose-dense paclitaxel once a week in combination with carboplatin every 3 weeks for advanced ovarian cancer: a phase 3, open-label, randomised controlled trial. Lancet 374(9698):1331, 2009

Kaufman B, Shapira-Frommer R, Schmutzler RK, et al: Olaparib monotherapy in patients with advanced cancer and a germline BRCA1/2 mutation. J Clin Oncol 33(3):244, 2015

Khuri FR: Weighing the hazards of erythropoiesis stimulation in patients with cancer. N Engl J Med 356(24):2445, 2007

Kris MG, Hesketh PJ, Somerfield MR, et al: American Society of Clinical Oncology guideline for antiemetics in oncology: update 2006. J Clin Oncol 24(18):1, 2006

Ledermann J, Harter P, Gourley C, et al: Olaparib maintenance therapy in patients with platinum-sensitive relapsed serous ovarian cancer: a preplanned retrospective analysis of outcomes by BRCA status in a randomised phase 2 trial. Lancet Oncol 15(8):852, 2014

Liu JF, Barry WT, Birrer M, et al: Combination cediranib and olaparib versus olaparib alone for women with recurrent platinum-sensitive ovarian cancer: a randomised phase 2 study. Lancet Oncol 15(11):1207, 2014

Long HJ III, Bundy BN, Grendys EC Jr., et al: Randomized phase III trial of cisplatin with or without topotecan in carcinoma of the uterine cervix: a Gynecologic Oncology Group Study. J Clin Oncol 23(21):4626, 2005

Mackay HJ, Buckanovich RJ, Hirte H, et al: A phase II study single agent of aflibercept (VEGF Trap) in patients with recurrent or metastatic gynecologic carcinosarcomas and uterine leiomyosarcoma. A trial of the Princess Margaret Hospital, Chicago and California Cancer Phase II Consortia. Gynecol Oncol 125(1):136, 2012

Mancari R, Signorelli M, Gadducci A, et al: Adjuvant chemotherapy in stage I-II uterine leiomyosarcoma: a multicentric retrospective study of 140 patients. Gynecol Oncol 133(3):531, 2014

Markman M, Blessing J, Rubin SC, et al: Phase II trial of weekly paclitaxel (80 mg/m^2) in platinum and paclitaxel-resistant ovarian and primary peritoneal cancers: a Gynecologic Oncology Group study. Gynecol Oncol 101(3):436, 2006

Matulonis UA, Berlin S, Ivy P, et al: Cediranib, an oral inhibitor of vascular endothelial growth factor receptor kinases, is an active drug in recurrent epithelial ovarian, fallopian tube, and peritoneal cancer. J Clin Oncol 27(33):5601, 2009

Mileshkin L, Antill Y, Rischin D: Management of complications of chemotherapy. In Gershenson DM, McGuire WP, Gore M, et al (eds): Gynecologic Cancer Controversies in Management. Philadelphia, Elsevier, 2004, p 618

Park JY, Jin KL, Kim DY, et al: Surgical staging and adjuvant chemotherapy in the management of patients with adult granulosa cell tumors of the ovary. Gynecol Oncol 125(1):80, 2012

Peng C, Fan NC, Ligier M, et al: Expression and regulation of gonadotropin-releasing hormone (GnRH) and GnRH receptor messenger ribonucleic acids in human granulosa-luteal cells. Endocrinology 135(5):1740, 1994

Pujade-Lauraine E, Hilpert F, Weber B, et al: Bevacizumab combined with chemotherapy for platinum-resistant recurrent ovarian cancer: the AURELIA open-label randomized phase III trial. J Clin Oncol 32(13):1302, 2014

Rizzo JD, Somerfield MR, Hagerty KL, et al: Use of epoetin and darbepoetin in patients with cancer: 2007 American Society of Clinical Oncology/American Society of Hematology clinical practice guideline update. J Clin Oncol 26(1):132, 2008

Roila F, Hesketh PJ, Herrstedt J, et al: Prevention of chemotherapy- and radiotherapy-induced emesis: results of the 2004 Perugia International Antiemetic Consensus Conference. Ann Oncol 17:20, 2006

Slomovitz BM, Lu KH, Johnston T, et al: A phase 2 study of the oral mammalian target of rapamycin inhibitor, everolimus, in patients with recurrent endometrial carcinoma. Cancer 116(23):5415, 2010

Spannuth WA, Leath CA, III, Huh WK, et al: A Phase II trial of weekly topotecan for patients with secondary platinum-resistant recurrent epithelial ovarian carcinoma following the failure of second-line therapy. Gynecol Oncol 104(3):591, 2007

Tew WP, Colombo N, Ray-Coquard I, et al: Intravenous aflibercept in patients with platinum-resistant, advanced ovarian cancer: results of a randomized, double-blind, phase 2, parallel-arm study. Cancer 120(3):335, 2014

Tewari KS, Sill MW, Long HJ 3rd, et al: Improved survival with bevacizumab in advanced cervical cancer. N Engl J Med 370(8):734, 2014

Tinker AV, Gebski V, Fitzharris B, et al: Phase II trial of weekly docetaxel for patients with relapsed ovarian cancer who have previously received paclitaxel—ANZGOG 02-01. Gynecol Oncol 104(3):647, 2007

Tonia T, Mettler A, Robert N, et al: Erythropoietin or darbepoetin for patients with cancer. Cochrane Database Syst Rev 12:CD003407, 2012

Weinberg LE, Lurain JR, Singh DK, et al: Survival and reproductive outcomes in women treated for malignant ovarian germ cell tumors. Gynecol Oncol 121(2):285, 2011

CHAPTER 28

Principles of Radiation Therapy

To effectively incorporate radiation treatment into cancer care, clinicians must understand the fundamental concepts and vocabulary used in radiation oncology. Clinically, radiation therapy, often combined with chemotherapy, can be used as primary treatment for many gynecologic malignancies (Table 28-1). Additionally, radiation therapy may be recommended postoperatively if the probability of tumor recurrence is high. Radiation therapy is also used frequently in the relief of symptoms caused by metastasis of any gynecologic cancer.

RADIATION PHYSICS

Radiation therapy is the focused delivery of energy in tissue to accomplish controlled biologic damage. Radiation used in this therapy can occur as electromagnetic waves or particles.

■ Electromagnetic Radiation

Photons (x-rays) and *gamma rays* are the two types of electromagnetic radiation used for radiation therapy. Photons, used in *external beam therapy*, are produced when a stream of electrons collides with a high atomic number target (tungsten) located in the head of a linear accelerator (Fig. 28-1). In contrast, gamma rays originate from unstable atom nuclei and are emitted during decay of radioactive materials, also termed radionuclides, which are widely used in *brachytherapy*.

■ Particle Radiation

Whereas electromagnetic waves are defined by their wavelengths, particles are defined by their masses. For clinical use, particles include electrons, neutrons, protons, helium ions, heavy charged ions, and pi mesons. Except for electrons, which are available in all modern radiation oncology centers, and protons, other particles have limited clinical use. Proton facility numbers are expanding, with 14 facilities operating in the United States and 10 additional centers under construction.

Particles are produced by linear accelerators or other high-energy generators and are usually delivered by external beam. Of clinically used particles, *electrons* are negatively charged and deposit most of their energy near the surface. In contrast, heavy charged particles, such as *protons*, deposit most of their energy in the absorbing tissues as their velocity decreases, that is, near the end of the particle path (the Bragg peak effect). Because of this, a major advantage of proton therapy is the lack of an exiting dose through normal tissues. Proton therapy use for gynecologic malignancies is primarily investigational. But as an example, proton therapy can treat affected deep pelvic and paraaortic lymph nodes, while sparing unnecessary dosing and injury to anterolateral organs, such as the bowel and kidneys (Fig. 28-2).

■ Radiation Sources

Radionuclides

Also called radioisotopes, radionuclides undergo nuclear decay and can emit: (1) positively charged alpha particles, (2) negatively charged beta particles (electrons), and (3) gamma rays. Radionuclides commercially available are shown in Table 28-2. Cesium and iridium are commonly used in gynecologic brachytherapy.

Linear Accelerator

One of the main types of radiation-producing units is the linear accelerator, also called a *linac*. A linac can produce both photon and electron beams (see Fig. 28-1). In the *photon-therapy mode*, indicated for deep-seated tumors, the accelerated electron beam is guided to hit a metal target to produce photons. The unit used to describe the energy of a photon beam is MV (million volts). In the *electron-therapy mode*, indicated for superficial lesions, the electron beam strikes a lead scattering foil instead of the metal target. The unit for electron beam energy is expressed in MeV (million electron volts). Figure 28-3 displays a linac with three moveable components: gantry, treatment head, and couch. These components can all rotate 360 degrees, which allows multiple fields and angles to achieve optimal dose delivery to a tumor.

TABLE 28-1. Role of Radiation Therapy in the Management of Gynecologic Cancers

Intent	Site
Curative	Cervix, vulva, vagina, uterus
Adjunctive to surgery	Cervix, vulva, vagina, uterus
Palliative	Metastasis causing symptoms: bleeding, pain, obstruction

Electromagnetic Radiation Energy Deposition

When electromagnetic radiation is used in daily clinical practice, it contacts target tissues, and energy is transferred to those tissues. This transfer creates ions by dislodging electrons from atoms within these tissues. These electrons then collide with surrounding molecules to initiate radiation damage.

There are three mechanisms involved in energy transfer: (1) photoelectric effect, (2) Compton effect, and (3) pair production

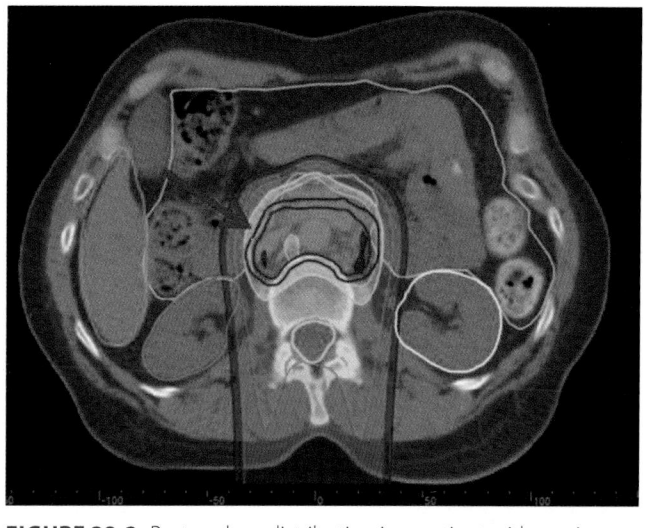

FIGURE 28-2 Proton dose distribution in a patient with cervical cancer receiving treatment to the paraaortic lymph nodes. The proton beam originates posteriorly and is directed anteriorly. The red arrow shows the target volume (*dark magenta outline*). The area anterior to this is bowel (*orange outline*), which is significantly spared from radiation.

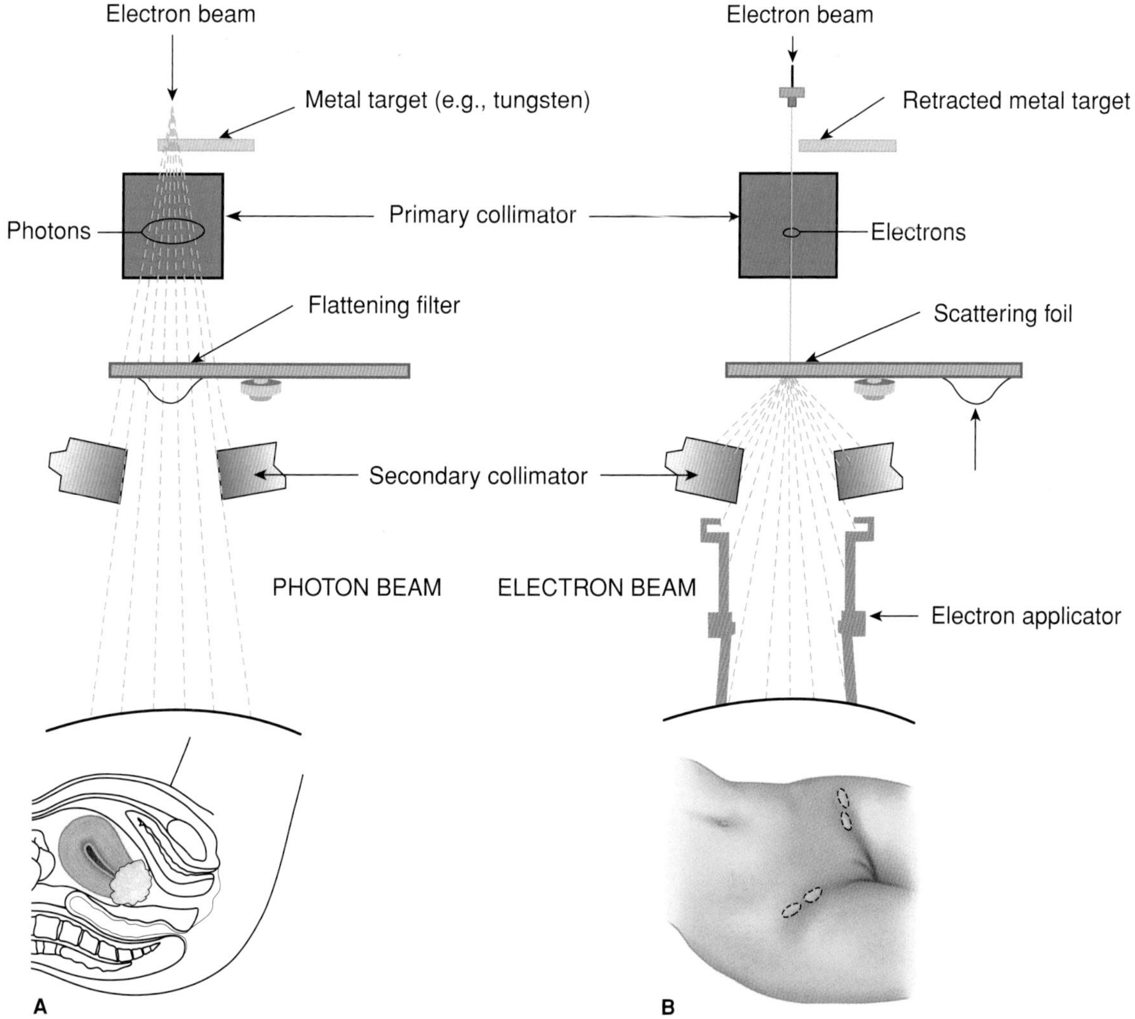

Electron beam

Metal target (e.g., tungsten)

Primary collimator

Photons

Flattening filter

Secondary collimator

PHOTON BEAM   ELECTRON BEAM

Electron beam

Retracted metal target

Electrons

Scattering foil

Electron applicator

A   **B**

FIGURE 28-1 Block diagram of a linear accelerator used to create external beam radiation. Either photon beams or electron beams may be produced. **A.** Photon beam therapy is suited for deep tumors such as the cervical cancer shown here. Beam energy is measured in million volts (MV). **B.** Electron beam therapy is indicated for superficial lesions such as inguinal lymph nodes. Beam energy is measured in million electron volts (MeV).

TABLE 28-2. Physical Properties and Clinical Use of Selected Radionuclides

Element	Radiation Energy (MeV)	Half-Life	Clinical Use
Cesium-137	0.6	30 years	Brachytherapy
Iridium-192	0.4	74 days	Brachytherapy
Cobalt-60	1.2	5 years	Brachytherapy
Iodine-125	0.028	60 days	Brachytherapy
Phosphorus-32	1.7	14 days	Intraperitoneal instillation
Gold-196	0.4	2.7 days	Intraperitoneal instillation
Strontium-89	1.4	51 days	Diffuse bone metastasis

MeV = million electron volts.

(Fig. 28-4). Depending on the energy level of the incident radiation, one of these mechanisms will predominate. The *photoelectric effect* is dominant if the incident energy is low (less than 100 kV). The *Compton effect* dominates in mid- to high energy ranges (1 MV to 20 MV) and is the most important in clinical radiation therapy. Last, *pair production* occurs when a photon beam with very high energy (beyond 20 MV) strikes the electromagnetic field of the nucleus.

■ Depth-dose Curve

Controlled biologic damage is accomplished by greater selective radiation dose distribution within malignant tissue than within the surrounding, "innocent bystander" normal tissues. This is achieved by using radiation beams with differing physical properties to define the spatial distribution of an absorbed dose when these beams strike tissue. Ideally, an absorbed radiation dose is as conformal as possible. Perfect conformality is achieved when the targeted malignant tissue absorbs 100 percent of the prescribed dose and the adjacent normal tissues absorb 0 percent.

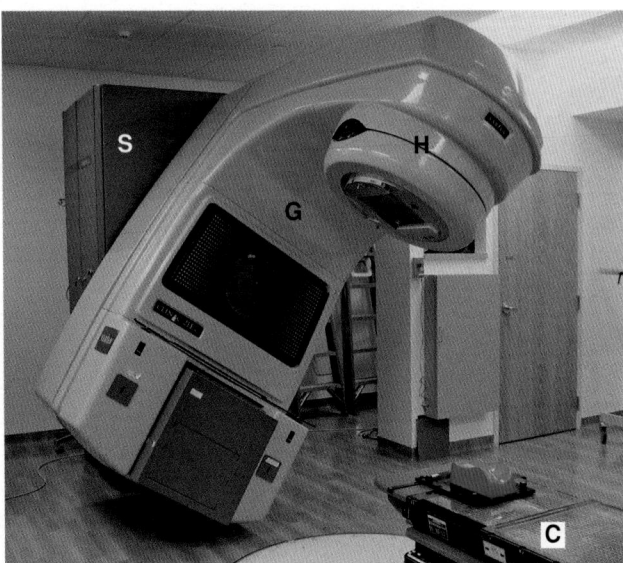

FIGURE 28-3 Linear accelerator currently in use at the University of Texas Southwestern Medical Center. The patient lies on the treatment couch (C). The gantry (G), couch, and head (H) can all rotate and allow radiation beams to reach target tissues through different angles. S = stand.

In practice, this cannot be obtained. However, both acute radiation side effects and the potential for late, delayed radiation complications can be minimized as the spatial radiation dose distribution approaches this ideal.

A *depth-dose curve* specifically illustrates the dose distribution of a given radiation beam as it penetrates tissues. Radiation oncologists rely on these curves when choosing a radiation beam with an appropriate energy to reach a given tumor. With electron beam therapy, the maximum dose lies close to the surface, and therefore, electron beam therapy is indicated for targets that are close to the skin surface, such as metastatic cancer to the inguinal lymph nodes. With high-energy photons, the maximum dose is deposited well below the surface. Beyond this point, the dose gradually tapers as energy is absorbed by the deep surrounding tissues. This explains the so called *skin-sparing effect* of high-energy photons. A patient with a pelvic malignancy is usually treated with at least 6-MV photon beams.

Dosimetry

This is the discipline of calculating the radiation dose absorbed by the patient. Dosimetric calculations are based on the depth-dose measurements of the radiation beams used to treat an actual patient. The dose distribution is usually displayed as a colorful map overlaid on the radiologic images of the patient (p. 616). These calculations *predict* the absorbed dose in a given situation.

■ Radiation Unit

Quantification of the absorbed radiation dose is essential as it correlates with the biologic effect of radiation. The current Standard International unit for absorbed dose is gray (Gy). One Gy equals 100 rad or 1 joule/kg. Clinically, the radiation doses for curative and palliative treatment are 70 to 85 Gy and 30 to 40 Gy, respectively.

RADIATION BIOLOGY

■ DNA Molecule as Target of Radiation Therapy's Biologic Effect

The DNA molecule is the target for the biologic effect of radiation on mammalian cells. DNA injuries involve its strands, bases, and cross-links, but the hallmark damage is breaking of single- and

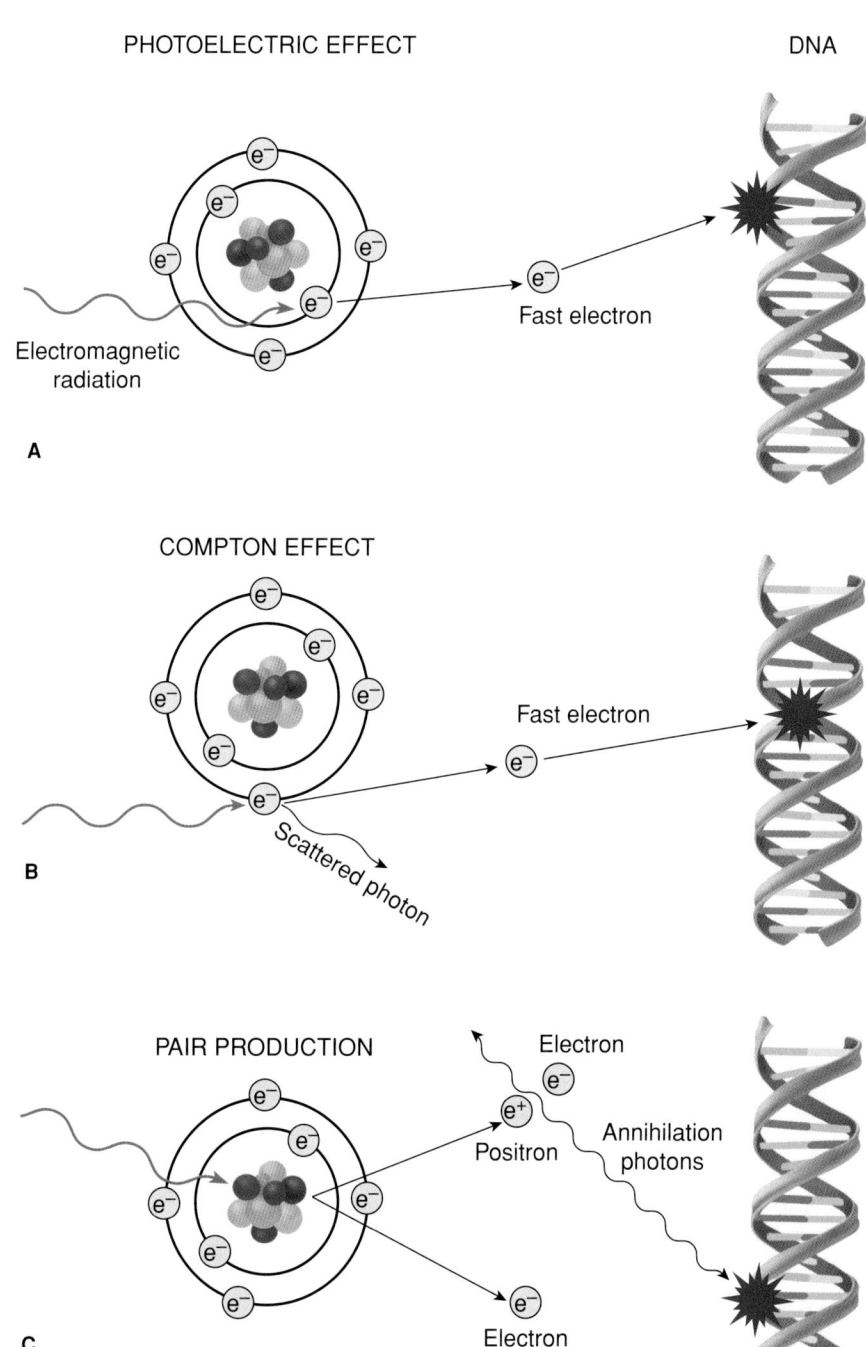

PHOTOELECTRIC EFFECT

Electromagnetic radiation

Fast electron

DNA

A

COMPTON EFFECT

Fast electron

Scattered photon

B

PAIR PRODUCTION

Electron

Positron

Annihilation photons

Electron

C

FIGURE 28-4 When electromagnetic radiation impacts target tissues, energy is transferred to those tissues. The three mechanisms involved in this energy transfer are the photoelectric effect, Compton effect, and pair production. Both photoelectric effect (A) and Compton effect (B) result in creation of fast electrons, which then initiate the biologic process of radiation damage. **A.** With photoelectric effect, radiation interacts with an inner orbital electron. **B.** With Compton effect, interaction occurs with an outer orbital electron. **C.** During pair production, impact of radiation on the atom's nuclear forces produces a positron-electron pair. When a positron later combines with a free electron in these tissues, two photons are created, which can then lead to radiation damage.

Direct versus Indirect Actions of Ionizing Radiation

Radiation can interact *directly* or *indirectly* with the atoms in the DNA molecule. Direct actions create ions that then initiate the biologic damage process. This *direct* effect is predominant with high linear energy transfer (LET) particles such as protons, fast neutrons, and heavy ions (Fig. 28-5). However, most DNA damage is caused indirectly, which is the predominant effect with low-LET particles such as photons. Indirect DNA damage occurs through an important chemical intermediate, the hydroxyl radical (OH·), which is highly reactive because of its unpaired electron.

Cell Death

The two main cell death pathways after radiation are *apoptosis* and *mitotic catastrophe*. Mitotic catastrophe is thought to be the most common mechanism of cell death after radiation exposure. With this, cells with damaged DNA enter mitosis prematurely, before DNA can be repaired, and die attempting to complete the next two to three mitotic cycles. Apoptosis, or programmed cell death, occurs after an intracellular stress, such as radiation-induced irreparable double-strand breaks. A series of events develop rapidly within hours, leading to cell membrane blebbing, apoptotic body formation in the cytoplasm, chromatin condensation, nuclear fragmentation, and DNA laddering (Okada, 2004).

Four R's of Radiation Biology: Repair, Reassortment, Repopulation, Reoxygenation

In classic radiation biology, there are four mechanisms by which cells respond to radiation. Cellular *repair* can be described by sublethal damage repair (SLDR) and potentially lethal damage repair (PLDR). SLDR occurs when a radiation dose is split into two or more fractions and a few hours separate the fractions. Cells have time to repair their damage, and their survival rate increases. The last process seen in SLDR is *repopulation*, which is the tissue's response to replenish the cell pool (Trott, 1999).

Following the initial repair of sublethal damage, *reassortment* begins. Within a tumor, proliferating cells are in different

most importantly double-stranded DNA. Double-strand breaks lead to DNA fragmentation when two or more breaks are formed and when cells attempt to repair these strand breaks. The DNA pieces may rejoin incorrectly, leading to gene translocation, mutation, or amplification and, ultimately, cell death.

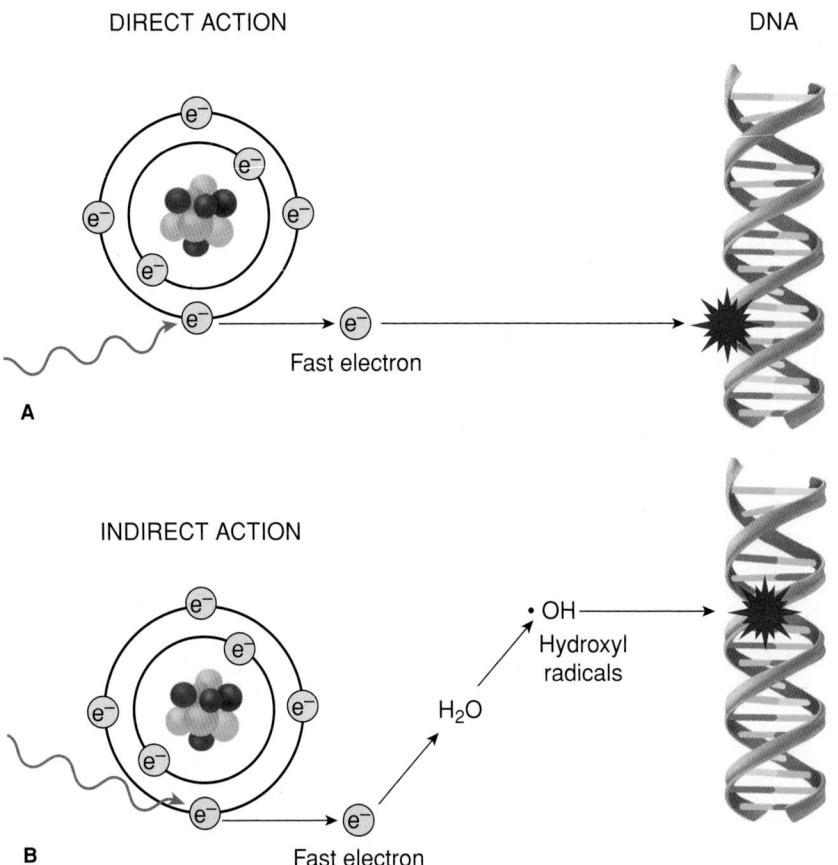

DIRECT ACTION

Fast electron

A

INDIRECT ACTION

• OH —
Hydroxyl
radicals

H_2O

Fast electron

B

FIGURE 28-5 Direct and indirect actions of radiation. **A.** Fast electrons may directly strike DNA to create damage. **B.** Alternatively, a fast electron may interact with water to create a hydroxyl radical, which subsequently interacts with DNA to cause injury.

DNA

The alpha/beta ratio reflects the response of normal tissues to radiation. *Early-responding tissue*s have a high alpha/beta ratio and will manifest reactions to radiation within a few days to weeks after treatment. Examples are tissues with high proliferation rates such as bone marrow, reproductive organs, and gastrointestinal tract mucosa. Preventatively, by administering multiple small radiation dose fractions, there is more sublethal damage repair, and early acute reactions can be decreased.

In contrast, *late-responding* tissues show clinical reactions only weeks to months after completion of a radiation therapy course. Examples are the lung, kidney, spinal cord, and brain. These tissues have a low alpha/beta ratio and are slow to respond. More time is needed to repair sublethal damage, and thus high-dose per fraction radiation therapy can easily lead to severe late complications.

RADIATION ONCOLOGY PRACTICE

The expertise of the radiation oncologist who is designing and monitoring a course of radiation treatment is paramount. Radiation oncology is as inherently "operator dependent" as surgical oncology. The radiation oncologist carves out, en-bloc, a volume of cancerous tissue, its local extensions, and its

phases of the cell cycle (Fig. 27-1, p. 593). Cells in mitosis (M) and G_2 are most sensitive to radiation. Conversely, cells in G_1 and S (DNA synthesis) phases are less sensitive (Pawlik, 2004). When exposed to radiation, those cells that are in the G_2/M phase are killed. During reassortment, surviving cell populations restart their progression through the mitotic cycle.

The fourth "R" of radiation biology theory is *reoxygenation*. A tumor cell population is composed of oxygenated and hypoxic components. Cells located within 100 microns of blood capillaries are oxygenated, and beyond 100 microns, cells are hypoxic. After radiation, the oxygenated cells are killed by chemical intermediates described earlier. Following cell death, the tumor shrinks and allows hypoxic cells to be positioned within the oxygen diffusion range of blood capillaries and become oxygenated.

■ Linear-quadratic Theory and the Alpha/Beta Ratio

For low-LET radiation, the linear-quadratic curve has been adopted to explain the relationship between the fraction of cells surviving a given dose of radiation (Fig. 28-6). The initial linear (alpha) portion of the curve shows that the probability of cell death is proportional to the radiation dose. In the higher-dose region, the curved quadratic (beta) portion indicates that the probability of cell death is proportional to the *square* of the dose.

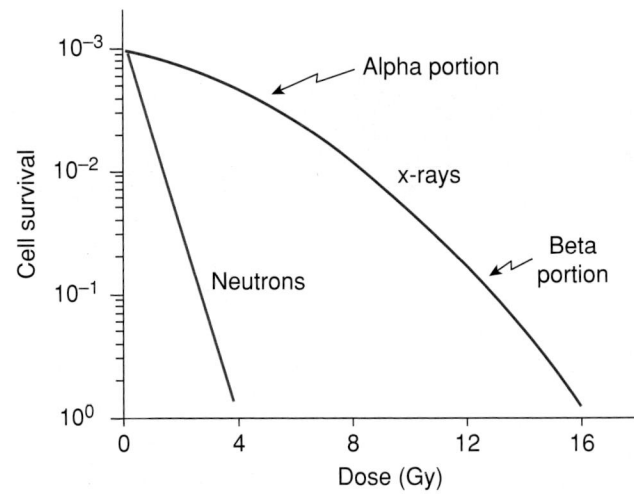

FIGURE 28-6 Linear quadratic mammalian cell survival curve. The cell survival is plotted on a logarithmic scale. The dose (in Gy) is on a linear scale. The typical cell survival curves with low-LET (linear energy transfer) (*blue curve*) and with high-LET radiation (*red line*) are shown. With low-LET x-ray doses, the alpha (linear) portion of the curve is flat and shows that cell survival is proportional to the dose. However, as the dose increases, the beta (quadratic) portion bends, which implies that cell survival is proportional to the dose squared. In contrast, with high-LET radiation, such as neutrons, the survival curve is straight.

regional lymphatics similar to radical surgical resection, while accommodating the patient's comorbidities, general health status, and surrounding normal tissue quality.

As cancer management is frequently multimodal, superior treatment outcomes are highly dependent on clear communication between radiation oncologists and their colleagues in surgical and medical oncology. Optimal integration of diagnostic imaging and histologic evaluation is also vital to planning and implementing potentially curative radiation therapy. As such, early involvement of the radiation oncologist in patient evaluation and counseling enhances the probability of effective and coordinated cancer care.

■ Radiation Fractionation Schemes

Parameters that affect the efficacy and safety of a radiation course include the total radiation dose applied, the size of each radiation "fraction" (treatment), the time between treatments ("fractionation schedule"), and the elapsed time to deliver the total prescribed dose.

Standard Fractionation

Successful eradication of a localized cancer requires that the cancer cells be killed more rapidly and efficiently than surviving cancer cells can proliferate and repopulate. Because of the inevitable exposure of some normal tissues to substantial radiation, there are limits to the total radiation dose that can be prudently administered to a given target volume. In general, delivery of this dose over the shortest feasible elapsed time will maximize efficacy. Accomplishing this objective is limited by the known deleterious consequences of a high dose per fraction on normal tissues. As noted, this can result in delayed radiation injury expressed months or years after therapy completion. For this reason, radiation delivered with curative intent is generally administered in daily treatments (Monday through Friday) of 1.8 Gy to 2.0 Gy. Cumulative doses range from 45 Gy to treat microscopic disease to 70 Gy or more to treat gross disease. This concern for delayed injury is lessened when short courses of radiation are administered with palliative intent, often in dose fractions of 2.5 Gy to 4.0 Gy.

Altered Fractionation

Regimens involving treatments given more than once a day are reserved for selected cases. In such instances, increased local tumor control and decreased long-term complications may be achieved by manipulating both fraction size and overall treatment time. This manipulation leads to a variety of altered fractionations. Two major strategies have been employed, namely, hyperfractionation and accelerated treatment.

With *hyperfractionation*, the reduction of late damage to normal tissues is sought, and accordingly, a smaller dose per fraction is given. Two or more fractions are administered each day, typically 6 hours apart to provide an interval for normal tissue repair.

Accelerated fractionation entails shortening the treatment duration with or without a decrease in total dose to overcome tumor cell repopulation. The usual weekend break is either shortened or eliminated. With accelerated treatment, however, severe acute reactions are frequent.

Altered fractionation has been studied in gynecologic cancers. Radiation Therapy Oncology Group (RTOG) trials 88-05 and 92-10 were Phase II trials that investigated the use of twice-daily radiation and chemoradiation, respectively, in advanced cervical cancer. RTOG 88-05 showed similar local control, survival rates, and toxicity compared with historical controls. However, when chemotherapy and larger-field twice-daily radiation were added, there were unacceptable rates of late Grade 4 toxicity (Grigsby, 2001, 2002).

■ Radiation Therapy

External Beam Radiation Therapy

External beam radiation therapy is indicated when an area to be irradiated is large. For example, the fields needed to treat a locally advanced cervical cancer may cover the whole pelvis and occasionally, the paraaortic lymph nodes.

Conformal radiation therapy (CRT) describes a radiation treatment technique that maximizes tumor damage while minimizing injury to the surrounding normal tissues. To this goal, the radiation oncologist must know the precise extent of the cancer to be irradiated and its relationship to surrounding normal tissues. This process begins with a review of the patient's cancer imaging including computed tomography (CT), magnetic resonance (MR) imaging, and positron emission tomography (PET). Imaging, along with careful review of the patient's pathology and operative report, assists in defining the 3-dimensional (3-D) target (tumor or regions of potential microscopic tumor spread) and normal tissue volumes.

Next, a simulation is performed in a simulation suite to delineate the anticipated therapy fields prior to an actual treatment session. During this process, patient positioning, immobilization techniques, and treatment fields are defined. If feasible, radiation blocks are also planned to shield normal tissues. The patient is placed in the treatment position, and a CT scan of the area of interest is performed. Later, on each of the computer-based CT scan slices, the radiation oncologist carefully delineates the anatomic areas that will receive a tumoricidal dose. During this, four volumes are defined: (1) a gross tumor volume (GTV), which encompasses any gross disease; (2) a clinical target volume (CTV), which incorporates any areas at risk for microscopic tumor spread; (3) a planning target volume (PTV), which accounts for uncertainties in treatment planning or delivery such as patient motion or daily set-up error; and (4) a volume that defines the normal organs at risk (OAR), which will be exposed, albeit to a lesser radiation dose.

Once simulation is completed, a radiation dosimetrist employs a treatment planning software to develop an optimal plan, called dose optimization. This is often a reiterative process in which the physician and the dosimetrist will arrive at an acceptable option, which means an optimal arrangement of the radiation beams.

One tool that is particularly helpful in the radiation planning and optimization process is the dose volume histogram (DVH). This is a graphic summary of the entire dose distribution to the cancer and normal structures. Thus, the DVH provides information regarding whether the cancer will be adequately treated with a tumoricidal dose and whether surrounding

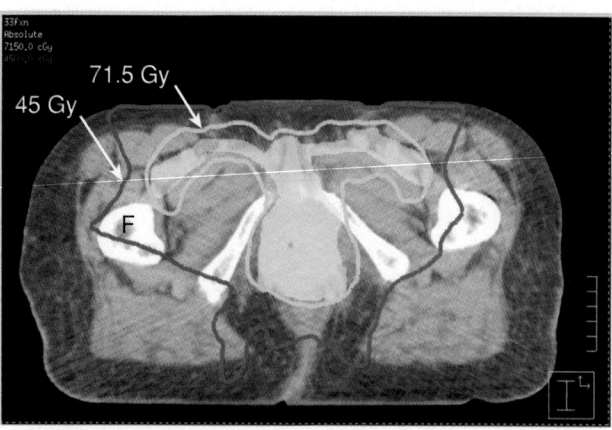

A

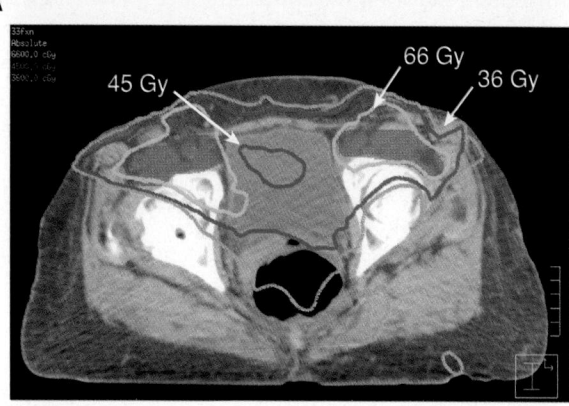

B

FIGURE 28-7 IMRT dose distribution in a patient with stage T4 N2 M0 cancer of the vulva. This technique allows for the delivery of tumoricidal doses to the vulva and inguinal nodes while minimizing that to normal tissues. **A.** The yellow area displays the actual vulvar cancer and inguinal lymph nodes. Doses to the vulva and femoral heads (F) are shown (*arrows*). The doses to the vulva and femoral heads are 71.5 Gy and 45 Gy, respectively. **B.** Pink shading displays the inguinal nodes. Doses to the inguinal nodes, bladder, and rectum are shown (*arrows*). The doses to the inguinal nodes, bladder, and rectum were 66 Gy, 45 Gy, and 36 Gy, respectively.

normal structures are minimally affected. In addition to the DVH, dose distributions are displayed as computer-generated radiation dose map images that are overlaid on the CT images (Fig. 28-7). This provides a visual dose-anatomy relationship. These dose distributions are produced for the radiation oncologist to review, adjust, and finally approve. The final chosen plan is reviewed by a radiation physicist who ensures that the physical and technical details can be implemented.

To further improve the conformality of the dose distribution, especially around concave targets, a more advanced 3D-CRT planning system, called *intensity-modulated radiation therapy (IMRT)*, can be used. As a result of this improved conformality, IMRT has the potential to decrease bowel and bladder toxicity during pelvic radiation therapy (Heron, 2003). IMRT modulates the intensity of radiation beams to be used with the help of dedicated computer software. For quality assurance, weekly or sometimes even daily imaging of the treated regions is performed to verify that treatment configurations are correct.

Stereotactic Body Radiation Therapy. Over the past decade, a novel external beam radiation therapy technique, *stereotactic body radiation therapy (SBRT)*, has become commonly used in sites such as the lung, liver, and spine. It uses a hypofractionated regimen of five or fewer fractions (10 to 20 Gy per fraction). Using *image-guided radiation therapy (IGRT)*, precise, safe SBRT has become possible through "real-time" approaches to overcome technical factors such as patient or organ motion and tumor size and shape changes during a treatment course.

Brachytherapy

Brachytherapy means treatment at a short distance. During this therapy, sealed or unsealed radioisotopes are inserted into the cancer or its immediate vicinity. Radiation doses fall sharply with increasing distances from the radioactive source. Thus, brachytherapy is indicated only for small tumor volumes (less than 3 to 4 cm). For this reason, brachytherapy is typically practiced after external beam radiation therapy has decreased a large tumor volume.

Brachytherapy may be intracavitary or interstitial. During *intracavitary brachytherapy*, applicators that hold sealed radioactive sources such as iridium-192 (^{192}Ir) are inserted into a body cavity such as the uterus. Alternatively, *interstitial brachytherapy* requires the placement of catheters or needles directly into the cancer and surrounding tissues.

Brachytherapy may be temporary or permanent. In *temporary brachytherapy*, the radioisotopes are removed from the patient after a period of time, ranging from minutes to days. All intracavitary and some interstitial implants are temporary. In *permanent brachytherapy*, the radioisotopes are left permanently to decay within the tissues.

Equipment. For routine gynecologic intracavitary implantation, standard equipment includes an applicator, called a *tandem*, which fits into the uterine cavity, and a pair of vaginal applicators, which are known as *ovoids* (Fig. 28-8). The tandem and ovoid device (T&O) is inserted under general anesthesia or conscious sedation. Following placement, radioactive sources can then be loaded into both the tandem and ovoids. In gynecologic oncology, brachytherapy with T&O is indicated for cervical cancer. For uterine cancer, vaginal brachytherapy with a cylinder is used to treat the vaginal apex or length of the

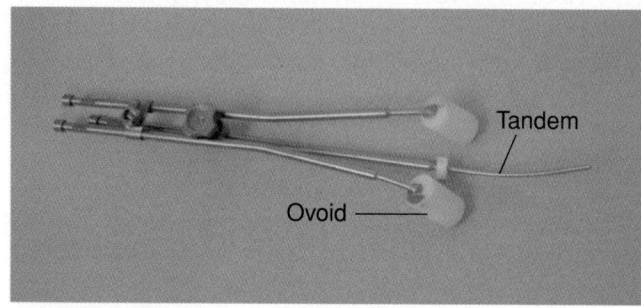

FIGURE 28-8 Typical tandem and ovoids used for cervical cancer brachytherapy. The long slender portion of the device (tandem) is inserted into the endometrial cavity, and white cylinders (ovoids) are positioned in the proximal vagina. Radioactive sources can be loaded into both the tandem and ovoid reservoirs.

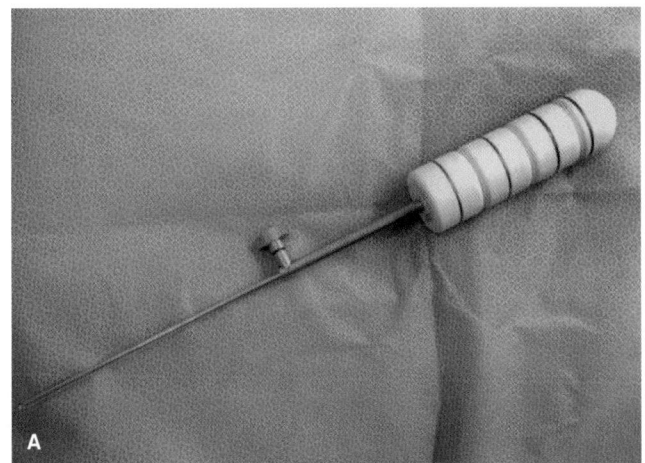

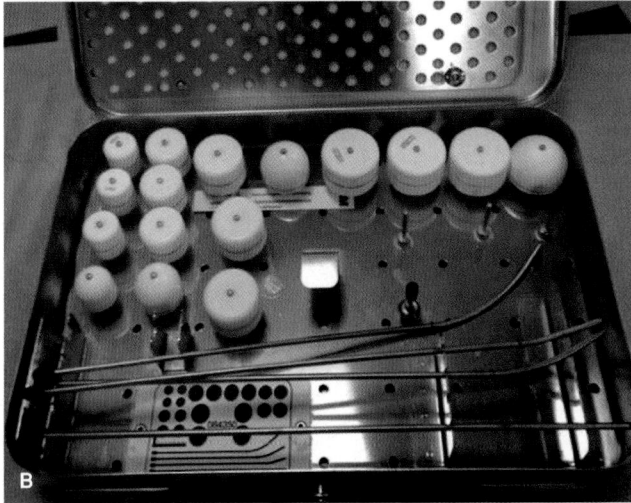

FIGURE 28-9 Typical cylinder **(A)** used for vaginal brachytherapy after surgery for uterine cancer. The cylinder is placed in the vagina and high-dose-rate brachytherapy is delivered. This treatment decreases the risk of vaginal cuff recurrences. **B.** The cylinder comes in different sizes to allow the most appropriate fit for the patient's anatomy. The largest possible diameter is preferred.

vagina, which is the most common site of disease recurrence after hysterectomy (Fig. 28-9).

For temporary interstitial implantation, flexible plastic catheters or metal needles are surgically placed into the target tissues and held in place by a perineal template. These are then afterloaded with ^{192}Ir seeds. Templates are suitable for patients with advanced cancers, suboptimal anatomy for T&O application, and selected recurrent cancers.

In addition to T&O, vaginal cylinder, and interstitial needles, physicians may choose to use a tandem and ring, split-ring, or tandem and cylinder. Appropriate brachytherapy applicator selection requires expertise, as applicator choice depends on patient anatomy and a specific device's dose distribution.

Manual versus Remote Afterloading. Once the brachytherapy instruments are in place, the radioactive sources are inserted. Historically, the sources were placed manually, however, this method increased hospital staff radiation exposure. Subsequently, a *remote afterloading* approach was developed and is commonly practiced today. This remote control system

delivers a single miniaturized iridium source from a protective safe through connecting cables to the holding devices previously inserted into the patient. Following treatment, the radioactive source is automatically retracted back into the safe.

Low Dose-rate versus High Dose-rate Brachytherapy. Traditionally, low dose-rate (LDR) brachytherapy is delivered over the course of many days and requires patient hospitalization. Over the past few decades, however, high dose-rate (HDR) brachytherapy has become more popular. With this technique, treatment is shortened to minutes. Low dose is defined as dose rates from 0.4 Gy to 2 Gy/hr, and high dose rate as rates higher than 12 Gy/hr. For example, with an intracavitary implant for cervical cancer and an LDR technique, a dose of 30 to 40 Gy is delivered continuously over several days. In contrast, with HDR, an equivalent dose can be delivered in 3 to 5 weekly fractions. The dose per fraction is 5 to 7 Gy and can be given in 10 to 20 minutes. Unlike LDR, HDR avoids lengthy inpatient hospitalization and minimizes patient immobility and thromboembolic events. Furthermore, long-term analysis shows similar local tumor control and late complication rates in patients treated for cervical cancer with both HDR and LDR (Arai, 1991; Hareyama, 2002; Wong, 2003).

■ Tumor Control Probability

With most epithelial cancers, the probability that radiation therapy will control a cancerous mass depends on the tumor's size and intrinsic radiosensitivity and on the radiation dose and delivery schedule. For example, within a given stage, large tumors are more difficult to control with radiation than smaller ones (Bentzen, 1996; Dubben, 1998).

Intrinsic Radiosensitivity

It is recognized that a tumor's radiosensitivity in general is determined by its pathologic type (Table 28-3). However, even cancers with a similar histology may have variable responses to radiation. This may be explained by heterogeneity within a given tumor and by the cancer cell's ability to repair radiation damage (Schwartz, 1988, 1996; Weichselbaum, 1992).

Treatment Time

When protracted time intervals are required to complete a fractionated radiation therapy course, tumor control probability decreases, especially in rapidly proliferating epithelial cancers. Thus, treatment breaks or delays for any reason are minimized. In a retrospective review of 209 patients with stage I to III cervical cancer treated with radiation therapy, the 5-year pelvic control and overall survival rates were better for those who

TABLE 28-3. Radiosensitivity of Some Selected Cancers

Sensitivity	Cancer Type
Highly sensitive	Lymphoma, dysgerminoma, small cell cancer, embryonal cancer
Moderately sensitive	Squamous carcinoma, adenocarcinoma
Poorly sensitive	Osteosarcoma, glioma, melanoma

completed the treatment in less than 55 days (87 percent and 65 percent, respectively) than for those who did so in more than 55 days (72 percent and 54 percent, respectively) (Petereit, 1995).

Tumor Hypoxia

Tumor hypoxia is a major factor leading to poor local tumor control and poor survival rates in patients with cervical cancer (Brizel, 1999; Nordsmark, 1996). The close relationship between tumor hypoxia, anemia, and angiogenesis was demonstrated in a study involving 87 patients with stage II, III, and IV cervical cancer treated with radiation only. Of these, patients with hemoglobin levels <11 g/dL and a median tumor oxygen tension pO_2 < 15 mm Hg had decreased 3-year survival rates (Dunst, 2003).

To overcome tumor hypoxia, many strategies have been devised and vary in efficacy. Of these, hyberbaric oxygen used in conjunction with radiation therapy in cervical cancer was not effective in clinical studies (Dische, 1999). An alternate method to increase oxygen delivery to tissues manipulates blood vessel hemodynamics with either inhaled carbogen (95-percent oxygen and 5-percent carbon dioxide) or nicotinamide (a vasoactive agent). This approach of *accelerated radiotherapy with carbogen and nicotinamide (ARCON)* improves tumor control in patients with anemia but is not commonly used (Janssens, 2014).

Another approach to minimize tumor hypoxia effects employs *bioreductive agents*. This family of hypoxic cell sensitizers selectively kills hypoxic cells. Earlier findings with one of these, tirapazamine (TPZ), was encouraging. However, results of a Gynecologic Oncology Group (GOG) phase III trial that evaluated TPZ, cisplatin, and radiation therapy compared with cisplatin and radiation show no improvement in survival or tumor control rates for patients with cervical cancers (DiSilvestro, 2014).

Last, to ensure adequate oxygen carrying capacity, a hemoglobin level of at least 12 g/dL is desirable in patients receiving radiation therapy. To this goal, transfusion ameliorates tumor hypoxia and increases radiation response. In a study of 204 women with cervical cancer who were treated with radiation, those who were transfused to maintain a hemoglobin level >11 g/dL had a similar 5-year disease-free survival rate (71 percent) compared with a group of women who never required transfusion. The disease-free survival rate was only 26 percent for those with persistent anemia (Kapp, 2002). The use of erythropoietin to maintain hemoglobin above 12 g/dL was also tested in a randomized trial of patients with cervical cancer receiving chemotherapy and radiation. This trial closed early due to concerns of increased thromboembolic events with the use of erythropoietin (Thomas, 2008).

■ Combination of Ionizing Radiation and Chemotherapy

Radiation is often combined with chemotherapy, surgery, or both to increase local disease control and decrease distant metastasis. Radiation therapy and chemotherapy can be administered in a concurrent or alternating fashion to maximize tumoricidal effects and minimize overlapping toxicities and complications (Steel, 1979). This practice is supported by results from many controlled studies involving cervical and other cancers.

In the management of gynecologic cancers, platinum compounds are most commonly used with radiation therapy. Both radiation and cisplatin cause single- and double-strand DNA breaks and base damage. Although most lesions are repaired, if a cisplatin-induced DNA adduct lies close to a radiation-induced single-strand break, then the damage is irreparable and leads to cell death (Amorino, 1999; Begg, 1990). Since the late 1990s, the standard treatment for newly diagnosed locally advanced cervical cancer has been radiation therapy and cisplatin (Keys, 1999; Morris, 1999; Rose, 1999).

Nucleoside analogues such as fludarabine and gemcitabine are also used to enhance the effects of radiation-induced cell killing. These agents inhibit DNA synthesis by blocking cells at the G_1/S checkpoint. The remaining cell population is synchronized at the G_2/M junction, the most radiation-sensitive phase of the cell cycle. Clinically, in a Phase III study of cervical cancer patients, the progression-free survival and overall survival rates improved in patients randomized to receive gemcitabine plus cisplatin and radiation followed by adjuvant gemcitabine compared with concurrent cisplatin and radiation alone (Duenãs-González, 2009). However, inclusion of gemcitabine is still considered investigational for cervical cancer treatment.

Taxanes, such as paclitaxel and docetaxel, enhance the effects of radiation by causing microtubule dysfunction and blocking cells at the G_2/M junction (Mason, 1999). Taxanes have been administered with platinum agents and radiation therapy in small nonrandomized trials involving patients with locally advanced cervical cancer (Lee, 2007).

■ Combination of Radiation Therapy and Surgery

Radiation therapy can be given before, after, or at the time of surgery. With this combination, surgical resection and its associated morbidity can often be minimized. For example, the combination of radiation and surgery in locally advanced vulvovaginal cancer can allow surgeons to avoid extensive surgery such as pelvic exenteration (Boronow, 1982).

Preoperative adjuvant radiation may offer several advantages for tumor control. First, primary cancers tend to locally infiltrate surrounding normal tissues with microscopic extension. Accordingly, radiation can be delivered prior to surgery to decrease the potential for locoregional and distant tumor dissemination and the likelihood of positive surgical margins. To sterilize areas of subclinical infiltration, doses of 40 to 50 Gy administered over 4 to 5 weeks are required. Although preoperative radiation therapy is not expected to render the main tumor mass cancer-free at the time of surgery, it is common to find no evidence of cancer in the surgical specimen. Second, in patients who present with unresectable cancers, preoperative radiation therapy can transform them into suitable candidates for a surgical attempt (Montana, 2000). Surgery is usually delayed 4 to 6 weeks after radiation completion. By then, the acute radiation reactions have subsided, and pathologic interpretation of the resected specimen is easier.

Two studies by the GOG (GOG 71 and 123) have investigated preoperative radiation and chemoradiation, respectively, in patients with bulky stage IB cervical cancer (Keys, 1999,

2003). In both trials, the pathologic complete response rate, defined as no residual disease in a resected specimen, approximated 50 percent.

Postoperatively, a high probability for local recurrence may often be predicted by factors such as positive margins, lymph node metastases, lymphovascular invasion, and high-grade disease. In these cases, postoperative radiation therapy may be beneficial and is ideally delivered 3 to 6 weeks following surgery. This delay allows initial wound healing (Sedlis, 1999). The radiation fields should encompass the operative bed due to the possibility of tumor contamination at the time of surgery and adjacent areas that are at risk for tumor dissemination.

Postoperative radiation is employed in the treatment of many gynecologic malignancies. For cervical cancer, postoperative radiation is recommended in those with lymphovascular invasion, deep stromal invasion, or large tumor size (Sedlis, 1999). Postoperative chemoradiation is offered if positive parametria, positive margins, or positive lymph nodes are found. The addition of cisplatin and 5-fluorouracil to radiation in cervical cancer patients with these high-risk features has been shown to improve survival and tumor control (Peters, 2000).

For uterine cancer, postoperative radiation is frequently used for patients with stage IB or greater disease. Several large randomized controlled trials have demonstrated significant improvements in local control in patients with intermediate-risk endometrial adenocarcinoma who receive adjuvant pelvic radiation (ASTEC/EN.5 Study Group, 2009; Creutzberg, 2011; Keys, 2004). Intermediate risk includes older age, lymphovascular invasion, deep myometrial invasion, or intermediate- or high-grade disease. Patients with fewer risk factors can often be treated with vaginal brachytherapy alone. Vaginal brachytherapy treats the vaginal apex, where approximately 75 percent of recurrences are located. A randomized trial showed similar vaginal and pelvic tumor control rates with fewer side effects when vaginal brachytherapy alone was compared with pelvic external beam radiation therapy (Nout, 2010).

Intraoperative radiation therapy (IORT) is infrequently elected. It may be delivered either by interstitial brachytherapy or by an electron beam produced by a dedicated linear accelerator installed in the operating room. A single dose of 10 to 20 Gy is typically directed to the area at risk for recurrence or suspected of harboring residual cancer (Gemignani, 2001).

■ Normal Tissue Response to Radiation Therapy

In general, radiation therapy is less well tolerated if: (1) the irradiated tissue volume is large, (2) the radiation dose is high, (3) the dose per fraction is large, and (4) the patient's age is advanced. Furthermore, the radiation damage to normal tissues can be exacerbated by factors such as prior surgery, concurrent chemotherapy, infection, diabetes mellitus, hypertension, and inflammatory bowel disease.

In general, if tissues with a rapid proliferation rate such as epithelium of the small intestine or oral cavity are irradiated, acute clinical symptoms develop within a few days to weeks. This contrasts with muscular, renal, and neural tissues, which have low proliferation rates and may not display signs of radiation

damage for months to years after treatment. To avoid serious complications, radiation oncologists must use published tolerance doses for normal tissues as a guide and rely on their own clinical experience. For example, to avoid severe rectal and bladder complications in patients with cervical cancer, doses of no more than 65 Gy and 70 Gy are recommended to the rectum and bladder, respectively (Milano, 2007).

Epithelium and Parenchyma

Atrophy is the most consistent sequela of radiation therapy. It affects all lining epithelia—including skin and the epithelia of the gastrointestinal, respiratory and genitourinary tracts and of the endocrine glands. Additionally, necrosis and ulceration may develop. Within the submucosa and deep soft tissues, fibrosis frequently follows radiation therapy, leading to tissue contracture and stenosis (Fajardo, 2005).

Of vascular structures, the capillary is the most radiosensitive, and ischemia results from endothelial damage, capillary wall rupture, loss of capillary segments, and reduction of microvascular networks. In large arteries, atheroma-like calcifications develop (Friedlander, 2003; Zidar, 1997).

Skin

Four general types of skin reactions may follow radiation therapy. In order of increasing severity, they include erythema, dry desquamation, moist desquamation, and skin necrosis. For many women during a 6 to 7 week radiation therapy course, the first three of these reactions are common. Within 2 weeks following radiation exposure, the skin develops mild erythema. By the fourth week, the redness becomes more pronounced and dry desquamation may begin. After 5 to 6 weeks, moist desquamation may follow. This involves epidermal sloughing, followed by serum and blood oozing through denuded skin. This reaction is mostly pronounced in skin folds, such as the inguinal, axillary, and inframammary creases.

Preventatively, throughout and after a radiation course, the skin is kept clean and aerated. For dry desquamation, ointments or aloe vera-containing creams promote dermal hydration with an emollient effect. During the moist desquamation phase, skin treatment may include moisturizers (e.g., Biafine), sitz baths, and silver sulfadiazine-containing, nonadhering dressings for weeping areas. Importantly, individuals are instructed to avoid applying heating pads, soaps, or alcohol-based lotions to irradiated skin.

Regeneration of the epithelium starts soon after radiation treatment and is usually complete in 4 to 6 weeks. Months later, areas of skin hyper- and hypopigmentation can be seen. The skin may remain atrophied, thin, and dry, and telangiectasias may be visible.

Vagina

Radiation therapy directed to the pelvis frequently leads to acute vaginal mucositis. Although mucosal ulceration is rare, discharge is present in most cases. For these women, a dilute hydrogen peroxide and water solution used at the vulva provides symptomatic relief.

In contrast to acute changes, delayed reactions to radiation may include atrophic vaginitis, formation of vaginal synechiae or telangiectasia, and most commonly, vaginal stricture. Less frequently, rectovaginal or vesicovaginal fistulas may develop after radiation therapy, especially with advanced-stage cancers. Of these delayed reactions, Grade 3 vaginal stricture is defined by the Common Terminology Criteria for Adverse Events (CTCAE) as "vaginal narrowing and/or shortening interfering with the use of tampons, sexual activity or physical examination" (National Cancer Institute, 2009). Preventatively, vaginal stricture or synechiae may be avoided if intercourse is resumed following treatment or if women are instructed regarding dilator use. Dilators are inserted vaginally by the patient daily for 10 seconds, and this schedule continues from radiation therapy completion until the first follow-up visit at 6 weeks. At this point, weekly insertion or intercourse is recommended. Increased severe late vaginal toxicity is associated with poor dilator compliance, concurrent chemotherapy, and age >50 (Gondi, 2012). Importantly, stricture prevention also aids the ability to complete thorough vaginal examinations for cancer surveillance.

For women who remain sexually active following radiation therapy, water-based *lubricants* (e.g., Astroglide or K-Y Jelly) may be of benefit during intercourse but have no sustained effects. For chronic vaginal dryness, *vaginal moisturizers* may prove superior. Moisturizers (e.g., Replens and K-Y Silk-E) can be used daily or several times weekly to maintain moist vaginal tissues. Alternatively, topical estrogen cream (e.g., Premarin cream) may improve atrophic symptoms in those who are estrogen candidates (Table 22-5, p. 505).

Despite these products, persistent adverse vaginal changes affect sexual dysfunction. In a study of 118 women treated for cervical cancer, 63 percent of those who engaged in sexual activities before radiation therapy continued to do so following treatment, although less frequently (Jensen, 2003). In a comparison of women treated with radiation versus radical hysterectomy and lymph node dissection for cervical cancer, women treated with radiation reported significantly lower sexual dysfunction scores than patients undergoing surgery (Frumovitz, 2005).

Ovary and Pregnancy Outcomes

The effects of radiation on ovarian function depend on radiation dose and patient age. For example, a dose of 4 Gy may sterilize 30 percent of young women, but 100 percent of those older than 40. In addition, fractionated radiation therapy appears to be more damaging. Ash (1980) noted that after 10 Gy given in 1 fraction, 27 percent of the women recovered ovarian function compared with only 10 percent of those receiving 12 Gy over 6 days. In patients with gynecologic cancers who receive pelvic radiation therapy, symptoms of ovarian failure mirror those of natural menopause, and symptom treatment is similar in those who are candidates (Chap. 22, p. 494).

To minimize radiation exposure to the ovaries of premenopausal women, the gonads may be surgically repositioned, termed *transposition,* out of the radiation fields. A review of prepubescent and adolescent girls undergoing transposition prior to pelvic radiation demonstrated long-term ovarian preservation rates ranging from 33 to 92 percent. However, only 11 of 347 women (3 percent) achieved pregnancy (Irtan, 2013). Moreover, among female childhood-cancer survivors who received abdominal irradiation, higher spontaneous abortion rates and lower first-born birthweights were observed compared with cancer survivors who were not irradiated (Hawkins, 1989).

Bladder

Most patients receiving pelvic radiation note some acute cystitis symptoms within 2 to 3 weeks of beginning treatment. Although urinary frequency, spasm, and pain develop commonly, hematuria is rare. Typically, phenazopyridine hydrochloride (Pyridium) or fluid ad lib promptly relieves symptoms. Antibiotics are prescribed when indicated. Major chronic complications following radiation therapy are infrequent and include bladder contracture and hematuria. For severe hematuria, bladder saline irrigation, transurethral cystoscopic fulguration, and temporary urinary diversion are proven techniques. Fistulas involving the bladder typically require urinary diversion.

Small Bowel

The small bowel is particularly vulnerable to acute early damage from radiation therapy. After a single dose of 5 to 10 Gy, crypt cells are destroyed, and villi become denuded. An acute malabsorption syndrome ensues to cause nausea, diarrhea, vomiting, and cramping. Adequate fluid intake and a low-lactose, low-fat, and low-fiber diet is recommended. Additionally, antinausea and antidiarrheal medications may be warranted (Tables 25-6, p. 570, and 42-7, p. 914). Bowel antispasmodics with sedatives (e.g., Donnatal) are also particularly helpful.

Patients are warned about the late, chronic nature of radiation-induced enteritis. Intermittent diarrhea, crampy abdominal pain, nausea, and vomiting, which in combination may mimic a low-grade bowel obstruction, can develop. Patients are at increased risk if there is comorbidity such as obesity, inflammatory conditions of the pelvis or bowel, prior abdominal surgeries, or small-vessel diseases resulting from diabetes or hypertension.

Preventatively, several types of devices have been surgically inserted to displace the small bowel from the pelvis. These have included saline-filled tissue expanders, omental slings, and absorbable mesh (Hoffman, 1998; Martin, 2005; Soper, 1988). Furthermore, defining the areas at risk with surgical clips and careful radiation therapy planning, including the use of IMRT, may minimize bowel toxicity (Portelance, 2001). Consideration of dose constraints can further minimize injury. Studies show that irradiating a volume larger than 15 cm^3 or a point dose greater than 55 Gy is associated with a significant risk of small bowel damage (Stanic, 2013; Verma, 2014). Radiation treatment with patients prone can also limit the small bowel dose (Adli, 2003). In contrast, trials incorporating radiation protectors, such as amifostine, have been unsuccessful (Small, 2011).

Rectosigmoid

Commonly, within a few weeks after radiation therapy initiation, patients may develop diarrhea, tenesmus, and mucoid discharge, which can be bloody. In these cases, antidiarrheal medications, low-residue diet, steroid-retention or sucralfate enemas, and hydration are management mainstays. Alternatively, rectal bleeding may be seen months to years after radiation therapy. Hemorrhage can at times be severe and require blood transfusion. Moreover, invasive procedures may be needed to control bleeding neovasculature. These include the topical application of 4-percent formalin, cryotherapy, and vessel coagulation with laser (Kantsevoy, 2003; Konishi, 2005; Smith, 2001; Ventrucci, 2001). During the evaluation of late-onset rectal bleeding, barium enema is often indicated. The study usually reveals narrowing of the rectosigmoid lumen and wall thickening. In cases of severe obstruction, resection of the involved colonic segment is necessary. In addition, rectovaginal fistulas may result from radiation therapy (Chap. 25, p. 573). Small fistulas may heal over many months following a diverting colostomy.

Brachytherapy, in addition to external beam radiation, can further escalate rectal toxicity. The D2cc metric (minimum dose to the most irradiated contiguous volume of 2 cc) is commonly used to evaluate the rectal dose in brachytherapy and has been associated with increased Grade 2 to 4 rectal toxicities when more than 62 Gy are delivered (Lee, 2012). This metric was developed as part of the GEC-ESTRO (Groupe Européen de Curiethérapie—European Society of Therapeutic Radiation Oncology) guidelines, which provide dose-reporting parameters for the bladder, rectum, and sigmoid colon using 3-D image-based treatment planning (Potter, 2006).

Kidney

Manifestations of acute radiation nephropathy typically appear 6 to 12 months after radiation exposure. Affected patients develop hypertension, edema, anemia, microscopic hematuria, proteinuria, and decreased creatinine clearance (Luxton, 1964). Although deteriorating renal function is occasionally reversible, it usually worsens and leads to chronic nephropathy. Patients receiving concurrent radiation and chemotherapy require special consideration, because of the nephrotoxicity associated with many chemotherapeutics.

Bone

Radiation-induced insufficiency fractures are not infrequent following pelvic radiation. They develop in weakened bone and typically manifest as pain. The sacroiliac joint is most commonly involved (Cooper, 1985). Rates are higher in patients receiving definitive radiation therapy, and in a large series of 557 patients with cervical cancer, 20 percent developed insufficiency fractures over 5 years (Oh, 2008). In a more recent series of 222 patients receiving postoperative pelvic radiation therapy, only 5 percent developed pelvic insufficiency fractures at a median time of 11.5 months after radiation therapy completion (Shih, 2013). The fracture rate was higher in patients with osteoporosis (16 percent), in those on hormone replacement therapy (15 percent), and in patients with a lower body mass index. Treatment for a pelvic insufficiency fracture is conservative and consists of pain management and rest, with most patients becoming symptom free by 20 months.

Hematologic Toxicity

Radiation therapy can significantly deplete bone marrow hematopoietic stem cells that include erythrocyte, leukocyte, and platelet precursors. These effects are exacerbated by combined chemoradiation or by irradiation of large fields that contain a significant portion of bone marrow. Accordingly, there are thresholds at which radiation is held to prevent further bone

TABLE 28-4. Susceptibility of Selected Tissues to Radiation-Induced Cancer

Susceptibility	Tissues
High	Bone marrow, female breast, thyroid
Moderate	Bladder, colon, stomach, liver, ovary
Low	Bone, connective tissue, muscle, cervix, uterus, rectum

marrow suppression. For example, if platelet levels measure $<35,000 \times 10^9/L$ and leukocyte counts are $<1.0 \times 10^9/L$, then radiation may be held until these values rise. For anemia, transfusion is recommended (p. 618). To spare bone marrow injury, IMRT may be beneficial (Klopp, 2013).

■ Radiation-induced Carcinogenesis

A secondary cancer may develop as a result of prior radiation therapy. The accepted criteria for the diagnosis of radiation-induced cancer require that the cancer be located within the previously irradiated region and that its pathology differ from that of the original malignancy. Additionally, there should be a latent period of at least a few years. In the updated analysis of the Post-Operative Radiation Therapy in Endometrial Carcinoma (PORTEC-1) trial, which compared postoperative adjuvant pelvic radiation against observation, the secondary cancer rates at 15 years were 22 percent in the radiation group compared with 16 percent in the observation group. However, this difference did not reach statistical significance (Creutzberg, 2011).

Development of a secondary radiation-induced cancer depends on factors such as patient age at exposure, radiation dose, and susceptibility of specific tissue types to radiation-induced carcinogenesis (Table 28-4). In general, those receiving higher radiation doses and those exposed at an earlier age have increased risks for second malignancies. The latency of secondary tumor development also varies depending on the type of second malignancy. For example, the latent period between radiation exposure and the clinical appearance of leukemia is less than 10 years, whereas solid tumors may not develop for decades. The most common example is development of uterine sarcoma years after pelvic radiation for treatment of cervical cancer (Mark, 1996). Preventatively, irradiation of smaller fields with advanced technologies such as IMRT compared with larger field 2-D external beam radiation may reduce the incidence of radiation-induced malignancies (Herrera, 2014).

REFERENCES

Adli M, Mayr NA, Kaiser HS et al: Does prone positioning reduce small bowel dose in pelvic radiation with intensity-modulated radiotherapy for gynecologic cancer? Int J Radiat Oncol Biol Phys 57(1):230, 2003
Amorino GP, Freeman ML, Carbone DP, et al: Radiopotentiation by the oral platinum agent, JM216: role of repair inhibition. Int J Radiat Oncol Biol Phys 44(2):399, 1999
Arai T, Nakano T, Fukuhisa K, et al: Second cancer after radiation therapy for cancer of the uterine cervix. Cancer 67(2):398, 1991
Ash P: The influence of radiation on fertility in man. Br J Radiol 53:271, 1980
ASTEC/EN.5 Study Group: Adjuvant external beam radiotherapy in the treatment of endometrial cancer (MRC ASTEC and NCIC CTG EN.5

randomised trials): pooled trial results, systematic review and meta-analysis. Lancet 373:137, 2009

Begg AC: Cisplatin and radiation: interaction probabilities and therapeutic possibilities. Int J Radiat Oncol Biol Phys 19(5):1183, 1990

Bentzen, SM: Tumor volume and local control probability: clinical data and radiobiological interpretations. Int J Radiat Oncol Biol Phys 36(1):247, 1996

Boronow RC: Combined therapy as an alternative to exenteration for locally advanced vulvo-vaginal cancer: rationale and results. Cancer 49(6):1085, 1982

Brizel DM, Dodge RK, Clough RW, et al: Oxygenation of head and neck cancer: changes during radiotherapy and impact on treatment outcome. Radiother Oncol 53(2):113, 1999

Cooper KL, Beabout JW, Swee RG: Insufficiency fractures of the sacrum. Radiology 156:15, 1985

Creutzberg CL, Nout RA, Lybeert ML, et al: Fifteen-year radiotherapy outcomes of the randomized PORTEC-1 trial for endometrial carcinoma. Int J Radiat Oncol Biol Phys 81(4):631, 2011

Dische S, Saunders MI, Sealy R, et al: Carcinoma of the cervix and the use of hyperbaric oxygen with radiotherapy: a report of a randomised controlled trial. Radiother Oncol 53(2):93, 1999

DiSilvestro PA, Ali S, Craighead PS, et al: Phase III randomized trial of weekly cisplatin and irradiation versus cisplatin and tirapazamine and irradiation in stages IB2, IIA, IIB, IIIB, and IVA cervical carcinoma limited to the pelvis: a Gynecologic Oncology Group study. J Clin Oncol 32(5):458, 2014

Dubben HH: Tumor volume: a basic and specific response predictor in radiotherapy. Radiother Oncol 47(2):167, 1998

Dueñas-González A, Zarba JJ, Alcedo JC, et al: A phase III study comparing concurrent gemcitabine (Gem) plus cisplatin (Cis) and radiation followed by adjuvant Gem plus Cis versus concurrent Cis and radiation in patients with stage IIB to IVA carcinoma of the cervix. Abstract No. CRA5507. Presented at the 45th Annual Meeting of the American Society of Clinical Oncology. 1-2 June 2009

Dunst J, Kuhnt T, Strauss HG, et al: Anemia in cervical cancers: impact on survival, patterns of relapse, and association with hypoxia and angiogenesis. Int J Radiat Oncol Biol Phys 56(3):778, 2003

Fajardo LF: The pathology of ionizing radiation as defined by morphologic patterns. Acta Oncol 44(1):13, 2005

Friedlander AH, Freymiller EG: Detection of radiation-accelerated atherosclerosis of the carotid artery by panoramic radiography. A new opportunity for dentists. J Am Dent Assoc 134(10):1361, 2003

Frumovitz M, Sun CC, Schover LR, et al: Quality of life and sexual functioning in cervical cancer survivors. J Clin Oncol 23(30):7428, 2005

Gemignani ML, Alektiar KM, Leitai M, et al: Radical surgical resection and high-dose intraoperative radiation therapy (HDR-IORT) in patients with recurrent gynecologic cancers. Int J Radiat Oncol Biol Phys 50(3):687, 2001

Gondi V, Bentzen SM, Sklenar KL et al: Severe late toxicities following concomitant chemoradiotherapy compared to radiotherapy alone in cervical cancer: an inter-era analysis. Int J Radiat Oncol Biol Phys 84(4):973, 2012

Grigsby PW, Heydon K, Mutch DG et al: Long-term follow up of RTOG 92-10: cervical cancer with positive para-aortic lymph nodes. Int J Radiat Oncol Biol Phys 51(4):982, 2001

Grigsby P, Winter K, Komaki R et al: Long-term follow-up of RTOG 88-05: twice-daily external irradiation with brachytherapy for carcinoma of the cervix. Int J Radiat Oncol Biol Phys 54:51, 2002

Hareyama M, Sakata K, Oouchi A, et al: High-dose-rate versus low-dose-rate intracavitary therapy for carcinoma of the uterine cervix: a randomized trial. Cancer 94(1):117, 2002

Hawkins MM, Smith RA: Pregnancy outcomes in childhood cancer survivors: probable effects of abdominal irradiation. Int J Cancer 43(3):399, 1989

Heron DE, Gerszten K, Selvaraj RN, et al: Conventional 3D conformal versus intensity-modulated radiotherapy for the adjuvant treatment of gynecologic malignancies: a comparative dosimetric study of dose-volume histograms. Gynecol Oncol 91(1):39, 2003

Herrera FG, Cruz OS, Achtari C, et al: Long-term outcome and late side effects in endometrial cancer patients treated with surgery and postoperative radiation therapy. Ann Surg Oncol 21(7):2390, 2014

Hoffman JP, Sigurdson ER, Eisenberg BL: Use of saline-filled tissue expanders to protect the small bowel from radiation. Oncology 12(1):51, 1998

Irtan S, Orbach D, Helfre S, et al: Ovarian transposition in prepubescent and adolescent girls with cancer. Lancet Oncol 14:e601, 2013

Janssens GO, Rademakers SE, Terhaard CH, et al: Improved recurrence-free survival with ARCON for anemic patients with laryngeal cancer. Clin Cancer Res 20(5):1345, 2014

Jensen PT, Groenvold M, Klee MC, et al: Longitudinal study of sexual function and vaginal changes after radiotherapy for cervical cancer. Int J Radiat Oncol Biol Phys 56(4):937, 2003

Kantsevoy SV, Cruz-Correa MR, Vaughn CA, et al: Endoscopic cryotherapy for the treatment of bleeding mucosal vascular lesions of the GI tract: a pilot study. Gastrointest Endosc 57(3):403, 2003

Kapp KS, Poschauko J, Geyer E, et al: Evaluation of the effect of routine packed red blood cell transfusion in anemic cervix cancer patients treated with radical radiotherapy. Int J Radiat Oncol Biol Phys 54(1):58, 2002

Keys HM, Bundy BN, Stehman FB, et al: A comparison of weekly cisplatin during radiation therapy versus irradiation alone each followed by adjuvant hysterectomy in bulky stage IB cervical carcinoma: a randomized trial of the Gynecologic Oncology Group. N Engl J Med 340:1154, 1999

Keys HM, Bundy BN, Stehman FB et al: Radiation therapy with and without extrafascial hysterectomy for bulky stage IB cervical carcinoma: a randomized trial of the Gynecologic Oncology Group. Gynecol Oncol 89(3):343, 2003

Keys HM, Roberts JA, Brunetto VL, et al: A phase III trial of surgery with or without adjunctive external pelvic radiation therapy in intermediate risk endometrial adenocarcinoma: a Gynecologic Oncology Group study. 92:744, 2004

Klopp AH, Moughan J, Portelance L, et al: Hematologic toxicity in RTOG 0418: a phase 2 study of postoperative IMRT for gynecologic cancers. Int J Radiat Oncol Biol Phys 86(1):83, 2013

Konishi T, Watanabe T, Kitayama J, et al: Endoscopic and histopathologic findings after formalin application for hemorrhage caused by chronic radiation-induced proctitis. Gastrointest Endosc 61(1):161, 2005

Lee JL, Viswanathan AN: Predictors of toxicity after image-guided high-dose-rate interstitial brachytherapy for gynecologic cancer. Int J Radiat Oncol Biol Phys 84(5):1192, 2012

Lee MY, Wu HG, Kim K, et al: Concurrent radiotherapy with paclitaxel/carboplatin chemotherapy as a definitive treatment for squamous cell carcinoma of the uterine cervix. Gynecol Oncol 104(1):95, 2007

Luxton RW, Kunkler PB: Radiation nephritis. Acta Radiol Ther Phys Biol 66:169, 1964

Mark RJ, Poen J, Tran LM et al: Postirradiation sarcoma of the gynecologic tract. A report of 13 cases and a discussion of the risk of radiation-induced gynecologic malignancies. Am J Clin Oncol 19(1):59, 1996

Martin J, Fitzpatrick K, Horan G, et al: Treatment with a belly-board device significantly reduces the volume of small bowel irradiated and results in low acute toxicity in adjuvant radiotherapy for gynecologic cancer: results of a prospective study. Radiother Oncol 74(3):267, 2005

Mason KA, Kishi K, Hunter N, et al: Effect of docetaxel on the therapeutic ratio of fractionated radiotherapy in vivo. Clin Cancer Res 5:4191, 1999

Milano MT, Constine LS, Okunieff P: Normal tissue tolerance dose metrics for radiation therapy of major organs. Semin Radiat Oncol 17:131, 2007

Montana GS, Thomas GM, Moore DH, et al: Preoperative chemo-radiation for carcinoma of the vulva with N2/N3 nodes: a gynecologic oncology group study. Int J Radiat Oncol Biol Phys 48(4):1007, 2000

Morris M, Eifel PJ, Watkins EB, et al: Pelvic radiation with concurrent chemotherapy versus pelvic and para-aortic radiation for high risk cervical cancer: a randomized Radiation Therapy Oncology Group clinical trial. N Engl J Med 340:1137, 1999

National Cancer Institute: Common Terminology Criteria for Adverse Events v4.0. NCI, NIH, DHHS. May 29, 2009. NIH publication #09-7473

Nordsmark M, Overgaard M, Overgaard J: Pretreatment oxygenation predicts radiation response in advanced squamous cell carcinoma of the head and neck. Radiother Oncol 41(1):31, 1996

Nout RA, Smit VT, Putter H, et al: Vaginal brachytherapy versus pelvic external beam radiotherapy for patients with endometrial cancer of high-intermediate risk (PORTEC-2): an open-label, non-inferiority, randomised trial. Lancet 375:816, 2010

Oh D, Huh SJ, Nam H et al: Pelvic insufficiency fracture after pelvic radiotherapy for cervical cancer: analysis of risk factors. Int J Radiat Oncol Biol Phys 70(4):1183, 2008

Okada H, Mak TW: Pathways of apoptotic and non-apoptotic death in tumour cells. Nat Rev Cancer 4(8):592, 2004

Pawlik TM, Keyomarsi K: Role of cell cycle in mediating sensitivity to radiotherapy. Int J Radiat Oncol Biol Phys 59(4):928, 2004

Petereit DG, Sarkaria JN, Chappell R, et al: The adverse effect of treatment prolongation in cervical carcinoma. Int J Radiat Oncol Biol Phys 32(5):1301, 1995

Peters WA, Liu PY, Barrett RJ, et al: Concurrent chemotherapy and pelvic radiation therapy compared with pelvic radiation therapy alone as adjuvant therapy after radical surgery in high-risk early-stage cancer of the cervix. J Clin Oncol 18(8):1606, 2000

Portelance L, Chao KS, Grigsby PW, et al: Intensity-modulated radiation therapy (IMRT) reduces small bowel, rectum, and bladder doses in patients with cervical cancer receiving pelvic and para-aortic irradiation. Int J Radiat Oncol Biol Phys 51(1):261, 2001

Potter R, Haie-Meder C, Van Limbergen E, et al: Recommendations from gynaecological (GYN) GEC ESTRO working group (II): concepts and terms in 3D image-based treatment planning in cervix cancer brachytherapy-3D dose volume parameters and aspects of 3D image-based anatomy, radiation physics, radiobiology. Radiother Oncol 78(1):67, 2006

Rose PG, Bundy BN, Watkins EB, et al: Concurrent cisplatin-based chemoradiation improves progression free and overall survival in advanced cervical cancer: results of a randomized Gynecologic Oncology Group study. N Engl J Med 340:1144, 1999

Schwartz JL, Mustafi R, Beckett MA, et al: DNA double-strand break rejoining rates, inherent radiation sensitivity and human tumor response to radiotherapy. Br J Cancer 74(1):37, 1996

Schwartz JL, Rotmensch J, Giovanazzi S, et al: Faster repair of DNA double-strand breaks in radioresistant human tumor cells. Int J Radiat Oncol Biol Phys 15(4):907, 1988

Sedlis A, Bundy BN, Rotman MZ, et al: A randomized trial of pelvic radiation therapy versus no further therapy in selected patients with stage IB carcinoma of the cervix after radical hysterectomy and pelvic lymphadenectomy: a Gynecologic Oncology Group study. Gynecol Oncol 73(2)177, 1999

Shih KK, Folkert MR, Kollmeier MA, et al: Pelvic insufficiency fractures in patients with cervical and endometrial cancer treated with postoperative pelvic radiation. Gynecol Oncol 128(3):540, 2013

Small W, Winter K, Levenback C et al: Extended-field irradiation and intracavitary brachytherapy combined with cisplatin and amifostine for cervical cancer with positive para-aortic or high common iliac lymph nodes: results of arm II of RTOG 0116. Int J Gynecol Cancer 21(7):1266, 2011

Smith S, Wallner K, Dominitz JA, et al: Argon plasma coagulation for rectal bleeding after prostate brachytherapy. Int J Radiat Oncol Biol Phys 51(3):636, 2001

Soper JT, Clarke-Pearson DL, Creasman WT: Absorbable synthetic mesh (910-polyglactin) intestinal sling to reduce radiation-induced small bowel injury in patients with pelvic malignancies. Gynecol Oncol 29(3):283, 1988

Stanic S, Mayadev JS: Tolerance of the small bowel to therapeutic irradiation: a focus on late toxicity in patients receiving para-aortic nodal irradiation for gynecologic malignancies. Int J Gynecol Cancer 23(4):592, 2013

Steel GG, Peckham MJ: Exploitable mechanisms in combined radiotherapy-chemotherapy: the concept of additivity. Int J Radiat Oncol Biol Phys 5(1):85, 1979

Thomas G, Ali S, Hoebers FJ, et al: Phase III trial to evaluate the efficacy of maintaining hemoglobin levels above 12.0 g/dL with erythropoietin vs above 10.0 g/dL without erythropoietin in anemic patients receiving concurrent radiation and cisplatin for cervical cancer. Gynecol Oncol 108(2):317, 2008

Trott KR: The mechanisms of acceleration of repopulation in squamous epithelia during daily irradiation. Acta Oncol 38(2):153, 1999

Ventrucci M, Di Simone MP, Giulietti P, et al: Efficacy and safety of Nd:YAG laser for the treatment of bleeding from radiation proctocolitis. Dig Liver Dis 33(3):230, 2001

Verma J, Sulman EP, Jhingran A et al: Dosimetric predictors of duodenal toxicity after intensity modulated radiation therapy for treatment of the para-aortic nodes in gynecologic cancer. Int J Radiat Oncol Biol Phys 88(2):357, 2014

Weichselbaum RR, Beckett MA, Hallahan DE, et al: Molecular targets to overcome radioresistance. Semin Oncol 19(4 Suppl 11):14, 1992

Wong FC, Tung SY, Leung TW, et al: Treatment results of high-dose-rate remote afterloading brachytherapy for cervical cancer and retrospective comparison of two regimens. Int J Radiat Oncol Biol Phys 55(5):1254, 2003

Zidar N, Ferlunga D, Hvala A, et al: Contribution to the pathogenesis of radiation-induced injury to large arteries. J Laryngol Otol 111(10):988, 1997

Preinvasive Lesions of the Lower Genital Tract

Office gynecology frequently involves the diagnosis and management of preinvasive lower genital tract disease, most often involving the uterine cervix. Since widespread introduction of the Papanicolaou (Pap) test in the 1950s, cervical cancer screening has reduced the incidence of and mortality rate from invasive cervical cancer by more than 70 percent (Howlader, 2014). This is true despite a continued rise in the incidence of preinvasive lesions (Kurdgelashvili, 2013). Approximately 7 percent of U.S. women who undergo Pap testing will have an abnormal result (Wright, 2012). An abnormal screening test prompts further patient evaluation, usually with colposcopy and biopsy. Histologic results are more definitive and inform appropriate management.

LOWER GENITAL TRACT NEOPLASIA

In the lower genital tract (LGT), the term *intraepithelial neoplasia* refers to squamous epithelial lesions that are potential precursors of invasive cancer. These lesions demonstrate a range of histologic abnormality from mild to severe based on cytoplasmic, nuclear, and histologic changes. The severity of a squamous intraepithelial lesion is graded by the proportion of epithelium with abnormal cells from the basement membrane upward toward the surface. In the case of cervical intraepithelial neoplasia (CIN), abnormal cells confined to the lower third of the squamous epithelium are referred to as *mild dysplasia* or *CIN 1*, extending into the middle third as *moderate dysplasia* or *CIN 2,* into the upper third as *severe dysplasia* or *CIN 3*, and full-thickness involvement as *carcinoma in situ (CIS)* (Fig. 29-1). Squamous neoplasia of the vagina, vulva, perianal, and anal squamous epithelia (VaIN, VIN, PAIN, and AIN, respectively) are graded similarly with the caveat that VIN 1 is no longer recognized (p. 647). The natural history of these extracervical lesions is less understood than for CIN. In contrast, the cervical columnar epithelium does not demonstrate an analogous neoplastic disease spectrum because it is only one cell-layer thick. Histologic abnormalities are therefore limited to either *adenocarcinoma in situ (AIS)* or *adenocarcinoma.*

The concept of cervical neoplasia as a spectrum has come under question with increasing insight into human papillomavirus (HPV) infection. Mild squamous dysplasia is now recognized as evidence of HPV infection, most of which is transient and unlikely to progress. Moderate to severe dysplastic squamous lesions are considered to be true cancer precursors. Current cytology reporting reflects this two-tier concept (Solomon, 2002). In 1989, the Bethesda System nomenclature replaced CIN with *squamous intraepithelial lesion (SIL)*. Because cytologic and histologic changes of HPV infection and CIN 1 cannot be distinguished reliably and because of their like natural histories, they are categorized together as *low-grade squamous intraepithelial lesions (LSIL)*. Similarly, CIN 2, CIN 3, and CIS are difficult to distinguish, are truer cancer precursors, and are all designated as *high-grade squamous intraepithelial lesions (HSIL)*. The diagnostic distinction between LSIL and HSIL is more reliable, biologically plausible, and clinically meaningful than diagnoses using the CIN system. This two-tiered nomenclature is now recommended, and guidelines for the management of these lesions are grouped accordingly (Darragh, 2012).

ANATOMIC CONSIDERATIONS

◼ External Genitalia

Precancerous lesions of the female LGT are often multifocal, can involve any of its structures, and may appear similar to benign processes. For example, *micropapillomatosis labialis* is a benign anatomic variant characterized by minute epithelial projections on the inner labia minora (Fig. 29-2). This condition can be easily mistaken for HPV-related lesions, but true HPV lesions tend to be multifocal and asymmetric, and to have multiple papillations arising from a single base (Ferris, 2004). Micropapillomatosis often shows spontaneous regression, and treatment is not indicated (Bergeron, 1990).

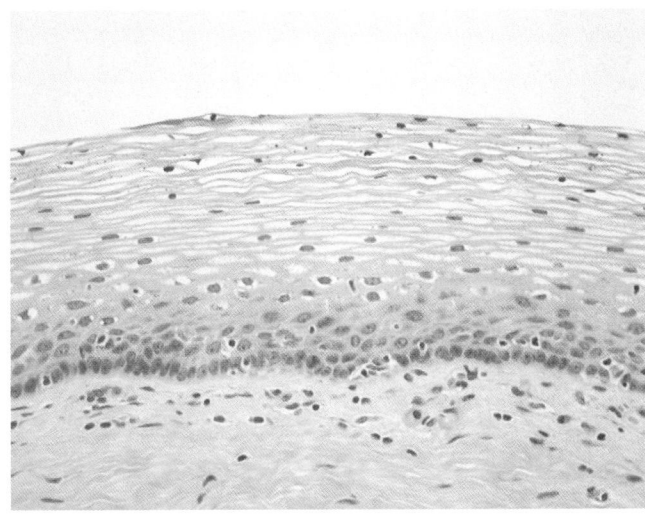

A

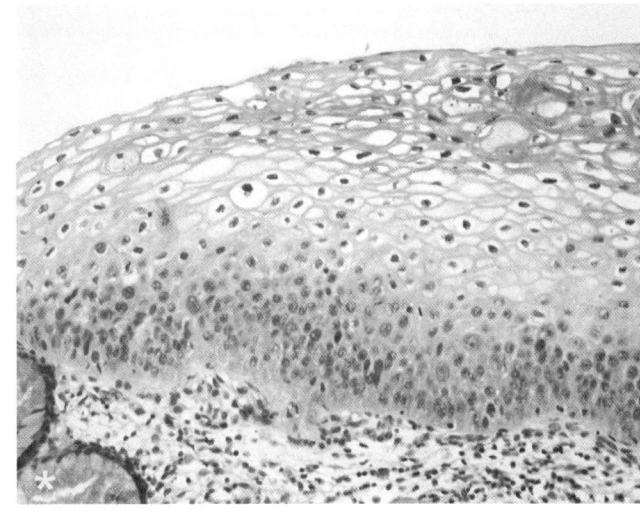

B

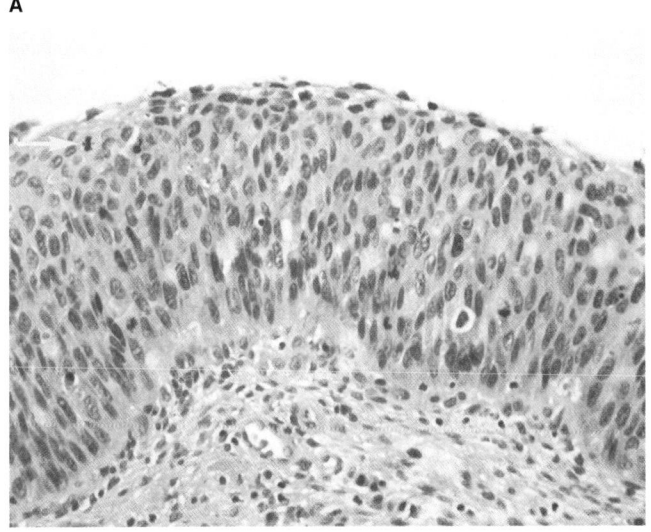

C

FIGURE 29-1 A. Normal ectocervical epithelium is a nonkeratinizing, stratified squamous epithelium. Mitoses are normally confined to the lower layers, namely, the basal and parabasal epithelial layers. **B.** Low-grade squamous intraepithelial lesion (LSIL). This biopsy's location at the transformation zone is indicated by the presence of both columnar epithelium (*asterisk*) and squamous epithelium. Low-grade SIL has a disordered proliferation of squamous cells and increased mitotic activity confined to the basal one third of the epithelium. Koilocytotic atypia, which is indicative of proliferative HPV infection, involves the more superficial epithelium. Koilocytosis is typified by nuclear enlargement, coarse chromatin, nuclear "wrinkling," and perinuclear halos. **C.** This high-grade SIL shows disordered, highly atypical squamous cells and increased mitotic activity involving the full thickness of the epithelium. Note the mitotic figure located close to epithelial surface (*yellow arrow*). (Used with permission from Dr. Kelley Carrick.)

Vagina

The vagina is lined by nonkeratinized squamous epithelium, and glands are absent. However, areas of columnar epithelium are occasionally found within the vaginal squamous mucosa, a condition termed *adenosis*. It is often attributable to in utero exposure to exogenous estrogen, particularly diethylstilbestrol (DES) (Trimble, 2001). These areas are red patches within the squamous epithelium and can be mistaken for ulcers or other lesions. With DES-related adenosis, careful palpation of the vagina is warranted in addition to visual inspection, as clear cell adenocarcinoma may be palpable before becoming visible.

Cervix

Squamocolumnar Junction

During embryogenesis, upward migration of stratified squamous epithelium from the urogenital sinus and vaginal plate is thought to replace müllerian epithelium (Ulfelder, 1976). This process usually terminates near the external cervical os, forming the original (congenital) squamocolumnar junction (SCJ). When visible on the ectocervix, the SCJ is a pink, smooth squamous epithelium juxtaposed against the red, velvety columnar epithelium

surrounding the external cervical os. Rarely, this migration is incomplete resulting in an SCJ in the upper vaginal fornices. This is a normal variant and also seen with in utero DES exposure.

The columnar epithelium is commonly referred to as "glandular." This is because it produces mucus, and its deep infoldings appear histologically similar to glandular tissue (Fig. 29-3). However, true glands, consisting of acini and ducts, are not present on the cervix (Ulfelder, 1976).

The location of the SCJ varies with age and hormonal status (Fig. 29-4). During the reproductive years, it everts outward onto the ectocervix, especially during adolescence, pregnancy, and with combination hormonal contraceptive use. It regresses into the endocervical canal during the natural process of squamous metaplasia and in low-estrogen states such as menopause, prolonged lactation, and long-term progestin-only contraceptive use.

Squamous Metaplasia

At puberty, the rise in estrogen levels leads to increased glycogenation of the LGT nonkeratinized squamous epithelium. In providing a carbohydrate source, glycogen allows vaginal flora to be dominated by lactobacilli, which produce lactic acid. The resultant acidic vaginal pH is the suspected stimulus for *squamous*

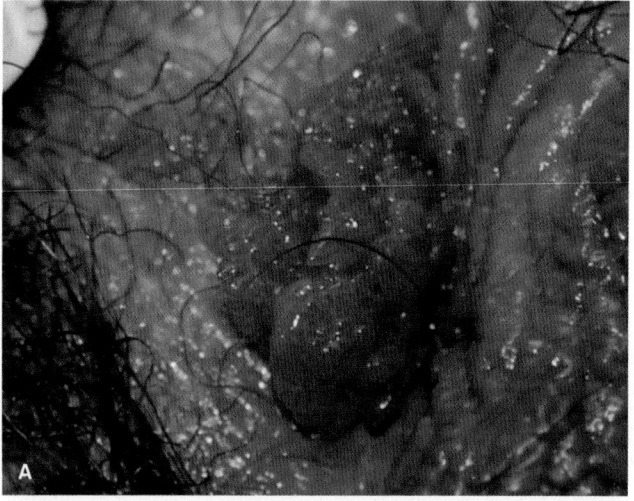

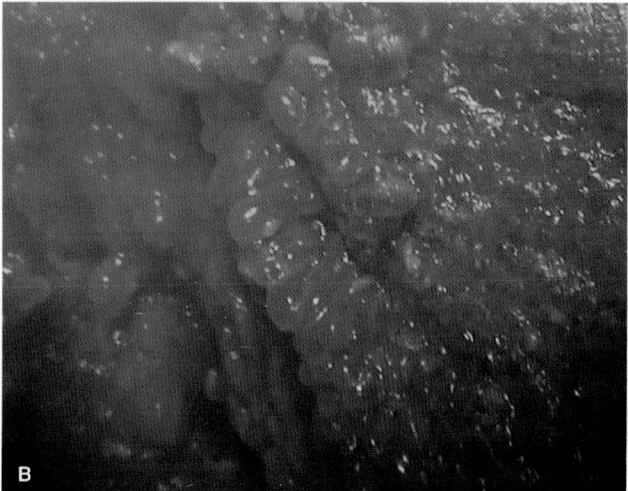

FIGURE 29-2 Benign lower genital tract lesions. **A.** Condylomata tend to be multifocal, asymmetric, and have multiple papillations arising from a single base. **B.** Micropapillomatosis labialis is a normal variant of vulvar anatomy encountered along the inner aspects of the labia minora and lower vagina. In contrast to condylomata, projections are uniform in size and shape and arise singly from their base attachments.

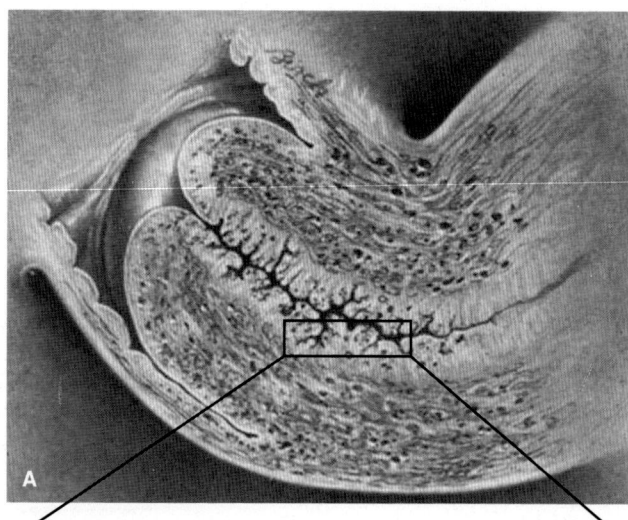

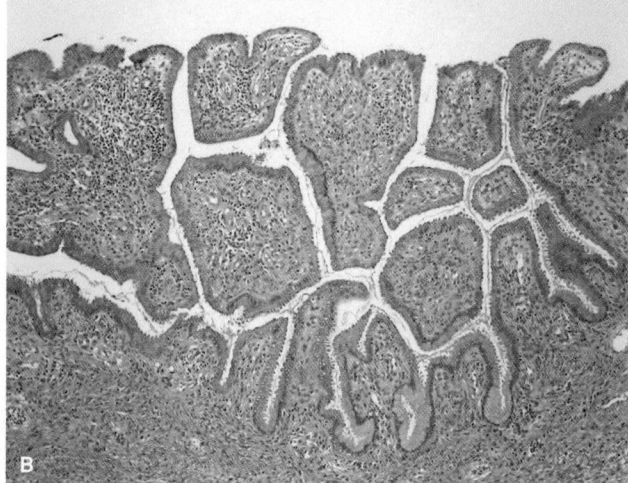

FIGURE 29-3 Endocervical anatomy. **A.** Sagittal view of the cervix. In this drawing, a portion of the endocervical canal is boxed. (Modified with permission from Eastman NJ, Hellman LM: Williams Obstetrics 12th ed., New York: Appleton-Century-Crofts, Inc; 1961.) **B.** The endocervix is lined by a simple columnar, mucin-secreting epithelium. Crypts and small exophytic projections appear pseudopapillary when viewed in cross section. (Used with permission from Dr. Kelley Carrick.)

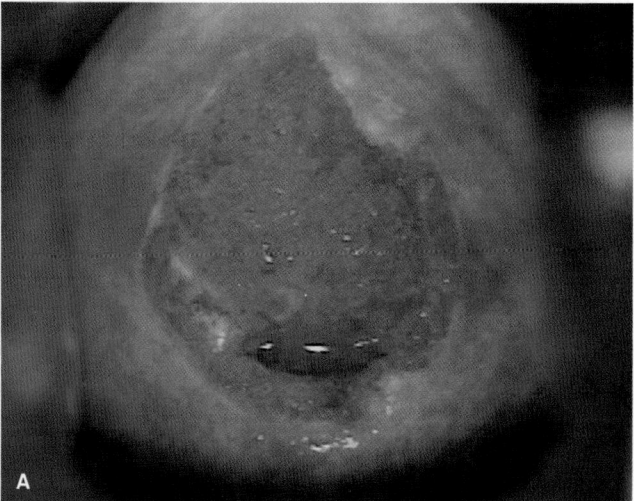

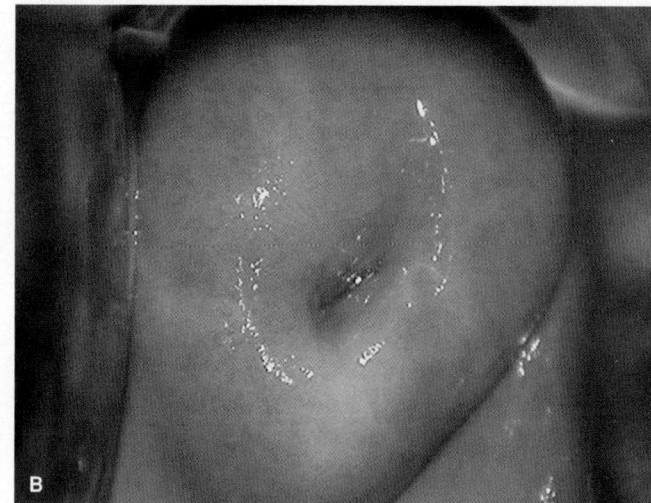

FIGURE 29-4 The location of the squamocolumnar junction (SCJ) is variable. **A.** The SCJ is located on the ectocervix and is fully visualized. **B.** The SCJ is located within the endocervical canal and is not visible.

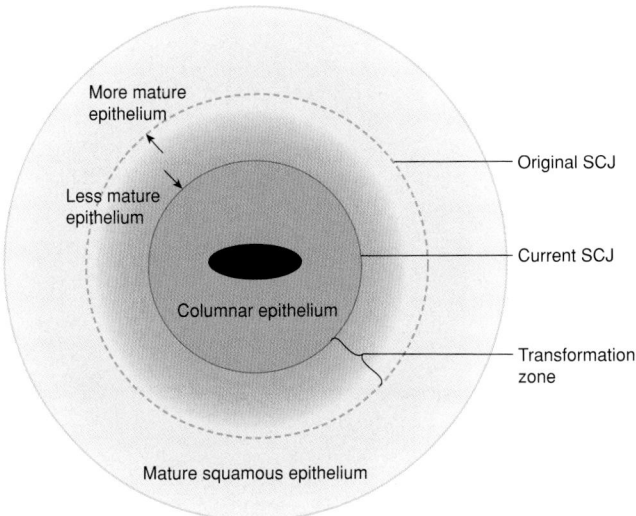

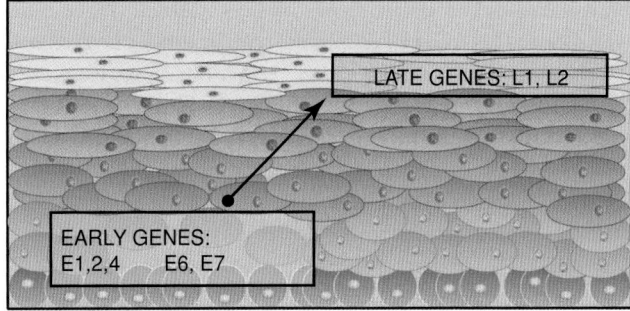

FIGURE 29-6 The human papillomavirus life cycle is completed in synchrony with squamous epithelium differentiation. Early genes, including the *E6* and *E7* oncogenes, are expressed most strongly within the basal and parabasal layers. The late genes encoding capsid proteins are expressed later in the superficial layers. Intact virus is shed during normal desquamation of superficial squames. Late genes are not strongly expressed in high-grade neoplastic lesions.

FIGURE 29-5 Schematic describing relevant cervical landmarks. The original squamocolumnar junction (SCJ) marks the terminal site of the upward migration of squamous epithelium during embryonic development. The SCJ location moves with age and hormonal status. With higher estrogen states, the SCJ everts outward. With low-estrogen states and with squamous metaplasia, the SCJ moves closer to the cervical os. The transformation zone consists of the band of squamous metaplasia lying between the original SCJ and new (current) SCJ. As the metaplastic epithelium matures, it moves outward relative to the newer, less mature areas of metaplasia and can become indistinguishable from the original squamous epithelium.

metaplasia, which is the normal replacement of columnar by squamous epithelium on the cervix. Relatively undifferentiated reserve cells underlying the cervical epithelia are the apparent precursors of the new metaplastic cells, which differentiate further into squamous epithelium. This normal process creates a progressively widening band of metaplastic and maturing squamous epithelium, termed the *transformation zone* (TZ), between the congenital (original) columnar epithelium and the squamous epithelium (Fig. 29-5).

Transformation Zone and Cervical Neoplasia

Nearly all cervical neoplasia, both squamous and columnar, develops within the TZ, usually adjacent to the new or current SCJ. Cervical reserve and immature metaplastic cells appear particularly vulnerable to the oncogenic effects of HPV and cocarcinogens (Stanley, 2010a). Squamous metaplasia is most active during adolescence and pregnancy. This may explain why early ages of first sexual activity and of first pregnancy are cervical cancer risk factors.

HUMAN PAPILLOMAVIRUS

■ Basic Virology

The causative role of HPV in nearly all cervical neoplasia and a significant proportion of vulvar, vaginal, and anal neoplasia is firmly established. HPV primarily infects human squamous or metaplastic epithelial cells. It is a double-stranded DNA virus with a protein capsid unique to each viral type. More than 150

genetically distinct HPV types have been identified, and of these, approximately 40 types infect the LGT (Doorbar, 2012).

The circular HPV genome consists of only nine identified open reading frames (Stanley, 2010a). In addition to one regulatory region, the six "early" (E) genes govern functions early in the viral life cycle, including DNA maintenance, replication, and transcription. Early genes are expressed in the lower squamous epithelial layers (Fig. 29-6). The two "late" genes encode the major (L1) and minor (L2) capsid proteins. These proteins are expressed in the superficial epithelial layers late in the viral life cycle and during the assemblage of new, infectious viral particles. Sequential HPV gene expression is synchronous with and dependent on squamous epithelial differentiation. Thus, completion of the viral life cycle takes place only within an intact, fully differentiating squamous epithelium (Doorbar, 2012). This makes it nearly impossible to culture HPV in vitro. HPV is a nonlytic virus, and therefore infectiousness depends on normal desquamation of infected epithelial cells. A new infection is initiated when the L1 and L2 capsid proteins bind to the epithelial basement membrane and/or basal cells, permitting entry of HPV viral particles into cells of a new host (Sapp, 2009).

Genital HPV is the most common sexually transmitted disease (STD) in the United States, and most sexually active adults are infected at some time (Dunne, 2014). Most incident HPV infections develop in women younger than 25 years. The point prevalence in U.S. females aged 14 to 59 years is 27 percent. It is highest in those aged 20 to 24 years (45 percent) and becomes less prevalent with increasing age (Dunne, 2007). Clinically, HPV types are classified as high-risk (HR) or low-risk (LR) based on their strength of association with cervical cancer. LR HPV types 6 and 11 cause nearly all genital warts, laryngeal papillomas, and a minority of subclinical HPV infections. LR HPV infections are rarely, if ever, oncogenic.

In contrast, persistent HR HPV infection is now viewed as required for the development of cervical cancer. HR HPV types, including 16, 18, 31, 33, 35, 45, and 58, along with a few less common types, account for approximately 95 percent of cervical cancer cases worldwide (Muñoz, 2003). HPV 16 is the most oncogenic, accounting for the largest percentage of

CIN 3 lesions (45 percent) and cervical cancers (55 percent) worldwide. It is also the dominant type in other HPV-related anogenital and oropharyngeal cancers (Schiffman, 2010; Smith, 2007). Although the prevalence of HPV 18 is much lower than that of HPV 16 in the general population, it is found in 13 percent of cervical squamous cell carcinomas, and in an even higher proportion of cervical adenocarcinomas and adenosquamous carcinomas (approximately 40 percent) (Bruni, 2010; Smith, 2007). Together, HPVs 16 and 18 account for approximately 70 percent of cervical cancers worldwide, 68 percent of squamous cell carcinomas, and 85 percent of adenocarcinomas (Bosch, 2008). HPV type 45 is the third most common found in cervical cancers (de Sanjose, 2010). HPV 16 accounts for more than 1 in 5 cervical HPV infections and is the most common HPV found among low-grade lesions and in women without neoplasia (Bruni, 2010; Herrero, 2000). Thus, HR HPV infection does not cause neoplasia in most infected women, and additional host, viral, and environmental factors determine progression to LGT neoplasia.

Transmission

The most important risk factors for the acquisition of genital HPV infection are the number of lifetime and recent sexual partners and early age at first sexual intercourse (Burk, 1996; Fairley, 1994; Franco, 1995). Genital HPV is transmitted by direct, usually sexual, contact with the genital skin, mucous membranes, or body fluids of an individual with either warts or subclinical HPV infection. The infectivity of inapparent (subclinical) HPV is assumed to be high. HPV is thought to access to the basal cell layer and basement membrane through microabrasions of the genital epithelium during sexual contact. Once infected, these basal cells may become a viral reservoir (Stanley, 2010b).

Cervical HR HPV infection generally requires penetrative intercourse. Oral-genital and hand-genital HPV transmissions are possible but are much less common than with genital-genital transmission (Winer, 2003). Women who have sex with women have rates of HR HPV positivity, abnormal cervical cytology, and high-grade cervical neoplasia similar to those of heterosexual women, but undergo cervical cancer screening less often. Women with or without past sexual experiences with men have a similar risk, implying that digital, oral, and perhaps object contact places them at risk of HR HPV infection (Marrazzo, 2000). Thus, all women who are sexually active should undergo cervical cancer screening according to current recommendations regardless of sexual orientation.

Genital HPV detection, including HR HPV, has been reported in apparently sexually naïve girls and young women (Doerfler, 2009; Winer, 2003). Nonetheless, genital warts that develop in children after infancy are always reason to consider the possibility of sexual abuse. HPV infection by nonsexual contact, autoinoculation, or fomite transfer appears possible. This is supported by reports of nongenital HPV types in a significant minority of pediatric and adolescent genital wart cases (Cohen, 1990; Obalek, 1990; Siegfried, 1997).

Congenital HPV infection from vertical transmission (mother to fetus or newborn) beyond transient skin colonization is rare. Conjunctival, laryngeal, vulvar, or perianal warts

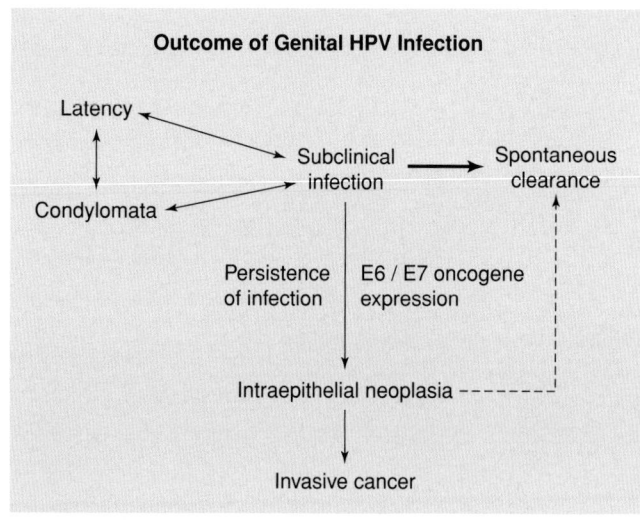

FIGURE 29-7 The natural history of genital human papillomavirus (HPV) infection varies between individuals and over time. Most infections are subclinical. Spontaneous resolution is the most common outcome. Neoplasia is the least common manifestation of HPV infection, developing as the result of persistent infection with integration of HPV DNA.

present at birth or that develop within 1 to 3 years of birth are most likely due to perinatal exposure to maternal HPV (Cohen, 1990). Infection is not linked to maternal genital warts or route of delivery (Silverberg, 2003; Syrjänen, 2010). Accordingly, cesarean delivery generally is not recommended for maternal HPV infection. Exceptions include cases of large genital warts that would obstruct delivery or might avulse and bleed with cervical dilation or vaginal delivery.

Infection Outcomes

Genital HPV infection causes variable outcomes (Fig. 29-7). These can be broadly grouped as latent or expressed infections. Infection expression may be productive, that is, creating infectious viral particles, or it may be neoplastic, causing preinvasive disease or malignancy. Most productive infections are subclinical, but a smaller percentage yields clinically apparent genital warts. Last, HPV infection can be transient or can become persistent. High-grade neoplasia (CIN 3 or worse) is the least common outcome of genital HPV infection, requiring HPV persistence.

Latent infection refers to that in which cells are infected, but HPV remains quiescent. There are no detectable tissue effects, as the virus is not actively replicating. The virus is present below detectable levels. Thus, it is uncertain whether apparent clearance of the HPV constitutes true eradication of HPV from infected tissues or whether it reflects latency.

Productive infections are characterized by viral life-cycle completion and plentiful production of infectious viral particles (Stanley, 2010a). Viral gene expression and assemblage are completed in synchrony with terminal squamous differentiation, concluding with desquamation of infected squames. These infections have little or no malignant potential because the HPV genome remains episomal and its oncogenes are expressed at very low levels (Durst, 1985; Stoler, 1996).

In both female and male genital tracts, productive HPV infections cause either visible genital warts (condyloma acuminata) or much more commonly, subclinical infections. Subclinical infections may be indirectly identified as low-grade cytologic, colposcopic, or histologic abnormalities. However, all these observational diagnoses are subjective and poorly reproducible. HPV testing more accurately reflects HPV infection but is limited to specific HPV types and viral loads.

With *neoplastic infection* (CIN 3 and cervical cancer), the circular HPV genome is disrupted and integrates at random locations into a host chromosome (Fig. 30-1, p. 659). Unrestrained transcription of the *E6* and *E7* oncogenes follows (Durst, 1985; Stoler, 1996). The E6 and E7 oncoproteins produced interfere with and accelerate degradation of p53 and pRb, which are key tumor suppressor proteins produced by the host (Fig. 30-2, p. 659). This leaves the infected cell vulnerable to malignant transformation by loss of cell-cycle control, cellular proliferation, and accumulation of DNA mutations over time (Doorbar, 2012).

In resultant preinvasive lesions, normal epithelial differentiation is disrupted and incomplete. The degree of disruption is used to grade histology as low-grade (encompassing HPV changes and CIN 1) or high-grade (CIN 2, CIN 3, and CIS). The average age at diagnosis of low-grade cervical disease is younger than that of high-grade lesions and invasive cancers. Thus, disease was thought to progress from milder- to higher-grade lesions over time. An alternative theory now proposes that low-grade lesions are generally acute, transient, and not oncogenic. High-grade lesions and cancers are monoclonal and arise de novo rather than from preexistent low-grade disease (Baseman, 2005; Kiviat, 1996).

The pathogenesis of HPV-related neoplasia at other anogenital sires is thought to be similar to that of the cervix. Genital HPV infection is usually multifocal and involves the cervix most often. Neoplasia at one site increases the risk of neoplasia elsewhere in the LGT (Spitzer, 1989).

Natural History of Infection

Infection with HPV, predominantly HR types, is very common soon after initiation of sexual activity (Brown, 2005; Winer, 2003). This infection often accompanies sexual debut and is not evidence of promiscuity (Collins, 2002).

Most HPV infection and related lesions, whether clinical or subclinical, spontaneously resolve, especially in adolescents and young women (Ho, 1998; Moscicki, 1998). Questions have been raised as to whether apparent clearance reflects true resolution or limited testing sensitivity (Winer, 2011). Several studies show that LR HPV infections resolve faster than those involving HR HPV (Moscicki, 2004; Schlecht, 2003; Woodman, 2001). Younger women frequently change HPV types, reflecting transience of infection and sequential reinfection by new partners rather than persistence (Ho, 1998; Rosenfeld, 1992). Simultaneous or sequential infection with multiple HPV types is common (Schiffman, 2010).

Persistent HR HPV infection is necessary for the development of cervical neoplasia. A minority of HPV infections become persistent, but most young women (65 percent) with

HPV 16/18 infections lasting more than 6 months will develop SIL (Trottier, 2009). The risk of progression to high-grade neoplasia increases with age, as HPV infection in older women is more likely to reflect persistence (Hildesheim, 1999). Cell-mediated immunity likely plays the largest role in HPV infection persistence and in progression or regression of benign and neoplastic lesions.

Infection Diagnosis

HPV infection is suspected based on clinical lesions or results of cytology, histology, and colposcopy, all of which are subjective and often inaccurate. Moreover, serology is unreliable and cannot distinguish past from current infection (Dillner, 1999). As noted, culture of HPV is not feasible. Thus, diagnosis is confirmed only by the direct detection of HPV nucleic acids by methods that include in situ hybridization, nucleic acid amplification testing (NAAT), polymerase chain reaction (PCR), or others (Molijn, 2005). Currently, four HR HPV tests are approved by the Food and Drug Administration (FDA) for clinical use, and all use NAAT to detect any of 13 or 14 HR HPV types. Two of these tests report specifically the presence of HPV 16 or HPV 18 to aid risk stratification and customized management. Due to clinical test limitations, a negative test result does not exclude HPV infection. Therefore, these tests are not indicated or useful for routine STD screening. LR HPV testing has no indication and can lead to inappropriate expense, further evaluation, and unnecessary treatment.

The clinical role of HR HPV testing for cervical cancer screening and for surveillance of SIL continues to evolve. It is not offered as a screen for HPV infection outside of current guidelines. Namely, appropriate clinical uses for HR HPV testing include: cotesting with cervical cytology screening in women aged 30 years or older, triage or surveillance of certain abnormal cytology results and untreated CIN, and posttreatment surveillance (Davey, 2014). One HR HPV test (cobas HPV Test) was recently FDA approved as a stand-alone screening test for cervical cancer for women 25 years of age and older (p. 634).

If typical genital warts are found in a young woman or if high-grade cervical neoplasia or invasive cancer is identified by cytology or histology, then HPV infection is assumed, and HPV testing is unnecessary. Because of high HPV prevalence in young women (less than age 25), HR HPV testing for cervical cancer screening is not recommended. HPV testing is not FDA approved for use in women after complete hysterectomy, and there are no guidelines for managing HPV test results in these women.

Infection Treatment

The indications to treat HPV-related LGT disease are symptomatic warts, high-grade neoplasia, or invasive cancer. No effective treatment resolves subclinical or latent HPV infection. Needless physical LGT damage may result from unrealistic attempts to eradicate HPV infections, which are usually self-limited. Encouragement of positive health behaviors and optimal management of immune compromise seems sensible. Treatment of cervical LSIL (HPV changes or CIN 1) is not necessary and is considered only after observation for at least 2 years.

Various treatment modalities are available for genital warts and are chosen according to lesion size, location, and number (Rosales, 2014). Mechanical removal or destruction, topical immunomodulators, and chemical or thermal coagulation can be used (Table 3-15, p. 71). Examination of a male partner does not benefit a female partner either by influencing reinfection or by altering the clinical course or treatment outcome for genital warts or LGT neoplasia (Centers for Disease Control and Prevention, 2010).

■ Infection Prevention

Behavior

Sexual abstinence, delaying coitarche, and limiting the number of sexual partners are logical strategies to avoid genital HPV infection and its adverse effects. However, evidence is lacking from trials of counseling and sexual practice modification. Condoms do not cover all potentially HPV-infected anogenital skin. Therefore, condoms may not be completely protective but are likely to reduce acquisition and transmission of HPV. Winer and associates (2003) conducted the first prospective study of male condom use and showed reductions in HPV infection rates in young women even if condoms were used inconsistently.

Vaccines

These offer the greatest promise for prevention and possibly reversal of its sequelae in those already infected. Local and humoral immunity likely protect against incident infection, and prophylactic vaccines elicit type-specific humoral antibody production that prevents new HPV infection by blocking its entry into host cells (Stanley, 2010b). They do not prevent transient HPV positivity or resolve preexistent infection. HPV vaccines have the potential to prevent malignancies at least six body sites that include cervix, vulva, vagina, penis, anal canal, and oropharynx.

Currently, three HPV vaccines are FDA approved for prevention of incident HPV infection and cervical neoplasia. They use recombinant technologies for the synthetic production of the L1 capsid proteins of each HPV type included in the vaccine. The resultant virus-like particles are highly immunogenic but are not infectious as they lack viral DNA (Stanley, 2010b).

Cervarix (HPV2) is a bivalent vaccine against HPVs 16 and 18. Gardasil (HPV4) is a quadrivalent vaccine against HPV types 6, 11, 16, and 18. HPV4 is being replaced by Gardasil 9 (HPV9), a nonavalent vaccine. HPV9 protects against all HPV types in HPV4 plus types 31, 33, 45, 52, and 58. Coverage of these additional HR HPV types will bring the theoretical percentage of cervical cancers prevented from 65 percent to approximately 80 percent. All three vaccines contain adjuvants that boost the immune response to vaccine antigens. They are administered in three intramuscular doses during a 6-month period. Specifically, the second dose is given 1 to 2 months after the first dose, and the third dose is given 6 months after the first dose. Prolongation of the dosing schedule does not appear to diminish immunogenicity. Optimal vaccination strategies administer these prior to sexual activity initiation, when the potential benefit is greatest. However, a history of prior sexual activity, HPV-related disease, or HPV-test positivity should not deter vaccine administration. Testing for HPV is not recommended prior to vaccination (American College of Obstetricians and Gynecologists, 2014a). The Advisory Committee on Immunization Practices (ACIP) currently recommends that HPV vaccine be administered routinely to girls aged 11 to 12 years (as early as age 9 years). Vaccination is also recommended for 13- to 26-year-old women not previously vaccinated (Markowitz, 2014; Petrosky, 2015). Vaccination can be given during lactation but is avoided during pregnancy (American College of Obstetricians and Gynecologists, 2014a). Immune compromised women are candidates to receive the vaccine and show high seroconversion rates despite the theoretical risk of a blunted immune response.

All three vaccines show nearly 100-percent efficacy in preventing incident infection and high-grade cervical neoplasia from HPV types included in the vaccines (Future II Study Group, 2007; Paavonen, 2009; Joura, 2015). HPV4 and HPV9 additionally protect against HPV types 6 and 11, which cause nearly all genital warts, laryngeal papillomatosis, and many low-grade cytologic abnormalities. HPV4 and HPV9 are approved for genital wart prevention in both males and females. They are also FDA approved for the prevention of vaginal, vulvar, and anal neoplasia. HPV2 does not prevent genital warts. It is not approved for extracervical LGT disease prevention, although theoretically it should.

HPV vaccines are highly immunogenic with maintenance of protection for at least 5 to 8 years after vaccination (Ferris, 2014; Harper, 2006). No evidence supports the need for later booster dosing. They have excellent safety profiles, are well-tolerated, and can be administered along with other recommended vaccinations.

Because HPV vaccines prevent most, but not all, HPV-related cervical cancers, cervical cancer screening should continue per current guidelines. Countries with high vaccination rates have seen dramatic reductions in anogenital warts, and reductions in Pap abnormalities and cervical neoplasia are expected (Ali, 2013). Despite suboptimal vaccination rates in the United States, HPV4 vaccine-type infections among U.S. adolescents have decreased by 56 percent since vaccine introduction in 2006 (Stokley, 2014).

CERVICAL INTRAEPITHELIAL NEOPLASIA

■ Risk Factors

Henk and associates (2010) estimated that 412,000 cases of CIN are diagnosed in the United State annually. Risk factors are similar to those of invasive cervical cancer, and CIN is most strongly related to persistent genital HR HPV infection and increasing age (Table 29-1) (Ho, 1995; Kjaer, 2002; Remmink, 1995).

The median age of cervical cancer diagnosis in the United States (late fifth decade) is approximately a decade later than for CIN. In an older woman, HPV infection is more likely to persist than resolve. Older age is linked with waning immune competence and also allows accumulation of genetic mutations over time that can lead to malignant cellular transformation.

TABLE 29-1. Risk Factors for Cervical Neoplasia

Demographic risk factors
Ethnicity (Latin American countries, U.S. minorities)
Low socioeconomic status
Increasing age

Behavioral risk factors
Early coitarche
Multiple sexual partners
Male partner with multiple prior sexual partners
Tobacco smoking
Dietary deficiencies

Medical risk factors
Cervical high-risk human papillomavirus infection
Exogenous hormones (combination hormonal
   contraceptives)
Parity
Immunosuppression
Inadequate screening

Additionally, adverse socioeconomic factors and decreased need for prenatal care and contraception cause older women to be screened less often.

Behavioral risk factors for CIN mirror those for HPV acquisition and include early onset of sexual activity, multiple sexual partners, and male partner promiscuity (Buckley, 1981; de Vet, 1994; Kjaer, 1991). After adjustments for HPV positivity and lower socioeconomic status, tobacco use also increases the preinvasive disease risk (Castle, 2004; Plummer, 2003).

Dietary deficiencies of certain vitamins such as A, C, E, beta carotene, and folic acid may alter cellular immunity to HPV infection. This may promote viral infection persistence and cervical neoplasia (Paavonen, 1990). However, in the United States, lack of association between dietary deficiencies and cervical disease may reflect the relatively sufficient nutritional status of even lower-income women (Amburgey, 1993).

Combination oral contraceptives (COCs) have been linked with an increased risk of cervical cancer in current users (International Collaboration of Epidemiological studies of Cervical Cancer, 2007). Possible mechanisms include increased persistence of HPV infection and oncogene expression (de Villiers, 2003). Conversely, multiple studies have failed to find an increased CIN risk in users of hormonal contraceptives or postmenopausal hormone therapy (Castle, 2005; Harris, 2009; Yasmeen, 2006). DES exposure in

utero appears to double the risk of developing high-grade cervical disease in addition to an increased risk of cervical and vaginal clear cell adenocarcinoma (Hoover, 2011).

Increasing parity has been correlated with cervical cancer risk, but it is unclear if this is related to earlier sexual activity, a progestin-exposure effect, or other factors. Immune suppression during pregnancy, hormonal influences on cervical epithelium, and physical trauma related to vaginal deliveries have all been suggested (Brinton, 1989; Muñoz, 2002).

Immunosuppressed women in general show increased risks for CIN and for greater lesion severity, multifocal lesion pattern, and lesions at multiple LGT sites. They also experience higher rates of treatment failure, persistence, and recurrence of LGT disease compared with those who are immunocompetent. Specifically, human immunodeficiency virus (HIV)-positive women have higher rates of abnormal Pap results and CIN compared with HIV-negative women (p. 651). Transplant recipients have an increased risk of developing a malignancy after transplantation, including neoplasms of the LGT and anal canal (Gomez-Lobo, 2009). Women on immunosuppressive medications for other disorders have higher rates of LGT neoplasia.

Inadequate screening is another risk factor. Of women diagnosed with cervical cancer in the United States, approximately 60 percent either have never been screened (50 percent) or have not had a Pap test during the previous 5 years (10 percent) (American College of Obstetricians and Gynecologists, 2012b). Lack of screening is a major contributor to higher rates of cervical cancer in socioeconomically disadvantaged women, particularly those of minority ethnicity, rural residence, or older age, and those who are recent immigrants (Benard, 2007).

■ Natural History

Preinvasive lesions can spontaneously regress, remain stable, or progress. The risk of progression to invasive cancer increases with the severity of CIN. Estimates of CIN progression, persistence, and regression are provided in a review by Ostor (1993) and shown in Table 29-2. Low-grade lesions are thought to be manifestations of acute HPV infection, and most spontaneously regress within a few years. High-grade lesions are less likely to do so. Castle and coworkers (2009b) calculated that approximately 40 percent of CIN 2 regresses spontaneously within 2 years. This is even more frequent (greater than 60 percent) in young, healthy women (Moscicki, 2010). CIN 2 is thought to be a mixture of low- and high-grade lesions that are difficult to distinguish histologically, rather than an intermediate step

TABLE 29-2. Natural History of Cervical Intraepithelial Neoplasia (CIN) Lesions

	Regression (%)	Persistence (%)	Progression to CIS (%)	Progression to Invasion (%)
CIN 1	57	32	11	1
CIN 2	43	35	22	5
CIN 3	32	<56	–	>12

CIS = carcinoma in situ.
Reproduced with permission from Ostor AG: Natural history of cervical intraepithelial neoplasia: a critical review. Int J Gynecol Pathol 1993 Apr;12(2):186–192.

in the progression from CIN 1 to CIN 3. The risk of progression to invasive cancer of biopsied but otherwise untreated CIN 3 lesions approximates 30 percent over 30 years (McCredie, 2008).

CERVICAL NEOPLASIA DIAGNOSIS

Cervical cancer screening ideally finds preinvasive lesions that can be eradicated or finds early-stage cervical cancer that can be treated successfully. Cervical cancer screening was previously limited to cervical cytology. But, during the past decade, HR HPV testing has also become an important screening tool.

In general, LGT preinvasive lesions are visible only with aided inspection. One exception is VIN, which is generally visible, palpable, or both. Only cervical lesions at either end of the neoplastic disease spectrum are grossly visible, namely, condylomata and invasive cancers. Accordingly, all symptoms suspicious for cervical neoplasia and grossly visible cervical lesions require prompt biopsy.

■ Cervical Cytology

Cervical cytologic screening is one of modern medicine's great success stories. It detects most cervical neoplasia during the typically prolonged premalignant or early occult invasive phases, when treatment outcomes are optimal. Conventional glass slides (traditionally called the *Pap smear*) and liquid-based Pap tests are considered equally acceptable for screening by all current guidelines (American College of Obstetricians and Gynecologists, 2012b; Saslow, 2012; U.S. Preventive Services Task Force, 2012).

Introduced in the 1940s, cervical cytology has never been evaluated in a randomized, controlled, or masked trial (Koss, 1989). However, countries with organized screening programs have consistently realized dramatic declines in both cervical cancer incidence and mortality rates. The Pap test's specificity is consistently high, approximating 98 percent. However, estimates of its sensitivity for detection of CIN 2 or worse are lower, are more variable, and range from 45 to 65 percent (Whitlock, 2011). This imperfect sensitivity is balanced by recommendations for repetitive screening throughout a woman's life. Although the incidence of cervical squamous carcinoma continues to decline, both the relative and absolute incidences of adenocarcinoma have increased, particularly in women younger than 50 (Herzog, 2007). Adenocarcinoma and adenosquamous carcinoma now account for at least 20 percent of cervical cancers. This increase may be due in part to the Pap test's lower sensitivity for detection of adenocarcinoma than for squamous cancers and their precursor lesions.

False-negative Pap test results may follow sampling error, in which abnormal cells are not present in the Pap test, or by screening error, in which the cells are present but missed or misclassified by the screener (Wilkinson, 1990). Mandated quality assurance measures and computerized slide-screening technologies address screening errors. Suboptimal management of abnormal results by providers and failure of patient follow up also contribute to avoidable cases of cervical cancer. Clinicians can maximize the benefit of screening by obtaining an optimal cytologic specimen and by adhering to current evidence-based guidelines for the management of abnormal test results.

Performing a Pap Test

Ideally, Pap tests are scheduled to avoid menstruation. Patients should abstain from vaginal intercourse, douching, vaginal tampon use, and intravaginal medicinal or contraceptive creams for a minimum of 24 to 48 hours before a test. Treatment of cervicitis or vaginitis prior to Pap testing is optimal. However, Pap testing is not deferred due to unexplained discharge or unscheduled bleeding, as these may be signs of cervical or other genital tract cancers.

As shown in Figure 21-9 (p. 488), the appearance of cervical squamous cells varies throughout the menstrual cycle and with hormonal status. Thus, clinical information aids accurate Pap interpretation and often includes: date of last menstrual period, current pregnancy, exogenous hormone use, menopausal status, complaints of abnormal bleeding, and prior abnormal Pap test results, CIN, or other LGT neoplasia. Additionally, intrauterine devices (IUDs) can cause reactive cellular changes, and their presence is noted. Full visualization of the cervix is essential for detection of gross lesions and SCJ identification. Speculum placement should be as comfortable as possible. A thin coating of water-based lubricant can be used on the outside of the speculum blades without compromising Pap test quality or interpretation (Griffith, 2005; Harmanli, 2010). Touching the cervix prior to performing a Pap test is avoided, as dysplastic epithelium may be inadvertently removed with minimal trauma. Discharge covering the cervix may be carefully absorbed by a large swab, with care not to contact the cervix. Vigorous blotting or rubbing may cause scant cellularity or a false-negative Pap test result. When indicated, additional sampling to detect other cervical or vaginal infection may follow Pap test collection.

Sampling of the transformation zone at the SCJ is paramount to the sensitivity of the Pap test. Techniques are adapted and sampling devices chosen according to SCJ location, which varies widely with age, obstetric trauma, and hormonal status. Women known or suspected of in utero DES exposure may also benefit from a separate Pap test of the upper vagina, as these women carry an additional risk for vaginal cancer.

Three types of plastic devices are commonly used to sample the cervix: the spatula, broom, and endocervical brush (also known as a cytobrush) (Fig. 29-8). A spatula predominantly samples the ectocervix. An endocervical brush samples the endocervical canal and is used in combination with a spatula. A broom samples both endo- and ectocervical epithelia simultaneously but can be supplemented by an endocervical brush. Wooden collection devices and cotton swabs are no longer recommended due to their inferior collection and release of cells.

A spatula is oriented to best fit the cervical contour, straddle the squamocolumnar junction, and sample the distal endocervical canal. A clinician firmly scrapes the cervical surface, completing at least one full rotation. After the spatula sample is obtained, the endocervical brush, with its conical shape and plastic bristles, is inserted into the endocervical canal only until the outermost bristles remain visible just within the external os. This prevents inadvertent sampling of lower uterine segment cells, which can be mistaken for atypical cervical cells. To avoid

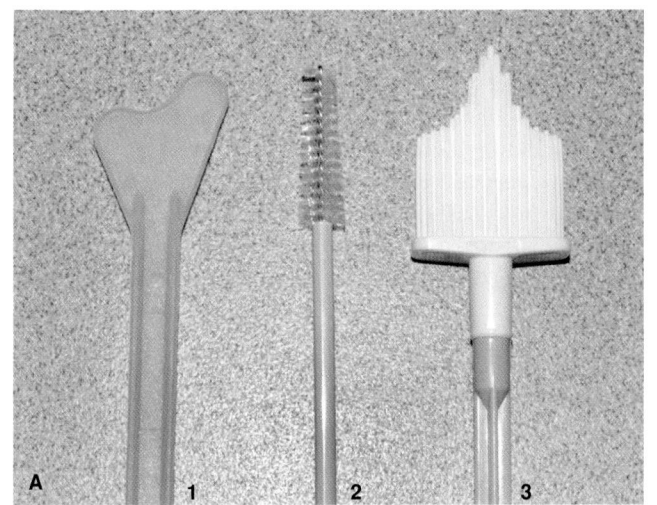

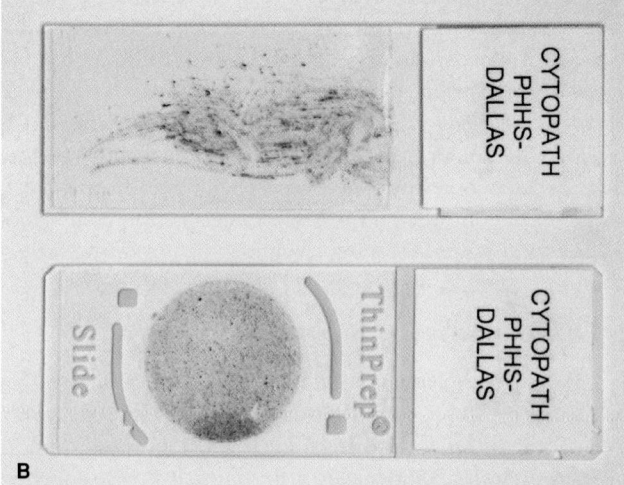

FIGURE 29-8 A. Cervical cytology collection devices: (1) Plastic spatula. (2) Endocervical brush. (3) Plastic broom. **B.** Pap preparations. Conventional cervical cytology is prepared by smearing collected cells directly onto a glass slide with the collection device followed by immediate fixation (*upper slide*). Liquid-based cytology involves transfer of collected cells from the collection device into a liquid transport medium with subsequent processing and transfer onto a glass slide. Cells are distributed over a smaller area, and debris, mucus, blood, and cell overlap are largely eliminated, allowing computer-assisted screening (*lower slide*). (Used with permission from Dr. Raheela Ashfaq.)

obscuring blood, the brush is rotated only one-quarter to one-half turn and is used after the ectocervix has been sampled. If the cervical canal is very wide, the brush is moved so as to contact all surfaces of the endocervical canal.

Broom devices have longer central bristles that are inserted into the endocervical canal. These longer bristles are flanked by shorter bristles that splay out over the ectocervix during rotation. Five rotations in the same direction are recommended. Reversing direction may cause loss of cellular material. Broom devices are favored for liquid-based Pap testing.

Cytology Collection

Conventional slide collection requires special care to avoid air drying artifact, a leading cause of poor slide quality. The spatula sample is held while the endocervical brush sampling immediately follows. The spatula sample is then quickly spread as evenly as possible over one half to two thirds of a glass slide (see Fig. 29-8). The endocervical brush is firmly rolled over the remaining area of the slide, after which fixation is quickly carried out by spraying from a distance of 10 to 12 inches or immersing the slide in fixative.

Currently, two liquid-based cytology (LBC) Pap tests are FDA approved. Sampling and cell transfer to a liquid medium is performed according to manufacturer specifications. SurePath allows for the use of all three device types but uses modified tips that are broken off and sent to the laboratory in the liquid medium. ThinPrep requires immediate and vigorous agitation of the chosen collection device(s) in the liquid medium, after which the device is discarded.

▪ HPV Testing

A role for HR HPV testing in cervical cancer screening is attractive due to its improved sensitivity for CIN 3 or cervical cancer and the objectivity of its results. However, strategies for incorporation of HPV testing must compensate for a decreased specificity, particularly in young women.

Cytology with HPV Cotesting

In 2003, the FDA first approved an HPV test for use with cytology for cervical cancer screening in women 30 years and older. The combination of HR HPV testing with cytology is referred to as *cotesting*. This strategy is not currently endorsed for women younger than 30 due to the high prevalence of HR HPV infection in this age group and the resultant lack of test specificity. HPV testing is usually performed from the residual LBC specimen after the cytology slide is prepared. Alternatively, a cervical sampling for HPV can be sent in a specific collection device separate from the cytology specimen. Testing is performed only for HR HPV types. As noted earlier, there is no clinical role for LR HPV testing (Castle, 2014; Thomsen, 2014).

The combination of HPV testing with cytology increases the sensitivity of a single screening test for high-grade neoplasia to nearly 100 percent and leads to earlier detection and management of HSIL (Ronco, 2010). The lack of sensitivity for cervical adenocarcinoma seen with traditional cytology testing also supports HPV testing use for primary screening (Castellsagué, 2006).

Due to a high negative predictive value for high-grade neoplasia, slow progression of new HPV infection to neoplasia, and increased cost, cotesting is repeated at 5-year intervals if both cytology and HPV test are negative. Clinical guidelines have been developed for management of abnormal cotest results (Saslow, 2012). If cytology is abnormal, current cytology management guidelines are followed (p. 636). Cytology-negative and HPV-positive test results will occur in less than 10 percent of screened patients (Castle, 2009a; Datta, 2008). In such cases, cotesting is repeated 12 months later. This is because the risk of high-grade neoplasia is less than that of a Pap test with an atypical squamous cell of undetermined significance (ASC-US) result, and most HPV infections will resolve during this time (Saslow, 2012). Colposcopy is recommended for persistently positive HPV DNA test results. An abnormal repeat cytology result is managed according to current guidelines regardless of concurrent HPV status.

An alternative strategy is now available for management of a negative cytology but a positive HR HPV test result. A reflex test specifically for HPVs 16 and 18, called *genotyping*, can be performed. If positive, immediate colposcopy is recommended (American College of Obstetricians and Gynecologists, 2012b; Saslow, 2012). This approach targets those at highest risk for significant disease, and evidence provides a sound basis for this strategy (Khan, 2005; Wright, 2015).

Primary HPV Testing

A growing body of evidence supports HR HPV testing alone without initial cytology as an option for primary cervical cancer screening (Castle, 2011; Cuzick, 2006; Dillner, 2013). In late 2014, the cobas HPV test was the first HPV test approved by the FDA for primary cervical cancer screening in women 25 years and older. This test gives simultaneous results for the presence or absence of HPVs 16 and 18 and for a group of 12 other oncogenic HPV types. This represents a profound paradigm shift in cervical cancer screening, in which Pap testing assumes a secondary role for the triage of HPV positive results.

HPV testing alone is approximately twice as sensitive (>90 percent) as a single Pap test and leads to earlier detection of high-grade neoplasias. The very high negative-predictive value of a single negative HPV test was shown by Sankaranarayanan (2009). During this 8-year study, a single round of HPV testing outperformed cytology, with no cervical cancer deaths within 8 years of a negative HR HPV test result. Recent evaluations show that cotesting does not perform any better than HPV testing alone (Dillner, 2013; Whitlock, 2011). However, specificity declines with HPV testing, particularly in younger women (Mayrand, 2007; Ronco, 2006, 2010). This could lead to excessive numbers of colposcopies, biopsies, and treatments. Triaging women with positive non-HPV16/18 HPV test results to reflex cytology is a viable counterbalance to the decreased specificity. Overall, this strategy is expected to result in more colposcopic referrals but yield higher and earlier HSIL detection rates.

Suggested interim guidelines for primary HPV test screening are recently published and will no doubt be debated and revised in coming years (Huh, 2015). These propose that screening with a HR HPV test can be used as an alternative to cytology alone or cotesting in women 25 years and older and at intervals no less than 3 years. Immediate colposcopy is recommended if HPV 16/18 is identified. If other HR HPV types are found, then triage to reflex cytology is proposed. Colposcopy is recommended for any cytologic abnormality. Importantly, as of mid-2015, major cervical cancer screening guidelines do not include this screening option.

■ Cervical Cancer Screening Guidelines

Perspective on Guidelines

Notably, *all* approved cervical cancer screening strategies, including the use of periodic cytology alone, dramatically reduce a woman's lifetime risk of developing or dying from cervical cancer. Since most women with positive HR HPV test results will not develop significant disease, the choice of screening strategy should be a shared decision by the provider and individual patient. Reviewed by the National Cancer Institute (2015a), the balance of benefits and harms of each screening strategy warrants careful consideration by both health care providers and health care policy agencies. With that perspective, guidelines are subsequently presented.

Evidence-based cervical cancer screening guidelines continue to evolve. In 2012, all major professional societies updated these. The American Cancer Society, the American Society for Colposcopy and Cervical Pathology, and the American Society for Clinical Pathology (ACS/ASCCP/ACP) jointly issued guidelines (Saslow, 2012). The U.S. Preventive Services Task Force (USPSTF) (Moyer, 2012) and the American College of Obstetricians and Gynecologists (2012b) each published guidelines as well. These three sets of guidelines agree with few exceptions and pertain only to average-risk women, that is, immunocompetent women with no history of HSIL or cervical cancer. All agree on the acceptability of both conventional and liquid-based Paps, the age of initiation and cessation of screening, screening intervals, and continued screening after HPV vaccination. Adherence to current guidelines should not preclude or delay other indicated gynecologic care. In particular, provision of contraception is never contingent on compliance with cervical cancer screening recommendations or the evaluation of cytologic abnormalities.

Screening Initiation

Cervical cancer screening ideally begins at age 21 in average-risk women. This is true regardless of sexual history, sexual orientation, or other risks. In young women, most Pap abnormalities represent transient HPV infection, and the spontaneous regression of even high-grade lesions is common (Moscicki, 2005). Most high-grade lesions are CIN 2 rather than CIN 3 in young women (Moscicki, 2008). Cervical cancer is exceedingly rare in adolescents and not as preventable by screening as for older women (Saslow, 2012). Additionally, treatment of high-grade CIN in adolescents is often followed by persistence of Pap abnormalities, and theoretically may have adverse reproductive consequences (Case, 2006; Moore, 2007).

Whether to begin screening earlier in the presence of significant immune compromise, as with HIV infection, use of immunosuppressive medications, and organ transplantation, is uncertain and not addressed by current guidelines. The Centers for Disease Control and Prevention (CDC) (2015) recommends initiation of screening soon after HIV diagnosis, even if before age 21, and repeat Pap testing in 6 months. As for other such conditions, clinician judgment is exercised, taking into consideration age and severity of immune compromise. In general, initial screening at age 21 seems reasonable (American College of Obstetricians and Gynecologists, 2012a).

Screening Interval and Strategy

Between ages 21 and 29, all guidelines recommend screening with cytology alone at 3-year intervals. Women aged 30 to 65 can continue screening with cytology alone at 3-year intervals or can begin cotesting at 5-year intervals. The risk of cancer is approximately the same using either strategy. USPSTF sees both strategies as equally effective, and cotesting is available to women wishing to extend their screening interval. However, both the ACS/ASCCP/ACP (Saslow, 2012) and American College of Obstetricians and Gynecologists (2012b) have deemed cotesting the preferred screening strategy in women 30 years and older. Women with HIV infection and other immune suppression should receive annual cytology screening (Centers for Disease Control and Prevention, 2015; American College of Obstetricians and Gynecologists, 2012a).

Screening Discontinuation

Screening may be stopped in women older than 65 if they have an average risk for cervical cancer and have undergone adequate screening, regardless of sexual history. Adequate screening is three consecutive, negative Pap results or two consecutive, negative cotest results in the prior 10 years, with the most recent within the past 5 years. Women with prior treatment for CIN 2, CIN 3, AIS, or cervical cancer should continue routine screening for at least 20 years, as they remain at increased long-term risk of cervical cancer (Saslow, 2012; Strander, 2007). It is uncertain when HIV-positive women can discontinue screening or whether this should continue annually and indefinitely for as long as there is reasonable life expectancy.

Posthysterectomy

Vaginal cancers are rare and account for less than 2 percent of cancers in women. All guidelines recommend against Pap screening in women who have undergone total hysterectomy for benign disease if there is no past history of high-grade CIN or cervical cancer. The absence of a cervix should be confirmed by examination or pathology report as many women are inaccurate in their reporting of hysterectomy type. Women who have undergone supracervical hysterectomy should continue routine screening. Recommendations for vaginal cytology after hysterectomy in women with histories of high-grade cervical neoplasia or cancer are less clear, as vaginal cancer is still rare, and screening is of uncertain benefit (Saslow, 2012). The American College of Obstetricians and Gynecologists (2012b) recommends cytology of the vaginal cuff every 3 years for 20 years after the initial posttreatment surveillance, which is generally a schedule of three Pap tests in the first 2 years posthysterectomy. HPV testing is not FDA-approved in the absence of a cervix but remains common. Evidence-based recommendations for managing vaginal HPV test results are nonexistent (Chappell, 2010). Such testing should be avoided.

■ The Bethesda System

Cervical cytology reporting is standardized by the Bethesda System nomenclature (National Cancer Institute Workshop, 1989; Nayar, 2015; Solomon, 2002). Clinically, the key elements reported are specimen adequacy and epithelial cell abnormalities (Tables 29-3 and 29-4). An overview of evidence-based guidelines for the initial management of cervical cytology abnormalities for nonpregnant women follows in the next paragraphs (American College of Obstetricians and Gynecologists, 2013; Massad, 2013). Full guidelines should be reviewed and applied on an individualized basis. Guidelines cannot address all clinical situations or prevent all cervical cancers.

TABLE 29-3. The 2014 Bethesda System Cytology Report Components

Specimen type
Conventional (Pap smear)
Liquid-based (Pap test)
Other

Specimen adequacy
Satisfactory for evaluation
Unsatisfactory for evaluation (reason specified)

General categorization (optional)
Negative for intraepithelial lesion or malignancy
Epithelial cell abnormality (see Table 29-4)
Other (see Interpretation/Results)

Interpretation/Results
Negative for intraepithelial lesion or malignancy
Epithelial cell abnormalities (see Table 29-4)
Nonneoplastic findings (optional)
    Cellular variations (atrophy, keratosis, metaplasia)
    Reactive cellular changes (inflammation, repair, radiation)
    Glandular cells status posthysterectomy
Organisms
    Trichomonas vaginalis
    Fungal organisms consistent with *Candida* spp
    Shift in flora suggestive of bacterial vaginosis
    Cellular changes consistent with herpes simplex virus
    Cellular changes consistent with cytomegalovirus
    Bacteria consistent with *Actinomyces* spp
    Other nonneoplastic findings (optional)
Other
    Endometrial cells in a woman ≥45 years of age
    Other malignant neoplasms (specified)

Adjunctive testing

Computer-assisted interpretation

Educational notes and comments (optional)

Adapted with permission from Nayar R, Wilbur DC: The Pap test and Bethesda 2014. Cancer Cytopathol 2015 May;123(5):271–281.

Specimen Adequacy

This is reported as *satisfactory* or *unsatisfactory* for evaluation and is based primarily on criteria for slide cellularity and the presence of obscuring blood or inflammation. The presence or absence of TZ components, that is, endocervical and/or squamous metaplastic cells, is also reported. A TZ component is not required for test adequacy. Although its presence is associated with increased detection of cytologic abnormalities, its absence is not associated with failure to diagnose CIN. Pap tests lacking TZ components are repeated in 3 years. For women 30 years and older, HPV testing is preferred and further testing is guided by results.

Unsatisfactory Pap tests are unreliable for the detection of cervical neoplasia and also for HR HPV by some HPV tests. Unsatisfactory Pap tests are repeated in 2 to 4 months. If atrophy or a specific infection is present, treatment before repeat cytology may be helpful. If the result is unsatisfactory again,

TABLE 29-4. The 2014 Bethesda System: Epithelial Cell Abnormalities

Squamous cell

Atypical squamous cells (ASC):
  of undetermined significance (ASC-US)
  cannot exclude HSIL (ASC-H)
Low-grade squamous intraepithelial lesion (LSIL)
High-grade squamous intraepithelial lesion (HSIL)
Squamous cell carcinoma

Glandular cell

Atypical glandular cells (AGC):
  Endocervical, endometrial, or not otherwise specified
Atypical glandular cells, favor neoplastic:
  Endocervical or not otherwise specified
Endocervical adenocarcinoma in situ (AIS)
Adenocarcinoma

Adapted with permission from Nayar R, Wilbur DC: The Pap test and Bethesda 2014. Cancer Cytopathol 2015 May;123(5):271–281.

colposcopy is recommended as this persistent result confers increased CIN risk. Rarely, obscuring blood or inflammation on cervical cytology may indicate invasive cancer. Therefore, unexplained vaginal discharge, abnormal bleeding, or abnormal physical findings should prompt immediate evaluation rather than waiting for repeat Pap testing.

Epithelial Cell Abnormality Management

A cytology report is a medical consultation that interprets a screening test and does not provide a diagnosis. A final diagnosis is determined clinically, often with results from histologic evaluation. Pap tests are interpreted as either being negative for intraepithelial lesion or malignancy (NILM) or demonstrating one or more epithelial cell abnormalities.

Atypical Squamous Cells of Undetermined Significance. The most common cytologic abnormality is ASC-US. This term indicates cells that suggest SIL but do not fulfill all the criteria. An ASC-US result often precedes the diagnosis of CIN 2 or 3, but this risk approximates only 5 to 10 percent. Cancer is found in only 1 to 2 per thousand (Solomon, 2002).

Management of ASC-US without HPV cotesting is repeat cytology in 1 year, and this is preferred for women aged 21 to 24. If the repeat Pap test result is abnormal, colposcopy is recommended. Reflex HPV testing is preferred in women 25 years and older and acceptable in those age 21 to 24 years. *Reflex testing* refers to HPV testing in response to a specific result and is not performed if cytology is negative. With an ASC-US Pap result, reflex HPV testing is a good discriminator of those with high-grade CIN and those without. ASC-US, HPV-positive test results have a risk profile similar to LSIL results and thus are evaluated with colposcopy. ASC-US, HPV-negative results are followed up with a cotest in 3 years or with cytology alone in women under age 25.

Low-grade Squamous Intraepithelial Lesion. LSIL encompasses the cytologic features of HPV infection and

CIN 1 but carries a 15 to 30 percent risk of CIN 2 or 3, similar to ASC-US, HPV-positive. Therefore, colposcopy is generally indicated for LSIL cytology.

Specifically, for LSIL with no HPV testing or with HPV-positive results, colposcopy is indicated in women aged 25 years and older. If a negative HPV test result is obtained due to cotesting, a repeat cotest in 1 year is preferred, but colposcopy is acceptable. Reflex HPV testing with an LSIL result is not useful in reproductive-aged women, as 75 to 85 percent will test positive for HR HPV. In women aged 21 to 24 years with an LSIL result, cytology follow-up is preferred to immediate colposcopy due to high rates of resolution. For postmenopausal women with LSIL and no HPV cotest, options include repeat cytology at 6 and 12 months, HPV testing, or colposcopy.

Atypical Squamous Cells, Cannot Exclude HSIL. Five to 10 percent of ASC is designated as atypical squamous cells, cannot exclude HSIL (ASC-H). This finding should not be confused with ASC-US. ASC-H describes cellular changes that do not fulfill criteria for HSIL cytology, but a high-grade lesion cannot be excluded. Histologic HSIL is found in upward of 25 percent of these cases, which is a higher rate than seen with ASC-US or LSIL. Thus, colposcopy is indicated regardless of age or concurrent HPV test result. Reflex HPV testing is not helpful due to a high rate of HPV-positivity. If colposcopy is inadequate, a diagnostic excision procedure is recommended.

High-grade Squamous Intraepithelial Lesion. HSIL cytology encompasses features of CIN 2 and CIN 3 (Fig. 29-9). It carries an elevated risk of underlying histologic HSIL (at least 70 percent) or invasive cancer (1 to 2 percent) (Kinney, 1998). Colposcopic evaluation is warranted for all HSIL cytology regardless of age or HPV status. Alternative management of HSIL cytology in women 25 years and older includes immediate loop electrosurgical excision procedure (LEEP), which is referred to as a *see-and-LEEP* approach. This strategy is reasonable because colposcopy may miss a high-grade lesion, and most HSIL cytologies eventually result in excision for diagnosis or treatment. Inadequate colposcopy should prompt excision unless initial biopsies show invasive cancer.

Glandular Cell Abnormalities. This group includes atypical glandular cells (AGC); AGC, favor neoplasia; and AIS. This category carries an increased risk of neoplasia (Zhao, 2009). Paradoxically, squamous neoplasia is more frequently diagnosed than glandular neoplasia upon evaluation of AGC cytology (Schnatz, 2006). There is also an elevated risk of endometrial and other reproductive tract cancers and cancers at other sites such as breast and colon. Approximately half of the neoplasia diagnosed subsequent to an AGC Pap is endometrial.

Accordingly, initial evaluation of a glandular abnormality includes colposcopy and endocervical sampling. It also includes endometrial sampling in patients 35 years and older or in younger women with risk factors for endometrial disease, which include abnormal bleeding or history suggesting chronic anovulation. If atypical endometrial cells are specified in the report, then initial endometrial and endocervical sampling is acceptable with subsequent colposcopy if these are negative.

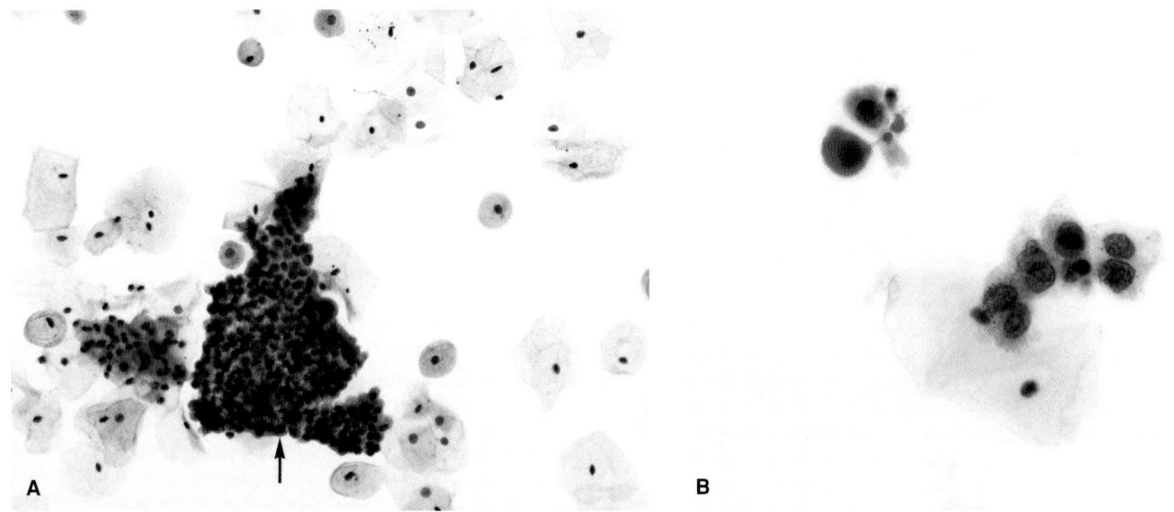

FIGURE 29-9 A. Normal Pap test. A fragment of benign endocervical epithelium with the characteristic "honeycomb" appearance conferred by the presence of cytoplasmic mucin is seen (*arrow*). Benign parabasal, intermediate, and superficial squamous cells are present in the background. **B.** Pap test reflecting high-grade squamous intraepithelial lesion. The dysplastic squamous cells have nuclear membrane irregularities and coarse chromatin. The increased nuclear to cytoplasmic size ratio would classify this as a moderate squamous dysplasia (CIN 2). (Used with permission from Ann Marie West, MBA, CT[ASCP].)

Reflex HPV testing is not recommended for the triage of glandular cytologic abnormalities. Indeed, a negative reflex HPV test result may dissuade appropriate evaluation of AGC cytology. However, HPV testing at the initial evaluation of AGC may help distinguish cervical from endometrial disease (Castle, 2010; de Oliveira, 2006).

If initial evaluation of glandular cytologic abnormalities is negative, management and surveillance are generally aggressive due to the significant risk of occult disease. Current guidelines should be followed (American College of Obstetricians and Gynecologists, 2013; Massad, 2013). Diagnostic excision is indicated following AGC, favor neoplasia and AIS Paps if initial evaluation does not result in a cancer diagnosis.

Carcinoma. Cytologies suspicious for squamous cell carcinoma or adenocarcinoma carry the highest risk of invasive cancer and are evaluated promptly. If initial evaluation fails to reveal invasive cancer, a diagnostic excision procedure is indicated.

Pregnancy. Pregnant patients 21 years and older are screened and their abnormal cytologies managed according to guidelines for the general population. However, deferred evaluation of ASC-US and LSIL cytologies until at least 6 weeks postpartum is acceptable (Massad, 2013). When indicated, the goal of colposcopy is to exclude invasive cancer. Colposcopy and ectocervical biopsy are safe and accurate during pregnancy (Economos, 1993). Endocervical and endometrial sampling are not performed during pregnancy to avoid amnionic membrane rupture and infection. Preinvasive neoplasia is not treated but rather is reevaluated postpartum. This is because lesion progression is typically slow and lesion grade may change during delivery and puerperal remodeling (Yost, 1999). Although cervical conization is infrequently performed during pregnancy, indications for this are discussed in Chapter 30 (p. 675).

Nonneoplastic Findings

Certain nonneoplastic findings may be reported, and these include findings consistent with, but not conclusively diagnos-

tic of, certain organisms. These findings include *Trichomonas vaginalis*, *Candida* species, *Actinomyces* species, herpes simplex virus, or shift in flora consistent with bacterial vaginosis. Sensitivity is generally limited, and accuracy of diagnosis varies (Fitzhugh, 2008). For this reason, confirmatory tests or clinical correlation should dictate any actions related to these findings. Other nonneoplastic findings are reactive changes associated with inflammation or repair, radiation changes, atrophy, and posthysterectomy benign glandular cells. None of these require a clinical response.

Benign endometrial cells seen in the cervical cytology of a postmenopausal woman confer an increased risk of endometrial hyperplasia and cancer. Because menstrual history and menopausal status are often unknown to the cytologist, benign endometrial cells are reported on cervical cytology for all women 45 years and older (Nayar, 2015). Premenopausal women do not require endometrial evaluation in the absence of abnormal bleeding.

◼ Colposcopy

Preparation

This outpatient procedure examines the lower anogenital tract with a binocular microscope affixed to a stand and requires skills that encompass colposcopic terminology, lesion identification and grading, and biopsy techniques. Its primary goal is to identify invasive or preinvasive neoplastic lesions for directed biopsy and subsequent management. It remains the gold standard evaluation of patients with abnormal cervical cytology. However, its sensitivity, interobserver agreement, and reproducibility are less than previously thought. Sensitivity estimates range between 50 and 80 percent (American College of Obstetricians and Gynecologists, 2013; Ferris, 2005; Jeronimo, 2007). This highlights the need for further evaluation or surveillance when initial colposcopy fails to reveal high-grade neoplasia.

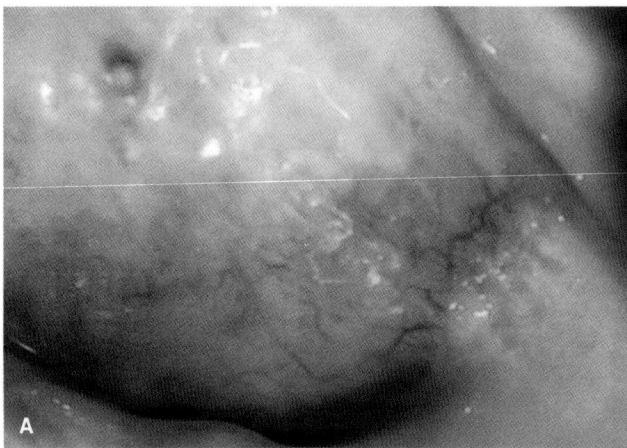

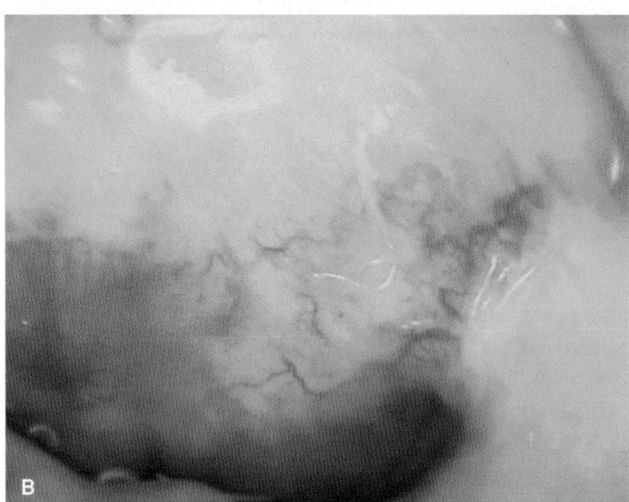

FIGURE 29-10 Evaluation of surface vessels. **A.** Benign surface vessels viewed through a colposcope using usual white light source. **B.** Use of a blue-green (red-free) light filter provides higher contrast and definition of vascular patterns.

There are many styles of colposcopes, but they all operate similarly. The colposcope contains a stereoscopic lens or digital imaging system that has magnification settings ranging from 3- to 20-fold. Its stand allows positioning, and a high-intensity light provides illumination. A green (red-free) light filter adds contrast to aid vascular pattern evaluations (Fig. 29-10).

Prior to colposcopic examination, a woman's medical history and record are reviewed and indications for colposcopy confirmed (Table 29-5). Urine pregnancy testing is performed if clinically indicated. Colposcopic examination is optimally timed to avoid menses. However, it is not delayed in the patient with a visible lesion, abnormal bleeding, or poor appointment compliance. In cases of severe cervicitis or other pelvic infection, treatment may be indicated before performing biopsies or endocervical curettage. Notably, abnormal cervical discharge in the absence of an identified pathogen may be a cancer indicator. A Pap test performed at the time of colposcopy is of questionable value, may obscure colposcopic findings, and should be performed on an individualized basis.

Solutions may aid colposcopic examination and are applied by gently dabbing a saturated swab or sponge or by spray-bottle misting so as not to traumatize the cervical epithelium. High-

TABLE 29-5. Clinical Considerations Directing Colposcopy
Clinical objectives
Provide a magnified view of LGT
Identify cervical squamocolumnar junction
Detect lesions suspicious for neoplasia
Direct lesion biopsy
Monitor patients with current or past LGT neoplasia
Clinical indications
Grossly visible LGT lesion
Abnormal cervical cancer screening
In utero diethylstilbestrol exposure
Contraindications: none
Relative contraindications
Upper or lower reproductive tract infection
Uncontrolled severe hypertension
Uncooperative or overly anxious patient

LGT = lower genital tract.

grade cervical lesions are particularly fragile. To begin, normal saline can help remove cervical mucus and allows initial assessment of vascular patterns and surface contours. Abnormal vessels, especially when viewed with green-filtered light, may be more prominent before acetic acid application.

Acetic acid in a 3- to 5-percent solution is a mucolytic agent thought to exert its effect by reversibly clumping nuclear chromatin. This causes neoplastic lesions to assume a thicker density and hues of white depending on the degree of abnormal nuclear density. Applying acetic acid to abnormal epithelium results in the *acetowhite change* characteristic of neoplastic lesions and of some benign conditions. Several minutes may be needed for this effect to become fully developed.

Dilute Lugol iodine solution stains mature squamous epithelial cells a dark purple-brown color in estrogenized women as a result of high cellular glycogen content. Due to incomplete cellular differentiation, dysplastic cells have lower glycogen content, fail to fully stain, and appear various shades of yellow (Fig. 29-11). This solution is particularly useful when abnormal tissue cannot be found using acetic acid alone. It is also used to define the limits of the active TZ, as immature squamous metaplasia does not stain as strongly as mature (fully differentiated) squamous epithelium. Lugol solution should not be used in patients allergic to iodine, radiographic contrast, or shellfish.

Examination

Two major components of colposcopic examination are general assessment and specific colposcopic findings. Careful description of these aids diagnosis and management of abnormalities. For this, standard colposcopic terminology used in the United States differs somewhat from that proposed by the International Federation for Cervical Pathology and Colposcopy (IFCPC) (Bornstein, 2012).

General colposcopic assessment has three components: cervical visualization, SCJ visibility, and TZ classification. First,

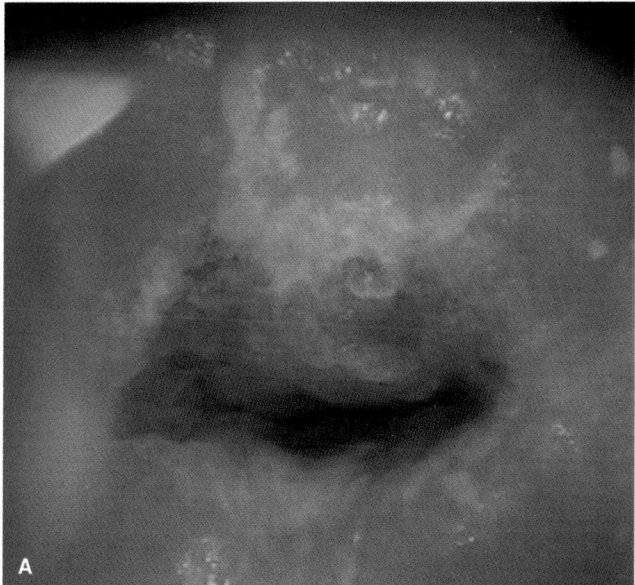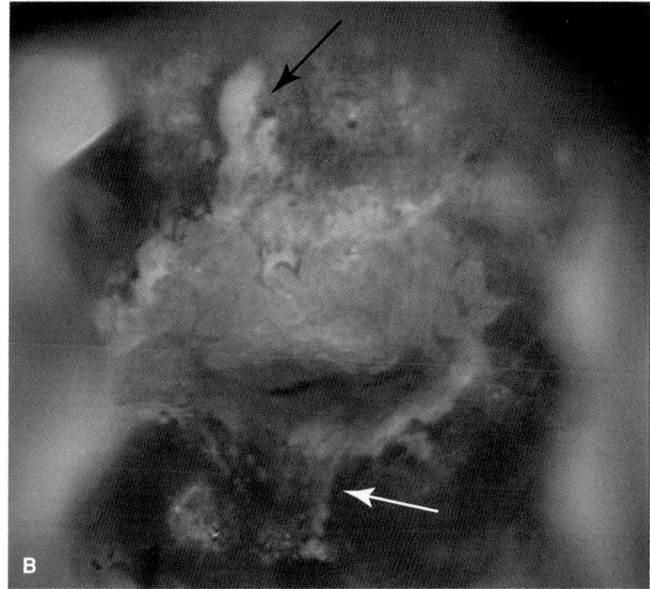

FIGURE 29-11 Solutions used for colposcopy. **A.** Cervix after application of acetic acid. Several areas of acetowhite change adjacent to the squamocolumnar junction are apparent. **B.** Same cervix after application of Lugol iodine solution. Nonstaining of the lesions at the 10 to 11 o'clock positions is seen (*black arrow*), while there is partial iodine uptake of acetowhite areas along the posterior SCJ (*white arrow*).

every examination is characterized by whether the cervix is fully seen or whether the evaluation is limited by inflammation, bleeding, scarring, or other obscuring causes. The IFCPC labels full cervix visualization as "adequate" and otherwise as "inadequate." However, current guidelines for management of abnormal cervical cytology and precancers issued by the ASCCP and standard U.S. practice reserve these descriptors for visibility of the SCJ and any lesions present (Massad, 2013).

Second, SCJ visibility is important, as nearly all cervical neoplasia is located within the TZ and at or adjacent to the SCJ. Within a neoplastic lesion, the most severe disease tends to be at the proximal (cephalad or upper) limit of the lesion. Therefore, the ability to see the entire SCJ and the upper limits of all lesions is essential to exclude invasive cancer and to determine disease severity. The IFCPC terminology characterizes the SCJ separately as completely, partially, or not visible. Current ASCCP guidelines define full visualization of both the SCJ and upper limits of all lesions present as "adequate." Otherwise, the examination is "inadequate" (Fig. 29-12). Finally, the IFCPC classifies the TZ location as types 1, 2, or 3. A type 1 TZ is entirely ectocervical and visible; a type 2 has an endocervical component that is fully visible; and a type 3 TZ has an endocervical component that cannot be completely visualized. Types 2 and 3 may have ectocervical TZ components of varying extent. If treatment is indicated, the size and location of the SCJ, TZ, and visible lesions are important determinants of the modality chosen.

Lesion Grading

Colposcopically, normal squamous epithelium of the cervix appears as a featureless, smooth, pale-pink surface. Blood vessels lie below this layer and therefore are not visible or are seen only as a fine capillary network. The mucin-secreting columnar epithelium appears red due to its thinness and the close proximity of blood vessels to the surface. It has a polypoid appearance due

to infoldings that form peaks and clefts (see Fig. 29-3). Against this normal colposcopic landscape, colposcopists discern abnormal tissue and choose for biopsy the sites most likely to harbor the most severe neoplasia. Several colposcopic grading systems quantify lesion qualities to improve diagnostic accuracy (Coppleson, 1993; Reid, 1985). Best known, the Reid Colposcopic Index is based on four lesion features, which are margin, color, vascular pattern, and Lugol solution staining. Each category is scored from 0 to 2, and the summation provides a numeric index that correlates with histology (Table 29-6).

The IFCPC has proposed a standardized nomenclature for lesion grading and recommends that it replace prior

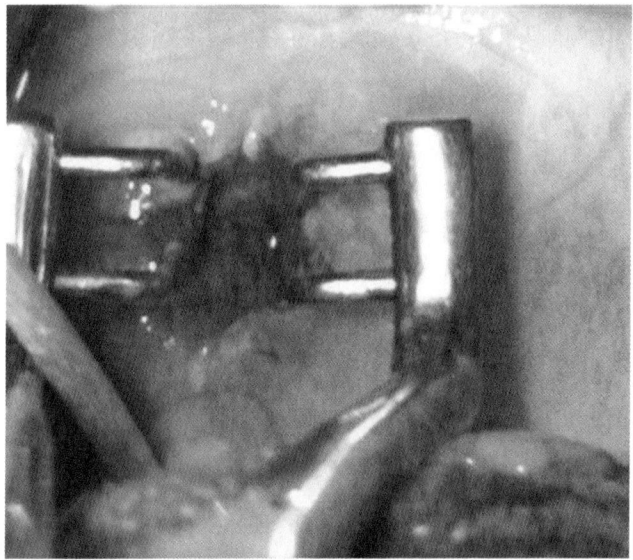

FIGURE 29-12 In colposcopic cases in which the squamocolumnar junction is initially inadequately seen, an endocervical speculum can aid in viewing the endocervical canal.

TABLE 29-6. Reid Colposcopic Index

Colposcopic Sign	Zero Points	1 Point	2 Points
Margin	Condylomatous Micropapillary Feathery Satellite lesions	Smooth Straight	Rolled Peeling Internal border
Color: acetowhitening	Shiny Snowy Translucent Transient	Duller white	Dull white Gray
Vessels	Fine patterns Uniform caliber and patterns	Absent	Coarse patterns Dilated with variable caliber and intercapillary distances
Iodine staining	Positive	Partial	Negative

Modified with permission from Reid R, Scalzi P: Genital warts and cervical cancer. VII. An improved colposcopic index for differentiating benign papillomaviral infections from high-grade cervical intraepithelial neoplasia. Am J Obstet Gynecol 1985 Nov 15;153(6):611–618.

terminologies (Bornstein, 2012). Lesions with low-grade characteristics are labeled grade 1 (minor) lesions, whereas higher-grade characteristics are grade 2 (major) findings.

Of Reid index features, lesion margins and color are best assessed following application of acetic acid. The color or degree of whiteness obtained, rapidity and duration of acetowhitening, and sharpness of lesion borders are observed. Grade 2 (major or high-grade) lesions demonstrate a more persistent, duller shade of white, whereas grade 1 (minor or low-grade) lesions are translucent or bright white and fade quickly. Generally, grade 1 lesions have feathery or irregular "geographic" margins, whereas grade 2 lesions have straighter, sharper outlines (Figs. 29-13 and 29-14). Other lesion features suggestive of a high-grade lesions are: internal borders (inner border sign), an opaque protuberance within a lesion (ridge sign), and cuffed crypt openings.

Abnormal vascular patterns include punctation, mosaicism, and atypical vessels. Punctate and mosaic patterns are graded on the basis of vessel caliber, intercapillary distance, and the uniformity of each of these. Fine punctation and mosaicism, which are created by narrow vessels and short, uniform intercapillary distances, typify low-grade (grade 1) lesions. A coarse pattern results from wider and more variable vessel diameters and spacing and indicates high-grade (grade 2) abnormalities. Atypical vessels are irregular in caliber, shape, course, and arrangement and raise suspicion for invasive cancer (Fig. 29-15).

■ Biopsy

Ectocervical Biopsy

Under direct colposcopic visualization, suspicious lesions are biopsied using cervical biopsy forceps (Fig. 29-16). Generally, cervical biopsy does not require an anesthetic. Thickened Monsel solution (ferric subsulfate) or a silver nitrate applicator are applied with pressure to the biopsy site, providing hemostasis if needed. Heavier bleeding is rare and can be controlled with direct pressure or brief vaginal packing.

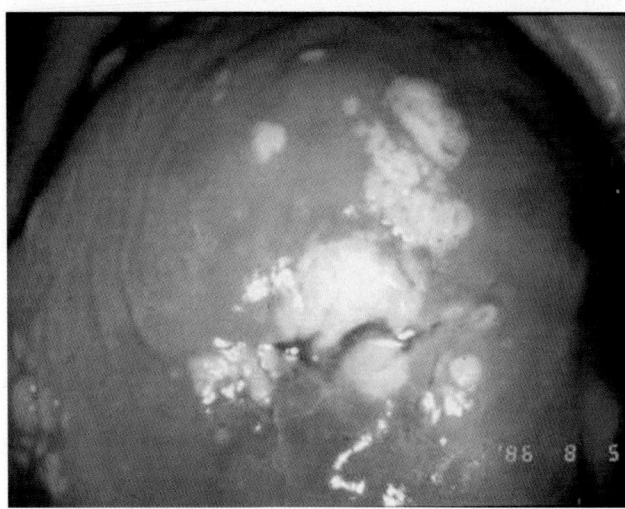

FIGURE 29-13 Low-grade squamous intraepithelial lesion (LSIL). After 5-percent acetic acid application, LSIL is often multifocal and bright white with irregular borders.

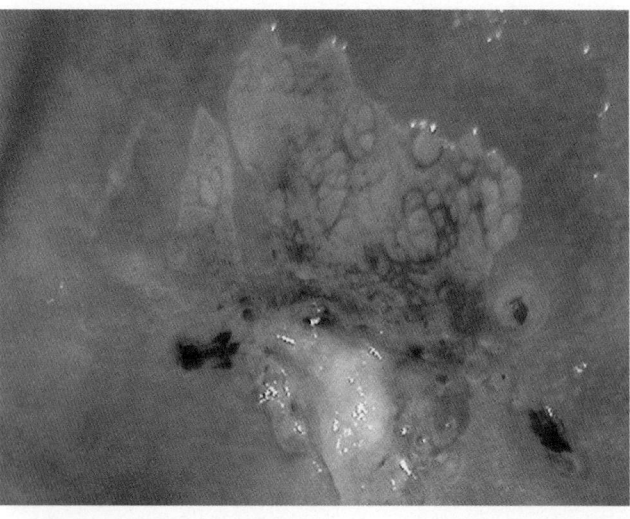

FIGURE 29-14 High-grade squamous intraepithelial lesion (HSIL). After 5-percent acetic acid application, HSIL demonstrates off-white dull color and coarse vascular pattern.

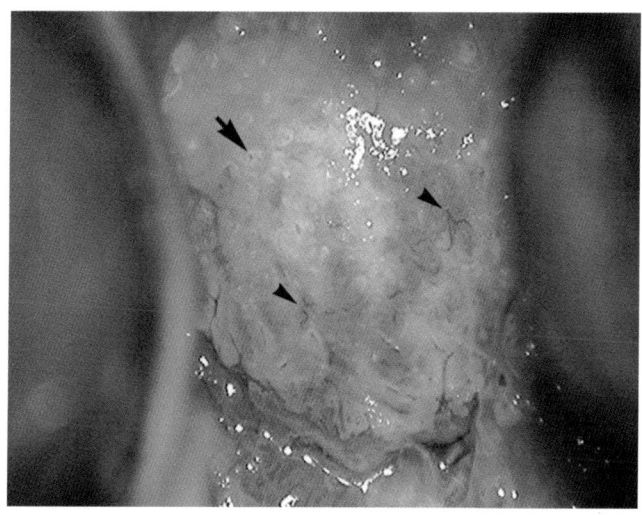

FIGURE 29-15 Colposcopy shows a large high-grade lesion with cuffed crypt openings (*arrow*) and atypical vessels (*arrowheads*) that are worrisome for invasive cancer.

Traditionally, biopsies have been limited to the most severe-appearing lesions. However, two studies have shown that colposcopically directed biopsy detects only 60 to 70 percent of high-grade disease. Disease detection rates increase with the addition of random biopsies of normal-appearing epithelium and with the total number of biopsies taken (Gage, 2006; Pretorius, 2004; Zuchna, 2010)). The American College of Obstetricians and Gynecologists (2013) recommends biopsy of all acetowhite lesions regardless of colposcopic impression, and repeat colposcopic evaluation is suggested for persistent low-grade cytologic abnormalities or HPV-positive results to counter the imperfect detection of HSIL by colposcopy.

Endocervical Sampling

For nonpregnant patients, endocervical sampling by curettage or brushing evaluates the endocervical canal epithelium that lies beyond the colposcope's view. Endocervical sampling is currently recommended during colposcopy in the following situations

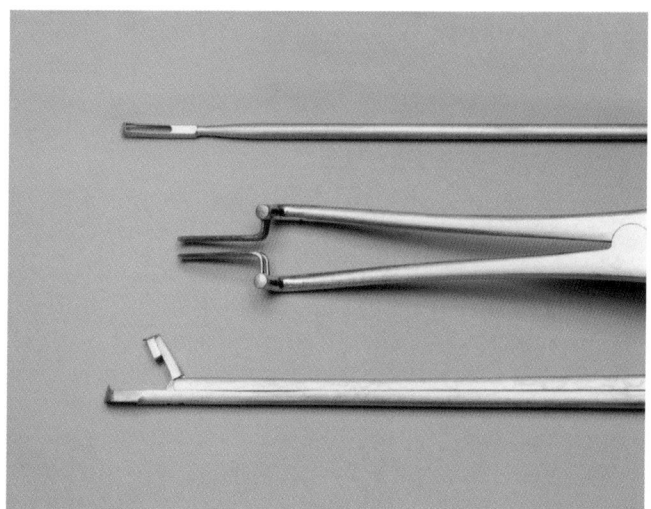

FIGURE 29-16 Tools used for cervical evaluation and biopsy. From top to bottom: endocervical curette, endocervical speculum, and cervical biopsy forceps.

(American College of Obstetricians and Gynecologists, 2013; Massad, 2013):

- Colposcopy is inadequate, or colposcopy is adequate but no lesion is identified. Endocervical sampling is acceptable in other cases at provider discretion.
- Initial evaluation of ASC-H, HSIL, AGC, or AIS cytology test results.
- Surveillance 4 to 6 months after excisional therapy if specimen margins are positive for HSIL.
- Surveillance after conization for AIS has been performed in women wishing fertility preservation. Negative endocervical curettage results add reassurance to this management (Schorge, 2003).

Endocervical sampling can be performed by either curettage or brushing. Endocervical curettage is performed by introducing an endocervical curette 1 to 2 cm into the cervical canal (see Fig. 29-16). The length and circumference of the canal is firmly curetted, carefully avoiding sampling of the ectocervix or the lower uterine segment. Endocervical scrapings admixed with cervical mucus are then removed using a ring forceps or cytobrush and included with the curettage specimen. Alternatively, vigorous brushing with a cytobrush may be used to obtain an endocervical tissue specimen. Endocervical brushing is more sensitive than curettage, but grading of any dysplasia present is more difficult. Endocervical sampling is often the most uncomfortable part of a colposcopic evaluation, and cramping is common.

CERVICAL INTRAEPITHELIAL NEOPLASIA MANAGEMENT

Evidence-based guidelines for the management of women with biopsy-confirmed CIN were developed by the ASCCP and updated in 2012 (Massad, 2013). These continue to use the CIN nomenclature since outcome data stratified by the newer SIL terminology are not yet available. Management of CIN involves either observation or treatment. Goals are to diagnose occult invasive cancer, detect progression of minor abnormalities, and treat high-grade dysplasia to decrease cancer risk. Detection and prevention of invasive cervical cancer, a relatively rare outcome, must be balanced against the potential harms of excessive testing and overtreatment that include procedure-related morbidities, possible adverse reproductive outcomes, and psychologic stress.

Special populations considered include women age 21 to 25 years and pregnant women. Immunosuppressed women are no longer considered a special population and can now be managed in accordance with general guidelines. However, the CDC (2010) and American College of Obstetricians and Gynecologists (2013) still question HPV testing for ASC-US triage and surveillance of HIV-positive women.

In general, women with higher grades of Pap abnormality and CIN, inadequate colposcopic examinations, abnormal endocervical samplings, and age older than 24 years are considered at higher risk of invasive cancer and are managed more aggressively. An overview of current CIN management guidelines for nonpregnant patients is presented here, but providers should consult comprehensive recommendations (American College of Obstetricians and Gynecologists, 2013; Massad, 2013). Guidelines are complex and are applied on an individualized basis, as they cannot address all clinical scenarios or individual patient situations. No guidelines can prevent all cases of cervical cancer.

CIN 1

CIN 1 exhibits a high rate of spontaneous regression. This diagnosis is poorly reproducible and thus unreliable. For this reason, CIN 1 is no longer treated aggressively. When diagnosed after a "lesser" cytologic abnormality such ASC-US, LSIL, or a negative Pap with either an HPV 16/18 genotype-positive or a persistent HR HPV-positive result, it can be observed indefinitely. Treatment is acceptable only if CIN 1 persists for more than 2 years regardless of colposcopic examination adequacy or presence of CIN 1 in an endocervical sampling. Treatment of CIN 1 in women under age 25 years is not recommended, even if persistent.

Observation consists of a cotest 12 months after CIN 1 diagnosis. If this is negative, resumption of routine screening is recommended 3 years later. In women age 21 to 25 years, observation with cytology alone at 12 months and 24 months is recommended instead of cotesting due to high rates of HPV positivity in this population. If CIN 1 is detected only in the endocervical sampling, sampling is repeated in 1 year in addition to other recommended surveillance. Abnormal surveillance results are followed by repeat colposcopy. Persistent CIN 1 may be treated by ablation or excision provided the colposcopic examination is adequate and endocervical sampling lacks HSIL (CIN 2/3) or ungraded CIN. If these criteria are not met, excision is recommended and ablation is unacceptable.

CIN 1 diagnosed after an ASC-H or HSIL Pap test result carries a higher risk of occult high-grade CIN. In women age 25 years or older with an adequate colposcopic examination, either a diagnostic excision or observation with cotesting at 12 and 24 months is acceptable. If colposcopy is inadequate, a diagnostic excision is indicated. Women age 21 to 24 years with CIN 1 diagnosed after a high-grade Pap abnormality can be monitored by colposcopic evaluation and cytology at 6-month intervals provided the colposcopic examination is adequate and endocervical samplings negative. Otherwise, excision is recommended. Persistent unexplained HSIL cytology results after 24 months of observation warrant an excision procedure.

CIN 2 and CIN 3

Generally, treatment is recommended for CIN 2 or 3 due to its significant malignant potential and the efficacy of treatment in preventing progression. Either ablation or excision is acceptable and is chosen according to individual patient, cervical TZ, and lesion characteristics.

When CIN 2/3 or ungraded CIN is found in an endocervical sampling or with an inadequate colposcopic examination, a diagnostic excision is needed to exclude occult invasive cancer. An unequivocal histologic diagnosis of CIN 3 is treated, not observed, regardless of age or reproductive history. Recurrence or persistence is treated with repeat excision, not ablation. Hysterectomy as primary therapy is unacceptable. It may be indicated if repeat excision is needed but not anatomically feasible or if high-grade CIN recurs or persists.

For young women, particularly of low parity, with CIN 2 or CIN 2/3 (HSIL, not otherwise specified) either observation or treatment are acceptable if colposcopy is adequate. In this context, "young women" refers to those individuals for whom the possible risk to future pregnancies from treatment outweighs the risk of progression to malignancy, although either of these is difficult to quantify. No upper age limit is recommended. Observation consists of repeat cytology and colposcopy at 6-month intervals. Observation of CIN 2 is preferred to treatment in younger women. If colposcopy is inadequate, CIN 3 is specified, or CIN 2 or CIN 2/3 persists at 24 months, then treatment is recommended.

Adenocarcinoma in Situ

Adenocarcinoma in situ (AIS) of the cervix, although uncommon, is increasing in incidence and typically diagnosed at a younger age (Herzog, 2007). Exclusion of invasive cancer and removal of all affected tissue are primary clinical goals. Management differs somewhat from that of CIN2/3 because AIS and adenocarcinoma are not easily identified colposcopically. Lesions can be multifocal, located deep within endocervical clefts, and extend farther into the endocervical canal (Massad, 2013). Diagnostic excision is required to exclude invasive cancer with maximum certainty. For nonpregnant women, excision is complemented by endocervical curettage. Choice of excision modality should favor an intact specimen with the most interpretable margins. Cold-knife conization is thus favored by many, but guidelines do not explicitly favor it over LEEP. If used, loop excision should be large enough to obviate the need for a second, deeper pass and should minimize cautery artifact. If there is no invasive cancer in the excision specimen, simple hysterectomy is recommended in women who have completed childbearing.

Women with AIS who strongly desire fertility preservation can be managed conservatively after an excision procedure. Individuals are counseled regarding the significant ongoing risk even with negative excision margins and endocervical sampling. The risk of residual AIS is reported to be as high as 80 percent in patients with positive margins (Krivak, 2001). Accordingly, repeat excision is advisable if hysterectomy is not planned. Close, long-term surveillance is recommended until hysterectomy is performed (Massad, 2013).

Postcolposcopy Surveillance without Treatment

When colposcopy fails to reveal high-grade CIN or there is spontaneous regression of high-grade CIN in young women, further surveillance is indicated given the significant false-negative rate of colposcopy and an increased risk of developing CIN in the future. This involves repeat cytology, HPV testing, or colposcopy alone or in combination depending on the original abnormal cytology result and age of the patient. Early surveillance generally is either cytology or cotest once or twice at 1-year intervals. Return to routine screening or an additional cotest generally occurs 3 years later. Exceptions are AGC, favor neoplasia and AIS Pap test results. These are always followed by excision unless invasive cancer is diagnosed during initial colposcopic examination and biopsy.

CERVICAL INTRAEPITHELIAL NEOPLASIA TREATMENT

Current treatment of CIN is limited to ablation or excision procedures encompassing the entire TZ. Unlike ablation, excision provides a histologic specimen for evaluation of excised margins and further assurance that invasive cancer is not present. Any treatment should reach a depth of 5 to 7 mm from the surface to treat CIN adequately. Excess depth is avoided to minimize potential adverse consequences. Treatment using topical agents or therapeutic vaccines remains investigational. Selection of treatment modality is individualized. Salient factors include patient age, parity, size and severity of lesions, cervix contour, prior CIN treatment, and coexisting medical conditions. Treatment selection also depends on an operator's experience and available equipment. No clear evidence shows any treatment technique to be superior, and surgical treatments have an approximate 90-percent success rate (Martin-Hirsch, 2013). A review of clinical considerations is provided by Khan and Smith-McKune (2014).

■ Ablation

In general, ablation of the TZ is effective for noninvasive ectocervical disease. Before ablation, evidence of glandular neoplasia or invasive cancer is excluded with the greatest certainty possible. Namely, cytology, histology, and colposcopic impression should be concordant; colposcopic examination must be adequate; and endocervical sampling should be negative for high-grade or ungraded CIN. Ablation should not be used after prior therapy, for an unexplained glandular cytologic abnormality, or for AIS. The most commonly used ablative treatment modalities are cryosurgery and carbon dioxide (CO_2) laser, and both techniques are illustrated in the atlas (Chap. 43, p. 989). Before the introduction of LEEP, when cold knife conization was the only excision option, these ablative techniques were used more commonly. The relative decreased morbidity and ease of performing loop excision compared with cold knife conization and the trends toward observation of CIN 1 and of some CIN 2 and CIN 2/3 lesions in young women has led to decreased use of ablative procedures.

Cryosurgery is an ablative method that delivers a refrigerant gas, usually nitrous oxide, to a metal probe that freezes tissue on contact. Cryonecrosis is achieved by crystallizing intracellular water. This treatment is most appropriate for lesions and TZ lying entirely on the ectocervix, for a smooth cervical surface without deep crevices, and for CIN limited to two quadrants of the cervix (Table 29-7). Cryosurgery is generally not favored for the treatment of CIN 3 due to higher rates of disease persistence following treatment and lack of a histologic specimen to exclude occult invasive cancer (Martin-Hirsch, 2013). Moreover, cryosurgery and other ablative techniques are not favored for HIV-positive women with CIN due to higher failure rates (Spitzer, 1999). Less evidence suggests subsequent adverse

TABLE 29-7. Cryosurgery: Clinical Characteristics

Advantages
Favorable safety profile
Outpatient procedure
No anesthetic requirements
Ease of procedure
Low-cost equipment with minimal maintenance
Bleeding complications rare
No proven adverse reproductive effects
Acceptable primary cure rate

Disadvantages
No tissue specimen for histopathology evaluation
Cannot treat lesions with unfavorable sizes or shapes
Uterine cramping
Potential for vasovagal reaction
Profuse vaginal discharge postprocedure
Cephalad migration of squamocolumnar junction

Data from Martin-Hirsch PL, Paraskevaidis E, Bryant A: Surgery for cervical intraepithelial neoplasia. Cochrane Database Syst Rev 2013 Dec 4;12:CD001318.

effects on pregnancy outcome with cryotherapy than with loop excision. Thus, cryotherapy may be underused (Khan, 2014).

CO_2 laser is another ablative option and is delivered using colposcopic guidance with a micromanipulator. Cervical tissue is vaporized to a depth of 5 to 7 mm. Laser ablation is appropriate for CIN lesions associated with an adequate colposcopic examination. It is well suited for large, irregularly shaped CIN lesions of all grades and for condylomatous and preinvasive lesions at other LGT sites. If the cervical lesion extends onto the vagina, laser ablation may help customize removal of the entire lesion with favorable depth control. Laser ablation can also be augmented by laser or loop excision of central tissue for cases in which an ectocervical lesion extends into the endocervical canal or in which colposcopy is inadequate (American College of Obstetricians and Gynecologists, 2013).

■ Excision

Clinical scenarios with the highest risk of occult invasive cancer but without definitive histologic confirmation are evaluated further with an excision procedure. These include high-grade cytologic abnormalities with discordant (negative or low-grade) biopsy results or with inadequate colposcopy; AGC, favor neoplasia or AIS cytology; AIS histology; and endocervical sampling indicating ungraded or high-grade CIN or glandular neoplasia. With glandular cytologic abnormalities or AIS, an excisional modality that provides an intact specimen with the most interpretable margins should be chosen (Massad, 2013). Excision is indicated for recurrence of high-grade CIN after treatment due to the increased risk for occult invasive cancer (Paraskevaidis, 1991). Diagnostic excision refers to situations in which invasive cancer has not been excluded by the criteria needed before an ablation is performed. A therapeutic excision refers to one performed when these criteria have been met.

Excisional treatment modalities include LEEP, cold-knife conization (CKC), and laser conization, which are all illustrated in the atlas (p. 992). Excisional procedures are associated with operative and long-term risks that include subsequent cervical stenosis and adverse pregnancy outcomes. For decades, CKC has been associated with cervical incompetence and preterm birth. The relationship between preterm birth and LEEP remains uncertain. Although some studies show LEEP to be an independent risk factor for preterm birth and premature rupture of membranes, others do not (Jakobsson, 2009; Kyrgiou, 2006; Sadler, 2004; Samson, 2005; Werner, 2010). An important confounder is the increased risk of preterm birth in women with cervical neoplasia compared with the general population even if they have not undergone an excisional procedure (Bruinsma, 2007; Conner, 2014; Shanbhag, 2009). This indicates that CIN and preterm birth have overlapping risk factors, making the contribution of treatment to this risk difficult to ascertain and controversial.

Of options, LEEP uses a thin wire on an insulated handle through which an electrical current is passed. This creates an instrument that can simultaneously cut and coagulate tissue, ideally during direct colposcopic visualization. Because LEEP can be performed using local anesthesia, it has become the primary outpatient treatment modality for high-grade cervical lesions, including those that extend into the endocervical canal (Table 29-8). LEEP provides a tissue specimen with margins that can be histologically assessed. Additionally, the size and shape of tissue excision can be customized by varying loop sizes and the order in which loops are used. This helps conserve cervical stroma volume.

Cold-knife conization is surgery that uses sharp excision to remove the cervical TZ and CIN lesion. It is performed in an operating room under general or regional anesthesia (Table 29-9). CKC is often preferred to LEEP for patients at highest risk for invasive cancer. These indications include cervical cytology suspicious for invasive cancer, patients older than 35 with CIN 3 or CIS, large high-grade lesions, and glandular neoplasia.

CO_2 laser conization allows precise tailoring of the cone shape to minimize stromal excision and yields less blood loss. Disadvantages are its expense, some thermal compromise of specimen margins, and special training requirements. This procedure can be performed under local, regional, or general anesthesia.

TABLE 29-8. Loop Electrosurgical Excision Procedure: Clinical Characteristics

Advantages
Favorable safety profile
Ease of procedure
Outpatient procedure using local anesthesia
Low-cost equipment
Tissue specimen for histopathology evaluation

Disadvantages
Thermal damage may obscure specimen margin status
Special training required
Risk of postprocedure bleeding
Theoretical risk of vapor plume inhalation

TABLE 29-9. Cold-Knife Conization Clinical Characteristics

Advantages
Anesthetized patient
Tissue specimen without margin compromise
Enhanced patient support if hemorrhage is encountered
Variety of instruments to individualize conization

Disadvantages
Potential for hemorrhage
Lengthier procedure
Postoperative discomfort
General or regional anesthesia required
Operating room setting
High cost
Larger volume of cervical stroma removed
Increased risk of adverse reproductive outcomes

Surveillance after Treatment

Additional surveillance is required to assess treatment success (American College of Obstetricians and Gynecologists, 2013; Massad, 2013). Patients who have undergone a cervical excision with margins negative for HSIL or who have undergone an ablative procedure may be followed with cotesting 1 year later or serial cotesting at 12 and 24 months depending on whether the original abnormal cytology or biopsies showed low- or high-grade changes. Additional cytology or cotesting again at 3 years is recommended before returning to routine screening. After treatment of HSIL, routine screening should continue for at least 20 years due to a persistently increased risk of cervical neoplasia, even if screening extends beyond age 65.

If excision margins or endocervical curettage performed immediately after an excision are positive for CIN 2 or CIN 3, then surveillance with repeat cytology and endocervical sampling 4 to 6 months later is preferred. Repeat excision is acceptable. Repeat diagnostic excision is indicated for special circumstances such as AIS or microinvasive carcinoma at the excision margins.

Hysterectomy

Hysterectomy is unacceptable as primary therapy for CIN (American College of Obstetricians and Gynecologists, 2013; Massad, 2013). However, it may be considered when treating recurrent high-grade cervical disease if childbearing has been completed or when a repeat cervical excision is strongly indicated but not technically feasible. Although hysterectomy provides the lowest CIN recurrence rate, invasive cancer must always be excluded beforehand. The choice of either a vaginal or abdominal approach is directed by other clinical factors. Hysterectomy is the preferred treatment of AIS when future fertility is not desired.

Even with negative cervical margins, hysterectomy performed for CIN 2 or worse is not completely protective. Patients, particularly those who are immunosuppressed, are at risk for recurrent disease and require postoperative interval cytologic screening of the vaginal cuff as described on page 635.

VAGINAL PREINVASIVE LESIONS

Pathophysiology

Vaginal cancer is a rare malignancy comprising only 1 to 2 percent of gynecologic cancers. Nearly 50 percent of cases are diagnosed in women aged 70 years and older (Kosary, 2007). Approximately 90 percent of vaginal cancers are squamous cell carcinomas. These appear to develop slowly from precancerous epithelial changes, called vaginal intraepithelial neoplasia (VaIN), in a fashion similar to cervical cancer from CIN.

VaIN demonstrates histopathology similar to CIN and VIN. It is rarely found as a primary lesion and most often develops as an extension of CIN, mainly in the upper third of the vagina (Diakomanolis, 2002; Hoffman, 1992a). Unlike the cervix, the vagina lacks a TZ susceptible to HPV-induced neoplasia. However, HPV may gain entry from vaginal mucosal abrasions and reparative metaplastic squamous cell activity (Woodruff, 1981). In one review, investigators found HPV DNA in up to 98 percent of VaIN lesions and in three quarters of vaginal cancers. HPV 16 is the most common type (Alemany, 2014). Thus, HPV vaccination against HPV types 16 and 18 has the potential to also prevent vaginal cancers (Smith, 2009).

The natural history of VaIN is less understood than that of CIN, although their similar risk factors suggest a similar etiology. Cervical and vulvar neoplasia increase the risk for VaIN and vaginal squamous cancer. Women treated for CIN 3 are at increased risk of developing both cervical and vaginal cancers, and this risk accelerates in those older than 60 (Strander, 2014). Moreover, a retrospective study suggests that hysterectomy is not definitive therapy for high-grade neoplasia, as researchers have found a subsequent high-grade VaIN recurrence rate greater than 7 percent (Schockaert, 2008).

Diagnosis

Generally, VaIN is asymptomatic. If present, symptoms may include spotting, discharge, and odor. Abnormal cytology is often the first indication of VaIN. Subsequent examination of the vagina with a colposcope, termed *vaginoscopy*, frequently identifies a lesion for biopsy. Prior to visual evaluation, careful palpation of the vagina is advisable, particularly if the patient has undergone hysterectomy for high-grade cervical neoplasia. In such cases, invasive cancer may present as a nodular lesion buried within the vaginal cuff before it becomes visible.

During vaginoscopy, inspecting the entire vagina using a colposcope can be challenging because of a large surface area, rugation, and surfaces parallel to the colposcope's visual axis. Particular attention is paid to the upper third of the vagina due to the common etiology of VaIN as an extension of CIN. After hysterectomy for high-grade CIN, abnormal vaginal cytology should prompt careful inspection of the vaginal cuff. By applying 3- to 5-percent acetic acid to the vaginal mucosa, acetowhite changes consistent with HPV infection or neoplasia are identified (Fig. 29-17). Vascular patterns are less common in VaIN lesions than with CIN, but coarse punctation and even atypical vessels may be seen in high-grade and invasive lesions. High-grade VaIN tends to demonstrate flat, dense acetowhitening with sharply demarcated borders. Half-strength Lugol

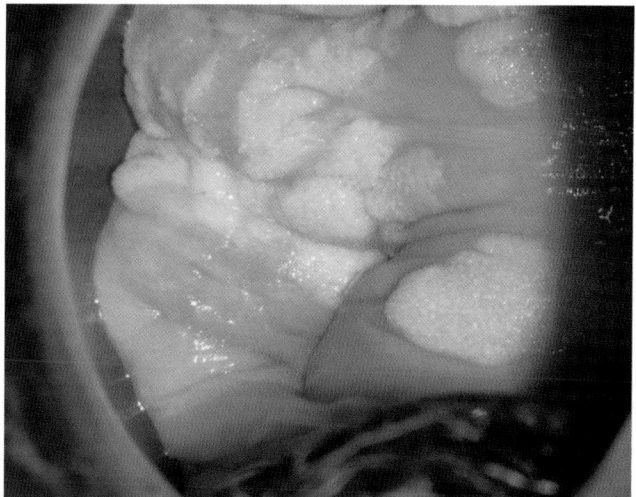

FIGURE 29-17 Vaginoscopy showing multifocal acetowhite human papillomavirus (HPV) lesions after application of 5-percent acetic acid.

solution applied to the vagina further delineates abnormal areas. Similar to cervical dysplasia, strongly nonstaining areas most likely contain abnormal epithelium. Iodine staining aids biopsy site selection, and areas with the least staining and straightest lesion margins are preferred. Biopsy may be obtained by means of a cervical biopsy forceps, and an Emmett hook can be used to elevate and stabilize vaginal tissue if needed. Local anesthesia is usually not necessary for biopsies of the upper third of the vagina but may be needed for more distal biopsies. The vaginal tissue is grasped and lifted to limit the biopsy depth. Menopausal women may have significant thinning of the vaginal mucosa, and biopsy is done with greater care or with a smaller biopsy forceps to avoid perforation of the vaginal wall. Hemostasis is achieved using silver nitrate applicators or Monsel paste. Vaginal lesion size, location, and specific biopsy sites are carefully documented for future management and surveillance.

Management

Like high-grade CIN, high-grade VaIN is believed to be a precancerous lesion and generally warrants eradication (Punnonen, 1989; Rome, 2000). Because vaginal neoplasia is uncommon, most management strategies are derived from small, retrospective, and statistically underpowered studies. Management of VaIN depends on the grade of neoplasia and may include observation, excision, ablation, topical antineoplastics, or rarely, radiation therapy. Each treatment method has advantages and disadvantages, and none has proven superior efficacy. Management strategies are determined by lesion size, number, and location; histologic diagnosis; and comprehensive patient counseling.

Low-Grade VaIN

In a long-term study of 132 patients with VaIN, Rome and associates (2000) found that an observational approach after biopsy resulted in VaIN 1 regression in seven of eight patients (88 percent). No VaIN 1 lesion progressed to high-grade VaIN or invasive cancer. Vaginal LSIL often represents atrophy or a transient HPV infection. Spontaneous regression is common, and observation is preferable in most cases. Aggressive treatment is avoided. Although no evidence-based guidelines are available, surveillance similar to that for low-grade CIN with repeat cytology with or without vaginoscopy every 6 to 12 months seems reasonable until abnormalities resolve or progress to HSIL.

High-grade VaIN

Observation of VaIN 2 may be considered in selected patients, but the safety of this approach is not established. Treatment choice for patients with high-grade VaIN is influenced by several factors including the location and number of lesions, the patient's sexual activity status, vaginal length, prior radiation therapy, previous treatment modalities in patients with recurrent VaIN, and clinician experience. Potential adverse effects of treatment on subsequent quality of life such as pain, difficulties with sexual intercourse, and scarring are always considered when choosing a therapeutic modality.

Wide local excision of a high-grade unifocal lesion or partial vaginectomy for multifocal lesions may be used. Hoffman (1992a) found that nine of 32 patients (28 percent) with prior hysterectomy and VaIN 3 had occult invasive cancer in the vaginal cuff. Therefore, surgical excision is considered for high-grade lesions involving the vaginal cuff, particularly if any thickening or nodularity of vaginal apex suggests occult invasive disease. Excisional procedures have the advantage of providing a surgical specimen for which resected-margin status can be determined and the presence of invasive vaginal cancer excluded. Partial vaginectomy is surgically challenging but has the highest cure rate and fewest recurrences for high-grade disease (Dodge, 2001). Wide local excision carries less morbidity than vaginectomy, but both procedures may be complicated by bladder or rectal injury and hemorrhage. In addition, subsequent vaginal scarring and stenosis may compromise vaginal intercourse or cause dyspareunia. Sharp dissection is favored for local excision and for partial vaginectomy. Laser causes significant thermal damage to the tissue specimen and generally is not recommended for excision of vaginal mucosa. Loop excision has poor depth control and carries a substantial risk of thermal damage to underlying pelvic structures, including the bladder and bowel. LEEP should not be used for vaginal surgery.

CO$_2$ laser ablation is an option for lesions not concerning for invasive disease. It is well suited for eradication of multifocal lesions and causes less scarring and blood loss than tissue excision. Rarely, excessive bleeding and thermal damage to the bladder and bowel can occur. In one study, investigators monitored 21 patients after high-grade VaIN CO$_2$ laser ablation and found that 14 percent had persistent disease requiring retreatment. One patient progressed to invasive carcinoma, which underscores the importance of long-term surveillance (Perrotta, 2013). A broader explanation of laser ablation techniques is found in Section 43-26 (p. 991).

Topical therapy, as with ablative procedures, is suitable if there is no suspicion of invasive disease by cytology, vaginoscopy, or histology. Persistent VaIN 2 and selected VaIN 3 lesions may be medically treated using 5-percent fluorouracil (5-FU) cream "off-label," as it is not FDA approved for this specific indication (Krebs, 1989). Its efficacy is unproven in large, randomized trials, and studies with small numbers of patients have demonstrated mixed results. Treatment regimens vary widely. One

dosing schedule calls for a 3-mL dose of cream placed in the vaginal vault by plastic vaginal applicator every other day for 3 days during the first week of treatment and once weekly thereafter for up to 10 weeks. 5-FU cream is often associated with a robust inflammatory reaction that can include vaginal burning and vulvar irritation. To minimize leakage onto the vulva, it is best applied intravaginally at bedtime, when a recumbent position will be maintained for hours. Additionally, an occlusive, water-resistant ointment can be used to protect the vulva. Protective gloves are worn when handling 5-FU cream, and measures are taken to avoid 5-FU contact by sexual partners. Patients selected for this treatment require thorough counseling, effective contraception as needed, consent for off-label medication use, and close monitoring for excessive inflammation and ulceration, which can lead to vaginal or vulvar scarring and loss of function.

Radiation therapy has a very limited role for treatment of high-grade VaIN. It carries a significant risk of serious morbidity and is reserved for select cases. In a review of 136 cases of vaginal carcinoma in situ, radiation therapy was used in 27 patients, and a 100-percent cure rate was noted. However, 63 percent developed significant complications including vaginal stenosis, adhesions, ulceration, necrosis, and fistula formation (Benedet, 1984). Furthermore, radiation treatment compromises subsequent cytologic, colposcopic, and histologic interpretation. Disease recurrence often necessitates radical surgery.

■ Prognosis

In a study of 132 patients treated for high-grade VaIN, excision and CO$_2$ laser ablation had similar cure rates of 69 percent. Topical 5-FU cream was curative in 46 percent of cases (Rome, 2000). Patients with any grade of vaginal neoplasia require long-term monitoring, as the persistence and recurrence rate for high-grade disease is significant. Currently, no evidence-based guidelines are available for posttreatment surveillance of VaIN. Monitoring includes collection of vaginal cytology and performance of vaginoscopy approximately 2 to 4 months after treatment is completed. Continued surveillance with periodic cytology with or without vaginoscopy at 6- to 12-month intervals for several years thereafter seems prudent. Long-term cytologic screening is needed thereafter.

VULVAR PREINVASIVE LESIONS

■ Pathophysiology

Vulvar cancer is rare. In 2015, vulvar cancer made up less than 5 percent of all gynecologic cancers and less than 0.6 percent of all cancers in the U.S. women (American Cancer Society, 2015). Ninety percent of vulvar cancer is squamous and in some cases may develop slowly from VIN (Fig. 29-18) (Judson, 2006). However, compared with CIN, VIN less often progresses to high-grade disease and cancer. The incidence of vulvar carcinoma in situ has increased significantly over the past several decades. This trend is particularly pronounced in younger women and is thought to be linked to the increased incidence of STDs, including HPV (Howe, 2001). Jones and coworkers (2005) reported that the mean age of women with VIN has decreased from 50 to 39 years since 1980.

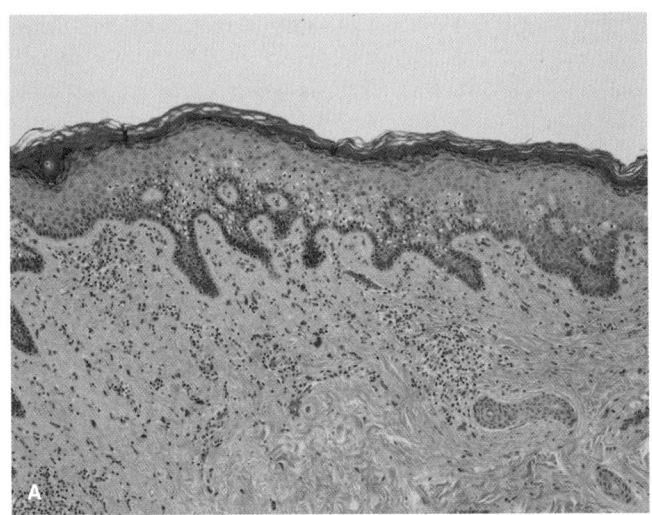 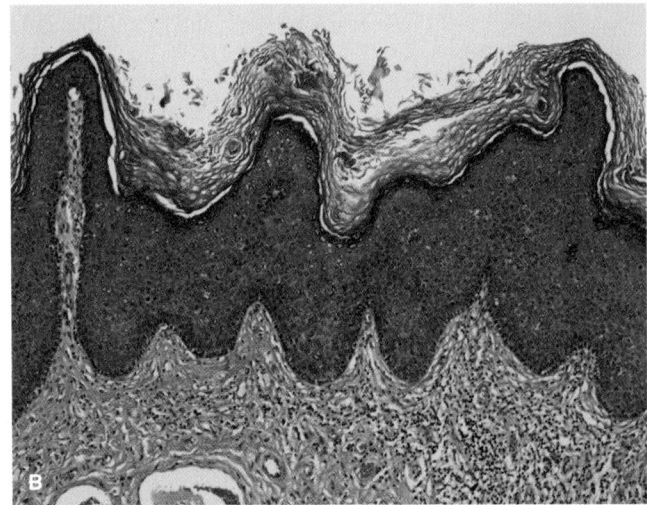

FIGURE 29-18 A. Normal vulvar histology. The squamous epithelium contains cells that show increasing cytoplasm as cells mature from the base to surface. In nondysplastic squamous epithelium, nuclei appear orderly and are devoid of atypical features such as nuclear membrane irregularities, chromatin coarseness, and pleomorphism. Mitoses are usually confined to the basal cell layers. **B.** High-grade squamous intraepithelial lesion (HSIL), usual type. In this example of HSIL/VIN 3 (usual type), the dysplastic squamous epithelium shows virtually no maturation from base to surface, as evidenced by a high nucleus-to-cytoplasm ratio in cells in all epithelial layers. The nuclei are crowded and disorderly. Although not appreciable at this medium power (10×), the epithelium showed increased mitoses and mitoses high in the epithelium. This particular example has a papillomatous surface, a common finding in vulvar HSIL lesions. (Used with permission from Dr. Kelley Carrick.)

Although HPV DNA has been found in up to 80 percent of VIN lesions, HPV is less commonly associated with vulvar cancers, and rates range between 15 and 80 percent (Del Pino, 2013). The progression of vulvar carcinoma in situ to invasive cancer has been strongly suggested, although not confirmed conclusively. Therefore, VIN 3 lesions are generally treated (van Seters, 2005).

■ Classification

Terminology for squamous VIN was introduced by the International Society for the Study of Vulvar Disease (ISSVD) in 1986. Under this classification, VIN grades 1, 2, and 3 were defined by abnormal cellular changes found to varying thicknesses within the squamous epithelium, similar to CIN (Wilkinson, 1986). In 2004, classification of VIN was simplified by the ISSVD (Sideri, 2005). The older designation of VIN 1 has been eliminated, whereas VIN 2 and 3 categories have been combined. This redefinition reflects whether lesions are likely to be premalignant and thus whether lesions require therapy. The VIN 1 category was eliminated because evidence is lacking that such lesions are cancer precursors. These lesions likely represent benign reactive changes or HPV effect usually caused by low-risk HPV types 6 and 11 (Smith, 2009; Srodon, 2006). Since the histologic distinction between VIN 2 and VIN 3 is not reliably reproducible, they are now combined under the term *VIN* (Table 29-10). Most recently, use of LSIL and HSIL terminology similar to other anogenital sites has been recommended for vulvar lesions (Darragh, 2012).

VIN is now categorized as *usual type (uVIN)*, *differentiated type (dVIN)*, or *unclassified type*. Of these, uVIN encompasses most former VIN 2, VIN 3, and vulvar CIS lesions. uVIN lesions can be subcategorized histologically as warty

(condylomatous), basaloid, or mixed and are associated with oncogenic HPV infection. HPV 16 is the most prevalent HPV type found in VIN 2/3 and vulvar cancer (Smith, 2009). In general, HPV-related high-grade VIN lesions histologically resemble high-grade CIN and tend to be multicentric (Feng, 2005; Haefner, 1995).

The entire lower genital tract is vulnerable to HPV infection. Therefore, risk factors for uVIN are similar to those for VaIN and CIN. Accordingly, uVIN risk is strongly associated with multiple sexual partners, STDs, and tobacco smoking, particularly in younger women (Hoffman, 1992b; Jones, 2005). It is

TABLE 29-10. Vulvar Intraepithelial Neoplasia (VIN): Terminology and Characteristics

VIN Type	Clinical Presentation and Risk Factors

VIN, usual type
  Warty
  Basaloid
  Mixed
	Formerly VIN 2, VIN 3, vulvar CIS
	Younger women
	Multicentric disease
	Oncogenic HPV infection
	Smoking, other STDs, immunosuppression

VIN, differentiated type	2–10% of former VIN 3 lesions Older, postmenopausal women Oncogenic HPV infection uncommon
VIN, unclassified type	Rare pagetoid lesions

CIS = carcinoma in situ; HPV = human papillomavirus; STD = sexually transmitted disease.

also seen as part of multifocal LGT neoplasia in immune compromised women.

In contrast, dVIN is less common and accounts for only 2 to 10 percent of all VIN cases (Hart, 2001). Such lesions tend to be unifocal and are typically found in older, nonsmoking, postmenopausal women in their sixth and seventh decade. Infection with oncogenic HPV is uncommon and probably does not play a role in the genesis of these lesions. Instead, they tend to be associated with chronic inflammatory skin conditions or p53 inactivation mutations (Del Pino, 2013). However, dVIN is more likely to progress to squamous cell carcinoma than uVIN. One study noted that progression of dVIN to vulvar squamous cell carcinoma was five times higher than for uVIN (van de Nieuwenhof, 2009). The pathologic diagnosis of dVIN is difficult and interobserver agreement is low. If clinical findings warrant, review by an experienced gynecologic pathologist may be helpful (van den Einden, 2013).

Rare pagetoid types of VIN 2 and 3 cannot be classified in any of the foregoing categories. These are termed *VIN, unclassified type* (Sideri, 2005).

■ Diagnosis

Clinical Findings

VIN may be asymptomatic and discovered with routine gynecologic examinations or during evaluation of abnormal cervical or vaginal cytology. When present, signs and symptoms (itching, burning, pain) may affect a patient's sexual functioning and quality of life. Whereas high-grade lesions of the cervix and vagina are generally invisible without acetic acid application and use of a colposcope, clinically significant VIN lesions are usually visible without the aid of special techniques. Lesions vary widely in appearance but are usually sharply demarcated (Del Pino, 2013). They may be white, hyperkeratotic plaques; hyperpigmented lesions; or areas of erythema. Lesions may be raised or flat. uVIN is associated with HPV-related lesions or neoplasia elsewhere in the anogenital tract. Often, lesions appear bulky, resemble condylomata, and are multifocal with extensive involvement of the perineum and adjacent skin (Fig. 29-19).

dVIN is generally unifocal and may be associated with lichen sclerosus or lichen simplex chronicus of the adjacent skin. A lesion may appear as an ulcer, warty papule, or hyperkeratotic plaque.

To avoid diagnostic delay, most focal vulvar lesions are biopsied, particularly lesions that are irregularly or darkly pigmented, asymmetric, large, elevated, roughened, nodular, or ulcerated. Ulceration, surrounding induration, or inguinal adenopathy raises suspicion for invasive cancer. Other scenarios suspicious for VIN include enlarging lesions, warty lesions in postmenopausal or immune compromised women, and warts that are atypical in appearance or persist despite topical therapies (American College of Obstetricians and Gynecologists, 2014b).

Vulvoscopy

Histologic confirmation is necessary before high-grade VIN is managed. Selection of the best location to biopsy is aided by magnification of the vulva, perineum, and perianal skin, usually with a colposcope. This examination is termed *vulvoscopy.* Alternatively, any good light source and a handheld magnifying lens can be used.

Vulvar epithelial changes are enhanced by applying a 3- to 5-percent acetic-acid-soaked gauze pad to the vulva for 5 minutes prior to examination. This is usually well tolerated but may cause pain or burning in the presence of vulvar irritation, ulceration, or fissures. Acetic acid accentuates the surface topography of lesions and may reveal acetowhite lesions not seen grossly. Pigmented VIN lesions tend to turn a dusky gray due to hyperkeratosis. Vascular patterns are generally not seen, but high-grade VIN rarely may demonstrate coarse punctation. Normal vulvar tissue, particularly the inner, posterior labia minora, may turn diffusely acetowhite and should not be treated based on this appearance.

As an alternative, 1-percent toluidine blue, a nuclear stain, may help define the best site for biopsy or for surgery margins (Joura, 1998). Its use is technically more challenging, and results are fraught with both false positives and false negatives. Therefore, its use has been largely abandoned.

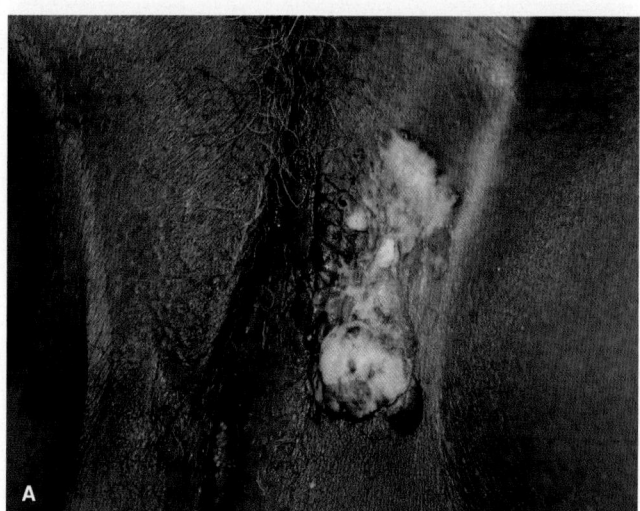
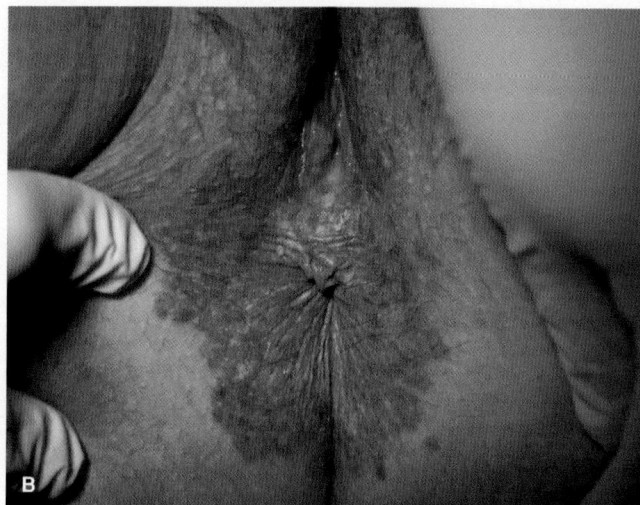

FIGURE 29-19 A. Bulky lesion of vulvar intraepithelial neoplasia (VIN), differentiated type. **B.** Extensive perineal and perianal extension of VIN, usual type.

The most abnormal-appearing areas are biopsied, although necrotic areas often yield nondiagnostic findings and are avoided if possible. Biopsies measuring up to 6 mm in diameter can be obtained using a Keyes punch after provision of a local anesthetic injection (Fig. 4-2, p. 88). Topical anesthetics can be applied several minutes prior to injection of local anesthesia to decrease discomfort. If lesions are close to the clitoral hood, general anesthesia is often warranted due to increased pain with injection of local anesthesia and increased vascularity. Biopsy sites measuring 4 mm or greater occasionally require suturing for hemostasis or cosmetic closure, especially on mucosal surfaces that stretch.

■ Management

VIN 1

As noted, the progression of VIN 1 to VIN 3 has not been established, and the VIN 1 category has been eliminated entirely. Thus, lesions reported as VIN 1 are not treated, but instead reassessed annually in patients at risk for high-grade VIN. Reassessment may include gross inspection or vulvoscopy and biopsy as clinically indicated if high-grade neoplasia is suspected.

VIN 2 and 3

With rare exception, high-grade VIN is treated (American College of Obstetricians and Gynecologists, 2014b). Standard treatment of high-grade lesions of the vulva consists of local destruction or excision. Medical management is currently limited (Pepas, 2011). VIN involving the hair-bearing areas of the vulva (external to Hart line) may extend deeper into pilosebaceous units, whereas mucosal lesions tend to be more superficial (Wright, 1992). VIN involves the pilosebaceous units in up to two thirds of cases, but rarely exceeds 2.5 mm in depth from the epidermal surface (Shatz, 1989). This is important for disease management, particularly if ablative procedures are considered. Regardless of the modality selected, treatment side effects are common and can include vulvar discomfort, poor wound healing, infection, and scarring that may result in chronic pain or dyspareunia. Thus, treatment objectives include: (1) improving patient symptoms, (2) preserving the appearance and function of the vulva, and (3) excluding and preventing invasive disease.

Wide local excision (WLE) with a surgical margin of at least 5 mm of normal tissue is preferred for large VIN lesions in which the possibility of invasive carcinoma cannot be excluded. Because disease recurrence is related to surgical margin status, frozen section histology of the specimen margins is advantageous (Friedrich, 1980; Jones, 2005). Hopkins (2001) reported disease recurrence rates of 20 percent for cases with negative surgical margins but 40 percent for those with positive margins. WLE can be disfiguring and may require plastic surgical techniques or skin grafting to minimize anatomic distortion, pain, and loss of function. Moreover, due to disease location, some patients are best treated by combined excisional and ablative procedures.

Laser ablation of VIN provides good cosmetic results, and the depth of tissue destruction can be adjusted for hair-bearing areas. However, CO_2 lesion ablation does not allow evaluation of a surgical specimen. Therefore, invasive carcinoma must be excluded beforehand by adequate biopsy. Laser is generally less disfiguring than WLE but can result in prolonged, painful healing. Preoperative counseling regarding anticipated postoperative results mirrors that for WLE. VIN recurrence has been reported more commonly following laser vaporization than after WLE (Herod, 1996). However, Hoffman (1992b) reported that 15 of 18 patients (83 percent) with VIN 3 remained free of recurrent disease after CO_2 laser ablation.

Cavitational ultrasonic surgical aspiration (CUSA) may be used to treat VIN confined solely to non-hair-bearing vulvar skin. Ultrasound is used to cause cavitation and disruption of affected tissue, which is then aspirated and collected (Section 43-28, p. 996). CUSA offers the advantages of laser, less scarring and pain than WLE, while additionally providing a pathologic specimen (von Gruenigen, 2007). However, the tissue specimen is fragmented and lacks the diagnostic accuracy of surgically excised tissue. Miller (2002) evaluated CUSA in 37 patients with VIN 2/3. They found an overall recurrence rate of 35 percent within a mean of 33 months.

Topical therapy can be considered if there is no concern for invasive cancer, the patient is able to self-administer the topical medication correctly, and the importance of compliance to follow-up is understood. No topical agent is FDA-approved specifically for the treatment of VIN. Cidofovir cream must be compounded. 5-FU is potentially caustic and teratogenic and is not a first-line choice for VIN treatment (National Cancer Institute, 2015b). The clinical efficacy of these two agents has not been demonstrated in clinical trials, and they are generally no longer used (American College of Obstetricians and Gynecologists, 2014b). Topical imiquimod (off-label) has garnered the most interest. It has lower toxicity, and numerous studies including two randomized controlled trials have reported favorable regression rates of high-grade VIN (Mahto, 2010; van Seters, 2008). A phase II study on the use of imiquimod in treating VIN 2/3 found a response rate of 77 percent and 20 percent recurrence rate compared with a recurrence rate of 53 percent in a surgically treated cohort (Le, 2007). The use of topical imiquimod for the treatment of lower genital tract neoplasia was recently reviewed by de Witte and colleagues (2015).

■ Prognosis and Prevention

Case reports exist describing the invasive potential of untreated, high-grade VIN (Jones, 2005). Jones and associates (1994) reviewed the outcome of 113 patients with VIN 3. They found that 87 percent of untreated patients progressed to vulvar cancer, whereas only 3.8 percent of treated patients progressed to invasive carcinoma. It is currently not possible to predict high-grade VIN lesion behavior. Regardless of the treatment modality chosen, recurrence is common (up to 50 percent), particularly in patients with multifocal disease or immune compromise. Indefinite surveillance for multifocal LGT disease is recommended. Moreover, some consider high-grade VIN to be an indication for colposcopic evaluation of the cervix and vagina regardless of normal cervical cytology. Posttreatment surveillance consists of careful vulvar reevaluation at 6 and 12 months and annual vulvar inspection thereafter (American College of Obstetricians and Gynecologists, 2014b).

For prevention, prophylactic HPV vaccination against types 16 and 18 has the potential to prevent approximately one third of vulvar cancers (Smith, 2009). Smoking cessation and optimization of compromised immune status are also important strategies.

ANAL INTRAEPITHELIAL NEOPLASIA

Pathophysiology

In 2015, 4630 new anal cancers and 610 anal cancer deaths are predicted for U.S. women, and this cancer's incidence and mortality rates have risen since 1975 (American Cancer Society, 2015). Anal cancer is strongly associated with anal intraepithelial neoplasia (AIN) (Palefsky, 1994). Studies also continue to suggest an association between high-risk cervical HPV infection, abnormal anal cytology, and anal cancer (Lamme, 2014; Sehnal, 2014; Valari, 2011). Santoso and associates (2010) reported a 12-percent prevalence of biopsy-proven AIN in a group of women with HPV-related disease. As with cervical cancers, HPV types 16 and 18 are the principal etiologic agents (Zbar, 2002).

Little is known of the natural history of anal HPV infection and its progressive potential in women, but it is suspected to behave similarly to cervicovaginal lesions. Cervical and anal lesions generally are manifested at or near their respective squamocolumnar epithelial junctions, which is called the *transition zone* in the anal canal (Goldstone, 2001). Anal disease is classified by the same cytologic and histologic nomenclature used to describe cervical disease. Thus, AIN 1, 2, and 3 correspond to mild, moderate, and severe dysplasia, respectively (Fig. 29-20). The newer nomenclature for squamous neoplasia throughout the anogenital tract replaces AIN 1 with anal LSIL, and AIN 2/3 with anal HSIL (Darragh, 2012).

Risk factors for AIN include anal HPV infection, receptive anal intercourse, tobacco smoking, and history of other STDs, including HIV. Anal cancer and its likely precursor, AIN 3, are increasing at higher rates in the HIV-positive compared with the HIV-negative population (Heard, 2015; Tandon, 2010).

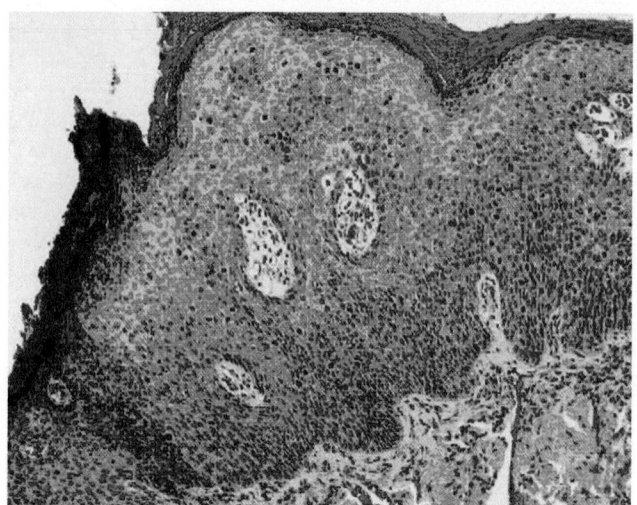

FIGURE 29-20 High-grade anal intraepithelial neoplasia (AIN) histology. (Used with permission from Dr. Raheela Ashfaq.)

Diagnosis

Currently, neither the American College of Obstetricians and Gynecologists nor the USPSTF provides screening recommendations for AIN in women. Potential approaches include periodic testing with anal cytology, HPV testing, or anoscopy, or a combination of these. Some suggest that annual cervical and anal cytology should be offered to all HIV-positive women, but only if the infrastructure necessary to evaluate and manage abnormal cytology results and precancerous lesions is available (Palefsky, 2005; Panther, 2005). For the generalist, patients may be referred to tertiary care centers or colorectal surgeons.

Anal cytology as a screening test has uncertain efficacy for AIN and anal cancer (Nahas, 2009; Santoso, 2010). If used, anal cytology may be more sensitive using liquid-based preparations than conventional glass slides (Friedlander, 2004; Sherman, 1995). Sampling is obtained by inserting a Dacron swab or endocervical brush moistened with water or a small amount of water-based lubricant approximately 5 cm into the anal canal, presumed above the anal transformation zone. The device is then withdrawn with a twirling motion while applying lateral pressure to the anal canal walls. The swab is then either swirled in the cytology solution to release exfoliated cells or smeared on a glass slide and fixed with isopropyl alcohol as with cervical cytology. Nothing per rectum is recommended 24 hours prior to an anal cytology test. Anal cytology may be reported using terminology analogous to the Bethesda 2001 nomenclature for cervical cytology.

High-resolution anoscopy uses illumination and magnification provided by a colposcope. Anoscopy is more challenging to perform than colposcopy for both patient and the provider, and special training is recommended. Acetic acid is applied to evaluate the anal canal in a manner similar to colposcopy (Fig. 29-21) (Jay, 1997). Anal neoplasia demonstrates colposcopic features similar to those of CIN, and analogous lesion grading and terminology are used. Biopsies are directed at the most abnormal areas. Some consider high-resolution anoscopy to be the gold standard for diagnosing AIN, but its role for primary screening or for the evaluation of abnormal anal cytology is not yet defined. It is presently available in a limited number of health centers.

Management

The benefits of screening for, identification of, and eradication of anal cancer precursor lesions are currently under investigation, and clinical guidelines are not yet unavailable. Some suggest that eradication of high-grade anal lesions may decrease the incidence of invasive anal cancer (Santoso, 2010). However, in contrast to cervical neoplasia, the protective effect of treating precursor lesions of the anal canal remains unproven (Williams, 1994; Scholefield, 2005). Thus, decisions regarding screening for and managing AIN should be shared by provider and patient on an individual basis. Abnormal anal cytology is best evaluated with high-resolution anoscopy. High-grade AIN lesions are referred to appropriate specialists for possible excision or ablative procedures.

Treatment is restricted to locally ablative or excisional procedures that eliminate individual high-grade intraepithelial lesions. Unlike the cervix, the entire anal squamocolumnar junction cannot be destroyed or removed due to potential morbidity.

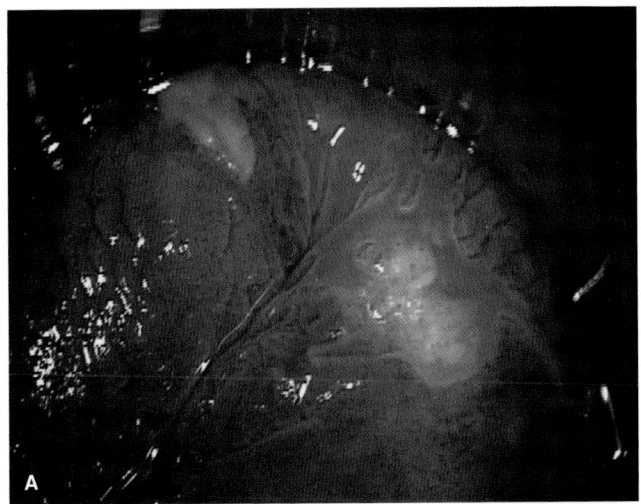

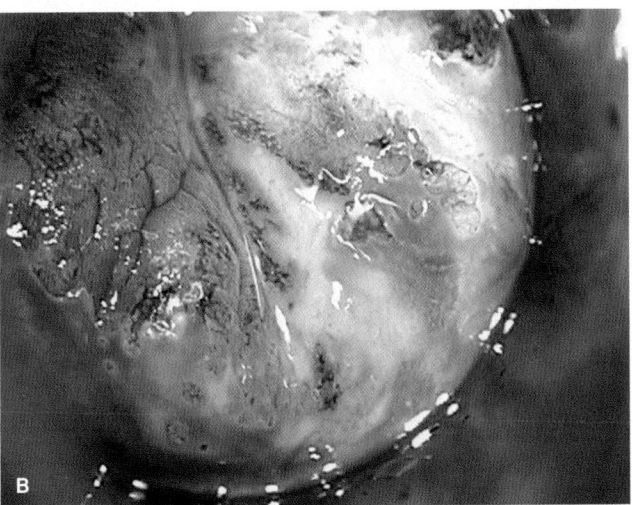

FIGURE 29-21 A. Translucent acetowhite lesion of low-grade anal intraepithelial neoplasia (AIN). **B.** Dense acetowhite lesion of high-grade AIN. (Used with permission from Naomi Jay, RN NP PhD.)

Biopsy-proven high-grade AIN lesions can be ablated using CO_2 laser or electrosurgical coagulation performed under general anesthesia, or infrared coagulation as an office procedure (Chang, 2002; Goldstone, 2005). Cryoablation and topically applied 85-percent trichloroacetic acid are other alternatives. Finally, as prevention, the FDA (2010) has approved both the quadrivalent (Gardasil) and nonavalent HPV (Gardasil 9) vaccines for the prevention of anal cancer and precancerous lesions associated with HPV types 6, 11, 16, and 18 in both males and females.

HIV-INFECTED PATIENTS

HIV-infected women have a high burden of HPV-associated anogenital disease. In this population, up to 60 percent of Pap tests are abnormal, and up to 40 percent have colposcopic evidence of dysplasia. Compared with rates in HIV-uninfected women, HIV-infected women show higher rates of both CIN and VIN (Ellerbrock, 2000; Spitzer, 1999; Wright, 1994). Moreover, abnormal cervical cytology and/or cervical HPV results increase risks for anal HPV infection and anal neoplasia (Tandon, 2010; Heard, 2015). The risks of all HPV-associated

cancers of the vulva, vagina, and anus appear to increase during the period from 5 years before to 5 years after HIV seroconversion (Chaturvedi, 2009).

HIV infection influences LGT disease prognosis. For example, during the early years of the acquired immunodeficiency disease (AIDS) epidemic, Maiman and colleagues (1990) observed 100-percent mortality rates in HIV-positive women with cervical cancer compared with only 37 percent of HIV-negative women in a study cohort. Because of the increased risk of cervical cancer and poorer prognosis, cervical cancer was designated as an AIDS-defining condition. Fortunately, HIV-infected women who receive regular screening and recommended follow-up for CIN experience the same incidence of invasive cervical cancer as do HIV-negative women (Massad, 2009).

Because of a significantly higher risk of developing SIL, cervical cytologic screening is obtained every 6 months for the first year after an HIV infection diagnosis (Centers for Disease Control and Prevention, 2015). Thereafter, indefinite annual screening is recommended (American College of Obstetricians and Gynecologists, 2012a; Kaplan, 2009). In addition, women with HIV may benefit from anal Pap screening (Palefsky, 2001). However, evidence-based screening recommendations for AIN and anal cancer are not yet available. Women with HIV infection are routinely questioned about anorectal symptoms such as pain or bleeding and provided periodic digital rectal examinations.

The 2012 Consensus Guidelines recommend that Pap test abnormalities, including ASC-US, in HIV-positive women be managed as in the general population (Massad, 2013). However, the Centers for Disease Control and Prevention has questioned the utility of HPV testing for the triage of ASC-US in this group and thus recommends that all HIV-positive women with ASC-US results be referred for colposcopy (Kaplan, 2009). Because HIV-positive women with CIN are often found to have extensive, multifocal dysplastic epithelial disease, any colposcopic examination includes inspection of the entire LGT (Hillemanns, 1996; Tandon, 2010).

HIV-positive women are at higher risk of disease persistence, recurrence, and progression after CIN or VIN treatment, and poorer outcomes appear to correlate with degree of immune suppression. Cryotherapy for CIN has a particularly high failure rate among treatment methods (Korn, 1996; Spitzer, 1999). Additionally, ablative modalities have an increased risk of obscuring occult invasive cancer in high-grade lesions. Cervical excisional procedures including loop excision and cold-knife conization provide histologic confirmation and margins for evaluation. Although excisional therapy is effective for eradicating CIN in immune competent patients, the same treatment may be effective only in preventing progression to cancer in HIV-infected women (Heard, 2005).

The therapeutic impact of highly active antiretroviral therapy (HAART) on HPV infection is poorly understood, and results are conflicting (Heard, 2004). To date, HAART has not been shown consistently to improve the natural history of HPV-related diseases. In fact, anal cancer rates in HIV-infected individuals have continued to increase over the past decade (De Vuyst, 2008; Tandon, 2010). Indeed, if HAART does not alter the incidence or progression of HPV-related disease, individuals on

HAART may gain sufficient longevity to develop HPV-related epithelial cancers (de Sanjose, 2002).

REFERENCES

Alemany L, Saunier M, Tinoco L, et al: Large contribution of human papillomavirus in vaginal neoplastic lesions: a worldwide study in 597 samples. Eur J Cancer 50(16):2846, 2014

Ali H, Donovan B, Wand H, et al: Genital warts in young Australians five years into national human papillomavirus vaccination programme: national surveillance data. BMJ 346:f2032, 2013

Amburgey CF, VanEenwyk J, Davis FG, et al: Undernutrition as a risk factor for cervical intraepithelial neoplasia: a case-control analysis. Nutr Cancer 20(1):51, 1993

American Cancer Society: Estimated number of new cancer cases and deaths by sex, US, 2015. Available at: http://www.cancer.org/acs/groups/content/@editorial/documents/document/acspc-044514.pdf. Accessed April 9, 2015

American College of Obstetricians and Gynecologists: Gynecologic care for women with human immunodeficiency virus. Practice Bulletin No. 117, December 2010, Reaffirmed 2012a

American College of Obstetricians and Gynecologists: Human papillomavirus vaccination. Committee Opinion No. 588, March 2014a

American College of Obstetricians and Gynecologists: Management of abnormal cervical cancer screening results and cervical cancer precursors. Practice Bulletin No. 140, December, 2013

American College of Obstetricians and Gynecologists: Management of vulvar intraepithelial neoplasia. Committee Opinion No. 509, November 2011, Reaffirmed 2014b

American College of Obstetricians and Gynecologists: Screening for cervical cancer. Practice Bulletin No. 131, November 2012b

Baseman JG, Koutsky LA: The epidemiology of human papillomavirus infections. J Clin Virol 32(Suppl 1):S16, 2005

Benard VB, Coughlin SS, Thompson T, et al: Cervical cancer incidence in the United States by area of residence, 1998-2001. Obstet Gynecol 110:681, 2007

Benedet JL, Sanders BH: Carcinoma in situ of the vagina. Am J Obstet Gynecol 148(5):695, 1984

Bergeron C, Ferenczy A, Richart RM, et al: Micropapillomatosis labialis appears unrelated to human papillomavirus. Obstet Gynecol 76(2):281, 1990

Bornstein J, Bentley J, Bösze P, et al. 2011 colposcopic terminology of the International Federation for Cervical Pathology and Colposcopy. Obstet Gynecol 120(3):166, 2012

Bosch FX, Burchell AN, Schiffman M, et al: Epidemiology and natural history of human papillomavirus infections and type-specific implications in cervical neoplasia. Vaccine 265:K1, 2008

Brinton LA, Reeves WC, Brenes MM, et al: Parity as a risk factor for cervical cancer. Am J Epidemiol 130:486, 1989

Brown DR, Shew ML, Qadadri B, et al: A longitudinal study of genital human papillomavirus infection in a cohort of closely followed adolescent women. J Infect Dis 191(2):182, 2005

Bruinsma F, Lumley J, Tan J, et al: Precancerous changes in the cervix and risk of subsequent preterm birth. BJOG 114:70, 2007

Bruni L, Diaz M, Castellsagué X, et al: Cervical human papillomavirus prevalence in 5 continents: meta-analysis of 1 million women with normal cytological findings. J Infect Dis 202(12):1789, 2010

Buckley JD, Harris RW, Doll R, et al: Case-control study of the husbands of women with dysplasia or carcinoma of the cervix uteri. Lancet 2(8254):1010, 1981

Burk RD, Ho GY, Beardsley L, et al: Sexual behavior and partner characteristics are the predominant risk factors for genital human papillomavirus infection in young women. J Infect Dis 174(4):679, 1996

Case AS, Rocconi RP, Straughn JM Jr, et al: Cervical intraepithelial neoplasia in adolescent women. Obstet Gynecol 108:1369, 2006

Castellsagué X, Diaz M, de Sanjosé S, et al: Worldwide human papillomavirus etiology of cervical adenocarcinoma and its cofactors: implications for screening and prevention. J Natl Cancer Inst 98:303, 2006

Castle PE: Beyond human papillomavirus: the cervix, exogenous secondary factors, and the development of cervical precancer and cancer. J Low Genit Tract Dis 8(3):224, 2004

Castle PE, Fetterman B, Poitras N, et al: Five-year experience of human papillomavirus DNA and Papanicolaou test cotesting. Obstet Gynecol 113:595, 2009a

Castle PE, Fetterman B, Poitras N, et al: Relationship of atypical glandular cell cytology, age, and human papillomavirus detection to cervical and endometrial cancer risks. Obstet Gynecol 115:243, 2010

Castle PE, Hunt WC, Langsfeld E, et al: Three-year risk of cervical precancer and cancer after the detection of low-risk human papillomavirus genotypes targeted by a commercial test. Obstet Gynecol 123:49, 2014

Castle PE, Schiffman M, Wheeler CM, et al: Evidence for frequent regression of cervical intraepithelial neoplasia-grade 2. Obstet Gynecol 113:18, 2009b

Castle PE, Stoler MH, Wright TC, et al: Performance of carcinogenic human papillomavirus (HPV) testing and HPV16 or HPV18 genotyping for cervical cancer screening of women aged 25 years and older: a subanalysis of the ATHENA study. Lancet Oncol 12:880, 2011

Castle PE, Walker JL, Schiffman M, et al: Hormonal contraceptive use, pregnancy and parity, and the risk of cervical intraepithelial neoplasia 3 among oncogenic HPV DNA-positive women with equivocal or mildly abnormal cytology. Int J Cancer 117(6):1007, 2005

Centers for Disease Control and Prevention: Sexually transmitted diseases treatment guidelines, 2010. MMWR 59(12):1, 2010

Centers for Disease Control and Prevention: Sexually transmitted diseases treatment guidelines, 2015. MMWR 64(3):1, 2015

Chang GJ, Berry JM, Jay N, et al: Surgical treatment of high-grade anal squamous intraepithelial lesions: a prospective study. Dis Colon Rectum 45(4):453, 2002

Chappell CA, West AM, Kabbani W, et al: Off-label high-risk HPV DNA testing of vaginal ASC-US and LSIL cytologic abnormalities at Parkland Hospital. J Low Genit Tract Dis 14(4):352, 2010

Chaturvedi AK, Madeleine MM, Biggar RJ: et al: Risk of human papillomavirus-associated cancers among persons with AIDS. J Natl Cancer Inst 101(16):1120, 2009

Cohen BA, Honig P, Androphy E: Anogenital warts in children. Clinical and virologic evaluation for sexual abuse. Arch Dermatol 126(12):1575, 1990

Collins S, Mazloomzadeh S, Winter H, et al: High incidence of cervical human papillomavirus infection in women during their first sexual relationship. BJOG 109(1):96, 2002

Conner SN, Frey H, Cahill AG, et al: Loop electrosurgical excision procedure and risk of preterm birth: a systematic review and meta-analysis. Obstet Gynecol 123(4):752, 2014

Coppleson M, Dalrymple JC, Atkinson KH: Colposcopic differentiation of abnormalities arising in the transformation zone. Obstet Gynecol Clin North Am 20(1):83, 1993

Cuzick J, Clavel C, Petry KU, et al: Overview of the European and North American studies on HPV testing in primary cervical cancer screening. Int J Cancer 119:1095, 2006

Darragh TM, Colga TJ, Cox JT, et al: The lower anogenital squamous terminology standardization project for HPV-associated lesions: background and consensus recommendations from the College of American Pathologists and the American Society for Colposcopy and Cervical Pathology. J Low Genit Tract Dis 16(3):205, 2012

Datta SD, Koutsky LA, Ratelle S, et al: Human papillomavirus infection and cervical cytology in women screened for cervical cancer in the United States, 2003-2005. Ann Intern Med 148:493, 2008

Davey DD, Goulart R, Nayar, et al: Statement on human papillomavirus DNA test utilization. Am J Clin Pathol 141:459, 2014

Del Pino M, Rodriguez-Carunchio L, Ordi J: Pathways of vulvar intraepithelial neoplasia and squamous cell carcinoma. Histopathology 62(1):161, 2013

de Oliveira ER, Derchain SF, Sarian LO, et al: Prediction of high-grade cervical disease with human papillomavirus detect in women with glandular and squamous cytologic abnormalities. Int J Gynecol Cancer 16:1055, 2006

de Sanjose S, Palefsky J: Cervical and anal HPV infections in HIV positive women and men. Virus Res 89(2):201, 2002

de Sanjose S, Quint WG, Alemany L, et al: Human papillomavirus genotype attribution in invasive cancer: a retrospective cross-sectional worldwide study. Lancet Oncol 11(11):1048, 2010

de Vet HC, Sturmans F: Risk factors for cervical dysplasia: implications for prevention. Public Health 108(4):241, 1994

de Villiers EM: Relationship between steroid hormone contraceptives and HPV, cervical intraepithelial neoplasia and cervical carcinoma. Int J Cancer 103(6):705, 2003

De Vuyst H, Lillo F, Broutet N, et al: HIV, human papillomavirus, and cervical neoplasia and cancer in the era of highly active antiretroviral therapy. Eur J Cancer Prev 17:545, 2008

de Witte CJ, van de Sande AJ, van Beekhuizen HJ, et al: Imiquimod in cervical, vaginal, and vulvar intraepithelial neoplasia: a review. Gynecol Oncol 139(2):377, 2015

Diakomanolis E, Stefanidis K, Rodolakis A, et al: Vaginal intraepithelial neoplasia: report of 102 cases. Eur J Gynaecol Oncol 23(5):457, 2002

Dillner J: Primary human papillomavirus testing in organized cervical screening. Curr Opin Obstet Gynecol 25:11, 2013

Dillner J: The serological response to papillomaviruses. Semin Cancer Biol 9(6):423, 1999

Dodge JA, Eltabbakh GH, Mount SL, et al: Clinical features and risk of recurrence among patients with vaginal intraepithelial neoplasia. Gynecol Oncol 83(2):363, 2001

Doerfler D, Bernhaus A, Kottmel A, et al: Human papilloma virus infection prior to coitarche. Am J Obstet Gynecol 200:487.e1, 2009

Doorbar J, Quint W, Banks L, et al: The biology and life-cycle of human papillomaviruses. Vaccine 30(Suppl 5):F55, 2012

Dunne EF, Markowitz LE, Saraiya M, et al: CDC Grand Rounds: reducing the burden of HPV-associated cancer and disease. MMWR 63(4):69, 2014

Dunne EF, Unger ER, Sternberg M, et al: Prevalence of HPV infection among females in the United States. JAMA 297:813, 2007

Durst M, Kleinheinz A, Hotz M, et al: The physical state of human papillomavirus type 16 DNA in benign and malignant genital tumours. J Gen Virol 66(Pt 7):1515, 1985

Economos K, Perez Veridiano N, Delke I, et al: Abnormal cervical cytology in pregnancy: a 17-year experience. Obstet Gynecol 81(6):915, 1993

Ellerbrock TV, Chiasson MA, Bush TJ, et al: Incidence of cervical squamous intraepithelial lesions in HIV-infected women. JAMA 283(8):1031, 2000

Fairley CK, Chen S, Ugoni A, et al: Human papillomavirus infection and its relationship to recent and distant sexual partners. Obstet Gynecol 84(5):755, 1994

Feng Q, Kiviat NB: New and surprising insights into pathogenesis of multicentric squamous cancers in the female lower genital tract. J Natl Cancer Inst 97:1798, 2005

Ferris DG, Cox JT, O'Connor DM: The biology and significance of human papillomavirus infection. In Haefner HK, Krumholz BA, Massad LS (eds): Modern Colposcopy. Dubuque, Kendall/Hunt Publishing Company, 2004, p 454

Ferris DG, Litaker M: Interobserver agreement for colposcopy quality control using digitized colposcopic images during the ALTS trial. J Low Genit Tract Dis 9(1):29, 2005

Ferris D, Samakoses R, Block SL, et al: Long-term study of a quadrivalent human papillomavirus vaccine. Pediatrics 134:e657, 2014

Fitzhugh VA, Heller DS: Significance of a diagnosis of microorganisms on Pap smear. J Low Genit Tract Dis 12(1):40, 2008

Food and Drug Administration: Gardasil approved to prevent anal cancer. FDA News Release, December 22, 2010

Franco EL, Villa LL, Ruiz A, et al: Transmission of cervical human papillomavirus infection by sexual activity: differences between low and high oncogenic risk types. J Infect Dis 172(3):756, 1995

Friedlander MA, Stier E, Lin O: Anorectal cytology as a screening tool for anal squamous lesions: cytologic, anoscopic, and histologic correlation. Cancer 102(1):19, 2004

Friedrich EG Jr, Wilkinson EJ, Fu YS: Carcinoma in situ of the vulva: a continuing challenge. Am J Obstet Gynecol 136(7):830, 1980

Future II Study Group: Quadrivalent vaccine against human papillomavirus to prevent high-grade cervical lesions. N Engl J Med 356(19):1915, 2007

Gage JC, Anson VW, Abbey K, et al: Number of cervical biopsies and sensitivity of colposcopy. Obstet Gynecol 108(2):264, 2006

Goldstone SE, Kawalek AZ, Huyett JW: Infrared coagulator: a useful tool for treating anal squamous intraepithelial lesions. Dis Colon Rectum 48(5):1042, 2005

Goldstone SE, Winkler B, Ufford LJ, et al: High prevalence of anal squamous intraepithelial lesions and squamous-cell carcinoma in men who have sex with men as seen in a surgical practice. Dis Colon Rectum 44(5):690, 2001

Gomez-Lobo V: Gynecologic care of the transplant recipient. Postgrad Obstet Gynecol 29(10):1, 2009

Griffith WF, Stuart GS, Gluck KL, et al: Vaginal speculum lubrication and its effects on cervical cytology and microbiology. Contraception 72:60, 2005

Haefner HK, Tate JE, McLachlin CM, et al: Vulvar intraepithelial neoplasia: age, morphological phenotype, papillomavirus DNA, and coexisting invasive carcinoma. Hum Pathol 26(2):147, 1995

Harmanli O, Jones KA: Using lubrication for speculum insertion. Obstet Gynecol 116(No. 2, Part 1):415, 2010

Harper DM, Franco EL, Wheeler CM, et al: Sustained efficacy up to 4.5 years of a bivalent L1 virus-like particle vaccine against human papillomavirus types 16 and 18: follow-up from a randomised control trial. Lancet 367(9518):1247, 2006

Harris TG, Miller L, Kulasingam SL, et al: Depot-medroxyprogesterone acetate and combined oral contraceptive use and cervical neoplasia among women with oncogenic human papillomavirus infection. Am J Obstet Gynecol 200:489.e1, 2009

Hart WR: Vulvar intraepithelial neoplasia: historical aspects and current status. Int J Gynecol Pathol 20(1):16, 2001

Heard I, Etienney I, Potard V, et al: High prevalence of anal human papillomavirus-associated cancer precursors in a contemporary cohort of asymptomatic HIV-infected women. Clin Infect Dis 60(10):1559, 2015

Heard I, Palefsky JM, Kazatchkine MD: The impact of HIV antiviral therapy on human papillomavirus (HPV) infections and HPV-related diseases. Antivir Ther 9(1):13, 2004

Heard I, Potard V, Foulot H, et al: High rate of recurrence of cervical intraepithelial neoplasia after surgery in HIV-positive women. J Acquir Immune Defic Syndr 39(4):412, 2005

Henk HJ, Insigna RP, Singhal PK, Darkow T: Incidence and costs of cervical intraepithelial neoplasia in a US commercially insured population. Low Genit Tract Dis 4(1):29, 2010

Herod JJ, Shafi MI, Rollason TP, et al: Vulvar intraepithelial neoplasia: long term follow up of treated and untreated women. BJOG 103(5):446, 1996

Herrero R, Hildesheim A, Bratti C, et al: Population-based study of human papillomavirus infection and cervical neoplasia in rural Costa Rica. J Natl Cancer Inst 92(6):464, 2000

Herzog TJ, Monk BJ: Reducing the burden of glandular carcinomas of the uterine cervix. Am J Obstet Gynecol 197(6):566, 2007

Hildesheim A, Hadjimichael O, Schwartz PE, et al: Risk factors for rapid-onset cervical cancer. Am J Obstet Gynecol 180(3 Pt 1):571, 1999

Hillemanns P, Ellerbrock TV, McPhillips S, et al: Prevalence of anal human papillomavirus infection and anal cytologic abnormalities in HIV-seropositive women. AIDS 10(14):1641, 1996

Ho GY, Bierman R, Beardsley L, et al: Natural history of cervicovaginal papillomavirus infection in young women. N Engl J Med 338(7):423, 1998

Ho GY, Burk RD, Klein S, et al: Persistent genital human papillomavirus infection as a risk factor for persistent cervical dysplasia. J Natl Cancer Inst 87(18):1365, 1995

Hoffman MS, DeCesare SL, Roberts WS, et al: Upper vaginectomy for in situ and occult, superficially invasive carcinoma of the vagina. Am J Obstet Gynecol 166(1 Pt 1):30, 1992a

Hoffman MS, Pinelli DM, Finan M, et al: Laser vaporization for vulvar intraepithelial neoplasia III. J Reprod Med 37(2):135, 1992b

Hoover RN, Hyer M, Pfeiffer RM, et al: Adverse health outcomes in women exposed in utero to diethylstilbestrol. N Engl J Med 365 (14): 1304, 2011

Hopkins MP, Nemunaitis-Keller J: Carcinoma of the vulva. Obstet Gynecol Clin North Am 28(4):791, 2001

Howe HL, Wingo PA, Thun MJ, et al: Annual report to the nation on the status of cancer (1973 through 1998), featuring cancers with recent increasing trends. J Natl Cancer Inst 93(11):824, 2001

Howlader N, Noone AM, Krapcho M, et al: SEER Cancer Statistics Review, 1975-2011. Bethesda, National Cancer Institute, 2014

Huh WK, Ault KA, Chelmow D, et al: Use of high-risk human papillomavirus testing for cervical cancer screening: interim clinical guidance. Obstet Gynecol 125(2):330, 2015

International Collaboration of Epidemiological Studies of Cervical Cancer: Cervical cancer and hormonal contraceptives: collaborative reanalysis of individual data for 16573 women with cervical cancer and 35509 women without cervical cancer from 24 epidemiological studies. Lancet 370:1609, 2007

Jakobsson M, Gissler M, Paavonen J, et al: Loop electrosurgical excision procedure and the risk for preterm birth. Obstet Gynecol 114:504, 2009

Jay N, Berry JM, Hogeboom CJ, et al: Colposcopic appearance of anal squamous intraepithelial lesions: relationship to histopathology. Dis Colon Rectum 40(8):919, 1997

Jeronimo J, Massad LS, Castle PE, et al: Interobserver agreement in the evaluation of digitized cervical images. Obstet Gynecol 110:833, 2007

Jones RW, Rowan DM: Vulvar intraepithelial neoplasia III: a clinical study of the outcome in 113 cases with relation to the later development of invasive vulvar carcinoma. Obstet Gynecol 84(5):741, 1994

Jones RW, Rowan DM, Stewart AW: Vulvar intraepithelial neoplasia: aspects of the natural history and outcome in 405 women. Obstet Gynecol 106(6):1319, 2005

Joura EA, Giuliano AR, Iversen OE, et al: A 9-valent HPV vaccine against infection and intraepithelial neoplasia in women. Broad Spectrum HPV Vaccine Study. N Engl J Med 372(8):711, 2015

Joura EA, Zeisler H, Losch A, et al: Differentiating vulvar intraepithelial neoplasia from nonneoplastic epithelial disorders. The toluidine blue test. J Reprod Med 43(8):671, 1998

Judson PL, Habermann EB, Baxter NN, et al: Trends in the incidence of invasive and in situ vulvar carcinoma. Obstet Gynecol 107:1018, 2006

Kaplan JE, Benson C, Holmes KH, et al: Guidelines for prevention and treatment of opportunistic infections in HIV-infected adults and adolescents. MMWR Recomm Rep 58(4):1, 2009

Khan MJ, Castle PE, Lorincz AT, et al: The elevated 10-year risk of cervical precancer and cancer in women with human papillomavirus (HPV) type 16 or 18 and the possible utility of type-specific HPV testing in clinical practice. J Natl Cancer Inst 97:1072, 2005

Khan MJ, Smith-McCune KK: Treatment of cervical precancers: back to basics. Obstet Gynecol 123(6):1339, 2014

Kinney WK, Manos MM, Hurley LB, et al: Where's the high-grade cervical neoplasia? The importance of minimally abnormal Papanicolaou diagnoses. Obstet Gynecol 91(6):973, 1998

Kiviat N: Natural history of cervical neoplasia: overview and update. Am J Obstet Gynecol 175(4 Pt 2):1099, 1996

Kjaer SK, de Villiers EM, Dahl C, et al: Case-control study of risk factors for cervical neoplasia in Denmark. I: role of the "male factor" in women with one lifetime sexual partner. Int J Cancer 48(1):39, 1991

Kjaer SK, van den Brule AJ, Paull G, et al: Type specific persistence of high risk human papillomavirus (HPV) as indicator of high grade cervical squamous intraepithelial lesions in young women: population based prospective follow up study. BMJ 325(7364):572, 2002

Korn AP, Abercrombie PD, Foster A: Vulvar intraepithelial neoplasia in women infected with human immunodeficiency virus-1. Gynecol Oncol 61:384, 1996

Kosary C: Cancer of the vagina. In Ries LAG, Young JL, Keel GE, et al (eds): SEER Survival Monograph: Cancer Survival Among Adults: U.S. SEER Program, 1988-2001, Patient and Tumor Characteristics. NIH Publication No. 07-6215, Bethesda, 2007

Koss LG: The Papanicolaou test for cervical cancer detection. A triumph and a tragedy. JAMA 261(5):737, 1989

Krebs HB: Treatment of vaginal intraepithelial neoplasia with laser and tropical 5-fluorouracil. Obstet Gynecol 73(4):657, 1989

Krivak TC, Rose GS, McBroom JW, et al: Cervical adenocarcinoma in situ: a systematic review of therapeutic options and predictors of persistent or recurrent disease. Obstet Gynecol Surv 56(9):567, 2001

Kurdgelashvili G, Dores GM, Srour SA, et al: Incidence of potentially human papillomavirus-related neoplasms in the United States, 1978 to 2007. Cancer 119(12):2291, 2013

Kyrgiou M, Koliopoulos G, Martin-Hirsch P, et al: Obstetric outcomes after conservative treatment for intraepithelial or early invasive cervical lesions: systematic review and meta-analysis. Lancet 367:489, 2006

Lamme J, Pattaratornkosohn T, Mercado-Abadie J, et al: Concurrent anal human papillomavirus and abnormal anal cytology in women with known cervical dysplasia. Obstet Gynecol 124(2Pt 1), 242, 2014

Le T, Menard C, Hicks-Boucher W, et al: Final results of a phase 2 study using continuous 5% imiquimod cream application in the primary treatment of high-grade vulva intraepithelial neoplasia. Gynecol Oncol 106(3):579, 2007

Mahto M, Nathan M, O'Maony C: More than a decade on: review of the use of imiquimod in lower anogenital intraepithelial neoplasia. Int J STD AIDS 21:8, 2010

Maiman M, Fruchter RG, Serur E, et al: Human immunodeficiency virus infection and cervical neoplasia. Gynecol Oncol 38:377, 1990

Markowitz LE, Dunne EF, Saraiya M, et al: Human papillomavirus vaccination: recommendations of the Advisory Committee on Immunization Practices (ACIP). MMWR 63(RR-05):1, 2014

Marrazzo JM, Stine K, Koutsky LA: Genital human papillomavirus infection in women who have sex with women: a review. Am J Obstet Gynecol 183(3):770, 2000

Martin-Hirsch PL, Paraskevaidis E, Bryant A: Surgery for cervical intraepithelial neoplasia. Cochrane Database Syst Rev 6:CD001318, 2013

Massad LS, Einstein MH, Huh WK, et al: 2012 Updated consensus guidelines for the management of abnormal cervical cancer screening tests and cancer precursors. J Low Genit Tract Dis 17(5):S1, 2013

Massad LS, Seaberg EC, Watts DH, et al: Long-term incidence of cervical cancer in women with human immunodeficiency virus. Cancer 115:524, 2009

Mayrand MH, Duarte-Franco E, Rodrigues I, et al: Human papillomavirus DNS versus Papanicolaou screening tests for cervical cancer. N Engl J Med 357(16):1579, 2007

McCredie MRE, Sharples KJ, Paul C, et al: Natural history of cervical neoplasia and risk of invasive cancer in women with cervical intraepithelial neoplasia 3: a retrospective cohort study. Lancet Oncol 9(5):425, 2008

Miller BE: Vulvar intraepithelial neoplasia treated with cavitational ultrasonic surgical aspiration. Gynecol Oncol 85(1):114, 2002

Molijn A, Kleter B, Quint W, et al: Molecular diagnosis of human papillomavirus (HPV) infections. J Clin Virol 32(Suppl 1):S43, 2005

Moore K, Cofer A, Elliot L, et al: Adolescent cervical dysplasia: histologic evaluation, treatment, and outcomes. Am J Obstet Gynecol 197:141.e1, 2007

Moyer VA: Screening for cervical cancer: U.S. Preventive Services Task Force recommendation statement. Ann Intern Med 156:880, 2012

Moscicki AB: Impact of HPV infection in adolescent populations. J Adolesc Health 37:S3, 2005

Moscicki AB, Ma Y, Wibbelsman C, et al: Rate of and risks for regression of cervical intraepithelial neoplasia 2 in adolescents and young women. Obstet Gynecol l16(6):1373, 2010

Moscicki AB, Ma Y, Wibbelsman C, et al: Risks for cervical intraepithelial neoplasia 3 among adolescents and young women with abnormal cytology. Obstet Gynecol 112:1335, 2008

Moscicki AB, Shiboski S, Broering J, et al: The natural history of human papillomavirus infection as measured by repeated DNA testing in adolescent and young women. J Pediatr 132(2):277, 1998

Moscicki AB, Shiboski S, Hills NK, et al: Regression of low-grade squamous intra-epithelial lesions in young women. Lancet 364(9446):1678, 2004

Muñoz N, Bosch FX, de Sanjose S, et al: Epidemiologic classification of human papillomavirus types associated with cervical cancer. N Engl J Med 348(6):518, 2003

Muñoz N, Franceschi S, Bosetti C, et al: Role of parity and human papillomavirus in cervical cancer: the IARC multicentric case-control study. Lancet 359:1093, 2002

Nahas CS, da Silva Filho EV, Segurado AA, et al: Screening anal dysplasia in HIV-infected patients: is there an agreement between anal Pap smear and high-resolution anoscopy-guided biopsy? Dis Colon Rectum 52:1854, 2009

National Cancer Institute: Cervical cancer screening PDQ®. 2015a. Available at: http://cancer.gov/cancertopics/pdq/screening/cervical/HealthProfessional. Accessed April 9, 2015

National Cancer Institute: Vulvar cancer treatment PDQ®. 2015b. Available at: http://www.cancer.gov/cancertopics/pdq/treatment/vulvar/HealthProfessional. Accessed April 9, 2015

National Cancer Institute Workshop: The 1988 Bethesda system for reporting cervical/vaginal cytological diagnoses. JAMA 262(7):931, 1989

Nayar R, Wilbur DC: The Pap test and Bethesda 2014. Cancer Cytopathol 123(5):271, 2015

Obalek S, Jablonska S, Favre M, et al: Condylomata acuminata in children: frequent association with human papillomaviruses responsible for cutaneous warts. J Am Acad Dermatol 23(2 Pt 1):205, 1990

Ostor AG: Natural history of cervical intraepithelial neoplasia: a critical review. Int J Gynecol Pathol 12(2):186, 1993

Paavonen J, Koutsky LA, Kiviat N: Cervical neoplasia and other STD related genital and anal neoplasias. In Holmes KK, Mardh PA, Sparling PG, et al (eds): Sexually Transmitted Diseases, 2nd ed. New York, McGraw-Hill, 1990, p 561

Paavonen J, Naud P, Salmerón J, et al: Efficacy of human papillomavirus (HPV)-16/18 AS04-adjuvanted vaccine against cervical infection and precancer caused by oncogenic HPV types (PATRICIA): final analysis of a double-blind, randomized study in young women. Lancet 374:301, 2009

Palefsky JM: Anal human papillomavirus infection and anal cancer in HIV-positive individuals: an emerging problem. AIDS 8:283, 1994

Palefsky JM, Holly EA, Efirdc JT, et al: Anal intraepithelial neoplasia in the highly active antiretroviral therapy era among HIV-positive men who have sex with men. AIDS 19(13):1407, 2005

Palefsky JM, Holly EA, Ralston ML, et al: Prevalence and risk factors for anal human papillomavirus infection in human immunodeficiency virus (HIV)-positive and high-risk HIV-negative women. J Infect Dis 183(3):383, 2001

Panther LA, Schlecht HP, Dezube BJ: Spectrum of human papillomavirus-related dysplasia and carcinoma of the anus in HIV-infected patients. AIDS Read 15(2):79, 2005

Pepas L, Kaushik S, Bryant A, et al: Medical interventions for high grade vulvar intraepithelial neoplasia. Cochrane Database Syst Rev 4:CD007924, 2011

Paraskevaidis E, Jandial L, Mann E, et al: Pattern of treatment failure following laser for cervical intraepithelial neoplasia: implications for follow-up protocol. Obstet Gynecol 78:80, 1991

Perrotta M, Marchitelli CE, Velazco AF, et al: Use of CO_2 laser vaporization for the treatment of high-grade vaginal intraepithelial neoplasia. J Low Genit Tract Dis 17(1):23, 2013

Petrosky E, Bocchini JA, Harri S, et al: Use of 9-valent human papillomavirus (HPV) vaccine: updated HPV vaccination recommendations of the advisory committee on immunization practices. MMWR 64(11):w300, 2015

Plummer M, Herrero R, Franceschi S, et al: Smoking and cervical cancer: pooled analysis of the IARC multi-centric case-control study. Cancer Causes Control 14(9):805, 2003

Pretorius RG, Zhang WH, Belinson JL, et al: Colposcopically directed biopsy, random cervical biopsy, and endocervical curettage in the diagnosis of cervical intraepithelial neoplasia II or worse. Am J Obstet Gynecol 191:430, 2004

Punnonen R, Kallioniemi OP, Mattila J, et al: Primary invasive and in situ vaginal carcinoma. Flow cytometric analysis of DNA aneuploidy and cell proliferation from archival paraffin-embedded tissue. Eur J Obstet Gynecol Reprod Biol 32(3):247, 1989

Reid R, Scalzi P: Genital warts and cervical cancer. VII. An improved colposcopic index for differentiating benign papillomaviral infections from high-grade cervical intraepithelial neoplasia. Am J Obstet Gynecol 153(6):611, 1985

Remmink AJ, Walboomers JM, Helmerhorst TJ, et al: The presence of persistent high-risk HPV genotypes in dysplastic cervical lesions is associated with progressive disease: natural history up to 36 months. Int J Cancer 61(3):306, 1995

Rome RM, England PG: Management of vaginal intraepithelial neoplasia: a series of 132 cases with long-term follow-up. Int J Gynecol Cancer 10:382, 2000

Ronco G, Giorgi-Rossi P, Carozzi F, et al: Efficacy of human papillomavirus testing for the detection of invasive cervical cancers and cervical intraepithelial neoplasia: a randomized controlled trial. Lancet Oncol 11:249, 2010

Ronco G, Segnan N, Giorgi-Rossi P, et al: Human papillomavirus testing and liquid-based cytology: results at recruitment from the new technologies for cervical cancer randomized controlled trial. J Natl Cancer Inst 98(11):765, 2006

Rosales R, Rosales C: Immune therapy for human papillomavirus-related cancers. World J Clin Oncol 5(5):1002, 2014

Rosenfeld WD, Rose E, Vermund SH, et al: Follow-up evaluation of cervicovaginal human papillomavirus infection in adolescents. J Pediatr 121(2):307, 1992

Sadler L, Saftlas A, Wang W, et al: Treatment for cervical intraepithelial neoplasia and risk of preterm delivery. JAMA 291:2100, 2004

Samson SL, Bentley JR, Fahey TJ, et al: The effect of loop electrosurgical excision procedure on future pregnancy outcome. Obstet Gynecol 105:325, 2005

Sankaranarayanan R, Nene BM, Shastri SS, et al: Screening for cervical cancer in rural India. N Engl J Med 360:1385, 2009

Santoso J, Long M, Crigger M, et al: Anal intraepithelial neoplasia in women with genital intraepithelial neoplasia. Obstet Gynecol 116(3):578, 2010

Sapp M, Bienkowska-Haba M: Viral entry mechanisms: human papillomavirus and a long journey from extracellular matrix to the nucleus. FEBS J 276:7206, 2009

Saslow D, Solomon D, Lawson HW, et al: American Cancer Society, American Society for Colposcopy and Cervical Pathology, and American Society for Clinical Pathology screening guidelines for the prevention and early detection of cervical cancer. CA Cancer 62(3):147, 2012

Schiffman M, Wentzensen N: From human papillomavirus to cervical cancer. Obstet Gynecol 116(1):177, 2010

Schlecht NF, Platt RW, Duarte-Franco E, et al: Human papillomavirus infection and time to progression and regression of cervical intraepithelial neoplasia. J Natl Cancer Inst 95(17):1336, 2003

Schnatz PF, Guile M, O'Sullivan DM, et al: Clinical significance of atypical glandular cells on cervical cytology. Obstet Gynecol 107:701, 2006

Schockaert S, Poppe W, Arbyn M, et al: Incidence of vaginal intraepithelial neoplasia after hysterectomy for cervical intraepithelial neoplasia: a retrospective study. Am J Obstet Gynecol 199:113.e1, 2008

Scholefield JH, Castle MT, Watson NF: Malignant transformation of high-grade anal intraepithelial neoplasia. Br J Surg 92(9):1133, 2005

Schorge JO, Lea JS, Ashfaq R: Postconization surveillance of cervical adenocarcinoma in situ: a prospective trial. J Reprod Med 48(10):751, 2003

Sehnal B, Dusek L, Cibula D, et al: The relationship between the cervical and anal HPV infection in women with cervical intraepithelial neoplasia. J Clin Virol 59(1):18, 2014

Shanbhag S, Clark H, Timmaraju V, et al: Pregnancy outcome after treatment for cervical intraepithelial neoplasia. Obstet Gynecol 114:727, 2009

Shatz P, Bergeron C, Wilkinson EJ, et al: Vulvar intraepithelial neoplasia and skin appendage involvement. Obstet Gynecol 74(5):769, 1989

Sherman ME, Friedman HB, Busseniers AE, et al: Cytologic diagnosis of anal intraepithelial neoplasia using smears and cytyc thin-preps. Mod Pathol 8(3):270, 1995

Sideri M, Jones RW, Wilkinson EJ, et al: Squamous vulvar intraepithelial neoplasia: 2004 modified terminology, ISSVD Vulvar Oncology Subcommittee. J Reprod Med 50(11):807, 2005

Siegfried EC, Frasier LD: Anogenital warts in children. Adv Dermatol 12:141, 1997

Silverberg MJ, Thorsen P, Lindeberg H, et al: Condyloma in pregnancy is strongly predictive of juvenile-onset recurrent respiratory papillomatosis. Obstet Gynecol 101(4):645, 2003

Smith JS, Backes DM, Hoots BE, et al: Human papillomavirus type-distribution in vulvar and vaginal cancers and their associated precursors. Obstet Gynecol 113(4):917, 2009

Smith JS, Lindsay L, Hoots B, et al: Human papillomavirus type distribution in invasive cervical cancer and high-grade cervical lesions: a meta-analysis update. Int J Cancer 121:621, 2007

Solomon D, Davey D, Kurman R, et al: The 2001 Bethesda System: terminology for reporting results of cervical cytology. JAMA 287(16):2114, 2002

Spitzer M: Lower genital tract intraepithelial neoplasia in HIV-infected women: guidelines for evaluation and management. Obstet Gynecol Surv 54(2):131, 1999

Spitzer M, Krumholz BA, Seltzer VL: The multicentric nature of disease related to human papillomavirus infection of the female lower genital tract. Obstet Gynecol 73(3 Pt 1):303, 1989

Srodon M, Stoler MH, Baber GB, et al: The distribution of low and high-risk HPV types in vulvar and vaginal intraepithelial neoplasia (VIN and VaIN). Am J Surg Pathol 30:1513, 2006

Stanley M: Pathology and epidemiology of HPV infection in females. Gynecol Oncol 117:S5, 2010a

Stanley M: Prospects for new human papillomavirus vaccines. Curr Opin Infect Dis 23:70, 2010b

Stokley S, Jeyarajah J, Yankey D, et al: Human papillomavirus coverage among adolescents, 2007–2013, and post-licensure vaccine safety monitoring, 2006–2014—United States. MMWR 63(29):620, 2014

Stoler MH: A brief synopsis of the role of human papillomaviruses in cervical carcinogenesis. Am J Obstet Gynecol 175(4 Pt 2):1091, 1996

Strander B, Andersson-Ellström A, Milson L, et al: Risk of invasive cancer after treatment for cervical intraepithelial neoplasia grade 3: population based cohort study. BMJ 335:1077, 2007

Strander B, Hällgren J, Sparén P: Effect of ageing on cervical or vaginal cancer in Swedish women previously treated for cervical intraepithelial neoplasia 3: population based cohort study of long term incidence and mortality. BMJ 348:17361, 2014

Syrjänen S: Current concepts on human papillomavirus infections in children. APMIS 118(6-7):494, 2010

Tandon R, Baranoski AS, Huang F, et al: Abnormal anal cytology in HIV-infected women. Am J Obstet Gynecol 203:21.e1, 2010

Thomsen LT, Frederiksen K, Munk C, et al: High-risk and low-risk human papillomavirus and the absolute risk of cervical intraepithelial neoplasia or cancer. Obstet Gynecol 123:57, 2014

Trimble EL: A guest editorial: update on diethylstilbestrol. Obstet Gynecol Surv 56(4):187, 2001

Trottier H, Mahmud SM, Lindsay L, et al: Persistence of an incident human papillomavirus infection and timing of cervical lesions in previously unexposed young women. Cancer Epidemiol Biomarkers Prev 18(3):854, 2009

U.S. Preventive Services Task Force: Final recommendation statement: cervical cancer: screening, March 2012. Available at: http://www.uspreventiveservicestaskforce.org/Page/Document/RecommendationStatementFinal/cervical-cancer-screening. Accessed April 9, 2015

Ulfelder H, Robboy SJ: The embryologic development of the human vagina. Am J Obstet Gynecol 126(7):769, 1976

Valari O, Koliopoulos G, Karakitsos P, et al: Human papillomavirus DNA and mRNA positivity of the anal canal in women with lower genital tract HPV lesions; predictors and clinical implications. Gynecol Oncol 122:505, 2011

van de Nieuwenhof HP, Massuger LF, van der Avoort I, et al: Vulvar squamous cell carcinoma development after diagnosis of VIN increases with age. Eur J Cancer 45(5):851, 2009

van den Einden LC, de Hullu JA, Massuger LF, et al: Interobserver variability and the effect of education in the histopathological diagnosis of differentiated vulvar intraepithelial neoplasia. Mod Pathol 26:874, 2013

van Seters M, van Beurden M, de Craen AJ: Is the assumed natural history of vulvar intraepithelial neoplasia III based on enough evidence? A systematic review of 3322 published patients. Gynecol Oncol 97(2):645, 2005

van Seters M, van Beurden M, ten Kate FJ, et al: Treatment of vulvar intraepithelial neoplasia with topical imiquimod. N Engl J Med 358:1465, 2008

von Gruenigen VE, Gibbons HE, Gibbins K, et al: Surgical treatments for vulvar and vaginal dysplasia. Obstet Gynecol 109:942, 2007

Werner CL, Lo JY, Heffernan T, et al: Loop electrosurgical excision procedure and risk of preterm birth. Obstet Gynecol 115:605, 2010

Whitlock EP, Vesco KK, Eder M, et al: Liquid-based cytology and human papillomavirus testing to screen for cervical cancer: a systematic review for the U.S. Preventive Services Task Force. Ann Intern Med 155:687, 2011

Wilkinson EJ: Pap smears and screening for cervical neoplasia. Clin Obstet Gynecol 33(4):817, 1990

Wilkinson EJ, Kneale B, Lynch PJ: Report of the ISSVD Terminology Committee. J Reprod Med 31:973, 1986

Williams AB, Darragh TM, Vranizan K, et al: Anal and cervical human papillomavirus infection and risk of anal and cervical epithelial abnormalities in human immunodeficiency virus-infected women. Obstet Gynecol 83(2):205, 1994

Winer RL, Hughes JP, Feng Q, et al: Early natural history of incident, type-specific human papillomavirus infections in newly sexually active young women. Cancer Epidemiol Biomarkers Prev 20(4):699, 2011

Winer RL, Lee SK, Hughes JP, et al: Genital human papillomavirus infection: incidence and risk factors in a cohort of female university students. Am J Epidemiol 157(3):218, 2003

Woodman CB, Collins S, Winter H, et al: Natural history of cervical human papillomavirus infection in young women: a longitudinal cohort study. Lancet 357(9271):1831, 2001

Woodruff JD: Carcinoma in situ of the vagina. Clin Obstet Gynecol 24(2):485, 1981

Wright TC, Ellerbrock TV, Chiasson MA, et al: Cervical intraepithelial neoplasia in women infected with human immunodeficiency virus: prevalence, risk factors, and validity of Papanicolaou smears. New York Cervical Disease Study. Obstet Gynecol 84(4):591, 1994

Wright TC, Stoler MH, Behrens CM, et al: Primary cervical cancer screening with human papillomavirus: end of study results from the ATHENA study using HPV as the first-line screening test. Gynecol Oncol 136(2):189, 2015

Wright TC, Stoler MH, Behrens CM, et al: The ATHENA human papillomavirus study: design, methods, and baseline results. Am J Obstet Gynecol 206:46e1, 2012

Wright VC, Chapman W: Intraepithelial neoplasia of the lower female genital tract: etiology, investigation, and management. Semin Surg Oncol 8:180, 1992

Yasmeen S, Romano PS, Pettinger M, et al: Incidence of cervical cytological abnormalities with aging in the Women's Health Initiative. Obstet Gynecol 108:410, 2006

Yost NP, Santoso JT, McIntire DD, et al: Postpartum regression rates of antepartum cervical intraepithelial neoplasia II and III lesions. Obstet Gynecol 93(3):359, 1999

Zbar AP, Fenger C, Efron J, et al: The pathology and molecular biology of anal intraepithelial neoplasia: comparisons with cervical and vulvar intraepithelial carcinoma. Int J Colorectal Dis 17(4):203, 2002

Zhao C, Florea A, Onisko A, et al: Histologic follow-up results in 662 patients with Pap test findings of atypical glandular cells: results from a large academic women's hospital laboratory employing sensitive screening methods. Gynecol Oncol 114:383, 2009

Zuchna C, Hager M, Tringler B, et al: Diagnostic accuracy of guided cervical biopsies: a prospective multicenter study comparing the histopathology of simultaneous biopsy and cone specimen. Am J Obstet Gynecol 203:321.e1, 2010

CHAPTER 30

Cervical Cancer

Cervical cancer is the most common gynecologic cancer in women worldwide. Most of these cancers stem from infection with the human papillomavirus (HPV), although other host factors affect neoplastic progression following initial infection. Compared with other gynecologic malignancies, cervical cancer develops in a younger population. Thus, screening for this neoplasia typically begins in young adulthood.

Most early cancers are asymptomatic. Thus, diagnosis usually follows histologic evaluation of biopsies taken during colposcopic examination or from a grossly abnormal cervix. This cancer is staged clinically, and this in turn directs treatment. In general, early-stage disease is effectively eradicated surgically. For advanced disease, chemoradiation is primarily selected. As expected, disease prognosis differs with tumor stage, and stage is the most important indicator of long-term survival.

Prevention lies mainly in identifying and treating women with high-grade dysplasia, and in HPV vaccination. Accordingly, as detailed in Chapter 29, regular screening is recommended and

HPV vaccination is encouraged to lower rates of cervical cancer in the future.

INCIDENCE

Worldwide, cervical cancer is common, and it ranks fourth among all malignancies for women (World Health Organization, 2012). In general, higher incidences are found in developing countries, and these countries contribute 85 percent of reported cases annually. Mortality rates are similarly higher in these populations (Torre, 2015). This incidence and survival disparity highlights successes achieved by long-term cervical cancer screening programs.

In the United States, cervical cancer is the third most common gynecologic cancer and the 11th most common solid malignant neoplasm among women. Women have a 1 in 132 lifetime risk of developing this cancer. In 2015, the American Cancer Society estimated 12,900 new cases and 4100 deaths from this malignancy (Siegel, 2015). Of U.S. women, black women and those in lower socioeconomic groups have the highest age-adjusted cervical cancer death rates, and Hispanic women have the highest incidence rates (Table 30-1). This trend is thought to stem mainly from financial and cultural characteristics affecting access to screening and treatment. The age at which cervical cancer develops is in general earlier than that of other gynecologic malignancies, and the median age at diagnosis is 49 years (Howlader, 2014).

RISKS

In addition to demographic differences, other risks may alter HPV acquisition or action. Notably, the greatest risk is the lack of regular cervical cancer screening (Abed, 2006; Leyden, 2005). Most communities adopting such screening have documented decreased incidences of this cancer (Jemal, 2006).

HPV is the primary etiologic infectious agent associated with cervical cancer (Ley, 1991; Schiffman, 1993). Although other sexually transmitted factors, including herpes simplex virus 2, may play a concurrent causative role, 99.7 percent of cervical cancers are associated with an oncogenic HPV subtype (Walboomers, 1999). In one study, 57 percent of invasive cervical cancer cases were attributable to HPV serotype 16. Serotype 18 was associated with 16 percent of invasive disease cases (Li, 2010). Each of these serotypes can lead to either squamous cell carcinoma or adenocarcinoma of the cervix. However, HPV 16 is more commonly associated with squamous cell carcinoma of the cervix, whereas HPV 18 is a risk factor for cervical adenocarcinoma (Bulk, 2006).

TABLE 30-1. Cervical Cancer Age-Adjusted Incidence and Death Rates (per 100,000 women per year)

	All Races	White	Black	Asian American & Pacific Islander	American Indian & Alaskan Native	Hispanic
Incidence	7.8	7.8	9.4	6.4	7.6	10.2
Death	2.3	2.1	4.1	1.8	3.4	2.8

Based on cases diagnosed during 2007 through 2011 from 18 geographic areas in the Surveillance, Epidemiology and End Results (SEER) Program.
Data from Howlader N, Noone AM, Krapcho M, et al: SEER Cancer Statistics Review, 1975-2011, National Cancer Institute. 2014.

Of other risks, lower educational attainment, older age, obesity, smoking, and neighborhood poverty are independently related to lower rates of cervical cancer screening. Specifically, those living in impoverished neighborhoods have limited access to testing and may benefit from screening outreach programs (Datta, 2006).

Cigarette smoking, both active and passive, increases cervical cancer risk. Among HPV-infected women, current and former smokers have a two- to threefold increased incidence of high-grade squamous intraepithelial lesion (HSIL) or invasive cancer. Passive smoking is also associated with increased risk, but to a lesser extent (Trimble, 2005). The mechanism underlying the association between smoking and this cancer is unclear, but smoking may alter HPV infection in those who smoke. For example, "ever smoking" has been associated with reduced clearance of high-risk HPV (Koshiol, 2006; Plummer, 2003). Tobacco smoke may also alter viral oncoprotein expression in cells in which the HPV is not integrated into the host genome (Wei, 2014).

Parity has a significant association with cervical cancer. Specifically, women with seven prior full-term pregnancies have an approximately fourfold risk, and those with one or two have a twofold risk compared with nulliparas (Muñoz, 2002).

Long-term *combination oral contraceptive (COC)* use is another risk. In women who are positive for cervical HPV DNA and who use COCs, cervical carcinoma rates increase by up to fourfold compared with women who are HPV-positive and never users (Moreno, 2002). Additionally, current COC users and women who are within 9 years of use have a significantly higher risk of developing both squamous cell and adenocarcinoma of the cervix (International Collaboration of Epidemiological Studies of Cervical Cancer, 2006). Encouragingly, the relative risk to COC users appears to decline after cessation. Data from 24 epidemiologic studies showed that by 10 or more years following COC cessation, cervical cancer risk returns to that of never users (International Collaboration of Epidemiological Studies of Cervical Cancer, 2007).

Sexual activity logically has an association as HPV is sexually transmitted. Having more than six lifetime sexual partners elevates the relative risk of cervical cancer. Similarly, an early age of first intercourse before age 20 confers an increased risk of developing this malignancy. Intercourse after age 21 only shows a trend toward an elevated risk. Moreover, abstinence from sexual activity and barrier protection during sexual intercourse decrease cervical cancer incidence (International Collaboration of Epidemiological Studies of Cervical Cancer, 2006).

Immunosuppressed women have an increased risk of developing cervical cancer. Cervical cancer is an acquired immune deficiency syndrome (AIDS)-defining illness. The standardized incidence ratio (SIR) of developing this cancer in HIV-infected women is 5.82. For transplant recipients the SIR is 2.013 for this malignancy (Grulich, 2007). Women with autoimmune diseases who use immunosuppressants do not appear to have an increased cervical cancer risk, except for azathioprine users (Dugue, 2015).

PATHOPHYSIOLOGY

■ Tumorigenesis

Most women readily clear HPV, but those with persistent infection may develop preinvasive dysplastic cervical lesions. From such lesions, squamous cell carcinoma of the cervix typically arises at the squamocolumnar junction (Bosch, 2002). In general, progression from dysplasia to invasive cancer requires several years, although times can vary widely. The molecular alterations involved with cervical carcinogenesis are complex and not fully understood. Carcinogenesis currently is suspected to result from the interactive effects among environmental insults, host immunity, and somatic-cell genomic variations (Helt, 2002; Jones, 1997, 2006; Wentzensen, 2004).

Increasing evidence suggests that HPV oncoproteins may be a critical component of continued cancer cell proliferation (Mantovani, 1999; Munger, 2001). Unlike low-risk serotypes, oncogenic HPV serotypes can integrate into human DNA (Fig. 30-1). As a result, with infection, oncogenic HPV's early replication proteins E1 and E2 enable the virus to replicate within cervical cells. These proteins are expressed at high levels early in HPV infection. They can lead to cytologic changes detected as low-grade squamous intraepithelial (LSIL) cytologic findings on Pap smears.

Amplification of viral replication and subsequent transformation of normal cells into tumor cells may follow (Mantovani, 1999). Specifically, the viral gene products E6 and E7 oncoproteins are implicated in this transformation (Fig. 30-2). E7 protein binds to the retinoblastoma (Rb) tumor suppressor protein, whereas E6 binds to the p53 tumor suppressor protein. In both instances, binding leads to degradation of these suppressor proteins. The E6 effect of p53 degradation is well studied and linked with the proliferation and immortalization of cervical cells (Jones, 1997, 2006; Mantovani, 1999; Munger, 2001).

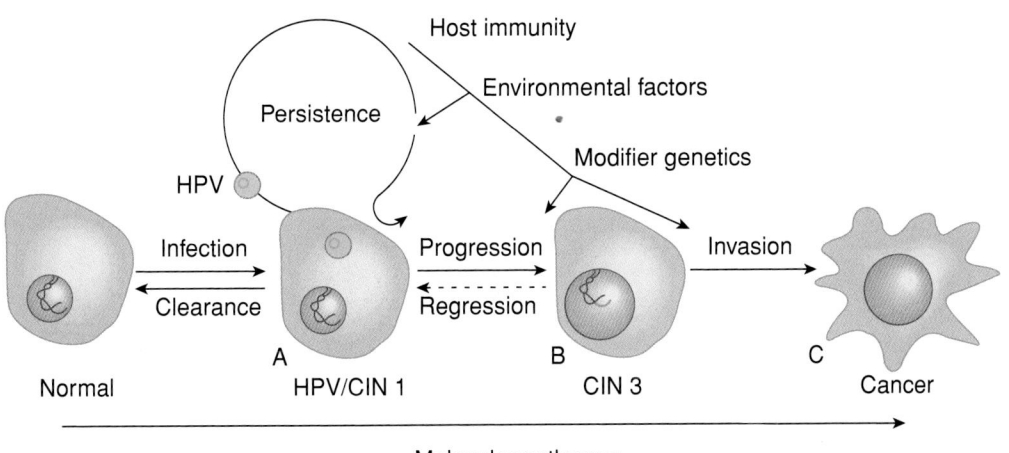

FIGURE 30-1 Critical end points lie on the spectrum of cervical dysplasia. **A.** This initial point is the cell at risk due to active HPV infection. The HPV genome (*blue ring*) exists as a plasmid, separate from the host DNA. **B.** The clinically relevant preinvasive lesion, cervical intraepithelial neoplasia 3 (CIN 3) or carcinoma in situ (CIS), is an intermediate stage in cervical cancer development. The HPV genome has become integrated into the host DNA, resulting in increased proliferative ability. **C.** Interactive effects between environmental insults, host immunity, and somatic cell genomic variations lead to invasive cervical cancer.

■ Tumor Spread

Following tumorigenesis, the pattern of local growth may be exophytic if a cancer arises from the ectocervix, or may be endophytic if it arises from the endocervical canal (Fig. 30-3). Lesions lower in the canal and on the ectocervix are more likely to be clinically visible during physical examination. Alternatively, growth may be infiltrative, and in these cases, ulcerated lesions are common if necrosis accompanies this growth. As primary

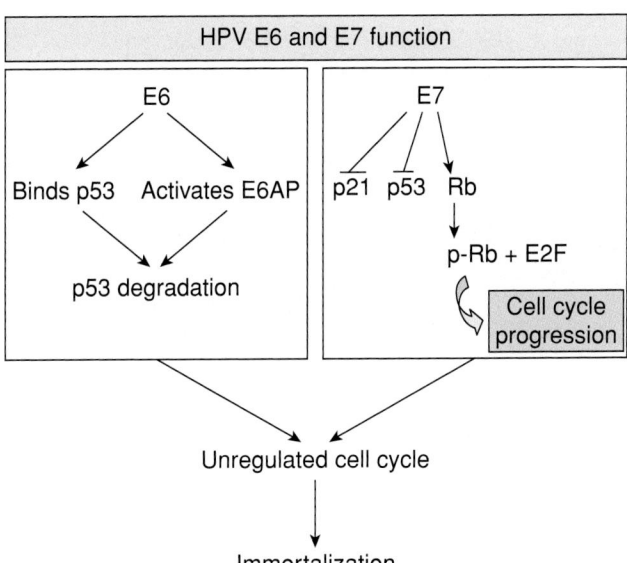

FIGURE 30-2 Effects of E6 and E7 oncoproteins. On the left, viral oncoprotein E6 directly binds p53 and also activates E6AP to degrade p53 tumor suppressor protein. On the right, E7 oncoprotein phosphorylates retinoblastoma tumor suppressor protein, resulting in release of E2F transcription factors, which are involved in cell cycle progression. E7 also downregulates p21 tumor suppressor protein production and subverts p53 function. The cumulative effect of E6 and E7 oncoproteins eventually results in cell cycle alteration, promoting uncontrolled cell proliferation.

lesions enlarge and lymphatic involvement progresses, local invasion increases and will eventually become extensive.

Lymphatic Spread

Lymph Node Groups. The pattern of tumor spread typically follows cervical lymphatic drainage. Thus, familiarity with this drainage aids understanding the surgical steps of radical hysterectomy performed for this cancer (Section 46-1, p. 1134). The cervix has a rich network of lymphatics, which follow the course of the uterine artery (Fig. 30-4). These channels drain principally into the paracervical and parametrial lymph nodes. These lymph nodes are clinically important and thus are removed as part of parametrial resection during radical hysterectomy. From the parametrial and paracervical nodes, lymph subsequently flows into the obturator lymph nodes and into the internal, external, common iliac lymph nodes, and ultimately the paraaortic lymph nodes. Accordingly, pelvic and common iliac lymph nodes are also traditionally removed concurrently with radical hysterectomy. In contrast, lymphatic channels from the posterior cervix course through the rectal pillars and the uterosacral ligaments to the rectal lymph nodes. These nodes are also encountered and are removed during the extended resection of the uterosacral ligaments that is characteristic of radical hysterectomy.

Lymphovascular Space Involvement. As tumor invades deeper into the stroma, it enters blood capillaries and lymphatic channels (Fig. 30-5). Termed *lymphovascular space involvement* (LVSI), this type of invasive growth is not included in the clinical staging of cervical cancer. However, its presence is regarded as a poor prognostic indicator, especially in early-stage cervical cancers. Thus, the presence of LVSI often requires tailoring the planned surgical procedure and adjuvant radiation treatment.

Local and Distant Tumor Extension

With extension through the parametria to the pelvic sidewall, ureteral blockage frequently develops, resulting in hydronephrosis

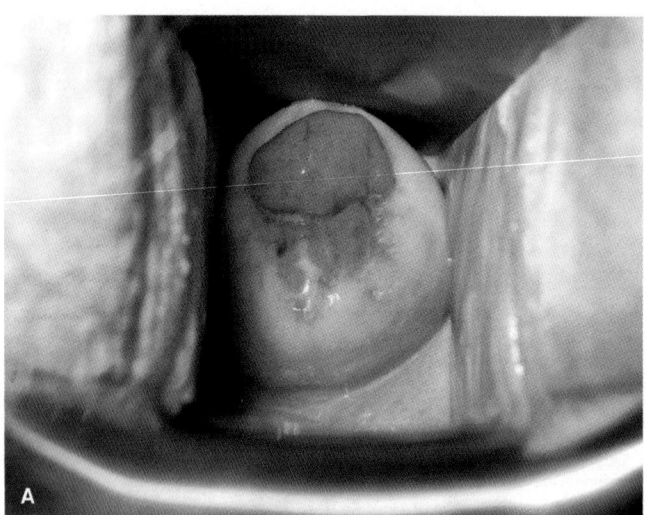
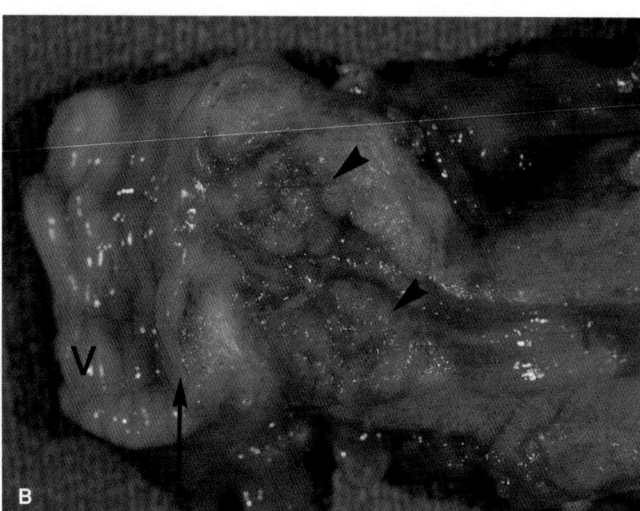

FIGURE 30-3 Cervical adenocarcinoma. **A.** Invasive cancer originating from the endocervix. (Photograph contributed by Dr. David Miller.) **B**. Exophytic growth of cervical adenocarcinoma into the endocervical canal (*arrowheads*). In this radical hysterectomy specimen, proximal vagina (V) is excised with the cervix, and an arrow marks the ectocervix.

(Fig. 30-6). Additionally, the bladder may be invaded by direct tumor extension through the vesicouterine ligaments (bladder pillars). The rectum is invaded less often because it is anatomically separated from cervix by the posterior cul-de-sac. Distant metastasis results from hematogenous dissemination, and the lungs, ovaries, liver, and bone are the most frequently affected.

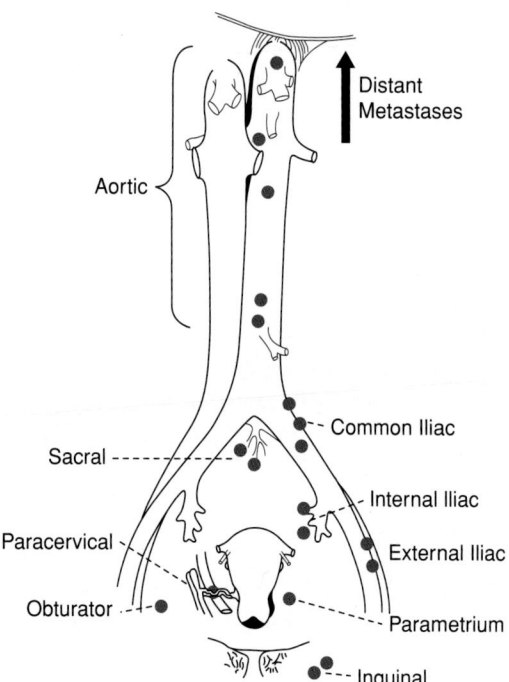

FIGURE 30-4 Lymphatic drainage of the cervix. The parametrial lymph nodes are removed as part of the radical hysterectomy. Lymph node dissection for cervical cancer includes removal of pelvic lymph nodes (from the external iliac artery and vein, internal iliac artery, and the common iliac artery) with or without a paraaortic lymph node dissection to the level of the inferior mesenteric artery. (Reproduced with permission from Henriksen E: The lymphatic spread of carcinoma of the cervix and of the body of the uterus; a study of 420 necropsies, Am J Obstet Gynecol 1949 Nov;58(5):924–942.)

HISTOLOGIC TYPES

■ Squamous Cell Carcinoma

The two most common histologic subtypes of cervical cancer are squamous cell and adenocarcinoma (Table 30-2). Of these, squamous cell tumors predominate, comprise about 70 percent of all cervical cancers, and arise from the ectocervix. Over the past 30 years, the incidence of squamous cell cancers has declined, whereas that of cervical adenocarcinoma has risen. These changes may be attributed to an improved method of screening for early squamous lesions of the cervix and an increase in HPV prevalence (Vizcaino, 2000). Squamous cell carcinomas can be subdivided into keratinizing and nonkeratinizing carcinomas (Fig. 30-7).

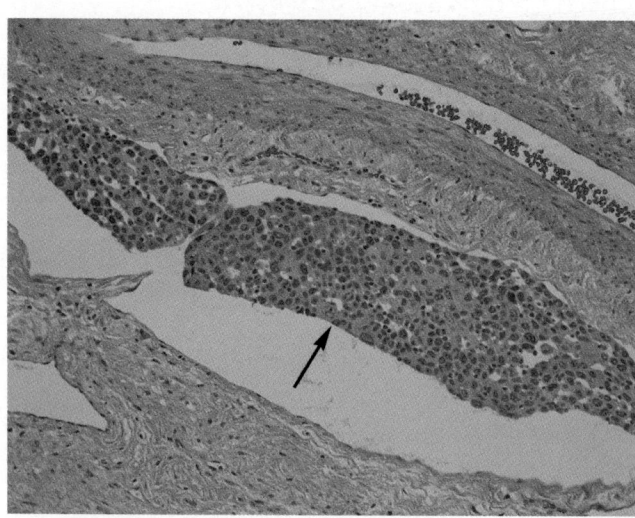

FIGURE 30-5 Photomicrograph of lymphovascular space involvement. A large lymphatic channel is plugged with squamous cell carcinoma (*arrow*). (Used with permission from Dr. Raheela Ashfaq.)

TABLE 30-2. Histologic Subtypes of Cervical Cancer

Squamous
Keratinizing
Nonkeratinizing
Papillary

Adenocarcinoma
Mucinous
  Endocervical
  Intestinal
  Minimal deviation
  Villoglandular
Endometrioid
Serous
Clear cell
Mesonephric

Mixed cervical carcinoma
Adenosquamous
Glassy cell

Neuroendocrine cervical tumor
Large cell neuroendocrine
Small cell neuroendocrine

Others
Sarcoma
Lymphoma
Melanoma

Squamous cell carcinomas represent 75% of all cervical cancer, and adenocarcinomas account for 20–25% of cervical cancers. The other cell types are rare.

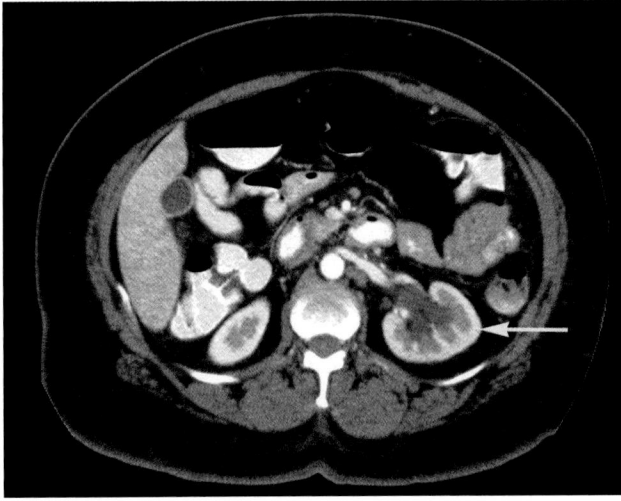

FIGURE 30-6 Computed tomography (CT) scan reveals hydrone-phrosis (*arrow*) caused by tumor compression of the left ureter.

■ **Adenocarcinomas**

Adenocarcinomas are a group of cervical cancers composed of the subtypes listed in Table 30-2. In contrast to squamous cell cervical carcinoma, adenocarcinomas make up 25 percent of cervical cancers and arise from the endocervical mucus-producing columnar cells. Because of this origin within the endocervix, adenocarcinomas are often occult and may be advanced before becoming clinically evident. They often give the cervix a palpable barrel shape during pelvic examination.

Adenocarcinomas exhibit various histologic patterns composed of diverse cell types. Of these, *mucinous adenocarcinomas* are the most common and are subdivided as shown in Table 30-2. The mucinous endocervical type retains resemblance to normal endocervical tissue (Fig. 30-8). The intestinal type resembles intestinal cells and may include goblet cells. *Minimal deviation adenocarcinoma,* also known as adenoma malignum,

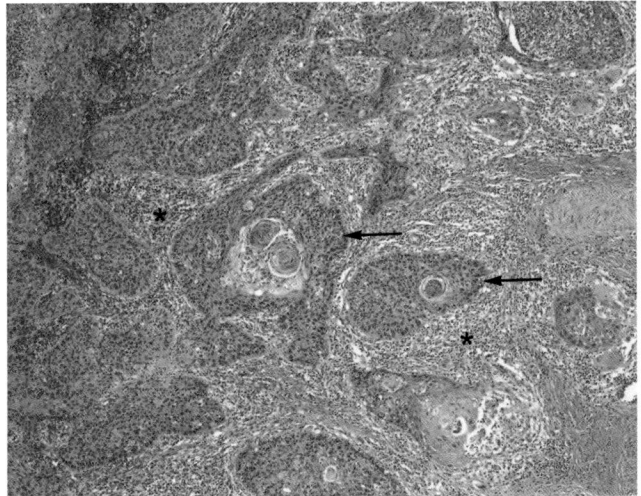

FIGURE 30-7 Squamous cell cervical cancer. Irregular nests of malignant cells (*arrows*) show eosinophilic keratin pearls at their center, which is a classic diagnostic feature. These nests invade the stroma accompanied by a brisk lymphocytic response (*asterisks*). (Used with permission from Dr. Raheela Ashfaq.)

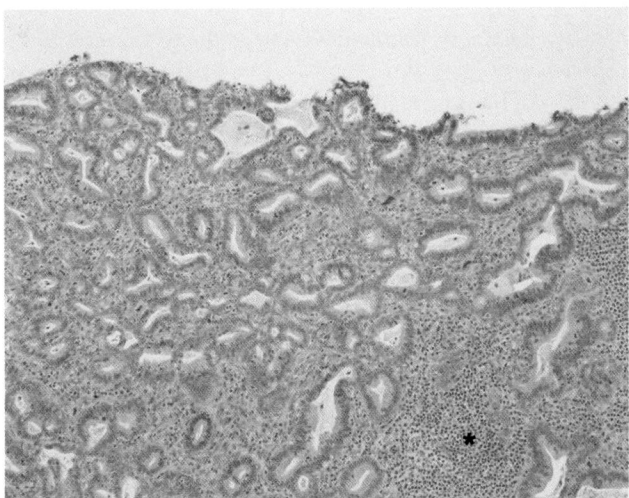

FIGURE 30-8 This invasive cervical adenocarcinoma is characterized by columnar cells with moderate nuclear atypia and mitotic activity. Tumor cells form glands that resemble native endocervical glands but invade the stroma haphazardly. A chronic inflammatory infiltrate is present on the right (*asterisk*).

is characterized by cytologically bland glands that are abnormal in size and shape. These tumors contain an increased number of glands positioned at a deeper level than normal endocervical glands. Women with Peutz-Jeghers syndrome are at increased risk of developing adenoma malignum. *Villoglandular adenocarcinomas* are made up of surface papillae.

Endometrioid adenocarcinomas are the second most frequently identified and display glands resembling those of the endometrium. *Serous carcinoma* is identical to serous carcinomas of the ovaries or uterus and is rare. *Clear cell adenocarcinoma* accounts for less than 5 percent of cervical adenocarcinomas and is named for its clear cytoplasm (Jaworski, 2009). Rarely, adenocarcinomas arise in mesonephric remnants in the cervix and are termed *mesonephric adenocarcinomas*.

Prognosis Comparison

Evidence describing the prognosis of squamous cell carcinoma compared with that of adenocarcinoma is contradictory. For stage IB and IIA cervical cancer, one study showed a statistically significant lower overall survival rate in those with adenocarcinoma compared with women with squamous cell carcinoma (Landoni, 1997). However, the Gynecologic Oncology Group (GOG) found in a subsequent study that overall survival rates in women with stage IB squamous and adenocarcinomas of the cervix are similar (Look, 1996).

For advanced-stage (stage IIB to IVA) cancers, evidence suggests that cervical adenocarcinomas may portend a poorer overall survival rate compared with similarly staged squamous cell carcinomas (Eifel, 1990; Lea, 2002). The 2006 International Federation of Obstetricians and Gynecologists (FIGO) annual report, which reported on more than 11,000 squamous carcinomas and 1613 adenocarcinomas, demonstrated that women with adenocarcinomas have worse overall survival rates at every stage compared with those with squamous cell carcinoma (Quinn, 2006). In sum, evidence suggests that adenocarcinoma of the cervix is a high-risk cell type.

■ Other Tumor Types

Mixed cervical carcinomas are rare. Of these, *adenosquamous carcinomas* do not differ grossly from adenocarcinomas of the cervix. The squamous component is poorly differentiated and shows little keratinization. *Glassy cell carcinoma* describes a form of poorly differentiated adenosquamous carcinoma in which cells display cytoplasm with a ground-glass appearance.

Neuroendocrine tumors of the cervix include large cell and small cell tumors. These rare malignancies are highly aggressive, and even early-stage cancers have a relatively low disease-free survival rate despite treatment with radical hysterectomy and adjuvant chemotherapy (Albores-Saavedra, 1997; Viswanathan, 2004). Often, neuroendocrine markers, including chromogranin, synaptophysin, and CD56, are used to confirm the diagnosis. Uncommonly, endocrine and paraendocrine tumors are associated with these neuroendocrine tumors.

Of other rare types, the cervix may be the site of sarcomas, malignant lymphomas, and melanomas. Cervical leiomyosarcomas and cervical stromal sarcomas have a poor prognosis, similar to that for uterine sarcomas. Melanomas often present as ulcerated blue or black nodules and also have a poor prognosis.

DIAGNOSIS

■ Symptoms

Some women diagnosed with this cancer are asymptomatic. In others, early-stage cervical cancer may create a watery, blood-tinged vaginal discharge. Intermittent vaginal bleeding that follows coitus or douching can also be noted. As a malignancy enlarges, bleeding typically intensifies, and occasionally, a woman presents with uncontrolled hemorrhage from a tumor bed. In such cases, bleeding can often be controlled with a combination of Monsel paste (ferric subsulfate) and vaginal packing. Topical acetone can also be used to obtain hemostasis, especially in cases refractory to Monsel paste (Patsner, 1993). Burning from acetone makes it a less desirable choice than Monsel paste. With vaginal packing, the patient ideally remains at bed rest, and a Foley catheter is concurrently inserted to drain the bladder. The pack may interfere with normal voiding, and the catheter also allows for accurate monitoring of urine output during volume repletion. If bleeding continues, emergent radiation can be delivered. Alternatively, internal iliac artery embolization or ligation can be performed in cases of refractory hemorrhage. However, caution is used for these latter two options, as tumor oxygenation is decreased if these blood supplies are occluded. Radiation therapy is a primary component of advanced-stage cancer, and as noted in Chapter 28 (p. 613), radiation's effects are diminished in low-oxygen environments and can translate into worsening disease-specific survival rates (Kapp, 2005). In those with significant bleeding, hemodynamic support of the patient follows that described in Chapter 40 (p. 864).

■ Physical Examination

Most women with this cancer have normal general physical examination findings. In those with suspected cervical cancer, a thorough external genital and vaginal examination is performed. Because HPV is a shared risk factor for cervical, vaginal, vulvar, and anal cancers, concomitant lesions are sought. With speculum examination, the cervix may appear grossly normal if cancer is microinvasive. Visible disease displays varied appearances. Lesions may be an exophytic or endophytic growth; a polypoid mass, papillary tissue, or barrel-shaped cervix; a cervical ulceration or granular mass; or necrotic tissue. A watery, purulent, or bloody discharge can also be seen. For this reason, cervical cancer may mirror the appearance of a cervical leiomyoma, cervical polyp, vaginitis, cervical eversion, cervicitis, threatened abortion, placenta previa, cervical pregnancy, condyloma acuminata, herpetic ulcer, chancre, or a prolapsing uterine leiomyoma, polyp, or sarcoma.

During bimanual examination, a clinician may palpate an enlarged uterus resulting from tumor invasion and growth. Alternatively, hematometra or pyometra may expand the endometrial cavity following obstruction of fluid egress by a primary cervical cancer. In this case, the uterus may feel enlarged and boggy. Advanced cervical cancer cases can extend into the vagina, and disease extent can be appreciated during anterior vaginal wall palpation or during rectovaginal examination. With posterior spread, palpation of the rectovaginal septum between the index and middle finger of an examiner's hand reveals a thick, hard, irregular septum. The proximal posterior vaginal wall is most commonly invaded. In addition, during digital rectal examination, parametrial, uterosacral, and pelvic sidewall involvement can be appreciated. Either one or both parametria may be invaded, and involved tissues feel thick, irregular, firm, and less mobile. A fixed mass indicates that tumor has probably extended to the pelvic sidewalls. However, a central lesion can become as large as 8 to 10 cm in diameter before reaching the sidewall.

With advancing disease, enlarged supraclavicular or inguinal lymphadenopathy suggest lymphatic tumor spread. Lower extremity edema and low back pain, often radiating down the posterior leg, may reflect compression of the sciatic nerve root, lymphatics, veins, or ureter by an expanding tumor. With ureteral obstruction, hydronephrosis and uremia can follow and may occasionally be the initial presenting finding. In these cases, ureteral stenting or percutaneous nephrostomy tube insertion are usually required. Kidney function is ideally preserved for chemotherapy. Additionally, with tumor invasion into the bladder or rectum, hematuria and/or vesicovaginal or rectovaginal fistula may be found.

■ Papanicolaou Test and Cervical Biopsy

Histologic evaluation of cervical biopsy is the primary tool to diagnose cervical cancer. Although Papanicolaou (Pap) tests are performed extensively to screen for this cancer, this test does not always detect cervical cancer. Specifically, Pap testing has only a 53- to 80-percent sensitivity for detecting high-grade lesions on any given single test (Agorastos, 2015; Benoit, 1984; Soost, 1991). Thus, the preventive power of Pap testing lies in regular serial screening (Fig. 30-9). Moreover, in women who have stage I cervical cancer, only 30 to 50 percent of single cytologic smears obtained are read as positive for cancer (Benoit, 1984). Hence, Pap testing alone for evaluation of a suspicious lesion is discouraged. Instead, these lesions are directly biopsied with Tischler biopsy forceps or a Kevorkian curette (Fig. 29-16, p. 641). When possible, biopsies are taken from the tumor periphery, as central

portions often contain only necrotic tissue, which will fail to yield a diagnosis. Moreover, biopsies ideally include underlying stroma, so that invasion, if present, can be assessed.

If abnormal Pap test findings are noted, colposcopy is often performed, and adequate cervical and endocervical biopsies are obtained. In some cases, cold knife conization is needed for this. Indications for colposcopy and conization are outlined in Chapter 29, and cervical punch biopsies or conization specimens are the most accurate for allowing assessment of cervical cancer invasion. Both sample types typically contain underlying stroma and enable differentiation between invasive and in situ carcinomas. For this determination, conization specimens provide a larger tissue sample and are most helpful.

STAGING

Cervical cancers are staged clinically. Allowable components of staging include cold-knife conization, pelvic examination under anesthesia, cystoscopy, proctoscopy, chest radiograph, and intravenous pyelogram (or this portion of the computed tomography [CT] scan can be used). Table 30-3 lists these and also contains radiologic and laboratory tools that are not included in formal staging but may contribute additional information. Bullous edema is not sufficient for the diagnosis of bladder involvement, and this involvement must be biopsy proven. Lymph node metastasis does not change the clinical stage. The staging system widely used for cervical cancer is that developed by the FIGO in collaboration with the World Health Organization (WHO) and the International Union Against Cancer (UICC). This staging was updated in 2009 and is detailed in Table 30-4 and Figure 30-10. In this chapter, *early-stage disease* refers to FIGO stages I through IIA. The term *advanced-stage disease* describes stages IIB and higher.

Within each oncology chapter of this text, staging of each cancer type (cervix, vulva, vagina, uterus, ovary) will be presented. FIGO classification is used for gynecologic cancers.

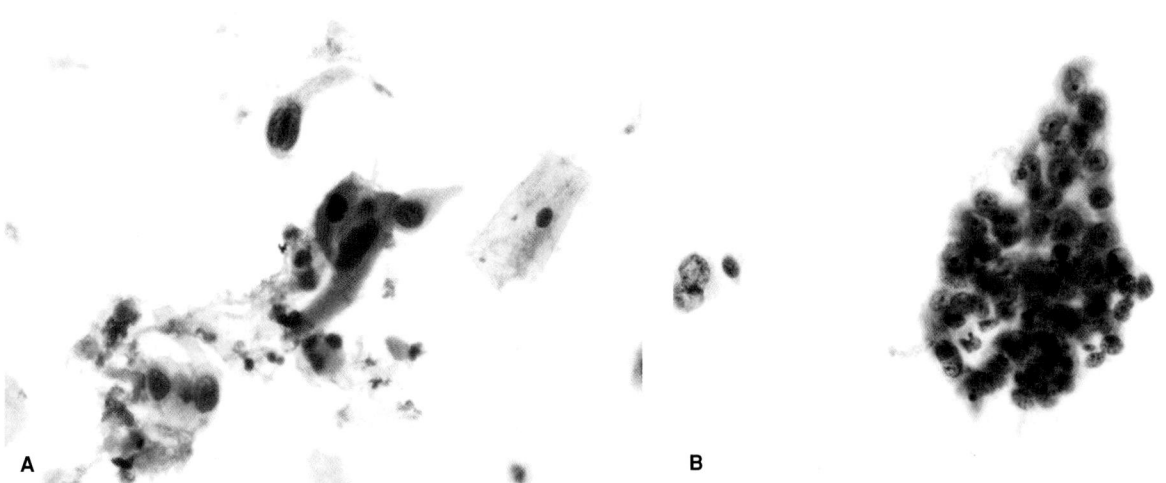

FIGURE 30-9 A. Pap smear, squamous cell carcinoma. Some show spindled tumor cells and/or cytoplasmic keratinization, as evidenced by dense orangeophilic cytoplasm. **B.** Pap smear, endocervical adenocarcinoma. This shows malignant cytologic features including nuclear pleomorphism, nuclear membrane abnormalities, and nucleolar prominence. Cytoplasm tends to be more delicate than in squamous carcinoma and may contain mucin. (Photographs contributed by Ann Marie West, MBA, CT[ASCP].)

TABLE 30-3. Testing Used During Cervical Cancer Evaluation

Testing	To Identify:
Laboratory	
CBC	Anemia
Urinalysis	Hematuria
Chemistry profile	Electrolyte abnormality
Liver function	Liver metastasis
Creatinine/BUN	Renal impairment or obstruction
Radiologic	
Chest radiograph	Lung metastasis
Intravenous pyelogram	Hydronephrosis
CT scan (abdominopelvic)	Nodal or distant organ metastasis; hydronephrosis
MR imaging	Local parametrial invasion; nodal metastasis
PET scan	Nodal or distant organ metastasis
Procedural	
Cystoscopy	Bladder tumor invasion
Proctoscopy	Rectal tumor invasion
EUA	Extent of pelvic tumor spread; clinical staging

BUN = blood urea nitrogen; CBC = complete blood count; CT = computed tomography; EUA = examination under anesthesia; MR = magnetic resonance; PET = positron emission tomography.

TABLE 30-4. Clinical Stages of Cervical Cancer (FIGO, Revised 2009)

Stage	Characteristics
0	**Carcinoma in situ, cervical intraepithelial lesion (CIN) 3**
I	**Carcinoma is strictly confined to cervix (extension to corpus should be disregarded)**
IA	Microscopic lesion, invasion is limited to measured stromal invasion with a maximum depth of 5 mm and no wider than 7 mm
IA1	Measured invasion of stroma no greater than 3 mm in depth and no wider than 7 mm
IA2	Measured invasion of stroma greater than 3 mm and no greater than 5 mm in depth and no wider than 7 mm
IB	Clinical lesions confined to the cervix or preclinical lesions greater than IA
IB1	Clinical lesions no greater than 4 cm in size
IB2	Clinical lesions greater than 4 cm in size
II	**Carcinoma extends beyond cervix but has not extended to pelvic wall; it involves vagina, but not as far as the lower third**
IIA	No obvious parametrial invasion
IIA1	Clinical lesions no greater than 4 cm in size
IIA2	Clinical lesions greater than 4 cm in size
IIB	Obvious parametrial involvement
III	**Carcinoma has extended to the pelvic wall; on rectal examination there is no cancer-free space between tumor and pelvic wall; tumor involves lower third of vagina; all cases with hydronephrosis or nonfunctioning kidney should be included, unless they are known to be due to another cause**
IIIA	No extension to pelvic wall, but involvement of lower third of vagina
IIIB	Extension to pelvic wall, or hydronephrosis or nonfunctioning kidney due to tumor
IV	**Carcinoma has extended beyond true pelvis or has clinically involved mucosa of bladder or rectum**
IVA	Spread of growth to adjacent pelvic organs
IVB	Spread to distant organs

FIGO = International Federation of Obstetricians and Gynecologists.
Modified with permission from Pecorelli S: Revised FIGO staging for carcinoma of the vulva, cervix, and endometrium. Int J Gynaecol Obstet 2009 May;105(2):103–104.

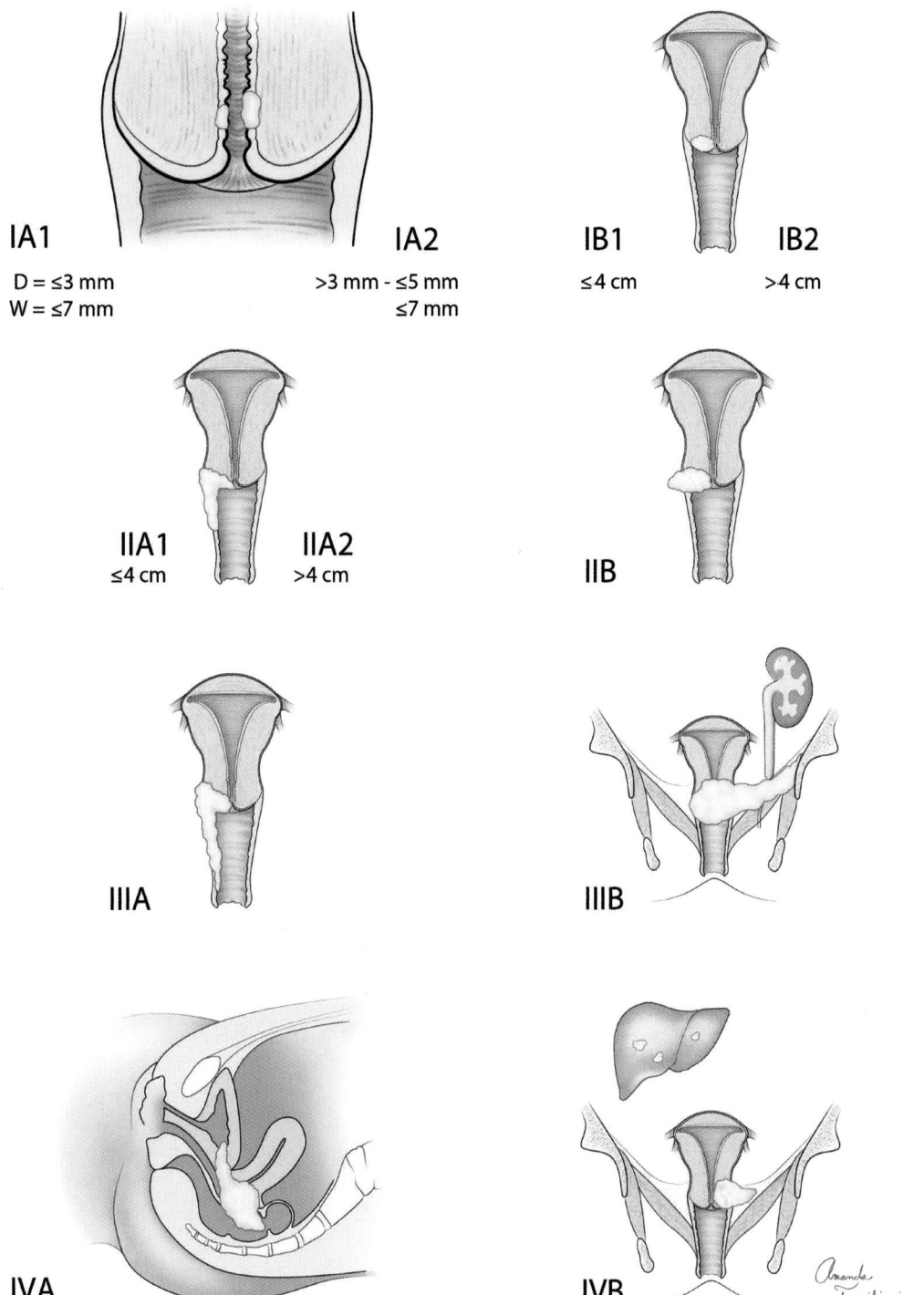

FIGURE 30-10 The International Federation of Gynecologists and Obstetricians (FIGO) stages of cervical cancer. D = depth; W = width.

In contrast, the American Joint Committee on Cancer (AJCC) developed the *TNM Staging System,* which is based on the extent of the tumor (T), the extent of spread to the lymph nodes (N), and the presence of metastasis (M). Breast cancer is staged with this latter system, as shown in Table 12-5 (p. 290).

RADIOLOGIC IMAGING

As discussed, cervical cancer is staged clinically, and accurate evaluation is critical to appropriate treatment planning. For example, early-stage tumors may be treated surgically, whereas more advanced tumors require radiation and/or chemotherapy. Although imaging does not affect assignment of stage (except lung metastases seen on chest radiograph and hydronephrosis seen on CT scan), imaging results can tailor treatment for an individual. In addition, lymph node metastases, although not included in the FIGO system, worsen patient prognosis and may be identified with imaging. Thus, radiologic tools such as CT scanning, magnetic resonance (MR) imaging, or positron emission tomography (PET) scanning are commonly used as adjuncts in initial cervical cancer evaluation. However, no uniform approach to the use of these has been developed.

Magnetic Resonance Imaging

For defining anatomy, this high-resolution imaging tool offers superior contrast resolution at soft-tissue interfaces. Thus, MR imaging effectively measures tumor size, delineates cervical tumor boundaries, and identifies surrounding bladder, rectal, or parametrial invasion. Unfortunately, MR imaging is less accurate for diagnosing microscopic or deep cervical stromal invasion or identifying minimal parametrial extension (Mitchell, 2006). These particular distinctions are important as both stromal and parametrial invasion may affect suitability for a given planned treatment. In addition, false-negative findings occur with small volumes of disease and with tissue foci in which cancer cannot be differentiated from scar or necrosis. In these cases, PET scanning identifies metabolic rather than anatomic changes and can be a complementary tool.

For primary cervical cancer, MR imaging is superior to CT for determining carcinoma size, local tumor extension, and lymph node involvement (Bipat, 2003; Mitchell, 2006; Subak, 1995). MR imaging is often preferred for patients being considered for fertility-sparing radical trachelectomy (Abu-Rustum, 2008; Olawaiye, 2009). Overall, however, both MR imaging and CT perform similarly in cervical cancer (Hricak, 2005).

Computed Tomography

This is the most widely used imaging tool for the assessment of nodal involvement and distant metastatic disease. It offers high-resolution depiction of anatomy, especially when used with contrast. CT scanning is not a component of FIGO staging. However, it is obtained in many women with cervical cancer to evaluate tumor size and bulky extension beyond the cervix. CT can also aid detection of enlarged lymph nodes, ureteral obstruction, or distant metastasis (Follen, 2003).

However, CT has limitations similar to MR imaging. CT is not accurate for assessing subtle parametrial invasion or deep cervical stromal invasion because of its poor soft-tissue contrast resolution. CT is also limited by its inability to detect small-volume metastatic involvement in normal-size lymph nodes. Moreover, internal node architecture is often poorly defined. This makes distinction between reactive node hyperplasia and true metastatic disease difficult.

Positron Emission Tomography

This nuclear medicine imaging technique creates an image of functional processes within the body. With FDG-PET, a radiolabeled analogue of glucose, fluorodeoxyglucose (FDG), is injected intravenously and is taken up by metabolically active cells such as tumor cells. PET provides a poor depiction of detailed anatomy, thus scans are frequently read side-by-side with CT scans. The combination allows correlation of metabolic and anatomic data. As a result, current PET scanners are now commonly integrated with CT scanners, and the two scans can be performed during the same session (Fig. 2-33, p. 46).

FDG-PET is superior to CT or MR imaging for lymph node metastasis identification (Belhocine, 2002; Havrilesky, 2005;

Selman, 2008). However, PET is insensitive for lymphatic metastasis <5 mm. Moreover, its role in early-stage smaller, resectable tumors is limited (Sironi, 2006; Wright, 2005). PET scans can be useful in planning radiation treatment fields and also in identifying those patients who have distant metastatic disease and are candidates for palliative chemotherapy rather than curative-intent chemoradiotherapy.

LYMPH NODE DISSECTION

As noted, cervical cancer is staged clinically and not surgically. However, surgical evaluation of retroperitoneal pelvic and para-aortic lymph nodes offers accurate metastasis detection that is superior to radiologic imaging (Goff, 1999). As a result, lymph node dissection may modify a patient's primary treatment strategy based on the level of nodal disease. For example, radiation fields may be altered to ensure that patients with negative paraaortic lymph nodes are not overtreated with extended-field radiation and that patients with positive paraaortic lymph nodes are not undertreated. Potential candidates include patients with positive or suspected positive pelvic nodes undergoing chemoradiation treatment. Supporting studies show that if positive pelvic/paraaortic nodes are identified, patients may receive a significant survival benefit from extended chemotherapy and/or extended field radiation therapy (Hacker, 1995; Holcomb, 1999; Leblanc, 2007).

In addition, tumor-laden nodes may be debulked. Several studies report similar disease-free survival rates for patients whose macroscopic nodal disease is resected compared with women with microscopic nodal disease (Cosin, 1998; Downey, 1989; Hacker, 1995). That said, there is virtually no long-term survival for patients with unresectable bulky paraaortic lymph nodes.

During lymphadenectomy, most experts recommend lymph node dissection in the common iliac and paraaortic region and resection of macroscopic lymph nodes (Querleu, 2000). Traditional laparotomy and minimally invasive surgery (MIS) approaches have been compared. Although diagnostically equivalent, laparoscopic approaches offer postoperative MIS advantages. In addition, laparoscopic lymph node dissection has been associated with significantly less radiation morbidity than that with radiation following laparotomic approaches (Vasilev, 1995).

Despite these suggested benefits, some experts argue that the benefits of surgical staging, if any, are minimal. These studies estimate only a 4- to 6-percent survival benefit after aggressive surgical debulking of retroperitoneal lymph nodes (Kupets, 2002; Petereit, 1998).

PROGNOSIS

The significance of tumor burden on survival is well demonstrated, whether measured by FIGO stage, centimeter size, or surgical staging (Stehman, 1991). Of these definers, FIGO stage is the most significant prognostic factor (Table 30-5). However, within each stage distribution, lymph node involvement also becomes an important modifier in determining prognosis. For example, in early-stage cervical cancer (stages I through IIA), nodal metastases are an independent predictor of survival (Delgado, 1990; Tinga, 1990). One GOG study demonstrated

TABLE 30-5. Cervical Cancer Survival Rates According to Stage

Stage	5-Year Survival
IA	100%
IB	88%
IIA	68%
IIB	44%
III	18–39%
IVA	18–34%

Data from from Grigsby, 1991; Komaki, 1995; Webb, 1980.

a 3-year survival rate of 86 percent for women with early-stage cervical cancer and negative pelvic lymph nodes, compared with a 3-year survival rate of 74 percent in patients who had one or more positive lymph nodes (Delgado, 1990).

In addition, the number of nodal metastases is predictive. Studies demonstrate significantly higher 5-year survival rates in those with one positive lymph node compared with rates in women with multiple involved nodes (Tinga, 1990). In advanced-stage (stage IIB through IV) cervical cancer, lymph node metastases also worsen prognosis. In general, microscopic nodal involvement has a better prognosis than macroscopic nodal disease (Cosin, 1998; Hacker, 1995).

EARLY-STAGE PRIMARY DISEASE TREATMENT

■ Stage IA

The term *microinvasive cervical cancer* identifies this subgroup of small tumors. By definition, these tumors are not visible to the naked eye. Specifically, as seen in Table 30-4, criteria for stage IA tumors limit invasion depth to no greater than 5 mm and lateral spread to no wider than 7 mm. Microinvasive cervical cancer carries a minor risk of lymph node involvement and excellent prognosis following treatment. A retrospective study compared tumors with horizontal spread ≤7 mm and those with >7 mm spread. Higher rates of pelvic lymph node metastasis and recurrence rates were noted as tumor spread further than 7 mm (Takeshima, 1999).

Stage IA tumors are further divided into IA1 and IA2. These cancers are subdivided to reflect increasing depth and width of invasion and increasing risks for lymph node involvement.

Stage IA1

These microinvasive tumors invade no deeper than 3 mm, spread no wider than 7 mm, and are associated with the lowest risk for lymph node metastasis. Squamous cervical cancers with stromal invasion less than 1 mm have a 1-percent risk of nodal metastasis, and those with 1 to 3 mm of stromal invasion carry a 1.5-percent risk. Of 4098 women studied with this tumor stage, less than 1 percent died of disease following surgery (Ostor, 1995). Because of the low risk of spread into the parametrial or uterosacral nodes, these lesions may be

effectively treated with cervical conization alone (Table 30-6) (Keighley, 1968; Kolstad, 1989; Morris, 1993; Ostor, 1994). However, a total extrafascial hysterectomy (type I hysterectomy) is preferred for women who have completed childbearing. Hysterectomy types are described in Table 30-7.

In stage IA1 microinvasive cancers, the presence of LVSI increases the risk of lymph node metastasis and cancer recurrence to approximately 5 percent. Accordingly, at our institution, these cases are traditionally managed with modified radical hysterectomy (type II hysterectomy) and pelvic lymphadenectomy. Radical trachelectomy with pelvic lymph node dissection can be considered in women desiring fertility preservation (Olawaiye, 2009). This is described on page 670.

Adenocarcinomas are typically diagnosed at a more advanced stage than squamous cell cervical cancers. Thus, microinvasive adenocarcinomas present a unique management dilemma, due to sparse data regarding this tumor stage. However, based on evaluation of Surveillance Epidemiology and End Result (SEER) data provided by the National Cancer Institute, the incidence of lymph node involvement is similar to that with squamous cancers (Smith, 2002; Spoozak, 2012). Of microinvasive cervical adenocarcinomas, 59 cases managed with uterine preservation and conization have been reported in the literature (Baalbergen, 2011; Bisseling, 2007; Ceballos, 2006; McHale, 2001; Reynolds, 2010; Schorge, 2000; Yahata, 2010). Of these cases, following conization, no recurrences were identified during surveillance in women without LVSI. According to SEER data, the 5-year overall survival for women with stage IA1 adenocarcinoma treated with conization is 98 percent (Spoozak, 2012).

Stage IA2

These microinvasive cervical lesions have 3 to 5 mm of stromal invasion, have a 7-percent risk of lymph node metastasis, and carry a >4-percent risk of disease recurrence. In this group of women, the safety of conservative therapy is yet to be proven. Thus, for this degree of invasion, radical hysterectomy and pelvic lymphadenectomy is recommended.

For fertility preservation, stage IA2 squamous cervical lesions may be treated with radical trachelectomy and lymphadenectomy. A nonabsorbable cerclage may be placed concurrently with such radical trachelectomy to improve cervical competence during pregnancy. These procedures have high cure rates, and successful pregnancies have been reported. If women are carefully selected for age <45 years, smaller tumor size (<2 cm), and negative nodal involvement, then reported recurrence rates are similar to those of radical hysterectomy (Burnett, 2003; Covens, 1999a,b; Gien, 2010; Olawaiye, 2009). Some experts will offer radical trachelectomy to patients with tumors up to 4 cm (stage IB1). However, prior to surgery, approximately one third of patients with this tumor stage will instead be found to need radical hysterectomy or adjuvant chemoradiation due to intermediate- or high-risk features (Abu-Rustum, 2008; Gien, 2010). Preoperative MR imaging to evaluate the parametria and/or CT scan to evaluate extracervical disease is recommended in these cases. If tumor has extended proximally past the internal cervical os, then trachelectomy is contraindicated. Although this technique is promising, it carries a learning curve, and further studies to validate its efficacy are needed.

TABLE 30-6. General Treatment for Primary Invasive Cervical Carcinoma[a]

Cancer Stage	Treatment
IA1[b]	Simple hysterectomy preferred if childbearing completed ***or*** Cervical conization
IA1[b] (with LVSI)	Modified radical hysterectomy and pelvic lymphadenectomy ***or*** Radical trachelectomy and pelvic lymphadenectomy for selected patients desiring fertility
IA2[b,c]	Radical hysterectomy and pelvic lymphadenectomy ***or*** Radical trachelectomy and pelvic lymphadenectomy for selected patients desiring fertility
IB1[c] Some IB2 IIA1	Radical hysterectomy and pelvic lymphadenectomy or radical trachelectomy and pelvic lymphadenectomy for selected patients desiring fertility ***or*** Chemoradiation
Bulky IB2 IIA2	Chemoradiation
IIB to IVA	Chemoradiation ***or*** Rarely, pelvic exenteration[d]
IVB	Palliative chemotherapy ***and/or*** Palliative radiotherapy ***OR*** Supportive care (hospice)

[a]For individual patients, recommendations for treatment can vary, depending on the clinical circumstances.
[b]Intracavitary brachytherapy may be selected for nonsurgical candidates.
[c]Some institutions perform modified (type II) radical hysterectomy and pelvic lymphadenectomy for stage IA2 lesions and smaller stage IB tumors.
[d]A patient with stage IVA lesion with a fistula may be a candidate for a pelvic exenteration.

In addition to stage IA1 tumors, some centers are evaluating the safety of conization or extrafascial hysterectomy for a broader group of women with early-stage cervical cancer, since parametrial involvement in microinvasive cervical cancer is rare (Hou, 2011). One study, which included 51 women with stage IA1 to stage IB1 cervical cancer, demonstrated no recurrences at a median surveillance of 21 months for women treated with conization or extrafascial hysterectomy and no nodal dissection (Bouchard-Fortier, 2014). Two women received adjuvant chemoradiation based on specimen histologic analysis results. In addition, SEER data that included 3987 women with microinvasive cervical cancer showed similar survival rates for women with adenocarcinoma treated with conization compared with hysterectomy. However, women with squamous cell carcinoma undergoing hysterectomy had improved survival rates compared with women undergoing conization (Spoozak, 2012).

Alternatively, patients with microinvasive carcinoma (stages IA1 and IA2) can be treated with intracavitary brachytherapy alone with excellent results (Grigsby, 1991; Hamberger, 1978). Potential candidates for vaginal brachytherapy include women who are elderly or who are not surgical candidates due to comorbid medical disease.

Hysterectomy

Women with FIGO stage IA2 through IIA cervical cancer, that is, those without obvious parametrial involvement, may be selected for radical hysterectomy with pelvic lymph node dissection and with or without paraaortic lymph node dissection. Surgery is appropriate for those who are physically able to tolerate an aggressive surgical procedure, those who wish to avoid the long-term effects of radiation therapy, and/or those who have contraindications to pelvic radiotherapy. Typical candidates include young patients who desire ovarian preservation and retention of a functional, nonirradiated vagina.

Historically, there are five types of hysterectomy, as described by Piver and colleagues (1974). However, hysterectomy techniques used clinically today vary depending on the degree of surrounding tissue that is resected and are categorized as type I, II, or III (see Table 30-7).

Type I hysterectomy, also known as an *extrafascial hysterectomy* or *simple hysterectomy*, removes the uterus and cervix, but does not require excision of the parametrium or paracolpium. It is appropriately selected for benign gynecologic pathology, preinvasive cervical disease, and stage IA1 cervical cancer.

TABLE 30-7. Tissues Resected During Simple and Extended Hysterectomy

Procedure[b]	Type[c]	Involved Tissues[a]			
		Parametria & Paracolpos	Uterine Vessels	Uterosacral Ligament	Vagina
Simple hysterectomy	I	Preserve	Ligate at uterine isthmus	Transect at uterine insertion	Preserve
Modified radical hysterectomy	II	Removed medial to ureter	Ligate at level of ureter	Transect midway between uterus & rectum	Remove 1–2 cm
Radical abdominal hysterectomy	III	Removed medial to uterine vessel origin	Ligate at origin from internal iliac vessels	Transect near rectum[d]	Remove ≥2 cm
Type	IV[e]	Removed medial to uterine vessel origin	Ligate at origin from internal iliac vessels; ligate superior vesical artery	Transect near rectum	Remove 3/4ths
Type	V[e,f]	Removed medial to uterine vessel origin	Ligate at origin from internal iliac vessels; ligate superior vesical artery	Transect near rectum	Remove 3/4ths
Radical vaginal hysterectomy		Removed medial to ureter	Ligate at level of ureter	Partially removed	Remove ≥2 cm
Radical vaginal trachelectomy		Partially removed	Ligate descending cervicovaginal branch	Transect midway between uterus & rectum	Remove 1–2 cm
Radical abdominal trachelectomy		Removed medial to uterine vessel origin	Ligate at origin from internal iliac vessels	Transect near rectum	Remove ≥2 cm

[a]Pelvic lymph node dissection accompanies all except simple hysterectomy.
[b]Hysterectomy includes corpus and cervix removal. For all procedures, unaffected ovaries may remain in premenopausal women, but entire adnexa are usually removed in postmenopausal patients.
[c]Rutledge classification of extended hysterectomy (Piver, 1974).
[d]Although Piver, 1974, described resection of the entire uterosacral ligament, this is not done in practice today due to the high incidence of postoperative urinary retention. Instead, the uterosacral ligaments are divided near the rectum.
[e]Although described by Piver, 1974, these procedures are currently not used clinically.
[f]With Type V, the bladder and proximal ureter are removed.

Type II hysterectomy, also known as *modified radical hysterectomy*, removes the cervix, proximal vagina, and parametrial and paracervical tissue. This hysterectomy is well suited for tumors in patients with stage IA1 cervical cancer who have positive margins following conization and have insufficient cervix to repeat conization. This hysterectomy is also appropriate for patients with stage IA1 cervical cancer with LVSI. Some institutions perform type II hysterectomies in women with stage IA2 tumors and smaller stage IB tumors with good outcomes (Landoni, 2001).

Type III hysterectomy, also known as *radical hysterectomy*, requires greater resection of the parametria. Its goal is to remove microscopic disease that has extended into the parametrium, paracolpium, and around the uterosacral ligaments. To summarize surgical steps, the uterine arteries are ligated at their origin from the internal iliac arteries near the pelvic sidewall, and all tissue medial to this origin, that is, the parametrium, is resected (Fig. 30-11) (Section 46-1, p. 1134). The ureters are completely dissected from their beds and moved laterally for protection during wide excision of the parametrium and

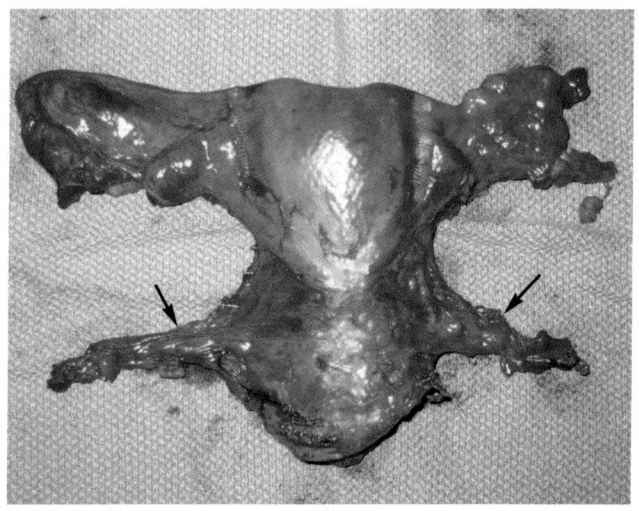

FIGURE 30-11 Gross surgical specimen following radical hysterectomy. The specimen includes the uterus, parametria (*arrows*), adnexa, and 2 cm of proximal vagina.

paracolpium. The bladder and rectum are mobilized caudally and off the vagina to permit resection of ≥2 cm of proximal vagina. The uterosacral ligaments are clamped at their midpoint. This procedure is performed for stage IA2, stage IB1, stage IIA1, and for some stage IB2 lesions, and for patients with relative contraindications to radiation. These contraindications include diabetes, pelvic inflammatory disease, hypertension, collagen disease, inflammatory bowel disease, or adnexal masses.

The approach for type I, II, and III hysterectomies can be abdominal, laparoscopic, robot-assisted, or vaginal, depending on patient characteristics and surgeon experience. Advantages of MIS include less blood loss and shorter hospital stay. Intra- and postoperative complications are similar regardless of approach (Ramirez, 2008). Long-term follow-up of patients undergoing laparoscopic radical hysterectomy demonstrates excellent overall survival rates (Lee, 2010).

Radical Trachelectomy

This surgical option can preserve fertility in selected young women with cervical cancer, and the cancer stages appropriate for radical trachelectomy mirror those for radical hysterectomy. Compared with radical hysterectomy, radical trachelectomy is less often performed.

Radical trachelectomy was originally completed vaginally, as described by Dargent (2000), but an abdominal approach is now used more commonly (Abu-Rustum, 2006). The abdominal approach allows for a larger resection of the parametria and is suitable for patients with larger tumors (>2 cm). With radical trachelectomy, steps of radical hysterectomy proceed and thus the uterine vessels are ligated, the parametria is resected, ureterolysis is completed, the bladder and rectum are mobilized, and the upper vagina is resected. To remove the cervix, the uterus is incised at or just below the level of the internal os, with the goal to leave 5 mm of endocervix still attached to the uterus. At this remaining endocervical margin, a thin tissue sample is sharply excised, termed a *shave margin*, and sent for frozen section. If cancer is absent in this specimen, then reconstruction may proceed. For this, a cerclage using permanent suture is placed, and the knot is tied posteriorly. The uterus is then stitched to the vagina using absorbable sutures. From each side, the corpus ultimately retains blood supply through the uterine branch of the ovarian artery.

Following radical trachelectomy, women continue to menstruate, and conception can occur naturally. However, cervical stenosis may develop, and thus intrauterine insemination or in vitro fertilization is often needed. Pregnancies are frequently complicated by second-trimester loss and higher rates of preterm birth (Plante, 2005; Shepherd, 2008). In a review of 485 women for whom a radical abdominal trachelectomy was planned, 47 cases (10 percent) were converted to radical hysterectomy. Another 25 women required adjuvant therapy based on final pathologic specimen findings. Thus, 413 women (85 percent) retained fertility. In this fertile cohort, there were 75 pregnancies, 18 miscarriages, 47 deliveries (19 term, 12 preterm, 16 not stated), and 10 women were pregnant at the time of publication (Pareja, 2013). Cesarean delivery with a classical incision is recommended.

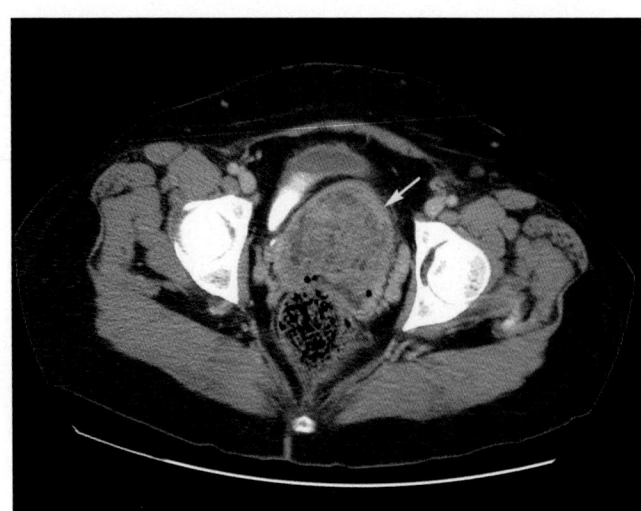

FIGURE 30-12 Computed tomography (CT) scan of stage IB2 cervical cancer (*arrow*).

■ Stage IB to IIA

Stage IB lesions are defined as those extending past the limits of microinvasion yet still confined to the cervix. This stage is subcategorized either as IB1 if tumors measure ≤4 cm or as IB2 if they measure >4 cm (Fig. 30-12).

Stage II cancers extend outside the cervix. They may invade the upper vagina and the parametria but do not reach the pelvic sidewalls. Stage IIA tumors have no parametrial involvement but do extend vaginally as far as the proximal two thirds of the vagina. Stage IIA is further subdivided into stage IIA1 for tumor size ≤4 cm and IIA2 for tumor size >4 cm. Stage IIB cancer may invade the vagina to a similar extent and also invade the parametria.

Treatment

Stage IB to IIA cancers do not extend into the parametria and thus can be managed with either surgery or chemoradiation. In a prospective study of primary therapy, 393 women were randomly assigned to undergo radical hysterectomy and pelvic lymphadenectomy or receive primary radiation therapy. Five-year overall survival and disease-free survival rates were statistically equivalent (83 percent and 74 percent, respectively). Patients who underwent radical surgery followed by radiation had the worst morbidity (Landoni, 1997).

Because chemoradiation and surgery are both viable options, the optimum treatment for each woman ideally assesses clinical factors such as menopausal status, age, concurrent medical illness, tumor histology, and cervical diameter. For stage IB1 and IIA1 cervical cancers, it is left to the physician's discretion and patient preference as to which treatment modality is preferred. Our general approach to patients with bulky stage IB2 or stage II cervical cancers, that is, those measuring >4 cm, is to manage them primarily with chemoradiation, in a similar fashion to advanced-stage cervical cancers.

In general, radical hysterectomy for stage IB through IIA tumors is usually selected for premenopausal women who wish to preserve ovarian function and for women who have concerns about altered sexual functioning following radiotherapy. Age and weight are not contraindications to surgery. However, in general, older women may have longer hospital stays, and heavier women can have longer operative time, greater blood loss, and higher rates of wound complications. Surgery is contraindicated in patients with severe cardiac or pulmonary disease.

In those electing surgery, oophorectomy may be deferred in younger women. One GOG study evaluated tumor spread to the ovary in those with IB tumors electing radical hysterectomy without adnexectomy. Ovarian metastases were identified in only 0.5 percent of 770 women with stage IB squamous cell cancers and in 2 percent of those with adenocarcinomas (Sutton, 1992). For those electing ovarian preservation, ovarian transposition, accomplished by oophoropexy of the ovary into the upper abdomen, can be performed during radical hysterectomy. This repositioning helps preserve ovarian function, in case postoperative pelvic radiation is indicated. In addition, to reduce complications from radiotherapy that might be needed following radical hysterectomy, a surgeon may perform an omental J-flap. Namely, after surgery, the small bowel may become fixed in the pelvis by adhesions, which renders it vulnerable to radiation damage. The omental J-flap can fill the pelvis to reduce this adhesion risk and is described in Section 46-14 (p. 1186).

Systematic lymphadenectomy can lead to complications such as lymphocyst and lymphedema. Therefore, in women with cervical cancer, sentinel lymph node mapping to assess lymphatic spread while avoiding extensive nodal resection is attractive. As a review, the sentinel node is the first node(s) receiving lymphatic drainage from a given tumor. To find this node, either blue dye or a technetium radioactive tracer or both are separately injected preoperatively into the cervix. At surgery, the sentinel node is stained blue and emits radioactivity discernible by Geiger counter. From a metaanalysis including 67 studies, the pooled sentinel node detection rate was 89 percent and sensitivity was 90 percent. Both were highest in women injected with both radiotracer and blue dye. Smaller tumor size (<2 cm) and early-stage diseases were associated with the highest sensitivity and detection rate. At this time, sentinel node for cervical cancer remains experimental (Kadkhodayan, 2015).

Weighing Surgical and Radiotherapy Complications

Complications for early-stage cervical cancer radical surgery include ureteral stricture, ureterovaginal fistula, vesicovaginal fistula, bladder dysfunction, constipation, wound breakdown, lymphocyst, and lymphedema. The risk of venous thromboembolism warrants chemoprophylaxis and/or sequential compression devices as outlined in Table 39-8 (p. 836). If radiotherapy is added as an adjuvant to surgery, the risk of many of these is increased.

On the other hand, radiation therapy also carries long-term complications described in Chapter 28 (p. 619). Of these, altered sexual function secondary to a shortened vagina, dyspareunia, psychological factors, and vaginal stenosis are common. Late urinary and bowel complications such as fistula formation, enteritis, proctitis, and bowel obstruction may also develop following radiotherapy.

Positive Pelvic Lymph Nodes

Approximately 15 percent of patients with stage I through IIA cervical cancers will have positive pelvic nodes. Risk factors for lymph node involvement include those listed in Table 30-8. Of those with involved nodes, 50 percent will have grossly positive pelvic nodes intraoperatively. In most cases involving grossly

TABLE 30-8. Percentage of Cases with Positive Pelvic Lymph Nodes by Pathologic Factors[a]

Factor	(%)	p value
Histologic grade		0.01
1	9.7	
2	13.9	
3	21.8	
Keratinizing/cell size		0.6
Large cell nonkeratinizing	14.5	
Large cell keratinizing	17.2	
Small cell/other	17.6	
Depth of invasion		0.0001
≤5 mm	3.4	
6–10 mm	15.1	
11–15 mm	22.2	
16–20 mm	38.8	
21+ mm	22.6	
Stromal invasion		0.0001
Inner third	4.5	
Middle third	13.3	
Outer third	26.4	
Uterine extension		0.2
Negative	14.6	
Positive	21.6	
Surgical margins		0.4
Negative	15.2	
Positive	25.0	
Parametrial extension		0.0001
Negative	13.5	
Positive	43.2	
LVSI		0.0001
Negative	8.2	
Positive	25.4	

[a]Patients with squamous cell carcinoma, no gross disease beyond the uterus and cervix, and negative aortic nodes. LVSI = lymphovascular space involvement.
Data from Delgado G, Bundy B, Zaino R, et al: Prospective surgical-pathological study of disease-free interval in patients with stage IB squamous cell carcinoma of the cervix: a Gynecologic Oncology Group study. Gynecol Oncol 1990 Sep;38(3):352–357.

positive nodes, radical hysterectomy is abandoned. After recovering from surgery, whole-pelvic radiation and brachytherapy with concomitant chemotherapy is administered. The 50 percent of patients with involved nodes not grossly identified intraoperatively are considered to be at high risk of recurrence following their radical hysterectomy. As described subsequently, these women require postoperative adjuvant chemoradiation therapy.

Recurrence Risk

For women who have completed radical surgery for early-stage cervical cancer, the GOG has defined risk factors to help identify women for tumor recurrence. *Intermediate risk* describes those who on average would have a 30-percent risk of cancer recurrence within 3 years. Factors included in this model are depth of tumor invasion, clinical tumor diameter, and LVSI.

To determine appropriate treatment, patients with these intermediate-risk factors have been studied. In one trial, women were randomly assigned to receive pelvic radiation therapy following radical hysterectomy or to undergo radical hysterectomy and observation. A nearly 50-percent reduced risk of recurrence was found in those who received postoperative adjuvant radiation therapy (Sedlis, 1999). However, this adjuvant radiation does not prolong overall survival. Notably, these patients did not receive chemoradiation. In our practice, these intermediate-risk patients are counseled regarding their recurrence risk and offered the option of adjuvant chemoradiation therapy. A GOG clinical trial (GOG #263) that is assessing chemoradiation in this patient population is ongoing.

A *high-risk* category of early-stage cervical cancer patients who underwent radical surgery has also been described. High-risk is defined as a 50- to 70-percent risk of recurrence within 5 years. These women have positive lymph nodes, positive surgical margins, or microscopically positive parametria (Peters, 2000). This group is routinely offered adjuvant radiation therapy. Moreover, the GOG demonstrated that the addition of concurrent chemotherapy significantly prolongs disease-free and overall survival rates in this group of women with high-risk early-stage cancer (Peters, 2000).

Adjuvant Hysterectomy Following Primary Radiation

Treating bulky stage I (IB2) cervical cancers with adjuvant hysterectomy after radiation therapy has been evaluated. Adjuvant hysterectomy reduces locoregional relapse but does not contribute to an overall improvement in survival rates. However, initial lesion size may affect efficacy. In one study, those with tumors measuring <7 cm who underwent postradiation hysterectomy survived longer than did women with equivalent tumors in the radiation-only regimen group. In contrast, those with lesions ≥7 cm who underwent postradiation hysterectomy fared worse than their counterparts receiving only radiotherapy (Keys, 2003).

Early-stage Cervical Adenocarcinoma

These cancers may be more radioresistant than squamous cell cervical carcinomas. Although some prefer radical hysterectomy to radiotherapy, studies suggest equivalent survival rates with either (Eifel, 1991, 1995; Hopkins, 1988; Nakano, 1995). However, larger lesions may not regress if managed by radiation alone (Leveque, 1998; Silver, 1998). The centers of bulky tumors may be less radiosensitive due to relative cellular hypoxia. This effect underscores the advantages of radical hysterectomy for women with stage I cervical adenocarcinoma.

ADVANCED-STAGE PRIMARY DISEASE TREATMENT

▪ Stages IIB through IVA

Advanced-stage cervical cancers extend past the confines of the cervix and often involve adjacent organs and retroperitoneal lymph nodes. If untreated, these tumors progress rapidly. Treatment for these tumors is individualized, yet most advanced-stage tumors have a poor prognosis and 5-year survival rates are <50 percent.

Radiation Therapy

This modality forms the cornerstone of advanced-stage cervical cancer management. Both external beam pelvic radiation and brachytherapy are typically delivered (Chap. 28, p. 615). Of these, external beam radiation usually precedes intracavitary radiation, which is one form of brachytherapy. External beam radiation is commonly administered in 25 fractions during 5 weeks (40 to 50 Gy). During evaluation, if paraaortic nodal metastases are found, then extended-field radiation can be added to treat these affected lymph nodes.

During brachytherapy, bowel and bladder are packed away from the intracavitary source using vaginal packing during tandem insertion to limit radiation to these organs. Treatment is often prescribed to point A, that is, a point 2 cm lateral and 2 cm superior to the external cervical os, and to point B, which is a point 3 cm lateral to point A. Side effects during and following radiation therapy are common, and these are discussed in Chapter 28 (p. 619).

Chemoradiation

Current evidence indicates that chemotherapy given concurrently with radiation therapy significantly improves overall and disease-free survival rates of women with cervical cancer. Chemoradiation is also associated with superior survival rates compared with pelvic and extended-field paraaortic region irradiation alone (Morris, 1999). After five trials demonstrated improved survival rates, it is now recommended that cisplatin-based chemotherapy should be considered in women undergoing radiation for cervical cancer (Keys, 1999; Morris, 1999; Peters, 2000; Rose, 1999; Whitney, 1999).

Of chemotherapy agents, cisplatin-containing regimens have been associated with the best survival rates (Rose, 1999; Whitney, 1999). The characteristics of this agent are described in Chapter 27 (p. 602), and Figure 30-13 describes its

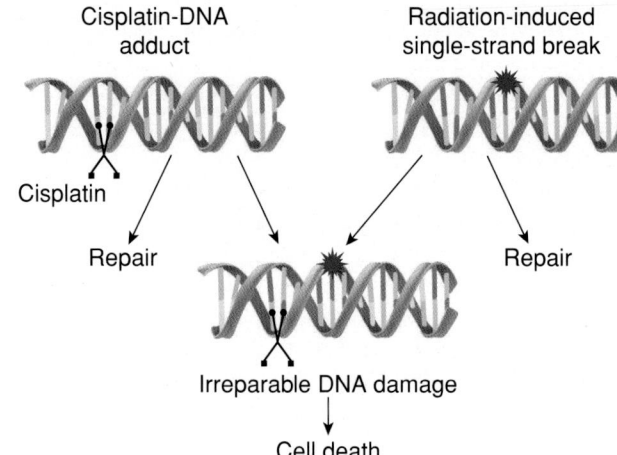

FIGURE 30-13 Cisplatin can bind covalently to DNA bases. Radiation therapy may create single-strand breaks. If occurring alone, each damaging event is likely to be repaired. However, if both occur in close proximity, irreparable damage can lead to cell death.

tumoricidal action. Nonplatinum regimens also have activity but have not been directly compared with cisplatin-containing regimens (Vale, 2008). At our institution, cisplatin is given weekly for 5 weeks. It is administered concurrently with external beam radiation and with brachytherapy. Unfortunately, the recurrence risk remains as high as 40 percent after chemoradiation given for curative intent (Chemoradiotherapy for Cervical Cancer Meta-Analysis Collaboration, 2009). Therefore, a large international randomized Phase III trial is currently evaluating whether the addition of adjuvant chemotherapy after completion of chemoradiation improves overall survival rates for women with stage IB1 with positive nodes and for those with stage IB2 through IVA disease.

Pelvic Exenteration for Primary Disease

This ultraradical surgery encompasses removal of the bladder, rectum, uterus, fallopian tubes and ovaries (if present), vagina, and surrounding tissues (Section 46-4, p. 1149). Primary exenteration may be considered for women with stage IVA cancer, that is, with direct tumor invasion into bladder and/or bowel but without distant spread. Exenteration is rarely performed for this indication, yet for suitable candidates, the survival rate can reach 30 percent (Million, 1972; Upadhyay, 1988).

■ Stage IVB

Patients with stage IVB disease have a poor prognosis and are treated with a goal of palliation. Pelvic radiation is administered to control vaginal bleeding and pain. Systemic chemotherapy is offered to palliate symptoms and prolong overall survival. The chemotherapy regimens used in this group of women are similar to those used in the setting of recurrent cancer.

SURVEILLANCE

■ Following Radiotherapy

Women who receive radiotherapy are closely monitored to assess their response. Tumors may be expected to regress for up to 3 months after therapy. Pelvic examination and/or radiologic scanning should document progressive shrinkage of the cervical mass. The rectovaginal examination is used to detect nodularity in the ligaments and parametria. If disease progresses locally after this interval, prognosis is poor. Pelvic exenteration may sometimes be indicated for this clinical setting.

In general, patients are seen at 3-month intervals for 2 years, then every 6 months until 5 years have passed from treatment, and then annually. At each visit, in addition to pelvic examination, a thorough manual nodal survey includes neck, supraclavicular, axillary, and inguinal lymph nodes. A cervical or vaginal cuff Pap test is also collected annually for 20 years after treatment completion. Findings of high-grade squamous intraepithelial lesions with screening should prompt colposcopic evaluation and biopsy of suspicious lesions. If recurrent cancer is diagnosed from these biopsies, then CT imaging is performed.

Once radiotherapy is completed, patients are encouraged to use a vaginal dilator or have vaginal intercourse three times per week. This helps keep the vagina patent, aids pelvic examination

and Pap testing in the future, and ensures that the patient can remain sexually active if desired. Otherwise, radiation may result in vaginal fibrosis, leading to a shortened, nonfunctional vagina. The use of a water-based lubricant is also recommended.

■ Following Surgery

After a radical hysterectomy, 80 percent of recurrences are detected within the subsequent 2 years. During patient surveillance, an abnormal pelvic mass or abnormal pelvic examination finding typically prompts CT scanning of the abdomen and pelvis. Findings include cervical or vaginal lesion, rectovaginal nodularity, pain radiating down the posterior thigh, or new-onset lower extremity edema. Pelvic recurrences after radical hysterectomy, if diagnosed early, can be treated with radiation therapy. The same schedule of visits and Pap testing as just outlined for surveillance following radiotherapy is then recommended.

■ Hormone Therapy

Cervical cancer is not estrogen-dependent and thus hormone therapy is not contraindicated to treat menopausal symptoms, taking into account the risks and benefits discussed in Chapter 22 (p. 494). Moreover, hormone therapy is strongly considered for any premenopausal patient undergoing radiation treatment for cervical cancer until the average age of menopause. This is because radiation doses given for cervical cancer lead to menopause. Ovaries previously transposed out of the pelvic radiation field may be exceptions. Either systemic or vaginal forms are suitable. Estrogen alone is used if the uterus has been surgically removed, whereas combination hormonal therapy is given if the uterus remains.

SECONDARY DISEASE

This is defined as either persistent or recurrent cancer. *Persistent disease* is cervical cancer that has not completely regressed within 3 months of finishing radiotherapy. *Recurrent disease* is defined as a new lesion after primary therapy completion and initial regression.

Treatment of persistent or recurrent disease depends on its location and extent. The intent in these cases is usually palliative. However, in certain instances, a woman may qualify for pelvic radiation if she previously had not received this treatment. Alternatively, a woman may be a candidate for curative-intent surgery. Metastatic cervical cancer is not curable. In this setting, the goal of chemotherapy is to maximize existing patient quality of life and prolong survival.

■ Pelvic Exenteration for Secondary Disease

When curative-intent surgery is contemplated, local disease should be biopsy proven. Clinically, a patient may be considered for pelvic exenteration if the triad of lower extremity edema, back pain, and hydronephrosis are absent. If present, these suggest disease extension to the pelvic sidewalls, which would contraindicate surgery. In addition, regional and distant metastasis should be excluded by both physical examination and radiologic imaging, which typically is a PET/CT scan.

TABLE 30-9. Combination Chemotherapy Regimens and Response Rates of Cervical Cancer

Study	Chemotherapy Agents	Response Rates (%)	Progression-free Survival (months)	Overall Survival (months)
Moore, 2004	Cisplatin vs.	19	2.8	8.8
	Cisplatin and paclitaxel	36	4.8	9.7
Long, 2005	Cisplatin vs.	13	2.9	6.5
	Cisplatin and topotecan	27	4.6	9.4
Morris, 2004	Cisplatin and vinorelbine	30	5.5	—
Brewer, 2006	Cisplatin and gemcitabine	22	2.1	—
Monk, 2009	Cisplatin and paclitaxel vs.	29	5.8	12.9
	Cisplatin and vinorelbine vs.	26	4	
	Cisplatin and gemcitabine vs.	22	4.7 }	10–10.3
	Cisplatin and topotecan	23	4.6)	
Tewari, 2014	Cisplatin and paclitaxel ±	45	7.6	14.3
	bevacizumab vs.	50		17.5
	Topotecan and paclitaxel ±	27	5.7	12.7
	bevacizumab	47		16.2

Pelvic exenteration begins with exploratory laparotomy, biopsies of suspicious lesions, and paraaortic lymph node evaluation. Exenteration is completed only if no disease is found in frozen section specimens sampled at the beginning of the surgery. A complete surgical description of this procedure is found in Section 46-4 (p. 1149).

Alternatively, in highly selected patients, radical hysterectomy may be considered as an alternative to pelvic exenteration (Coleman, 1994). In these circumstances, women should have small cervical recurrences measuring less than 2 cm and have disease-free pelvic lymph nodes both prior to and during surgery.

With either operation, intraoperative and postoperative complications can be significant. Reported 5-year survival rates approximate 50 percent. Most recurrences occur in the first 2 years postoperatively (Berek, 2005; Goldberg, 2006).

■ Radiotherapy or Chemotherapy for Secondary Disease

Patients with central or limited peripheral recurrences who are radiotherapy naïve are candidates for curative-intent chemoradiation treatment. In these groups, survival rates of 30 to 70 percent have been reported (Ijaz, 1998; Ito, 1997; Lanciano, 1996; Potter, 1990).

Antineoplastic drugs are used to palliate both disease and symptoms of advanced, persistent, or recurrent cervical cancer (Table 30-9). Cisplatin is considered the single most active cytotoxic agent in this setting (Thigpen, 1995). Overall, response duration to cisplatin is 4 to 6 months, and survival in such women only approximates 7 months (Vermorken, 1993). A four-arm prospective randomized study demonstrated that the combinations of cisplatin with topotecan, vinorelbine, or gemcitabine are not superior to the combination of cisplatin and paclitaxel (Monk, 2009). Most recently, a randomized study evaluated adding bevacizumab to combination chemotherapy. Bevacizumab (Avastin) is a monoclonal antibody targeting vascular endothelial growth factor (VEGF). This addition increased the median overall survival length by 3.7 months (see Table 30-9) (Tewari, 2014).

PALLIATIVE CARE

Palliative chemotherapy is administered only if this treatment does not significantly lower patient quality of life and is balanced against the benefits of supportive care. Women with persistent nausea and vomiting from tumor-associated ileus may benefit from a gastrostomy tube. Bowel obstruction can be managed surgically, provided a patient is an appropriate surgical candidate. Percutaneous nephrostomy tubes may be placed for urinary fistulas or urinary tract obstruction.

Pain management forms the basis of palliation, and an extensive list of pain medications is found in Table 42-2 (p. 910). Cervical cancer patients can experience significant pain, and this is assessed at each visit. Many will require narcotics. If a patient has been using opioids and is hospitalized for inadequate pain control, then patient-controlled analgesia is considered. The total dose that controls the pain in a 24-hour period is determined. This dose can then be converted an equivalent dose of long-acting opioids. To allow for incomplete cross-tolerance between narcotics, the dose should be decreased by 25 to 50 percent. A supplemental short-acting opioid can be available for breakthrough pain and is typically prescribed at a dose that is 10 to 20 percent of the long-acting total daily dose and given at appropriate intervals. Narcotics can constipate, and patients using these are given a bowel regimen. This can be individualized, and suitable agents are listed in Table 25-6 (p. 570). In particular, a combination of stool softeners (docusate sodium) plus laxative (senna) plus polyethylene glycol is often effective.

We recommend discussion of medical directives if a patient has adequate mental capability. Often, such discussion is conducted over time, giving a woman an opportunity to understand the severity and progression of her disease. Home hospice is an invaluable part of terminal care for most of these women, who require intensive pain management and considerable assistance with daily living activities.

MANAGEMENT DURING PREGNANCY

Survival rates between pregnant and nonpregnant women with cervical cancer do not differ when matched by age, stage, and year of diagnosis. Overall survival rates are slightly better for cervical cancer in pregnancy, because an increased proportion of patients have stage I disease.

■ Diagnosis

A Pap test is recommended for all pregnant patients older than 21 at the initial prenatal visit. Additionally, clinically suspicious lesions are directly biopsied. If Pap test results reveal HSIL, adenocarcinoma in situ (AIS), or suspected malignancy, then colposcopy is performed and biopsies are obtained. However, endocervical curettage is excluded to prevent amnionic sac rupture.

If Pap testing indicates malignant cells and colposcopy-directed biopsy fails to confirm malignancy, then diagnostic conization may be necessary. Many experts recommend delaying conization until the second trimester due to concern about pregnancy loss, however, median blood loss during excisional procedures increases with gestational age, especially in the third trimester. In pregnant patients, a loop electrosurgical excision procedure (LEEP) does not appear to offer an advantage compared with cold-knife conization. Moreover, one study found a surgical complication rate of 25 percent with LEEP in pregnancy, and 47 percent of the women had persistent or recurrent disease (Robinson, 1997).

■ Stages I and II Cancer in Pregnancy

Women with microinvasive squamous cell cervical carcinoma found during conization that measures ≤3 mm and contains no LVSI (stage IA1) may deliver vaginally and be reevaluated 6 weeks postpartum. Moreover, for those with stage IA or IB disease, studies find no increased maternal risk if treatment is intentionally delayed to optimize fetal maturity regardless of the trimester in which the cancer was diagnosed. Given the outcomes, a planned treatment delay is generally acceptable for women who are 20 or more weeks' gestational age at diagnosis with stage I disease and who desire to continue their pregnancy. However, a patient may be able to delay from earlier gestational ages if she wishes. For women who wish to continue pregnancy, pelvic lymph node dissection can be performed in pregnancy in the first and second trimester via MIS (Vercellino, 2014). Women with positive nodes may elect to be treated with definitive treatment, rather than delay treatment, or may opt for neoadjuvant chemotherapy during pregnancy or for early delivery. For women who have a previable gestation and who desire definitive treatment of early-stage disease, a radical hysterectomy with the fetus in situ and lymphadenectomy can be performed. For patients with stage IA2 through IIA1, a cesarean section via a classical uterine incision may be performed at term, followed immediately by radical hysterectomy and lymph node dissection. Notably, a classical cesarean incision minimizes the risk of cutting through tumor in the lower uterine segment, which can cause serious blood loss and result in tumor spread.

■ Advanced Cervical Cancer in Pregnancy

Women with advanced cervical cancer diagnosed prior to fetal viability are offered primary chemoradiation. Spontaneous abortion of the fetus tends to follow whole-pelvis radiation therapy. For women who decline pregnancy termination, systemic chemotherapy can be administered. Cisplatin with vincristine or with paclitaxel can be administered in pregnancy. Congenital anomalies, growth restriction, and preterm delivery do not appear to be increased in fetuses of women who receive chemotherapy after the first trimester (Cardonick, 2010). If cancer is diagnosed after fetal viability is reached and a delay until fetal pulmonary maturity is elected, then a classical cesarean delivery is performed. Chemoradiation is administered after uterine involution. For patients with advanced disease and treatment delay, pregnancy may impair prognosis. A woman who elects to delay treatment, to provide quantifiable benefit to her fetus, will have to accept an undefined risk of disease progression.

REFERENCES

Abed Z, O'Leary M, Hand K, et al: Cervical screening history in patients with early stage carcinoma of the cervix. Ir Med J 99:140, 2006

Abu-Rustum NR, Neubauer N, Sonoda Y, et al: Surgical and pathologic outcomes of fertility-sparing radical abdominal trachelectomy for FIGO stage IB1 cervical cancer. Gynecol Oncol 111:261, 2008

Abu-Rustum NR, Sonoda Y, Black D, et al: Fertility-sparing radical abdominal trachelectomy for cervical carcinoma: technique and review of the literature. Gynecol Oncol 103:807, 2006

Agorastos T, Chatzistamatiou K, Katsamagkas T, et al: Primary screening for cervical cancer based on high-risk human papillomavirus (HPV) detection and HPV 16 and HPV 18 genotyping, in comparison to cytology. PLoS One 10:1, 2015

Albores-Saavedra J, Gersell D, Gilks CB, et al: Terminology of endocrine tumors of the uterine cervix: results of a workshop sponsored by the College of American Pathologists and the National Cancer Institute. Arch Pathol Lab Med 121:34, 1997

Baalbergen A, Smedts F, Helmerhorst TJ: Conservative therapy in microinvasive adenocarcinoma of the uterine cervix is justified. An analysis of 59 cases and a review of the literature. Int J Gynecol Cancer 21:1620, 2011

Belhocine T, Thille A, Fridman V, et al: Contribution of whole-body ¹⁸FDG PET imaging in the management of cervical cancer. Gynecol Oncol 87:90, 2002

Benoit AG, Krepart GV, Lotocki RJ: Results of prior cytologic screening in patients with a diagnosis of stage I carcinoma of the cervix. Am J Obstet Gynecol 148:690, 1984

Berek JS, Howe C, Lagasse LD, et al: Pelvic exenteration for recurrent gynecologic malignancy: survival and morbidity analysis of the 45-year experience at UCLA. Gynecol Oncol 99:153, 2005

Bipat S, Glas AS, van der Velden J, et al: Computed tomography and magnetic resonance imaging in staging of uterine cervical carcinoma: a systemic review. Gynecol Oncol 91:59, 2003

Bisseling KCHM, Bekkers RLM, Rome RM, et al: Treatment of microinvasive adenocarcinoma of the uterine cervix: a retrospective study and review of the literature. Gynecol Oncol 107:424, 2007

Bosch FX, Munoz N: The viral etiology of cervical cancer. Virus Res 89:183, 2002

Bouchard-Fortier G, Reade CJ, Covens A: Non-radical surgery for small early-stage cervical cancer. Is it time? Gynecol Oncol 132:624, 2014

Brewer CA, Blessing JA, Nagourney RA, et al: Cisplatin plus gemcitabine in previously treated squamous cell carcinoma of the cervix: a phase II study of the Gynecologic Oncology Group. Gynecol Oncol 100(2):385, 2006

Bulk S, Berkhof J, Bulkmans NWJ, et al: Preferential risk of HPV16 for squamous cell carcinoma and of HPV18 for adenocarcinoma of the cervix compared to women with normal cytology in the Netherlands. Br J Cancer 94:171, 2006

SECTION 4

Burnett AF, Roman LD, O'Meara AT, et al: Radical vaginal trachelectomy and pelvic lymphadenectomy for preservation of fertility in early cervical carcinoma. Gynecol Oncol 88:419, 2003

Cardonick E, Usmani A, Ghaffar S: Perinatal outcomes of a pregnancy complicated by cancer, including neonatal follow-up after in utero exposure to chemotherapy. Am J Clin Oncol 33:221, 2010

Ceballos KM, Shaw D, Daya D: Microinvasive cervical adenocarcinoma (FIGO stage IA tumors), results of surgical staging and outcome analysis. Am J Surg Pathol 30:370, 2006

Chemoradiotherapy for Cervical Cancer Meta-Analysis Collaboration: Reducing uncertainties about the effects of chemoradiotherapy for cervical cancer: a systematic review and meta-analysis of individual patient data from 18 randomized trials. J Clin Oncol 26:5802, 2008

Coleman RL, Keeney ED, Freedman RS, et al: Radical hysterectomy for recurrent carcinoma of the uterine cervix after radiotherapy. Gynecol Oncol 55:29, 1994

Cosin JA, Fowler JM, Chen MD, et al: Pretreatment surgical staging of patients with cervical carcinoma: the case for lymph node debulking. Cancer 82:2241, 1998

Covens A, Kirby J, Shaw P, et al: Prognostic factors for relapse and pelvic lymph node metastases in early stage I adenocarcinoma of the cervix. Gynecol Oncol 74:423, 1999a

Covens A, Shaw P, Murphy J, et al: Is radical trachelectomy a safe alternative to radical hysterectomy for patients with stage IA-B carcinoma of the cervix? Cancer 86:2273, 1999b

Dargent D, Martin X, Saccetoni A, et al: Laparoscopic vaginal radical trachelectomy. Cancer 88:1877, 2000

Datta GD, Colditz GA, Kawachi I, et al: Individual-, neighborhood-, and state-level socioeconomic predictors of cervical carcinoma screening among U.S. black women: a multilevel analysis. Cancer 106:664, 2006

Delgado G, Bundy B, Zaino R, et al: Prospective surgical-pathological study of disease-free interval in patients with stage IB squamous cell carcinoma of the cervix: a Gynecologic Oncology Group study. Gynecol Oncol 38:352, 1990

Downey GO, Potish RA, Adock LL, et al: Pretreatment surgical staging in cervical carcinoma: therapeutic efficacy of pelvic lymph node resection. Am J Obstet Gynecol 160:1055, 1989

Dugue P, Rebolj M, Hallas J, et al: Risk of cervical cancer in women with autoimmune diseases, in relation with their use of immunosuppressants and screening: population-based cohort study. Int J Cancer 136:E711, 2015

Eifel PJ, Burke TW, Delclos L, et al: Early stage I adenocarcinoma of the uterine cervix: treatment results in patients with tumors less than or equal to 4 cm in diameter. Gynecol Oncol 41:199, 1991

Eifel PJ, Burke TW, Morris M, et al: Adenocarcinoma as an independent risk factor for disease recurrence in patients with stage IB cervical carcinoma. Gynecol Oncol 59:38, 1995

Eifel PJ, Morris M, Oswald MJ, et al: Adenocarcinoma of the uterine cervix. Prognosis and patterns of failure in 367 cases. Cancer 65:2507, 1990

Follen M, Levenback CF, Iyer RB, et al: Imaging in cervical cancer. Cancer 98(9S):2028, 2003

Gien LT, Covens A: Fertility-sparing options for early stage cervical cancer. Gynecol Oncol 117:350, 2010

Goff BA, Muntz HG, Paley PJ, et al: Impact of surgical staging in women with locally advanced cervical cancer. Gynecol Oncol 74:436, 1999

Goldberg GL, Sukumvanich P, Einstein MH, et al: Total pelvic exenteration: the Albert Einstein College of Medicine/Montefiore Medical Center experience (1987 to 2003). Gynecol Oncol 101:261, 2006

Grigsby PW, Perez CA: Radiotherapy alone for medically inoperable carcinoma of the cervix: stage IA and carcinoma in situ. Int J Radiat Oncol Biol Phys 21:375, 1991

Grulich AE, van Leeuwen MT, Falster MO, et al: Incidence of cancers in people with HIV/AIDS compared with immunosuppressed transplant recipients: a meta-analysis. Lancet 370:59, 2007

Hacker NF, Wain GV, Nicklin JL: Resection of bulky positive lymph nodes in patients with cervical carcinoma. Int J Gynecol Cancer 5:250, 1995

Hamberger AD, Fletcher GH, Wharton JT: Results of treatment of early stage I carcinoma of the uterine cervix with intracavitary radium alone. Cancer 41:980, 1978

Havrilesky LJ, Kulasingam SL, Matchar DB, et al: FDG-PET for management of cervical and ovarian cancer. Gynecol Oncol 97: 183, 2005

Helt AM, Funk JO, Galloway DA: Inactivation of both the retinoblastoma tumor suppressor and p21 by the human papillomavirus type 16 E7 oncoprotein is necessary to inhibit cell cycle arrest in human epithelial cells. J Virol 76:10559, 2002

Henriksen E: The lymphatic spread of carcinoma of the cervix and of the body of the uterus; a study of 420 necropsies. Am J Obstet Gynecol 58(5):924, 1949

Holcomb K, Abulafia O, Matthews RP, et al: The impact of pretreatment staging laparotomy on survival in locally advanced cervical carcinoma. Eur J Gynaecol Oncol 20:90, 1999

Hopkins MP, Schmidt RW, Roberts JA, et al: The prognosis and treatment of stage I adenocarcinoma of the cervix. Obstet Gynecol 72:915, 1988

Hou J, Goldberg GL, Qualls CR, et al: Risk factors for poor prognosis in microinvasive adenocarcinoma of the uterine cervix (IA1 and IA2): a pooled analysis. Gynecol Oncol 121:135, 2011

Howlader N, Noone AM, Krapcho M, et al: SEER Cancer Statistics Review, 1975-2011, National Cancer Institute. 2014. Available at: http://seer.cancer.gov/csr/1975_2011/. Accessed April 12, 2015

Hricak H, Gatsonis C, Chi, et al: Role of imaging in pretreatment evaluation of early invasive cervical cancer: results of the intergroup study American College of Radiology Imaging Network 6651–Gynecologic Oncology Group 183. J Clin Oncol 23:9329, 2005

Ijaz T, Eifel PJ, Burke T, et al: Radiation therapy of pelvic recurrence after radical hysterectomy for cervical carcinoma. Gynecol Oncol 70:241, 1998

International Collaboration of Epidemiological Studies of Cervical Cancer: Comparison of risk factors for invasive squamous cell carcinoma and adenocarcinoma of the cervix: collaborative reanalysis of individual data on 8,097 women with squamous cell carcinoma and 1,374 women with adenocarcinoma from 12 epidemiological studies. Int J Cancer 120:885, 2006

International Collaboration of Epidemiological Studies of Cervical Cancer, Appleby P, Beral V, et al: Cervical cancer and hormonal contraceptives: collaborative reanalysis of individual data for 16,573 women with cervical cancer and 35,509 women without cervical cancer from 24 epidemiological studies. Lancet 370(9599):1609, 2007

Ito H, Shigematsu N, Kawada T, et al: Radiotherapy for centrally recurrent cervical cancer of the vaginal stump following hysterectomy. Gynecol Oncol 67:154, 1997

Jaworski RC, Roberts JM, Robboy SJ, et al: Cervical glandular neoplasia. In Robboy SJ, Mutter GL, Prat J, et al (eds): Robboy's Pathology of the Female Reproductive Tract, 2nd ed. Churchill Livingstone Elsevier, 2009, p 273

Jemal A, Siegel R, Ward E, et al: Cancer statistics, 2006. CA Cancer J Clin 56: 106, 2006

Jones DL, Munger K: Analysis of the p53-mediated G1 growth arrest pathway in cells expressing the human papillomavirus type 16 E7 oncoprotein. J Virol 71:2905, 1997

Jones EE, Wells SI: Cervical cancer and human papillomaviruses: inactivation of retinoblastoma and other tumor suppressor pathways. Curr Mol Med 6:795, 2006

Kadkhodayan S, Hasanzadeh M, Treglia G, et al: Sentinel node biopsy for lymph nodal staging of uterine cervix cancer: a systematic review and meta-analysis of the pertinent literature. Eur J Surg Oncol 41:1, 2015

Kapp KS, Poschauko J, Tauss J, et al: Analysis of the prognostic impact of tumor embolization before definitive radiotherapy for cervical carcinoma. Int J Radiat Oncol Biol Phys 62:1399, 2005

Keighley E: Carcinoma of the cervix among prostitutes in a women's prison. Br J Vener Dis 44:254, 1968

Keys HM, Bundy BN, Stehman FB, et al: Cisplatin, radiation and adjuvant hysterectomy compared with radiation and adjuvant hysterectomy for bulky stage IB cervical carcinoma. N Engl J Med 340: 1154, 1999

Keys HM, Bundy BN, Stehman FB, et al: Radiation therapy with and without extrafascial hysterectomy for bulky stage IB cervical carcinoma: a randomized trial of the Gynecologic Oncology Group. Gynecol Oncol 89:343, 2003

Kolstad P: Follow-up study of 232 patients with stage Ia1 and 411 patients with stage Ia2 squamous cell carcinoma of the cervix (microinvasive carcinoma). Gynecol Oncol 33:265, 1989

Komaki R, Brickner TJ, Hanlon AL, et al: Long-term results of treatment of cervical carcinoma in the United States in 1973, 1978, and 1983: Patterns of Care Study (PCS). Int J Radiat Oncol Biol Phys 31:973, 1995

Koshiol J, Schroeder J, Jamieson DJ, et al: Smoking and time to clearance of human papillomavirus infection in HIV-seropositive and HIV-seronegative women. Am J Epidemiol 164:176, 2006

Kupets R, Thomas GM, Covens A: Is there a role for pelvic lymph node debulking in advanced cervical cancer? Gynecol Oncol 87:163, 2002

Lanciano R: Radiotherapy for the treatment of locally recurrent cervical cancer. J Natl Cancer Inst Monogr 21:113, 1996

Landoni F, Maneo A, Colombo A, et al: Randomised study of radical surgery versus radiotherapy for stage Ib-IIa cervical cancer. Lancet 350:535, 1997

Landoni F, Maneo A, Cormio G, et al: Class II versus class III radical hysterectomy in stage IB-IIA cervical cancer: a prospective randomized study. Gynecol Oncol 80:3, 2001

Lea JS, Sheets EE, Wenham RM, et al: Stage IIB-IVB cervical adenocarcinoma: prognostic factors and survival. Gynecol Oncol 84:115, 2002

Leblanc E, Narducci F, Frumovitz, et al: Therapeutic value of pretherapeutic laparoscopic staging of locally advanced cervical carcinoma. Gynecol Oncol 105:304, 2007

Lee CL, Wu KY, Juang KG, et al: Long-term survival outcomes of laparoscopically assisted radical hysterectomy in treating early-stage cervical cancer. Am J Obstet Gynecol 203:165.e1, 2010

Leveque J, Laurent JF, Burtin F, et al: Prognostic factors of the uterine cervix adenocarcinoma. Eur J Obstet Gynecol Reprod Biol 80:209, 1998

Ley C, Bauer HM, Reingold A, et al: Determinants of genital human papillomavirus infection in young women. J Natl Cancer Inst 83:997, 1991

Leyden WA, Manos MM, Geiger AM, et al: Cervical cancer in women with comprehensive health care access: attributable factors in the screening process. J Natl Cancer Inst 97:675, 2005

Li N, Franceschi S, Howell-Jones R, et al: Human papillomavirus type distribution in 30,848 invasive cervical cancers worldwide: variation by geographical region, histological type and year of publication. Int J Cancer, 2010

Long HJ III, Bundy BN, Grendys EC Jr, et al: Randomized phase III trial of cisplatin with or without topotecan in carcinoma of the uterine cervix: a Gynecologic Oncology Group study. J Clin Oncol 23(21):4626, 2005

Look KY, Brunetto VL, Clarke-Pearson DL, et al: An analysis of cell type in patients with surgically staged stage IB carcinoma of the cervix: a Gynecologic Oncology Group study. Gynecol Oncol 63:304, 1996

Mantovani F, Banks L: Inhibition of E6 induced degradation of p53 is not sufficient for stabilization of p53 protein in cervical tumour derived cell lines. Oncogene 18:3309, 1999

McHale MT, Le TD, Burger RA, et al: Fertility sparing treatment for in situ and early invasive adenocarcinoma of the cervix. Obstet Gynecol 98:726, 2001

Million RR, Rutledge F, Fletcher GH: Stage IV carcinoma of the cervix with bladder invasion. Am J Obstet Gynecol 113:239, 1972

Mitchell DG, Snyder B, Coakley F, et al: Early invasive cervical cancer: tumor delineation by magnetic resonance imaging, computed tomography, and clinical examination, verified by pathologic results, in the ACRIN 6651/GOG 183 intergroup study. J Clin Oncol 24:5687, 2006

Monk BJ, Sill MW, McMeekin DS, et al: Phase III trial of four cisplatin-containing doublet combinations in stage IVB, recurrent, or persistent cervical carcinoma: a Gynecologic Oncology Group study. J Clin Oncol 27:1, 2009

Moore DH, Blessing JA, McQuellon RP, et al: Phase III study of cisplatin with or without paclitaxel in stage IVB, recurrent, or persistent squamous cell carcinoma of the cervix: a Gynecologic Oncology Group study. J Clin Oncol 22(15):3113, 2004

Moreno V, Bosch FX, Muñoz N, et al: Effect of oral contraceptives on risk of cervical cancer in women with human papillomavirus infection: the IARC multicentric case-control study. Lancet 359:1085, 2002

Morris M, Blessing JA, Monk BJ, et al: Phase II study of cisplatin and vinorelbine in squamous cell carcinoma of the cervix: a Gynecologic Oncology Group study. J Clin Oncol 22(16):3340, 2004

Morris M, Eifel PJ, Lu J, et al: Pelvic radiation with concurrent chemotherapy compared with pelvic and para-aortic radiation for high-risk cervical cancer. N Engl J Med 340:1137, 1999

Morris M, Mitchell MF, Silva EG, et al: Cervical conization as definitive therapy for early invasive squamous carcinoma of the cervix. Gynecol Oncol 51:193, 1993

Munger K, Basile JR, Duensing S, et al: Biological activities and molecular targets of the human papillomavirus E7 oncoprotein. Oncogene 20:7888, 2001

Muñoz N, Franceschi S, Bosetti C, et al: Role of parity and human papillomavirus in cervical cancer: the IARC multicentric case-control study. Lancet 359:1093, 2002

Nakano T, Arai T, Morita S, et al: Radiation therapy alone for adenocarcinoma of the uterine cervix. Int J Radiat Oncol Biol Phys 32:1331, 1995

Olawaiye A, Del Carmen M, Tambouret R, et al: Abdominal radical trachelectomy: success and pitfalls in a general gynecologic oncology practice. Gynecol Oncol 112:506, 2009

Ostor AG: Pandora's box or Ariadne's thread? Definition and prognostic significance of microinvasion in the uterine cervix. Squamous lesions. Pathol Annu 30(Pt 2):103, 1995

Ostor AG, Rome RM: Micro-invasive squamous cell carcinoma of the cervix: a clinico-pathologic study of 200 cases with long-term follow-up. Int J Gynecol Cancer 4:257, 1994

Pareja R, Rendon GJ, Sanz-Lomana CM, et al: Surgical, oncological, and obstetrical outcomes after abdominal radical trachelectomy: a systematic literature review. Gynecol Oncol 131:77, 2013

Patsner B: Topical acetone for control of life-threatening vaginal hemorrhage from recurrent gynecologic cancer. Eur J Gynaecol Oncol 14:33, 1993

Pecorelli S: Revised FIGO staging for carcinoma of the vulva, cervix, and endometrium. Int J Gynaecol Obstet 105(2):103, 2009

Petereit DG, Hartenbach EM, Thomas GM: Para-aortic lymph node evaluation in cervical cancer: the impact of staging upon treatment decisions and outcome. Int J Gynecol Cancer 8:353, 1998

Peters WA III, Liu PY, Barrett RJ, et al: Concurrent chemotherapy and pelvic radiation therapy compared with pelvic radiation therapy alone as adjuvant therapy after radical surgery in high-risk early-stage cancer of the cervix. J Clin Oncol 18:1606, 2000

Piver MS, Rutledge F, Smith JP: Five classes of extended hysterectomy for women with cervical cancer. Obstet Gynecol 44(2):265, 1974

Plante M, Renaud MC, Hoskins IA, et al: Vaginal radical trachelectomy: a valuable fertility-preserving option in the management of early-stage cervical cancer. A series of 50 pregnancies and review of the literature. Gynecol Oncol 98(1):3, 2005

Plummer M, Herrero R, Franceschi S, et al: Smoking and cervical cancer: pooled analysis of the IARC multi-centric case-control study. Cancer Causes Control 14:805, 2003

Potter ME, Alvarez RD, Gay FL, et al: Optimal therapy for pelvic recurrence after radical hysterectomy for early-stage cervical cancer. Gynecol Oncol 37:74, 1990

Querleu D, Dargent D, Ansquer Y, et al: Extraperitoneal endosurgical aortic and common iliac dissection in the staging of bulky or advanced cervical carcinomas. Cancer 88:1883, 2000

Quinn MA, Benedet JL, Odicino F, et al: Carcinoma of the cervix uteri. Int J Gynecol Obstet 95(suppl 1):S43, 2006

Ramirez PT, Soliman PT, Schmeler KM, et al: Laparoscopic and robotic techniques for radical hysterectomy in patients with early-stage cervical cancer. Gynecol Oncol 110:S21, 2008

Reynolds EA, Tierney K, Keeney GL, et al: Analysis of outcomes of microinvasive adenocarcinoma of the uterine cervix by treatment type. Obstet Gynecol 116:1150, 2010

Robinson WR, Webb S, Tirpack J, et al: Management of cervical intraepithelial neoplasia during pregnancy with LOOP excision. Gynecol Oncol 64:153, 1997

Rose PG, Adler LP, Rodriguez M, et al: Positron emission tomography for evaluating para-aortic nodal metastasis in locally advanced cervical cancer before surgical staging: a surgicopathologic study. J Clin Oncol 17:41, 1999

Schiffman MH, Bauer HM, Hoover RN, et al: Epidemiologic evidence showing that human papillomavirus infection causes most cervical intraepithelial neoplasia. J Natl Cancer Inst 85:958, 1993

Schorge JO, Lee KR, Sheets EE: Prospective management of stage IA(1) cervical adenocarcinoma by conization alone to preserve fertility: a preliminary report. Gynecol Oncol 78:217, 2000

Sedlis A, Bundy BN, Rotman MZ, et al: A randomized trial of pelvic radiation therapy versus no further therapy in selected patients with stage IB carcinoma of the cervix after radical hysterectomy and pelvic lymphadenectomy: a Gynecologic Oncology Group Study. Gynecol Oncol 73:177, 1999

Selman TJ, Mann C, Zamora J, et al: Diagnostic accuracy of tests for lymph node status in primary cervical cancer: a systematic review and meta-analysis. CMAJ 178:855, 2008

Shepherd JH, Milliken DA: Conservative surgery for carcinoma of the cervix. Clin Oncol 20:395, 2008

Siegel RL, Miller KD, Jemal A: Cancer statistics, 2015. CA Cancer J Clin 65(1):5, 2015

Silver DF, Hempling RE, Piver MS, et al: Stage I adenocarcinoma of the cervix: does lesion size affect treatment options and prognosis?. Am J Clin Oncol 21:431, 1998

Sironi S, Buda A, Picchio M, et al: Lymph node metastasis in patients with clinical early-stage cervical cancer: detection with integrated FDG PET/CT. Radiology 238:272, 2006

Smith HO, Qualls CR, Romero AA, et al: Is there a difference in survival for IA1 and IA2 adenocarcinoma of the uterine cervix? Gynecol Oncol 85:229, 2002

Soost HJ, Lange HJ, Lehmacher W, et al: The validation of cervical cytology. Sensitivity, specificity and predictive values. Acta Cytol 35:8, 1991

Spoozak L, Lewin S, Burke WM, et al: Microinvasive adenocarcinoma of the cervix. Am J Obstet Gynecol 206:80, 2012

Stehman FB, Bundy BN, DiSaia PJ, et al: Carcinoma of the cervix treated with radiation therapy. I. A multivariate analysis of prognostic variables in the Gynecologic Oncology Group. Cancer 67:2776, 1991

Subak LL, Hricak H, Powell CB, et al: Cervical carcinoma: computed tomography and magnetic resonance imaging for preoperative staging. Obstet Gynecol 86:43, 1995

Sutton GP, Bundy BN, Delgado G, et al: Ovarian metastases in stage IB carcinoma of the cervix: a Gynecologic Oncology Group study. Am J Obstet Gynecol 166(1 Pt 1):50, 1992

Takeshima N, Yanoh K, Tabata T, et al: Assessment of the revised International Federation of Gynecology and Obstetrics staging for early invasive squamous cervical cancer. Gynecol Oncol 74:165, 1999

Tewari KS, Sill MW, Long HJ, et al: Improved survival with bevacizumab in advanced cervical cancer. N Engl J Med 370:734, 2014

Thigpen JT, Vance R, Puneky L, et al: Chemotherapy as a palliative treatment in carcinoma of the uterine cervix. Semin Oncol 22(2 Suppl 3):16, 1995

Tinga DJ, Timmer PR, Bouma J, et al: Prognostic significance of single versus multiple lymph node metastases in cervical carcinoma stage IB. Gynecol Oncol 39:175, 1990

Torre LA, Bray F, Siegel RL, et al: Global cancer statistics, 2012. CA Cancer J Clin 65:87, 2015

Trimble CL, Genkinger JM, Burke AE, et al: Active and passive cigarette smoking and the risk of cervical neoplasia. Obstet Gynecol 105:174, 2005

Upadhyay SK, Symonds RP, Haelterman M, et al: The treatment of stage IV carcinoma of cervix by radical dose radiotherapy. Radiother Oncol 11:15, 1988

Vale C, Chemoradiotherapy for Cervical Cancer Meta-Analysis Collaboration: Reducing uncertainties about the effects of chemoradiotherapy for cervical cancer: a systematic review and meta-analysis of individual patient data from 18 randomized trials. J Clin Oncol 26:5802, 2008

Vasilev SA, McGonigle KF: Extraperitoneal laparoscopic paraaortic lymph node dissection: development of a technique. J Laparoendosc Surg 5:85, 1995

Vercellino GF, Koehler C, Erdemoglu E, et al: Laparoscopic pelvic lymphadenectomy in 32 pregnant patients with cervical cancer: rationale, description of the technique, and outcome. Int J Gynecol Cancer 24:364, 2014

Vermorken JB: The role of chemotherapy in squamous cell carcinoma of the uterine cervix: a review. Int J Gynecol Cancer 3:129, 1993

Viswanathan AN, Deavers MT, Jhingran A, et al: Small cell neuroendocrine carcinoma of the cervix: outcome and patterns of recurrence. Gynecol Oncol 93:27, 2004

Vizcaino AP, Moreno V, Bosch FX, et al: International trends in incidence of cervical cancer: II. Squamous-cell carcinoma. Int J Cancer 86:429, 2000

Walboomers JN, Jacons MV, Manos M, et al: Human papillomavirus is a necessary cause of invasive cervical cancer worldwide. J Pathol 189:12, 1999

Webb MJ, Symmonds RE: Site of recurrence of cervical cancer after radical hysterectomy. Am J Obstet Gynecol 138(7 Pt 1):813, 1980

Wei L, Griego AM, Chu M, et al: Tobacco exposure results in increased E6 and E7 oncogene expression, DNA damage and mutation rates in cells maintaining episomal human papillomavirus 16 genomes. Carcinogenesis 35:2372, 2014

Wentzensen N, Vinokurova S, von Knebel DM: Systematic review of genomic integration sites of human papillomavirus genomes in epithelial dysplasia and invasive cancer of the female lower genital tract. Cancer Res 64:3878, 2004

Whitney CW, Sause W, Bundy BN, et al: Randomized comparison of fluorouracil plus cisplatin versus hydroxyurea as an adjunct to radiation therapy in stage IIB-IVA carcinoma of the cervix with negative para-aortic lymph nodes: a Gynecologic Oncology Group and Southwest Oncology Group study. J Clin Oncol 17:1339, 1999

World Health Organization: GLOBOCAN 2012: Estimated Cancer Incidence, Mortality and Prevalence Worldwide in 2012. Available at: http://globocan.iarc.fr. Accessed January 27, 2015

Wright JD, Dehdashti F, Herzog TJ, et al: Preoperative lymph node staging of early-stage cervical carcinoma by [18F]-fluoro-2-deoxy-d-glucose-positron emission tomography. Cancer 104:2484, 2005

Yahata T, Nishino K, Kashmima K, et al: Conservative treatment of stage IA1 adenocarcinoma of the uterine cervix with a long-term follow-up. Int J Gynecol Cancer 20:1063, 2010

CHAPTER 31

Vulvar Cancer

Vulvar cancers comprise only about 4 percent of all gynecologic malignancies. Most vulvar cancers are diagnosed at an early stage (I and II). Advanced disease is found mainly in older women, perhaps due to clinical and behavioral barriers that lead to diagnostic delays. Thus, biopsy of any abnormal vulvar lesion is imperative to help diagnose this cancer early.

In the United States, vulvar cancers carry a comparatively good prognosis with a 5-year relative survival rate of 78 percent (Stroup, 2008). For resectable disease, traditional therapy includes radical excision of the vulva plus inguinal lymphadenectomy or plus sentinel lymph node biopsy. For advanced stages, chemoradiation may be used either primarily or as an adjunct to surgery to aid tumor control. All of these treatments can result in extensive short- and long-term morbidity and dramatic anatomic and functional deformity. Accordingly, vulvar cancer management recently has trended toward more conservative surgery that preserves oncologic outcome, lessens morbidity, and improves psychosexual well-being.

RELEVANT ANATOMY

The *vulva* includes the mons pubis, labia majora and minora, clitoris, vestibule, vestibular bulbs, Bartholin glands, lesser vestibular glands, paraurethral glands, and the urethral and vaginal openings. Lateral margins of the vulva are the labiocrural folds (Fig. 38-25, p. 818). Vulvar cancer may involve any of these external structures and typically arises within the covering squamous epithelium. Unlike the cervix, the vulva lacks an identifiable transformation zone. That said, squamous neoplasia arises predominantly on the vestibule at the border between the vulvar keratinized stratified squamous epithelium, which lies laterally, and the nonkeratinized squamous mucosa, which lies medially. This demarcation line is termed Hart line.

Deep to the vulva are the superficial and deep urogenital triangle compartments. The superficial space lies between Colles fascia (superficial perineal fascia) and the perineal membrane (deep perineal fascia) (Fig. 38-26 p. 819). Within this space lie the ischiocavernosus, bulbospongiosus, and transverse perineal muscles and the highly vascular vestibular bulb and clitoral crus. During radical vulvectomy, dissection is carried to the depth of the perineal membrane. As a result, contents of this superficial urogenital triangle compartment that lie beneath the mass are removed during tumor excision.

The lymphatics of the vulva and distal third of the vagina typically drain into the superficial inguinal node group (Fig. 38-29, p. 823). From here, lymph travels through the deep femoral lymphatics and the node of Cloquet to the pelvic nodal groups. Importantly, lymph can also drain directly from the clitoris and upper labia to the deep femoral nodes (Way, 1948). Vulvar lymphatics cross at the mons pubis and the posterior fourchette but do not cross the labiocrural folds (Morley, 1976). Thus, lesions found within 2 cm of the midline may spread to lymph nodes on either side. In contrast, lateral lesions rarely send metastases to contralateral nodes. This anatomy point influences the decision for ipsilateral or bilateral node dissection, as discussed later.

The superficial inguinal nodes cluster within the femoral triangle formed by: the inguinal ligament, sartorius muscle, and adductor longus muscle. The deep femoral nodes lie within the borders of the fossa ovalis and just medial to the femoral vein. An *inguinofemoral lymphadenectomy* typically refers to removal of both superficial inguinal and deep femoral lymph nodes (Levenback, 1996).

EPIDEMIOLOGY

In the United States, women have a 1 in 333 chance of developing this cancer at some point. In 2014, approximately 4850 new vulvar cancers and 1030 cancer deaths were predicted (National Cancer Institute, 2014). The age-adjusted incidence of invasive vulvar tumors in the United States has trended upward during the past three decades due to an aging population and greater longevity of human immunodeficiency virus (HIV)-infected women. This increase persists among all age groups and all geographic areas (Bodelon, 2009). Specifically, the age-adjusted incidence of vulvar carcinoma in situ (CIS)

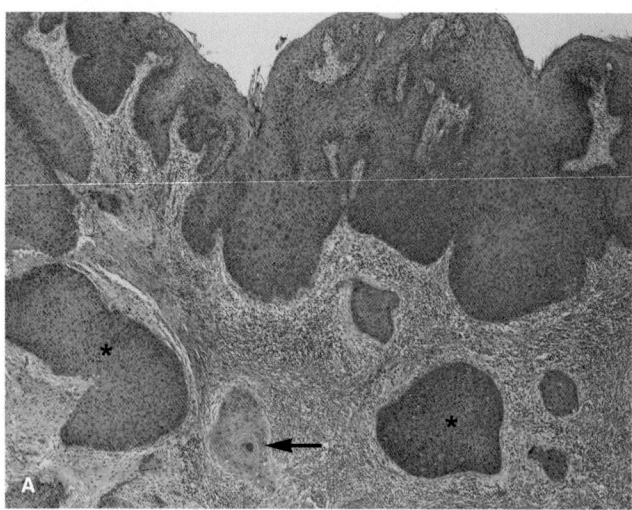
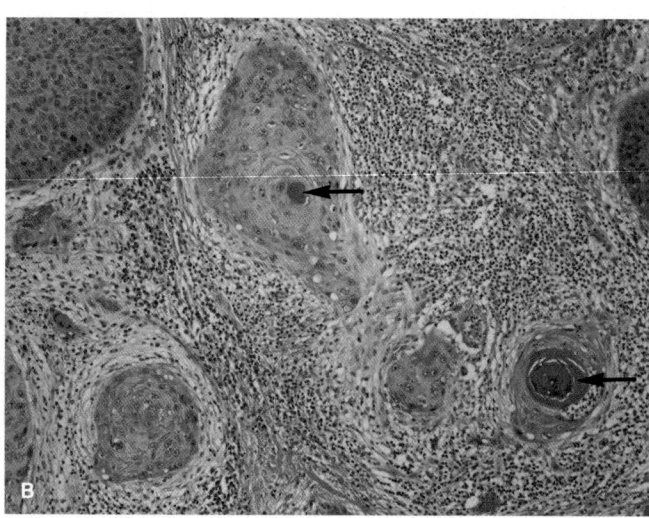

FIGURE 31-1 Vulvar squamous cell carcinoma. **A.** Low-power view. The surface epithelium shows high-grade squamous dysplasia. Nests of invasive squamous cell carcinoma (*arrow*) are present. A brisk chronic inflammatory infiltrate is present as is often the case with invasive squamous cell carcinoma. Portions of the surface epithelium extend deep and are cut tangentially (*asterisks*), giving the false impression of invasive tumor at these sites. **B.** Tumor shows classic diagnostic features of invasive squamous cell carcinoma that include a squamoid appearance, intercellular bridges, and brightly eosinophilic keratin pearls (*arrows*). Nests of invasive tumor are surrounded by chronic inflammation. (Used with permission from Dr. Kelley Carrick.)

has increased by 3.5 percent per year, whereas that of invasive cancers has risen by 1 percent yearly (Jemal, 2010).

Of vulvar tumors, approximately 90 percent are squamous cell carcinoma (Fig. 31-1). Malignant melanoma is the second most common, but rare histologic subtypes may also be encountered (Table 31-1).

RISK FACTORS

Age is a prominent factor and positively correlates with this cancer. Less than 20 percent of affected women are younger than

TABLE 31-1. Vulvar Cancer Histologic Subtypes

Vulvar carcinomas
Squamous cell carcinoma
Adenocarcinoma
Carcinoma of Bartholin gland
   Adenocarcinoma
   Squamous carcinoma
   Transitional cell
Vulva Paget disease
Merkel cell tumors
Verrucous carcinoma
Basal cell carcinoma

Vulvar malignant melanoma

Vulvar sarcoma
Leiomyosarcoma
Malignant fibrous histiocytoma
Epithelial sarcoma
Malignant rhabdoid tumor

Metastatic cancers to vulva

Yolk sac tumors

50 years, and more than half of cases develop in women older than 70. Survival rates also differ by age. Kumar and associates (2009) described a hazard ratio of nearly 4 for death in women older than 50 years compared with younger women. Last, vulvar cancer pathology can be divided into two distinct age-dependent profiles. Those that develop in younger women (<55 years) tend to have the same risk profile as other anogenital cancers. These cancers are usually described histologically as basaloid or warty and are linked with human papillomavirus (HPV) in 50 percent of cases. In contrast, older affected women typically are nonsmokers and lack a history of prior sexually transmitted infections. Their cancers are largely keratinizing, and HPV DNA is found in only 15 percent (Canavan, 2002; Madeleine, 1997). Such HPV-independent vulvar cancers have been associated with lichen sclerosus and with genetic alterations such as mutations in *p53*. This tumor suppressor gene normally modulates cell death, and its mutation can be carcinogenic.

Infection with high-risk HPV serotypes is another vulvar cancer risk. Serotype 16 predominates, although HPV serotypes 18, 31, 33, and 45 are also reported. Although HPV is implicated in many vulvar cancers, stronger correlations are noted between HPV infection and preinvasive vulvar lesions (Hildesheim, 1997). Specifically, HPV DNA is detected in 50 to 70 percent of invasive lesions but is seen in >90 percent of vulvar intraepithelial neoplasia (VIN) lesions (Gargano, 2012). HPV becomes a stronger contributor when combined with other cofactors such as smoking or herpes simplex virus (HSV) infection (Madeleine, 1997). Women who have smoked and have a history of HPV genital warts have a 35–fold increased risk for developing vulvar cancer compared with women without these predispositions (Brinton, 1990; Kirschner, 1995). For these reasons, prophylactic vaccination against high-risk HPV may ultimately reduce vulvar cancer incidence. A full discussion of HPV and VIN is found in Chapter 29 (p. 646)

Herpes simplex virus infection is also linked with vulvar cancer in several studies (Hildesheim, 1997; Madeleine, 1997). As noted, the association is more prominent when coupled with other cofactors such as smoking. Thus, the causal link between HSV alone and vulvar cancer is not considered conclusive.

Chronic immunosuppression can predispose to vulvar cancer. For example, transplant patients have a high incidence. In this group, vulvar cancer develops at a much younger age than in the general population, and more than 50 percent have a prior history of condyloma acuminata (Penn, 2002). With HIV, vulvar cancer rates are also increased (Elit, 2005; Frisch, 2000). And, of the increased high-grade VIN and invasive vulvar carcinoma incidence noted in younger women, HIV-infected patients make up the majority (Casolati, 2003). A possible explanation for this is the association of HIV and high-risk HPV subtypes. However, vulvar cancer is not yet considered an acquired immunodeficiency syndrome (AIDS)-defining malignancy. Because of these links with vulvar cancer, we recommend that all immunocompromised women undergo thorough vulvar inspection and, when indicated, vulvoscopy and biopsy.

Lichen sclerosus is a chronic vulvar inflammatory disease and is related to vulvar cancer development. Keratinocytes affected by lichen sclerosus show a proliferative phenotype and can exhibit markers of neoplastic progression. As such, lichen sclerosus may be a precursor lesion in some invasive squamous vulvar cancers (Rolfe, 2001). Vulvar cancers coexistent with lichen sclerosus tend to develop in older women, predominate in near the clitoris, and lack association with VIN 3.

Last, progression from *VIN 3* to invasive cancer is suspected. Several reports demonstrate that in a small percentage of women older than 30 years, untreated lesions can progress to invasive cancer within a mean of 4 years (Jones, 2005; van Seters, 2005). Although this progression cannot be conclusively validated, we recommend that patients with moderate and severe vulvar dysplasias receive early definitive treatment (Chap. 29, p. 649).

DIAGNOSIS

◼ Symptoms

Women with VIN and vulvar cancer commonly present with pruritus and a visible lesion (Fig. 31-2). However, pain, bleeding, ulceration, or inguinal mass may be other complaints (Fig. 31-3). Manifestations can persist for weeks or months before diagnosis, as many patients may be embarrassed or may not recognize the significance of their symptoms.

◼ Lesion Evaluation

Lesions may be raised, ulcerated, pigmented, or warty, but in younger women with multifocal disease, a well-defined mass is not always present. Importantly, other clinical entities may present similarly and include preinvasive neoplasia (VIN), infection, chronic inflammatory disease, and granulomatous disease. Thus, the goal of evaluation is to obtain an accurate and definitive pathologic diagnosis.

For this, colposcopic examination of the vulva, termed *vulvoscopy,* can direct biopsy site selection. To begin, the vulva is soaked with 3-percent acetic acid for 5 minutes to allow

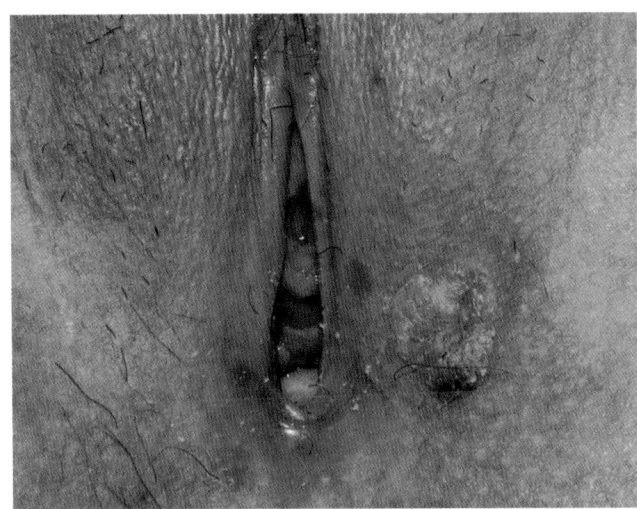

FIGURE 31-2 Early-stage squamous cell cancer of the vulva.

adequate penetration into the keratin layer. This aids identification of acetowhite areas and abnormal vascular patterns, which are characteristics of vulvar neoplasia. The entire vulva and perianal skin are systematically examined. We recommend obtaining multiple biopsies, as illustrated in Figure 4-2 (p. 88), from the most suspicious raised or dyspigmented skin. Specimens removed with a Keyes punch should be approximately 4 mm thick to include the surface epithelial lesion and the underlying stroma. This permits evaluation for invasion and depth of invasion. Concurrent colposcopic examination of the cervix and vagina and careful evaluation of the perianal area are recommended to diagnose any synchronous lesions or associated neoplasm of the lower genital tract.

◼ Cancer Patient Evaluation

Following histologic diagnosis, a patient with vulvar cancer is assessed for the clinical extent of disease and for comorbid conditions. Thus, detailed physical examination includes measurement

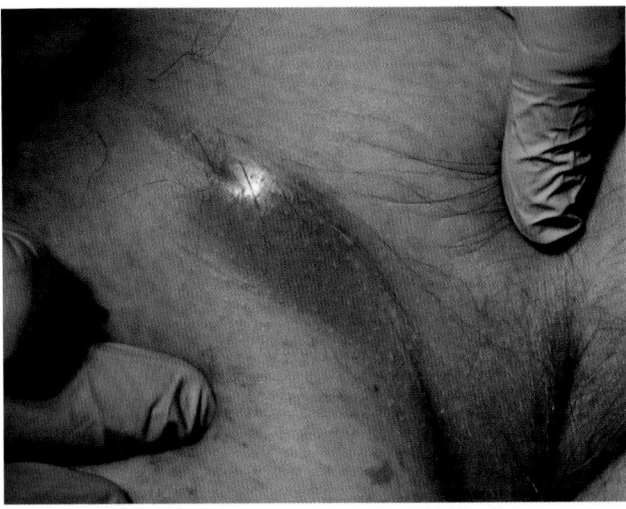

FIGURE 31-3 Enlarged inguinal lymph node containing metastatic squamous cell vulvar cancer. (Used with permission from Dr. William Griffith.)

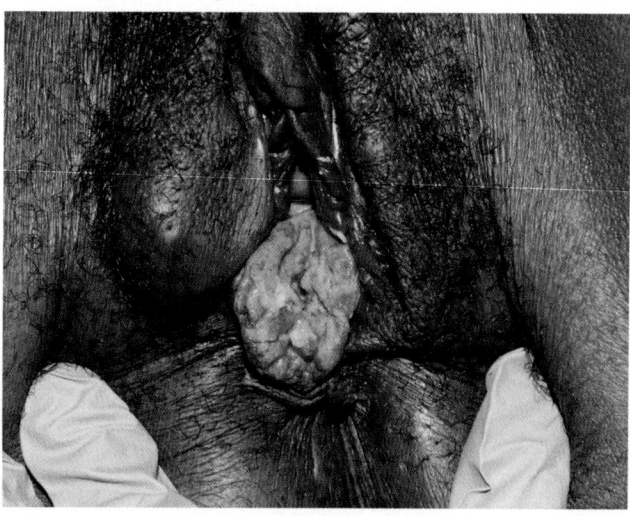

FIGURE 31-4 Photograph of invasive vulvar cancer.

of the primary tumor and evaluation of cancer extension into other genitourinary system compartments, the anal canal, the bony pelvis, and inguinal lymph nodes. At our institution, if a thorough physical examination is not possible because of patient discomfort or disease extent, an examination under anesthesia is performed. This may be coupled with cystourethroscopy, proctosigmoidoscopy, or both if suspicion of tumor invasion into the urethra, bladder, or anal canal is high (Fig. 31-4).

Women with small tumors and clinically negative groin nodes require few additional diagnostic studies other than those

needed for surgical preparation (Chap. 39, p. 825). Although not a formal part of surgical tumor staging, preoperative imaging may complement staging in those with larger tumors or with clinically suspected metastatic disease. In such cases, a chest radiograph and computed tomography (CT), positron emission tomography (PET), or magnetic resonance (MR) imaging of the abdomen and pelvis provide information regarding disease extent or metastases that may modify preoperative planning.

■ Staging Systems

The International Federation of Gynecology and Obstetrics (FIGO) advocates surgical staging of patients with vulvar cancer that is based on a tumor, nodal, metastatic (TNM) classification. Thus, staging involves: (1) primary tumor resection to obtain tumor dimensions and (2) dissection of superficial and deep inguinofemoral lymph nodes to evaluate tumor spread (Pecorelli, 2009). This system is used to direct treatment and predict prognosis (Van der Steen, 2010). Table 31-2 and Figure 31-5 describe FIGO staging and American Joint Committee on Cancer (AJCC) staging criteria for all vulvar cancer types except melanoma. This cancer's staging is discussed separately on page 688. The general nuanced differences between FIGO and AJCC systems are described in Chapter 30 (p. 663).

PROGNOSIS

Overall survival rates of women with squamous cell carcinoma of the vulva are relatively good. Five-year survival rates of 75

TABLE 31-2. Invasive Vulvar Cancer Staging

TNM[a]	Stage[b]	Characteristics
	I	**Tumor confined to the vulva**
T1a	IA	Lesions ≤2 cm in size, confined to the vulva or perineum and with stromal invasion ≤1.0 mm[c], no nodal metastasis
T1b	IB	Lesions >2 cm in size or with stromal invasion >1.0 mm[c], confined to the vulva or perineum, with negative nodes
T2	**II**	**Tumor of any size with extension to adjacent perineal structures (1/3 lower urethra, 1/3 lower vagina, anus) with negative nodes**
	III	**Tumor of any size with or without extension to adjacent perineal structures (1/3 lower urethra, 1/3 lower vagina, anus) with positive inguinofemoral lymph nodes**
N1b	IIIA	(i) With 1 lymph node metastasis (≥5 mm), or
N1a		(ii) 1–2 lymph node metastasis(es) (<5 mm)
N2b	IIIB	(i) With 2 or more lymph node metastases (≥5 mm), or
N2a		(ii) 3 or more lymph node metastases (<5 mm)
N2c	IIIC	With positive nodes with extracapsular spread
	IV	**Tumor invades other regional (2/3 upper urethra, 2/3 upper vagina), or distant structures**
T3	IVA	Tumor invades any of the following:
		(i) upper urethral and/or vaginal mucosa, bladder mucosa, rectal mucosa, or fixed to pelvic bone, or
		(ii) fixed or ulcerated inguinofemoral lymph nodes
M1	IVB	Any distant metastasis including pelvic lymph nodes

[a]American Joint Commission on Cancer staging that reflects tumor, nodes, and metastases (TNM).
[b]International Federation of Gynecology and Obstetrics (FIGO) staging.
[c]The *depth of invasion* is defined as the measurement of the tumor from the epithelial-stromal junction of the adjacent most superficial dermal papilla to the deepest point of invasion.

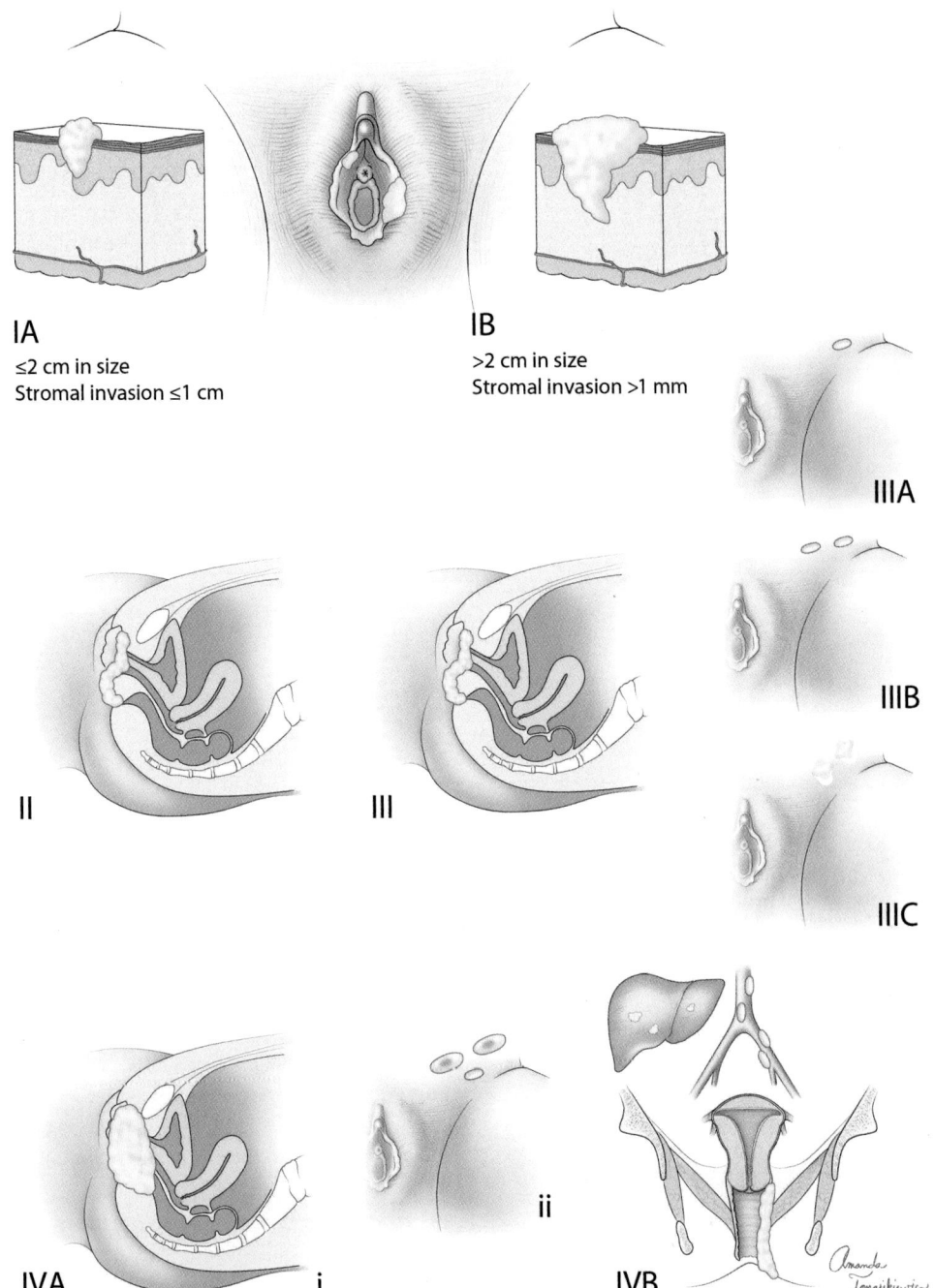

IA
≤2 cm in size
Stromal invasion ≤1 cm

IB
>2 cm in size
Stromal invasion >1 mm

IIIA

IIIB

IIIC

II

III

IVA   **i**   **IVB**   **ii**

FIGURE 31-5 FIGO (International Federation of Gynecology and Obstetrics) staging of invasive vulvar cancer.

to 90 percent are routinely cited for stage I and II disease. As anticipated, 5-year survival rates for higher stages are poorer, and rates of 54 percent for stage III and 16 percent for stage IVB are reported (American Cancer Society, 2015). Apart from FIGO stage, other important prognostic factors include lymph node metastasis, lesion size, depth of invasion, resected-margin status, and lymphatic vascular space involvement (LVSI) (Table 31-3).

Of these, *lymph node metastasis* is the single most important vulvar cancer predictor, since inguinal node metastasis reduces long-term survival rates by 50 percent (Farias-Eisner, 1994; Figge, 1985). Nodal status is determined by surgical resection and histologic evaluation. Among patients with nodal metastasis,

other factors further predict poor prognosis. These include a high number of involved lymph nodes, large nodal metastasis size, extracapsular invasion, and fixed or ulcerated nodes (Homesley, 1991; Origoni, 1992).

Tumor diameter also influences survival rates. But this stems mainly from the positive correlation between lesion size and nodal metastasis rates (Homesley, 1993).

Depth of invasion is another prognostic element. As shown in Figure 31-6, this depth is measured from the basement membrane to the deepest point of invasion (Kurman, 2014). Tumors with a depth of invasion <1 mm carry little or no risk of inguinal lymph node metastasis. However, increased nodal metastasis rates positively correlate with greater invasion rates.

TABLE 31-3. Prognostic Predictors and Clinical Effects

Depth of Invasion (mm)	Positive Nodes (%)
1	3
2	9
3	19
4	31
5	33
≥5	48

Tumor Diameter (cm)	5-Year Survival (%)
0–1	90
1–2	89
2–3	83
3–4	63
>4	44

Adapted with permission from Homesley HD, Bundy BN, Sedlis A, et al: Prognostic factors for groin node metastasis in squamous cell carcinoma of the vulva (a Gynecologic Oncology Group study). Gynecol Oncol 1993 Jun;49(3):279–283.

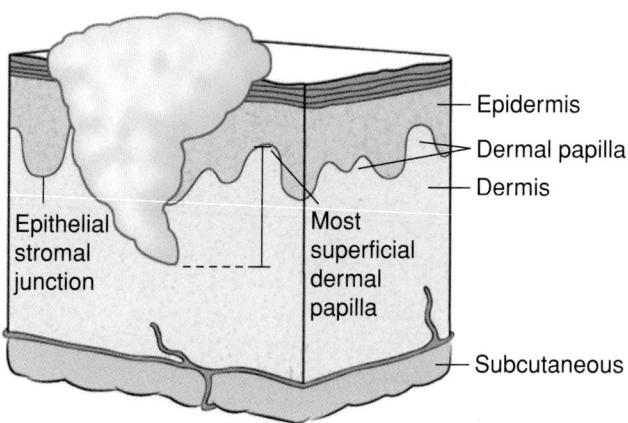

FIGURE 31-6 Histologic measurement of invasive vulvar cancer. Depth of invasion is measured from the junction between the epithelium and stroma of the most superficial dermal papilla to the greatest depth of tumor invasion.

Surgical margins that are tumor-free decrease local tumor recurrence rates, and traditionally a 1- to 2-cm tumor-free margin is desired. More specifically, two large retrospective series demonstrated that a tumor-free surgical margin ≥8 mm yielded a high rate of local control. In contrast, if tumor was found within this 8-mm margin, the recurrence rate was 23 to 48 percent (Chan, 2007; Heaps, 1990). Hence, when lesions are close to the clitoris, anus, urethra, or vagina, a 1-cm surgical tumor-free margin may be used to preserve important anatomy yet still provide optimal resection.

Lymphatic vascular space invasion (LVSI) describes histologic identification of tumor cells within lymphatic vessels and is a predictor of early disease recurrence (Preti, 2005). LVSI is also associated with a higher frequency of lymph node metastasis and a lower overall 5-year survival rate (Hoskins, 2000).

TREATMENT

■ Surgery

For vulvar cancer treatment, surgery is often an integral part. Potential procedures, in increasing order of radicality, include wide local excision (WLE), radical partial vulvectomy, and radical complete vulvectomy.

Of these, *wide local excision* is appropriate only for microinvasive tumors (stage IA) of the vulva. With this excision, also termed *simple partial vulvectomy*, 1-cm surgical margins are obtained around the lesion. Deep surgical margins measuring 1 cm are also preferred. This deep margin usually corresponds to Colles fascia (Fig. 38-25, p. 818).

With *radical partial vulvectomy* (Section 46-25, p. 1210), tumor-containing portions of the vulva are completely removed, wherever they are located. Skin margins are 1 to 2 cm, and excision extends deep to the perineal membrane (Fig. 31-7). Radical

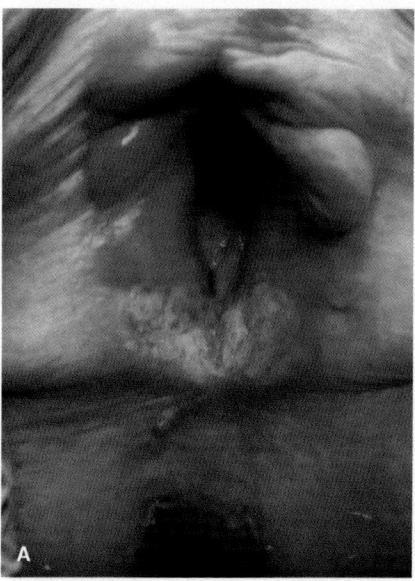
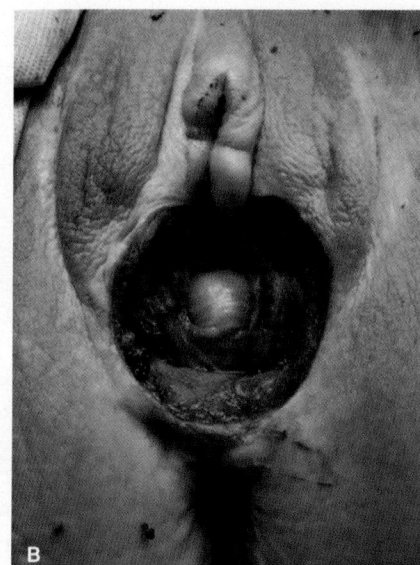
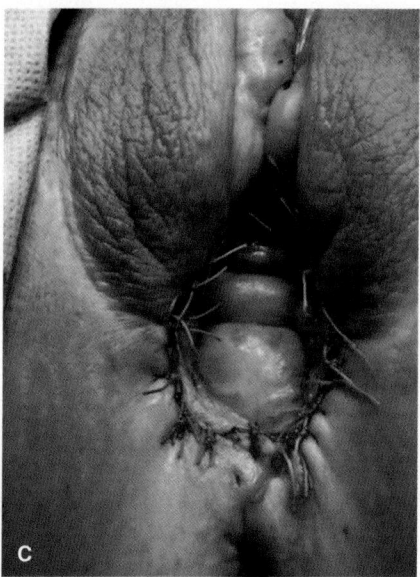

FIGURE 31-7 A. Vulvar cancer following radiation therapy and in preparation for surgical excision. **B.** Radical partial vulvectomy. **C.** Final surgical closure. (Used with permission from Dr. David Miller.)

partial vulvectomy is typically reserved for unifocal lesions that are clinically confined to the labia majora, labia minora, mons, vestibule, and/or perineum and that have limited involvement of the adjacent urethra, vagina, and/or anus. Moreover, only patients with a solitary tumor that is not too large or too extensive and with an otherwise normal vulva are considered for this vulva-conserving surgery.

Radical total vulvectomy (Section 46-26, p. 1213) is a complete dissection of vulvar tissue to the level of the perineal membrane and the periosteum of the pubic rami or symphysis. Adequate margins will generally require an incision in the labiocrural fold that extends down to the fourchette and up over the mons pubis. All intervening subcutaneous tissue is excised. Lesions involving or adjacent to the clitoris may require wider margins cephalad to the mons. Such radical resections are performed for large midline or multifocal vulvar cancers. Flap reconstruction is occasionally needed and described in Section 46-28 (p. 1219). Contraindications to a radical complete vulvectomy include poor surgical risk, poor patient compliance, and metastatic disease beyond regional lymph nodes.

Of the three procedures shown in Figure 31-8, the en bloc incision, colloquially termed the *butterfly* or *longhorn* incision, has largely been abandoned. It has survival rates equivalent to radical complete vulvectomy but carries significantly greater morbidity.

Inguinofemoral Lymphadenectomy

This procedure is usually an integral part of surgical cancer staging and accompanies radical partial or radical complete vulvectomy. It is recommended for all vulvar squamous carcinomas that invade deeper than 1 mm on initial biopsy or have a tumor diameter >2 cm regardless of invasion depth (stages IB-IVA). To maximize metastatic disease detection and staging accuracy, surgical evaluation of the groin nodes is recommended. Traditionally, both the superficial inguinal and deep femoral lymph nodes have been removed for evaluation of metastatic disease (Gordinier, 2003). Moreover, lymph nodes may be excised unilaterally or bilaterally. Traditionally, an ipsilateral inguinofemoral lymphadenectomy is performed for a "lateralized" vulvar lesion, namely, one that lies >2 cm beyond the midline. Bilateral node excision is recommended for all lesions within 2 cm of the midline. Aside from acquiring staging information, inguinofemoral lymphadenectomy may also be used to debulk large, cancerous lymph nodes.

Entire steps for lymphadenectomy are described and illustrated in Section 46-27 (p. 1216). To summarize, the superficial inguinal lymph nodes lie within the fatty tissue caudal to the inguinal ligament and superficial to the thigh's fascia lata. This node-containing tissue is dissected free to reach the fossa ovalis. Here, deep femoral nodes are excised from their location medial to and alongside the femoral vein. For these deep nodes, a modified approach preserves the cribriform fascia (portion of fascia lata overlying the fossa ovalis) by removing the deep femoral nodes through the cribriform fascia's perforations. This modification yields cancer recurrence rates comparable to those obtained following classic inguinofemoral node dissection (Bell, 2000; Hacker, 1983). Advantageously, complication rates of wound breakdown, infection, and lymphedema are significantly

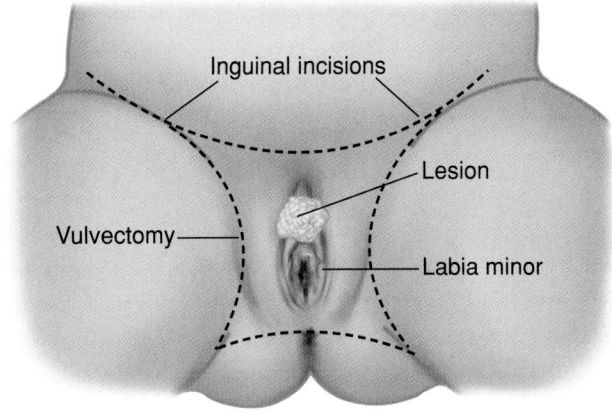

A

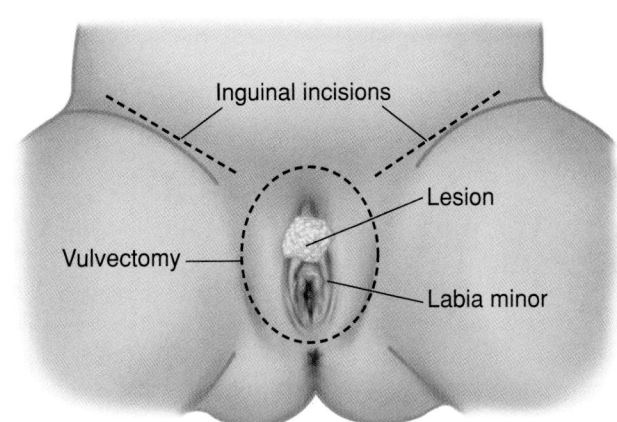

B

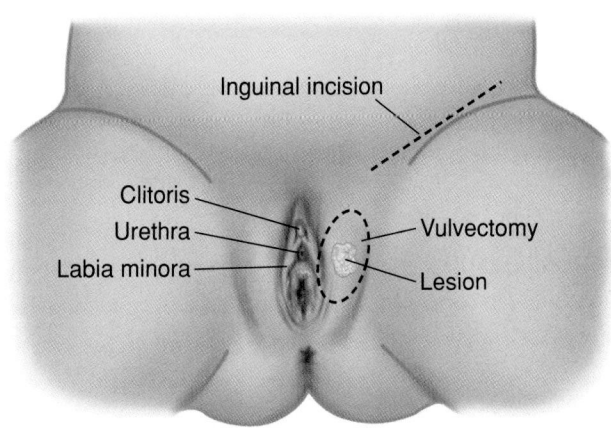

C

FIGURE 31-8 Types of vulvectomy used in the treatment of vulvar cancer. **A.** En bloc radical vulvectomy with bilateral inguinofemoral lymphadenectomy. **B.** Radical complete vulvectomy with bilateral inguinofemoral lymphadenectomy. **C.** Radical partial vulvectomy with ipsilateral inguinofemoral lymphadenectomy.

decreased (Table 31-4). However, a classic inguinofemoral node dissection on occasion is required to reach these deep femoral lymph nodes. In such cases, the cribriform fascia is transected, lymph nodes are removed, and the sartorius muscle can then be transposed over the femoral vessels. This transposition may reduce the risk of postoperative erosion into the skeletonized femoral vessels if superficial wound dehiscence occurs. However,

TABLE 31-4. Postoperative Complications of Inguinofemoral Lymphadenectomy

Complication	No. of Events	Percent of Groins
Lymphedema	13	14.0
Lymphocele	11	11.8
Groin infection	7	7.5
Groin necrosis	2	2.2
Groin separation	7	7.5

Reproduced with permission from Bell JG, Lea JS, Reid GC: Complete groin lymphadenectomy with preservation of the fascia lata in the treatment of vulvar carcinoma, Gynecol Oncol 2000 May;77(2):314–318.

this transposition does not reduce overall postoperative wound morbidity rates (Judson, 2004; Rouzier, 2003).

Surgical evaluation of the groin nodes has been reported to confer a superior prognosis compared with primary groin irradiation. A phase III randomized controlled trial conducted by the Gynecologic Oncology Group (GOG) showed that patients undergoing primary groin dissection experienced significantly fewer groin recurrences and a better prognosis compared with women receiving groin irradiation (Stehman, 1992b). Furthermore, limiting node dissection to only the superficial inguinal nodes also confers a higher groin recurrence rate compared with historical controls undergoing removal of both superficial and deep nodes (Stehman, 1992a). Higher than acceptable groin recurrence rates have also been described for patients who received primary groin irradiation (Manavi, 1997; Perez, 1993). Thus, in general, both deep and superficial inguinal lymph node removal is recommended to allow for thorough evaluation for nodal metastasis. But, because of groin dissection morbidity, this advantage has been challenged for those with early-stage disease and clinically negative nodes. Namely, recent evidence supports the use of sentinel lymph node biopsy in vulvar lesions <4 cm in diameter and assures a low false-negative rate of undetected nodal metastasis.

Sentinel Lymph Node Biopsy

As another less morbid option, selective dissection of a solitary node or nodes, termed *sentinel lymph node biopsy (SLNB)*, dramatically reduces surgical morbidity yet adequately assesses nodal involvement. Physiologically, the first lymph node to receive tumor lymphatic drainage is termed the *sentinel lymph node*. Thus, a sentinel lymph node devoid of disease implies absent lymph node metastases within the entire lymph node basin. SLNB is not performed if groin node metastases are clinically suspected.

Currently, both lymphoscintigraphy and isosulfan blue dye techniques are recommended when performing SLNB for vulvar cancer (Levenback, 2008). To begin, intraoperative lymphatic mapping is accomplished by injecting radionuclide intradermally at the tumor border that lies closest to the ipsilateral groin. For midline tumors, both sides of the tumor are injected. A handheld gamma counter aids attempts to identify the sentinel node subcutaneously, and the skin is marked by pen over the strongest signal. Next, isosulfan blue dye is injected at the same tumor border. Last, the groin skin over the prior pen mark is incised approximately 5 minutes later (Fig. 31-9). The tracer and dye are taken up by the specific node that drains the tumor site first. The handheld gamma counter signal may assist in localizing the sentinel node, and/or it can be visually identified by its blue color. Once identified, it is separated and excised from the other nodes within that regional group.

Several studies have confirmed the accuracy of SLNB to predict vulvar cancer metastasis in the inguinal lymph nodes. One multicenter trial by the GOG reported the sensitivity of this technique was >90 percent and the false negative rate was 2 percent for tumors measuring <4 cm. Patients with tumors measuring ≥2 cm and invading to a depth >1 mm and with clinically negative nodes were included in the study (Levenback, 2012). SLNB for patients with a vulvar lesion that does not involve midline structures but that also does not meet the definition of a lateralized lesion is appealing as it potentially avoids unnecessary groin exploration on one side (Coleman, 2013).

A second study, the GROningen International Study on Sentinel nodes in Vulvar cancer (GROINSS-V), evaluated SLNB for patients with squamous cell cancer of the vulva measuring <4 cm. It too confirmed the predictive value of SLNB. Moreover, this study concluded that the risk of metastasis to additional inguinal lymph nodes increases with sentinel-node metastasis

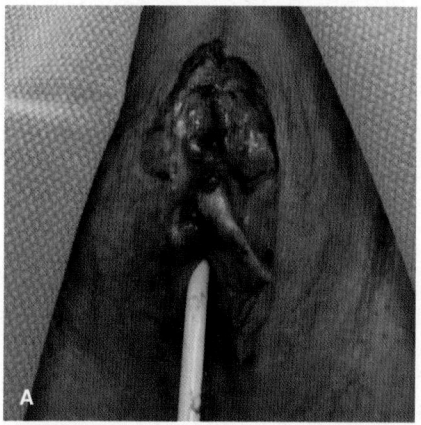
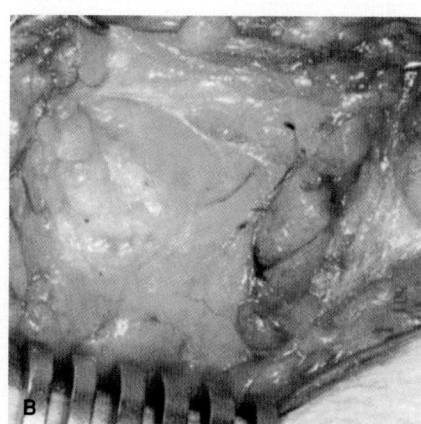
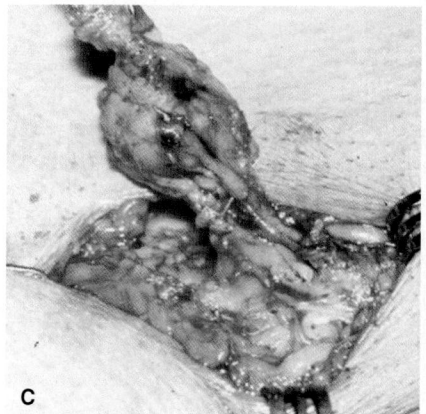

FIGURE 31-9 Sentinel lymph node evaluation. **A.** Blue dye and radiotracer are injected at the tumor periphery. **B.** Blue dye is taken up by the specific node that drains the tumor site. **C.** This sentinel node can be visually identified, separated from the other nodes within the regional group, and removed for evaluation.

size (Oonk, 2010; Van der Zee, 2008). Last, one ongoing prospective study (GROINSS-V-II) is observing early-stage vulvar cancer patients with a sentinel node metastasis measuring ≤2 mm to see if complete inguinofemoral lymphadenectomy can be safely replaced by adjuvant radiotherapy following vulvectomy.

■ Microinvasive Tumors (Stage IA)

Within the FIGO system, stage I vulvar cancers are divided into two categories. Stage IA lesions measure ≤2 cm in diameter, are confined to the vulva or perineum, and display stromal invasion ≤1 mm. These lesions, termed *microinvasive cancers*, reflect a subpopulation in which the risk of inguinal metastasis is negligible (Binder, 1990; Donaldson, 1981; Hacker, 1984). Women with microinvasive stage IA tumors tend to be younger and have multifocal disease associated with HPV. For probable cure, these patients can undergo wide local excision with a 1-cm margin. Lymphadenectomy is not indicated because associated lymph node metastasis is rare.

■ Stage IB–II

Patients with early-stage vulvar cancer typically present with T1B and T2 lesions (stage IB and II) of the vulva and clinically negative groin nodes. For stage IB lesions, radical resection of the primary tumor and inguinofemoral lymphadenectomy is recommended. If adequate margins and dissection to the perineal membranes can be achieved, then radical partial vulvectomy offers similar recurrence rates but less morbidity than radical complete vulvectomy (Tantipalakorn, 2009). Because 20 to 30 percent of women with T1 and T2 disease will have diseased nodes, SLNB and/or inguinofemoral lymphadenectomy is performed. As described on page 685, lesion laterality and clinical impression regarding groin involvement guides the decision to perform ipsilateral or bilateral groin dissection.

Stage II cancers are most often managed with a larger radical partial excision. For example, a 4-cm lesion involving the clitoral hood may be managed by an anterior hemivulvectomy and bilateral inguinofemoral lymphadenectomy. Again, reported experience with conservative surgery suggests identical local recurrence rates if 1- to 2-cm surgical margins are achieved (Burke, 1995; Farias–Eisner, 1994; Tantipalakorn, 2009). Occasionally, a radical complete vulvectomy may be required, depending on tumor size and location.

■ Stage III

By definition, stage III vulvar cancers include node-positive tumors. Affected patients have T1 or T2 vulvar lesions with regional nodal spread that is not fixed or ulcerated. Most patients with clinically negative nodes have typically undergone a radical partial or complete vulvectomy and inguinofemoral lymphadenectomy. However, in cases where groin nodes are grossly positive and resectable, "nodal debulking" is performed but further nodal dissection is forfeited. This allows adjuvant radiotherapy to treat any residual microscopic disease yet minimize additional groin dissection morbidity. In practice, most women with stage III vulvar cancer are treated with adjuvant radiation therapy directed to both groins and the pelvis.

Efficacy for this was shown in a randomized GOG trial of 114 patients with invasive squamous cell carcinoma of the vulva and diseased groin nodes. Adjuvant radiation to both groins and the pelvic midplane proved superior to extended pelvic node resection. However, 12 percent of women completing radiotherapy still relapsed in the groin and pelvis, and 8.5 percent at distant sites (Homesley, 1986; Kunos, 2009).

Nodal metastasis does not increase the risk of recurrence on the vulva. Hence, adjuvant radiation to the vulva is the treating physician's decision and guided by margin status, tumor size, and LVSI.

The addition of platinum-based chemotherapy concurrent with radiation therapy stems from treatment of cervical cancer. Also, extrapolation of apparent efficacy in phase II trials of more locally advanced vulvar cancer suggests a role for this for postoperative patients with lymph node metastases (Moore, 1998, 2012). To improve control in both inguinal and pelvic lymph nodes and survival rates, a randomized phase III trial (GOG protocol #185) is currently comparing adjuvant radiation therapy and the combination of radiation plus weekly cisplatin chemotherapy in vulvar cancer patients with positive nodes.

■ Stage IVA

These locally advanced vulvar cancers involve the proximal urethra, proximal vagina, bladder or rectal mucosa, or pelvic bone and may or may not have affected inguinal lymph nodes. With stage IVA vulvar cancers, women occasionally can be treated with radical primary surgery. Much more often, tumor size and location necessitate some form of exenterative surgical procedure to remove the entire lesion with adequate margins. Such unresectable, locally advanced vulvar cancers can be effectively treated with neoadjuvant chemoradiation to drastically minimize the surgical resection required. Two Phase II studies conducted by the GOG have demonstrated the feasibility of this approach using cisplatin regimens (Moore, 1998, 2012). An on-going Phase II trial is currently evaluating the efficacy of cisplatin, gemcitabine, and intensity-modulated radiation therapy (IMRT) for primary treatment of locally advanced squamous cell carcinoma of the vulva. As described in Chapter 28 (p. 616), IMRT offers greater sculpting of radiation delivery to minimize toxicity.

Our current practice is to offer preoperative cisplatin-based chemoradiation to women with inoperable primary tumors or with extensive lesions that would require pelvic exenteration. In cases without fixed groin nodes, pretreatment inguinofemoral lymphadenectomy is performed to determine the need for groin irradiation. If groin nodes are fixed or ulcerated, then primary chemoradiation is administered.

If residual disease remains on the vulva following chemoradiation, then local resection is indicated. If there has been complete clinical response, the primary tumor site undergoes excisional biopsy to confirm pathologic response. Unresected groins that are clinically or radiographically positive 8 weeks after surgery are biopsied by fine-needle aspiration (FNA). If the FNA is positive, a targeted excision of the groin is performed.

In contrast, for stage IVB vulvar cancer, treatment is individualized. A multimodality approach is used to achieve palliation.

SURVEILLANCE

After completing primary treatment, all patients receive thorough physical examination, including inguinal lymph node palpation and pelvic examination every 3 months for the first 2 to 3 years. Surveillance examinations are then scheduled every 6 months to complete a total of 5 years. Thereafter, disease-free women may be seen annually. Vulvoscopy and biopsies are performed if concerning areas are noted during history or physical examination. Radiologic imaging and biopsies to diagnose possible tumor recurrence are performed as indicated.

RECURRENT DISEASE

■ Vulvar Recurrences

In a woman with suspected recurrence, careful evaluation is completed to define the disease extent. Local vulvar recurrences are most common, and surgical reexcision is usually the best option. Radical partial vulvectomy is appropriate for smaller lesions. For large central recurrences involving the urethra, vagina, or rectum, a total pelvic exenteration with reconstructive surgery may be required (Section 46-4, p. 1149). With exenteration, to maintain sexual function, vaginal reconstruction can be completed at the time of surgery or after a short postoperative interval (Section 46-9, p. 1165). Radiated tissue often has a poor blood supply. Thus, vulvar recurrences in a previously radiated field typically require myocutaneous flaps for reconstruction after surgical resection. Last, for patients who are not surgical candidates and are radiation naïve to the vulva, external beam radiation combined with interstitial brachytherapy can be an option.

■ Distant Recurrences

Inguinal lymph node recurrences are virtually always associated with ultimately fatal disease, and few women are alive at the end of the first year following this diagnosis. Women with pelvic or distant metastases can be offered palliative chemotherapy. Combination platinum-based chemotherapy has modest activity in recurrent vulvar cancers (Cunningham, 1997; Moore, 1998). Platinum-based regimens (e.g., cisplatin/paclitaxel) as recommended for advanced cervical cancer might be considered for vulvar cancer if palliative chemotherapy is indicated.

MANAGEMENT DURING PREGNANCY

Squamous cell cancer of the vulva diagnosed and surgically treated during pregnancy is rare, and an incidence of 1 per 20,000 deliveries has been reported (DiSaia, 1997). Nevertheless, any suspicious lesion is evaluated, even during pregnancy.

Radical complete or partial vulvectomy and inguinofemoral lymphadenectomy can be performed when indicated after the first trimester. During the third trimester, markedly increased genital vasculature can increase surgical morbidity. In general, if a diagnosis is made during the late third trimester, lesions may be removed by wide local excision, and definitive surgery completed postpartum. In cases diagnosed at delivery, definitive surgery is performed typically 2 to 3 weeks postpartum.

The mode of delivery following cancer surgery is heavily influenced by the state of the postsurgical vulva. In instances of vaginal stenosis, significant fibrosis, or tumor involvement, a cesarean delivery is recommended, otherwise vaginal delivery is appropriate.

VERRUCOUS CARCINOMA

This rare variant of squamous cell carcinoma constitutes less than 1 percent of all vulvar cancers. Its etiology is unknown, but HPV genome has been found in some of these tumors. Verrucous carcinomas are locally invasive and rarely metastasize. Most women have a cauliflower-shaped vulvar mass that usually elicits pruritus or pain. Surgery is preferred, and most tumors are excised by wide local excision that ensures a 1-cm surrounding margin. Inadequate margins risk local recurrence. Verrucous carcinomas are resistant to radiotherapy and may undergo anaplastic transformation to become more aggressive and invasive. Enlarged groin lymph nodes are evaluated preoperatively by FNA because they usually are inflammatory.

MELANOMA

■ Clinical Presentation and Staging

Melanoma is the second most common vulvar cancer and accounts for 10 percent of all vulvar malignancies. Vulvar melanoma disproportionately affects the elderly and develops more commonly among whites than other races. Vulvar melanoma has an overall poor prognosis, and 5-year survival rates range from 8 to 55 percent (Evans, 1994; Piura, 1992).

Malignant vulvar melanomas most commonly arise from the labia minora, labia majora, or clitoris (Fig. 31-10) (Moore, 1998; Woolcott, 1988). Some benign pigmented lesions can also be found here and include lentigo simplex, vulvar melanosis, acanthosis nigricans, seborrheic keratosis, and nevi (Chap. 4, p. 95). Last, pigmented vulvar neoplasia may be VIN, squamous cell carcinoma, or Paget disease. Thus, tissue sampling is mandatory, and immunohistochemical studies or electron

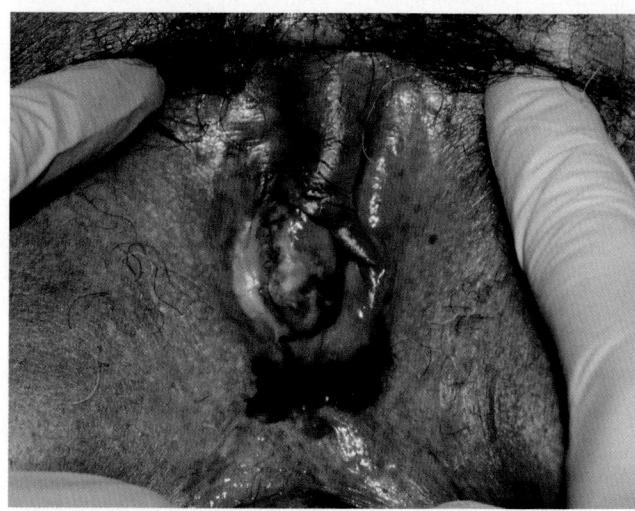

FIGURE 31-10 Vulvar melanoma. (Used with permission from Dr. William Griffith.)

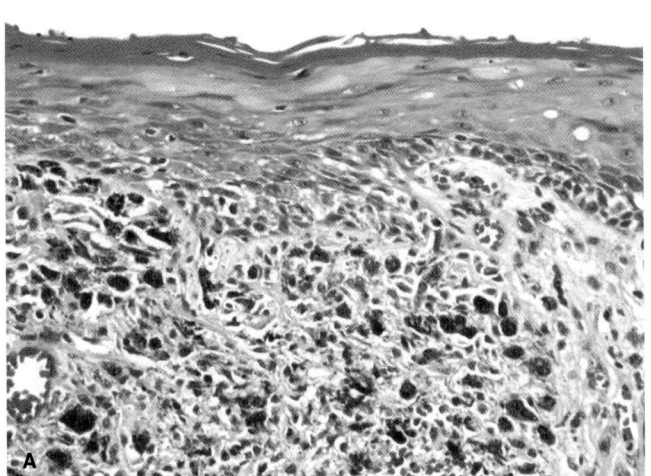
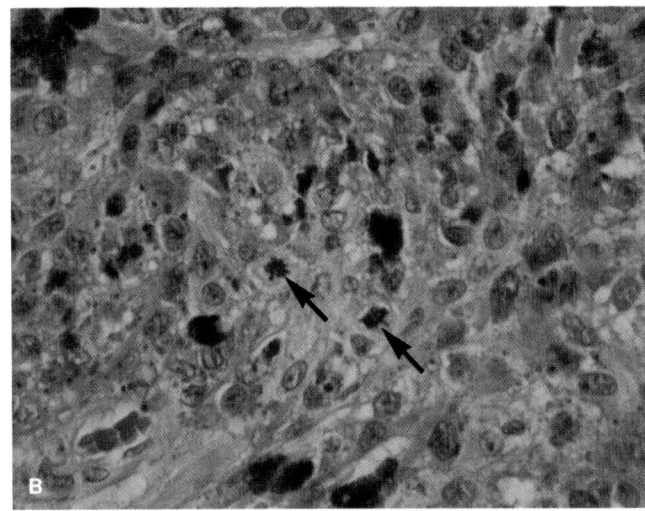

FIGURE 31-11 Photomicrographs of vulvar melanoma. **A.** Medium-power view. Atypical, hyperchromatic melanoma cells are identified within the basal portion of the surface epithelium. Melanoma cells containing intracytoplasmic melanin pigment invade subepithelial stroma in a broad swathe. **B.** High-power view. The malignant melanoma cells in this case have occasionally prominent nucleoli, abundant intracytoplasmic melanin pigment, and frequent mitoses including abnormal mitoses (*arrows*). (Used with permission from Dr. Kelley Carrick.)

microscopy can help clarify the diagnosis (Fig. 31-11). Three histologic subtypes of vulvar melanoma have been described: superficial spreading melanoma (SS), nodular melanoma (NM), and acral lentiginous melanoma (AL).

Vulvar melanomas have been staged by several microstaging systems that include the Chung, the Clark, and the Breslow systems and by the macroscopic systems published by FIGO and AJCC (Table 31-5). Of these, the AJCC stage and Breslow thickness are major predictors of overall survival and are used most often. Breslow thickness measures in millimeters the thickest portion of the lesion from the intact epithelium's most superficial surface to the deepest point of invasion (Moxley, 2011; Verschraegen, 2001).

■ Treatment

Surgery

Vulvar melanoma has limited response to both chemotherapy and radiotherapy. Thus, excision is the single best definitive therapy. Conservative surgery, such as wide local excision or a radical partial vulvectomy, is preferred as radical surgery appears to offer no greater survival advantage (Irvin, 2001; Verschraegen, 2001).

Nodal metastasis is a major predictor of prognosis. The incidence of occult inguinal lymph node metastases is <5 percent for thin melanomas measuring <1 mm thickness, but >70 percent for lesions >4 mm (Hoskins, 2000). Women with clinically positive groin lymph nodes should undergo inguino-femoral lymphadenectomy if possible, as surgical removal of regional disease is the most effective method of control. In patients with clinically negative groins, the decision to perform inguinofemoral lymphadenectomy or SLNB is influenced by lesion thickness. Primary lesions that warrant inguinofemoral node evaluation are those that have a Breslow thickness >1 mm. Other high-risk candidate lesions are lesions <1 mm thick but showing ulceration, a mitotic rate >1 per mm^2, or

LVSI, and those lesions with ambiguous thickness due to a biopsy's positive deep margin (Lens, 2002b). At our institution, we encourage women with clinically negative groins to first undergo SLNB. If diseased nodes are detected, then an inguinofemoral lymphadenectomy can be considered.

Adjuvant Therapy

Women may be considered for adjuvant therapy if their primary vulvar melanoma poses a great risk for disease recurrence. Factors include lesions that are 2 to 4 mm thick and ulcerated, deep primary tumors, positive nodes, or other high-risk features.

Of options, in certain patients with regional cutaneous melanoma involving other body surfaces, adjuvant alpha interferon (IFN-α) increases both progression-free and overall survival rates (Lens, 2002a). At our institution, however, we strongly advocate enrollment in a trial for such patients, recognizing that interferon regimens have considerable toxicity and offer limited benefit.

Adjuvant radiation therapy also shows some promise to reduce locoregional recurrence rates (Ballo, 2005). The National Comprehensive Cancer Network (NCCN) guidelines for treatment of positive resection margins or macroscopically positive fully resected nodal basins include radiotherapy to the affected areas.

Metastatic Disease

Metastatic melanoma is challenging to treat, and 5-year survival rates are <20 percent (Sugiyama, 2007). Resection of distant metastases can be considered for selected patients in whom a survival benefit might be expected compared with medical treatment.

For systemic therapy, several options are available. Preferred regimens include ipilimumab, vemurafenib, or high-dose interleukin-2 (HD IL-2). Of these, HD IL-2 (Proleukin) was approved by the Food and Drug Administration (FDA) in 1998 for metastatic melanoma and benefits a small patient

TABLE 31-5. Melanoma Staging

Staging	Class	Thickness (mm)	Tumor Ulceration Status/Mitoses
IA	T1a, N0, M0	≤1	a: Without ulceration and mitosis <1/ mm^2
IB	T1b, "		b: With ulceration or mitosis ≥1/ mm^2
	T2a, "	1.01–2.0	a: Without ulceration
IIA	T2b, "		b: With ulceration
	T3a, "	2.01–4.0	a: Without ulceration
IIB	T3b, "		b: With ulceration
	T4a, "	>4.0	a: Without ulceration
IIC	T4b, "		b: With ulceration

Staging	Class	Lymph Node (No.)	Nodal Metastatic Burden
IIIA	T1-4a, N1a, M0	1	a: Micrometastasis
	T1-4a, N2a, "	2–3	a: Micrometastasis
IIIB	T1-4b, N1a, '	1	a: Micrometastasis
	T1-4b, N2a, "	2–3	a: Micrometastasis
	T1-4a, N1b, "	1	b: Macrometastasis
	T1-4a, N2b, "	2–3	b: Macrometastasis
	T1-4a, N2c, "	2–3	c: In transit metastasis only
IIIC	T1-4b, N1b, "	1	b: Macrometastasis
	T1-4b, N2b, "	2–3	b: Macrometastasis
	T1-4b, N2c, "	2–3	c In transit metastasis only
	Any T, N3, "	>4	

Staging	Class	Distant Metastasis Site
IV	Any T or N, M1a	Distant skin, subQ, or node
	Any T or N, M1b	Lung
	Any T or N, M1c	Other viscera

SubQ = subcutaneous.
Reproduced with permission from Balch CM, Gershenwald JE, Soong S, et al: Final version of 2009 AJCC melanoma staging and classification. J Clin Oncol 2009 Dec 20;27(36):6199–6206.

subset. Based on these findings, other novel immunotherapeutic approaches have subsequently been investigated.

One novel approach involves T-cell mechanisms that self-regulate T-cell activation through expression of *cytotoxic T-lymphocyte-associated antigen 4 (CTLA-4)*. Ipilimumab is a fully human monoclonal antibody that blocks CTLA-4, thereby increasing T-cell activity and promoting antitumor actions. Ipilimumab (Yervoy) received FDA approval for treatment of metastatic melanoma in March 2011. Although the response rate and overall survival rates with ipilimumab are modest, therapy toxicities, which include immune-related enterocolitis, hepatitis, and dermatitis, are manageable.

In addition, recognition of other key molecular mutations that drive melanoma tumorigenesis has led to promising agents that selectively inhibit the actions of these mutations. Namely, *BRAF* and *c-KIT* mutations may be found in these tumors, and women with melanoma often have their tumors tested for these mutations. Vemurafenib (Zelboraf), a BRAF inhibitor, was approved by the FDA for treatment of metastatic or unresectable melanoma that exhibits the *BRAF* mutation (Robert, 2011). Imatanib (Gleevec) may be used for tumors with the *c-KIT* mutation.

Last, *biochemotherapy* refers to regimens that combine cytotoxic agents with IFN-α and/or HD IL-2. Biochemotherapy may provide a palliative benefit in patients who are symptomatic and/or have rapidly progressive disease. However, the lack of survival benefit with biochemotherapy suggests that alternative therapies should be considered.

BASAL CELL CARCINOMA

Basal cell carcinoma (BCC) of the vulva accounts for <2 percent of all vulvar cancers and is most commonly found in elderly women (DiSaia, 1997). Lesions typically arise on the labia majora, are characterized by poor pigmentation and pruritus, and often mimic eczema, psoriasis, or intertrigo. As a result, correct diagnosis is often delayed due to treatment for other presumed inflammatory or infectious dermatoses.

Although ultraviolet radiation is thought to be the primary risk factor for BCC on sun-exposed areas, its development on sun-protected areas raises the possibility of other, yet undefined, etiologies. Some suggest that local trauma and advancing age may contribute at these sites (LeSueur, 2003; Wermuth, 1970).

Basal cell carcinoma is removed by radical partial vulvectomy using a minimum surgical margin of 1 cm. Lymphatic or distant spread is rare, but inguinofemoral lymphadenectomy or SLNB is considered for clinically suspicious nodes. However, disease may locally recur, particularly in tumors removed with suboptimal margins. Most basal cell carcinomas of the vulva are indolent

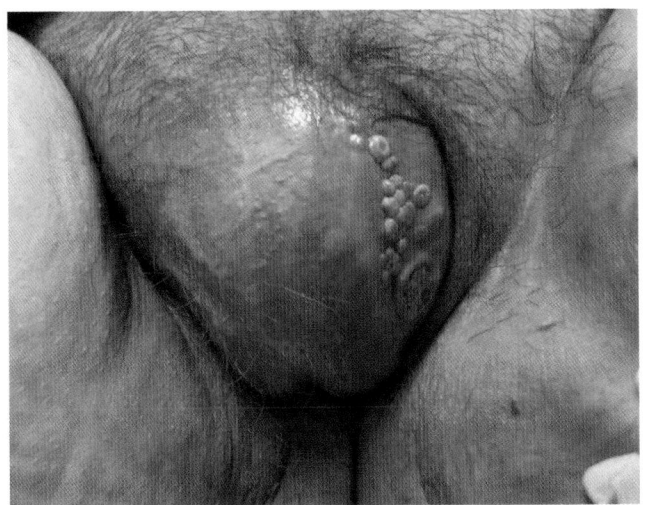

FIGURE 31-12 Vulvar epithelioid sarcoma.

and locally invasive, but rarely metastatic. If surgery is contra-indicated, then primary radiation therapy can be considered. Local immunomodulators such as imiquimod can be selected for patients who are inappropriate surgical candidates. Because surgery is the recommended treatment, any other treatment modalities will warrant close observation to detect cancer progression.

VULVAR SARCOMA

Sarcoma of the vulva is rare, and leiomyosarcoma, malignant fibrous histiocytoma, epithelioid sarcoma, and malignant rhab-doid tumor are the more frequently encountered histologic types. Of these, leiomyosarcoma appears to be most common. Tumors typically develop as isolated masses on labia majora, clitoris, or Bartholin gland (Fig. 31-12). Unlike squamous cell carcinoma, the age of affected women is significantly broader and varies between histologic types.

The outcome of vulvar sarcomas is influenced by size, degree of mitotic activity, and level of infiltration. That is, disease associated with lesions >5 cm in diameter, with infiltrating margins, with extensive necrosis, and with more than five mitoses per 10 high-power fields is most likely to recur after surgical resection (Magné, 2011).

Hematogenous metastasis is the most frequent route of tumor dissemination. Radical partial or complete vulvectomy or pelvic exenteration is recommended if total surgical resection is possible. Removal of inguinofemoral lymph nodes is performed if nodes are large and/or symptomatic. Adjuvant radiation, che-motherapy or both can be considered depending on risk factors for recurrence. Neoadjuvant chemotherapy and/or radiotherapy are considerations for unresectable vulvar sarcomas.

BARTHOLIN GLAND CARCINOMA

Primary malignant tumors arising from the Bartholin gland can be adenocarcinomas, squamous cell carcinomas, or transitional cell carcinomas. The incidence of Bartholin gland carcinomas peaks in women in their mid-60s. Soft, distensible tissue normally surrounds these glands, and tumors may reach considerable

size before patients develop symptoms. Dyspareunia is a common first complaint. Bartholin gland enlargement in a woman older than 40 years and recurrent cysts or abscesses warrant a biopsy or excision. Similarly, all solid masses require FNA or biopsy to establish a definitive diagnosis.

Bartholin gland carcinomas tend to spread into the ischio-rectal fossa and have a propensity for lymphatic spread into the inguinal and pelvic lymph nodes. Therapy for most early cancer stages includes a radical partial vulvectomy with inguinofemo-ral lymphadenectomy. Decisions to perform ipsilateral or bilat-eral groin dissection follow the same criteria as for squamous cell tumors. Postoperative chemoradiation has been shown to reduce the likelihood of local recurrence for all stages. If the initial lesion impinges on the rectum or anal sphincter, preop-erative chemoradiation can be used to avoid extensive surgery.

VULVAR PAGET DISEASE

Extramammary Paget disease is a heterogeneous group of intraepithelial neoplasias and when present on the vulva, appears as an eczematoid, red, weeping area (Fig. 31-13). These are often localized to the labia majora, perineal body, or cli-toris. This disease typically develops in older white women and accounts for approximately 2 percent of all vulvar tumors. Vulvar Paget disease is accompanied by invasive Paget disease or adenocarcinoma of the vulva in 10 to 20 percent of cases (Hoskins, 2000). Moreover, 20 percent of patients with extra-mammary Paget disease will have a carcinoma at another non-vulvar location (Pang, 2010; Wilkinson, 2002).

A histologic classification proposed by Wilkinson and Brown (2002) includes: (1) primary vulvar cutaneous Paget disease, (2) Paget disease as an extension of transitional cell carcinoma of the bladder or urethra, and (3) Paget disease as an extension of an associated adjacent primary cancer such vulvar, anal, or rec-tal cancers. The histologic differentiation of these Paget disease types is important because the specific diagnosis significantly influences treatment selection.

Of these, primary cutaneous vulvar Paget disease displays slow growth. Diseased areas ideally are resected by wide local excision with a 1- to 2-cm margin. In contrast to VIN 3 treat-ment, margins are frequently positive, and disease recurrence is common regardless of the surgical margin status (Black, 2007). If invasive disease is suspected, radical partial vulvectomy is warranted by extending the deep margins to the perineal mem-brane. The latter is frequently accompanied with an ipsilateral or bilateral inguinofemoral lymphadenectomy.

Recurrent Paget disease is common, and long-term surveil-lance is prudent since repeat surgical excision is often necessary. Moreover, screening and surveillance for tumors at nongyneco-logic sites is considered and includes evaluation of the breasts and the gastrointestinal and genitourinary tracts. A detailed dis-cussion of Paget disease of the breast is presented in Chapter 12 (p. 285).

CANCER METASTATIC TO THE VULVA

Metastatic tumors make up approximately 8 percent of all vulvar cancers. Tumors may extend from primary cancers of

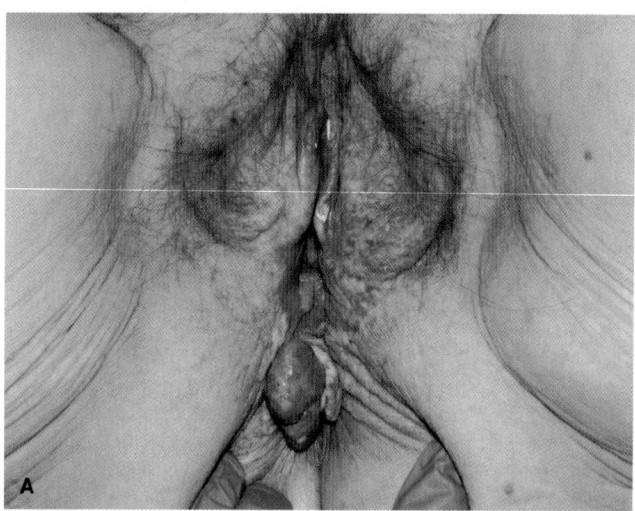
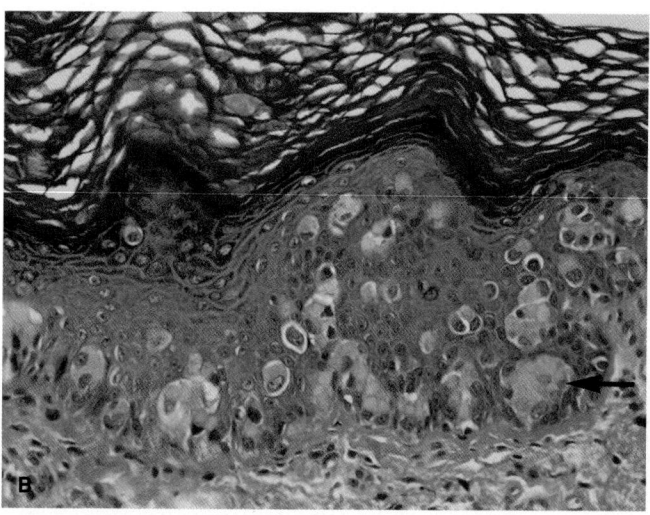

FIGURE 31-13 A. Vulvar Paget disease involving the labia bilaterally, perineum, perianus, and solid right perianal mass. (Used with permission from Dr. Claudia Werner.) **B.** Photomicrograph of primary cutaneous vulvar Paget disease. This is characterized microscopically by the presence of relatively large atypical cells with prominent nucleoli and abundant delicate cytoplasm (*arrow*). These cells are disposed singly or in clusters at various levels within the epithelium. The neoplastic cells are most often confined to the epithelium and would in these instances be classified as an adenocarcinoma in situ. (Used with permission from Dr. Kelley Carrick.)

the bladder, urethra, vagina, or rectum. Less proximate cancers include those from the breast, kidney, lung, stomach, and gestational choriocarcinoma (Wilkinson, 2011).

REFERENCES

American Cancer Society: Vulvar cancer. 2015. Available at: http://www.cancer.org/cancer/vulvarcancer/detailedguide/vulvar-cancer-key-statistics. Accessed January 21, 2015

Balch CM, Gershenwald JE, Soong S, et al: Final version of 2009 AJCC melanoma staging and classification. J Clin Oncol 27(36):6199, 2009

Ballo MT, Garden AS, Myers JN, et al: Melanoma metastatic to cervical lymph nodes: can radiotherapy replace formal dissection after local excision of nodal disease? Head Neck 27(8):718, 2005

Bell JG, Lea JS, Reid GC: Complete groin lymphadenectomy with preservation of the fascia lata in the treatment of vulvar carcinoma. Gynecol Oncol 77:314, 2000

Binder SW, Huang I, Fu YS, et al: Risk factors for the development of lymph node metastasis in vulvar squamous cell carcinoma. Gynecol Oncol 37:9, 1990

Black D, Tornos C, Soslow RA, et al: The outcomes of patients with positive margins after excision for intraepithelial Paget's disease of the vulva. Gynecol Oncol 104:547, 2007

Bodelon C, Madeleine MM, Voigt LF, et al: Is the incidence of invasive vulvar cancer increasing in the United States? Cancer Causes Control 20:1779, 2009

Brinton LA, Nasca PC, Mallin K, et al: Case-control study of cancer of the vulva. Obstet Gynecol 75:859, 1990

Burke TW, Levenback C, Coleman RL, et al: Surgical therapy of T1 and T2 vulvar carcinoma: further experience with radical wide excision and selective inguinal lymphadenectomy. Gynecol Oncol 57:215, 1995

Canavan TP, Cohen D: Vulvar cancer. Am Fam Physician 66(7):1269, 2002

Casolati E, Agarossi A, Valieri M, et al: Vulvar neoplasia in HIV positive women: a review. Med Wieku Rozwoj 7(4 Pt 1):487, 2003

Chan JK, Sugiyama V, Pham H, et al: Margin distance and other clinicopathologic prognostic factors in vulvar carcinoma: a multivariate analysis. Gynecol Oncol 104:636, 2007

Coleman RL, Ali S, Levenback CF, et al: Is bilateral lymphadenectomy for midline squamous carcinoma of the vulva always necessary? An analysis from Gynecologic Oncology Group (GOG) 173. Gynecol Oncol 128(2):155, 2013

Cunningham MJ, Goyer RP, Gibbons SK, et al: Primary radiation, cisplatin, and 5-fluorouracil for advanced squamous carcinoma of the vulva. Gynecol Oncol 66:258, 1997

DiSaia PJ, Creasman WT (eds): Invasive cancer of the vulva. In Clinical Gynecologic Oncology, 5th ed. St. Louis, Mosby–Year Book, 1997, pp 202, 229

Donaldson ES, Powell DE, Hanson MB, et al: Prognostic parameters in invasive vulvar cancer. Gynecol Oncol 11:184, 1981

Elit L, Voruganti S, Simunovic M: Invasive vulvar cancer in a woman with human immunodeficiency virus: case report and review of the literature. Gynecol Oncol 98:151, 2005

Evans RA: Review and current perspectives of cutaneous malignant melanoma. J Am Coll Surg 179:764, 1994

Farias-Eisner R, Cirisano FD, Grouse D, et al: Conservative and individualized surgery for early squamous carcinoma of the vulva: the treatment of choice for stage I and II (T1–2N0–1M0) disease. Gynecol Oncol 53:55, 1994

Figge DC, Tamimi HK, Greer BE: Lymphatic spread in carcinoma of the vulva. Am J Obstet Gynecol 152:387, 1985

Frisch M, Biggar RJ, Goedert JJ: Human papillomavirus-associated cancers in patients with human immunodeficiency virus infection and acquired immunodeficiency syndrome. J Natl Cancer Inst 92:1500, 2000

Gargano, JW, Wilkinson EJ, et al: Prevalence of human papilloma virus types in invasive vulvar cancers and vulvar intraepithelial neoplasia 3 in the United States before vaccine introduction. J Low Genit Tract Dis 16(4):471, 2012

Gordinier ME, Malpica A, Burke TW, et al: Groin recurrence in patients with vulvar cancer with negative nodes on superficial inguinal lymphadenectomy. Gynecol Oncol 90:625, 2003

Hacker NF, Berek JS, Lagasse LD, et al: Individualization of treatment for stage I squamous cell vulvar carcinoma. Obstet Gynecol 63:155, 1984

Hacker NF, Berek JS, Lagasse LD, et al: Management of regional lymph nodes and their prognostic influence in vulvar cancer. Obstet Gynecol 61(4):408, 1983

Heaps JM, Fu YS, Montz FJ, et al: Surgical-pathologic variables predictive of local recurrence in squamous cell carcinoma of the vulva. Gynecol Oncol 38(3):309, 1990

Hildesheim A, Han CL, Brinton LA, et al: Human papillomavirus type 16 and risk of preinvasive and invasive vulvar cancer: results from a seroepidemiological case-control study. Obstet Gynecol 90:748, 1997

Homesley HD, Bundy BN, Sedlis A, et al: Assessment of current International Federation of Gynecology and Obstetrics staging of vulvar carcinoma relative to prognostic factors for survival (a Gynecologic Oncology Group study). Am J Obstet Gynecol 164(4):997, 1991

Homesley HD, Bundy BN, Sedlis A, et al: Prognostic factors for groin node metastasis in squamous cell carcinoma of the vulva (a Gynecologic Oncology Group study). Gynecol Oncol 49(3):279, 1993

Homesley HD, Bundy BN, Sedlis A, et al: Radiation therapy versus pelvic node resection for carcinoma of the vulva with positive groin nodes. Obstet Gynecol 68:733, 1986

Hoskins WJ, Perez CA, Young RC (eds): Vulva. In Principles and Practice of Gynecologic Oncology, 3rd ed. Philadelphia, Lippincott Williams & Wilkins, 2000, p 665

Irvin WP Jr, Legallo RL, Stoler MH, et al: Vulvar melanoma: a retrospective analysis and literature review. Gynecol Oncol 83:457, 2001

Jemal A, Siegel R, Xu J, et al: Cancer statistics, 2010. CA Cancer J Clin 60(5):277, 2010

Jones RW, Rowan DM, Stewart AW: Vulvar intraepithelial neoplasia: aspects of the natural history and outcome in 405 women. Obstet Gynecol 106:1319, 2005

Judson PL, Jonson AL, Paley PJ, et al: A prospective, randomized study analyzing Sartorius transposition following inguinal-femoral lymphadenectomy. Gynecol Oncol 95:226, 2004

Kirschner CV, Yordan EL, De Geest K, et al: Smoking, obesity, and survival in squamous cell carcinoma of the vulva. Gynecol Oncol 56:79, 1995

Kumar S, Shah JP, Bryant CS, et al: A comparison of younger vs older women with vulvar cancer in the United States. Am J Obstet Gynecol 200(5):e52, 2009

Kunos C, Simpkins F, Gibbons H, et al: Radiation therapy compared with pelvic node resection for node-positive vulvar cancer: a randomized controlled trial. Obstet Gynecol 114:537, 2009

Kurman RJ, Carcangiu ML, Herrington CS, et al (eds): WHO Classification of Tumours of Female Reproductive Organs, 4th ed. Lyon, International Agency for Research on Cancer, 2014, p 231

Lens MB, Dawes M: Interferon alfa therapy for malignant melanoma: a systematic review of randomized controlled trials. J Clin Oncol 20(7):1818, 2002a

Lens MB, Dawes M, Goodacre T, et al: Excision margins in the treatment of primary cutaneous melanoma: a systematic review of randomized controlled trials comparing narrow vs wide excision. Arch Surg 137(10):1101, 2002b

LeSueur BW, DiCaudo DJ, Connolly SM: Axillary basal cell carcinoma. Dermatol Surg 29:1105, 2003

Levenback C: Update on sentinel lymph node biopsy in gynecologic cancers. Gynecol Oncol 111(2 Suppl):S42, 2008

Levenback C, Morris M, Burke TW, et al: Groin dissection practices among gynecologic oncologists treating early vulvar cancer. Gynecol Oncol 62(1):73, 1996

Levenback CF, Ali S, Coleman RL, et al: Lymphatic mapping and sentinel lymph node biopsy in women with squamous cell carcinoma of the vulva: a gynecologic oncology group study. J Clin Oncol 30(31):3786, 2012

Madeleine MM, Daling JR, Carter JJ, et al: Cofactors with human papillomavirus in a population-based study of vulvar cancer. J Natl Cancer Inst 89:1516, 1997

Magné N, Pacaut C, Auberdiac P, et al: Sarcoma of vulva, vagina and ovary. Best Pract Res Clin Obstet Gynaecol 25(6):797, 2011

Manavi M, Berger A, Kucera E, et al: Does T1, N0-1 vulvar cancer treated by vulvectomy but not lymphadenectomy need inguinofemoral radiation? Int J Radiat Oncol Biol Phys 38(4):749, 1997

Moore D, Ali S, Barnes M, et al: A phase II trial of radiation therapy and weekly cisplatin chemotherapy for the treatment of locally advanced squamous cell carcinoma of the vulva: a Gynecologic Oncology Group study. Gynecol Oncol 124(3):529, 2012

Moore DH, Thomas GM, Montana GS, et al: Preoperative chemoradiation for advanced vulvar cancer: a phase II study of the Gynecologic Oncology Group. Int J Radiat Oncol Biol Phys 42:79, 1998

Morley GW: Infiltrative carcinoma of the vulva: results of surgical treatment. Am J Obstet Gynecol 124:874, 1976

Moxley KM, Fader AN, Rose PG, et al: Malignant melanoma of the vulva: an extension of cutaneous melanoma? Gynecol Oncol 122(3):612, 2011

National Cancer Institute: Surveillance, epidemiology, and end results (SEER) program. SEER stat fact sheets: vulvar cancer, 2014. Available at: http://seer.cancer.gov/statfacts/html/vulva.html. Accessed January 16, 2015

Oonk MH, van Hemel BM, Hollema H, et al: Size of sentinel-node metastasis and chances of non-sentinel-node involvement and survival in early stage vulvar cancer: results from GROINSS-V, a multicentre observational study. Lancet Oncol 11:646, 2010

Origoni M, Sideri M, Garsia S, et al: Prognostic value of pathological patterns of lymph node positivity in squamous cell carcinoma of the vulva stage III and IVA FIGO. Gynecol Oncol 45:313, 1992

Pang J, Assaad D, Breen, D et al: Extramammary Paget disease: review of patients seen in a non-melanoma skin cancer clinic. Curr Oncol 17(5):43, 2010

Pecorelli S: Revised FIGO staging for carcinoma of the vulva, cervix, and endometrium. Int J Gynaecol Obstet 105(2):103, 2009

Penn I: Cancers in renal transplant recipients. Adv Ren Replace Ther 7(2):147, 2000

Perez CA, Grigsby PW, Galakatos A, et al: Radiation therapy in management of carcinoma of the vulva with emphasis on conservation therapy. Cancer 71(11):3707, 1993

Piura B, Egan M, Lopes A, et al: Malignant melanoma of the vulva: a clinicopathologic study of 18 cases. J Surg Oncol 50:234, 1992

Preti M, Rouzier R, Mariani L, et al: Superficially invasive carcinoma of the vulva: diagnosis and treatment. Clin Obstet Gynecol 48:862, 2005

Robert C, Thomas L, Bondarenko I, et al: Ipilimumab plus dacarbazine for previously untreated metastatic melanoma. N Engl J Med 364(26):2517, 2011

Rolfe KJ, Crow JC, Benjamin E, et al: Cyclin D1 and retinoblastoma protein in vulvar cancer and adjacent lesions. Int J Gynecol Cancer 11:381, 2001

Rouzier R, Haddad B, Dubernard G, et al: Inguinofemoral dissection for carcinoma of the vulva: effect of modifications of extent and technique on morbidity and survival. J Am Coll Surg 196:442, 2003

Stehman FB, Bundy BN, Dvoretsky PM, et al: Early stage I carcinoma of the vulva treated with superficial inguinal lymphadenectomy and modified excision hemivulvectomy: a prospective study of the Gynecologic Oncology Group. Obstet Gynecol 79:490, 1992a

Stehman FB, Bundy BN, Thomas G, et al: Groin dissection versus groin radiation in carcinoma of the vulva: a Gynecologic Oncology Group study. Int J Radiat Oncol Biol Phys 24(2):389, 1992b

Stehman FB, Look KY: Carcinoma of the vulva. Obstet Gynecol 107(3):719, 2006

Stroup AM, Harlan LC, Trimble EL: Demographic, clinical, and treatment trends among women diagnosed with vulvar cancer in the United States. Gynecol Oncol 108(3):577, 2008

Sugiyama VE, Chan JK, Shin JY, et al: Vulvar melanoma: a multivariable analysis of 644 patients. Obstet Gynecol 110:296, 2007

Tantipalakorn C, Robertson G, Marsden DE, et al: Outcome and patterns of recurrence for International Federation of Gynecology and Obstetrics (FIGO) stages I and II squamous cell vulvar cancer. Obstet Gynecol 113(4):895, 2009

Van der Steen S, de Nieuwenhof HP, Massuger L, et al: New FIGO staging system of vulvar cancer indeed provides a better reflection of prognosis. Gynecol Oncol 119(3):520, 2010

Van der Zee AG, Oonk MH, De Hullu JA, et al: Sentinel node dissection is safe in the treatment of early-stage vulvar cancer. J Clin Oncol 26:884, 2008

van Seters M, van Beurden M, de Craen AJ: Is the assumed natural history of vulvar intraepithelial neoplasia III based on enough evidence? A systematic review of 3322 published patients. Gynecol Oncol 97:645, 2005

Verschraegen CF, Benjapibal M, Supakarapongkul W, et al: Vulvar melanoma at the M. D. Anderson Cancer Center: 25 years later. Int J Gynecol Cancer 11:359, 2001

Way S: The anatomy of the lymphatic drainage of the vulva and its influence on the radical operation for carcinoma. Ann R Coll Surg Engl 3(4):187, 1948

Wermuth BM, Fajardo LF: Metastatic basal cell carcinoma: a review. Arch Pathol 90:458, 1970

Wilkinson EJ: Premalignant and malignant tumors of the vulva. In Kurman RJ, Ellenson LH, Ronnett BM (eds): Blaustein's Pathology of the Female Genital Tract, New York, Springer, 2011, p 95

Wilkinson EJ, Brown HM: Vulvar Paget disease of urothelial origin: a report of three cases and a proposed classification of vulvar Paget disease. Hum Pathol 33(5):549, 2002

Woolcott RJ, Henry RJ, Houghton CR: Malignant melanoma of the vulva: Australian experience. J Reprod Med 33:699, 1988

CHAPTER 32

Vaginal Cancer

Cancer found in the vagina is most likely metastatic disease. Primary vaginal carcinoma is rare and makes up only 3 percent of all gynecologic malignancies (Siegel, 2015). This low incidence reflects the infrequency with which primary carcinoma arises in the vagina and the strict criteria for its diagnosis. According to International Federation of Gynecology and Obstetrics (FIGO) staging criteria, a vaginal lesion that involves adjacent organs such as the cervix or vulva, by convention, is deemed primary cervical or vulvar, respectively (Pecorelli, 1999). The most common histologic type of primary vaginal cancer is squamous cell carcinoma, followed by adenocarcinoma (Platz, 1995).

RELEVANT ANATOMY

During embryogenesis, the müllerian ducts fuse caudally to form the uterovaginal canal (Chap. 18, p. 404). The canal's distal portion forms the proximal vagina, whereas the distal vagina arises from the urogenital sinus. The uterovaginal canal is lined by columnar epithelium, which is subsequently replaced by squamous cells migrating cephalad from the urogenital sinus. These squamous cells stratify, and the vaginal epithelium matures and thickens. Underlying this epithelium, muscularis and adventitial layers surround the vaginal tube.

With vaginal cancer, local extension and lymphatic invasion are common patterns of spread. The lymphatic channels that drain the vagina form extensive, complex, and variable anastomoses. As a result, any node in the pelvis, groin, or anorectal area may drain any part of the vagina. Of these, the external, internal, and common iliac lymph nodes are the primary sites of vaginal lymphatic drainage. Thus, pelvic lymphadenectomy, which samples these nodal groups, is commonly performed during primary surgical excision of proximally located vaginal cancers. Alternatively, lymphatic vessels of the posterior vagina may empty into the inferior gluteal, presacral, or perirectal

nodes, and those of the vagina's distal third may drain to the superficial and deep inguinal lymph nodes (Frank, 2005).

Hematogenous spread of vaginal cancer is less frequent, and venous drainage consists of the uterine, pudendal, and rectal veins, which drain into the internal iliac vein. Arterial blood supply to the vagina comes primarily from internal iliac artery branches, which include the uterine, vaginal, middle rectal, and internal pudendal arteries (Fig. 38-12, p. 805).

INCIDENCE

According to estimates for 2015, 4070 new cases of vaginal cancer will be diagnosed in the United States, and there will be 910 deaths (Siegel, 2015). The overall incidence is 0.45 cases per 100,000 women but is notably lower in whites (0.42 cases) compared with black and Hispanic women (0.73 and 0.56 cases, respectively). Vaginal cancer rates increase with age and peak among women ≥80 years. The median age at diagnosis is 58 (Watson, 2009). Of histologic forms, squamous cell carcinoma accounts for 70 to 80 percent of all primary vaginal cancer cases (Beller, 2003; Platz, 1995).

SQUAMOUS CELL CARCINOMA

■ Risks

Squamous cell cancer of the vagina arises within its stratified nonkeratinized epithelium (Fig. 32-1). As with other cancers of the lower reproductive tract, human papillomavirus (HPV) has been closely linked with squamous cell vaginal cancer (Chap. 30, p. 658). A systematic review found an HPV prevalence of 65 percent in samples from invasive vaginal cancer, and a 93-percent prevalence in high-grade vaginal dysplasia lesions. HPV 16 was the most common type and was present in 55 percent of vaginal cancer samplings (Smith, 2009). A retrospective cross-sectional study involving 31 countries found similar results (Alemany, 2014).

Because of this association with HPV infection, vaginal in situ and invasive squamous cell carcinomas share risk factors similar to those for cervical cancer. Some of these include multiple lifetime sexual partners, early age at first intercourse, and current cigarette smoking. Women with a vulvar or cervical cancer history are also at increased risk. This last association may stem from the field effect of HPV affecting multiple lower genital tract epithelia or may result from direct tumor spread.

Vaginal intraepithelial neoplasia (VaIN) is a precursor to invasive vaginal cancer, and approximately 2 to 3 percent of patients with VaIN will progress to invasive cancer (Dodge,

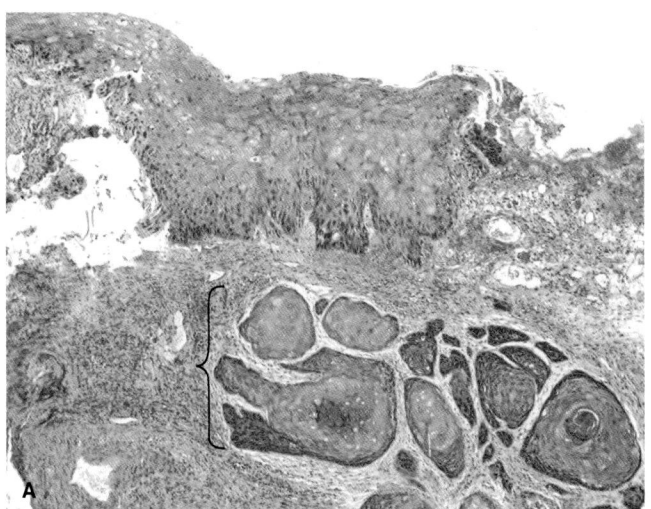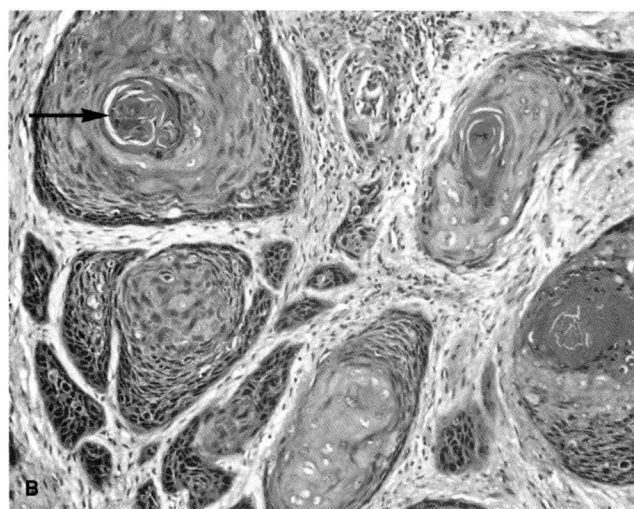

FIGURE 32-1 Sections showing invasive squamous cell carcinoma of the vagina. **A.** Invasive, well-differentiated squamous cell carcinoma of the vagina (*bracket*) invading the subepithelial stroma (×4). **B.** Invasive, well-differentiated squamous cell carcinoma of the vagina (×10). Invasive tumor is composed of irregular nests of malignant squamous cells with keratin pearls (*arrow*) and intercellular bridges. (Used with permission from Dr. Kelley Carrick.)

2001; Ratnavelu, 2013). The quadrivalent HPV vaccine is effective in preventing VaIN 2 and 3 associated with HPV 16 or 18 (Joura, 2007). It is possible that use of this vaccine will decrease invasive vaginal cancer rates in the future.

Diagnosis

Vaginal bleeding is the most common complaint associated with vaginal cancer, although pelvic pain and vaginal discharge also may be noted. Less frequently, lesions involving the anterior vaginal wall may lead to dysuria, hematuria, or urgency. Alternatively, constipation may result from posterior wall masses. Most vaginal cancers develop in the upper third of the vagina. Moreover, of those with cancers, women who have had a prior hysterectomy are significantly more likely to have lesions in the upper vagina (70 percent) than those without prior hysterectomy (36 percent) (Chyle, 1996).

During pelvic evaluation in all women, the vagina is inspected as the speculum is inserted or removed. If a gross lesion is found, vaginal cancer usually can be diagnosed by punch biopsy in the office. Biopsy may be obtained with Tischler biopsy forceps (Fig. 29-16, p. 641). An Emmett hook, one type of skin hook, may be useful to elevate and stabilize vaginal tissue during biopsy. Monsel paste is applied as needed for hemostasis. If a gross lesion is not detectable, vaginoscopy can guide directed biopsy. Bimanual examination assists in determining the tumor size, and rectovaginal examination is especially important for posterior wall lesions.

Once cancer is diagnosed, no specific laboratory testing other than that used generally for preoperative preparation such as complete blood count and serum chemistry panel is required.

Staging and Classification

Vaginal cancer staging is similar to that for cervical cancer and is completed clinically by physical examination and with the

assistance of cystourethroscopy and/or proctosigmoidoscopy depending on tumor location. Chest radiography aids the search for metastatic disease (Table 32-1 and Table 32-2). If needed, general anesthesia can permit a more detailed pelvic examination for accurate staging. Proctosigmoidoscopy to a depth of at least 15 cm can detect local bowel invasion, whereas cystourethroscopy assists identification of bladder or urethral involvement.

Computed tomography (CT) scanning, magnetic resonance (MR) imaging, and fluorodeoxyglucose-positron emission tomography (FDG-PET) may also be useful in treatment planning but are not classically used to determine disease stage. CT scanning can delineate the size and extent of many tumors (Fig. 32-2). However, if the extent of cancer expansion is unclear, MR imaging is the most useful radiologic tool available to visualize the vagina due to its superior soft tissue resolution. FDG-PET can also be selected to evaluate lymph node involvement and distant metastases. In one study, FDG-PET was more sensitive than CT for detection of abnormal lymph nodes (Lamoreaux, 2005).

TABLE 32-1. Vaginal Cancer Evaluation

Vaginal biopsy
Physical examination
Endocervical curettage
Endometrial biopsy
Cystourethroscopy
Proctosigmoidoscopy
Chest radiograph
Abdominopelvic CT scan, MR imaging, or PET CT[a]

[a]Useful for treatment planning but not used to assign FIGO stage.
CT = computed tomography; MR = magnetic resonance; PET = positron emission tomography.

TABLE 32-2. FIGO Staging Classification of Vaginal Cancer

Stage	Characteristics
I	The carcinoma is limited to the vaginal wall
II	The carcinoma has involved the subvaginal tissue but has not extended to the pelvic wall
III	The carcinoma has extended to the pelvic wall
IV	The carcinoma has extended beyond the true pelvis or has involved the mucosa of the bladder or rectum; bullous edema as such does not permit a case to be allotted to stage IV
IVA	Tumor invades bladder and/or rectal mucosa and/or direct extension beyond the true pelvis
IVB	Spread to distant organs

FIGO = International Federation of Gynecology and Obstetrics.
FIGO Committee on Gynecologic Oncology, 2009.

■ Prognosis

The prognosis of vaginal squamous cell carcinoma has improved since the 1950s, when the 5-year survival rate was only 18 percent. Advances in radiation technology and earlier diagnosis are largely responsible for the improved 5-year survival rate, which now ranges from 45 to 68 percent for all stages (Ghia, 2011; Hellman, 2006).

The prognosis of vaginal squamous cell carcinoma depends primarily on FIGO stage (Fig. 32-3 and Table 32-2) (Frank, 2005; Peters, 1985). Other factors associated with poor prognosis include larger tumor size, adenocarcinoma cell type, and older age (Hellman, 2006; Tjalma, 2001; Tran, 2007). The 5-year disease-specific survival rate is 85 to 92 percent for women with stage I disease, 68 to 78 percent for those with stage II, and 13 to 58 percent for those with stage III or IV (Fig. 32-4) (Frank, 2005; Tran, 2007).

■ Treatment

Stage I

Because of vaginal cancer's rarity, data are limited to guide evidence-based treatment. Therefore, therapy is individualized and based on factors such as tumor type, stage, location, and size.

For stage I disease, both surgery and radiotherapy are options. However, surgery is preferred for most if negative surgical margins can be achieved. Surgery includes radical vaginectomy, radical hysterectomy (for women with an intact uterus), and pelvic lymphadenectomy for most tumors located in the upper third of the vaginal vault. A review of the National Cancer Data Base showed that women with stage I disease treated

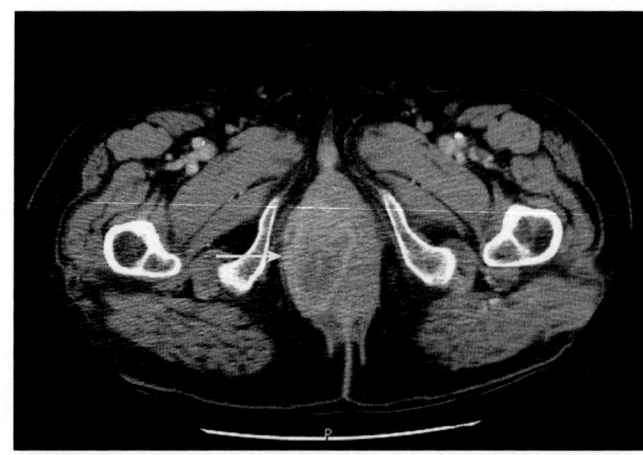

FIGURE 32-2 Computed tomography (CT) scan reveals size and extent of vaginal mass (*arrow*).

with surgery alone had a significantly improved 5-year survival rate compared with those treated with radiation (90 percent versus 63 percent) (Creasman, 1998). However, other reports have found no significant difference in disease-free survival rates in women with stage I disease treated with surgery compared

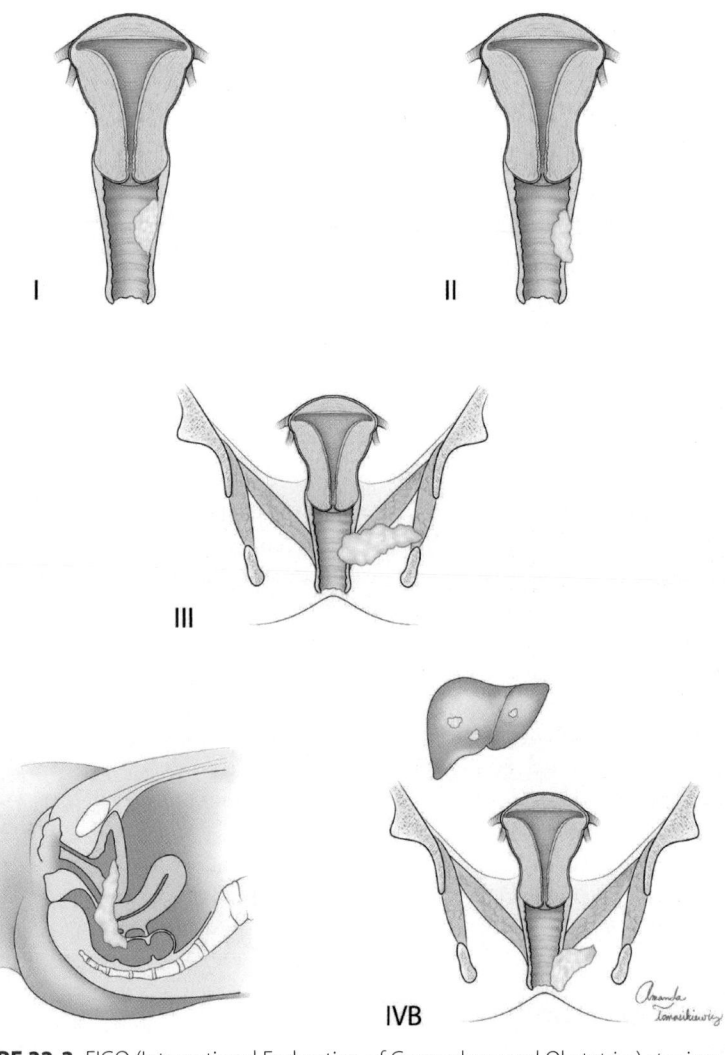

FIGURE 32-3 FIGO (International Federation of Gynecology and Obstetrics) staging of vaginal cancer.

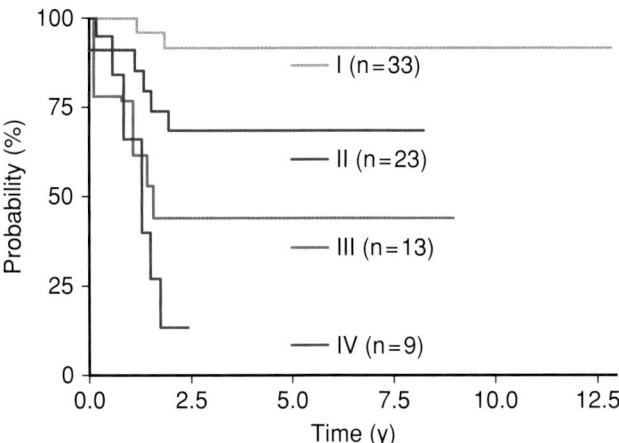

FIGURE 32-4 Disease-specific survival stratified by International Federation of Gynecology and Obstetrics (FIGO) stage. (Reproduced with permission from Tran PT, Su Z, Lee P, et al: Prognostic factors for outcomes and complications for primary squamous cell carcinoma of the vagina treated with radiation. Gynecol Oncol 2007 Jun;105(3):641–649.)

with radiation alone (Stock, 1995). Radiotherapy may be delivered by external beam, with or without brachytherapy. Further, brachytherapy alone has been used successfully to treat selected small stage I lesions (Nori, 1983; Perez, 1999; Reddy, 1991).

Stage II

Depending on circumstances and the treating clinician, primary surgery or radiation may be selected for stage II cancers. Stock and colleagues (1995) found a significant survival advantage at 5 years in those with stage II disease treated with surgery compared with those treated with radiation (62 percent versus 53 percent). Review of the National Cancer Data Base showed that the 5-year survival rate for women with stage II disease treated with surgery alone was 70 percent; with radiotherapy alone, 57 percent; and with a combination of surgery and radiotherapy, 58 percent (Creasman, 1998). However, other researchers have found no survival advantage from surgery compared with radiotherapy in stage II disease (Davis, 1991; Rubin, 1985).

Radiation is generally recommended if negative margins cannot be achieved surgically due to tumor location or size or to patient comorbidities that preclude surgery. If primary radiation is administered for stage II disease, a combination of external beam radiation and brachytherapy is the most common regimen. External beam radiation generally is given first, and depending on tumor response, brachytherapy is tailored to remaining disease. As discussed subsequently, adjuvant chemotherapy is often administered during radiation therapy.

Stage III and IVA

For advanced disease, external beam radiation alone or in combination with brachytherapy is usually administered (Frank, 2005). Concurrent chemotherapy with cisplatin as a radiation sensitizer is generally also recommended.

Stage IVB

Metastatic vaginal cancer is not curable, and treatment may include systemic chemotherapy or supportive hospice care. The most common sites of distant spread include liver, lung, and bone.

The choice of chemotherapeutic agents is commonly extrapolated from cervical cancer data. For example, bevacizumab (Avastin) was approved by the Food and Drug Administration (FDA) in 2014 as a treatment for metastatic cervical cancer, in combination with paclitaxel and either cisplatin or topotecan. The addition of bevacizumab to these chemotherapy combinations improved overall survival length by approximately 4 months in women with metastatic cervical cancer (Tewari, 2014).

Chemoradiation

The numbers of women with vaginal cancer have been too small to make a prospective, randomized trial feasible. However, concurrent chemotherapy with cisplatin can be considered to benefit those with locally advanced vaginal cancer because of its proven efficacy in cervical cancer treatment. The characteristics of this agent are described in Chapter 27 (p. 602) and Figure 30-13 (p. 672). In a small series of vaginal cancer cases, adjuvant chemotherapy provided a 10- to 33-percent decline in the total radiation dose delivered (Dalrymple, 2004). Although not intending to show an improved survival rate with chemoradiation, the authors found that local control of tumor growth and survival rates were comparable with those who had received higher radiation doses alone. Smaller total radiation doses may lead to lower rates of vaginal stenosis and fistula formation.

In a Surveillance Epidemiology and End Result (SEER) database analysis of 326 patients with vaginal cancer treated with external beam radiation and/or brachytherapy between 1991 and 2005, a notable increase in sensitizing chemotherapy use was observed after the 1999 National Cancer Institute announcement confirmed the efficacy of chemoradiation in cervical cancer. Despite this increased use, the authors did not observe any survival advantage among those vaginal cancer patients who received chemoradiation compared with radiation alone (Ghia, 2011).

A recent phase II trial, which included 22 cervical cancer patients and three with stage II–IV vaginal cancer, demonstrated a 96-percent response rate for women given weekly cisplatin, radiation, and triapine, a ribonucleotide reductase inhibitor (Kunos, 2013). Larger studies are planned in cervical cancer patients.

Chemotherapy

In general, chemotherapy alone is ineffective to treat vaginal cancer, although data are limited. The Gynecologic Oncology Group (GOG) performed a Phase II trial evaluating 50 mg/m^2 doses of cisplatin given every 3 weeks for advanced or recurrent vaginal cancer in 26 patients. Only one woman with squamous cell carcinoma achieved a complete response. Five of 16 patients with squamous cell carcinoma had stable disease, and 10 had cancer progression. Based on this trial, single-agent cisplatin is considered to have insignificant activity at that dose and schedule (Thigpen, 1986). To date, this has been the only prospective GOG trial evaluating chemotherapy alone for vaginal cancer.

Radiation Therapy

Radiation to the primary tumor usually involves pelvic external beam with or without brachytherapy, and often concurrent platinum-based sensitizing chemotherapy depending on the stage and other factors described above. Additionally, groin radiation is effective in patients with palpable nodal metastases.

Moreover, elective irradiation may be delivered to clinically negative inguinal lymph nodes if the distal third of the vagina is involved. In a retrospective review, Perez and colleagues (1999) found that of 100 women who did not receive groin radiation, if disease was confined to the upper two thirds of the vagina, then none developed groin metastases. However, 10 percent of patients with lower-third primary tumors and 5 percent with tumors involving the entire length of the vagina developed inguinal node metastases.

■ Surveillance

Treatment failures usually develop within 2 years of primary therapy completion. Thus, patients are typically examined every 3 months for the first 2 years and then every 6 months until 5 years of surveillance is completed (Pingley, 2000; Rubin, 1985). After 5 years following treatment, women can be seen annually. A Pap smear and pelvic examination with careful attention to the inguinal and scalene nodes are performed. Surveillance with CT or MR imaging is at the clinician's discretion.

■ Recurrent Disease

Disease recurrence should be confirmed by biopsy if further treatment is planned. Therapeutic options in women with central pelvic recurrence who have had prior pelvic radiation are limited. Pelvic exenteration can be considered if a patient is psychologically and medically fit to undergo radical surgery associated with high morbidity (Chap. 46, p. 1149). It is attempted only in those whose disease is limited to the central pelvis. Therefore, clinicians are alert to the triad of sciatic pain, leg edema, and hydronephrosis, which suggests pelvic sidewall disease. These women are not surgical candidates but can be managed with chemoradiation or with chemotherapy alone for women previously irradiated.

Survival after relapse is poor. In a review of 301 patients, 5-year survival was 20 percent for local recurrence and 4 percent for metastatic disease recurrence (Chyle, 1996).

ADENOCARCINOMA

Primary adenocarcinoma of the vagina is rare, making up only 13 percent of all vaginal cancers (Platz, 1995). Histologic types include clear cell, endometrioid, mucinous, and serous carcinoma, and these may arise in endometriosis foci, in areas of vaginal adenosis, in periurethral glands, or in wolffian duct remnants. *Adenosis* in the vagina is defined by subepithelial glandular structures lined by mucinous columnar cells that resemble endocervical cells (Sandberg, 1965). These represent residual glands of müllerian origin. Clinically, adenosis appears as red granular spots or patches and does not stain following Lugol solution application. Vaginal adenosis is a condition common in females exposed in utero to diethylstilbestrol (DES) (Chap. 18, p. 423).

More commonly, vaginal adenocarcinoma is metastatic disease, typically from a lesion higher in the genital tract. Disease is frequently metastatic from the endometrium, although it also may originate from the cervix or ovary (Saitoh, 2005). In addition, adenocarcinoma metastases from the breast, pancreas, kidney, and colon also have been identified in the vagina.

Treatment is similar to that for squamous cell carcinoma. Thus, surgery, radiation, or a combination of both can be used. Primary vaginal adenocarcinoma in general is more aggressive than squamous cell carcinoma. In one series of 30 patients, it was associated with local and metastatic relapse rates that were more than double those for squamous cell carcinoma (Chyle, 1996).

■ Clear Cell Adenocarcinoma

Of primary vaginal adenocarcinomas, the clear cell type is most closely associated with DES exposure. In the United States starting around 1940, DES was used off-label to prevent miscarriage. In 1971, clear cell adenocarcinoma of the vagina was linked to in utero DES exposure, and subsequently, pregnancy became a contraindication to DES use. Despite this, an estimated 1 to 4 million women used this synthetic estrogen and approximately 0.01 percent of females exposed in utero developed vaginal clear cell adenocarcinoma (Melnick, 1987). Most DES-exposed patients with vaginal cancer were born between 1951 and 1953, when the drug was prescribed most frequently. The median age at diagnosis of vaginal clear cell carcinoma in the United States is 19 years.

However, in the Netherlands, a bimodal distribution of vaginal clear cell carcinoma has been observed—the first peak occurring with a mean age of 26 years and the second at 71 years. The younger group had all been exposed in utero to DES, whereas the older group, born before 1947, had not been exposed (Hanselaar, 1997). It remains to be seen if the incidence of vaginal clear cell carcinoma will rise as the DES-exposed population ages.

Treatment is similar to that for squamous cell carcinoma of the vagina. The 5-year survival rate for 219 women with stage I vaginal clear cell adenocarcinoma was 92 percent and was equivalent regardless of therapy mode (Senekjian, 1987). The reported 5-year survival for 76 patients with stage II disease was 83 percent (Senekjian, 1988). A smaller study from MD Anderson shows worse pelvic control (31 versus 81 percent) and worse 5-year overall survival rate (34 versus 58 percent) for women with primary adenocarcinoma of the vagina not associated with DES exposure compared with squamous cell carcinoma of the vagina. Five-year survival rates for non-DES-associated vaginal cancer were 80 percent for stage I disease, 34 percent for stage II, 26 percent for stage III, and no survivors with stage IV disease (Frank, 2007).

MESENCHYMAL TUMORS

■ Embryonal Rhabdomyosarcoma

This is the most common malignancy of the vagina in infants and children, and most embryonal rhabdomyosarcomas are the sarcoma botryoides subtype. This rare tumor develops almost exclusively in girls younger than 5 years, although vaginal and cervical sarcoma botryoides have been reported in females aged 15 to 20 years (Copeland, 1985). In infants and children, sarcoma botryoides usually is found in the vagina; in reproductive-aged women, within the cervix; and after menopause, within the uterus. Its name, derived from the Greek word *botrys,* which means "bunch of grapes," describes its appearance (Fig. 32-5).

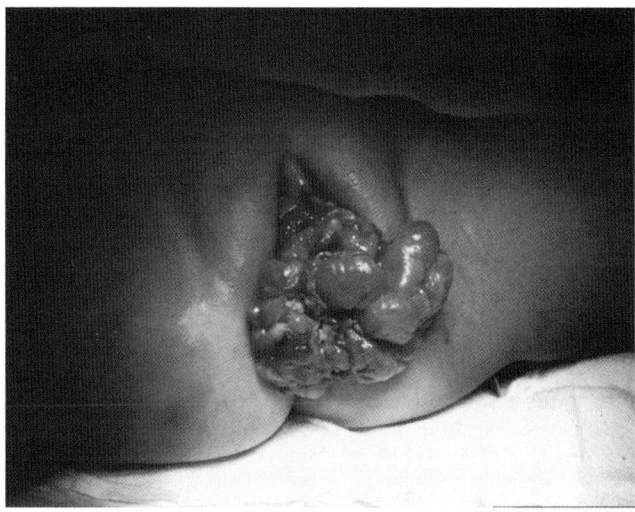

FIGURE 32-5 Sarcoma botryoides protruding through the vaginal introitus. (Reproduced with permission from the North American Society for Pediatric and Adolescent Gynecology.)

The gross specimen can exhibit multiple polyp-like structures or can be a solitary growth with a nodular, cystic, or pedunculated appearance (Hilgers, 1970). Although this distinctive appearance may guide diagnosis, the classic histologic finding of this tumor is the rhabdomyoblast. Typical complaints include bleeding or a vaginal mass.

Embryonal rhabdomyosarcomas have a poor prognosis, but sarcoma botryoides is the easiest to treat and has the best chance of cure. It may be that its superficial location allows earlier detection (Copeland, 1985). Childhood sarcoma botryoides treatment has dramatically changed. It has gradually shifted away from radical pelvic exenteration surgery and toward primary chemotherapy plus adjuvant conservative surgery to excise residual tumor (Andrassy, 1995, 1999; Hays, 1981, 1985).

■ Leiomyosarcoma

This is the most common type of vaginal sarcoma in adults. However, it makes up no more than 1 percent of vaginal malignancies, and only 140 cases have been described in the literature to date (Ahram, 2006; Khosla, 2014; Suh, 2008). The age of affected individuals is broad, but most are older than 40 years (Zaino, 2011). Because of the small number of these tumors, their epidemiology has not been widely studied, and few risk factors have been identified. However, patients previously treated with pelvic radiotherapy for cervical cancer appear to be at risk.

Affected women most often complain of an asymptomatic vaginal mass, but other symptoms mirror those of their squamous cell counterpart. Any wall of the vagina may be affected, but most tumors develop posteriorly (Ahram, 2006). Microscopically, tumors resemble uterine leiomyosarcoma (Fig. 34-2, p. 725). Tumors spread by local invasion and hematogenous dissemination.

Surgical resection with negative margins is the preferred primary treatment. The benefit of adjuvant radiation is unclear due to a lack of controlled trials. However, some clinicians recommend adjuvant radiation for those with high-grade tumor or local recurrence (Curtin, 1995).

MELANOMA

Primary malignant melanoma in the vagina is rare, accounting for less than 3 percent of all vaginal cancers. In women, only 1.6 percent of melanomas are genital. The most common site is the vulva (70 percent), followed by the vagina (21 percent) and the cervix (9 percent) (Miner, 2004). Using data from the SEER database, the incidence of vaginal melanoma is between 0.26 and 0.46 per 1 million women per year (Hu, 2010; Weinstock, 1994). Both U.S. and Swedish studies have shown the mean age at diagnosis to be 66 years (Ragnarsson-Olding, 1993; Reid, 1989).

The most frequent presenting symptoms include vaginal bleeding, discharge, and vaginal mass (Fig. 32-6) (Gupta, 2002; Reid, 1989). Most are located in the distal vagina (Frumovitz, 2010; Xia, 2014). Vaginal melanoma is often detected late, and this may be largely responsible for poor treatment outcomes.

With a reported 5-year survival rate ranging from 10 to 20 percent, the prognosis is among the worst of vaginal malignancies (Ragnarsson-Olding, 1993; Weinstock, 1994; Xia, 2014). Although survival rates are significantly better for those with vaginal lesions measuring <3 cm, FIGO staging of vaginal melanomas does not accurately predict survival (Reid, 1989). Thus, staging criteria specific to melanoma are used. Cutaneous melanomas at other body sites are staged by microstaging systems, including the Chung, the Clark, and the Breslow systems, which use criteria such depth of invasion, tumor size, and tumor thickness (Chap. 31, p. 688). However, Clark levels are not applicable to vaginal melanoma because the typical microscopic skin landmarks used are not present. Therefore, staging is based on tumor thickness, as described by Breslow or Chung.

Treatment is extrapolated from cutaneous melanomas, due to the rarity of vaginal melanoma. Surgery is preferred, when feasible. Although some advocate radical surgery, including exenteration, growing evidence shows that wide local excision has similar survival rates and less morbidity (Buchanan, 1998; Xia, 2014). However, the recommended clinical surgical margin for a melanoma with a Breslow thickness ≤1 mm is 1 cm; a thickness 1 to 2 mm warrants a 1- to 2-cm margin; and a thickness

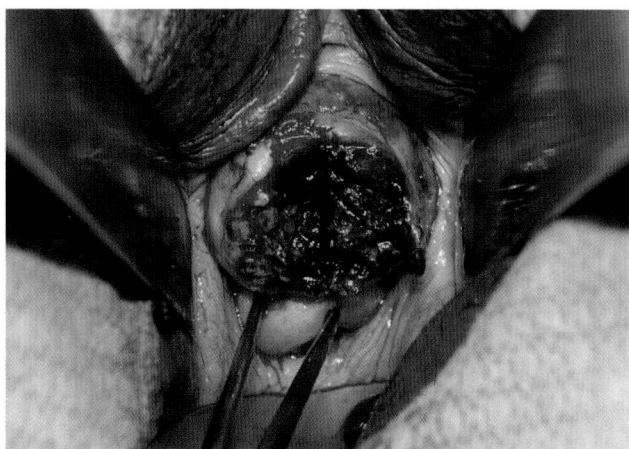

FIGURE 32-6 Vaginal melanoma of the anterior vaginal wall. Below the mass, a tenaculum can be seen on the uninvolved cervix. (Used with permission from Drs. Siobhan Kehoe and Dustin Manders.)

>2 mm requires a 2-cm margin (National Comprehensive Cancer Network, 2014). One study demonstrated a survival benefit to the wide local excision approach (Frumovitz, 2010). However, because of their size or location, many vaginal melanomas are not amenable to this less radical approach.

Melanomas generally are thought to be radioresistant. However, radiation therapy in one series was found to provide local tumor control in women who had surgically unresectable disease (Miner, 2004).

Treatment of advanced and metastatic cutaneous melanoma has progressed, and multiple targeted biologic agents are now available. Mutations in the *BRAF* and *KIT* oncogenes have been found in cutaneous and mucosal melanomas, and women with vaginal melanoma have their tumor tested for these mutations (Leitao, 2014). Options for those with $BRAF^{V600E}$ mutations include vemurafenib, dabrafenib, and trametinib (Chapman, 2011; Flaherty, 2012a,b; Hauschild, 2012; Sosman, 2012). Imatanib may be used for tumors with the *c-KIT* mutation (Carvajal, 2011). Ipilimumab is a monoclonal antibody that promotes T-cell activation, which in turn produces antitumor effects. Its use in patients with metastatic melanoma improves overall survival rates (Hodi, 2010). Recently, the monoclonal antibodies pembrolizumab and nivolumab, which target programmed death 1 protein (PD-1), have been compared with and also combined with ipilimumab for advanced melanoma. The anti-PD-1 immunotherapy drugs are now preferred for the treatment of advanced melanoma, as they offer increased progression-free survival rates, objective-response rates, but fewer serious adverse events than ipilimumab monotherapy (Postow, 2015; Robert, 2015).

REFERENCES

Ahram J, Lemus R, Schiavello HJ: Leiomyosarcoma of the vagina: case report and literature review. Int J Gynecol Cancer 16:884, 2006

Alemany L, Saunier M, Tinoco L, et al: Large contribution of human papillomavirus in vaginal neoplastic lesions: a worldwide study in 597 samples. Eur J Cancer 50(16):2846, 2014

Andrassy RJ, Hays DM, Raney RB, et al: Conservative surgical management of vaginal and vulvar pediatric rhabdomyosarcoma: a report from the Intergroup Rhabdomyosarcoma Study III. J Pediatr Surg 30:1034, 1995

Andrassy RJ, Wiener ES, Raney RB, et al: Progress in the surgical management of vaginal rhabdomyosarcoma: a 25-year review from the Intergroup Rhabdomyosarcoma Study Group. J Pediatr Surg 34:731, 1999

Beller U, Maisonneuve P, Benedet JL, et al: Carcinoma of the vagina. Int J Gynaecol Obstet 83 Suppl 1):27, 2003

Buchanan DJ, Schlaerth J, Kurosaki T: Primary vaginal melanoma: thirteen-year disease-free survival after wide local excision and review of recent literature. Am J Obstet Gynecol 178:1177, 1998

Carvajal RD, Antonescu CR, Wolchok JD, et al: KIT as a therapeutic target in metastatic melanoma. JAMA 395:2327, 2011

Chapman PB, Hauschild A, Robert C, et al: Improved survival with vemurafenib in melanoma with BRAF V600E mutation. N Engl J Med 364:2507, 2011

Chyle V, Zagars GK, Wheeler JA, et al: Definitive radiotherapy for carcinoma of the vagina: outcome and prognostic factors. Int J Radiat Oncol Biol Phys 35:891, 1996

Copeland LJ, Gershenson DM, Saul PB, et al: Sarcoma botryoides of the female genital tract. Obstet Gynecol 66:262, 1985

Creasman WT, Phillips JL, Menck HR: The National Cancer Data Base report on cancer of the vagina. Cancer 83:1033, 1998

Curtin JP, Saigo P, Slucher B, et al: Soft-tissue sarcoma of the vagina and vulva: a clinicopathologic study. Obstet Gynecol 86:269, 1995

Dalrymple JL, Russell AH, Lee SW, et al: Chemoradiation for primary invasive squamous carcinoma of the vagina. Int J Gynecol Cancer 14:110, 2004

Davis KP, Stanhope CR, Garton GR, et al: Invasive vaginal carcinoma: analysis of early-stage disease. Gynecol Oncol 42:131, 1991

Dodge JA, Eltabbakh GH, Mount SL, et al: Clinical features and risk of recurrence among patients with vaginal intraepithelial neoplasia. Gynecol Oncol 83:363, 2001

FIGO Committee on Gynecologic Oncology: Current FIGO staging for cancer of the vagina, fallopian tube, ovary, and gestational trophoblastic neoplasia. Int J Gynaecol Obstet 105(1):3, 2009

Flaherty KT, Infante JR, Daud A, et al: Combined BRAF and MEK inhibition in melanoma with BRAF V600 mutations. N Engl J Med 367:1694, 2012a

Flaherty KT, Robert C, Hersey P, et al: Improved survival with MEK inhibition in BRAF-mutated melanoma. N Engl J Med 367:107, 2012b

Frank SJ, Deavers MT, Jhingran A, et al: Primary adenocarcinoma of the vagina not associated with diethylstilbestrol (DES) exposure. Gynecol Oncol 105:470, 2007

Frank SJ, Jhingran A, Levenback C, et al: Definitive radiation therapy for squamous cell carcinoma of the vagina. Int J Radiat Oncol Biol Phys 62:138, 2005

Frumovitz M, Etcheparevorda M, Sun CC, et al: Primary malignant melanoma of the vagina. Obstet Gynecol 116:1358, 2010

Ghia AJ, Gonzalez VJ, Tward JD, et al: Primary vaginal cancer and chemoradiotherapy: a patterns-of-care analysis. Int J Gynecol Cancer 21:378, 2011

Gupta D, Malpica A, Deavers MT, et al: Vaginal melanoma: a clinicopathologic and immunohistochemical study of 26 cases. Am J Surg Pathol 26:1450, 2002

Hanselaar A, van Loosbroek M, Schuurbiers O, et al: Clear cell adenocarcinoma of the vagina and cervix: an update of the central Netherlands registry showing twin age incidence peaks. Cancer 79:2229, 1997

Hauschild A, Grob JJ, Demidov LV, et al: Dabrafenib in BRAF-mutated metastatic melanoma: a multicenter, open-label, phase 3 randomised controlled trial. Lancet 380:358, 2012

Hays DM, Raney RB Jr, Lawrence W Jr, et al: Rhabdomyosarcoma of the female urogenital tract. J Pediatr Surg 16:828, 1981

Hays DM, Shimada H, Raney RB Jr, et al: Sarcomas of the vagina and uterus: the Intergroup Rhabdomyosarcoma Study. J Pediatr Surg 20:718, 1985

Hellman K, Lundell M, Silfversward C, et al: Clinical and histopathologic factors related to prognosis in primary squamous cell carcinoma of the vagina. Int J Gynecol Cancer 16:1201, 2006

Hilgers RD, Malkasian GD Jr, Soule EH: Embryonal rhabdomyosarcoma (botryoid type) of the vagina: a clinicopathologic review. Am J Obstet Gynecol 107:484, 1970

Hodi FS, O'Day SJ, McDermott DF, et al: Improved survival with ipilimumab in patients with metastatic melanoma. N Engl J Med 363:711, 2010

Hu DN, Yu GP, McCormick SA: Population-based incidence of vulvar and vaginal melanoma in various races and ethnic groups with comparisons to other site-specific melanomas. Melanoma Res 20(2):153, 2010

Joura EA, Leodolter S, Hernandez-Avila M, et al: Efficacy of a quadrivalent prophylactic human papillomavirus (types 6, 11, 16, and 18) L1 virus-like-particle vaccine against high-grade vulval and vaginal lesions: a combined analysis of three randomized clinical trials. Lancet 369(9574):1693, 2007

Khosla D, Patel FD, Kumar R, et al: Leiomyosarcoma of the vagina: a rare entity with comprehensive review of the literature. Int J Appl Basic Med Res 4:128, 2014

Kunos CA, Radivoyevitch T, Waggoner S, et al: Radiochemotherapy plus 3-aminopyridine-2-carboxaldehyde thiosemicarbazone (3-AP, NSC #663249) in advanced-stage cervical and vaginal cancers. Gynecol Oncol 130:75, 2013

Lamoreaux WT, Grisby PW, Dehdashti F, et al: FDG-PET evaluation of vaginal carcinoma. Int J Radiat Oncol Biol Phys 62:733, 2005

Leitao MM: Management of vulvar and vaginal melanomas: current and future strategies. Am Soc Clin Oncol Educ Book 2014:e277, 2014

Melnick S, Cole P, Anderson D, et al: Rates and risks of diethylstilbestrol-related clear-cell adenocarcinoma of the vagina and cervix: an update. N Engl J Med 316:514, 1987

Miner TJ, Delgado R, Zeisler J, et al: Primary vaginal melanoma: a critical analysis of therapy. Ann Surg Oncol 11:34, 2004

National Comprehensive Cancer Network: NCCN guidelines versions 4.2014 Melanoma. Available at http://www.nccn.org/professionals/physician_gls/pdf/melanoma.pdf. Accessed October 7, 2014

Nori D, Hilaris BS, Stanimir G, et al: Radiation therapy of primary vaginal carcinoma. Int J Radiat Oncol Biol Phys 9:1471, 1983

North American Society for Pediatric and Adolescent Gynecology: The PediGYN Teaching Slide Set. Philadelphia, 2001, Slide 124

Pecorelli S, Benedet JL, Creasman WT, et al: FIGO staging of gynecologic cancer. 1994–1997 FIGO Committee on Gynecologic Oncology. International Federation of Gynecology and Obstetrics. Int J Gynaecol Obstet 65:243, 1999

Perez CA, Grigsby PW, Garipagaoglu M, et al: Factors affecting long-term outcome of irradiation in carcinoma of the vagina. Int J Radiat Oncol Biol Phys 44:37, 1999

Peters WA III, Kumar NB, Morley GW: Carcinoma of the vagina: factors influencing treatment outcome. Cancer 55:892, 1985

Pingley S, Shrivastava SK, Sarin R, et al: Primary carcinoma of the vagina: Tata Memorial Hospital experience. Int J Radiat Oncol Biol Phys 46:101, 2000

Platz CE, Benda JA: Female genital tract cancer. Cancer 75:270, 1995

Postow MA, Chesney J, Pavlick AC, et al: Nivolumab and ipilimumab versus ipilmumab in untreated melanoma. N Engl J Med 372:2006, 2015

Ragnarsson-Olding B, Johansson H, Rutqvist LE, et al: Malignant melanoma of the vulva and vagina: trends in incidence, age distribution, and long-term survival among 245 consecutive cases in Sweden 1960–1984. Cancer 71:1893, 1993

Ratnavelu N, Patel A, Fisher AD, et al: High-grade vaginal intraepithelial neoplasia: can we be selective about who we treat? BJOG 120:887, 2013

Reddy S, Saxena VS, Reddy S, et al: Results of radiotherapeutic management of primary carcinoma of the vagina. Int J Radiat Oncol Biol Phys 21:1041, 1991

Reid GC, Schmidt RW, Roberts JA, et al: Primary melanoma of the vagina: a clinicopathologic analysis. Obstet Gynecol 74:190, 1989

Robert C, Schachter J, Long GV, et al: Pembrolizumab versus ipilimumab in advanced melanoma. N Engl J Med 372:2521, 2015

Rubin SC, Young J, Mikuta JJ: Squamous carcinoma of the vagina: treatment, complications, and long-term follow-up. Gynecol Oncol 20:346, 1985

Saitoh M, Hayasaka T, Ohmichi M, et al: Primary mucinous adenocarcinoma of the vagina: possibility of differentiating from metastatic adenocarcinomas. Pathol Int 55:372, 2005

Sandberg EC, Danielson RW, Cauwet RW, et al: Adenosis vaginae. Am J Obstet Gynecol 93:209, 1965

Senekjian EK, Frey KW, Anderson D, et al: Local therapy in stage I clear cell adenocarcinoma of the vagina. Cancer 60:1319, 1987

Senekjian EK, Frey KW, Stone C, et al: An evaluation of stage II vaginal clear cell adenocarcinoma according to substages. Gynecol Oncol 31:56, 1988

Siegel R, Ma J, Zou Z, et al: Cancer statistics. CA Cancer J Clin 65:5, 2015

Smith JS, Backes DM, Hoots BE, et al: Human papillomavirus type-distribution in vulvar and vaginal cancer and their associated precursors. Obstet Gynecol 113:917, 2009

Sosman JA, Kim KB, Schuchter L, et al: Survival in BRAF V600-mutant advanced melanoma treated with vemurafenib. N Engl J Med 366:707, 2012

Stock RG, Chen AS, Seski J: A 30-year experience in the management of primary carcinoma of the vagina: analysis of prognostic factors and treatment modalities. Gynecol Oncol 56:45, 1995

Suh MJ, Park DC: Leiomyosarcoma of the vagina: a case report and review from the literature. J Gynecol Oncol 4:261, 2008

Tewari KS, Sill MW, Long HJ, et al: Improved survival with bevacizumab in advanced cervical cancer. N Engl J Med 370(8):734, 2014

Thigpen JT, Blessing JA, Homesley HD, et al: Phase II trial of cisplatin in advanced or recurrent cancer of the vagina: a Gynecologic Oncology Group Study. Gynecol Oncol 23:101, 1986

Tjalma WA, Monaghan JM, de Barros Lopes A, et al: The role of surgery in invasive squamous carcinoma of the vagina. Gynecol Oncol 81:360, 2001

Tran PT, Su Z, Lee P, et al: Prognostic factors for outcomes and complications for primary squamous cell carcinoma of the vagina treated with radiation. Gynecol Oncol 105:641, 2007

Watson M, Saraiya M, Wu X: Update of HPV-associated female genital cancers in the United States, 1999–2004. J Womens Health 18:1731, 2009

Weinstock MA: Malignant melanoma of the vulva and vagina in the United States: patterns of incidence and population-based estimates of survival. Am J Obstet Gynecol 171:1225, 1994

Xia L, Han D, Yang W, et al: Primary malignant melanoma of the vagina. A retrospective clinicopathologic study of 44 cases. Int J Gynecol Cancer 24:149, 2014

Zaino RJ, Nucci M, Kurman RJ: Diseases of the vagina. In Kurman RJ, Ellenson LH, Ronnett BM (eds): Blaustein's Pathology of the Female Genital Tract, 6th ed. New York, Springer, 2011, p 137

CHAPTER 32

CHAPTER 33

Endometrial Cancer

In the United States, endometrial cancer is the most common gynecologic malignancy. Risk factors include obesity and advancing age. As these factors are now more prevalent, the incidence of endometrial cancer continues to increase. Fortunately, patients usually seek medical attention early due to vaginal bleeding, and endometrial biopsy leads quickly to diagnosis. The primary treatment is hysterectomy with bilateral salpingo-oophorectomy (BSO) and staging lymphadenectomy for most women. Three quarters will have stage I disease that is curable by surgery alone. Patients with more advanced disease typically require postoperative combination chemotherapy, radiotherapy, or both.

EPIDEMIOLOGY AND RISK FACTORS

In the United States, women have a 3-percent lifetime risk of developing endometrial cancer. Although an estimated 54,870 new cases were diagnosed, only 10,170 deaths are expected in 2015. As noted, most patients are diagnosed early and subsequently cured. As a result, endometrial cancer is the fourth leading cause of cancer, but the seventh leading cause of cancer deaths among women (Siegel, 2015).

Endometrial adenocarcinomas are categorized as type I or type II based on histology. Type I, that is, endometrioid type, makes up 80 to 90 percent of all cases (Felix, 2010). The other 10 to 20 percent are type II cancers, namely, the non-endometrioid histologic types that include serous and clear cell adenocarcinomas. Risk factors for developing endometrial cancer are numerous (Table 33-1). Risks specifically for type I cancers are associated with an excess-estrogen environment.

Of these, *obesity* is the most common cause of endogenous overproduction of estrogen. Excessive adipose tissue increases peripheral aromatization of androstenedione to estrone. In premenopausal women, elevated estrone levels trigger abnormal feedback in the hypothalamic-pituitary-ovarian axis. The clinical result is oligo- or anovulation. In the absence of ovulation, the endometrium is exposed to virtually continuous estrogen stimulation without subsequent progestational effect and without menstrual withdrawal bleeding.

Unopposed estrogen therapy is the next most important potential inciting factor. Fortunately, the malignant potential of continuously administered estrogen was recognized more than three decades ago (Smith, 1975). Currently, it is rare to encounter a woman with a uterus who has taken unopposed estrogen for years. Instead, combined estrogen plus progestin hormonal replacement therapy (combination HRT) is routinely prescribed for postmenopausal women with a uterus to reduce estrogen-related endometrial cancer risk (Strom, 2006). Moreover, in one study, the endometrial cancer risk was lower in women taking continuous combination HRT for greater than 6 months compared with those women who had never taken HRT (Phipps, 2011).

Menstrual and reproductive influences are commonly associated with endometrial cancer. For example, early age at menarche or late age of menopause are both associated with increased risk (Wernli, 2006). Classically, women with polycystic ovarian syndrome (PCOS) are anovulatory and thus also have an increased risk of developing this cancer (Fearnley, 2010; Pillay, 2006).

Environment is implicated in endometrial cancer in several ways. Women in Western and developed societies have a much higher incidence (Parkin, 2005). Obvious confounding variables within these populations, such as obesity and low parity, account for much of this effect. However, a possible role for nutrition—especially a diet with a high animal-fat content—is another explanation (Goodman, 1997). Immigrant populations tend to assume the risks of native populations within one or two generations, highlighting the importance of environmental influences (Liao, 2003).

Older age is linked with endometrial cancer development. The average age at diagnosis is the early 60s, and overall,

TABLE 33-1. Factors Affecting Endometrial Cancer Risk

Obesity
Polycystic ovarian syndrome
Long-term, high-dose unopposed menopausal estrogens
Early age of menarche
Late age of natural menopause
Infertility
Nulliparity
Menstrual irregularities
North America or northern Europe residence
Higher education or income level
White race
Older age
Tamoxifen, high cumulative doses
DM, CHTN, or gallbladder disease
Long-term COC use
Cigarette smoking

CHTN = chronic hypertension; COCs = combination oral contraceptives; DM = diabetes mellitus.

approximately 80 percent of these cancers are diagnosed in postmenopausal women older than 55 years (Madison, 2004; Schottenfeld, 1995). Approximately 8 percent of endometrial cancers develop in patients younger than 45 years (Howlader, 2014). Of note, Nevadunsky and associates (2014) found that the age at diagnosis of endometrioid cancer decreased linearly with increasing body mass index (BMI).

Family history is another risk for endometrial cancer. Endometrial cancer is the most common extracolonic manifestation in Lynch syndrome (hereditary nonpolyposis colorectal cancer [HNPCC]) (Hemminki, 2005). This autosomal-dominant syndrome results primarily from mutations in the mismatch repair genes. The mismatch-repair genes associated with Lynch are *MLH1, MSH2, MSH6,* and *PMS2* (Bansal, 2009). Gene mutation prevents repair of base mismatches, which are commonly produced during DNA replication. Inactivity of this DNA repair system leads to mutations that can promote carcinogenesis. Mutation carriers have a risk of developing endometrial cancer that ranges from 40 to 60 percent. Among affected women, the endometrial cancer risk actually exceeds that for colorectal cancer and often develops at a young age (Aarnio, 1999; Delin, 2004). Of endometrial cancer cases, 2 to 5 percent are attributable to Lynch syndrome (Hampel, 2006). In general, most familial cases develop in premenopausal women (Gruber, 1996).

Women who carry mutations in *BRCA1* and *BRCA2* genes are at increased risk for breast and ovarian cancer. They may also have a slightly elevated risk for endometrial cancer, but only because associated breast cancers are often treated with tamoxifen (Beiner, 2007; Thai, 1998).

Tamoxifen causes a two- to threefold higher risk of developing endometrial cancer by its modest "unopposed" estrogenic effect on the endometrium (Chap. 27, p. 603). The increased risk of endometrial cancer affects postmenopausal women almost exclusively, and cancer rates increase linearly with the

duration and cumulative dose of tamoxifen therapy (Fisher, 1998; van Leeuwen, 1994). Accordingly, women taking tamoxifen are counseled regarding this endometrial risk and should report vaginal spotting, bleeding, or discharge. That said, unless a tamoxifen-treated patient has such symptoms or is identified to be at otherwise high risk for endometrial cancer, routine endometrial surveillance does not increase early detection rates (American College of Obstetricians and Gynecologists, 2014c).

Coexisting medical conditions such as diabetes mellitus, hypertension, and gallbladder disease are more commonly associated with endometrial cancer (Morimoto, 2006; Soliman, 2005). In general, these are frequent sequelae of obesity and an environment of chronic excess estrogen.

In contrast, *combination oral contraceptive* (COC) use for at least 1 year confers as much as a 30- to 50-percent reduced risk of endometrial cancer, and risk reduction extends for 10 to 20 years (Dossus, 2010; Stanford, 1993). This most likely derives from a chemopreventive effect on the endometrium provided by the progestin component (Maxwell, 2006). Logically, progesterone intrauterine devices (IUDs) also confer long-term endometrial cancer protection (Tao, 2006). Moreover, similar protective effects have been found with inert and copper IUD types (Felix, 2015).

Smokers have a lower risk of developing endometrial cancer. The biologic mechanism is multifactorial but in part involves lower circulating estrogen levels from weight reduction, earlier age at menopause, and altered hormonal metabolism. Both current and past smoking have a long-lasting influence (Viswanathan, 2005).

ENDOMETRIAL HYPERPLASIA

Most endometrial cancers arise following progression of histologically distinguishable hyperplastic lesions. In fact, endometrial hyperplasia is the only known direct precursor of invasive disease. Endometrial hyperplasia is defined as endometrial thickening with proliferation of irregularly sized and shaped glands and an increased gland-to-stroma ratio (Fig. 33-1) (Ellenson, 2011b). In the absence of such thickening, lesions are best designated as *disorderly proliferative endometrium* or *focal glandular crowding*.

■ Classification

Endometrial hyperplasia represents a continuum of histopathologic findings. The classification system used by the World Health Organization (WHO) and International Society of Gynecological Pathologists designates four different types with varying malignant potential (Table 33-2) (Kurman, 1985, 2014). Hyperplasias are classified as *simple* or *complex,* based on the absence or presence of architectural abnormalities of the endometrial glands. Abnormalities include gland crowding and complexity (see Fig. 33-1). Most importantly, hyperplasias are additionally labeled as *atypical* if they demonstrate nuclear atypia of the endometrial gland cells. Atypical endometrial hyperplasias are clearly associated with the subsequent development of adenocarcinoma. Simple atypical hyperplasia is a relatively uncommon diagnosis. In general, most have a complex architecture.

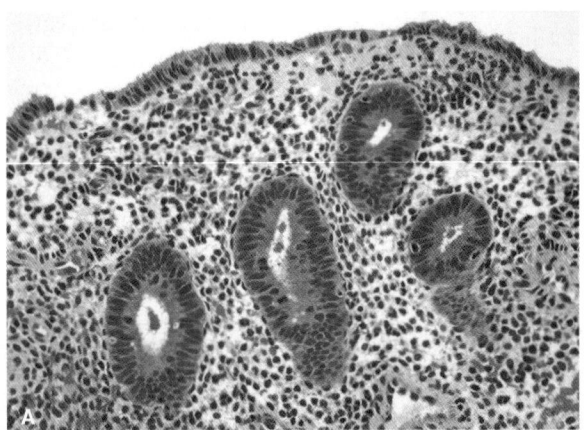

Normal proliferative endometrium

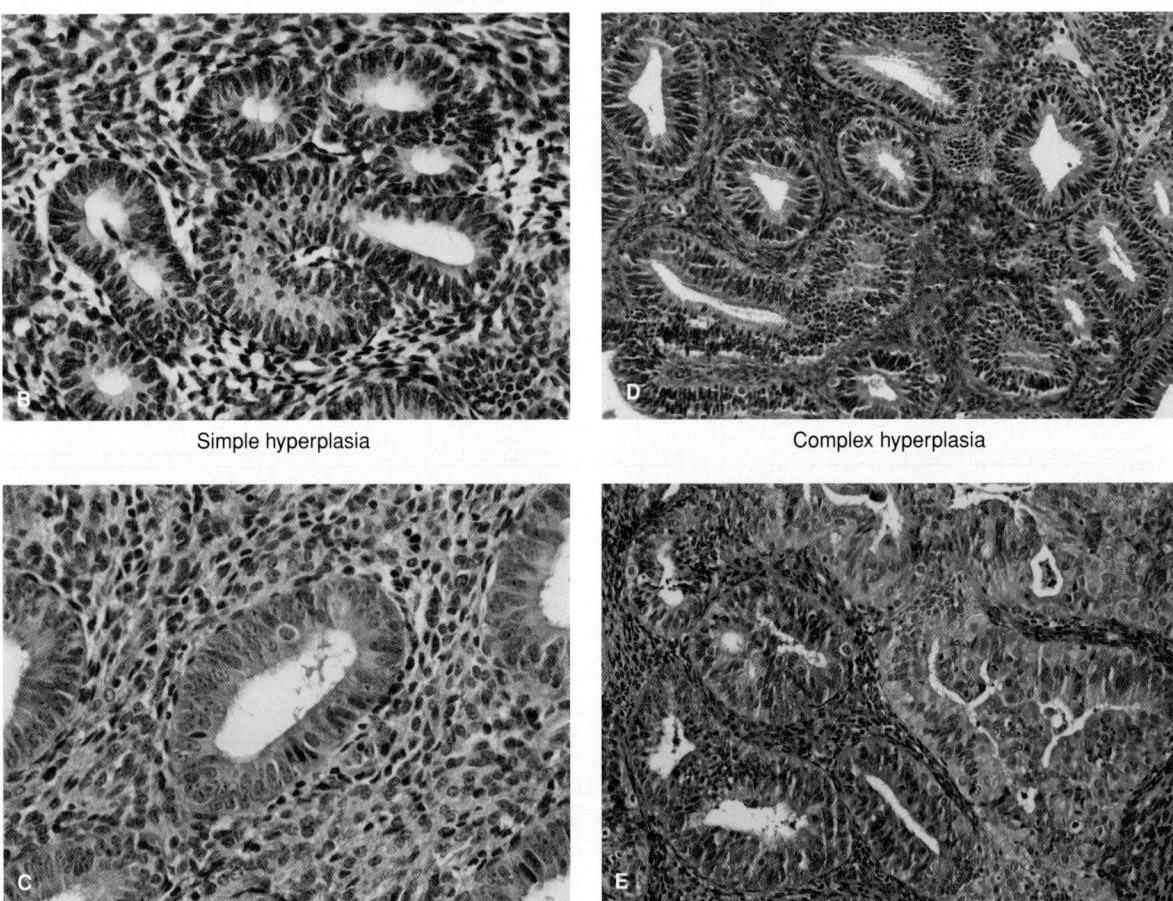

Simple hyperplasia

Complex hyperplasia

Simple hyperplasia with atypia

Complex hyperplasia with atypia

FIGURE 33-1 A. This high-power view of normal proliferative endometrium shows regularly spaced glands composed of stratified columnar epithelium with bland, slightly elongate nuclei. **B.** In simple hyperplasia, glands are modestly crowded and typically display normal tubular shape or mild gland-shape abnormalities. Nuclei are bland. **C.** In this case of simple hyperplasia with atypia, glands are only mildly crowded. Occasional glands show nuclear atypia characterized by nuclear rounding and visible nucleoli. **D.** In complex hyperplasia, glands are more markedly crowded. Some specimens show architectural abnormalities such as papillary infoldings, although the gland profiles in this case are fairly regular. **E.** In complex hyperplasia with atypia, glands are markedly crowded and some have papillary infoldings. Nuclei show variable atypia. (Used with permission from Dr. Kelley Carrick.)

Although endometrial hyperplasias are formally classified in these four different groups, they tend to be morphologically heterogeneous, both within and between individual patients. This histologic diversity explains why only a small number of conserved features are useful as diagnostic criteria. As a result, reproducible scoring of cytologic atypia is often challenging, particularly with a small amount of tissue from a biopsy sample.

Endometrial intraepithelial neoplasia (EIN) is a term introduced to more accurately distinguish the two very different clinical categories of hyperplasia: (1) normal polyclonal endometria diffusely responding to an abnormal hormonal environment and (2) intrinsically proliferative monoclonal lesions that arise focally and confer an elevated risk of adenocarcinoma (Mutter, 2000). This nomenclature emphasizes the malignant potential

TABLE 33-2. World Health Organization Classification of Endometrial Hyperplasia

Types	Progressing to Cancer (%)
Simple hyperplasia	1
Complex hyperplasia	3
Simple atypical hyperplasia	8
Complex atypical hyperplasia	29

Data from Kurman RJ, Kaminski PF, Norris HJ: The behavior of endometrial hyperplasia. A long-term study of "untreated" hyperplasia in 170 patients. Cancer 1985 Jul 15;56(2):403–412.

of endometrial precancers and is in keeping with similar precedents in the cervix (CIN [cervical intraepithelial neoplasia]), vagina (VaIN), and vulva (VIN) (Chap. 29, p. 624).

Using this system, anovulatory or prolonged estrogen-exposed endometria without atypia are generally designated as *endometrial hyperplasias*. In contrast, EIN is used to describe all endometria delineated as premalignant by a combination of three morphometric features. The qualities reflect glandular volume, architectural complexity, and cytologic abnormality. The EIN classification system is a more accurate and reproducible way to predict progression to cancer (Baak, 2005; Hecht, 2005). This classification is endorsed by the Society of Gynecologic Oncology and American College of Obstetricians and Gynecologists (2015) but has not been universally implemented.

■ Clinical Features and Diagnosis

The risks for developing endometrial hyperplasia generally mirror those for invasive carcinoma (Anastasiadis, 2000; Ricci, 2002). Two thirds of women present with postmenopausal bleeding (Horn, 2004). However, premenopausal women with abnormal uterine bleeding (AUB) are also evaluated as described in Chapter 8 (p. 182).

As hyperplasia is a histologic diagnosis, a Pipelle office endometrial biopsy (EMB) or outpatient dilatation and curettage (D & C) are suitable choices for endometrial sampling. The American College of Obstetricians and Gynecologists (2014a) recommends such sample for women older than 45 years with AUB. EMB is also considered for those younger than 45 with chronic excess estrogen exposure (exogenous or endogenous), failed medical management, and persistent AUB.

In those with AUB, transvaginal sonography to measure endometrial thickness is also a feasible method for predicting endometrial hyperplasia (Granberg, 1991; Jacobs, 2011). In postmenopausal women, endometrial stripe thickness measurements ≤4 mm are associated with bleeding that is attributed to endometrial atrophy (American College of Obstetricians and Gynecologists, 2013). Postmenopausal women with a thicker endometrium warrant biopsy. Sonography may also identify abnormal echostructural changes in the endometrium. Cystic endometrial changes suggest polyps, homogeneously thickened endometrium may indicate hyperplasia, and a heterogeneous structural pattern is suspicious for malignancy (Figs. 33-2 and 33-3). However, these sonographic findings show great overlap and cannot be used alone.

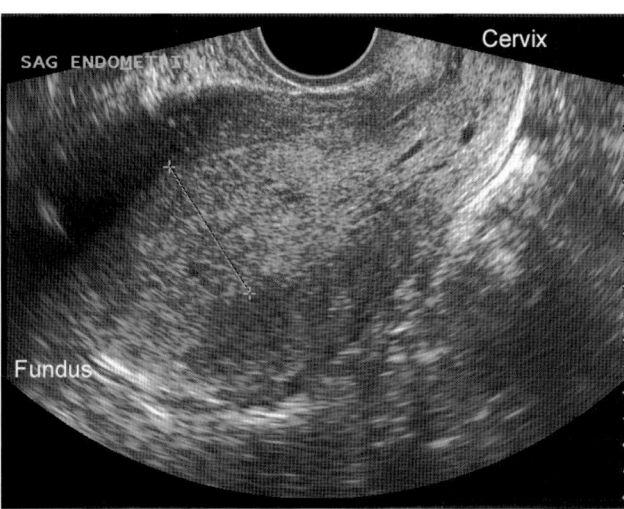

FIGURE 33-2 Transvaginal sonographic image of a uterus. In this sagittal view, the markedly thickened endometrium, which is measured by the calipers, suggests endometrial hyperplasia. (Used with permission from Dr. Elysia Moschos.)

For premenopausal women, transvaginal sonography is often performed to exclude structural sources of abnormal bleeding. Similarly, researchers have attempted to create endometrial thickness guidelines. However, endometrial thicknesses can vary considerably among premenopausal women during normal menstrual cycling. From studies, suggested evidence-based abnormal thresholds range from >4 mm to >16 mm (Breitkopf, 2004; Goldstein, 1997; Shi, 2008). Thus, consensus for an endometrial thickness threshold has not been established for this group. That said, in reproductive-aged women with a thick endometrium combined with other hyperplasia risk factors, EMB may be prudent.

Of other tools, hysteroscopy is more sensitive for focal endometrial lesions. Hyperplastic endometrium is grossly indistinct,

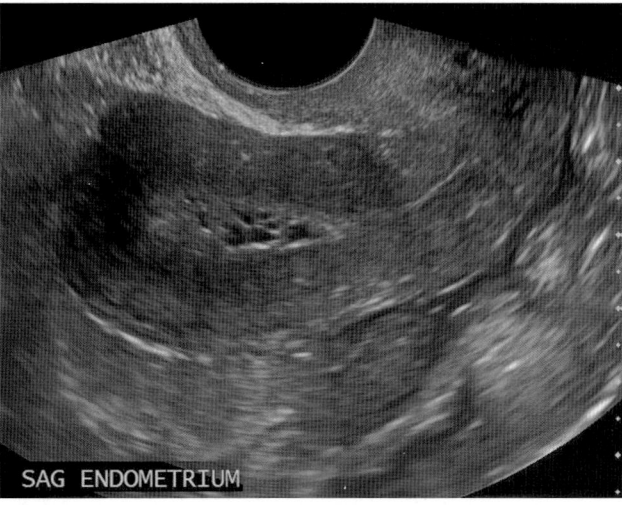

FIGURE 33-3 Transvaginal sagittal image of the endometrium from a 38-year-old woman with chronic oligomenorrhea. The abnormal endometrium is thickened, echogenic, and heterogeneous in echotexture and contains tiny cystic foci. Biopsy revealed grade 1 endometrioid adenocarcinoma, which was confirmed at surgery. (Used with permission from Dr. Elysia Moschos.)

and thus hysteroscopy has poor sensitivity for this diagnosis (Ben Yehuda, 1998; Garuti, 2006).

Occasionally, an adnexal mass may be palpable during examination and in most cases is a benign ovarian cyst. However, any solid features noted during transvaginal sonography raises the possibility of a coexisting ovarian granulosa cell tumor. These tumors produce excess estrogen that results in up to a 30-percent risk of endometrial hyperplasia or less commonly, endometrial carcinoma (Chap. 36, p. 770) (Ayhan, 1994).

■ Treatment

Management of women with endometrial hyperplasia mainly depends on a patient's age, comorbid risks for surgery, desire for fertility, and specific histologic features such as cytologic atypia. Traditional treatment has been surgery. Hormonal therapy is another option and includes oral or injectable progestins or the progestin (levonorgestrel-releasing) IUD.

There is some inconsistency of diagnosis and uncertainty in predicting the stability of individual lesions. Specifically, several studies have documented low reproducibility for WHO classifications of endometrial hyperplasia (Allison, 2008; Sherman, 2008; Zaino, 2006). In addition, there is no way to anticipate which types will involute with progestin therapy. However, as long as an endometrial sample is representative and a provider has no reason to suspect a coexisting invasive carcinoma, the decision to treat endometrial hyperplasia through hormonal or surgical means relies on clinical judgment.

Nonatypical Endometrial Hyperplasia

Premenopausal Women. Nonatypical lesions may spontaneous regress without therapy. However, progestins are generally used to address the underlying etiology, that is, chronic anovulation and excess estrogen (Terakawa, 1997). Premenopausal women with nonatypical endometrial hyperplasia typically require a 3- to 6-month course of low-dose progestin therapy. Cyclic medroxyprogesterone acetate (MPA) (Provera) given orally for 12 to 14 days each month at a dose of 10 to 20 mg daily is commonly used. Continuous daily dosing with MPA 10 mg is suitable and may be more effective than cyclic administration in reversing hyperplastic changes. Another frequently used option is COC pills for those without contraindications. The levonorgestrel-releasing IUD is also effective (Gallos, 2010; Ørbo, 2014; Scarselli, 2011).

In general, follow-up endometrial biopsy is performed to document regression. In those with an IUD, endometrial biopsy can be performed without device removal. After regression, a key point is to continue endometrial protection. Thus, once hyperplastic changes resolve, patients are continued on progestins and observed until menopause. Additional endometrial sampling is required for new bleeding.

Postmenopausal Women. Postmenopausal women with nonatypical endometrial hyperplasia may also be treated with low-dose oral cyclic MPA or a continuous 10-mg daily regimen. However, it is particularly important in older women to be confident that the sample obtained is adequate for excluding cytologic atypia. D & C may be indicated in some circumstances, especially if the tissue from Pipelle sampling is scant or if recurrent bleeding is noted.

In most cases, a form of progestin therapy is used to treat endometrial hyperplasia without atypia. But, affected postmenopausal patients who have a contraindication to progestin therapy or who cannot tolerate the therapy can be expectantly managed. Complex hyperplasia without atypia is usually treated chronically with progestins. With either complex or simple hyperplasia without atypia, office endometrial biopsy is recommended every 3 to 6 months until lesion resolution is achieved.

Response to Progestins. In cases of endometrial hyperplasia without atypia, the risk of progression to endometrial cancer is low (1 to 3 percent). The overall clinical and pathologic regression rates to progestin therapy range from 70 to 80 percent for nonatypical endometrial hyperplasia (Rattanachaiyanont, 2005; Reed, 2009). Patients with persistent disease on repeated biopsy may be switched to a higher-dose regimen such as MPA, 40 to 100 mg orally daily. Also, megestrol acetate (Megace), 160 mg daily or 80 mg twice daily, is suitable. It can be increased even up to 160 mg twice daily if no regression is initially achieved. Again, a clinician must confirm that hormonal ablation has occurred by resampling the endometrium after a suitable therapeutic interval, usually 3 to 6 months. Hysterectomy may also be considered for lesions that are refractory to medical management.

If surgery is selected, a minimally invasive surgery (MIS) approach is considered, and options are laparoscopic, robotic, or vaginal hysterectomy. In cases in which hyperplasia has been proven or is suspected, the uterus is removed in toto and without morcellation, which might disseminate the lesion. Because the lesion may extend into the lower uterine segment or upper endocervix, supracervical hysterectomy is not appropriate for women undergoing hysterectomy for treatment of endometrial hyperplasia.

Atypical Endometrial Hyperplasia

Hysterectomy is the preferred treatment for women with atypical endometrial hyperplasia because the risk of progression to cancer over time approximates 29 percent. There is also a high rate of finding concurrent invasive malignancy coexistent with the atypical hyperplasia (Horn, 2004; Trimble, 2006). In postmenopausal women, a hysterectomy with removal of both tubes and ovaries is recommended.

In premenopausal women who have completed childbearing, hysterectomy is performed for atypical hyperplasia. Risk-reducing salpingectomy is encouraged to potentially lower cancer risk that arises from the fallopian tubes (American College of Obstetricians and Gynecologists, 2015d). For premenopausal women, removal of the ovaries is optional. The deciding factors mirror those for women contemplating BSO for other benign indications and are outlined fully in Section 43-12 (p. 951).

Premenopausal women who strongly wish to preserve fertility can be treated with progestins (Trimble, 2012). High-dose progestin therapy, megestrol acetate 80 mg orally twice daily, is an option for motivated patients who will be compliant with surveillance (Randall, 1997). The IUD that releases 20 μg of intrauterine levonorgestrel daily (Mirena) is also suitable (Ørbo, 2014). Poor surgical candidates may also warrant an attempt at hormonal ablation with progestins. Resolution of the hyperplasia must be confirmed by serial endometrial biopsies every 3 months until response is documented. Otherwise, hysterectomy is recommended. Following hyperplasia resolution, surveillance and progestins continue long-term due to the potential for eventual progression to carcinoma (Rubatt, 2005). Once fertility is complete, hysterectomy is again recommended.

The Gynecologic Oncology Group (GOG) performed a prospective cohort study of 289 patients who had a diagnosis of atypical endometrial hyperplasia. Participants underwent hysterectomy within 3 months of their biopsy, and 43 percent were found to have a concurrent endometrial carcinoma (Trimble, 2006). Suh-Burgmann and associates (2009) found a similarly high number of 48 percent. Results demonstrate the difficulty in attaining an accurate diagnosis before hysterectomy and the potential risks of conservative hormonal treatment.

Generalists in obstetrics and gynecology who perform hysterectomy for atypical endometrial hyperplasia should recognize the possibility of a coexisting invasive malignancy and the possible need for surgical staging. At a minimum, peritoneal washings are obtained prior to performing a hysterectomy. In addition, the uterus should be opened and examined in the operating room. From this, a frozen section analysis can be performed to search for concurrent cancer and determine grade and depth of invasion if found. Any suspicion for myometrial invasion is an appropriate indication for intraoperative consultation with a gynecologic oncologist.

ENDOMETRIAL CANCER

■ Pathogenesis

Endometrial cancer is a biologically and histologically diverse group of neoplasms characterized by a dualistic model of pathogenesis. As noted, type I endometrioid adenocarcinomas comprise most cases. They are estrogen-dependent, low grade, and derived from atypical endometrial hyperplasia. In contrast, type II cancers are serous or clear cell histology, have no precursor lesion, and portend a more aggressive clinical course (Table 33-3). The morphologic and clinical differences are paralleled by genetic distinctions. Namely, type I and II tumors carry mutations of independent sets of genes (Bansal, 2009; Hecht, 2006). The two pathways of endometrial cancer pathogenesis have significant overlap and thus result in a spectrum of histologic features.

TABLE 33-3. Type I and II Endometrial Carcinoma: Distinguishing Features

Feature	Type I	Type II
Chronic estrogen	Present	Absent
Menopause status	Pre-/peri-	Post-
Hyperplasia	Present	Absent
Race	White	Black
Grade	Low	High
Invasion[a]	Minimal	Deep
Behavior	Stable	Aggressive
Subtypes	Endometrioid	Serous
		Clear cell

[a]Myometrial invasion.
Data from Kurman RJ: Blaustein's Pathology of the Female Genital Tract. 4th edition. Berlin: Springer-Verlag; 1994.

■ Prevention

Education can be effective prevention, as many endometrial cancer risks are alterable. Women with PCOS may benefit from weight loss and chronic progestin supplementation (Chap. 17, p. 397). Assessing and managing obesity as described in Chapter 1 may also lower risks.

For women at average risk or increased risk, routine screening of hyperplasia or endometrial cancer is not advocated. Instead, at the onset of menopause, women are counseled on the risks and symptoms of endometrial cancer and strongly encouraged to report unexpected bleeding or spotting to their provider. One screening exception is the woman with Lynch syndrome. For these individuals, EMB is recommended every 1 to 2 years beginning at age 30 to 35 years (American College of Obstetricians and Gynecologists, 2014b; Smith, 2015).

Genetic testing criteria have been published to identify the individual with Lynch syndrome (Table 33-4) (Lancaster, 2015). Lynch syndrome cancers include colon, endometrium, small bowel, renal pelvis and ureter, and ovary, among others (Vasen, 1999). Referral for genetic counseling can further clarify which patients may benefit from specific germline testing (Balmana, 2006; Chen, 2006). Endometrial cancer is the most common "sentinel cancer," thus, obstetrician-gynecologists play a pivotal role in the identification of women with Lynch syndrome (Lu, 2005).

Since women with Lynch syndrome have such a high lifetime risk of developing endometrial cancer (40 to 60 percent),

TABLE 33-4. Lynch Syndrome Genetic Screening Recommendations

Patients with endometrial or colorectal cancer and tumor evidence of:
  Microsatellite instability or
  DNA mismatch repair protein loss

First-degree relative with endometrial or colorectal cancer who was diagnosed:
  Before age 60 years or
  Is at risk for Lynch syndrome based on personal and medical history

First- or second-degree relative with a known DNA mismatch repair gene mutation

Reproduced with permission from Lancaster JM, Powell CB, Chen LM, et al: Society of Gynecologic Oncology statement on risk assessment for inherited gynecologic cancer predispositions, Gynecol Oncol 2015 Jan;136(1):3–7.

prophylactic hysterectomy is recommended once affected women reach the early to mid 40s. In a cohort of 315 HNPCC-mutation carriers, Schmeler and coworkers (2006) confirmed the benefit of this approach by reporting a 100-percent endometrial cancer risk reduction. In general, BSO is also performed due to the 9- to 12-percent lifetime risk of ovarian cancer. Prior to hysterectomy, colon cancer screening with colonoscopy should be up to date (American College of Obstetrician and Gynecologists, 2014b).

■ Diagnosis

Signs and Symptoms

Early diagnosis of endometrial cancer is almost entirely dependent on the prompt recognition and evaluation of irregular vaginal bleeding. In premenopausal women, a clinician must maintain a high index of suspicion for a history of prolonged, heavy menstruation or intermenstrual spotting, because many other benign disorders give rise to similar symptoms (Table 8-1, p. 181). Postmenopausal bleeding is particularly worrisome, leading to a 5- to 10-percent likelihood of diagnosing endometrial carcinoma (Gredmark, 1995; Iatrakis, 1997). Abnormal vaginal discharge may be another symptom in older women.

Unfortunately, some patients do not seek medical attention despite months or years of heavy, irregular bleeding. In more advanced disease, pelvic pressure and pain may reflect uterine enlargement or extrauterine tumor spread. Patients with serous or clear cell tumors often present with signs and symptoms suggestive of advanced epithelial ovarian cancer that include pelvic pain or pressure, bloating, early satiety, and increasing abdominal girth (Chap. 35, p. 741).

Papanicolaou Test

Pap testing is not an indicated test to diagnose endometrial cancer, and 50 percent of women with endometrial cancer will have normal findings (Gu, 2001). Liquid-based cytology appears to increase the detection of glandular abnormalities, but not enough to cause a shift in clinical practice (Guidos, 2000; Schorge, 2002). However, some findings from Pap testing should prompt further investigation. Benign endometrial cells are occasionally recorded on a routine Pap test report in women 45 years or older. In premenopausal women, this is often a finding of limited importance, especially if a test is obtained following menses. However, postmenopausal women with such findings have a 3- to 5-percent risk of endometrial cancer (Simsir, 2005). In those using HRT, the prevalence of benign endometrial cells on smears is increased, and the associated risk of malignancy is less (1 to 2 percent) (Mount, 2002). Although endometrial biopsy is considered in asymptomatic postmenopausal women if this finding is reported, most patients ultimately diagnosed with hyperplasia or cancers also have concomitant abnormal bleeding (Ashfaq, 2001).

In contrast, *atypical* glandular cells found during Pap testing carry higher risks for underlying cervical or endometrial neoplasia. Accordingly, evaluation of a glandular abnormality includes colposcopy and endocervical curettage (ECC). It may

also include endometrial sampling in nonpregnant patients older than 35 years or in those younger if there is a history of abnormal bleeding, if risk factors for endometrial disease are noted, or if the cytology specifies that the atypical glandular cells are of endometrial origin.

Endometrial Sampling

Office Pipelle biopsy is preferred for the initial evaluation of women with bleeding suspicious for malignancy (Feldman, 1993). However, if sampling techniques fail to provide sufficient diagnostic information or if abnormal bleeding persists, D & C may be required to clarify the diagnosis.

The American College of Obstetricians and Gynecologists (2015b) considers hysteroscopy acceptable for AUB evaluation in those without suspected advanced-stage uterine or cervical cancer. However, hysteroscopy is more sensitive for focal endometrial lesions and thus has proved less helpful in diagnosing early endometrial cancer. In those cases in which hysteroscopy is used to evaluate abnormal bleeding and in which cancer is ultimately diagnosed, an increased incidence of positive peritoneal cytology has been noted during subsequent staging surgery (Obermair, 2000; Polyzos, 2010; Zerbe, 2000). Although the risk of peritoneal contamination by cancer cells may be increased by retrograde efflux of hysteroscopic media, patient prognosis overall does not appear to be worsened (Cicinelli, 2010; Revel, 2004).

Laboratory Testing

The only clinically useful tumor marker in the management of endometrial cancer is a serum CA125 level. Preoperatively, an elevated level indicates the possibility of more advanced disease (Powell, 2005). In practice, it is most useful in patients with advanced disease or serous subtypes to assist in monitoring response to therapy or during posttreatment surveillance. However, even in this setting, its utility in the absence of other clinical findings is limited (Price, 1998).

Imaging Studies

In general, for women with a well-differentiated type I endometrioid tumor, chest radiography is the only required preoperative imaging study. All other preoperative testing is directed toward general surgical preparation (Chap. 39, p. 825).

Computed tomography (CT) or magnetic resonance (MR) imaging is usually not necessary (American College of Obstetricians and Gynecologists, 2015c). However, CT scanning can be obtained preoperatively in cases with higher-grade lesions to assess for lymph node involvement or metastatic disease. MR imaging can occasionally help distinguish an endometrial cancer with cervical extension from a primary endocervical adenocarcinoma (Nagar, 2006). Moreover, women with serous features or other high-risk histology on preoperative biopsy and those with physical examination findings suggesting advanced disease are most appropriate for abdominopelvic CT scanning (Fig. 33-4). In these cases, advance knowledge of intraabdominal disease may help guide surgery and treatment. MR imaging is also recommended for women who are considering fertility-sparing management

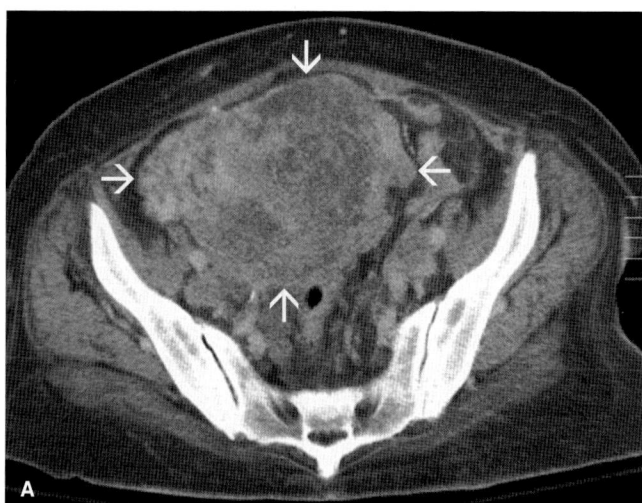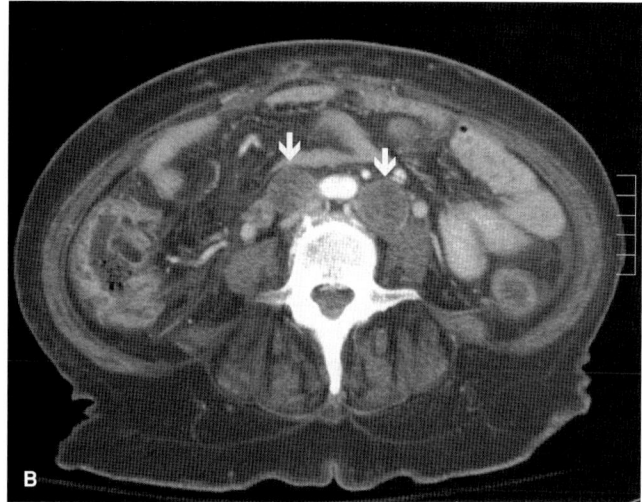

FIGURE 33-4 Computed tomographic (CT) images in the axial plane of a 61-year-old woman with endometrial cancer. **A.** Massively enlarged and inhomogeneous uterus (*arrows*) in the upper pelvis. **B.** At the level of the aortic bifurcation, enlarged lymph nodes are seen bilaterally (*arrows*), consistent with lymph node involvement. (Used with permission from Dr. Diane Twickler.)

with hormonal therapy, since it may not be an option if deep invasion is found.

Role of the Generalist

Although most endometrial cancers are cured by hysterectomy and BSO, primary management by gynecologic oncologists has advantages. It is an efficient use of health care resources, minimizes potential morbidity, is more likely to lead to staging, and improves the survival of patients with high-risk disease (Chan, 2011; Roland, 2004). Therefore, preoperative consultation is generally advisable for any patient with endometrial cancer who is being prepared for surgery by a generalist in obstetrics and gynecology. Postoperatively, a gynecologic oncologist should be consulted if cervical extension, extrauterine disease, or positive peritoneal washing cytology was found during surgery.

If treated by an oncologist, early-stage patients treated by surgery alone will return in many cases to their primary obstetrician-gynecologist for surveillance. Consultation is again recommended if recurrent disease is later suspected or identified.

When an endometrial cancer is unexpectedly diagnosed after hysterectomy performed by a generalist for other indications, consultation is also recommended. Possible therapeutic options include no further therapy and surveillance only, reoperation to complete surgical staging, or radiotherapy to prevent local recurrence. In general, the survival advantages of staging must be weighed against the complications from another surgical procedure (American College of Obstetricians and Gynecologists, 2015c). Fortunately, the advent of laparoscopic and robotic delayed staging offers the potential for less morbidity (Spirtos, 2005).

Pathology

The spectrum of aggressiveness within the histopathologic types of endometrial cancer is broad (Table 33-5). Most patients have endometrioid adenocarcinomas that behave indolently. However, some will have an unfavorable histology that portends

a much more aggressive tumor. In addition, the degree of tumor differentiation is an important predictor of disease spread.

Histologic Grade

The most widely used grading system for endometrial carcinoma is the three-tiered International Federation of Gynecology and Obstetrics (FIGO) system (Table 33-6). Grade 1 lesions typically are indolent with little propensity to spread outside the uterus or recur. Grade 2 tumors have an intermediate prognosis. Grade 3 cancers pose an increased potential for myometrial invasion and nodal metastasis.

Histologic grading is primarily determined by the tumor's architectural growth pattern (Zaino, 1994). However, there are a few exceptions, and the optimal method for determining grade is somewhat controversial. Nuclear atypia that is inappropriately advanced relative to the architectural grade raises a grade 1 or 2 tumor by one level. For example, a grade 2 lesion based on architectural features may be increased to a grade 3 lesion if significant nuclear atypia is present (Zaino, 1995). Nuclear grading based on the FIGO system is also used for all serous and clear cell adenocarcinomas (Pecorelli, 1999).

TABLE 33-5. Classification of Endometrial Carcinoma
Endometrioid adenocarcinoma
Squamous differentiation
Villoglandular
Secretory
Mucinous carcinoma
Serous carcinoma
Clear cell carcinoma
Mixed cell carcinoma
Neuroendocrine tumor
Undifferentiated carcinoma
Squamous cell carcinoma
Others

TABLE 33-6. Histopathologic Criteria for Assessing Grade

Grade	Definition
1	≤5% of a nonsquamous or nonmorular solid growth pattern
2	6–50% of a nonsquamous or nonmorular solid growth pattern
3	>50% of a nonsquamous or nonmorular solid growth pattern

Data from Pecorelli S, Benedet JL, Creasman WT, et al: FIGO staging of gynecologic cancer. 1994–1997 FIGO Committee on Gynecologic Oncology. Int J Gynaecol Obstet 1999 Jan;64(1):5–10.

Histologic Type

Endometrioid Adenocarcinoma. This is the most common histologic type of endometrial cancer and accounts for more than 75 percent of cases. This type I tumor characteristically contains glands that resemble those of the normal endometrium (Fig. 33-5). The concomitant presence of hyperplastic endometrium correlates with a low-grade tumor and a lack of myometrial invasion. However, when the glandular component decreases and is replaced by solid nests and sheets of cells, the tumor is classified as a higher grade (Kurman, 2014). In addition, an atrophic endometrium is more frequently associated with high-grade lesions that have a greater potential to metastasize (Kurman, 1994).

Endometrioid adenocarcinomas may also display variant forms. These include endometrioid adenocarcinoma with squamous differentiation or with villoglandular or secretory types

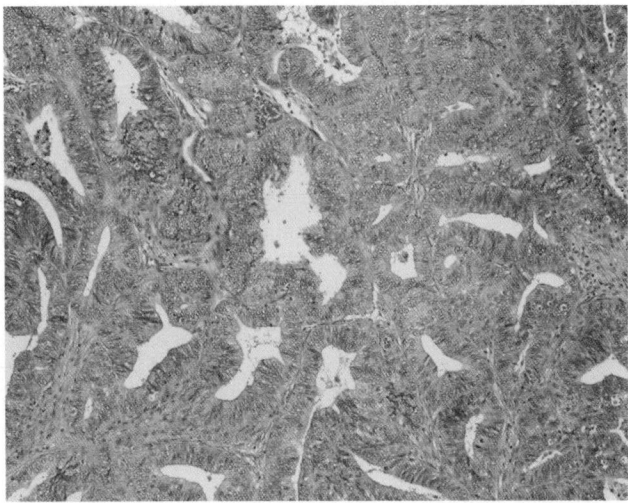

FIGURE 33-5 Endometrioid adenocarcinomas are composed of neoplastic glands resembling those of the normal endometrium. Cells are typically tall columnar with mild to moderate nuclear atypia. They form glands that are abnormally crowded or "back-to-back." Gland cribriforming, confluence, and villous structures are also common. It is these architectural forms, with the associated disappearance of intervening stroma, that distinguish well-differentiated endometrioid adenocarcinoma from complex hyperplasia. (Used with permission from Dr. Kelley Carrick.)

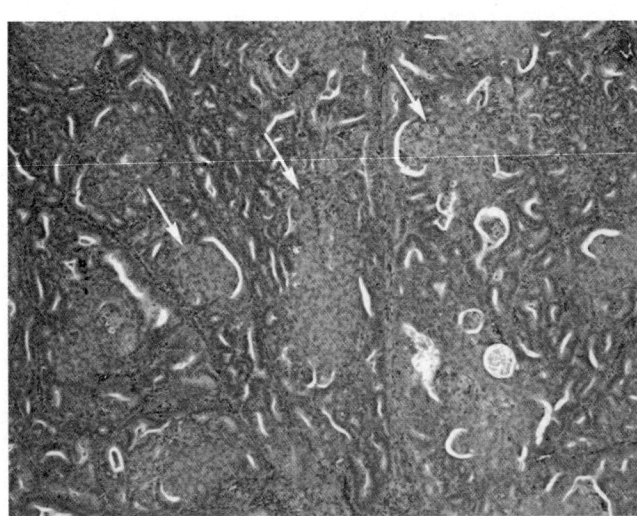

FIGURE 33-6 Endometrioid adenocarcinomas may show foci of squamous differentiation, which may be focal or relatively prominent. The squamous elements can have obvious squamous features such as keratinization or intercellular bridges or may be represented by less well-differentiated squamous morules (*white arrows*), as in this example. (Used with permission from Dr. Raheela Ashfaq.)

(Fig. 33-6). In general, the biologic behavior of these variant tumors reflects that of classic endometrioid adenocarcinoma.

Serous Carcinoma. Accounting for 5 to 10 percent of endometrial cancers, serous carcinoma typifies the highly aggressive type II tumors that arise from the atrophic endometrium of older women (Jordan, 2001). There is typically a complex pattern of papillary growth, and cells demonstrate marked nuclear atypia (Fig. 33-7). Commonly referred to as uterine papillary serous carcinoma (UPSC), its histologic appearance resembles epithelial ovarian cancer, and psammoma bodies are seen in 30 percent of cases (Kurman, 2014).

Grossly, the tumor is exophytic with a papillary appearance emerging from a small, atrophic uterus. These tumors may occasionally be confined within a polyp and have no evidence for spread (Carcangiu, 1992). However, UPSC has a known propensity for myometrial and lymphatic invasion. Intraperitoneal spread, such as omental caking, which is unusual for typical endometrioid adenocarcinoma, is also common even when myometrial invasion is minimal or absent (Fig. 33-8) (Sherman, 1992). As a result, it may be impossible to distinguish UPSC from epithelial ovarian cancer during surgery. Like ovarian carcinoma, these tumors usually secrete CA125. Thus, serial serum measurements can be useful marker to monitor disease postoperatively. UPSC is an aggressive cell type, and women with mixed endometrial cancers containing as little as 25 percent of UPSC have the same survival as those with pure uterine serous carcinoma (Ellenson, 2011a).

Clear Cell Carcinoma. Fewer than 5 percent of endometrial cancers are clear cell variants, but this is the other major type II tumor (Abeler, 1991). The microscopic appearance may be predominantly solid, cystic, tubular, or papillary. Most frequently, it consists of a mixture of two or more of these patterns (Fig. 33-9).

Endometrial clear cell adenocarcinomas are similar to those arising in the ovary, vagina, and cervix. Grossly, there are no characteristic features, but like UPSC, they tend to

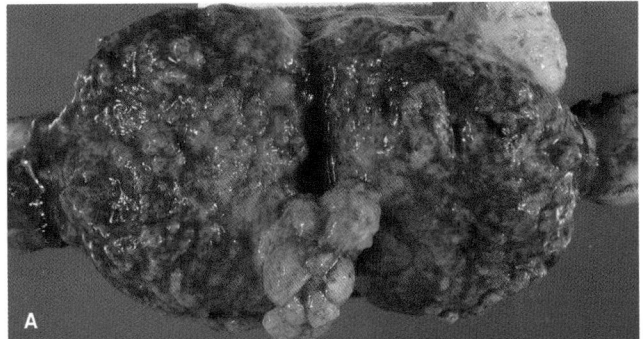

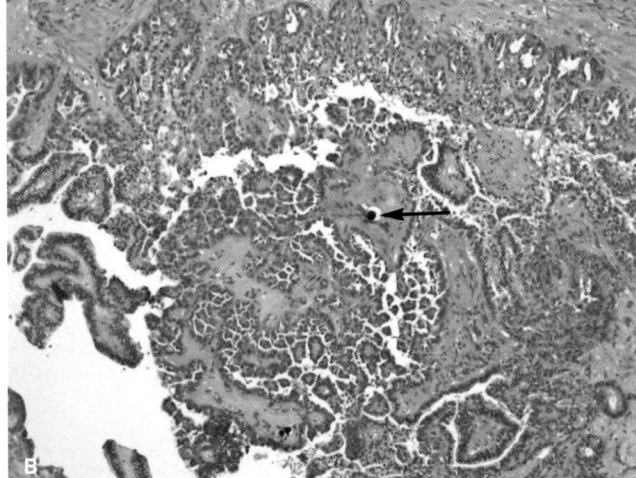

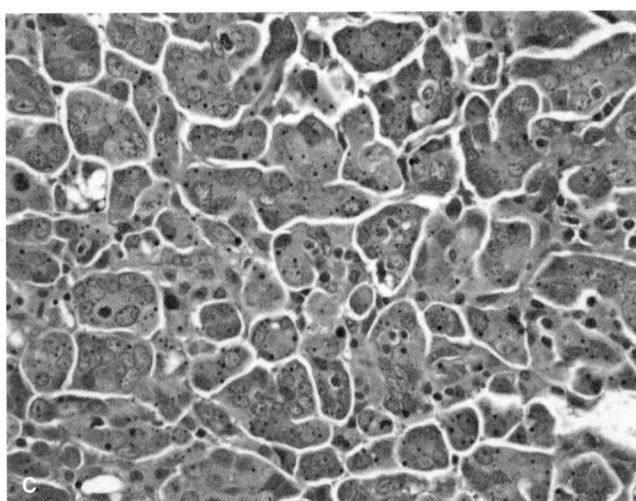

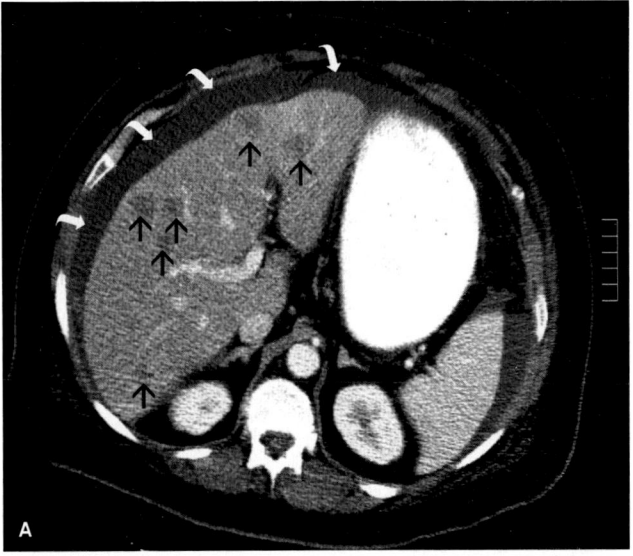

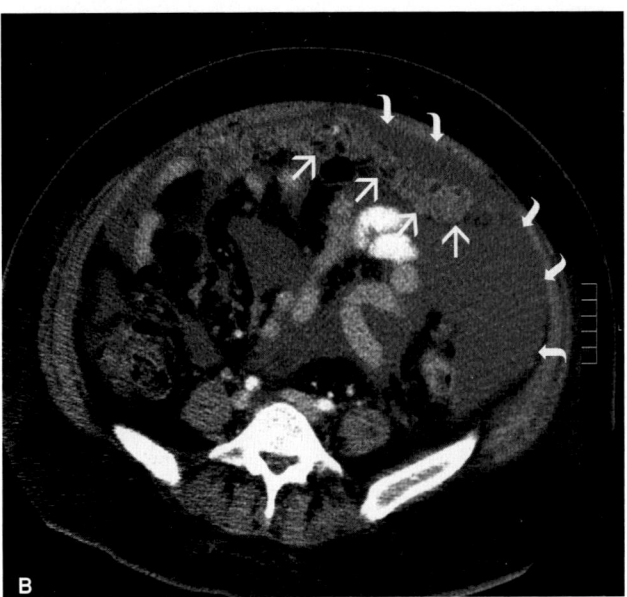

FIGURE 33-8 Computed-tomographic (CT) images of liver metastases, ascites, and omental caking in a 51-year-old woman with endometrial cancer. **A.** *Black arrows* demarcate multiple low-density areas in the liver that are consistent with metastases, and ascites (*curved, white arrows*) surrounding the liver. **B.** A more caudal image reveals omental caking (*white arrows*), surrounded by massive ascites (*curved, white arrows*).

FIGURE 33-7 Uterine papillary serous carcinoma. **A.** Uterine specimen. (Used with permission from Dr. Raheela Ashfaq.) **B.** This tumor is typically characterized by a papillary architecture. Psammoma bodies, which are concentrically laminated calcifications (*arrow*), may be present. **C.** Cells are typically rounded as opposed to columnar. They have high-grade nuclear features including relatively large, pleomorphic nuclei; prominent nucleoli; and frequent, abnormal mitoses. Multinucleate tumor cells are also common. (Used with permission from Dr. Kelley Carrick.)

be high-grade, deeply invasive tumors. Patients are often diagnosed with advanced disease and have a poor prognosis (Hamilton, 2006).

Mucinous Carcinoma. One to 2 percent of endometrial cancers have a mucinous appearance that forms more than half of the tumor. However, many endometrioid adenocarcinomas will have this as a focal component (Ross, 1983). Typically, mucinous tumors have a glandular pattern with uniform columnar cells and minimal stratification (Fig. 33-10). Almost all are stage I grade 1 lesions and carry a good prognosis (Melhem, 1987). Since endocervical epithelium merges with the lower uterine segment, the main diagnostic dilemma is

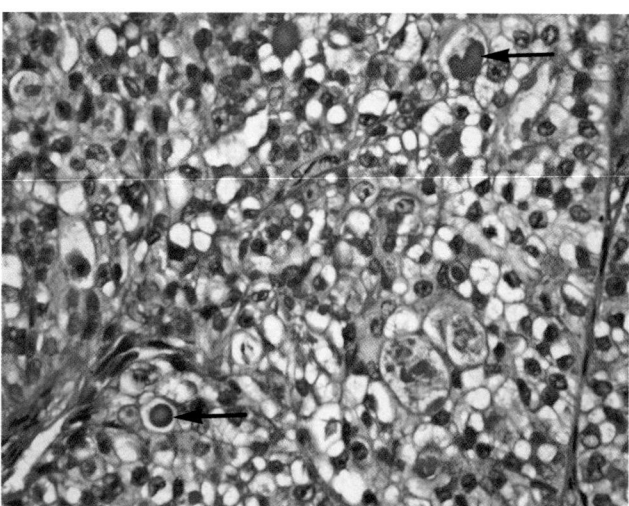

FIGURE 33-9 Clear cell adenocarcinomas are composed of cells with clear to eosinophilic granular cytoplasm. Cells are arranged in papillae, sheets, tubulocystic structures, or most often, some combination of these. Eosinophilic hyaline globules (*arrows*) are a common feature. In this example, nuclei are moderately pleomorphic, with nucleolar prominence. (Used with permission from Dr. Kelley Carrick.)

differentiating this tumor from a primary cervical adenocarcinoma. Immunostaining may be helpful, and MR imaging may further clarify the most likely site of origin. In general, to define anatomy, MR imaging is preferable to CT scanning as MR offers superior contrast resolution at soft-tissue interfaces.

Mixed Carcinoma, Undifferentiated Carcinoma, and Rare Types. An endometrial cancer may demonstrate combinations of two or more pure types. To be classified as a mixed carcinoma, a component must make up at least 10 percent of the tumor. Except for serous and clear cell histology, the combination of other types usually has no clinical significance. As a result, mixed carcinoma usually refers to an admixture of a type I (endometrioid adenocarcinoma and its variants) and a type II carcinoma (Kurman, 2014).

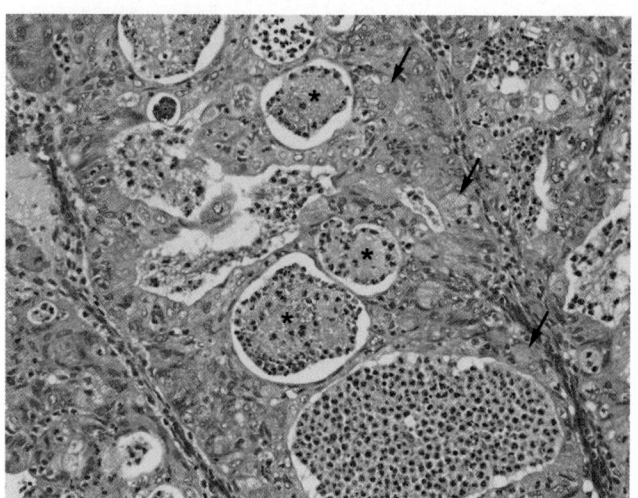

FIGURE 33-10 Mucinous adenocarcinoma of the endometrium has tumor cells containing intracytoplasmic mucin (*arrows*). Tumor cells form sheets and cribriform structures (*asterisks*), which in this example contain bluish mucin and numerous neutrophils. (Used with permission from Dr. Kelley Carrick.)

Undifferentiated carcinoma lacks architectural differentiation and is characterized by medium-sized, monotonous epithelial cells growing in solid sheets without a pattern (Silva, 2007). These represent 1 to 2 percent of endometrial cancers. Overall, the prognosis is worse than in patients with poorly differentiated endometrioid adenocarcinomas (Altrabulsi, 2005).

Of rare histologic types, fewer than 100 cases of *squamous cell carcinoma* of the endometrium have been reported. Diagnosis requires exclusion of an adenocarcinoma component and no connection with the squamous epithelium of the cervix (Varras, 2002). Typically, the prognosis is poor (Goodman, 1996). *Transitional cell carcinoma* of the endometrium is also rare, and metastatic disease from the bladder or ovary must be excluded during diagnosis (Ahluwalia, 2006).

Patterns of Spread

Endometrial cancers have several different potential ways to spread beyond the uterus (Morrow, 1991). Type I endometrioid tumors and their variants most commonly spread, in order of frequency, by: (1) direct extension, (2) lymphatic metastasis, (3) hematogenous dissemination, and (4) intraperitoneal exfoliation. Type II serous and clear cell carcinomas have a particular propensity for extrauterine disease, in a pattern that closely resembles epithelial ovarian cancer. In general, the various patterns of spread are interrelated and often develop simultaneously.

Invasion of the endometrial stroma and exophytic expansion within the uterine cavity follows initial growth of an early cancer. Over time, the tumor invades the myometrium and may ultimately perforate the serosa (Table 33-7). Tumors situated in the lower uterine segment tend to involve the cervix early, whereas those in the upper corpus tend to extend to the fallopian tubes or serosa. Advanced regional growth may lead to direct invasion into adjacent pelvic structures, including the bladder, large bowel, vagina, and broad ligament.

Lymphatic channel invasion and metastasis to the pelvic and paraaortic nodal chains can follow tumor penetration of the myometrium (Table 33-8). The lymphatic network draining the uterus is complex, and patients can have metastases to any single nodal group or combination of groups (Burke, 1996). This haphazard pattern is in contrast to cervical cancer, in which lymphatic spread usually follows

TABLE 33-7. Correlation of Histologic Grade and Depth of Myometrial Invasion in Stage I Patients (n = 5,095)

Myometrial Invasion	Grade		
	1	2	3
None	29%	11%	15%
≤50%	51%	59%	46%
>50%	20%	30%	39%

Data from Creasman WT, Odicino F, Maisonneuve P, et al: Carcinoma of the corpus uteri. FIGO 26th Annual Report on the Results of Treatment in Gynecological Cancer, Int J Gynaecol Obstet. 2006 Nov;95 Suppl 1:S105–S143.

TABLE 33-8. Correlation of Histologic Grade and Depth of Myometrial Invasion with Risk of Nodal Metastases

Myometrial Invasion	Pelvic Lymph Nodes			Paraaortic Lymph Nodes		
	G1	G2	G3	G1	G2	G3
None	1%	7%	16%	<1%	2%	5%
≤50%	2%	6%	10%	<1%	2%	4%
>50%	11%	21%	37%	2%	6%	13%

G = histologic grade.
Data from Creasman WT, Odicino F, Maisonneuve P, et al: Carcinoma of the corpus uteri. FIGO 26th Annual Report on the Results of Treatment in Gynecological Cancer, Int J Gynaecol Obstet. 2006 Nov;95 Suppl 1:S105–S143.

a stepwise progression from pelvic to paraaortic to scalene nodal groups.

Hematogenous dissemination most commonly results in metastases to the lung and less commonly to the liver, brain, bone, and other sites. Deep myometrial invasion is the strongest predictor of this pattern of spread (Mariani, 2001a).

Retrograde transtubal transport of exfoliated endometrial cancer cells carries malignant cells to the peritoneal cavity. Serosal perforation of the tumor is another possible pathway. Most types of endometrial cancer cells found in the peritoneal cavity disappear within a short time and have low malignant potential (Hirai, 2001). Alternatively, in the presence of other high-risk features, such as adnexal metastases or serous histology, widespread intraabdominal disease may result.

Port-site metastasis is a rare but possible method of cancer spread. Martínez and coworkers (2010) evaluated nearly 300 laparoscopic staging procedures for endometrial cancer. Port-site metastases complicated 0.33 percent of cases. Similarly, cancer dissemination following specimen morcellation has been reported (Graebe, 2015).

■ Treatment

Surgical Management

Patients with endometrial cancer should undergo hysterectomy, BSO, and surgical staging (including pelvic washings and lymphadenectomy) using the revised FIGO system (Table 33-9 and Fig. 33-11) (Mutch, 2009). For optimal patient management, the histopathologic description of the preoperative biopsy findings is carefully reviewed. Almost three quarters of patients are stage I at diagnosis (Table 33-10). Only a few circumstances contraindicate primary surgery and include a desire to preserve fertility, massive obesity, high operative risk, and clinically unresectable disease. In general, an extrafascial hysterectomy, also known as type I or simple hysterectomy, is sufficient. However, radical hysterectomy (type III hysterectomy) may be preferable for patients with clinically obvious cervical extension of endometrial cancer (Cornelison, 1999; Mariani, 2001b). Differences in these hysterectomy types are outlined in Table 30-7 (p. 669). Vaginal hysterectomy with or without BSO is another option for women who cannot undergo systematic surgical staging

TABLE 33-9. International Federation of Gynecology and Obstetrics (FIGO) Surgical Staging System for Endometrial Cancer

Stage[a]	Characteristics
I	**Tumor confined to the corpus uteri**
IA	No or less than half myometrial invasion
IB	Invasion equal to or more than half of the myometrium
II	**Tumor invades cervical stroma, but does not extend beyond the uterus[b]**
III	**Local and/or regional spread of the tumor**
IIIA	Tumor invades the serosa of the corpus uteri and/or adnexae[c]
IIIB	Vaginal and/or parametrial involvement[c]
IIIC	Metastases to pelvic and/or paraaortic lymph nodes[c]
IIIC1	Positive pelvic nodes
IIIC2	Positive paraaortic lymph nodes with or without positive pelvic lymph nodes
IV	**Tumor invades bladder and/or bowel mucosa, and/or distant metastases**
IVA	Tumor invasion of bladder and/or bowel mucosa
IVB	Distant metastases, including intraabdominal metastases and/or inguinal lymph nodes

[a]Either G1, G2, or G3. G = histologic grade.
[b]Endocervical glandular involvement only should be considered as stage I and no longer as stage II.
[c]Positive cytology has to be reported separately without changing the stage.
Reproduced with permission from Pecorelli S: Revised FIGO staging for carcinoma of the vulva, cervix, and endometrium, Int J Gynaecol Obstet. 2009 May;105(2):103–104.

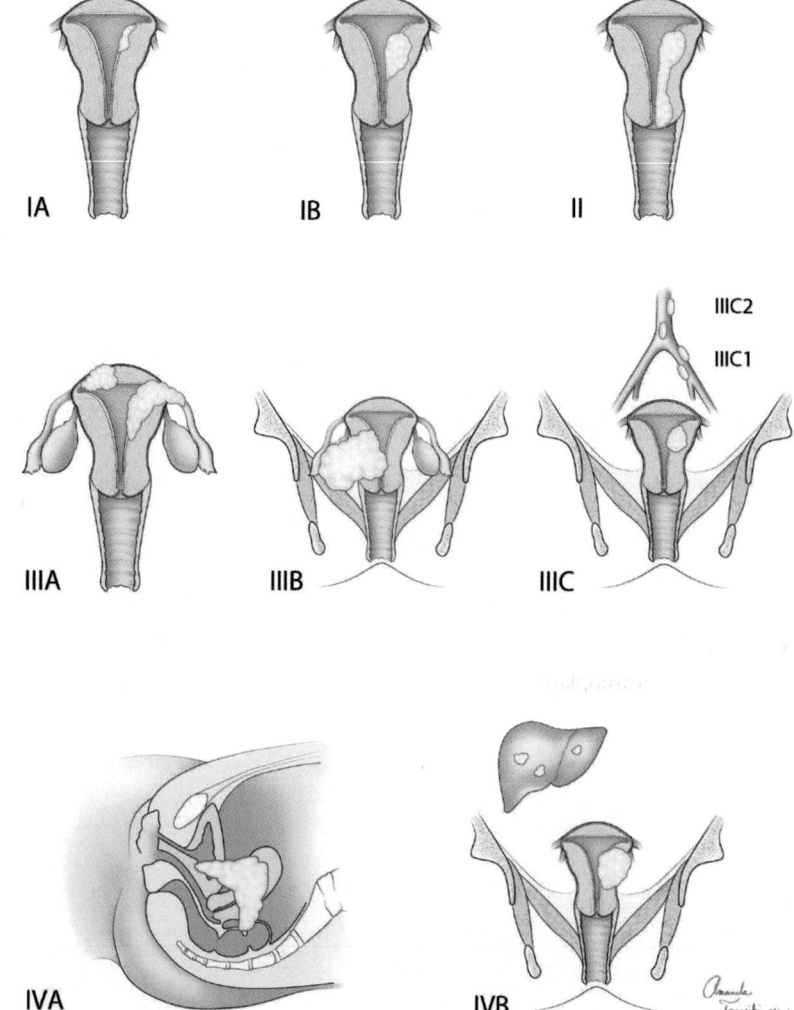

FIGURE 33-11 International Federation of Gynecology and Obstetrics (FIGO) staging of endometrial cancer.

due to comorbidities (American College of Obstetricians and Gynecologists, 2015c). Previously, laparotomy had been the standard approach. However, laparoscopic and robotic surgical staging are increasingly used for endometrial cancer that appears clinically confined to the uterus. Such MIS staging is safe, feasible, and now recommended (Walker, 2009).

Regardless of approach, upon entering the peritoneal cavity, washings are obtained by pouring 50 to 100 mL of sterile

TABLE 33-10. Distribution of Endometrial Cancer by FIGO Stage (n = 5281 patients)

FIGO stage	%
I	73
II	11
III	13
IV	3

Data from Creasman WT, Odicino F, Maisonneuve P, et al: Carcinoma of the corpus uteri. FIGO 26th Annual Report on the Results of Treatment in Gynecological Cancer, Int J Gynaecol Obstet. 2006 Nov;95 Suppl 1:S105–S143.

saline into the pelvis and collecting it for cytologic assessment. Retrieval of ascitic fluid is an acceptable alternative, but ascites is infrequently encountered. Next, a thorough intraabdominal and pelvic exploration is performed, and suspicious lesions are biopsied or excised. These preliminary procedures are followed by hysterectomy and BSO. The uterus is opened away from the operating table, and the depth of myometrial penetration may be determined by intraoperative gross examination or microscopic frozen section analysis (Sanjuan, 2006; Vorgias, 2002).

As noted, the risk of lymph node metastasis correlates with the tumor grade and depth of invasion into the myometrium. Historically, the combination of preoperative biopsy grade and intraoperative assessment of the depth of myometrial invasion were the two factors that surgeons used to determine whether to proceed with pelvic and paraaortic lymph node dissection. The inaccuracy of this approach has been reported (Eltabbakh, 2005; Leitao, 2008; Papadia, 2009). In addition, the depth of myometrial invasion determined in the operative room is often inaccurate (Frumovitz, 2004a,b).

Following hysterectomy and BSO, concurrent lymphadenectomy allows detection of positive nodes to guide appropriate treatment. Some retrospective studies have shown improved survival rates in patients who had undergone an adequate lymph node dissection (Kilgore, 1995; Todo, 2010). However, the advantage appears to be confined to those in high-risk groups. Thus, although still with some controversy, complete surgical staging with pelvic and paraaortic lymphadenectomy is recommended for patients with high-risk grade 1 endometrioid cancer and any case of grade 2, grade 3 or type II cancers. Lymph nodal staging for cases of low-risk grade 1 endometrioid cancer also is debated (Miller, 2006). Authors in two randomized trials reported no improvement in disease-free or overall survival rates after lymphadenectomy in patients with early-stage disease (Benedetti Panici, 2008; Kitchener, 2009). However, these trials were criticized because lymph node counts were low and lymph node status did not dictate treatment, as many patients received postoperative radiation regardless of their lymph node status. Moreover, concern exists that omitting lymphadenectomy may lead to missed metastatic disease and subsequent insufficient postoperative treatment. In addition, microscopic nodal disease may be unknowingly resected during lymphadenectomy and prevent future relapse.

Distinct from the above discussion, any suspicious pelvic or paraaortic lymph nodes should be removed and histologically evaluated. Excision of grossly involved lymph nodes leads to a survival advantage (Havrilesky, 2005).

Those patients with serous or clear cell features on preoperative biopsy should have extended surgical staging with an infracolic omentectomy and bilateral peritoneal biopsies of the pelvis, pericolic gutter, and diaphragm (Bristow, 2001a). As in ovarian cancer, a surgeon is also prepared to resect any metastases (Bristow, 2000).

Sentinel lymph node evaluation, as done in vulvar and breast cancers, is being investigated and may become a useful technique in endometrial cancer (Abu-Rustum, 2009). The practice does vary but usually involves injecting the ectocervix prior to surgery at the 3, 6, 9 and 12 o'clock positions with technetium sulfur colloid. Subsequent lymphoscintigraphy guides one to the sentinel lymph nodes. At the time of surgery, the cervix is also injected with lymphazurin or isosulfan blue at the 3 and 9 o'clock position. The radioactive and blue nodes are then identified (Frati, 2015). Although investigational, sentinel lymph node evaluation is appealing in that it reduces the potential side effects associated with complete lymphadenectomy, including lymphedema and lymphocyst formation, longer operating times, and increased blood loss. The sensitivity of sentinel lymph node mapping appears acceptable in small series, and a prospective study is being considered by the GOG.

As noted, an MIS approach is acceptable for suitable candidates undergoing hysterectomy and staging for endometrial cancer (Childers, 1994; Spirtos, 2005). The GOG LAP2 study was the first multicenter randomized trial of laparoscopy to address this. In the trial, conventional surgery including pelvic/paraaortic lymphadenectomy was compared with the same steps completed laparoscopically for clinical stage I and IIA endometrial carcinoma. Investigators found laparoscopic staging to be feasible and safe (Walker, 2009). Laparoscopy was completed without conversion in 74 percent of patients randomized to MIS. Advantageously, compared with those undergoing laparotomy, patients undergoing laparoscopy had similar rates of intraoperative injuries (9 versus 8 percent), fewer moderate to severe complications (14 versus 21 percent), shorter hospital stays (median 3 versus 4 days), and better quality of life at 6 weeks postoperatively. However, laparoscopic staging was linked with longer operative times (Kornblith, 2009; Walker, 2009). Long-term treatment success is not compromised with laparoscopic staging, and overall survival and recurrence rates in early reports are similar to those for a traditional abdominal approach (Ghezzi, 2010; Magrina, 1999; Walker, 2012; Zullo, 2009).

Robot-assisted laparoscopic staging of endometrial cancer has been embraced by many gynecologic oncologists to overcome MIS technical challenges, especially in obese patients. Early evidence shows it to be feasible and safe (Hoekstra, 2009). Compared with a laparoscopic approach for endometrial cancer staging, both major complication rates and mean number of lymph nodes removed are similar. The robotic approach results in less blood loss (Cardenas-Goicoechea, 2010; Seamon, 2009).

As described in Chapter 41 (p. 874), not all women are candidates for MIS. Limiting factors can include extensive adhesive disease, a large bulky uterus, morbid obesity, cardiopulmonary disease, and other patient comorbidities. Importantly, morcellation is avoided in cancer cases to prevent disease spread.

Surveillance

Most surgically treated patients can simply be followed by pelvic examination every 3 to 6 months for the first 2 years and then every 6 to 12 months thereafter (National Comprehensive Cancer Network, 2015). Pap testing is not a mandatory part of surveillance, as an asymptomatic vaginal recurrence is identified in less than 1 percent of patients (Bristow, 2006a; Cooper, 2006).

Women who have more advanced cancer that requires postoperative radiation or chemotherapy or both warrant more aggressive monitoring. Serum CA125 measurements may be valuable, particularly for UPSC, if the level was elevated prior to treatment. Intermittent imaging using CT scanning or MR imaging may also be indicated. In general, the pattern of recurrent disease depends on the original sites of metastasis and the treatment received.

Chemotherapy

Only three cytotoxic drugs with definite activity for endometrial cancer have been identified. Paclitaxel (Taxol), doxorubicin (Adriamycin), and cisplatin (Platinol) form TAP chemotherapy, which is one of the adjuvant treatment options for advanced endometrial cancer following surgery. In one GOG trial of 273 women (protocol #177), administration of seven courses of TAP was superior to doxorubicin plus cisplatin, but toxicity was increased—particularly peripheral neuropathy (Fleming, 2004). A less toxic alternative to TAP chemotherapy is paclitaxel plus carboplatin. Routinely used for ovarian cancer, this regimen is effective in advanced-stage endometrial cancer (Hoskins, 2001; Sovak, 2006, 2007). One GOG trial (protocol #209) compared TAP and the regimen of carboplatin plus paclitaxel. Results demonstrated that carboplatin plus paclitaxel was not inferior to TAP in terms of progression-free and overall survival rates. The toxicity profile favored carboplatin plus paclitaxel, and this regimen is generally used at our institution (Miller, 2012).

In practice, cytotoxic chemotherapy is frequently combined, sequenced, or sandwiched with radiotherapy in patients with advanced endometrial cancer following surgery. To reduce toxicity, directed pelvic or paraaortic radiation is usually employed rather than whole abdominal irradiation (Homesley, 2009; Miller, 2009).

Targeted Therapy

In some cases, current therapies fail to provide long-term disease control, and thus novel treatments are being investigated for endometrial cancer. Bevacizumab (Avastin), a vascular endothelial growth factor (VEGF) inhibitor, blocks angiogenesis. In a phase II trial for recurrent/persistent endometrial cancer, this targeted agent showed some salutary action, but further study is needed (Aghajanian, 2011). Another pathway, the fibroblast growth factor receptor pathway, is a potential target (Lee, 2014). The mTOR pathway is an additional target, as mutations in this pathway may lead to endometrial cancer. The GOG (protocol #0286B) is currently studying metformin with chemotherapy for the treatment of advanced/recurrent endometrial cancer. Early data show that metformin inhibits cell proliferation in endometrial cancer cell lines and that this effect is partially mediated through mTOR pathway inhibition. In addition, treatment with metformin in combination with paclitaxel resulted in a synergistic antiproliferative effect in these cell lines.

Radiation

Primary Radiation Therapy. This option rather than surgery is selected rarely and mainly for exceptionally poor surgical candidates. Intracavitary brachytherapy such as Heyman capsules with or without external beam pelvic radiation is the typical method (Chap. 28, p. 616). In general, the survival rate is 10 to 15 percent lower than that with surgical treatment (Chao, 1996; Fishman, 1996). These poor results suggest that a careful preoperative evaluation and appropriate consultation should be completed before any woman is denied the benefits of hysterectomy (American College of Obstetricians and Gynecologists, 2015c).

Adjuvant Radiation Therapy. In general, this option is offered after staging surgery to women at risk for endometrial cancer recurrence. Those with low-risk early-stage cancer are typically adequately treated with surgery, may not benefit from adjuvant therapy, and usually simply begin surveillance. The use of radiation in early-stage disease has been evaluated in three major trials, all of which demonstrated that adjuvant radiation improved local disease control and recurrence-free survival rates but did not decrease the rate of distant metastases or improve overall survival rates at 5 years (Aalders, 1980; Creutzberg, 2001, 2004; Keys, 2004).

However, in one of these trials, the recurrence-rate reduction was particularly evident in a high-intermediate risk subgroup of women: (1) with three risk factors (grade 2 or 3 tumors, lymphovascular invasion, and invasion of the outer third of the myometrium); (2) with age >50 years and two of these risk factors; and (3) with age >70 years and one risk factor (Keys, 2004). These elements have found their way into both clinical management and the design of more contemporary trials. Therefore, adjuvant radiation is usually offered to patients with high-intermediate risk stage I uterine cancers. However, because of the results of subsequent trials, the type of radiation offered is vaginal brachytherapy. The PORTEC-2 trial showed that vaginal brachytherapy was equivalent to whole pelvic radiation in those patients with high-intermediate risk endometrial cancer (Nout, 2010). Of note, local radiation can reduce the risk of local recurrence but does not improve overall survival rates.

For women with stage II endometrial cancer, the efficacy of postoperative radiotherapy is even harder to decipher. Most data derive from retrospective, single-institution experiences, and evidence supports external beam pelvic radiation, vaginal brachytherapy, both, or no further treatment (Cannon, 2009; Elshaikh, 2015; Rittenberg, 2005). As such, there is no standard approach, and most patients are treated individually based on coexisting risk factors (Feltmate, 1999).

For most women with stage III endometrial cancer, chemotherapy and/or tumor-directed postoperative external beam radiation is indicated (Barrena-Medel, 2009; Homesley, 2009). Most commonly, radiation therapy is specifically directed at pelvic disease but may extend to the paraaortic area if metastases are detected. Currently, results are pending from a randomized trial that compares chemoradiation and chemotherapy (carboplatin and paclitaxel) for advanced endometrial cancer (protocol #258). Few patients with stage IV disease are candidates for radiotherapy with curative intent. Infrequently, a locally confined stage IVA tumor may be an exception. With stage IV disease, intraperitoneal metastases most often lie outside a tolerated radiation field. Therefore, whole abdominal irradiation is not generally preferable to chemotherapy (Randall, 2006). As a result, the role of radiotherapy is generally palliative in these

women (Goff, 1994). Chemotherapy is a reasonable option for patients with advanced endometrial cancer.

Hormonal Therapy

Cancer Treatment. One of the unique characteristics of endometrial cancer is its hormonal responsiveness. Thus, for women who are not surgical candidates, continuous chronic progestin treatment or a levonorgestrel-releasing IUD can be primary treatment (Dhar, 2005; Montz, 2002). Also, in young premenopausal patients who desire fertility, similar primary progestin therapy can be used to reverse pathology.

As adjuvant therapy, single-agent high-dose progestins also have activity in women with advanced or recurrent disease (Lentz, 1996; Thigpen, 1999). Tamoxifen upregulates progesterone-receptor expression and is postulated to thereby improve progestin therapy efficacy. Clinically, high response rates have been noted with tamoxifen used adjunctively with progestin therapy (Fiorica, 2004; Whitney, 2004). In general, toxicity is low, but this combination is most often used for recurrent disease.

Estrogen Replacement Therapy. Due to the presumed role of excess estrogen in endometrial cancer development, estrogen supplementation following endometrial cancer treatment is often met with concern for stimulating malignancy recurrence. However, this effect has not been observed (Suriano, 2001). The GOG attempted to determine the risk of estrogen replacement therapy in endometrial cancer survivors by randomly assigning 1236 women who had undergone surgery for stage I and II endometrial cancer to receive either estrogen or placebo. Although the study did not meet its enrollment goals, the low recurrence rate (2 percent) was promising (Barakat, 2006). Women should be individually counseled regarding risks and benefits before beginning posttreatment estrogen replacement for menopausal symptoms.

Uterine Papillary Serous Carcinoma Management

This most aggressive type of endometrial carcinoma is uncommon, and thus, randomized trials are difficult to perform. As a result, most data are single-institution, retrospective analyses. Treatment is usually individualized but is often different from typical endometrioid adenocarcinoma.

If a preoperative biopsy demonstrates serous features, comprehensive surgical staging for UPSC is recommended. This includes total hysterectomy, BSO, peritoneal washings, pelvic/paraaortic lymph node dissection, infracolic omentectomy, and peritoneal biopsies (Chan, 2003). Even noninvasive disease is often widely metastatic (Gehrig, 2001). Fortunately, patients tend to have a good prognosis if surgical staging confirms that disease is confined to the uterus (stage I/II) (Grice, 1998).

Occasionally, no residual UPSC is evident on the hysterectomy specimen, or the tumor minimally involves the tip of a polyp. These women with surgical stage IA can safely be observed. However, all other patients with stage I disease are considered for adjuvant treatment. For this, one effective strategy is postoperative paclitaxel and carboplatin chemotherapy for three to six cycles combined with concomitant vaginal brachytherapy (Dietrich, 2005; Kelly, 2005). However, some data suggest an intrinsic radioresistance for UPSC tumors (Martin, 2005). In addition, based on the largest reported retrospective review of surgical stage I patients, Huh and coworkers (2003) questioned the benefit of any radiation therapy.

Women with stage II UPSC are more likely to benefit from pelvic radiotherapy with or without chemotherapy following surgery. Those having stage III disease are especially prone to have recurrent disease at distant sites. Accordingly, paclitaxel and carboplatin is considered in addition to tumor-directed radiotherapy after surgery (Bristow, 2001a; Slomovitz, 2003).

In practice, many patients will have stage IVB disease. Aggressive surgical cytoreduction is perhaps most important, because one of the strongest predictors of overall survival is the amount of residual disease. Postoperatively, at least six cycles of paclitaxel and carboplatin chemotherapy are indicated (Barrena-Medel, 2009; Bristow, 2001b; Moller, 2004). Enrollment in a clinical trial is strongly considered for cases of advanced uterine cancer.

Fertility-sparing Management

Hormonal therapy without hysterectomy is an option in carefully selected young women with endometrial cancer who desperately wish to preserve their fertility. Currently, patients considering fertility-sparing treatment are recommended to undergo a diagnostic hysteroscopy, sampling by D & C, and imaging to exclude deep myometrial invasion or extrauterine disease (Burke, 2014). Careful selection is also aided by a reproductive endocrinology consultation that clarifies the patient's posttreatment conception chances. Importantly, many of the biologic processes that lead to endometrial cancer also contribute to decreased fertility. In general, this strategy should apply only to those with grade 1 (type I tumor) adenocarcinomas and with no imaging evidence of myometrial invasion. Rarely, women with grade 2 lesions may be considered candidates, although it may advisable to further assess their disease laparoscopically (Morice, 2005). The aim of hormonal treatment is to reverse the lesion. However, any type of medical management obviously involves inherent risk that a patient must be willing to accept (Yang, 2005).

Progestins are most commonly used for conservative treatment. Oral megestrol acetate, 160 mg given daily or 80 mg twice daily, can promote cancer regression. Alternatively, oral or intramuscular MPA may be delivered at varying doses (Gotlieb, 2003). The levonorgestrel-releasing IUD is another acceptable option. Combining progestin therapy with tamoxifen or with gonadotropin-releasing hormone agonists is less frequently done (Wang, 2002). Regardless of the hormonal agent, recurrence rates are high during long-term observation (Gotlieb, 2003; Niwa, 2005). Despite the feasibility of this option, dosages, therapy duration, and surveillance schedules are not specifically defined.

Women receiving fertility-sparing management are carefully monitored by repeated endometrial biopsy or D & C every 3 months to assess treatment efficacy. Evidence for persistence often prompts a change in agent or a dosage increase. Hysterectomy and operative staging is recommended if a lesion fails to regress with hormonal therapy or if disease progression is suspected.

Delivery of a healthy infant is a reasonable expectation for those patients who respond to treatment and have normal histologic findings in surveillance endometrial samplings. However, assisted reproductive technologies may be required to achieve pregnancy in some cases. Postpartum, patients are again regularly monitored for recurrent endometrial adenocarcinoma (Ferrandina, 2005). In general, women should undergo hysterectomy at completion of childbearing or whenever the preservation of fertility is no longer desired.

TABLE 33-11. Poor Prognostic Variables in Endometrial Cancer

Advanced surgical stage
Older age
Histologic type: UPSC or clear cell adenocarcinoma
Advanced tumor grade
Presence of myometrial invasion
Presence of lymphovascular space invasion
Peritoneal cytology positive for cancer cells
Increased tumor size
High tumor expression levels of ER and PR

ER = estrogen receptor; PR = progesterone receptor; UPSC = uterine papillary serous carcinoma.

◼ Prognostic Factors

Many clinical and pathologic factors influence the likelihood of endometrial cancer recurrence and survival (Table 33-11) (Lurain, 1991; Schink, 1991). Of these, FIGO surgical stage is the most important overriding variable because it incorporates many of the most important risk factors (Table 33-12). Metastatic disease to the adnexa, pelvic/paraaortic lymph nodes, and peritoneal surfaces is reflected by the FIGO stage.

◼ Recurrent Disease

Patients with recurrent endometrial cancer typically require individualized treatment. In general, the site of relapse is the most important predictor of survival. Depending on the circumstances, surgery, radiation, chemotherapy, or a combination of these may be the best strategy. The most curable scenario is an isolated relapse at the vaginal apex in a previously unradiated patient. These women are usually effectively treated by external beam pelvic radiotherapy. In patients who were previously irradiated, exenteration is often the only curative option (Section 46-4, p. 1149) (Barakat, 1999; Morris, 1996). Nodal recurrences or isolated pelvic disease is more likely to result in further disease progression, regardless of treatment modality. However, either is often an appropriate indication for external

TABLE 33-12. Endometrial Cancer 5-year Survival Rates for Each Surgical Stage (n = 5562 patients)

Stage	Survival (%)	Stage	Survival (%)
IA	91	IIIA	60
IB	88	IIIB	41
IC	81	IIIC	32
IIA	77	IVA	20
IIB	67	IVB	5

Data from Creasman WT, Odicino F, Maisonneuve P, et al: Carcinoma of the corpus uteri. FIGO 26th Annual Report on the Results of Treatment in Gynecological Cancer, Int J Gynaecol Obstet. 2006 Nov;95 Suppl 1:S105–S143.

beam radiotherapy in those not previously irradiated. Salvage cytoreductive surgery may also be beneficial in selected patients (Awtrey, 2006; Bristow, 2006b).

Widely disseminated endometrial cancer or a relapse not amenable to radiation or surgery is an indication for systemic chemotherapy (Barrena-Medel, 2009). Patients are ideally enrolled in an experimental trial due to the limited duration of response with current salvage regimens and the urgent need for more effective therapy. Paclitaxel and carboplatin is an active combination for recurrent disease and found not to be inferior to TAP (Miller, 2012). Progestin therapy with or without tamoxifen is a less toxic option that is particularly useful in selected cases (Fiorica, 2004; Whitney, 2004). In general, effective palliation of women with incurable, recurrent endometrial cancer requires an ongoing dialogue to achieve the optimal balance between symptomatic relief and treatment toxicity.

REFERENCES

Aalders J, Abeler V, Kolstad P, et al: Postoperative external irradiation and prognostic parameters in stage I endometrial carcinoma: clinical and histopathologic study of 540 patients. Obstet Gynecol 56(4):419, 1980

Aarnio M, Sankila R, Pukkala E, et al: Cancer risk in mutation carriers of DNA-mismatch-repair genes. Int J Cancer 81(2):214, 1999

Abeler VM, Kjorstad KE: Clear cell carcinoma of the endometrium: a histopathological and clinical study of 97 cases. Gynecol Oncol 40(3):207, 1991

Abu-Rustum NR, Khoury-Collado F, Pandit-Taskar N, et al: Sentinel lymph node mapping for grade 1 endometrial cancer: is it the answer to the surgical staging dilemma? Gynecol Oncol 113(2):163, 2009

Aghajanian C, Sill MW, Darcy KM, et al: Phase II trial of bevacizumab in recurrent or persistent endometrial cancer: a Gynecologic Oncology Group study. J Clin Oncol 29(16):2259, 2011

Ahluwalia M, Light AM, Surampudi K, et al: Transitional cell carcinoma of the endometrium: a case report and review of the literature. Int J Gynecol Pathol 25(4):378, 2006

Allison KH, Reed SD, Voigt LF, et al: Diagnosing endometrial hyperplasia: why is it so difficult to agree? Am J Surg Pathol 32(5):691, 2008

Altrabulsi B, Malpica A, Deavers MT, et al: Undifferentiated carcinoma of the endometrium. Am J Surg Pathol 29(10):1316, 2005

American College of Obstetricians and Gynecologists: Diagnosis of abnormal uterine bleeding in reproductive-aged women. Practice Bulletin No. 128, July 2012, Reaffirmed 2014a

American College of Obstetricians and Gynecologists: Endometrial intraepithelial neoplasia. Committee Opinion No. 631, 2015a

American College of Obstetricians and Gynecologists: Hysteroscopy. Technology Assessment No. 7, June 2011, Reaffirmed 2015b

American College of Obstetricians and Gynecologists: Lynch syndrome. Practice Bulletin No. 147, November 2014b

American College of Obstetricians and Gynecologists: Management of endometrial cancer. Practice Bulletin No. 149, April 2015c

American College of Obstetricians and Gynecologists: Salpingectomy for ovarian cancer prevention. Committee Opinion No. 620, January 2015d

American College of Obstetricians and Gynecologists: Tamoxifen and uterine cancer. Committee Opinion No. 601, June 2014c

American College of Obstetricians and Gynecologists: The role of transvaginal ultrasonography in the evaluation of postmenopausal bleeding. Committee Opinion No. 440, August 2009, Reaffirmed 2013

Anastasiadis PG, Skaphida PG, Koutlaki NG, et al: Descriptive epidemiology of endometrial hyperplasia in patients with abnormal uterine bleeding. Eur J Gynaecol Oncol 21(2):131, 2000

Ashfaq R, Sharma S, Dulley T, et al: Clinical relevance of benign endometrial cells in postmenopausal women. Diagn Cytopathol 25(4):235, 2001

Awtrey CS, Cadungog MG, Leitao MM, et al: Surgical resection of recurrent endometrial carcinoma. Gynecol Oncol 102(3):480, 2006

Ayhan A, Tuncer ZS, Tuncer R, et al: Granulosa cell tumor of the ovary. A clinicopathological evaluation of 60 cases. Eur J Gynaecol Oncol 15(4):320, 1994

Baak JP, Mutter GL, Robboy S, et al: The molecular genetics and morphometrybased endometrial intraepithelial neoplasia classification system predicts disease progression in endometrial hyperplasia more accurately than the 1994 World Health Organization classification system. Cancer 103(11):2304, 2005

Balmana J, Stockwell DH, Steyerberg EW, et al: Prediction of MLH1 and MSH2 mutations in Lynch syndrome. JAMA 296(12):1469, 2006

Bansal N, Yendluri V, Wenham RM: The molecular biology of endometrial cancers and the implications for pathogenesis, classification, and targeted therapies. Cancer Control 16(1):8, 2009

Barakat RR, Bundy BN, Spirtos NM, et al: Randomized double-blind trial of estrogen replacement therapy versus placebo in stage I or II endometrial cancer: a Gynecologic Oncology Group Study. J Clin Oncol 24(4):587, 2006

Barakat RR, Goldman NA, Patel DA, et al: Pelvic exenteration for recurrent endometrial cancer. Gynecol Oncol 75(1):99, 1999

Barrena Medel NI, Bansal S, Miller DS, et al: Pharmacotherapy of endometrial cancer. Expert Opin Pharmacother 10(12):1939, 2009

Beiner ME, Finch A, Rosen B, et al: The risk of endometrial cancer in women with BRCA1 and BRCA2 mutations. A prospective study. Gynecol Oncol 104(1):7, 2007

Ben Yehuda OM, Kim YB, Leuchter RS: Does hysteroscopy improve upon the sensitivity of dilatation and curettage in the diagnosis of endometrial hyperplasia or carcinoma? Gynecol Oncol 68:4, 1998

Benedetti Panici P, Basile S, Maneschi F, et al: Systematic pelvic lymphadenectomy vs. no lymphadenectomy in early stage endometrial carcinoma: randomized clinical trial. J Natl Cancer Inst 100:1707, 2008

Breitkopf DM, Frederickson RA, Snyder RR: Detection of benign endometrial masses by endometrial stripe measurement in premenopausal women. Obstet Gynecol 104(1):2004

Bristow RE, Asrari F, Trimble EL, et al: Extended surgical staging for uterine papillary serous carcinoma: survival outcome of locoregional (stage I–III) disease. Gynecol Oncol 81(2):279, 2001a

Bristow RE, Duska LR, Montz FJ: The role of cytoreductive surgery in the management of stage IV uterine papillary serous carcinoma. Gynecol Oncol 81(1):92, 2001b

Bristow RE, Purinton SC, Santillan A, et al: Cost-effectiveness of routine vaginal cytology for endometrial cancer surveillance. Gynecol Oncol 103(2):709, 2006a

Bristow RE, Santillan A, Zahurak ML, et al: Salvage cytoreductive surgery for recurrent endometrial cancer. Gynecol Oncol 103(1):281, 2006b

Bristow RE, Zerbe MJ, Rosenshein NB, et al: Stage IVB endometrial carcinoma: the role of cytoreductive surgery and determinants of survival. Gynecol Oncol 78(2):85, 2000

Burke TW, Levenback C, Tornos C, et al: Intraabdominal lymphatic mapping to direct selective pelvic and paraaortic lymphadenectomy in women with high-risk endometrial cancer: results of a pilot study. Gynecol Oncol 62(2):169, 1996

Burke WM, Orr J, Leitao M, et al: Endometrial cancer: a review and current management strategies: part II. Gynecol Oncol 134(2):393, 2014

Cannon GM, Geye H, Terakedis BE, et al: Outcomes following surgery and adjuvant radiation in stage II endometrial adenocarcinoma. Gynecol Oncol 113(2):176, 2009

Carcangiu ML, Chambers JT: Uterine papillary serous carcinoma: a study on 108 cases with emphasis on the prognostic significance of associated endometrioid carcinoma, absence of invasion, and concomitant ovarian carcinoma. Gynecol Oncol 47(3):298, 1992

Cardenas-Goicoechea J, Adams S, Bhat SB, et al: Surgical outcomes of robotic-assisted surgical staging for endometrial cancer are equivalent to traditional laparoscopic staging at a minimally invasive surgical center. Gynecol Oncol 117(2):224, 2010

Chan JK, Loizzi V, Youssef M, et al: Significance of comprehensive surgical staging in noninvasive papillary serous carcinoma of the endometrium. Gynecol Oncol 90(1):181, 2003

Chan JK, Sherman AE, Kapp DS, et al: Influence of gynecologic oncologists on the survival of patients with endometrial cancer. J Clin Oncol 29(7):832, 2011

Chao CK, Grigsby PW, Perez CA, et al: Medically inoperable stage I endometrial carcinoma: a few dilemmas in radiotherapeutic management. Int J Radiat Oncol Biol Phys 34(1):27, 1996

Chen S, Wang W, Lee S, et al: Prediction of germline mutations and cancer risk in the Lynch syndrome. JAMA 296(12):1479, 2006

Childers JM, Spirtos NM, Brainard P, et al: Laparoscopic staging of the patient with incompletely staged early adenocarcinoma of the endometrium. Obstet Gynecol 83(4):597, 1994

Cicinelli E, Tinelli R, Colafiglio G, et al: Risk of long-term pelvic recurrences after fluid minihysteroscopy in women with endometrial carcinoma: a controlled randomized study. Menopause 17(3):511, 2010

Cooper AL, Dornfeld-Finke JM, Banks HW, et al: Is cytologic screening an effective surveillance method for detection of vaginal recurrence of uterine cancer? Obstet Gynecol 107(1):71, 2006

Cornelison TL, Trimble EL, Kosary CL: SEER data, corpus uteri cancer: treatment trends versus survival for FIGO stage II, 1988–1994. Gynecol Oncol 74(3):350, 1999

Creasman W, Odicino F, Maisonneuve P, et al: FIGO Annual Report on the Results of Treatment in Gynaecological Cancer. 1998

Creasman W, Odicino F, Maisonneuve P, et al: FIGO Annual Report on the Results of Treatment in Gynecological Cancer. 2006

Creutzberg CL, van Putten WL, Koper PC, et al: The morbidity of treatment for patients with Stage I endometrial cancer: results from a randomized trial. Int J Radiat Oncol Biol Phys 51(5):1246, 2001

Creutzberg CL, van Putten WL, Warlam-Rodenhuis CC, et al: Outcome of high-risk stage IC, grade 3, compared with stage I endometrial carcinoma patients: the Postoperative Radiation Therapy in Endometrial Carcinoma Trial. J Clin Oncol 22(7):1234, 2004

Delin JB, Miller DS, Coleman RL: Other primary malignancies in patients with uterine corpus malignancy. Am J Obstet Gynecol 190:1429, 2004

Dhar KK, NeedhiRajan T, Koslowski M, et al: Is levonorgestrel intrauterine system effective for treatment of early endometrial cancer? Report of four cases and review of the literature. Gynecol Oncol 97(3):924, 2005

Dietrich CS III, Modesitt SC, DePriest PD, et al: The efficacy of adjuvant platinum-based chemotherapy in stage I uterine papillary serous carcinoma (UPSC). Gynecol Oncol 99(3):557, 2005

Dossus L, Allen N, Kaaks R, et al: Reproductive risk factors and endometrial cancer: the European Prospective Investigation into Cancer and Nutrition. Int J Cancer 127(2):442, 2010

Ellenson LH, Ronnett BM, Kurman RJ: Precursor lesions of endometrial carcinoma. In Kurman RJ, Ellenson LH, Ronnett BM (eds): Blaustein's Pathology of the Female Genital Tract, New York, Springer, 2011a, p 360

Ellenson LH, Ronnett BM, Soslow RA: Endometrial cancer. In Kurman RJ, Ellenson LH, Ronnett BM (eds): Blaustein's Pathology of the Female Genital Tract, New York, Springer, 2011b, p 422

Elshaikh MA, Al-Wahab Z, Mahdi H, et al: Recurrence patterns and survival endpoints in women with stage II uterine endometrioid carcinoma: a multi-institution study. Gynecol Oncol 136(2):235, 2015

Eltabbakh GH, Shamonki J, Mount SL: Surgical stage, final grade, and survival of women with endometrial carcinoma whose preoperative endometrial biopsy shows well-differentiated tumors. Gynecol Oncol 99(2):309, 2005

Fearnley EJ, Marquart L, Spurdle AB, et al: Polycystic ovary syndrome increases the risk of endometrial cancer in women aged less than 50 years: an Australian case-control study. Cancer Causes Control 12:2303, 2010

Feldman S, Berkowitz RS, Tosteson AN: Cost-effectiveness of strategies to evaluate postmenopausal bleeding. Obstet Gynecol 81(6):968, 1993

Felix AS, Gaudet MM, La Vecchia C, et al: Intrauterine devices and endometrial cancer risk: a pooled analysis of the Epidemiology of Endometrial Cancer Consortium. Int J Cancer 136(5):E410, 2015

Felix AS, Weissfeld JL, Stone RA, et al: Factors associated with Type I and Type II endometrial cancer. Cancer Causes Control 21(11):1851, 2010

Feltmate CM, Duska LR, Chang Y, et al: Predictors of recurrence in surgical stage II endometrial adenocarcinoma. Gynecol Oncol 73(3):407, 1999

Ferrandina G, Zannoni GF, Gallotta V, et al: Progression of conservatively treated endometrial carcinoma after full term pregnancy: a case report. Gynecol Oncol 99(1):215, 2005

FIGO Committee on Gynecologic Oncology: Revised FIGO staging for carcinoma of the vulva, cervix, and endometrium. Int J Gynaecol Obstet 105(2):103, 2009

Fiorica JV, Brunetto VL, Hanjani P, et al: Phase II trial of alternating courses of megestrol acetate and tamoxifen in advanced endometrial carcinoma: a Gynecologic Oncology Group study. Gynecol Oncol 92(1):10, 2004

Fisher B, Costantino JP, Wickerham DL, et al: Tamoxifen for prevention of breast cancer: report of the National Surgical Adjuvant Breast and Bowel Project P-1 Study. J Natl Cancer Inst 90(18):1371, 1998

Fishman DA, Roberts KB, Chambers JT, et al: Radiation therapy as exclusive treatment for medically inoperable patients with stage I and II endometrioid carcinoma with endometrium. Gynecol Oncol 61(2):189, 1996

Fleming GF, Brunetto VL, Cella D, et al: Phase III trial of doxorubicin plus cisplatin with or without paclitaxel plus filgrastim in advanced endometrial carcinoma: a Gynecologic Oncology Group Study. J Clin Oncol 22(11):2159, 2004

Frati A, Ballester M, Dubernard G, et al: Contribution of lymphoscintigraphy for sentinel lymph node biopsy in women with early stage endometrial cancer: results of the SENTI-ENDO Study. Ann Surg Oncol 22(6):1980, 2015

Frumovitz M, Singh DK, Meyer L, et al: Predictors of final histology in patients with endometrial cancer. Gynecol Oncol 95(3):463, 2004a

Frumovitz M, Slomovitz BM, Singh DK, et al: Frozen section analyses as predictors of lymphatic spread in patients with early-stage uterine cancer. J Am Coll Surg 199(3):388, 2004b

Gallos ID, Shehmar M, Thangaratinam S, et al: Oral progestogens vs levonorgestrel-releasing intrauterine system for endometrial hyperplasia: a systematic review and metaanalysis. Am J Obstet Gynecol 203(6):547.e1, 2010

Garuti G, Mirra M, Luerti M: Hysteroscopic view in atypical endometrial hyperplasias: a correlation with pathologic findings on hysterectomy specimens. J Minim Invasive Gynecol 13(4):325, 2006

Gehrig PA, Groben PA, Fowler WC Jr, et al: Noninvasive papillary serous carcinoma of the endometrium. Obstet Gynecol 97(1):153, 2001

Ghezzi F, Cromi A, Uccella S, et al: Laparoscopic versus open surgery for endometrial cancer: a minimum 3-year follow-up study. Ann Surg Oncol 17(1):271, 2010

Goff BA, Goodman A, Muntz HG, et al: Surgical stage IV endometrial carcinoma: a study of 47 cases. Gynecol Oncol 52(2):237, 1994

Goldstein SR, Zeltser I, Horan CK, et al: Ultrasonography-based triage for perimenopausal patients with abnormal uterine bleeding. Am J Obstet Gynecol 177(1):102, 1997

Goodman A, Zukerberg LR, Rice LW, et al: Squamous cell carcinoma of the endometrium: a report of eight cases and a review of the literature. Gynecol Oncol 61(1):54, 1996

Goodman MT, Hankin JH, Wilkens LR, et al: Diet, body size, physical activity, and the risk of endometrial cancer. Cancer Res 57(22):5077, 1997

Gotlieb WH, Beiner ME, Shalmon B, et al: Outcome of fertility-sparing treatment with progestins in young patients with endometrial cancer. Obstet Gynecol 102(4):718, 2003

Graebe K, Garcia-Soto A, Aziz M, et al: Incidental power morcellation of malignancy: a retrospective cohort study. Gynecol Oncol 136(2):274, 2015

Granberg S, Wikland M, Karlsson B, et al: Endometrial thickness as measured by endovaginal ultrasonography for identifying endometrial abnormality. Am J Obstet Gynecol 164:47, 1991

Gredmark T, Kvint S, Havel G, et al: Histopathological findings in women with postmenopausal bleeding. BJOG 102(2):133, 1995

Grice J, Ek M, Greer B, et al: Uterine papillary serous carcinoma: evaluation of long-term survival in surgically staged patients. Gynecol Oncol 69(1):69, 1998

Gruber SB, Thompson WD: A population-based study of endometrial cancer and familial risk in younger women. Cancer and Steroid Hormone Study Group. Cancer Epidemiol Biomarkers Prev 5(6):411, 1996

Gu M, Shi W, Barakat RR, et al: Pap smears in women with endometrial carcinoma. Acta Cytol 45(4):555, 2001

Guidos BJ, Selvaggi SM: Detection of endometrial adenocarcinoma with the ThinPrep Pap test. Diagn Cytopathol 23(4):260, 2000

Hamilton CA, Cheung MK, Osann K, et al: Uterine papillary serous and clear cell carcinomas predict for poorer survival compared to grade 3 endometrioid corpus cancers. Br J Cancer 94(5):642, 2006

Hampel H, Frankel W, Panescu J, et al: Screening for Lynch syndrome (hereditary nonpolyposis colorectal cancer) among endometrial cancer patients. Cancer Res 66(15):7810, 2006

Havrilesky LJ, Cragun JM, Calingaert B, et al: Resection of lymph node metastases influences survival in stage IIIC endometrial cancer. Gynecol Oncol 99(3):689, 2005

Hecht JL, Ince TA, Baak JP, et al: Prediction of endometrial carcinoma by subjective endometrial intraepithelial neoplasia diagnosis. Mod Pathol 18(3):324, 2005

Hecht JL, Mutter GL: Molecular and pathologic aspects of endometrial carcinogenesis. J Clin Oncol 24(29):4783, 2006

Hemminki K, Bermejo JL, Granstrom C: Endometrial cancer: population attributable risks from reproductive, familial and socioeconomic factors. Eur J Cancer 41(14):2155, 2005

Hirai Y, Takeshima N, Kato T, et al: Malignant potential of positive peritoneal cytology in endometrial cancer. Obstet Gynecol 97(5 Pt 1):725, 2001

Hoekstra AV, Jairam-Thodla A, Rademaker A, et al: The impact of robotics on practice management of endometrial cancer: transitioning from traditional surgery. Int J Med Robot 5(4):392, 2009

Homesley HD, Filiaci V, Gibbons SK et al: A randomized phase III trial in advanced endometrial carcinoma of surgery and volume directed radiation followed by cisplatin and doxorubicin with or without paclitaxel: a Gynecologic Oncology Group study. Gynecol Oncol 112:543, 2009

Horn LC, Schnurrbusch U, Bilek K, et al: Risk of progression in complex and atypical endometrial hyperplasia: clinicopathologic analysis in cases with and without progestogen treatment. Int J Gynecol Cancer 14(2):348, 2004

Hoskins PJ, Swenerton KD, Pike JA, et al: Paclitaxel and carboplatin, alone or with irradiation, in advanced or recurrent endometrial cancer: a phase II study. J Clin Oncol 19(20):4048, 2001

Howlader N, Noone AM, Krapcho M, et al: SEER Cancer Statistics Review, 1975-2011, National Cancer Institute. 2014. Available at: http://seer.cancer.gov/csr/1975_2011/. Accessed April 12, 2015

Huh WK, Powell M, Leath CA III, et al: Uterine papillary serous carcinoma: comparisons of outcomes in surgical Stage I patients with and without adjuvant therapy. Gynecol Oncol 91(3):470, 2003

Iatrakis G, Diakakis I, Kourounis G, et al: Postmenopausal uterine bleeding. Clin Exp Obstet Gynecol 24(3):157, 1997

Jacobs I, Gentry-Maharaj A, Burnell M, et al: Sensitivity of transvaginal ultrasound screening for endometrial cancer in postmenopausal women: a case-control study within the UKCTOCS cohort. Lancet Oncol 12(1):38, 2011

Jordan LB, Abdul-Kader M, Al Nafussi A: Uterine serous papillary carcinoma: histopathologic changes within the female genital tract. Int J Gynecol Cancer 11(4):283, 2001

Kelly MG, O'Malley DM, Hui P, et al: Improved survival in surgical stage I patients with uterine papillary serous carcinoma (UPSC) treated with adjuvant platinum-based chemotherapy. Gynecol Oncol 98(3):353, 2005

Keys HM, Roberts JA, Brunetto VL, et al: A phase III trial of surgery with or without adjunctive external pelvic radiation therapy in intermediate risk endometrial adenocarcinoma: a Gynecologic Oncology Group study. Gynecol Oncol 92(3):744, 2004

Kilgore LC, Partridge EE, Alvarez RD, et al: Adenocarcinoma of the endometrium: survival comparisons of patients with and without pelvic node sampling. Gynecol Oncol 56(1):29, 1995

Kitchener H, Swart AM, Qian Q, et al: Efficacy of systematic pelvic lymphadenectomy in endometrial cancer (MRC ASTEC trial): a randomized study. Lancet 373:125, 2009

Kornblith AB, Huang HQ, Walker JL, et al: Quality of life of patients with endometrial cancer undergoing laparoscopic International Federation of Gynecology and Obstetrics staging compared with laparotomy: a Gynecologic Oncology Group study. J Clin Oncol 27(32):5337, 2009

Kurman RJ, Carcangiu ML, Herrington CS, et al (eds): WHO Classification of Tumours of Female Reproductive Organs, 4th ed. Lyon, International Agency for Research on Cancer, 2014

Kurman RJ, Kaminski PF, Norris HJ: The behavior of endometrial hyperplasia. A long-term study of "untreated" hyperplasia in 170 patients. Cancer 56(2):403, 1985

Kurman RJ, Norris HJ: Endometrial hyperplasia and related cellular changes. In Kurman RJ (ed): Blaustein's Pathology of the Female Genital Tract. 1994, p 411

Lancaster JM, Powell CB, Chen LM, et al: Society of Gynecologic Oncology statement on risk assessment for inherited gynecologic cancer predispositions. Gynecol Oncol 136(1):3, 2015

Lee PS, Secord AA: Targeted molecular pathways in endometrial cancer: a focus on the FGFR pathway. Cancer Treat Rev 40(4):507, 2014

Leitao MM, Kehoe S, Barakat RR, et al: Accuracy of preoperative endometrial sampling diagnosis of FIGO grade 1 endometrial adenocarcinoma. Gynecol Oncol 111:244, 2008

Lentz SS, Brady MF, Major FJ, et al: High-dose megestrol acetate in advanced or recurrent endometrial carcinoma: a Gynecologic Oncology Group Study. J Clin Oncol 14(2):357, 1996

Liao CK, Rosenblatt KA, Schwartz SM, et al: Endometrial cancer in Asian migrants to the United States and their descendants. Cancer Causes Control 14(4):357, 2003

Lu KH, Dinh M, Kohlmann W, et al: Gynecologic cancer as a "sentinel cancer" for women with hereditary nonpolyposis colorectal cancer syndrome. Obstet Gynecol 105(3):569, 2005

Lurain JR, Rice BL, Rademaker AW, et al: Prognostic factors associated with disease recurrence in clinical stage I adenocarcinoma of the endometrium. Obstet Gynecol 78:63, 1991

Madison T, Schottenfeld D, James SA, et al: Endometrial cancer: socioeconomic status and racial/ethnic differences in stage at diagnosis, treatment, and survival. Am J Public Health 94(12):2104, 2004

Magrina JF, Mutone NF, Weaver AL, et al: Laparoscopic lymphadenectomy and vaginal or laparoscopic hysterectomy with bilateral salpingo-oophorectomy for endometrial cancer: morbidity and survival. Am J Obstet Gynecol 181(2):376, 1999

Mariani A, Webb MJ, Keeney GL, et al: Hematogenous dissemination in corpus cancer. Gynecol Oncol 80(2):233, 2001a

Mariani A, Webb MJ, Keeney GL, et al: Role of wide/radical hysterectomy and pelvic lymph node dissection in endometrial cancer with cervical involvement. Gynecol Oncol 83(1):72, 2001b

Martin JD, Gilks B, Lim P: Papillary serous carcinoma—a less radio-sensitive subtype of endometrial cancer. Gynecol Oncol 98(2):299, 2005

Martínez A, Querleu D, Leblanc E, et al: Low incidence of port-site metastases after laparoscopic staging of uterine cancer. Gynecol Oncol 118(2):145, 2010

Maxwell GL, Schildkraut JM, Calingaert B, et al: Progestin and estrogen potency of combination oral contraceptives and endometrial cancer risk. Gynecol Oncol 103(2):535, 2006

Melhem MF, Tobon H: Mucinous adenocarcinoma of the endometrium: a clinico-pathological review of 18 cases. Int J Gynecol Pathol 6(4):347, 1987

Miller D, Filiaci V, Fleming G, et al: Randomized phase III noninferiority trial of first line chemotherapy for metastatic or recurrent endometrial carcinoma: a GOG study. Abstract 771. Gynecol Oncol 125(3):771, 2012

Miller DS: Advanced endometrial cancer: is lymphadenectomy necessary or sufficient? Gynecol Oncol 101(2):191, 2006

Miller DS, Fleming G, Randall ME: Chemo- and radiotherapy in adjuvant management of optimally debulked endometrial cancer. J Natl Compr Cancer Netw 7(5):535, 2009

Moller KA, Gehrig PA, Van Le L, et al: The role of optimal debulking in advanced stage serous cancer of the uterus. Gynecol Oncol 94(1):170, 2004

Montz FJ, Bristow RE, Bovicelli A, et al: Intrauterine progesterone treatment of early endometrial cancer. Am J Obstet Gynecol 186(4):651, 2002

Morice P, Fourchotte V, Sideris L, et al: A need for laparoscopic evaluation of patients with endometrial carcinoma selected for conservative treatment. Gynecol Oncol 96(1):245, 2005

Morimoto LM, Newcomb PA, Hampton JM, et al: Cholecystectomy and endometrial cancer: a marker of long-term elevated estrogen exposure? Int J Gynecol Cancer 16(3):1348, 2006

Morris M, Alvarez RD, Kinney WK, et al: Treatment of recurrent adenocarcinoma of the endometrium with pelvic exenteration. Gynecol Oncol 60(2):288, 1996

Morrow CP, Bundy BN, Kurman RJ, et al: Relationship between surgical-pathological risk factors and outcome in clinical stage I and II carcinoma of the endometrium: a Gynecologic Oncology Group study. Gynecol Oncol 40(1):55, 1991

Mount SL, Wegner EK, Eltabbakh GH, et al: Significant increase of benign endometrial cells on Papanicolaou smears in women using hormone replacement therapy. Obstet Gynecol 100(3):445, 2002

Mutch DG: The new FIGO staging system for cancers of the vulva, cervix, endometrium and sarcomas. Gynecol Oncol 115(3):325, 2009

Mutter GL: Endometrial intraepithelial neoplasia (EIN): will it bring order to chaos? The Endometrial Collaborative Group. Gynecol Oncol 76(3):287, 2000

Nagar H, Dobbs S, McClelland HR, et al: The diagnostic accuracy of magnetic resonance imaging in detecting cervical involvement in endometrial cancer. Gynecol Oncol 103(2):431, 2006

National Comprehensive Cancer Network: Uterine neoplasms, Version 1.2015. In NCCN Clinical Practice Guidelines in Oncology. National Comprehensive Cancer Network, 2015

Nevadunsky NS, Van Arsdale A, Strickler HD, et al: Obesity and age at diagnosis of endometrial cancer. Obstet Gynecol 124(2 Pt 1):300, 2014

Niwa K, Tagami K, Lian Z, et al: Outcome of fertility-preserving treatment in young women with endometrial carcinomas. BJOG 112(3):317, 2005

Nout RA, Smit VT, Putter H, et al: Vaginal brachytherapy versus pelvic external beam radiotherapy for patients with endometrial cancer of high-intermediate risk (PORTEC-2): an open-label, non-inferiority, randomised trial. Lancet 375(9717):816, 2010

Obermair A, Geramou M, Gucer F, et al: Does hysteroscopy facilitate tumor cell dissemination? Incidence of peritoneal cytology from patients with early stage endometrial carcinoma following dilatation and curettage (D & C) versus hysteroscopy and D & C. Cancer 88(1):139, 2000

Ørbo A, Vereide A, Arnes M, et al: Levonorgestrel-impregnated intrauterine device as treatment for endometrial hyperplasia: a national multicentre randomised trial. BJOG 121(4):477, 2014

Papadia A, Azioni G, Brusaca B, et al: Frozen section underestimates the need for surgical staging in endometrial cancer patients. Int J Gynecol Cancer 19(9):1570, 2009

Parkin DM, Bray F, Ferlay J, et al: Global cancer statistics, 2002. CA Cancer J Clin 55(2):74, 2005

Pecorelli S, Benedet JL, Creasman WT, et al: FIGO staging of gynecologic cancer. 1994-1997 FIGO Committee on Gynecologic Oncology. Int J Gynaecol Obstet 64(1):5, 1999

Phipps AI, Doherty JA, Voigt LF, et al: Long-term use of continuous-combined estrogen-progestin hormone therapy and risk of endometrial cancer. Cancer Causes Control 22(12):1639, 2011

Pillay OC, Te Fong LF, Crow JC, et al: The association between polycystic ovaries and endometrial cancer. Hum Reprod 21(4):924, 2006

Polyzos NP, Mauri D, Tsioras S, et al: Intraperitoneal dissemination of endometrial cancer cells after hysteroscopy: a systematic review and meta-analysis. Int J Gynecol Cancer 20(2):261, 2010

Powell JL, Hill KA, Shiro BC, et al: Preoperative serum CA-125 levels in treating endometrial cancer. J Reprod Med 50(8):585, 2005

Price FV, Chambers SK, Carcangiu ML, et al: CA 125 may not reflect disease status in patients with uterine serous carcinoma. Cancer 82(9):1720, 1998

Randall ME, Filiaci VL, Muss H, et al: Randomized phase III trial of whole-abdominal irradiation versus doxorubicin and cisplatin chemotherapy in advanced endometrial carcinoma: a Gynecologic Oncology Group Study. J Clin Oncol 24(1):36, 2006

Randall TC, Kurman RJ: Progestin treatment of atypical hyperplasia and well-differentiated carcinoma of the endometrium in women under age 40. Obstet Gynecol 90(3):434, 1997

Rattanachaiyanont M, Angsuwathana S, Techatrisak K, et al: Clinical and pathological responses of progestin therapy for non-atypical endometrial hyperplasia: a prospective study. J Obstet Gynaecol Res 31(2):98, 2005

Reed SD, Voigt LF, Newton KM, et al: Progestin therapy of complex endometrial hyperplasia with and without atypia. Obstet Gynecol 113(3):655, 2009

Revel A, Tsafrir A, Anteby SO, et al: Does hysteroscopy produce intraperitoneal spread of endometrial cancer cells? Obstet Gynecol Surv 59:280, 2004

Ricci E, Moroni S, Parazzini F, et al: Risk factors for endometrial hyperplasia: results from a case-control study. Int J Gynecol Cancer 12(3):257, 2002

Rittenberg PV, Lotocki RJ, Heywood MS, et al: Stage II endometrial carcinoma: limiting post-operative radiotherapy to the vaginal vault in node-negative tumors. Gynecol Oncol 98(3):434, 2005

Roland PY, Kelly FJ, Kulwicki CY, et al: The benefits of a gynecologic oncologist: a pattern of care study for endometrial cancer treatment. Gynecol Oncol 93(1):125, 2004

Ross JC, Eifel PJ, Cox RS, et al: Primary mucinous adenocarcinoma of the endometrium. A clinicopathologic and histochemical study. Am J Surg Pathol 7(8):715, 1983

Rubatt JM, Slomovitz BM, Burke TW, et al: Development of metastatic endometrial endometrioid adenocarcinoma while on progestin therapy for endometrial hyperplasia. Gynecol Oncol 99(2):472, 2005

Sanjuan A, Cobo T, Pahisa J, et al: Preoperative and intraoperative assessment of myometrial invasion and histologic grade in endometrial cancer: role of magnetic resonance imaging and frozen section. Int J Gynecol Cancer 16(1):385, 2006

Scarselli G, Bargelli G, Taddei GL, et al: Levonorgestrel-releasing intrauterine system (LNG-IUS) as an effective treatment option for endometrial hyperplasia: a 15-year follow-up study. Fertil Steril 95(1):420, 2011

Schink JC, Rademaker AW, Miller DS, et al: Tumor size in endometrial cancer. Cancer 67(11):2791, 1991

Schmeler KM, Lynch HT, Chen LM, et al: Prophylactic surgery to reduce the risk of gynecologic cancers in the Lynch syndrome. N Engl J Med 354(3):261, 2006

Schorge JO, Hossein SM, Hynan L, et al: ThinPrep detection of cervical and endometrial adenocarcinoma: a retrospective cohort study. Cancer 96(6):338, 2002

Schottenfeld D: Epidemiology of endometrial neoplasia. J Cell Biochem Suppl 23:151, 1995

Seamon LG, Cohn DE, Henretta MS, et al: Minimally invasive comprehensive surgical staging for endometrial cancer: robotics or laparoscopy? Gynecol Oncol 113(1):36, 2009

Sherman ME, Bitterman P, Rosenshein NB, et al: Uterine serous carcinoma. A morphologically diverse neoplasm with unifying clinicopathologic features. Am J Surg Pathol 16(6):600, 1992

Sherman ME, Ronnett BM, Ioffe OB, et al: Reproducibility of biopsy diagnoses of endometrial hyperplasia: evidence supporting a simplified classification. Int J Gynecol Pathol 27(3):318, 2008

Shi AA, Lee SI: Radiological reasoning: algorithmic workup of abnormal vaginal bleeding with endovaginal sonography and sonohysterography. AJR 191(6 Suppl):S68, 2008

Siegel RL, Miller KD, Jemal A: Cancer statistics, 2015. CA Cancer J Clin 65(1):5, 2015

Silva EG, Deavers MT, Malpica A: Undifferentiated carcinoma of the endometrium: a review. Pathology 39(1):134, 2007

Simsir A, Carter W, Elgert P, et al: Reporting endometrial cells in women 40 years and older: assessing the clinical usefulness of Bethesda 2001. Am J Clin Pathol 123(4):571, 2005

Slomovitz BM, Burke TW, Eifel PJ, et al: Uterine papillary serous carcinoma (UPSC): a single institution review of 129 cases. Gynecol Oncol 91(3):463, 2003

Smith DC, Prentice R, Thompson DJ, et al: Association of exogenous estrogen and endometrial carcinoma. N Engl J Med 293 (23):1164, 1975

Smith RA, Manassaram-Baptiste D, Brooks D, et al: Cancer screening in the United States, 2015: a review of current American Cancer Society guidelines and current issues in cancer screening. CA Cancer J Clin 65(1):30, 2015

Soliman PT, Oh JC, Schmeler KM, et al: Risk factors for young premenopausal women with endometrial cancer. Obstet Gynecol 105(3):575, 2005

Sovak MA, Dupont J, Hensley ML, et al: Paclitaxel and carboplatin in the treatment of advanced or recurrent endometrial cancer: a large retrospective study. Int J Gynecol Cancer 17(1):197, 2007

Sovak MA, Hensley ML, Dupont J, et al: Paclitaxel and carboplatin in the adjuvant treatment of patients with high-risk stage III and IV endometrial cancer: a retrospective study. Gynecol Oncol 103(2):451, 2006

Spirtos NM, Eisekop SM, Boike G, et al: Laparoscopic staging in patients with incompletely staged cancers of the uterus, ovary, fallopian tube, and primary peritoneum: a Gynecologic Oncology Group (GOG) study. Am J Obstet Gynecol 193(5):1645, 2005

Stanford JL, Brinton LA, Berman ML, et al: Oral contraceptives and endometrial cancer: do other risk factors modify the association? Int J Cancer 54(2):243, 1993

Strom BL, Schinnar R, Weber AL, et al: Case-control study of postmenopausal hormone replacement therapy and endometrial cancer. Am J Epidemiol 164(8):775, 2006

Suh-Burgmann E, Hung YY, Armstrong MA: Complex atypical endometrial hyperplasia: the risk of unrecognized adenocarcinoma and value of preoperative dilation and curettage. Obstet Gynecol 114(3):523, 2009

Suriano KA, McHale M, McLaren CE, et al: Estrogen replacement therapy in endometrial cancer patients: a matched control study. Obstet Gynecol 97(4):555, 2001

Tao MH, Xu WH, Zheng W, et al: Oral contraceptive and IUD use and endometrial cancer: a population-based case-control study in Shanghai, China. Int J Cancer 119(9):2142, 2006

Terakawa N, Kigawa J, Taketani Y, et al: The behavior of endometrial hyperplasia: a prospective study. Endometrial Hyperplasia Study Group. J Obstet Gynaecol Res 23(3):223, 1997

Thai TH, Du F, Tsan JT, et al: Mutations in the BRCA1-associated ring domain (BARD1) gene in primary breast, ovarian and uterine cancers. Hum Mol Genet 7(2):195, 1998

Thigpen JT, Brady MF, Alvarez RD, et al: Oral medroxyprogesterone acetate in the treatment of advanced or recurrent endometrial carcinoma: a dose-response study by the Gynecologic Oncology Group. J Clin Oncol 17(6):1736, 1999

Todo Y, Kato H, Kaneuchi M, et al: Survival effect of para-aortic lymphadenectomy in endometrial cancer (SEPAL study): a retrospective cohort analysis. Lancet 375(9721):1165, 2010

Trimble CL, Kauderer J, Zaino R, et al: Concurrent endometrial carcinoma in women with a biopsy diagnosis of atypical endometrial hyperplasia: a Gynecologic Oncology Group study. Cancer 106(4):812, 2006

Trimble CL, Method M, Leitao M, et al: Management of endometrial precancers. Obstet Gynecol 120(5):1160, 2012

van Leeuwen FE, Benraadt J, Coebergh JW, et al: Risk of endometrial cancer after tamoxifen treatment of breast cancer. Lancet 343(8895):448, 1994

Varras M, Kioses E: Five-year survival of a patient with primary endometrial squamous cell carcinoma: a case report and review of the literature. Eur J Gynaecol Oncol 23(4):327, 2002

Vasen HF, Watson P, Mecklin JP, et al: New clinical criteria for hereditary nonpolyposis colorectal cancer (HNPCC, Lynch syndrome) proposed by the International Collaborative Group on HNPCC. Gastroenterology 116(6):1453, 1999

Viswanathan AN, Feskanich D, De Vivo I, et al: Smoking and the risk of endometrial cancer: results from the Nurses' Health Study. Int J Cancer 114(6):996, 2005

Vorgias G, Hintipas E, Katsoulis M, et al: Intraoperative gross examination of myometrial invasion and cervical infiltration in patients with endometrial cancer: decision-making accuracy. Gynecol Oncol 85(3):483, 2002

Walker JL, Piedmonte MR, Spirtos, NM, et al: Laparoscopy compared with laparotomy for comprehensive surgical staging of uterine cancer: Gynecologic Oncology Group Study (LAP2). J Clin Oncol 27(32):5331, 2009

Walker JL, Piedmonte MR, Spirtos NM, et al: Recurrence and survival after random assignment to laparoscopy versus laparotomy for comprehensive surgical staging of uterine cancer: Gynecologic Oncology Group LAP2 Study. J Clin Oncol 30(7):695, 2012

Wang CB, Wang CJ, Huang HJ, et al: Fertility-preserving treatment in young patients with endometrial adenocarcinoma. Cancer 94(8):2192, 2002

Wernli KJ, Ray RM, Gao DL, et al: Menstrual and reproductive factors in relation to risk of endometrial cancer in Chinese women. Cancer Causes Control 17(7):949, 2006

Whitney CW, Brunetto VL, Zaino RJ, et al: Phase II study of medroxyprogesterone acetate plus tamoxifen in advanced endometrial carcinoma: a Gynecologic Oncology Group study. Gynecol Oncol 92(1):4, 2004

Yang YC, Wu CC, Chen CP, et al: Reevaluating the safety of fertility-sparing hormonal therapy for early endometrial cancer. Gynecol Oncol 99(2):287, 2005

Zaino RJ, Kauderer J, Trimble CL, et al: Reproducibility of the diagnosis of atypical endometrial hyperplasia: a Gynecologic Oncology Group study. Cancer 106(4):804, 2006

Zaino RJ, Kurman RJ, Diana KL, et al: The utility of the revised International Federation of Gynecology and Obstetrics histologic grading of endometrial adenocarcinoma using a defined nuclear grading system. A Gynecologic Oncology Group study. Cancer 75(1):81, 1995

Zaino RJ, Silverberg SG, Norris HJ, et al: The prognostic value of nuclear versus architectural grading in endometrial adenocarcinoma: a Gynecologic Oncology Group study. Int J Gynecol Pathol 13(1):29, 1994

Zerbe MJ, Zhang J, Bristow RE, et al: Retrograde seeding of malignant cells during hysteroscopy in presumed early endometrial cancer. Gynecol Oncol 79(1):55, 2000

Zullo F, Palomba S, Falbo A, et al: Laparoscopic surgery vs laparotomy for early stage endometrial cancer: long-term data of a randomized controlled trial. Am J Obstet Gynecol 200(3):296.e1, 2009

CHAPTER 34

Uterine Sarcoma

Malignant tumors of the uterine corpus are broadly divided into three main types: carcinomas, sarcomas, and carcinosarcomas. Although the latter two categories are rarely encountered, they tend to behave more aggressively and contribute to a disproportionately higher number of uterine cancer deaths. Pure sarcomas differentiate toward smooth muscle (leiomyosarcoma) or toward endometrial stroma (endometrial stromal tumors). Carcinosarcomas are mixed tumors demonstrating both epithelial and stromal components. These have also been known as malignant mixed müllerian tumor (MMMT). In general, uterine sarcomas and carcinosarcomas grow quickly, lymphatic or hematogenous spread occurs early, and the overall prognosis is poor. However, there are several notable exceptions among these tumors.

EPIDEMIOLOGY AND RISK FACTORS

Sarcomas account for approximately 3 to 8 percent of all malignancies of the uterine corpus (Brooks, 2004; D'Angelo, 2010; Major, 1993). Historically, uterine sarcomas included carcinosarcomas, accounting for 40 percent of cases; leiomyosarcomas, 40 percent; endometrial stromal sarcomas, 10 to 15 percent; and undifferentiated sarcomas, 5 to 10 percent. In 2009, the International Federation of Gynecology and Obstetrics (FIGO) reclassified carcinosarcomas as a metaplastic form of endometrial carcinoma. Despite this, carcinosarcomas are still commonly included in most retrospective studies of uterine sarcomas and in the 2014 World Health Organization (WHO) classification (Greer, 2015; Kurman, 2014; McCluggage, 2002).

Because of their infrequency, uterine sarcomas and carcinosarcomas have few identified risk factors. These include chronic excess estrogen exposure, tamoxifen use, African American race, and prior pelvic radiation. In contrast, combination oral contraceptive pill use and smoking appear to lower risks for some of these tumors (Felix, 2013).

PATHOGENESIS

Leiomyosarcomas have a monoclonal origin, and although commonly believed to arise from benign leiomyomas, for the most part they do not. Instead, they appear to develop de novo as solitary lesions (Zhang, 2006). Supporting this theory, leiomyosarcomas have molecular pathways distinct from those of leiomyomas or normal myometrium (Quade, 2004; Skubitz, 2003). They are, however, often found in proximity to leiomyomas.

Endometrial stromal tumors (ESS) have heterogeneous chromosomal aberrations (Halbwedl, 2005). However, the pattern of rearrangements is clearly nonrandom, and chromosomal arms 6p and 7p are frequently involved (Micci, 2006). Translocations involving several chromosomes and the resultant fusion proteins are thought to be involved in ESS pathogenesis (Lee, 2012; Panagopoulos, 2012).

Uterine carcinosarcomas are monoclonal, biphasic neoplasms. Namely, they are composed of separate but admixed malignant epithelial and malignant stromal elements (D'Angelo, 2010; Wada, 1997). Both the carcinoma and sarcoma components are thought to arise from a common epithelial progenitor cell. Acquisition of any number of genetic mutations, including defects in *p53* and DNA mismatch repair genes, may be sufficient to trigger tumorigenesis (Liu, 1994). These early molecular defects will be shared by both components as the tumor undergoes divergent carcinomatous and sarcomatous differentiation. Thereafter, acquired molecular defects will be discordant between the two components (Taylor, 2006). This genetic progression and subsequent diversion parallels the varying phenotypes observed in these tumors (Fujii, 2000).

DIAGNOSIS

■ Signs and Symptoms

As in endometrial cancer, abnormal vaginal bleeding is the most frequent symptom for uterine sarcomas and carcinosarcomas (Gonzalez-Bosquet, 1997). Pelvic or abdominal pain is also common. Up to one third of women will describe significant discomfort that may result from passage of clots, rapid uterine enlargement, or prolapse of a sarcomatous polyp through

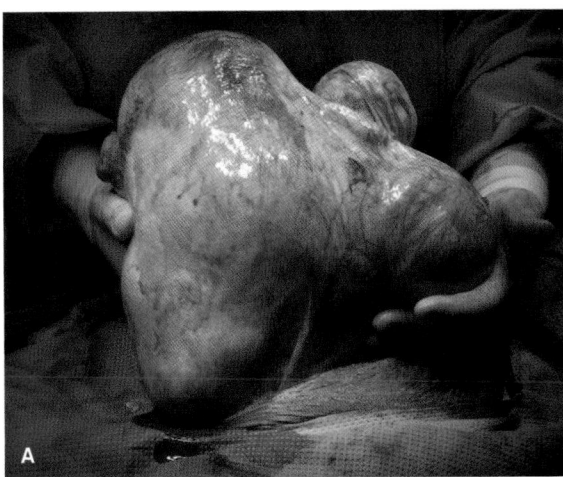 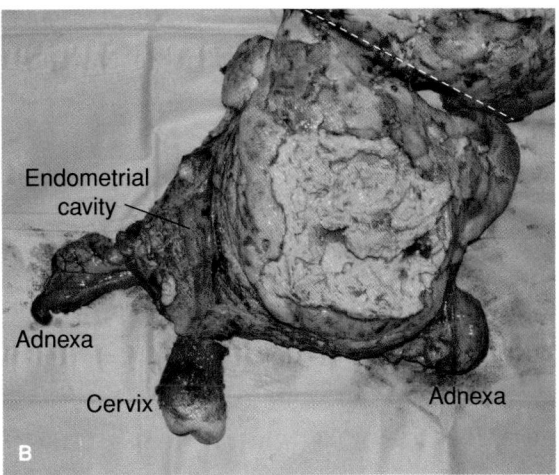

FIGURE 34-1 Leiomyosarcoma. **A.** Intraoperative photograph of an enlarged uterus before hysterectomy. **B.** Surgical specimen has been bisected and remains joined at the fundus. The other half of the specimen lies above the white dashed line and out of view. The large tumor lies to the right of the endometrial cavity. It has central necrosis seen as yellow amorphous debris with the tumor borders. (Used with permission from Dr. Martha Rac.)

an effaced cervix (De Fusco, 1989). In addition, a profuse, foul-smelling discharge may be obvious, and gastrointestinal and genitourinary complaints are also frequent. Importantly, degenerating leiomyomas with necrosis can mimic these same signs and symptoms.

With rapid growth, a uterus may extend out of the pelvis into the mid- or upper abdomen (Fig. 34-1). Fortunately, the incidence of malignancy in such cases is low (<0.5 percent), and in most instances, benign enlarging leiomyomas are found (Leibsohn, 1990; Parker, 1994). Although uterine leiomyosarcomas do tend to grow quickly, no criteria define what constitutes significant growth. Despite these often-dramatic presentations, many women with uterine sarcoma and carcinosarcoma will have few symptoms other than abnormal vaginal bleeding and a seemingly normal uterus on physical examination.

▧ Endometrial Sampling

The sensitivity of an office endometrial biopsy or dilatation and curettage (D & C) to detect sarcomatous elements is lower than that for endometrial carcinomas. Specifically, with leiomyosarcoma, symptomatic women receive a correct preoperative diagnosis in only 25 to 50 percent of cases. This inability to accurately sample the tumor is probably related to the origin of these neoplasms in the myometrium rather than the endometrium. Similarly, endometrial stromal nodules and endometrial stromal sarcomas may be undetectable by Pipelle biopsy, especially if the neoplasm is intramural (Yang, 2002). With carcinosarcoma, sampling will more often lead to a correct diagnosis, although in many cases only the carcinomatous features are evident. The reverse is also true, and occasionally a uterine carcinosarcoma is suspected based on endometrial biopsy findings, but no sarcomatous features are found within the hysterectomy specimen.

▧ Laboratory Testing

Elevated preoperative serum cancer antigen 125 (CA125) levels may indicate extrauterine disease and deep myometrial invasion in patients with carcinosarcoma. After surgery, CA125

measurement may be a somewhat useful marker to monitor disease response (Huang, 2007).

▧ Imaging Studies

Imaging studies are often helpful if sarcoma is diagnosed before hysterectomy. In most cases, a computed tomography (CT) scan of the abdomen and pelvis is routinely performed. This serves at least two purposes. First, sarcomas often violate normal soft tissue planes in the pelvis, and therefore, unresectable tumors may be identified preoperatively. Second, extrauterine metastases may be found. In either case, treatment may be altered based on radiographic findings.

If a diagnosis is still in question, magnetic resonance (MR) imaging helps distinguish uterine sarcoma from a benign "mimic" (Kido, 2003). As a diagnostic tool for sarcoma, sonography is far less helpful. Positron emission tomography (PET) scanning is most effective in the setting of recurrent uterine sarcoma but offers little advantage compared with CT or MR imaging (Sharma, 2012).

▧ Role of the Generalist

Preoperative consultation with a gynecologic oncologist is recommended for any patient with a biopsy suggesting uterine sarcoma or carcinosarcoma. The potential for intraabdominal metastases and disruption of tissue planes within the pelvis increases the technical difficulty and surgical risks. The approach to staging is subtly dissimilar to that of endometrial carcinomas. For example, due to the low rate of metastasis, only sampling nodes suspicious for leiomyosarcomas may be appropriate instead of performing complete pelvic and paraaortic lymphadenectomy (Leitao, 2003; Major, 1993). Moreover, ovarian preservation may be suitable with certain sarcomas because of their low risk for spread to the adnexa (Kapp, 2008; Li, 2005). In general, a treatment plan is best organized preoperatively, if possible.

Many uterine sarcomas and carcinosarcomas are not diagnosed until surgery or several days later when a pathology report is available. As a result, unstaged cases are common, and a gynecologic oncologist is consulted at the earliest feasible time. If the diagnosis is made postoperatively, the criteria to recommend surveillance only, reoperation, or radiotherapy vary widely and depend on the sarcoma type and other clinical circumstances. Generally, these options are less straightforward than in typical endometrial carcinomas, largely due to the rarity of these tumors and the comparatively limited data supporting one strategy over another.

With adoption of minimally invasive surgery (MIS), gynecologists are faced with uterine or myoma extraction through small incisions. Tissue fragmentation using power morcellation is one approach, but morcellation and dispersion of uterine or cervical cancers are concerns. In general, encountering unexpected sarcoma during surgery for presumed benign disease is rare, and rates range from 0.09 to 0.6 percent (Lieng, 2015; Lin, 2015). These investigators also found no clear preoperative risk factors. However, if a patient undergoes inadvertent morcellation and dispersion of an occult sarcoma, it may worsen her prognosis (Perri, 2009). In 2014, the Food and Drug Administration warned that power morcellator use should be curtailed in patients who are peri- or postmenopausal or who are candidates for en bloc removal through the vagina or a minilaparotomy. Moreover, if uncontained intraperitoneal morcellation is selected, patients should be aware of the risks that it poses.

PATHOLOGY

Uterine mesenchymal tumors are classified broadly into pure and mixed tumors (Table 34-1). Also, the term *homologous* denotes tissues normally found in the uterus and *heterologous* refers to tissue foreign to the uterus. Pure sarcomas are virtually all homologous and differentiate into mesenchymal tissue that is normally present within the uterus, such as smooth muscle (leiomyosarcoma) or stromal tissue within the endometrium (endometrial stromal tumors). Pure heterologous sarcomas, such as chondrosarcoma, are rare.

Mixed sarcomas contain a malignant mesenchymal component admixed with an epithelial element. If the epithelial element is also malignant, the tumor is termed *carcinosarcoma*. If the epithelial element is benign, the term *adenosarcoma* is used. Carcinosarcomas can be either homologous or heterologous, reflecting the pluripotentiality of the uterine primordium.

■ Leiomyosarcoma

Leiomyosarcomas account for 1 to 2 percent of all uterine malignancies. In a Surveillance, Epidemiology, and End Results (SEER) database study of 1396 patients, the median age at presentation was 52 years. Most tumors (68 percent) were stage I at the time of diagnosis, and stage II (3 percent), stage III (7 percent), and stage IV cancer (22 percent) formed the remainder (Kapp, 2008).

The histologic criteria for diagnosing leiomyosarcoma are somewhat controversial but include the frequency of mitotic figures, extent of nuclear atypia, and presence of coagulative tumor cell necrosis (Fig. 34-2). In reading Table 34-2, each row illustrates combinations of histologic findings that may be found in leiomyosarcomas. In most cases, the mitotic index exceeds 15 mitotic figures total when 10 high-power fields are examined, moderate to severe cytologic atypia is seen, and tumor cell

TABLE 34-1. World Health Organization Histological Classification of Mesenchymal Tumors of the Uterus

Mesenchymal tumors
Leiomyoma
  Cellular leiomyoma
  Leiomyoma with bizarre nuclei
  Mitotically active leiomyoma
  Hydropic leiomyoma
  Apoplectic leiomyoma
  Lipomatous leiomyoma (lipoleiomyoma)
  Epithelioid leiomyoma
  Myxoid leiomyoma
  Dissecting (cotyledonoid) leiomyoma
  Diffuse leiomyomatosis
  Intravenous leiomyomatosis
  Metastasizing leiomyoma
Smooth muscle tumor of uncertain malignant potential
Leiomyosarcoma
  Epithelial leiomyosarcoma
  Myxoid leiomyosarcoma
Endometrial stromal and related tumors
  Endometrial stromal nodule
  Low grade endometrial stromal sarcoma
  High grade endometrial stromal sarcoma
  Undifferentiated endometrial sarcoma
  Uterine tumor resembling ovarian sex cord tumor
Miscellaneous mesenchymal tumors
  Rhabdomyosarcoma
  Perivascular epithelioid cell tumor
    Benign
    Malignant
Others

Mixed epithelial and mesenchymal tumors
Adenomyoma
Atypical polypoid adenomyoma
Adenofibroma
Adenosarcoma
Carcinosarcoma (malignant müllerian mixed tumor, metaplastic carcinoma)

Adapted with permission from Kurman RJ, Carcangiu ML, Herrington CS, et al (eds): WHO Classification of Tumours of Female Reproductive Organs, 4th ed. Lyon, International Agency for Research on Cancer, 2014.

necrosis is prominent (Hendrickson, 2003; Zaloudek, 2011). Occasionally, a leiomyosarcoma will be reported as low-, intermediate-, or high-grade, but the overall utility of grading is controversial, and no universally accepted grading system exists.

■ Smooth Muscle Tumor of Uncertain Malignant Potential (STUMP)

Tumors that show some worrisome histologic features, such as necrosis or nuclear atypia, but that cannot be diagnosed reliably as benign or malignant based on generally applied criteria fall into this category. The diagnosis should be used sparingly and

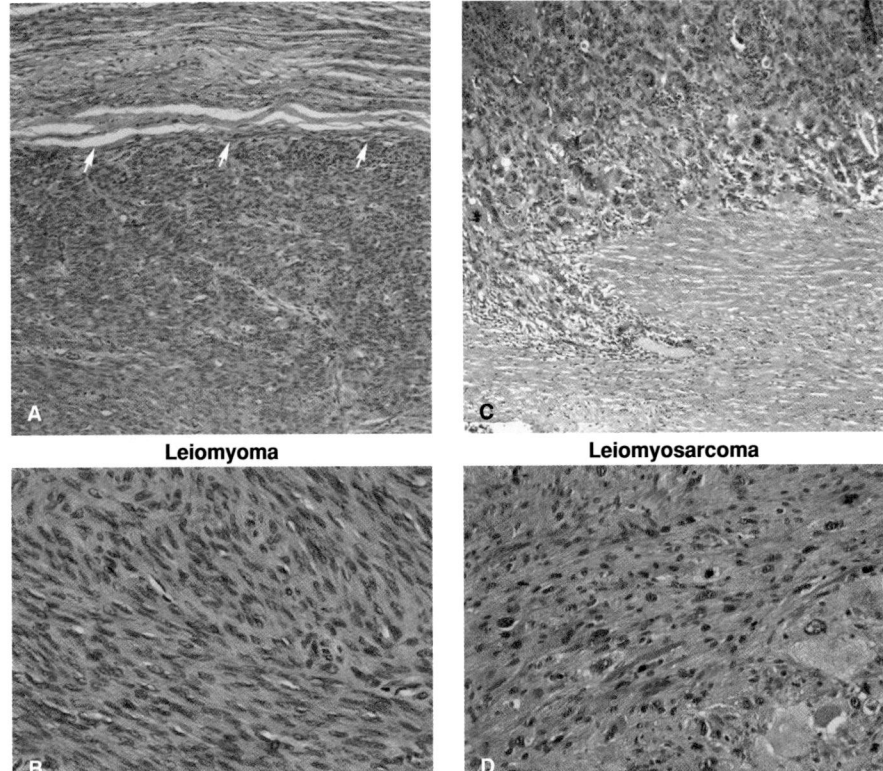

Leiomyoma

Leiomyosarcoma

FIGURE 34-2 Leiomyoma (**A, B**) and leiomyosarcoma (**C, D**). A. Leiomyomas tend to be well-circumscribed masses. This leiomyoma shows a well-demarcated interface (*arrows*) with the less cellular myometrium above it. B. Although leiomyomas may have variable histologic features, most are composed of bland spindled cells with blunt-ended nuclei and limited mitotic activity. C. Leiomyosarcoma is a malignant smooth muscle neoplasm that may differ markedly in its microscopic appearance from case to case. Generally, leiomyosarcoma shows some combination of coagulative tumor necrosis, increased mitotic activity, and/or nuclear atypia. This example has marked nuclear atypia and pleomorphism and an infiltrative growth pattern at its periphery. This differs from the usually smooth, pushing border of typical leiomyomas. D. This particular example has moderate to marked nuclear atypia. (Used with permission from Drs. Kelley Carrick and Raheela Ashfaq.)

of all uterine sarcomas. In a SEER database study of 831 patients, the median age at diagnosis was 52 years (Chan, 2008). Although constituting a wide morphologic spectrum, endometrial stromal tumors are composed exclusively of cells that resemble the endometrial stroma, and this category includes both benign stromal nodules and malignant stromal tumors (see Table 34-1).

Historically, there has been controversy in subdividing these tumors. The division of endometrial stromal sarcomas into low-grade and high-grade categories has fallen out of favor. In its place, the designation *endometrial stromal sarcoma* is now best restricted to neoplasms that were formerly referred to as low-grade. Alternatively, the term *high-grade undifferentiated sarcoma* is believed to more accurately reflect those tumors without recognizable evidence of a definite endometrial stromal phenotype. These lesions are almost invariably high grade and often resemble the mesenchymal component of a uterine carcinosarcoma (Oliva, 2000). In this revised classification, the distinctions are not determined by mitotic count but by features such as nuclear pleomorphism and necrosis (Evans, 1982; Hendrickson, 2003).

Endometrial Stromal Nodule

Representing less than a quarter of tumors in the endometrial stromal tumor group, these rare nodules are benign, characterized by a well-delineated margin, and composed of neoplastic cells that resemble proliferative-phase endometrial stromal cells. Grossly, the tumor is a solitary, round or oval, fleshy nodule measuring a few centimeters. Histologically, they are distinguished from endometrial stromal sarcomas by their lack of myometrial infiltration (Dionigi, 2002). Because these nodules are benign, myomectomy is an appropriate option. However, because differentiation between endometrial stromal sarcoma and this benign lesion cannot be determined clinically, it is important to remove the entire nodule. Thus, for large lesions, hysterectomy may be required (Hendrickson, 2003).

is reserved for smooth muscle neoplasms whose appearance is ambiguous (Hendrickson, 2003).

■ Endometrial Stromal Tumors

Significantly less common than leiomyosarcomas, the group of endometrial stromal tumors comprise fewer than 10 percent

TABLE 34-2. Diagnostic Criteria for Uterine Leiomyosarcoma

Coagulative Tumor Cell Necrosis	Mitotic Index[a]	Degree of Atypia
Present	≥10 MF/10 HPF	None
Present	Any	Diffuse, significant
Absent	≥10 MF/10 HPF	Diffuse, significant

[a]MF/10 HPF = the total number of mitotic figures (MF) counted when 10 high-powered fields (HPF) are examined. Adapted with pemission from Tavassoli FA, Devilee P (eds): World Health Organization Classification of Tumours. World Health Organization, 2003.

Endometrial Stromal Sarcoma

The precise frequency of these tumors is difficult to estimate because they are excluded from some reports and included in others, and the terminology used has been inconsistent. In general, endometrial stromal sarcomas (formerly called low grade) are thought to be the most frequently encountered stromal tumor variant and are twice as common as high-grade undifferentiated sarcomas.

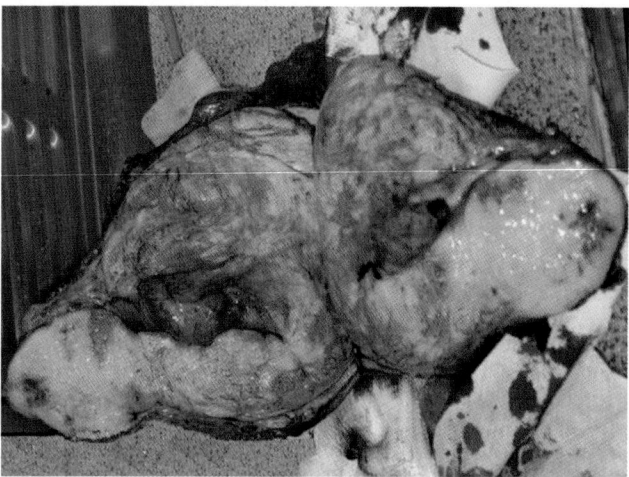

FIGURE 34-3 Endometrial stromal sarcoma. The surgical specimen has been bisected and remains joined at the fundus.

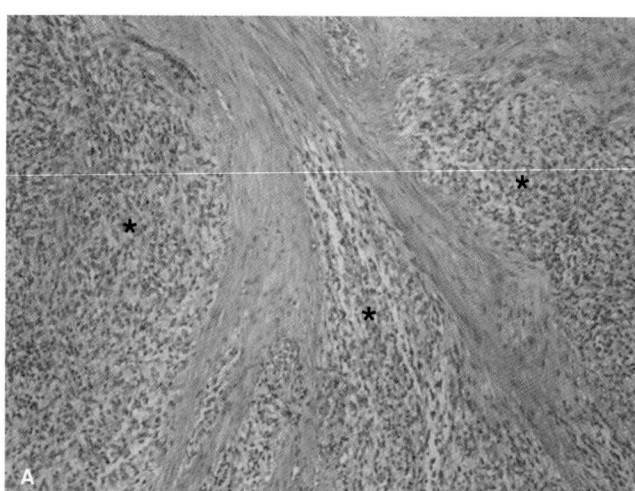

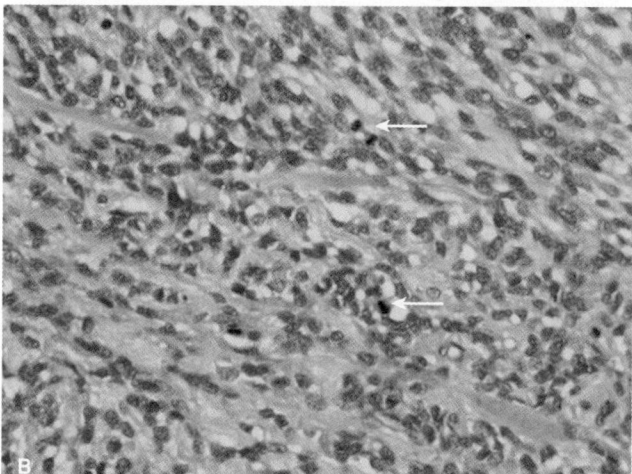

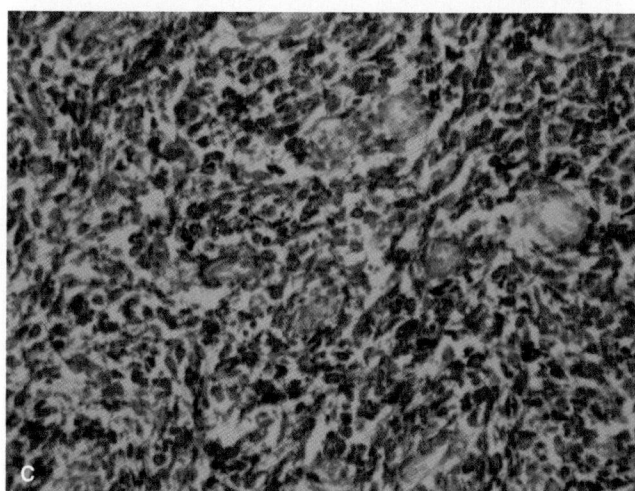

Typically, they extensively invade the myometrium and extend to the serosa in approximately half of cases (Fig. 34-3). Less often, they present as a solitary well-delineated, predominantly intramural mass that is difficult to grossly distinguish from an endometrial stromal nodule. Microscopically, endometrial stromal sarcomas resemble the stromal cells of proliferative-phase endometrium (Fig. 34-4).

Metastases are rarely detected prior to the diagnosis of the primary lesion. However, permeation of the lymphatic and vascular channels is characteristic. In up to one third of cases, extrauterine extension is present, often appearing as "worm-like" plugs of tumor within the vessels of the broad ligament and adnexa. At operation, this may resemble intravenous leiomyomatosis or a broad ligament leiomyoma, both described in Chapter 9 (p. 204). Frozen section analysis can usually make the distinction.

High-grade Undifferentiated Sarcoma

Compared with endometrial stromal sarcomas, these tumors tend to be larger and more polypoid, often filling the uterine cavity. Instead of an infiltrating pattern, high-grade undifferentiated sarcomas displace the myometrium more destructively, leading to prominent hemorrhage and necrosis.

Microscopically, the cells are larger and more pleomorphic. The presence of marked cellular atypia is characteristic. Typically, there are more than 10 mitoses per 10 high-power fields, but frequently there are more than 20 in the most active areas. These tumors lack specific differentiation and bear no histologic resemblance to endometrial stroma (Hendrickson, 2003; Zaloudek, 2011).

■ Carcinosarcoma

Accumulating clinical and pathologic evidence suggests that carcinosarcomas actually represent endometrial carcinomas that have undergone clonal evolution, resulting in the acquisition of sarcomatous features. In principle, these tumors are metaplastic carcinomas. Clinically, their pattern of spread more closely mirrors that of aggressive endometrial carcinomas than that of

FIGURE 34-4 Endometrial stromal sarcoma (ESS), same patient as in Figure 34-3. **A.** ESS is composed of cells morphologically similar to proliferative phase endometrial stromal cells. In this low-power view that involved the corpus and cervix, irregular tongues of tumor (*asterisks*) are seen dissecting into the cervical stroma. **B.** The tumor cells are spindled and relatively bland, similar to normal endometrial proliferative phase stroma. Two mitoses are identified in this single medium-power field (*white arrows*). **C.** Endometrial stroma marks positively with CD10, as does ESS. A battery of immunostains, including CD10, may be used to help distinguish ESS from other spindle cell neoplasms. (Used with permission from Dr. Kelley Carrick.)

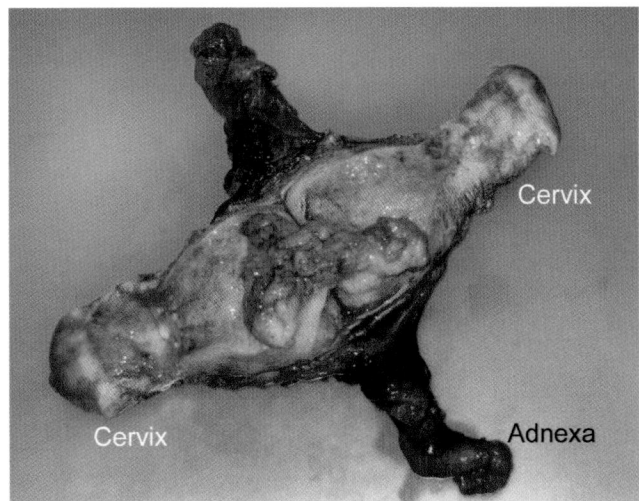

FIGURE 34-5 Carcinosarcoma. Photograph of the surgical specimen after it has been bisected and remains joined at the fundus.

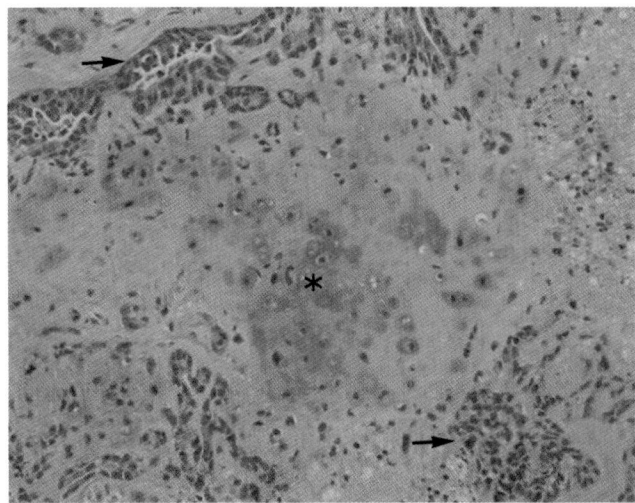

FIGURE 34-7 Carcinosarcoma with heterologous elements. In this carcinosarcoma with cartilaginous differentiation, malignant glands are present at the periphery (*arrows*). Centrally is a focus of malignant cartilage (*asterisk*), with its characteristic lacunae embedded within a bluish chondroid matrix. (Used with permission from Dr. Kelley Carrick.)

sarcomas. In addition, metastases usually show carcinomatous elements, with or without sarcomatous differentiation.

However, by convention, carcinosarcomas are usually grouped with uterine sarcomas, accounting for 2 to 3 percent of all uterine malignancies. Patients are often older, having an average age of 65 years. Fewer than 5 percent are diagnosed in women younger than 50. At the time of diagnosis, most cancers (40 percent) are stage I. Stage II (10 percent), stage III (25 percent), and stage IV disease (25 percent) make up the remainder (Sartori, 1997; Vaidya, 2006).

Grossly, the tumor is sessile or polypoid, bulky, necrotic, and often hemorrhagic (Fig. 34-5). It often fills the endometrial cavity and deeply invades the myometrium. On occasion, a large tumor protrudes through the external cervical os and fills the vaginal vault.

Microscopically, carcinosarcomas have an admixture of epithelial and mesenchymal differentiation. The malignant epithelial element is typically an adenocarcinoma of endometrioid type, but serous, clear cell, mucinous, squamous cell, and undifferentiated carcinoma are also common (Fig. 34-6). Mesenchymal components can be homologous, usually resembling endometrial stromal sarcomas or fibrosarcomas. Alternatively, heterologous mesenchymal differentiation can be found in association with areas of endometrial stromal or undifferentiated sarcomas. Most commonly, rhabdomyosarcoma or chondrosarcoma compose these cases of heterologous mesenchymal differentiation (Fig. 34-7). Although interesting,

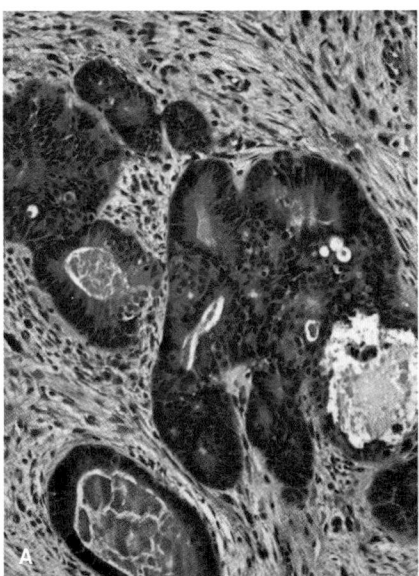

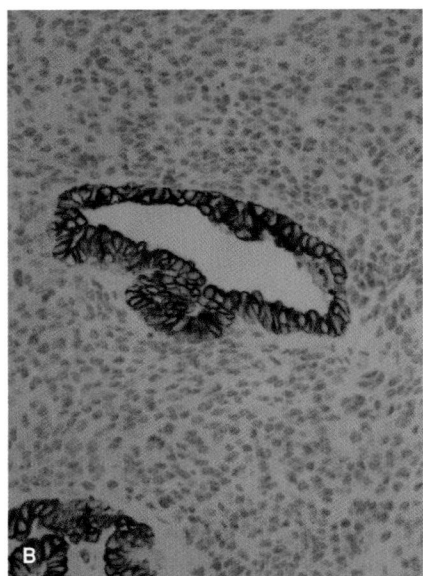

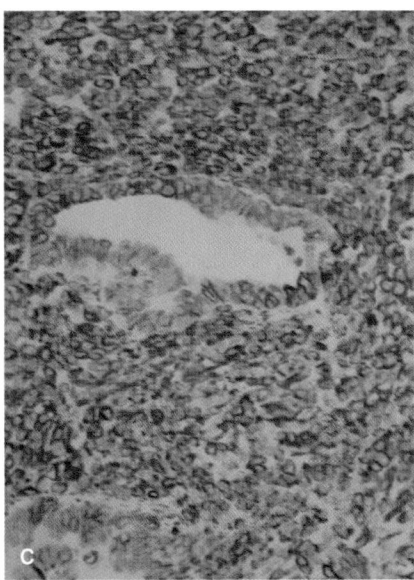

FIGURE 34-6 A. Carcinosarcoma is a biphasic malignant neoplasm composed of both carcinomatous and sarcomatous elements. In this example, malignant endometrioid-type glands are present within an atypical spindled stroma. **B.** Immunohistochemical stain for cytokeratin marks the epithelial component but not the stromal component. **C.** Conversely, an immunohistochemical stain for vimentin (a mesenchymal marker) stains the sarcomatous component. (Used with permission from Dr. Raheela Ashfaq.)

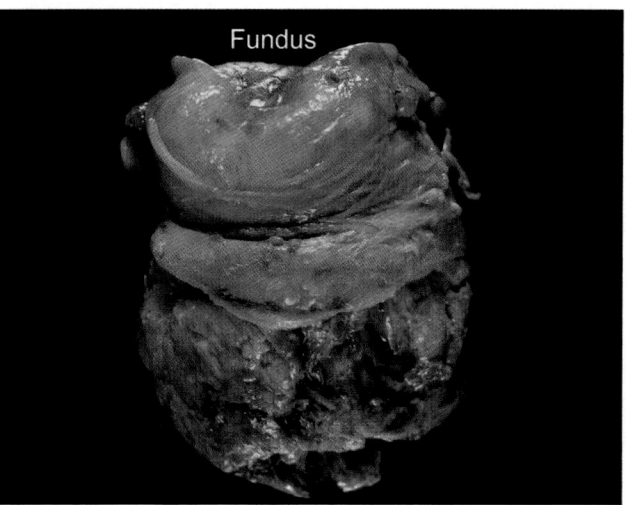

FIGURE 34-8 Gross uterine specimen with adenosarcoma.

there is no clinical importance to designating a uterine carcinosarcoma as homologous or heterologous (McCluggage, 2003).

■ Adenosarcoma

This rare, biphasic neoplasm is characterized by a benign epithelial component and a sarcomatous mesenchymal component. Tumors may develop in women of all ages. Grossly, adenosarcomas grow as exophytic polypoid masses that extend into the uterine cavity (Fig. 34-8). Rarely, they may arise in the myometrium, presumably from adenomyosis. Microscopically, isolated glands are dispersed throughout the mesenchymal component and are often dilated or compressed into thin slits (Fig. 34-9). Typically, the mesenchymal component resembles an endometrial stromal sarcoma or fibrosarcoma and contains varying amounts of fibrous tissue and smooth muscle. In general, these are considered low-grade tumors with mild atypia and relatively few mitotic figures. However, 10 percent have a more malignant behavior due to one-sided proliferation of the sarcomatous, often high-grade, component. These adenosarcomas are designated as having "sarcomatous overgrowth," and patients have a poor prognosis, similar to that of carcinosarcomas (Krivak, 2001; McCluggage, 2003).

PATTERNS OF SPREAD

Uterine sarcomas generally fall into two categories of malignant behavior. Leiomyosarcomas, high-grade undifferentiated sarcomas, and carcinosarcomas are consistently characterized by an aggressive growth pattern and rapid disease progression despite treatment. In contrast, endometrial stromal sarcomas and adenosarcomas have an indolent growth pattern with long disease-free intervals. All of these tumors invade, to some degree, by direct extension.

Leiomyosarcomas have a propensity for hematogenous dissemination. Lung metastases are particularly common, and more than half of patients will have distant spread if diagnosed with recurrent disease. To a lesser extent, leiomyosarcomas metastasize via lymphatic channels (Leitao, 2003). In a clinicopathologic Gynecologic Oncology Group (GOG) study, fewer than 5 percent of clinical stage I and II patients had nodal involvement (Major, 1993).

The opposite is true for carcinosarcomas, in which one third of patients with clinically stage I tumors will have nodal metastases (Park, 2010). Thus, comprehensive pelvic and paraaortic lymphadenectomy is particularly important (Temkin, 2007). Extraabdominal spread is less common, and most recurrences are found in the pelvis or abdomen.

STAGING

Uterine sarcomas are surgically staged. Formerly, most clinicians used the FIGO surgical staging system for endometrial cancer to stage uterine sarcomas. However, beginning in 2009, only carcinosarcomas share the same staging criteria as endometrial carcinomas (Table 33-9, p. 713). Endometrial

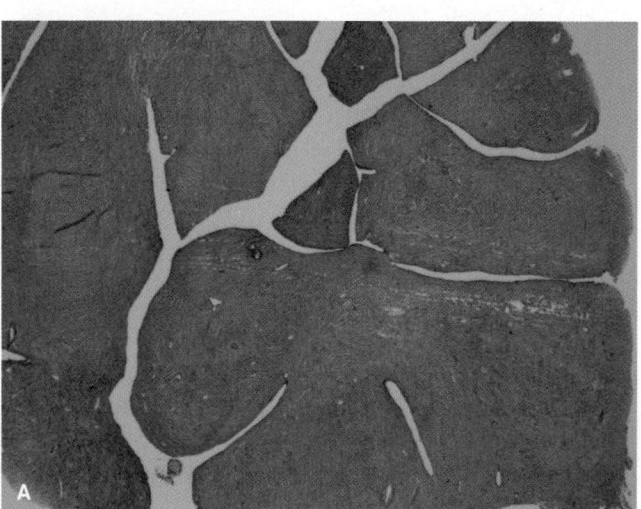
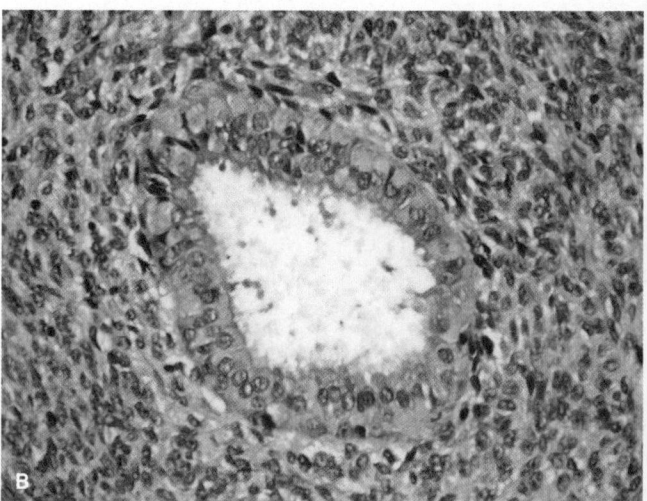

FIGURE 34-9 Adenosarcoma. **A.** A broad-based villous architecture is seen typically. **B.** Normal endometrial glands are surrounded by a cellular stroma consisting of a low-grade sarcoma. In this case, an endometrial stromal sarcoma is the sarcoma component. (Used with permission from Dr. Raheela Ashfaq.)

TABLE 34-3. FIGO Staging for Uterine Sarcomas (Leiomyosarcomas, Endometrial Stromal Sarcomas, Adenosarcomas, and Carcinosarcomas)

Stage	Characteristics
Leiomyosarcomas	
I	**Tumor limited to uterus**
IA	<5 cm
IB	>5 cm
II	**Tumor extends to the pelvis**
IIA	Adnexal involvement
IIB	Tumor extends to extrauterine pelvic tissue
III	**Tumor invades abdominal tissues (not just protruding into the abdomen)**
IIIA	One site
IIIB	>One site
IIIC	Metastasis to pelvic and/or paraaortic lymph nodes
IV	
IVA	Tumor invades bladder and/or rectum
IVB	Distant metastasis
Adenosarcomas and endometrial stromal sarcomas[a]	
I	**Tumor limited to uterus**
IA	Tumor limited to endometrium/endocervix with no myometrial invasion
IB	Less than or equal to half myometrial invasion
IC	More than half myometrial invasion
II	**Tumor extends to the pelvis**
IIA	Adnexal involvement
IIB	Tumor extends to extrauterine pelvic tissue
III	**Tumor invades abdominal tissues (not just protruding into the abdomen)**
IIIA	One site
IIIB	>One site
IIIC	Metastasis to pelvic and/or paraaortic lymph nodes
IV	
IVA	Tumor invades bladder and/or rectum
IVB	Distant metastasis

Carcinosarcomas
Carcinosarcomas should be staged as carcinomas of the endometrium (Table 33-9, p. 713).

[a]Note: Simultaneous tumors of the uterine corpus and ovary/pelvis in association with ovarian/pelvic endometriosis should be classified as independent primary tumors.
FIGO = International Federation of Gynecology and Obstetrics.

stromal sarcomas and adenosarcomas share new criteria, whereas leiomyosarcomas have a different system for stage I (Table 34-3 and Fig. 34-10).

TREATMENT OF EARLY-STAGE DISEASE (STAGES I AND II)

■ Surgery

The highest chance of cure is achieved by complete surgical resection of a sarcoma that is confined to the uterus. In general, laparotomy is performed due to the typical features of sarcomas, which include uterine enlargement, parametrial extension,

and tumor metastasis. Laparoscopic or vaginal approaches have not yet been shown to yield equivalent outcomes.

The staging laparotomy described for endometrial cancer in Chapter 33 (p. 713) can be revised to incorporate the unique spread patterns of uterine sarcomas. For instance, peritoneal washings may be easily obtained upon opening the abdomen but are not part of the staging system and have limited value (Kanbour, 1989). Exploration is particularly important to assess the abdomen for unresectable or widely metastatic disease that might indicate a need to abort the procedure. As in endometrial carcinomas, some evidence shows benefit from aggressive cytoreductive surgery (Dinh, 2004; Leath, 2007; Thomas, 2009).

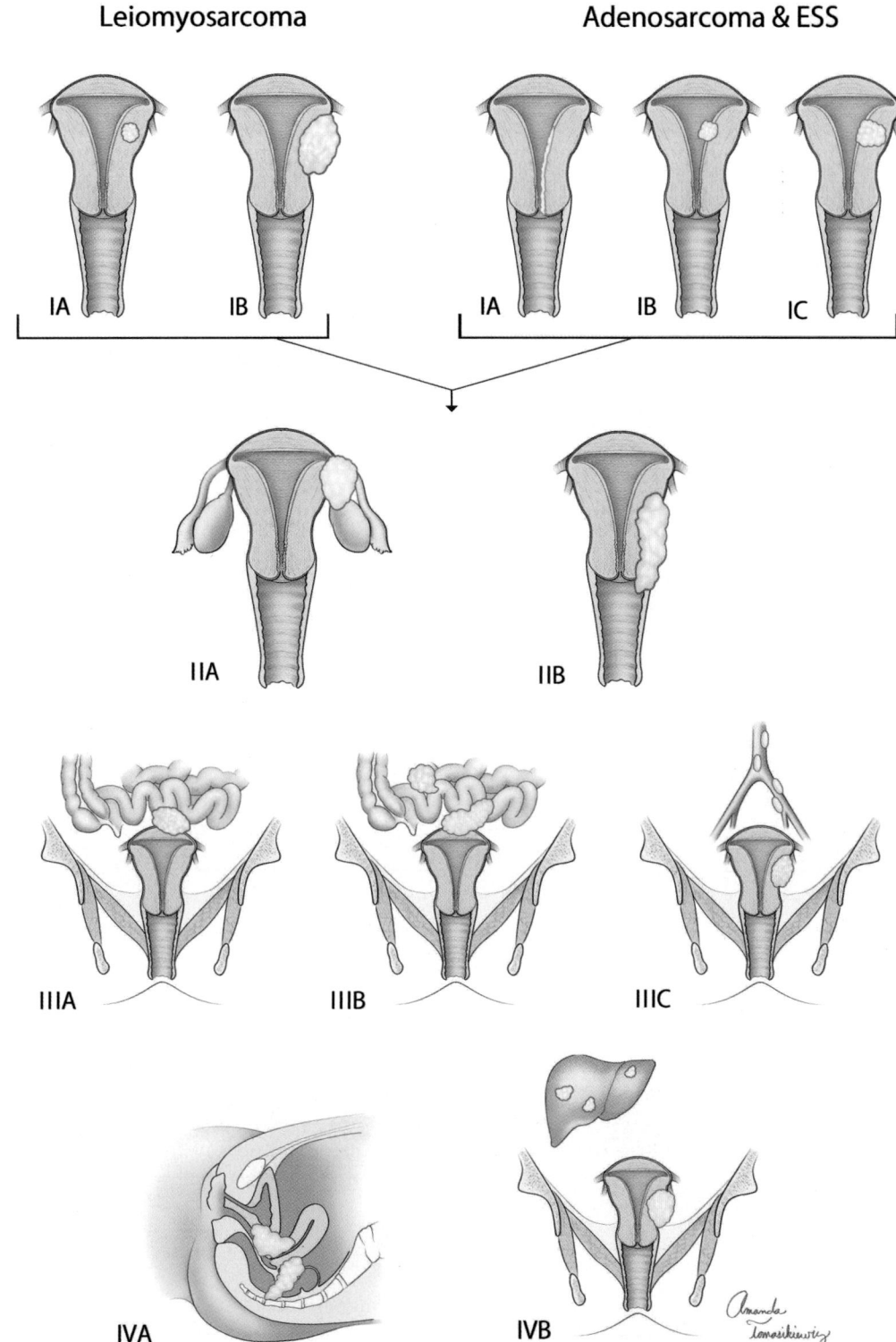

Leiomyosarcoma

Adenosarcoma & ESS

FIGURE 34-10 FIGO staging of leiomyosarcoma and that for adenosarcoma and endometrial stromal sarcoma (ESS).

With *uterine leiomyosarcoma*, all patients should undergo a hysterectomy, if feasible. A modified radical or radical procedure may be occasionally required if there is parametrial infiltration. In the absence of other gross disease, fewer than 5 percent will have ovarian or nodal metastases. Ovarian preservation is therefore an option for premenopausal women. In addition, lymph node dissection is reserved for patients with clinically suspicious nodes (Kapp, 2008; Leitao, 2003; Major, 1993). For STUMP, hysterectomy alone is sufficient.

Endometrial stromal tumors and *adenosarcomas* are also best treated by hysterectomy. Again, a more radical procedure may be required to encompass local disease. Preservation of the ovaries is generally accepted for endometrial stromal sarcomas or adenosarcomas in the absence of extrauterine disease (Chan,

2008; Li, 2005; Shah, 2008). However, bilateral salpingo-oophorectomy (BSO) is indicated for high-grade undifferentiated sarcomas (Leibsohn, 1990). Unlike leiomyosarcoma, lymph node dissection is typically more informative. Although nodal metastases are most often identified in patients with obvious extrauterine disease, they do occur in 5 to 10 percent of patients with no evidence for intraabdominal spread (Dos Santos, 2011; Goff, 1993; Signorelli, 2010).

For *uterine carcinosarcoma*, hysterectomy and BSO are mandatory. Lymph node metastases will be found in up to one third of patients with clinical stage I disease, and thus, comprehensive lymphadenectomy should be performed as for poorly differentiated endometrial cancers (Major, 1993; Nemani, 2008; Park, 2010; Temkin, 2007). Typically, disease spread is histologically consistent with the carcinomatous element of this mixed tumor. Because this component may be serous or clear cell, extended surgical staging with infracolic omentectomy and random peritoneal biopsies is also advisable (Greer, 2015).

Surveillance

In women with early-stage uterine sarcoma, adjuvant treatment is routinely employed but has not been demonstrated to improve survival rates (Greer, 2015; Reed, 2008). Thus, because the recurrence rate for the clinically aggressive types is excessive, enrollment in an experimental clinical trial should be carefully considered, if available. In practice, many patients receive postoperative radiation with or without chemotherapy.

After surgery, menopausal symptoms such as hot flushes may be treated as appropriate for uterine leiomyosarcomas, high-grade undifferentiated sarcomas, and adenosarcomas. However, although it is considered safe to preserve the ovaries in a premenopausal woman with endometrial stromal sarcoma, the use of estrogen replacement therapy has been associated with disease progression and is avoided (Chu, 2003; Pink, 2006). Similar caution is warranted for patients with uterine carcinosarcoma.

Surgically treated patients with uterine sarcoma should have a physical examination every 3 months for the first 2 years and then at 6- to 12-month intervals thereafter. Most recurrences will be distant, and thus Pap tests are largely irrelevant. In addition, serum CA125 levels are not routinely recommended, unless initially elevated prior to surgery. Depending on the type of sarcoma, a chest radiograph or CT imaging is performed every 6 to 12 months for 2 years, then annually. When clinically indicated, intermittent CT or MR imaging may also be helpful (Greer, 2015).

Adjuvant Radiation

Approximately half of patients with stage I disease who are observed without adjuvant therapy will relapse (Leath, 2009). Due to the rarity of these tumors and limited data to support a consistent approach, the use of postoperative therapy is usually individualized.

The role of postoperative radiotherapy for nonmetastatic disease is controversial. Prior retrospective studies of adjuvant external beam pelvic radiotherapy suggested reduced pelvic recurrence rates for carcinosarcoma, leiomyosarcoma, and endometrial stromal sarcoma (Callister, 2004; Hornback,

1986; Mahdavi, 2009; Malouf, 2010). However, results from a prospective trial that randomly assigned 224 women over 13 years with all subtypes of surgical stage I or II uterine sarcomas to receive either pelvic radiation or no further treatment have been reported. Although a reduced rate of pelvic relapse for those with carcinosarcomas was noted, no benefit was gained for those with leiomyosarcomas and no significant increase in survival rates for either group. Unfortunately, the number of patients with endometrial stromal sarcoma was too small to permit analysis (Reed, 2008).

Pelvic radiation does not prevent distant recurrences and has yet to be shown to improve survival rates (Nemani, 2008). In many circumstances, vaginal brachytherapy may be an alternative, especially if paired with systemic chemotherapy (Greer, 2015). Whole abdominal radiotherapy (WAR) has been proposed as a more definitive option. In one randomized phase III study of 232 patients with stage I-IV carcinosarcoma, WAR was compared with ifosfamide and cisplatin chemotherapy. Although no survival advantage was demonstrated, the observed differences favored the use of combination chemotherapy in future trials (Wolfson, 2007).

Adjuvant Chemotherapy

There is no proven survival benefit for using adjuvant chemotherapy in patients with stage I uterine sarcoma (Omura, 1985). However, because most patients will recur distantly, adjuvant systemic treatment is frequently used. For leiomyosarcomas, completely resected stage I and II disease treated with doxorubicin and ifosfamide was not associated with a significantly improved disease-free or overall survival benefit (Mancari, 2014). In high-grade undifferentiated sarcomas and carcinosarcomas, chemotherapy regimens used for more advanced disease may be considered. For stages I and II endometrial stromal sarcoma and adenosarcoma, observation is recommended (Greer, 2015).

Fertility-sparing Management

Rarely, young patients may desire to delay definitive hysterectomy after a fertility-sparing "myomectomy" demonstrates sarcomatous features on the final pathology report (Lissoni, 1998; Yan, 2010). Although expectant management following tumor resection can result in successful pregnancies in select patients, it is risky not to perform a hysterectomy, and eventually all such women should undergo hysterectomy (Lissoni, 1998). Most patients, even those with negative margins, should be counseled regarding definitive surgery and ovarian preservation during surgery for clinical stage I uterine leiomyosarcomas or endometrial stromal sarcomas. Egg retrieval, assisted reproductive technologies, and pregnancy surrogacy would still be possible. For more advanced disease, fertility-sparing management is not a reasonable option.

TREATMENT OF ADVANCED (STAGES III AND IV) OR RECURRENT DISEASE

Patients with advanced or recurrent uterine sarcoma generally have a dismal prognosis. For advanced-stage disease, upfront surgery with maximal effort to completely remove all visible disease (similar in approach to advanced ovarian cancer) is considered standard. This is generally followed by adjuvant chemotherapy. Neoadjuvant chemotherapy can be considered for patients whose disease is considered unresectable or who are medically unfit for surgery.

For recurrent disease, secondary cytoreductive surgery may be feasible in some circumstances (Giuntoli, 2007). Palliative radiation may also have a role, depending on the site and distribution of the tumor. In general, uterine sarcomas have a propensity for relapse at distant sites, and chemotherapy is more useful. Since current treatment options have only modest efficacy, patients are encouraged to enroll in experimental clinical trials.

■ Leiomyosarcoma

Doxorubicin is considered the most active single agent (Miller, 2000; Omura, 1983). However, treatment with the combination of gemcitabine and docetaxel currently has the highest proven response rate (36 percent) (Hensley, 2008). Addition of bevacizumab to this regimen was not beneficial (Hensley, 2015).

For late recurrences of leiomyosarcoma, surgery must be individualized. Five-year survival rates of 30 to 50 percent have been reported following pulmonary resection for lung metastases. Local and regional recurrences may also be amenable to surgical resection (Giuntoli, 2007).

■ Endometrial Stromal Tumors

Surgical resection may be feasible for some patients with recurrent endometrial stromal sarcoma, but hormonal therapy is particularly useful. In general, these tumors are estrogen- and progesterone-receptor (ER/PR) positive (Sutton, 1986). Progestins such as megestrol acetate and medroxyprogesterone acetate are most commonly used either postoperatively for advanced-stage disease or for relapses (Reich, 2006). Using this strategy, complete responses are often possible. Aromatase inhibitors and gonadotropin-releasing hormone (GnRH) agonists have also demonstrated activity (Burke, 2004; Leunen, 2004).

High-grade undifferentiated sarcomas do not exhibit the same level of sensitivity to hormonal agents, primarily because they are usually ER/PR negative. Advanced disease or recurrences of these rare tumors are also typically not amenable to surgical resection, although palliative radiation may have some utility. Systemic chemotherapy is usually the only option, and ifosfamide is the only cytotoxic drug with proven activity (Sutton, 1996).

■ Carcinosarcoma

Ifosfamide is the most active single agent for carcinosarcoma. The combination of ifosfamide and paclitaxel is the current preferred treatment for advanced or recurrent uterine carcinosarcoma (Galaal, 2011). In a recent phase III GOG trial randomizing 179 patients, this regimen demonstrated a superior response rate (45 versus 29 percent) and survival advantage compared with ifosfamide alone (protocol #161) (Homesley, 2007). The combination of carboplatin and paclitaxel is also active and is being compared with ifosfamide and paclitaxel in an ongoing GOG trial (protocol #261) (King, 2009; Powell, 2010).

TABLE 34-4. Overall Survival Rates of Women with Uterine Sarcomas (All Stages)

Type	5-Year Survival
Carcinosarcoma	35%
Leiomyosarcoma	25%
Endometrial stromal tumors	
Endometrial stromal sarcoma	60%
High-grade undifferentiated sarcoma	25%

Data from Acharya S, Hensley ML, Montag AC, et al: Rare uterine cancers, Lancet Oncol 2005 Dec;6(12):961–71.

SURVIVAL AND PROGNOSTIC FACTORS

In general, women with uterine sarcoma have a poor prognosis (Table 34-4). In a study of 141 women followed for a median of 3 years, 74 percent died of disease progression. FIGO stage is the most important independent variable associated with survival (Livi, 2003). Other poor prognostic factors across all subtypes include older age, African-American race, and lack of primary surgery (Chan, 2008; Kapp, 2008; Nemani, 2008).

Tumor histology is the other main predictor of outcome. Leiomyosarcomas have the worst prognosis and are followed by carcinosarcoma and the group of endometrial stromal tumors (Livi, 2003). Endometrial stromal sarcomas and uterine adenosarcomas without sarcomatous overgrowth are the two notable exceptions. Patients with these tumors tend to have a good prognosis due to their indolent growth (Pautier, 2000; Verschraegen, 1998).

REFERENCES

Acharya S, Hensley ML, Montag AC, et al: Rare uterine cancers. Lancet Oncol 6(12):961, 2005

Brooks SE, Zhan M, Cote T, et al: Surveillance, epidemiology, and end results analysis of 2677 cases of uterine sarcoma 1989-1999. Gynecol Oncol 93(1):204, 2004

Burke C, Hickey K: Treatment of endometrial stromal sarcoma with a gonadotropin-releasing hormone analogue. Obstet Gynecol 104(5 Pt 2):1182, 2004

Callister M, Ramondetta LM, Jhingran A, et al: Malignant mixed Mullerian tumors of the uterus: analysis of patterns of failure, prognostic factors, and treatment outcome. Int J Radiat Oncol Biol Phys 58(3):786, 2004

Chan JK, Kawar NM, Shin JY, et al: Endometrial stromal sarcoma: a population-based analysis. Br J Cancer 99:1210, 2008

Chu MC, Mor G, Lim C, et al: Low-grade endometrial stromal sarcoma: hormonal aspects. Gynecol Oncol 90(1):170, 2003

D'Angelo E, Prat J: Uterine sarcomas: a review. Gynecol Oncol 116:131, 2010

De Fusco PA, Gaffey TA, Malkasian GD Jr, et al: Endometrial stromal sarcoma: review of Mayo Clinic experience, 1945-1980. Gynecol Oncol 35(1):8, 1989

Dinh TA, Oliva EA, Fuller AF Jr, et al: The treatment of uterine leiomyosarcoma. Results from a 10-year experience (1990-1999) at the Massachusetts General Hospital. Gynecol Oncol 92:648, 2004

Dionigi A, Oliva E, Clement PB, et al: Endometrial stromal nodules and endometrial stromal tumors with limited infiltration: a clinicopathologic study of 50 cases. Am J Surg Pathol 26(5):567, 2002

Dos Santos LA, Garg K, Diaz JP, et al: Incidence of lymph node and adnexal metastasis in endometrial stromal sarcoma. Gynecol Oncol 121(2):319, 2011

Evans HL: Endometrial stromal sarcoma and poorly differentiated endometrial sarcoma. Cancer 50(10):2170, 1982

Felix AS, Cook LS, Gaudet MM, et al: The etiology of uterine sarcomas: a pooled analysis of the epidemiology of endometrial cancer consortium. Br J Cancer 108(3):727, 2013

Food and Drug Administration: UPDATED laparoscopic uterine power morcellation in hysterectomy and myomectomy: FDA safety communication. 2014. Available at: http://www.fda.gov/medicaldevices/safety/ucm424443. htm. Accessed March 9, 2015

Fujii H, Yoshida M, Gong ZX, et al: Frequent genetic heterogeneity in the clonal evolution of gynecological carcinosarcoma and its influence on phenotypic diversity. Cancer Res 60(1):114, 2000

Galaal K, van der Heijden E, Godfrey K, et al: Adjuvant radiotherapy and/or chemotherapy after surgery for uterine carcinosarcoma. Cochrane Database Syst Rev 2:CD006812, 2013

Giuntoli RL, Garrett-Mayer E, Bristow RE, et al: Secondary cytoreduction in the management of recurrent uterine leiomyosarcoma. Gynecol Oncol 106(1):82, 2007

Goff BA, Rice LW, Fleischhacker D, et al: Uterine leiomyosarcoma and endometrial stromal sarcoma: lymph node metastases and sites of recurrence. Gynecol Oncol 50(1):105, 1993

Gonzalez-Bosquet E, Martinez-Palones JM, Gonzalez-Bosquet J, et al: Uterine sarcoma: a clinicopathological study of 93 cases. Eur J Gynaecol Oncol 18(3): 192, 1997

Greer BE, Koh WJ, Abu-Rustum NR, et al: Uterine neoplasms. NCCN Clinical Practice Guidelines in Oncology. Version 2. 2015. Available at: www.nccn.org. Accessed April 24, 2015

Halbwedl I, Ullmann R, Kremser ML, et al: Chromosomal alterations in low-grade endometrial stromal sarcoma and undifferentiated endometrial sarcoma as detected by comparative genomic hybridization. Gynecol Oncol 97(2):582, 2005

Hendrickson MR, Tavassoli FA, Kempson RL, et al: Tumors of the uterine corpus [Mesenchymal tumors and related lesions]. In Tavassoli FA, Devilee P (eds): World Health Organization Classification of Tumours. 2003, p 233

Hensley ML, Blessing JA, Mannel R, et al: Fixed-dose rate gemcitabine plus docetaxel as first-line therapy for metastatic uterine leiomyosarcoma: a Gynecologic Oncology Group phase II trial. Gynecol Oncol 109:329, 2008

Hensley ML, Miller DS, O'Malley DM, et al: Randomized phase III trial of gemcitabine plus docetaxel plus bevacizumab or placebo as first line treatment for metastatic uterine leiomyosarcoma: an NRG Oncology/ Gynecologic Oncology Group study. J Clin Oncol 33(10):1180, 2015

Homesley HD, Filiaci V, Markman M, et al: Phase III trial of ifosfamide with or without paclitaxel in advanced uterine carcinosarcoma: a Gynecologic Oncology Group Study. J Clin Oncol 25:526, 2007

Hornback NB, Omura G, Major FJ: Observations on the use of adjuvant radiation therapy in patients with stage I and II uterine sarcoma. Int J Radiat Oncol Biol Phys 12(12):2127, 1986

Huang GS, Chiu LG, Gebb JS, et al: Serum CA125 predicts extrauterine disease and survival in uterine carcinosarcoma. Gynecol Oncol 107:513, 2007

Kanbour AI, Buchsbaum HJ, Hall A, et al: Peritoneal cytology in malignant mixed mullerian tumors of the uterus. Gynecol Oncol 33(1):91, 1989

Kapp DS, Shin JY, Chan JK: Prognostic factors and survival in 1396 patients with uterine leiomyosarcomas: emphasis on impact of lymphadenectomy and oophorectomy. Cancer 112(4):820, 2008

Kido A, Togashi K, Koyama T, et al: Diffusely enlarged uterus: evaluation with MR imaging. Radiographics 23(6):1423, 2003

King LP, Miller DS: Recent progress: gynecologic oncology group trials in uterine corpus tumors. Rev Recent Clin Trials 4(2):70, 2009

Krivak TC, Seidman JD, McBroom JW, et al: Uterine adenosarcoma with sarcomatous overgrowth versus uterine carcinosarcoma: comparison of treatment and survival. Gynecol Oncol 83(1):89, 2001

Kurman RJ, Carcangiu ML, Herrington CS, et al (eds): WHO Classification of Tumours of Female Reproductive Organs, 4th ed. Lyon, International Agency for Research on Cancer, 2014

Leath CA III, Huh WK, Hyde J Jr, et al: A multi-institutional review of outcomes of endometrial stromal sarcoma. Gynecol Oncol 105:630, 2007

Leath CA III, Numnum TM, Kendrick JE, et al: Patterns of failure for conservatively managed surgical stage I uterine carcinosarcoma: implications for adjuvant therapy. Int J Gynecol Cancer 19:888, 2009

Lee CH, Ou WB, Mariño-Enriquez A, et al: 14-3-3 fusion oncogenes in high-grade endometrial stromal sarcoma. Proc Natl Acad Sci USA 109(3):929, 2012

Leibsohn S, d'Ablaing G, Mishell DR, et al: Leiomyosarcoma in a series of hysterectomies performed for presumed uterine leiomyomas. Am J Obstet Gynecol 162(4):968, 1990

Leitao MM, Sonoda Y, Brennan MF, et al: Incidence of lymph node and ovarian metastases in leiomyosarcoma of the uterus. Gynecol Oncol 91(1):209, 2003

Leunen M, Breugelmans M, De Sutter P, et al: Low-grade endometrial stromal sarcoma treated with the aromatase inhibitor letrozole. Gynecol Oncol 95(3):769, 2004

Li AJ, Giuntoli RL, Drake R, et al: Ovarian preservation in stage I low-grade endometrial stromal sarcomas. Obstet Gynecol 106(6):1304, 2005

Lieng M, Berner E, Busund B: Risk of morcellation of uterine leiomyosarcomas in laparoscopic supracervical hysterectomy and laparoscopic myomectomy, a retrospective trial including 4791 women. J Minim Invasive Gynecol 22(3): 410, 2015

Lin K, Hechanova M, Richardson DL, et al: Risk of occult uterine sarcoma in women undergoing hysterectomy for benign indications. Abstract presented at American Congress of Obstetricians and Gynecologists Annual Clinic and Scientific Meeting. San Francisco, 2-6 May 2015

Lissoni A, Cormio G, Bonazzi C, et al: Fertility-sparing surgery in uterine leiomyosarcoma. Gynecol Oncol 70(3):348, 1998

Liu FS, Kohler MF, Marks JR, et al: Mutation and overexpression of the p53 tumor suppressor gene frequently occurs in uterine and ovarian sarcomas. Obstet Gynecol 83(1):118, 1994

Livi L, Paiar F, Shah N, et al: Uterine sarcoma: twenty-seven years of experience. Int J Radiat Oncol Biol Phys 57(5):1366, 2003

Mahdavi A, Monk BJ, Ragazzo J, et al: Pelvic radiation improves local control after hysterectomy for uterine leiomyosarcoma: a 20-year experience. Int J Gynecol Cancer 19:1080, 2009

Major FJ, Blessing JA, Silverberg SG, et al: Prognostic factors in early-stage uterine sarcoma. A Gynecologic Oncology Group study. Cancer 71(4 Suppl): 1702, 1993

Malouf GG, Duclos J, Rey A, et al: Impact of adjuvant treatment modalities on the management of patients with stage I-II endometrial stromal sarcoma. Ann Oncol 21:2102, 2010

Mancari R, Signorelli M, Gadducci A, et al: Adjuvant chemotherapy in stage I-II uterine leiomyosarcoma: a multicentric retrospective study of 140 patients. Gynecol Oncol 133(3):531, 2014

McCluggage WG: Uterine carcinosarcomas (malignant mixed Mullerian tumors) are metaplastic carcinomas. Int J Gynecol Cancer 12:687, 2002

McCluggage WG, Haller U, Kurman RJ, et al: Tumors of the uterine corpus [Mixed epithelial and mesenchymal tumors]. In Tavassoli FA, Devilee P (eds): World Health Organization Classification of Tumours. 2003, p 245

Micci F, Panagopoulos I, Bjerkehagen B, et al: Consistent rearrangement of chromosomal band 6p21 with generation of fusion genes JAZF1/PHF1 and EPC1/PHF1 in endometrial stromal sarcoma. Cancer Res 66(1):107, 2006

Miller DS, Blessing JA, Kilgore LC, et al: Phase II trial of topotecan in patients with advanced, persistent, or recurrent uterine leiomyosarcomas: a Gynecologic Oncology Group Study. Am J Clin Oncol 23(4):355-7, 2000

Nemani D, Mitra N, Guo M, et al: Assessing the effects of lymphadenectomy and radiation therapy in patients with uterine carcinosarcoma: a SEER analysis. Gynecol Oncol 111:82, 2008

Oliva E, Clement PB, Young RH: Endometrial stromal tumors: an update on a group of tumors with a protean phenotype. Adv Anat Pathol 7(5):257, 2000

Omura GA, Blessing JA, Major F, et al: A randomized clinical trial of adjuvant adriamycin in uterine sarcomas: a Gynecologic Oncology Group Study. J Clin Oncol 3(9):1240, 1985

Omura GA, Major FJ, Blessing JA, et al: A randomized study of adriamycin with and without dimethyl triazenoimidazole carboxamide in advanced uterine sarcomas. Cancer 52(4):626, 1983

Panagopoulos I, Micci F, Thorsen J, et al: Novel fusion of MYST/ESA1-associated factor 6 and PHF1 in endometrial stromal sarcoma. PLoS One 7(6):e39354, 2012

Park JY, Kim DY, Kim JH, et al: The role of pelvic and/or para-aortic lymphadenectomy in surgical management of apparently early carcinosarcoma of uterus. Ann Surg Oncol 17:861, 2010

Parker WH, Fu YS, Berek JS: Uterine sarcoma in patients operated on for presumed leiomyoma and rapidly growing leiomyoma. Obstet Gynecol 83(3):414, 1994

Pautier P, Genestie C, Rey A, et al: Analysis of clinicopathologic prognostic factors for 157 uterine sarcomas and evaluation of a grading score validated for soft tissue sarcoma. Cancer 88(6):1425, 2000

Perri T, Korach J, Sadetzki S, et al: Uterine leiomyosarcoma: does the primary surgical procedure matter? Int J Gynecol Cancer 19:257, 2009

Pink D, Lindner T, Mrozek A, et al: Harm or benefit of hormonal treatment in metastatic low-grade endometrial stromal sarcoma: single center experience with 10 cases and review of the literature. Gynecol Oncol 101(3):464, 2006

Powell MA, Filiaci VL, Rose PG, et al: Phase II evaluation of paclitaxel and carboplatin in the treatment of carcinosarcoma of the uterus: a Gynecologic Oncology Group study. J Clin Oncol 28(16):2727, 2010

Quade BJ, Wang TY, Sornberger K, et al: Molecular pathogenesis of uterine smooth muscle tumors from transcriptional profiling. Genes Chromosomes Cancer 40(2):97, 2004

Reed NS, Mangioni C, Malmstrom H, et al: Phase III randomised study to evaluate the role of adjuvant pelvic radiotherapy in the treatment of uterine sarcomas stages I and II: a European Organisation for Research and Treatment of Cancer Gynaecological Cancer Group Study (protocol 55874). Eur J Cancer 44:808, 2008

Reich O, Regauer S: Survey of adjuvant hormone therapy in patients after endometrial stromal sarcoma. Eur J Gynaecol Oncol 27(2):150, 2006

Sartori E, Bazzurini L, Gadducci A, et al: Carcinosarcoma of the uterus: a clinicopathological multicenter CTF study. Gynecol Oncol 67:70, 1997

Shah JP, Bryant CS, Kumar S, et al: Lymphadenectomy and ovarian preservation in low-grade endometrial stromal sarcoma. Obstet Gynecol 112:1102, 2008

Sharma P, Kumar R, Singh H, et al: Role of FDG PET-CT in detecting recurrence in patients with uterine sarcoma: comparison with conventional imaging. Nucl Med Commun 33(2):185, 2012

Signorelli M, Fruscio R, Dell-Anna T, et al: Lymphadenectomy in uterine low-grade endometrial stromal sarcoma: an analysis of 19 cases and a literature review. Int J Gynecol Cancer 20:1363, 2010

Skubitz KM, Skubitz APN: Differential gene expression in leiomyosarcoma. Cancer 98(5):1029, 2003

Sutton G, Blessing JA, Park R, et al: Ifosfamide treatment of recurrent or metastatic endometrial stromal sarcomas previously unexposed to chemotherapy: a study of the Gynecologic Oncology Group. Obstet Gynecol 87(5 Pt 1): 747, 1996

Sutton GP, Stehman FB, Michael H, et al: Estrogen and progesterone receptors in uterine sarcomas. Obstet Gynecol 68(5):709, 1986

Taylor NP, Zighelboim I, Huettner PC, et al: DNA mismatch repair and TP53 defects are early events in uterine carcinosarcoma tumorigenesis. Mod Pathol 19(10):1333, 2006

Temkin SM, Hellmann M, Lee YC, et al: Early-stage carcinosarcoma of the uterus: the significance of lymph node count. Int J Gynecol Cancer 17:215, 2007

Thomas MB, Keeney GL, Podratz KC, et al: Endometrial stromal sarcoma: treatment and patterns of recurrence. Int J Gynecol Cancer 19:253, 2009

Vaidya AP, Horowitz NS, Oliva E, et al: Uterine malignant mixed müllerian tumors should not be included in studies of endometrial carcinoma. Gynecol Oncol 103:684, 2006

Verschraegen CF, Vasuratna A, Edwards C, et al: Clinicopathologic analysis of mullerian adenosarcoma: the M.D. Anderson Cancer Center experience. Oncol Rep 5 (4):939, 1998

Wada H, Enomoto T, Fujita M, et al: Molecular evidence that most but not all carcinosarcomas of the uterus are combination tumors. Cancer Res 57(23):5379, 1997

Wolfson AH, Brady MF, Rocereto T, et al: A gynecologic oncology group randomized phase III trial of whole abdominal irradiation (WAI) vs. cisplatin-ifosfamide and mesna (CIM) as post-surgical therapy in stage I-IV carcinosarcoma (CS) of the uterus. Gynecol Oncol 107:177, 2007

Yan L, Tian Y, Zhao X: Successful pregnancy after fertility-preserving surgery for endometrial stromal sarcoma. Fertil Steril 93:269.e1, 2010

Yang GC, Wan LS, Del Priore G: Factors influencing the detection of uterine cancer by suction curettage and endometrial brushing. J Reprod Med 47(12):1005, 2002

Zaloudek C, Hendrickson MR, Soslow RA: Mesenchymal tumors of the uterus. In Kurman RJ, Ellenson LH, Ronnett BM (eds): Blaustein's Pathology of the Female Genital Tract, 6th ed. New York, Springer, 2011, p 453

Zhang P, Zhang C, Hao J, et al: Use of X-chromosome inactivation pattern to determine the clonal origins of uterine leiomyoma and leiomyosarcoma. Hum Pathol 37(10):1350, 2006

CHAPTER 35

Epithelial Ovarian Cancer

In the United States, ovarian cancer accounts for more deaths than all other gynecologic malignancies combined. Worldwide each year, more than 225,000 women are diagnosed, and 140,000 women die from this disease (Jemal, 2011). Of these, epithelial ovarian carcinomas make up 90 to 95 percent of all cases, including the more indolent low-malignant-potential (borderline) tumors (Quirk, 2005). The remainder includes germ cell and sex cord-stromal tumors, which are described in Chapter 36 (p. 760). Due to the similarities of primary peritoneal carcinomas and fallopian tube cancers, they are included within this section for simplicity.

Approximately one quarter of patients will have stage I disease and an excellent long-term survival rate. However, there are no effective screening tests for ovarian cancer and few notable early symptoms. As a result, two thirds of patients have advanced disease when they are diagnosed. Aggressive debulking surgery, followed by platinum-based chemotherapy, usually results in clinical remission. However, up to 80 percent of these women will develop a relapse that eventually leads to disease progression and death.

EPIDEMIOLOGY AND RISK FACTORS

One in 78 American women (1.3 percent) will develop ovarian cancer during her lifetime. Because the incidence has slowly declined since the early 1990s, ovarian cancer is now the ninth leading cause of cancer in women. In 2015, 21, 290 new cases and 14,180 deaths are expected, and ovarian cancer remains the fifth leading cause of cancer-related death (Siegel, 2015). Overall, the average age at diagnosis is in the early 60s.

Numerous reproductive, environmental, and genetic risk factors have been associated with ovarian cancer (Table 35-1). The most important is a *family history* of breast or ovarian cancer, and approximately 10 percent of patients have an inherited genetic predisposition. For the other 90 percent with no identifiable genetic link for their ovarian cancer, most risks are related to a pattern of uninterrupted ovulatory cycles during the reproductive years (Pelucchi, 2007). Repeated stimulation of the ovarian surface epithelium is hypothesized to lead to malignant transformation (Schildkraut, 1997).

Nulliparity is associated with long periods of repetitive ovulation, and patients without children have double the risk of developing ovarian cancer (Purdie, 2003). Among nulliparous women, those with a history of infertility have an even higher risk. Although the reasons are unclear, it is more likely to be an inherent ovarian predisposition rather than an iatrogenic effect of ovulation-inducing drugs. For example, women treated for infertility who successfully achieve a live birth do not have an increased risk of

TABLE 35-1. Risk Factors for Developing Epithelial Ovarian Cancer

Nulliparity
Early menarche
Late menopause
White race
Increasing age
Residence in North America and Northern Europe
Family history
Personal history of breast cancer
Ethnic background (European Jewish, Icelandic, Hungarian)
Postmenopausal hormone therapy
Pelvic inflammatory disease

Modified with permission from Schorge JO, Modesitt SC, Coleman RL, et al: SGO White Paper on ovarian cancer: etiology, screening and surveillance, Gynecol Oncol. 2010 Oct;119(1):7–17.

TABLE 35-2. Women Who Should Undergo Genetic Testing

Epithelial ovarian cancer[a] at any age
Breast cancer diagnosed at age 45 or younger
Breast cancer with two distinct and sequential primaries, first one diagnosed at age 50 or younger
Breast cancer that is triple-negative diagnosed at age 60 or younger
Breast cancer at any age, with at least one close relative[b] diagnosed at age 50 or younger
Breast cancer diagnosed at any age, with two or more close relatives with breast cancer; one close relative with epithelial ovarian cancer; or two close relatives with pancreatic cancer or aggressive prostate cancer
Breast cancer, with a close male relative with breast cancer at any age
Breast cancer and Ashkenazi Jewish ancestry
Individuals from a family with a known deleterious *BRCA1* or *BRCA2* mutation

[a]Throughout table, peritoneal and fallopian tube cancer are considered as part of the spectrum of the Hereditary Breast/Ovarian Cancer syndrome.
[b]Throughout table, *close relative* is defined as a first-, second-, or third-degree relative (i.e., mother, sister, daughter, aunt, niece, grandmother, granddaughter, first cousin, great grandmother, great aunt).
Adapted with permission from Lancaster JM, Powell CB, Chen LM, et al: Society of Gynecologic Oncology statement on risk assessment for inherited gynecologic cancer predispositions. Gynecol Oncol 2015 Jan;136(1):3–7.

ovarian cancer (Rossing, 2004). In general, risks decrease with each live birth, eventually plateauing in women delivering five times (Hinkula, 2006). One theory suggests that pregnancy may induce premalignant ovarian cell shedding (Rostgaard, 2003).

Early menarche and *late menopause* are also associated risks. In contrast, breastfeeding has a protective effect, perhaps by prolonging amenorrhea (Yen, 2003). Presumably by also preventing ovulation, long-term combination oral contraceptive use reduces the risk of ovarian cancer by 50 percent. The duration of protection lasts up to 25 years after the last use (Riman, 2002). In contrast, hormone replacement therapy after menopause has an elevated associated risk (Lacey, 2006; Mørch, 2009).

White women have the highest incidence of ovarian cancer among all racial and ethnic groups (Quirk, 2005). Compared with that of black and Hispanic women, the risk is elevated by 30 to 40 percent (Goodman, 2003). Although exact reasons are unknown, racial discrepancies in parity and rates of gynecologic surgery may account for some of the differences.

Tubal ligation and *hysterectomy* are each associated with a substantial reduction in risk (Rice, 2014). Theoretically, any gynecologic procedure that precludes irritants from reaching the ovaries via ascension from the lower genital tract might plausibly exert a similar protective effect. In turn, women who regularly use perineal talc may possibly have an elevated risk (Gertig, 2000; Houghton, 2014; Rosenblatt, 2011).

Age is another risk, and the overall incidence of ovarian cancer rises with age up to the mid-70s and then declines slightly among women beyond 80 years (Goodman, 2003). In general, aging allows an extended period to accumulate random genetic alterations within the ovarian surface epithelium.

Women *residing in North America, Northern Europe, or any industrialized Western country* have a higher ovarian cancer risk. Globally, the incidence varies greatly, but developing countries and Japan have the lowest rates (Jemal, 2011). Regional dietary habits may be partly responsible (Kiani, 2006). For example, consumption of foods low in fat but high in fiber, carotene, and vitamins appears protective (Zhang, 2004).

A *family history* of ovarian cancer in a first-degree relative, that is, a mother, daughter, or sister, triples a woman's lifetime risk. The

risks further escalate with two or more afflicted first-degree relatives, or with other individuals with premenopausal breast cancer. If a family history is mainly composed of colon cancer, clinicians may consider Lynch syndrome, also known as *hereditary nonpolyposis colorectal cancer* (HNPCC). Patients with this syndrome have a high lifetime risk of colon cancer (85 percent) and ovarian cancer (10 to 12 percent). Because the predominant gynecologic malignancy is endometrial cancer (40 to 60 percent lifetime risk), HNPCC is described in more detail in Chapter 33 (p. 703).

Hereditary Breast and Ovarian Cancer

Genetic Screening

More than 90 percent of inherited ovarian cancers result from germline mutations in the *BRCA1* or *BRCA2* genes. Thus, any patient with a personal history of epithelial ovarian cancer or breast cancer in certain circumstances, or from a family with a known deleterious mutation, should undergo testing (Table 35-2) (Daly, 2014).

Typically, a patient is referred to a certified genetic counselor, and a comprehensive pedigree is constructed first. Then, risk assessment is performed using one of several validated population models. These include the BRCAPRO and Tyrer-Cuzick programs, which are available, respectively, at: http://www4.utsouthwestern.edu/breasthealth/cagene/default.asp, and by contacting the International Breast Cancer Intervention Study (IBIS) at ibis@cancer.org.uk. These models and their associated software allow quantification of an individual's risk for carrying a germline deleterious mutation of the *BRCA1* and *BRCA2* genes (Euhus, 2002; James, 2006; Parmigiani, 2007). However, assessment of family history, even by a validated model, cannot effectively target testing to a high-risk ovarian cancer patient population, which strongly supports the recommendation to offer *BRCA1/BRCA2* genetic testing to all patients with high-grade serous ovarian cancer regardless of family history (Daniels, 2014; Norquist, 2013).

BRCA1 and *BRCA2* Genes

These are two tumor-suppressor genes, whose protein products are BRCA1 and BRCA2. These two proteins interact with

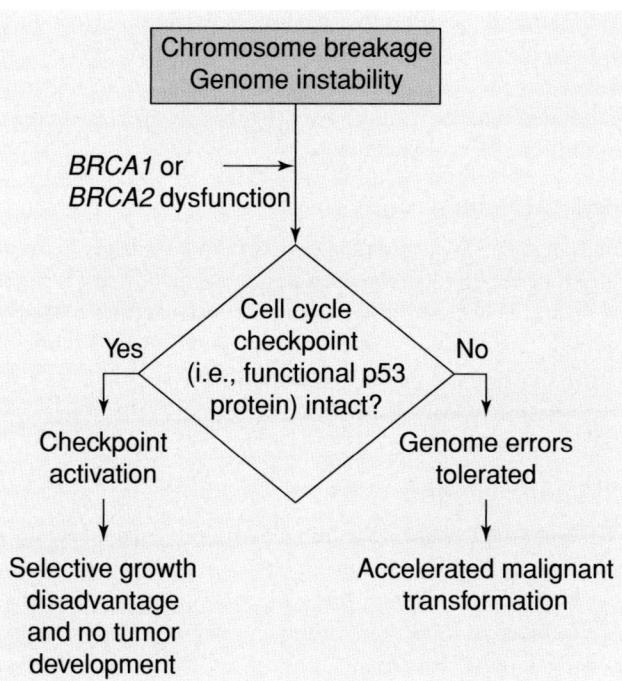

FIGURE 35-1 Diagram describing the role of the *BRCA* mutation in tumor development. Cells with damaged DNA are frequently blocked at checkpoints along the cell cycle and thereby prohibited from moving to the mitotic phase. If these checkpoints are non-functional, then these genomic errors may be tolerated and lead to malignant transformation. (Reproduced with permission from Scully R, Livingston DM: In search of the tumour-suppressor functions of BRCA1 and BRCA2, Nature 2000 Nov 23;408(6811):429–432.)

recombination/DNA repair proteins to preserve intact chromosomal structure. Mutations of *BRCA1* and *BRCA2* genes lead to BRCA1 and BRCA2 protein dysfunction, which results in genetic instability and subjects cells to a higher risk of malignant transformation (Fig. 35-1) (Deng, 2006; Scully, 2000).

The *BRCA1* gene is located on chromosome 17q21. Patients with a proven mutation have a dramatically elevated risk of developing ovarian cancer (39 to 46 percent). *BRCA2* is located on chromosome 13q12 and in general is less likely to lead to ovarian cancer (12 to 20 percent). The estimated lifetime risk of breast cancer with a *BRCA1* or *BRCA2* mutation is 65 to 74 percent (American College of Obstetricians and Gynecologists, 2013; Chen, 2006; Risch, 2006). Both genes are inherited in an autosomal dominant fashion, but with variable penetrance. In essence, a carrier has a 50:50 chance of passing the gene to a son or daughter, but it is uncertain whether an individual with the gene mutation will actually develop breast or ovarian cancer. As a result, manifestations of *BRCA1* or *BRCA2* mutations can appear to skip generations.

Genetic Testing

Ideally, genetic testing identifies women with deleterious *BRCA1* and *BRCA2* mutations, leads to intervention with prophylactic surgery, and thereby prevents ovarian cancer. Three distinct results are possible with this testing. A "positive" test suggests the presence of a deleterious mutation. The most common are the three "Jewish founder" mutations: 185delAG or 5382insC in *BRCA1* and 6174delT in *BRCA2*. Each of these "frameshift" mutations significantly alters the downstream amino acid sequence, resulting in alteration of the BRCA1 or BRCA2 tumor suppressor protein. As suggested, these three specific mutations are thought to have originated from within the Ashkenazi population thousands of years ago. Although Jewish founder mutations are most common, any frameshift mutation within the *BRCA* genes may result in a deleterious predisposition to developing breast and ovarian cancer.

Second, "variants of uncertain clinical significance" may actually be pathogenic (true mutations) or just polymorphisms (normal variants found in at least 1 percent of alleles in the general population). These unclassified variants are common, representing approximately one third of *BRCA1* test results and half of those for *BRCA2*. Most are missense mutations, which result in a single amino acid change in the protein, without a frameshift. Given the prognostic uncertainty and high rate of reclassification, individualized counseling and directing efforts toward surveillance, chemoprevention, or salpingectomy are recommended (Garcia, 2014).

The third potential and most reassuring genetic test result is "negative." However, due to the large size of the *BRCA1* and *BRCA2* genes, the false-negative rate is 5 to 10 percent. To capture additional, otherwise undetected mutations, reflex testing of large genomic rearrangements is available for high-risk patients (Palma, 2008).

PREVENTION

■ Ovarian Cancer Screening

In addition to genetic testing, other screening strategies for ovarian cancer have been evaluated. However, despite enormous effort, there is no proof that routine screening with serum markers, sonography, or pelvic examinations decreases mortality rates (American College of Obstetricians and Gynecologists, 2013; Morgan, 2014; Schorge, 2010a). Hundreds of possible markers have been identified, yet no test currently available approaches sufficient levels of accuracy (American College of Obstetricians and Gynecologists, 2011).

High-risk Women

For the most part, screening strategies are directed at *BRCA1* or *BRCA2* carriers, in addition to women with a strong family history of breast and ovarian cancer. Most commonly, cancer antigen 125 (CA125) level measurements and/or transvaginal sonography have been tested, albeit with marginal success. Thus, in *BRCA1* or *BRCA2* mutation carriers who do not wish to undergo prophylactic surgery, a screening strategy that combines thorough pelvic examination, transvaginal sonographic evaluation, and CA125 blood testing may be offered (American College of Obstetricians and Gynecologists, 2013).

CA125 is a glycoprotein that is not produced by normal ovarian epithelium but that may be produced by both benign and malignant ovarian tumors. CA125 is synthesized within affected ovarian epithelial cells and often secreted into cysts. In benign tumors, excess antigen is released into and may accumulate within cyst fluid. Hypothetically, abnormal tissue architecture associated with malignant tumors allows antigen release into the vascular circulation (Verheijen, 1999).

Alone, CA125 is not a useful marker for detecting ovarian cancer. However, a more sensitive *Risk of Ovarian Cancer*

Algorithm (ROCA) has been developed and is based on the slope of serial CA125 measurements drawn at regular intervals (Skates, 2003). If a ROCA score exceeds a 1-percent risk of having ovarian cancer, patients then undergo transvaginal sonography to determine whether additional intervention is warranted. This strategy is currently being studied in a prospective, international trial of 2605 high-risk women who initially chose to undergo either risk-reducing salpingo-oophorectomy or screening alone (Greene, 2008).

General Population

Because no sufficiently accurate early detection tests are currently available, routine screening for women at average risk is not recommended (Moyer, 2012). For example, in the United States' prospective Prostate, Lung, Colorectal and Ovarian (PLCO) Trial of screening versus usual care, 34,261 women without prior oophorectomy were randomly assigned to annual CA125 level measurement and transvaginal sonographic examination. Of those with an abnormal screen, approximately 1 percent had invasive ovarian cancer, demonstrating a relatively low predictive value of both tests (Buys, 2005, 2011; Partridge, 2009).

To evaluate the efficacy, cost, morbidity, compliance, and acceptability of ROCA-based CA125 screening and study-directed sonography, a randomized trial of 202,638 patients was conducted. In The United Kingdom Collaborative Trial of Ovarian Cancer Screening (UKCTOCS), asymptomatic, average-risk postmenopausal women aged 50 to 74 years were randomly assigned to no treatment, to annual CA125 screening with transvaginal sonography as a second-line test if indicated by ROCA interpretation, or to annual screening with transvaginal sonography. The ROCA-directed approach demonstrated a 35-percent positive-predictive value, more than 10 times higher than annual sonography (3 percent). Although in this study ROCA-directed sonography was shown to be feasible, the results of ongoing screening to determine whether there is any meaningful effect on mortality rates will be available in 2015 (Menon, 2009, 2014). Despite most major professional and government groups recommending against it, approximately a third of U.S. physicians continue to order CA125 or sonography to screen for ovarian cancer (Baldwin, 2012).

New Biomarkers and Proteomics

To identify a more accurate screening test for early ovarian cancer detection, various potential biomarkers have been described. Dozens have been evaluated alone and in combination with CA125 (Cramer, 2011; Yurkovetsky, 2010).

One example, based on a preliminary study published in 2002, suggested that proteomics may help detect early-stage ovarian cancer (Petricoin, 2002). By profiling the patterns of thousands of proteins with a high degree of sensitivity and specificity, it was hoped that an accurate test, such as OvaCheck, would reliably distinguish those with early ovarian cancer from unaffected women.

Another entry, the OvaSure blood test, has also generated enthusiasm. Based on the simultaneous evaluation of six analytes (leptin, osteopontin, insulin-like growth factor-II, macrophage inhibitory factor, and CA125), it was reported to yield high sensitivity and specificity for ovarian cancer (Mor, 2005; Visintin, 2008).

Importantly, prospective clinical trials must be designed and completed before any of these new diagnostic tests can be offered outside of a trial. Unfortunately, neither proteomics nor any other screening strategy is currently near implementation into routine clinical practice.

Physical Examination

In general, pelvic examination only occasionally detects ovarian cancer, generally when the disease is already in advanced stages. In asymptomatic women, there is no evidence that it lowers mortality or morbidity rates as a screening test (Bloomfield, 2014). As a result, bimanual examination was not even included as a screening modality in either the PLCO or UKCTOCS trials.

Chemoprevention

Oral contraceptive use is associated with a 50-percent decreased risk of developing ovarian cancer. However, there is a short-term increased risk of developing breast cancer and cervical cancer that should be considered when counseling patients (International Collaboration of Epidemiological Studies of Cervical Cancer, 2006, 2007; National Cancer Institute, 2014a).

Prophylactic Surgery

The only proven way to directly prevent ovarian cancer is surgical removal. In *BRCA1* or *BRCA2* carriers, prophylactic bilateral salpingo-oophorectomy (BSO) may be performed either upon completion of childbearing or by age 40 years (American College of Obstetricians and Gynecologists, 2013, 2014). In these patients, the procedure is approximately 90-percent effective in preventing epithelial ovarian cancer (Kauff, 2002; Rebbeck, 2002). Prophylactic BSO reduces the risk of developing breast cancer by 50 percent (Rebbeck, 2002). Predictably, the protective effect is strongest among premenopausal women (Kramer, 2005). In women with HNPCC, the ovarian cancer risk reduction approaches 100 percent (Schmeler, 2006). Yet, significant adverse consequences accompany premature menopause. Moreover, recent studies suggest that a substantial proportion of "ovarian cancers" in high-risk women actually arise from precursor lesions located in the distal fallopian tube. Thus, prophylactic salpingectomy followed later by postmenopausal oophorectomy may be a safe alternative (Holman, 2014; Kwon, 2013; Perets, 2013). Surgical excision ideally removes the entire tube from fimbria to uterotubal junction, but the interstitial portion within the myometrium remains.

The term *prophylactic* implies that the tubes and ovaries are normal at the time of removal. However, approximately 4 to 5 percent of *BRCA* mutation carriers undergoing prophylactic BSO will have an otherwise undetected, often microscopic, cancer at the time of surgery (Sherman, 2014). In fact, the distal fallopian tube seems to be the dominant site of origin for occult malignancies detected during risk-reducing surgery (Callahan, 2007). To account for this possibility, cytologic washings, peritoneal biopsies, and an omental sample may be routinely collected during surgery. When submitting the final surgical specimen, the pathology requisition should clearly state that the BSO was performed for a prophylactic indication. In these cases, the ovaries and tubes, especially the fimbria, undergo more intensive scrutiny and are serially microsectioned to identify occult disease. Using a rigorous operative and pathologic protocol such as this can significantly increase the detection rate of occult tubal or ovarian malignancy in *BRCA* mutation carriers (Powell, 2005). Typically, the excision, washings, and biopsies can all be completed by laparoscopic surgery.

Prophylactic BSO in young women will induce premature menopause and its associated effects of vasomotor and urogenital symptoms, decline in sexual interest, and osteoporosis (National Cancer Institute, 2014a). Estrogen replacement therapy is commonly used to alleviate these symptoms but may be less effective than is often assumed (Madalinska, 2006). Overall, mainly due to the favorable impact in reducing cancer worries, prophylactic BSO does not adversely affect quality of life (Madalinska, 2005).

In women with the HNPCC syndrome, hysterectomy is mandatory when performing prophylactic BSO because of coexisting endometrial cancer risks. In *BRCA* mutation carriers, it should not be recommended routinely (Vyarvelska, 2014). Few reports have suggested a meaningful association between *BRCA* mutations and an increased risk of endometrial cancer. Mainly, these develop in patients taking tamoxifen for breast cancer treatment or breast cancer chemoprevention (Beiner, 2007).

In low-risk patients who are not *BRCA* carriers, risk-reducing salpingectomy is now also considered in those undergoing hysterectomy or permanent sterilization, in hopes of preventing pelvic serous cancers (Creinin, 2014; Lessard-Anderson, 2014; McAlpine, 2014; Morelli, 2013). This consideration has been endorsed by both the Society of Gynecologic Oncology (2013) and the American College of Obstetricians and Gynecologists (2015). Pathologic specimen processing in low-risk women includes representative sections of the tube, any suspicious lesions, and entire sectioning of the fimbriae. Neither organization specifies pelvic washing collection in this low-risk population.

LOW-MALIGNANT-POTENTIAL TUMORS

■ Pathology

Ten to 15 percent of epithelial ovarian cancers have histologic and biologic features that are intermediate between clearly benign cysts and frankly invasive carcinomas. In general, these low-malignant-potential (LMP) tumors, also termed *borderline tumors*, are associated with risk factors that are similar to those for epithelial ovarian cancer (Huusom, 2006). Typically, they are not considered part of any of the hereditary breast-ovarian cancer syndromes. Although LMP tumors may develop at any age, on average, patients are in their mid-40s, which is 15 years younger than women with invasive ovarian carcinoma. For various reasons, their diagnosis and optimal management are frequently problematic.

Histologically, LMP tumors are distinguished from benign cysts by having at least two of the following features: nuclear atypia, epithelial stratification, microscopic papillary projections, cellular pleomorphism, or mitotic activity (Fig. 35-2). Unlike invasive carcinomas, LMP tumors lack stromal invasion. However, up to 10 percent of LMP tumors will exhibit areas of *microinvasion*, defined as foci measuring <3 mm in diameter and forming <5 percent of the tumor (Buttin, 2002). Due to

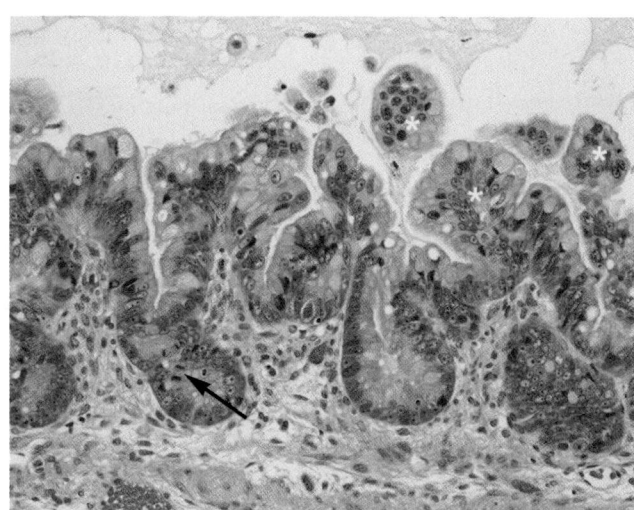

FIGURE 35-2 Mucinous borderline tumor. These tumors are distinguished from benign mucinous cystadenomas by the presence of epithelial proliferation and nuclear atypia. This example of a mucinous borderline tumor has mild to moderate nuclear atypia as evidenced by limited nuclear pleomorphism and visible nucleoli. A mitotic figure is also seen (*arrow*). Epithelial proliferation is indicated by epithelial tufts (*asterisks*), which are unsupported by fibrovascular cores. (Used with permission from Dr. Kelley Carrick.)

the subtle nature of many of these findings, it is challenging to diagnose an LMP tumor with certainty based on frozen section specimen analysis.

■ Clinical Features

Ovarian LMP tumors present similar to other adnexal masses. Patients may have pelvic pain, distention, or increasing abdominal girth. Alternatively, an asymptomatic mass may be palpated during routine pelvic examination. These tumors are occasionally detected as an incidental finding during routine obstetric sonographic examination or at the time of cesarean delivery.

As with other ovarian tumors, size varies widely. Preoperatively, there is no pathognomonic sonographic appearance, and serum CA125 levels are nonspecific. Depending on the clinical setting, computed tomography (CT) scanning may be indicated to exclude ascites or omental caking, which would suggest a more typical ovarian cancer. Regardless, any woman with a suspicious adnexal mass should have it removed.

■ Treatment

Surgery is the cornerstone management for LMP tumors. The operative plan will vary, depending on circumstances, and patients are carefully counseled beforehand. All women should be prepared for complete ovarian cancer surgical staging or debulking, if necessary. In many cases, a laparoscopic approach is appropriate. If laparotomy is planned, then a vertical incision is selected to allow access to the upper abdomen and paraaortic nodes, if needed, for cancer staging.

During surgery, peritoneal washings are immediately collected upon entrance into the abdomen, followed by exploration. The ovarian mass is removed intact and submitted for pathologic consultation and frozen section evaluation. However, it is almost impossible to know with certainty whether a patient

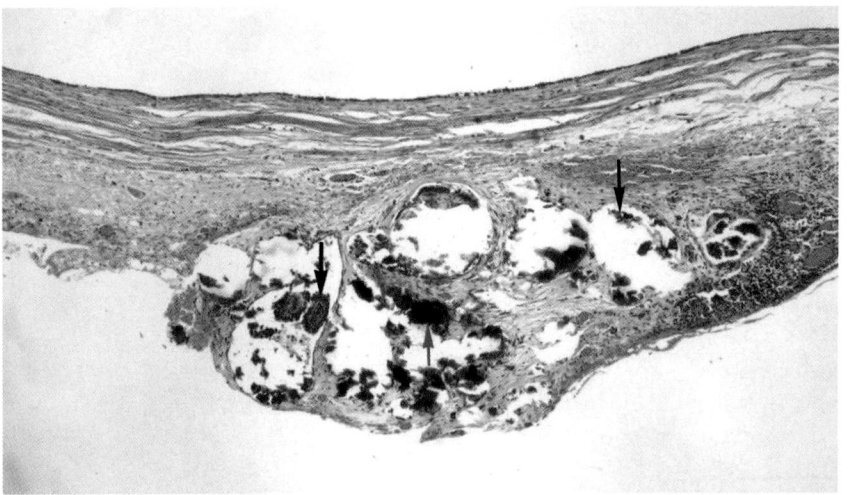

FIGURE 35-3 Noninvasive implant from patient with ovarian serous borderline tumor. A noninvasive implant does not have destructive invasion of the underlying tissue. In this noninvasive implant, proliferative serous-type epithelium (*black arrows*) and psammoma bodies (*blue arrow*) typical of serous proliferations appear to adhere to the peritoneal tissue, but do not invade it. Psammoma bodies are fragmented in this tissue, as calcified material often shatters when sectioned if not decalcified prior to sectioning. (Used with permission from Dr. Raheela Ashfaq.)

has a benign adnexal mass, LMP tumor, or invasive ovarian cancer until final histologic slides have been reviewed (Houck, 2000; Tempfer, 2007). Accordingly, in those with LMP diagnosed intraoperatively, premenopausal women who have not completed childbearing may undergo fertility-sparing surgery with preservation of the uterus and contralateral ovary (Park, 2009; Zanetta, 2001). This is a reasonable approach even if the final diagnosis shows invasive stage I cancer (Schilder, 2002). Alternatively, postmenopausal women should undergo hysterectomy with BSO.

Limited staging biopsies of the peritoneum and omentum are considered, although they rarely contain microscopic foci of metastatic LMP unless the tissues appear abnormal (Kristensen, 2014). Additionally, the appendix is also examined and potentially removed, especially if the tumor has mucinous histology (Timofeev, 2010). In the absence of enlarged nodes or a frozen section suggestive of frankly invasive disease, routine pelvic and paraaortic lymph node dissection may not be necessary (Rao, 2004).

LMP tumors are staged with the same FIGO criteria used for invasive ovarian cancer (p. 748). For the most part, surgical staging has limited value in altering the prognosis of those with LMP tumors unless invasive cancer is ultimately diagnosed (Wingo, 2006). Although 97 percent of gynecologic oncologists advocate comprehensive surgical staging of LMP tumors, in current practice it is performed in only 12 percent of patients (Lin, 1999; Menzin, 2000). This disparity stems from the fact that often the diagnosis is not suspected intraoperatively, no frozen section is requested or it is inaccurate, and a clinician is alerted only when the final pathology report has been completed. In this circumstance, consultation with a gynecologic oncologist is recommended, but comprehensive surgical restaging is not necessarily required if the tumor appears confined to a single ovary (Zapardiel, 2010). However, if a cystectomy has

been performed, the risk of residual disease should prompt a discussion regarding removal of the entire adnexa with washings and limited staging (Poncelet, 2006).

For patients with stage II-IV disease, usually demonstrated by noninvasive implants (Fig. 35-3) or nodal metastases, the utility of adjuvant chemotherapy is speculative (Shih, 2010; Sutton, 1991). The most worrisome finding is invasive peritoneal implants. In general, these patients are treated like those with typical epithelial ovarian carcinoma, including debulking and postoperative chemotherapy (Leary, 2014).

■ Prognosis

The prognosis is excellent for patients with ovarian LMP tumors. Five-year survival rates range from 96 to 99 percent for stages I-III, whereas it reaches 77 percent for stage IV disease (Trimble, 2002). Overall, more than 80 percent have stage I disease, and if treated by hysterectomy and BSO, stage I tumors rarely, if ever, recur (du Bois, 2013). In fact, such women have an overall survival similar to the general population (Hannibal, 2014). Fertility-sparing surgery is associated with up to a 15-percent risk of relapse, usually in the contralateral ovary, but remains highly curable by reoperation and resection (Park, 2009; Rao, 2005).

Approximately 15 percent of LMP tumors have stage II and III disease, almost invariably of serous histology. Stage IV ovarian LMP tumors account for fewer than 5 percent of diagnoses and have the worst prognosis (Trimble, 2002). For these advanced-stage tumors, the most reliable prognostic indicators are the presence of invasive peritoneal implants or residual disease after surgery (Morice, 2014; Seidman, 2000).

Due to the indolent nature of these tumors, symptomatic recurrence often takes place years or even decades after diagnosis (Silva, 2006). Approximately 70 percent of relapses have only LMP histology. Malignant transformation into an invasive ovarian cancer develops in the other 30 percent. Most of these are low-grade carcinomas, but approximately one third will have high-grade features, which adversely affects prognosis (du Bois, 2013; Harter, 2014). As in primary ovarian LMP tumors, complete surgical excision is the most effective therapy for recurrent disease (Crane, 2015). Chemotherapy is reserved for patients with invasive features, but low-grade tumors tend to be particularly resistant to standard agents, such as carboplatin and paclitaxel. Typically, multiple different regimens are used, including hormonal therapy (Gourley, 2014).

EPITHELIAL OVARIAN CANCER

■ Pathogenesis

There are at least three distinct tumorigenic pathways to account for the heterogeneity of epithelial ovarian cancer. First, relatively few cases seem to arise from an accumulation

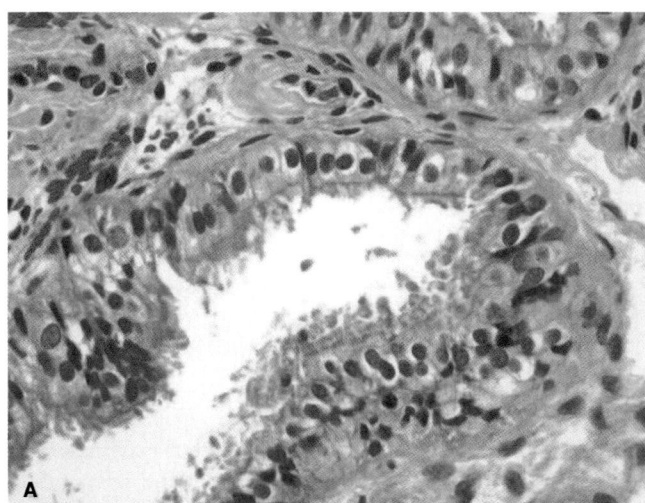 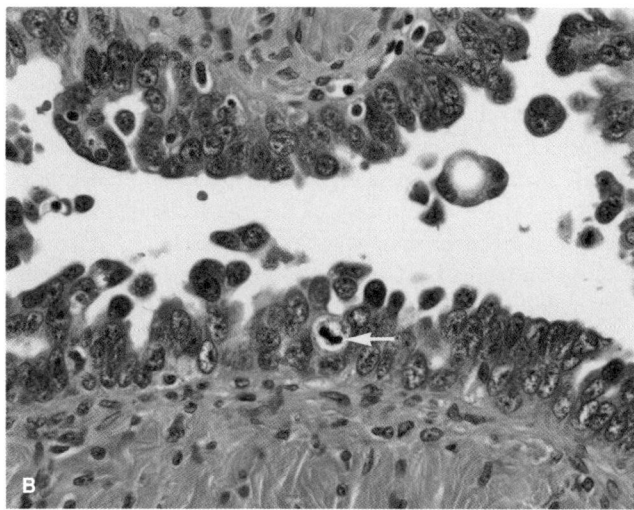

FIGURE 35-4 A. Normal fallopian tube epithelium is composed of three cell types—ciliated cells, secretory cells, and intercalary cells. **B.** Serous carcinoma in situ of the fallopian tube. The cells of serous carcinoma lining this tube are markedly atypical, with nuclear pleomorphism, chromatin coarseness, loss of nuclear polarity, mitotic activity (*arrow*), and epithelial proliferation/tufting. (Used with permission from Dr. Kelley Carrick.)

of genetic alterations that leads to malignant transformation of benign cysts to LMP tumors and ultimate progression to invasive ovarian carcinoma (Makarla, 2005). Typically, these invasive tumors are low-grade and clinically indolent, and K-*ras* oncogenic mutations occur early. The *ras* family of oncogenes includes K-*ras*, H-*ras*, and N-*ras*. Their protein products participate in cell cycle regulation and cell proliferation control. As such, *ras* mutations are implicated in carcinogenesis by their inhibition of cellular apoptosis and promotion of cellular proliferation (Mammas, 2005).

Second, at least 10 percent of epithelial ovarian carcinomas, invariably high-grade serous tumors, result from an inherited predisposition. Women born with a *BRCA* gene mutation require only one "hit" to the other normal copy (allele) to "knock out" the BRCA tumor-suppressor gene product. As a result, BRCA-related cancers develop approximately 15 years before sporadic cases. Current data suggests that serous tubal intraepithelial carcinoma (STIC) is a precursor condition for a significant percentage of serous carcinomas, which were formerly thought to arise spontaneously on the ovarian or peritoneal surface (Fig. 35-4) (Levanon, 2008; Medeiros, 2006; Perets, 2013). Thereafter, BRCA-related serous cancers appear to have a unique molecular pathogenesis, requiring p53 inactivation to progress (Buller, 2001; Landen, 2008; Schorge, 2000). *p53* is a tumor suppressor gene. Its protein product prohibits cells from entering subsequent stages of cell division and thereby halts uncontrolled tumor cell replication. Mutations in *p53* are linked with various cancers. In fact, loss of BRCA and p53 protein function has been detected prior to invasion, further supporting its importance as an early triggering event (Werness, 2000).

Third, most carcinomas appear to originate de novo from ovarian surface epithelial cells that are sequestered in cortical inclusion cysts (CICs) within the ovarian stroma. Numerous inciting events and subsequent pathways have been proposed. For example, cyclic repair of the ovarian surface during long periods of repetitive ovulation requires abundant cellular proliferation. In these women, spontaneous *p53* mutations arising during the DNA synthesis that accompanies this proliferation appear to play a primary carcinogenetic role (Schildkraut, 1997). Ultimately, the replicative stress and DNA damage transforms the entrapped surface epithelial cells within CICs into any of the histologic ovarian cancer variants (Levanon, 2008).

■ Diagnosis

Symptoms and Physical Findings

Ovarian cancer is typically portrayed as a "silent" killer that lacks appreciable early signs or symptoms. This is a misconception. Actually, patients are often symptomatic for several months before the diagnosis, even with early-stage disease (Goff, 2000). The difficulty is distinguishing these symptoms from those that normally occur in women.

In general, persistent symptoms that are more severe or frequent than expected and have a recent onset warrant further diagnostic investigation. Commonly, increased abdominal size, bloating, urinary urgency, and pelvic pain are reported. Additionally, fatigue, indigestion, inability to eat normally, constipation, and back pain may be noted (Goff, 2004). Abnormal vaginal bleeding occurs rarely. Occasionally, patients may present with nausea, vomiting, and a partial bowel obstruction if carcinomatosis is particularly widespread. Unfortunately, many women and clinicians are quick to attribute most symptoms to menopause, aging, dietary changes, stress, depression, or functional bowel problems, and diagnosis is often delayed.

A pelvic or pelvic-abdominal mass is palpable in most patients with ovarian cancer during bimanual evaluation. Malignant tumors tend to be solid, nodular, and fixed, but there are no classic findings that distinguish these growths from benign tumors. Paradoxically, a huge mass filling the pelvis and abdomen more often represents a benign or borderline tumor. To aid surgical planning, a rectovaginal examination is also performed. For example, a woman with cancer involving the rectovaginal septum may need to be positioned in dorsal lithotomy to perform a low anterior colon resection as a part of tumor excision.

The presence of a fluid wave, or less commonly, flank bulging, suggests the presence of significant ascites. In a woman with a pelvic mass and ascites, the diagnosis is ovarian cancer until proven otherwise. However, ascites without an identifiable pelvic mass suggests the possibility of cirrhosis or other primary malignancies such as gastric or pancreatic cancers. In advanced disease, examination of the upper abdomen usually reveals a central mass signifying omental caking.

Auscultation of the chest is also important, since patients with malignant pleural effusions may not be overtly symptomatic. The remainder of the examination includes palpation of the peripheral nodes in addition to a general physical assessment.

Laboratory Testing

A routine complete blood count and metabolic panel often demonstrates a few characteristic features. Of affected women, 20 to 25 percent will present with thrombocytosis (platelet count $>400 \times 10^9$/L) (Li, 2004). Malignant ovarian cells releasing cytokines are believed to increase platelet production rates. Hyponatremia, typically ranging between 125 and 130 mEq/L, is another common finding. In these patients, tumor secretion of a vasopressin-like substance can cause a clinical picture suggesting a syndrome of inappropriate antidiuretic hormone (SIADH).

The serum CA125 level is integral to epithelial ovarian cancer management. In 90 percent of women presenting with malignant nonmucinous tumors, CA125 levels are elevated. However, there are caveats during adnexal mass evaluation. Half of stage I ovarian cancers will have a normal CA125 measurement (false-negative). Also, an elevated value (false-positive) may be associated with various common benign indications such as pelvic inflammatory disease, endometriosis, leiomyomas, pregnancy, and even menstruation. Thus, in postmenopausal women with a pelvic mass, a CA125 measurement may better predict a higher likelihood of malignancy (Im, 2005).

Another marker, the human epididymal protein 4 (HE4) tumor marker, is approved by the U.S. Food and Drug Administration (FDA), along with CA125, when used in the Risk of Ovarian Malignancy Algorithm (ROMA) to determine the likelihood of finding malignancy at surgery in women with an adnexal mass. The ROMA score is derived from the results of both blood tests, plus menopausal status (Moore, 2009, 2010).

OVA1 is another biomarker blood test panel that may be used for the preoperative triage of women with an identified ovarian mass when surgery is planned (Ueland, 2011; Ware Miller, 2011). Scores ≥5.0 in premenopausal and scores ≥4.4 in postmenopausal women suggest a need for gynecologic oncologist consultation. Importantly, this test is not a screening tool and is reserved for those with a known surgical mass to aid preoperative triage (Vermillion Inc, 2012; Zhang, 2010). Validation studies evaluating ROMA and OVA1 are limited, and their role in preoperative triage is yet to be clearly defined. As a result, they are not necessarily recommended for determining the status of an undiagnosed pelvic mass (Morgan, 2014). Last, when a mucinous ovarian tumor is identified, serum tumor markers that may be better indicators of disease are cancer antigen 19-9 (CA19-9) and carcinoembryonic antigen (CEA).

Imaging

Transvaginal sonography is typically the most useful imaging test to differentiate benign tumors and early-stage ovarian cancers (Chap. 2, p. 33). In general, malignant tumors are multiloculated, solid or echogenic, and large (>5 cm), and they have thick septa with areas of nodularity (Fig. 35-5A). Other features may include papillary projections or neovascularization—demonstrated by adding color Doppler (Figs. 35-5B and 35-5C). Although several presumptive models have been described in an attempt to distinguish benign masses from ovarian cancers preoperatively, none have been universally implemented (Timmerman, 2005; Twickler, 1999).

In patients with advanced disease, sonography is less helpful. The pelvic sonogram may be particularly difficult to interpret if a large mass encompasses the uterus, adnexa, and surrounding structures. Ascites, if present, is easily detected, but in general, abdominal sonography has limited use.

Of *radiographic tests*, patients with suspected ovarian cancer should have a chest radiograph to detect pulmonary effusions or infrequently, pulmonary metastases. Rarely, a barium enema is clinically helpful in excluding diverticular disease or colon cancer or in identifying ovarian cancer involvement of the rectosigmoid.

Computed tomography (CT) scanning has a primary role in treatment planning for women with advanced ovarian cancer. Preoperatively, implants in the liver, retroperitoneum, omentum, or other intraabdominal site are detected to thereby guide surgical cytoreduction or demonstrate obviously unresectable disease (Fig. 35-6) (Suidan, 2014). However, CT is not particularly reliable in detecting intraperitoneal disease smaller than 1 to 2 cm in diameter. Moreover, CT scanning accuracy is poor for differentiating a benign ovarian mass from a malignant tumor when disease is limited to the pelvis. In these cases, transvaginal sonography is superior. Other radiologic studies such as magnetic resonance (MR) imaging, bone scans, and positron emission tomography (PET) in general provide limited additional information preoperatively.

Paracentesis

A woman with a pelvic mass and ascites can usually be assumed to have ovarian cancer until surgically proven otherwise. Thus, few patients require diagnostic paracentesis. Moreover, this procedure is typically avoided diagnostically as cytologic results are usually nonspecific and abdominal wall metastases may form at the needle entry site (Kruitwagen, 1996). However, paracentesis may be indicated for those with ascites in the *absence* of a pelvic mass.

Aside from diagnosis, paracentesis may also relieve volume-related symptoms in those with large accumulations. This may be done at the bedside, using connector tubing and vacuum bottles, or completed by an interventional radiologist. Relative dehydration is common afterward and manifest by thirst, oliguria, and short-term creatinine level rise, which all correct with normal oral intake.

■ Role of the Generalist

Using the currently available diagnostic modalities, clinicians often face tremendous difficulty in distinguishing benign from

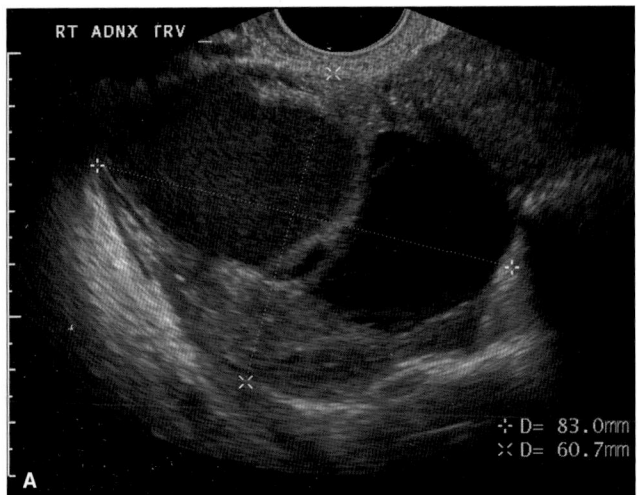

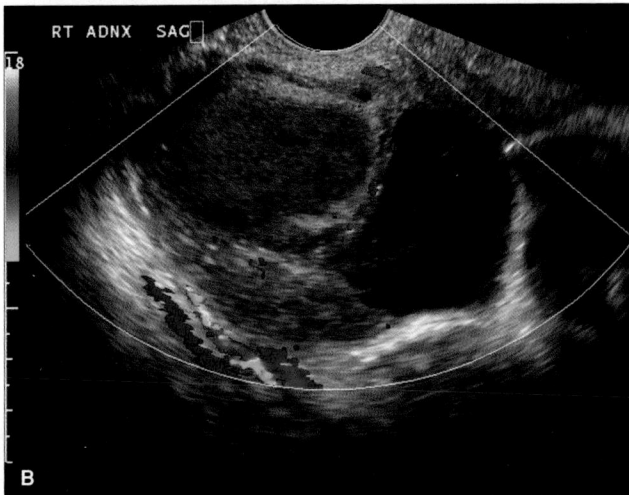

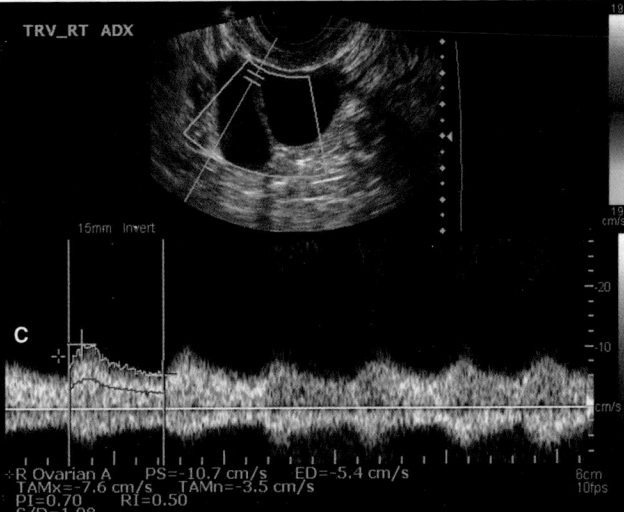

FIGURE 35-5 Sonograms of an ovarian cyst. **A.** Transvaginal sonogram depicts a complex ovarian mass (*calipers*). Cystic and solid components and a thick intracystic septum are seen. These findings increase clinical concern for malignancy. **B.** Color Doppler transvaginal sonogram shows neovascularization within this ovarian tumor. **C.** Transvaginal Doppler study of ovarian mass vessels reveals decreased impedance. (Used with permission from Dr. Diane Twickler.)

malignant. However, ascites or evidence of metastases should prompt consultation with an oncologist (American College of Obstetricians and Gynecologists, 2011). Additionally, premenopausal women with elevated CA125 levels (i.e., >200 U/mL) or an OVA1 score ≥5.0 and postmenopausal women with any CA125 level elevation or an OVA1 score ≥4.4 are at higher risk.

Ideally, for patients with suspicious adnexal masses, surgery is performed in a hospital with a pathologist able to reliably interpret an intraoperative frozen section. At minimum, samples for peritoneal cytology are obtained when the abdomen is entered. The mass is then removed intact through an incision that permits thorough staging and resection of possible metastatic sites (American College of Obstetricians and Gynecologists, 2011).

If malignancy is diagnosed, then surgical staging is completed. However, in a study of more than 10,000 women with ovarian cancer, almost half of those with early-stage disease did not undergo the recommended surgical procedures (Goff, 2006). Surgeons should be prepared to appropriately stage and potentially debulk ovarian cancer or have a gynecologic oncologist immediately available. This type of careful planning has been shown to achieve the best possible surgical result and improve survival rates (Earle, 2006; Engelen, 2006; Mercado, 2010). Moreover, since broader resources are usually available, patients cared for at high-volume hospitals also tend to have better outcomes (Bristow, 2010).

For women with malignancy identified only postoperatively or intraoperatively and without adequate staging, management will vary. Women with suspected early-stage disease may be restaged laparoscopically. Those with advanced disease may undergo a second laparotomy to obtain optimal tumor debulking (Grabowski, 2012). However, if extensive disease is found at the initial surgery, then chemotherapy may be selected first and followed later by laparotomy to obtain optimal interval cytoreduction.

At some point during postoperative surveillance, many women with early-stage disease, depending on the diagnosis, will return to their referring physician. Monitoring for relapse is often coordinated between the gynecologic oncologist and generalist in obstetrics and gynecology, especially if no chemotherapy is required following surgery.

■ Pathology

Although epithelial ovarian cancer is often considered a single entity, the different histologic types vary in their behavior (Table 35-3). Sometimes, two or more cell types are mixed. Within each histologic type, tumors are further categorized as benign, borderline (low malignant potential), or malignant.

Mainly in early-stage disease, grade is an important prognostic factor that affects treatment planning (Morgan, 2014). Unfortunately, no grading system for epithelial ovarian carcinoma is universally accepted. Instead, numerous different schemata, most based on architecture and/or nuclear pleomorphism, are currently used. In general, tumors are classified as grade 1 (well-differentiated), grade 2 (moderately differentiated), and grade 3 (poorly differentiated) lesions (Pecorelli, 1999).

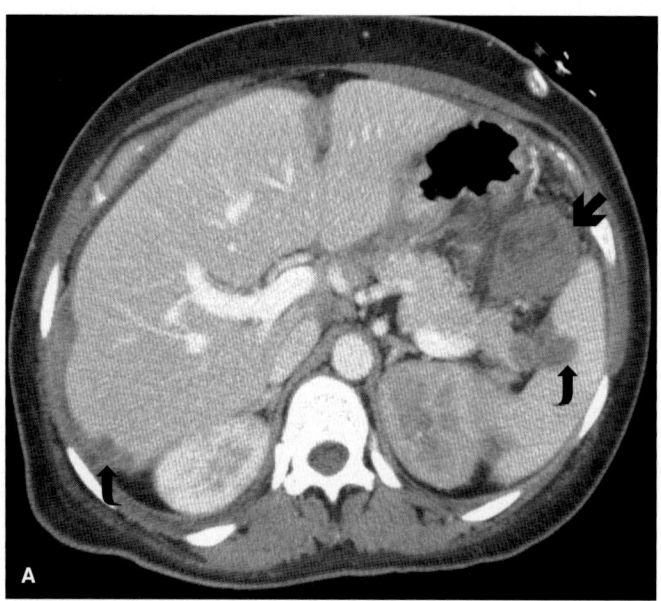 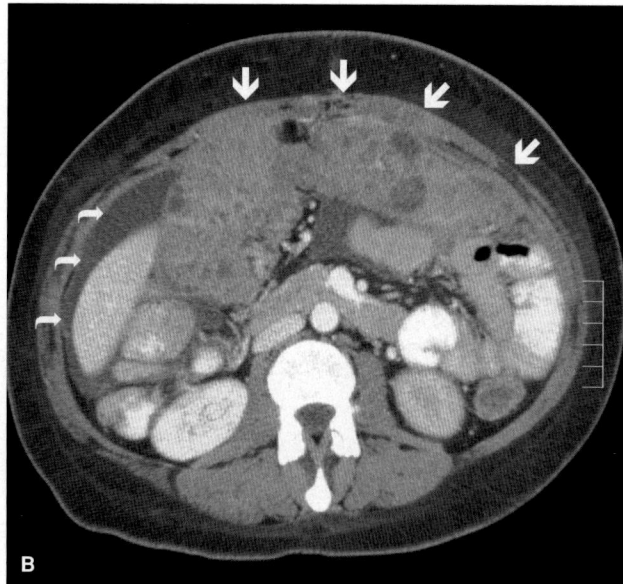

FIGURE 35-6 Computed tomographic scans in a woman with ovarian cancer. **A.** Axial CT scan at the level of the liver and spleen reveals metastatic lesions in the spleen and liver (*curved arrows*) and a bulky lesion at the splenorenal ligament (*arrow*). **B.** More caudal axial CT reveals ascites (*curved arrows*) and marked omental caking (*arrows*). (Used with permission from Dr. Diane Twickler.)

Grossly, there are no distinguishing features among the types of epithelial ovarian cancer. In general, each has solid and cystic areas of varying sizes (Fig. 35-7).

Serous Tumors

More than 50 percent of all epithelial ovarian cancers have serous histology. Microscopically, in well-differentiated tumors, cells may resemble fallopian tube epithelium, whereas in poorly differentiated tumors, anaplastic cells with severe nuclear atypia predominate (Fig. 35-8). During frozen section analysis, psammoma bodies are essentially pathognomonic of an ovarian-type serous carcinoma. Often, these tumors contain various other cell types as a minor component (<10 percent) that may cause diagnostic problems but do not influence outcome (Lee, 2003).

TABLE 35-3. World Health Organization Histological Classification of Ovarian Carcinoma

Serous adenocarcinoma
Mucinous adenocarcinoma
Endometrioid adenocarcinoma
Clear cell adenocarcinoma
Malignant Brenner tumor
Mixed epithelial and mesenchymal
   Adenosarcoma
   Carcinosarcoma
Squamous cell carcinoma
Mixed carcinoma
Undifferentiated carcinoma
Small cell carcinoma

Adapted with permission from Kurman RJ, Carcangiu ML, Herrington CS, et al (eds): WHO Classification of Tumours of Female Reproductive Organs, 4th ed. Lyon, International Agency for Research on Cancer, 2014.

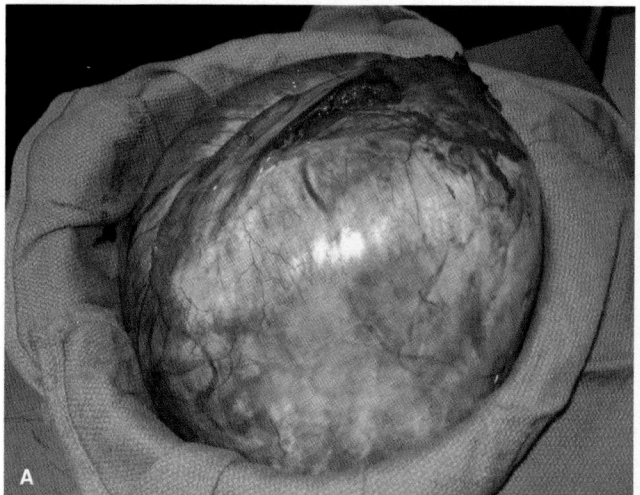

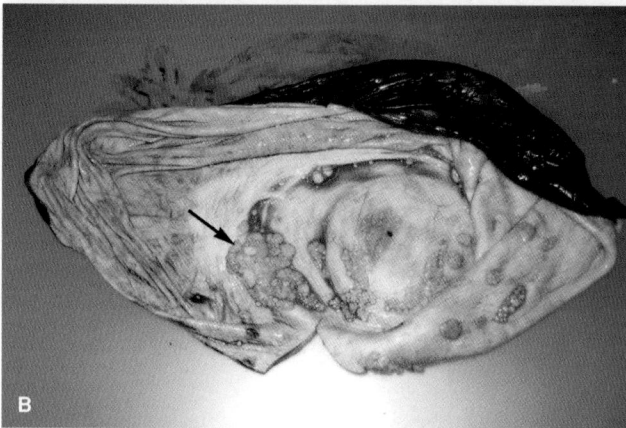

FIGURE 35-7 A. Excised cystic ovarian mass. Note the fallopian tube stretched over the top of the ovarian capsule. **B.** Opened tumor reveals the inner cyst wall and scattered papillary tumor growth (*arrow*). (Photographs contributed by Dr. David Miller.)

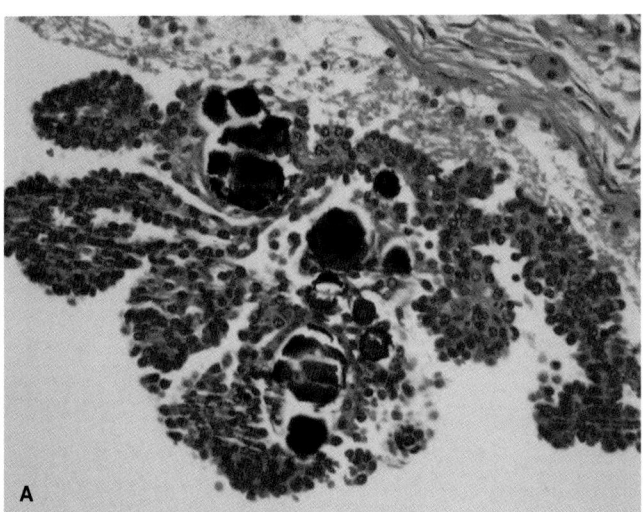 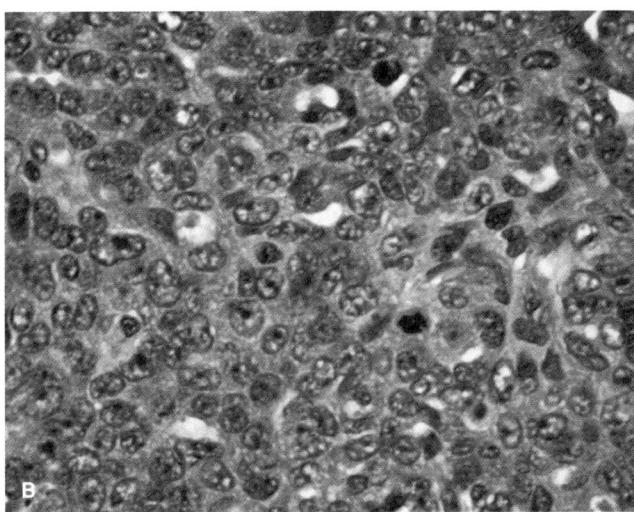

FIGURE 35-8 Serous carcinomas vary in regard to their degree of differentiation, as manifested by their architecture, degree of cytologic atypia and pleomorphism, and mitotic rate. **A.** In this relatively well-differentiated example of serous carcinoma, serous-type cells with moderate nuclear atypia form papillae and project into a cystic space. Numerous psammoma bodies, which are extracellular round laminar eosinophilic collections of calcium, are seen here. **B.** In this less well-differentiated example of serous carcinoma, moderately to markedly atypical cells form sheets, as opposed to the glands and papillae formed by better-differentiated tumors. (Used with permission from Dr. Kelley Carrick.)

Endometrioid Tumors

Endometrioid adenocarcinomas compose 15 to 20 percent of epithelial ovarian cancers and are the second most common histologic type (Fig. 35-9). The lower frequency results largely because poorly differentiated endometrioid and serous tumors cannot be easily distinguished and such cases are usually classified as serous. As a result, well-differentiated endometrioid tumors are proportionally more common, which may also explain their overall relatively good prognosis.

In 15 to 20 percent of cases, uterine endometrial adenocarcinoma coexists. This is usually regarded as a synchronous

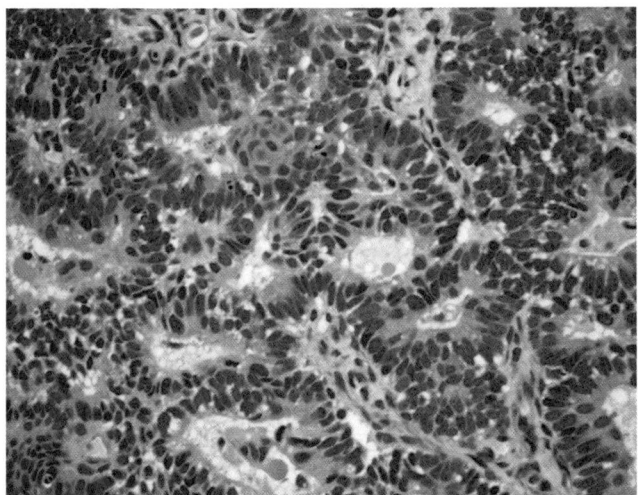

FIGURE 35-9 Ovarian endometrioid adenocarcinomas are morphologically similar to their more common counterparts arising in the endometrium. Better-differentiated tumors like this one have glands resembling proliferative endometrial glands, which grow in a confluent pattern. More poorly differentiated tumors have a variable percentage of solid growth and/or increased nuclear atypia. Like their endometrial counterparts, these tumors may show squamous differentiation. (Used with permission from Dr. Raheela Ashfaq.)

tumor, but metastasis from one site to the other is difficult to exclude (Soliman, 2004). A müllerian "field effect" is theorized to account for these independently developing, histologically similar tumors. In addition, many such patients are noted to have pelvic endometriosis.

Malignant mixed müllerian tumor, now preferably termed carcinosarcoma, by definition contains malignant epithelial and mesenchymal elements. It represents <1 percent of ovarian cancers, carries a poor prognosis, and is histologically similar to uterine primary tumors (Rauh-Hain, 2011).

Mucinous Tumors

Mucinous adenocarcinomas compose 5 to 10 percent of true epithelial ovarian cancers. The frequency is usually overestimated because many are undetected primary intestinal cancers from the appendix or colon. Well-differentiated ovarian mucinous tumors closely resemble mucin-secreting adenocarcinomas of intestinal or endocervical origin (Fig. 35-10). Histologically, the distinction may be impossible without clinical correlation (Lee, 2003). Advanced-stage mucinous ovarian carcinomas are rare, tend to be resistant to platinum chemotherapy, and have a prognosis significantly worse than that for serous tumors (Zaino, 2011).

Pseudomyxoma Peritonei. This clinical term describes the rare finding of abundant mucoid or gelatinous material in the pelvis and abdominal cavity, surrounded by thin fibrous capsules. An ovarian mucinous carcinoma with ascites rarely results in this condition, and evidence suggests that ovarian mucinous tumors associated with pseudomyxoma peritonei are almost all metastatic rather than primary. As a result, appendiceal or other intestinal sites of origin should be excluded (Ronnett, 1997). The primary appendiceal tumor may be small relative to the ovarian tumor(s) and may not be appreciated macroscopically. Thus, removal and thorough histologic examination of the appendix is indicated in all cases of pseudomyxoma peritonei.

If the peritoneal epithelial cells are benign or borderline-appearing, the condition is referred to as *disseminated peritoneal adenomucinosis*. Affected patients have a benign or protracted, indolent clinical course (Ronnett, 2001). If the peritoneal epithelial cells appear malignant, the clinical course is invariably fatal.

Clear Cell Adenocarcinoma

Comprising 5 to 10 percent of epithelial ovarian cancers, clear cell adenocarcinomas are most frequently associated with pelvic endometriosis. These tumors appear similar to clear cell carcinomas that develop sporadically in the uterus, vagina, and cervix. Typically, tumors are confined to the ovary and generally are cured by surgery alone. However, the 20 percent presenting with advanced disease tend to be platinum resistant and carry a worse prognosis than serous carcinoma (Al-Barrak, 2011).

Microscopically, both clear and "hobnail" cells are characteristic (Fig. 35-11). In clear cells, the visibly clear cytoplasm results from the dissolution of glycogen as the tissue specimen is histologically prepared. Hobnail cells have bulbous nuclei that protrude far into the cystic lumen beyond the apparent cytoplasmic limits of the cell (Lee, 2003).

Transitional Cell Tumors

Of these, the rare *malignant Brenner tumor* characteristically has poorly differentiated transitional cell carcinoma coupled with foci of benign or borderline Brenner tumor. Microscopically, the transitional cell component resembles carcinomas arising from the urinary tract, often with squamous differentiation. Brenner tumors classically have a dense, abundant fibrous stroma with embedded nests of transitional epithelium.

Transitional cell carcinoma accounts for fewer than 5 percent of ovarian cancers. These tumors lack a demonstrable Brenner component. Patients with transitional cell carcinoma have a

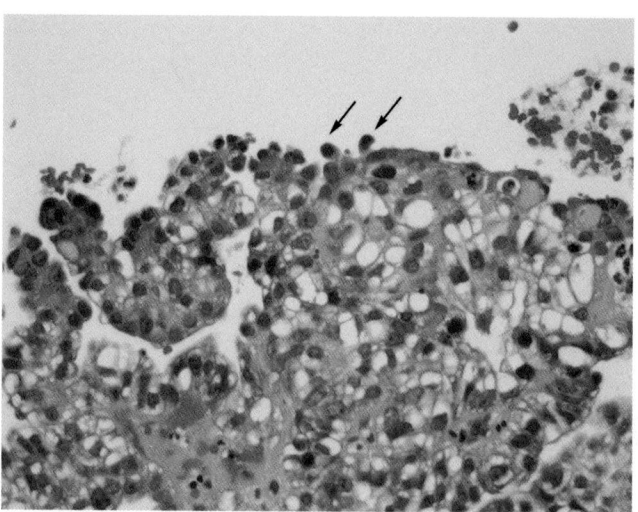

FIGURE 35-11 Clear cell adenocarcinoma is typically composed of cells with clear to eosinophilic cytoplasm that are arranged in cysts, tubules, papillae, and/or sheets. In the ovary, it looks similar to its counterparts in the endometrium and cervix/vagina. In this example, hobnail cells are marked by the arrows. (Used with permission from Dr. Kelley Carrick.)

worse prognosis than those with malignant Brenner tumors, but a better prognosis than those with other histologic types of epithelial ovarian cancer (Guseh, 2014). Microscopically, transitional cell carcinoma resembles a primary bladder carcinoma but has an immunoreactive pattern consistent with ovarian origin (Lee, 2003). Thus, transitional cell carcinoma is now considered a high-grade form of serous carcinoma.

Other Histologic Types

Of these, primary squamous cell carcinoma of the ovary is rare. This is the newest category to be recognized and typically carries a poor prognosis for most with advanced disease (Park, 2010). More commonly, squamous cell carcinomas arise from mature cystic teratomas (dermoid cysts) and are classified as malignant ovarian germ cell tumors (Pins, 1996). In other cases, ovarian endometrioid variants may have extensive squamous differentiation, or alternatively, metastases from a cervical primary are present.

Mixed carcinoma describes an ovarian cancer that contains more than 10 percent of a second cell type. Common combinations include mixed clear cell/endometrioid or serous/endometrioid adenocarcinomas.

Undifferentiated carcinomas are rare epithelial ovarian tumors that are too poorly differentiated to be classified into any of the müllerian types previously described. Microscopically, the cells are arranged in solid groups or sheets with numerous mitotic figures and marked cytologic atypia. Typically, foci of müllerian carcinoma, usually serous, are found within the tumor. Overall, undifferentiated carcinomas of the ovary have a poor prognosis compared with the other histologic types (Silva, 1991).

Small cell carcinomas are rare, extremely malignant, and consist of two subgroups. Most patients have a *hypercalcemic type*, which typically develops in young women. Nearly all tumors are unilateral, and two thirds are associated with elevated serum calcium levels that resolve postoperatively (Young, 1994). Recent

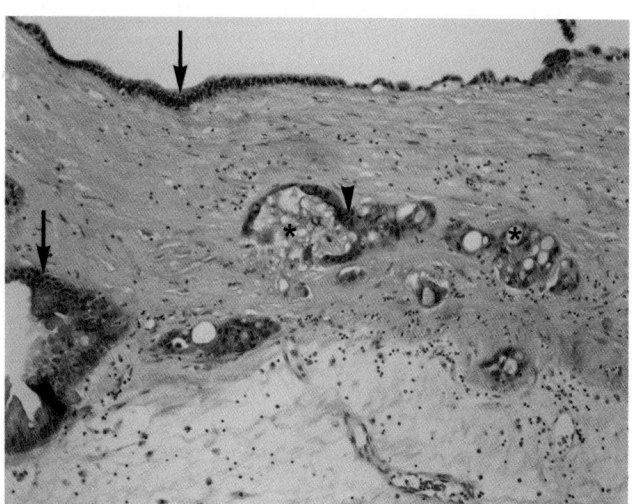

FIGURE 35-10 This mucinous carcinoma arose within a 15-cm mucinous cystadenoma. Benign mucinous-type epithelium lining cystic spaces of the background cystadenoma is seen (*arrows*). A carcinomatous component (*arrowhead*) invades the stroma in a haphazard fashion at the center of the photomicrograph. The malignant cells are arranged in clusters and poorly formed glands, which have intracytoplasmic and intraluminal mucin (*asterisks*). (Used with permission from Dr. Kelley Carrick.)

TABLE 35-4. Criteria for Diagnosing Primary Peritoneal Carcinoma When Ovaries Are Present

Both ovaries must be normal in size or enlarged by a benign process
The involvement in the extraovarian sites must be greater than the involvement on the surface of either ovary
The ovarian tumor involvement must be either nonexistent, confined to the ovarian surface epithelium without stromal
invasion, or involving the cortical stroma with tumor size less than 5 × 5 mm

data suggest these highly lethal tumors arise via a specific mutation in the *SMARCA4* gene (Jelinic, 2014). The *pulmonary type* resembles oat-cell carcinoma of the lung and develops in older women. Half of these women have bilateral ovarian disease (Eichhorn, 1992). In general, patients with small cell carcinoma die within 2 years from rapid disease progression.

Primary Peritoneal Carcinoma

Up to 15 percent of "typical" epithelial ovarian cancers are actually primary peritoneal carcinomas that develop de novo from the lining of the pelvis and abdomen. In some cases, especially among *BRCA1* mutation carriers, independent malignant transformation occurs at multiple peritoneal sites simultaneously (Schorge, 1998). However, more recent data suggest that nearly half of presumed cases actually arise in the tubal fimbria (Carlson, 2008).

Clinically and histologically, these tumors are virtually indistinguishable from epithelial ovarian cancer. However, primary peritoneal carcinoma may develop in a woman years after undergoing BSO. If ovaries are still present, several criteria are required to make the diagnosis (Table 35-4). By far the most common variant is papillary serous, but any of the other histologic types are possible. In general, the staging, treatment, and prognosis of primary peritoneal carcinoma are the same as for epithelial ovarian cancer (Mok, 2003). The differential diagnosis mainly includes malignant mesothelioma.

Fallopian Tube Carcinoma

Historically, this carcinoma was assumed to be rarer than epithelial ovarian cancer. However, the fallopian tube fimbria have recently been identified as an origin for many high-grade pelvic serous carcinomas that were previously assumed to arise from the ovary or peritoneum (Fig. 35-12) (Levanon, 2008).

Clinically, this fallopian tube carcinoma is similar to epithelial ovarian cancer. For the most part, risk factors, histologic types, surgical staging, pattern of spread, treatment, and prognosis are comparable. To be considered a primary fallopian tube carcinoma, the tumor must be located macroscopically within the tube or its fimbriated end. Additionally, the uterus and ovary must not contain carcinoma, or if they do, it must be clearly different from the fallopian tube lesion (Alvarado-Cabrero, 2003).

Secondary Tumors

Malignant tumors that metastasize to the ovary are almost invariably bilateral. The term *Krukenberg tumor* refers to a metastatic mucinous/signet ring cell adenocarcinoma of the ovaries that typically originates from primary tumors of the intestinal tract, characteristically the stomach (Fig. 35-13). Ovarian metastases

often represent a late disseminated stage of the disease in which other hematogenous metastases are also found (Prat, 2003).

Patterns of Spread

In general, epithelial ovarian cancers predominantly metastasize by *exfoliation*. Malignant cells are first released into the peritoneal

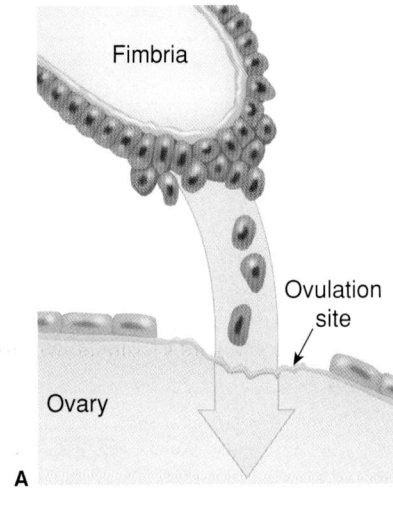

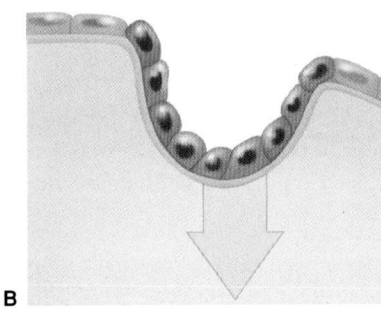

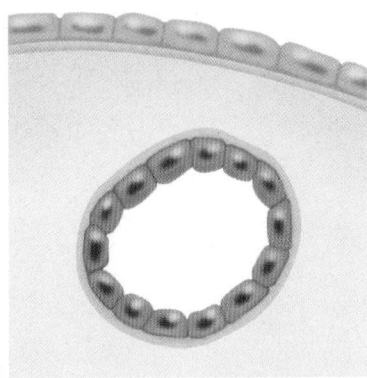

FIGURE 35-12 A. Epithelial cells from the fimbria are released and implant on the denuded surface of the ovary at the site of ovulation. **B & C.** Subsequently, an inclusion cyst is formed.

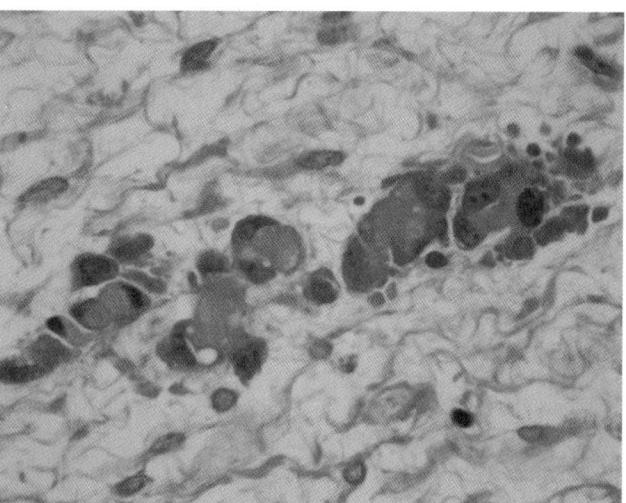

FIGURE 35-13 Krukenberg tumor. This metastatic, poorly differentiated adenocarcinoma is characterized by singly disposed cells with an intracytoplasmic mucin globule that displaces the nucleus to the cell periphery, producing a signet-ring-like cytomorphology. (Used with permission from Dr. Raheela Ashfaq.)

cavity when the tumor penetrates through the ovarian capsule surface. By following the normal circulation of peritoneal fluid, cells may then develop into implants anywhere in the abdomen. A unique characteristic of ovarian cancer is that metastatic tumors do not usually infiltrate visceral organs, but exist as surface implants. As a result, aggressive debulking is possible with reasonable morbidity.

Due to its marked vascularity, the omentum is the most frequent location to support metastatic disease and is often extensively involved with tumor (Fig. 35-14). Nodules are also commonly present on the undersurface of the right hemidiaphragm and small bowel serosa, but all intraperitoneal surfaces are at risk.

Lymphatic dissemination is the other primary mode of spread. Malignant cells move through channels that follow the ovarian blood supply along the infundibulopelvic ligament

and that terminate in paraaortic lymph nodes up to or above the level of the renal vessels. Other lymphatics pass laterally through the broad ligament and parametrium to the external iliac, obturator, and internal iliac nodal chains. Infrequently, metastases can also follow the round ligament to the inguinal nodes (Lee, 2003).

Direct extension of a progressively enlarging ovarian cancer may create confluent tumor involvement of the pelvic peritoneum and adjacent structures, including the uterus, rectosigmoid colon, and fallopian tubes. Usually, this is associated with significant induration of the surrounding tissues.

In advanced disease, several liters of ascites may collect. Either increased production of carcinomatous fluid or decreased clearance by obstructed lymphatic channels are purported causes. Similarly, by traversing the diaphragm, a malignant pleural effusion may develop, almost invariably on the right.

Hematogenous spread is atypical. In most cases, metastases to the liver or lung parenchyma, brain, or kidneys are observed in patients with recurrent, end-stage disease, and not at initial diagnosis.

■ Staging

Ovarian cancer is surgically staged, and stage is assigned according to findings before tumor removal and debulking (Fig. 35-15). The International Federation of Gynecology and Obstetrics (FIGO) stages reflect the typical patterns of ovarian cancer spread (Table 35-5) (Prat, 2014). Even if a tumor appears clinically confined to the ovary, in many cases it will have detectable metastases. Therefore, accurate surgical staging is crucial to guide treatment. Approximately one third of patients have surgical stage I or II disease (Table 35-6).

■ Management of Early-stage Ovarian Cancer

Surgical Staging

If a malignancy appears clinically confined to the ovary, surgical removal and comprehensive staging is performed. Typically, the abdominal incision must be adequate to identify and resect any disease that may have been missed during physical examination or imaging. The operation begins by aspirating free ascitic fluid or collecting peritoneal washings. This is followed by inspection and palpation of all peritoneal surfaces. Next, an extrafascial hysterectomy and BSO are performed. In the absence of gross extraovarian disease, the infracolic omentum should be removed or at least biopsied (Section 46-14, p. 1186). Additionally, random peritoneal biopsies or scrapings are obtained, ideally near the diaphragms (Lee, 2014; Timmers, 2010). The most prognostically important step, a pelvic and infrarenal paraaortic lymphadenectomy, is also completed (Sections 46-11, p. 1172) (Chan, 2007; Cress, 2011; Whitney, 2011).

Laparoscopic staging is particularly valuable as a primary treatment in women who have an apparent stage I ovarian cancer. Alternatively, unstaged patients may have their staging completed laparoscopically. In general, for minimally invasive staging, all of the required procedures can be safely performed (Chi, 2005). The main putative benefits are a shorter hospital stay and quicker recovery (Tozzi, 2004). However, nodal

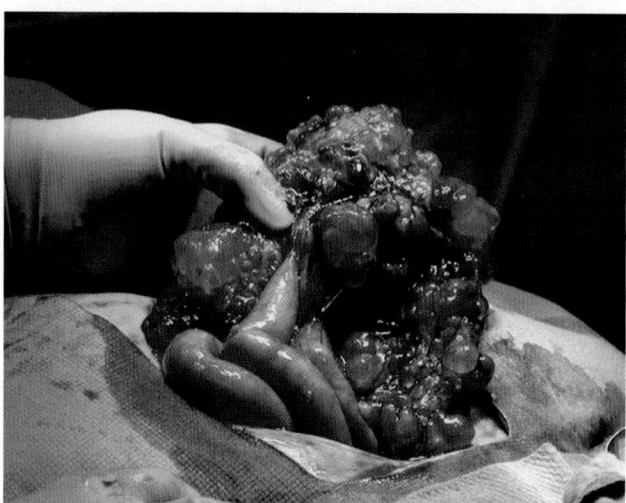

FIGURE 35-14 Photograph showing omental caking caused by tumor invasion.

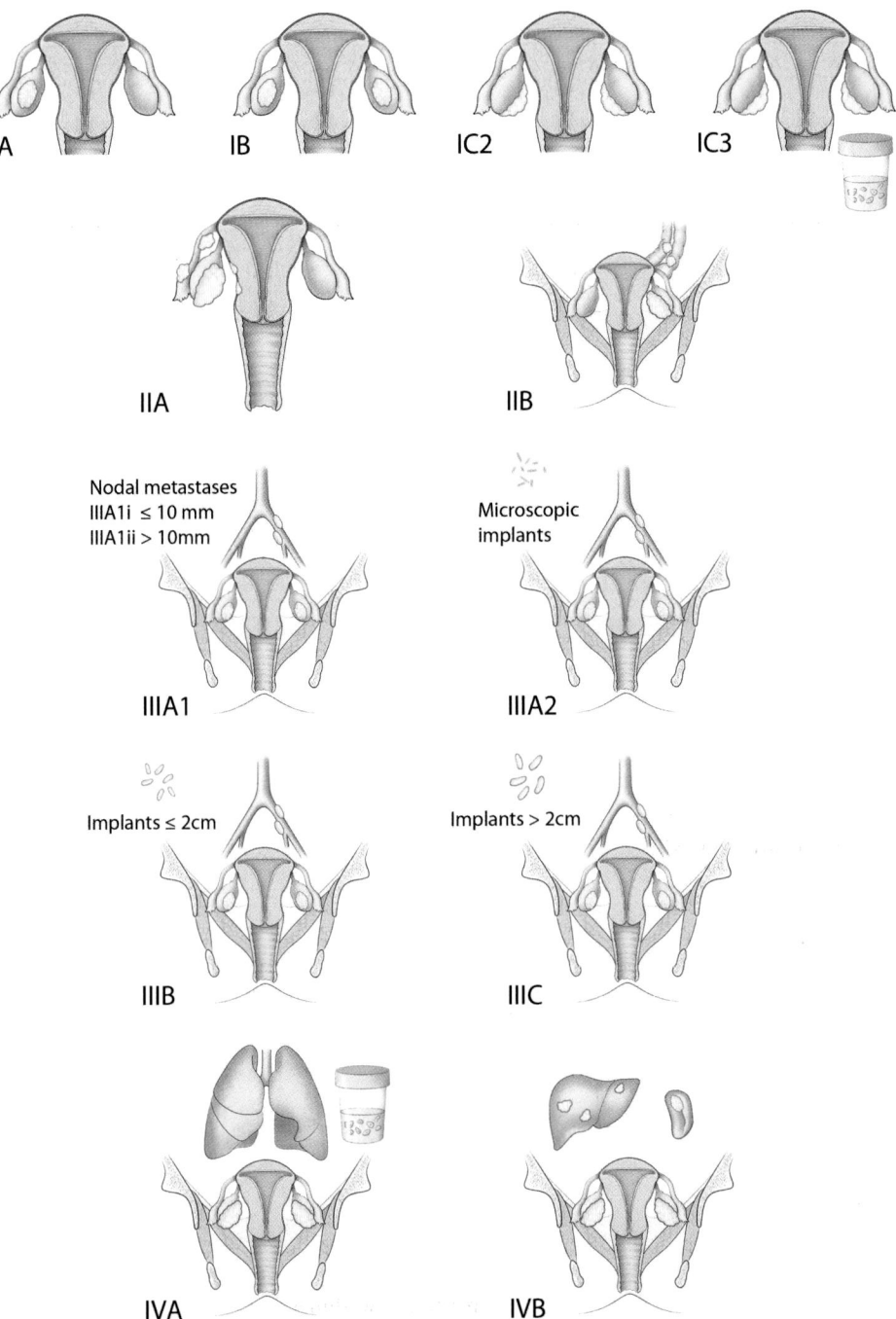

IA   IB   IC2   IC3

IIA   IIB

Nodal metastases
IIIA1i ≤ 10 mm
IIIA1ii > 10mm

Microscopic
implants

IIIA1   IIIA2

Implants ≤ 2cm   Implants > 2cm

IIIB   IIIC

IVA   IVB

FIGURE 35-15 International Federation of Gynecology and Obstetrics (FIGO) staging for ovarian cancer.

counts may be inferior, and required exploration of the abdomen during staging is unavoidably limited.

Fertility-sparing Management

Approximately 10 percent of epithelial ovarian cancers develop in women younger than 40 years. In selected cases, fertility-sparing surgery may be an option if disease appears confined to one ovary. Although many patients will be up-staged as a result of the operative findings, those with surgical stage I disease have an excellent long-term survival following unilateral adnexectomy. In some cases, postoperative chemotherapy may be required, but patients will usually retain their ability to conceive and

ultimately carry a pregnancy to term (Schilder, 2002).

Postsurgical Management

In women with stage IA or IB, grade 1 or 2 epithelial ovarian carcinoma, observation without further treatment following surgery is appropriate (Young, 1990). However, one third of patients who appear to have disease confined to the ovary will be "up-staged" by surgical staging and require postoperative chemotherapy.

Women with stage IA or IB, grade 3 epithelial ovarian cancer and all stage IC and II tumors are treated with carboplatin (Paraplatin) and paclitaxel (Taxol) chemotherapy (Morgan, 2014; Trimbos, 2003). In a Phase III Gynecologic Oncology Group (GOG) trial (protocol #157), women with early-stage disease were randomly assigned to either three or six cycles of this combination. Overall, three cycles resulted in a relapse rate comparable to that for six cycles but caused less toxicity (Bell, 2006). However, in a subanalysis of patients in this study who had serous tumors, treatment with six cycles decreased the relapse risk (Chan, 2010a).

Despite chemotherapy, more than 20 percent of women with early-stage disease develop recurrences within 5 years. In response, the GOG conducted a randomized Phase III trial of postoperative carboplatin and paclitaxel chemotherapy followed by observation or weekly paclitaxel for 24 weeks (protocol #175). Unfortunately, no benefit to maintenance paclitaxel was observed for early-stage patients (Mannel, 2011).

Surveillance

After treatment completion, women with early-stage ovarian cancer may be followed every 2 to 4 months for the first 2 years, then twice yearly for an additional 3 years, and then annually. At each visit, complete physical and pelvic examinations are performed. In addition, a serum CA125 level may be indicated if it was initially elevated (Morgan, 2014). However, a multi-institutional European trial evaluated the utility of CA125 levels for ovarian cancer monitoring after primary therapy completion.

TABLE 35-5. FIGO Staging of Carcinoma of the Ovary, Fallopian Tube, and Primary Peritoneal Carcinoma

Stage	Characteristics
I	**Tumor confined to ovaries (or to fallopian tubes)[a]**
IA	Tumor limited to 1 ovary (or 1 tube); capsule intact, no tumor on surface, negative washings
IB	Tumor involves both ovaries (or both tubes), otherwise like IA
IC1	Tumor limited to 1 or both ovaries (or tubes), with surgical spill
IC2	Tumor limited to 1 or both ovaries (or tubes), with capsule rupture before surgery or tumor on ovarian surface
IC3	Tumor limited to 1 or both ovaries (or tubes), with malignant cells in ascites or peritoneal washings
II	**Tumor involves 1 or both ovaries (or 1 or both tubes)[a] with pelvic extension (below the pelvic brim) or primary peritoneal cancer**
IIA	Extension and/or implants on uterus and/or fallopian tubes (and/or ovaries)
IIB	Extension to other pelvic intraperitoneal tissues
III	**Tumor involves 1 or both ovaries (or 1 or both tubes)[a] with cytologically or histologically confirmed spread to the peritoneum outside the pelvis and/or metastasis to retroperitoneal lymph nodes**
IIIA1	Positive retroperitoneal lymph nodes only
(i)	Metastasis ≤10 mm
(ii)	Metastasis >10 mm
IIIA2	Microscopic, extrapelvic (above the brim) peritoneal involvement ± positive retroperitoneal nodes
IIIB	Macroscopic, extrapelvic, peritoneal metastasis ≤2 cm ± positive retroperitoneal nodes. Includes extension to capsule of liver/spleen
IIIC	Macroscopic, extrapelvic, peritoneal metastasis >2 cm ± positive retroperitoneal nodes. Includes extension to capsule of liver/spleen
IV	**Distant metastasis excluding peritoneal metastasis**
IVA	Pleural effusion with positive cytology
IVB	Hepatic and/or splenic parenchymal metastasis, metastasis to extraabdominal organs (including inguinal lymph nodes and lymph nodes outside of the abdominal cavity)

[a]Content in parentheses referring to tubes pertains to fallopian tube carcinoma.
FIGO = International Federation of Gynecology and Obstetrics.
Data from Prat J and FIGO Committee on Gynecologic Oncology: Staging classification for cancer of the ovary, fallopian tube, and peritoneum, Int J Gynaecol Obstet. 2014 Jan;124(1):1–5.

Women with relapsed ovarian cancer did not live longer by starting chemotherapy earlier based on a rising CA125 level compared with delaying treatment until symptoms developed. The group monitored with CA125 tests received 5 more months of chemotherapy overall, whereas women who were diagnosed and treated later for clinically evident recurrence had higher quality-of-life measures (Rustin, 2010).

TABLE 35-6. Distribution of Epithelial Ovarian Cancer by FIGO Stage (n = 4825 patients)

FIGO Stage	Percent
I	28
II	8
III	50
IV	13

FIGO = International Federation of Gynecology and Obstetrics.
Data from Heintz APM, Odicino F, Maisonneuve P, et al: Carcinoma of the ovary. FIGO 26th Annual Report on the Results of Treatment in Gynecological Cancer, Int J Obstet Gynecol 92006 Nov;95 Suppl 1:S161–S92.

Whether suspected by examination, CA125 level elevation, or new symptoms, recurrent disease must be confirmed with the aid of imaging. Of modalities, CT is initially most helpful to identify intraperitoneal disease.

■ Management of Advanced Ovarian Cancer

Approximately two thirds of patients will have stage III-IV disease, and sequenced multimodality therapy offers the most successful outcomes (Earle, 2006). Ideally, surgical cytoreduction is initially performed to remove all gross disease and is followed by six courses of platinum-based chemotherapy. However, some women are not appropriate candidates for primary surgery due to their medical condition, and others will have unresectable tumor. Additionally, one randomized trial concluded that initial treatment with chemotherapy followed by interval debulking surgery might achieve equivalent results (Vergote, 2010). To effectively balance all clinical factors, each patient is individually assessed before initiating treatment.

Primary Cytoreductive Surgery

Residual Disease. Since the initial report by Griffiths (1975) suggested the clinical benefits of debulking, its value has been largely assumed. Numerous retrospective studies have subsequently supported the apparent survival advantage in women with advanced ovarian cancer. For subsequent decades, a cytoreductive effort was considered "optimal" if less than or equal to *1 cm residual disease* could be achieved. Specifically, 1 cm residual disease describes a surgical result in which none of any remaining areas of tumor individually measures greater than 1 cm. However, the assessment of gross remaining disease is entirely subjective, and often inaccurate due to tissue induration or other factors (Chi, 2007). Perhaps due to the inability to reliably quantify remaining disease, a subanalysis of accumulated data from several prospective GOG trials was completed. It demonstrated for those with stage III ovarian cancer that patients with 0.1 to 1.0 cm residual had only marginally improved overall survival compared with patients with greater than 1 cm. In fact, dramatic survival benefit was only achieved with complete resection (Winter, 2007). Based on these findings and other similar reports, a growing consensus supports that optimal debulking should be defined as no gross residual disease (Chang, 2012; Schorge, 2014).

Several reasons substantiate beliefs that ovarian cancer implant resection prolongs survival. First, surgery removes large volumes of chemoresistant tumor cell clones. Second, excision of necrotic tissue improves drug delivery to remaining well-vascularized cells. Third, small residual tumor implants should be faster growing and therefore more susceptible to chemotherapy. Fourth, smaller cancer cell populations should require fewer chemotherapy cycles, which lowers chances of chemoresistance. Finally, removal of bulky disease potentially enhances the immune system.

Whether any of these supposed advantages to debulking are actually clinically relevant is debatable (Covens, 2000). However, because of the presumed benefits, primary surgical cytoreduction is generally performed whenever an optimal result is clinically feasible. Yet, physical examination and imaging findings alone inherently limit the ability to accurately predict surgical success. As a result, preoperative laparoscopic evaluation is being studied as a method for patient triage (Fagotti, 2005, 2013; Morgan, 2014). However, since the goal is the maximal resection of the primary ovarian cancer and all metastatic disease, laparoscopic or robotic surgery has a limited role in debulking (Magrina, 2011; Nezhat, 2010). Typically, various procedures are required to achieve minimal residual disease, as described subsequently.

Surgical Approach to Cytoreductive Surgery. In general, a vertical incision is recommended to provide access to the entire abdomen. Women with advanced disease do not require peritoneal washings or cytologic assessment of fluid, but often several liters of ascites will need to be evacuated to improve visualization. Next, the abdomen is carefully explored to quickly determine if optimal debulking is feasible. It is preferable to perform a limited surgical procedure rather than extensive debulking if it is obvious that bulky tumors will be left behind. If hysterectomy and BSO is not possible, a biopsy of the ovary and sampling of the endometrium by dilatation and curettage is performed to confirm an ovarian primary and exclude the possibility of widely metastatic uterine papillary serous carcinoma. However, if disease is resectable, then surgery should begin with the least complicated procedure.

Often, an infracolic omentectomy can be easily performed and extended (i.e., gastrocolic), as needed, to encompass the disease. A frozen section analysis can then be requested to confirm the presumed diagnosis of epithelial ovarian cancer. The

pelvis is assessed next. Usually, an extrafascial type I abdominal hysterectomy and BSO is sufficient. However, when the tumor is confluent or invading the rectosigmoid, an en bloc resection, low anterior resection, or modified posterior pelvic exenteration may be required. These and other surgeries mentioned in this section are described and illustrated in Chapter 46 (p. 1134).

Patients with abdominal tumor nodules measuring <2 cm (apparent stage IIIB) should have bilateral pelvic and paraaortic node lymphadenectomy to provide the most accurate surgical staging. In patients with stage IV disease and those with abdominal tumor nodules at least 2 cm (already stage IIIC disease), nodal dissection is not necessarily required for staging purposes (Whitney, 2011). However, if it is not performed, a significant percentage of otherwise completely resected patients may not benefit from removal of unrecognized macroscopic nodal disease (Eisenkop, 2001). Systematic lymphadenectomy in advanced ovarian cancer appears to benefit mainly those patients with complete intraperitoneal debulking (du Bois, 2010; Panici, 2005).

Optimal surgical cytoreduction may also require various other radical procedures, including splenectomy, diaphragm stripping/resection, and small or large bowel resection (Aletti, 2006; McCann, 2011). Surgically aggressive centers experienced in such techniques report higher rates of achieving minimal residual disease that correspond to better outcomes (Aletti, 2009; Chi, 2009a; Wimberger, 2007). For diagnostic purposes and since it is a frequent site of disease, an appendectomy is also commonly included (Timofeev, 2010).

Neoadjuvant Chemotherapy and Interval Cytoreductive Surgery

Many women do not undergo initial optimal surgical debulking. In some of these cases, imaging studies may suggest unresectable disease. Other patients may be too medically compromised, may not have received initial care by a gynecologic oncologist, or may have large-volume "suboptimal" residual disease despite attempted debulking. In such circumstances, three to four courses of chemotherapy are used to shrink disease before attempting an "interval" cytoreductive surgery.

Such neoadjuvant chemotherapy with an interval procedure is associated with less perioperative morbidity, increased rates of optimal cytoreduction, and similar survival rates, but had never been directly compared with primary debulking until more recently (Hou, 2007; Kang, 2009). Vergote and colleagues (2010) reported results of a randomized phase III trial of 634 patients with stage IIIC or IV epithelial ovarian cancer, many of whom had extensive upper abdominal disease. In that study, neoadjuvant chemotherapy followed by interval debulking was *not* inferior to primary cytoreductive surgery. Since fewer than half of the primary surgery patients had debulking to 1 cm residual disease, the survival rates of both groups were comparable to those in other chemotherapy trials of patients with large-volume residual disease (Ozols, 2003). As many expert centers in the United States routinely incorporate ultraradical procedures to achieve complete resection, it is reasonable to think that a more aggressive cytoreductive attempt might have led to a better outcome for the group randomized to surgery (Chi, 2012). Although this remains unproven, the strongest variable predicting overall survival was debulking to microscopic residual disease, whether performed as primary treatment or after three cycles of chemotherapy (Vergote, 2010). Thus, the benefits of interval debulking mainly occur in patients who have very advanced, unresectable disease or who did not initially have a maximal surgical effort by a gynecologic oncologist (Rose, 2004; Tangjitgamol, 2009; van der Burg, 1995).

Adjuvant Chemotherapy

Intravenous Chemotherapy. Advanced ovarian cancer is considered to be relatively sensitive to cytotoxic agents. Largely due to recent advances in identifying active drugs, survival duration among patients has increased over the past two decades. Despite such improvements, fewer than 20 percent of those requiring chemotherapy will be cured. This is largely due to clinically occult residual chemoresistant tumor cells.

Platinum-based chemotherapy is the foundation for systemic treatment of most epithelial ovarian cancer types, although alternative regimens are currently being studied for advanced mucinous and clear cell carcinomas because of their known resistance. In two large collaborative group trials (GOG protocol #158 and Arbeitsgemeinschaft Gynäkologische Onkologie [AGO] protocol OVAR-3), the combination of carboplatin and paclitaxel was easier to administer, similarly efficacious, and less toxic than a cisplatin/paclitaxel regimen (du Bois, 2003; Ozols, 2003). As a result, the most widely used intravenous (IV) regimen in the United States is six courses of carboplatin and paclitaxel. If additional cycles are required to achieve clinical remission, this suggests relative tumor chemoresistance and usually leads to an earlier relapse. In Europe, single-agent carboplatin is often used. This preference is based on two large Phase III trials of the International Collaborative Ovarian Neoplasm (ICON) Group, which did not detect a survival advantage for combination chemotherapy (The ICON Collaborators, 1998; The ICON Group, 2002).

Although the carboplatin and paclitaxel regimen is undoubtedly effective, other modifications have been studied. For instance, the addition of a third cytotoxic agent was postulated to further improve outcome. Unfortunately, none of the experimental regimens demonstrated superiority compared with the control group (Bookman, 2009). Addition of the biologic agent bevacizumab (Avastin) during primary chemotherapy, followed by use as maintenance therapy, has been shown to provide only a modest improvement in progression-free survival (GOG protocol #218 and ICON-7) (Burger, 2011; Perren, 2011). Finally, administering paclitaxel in a dose-dense weekly schedule may have some advantages but at the cost of additional toxicity (Katsumata, 2009). The GOG conducted a definitive phase III trial comparing dose-dense paclitaxel with carboplatin versus every-3-week paclitaxel and carboplatin. In addition, suboptimally debulked patients in both groups received optional bevacizumab (protocol #262). The results are not yet available.

Intraperitoneal Chemotherapy. In 2006, the National Cancer Institute issued a rare Clinical Announcement encouraging the use of intraperitoneal (IP) chemotherapy. This coincided with the publication of results from a Phase III GOG trial (protocol #172) of optimally debulked stage III ovarian cancer patients who were randomly assigned to receive either IV or combination IV/IP paclitaxel and cisplatin chemotherapy

TABLE 35-7. Intraperitoneal Chemotherapy Regimen for Ovarian Cancer

Day 1	Paclitaxel 135 mg/m^2 IV over 24 hour
Day 2	Cisplatin 75 to 100 mg/m^2 intraperitoneal
Day 8	Paclitaxel 60 mg/m^2 intraperitoneal

©National Comprehensive Cancer Network, Inc., 2014. Ovarian cancer, including fallopian tube cancer and primary peritoneal cancer, version 3.2014.

(Table 35-7). The median duration of overall survival was 66 months in the IV/IP group compared with 50 months in the IV group (Armstrong, 2006). By comparison, survival in both groups far exceeded patients treated in the Vergote trial (29 to 30 months median survival), described on page 751 (Vergote, 2010). Despite this dramatic improvement in survival, many clinicians still remain unconvinced of its efficacy and do not routinely recommend IP chemotherapy (Gore, 2006).

The theoretical advantages of IP chemotherapy are dramatic. In general, epithelial ovarian cancer mainly spreads along peritoneal surfaces. In postoperative patients with minimal residual disease, a much higher dose of chemotherapy can be achieved at the tumor site by administration directly into the abdomen (Alberts, 1996; Markman, 2001).

Obviously, not every woman with advanced ovarian cancer is an appropriate candidate for IP chemotherapy. Stage IV patients and those with large-volume residual disease are theoretically least likely to benefit. In addition, toxicity is generally higher with IP therapy, catheter-related problems are common, and the true long-term survival advantage remains controversial (Walker, 2006). Regardless, IP therapy should certainly be considered for low-volume, optimally debulked disease (Morgan, 2014). However, the choice to receive or not receive IP chemotherapy should ultimately be a decision made by an informed patient (Alberts, 2006).

In light of the National Cancer Institute clinical announcement and ensuing debate, newer IP regimens are currently being tested. One current randomized phase III GOG trial (protocol #252) compared: (1) dose-dense paclitaxel and IV carboplatin, (2) dose-dense paclitaxel and IP carboplatin, and (3) a modified GOG protocol #172 IP cisplatin regimen. All groups received concurrent bevacizumab followed by maintenance bevacizumab. It is anticipated that when these data are published, they will shape future applications of ovarian cancer IP therapy.

Management of Patients in Remission

In most women with advanced ovarian cancer, the combination of surgery and platinum-based chemotherapy will result in clinical remission (normal examination, CA125 levels, and CT scan findings). However, up to 80 percent will eventually relapse and die from disease progression. Lower CA125 levels, that is, single-digit values, are generally associated with longer time until relapse and better survival rates (Juretzka, 2007). Since most patients achieving remission will have residual, clinically occult drug-resistant cells, several options are appropriate to consider and include surveillance, second-look surgery, maintenance chemotherapy, and abdominal radiotherapy. Unfortunately, there is no solid proof that any intervention is beneficial.

First, surveillance after treatment completion may include regular examinations and CA125 levels, as in early-stage disease. In those with new symptoms, physical findings, or rising CA125 titers, imaging may be indicated. In general, clinicians should maintain a heightened suspicion for relapse.

Another option, *second-look surgery*, is the "gold standard" to identify residual disease at treatment completion. For numerous reasons, mainly a lack of proven clinical benefit, this is not routinely performed. Instead, a second-look laparotomy or laparoscopy primarily serves as a useful early end point in assessing the treatment effectiveness within an experimental protocol. Otherwise, no prospective clinical trials have demonstrated a survival advantage. Second-look surgery does have prognostic value, since a procedure that reveals no recurrent disease is associated with an improved survival rate.

A third option is *maintenance chemotherapy*, also termed *consolidation therapy*. There is limited evidence to suggest any advantage for additional treatment in women who achieve clinical remission after six courses of platinum-based chemotherapy. However, due to the known high rate of recurrence, several agents have been tested as maintenance therapy, in randomized studies. Of these, monthly paclitaxel for 12 cycles was observed to extend progression-free survival by 7 months compared with only three courses of treatment. However, cumulative toxicity, most notably neuropathy, was substantial and resulted in frequent dose reductions. Unfortunately, the trial did not demonstrate improved overall survival rates among patients receiving prolonged maintenance therapy (Markman, 2003, 2009). To determine whether lower-dose paclitaxel or CT-2103 (Xyotax) could reduce the death rate compared with no maintenance therapy, the GOG is currently conducting a Phase III trial of women with advanced ovarian cancer who achieved clinical remission after standard platinum-based chemotherapy (protocol #212).

Bevacizumab, an antiangiogenic agent, has also been studied as maintenance therapy in several phase III trials. In GOG protocol #218 and the Gynecologic InterGroup Trial (ICON-7) studies noted earlier (p. 752), when bevacizumab was combined with paclitaxel and carboplatin, then continued alone for a year of maintenance therapy, it demonstrated only a 2- to 4-month prolongation of progression-free survival, but no overall survival benefit. Of added interest, when maintenance bevacizumab was stopped, several patients experienced relapse soon after (Burger, 2011; Perren, 2011). Therefore, current trials allow maintenance bevacizumab to be continued indefinitely or until there is evidence for disease progression.

Pazopanib, an oral multikinase inhibitor of vascular endothelial growth factor receptor (VEGFR), has also shown some promise as maintenance therapy. In a Phase III trial, patients receiving pazopanib had a 5.6-month improvement in progression-free survival compared with placebo, but with significant toxicity and lack of overall survival benefit (du Bois, 2014).

A fourth option, *radiation therapy*, is rarely used in the United States for patients in remission after primary therapy. Whole abdominal radiotherapy has unproven benefit, and fears of excessive toxicity such as radiation enteritis are a concern (Sorbe, 2003). However, the long-term effectiveness of this consolidation strategy is comparable to that achieved in women treated with other modalities.

TABLE 35-8. Epithelial Ovarian Cancer 5-Year Survival Rates

Stage	5-Year Survival (%)
Localized (confined to primary site)	92
Regional (spread to regional nodes)	72
Distant (cancer has metastasized)	27
Unknown (unstaged)	22

Reproduced with permission from National Cancer Institute: Ovarian epithelial cancer treatment (PDQ), 2014b. Available at: www.cancer.gov/cancertopics/pdq/treatment/ovarianepithelial/healthprofessional. Accessed January 12, 2015.

Prognostic Factors

The overall 5-year survival rate of all stages of epithelial ovarian cancer approximates 45 percent, far lower than uterine (84 percent) or cervical cancer (73 percent) (National Cancer Institute, 2014b). Survival rates mirror the assigned FIGO stage and largely depend on whether the disease has metastasized or not (Table 35-8). Additional prognostic factors are shown in Table 35-9). Interestingly, BRCA mutation carriers have a better prognosis, chiefly due to increased platinum sensitivity (Alsop, 2012; Lacour, 2011). However, even with favorable prognostic factors and despite recent innovations, most patients will ultimately relapse.

Management of Recurrent Ovarian Cancer

Gradual elevation of the CA125 level is usually the first sign of relapse. Tamoxifen may be administered when there is only "biochemical" evidence for disease progression, because it has some activity in treating recurrent disease and toxicity is minimal (Hurteau, 2010). Alternatively, patients may be offered participation in a clinical trial, started on conventional cytotoxic chemotherapy, or observed until clinical symptoms arise. Without treatment, the recurrence will usually become clinically obvious within 2 to 6 months. Almost invariably, the tumor will be located somewhere within the abdomen. Women who progress during primary chemotherapy are classified as having "platinum-refractory" disease and have a dismal prognosis. Those who relapse within 6 months of therapy have

TABLE 35-9. Most Important Favorable Prognostic Factors for Ovarian Cancer

Younger age
Good performance status
Cell type other than mucinous and clear cell
Well-differentiated tumor
Smaller disease volume prior to surgical debulking
No ascites
Smaller residual tumor after primary cytoreductive surgery

Reproduced with permission from National Cancer Institute: Ovarian epithelial cancer treatment (PDQ), 2014b. Available at: www.cancer.gov/cancertopics/pdq/treatment/ovarianepithelial/healthprofessional. Accessed January 12, 2015.

"platinum-resistant" ovarian cancer and a somewhat prolonged survival. In general, patients in either category are treated with palliative single-agent nonplatinum chemotherapy. For this, participation in an experimental clinical trial is offered whenever possible. Otherwise, response rates typically range from 5 to 15 percent using FDA-approved conventional cytotoxic drugs such as paclitaxel, pegylated liposomal doxorubicin (Doxil), docetaxel (Taxotere), topotecan (Hycamtin), or gemcitabine (Gemzar). Recently, bevacizumab in combination with weekly paclitaxel, doxorubicin, or topotecan was shown to provide a 27-percent response rate, which more than doubled the rate with single-agent chemotherapy alone in patients with platinum-resistant disease (Pujade-Lauraine, 2014). As a result, bevacizumab is now FDA-approved for this indication.

Women who relapse more than 6 to 12 months after primary therapy completion are considered "platinum-sensitive." These patients, especially those in prolonged remission beyond 18, 24, or 36 months, are usually treated with a platinum-based combination. Carboplatin combined with either paclitaxel or gemcitabine has demonstrated modest superiority compared with carboplatin alone (Parmar, 2003; Pfisterer, 2006). Moreover, in one randomized phase III trial, the novel combination of carboplatin and pegylated liposomal doxorubicin was superior to carboplatin and paclitaxel (Pujade-Lauraine, 2010). Of interest, although patients with primary early-stage ovarian cancer have a more favorable overall prognosis, survival after relapse is comparable to those who recurred after treatment of advanced-stage disease (Chan, 2010b).

Secondary Cytoreductive Surgery

Although patient selection is somewhat arbitrary, the best candidates for secondary cytoreductive surgery have: (1) platinum-sensitive disease, (2) a prior prolonged disease-free interval, (3) a solitary-site recurrence, and (4) no ascites (Chi, 2006). To achieve a maximal survival benefit, debulking must result in minimal residual disease (Harter, 2006; Schorge, 2010b). However, approximately half of patients will be explored without achieving this goal.

The overall survival benefit of this approach is currently being studied in a Phase III GOG trial (protocol #213). This randomizes surgical candidates with platinum-sensitive relapsed disease to secondary debulking or not, followed by carboplatin and paclitaxel with or without additional bevacizumab. Of patients enrolled in this study, only 15 to 20 percent have thus far been considered surgical candidates.

Salvage Chemotherapy

In general, most relapsed ovarian cancer patients will end up receiving multiple sequential courses of chemotherapy (Morgan, 2014). Regardless of which regimen is selected initially, reevaluation usually follows two to four cycles of chemotherapy (depending on the agent) to determine the clinical benefit (Morgan, 2014). Typically, a CA125 level decline with or without confirmation of tumor shrinkage by CT provides sufficient reassurance to continue therapy. Nonresponders are changed to a different regimen. Patients with a germline *BRCA1* or *BRCA2* gene mutation who develop resistance to platinum may benefit from targeted therapy with olaparib (Lynparza), now FDA-approved for this indication (Chap. 27, p. 605) (Kaufman, 2015). However, at some point, usually after multiple agents have been tried, treatment will no longer be efficacious, which should prompt a discussion about further goals of care.

It would seem plausible that targeting therapy for an individual patient's disease might be more effective than empiric drug selection. In vitro chemosensitivity testing is occasionally used for this purpose. In principle, different agents are tested against the patient's tumor, and the chemotherapeutic drug demonstrating the best response should result in a better outcome. Unfortunately, this approach lacks demonstrable efficacy and is not recommended outside of a clinical trial (Burstein, 2011; Morgan, 2014).

■ Palliation of End-stage Ovarian Cancer

At some point, patients with recurrent disease will develop worsening symptoms that warrant reevaluation of their overall treatment strategy. Of these, intermittent episodes of partial small and large bowel obstruction are common during treatment.

Bowel obstruction that does not resolve with nasogastric suction can be managed in two very different ways. Patients at first relapse or early in their course may warrant an aggressive approach that includes chemotherapy with or without surgical intervention and incorporates total parenteral nutrition. A colostomy, ileostomy, or intestinal bypass will often relieve symptoms (Chi, 2009b). Unfortunately, a satisfactory surgical result is sometimes impossible due to disease burden, and multiple sites of partial or complete obstruction. In addition, successful palliation is rarely achieved when the transit time is prolonged due to diffuse peritoneal carcinomatosis or when anatomy requires a bypass that results in the short bowel syndrome. Further, recovery may be complicated by an enterocutaneous fistula, reobstruction, or other morbid event (Pothuri, 2004). For patients with a refractory bowel obstruction due to progressive disease despite multiple lines of chemotherapy, the best approach is usually placement of a palliative gastrostomy tube, IV hydration, and hospice care. The final decision regarding how to proceed should be based on a frank discussion. Topics include treatment options, the natural history of progressive ovarian cancer, and the realistic improbability of further disease response by switching to a different therapy.

Another common scenario is a woman with symptomatic, rapidly reaccumulating ascitic fluid. This may be alleviated by repeated paracenteses or by placement of an indwelling peritoneal catheter (Pleurx), which can be self-drained as needed. Similarly, a refractory malignant pleural effusion can usually be managed by thoracentesis, indwelling pleural catheter placement, or pleurodesis. With the last, irritants are instilled into the pleural space to incite adhesions that obliterate the space.

Although these procedures and others may be appropriate in selected patients, the inability to halt disease progression should be acknowledged. In addition, any intervention has the potential to result in an unanticipated, catastrophic complication. Overall, palliative procedures are most compassionately used when incorporated into the overall treatment plan. For example, in a woman with stable disease and normal renal function, tumor-induced ureteral compression and hydronephrosis does not necessarily require stent placement or a nephrostomy tube.

All patients deserve a positive, hopeful, but honest approach to the management of progressive, incurable disease. Often, there are unrealistic expectations regarding the benefit of palliative chemotherapy, but emotionally it may be preferable to the idea of "giving up" (Doyle, 2001). There is no substitute for mutual trust in the doctor–patient relationship when making sound decisions aimed at improving the quality of life of women with end-stage ovarian cancer.

REFERENCES

Al-Barrak J, Santos JL, Tinker A, et al: Exploring palliative treatment outcomes in women with advanced or recurrent ovarian clear cell carcinoma. Gynecol Oncol 122(1):107, 2011

Alberts DS, Liu PY, Hannigan EV, et al: Intraperitoneal cisplatin plus intravenous cyclophosphamide versus intravenous cisplatin plus intravenous cyclophosphamide for stage III ovarian cancer. N Engl J Med 335:1950, 1996

Alberts DS, Markman M, Muggia F, et al: Proceedings of a GOG workshop on intraperitoneal therapy for ovarian cancers. Gynecol Oncol 103(3):738, 2006

Aletti GD, Dowdy SC, Gostout BS, et al: Quality improvement in the surgical approach to advanced ovarian cancer: the Mayo Clinic experience. J Am Coll Surg 208:614, 2009

Aletti GD, Dowdy SC, Podratz KC, et al: Surgical treatment of diaphragm disease correlates with improved survival in optimally debulked advanced stage ovarian cancer. Gynecol Oncol 100:283, 2006

Alsop K, Fereday S, Meldrum C, et al: BRCA mutation frequency and patterns of treatment response in BRCA mutation-positive women with ovarian cancer: a report from the Australian Ovarian Cancer Study Group. J Clin Oncol 30(21):2654, 2012

Alvarado-Cabrero I, Cheung A, Caduff R: Tumours of the fallopian tube and uterine ligaments [Tumours of the fallopian tube]. In Tavassoli FA, Devilee P (eds): World Health Organization Classification of Tumours. Geneva, WHO, 2003, p 206

American College of Obstetricians and Gynecologists: Elective and risk-reducing salpingo-oophorectomy. Practice Bulletin No. 89, January 2008, Reaffirmed 2014

American College of Obstetricians and Gynecologists: Hereditary breast and ovarian cancer syndrome. Practice Bulletin No. 103, April 2009, Reaffirmed 2013

American College of Obstetricians and Gynecologists: Salpingectomy for ovarian cancer prevention. Committee Opinion No. 620, January 2015

American College of Obstetricians and Gynecologists: The role of the generalist obstetrician-gynecologist in the early detection of ovarian cancer. Committee Opinion No. 477, March 2011

Armstrong DK, Bundy B, Wenzel L, et al: Intraperitoneal cisplatin and paclitaxel in ovarian cancer. N Engl J Med 354:34, 2006

Baldwin LM, Trivers KF, Matthews B, et al: Vignette-based study of ovarian cancer screening: do U.S. physicians report adhering to evidence-based recommendations? Ann Intern Med 156(3):182, 2012

Beiner ME, Finch A, Rosen B, et al: The risk of endometrial cancer in women with BRCA1 and BRCA2 mutations: a prospective study. Gynecol Oncol 104(1):7, 2007

Bell J, Brady MF, Young RC, et al: Randomized phase III trial of three versus six cycles of adjuvant carboplatin and paclitaxel in early stage epithelial ovarian carcinoma: a Gynecologic Oncology Group study. Gynecol Oncol 102:432, 2006

Bloomfield HE, Olson A, Greer N, et al: Screening pelvic examinations in asymptomatic, average-risk adult women: an evidence report for a clinical practice guideline from the American College of Physicians. Ann Intern Med 161(1):46, 2014

Bookman MA, Brady MF, McGuire WP, et al: Evaluation of new platinum-based treatment regimens in advanced-stage ovarian cancer: a phase III trial of the Gynecologic Cancer Intergroup. J Clin Oncol 27:1419, 2009

Bristow RE, Palis BE, Chi DS, et al: The National Cancer Database report on advanced-stage epithelial ovarian cancer: impact of hospital surgical case volume on overall survival and surgical treatment paradigm. Gynecol Oncol 118:262, 2010

Buller RE, Lallas TA, Shahin MS, et al: The p53 mutational spectrum associated with BRCA1 mutant ovarian cancer. Clin Cancer Res 7:831, 2001

Burger RA, Brady MF, Bookman MA, et al: Incorporation of bevacizumab in the primary treatment of ovarian cancer. N Engl J Med 365(26):2473, 2011

Burstein HJ, Mangu PB, Somerfield MR, et al: American Society of Clinical Oncology clinical practice guideline update on the use of chemotherapy sensitivity and resistance assays. J Clin Oncol 29(24):3328, 2011

Buttin BM, Herzog TJ, Powell MA, et al: Epithelial ovarian tumors of low malignant potential: the role of microinvasion. Obstet Gynecol 99:11, 2002

Buys SS, Partridge E, Black A, et al: Effect of screening on ovarian cancer mortality: the Prostate, Lung, Colorectal and Ovarian (PLCO) Cancer Screening Randomized Controlled Trial. JAMA 305(22):2295, 2011

Buys SS, Partridge E, Greene MH, et al: Ovarian cancer screening in the Prostate, Lung, Colorectal and Ovarian (PLCO) cancer screening trial: findings from the initial screen of a randomized trial. Am J Obstet Gynecol 193:1630, 2005

Callahan MJ, Crum CP, Medeiros F, et al: Primary fallopian tube malignancies in BRCA-positive women undergoing surgery for ovarian cancer risk reduction. J Clin Oncol 25:3985, 2007

Carlson JW, Miron A, Jarboe EA, et al: Serous tubal intraepithelial carcinoma: its potential role in primary peritoneal serous carcinoma and serous cancer prevention. J Clin Oncol 26:4160, 2008

Chan JK, Munro EG, Cheung MK, et al: Association of lymphadenectomy and survival in stage I ovarian cancer patients. Obstet Gynecol 109:12, 2007

Chan JK, Tian C, Fleming GF, et al: The potential benefit of 6 vs. 3 cycles of chemotherapy in subsets of women with early-stage high-risk epithelial ovarian cancer: an exploratory analysis of a Gynecologic Oncology Group study. Gynecol Oncol 116:301, 2010a

Chan JK, Tian C, Teoh D, et al: Survival after recurrence in early-stage high-risk epithelial ovarian cancer: a Gynecologic Oncology Group study. Gynecol Oncol 116:307, 2010b

Chang SJ, Bristow RE: Evolution of surgical treatment paradigms for advanced-stage ovarian cancer: redefining "optimal" residual disease. Gynecol Oncol 125(2):483, 2012

Chen S, Iversen ES, Friebel T, et al: Characterization of BRCA1 and BRCA2 mutations in a large United States sample. J Clin Oncol 24:863, 2006

Chi DS, Abu-Rustum NR, Sonoda Y, et al: The safety and efficacy of laparoscopic surgical staging of apparent stage I ovarian and fallopian tube cancers. Am J Obstet Gynecol 192:1614, 2005

Chi DS, Eisenhauer EL, Zivanovic O, et al: Improved progression-free and overall survival in advanced ovarian cancer as a result of a change in surgical paradigm. Gynecol Oncol 114:26, 2009a

Chi DS, McCaughty K, Diaz JP, et al: Guidelines and selection criteria for secondary cytoreductive surgery in patients with recurrent, platinum-sensitive epithelial ovarian carcinoma. Cancer 106:1933, 2006

Chi DS, Musa F, Dao F, et al: An analysis of patients with bulky advanced stage ovarian, tubal, and peritoneal carcinoma treated with primary debulking surgery (PDS) during an identical time period as the randomized EORTC-NCIC trial of PDS vs neoadjuvant chemotherapy (NACT). Gynecol Oncol 124(1):10, 2012

Chi DS, Phaeton R, Miner TJ, et al: A prospective outcomes analysis of palliative procedures performed for malignant intestinal obstruction due to recurrent ovarian cancer. Oncologist 14:835, 2009b

Chi DS, Ramirez PT, Teitcher JB, et al: Prospective study of the correlation between postoperative computed tomography scan and primary surgeon assessment in patients with advanced ovarian, tubal, and peritoneal carcinoma reported to have undergone primary surgical cytoreduction to residual disease 1 cm or less. J Clin Oncol 25(31):4946, 2007

Covens AL: A critique of surgical cytoreduction in advanced ovarian cancer. Gynecol Oncol 78:269, 2000

Cramer DW, Bast RC Jr, Berg CD, et al: Ovarian cancer biomarker performance in prostate, lung, colorectal, and ovarian cancer screening trial specimens. Cancer Prev Res 4:65, 2011

Crane EK, Sun CC, Ramirez PT, et al: The role of secondary cytoreduction in low-grade serous ovarian cancer or peritoneal cancer. Gynecol Oncol 136(1):25, 2015

Creinin MD, Zite N: Female tubal sterilization: the time has come to routinely consider removal. Obstet Gynecol 124(3):596, 2014

Cress RD, Bauer K, O'Malley CD, et al: Surgical staging of early stage epithelial ovarian cancer: results from the CDC-NPCR ovarian patterns of care study. Gynecol Oncol 121:94, 2011

Daly MB, Pilarski R, Axilbund JE, et al: Genetic/familial high-risk assessment: breast and ovarian, version 1.2014. J Natl Compr Canc Netw 12(9):1326, 2014

Daniels MS, Babb SA, King RH, et al: Underestimation of risk of a BRCA1 or BRCA2 mutation in women with high-grade serous ovarian cancer by BRCAPRO: a multi-institution study. J Clin Oncol 32(12):1249, 2014

Deng CX: BRCA1: cell cycle checkpoint, genetic instability, DNA damage response and cancer evolution. Nucleic Acids Res 34:1416, 2006

Doyle C, Crump M, Pintilie M, et al: Does palliative chemotherapy palliate? Evaluation of expectations, outcomes, and costs in women receiving chemotherapy for advanced ovarian cancer. J Clin Oncol 19:1266, 2001

du Bois A, Ewald-Riegler N, de Gregorio N, et al: Borderline tumours of the ovary: a cohort study of the Arbeitsgemeinschaft Gynäkologische Onkologie (AGO) Study Group. Eur J Cancer 49(8):1905, 2013 du Bois A, Floquet A, Kim JW, et al: Incorporation of pazopanib in maintenance therapy of ovarian cancer. J Clin Oncol 32(30):3374, 2014

du Bois A, Luck HJ, Meier W, et al: A randomized clinical trial of cisplatin/paclitaxel versus carboplatin/paclitaxel as first-line treatment of ovarian cancer. J Natl Cancer Inst 95:1320, 2003

du Bois A, Reuss A, Harter P, et al: Potential role of lymphadenectomy in advanced ovarian cancer: a combined exploratory analysis of three prospectively randomized phase III multicenter trials. J Clin Oncol 28:1733, 2010

Earle CC, Schrag D, Neville BA, et al: Effect of surgeon specialty on processes of care and outcomes for ovarian cancer patients. J Natl Cancer Inst 98:172, 2006

Eichhorn JH, Young RH, Scully RE: Primary ovarian small cell carcinoma of pulmonary type: a clinicopathologic, immunohistologic, and flow cytometric analysis of 11 cases. Am J Surg Pathol 16:926, 1992

Eisenkop SM, Spirtos NM: The clinical significance of occult macroscopically positive retroperitoneal nodes in patients with epithelial ovarian cancer. Gynecol Oncol 82:143, 2001

Engelen MJ, Kos HE, Willemse PH, et al: Surgery by consultant gynecologic oncologists improves survival in patients with ovarian carcinoma. Cancer 106:589, 2006

Euhus DM, Smith KC, Robinson L, et al: Pretest prediction of BRCA1 or BRCA2 mutation by risk counselors and the computer model BRCAPRO. J Natl Cancer Inst 94:844, 2002

Fagotti A, Fanfani F, Ludovisi M, et al: Role of laparoscopy to assess the chance of optimal cytoreductive surgery in advanced ovarian cancer: a pilot study. Gynecol Oncol 96(3):729, 2005

Fagotti A, Vizzielli G, De Iaco P, et al: A multicentric trial (Olympia-MITO 13) on the accuracy of laparoscopy to assess peritoneal spread in ovarian cancer. Am J Obstet Gynecol 209(5):462.e1, 2013

Garcia C, Lyon L, Littell RD, et al: Comparison of risk management strategies between women testing positive for a BRCA variant of unknown significance and women with known BRCA deleterious mutations. Genet Med 16(12):896, 2014

Gertig DM, Hunter DJ, Cramer DW, et al: Prospective study of talc use and ovarian cancer. J Natl Cancer Inst 92:249, 2000

Goff BA, Mandel L, Muntz HG, et al: Ovarian carcinoma diagnosis. Cancer 89:2068, 2000

Goff BA, Mandel LS, Melancon CH, et al: Frequency of symptoms of ovarian cancer in women presenting to primary care clinics. JAMA 291:2705, 2004

Goff BA, Matthews BJ, Wynn M, et al: Ovarian cancer: patterns of surgical care across the United States. Gynecol Oncol 103:383, 2006

Goodman MT, Howe HL, Tung KH, et al: Incidence of ovarian cancer by race and ethnicity in the United States, 1992–1997. Cancer 97:2676, 2003

Gore M, du Bois A, Vergote I: Intraperitoneal chemotherapy in ovarian cancer remains experimental. J Clin Oncol 24:4528, 2006

Gourley C, Farley J, Provencher DM, et al: Gynecologic Cancer InterGroup (GCIG) consensus review for ovarian and primary peritoneal low-grade serous carcinomas. Int J Gynecol Cancer 24(9 Suppl 3):S9, 2014

Grabowski JP, Harter P, Hils R, et al: Outcome of immediate re-operation or interval debulking after chemotherapy at a gynecologic oncology center after initially incomplete cytoreduction of advanced ovarian cancer. Gynecol Oncol 126(1):54, 2012

Greene MH, Piedmonte M, Alberts D, et al: A prospective study of risk-reducing salpingo-oophorectomy and longitudinal CA-125 screening among women at increased genetic risk of ovarian cancer: design and baseline characteristics: a Gynecologic Oncology Group study. Cancer Epidemiol Biomarkers Prev 17:594, 2008

Griffiths CT: Surgical resection of tumor bulk in the primary treatment of ovarian carcinoma. Natl Cancer Inst Monogr 42:101, 1975

Guseh SH, Rauh-Hain JA, Tambouret RH, et al: Transitional cell carcinoma of the ovary: a case-control study. Gynecol Oncol 132(3):649, 2014

Hannibal CG, Vang R, Junge J, et al: A nationwide study of serous "borderline" ovarian tumors in Denmark 1978-2002: centralized pathology review and overall survival compared with the general population. Gynecol Oncol 134(2):267, 2014

Harter P, Bois A, Hahmann M, et al: Surgery in recurrent ovarian cancer: the Arbeitsgemeinschaft Gynaekologische Onkologie (AGO) DESKTOP OVAR Trial. Ann Surg Oncol 13:1702, 2006

Harter P, Gershenson D, Lhomme C, et al: Gynecologic Cancer InterGroup (GCIG) consensus review for ovarian tumors of low malignant potential (borderline ovarian tumors). Int J Gynecol Cancer 24(9 Suppl 3):S5, 2014

Heintz APM, Odicino F, Maisonneuve P, et al: Carcinoma of the ovary. In FIGO annual report on the results of treatment in gynaecological cancer. Int J Obstet Gynecol 95(Suppl 1):S161, 2006

Hinkula M, Pukkala E, Kyyronen P, et al: Incidence of ovarian cancer of grand multiparous women: a population-based study in Finland. Gynecol Oncol 103:207, 2006

Holman LL, Friedman S, Daniels MS, et al: Acceptability of prophylactic salpingectomy with delayed oophorectomy as risk-reducing surgery among BRCA mutation carriers. Gynecol Oncol 133(2):283, 2014

Hou JY, Kelly MG, Yu H, et al: Neoadjuvant chemotherapy lessens surgical morbidity in advanced ovarian cancer and leads to improved survival in stage IV disease. Gynecol Oncol 105:211, 2007

Houck K, Nikrui N, Duska L, et al: Borderline tumors of the ovary: correlation of frozen and permanent histopathologic diagnosis. Obstet Gynecol 95:839, 2000

Houghton SC, Reeves KW, Hankinson SE, et al: Perineal powder use and risk of ovarian cancer. J Natl Cancer Inst 106(9):1, 2014

Hurteau JA, Brady MF, Darcy KM, et al: Randomized phase III trial of tamoxifen versus thalidomide in women with biochemical-recurrent-only epithelial ovarian, fallopian tube or primary peritoneal carcinoma after a complete response to first-line platinum/taxane chemotherapy with an evaluation of serum vascular endothelial growth factor (VEGF): a Gynecologic Oncology Group study. Gynecol Oncol 119:444, 2010

Huusom LD, Frederiksen K, Hogdall EV, et al: Association of reproductive factors, oral contraceptive use and selected lifestyle factors with the risk of ovarian borderline tumors: a Danish case-control study. Cancer Causes Control 17:821, 2006

Im SS, Gordon AN, Buttin BM, et al: Validation of referral guidelines for women with pelvic masses. Obstet Gynecol 105:35, 2005

International Collaboration of Epidemiological Studies of Cervical Cancer: Comparison of risk factors for invasive squamous cell carcinoma and adenocarcinoma of the cervix: collaborative reanalysis of individual data on 8,097 women with squamous cell carcinoma and 1,374 women with adenocarcinoma from 12 epidemiological studies. Int J Cancer 120:885, 2006

International Collaboration of Epidemiological Studies of Cervical Cancer, Appleby P, Beral V, et al: Cervical cancer and hormonal contraceptives: collaborative reanalysis of individual data for 16,573 women with cervical cancer and 35,509 women without cervical cancer from 24 epidemiological studies. Lancet 370(9599):1609, 2007

James PA, Doherty R, Harris M, et al: Optimal selection of individuals for BRCA mutation testing: a comparison of available methods. J Clin Oncol 24:707, 2006

Jelinic P, Mueller JJ, Olvera N, et al: Recurrent SMARCA4 mutations in small cell carcinoma of the ovary. Nat Genet 46(5):424, 2014

Jemal A, Bray F, Center MM, et al: Global cancer statistics. CA Cancer J Clin 61:69, 2011

Juretzka MM, Barakat RR, Chi DS, et al: CA-125 level as a predictor of progression-free survival and overall survival in ovarian cancer patients with surgically defined disease status prior to the initiation of intraperitoneal consolidation therapy. Gynecol Oncol 104(1):176, 2007

Kang S, Nam BH: Does neoadjuvant chemotherapy increase optimal cytoreduction rate in advanced ovarian cancer? Meta-analysis of 21 studies. Ann Surg Oncol 16:2315, 2009

Katsumata N, Yasuda M, Takahashi F, et al: Dose-dense paclitaxel once a week in combination with carboplatin every 3 weeks for advanced ovarian cancer: a phase 3, open-label, randomized controlled trial. Lancet 374:1331, 2009

Kauff ND, Satagopan JM, Robson ME, et al: Risk-reducing salpingo-oophorectomy in women with a BRCA1 or BRCA2 mutation. N Engl J Med 346:1609, 2002

Kaufman B, Shapira-Frommer R, Schmutzler RK, et al: Olaparib monotherapy in patients with advanced cancer and a germline BRCA1/2 mutation. J Clin Oncol 33(3):244, 2015

Kiani F, Knutsen S, Singh P, et al: Dietary risk factors for ovarian cancer: the Adventist Health Study (United States). Cancer Causes Control 17:137, 2006

Kramer JL, Velazquez IA, Chen BE, et al: Prophylactic oophorectomy reduces breast cancer penetrance during prospective, long-term follow-up of BRCA1 mutation carriers. J Clin Oncol 23:8629, 2005

Kristensen GS, Schledermann D, Mogensen O, et al: The value of random biopsies, omentectomy, and hysterectomy in operations for borderline ovarian tumors. Int J Gynecol Cancer 24(5):874, 2014

Kruitwagen RF, Swinkels BM, Keyser KG, et al: Incidence and effect on survival of abdominal wall metastases at trocar or puncture sites following laparoscopy or paracentesis in women with ovarian cancer. Gynecol Oncol 60:233, 1996

Kurman RJ, Carcangiu ML, Herrington CS, et al (eds): WHO Classification of Tumours of Female Reproductive Organs, 4th ed. Lyon, International Agency for Research on Cancer, 2014

Kwon JS, Tinker A, Pansegrau G, et al: Prophylactic salpingectomy and delayed oophorectomy as an alternative for BRCA mutation carriers. Obstet Gynecol 121(1):14, 2013

Lacey JV Jr, Brinton LA, Leitzmann MF, et al: Menopausal hormone therapy and ovarian cancer risk in the National Institutes of Health–AARP Diet and Health Study cohort. J Natl Cancer Inst 98:1397, 2006

Lacour RA, Westin SN, Meyer LA, et al: Improved survival in non-Ashkenazi Jewish ovarian cancer patients with BRCA1 and BRCA2 gene mutations. Gynecol Oncol 121:358, 2011

Lancaster JM, Powell CB, Chen LM, et al: Society of Gynecologic Oncology statement on risk assessment for inherited gynecologic cancer predispositions. Gynecol Oncol 136(1):3, 2015

Landen CN Jr, Birrer MJ, Sood AK: Early events in the pathogenesis of epithelial ovarian cancer. J Clin Oncol 26:995, 2008

Leary A, Petrella MC, Pautier P, et al: Adjuvant platinum-based chemotherapy for borderline serous ovarian tumors with invasive implants. Gynecol Oncol 132(1):23, 2014

Lee JY, Kim HS, Chung HH, et al: The role of omentectomy and random peritoneal biopsies as part of comprehensive surgical staging in apparent early-stage epithelial ovarian cancer. Ann Surg Oncol 21(8):2762, 2014

Lee KR, Tavassoli FA, Prat J, et al: Tumours of the ovary and peritoneum [Surface epithelial-stromal tumours]. In Tavassoli FA, Devilee P (eds): World Health Organization Classification of Tumours. Geneva, WHO, 2003, p 117

Lessard-Anderson CR, Handlogten KS, Molitor RJ, et al: Effect of tubal sterilization technique on risk of serous epithelial ovarian and primary peritoneal carcinoma. Gynecol Oncol 135(3):423, 2014

Levanon K, Crum C, Drapkin R: New insights into the pathogenesis of serous ovarian cancer and its clinical impact. J Clin Oncol 26:5284, 2008

Li AJ, Madden AC, Cass I, et al: The prognostic significance of thrombocytosis in epithelial ovarian carcinoma. Gynecol Oncol 92:211, 2004

Lin HW, Tu YY, Lin SY, et al: Risk of ovarian cancer in women with pelvic inflammatory disease: a population-based study. Lancet Oncol 12(9):900, 2011

Lin PS, Gershenson DM, Bevers MW, et al: The current status of surgical staging of ovarian serous borderline tumors. Cancer 85:905, 1999

Madalinska JB, Hollenstein J, Bleiker E, et al: Quality-of-life effects of prophylactic salpingo-oophorectomy versus gynecologic screening among women at increased risk of hereditary ovarian cancer. J Clin Oncol 23:6890, 2005

Madalinska JB, van Beurden M, Bleiker EM, et al: The impact of hormone replacement therapy on menopausal symptoms in younger high-risk women after prophylactic salpingo-oophorectomy. J Clin Oncol 24:3576, 2006

Magrina JF, Zanagnolo V, Noble BN, et al: Robotic approach for ovarian cancer: perioperative and survival results and comparison with laparoscopy and laparotomy. Gynecol Oncol 121:100, 2011

Makarla PB, Saboorian MH, Ashfaq R, et al: Promoter hypermethylation profile of ovarian epithelial neoplasms. Clin Cancer Res 11:5365, 2005

Mammas IN, Zafiropoulos A, Spandidos DA: Involvement of the ras genes in female genital tract cancer. Int J Oncol 26:1241, 2005

Mannel RS, Brady MF, Kohn EC, et al: A randomized phase III trial of IV carboplatin and paclitaxel × 3 courses followed by observation versus weekly maintenance low-dose paclitaxel in patients with early-stage ovarian carcinoma: a Gynecologic Oncology Group study. Gynecol Oncol 122(1):89, 2011

Markman M, Bundy BN, Alberts DS, et al: Phase III trial of standard-dose intravenous cisplatin plus paclitaxel versus moderately high-dose carboplatin followed by intravenous paclitaxel and intraperitoneal cisplatin in small-volume stage III ovarian carcinoma: an intergroup study of the Gynecologic Oncology Group, Southwestern Oncology Group, and Eastern Cooperative Oncology Group. J Clin Oncol 19:1001, 2001

Markman M, Liu PY, Moon J, et al: Impact on survival of 12 versus 3 monthly cycles of paclitaxel (175 mg/m^2) administered to patients with advanced ovarian cancer who attained a complete response to primary platinum-paclitaxel: follow-up of a Southwest Oncology Group and Gynecologic Oncology Group phase III trial. Gynecol Oncol 114(2):195, 2009

Markman M, Liu PY, Wilczynski S, et al: Phase III randomized trial of 12 versus 3 months of maintenance paclitaxel in patients with advanced ovarian cancer after complete response to platinum and paclitaxel-based chemotherapy: a Southwest Oncology Group and Gynecologic Oncology Group trial. J Clin Oncol 21:2460, 2003

McAlpine JN, Hanley GE, Woo MM, et al: Opportunistic salpingectomy: uptake, risks, and complications of a regional initiative for ovarian cancer prevention. Am J Obstet Gynecol 210(5):471.e1, 2014

McCann CK, Growdon WB, Munro EG, et al: Prognostic significance of splenectomy as part of initial cytoreductive surgery in ovarian cancer. Ann Surg Oncol 18(10):2912, 2011

Medeiros F, Muto MG, Lee Y, et al: The tubal fimbria is a preferred site for early adenocarcinoma in women with familial ovarian cancer syndrome. Am J Surg Pathol 30(2):230, 2006

Menon U, Gentry-Maharaj A, Hallett R, et al: Sensitivity and specificity of multimodal and ultrasound screening for ovarian cancer, and stage distribution of detected cancers: results of the prevalence screen of the UK Collaborative Trial of Ovarian Cancer Screening (UKCTOCS). Lancet Oncol 10:327, 2009

Menon U, Griffin M, Gentry-Maharaj A: Ovarian cancer screening—current status, future directions. Gynecol Oncol 132(2):490, 2014

Menzin AW, Gal D, Lovecchio JL: Contemporary surgical management of borderline ovarian tumors: a survey of the Society of Gynecologic Oncologists. Gynecol Oncol 78:7, 2000

Mercado C, Zingmond D, Karlan BY, et al: Quality of care in advanced ovarian cancer: the importance of provider specialty. Gynecol Oncol 117:18, 2010

Mok SC, Schorge JO, Welch WR, et al: Tumours of the ovary and peritoneum [Peritoneal tumours]. In Tavassoli FA, Devilee P (eds): World Health Organization Classification of Tumours. Geneva, WHO, 2003, p 197

Moore RG, Jabre-Raughley M, Brown AK, et al: Comparison of a novel multiple marker assay vs the Risk of Malignancy Index for the prediction of epithelial cancer in patients with a pelvic mass. Am J Obstet Gynecol 203(3):228.e1, 2010

Moore RG, McMeekin DS, Brown AK, et al: A novel multiple marker bioassay utilizing HE4 and CA125 for the prediction of ovarian cancer in patients with a pelvic mass. Gynecol Oncol 112(1):40, 2009

Mor G, Visintin I, Lai Y, et al: Serum protein markers for early detection of ovarian cancer. Proc Natl Acad Sci USA 102:7677, 2005

Mørch LS, Løkkegaard E, Andreasen AH, et al: Hormone therapy and ovarian cancer. JAMA 302(3):298, 2009

Morelli M, Venturella R, Mocciaro R, et al: Prophylactic salpingectomy in premenopausal low-risk women for ovarian cancer: primum non nocere. Gynecol Oncol 129(3):448, 2013

Morgan RJ Jr, Armstrong DK, Alvarez RD, et al: Ovarian cancer, including fallopian tube cancer and primary peritoneal cancer, 3.2014. NCCN Clinical Practice Guidelines in Oncology. Available at: http://www.nccn.org/professionals/physician_gls/f_guidelines.asp. Accessed January 12, 2015

Morice P, Uzan C, Fauvet R, et al: Borderline ovarian tumour: pathological diagnostic dilemma and risk factors for invasive or lethal recurrence. Lancet Oncol 13(3):e103, 2012

Moyer VA, U.S. Preventive Services Task Force: Screening for ovarian cancer: U.S. Preventive Services Task Force reaffirmation recommendation statement. Ann Intern Med 157(12):900, 2012

National Cancer Institute: National Cancer Institute issues clinical announcement for preferred method of treatment for advanced ovarian cancer. January 4, 2006. Available at: http://www.cancer.gov/newscenter/newsfromnci/2006/ipchemotherapyrelease. Accessed January 12, 2015

National Cancer Institute: Ovarian cancer prevention (PDQ), 2014a. Available at: http://www.cancer.gov/cancertopics/pdq/prevention/ovarian/HealthProfessional. Accessed January 12, 2015

National Cancer Institute: Ovarian epithelial cancer treatment (PDQ), 2014b. Available at: www.cancer.gov/cancertopics/pdq/treatment/ovarianepithelial/healthprofessional. Accessed January 12, 2015

Nezhat FR, DeNoble SM, Liu CS, et al: The safety and efficacy of laparoscopic surgical staging and debulking of apparent advanced stage ovarian, fallopian tube, and primary peritoneal cancers. JSLS 14:155, 2010

Norquist BM, Pennington KP, Agnew KJ, et al: Characteristics of women with ovarian carcinoma who have BRCA1 and BRCA2 mutations not identified by clinical testing. Gynecol Oncol 128(3):483, 2013

Ozols RF, Bundy BN, Greer BE, et al: Phase III trial of carboplatin and paclitaxel compared with cisplatin and paclitaxel in patients with optimally resected stage III ovarian cancer: a Gynecologic Oncology Group study. J Clin Oncol 21:3194, 2003

Palma MD, Domchek SM, Stopfer J, et al: The relative contribution of point mutations and genomic rearrangements in BRCA1 and BRCA2 in high-risk breast cancer families. Cancer Res 68(17):7006, 2008

Panici PB, Maggioni A, Hacker N, et al: Systematic aortic and pelvic lymphadenectomy versus resection of bulky nodes only in optimally debulked advanced ovarian cancer: a randomized trial. J Natl Cancer Inst 97:560, 2005

Park JY, Kim DY, Kim JH, et al: Surgical management of borderline ovarian tumors: the role of fertility-sparing surgery. Gynecol Oncol 113:75, 2009

Park JY, Song JS, Choi G, et al: Pure primary squamous cell carcinoma of the ovary: a report of two cases and review of the literature. Int J Gynecol Pathol 29:328, 2010

Parmar MK, Ledermann JA, Colombo N, et al: Paclitaxel plus platinum-based chemotherapy versus conventional platinum-based chemotherapy in women with relapsed ovarian cancer: the ICON4/AGO-OVAR-2.2 trial. Lancet 361:2099, 2003

Parmigiani G, Chen S, Iversen Jr ES, et al: Validity of models for predicting BRCA1 and BRCA2 mutations. Ann Intern Med 147:441, 2007

Partridge E, Kreimer AR, Greenlee RT, et al: Results from four rounds of ovarian cancer screening in a randomized trial. Obstet Gynecol 113:775, 2009

Pecorelli S, Benedet JL, Creasman WT, et al: FIGO staging of gynecologic cancer, 1994–1997. FIGO Committee on Gynecologic Oncology,

International Federation of Gynecology and Obstetrics. Int J Gynaecol Obstet 65:243, 1999

Pelucchi C, Galeone C, Talamini R, et al: Lifetime ovulatory cycles and ovarian cancer risk in 2 Italian case-control studies. Am J Obstet Gynecol 196(1):83.e1, 2007

Perets R, Wyant GA, Muto KW, et al: Transformation of the fallopian tube secretory epithelium leads to high-grade serous ovarian cancer in Brca;Tp53;Pten models. Cancer Cell 24(6):751, 2013

Perren TJ, Swart AM, Pfisterer J, et al: A phase 3 trial of bevacizumab in ovarian cancer. N Engl J Med 365(26):2484, 2011

Petricoin EF, Ardekani AM, Hitt BA, et al: Use of proteomic patterns in serum to identify ovarian cancer. Lancet 359:572, 2002

Pfisterer J, Plante M, Vergote I, et al: Gemcitabine plus carboplatin compared with carboplatin in patients with platinum-sensitive recurrent ovarian cancer: an intergroup trial of the AGO-OVAR, the NCIC CTG, and the EORTC GCG. J Clin Oncol 24:4699, 2006

Pins MR, Young RH, Daly WJ, et al: Primary squamous cell carcinoma of the ovary. Report of 37 cases. Am J Surg Pathol 20:823, 1996

Poncelet C, Fauvet R, Boccara J, et al: Recurrence after cystectomy for borderline ovarian tumors: results of a French multicenter study. Ann Surg Oncol 13:565, 2006

Pothuri B, Meyer L, Gerardi M, et al: Reoperation for palliation of recurrent malignant bowel obstruction in ovarian carcinoma. Gynecol Oncol 95:193, 2004

Powell CB, Kenley E, Chen LM, et al: Risk-reducing salpingo-oophorectomy in *BRCA* mutation carriers: role of serial sectioning in the detection of occult malignancy. J Clin Oncol 23:127, 2005

Prat J, FIGO Committee on Gynecologic Oncology: Staging classification for cancer of the ovary, fallopian tube, and peritoneum. Int J Gynaecol Obstet 124(1):1, 2014

Prat J, Morice P: Tumours of the ovary and peritoneum [Secondary tumours of the ovary]. In Tavassoli FA, Devilee P (eds): World Health Organization Classification of Tumours. Geneva, WHO, 2003, p 193

Pujade-Lauraine E, Hilpert F, Weber B, et al: Bevacizumab combined with chemotherapy for platinum-resistant recurrent ovarian cancer: the AURELIA open-label randomized phase III trial. J Clin Oncol 32(13):1302, 2014

Pujade-Lauraine E, Wagner U, Aavall-Lundqvist E, et al: Pegylated liposomal doxorubicin and carboplatin compared with paclitaxel and carboplatin for patients with platinum-sensitive ovarian cancer in late relapse. J Clin Oncol 28:3323, 2010

Purdie DM, Bain CJ, Siskind V, et al: Ovulation and risk of epithelial ovarian cancer. Int J Cancer 104:228, 2003

Quirk JT, Natarajan N: Ovarian cancer incidence in the United States, 1992–1999. Gynecol Oncol 97:519, 2005

Rao GG, Skinner E, Gehrig PA, et al: Surgical staging of ovarian low malignant potential tumors. Obstet Gynecol 104:261, 2004

Rao GG, Skinner EN, Gehrig PA, et al: Fertility-sparing surgery for ovarian low malignant potential tumors. Gynecol Oncol 98:263, 2005

Rauh-Hain JA, Growdon WB, Rodriguez N, et al: Carcinosarcoma of the ovary: a case-control study. Gynecol Oncol 121(3):477, 2011

Rebbeck TR, Lynch HT, Neuhausen SL, et al: Prophylactic oophorectomy in carriers of *BRCA1* or *BRCA2* mutations. N Engl J Med 346:1616, 2002

Rice MS, Hankinson SE, Tworoger SS: Tubal ligation, hysterectomy, unilateral oophorectomy, and risk of ovarian cancer in the Nurses' Health Studies. Fertil Steril 102(1):192, 2014

Riman T, Dickman PW, Nilsson S, et al: Risk factors for invasive epithelial ovarian cancer: results from a Swedish case-control study. Am J Epidemiol 156:363, 2002

Risch HA, McLaughlin JR, Cole DE, et al: Population *BRCA1* and *BRCA2* mutation frequencies and cancer penetrances: a kin-cohort study in Ontario, Canada. J Natl Cancer Inst 98:1694, 2006

Ronnett BM, Shmookler BM, Sugarbaker PH, et al: Pseudomyxoma peritonei: new concepts in diagnosis, origin, nomenclature, and relationship to mucinous borderline (low malignant potential) tumors of the ovary. Anat Pathol 2197, 1997

Ronnett BM, Yan H, Kurman RJ, et al: Patients with pseudomyxoma peritonei associated with disseminated peritoneal adenomucinosis have a significantly more favorable prognosis than patients with peritoneal mucinous carcinomatosis. Cancer 92:85, 2001

Rose PG, Nerenstone S, Brady MF, et al: Secondary surgical cytoreduction for advanced ovarian carcinoma. N Engl J Med 351:2489, 2004

Rosenblatt KA, Weiss NS, Cushing-Haugen KL, et al: Genital powder exposure and the risk of epithelial ovarian cancer. Cancer Causes Control 22:737, 2011

Rossing MA, Tang MT, Flagg EW, et al: A case-control study of ovarian cancer in relation to infertility and the use of ovulation-inducing drugs. Am J Epidemiol 160:1070, 2004

Rostgaard K, Wohlfahrt J, Andersen PK, et al: Does pregnancy induce the shedding of premalignant ovarian cells? Epidemiology 14:168, 2003

Rustin GJS, van der Burg MEL, Griffin CL, et al: Early versus delayed treatment of relapsed ovarian cancer (MRC OV05/EORTC 55955): a randomized trial. Lancet 376:1155, 2010

Schilder JM, Thompson AM, DePriest PD, et al: Outcome of reproductive age women with stage IA or IC invasive epithelial ovarian cancer treated with fertility-sparing therapy. Gynecol Oncol 87:1, 2002

Schildkraut JM, Bastos E, Berchuck A: Relationship between lifetime ovulatory cycles and overexpression of mutant *p53* in epithelial ovarian cancer. J Natl Cancer Inst 89:932, 1997

Schmeler KM, Lynch HT, Chen LM, et al: Prophylactic surgery to reduce the risk of gynecologic cancers in the Lynch syndrome. N Engl J Med 354:261, 2006

Schorge JO, Clark RM, Lee SI, et al: Primary debulking surgery for advanced ovarian cancer: are you a believer or a dissenter? Gynecol Oncol 135(3):595, 2014

Schorge JO, Modesitt SC, Coleman RL, et al: SGO White Paper on ovarian cancer: etiology, screening and surveillance. Gynecol Oncol 119:7, 2010a

Schorge JO, Muto MG, Lee SJ, et al: *BRCA1*-related papillary serous carcinoma of the peritoneum has a unique molecular pathogenesis. Cancer Res 60:1361, 2000

Schorge JO, Muto MG, Welch WR, et al: Molecular evidence for multifocal papillary serous carcinoma of the peritoneum in patients with germline *BRCA1* mutations. J Natl Cancer Inst 90:841, 1998

Schorge JO, Wingo SN, Bhore R, et al: Secondary cytoreductive surgery for platinum-sensitive ovarian cancer. Int J Gynaecol Obstet 108:123, 2010b

Scully R, Livingston DM: In search of the tumour-suppressor functions of *BRCA1* and *BRCA2*. Nature 408:429, 2000

Seidman JD, Kurman RJ: Ovarian serous borderline tumors: a critical review of the literature with emphasis on prognostic indicators. Hum Pathol 31:539, 2000

Sherman ME, Piedmonte M, Mai PL, et al: Pathologic findings at risk-reducing salpingo-oophorectomy: primary results from Gynecologic Oncology Group Trial GOG-0199. J Clin Oncol 32(29):3275, 2014

Shih KK, Zhou QC, Aghajanian C, et al: Patterns of recurrence and role of adjuvant chemotherapy in stage II-IV serous ovarian borderline tumors. Gynecol Oncol 119:270, 2010

Siegel RL, Miller KD, Jemal A: Cancer statistics, 2015. CA Cancer J Clin 65(1):5, 2015

Silva EG, Gershenson DM, Malpica A, et al: The recurrence and the overall survival rates of ovarian serous borderline neoplasms with noninvasive implants is time dependent. Am J Surg Pathol 30:1367, 2006

Silva EG, Tornos C, Bailey MA, et al: Undifferentiated carcinoma of the ovary. Arch Pathol Lab Med 115:377, 1991

Skates SJ, Menon U, MacDonald N, et al: Calculation of the risk of ovarian cancer from serial CA-125 values for preclinical detection in postmenopausal women. J Clin Oncol 21:206, 2003

Society of Gynecologic Oncology: SGO clinical practice statement: salpingectomy for ovarian cancer prevention. November 2013. Available at: https://www.sgo.org/clinical-practice/guidelines/sgo-clinical-practice-statement-salpingectomy-for-ovarian-cancer-prevention/. Accessed January 11, 2015

Soliman PT, Slomovitz BM, Broaddus RR, et al: Synchronous primary cancers of the endometrium and ovary: a single institution review of 84 cases. Gynecol Oncol 94:456, 2004

Sorbe B: Consolidation treatment of advanced (FIGO stage III) ovarian carcinoma in complete surgical remission after induction chemotherapy: a randomized, controlled, clinical trial comparing whole abdominal radiotherapy, chemotherapy, and no further treatment. Int J Gynecol Cancer 13:278, 2003

Suidan RS, Ramirez PT, Sarasohn DM, et al: A multicenter prospective trial evaluating the ability of preoperative computed tomography scan and serum CA-125 to predict suboptimal cytoreduction at primary debulking surgery for advanced ovarian, fallopian tube, and peritoneal cancer. Gynecol Oncol 134(3):455, 2014

Sutton GP, Bundy BN, Omura GA, et al: Stage III ovarian tumors of low malignant potential treated with cisplatin combination therapy: a Gynecologic Oncology Group study. Gynecol Oncol 41:230, 1991

Tangjitgamol S, Manusirivithaya S, Laopaiboon M, et al: Interval debulking surgery for advanced epithelial ovarian cancer. Cochrane Database Syst Rev 2:CD006014, 2009

Tempfer CB, Polterauer S, Bentz EK, et al: Accuracy of intraoperative frozen section analysis in borderline tumors of the ovary: a retrospective analysis of 96 cases and review of the literature. Gynecol Oncol 107:248, 2007

The ICON Collaborators: ICON2: Randomised trial of single-agent carboplatin against three-drug combination of CAP (cyclophosphamide, doxorubicin, and cisplatin) in women with ovarian cancer. International Collaborative Ovarian Neoplasm Study. Lancet 352:1571, 1998

The ICON Group: Paclitaxel plus carboplatin versus standard chemotherapy with either single-agent carboplatin or cyclophosphamide, doxorubicin, and cisplatin in women with ovarian cancer: the ICON3 randomised trial. Lancet 360:505, 2002

Timmerman D, Testa AC, Bourne T, et al: Logistic regression model to distinguish between the benign and malignant adnexal mass before surgery: a multicenter study by the International Ovarian Tumor Analysis Group. J Clin Oncol 23:8794, 2005

Timmers PJ, Zwinderman K, Coens C, et al: Lymph node sampling and taking of blind biopsies are important elements of the surgical staging of early ovarian cancer. Int J Gynecol Cancer 20:1142, 2010

Timofeev J, Galgano MT, Stoler MH, et al: Appendiceal pathology at the time of oophorectomy for ovarian neoplasms. Obstet Gynecol 116:1348, 2010

Tozzi R, Kohler C, Ferrara A, et al: Laparoscopic treatment of early ovarian cancer: surgical and survival outcomes. Gynecol Oncol 93:199, 2004

Trimble CL, Kosary C, Trimble EL: Long-term survival and patterns of care in women with ovarian tumors of low malignant potential. Gynecol Oncol 86:34, 2002

Trimbos JB, Parmar M, Vergote I, et al: International Collaborative Ovarian Neoplasm trial 1 and Adjuvant ChemoTherapy in Ovarian Neoplasm trial: Two parallel randomized phase III trials of adjuvant chemotherapy in patients with early-stage ovarian carcinoma. J Natl Cancer Inst 95:105, 2003

Twickler DM, Forte TB, Santos-Ramos R, et al: The ovarian tumor index predicts risk for malignancy. Cancer 86:2280, 1999

Ueland FR, Desmone CP, Seamon LG, et al: Effectiveness of a multivariate index assay in the preoperative assessment of ovarian tumors. Obstet Gynecol 117(6):1289, 2011

van der Burg ME, van Lent M, Buyse M, et al: The effect of debulking surgery after induction chemotherapy on the prognosis in advanced epithelial ovarian cancer. Gynecological Cancer Cooperative Group of the European Organization for Research and Treatment of Cancer. N Engl J Med 332:629, 1995

Vergote I, Trope CG, Amant F, et al: Neoadjuvant chemotherapy or primary surgery in stage IIIC or IV ovarian cancer. N Engl J Med 363:943, 2010

Verheijen RH, Mensdorff-Pouilly S, van Kamp GJ, et al: CA-125: fundamental and clinical aspects. Semin Cancer Biol 9:117, 1999

Vermillion Inc: OVA1 instructions for use: executive summary. Austin, Vermillion Inc, July 15, 2012

Visintin I, Feng Z, Longton G, et al: Diagnostic markers for early detection of ovarian cancer. Clin Cancer Res 14:1065, 2008

Vyarvelska I, Rosen B, Narod SA: Should hysterectomy complement prophylactic salpingo-oophorectomy in BRCA1 and BRCA2 mutation carriers? Gynecol Oncol 134(2):219, 2014

Walker JL, Armstrong DK, Huang HQ, et al: Intraperitoneal catheter outcomes in a phase III trial of intravenous versus intraperitoneal chemotherapy in optimal stage III ovarian and primary peritoneal cancer: a Gynecologic Oncology Group study. Gynecol Oncol 100:27, 2006

Ware Miller R, Smith A, DeSimone CP, et al: Performance of the American College of Obstetricians and Gynecologists' ovarian tumor referral guidelines with a multivariate index assay. Obstet Gynecol 117(6):1298, 2011

Werness BA, Parvatiyar P, Ramus SJ, et al: Ovarian carcinoma in situ with germline BRCA1 mutation and loss of heterozygosity at BRCA1 and TP53. J Natl Cancer Inst 92:1088, 2000

Whitney CW: Gynecologic Oncology Group Surgical Procedures Manual. Gynecologic Oncology Group. 2011. Available at: https://gogmember.gog.org/manuals/pdf/surgman.pdf. Accessed February 24, 2015

Wimberger P, Lehmann N, Kimmig R, et al: Prognostic factors for complete debulking in advanced ovarian cancer and its impact on survival. An exploratory analysis of a prospectively randomized phase III study of AGO-OVAR. Gynecol Oncol 106:69, 2007

Wingo SN, Knowles LM, Carrick KS, et al: Retrospective cohort study of surgical staging for ovarian low malignant potential tumors. Am J Obstet Gynecol 194:e20, 2006

Winter WE 3rd, Maxwell GL, Tian C, et al: Prognostic factors for stage III epithelial ovarian cancer: a Gynecologic Oncology Group Study. J Clin Oncol 25(24):3621, 2007

Yen ML, Yen BL, Bai CH, et al: Risk factors for ovarian cancer in Taiwan: a case-control study in a low-incidence population. Gynecol Oncol 89:318, 2003

Young RC, Walton LA, Ellenberg SS, et al: Adjuvant therapy in stage I and stage II epithelial ovarian cancer: results of two prospective, randomized trials. N Engl J Med 322:1021, 1990

Young RH, Oliva E, Scully RE: Small cell carcinoma of the ovary, hypercalcemic type: a clinicopathological analysis of 150 cases. Am J Surg Pathol 18:1102, 1994

Yurkovetsky Z, Skates S, Lomakin A, et al: Development of a multimarker assay for early detection of ovarian cancer. J Clin Oncol 28:2159, 2010

Zaino RJ, Brady MF, Lele SM, et al: Advanced stage mucinous adenocarcinoma of the ovary is both rare and highly lethal: a Gynecologic Oncology Group study. Cancer 117:554, 2011

Zanetta G, Rota S, Chiari S, et al: Behavior of borderline tumors with particular interest to persistence, recurrence, and progression to invasive carcinoma: a prospective study. J Clin Oncol 19:2658, 2001

Zapardiel I, Rosenberg P, Peiretti M, et al: The role of restaging borderline ovarian tumors: single institution experience and review of the literature. Gynecol Oncol 119:274, 2010

Zhang M, Lee AH, Binns CW: Reproductive and dietary risk factors for epithelial ovarian cancer in China. Gynecol Oncol 92:320, 2004

Zhang Z, Chan DW: The road from discovery to clinical diagnostics: lessons learned from the first FDA-cleared in vitro diagnostic multivariate index assay of proteomic biomarkers. Cancer Epidemiol Biomarkers Prev 19(12):2995, 2010

CHAPTER 36

Ovarian Germ Cell and Sex Cord-Stromal Tumors

Three major categories account for virtually all malignant ovarian tumors. Organization of these groups is based on the anatomic structures from which the tumors originate (Fig. 36-1). Epithelial ovarian cancers account for 90 to 95 percent of malignant ovarian tumors (Chap. 35, p. 735). Germ cell and sex cord-stromal ovarian tumors account for the remaining 5 to 10 percent and have unique qualities that require a special management approach (Quirk, 2005).

MALIGNANT OVARIAN GERM CELL TUMORS

Germ cell tumors arise from the ovary's germinal elements and make up one third of all ovarian neoplasms. The mature cystic teratoma, also called *dermoid cyst,* is by far the most common subtype. This accounts for 95 percent of all germ cell tumors, is clinically benign, and discussed in Chapter 9 (p. 219). In contrast, malignant germ cell tumors compose 2 to 3 percent of malignant ovarian cancers in Western countries and include *dysgerminoma, yolk sac tumor, immature teratoma,* and other less common types.

Three features distinguish malignant germ cell tumors from epithelial ovarian cancers. First, individuals typically present at a younger age, usually in their teens or early 20s. Second, most have stage I disease at diagnosis. Third, prognosis is excellent—even for those with advanced disease—due to exquisite tumor chemosensitivity. Fertility-sparing surgery is the primary treatment for women seeking future pregnancy, although most will require postoperative chemotherapy.

■ Epidemiology

The age-adjusted incidence rate of malignant ovarian germ cell tumors in the United States is much lower (0.4 per 100,000 women) than that of epithelial ovarian carcinomas (15.5) (Quirk, 2005). Smith and associates (2006) analyzed 1262 cases of malignant ovarian germ cell from 1973 to 2002 and observed that incidence rates have declined 10 percent during the past 30 years. Unlike a significant proportion of epithelial ovarian carcinomas, malignant germ cell tumors are not generally considered heritable, although rare familial cases are reported (Galani, 2005; Stettner, 1999).

These tumors are the most common ovarian malignancies diagnosed during childhood and adolescence, although only 1 percent of all ovarian cancers develop in these age groups. At age 20, however, the incidence of epithelial ovarian carcinoma begins to rise and exceeds that of germ cell tumors (Young, 2003).

■ Diagnosis
Patient Findings

The signs and symptoms associated with these tumors vary, but in general, most originate from tumor growth and the hormones they produce. Subacute abdominal pain is the presenting symptom in 85 percent of patients and reflects rapid growth of a large, unilateral tumor undergoing capsular distention, hemorrhage, or necrosis. In 10 percent of cases, cyst rupture, torsion, or intraperitoneal hemorrhage leads to an acute abdomen (Gershenson, 2007a). In more advanced disease, ascites may develop and cause abdominal distention. Because of the hormonal changes that frequently accompany these tumors, menses can become heavy or irregular. Although most individuals note one or more of these symptoms, one quarter of individuals are asymptomatic, and a pelvic mass is noted unexpectedly during physical or sonographic examination (Curtin, 1994).

Individuals typically seek care within 1 month of the onset of abdominal complaints, although some note subtle waxing and waning of symptoms for more than a year. Vague pelvic symptoms are common during adolescence due to initiation of ovulation and menstrual cramping. As a result, early symptoms may be missed. Moreover, girls may be silent about changes to their normal pattern, fearful of their significance. Most young women with these tumors are nulligravidas with normal periods, but as discussed later, dysgenetic gonads is a known risk factor for development of these tumors (Brown, 2014b). Therefore, adolescents who present with pelvic masses and delayed menarche should be evaluated for gonadal dysgenesis (Chap. 16, p. 373).

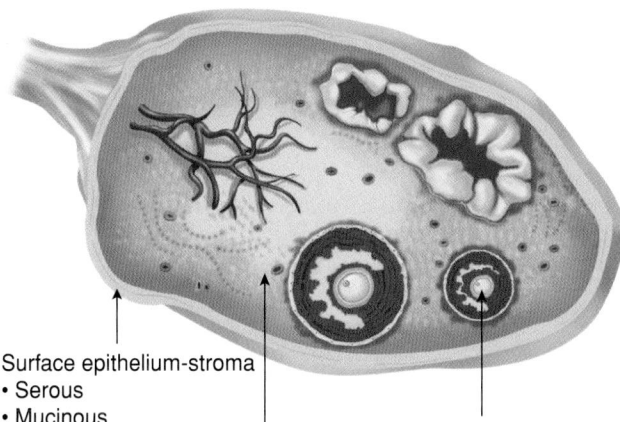

FIGURE 36-1 Origins of the three main types of ovarian tumors. (Adapted with permission from Chen VW, Ruiz B, Killeen JL, et al: Pathology and classification of ovarian tumors, Cancer 2003 May 15;97(10 Suppl):2631–42.)

Surface epithelium-stroma
• Serous
• Mucinous
• Endometrioid
• Clear cell
• Transitional cell

Sex cord-stroma
• Granulosa cell
• Thecoma
• Fibroma
• Sertoli cell
• Sertoli-Leydig
• Steroid

Germ cells
• Dysgerminoma
• Yolk sac
• Embryonal carcinoma
• Choriocarcinoma
• Teratoma

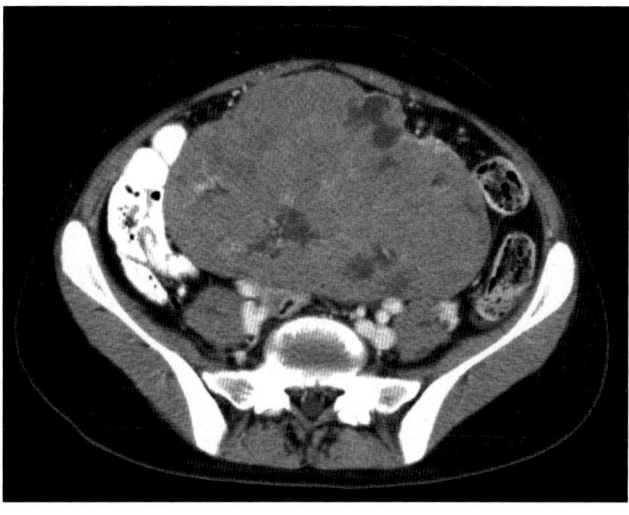

FIGURE 36-2 Computed tomographic (CT) scan of a germ cell tumor.

Distinguishing physical findings are typically lacking in individuals with malignant germ cell tumors. A palpable mass on pelvic examination is the most common. In children and adolescents, however, completing a comprehensive pelvic or transvaginal sonographic examination can be difficult and can lead to diagnostic delay. Accordingly, premenarchal patients may require examination under anesthesia to adequately assess a suspected adnexal tumor. The remainder of the physical examination searches for signs of ascites, pleural effusion, and organomegaly.

Laboratory Testing

In patients with a suspected malignant germ cell tumor, serum human chorionic gonadotropin (hCG) and alpha-fetoprotein (AFP) tumor markers, complete blood count, and liver function tests are drawn before treatment. Alternatively, the appropriate tumor markers may be ordered in the operating room if the diagnosis was not previously suspected (Table 36-1). Preoperative karyotyping of young women with primary amenorrhea

TABLE 36-1. Serum Tumor Markers in Malignant Ovarian Germ Cell Tumors

Histology	AFP	hCG
Dysgerminoma	−	±
Yolk sac tumor	+	−
Immature teratoma	±	−
Choriocarcinoma	−	+
Embryonal carcinoma	+	+
Mixed germ cell tumor	±	±
Polyembryoma	±	±

AFP = alpha-fetoprotein; hCG = human chorionic gonadotropin.

and a suspected germ cell tumor can clarify whether both ovaries should be removed, as in the case of individuals with gonadal dysgenesis (Hoepffner, 2005).

Imaging

Early symptoms can be misinterpreted as those of pregnancy, and acute pain may be confused with appendicitis. Finding an adnexal mass is the first diagnostic step. In most cases, sonography can adequately display those qualities that typically characterize benign and malignant ovarian masses (Chap. 9, p. 217). Functional ovarian cysts are vastly more common in young women. Once these hypoechoic smooth-walled cysts are identified by sonography, they may be observed. Mature cystic teratomas (dermoid cysts) usually display characteristic features when imaged with sonography or computed tomography (CT) (Chap. 9, p. 220). In contrast, the appearance of malignant germ cell tumors differs, and a multilobulated complex ovarian mass is typical (Fig. 36-2). Moreover, prominent blood flow in the fibrovascular septa may be seen using color flow Doppler sonography and suggests the likelihood of malignancy (Kim, 1995). Additional preoperative CT or magnetic resonance (MR) imaging may be indicated based on clinical suspicion. Chest radiography is warranted upon diagnosis to search for tumor metastases in the lungs or mediastinum.

Diagnostic Procedures

Surgical resection is generally required for definitive tissue diagnosis, staging, and treatment. The surgeon should request a frozen section analysis to confirm the diagnosis, but discrepancies between frozen section interpretations and the final paraffin histology are commonplace (Kusamura, 2000). In addition, specific immunostaining is often required to resolve equivocal cases (Cheng, 2004; Ramalingam, 2004; Ulbright, 2005). In contrast, a sonographically or CT-guided percutaneous biopsy has a very limited role in the management of select patients with an ovarian mass suspicious for malignancy.

■ Role of the Generalist

Most patients will initially be seen by a generalist gynecologist. Initial symptoms may point to the more common functional ovarian cyst. Persistent symptoms or an enlarging pelvic mass, however, should prompt sonographic evaluation. If a complex ovarian mass with solid features is noted in this young age group, then measurement of serum hCG and AFP levels and referral to a gynecologic oncologist for primary surgical management should ensue.

If a specialist is unavailable or the diagnosis is not anticipated beforehand, intraoperative decision making is crucial to adequately treat the patient without compromising future fertility. Peritoneal washings are obtained and set aside before proceeding with dissection of any suspicious adnexal mass. These can be discarded later if malignancy is excluded. Initially, the decision to perform cystectomy or oophorectomy depends on the clinical circumstances (Chap. 9, p. 216). In general, the entire adnexa should be removed once a malignant ovarian germ cell tumor is diagnosed. A generalist gynecologist should request intraoperative assistance with staging from a gynecologic oncologist or refer the patient postoperatively if a specialist is not immediately available. At minimum, the abdomen should be explored. Palpation of the omentum and upper abdomen and inspection of the pelvis—especially the contralateral ovary—is easy to perform and document.

■ Pathology

Classification

The modified World Health Organization (WHO) classification of ovarian germ cell tumors is presented in Table 36-2. These tumors are composed of several histologically different tumor types derived from primordial germ cells of the embryonic gonad. There are two major categories: primitive malignant germ

TABLE 36-2. Modified WHO Classification of Ovarian Germ Cell Tumors

Germ cell tumors
Dysgerminoma
Yolk sac tumor (endodermal sinus tumor)
Embryonal carcinoma
Nongestational choriocarcinoma
Mature teratoma
　Solid
　Cystic(dermoid cyst)
Immature teratoma
Mixed germ cell tumor

Monodermal teratoma and highly specialized types arising from a mature cystic teratoma
Thyroid tumors (struma ovarii: benign or malignant)
Carcinoids
Neuroectodermal tumors
Carcinomas (squamous cell or adeno-)
Sebaceous tumors

WHO = World Health Organization.
Adapted with permission from Kurman RJ, Carcangiu ML, Herrington CS, et al (eds): WHO Classification of Tumours of Female Reproductive Organs, 4th ed. Lyon, International Agency for Research on Cancer, 2014.

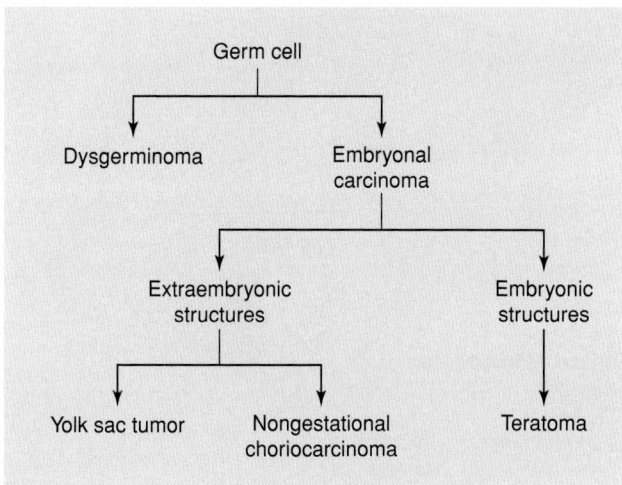

FIGURE 36-3 Differentiation pathway of germ cell tumors.

cell tumors (dysgerminomas) and teratomas, almost all of which are accounted for by mature cystic teratomas (dermoid cysts).

Histogenesis

Primitive germ cells migrate from the wall of the yolk sac to the gonadal ridge (Fig. 18-1, p. 405). As a result, most germ cell tumors arise in the gonad. Rarely, these tumors may develop primarily in extragonadal sites such as the central nervous system, mediastinum, or retroperitoneum (Hsu, 2002).

Ovarian germ cell tumors have a variable pattern of differentiation (Fig. 36-3). Dysgerminomas are primitive neoplasms that do not have the potential for further differentiation. Embryonal carcinomas are composed of multipotential cells that are capable of further differentiation. This lesion is the precursor of several other types of extraembryonic (yolk sac tumor, choriocarcinoma) or embryonic (teratoma) germ cell tumors. The process of differentiation is dynamic, and the resulting neoplasms may be composed of different elements that show various stages of development (Teilum, 1965).

Dysgerminoma

Because their incidence has declined by approximately 30 percent over the past few decades, dysgerminomas currently account for only approximately one third of all malignant ovarian germ cell tumors (Chan, 2008; Smith, 2006). Dysgerminomas are the most common ovarian malignancy detected during pregnancy. This is believed to be an age-related coincidence, however, and not due to some particular characteristic of gestation.

Five percent of dysgerminomas are discovered in phenotypic females with karyotypically abnormal gonads, specifically, with the presence of a normal or abnormal Y-chromosome (Morimura, 1998). Commonly, this group includes those with Turner syndrome mosaicism (45,X/46,XY) and with Swyer syndrome (46,XY, pure gonadal dysgenesis) (Chap. 16, p. 373). The dysgenetic gonads of these individuals often contain gonadoblastomas, which are benign germ cell neoplasms. These tumors may regress or alternatively may undergo malignant transformation, most commonly to dysgerminoma. Because approximately 40 percent of gonadoblastomas in these individuals undergo malignant transformation, both ovaries should be removed (Brown, 2014b; Hoepffner, 2005; Pena-Alonso, 2005).

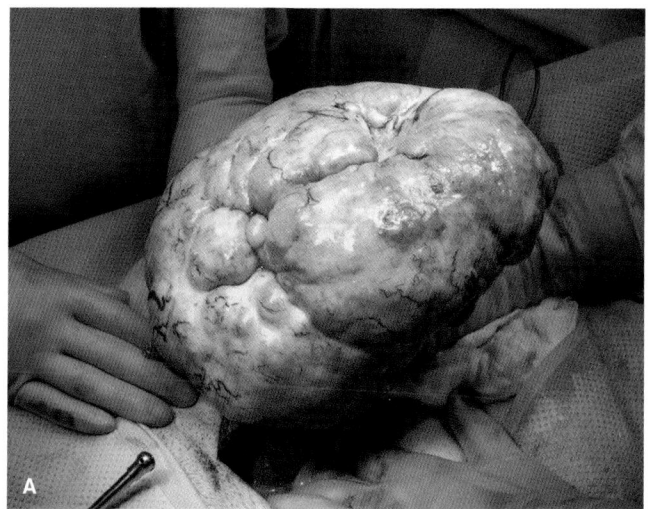
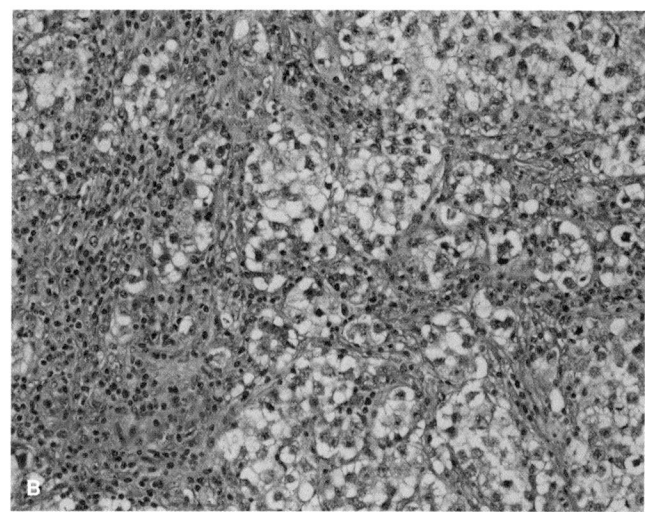

FIGURE 36-4 Dysgerminoma. **A.** Intraoperative photograph. **B.** Dysgerminoma is characterized microscopically by a relatively monotonous population of cells resembling primordial germ cells, with a central rounded or square-edged nucleus and abundant clear, glycogen-rich cytoplasm. As in this case, the tumor often contains fibrous septa, seen here as eosinophilic strands, which are infiltrated by chronic inflammatory cells including lymphocytes, macrophages, and occasional plasma cells. (Used with permission from Dr. Kelley Carrick.)

Dysgerminomas are the only germ cell malignancy with a significant rate of bilateral ovarian involvement—15 to 20 percent. Half of patients with bilateral lesions will have grossly obvious disease, whereas cancer in the remainder will only be detected microscopically. Five percent of women have elevated serum hCG levels due to intermingled syncytiotrophoblast. Similarly, serum lactate dehydrogenase (LDH) and the isoenzymes LDH-1 and LDH-2 may also be useful in monitoring individuals for disease recurrence (Pressley, 1992; Schwartz, 1988).

Dysgerminomas have a variable gross appearance, but in general are solid, pink to tan to cream-colored lobulated masses (Fig. 36-4). Microscopically, there is a monotonous proliferation of large, rounded, polyhedral clear cells that are rich in cytoplasmic glycogen and contain uniform central nuclei with one or a few prominent nucleoli. The tumor cells closely resemble the primordial germ cells of the embryo and are histologically identical to seminoma of the testis.

The standard treatment of dysgerminoma usually involves fertility-sparing surgery with unilateral salpingo-oophorectomy (USO). In some extenuating circumstances, ovarian cystectomy may be considered (Vicus, 2010). Surgical staging is generally extrapolated from epithelial ovarian cancer, but lymphadenectomy is particularly important (Chap. 35, p. 748). Of the malignant germ cell tumors, dysgerminoma has the highest rate of nodal metastases, approximately 25 to 30 percent (Kumar, 2008). Although staging deviations do not adversely affect survival, comprehensive staging allows a safe observation strategy for stage IA tumors (Billmire, 2004; Palenzuela, 2008).

Preservation of the contralateral ovary leads to "recurrent" dysgerminoma in 5 to 10 percent of retained gonads during the next 2 years. This finding in many cases is thought to reflect the high rate of clinically occult disease in the remaining ovary rather than true recurrence. Indeed, at least 75 percent of recurrences develop within the first year of diagnosis (Vicus, 2010). Other common recurrence sites are within the peritoneal cavity or retroperitoneal lymph nodes. Despite this significant incidence of recurrent disease, a conservative surgical approach does not adversely affect long-term survival because of this cancer's sensitivity to chemotherapy (Liu, 2013).

Dysgerminomas have the best prognosis of all malignant ovarian germ cell tumor variants. Two thirds are stage I at diagnosis, and the 5-year disease-specific survival rate approximates 99 percent (Table 36-3). Even those with advanced disease have high survival rates following chemotherapy. For example, those with stage II-IV disease have a greater than 98-percent survival rate with platinum-based agents (Chan, 2008).

TABLE 36-3. Stage at Diagnosis and 5-Year Survival of Common Malignant Ovarian Germ Cell Tumors

	Dysgerminoma	Yolk Sac Tumor	Immature Teratoma
Stage			
I	66%	61%	72%
II–IV	34%	39%	28%
Survival			
Stage I	99%	93%	98%
Stage II–IV	>98%	64–91%	73–88%

Sources for survival figures are referenced within the text.

Yolk Sac Tumors

These tumors account for 10 to 20 percent of all malignant ovarian germ cell tumors. These lesions were previously called endodermal sinus tumors, but the terminology has been revised. One third of individuals are premenarchal at the time of initial presentation. Involvement of both gonads is rare, and the other ovary is usually involved with metastatic disease only when there are other metastases in the peritoneal cavity.

Grossly, these tumors form solid masses that are more yellow and friable than dysgerminomas. They are often focally necrotic and hemorrhagic, with cystic degeneration and rupture. The microscopic appearance of yolk sac tumors is often diverse. The most common appearance, the reticular pattern, reflects extraembryonic differentiation, with the formation of a network of irregular anastomosing spaces that are lined by primitive epithelial cells. *Schiller-Duval bodies* are pathognomonic when present (Fig. 36-5). These characteristics have a single papilla, which is lined by tumor cells and contains a central vessel. Alpha-fetoprotein is commonly produced. As a result, yolk sac tumors usually contain cells that stain immunohistochemically for AFP, and serum levels can serve as a reliable tumor marker in posttreatment surveillance.

Yolk sac tumors are the deadliest malignant ovarian germ cell tumor type. As a result, all patients are treated with chemotherapy regardless of stage. Fortunately, more than half present with stage I disease, corresponding to a 5-year disease-specific survival rate of approximately 93 percent (Chan, 2008). Disadvantageously, yolk sac tumors have a greater propensity for rapid growth, peritoneal spread, and distant hematogenous dissemination to the lungs. Accordingly, individuals with stage II-IV disease have a 5-year survival rate ranging from 64 to 91 percent. Of tumor recurrences, most will occur within the first year, and treatment is usually ineffective (Cicin, 2009).

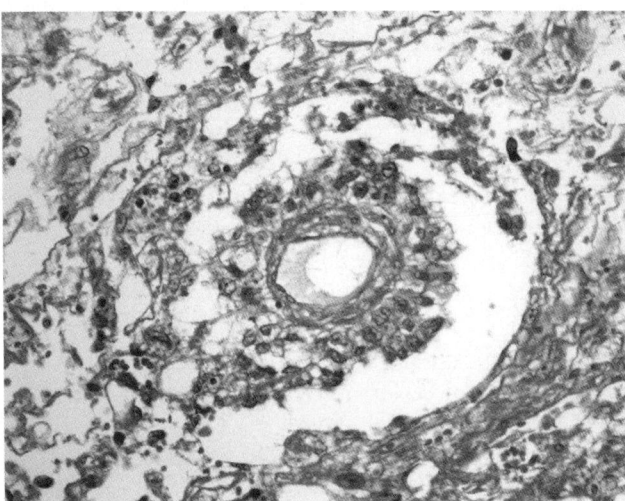

FIGURE 36-5 Schiller-Duval body. This structure consists of a central capillary surrounded by tumor cells, present within a cystic space that may be lined by flat to cuboidal tumor cells. When present, the Schiller-Duval body is pathognomonic for yolk sac tumor, although they are conspicuous in only a minority of cases. In any given case, Schiller-Duval bodies may be few in number, absent, or have atypical morphologic features. (Used with permission from Dr. Kelley Carrick.)

Other Primitive Germ Cell Tumors

The rarest subtypes of nondysgerminomatous tumors are typically mixed with other more common variants and usually are not found in pure form.

Embryonal Carcinoma. Patients diagnosed with embryonal carcinoma are characteristically younger, with a mean age of 14 years, than those having other types of germ cell tumors. Epithelial cells resembling those of the embryonic disc form these primitive tumors. The solid disorganized sheets of large anaplastic cells, glandlike spaces, and papillary structures are distinctive and allow easy identification of these rare tumors (Ulbright, 2005). Although dysgerminomas are the most common germ cell tumor resulting from malignant transformation of gonadoblastomas in individuals with dysgenetic gonads, occasionally embryonal "testicular" tumors may also originate (LaPolla, 1990). Embryonal carcinomas typically produce hCG, and 75 percent also secrete AFP.

Polyembryoma. These rare tumors characteristically contain many embryolike bodies. Each has a small central "germ disc" positioned between two cavities, one mimicking an amnionic cavity and the other a yolk sac. Syncytiotrophoblast giant cells are frequent, but elements other than the embryoid bodies should constitute less than 10 percent of the tumor for the "polyembryoma" designation to be used. Conceptually, these tumors may be viewed as a bridge between the primitive (dysgerminoma) and differentiated (teratoma) germ cell tumor types. For this reason, polyembryomas are often considered to be the most immature of all teratomas (Ulbright, 2005). Serum AFP or hCG levels or both may be elevated in these individuals due to the yolk sac and syncytial components, respectively (Takemori, 1998).

Choriocarcinoma. Primary ovarian choriocarcinoma arising from a germ cell appears similar to gestational choriocarcinoma with ovarian metastases, which is discussed in Chapter 37 (p. 785). The distinction is important because nongestational tumors have a poorer prognosis (Corakci, 2005). The detection of other germ cell components indicates nongestational choriocarcinoma, whereas a concomitant or proximate pregnancy suggests a gestational form (Ulbright, 2005). Clinical manifestations are common and result from high hCG levels produced by these rare tumors. These elevated levels may induce sexual precocity in prepubertal girls or heavy, irregular bleeding in reproductive-aged women (Oliva, 1993).

Mixed Germ Cell Tumors

Ovarian germ cell tumors have a mixed pattern of cellular differentiation in 25 to 30 percent of cases, although the incidence of these tumors has also declined by approximately 30 percent over the past few decades (Smith, 2006). Dysgerminoma is the most common component and is typically seen with yolk sac tumor or immature teratoma or both. The frequency of bilateral ovarian involvement depends on the presence or absence of a dysgerminoma component and increases when it is present. However, treatment and prognosis are determined by the nondysgerminomatous component (Low, 2000). For this reason, elevated serum hCG and particularly AFP levels in a woman with a presumed pure dysgerminoma should prompt a search for other germ cell components by a more extensive histologic evaluation (Aoki, 2003).

Immature Teratomas

Due to a 60-percent increased incidence during the past few decades, immature teratomas are now the most common variant and account for 40 to 50 percent of all malignant ovarian germ cell tumors (Chan, 2008; Smith, 2006). They are composed of tissues derived from the three germ layers: ectoderm, mesoderm, and endoderm. The presence of immature or embryonal structures, however, distinguishes these tumors from the much more common and benign mature cystic teratoma (dermoid cyst). Bilateral ovarian involvement is rare, but 10 percent have a mature teratoma in the contralateral ovary. Tumor markers are often not elevated unless the immature teratoma is mingled with other germ cell tumor types. Alpha-fetoprotein, cancer antigen 125 (CA125), CA19-9, and carcinoembryonic antigen (CEA) may be helpful in some cases (Li, 2002).

With gross external inspection, these tumors are large, rounded or lobulated, soft or firm masses. They frequently perforate the ovarian capsule and invade locally. The most frequent site of dissemination is the peritoneum and much less commonly the retroperitoneal lymph nodes. With local invasion, surrounding adhesions commonly form and are thought to explain the lower rates of torsion with this tumor compared with that of its benign mature counterpart (Cass, 2001). On cut surface, the interior is typically solid with intermittent cystic areas, but occasionally the reverse is seen, with solid nodules present only in the cyst wall (Fig. 36-6). Solid parts may correspond to the immature elements, cartilage, bone, or a combination of these. Cystic areas are filled with hair and with serous fluid, mucinous fluid, or sebum.

Microscopic examination reveals a disorderly mixture of tissues. Of the immature elements, neuroectodermal tissues almost always predominate and are arranged as primitive tubules and sheets of small, round, malignant cells that may be associated with glia formation. The diagnosis is usually difficult to confirm during frozen section analysis, and most tumors are confirmed only on final pathologic review (Pavlakis, 2009). Tumors are graded 1 to 3 primarily by the amount of immature neural tissue they contain. O'Connor and Norris (1994) analyzed 244 immature teratomas and noted significant inconsistencies in grade assignment by different observers. For this reason, they proposed changing the system to two grades: low (previous grades 1 and 2) and high (previous grade 3). This practice, however, has not been universally accepted.

In general, survival is predicted most accurately by stage and by histologic grade of the tumor. For example, almost three quarters of immature teratomas are stage I at diagnosis and have a 5-year survival rate of 98 percent (Chan, 2008). Those with stage IA grade 1 immature teratomas have an excellent prognosis and do not require adjuvant chemotherapy (Bonazzi, 1994; Marina, 1999). Patients with stage II-IV disease have a 5-year survival rate ranging from 73 to 88 percent (Chan, 2008).

Unilateral salpingo-oophorectomy is the standard care for these and other malignant germ cell tumors in reproductive-aged women. Beiner and colleagues (2004), however, treated eight women with early-stage immature teratoma with ovarian cystectomy and adjuvant chemotherapy and noted no recurrences.

Immature teratomas may be associated with mature tissue implants studding the peritoneum that do not increase the stage of the tumor or diminish the prospect of survival. However, these implants of mature teratomatous elements, even though benign, are resistant to chemotherapy and can enlarge during or after chemotherapy. Termed the *growing teratoma syndrome,* these implants require second-look surgery and resection to exclude recurrent malignancy (Zagame, 2006).

Malignant Transformation of Mature Cystic Teratomas (Dermoid Cysts)

These rare tumors are the only germ cell variants that typically develop in postmenopausal women. Malignant areas are

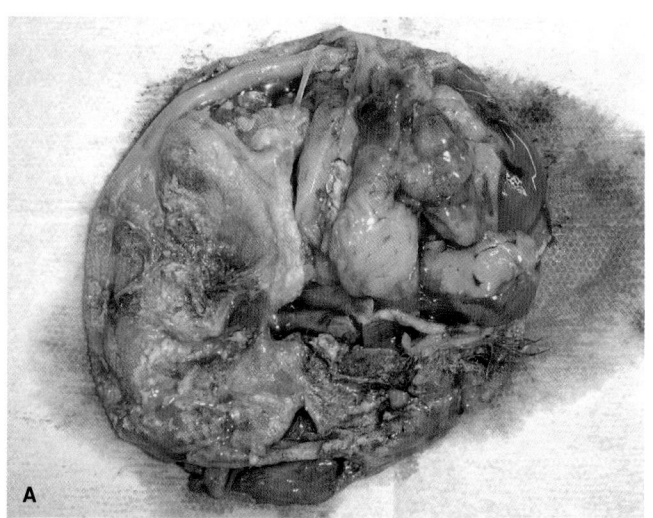
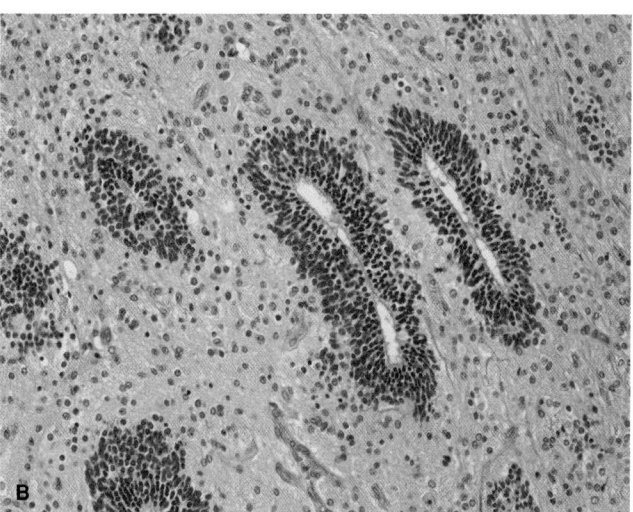

FIGURE 36-6 Immature teratoma. **A.** This opened surgical specimen shows characteristic solid and cystic architecture. As in mature teratomas, hair and other skin elements are often found. **B.** Immature teratomas contain a disorderly mixture of mature and immature tissues derived from the three germ cell layers—ectoderm, mesoderm, and endoderm. Of the immature elements, immature neuroepithelium is the most common. Here, immature neuroepithelial cells arranged in rosettes lie within a background of mature neural tissue. (Used with permission from Dr. Kelley Carrick.)

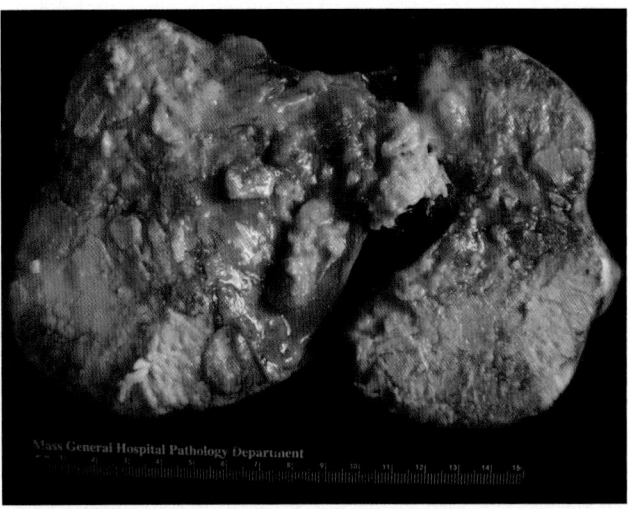

FIGURE 36-7 This opened surgical specimen reveals squamous cell carcinoma malignant transformation within a mature cystic teratoma.

usually found as small nodules in the cyst wall or a polypoid mass within the lumen after removal of the entire mature cystic teratoma (Pins, 1996). Squamous cell carcinoma is most common and is found in approximately 1 percent of mature cystic teratomas (Fig. 36-7). Platinum-based chemotherapy with or without pelvic radiation is most often used for adjuvant treatment of early-stage disease (Dos Santos, 2007). However, regardless of treatment received, patients with advanced disease do poorly (Gainford, 2010).

Other uncommon types of malignant features may include basal-cell carcinomas, sebaceous tumors, malignant melanomas, adenocarcinomas, sarcomas, and neuroectodermal tumors. Moreover, endocrine-type neoplasms such as struma ovarii (teratoma composed mainly of thyroid tissue) and carcinoid may also be found within mature cystic teratomas.

■ Treatment

Surgery

A vertical abdominal incision is traditionally recommended if ovarian malignancy is suspected. However, increasingly, investigators with advanced endoscopic skills have noted laparoscopy to be a safe and effective alternative for women with smaller ovarian masses and apparent stage I disease (Shim, 2013).

If present, ascites is evacuated and sent for cytologic evaluation. Otherwise, washings of the pelvis and paracolic gutters are collected for analysis prior to manipulation of the intraperitoneal contents. The entire peritoneal cavity is systematically inspected. The ovaries are assessed for size, tumor involvement, capsular rupture, external excrescences, and adherence to surrounding structures.

Fertility-sparing USO is performed in all reproductive-aged women diagnosed with malignant ovarian germ cell tumors, as this conservative approach in general does not adversely affect survival (Chan, 2008; Lee, 2009). Following USO, blind biopsy or wedge resection of a normal-appearing contralateral ovary is not recommended. For those who have completed childbearing, hysterectomy with bilateral salpingo-oophorectomy

(BSO) is appropriate (Brown, 2014b). In either case, following removal of the affected ovary, surgical staging by laparotomy or laparoscopy proceeds as previously described for epithelial ovarian cancer (Chap. 35, p. 748) (Gershenson, 2007a). Because of tumor dissemination patterns, lymphadenectomy is most important for dysgerminomas, whereas staging peritoneal and omental biopsies are particularly valuable for yolk sac tumors and immature teratomas (Kleppe, 2014).

Cytoreductive surgery is recommended for advanced-stage malignant ovarian germ cell tumors if it can be accomplished with minimal residual disease (Bafna, 2001; Nawa, 2001; Suita, 2002). The same general principles for debulking are applied as described for epithelial ovarian cancer. Because of the exquisite chemosensitivity of most malignant germ cell tumors, however, neoadjuvant chemotherapy is a reasonable option for patients thought to be unresectable (Talukdar, 2014).

Many women will be referred to an oncologist after USO for a tumor that was clinically confined to the excised ovary. For such patients, if initial surgical staging was incomplete, options may include a second surgery to complete primary staging, regular surveillance, or adjuvant chemotherapy. Unfortunately, few data support a preferred approach. Because of its minimally invasive qualities, laparoscopy is a particularly attractive option for delayed surgical staging following primary excision and has been shown to accurately detect those women who require chemotherapy (Leblanc, 2004). Surgical staging following primary excision, however, is less important for scenarios in which chemotherapy will be administered regardless of surgical findings such as clinical stage I yolk sac tumors and high-grade clinical stage I immature teratomas (Stier, 1996). In such patients, reassurance of no abnormalities by CT imaging is often sufficient prior to proceeding with adjuvant chemotherapy (Gershenson, 2007a).

Surveillance

Patients with malignant ovarian germ cell tumors are followed by careful clinical, radiologic, and serologic surveillance every 3 months for the first 2 years after therapy completion (Dark, 1997). Ninety percent of recurrences develop within this time frame (Messing, 1992). Second-look surgery at the completion of therapy is not necessary in women with completely resected disease or in those individuals with advanced tumor that does not contain teratoma. However, incompletely resected immature teratoma is the one circumstance among all types of ovarian cancer in which patients clearly benefit from second-look surgery and excision of chemorefractory tumor (Culine, 1996; Rezk, 2005; Williams, 1994).

Chemotherapy

Stage IA dysgerminomas and stage IA grade 1 immature teratomas do not require additional chemotherapy. More advanced disease and all other histologic types of malignant ovarian germ cell tumors have historically been treated with combination chemotherapy after surgery (Suita, 2002; Tewari, 2000). However, there is a strong trend toward exploring the feasibility of surgery followed by close surveillance in pediatric and adolescent girls (Billmire, 2014). Because chemotherapy remains effective when used at the time of relapse, some investigators are attempting to identify additional low-risk, early-stage subgroups that may be observed postoperatively and thereby avoid treatment-related toxicity (Bonazzi, 1994; Cushing, 1999; Dark, 1997). However, before this strategy can be incorporated into general practice, additional large studies are needed.

The standard regimen is a 5-day course of bleomycin, etoposide, and cisplatin (BEP) given every 3 weeks (Gershenson, 1990; Williams, 1987). Modified 3-day BEP combinations are also safe and effective (Chen, 2014; Dimopoulos, 2004). Carboplatin and etoposide, given in three cycles, has shown promise as an alternative for selected patients (Williams, 2004). For women with incompletely resected disease, at least four courses of BEP are usually recommended (Williams, 1991).

Radiation

Chemotherapy has replaced radiation as the preferred adjuvant treatment for all types of malignant ovarian germ cell tumors. This transition was prompted primarily by the exquisite sensitivity of these tumors to either modality, but higher likelihood of retained ovarian function using chemotherapy (Solheim, 2015). Patients treated with radiotherapy are also much more likely to develop a second cancer within 10 years (Solheim, 2014). Occasional situations may still exist in which radiotherapy is considered, such as palliation of a germ cell tumor that has demonstrated resistance to chemotherapy.

Relapse

At least four courses of BEP chemotherapy is the preferred treatment for recurrent ovarian germ cell tumors in women initially managed with surgery alone. Patients who achieved a sustained clinical remission of greater than 6 months after completing BEP or another platinum-based chemotherapy regimen may be treated again with BEP. Because their tumors are generally more responsive, these "platinum-sensitive" patients have a much better prognosis. However, women who do not achieve remission with BEP chemotherapy or relapse within a few months (fewer than 6) are considered "platinum-resistant," and treatment options are limited. Chemorefractory cases with dysgerminoma or immature teratoma appear to have a better outcome than other subtypes, and surgical salvage aimed at achieving no residual disease may benefit some patients (Li, 2007). Another option for this group is vincristine, dactinomycin, and cyclophosphamide (VAC) (Gershenson, 1985). Other potentially active drugs include paclitaxel, gemcitabine, and oxaliplatin (Hinton, 2002; Kollmannsberger, 2006).

Second-look procedures with surgical debulking have a limited role because of the inherent chemosensitivity of these recurrent tumors. Chemorefractory immature teratomas are notable exceptions (Munkarah, 1994). Growth or persistence of a tumor after chemotherapy does not necessarily imply progression of malignancy, but these masses should still be resected (Geisler, 1994).

■ Prognosis

Malignant ovarian germ cell tumors have an excellent overall prognosis (see Table 36-3) (Solheim, 2013, 2014). Moreover, the number of cases with distant and unstaged disease has dramatically declined, suggesting that germ cell tumors are being diagnosed earlier. In addition, the survival rates have significantly improved for all subtypes, especially with the demonstrated efficacy of cisplatin-based combination therapy (Smith, 2006). Histologic cell type, elevated serum marker levels, surgical stage, and the amount of residual disease at initial surgery are the major variables affecting prognosis (Murugaesu, 2006; Smith, 2006). Typically, pure dysgerminomas recur within 2 years and are highly treatable (Vicus, 2010). However, for nondysgerminomatous tumors, outcome after relapse is poor, and fewer than 10 percent of patients achieve long-term survival (Murugaesu, 2006).

Most women treated with fertility-sparing surgery, with or without chemotherapy, will resume normal menses and are able to conceive and bear children (Gershenson, 2007b; Zanetta, 2001). In addition, none of the reported studies has noted an increased rate of birth defects or spontaneous abortion in those treated with chemotherapy (Brewer, 1999; Low, 2000; Tangir, 2003; Zanetta, 2001).

■ Management During Pregnancy

Persistent adnexal masses are detected in 1 to 2 percent of all pregnancies. These neoplasms are usually seen during routine obstetric sonographic examination, but occasionally a dramatically elevated maternal serum alpha-fetoprotein (MSAFP) level is the presenting sign of a malignant germ cell tumor (Horbelt, 1994; Montz, 1989). Mature cystic teratomas (dermoid cysts) make up one third of tumors resected during pregnancy. In contrast, dysgerminomas account for only 1 to 2 percent of such neoplasms but still are the most common ovarian malignancy during pregnancy. Development of other germ cell tumors is rare (Shimizu, 2003).

Initial surgical management including surgical staging is the same as for the nonpregnant woman (Horbelt, 1994; Zhao, 2006). Fortunately, very few patients have advanced disease necessitating radical dissection for cytoreduction. The decision to administer chemotherapy during pregnancy is controversial. Malignant ovarian germ cell tumors have the propensity to grow rapidly, and delaying treatment until after delivery is potentially hazardous. Treatment with BEP appears to be safe during pregnancy, but some reports have speculated that fetal complications are possible (Elit, 1999; Horbelt, 1994). For this reason, some advocate postponing treatment until the puerperium (Shimizu, 2003). Unfortunately, there are no results from large studies to resolve this dilemma. Although BEP administration may be delayed until the puerperium for completely resected dysgerminomas, patients with nondysgerminomatous tumors (mainly yolk sac tumors and immature teratomas) and incompletely resected disease warrant strong consideration of chemotherapy during pregnancy.

OVARIAN SEX CORD-STROMAL TUMORS

Sex cord-stromal tumors (SCSTs) are a heterogeneous group of rare neoplasms that originate from the ovarian matrix. Cells within this matrix have the potential for hormone production, and nearly 90 percent of hormone-producing ovarian tumors are SCSTs. As a result, individuals with these tumors typically present with signs and symptoms of estrogen or androgen excess.

Surgical resection is the primary treatment, and SCSTs are generally confined to one ovary at the time of diagnosis. Moreover, most have an indolent growth pattern and low malignant potential. For these reasons, few patients ever require platinum-based chemotherapy. Although recurrent disease often responds poorly to treatment, patients may live for many years because of characteristically slow tumor progression.

The overall prognosis of ovarian SCSTs is excellent—primarily due to early-stage disease at diagnosis and curative surgery. The scarcity of these tumors, however, limits the understanding of their natural history, treatment, and prognosis.

■ Epidemiology

SCSTs account for 3 to 5 percent of ovarian malignancies (Ray-Coquard, 2014). These tumors are more than twice as likely to develop in black women for reasons that are unclear (Quirk, 2005). In contrast with epithelial ovarian cancers or malignant germ cell tumors, ovarian SCSTs typically affect women of all ages. This range contains a unique bimodal distribution that reflects inherent tumor heterogeneity. For example, juvenile granulosa cell tumors, Sertoli-Leydig cell tumors, and sclerosing stromal tumors are found predominantly in prepubertal girls and women within the first three decades of life (Schneider, 2005). Adult granulosa cell tumors commonly develop in older women, at an average age in the mid-50s (van Meurs, 2013).

There are no proven risk factors for SCSTs. However, in a hypothesis-generating case-control study, Boyce and coworkers (2009) observed that obesity as a hyperestrogenic state was independently associated, whereas parity, smoking, and oral contraceptive use were protective.

The etiology of SCSTs is largely unknown. However, a single, recurrent *FOXL2* gene mutation (402C>G) is present in virtually all adult-type granulosa cell tumors. Thus, mutant *FOXL2* appears to be a highly specific event in the pathogenesis of these rare tumors (Schrader, 2009; Shah, 2009). The other major finding is that women with a germline *DICER1* mutation are predisposed to developing SCSTs (Heravi-Moussavi, 2012). Otherwise, there is no known inherited predisposition for the development of these tumors, and familial cases are rare (Stevens, 2005). However, ovarian SCSTs do develop in association with several defined hereditary disorders at a frequency that exceeds mere chance. Associated disorders include Ollier disease, which is characterized by multiple benign but disfiguring cartilaginous neoplasms, and Peutz-Jeghers syndrome, characterized by intestinal hamartomatous polyps (Stevens, 2005).

■ Diagnosis

Patient Findings

Isosexual precocious puberty is the presenting sign in more than 80 percent of prepubertal girls ultimately diagnosed with an ovarian SCST (Kalfa, 2005). Adolescents often report secondary amenorrhea. As a result, these young individuals presenting with endocrinologic symptoms tend to be diagnosed at earlier stages. Abdominal pain and distention are other common complaints in this age group (Schneider, 2003a).

In adult women, heavy, irregular bleeding and postmenopausal bleeding are the most frequent symptoms. In addition,

TABLE 36-4. Tumor Markers for Ovarian Sex Cord-Stromal Tumors with Malignant Potential

Granulosa cell tumors (adult and juvenile)	Inhibin A and B; estradiol (not as reliable)
Sertoli-Leydig cell tumors	Inhibin A and B; occasionally alpha-fetoprotein
Sex cord tumor with annular tubules	Inhibin A and B
Steroid cell tumors not otherwise specified	Steroid hormones elevated pretreatment

mild hirsutism that rapidly progresses to frank virilization should prompt evaluation to exclude these tumors. The classic presentation is a postmenopausal woman with rapidly evolving stigmata of androgen excess and a complex adnexal mass. Abdominal pain or a mass palpable by the patient herself are other telling signs and symptoms (Chan, 2005).

The size of SCSTs varies widely, but most women have a palpable abdominal or pelvic mass during examination regardless of their age. A fluid wave and other physical findings suggestive of advanced disease, however, are rare.

Laboratory Testing

Elevated circulating levels of testosterone or androstenedione or both are strongly suggestive of an ovarian SCST in a woman with signs and symptoms of virilization. Clinical hyperandrogenism is more likely to be idiopathic or related to polycystic ovarian syndrome, but serum testosterone levels >150 g/dL or dehydroepiandrosterone sulfate (DHEAS) levels >8000 g/L strongly suggest the possibility of an androgen-secreting tumor (Carmina, 2006). In most instances, tumor marker studies are not obtained preoperatively, because the diagnosis of ovarian SCST is often not suspected. When the diagnosis is confirmed, the appropriate tumor markers may be drawn during or following surgery (Table 36-4).

Imaging

The gross appearances of SCSTs range from large multicystic masses to small solid masses—effectively precluding a specific radiologic diagnosis. Granulosa cell tumors often sonographically demonstrate semisolid features but are not reliably discernible from epithelial tumors (Fig. 36-8) (Sharony, 2001). In addition, the endometrium may be thickened from increased tumor estrogen production. Although CT or MR imaging has been used to clarify indeterminate sonograms, there is no definitive radiologic study to diagnose these tumors (Jung, 2005).

Diagnostic Procedures

Patients with an ovarian mass suspicious for malignancy based on clinical and sonographic findings require surgical resection for definitive tissue diagnosis, staging, and treatment. Sonographically or CT-guided percutaneous biopsy has no role. Moreover, diagnostic laparoscopy or laparotomy with visual assessment of the adnexal mass alone is inadequate. Thus, excision and pathologic evaluation are necessary. Following removal, ovarian SCSTs can usually be distinguished histologically from germ cell tumors, epithelial ovarian cancers, or other spindle-cell neoplasms by immunostaining for inhibin (Cathro, 2005; Schneider, 2005).

Role of the Generalist

Preoperatively, patients with a potentially malignant ovarian SCST are ideally referred to a gynecologic oncologist for evaluation. Most ovarian SCSTs, however, are diagnosed by generalist gynecologists following resection of a seemingly benign but complex mass in a woman with a CA125 level that is typically normal, if known beforehand. The initial surgery is often performed in a community-based hospital and without adequate staging. In this setting, prior to referral, histologic results should be reviewed and confirmed by an experienced pathologist. Following referral to a gynecologic oncologist, surgical staging may be indicated.

Pathology
Classification

Ovarian SCSTs arise from sex cord and mesenchymal cells of the embryonic gonad (Chap. 18, p. 407). Granulosa and Sertoli cells develop from the sex cords and thus from the coelomic epithelium. In contrast, theca cells, Leydig cells, and fibroblasts are derived from the mesenchyme. The primitive gonadal stroma possesses sexual bipotentiality. Therefore, developing tumors may be composed of a male-directed cell type (Sertoli or Leydig cell) or a female-directed cell type (granulosa or theca cell). Although distinct categories of SCSTs have been defined, mixed tumors are relatively common (Table 36-5). For example, ovarian granulosa cell tumors may have admixed Sertoli components. Similarly, tumors that are predominantly Sertoli or

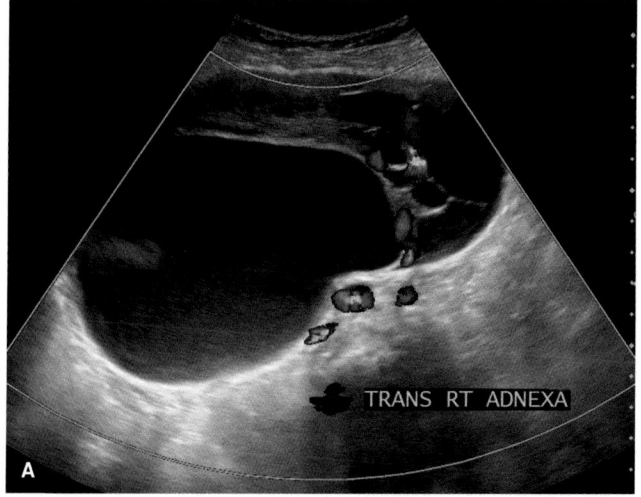
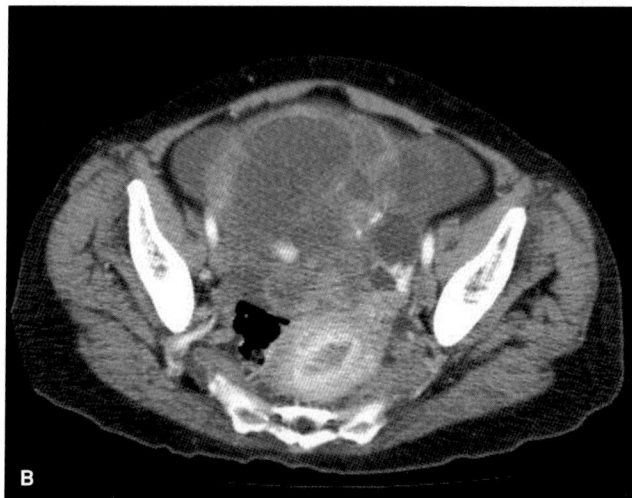
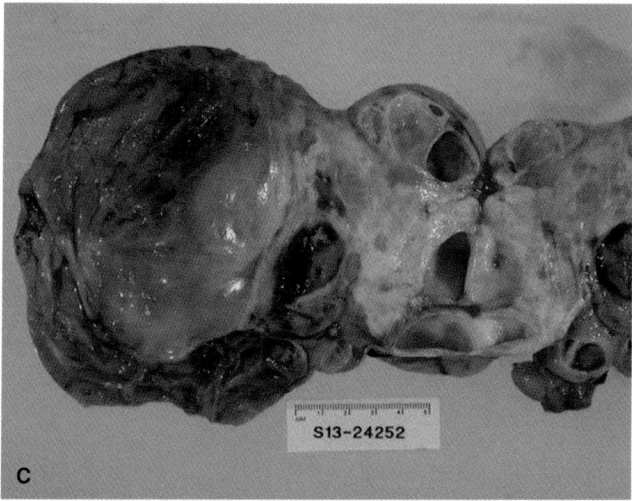

FIGURE 36-8 Adult granulosa cell tumor. **A.** Abdominal sonography displays a large adnexal mass with solid and cystic areas. With application of color Doppler, thick vascular septa are seen. **B.** Computed tomographic (CT) scan of the same tumor. **C.** The tumor was opened after excision, and again its mixed architecture is noted. (Used with permission from Dr. Christa Nagel.)

TABLE 36-5. Modified WHO Classification of Ovarian Sex Cord-Stromal Tumors

Pure stromal tumors
Fibroma/fibrosarcoma
Thecoma
Sclerosing stromal tumor
Leydig cell tumor
Steroid cell tumor

Pure sex cord tumors
Granulosa cell tumor
  Adult type
  Juvenile type
Sertoli cell tumor
Sex cord tumor with annular tubules

Mixed sex cord-stromal tumors
Sertoli-Leydig cell tumors
Sex cord-stromal tumors, NOS

NOS = not otherwise specified; WHO = World Health Organization.
Adapted with permission from Kurman RJ, Carcangiu ML, Herrington CS, et al (eds): WHO Classification of Tumours of Female Reproductive Organs, 4th ed. Lyon, International Agency for Research on Cancer, 2014.

Sertoli-Leydig cells may contain minor granulosa cell elements. These mixed tumors are believed to arise from a common lineage with variable differentiation and do not represent two concurrent separate entities (McKenna, 2005; Vang, 2004).

Histologic Grading

Ovarian granulosa cell tumors are universally considered to have malignant potential, but most other SCST subtypes do not have definitive criteria for clearly defining benign and malignant. Attempts to grade these tumors using nuclear characteristics or mitotic activity counts have produced inconsistent results (Chen, 2003).

Patterns of Growth and Spread

The natural history of SCSTs in general differs greatly from that of epithelial ovarian carcinomas. For example, most of these tumors have low malignant potential. They are typically unilateral and remain localized, retain hormone-secreting functions, and infrequently relapse. Recurrences tend to be late and usually develop in the abdomen or pelvis (Abu-Rustum, 2006). Bone metastases are rare (Dubuc-Lissoir, 2001).

Granulosa Cell Tumors

Adult Granulosa Cell Tumors. Seventy percent of ovarian SCSTs are granulosa cell tumors (Colombo, 2007). These tumors are formed by cells believed to arise from those surrounding the germinal cells within ovarian follicles. There are two clinically and histologically distinct types: the adult form, which makes up 95 percent of cases, and the juvenile type, accounting for 5 percent.

With adult granulosa cell tumor, most women are diagnosed after age 30, and the average age approximates 55 years. Heavy, irregular menstrual bleeding and postmenopausal bleeding are common and reflect prolonged exposure of the endometrium to estrogen. Related to this estrogen excess, coexisting pathology such as endometrial hyperplasia or adenocarcinoma has been found in 25 to 30 percent of patients with adult granulosa cell tumor (van

Meurs, 2013). Similarly, breast enlargement and tenderness are frequent associated complaints, and secondary amenorrhea has been reported (Kurihara, 2004). Alternatively, symptoms may stem from the mass of the ovary rather than from hormones produced (Ray-Coquard, 2014). An enlarging and potentially hemorrhagic tumor can cause abdominal pain and distention. Acute pelvic pain may suggest adnexal torsion, or tumor rupture with hemoperitoneum can mimic ectopic pregnancy.

During surgery, if an adult granulosa cell tumor is confirmed, tumor markers may be requested. Of these, inhibin B seems to be more accurate than inhibin A, frequently being elevated months before clinical detection of recurrence (Mom, 2007). The diagnostic value of these markers, however, is often hampered by their physiologically broad normal ranges (Schneider, 2005). Estradiol also has limited use in surveillance. This is particularly true for the younger patient wishing to preserve fertility and having the contralateral ovary left in situ.

Grossly, adult granulosa cell tumors are large and multicystic and often exceed 10 to 15 cm in diameter (see Fig. 36-8). The surface is frequently edematous and unusually adhered to other pelvic organs. For this reason, more extensive dissection is typically required than for epithelial ovarian cancers or malignant germ cell tumors. During excision, inadvertent rupture and intraoperative bleeding from the tumor itself is also common.

The interior of the tumor is highly variable. Solid components may predominate with large areas of hemorrhage and necrosis. Alternatively, it can be cystic, with numerous locules filled with serosanguinous or gelatinous fluid (Colombo, 2007). Microscopic examination shows predominately granulosa cells with pale, grooved, "coffee bean" nuclei. The characteristic microscopic feature is the *Call-Exner body*—a rosette arrangement of cells around an eosinophilic fluid space (Fig. 36-9).

Adult granulosa cell tumors are low-grade malignancies that typically demonstrate indolent growth. Ninety-five percent are unilateral, and 70 to 90 percent are stage I at diagnosis (Table 36-6). The 5-year survival for patients with stage I disease is 90 to 95 percent (Colombo, 2007; Zhang, 2007). However, 15 to

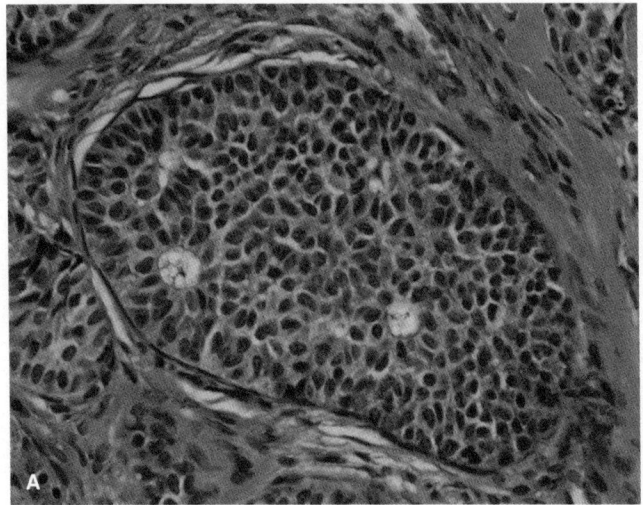 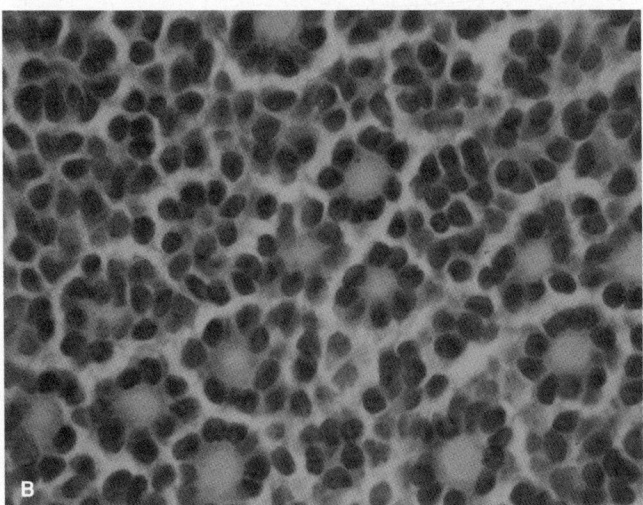

FIGURE 36-9 Adult granulosa cell tumor. **A.** Cells are typically crowded and contain scant, pale cytoplasm. Their elongated nuclei may have a longitudinal fold or groove that gives them a "coffee bean" appearance. **B.** Call-Exner bodies are identified by their rosette appearance. (Used with permission from Dr. Raheela Ashfaq.)

TABLE 36-6. Stage and Survival of Common Ovarian Sex Cord-Stromal Tumors

	Adult Granulosa Cell	Sertoli-Leydig Cell
Stage at diagnosis		
I	70–90%	97%
II–IV	10–20%	2–3%
Five-year survival		
Stage I	90–95%	90–95%
Stage II–IV	30–50%	10–20%

Sources for survival figures are referenced within the text.

25 percent of stage I tumors will eventually relapse. The median time to recurrence is 5 to 6 years, but may be several decades (Abu-Rustum, 2006; East, 2005). Advantageously, these indolent tumors usually progress slowly thereafter, and the median length of survival after relapse is another 6 years. Advanced tumor stage and residual disease are poor prognostic factors (Al Badawi, 2002; Sehouli, 2004). Patients with stage II-IV tumors have a 5-year survival rate of 30 to 50 percent (Malmstrom, 1994; Miller, 1997; Piura, 1994). Cellular atypia and mitotic count may help in determining the prognosis but are difficult to reproducibly quantify (Miller, 2001).

Juvenile Granulosa Cell Tumors. These rare neoplasms develop primarily in children and young adults, and approximately 90 percent are diagnosed before puberty (Colombo, 2007). The mean age at diagnosis is 13 years, but patient ages range from newborn to 67 years (Young, 1984). Juvenile granulosa cell tumors are sometimes associated with Ollier disease or with Maffucci syndrome, which is characterized by endochondromas and hemangiomas (Young, 1984; Yuan, 2004).

In affected females, estrogen, progesterone, and testosterone levels may be elevated and lead to suppression of gonadotropins. As a result, menstrual irregularities or amenorrhea are common. Prepubertal girls typically display isosexual precocious puberty, which is characterized by breast enlargement and development of pubic hair, vaginal secretions, and other secondary sexual characteristics. These tumors infrequently secrete androgens, but in such cases may induce virilization. Despite these endocrinologic signs, a delayed diagnosis of juvenile granulosa cell tumors in pre- and postpubertal girls is common and associated with a higher risk of peritoneal tumor spread (Kalfa, 2005).

In addition to hormonal changes, individuals may display tumor effects. For example, older patients usually seek medical attention for abdominal pain or swelling. Preoperative rupture with resulting hemoperitoneum may create acute abdominal symptoms in 5 to 10 percent of cases (Colombo, 2007). Ascites is present in 10 percent (Young, 1984).

Juvenile granulosa cell tumors are grossly similar to the adult-type tumor and display variable solid and cystic components. They can attain significant size and have an average diameter of approximately 12 cm. Microscopically, cytologic features that distinguish these tumors from the adult type are their rounded, hyperchromatic nuclei without "coffee-bean"

grooves. Call-Exner bodies are rare, but often there is a theca cell component (Young, 1984).

Prognosis is excellent, and the 5-year survival rate is 95 percent. Similar to adult-type tumors, 95 percent of juvenile granulosa cell tumors are unilateral and stage I at diagnosis (Young, 1984). However, the juvenile type is more aggressive in advanced stages, and the time to relapse and death is much shorter. Recurrences typically develop within 3 years and are highly lethal. Later recurrences are unusual (Frausto, 2004).

Thecoma-Fibroma Group

Thecomas. These are relatively common SCSTs and are rarely malignant. Thecomas are unique because they typically develop in postmenopausal women in their mid-60s and develop infrequently before age 30. These solid tumors are among the most hormonally active of the SCSTs and usually produce excess estrogen. As a result, the primary signs and symptoms are abnormal vaginal bleeding or pelvic mass or both. Many women also present with concurrent endometrial hyperplasia or adenocarcinoma (Aboud, 1997). These tumors are composed of lipid-laden stromal cells that are occasionally luteinized. Half of these luteinized thecomas are either hormonally inactive or androgenic with the potential for inducing masculinization.

Thecomas are solid tumors whose cells resemble the theca cells that normally surround the ovarian follicles (Chen, 2003). Because of this texture, these tumors appear sonographically as solid adnexal masses and may mimic extrauterine leiomyomas.

Bilateral ovarian involvement and extraovarian spread are rare. Fortunately, ovarian thecomas are clinically benign, and surgical resection is curative.

Fibromas-Fibrosarcomas. Fibromas are also relatively common, hormonally inactive SCST variants that usually occur in perimenopausal and menopausal women (Chechia, 2008). These solid, generally benign ovarian neoplasms arise from the spindled stromal cells that form collagen. Most fibromas are found incidentally during pelvic or sonographic examination. They are round, oval, or lobulated solid tumors associated with free fluid or less commonly, with frank ascites and possess minimal to moderate vascularization (Paladini, 2009).

Perhaps 1 percent of women present with *Meigs syndrome,* which is a triad of pleural effusion, ascites, and a solid ovarian mass (Siddiqui, 1995). Pleural effusions are usually right-sided, and these, as well as accompanying ascites, are typically transudative and resolve after tumor resection (Majzlin, 1964). Despite this association of ascites with benign fibromas, when ascites and a pelvic mass coexist, evaluation is based on an assumption of malignancy.

The prognosis following excision of fibromas is that for any benign tumor. However, 10 percent will demonstrate increased cellularity and varying degrees of pleomorphism and mitotic activity that indicate a tumor better characterized as having low malignant potential. In 1 percent of cases, malignant transformation to fibrosarcoma is found.

Sclerosing Stromal Tumors. These tumors are rare and account for less than 5 percent of SCSTs. The average patient age is approximately 20 years, and 80 percent develop before age 30. Sclerosing stromal tumors are clinically benign and typically unilateral. Menstrual irregularities and pelvic pain are both frequent symptoms (Marelli, 1998). Ascites is seldom encountered (unlike fibromas), and sclerosing stromal tumors are hormonally inactive (unlike thecomas). Tumor size ranges from microscopic to 20 cm. Histologically, the presence of pseudolobulation of cellular areas separated by edematous connective tissue, increased vascularity, and prominent areas of sclerosis are distinguishing features.

Sertoli-Stromal Cell Tumors

Sertoli Cell Tumors. Ovarian Sertoli cell tumors are rare and account for less than 5 percent of all SCSTs. The mean patient age at diagnosis is 30 years, but ages range from 2 to 76 years. One quarter of patients present with estrogenic or androgenic manifestations, but most tumors are clinically nonfunctional.

Sertoli cell tumors are typically unilateral, solid, and yellow and measure 4 to 12 cm in diameter. Derived from the cell type that gives rise to the seminiferous tubules, these tumor cells often organize into histologically characteristic tubules (Young, 2005). Sertoli cell tumors, however, may also mimic many different tumors, and immunostaining in these cases is invaluable to confirm the diagnosis.

More than 80 percent are stage I at diagnosis, and most are clinically benign. Moderate cytologic atypia, brisk mitotic activity, and tumor cell necrosis are indicators of greater malignant potential and are found in 10 percent of individuals with stage I disease and most of those with stage II-IV tumors. The risk of recurrence is higher when these features are identified (Oliva, 2005).

Sertoli-Leydig Cell Tumors. Sertoli-Leydig cell tumors comprise only 5 to 10 percent of ovarian SCSTs (Zhang, 2007). Their incidence mirrors that of Sertoli cell tumors, and the average age is 25 years. Although Sertoli-Leydig cell tumors have been identified in children and postmenopausal females, more than 90 percent develop during the reproductive years.

These tumors frequently produce sex-steroid hormones, most commonly androgens. As a result, frank virilization develops in one third of affected women, and another 10 percent have clinical manifestations of androgen excess (Young, 1985). Menstrual disorders are also common. Accordingly, Sertoli-Leydig cell tumors are suspected preoperatively in a patient with a unilaterally palpable adnexal mass and with androgenic manifestations. For these women, an elevated serum testosterone-to-androstenedione ratio further suggests the diagnosis.

Although these hormonal effects frequently develop, one half of patients will have nonspecific abdominal mass symptoms as their only presenting complaint. Associated ascites is infrequent (Outwater, 2000). Thyroid abnormalities also coexist with Sertoli-Leydig cell tumors at a frequency that exceeds mere chance.

These tumors tend to be large at the time of excision with an average diameter greater than 10 cm, but ranges from 1 to 50 cm have been reported. In most cases, Sertoli-Leydig cell tumors appear yellow and lobulated. Tumors can be solid, partially cystic, or completely cystic, and they may or may not have polypoid or vesicular structures in their interior (Fig. 36-10).

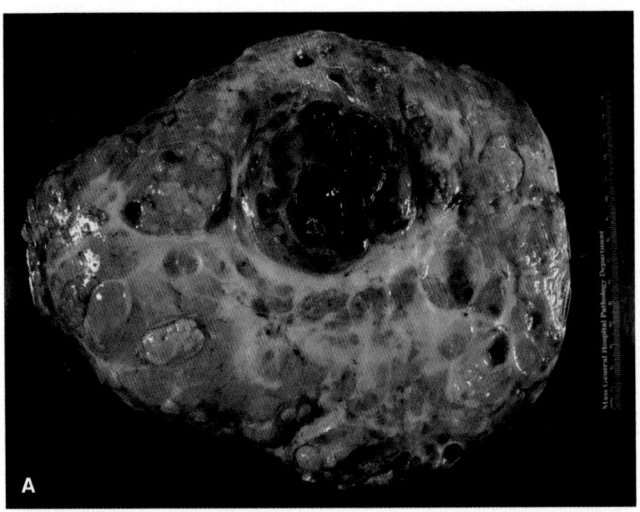

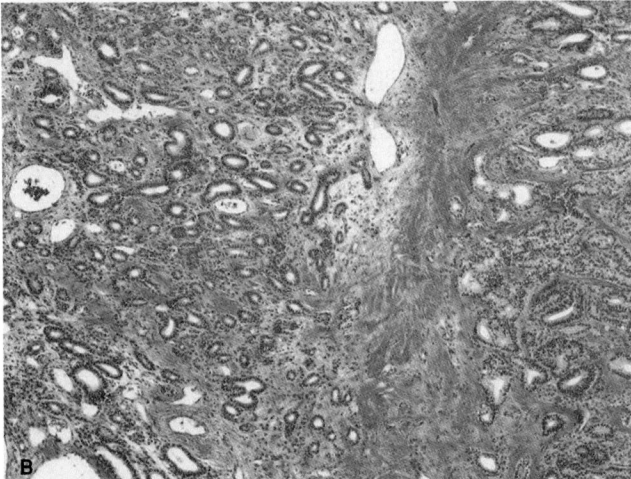

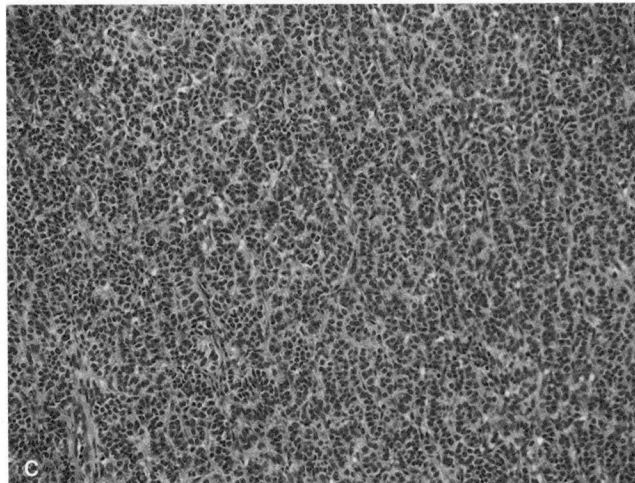

FIGURE 36-10 Sertoli-Leydig cell tumor (SLCT). **A.** SLCTs show variable gross features depending on the degree of differentiation and presence of heterologous elements. This opened surgical specimen has a predominantly solid cut surface with focal cysts, variegated yellow-brown color, and foci of hemorrhage. **B.** Well-differentiated SLCT composed of hollow tubules admixed with clusters of mature Leydig cells. **C.** This intermediate differentiated SLCT contains solid tubules, which are thought to resemble those of the fetal testis. (Used with permission from Dr. Katja Gwin.)

Microscopically, these morphologically diverse tumors contain cells resembling epithelial and stromal testicular cells in varying proportions. The five subtypes of differentiation (well, intermediate, poor, retiform, and heterologous) have considerable overlap. Well-differentiated tumors are all clinically benign (Chen, 2003; Young, 2005).

Overall, 15 to 20 percent of Sertoli-Leydig cell tumors are clinically malignant. Prognosis depends predominantly on the stage and degree of tumor differentiation in these malignant variants. For example, Young and Scully (1985) performed a clinicopathologic analysis of 207 cases and identified stage I disease in 97 percent. The 5-year survival rate for patients with stage I disease exceeds 90 percent (Zaloudek, 1984). Malignant features were observed in approximately 10 percent of tumors with intermediate differentiation and in 60 percent of poorly differentiated tumors. Retiform and heterologous elements are seen only in intermediate or poorly differentiated Sertoli-Leydig cell tumors and typically are associated with poorer prognosis. Overall, the 2 to 3 percent of patients with stage II-IV disease have a dismal prognosis (Young, 1985).

Sex Cord Tumors with Annular Tubules

This tumor accounts for 5 percent of SCSTs and is characterized by ring-shaped tubules and distinctive cellular elements that are histologically intermediate between Sertoli-cell and granulosa cell tumors. There are two clinically distinct types. One third are clinically benign and develop in patients with Peutz-Jeghers syndrome (PJS). These tumors are typically small, multifocal, calcified, bilateral, and diagnosed incidentally. Fifteen percent of PJS-associated cases will also develop adenoma malignum of the cervix, which is a rare, extremely well-differentiated adenocarcinoma. In contrast, two thirds of tumors are not associated with PJS. These masses are usually larger, unilateral, and symptomatic and carry a clinical malignancy rate of 15 to 20 percent (Young, 1982).

Steroid Cell Tumors

Fewer than 5 percent of SCSTs are steroid cell tumors. The average age at diagnosis is the mid-20s, but patients can present at virtually any age. These tumors are composed entirely or predominantly of cells that resemble steroid hormone-secreting cells and are categorized according to the histologic composition of these cells.

Stromal luteomas are clinically benign tumors that by definition lie completely within the ovarian stroma. They are usually seen in postmenopausal women. Estrogenic effects are common, but occasional individuals have androgenic manifestations.

Leydig cell tumors are also benign and typically are seen in postmenopausal women. They are distinguished microscopically by rectangular, crystal-like cytoplasmic inclusions, termed crystals of Reinke. Leydig cells secrete testosterone, and these tumors are usually associated with androgenic effects.

Steroid cell tumors not otherwise specified (NOS) are the most common subtype within this group and typically present in younger reproductive-aged women. Some of these cases may represent large stromal luteomas that have grown to reach the ovarian surface or Leydig-cell tumors in which Reinke crystals cannot be identified. These tumors are typically associated with androgen excess, but estrogen or cortisol overproduction (i.e., Cushing syndrome) has also been reported. One third of steroid cell tumors NOS are clinically malignant and have a dismal prognosis (Oliva, 2005).

Unclassified Sex Cord-Stromal Tumors

Unclassified tumors account for 5 percent of SCSTs and have no clearly predominant pattern of testicular (Sertoli cells) or ovarian (granulosa cells) differentiation. These ill-defined tumors are especially common during pregnancy due to alterations in their usual clinical and pathologic features (Young, 2005). They may be estrogenic, androgenic, or nonfunctional. The prognosis is similar to that of granulosa cell tumors and Sertoli-Leydig cell tumors of similar degrees of differentiation.

Gynandroblastomas

These are the rarest type of ovarian SCST. Patients present at a mean age of 30 years and typically have menstrual irregularities or evidence of hormonal excess. The tumors are characterized by intermingled granulosa cells and tubules of Sertoli cells. Theca or Leydig cells or both may also be present in varying degrees. Gynandroblastomas have low malignant potential, and only one death has been reported (Martin-Jimenez, 1994).

■ Treatment
Surgery

The mainstay of treatment for patients with an ovarian SCST is complete surgical resection. This group shows relative insensitivity to adjuvant chemotherapy or radiation. Thus, operative goals are to establish a definitive tissue diagnosis, determine the extent of disease, and also remove all grossly visible tumors in those infrequent patients with advanced-stage disease. Moreover, during preoperative planning, clinicians should consider the patient's age and desire for future fertility. Hysterectomy with BSO is performed for those who have completed childbearing, whereas fertility-sparing USO with preservation of the uterus and remaining ovary may be appropriate in the absence of obvious disease spread to these organs (Zanagnolo, 2004). Endometrial sampling is performed, especially if fertility-sparing surgery is planned in women with granulosa cell tumors or thecomas. This is because many of these patients will have coexisting endometrial hyperplasia or adenocarcinoma that may affect the decision for hysterectomy.

Minimally invasive laparoscopic surgery has a variety of relevant applications. For some, the diagnosis of SCST may not be discovered until the mass is laparoscopically removed and sent for frozen section analysis. Laparoscopic surgical staging can then proceed. When the diagnosis is not made until the final pathology report is confirmed postoperatively, laparoscopic staging may be proposed to determine whether metastatic disease is present. This can reduce the morbidity of a second operation (Shim, 2013).

Surgical staging is essential to determine the extent of disease and the need for adjuvant therapy in most individuals with potentially malignant SCST subtypes (Fig. 36-11). That said, only approximately 20 percent of cases have complete staging (Abu-Rustum, 2006; Brown, 2009). More recent data suggest

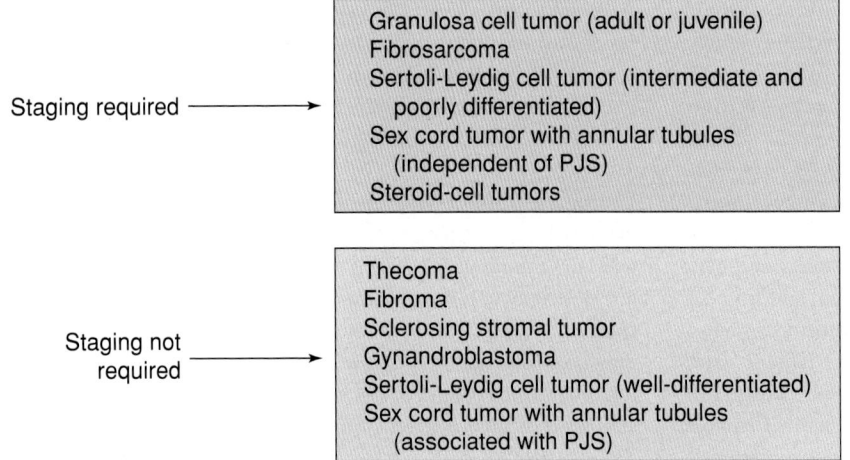

Staging required ———→
- Granulosa cell tumor (adult or juvenile)
- Fibrosarcoma
- Sertoli-Leydig cell tumor (intermediate and poorly differentiated)
- Sex cord tumor with annular tubules (independent of PJS)
- Steroid-cell tumors

Staging not required ———→
- Thecoma
- Fibroma
- Sclerosing stromal tumor
- Gynandroblastoma
- Sertoli-Leydig cell tumor (well-differentiated)
- Sex cord tumor with annular tubules (associated with PJS)

FIGURE 36-11 Staging of sex cord-stromal tumors. PJS = Peutz-Jeghers syndrome.

that, due to surface and hematogenous routes of spread, the standard ovarian cancer procedure can be modified. Pelvic washings, exploration of the abdomen, peritoneal biopsies, and partial omentectomy remain important. However, the utility of routine pelvic and paraaortic lymphadenectomy has been increasingly challenged. In a study of 262 ovarian SCSTs, none of the 58 patients undergoing nodal dissection had positive nodes (Brown, 2009). Additionally, performing a lymphadenectomy has not been shown to improve survival rates in those with SCSTs (Chan, 2007).

Surgical removal of hormone-producing SCSTs results in an immediate drop in elevated preoperative sex-steroid hormone levels. Physical manifestations of these elevated levels, however, partially or completely resolve more gradually.

Surveillance

In general, women with stage I ovarian SCSTs have an excellent prognosis following surgery alone and usually can be followed at regular intervals without the need for further treatment (Schneider, 2003a). Surveillance includes a general physical and pelvic examination, serum marker level testing, and imaging as clinically indicated.

Chemotherapy

The decision to administer postoperative therapy depends on various factors (Fig. 36-12). Although typically treated solely with surgery, malignant stage I ovarian SCSTs may require adjuvant chemotherapy when large tumor size, high mitotic index, capsular excrescences, tumor rupture, incomplete staging, or equivocal pathology results are noted. Women with one or more of these suspicious features are thought to be at higher risk of relapse and are considered for platinum-based chemotherapy (Schneider, 2003b). In addition,

stage II-IV disease warrants postoperative treatment. In general, SCSTs display less sensitivity to chemotherapy than other ovarian malignancies, but most women at high risk for disease progression can be treated successfully with adjuvant platinum-based chemotherapy (van Meurs, 2014).

The 5-day bleomycin, etoposide, and cisplatin (BEP) regimen is the most widely used first-line chemotherapy combination (Gershenson, 1996; Homesley, 1999). For completely resected disease, three courses given every 3 weeks are sufficient. Four cycles are recommended for patients with incompletely resected tumor (Homesley, 1999). In addition to BEP, taxanes have demonstrated activity against ovarian SCSTs, and combination paclitaxel and carboplatin chemotherapy shows promising results (Brown, 2004, 2005). To determine the most effective regimen, a prospective randomized study is currently underway, comparing paclitaxel and carboplatin to BEP in those with newly diagnosed ovarian SCSTs (GOG protocol #264). Unfortunately, the relative scarcity of women who have ovarian SCST and receive chemotherapy limits the ability to conduct large randomized studies.

Radiation

Postoperative radiation therapy currently has a limited role in the management of ovarian SCSTs. There is some evidence indicating a prolonged survival in at least some women with newly diagnosed disease who received whole-abdominal radiotherapy (Wolf, 1999). However, chemotherapy is usually the

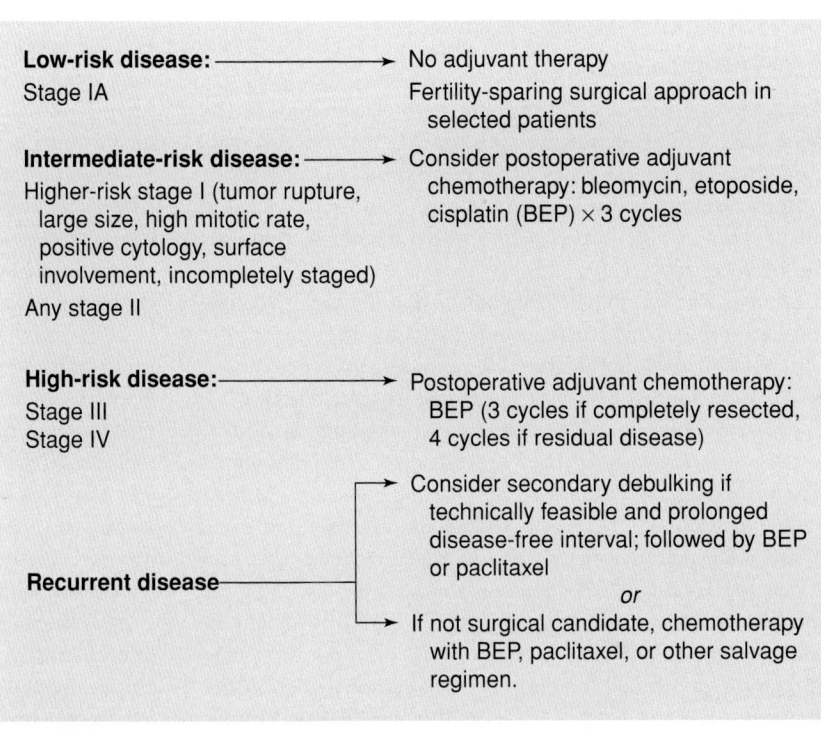

Low-risk disease: ———→ No adjuvant therapy
Stage IA   Fertility-sparing surgical approach in selected patients

Intermediate-risk disease: ———→ Consider postoperative adjuvant chemotherapy: bleomycin, etoposide, cisplatin (BEP) × 3 cycles
Higher-risk stage I (tumor rupture, large size, high mitotic rate, positive cytology, surface involvement, incompletely staged)
Any stage II

High-risk disease: ———→ Postoperative adjuvant chemotherapy: BEP (3 cycles if completely resected, 4 cycles if residual disease)
Stage III
Stage IV

Recurrent disease ———→ Consider secondary debulking if technically feasible and prolonged disease-free interval; followed by BEP or paclitaxel
or
If not surgical candidate, chemotherapy with BEP, paclitaxel, or other salvage regimen.

FIGURE 36-12 Postoperative treatment of sex cord-stromal tumors.

primary postoperative treatment because it is generally better tolerated, more widely accessible, and easier to administer. Radiation is best reserved for palliation of local symptoms (Dubuc-Lissoir, 2001).

Relapse

The management of recurrent ovarian SCST depends on the clinical circumstances. Secondary surgical debulking is strongly considered due to the indolent growth pattern, the typically long disease-free interval after initial treatment, and the inherent insensitivity to chemotherapy (Crew, 2005; Powell, 2001). Platinum-based combination chemotherapy is the primary treatment chosen for recurrent disease with or without surgical debulking (Uygun, 2003). Of regimens, BEP is most frequently administered because it has the highest known response rate (Homesley, 1999). Paclitaxel is another promising agent that was evaluated as a single agent in a phase II Gynecologic Oncology Group trial (GOG protocol #187).

There is no standard treatment for women who have progressive disease despite aggressive surgery and platinum-based chemotherapy. Bevacizumab (Avastin) demonstrated a 17-percent response rate in a Phase II trial (GOG protocol #251) (Brown, 2014a). Vincristine, actinomycin D, and cyclophosphamide (VAC) regimen has limited activity (Ayhan, 1996; Zanagnolo, 2004). Hormonal therapy is minimally toxic, but the clinical experience with this approach is extremely limited (Hardy, 2005). Medroxyprogesterone acetate and the gonadotropin-releasing hormone (GnRH) agonist leuprolide acetate (Lupron) have each demonstrated activity in halting the growth of recurrent ovarian SCSTs (Fishman, 1996; Homesley, 1999). GnRH antagonists, however, may not be as effective (Ameryckx, 2005).

In addition to traditional drugs, discovery of the *FOXL2* 402C>G mutation occurring exclusively in all adult granulosa cell tumors may lead to the development of targeted therapies for women with advanced or recurrent disease. Currently, FOXL2 as a transcription factor does not represent a pharmacologic target. Further insights into its function and downstream effects may identify molecular alterations in these tumors that can be targeted (Kobel, 2009).

■ Prognosis

In general, ovarian SCSTs portend a much better prognosis than epithelial ovarian carcinomas chiefly because most women with SCSTs are diagnosed with stage I disease. Stage II-IV tumors are rare, but women with these cancers have a poor prognosis similar to their counterparts with epithelial disease. Unfortunately, improvements in survival rates have not been observed in ovarian SCSTs during the past few decades (Chan, 2006).

Of the clinical factors affecting prognosis, surgical stage and residual disease are the most important (Lee, 2008; Zanagnolo, 2004). Further, in a Surveillance, Epidemiology and End Results (SEER) database study, Zhang and colleagues (2007) performed a multivariate analysis of 376 women with SCSTs. They concluded that age younger than 50 years was also an independent predictor of an improved survival rate.

■ Management During Pregnancy

Ovarian SCSTs are rarely detected during pregnancy (Okada, 2004). In a California population-based study of more than 4 million obstetric patients, one granulosa cell tumor was diagnosed among 202 women with an ovarian malignancy (Leiserowitz, 2006). Granulosa cell tumors are most common, but only 10 percent are diagnosed during pregnancy (Hasiakos, 2006). One third of pregnant women with SCSTs are incidentally diagnosed at cesarean delivery, one third has abdominal pain or swelling, and the remainder may present with hemoperitoneum, virilization, or vaginal bleeding (Young, 1984). Surgical management should be the same as for the nonpregnant woman. For most, conservative management with USO and staging is the primary procedure, but hysterectomy and BSO may be indicated in selected circumstances (Young, 1984). Postoperative chemotherapy is typically withheld until after delivery because SCSTs have an indolent growth pattern.

REFERENCES

Aboud E: A review of granulosa cell tumours and thecomas of the ovary. Arch Gynecol Obstet 259:161, 1997

Abu-Rustum NR, Restivo A, Ivy J, et al: Retroperitoneal nodal metastasis in primary and recurrent granulosa cell tumors of the ovary. Gynecol Oncol 103:31, 2006

Al Badawi IA, Brasher PM, Ghatage P, et al: Postoperative chemotherapy in advanced ovarian granulosa cell tumors. Int J Gynecol Cancer 12:119, 2002

Ameryckx L, Fatemi HM, De Sutter P, et al: GnRH antagonist in the adjuvant treatment of a recurrent ovarian granulosa cell tumor: a case report. Gynecol Oncol 99:764, 2005

Aoki Y, Kase H, Fujita K, et al: Dysgerminoma with a slightly elevated alpha-fetoprotein level diagnosed as a mixed germ cell tumor after recurrence. Gynecol Obstet Invest 55:58, 2003

Ayhan A, Tuncer ZS, Hakverdi AU, et al: Sertoli–Leydig cell tumor of the ovary: a clinicopathologic study of 10 cases. Eur J Gynaecol Oncol 17:75, 1996

Bafna UD, Umadevi K, Kumaran C, et al: Germ cell tumors of the ovary: is there a role for aggressive cytoreductive surgery for nondysgerminomatous tumors? Int J Gynecol Cancer 11:300, 2001

Beiner ME, Gotlieb WH, Korach Y, et al: Cystectomy for immature teratoma of the ovary. Gynecol Oncol 93:381, 2004

Billmire D, Vinocur C, Rescorla F, et al: Outcome and staging evaluation in malignant germ cell tumors of the ovary in children and adolescents: an intergroup study. J Pediatr Surg 39:424, 2004

Billmire DF, Cullen JW, Rescorla FJ, et al: Surveillance after initial surgery for pediatric and adolescent girls with stage I ovarian germ cell tumors: report from the Children's Oncology Group. J Clin Oncol 32(5):465, 2014

Bonazzi C, Peccatori F, Colombo N, et al: Pure ovarian immature teratoma, a unique and curable disease: 10 years' experience of 32 prospectively treated patients. Obstet Gynecol 84:598, 1994

Boyce EA, Costaggini I, Vitonis A, et al: The epidemiology of ovarian granulosa cell tumors: a case-control study. Gynecol Oncol 115:221, 2009

Brewer M, Gershenson DM, Herzog CE, et al: Outcome and reproductive function after chemotherapy for ovarian dysgerminoma. J Clin Oncol 17:2670, 1999

Brown J, Brady WE, Schink J, et al: Efficacy and safety of bevacizumab in recurrent sex cord-stromal ovarian tumors: results of a phase 2 trial of the Gynecologic Oncology Group. Cancer 120(3):344, 2014a

Brown J, Friedlander M, Backes FJ, et al: Gynecologic Cancer Intergroup (GCIG) consensus review for ovarian germ cell tumors. Int J Gynecol Cancer 24(9 Suppl 3):S48, 2014b

Brown J, Shvartsman HS, Deavers MT, et al: The activity of taxanes compared with bleomycin, etoposide, and cisplatin in the treatment of sex cord-stromal ovarian tumors. Gynecol Oncol 97:489, 2005

Brown J, Shvartsman HS, Deavers MT, et al: The activity of taxanes in the treatment of sex cord-stromal ovarian tumors. J Clin Oncol 22:3517, 2004

Brown J, Sood AK, Deavers MT, et al: Patterns of metastasis in sex cord-stromal tumors of the ovary: can routine staging lymphadenectomy be omitted? Gynecol Oncol 113:86, 2009

Carmina E, Rosato F, Janni A, et al: Extensive clinical experience: relative prevalence of different androgen excess disorders in 950 women referred because of clinical hyperandrogenism. J Clin Endocrinol Metab 91:2, 2006

Cass DL, Hawkins E, Brandt ML, et al: Surgery for ovarian masses in infants, children, and adolescents: 102 consecutive patients treated in a 15-year period. J Pediatr Surg 36:693, 2001

Cathro HP, Stoler MH: The utility of calretinin, inhibin, and WT1 immunohistochemical staining in the differential diagnosis of ovarian tumors. Hum Pathol 36:195, 2005

Chan JK, Cheung MK, Husain A, et al: Patterns and progress in ovarian cancer over 14 years. Obstet Gynecol 108:521, 2006

Chan JK, Munro EG, Cheung MK, et al: Association of lymphadenectomy and survival in stage I ovarian cancer patients. Obstet Gynecol 109:12, 2007

Chan JK, Tewari KS, Waller S, et al: The influence of conservative surgical practices for malignant ovarian germ cell tumors. J Surg Oncol 98:111, 2008

Chan JK, Zhang M, Kaleb V, et al: Prognostic factors responsible for survival in sex cord stromal tumors of the ovary: a multivariate analysis. Gynecol Oncol 96:204, 2005

Chechia A, Attia L, Temime RB, et al: Incidence, clinical analysis, and management of ovarian fibromas and fibrothecomas. Am J Obstet Gynecol 199:473e1, 2008

Chen CA, Lin H, Weng CS, et al: Outcome of 3-day bleomycin, etoposide and cisplatin chemotherapeutic regimen for patients with malignant ovarian germ cell tumours: a Taiwanese Gynecologic Oncology Group study. Eur J Cancer 50(18):3161, 2014

Chen VW, Ruiz B, Killeen JL, et al: Pathology and classification of ovarian tumors. Cancer 97:2631, 2003

Cheng L, Thomas A, Roth LM, et al: OCT4: a novel biomarker for dysgerminoma of the ovary. Am J Surg Pathol 28:1341, 2004

Cicin I, Saip P, Guney N, et al: Yolk sac tumours of the ovary: evaluation of clinicopathological features and prognostic factors. Eur J Obstet Gynecol Reprod Biol 146:210, 2009

Colombo N, Parma G, Zanagnolo V, et al: Management of ovarian stromal cell tumors. J Clin Oncol 25:2944, 2007

Corakci A, Ozeren S, Ozkan S, et al: Pure nongestational choriocarcinoma of ovary. Arch Gynecol Obstet 271:176, 2005

Crew KD, Cohen MH, Smith DH, et al: Long natural history of recurrent granulosa cell tumor of the ovary 23 years after initial diagnosis: a case report and review of the literature. Gynecol Oncol 96:235, 2005

Culine S, Lhomme C, Michel G, et al: Is there a role for second-look laparotomy in the management of malignant germ cell tumors of the ovary? Experience at Institut Gustave Roussy. J Surg Oncol 62:40, 1996

Curtin JP, Morrow CP, D'Ablaing G, et al: Malignant germ cell tumors of the ovary: 20-year report of LAC-USC Women's Hospital. Int J Gynecol Cancer 4:29, 1994

Cushing B, Giller R, Ablin A, et al: Surgical resection alone is effective treatment for ovarian immature teratoma in children and adolescents: a report of the Pediatric Oncology Group and the Children's Cancer Group. Am J Obstet Gynecol 181:353, 1999

Dark GG, Bower M, Newlands ES, et al: Surveillance policy for stage I ovarian germ cell tumors. J Clin Oncol 15:620, 1997

Dimopoulos MA, Papadimitriou C, Hamilos G, et al: Treatment of ovarian germ cell tumors with a 3-day bleomycin, etoposide, and cisplatin regimen: a prospective multicenter study. Gynecol Oncol 95:695, 2004

Dos Santos L, Mok E, Iasonos A, et al: Squamous cell carcinoma arising in mature cystic teratoma of the ovary: a case series and review of the literature. Gynecol Oncol 105:321, 2007

Dubuc-Lissoir J, Berthiaume MJ, Boubez G, et al: Bone metastasis from a granulosa cell tumor of the ovary. Gynecol Oncol 83:400, 2001

East N, Alobaid A, Goffin F, et al: Granulosa cell tumour: a recurrence 40 years after initial diagnosis. J Obstet Gynaecol Can 27:363, 2005

Elit L, Bocking A, Kenyon C, et al: An endodermal sinus tumor diagnosed in pregnancy: case report and review of the literature. Gynecol Oncol 72:123, 1999

Fishman A, Kudelka AP, Tresukosol D, et al: Leuprolide acetate for treating refractory or persistent ovarian granulosa cell tumor. J Reprod Med 41:393, 1996

Frausto SD, Geisler JP, Fletcher MS, et al: Late recurrence of juvenile granulosa cell tumor of the ovary. Am J Obstet Gynecol 1:366, 2004

Gainford MC, Tinker A, Carter J, et al: Malignant transformation within ovarian dermoid cysts: an audit of treatment received and patient outcomes. An Australia New Zealand Gynaecological Oncology Group (ANZGOG) and Gynaecologic Cancer Intergroup (GCIG) study. Int J Gynecol Cancer 20:75, 2010

Galani E, Alamanis C, Dimopoulos MA: Familial female and male germ cell cancer: a new syndrome? Gynecol Oncol 96:254, 2005

Geisler JP, Goulet R, Foster RS, et al: Growing teratoma syndrome after chemotherapy for germ cell tumors of the ovary. Obstet Gynecol 84:719, 1994

Gershenson DM: Management of ovarian germ cell tumors. J Clin Oncol 25:2938, 2007a

Gershenson DM, Copeland LJ, Kavanagh JJ, et al: Treatment of malignant nondysgerminomatous germ cell tumors of the ovary with vincristine, dactinomycin, and cyclophosphamide. Cancer 56:2756, 1985

Gershenson DM, Miller AM, Champion VL, et al: Reproductive and sexual function after platinum-based chemotherapy in long-term ovarian germ cell tumor survivors: a Gynecologic Oncology Group study. J Clin Oncol 25:2792, 2007b

Gershenson DM, Morris M, Burke TW, et al: Treatment of poor-prognosis sex cord–stromal tumors of the ovary with the combination of bleomycin, etoposide, and cisplatin. Obstet Gynecol 87:527, 1996

Gershenson DM, Morris M, Cangir A, et al: Treatment of malignant germ cell tumors of the ovary with bleomycin, etoposide, and cisplatin. J Clin Oncol 8:715, 1990

Hardy RD, Bell JG, Nicely CJ, et al: Hormonal treatment of a recurrent granulosa cell tumor of the ovary: case report and review of the literature. Gynecol Oncol 96:865, 2005

Hasiakos D, Papakonstantinou K, Goula K, et al: Juvenile granulosa cell tumor associated with pregnancy: report of a case and review of the literature. Gynecol Oncol 100(2):426, 2006

Heravi-Moussavi A, Anglesio MS, Cheng SW, et al: Recurrent somatic DICER1 mutations in nonepithelial ovarian cancers. N Engl J Med 366(3):234, 2012

Hinton S, Catalano P, Einhorn LH, et al: Phase II study of paclitaxel plus gemcitabine in refractory germ cell tumors (E9897): a trial of the Eastern Cooperative Oncology Group. J Clin Oncol 20:1859, 2002

Hoepffner W, Horn LC, Simon E, et al: Gonadoblastomas in 5 patients with 46,XY gonadal dysgenesis. Exp Clin Endocrinol Diabetes 113:231, 2005

Homesley HD, Bundy BN, Hurteau JA, et al: Bleomycin, etoposide, and cisplatin combination therapy of ovarian granulosa cell tumors and other stromal malignancies: a Gynecologic Oncology Group study. Gynecol Oncol 72:131, 1999

Horbelt D, Delmore J, Meisel R, et al: Mixed germ cell malignancy of the ovary concurrent with pregnancy. Obstet Gynecol 84:662, 1994

Hsu YJ, Pai L, Chen YC, et al: Extragonadal germ cell tumors in Taiwan: an analysis of treatment results of 59 patients. Cancer 95:766, 2002

Jung SE, Rha SE, Lee JM, et al: CT and MRI findings of sex cord–stromal tumor of the ovary. AJR 185:207, 2005

Kalfa N, Patte C, Orbach D, et al: A nationwide study of granulosa cell tumors in pre- and postpubertal girls: missed diagnosis of endocrine manifestations worsens prognosis. J Pediatr Endocrinol Metab 18:25, 2005

Kim SH, Kang SB: Ovarian dysgerminoma: color Doppler ultrasonographic findings and comparison with CT and MR imaging findings. J Ultrasound Med 14:843, 1995

Kleppe M, Amkreutz LC, Van Gorp T, et al: Lymph-node metastasis in stage I and II sex cord stromal and malignant germ cell tumours of the ovary: a systematic review. Gynecol Oncol 133(1):124, 2014

Kobel M, Gilks CB, Huntsman DG: Adult-type granulosa cell tumors and FOXL2 mutation. Cancer Res 69:9160, 2009

Kollmannsberger C, Nichols C, Bokemeyer C: Recent advances in management of patients with platinum-refractory testicular germ cell tumors. Cancer 106(6):1217, 2006

Kumar S, Shah JP, Bryant CS, et al: The prevalence and prognostic impact of lymph node metastasis in malignant germ cell tumors of the ovary. Gynecol Oncol 110:125, 2008

Kurihara S, Hirakawa T, Amada S, et al: Inhibin-producing ovarian granulosa cell tumor as a cause of secondary amenorrhea: case report and review of the literature. J Obstet Gynaecol Res 30:439, 2004

Kurman RJ, Carcangiu ML, Herrington CS, et al (eds): WHO Classification of Tumours of Female Reproductive Organs, 4th ed. Lyon, International Agency for Research on Cancer, 2014

Kusamura S, Teixeira LC, dos Santos MA, et al: Ovarian germ cell cancer: clinicopathologic analysis and outcome of 31 cases. Tumori 86:450, 2000

LaPolla JP, Fiorica JV, Turnquist D, et al: Successful therapy of metastatic embryonal carcinoma coexisting with gonadoblastoma in a patient with 46,XY pure gonadal dysgenesis (Swyer's syndrome). Gynecol Oncol 37:417, 1990

Leblanc E, Querleu D, Narducci F, et al: Laparoscopic restaging of early stage invasive adnexal tumors: a 10-year experience. Gynecol Oncol 94:624, 2004

Lee KH, Lee IH, Kim BG, et al: Clinicopathologic characteristics of malignant germ cell tumors in the ovaries of Korean women: a Korean Gynecologic Oncology Group Study. Int J Gynecol Cancer 19:84, 2009

Lee YK, Park NH, Kim JW, et al: Characteristics of recurrence in adult-type granulosa cell tumor. Int J Gynecol Cancer 18:642, 2008

Leiserowitz GS, Xing G, Cress R, et al: Adnexal masses in pregnancy: how often are they malignant? Gynecol Oncol 101(2):315, 2006

Li H, Hong W, Zhang R, et al: Retrospective analysis of 67 consecutive cases of pure ovarian immature teratoma. Chin Med J (Engl) 115:1496, 2002

Li J, Yang W, Wu X: Prognostic factors and role of salvage surgery in chemorefractory ovarian germ cell malignancies: a study in Chinese patients. Gynecol Oncol 105:769, 2007

Liu Q, Ding X, Yang J, et al: The significance of comprehensive staging surgery in malignant ovarian germ cell tumors. Gynecol Oncol 131(3):551, 2013

Low JJ, Perrin LC, Crandon AJ, et al: Conservative surgery to preserve ovarian function in patients with malignant ovarian germ cell tumors: a review of 74 cases. Cancer 89:391, 2000

Majzlin G, Stevens FL: Meigs' syndrome. Case report and review of literature. J Int Coll Surg 42:625, 1964

Malmstrom H, Hogberg T, Risberg B, et al: Granulosa cell tumors of the ovary: prognostic factors and outcome. Gynecol Oncol 52:50, 1994

Marelli G, Carinelli S, Mariani A, et al: Sclerosing stromal tumor of the ovary: report of eight cases and review of the literature. Eur J Obstet Gynecol Reprod Biol 76:85, 1998

Marina NM, Cushing B, Giller R, et al: Complete surgical excision is effective treatment for children with immature teratomas with or without malignant elements: a Pediatric Oncology Group/Children's Cancer Group Intergroup study. J Clin Oncol 17:2137, 1999

Martin-Jimenez A, Condom-Munro E, Valls-Porcel M, et al: [Gynandroblastoma of the ovary: review of the literature.] French. J Gynecol Obstet Biol Reprod (Paris) 23:391, 1994

McKenna M, Kenny B, Dorman G, et al: Combined adult granulosa cell tumor and mucinous cystadenoma of the ovary: granulosa cell tumor with heterologous mucinous elements. Int J Gynecol Pathol 24:224, 2005

Messing MJ, Gershenson DM, Morris M, et al: Primary treatment failure in patients with malignant ovarian germ cell neoplasms. Int J Gynecol Cancer 2:295, 1992

Miller BE, Barron BA, Dockter ME, et al: Parameters of differentiation and proliferation in adult granulosa cell tumors of the ovary. Cancer Detect Prev 25:48, 2001

Miller BE, Barron BA, Wan JY, et al: Prognostic factors in adult granulosa cell tumor of the ovary. Cancer 79:1951, 1997

Mom CH, Engelen MJ, Willemse PH, et al: Granulosa cell tumors of the ovary: the clinical value of serum inhibin A and B levels in a large single center cohort. Gynecol Oncol 105:365, 2007

Montz FJ, Horenstein J, Platt LD: The diagnosis of immature teratoma by maternal serum alpha-fetoprotein screening. Obstet Gynecol 73:522, 1989

Morimura Y, Nishiyama H, Yanagida K, et al: Dysgerminoma with syncytiotrophoblastic giant cells arising from 46,XX pure gonadal dysgenesis. Obstet Gynecol 92:654, 1998

Munkarah A, Gershenson DM, Levenback C, et al: Salvage surgery for chemorefractory ovarian germ cell tumors. Gynecol Oncol 55:217, 1994

Murugaesu N, Schmid P, Dancey G, et al: Malignant ovarian germ cell tumors: identification of novel prognostic markers and long-term outcome after multimodality treatment. J Clin Oncol 24:4862, 2006

Nawa A, Obata N, Kikkawa F, et al: Prognostic factors of patients with yolk sac tumors of the ovary. Am J Obstet Gynecol 184:1182, 2001

O'Connor DM, Norris HJ: The influence of grade on the outcome of stage I ovarian immature (malignant) teratomas and the reproducibility of grading. Int J Gynecol Pathol 13:283, 1994

Okada I, Nakagawa S, Takemura Y, et al: Ovarian thecoma associated in the first trimester of pregnancy. J Obstet Gynaecol Res 30:368, 2004

Oliva E, Alvarez T, Young RH: Sertoli cell tumors of the ovary: a clinicopathologic and immunohistochemical study of 54 cases. Am J Surg Pathol 29:143, 2005

Oliva E, Andrada E, Pezzica E, et al: Ovarian carcinomas with choriocarcinomatous differentiation. Cancer 72:2441, 1993

Outwater EK, Marchetto B, Wagner BJ: Virilizing tumors of the ovary: imaging features. Ultrasound Obstet Gynecol 15:365, 2000

Paladini D, Testa A, Van Holsbeke C, et al: Imaging in gynecological disease (5): clinical and ultrasound characteristics in fibroma and fibrothecoma of the ovary. Ultrasound Obstet Gynecol 34:188, 2009

Palenzuela G, Martin E, Meunier A, et al: Comprehensive staging allows for excellent outcome in patients with localized malignant germ cell tumor of the ovary. Ann Surg 248:836, 2008

Pavlakis K, Messini I, Vrekoussis T, et al: Intraoperative assessment of epithelial and non-epithelial ovarian tumors: a 7-year review. Eur J Gynaecol Oncol 30:657, 2009

Pena-Alonso R, Nieto K, Alvarez R, et al: Distribution of Y-chromosome-bearing cells in gonadoblastoma and dysgenetic testis in 45,X/46,XY infants. Mod Pathol 18:439, 2005

Pins MR, Young RH, Daly WJ, et al: Primary squamous cell carcinoma of the ovary: report of 37 cases. Am J Surg Pathol 20:823, 1996

Piura B, Nemet D, Yanai-Inbar I, et al: Granulosa cell tumor of the ovary: a study of 18 cases. J Surg Oncol 55:71, 1994

Powell JL, Connor GP, Henderson GS: Management of recurrent juvenile granulosa cell tumor of the ovary. Gynecol Oncol 81:113, 2001

Pressley RH, Muntz HG, Falkenberry S, et al: Serum lactic dehydrogenase as a tumor marker in dysgerminoma. Gynecol Oncol 44:281, 1992

Quirk JT, Natarajan N: Ovarian cancer incidence in the United States, 1992–1999. Gynecol Oncol 97:519, 2005

Ramalingam P, Malpica A, Silva EG, et al: The use of cytokeratin 7 and EMA in differentiating ovarian yolk sac tumors from endometrioid and clear cell carcinomas. Am J Surg Pathol 28:1499, 2004

Ray-Coquard I, Brown J, Harter P, Gynecologic Cancer InterGroup (GCIG) consensus review for ovarian sex cord stromal tumors. Int J Gynecol Cancer 24(9 Suppl 3):S42, 2014

Rezk Y, Sheinfeld J, Chi DS: Prolonged survival following salvage surgery for chemorefractory ovarian immature teratoma: a case report and review of the literature. Gynecol Oncol 96:883, 2005

Schneider DT, Calaminus G, Harms D, et al: Ovarian sex cord–stromal tumors in children and adolescents. J Reprod Med 50:439, 2005

Schneider DT, Calaminus G, Wessalowski R, et al: Ovarian sex cord–stromal tumors in children and adolescents. J Clin Oncol 21:2357, 2003a

Schneider DT, Janig U, Calaminus G, et al: Ovarian sex cord–stromal tumors: a clinicopathological study of 72 cases from the Kiel Pediatric Tumor Registry. Virchows Arch 443:549, 2003b

Schrader KA, Gorbatcheva B, Senz J, et al: The specificity of the FLXL2 c.402G>G somatic mutation: a survey of solid tumors. PLoS One 4(11): e7988, 2009

Schwartz PE, Morris JM: Serum lactic dehydrogenase: a tumor marker for dysgerminoma. Obstet Gynecol 72:511, 1988

Sehouli J, Drescher FS, Mustea A, et al: Granulosa cell tumor of the ovary: 10 years follow-up data of 65 patients. Anticancer Res 24:1223, 2004

Shah SP, Kobel M, Senz J, et al: Mutation of FOXL2 in granulosa-cell tumors of the ovary. N Engl J Med 360:2719, 2009

Sharony R, Aviram R, Fishman A, et al: Granulosa cell tumors of the ovary: do they have any unique ultrasonographic and color Doppler flow features? Int J Gynecol Cancer 11:229, 2001

Shim SH, Kim DY, Lee SW, et al: Laparoscopic management of early-stage malignant nonepithelial ovarian tumors: surgical and survival outcomes. Int J Gynecol Cancer 23(2):249, 2013

Shimizu Y, Komiyama S, Kobayashi T, et al: Successful management of endodermal sinus tumor of the ovary associated with pregnancy. Gynecol Oncol 88:447, 2003

Siddiqui M, Toub DB: Cellular fibroma of the ovary with Meigs' syndrome and elevated CA-125: a case report. J Reprod Med 40:817, 1995

Smith HO, Berwick M, Verschraegen CF, et al: Incidence and survival rates for female malignant germ cell tumors. Obstet Gynecol 107:1075, 2006

Solheim O, Gershenson DM, Tropé CG, Prognostic factors in malignant ovarian germ cell tumors (The Surveillance, Epidemiology and End Results experience 1978–2010). Eur J Cancer 50(11):1942, 2014

Solheim O, Kaern J, Tropé CG, et al: Malignant ovarian germ cell tumors: presentation, survival and second cancer in a population based Norwegian cohort (1953–2009). Gynecol Oncol 131(2):330, 2013

Solheim O, Tropé CG, Rokkones E, et al: Fertility and gonadal function after adjuvant therapy in women diagnosed with a malignant ovarian germ cell tumor (MOGCT) during the "cisplatin era." Gynecol Oncol 136(2):224, 2015

Stettner AR, Hartenbach EM, Schink JC, et al: Familial ovarian germ cell cancer: report and review. Am J Med Genet 84:43, 1999

Stevens TA, Brown J, Zander DS, et al: Adult granulosa cell tumors of the ovary in two first-degree relatives. Gynecol Oncol 98:502, 2005

Stier EA, Barakat RR, Curtin JP, et al: Laparotomy to complete staging of presumed early ovarian cancer. Obstet Gynecol 87:737, 1996

Suita S, Shono K, Tajiri T, et al: Malignant germ cell tumors: clinical characteristics, treatment, and outcome. A report from the study group for Pediatric Solid Malignant Tumors in the Kyushu Area, Japan. J Pediatr Surg 37:1703, 2002

Takemori M, Nishimura R, Yamasaki M, et al: Ovarian mixed germ cell tumor composed of polyembryoma and immature teratoma. Gynecol Oncol 69:260, 1998

Talukdar S, Kumar S, Bhatla N, et al: Neo-adjuvant chemotherapy in the treatment of advanced malignant germ cell tumors of ovary. Gynecol Oncol 132(1):28, 2014

Tangir J, Zelterman D, Ma W, et al: Reproductive function after conservative surgery and chemotherapy for malignant germ cell tumors of the ovary. Obstet Gynecol 101:251, 2003

Teilum G: Classification of endodermal sinus tumour (mesoblastoma vitellinum) and so-called "embryonal carcinoma" of the ovary. Acta Pathol Microbiol Scand 64:407, 1965

Tewari K, Cappuccini F, DiSaia PJ, et al: Malignant germ cell tumors of the ovary. Obstet Gynecol 95:128, 2000

Ulbright TM: Germ cell tumors of the gonads: a selective review emphasizing problems in differential diagnosis, newly appreciated, and controversial issues. Mod Pathol 18 (Suppl 2):S61, 2005

Uygun K, Aydiner A, Saip P, et al: Clinical parameters and treatment results in recurrent granulosa cell tumor of the ovary. Gynecol Oncol 88:400, 2003

van Meurs HS, Bleeker MC, van der Velden J, et al: The incidence of endometrial hyperplasia and cancer in 1031 patients with a granulosa cell tumor of the ovary: long-term follow-up in a population-based cohort study. Int J Gynecol Cancer 23(8):1417, 2013

van Meurs HS, Buist MR, Westermann AM, et al: Effectiveness of chemotherapy in measurable granulosa cell tumors: a retrospective study and review of literature. Int J Gynecol Cancer 24(3):496, 2014

Vang R, Herrmann ME, Tavassoli FA: Comparative immunohistochemical analysis of granulosa and Sertoli components in ovarian sex cord–stromal tumors with mixed differentiation: potential implications for derivation of Sertoli differentiation in ovarian tumors. Int J Gynecol Pathol 23:151, 2004

Vicus D, Beiner ME, Klachook S, et al: Pure dysgerminoma of the ovary 35 years on: a single institutional experience. Gynecol Oncol 117:23, 2010

Williams SD, Birch R, Einhorn LH, et al: Treatment of disseminated germ cell tumors with cisplatin, bleomycin, and either vinblastine or etoposide. N Engl J Med 316:1435, 1987

Williams SD, Blessing JA, DiSaia PJ, et al: Second-look laparotomy in ovarian germ cell tumors: the Gynecologic Oncology Group experience. Gynecol Oncol 52:287, 1994

Williams SD, Blessing JA, Hatch KD, et al: Chemotherapy of advanced dysgerminoma: trials of the Gynecologic Oncology Group. J Clin Oncol 9:1950, 1991

Williams SD, Kauderer J, Burnett AF, et al: Adjuvant therapy of completely resected dysgerminoma with carboplatin and etoposide: a trial of the Gynecologic Oncology Group. Gynecol Oncol 95:496, 2004

Wolf JK, Mullen J, Eifel PJ, et al: Radiation treatment of advanced or recurrent granulosa cell tumor of the ovary. Gynecol Oncol 73:35, 1999

Young JL Jr, Cheng WX, Roffers SD, et al: Ovarian cancer in children and young adults in the United States, 1992–1997. Cancer 97:2694, 2003

Young RH: Sex cord–stromal tumors of the ovary and testis: their similarities and differences with consideration of selected problems. Mod Pathol 18:S81, 2005

Young RH, Dudley AG, Scully RE: Granulosa cell, Sertoli–Leydig cell, and unclassified sex cord–stromal tumors associated with pregnancy: a clinicopathological analysis of thirty-six cases. Gynecol Oncol 18:181, 1984

Young RH, Scully RE: Ovarian Sertoli–Leydig cell tumors: a clinicopathological analysis of 207 cases. Am J Surg Pathol 9:543, 1985

Young RH, Welch WR, Dickersin GR, et al: Ovarian sex cord tumor with annular tubules: review of 74 cases including 27 with Peutz-Jeghers syndrome and four with adenoma malignum of the cervix. Cancer 50:1384, 1982

Yuan JQ, Lin XN, Xu JY, et al: Ovarian juvenile granulosa cell tumor associated with Maffucci's syndrome: case report. Chin Med J 117:1592, 2004

Zagame L, Pautier P, Duvillard P, et al: Growing teratoma syndrome after ovarian germ cell tumors. Obstet Gynecol 108:509, 2006

Zaloudek C, Norris HJ: Sertoli-Leydig tumors of the ovary: a clinicopathologic study of 64 intermediate and poorly differentiated neoplasms. Am J Surg Pathol 8:405, 1984

Zanagnolo V, Pasinetti B, Sartori E: Clinical review of 63 cases of sex cord stromal tumors. Eur J Gynaecol Oncol 25:431, 2004

Zanetta G, Bonazzi C, Cantu M, et al: Survival and reproductive function after treatment of malignant germ cell ovarian tumors. J Clin Oncol 19:1015, 2001

Zhang M, Cheung MK, Shin JY, et al: Prognostic factors responsible for survival in sex cord stromal tumors of the ovary—an analysis of 376 women. Gynecol Oncol 104:396, 2007

Zhao XY, Huang HF, Lian LJ, et al: Ovarian cancer in pregnancy: a clinicopathologic analysis of 22 cases and review of the literature. Int J Gynecol Cancer 16:8, 2006

CHAPTER 37

Gestational Trophoblastic Disease

Gestational trophoblastic disease (GTD) refers to a spectrum of interrelated but histologically distinct tumors originating from the placenta (Table 37-1). These diseases are characterized by a reliable tumor marker, which is the β-subunit of human chorionic gonadotropin (β-hCG), and have varied tendencies for local invasion and spread.

Gestational trophoblastic neoplasia (GTN) refers to the subset of GTD that develops malignant sequelae. These tumors require formal staging and typically respond favorably to chemotherapy. Most commonly, GTN develops after a molar pregnancy but may follow any gestation. The prognosis for most GTN cases is

---

TABLE 37-1. Modified WHO Classification of GTD

Molar pregnancies
Hydatidiform mole
  Complete
  Partial
Invasive mole

Trophoblastic tumors
Choriocarcinoma
Placental site trophoblastic tumor
Epithelioid trophoblastic tumor

GTD = gestational trophoblastic disease; WHO = World Health Organization.
Modified with permission from Kurman RJ, Carcangiu ML, Herrington CS, et al (eds): WHO Classification of Tumours of Female Reproductive Organs, 4th ed. Lyon, International Agency for Research on Cancer, 2014.

---

excellent, and patients are routinely cured, even with widespread metastases. The outlook for preservation of fertility and for successful subsequent pregnancy outcomes is equally bright (Vargas, 2014; Wong, 2014). Accordingly, although GTD is uncommon, because the opportunity for cure is great, clinicians should be familiar with its presentation, diagnosis, and management.

EPIDEMIOLOGY AND RISK FACTORS

The incidence of GTD has remained fairly constant at approximately 1 to 2 per 1000 deliveries in North America and Europe (Drake, 2006; Loukovaara, 2005; Lybol, 2011). Although historically higher incidence rates have been reported in parts of Asia, some of this disparity may reflect discrepancies between population-based and hospital-based data collection (Chong, 1999; Kim, 2004; Matsui, 2003). Improved socioeconomic conditions and dietary changes may be partly responsible as well. That said, certain Southeast Asian populations as well as Hispanics and Native Americans living in the United States do have increased incidences (Drake, 2006; Smith, 2003; Tham, 2003).

Maternal age at the upper and lower extremes carries a higher risk of GTD (Altman, 2008; Loukovaara, 2005). This association is much greater for complete moles, whereas the risk of partial molar pregnancy varies relatively little with age. Moreover, compared with the risk in those aged 15 years or younger, the degree of risk is much greater for women 45 years (1 percent) or older (17 percent at age 50) (Savage, 2010; Sebire, 2002a). One explanation relates to ova from older women having higher rates of abnormal fertilization. Similarly, older paternal age has been associated with increased risk (La Vecchia, 1984; Parazzini, 1986).

A history of prior unsuccessful pregnancies also increases the risk of GTD. For example, previous spontaneous abortion at least doubles the risk of molar pregnancy (Parazzini, 1991). More significantly, a personal history of GTD increases the risk of developing a molar gestation in a subsequent pregnancy at least 10-fold. The frequency in a subsequent conception is approximately 1 percent, and most cases mirror the same type of mole as the preceding pregnancy (Garrett, 2008; Sebire, 2003). Furthermore, following two episodes of molar pregnancy, 23 percent of later conceptions result in another molar gestation (Berkowitz, 1998). For this reason, women with a prior history of GTD should undergo first-trimester sonographic examination in subsequent pregnancies. Familial molar pregnancies, however, are rare (Fallahian, 2003).

Of other risk factors, combination oral contraceptive (COC) pill use has been associated with an increased risk of GTD. Specifically, prior COC use approximately doubles the risk, and longer duration of use also correlates positively with risk (Palmer, 1999; Parazzini, 2002). Moreover, women who

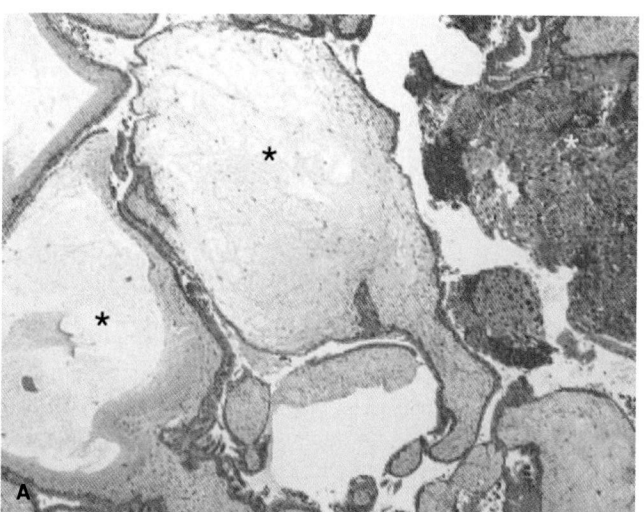
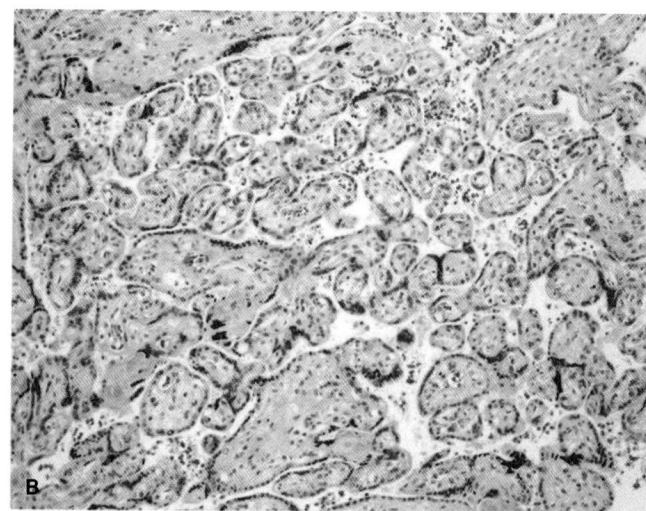

FIGURE 37-1 A. Complete hydatidiform mole. These moles classically have swollen enlarged villi, some of which show cistern formation, that is, central cavitation within the large villi (*black asterisks*). Seen diffusely throughout the placenta, these villous changes create the vesicles noted grossly in complete moles (see Fig. 37-3). Complete moles also typically show trophoblastic proliferation (*yellow asterisk*), which may be focal or widespread. (Used with permission from Dr. Erika Fong.) **B.** Normal term placenta showing smaller, nonedematous villi and absence of trophoblastic proliferation. (Used with permission from Dr. Kelley Carrick.)

used COCs during the cycle in which they conceived have a higher risk in some but not all studies (Costa, 2006; Palmer, 1999). Many of these associations, however, are weak and could be explained by confounding factors other than causality (Parazzini, 2002).

Some epidemiologic characteristics differ markedly between complete and partial moles. For example, vitamin A deficiency and low dietary intake of carotene are associated only with an increased risk of complete moles (Berkowitz, 1985, 1995; Parazzini, 1988). Partial moles have been linked to higher educational levels, smoking, irregular menstrual cycles, and obstetric histories in which only male infants are among the prior live births (Berkowitz, 1995; Parazzini, 1986).

HYDATIDIFORM MOLE (MOLAR PREGNANCY)

Hydatidiform moles are abnormal pregnancies characterized histologically by aberrant changes within the placenta. Classically, the chorionic villi in these placenta show varying degrees of trophoblast proliferation and edema of the stroma within villi (Fig. 37-1). Hydatidiform moles are categorized as either *complete hydatidiform moles* or *partial hydatidiform moles* (Table 37-2). Chromosomal abnormalities play an integral role in hydatidiform mole development.

■ Complete Hydatidiform Mole

These molar pregnancies differ from partial moles with regard to their karyotype, their histologic appearance, and their clinical presentation. First, complete moles typically have a diploid karyotype, and 85 to 90 percent of cases are 46,XX. The chromosomes, however, in these pregnancies are entirely of paternal origin, and thus, the diploid set is described as *diandric*. Specifically, complete moles are formed by *androgenesis*, in which the ovum is fertilized by a haploid sperm that then duplicates its own chromosomes after meiosis (Fig. 37-2) (Fan, 2002; Kajii, 1977). The ovum fails to contribute chromosomes. Most of these moles are 46,XX, but dispermic fertilization of a single ovum, that is, simultaneous fertilization by two sperm, can produce a 46,XY karyotype (Lawler, 1987). Although

TABLE 37-2. Features of Hydatidiform Moles		
Feature	**Complete Mole**	**Partial Mole**
Karyotype	46,XX or 46,XY	69,XXX or 69,XXY
Pathology		
Fetus/embryo	Absent	Present
Villous edema	Diffuse	Focal
Trophoblastic proliferation	Can be marked	Focal and minimal
p57Kip2 immunostaining	Negative	Positive
Clinical presentation		
Typical diagnosis	Molar gestation	Missed abortion
Postmolar malignant sequelae	15%	4–6%

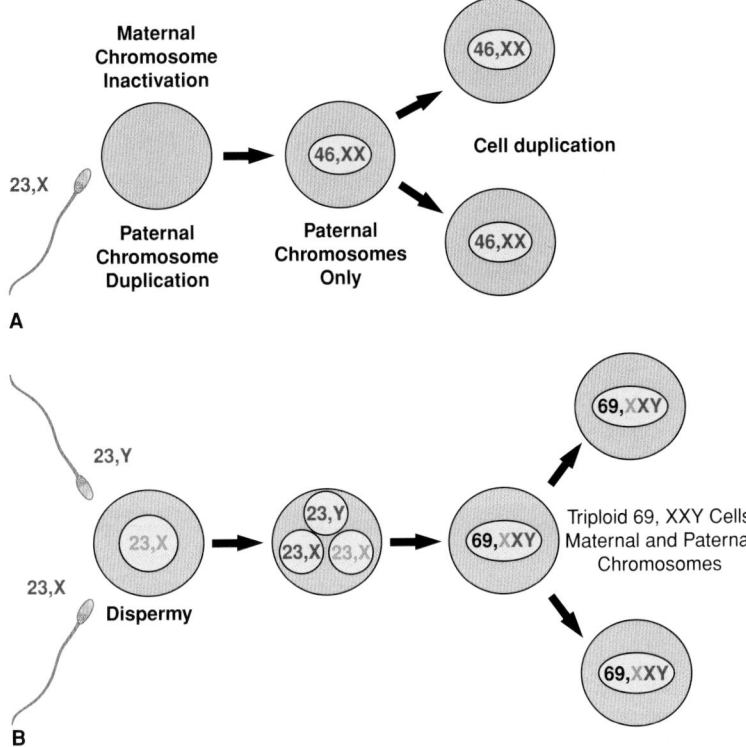

A

B

FIGURE 37-2 A. A 46,XX complete mole may be formed if a 23,X-bearing haploid sperm penetrates a 23,X-containing haploid egg whose genes have become "inactive." Paternal chromosomes then duplicate to create a 46,XX diploid chromosomal complement solely of paternal origin. Alternatively, this same type of inactivated egg can be fertilized independently by two sperm, either 23,X- or 23,Y-bearing, to create a 46,XX or 46,XY chromosomal complement, again of paternal origin only. **B.** Partial moles may be formed if two sperm, either 23,X- or 23,Y-bearing, both fertilize a 23,X-containing haploid egg, whose genes have not been inactivated. The resulting fertilized egg is triploid. Alternatively, a similar haploid egg may be fertilized by an unreduced diploid 46,XY sperm.

nuclear DNA is entirely paternal, mitochondrial DNA remains maternal in origin (Azuma, 1991).

Microscopically, complete moles display enlarged, edematous villi and abnormal trophoblastic proliferation. These changes diffusely involve the entire placenta (see Fig. 37-1). Macroscopically, these changes transform the chorionic villi into clusters of vesicles with variable dimensions. Indeed, the name *hydatidiform mole* literally stems from this "bunch of grapes" appearance. In these pregnancies, no fetal tissue or amnion is produced. As a result, this mass of placental tissue completely fills the endometrial cavity (Fig. 37-3).

Clinically, the presentation of a complete mole has changed considerably. In the 1960s and 1970s, more than half of affected patients had anemia and uterine sizes in excess of that predicted for their gestational age. In addition, hyperemesis gravidarum, preeclampsia, and theca-lutein cysts developed in approximately one quarter of women (Soto-Wright, 1995). As described in Chapter 9 (p. 219), theca-lutein cysts develop with prolonged exposure to luteinizing hormone (LH) or β-hCG (Fig. 37-4). These cysts range in size from 3 to 20 cm, and most regress with falling β-hCG titers after molar evacuation. If such cysts are present, and especially if they are bilateral, the risk of postmolar GTN is increased.

Complete moles, however, infrequently present today with these traditional signs and symptoms (Mangili, 2008). As a result of β-hCG testing and sonography, the mean gestational age at evacuation currently approximates 12 weeks, compared with 16 to 17 weeks in the 1960s and 1970s (Drake, 2006; Soto-Wright, 1995). A large proportion of patients are asymptomatic at diagnosis (Joneborg, 2014). For the remainder, vaginal bleeding remains the most common presenting symptom, and β-hCG levels are often greater than expected. One quarter of women will present with uterine size greater than dates, but the incidence of anemia is less than 10 percent. Moreover, hyperemesis gravidarum, preeclampsia, and symptomatic theca-lutein cysts are now rare (Soto-Wright, 1995). Currently, these sequelae typically develop chiefly in patients without early prenatal care who present with a more advanced gestational age and markedly elevated serum β-hCG levels. Last, plasma thyroxine levels are often increased in women with complete moles, but clinical hyperthyroidism is infrequent. In these circumstances, serum free thyroxine levels are elevated as a consequence of the thyrotropin-like effect of β-hCG (Chap. 15, p. 335).

■ Partial Hydatidiform Mole

These moles differ from complete hydatidiform moles clinically, genetically, and histologically. The degree and extent of trophoblastic proliferation and villous edema are decreased compared with those of complete moles. Moreover, most partial moles contain fetal tissue and amnion, in addition to placental tissues.

As a result, patients with partial moles typically present with signs and symptoms of an incomplete or missed abortion. Many women will have vaginal bleeding. However, because trophoblastic proliferation is slight and only focal, uterine enlargement in excess of gestational

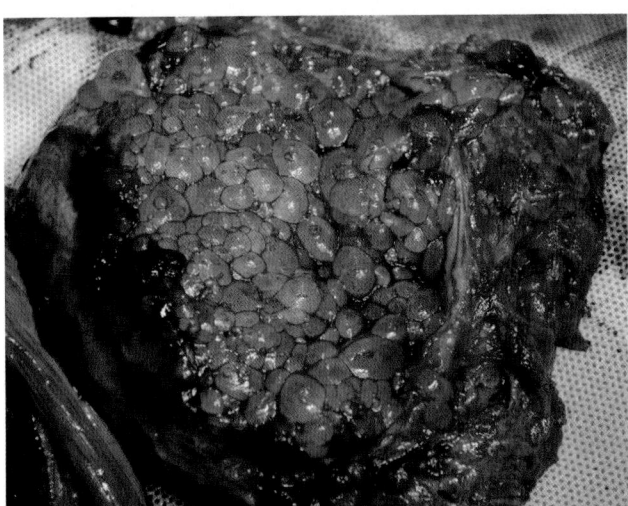

FIGURE 37-3 Photograph of a complete hydatidiform mole. Note the grapelike fluid-filled clusters of chorionic villi. (Used with permission from Dr. Sasha Andrews.)

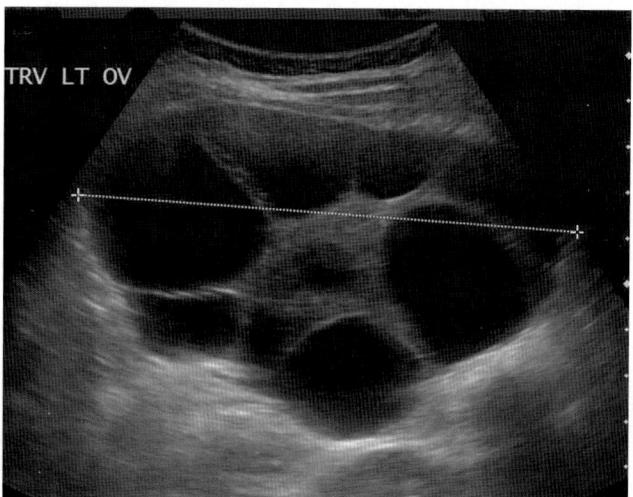

FIGURE 37-4 Transvaginal sonogram of multiple theca-lutein cysts within one ovary of a woman with a complete molar pregnancy. Bilateral, multiple simple cysts are characteristic findings.

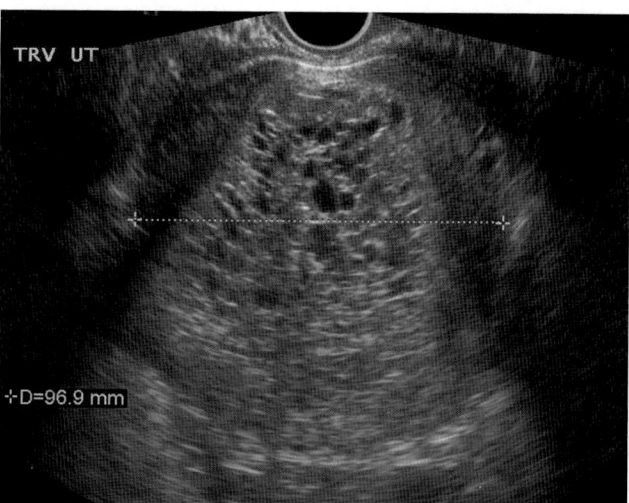

FIGURE 37-5 Transverse sonographic view of a uterus with a complete hydatidiform mole. The classic "snowstorm" appearance is created by the multiple placental vesicles. The mole completely fills this uterine cavity, and calipers are placed on the outer uterine borders.

age is uncommon. Similarly, preeclampsia, theca-lutein cysts, hyperthyroidism, or other dramatic clinical features are rare. Preevacuation β-hCG levels are typically much lower than those for complete moles and often do not exceed 100,000 mIU/mL. For this reason, partial moles are often not identified until after a histologic review of a curettage specimen.

Partial moles have a triploid karyotype (69,XXX, 69,XXY, or less commonly 69,XYY) that is composed of one maternal and two paternal haploid sets of chromosomes (see Fig. 37-2) (Lawler, 1991). The coexisting fetus present with a partial mole is nonviable and typically has multiple malformations with abnormal growth (Jauniaux, 1999).

▪ Diagnosis

Clinical Assessment

In reproductive-aged women with vaginal bleeding, diagnoses may include gynecologic causes of bleeding and complications of first-trimester pregnancy. The trophoblast of molar pregnancies produce β-hCG, and elevated hormone levels reflect their proliferation. Accordingly, initial urine or serum β-hCG measurement and transvaginal sonography are invaluable in guiding evaluation. Because of these, first-trimester diagnosis of hydatidiform mole is now common.

Although β-hCG levels are helpful, the diagnosis of molar pregnancy is more frequently found sonographically. Most first-trimester complete moles demonstrate a complex, echogenic, intrauterine mass containing many small cystic spaces, which reflect swollen chorionic villi. Fetal tissues and amnionic sac are absent (Fig. 37-5) (Benson, 2000). In contrast, sonographic features of a partial molar pregnancy include a thickened, hydropic placenta with a concomitant fetus (Zhou, 2005).

However, there are diagnostic limitations. For example, β-hCG levels in early molar pregnancies may not always be elevated in the first trimester (Lazarus, 1999). Moreover, sonography can lead to a false-negative diagnosis if performed at very early gestational ages, before the chorionic villi have attained their characteristic vesicular pattern. Studies show that only 20 to 30 percent of patients may have sonographic evidence to indicate a partial mole

(Johns, 2005; Lindholm, 1999; Sebire, 2001). Consequently, diagnosis in early gestations is usually difficult. Often, the diagnosis commonly is not made until after histologic review of the abortal specimen. In unclear cases with a live fetus and a desired pregnancy, fetal karyotyping to identify a triploid fetal chromosomal pattern can clarify the diagnosis and management.

Histopathology

The histopathologic changes typical of hydatidiform moles are listed in Table 37-2. But, in early pregnancy, it may be difficult to distinguish among these and a hydropic abortus. Hydropic abortuses are pregnancies formed by the traditional union of one haploid egg and one haploid sperm but are pregnancies that have failed. Their placentas display *hydropic degeneration,* in which villi are edematous and swollen, and thus mimic some villous features of hydatidiform moles (Fig. 37-6). Although no single criterion distinguishes these three, complete moles generally have two prominent features: (1) trophoblastic proliferation and (2) hydropic villi. In gestations younger than 10 weeks, however, hydropic villi may not be apparent, and molar stroma may still be vascular (Paradinas, 1997). As a result, identification of early complete moles must rely on more subtle histologic abnormalities, supplemented by immunohistochemical and molecular diagnostic techniques. Partial moles are optimally diagnosed when three or four major diagnostic criteria are demonstrated: (1) two populations of villi, (2) enlarged, irregular, dysmorphic villi (with trophoblast inclusions), (3) enlarged, cavitated villi (≥3 to 4 mm), and (4) syncytiotrophoblast hyperplasia/atypia (Chew, 2000). Good diagnostic reproducibility can still be achieved in most circumstances using these histologic distinctions of complete and partial mole.

Ancillary Techniques

Histopathologic evaluation can be enhanced by immunohistochemical staining for *p57* expression and by molecular genotyping. p57KIP2 is a nuclear protein whose gene is paternally imprinted and maternally expressed. This means that the gene product is produced only in tissues containing a maternal

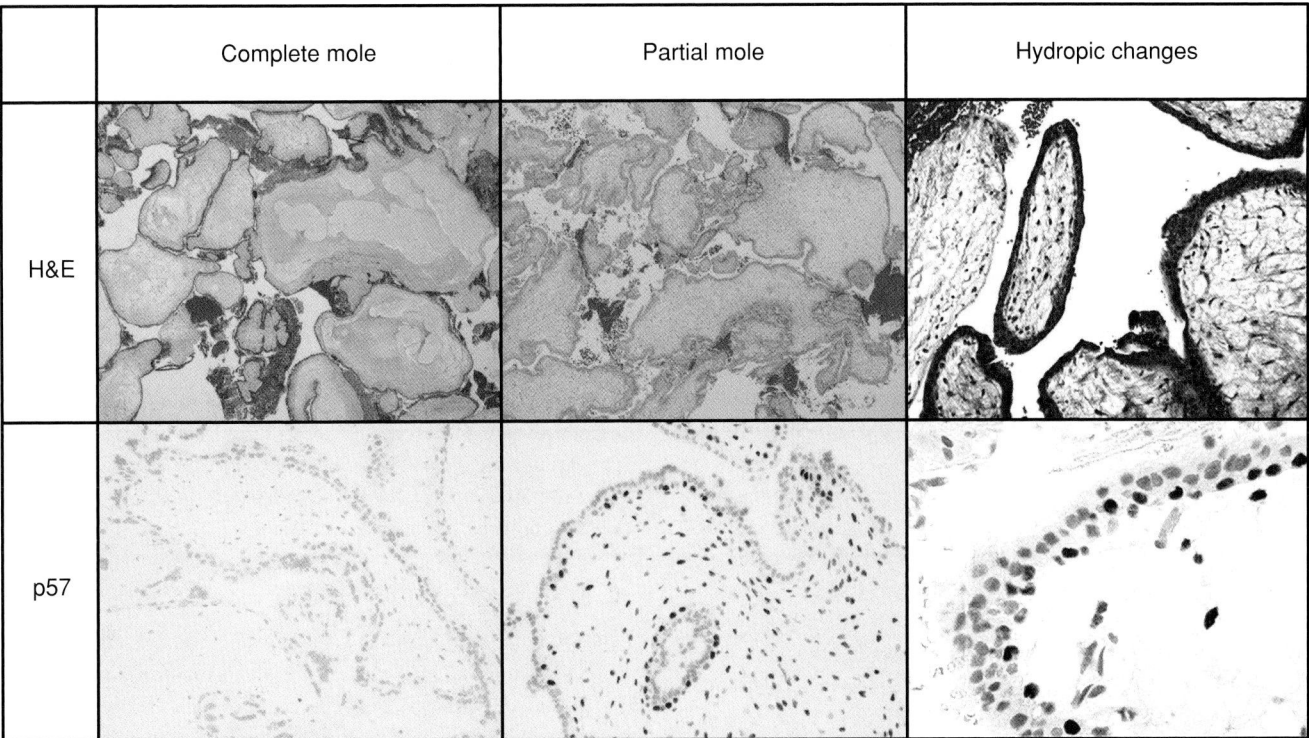

	Complete mole	Partial mole	Hydropic changes
H&E			
p57			

FIGURE 37-6 Composite diagram of differences among normal hydropic abortuses and partial or complete hydatidiform moles. The first row shows typical appearances after hematoxylin and eosin (H&E) staining. The second row shows results after p57 staining. p57 is a nuclear protein whose gene product is produced only in tissues containing a maternal allele. After immunostaining for p57, note the positive (brown) staining in the villi of the partial hydatidiform mole and normal hydropic abortus. This contrasts to the absent staining for p57 in the complete mole (only blue counterstain is seen). (Used with permission from Drs. Kelley Carrick and Raheela Ashfaq.)

allele. Because complete moles contain only paternal genes, the p57KIP2 protein is absent in complete moles, and tissues do not pick up this stain (Merchant, 2005). In contrast, this nuclear protein is strongly expressed in normal placentas, in spontaneous pregnancy losses with hydropic degeneration, and in partial hydatidiform moles (Castrillon, 2001). Accordingly, immunostaining for p57KIP2 is an effective means to isolate complete mole from the diagnostic list. For distinction of a partial mole from a nonmolar hydropic abortus, both of which express *p57*, molecular genotyping can be used. Molecular genotyping determines the parental source of polymorphic alleles. Thereby, it can distinguish among a diploid diandric genome (complete mole), a triploid diandric-monogynic genome (partial mole), or biparental diploidy (nonmolar abortus) (Ronnett, 2011).

■ Treatment

Suction curettage is the preferred method of evacuation regardless of uterine size in patients who wish to remain fertile (American College of Obstetricians and Gynecologists, 2014; Tidy, 2000). Nulliparous women are not given prostanoids to ripen the cervix since these drugs can induce uterine contractions and might increase the risk of trophoblastic embolization to the pulmonary vasculature (Seckl, 2010). Hysterectomy is rarely recommended unless the patient wishes surgical sterilization or is approaching menopause (Elias, 2010). Symptomatic theca-lutein ovarian cysts are an unusual finding and tend to regress after molar evacuation. In extreme cases, these may be aspirated, but oophorectomy is not performed except when torsion leads to extensive ovarian infarction (Mungan, 1996).

Prior to surgery, patients are evaluated for associated medical complications. Fortunately, thyroid storm from untreated hyperthyroidism, respiratory insufficiency from trophoblastic emboli, and other severe coexisting conditions are rare. Because of the tremendous vascularity of these placentas, blood products should be available prior to the evacuation of larger moles, and adequate infusion lines established.

At the beginning of the evacuation, the cervix is dilated to admit a 10- to 12-mm plastic suction curette. As aspiration of molar tissues ensues, intravenous oxytocin is given. At our institution, 20 units of synthetic oxytocin (Pitocin) are mixed with 1 L of crystalloid and infused at rates to achieve uterine contraction. In some cases, intraoperative sonography may be indicated to help reduce the risk of uterine perforation and assist in confirming complete evacuation. Finally, a thorough, gentle curettage is performed.

Following curettage, because of the possibility of partial mole and its attendant fetal tissue, Rh immune globulin is given to nonsensitized Rh D-negative women. Rh immune globulin, however, may be withheld if the diagnosis of complete mole is certain (Fung Kee, 2003).

■ Postmolar Surveillance

Gestational trophoblastic neoplasia develops after evacuation in 15 percent of patients with complete moles (Golfier, 2007; Wolfberg, 2004). Despite the trend of diagnosing these abnormal pregnancies at earlier gestational ages, this incidence has not declined (Seckl, 2004). Of those women who develop GTN, three quarters have locally invasive molar disease and the remaining one quarter develop metastases. In contrast, GTN develops in only 4 to 6 percent of patients with partial moles following evacuation (Feltmate, 2006; Lavie, 2005). Malignant transformation into metastatic choriocarcinoma does occur after partial mole evacuation, but this is rare (0.1 percent) (Cheung, 2004; Seckl, 2000).

No pathologic or clinical features at presentation accurately predict which patients will ultimately develop GTN. Because of the trophoblastic proliferation that characterizes these neoplasms, serial serum β-hCG levels following molar evacuation can be used to effectively monitor patients for GTN development. Therefore, postmolar surveillance with serial quantitative serum β-hCG levels is the standard. Titers are monitored following uterine evacuation at least every 1 to 2 weeks until they become undetectable.

After undetectable β-hCG levels are achieved, subsequent monthly levels are drawn during 6 months of surveillance for all patients with a molar gestation (Sebire, 2007). However, poor compliance with prolonged monitoring has been reported—especially among indigent women and certain ethnic groups in the United States (Allen, 2003; Massad, 2000). A single blood sample demonstrating an undetectable level of β-hCG following molar evacuation is sufficient to exclude the possibility of progression to GTN in most patients. Thus, some women, especially those with a partial mole, may be safely discharged from routine surveillance once an undetectable value is achieved (Lavie, 2005; Wolfberg, 2004). Shortened surveillance could enable women to attempt a subsequent pregnancy sooner. However, GTN may still rarely develop after an hCG level has returned to normal, potentially leading to increased morbidity (Kerkmeijer, 2007; Sebire, 2007).

When pregnancies occur during the monitoring period, the resulting normal β-hCG production can hinder detection of postmolar progression to GTN (Allen, 2003). But other than complicating the monitoring schedule, these pregnancies fortunately are otherwise uneventful (Tuncer, 1999). To prevent difficulties with interpretation, women are encouraged to use effective contraception until achieving a β-hCG titer <5 mIU/mL or below the individual assay's threshold. COC use decreases the likelihood of pregnancy compared with less effective barrier contraception and does not increase the risk of GTN (Costa, 2006; Gaffield, 2009). Injectable medroxyprogesterone acetate is particularly useful when poor compliance is anticipated (Massad, 2000). In contrast, intrauterine devices are not inserted until the β-hCG level is undetectable because of the risk of uterine perforation if an invasive mole is present.

■ Prophylactic Chemotherapy

At the time of molar evacuation, chemotherapy can be administered to help prevent GTN development in high-risk patients who are unlikely to be compliant or for whom β-hCG surveillance is not available. In clinical practice, however, correctly categorizing a woman as high-risk for GTN development is difficult, as no combination of risk factors is universally accepted. Typical patients have complete moles and multiple risk factors, such as age >40 years, previous history of molar pregnancy, or

an excessively high β-hCG titer prior to evacuation. That said, few women are ultimately assigned to this group. Moreover, due to the risks of increased drug resistance, delayed treatment of GTN, and toxic side effects, this practice cannot currently be recommended (American College of Obstetricians and Gynecologists, 2014; Fu, 2012). Prophylactic chemotherapy is not routinely offered in the United States and Europe.

However, a single dose of dactinomycin has been shown to reduce the incidence of postmolar GTN in certain populations. For example, in one randomized trial, 60 Thai women who had high-risk complete moles were assigned to receive either prophylactic dactinomycin or placebo at the time of evacuation (Limpongsanurak, 2001). Adjuvant chemotherapy reduced the incidence of GTN from 50 percent to 14 percent, but toxicity was significant. As a result, prophylactic chemotherapy is generally used only in those countries with limited resources to reliably monitor patients after evacuation (Uberti, 2009).

■ Ectopic Molar Pregnancy

The true incidence of GTD developing outside the uterine cavity approximates 1.5 per 1 million births (Gillespie, 2004). More than 90 percent of suspected cases will reflect an overdiagnosis of florid extravillous trophoblastic proliferation in the fallopian tube (Burton, 2001; Sebire, 2005b). As with any ectopic pregnancy, initial management usually involves surgical removal of the conceptus and histopathologic evaluation.

■ Coexistent Fetus

At times, a twin pregnancy can consist of a hydatidiform mole and a coexisting fetus. The estimated incidence is 1 per 20,000 to 100,000 pregnancies (Fig. 37-7). Sebire and associates (2002b) described the outcome of 77 twin pregnancies, each composed of a complete mole and a healthy cotwin. Of this group, 24 women chose to have an elective termination, and 53 continued their pregnancies. Twenty-three gestations spontaneously aborted at less than 24 weeks, two were terminated due to severe preeclampsia, and 28 pregnancies lasted at least 24 weeks—resulting in 20 live births. The authors demonstrated that coexisting complete moles and healthy cotwin pregnancies have a high risk of spontaneous abortion, but approximately 40 percent result in live births. The risk of progression to GTN was 16 percent in first-trimester terminations and not significantly higher (21 percent) in women who continued their pregnancies. Because the risk of malignancy is unchanged with advancement of gestational age, pregnancy continuation may be allowed, provided that severe maternal complications are controlled and fetal growth is normal. Importantly, these cases should be distinguished early from a single partial molar pregnancy with its abnormal associated fetus. Fetal karyotyping to confirm a normal fetal chromosomal pattern is also recommended (Marcorelles, 2005; Matsui, 2000).

GESTATIONAL TROPHOBLASTIC NEOPLASIA

This term primarily encompasses pathologic entities that are characterized by aggressive invasion of the endometrium and

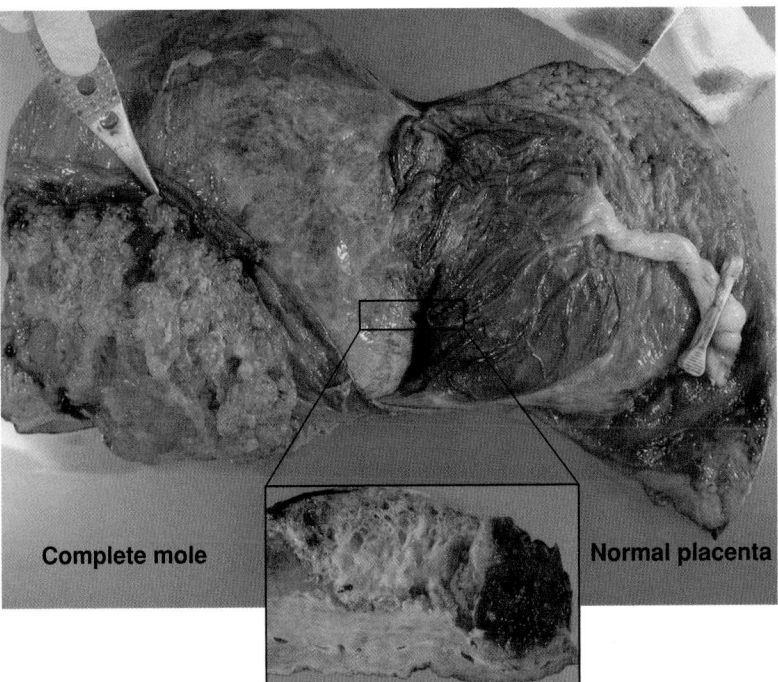

FIGURE 37-7 Photograph of placentas from a twin pregnancy with one normal twin and with a complete mole. The complete mole (*left*) shows the characteristic vesicular structure. The placenta on the *right* appears grossly normal. A transverse section through the border between these two is shown (*inset*). (Used with permission from Drs. April Bleich and Brian Levenson.)

myometrium by trophoblast cells. Histologic categories include common tumors such as the invasive mole and gestational choriocarcinoma, as well as the rare placental-site trophoblastic tumor and epithelioid trophoblastic tumor. Although these histologic types have been characterized, in most cases of GTN, no tissue is available for pathologic study. Instead, GTN is diagnosed based on elevated β-hCG levels and managed clinically.

Gestational trophoblastic neoplasia typically develops with or follows some form of pregnancy. Most cases follow a hydatidiform

mole. Rarely, GTN develops after a live birth, miscarriage, or termination. Occasionally, the antecedent gestation cannot be confirmed with certainty. Many of the reported nonmolar cases may actually represent disease originating from an unrecognized early mole (Sebire, 2005a).

■ Histologic Classification

Invasive Mole

This common manifestation of GTN is characterized by whole chorionic villi that accompany excessive trophoblastic overgrowth and invasion (Fig. 37-8). These tissues penetrate deep into the myometrium, sometimes to involve the peritoneum, adjacent parametrium, or vaginal vault. Such moles are locally invasive but generally lack the pronounced tendency to develop widespread metastases typical of choriocarcinoma. Invasive moles originate almost exclusively from a complete or a partial hydatidiform mole (Sebire, 2005a).

Gestational Choriocarcinoma

This extremely malignant tumor contains sheets of anaplastic trophoblast and prominent hemorrhage, necrosis, and vascular invasion (see Fig. 37-8). However, formed villous structures are characteristically absent. Gestational choriocarcinoma initially invades the endometrium and myometrium but tends to develop early blood-borne systemic metastases (Fig. 37-9).

Most cases develop following evacuation of a molar pregnancy, but these tumors may also follow a nonmolar pregnancy. Specifically, gestational choriocarcinoma develops in approximately 1 in 30,000 nonmolar pregnancies. Two thirds of such cases follow term pregnancies, and one third develop after a spontaneous abortion or pregnancy termination. One

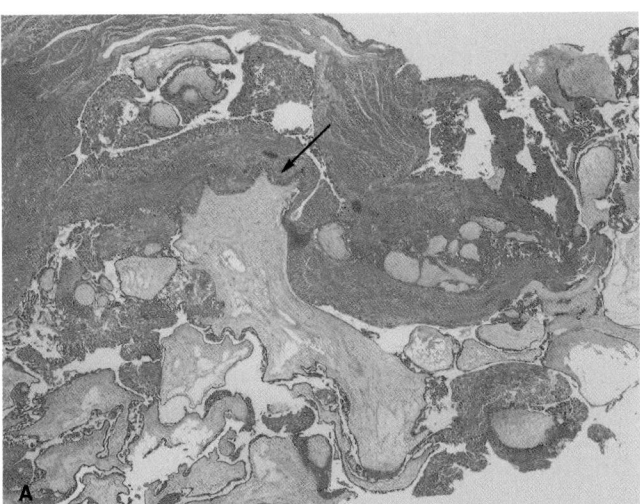

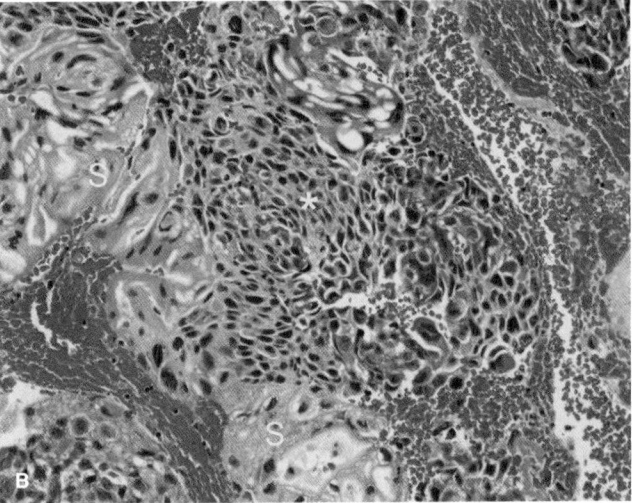

FIGURE 37-8 A. An invasive mole contains whole villi that invade locally. The arrow marks one villus invading deeply into the adjacent myometrium. (Used with permission from Dr. Ona Faye-Peterson.) **B.** Choriocarcinoma is a biphasic tumor characterized by intermediate trophoblast and cytotrophoblast (*asterisk*), intimately admixed with multinucleate syncytiotrophoblast (*S*). Choriocarcinoma is a vascular tumor, typically with prominent hemorrhage, as evidenced by the abundant blood in the background. (Used with permission from Dr. Kelley Carrick.)

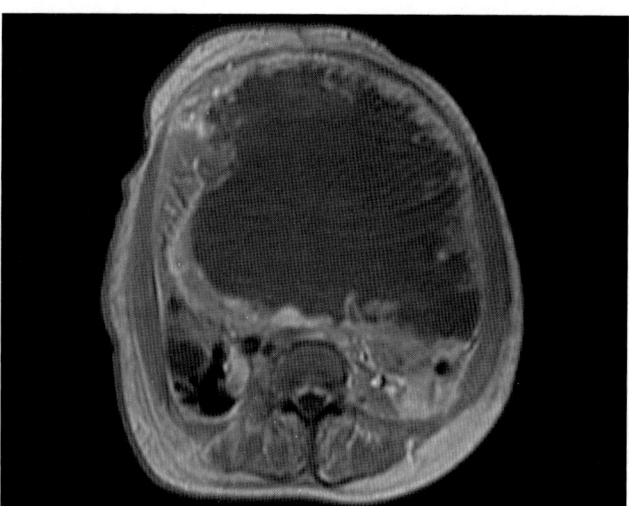

FIGURE 37-9 Computed-tomography (CT) scan of choriocarcinoma invading the uterus.

review of 100 patients with nonmolar gestational choriocarcinoma reported that 62 presented after a live birth, 6 after a live birth preceded by a molar pregnancy, and 32 after a nonmolar abortion (Tidy, 1995). Vaginal bleeding was the most common symptom in all groups. For this reason, abnormal bleeding for more than 6 weeks following any pregnancy warrants evaluation with β-hCG testing to exclude a new pregnancy or GTN.

When choriocarcinoma is diagnosed after a live birth, the antecedent pregnancy usually proceeded normally to term. One case series collected between 1964 and 1996 showed that in 89 percent of cases, the preceding pregnancy had produced an uncomplicated live birth (Rodabaugh, 1998). Hydrops, while a notable complication in the remaining fetuses in this earlier series, was not observed in a more recent cohort compiled between 1996 and 2011 (Diver, 2013). Occasionally, unanticipated choriocarcinoma is detected in an otherwise normal-appearing placenta at delivery. More commonly, however, the diagnosis of choriocarcinoma is delayed for months due to subtle signs and symptoms. Most patients present with intermenstrual bleeding, and high β-hCG levels are detected (Lok, 2006). Less frequently, the diagnosis is made in an asymptomatic woman by an incidental positive pregnancy test (Diver, 2013). In part because of the typical delay to diagnosis, choriocarcinomas following term pregnancies are associated with high-risk features and a higher mortality rate than GTN following nonmolar abortions. Death rates range from 10 to 15 percent (Diver, 2013; Lok, 2006; Rodabaugh, 1998; Tidy, 1995).

In contrast to this gestational choriocarcinoma, primary "nongestational" choriocarcinoma is an ovarian germ cell tumor (Chap. 36, p. 764). Although rare, ovarian choriocarcinoma has a histologic appearance identical to that of gestational choriocarcinoma. It is in part distinguished by the lack of a preceding pregnancy (Lee, 2009).

Placental-site Trophoblastic Tumor

This tumor consists predominantly of intermediate trophoblasts at the placental site. It is a rare GTN variant with unique disease behavior. Placental-site trophoblastic tumor (PSTT) can follow

any type of pregnancy but develops most commonly following a term gestation (Papadopoulos, 2002). Typically, patients have irregular bleeding months or years after the antecedent pregnancy, and the diagnosis is not entertained until endometrial sampling has been performed (Feltmate, 2001). PSTT tends to infiltrate only within the uterus, disseminates late in its course, and produces low β-hCG levels (van Trommel, 2013). Of interest, an elevated proportion of free β-subunit can help to discriminate it from other GTN types if the endometrial biopsy is equivocal (Cole, 2008; Harvey, 2008). When this tumor does spread, the pattern mirrors that of gestational choriocarcinoma. Metastases often spread to the lungs, liver, or vagina (Baergen, 2006).

Hysterectomy is the primary treatment for nonmetastatic PSTT due to its relative insensitivity to chemotherapy. In particularly motivated patients, fertility-sparing procedures have mixed results (Feltmate, 2001; Machtinger, 2005; Papadopoulos, 2002; Taylor, 2013b).

Metastatic PSTT has a much poorer prognosis than its postmolar GTN counterparts. As a result, aggressive combination chemotherapy is indicated. EMA/EP regimens of etoposide, methotrexate, and dactinomycin (actinomycin D) that alternate with etoposide and cisplatin (Platinol) are considered the most effective (Newlands, 2000). Radiation, however, may also have a role. The overall 10-year survival is 70 percent, but patients with metastases, especially stage IV disease, have a much poorer prognosis (Hassadia, 2005; Hyman, 2013; Schmid, 2009).

Epithelioid Trophoblastic Tumor

This rare trophoblastic tumor is distinct from gestational choriocarcinoma and PSTT. The preceding pregnancy event may be remote, or in some cases, a prior gestation cannot be confirmed (Palmer, 2008). Epithelioid trophoblastic tumor develops from neoplastic transformation of chorionic-type intermediate trophoblast. Microscopically, this tumor resembles PSTT, but the cells are smaller and display less nuclear pleomorphism. Grossly, epithelioid trophoblastic tumor grows in a nodular fashion rather than the infiltrative pattern of PSTT (Shih, 1998). Hysterectomy is again the primary treatment due to presumed chemoresistance and since the diagnosis is usually confirmed in advance by endometrial biopsy. More than one third of patients will present with metastatic disease and demonstrable chemoresistance to multiagent therapy, which portends a poor prognosis (Davis, 2015; Palmer, 2008).

■ Diagnosis

Most GTN cases are clinically diagnosed, using β-hCG evidence to identify persistent trophoblastic tissue (Table 37-3). Tissue is infrequently available for pathologic diagnosis, unless a diagnosis of placental-site or nongestational tumor is being considered. As a result, most centers in the United States diagnose GTN on the basis of rising β-hCG values or a persistent plateau of β-hCG values for at least 3 weeks. Unfortunately, uniformity is lacking in the definition of a persistent plateau. Additionally, the diagnostic criteria are less stringent in the United States than in Europe. This is partly because of concern that some patients may be lost to follow-up if stricter criteria are used.

TABLE 37-3. FIGO Criteria for Gestational Trophoblastic Neoplasia Diagnosis

β-hCG level plateau persists in four measurements during a period of 3 weeks or longer (days 1, 7, 14, and 21)
β-hCG level rise in 3 weekly consecutive measurements or longer, over a period of 2 weeks or more (days 1, 7, and 14)
β-hCG level remains elevated for 6 months or more
Histologic diagnosis of choriocarcinoma

β-hCG = beta human chorionic gonadotropin; FIGO = International Federation of Gynecology and Obstetrics.
Data from FIGO Oncology Committee: FIGO staging for gestational trophoblastic neoplasia 2000. Int J Gynaecol Obstet 2002 Jun;77(3):285–287.

When serologic criteria for GTN are met, a new intrauterine pregnancy is excluded using β-hCG levels that are correlated with sonographic findings. This is done especially if there has been a long delay in monitoring of serial β-hCG levels or non-compliance with contraception or both.

■ Assessment

Patients with GTN undergo a thorough pretreatment assessment to determine disease extent. The initial evaluation may be limited to pelvic examination, chest radiograph, and pelvic sonography or abdominopelvic computed tomography (CT) scanning. Although approximately 40 percent of patients will have micrometastases not otherwise visible on chest radiography, chest CT is not needed because these small lesions do not affect outcome (Darby, 2009; Garner, 2004). However, pulmonary lesions identified on chest radiograph should prompt CT of the chest and magnetic resonance (MR) imaging of the brain. Fortunately, central nervous system involvement is rare in the absence of neurologic symptoms or signs (Price, 2010). Positron emission tomography (PET) may occasionally be useful to evaluate occult choriocarcinoma or relapse from previously treated GTN when conventional imaging is equivocal or fails to identify metastatic disease (Dhillon, 2006; Numnum, 2005).

■ Staging

Gestational trophoblastic neoplasia is anatomically staged based on a system adopted by the International Federation of Gynecology and Obstetrics (FIGO) (Table 37-4 and Fig. 37-10). Patients at low risk for therapeutic failure are distinguished from those at high risk by using the modified prognostic scoring system of the World Health Organization (WHO) (Table 37-5). About 95 percent of patients will have a WHO score of 0 to 6 and will be considered to have low-risk disease (Sita-Lumsden, 2012). The remainder will have a score of 7 or higher and be assigned to the high-risk GTN group. For the most accurate description of affected patients, the Roman numeral corresponding to FIGO stage is separated by a colon from the sum of the risk factor scores, for example, stage II:4 or stage IV:9. This description best reflects disease behavior (Ngan, 2004). Women with high-risk scores are more likely to have tumors that are resistant to single-agent chemotherapy. They are therefore treated initially with combination chemotherapy. Although patients with stage I disease infrequently have a high-risk score, those with stage IV disease invariably have a high-risk score. Women diagnosed with FIGO stage I, II, or III GTN have a survival rate approaching 100 percent (Lurain, 2010).

Nonmetastatic Disease

Invasive moles arising from complete molar gestations make up most nonmetastatic GTN cases. Approximately 12 percent of complete moles develop locally invasive disease after evacuation, compared with only 4 to 6 percent of partial moles. Epithelioid trophoblastic tumor and PSTT are other rare causes of nonmetastatic GTN. Locally invasive trophoblastic tumors may perforate the myometrium and lead to intraperitoneal bleeding (Mackenzie, 1993). Alternatively, vaginal hemorrhage can follow tumor erosion into uterine vessels, or necrotic tumor may involve the uterine wall and serve as a nidus for infection. Fortunately, the prognosis is typically excellent for all types of nonmetastatic disease despite these possible manifestations.

Metastatic Disease

Choriocarcinomas originating from complete molar gestations account for most cases of metastatic GTN. Three to 4 percent of complete moles develop metastatic choriocarcinoma after evacuation. This event is rare following any other type of molar or nonmolar gestation. Choriocarcinomas have a propensity for distant spread and should be suspected in any woman of reproductive age with metastatic disease from an unknown primary (Tidy, 1995). Moreover, because of this tendency,

TABLE 37-4. FIGO Anatomic Staging of GTN

Stage	Characteristics
I	Disease confined to the uterus
II	GTN extends outside of the uterus but is limited to the genital structures (adnexa, vagina, broad ligament)
III	GTN extends to the lungs, with or without known genital tract involvement
IV	All other metastatic sites

FIGO = International Federation of Gynecology and Obstetrics; GTN = gestational trophoblastic neoplasia.
Reproduced with permission from FIGO Committee on Gynecologic Oncology: Current FIGO staging for cancer of the vagina, fallopian tube, ovary, and gestational trophoblastic neoplasia. Int J Gynaecol Obstet 2009 Apr;105(1):3–4.

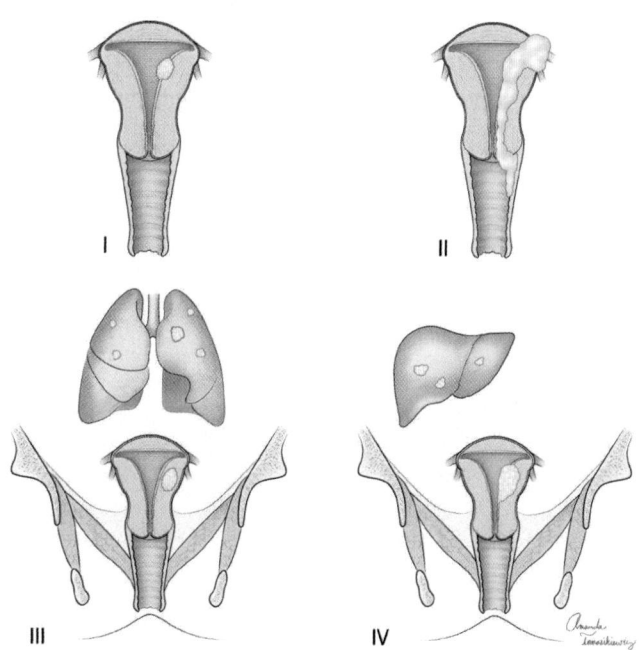

FIGURE 37-10 International Federation of Gynecology and Obstetrics (FIGO) staging of gestational trophoblastic neoplasia.

chemotherapy is indicated whenever choriocarcinoma is diagnosed histologically.

Although many patients are largely asymptomatic, metastatic GTN is highly vascular and prone to severe hemorrhage either spontaneously or during biopsy. Heavy menstrual bleeding is a common presenting symptom. The most common sites of spread are the lungs (80 percent), vagina (30 percent), pelvis (20 percent), liver (10 percent), and brain (10 percent) (Fig. 37-11). Patients with pulmonary metastases typically have asymptomatic lesions identified on routine chest radiograph and infrequently present with cough, dyspnea, hemoptysis, pleuritic chest pain, or signs of pulmonary hypertension (Seckl, 1991). In patients with early development of respiratory failure that requires intubation, the overall outcome is poor. Hepatic

or cerebral involvement is encountered almost exclusively in patients who have had an antecedent nonmolar pregnancy and a protracted delay in tumor diagnosis (Newlands, 2002; Savage, 2015b). These women may present with associated hemorrhagic events. Virtually all patients with hepatic or cerebral metastases have concurrent pulmonary or vaginal involvement or both. Great caution is used in attempting excision of any metastatic disease site due to the risk of profuse hemorrhage. Thus, this practice is almost uniformly avoided except in extenuating circumstances of life-threatening brainstem herniation or chemotherapy-resistant disease.

■ Treatment
Surgery

Most patients diagnosed with postmolar GTN have persistent tumor confined to the endometrial cavity and are treated primarily with chemotherapeutic agents. Repeat dilatation and curettage is generally avoided to prevent morbidity and mortality caused by uterine perforation, hemorrhage, infection, uterine adhesions, and anesthetic complications (American College of Obstetricians and Gynecologists, 2014). Accordingly, second evacuations are not typically performed in the United States unless patients have persistent uterine bleeding and substantial amounts of retained molar tissue. Repeat uterine curettage is a more standard part of postmolar GTN management in Europe. This practice reduces both the number of patients needing any further treatment and the number of courses in those who do require chemotherapy (Pezeshki, 2004; van Trommel, 2005). A second evacuation followed by continued surveillance, however, is a less attractive option, even for poorly compliant patients, than single-agent chemotherapy (Allen, 2003; Massad, 2000).

Hysterectomy may play several roles in GTN treatment. First, it may be performed to primarily treat PSTT, epithelioid trophoblastic tumors, or other chemotherapy-resistant disease. Second, severe uncontrollable vaginal or intraabdominal bleeding may necessitate hysterectomy as an emergency procedure (Clark, 2010). Because of these more extreme indications,

TABLE 37-5. Modified WHO Prognostic Scoring System as Adapted by FIGO

Scores	0	1	2	4
Age (yr)	<40	≥40	—	—
Antecedent pregnancy	Mole	Abortion	Term	—
Interval months from index pregnancy	<4	4–6	7–12	>12
Pretreatment serum β-hCG (mIU/mL)	$<10^3$	$10^3–<10^4$	$10^4–<10^5$	$≥10^5$
Largest tumor size (including uterus)	<3 cm	3–4 cm	≥5 cm	—
Site of metastases	—	Spleen, kidney	GI	Liver, brain
Number of metastases	—	1–4	5–8	>8
Previous failed chemotherapy drugs	—	—	1	≥2

Low risk = WHO score of 0 to 6; high risk = WHO score of ≥7.
β-hCG = beta human chorionic gonadotropin; FIGO = International Federation of Gynecology and Obstetrics; GI = gastrointestinal; WHO = World Health Organization.
Reproduced with permission from FIGO Committee on Gynecologic Oncology: Current FIGO staging for cancer of the vagina, fallopian tube, ovary, and gestational trophoblastic neoplasia. Int J Gynaecol Obstet 2009 Apr;105(1):3–4.

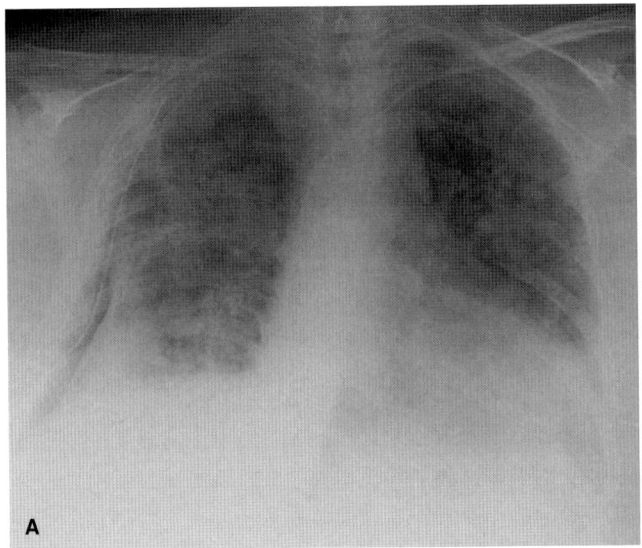

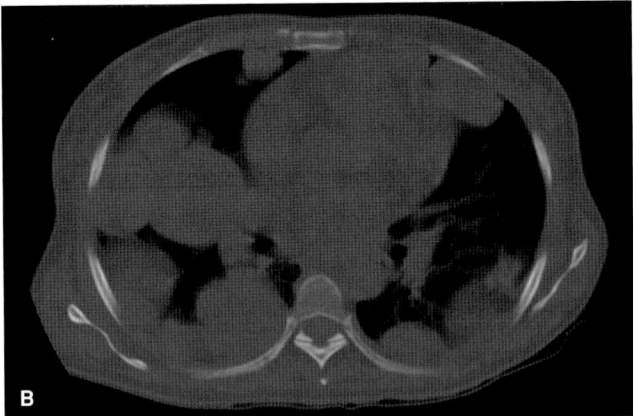

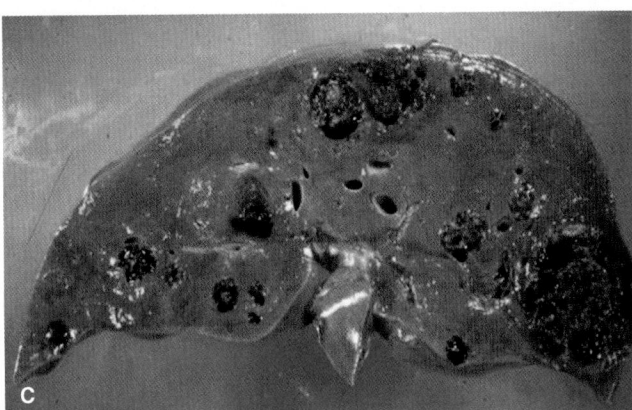

FIGURE 37-11 Common sites of gestational trophoblastic neoplasia metastasis. **A.** Chest radiography demonstrates widespread metastatic lesions. (Used with permission from Dr. Michael G. Connor.) **B.** Computed-tomography (CT) scan of metastatic disease to the lung. **C.** Autopsy specimen shows multiple hemorrhagic hepatic metastases. (Used with permission from Dr. Michael G. Connor.)

most women undergoing hysterectomy have elevated pretreatment risk scores, unusual pathology, and higher mortality rates (Pisal, 2002). Finally, adjuvant hysterectomy decreases the total dose of chemotherapy needed to achieve clinical remission in low-risk GTN. Patients with disease apparently confined to the uterus who do not desire future fertility should

be counseled about this option (Suzuka, 2001). However, the risk of GTN persistence after hysterectomy remains approximately 3 to 5 percent, and these patients should be monitored postoperatively (American College of Obstetricians and Gynecologists, 2014).

Residual lung metastases may persist in 10 to 20 percent of patients achieving clinical remission of GTN after chemotherapy completion. These patients do not appear to have an increased risk of relapse compared with those having normal chest radiographs or CT scans. Thus, thoracotomy is not usually necessary unless remission cannot otherwise be achieved (Powles, 2006). In general, the optimal patient to be counseled for thoracotomy will have stage III GTN, a preoperative β-hCG level <1500 mIU/mL, and a solitary lung nodule resistant to chemotherapy (Cao, 2009; Fleming, 2008).

Chemotherapy for Low-Risk GTN

Methotrexate. Most patients with hydatidiform mole who develop GTN are at low risk of chemotherapy resistance (score 0-6) (Seckl, 2010). Single-agent methotrexate is the most common treatment, and complete response rates range from 67 to 81 percent for variations of the two most common intramuscular (IM) methotrexate regimens (Table 37-6). Although bundled as low-risk disease, the highest cure rates occur in patients with the lowest WHO scores (0-1), and rates decline proportionally as WHO scores rise (Sita-Lumsden, 2012). Thus, patients with a WHO score of 6 should at least be considered for upfront combination therapy (Taylor, 2013a). Overall, 19 to 33 percent of women develop methotrexate resistance and are switched to other agents, described subsequently.

With methotrexate, the Gynecologic Oncology Group (GOG) conducted a prospective cohort dose-escalation study (protocol #79) of weekly administration that established a maximum dose of 50 mg/m^2 with minimal toxicity (Homesley, 1988, 1990). This regimen is continued weekly until β-hCG levels are undetectable, and then two or three additional weekly doses are given (Lybol, 2012). Alternatively, Charing Cross Hospital and University of Sheffield investigators currently use an 8-day alternating regimen of 50 mg IM methotrexate on treatment days 1, 3, 5, and 7, and oral folinic acid, 7.5 to 15 mg taken orally on days 2, 4, 6, and 8. Treatment is repeated every 2 weeks (Taylor, 2013a).

As discussed more fully in Chapter 27 (p. 596), methotrexate is a folic acid antagonist that inhibits DNA synthesis. Mild stomatitis is the most common side effect, but other serosal symptoms, especially pleurisy, develop in up to one quarter of patients treated with low-dose methotrexate. Pericarditis, peritonitis, and pneumonitis are infrequent (Sharma, 1999). Toxicity develops more frequently with the more intense 8-day regimen compared with weekly administration. This is despite routine folinic acid "rescue," which is provided to protect normal mucosal and serosal cells (Chap. 27, p. 597) (Gleeson, 1993).

Dactinomycin. Dactinomycin is less frequently used for the primary treatment of low-risk disease due to toxicity concerns, but it has superior efficacy as a single agent (Alazzam, 2012a; Yarandi, 2008). In a prospective GOG trial (protocol #174) of low-risk GTN, patients were randomly assigned to biweekly

TABLE 37-6. Intramuscular Methotrexate Regimens for Treatment of Low-Risk GTN

Frequency	Dose	Population Studied	CR Rate (%)	Study
Weekly	30–50 mg/m^2	Nonmetastatic GTN	74–81	Homesley, 1988, 1990
	50 mg/m^2	Low-risk GTN	70	Kang, 2010
Days 1,3,5,7	50 mg/d	Low-risk GTN	67–72	Kang, 2010; Khan, 2003; McNeish, 2002
	1 mg/kg	Low-risk GTN	78	Chalouhi, 2009

CR = clinical remission (calculated for first-line treatment without needing alternative chemotherapy); GTN = gestational trophoblastic neoplasia.

"pulse" 1.25-mg dose dactinomycin or to weekly methotrexate, 30 mg/m^2. Among 215 eligible patients, a complete response was observed in 69 percent given dactinomycin and in 53 percent given methotrexate. However, advocates of methotrexate have speculated that the unexpectedly low efficacy of methotrexate observed in this study may be due to subtherapeutic dosing. Moreover, those randomized to dactinomycin were twice as likely to develop alopecia and were the only patients to develop grade 4 toxicity, defined in Chapter 27 (p. 605) (Osborne, 2008). As yet, no trials have directly compared pulse dactinomycin and the widely used 8-day methotrexate regimen. Since survival rates are so high, methotrexate is usually tried first because most clinicians consider it to be the least toxic.

Patients who do not respond to an initial single-agent chemotherapeutic regimen fail to have persistently dropping β-hCG levels. These women should have their score recalculated using the modified WHO prognostic scoring system. Most women will still be considered low-risk and may be switched to a single-agent second-line therapy. Methotrexate-resistant GTN often responds to dactinomycin (Chapman-Davis, 2012; Chen, 2004). The GOG demonstrated a 74-percent success rate in a Phase II trial (protocol #176) of pulse dactinomycin as salvage treatment in 38 patients with methotrexate-resistant GTN (Covens, 2006). Etoposide is less commonly used in this setting but is also effective (Mangili, 1996). Patients initially treated with pulse dactinomycin who develop resistant GTN may still be successfully treated with the 5-day course of dactinomycin (Kohorn, 2002). Alternatively, single-agent methotrexate or etoposide is often effective in these cases (Matsui, 2005).

Chemotherapy for High-Risk GTN

Approximately 5 percent of GTN patients present with high-risk disease and usually have numerous metastases months or years after the causative pregnancy. Such patients are likely to develop drug resistance to single-agent chemotherapy (Seckl, 2010). Etoposide, methotrexate, and dactinomycin (actinomycin D) alternating with cyclophosphamide and vincristine (Oncovin) (EMA/CO) chemotherapy is a well-tolerated and highly effective regimen for high-risk GTN. It is considered the preferred treatment for most high-risk disease. Bower and associates (1997) reported a 78-percent complete remission rate in 272 consecutive women. Similarly, other investigators have observed a 71- to 78-percent complete response rate with the EMA/CO regimen (Escobar, 2003; Lu, 2008).

Response rates are comparable whether patients are treated primarily or after failure of single-agent methotrexate and/or dactinomycin.

Patients with high-risk disease have an overall survival rate of 86 to 92 percent, although approximately one quarter become refractory to or relapse from EMA/CO (Bower, 1997; Escobar, 2003; Lu, 2008; Lurain, 2010). Secondary treatment usually involves platinum-based chemotherapy combined with possible surgical excision of resistant disease (Alazzam, 2012b). Newlands and colleagues (2000) reported an 88-percent survival rate among 34 patients by replacing the cyclophosphamide and vincristine component with etoposide and cisplatin (EMA/EP). EMA/EP is an effective option in patients resistant to EMA/CO, but paclitaxel (Taxol) plus cisplatin alternating with paclitaxel plus etoposide (TP/TE) has comparable efficacy and appears less toxic (Patel, 2010; Wang, 2008). Bleomycin, etoposide, and cisplatin (BEP) is another potentially effective regimen (Lurain, 2005).

High-risk patients with a large disease burden are at risk for early death with standard EMA/CO due to tumor-lysis related hemorrhage and clinical deterioration. In these selected circumstances, "induction low-dose etoposide-cisplatin" appears to reduce the mortality risk 10-fold (Alifrangis, 2013).

Brain Metastases

Patients with cerebral metastases may present with seizures, headaches, or hemiparesis (Newlands, 2002). Occasionally, they are moribund on arrival after not recognizing the significance of their symptoms or following an extended delay in diagnosis. In such extenuating circumstances, emergency craniotomy may be indicated to stabilize the patient and is followed by critical care support throughout the active phase of treatment (Savage, 2015b). In experienced centers, virtually all GTN-related deaths occur in stage IV patients with WHO risk scores of 12 or more (Lurain, 2010).

Fortunately, the cure rate for those with brain metastases is high if neurologic deterioration does not occur within the first weeks after diagnosis. The sequence of aggressive multimodality therapy is controversial but may include chemotherapy, surgery, and radiation. Savage and coworkers (2015b) reported an 85-percent survival rate among 27 patients treated from 1991 to 2013 by EMA/CO or EMA/EP with an enhanced intravenous dose (1 g/m^2) of methotrexate combined with intrathecal methotrexate until β-hCG levels were undetectable. Whole-brain radiation therapy can also be an efficacious adjunct to combination chemotherapy and surgery but can induce permanent intellectual impairment (Cagayan, 2006; Schechter, 1998).

■ Posttreatment

Surveillance

Monitoring of patients with low-risk GTN consists of weekly β-hCG measurements until the level is undetectable for 3 consecutive weeks. This is followed by monthly titers until the level is undetectable for 12 months. Patients with high-risk disease are followed for 24 months due to the greater risk of late relapse. Patients are encouraged to use effective contraception, as outlined earlier, during the entire surveillance period.

Treatment Sequelae

Despite the favorable prognosis, patients and their partners carry pregnancy concerns for a protracted time (Wenzel, 1992). Sexual dysfunction is an underreported complication (Cagayan, 2008). These and other potential sequelae highlight the importance of a multidisciplinary approach to management (Ferreira, 2009).

Although patients may expect a normal reproductive outcome after achieving remission from GTD, some evidence suggests that adverse maternal outcomes and spontaneous abortion occur more frequently among those who conceive within 6 months of chemotherapy completion (Braga, 2009). Women having a pregnancy affected by a histologically confirmed complete or partial mole may be counseled that the risk of a repeat mole in a subsequent pregnancy approximates 1 percent (Garrett, 2008). Most will be of the same type of mole as the preceding pregnancy (Sebire, 2003). Women who become pregnant within 12 months postchemotherapy for GTN can be reassured of a likely favorable outcome, although the safest option is still to delay pregnancy for the full year (Williams, 2014). Pregnancy after combination EMA/CO chemotherapy for GTN also has a high probability of success and favorable outcome (Lok, 2003). All major cytotoxic treatments except methotrexate increase the risk of early menopause (Savage, 2015a).

In some cases, secondary tumors can develop as a result of cancer treatment. Etoposide-based combination chemotherapy has been associated with an increased risk of leukemia, colon cancer, melanoma, and breast cancer up to 25 years after treatment for GTN. An overall 50-percent excess risk was observed (Rustin, 1996). Etoposide is therefore reserved to treat patients who are likely to be resistant to single-agent chemotherapy and, in particular, those with high-risk metastatic disease.

Quiescent Gestational Trophoblastic Disease

Patients with persistent mild elevations (usually ≤50 mIU/mL) of true β-hCG may have a dormant premalignant condition if no tumor is identified by physical examination or imaging studies (Khanlian, 2003). In this instance, phantom β-hCG, described next, should also be conclusively excluded as a possibility. The low β-hCG titers may persist for months or years before disappearing. Chemotherapy and surgery usually have no effect. Hormonal contraception may be helpful in lowering titers to an undetectable level, but patients are closely monitored since metastatic GTN may eventually develop (Khanlian, 2003; Kohorn, 2002; Palmieri, 2007).

■ Phantom β-hCG

Occasionally, persistent mild elevations of serum β-hCG are detected that lead physicians to erroneously treat patients with cytotoxic chemotherapy or hysterectomy or both, when in reality no true β-hCG molecule or trophoblastic disease is present (Cole, 1998; Rotmensch, 2000). This "phantom" β-hCG reading results from heterophilic antibodies in the serum that interfere with the β-hCG immunoassay and cause a false-positive result.

Several steps can clarify the diagnosis. First, a urine pregnancy test can be performed. With phantom β-hCG, the heterophilic antibodies are not filtered or renally excreted. Thus, these test-altering antibodies will be absent from the urine, and urine testing will show true negative results for β-hCG. Importantly, to conclusively exclude trophoblastic disease by this method, the index serum β-hCG level must be significantly higher than the detection threshold of the urine test. Second, performing serial dilutions of the serum sample leads to a proportional decrease in the β-hCG level if β-hCG is truly present. However, phantom β-hCG measurements will be unchanged by dilution. In addition, if phantom β-hCG is suspected, some specialized laboratories may be able to block the heterophilic antibodies. Last, heterophilic antibodies will cause interference with one assay, but they may bind poorly to another assay's antibodies. Thus, switching β-hCG assay kits to one by a different manufacturer may accurately demonstrate the absence of true β-hCG (Cole, 1998; Olsen, 2001; Rotmensch, 2000).

REFERENCES

Alazzam M, Tidy J, Hancock BW, et al: First line chemotherapy in low risk gestational trophoblastic neoplasia. Cochrane Database Syst Rev 7:CD007102, 2012a

Alazzam M, Tidy J, Osborne R, et al: Chemotherapy for resistant or recurrent gestational trophoblastic neoplasia. Cochrane Database Syst Rev 12: CD008891, 2012b

Alifrangis C, Agarwal R, Short D, et al: EMA/CO for high-risk gestational trophoblastic neoplasia: good outcomes with induction low-dose etoposide-cisplatin and genetic analysis. J Clin Oncol 31(2):280, 2013

Allen JE, King MR, Farrar DF, et al: Postmolar surveillance at a trophoblastic disease center that serves indigent women. Am J Obstet Gynecol 188:1151, 2003

Altman AD, Bentley B, Murray S, et al: Maternal age-related rates of gestational trophoblastic disease. Obstet Gynecol 112:244, 2008

American College of Obstetricians and Gynecologists: Diagnosis and treatment of gestational trophoblastic disease. Practice Bulletin No. 53, June 2004, Reaffirmed 2014

Azuma C, Saji F, Tokugawa Y, et al: Application of gene amplification by polymerase chain reaction to genetic analysis of molar mitochondrial DNA: the detection of anuclear empty ovum as the cause of complete mole. Gynecol Oncol 40:29, 1991

Baergen RN, Rutgers JL, Young RH, et al: Placental site trophoblastic tumor: a study of 55 cases and review of the literature emphasizing factors of prognostic significance. Gynecol Oncol 100:511, 2006

Benson CB, Genest DR, Bernstein MR, et al: Sonographic appearance of first trimester complete hydatidiform moles. Ultrasound Obstet Gynecol 16:188, 2000

Berkowitz RS, Bernstein MR, Harlow BL, et al: Case-control study of risk factors for partial molar pregnancy. Am J Obstet Gynecol 173:788, 1995

Berkowitz RS, Cramer DW, Bernstein MR, et al: Risk factors for complete molar pregnancy from a case-control study. Am J Obstet Gynecol 152:1016, 1985

Berkowitz RS, Im SS, Bernstein MR, et al: Gestational trophoblastic disease: subsequent pregnancy outcome, including repeat molar pregnancy. J Reprod Med 43:81, 1998

Bower M, Newlands ES, Holden L, et al: EMA/CO for high-risk gestational trophoblastic tumors: results from a cohort of 272 patients. J Clin Oncol 15: 2636, 1997

Braga A, Maesta I, Michelin OC, et al: Maternal and perinatal outcomes of first pregnancy after chemotherapy for gestational trophoblastic neoplasia in Brazilian women. Gynecol Oncol 112:568, 2009

Burton JL, Lidbury EA, Gillespie AM, et al: Overdiagnosis of hydatidiform mole in early tubal ectopic pregnancy. Histopathology 38:409, 2001

Cagayan MS: Sexual dysfunction as a complication of treatment of gestational trophoblastic neoplasia. J Reprod Med 53:595, 2008

Cagayan MS, Lu-Lasala LR: Management of gestational trophoblastic neoplasia with metastasis to the central nervous system: a 12-year review at the Phillippe General Hospital. J Reprod Med 51:785, 2006

Cao Y, Xiang Y, Feng F, et al: Surgical resection in the management of pulmonary metastatic disease of gestational trophoblastic neoplasia. Int J Gynecol Cancer 19:798, 2009

Castrillon DH, Sun D, Weremowicz S, et al: Discrimination of complete hydatidiform mole from its mimics by immunohistochemistry of the paternally imprinted gene product p57KIP2. Am J Surg Pathol 25:1225, 2001

Chalouhi GE, Golfier F, Soignon P, et al: Methotrexate for 2000 FIGO low-risk gestational trophoblastic neoplasia patients: efficacy and toxicity. Am J Obstet Gynecol 200(6):643.e1, 2009

Chapman-Davis E, Hoekstra AV, Rademaker AW, et al: Treatment of non-metastatic and metastatic low-risk gestational trophoblastic neoplasia: factors associated with resistance to single-agent methotrexate chemotherapy. Gynecol Oncol 125(3):572, 2012

Chen LM, Lengyel ER, Bethan PC: Single-agent pulse dactinomycin has only modest activity for methotrexate-resistant gestational trophoblastic neoplasia. Gynecol Oncol 94:204, 2004

Cheung AN, Khoo US, Lai CY, et al: Metastatic trophoblastic disease after an initial diagnosis of partial hydatidiform mole: genotyping and chromosome in situ hybridization analysis. Cancer 100:1411, 2004

Chew SH, Perlman EJ, Williams R, et al: Morphology and DNA content analysis in the evaluation of first trimester placentas for partial hydatidiform mole (PHM). Hum Pathol 31:914, 2000

Chong CY, Koh CF: Hydatidiform mole in Kandang Kerbau Hospital: a 5-year review. Singapore Med J 40:265, 1999

Clark RM, Nevadunsky NS, Ghosh S, et al: The evolving role of hysterectomy in gestational trophoblastic neoplasia at the New England Trophoblastic Disease Center. J Reprod Med 5:194, 2010

Cole LA: Phantom hCG and phantom choriocarcinoma. Gynecol Oncol 71:325, 1998

Cole LA, Khanlian SA, Muller CY: Blood test for placental site trophoblastic tumor and nontrophoblastic malignancy for evaluating patients with low positive human chorionic gonadotropin results. J Reprod Med 53:457, 2008

Costa HL, Doyle P: Influence of oral contraceptives in the development of post-molar trophoblastic neoplasia—a systematic review. Gynecol Oncol 100:579, 2006

Covens A, Filiaci VL, Burger RA, et al: Phase II trial of pulse dactinomycin as salvage therapy for failed low-risk gestational trophoblastic neoplasia: a Gynecologic Oncology Group study. Cancer 107(6):1280, 2006

Darby S, Jolley I, Pennington S: Does chest CT matter in the staging of GTN? Gynecol Oncol 112:155, 2009

Davis MR, Howitt BE, Quade BJ, et al: Epithelioid trophoblastic tumor: a single institution case series at the New England Trophoblastic Disease Center. Gynecol Oncol 137(3):456, 2015

Dhillon T, Palmieri C, Sebire NJ, et al: Value of whole body [18]FDG-PET to identify the active site of gestational trophoblastic neoplasia. J Reprod Med 51:979, 2006

Diver E, May T, Vargas R, et al: Changes in clinical presentation of post-term choriocarcinoma at the New England Trophoblastic Disease Center in recent years. Gynecol Oncol 130(3):483, 2013

Drake RD, Rao GG, McIntire DD, et al: Gestational trophoblastic disease among Hispanic women: a 21-year hospital-based study. Gynecol Oncol 103(1):81, 2006

Elias KM, Goldstein DP, Berkowitz RS: Complete hydatidiform mole in women older than age 50. J Reprod Med 55:208, 2010

Escobar PF, Lurain JR, Singh DK, et al: Treatment of high-risk gestational trophoblastic neoplasia with etoposide, methotrexate, actinomycin D, cyclophosphamide, and vincristine chemotherapy. Gynecol Oncol 91:552, 2003

Fallahian M: Familial gestational trophoblastic disease. Placenta 24:797, 2003

Fan JB, Surti U, Taillon-Miller P, et al: Paternal origins of complete hydatidiform moles proven by whole genome single-nucleotide polymorphism haplotyping. Genomics 79:58, 2002

Feltmate CM, Genest DR, Wise L, et al: Placental site trophoblastic tumor: a 17-year experience at the New England Trophoblastic Disease Center. Gynecol Oncol 82:415, 2001

Feltmate CM, Growdon WB, Wolfberg AJ, et al: Clinical characteristics of persistent gestational trophoblastic neoplasia after partial hydatidiform molar pregnancy. J Reprod Med 51:902, 2006

Ferreira EG, Maesta I, Michelin OC, et al: Assessment of quality of life and psychologic aspects in patients with gestational trophoblastic disease. J Reprod Med 54:239, 2009

FIGO Committee on Gynecologic Oncology: Current FIGO staging for cancer of the vagina, fallopian tube, ovary, and gestational trophoblastic neoplasia. Int J Gynaecol Obstet 105:3, 2009

FIGO Oncology Committee: FIGO staging for gestational trophoblastic neoplasia 2000. Int J Gynaecol Obstet 77:285, 2002

Fleming EL, Garrett L, Growdon WB, et al: The changing role of thoracotomy in gestational trophoblastic neoplasia at the New England Trophoblastic Disease Center. J Reprod Med 53:493, 2008

Fu J, Fang F, Xie L, et al: Prophylactic chemotherapy for hydatidiform mole to prevent gestational trophoblastic neoplasia. Cochrane Database Syst Rev 10:CD007289, 2012

Fung Kee FK, Eason E, Crane J, et al: Prevention of Rh alloimmunization. J Obstet Gynaecol Can 25:765, 2003

Gaffield ME, Kapp N, Curtis KM: Combined oral contraceptive and intra-uterine device use among women with gestational trophoblastic disease. Contraception 80:363, 2009

Garner EI, Garrett A, Goldstein DP, et al: Significance of chest computed tomography findings in the evaluation and treatment of persistent gestational trophoblastic neoplasia. J Reprod Med 49:411, 2004

Garrett LA, Garner EI, Feltmate CM, et al: Subsequent pregnancy outcomes in patients with molar pregnancy and persistent gestational trophoblastic neoplasia. J Reprod Med 53(7):481, 2008

Gillespie AM, Lidbury EA, Tidy JA, et al: The clinical presentation, treatment, and outcome of patients diagnosed with possible ectopic molar gestation. Int J Gynecol Cancer 14:366, 2004

Gleeson NC, Finan MA, Fiorica JV, et al: Nonmetastatic gestational trophoblastic disease: weekly methotrexate compared with 8-day methotrexate-folinic acid. Eur J Gynaecol Oncol 14:461, 1993

Golfier F, Raudrant D, Frappart L, et al: First epidemiological data from the French Trophoblastic Disease Reference Center. Am J Obstet Gynecol 196:172.e1, 2007

Harvey RA, Pursglove HD, Schmid P, et al: Human chorionic gonadotropin free beta-subunit measurement as a marker of placental site trophoblastic tumors. J Reprod Med 53:643, 2008

Hassadia A, Gillespie A, Tidy J, et al: Placental site trophoblastic tumour: clinical features and management. Gynecol Oncol 99:603, 2005

Homesley HD, Blessing JA, Rettenmaier M, et al: Weekly intramuscular methotrexate for nonmetastatic gestational trophoblastic disease. Obstet Gynecol 72:413, 1988

Homesley HD, Blessing JA, Schlaerth J, et al: Rapid escalation of weekly intramuscular methotrexate for nonmetastatic gestational trophoblastic disease: a Gynecologic Oncology Group study. Gynecol Oncol 39:305, 1990

Hyman DM, Bakios L, Gualtiere G, et al: Placental site trophoblastic tumor: analysis of presentation, treatment, and outcome. Gynecol Oncol 129(1):58, 2013

Jauniaux E: Partial moles: from postnatal to prenatal diagnosis. Placenta 20:379, 1999

Johns J, Greenwold N, Buckley S, et al: A prospective study of ultrasound screening for molar pregnancies in missed miscarriages. Ultrasound Obstet Gynecol 25:493, 2005

Joneborg U, Marions L. Current clinical features of complete and partial hydatidiform mole in Sweden. J Reprod Med 59(1–2):51, 2014

Kajii T, Ohama K: Androgenetic origin of hydatidiform mole. Nature 268:633, 1977

Kang WD, Choi HS, Kim SM: Weekly methotrexate (50 mg/m^2) without dose escalation as a primary regimen for low-risk gestational trophoblastic neoplasia. Gynecol Oncol 117(3):477, 2010

Kerkmeijer LG, Wielsma S, Massuger LF, et al: Recurrent gestational trophoblastic disease after hCG normalization following hydatidiform mole in The Netherlands. Gynecol Oncol 106:142, 2007

Khan F, Everard J, Ahmed S, et al: Low-risk persistent gestational trophoblastic disease treated with low-dose methotrexate: efficacy, acute and long-term effects. Br J Cancer 89:2197, 2003

Khanlian SA, Smith HO, Cole LA: Persistent low levels of human chorionic gonadotropin: a premalignant gestational trophoblastic disease. Am J Obstet Gynecol 188:1254, 2003

Kim SJ, Lee C, Kwon SY, et al: Studying changes in the incidence, diagnosis and management of GTD: the South Korean model. J Reprod Med 49:643, 2004

Kohorn EI: Persistent low-level "real" human chorionic gonadotropin: a clinical challenge and a therapeutic dilemma. Gynecol Oncol 85:315, 2002

Kurman RJ, Carcangiu ML, Herrington CS, et al (eds): WHO Classification of Tumours of Female Reproductive Organs, 4th ed. Lyon, International Agency for Research on Cancer, 2014

La Vecchia C, Parazzini F, Decarli A, et al: Age of parents and risk of gestational trophoblastic disease. J Natl Cancer Inst 73:639, 1984

Lavie I, Rao GG, Castrillon DH, et al: Duration of human chorionic gonadotropin surveillance for partial hydatidiform moles. Am J Obstet Gynecol 192:1362, 2005

Lawler SD, Fisher RA: Genetic studies in hydatidiform mole with clinical correlations. Placenta 8:77, 1987

Lawler SD, Fisher RA, Dent J: A prospective genetic study of complete and partial hydatidiform moles. Am J Obstet Gynecol 164:1270, 1991

Lazarus E, Hulka C, Siewert B, et al: Sonographic appearance of early complete molar pregnancies. J Ultrasound Med 18:589, 1999

Lee KH, Lee IH, Kim BG, et al: Clinicopathologic characteristics of malignant germ cell tumors in the ovaries of Korean women: a Korean Gynecologic Oncology Group Study. Int J Gynecol Cancer 19:84, 2009

Limpongsanurak S: Prophylactic actinomycin D for high-risk complete hydatidiform mole. J Reprod Med 46:110, 2001

Lindholm H, Flam F: The diagnosis of molar pregnancy by sonography and gross morphology. Acta Obstet Gynecol Scand 78:6, 1999

Lok CA, Ansink AC, Grootfaam D, et al: Treatment and prognosis of post term choriocarcinoma in The Netherlands. Gynecol Oncol 103:698, 2006

Lok CA, van der Houwen C, ten Kate-Booij MJ, et al: Pregnancy after EMA/CO for gestational trophoblastic disease: a report from The Netherlands. BJOG 110:560, 2003

Loukovaara M, Pukkala E, Lehtovirta P, et al: Epidemiology of hydatidiform mole in Finland, 1975 to 2001. Eur J Gynaecol Oncol 26:207, 2005

Lu WG, Ye F, Shen YM, et al: EMA-CO chemotherapy for high-risk gestational trophoblastic neoplasia: a clinical analysis of 54 patients. Int J Gynecol Cancer 18:357, 2008

Lurain JR, Nejad B: Secondary chemotherapy for high-risk gestational trophoblastic neoplasia. Gynecol Oncol 97:618, 2005

Lurain JR, Singh DK, Schink JC: Management of metastatic high-risk gestational trophoblastic neoplasia: FIGO stage II-IV: risk factor score > or = 7. J Reprod Med 55:199, 2010

Lybol C, Sweep FC, Harvey R, et al: Relapse rates after two versus three consolidation courses of methotrexate in the treatment of low-risk gestational trophoblastic neoplasia. Gynecol Oncol 125(3):576, 2012

Lybol C, Thomas CM, Bulten J, et al: Increase in the incidence of gestational trophoblastic disease in The Netherlands. Gynecol Oncol 121(2):334, 2011

Machtinger R, Gotlieb WH, Korach J, et al: Placental site trophoblastic tumor: outcome of five cases including fertility-preserving management. Gynecol Oncol 96:56, 2005

Mackenzie F, Mathers A, Kennedy J: Invasive hydatidiform mole presenting as an acute primary haemoperitoneum. BJOG 100:953, 1993

Mangili G, Garavaglia E, Cavoretto P, et al: Clinical presentation of hydatidiform mole in northern Italy: has it changed in the last 20 years? Am J Obstet Gynecol 2008 198(3):302.e1–4, 2008

Mangili G, Garavaglia E, Frigerio L, et al: Management of low-risk gestational trophoblastic tumors with etoposide (VP16) in patients resistant to methotrexate. Gynecol Oncol 61:218, 1996

Marcorelles P, Audrezet MP, Le Bris MJ, et al: Diagnosis and outcome of complete hydatidiform mole coexisting with a live twin fetus. Eur J Obstet Gynecol Reprod Biol 118:21, 2005

Massad LS, Abu-Rustum NR, Lee SS, et al: Poor compliance with postmolar surveillance and treatment protocols by indigent women. Obstet Gynecol 96:940, 2000

Matsui H, Iitsuka Y, Yamazawa K, et al: Changes in the incidence of molar pregnancies: a population-based study in Chiba Prefecture and Japan between 1974 and 2000. Hum Reprod 18:172, 2003

Matsui H, Sekiya S, Hando T, et al: Hydatidiform mole coexistent with a twin live fetus: a national collaborative study in Japan. Hum Reprod 15:608, 2000

Matsui H, Suzuka K, Yamazawa K, et al: Relapse rate of patients with low-risk gestational trophoblastic tumor initially treated with single-agent chemotherapy. Gynecol Oncol 96:616, 2005

McNeish IA, Strickland S, Holden L, et al: Low-risk persistent gestational trophoblastic disease: outcome after initial treatment with low-dose methotrexate and folinic acid from 1992 to 2000. J Clin Oncol 20:1838, 2002

Merchant SH, Amin MB, Viswanatha DS, et al: p57KIP2 immunohistochemistry in early molar pregnancies: emphasis on its complementary role in the differential diagnosis of hydropic abortuses. Hum Pathol 36:180, 2005

Mungan T, Kuscu E, Dabakoglu T, et al: Hydatidiform mole: clinical analysis of 310 patients. Int J Gynaecol Obstet 52:233, 1996

Newlands ES, Holden L, Seckl MJ, et al: Management of brain metastases in patients with high-risk gestational trophoblastic tumors. J Reprod Med 47:465, 2002

Newlands ES, Mulholland PJ, Holden L, et al: Etoposide and cisplatin/etoposide, methotrexate, and actinomycin D (EMA) chemotherapy for patients with high-risk gestational trophoblastic tumors refractory to EMA/cyclophosphamide and vincristine chemotherapy and patients presenting with metastatic placental site trophoblastic tumors. J Clin Oncol 18:854, 2000

Ngan HY: The practicability of FIGO 2000 staging for gestational trophoblastic neoplasia. Int J Gynecol Cancer 14:202, 2004

Numnum TM, Leath CA III, Straughn JM Jr, et al: Occult choriocarcinoma discovered by positron emission tomography/computed tomography imaging following a successful pregnancy. Gynecol Oncol 97:713, 2005

Olsen TG, Hubert PR, Nycum LR: Falsely elevated human chorionic gonadotropin leading to unnecessary therapy. Obstet Gynecol 98:843, 2001

Osborne R, Filiaci V, Schink J, et al: A randomized phase III trial comparing weekly parenteral methotrexate and "pulsed" dactinomycin as primary management for low-risk gestational trophoblastic neoplasia: a Gynecologic Oncology Group study. Gynecol Oncol 108:S2, 2008

Palmer JE, Macdonald M, Wells M, et al: Epithelioid trophoblastic tumor: a review of the literature. J Reprod Med 53:465, 2008

Palmer JR, Driscoll SG, Rosenberg L: Oral contraceptive use and risk of gestational trophoblastic tumors. J Natl Cancer Inst 91:635, 1999

Palmieri C, Dhillon T, Fisher RA, et al: Management and outcome of healthy women with a persistently elevated beta-hCG. Gynecol Oncol 106:35, 2007

Papadopoulos AJ, Foskett M, Seckl MJ, et al: Twenty-five years' clinical experience with placental site trophoblastic tumors. J Reprod Med 47:460, 2002

Paradinas FJ, Fisher RA, Browne P, et al: Diploid hydatidiform moles with fetal red blood cells in molar villi: 1. Pathology, incidence, and prognosis. J Pathol 181:183, 1997

Parazzini F, Cipriani S, Mangili G, et al: Oral contraceptives and risk of gestational trophoblastic disease. Contraception 65:425, 2002

Parazzini F, La Vecchia C, Mangili G, et al: Dietary factors and risk of trophoblastic disease. Am J Obstet Gynecol 158:93, 1988

Parazzini F, La Vecchia C, Pampallona S: Parental age and risk of complete and partial hydatidiform mole. BJOG 93:582, 1986

Parazzini F, Mangili G, La Vecchia C, et al: Risk factors for gestational trophoblastic disease: a separate analysis of complete and partial hydatidiform moles. Obstet Gynecol 78:1039, 1991

Patel SM, Desai A: Management of drug resistant gestational trophoblastic neoplasia. J Reprod Med 55:296, 2010

Pezeshki M, Hancock BW, Silcocks P, et al: The role of repeat uterine evacuation in the management of persistent gestational trophoblastic disease. Gynecol Oncol 95:423, 2004

Pisal N, North C, Tidy J, et al: Role of hysterectomy in management of gestational trophoblastic disease. Gynecol Oncol 87:190, 2002

Powles T, Savage P, Short D, et al: Residual lung lesions after completion of chemotherapy for gestational trophoblastic neoplasia: should we operate? Br J Cancer 94:51, 2006

Price JM, Hancock BW, Tidy J, et al: Screening for central nervous system disease in metastatic gestational trophoblastic neoplasia. J Reprod Med 55:301, 2010

Rodabaugh KJ, Bernstein MR, Goldstein DP, et al: Natural history of postterm choriocarcinoma. J Reprod Med 43:75, 1998

Ronnett BM, DeScipio C, Murphy KM. Hydatidiform moles: ancillary techniques to refine diagnosis. Int J Gynecol Pathol 30(2):101, 2011

Rotmensch S, Cole LA: False diagnosis and needless therapy of presumed malignant disease in women with false-positive human chorionic gonadotropin concentrations. Lancet 355:712, 2000

Rustin GJ, Newlands ES, Lutz JM, et al: Combination but not single-agent methotrexate chemotherapy for gestational trophoblastic tumors increases the incidence of second tumors. J Clin Oncol 14:2769, 1996

Savage P, Cooke R, O'Nions J, et al: Effects of single-agent and combination chemotherapy of gestational trophoblastic tumors on risks of second malignancy and early menopause. J Clin Oncol 33(5):472, 2015a

Savage P, Kelpanides I, Tuthill M, et al: Brain metastases in gestational trophoblast neoplasia: an update on incidence, management and outcome. Gynecol Oncol 137(1):73, 2015b

Savage P, Williams J, Wong SL, et al: The demographics of molar pregnancies in England and Wales from 2000–2009. J Reprod Med 5:341, 2010

Schechter NR, Mychalczak B, Jones W, et al: Prognosis of patients treated with whole-brain radiation therapy for metastatic gestational trophoblastic disease. Gynecol Oncol 68:183, 1998

Schmid P, Nagai Y, Agarwal R, et al: Prognostic markers and long-term outcome of placental-site trophoblastic tumors: a retrospective observational study. Lancet 374:48, 2009

Sebire NJ, Fisher RA, Foskett M, et al: Risk of recurrent hydatidiform mole and subsequent pregnancy outcome following complete or partial hydatidiform molar pregnancy. BJOG 110:22, 2003

Sebire NJ, Foskett M, Fisher RA, et al: Persistent gestational trophoblastic disease is rarely, if ever, derived from nonmolar first-trimester miscarriage. Med Hypoth 64:689, 2005a

Sebire NJ, Foskett M, Fisher RA, et al: Risk of partial and complete hydatidiform molar pregnancy in relation to maternal age. BJOG 109:99, 2002a

Sebire NJ, Foskett M, Paradinas FJ, et al: Outcome of twin pregnancies with complete hydatidiform mole and healthy cotwin. Lancet 359:2165, 2002b

Sebire NJ, Foskett M, Short D, et al: Shortened duration of human chorionic gonadotrophin surveillance following complete or partial hydatidiform mole: evidence for revised protocol of a UK regional trophoblastic disease unit. BJOG 114:760, 2007

Sebire NJ, Lindsay I, Fisher RA, et al: Overdiagnosis of complete and partial hydatidiform mole in tubal ectopic pregnancies. Int J Gynecol Pathol 24:260, 2005b

Sebire NJ, Rees H, Paradinas F, et al: The diagnostic implications of routine ultrasound examination in histologically confirmed early molar pregnancies. Ultrasound Obstet Gynecol 18:662, 2001

Seckl MJ, Dhillon T, Dancey G, et al: Increased gestational age at evacuation of a complete hydatidiform mole: does it correlate with increased risk of requiring chemotherapy? J Reprod Med 49:527, 2004

Seckl MJ, Fisher RA, Salerno G, et al: Choriocarcinoma and partial hydatidiform moles. Lancet 356:36, 2000

Seckl MJ, Rustin GJS, Newlands ES, et al: Pulmonary embolism, pulmonary hypertension, and choriocarcinoma. Lancet 338:1313, 1991

Seckl MJ, Sebire NJ, Berkowitz RS: Gestational trophoblastic disease. Lancet 376:717, 2010

Sharma S, Jagdev S, Coleman RE, et al: Serosal complications of single-agent low-dose methotrexate used in gestational trophoblastic diseases: first reported case of methotrexate-induced peritonitis. Br J Cancer 81:1037, 1999

Shih IM, Kurman RJ: Epithelioid trophoblastic tumor: a neoplasm distinct from choriocarcinoma and placental site trophoblastic tumor simulating carcinoma. Am J Surg Pathol 22:1393, 1998

Sita-Lumsden A, Short D, Lindsay I, et al: Treatment outcomes for 618 women with gestational trophoblastic tumours following a molar pregnancy at the Charing Cross Hospital, 2000–2009. Br J Cancer 107(11):1810, 2012

Smith HO, Hilgers RD, Bedrick EJ, et al: Ethnic differences at risk for gestational trophoblastic disease in New Mexico: a 25-year population-based study. Am J Obstet Gynecol 188:357, 2003

Soto-Wright V, Bernstein M, Goldstein DP, et al: The changing clinical presentation of complete molar pregnancy. Obstet Gynecol 86:775, 1995

Suzuka K, Matsui H, Iitsuka Y, et al: Adjuvant hysterectomy in low-risk gestational trophoblastic disease. Obstet Gynecol 97:431, 2001

Taylor F, Grew T, Everard J, et al: The outcome of patients with low risk gestational trophoblastic neoplasia treated with single agent intramuscular methotrexate and oral folinic acid. Eur J Cancer 49(15):3184, 2013a

Taylor JS, Viera L, Caputo TA, et al: Unsuccessful planned conservative resection of placental site trophoblastic tumor. Obstet Gynecol 121(2 Pt 2 Suppl 1):465, 2013b

Tham BW, Everard JE, Tidy JA, et al: Gestational trophoblastic disease in the Asian population of northern England and North Wales. BJOG 110:555, 2003

Tidy JA, Gillespie AM, Bright N, et al: Gestational trophoblastic disease: a study of mode of evacuation and subsequent need for treatment with chemotherapy. Gynecol Oncol 78:309, 2000

Tidy JA, Rustin GJ, Newlands ES, et al: Presentation and management of choriocarcinoma after nonmolar pregnancy. BJOG 102:715, 1995

Tuncer ZS, Bernstein MR, Goldstein DP, et al: Outcome of pregnancies occurring within 1 year of hydatidiform mole. Obstet Gynecol 94:588, 1999

Uberti EM, Fajardo MD, da Cunha AG, et al: Prevention of postmolar gestational trophoblastic neoplasia using prophylactic single bolus dose of actinomycin D in high-risk hydatidiform mole: a simple, effective, secure and low-cost approach without adverse effects on compliance to general follow-up or subsequent treatment. Gynecol Oncol 114:299, 2009

van Trommel NE, Lok CA, Bulten H, et al: Long-term outcome of placental site trophoblastic tumor in The Netherlands. J Reprod Med 58(5–6):224, 2013

van Trommel NE, Massuger LF, Verheijen RH, et al: The curative effect of a second curettage in persistent trophoblastic disease: a retrospective cohort survey. Gynecol Oncol 99:6, 2005

Vargas R, Barroilhet LM, Esselen K, et al: Subsequent pregnancy outcomes after complete and partial molar pregnancy, recurrent molar pregnancy, and gestational trophoblastic neoplasia: an update from the New England Trophoblastic Disease Center. J Reprod Med 59(5–6):188, 2014

Wang J, Short D, Sebire NJ, et al: Salvage chemotherapy of relapsed or high-risk gestational trophoblastic neoplasia (GTN) with paclitaxel/cisplatin alternating with paclitaxel/etoposide (TP/TE). Ann Oncol 19:1578, 2008

Wenzel L, Berkowitz R, Robinson S, et al: The psychological, social, and sexual consequences of gestational trophoblastic disease. Gynecol Oncol 46:74, 1992

Williams J, Short D, Dayal L, et al: Effect of early pregnancy following chemotherapy on disease relapse and fetal outcome in women treated for gestational trophoblastic neoplasia. J Reprod Med 59(5–6):248, 2014

Wolfberg AJ, Feltmate C, Goldstein DP, et al: Low risk of relapse after achieving undetectable hCG levels in women with complete molar pregnancy. Obstet Gynecol 104:551, 2004

Wong JM, Liu D, Lurain JR: Reproductive outcomes after multiagent chemotherapy for high-risk gestational trophoblastic neoplasia. J Reprod Med 59(5–6):204, 2014

Yarandi F, Eftekhar Z, Shojaei H, et al: Pulse methotrexate versus pulse actinomycin D in the treatment of low-risk gestational trophoblastic neoplasia. Int J Gynaecol Obstet 103:33, 2008

Zhou Q, Lei XY, Xie Q, et al: Sonographic and Doppler imaging in the diagnosis and treatment of gestational trophoblastic disease: a 12-year experience. J Ultrasound Med 24:15, 2005

SECTION 5
ASPECTS OF GYNECOLOGIC SURGERY

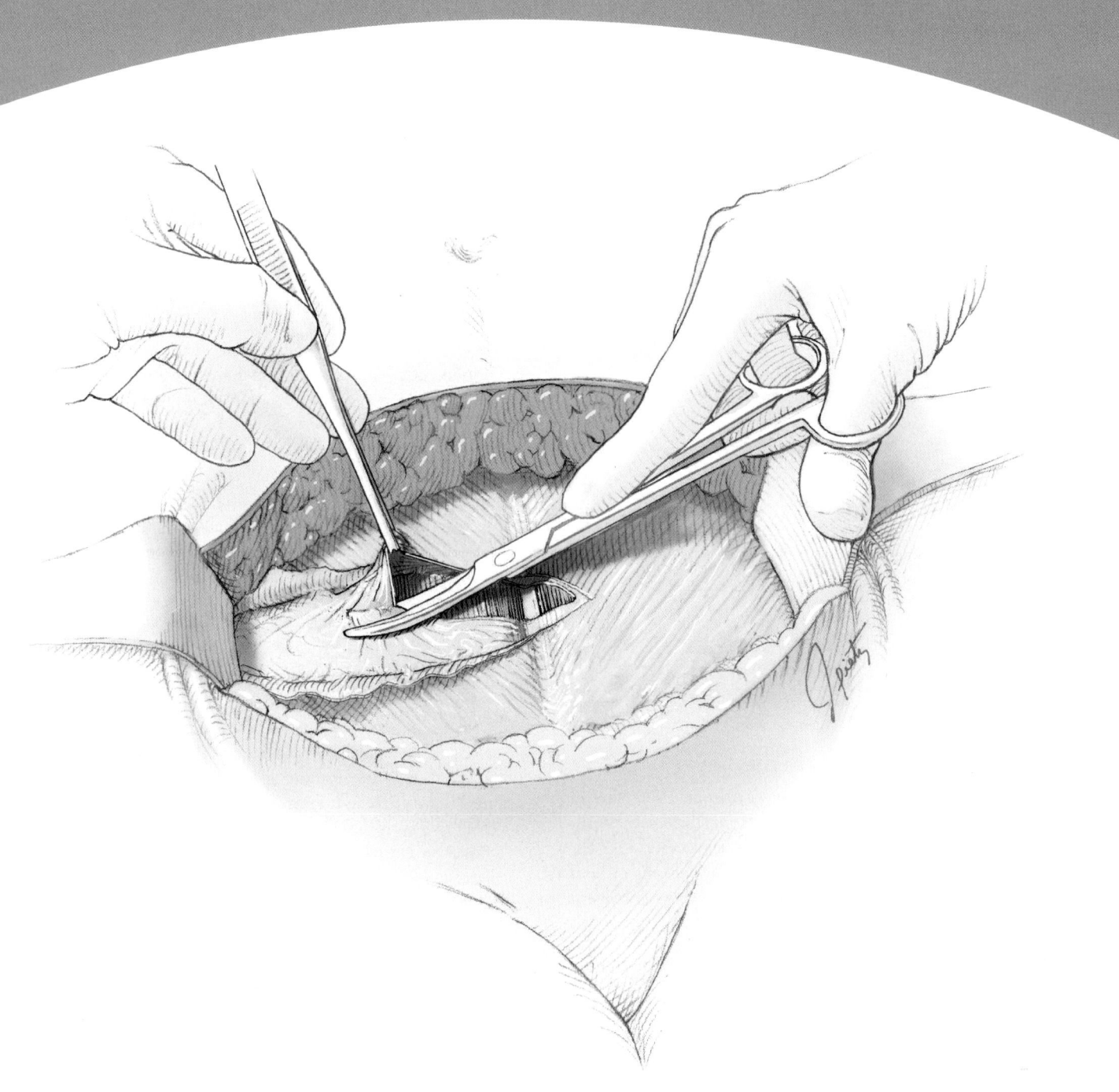

CHAPTER 38

Anatomy

ANTERIOR ABDOMINAL WALL

The anterior abdominal wall provides core support to the human torso, confines abdominal viscera, and contributes muscular action for functions such as respiration and elimination. In gynecology, an understanding of the layered structure of the anterior abdominal wall is needed to effectively enter the peritoneal cavity for surgery without neurovascular complications.

■ Skin and Subcutaneous Layer

Within the skin, the term *Langer lines* describes the orientation of dermal fibers. In the anterior abdominal wall, they are arranged primarily transversely (Fig. 38-1). As a result, vertical skin incisions sustain more lateral tension and thus in general, develop wider scars compared with transverse skin incisions.

The subcutaneous layer lies deep to the skin. In the anterior abdominal wall, this layer is separated into a superficial, predominantly fatty layer known as *Camper fascia* and a deeper, more membranous layer known as *Scarpa fascia* (Fig. 38-2). Camper and Scarpa fasciae are not discrete layers but represent a continuum. If traced caudally, scarpa fascia is continuous with Colles fascia in the perineum.

Clinically, Scarpa fascia is better developed in the lower abdomen and during surgery can be best identified in the lateral portions of a low transverse incision, just superficial to the rectus fascia. In contrast, this fascia is rarely recognized during midline incisions.

■ Rectus Sheath

The *external oblique*, *internal oblique*, and *transversus abdominis muscles* (flank muscles) all contain a lateral muscular portion and medial fibrous aponeurotic portion. All of their aponeuroses conjoin, and these layers create the rectus sheath (see Fig. 38-2). In the midline, the aponeurotic layers fuse to create the linea alba. In the lower abdomen, transition from the muscular to the aponeurotic component of the external oblique muscle takes place along a vertical line through the anterior superior iliac spine. Transition from muscle to aponeurosis for the internal oblique and transversus abdominis muscles takes place at a more medial site. Accordingly, during low transverse incisions, muscle fibers of the internal oblique muscle are often noted below the aponeurotic layer of the external oblique muscle.

The anatomy of the rectus sheath above and below the *arcuate line* has significance (see Fig. 38-2). This horizontal line defines the level at which the rectus sheath passes only anterior to the rectus abdominis muscle, and this line typically lies midway between the umbilicus and pubic symphysis. Cephalad to the arcuate line, the rectus sheath lies both anterior and posterior to the rectus abdominis muscle. At this level, the anterior rectus sheath is formed by the aponeurosis of the external oblique muscle and the split aponeurosis of the internal oblique muscle. The posterior rectus sheath is formed by the split aponeurosis of the internal oblique muscle and aponeurosis of the transversus abdominis muscle. Caudad to the arcuate line, all aponeurotic layers pass anterior to the rectus abdominis muscle. Thus, in the lower abdomen, the posterior surface of the rectus abdominis muscle is in direct contact with the transversalis fascia, described next.

Surgically, because the aponeuroses of the internal oblique and transversus abdominis muscles in the lower abdomen fuse, only two layers are identified during low transverse fascial incisions. In contrast, during midline vertical incision, only one fascial layer, namely, the linea alba, is encountered.

Similar to skin fibers, the flank muscle and rectus sheath fibers are oriented primarily transversely. Thus, suture lines placed in a vertical fascial incision must withstand more tension than those in a transverse incision. As a result, vertical fascial incisions are more prone to dehiscence and hernia formation. In addition to incisional hernias, ventral wall hernias are most common along the linea alba. Another type of anterior abdominal wall hernia, the Spiegelian hernia, is rare and forms at the lateral rectus abdominis border, typically at the level of the arcuate line (Fig. 11-8, p. 267).

■ Transversalis Fascia

This thin fibrous tissue layer lies between the inner surface of the transversus abdominis muscle and preperitoneal fat. Thus,

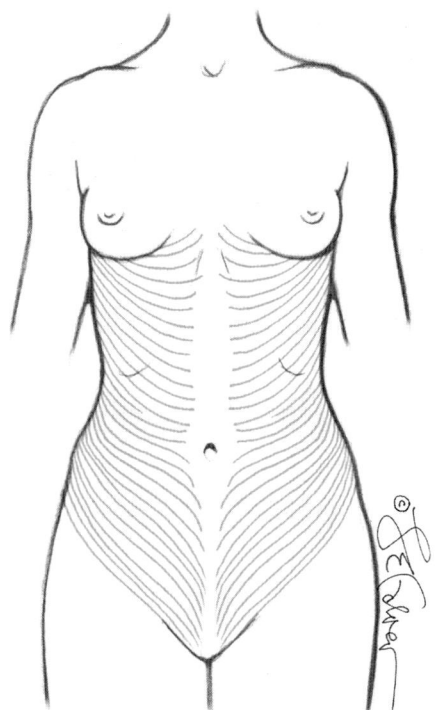

FIGURE 38-1 Langer lines of skin tension.

it serves as part of the general fascial layer that lines the abdominal cavity (see Fig. 38-2) (Memon, 1999). Inferiorly, the transversalis fascia blends with the periosteum of the pubic bones.

Surgically, this fascia is best recognized as the layer bluntly or sharply dissected off the anterior surface of the bladder during entry into the abdominal cavity. This is the layer of tissue that is last penetrated to gain extraperitoneal entry into the retropubic space (p. 813).

■ Peritoneum

The peritoneum that lines the inner surface of the abdominal walls is termed *parietal peritoneum*. In the anterior abdominal wall, there are five elevations of parietal peritoneum that are raised by different structures (see Fig. 38-2). All five converge toward the umbilicus and are known as *umbilical ligaments*.

The single *median umbilical ligament* is formed by the *urachus*, an obliterated tube that extends from the apex of the bladder to the umbilicus. In fetal life, the urachus, which is a fibrous remnant of the allantois, extends from the umbilical cord to the urogenital sinus, which gives rise to the bladder. The paired *medial umbilical ligaments* are formed by the obliterated umbilical arteries that connected the internal iliac arteries to the umbilical cord in fetal life. The paired *lateral umbilical ligaments* contain the patent inferior epigastric vessels. The initial course of

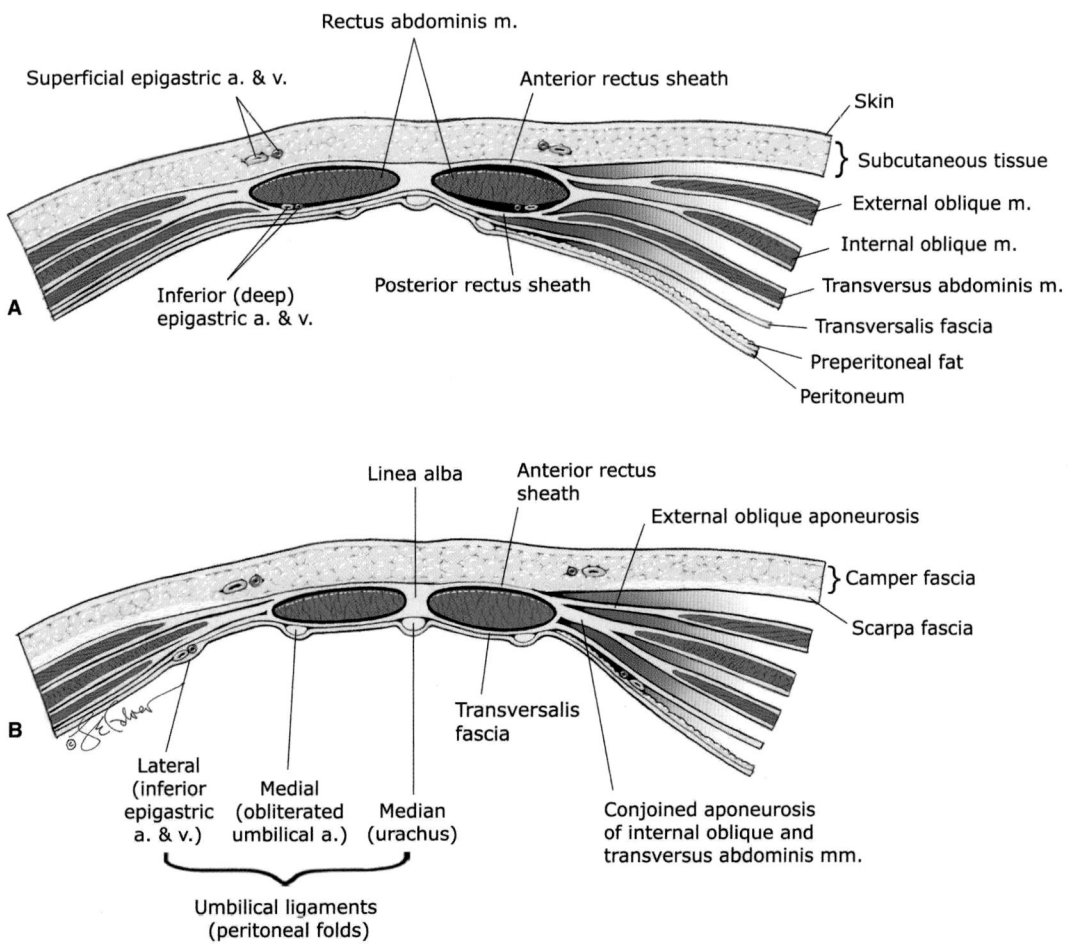

FIGURE 38-2 Transverse sections of the anterior abdominal wall above **(A)** and below **(B)** the arcuate line.

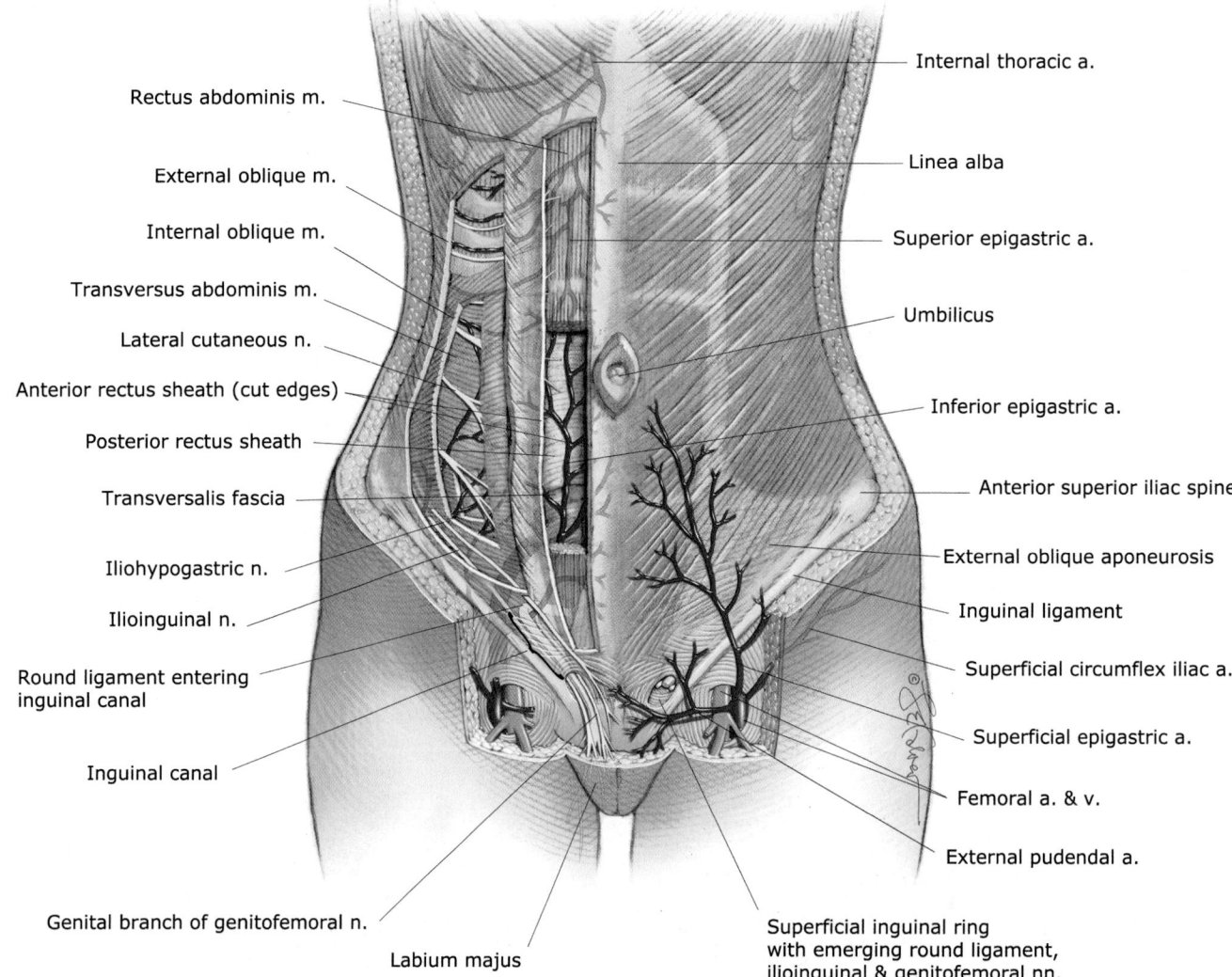

FIGURE 38-3 Anterior abdominal wall anatomy.

these vessels is just medial to the round ligament as the ligament enters the deep inguinal ring (Fig. 38-3).

Surgically, transection of a patent urachus can result in extravasation of urine into the abdominal cavity. In addition, the differential diagnosis of a midline anterior abdominal wall cyst includes urachal cyst, urachal sinus, and urachal diverticulum.

The umbilical ligaments serve as valuable laparoscopic landmarks. First, the inferior epigastric vessels can be injured during accessory trocar placement (Hurd, 1994; Rahn, 2010). Thus, direct visualization of the lateral umbilical folds can prevent injury to these vessels during laparoscopic port placement. Second, the medial umbilical ligaments, if followed proximally, can guide a surgeon to the internal iliac artery and then to the uterine arteries. The medial umbilical ligament also forms the medial border of the paravesical space, which is developed during radical hysterectomy to isolate the parametrium.

■ Blood Supply
Femoral Branches

The *superficial epigastric, superficial circumflex iliac,* and *external pudendal arteries* arise from the femoral artery just below the

inguinal ligament in the femoral triangle, which is bordered by this ligament, the sartorius muscle, and the adductor longus muscle (p. 823). These vessels supply the skin and subcutaneous layers of the anterior abdominal wall and mons pubis. The superficial epigastric vessels course diagonally toward the umbilicus, similar to the inferior "deep" epigastric vessels.

Surgically, during low transverse skin incision creation, the superficial epigastric vessels can usually be identified halfway between the skin and the rectus fascia, several centimeters from the midline. During laparoscopic procedures in thin patients, these vessels can be identified by transillumination (Chap. 41, p. 895).

The external pudendal vessels form rich anastomoses with their contralateral equivalents and with other superficial branches. These anastomoses account for the extensive bleeding often encountered with incisions made in the mons pubis area such as for retropubic midurethral sling incisions.

External Iliac Branches

The *inferior "deep" epigastric vessels* and *deep circumflex iliac vessels* are branches of the external iliac vessels (see Fig. 38-3). They supply the muscles and fascia of the anterior abdominal wall.

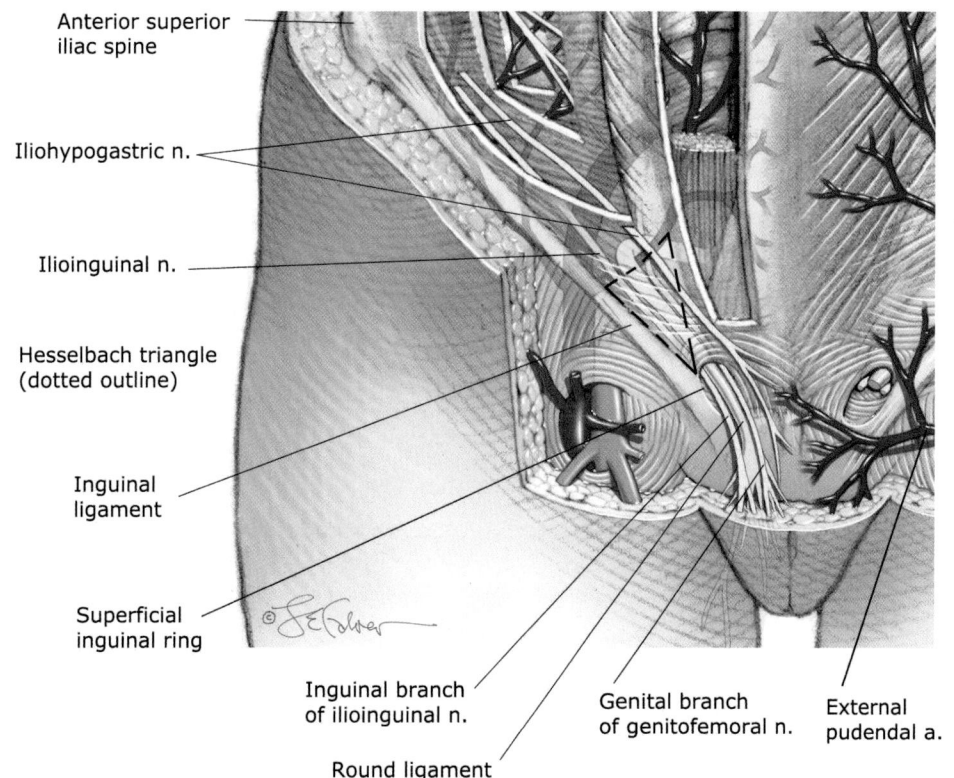

Anterior superior
iliac spine

Iliohypogastric n.

Ilioinguinal n.

Hesselbach triangle
(dotted outline)

Inguinal
ligament

Superficial
inguinal ring

Inguinal branch
of ilioinguinal n.

Round ligament

Genital branch
of genitofemoral n.

External
pudendal a.

FIGURE 38-4 Inguinal and upper thigh anatomy.

The inferior epigastric vessels initially course lateral to, then posterior to the rectus abdominis muscle, which they supply. They then pass anterior to the posterior rectus sheath and course between the sheath and the rectus muscles (see Figs. 38-2 and 38-3). Near the umbilicus, the inferior epigastric vessels anastomose with the superior epigastric artery and veins, which are branches of the internal thoracic vessels.

Hesselbach triangle is the region in the anterior abdominal wall bounded inferiorly by the inguinal ligament, medially by the lateral border of the rectus muscles, and laterally by the inferior epigastric vessels (Fig. 38-4). Direct hernias protrude through the abdominal wall within Hesselbach triangle. In contrast, indirect hernias protrude into the deep inguinal ring lying lateral to this triangle.

Surgically, low transverse abdominal incisions that extend beyond the lateral margins of the rectus muscles can lead to inferior epigastric vessel laceration with severe hemorrhage or anterior abdominal wall hematoma formation. These vessels should be identified and ligated when performing a Maylard incision. As another surgical landmark, the deep circumflex iliac vein serves as the caudal border during pelvic lymph node dissection.

■ Innervation

The anterior abdominal wall is innervated by the abdominal extensions of the intercostal nerves (T7-11), the subcostal nerve (T12), and the iliohypogastric and the ilioinguinal nerves (L1) (see Fig. 38-3). The T10 dermatome approximates the level of the umbilicus. Of these, the iliohypogastric nerve provides sensation to the skin over the suprapubic area. The ilioinguinal nerve supplies the skin of the lower abdominal wall and

upper portion of the labia majora and medial portion of the thigh through its inguinal branch (see Fig. 38-4). At a site 2 to 3 cm medial to the anterior superior iliac spine, these two nerves pierce through the internal oblique muscle and course superficial to it and toward the midline (Whiteside, 2003).

Clinically, the ilioinguinal and iliohypogastric nerves can be entrapped during closure of low transverse incisions, especially if incisions extend beyond the lateral borders of the rectus abdominis muscle. They may also be wounded by lower abdominal insertion of accessory trocars. The risk of iliohypogastric and ilioinguinal nerve injury can be minimized if lateral trocars are placed superior to the anterior superior iliac spines and if low transverse fascial incisions are not extended beyond the lateral borders of the rectus muscle (Rahn, 2010).

BONY PELVIS

■ Pelvic Bones and Joints

The *sacrum*; the *coccyx;* and two hip bones, termed the *innominate bones* form the bony pelvis (Fig. 38-5). The innominate bones consist of the *ilium, ischium,* and *pubis,* which fuse at the *acetabulum,* a cup-shaped structure that articulates with the femoral head. The ilium articulates with the sacrum posteriorly at the sacroiliac joint, and the pubic bones articulate with each other anteriorly at the symphysis pubis. The sacroiliac joint is a synovial joint that connects the articular surfaces of the sacrum and ilium. This joint and its ligaments contribute significantly to the stability of the bony pelvis. The symphysis pubis is a cartilaginous joint, which connects the articular surfaces of the pubic bones by way of a fibrocartilaginous disc. The ischial

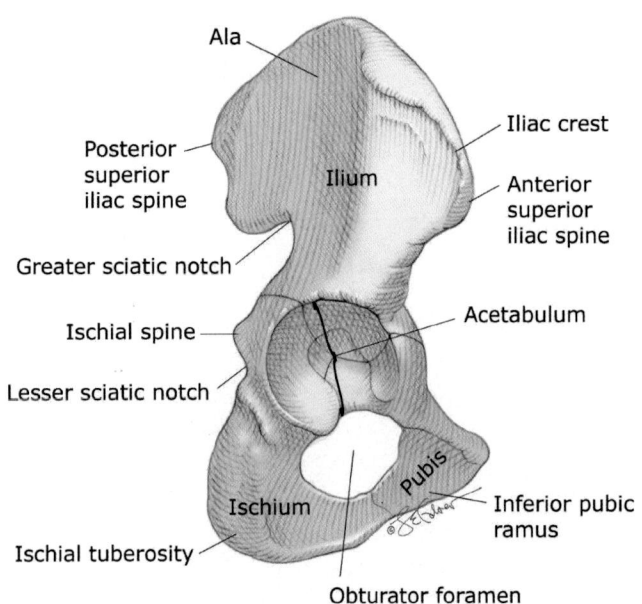

FIGURE 38-5 Right os coxae.

spines are clinically important bony prominences that project posteromedially from the medial surface of the ischium approximately at the level of the fifth sacral vertebra (S5).

■ Pelvic Openings

The posterior, lateral, and inferior walls of the pelvis have several openings through which many important structures pass. The large *obturator foramen* between the ischium and pubis is filled almost completely by the obturator membrane. In the superior portion of this membrane, a small aperture known as the *obturator canal* allows passage of the obturator neurovascular bundle into the medial (adductor) compartment of the thigh (Fig. 38-6).

The posterolateral walls of the pelvis are not covered by bone. Instead, two important accessory ligaments, the *sacrospinous* and *sacrotuberous ligaments*, divide the greater and lesser sciatic notches of the ischium into the *greater sciatic foramen* and *lesser sciatic foramen*. Through the greater sciatic foramen, the

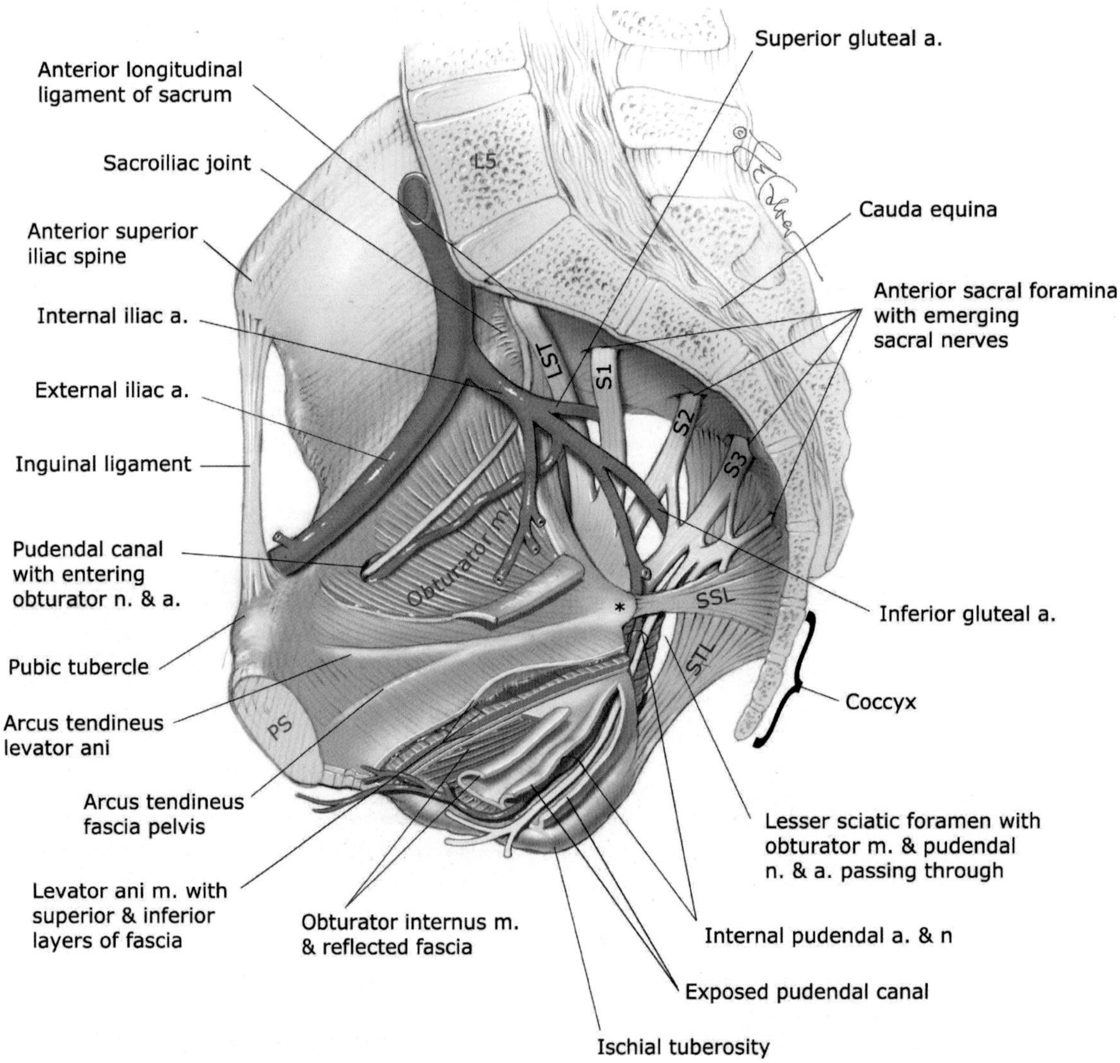

FIGURE 38-6 Bones, ligaments, and openings of the pelvic walls and associated structures. Note the obturator internus muscle extending below the levator ani muscle and then exiting through the lesser sciatic foramen to insert into the lateral femoral trochanter. Ischial spine is marked by an asterisk. L5 = fifth lumbar vertebra; LST = lumbosacral trunk; PS = pubic symphysis; S1–S3 = first through third sacral nerves; SSL = sacrospinous ligament; STL = sacrotuberous ligament.

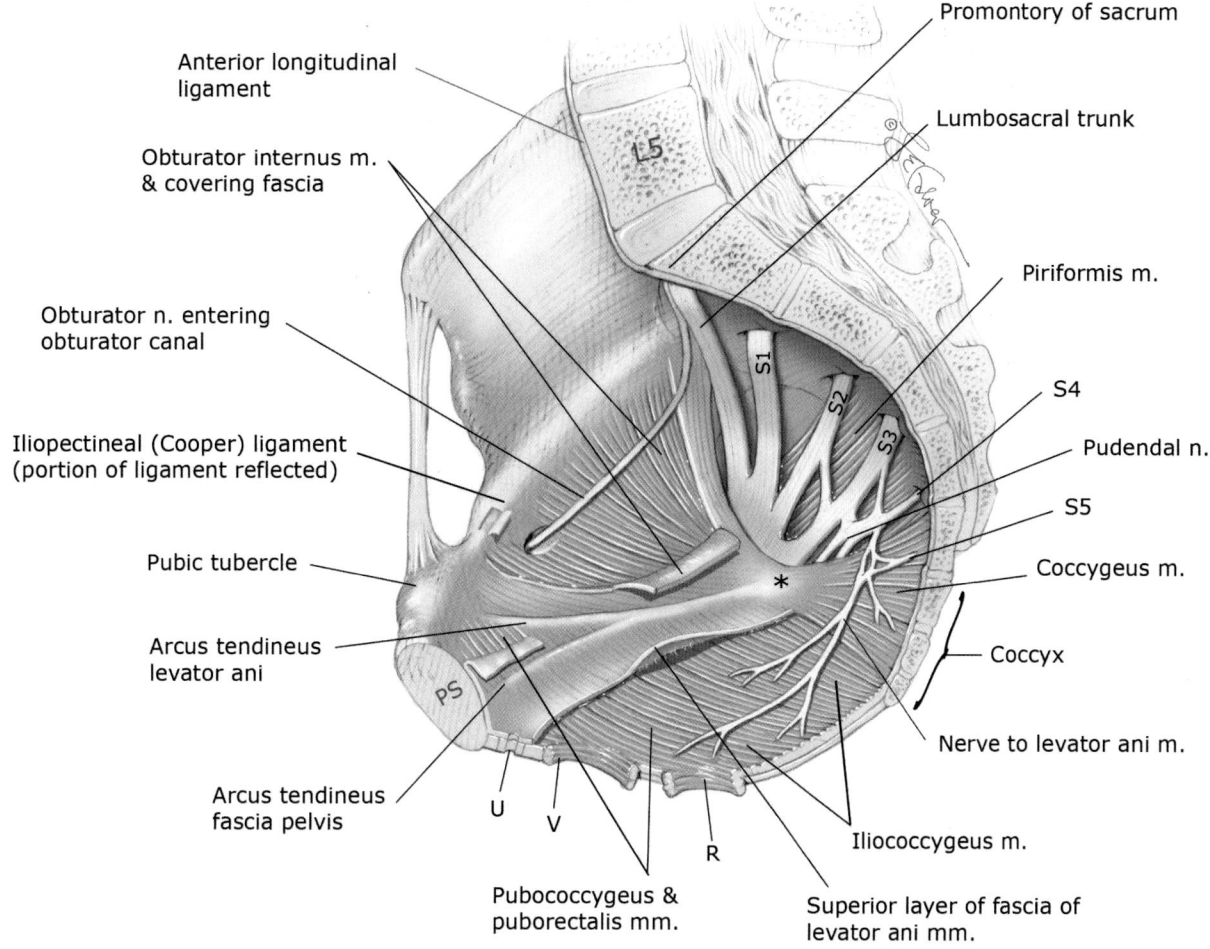

Promontory of sacrum

Anterior longitudinal
ligament

Lumbosacral trunk

Obturator internus m.
& covering fascia

Piriformis m.

Obturator n. entering
obturator canal

S1

S2

S3

S4

Pudendal n.

Iliopectineal (Cooper) ligament
(portion of ligament reflected)

S5

Pubic tubercle

Coccygeus m.

Arcus tendineus
levator ani

Coccyx

Arcus tendineus
fascia pelvis

Nerve to levator ani m.

U   V

Iliococcygeus m.

R

Superior layer of fascia of
levator ani mm.

Pubococcygeus &
puborectalis mm.

PS

FIGURE 38-7 Muscles and fascia of the pelvic walls and pelvic floor innervation. Ischial spine is marked by an asterisk. L5 = fifth lumbar vertebra; PS = pubic symphysis; R = rectum; S1–S5 = first through fifth sacral nerves; U = urethra; V = vagina.

piriformis muscle, internal pudendal and superior and inferior gluteal vessels, sciatic and pudendal nerve, and other branches of the sacral nerve plexus pass in close proximity to the ischial spines. Surgically, this anatomy is critical to avoid neurovascular injury during sacrospinous fixation procedures and when administering pudendal nerve blockade (Roshanravan, 2007).

The internal pudendal vessels, pudendal nerve, and obturator internus tendon pass through the lesser sciatic foramen. Posteriorly, four pairs of pelvic sacral foramina allow passage of the anterior divisions of the first four sacral nerves and lateral sacral arteries and veins.

■ Ligaments

The ligaments of the pelvis vary in composition and function. They range from connective tissue structures that support the bony pelvis and pelvic organs to smooth muscle and loose areolar tissue that add no significant support. The *sacrospinous, sacrotuberous,* and *anterior longitudinal ligaments* of the sacrum consist of dense connective tissue that joins bony structures and contributes significantly to bony pelvis stability (see Fig. 38-6).

The round and broad ligaments consist of smooth muscle and loose areolar tissue, respectively. Although they connect the uterus and adnexa to the pelvic walls, they do not contribute to

the support of these organs. In contrast, the cardinal and uterosacral ligaments do aid pelvic organ support and are discussed later (p. 808).

Clinically, the sacrospinous and anterior longitudinal ligament serve as suture fixation sites in suspensory procedures used to correct pelvic organ prolapse. The iliopectineal ligament, also termed Cooper ligament, is a thickening in the pubic bone periosteum, which is often used to anchor sutures in retropubic bladder neck suspension procedures (Fig. 38-7).

PELVIC WALL MUSCLES AND FASCIA

The posterior, lateral, and inferior walls of the pelvis are partially covered by striated muscles and their investing layers of fasciae (see Fig. 38-7). The *piriformis muscle* arises from the anterior and lateral surface of the sacrum and partially fills the posterolateral pelvic walls. It exits the pelvis through the greater sciatic foramen, attaches to the greater trochanter of the femur, and functions as an external or lateral hip rotator. Clinically, stretch injury to the piriformis muscle may cause persistent hip pain that can be confused with other hip or pelvic pathology.

The obturator internus muscle partially fills the sidewalls of the pelvis. This muscle arises from the pelvic surfaces of the ilium and ischium and from the obturator membrane. It exits

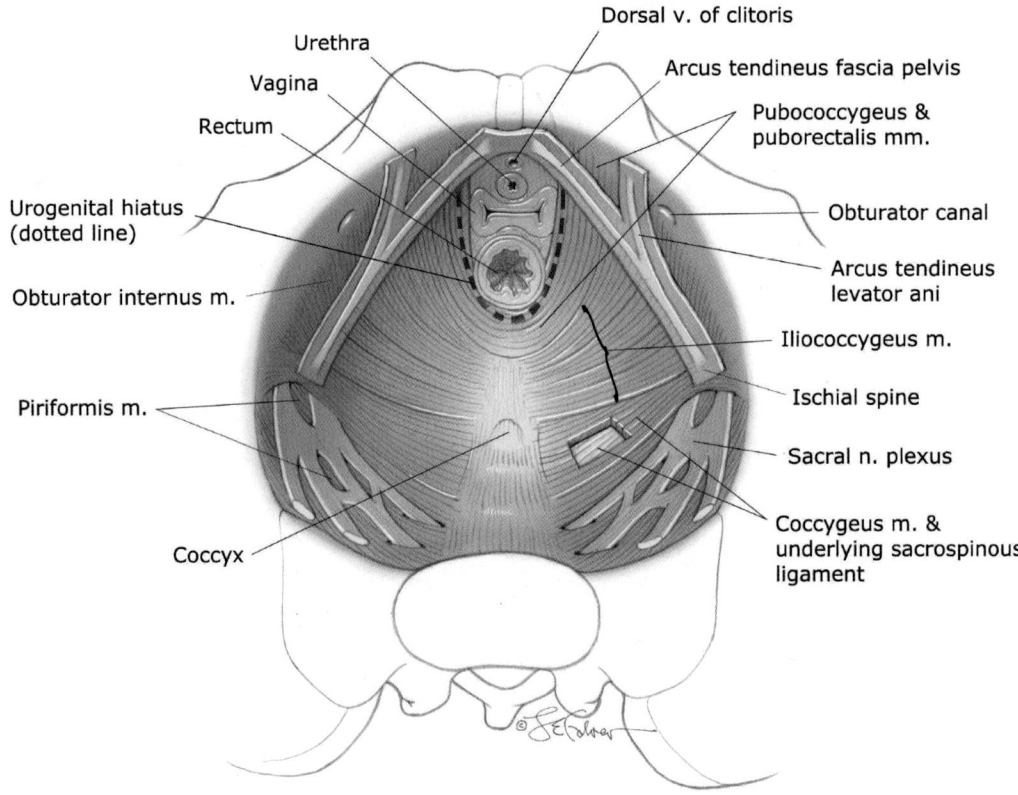

FIGURE 38-8 Superior view of pelvic floor and pelvic wall muscles.

the pelvis through the lesser sciatic foramen, attaches to the greater trochanter of the femur, and also functions as an external hip rotator.

The fascia that invests striated muscles is termed *parietal fascia*. Pelvic parietal fascia provides muscle attachment to the bony pelvis and serves as anchoring points for *visceral fascia*, also termed *endopelvic fascia*. The *arcus tendineus levator ani* is a condensation of parietal fascia covering the medial surface of the obturator internus muscle (see Fig. 38-7 and Fig. 38-8). This structure serves as the point of origin for parts of the very important levator ani muscle. Also shown is the *arcus tendineus fascia pelvis*, a condensation of parietal fascia covering the medial aspects of the obturator internus and levator ani muscles. It serves as the lateral point of attachment of the anterior vaginal wall.

PELVIC FLOOR

The muscles that span the pelvic floor are collectively known as the *pelvic diaphragm* (see Figs. 38-7, 38-8, and Fig. 38-9). This diaphragm consists of the levator ani and coccygeus muscles, along with their superior and inferior investing fascial layers. Inferior to the pelvic diaphragm, the perineal membrane and perineal body also contribute to the pelvic floor (p. 820). The *urogenital hiatus* is the U-shaped opening in the pelvic floor muscles through which the urethra, vagina, and rectum pass.

■ Levator Ani Muscles

These are the most important muscles in the pelvic floor and provide critical pelvic organ support (see Figs. 38-7 through

38-9). Physiologically, normal levator ani muscles maintain a constant state of contraction, thus providing a stable floor, which supports the weight of the abdominopelvic contents against intraabdominal forces.

The levator ani muscle is a complex unit, which consists of several muscle components with different origins and insertions and therefore different functions. The *pubococcygeus, puborectalis*, and *iliococcygeus muscles* are the three components. Of these, the pubococcygeus muscle is further divided into the *pubovaginalis, puboperinealis*, and *puboanalis muscles* according to their fiber attachments. Due to the significant attachments of the pubococcygeus muscle to the walls of the pelvic viscera, the term *pubovisceral muscle* is frequently used (Kerney, 2004; Lawson, 1974).

Pubococcygeus Muscle

The anterior ends of the pubococcygeus (pubovisceral muscle) arise on either side from the inner surface of the pubic bone. The *pubovaginalis* refers to the medial fibers that attach to the lateral walls of the vagina (see Fig. 38-9). Although there are no direct attachments of the levator ani muscles to the urethra in females, those fibers of the muscle that attach to the vagina are responsible for elevating the urethra during a pelvic muscle contraction and hence may contribute to urinary continence (DeLancey, 1990). The *puboperinealis* refers to the fibers that attach to the perineal body and draw this structure toward the pubic symphysis. The *puboanalis* refers to the fibers that attach to the anus at the intersphincteric groove between the internal and external anal sphincters. These fibers elevate the anus and, along with the rest of the pubococcygeus and puborectalis fibers, keep the urogenital hiatus narrowed (see Fig. 38-8).

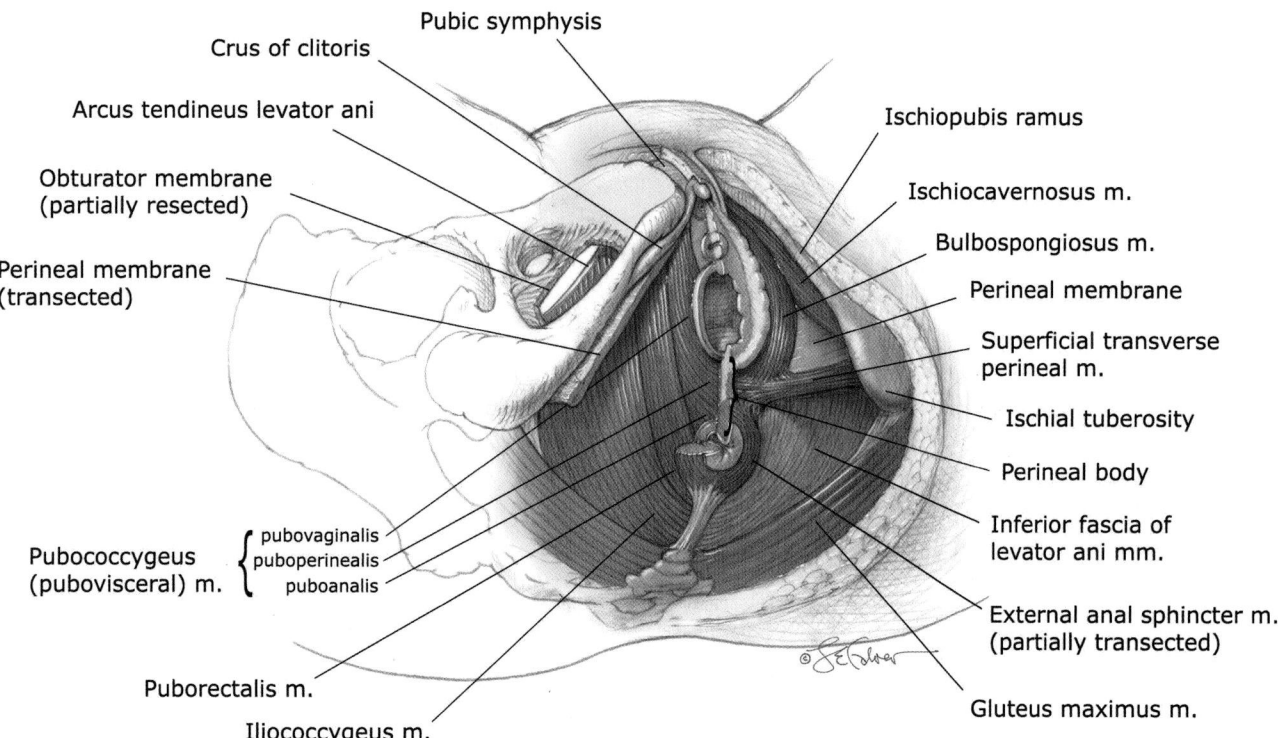

FIGURE 38-9 Inferior view of pelvic floor.

Puborectalis Muscle

The puborectalis represents the medial and inferior fibers of the levator ani muscle that arise on either side from the pubic bone and form a U-shaped sling behind the anorectal junction (Figs. 38-8 through 38-10). The action of the puborectalis draws the anorectal junction toward the pubis, contributing to the anorectal angle. This muscle is considered part of the anal sphincter complex and may contribute to fecal continence (Chap. 25, p. 561).

Iliococcygeus Muscle

This muscle is the most posterior and thinnest part of the levator ani muscle and has a primarily supportive role. It arises laterally from the arcus tendineus levator ani and the ischial spines (see Figs. 38-7 through 38-10). Muscle fibers from one side join those from the opposite side in the midline between the anus and the coccyx. This meeting line is termed the *iliococcygeal* or *anococcygeal raphe*. In addition to the iliococcygeus muscle, some fibers of the pubococcygeus muscle pass behind the rectum and attach to the coccyx. These muscle fibers course cephalad or deep to the iliococcygeus muscle and may also contribute to the anococcygeal raphe. The *levator plate* is the clinical term used to describe the anococcygeal raphe (see Fig. 38-10). This portion of the levator muscles forms a supportive shelf on which the rectum, upper vagina, and uterus rest.

The levator plate in women with normal support has a mean angle of 44 degrees relative to a horizontal reference line during Valsalva, although earlier studies suggested no elevation (Berglas, 1953; Hsu, 2006). During Valsalva, women with prolapse have a statistically greater levator plate angle compared with controls. This larger angle moderately correlates with larger levator hiatus length and greater displacement of the perineal body in women with prolapse compared with controls.

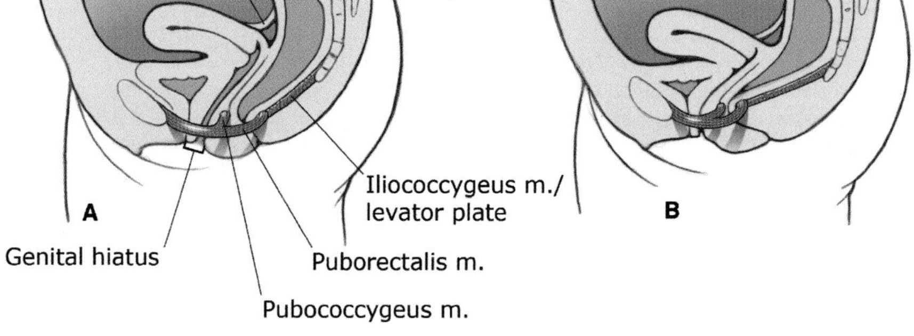

FIGURE 38-10 Pelvic organs and pelvic floor muscle and connective tissue interaction at rest (**A**) and with increasing intraabdominal pressure (**B**).

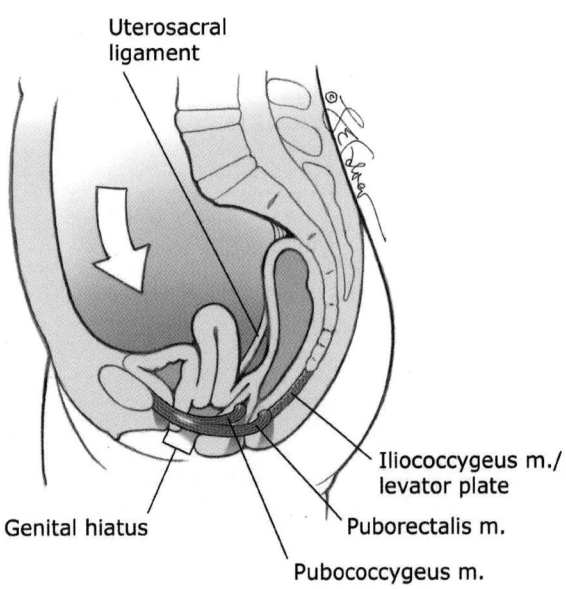

FIGURE 38-11 Pelvic floor muscles and connective tissue interaction in setting of pelvic organ prolapse.

With this in mind, one theory suggests that levator plate support prevents excessive tension or stretching of the connective tissue pelvic ligaments and fasciae (Paramore, 1908). Neuromuscular injury to the levator muscles may lead to eventual sagging or vertical inclination of the levator plate and opening of the urogenital hiatus. Consequently, the vaginal axis becomes more vertical, and the cervix is oriented over the opened hiatus (Fig. 38-11). The mechanical effect of this change is to increase strain on connective tissues that support the pelvic viscera. Increased urogenital hiatus size has been shown to correlate with increased prolapse severity (DeLancey, 1998).

■ Pelvic Floor Innervation

The pelvic diaphragm muscles are primarily innervated by direct somatic efferents from the second through the fifth sacral nerve roots (S2-5) (see Fig. 38-7) (Barber, 2002; Roshanravan, 2007).

Traditionally, a dual innervation has been described. The pelvic or superior surface of the muscles is supplied by direct efferents from S2-5, collectively known as the nerve to the levator ani muscle. The perineal or inferior surface is supplied by pudendal nerve branches. This latter relationship has been challenged, and investigators suggest that the pudendal nerve does not contribute to levator muscle innervation (Barber, 2002). Pudendal branches do, however, innervate parts of the

striated urethral sphincter and external anal sphincter muscles (p. 822). Such separate innervation may explain why some women develop pelvic organ prolapse and others develop urinary or fecal incontinence (Heit, 1996).

■ Pelvic Connective Tissue

Subperitoneal perivascular connective tissue and loose areolar tissue are found throughout the pelvis. This tissue connects the pelvic viscera to the pelvic walls and is termed *visceral* or *endopelvic "fascia."* Recall that visceral fascia differs from parietal fascia, which invests most striated muscles (Table 38-1). Visceral fascia is intimately associated with the walls of the viscera and cannot be dissected in the same way that parietal fascia can be separated from its skeletal muscle.

Condensations of visceral connective tissue that have assumed special supportive roles have been given different names. Some examples include the cardinal and uterosacral ligaments and the vesicovaginal and rectovaginal fascia. These are described further in later sections.

PELVIC BLOOD SUPPLY

The pelvic organs are supplied by the visceral branches of the internal iliac (hypogastric) artery and by direct branches from the abdominal aorta (Fig. 38-12). Clinically, the internal iliac artery can be separated into an anterior and posterior division in the area of the greater sciatic foramen (see Fig. 38-6). Each division has three parietal branches that supply nonvisceral structures. The *iliolumbar, lateral sacral,* and *superior gluteal arteries* are the three parietal branches of the posterior division. The *internal pudendal, obturator,* and *inferior gluteal arteries* are parietal branches that most commonly arise from the anterior division. The remaining branches of the anterior division supply pelvic viscera (bladder, uterus, vagina, and rectum). These include the *uterine, vaginal,* and *middle rectal arteries* and the *superior vesical arteries.* The superior vesical arteries commonly arise from the patent part of the umbilical arteries (Table 38-2). Internal iliac branches that supply the inferior and middle portions of the bladder are present in women, but their origin is highly variable. The middle rectal arteries are generally very small-caliber vessels but may be absent. They usually contribute to posterior vaginal wall blood supply.

The two most important direct branches of the aorta that contribute to pelvic organ blood supply are the superior rectal and ovarian arteries. The *superior rectal artery,* which is the terminal branch of the inferior mesenteric artery, anastomoses with the middle rectal arteries, thus contributing blood supply to the

TABLE 38-1. Differences between Visceral and Parietal Fascia of the Pelvic Floor Muscles

	Type of Fascia	
Characteristic	**Visceral or Endopelvic**	**Parietal**
Histologic	Loose arrangements of collagen, elastin, and adipose tissue	Organized collagen arrangements
Function	Allows expansion and contraction of invested structures	Provides muscle attachment to bones
Supportive role	Condensations lend some support to invested organs; encases neurovascular structures	Invests muscles to provide pelvic floor stability and function
Tensile strength	Elastic	Rigid

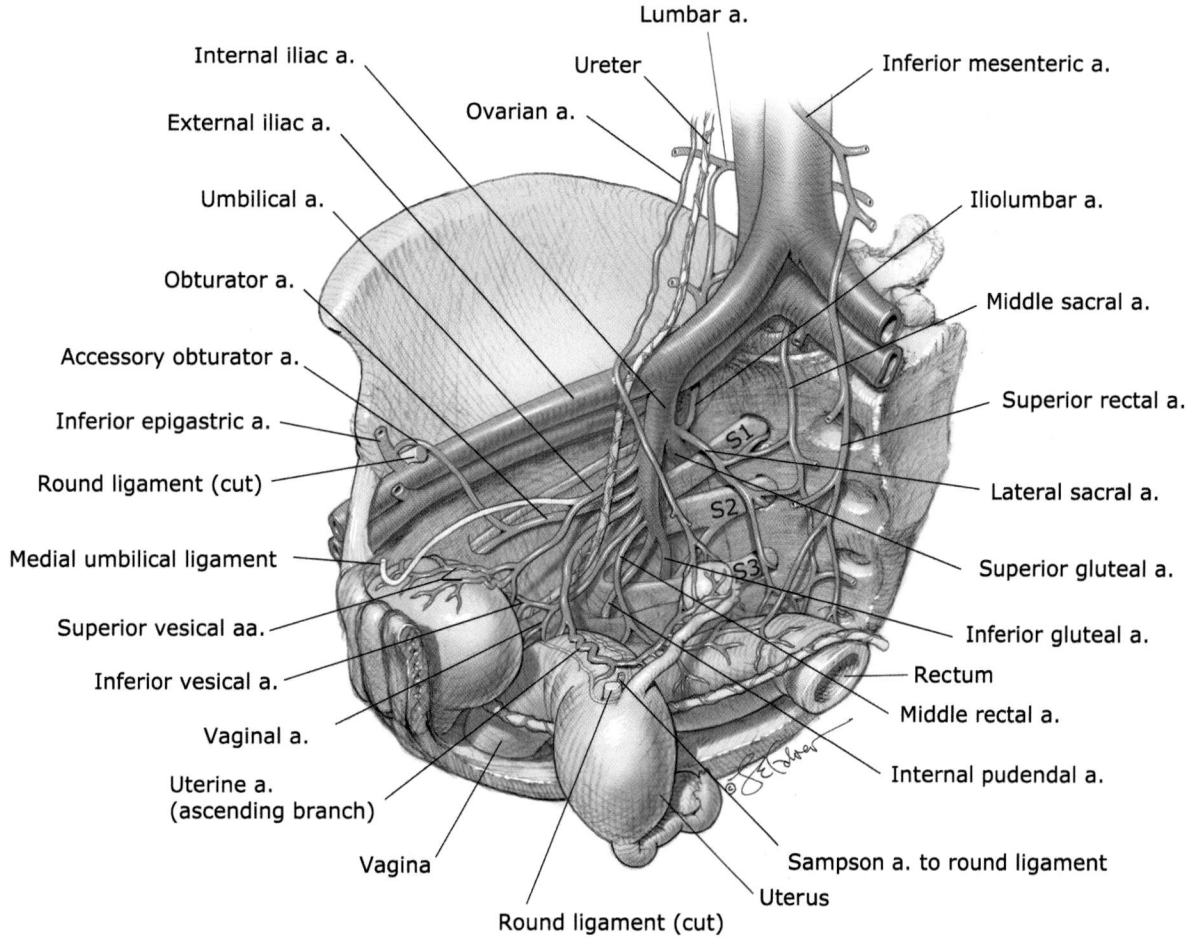

Lumbar a.

Internal iliac a.

Ureter

Ovarian a.

Inferior mesenteric a.

External iliac a.

Umbilical a.

Iliolumbar a.

Obturator a.

Middle sacral a.

Accessory obturator a.

Superior rectal a.

Inferior epigastric a.

S1

Round ligament (cut)

S2

Lateral sacral a.

Medial umbilical ligament

S3

Superior gluteal a.

Superior vesical aa.

Inferior gluteal a.

Inferior vesical a.

Rectum

Vaginal a.

Middle rectal a.

Uterine a.
(ascending branch)

Internal pudendal a.

Vagina

Sampson a. to round ligament

Uterus

Round ligament (cut)

FIGURE 38-12 Pelvic arteries. In this image, the uterus and rectum are reflected to the left.

TABLE 38-2. Pelvic Blood Supply			
Internal Iliac Artery[a]			
Anterior Division		**Posterior Division**	
Parietal Branches	**Visceral Branches**	**Parietal Branches**	**Visceral Branches**
Obturator	Superior vesical (from patent	Iliolumbar	None
Internal pudendal	segment of umbilical)	Lateral sacral	
Inferior gluteal	Uterine	Superior gluteal	
	Vaginal		
	Middle rectal		
	Middle & inferior vesicals (±)		
Direct Branches of Aorta			
Parietal Branches		**Visceral Branches**	
Middle sacral		Ovarian	
		Superior rectal (terminal branch of inferior mesenteric)	
Aortic to Internal Iliac Artery Anastomoses			
Ovarian to uterine		Middle sacral to lateral sacral	
Superior rectal to middle rectal		Lumbar to iliolumbar	

[a]Note that great variability exists in the origin and distribution of internal iliac branches.

rectum and vagina. The *ovarian arteries* arise directly from the aorta just inferior to the renal vessels and anastomose with the ascending branch of the uterine artery. These anastomoses contribute to the blood supply of the uterus and adnexa. Other important anastomoses between the aorta and internal iliac arteries include anastomoses between the middle sacral and lateral sacral arteries and anastomoses between the lumbar and iliolumbar arteries.

PELVIC INNERVATION

Nerve supply to the visceral structures in the pelvis (bladder, urethra, vagina, uterus, adnexa, and rectum) arises from the autonomic nervous system. The two most important components of this system in the pelvis include the *superior* and *inferior hypogastric plexuses*. The superior hypogastric plexus, also known as the *presacral nerve*, is an extension of the aortic plexus found below the aortic bifurcation (Fig. 38-13). This plexus primarily contains sympathetic fibers and sensory afferent fibers from the uterus.

The superior hypogastric plexus terminates by dividing into the hypogastric nerves. These nerves join parasympathetic efferents from the second through the fourth sacral nerve roots (pelvic splanchnic nerves) to form the *inferior hypogastric plexus*, also known as the *pelvic plexus*. In addition, the inferior hypogastric plexus generally receives contributions from the sacral sympathetic trunk.

With variability, fibers of the inferior hypogastric plexus accompany the branches of the internal iliac artery to the pelvic viscera. Accordingly, they are divided into three portions: the vesical, uterovaginal (Frankenhäuser ganglion), and middle rectal plexuses. Extensions of the inferior hypogastric plexus reach the perineum along the vagina and urethra to innervate the clitoris and vestibular bulbs.

Clinically, the sensory afferent fibers contained within the superior hypogastric plexus are targeted in presacral neurectomy, a surgical procedure performed to treat central pelvic pain (Chap. 11, p. 260). Although visceral and sexual dysfunction has been reported following complete interruption of the superior hypogastric plexus, contributions from the sacral sympathetic trunk may offset interruption of this sympathetic component to the inferior hypogastric plexus. Injury to the branches of the inferior hypogastric plexus during cancer debulking or other extensive pelvic surgeries can lead to varying degrees of voiding, sexual, and defecatory dysfunction.

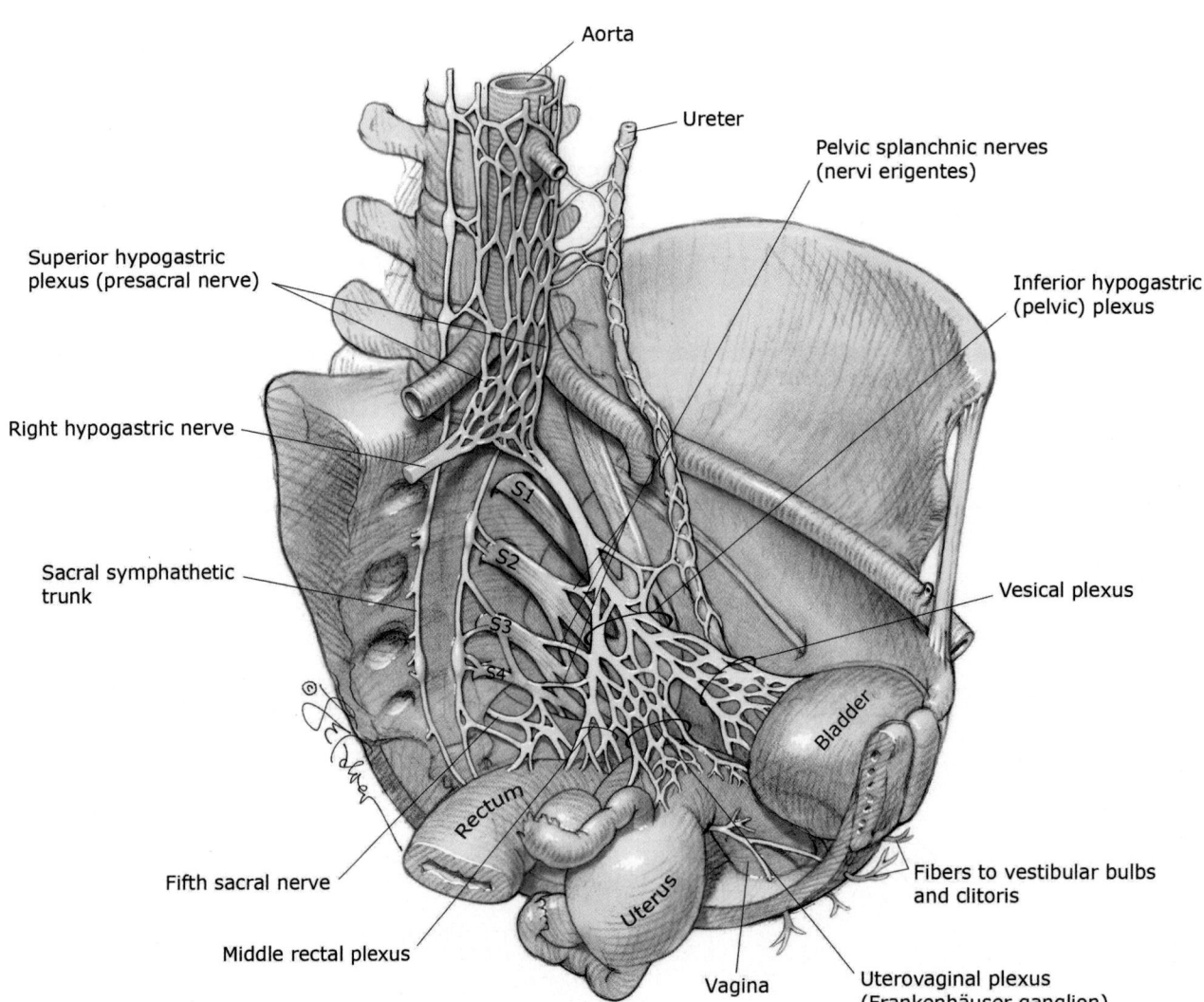

FIGURE 38-13 Pelvic autonomic nerves. Superior and inferior hypogastric plexuses. S1–S4 = first through fourth sacral nerves.

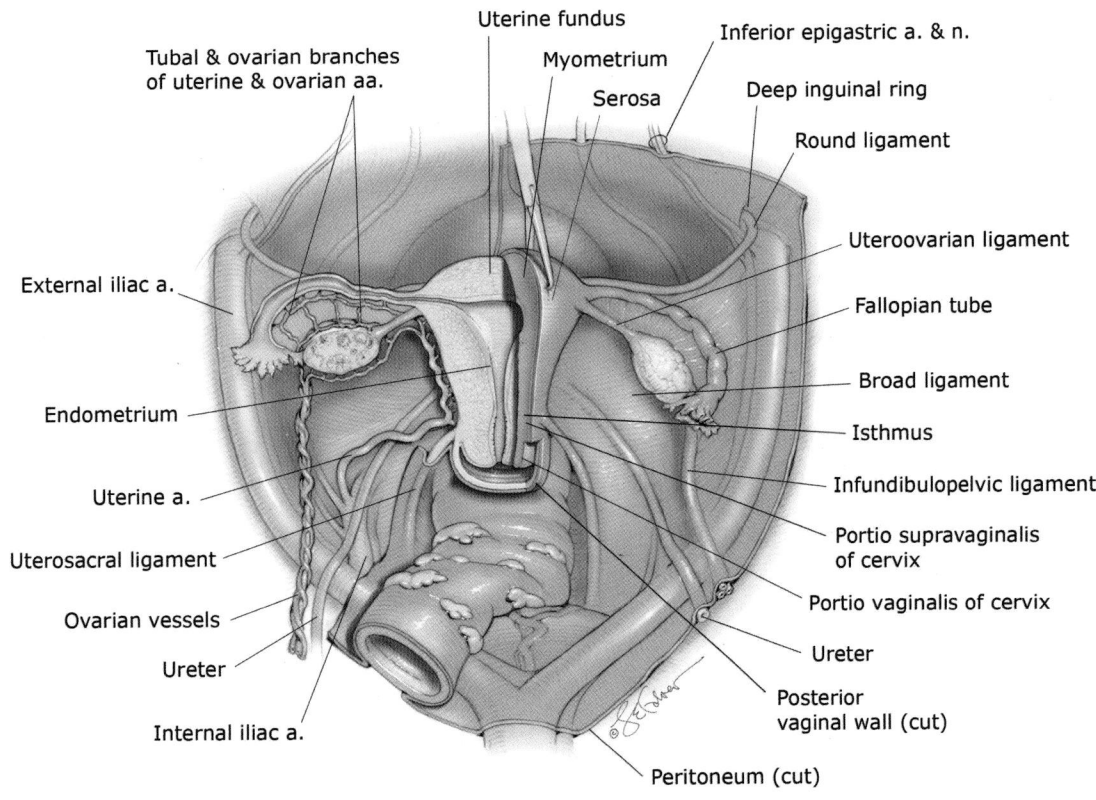

Tubal & ovarian branches
of uterine & ovarian aa.

Uterine fundus

Myometrium

Serosa

Inferior epigastric a. & n.

Deep inguinal ring

Round ligament

Uteroovarian ligament

Fallopian tube

Broad ligament

Isthmus

Infundibulopelvic ligament

Portio supravaginalis
of cervix

Portio vaginalis of cervix

Ureter

Posterior
vaginal wall (cut)

External iliac a.

Endometrium

Uterine a.

Uterosacral ligament

Ovarian vessels

Ureter

Internal iliac a.

Peritoneum (cut)

FIGURE 38-14 Uterus, adnexa, and associated anatomy.

PELVIC VISCERA

■ Uterus

The uterus is a fibromuscular hollow organ situated between the bladder and the rectum. The uterus is divided into two portions: an upper muscular body, the *corpus*, and a lower fibrous *cervix* (Fig. 38-14). The transition between the corpus and the cervix is known as the *uterine isthmus*. This also marks the transition from endocervical canal to endometrial cavity. The portion of the corpus that extends above the entry level of the fallopian tubes into the endometrial cavity is known as the *fundus*.

The shape, weight, and dimensions of the uterus vary according to parity and estrogen stimulation. Before menarche and after menopause, the corpus and cervix are approximately equal in size, but during the reproductive years, the uterine corpus is significantly larger than the cervix. In the adult, nonpregnant woman, the uterus measures approximately 7 cm in length and 5 cm in width at the fundus.

Endometrium and Serosa

The uterus consists of an inner mucosal layer called the *endometrium*, which surrounds the endometrial cavity, and a thick muscular wall known as the *myometrium*. The endometrium consists of columnar epithelium and specialized stroma. The superficial portion of the endometrium undergoes cyclic changes with the menstrual cycle.

The spiral arterioles located in the endometrium undergo hormonally mediated constriction or spasm that promotes shedding of the superficial portion of the endometrium with each menstrual cycle. The deeper basalis layer of the endometrium is preserved after this shedding and is responsible for regeneration of a new superficial layer.

Peritoneal serosa overlies the uterus, except at two sites. First, the anterior portion of the cervix is covered by the bladder. Second, the lateral portions of the corpus and cervix attach to the broad and cardinal ligaments.

Cervix

The uterine cervix begins caudal to the uterine isthmus and is approximately 3 cm in length. The wall of the cervix consists primarily of fibrous tissue and a smaller amount of smooth muscle. The smooth muscle is found on the cervical wall periphery and serves as the attachment point for the cardinal and uterosacral ligaments and for the fibromuscular walls of the vagina.

The attachments of the vaginal walls to the outer cervix divide it into a vaginal part known as the *portio vaginalis* and a supravaginal part known as the *portio supravaginalis* (see Fig. 38-14). The portio vaginalis is covered by nonkeratinizing squamous epithelium.

The endocervical canal is lined by columnar, mucus-secreting epithelium. The lower border of the canal, called the external cervical os, contains a transition from the squamous epithelium of the portio vaginalis to the columnar epithelium of the cervical canal. The exact location of this transition, termed the *squamocolumnar junction,* varies depending on hormonal status (Fig. 29-5, p. 625). At the upper border of the endocervical canal is the internal cervical os, where the narrow cervical canal becomes continuous with the wider endometrial cavity.

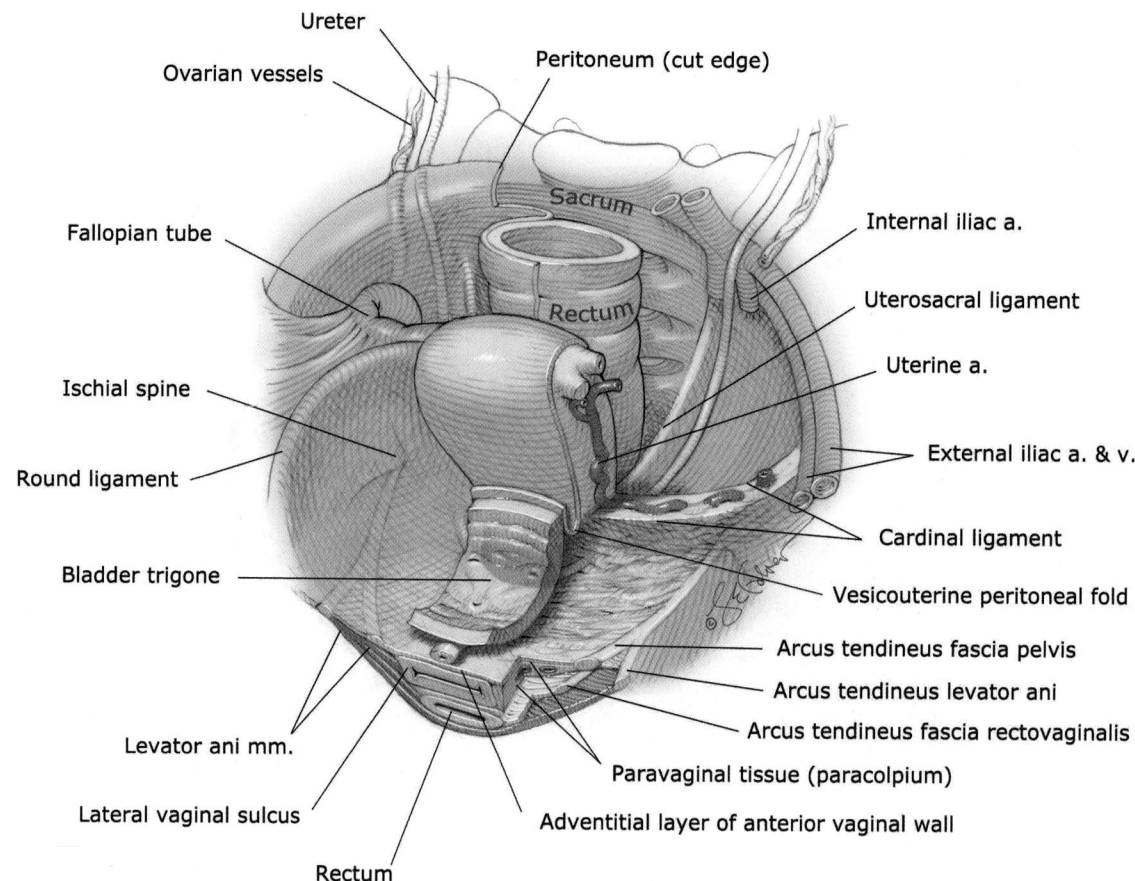

Ureter
Ovarian vessels
Peritoneum (cut edge)
Sacrum
Rectum
Fallopian tube
Internal iliac a.
Uterosacral ligament
Uterine a.
Ischial spine
External iliac a. & v.
Round ligament
Cardinal ligament
Vesicouterine peritoneal fold
Bladder trigone
Arcus tendineus fascia pelvis
Arcus tendineus levator ani
Arcus tendineus fascia rectovaginalis
Levator ani mm.
Paravaginal tissue (paracolpium)
Lateral vaginal sulcus
Adventitial layer of anterior vaginal wall
Rectum

FIGURE 38-15 Pelvic viscera and their connective tissue support. Relationship of the urethra, bladder trigone, and distal ureter to the anterior vaginal wall and to the uterine cervix.

Uterine Support

The main support of the uterus and cervix is provided by the levator ani muscles and the connective tissue that attaches the outer cervix to the pelvic walls. The connective tissue that attaches lateral to the uterus and cervix on each side is called the *parametrium* and continues caudad along the vagina as the *paracolpium*. The parametrium consists of what is clinically known as the *cardinal ligament* and *uterosacral ligament* (Fig. 38-15).

The cardinal ligaments, also termed *transverse cervical ligaments* or *Mackenrodt ligaments*, consist primarily of perivascular connective tissue (Range, 1964). They attach to the posterolateral pelvic walls near the origin of the internal iliac artery and surround the vessels supplying the uterus and vagina.

The uterosacral ligaments insert broadly into the posterior pelvic walls and sacrum and form the lateral boundaries of the cul-de-sac of Douglas. These ligaments originate from the posterior inferior surface of the cervix, but may also originate, in part, from the proximal posterior vagina (Umek, 2004). They consist primarily of smooth muscle and contain some pelvic autonomic nerves (Campbell, 1950; Ripperda, 2015).

Clinically, during pelvic reconstructive surgeries that use the uterosacral ligaments as attachment sites for the vaginal apex, surrounding structures are especially vulnerable (Wieslander, 2007). Namely, the rectum lies medial to the uterosacral ligaments. The ureter, pelvic sidewall vessels, and sacral nerves run lateral to and close to these ligaments.

Round Ligaments

These ligaments are smooth muscle extensions of the uterine corpus and represent the homologue of the gubernaculum testis. The round ligaments arise from the lateral aspect of the corpus just below and anterior to the origin of the fallopian tubes. They extend laterally to the pelvic sidewall (see Fig. 38-14). They enter the retroperitoneal space and pass lateral to the inferior epigastric vessels before entering the inguinal canal through the internal inguinal ring. After coursing through the inguinal canal, the round ligaments exit through the external inguinal ring to terminate in the subcutaneous tissue of the labia majora (see Fig. 38-4). The round ligaments do not significantly contribute to uterine support. They receive their blood supply from a small branch of the uterine or ovarian artery known as *Sampson artery*.

Clinically, the location of the round ligament anterior to the fallopian tube can assist a surgeon during tubal sterilization through a minilaparotomy incision. This may be especially true if pelvic adhesions limit tubal mobility and thus hinder identification of fimbria prior to tubal ligation.

Division of the round ligament is typically an initial step in abdominal and laparoscopic hysterectomy. Its transection opens the broad ligament leaves and provides access to the pelvic sidewall retroperitoneum. This access allows direct visualization of the ureter and permits isolation of the uterine artery for safe ligation.

Broad Ligaments

These ligaments are double layers of peritoneum that extend from the lateral walls of the uterus to the pelvic walls (see Fig. 38-14). Within the upper portion of these two layers, the fallopian tube, the ovarian ligament, and round ligament are found. Each of these has its separate mesentery, called the *mesosalpinx, mesovarium,* and *mesoteres,* respectively, which carry nerves and vessels to these structures. At the lateral border of the fallopian tube and the ovary, the broad ligament ends where the infundibulopelvic ligament, described later on this page, blends with the pelvic wall. The cardinal and distal uterosacral ligaments lie within the lower portion or "base" of the broad ligament.

Uterine Blood Supply

The blood supply to the uterine corpus arises from the ascending branch of the uterine artery and from the medial or uterine branch of the ovarian artery (see Figs. 38-14 and 38-15). The uterine artery may originate directly from the internal iliac artery, or it may have a common origin with the internal pudendal or with the vaginal artery (see Fig. 38-12). The uterine artery approaches the uterus in the area of the uterine isthmus. Here, the uterine artery courses over the ureter and provides a small branch to it. Several uterine veins course along the side of the artery and are variably found over or under the ureter. The uterine artery then divides into a larger ascending and a smaller descending branch that course alongside the uterus and cervix, respectively. These vessels connect on the lateral border of the uterus but form an anastomotic arterial arcade that supplies the uterine walls (Fig. 8-3, p. 182). The cervix is supplied by the descending or cervical branch of the uterine artery and by ascending branches of the vaginal artery.

Clinically, because the uterus receives dual blood supply from both ovarian and uterine vessels, some surgeons during myomectomy place tourniquets at both the infundibulopelvic ligament and uterine isthmus. This decreases blood flow from the ovarian and uterine arteries, respectively.

Uterine Lymphatic Drainage

Lymphatic drainage of the uterus is primarily to the obturator and internal and external iliac nodes (Fig. 38-16). However, some lymphatic channels from the uterine corpus may pass along the round ligaments to the superficial inguinal nodes, and others may extend along the uterosacral ligaments to the lateral sacral nodes.

Uterine Innervation

The uterus is innervated by fibers of the uterovaginal plexus, also known as Frankenhäuser ganglion. These fibers travel along the uterine arteries and are found in the connective tissue of the cardinal ligaments (see Fig. 38-13).

■ Ovaries and Fallopian Tubes

Ovaries

The ovaries and fallopian tubes constitute the *uterine adnexa*. The size and hormonal activity of the ovaries are dependent on age, stage of the menstrual cycle, and exogenous hormonal suppression. During reproductive years, the ovaries measure 2.5 to

5 cm in length, 1.5 to 3 cm in thickness, and 0.7 to 1.5 cm in width.

The ovaries consist of an *outer cortex* and an *inner medulla.* The ovarian cortex is made up of a specialized stroma punctuated with follicles, corpora lutea, and corpora albicantia. A single layer of mesothelial cells covers this cortex as a surface epithelium. The medullary portion of the ovary primarily consists of fibromuscular tissue and blood vessels. Vessels and nerves enter the medulla at the *hilum*, which is a depression along the mesenteric border of the ovary. The medial aspect of the ovary is connected to the uterus by the *uteroovarian ligament* (see Fig. 38-14). Laterally, each ovary is attached to the pelvic wall by an *infundibulopelvic ligament*, also termed *suspensory ligament* of the ovary, which contains the ovarian vessels and nerves.

The blood supply to the ovaries comes from the *ovarian arteries*, which arise from the anterior surface of the abdominal aorta just below the origin of the renal arteries and from the ovarian branches of the uterine arteries (see Fig. 38-16). The *ovarian veins* follow the same retroperitoneal course as the arteries. The right ovarian vein drains into the inferior vena cava, and the left ovarian vein drains into the left renal vein.

Lymphatic drainage of the ovaries follows the ovarian vessels to the lower abdominal aorta, where they drain into the paraaortic nodes. For their innervation, the ovaries are supplied by extensions of the renal plexus that course along the ovarian vessels in the infundibulopelvic ligament and variably by contributions of the inferior hypogastric plexus.

Fallopian Tubes

The fallopian tubes are tubular structures that measure 7 to 12 cm in length (see Fig. 38-14). Each tube has four identifiable portions. The *interstitial portion* passes through the body of the uterus at the region known as the *cornua*. The *isthmic portion* begins adjacent to the uterine corpus. It consists of a narrow lumen and a thick muscular wall. The *ampullary portion* is recognized as the lumen of the isthmic portion of the tube widens. In addition, this segment has a more convoluted mucosa. The *fimbriated portion* is the distal continuation of the ampullary segment. The fimbriated end has many frondlike projections that provide a wide surface area for ovum pickup. The *fimbria ovarica* is the extension that contacts the ovary.

The ovarian artery runs along the ovary's hilum and sends several branches through the mesosalpinx to supply the fallopian tubes (see Fig. 38-14). The venous plexus, lymphatic drainage, and nerve supply of the fallopian tubes follow a similar course to that of the ovaries.

■ Vagina

The vagina is a hollow viscus whose shape is determined by the structures that surround it and by the attachments of its lateral walls to the pelvic walls. The distal portion of the vagina is constricted by the action of the levator ani muscles (see Fig. 38-10). Above the pelvic floor, the vaginal lumen is more capacious and distensible. In the standing or anatomic position, the apex of the vagina is directed posteriorly toward the ischial spines, and the upper two thirds of the vaginal tube lie almost parallel to the plane of the levator plate. Although variable, the average

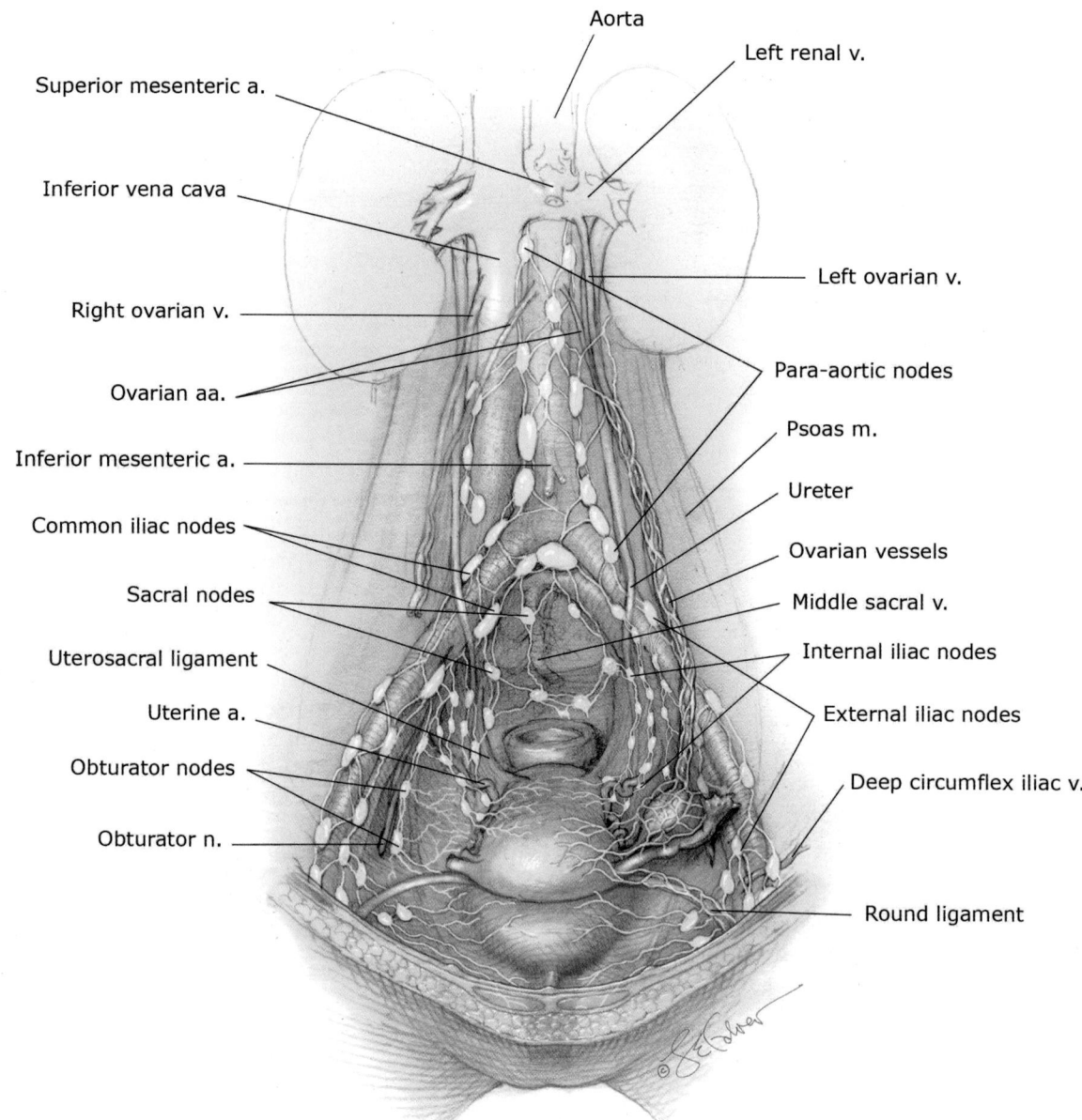

FIGURE 38-16 Pelvic lymph nodes and the course of the ureter and ovarian vessels.

length of the anterior vaginal wall is 7 cm and that of the posterior wall is 9 cm. The recesses within the vaginal lumen in front of and behind the cervix are known as the *anterior fornix* and *posterior fornix*, respectively (Fig. 38-17). The vaginal walls consist of three layers: (1) adjacent to the lumen, a layer of nonkeratinized squamous epithelium with an outer lamina propria; (2) a muscular layer of smooth muscle, collagen, and elastin; and (3) an outer adventitial layer of collagen and elastin (Weber, 1995, 1997). These latter two form the fibromuscular component of the vagina.

The vagina lies between the bladder and rectum and, along with its connections to the pelvic walls, provides support to these structures (see Figs. 38-15 and 38-17). The vagina is separated from the bladder anteriorly and the rectum posteriorly by the vaginal adventitia. The lateral continuation of this adventitial layer contributes the paravaginal tissue that attaches the walls of the vagina to the pelvic walls. This paravaginal tissue constitutes the paracolpium. This tissue consists of loose areo-

lar and fatty tissue containing blood vessels, lymphatics, and nerves. The anterior fibromuscular vaginal wall and its paravaginal attachments to the arcus tendineus fascia pelvis represent the layer that supports the bladder and urethra and is clinically referred to as pubovesicocervical fascia (see Fig. 38-15).

The lateral attachments of the posterior vaginal walls are to the fascia covering the upper surface of the levator ani muscles. The posterior vaginal wall and its connective tissue attachments to the sidewall support the rectum. This layer is clinically known as the rectovaginal fascia or fascia of Denonvilliers. However, similar to microscopic findings of the anterior vaginal wall, histologic studies have failed to show a separate layer between the posterior wall of the vagina and the rectum except in the distal 3 to 4 cm. Here, the dense fibromuscular tissue of the perineal body separates these structures (DeLancey, 1999).

Surgically, dissections in the anterior vaginal wall or in the posterior vaginal wall separate portions of the vaginal muscularis from the epithelium for surgeries such as anterior and posterior

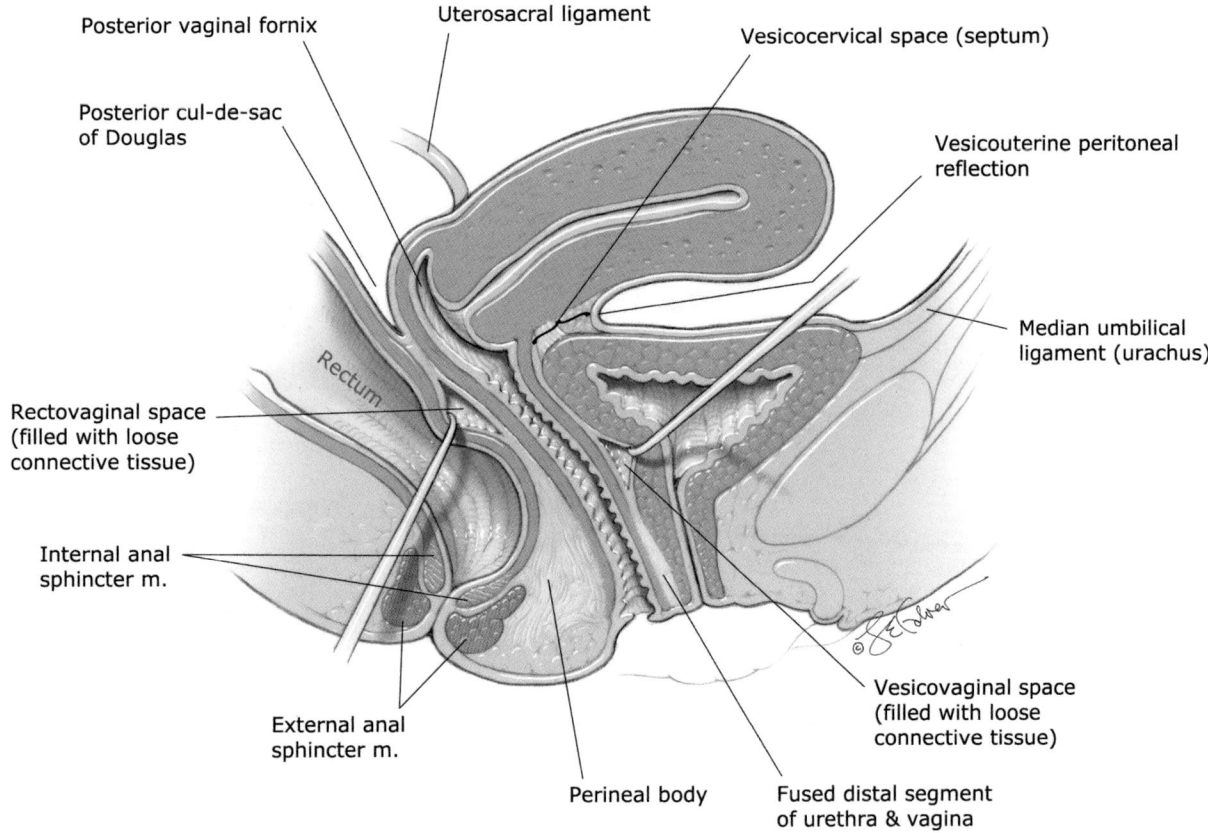

Posterior vaginal fornix   Uterosacral ligament   Vesicocervical space (septum)

Posterior cul-de-sac of Douglas

Vesicouterine peritoneal reflection

Rectum

Median umbilical ligament (urachus)

Rectovaginal space (filled with loose connective tissue)

Internal anal sphincter m.

External anal sphincter m.

Perineal body

Fused distal segment of urethra & vagina

Vesicovaginal space (filled with loose connective tissue)

FIGURE 38-17 Surgical cleavage planes and vaginal wall layers.

colporrhaphy. In contrast, posterior or anterior access to the coccygeus-sacrospinous ligament complex is accomplished by incising the full thickness of the anterior or posterior fibromuscular wall of the vagina, respectively. This deeper dissection allows access to the vesicovaginal or rectovaginal space and lateral dissection from these spaces allows access to the pararectal space. Because there is no true histologic "fascial" layer between the vagina and the bladder and between the vagina and the rectum, some recommend that terms such as "pubocervical/pubovesical fascia" or "rectovaginal fascia" be abandoned. They propose that these be replaced by more accurate descriptive terms such as *vaginal muscularis* or *fibromuscular layer of the anterior and posterior vaginal walls.*

Vesicocervical and Vesicovaginal "Potential" Spaces

The *vesicocervical space* begins below the vesicouterine peritoneal fold or reflection, which represents the loose attachments of the peritoneum in the anterior cul-de-sac (see Figs. 38-17 and 38-18). The vesicocervical space continues down as the *vesicovaginal space*, which extends to the junction of the proximal and middle thirds of the urethra. Below this point, the urethra and vagina fuse.

Clinically, during an abdominal hysterectomy or cesarean delivery, surgeons easily lift and incise the vesicouterine peritoneal fold to create a bladder flap and then open the vesicocervical space. For vaginal hysterectomy, the distance between the anterior vaginal fornix and the anterior cul-de-sac peritoneum

spans several centimeters. Thus, to successfully enter the peritoneal cavity anteriorly, proper identification and sharp dissection of the loose connective tissue that lies within the vesicovaginal and then vesicocervical spaces is necessary (see Fig. 38-17) (Balgobin, 2011).

Rectovaginal Space

This is adjacent to the posterior surface of the vagina. It extends from the cul-de-sac of Douglas down to the superior border of the perineal body, which extends 2 to 3 cm cephalad to the hymeneal ring (see Figs. 38-17 and 38-18). Rectal pillars, also known as the deep uterosacral or rectouterine ligaments, are fibers of the cardinal-uterosacral ligament complex that extend down from the cervix and attach to the upper portion of the posterior vaginal wall. These fibers connect the vagina to the lateral walls of the rectum and to the sacrum. These pillars also separate the midline rectovaginal space from the more lateral pararectal spaces.

Clinically, the rectovaginal space contains loose areolar tissue and is easily opened with finger dissection during abdominal surgery (see Fig. 38-18). Perforation of the rectal pillar fibers allows access to the sacrospinous ligaments used in vaginal suspension procedures.

The posterior cul-de-sac peritoneum extends down the posterior vaginal wall 2 to 3 cm inferior to the posterior vaginal fornix (Kuhn, 1982). Thus, during vaginal hysterectomy, in contrast to anterior peritoneal cavity entry, entering the peritoneal cavity posteriorly is readily done by incising the vaginal wall in the area of the posterior fornix (see Fig. 38-17).

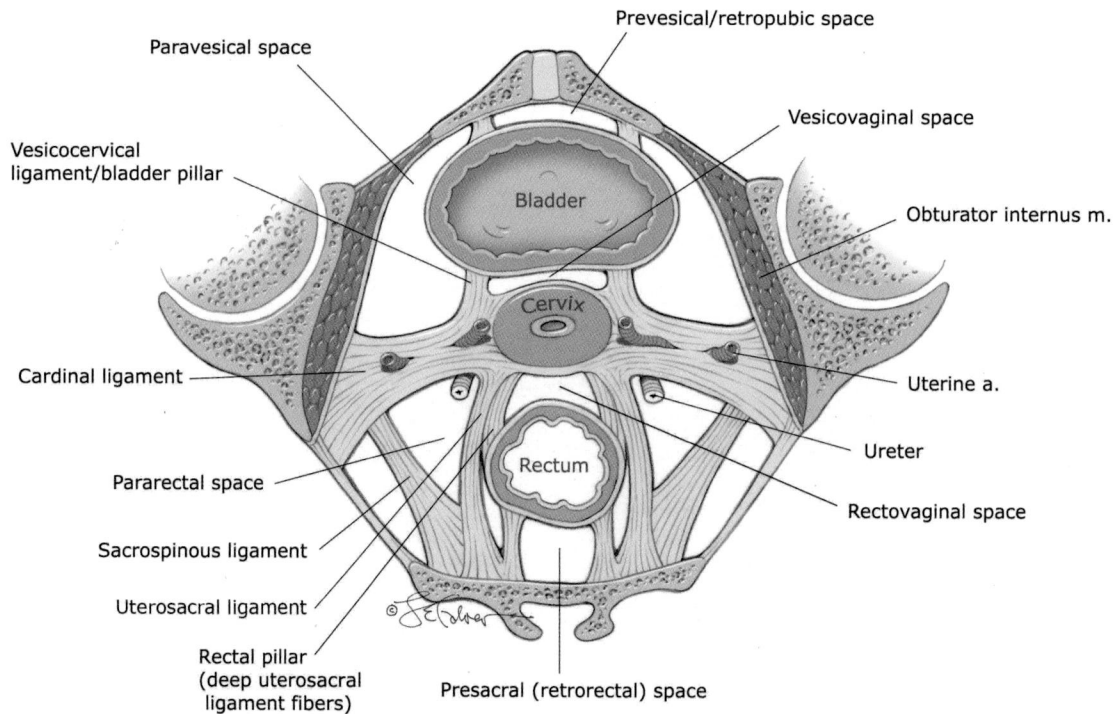

FIGURE 38-18 Connective tissue and surgical spaces of the pelvis.

Vaginal Support

The main support of the vagina is provided by the levator ani muscles and the connective tissue that attaches the lateral walls of the vagina to the pelvic walls. These attachments are the cardinal and uterosacral ligaments. Although the visceral connective tissue in the pelvis is continuous and interdependent, DeLancey (1992) has described three levels of vaginal connective tissue support that help explain pelvic support dysfunction.

For upper vaginal support, the parametrium continues caudally down the vagina as the paracolpium (see Fig. 38-15). This tissue attaches the upper vagina to the pelvic wall, suspending it over the pelvic floor. These attachments are known as *level I support* or *suspensory axis* and provide connective tissue support to the vaginal apex after hysterectomy. In the standing position, level I support fibers are vertically oriented. Clinical manifestations of level I support defects include uterine prolapse or posthysterectomy vaginal vault prolapse.

For midvaginal support, the lateral walls of the vagina's midportion are attached to the pelvic walls on each side by visceral connective tissue known as endopelvic fascia. These lateral attachments of the vaginal walls blend into the arcus tendineus fascia pelvis and to the medial aspect of the levator ani muscles, and in doing so create the anterior and posterior lateral vaginal sulci (see Fig. 38-15). These grooves run along the vaginal sidewalls and give the vagina an "H" shape when viewed in cross section. As noted earlier, the arcus tendineus fascia pelvis covers the medial aspect of the obturator internus and levator ani muscles. It spans from the inner and lower surface of the pubic bones to the ischial spines (see Figs. 38-7 and 38-15).

Attachment of the anterior vaginal wall to the levator ani muscles is responsible for the bladder neck elevation noted with cough or Valsalva maneuver (see Fig. 38-10). Thus, these midvaginal attachments may have significance for stress urinary continence and are referred to as *level II support* or the *attachment axis*. Clinical manifestations of level II support defects include anterior and posterior vaginal wall prolapse and stress urinary incontinence.

For distal vaginal support, the distal third of the vagina is directly attached to its surrounding structures (see Fig. 38-9). Anteriorly, the vagina is fused with the urethra. Laterally it attaches to the pubovaginalis muscle and perineal membrane, and posteriorly to the perineal body. These vaginal attachments are referred to as *level III support* or the *fusion axis* and are considered the strongest of the vaginal support components. Clinically, failure of this level of support can result in distal rectoceles or perineal descent. Anal incontinence may also result if the perineal body is absent, as may follow obstetric trauma.

Vaginal Blood Supply, Lymphatics, and Innervation

The main blood supply to the vagina arises from the descending or cervical branch of the uterine artery and from the vaginal artery, a branch of the internal iliac artery (see Fig. 38-12). These vessels form an anastomotic arcade along the lateral sides of the vagina at the level of the vaginal sulci. They also anastomose with the contralateral vessels at points on the anterior and posterior walls of the vagina. Additionally, the middle rectal artery from the internal iliac artery contributes to the posterior vaginal wall supply. The distal walls of the vagina also receive contributions from the internal pudendal artery (p. 822). Lymphatic drainage of the upper two thirds of the vagina is similar to that of the uterus as described on page 809. The distal part of the vagina drains with the vulvar lymphatics to the inguinal nodes. A more detailed description of the vulvar lymphatics is presented on page 822. Last, vaginal innervation

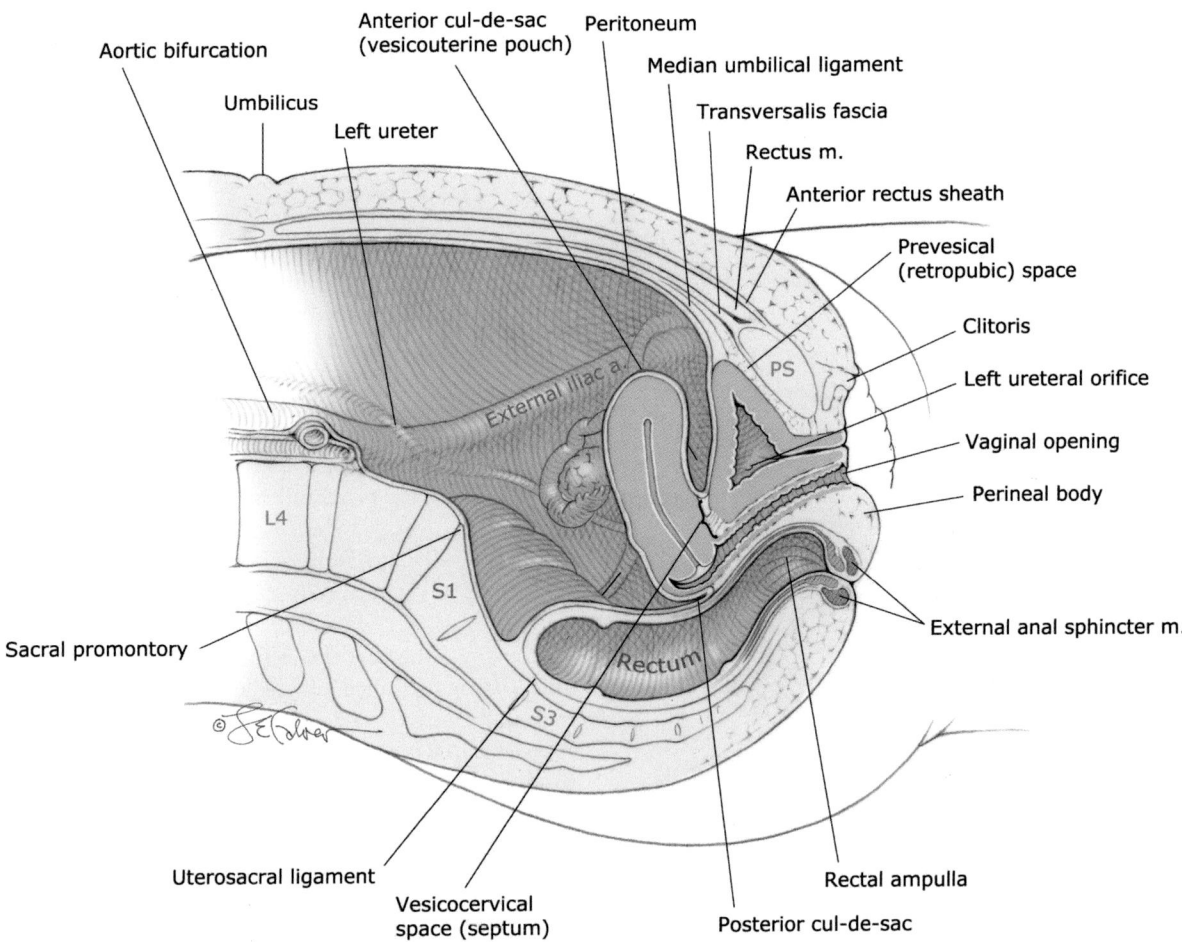

Aortic bifurcation

Umbilicus

Left ureter

Anterior cul-de-sac
(vesicouterine pouch)

Peritoneum

Median umbilical ligament

Transversalis fascia

Rectus m.

Anterior rectus sheath

Prevesical
(retropubic) space

Clitoris

Left ureteral orifice

Vaginal opening

Perineal body

External iliac a.

PS

L4

S1

S3

Sacral promontory

Rectum

External anal sphincter m.

Uterosacral ligament

Vesicocervical
space (septum)

Posterior cul-de-sac

Rectal ampulla

FIGURE 38-19 Midsagittal view of pelvic structures and associated anatomy. L4 = fourth lumbar vertebra; PS = pubic symphysis; S1, S3 = first and third sacral vertebrae.

comes from inferior extensions of the uterovaginal plexus, a component of the inferior hypogastric plexus (see Fig. 38-13).

Lower Urinary Tract Structures

Bladder

The bladder is a hollow organ that stores and evacuates urine (Fig. 38-19). Anteriorly, the bladder rests against the inner surface of the pubic bones and then, as it fills, also against the anterior abdominal wall. Posteriorly, it rests against the vagina and cervix. Anteroinferiorly and laterally, the bladder contacts the loose connective and fatty tissue that fills the retropubic space, and here, the bladder lacks a peritoneal covering. The reflection of the bladder onto the abdominal wall is triangular, and the triangle apex is continuous with the median umbilical ligament.

Clinically, an intentional cystotomy can be made to confirm patency of the ureteral orifices, to assist with surgical dissection, or to place ureteral stents. The incision is ideally placed in the retropubic extraperitoneal portion of the bladder close to the apex. This avoids direct contact between the abdominopelvic viscera and the cystotomy site and minimizes the risk of fistula formation.

The bladder wall consists of coarse bundles of smooth muscle known as the *detrusor muscle*, which extends into the upper part of the urethra. Although separate layers of the detrusor are described, they are not as well defined as the layers of other viscous structures (Fig. 23-1, p. 517). The innermost layer of the bladder wall is plexiform, which can be seen from the pattern of trabeculations noted during cystoscopy. The mucosa of the bladder consists of transitional epithelium and underlying lamina propria. A submucosal layer intervenes between this mucosa and the detrusor muscle.

The bladder is divided into a *dome* and a *base* approximately at the level of the ureteral orifices. The dome is thin walled and distensible, whereas the base is thicker and undergoes less distention during filling (see Fig. 38-15). The bladder base consists of the *vesical trigone* and the *detrusor loops*. These loops are two U-shaped bands of fibers found at the *vesical neck*, where the urethra enters the bladder wall. Ureteral orifices lie within the trigone and empty here into the bladder. The pelvic ureter courses in the pelvic sidewall retroperitoneum and is discussed on page 816.

The blood supply to the bladder arises from the superior vesical arteries, which are branches of the patent portion of the umbilical artery. Other contributors are the middle and inferior vesical arteries, which, when present, often arise from either the internal pudendal or the vaginal arteries (see Fig. 38-12). The nerve supply to the bladder arises from the vesical plexus, a component of the inferior hypogastric plexus (see Fig. 38-13).

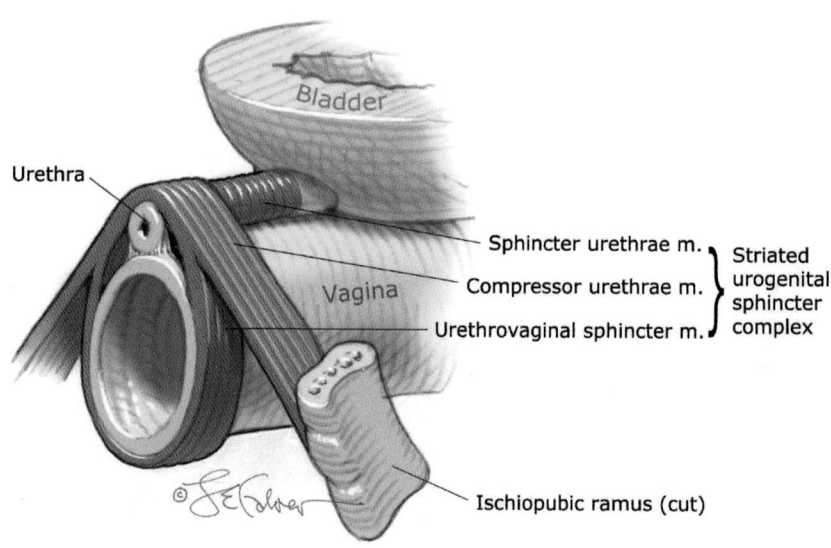

FIGURE 38-20 Urethra and associated muscles.

Urethra

The female urethra measures 3 to 4 cm in length. The urethral lumen begins at the internal urinary meatus within the bladder, and then courses through the bladder base for less than a centimeter. This region where the urethral lumen traverses the bladder base is called the *bladder neck*. The distal two thirds of the urethra are fused with the anterior vaginal wall.

The walls of the urethra begin outside the bladder wall. They consist of two layers of smooth muscle, an inner longitudinal and an outer circular, which are in turn surrounded by a circular layer of skeletal muscle referred to as the *sphincter urethrae* or *rhabdosphincter* (Fig. 38-20). Approximately at the junction of the middle and lower third of the urethra, and just above or deep to the perineal membrane, two strap skeletal muscles called the *urethrovaginal sphincter* and *compressor urethrae* are found. These muscles were previously known as the *deep transverse perineal muscles* in females. Together with the sphincter urethrae, they constitute the *striated urogenital sphincter complex.* Together, these three muscles function as a unit and have a complex and controversial innervation. Their fibers act cumulatively to supply constant tonus and to provide emergency reflex activity mainly in the distal half of the urethra to sustain continence.

Distal to the depth of the perineal membrane, the walls of the urethra consist of fibrous tissue, serving as the nozzle that directs the urine stream. The urethra has a prominent submucosal layer that is lined by hormonally sensitive stratified squamous epithelium (Fig. 23-8, p. 520). Within the submucosal layer on the dorsal (vaginal) surface of the urethra is a group of glands known as the paraurethral glands, which open into the urethral lumen (Fig. 26-3, p. 583). Duct openings of the two most prominent glands, termed Skene glands, are seen on the inner surface of the external urethral orifice (p. 818).

The urethra receives its blood supply from branches of the inferior vesical/vaginal and internal pudendal arteries. Although still controversial, the pudendal nerve is believed to innervate the most distal part of the striated urogenital sphincter complex. Somatic efferent branches from S2–S4 that course along the

inferior hypogastric plexus variably innervate the sphincter urethrae. An additional discussion of lower urinary tract innervation is found in Chapter 23 (p. 516).

Clinically, chronic infection of the paraurethral glands can lead to urethral diverticula. Due to the multiple openings of these glands along the length of the urethra, diverticula may develop at various sites along the urethra.

■ Rectum

The rectum is continuous with the sigmoid colon approximately at the level of the third sacral vertebra (see Fig. 38-19). It descends on the anterior surface of the sacrum for approximately 12 cm and ends in the anal canal after passing through the levator hiatus. The anterior and lateral portions of the proximal two thirds of the rectum are covered by peritoneum. The peritoneum is then reflected onto the posterior vaginal wall to form the posterior *cul-de-sac of Douglas*, also termed *rectouterine pouch*. In women, the cul-de-sac is located approximately 5 to 6 cm from the anal orifice and can be palpated manually during rectal or vaginal examination. At its commencement, the rectal wall is similar to that of the sigmoid, but near its termination it becomes dilated to form the rectal ampulla, which begins below the posterior cul-de-sac peritoneum.

The rectum contains several, usually three, transverse folds called the *plicae transversales recti*, also termed valves of Houston (Fig. 38-21). The largest and most constant of these folds is located anteriorly and to the right, approximately 8 cm from the anal orifice. These folds may contribute to fecal continence by supporting fecal matter above the anal canal. Clinically, in the empty state, the transverse rectal folds overlap each other, making it difficult at times to manipulate an examining finger or endoscopy tube past this level.

RETROPERITONEAL SURGICAL SPACES

■ Pelvic Sidewall

Several retroperitoneal spaces are important for the pelvic surgeon. Of these, the retroperitoneal space of the pelvic sidewalls contains the internal iliac vessels and pelvic lymphatics, pelvic ureter, and obturator nerve.

During surgery, entering the retroperitoneum at the pelvic sidewall can be used to identify the ureter (Fig. 38-22). Moreover, it is an essential step for many of the surgeries described in gynecologic oncology.

Vessels

The major pelvic vessels are shown in Figures 38-12, 38-14, and 38-22. The internal iliac and external iliac vessels and their corresponding lymph node groups lie within the pelvic sidewall retroperitoneal space (see Fig. 38-16).

Clinically, if severe hemorrhage is encountered during pelvic surgery, the internal iliac artery may be ligated to decrease the

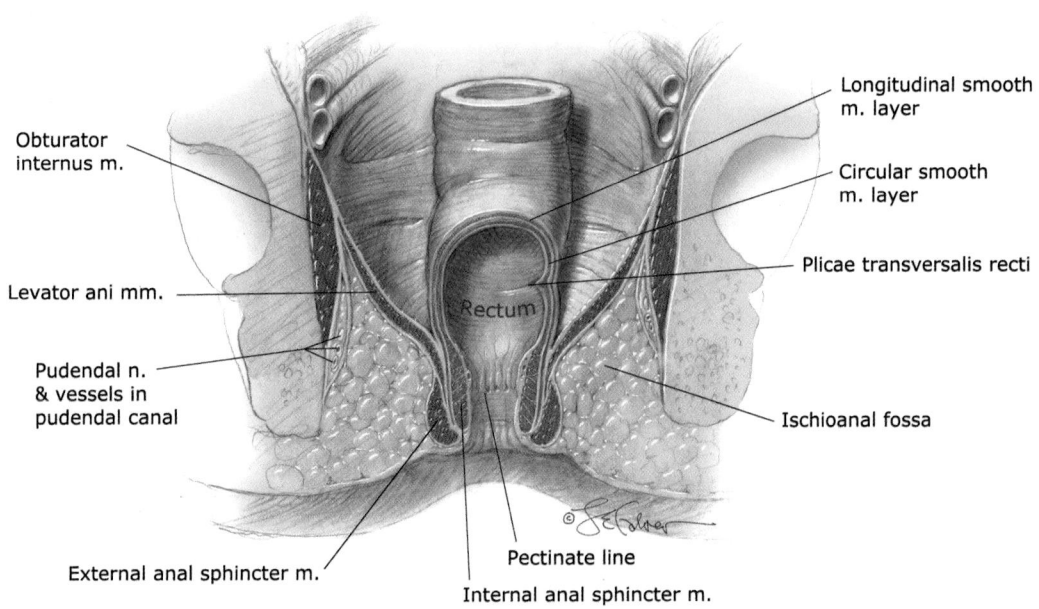

Obturator
internus m.

Levator ani mm.

Pudendal n.
& vessels in
pudendal canal

Longitudinal smooth
m. layer

Circular smooth
m. layer

Plicae transversalis recti

Rectum

Ischioanal fossa

External anal sphincter m.

Pectinate line

Internal anal sphincter m.

FIGURE 38-21 Ischioanal fossa and anal sphincter complex.

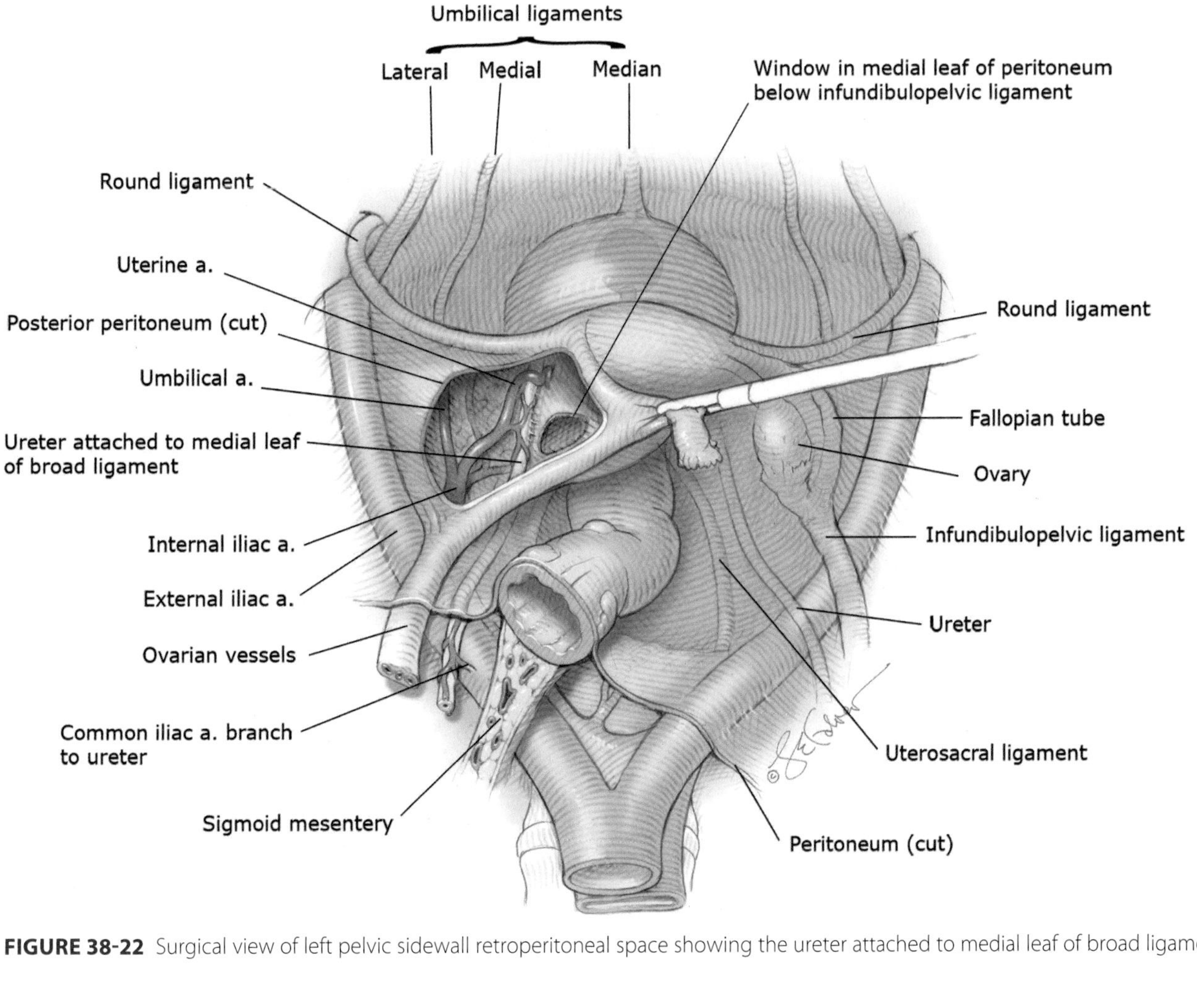

Umbilical ligaments

Lateral   Medial   Median

Round ligament

Uterine a.

Posterior peritoneum (cut)

Umbilical a.

Ureter attached to medial leaf
of broad ligament

Internal iliac a.

External iliac a.

Ovarian vessels

Common iliac a. branch
to ureter

Sigmoid mesentery

Window in medial leaf of peritoneum
below infundibulopelvic ligament

Round ligament

Fallopian tube

Ovary

Infundibulopelvic ligament

Ureter

Uterosacral ligament

Peritoneum (cut)

FIGURE 38-22 Surgical view of left pelvic sidewall retroperitoneal space showing the ureter attached to medial leaf of broad ligament.

pulse pressure to pelvic organs. When this vessel is dissected, the ureter is also identified and avoided. The internal iliac artery is ligated distal to the origin of its posterior division branches. This helps to prevent significant devascularization of the gluteal muscles. These posterior division branches generally arise from the posterolateral wall of the internal iliac artery at a site 3 to 4 cm from its origin off the common iliac artery (Bleich, 2007).

Pelvic Ureter

As the ureter enters the pelvis, it crosses over the bifurcation of the common iliac artery or the proximal portion of the external iliac artery and passes just medial to the ovarian vessels (see Fig. 38-15). It descends into the pelvis attached to the medial leaf of the pelvic sidewall peritoneum. Along this course, the ureter lies medial to the internal iliac branches and anterolateral to the uterosacral ligaments (see Figs. 38-14, 38-15, and 38-22). The ureter then traverses through the cardinal ligament approximately 1 to 2 cm lateral to the cervix. Near the level of the uterine isthmus, it courses below the uterine artery ("water under the bridge"). It then travels anteromedially toward the bladder base (see Fig. 38-15). In this path, it runs close to the upper third of the anterior vaginal wall (Rahn, 2007). Finally, the ureter enters the bladder and travels obliquely for approximately 1.5 cm before opening at the ureteral orifices.

The pelvic ureter receives blood supply from the vessels it passes: the common iliac, internal iliac, uterine, and superior vesical vessels. The ureter's course runs medial to these vessels, and thus its blood supply reaches the ureter from lateral sources. This is important during ureteral isolation. In contrast, the abdominal part of the ureter courses lateral to major vessels and accordingly, it receives most of its blood supply from medially located vessels. Vascular anastomoses on the connective tissue sheath enveloping the ureter form a longitudinal network of vessels.

Clinically, because of the pelvic ureter's proximity to many structures encountered during gynecologic surgery, emphasis is placed on its precise intraoperative identification. Most ureters are injured during gynecologic surgery for benign disease. More than 50 percent of these injuries are not diagnosed intraoperatively (Ibeanu, 2009). The most common sites of injury include: (1) the pelvic brim area during infundibulopelvic ligament clamping; (2) the isthmic region during uterine artery ligation, (3) the pelvic sidewall during uterosacral ligament suturing, and (4) the lateral vaginal apex during vaginal cuff clamping or suturing.

■ Presacral Space

This retroperitoneal space lies between the rectosigmoid/posterior abdominal wall peritoneum and the sacrum (Figs. 38-18 and 38-23). It begins below the aortic bifurcation and extends

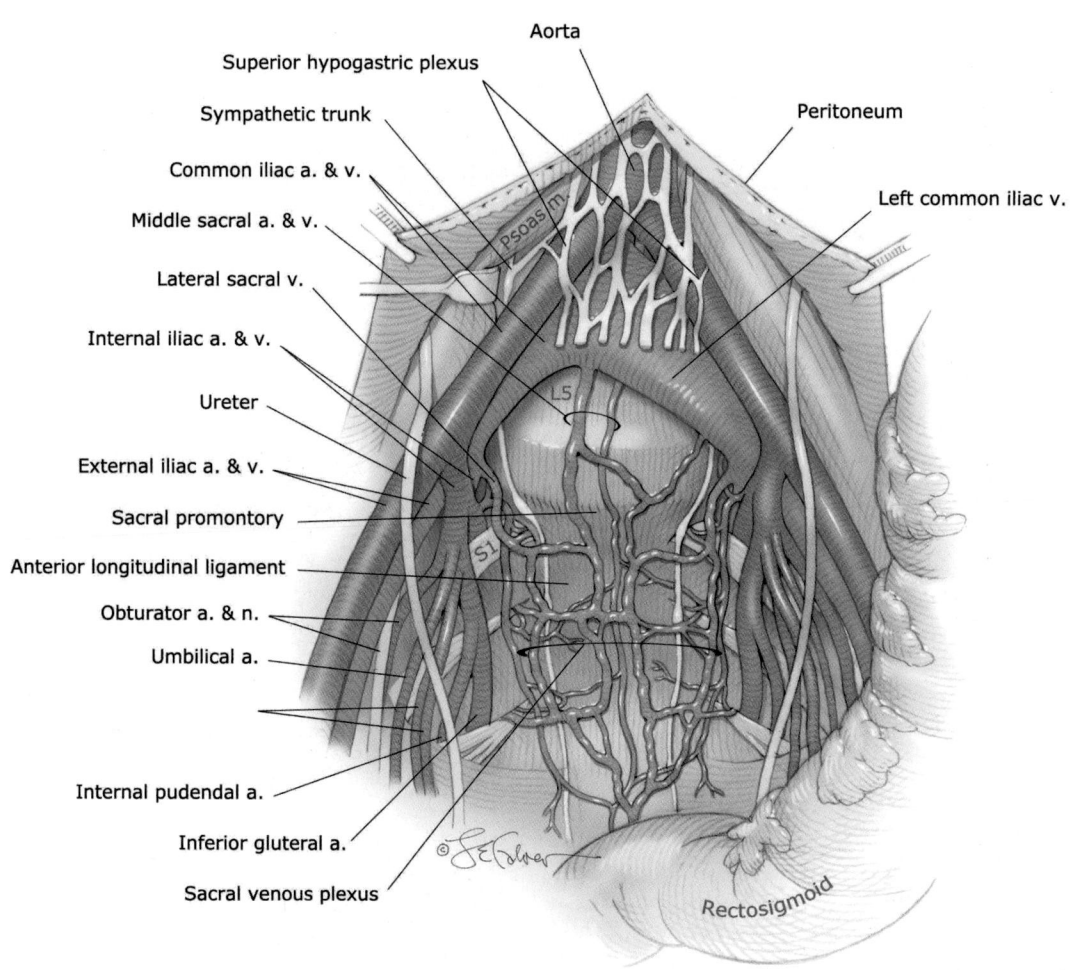

FIGURE 38-23 Presacral space. L5 = fifth lumbar vertebra; S1 = first sacral nerve.

inferiorly to the pelvic floor. Laterally, this space is bounded by the internal iliac vessels and branches and by the fascia that covers the piriformis muscle and sacral nerves. Contained within the loose areolar and connective tissue of this space are the superior hypogastric plexus, hypogastric nerves, and portions of the inferior hypogastric plexus (see Figs. 38-14 and 38-23). The sacral lymph node group is also found here (see Fig. 38-16). In addition, the sacral sympathetic trunk, a continuation of the lumbar trunk, lies against the sacrum's ventral surface and medial to the sacral foramina.

The presacral space contains an extensive and intricate venous plexus, termed the *sacral venous plexus*. This plexus is formed primarily by the anastomoses of the middle and lateral sacral veins on the anterior surface of the sacrum. The *middle sacral vein* commonly drains from this plexus into the left common iliac vein, whereas each *lateral sacral vein* opens into its respective internal iliac vein. Ultimately, these vessels drain into the caval system. The sacral venous plexus also receives contributions from the *lumbar veins* of the posterior abdominal wall and from the *basivertebral veins* that pass through the pelvic sacral foramina. The *middle sacral artery*, which courses in proximity to the *middle sacral vein*, arises from the posterior and distal part of the abdominal aorta.

In studies of presacral space vascular anatomy, the left common iliac vein was the closest major vessel identified both cephalad and lateral to the midsacral promontory. The average distance of the left common iliac vein from the midsacral promontory is 2.7 cm (range 0.9–5.2 cm) (Good, 2013b; Wieslander, 2006).

Surgically, the presacral space is most commonly entered to perform abdominal sacrocolpopexy or presacral neurectomy.

Importantly, during these procedures, bleeding from the sacral venous plexus may be difficult to control as the veins may retract into the sacral foramina. For sacrocolpopexy, the sacral promontory's midpoint is an important landmark, and the right ureter, right common iliac artery, and left common iliac vein are found within 3 cm of the midsacral promontory (Good, 2013b; Weislander, 2007). Moreover, the first sacral nerve can be expected approximately 3 cm from the upper surface of the sacrum and 1.5 cm from the midline (Good, 2013b). In supine women, the most prominent presacral space structure is the L5–S1 disc, which extends approximately 1.5 cm cephalad to the "true" sacral promontory (Good, 2013a). Awareness of a 60-degree average drop between the anterior surfaces of L5 and S1 vertebrae assists intraoperative localization of the promontory.

■ Prevesical Space

This space is also called the retropubic space or *space of Retzius*. During laparotomy, if an extraperitoneal approach is selected, this space can be entered by perforating the transversalis fascial layer of the anterior abdominal wall (see Fig. 38-19). If an intraperitoneal approach is chosen, then only the anterior abdominal wall peritoneum is incised to access this space. The prevesical space is bounded by the bony pelvis and muscles of the pelvic wall anteriorly and laterally and by the anterior abdominal wall ventrally (see Figs. 38-18, 38-19, and Fig. 38-24). The bladder and proximal urethra lie posterior within this space. Attachments of the paravaginal connective tissue to the arcus tendineus fascia pelvis constitute the posterolateral limit of the space and separate this space from the vesicovaginal and vesicocervical spaces.

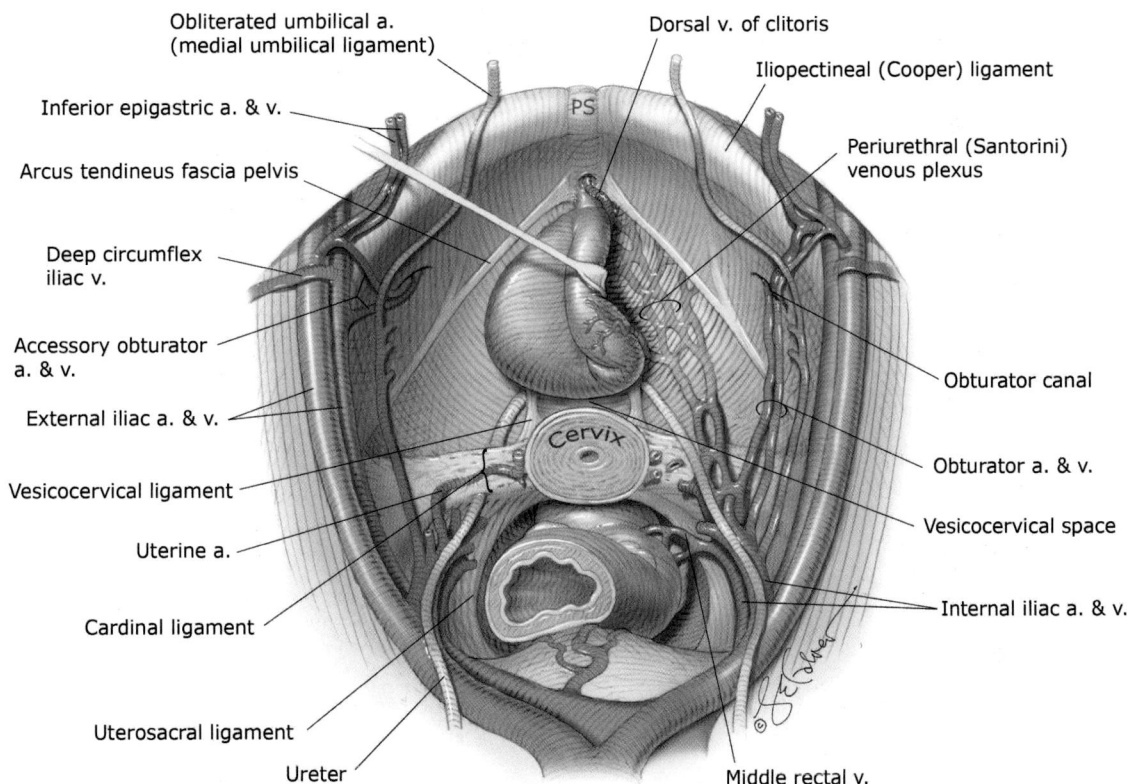

FIGURE 38-24 Retropubic space. PS = pubic symphysis.

There are several vessels and nerves in this space. The *dorsal vein of the clitoris* passes under the lower border of the pubic symphysis and drains into the *periurethral-perivesical venous plexus,* also termed the *plexus of Santorini* (Pathi, 2009). The *obturator neurovascular bundle* courses along the lateral pelvic walls and enters the obturator canal to reach the medial compartment of the thigh. The autonomic nerve branches that supply the bladder and urethra course on the lateral borders of these structures. Additionally, in most women, accessory obturator vessels that arise from or open into the inferior epigastric or external iliac vessels are found crossing the superior pubic rami and connecting with the obturator vessels near the obturator canal. Clinically, the obliterated umbilical or the superior vesical arteries are used to describe the medial boundary of the paravesical space. The paravesical space represents the lateral boundaries of the prevesical space (see Fig. 38-18).

Surgically, injury to the obturator neurovascular bundle or accessory obturator vessels is most often associated with pelvic lymph node dissection, paravaginal defect repair, and pelvic fractures. The obturator canal is found approximately 5 to 6 cm from the midline of the pubic symphysis, and 1 to 2 cm below the upper margin of the iliopectineal ligament (Drewes, 2005).

Bleeding from the periurethral-perivesical venous plexus is often encountered while placing sutures or passing needles into this space during retropubic bladder neck suspensions and midurethral retropubic procedures, respectively. This venous ooze usually stops when pressure is applied or sutures are tied.

In a cadaver study, proximal paravaginal defect repair sutures placed at the level of the ischial spines were found an average of 2.3 cm away from the ureter but as close as 5 mm (Rahn, 2007). This further highlights the value of intraoperative cystoscopy during retropubic surgeries.

VULVA AND PERINEUM

■ Vulva

The external female genitalia, collectively known as the *vulva*, lie on the pubic bones and extend posteriorly. Structures included are the mons pubis, labia majora and minora, clitoris, vestibule, vestibular bulbs, greater vestibular glands (Bartholin glands), lesser vestibular glands, Skene and paraurethral glands, and the urethral and vaginal orifices (Fig. 38-25). The embryologic development and homologues of these structures can be found in Table 18-1 (p. 404).

Mons Pubis and Labia Majora

The *mons pubis*, also called the *mons veneris*, is the rounded fat pad that lies ventral to the pubic symphysis. The labia majora are two prominent folds that extend from the mons pubis toward the perineal body posteriorly. Skin over the mons pubis and labia majora contains hair and has a subcutaneous layer similar to that of the anterior abdominal wall. The subcutaneous layer consists of a superficial fatty layer similar to Camper fascia, and a deeper membranous layer, *Colles fascia* (see Fig. 38-25). Also known as the *superficial perineal fascia*, Colles fascia is similar to and continuous with Scarpa fascia of the anterior abdominal wall.

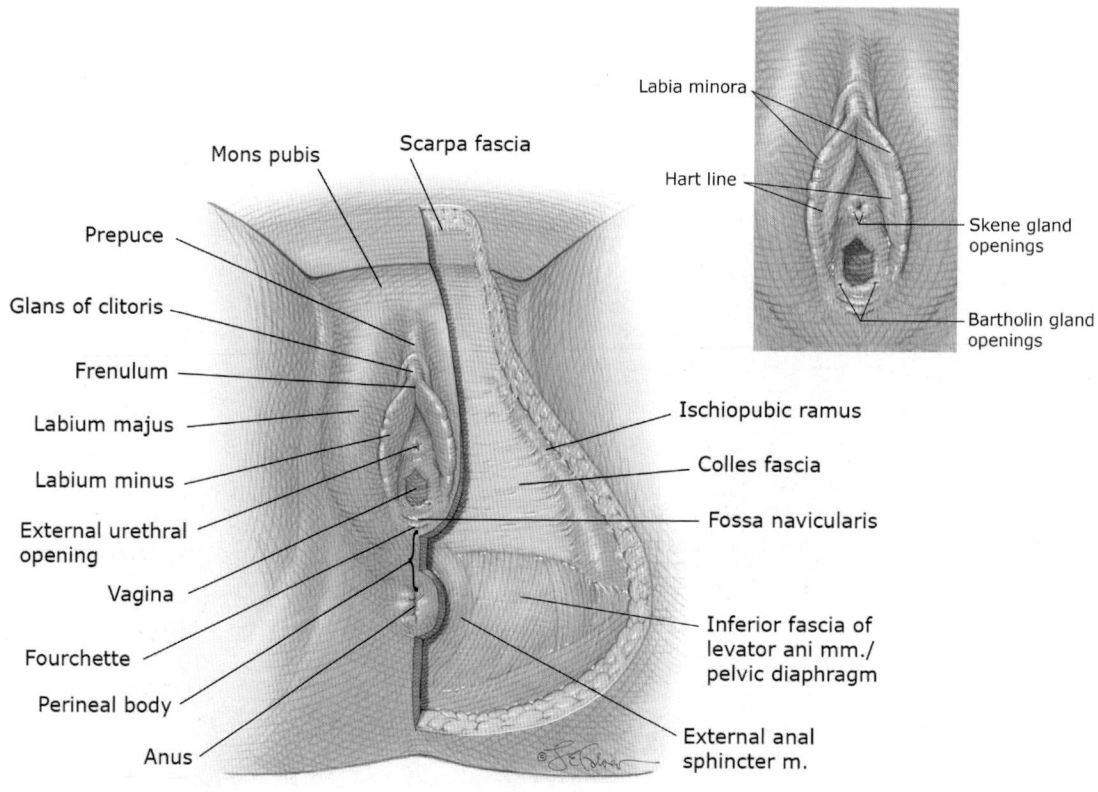

FIGURE 38-25 Vulvar structures and subcutaneous layer of anterior perineal triangle. Note the continuity of Colles and Scarpa fasciae. Inset: Vestibule boundaries and openings onto vestibule.

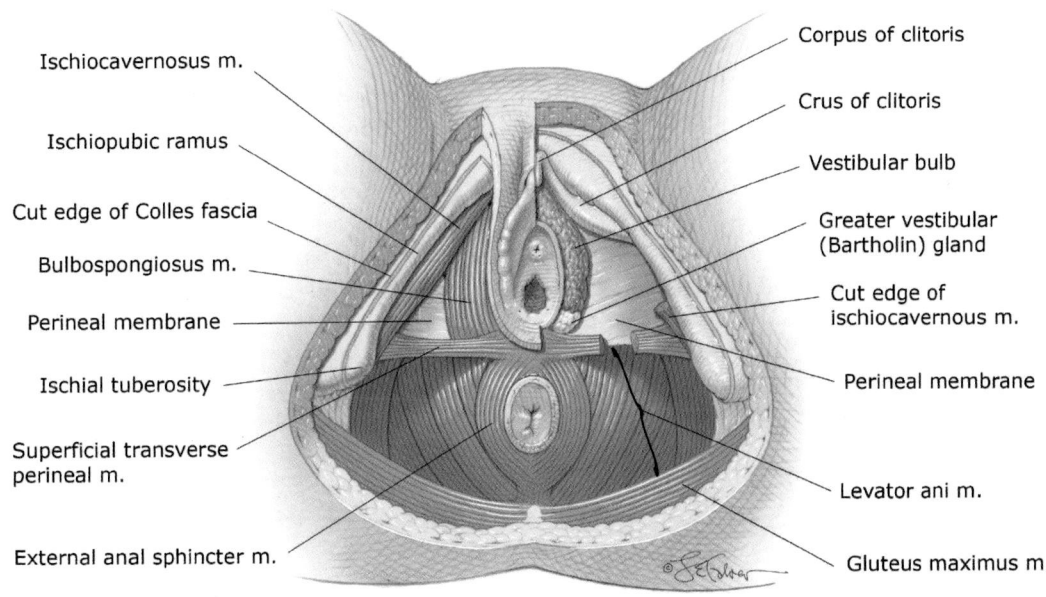

FIGURE 38-26 Anterior (superficial space of anterior triangle) and posterior perineal triangles. On the image's left are the structures noted after removal of Colles fascia. On the image's right are the structures noted after removal of the superficial perineal muscles.

The round ligament and obliterated *processus vaginalis*, which is also termed the *canal of Nuck*, exit the inguinal canal and attach to the adipose tissue or skin of the labia majora.

Clinically, Colles fascia attaches firmly to the ischiopubic rami laterally and the perineal membrane posteriorly. These attachments prevent the spread of fluid, blood, or infection from the superficial perineal space to the thighs or posterior perineal triangle. Anteriorly, Colles fascia has no attachments to the pubic rami, and it is therefore continuous with the lower anterior abdominal wall (see Fig. 38-25). This continuity may allow the spread of fluid, blood, and infection between these compartments.

Clinically, a mass found in one labium majus may be a leiomyoma arising from the distal round ligament, a persistent processus vaginalis, or breast tissue along the distal milk line. An indirect inguinal hernia may also reach the labium majus by passing through the deep inguinal ring and inguinal canal.

Labia Minora

These two cutaneous folds lie between the labia majora (see Fig. 38-25). Anteriorly, each labium minus bifurcates to form two folds that surround the glans of the clitoris. The prepuce is the anterior fold that overlies the glans, and the frenulum is the fold that passes below the clitoris. Posteriorly, the labia minora end at the fourchette.

In contrast to the skin that overlies the labia majora, the skin of the labia minora does not contain hair. Also, the subcutaneous tissue is devoid of fat and consists primarily of loose connective tissue. This latter attribute allows mobility of the skin during sex and accounts for the ease of dissection with vulvectomy.

Clinically, labia minora are typically symmetric, but their size and shape can vary widely between women. In some, these winglike structures are pendulous and can be drawn into the vagina during coitus. If associated with dyspareunia in this setting, the labia can be surgically reduced. Moreover, chronic dermatologic diseases such as lichen sclerosus may lead to significant atrophy or disappearance of the labia minora.

Clitoris

This is the female erectile structure homologous to the penis. It consists of a glans, a body, and two crura. The glans contains many nerve endings and is covered by a thinly keratinized stratified squamous epithelium. The body measures approximately 2 cm and is connected to the pubic ramus by the crura (Fig. 38-26).

Vaginal Vestibule

This is the area between the two labia minora. It is bounded laterally by the line of Hart and medially by the hymeneal ring. Hart line represents the demarcation between the skin and mucous membrane on the inner surface of the labia minora. The vestibule extends from the clitoris anteriorly to the fourchette posteriorly (see Fig. 38-25 inset). It contains the openings of the urethra; vagina; greater vestibular glands, also known as Bartholin glands; and Skene glands, which are the largest pair of paraurethral glands. It also contains the numerous openings of the lesser vestibular glands. A shallow vestibular depression known as the navicular fossa lies between the vaginal orifice and the fourchette.

Clinically, localized vulvar dysesthesia—also termed vulvar vestibulitis—is characterized by pain with vaginal penetration, localized point tenderness, and erythema of the vestibular mucosa. In other women, when choosing incision sites for Bartholin gland drainage or marsupialization, Hart line is clinically relevant. That is, in attempts to recreate near-normal gland duct anatomy following these procedures, incisions placed external to Hart line are avoided (Kaufman, 1994).

Vestibular Bulbs

These are homologues to the male penile bulb and corpus spongiosum. They are two elongated, approximately 3-cm long, richly vascular erectile masses that surround the vaginal orifice (see Fig. 38-26). Their posterior ends are in contact with the Bartholin glands. Their anterior ends are joined to one another and to the clitoris. Their deep surfaces are in contact with the perineal membrane, and their superficial surfaces are partially covered by the bulbospongiosus muscles.

Clinically, the proximity of the Bartholin glands to the vestibular bulbs accounts for the significant bleeding often encountered with Bartholin gland excision (Section 43-20, p. 975). Following vulvar trauma, laceration of these bulbs or the clitoral crus may lead to sizable hematomas.

Bartholin Glands

These are the homologues of the male bulbourethral or Cowper glands. They are in contact with and often overlapped by the posterior ends of the vestibular bulbs (see Fig. 38-26). Each gland is connected to the vestibule by an approximately 2-cm long duct. The ducts open in the groove between the hymen and the labia minora—the vestibule—at approximately 5 and 7 o'clock positions.

The glands contain columnar cells that secrete clear or whitish mucus with lubricant properties. These glands are stimulated by sexual arousal. Contraction of the bulbospongiosus muscle, which covers the superficial surface of the gland, expresses gland secretions.

Clinically, obstruction of the Bartholin ducts by proteinaceous material or by inflammation from infection can lead to cysts of variable sizes. An infected cyst can lead to an abscess, which typically requires surgical drainage. Symptomatic or recurrent cysts may require marsupialization or gland excision.

◼ Perineum

The *perineum* is the diamond-shaped area between the thighs (see Fig. 38-25). It is bounded deeply by the inferior fascia of the pelvic diaphragm and superficially by the skin between the thighs. The anterior, posterior, and lateral boundaries of the perineum are the same as those of the bony pelvic outlet: the pubic symphysis anteriorly, ischiopubic rami and ischial tuberosities anterolaterally, coccyx posteriorly, and sacrotuberous ligaments posterolaterally. An arbitrary line joining the ischial tuberosities divides the perineum into the anterior or *urogenital triangle,* and a posterior or *anal triangle.*

Anterior (Urogenital) Triangle

Structures that comprise the vulva or external female genitalia lie in the anterior triangle of the perineum. The base or posterior border of this triangle is the *interischial line,* which usually overlies the *superficial transverse perineal muscles* (see Fig. 38-26).

The anterior perineal triangle can be further divided into a *superficial* and a *deep pouch* or *space* by the *perineal membrane.* The superficial perineal space lies superficial to the perineal membrane, and the deep space lies above or deep to the membrane.

Superficial Space. This space of the anterior triangle is an enclosed compartment that lies between Colles fascia and the perineal membrane. It contains the ischiocavernosus, bulbospongiosus, and superficial transverse perineal muscles; Bartholin glands; vestibular bulbs; clitoris; and branches of the pudendal vessels and nerve. The urethra and vagina traverse this space.

The *ischiocavernosus muscle* attaches to the medial aspect of the ischial tuberosities posteriorly and the ischiopubic rami laterally. Anteriorly, it attaches to the crus of the clitoris. This muscle may help maintain clitoral erection by compressing the crus of the clitoris, thus retarding venous drainage.

The *bulbospongiosus muscle,* also known as the bulbocavernosus muscle, covers the superficial portion of the vestibular bulbs and Bartholin glands. These muscles attach to the body of the clitoris anteriorly and the perineal body posteriorly. The muscles act to constrict the vaginal lumen, contributing to the release of Bartholin gland secretions. They may also contribute to clitoral erection by compressing the deep dorsal vein of the clitoris. The bulbospongiosus muscle, along with the ischiocavernosus muscle, acts to pull the clitoris downward.

The *superficial transverse perineal muscles* are narrow strips that attach to the ischial tuberosity laterally and the perineal body medially. They may be attenuated or even absent, but when present, they contribute to the perineal body.

Deep Perineal Space. This pouch lies deep or superior to the perineal membrane (Fig. 38-27). In contrast to the superficial space, which is a closed compartment, the deep space is continuous superiorly with the pelvic cavity. It contains the compressor urethrae and urethrovaginal sphincter muscles, parts of the urethra and vagina, branches of the internal pudendal artery, and the dorsal nerve and vein of the clitoris.

Perineal Membrane (Urogenital Diaphragm). Traditionally, a trilaminar, triangular urogenital diaphragm has been described as the main component of the deep perineal space. According to this concept, the urogenital diaphragm consisted of the deep transverse perineal muscles and sphincter urethrae muscles between the perineal membrane (inferior fascia of the urogenital diaphragm) and a superior layer of fascia (superior fascia of the urogenital diaphragm). However, the term *diaphragm* is used to describe a closed compartment. As described earlier, the deep perineal space is an open compartment. It is bounded inferiorly by the perineal membrane and extends up into the pelvis (Oelrich, 1980, 1983). As a result, when describing perineal anatomy, the terms *urogenital diaphragm* or *inferior fascia of the urogenital diaphragm* are misnomers and have been replaced by the anatomically correct term, *perineal membrane.*

The perineal membrane constitutes the deep boundary of the superficial perineal space (see Fig. 38-27). It attaches laterally to the ischiopubic rami, medially to the distal third of the urethra and vagina, and posteriorly to the perineal body. Anteriorly, it attaches to the arcuate ligament of the pubis. In this area, the perineal membrane is particularly thick and is often referred to as the *pubourethral ligament.*

The perineal membrane consists of two histologically and probably functionally distinct portions that span the opening of the anterior pelvic triangle (Stein, 2008). The dorsal or posterior portion is a dense fibrous tissue sheet that attaches laterally to the ischiopubic rami and medially to the distal third of the vagina and to the perineal body (see Fig. 38-27). The ventral or anterior portion of the perineal membrane is intimately associated with the compressor urethrae and urethrovaginal sphincter

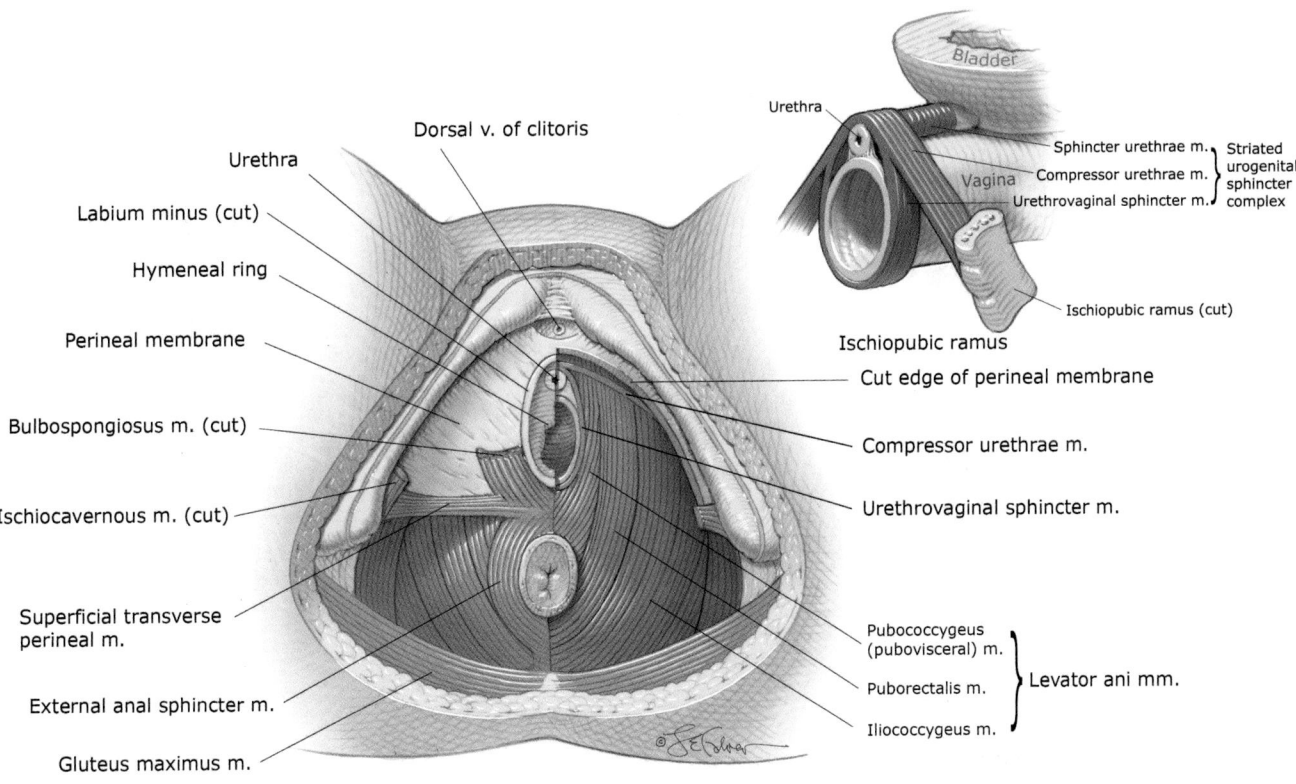

Dorsal v. of clitoris

Urethra

Labium minus (cut)

Hymeneal ring

Perineal membrane

Bulbospongiosus m. (cut)

Ischiocavernous m. (cut)

Superficial transverse
perineal m.

External anal sphincter m.

Gluteus maximus m.

Bladder

Urethra

Sphincter urethrae m. ⎫ Striated
Compressor urethrae m. ⎬ urogenital
Urethrovaginal sphincter m. ⎭ sphincter complex

Vagina

Ischiopubic ramus (cut)

Ischiopubic ramus

Cut edge of perineal membrane

Compressor urethrae m.

Urethrovaginal sphincter m.

Pubococcygeus
(pubovisceral) m. ⎫
Puborectalis m. ⎬ Levator ani mm.
Iliococcygeus m. ⎭

FIGURE 38-27 Deep space of anterior perineal triangle. On the image's right lie structures noted after removal of the perineal membrane. Also shown are all structures that attach to perineal body: bulbospongiosus, superficial transverse perineal, external anal sphincter, and puboperinealis muscles, perineal membrane, and urethrovaginal sphincter. Inset: Striated urogenital sphincter muscles.

muscles, previously called the deep transverse perineal muscles in the female (see Fig. 38-27 inset). Moreover, the ventral portion of the perineal membrane is continuous with the insertion of the arcus tendineus fascia pelvis to the pubic bones (see Fig. 38-20). The deep or superior surface of the perineal membrane appears to have direct connections to the levator ani muscles, and the superficial or inferior surface of the membrane fuses with the vestibular bulb and clitoral crus.

Clinically, the perineal membrane attaches to the lateral walls of the vagina approximately at level of the hymen. It provides support to the distal vagina and urethra by attaching these structures to the bony pelvis. In addition, its attachments to the levator ani muscles suggest that the perineal membrane may play an active role in support.

Posterior (Anal) Triangle

This triangle contains the ischioanal fossa, anal canal, anal sphincter complex, and branches of the internal pudendal vessels and pudendal nerve (Figs. 38-21, 38-27, and Fig. 38-28). It is bounded deeply by the fascia overlying the inferior surface of the levator ani muscles, and laterally by the fascia overlying the medial surface of the obturator internus muscles. A splitting of the obturator internus fascia in this area is known as the *pudendal* or *Alcock canal* (see Figs. 38-6 and 38-21). This canal allows passage of the internal pudendal vessels and pudendal nerve before these structures split into terminal branches to supply the structures of the vulva and perineum (see Fig. 38-28).

The *ischioanal* or *ischiorectal fossa* fills most of the anal triangle (see Figs. 38-21 and 38-28). It contains adipose tissue

and occasional blood vessels. The anal canal and anal sphincter complex lie in the center of this fossa. The ischioanal fossa is bounded superomedially by the inferior fascia of the levator muscles; anterolaterally by the fascia covering the medial surface of the obturator internus muscles and the ischial tuberosities; and posterolaterally by the lower border of the gluteus maximus muscles and sacrotuberous ligaments. At a superficial level, the ischioanal fossa is bounded anteriorly by the superficial transverse perineal muscles. At a superior or deeper level, there is no fascial boundary between the fossa and the tissues deep to the perineal membrane. Posterior to the anus, the contents of the fossa are continuous across the midline except for the attachments of the external anal sphincter fibers to the coccyx. This continuity of the ischioanal fossa across perineal compartments allows fluid, infection, and malignancy to spread from one side of the anal canal to the other, and also into the anterior perineal compartment deep to the perineal membrane.

The anal sphincter complex consists of two sphincters and the puborectalis muscle. The external anal sphincter consists of striated muscle that surrounds the distal anal canal. It consists of a superficial and a deep portion. The more superficial fibers lie caudal to the internal sphincter and are separated from the anal epithelium only by submucosa. The deep fibers blend with the lowest fibers of the puborectalis muscle. The external sphincter is primarily innervated by the inferior rectal branch of the pudendal nerve. The external anal sphincter is responsible for the squeeze pressure of the anal canal.

The internal anal sphincter is the thickening of the circular smooth muscle layer of the anal wall (see Fig. 38-21). It

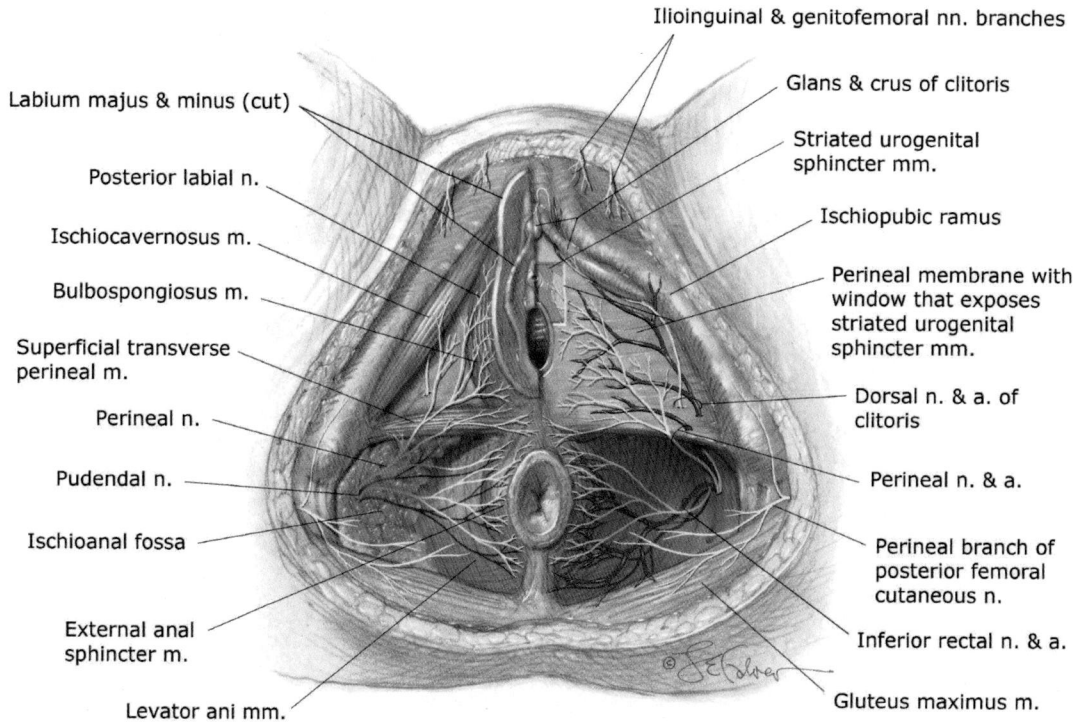

Ilioinguinal & genitofemoral nn. branches

Glans & crus of clitoris

Striated urogenital
sphincter mm.

Ischiopubic ramus

Perineal membrane with
window that exposes
striated urogenital
sphincter mm.

Dorsal n. & a. of
clitoris

Perineal n. & a.

Perineal branch of
posterior femoral
cutaneous n.

Inferior rectal n. & a.

Gluteus maximus m.

Labium majus & minus (cut)

Posterior labial n.

Ischiocavernosus m.

Bulbospongiosus m.

Superficial transverse
perineal m.

Perineal n.

Pudendal n.

Ischioanal fossa

External anal
sphincter m.

Levator ani mm.

FIGURE 38-28 Pudendal nerve and vessels. Nerve supply to striated urogenital sphincter and external anal sphincter muscles.

is under the control of the autonomic nervous system and is responsible for approximately 80 percent of the resting pressure of the anal canal.

As noted earlier, the puborectalis muscle comprises the medial portion of the levator ani muscle that arises on either side from the inner surface of the pubic bones. It passes behind the rectum and forms a sling behind the anorectal junction, contributing to the anorectal angle and possibly to fecal continence (see Figs. 38-9, 38-10, and 38-27).

Perineal Body

This fibromuscular tissue mass lies between the distal part of the posterior vaginal wall and the anus. It is formed by the attachment of several structures. Inferiorly or superficially, the structures that attach to and contribute to the perineal body include the bulbospongiosus, superficial transverse perineal, and external anal sphincter muscles (see Fig. 38-26). Structures that attach at a superior or deeper level are the perineal membrane, levator ani muscles and covering fascia, urethrovaginal sphincter muscles, and distal part of the posterior vaginal wall (see Fig. 38-27). The anterior-to-posterior and the superior-to-inferior extents of the perineal body each measure approximately 2 to 4 cm (see Fig. 38-17).

Clinically, during vaginal laceration repairs and with pelvic reconstructive procedures, particular attention is given to perineal body reconstruction. As noted on page 812, the distal support provided by the perineal body helps prevent pelvic organ prolapse and other pelvic floor dysfunction.

■ Blood Supply, Lymphatics, and Innervation
Blood Vessels

The external pudendal artery is a branch of the femoral artery and supplies the skin and subcutaneous tissue of the mons

pubis (see Fig. 38-3). The internal pudendal artery is a terminal branch of the internal iliac artery (see Fig. 38-6). It exits the pelvis through the greater sciatic foramen, passes behind the ischial spines, and reenters the perineum through the lesser sciatic foramen. It then has a variable course through the pudendal or Alcock canal, and then divides into terminal branches. These are the inferior rectal, perineal, and clitoral arteries (see Fig. 38-28). Branches to the perineum sometimes arise from the pudendal artery before it exits the pelvis. These vessels are called accessory pudendal arteries. Other accessory vessels may also arise directly from the anterior or posterior division of the internal iliac artery.

The veins that drain the structures of the vulva and perineum have courses and names similar to those of the arteries. Venous blood from the vestibular bulbs and other structures, with the exception of the erectile tissue of the clitoris, drains into the internal pudendal veins. The erectile tissue drains into the dorsal vein of the clitoris (see Fig. 38-27). This vein courses backward into the pelvis and terminates in the periurethral–perivesical venous plexus (see Fig. 38-24). The venous plexus that drains the rectum and anal canal empties into the superior, middle, and inferior rectal veins. The superior rectal vein drains into the inferior mesenteric vein, a tributary of the portal vein. The middle rectal vein drains into the internal iliac vein. The inferior rectal vein drains into the internal pudendal and then the internal iliac vein.

Lymphatic Drainage

Structures of the vulva and perineum drain into the inguinal lymph nodes, which are located below the inguinal ligament in the upper anterior and medial thigh (Fig. 38-29). There are 10 to 20 inguinal nodes, which are divided into a superficial and a deep group. Nodes of the superficial inguinal group are

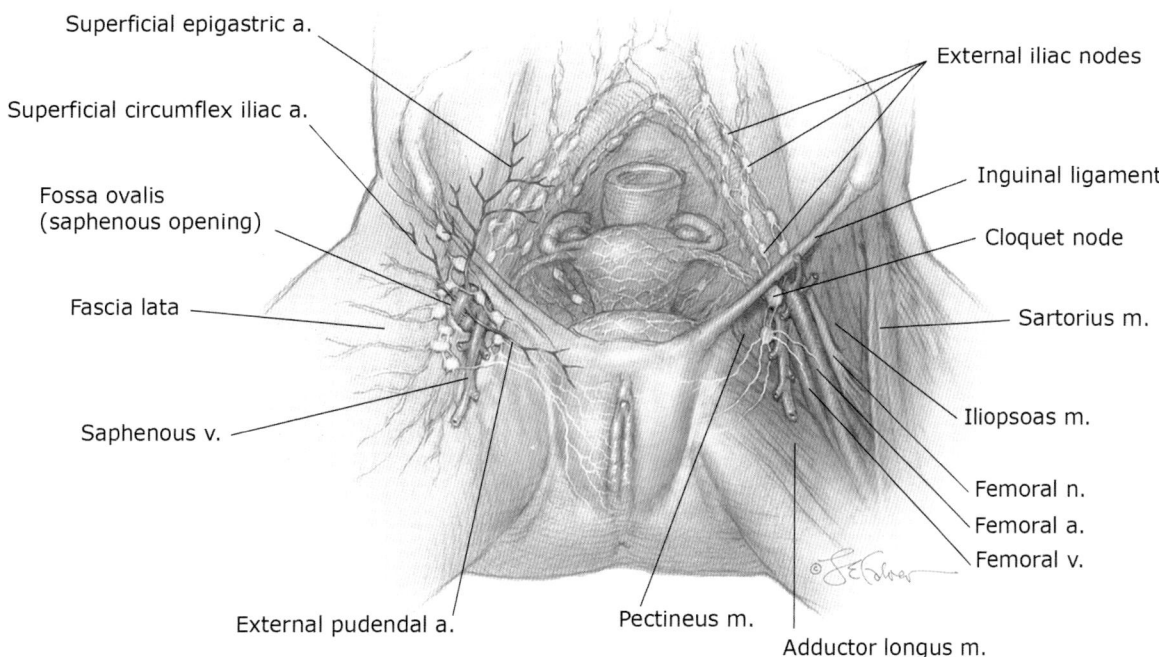

Superficial epigastric a.

Superficial circumflex iliac a.

Fossa ovalis
(saphenous opening)

Fascia lata

Saphenous v.

External iliac nodes

Inguinal ligament

Cloquet node

Sartorius m.

Iliopsoas m.

Femoral n.
Femoral a.
Femoral v.

External pudendal a.   Pectineus m.

Adductor longus m.

FIGURE 38-29 Inguinal lymph nodes and contents of femoral triangle. Superficial inguinal nodes are shown on the image's left, and deep inguinal nodes appear on the image's right.

more numerous, and they are found in the membranous layer of the subcutaneous tissue of the anterior thigh, just superficial to the fascia lata.

The deep inguinal nodes vary from one to three in number and are located deep to the fascia lata in the femoral triangle. This triangle is bordered superiorly by the inguinal ligament, laterally by the medial border of the *sartorius muscle*, and medially by the medial border of the *adductor longus muscle*. The *iliopsoas* and *pectineus muscles* form its floor. From lateral to medial, the structures found in this triangle are the femoral nerve, artery, vein, and deep inguinal lymphatics. The femoral canal is the space that lies on the medial side of the femoral vein and that contains the deep inguinal nodes. The femoral ring is the abdominal opening of the femoral canal. The *fossa ovalis* or *saphenous opening* is an oval opening in the fascia lata and allows communication between superficial and deep inguinal nodes. Of the deep inguinal nodes, the highest one—*Cloquet node*—is located in the lateral part of the femoral ring. Efferent channels from the deep inguinal nodes pass through the femoral canal and femoral ring to the external iliac nodes. Lymphatics from the skin of the labia, clitoris, and remainder of the perineum drain into the superficial inguinal nodes. The glans and corpora cavernosa of the clitoris may drain directly to the deep inguinal nodes.

Surgically, sampling of the superficial, and sometimes also the deep, inguinal nodes is completed as one part of radical vulvectomy. Familiarity with the surrounding anatomy is essential.

Innervation

The inferior anal, perineal, and dorsal nerve of the clitoris are branches of the pudendal nerve and provide sensory and motor innervation to the perineum (see Fig. 38-28). The pudendal nerve is a branch of the sacral plexus and is formed by the anterior rami of the second through fourth sacral nerves (see Fig. 38-6).

It has a course and distribution similar to those of the internal pudendal artery. In addition, the perineal branches of the posterior femoral cutaneous nerve (S1-S3) supply the skin of the external genitalia and adjacent proximal medial surface of the thigh.

Clinically, pudendal nerve blocks can be performed transvaginally or transgluteally by injecting local anesthesia just medial and inferior to the ischial spine. Importantly, inadvertent injection of local anesthetic into the internal pudendal vessels may lead to seizure activity and other complications (Chap. 40, p. 842).

Postsurgical pain in the distribution of the dorsal nerve of the clitoris has been reported following midurethral sling procedures. However, anatomic studies show that this nerve courses superficial or caudal to the perineal membrane, and trocar and mesh placement during these procedures remains deep or cephalad to the membrane (Montoya, 2011; Rahn, 2006).

Clitoral erection requires parasympathetic visceral efferents derived from the pelvic plexus nerves, sometimes called *nervi erigentes*. These arise from the second to the fourth sacral spinal cord segments. They reach the perineum along the urethra and vagina, passing through the urogenital hiatus (see Fig. 38-13). Sympathetic fibers reach the perineum with the pudendal nerve.

REFERENCES

Balgobin S, Carrick KS, Montoya TI, et al: Surgical dimensions and histology of the vesicocervical space. 37th Annual SGS Scientific Meeting, San Antonio, Poster presentation, April 2011

Barber MD, Bremer RE, Thor KB, et al: Innervation of the female levator ani muscles. Am J Obstet Gynecol 187:64, 2002

Berglas B, Rubin IC: The study of the supportive structures of the uterus by levator myography. Surg Gynecol Obstet 97:677, 1953

Bleich AT, Rahn DD, Wieslander CK, et al: Posterior division of the internal iliac artery: anatomic variations and clinical applications. Am J Obstet Gynecol 197(6):658.e1, 2007

Campbell RM: The anatomy and histology of the sacrouterine ligaments. Am J Obstet Gynecol 59:1, 1950

DeLancey JO: Anatomic aspects of vaginal eversion after hysterectomy. Am J Obstet Gynecol 166:1717, 1992

DeLancey JO: Structural anatomy of the posterior pelvic compartment as it relates to rectocele. Am J Obstet Gynecol 180:815, 1999

DeLancey JO, Hurd WW: Size of the urogenital hiatus in the levator ani muscles in normal women and women with pelvic organ prolapse. Obstet Gynecol 91:364, 1998

DeLancey JO, Starr RA: Histology of the connection between the vagina and levator ani muscles: implications for the urinary function. J Reprod Med 35:765, 1990

Drewes PG, Marinis SI, Schaffer JI, et al: Vascular anatomy over the superior pubic rami in female cadavers. Am J Obstet Gynecol 193(6):2165, 2005

Good MM, Abele TA, Balgobin S, et al: L5-S1 discitis—can it be prevented? Obstet Gynecol 121:285, 2013a

Good MM, Abele TA, Balgobin S, et al: Vascular and ureteral anatomy relative to the midsacral promontory. Am J Obstet Gynecol 208:486.e1, 2013b

Heit M, Benson T, Russell B, et al: Levator ani muscle in women with genitourinary prolapse: indirect assessment by muscle histopathology. Neurourol Urodyn 15:17, 1996

Hsu Y, Summers A, Hussain HK, et al: Levator plate angle in women with pelvic organ prolapse compared to women with normal support using dynamic MR imaging. Am J Obstet Gynecol 194:1427, 2006

Hurd WW, Bud RO, DeLancey JO, et al: The location of abdominal wall blood vessels in relationship to abdominal landmarks apparent at laparoscopy. Am J Obstet Gynecol 171(3):642, 1994

Ibeanu OA, Chesson RR, Echols KT, et al: Urinary tract injury during hysterectomy based on universal cystoscopy. Obstet Gynecol 113:6, 2009

Kaufman RH: Cystic tumors. In Kaufman RH, Faro S (eds): Benign Diseases of the Vulva and Vagina. St Louis, Mosby, 1994, p 238

Kerney R, Sawhney R, DeLancey JO: Levator ani muscle anatomy evaluated by origin-insertion pairs. Obstet Gynecol 104:168, 2004

Kuhn RJ, Hollyock VE: Observations of the anatomy of the rectovaginal pouch and rectovaginal septum. Obstet Gynecol 59:445, 1982

Lawson JO: Pelvic anatomy: I. Pelvic floor muscles. Ann R Coll Surg Engl 54:244, 1974

Memon MA, Quinn TH, Cahill DR: Transversalis fascia: historical aspects and its place in contemporary inguinal herniorrhaphy. J Laparoendosc Adv Surg Tech A 9:267, 1999

Montoya TI, Calver L, Carrick KS, et al: Anatomic relationships of the pudendal nerve branches: assessment of injury risk with common surgical procedures. 37th Annual SGS Scientific Meeting, San Antonio, Oral presentation, April 2011

Oelrich T: The striated urogenital sphincter muscle in the female. Anat Rec 205:223, 1983

Oelrich TM: The urethral sphincter muscle in the male. Am J Anat 158:229, 1980

Paramore RH: The supports-in-chief of the female pelvic viscera. BJOG 13:391, 1908

Pathi SD, Castellanos ME, Corton MM: Variability of the retropubic space anatomy in female cadavers. Am J Obstet Gynecol 201(5):524.e1, 2009

Rahn DD, Bleich AT, Wai CY, et al: Anatomic relationships of the distal third of the pelvic ureter, trigone, and urethra in unembalmed female cadavers. Am J Obstet Gynecol 197:668.e1, 2007

Rahn DD, Marinis SI, Schaffer JI, et al: Anatomical path of the tension-free vaginal tape: reassessing current teachings. Am J Obstet Gynecology 195(6):1809, 2006

Rahn DD, Phelan JN, White AB, et al: Clinical correlates of anterior abdominal wall neurovascular anatomy in gynecologic surgery. Am J Obstet Gynecol 202:234.e1, 2010

Range RL, Woodburne RT: The gross and microscopic anatomy of the transverse cervical ligaments. Am J Obstet Gynecol 90:460, 1964

Ripperda CM, Jackson LA, Phelan JN, et al: Anatomic relationships of the pelvic autonomic nervous system in female cadavers: clinical applications to pelvic surgery. Oral presentation at AUGS Annual Scientific Meeting, 13-17 October, 2015

Roshanravan SM, Wieslander CK, Schaffer JI, et al: Neurovascular anatomy of the sacrospinous ligament region in female cadavers: implications in sacrospinous ligament fixation. Am J Obstet Gynecol 197(6):660.e1, 2007

Stein TA, DeLancey JO: Structure of the perineal membrane in females: gross and microscopic anatomy. Obstet Gynecol 111:686, 2008

Umek WH, Morgan DM, Ashton-Miller JA, et al: Quantitative analysis of uterosacral ligament origin and insertion points by magnetic resonance imaging. Obstet Gynecol 103(3):447, 2004

Weber AM, Walters MD: Anterior vaginal prolapse: review of anatomy and techniques of surgical repair. Obstet Gynecol 89:311, 1997

Weber AM, Walter MD: What is vaginal fascia? AUGS Q Rep 13, 1995

Whiteside JL, Barber MD, Walters MD, et al: Anatomy of ilioinguinal and iliohypogastric nerves in relation to trocar placement and low transverse incisions. Am J Obstet Gynecol 189:1574, 2003

Wieslander CK, Rahn DD, McIntire DD, et al: Vascular anatomy of the presacral space in unembalmed female cadavers. Am J Obstet Gynecol 195(6):1736, 2006

Wieslander CK, Roshanravan SM, Wai CY, et al: Uterosacral ligament suspension sutures: anatomic relationships in unembalmed female cadavers. Am J Obstet Gynecol 197:672.e1, 2007

CHAPTER 39

Preoperative Considerations

Each year, more than 30 million surgical procedures are performed. During these, nearly 1 million patients suffer a postoperative complication (Mangano, 2004). As surgeons, gynecologists assume responsibility for assessing a patient's clinical status to identify modifiable risk factors and prevent perioperative morbidity. However, clinicians should also be prepared to diagnose and manage such complications if they arise.

PREOPERATIVE PATIENT EVALUATION

A properly performed preoperative evaluation serves three important functions. It uncovers comorbidities that require further evaluation and improvement to avert perioperative complications. Second, evaluation allows effective use of operating room resources (Roizen, 2000). Finally, the surgeon is able to anticipate potential problems and devise an appropriate perioperative plan (Johnson, 2008).

In many cases, a thorough history and physical examination averts the need for medical consultation. However, if a poorly controlled or previously undiagnosed disease is discovered, consultation with an internist can be beneficial. Preoperative internal medicine consultation does not provide "medical clearance" but rather offers a risk assessment of a woman's current medical state. For consultation, a summary of the surgical illness is provided, and clear questions are posed to the consultant (Fleisher, 2009; Goldman, 1983). In addition, a complete his-

tory and physical examination and prior medical records that report already completed diagnostic testing should be available to the consulting physician. This can prevent unnecessary surgical delays and cost from redundant testing.

PULMONARY EVALUATION

■ Risk Factors for Pulmonary Complications

Common postoperative pulmonary morbidities include atelectasis, pneumonia, and exacerbation of chronic lung diseases. Incidences of such complications following surgery are estimated to be between 20 and 70 percent (Bernstein, 2008; Brooks-Brunn, 1997; Qaseem, 2006).

Risks for pulmonary complications fall into one of two major categories: procedure-related and patient-related. Of procedure-related risks, upper abdominal incisions as they approach the diaphragm can worsen pulmonary function through three mechanisms, shown in Figure 39-1. Resulting poor diaphragmatic movement can produce persistent declines in vital capacity and in functional residual capacity. These predispose to atelectasis (Warner, 2000). Surgery duration is another procedure-associated factor. Operations in which patients receive general anesthesia for longer than 3 hours are associated with nearly double the rate of postoperative pulmonary complications. Finally, emergency surgery remains a significant independent risk. Although these factors are largely unmodifiable, an appreciation of their sequelae should prompt increased postoperative vigilance.

Of patient-associated factors, *age* plays a role. Individuals older than 60 years are at increased risk for developing postoperative pulmonary complications. After patients are stratified for comorbidities, those between 60 and 69 years have a two-fold increased risk. In those older than 70 years, risk rises threefold (Qaseem, 2006). Importantly, for at-risk patients, baseline cognition should be documented and postoperative sensorium monitored, as changes may be an early indicator of pulmonary function compromise.

Smoking, specifically a greater than 20-pack-year smoking history, confers a high incidence of postoperative pulmonary complications. Fortunately, this risk can be reduced with smoking abstinence before surgery. Preoperative cessation for at least 6 to 8 weeks offers significant improvement in lung function and reversal of smoking-related immune impairment (Akrawi, 1997; Buist, 1976). Other short-term benefits may be related to reduced nicotine and carboxyhemoglobin levels, improved mucociliary function, decreased upper airway hypersensitivity, and improved wound healing (Møller, 2002; Nakagawa, 2001). Patients with a 6-month or longer history of smoking cessation have complication risks similar to those who have never

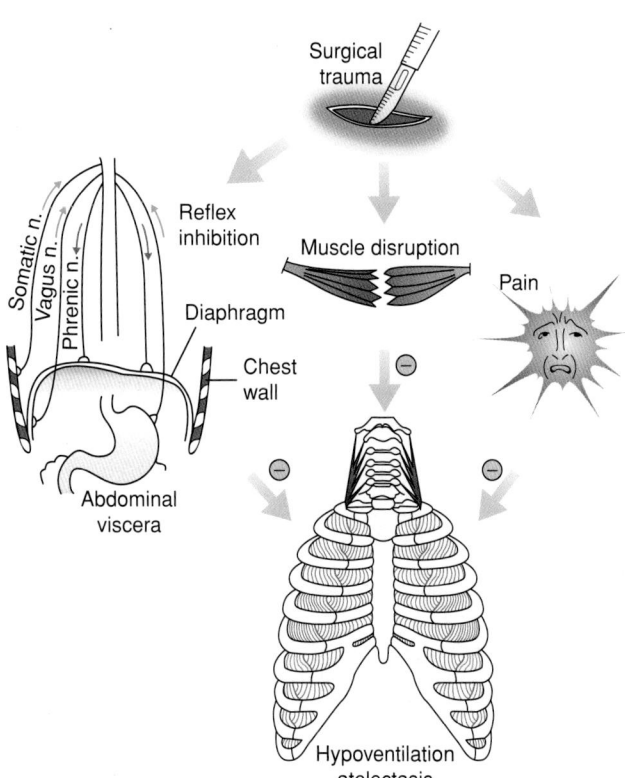

FIGURE 39-1 Surgical factors producing respiratory muscle dysfunction. These factors can reduce lung volumes and produce hypoventilation and atelectasis. (Reproduced with permission from Warner DO: Preventing postoperative pulmonary complications: the role of the anesthesiologist. Anesthesiology 2000 May;92(5):1467–1472.)

smoked. Moreover, patients often see surgery as an opportunity for positive change (Shi, 2010). Brief interventions offered in close proximity to surgery may have small benefit on long-term smoking behavior (Thomsen, 2014). Education alone may prompt successful behavior modification. For others, agents to assist with smoking cessation can be found in Table 1-4, (p. 11).

In *chronic obstructive pulmonary disease (COPD),* inflammatory mediators may account for the intra- and extrapulmonary complications observed in affected patients (Maddali, 2008). Simple COPD optimization may not reduce the incidence of postoperative pulmonary complications. However, postoperative physiotherapy and incentive spirometry with inspiratory muscle training reduce complication rates (Agostini, 2010).

Obesity can decreases chest wall compliance and functional residual capacity and predispose patients with a body mass index (BMI) ≥ 30 kg/m^2 to intra- and postoperative atelectasis (Agostini, 2010; Zerah, 1993). Eichenberger and colleagues (2002) observed that pulmonary changes in these patients may persist for more than 24 hours and require aggressive postoperative lung expansion. Moreover, in obese patients undergoing laparoscopy, these pulmonary parameters are further compromised by increased intraabdominal pressures from pneumoperitoneum, as described in Chapter 41 (p. 874).

Asthma, if well-controlled, is not a risk factor for postoperative pulmonary complications. Warner and coworkers (1996) reported that rates of bronchospasm were less than 2 percent in asthmatic patients.

◼ Diagnostic Evaluation
History and Physical Examination

Elements in a pulmonary review of systems that may serve as harbingers of underlying disease include poor exercise tolerance, chronic cough, and otherwise unexplained dyspnea (Smetana, 1999). Examination findings of decreased breath sounds, dullness to percussion, rales, wheezes, rhonchi, and a prolonged expiratory phase can carry a nearly sixfold increase in pulmonary complications (Straus, 2000).

Pulmonary Function Tests (PFTs) and Chest Radiography

In general, pulmonary function tests (PFTs) offer little information during preoperative pulmonary assessment of patients undergoing nonthoracic procedures. Outside of diagnosing COPD, PFTs are not superior to a thorough history and physical examination (Johnson, 2008; Qaseem, 2006). However, if the etiology of pulmonary symptoms remains unclear after clinical examination, then PFTs may provide information to alter perioperative management.

Chest radiography is not routinely obtained preoperatively. Compared with a clinical history and physical examination, preoperative chest radiographs rarely provide evidence to modify therapy (Archer, 1993). The American College of Radiology (2011) recommends that patients with new or exacerbated cardiopulmonary symptoms or those older than 70 years with chronic cardiopulmonary disease as suitable candidates for imaging. Although not exhaustive, conditions for which radiography may be reasonable include acute or chronic cardiovascular or pulmonary disease, cancer, American Society of Anesthesiologist (ASA) status >3, heavy smoking, immunosuppression, recent chest radiation therapy, and recent emigration from areas with endemic pulmonary disease.

Biochemical Markers

The National Veterans Administration Surgical Quality Improvement Program reported that serum albumin levels less than 3.5 g/dL were significantly associated with increased perioperative pulmonary morbidity and mortality rates (Arozullah, 2000; Lee, 2009). For each 1 mg/dL decline in serum albumin concentration, the odds of mortality are increased by 137 percent and morbidity by 89 percent (Vincent, 2004). Serum albumin's association with morbidity and mortality may be due to confounding comorbidity, and thus it is a marker of malnutrition and disease (Goldwasser, 1997). Although a serum albumin level is not routinely recommended for gynecologic procedures, the information may be predictive in the elderly or in those with multiple comorbidities. Moreover, serum blood urea nitrogen (BUN) levels greater than 21 mg/dL similarly correlate with increased morbidity and mortality rates, but not to the same degree as serum albumin levels.

Preoperative Pulmonary Guidelines

The ASA Classification was created to help predict perioperative mortality rates. It also serves to assess risks for cardiovascular and pulmonary complications (Wolters, 1996). Table 39-1 summarizes the ASA categories and associated rates of postoperative pulmonary complications (Qaseem, 2006).

TABLE 39-1. American Society of Anesthesiologists (ASA) Classification

ASA Class	Class Definition	Rates of PPCs by Class (%)
I	Normally healthy patient	1.2
II	With mild systemic disease	5.4
III	With systemic disease that is not incapacitating	11.4
IV	With an incapacitating systemic disease that is a constant threat to life	10.9
V	Moribund patient who is not expected to survive for 24 hours with or without operation	NA

NA = not applicable; PPCs = postoperative pulmonary complications.
Modified with permission from Qaseem A, Snow V, Fitterman N, et al: Risk assessment for and strategies to reduce perioperative pulmonary complications for patients undergoing noncardiothoracic surgery: a guideline from the American College of Physicians. Ann Intern Med 2006 Apr 18;144(8):575–580.

■ Postoperative Prevention

Lung Expansion Modalities

Techniques aimed at reducing anticipated postoperative decreases in lung volume can be simple and include deep breathing exercises, incentive spirometry, and early ambulation. In conscious and cooperative patients, deep breathing effectively improves lung compliance and gas distribution (Chumillas, 1998; Ferris, 1960; Thomas, 1994). With these exercises, a woman is asked to take five sequential deep breaths every hour while awake and hold each for 5 seconds. An incentive spirometer can be added to provide direct visual feedback of her efforts. Last, early ambulation can enhance lung expansion and provide some protection against venous thromboembolism. Meyers and associates (1975) demonstrated an increase in functional residual lung capacity of up to 20 percent by simply maintaining an upright posture. Alternatively, formal respiratory physiotherapy may include chest physical therapy in the form of percussion, clapping, or vibration; intermittent positive-pressure breathing (IPPB); and continuous positive airway pressure (CPAP).

The simple and the more formal prophylactic methods are all effective in preventing postoperative pulmonary morbidity, and no method is superior to another. Thomas and colleagues (1994) performed a metaanalysis to compare incentive spirometry (IS), IPPB, and deep-breathing exercises (DBE). In comparison with no therapy, IS and DBE are superior in preventing postoperative pulmonary complications, and greater than 50-percent reductions were observed. In addition, no significant differences were noted comparing IS to DBE, IS to IPPB, and DBE to IPPB (Thomas, 1994). However, chest physical therapy, IPPB, and CPAP are more expensive and labor intensive (Pasquina, 2006). Accordingly, these methods are typically reserved for patients who are unable to perform simpler effort-dependent therapies.

Nasogastric Decompression

Postoperatively, nasogastric tubes (NGTs) are often placed for gastric decompression. However, nasogastric intubation bypasses normal upper and lower respiratory tract mucosal defenses and exposes patients to risks for nosocomial sinusitis and pneumonia. Routine use of NGT after surgery is associated with increased cases of pneumonia, atelectasis, and aspiration compared with selective use (Cheatham, 1995). Indications for selective use might include symptomatic abdominal distention or postoperative nausea and vomiting from suspected ileus. Accordingly, the choice to implement NGT drainage is balanced against respiratory risks.

CARDIAC EVALUATION

■ Risk Factors for Cardiac Complications

Coronary artery disease (CAD) is a leading cause of death in developed countries and contributes significantly to perioperative cardiac complication rates in patients undergoing procedures (Stepp, 2005; Williams, 2009). Accordingly, much of cardiac risk assessment focuses on CAD and is described on page 828.

For *congestive heart failure (CHF)*, a cardiologist may employ strategies to maximize hemodynamic function, such as preoperative coronary revascularization or perioperative medical therapy. With CHF, diuretics are commonly used. However, perioperatively, restraining their use will usually avoid intraoperative hypovolemia and related hypotension. But, if fluid resuscitation is needed, it ideally is gradual and limited to avoid volume overload.

Arrhythmias are usually symptoms of underlying cardiopulmonary disease or electrolyte abnormalities. Accordingly, preoperative management focuses on correcting the primary process. However, if pacemakers and implantable cardioverter-defibrillators (ICDs) are required for arrhythmia treatment prior to surgery, they are typically placed for the same indications as in nonoperative circumstances (Gregoratos, 2002). For those with pacemakers in place, electrosurgery can create electromagnetic interference even during noncardiac surgical and endoscopic procedures. Although encountered less frequently with newer devices, such interference can lead to pacing failure or complete system malfunction (Cheng, 2008). Thus, current guidelines recommend that all systems be evaluated by an appropriately trained physician before and after any invasive procedure (Fleisher, 2009). In addition, as discussed in Chapter 40 (p. 859), intraoperative efforts strive to minimize the chance for electromagnetic interference from electrosurgery. Practices include selecting bipolar electrosurgery if possible, using short intermittent bursts of electric current at the lowest possible energy levels, maximizing the distance between the current source and cardiac device, and placing the grounding pad in a position to minimize current flow toward the device.

Hypertension is not predictive of perioperative cardiac events and should not postpone surgery (Goldman, 1979; Weksler, 2003). Exceptions for elective procedures might include systolic blood pressures >180 mm Hg and diastolic blood pressures >110 mm Hg. If possible, to lower postoperative cardiac complications related to hypertension, blood pressure is lowered several months prior to an anticipated procedure (Fleisher, 2002). Preoperatively, patients on angiotensin-converting enzyme inhibitors and angiotensin-receptor antagonists have

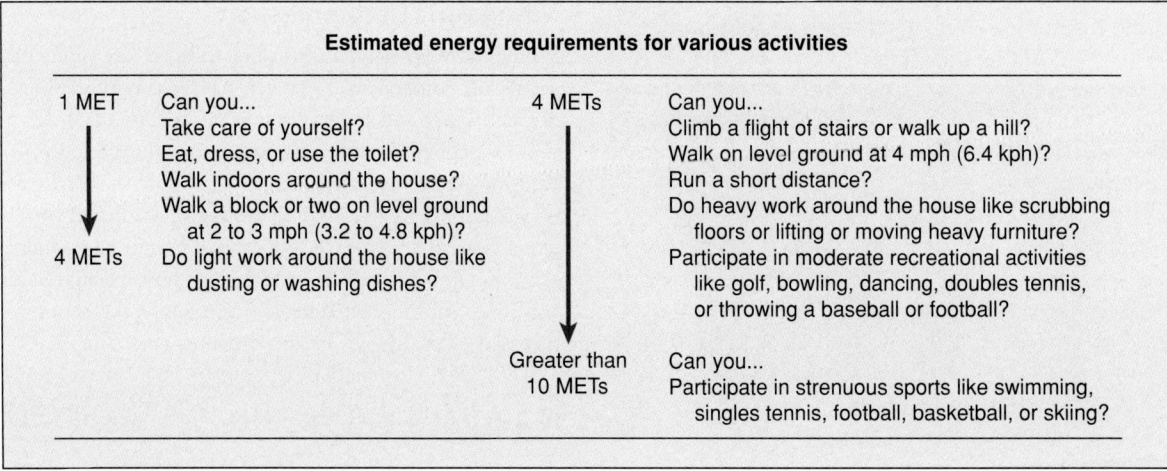

FIGURE 39-2 Questions used to assess functional capacity. METs are used in the algorithm in Figure 39-3. CAD = coronary artery disease; kph = kilometers per hour; MET = metabolic equivalent; mph = miles per hour. (Reproduced with permission from Fleisher LA, Beckman JA, Brown KA, et al: 2009 ACCF/AHA focused update on perioperative beta blockade incorporated into the ACC/AHA 2007 guidelines on perioperative cardiovascular evaluation and care for noncardiac surgery: a report of the American College of Cardiology Foundation/American Heart Association Task Force on Practice Guidelines. Circulation 2009 Nov 24;120(21):e169–e276.)

their morning dose held to reduce the risk of immediate post-induction hypotension (Comfere, 2005). In all patients with hypertension, avoiding hypo- or hypertension intraoperatively with careful postoperative monitoring is recommended. Importantly, intravascular volume expansion, pain, and agitation may exacerbate postoperative hypertension.

Valvular heart disease is a less frequently encountered cardiac comorbidity. Of these, aortic stenosis carries the highest independent factor for perioperative complications (Kertai, 2004). For other lesions, the degree of heart failure and associated cardiac arrhythmias are the best indicators of risk. If cardiac sounds are suggestive of valvular disease, echocardiography will assist in defining the abnormality. Importantly, endocarditis prophylaxis for valvular lesions during gastrointestinal (GI) or genitourinary (GU) procedures is no longer recommended by the American Heart Association (Nishimura, 2014). The transient enterococcal bacteremia caused by these procedures has not been irrefutably correlated to infective endocarditis.

■ Diagnostic Evaluation
History and Physical Examination

As with pulmonary disease, history and physical examination can effectively identify or characterize cardiac disease. One questioning strategy is outlined in Figure 39-2. During physical examination, surgeons observe for dependent edema or jugular venous distention, whereas chest palpation searches for the point of maximum impulse and possible thrills. Auscultation of carotid arteries should exclude bruits, and listening at cardiac points investigates cardiac rate, regularity, and extra heart sounds.

Cardiac Testing

Of preoperative cardiac tests, 12-lead electrocardiogram (ECG) and chest radiograph are commonly considered. According to the American College of Cardiology and the American Heart Association (ACC/AHA), ECG is reasonable for patients with known coronary heart disease, significant arrhythmia, peripheral arterial disease, cerebrovascular disease, or other significant struc-

tural heart disease. ECG is not recommended for those undergoing low-risk surgeries. For asymptomatic patients without known coronary heart disease, ECG may be considered, but again is not useful in those undergoing low-risk procedures (Fleisher, 2014). Indications for preoperative chest radiography are limited and discussed on page 826. Other testing is usually ordered by a consulting cardiologist and often directed by guidelines discussed next.

Preoperative Cardiac Guidelines

Preoperative guidelines have been developed by several groups to help predict perioperative cardiac complications and direct perioperative care. The two most prominent are: (1) those jointly developed by the ACC/AHA and (2) the Revised Cardiac Risk Index (RCRI) (Fleisher, 2014; Lee, 1999).

Of the two, ACC/AHA guidelines provide a stepwise strategy to assess three major considerations—clinical predictors, surgery-specific risk, and functional capacity—to ascertain the need for cardiac testing (Fig. 39-3). In general, for gynecologic surgery, cardiac complication risks are greatest with major emergency procedures and operations associated with large intravascular fluid shifts. In contrast, lowest risks are found with planned, brief endoscopic procedures.

The Revised Cardiac Risk Index is an easy assessment of clinical predictors. It has been tested extensively and offers accurate estimates of cardiac risk (Lee, 1999). The major difference between the RCRI and the ACC/AHA guidelines is the incorporation of exercise capacity in the ACC/AHA tool. Creators of the RCRI suggest that cardiac risk may be overestimated by a patient's noncardiac limitations in exercise function, such as musculoskeletal pain. Thus, these investigators place greater emphasis on cardiac and vascular disease markers.

■ Prevention Strategies
Perioperative Beta-blockers

Preoperative beta-blocker use to reduce in-hospital mortality rates were advocated as a result of the Dutch Echocardiographic Cardiac Risk Evaluation Applying Stress Echocardiography

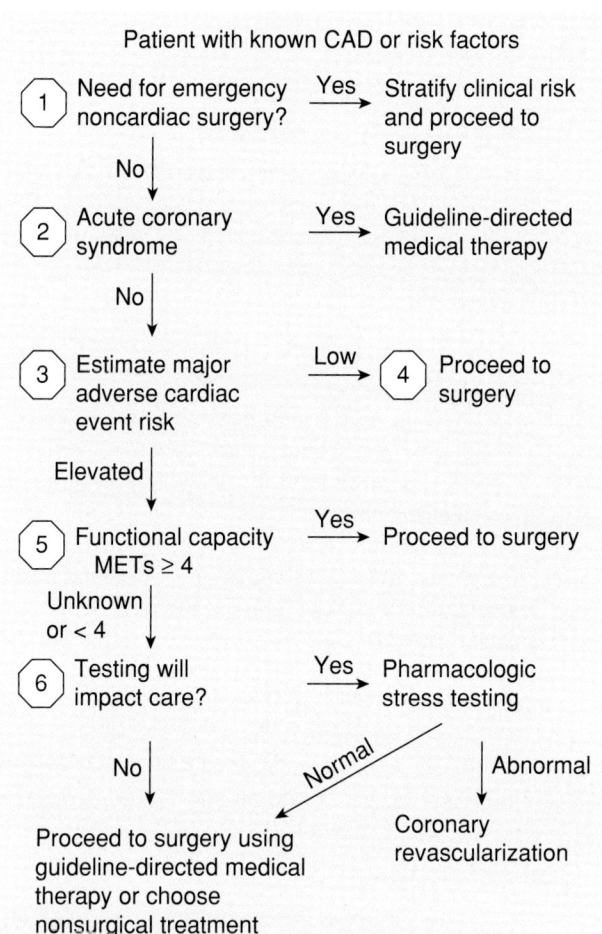

Patient with known CAD or risk factors

1. Need for emergency noncardiac surgery? — Yes → Stratify clinical risk and proceed to surgery

No ↓

2. Acute coronary syndrome — Yes → Guideline-directed medical therapy

No ↓

3. Estimate major adverse cardiac event risk — Low → 4. Proceed to surgery

Elevated ↓

5. Functional capacity METs ≥ 4 — Yes → Proceed to surgery

Unknown or < 4 ↓

6. Testing will impact care? — Yes → Pharmacologic stress testing

No ↓   Normal ↙   ↓ Abnormal

Proceed to surgery using guideline-directed medical therapy or choose nonsurgical treatment   Coronary revascularization

FIGURE 39-3 Stepwise approach to perioperative cardiac assessment in those with coronary artery disease (CAD). MET = metabolic equivalent. (Adapted with permission from Fleisher LA, Fleischmann KE, Auerbach AD, et al: 2014 ACC/AHA Guideline on Perioperative Cardiovascular Evaluation and Management of Patients Undergoing Noncardiac Surgery: a Report of the American College of Cardiology/American Heart Association Task Force on Practice Guidelines, J Am Coll Cardiol 2014 Dec 9;64(22):e77–137.)

(DECREASE) family of studies. Unfortunately, fictitious databases and errant methods led to a discounting of these results (Erasmus Medical Centre, 2012). Subsequently, Bouri and colleagues (2014) conducted a metaanalysis of the available secure data from randomized controlled trials assessing the value of perioperative beta-blockade. They found the use of beta-blockers caused a statistically significant increase in all-cause mortality rates by 27 percent. Despite a reduction in non-fatal myocardial infarctions, rates of stroke and hypotension increased significantly. These new findings challenge the current AHA guidelines recommending beta-blockade in targeted high-risk patients and even suggest that they may benefit the least (Poldermans, 2009).

Coronary Revascularization

Diagnostic cardiac catheterization is considered in high-risk cardiac patients if noninvasive stress testing suggests advanced disease. In such cases, revascularization through coronary artery bypass grafting (CABG) or percutaneous coronary interventions offer comparable benefits perioperatively (Hassan, 2001).

Anemia

This has been shown to be an independent risk factor for congestive heart failure (Kannel, 1987). A study by Silverberg and associates (2001) found that correction of even mild anemia (Hgb <12.5 percent) offered significant improvements in cardiac function. Iron therapy is not a substitution for appropriate cardiac disease treatment, but extrapolated data suggest that maintaining a hemoglobin level above 10 percent is important and reduces perioperative morbidity and mortality rates for those with cardiac disease.

HEPATIC EVALUATION

The rising incidence of hepatic disease has similarly increased the number of patients with hepatic dysfunction. Perioperative care must address this impairment, as the liver plays a central role in drug metabolism; synthesis of proteins, glucose, and coagulation factors; and excretion of endogenous compounds.

Patients with suspected disease are queried regarding family histories of jaundice or anemia, recent travel history, exposure to alcohol or other hepatotoxins, and medication use (Suman, 2006). Physical findings include jaundice, scleral icterus, spider angiomas, ascites, hepatomegaly, asterixis, and cachexia.

If underlying liver disease is known or suspected, hepatic function is assessed. In addition, prothrombin time (PT), partial thromboplastin time (PTT), serum albumin level, and a serum chemistry panel are valuable adjuncts.

Of liver diseases, acute and chronic hepatitis are commonly encountered. With acute hepatitis, regardless of the cause, high associated perioperative mortality rates have been documented by multiple investigators. For this reason, primary management involves supportive care and delay of elective surgery until the acute process has subsided (Patel, 1999). In those with chronic hepatitis, hepatic dysfunction is variable. Compensated disease carries a low risk of perioperative complications (Sirinek, 1987). However, in patients with cirrhosis, the Child-Pugh score is a useful tool to predict survival after abdominal surgery. Clinical measures include serum total bilirubin and albumin levels, international normalized ratio (INR) values, and severity of associated ascites and encephalopathy. Approximate mortality risks based on Child-Pugh class are class A—10 percent; class B—30 percent; and class C—70 percent (Mansour, 1997).

RENAL EVALUATION

The kidney is involved with metabolic waste excretion, erythropoietin production, and fluid and electrolyte balance. Accordingly, patients with known renal insufficiency typically have serum electrolytes, renal function, and complete blood count (CBC) evaluated prior to surgery. Chronic anemia due to renal insufficiency will typically require preoperative administration of erythropoietin or perioperative transfusion depending on the procedure planned and degree of anemia. Dialysis patients require intensive pre- and postoperative surveillance for signs of electrolyte abnormalities and fluid overload. Ideally, these patients' volume status and electrolytes (potassium in particular) are optimized by performing dialysis the day prior to surgery. Additionally, further renal insult is averted by avoiding nephrotoxic agents. Pharmacokinetic consultation may be warranted to adjust other medication dosages as serum levels in these patients may be unpredictable postoperatively.

HEMATOLOGIC EVALUATION

Anemia

This is frequently encountered in preoperative gynecologic surgery evaluation. In the absence of a clear etiology, evaluation serves to potentially correct reversible causes. Queries focus on signs of symptomatic anemia such as fatigue, dyspnea with exertion, and palpitations. Inquiry also seeks to identify risk factors for underlying cardiovascular disease as anemia is less well tolerated in these individuals. The physical examination incorporates thorough pelvic and rectal examination, stool guaiac screening, and urinalysis.

With chronic anemia, erythrocyte indices derived from a CBC reflect a microcytic, hypochromic anemia and show decreases is mean corpuscular volume (MCV), mean corpuscular hemoglobin (MCH), and mean corpuscular hemoglobin concentration (MCHC). Moreover, in classic iron-deficiency anemia from chronic blood loss, an elevated platelet count and decreased reticulocyte count can be seen. In those for whom the cause of anemia is unclear, those with profound anemia, or those who fail to improve with oral iron therapy, addition testing is prudent. Iron studies, vitamin B_{12}, and folate levels are often indicated. Iron-deficiency anemia produces low serum ferritin and iron levels, elevated total iron-binding capacity, and normal vitamin B_{12} and folate levels.

Several pharmacologic options are available for preoperative iron supplementation. For oral intake, ferrous sulfate (Feosol, Slow Fe), ferrous gluconate (Fergon), ferrous fumarate (Ircon, Fero-Sequels), and iron polysaccharide (Ferrex) are available. Importantly, each of the ferrous salts has a different content of *elemental iron*. In general, therapy to correct iron deficiency ideally provides 150 to 200 mg of elemental iron daily. Thus, common and equivalent oral replacement regimens include ferrous sulfate, 325 mg tablet (contains 65 mg elemental iron), or ferrous fumarate, 200 mg tablet (contains 64 mg elemental iron), three times daily. Okuyama and associates (2005) found that provision of 200 mg of elemental iron 2 weeks preoperatively significantly reduced the need for intraoperative transfusion. Constipation is the primary source of preparation intolerance and can be improved with dietary changes, bulk laxatives, and stool softeners (Table 25-6, p. 570).

In addition to oral forms, several Food and Drug Administration (FDA)-approved intravenous (IV) iron preparations are currently available. These include ferric gluconate (Ferrlecit), iron sucrose (Venofer), ferumoxytol (Feraheme), ferric carboxymaltose (Injectafer), and low-molecular-weight iron dextran (INFeD) (DeLoughery, 2014). The newer preparations have a much lower risk of anaphylactic reactions and are considered safe (Shander, 2010). The hemoglobin effects can be seen as quickly as 1 week after the first dose. For most women, iron therapy administered orally is effective to correct anemia. However, these IV forms may be most appropriate for women with poor absorption secondary to gastrointestinal disease, those with chronic renal disease, or those with an intolerance or lack of response to oral iron.

In women with acute bleeding, transfusion may be required perioperatively. The decision to transfuse depends in part on a patient's cardiac status. A full discussion of resuscitation is found in Chapter 40 (p. 864).

Autologous Blood Donation

Fear of infection from allogeneic blood transfusions has led to development of autologous transfusion practices. Two of the most popular options include preoperative autologous donation and salvage autologous transfusions. Both are discussed in detail in Chapter 40 (p. 859) (Vanderlinde, 2002).

Coagulopathies

Coagulopathies are generally grouped into two categories—inherited or acquired. Of acquired forms, a careful review of systems and complete medication list, including herbal preparations, may highlight potential causes. In either form, disorders involving platelets or clotting factors can be identified with a careful history and physical examination. A personal history of easy bruising, unexpected amounts of bleeding with minor injury, or lifelong menorrhagia alert a clinician to the possibility of coagulopathy. Screening for coagulopathies is outlined in Chapter 8 (p. 192), and the specifics of replacement are described in Chapter 40 (p. 867). In general, for those undergoing procedures, a transfusion threshold of ≤50,000/μL is used, and for major surgery, ≤100,000/μL (James, 2011).

Oral Anticoagulation

In patients who take anticoagulants following a venous thromboembolism (VTE), the timing of surgery can often lower the risk of postoperative VTE. After an acute VTE, the recurrence risk without anticoagulation is between 40 and 50 percent. However, the risk of recurrent disease drops significantly after 3 months of warfarin therapy. Moreover, a delay in surgery and continued warfarin therapy for an additional 2 to 3 months (6 months total) drops the recurrence risk to 5 to 10 percent and avoids a need for preoperative heparin (Kearon, 1997; Levine, 1995). Thus, in those with recent VTE, a surgical delay, if feasible, may be advantageous and should be considered. When surgery must proceed, protocols for anticoagulant management are described next.

Preoperative Management

Women with atrial fibrillation, mechanical heart valve, or recent VTE are at increased risk for VTE. As a result, chronic oral warfarin therapy is typically prescribed. For these patients, a surgeon must compromise between the need for anticoagulation and risk of surgical bleeding complications. The American College of Obstetricians and Gynecologists (2014b) has summarized recommendations to address this balance (Table 39-2). In general, anticoagulation is typically halted prior to surgery and started shortly postoperatively. Unfortunately, the effects of warfarin reverse slowly. Thus, patients are often transitioned or "bridged" to heparin, which can be stopped and restarting more readily. Both low-molecular-weight heparin (LMWH) and unfractionated heparin (UFH) are options (Table 39-3). Of LWMH choices, enoxaparin (Lovenox) is commonly selected. During bridging, warfarin is stopped several days before surgery, and heparin is begun (Douketis, 2012; White,

CHAPTER 39

TABLE 39-2. Perioperative Management of Patients on Chronic Antithrombotic Therapy

Condition	Bleeding Risk	High VTE Risk	Moderate VTE Risk	Low VTE Risk
Prior VTE	High	Protocol A	Protocol C	Protocol C
	Moderate	Protocol A	Protocol B or C Consider mechanical prophylaxis	Protocol C
Atrial fibrillation	High	Protocol A	Protocol C or B	Protocol C or B
	Moderate	Protocol A	Protocol A or B	Protocol B or C
Mechanical heart valve	High	Protocol A	Protocol A or B	Protocol C
	Moderate	Protocol A	Protocol A	Protocol C or B

Protocol A: Use bridging therapy with therapeutic-dose low-molecular-weight heparin (LMWH) or unfractionated heparin (UFH). Therapeutic-dose enoxaparin is 1 mg/kg subcutaneously (SC) twice daily or 1.5 mg/kg once daily. Therapeutic-dose intravenous (IV) UFH is 80 units/kg IV push, then 18 units/kg/hr.

Protocol B: Use bridging therapy with low-dose LMWH or low-dose UFH. Low-dose enoxaparin is 30 mg twice SC daily or 40 mg once SC daily. Low-dose UFH is 5000–7500 units SC twice daily.

Protocol C: Stop long-term anticoagulation therapy. Do not use bridging therapy. Restart long-term anticoagulation after surgery. Use mechanical prophylaxis with an intermittent compression device during surgery and until long-term anticoagulation is therapeutic.

[a]Protocol steps for warfarin bridging are found in Table 39-3.

VTE = venous thromboembolism.

Data from Committee opinion no 610: chronic antithrombotic therapy and gynecologic surgery, Obstet Gynecol 2014 Oct;124(4):856–862.

1995). In those with a therapeutic INR (between 2.0 and 3.0), approximately 5 to 6 days are required for this ratio to reach 1.5. Once this is achieved, surgery can safely proceed. During bridging therapy, the last dose of LMWH is administered 24 hours prior to surgery. With UFH, therapy is halted 4 to 6 hours prior to surgery (Douketis, 2012).

Unfortunately, emergency surgery may not allow time for such bridging. In these cases, warfarin is halted, and vitamin K is provided. This vitamin promotes factor synthesis, and in urgent cases, a 5- to 10-mg IV dose is suitable (Holbrook, 2012). To minimize the anaphylactic risk, vitamin K is mixed in a minimum 50 mL of IV fluid and administered over at least 20 minutes. Vitamin K requires 4 to 6 hours to achieve clinical effects. Thus, fresh frozen plasma (FFP) may be added at a dose of 15 mL/kg, and each FFP unit has a volume of 200 to 250 mL. Prothrombin complex concentrate (PCC) is a human-derived product containing factors II, IX, and X. PCC does not require thawing and may be used in place of FFP (Ageno, 2012).

TABLE 39-3. Anticoagulant Management

Bridging protocol for warfarin

5 days before surgery	Stop warfarin; start LMWH or UFH
	Stop LMWH 24 hours before surgery or stop UFH at least 4–6 hours before surgery
1 day before surgery	Check INR. If INR >1.5, give 1–2 mg of oral vitamin K
	Recheck INR
Surgery day	Start LMWH or UFH 12–24 hours after surgery, if bleeding risk is low
1 day after surgery	Start warfarin
5 days after surgery	Stop LMWH or UFH once INR is >2. Continue warfarin

Protocol for direct oral anticoagulant

1–2 days before surgery	Stop agent: dabigatran 2 days prior; apixaban and rivaroxaban 1 day prior
1 day after surgery	Start agent

Protocol for antiplatelet agents

7 days before surgery	Stop aspirin or clopidogrel
1 day after surgery	Start agent 12–24 hours after surgery

INR = international normalized ratio; LMWH = low-molecular-weight heparin; UFH = unfractionated heparin.

Data from Committee opinion no 610: chronic antithrombotic therapy and gynecologic surgery, Obstet Gynecol 2014 Oct;124(4):856-862; Douketis J, Bell AD, Eikelboom J, et al: Approach to the new oral anticoagulants in family practice: Part 2: addressing frequently asked questions, Can Fam Physician 2014 Nov;60(11):997–1001.

Although warfarin antagonizes all vitamin K-dependent clotting factors, newer *direct oral anticoagulants (DOACs)* inhibit specific factors. The three currently licensed medications are dabigatran (Pradaxa), which targets factor IIa (thrombin), and rivaroxaban (Xarelto) and apixaban (Eliquis), which target factor Xa. Because of their recent introduction, few studies provide recommendations for their perioperative management (Kozek-Langenecker, 2014). The pharmacologic half-life is 14 hours for dabigatran and 9 hours for rivaroxaban and apixaban (Schaden, 2010). Thus, in women with normal preoperative creatinine clearance, stopping rivaroxaban and apixaban 24 hours prior to surgery and halting dabigatran 48 hours prior to surgery is reasonable. The withdrawal time is doubled if the creatinine clearance is <50 mL/min or the risk of perioperative bleeding is high (Ortel, 2012).

For the DOACs, global coagulation tests such as INR, PT, and activated partial thromboplastin time (aPTT) less reliably reflect coagulant activity. For the factor Xa inhibitors rivaroxaban and apixaban, anti-factor Xa assays can be used to measure their activity. For dabigatran, an aPTT >90 seconds and an INR >2 suggest possible overdosing (Lindahl, 2011). Also for dabigatran, thrombin time testing is more sensitive and normal values exclude significant anticoagulant effect. However, the turnaround time with this specific test can be long.

For emergent surgery, the DOACs have no antidote, and management of life-threatening bleeding remains empirical. Fortunately, anticoagulant effects rapidly dissipate because of the drugs' short half-lives. Indirect evidence suggests that recombinant factor VIIa (NovoSeven) or a prothrombin complex concentrate may be helpful (Ageno, 2012).

Last, antiplatelet agents such as aspirin and clopidogrel (Plavix) may increase surgical bleeding. These are generally stopped 7 days prior to surgery (American College of Obstetricians and Gynecologists, 2014b).

Postoperative Management

After surgery, heparin, either UFH or LMWH, is restarted 12 to 24 hours after major surgery (see Table 39-3). Oral warfarin therapy is started concurrently as several days are required to regain therapeutic levels (Harrison, 1997; White, 1994). Once the INR ranges between 2 and 3, then heparin is discontinued. DOACs are typically restarted 24 hours following surgery. Antiplatelet agents may be resumed 12 to 24 hours following surgery. In all cases, agents are begun only after surgical hemostasis is confirmed.

ENDOCRINE EVALUATION

Hyperthyroidism and Hypothyroidism

The pathophysiologic stress of surgery can exacerbate endocrine conditions such as thyroid dysfunction, diabetes mellitus, and adrenal insufficiency. Of these, both hyper- and hypothyroidism have anesthetic and metabolic derangements unique to each disease state. Nevertheless, management goals for each aim to achieve a euthyroid state before surgery.

Hyperthyroidism carries the risk of developing thyroid storm perioperatively. Moreover, airway compromise is a risk in those with goiter. Thus, during physical examination, tracheal deviation is sought. In addition to thyroid function tests, an ECG and serum electrolyte levels can help predict signs of preexisting metabolic stress. Patients are encouraged to maintain their usual medications at prescribed dosages until the day of surgery.

Newly diagnosed hypothyroidism generally does not require preoperative therapy other than thyroid hormone replacement. Exceptions include cases of severe disease with signs of cardiac depression, electrolyte irregularities, and hypoglycemia.

Diabetes Mellitus

Long-term complications of diabetes mellitus may include vascular, neurologic, cardiac, and renal dysfunction. Thus, a vigilant preoperative risk assessment for these in affected women is essential. In addition, increased postoperative morbidity rates have been linked with poor preoperative glycemic control. Specifically, glucose levels >200 mg/dL and hemoglobin A_{1c} levels >7 are both associated with significantly increased rates of postoperative wound infection (Dronge, 2006; Trick, 2000).

At minimum, diabetic patients undergoing major surgical procedures benefit from three diagnostic tests—serum electrolyte levels, urinalysis, and ECG. These screen for metabolic disturbances, undiagnosed nephropathy, and unrecognized cardiac ischemia, respectively.

In general, stress induced by surgery and anesthesia elevates catecholamine levels, relative insulin deficiency, and hyperglycemia (Devereaux, 2005). Although glycemic responses vary with surgery, overt hyperglycemia is avoided to minimize postoperative complications related to dehydration, electrolyte abnormalities, diminished wound healing, and even ketoacidosis in type 1 diabetics (Jacober, 1999). However, fluctuations in oral intake and metabolic needs make optimal glycemic control labor intensive. Moreover, clear evidence for glucose targets are lacking. As a result, most providers aim for glucose readings below 200 mg/dL (Table 39-4) (Finney, 2003; Garber, 2004; Hoogwerf, 2006). Table 39-5 and Figure 39-4 summarize perioperative recommendations set forth by Jacober and coworkers (1999) based on disease severity.

Adrenal Insufficiency

Inadequacy of the hypothalamic-pituitary-adrenal (HPA) axis due to secondary suppression from chronic steroid use can lead to perioperative hypotension. Despite this physiologic understanding, controversy surrounds perioperative corticosteroid supplementation.

Corticosteroid users who undergo minor surgical procedures or who use lower doses are generally assumed not to be at risk for adrenal suppression, and additional corticosteroid therapy is not recommended. The value of perioperative supplementation remains an area of chronic debate (Bromberg, 1991; Marik, 2008). Systematic reviews of the literature regarding perioperative supplemental doses of corticosteroids find no evidence to support additional supratherapeutic "stress doses." Instead, patients should continue their usual daily dose (Kelly, 2013; Marik, 2008). Close hemodynamic monitoring is performed to look for volume-refractory hypotension, at which time stress-dose corticosteroids are initiated for presumed secondary

TABLE 39-4. Sliding-Scale Insulin Order Example[a]

Blood Glucose, mmol/L (mg/dL)[b]	Increment Formula	Calculation	Short-Acting Insulin, units
0–11.0 (0–200)	0	0	0
11.1–14.0 (201–250)	1 × (TDI/30)	1 × (120/30)	4
14.1–17.0 (251–300)	2 × (TDI/30)	2 × (120/30)	4
17.1–20.0 (301–350)	3 × (TDI/30)	3 × (120/30)	12
20.1–23.0 (251–400)	4 × (TDI/30)	1 × (120/30)	16
23.1–26.0 (401–450)	5 × (TDI/30)	5 × (120/30)	20
>26.0 (>450)	Call physician	Call physician	Call physician

[a]Example uses a preoperative total daily insulin dose (TDI) of 120 units.
[b]For convenience, conversions of millimoles per liter to milligrams per deciliter are approximate.
Reproduced with permission from Jacober SJ, Sowers JR: An update on perioperative management of diabetes. Arch Intern Med 1999 Nov 8;159(20):2405–2411.

adrenal insufficiency. Of note, Marik and Varon (2008) observed that patients receiving corticosteroids due to *primary* hypothalamic-pituitary-adrenal axis disease require stress doses in the perioperative period. One regimen is hydrocortisone, 100 mg administered IV every 8 hours and titrated to reduced doses as the patient improves.

DIAGNOSTIC TESTING GUIDELINES

In the absence of a clinical indication, a rote panel of preoperative tests does not enhance the safety or quality of care. Roizen and colleagues (2000) noted that nearly half of abnormalities found on routine preoperative testing were ignored by clinicians. Moreover, multiple studies have documented the inefficiency of hematologic tests for obtaining clinically significant diagnoses (Kaplan, 1985; Korvin, 1975). Most importantly, diagnostic testing has not been shown to outperform a clinical history and physical examination (Rucker, 1983). Thus, in the absence of changes in clinical status, diagnostic tests found to be normal 4 to 6 months prior to surgery may be used as "preoperative tests." In patients managed this way, MacPherson and coworkers (1990) found that fewer than 2 percent had significant changes during the course of 4 months.

Codified guidelines for preoperative testing have not been crafted in the United States. However, in the United Kingdom, the National Institute for Health and Clinical Excellence (NICE) has indications for such testing. Complete documents are available at: http://www.nice.org.uk/guidance/cg3.

INFORMED CONSENT

Obtaining informed consent is a process and not merely a medical record document (Lavelle-Jones, 1993; Nandi, 2006). This conversation between a clinician and patient enhances a woman's awareness of her diagnosis and contains a discussion of medical and surgical care alternatives, procedure goals and limitations, and surgical risks. Multimedia decision support tools, such as photographs, pamphlets, and educational videos, can augment the discussion (Coulter, 2007; Stacey, 2014). When informed consent cannot be obtained from the patient, an independent surrogate should be identified to represent the patient's best interest and wishes (American College of Obstetricians and Gynecologists, 2012). Ultimately, written documentation of the entire process serves as a historical record of a patient's understanding and agreement within the medical records.

Despite a clinician's recommendations, an informed patient may decline a particular intervention. A woman's decision-making autonomy must be respected, and a clinician documents informed refusal in the medical record. Appropriate documentation includes: (1) a patient's refusal to consent to the recommended intervention, (2) notation that the value of the intervention has been explained to the patient, (3) a

TABLE 39-5. Perioperative Management of Diabetes Mellitus by Disease Type

Disease	Preoperative Management	Postoperative Management
Type 2 DM treated with diet alone	No additional care with PRN subcutaneous regular insulin for AM hyperglycemia	PRN subcutaneous regular insulin
Type 2 DM treated with oral hypoglycemic agents	Discontinue all agents on the day of surgery	Supplemental subcutaneous insulin until return of normal diet, at which time preoperative therapy can be reinstituted
Type 1 or 2 DM treated with insulin	See Figure 39-3	Sliding-scale insulin (see Table 39-4)

DM = diabetes mellitus; PRN = as needed.
Data from Jacober SJ, Sowers JR: An update on perioperative management of diabetes. Arch Intern Med 1999 Nov 8;159(20):2405–2411.

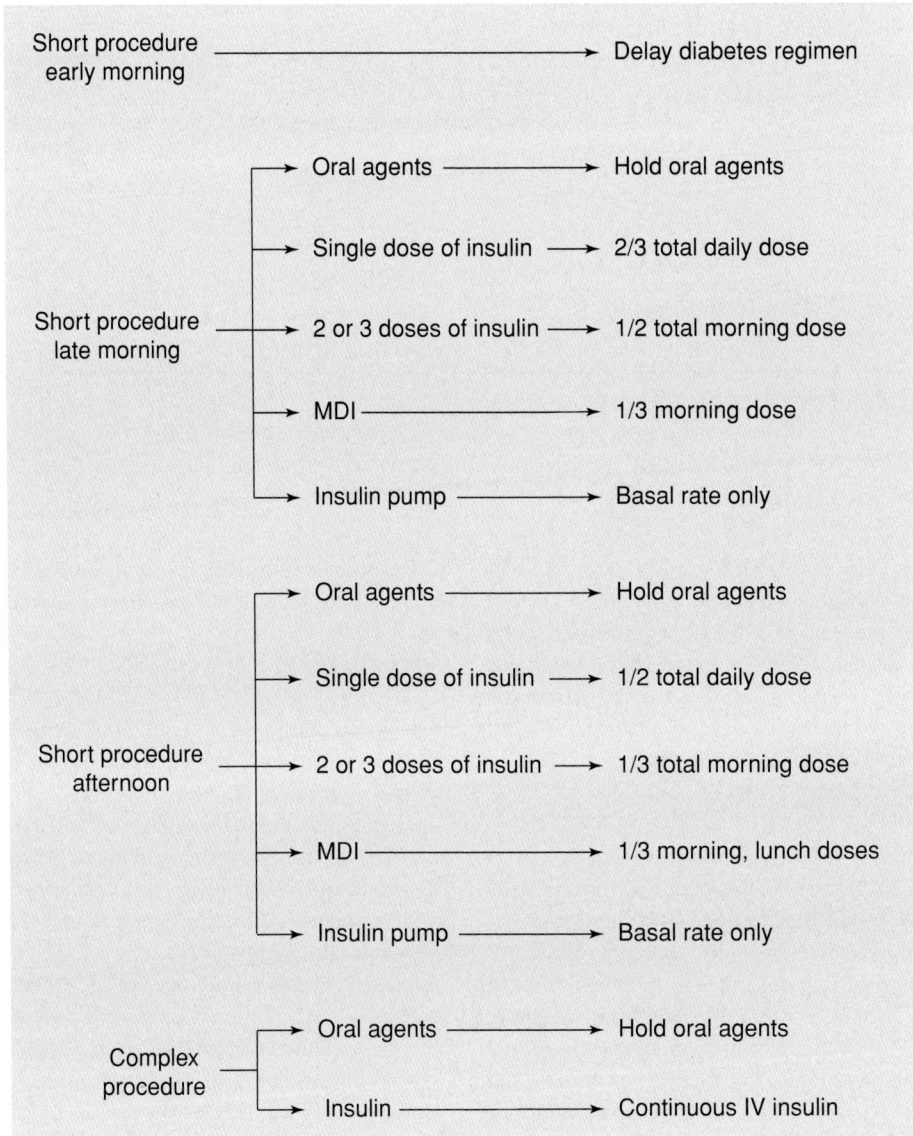

FIGURE 39-4 Perioperative management recommendations for surgical patients with diabetes mellitus. IV = intravenous; MDI = multiple doses of short-acting insulin. (Reproduced with permission from Jacober SJ, Sowers JR: An update on perioperative management of diabetes. Arch Intern Med 1999 Nov 8;159(20):2405–2411.)

patient's reasons for refusal, and (4) a statement describing the health consequences as described to the patient.

INFECTION PROPHYLAXIS

Appropriate antibiotic prophylaxis can significantly reduce hospital-acquired infections following gynecologic surgery. Selection recommendations are summarized in Table 39-6. Decisions regarding the choice, timing, and duration of antibiotic prophylaxis are guided by the intended procedure and the anticipated organisms to be encountered (Chap. 3, p. 76). Typically, a single dose of antibiotics is given at anesthesia induction. Additional doses are considered in cases with blood loss >1500 mL or with duration longer than 3 hours. For obese individuals, a higher antibiotic dose is suggested (American College of Obstetricians and Gynecologists, 2014a). Recommendations do not support subacute bacterial endocarditis prophylaxis prior to GI or GU surgeries, as noted on page 828.

GASTROINTESTINAL BOWEL PREPARATION

Mechanical bowel preparation was previously advocated if the risk for colon injury was high. This supposedly prevented bowel anastomosis leaks from passage of hard feces and reduced fecal and bacterial loads to lower wound infection rates (Barker, 1971; Nichols, 1971).

Multiple studies, however, question routine mechanical bowel preparation (Duncan, 2009; Platell, 1997). Güenaga and coworkers (2011) performed a review of trials to determine the effectiveness of such preparation on morbidity and mortality rates in colorectal surgery. They found no evidence to support the perceived benefit from mechanical bowel preparation. Similar results have been found with laparoscopic surgery and pelvic floor procedures (Ballard, 2014; Muzii, 2006). Moreover, bowel preparation does not decrease microbial contamination of the peritoneal cavity and subcutis after elective open colon surgery (Fa-Si-Oen, 2005).

TABLE 39-6. Antimicrobial Prophylactic Regimens by Procedure[a]

Procedure	Antibiotic	Dose (single dose)
Hysterectomy	1. Cefazolin[b]	1 g or 2 g[c] IV
Urogynecology procedures	2. Clindamycin[d] **PLUS**	600 mg IV
	Gentamicin **or**	1.5 mg/kg IV
	Quinolone[e] **or**	400 mg IV
	Aztreonam	1g IV
	3. Metronidazole[d] **PLUS**	500 mg IV
	Gentamicin **or**	1.5 mg/kg IV
	Quinolone[e]	400 mg IV
Laparoscopy[f]: diagnostic or operative	None	
Laparotomy	None	
Hysteroscopy: diagnostic or operative	None	
Hysterosalpingogram or chromotubation	Doxycycline[g]	100 mg orally, twice daily
IUD insertion	None	
Endometrial biopsy	None	
Induced abortion dilatation and evacuation	Doxycycline	100 mg orally 1 hour before and 200 mg orally after surgery **or**
	Metronidazole	500 mg orally twice daily for 5 d
Urodynamics	None	

[a]A convenient time to administer antibiotic prophylaxis is just before anesthesia induction.
[b]Acceptable alternatives include cefotetan, cefoxitin, cefuroxime, or ampicillin-sulbactam.
[c]A 2-g dose is recommended in women with a body mass index >35 or weight >100 kg or 220 lb.
[d]Antimicrobial agents of choice in women with a history of immediate hypersensitivity to penicillin.
[e]Ciprofloxacin, levofloxacin, or moxifloxacin.
[f]For total laparoscopic hysterectomy, prophylaxis is given.
[g]If patient has a history of pelvic inflammatory disease or procedure demonstrates dilated fallopian tubes. No prophylaxis is indicated for a study without dilated tubes.
IV = intravenously; IUD = intrauterine device.
Reproduced with permission from ACOG Committee on Practice Bulletins–Gynecology: ACOG practice bulletin No. 104: antibiotic prophylaxis for gynecologic procedures, Obstet Gynecol. 2009 May;113(5):1180–1189.

Although its routine use should be limited, mechanical bowel preparation may be elected for certain advanced laparoscopic surgeries or for female pelvic reconstructive procedures involving the posterior vaginal wall and anal sphincter. In these cases, evacuation of rectal stool provides additional operating space and undistorted anatomy. Moreover, following sphincteroplasty, preoperative evacuation typically delays stooling and allows initial healing. Various regimens exist: (1) low-residue or clear liquid diets the day(s) prior to surgery, (2) oral cathartics such as 240 mL of senna extract (Senokot, X-Prep) or 240 mL of magnesium citrate, (3) sodium phosphate enemas (Fleet), (4) oral phosphates (Visicol, Fleet Phospho-soda), or (5) oral polyethylene glycol (PEG) solutions (GoLYTELY, NuLYTELY, HalfLytely).

THROMBOEMBOLISM PREVENTION

Prophylaxis against VTE ranks in the top 10 patient safety practices recommended by the Agency for Healthcare Research and Quality (AHRQ) and the National Quality Forum (Kaafarani, 2011). In the United States alone, the annual incidence of deep-vein thrombosis (DVT) and pulmonary thromboembolism are estimated to approach 600,000, with more than 100,000 deaths each year (Beckman, 2010). Ten to 30 percent of those diagnosed with VTE die within 1 month of diagnosis. National recommendations for prophylaxis against VTE follow a risk-based approach. The Caprini score is a tool validated using a large sample of general, vascular, and urologic surgery patients (Table 39-7) (Gould, 2012). Despite not being validated in gynecologic surgery, the patient populations are similar enough

TABLE 39-7. Caprini Risk Assessment Model

1 Point	2 Points	3 Points	5 Points
Age 41–60 yr	Age 61–74 yr	Age ≥75 yr	Stroke <1 month
Minor surgery	Arthroscopic surgery	Prior VTE	Elective arthroplasty
BMI >25 kg/m²	Major laparotomy (>45 min)	Family history of VTE	Hip, pelvis, or leg fracture
Swollen legs	Laparoscopy (>45 min)	Factor V Leiden	Acute spinal cord injury
Varicose veins	Malignancy	Prothrombin 20210A	<1 month
Pregnancy or postpartum	Bed rest >72 hr	Lupus anticoagulant	
Recurrent spontaneous abortion	Immobilizing plaster cast	Anticardiolipin antibodies	
COC or HRT use	Central venous access	Elevated serum homocysteine	
Sepsis <1 month		Heparin-induced	
Serious lung disease <1 month		thrombocytopenia	
Abnormal pulmonary function		Other thrombophilia	
Acute myocardial infarction			
CHF <1 month			
Inflammatory bowel disease			
Bed rest			

BMI = body mass index; CHF = congestive heart failure; COC = combination oral contraceptive; HRT = hormone replacement therapy; VTE = venous thromboembolism.
Reproduced with permission from Gould MK, Garcia DA, Wren SM, et al: Prevention of VTE in nonorthopedic surgical patients: Antithrombotic Therapy and Prevention of Thrombosis, 9th ed: American College of Chest Physicians Evidence-Based Clinical Practice Guidelines. Chest 2012 Feb;141(2 Suppl):e227S–2277S.

that extrapolation is reasonable. Caprini scores of 0–1 points categorize a patient as "very low risk," 2 points reflect "low risk," 3–4 points confer "moderate risk," and ≥5 points places patients at "high risk." These points are transferable to Table 39-8.

Thrombophilias

Of VTE risk factors, thrombophilias are inherited or acquired deficiencies of inhibitory proteins of the coagula-

tion cascade. These can lead to hypercoagulability and recurrent VTE.

Of these heritable coagulopathies, *antithrombin deficiency*, although rare, is the most thrombogenic. Thrombin is produced by the enzymatic cleavage of prothrombin (Fig. 39-5). Thrombin converts fibrinogen to an active form that assembles into fibrin for clot formation. Antithrombin, previously known as antithrombin III, binds to and inactivates thrombin and the

TABLE 39-8. Thromboprophylaxis based on VTE and Bleeding Risks

Risk of VTE (Caprini score)[a]	Risk & Consequences of Major Bleeding Complications	
	Average Bleeding Risk	**High Bleeding Risk or Severe Consequences**
Very low (0–1)	No specific prophylaxis	
Low (2)	Mechanical prophylaxis (IPC preferred)	
Moderate (3–4)	LDUH, LMWH, or MP (IPC preferred)	Mechanical prophylaxis (IPC preferred)
High (≥5)	LDUH *or* LMWH *PLUS* MP (CS or IPC)	
High-risk, cancer surgery	Same as high risk *PLUS* extended LMWH prophylaxis	MP (IPC preferred), until bleeding risk subsides and pharmacologic prophylaxis can be added
High-risk, heparin NA or CI	Fondaparinux or low-dose ASA *or* MP (IPC preferred) *or* both	

[a]Calculation of Caprini score is found in Table 39-7

ASA = aspirin; CI = contraindicated; CS = compression stockings; LDUH = low-dose unfractionated heparin; LMWH = low-molecular-weight heparin; IPC = intermittent pneumatic compression; MP = mechanical prophylaxis; NA = not available; VTE = venous thromboembolism.
Reproduced with permission from Gould MK, Garcia DA, Wren SM, et al: Prevention of VTE in nonorthopedic surgical patients: Antithrombotic Therapy and Prevention of Thrombosis, 9th ed: American College of Chest Physicians Evidence-Based Clinical Practice Guidelines. Chest 2012 Feb;141(2 Suppl):e227S–2277S.

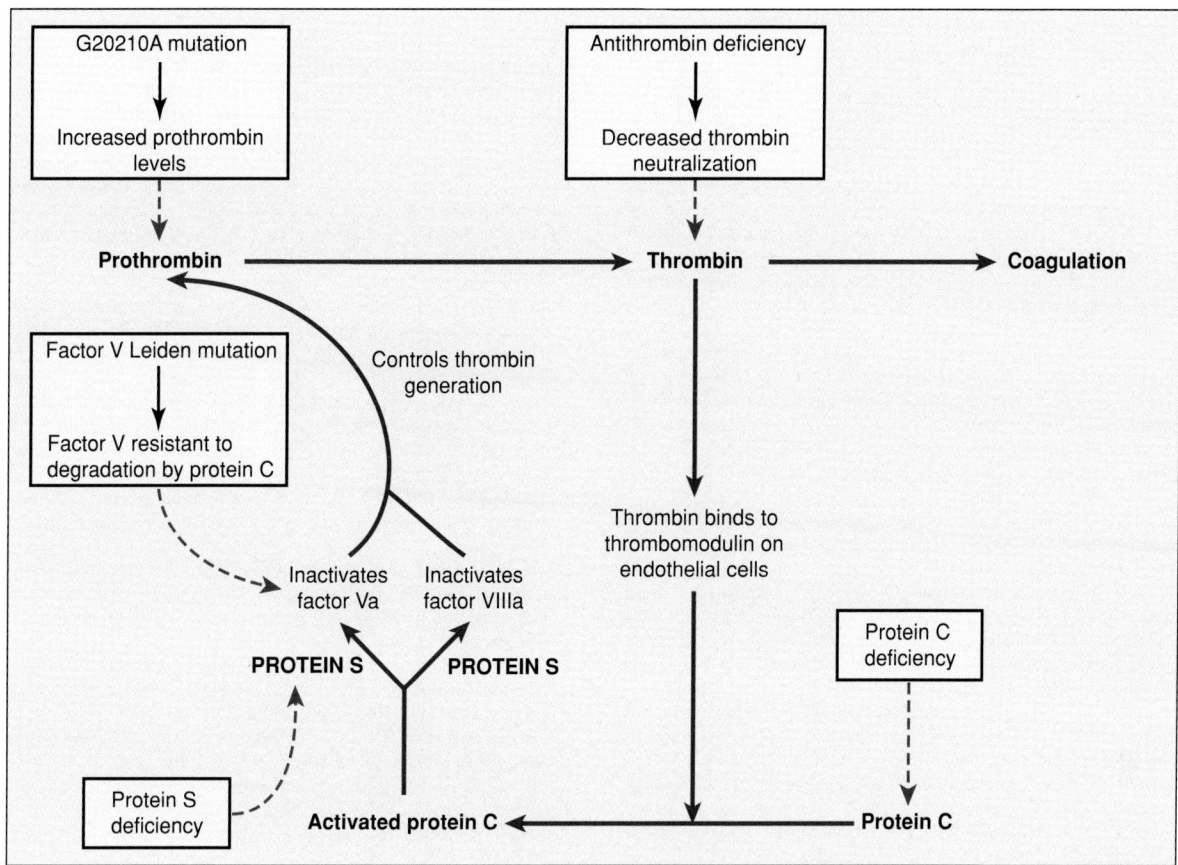

FIGURE 39-5 Points of the coagulation cascade affected by some of the thrombophilias.

activated coagulation factors IXa, Xa, XIa, and XIIa. If thrombin is not inactivated, then coagulation is favored.

Protein C and *protein S deficiencies* are other thrombophilias. When thrombin is bound to thrombomodulin on intact endothelium, its procoagulant activities are neutralized. In this bound state, thrombin also activates protein C, a natural anticoagulant. Protein C and its cofactor, protein S, limit coagulation, in part, by inactivating factors Va and VIIIa.

Activated protein C resistance (Factor V Leiden mutation) is the most prevalent thrombophilia and is caused by a single mutation in the factor V gene. The mutation makes FVa resist to degradation by activated protein C. The unimpeded abnormal factor V protein retains its procoagulant activity and predisposes to thrombosis.

Prothrombin G20210A mutation is a thrombophilia stemming from a prothrombin gene missense mutation that leads to excessive prothrombin accumulation. This may then be converted to thrombin to create a hypercoagulable state.

Guidelines to direct thrombophilia testing are lacking in the United States, and those of other international groups are incongruous (De Stefano, 2013). The UK-based NICE guidelines (2012) recommend screening patients who have an unprovoked VTE but not those with a provoked VTE. They also recommend against screening asymptomatic first-degree relatives of a known thrombophilia patient who experienced a VTE.

Hormone Discontinuation

Of risks, hormone use is one factor that can be modified prior elective surgery. Combined oral contraceptive pills (COCs) induce hypercoagulable changes that are reversed if COCs are

stopped at least 6 weeks prior to surgery (Robinson, 1991; Vessey, 1986). To balance the risk of unintended pregnancy in women halting COCs, a suitable alternative is recommended with clear instructions on use. In the decision to halt COCs prior to surgery, the risk of VTE in an individual must be weighed against the risk of unintended pregnancy. In those undergoing major surgery and COC continuation, heparin prophylaxis is considered (American College of Obstetricians and Gynecologists, 2013).

Postmenopausal hormone replacement therapy (HRT) may slightly increase the incidence of postsurgical VTE but not to the same degree as the surgical procedure itself (Ueng, 2010). Thus, women are appropriately counseled on this additional postoperative risk, but the value and duration of HRT cessation to negate this increased risk is unclear.

Prophylaxis Options

Various options for VTE prevention exist. Early ambulation, although encouraged after surgery, is not regarded as a primary strategy for VTE prophylaxis (Michota, 2006). Graded compression stockings (T.E.D. hose) prevent pooling of blood in the calves. If these are used alone and fitted properly, DVT rates are reduced 50 percent. If used in conjunction with other methods of prophylaxis, additional benefit is achieved (Amaragiri, 2000). Intermittent pneumatic compression (IPC) primarily works by improving venous flow. It appears to be effective in moderate- and high-risk patients, if initiated prior to the induction of anesthesia and continued until patients are fully ambulating (Clarke-Pearson, 1993; Gould, 2012). Pharmacologic methods of VTE prophylaxis include low-dose

UFH, LMWH, and DOACs. Table 39-8 summarizes appropriate treatment strategies based on risk status.

REFERENCES

Ageno W, Gallus AS, Wittkowsky A, et al: Oral anticoagulant therapy: Antithrombotic Therapy and Prevention of Thrombosis, 9th ed: American College of Chest Physicians Evidence-Based Clinical Practice Guidelines. Chest 141(2 Suppl):e44S, 2012

Agostini P, Cieslik H, Rathinam S, et al: Postoperative pulmonary complications following thoracic surgery: are there any modifiable risk factors? Thorax 65(9):815, 2010

Akrawi W, Benumof JL: A pathophysiological basis for informed preoperative smoking cessation counseling. J Cardiothorac Vasc Anesth 11(5):629, 1997

Amaragiri SV, Lees TA: Elastic compression stockings for prevention of deep vein thrombosis. Cochrane Database Syst Rev 3:CD001484, 2000

American College of Obstetricians and Gynecologists: Antibiotic prophylaxis for gynecologic procedures. Practice Bulletin No. 104, May 2009, Reaffirmed 2014a

American College of Obstetricians and Gynecologists: Chronic antithrombotic therapy and gynecologic surgery. Committee Opinion No. 610, October 2014b

American College of Obstetricians and Gynecologists: Informed consent. Committee Opinion No. 439, August 2009, Reaffirmed 2012

American College of Obstetricians and Gynecologists: Prevention of deep vein thrombosis and pulmonary embolism. Practice Bulletin No. 84, August 2007, Reaffirmed 2013

American College of Radiology: ACR appropriateness criteria: Routine admission and preoperative chest radiography. Reston, American College of Radiology, 2000, Reaffirmed 2011

Archer C, Levy AR, McGregor M: Value of routine preoperative chest x-rays: a meta-analysis. Can J Anaesth 40:1022, 1993

Arozullah AM, Daley J, Henderson WG, et al: Multifactorial risk index for predicting postoperative respiratory failure in men after major noncardiac surgery. The National Veterans Administration Surgical Quality Improvement Program. Ann Surg 232:242, 2000

Ballard AC, Parker-Autry CY, Markland AD, et al: Bowel preparation before vaginal prolapse surgery: a randomized controlled trial. Obstet Gynecol 123(2 Pt 1):232, 2014

Barker K, Graham NG, Mason MC, et al: The relative significance of preoperative oral antibiotics, mechanical bowel preparation, and preoperative peritoneal contamination in the avoidance of sepsis after radical surgery for ulcerative colitis and Crohn's disease of the large bowel. Br J Surg 58:270, 1971

Beckman MG, Hooper WC, Critchley SE, et al: Venous thromboembolism: a public health concern. Am J Prev Med 38(4 Suppl):S495, 2010

Bernstein WK, Deshpande S: Preoperative evaluation for thoracic surgery. Semin Cardiothorac Vasc Anesth 12(2):109, 2008

Bouri S, Shun-Shin MJ, Cole GD, et al: Meta-analysis of secure randomised controlled trials of β-blockade to prevent perioperative death in non-cardiac surgery. Heart 100(6):456, 2014

Bromberg JS, Alfrey EJ, Barker CF, et al: Adrenal suppression and steroid supplementation in renal transplant recipients. Transplantation 51:385, 1991

Brooks-Brunn JA: Predictors of postoperative pulmonary complications following abdominal surgery. Chest 111:564, 1997

Buist AS, Sexton GJ, Nagy JM, et al: The effect of smoking cessation and modification on lung function. Am Rev Respir Dis 114(1):115, 1976

Cheatham ML, Chapman WC, Key SP, et al: A meta-analysis of selective versus routine nasogastric decompression after elective laparotomy. Ann Surg 221:469, 1995

Cheng A, Nazarian S, Spragg DD, et al: Effects of surgical and endoscopic electrocautery on modern-day permanent pacemaker and implantable cardioverter-defibrillator systems. Pacing Clin Electrophysiol 31(3):344, 2008

Chumillas S, Ponce JL, Delgado F, et al: Prevention of postoperative pulmonary complications through respiratory rehabilitation: a controlled clinical study. Arch Phys Med Rehabil 79:5, 1998

Clarke-Pearson DL, Synan IS, Dodge R, et al: A randomized trial of low-dose heparin and intermittent pneumatic calf compression for the prevention of deep venous thrombosis after gynecologic oncology surgery. Am J Obstet Gynecol 168:1146, 1993

Comfere T, Sprung J, Kumar M, et al: Angiotensin system inhibitors in a general surgical population. Anesth Analg 100(3):636, 2005

Coulter A, Ellins J: Effectiveness of strategies for informing, educating, and involving patients. BMJ 335(7609):24, 2007

Cunningham FG, Leveno KL, Bloom SL, et al (eds): Thromboembolic disorders. In Williams Obstetrics, 24th ed. New York, McGraw-Hill, 2014, p 1030

DeLoughery TG: Microcytic anemia. N Engl J Med 371(14):1324, 2014

De Stefano V, Rossi E: Testing for inherited thrombophilia and consequences for antithrombotic prophylaxis in patients with venous thromboembolism and their relatives. A review of the Guidelines from Scientific Societies and Working Groups. Thromb Haemost 110(4):697, 2013

Devereaux PJ, Goldman L, Cook DJ, et al: Perioperative cardiac events in patients undergoing noncardiac surgery: a review of the magnitude of the problem, the pathophysiology of the events and methods to estimate and communicate risk. CMAJ 173(6):627, 2005

Douketis J, Bell AD, Eikelboom J, et al: Approach to the new oral anticoagulants in family practice: Part 2: addressing frequently asked questions. Can Fam Physician 60(11):997, 2014

Douketis JD, Spyropoulos AC, Spencer FA, et al: Perioperative management of antithrombotic therapy: Antithrombotic Therapy and Prevention of Thrombosis, 9th ed: American College of Chest Physicians Evidence-Based Clinical Practice Guidelines. Chest 141(2 Suppl):e326S, 2012

Dronge AS, Perkal MF, Kancir S, et al: Long-term glycemic control and postoperative infectious complications. Arch Surg 141:375, 2006

Duncan JE, Quietmeyer CM: Bowel preparation: current status. Clin Colon Rectal Surg 22(1):14, 2009

Eichenberger A, Proietti S, Wicky S, et al: Morbid obesity and postoperative pulmonary atelectasis: an underestimated problem. Anesth Analg 95:1788, 2002

Erasmus Medical Centre: Report on the 2012 follow-up investigation of possible breaches of academic integrity. 2012. Available at: http://cardiobrief.files.wordpress.com/2012/10/integrity-report-2012–10-english-translation.pdf. Accessed January 13, 2015

Fa-Si-Oen P, Roumen R, Buitenweg J, et al: Mechanical bowel preparation or not? Outcome of a multicenter, randomized trial in elective open colon surgery. Dis Colon Rectum 48:1509, 2005

Ferris BG Jr, Pollard DS: Effect of deep and quiet breathing on pulmonary compliance in man. J Clin Invest 39:143, 1960

Finney SJ, Zekveld C, Elia A, et al: Glucose control and mortality in critically ill patients. JAMA 290:2041, 2003

Fleisher LA: Preoperative evaluation of the patient with hypertension. JAMA 287:2043, 2002

Fleisher LA, Beckman JA, Brown KA, et al: 2009 ACCF/AHA focused update on perioperative beta blockade incorporated into the ACC/AHA 2007 guidelines on perioperative cardiovascular evaluation and care for noncardiac surgery: a report of the American College of Cardiology Foundation/American Heart Association Task Force on Practice Guidelines. Circulation 120(21):e169, 2009

Fleisher LA, Fleischmann KE, Auerbach AD, et al: 2014 ACC/AHA Guideline on Perioperative Cardiovascular Evaluation and Management of Patients Undergoing Noncardiac Surgery: a Report of the American College of Cardiology/American Heart Association Task Force on Practice Guidelines. J Am Coll Cardiol 64(22):e77, 2014

Garber AJ, Moghissi ES, Bransome ED Jr, et al: American College of Endocrinology position statement on inpatient diabetes and metabolic control. Endocr Pract 10:77, 2004

Goldman L, Caldera DL: Risks of general anesthesia and elective operation in the hypertensive patient. Anesthesiology 50:285, 1979

Goldman L, Lee T, Rudd P: Ten Commandments for effective consultations. Arch Intern Med 143:1753, 1983

Goldwasser P, Feldman J: Association of serum albumin and mortality risk. J Clin Epidemiol 50:693, 1997

Gould MK, Garcia DA, Wren SM, et al: Prevention of VTE in nonorthopedic surgical patients: Antithrombotic Therapy and Prevention of Thrombosis, 9th ed: American College of Chest Physicians Evidence-Based Clinical Practice Guidelines. Chest 141(2 Suppl):e227S, 2012

Gregoratos G, Abrams J, Epstein AE, et al: ACC/AHA/NASPE 2002 guideline update for implantation of cardiac pacemakers and antiarrhythmia devices: summary article: a report of the American College of Cardiology/American Heart Association Task Force on Practice Guidelines (ACC/AHA/NASPE Committee to Update the 1998 Pacemaker Guidelines). Circulation 106: 2145, 2002

Güenaga KF, Matos D, Wille-Jørgensen P, et al: Mechanical bowel preparation for elective colorectal surgery. Cochrane Database Syst Rev 9:CD001544, 2011

Harrison L, Johnston M, Massicotte MP, et al: Comparison of 5-mg and 10-mg loading doses in initiation of warfarin therapy. Ann Intern Med 126: 133, 1997

Hassan SA, Hlatky MA, Boothroyd DB, et al: Outcomes of noncardiac surgery after coronary bypass surgery or coronary angioplasty in the Bypass Angioplasty Revascularization Investigation (BARI). Am J Med 110:260, 2001

Hlatky MA, Boineau RE, Higginbotham MB, et al: A brief self-administered questionnaire to determine functional capacity (the Duke Activity Status Index). Am J Cardiol 64(10):651, 1989

Holbrook A, Schulman S, Witt DM, et al: Evidence-based management of anticoagulant therapy: Antithrombotic Therapy and Prevention of Thrombosis, 9th ed: American College of Chest Physicians Evidence-Based Clinical Practice Guidelines. Chest 141(2 Suppl):e152S, 2012

Hoogwerf BJ: Perioperative management of diabetes mellitus: how should we act on the limited evidence? Cleve Clin J Med 73(Suppl 1):S95, 2006

Jacober SJ, Sowers JR: An update on perioperative management of diabetes. Arch Intern Med 159:2405, 1999

James AH, Kouides PA, Abdul-Kadir R, et al: Evaluation and management of acute menorrhagia in women with and without underlying bleeding disorders: consensus from an international expert panel. Eur J Obstet Gynecol Reprod Biol 158(2):124, 2011

Johnson BE, Porter J: Preoperative evaluation of the gynecologic patient: considerations for improved outcomes. Obstet Gynecol 111(5):1183, 2008

Kaafarani HMA, Borzecki AM, Itani KMF, et al: Validity of selected patient safety indicators: opportunities and concerns. J Am Coll Surg 212(6):924, 2011

Kannel WB: Epidemiology and prevention of cardiac failure: Framingham Study insights. Eur Heart J 8:23, 1987

Kaplan EB, Sheiner LB, Boeckmann AJ, et al: The usefulness of preoperative laboratory screening. JAMA 253:3576, 1985

Kearon C, Hirsh J: Management of anticoagulation before and after elective surgery. N Engl J Med 336:1506, 1997

Kelly KN, Domajnko B: Perioperative stress-dose steroids. Clin Colon Rectal Surg 26(3):163, 2013

Kertai MD, Bountioukos M, Boersma E, et al: Aortic stenosis: an underestimated risk factor for perioperative complications in patients undergoing noncardiac surgery. Am J Med 116:8, 2004

Korvin CC, Pearce RH, Stanley J: Admissions screening: clinical benefits. Ann Intern Med 83:197, 1975

Kozek-Langenecker SA: Perioperative management issues of direct oral anticoagulants. Semin Hematol 51(2):112, 2014

Lavelle-Jones C, Byrne DJ, Rice P, et al: Factors affecting quality of informed consent. Br Med J 306:885, 1993

Lee HP, Chang YY, Jean YH, et al: Importance of serum albumin level in the preoperative tests conducted in elderly patients with hip fracture. Injury 40(7):756, 2009

Lee TH, Marcantonio ER, Mangione CM, et al: Derivation and prospective validation of a simple index for prediction of cardiac risk of major noncardiac surgery. Circulation 100:1043, 1999

Levine MN, Hirsh J, Gent M, et al: Optimal duration of oral anticoagulant therapy: a randomized trial comparing four weeks with three months of warfarin in patients with proximal deep vein thrombosis. Thromb Haemost 74:606, 1995

Lindahl TL, Baghaei F, Blixter IF, et al: Effects of the oral, direct thrombin inhibitor dabigatran on five common coagulation assays. Thromb Haemost 105(2):371, 2011

Macpherson DS, Snow R, Lofgren RP: Preoperative screening: value of previous tests. Ann Intern Med 113:969, 1990

Maddali MM: Chronic obstructive lung disease: perioperative management. Middle East J Anesthesiol 19(6):1219, 2008

Mangano DT: Perioperative medicine: NHLBI working group deliberations and recommendations. J Cardiothorac Vasc Anesth 18:1, 2004

Mansour A, Watson W, Shayani V, et al: Abdominal operations in patients with cirrhosis: still a major surgical challenge. Surgery 122(4):730, 1997

Marik PE, Varon J: Requirement of perioperative stress doses of corticosteroids: a systematic review of the literature. Arch Surg 143(12):1222, 2008

Meyers JR, Lembeck L, O'Kane H, et al: Changes in functional residual capacity of the lung after operation. Arch Surg 110:576, 1975

Michota FA Jr: Preventing venous thromboembolism in surgical patients. Cleve Clin J Med 73:S88, 2006

Møller AM, Villebro N, Pedersen T, et al: Effect of preoperative smoking intervention on postoperative complications: a randomised clinical trial. Lancet 359:114, 2002

Muzii L, Bellati F, Zullo MA, et al: Mechanical bowel preparation before gynecologic laparoscopy: a randomized, single-blind, controlled trial. Fertil Steril 85:689, 2006

Nakagawa M, Tanaka H, Tsukuma H, et al: Relationship between the duration of the preoperative smoke-free period and the incidence of postoperative pulmonary complications after pulmonary surgery. Chest 120:705, 2001

Nandi PL: Ethical aspects of clinical practice. Arch Surg 135:22, 2000

National Institute for Health and Clinical Excellence: Venous thromboembolic diseases: the management of venous thromboembolic diseases and the role of thrombophilia testing. Clinical Guideline 144. London, 2012

Nichols RL, Condon RE: Preoperative preparation of the colon. Surg Gynecol Obstet 132:323, 1971

Nishimura RA, Otto CM, Bonow RO, et al: 2014 AHA/ACC Guideline for the Management of Patients With Valvular Heart Disease: a report of the American College of Cardiology/American Heart Association Task Force on Practice Guidelines. Circulation 129(23):e521, 2014

Okuyama M, Ikeda K, Shibata T, et al: Preoperative iron supplementation and intraoperative transfusion during colorectal cancer surgery. Surg Today 35(1):36, 2005

Ortel TL: Perioperative management of patients on chronic antithrombotic therapy. Blood 120(24):4699, 2012

Pasquina P, Tramer MR, Granier JM, et al: Respiratory physiotherapy to prevent pulmonary complications after abdominal surgery: a systematic review. Chest 130:1887, 2006

Patel T: Surgery in the patient with liver disease. Mayo Clin Proc 74:593, 1999

Platell C, Hall JC: Atelectasis after abdominal surgery. J Am Coll Surg 185:584, 1997

Poldermans D, Devereaux PJ: The experts debate: perioperative beta-blockade for noncardiac surgery—proven safe or not? Cleve Clin J Med 76 (Suppl 4):S84, 2009

Qaseem A, Snow V, Fitterman N, et al: Risk assessment for and strategies to reduce perioperative pulmonary complications for patients undergoing non-cardiothoracic surgery: a guideline from the American College of Physicians. Ann Intern Med 144:575, 2006

Robinson GE, Burren T, Mackie IJ, et al: Changes in haemostasis after stopping the combined contraceptive pill: implications for major surgery. Br Med J 302:269, 1991

Roizen MF: More preoperative assessment by physicians and less by laboratory tests. N Engl J Med 342:204, 2000

Rucker L, Frye EB, Staten MA: Usefulness of screening chest roentgenograms in preoperative patients. JAMA 250:3209, 1983

Schaden E, Kozek-Langenecker SA: Direct thrombin inhibitors: pharmacology and application in intensive care medicine. Intensive Care Med 36(7):1127, 2010

Shander A, Spence RK, Auerbach M: Can intravenous iron therapy meet the unmet needs created by the new restrictions on erythropoietic stimulating agents? Transfusion 50(3):719, 2010

Shi Y, Warner DO: Surgery as a teachable moment for smoking cessation. Anesthesiology 112(1):102, 2010

Silverberg DS, Wexler D, Sheps D, et al: The effect of correction of mild anemia in severe, resistant congestive heart failure using subcutaneous erythropoietin and intravenous iron: a randomized, controlled study. J Am Coll Cardiol 37:1775, 2001

Sirinek KR, Burk RR, Brown M, et al: Improving survival in patients with cirrhosis undergoing major abdominal operations. Arch Surg 122:271, 1987

Smetana GW: Preoperative pulmonary evaluation. N Engl J Med 340:937, 1999

Stacey D, Légaré F, Col NF, et al: Decision aids for people facing health treatment or screening decisions. Cochrane Database Syst Rev 1:CD001431, 2014

Stepp KJ, Barber MD, Yoo EH, et al: Incidence of perioperative complications of urogynecologic surgery in elderly women. Am J Obstet Gynecol 192(5):1630, 2005

Straus SE, McAlister FA, Sackett DL, et al: The accuracy of patient history, wheezing, and laryngeal measurements in diagnosing obstructive airway disease. CARE-COAD1 Group. Clinical Assessment of the Reliability of the Examination—Chronic Obstructive Airways Disease. JAMA 283:1853, 2000

Suman A, Carey WD: Assessing the risk of surgery in patients with liver disease. Cleve Clin J Med 73(4):398, 2006

Thomas JA, McIntosh JM: Are incentive spirometry, intermittent positive pressure breathing, and deep breathing exercises effective in the prevention of postoperative pulmonary complications after upper abdominal surgery? A systematic overview and meta-analysis. Phys Ther 74:3, 1994

Thomsen T, Villebro N, Møller AM: Interventions for preoperative smoking cessation. Cochrane Database Syst Rev 3:CD002294, 2014

Trick WE, Scheckler WE, Tokars JI, et al: Modifiable risk factors associated with deep sternal site infection after coronary artery bypass grafting. J Thorac Cardiovasc Surg 119:108, 2000

Ueng J, Douketis JD: Prevention and treatment of hormone-associated venous thromboembolism: a patient management approach. Hematol Oncol Clin North Am 24(4):683, 2010

Vanderlinde ES, Heal JM, Blumberg N: Autologous transfusion. Br Med J 324:772, 2002

Vessey M, Mant D, Smith A, et al: Oral contraceptives and venous thromboembolism: findings in a large prospective study. Br Med J (Clin Res Ed) 292:526, 1986

Vincent JL, Navickis RG, Wilkes MM: Morbidity in hospitalized patients receiving human albumin: a meta-analysis of randomized, controlled trials. Crit Care Med 32(10):2029. 2004

Warner DO: Preventing postoperative pulmonary complications: the role of the anesthesiologist. Anesthesiology 92:1467, 2000

Warner DO, Warner MA, Barnes RD, et al: Perioperative respiratory complications in patients with asthma. Anesthesiology 85:460, 1996

Weksler N, Klein M, Szendro G, et al: The dilemma of immediate preoperative hypertension: to treat and operate or to postpone surgery? J Clin Anesth 15:179, 2003

White RH, McKittrick T, Hutchinson R, et al: Temporary discontinuation of warfarin therapy: changes in the international normalized ratio. Ann Intern Med 122:40, 1995

Williams FM, Bergin JD: Cardiac screening before noncardiac surgery. Surg Clin North Am 89(4):747, 2009

Wolters U, Wolf T, Stutzer H, et al: ASA classification and perioperative variables as predictors of postoperative outcome. Br J Anaesth 77:217, 1996

Zerah F, Harf A, Perlemuter L, et al: Effects of obesity on respiratory resistance. Chest 103:1470, 1993

Intraoperative Considerations

Gynecologic surgery is used to treat a broad spectrum of underlying pathology. As a result, the list of surgical procedures is extensive, but in general, techniques maximize tissue healing and patient recovery. Successful outcomes depend on appropriate patient and procedure selection, sound intraoperative technique, and preparation for possible complications.

ANESTHESIA SELECTION

Many anesthetic options are available for patients undergoing gynecologic procedures and include general anesthesia, regional analgesia, or local paracervical blockade with or without conscious sedation. These anesthetic techniques are provided by clinicians who are skilled with their placement and capable of managing their side effects. Thus, paracervical blockade and intravenous sedation may be provided by gynecologists. General and regional anesthesia typically are delivered and managed by anesthesiology staff.

Anesthesia selection for gynecologic surgery is complex and influenced by the procedure planned, extent of disease, patient comorbidities, and personal preferences of the patient, anesthesiologist, and surgeon. Last, the providing hospital or clinic may further define options based on their practicing norms and availability of personnel or equipment. For example, an outpatient gynecology clinic may be equipped to provide paracervical blockade or intravenous conscious sedation, but may lack sophisticated equipment or expertise required for regional or general anesthesia.

In all cases, both the anesthesia provider and the surgeon communicate regarding patient and surgery progress and are prepared for potential problems. Difficult patient intubation may complicate general anesthesia, and regional anesthetic procedures may lead to higher than anticipated levels of blockade and respiratory muscle dysfunction. Cases using paracervical blockade may be complicated by inadequate levels of anesthesia, or conversely by anesthetic toxicity. Conscious sedation may also fail to provide adequate analgesia, or alternatively may lead to respiratory depression. Thus, no procedure is free of risk, and contingency plans for each should be in place.

■ Paracervical Block

Paracervical block is used most commonly during first-trimester pregnancy evacuation but also may be selected for cervical ablative or excisional procedures, transvaginal sonographically guided oocyte retrieval, and in-office hysteroscopy. Some studies have also described preemptive analgesia with paracervical block for vaginal hysterectomy (Long, 2009; O'Neal, 2003). Paracervical blockade is often combined with nonsteroidal antiinflammatory drugs (NSAIDs) or intravenous conscious sedation or both. Conscious sedation may be achieved with several agents, but intravenous midazolam (Versed) and fentanyl (Sublimaze) is a frequent combination (Lichtenberg, 2001).

Technique

The cervix, vagina, and uterus are richly supplied by nerves of the uterovaginal plexus (Fig. 38-13, p. 806). Also known as *Frankenhäuser plexus*, this plexus lies within the connective tissue lateral to the uterosacral ligaments. For this reason, paracervical injections are most effective if placed immediately lateral to the insertion of the uterosacral ligaments into the uterus (Rogers, 1998). Thus, divided doses are given at the 4 and 8 o'clock positions at the cervical base (Fig. 40-1).

In most cases, total doses of 10 mL of 0.25-percent bupivacaine, 1-percent mepivacaine, or 1- or 2-percent lidocaine may be administered (Cicinelli, 1998; Hong, 2006; Lau, 1999). However, specific calculation of a maximum safe dose for each patient before injection is recommended (Dorian, 2015). The toxic dose of lidocaine approximates 4.5 mg/kg (Table 40-1). For a 50-kg woman, this would equal 225 mg. Thus, if a

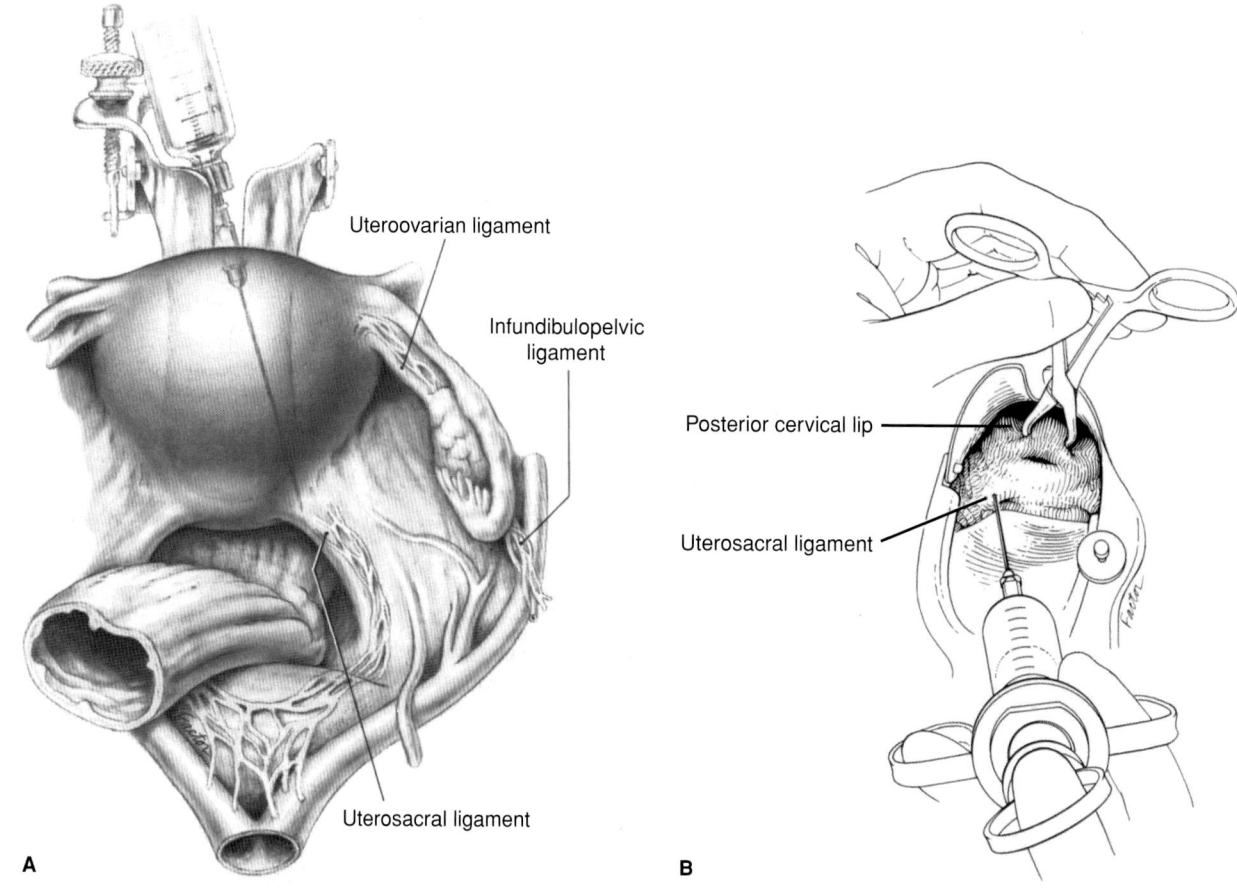

FIGURE 40-1 Paracervical blockade. **A.** Abdominal view of a paracervical block. Local anesthetic is infiltrated near sensory innervation of the cervix, which lies near the uterosacral ligament. **B.** Vaginal view of the injection of local anesthetics into the cervical base at 4 and 8 o'clock. (Reproduced with permission from Penfield JA: Gynecologic Surgery under Local Anesthesia. Baltimore: Urban and Schwarzenberg; 1986.)

1-percent lidocaine solution is used, the calculated allowed amount would be: 225 mg ÷ 10 mg/mL = 22.5 mL. Of note, for any drug solution, 1-percent = 10 mg/mL.

Anesthesia is presumed to result from pharmacologic nerve conduction blockade by the local anesthetic agent (Chanrachakul, 2001). The injection itself may have an immediate anesthetic effect by swelling surrounding tissue and exerting mechanical pressure on nerves to disrupt neural transmission (Phair, 2002; Wiebe, 1995). Addition of epinephrine to these solutions leads to local vasoconstriction, which enhances analgesia quality, prolongs duration of action, and decreases toxicity.

Thus, higher maximum doses may be used. Return of neural function is spontaneous as the drug is metabolized.

In general, increased doses of local anesthetics may lead to clinically significant conduction blockade within the central nervous system (CNS) and heart. Signs range from drowsiness, tinnitus, perioral tingling, and visual disturbances to confusion, seizure, coma, and ventricular arrhythmia. Monitoring patients for the subtle symptoms of CNS toxicity is important because the therapeutic-to-toxic ratios are often narrow with these agents.

When toxicity develops, cardiac effects are potentiated by acidosis, hypercapnia, and hypoxia. Thus, treatment typically

TABLE 40-1. Characteristics of Local Anesthetics

Drug (Brand name)	Available Concentrations (%)	Maximum Dose (mg/kg)	Maximum Dose with Epinephrine (mg/kg)	Duration (hr)
Moderate-duration				
Lidocaine (Xylocaine)	0.5, 1, 2	4.5	7	0.5–1
Mepivicaine (Carbocaine)	1, 1.5, 2	4	7	0.75–1.5
Prilocaine (Citanest)	0.5, 1	7	8.5	0.5–1.5
Long-duration				
Bupivacaine (Marcaine)	0.25, 0.5, 0.75	2.5	3	2–4
Etidocaine (Duranest)	0.5, 1	4	5.5	2–3

includes intravenous access, adequate oxygenation, and seizure control. A benzodiazepine such as diazepam (Valium) given intravenously is effective anticonvulsant therapy (Naguib, 1998). For treatment, diazepam, 2 mg/min, is administered until seizures stop or a total dose of 20 mg is delivered.

■ Intrauterine Instillation

Injection of local anesthetic solutions through a catheter into the uterine cavity has been reported to safely lower pain scores in women undergoing in-office hysteroscopy or endometrial biopsy (Cicinelli, 1997; Trolice, 2000). The presumed mechanism is anesthetic blockade of nerve endings within the endometrial mucosa. Studies have used 5-mL doses of 2-percent lidocaine or of 2-percent mepivacaine. For first-trimester abortion procedures, Edelman and coworkers (2004, 2006) evaluated instillation of 5 mL of 4-percent lidocaine combined with paracervical blockade. However, for this indication, a significant number of women reported symptoms attributed to lidocaine toxicity.

■ Postoperative Pain

Anesthesiologists are employing multimodal strategies intraoperatively to reduce postoperative pain. Gabapentin and ketorolac are now in common use (Alayed, 2014; De Oliveira, 2012). The transversus abdominis plane (TAP) block has been studied in abdominal and laparoscopic hysterectomy with promising results (Carney, 2008; De Oliveira, 2014). The surgeon may also improve postoperative analgesia by implanting suprafascial wound soaker catheters to administer local anesthesia (Iyer, 2010; Kushner, 2005). Additionally, local infiltrative analgesia, using a long-acting medication such as liposomal bupivacaine, may be injected into the incision by the surgeon (Barrington, 2013).

SURGICAL SAFETY

Communication between all members of the team is vital to the success of an operation and avoidance of patient harm. The Joint Commission established the *Universal Protocol for Preventing Wrong Site, Wrong Procedure, and Wrong Person Surgery* (Joint Commission, 2009). This protocol encompasses three components: (1) preprocedural verification of all relevant documents, (2) marking the operative site, and (3) completion of a "time out" prior to procedure initiation. The "time out" requires attention of the entire team to assess that patient, site, and procedure are correctly identified. Important interactions also include introduction of the patient care team members, verification of prophylactic antibiotics, anticipated procedure length, and communication of anticipated complications such as potential for large blood loss. Additionally, requests for special instrumentation are addressed preoperatively to prevent potential patient compromise that may accompany lacking an instrument at the time it is needed. Breakdowns in communication are common across pre-, intra-, and postoperative phases of care and are linked to adverse events and patient harm (Greenberg, 2007; Nagpal, 2010). Specifically, the transfer of a patient to a new care team or new location has been identified

as a time particularly vulnerable to communication breakdowns (Greenberg, 2007).

SURGICAL ASSISTANT

A gynecology resident may sometimes feel that the role of assistant is unimportant. However, an experienced surgeon knows the critical difference that good assistance can provide. Assistants should anticipate surgeon needs and aid smooth progress of the operation. Therefore, an assistant must be familiar with the planned procedure's steps, relevant anatomy, and clinical patient details.

Maintaining exposure by proper retraction and keeping the operative field clear of obstruction are primary functions. Laparotomy sponge or suction use is timed to avoid interfering with the surgeon, and a sponge is used to blot rather than wipe. Immediate pressure is placed on bleeding surfaces until the situation can be assessed systematically. Clamps are released slowly to avoid tissue slippage. Attention must be fixed on the procedure. Thus, if music or conversation is distracting, they are avoided.

NERVE INJURY PREVENTION

Anesthetized patients who undergo prolonged gynecologic procedures are at risk for peripheral neuropathy of their upper or lower extremities. These neuropathies are uncommon, and cited incidences approximate 2 percent of gynecologic cases (Cardosi, 2002). Neurologic deficits typically are mild, transient, and resolve spontaneously. Infrequently, prolonged or permanent disability may result.

During gynecologic surgery, lower extremity injuries can involve nerves of the lumbosacral plexus. Mechanisms of injury include surgical nerve transection, rupture following increased stretch, or nerve ischemia. Ischemia may result from compression of perineural vessels during prolonged or pronounced nerve stretch or compression. Although any patient may develop postoperative neuropathy, higher rates are noted in patients who smoke, who have anatomic abnormalities, or who are thin, diabetic, or alcoholic. Use of self-retaining retractors and prolonged surgical duration are additional factors (Warner, 2000).

Symptoms reflect functional loss of the affected nerve. Motor loss typically manifests as muscle weakness, whereas sensory loss may be noted as anesthesia, paresthesia, or pain in the nerve's sensory distribution (Fig. 40-2 and Table 40-2). Therefore, a detailed neurologic examination allows clinical identification of most peripheral neuropathies. Electrodiagnostic testing is indicated if motor function is diminished (Knockaert, 1996). Generally, electromyography is most useful after a 2- to 3-week delay to permit denervational changes to fully develop within affected muscles (Winfree, 2005).

Treatment will vary depending on whether motor or sensory function is affected. If motor function is impaired, neurologic consultation is typically warranted. Physical therapy begins immediately to minimize contracture and muscle atrophy. Alternatively, for those with only mild sensory losses, observation for return of function is reasonable. For those with pain, treatments may include oral analgesics, gabapentin, biofeedback, and serial trigger point injection with local anesthetics.

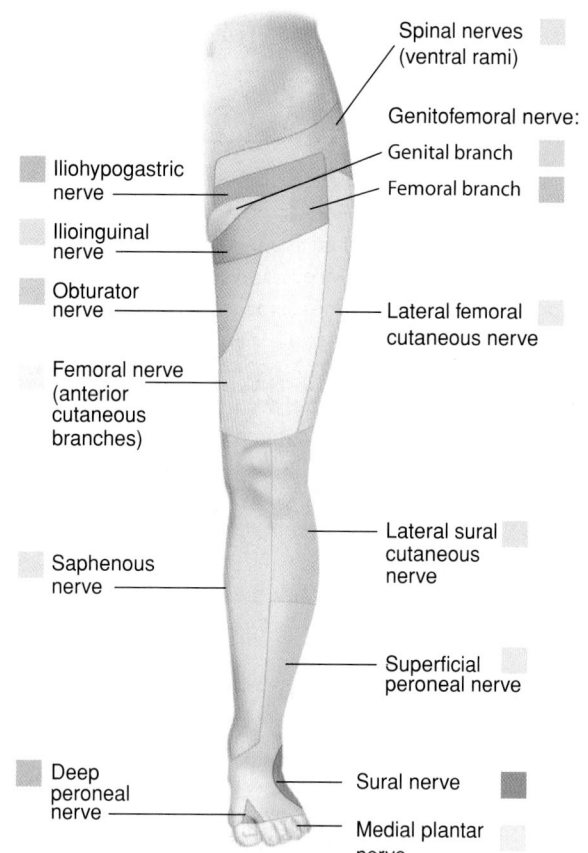

FIGURE 40-2 Peripheral nerves and their corresponding areas of sensory innervation.

■ Laparotomy

Femoral Nerve

This nerve perforates the psoas muscle early in its course and passes medially beneath the inguinal ligament before exiting the pelvis. It then enters the femoral triangle to lie lateral to the femoral artery and vein. This nerve can be compressed

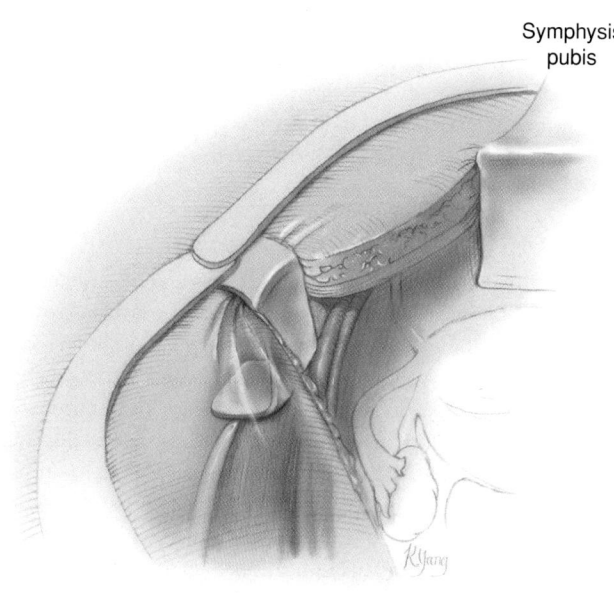

FIGURE 40-3 If poorly positioned, the lateral blade of a self-retaining retractor can press against the femoral nerve lying atop the psoas muscle.

anywhere along its course but is particularly susceptible within the body of the psoas muscle and at the inguinal ligament. Improper placement of a self-retaining retractor is the most common cause of surgical femoral nerve injury, and rates following abdominal hysterectomy may reach 10 percent (Fig. 40-3) (Goldman, 1985; Kvist-Poulsen, 1982). In affected women, the patellar reflex is usually absent in addition to impaired sensory and motor function.

In prevention, lateral retractor blades are selected and positioned such that only the rectus abdominis muscle and not the psoas muscle is retracted (Chen, 1995). The retractor blades are evaluated when placed, to confirm that they are not resting on the psoas muscle. For thin patients, folded laparotomy towels may be placed between the retractor

TABLE 40-2. The Lumbosacral Plexus Nerve Plexus (L1-S4)			
Nerve	**Origin**	**Motor Function**	**Sensory Function**
Ilioinguinal	L1	None	Inferior abdominal wall, mons pubis, labia majora
Iliohypogastric	L1	None	Inferior abdominal wall, upper lateral gluteal region
Genitofemoral	L1–2	None	Labia majora, anterior superior thigh
Femoral	L2–3	None	Anterolateral thigh
Cutaneous femoral	L2–4	Hip flexion, adduction; knee extension	Anterior and inferomedial thigh, medial calf
Obturator	L2–4	Thigh adduction, lateral rotation	Superomedial thigh
Pudendal	S2–4	Muscles of perineum; external anal and urethral sphincters	Perineum
Sciatic	L4-S3		
Common peroneal	L4-S2	Knee flexion; foot dorsiflexion, eversion; toe extension	Lateral calf, foot dorsum
Tibial	L4-S3	Thigh extension; knee flexion; foot plantar flexion, inversion	Foot plantar surface, toes

rim and skin to elevate blades away from the psoas muscle. Importantly, a small percentage of cases occur when a retractor has not been used.

Genitofemoral and Lateral Femoral Cutaneous Nerve

The genitofemoral nerve pierces the medial border of the psoas muscle and traverses below the peritoneum on this muscle's surface. Similar to the femoral nerve, the genitofemoral nerve may suffer injury during psoas muscle compression (Murovic, 2005). In addition, this nerve may be injured during removal of a large pelvic mass adhered to the sidewall or during pelvic lymph node dissection (Irvin, 2004).

The lateral femoral cutaneous nerve appears at the lateral border of the psoas major muscle just above the crest of the ilium. It courses obliquely across the anterior surface of the iliacus muscle and dips beneath the inguinal ligament laterally as the nerve exits the pelvis. This nerve may also be compressed or be injured during dissections (Aszmann, 1997). Painful neuropathy specifically involving the lateral femoral cutaneous nerve carries the specific name *meralgia paresthetica*.

■ Transverse Incisions

Nerve injury during transverse abdominal entry is common and typically involves the ilioinguinal and iliohypogastric nerves or less frequently, genitofemoral nerve branches. The ilioinguinal and iliohypogastric nerves emerge through the internal oblique muscle approximately 2 to 3 cm inferomedial to the anterosuperior iliac spine (Whiteside, 2003). The iliohypogastric nerve extends a lateral branch to innervate the lateral gluteal skin. An anterior branch reaches horizontally toward the midline and runs deep to the external oblique muscle. Near the midline, this nerve perforates the external oblique muscle and becomes cutaneous to innervate the superficial tissues and skin in the region above the symphysis pubis. The ilioinguinal nerve extends medially to enter the inguinal canal and innervates the lower abdomen, labia majora, and upper thigh.

These are sensory nerves, and fortunately, most skin anesthesia or paresthesias that follow their injury resolves with time. Accordingly, injuries frequently are underreported by both patients and clinicians. Less often, pain can begin immediately or many years later and is usually sharp and episodic and radiates to the upper thigh, labia, or upper gluteal region. Later, sensations may become chronic and burning, as described in Chapter 11 (p. 249). To avoid compromising these nerves, a surgeon ideally avoids extending the fascial incision beyond the lateral border of the rectus abdominis muscles (Rahn, 2010).

■ Pelvic Sidewall Dissection

The obturator nerve pierces the medial border of the psoas muscle and extends anteriorly along the lesser wall of the pelvis. The obturator nerve exits through the obturator foramen. Lymph node dissection, tumor excision, or endometriosis resection performed at the pelvic sidewall may injure the obturator or genitofemoral nerves. Moreover, the obturator nerve also can be injured during dissection within the space of Retzius during some urogynecologic procedures.

■ Dorsal Lithotomy

This surgical position is used for vaginal, laparoscopic, and hysteroscopic surgeries. It is modified and described as standard or low lithotomy positions (Fig. 40-4). Dorsal lithotomy may be associated with injury to several nerves derived from the lumbosacral plexus, including the femoral, sciatic, and peroneal nerves. For example, compression and ischemic injury of the femoral nerve beneath the rigid inguinal ligament can follow prolonged sharp flexion, abduction, and external hip rotation in dorsal lithotomy (Fig. 40-5) (Ducic, 2005; Hsieh, 1998). Ideal positioning as shown can minimize these injuries.

The sciatic nerve, derived from the lower sacral plexus, exits the pelvis through the greater sciatic foramen. It extends down the posterior thigh and branches into the tibial nerve and common peroneal nerve above the popliteal fossa. The sciatic and common peroneal nerves are anatomically fixed at the sciatic notch and head of the fibula, respectively. For this reason, sciatic nerve injury may reflect impaired function of the entire sciatic nerve or only the common peroneal division. Sciatic nerve stretch injury can develop if a patient's hips are placed in sharp flexion or pronounced external rotation or both. Moreover, even an appropriately positioned patient may be injured if a surgical assistant during vaginal surgery leans against the thigh and creates extreme hip flexion.

The common peroneal nerve, now termed the *common fibular nerve,* originates above the popliteal fossa and crosses the lateral head of the fibula before it descends down the lateral calf. At the lateral fibular head, this nerve is at risk for compression against leg stirrups. Therefore, the addition of cushioned padding or patient positioning that avoids pressure at this point is warranted (Philosophe, 2003).

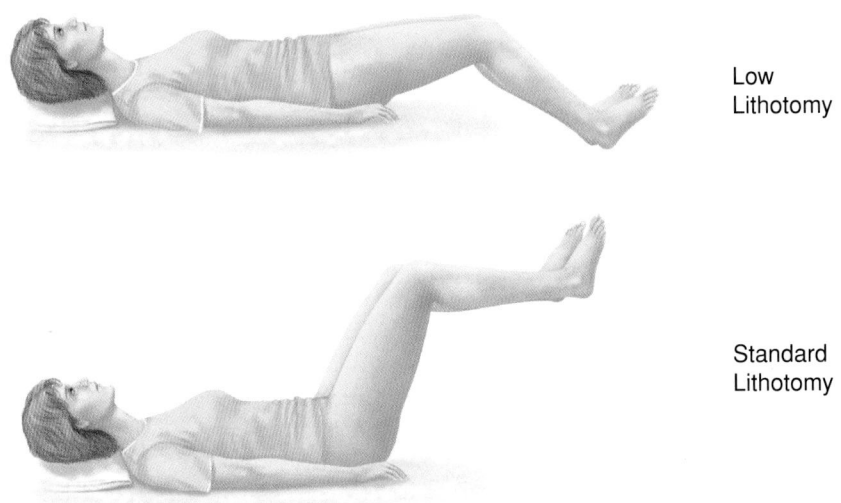

Low Lithotomy

Standard Lithotomy

FIGURE 40-4 Lithotomy positions used in gynecologic surgery.

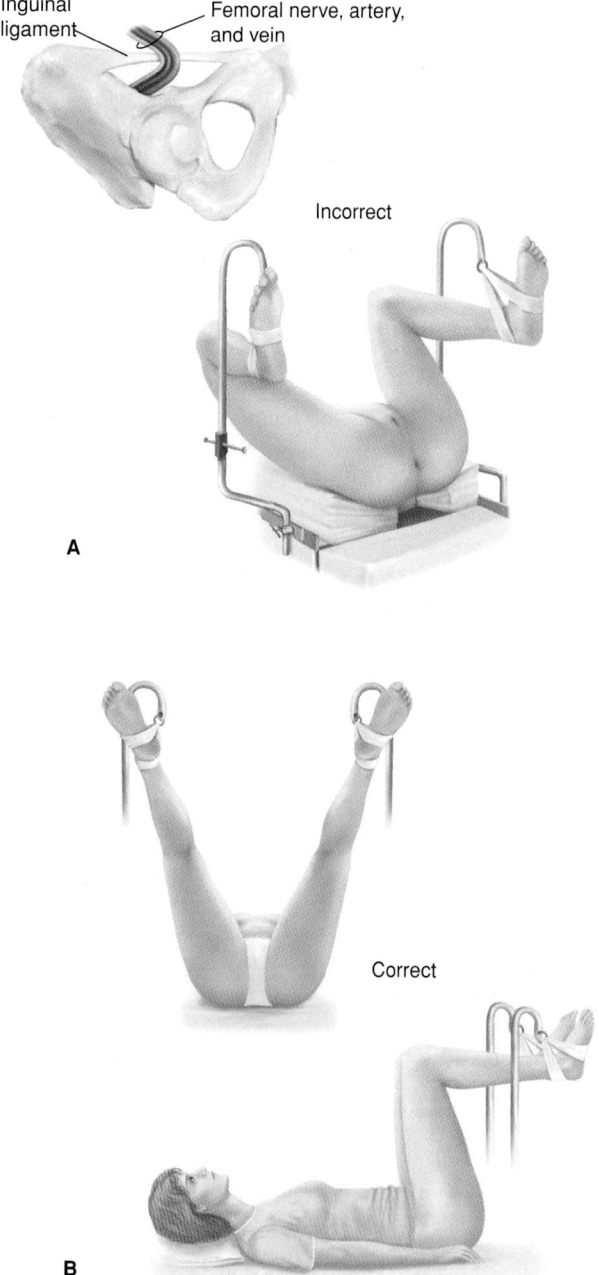

FIGURE 40-5 Lithotomy positioning. **A.** Hyperflexion of the hip can lead to compression of the femoral nerve against the inguinal ligament. (Redrawn from Anderton, 1988.) **B.** Ideal dorsal lithotomy positioning with limited hip flexion, abduction, and external rotation. (Adapted with permission from Irvin W, Andersen W, Taylor P, et al: Minimizing the risk of neurologic injury in gynecologic surgery. Obstet Gynecol 2004 Feb;103(2):374–382.)

▇ Brachial Plexus

This plexus derives from the ventral rami of C5-T1, traverses the neck and axilla, and supplies the arm and shoulder. Positioning injuries can follow hyperextension of the upper extremity, for example, when the arm is positioned at an angle to the body that exceeds 90 degrees. Additionally, even in situations in which the arm has been positioned appropriately, inadvertently leaning against the arm or placing the patient in steep Trendelenburg position may push the extremity into hyperextension. With

injury, either motor or sensory function can be lost (Warner, 1998). Peripheral ulnar neuropathies can also develop by external compression if the arm is placed at the patient's side. Padding the elbow may help avoid this (Warner, 1998).

SURGICAL INCISIONS

In women for whom laparotomy is selected, an ideal abdominal incision allows rapid entry, affords adequate exposure, permits early ambulation, promotes strong wound healing, does not compromise pulmonary function, and maximizes cosmetic results. These criteria form the foundation in choosing the best incision for each patient. In gynecology, opening the abdomen typically is achieved using a midline vertical incision or one of three low transverse incisions, the Pfannenstiel, Cherney, or Maylard incisions.

▇ Midline Vertical Incision

This incision is used frequently if access to the upper abdomen and generous operating space are required. It can be extended up and above the umbilicus and thus is preferred when the preoperative diagnosis is uncertain. Moreover, simple midline anatomy allows quick entry into the abdomen and low rates of neurovascular injury to the anterior abdominal wall (Greenall, 1980; Lacy, 1994). Moreover, because of decreased midline vascularity, Nygaard and Squatrito (1996) recommend this incision in patients who have coagulopathy, decline transfusion, or are administered systemic anticoagulation.

Its greatest disadvantage stems from increased tension on the incision when abdominal muscles contract. For this reason, compared with transverse incisions, midline vertical incisions are associated with higher rates of fascial dehiscence and hernia formation and poorer cosmetic results (Grantcharov, 2001; Kisielinski, 2004). Additionally, patients who have repeat vertical incisions for gynecologic indications tend to develop more adhesive disease than with low transverse incisions (Brill, 1995).

▇ Transverse Incisions

These incisions are used commonly in benign gynecologic surgery, provide several advantages, and are illustrated in the atlas (p. 929). They follow Langer lines of skin tension and thus offer superior cosmetic results. They also carry low rates of incisional hernia (Luijendijk, 1997). Moreover, their placement in the lower abdomen is associated with decreased postoperative pain and improved pulmonary function compared with midline vertical incisions. Of low transverse incisions, Pfannenstiel incision is typically the simplest to perform, and for this reason, it is selected most often.

Despite these advantages, transverse incisions have limitations. These incisions limit access to the upper abdomen and offer smaller operating space compared with midline incisions. This is especially true of the Pfannenstiel incision and results from narrowing of the surgical field by intact rectus abdominis muscle bellies, which straddle the incision.

Consequently, Cherney and Maylard incisions were developed to overcome this restriction, and to some degree, they do improve exposure. The Cherney incision releases the rectus abdominis muscle at its inferior tendinous insertion. This approach affords greater exposure of pelvic organs and access to the space of Retzius. The Cherney incision may also be used if a Pfannenstiel incision has already been initiated, but then additional exposure is required.

The Maylard incision transects the rectus abdominis muscle and provides substantial operative space. However, it is technically more difficult because isolation and ligation of the inferior epigastric arteries are required. The incision is used infrequently because of concerns regarding operative pain, decreased abdominal wall strength, longer operating times, and increased febrile morbidity. Randomized studies, however, have not supported these concerns (Ayers, 1987; Giacalone, 2002). This incision is avoided in patients whose superior epigastric vessels have been interrupted and in those with significant peripheral vascular disease who may rely on the inferior epigastric arteries for lower-extremity collateral blood supply.

◼ Incision Creation

Entry into the abdomen begins with scalpel incision of the skin, and scars are excised to improve wound healing and cosmetic results. Although an electrosurgical blade may be used to incise the skin, faster healing and improved appearance in general follow scalpel incision (Hambley, 1988; Singer, 2002b).

For the remaining layers, scalpel or electrosurgical blade may be selected, with no differences in short- or long-term wound healing with either (Franchi, 2001). However, in evaluating surgical bleeding and postoperative pain, Jenkins (2003), in his review, noted an advantage with electrosurgical blade use. Regardless of type of incision or instrument used, adherence to proper technique is emphasized: obtaining meticulous hemostasis, minimizing devitalized tissue, and avoiding dead space creation.

WOUND CLOSURE

Following laparotomy, closure of a laparotomy incision must address the peritoneum, fascia, subcutaneous layer, and skin. Wound closure may be broadly categorized as either primary or secondary. With primary closure, materials are used to approximate tissue layers. In closure by secondary intention, wound layers remain open and heal by a combination of contraction, granulation, and epithelialization. Secondary closure is used infrequently in gynecologic surgery and typically is indicated if tissues planned for closure contain significant infection. The option of delayed primary closure is also available in these situations once infection has cleared.

Optimal closure of a laparotomy incision is the subject of much debate. Most data stem from general surgery and gynecologic oncology studies on midline abdominal incision closure and from research on cesarean delivery techniques. Ideally, closure avoids wound infection, adhesion formation, dehiscence, and hernia or sinus tract formation; minimizes patient discomfort; yet preserves cosmesis to the extent possible.

◼ Peritoneum and Fascia

The peritoneum provides no abdominal wall strength, and closure of this layer has been suggested to prevent adhesions between the anterior abdominal wall and adjacent organs.

However, evidence is conflicting, and several studies have shown that nonclosure of the peritoneum compared with closure decreases operating time without increasing adhesion formation, wound complications, or infection (Franchi, 1997; Gupta, 1998; Tulandi, 1988). However, few well-done randomized controlled trials have assessed long-term adhesion formation. Accordingly, closure of the visceral or parietal peritoneum is often provider dependent. Without closure, this layer typically regenerates within days following surgery (Lipscomb, 1996).

Thus in many cases, the first tissue closed is fascia. Many studies have supported the use of a continuous running-stitch closure of abdominal incisions compared with interrupted closure of the fascia (Colombo, 1997; Orr, 1990; Shepherd, 1983). Continuous closure usually is faster and associated with comparable rates of dehiscence, wound infection, and hernia formation. Suture material selection tends to favor delayed-absorbable suture compared with nonabsorbable. Delayed-absorbable sutures appear to afford adequate wound support yet lead to less pain and lower rates of sinus tract formation (Carlson, 1995; Leaper, 1977; Wissing, 1987). However, nonabsorbable suture is considered if a hernia is identified or if the incision has cut through previously placed mesh. A 0-gauge or no. 1 suture is suitable for closure of most fascial incisions. Sutures are placed approximately 1 cm apart and 1.2 to 1.5 cm from the fascial edge. Little additional security is attained beyond 1.5 cm (Campbell, 1989). Stitches ideally appose fascial edges and allow tissues to swell postoperatively without cutting through fascia or causing avascular necrosis.

◼ Subcutaneous Adipose Layer and Skin

Collections of blood and fluid serve as potential accelerants to bacterial growth. For this reason, to decrease rates of hematoma or seroma, investigators have evaluated subcutaneous layer suture closure or drains. In those with layers less than 2 cm thick, most studies have found no advantage to either practice. However, wound infection and fat thickness are the greatest risk factors for subcutaneous layer dehiscence (Soper, 1971; Vermillion, 2000). For patients with subcutaneous layers 2 cm or more thick, closing the subcutaneous layer is effective prevention (Gallup, 1996; Guvenal, 2002; Naumann, 1995). The ideal suture and technique for closure of this layer are unknown, but efforts ideally close dead space yet minimize suture burden and inflammatory reaction. A 2-0 gauge plain gut suture is one suitable choice.

Skin may be closed effectively with staples, subcuticular suturing, wound tape, or tissue adhesive. Thus, in most instances, surgeon preference influences closure method. Technically, the incision line is approximated without skin tension, and subcutaneous adipose or deep dermal suturing may assist with carrying tension loads.

Of options, the running subcuticular suture is placed by taking horizontal bites through the dermis on alternating sides of the wound using absorbable suture (Fig. 40-6). Delayed-absorbable material such as polyglactin (Vicryl) or poliglecaprone (Monocryl) in a fine gauge, such as 3-0 or 4-0, is suitable. Advantages include decreased cost, effective skin approximation, and no required suture removal. However, this method

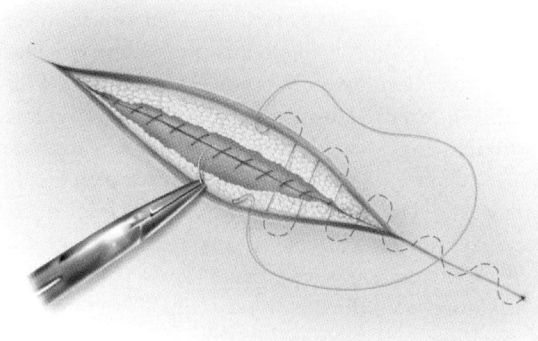

FIGURE 40-6 During subcuticular suturing, stitches are placed with a needle horizontal to the dermis. Suturing is advanced by sequentially piercing just below the dermis on alternating sides. The spot where the first stitch exits the subcutis marks the site along the wound length that the needle should enter on the opposite side.

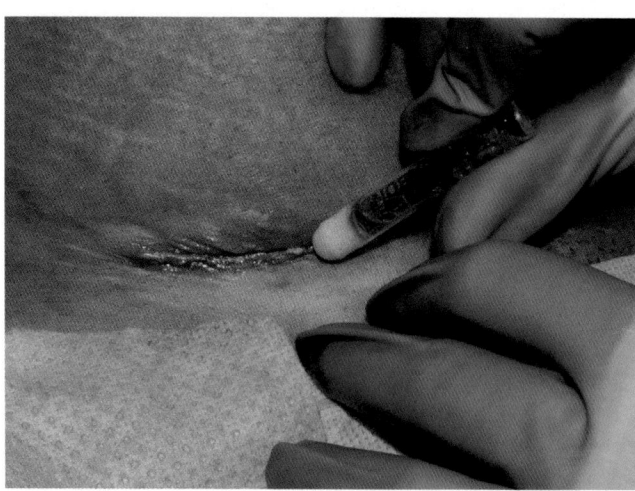

FIGURE 40-7 Application of topical skin adhesive to incision. Adhesive should be placed over apposed skin edges. Application should extend out approximately 0.5 cm laterally from the incision. (Used with permission from Dr. Christine Wan.)

typically requires the greatest amount of time and technical expertise.

Automatic stapling devices are favored because of their fast application and secure wound closure. However, they do not allow as meticulous a closure as sutures, and wounds requiring accurate approximation of tissue are not ideal candidates for staple closure (Singer, 1997). Staples may be uncomfortable, may be associated with discomfort during removal, and require the patient to return for staple removal.

Before stapling, the wound edges are everted, preferably by a second operator. If the edges of a wound invert or if one edge rolls under the opposite side, a poorly formed, deep, noticeable scar will result. Additionally, pressing too hard against the skin surface with the stapler is avoided to prevent placing the staple too deep and causing ischemia within the staple loop. When placed properly, the crossbar of the staple is elevated a few millimeters above the skin surface (Lammers, 2004). Staples are removed in a timely fashion to avoid leaving "track mark" scarring.

Of topical skin adhesives, octyl-2-cyanoacrylate (Dermabond) is applied as a liquid and polymerizes to a firm, pliable film that binds to the epithelium and bridges wound edges (Fig. 40-7). It can be used for closure of skin incisions that carry minimal tension such as laparoscopy trocar or transverse laparotomy incisions, or as an adjunct protective layer in larger incisions. Tissue adhesives achieve results similar to those for traditional sutures (Blondeel, 2004; Singer, 2002a).

Following approximation of deeper incision layers, the adhesive is applied in three thin layers above apposed skin edges. The adhesive extends at least ½ cm on each side of the apposed wound edges. Placement of the liquid between skin edges is avoided because the adhesive may retard healing (Quinn, 1997). Although 30 seconds between layers for drying is required, application is fast. Moreover, adhesives create their own dressing and appear to afford some antibacterial protection (Bhende, 2002). The adhesive sloughs in 7 to 10 days. Showering and gentle washing of the site are allowed, but swimming is discouraged. Petroleum-based products on the wound can decrease adhesive tensile strength and are avoided.

The primary indication for tape closure is a superficial straight laceration under little tension. Thus, closure of laparoscopy trocar sites or laparotomy incisions in which deep layer closure has brought skin edges into close proximity are suitable cases. Moreover, skin edges ideally are thoroughly dry for proper adhesion. Thus, tape may not be appropriate for a wet or oozing wound, for concave surfaces such as the umbilicus, for areas of significant tissue tension, or for areas of marked tissue laxity.

Tape closure is fast, inexpensive, and associated with high patient satisfaction scores. Tapes typically are removed by the patient 7 to 10 days following surgery. They may also be used after staple removal to provide additional strength, as wounds have regained only approximately 3 percent of their final strength at 1 week. Adhesive tape strips are applied in a parallel, nonoverlapping fashion after coating the entire application area with adjuvant adhesive such as tincture of benzoin (Katz, 1999). Importantly, skin blistering may develop if tape is stretched excessively taut across the wound (Lammers, 2004; Rodeheaver, 1983).

INSTRUMENTS

Scalpel and Blades

Surgical instruments have been designed to extend the capability of a surgeon's hands and thus are crafted to retract, cut, grasp, and clear the operative field. Tissue types encountered in gynecologic surgery vary, and accordingly, so too do the size, fineness, and strength of the tools used.

Of these tools, typical surgical blades used in gynecologic surgery are pictured in Figure 40-8 and include number 10, 11, 15, and 20 blades. Function follows form, and larger blades are used for coarser tissues or larger incisions, whereas a no. 15 blade is selected for finer incisions. The acute angle and pointed tip of a no. 11 blade can easily incise tough-walled abscesses for drainage, such as those of the Bartholin gland duct.

With a correct scalpel grasp, a surgeon can direct blade movement. Fingers may be positioned either to straddle the scalpel, termed the "power grip," "violin grip," or "bow grip,"

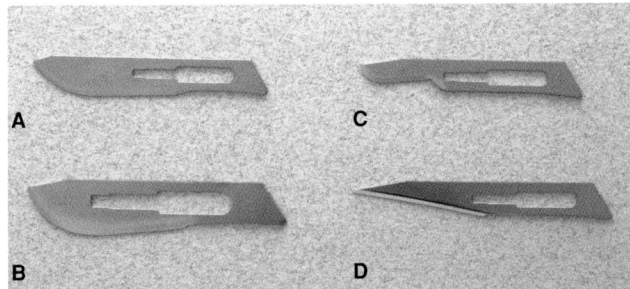

FIGURE 40-8 Photograph of surgical blades commonly used in gynecology. **A.** No. 10. **B.** No. 20. **C.** No. 15. **D.** No. 11.

which maximizes the use of the knife belly. Alternatively, the scalpel is held like a pencil, termed the "pencil grip" or "precision grip" (Fig. 40-9). With the no. 10 and no. 20 blades, the scalpel is held at a 20- to 30-degree angle to the skin and drawn firmly along the skin toward the surgeon using the arm with minimal wrist and finger movement. This motion aids cutting with the full length of the scalpel belly and avoids burying the tip. The initial incision penetrates the dermis, and the scalpel remains perpendicular to the surface to prevent skin edge beveling. Firm and symmetrical lateral skin traction keeps the incision straight and helps avoid multiple tracks and irregular skin edges.

The no. 15 and 11 blades, in contrast, are typically held using the pencil grip to make fine, precise incisions. With the no. 15 blade, the scalpel is held approximately 45 degrees to the skin surface. Fine knife dissection is best controlled using the fingers, and the heel of the hand can be stabilized on adjacent tissue. The no. 11 blade scalpel is ideal for stab incisions and is held upright at nearly 90 degrees to the surface. Creating tension at the skin surface is important as it reduces the amount of force required for penetration. Omission of this can result in

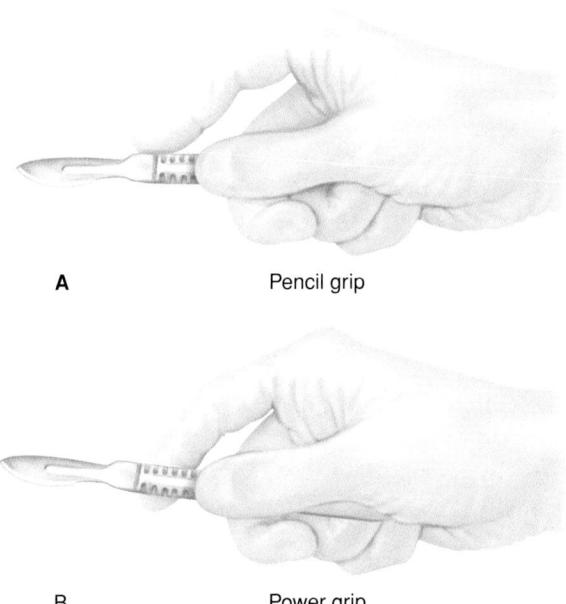

FIGURE 40-9 Scalpel grips. **A.** Scalpel is held as one would a pencil, and movement is directed by the thumb and index finger. **B.** Scalpel is held between the thumb and third finger. The end of the blade is forced up against the thenar muscles of the hand.

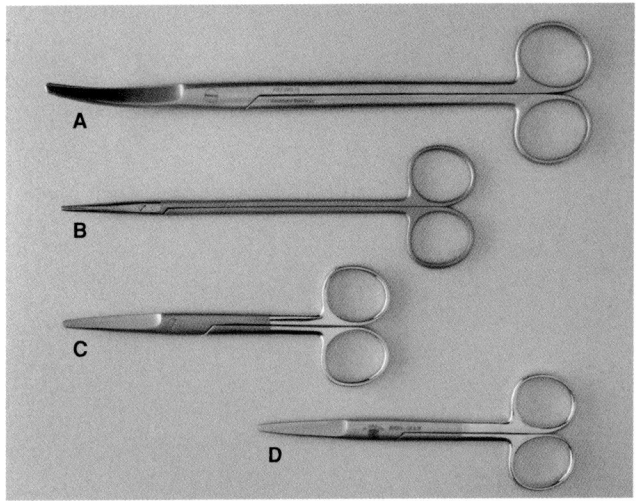

FIGURE 40-10 Scissors. **A.** Jorgenson. **B.** Metzenbaum. **C.** Curved Mayo. **D.** Straight Mayo. (Used with permission from U.S. Surgitech, Inc.)

uncontrolled penetration of underlying structures. To lengthen the incision, a gentle in-and-out sawing motion is used.

Scissors

These are used commonly to divide tissues, and modification in blade shape and size allows their use across various tissue textures (Fig. 40-10). For correct positioning, the thumb and fourth finger are placed within the instrument's rings, and the index finger is set against the crosspiece of the scissors for greater control. This "tripod" grip allows maximum shear, torque, and closing forces to be applied and provides superior stability and control. In general, surgeons cut away from themselves and from dominant to nondominant sides.

The fine blades of Metzenbaum or iris scissors are used routinely to dissect or define natural tissue planes such as dividing thin adhesions or incising peritoneum or vaginal epithelium. During dissection, traction on opposing poles of the tissue to be dissected typically simplifies the process, and a small nick is often necessary to enter the correct tissue plane. The blades are closed and inserted between planes, following the natural curves of tissues being dissected (Fig. 40-11). The blades are opened and then withdrawn. After turning both wrist and blades 90 degrees, the surgeon reinserts the lower blade, and tissues are divided. When dissecting around a curve, the scissors follow the natural curve of the structure. Dissection proceeds in the same plane to avoid burrowing into the structure or deviating away and toward unintended adjacent tissues.

For thicker tissues, sturdier scissors such as curved Mayo scissors are used. Similarly, Jorgenson scissors have thick blades and tips that are curved at a 90-degree angle. These are used commonly to separate the vagina and uterus during the final steps of hysterectomy. Suture-cutting scissors have blunt, flat blades and are reserved for this function to avoid dulling tissue scissors.

Needle Holders

These may be straight or curved, and commonly, one with straight, blunt jaws is chosen during routine tissue approximation

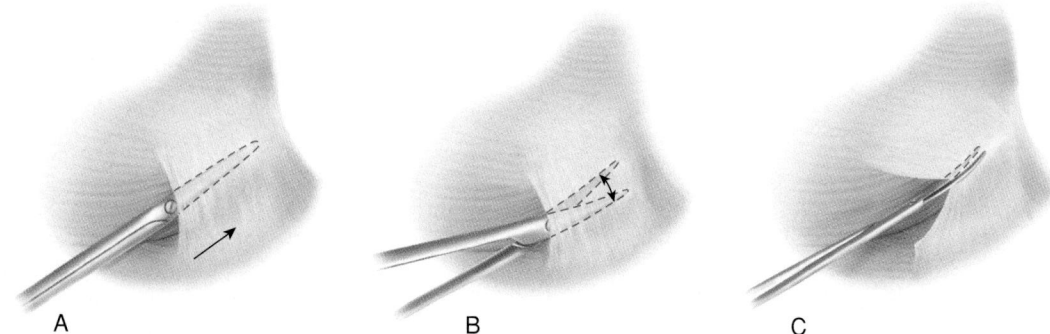

A   B   C

FIGURE 40-11 Plane dissection. **A.** During development of tissue planes, the tips of closed Metzenbaum scissors are placed at the border between two tissues, and forward pressure is applied to advance the tips. **B.** Scissors are spread to expand the tissue plane. **C.** The scissors are retracted and rotated 90 degrees. The lower blade is reinserted into the newly created tissue plane, and tissues are divided.

and pedicle ligation. Needles ideally pierce tissues perpendicularly. Thus, in most cases, the needle holder grasps a needle at a right angle and at a site approximately two-thirds from the needle tip.

Alternatively, some needle holders, such as the Heaney needle holder, are curved and aid needle placement in confined or angled areas. If a curved holder is used, the needle is grasped similarly, and the inner curve of the holder typically faces the needle swage (Fig. 40-12).

Traditionally, the needle holder is held with the thumb and fourth finger in the rings. The greatest advantage of this grip is the precision afforded. The spring tension of the handles is relieved from the lock in a controlled fashion, thereby releasing and regrasping the needle more precisely. Alternatively, with the "palmar grip," the needle holder is held between the ball of the thumb and the remaining fingers, and no fingers enter the instrument rings. This grip allows a simple rotating motion for driving curved needles through an arc. Its greatest advantage is the time saved during continuous suturing, as the needle can be released, regrasped, and redirected efficiently without replacing fingers into the instrument rings. Disadvantageously, this grip has the potential to lack precision during needle release. When

unlocking the needle driver, release of the spring lock should be smooth and gradual. This avoids an abrupt release, which may suddenly pop the handles apart with potential for awkwardness, loss of needle control, and tissue injury.

■ Tissue Forceps

Forceps function to hold tissue during cutting, retract tissue for exposure, stabilize tissue during suturing, extract needles, grasp vessels for electrosurgical coagulation, pass ligatures around hemostats, and pack sponges. Forceps are held so that one blade functions as an extension of the thumb and the other as an extension of the opposing fingers. Alternate grips may appear awkward and limit the full range of wrist motion, leading to suboptimal instrument use.

Heavy-toothed forceps, such as the Potts-Smith single-toothed forceps, Bonney forceps, and Ferriss-Smith forceps, are used when a firm grasp is more important than gentle tissue handling (Fig. 40-13A). These tools are often used to hold fascia for abdominal wound closure.

Light-toothed forceps, such as the single-toothed Adson, concentrate force on a tiny area and give more holding power with less tissue destruction. These are used for more delicate work on moderately dense tissue such as skin. Nontoothed forceps, also known as smooth forceps, exert their grip through serrations on the opposing tips (Fig. 40-13B). They are typically used for delicate tissue handling and provide some holding power with minimal injury. DeBakey forceps are another type of smooth forceps originally designed as vascular forceps but can be occasionally used for other delicate tissues. In contrast, the broader, shallow-grooved tips of Russian forceps and Singley forceps may be preferred if a broader or thicker area of tissue is manipulated.

■ Retractors

Abdominal Surgery Retractors

Clear visualization is essential during surgery, and retractors conform to body and organ angles to allow tissues to be pulled back from an operative field. In gynecology, retractors may be grouped broadly as self-retaining or handheld and as vaginal or abdominal.

During abdominal surgery, retractors that by themselves hold abdominal wall muscles apart, termed *self-retaining*, are used commonly. Styles such as the Kirschner and O'Connor-O'Sullivan

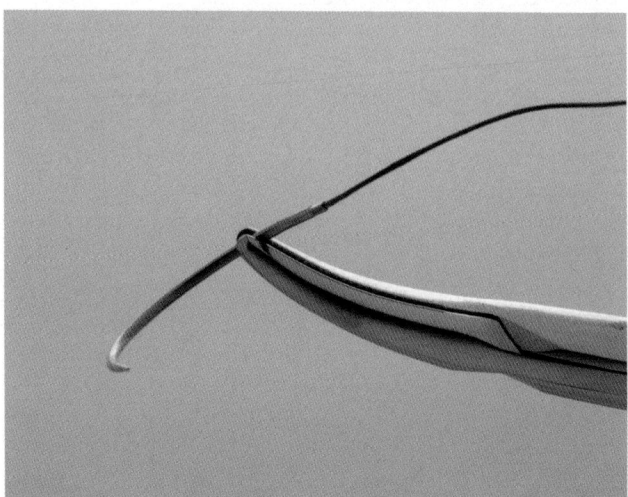

FIGURE 40-12 Correct grasp of a needle using a curved needle holder. The curve of the tip faces the needle swage. (Used with permission from U.S. Surgitech, Inc.)

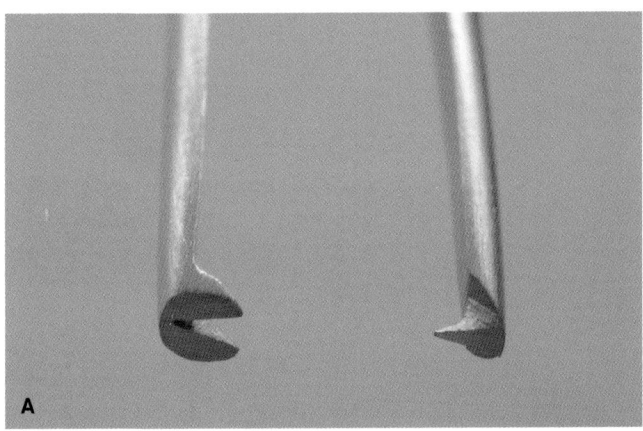

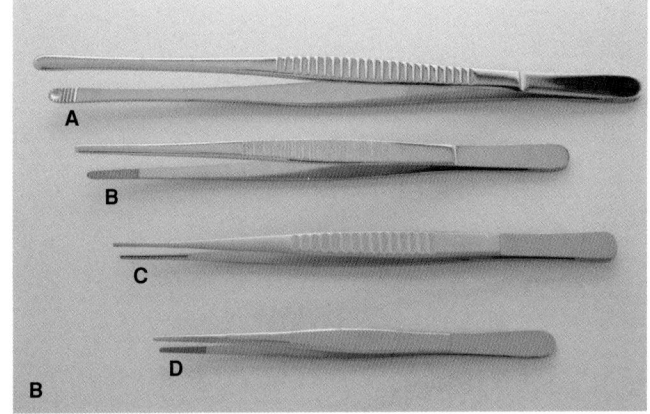

FIGURE 40-13 Forcep types. **A.** Tip of toothed forceps allows a firm tissue grasp. **B.** Smooth tissue forceps. *A*, Russian. *B*, Dressing. *C*, DeBakey. *D*, Short smooth. (Used with permission from U.S. Surgitech, Inc.)

contain four broad, gently curved blades and retract in four directions. Blades pull the bladder caudally and the anterior abdominal wall muscles laterally and cephalad. The Balfour retractor retracts in three directions but can be made to retract in four with the addition of an upper arm attachment. Alternatively, ring-shaped retractors such as the Bookwalter and Denis Browne styles offer greater variability in the number and positioning of retractor blades. However, these styles usually require more time to assemble and place. With all of these retractors, deep or shallow blades can be attached to the outer metal frame according to the abdominal cavity depth. As discussed earlier, blades should be shallow enough to avoid femoral nerve compression.

In addition to these metal bladed styles, several disposable retractors consist of two equal-sized plastic rings connected by a cylindrical plastic sheath. One ring collapses into a canoe shape that can be threaded through the incision and into the abdomen. Once inside the abdomen, it springs again to its circular form. The second ring remains outside. Between these rings, the plastic sheath spans the thickness of the abdominal wall and creates 360-degree retraction. As shown in Figure 44-8.7, Alexis or Mobius brands can be ideal for minilaparotomy, but sizes are also available for laparotomy.

Handheld retractors may be used in addition to or in place of self-retaining styles. These instruments allow retraction in only one direction but can be placed and repositioned quickly. The Richardson retractor has a sturdy, shallow right-angled blade that can hook around an incision for abdominal wall retraction (Fig. 40-14). Alternatively, Deaver retractors have a gentle arching shape and conform easily to the curve of the anterior abdominal wall. Compared with Richardson retractors, they offer increased blade depth and are often used to retract bowel, bladder, or anterior abdominal wall muscles. A Harrington retractor, also called a *sweetheart retractor,* has a broader tip that also effectively holds back bowel.

In certain instances, such as during suturing of the vaginal cuff, a thin, deep retractor blade, termed a *malleable retractor,* may be required to retract or protect surrounding organs. Also called a *ribbon retractor,* this tool is a long, relatively flexible metal strip that can be bent to conform to various body contours for effective retraction. Narrow and wider sizes are available. These also may be used to cover and protect underlying bowel from needle-stick injury during abdominal wall closure.

For smaller incisions, the preceding retractors are too large, and those with smaller blades such as the Army-Navy retractor or S-retractor are selected. S-retractors offer thinner, deeper blades, whereas the sturdier blades of the Army-Navy style allow stronger retraction (Fig. 40-15). A Weitlaner self-retaining retractor may also be used for minilaparotomy incisions.

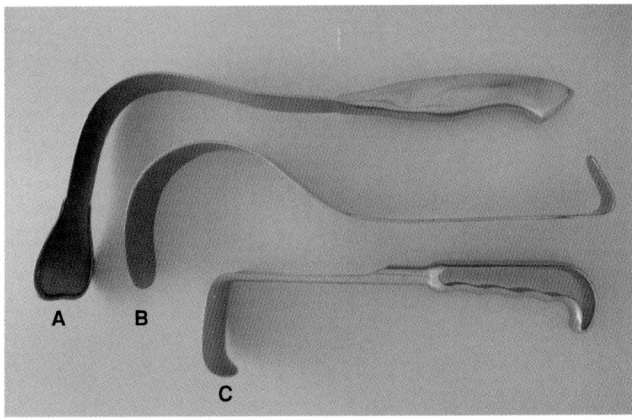

FIGURE 40-14 Long handheld abdominal retractors. **A.** Harrington. **B.** Deaver. **C.** Richardson. (Used with permission from U.S. Surgitech, Inc.)

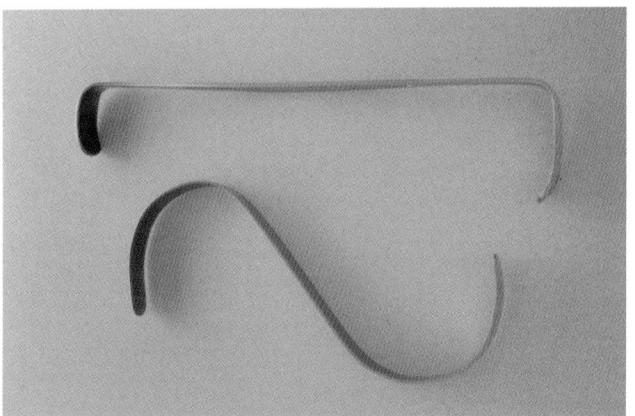

FIGURE 40-15 Short handheld abdominal retractors. Army-Navy (*above*). S-retractor (*below*). (Used with permission from U.S. Surgitech, Inc.)

SECTION 5

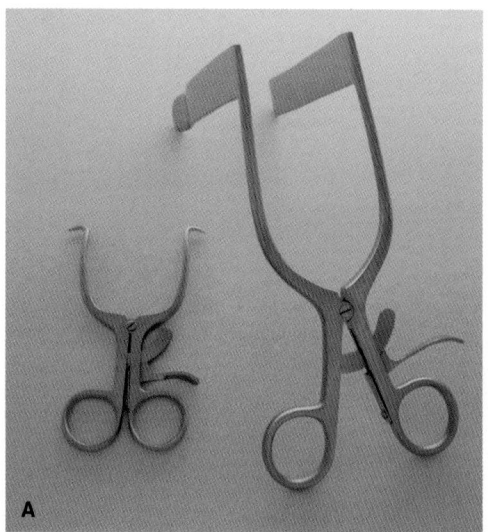

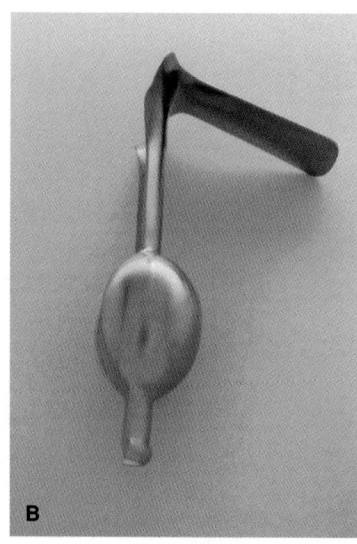

FIGURE 40-16 Vaginal self-retaining retractors. **A.** Gelpi retractor (*left*). Rigby retractor (*right*). **B.** Auvard weighted vaginal speculum. (Used with permission from U.S. Surgitech, Inc.)

Vaginal Surgery Retractors

The vaginal walls can be separated using several self-retaining models. The Gelpi retractor has two narrow teeth that are placed distally against opposing lateral vaginal walls and is most appropriate for perineal procedures (Fig. 40-16A). The Rigby retractor, with its longer blades, effectively separates lateral vaginal walls, whereas a Graves speculum, shown in Figure 1-6 (p. 5), holds apart anterior and posterior walls. An Auvard weighted speculum contains a long, single blade and ballasted end, which uses gravity to pull the posterior vaginal wall downward (Fig. 40-16B).

The degree of retraction offered by vaginal self-retaining retractors, however, at times may be limited. Therefore, handheld retractors are often required to augment or replace these instruments. Handheld retractors used in vaginal surgery include the Heaney right-angle retractor, the narrow Deaver retractor, and the Breisky-Navratil retractor (Figs. 40-17). Additionally, during vaginal procedures, the cervix often must be manipulated. Lahey thyroid clamps offer a secure grip dur-

ing vaginal hysterectomy, but their several sharp teeth can cause significant trauma. These are therefore less than ideal in patients in whom the cervix will remain. In these patients, in whom curettage or laparoscopy is performed, a single-toothed tenaculum can afford a firm grip but with less cervical damage (Fig. 40-18).

■ Tissue Clamps

Retraction is a fundamental requirement during most gynecologic surgery. As a result, various shapes, sizes, and strengths of clamps have been created to manipulate the different tissues encountered. For example, the smooth, cupped jaws of a Babcock clamp are ideal for gentle elevation of fallopian tubes, whereas the serrated teeth of the Allis and Allis-Adair clamps can provide a fine, firm grip on covering epithelia or serosa during dissection (Fig. 40-19).

Clamps are also used to occlude vascular and tissue pedicles during organ excision. Hemostats and Mixter right-angle clamps have small, slender jaws with fine inner transverse ridges to atraumatically grasp delicate tissue, especially vessels (Fig. 40-20).

Heavier clamps are required to grasp and manipulate stiffer tissues such as fascia and include Pean (also termed Kelly) and Kocher (also termed Ochsner) clamps. These clamps have finely spaced transverse grooves along their inner jaws to minimize tissue slippage. They may be straight or curved to fit tissue contours and like Kocher clamps, may contain a set of interlocking teeth at the tip for additional grip security. Another choice, the ring forceps, has large open circular jaws with fine transverse grooves. These effectively grasp broad, flat surfaces. Additionally, a folded gauze sponge can be placed between its jaws and used to absorb blood from the operative field or gently retract tissues.

Ligaments that support the uterus and vagina are fibrous and vascular. Thus, a sturdy clamp that resists tissue slippage

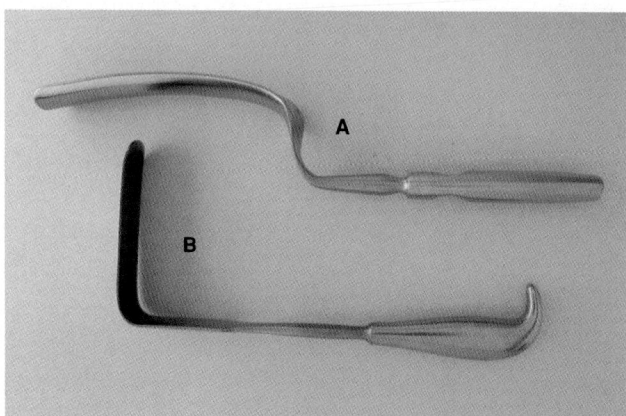

FIGURE 40-17 Vaginal handheld retractors. **A.** Breisky-Navratil retractor. **B.** Right-angle retractor. (Used with permission from U.S. Surgitech, Inc.)

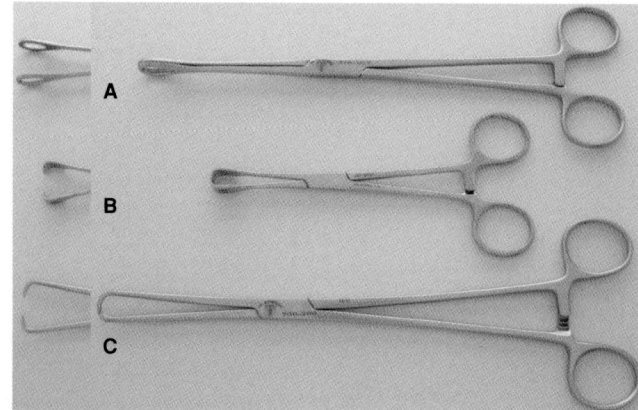

FIGURE 40-18 Clamps shown both open (*left*) and closed (*right*). **A.** Ring forceps. **B.** Lahey-thyroid clamp. **C.** Single-toothed tenaculum. (Used with permission from U.S. Surgitech, Inc.)

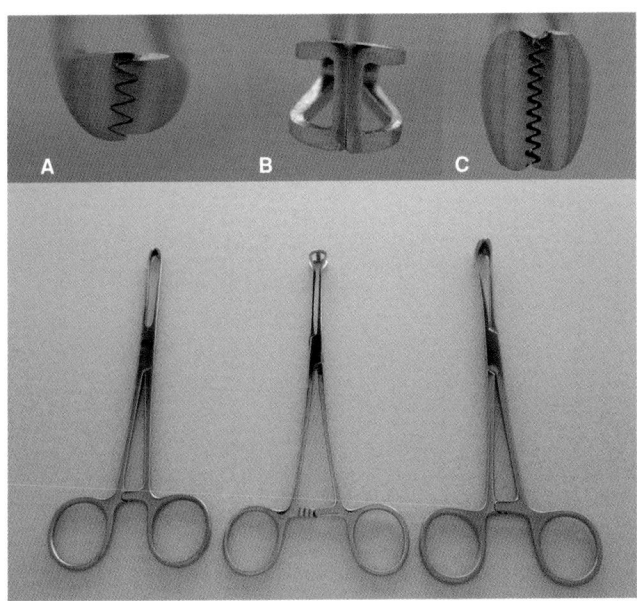

FIGURE 40-19 Tissue clamps. **A.** Allis. **B.** Babcock. **C.** Allis-Adair. (Used with permission from U.S. Surgitech, Inc.)

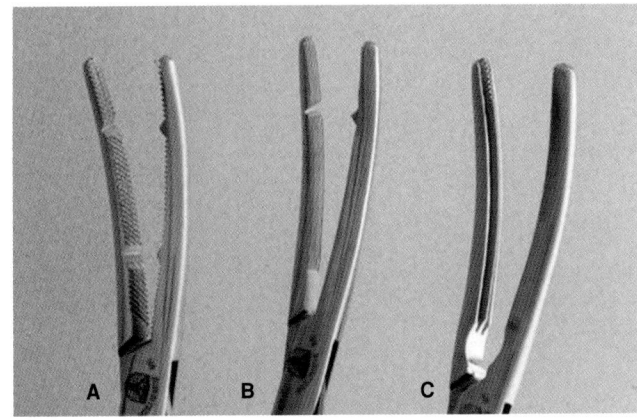

FIGURE 40-21 Heavy tissue clamps. **A.** Heaney. **B.** Heaney-Ballantine. **C.** Zeppelin. (Used with permission from U.S. Surgitech, Inc.)

from its jaws is required during hysterectomy. Several clamps, including Heaney, Ballantine, Rogers, Zeppelin, and Masterson clamps, among others, are effective (Fig. 40-21). The thick, durable jaws of these clamps carry deep, finely spaced grooves or serrations arranged either transversely or longitudinally for secure tissue grasping. Additionally, some contain a set of interlocking teeth at the tip or heel or both. Although this modification improves grip, it also may increase tissue trauma. More acutely angled clamps are typically selected when available operating space is cramped.

Securing tissue pedicles may be accomplished using a variety of suturing techniques (Fig. 40-22). A single tie alone may be placed around the pedicle. In addition, a second distal trans-

fixing suture can be placed to minimize dislodgement of the suture by vessel pulse pressures or pedicle manipulation.

■ Suction Tips

During gynecologic surgery, bleeding, peritoneal fluids, pus, ovarian cyst contents, and irrigants may obscure the operating field. Accordingly, choice of suction tip typically is dictated by the type and amount of fluid encountered. Adson and Frazier

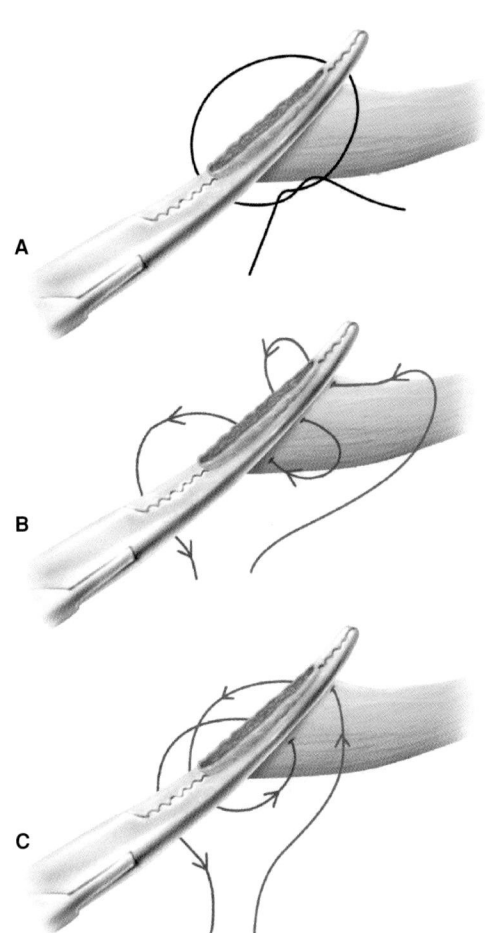

FIGURE 40-22 Different pedicle ligation techniques. All are transfixing ligatures except for **(A)**. (Used with permission from U.S. Surgitech, Inc.)

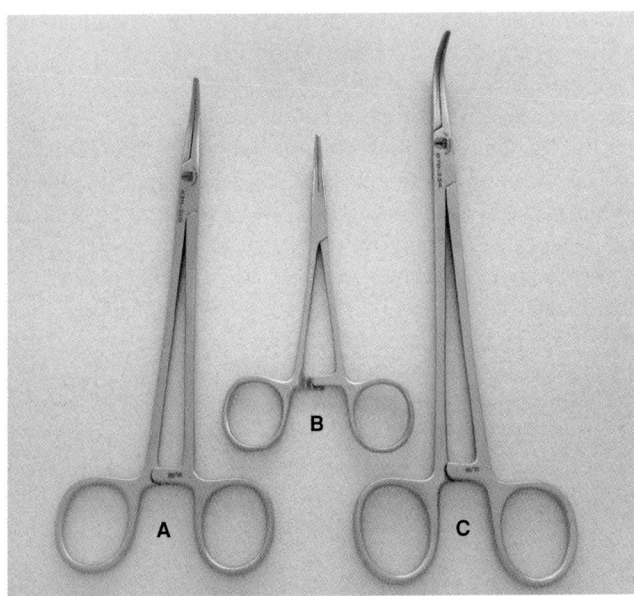

FIGURE 40-20 Vascular clamps. **A.** Tonsil. **B.** Hemostat. **C.** Mixter right-angle clamp. (Used with permission from U.S. Surgitech, Inc.)

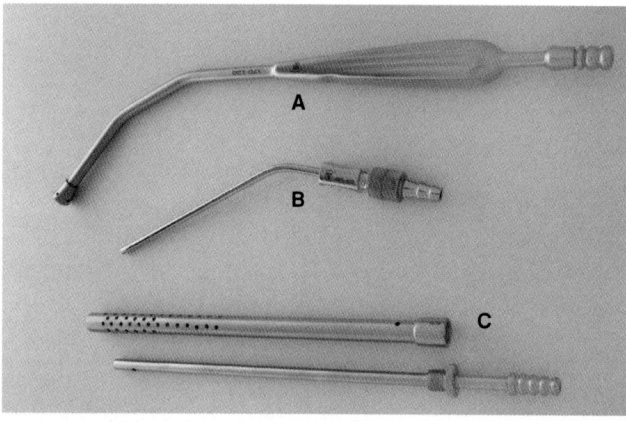

FIGURE 40-23 Suction tips. **A.** Yankauer. **B.** Frazier. **C.** Poole. (Used with permission from U.S. Surgitech, Inc.)

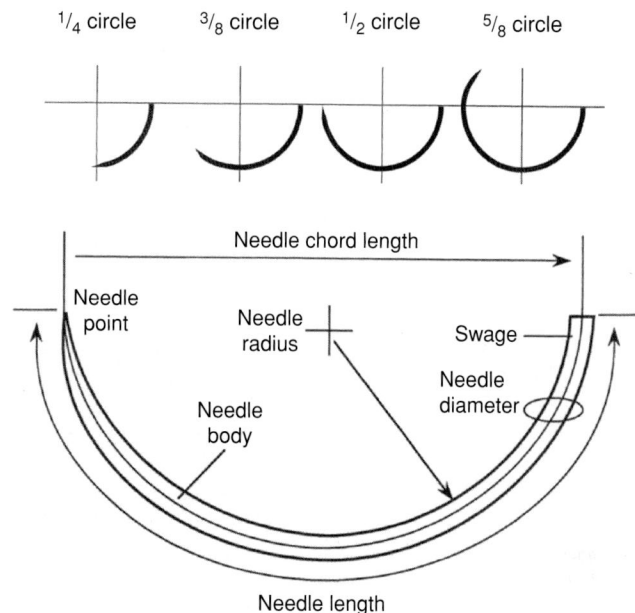

FIGURE 40-24 Various needle configurations and characteristics of a curved surgical needle.

suction tips are fine bore and are useful in shallow or confined areas and when little bleeding is noted (Fig. 40-23).

Alternatively, a Yankauer suction tip offers a midrange-sized tip and is used commonly in general gynecology cases. However, if a larger volume of fluid or blood is expected, then a Poole suction tip may be desired. Its multiple pores allow continued suction even if some are obstructed with clot or tissue. In addition to removing large volumes of fluid quickly, this suction tip's sieved sheath may be removed. The thinner-bore inner suction cannula can then be used for finer suctioning. Larger-bore Karman suction cannulas are used for products of conception evacuation and are discussed in Section 43-16 (p. 966).

NEEDLES, SUTURES, AND KNOTS

These are foundational tools of tissue approximation, vessel ligation, and wound closure. They are crafted in various strengths, shapes, and sizes to meet surgical needs. Appropriate selection can profoundly affect wound healing and patient recovery. Thus, surgeons should be familiar with their characteristics and most appropriate applications.

■ Needles

The ideal surgical needle pierces tissue with ease, with minimal tissue damage, and without bending or breaking. Tissues differ in their density and location, and thus needles are designed with variable sizes, shapes, and tips. The anatomy of a needle is simple: each contains a tip, body, and site of suture attachment (Fig. 40-24). For most gynecologic cases, the suture and needle used are attached as a continuous unit, which is described as *swaged*. This contrasts with needles that have eyes for suture threading. Swaged needles may be firmly secured to the suture and require cutting at the end of suturing. Alternatively, *controlled-release,* or "pop-off," swaged needles detach from the suture with a brisk tug. Controlled-release needles are often used when securing vascular pedicles or placing interrupted sutures. Continuous running suturing typically requires a swaged needle without the controlled-release feature.

In certain urogynecologic procedures, such as abdominal sacrocolpopexy, a *double-armed suture* is often chosen. This

suture contains identical swaged needles at each of its ends. This design enables surgeons to suture distant tissues with different ends of the suture before approximating them.

Descriptors of needle size and shape are noted in Figure 40-24. Of these, needle radius, circle configuration, and gauge more frequently influence surgical selection. For example, a needle should be large enough to pass completely through the tissue and exit far enough to allow the needle holder to be repositioned on the end of the needle at a safe distance from the tip. Repeated grasping of the needle tip leads to a dulled tip. A dulled tip subsequently leads to difficult tissue penetration and greater tissue trauma.

For thicker tissues, a larger radius and gauge are warranted. For confined surgical spaces, a needle with smaller radius and greater circle configuration typically is required. Thus, for most gynecologic procedures, a three-eighths or one-half circle configuration is used. For some urogynecologic operations, a five-eighths circle configuration is preferred.

The tip should allow passage of the needle through tissue with the smallest amount of tissue damage. Those with tapered points are used for suturing thin tissues, such as peritoneum (Fig. 40-25). Alternatively, cutting needles are preferred for denser tissue such as fascia and ligaments. Cutting points have sharp edges laterally and a third sharp edge extending either toward or away from the needle's inner curve. A conventional cutting needle features the third cutting edge on the inside curve and provides shallower tissue bites. In contrast, reverse cutting needles have the third cutting edge directed away from the inner curve of the needle and are used for particularly tough tissues.

■ Sutures

Sutures maximize wound healing and tissue support and are categorized by their biologic or synthetic derivation, their

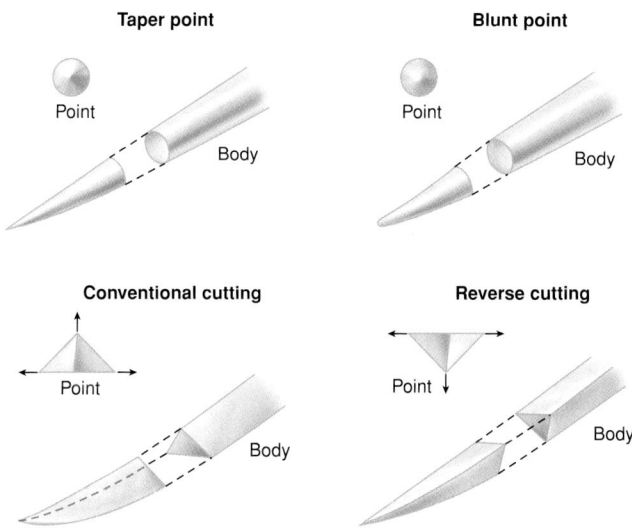

FIGURE 40-25 Configurations of various needle tips and bodies.

TABLE 40-4. Suture Designation

U.S.P. Designation	Synthetic absorbable diameter (mm)
5	0.7
4	0.6
3	0.6
2	0.5
1	0.4
0	0.35
2–0	0.3
3–0	0.2
4–0	0.15
5–0	0.1

filamentous structure, and their ability to be degraded and reabsorbed (Table 40-3). Other qualities are described in the subsequent paragraphs.

Sutures such as catgut, silk, linen, and cotton are derived from biologic sources. As a group, biologic sutures produce the greatest tissue reaction and have the lowest tensile strength profile. Accordingly, most suture materials currently used in gynecologic surgery are synthetic.

Of synthetic materials, the number of strands that make up a given suture defines it as either *monofilament* or *multifilament*. Monofilament suture is constructed as a single strand, whereas multifilament suture contains multiple strands that are braided or twisted. Monofilament sutures have lower friction coefficients and therefore pull more easily through tissues, and as a result, they create less tissue injury. As a group, they tend to incite less tissue reaction. Moreover, braid crevices are absent, and bacteria therefore are less likely to adhere (Bucknall, 1983; Sharp, 1982). However, monofilament sutures are in general less pliant for knot tying and, if nicked by instruments, are more prone to break.

The diameter of a suture reflects its size and is measured in tenths of a millimeter (Table 40-4). A midpoint diameter size is designated as 0, and as suture diameter increases above this, arabic numbers are assigned. For example, no. 1 catgut is thicker than 0-gauge catgut. As suture diameter decreases from this midpoint, 0s are added. By convention, an arabic number followed by a 0 also may be used to reflect the total number of 0s. For example, 3-0 suture also may be represented as 000. Moreover, 3-0 suture is greater in diameter than 4-0 (0000) suture.

Ideally, the appropriate suture caliber is fine enough to limit tissue damage during placement and minimize subsequent tissue reaction yet provide ample tensile strength to support and approximate involved tissues. Defined as the amount of weight necessary to break a suture divided by its cross-sectional area, *tensile strength* is an important characteristic for suture selection. The tensile strength of material chosen should approximate the strength of the tissues being sutured.

Tensile strength is lost at different rates among suture types. Materials that have lost most of their tensile strength by 60 days following surgery are considered to be *absorbable* (Bennett, 1988).

TABLE 40-3. Specific Suture Material Characteristics

Type	Configuration	Tensile Strength	Handling	Knot Security	Reactivity
Nonabsorbable					
Silk	Braided	Good	Good	Good	High
Nylon	Monofilament	High	Fair	Fair	Low
Prolene	Monofilament	Good	Poor	Poor	Low
Mersilene	Braided synthetic	High	Good	Good	Moderate
Ethibond	Braided, coated	High	Fair	Fair	Moderate
Absorbable					
Gut (plain)	Twisted	Poor	Fair	Poor	Low
Chromic (gut)	Twisted	Poor	Fair	Poor	High
Dexon	Braided	Good	Good	Good	Low
Vicryl	Braided	Good	Good	Fair	Low
PDS II	Monofilament	Good	Fair	Poor	Low
Monocryl	Monofilament	Fair	Good	Good	Low

Absorbable suture is destroyed enzymatically or hydrolyzed, whereas nonabsorbable suture persists and ultimately is encapsulated. Ideally, absorbable suture material remains throughout wound healing but no longer. Logically, individual tissue healing characteristics typically dictate whether short- or long-term sutures are required. Accordingly, nonabsorbable material plays a greater role in pelvic floor reconstruction procedures, whereas absorbable suture is used routinely in general gynecologic surgery.

All sutures, when placed within tissue, will incite inflammation. This response mirrors the total amount of suture placed and the suture's chemical composition (Edlich, 1973). In general, lower inflammatory responses are elicited by monofilament structure compared with multifilament, and synthetically derived compared with natural fiber (Sharp, 1982).

The ease of fluid to wick from the wet end of a suture to its dry end defines its *capillarity*. A suture's *fluid absorption ability* describes the amount of fluid it absorbs when immersed. Both properties are presumed to have an impact on the access of contaminating bacteria. Increased capillarity and fluid absorption ability greatly increase the amount of bacteria similarly absorbed (Blomstedt, 1977). In general, multifilament sutures, even those with coatings, display greater capillarity compared with synthetic monofilament sutures (Geiger, 2005).

The ability of a material to return to its prior length following stretch defines its *elasticity*. For tissues in which swelling or movement is expected postoperatively, a suture with increased elasticity is preferred because it will stretch rather than cut into approximated tissues. *Memory* defines the ability of material to return to original form following deformation. Sutures with greater memory tend to untie more easily during knot tying.

■ Knots

The surgical knot is the weakest link in a tied suture loop, and the force necessary to break a knotted suture is less than that to break an individual suture strand. Knot failure can lead to serious complications such as bleeding, hernias, and wound dehiscence (Batra, 1993; Trimbos, 1984). Thus, an understanding of knots is essential.

A surgical knot consists of: a loop, which maintains tissue apposition, and a knot, composed of several throws snugged against each other. A single throw is formed when one strand is wrapped around the other one time, and when wrapped twice, a double throw is created (Zimmer, 1991). This double weave forms the basis of a surgeon's knot. In characterizing knots, each throw is given a numerical description, in which single throws are designated as number 1, and double throws as number 2. If successive throws are identical, a multiplication sign is placed between the numbers. If throws mirror one another, then an equal sign is used. Thus, a square knot is described as 1 = 1; granny knot, 1 × 1; and square surgeon's knot, 2 = 1 (Fig. 40-26). Alternative nomenclature schemes exist, but understanding the basic principles of knot construction is more clinically relevant than these descriptive definitions (Dinsmore, 1995).

Flat and Sliding Knots

Surgical knots can have flat or sliding configurations. Flat configurations include square, granny, and surgeon's knots.

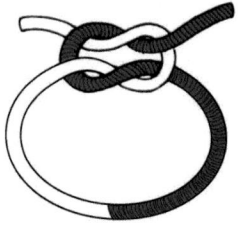
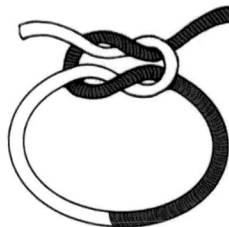
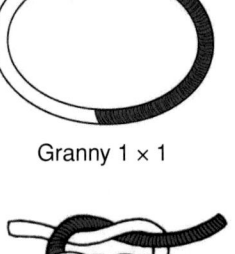
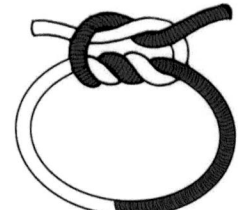
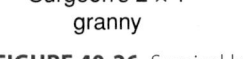

Granny 1 × 1   Square 1 = 1

Surgeon's 2 × 1 granny   Surgeon's 2 = 1 square

FIGURE 40-26 Surgical knots.

To construct a flat square knot, forehanded and backhanded throws are alternated, and the suture strands are pulled with equal tension in opposite directions but in the same plane. In addition, the suture strands or the hands may have to cross with each throw to ensure that the knot lies flat.

In contrast, sliding knots, also termed slip knots, are characterized as identical, nonidentical, and parallel. They are created when unequal tension is applied to the strands, such as during one-hand knot tying. Sliding knots are useful in situations when flat square knotting is difficult or cumbersome, such as in the deep pelvis or vagina (Ivy, 2004b). In general, sliding knots have been shown to have a higher failure rate than that of flat knots (Hurt, 2005; Schubert, 2002).

Identical sliding knots are created by holding one strand constantly under tension and repeating identical tying maneuvers with the other hand. Unfortunately, these identical sliding knots carry a high failure rate and are not recommended for general use (Schubert, 2002; Trimbos, 1984, 1986). *Nonidentical sliding knots* are formed when a suture strand is held under constant tension, and one hand alternates forehanded and backhanded tying around this strand (Trimbos, 1986). This knot is the most frequent and practical knot used for vaginal surgery. Although these knots can unravel, additional throws can greatly improve their security (Ivy, 2004a; Trimbos, 1984; van Rijjsel, 1990). A loop-to-strand variation of the nonidentical sliding knot is performed by holding the final loop of a continuous suture line taut, while alternate throws are made around the loop with the remaining single strand. Scant data support the security of this knot type in gynecologic surgery. When completed with monofilament suture, these knots carry high failure rates (Hurt, 2005).

Finally, with a *parallel sliding knot*, the suture strand under tension is alternated with each throw, causing alternate throws to slide down the other strand each time. Existing studies show this knot to be strong and reliable (Ivy, 2004b; Trimbos, 1986).

Surgical Knot Effectiveness

The effectiveness of surgical knots depends mainly on two parameters: initial loop security and knot security. *Loop security* describes the ability to maintain a tight suture loop around the tissue as the initial knot throws are placed (Lo, 2004). Suture loops that are initially loose will fail to secure tissues no matter how tightly the knot is tied and will result in ineffective knots, colloquially termed "air knots" (Burkhart, 1998). Three ways to optimize loop security include: maintenance of tension on both strands during tying, use of an initial surgeon's throw, and slip knots (Anderson, 1980). If slip knots are placed initially, they can be converted to square knots or reinforced with a square knot once the pedicle or vessel is secured. Importantly, upward tension on both strands deep within a body cavity should be limited. Excessive force can avulse the pedicle or cause the suture loop to pull completely off.

For *knot security*, the tension with which a given throw is tied is the most important. A knot laid down tightly under great tension is less likely to slip than a knot with the same configuration but with more throws tied loosely (Gunderson, 1987).

The number and type of knots required to secure various suture materials vary. Qualities such as elasticity and memory often direct these recommendations. In general, multifilament sutures are easier to handle and display less memory, whereas synthetic monofilament suture or multifilament sutures with coatings have increased memory and may hold a knot poorly. For most sutures, four to six throws appears to be adequate, but the exact number depends on the type of suture and whether a flat or sliding knot is formed. Up to a point, additional throws provide more security to a knot, but this benefit must be balanced against the corresponding elevated infection risk from increased knot volume (van Rijssel, 1990).

ELECTROSURGERY

Semantically, *electrosurgery* differs from *electrocautery*, although the terms are often incorrectly interchanged. With electrocautery, electric current passes through a metal object, such as a wire loop, with internal resistance. Passage of current heats the loop, which then may be used surgically. The flow of current is limited to the metal being heated, and no current enters the patient. In contrast, electrosurgery directs the flow of current to the tissues themselves and produces localized tissue heating and destruction. As a result, electric current must pass through tissues to produce the desired effect (Amaral, 2005). The electrosurgical circuit contains four main parts: the generator, the active electrode, the patient, and the return electrode. Electrosurgery may be broadly categorized as monopolar or bipolar depending on the proximity of these two electrodes.

■ Monopolar Electrosurgery

Electric current is the flow of electrons through a circuit (Fig. 40-27). *Voltage* is the force that drives those charges around the circuit. *Impedance* is the combination of resistance, inductance, and capacitance that alternating current meets along the way (Morris, 2006). In monopolar electrosurgery, the return electrode in clinical use is the grounding pad. Current

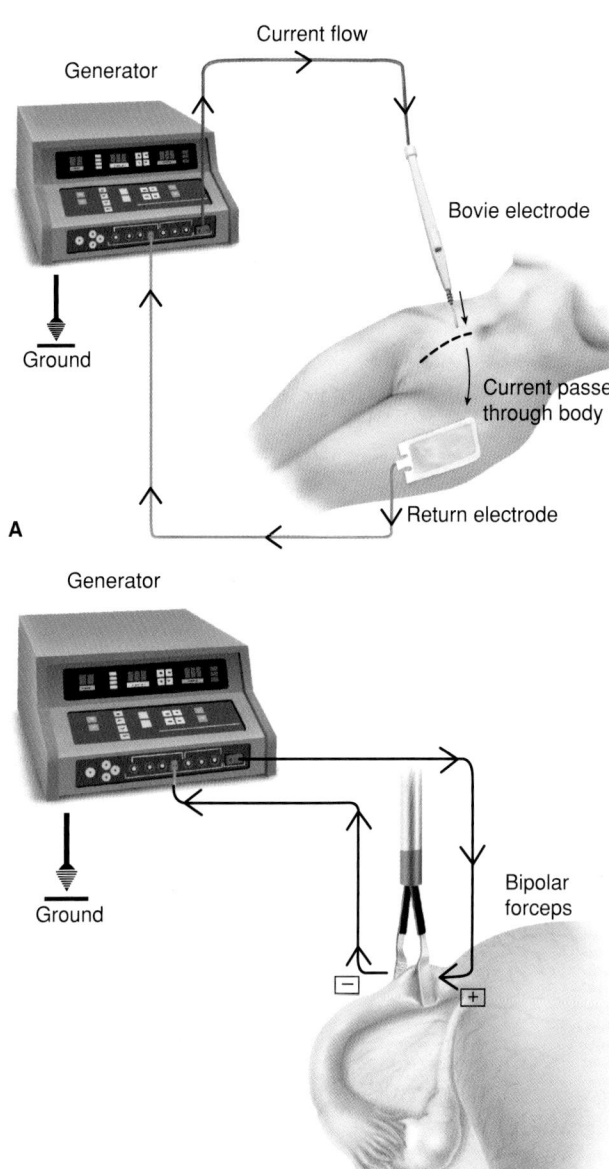

FIGURE 40-27 Circuits in electrosurgery. **A.** Monopolar electrosurgical circuit. **B.** Bipolar electrosurgical circuit.

therefore flows: (1) from the generator, which is the source of voltage, (2) through the electrosurgical tip to the patient, the source of impedance, and then (3) onto the grounding pad, where it is dispersed. Current leaves the pad to return to the generator, and the circuit is completed (Deatrick, 2015). In electrosurgery, tissue impedance converts electric current into thermal energy that causes tissue temperatures to rise. It is these thermal increases that create electrosurgery's tissue effects.

Surgical Effects

Differing tissue effects are created by altering the manner in which current is produced and delivered. First, altering the current wave pattern can affect tissue temperatures. For example, the high-frequency continuous sinusoidal waveform produced with cutting current creates higher tissue temperatures than that with coagulation current (Fig. 40-28). Second, the extent

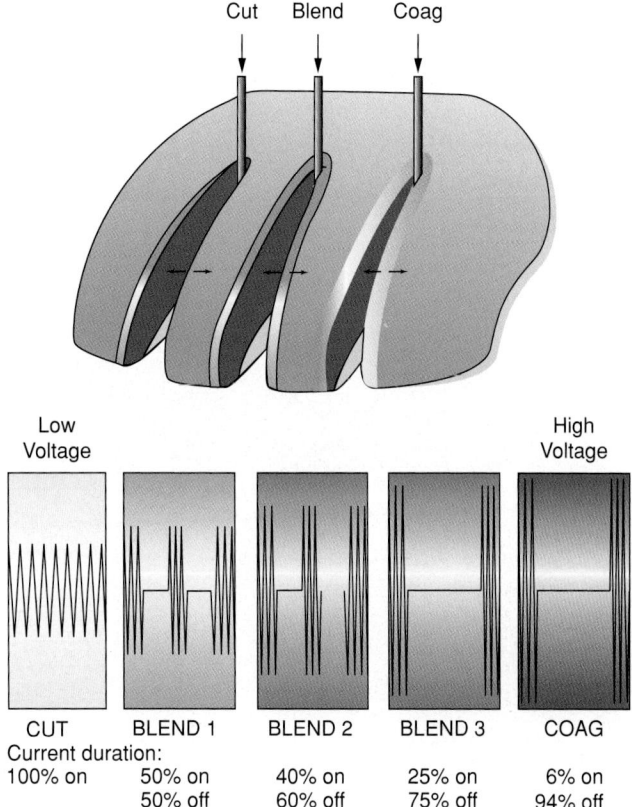

FIGURE 40-28 Tissue effects vary with cutting, blended, and coagulation currents. There is more lateral thermal damage with a pure coagulation current compared with a pure cutting or blended current. The duration of applied energy varies between current types.

to which current is spread over an area, also termed *current density,* alters the rate of heat generation (Fig. 40-29). Thus, if current is concentrated onto a small area, such as a needle-tip electrode, greater tissue temperatures are generated than if delivered over a wider area, such as an electrosurgical blade. In addition to current density, voltage can alter tissue effects. As voltage increases, the degree of thermal tissue damage similarly increases. And finally, the qualities and impedance of the tissues themselves affect energy transfer and heat dissipation. For example, water has low electrical impedance and liberates little heat, whereas skin with its greater impedance generates significantly higher tissue temperatures (Amaral, 2005).

With electrosurgical cutting, a continuous sine wave of current is produced. The flow of high-frequency current typically is concentrated through an electrosurgical needle or blade and meets tissue impedance. Sparks are created between the tissue and electrode, intense heat is produced, cellular water vaporizes, and cells in the immediate area burst. Tissues are cut cleanly, and there is minimal coagulum production. As a result, few vessels are sealed, and minimal hemostasis accompanies electrosurgical cutting.

In contrast, coagulation current does not produce a constant waveform. Less heat is produced than with cutting current. However, tissue temperature still rises sufficiently to denature protein and disrupt normal cellular architecture. Cells are not vaporized instantly, and cellular debris remains associated with

wound edges. This coagulum seals smaller blood vessels and controls local bleeding (Singh, 2006).

Variations in the percentage of time that current is flowing can create electrosurgical effects that contain both cutting and coagulating features. Such *blended currents* are used commonly in gynecologic surgery. In most cases, selection of specific percentages of cutting and coagulation current is affected by surgeon preference and type of tissues encountered. Thinner vascular tissue may be best suited for a blend with less active current time, whereas denser avascular tissues may require a greater percentage of active current.

Patient Grounding

As discussed earlier, current is concentrated at the electrode tip and enters the patient at a small site. Current follows the path of least resistance and exits the body through a grounding pad that is designed to have a large surface area, high conductivity, and low resistance. Dissipation across this large surface area allows current to leave the body without generating significant tissue temperatures at the exit site.

However, patient burns may result if current is concentrated through a return electrode. Clinically, this may occur if a grounding pad is partially dislodged. In this setting, the surface area is decreased, and the exiting current concentration and the tissue temperatures at the exit site rise. In addition, patient jewelry, metal candy cane stirrups, or other surfaces with high conductivity and low resistance may serve as a return electrode. In such cases, patients may be burned by concentrated current exiting through these small contact sites. Ideally, grounding

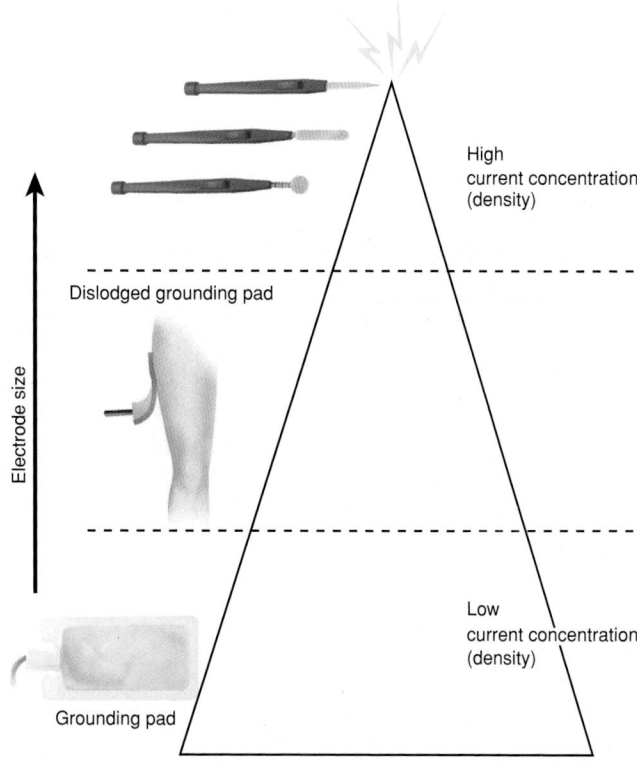

FIGURE 40-29 Current concentration and its effects. Thermal energy and risk for tissue injury diminish as current density decreases and electrode area increases.

pads are firmly adhered to a relatively flat body surface that is near the operative field. Thus, in most gynecology procedures, grounding pads are placed along the lateral upper thigh.

Patients with pacemakers, implantable cardioverter-defibrillators (ICDs), or other electrical implants require special precautions. Stray electrosurgical current may be interpreted as an intracardiac signal by an implanted device and lead to pacing changes. In addition, myocardial electrical burns may result from conduction of current through the pacing electrode rather than through the grounding pad (Pinski, 2002). Accordingly, for patients with these devices, preventive recommendations include pre- and postoperative cardiology consultation; use of minimal monopolar electrosurgical current settings or substitution with bipolar electrosurgery or harmonic scalpel; continuous cardiac monitoring; contingency plans for arrhythmias; and close proximity of active and return electrodes (Crossley, 2011).

◼ Bipolar Electrosurgery

This form of electrosurgery differs from monopolar electrosurgery in that the tip of a bipolar device contains both an active electrode and a return electrode. For this reason, a distant grounding return pad is not required. Coagulation current is concentrated on tissues grasped between the electrodes, and tissue must remain between them. If tissue slips from between the tips, then active and return electrodes contact and create a short circuit. Coagulation will not occur (Michelassi, 1997). Bipolar electrosurgery uses only coagulation current and lacks cutting capability. However, it is useful for vessels coagulation and also is used during laparoscopic sterilization to coagulate fallopian tubes (Section 44-2, p. 1007).

◼ Argon Beam Coagulation

With argon beam coagulation (ABC), radiofrequency energy is transferred to tissues through a jet of inert argon gas to create noncontact monopolar electrothermal coagulation. Additionally, the gas jet clears blood and tissue debris during coagulation. Advantages of ABC include the ability to coagulate broad surface areas and larger vessels (Beckley, 2004). In gynecologic surgery, ABC is used most often during ovarian staging cases in which extensive debulking may be required.

ULTRASONIC ENERGY

Sound waves are mechanical waves that transport energy through a medium. Those above audible range are described as *ultrasound* or *ultrasonic*. In medicine, ultrasound waves that are applied at low levels such as those used in diagnostic sonography are harmless. However, if higher power levels are used, then mechanical energy transferred to the affected tissues is strong enough to produce cutting, coagulation, or tissue cavitation.

Of tools, the ultrasonic scalpel, also known as a *Harmonic scalpel*, has a tip that vibrates at high frequency. This allows the surgical device to be used effectively for both cutting and coagulating during laparotomy or laparoscopy (Gyr, 2001; Wang, 2000). The vibrating tip transfers mechanical energy to tissues. Mechanical energy breaks hydrogen bonds and generates

heat within tissues to denature protein and form a sticky coagulum that produces hemostasis. A balance between cutting and coagulation is controlled by three factors: power levels, tissue tension, and blade sharpness. Higher power level, greater tissue tension, and a sharp blade will lead to cutting. Lower power, decreased tissue tension, and a blunt blade will create slower cutting and greater hemostasis (Sinha, 2003).

Used most commonly in laparoscopic surgery, the ultrasonic scalpel serves as an alternative to suture ligation, electrosurgical coagulation, laser, and stapling or clipping devices. However, only a few studies have compared the clinical effectiveness of this method with other methods of hemostasis (Kauko, 1998).

Cavitational ultrasonic surgical aspiration (CUSA) is another ultrasound-based tool. The ultrasonic surgical aspirator handpiece contains three main components: a high-frequency vibrator, which transfers the ultrasonic energy to tissues; irrigation tubing, which directs cooling saline to the tip; and a suction system, which draws tissue up to the tip for contact with the vibrator and which also clears away tissue fragments and irrigant. Ultrasound energy can be used to raise tissue temperatures dramatically and thereby disrupt tissue architecture by a process termed *cavitation*. For cavitation, the CUSA tip produces mechanical waves that create heat and vapor pockets around cells in tissues with high water content such as adipose, muscle, and carcinoma. Collapse of these pockets leads to disruption of cell architecture (Jallo, 2001). Affected tissues are removed subsequently by suction aspiration. However, tissues containing less water and higher contents of collagen and elastic fibers, such as blood vessels, nerves, ureters, and serosa, are more resistant to damage (van Dam, 1996).

In gynecology, CUSA has a limited surgical role. It may be used effectively in the treatment of vulvar intraepithelial neoplasia and bulky condyloma acuminata (Section 43-28, p. 996). It can also speed cytoreductive ovarian cancer surgery (Aletti, 2006; Deppe, 1988; Robinson, 2000; van Dam, 1996).

MANAGEMENT OF HEMORRHAGE

◼ Autologous Donation and Cell Salvage

Although the risk of hemorrhage accompanies most gynecologic procedures, certain factors are associated with higher rates of bleeding and are assessed prior to surgery. Specifically, obesity, the presence of a large pelvic mass, adhesions such as those from endometriosis or pelvic inflammatory disease, cancer or prior radiation, and coagulation dysfunction have been linked with an increased risk of hemorrhage. For those identified to be at risk, intraoperative red cell salvage or preoperative autologous blood donation can be considered.

Red blood cell (RBC) salvage machines (Autolog; Cell Saver) collect, filter, and centrifuge blood lost during surgery. RBCs are heavier and are separated from plasma and smaller blood components during centrifugation and are then reinfused into the patient. Anticoagulants such as heparin or citrate are added to prevent clotting (Karger, 2005). Salvage efficiencies approximate 60 percent with good technique. However, vacuum levels, suction tip size, and thoroughness of salvaging efforts can affect this value. For example, turbulence destroys RBCs. Thus, suction

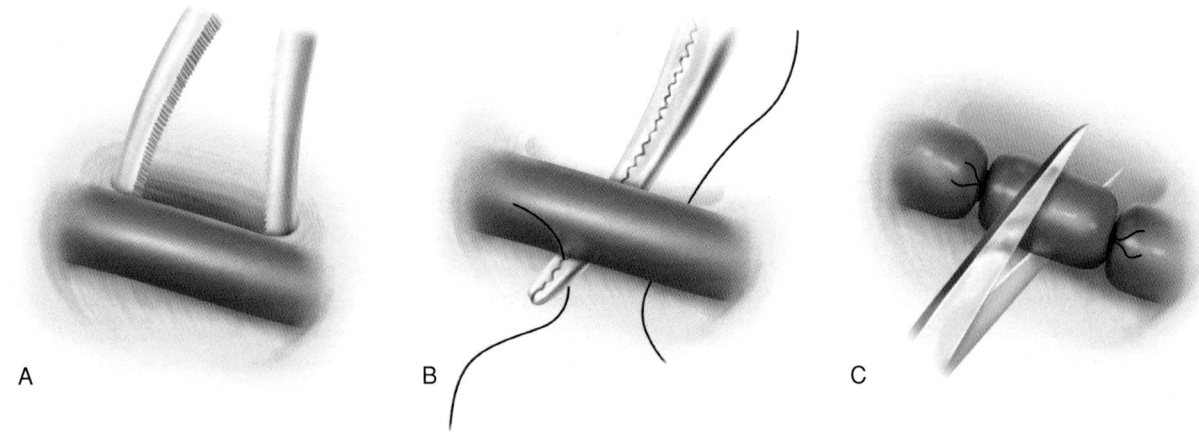

FIGURE 40-30 Steps in vessel isolation, ligation and transection. **A.** During vessel isolation, a clamp tip can be opened and closed parallel to the side of the vessel to dissect away loose surrounding tissue. **B.** The tip of the clamp is insinuated beneath the vessel, and the jaws are opened and elevated. A suture ligature can then be grasped and pulled beneath the vessel. **C.** Two sutures are placed around the vessel, and it is transected between these ligation points.

tips with greater diameters and lower suction force can minimize hemolysis (Waters, 2005). Additionally, laparotomy sponges can be rinsed in sterile saline to maximize RBC removal. The RBC-containing saline then is suctioned into the salvage device for processing. The filtering systems in these devices have limitations. Accordingly, RBC salvage is not appropriate for contaminated cases or those in which malignancy, hemostatic agents, or amnionic fluid may be present (Waters, 2004).

Another approach for cases with expected hemorrhage involves preoperative autologous donation. Thus, to avoid potential transfusion reaction or blood-borne infection, a patient may elect to donate her own blood for personal use approximately once a week for 3 to 5 weeks preceding surgery. Patient hemoglobin levels should be greater than 11.0 g/dL before each donation. Moreover, units are not collected within 72 hours before surgery. This allows intravascular volume to be replenished by the patient and units to be processed by the blood bank (Goodnough, 2005). Disadvantageously, this process has been associated with preoperative anemia secondary to donation, more liberal transfusion, transfusion reaction following clerical error, volume overload, and bacterial contamination of blood products during processing (Henry, 2002; Kanter, 1996, 1999).

Improved blood banking safety has accompanied a decline in preoperative autologous donation (Brecher, 2002). Moreover, for most gynecologic cases, the risk of transfusion is low. For these reasons, autologous donation typically is reserved for selected instances in which the risk of transfusion is significant, such as radical hysterectomy or surgery for patients with coagulopathies. Additionally, patients with rare blood phenotypes in whom acquisition of compatible blood may be difficult may benefit from autologous donation.

▪ Proper Surgical Method

In many instances, proper surgical technique can minimize vascular injury and hemorrhage. Thus, prior to ligation, vessels ideally have excess connective tissue removed sharply in a process called *skeletonizing*. Additionally, tissue clamps selected for grasping a vascular pedicle are large enough to contain the

entire pedicle in the distal portion of the clamp. Large pedicles that force excess tissue toward the clamp's heel carry greater risk of tissue slipping from the heel and bleeding. Once secure, sutures placed on vascular pedicles are not to be used for traction because the risk of avulsing the suture or vessel increases.

Tying an intact vessel at two places along its length before tissue cutting is considered in certain situations. This technique may be appropriate if a vessel is on tension or if space for a clamp is limited, such as when the ureter or bowel is in close proximity. A window is created below the vessel and ties are passed beneath the vessel before doubly ligating and dividing it (Fig. 40-30).

▪ Steps of Hemorrhage Management

A methodical approach to intraoperative hemorrhage is critical to minimize patient morbidity. If an isolated vessel is clearly identified, then grasping it with a hemostat, vascular clamp, or fine forceps may allow ligation, electrosurgical coagulation, or vascular clip application.

In contrast, venous bleeding in the pelvis is typically from a venous plexus and rarely stems from a single vessel. A pelvic venous plexus contains thin-walled veins. Accordingly, indiscriminate clamping, suturing, clipping, and electrosurgical coagulation can cause further laceration and bleeding. However, if other vulnerable structures have been retracted and protected, a few shallow stitches that incorporate the bleeding area can be placed using fine absorbable suture.

If these initial efforts are unsuccessful and significant hemorrhage continues, the bleeding site is compressed with fingertips, sponge stick, or laparotomy sponges. Anesthesia staff is informed of events to allow for additional monitoring. Nursing staff is also informed as additional resources may be required, such as specialized instruments, suture, clips, and blood products. Fluid resuscitation is individualized depending on the degree of hemorrhage and other patient factors described later.

Adequate exposure typically aids control of bleeding. The operative field is assessed and increased as needed by extending a vertical incision cephalad, converting a Pfannenstiel incision to a Cherney incision, adding retractors, or converting a vaginal or laparoscopic approach to laparotomy. A second suctioning system may be required, and appropriate suture or clips are made available before removing pressure. Additional dissection of avascular planes around the bleeding site may improve isolation and ligation of a lacerated vessel. Furthermore, nearby vulnerable structures such as the bladder, ureter, or other vessels are identified and protected. After these steps, the surgeon may remove the tamponading pressure to assess the location, amount, and character of bleeding and to formulate the most appropriate technique for controlling it.

Vessel Ligation

As noted, bleeding vessels may be tied, clipped, or coagulated. Advantages to suture ligation include low cost and effectiveness over a broad range of vessel diameters. However, knot tying in general is time-consuming, is difficult in narrow spaces, and can be associated with ligature slippage or breakage. Small vessels may be ligated by a free-tie suture placed around the heel and tip of a vascular clamp and then secured with knots (see Fig. 40-23A). Alternatively, surgeons often prefer to secure larger vascular pedicles with two separate sutures. The first ligature is a free tie placed around the toe and heel of a vascular clamp and tied. The second ligature is distal to the first and typically incorporates a bite through the tissue pedicle (see Fig. 40-23B, C). Such *transfixion* of the ligature to the pedicle decreases the risk that it will slip off the pedicle's end. Importantly, this second ligature is placed distal to the first to avert hematoma formation if a vessel is pierced during transfixion.

Alternatively, titanium clips seal vessels by direct compression. They are used more commonly during gynecologic oncology cases and offer the advantage of speed. However, clips are expensive, require surgical dissection of the vessel prior to application, and may dislodge from a vessel. Their use in routine gynecology is limited by these factors and surgeon preference.

Electrical and ultrasound energy also may be used to seal vessels. Ultrasonic coagulating shears (Autosonix; Harmonic scalpel; Sonosurg) and electrosurgical bipolar vessel sealing clamps (Enseal; LigaSure) transfer energy that denatures vascular collagen and elastin. Some of these seal vessels up to 7 mm in diameter (Heniford, 2001). Thermal spread for these devices is comparable and averages 2.5 mm (Harold, 2003). These tools are particularly useful for laparoscopic surgeries, in which knot tying is time-consuming.

Local Topical Hemostats

These topical products may be placed on bleeding sites where ligature or vessel coagulation is not possible or has been ineffective. They are most effective in controlling low-pressure bleeding, such as from veins, capillaries, and small arteries. Commercially available materials are categorized as mechanical hemostats, active hemostats, flowable hemostats, and fibrin sealants (Table 40-5). Some liquid hemostats deliver topical thrombin or thrombin

TABLE 40-5. Topical Hemostatic Agents

Type of Agent	Brand Name	Material
Mechanical Hemostats		
Oxidized, regenerated methylcellulose	Surgicel	Flat loose woven fabric
	Surgicel Fibrillar	Flat peelable layers and tufts
	Surgicel Nu-knit	Flat loose woven fabric
	Surgicel SNoW	Flat nonwoven fabric
Porcine gelatin	Surgifoam	Powder or flat sponge
	Gelfoam	Powder or flat sponge
	Surgiflo[a]	Powder
Bovine collagen	Avitene	Powder, sheet, or flat sponge
	Instat	Powder
Active Hemostats		
Bovine thrombin	Thrombin-JMI	Liquid spray
Bovine thrombin + gelatin	Thrombi-Gel	Flat sponge
Bovine thrombin + methylcellulose	Thrombi-Pad	Flat sheet
Human thrombin	Evithrom[a]	Liquid
Recombinant thrombin	Recothrom	Liquid
Flowable Hemostats		
Bovine gelatin + human thrombin	FloSeal Matrix	Liquid
Porcine gelatin + Human thrombin	Surgiflo + Evithrom	Liquid
Fibrin Sealants		
Human thrombin, fibrinogen, plasminogen	Tisseel	Spray or drip application
Human thrombin, fibrinogen	Evicel	Spray or drip application

[a]Surgiflo and Evithrom can be combined to form flowable hemostat.

plus fibrinogen and thereby induce clot formation. Others provide combined effects that, in sum, create direct pressure against wound surfaces, entrap platelets, promote platelet aggregation, and serve as a scaffold on which clot can organize.

Although effective, these agents do have disadvantages. They should not be introduced intravascularly or used with RBC salvage machines. Packing agents tightly into bony foramina is avoided because these agents can swell and cause neurologic dysfunction or pressure necrosis. Moreover, they are not placed within skin edges because they may retard edge reapproximation. They may serve as an infection nidus and thus may not be appropriate in grossly infected tissue (Baxter Healthcare, 2014; Pfizer, 2014). Few data support the use of one agent over another. Selection typically is dictated by surgeon preference and availability in the operating room.

Tranexamic Acid

Intravenous administration of tranexamic acid, an effective antifibrinolytic, has been widely investigated in trauma surgery (Hunt, 2015). It is a synthetic lysine derivative, which blocks the conversion of plasminogen to plasmin, as illustrated in Figure 8-12 (p. 196). Massive hemorrhage may be complicated by coagulopathy and uncontrollable microvascular hemorrhage. Tranexamic acid, 1 g given intravenously, may be of benefit in this setting in concert with pelvic pressure and blood component administration.

Pelvic Artery Embolization or Pelvic Packing

As described in Chapter 9 (p. 209), embolization similar to that used to treat symptomatic leiomyomas can be used to occlude either the internal iliac artery or the uterine artery. This technique has been described in the management of hemorrhage in both gynecologic and obstetric cases.

In other cases, for patients with persistent heavy bleeding despite attempts at control, pelvic packing with gauze and termination of the operation may be warranted. Rolls of gauze are packed against the bleeding site to provide constant local pressure. Typically, 24 to 48 hours later, if the patient is stable and bleeding appears to have stopped clinically, packing is removed. Some surgeons recommend leaving one end of the gauze outside the wound. After administration of general anesthesia, packing is pulled slowly through a small opening left in the incision. Alternatively, entire gauze rolls may be packed into the abdomen and removed during a second laparotomy (Newton, 1988).

Internal Iliac Artery Ligation

The internal iliac artery, also called the *hypogastric artery,* contains anterior and posterior divisions. Its anterior division supplies blood to central pelvic viscera (Fig. 38-12, p. 805). Occlusion of the internal iliac artery decreases mean blood flow by 48 percent in branches distal to ligation, which in many cases slows hemorrhage sufficiently to allow identification of specific bleeding sites (Burchell, 1968). Fortunately, the female pelvis has extensive collateral circulation, and the internal iliac artery shares arterial anastomoses with branches of the aorta, external iliac artery, and femoral artery. For this reason, ligation of the internal iliac's anterior division can be performed without compromise to pelvic organ viability. Several studies

have described normal postligation fertility in these women (Demirci, 2005; Nizard, 2003).

To perform ligation, the round ligament is divided, and the pelvic sidewall peritoneum lateral to the infundibulopelvic ligament is incised cephalad. Identification of the internal iliac artery is essential because ligation of the common or external iliac arteries will have vascular consequences to the lower extremity. Once the internal iliac artery is located, a Mixter right-angle clamp is placed under the vessel at a point 2 to 3 cm distal to the bifurcation of the common iliac artery. Two free ties of no. 1 or 0 absorbable suture are passed beneath the artery and then secured (Fig. 40-31). The artery is ligated but not transected. If the internal iliac is ligated at this site, its posterior division theoretically should be spared (Bleich, 2007). Care is required in passing instruments beneath the artery because the thin-walled internal iliac vein is easily lacerated.

◼ Specific Sites of Bleeding
Infundibulopelvic Ligament

During or after ligation of this vascular pedicle, a lacerated ovarian vessel may retract into the retroperitoneum to create a hematoma. In most cases, isolation of the bleeding vessel is required to halt hematoma expansion. For this, the pelvic sidewall peritoneum lateral to the ureter and the hematoma is opened, and the incision is extended cephalad to the upper pole of the hematoma. The incision in the peritoneum may be carried up the white line of Toldt. This line, found on the right and the left, is the peritoneum's posterior reflection over the mesenteric attachment site of the ascending or descending colon to the posterior abdominal wall. The upper pole of the hematoma is identified by a return to normal vessel caliber above the hematoma. The ovarian vessels are identified, and a closed Mixter right-angle clamp is placed beneath them. A tie on a pass then is threaded beneath and used to ligate these vessels. If large, the hematoma then is evacuated to minimize infection risk (Tomacruz, 2001). In rare cases in which vascular or ureteral anatomy is unclear, an ovarian artery may require ligation as proximal as its aortic origin below the renal arteries (Masterson, 1995).

Space of Retzius and Presacral Venous Plexus

The space of Retzius, also called the retropubic space, is often entered during urogynecologic procedures and contains important vascular structures such as the venous plexus of Santorini, the obturator vessels, and the aberrant obturator vessel (Fig. 38-24, p. 817). Approximately 2 percent of tension-free vaginal tape procedures are complicated by bleeding in this space (Kolle, 2005; Kuuva, 2002). In most instances, bleeding is controlled with pressure or suturing.

In contrast, the presacral venous plexus can be lacerated by dissection or suturing during sacrocolpopexy (Fig. 38-23, p. 816). Cut vessels may retract into the vertebral bone, and problematic bleeding can follow. Management is described in full in Section 45-17 (p. 1099).

Major Pelvic Vessels

High-volume pelvic vessels include the internal, external, and common iliac vessels, the inferior vena cava, and aorta. These

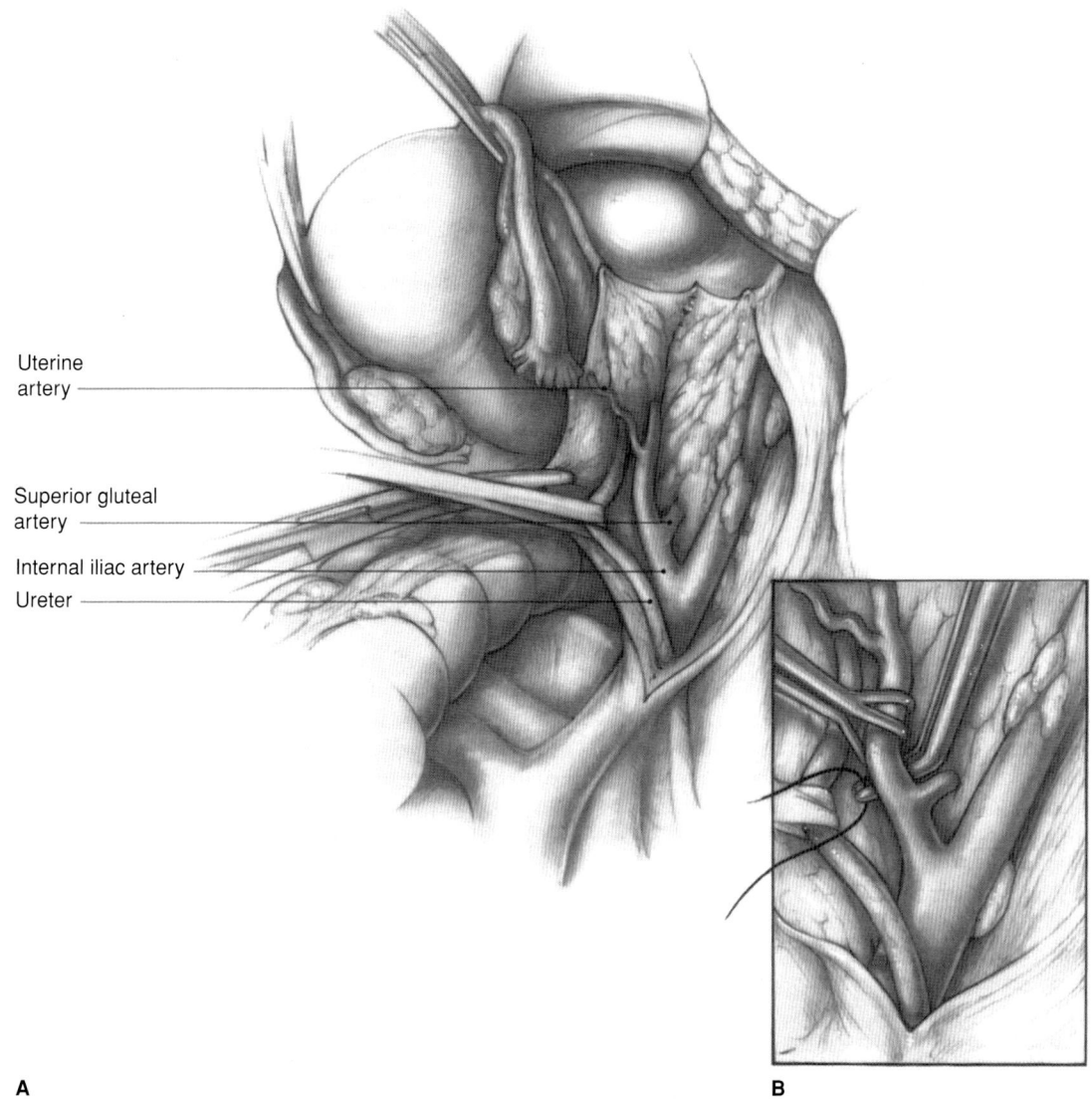

Uterine
artery

Superior gluteal
artery

Internal iliac artery

Ureter

A

B

FIGURE 40-31 Internal iliac artery ligation. After opening the retroperitoneal space, the ureter is identified and retracted medially. **Inset.** The internal iliac artery is identified and gently elevated with a Babcock clamp. A Mixter right-angle clamp is placed beneath the artery to receive a free tie for ligation. (Reproduced with permission from Cunningham FG, Vandorsten JP, Gilstrap LC: Operative Obstetrics, 2nd ed. New York: McGraw-Hill; 2002.)

may be lacerated during tumor removal, endometriosis excision, or laparoscopic trocar placement.

Initially following large vessel injury, pressure is applied for several minutes. Although gynecologic surgeons may attempt to repair these injuries, excessive delay in obtaining vascular surgery assistance often leads to greater blood loss (Oderich, 2004). Therefore, in many instances, pressure is applied, a vascular surgeon is consulted for repair, blood products are made available, and exposure is maximized. If a large vessel is punctured by a trocar or needle during laparoscopic entry, the instrument should remain in place to act as a plug while preparations for repair are made.

As discussed earlier, internal iliac artery ligation does not lead to ischemia of central pelvic organs due to collateral blood supply. However, injury to the external or common iliac arteries requires repair to maintain blood supply to the lower extremity. Consultation with a vascular surgeon may be indicated depending on the degree of laceration and surgeon skill. Maneuvers

that may extend the injury are avoided until appropriate assistance is available.

If repair is undertaken, familiarity with this vascular anatomy is essential. On the left, the common and external iliac arteries remain lateral to their respective veins. On the right, however, the common iliac artery runs medial to the vein.

These arteries can be repaired by placing vascular clamps 2 to 3 cm proximal and distal to the tear, then closing the defect with a continuous suture line using monofilament synthetic 5-0 suture (Gostout, 2002; Tomacruz, 2001). The proximal clamp is removed first to allow air and debris to exit the suture line, and then the distal clamp is removed.

Parametrial and Paravaginal Vessels

During obstetric and gynecologic surgery, vessels supplying the uterus and vagina, especially venous plexuses, can be lacerated. At times, bleeding may not be easily identified and controlled by direct pressure, suturing, or clips. In these extreme situations, ligation of the internal iliac artery, which is a main source of blood supply to the pelvis, may decrease pooling of blood and afford a better opportunity to find a bleeding source. Alternatively, if resources are available, pelvic artery embolization is effective in controlling pelvic hemorrhage. Despite these techniques, in rare persistent situations, pelvic packing and termination of surgery may be indicated.

FLUID RESUSCITATION AND BLOOD TRANSFUSION

The intraoperative and immediate postoperative periods are viewed as resuscitative phases, with a goal of attaining relative euvolemia. With acute hemorrhage, priorities include control of additional losses and replacement of sufficient intravascular volume for tissue perfusion and oxygenation. In hypoperfused areas, progressive failure of oxidative metabolism with lactate production leads to worsening systemic metabolic acidosis and eventual organ damage. To avoid these effects, resuscitation begins with an assessment of the patient's clinical status, calculation of total blood volume, and estimation of blood loss.

■ Clinical Assessment

Total blood volume for an adult approximates 70 mL/kg, and thus a 50-kg woman's calculated blood volume is 3500 mL. Of this volume, 15 percent can be lost by most patients with no changes in arterial pressure or heart rate. A 15-percent blood loss can be roughly calculated by multiplication of a patient's weight in kilograms by 10. Thus, for a 50-kg woman, a 15-percent loss approximates 500 mL.

With losses of 15 to 30 percent (500 to 1000 mL for a 50-kg woman), tachycardia and narrowing of the pulse pressure are seen (Table 40-6). Peripheral vasoconstriction leads to pale, cool extremities and poor capillary refill. In unanesthetized patients,

there may be mild confusion or lethargy. In most women with normal preoperative hemoglobin levels, this amount of blood loss requires fluid volume replacement, but RBC transfusion typically is not required. Greater losses, however, lead to worsening perfusion, hypotension, and tachycardia. In these cases, blood transfusion in combination with fluid resuscitation typically is indicated (Murphy, 2001).

During surgery, blood collects in suction canisters and laparotomy sponges. Although calculations from these sources provide surgeons with an approximation, blood loss estimates typically are low, and inaccuracy increases as the length and extent of a procedure increases (Bose, 2006; Santoso, 2001). Additionally, a hematocrit may be measured to assess hemorrhage. However, hematocrit values typically lag true losses, and values may reflect only the degree of hemorrhage. For example, following a blood loss of 1000 mL, hematocrit levels typically fall only 3 volume percent in the first hour but usually show an 8 volume percent drop at 72 hours (Schwartz, 2006). Hemorrhage leads to global tissue hypoxia, anaerobic metabolism, and lactate production. Thus, elevated serum lactate levels can be a helpful marker. Blood gas analysis can also provide a rapid estimate of the serum base deficit. Hemorrhage severity can be predicted using the following stratification of these base deficits: 2 to −5 (mild hemorrhage), −6 to −14 (moderate hemorrhage), and −15 or less (severe hemorrhage). If patients continue to have dropping base deficits despite aggressive resuscitation, ongoing hemorrhage is a concern (Davis, 1988).

■ Fluid Resuscitation

If hypovolemia is identified, fluid resuscitation begins with crystalloid solutions. If hypotension and tachycardia are present, rapid replacement is warranted, and 1 or 2 liters, as indicated, may be infused over several minutes. Normal saline and lactated Ringer solutions are the two crystalloids used

TABLE 40-6. Clinical Findings Associated with Increasing Severity of Hemorrhage

Hemorrhage Class	Class I	Class II	Class III	Class IV
Blood loss				
Percentage	<15	15–30	30–40	>40
Volume (mL)	750	800–1500	1500–2000	>2000
Blood pressure				
Systolic	Unchanged	Normal	Reduced	Very low
Diastolic	Unchanged	Raised	Reduced	Very low, unrecordable
Pulse (beats/min)	Slight tachycardia	100–120	(thready)	>120 (thready)
Capillary refill	Normal	Slow (>2 sec)	Slow (>2 sec)	Undetectable
Respiratory rate	Normal	Normal	Tachypnea (>20/min)	Tachypnea (>20/min)
Urinary flow rate (mL/hr)	>30	20–30	10–20	0–10
Extremities	Normal color	Pale	Pale	Pale and cold
Complexion	Normal	Pale	Pale	Ashen
Mental state	Alert	Anxious or aggressive	Anxious, aggressive, or drowsy	Drowsy, confused, or unconscious

Reproduced with permission from Baskett PJ: ABC of major trauma. Management of hypovolaemic shock, BMJ 1990 Jun 2;300(6737):1453-7.

commonly, and their composition is described in Chapter 42 (p. 908). For moderate hemorrhage, both perform equally well as fluid replacements (Healey, 1998).

Although crystalloids have an immediate effect to expand intravascular volume, a portion will extravasate into extracellular tissues. Thus, in the setting of hemorrhage, crystalloid volume is administered in a 3:1 ratio to blood lost (Moore, 2004). Clinically, urine output of 0.5 mL/kg/per hour or 30 mL or more per hour, heart rate less than 100 beats per minute, and systolic blood pressure greater than 90 mm Hg may be used as general indicators of volume improvement. If rapid crystalloid infusion fails to correct hypotension or tachycardia, then RBC transfusion usually is prudent.

In addition to or as an alternative to crystalloid solutions, colloids may be used for volume expansion. These fluids have higher molecular weights than crystalloids. As a result, a greater portion remains intravascular and is not lost to extracellular extravasation. Despite this perceived advantage, studies comparing survival rates when crystalloids or colloids are administered find no superiority with colloids but greater expense (Perel, 2013).

Intraoperative fluid management strategies broadly fall into categories of liberal (sometimes thought of as fixed volume), restrictive, or goal directed. Of these, evidence from colorectal and trauma surgery is now more supportive of restrictive management. Less bowel edema, quicker return of bowel function, and fewer pulmonary complications are all purported benefits (Chappell, 2008; Joshi, 2005). Restrictive strategies generally use colloid to replace blood loss in a 1:1 ratio, unless red cell transfusion is indicated. Crystalloids are then used to replace urine and insensible losses 1:1. In contrast, liberal strategies rely on large volumes of crystalloid. Last, goal directed therapy refers to using a monitoring device (such as an arterial line) and administering fluids to achieve a goal (such as maximizing stroke volume). Patients with severe comorbid conditions undergoing major procedures may benefit from this strategy (Chappell, 2008).

■ Red Blood Cell Replacement

Clinical Assessment

The decision to administer RBCs is complex and must balance the risks of transfusion with needs for adequate tissue oxygenation. Assessment includes hemoglobin level, vital signs, patient age, risks for further blood loss, and underlying medical conditions, especially cardiac disease. These needs will vary depending on the clinical setting. Accordingly, no specific hemoglobin threshold dictates when RBCs are administered. Consensus guidelines suggest that in those without significant cardiac disease, transfusion to a hemoglobin level above 10 g/dL is rarely indicated (Carless, 2010). If hemoglobin levels acutely drop to 6 g/dL, transfusion almost always is required (Madjdpour, 2006). Hemoglobin levels between 6 and 10 g/dL are more problematic, and patient factors and risk for continued hemorrhage dictate therapy (American Society of Anesthesiologists, 2015). In one randomized study of 838 critically ill patients, one group of euvolemic patients received transfusion when their hemoglobin levels fell below 7 g/dL. These individuals

fared better than those transfused at an earlier threshold (hemoglobin below 10 g/dL), excepting those with significant cardiac disease (Hébert, 1999).

Transfusion

When the possible need for transfusion is present, an order for a *type and screen* informs blood bank personnel that blood products may be required and initiates two tests to characterize a patient's RBCs. The first evaluation, termed *typing*, mixes commercially available standardized controls with a patient's blood sample to determine her ABO type and Rh phenotype. The second test, or *screen*, combines a patient's plasma sample with control RBCs that express clinically significant RBC antigens. If a patient has formed antibodies to any of these specific RBC surface antigens, then agglutination or hemolysis of the sample is seen. However, if blood is needed immediately and a full screen is not possible, then ABO type-specific blood or O-negative blood may be used. Typing and screening require approximately 45 minutes for completion and are valid for 3 days in patients who do receive transfusion. In those who are not transfused, the validity is considerably longer and typically is determined by individual blood banks. Alternatively, an order to *type and crossmatch* blood products alerts blood bank personnel to designate specific units of blood solely for one individual's use. Those specific units are tested against the patient's for specific antigen reactions.

Previously, whole-blood transfusion was used commonly to provide RBCs, coagulation factors, and plasma proteins. This largely has been replaced by component therapy. Packed RBCs are the primary product used for most clinical situations and are prepared by removing most of the supernatant plasma during centrifugation. One unit of packed RBCs contains the same red cell mass as 1 unit of whole blood at approximately half the volume and twice the hematocrit (70 to 80 percent). One unit of packed RBCs raises the hematocrit approximately 3 volume percent in an adult or increases the hemoglobin level of a 70-kg individual by 1 g/dL (Table 40-7) (Gorgas, 2004). With severe hemorrhage that is anticipated to require ≥10 RBC units, massive transfusion protocols that combine units of packed RBCs, platelets, and plasma in 1:1:1 ratios are effective (McDaniel, 2014).

Complications

Despite numerous tests for compatibility, adverse reactions to blood products can develop. An acute or delayed hemolytic transfusion reaction, febrile nonhemolytic transfusion reaction, allergic reaction, infection, or associated lung injury are among these.

First, *acute hemolytic transfusion reaction* involves acute immune-mediated hemolysis usually from destruction of transfused RBCs by patient antibodies. This most commonly results from ABO incompatibility. Symptoms begin within minutes or hours of transfusion and may include chills, fever, urticaria, tachycardia, dyspnea, nausea and vomiting, hypotension, and chest and back pain. In addition, these reactions can lead to acute tubular necrosis or disseminated intravascular coagulopathy, and treatment is directed to these serious complications.

If acute hemolysis is suspected, transfusion is halted immediately. A sample of the patient's blood is sent with the remaining donor unit for evaluation in the blood bank. In patients

TABLE 40-7. Characteristics of Blood Components

Component	Volume, mL	Content	Clinical Response
PRBCs	180–200	RBCs	Increases Hb 1 g/dL and Hct 3%
Platelets			Increases platelet count:
Random-donor unit	50–70	5.5×10^{10} platelets	$5–10 \times 10^9$/L
Single-donor collection	200–400	3.0×10^{11} platelets	$>10 \times 10^9$/L within 1 hr and $>7.5 \times 10^9$/L within 24 hr posttransfusion
FFP	200–250	Coagulation factors, including fibrinogen, proteins C and S, antithrombin	Increases coagulation factors ~2%
Cryoprecipitate	10–15	Fibrinogen, factor VIII, vWF	Increases fibrinogen level 0.1 g/L

FFP = fresh-frozen plasma; Hct = hematocrit; Hb = hemoglobin; PRBCs = packed red blood cells; RBCs = red blood cells; vWF = von Willebrand factor.
Reproduced with permission from Kasper DL, Fauci AS, Longo DL, et al: Harrison's Principles of Internal Medicine, 19th ed. New York: McGraw-Hill; 2015.

with significant hemolysis, laboratory values will be altered. Specifically, serum haptoglobin levels will be lowered; serum lactate dehydrogenase and bilirubin levels will be increased; and serum and urine hemoglobin levels will be elevated. Serum creatinine and electrolyte levels and coagulation studies additionally are ordered. To prevent renal toxicity, diuresis is prompted with intravenous crystalloids and administration of furosemide or mannitol. Alkalinization of urine may prevent precipitation of hemoglobin within the renal tubules, and therefore, intravenous bicarbonate also may be given.

In contrast to acute hemolytic transfusion reaction, *delayed hemolytic transfusion* reactions may develop days or weeks later. Patients often lack acute symptoms, but lowered hemoglobin levels, fever, jaundice, and hemoglobinemia may be noted. Clinical intervention typically is not required in these cases.

Febrile nonhemolytic transfusion reaction is characterized by chills and a greater than 1°C rise in temperature and is the most common transfusion reaction. Blood transfusion typically is stopped to exclude a hemolytic reaction, and treatment is supportive. For patients with a previous history of febrile reaction, premedication with an antipyretic such as acetaminophen prior to transfusion is reasonable.

Last, an *allergic reaction* can follow an antibody-mediated response to donor plasma proteins. Urticaria alone may develop during transfusion and typically is not associated with serious sequelae. The transfusion does not need to be stopped, and treatment with an antihistamine, such as diphenhydramine (Benadryl) 50 mg orally or intramuscularly, usually suffices. Rarely, an anaphylactic reaction may complicate transfusion, and treatment follows that for classic anaphylaxis (Table 27-2, p. 596).

Infectious complications associated with packed RBC transfusion are uncommon. The risk for transmission of HIV and hepatitis B and C virus has diminished over the past decade, and bacterial contamination now stands as a greater infection risk. In addition, emerging infection concerns include transmission of West Nile virus, transfusion-transmitted virus (TTV), hepatitis G, Epstein-Barr virus, and Creutzfeldt-Jakob disease (Luban, 2005).

Transfusion-related acute lung injury (TRALI) is an infrequent but serious complication of blood component therapy that is similar clinically to acute respiratory distress syndrome (ARDS). Symptoms develop within 6 hours of transfusion and may include extreme respiratory distress, frothy sputum, hypotension, fever, and tachycardia. Noncardiogenic pulmonary edema with diffuse bilateral pulmonary infiltrates on chest radiography is characteristic (Toy, 2005). Treatment of TRALI is supportive and focuses on oxygenation and blood pressure support (Silliman, 2005; Swanson, 2006).

■ Platelet Replacement

For patients with moderate hemorrhage, RBC transfusion typically is sufficient, but for patients with severe hemorrhage, platelet transfusion also may be indicated. Platelets may be acquired from a single individual during plateletpheresis and are termed *single-donor platelets*. Alternatively, platelets may be derived from random units of whole blood and are referred to as *random-donor platelets*.

Fewer platelets are harvested from a unit of whole blood compared with the amount removed during donor plateletpheresis. Specifically, a single-donor platelet dose contains at least 3×10^{11} platelets in 250 to 300 mL of plasma, and this approximates the dose from six random-donor platelet concentrates. Each random-donor platelet concentrate contain 5.5×10^{10} platelets suspended in approximately 50 mL of plasma. Each concentrate transfused should raise the platelet count by 5 to 10×10^9/L, and the usual therapeutic dose is one platelet concentrate per 10 kg of body weight. Five to six concentrates provide a typical adult dose. Donor plasma must be compatible with recipient erythrocytes because a few RBCs are invariably transfused along with the platelets. Only platelets from D-negative donors should be given to D-negative recipients.

Surgical patients with bleeding usually require platelet transfusion if the platelet count is less than 50×10^9/L and rarely require therapy if it is greater than 100×10^9/L (American Society of Anesthesiologists, 2015). With counts between 50 and 100×10^9/L, the decision to provide platelet transfusion is based on a patient's risk for additional significant bleeding.

■ Factor Replacement

Fresh-frozen plasma (FFP) is one option for factor replacement and is prepared from whole blood or by plasmapheresis. It is stored frozen, and approximately 30 minutes are required for it to thaw. One unit contains all coagulation factors, including 2 to 5 mg/mL of fibrinogen in 250 mL of volume. Recommended FFP dosing is 15 mL/kg. Fresh-frozen plasma is used commonly as first-line hemostatic therapy in massive hemorrhage because it replaces multiple coagulation factors. It is considered in a bleeding woman with a fibrinogen level below 1.0 g/L or with abnormal prothrombin and partial thromboplastin times.

Another option, cryoprecipitate, is prepared from fresh-frozen plasma and contains fibrinogen, factor VIII, von Willebrand factor, factor XIII, and fibronectin. Cryoprecipitate was developed and used originally for treatment of hemophilia A and von Willebrand disease. However, specific factor concentrates are now available for these disorders, and thus, the clinical indications for cryoprecipitate are limited. Fresh-frozen plasma provides all coagulation factors and is favored in severe hemorrhage over cryoprecipitate. However, cryoprecipitate is an excellent source of fibrinogen and may be indicated if fibrinogen levels persist below 1.0 g/L despite administration of fresh-frozen plasma, such as in disseminated intravascular coagulopathy (DIC). The dose of cryoprecipitate is usually 2 mL/kg of body weight, and each unit contains approximately 15 mL volume. One unit typically increases the fibrinogen level by 10 mg/dL (Erber, 2006).

ADJACENT ORGAN SURGICAL INJURY

■ Lower Urinary Tract

Sound anatomic knowledge, adequate operating exposure, meticulous technique, and surgical experience are essential to avoid surrounding organ injury during pelvic surgery. The lower gastrointestinal and urinary tracts are closely related to the female reproductive organs, and disease processes, anatomic distortion, and adverse operating conditions can increase their injury risk.

Iatrogenic damage to the lower urinary tract is common, and up to 75 percent of ureter or bladder injuries sustained during gynecologic surgery occur during hysterectomy (Walters, 2007). Most injuries have no antecedent risk factors, but high-risk elements are ideally sought preoperatively. These include compromised visibility from large pelvic masses, hemorrhage, pregnancy, obesity, inadequate incision, suboptimal retraction, and poor lighting. Additionally, scarring or anatomic distortion from cervical and broad ligament leiomyomas, malignancy, endometriosis, pelvic organ prolapse, and prior pelvic infection, surgery, or radiation are risks (Brandes, 2004; Francis, 2002).

Patients who sustain surgical injury to the bladder or ureter suffer significantly greater morbidity. In one case-control study, women with injury to the lower urinary tract during abdominal hysterectomy had significantly greater operative time, estimated blood loss, blood transfusion rates, febrile morbidity, and postoperative stay length than their respective controls (Carley, 2002).

■ Bladder Injury

Cystotomy is common and complicates approximately 0.3 to 11 per 1000 benign gynecologic surgeries, especially urogyneco-

logic procedures and hysterectomy (Gilmour, 2006; Mathevet, 2001). In sum, depending on the procedure, the bladder may be at greater risk during: (1) initial abdominal entry when incising the anterior parietal peritoneum, (2) dissection within the space of Retzius, (3) vaginal epithelium dissection during anterior colporrhaphy, or (4) hysterectomy when dissecting in the vesicocervical space, entering the anterior vagina, or suturing the vaginal cuff. With hysterectomy, bladder injury traditionally has been associated more often with the vaginal hysterectomy, but some data suggest that laparoscopic procedures pose the greatest risk (Francis, 2002; Frankman, 2010; Harris, 1997). Preventatively, clear identification of the bladder, gentle retraction, meticulous surgical technique, sharp dissection, and maintenance of a drained bladder intraoperatively are standard principles.

Cystotomy is suspected if a Foley bulb, bloody urine, or urine leaking into the operative field is seen. During laparoscopy, the Foley bag may also distend with gas from the pneumoperitoneum. For diagnosis, retrograde instillation of sterile milk through a catheter confirms injury and delineates its full extent. This is superior to methylene blue and indigo carmine dyes, as infant formula does not stain surrounding tissues and is readily available. In addition, small defects can be difficult to identify and repair if the tissues surrounding the defect become dye stained. Prior to repair, cystoscopy is indicated for any bladder base injury to assess ureteral patency. In addition, the full extent of injury can be defined, and the bladder can be evaluated for additional injuries or intravesical sutures. If bladder distension cannot be maintained during cystoscopy or if the patient is not in dorsal lithotomy, the ureteral orifices can also be evaluated grossly through the cystotomy site. If the cystotomy is small, suprapubic teloscopy, which is described in Chapter 45, is also an option, or the cystotomy can be extended to allow evaluation.

Repair during the primary surgery is preferred and lowers risks of later vesicovaginal fistula formation. Principles of repair include injury delineation; wide mobilization of surrounding tissues; tension-free, multilayered, watertight closure; and adequate postoperative bladder drainage (Utrie, 1998). Suture identified in the bladder is cut, as persistence can lead to cystitis, stone formation, or both. Needle-stick and subcentimeter lacerations can be managed conservatively. Larger defects may be closed in two or three layers with a running stitch using 3-0 absorbable or delayed-absorbable suture (Fig. 40-32). The first layer inverts the mucosa into the bladder, and subsequent layers reapproximate the bladder muscularis and serosa. In the area of the trigone, the ureters are typically stented first, and the repair may be performed with interrupted sutures to avoid ureteral kinking (Popert, 2004). Postoperatively, continuous bladder drainage is continued for 7 to 10 days (Utrie, 1998). Evidence is conflicting regarding the use of prophylactic antibiotics for the expected duration of catheterization, and thus remains at the provider's discretion.

■ Urethral Injury

The female urethra is rarely injured during gynecologic surgery, but cystoscopy, urethral diverticulum repairs, antiincontinence operations, and possibly anterior colporrhaphy are at-risk procedures. Repair is completed with 3-0 or 4-0 absorbable suture in an interrupted fashion and in multiple layers, if possible. Similar to cystotomy, a Foley catheter is typically placed

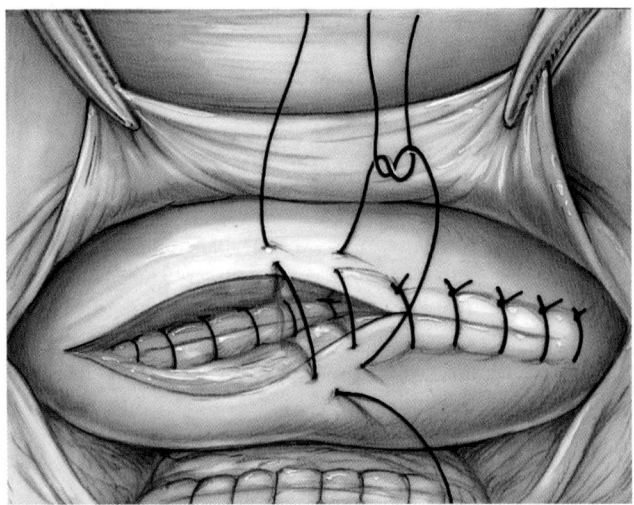

FIGURE 40-32 Cystotomy repair. The primary layer inverts the bladder mucosa with running or interrupted sutures of 3-0 delayed-absorbable or absorbable suture. Second and possibly a third layer approximate the bladder muscularis to reinforce the incision closure. (Reproduced with permission from Cunningham FG, Vandorsten JP, Gilstrap LC: Operative Obstetrics, 2nd ed. New York: McGraw-Hill; 2002.)

postoperatively for 7 to 10 days, with antibiotic prophylaxis provided at the surgeon's discretion (Francis, 2002).

■ Ureteral Injury

This is uncommon in benign gynecologic surgery, and the incidence approximates 0.2 to 7.3 per 1000 surgeries. For hysterectomy, the highest rate of ureteral injury is linked with laparoscopic hysterectomy, and the lowest with vaginal hysterectomy (Gilmour, 2006). Other associated procedures include operations for pelvic organ prolapse, incontinence, malignancy, or endometriosis (Patel, 2009; Utrie, 1998).

The ureter is 25 to 30 cm long, and its anatomy is described in Chapter 38 (p. 816). Gynecologic ureteral injury typically occurs in the distal third and includes transection, ligation, kinking, and crushing (Brandes, 2004; Utrie, 1998). Trauma to the outer sheath can also disrupt ureteral blood supply. Of these, the ureter more often is transected or kinked, and each accounts for approximately 40 percent of injuries. During hysterectomy, the most common trauma site is at the level of the uterine artery and accounts for 80 percent of injuries (Ibeanu, 2009). The ureter is also vulnerable near the pelvic brim during adnexectomy and at the distal uterosacral ligaments. Mechanisms of injury include clamping or suturing with the ureter poorly visualized. Thermal insult or devascularization may lead to stricture or leak.

Injury prevention measures include preoperative risk evaluation and if indicated, intravenous pyelography (IVP) or computed tomography (CT). Ureteral stenting assists with intraoperative recognition but does not necessarily prevent injury. As with bladder injury, the best prevention is sound intraoperative technique and direct visualization of the peristalsing ureter. Also, the ureter may be felt to "snap" if palpated and stretched along its course on the broad ligament's medial leaf. However, vessels, adipose tissue, and peritoneal folds can mimic this.

Diagnosis

Iatrogenic injury ideally is diagnosed early, as immediate repair is associated with improved outcomes and less patient morbidity (Neuman, 1991; Sakellariou, 2002). Damage may be seen directly or identified during intraoperative cystoscopy. Intravenous administration of indigo carmine or methylene blue can aid cystoscopic evaluation, with observation of blue-stained urine from the ureteral orifices. This is described fully in Section 45-1 of the atlas (p. 1057). However, use of the latter may increase given current indigo carmine shortages. With these dyes, blue effluent is usually seen in 5 to 10 minutes. Failure to see dye after 30 to 40 minutes mandates further evaluation with either IVP or ureteral catheterization. Unfortunately, normal-appearing findings at cystoscopy do not guarantee ureteral integrity, as nonobstructive, partially obstructive, or late ureteral injuries may be unrecognized.

Diagnosing injury shortly after surgery is challenging, as patient symptoms may be attributable to other causes. Thus, thorough patient evaluation and a high clinical suspicion are crucial. Renal damage may begin 24 hours after obstruction and can be irreversible in 1 to 6 weeks (Walter, 2002). Symptoms usually develop about 48 hours after surgery, and fever, abdominal pain, flank pain, and watery discharge may be among these. Findings can include leukocytosis, elevated blood urea nitrogen level, and ileus. Prolonged skin or vaginal drainage suggests a urinary leak, and high creatinine levels in these fluids are diagnostic of urine. Serum creatinine measurement may or may not be helpful. In one retrospective study of 187 patients, a 24-hour postoperative change <0.3 mg/dL from preoperative levels had a specificity of 98 percent and negative predictive value of 100 percent in confirming bilateral ureteral patency. Because an increase >0.2 mg/dL has been associated with obstruction, the authors recommended repeating a creatinine measurement and renal imaging for persistent elevation above this level (Walter, 2002). With elevated serum creatinine levels, calculation of the fractional excretion of sodium (FENa) or assessment of urine sodium levels may also help clarify the renal injury source as prerenal, intrarenal, or postrenal, as described in Chapter 42 (p. 916).

Sonography, CT, or magnetic resonance (MR) imaging will help identify hydronephrosis, urinoma, or abscess. Lack of contrast in the distal ureter on delayed CT images confirms total obstruction (Armenakas, 1999). IVP can also help localize injury. However, IV contrast can be nephrotoxic, and thus CT with contrast may be a less than ideal choice for those with already elevated creatinine levels. Retrograde pyelography with fluoroscopic guidance and attempted retrograde ureteral stent placement can be considered in cases where suspicion remains high, and IVP is contraindicated or has equivocal findings. All of these imaging modalities can be used to diagnose injury in both the early and late postoperative periods.

Treatment

The best repair method depends on the location, extent, time from surgery, and mechanism of injury. Expert assistance from a urogynecologist, gynecologic oncologist, or urologist may be prudent. The ureter can be repaired by stenting, reimplantation, or end-to-end reanastomosis. For low-grade sheath injuries from clamping or suturing, removal of the insult and stent placement may be sufficient. For incomplete obstruction or injury identified postoperatively, stenting alone can resolve injuries in up to 80 percent of cases. For more extensive injury, either reimplantation or reanastomosis is performed (Utrie, 1998).

Reimplantation, namely, *ureteroneocystotomy*, is preferred for injuries within 6 cm of the bladder. Uncommonly with this, if the ureter is short, a psoas hitch, that is, mobilizing the bladder and attaching it to the psoas muscle tendon, may be necessary to bridge the gap and relieve tension on the repair. An alternative to the psoas hitch is a Boari flap. In this procedure, the bladder ipsilateral to the injury is mobilized, and a pedicle of anterior bladder wall is fashioned into a tube to bridge to the ureter.

For injuries greater than 7 cm from the bladder, ureteral reanastomosis, that is, *ureteroureterostomy*, is preferred. Rarely, transureteroureterostomy is needed for a more proximal injury or one in which the bladder cannot be mobilized. With this procedure, the injured ureter is tunneled across and connected to the healthy ureter.

Little evidence guides the decision for reoperation in the early postoperative period. Intraoperatively, tissues are in their best condition, and the likelihood for successful repair is great. However, most iatrogenic injuries are recognized after a delay and tend to be complex (Brandes, 2004). In general, reexploration within the first few days appears to be well tolerated, leads to good outcomes, and is not technically difficult (Preston, 2000; Stanhope, 1991). Firm recommendations regarding reoperation beyond this early postoperative period are lacking, but reexploration 2 to 3 weeks after initial surgery is difficult due to inflammation, fibrosis, adhesions, hematoma, and distorted anatomy (Brandes, 2004).

For delayed diagnoses, retrograde stenting is unsuccessful in 50 to 95 percent of cases and recommended only for certain low-grade injuries (Brandes, 2004). Occasionally, an antegrade stent can be placed percutaneously, which will avoid the need for laparotomy, provided there is no ureteral leak or stricture. More extensive damage, such as complete transection, cannot be easily stented and is more appropriately repaired by definitive surgery. When diagnosis is significantly delayed, urinary diversion with a percutaneous nephrostomy (PCN) and later repair is preferred. For some low-grade lesions, such as ligation with absorbable suture, proximal urinary diversion by PCN may allow spontaneous healing without further surgery. In addition, PCN diversion may be used as a temporizing measure for patients temporarily unfit for surgery (Preston, 2000).

■ Universal Cystoscopy

Lower urinary tract injury is poorly detected by direct visualization, and rates range from 7 to 12 percent for ureteral trauma and approximate 35 percent for bladder damage (Vakili, 2005). To increase early diagnosis, universal intraoperative cystoscopy has been advocated, and detection rates are near 96 percent (Ibeanu, 2009; Vakili, 2005; Visco, 2001). Proponents argue that the procedure is cost-effective, carries minimal risk, and prevents both postoperative morbidity and liability. Opponents cite overall low rates of injury, imperfect detection rates, increased costs, credentialing problems, and a need for training

(Patel, 2009). Using a decision analysis model, one study estimated that routine cystoscopy was cost-effective when ureteral injury rates were above 1.5 percent for abdominal hysterectomy and 2 percent for vaginal and laparoscopically assisted hysterectomy (Visco, 2001).

Cystoscopy is currently indicated for urogynecologic procedures, but there are no strict recommendations for other routine gynecologic procedures, including hysterectomy (American College of Obstetricians and Gynecologists, 2013; Patel, 2009). At present, the decision remains at the surgeon's discretion. Some have elected selective cystoscopy, or cystoscopy restricted to patients with risk factors or when intraoperative events make injury more likely.

■ Bowel Injury

Injury to the bowel infrequently complicates gynecologic surgery, and rates are <1 percent (Harris, 1997; Makinen, 2001). A traumatic breach during dissection is the most common, particularly if the bowel wall is abnormally fixed by adhesions (Mathevet, 2001; Maxwell, 2004). Additional risks include reduced organ mobility from Crohn disease or diverticulitis, laparoscopic trocar or Veress needle insertion, diathermy use, and anterior abdominal wall entry during laparotomy.

For the gynecologic surgeon, prevention and injury recognition help avoid serious postoperative sequelae. Strict adherence to surgical principles with sharp dissection for adhesions, gentle tissue handling, adequate exposure, light retraction, and sparing use of diathermy near hollow organs is key. Entering through prior abdominal incisions, dissection proceeds methodically in layers. Alternatively, a separate incision or extension of the existing one to an area that has not been previously opened can be considered. After any extensive pelvic dissection, the bowel is systematically inspected along its entire length to detect serosal defects and unrecognized perforation. At suspected sites, the bowel is scrutinized for mucosal eversion and content leakage. Evaluation is gentle to avoid additional damage.

Management of enterotomy depends on the site and size of injury, surgeon skill, degree of blood supply compromise, and time of recognition. With the small intestines, serosal defects may be either left alone or reinforced with small-gauge absorbable suture (Maxwell, 2004). Short small-intestine enterotomies may be repaired in layers using fine absorbable suture. During repair, rubber-shod clamps are placed across the intestinal lumen on either side of the wound to prevent content spill. To avoid narrowing of the bowel lumen, the suture line should lie transverse to the normal axis of the intestine (Stanton, 1987). Postoperative antibiotics are typically not required.

Large-bowel injuries increase the risk of fecal peritonitis, sepsis, and poor wound healing. Serosal defects and small lacerations may be managed similarly to those of the small intestine. For more extensive injuries or fecal soiling that may require resection, diversion, or complicated repair, consultation with a gynecologic oncologist or colorectal surgeon is often indicated. Broad-spectrum antibiotic prophylaxis is provided for the next 24 hours in these cases. In general, for both small and large intestinal injuries, early feeding is acceptable and not associated with repair site complications (Fanning, 2001).

Rectal injury occurs most commonly during vaginal surgery, especially during posterior colpotomy or posterior colporrhaphy. These injuries are typically midline, extraperitoneal, and less than 2 cm. Postmenopausal status, prior posterior colporrhaphy, or pathology that obliterates the cul-de-sac or limits organ mobility increases injury risk (Hoffman, 1999; Mathevet, 2001). Prevention centers on careful examination under anesthesia to detect cul-de-sac fullness or uterine immobility, sharp dissection with the aid of a guiding rectal finger, and vasoconstricting agent use to reduce obscuring operative field bleeding.

Rectal injury may be extraperitoneal or intraperitoneal, and rectal examination will typically detect the injury and delineate its borders. Minor intraperitoneal injuries with minimal or no contamination can be repaired primarily in layers as described previously. Larger injuries with gross soiling may require expert consultation. Broad-spectrum antibiotic prophylaxis is provided for the next 24 hours in these cases.

Low extraperitoneal rectal injury during vaginal surgery in a healthy patient can be repaired primarily and rarely requires a diverting colostomy or abdominal repair. Repair is accomplished transvaginally using two to three layers of fine absorbable suture. The peritoneum may be used as an additional layer for injuries near the peritoneal reflection. During repair, a digit in the rectum exposes the defect, tissues surrounding the defect are mobilized, the site is copiously irrigated, and appropriate antibiotic prophylaxis is provided for 24 hours (Hoffman, 1999). In general, small (<2 cm) rectal injuries recognized and repaired at the time of vaginal surgery tend to heal well without complications or fistula formation (Mathevet, 2001). Diet can be advanced as tolerated, but a stool softener is recommended once the patient is taking solid foods (Hoffman, 1999).

REFERENCES

Alayed N, Alghanaim N, Tan X, et al: Preemptive use of gabapentin in abdominal hysterectomy: a systematic review and meta-analysis. Obstet Gynecol 123:1221, 2014

Aletti GD, Dowdy SC, Podratz KC, et al: Surgical treatment of diaphragm disease correlates with improved survival in optimally debulked advanced stage ovarian cancer. Gynecol Oncol 100(2):283, 2006

Amaral J: Electrosurgery and ultrasound for cutting and coagulating tissue in minimally invasive surgery. In Soper N, Swanstrom L, Eubanks W (eds): Mastery of Endoscopic and Laparoscopic Surgery. Philadelphia, Lippincott Williams & Wilkins, 2005, p 67

American College of Obstetricians and Gynecologists: The role of cystourethroscopy in the generalist obstetrician-gynecologist practice. Committee Opinion No. 372, July 2007, Reaffirmed 2013

American Society of Anesthesiologists: Practice guidelines for perioperative blood management: an updated report by the American Society of Anesthesiologists Task Force on Perioperative Blood Management. Anesthesiol 122(2):241, 2015

Anderson RM, Romfh RF: Technique in the Use of Surgical Tools. New York, Appleton-Century-Crofts, 1980

Anderton J, Keen R, Neave R: The lithotomy position. Positioning the Surgical Patient. London, Butterworths, 1988, p 20

Armenakas NA: Current methods of diagnosis and management of ureteral injuries. World J Urol 17:8, 1999

Aszmann OC, Dellon ES, Dellon AL: Anatomical course of the lateral femoral cutaneous nerve and its susceptibility to compression and injury. Plast Reconst Surg 100(3):600, 1997

Ayers JW, Morley GW: Surgical incision for cesarean section. Obstet Gynecol 70(5):706, 1987

Barrington J, Dalury D, Emerson R, et al: Improving patient outcomes through advanced pain management techniques in total hip and knee arthroplasty. Am J Orthop 42(10 Suppl):S1, 2013

Baskett PJ: ABC of major trauma. Management of hypovolaemic shock. BMJ 300(6737):1453, 1990

Batra EK, Franz DA, Towler MA, et al: Influence of surgeon's tying technique on knot security. J Appl Biomater 4:241, 1993

Baxter Healthcare: Floseal hemostatic matrix: instructions for use. Hayward, Baxter Healthcare, 2014

Beckley ML, Ghafourpour KL, Indresano AT: The use of argon beam coagulation to control hemorrhage: a case report and review of the technology. J Oral Maxillofacial Surg 62:615, 2004

Bennett RG: Selection of wound closure materials. J Am Acad Dermatol 18(4 Pt 1):619, 1988

Bhende S, Rothenburger S, Spangler DJ, et al: In vitro assessment of microbial barrier properties of Dermabond topical skin adhesive. Surg Infect 3(3):251, 2002

Bleich AT, Rahn DD, Wieslander CK, et al: Posterior division of the internal iliac artery: anatomic variations and clinical applications. Am J Obstet Gynecol 197(6):658.e1, 2007

Blomstedt B, Osterberg B, Bergstrand A: Suture material and bacterial transport. An experimental study. Acta Chirurg Scand 143(2):71, 1977

Blondeel PNV, Murphy JW, Debrosse D, et al: Closure of long surgical incisions with a new formulation of 2-octylcyanoacrylate tissue adhesive versus commercially available methods. Am J Surg 188(3):307, 2004

Bose P, Regan F, Paterson-Brown S: Improving the accuracy of estimated blood loss at obstetric haemorrhage using clinical reconstructions. BJOG 113(8):919, 2006

Brandes S, Coburn M, Armenakas N, et al: Consensus on genitourinary trauma: diagnosis and management of ureteric injury: an evidence-based analysis. BJUI 94:277, 2004

Brecher ME, Goodnough LT: The rise and fall of preoperative autologous blood donation. Transfusion 42(12):1618, 2002

Brill AI, Nezhat F, Nezhat C, et al: The incidence of adhesions after prior laparotomy: a laparoscopic appraisal. Obstet Gynecol 85:269, 1995

Bucknall TE: Factors influencing wound complications: a clinical and experimental study. Ann R Coll Surg Engl 65(2):71, 1983

Burchell RC: Physiology of internal iliac artery ligation. J Obstet Gynaecol Br Commonwealth 75(6):642, 1968

Burkhart SS, Wirth MA, Simonick M, et al: Loop security as a determinant of tissue fixation security. Arthroscopy 14:773, 1998

Campbell JA, Temple WJ, Frank CB, et al: A biomechanical study of suture pullout in linea alba. Surgery 106:888, 1989

Cardosi RJ, Cox CS, Hoffman MS: Postoperative neuropathies after major pelvic surgery. Obstet Gynecol 100(2):240, 2002

Carless PA, Henry DA, Carson JL, et al: Transfusion thresholds and other strategies for guiding allogeneic red blood cell transfusion. Cochrane Database Syst Rev 10:CD002042, 2010

Carley ME, McIntire D, Carley JM, et al: Incidence, risk factors and morbidity of unintended bladder or ureter injury during hysterectomy. Int Urogynecol J 13:18, 2002

Carlson MA, Condon RE: Polyglyconate (Maxon) versus nylon suture in midline abdominal incision closure: a prospective randomized trial. Am Surgeon 61(11):980, 1995

Carney J, McDonell J, Ochana A, et al: The transversus abdominis plane block provides effective postoperative analgesia in patients undergoing total abdominal hysterectomy. Anesth Analg 107:2056, 2008

Chanrachakul B, Likittanasombut P, Prasertsawat P, et al: Lidocaine versus plain saline for pain relief in fractional curettage: a randomized controlled trial. Obstet Gynecol 98(4):592, 2001

Chappell D, Jacob M, Hofmann-Kiefer K, et al: A rational approach to perioperative fluid management. Anesthesiology 109:723, 2008

Chen SS, Lin AT, Chen KK, et al: Femoral neuropathy after pelvic surgery. Urology 46(4):575, 1995

Cicinelli E, Didonna T, Ambrosi G, et al: Topical anaesthesia for diagnostic hysteroscopy and endometrial biopsy in postmenopausal women: a randomised placebo-controlled double-blind study. BJOG 104(3):316, 1997

Cicinelli E, Didonna T, Schonauer LM, et al: Paracervical anesthesia for hysteroscopy and endometrial biopsy in postmenopausal women: a randomized, double-blind, placebo-controlled study. J Reprod Med Obstet Gynecol 43(12):1014, 1998

Colombo M, Maggioni A, Parma G, et al: A randomized comparison of continuous versus interrupted mass closure of midline incisions in patients with gynecologic cancer. Obstet Gynecol 89(5 Pt 1):684, 1997

Crossley GH, Poole JE, Rozner MA, et al: The Heart Rhythm Society (HRS)/ American Society of Anesthesiologists (ASA) Expert Consensus Statement on the perioperative management of patients with implantable defibrillators, pacemakers and arrhythmia monitors: facilities and patient management. Heart Rhythm 8(7):1114, 2011

Davis JW, Shackford SR, Mackersie RC, et al: Base deficit as a guide to volume resuscitation. J Trauma 28:1464, 1988

Deatrick KB, Doherty GM: Power sources in surgery. In Doherty GM (ed): Current Surgical Diagnosis and Treatment, 14th ed. New York, McGraw-Hill Education, 2015

Demirci F, Ozdemir I, Safak A, et al: Comparison of colour Doppler indices of pelvic arteries in women with bilateral hypogastric artery ligation and controls. J Obstet Gynaecol 25(3):273, 2005

De Oliveira G Jr, Agarwal D, Benzon H: Perioperative single dose ketorolac to prevent postoperative pain: a meta-analysis of randomized trials. Anesth Analg 114:424, 2012

De Oliveira G Jr, Castro-Alves L, Nader A, et al: Transversus abdominis plane block to ameliorate postoperative pain outcomes after laparoscopic surgery: a meta-analysis of randomized controlled trials. Anesth Analg 118:454, 2014

Deppe G, Malviya VK, Malone JM Jr: Debulking surgery for ovarian cancer with the Cavitron Ultrasonic Surgical Aspirator (CUSA)—a preliminary report. Gynecol Oncol 31(1):223, 1988

Dinsmore RC: Understanding surgical knot security: a proposal to standardize the literature. J Am Coll Surg 180(6):689, 1995

Dorian R: Anesthesia of the surgical patient. In Brunicardi F, Andersen D, Billiar T, et al (eds): Schwartz's Principles of Surgery, 10th ed. New York, McGraw-Hill, 2015

Ducic I, Dellon L, Larson EE: Treatment concepts for idiopathic and iatrogenic femoral nerve mononeuropathy. Ann Plast Surg 55(4):397, 2005

Dunn DL: Wound Closure Manual. Somerville, Ethicon, 2004, pp 49, 53

Dzieczkowski JS, Anderson KC: Transfusion biology and therapy. In Longo DL, Fauci AS, Kasper DL, et al (eds): Harrison's Principles of Internal Medicine, 18th ed. New York, McGraw-Hill, 2012

Edelman A, Nichols MD, Leclair C, et al: Four percent intrauterine lidocaine infusion for pain management in first-trimester abortions. Obstet Gynecol 107(2 Pt 1):269, 2006

Edelman A, Nichols MD, Leclair C, et al: Intrauterine lidocaine infusion for pain management in first-trimester abortions. Obstet Gynecol 103(6):1267, 2004

Edlich RF, Panek PH, Rodeheaver GT, et al: Physical and chemical configuration of sutures in the development of surgical infection. Ann Surg 177(6):679, 1973

Erber WN, Perry DJ: Plasma and plasma products in the treatment of massive haemorrhage. Best Pract Res Clin Haematol 19(1):97, 2006

Fanning J, Andrews SA: Early postoperative feeding after major gynecologic surgery: evidence-based scientific medicine. Am J Obstet Gynecol 185(1):1, 2001

Franchi M, Ghezzi F, Benedetti-Panici PL, et al: A multicentre collaborative study on the use of cold scalpel and electrocautery for midline abdominal incision. Am J Surg 181(2):128, 2001

Franchi M, Ghezzi F, Zanaboni F, et al: Nonclosure of peritoneum at radical abdominal hysterectomy and pelvic node dissection: a randomized study. Obstet Gynecol 90(4 Pt 1):622, 1997

Francis SL, Magrina JF, Novicki D, et al: Intraoperative injuries of the urinary tract. J Gynecol Oncol 7:65, 2002

Frankman EA, Wang L, Bunker CH, et al: Lower urinary tract injury in women in the United States, 1979–2006. Am J Obstet Gynecol 202(5):495e1, 2010

Gallup DC, Gallup DG, Nolan TE: Use of a subcutaneous closed drainage system and antibiotics in obese gynecologic patients. Am J Obstet Gynecol 175:358, 1996

Geiger D, Debus ES, Ziegler UE, et al: Capillary activity of surgical sutures and suture-dependent bacterial transport: a qualitative study. Surg Infect 6(4):377, 2005

Giacalone PL, Daures JP, Vignal J, et al: Pfannenstiel versus Maylard incision for cesarean delivery: a randomized controlled trial. Obstet Gynecol 99(5 Pt 1):745, 2002

Gilmour DT, Das S, Flowerdew G: Rates of urinary tract injury from gynecologic surgery and the role of intraoperative cystoscopy. Obstet Gynecol 107(6):1366, 2006

Gilstrap LC 3rd: Management of postpartum hemorrhage. In Gilstrap LC, Cunningham FG, Vandorsten JP (eds): Operative Obstetrics, 2nd ed. McGraw-Hill, New York, 2002

Goldman JA, Feldberg D, Dicker D, et al: Femoral neuropathy subsequent to abdominal hysterectomy. A comparative study. Eur J Obstet Gynecol Reprod Biol 20(6):385, 1985

Goodnough LT: Autologous blood donation. Anesthesiol Clin North Am 23(2):263, 2005

Gorgas D: Transfusion therapy: blood and blood products. In Roberts J, Hedges J, Chanmugam AS, et al (eds): Clinical Procedures in Emergency Medicine. Philadelphia, WB Saunders, 2004

Gostout BS, Cliby WA, Podratz KC: Prevention and management of acute intraoperative bleeding. Clin Obstet Gynecol 45(2):481, 2002

Grantcharov TP, Rosenberg J: Vertical compared with transverse incisions in abdominal surgery. Eur J Surg 167(4):260, 2001

Greenall MJ, Evans M, Pollock AV: Midline or transverse laparotomy? A random controlled clinical trial. Part I: influence on healing. Br J Surg 67(3):188, 1980

Greenberg CC, Regenbogen SE, Studdert DM, et al: Patterns of communication breakdowns resulting in injury to surgical patients. J Am Coll Surg 204:533, 2007

Gunderson PE: The half-hitch knot: a rational alternative to the square knot. Am J Surg 54:538, 1987

Gupta JK, Dinas K, Khan KS: To peritonealize or not to peritonealize? A randomized trial at abdominal hysterectomy. Am J Obstet Gynecol 178(4):796, 1998

Guvenal T, Duran B, Kemirkoprulu N, et al: Prevention of superficial wound disruption in Pfannenstiel incisions by using a subcutaneous drain. Int J Gynecol Obstet 77:151, 2002

Gyr T, Ghezzi F, Arslanagic S, et al: Minimal invasive laparoscopic hysterectomy with ultrasonic scalpel. Am J Surg 181(6):516, 2001

Hambley R, Hebda PA, Abell E, et al: Wound healing of skin incisions produced by ultrasonically vibrating knife, scalpel, electrosurgery, and carbon dioxide laser. J Dermatol Surg Oncol 14(11):1213, 1988

Harold KL, Pollinger H, Matthews BD, et al: Comparison of ultrasonic energy, bipolar thermal energy, and vascular clips for the hemostasis of small-, medium-, and large-sized arteries. Surg Endosc 17(8):1228, 2003

Harris WJ: Complications of hysterectomy. Clin Obstet Gynecol 40(4):928, 1997

Healey MA, Davis RE, Liu FC, et al: Lactated Ringer's is superior to normal saline in a model of massive hemorrhage and resuscitation. J Trauma 45(5):894, 1998

Hébert PC, Wells G, Blajchman MA, et al: A multicenter, randomized, controlled clinical trial of transfusion requirements in critical care. Transfusion Requirements in Critical Care Investigators, Canadian Critical Care Trials Group. N Engl J Med 340(6):409, 1999

Heniford BT, Matthews BD, Sing RF, et al: Initial results with an electrothermal bipolar vessel sealer. Surg Endosc 15(8):799, 2001

Henry DA, Carless PA, Moxey AJ, et al: Pre-operative autologous donation for minimising perioperative allogeneic blood transfusion. Cochrane Database Syst Rev 2:CD003602, 2002

Hoffman MS, Lynch C, Lockhart J, et al: Injury of the rectum during vaginal surgery. Am J Obstet Gynecol 181:274, 1999

Hong JY, Kim J: Use of paracervical analgesia for outpatient hysteroscopic surgery: a randomized, double-blind, placebo-controlled study. Amb Surg 12(4):181, 2006

Hsieh LF, Liaw ES, Cheng HY, et al: Bilateral femoral neuropathy after vaginal hysterectomy. Arch Phys Med Rehabil 79(8):1018, 1998

Hunt BJ: The current place of tranexamic acid in the management of bleeding. Anaesthesia 70 (Suppl 1):50, 2015

Hurt J, Unger JB, Ivy JJ, et al: Tying a loop-to-strand suture: is it safe? Am J Obstet Gynecol 192:1094, 2005

Ibeanu OA, Chesson RR, Echols KT, et al: Urinary tract injury during hysterectomy based on universal cystoscopy. Obstet Gynecol 113:6, 2009

Irvin W, Andersen W, Taylor P, et al: Minimizing the risk of neurologic injury in gynecologic surgery. Obstet Gynecol 103(2):374, 2004

Ivy JJ, Unger JB, Hurt J, et al: The effect of number of throws on knot security with non-identical sliding knots. Am J Obstet Gynecol 191:1618, 2004a

Ivy JJ, Unger JB, Mukherjee D: Knot integrity with nonidentical and parallel sliding knots. Am J Obstet Gynecol 190:83, 2004b

Iyer C, Robertson D, Lenkovsky F, et al. Gastric bypass and on-Q pump: effectiveness of soaker catheter system on recovery of bariatric surgery patients. Surg Obes Relat Dis 6(2):181, 2010

Jallo GI: CUSA EXcel ultrasonic aspiration system. Neurosurgery 48(3):695, 2001

Jenkins TR: It's time to challenge surgical dogma with evidence-based data. Am J Obstet Gynecol 189(2):423, 2003

Joint Commission: Universal protocol for preventing wrong site, wrong procedure, and wrong person surgery. Oakbrook Terrace, Joint Commission, 2009

Joshi G: Intraoperative fluid restriction improves outcome after major elective gastrointestinal surgery. Anesth Analg 101:601, 2005

Kanter MH, van Maanen D, Anders KH, et al: A study of an educational intervention to decrease inappropriate preoperative autologous blood donation: its effectiveness and the effect on subsequent transfusion rates in elective hysterectomy. Transfusion 39(8):801, 1999

Kanter MH, van Maanen D, Anders KH, et al: Preoperative autologous blood donations before elective hysterectomy. JAMA 276(10):798, 1996

Karger R, Kretschmer V: Modern concepts of autologous haemotherapy. Transfus Apher Sci 32(2):185, 2005

Katz KH, Desciak EB, Maloney ME: The optimal application of surgical adhesive tape strips. Dermatol Surg 25(9):686, 1999

Kauko M: New techniques using the ultrasonic scalpel in laparoscopic hysterectomy. Curr Opin Obstet Gynecol 10(4):303, 1998

Kisielinski K, Conze J, Murken AH, et al: The Pfannenstiel or so called "bikini cut": still effective more than 100 years after first description. Hernia 8(3):177, 2004

Knockaert DC, Boonen AL, Bruyninckx FL, et al: Electromyographic findings in ilioinguinal-iliohypogastric nerve entrapment syndrome. Acta Clin Belg 51(3):156, 1996

Kolle D, Tamussino K, Hanzal E, et al: Bleeding complications with the tension-free vaginal tape operation. Am J Obstet Gynecol 193(6):2045, 2005

Kushner DM, LaGalbo R, Connor JP, et al: Use of a bupivacaine continuous wound infusion system in gynecologic oncology: a randomized trial. Obstet Gynecol 106(2):227, 2005

Kuuva N, Nilsson CG: A nationwide analysis of complications associated with the tension-free vaginal tape (TVT) procedure. Acta Obstet Gynecol Scand 81(1):72, 2002

Kvist-Poulsen H, Borel J: Iatrogenic femoral neuropathy subsequent to abdominal hysterectomy: incidence and prevention. Obstet Gynecol 60(4):516, 1982

Lacy PD, Burke PE, O'Regan M, et al: The comparison of type of incision for transperitoneal abdominal aortic surgery based on postoperative respiratory complications and morbidity. Eur J Vasc Surg 8(1):52, 1994

Lammers R, Trott A: Methods of wound closure. In Roberts J, Hedges J (eds): Clinical Procedures in Emergency Medicine. Philadelphia, WB Saunders, 2004, p 655

Lau WC, Lo WK, Tam WH, et al: Paracervical anaesthesia in outpatient hysteroscopy: a randomised double-blind placebo-controlled trial. BJOG 106(4):356, 1999

Leaper DJ, Pollock AV, Evans M: Abdominal wound closure: a trial of nylon, polyglycolic acid and steel sutures. Br J Surg 64(8):603, 1977

Lichtenberg ES, Paul M, Jones H: First trimester surgical abortion practices: a survey of National Abortion Federation members. Contraception 64(6):345, 2001

Lipscomb GH, Ling FW, Stovall TG, et al: Peritoneal closure at vaginal hysterectomy: a reassessment. Obstet Gynecol 87(1):40, 1996

Lo IK, Burkhart SS, Chan KC, et al: Arthroscopic knots: determining the optimal balance of loop security and knot security. Arthroscopy 20:489, 2004

Long JB, Elland RJ, Hentz JG, et al: Randomized trial of preemptive local analgesia in vaginal surgery. Int Urogynecol J Pelvic Floor Dysfunct 20(1):5, 2009

Luban NL: Transfusion safety: where are we today? Ann NY Acad Sci 1054:325, 2005

Lucci JA: Urologic and gastrointestinal injuries. In Gilstrap LC, Cunningham FG, Vandorsten JP (eds): Operative Obstetrics, 2nd ed. McGraw-Hill, New York, 2002

Luijendijk RW, Jeekel J, Storm RK, et al: The low transverse Pfannenstiel incision and the prevalence of incisional hernia and nerve entrapment. Ann Surg 225(4):365, 1997

Madjdpour C, Spahn DR, Weiskopf RB: Anemia and perioperative red blood cell transfusion: a matter of tolerance. Crit Care Med 34(5 Suppl):S102, 2006

Makinen J, Johansson J, Tomas C, et al: Morbidity of 10110 hysterectomies by type of approach. Hum Reprod 16(7):1473, 2001

Masterson B: Intraoperative hemorrhage. In Nichols D, DeLancey J (eds): Clinical Problems, Injuries and Complications of Gynecologic and Obstetric Surgery. Baltimore, Williams & Wilkins, 1995, p 14

Mathevet P, Valencia P, Cousin C, et al: Operative injuries during vaginal hysterectomy. Eur J Obstet Gynecol Reprod Biol 97:71, 2001

Maxwell DJ (ed): Surgical Techniques in Obstetrics and Gynecology. London, Churchill-Livingstone, 2004

McDaniel LM, Etchill EW, Raval JS, et al: State of the art: massive transfusion. Transfus Med 24(3):138, 2014

Michelassi F, Hurst R: Electrocautery, argon beam coagulation, cryotherapy, and other hemostatic and tissue ablative instruments. In Nyhus L, Baker R, Fischer J (eds): Mastery of Surgery. Boston, Little, Brown, and Company, 1997, p 234

Moore FA, McKinley BA, Moore EE: The next generation in shock resuscitation. Lancet 363(9425):1988, 2004

Morris ML: Electrosurgery in the gastroenterology suite: principles, practice, and safety. Gastroenterol Nurs 29(2):126, 2006

Murovic JA, Kim DH, Tiel RL, et al: Surgical management of 10 genitofemoral neuralgias at the Louisiana State University Health Sciences Center. Neurosurgery 56(2):298, 2005

Murphy MF, Wallington TB, Kelsey P, et al: Guidelines for the clinical use of red cell transfusions. Br J Haematol 113(1):24, 2001

Nagpal K, Vats A, Ahmed K, et al: A systematic quantitative assessment of risks associated with poor communication in surgical care. Arch Surg 145(6):582, 2010

Naguib M, Magboul MM, Samarkandi AH, et al: Adverse effects and drug interactions associated with local and regional anaesthesia. Drug Safety 18(4):221, 1998

Naumann RW, Hauth JC, Owen J, et al: Subcutaneous tissue approximation in relation to wound disruption after cesarean delivery in obese women. Obstet Gynecol 85:412, 1995

Neuman M, Eidelman A, Langer R, et al: Iatrogenic injuries to the ureter during gynecologic and obstetric operations. Surg Gynecol Obstet 173(4):268, 1991

Newton M: Intraoperative complications. In Newton M, Newton E (eds): Complications of Gynecologic and Obstetric Management. Philadelphia, WB Saunders, 1988, p 36

Nizard J, Barrinque L, Frydman R, et al: Fertility and pregnancy outcomes following hypogastric artery ligation for severe post-partum haemorrhage. Hum Reprod 18(4):844, 2003

Nygaard IE, Squatrito RC: Abdominal incisions from creation to closure. Obstet Gynecol Surv 51(7):429, 1996

Oderich GS, Panneton JM, Hofer J, et al: Iatrogenic operative injuries of abdominal and pelvic veins: a potentially lethal complication. J Vasc Surg 39(5):931, 2004

O'Neal MG, Beste T, Shackelford DP: Utility of preemptive local analgesia in vaginal hysterectomy. Am J Obstet Gynecol 189(6):1539, 2003

Orr JW Jr, Orr PF, Barrett JM, et al: Continuous or interrupted fascial closure: a prospective evaluation of No. 1 Maxon suture in 402 gynecologic procedures. Am J Obstet Gynecol 163(5 Pt 1):1485, 1990

Patel H, Bhatia N: Universal cystoscopy for timely detection of urinary tract injuries during pelvic surgery. Curr Opin Obstet Gynecol 21(5):415, 2009

Penfield JA: Gynecologic Surgery under Local Anesthesia. Baltimore, Urban and Schwarzenberg, 1986, p 48

Perel P, Roberts I, Ker K: Colloids versus crystalloids for fluid resuscitation in critically ill patients. Cochrane Database Syst Rev 2:CD000567, 2013

Pfizer: Gelfoam absorbable gelatin powder. Package Insert. Kalamazoo, Pfizer, 2014

Phair N, Jensen JT, Nichols MD: Paracervical block and elective abortion: the effect on pain of waiting between injection and procedure. Am J Obstet Gynecol 186(6):1304, 2002

Philosophe R: Avoiding complications of laparoscopic surgery. Fertil Steril 80(Suppl 4):30, 2003

Pinski SL, Trohman RG: Interference in implanted cardiac devices, part II. Pacing Clin Electrophysiol 25(10):1496, 2002

Popert R: Techniques from the urologists. In Maxwell DJ (ed): Surgical Techniques in Obstetrics and Gynaecology. Edinburgh, Churchill Livingstone, 2004, pp 189, 195

Preston JM: Iatrogenic ureteric injury: common medicolegal pitfalls. BJU Int 86(3):313, 2000

Quinn J, Wells G, Sutcliffe T, et al: A randomized trial comparing octylcyanoacrylate tissue adhesive and sutures in the management of lacerations. JAMA 277(19):1527, 1997

Rahn DD, Phelan JN, Roshanravan SM, et al: Anterior abdominal wall nerve and vessel anatomy: clinical implications for gynecologic surgery. Am J Obstet Gynecol 202:234.e1, 2010

Robinson JB, Sun CC, Bodurka-Bevers D, et al: Cavitational ultrasonic surgical aspiration for the treatment of vaginal intraepithelial neoplasia. Gynecol Oncol 78(2):235, 2000

Rodeheaver GT, Halverson JM, Edlich RF: Mechanical performance of wound closure tapes. Ann Emerg Med 12(4):203, 1983

Rogers R Jr: Basic pelvic neuroanatomy. In Steege J, Metzger D, Levy B (eds): Chronic Pelvic Pain: an Integrated Approach. Philadelphia, WB Saunders, 1998, p 31

Sakellariou P, Protopapas AG, Voulgaris Z, et al: Management of ureteric injuries during gynecological operations: 10 years experience. Eur J Obstet Gynecol Reprod Biol 101(2):179, 2002

Santoso JT, Dinh TA, Omar S, et al: Surgical blood loss in abdominal hysterectomy. Gynecol Oncol 82(2):364, 2001

Schubert DC, Unger JB, Mukherjee D, et al: Mechanical performance of knots using braided and monofilament absorbable sutures. Am J Obstet Gynecol 187:1438, 2002

Schwartz D, Kaplan K, Schwartz S: Hemostasis, surgical bleeding, and transfusion. In Brunicardi F, Anersen D, Billiar T, et al (eds): Schwartz's Principles of Surgery. New York, McGraw-Hill, 2006

Sharp WV, Belden TA, King PH, et al: Suture resistance to infection. Surg 91(1):61, 1982

Shepherd JH, Cavanagh D, Riggs D, et al: Abdominal wound closure using a nonabsorbable single-layer technique. Obstet Gynecol 61(2):248, 1983

Silliman CC, Ambruso DR, Boshkov LK: Transfusion-related acute lung injury. Blood 105(6):2266, 2005

Singer AJ, Hollander JE, Quinn JV: Evaluation and management of traumatic lacerations. N Engl J Med 337(16):1142, 1997

Singer AJ, Quinn JV, Clark RE, et al: Closure of lacerations and incisions with octylcyanoacrylate: a multicenter randomized controlled trial. Surgery 131(3):270, 2002a

Singer AJ, Quinn JV, Thode HC Jr, et al: Determinants of poor outcome after laceration and surgical incision repair. Plast Reconst Surg 110(2):429, 2002b

Singh S, Maxwell D: Tools of the trade. Best Pract Res Clin Obstet Gynaecol 20(1):41, 2006

Sinha UK, Gallagher LA: Effects of steel scalpel, ultrasonic scalpel, CO_2 laser, and monopolar and bipolar electrosurgery on wound healing in guinea pig oral mucosa. Laryngoscope 113(2):228, 2003

Soper DE, Bump RC, Hurt WG: Wound infection after abdominal hysterectomy: effect of the depth of subcutaneous tissue. Am J Obstet Gynecol 173(2):465, 1971

Stanhope CR, Wilson FO, Utz WJ, et al: Suture entrapment and secondary ureteral obstruction. Am J Obstet Gynecol 164(6 Pt 1):1513, 1991

Stanton SL: Intestinal injury and how to cope. In Principles of Gynaecological Surgery, Berlin, Springer, 1987, p 159

Swanson K, Dwyre DM, Krochmal J, et al: Transfusion-related acute lung injury (TRALI): current clinical and pathophysiologic considerations. Lung 184(3):177, 2006

Tomacruz RS, Bristow RE, Montz FJ: Management of pelvic hemorrhage. Surg Clin North Am 81(4):925, 2001

Toy P, Popovsky MA, Abraham E, et al: Transfusion-related acute lung injury: definition and review. Crit Care Med 33(4):721, 2005

Trimbos JB: Security of various knots commonly used in surgical practice. Obstet Gynecol 64:274, 1984

Trimbos JB, van Rijssel EJC, Klopper PJ: Performance of sliding knots in monofilament and multifilament suture material. Obstet Gynecol 68:425, 1986

Trolice MP, Fishburne C Jr, McGrady S: Anesthetic efficacy of intrauterine lidocaine for endometrial biopsy: a randomized double-masked trial. Obstet Gynecol 95(3):345, 2000

Tulandi T, Hum HS, Gelfand MM: Closure of laparotomy incisions with or without peritoneal suturing and second-look laparoscopy. Am J Obstet Gynecol 158(3 Pt 1):536, 1988

Utrie JW: Bladder and ureteral injury: prevention and management. Clin Obstet Gynecol 41(3):755, 1998

Vakili B, Chesson RR, Kyle BL, et al: The incidence of urinary tract injury during hysterectomy: a prospective analysis based on universal cystoscopy. Am J Obstet Gynecol 192(5):1599, 2005

van Dam PA, Tjalma W, Weyler J, et al: Ultraradical debulking of epithelial ovarian cancer with the ultrasonic surgical aspirator: a prospective randomized trial. Am J Obstet Gynecol 174(3):943, 1996

van Rijssel EJC, Trimbos JB, Booster MH: Mechanical performance of square knots and sliding knots in surgery: a comparative study. Am J Obstet Gynecol 162:93, 1990

Vermillion ST, Lamoutte C, Soper DE, et al: Wound infection after cesarean: effect of subcutaneous tissue thickness. Obstet Gynecol 95(6 Pt 1):923, 2000

Visco AG, Taber KH, Weidner AC, et al: Cost-effectiveness of universal cystoscopy to identify ureteral injury at hysterectomy. Obstet Gynecol 97(5 Pt 1):685, 2001

Walter AJ, Magtibay PM, Morse AN, et al: Perioperative changes in serum creatinine after gynecologic surgery. Am J Obstet Gynecol 186:1315, 2002

Walters MD, Karram MM (eds): Urogynecology and Reconstructive Pelvic Surgery, 3rd ed. Philadelphia, Mosby, 2007

Wang CJ, Yen CF, Lee CL, et al: Comparison of the efficacy of laparosonic coagulating shears and electrosurgery in laparoscopically assisted vaginal hysterectomy: preliminary results. Int Surg 85(1):88, 2000

Warner MA: Perioperative neuropathies. Mayo Clin Proc 73(6):567, 1998

Warner MA, Warner DO, Harper CM, et al: Lower extremity neuropathies associated with lithotomy positions. Anesthesiology 93(4):938, 2000

Waters JH: Indications and contraindications of cell salvage. Transfusion 44(12 Suppl):40S, 2004

Waters JH: Red blood cell recovery and reinfusion. Anesthesiol Clin North Am 23(2):283, 2005

Whiteside JL, Barber MD, Walters MD, et al: Anatomy of ilioinguinal and iliohypogastric nerves in relation to trocar placement and low transverse incisions. Am J Obstet Gynecol 189(6):1574, 2003

Wiebe ER, Rawling M: Pain control in abortion. Int J Gynecol Obstet 50(1):41, 1995

Winfree CJ: Peripheral nerve injury evaluation and management. Curr Surg 62(5):469, 2005

Wissing J, van Vroonhoven TJ, Schattenkerk ME, et al: Fascia closure after midline laparotomy: results of a randomized trial. Br J Surg 74(8):738, 1987

Zimmer CA, Thacker JG, Powell DM, et al: Influence of knot configuration and tying technique on the mechanical performance of sutures. J Emerg Med 9:107, 1991

CHAPTER 41

Minimally Invasive Surgery Fundamentals

Minimally invasive surgery (MIS) is characteristically performed through a small incision or no incision, and visualization is provided by endoscopes. Both laparoscopy and hysteroscopy are considered in this category. With laparoscopy, small abdominal incisions provide access to introduce an endoscope and surgical instruments into the abdomen. To increase operative space, a pneumoperitoneum is created. As such, laparoscopy provides a minimally invasive option for women undergoing intraabdominal gynecologic surgery. And, with its technology improvements, almost all major intraabdominal gynecologic procedures can now be performed with MIS.

Hysteroscopy uses an endoscope and uterine cavity distending medium to provide an internal view of the endometrial cavity. This tool permits both the diagnosis and operative treatment of intrauterine pathology.

FACTORS IN CHOOSING LAPAROSCOPY

In theory, laparoscopic surgery differs from laparotomy only by its mode of access to the operative field. However, inherent qualities can make some surgical steps more difficult. These include indirect palpation of tissue, counterintuitive motion, a finite number of ports for abdominal access, restricted movement, and replacement of normal 3-dimensional (3-D) vision by 2-dimensional (2-D) video images. In appropriately selected patients, the trade-off is a faster recovery, improved cosmesis, less postoperative pain, diminished adhesion formation, and at least equivalent surgical results (Ellström, 1998; Falcone, 1999; Lundorff, 1991; Mais, 1996; Nieboer, 2009). The decision to perform laparoscopy is based on several parameters. Primary among these are patient factors, availability of appropriate instrumentation, and surgeon skill.

■ Patient Factors

Laparoscopy using a pneumoperitoneum is contraindicated in very few clinical conditions, but these include acute glaucoma, retinal detachment, increased intracranial pressure, and some types of ventriculoperitoneal shunts. Thus, laparoscopy is appropriate for many, although modifications are warranted for certain clinical situations. Several are discussed subsequently.

Prior Surgeries

With laparoscopy, adhesive disease increases the risk of visceral and vascular injury during abdominal entry. Adhesions are also associated with higher conversion rates to laparotomy because long and tedious adhesiolysis may be completed by some surgeons more quickly with open surgical dissection techniques. Thus, during preoperative physical examination, a surgeon notes the location of previous surgical scars and ascertains the risk of possible intraabdominal adhesive disease (Table 41-1). Similarly, a history of endometriosis, pelvic inflammatory disease, or radiation treatment may predispose to adhesions. In addition, abdominal wall hernias or hernia repairs and any reparative mesh are identified and avoided during trocar insertion. If abnormal findings are found during this preoperative evaluation, plans for an alternative entry site are considered (p. 894).

Laparoscopic Physiology

Compared with traditional open laparotomy, laparoscopy produces several distinct cardiovascular and pulmonary physiologic changes. These result mainly from: (1) absorption across the peritoneum and into circulation of carbon dioxide (CO_2) used for insufflation, (2) increased intraabdominal pressure created by the pneumoperitoneum, and (3) head-down Trendelenburg positioning. These changes are typically tolerated by those in generally good health but may be less so in those with cardiovascular or pulmonary compromise. Thus for patient safety, surgeons should be familiar with these physiologic alterations.

During laparoscopy, a pneumoperitoneum is created, in most cases with CO_2. Absorption of this gas across the peritoneum can lead to systemic CO_2 accumulation and hypercarbia. In turn, hypercarbia produces sympathetic stimulation that raises systemic and pulmonary vascular resistance and increases blood pressure. If

TABLE 41-1. Frequency of Umbilical Adhesions Found at Laparoscopy in Women with and without Prior Abdominal Surgery

	Sample Size/ Prior Surgery	No Prior Surgery	Prior Laparoscopy	Prior Low Transverse Incision	Prior Vertical Midline Incision (VML)
Agarwala (2005)	918/ surgery	—	16%	22%	62%
Brill (1995)	360/ laparotomy	—	—	27%	55% with VML below umbilicus
					67% with VML above umbilicus
Audebert (2000)	814/laparoscopy	0.68%	1.6%	19.8%	51.7%
Sepilian (2007)	151/ laparoscopy	—	21%	—	—

hypercarbia is not cleared by compensatory ventilation, acidemia develops. From this, direct myocardial contractility depression and decreased cardiac output can follow (Ho, 1995; Reynolds, 2003; Sharma, 1996). Hypercarbia can also lead to tachycardia and arrhythmia. Less commonly, bradycardia can stem from vagal stimulation. This may follow pelvic organ manipulation, cervical stretching during uterine manipulator placement, or peritoneal stretching during pneumoperitoneum creation.

Insufflation of any gas elevates intraabdominal pressure. This increased pressure decreases flow in the inferior vena cava, causes blood pooling in the legs, and raises venous resistance. In sum, venous return to the heart is decreased, and thereby cardiac output is lowered. Increased intraabdominal pressure can also directly lower splanchnic blood flow.

Intraoperative pulmonary function may be challenged during laparoscopy. First, the diaphragm is displaced upward by intraabdominal pressure from the pneumoperitoneum. This can be accentuated by organs also being pushed cephalad against the diaphragm during Trendelenburg positioning. Moreover, insufflation pressures stiffen the diaphragm and chest wall. Together, these alterations lead to higher required airway pressures to achieve adequate mechanical ventilation. Also, as the diaphragm moves up, lung volume and functional residual capacity are diminished, which in turn reduces the reserve volume for oxygenation. Moreover, this lung volume decline favors a tendency for the lung to collapse, leading to atelectasis. This can create ventilation and perfusion mismatching and an increased alveolar-arterial oxygen gradient. In sum, all of these factors favor poorer oxygenation.

Urinary output commonly is diminished during laparoscopy. This may result from the lowered cardiac output, decreased splanchnic blood flow, direct renal parenchymal compression, or the release of renin, aldosterone, or antidiuretic hormone. Together, these lessen renal blood flow, reduce glomerular filtration rate, and diminish urine output. Importantly, renal function returns to normal following pneumoperitoneum decompression (Demyttenaere, 2007).

Health Conditions

Several coexistent medical disorders are particularly relevant when considering laparoscopy. These include cardiac and pulmonary disease, intestinal obstruction, hemoperitoneum and hemodynamic instability, and pregnancy. As just described, in those with severe cardiac or pulmonary disease, elevated intraabdominal pressures and steep Trendelenburg positioning may not be tolerated, as they decrease venous return and pulmonary reserve. Unfortunately, with laparoscopy, these techniques are often required for adequate visualization and instrument manipulation. In addition, CO_2 is used to distend the abdomen during laparoscopy. As noted, it is absorbed across the peritoneum into circulation, and hypercarbia may follow. Accordingly, in those with pulmonary or cardiovascular limitations, lowering intraabdominal pressures and flattening the degree of Trendelenburg are advantageous.

For a clinically stable patient with hemoperitoneum, laparoscopy is not contraindicated. Thus, ruptured ectopic pregnancies or a ruptured bleeding ovarian cyst may be treated via MIS. Although an unstable patient was previously considered a contraindication to laparoscopic surgery, many skilled surgeons feel they can safely and quickly enter the abdomen laparoscopically. That said, the lowered venous return and cardiac output must be factored into the decision to select laparoscopy for such patients.

Concurrent intestinal obstruction and its associated bowel distention may increase risks for bowel injury during abdominal entry. In these situations, open entry to gain initial abdominal access may be beneficial (p. 893). However, ischemic bowel may be poorly served by pneumoperitoneum-related diminished splanchnic blood flow.

Obesity

In the past, obesity had been considered a relative contraindication for gynecologic laparoscopy. First, adequate ventilation may be difficult. In general, obese patients display reduced lung compliance that is proportional to their body mass index (BMI). Moreover, abdominal wall adiposity lowers abdominal wall compliance, which in turn elevates the pneumoperitoneum pressure required for surgery. Also, fattier omentum and mesenteric fat add to the bulk forced against the diaphragm in Trendelenburg position. Other limitations include a thick subcutaneous layer that encumbers laparoscopic instrument motion. It can also hinder abdominal entry, and trocar tunneling during insertion is common. Just patient girth relative to surgeon arm length may limit instrument manipulation.

As possible fixes, placement of an extra ancillary port for adequate manipulation of omentum and bowel out of the operative field can be helpful. Coordination with the anesthesia team to find a comfortable degree of Trendelenburg for both successful operative manipulations and adequate ventilation is essential. Longer "bariatric" instruments can overcome many length limitations.

As a result, with a skilled surgeon, obese patients may actually benefit from MIS. In studies, healthy obese patients experience less pain, quicker recovery, and fewer postoperative complications such as wound infections and postoperative ileus after laparoscopy compared with laparotomy (Eltabbakh, 1999, 2000; Scribner, 2002). That said, certain operative parameters may be adversely affected in obese patients undergoing laparoscopy compared with normal-weight patients. Higher conversion rates to laparotomy, longer operating times, and longer hospitalizations have been noted (Chopin, 2009; Heinberg, 2004; Thomas, 2006). However, this has not been found by all investigators, and overall outcomes may be superior to an open abdominal approach (Camanni, 2010; O'Hanlan, 2003; Shah, 2015).

Pregnancy

Nonurgent conditions identified during pregnancy may often be delayed and addressed postpartum. However, laparoscopy may be performed during any trimester. Thus, familiarity with the superimposed physiologic changes of pregnancy can improve maternal and fetal safety (O'Rourke, 2006; Reynolds, 2003).

Perioperatively, a wedge can be placed beneath the mother's back on the right to create a left-lateral tilt and displace the uterus. For second- or third-trimester pregnancies, this can minimize the decreased venous return that results from pneumoperitoneum and from an enlarged uterus compressing pelvic veins and inferior vena cava. Also, rates of venous thromboembolism (VTE) are increased during pregnancy due to gestational hypercoagulability. Placing sequential compression stockings can help lower this risk.

Intraoperatively, steps involve avoiding placement of intracervical uterine manipulators, limiting insufflation pressures to 10 to 15 mm Hg, maintaining maternal end-tidal CO_2 levels between 32 and 34 mm Hg, moving trocar placement appropriately cephalad to avoid puncture of the gravid uterus, and limiting uterine manipulation (Pearl, 2011). Of note, the routine use of perioperative prophylactic tocolytics is not recommended in these cases. However, pre- and postoperative fetal heart rate assessment and contraction monitoring for more advanced gestations are typically implemented.

Underlying Pathology

For adnexal masses, myomectomy, and supracervical hysterectomy, operative planning must address appropriate specimen removal. As discussed later, options include endoscopic bags, morcellation, colpotomy, or minilaparotomy incisions (p. 896). To guide selection, specimen size and the risks for occult malignancy and abdominal tumor seeding are assessed. Importantly, for masses that are known or strongly suspected to be malignant, laparoscopy is avoided if patient outcome could be compromised by specimen rupture, seeding, or morcellation or by incomplete resection or staging.

■ Facility Factors

In addition to patient factors, a surgeon must also consider environmental factors. The availability of appropriate anesthesia care, surgical nursing, support staff, and proper instrumentation influences procedure selection. Advanced operative laparoscopy is a coordinated team effort that requires multiple simultaneous activities, overseen and directed by the surgeon.

PATIENT PREPARATION

■ Prophylaxis

Randomized clinical trials have demonstrated that prophylactic antibiotics significantly reduce postoperative infectious morbidity rates following abdominal or vaginal hysterectomy. During laparoscopic hysterectomy, the vagina is similarly opened. Thus, preoperative antibiotics are recommended, and selection can be aided by American College of Obstetricians and Gynecologists guidelines (2014) found in Table 39-6 (p. 835). Antibiotics are generally given at the induction of anesthesia. For other types of laparoscopic procedures, data do not support antibiotic prophylaxis for clean surgical cases, that is, those that do not enter the vagina, bowel, or urinary tract (Chap. 3, p. 75).

For thromboprophylaxis, the same principles used for other abdominal surgeries are applied to laparoscopic cases (American College of Obstetricians and Gynecologists, 2013). Specific to laparoscopy, pneumoperitoneum pressure may decrease venous return from the lower extremities (Caprini, 1994; Ido, 1995). Thus, for those in whom VTE prophylaxis is planned, preventative measures are administered early and prior to anesthesia induction. A complete list of VTE prophylaxis and guidelines for its use can be found in Table 39-8 (p. 836).

■ Preoperative Bowel Preparation

The benefits of routine mechanical bowel preparation are debatable, and thus plans for bowel preparation are individualized (Chap. 39, p. 834). If the risk of bowel injury and stool spillage is increased because of pelvic adhesions or advanced endometriosis, then bowel preparation may limit fecal contamination at the surgical site. Moreover, if proctosigmoidoscopy is planned, an appropriate bowel preparation allows adequate visualization.

■ Anesthesia Selection

Laparoscopy can be completed using general or regional anesthesia. In most cases, general anesthesia with endotracheal intubation is selected to provide: (1) adequate patient comfort, (2) controlled ventilation to correct hypercarbia, (3) muscle relaxation, (4) airway protection from regurgitation due to increased intraabdominal pressures, and (5) orogastric tube placement. Some studies suggest that injection of local anesthesia at port sites may diminish postoperative pain (Einarsson, 2004).

■ Consent

Laparoscopy itself is usually associated with little associated morbidity. Of major complications, the most common is organ injury caused by puncture or by electrosurgical tools and is described later. If these occur or if surgery is hindered by bleeding or adhesions, conversion to laparotomy may be necessary.

Overall, this risk of conversion is low, and logically, rates decline as surgeon experience accrues.

Minor complications of laparoscopy occur more frequently. These may include wound infection or hematoma, subcutaneous emphysema from CO_2 infiltration, vulvar edema, and postoperative peritoneal irritation from retained intraabdominal CO_2. Irritation stems from conversion of CO_2 to carbonic acid, which can be a direct irritant.

Puncture Injuries

Because sharp tools are used during laparoscopic entry, vessels and abdominal organs may be punctured. Risk factors have been identified and include intraabdominal adhesions, insufficient gastric emptying, full bladder, insufficient pneumoperitoneum, poor muscle relaxation, thin patient habitus, and unsuitable angle or force of tool insertion. As discussed later, several authors advocate an open entry method as a means to help lower puncture injury rates (Catarci, 2001; Hasson, 2000; Long, 2008).

Organ Injury

The organ most frequently injured during laparoscopy is bowel, and rates of 0.6 and 1.6 per 1000 cases are reported (Chapron, 1999; Harkki-Siren, 1997). Women with previous laparotomy have a higher incidence of abdominal adhesions and are at greatest risk for this complication.

Unfortunately, bowel injury sustained during laparoscopy is often missed intraoperatively. For example, in an observational study by Chandler and coworkers (2001), nearly 50 percent of both small- and large-bowel injuries were unrecognized for 24 hours or longer. Typically, these patients present with fever, abdominal pain, nausea, and vomiting within 48 hours of surgery (Li, 1997).

In laparoscopic cases, decompression of the stomach with an orogastric tube prior to obtaining laparoscopic access can lower the stomach puncture risk. Moreover, in those with suspected abdominal adhesive disease, several preventative steps can help avoid bowel injury. These include: (1) introduction of a microlaparoscope to scout for adhesions, (2) preoperative sonography using the visceral slide test to exclude bowel adhered to the anterior abdominal wall, and (3) an alternative site for primary trocar entry, for example in the left hypochondrium (Palmer point), rather than at the umbilicus.

Bladder puncture is uncommon with laparoscopy. Bladder decompression prior to and during surgery and careful placement of secondary trocars under direct visualization will prevent many injuries. However, with increased rates of laparoscopic hysterectomy, rates of bladder and ureteral damage have concurrently risen. These occur at the same surgical steps associated with urinary tract injury during abdominal hysterectomy.

Vascular or Nerve Injury

Major vascular injury associated with laparoscopy is rare and typically results during primary trocar insertion. Puncture rates are cited as 0.09 to 5 per 1000 cases, and characteristically, the terminal aorta, inferior vena cava, and iliac vessels, particularly the right common iliac artery, may be injured (Bergqvist, 1987; Catarci, 2001; Nordestgaard, 1995). Rarely, air embolism from gas insufflation following vessel puncture may occur.

Although infrequent, a significant number of deaths result from large vessel injury (Baadsgaard, 1989; Munro, 2002). Prevention may include use of the open entry technique or awareness of the angle and force of trocar entry. Despite these steps, if a large vessel is punctured, the wounding instrument is not removed because it may act as a vascular plug. Moreover, this tool is held stable to avoid extending the laceration. In most cases, laparotomy, direct manual pressure on the vessel, steps for hemodynamic resuscitation, and notification of a vascular surgeon should follow expeditiously.

In contrast, if the inferior epigastric artery is injured, several simple techniques can control hemorrhage. First, bipolar electrosurgical coagulation of the bleeding site may suffice in many cases. If this fails to control bleeding, a 14F Foley catheter can be threaded through the cannula of the wounding trocar or through the defect created by this trocar. The Foley balloon then is inflated and pulled upward to create direct pressure against the posterior surface of the anterior abdominal wall. At the skin surface, a Kelly clamp is placed perpendicular across the Foley catheter and parallel to the skin to hold the balloon firmly in place. The balloon and catheter can be removed approximately 12 hours later. Alternatively, sutures can be placed that traverse the skin, abdominal wall, and peritoneum; arch under the bleeding vessel; and exit the abdomen to directly ligate the vessel (Fig. 41-1). Similarly, the Carter-Thomason tool can be used to ligate both ends of this vessel.

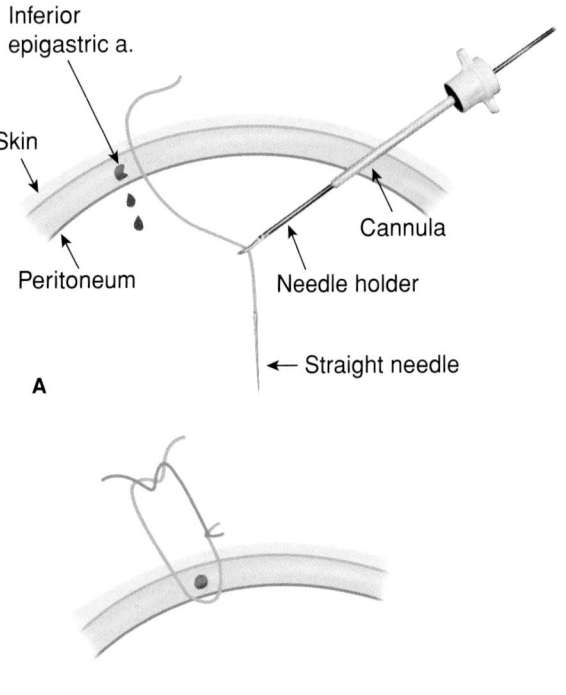

FIGURE 41-1 Ligation of lacerated inferior epigastric artery. **A.** Suture with an attached straight Keith needle is driven through the anterior abdominal wall lateral and caudal to the bleeding artery. This is performed using direct laparoscopic visualization to avoid organ injury. A laparoscopic needle driver regrasps the needle. **B.** The needle is then driven upward and through the anterior abdominal wall on the other side of the vessel. The suture loop is tied. This process is repeated cephalad to the bleeding vessel. This places sutures proximal and distal to the site of vessel laceration.

Nerve injury can follow in patients placed for extended periods in the dorsal lithotomy position with arms abducted. From this, injury to the common peroneal, femoral, lateral femoral cutaneous, obturator, sciatic, and ulnar nerves and to the brachial plexus is possible (Barnett, 2007). Specific injuries and prevention are described in Chapter 40 (p. 843). Attention paid to patient position and surgery duration prevent many of these complications.

Thermal Injury

Accidental burns may follow direct instrument contact or stray electric current. Fortunately, the risk of this complication is low. Prevention steps include keeping instrument tips within the visual field when electric current is applied, strict instrument maintenance to identify insulation defects, employment of bipolar coagulation or harmonic energy for hemostasis when feasible, and use of lower-voltage (cutting) current whenever possible to reduce the applied voltage (Wu, 2000).

Incisional Hernia

Incisional hernias are a potential long-term consequence of laparoscopy. The incidence approximates 1 percent but may rise in the future with increased use of larger trocars for operative laparoscopy and single-port umbilical techniques. Approximately one fourth of hernias are umbilical, and the remainder develop at secondary trocar sites (Lajer, 1997).

A major risk for incisional hernia is use of large trocars measuring ≥10 mm in diameter or port sites from which larger specimens are extracted. Preventatively, smaller trocar use when possible and fascial closure of larger trocars wound sites is advocated. The use of trocars with conical rather than pyramidal tips can also lower this incidence (Leibl, 1999). Finally, peritoneal tissue is ideally not drawn into the superficial layers of the wound when removing the cannulas (Boughey, 2003; Montz, 1994).

Trocar-site Metastasis

Rates of trocar-site cancer metastasis are low, and this complicates the clinical course of approximately 1 percent of patients in whom gynecologic malignancy is identified. Similarly, port-site seeding of other tissues such as endometriosis has been reported. Metastases are more frequent with ovarian cancer than other malignancies, and higher rates are seen with more advanced disease (Abu-Rustum, 2004; Childers, 1994; Zivanovic, 2008). Although most trocar-site metastases are associated with advanced stages of disease, metastasis has followed surgery for tumors of low malignant potential. As a result, the steps of laparoscopy itself have been evaluated as a risk for tumor spread to the trocar sites (Ramirez, 2004). Currently, no evidence-based consensus addresses prevention of this complication. Thus, the careful tissue extraction techniques described on page 896 are encouraged.

OPERATING ROOM ORGANIZATION

■ Operating Equipment

In laparoscopy, tool movement is limited compared with laparotomy, secondary to instrument angle restrictions and fixed ports (Berguer, 2001). Thus, room organization is essential, and equipment is positioned *before* the procedure begins. Also preoperatively, all instruments are checked and tested to confirm proper functioning.

Although equipment positioning may vary based on surgeon preference, the following is suggested to optimize efficiency and safety. The operating room table is centered in the room, and surgical lights lie directly above the operative field. Prior to surgery, this bed is checked to ensure it moves up and down and into steep Trendelenburg position. Obese patients may require a larger bariatric operating table.

Video monitors may be fixed to the ceiling with articulating arms or may be placed on portable stands. One monitor may suffice for simple procedures, however, two monitors provide easy viewing by the surgeon and assistant. When operating in the pelvis, the monitor is placed directly in front of the surgeon, and the surgeon, forearm-instrument axis, and video monitor are aligned in a straight line. Thus, placement of the video monitor for most gynecologic surgeries is near the patient's upper thigh (Fig. 41-2). For best surgeon ergonomics, monitor height is 10 to 20 degrees below eye level to prevent neck strain (van Det, 2009). Also, surgeons stand an appropriate distance and height relative to the operating table such that their arms

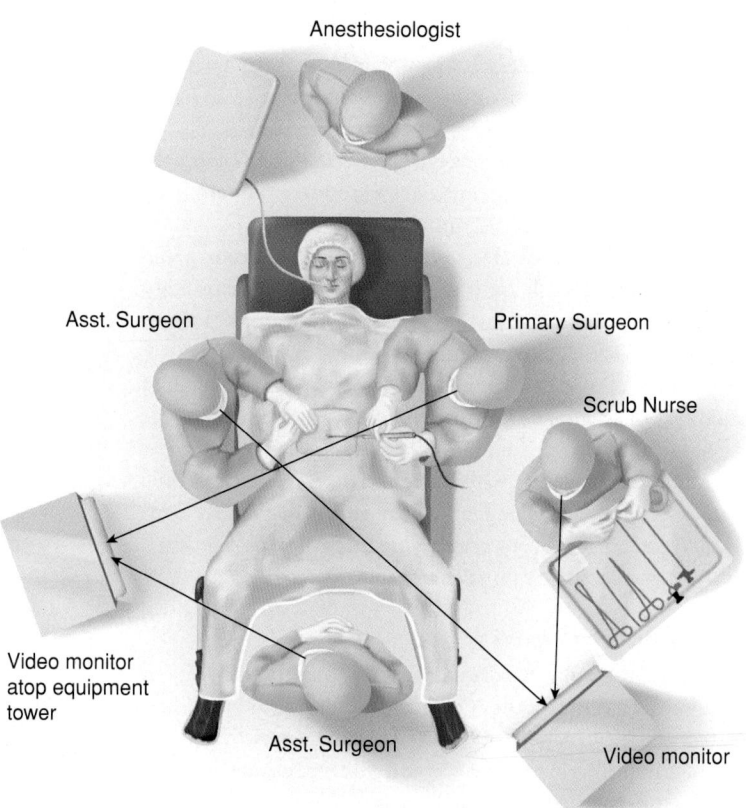

FIGURE 41-2 Operating room arrangement for laparoscopy.

are slightly abducted, their shoulders are inwardly rotated, and their elbows are extended from 90 to 120 degrees. This positioning can minimize surgeon fatigue. The scrub technician and Mayo stand generally are positioned on the side of the primary surgeon near the patient's leg. Here, instruments can be easily passed to both surgeons. The Mayo stand is organized with frequently used handheld instruments.

A dedicated cabinet or "tower" houses the laparoscopic light source, gas insufflator, and image capture equipment. The tower is positioned on the side opposite the primary surgeon such that he or she has an unobstructed view of equipment display panels. All insufflation tubing, camera, and light cords ideally exit the operating field from the same direction and connect to the equipment tower. Similarly, electrosurgical equipment and pedals are organized so that all these cords are aligned in one direction to reach a separate cart that houses these electrosurgical units. Pedals are oriented appropriately for the primary surgeon to comfortably reach without adjusting his body or moving his eyes from the monitor.

Patient Positioning

This is another essential component of safe laparoscopy. Following anesthesia induction, a patient is placed in low dorsal lithotomy position with the legs in booted support stirrups (see Fig. 41-2). To aid proper leg positioning, the stirrup brackets, which holster the stirrups, are attached to the table at the level of the patient hips. To prevent femoral nerve injury, the hips are positioned without sharp flexion or marked abduction or external hip rotation. The knees are not flexed more than 90 degrees and are appropriately positioned and padded to avoid common peroneal nerve compression. To avert slipping when in steep Trendelenburg position and to minimize lower back pressure, a patient can be placed directly on an antiskid material such as egg-crate or gel pad. With these, patient skin directly contacts the padding (Klauschie, 2010; Lamvu, 2004). If uterine manipulation is needed, the buttocks are placed slightly past the edge of the table.

Patient arms are tucked to the side in military position. This allows improved patient access and prevents upper extremity hyperextension, which can result in brachial plexus injury. The arms may be tucked using an extended draw sheet, which is placed under the gel pad. This relationship limits arm slippage, which can generate pressure against the brachial plexus. Even in obese patients, the use of antiskid material and arm tucking is useful in preventing slippage for long periods in steep Trendelenburg position (Klauschie, 2010). The arms are padded to avert compression of the ulnar and median nerves. Fingertips are facing the thighs, well-padded, and positioned away from the moving foot of the bed to prevent unintentional amputation. During arm positioning, finger oxygen monitors and intravenous access should not be dislodged.

Shoulder braces are padded brackets that are placed on the cephalic side of the operating room bed and arch around to the patient's acromion. Their goal is to brace the shoulder and prevent the head from slipping off the bed when in Trendelenburg position. If shoulder braces are required, we recommend tucking the arms in addition to using well-padded braces. However, due to the risk of nerve injury, the use of shoulder braces in general should be limited. Specifically, brachial plexus injury complicates 0.16 percent of gynecologic laparoscopic procedures. When shoulder braces are used, compression over the acromion may apply pressure that stretches the plexus. Moreover, lateral compression by braces may compress the humerus against the plexus. Both predispose to brachial plexus injury (Romanowski, 1993).

LAPAROSCOPIC INSTRUMENTS

Instrument Anatomy

Successful laparoscopic surgery relies on the use of appropriate surgical instruments. Most surgeons have designated preferences for certain types of graspers, dissectors, and cutting instruments. Many of these have been adapted and modified for laparoscopic surgery and undergo frequent updates. Moreover, new designs further aid retraction and dissection, thereby increasing the number of procedures that can be performed laparoscopically.

The components of a laparoscopic instrument include the hand grip, shaft, jaw, and tip (Fig. 41-3). In general, an instrument tip's diameter is concordant with its shaft diameter, and standard sizes fit through 5-mm or 10-mm diameter cannulas. Additionally, 3-mm, 8-mm, and 15-mm instrument diameters are available for many tips. The tip defines instrument function. Jaws may be double action or single action. With a single-action jaw, one tip is fixed, lies in the same axis as the shaft, and offers greater stability during the action performed. Double-action jaws have tips that move synchronously, and this jaw offers a wider angle in which to perform its function. Some jaws are now modified by a compression feature that allows full-length scissor blades to secure the tissue in the tip crux and then cut tissue with greater stability and precision.

Important instrument qualities are comfort and ease of use, which stem primarily from the hand grip shape, the instrument length, and its locking capability. Most laparoscopic instruments have a standard 33-cm length. Due to the popularity of bariatric MIS, extended instruments are now available for procedures in obese patients. Specifically, long Veress needles

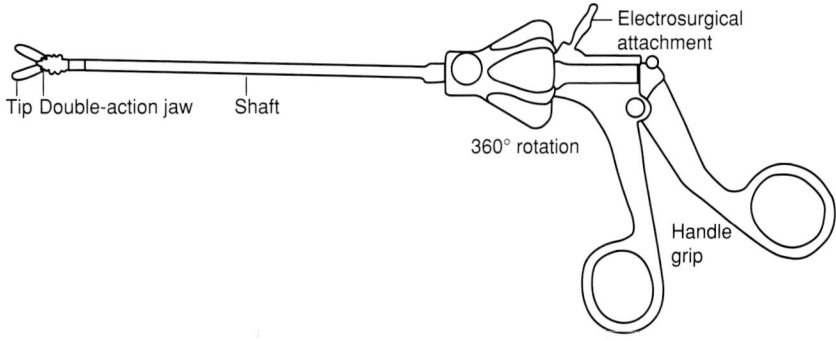

FIGURE 41-3 Parts of a typical laparoscopic instrument.

and trocars and longer instrument shaft lengths offer improved manipulation through a thickened pannus. Although permitting better access, these longer instruments are often more difficult to manipulate due to altered operating angles caused by the extended length.

In the hand grip, a locking feature allows a surgeon to hold tissue without maintaining constant pressure against the grip. This decreases hand fatigue. The ability to rotate an instrument tip 360 degrees is now preferred. This versatility allows access to additional anatomic spaces and decreases the need for uncomfortable surgeon hand or arm rotation.

Disposable versus Reusable

Many laparoscopic instruments are available in both reusable and disposable forms, each having its own advantages. The main advantage to reusable instruments is lowered expense. Analyses demonstrate that disposable instruments add significant cost compared with reusable ones (Campbell, 2003; Morrison, 2004). The main advantage to disposable instruments is the consistent tool sharpness and avoidance of lost instrument parts. For example, dull scissors may lead to longer operating times and ineffectual surgical technique. Corson and associates (1989) showed that reusable trocars, although sharpened at regular intervals, still required twice the force for entry compared with disposable trocars. As a compromise, modified trocar systems combine the strength of these two features. Namely, the cannula is reusable, whereas a disposable inner trocar offers a consistently sharper tip.

Manipulators
Atraumatic Manipulators

During laparoscopic surgery, abdominopelvic organs may be elevated, retracted, or placed on tension (Fig. 41-4). Most current instrument designs have incorporated safety considerations to minimize organ trauma yet allow effective manipulation. Of these, the blunt probe has an end that is modified to decrease the perforation risk to retracted tissues. It is used for exploration and retraction and is a preferred tool during diagnostic laparoscopy. Most blunt probes are stainless steel and are conductive of electric current. However, disposable probes constructed of nonconductive materials are available.

Graspers are divided into two main categories, atraumatic and those with toothed or serrated tips. Atraumatic graspers are used for exploration, gentle traction, and delicate tissue handing. The 5-mm diameter is a popular size, although 3-mm and 10-mm sizes are available. Most of these graspers have a double-action jaw, and the hand grip is typically nonlocking. Their gradually tapering curved tip permits the surgeon to define and separate tissue planes and is generally preferred for blunt dissection.

The Maryland clamp is an example of a curved blunt tip used for dissection and grasping. It compares to the pean, hemostat, or munion, which are used in open surgery. Additionally, it can double as a needle driver if needed. Although technically considered atraumatic, this clamp may crush delicate tissues such as the fallopian tube or bowel.

The alligator clamp is a blunt grasper with a long, wide tip that handles delicate tissues with minimal crush-injury risk. It is useful for manipulating bowel, larger vessels, or reproductive organs or for exploration of vascular compartments that may be easily punctured or lacerated. However, its ability to retract tissues under tension is limited due to its atraumatic characteristics.

The Babcock clamp is another atraumatic tip that handles delicate tissues with minimal crushing. Its surgical role is similar to that in open techniques. However, as with the alligator clamp, its ability to retract or grasp during applied tension is poor due to slippage.

Ideally, all of these clamps are included in a general laparoscopic surgical tray for most laparoscopic procedures. Figure 41-4 shows additional tips with similar characteristics. As seen, some tips have window openings and are described as fenestrated. These are useful for tissue elevation or retraction or for passing sutures during vessel ligation.

Traumatic Graspers

Graspers with tips that are serrated or toothed are used in procedures that involve resection and tissue approximation (Fig. 41-5). Generally, such tissues are placed on tension, and a strong hold is required. In addition, a locking hand grip is typically preferred to keep grasped tissues secured. Most of these instruments have double-action jaws to allow a wide tissue purchase. In situations in which greater grip and tension strength is required, however, a tip with a single-action jaw and locking hand grip may be preferred.

Toothed graspers have teeth at their tip's end. These are superior for tissue manipulation but function poorly as graspers for sutures or needles. One example is the

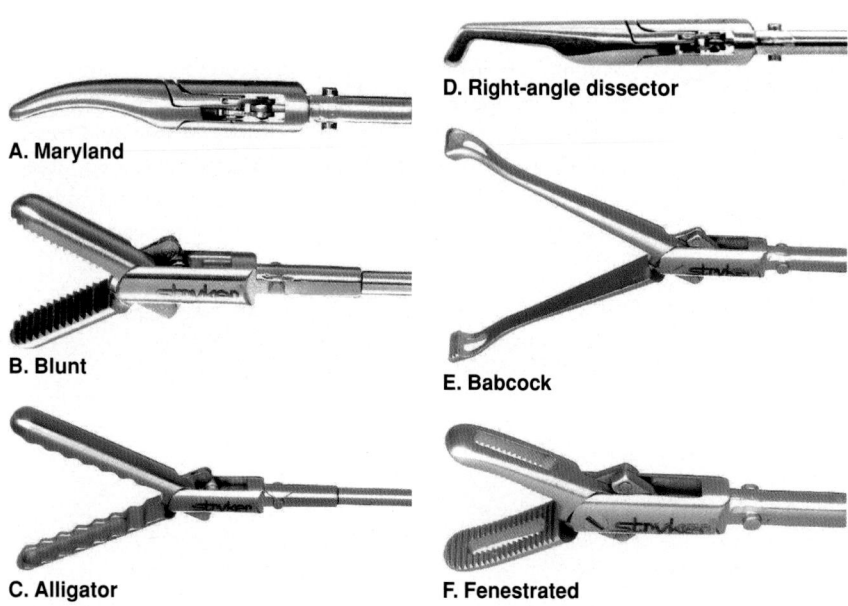

A. Maryland

B. Blunt

C. Alligator

D. Right-angle dissector

E. Babcock

F. Fenestrated

FIGURE 41-4 Laparoscopic atraumatic graspers. (Reproduced with permission from Stryker Endoscopy.)

Traumatic graspers   **Scissors**

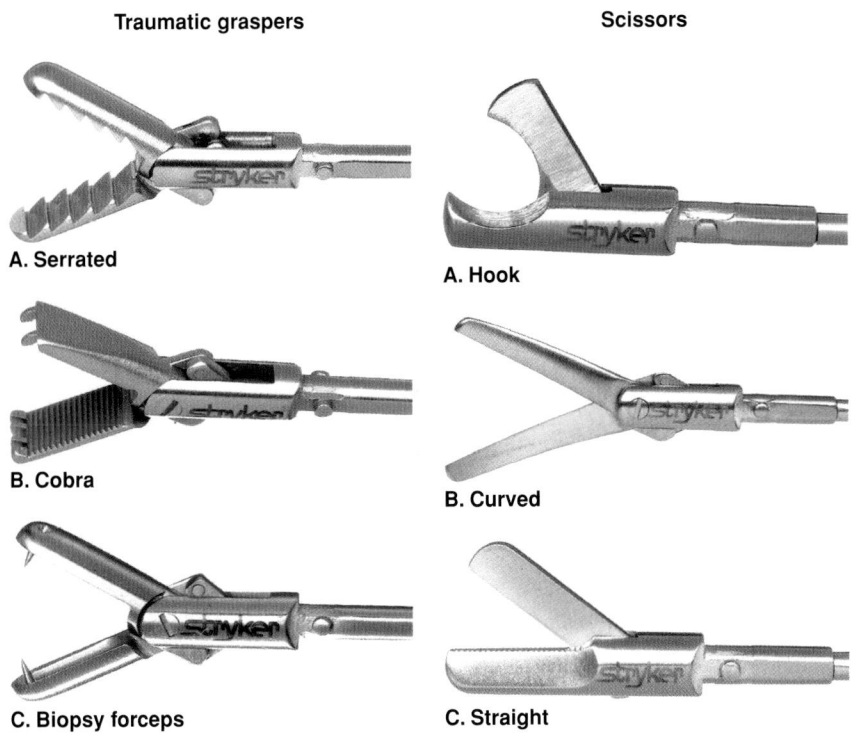

A. Serrated

B. Cobra

C. Biopsy forceps

A. Hook

B. Curved

C. Straight

FIGURE 41-5 Laparoscopic traumatic graspers (*left*) and scissors (*right*). (Reproduced with permission from Stryker Endoscopy.)

laparoscopic tenaculum. Single-tooth and double-tooth tenaculums are both available and effectively hold and retract dense, heavy tissue. The single-tooth tenaculum usually has a double-action jaw, whereas the double-tooth tenaculum is available with either a single- or double-action jaw. Both usually offer a locking hand grip. A tenaculum is traumatic and thus is generally used only on tissue to be resected or repaired. One common use is to grasp and remove tissue during morcellation.

The cobra grasper is a toothed instrument with a double-action jaw. It has short teeth on each side and is excellent for tissue retraction due to its strong grip strength. It is considered a traumatic grasper and is not used on delicate tissues.

Some of the toothed instruments are designed with less traumatic teeth and are selected when less tissue crushing is desired. For example, ovarian biopsy forceps provide adequate grasp with minimal tissue crushing. An appropriate setting might be ovarian cyst resection and subsequent ovarian repair. An Allis grasper has blunter teeth for grasping and holding tissue during resection. However, it provides less gripping strength than the cobra.

Serrated graspers are considered traumatic but are less damaging than toothed graspers. They offer a secure grip with minimal tissue damage and generally are used in repairs or tissue approximation. Because of their variety, a surgeon should be familiar with their grips and tissue effects to select the one that best fits the planned procedure. Serrated graspers may be fenestrated or nonfenestrated, may offer a locking hand grip, and may have single-action or double-action jaws.

A corkscrew tip probe is frequently used for marked retraction of more solid masses such as leiomyomas. It offers superior grip and strength but is limited by the trauma created as it is screwed into the tissue to be held. Additionally, surgeons are

mindful of the tip location when advancing it, as the downward force required to spiral the corkscrew tip may inadvertently perforate adjacent tissues. Despite this risk, this tool can be invaluable when manipulating solid, bulky leiomyomas or uteri.

Newer, small, 2-mm and 3-mm accessory manipulators have a trocar built around the instrument shaft. These can be placed percutaneously to augment surgical manipulation yet leave only a tiny residual abdominal wall scar. Of the two available designs, one is fully disposable and the other is reusable.

Uterine Manipulators

These devices were originally designed to offer manipulation of the uterus to create tension, expand operating space, or improve access to specific parts of the pelvis. The Hulka and the Sargis uterine manipulators are reusable stainless steel instruments that contain the following: a stiff blunt tip for insertion into the endocervical canal, a toothed tip that affixes to the cervical lip for stabilization, and a handle for vaginal placement (Fig. 41-6). For these manipulators, the cervix should to be patent to allow entry into the lower uterine cavity.

Uterine manipulators have become increasingly versatile and offer additional functions. The Cohen cannula manipulator has

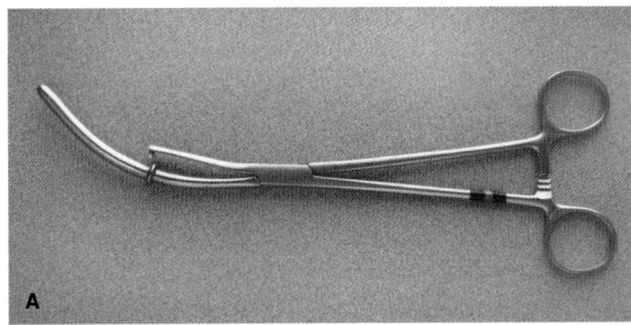

A

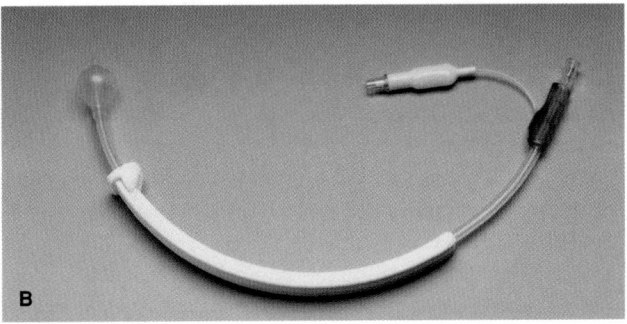

B

FIGURE 41-6 A. Hulka uterine manipulator. **B.** A balloon-type uterine manipulator. The deflated balloon tip is inserted into the endometrial cavity. The balloon is inflated to hold the stiff manipulator in place.

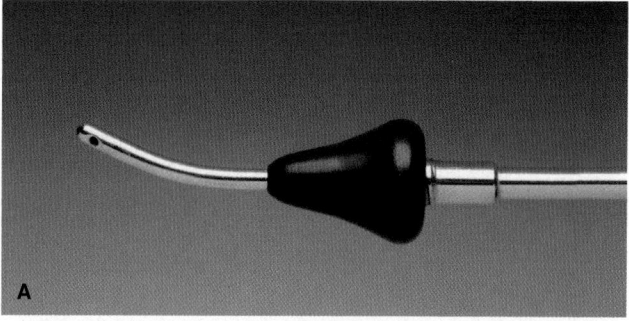

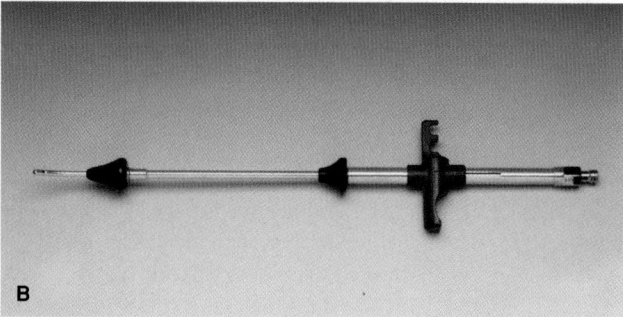

FIGURE 41-7 Cohen cannula. This device is used in conjunction with a separate tenaculum. The tenaculum is placed horizontally on the anterior cervical lip. **A.** The narrow cephalad tip of the cannula fits into the endocervical canal. The conical head abuts the external cervical os and limits insertion into the endometrial cavity. **B.** The caudad portion contains a crossbar into which the ratcheted handle of the cervical tenaculum fits.

a hard-rubber conical tip with a patent cannula for dye injection into the uterus, such as with chromotubation (Fig. 41-7). For placement, a single-tooth tenaculum is placed on the anterior cervical lip. The manipulator's conical tip wedges firmly against the cervix and thereby minimizes retrograde dye egress back through the os. The distal end of the Cohen manipulator then articulates with the crossbar that extends between the tenaculum's finger rings. Although commonly used, its range of motion is hindered by its straight shaft. Thus, the ability to dramatically flex a uterus anteriorly or posteriorly may be limited. The Rubin cannula manipulator is similar, with the same disadvantages. Greater flexion may be offered by the Hayden and Valtchev uterine manipulators. These have tip options, either conical or longer blunt intrauterine probes, which attach to a wristed joint at the distal end of the instrument shaft. This joint permits improved anteflexion and retroflexion. All of the manipulators just described affix to the cervical lip for stability. Thus, the risk of cervical trauma, although usually minimal, is disadvantageous.

Disposable uterine manipulators such as the Harris-Kronner Uterine Manipulator Injector (HUMI) or the Zinnati Uterine Manipulator Injector (ZUMI) also have a cannula for introducing dye to assess uterine and tubal patency (see Fig. 41-6). Rather than affixing to the cervix, an intracavitary balloon at the manipulator's uterine end is expanded similar to a Foley balloon once the manipulator is placed. This prevents the device from dislodging. Due to the length and firmness of the material used, these devices are advantageous for oversized uteri.

At times, a vaginal sponge stick is a practical manipulator for elevation and identification of pelvic structures. This may be selected by an advanced surgeon who wishes to eliminate the manipulator or chosen in cases in which the uterine fundus is absent. Last, newer manipulator designs have emerged to complement laparoscopic hysterectomy and are illustrated in Chapter 44 (p. 1034).

■ Scissors

These are integral to most laparoscopic procedures and are available in reusable and disposable models. Scissor tips vary depending on the type of dissection or resection needed (see Fig. 41-5). Scissors preferred for dissection commonly have a curved, somewhat blunted, tip that tapers similar to Metzenbaum scissors. This shape allows a surgeon to use standard techniques for tissue separation and resection with minimal trauma to the surrounding tissues (Chap. 40, p. 849). These curved blades may be smooth or slightly serrated. A serrated edge tends to hold tissue and minimize slippage prior to cutting. A smooth blade is preferred for sharp dissection, such as with adhesiolysis.

Straight scissors also come with smooth or serrated blades. They are used more for cutting and are less desired for dissection. Many straight scissors are designed with a single-action jaw, and some surgeons feel this offers better control.

Hooked scissors have a rounded, blunt tip and hooked blades. When initially approximated, the blades close around the tissue without cutting and then cut from the tip toward the hinge. This offers a controlled transection and is useful for partial transection of tissues. Moreover, its design allows a surgeon to confirm optimum placement before cutting. This type of scissors is commonly used for suture cutting.

■ Suction and Irrigation Devices

Successful laparoscopy requires a clear visual field. Thus, an effective and efficient suction and irrigation system is integral to procedures that require fluid or smoke removal (Fig. 41-8). Older systems were extremely slow and thereby prolonged operative time or failed to adequately clear a field with brisk bleeding. Newer motorized systems provide faster irrigation and evacuation, and motors usually have two speeds, which can be manually adjusted. The suction tips are available in 3-, 5-, and 10-mm diameters, thereby tailoring instrument capability

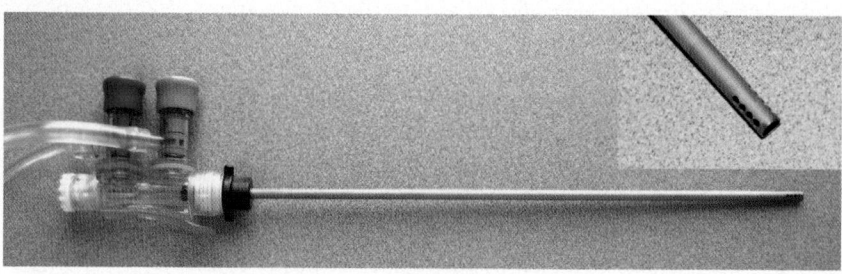

FIGURE 41-8 Suction-irrigator. Inset: Irrigator tip.

to the clinical setting. The latest generation systems also permit additional instruments to be placed through the hollow suction tip for concurrent monopolar electrosurgery. Newer models also have attachments to fluid management systems to monitor infused and extracted volumes.

When using a suction irrigation system, all of the suction holes are ideally submerged in the fluid to be removed. This avoids inadvertent insufflation gas removal, which then collapses the operative field. Additionally, the probe may cause suction damage to viscera, especially delicate structures such as tubal fimbria and bowel epiploica. To avoid damage, suction is used when there is a safe distance from vulnerable structures and with the assistance of another instrument to move these structures away from the suction tip.

■ Tissue Extraction

Morcellators

These tools cut excised tissues into smaller pieces, which can then be extracted. Available morcellators use either thin cutting blades or pulsatile kinetic energy. Bladed morcellators consist of a hollow large-bore shaft that contains razorlike blades to shave tissues into thin strips. One of these, the Storz Rotocut, is reusable but houses disposable stainless steel blades that are efficient in cutting through dense masses. Although bulkier and heavier than others, it is among the fastest and most effective. The Lina Morcellator has a built-in battery pack, is slower but more ergonomic, and is disposable. The MOREsolution morcellator offers a 2-cm-diameter blade, which is currently the largest and may be helpful for large masses. Another device, the Gynecare Morcellex, is currently unavailable due to a voluntary suspension of worldwide sales. Each mechanical morcellator has its advantages, and familiarity with these allows selection of the most suitable instrument for a given tissue.

Another morcellator, the PKS PlasmaSORD Bipolar Morcellator, is bladeless. Instead, it uses plasma kinetic energy, which is a form of pulsatile bipolar energy. It works well for hysterectomy and myomectomy specimen morcellation. However, it produces a large smoke plume, which reduces visibility and thereby increases operative time. Accordingly, cases with larger specimens may have extended operative times with this instrument compared with bladed instruments. However, no randomized studies support the superiority of one morcellator over another.

Endoscopic Retrieval Pouches

Endoscopic bags for tissue retrieval vary in size and vinyl strength. Some are free-standing sacs designed for manual introduction into the abdominal cavity through cannulas and are preferred for larger and denser masses. Once loaded, the sac is simply lifted through an appropriately sized abdominal wall incision.

Other types are manufactured as pouches attached to support arms at the end of a laparoscopic shaft to create a self-contained unit. As shown in Figure 41-9, the support arms open the sac. Once the mass is bagged, the arms and pouch are retracted and removed through the cannula. The cannula is then removed, bringing the bag to the incision where it is extracted.

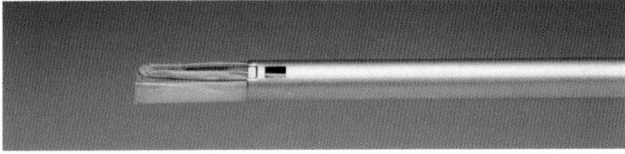
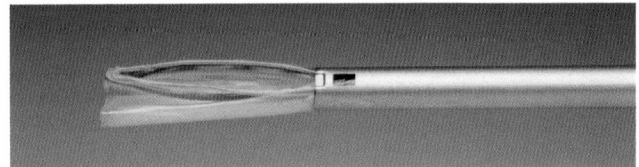
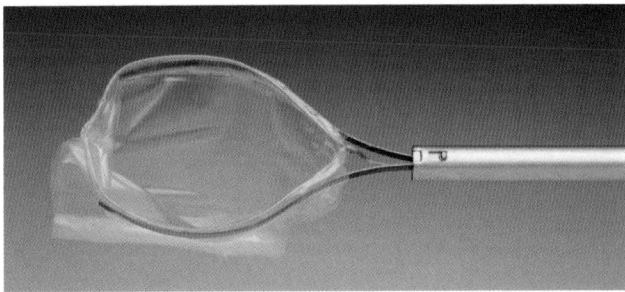

FIGURE 41-9 Endoscopic sac during progressing stages of deployment.

With either sac type, if a specimen does not compress or cannot be drained, the incision may require enlargement.

Self-retaining Retractors

Designed to complement MIS, nonmetal self-retaining retractors consist of two equal-sized plastic rings connected by a cylindrical plastic sheath. One ring collapses into a canoe shape that can be threaded through the incision and into the abdomen. Once inside the abdomen, it springs again into its circular form. The second ring remains exteriorized. Between these rings, the plastic sheath spans the thickness of the abdominal wall. To hold the retractor in place, a surgeon everts the exterior ring multiple times until the plastic sheath is tight against the skin and subcutaneous layers. This form creates 360-degree retraction. These disposable retractors maximize incision size because of their circular shape and by eliminating thick metal retractor blades within the wound opening. Brands include the Alexis and Mobius retractors, and available sizes range from extra small to extra large. In some studies, these retractors provide wound protection and lower wound infection rates (Horiuchi, 2007; Reid, 2010).

For MIS cases, these devices offer several functions. First, they retract minilaparotomy incisions to aid large specimen removal. Moreover, certain procedures, such as laparoscopic myomectomy, can also be completed through these incisions (Section 44-8, p. 1025). Second, concern about tissue dissemination has prompted development of retrieval bags that are coupled with these self-retaining retractors. For this, the retrieval bag is initially placed into the abdomen. The bag containing the excised specimen is then brought to the surface and is fanned open outside and around the minilaparotomy incision. The self-retaining circular retractor is then placed into the bag's interior and simultaneously opened within the incision. This creates a closed environment in which the specimen can be sharply morcellated manually with scissor or knife. Long-term data on safety and efficacy of this enclosed approach are not yet available.

■ Energy Systems in Minimally Invasive Surgery

Understanding principles and correct use of electrosurgical instruments is essential to safe laparoscopy. The same principles of electrosurgery in open surgery apply to laparoscopy (Chap. 40, p. 857). However, special considerations are necessary in a closed, minimally invasive environment. For example, the entire length of an instrument may extend past a surgeon's visual field, thus risking unintended electrosurgical burns. Fortunately, advances in instrumentation mitigate many of the physical constraints inherent to MIS.

Monopolar Electrosurgery

Monopolar instruments may be useful for tissue cutting, dissection, vaporization, and desiccation. Delivery of this energy is usually through scissors or needle point tip. Of these, monopolar scissors coagulate tissues within its jaws prior to incision. This is typically used for thin tissues and small vessels. In addition, closed blade tips can act simultaneously to cut tissue and achieve hemostasis. Monopolar energy delivered though a needle point tip is used for functions ranging from ovarian drilling to development of peritoneal planes during hydrodissection.

Unintended thermal injuries form the main risk with this energy type. With monopolar instruments, insulation failures, direct coupling, or capacitive coupling may each result in unintended, potentially serious electrosurgical burns. First, insulation failures are breaches in an instrument's insulation. This break provides an alternate pathway for current flow. When a monopolar instrument is activated, electric current may travel from the electrode through the insulation breach and discharge to any tissue in contact with this breach. This current flow may cause thermal damage to surrounding visceral and vascular structures without the surgeon ever being aware. Accordingly, before electrosurgical tools are used, systematic inspection should look for insulation cracks throughout their length, for aberrant or loose cord connections, and for assurance that a grounding pad is correctly placed on the patient.

Another monopolar effect is direct coupling, which occurs when an activated electrode contacts another metal object—either intentionally or unintentionally. This technique is frequently used during open surgery to achieve hemostasis of small vessels, such as when the electrosurgical blade tip is touched to a hemostat around a small vessel. However, in laparoscopy, unintentional direct coupling may occur when a metal instrument or object (such as a metal cannula) contacts an active monopolar instrument and thus provides an alternate and undesired current flow to surrounding viscera.

Another hazard with monopolar instruments is the risk of capacitive coupling. A capacitor is defined as two conductors separated by a nonconducting medium. During laparoscopy, an "inadvertent capacitor" can be created when a conductive active electrode (e.g., monopolar scissors) is surrounded by a nonconducting medium (insulation around the scissors) and is placed through another conductive medium (a metal cannula).

This capacitor creates an electrostatic field between the two conductors. When current is activated through one of the conductors, this in turn will induce a current in the second conductor. Capacitative coupling occurs when this system discharges current into other surrounding conductive material. In the case of an all-metal cannula, current can be dissipated throughout the abdominal wall. With hybrid cannula systems, in which a metal cannula is anchored by a plastic sleeve or collar, the capacitor that is created has no place to discharge. Stray current can then exit to adjacent tissue that is in contact with the metal portion of the cannula, thereby damaging nearby vascular or visceral structures. This risk can be reduced by avoiding hybrid cannulas and by selecting bipolar instruments. Moreover, the addition of an integrated shield on the electrode shaft of some monopolar instruments, which monitors for stray current, can prevent this complication.

Bipolar Electrosurgery

Bipolar energy is mainly used in laparoscopy for tissue desiccation and hemostasis. Many types of bipolar forceps are available for various uses (Fig. 41-10). The 3-mm paddle forceps are used for tubal coagulation during sterilization procedures. Flat-tip forceps desiccate larger vessels and tissue pedicles. Fine-tip, "microbipolar" forceps aid hemostasis near or on vulnerable structures such as the ureter, bowel, and fallopian tubes. Burns are less of a concern with bipolar energy because the currents used are typically lower. Currents, for the most part, also stay confined between the two closely approximated electrodes.

For hemostasis, energy is delivered to denature collagen and elastin in vessel walls and thus seal the vessel. During this process, the bipolar device uniformly compresses the tissue and provides internal monitoring to adjust energy delivery. When evaluating these devices, important considerations include thermal spread, ability to provide desired tissue effects, consistency of results, time required to achieve results, plume produced, and maximum vessel diameter that can be securely sealed (Lamberton, 2008; Newcomb, 2009).

Currently used advanced bipolar devices such as the LigaSure, Plasmakinetic (PK) Gyrus, and Enseal are multifunctional tools that can be used for both tissue desiccation and dissection. Each of these devices employs a low voltage to deliver energy to tissue and carry impedance feedback to the electrosurgical unit to locally regulate thermal tissue effects. These adaptations allow for reduced collateral injury from thermal spread, an improved tissue seal, less plume production, and diminished tissue sticking. Whereas the LigaSure delivers a continuous bipolar radiofrequency waveform, the PK delivers energy in a pulsed waveform. The Enseal system has a temperature-controlled feedback mechanism at its tip, which "locally" modulates energy delivery.

Ultrasonic Energy

The Harmonic scalpel, also known as an ultrasonic scalpel, uses ultrasonic energy, which is converted to mechanical energy at the active blade. Seen as the lower blade in Figure 41-10F, the active blade vibrates to deliver high-frequency ultrasonically generated frictional force, whereas the inactive upper arm holds tissues in apposition against the active blade. Alternatively, the active blade may be used alone. Either cutting or coagulating effects

Monopolar tools

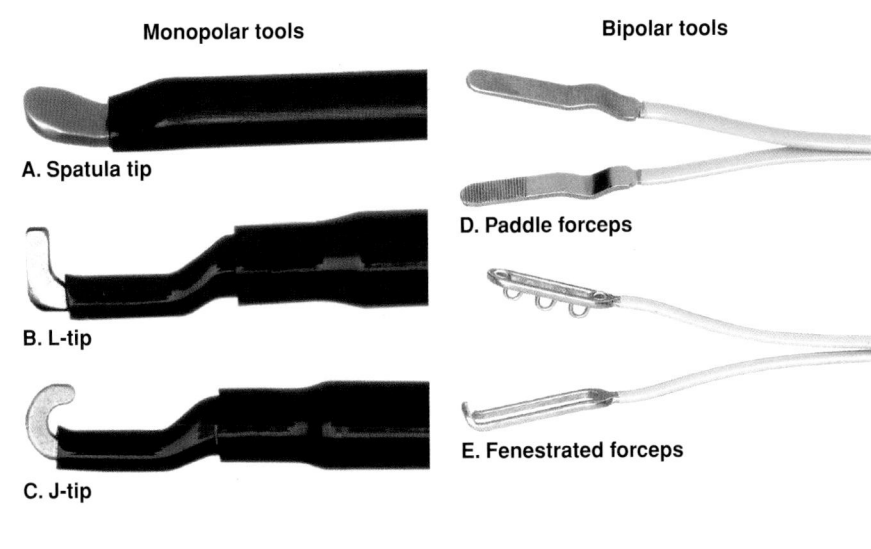

A. Spatula tip

B. L-tip

C. J-tip

Bipolar tools

D. Paddle forceps

E. Fenestrated forceps

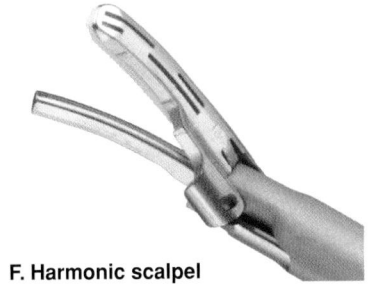

F. Harmonic scalpel

FIGURE 41-10 A-C. Laparoscopic monopolar tools. **D** and **E.** Bipolar tools. (Reproduced with permission from Stryker Endoscopy.) **F.** Laparoscopic Harmonic scalpel. (Reproduced with permission from Ethicon.)

can be achieved, and a balance between these two is created by controlling several factors: power levels, tissue tension, blade sharpness, and application time. Higher power level, greater tissue tension, and a sharp blade will lead to cutting. Lower power, decreased tissue tension, and a blunt blade will create slower cutting and greater hemostasis. Limitations of the Harmonic scalpel include limited ability to coagulate vessels larger than 5 mm and the requirement for the surgeon to balance the factors listed above (Bubenik, 2005; Lamberton, 2008).

Laser Energy

Lasers were widely used in laparoscopy in the 1980 through 1990s and include the CO_2, argon, KTP (potassium titanyl phosphate), the Nd-YAG (neodymium:yttrium-aluminum-garnet) lasers. These are generally used through an operative channel on the laparoscope or via a separate port. These lasers can cut, coagulate, and vaporize tissues and are employed for lysis of adhesions, tubal surgery, and endometriosis fulguration or resection. In the hands of skilled surgeons, lasers offer precision and control with minimal effect on surrounding tissue. Thus, a laser is able to work near or over sensitive structures such as bowel, bladder, ureters, and vessels. Disadvantages are its learning curve, expense, lack of portability, and smoke production.

Laparoscopic Leiomyoma Ablation

Myolysis describes leiomyoma puncture by energy-based probes that incite tissue necrosis and subsequent shrinkage. Of these,

bipolar energy and cryoablation have been used with varying degrees of success and thus have not gained widespread popularity with gynecologic surgeons.

The Acessa procedure instead uses monopolar energy combined with ultrasound guidance through laparoscopic instrumentation (Fig. 41-11). For this, a special ultrasound probe is placed during laparoscopy through a 10-mm lower abdominal port and directly contacts the uterus to localize myomas. This allows better myoma visualization by permitting views from several angles. A thick radiofrequency needle is inserted through a separate abdominal wall puncture site and then punctures each tumor serially under sonographic guidance. Once the needle is inserted into a myoma, a deployable electrode array housed within the needle is expanded within the tumor to deliver the destructive energy. Real-time laparoscopic and sonographic surveillance confirm that the electrodes remain within the mass. The outpatient Acessa procedure is typically performed in the operating suite with general anesthesia. Postoperative oral narcotics or nonsteroidal antiinflammatory drugs (NSAIDs) provide sufficient postoperative analgesia for most women (Galen, 2013).

With this approach, early evidence shows improved patient symptoms and a reintervention rate of 11 percent at 3 years (Berman, 2014). Other long-term data regarding outcomes are lacking, but current ongoing studies will add information.

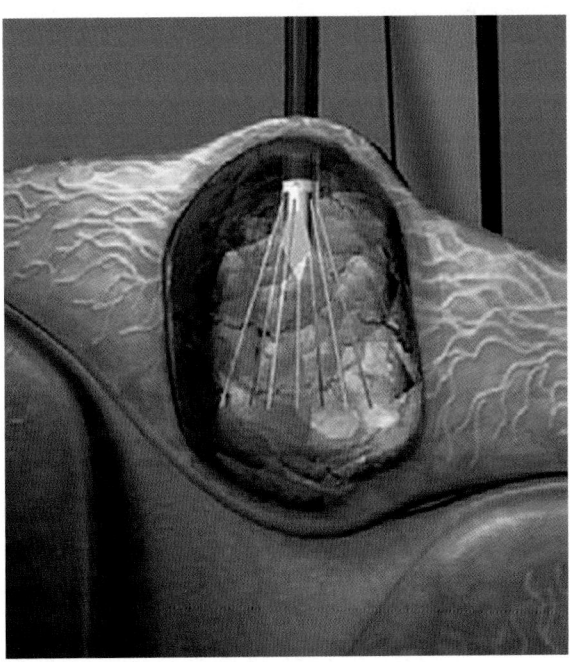

FIGURE 41-11 Acessa system for myolysis. Reproduced with permission of Halt Medical.

■ Laparoscopic Optics

Laparoscope Construction

Successful MIS requires excellent visual acuity provided by high-intensity light sources and laparoscopes with focused lenses. The modern-day rod lens system contains a series of lenses that are the diameter of the laparoscope cylinder. At the periphery of each lens are small scalloped grooves that permit light-carrying fibers to reach the endoscope end. This provides a well-lit image and minimal distortion. Uniquely, the space between lenses is filled with small, tightly packed glass rods. These rods fit exactly, which make them self-aligning to require no other structural support. Appropriate curvature and coatings to the rod ends and optimal glass type permit superb image quality—even with cylinder tubes measuring only 1 mm in diameter.

In addition to its main cylinder, a laparoscope contains an eyepiece, to which a camera can be affixed. The camera usually is an attachable springed plastic cap that can be clipped onto the eyepiece. The main cylinder also has an adapter on its exterior to attach the light-source cable. Laparoscope diameters range from 0.8 to 15 mm. In general, greater diameters offer superior optics but require a larger incision. This trade-off typically dictates laparoscope selection for a given procedure.

Differing from traditional straight-shaft endoscopes, operative laparoscopes have an eyepiece that branches off at a 45- or 90-degree angle from the straight operative shaft. This permits tools to be placed through the operative shaft, which are then seen by the endoscope. Instruments used are generally longer than instruments typically placed in accessory ports. Most instruments are 45 cm, which is considered bariatric length. Lasers are also frequently placed through the operative shaft and can allow for precise energy application.

Angles of View

Similar to hysteroscopes and cystoscopes, laparoscopes vary in their angle of view. The most common are 0-, 30-, and 45-degree laparoscopes, and each offers a different view of the peritoneal cavity. A 0-degree endoscope offers a forward view and is preferred by most gynecologists. This laparoscope is used in most diagnostic procedures or simple surgeries involving biopsies, simple adhesiolysis, and excision of small masses or organs such as an ovary, fallopian tube, or appendix.

In contrast, angled-view endoscopes provide a lateral and larger field of view. These are useful during cases with more complicated pathology such as dense adhesions that obstruct the traditional forward view. For example, during difficult dissection in which multiple instruments are in action, an angled-view laparoscope offers a panoramic view at a distance. This provides a surgical field in which all instruments in use can be seen.

Angled-view endoscopes also allow a lateral view of pathology. For example, if an angled-view laparoscope is placed at one pelvic sidewall and is directed to the opposite sidewall, a surgeon is provided a large lateral visual operating space. Moreover, angled views are valuable along the sides of organs. With a large myomatous uterus, it may be challenging to identify the uterine artery and cardinal ligaments. An angled-view laparoscope permits a surgeon to "slide" along the lateral border of the uterus to

reach these. Similar benefits are gained when operating in small spaces such as in the deep pelvis or space of Retzius.

Clearly, the 0-degree laparoscope is easier to master. However, the advantages for advanced procedures warrant the time needed to operate using an oblique view. Importantly, during orienting with an angled-view laparoscope, when the field of view is directed downward, the light cord attached to the endoscope is positioned up. Conversely, if the view is upward, the light cord will be positioned down. To maintain orientation when changing viewing polarity, the camera buttons remain facing upward, while the light cord rotates in relation to it.

Flexible Laparoscopes

The tips of these special laparoscopes are able to bend to a greater degree. As such, they can travel into smaller spaces or around corners. Whereas traditional fiberoptic laparoscopes contain fiber bundles that run the length of the endoscope, these flexible endoscopes house a camera chip at their end to transmit images as electrical signals. This results in less image distortion. This concept has also provided the option of dual camera technology, which uses two camera chips at the tip. As benefits, optics and opportunities for more advanced procedures are improved. Some newer models afford a 3-D view and are used for single-port laparoscopic approaches, in which there is traditionally less maneuverability (p. 894).

Lighting

Light is transmitted through the laparoscope from a light source via the light cable. Originally, endoscopic light was provided by incandescent lightbulbs, which produced little light and transmitted increased heat. Currently, a cold light source is used and provides a more intense beam. The term "cold light" describes the dissipation of heat along the length of the cable. Cold light sources use halogen, xenon, or halide modalities for the lamps. Despite heat dissipation, the light source still creates a hot tip at the distal laparoscope end. Thus, prolonged exposure of the tip to surgical drapes, patient skin, or internal organs is avoided. Thermal injuries have resulted from such exposure.

Light cables connect the light source to the endoscope. Of these, two types are available: fiberoptic and fluid filled. The fiberoptic cable contains multiple coaxial quartz fibers that transmit light with relatively little heat conduction. However, these cables suffer from fiber breakage and need to be serviced often. In contrast, fluid-filled cables transmit more light and conduct more heat than the fiber cables. They are stiffer and have decreased maneuverability. This coupled with difficulty in sterilization may make this type less preferred.

Once attached to a camera and light source, most laparoscopes must be adjusted to a "true white" to ensure that the colors in the viewing field are accurate. This is called *white balancing* and is performed at the procedure's beginning.

ROBOTIC SURGERY

One modern approach to MIS uses robotic assistance, and most abdominal gynecologic procedures can be completed with this technique. Similar to laparoscopy, robotic surgery uses abdominal ports to introduce instruments and a pneumoperitoneum to expand the operative field. One positive difference is the miniaturized and wristed articulating instrument tips that allow successful completion of complex procedures in tight operating spaces. The instrument tips mimic those used in open surgery and in laparoscopy and include graspers, needle drivers, and cutting instruments. Advanced video technology within an 8-mm laparoscope provides a high-definition and magnified view.

Of disadvantages, tactile feedback is lost with robotic surgery and forces a surgeon to use visual cues. This is a learned skill that carries a significant learning curve. However, surgeons experienced in advanced laparoscopic techniques adapt more quickly. Other disadvantages include extended initial set-up time needed during each case, physician training costs, and robot and instrument expenses.

◼ Robot

Currently, the only commercially available robot is the da Vinci system. As shown in Figure 41-12, one or two surgeon consoles are used to control robot arm movement. A separate cart stands at the surgical bedside and serves as the base for the four robotic arms. Of these arms, one controls the laparoscope, whereas the other arms hold robotic instruments. Procedures are performed using two or three of the instrument arms according to the procedure's needs and surgeon's preference. The second surgeon console is generally used for training. If port sites in addition to the basic four are needed, an assistant surgeon can also work at the patient bedside through one or two traditional laparoscopic accessory ports. These are generally placed in the right or left upper quadrants. Typically, 5- to 15-mm trocars are used for

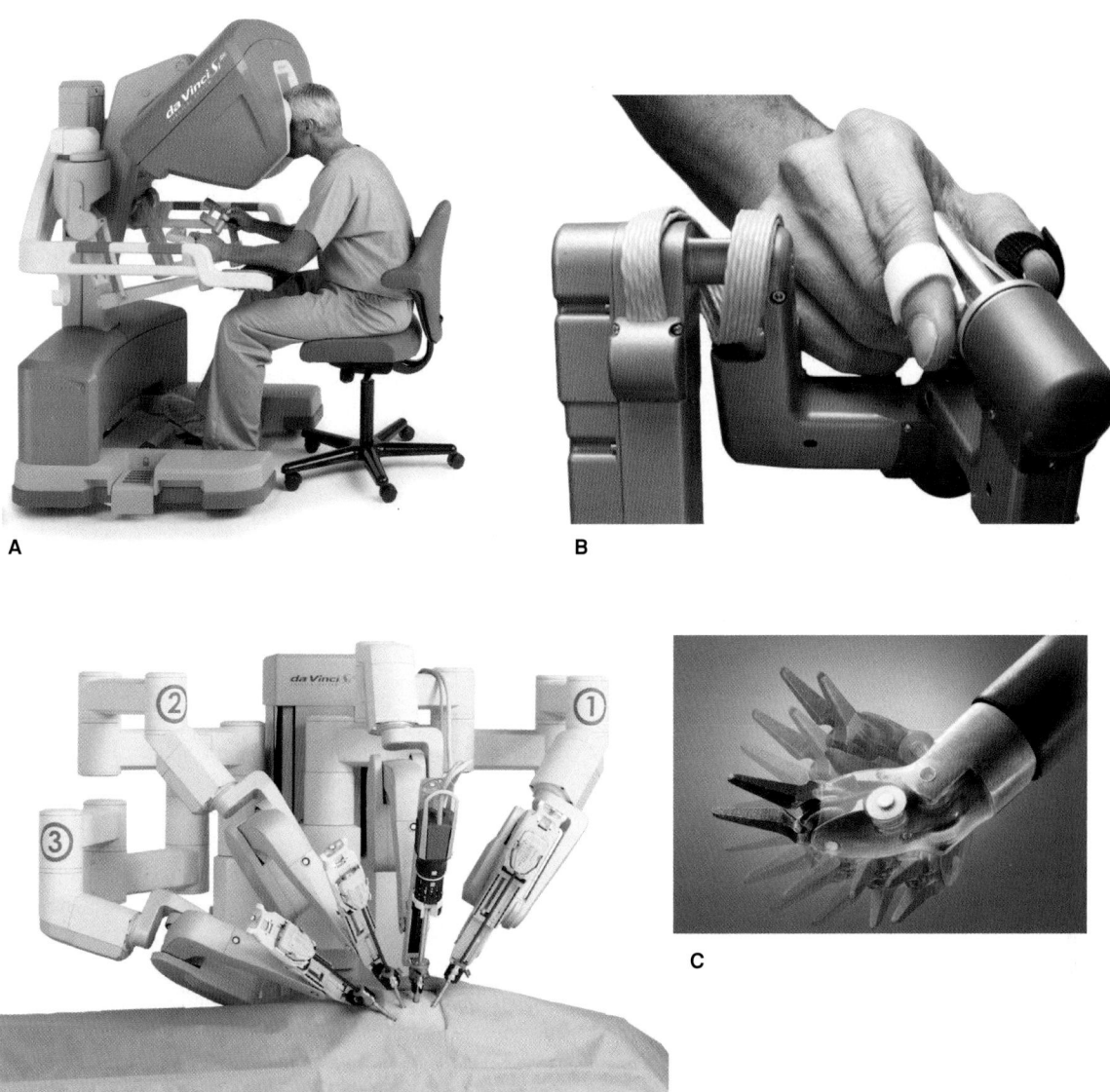

FIGURE 41-12 Da Vinci Surgical System. **A.** Operator console. **B.** A surgeon's finger movements are translated into robotic instrument movement. **C.** Wristed instruments provide a wide range of motion. **D.** Robot at operative bedside. (Reproduced with permission from Intuitive Surgical, Inc.)

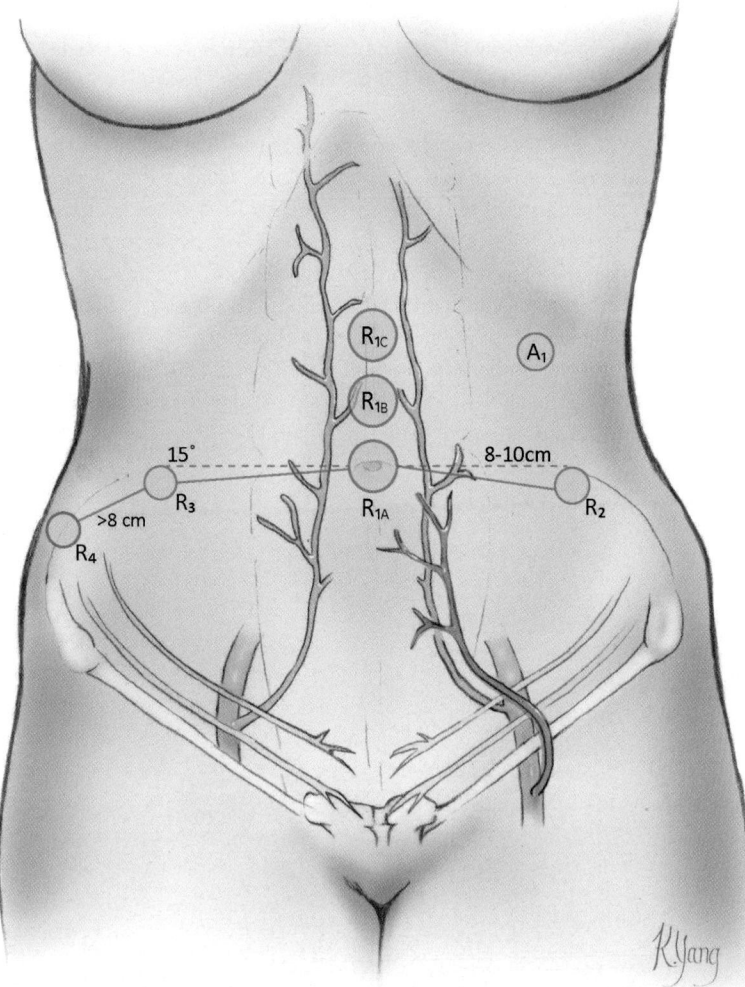

FIGURE 41-13 Typical port placements for robotic surgery. The R₁ port will house the laparoscope. Its site may be moved cephalad depending on the size of pelvic pathology as illustrated by R₁ₐ-R₁c. The other robot port sites are marked as R₂, R₃, and R₄. The assistant surgeon port site is marked as A₁. Here the superficial epigastric artery is shown arising from the femoral artery, whereas the inferior epigastric artery is a branch of the external iliac artery. The iliohypogastric and ilioinguinal nerves are also seen.

the accessory port(s), depending on the instruments required for a given procedure.

During port placement, initial abdominal entry and subsequent accessory trocars are inserted similar to laparoscopy (p. 889). Port placement for robotic surgery is unique in that ports must be placed with a minimum intervening distance of 8 cm. This keeps the robot arms from colliding with each other and with any accessory ports. As shown in Figure 41-13, the level of the laparoscope's port depends on the procedure, the complexity of the pathology, and previous patient surgeries. Importantly, a black ring around the cannula marks the depth to which a trocar is inserted. Insertion to this depth is essential to provide the robot arms the correct fulcrum to function optimally and lessens port-site tissue trauma.

Of newer modifications, reduced-port robotic surgery uses microtip percutaneous instruments to minimize the number of 8-mm ports. Its advantage is yet to be proven with randomized trials. As another modification, the Food and Drug Administration (FDA) has approved instrumentation for single-site robotic

surgery for certain gynecologic procedures. A fuller discussion of single-site laparoscopy is found on page 894.

■ Patient Selection

When selecting a robotic approach, both patient and procedure characteristics are considered. First, procedures that are currently performed efficiently by conventional laparoscopy should not be replaced by robotic surgery (American College of Obstetricians and Gynecologists, 2015). Rather, this modality is an alternative to laparotomy and thus may offer the patient a more rapid recovery and decreased postoperative morbidity. Second, patients chosen for this technique should be able to withstand conventional laparoscopic physiologic changes discussed earlier (p. 874). As with laparoscopy, a high patient BMI may limit the robotic approach but is not a contraindication and must have the joint effort of the anesthesiologist.

LAPAROSCOPIC ANATOMY

■ Anterior Abdominal Wall

The laparoscopic view of pelvic anatomy may differ slightly from laparotomy due to the effects of pneumoperitoneum, Trendelenburg positioning, and the translation of a 3-D reality into a 2-D image on the monitor.

When planning abdominal entry, key structures of the anterior abdominal wall are considered to avert neurovascular complications. Key landmarks include the umbilicus, anterior superior iliac spine, and pubic symphysis. Especially in the obese patient in whom a large pannus may alter anatomic relationships, bony landmarks are used to plan safe port placement.

The umbilicus is generally located at the level of the L3-L4 vertebrae, although it may lie above or below depending on habitus. In most patients, the aorta bifurcates at the union of L4-L5 vertebrae (Nezhat, 1998). However, in obese patients, the umbilicus tends to be caudal to this aortic bifurcation. In all patients, the left common iliac vein crosses the midline approximately 3 to 6 cm caudal to the aortic bifurcation, and the umbilicus is always cephalad to this point. The umbilicus is more caudal in heavier women. In normal-weight supine patients, these structures are considered during initial trocar entry at the umbilicus as they lie approximately 6 cm deep to the base of the umbilicus and may be closer in thinner patients (Hurd, 1992).

Accessory ports are placed under direct visualization of important anatomic structures including the bladder, bowel, and the inferior (deep) and superficial epigastric vessels. The inferior epigastric artery travels along the lateral third of the posterior surface of the rectus abdominis muscle and should be visualized intraperitoneally, running lateral to the medial umbilical ligaments (see Fig. 41-13). The superficial epigastric artery, a branch of the femoral artery, travels in the subcutaneous tissue in a path similar to that of the inferior epigastric vessels. The superficial epigastric artery may be identified by transillumination of the anterior abdominal wall with the laparoscope. Although it cannot be visualized, nerve supply of the anterior abdominal wall is also considered to avoid trauma during trocar placement. Both the ilioinguinal and iliohypogastric nerves can be lacerated during ancillary port placement. Steps to limit injury to these nerves and vessels are described on page 895.

Retroperitoneal Structures

Along the anterior abdominal wall, five prominent ligaments lie beneath the peritoneum and can be seen laparoscopically. These superficial intraperitoneal landmarks run cephalad to caudad and may be used to identify key anatomic structures in the retroperitoneum (Fig. 41-14). In the midline, the *median umbilical ligament* traverses from the bladder dome to the umbilicus and is the obliterated urachus.

Lateral to this lie the *medial umbilical folds*, which cover the obliterated umbilical arteries. Identification of the medial umbilical ligament is essential in the setting of a frozen pelvis and can provide access to the internal iliac artery. For this, the medial umbilical ligament is followed underneath the round ligament, through the broad ligament, to the superior vesicle artery, and finally to the internal iliac artery.

Running laterally to the medial umbilical folds and to the round ligaments are the *lateral umbilical folds*. These folds are formed by peritoneum overlying the inferior epigastric vessels before they enter the rectus sheath. Direct intraperitoneal visualization of the lateral umbilical folds will prevent injury to these vessels during port placement.

In the pelvic retroperitoneum, laparoscopy usually allows easy direct identification of the ureter and vessels of the pelvic sidewall. Moreover, the course of the pelvic ureter traveling from the pelvic brim, along the pelvic sidewall, and lateral to the cervix should routinely be appreciated with every laparoscopy to ensure normal peristalsis and caliber. To avoid injury to the ureter, its course is frequently confirmed during adnexal surgery, hysterectomy, and cases with adhesive disease.

ABDOMINAL ACCESS

The choice of entry site and method is influenced by factors that include body habitus, prior surgery, risk of encountering adhesive disease, intended procedure, surgeon skill, and the site, size, and type of pathology. Nearly half of all laparoscopic complications occur during abdominal entry, and nearly one quarter of these are undetected until the postoperative period (Bhoyrul, 2001; Chandler, 2001). Thus, entry carefully factors the above variables. Each of the methods discussed below may be beneficial in different situations, but all have potential risks. It has not been established which entry method is safest.

Umbilical Entry

The umbilicus is the most frequent entry site, although the left upper quadrant and subxiphoid area are others. The umbilicus is preferred for primary trocar placement because the subcutaneous and preperitoneal tissue layers are thinnest at the fused umbilical plate. Thus, the transumbilical approach is the shortest distance to the abdominal cavity, even in obese patients. From a cosmetic standpoint, the umbilical fossa also conceals the port-site scar.

Laparoscopic entry can be performed with an open or closed technique. With closed entry, either a Veress needle or laparoscopic trocar is used to pierce the fascia and peritoneum to gain abdominal entry. Closed entry techniques offer quick access to the abdominal cavity with a low risk of injury (Bonjer, 1997; Catarci, 2001). With open entry, the fascia is grasped with Allis clamps or peans and surgically incised. The peritoneum is then grasped and opened. Some authors advocate an open entry method as a way to lower puncture injury rates. However, metaanalyses fail to show that any of the following techniques are superior to the others (Ahmad, 2008; Vilos, 2007).

Closed Entry

During laparoscopic entry, surgeons appropriately assess patient habitus and their physical relationship to the supine patient. To diminish the downward thrust when placing the Veress needle and trocars, a surgeon adjusts the table height and uses a short stepstool if necessary. The aorta and its bifurcation lie beneath the umbilicus. To maximize the distance between the puncturing instrument and these vessels and avert vascular injury, premature Trendelenburg positioning is avoided, and the patient should lie flat. Moreover, to minimize visceral puncture during abdominal entry, the surgeon should empty the patient's bladder and confirm with the anesthesiologist that an orogastric tube has emptied the stomach. Palpation over these areas can confirm adequate decompression. The sacral promontory and aorta are also palpated, and a Veress needle or trocar with a length sufficient to reach the peritoneal cavity is selected. Finally, once all equipment is checked and correctly connected,

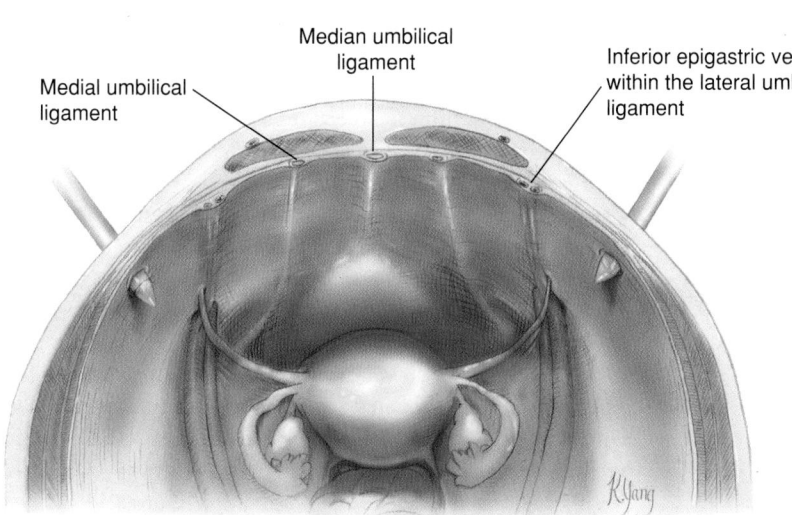

FIGURE 41-14 Umbilical ligaments relative to trocar placement.

Median umbilical ligament

Medial umbilical ligament

Inferior epigastric vessels within the lateral umbilical ligament the surgeon confirms with the anesthesiologist that the patient is fully paralyzed to prevent involuntary patient movement during abdominal entry.

Veress Needle Entry. The goal of this closed technique is to first create a pneumoperitoneum with a 14-gauge Veress needle. Once a pneumoperitoneum is created, the fascia and peritoneum are then secondarily punctured with a trocar. The pneumoperitoneum serves to tense the peritoneum and increases the distance of the viscera and retroperitoneal structures from the trocar entering the abdominal wall. These ideally help lower the risk of puncture injury during trocar insertion.

With all the closed methods, a skin incision appropriate to the trocar size is created, usually at the umbilicus. The incision can be either horizontal or vertical, is placed centrally within the umbilicus, and can be made with a no. 11 or 15 blade. Skin hooks or Allis clamps can aid in everting the umbilicus.

To begin, a Veress needle tip pierces through the fascia and peritoneum and enters the intraabdominal cavity to allow its insufflation with CO_2. During both Veress and trocar placement, many surgeons recommend abdominal wall elevation, either manually or with instruments such as towel clips (Fig. 41-15). A study using computed tomography images revealed that up to 8 cm can be added between the incision and retroperitoneum by elevation with towel clips (Shamiyeh,

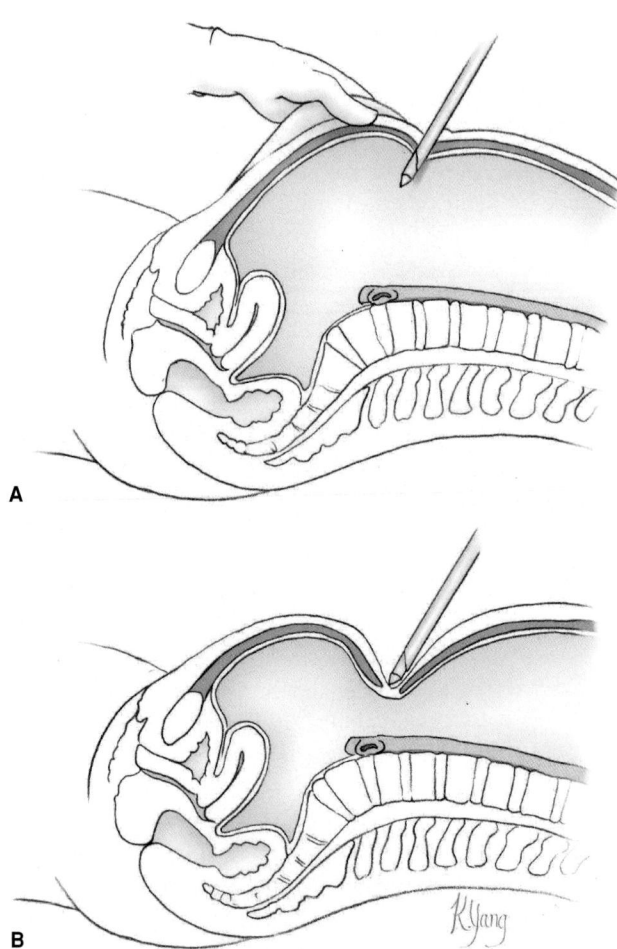

FIGURE 41-15 Primary trocar insertion. **A.** With anterior abdominal wall elevation. **B.** Without anterior abdominal wall elevation.

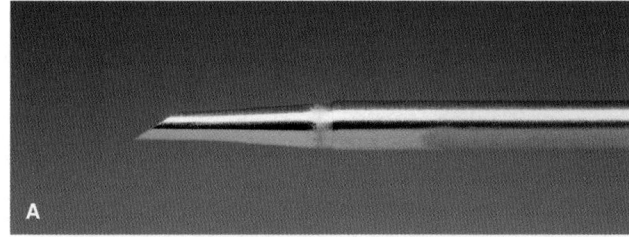

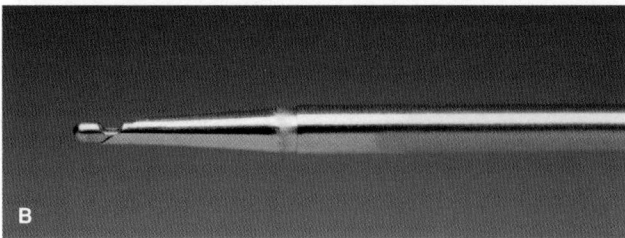

FIGURE 41-16 The Veress needle consists of a sharp outer needle (**A**), which houses a blunt-tipped, spring-loaded inner stylet (**B**).

2009). Abdominal wall elevation also provides a controlled countertension to the downward thrust of the Veress needle and subsequent trocar during insertion.

The Veress needle has a spring-loaded obturator (Fig. 41-16). As the device contacts the fascia, the obturator is pushed back, and the needle pierces the fascia and peritoneum. As soon as the tip enters the abdominal cavity, the obturator springs forward to prevent the needle from injuring abdominal viscera.

Prior to insertion, the Veress needle is checked for patency by flushing saline through the needle. The spring mechanism is also confirmed to function appropriately. The patient and operating table are flat, and the anterior abdominal wall is elevated. The Veress needle is inserted at a 45- to 90-degree angle depending on patient habitus and abdominal wall thickness. In patients with a normal BMI, angling the needle at a 45-degree angle permits abdominal entry yet minimizes the risk of great vessel injury (Fig. 41-17). With the Veress needle angled toward the hollow of the pelvis in the midline, there is a sensation of two "pops" as the tip of the needle penetrates the fascia and then the peritoneum. As shown in the figure, in overweight and obese individuals, smaller insertion angles are needed to successfully enter the abdomen.

Entry failures with this method usually stem from Veress needle tip placement into the preperitoneal space (Fig. 41-18). Flow of gas through the needle creates an extraperitoneal insufflation. This gaseous dissection of the peritoneum away from the anterior abdominal wall hinders the trocar in piercing the peritoneum. Instead, the trocar further stretches and pushes the peritoneum internally. Fortunately, this problem can often be overcome by a second attempt with the Veress needle above the umbilicus or by switching to an open entry technique (Fig. 41-19).

Preperitoneal insertion of the Veress needle is common and can lead to abandonment of the laparoscopic procedure. Thus, confirmation of correct needle placement in the peritoneal cavity is essential. For confirmation, a 10-mL syringe containing 5 mL of saline is attached to the hub of the inserted Veress needle. With aspiration, air bubbles should be seen in the syringe. If blood or bowel contents are aspirated, concern for vascular or

Normal   Overweight   Obese

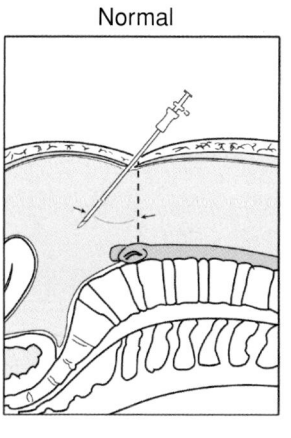 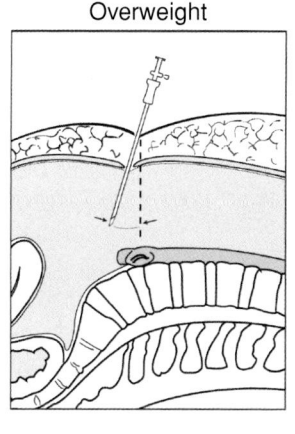 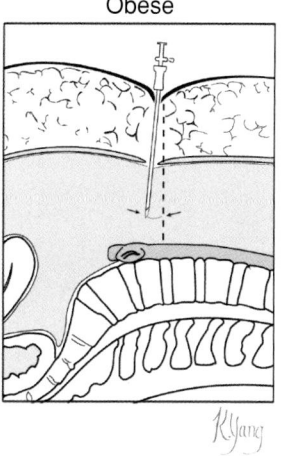

FIGURE 41-17 The appropriate angle needed for the Veress needle to enter the abdomen without injury to the aorta varies with the degree of body fat.

visceral injury should be high. In these cases, the needle is left in place to help localize the puncture site and act as a vascular plug as discussed on page 877.

After aspiration, saline is easily injected with no resistance. The surgeon should be unable to reaspirate this saline, which has dispersed into the abdominal cavity. Similarly, a hanging drop test can be used. With this, a few drops of saline are placed on the external open end of the Veress needle. If the needle tip is correctly inserted, the fluid drops disappear into the negative pressure of the abdominal cavity. If incorrect entry is suspected, the needle is withdrawn and checked for patency. Moving the Veress needle from side to side is avoided at this stage. Such movement can create rents in the omentum or injure bowel.

Once correct placement is confirmed by these methods, the CO_2 insufflation tubing can be attached to the needle. A low-volume flow of CO_2 is selected, and initial intraabdominal pressure recordings should be <8 mm Hg while the abdominal wall is manually lifted. If the pressure is elevated, the needle is immediately removed. The initial pressure is the most sensitive measurement of correct intraperitoneal Veress needle placement (Vilos, 2007). With the needle correctly inserted, pressure and gas flow may be increased. Simultaneously, the electronic insufflator parameters are closely monitored to ensure a steady increase in the pressure and continued flow. If the intraperitoneal pressure rises rapidly prior to insufflation of 1.5 to 2 L of gas, one again is concerned for preperitoneal insufflation.

During insufflation, the abdomen is observed for a uniform distention and dullness to percussion over the liver. Since the total volume required to appropriately insufflate an abdomen will vary depending on patient habitus, intraperitoneal pressure, rather than total volume of gas, is used to determine adequate peritoneal insufflation. During normal insufflation, pressures should not exceed 20 mm Hg. Such elevated pressure can lead to hemodynamic and pulmonary compromise. When an intraperitoneal pressure of 20 mm Hg is achieved, the Veress needle may be withdrawn, and the pneumoperitoneum should assist safe primary trocar insertion. This transiently elevated intraabdominal pressure provides a volumetric countertension for primary trocar insertion. However, once the primary trocar is inserted, the insufflation pressure is dropped to <15 mm Hg, or to the lowest pressure that allows the planned procedure to be adequately visualized and safely performed.

Although data from multiple studies are conflicting, it has been proposed that the use of humidified CO_2 for insufflation through out a case may have advantages. These include decreased postoperative pain, improved visualization from less lens fogging, and in animal studies, less de novo adhesion formation (Farley, 2004; Ott, 1998; Peng, 2009; Sammour, 2008).

Primary Trocar Placement. Once adequate insufflation is achieved, the primary trocar may then be placed. Trocars are

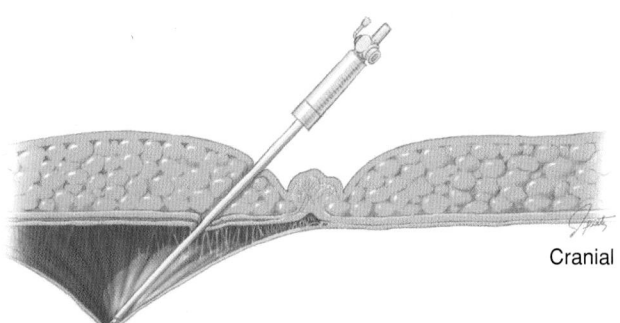

FIGURE 41-18 Veress needle tenting the peritoneal layer.

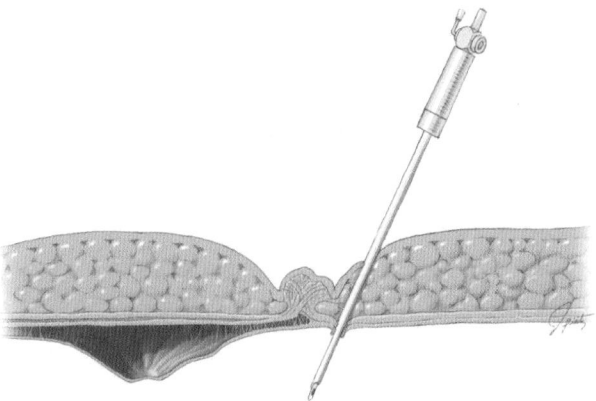

FIGURE 41-19 Veress needle replaced above the umbilicus.

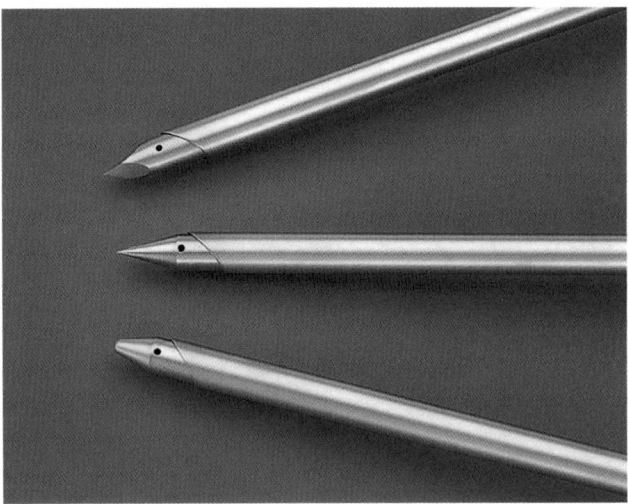

FIGURE 41-20 Trocars consist of outer cannula and inner obturator. The trocar is used to gain access to the abdomen. The obturator then is removed, and the cannula serves as a conduit through which to introduce instruments. Obturators may have a pyramidal (*top*), conical (*middle*), or blunt tip (*bottom*). (Reproduced with permission from Karl Storz America, Inc.)

used gain access to the abdominal cavity. First-generation trocars consist of a hollow, long, slender cannula that sheaths an inner obturator. Trocars typically range from 5 to 12 mm in diameter, and their tips may be conical, pyramidal, or blunt (Fig. 41-20).

Conical trocars are smooth except for their more pointed tip and have no cutting edges. They split the fascia rather than cut it and thus are preferred by some to lower risks of postoperative hernia formation and vessel injury (Hurd, 1995; Leibl, 1999). However, they require more penetration force to insert. In contrast, pyramidal trocars have sharp edges and tip and as a result, cut the fascia as they are inserted into the abdomen.

In the 1980s, trocars with retractable shields were introduced. Similar to the concept used with the Veress needle, a hollow plastic retractable shield covers the trocar tip both before and after the trocar pierces the abdominal wall. In this manner, the cutting edge is exposed only during its passage through the fascia. Despite theoretical advantages to these shielded trocars in preventing organ injury, studies have failed to show superiority of this design (Fuller, 2003).

Initial trocar entry is a blind procedure and is completed with the patient still supine and flat. The Veress needle is removed, and the trocar's tip is placed in the umbilical incision. The trocar handle is cupped in the palm of the dominant hand, and the same hand's index finger is extended along the trocar shaft to splint the trocar from too deep of insertion. The angle of trocar insertion should mirror that of the Veress needle. The anterior abdominal wall is elevated. With control and minimal downward force, the trocar punctures the fascia and underlying peritoneum and enters the abdominal cavity. After insertion, the trocar obturator is removed, and the cannula may be advanced slightly to ensure adequate placement into the peritoneal cavity. At this point, the laparoscope is inserted through the umbilical cannula to visually confirm safe and atraumatic entry.

VersaStep System. Similar to the Veress needle method, a VersaStep System may be used. This consists of a stretchable nylon sheath over a disposable Veress needle (Fig. 41-21). The first step of insertion is identical to Veress needle insertion and peritoneal insufflation. Once insufflation is complete, the Veress needle is removed, leaving the nylon sheath in situ. A trocar with a blunt inner obturator is inserted into the nylon sheath. Downward, gradual continuous pressure by the trocar causes the nylon sheath to stretch and accommodate as the trocar is advanced. The obturator is then removed, leaving only the nylon sheath and cannula as the operative port. The benefit of this system is that only a blunt trocar is used, thus potentially

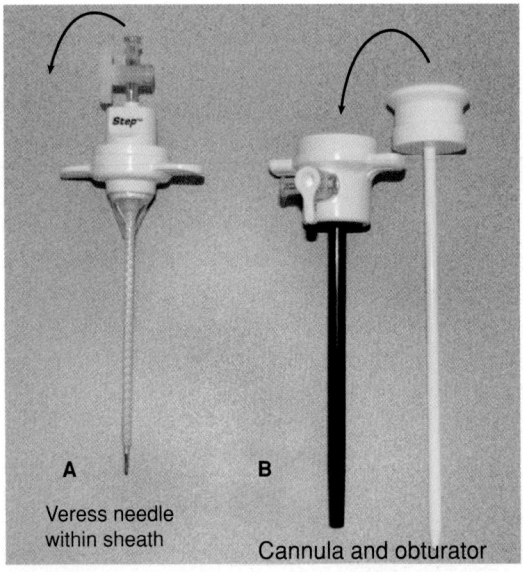
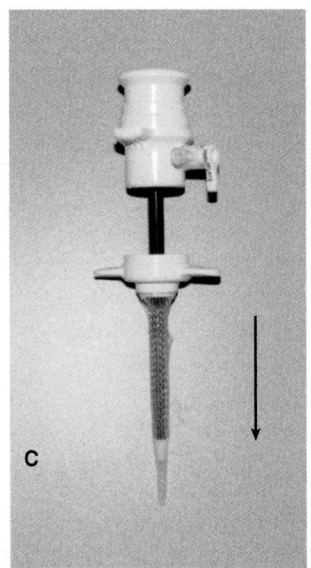
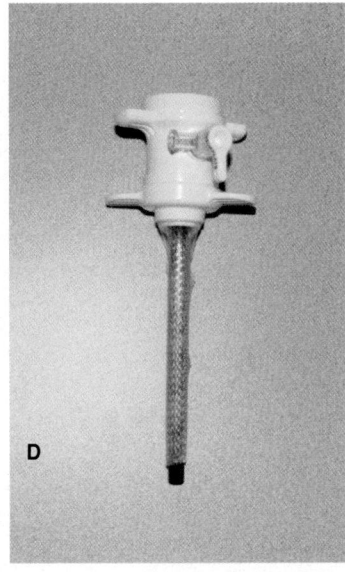

A Veress needle within sheath
B Cannula and obturator
C
D

FIGURE 41-21 VersaStep system. **A.** The Veress needle housed within a nylon sheath is placed as a traditional Veress needle would be. Once inserted intraabdominally, the Veress needle is removed and the sheath remains within the abdominal incision. **B.** Next, the white obturator is placed within the black cannula. **C.** Together, this trocar is threaded intraabdominally through the nylon sheath. **D.** Last, the obturator is removed. The black cannula is completely sheathed by the nylon sleeve and has gained access to the abdomen.

diminishing traumatic injuries from a cutting blade. Also, the conical dilator may create a smaller fascial defect.

Optical Access Trocar Entry. To reduce bowel injury risk at the time of primary trocar insertion, optical trocars were developed. These devices, in essence, combine the laparoscope and trocar into one tool. Importantly, the laparoscope should be focused once it is housed within the trocar and prior to insertion. During use, the optical trocar transmits images of the abdominal wall layers to the television monitor. These layers then are pierced under direct visualization by trocar tip advancement. If choosing an umbilical entry, the layers visualized, in sequence, should be the subcutaneous fat, the linea alba (fascia), preperitoneal fat, and peritoneum.

Optical entry methods can be used with and without the prior establishment of pneumoperitoneum. Despite the theoretical advantage of this type of trocar, major organ injury still has been reported. Moreover, no large studies have established its clinical superiority over other entry techniques (Sharp, 2002).

Direct Trocar Entry. Because of entry failures associated with preperitoneal insufflation, a direct trocar entry method may be preferred (Copeland, 1983; Dingfelder, 1978). For this, the abdominal wall is elevated and directly pierced with a trocar without prior insufflation. Comparative studies between Veress needle and direct trocar techniques show lower rates of entry failure with the direct method (Byron, 1993; Clayman, 2005; Gunenc, 2005). Moreover, investigators note comparable or lower associated minor complication rates with the direct entry method.

Open Umbilical Entry

To lower puncture injury rates with closed entry methods, an open entry technique was described by Hasson (1971, 1974). For this, a 1- to 2-cm transverse skin incision at the lower edge of the umbilicus is made while applying tension with fine-toothed forceps to its lateral borders. Skin edges are retracted laterally, and the subcutaneous layer is divided to expose the linea alba. This fascia is lifted and everted upward with two Allis clamps (Fig. 41-22). A 0.5- to 1-cm incision with scalpel

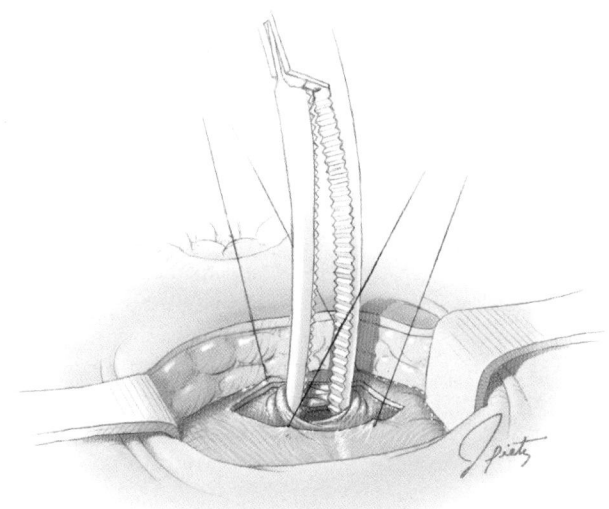

FIGURE 41-23 Peritoneal entry during open entry.

or scissors then transects the fascia. The Allis clamps are repositioned, one on each free fascial edge.

A hemostat or finger is used to bluntly open the peritoneum, and the end of an S-retractor is placed into the abdomen. The abdominal portion of the retractor is used to elevate the abdominal wall and shield the underlying organs as a stitch of 0-gauge delayed-absorbable suture is placed parallel on one side of the fascial opening (Fig. 41-23). This suture is not tied. This suturing step is repeated on the opposite fascial edge.

The distal, blunt end of the Hassan trocar then is inserted into the incision. The fascial tag sutures are pulled firmly upward and threaded into the suture holders found on either side of the cannula's proximal end (Fig. 41-24). The blunt obturator is removed, and the laparoscope is threaded through the cannula.

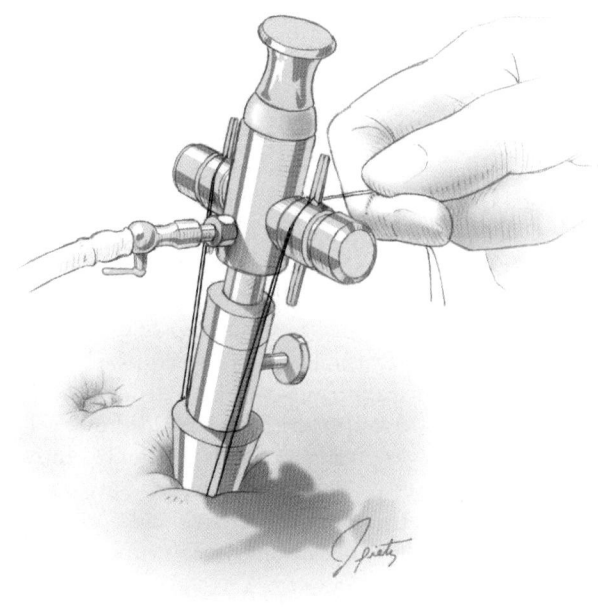

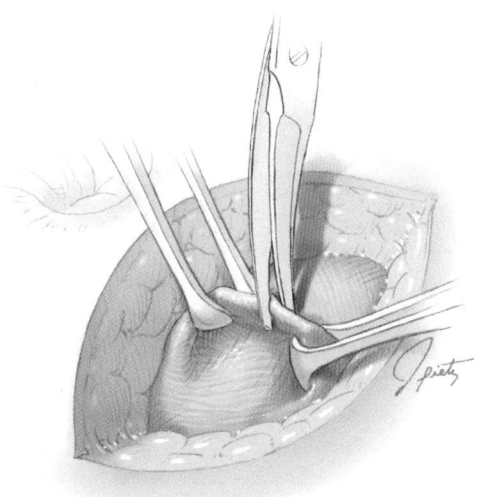

FIGURE 41-22 Fascial incision for open entry.

FIGURE 41-24 Primary trocar placement with open entry.

In a retrospective review of more than 5000 open entry procedures, Hasson and associates (2000) noted that minor and medium-risk complications developed at a rate of 0.5 percent. Moreover, in studies comparing open and closed techniques, open methods showed lower rates of entry failure and organ injury (Bonjer, 1997; Merlin, 2003). Open entry is recommended by many surgeons for patients with prior abdominal surgery, for those following a closed technique entry failure, for those with a large cystic mass, and for pediatric or pregnant patients (Madeb, 2004). This technique, however, is not foolproof, and organ injury, mainly bowel, has been described (Magrina, 2002). Typically, this method of entry takes longer than closed entry, and the pneumoperitoneum can be difficult to maintain in some cases due to air escape around the cannula.

■ Alternative Entry Sites
Anterior Abdominal Wall

At times, the umbilicus may be unsuitable for initial abdominal entry, and surgeons should develop comfort with entry at an alternative site. Of concerns, adhesive disease may tether bowel beneath the umbilicus and is suspected in women with prior intraabdominal surgery, infection, endometriosis, or malignancy (see Table 42-1). Similarly, surgical mesh placed during umbilical herniorrhaphy is also linked with adhesive disease, and entry at this site may also disrupt the hernia repair. Nonumbilical entry can also avoid inadvertent trauma to or rupture of a large intraabdominal mass or gravid uterus.

Nonumbilical anterior abdominal wall entry has been described at various locations. The left upper quadrant is most common, but the subxiphoid area is another. Both have the advantage of providing working ports at these sites once safe entry is achieved.

Of these, left upper quadrant entry is simple, has a low risk of complications, and usually is free of adhesions (Agarwala, 2005; Howard, 1997; Palmer, 1974). Although left upper quadrant access may be obtained at either Palmer point or the ninth intercostal space, the easy accessibility of Palmer point makes this a favored site. Palmer point is located 3 cm below the left costal margin in the midclavicular line. Organs in close proximity to this point are the stomach, left lobe of the liver, spleen, and retroperitoneal structures, which may be as close as 1.5 cm (Giannios, 2009; Tulikangas, 2000).

For entry at Palmer point, one ensures that the stomach is emptied using suction with an orogastric or nasogastric tube. Palpating the area will ensure adequate emptying and exclude incidental splenomegaly. A skin incision adequate for trocar insertion is made at Palmer point. With anterior abdominal wall elevation, the Veress needle is inserted in the skin incision at an angle slightly less than 90 degrees and is directed caudad to avoid liver injury. Initial intraabdominal pressure of <10 mm Hg indicates correct intraperitoneal placement. Once adequate insufflation is obtained, the Veress needle may be removed and a trocar inserted. Alternatively, direct trocar entry may be performed at Palmer point as well. We favor an optical access trocar to permit each layer of the anterior abdominal wall to be seen as it is penetrated (Vellinga, 2009).

For this, the anterior abdominal wall is elevated, and the trocar with laparoscope is placed into the skin incision. The trocar is directed at a 90-degree angle. During insertion, one should observe the following in sequence: subcutaneous fat, outer fascial layer, muscle layer, inner fascial layer, peritoneum, and finally, abdominal organs. Remember that above the level of the arcuate line, posterior rectus sheath fascia is present and is the inner fascial layer.

Natural Orifice Transluminal Endoscopic Surgery

This method uses existing natural orifices such as the vagina, stomach, bladder, and rectum to access the peritoneum. In addition, a transuterine approach has been described. Although infrequently used in current practice, interest is renewed in laparoscopic access through the posterior fornix. Proposed advantages of this method are improved access to organs, better cosmesis from elimination of an external scar, shorter hospitalizations, and possibly less postoperative pain and fewer postoperative complications.

■ Single-port Access Laparoscopy

Single-incision surgery is a laparoscopic approach in which a sole 2- to 3-cm incision accommodates a single larger port that concurrently houses multiple instruments. It is also known as single-incision laparoscopic surgery (SILS), laparoendoscopic single-site surgery (LESS), and single-port access (SPA). The proposed advantages of this method are improved cosmesis from a single port, which is usually buried in the umbilicus, and possibly faster return to normal activity. This is balanced against the longer incision that potentially has greater risks for postoperative pain, wound infection or dehiscence, and later incisional hernia. Moreover, single-incision surgery is technically more challenging than conventional laparoscopy due to instrument crowding at a single port, limited visualization, and loss of instrument triangulation (Uppal, 2011). *Triangulation* describes instruments converging on a focal point from lateral angles of origin. These angles create opposing forces, which are essential for effective tissue retraction, dissection, and resection. However, SPA has grown in popularity with advances in articulating instruments and flexible-tip endoscopes, which help deal with some of these challenges.

For laparoscopic SPA, several ports are popular. The SILS port (Covidien) is limited to umbilical placement and may not be suitable for large pathology that encroaches on the umbilicus. The Gelpoint (Applied Medical) may be inserted almost anywhere on the abdominal wall due to the variable depth of its self-retaining sheath attached between the two rigid loops (Fig. 41-25). Moreover, the gel dome lacks preset silos for the trocars, and thus allows any size trocar to be inserted in individualized groupings.

For robotic SPA, the Single Site port (da Vinci) is placed in the umbilicus and contains cannulas for the curved trocars used in this approach. This system is limited by the required port placement but offers an alternative for suitable candidates. Instrument choices and movement are more limited. For example, the traditional wristed models are not offered, but the longer curved trocars may offer sufficient triangulation.

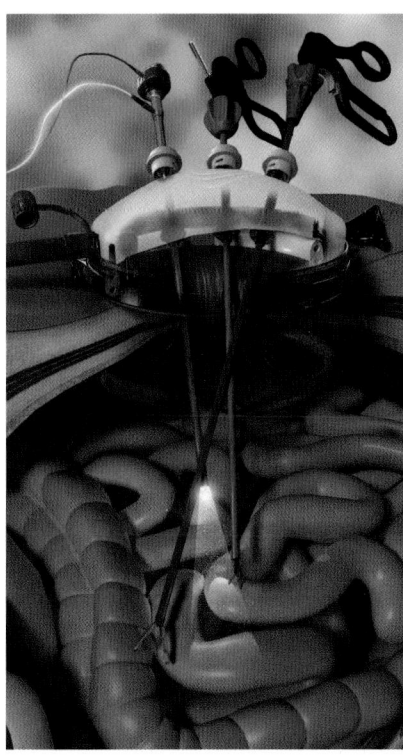

FIGURE 41-25 GelPOINT Advanced Access System. (Reproduced with permission from Applied Medical Resources Corporation.)

Gasless Laparoscopy

This variation of traditional laparoscopy addresses the physiologic disadvantages of pneumoperitoneum just described. With this method, an abdominal wall lift device elevates the abdominal wall to create the laparoscopic working space, and thus no gas is required. Additional advantages include the sustained visualization after colpotomy or with continuous suctioning. Despite advantages, drawbacks are a "tent-shaped" operating space, additional required incisions, and time needed for the lift device assembly. These currently limit its routine use, but gasless laparoscopy may still have value in high-risk patients with cardiorespiratory diseases (Cravello, 1999; Goldberg, 1997; Negrin Perez, 1999).

Accessory Port Placement

Once primary abdominal access is achieved, additional operative ports are needed to insert instruments. The number, location, and size of these cannulas will vary depending on the tools required and the laparoscopic procedure. For additional port placement, the patient is placed in Trendelenburg position to displace bowel from the pelvis and provide an unobstructed view. Ancillary trocars are always placed under direct laparoscopic visualization to minimize the puncture risk to anterior abdominal wall vessels or abdominal viscera. The camera is generally driven by the first assistant or in some cases by the second assistant to free two surgeons' hands for the actual operative tasks.

Appropriate ancillary port site selection is a key step in operative planning. Correct placement permits triangulation. Poorly placed ports may create instrument angles that lead to ineffective movement, surgeon fatigue, and iatrogenic complications.

Of sites, the suprapubic midline site is most frequently used. Prior to trocar insertion, the bladder is emptied, and the trocar is placed after identification of both the bladder and the urachus. For operative laparoscopy, placement of two lower quadrant ports lateral to the inferior epigastric vessels is also common. Their sites are individualized according to patient anatomy and pathology. Generally, larger pelvic masses require more cephalad placement.

During accessory port placement, transillumination of the anterior abdominal wall is useful to avoid puncture of the superficial epigastric vessels. In this process, the laparoscope, within the abdominal cavity, is placed directly against the peritoneal surface of the anterior wall. This light is seen externally as a red circular glow, and the superficial epigastric arteries are seen as dark vessels traversing it.

Unfortunately, the inferior epigastric arteries lie deep to the rectus abdominis muscle and are poorly seen with transillumination. These arteries, however, can be seen by direct laparoscopic visualization in most cases (Fig. 41-26) (Hurd, 2003). Also, anatomic landmarks can be used to limit vessel puncture risks. For example, Epstein and coworkers (2004) noted that the main stem of the inferior epigastric artery can be avoided if trocars are inserted within the lateral third of the distance between the midline and anterior superior iliac spine (ASIS). Rahn and colleagues (2010) noted that the inferior epigastric vessels were 3.7 cm from the midline at the level of the ASIS and were always lateral to the rectus abdominis muscle at a level 2 cm superior to the pubic symphysis.

Ideally, port placement will also minimize the risk of ilioinguinal and iliohypogastric nerve injury. Most injuries to these

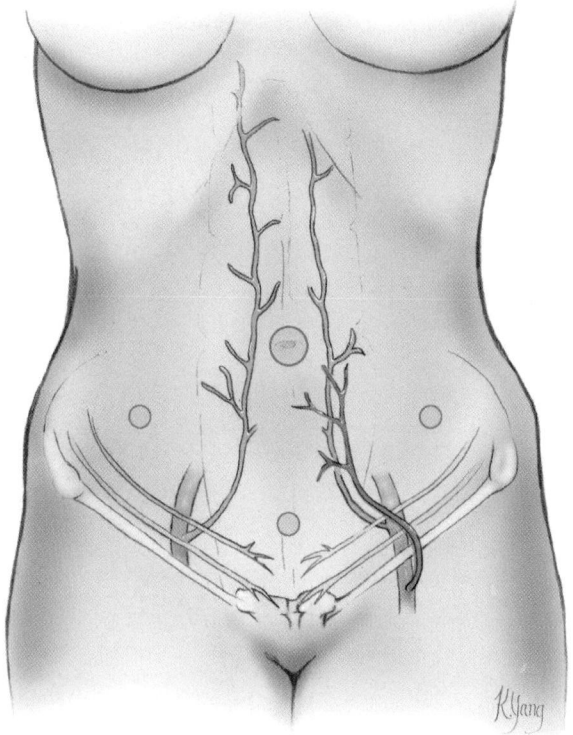

FIGURE 41-26 Common abdominal access sites include a primary entry site inferior to umbilicus and smaller accessory trocar sites in the lower abdomen.

nerves and to the inferior epigastric vessels can be averted by placing the accessory ports superior to the ASIS and >6 cm from the abdomen's midline (Rahn, 2010). Once all ports are positioned, the planned procedure is begun.

■ Tissue Extraction

Near the end of many MIS procedures, safe tissue extraction is an essential step. However, port-site seeding and inadvertent dissemination of both benign and malignant tissue during specimen fragmentation and extraction are risks. Several studies have described peritoneal leiomyomatosis, parasitic myomas, and de novo endometriosis following power morcellation of uteri and myomas (Kho, 2009; Milad, 2013; Sepilian, 2003). Moreover, morcellation of occult cancer may worsen patient prognosis. This may be particularly likely with uterine sarcoma, which has been a topic of debate (Park, 2011; Pritts, 2015).

Alternatives to power morcellation are varied. First, through minilaparatomy incisions ranging from 1 to 4 cm, myomas and uteri may be brought to the anterior abdominal wall (Fig. 44-8, p. 1025). Here, they can be hand morcellated with a scalpel or scissors and extracted (Alessandri, 2006; Panici, 2005).

Second, posterior colpotomy is safe and effective to open the cul-de-sac for bulky tissue removal (Ghezzi, 2012). As shown in Figure 41-27, a posterior colpotomy is created similar to that for vaginal hysterectomy. Namely, the cervix is lifted upward, and the vagina of the posterior fornix is stretched outward and downward to create tension. Curved Mayo scissors then incise the intervening vaginal wall and peritoneum to enter the abdomen via the posterior cul-de-sac. Once entry is confirmed, vaginal retractors can be placed for exposure. Alternatively, posterior colpotomy can be completed during laparoscopy. As

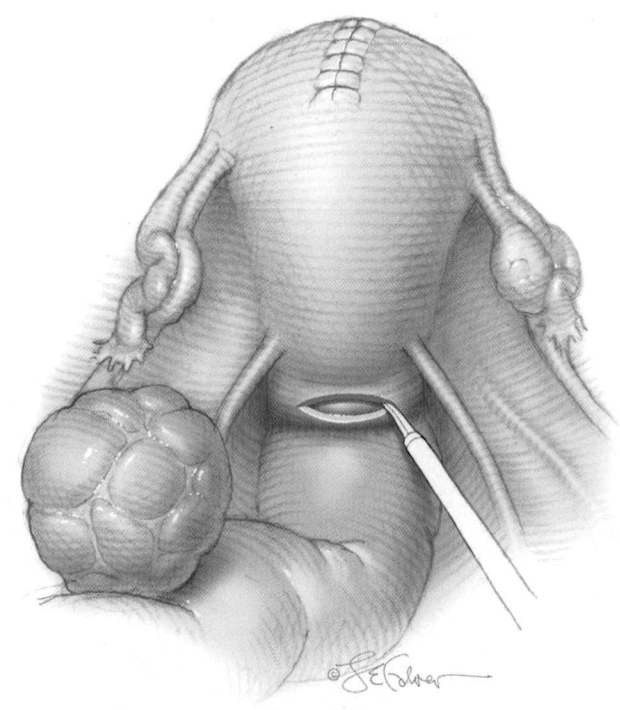

FIGURE 41-28 Posterior colpotomy incision from an abdominal approach.

Figure 41-28 illustrates, the uterosacral ligaments and ureters are first identified. A wide, blunt vaginal probe is inserted to elevate, accentuate, and stretch the posterior vaginal fornix for incision. Using an energy-based device, the vaginal wall is incised below the level of the cervix and between the uterosacral ligaments to create the posterior colpotomy incision. Whether through this opening or a minilaparatomy, the addition of a tissue retrieval bag during tissue extraction can create a closed environment for morcellation (Fig. 41-29). This reduces the

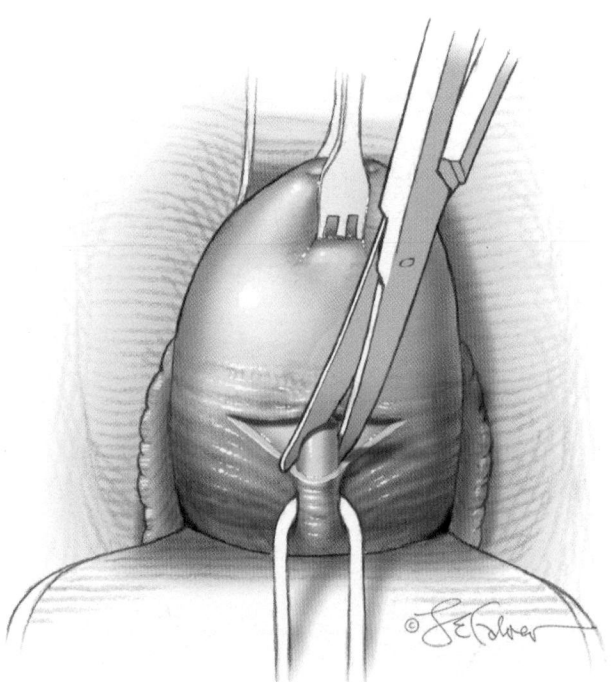

FIGURE 41-27 Posterior colpotomy incision from a vaginal approach.

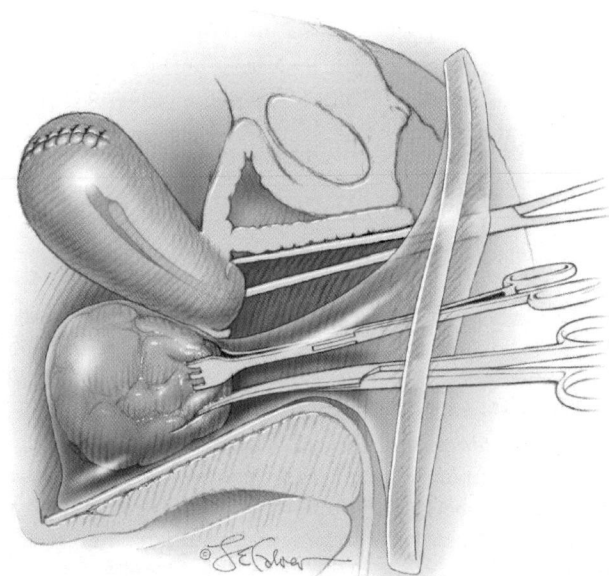

FIGURE 41-29 Through the posterior colpotomy, enclosed morcellation can be completed. In this instance, a large myoma is being sharply divided.

risk of inadvertent tissue dissemination during fragmentation, although long-term safety data are needed.

A third method, enclosed power morcellation, is still being studied. For this, a large endoscopic bag that can house the insufflation gas, conform to the abdominal cavity, and flatten against the intraperitoneal organs is introduced through a laparoscopic port. In the abdomen, it is unfolded to allow the specimen and gas to be contained. Depending on the pathology, the bag may be exteriorized through one abdominal port or incision, or may function during morcellation simply as a liner that catches any disseminated tissue (Einarsson, 2014). Following morcellation, the gas is released, and bag and tissue fragments are removed. Limitations of currently available retrieval bags involve the pouch size, the working aperture diameter, tensile strength, and permeability (Cohen, 2014).

■ Abdominal Entry Closure

The intraabdominal pressure produced by the pneumoperitoneum has an excellent hemostatic effect. Thus, at the end of cases, sites of potential bleeding are evaluated under a reduced pressure. A portion of the pneumoperitoneum is allowed to escape, and the intraabdominal pressure gauge is reset to 7 or 8 mm Hg. Vessels that need sealing will be seen and treated prior to procedure completion.

With surgery completed, CO_2 insufflation is halted, and the gas tubing is disconnected from the primary cannula. The gas ports on all cannulas are opened to deflate the abdominal cavity. To prevent diaphragmatic irritation from retained CO_2, manual pressure is placed on the abdomen to help expel remaining gas. Next, cannulas are removed under laparoscopic visualization. This allows evaluation for bleeding from punctured vessels that may have been tamponaded by the cannula or the pneumoperitoneum. These sites and other potential bleeding sites are reinspected as the pneumoperitoneum diminishes. Additionally, visualization prevents herniation of bowel or omentum up through the cannula track and into the anterior abdominal wall. Once all secondary cannulas are out, the laparoscope and then the primary cannula are removed.

Many surgeons recommend reapproximation of fascial defects at port sites to prevent anterior abdominal wall hernia formation. Although closure of the fascial defect does not obviate the risk of hernia formation, in general, most surgeons close ancillary ports sites ≥10 mm. The fascia can be closed by direct visualization with the assistance of S-retractors. The fascia is grasped with Allis clamps and then reapproximated with interrupted stitches of 0-gauge delayed-absorbable suture. Also, several laparoscopic closure devices (Carter-Thomason, EndoClose, and neoClose devices) are available. With these, fascial defects are reapproximated during direct laparoscopic visualization.

Skin incisions are closed with a subcuticular stitch of 4-0 gauge delayed-absorbable suture. Alternatively, the skin may be closed with cyanoacrylate tissue adhesive (Dermabond) or with skin tape (Steri-Strip Elastic) plus benzoin tincture (Chap. 40, p. 847).

Open Entry Incision Closure

During removal of the Hasson trocar, sutures originally placed in the fascia are unthreaded from the cannula. Each of these

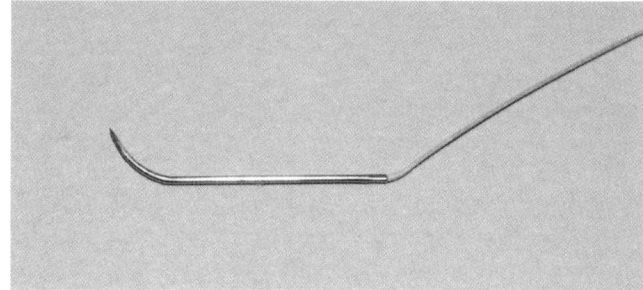

FIGURE 41-30 Ski needle.

sutures then is brought to the midline of the incision, and square knots are tied to close the fascial defect. The skin is reapproximated in a similar manner to that just described with closed abdominal entry.

SURGICAL BASICS

■ Tissue Approximation
Suturing Tools

Following tissue excision, reapproximation with suture is often needed. Subsequent knot tying may be performed using either inside the body, *intracorporeal*, or outside the body, *extracorporeal*, techniques. For these skills, a learning curve demands a time investment, not only in the operating room, but also with box trainers or simulators. Some newer devices can make these essential steps of surgery less challenging. Typically, selection is based on the procedure planned, surgeon preference, and reapproximation goals.

Needles for MIS suturing must pass through the placed ports. For this, the suture is grasped approximately 1 cm from the needle swage and passed through an appropriately sized cannula. Thus, the needle type chosen will depend on the size of available cannulas. One option, the ski needle, can pass through a narrow cannula (Fig. 41-30). Straight Keith needles can also be easily passed through cannulas of any size. However, their wide, flat arcs prohibit their use in tight anatomic spaces, which require a needle with a fuller arc. Conventional needle shapes and sizes often require higher-diameter ports.

Needle driver styles are also varied and are curved or straight and have either a smooth or finely serrated inner surface (Fig. 41-31). Driver tips are tapered to limit tissue trauma. They also have a single-action jaw to provide a stable needle grasp.

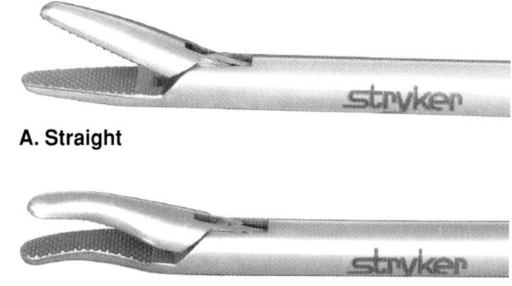

A. Straight

B. Curved

FIGURE 41-31 Laparoscopic needle driver. (Reproduced with permission from Stryker Endoscopy.)

To assist with needle grasping, some driver tips are designed to guide the needle into a correct driving position. Termed *self-righting*, these drivers may be less desirable for suturing in difficult-to-reach anatomic spaces. Here, the needle may need to be grasped by the driver at an oblique angle to achieve correct suture placement. Other needle driver features include a coaxial (rotating) handle and a locking grip. These hold the needle in place yet decrease hand strain. With suturing, the needle driver is held in the dominant hand, while the nondominant hand holds a tissue grasper. Alternatively, some surgeons prefer to use a second needle driver in the nondominant hand. This assists in grasping the tissue, retrieving the needle or sutures from the dominant hand, and providing countertraction when needed.

Disposable suturing devices render needle drivers unnecessary for tissue approximation. The Endo Stitch is a 10-mm-diameter instrument with a double-action jaw. A short, straight needle juts at a right angle from the inner surface of one tip. As the instrument tips are closed, the needle passes through the desired tissue. Then, with the tips still closed and with the flip of a handle toggle, the detachable needle is released from the first tip and reanchors at a right angle into the opposite tip. Instruments containing delayed-absorbable, barbed, or nonabsorbable suture are available. Also, the LSI suturing device is a 5-mm instrument with a hooked tip that passes a straight needle through the tissue. Both suturing tools have benefits and limitations, and familiarity with both is advantageous.

Sutures are broadly categorized as: (1) absorbable, delayed-absorbable, and permanent, (2) as monofilament or braided, (3) as natural or synthetic, and (4) as barbed or unbarbed. Suture selection depends primarily on the characteristics of tissues to be approximated and on the functional goals of reapproximation. Importantly, compared with traditional surgery, laparoscopic knot tying creates increased friction and suture fraying, and time between knot throws is longer. Thus, greater tensile strength and increased memory become more valued suture traits. For example, synthetic delayed-absorbable suture offers high tensile strength, less tissue reactivity, greater knot reliability, and easy handling for either intracorporeal or extracorporeal knot tying. Of filament types, although monofilament suture passes more smoothly through tissues, braided suture ties more easily and breaks less frequently. Last, the most common absorbable suture is catgut. However, compared with delayed-absorbable suture, this material provides less tensile strength and less knot security. Accordingly, catgut is less popular for MIS. If used, intracorporeal knot tying is generally preferred due to the significant fraying that occurs with this suture during extracorporeal tying.

For laparoscopy, narrow sutures in the 2-0 and 3-0 gauge range are preferred. This diameter provides suitable tensile strength to prevent suture breakage. Yet, it is thin enough to limit scarring from foreign-body reaction and to harbor fewer bacteria compared with thicker suture. However, for some procedures, such as vaginal cuff closure, the greater tensile strength provided by a 0-gauge suture is required.

Barbed sutures offer the unique ability to maintain tensile pressure on a continuous suture line. With this synthetic suture,

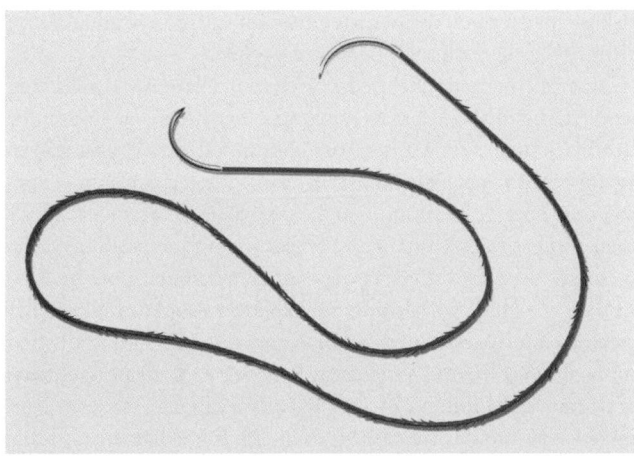

FIGURE 41-32 Barbed suture. (Reproduced with permission from Angiotech Pharmaceuticals, Inc.)

multiple barbs are evenly spaced around the suture's outer surface (Fig. 41-32). These barbs flatten as they pass through the tissues to be approximated but flare out once through to the other side. These flared barbs prevent suture from slipping back through the approximated tissues. As a result, the tissues remain joined with evenly distributed tissue tension (Greenberg, 2008). By its design, this suture obviates the need for knot tying. Available barbed-suture products include Quill, Stratafix, and V-Loc sutures.

Barbed suture may be uni- or bidirectional, and these differ in the direction that suturing can proceed. *Unidirectional suture* has a small preformed loop at the tail end, which serves as the knot for that end of the suture line. Suturing moves from the looped end in the other direction. *Bidirectional suture* has needles at each end. Suturing begins at the incision midpoint and can then progress in both directions along the incision. With either suture type, the tissue is approximated by cinching the final suture line or placing a suture loop in the opposite direction. No final knot is needed to secure the suture line, which is held in place by the barbs. Alternatively, an anchoring hemostatic clip may be placed to secure the suture line end. In general, barbed suture may be advantageous for myometrial reapproximation during laparoscopic myomectomy or for vaginal cuff closure during total laparoscopic hysterectomy. At completion of the running suture line, the suture is cut short to avoid puncture of adjacent tissue by a barb.

Knots

The length of suture will depend on the proposed suturing and knot tying. In general, 6 to 8 cm is needed for intracorporeal knot tying, and 24 to 36 cm for extracorporeal tying. Longer lengths are required for running stitches and for complicated knots compared with simple interrupted stitches.

Once tissues are approximated, the suture is tied by the intracorporeal or extracorporeal technique and then trimmed. Of the two, intracorporeal tying has a steeper learning curve because the surgeon must use laparoscopic instruments rather than fingers to loop the suture (Fig. 41-33). Extracorporeal knot tying is simpler for most surgeons because the suture is looped with fingers as in traditional tying. Each formed knot throw is

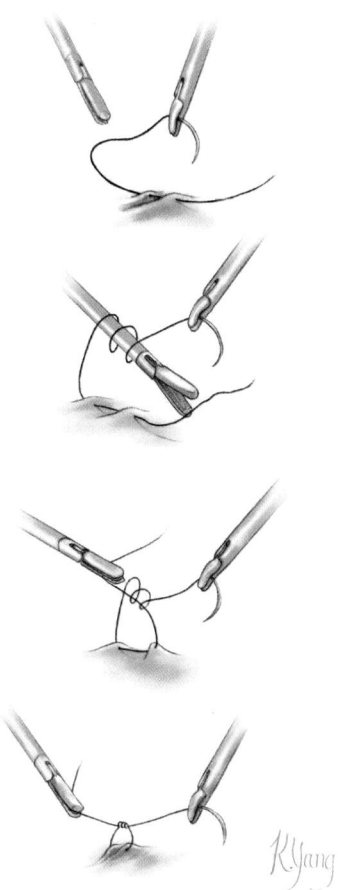

FIGURE 41-33 Intracorporeal knot tying.

then guided through a laparoscopic cannula and cinched with a knot pusher to create the knot (Fig. 41-34). Of suture types, stronger braided suture is preferred if the knot pusher is used because suture fraying is a side effect of this technique. Another disadvantage of extracorporeal knot tying compared with intracorporeal methods is that it often causes more tissue tension and can tear delicate tissues.

As an alternative to manual knot tying, disposable clips can be placed at the end of a suture line for security. Specifically, a hemoclip is a titanium V-shaped clip with arms that can be squeezed together during application. These clips were originally designed to compress vessels for hemostasis and are available in various sizes. At the end of a running suture line, hemoclips can also be placed across the suture tail to prevent stitch unraveling. If used for this purpose, two clips are advisable. More recent developments include the Lapra-Ty. This has a locking clip made of delayed-absorbable polydioxanone, which is also used in the suture brand PDS. Its ability to be absorbed and its lock are advantages, whereas its need for a 11- to 12-mm port may be disadvantageous in some settings. Also, these ties are only approved to anchor suture diameters greater

than 4-0 gauge. Another option is the 5-mm Ti-KNOT instrument. With this disposable device, a special titanium clip is placed around a single or a double strand of suture. With any of these alternatives to laparoscopic knot tying, the cost may be justified by the time saved in the operating room.

Stapling

In gynecologic surgery, vascular tissue is typically ligated first and then transected. Ligation may be achieved with electrosurgical tools described earlier, with stapling devices, or with suture loops. Linear staplers are mainly used for achieving anastomoses as in bowel surgery and are not frequently employed for gynecologic procedures. When selected in gynecologic laparoscopic surgery, they are chiefly used to ligate vascular pedicles, such as the infundibulopelvic ligament. Once fired, the stapler lays down three staggered double rows of staples while dividing tissue in between.

The staplers are available in 35- or 45-cm lengths and contain an end called the "anvil," which houses the staple cartridges. *Vascular cartridges* apply staples that are 1 mm high when closed. *Tissue cartridges* apply those that are 1.5 mm when closed and are suitable for thicker pedicles. Stapling provides hemostasis and gentle handling of tissue, which should lead to less necrosis and better healing.

Newer models have added articulating and rotating capabilities at the jaw. These attributes permit stapling at an angle. Most staples are titanium. However, newer angled staplers for the vaginal cuff use delayed-absorbable material such as Polyglactin 910 for their staples. A main limitation to stapler use is generally the price of the device and cartridges, which can be costly compared with suture. However, if operating time is reduced, these costs can be negligible.

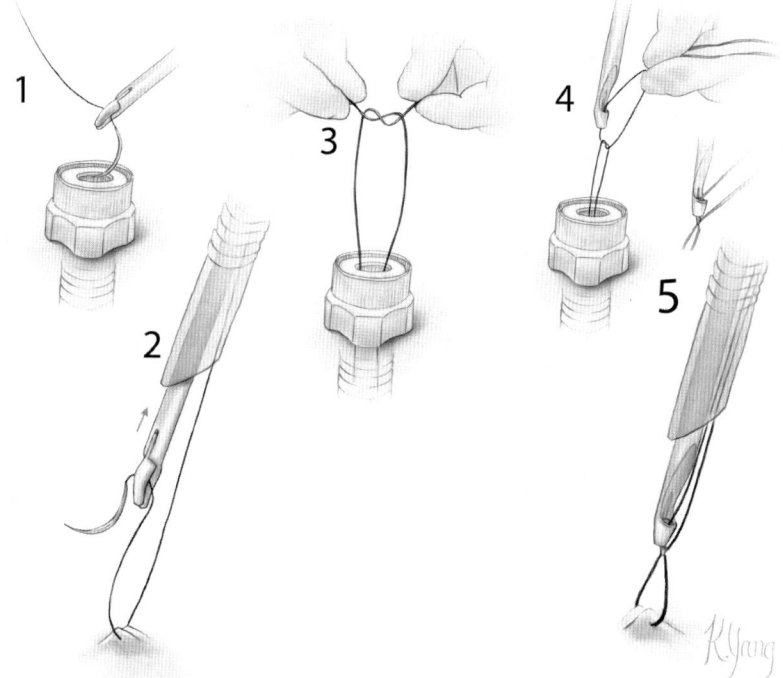

FIGURE 41-34 Extracorporeal knot typing.

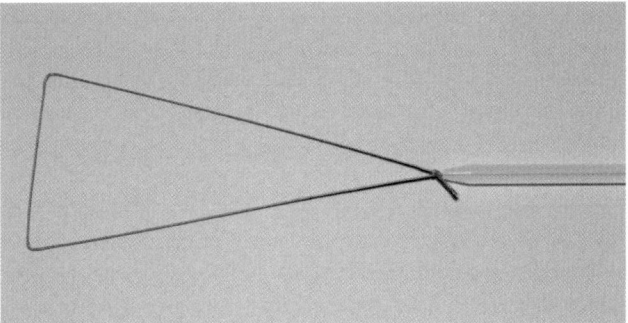

FIGURE 41-35 Laparoscopic suture loop.

Suture Loops

Preformed suture loops, such as the Endoloop, may also be used to ligate tissue pedicles (Fig. 41-35). This instrument has a length of suture housed within a stiff, 5-mm-diameter rod and has a pretied loop at the end. The loop is guided around the intended tissue pedicle by the stiff rod and then is cinched like a noose. The rod tip, similar to an index finger during manual knot tying, adds pressure to secure the knot in place. Loops of absorbable, delayed-absorbable, and permanent suture are available. Other types of knots that are pretied loops include the Roeder knot, Meltzer knot, and Tayside knot. These currently are not as popular as the square knot.

■ Laparoscopic Dissection Techniques

Pelvic adhesions are often lysed to reestablish normal anatomy and complete planned surgery. Some situations require the use of sharp dissection, especially if adhesions are not amenable to blunt tissue separation. For cutting fine adhesions, the tissue band may be placed on gentle stretch using an atraumatic grasper or blunt probe. Curved scissors with a dissecting tip or an energy modality (monopolar, bipolar, or harmonic) are frequently used.

If denser adhesions are found, they are divided in layers to prevent injury to adjacent adhered organs. Traction and countertraction aid in tissue plane identification. As the surgeon begins to separate tissues with tension, the plane of attachment may be identified, and the scissor tips create a small incision (Fig. 40-11, p. 850). The tip is then eased between the tissue layers to create an opening by spreading the blades outward. The initial snip carries the risk of injury to the underlying viscera or vessel and is made as shallow as possible. The use of energy sources in these situations is generally discouraged, as thermal injury may have a wider effect that may not be readily apparent. Conversely, a sharp cut is easier to identify and repair intraoperatively. The scissors used may be curved or straight depending on the contour of the pelvic organs. Once a plane is developed, wider and deeper strokes are used to complete tissue dissection.

Hydrodissection is another technique often used in MIS. With this, normal saline or other irrigation fluid is injected under pressure to separate tissue planes. For example, peritoneal endometriosis can be lifted and excised with greater ease and less trauma to retroperitoneal structures. Other uses include resection of cysts from an ovary, removal of ectopic products from a fallopian tube, or separation of tissue planes that might be obscured or in close proximity to vascular spaces or bowel.

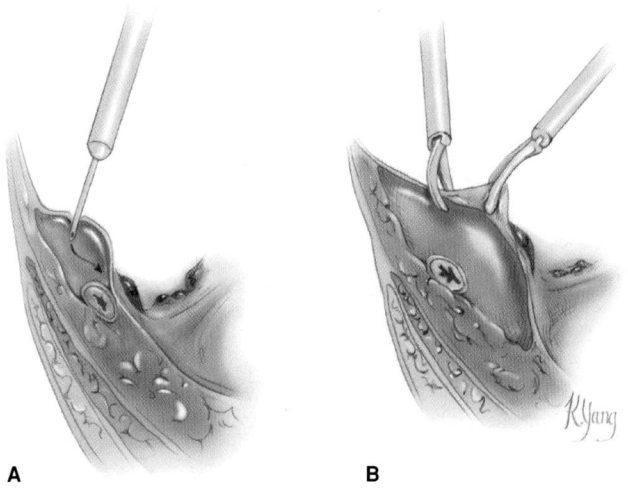

A   **B**

FIGURE 41-36 Hydrodissection to remove endometriotic implants on peritoneum that overlies the ureter, seen here in cross section. **A.** Needle insertion and fluid instillation. **B.** Peritoneal implant excision is completed without injury to the ureter.

As shown in Figure 41-36, an atraumatic grasper lifts the tissue at the junction point, and a needle tip is inserted with the bevel away from the structure to be protected. Irrigation fluid is injected and creates a balloon effect. Depending on the location, 5 to 30 mL of fluid is instilled. A suction-irrigation system also is helpful for this technique. With this instrument, once the peritoneum is incised, the suction tip is insinuated into the opening. Fluid is forced to gently separate the tissue planes (Fig. 44-4.2, p. 1014). Often, hydrodissection allows a surgeon to identify natural planes that might otherwise be obscured.

■ Hemostasis

As tissue planes are developed, bleeding is variably encountered. Requirements for vessel sealing differ according to vessel diameters. For small vessels, spot coagulation is suitable, and a monopolar tool is satisfactory and mimics the electrosurgical blade (Bovie) use in open procedures. For larger vessels, the bipolar or Harmonic technologies are preferred. Of these, the Harmonic grasper coagulates or denatures the vessel tissue and can seal vessels up to 5 mm in diameter. Advanced bipolar technologies achieve vessel sealing by desiccation and can effectively seal vessels ranging from 5 to 7 mm in diameter. When choosing a modality, the thermal spread of a device is considered. Last, microbipolar probes and needle-tip monopolar probes are useful for delicate tissues such as the fallopian tubes. The thermal spread is minimal, and the tip sizes are optimal for the small but friable vessels.

Liquid topical hemostatic agents have also gained popularity and have been adapted for laparoscopic use (Table 40-5, p. 861). When using a laparoscopic adaptor, a portion of the matrix may remain in the applicator cannula. Thus, to avoid retained and thus wasted sealant, a surgeon flushes the cannula following initial matrix application. For this, a plunger is included in many sealant kits, or a syringe filled with air may be used to force matrix through the cannula and onto the desired tissue. Alternatively, an oxidized regenerated cellulose fabric sheet (Surgicel) can be used.

HYSTEROSCOPIC PREOPERATIVE CONSIDERATIONS

Patient Evaluation

Hysteroscopy allows an endoscopic view of the endometrial cavity and tubal ostia for both the diagnosis and operative treatment of intrauterine pathology. The role of hysteroscopy in modern gynecology has expanded rapidly with development of more effective hysteroscopic instruments and smaller endoscopes, bringing many procedures into the office. Indications for hysteroscopy vary and include evaluation and in some cases, treatment of infertility, recurrent miscarriage, abnormal uterine bleeding, amenorrhea, and retained foreign bodies. With hysteroscopic techniques, abnormal bleeding can be treated with endometrial ablation, polypectomy, or submucous myomectomy. Infertility may be improved with resection of intrauterine adhesions or a septum. Additionally, obstructed tubal ostia may be unblocked or dilated. Alternatively, for those seeking sterilization, hysteroscopic tubal occlusion can serve as an effective and safe method of contraception.

Because the indications for hysteroscopy are varied, patient evaluations for specific disorders are discussed in their respective chapters. More generally, continuing pregnancy is an absolute contraindication to hysteroscopy and should be excluded with serum or urine β-human chorionic gonadotropin testing prior to surgery. In addition, cervicitis or pelvic infection is treated prior to hysteroscopy, and screening for *Neisseria gonorrhoeae* and *Chlamydia trachomatis* in those with risk factors is prudent (Table 1-1, p. 6). For those with abnormal bleeding and significant risks for endometrial cancer, preoperative endometrial Pipelle sampling is reasonable as seeding of the peritoneal cavity with cancer cells has been noted following hysteroscopy (Chap. 8, p. 187).

If diagnostic hysteroscopy is planned to locate and remove a foreign body, preoperative imaging is recommended, usually with transvaginal sonography. For example, in some cases, an intrauterine device (IUD) or retained fetal bone may have perforated the uterine wall, lie predominantly outside the uterus, and thus be best removed by laparoscopy.

Consent

The risk of complications for women undergoing hysteroscopy is low and cited at less than 1 to 3 percent (Hulka, 1993; Jansen, 2000; Propst, 2000). Complications are similar to those associated with dilatation and curettage and include uterine perforation, inability to sufficiently dilate the cervix, hemorrhage, cervical laceration, and postoperative endometritis. In addition, because either gas or liquid medium is required to distend the endometrial cavity during hysteroscopy, gas venous embolism and excessive intravascular fluid absorption are risks discussed later. In general, complication rates increase with the length and complexity of the procedure planned.

In the event of uterine perforation during hysteroscopy, diagnostic laparoscopy may be indicated for evaluation of the surrounding pelvic organs. Thus, patients are additionally consented and aware of the possible need for laparoscopy.

Patient Preparation

Infectious and venous thromboembolic (VTE) complications following hysteroscopic surgery are rare. Accordingly, preoperative antibiotics or VTE prophylaxis is typically not required (American College of Obstetricians and Gynecologists, 2013, 2014).

Endometrial Thickness

In premenopausal women, hysteroscopy is ideally performed in the early proliferative phase of the menstrual cycle, when the endometrium is relatively thin. This allows small masses to be identified and easily removed. Alternatively, agents that induce endometrial atrophy such as progestins, combination oral contraceptives, or gonadotropin-releasing hormone (GnRH) agonists have been administered individually prior to an anticipated surgery. Although these effectively thin the endometrium, many of these agents have disadvantages including expense, adverse side effects, and surgical delay while atrophy ensues.

Cervical Dilatation

For operative hysteroscopy, dilatation of the cervix is typically required to insert an 8- to 10-mm hysteroscope or resectoscope. To ease dilatation and lower the risk of uterine perforation, cervical preparation is considered. Misoprostol (Cytotec), a synthetic prostaglandin E_1 analogue, may be administered orally the night before and if desired, again the morning of surgery to aid cervical softening. Commonly used dosing options include 200 or 400 μg vaginally or 400 μg orally once 12 to 24 hours prior to surgery. Common side effects include cramping, uterine bleeding, or nausea. Thus, the need for softening is balanced against these side effects, especially bleeding that might limit endoscopic visualization.

If cervical stenosis is encountered intraoperatively, smaller caliber tools, such as a lacrimal duct probe, may be guided into the external cervical os to define the canal path. In these situations, transabdominal sonography may be helpful when done simultaneously with dilatation to help ensure proper placement (Christianson, 2008). Also, injection of intracervical dilute vasopressin can diminish the force required for cervical dilation (Phillips, 1997). Because the onset of action is rapid, this is especially helpful if stenosis was not anticipated preoperatively. As a potent vasoconstrictor, however, vasopressin is ideally avoided in those with serious hypertension and cardiovascular disease.

HYSTEROSCOPIC INSTRUMENTS

Rigid Hysteroscope

Hysteroscopy requires a hysteroscope, light source, uterine distention medium, and, in many cases, a video camera system. Most hysteroscopes consists of a 3- to 4-mm-diameter endoscope surrounded by an outer sheath. Smaller diameter hysteroscopes have been developed, although their use is limited by their decreased field of view and lower light intensity. Hysteroscopes are broadly classified as diagnostic or operative. Diagnostic hysteroscopes offer a small diameter, which provides an adequate endometrial cavity view yet requires minimal if any cervical dilatation. Operative hysteroscopes have sheaths that increase

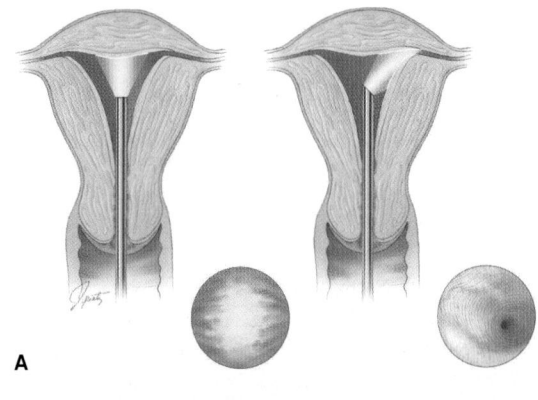

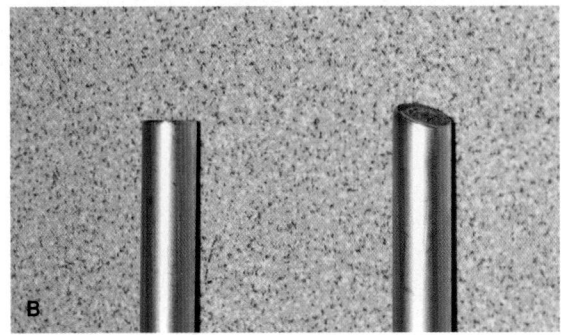

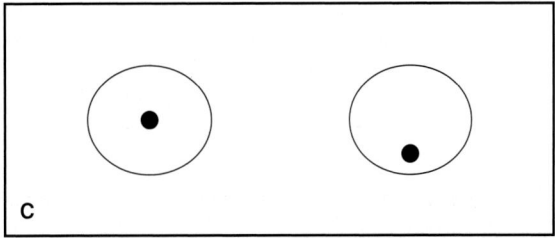

FIGURE 41-37 Differences between a 0-degree hysteroscope (*left*) and 30-degree hysteroscope (*right*). **A.** Intracavitary views **B.** A 30-degree endoscope has an angled tip. **C.** Views of the endocervical canal (*black dot*) during hysteroscope insertion.

the overall diameter and necessitate cervical dilation in most cases. Thus, cases requiring operative hysteroscopes are best managed under general or regional anesthesia in the operating room for patient comfort and safety.

Individual endoscopes offer specific angles of view. Although 0- through 70-degree angles (0, 12, 25, 30, and 70 degrees) are available, a 0- or 12-degree hysteroscope allows the easiest orientation within the uterine cavity for most procedures (Fig. 41-37). The 12-, 25-, 30-, and 70-degree angles provide additional lateral views, which are often required for complex operative procedures. There are also devices that have 90- to 110-degree angles of view, although these are infrequently used.

In general, the light source system used in hysteroscopy is the same type as for laparoscopy. However, the intensity is typically less than for most laparoscopic procedures. During assembly of the hysteroscope at the beginning of the procedure, the light source attaches directly to the endoscope.

An outer sheath surrounds the endoscope and directs fluid, and in some cases instruments, to the endometrial cavity. In directing fluid flow, sheaths are constructed to allow either

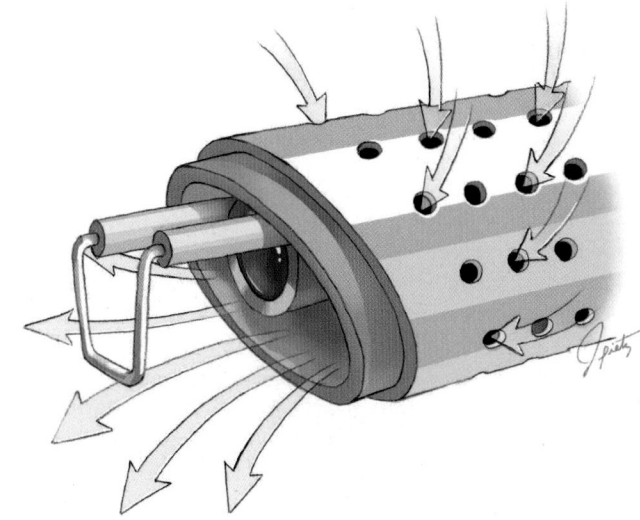

FIGURE 41-38 Distention medium flow through resectoscope.

unidirectional or bidirectional flow of distending media. Sheaths that allow continuous flow, that is, bidirectional inflow and outflow circulation of the distention medium, are most valuable in cases in which bleeding or large fluid volume deficits are expected (Fig. 41-38). This circulation helps clear blood from the operative field and assists with fluid volume deficit calculation. The type of tubing attached to the hysteroscope sheath is dictated by the fluid management system.

In operative hysteroscopes, the outer sheath also allows the use of semirigid, rigid, and flexible instruments. The basic set that will suffice for most cases includes biopsy forceps, grasping forceps, and scissors. Of these, biopsy forceps are somewhat sharp and cuplike. Grasping forceps permit removal of tissue or foreign bodies and may be toothed. Last, scissors can lyse adhesions, resect masses, or excise an intrauterine septum. Generally 5F in diameter and 34 to 40 cm long, these instruments are much smaller than the instruments used with the resectoscope. None of these requires special distention media or energy. Flexible electrodes used to vaporize tissue may also be passed through this sheath.

Bettochi Hysteroscope

This small, 4-mm-diameter rigid operative hysteroscope has a 5F (1.67 mm) operating channel that provides diagnostic and operative capability. Additionally, the hysteroscope diameter is oblong rather than circular, which conforms to the cervical canal's configuration (Bradley, 2009). Biopsy forceps, monopolar and bipolar electrosurgical scissors, bipolar needle-like tip, or delivery devices for transcervical sterilization can easily pass through this hysteroscope's working channel. The flow sheath has a small diameter yet permits sufficient flow to avoid compromised optical quality. These hysteroscopes are available in 0-degree and angled views.

Flexible Hysteroscope

These hysteroscopes have tips that can deflect over a range of 120 to 160 degrees. Although their optical view is less clear than that with rigid hysteroscopes, they offer easy maneuverability within irregularly shaped endometrial cavities. This can be helpful when tubal access is required or during lysis of adhesions. Additionally, flexible hysteroscopes cause less intraoperative pain than rigid ones and may benefit office procedures (Unfried, 2001).

■ Resectoscope

If resection of intrauterine tissues is planned, a resectoscope may be used. This tool consists of inner and outer sheaths. The inner sheath houses a 3- to 4-mm-diameter endoscope and a channel for fluid medium inflow. The 8- to 10-mm outer sheath contains an electrosurgical resection loop and allows fluid egress from the uterus through a series of small holes near the sheath's distal end. By means of a spring mechanism, the resection loop can be extended and then retracted to shave off contacted tissues. Through its central cannula, larger instruments that are energy-based for tissue resection can also be passed. These include the roller bar, roller ball, vaporizing electrodes (monopolar, bipolar, laser), hot scalpel, and motorized morcellator.

■ Hysteroscopic Morcellator

For resection of polyps, submucosal leiomyomas, septa, or synechiae, a hysteroscopic morcellator may be chosen. Hysteroscopic morcellators offer different tips depending on tissue type. For polyp resection, a rakelike tip is used. For resection of firmer tissue, a cutting tip is selected. Both tips contain a mechanized blade that fragments tissue. These tips are attached to a hollow cannula that evacuates the tissue fragments by suction to a collection receptacle. The morcellator fits through the working channel of a 9-mm or greater operative hysteroscopic cannula.

DISTENTION MEDIA

Because the anterior and posterior uterine walls lie in apposition, a distention medium is required to expand the endometrial cavity for viewing. Fluid media include saline, and low-viscous fluids, such as sorbitol, mannitol, and glycine solutions (Table 41-2). Historically, carbon dioxide was used for diagnostic hysteroscopy but is infrequently employed today. Each group has distinct advantages and properties. To expand the cavity, intrauterine pressures of these media must reach 45 to 80 mm Hg. Rarely is more than 100 mm Hg required. Moreover, because for most women, mean arterial pressure approximates 100 mm Hg, higher pressures can result in increased intravasation of media into the patient's circulation to create fluid volume overload.

TABLE 41-2. Hysteroscopic Media

Medium	Properties	Indications	Risks	Safety Measures
Gas				
Carbon dioxide	Colorless gas	Diagnostic	Gas embolism	Avoid Trendelenburg Keep flow <100 mL/min Intrauterine pressure <100 mm Hg
Electrolyte fluid				

0.9% saline	Isotonic
	380 mOsm/kg H_2O
		Diagnostic
		Operative w/
		  bipolar tools
			Volume overload	Plan to complete procedure at
				  750 mL deficit
				Stop procedure at 2.5 L deficit
				End earlier in patients with
				  comorbidities or elderly

Lactated Ringer	Isotonic 273 mOsm/kg H_2O	Same as above	Volume overload	Same as above
Electrolyte-poor fluid				

Sorbitol 3%	Hypoosmolar
	178 mOsm/kg H_2O
		Operative w/ monopolar
		  tools
			Volume overload
			Hyponatremia
			Hypoosmolality
			Hyperglycemia
				Plan to complete procedure at
				  750 mL deficit
				Stop procedure at 1–1.5L deficit
				End earlier in patients with
				  comorbidities or elderly

Mannitol 5%	Isoosmolar 280 mOsm/kg H_2O	Operative w/ monopolar tools	Volume overload Hyponatremia	Same as above
Glycine 1.5%	Hypoosmolar 200 mOsm /kg H_2O	Operative w/ monopolar tools	Volume overload Hyponatremia Hypoosmolality Hyperammonemia	Same as above

Data from Cooper, 2000; American Association of Gynecologic Laparoscopists, 2013; American College of Obstetricians and Gynecologists, 2011.

Carbon Dioxide

This gaseous distention medium, when used under pressure, tends to flatten the endometrium and provides excellent visibility. A continuous flow is necessary to replace any gas lost through the tubes, and typically flow rates of 40 to 50 mL/min are adequate. Rates higher than 100 mL/min are associated with increased risks for gas embolism and therefore discouraged. Specialized hysteroscopic machines, which limit maximum flow rates, should be used. Importantly, because *laparoscopic* insufflating machines can permit flow rates >1000 mL/min, these should not be used for hysteroscopy.

Disadvantages to CO_2 include its tendency, when mixed with blood or mucus, to form visually obstructive gas bubbles. Accordingly, prior to hysteroscope insertion, blood and mucus are carefully removed from the cervical os with a dry swab (Sutton, 2006). Similarly, use of CO_2 with thermal energy sources is avoided as smoke production prohibits adequate viewing. Because of these limitations, CO_2 is best used in cases in which minimal bleeding is anticipated, such as diagnostic hysteroscopy. The most serious complication associated with CO_2 use is venous gas embolism and is discussed on page 905.

Fluid Media

Bleeding is common with operative hysteroscopy procedures. Thus rather than CO_2, fluid media are typically selected because of their optical clarity and ability to mix with blood. The main risk of fluid distention media, however, involves increased fluid absorption and circulatory fluid volume overload. Volume overload may develop with any of the fluid media and results from various mechanisms. As examples, absorption across the endometrium, intravasation through surgically opened venous channels, and spill from the fallopian tubes with absorption by the peritoneum have all been suggested. Therefore, clinical settings in which procedures are long, increased distention pressures are used, or large tissue areas are resected all carry a greater risk.

Fluid distention media can be divided according to their viscosity and electrolyte status. In general, low-viscosity fluids are used in modern hysteroscopy. An appropriate medium is selected based on its compatibility with electrosurgical instrumentation.

Low-viscosity Electrolyte Fluids

Normal saline and lactated Ringer solutions are isotonic, electrolyte fluids. They are readily available in the operating room and are frequently used for diagnostic hysteroscopy. However, these fluids cannot be used with monopolar electrosurgery. Specifically, these solutions conduct current; thus, dissipate the energy; and thereby render the instrument useless.

These electrolyte-containing, isotonic fluids have lower associated risks of hyponatremia compared with hypoosmolar fluids, described in the next section. Still, rapid absorption can lead to pulmonary edema. In general, when using isotonic medium in a healthy patient, a surgeon should consider terminating the procedure when the fluid deficit nears 2500 mL (American Association of Gynecologic Laparoscopists, 2013; American College of Obstetricians and Gynecologists, 2011).

Low-viscosity, Electrolyte-poor Fluids

Of other available media, 1.5-percent glycine, 3-percent sorbitol, and 5-percent mannitol are all low-viscosity, electrolyte-poor fluids. Because they are nonconducting, these media are used for electrosurgery involving monopolar instruments. Unfortunately, these fluids can create volume overload with concurrent development of hyponatremia and hypoosmolality and the potential for cerebral edema and death (American College of Obstetricians and Gynecologists, 2011). Mechanistically, sorbitol is a six-carbon sugar and is metabolized following absorption. This effectively leaves free water in the intravascular space. Normal serum sodium levels are 135 to 145 mEq/L, and levels significantly below this may lead to seizure followed by respiratory arrest. In addition, hypokalemia and hypocalcemia can often develop concurrently. Five-percent mannitol, also a six-carbon sugar, is isoosmolar and so has diuretic properties but does not lead to serum osmolality changes (American Association of Gynecologic Laparoscopists, 2013).

In cases in which large fluid volume deficits are calculated, measurement of serum electrolyte levels is warranted. If a serum sodium level lower than 125 mEq/L is reached, postoperative care should be continued in a critical care setting. Treatment includes stimulation of diuresis with furosemide (Lasix), 20 to 40 mg given intravenously. Correction of hyponatremia is achieved with 3-percent sodium chloride, administered at a rate of 0.5 to 2 mL/kg/hr. In those with acute neurologic symptoms, 3-percent saline can instead be given in a 100-mL infusion over 30 minutes and repeated an additional two times if needed (Nagler, 2014; Verbalis, 2013). The goal of therapy is to reach a serum sodium level of 135 mEq/L within 24 hours. Overcorrection is avoided to prevent additional cerebral effects (Nagler, 2014; Verbalis, 2013). Consultation with an internal medicine specialist may be helpful.

To assist with intraoperative fluid volume calculation, most operative hysteroscopes contain continuous flow systems that allow fluid deficits to be calculated. Calculation of deficits is performed every 15 minutes during procedures. If a procedure has the potential for larger deficits, a Foley catheter is also warranted for urine output monitoring. Moreover, an ongoing communication with participating anesthesia staff regarding large fluid deficits is prudent. If deficits of a hypotonic solution reach 1000 mL, a surgeon should consider procedure termination, measure electrolytes, and give diuretics as indicated (American Association of Gynecologic Laparoscopists, 2013). At the end of every hysteroscopic procedure, a final deficit is determined, and this value is recorded in the operative note.

Hysteroscopic Electrosurgery

Many widely used hysteroscopic tissue resection or desiccation techniques rely on monopolar current. Because current is dissipated and is thus ineffective in electrolyte solutions, these techniques have typically required nonelectrolyte solutions such as sorbitol, mannitol, and glycine. However, as just discussed, these media can be associated with hyponatremia if fluid volume overload develops.

Alternatively, bipolar electrosurgery systems (Versapoint Bipolar Electrosurgery System and Karl Storz bipolar resectoscope) allow use of traditional hysteroscopic tools in a saline solution. The Versapoint system has attachments that include a loop resecting electrode and multiedged vaporizing electrode. There are also ball, spring, and twizzle tips that can be employed for vaporization, desiccation, and cutting. The Karl Storz resectoscope (22F) has a cutting loop, ball tip, and pointed coagulation electrode attachments.

HYSTEROSCOPIC COMPLICATIONS

Uterine Perforation

In addition to fluid overload, uterine perforation or bleeding may complicate hysteroscopy. The uterus may be perforated during uterine sounding, cervical dilatation, or hysteroscopic procedures. Fundal perforations created by sounds, dilators, or hysteroscopes can be managed conservatively, as the myometrium will typically contract around these defects. In contrast, lateral perforation may perforate the broad ligament or injure larger pelvic vessels; posterior perforation may injure the rectum; and those caused by electrosurgical tools may cause organ laceration or burn. Diagnostic laparoscopy is indicated in these cases. Similarly, anterior perforations should prompt cystoscopy to evaluate associated bladder injury.

Gas Embolization

If vessels are opened during cervical dilation or during endometrial or myometrial disruption, gas under pressure can be forced into the vasculature. Any undissolved portion can reach the lungs. CO_2 is many times more soluble in plasma than is room air, and it typically dissolves sufficiently during transit from the pelvis (Corson, 1988). As a result, pulmonary embolism is rare in diagnostic hysteroscopic cases using CO_2 (Brandner, 1999). In contrast, room air is poorly soluble in blood, and embolization can lead to rapid cardiovascular collapse. Signs and symptoms include chest pain, dyspnea, and hypotension. Anesthesia staff may note decreased end-tidal CO_2 levels, oxygen desaturation, dysrhythmias, or a "mill wheel" murmur (Groenman, 2008). To manage this emergency, the patient is placed in the left lateral decubitus position with the head tilted downward. This aids movement of the air from the right outflow tract to the apex of the right ventricle, where the embolus may be aspirated (American College of Obstetricians and Gynecologists, 2011).

Surgeons can minimize the risk of gas embolism by avoiding Trendelenburg positioning of the patient during hysteroscopy, ensuring that air bubbles are purged from all tubing prior to introduction of the hysteroscope into the uterus, maintaining intrauterine pressures <100 mm Hg, minimizing the effort needed to dilate the cervix, avoiding deep myometrial resections, and limiting multiple removals and reinsertions of the hysteroscope in and out of the uterine cavity.

Hemorrhage

Heavy bleeding may develop during or following resection procedures. Although hysteroscopic electrosurgical electrodes may be used to contact and coagulate smaller vessels, these may be less effective for larger ones. If heavy bleeding is encountered and is refractory to electrosurgical coagulation, termination of the procedure may be indicated. A Foley catheter balloon can be placed into the endometrial cavity and inflated incrementally with 5 to 10 mL of saline until moderate resistance to catheter tension is noted. An attached collection bag can be used to document blood loss and bleeding cessation. After several hours, the catheter may be removed.

REFERENCES

Abu-Rustum NR, Rhee EH, Chi DS, et al: Subcutaneous tumor implantation after laparoscopic procedures in women with malignant disease. Obstet Gynecol 103(3):480, 2004

Agarwala N, Liu CY: Safe entry techniques during laparoscopy: left upper quadrant entry using the ninth intercostal space—a review of 918 procedures. J Minim Invasive Gynecol 12(1):55, 2005

Ahmad G, Duffy JM, Phillips K, et al: Laparoscopic entry techniques. Cochrane Database Syst Rev 2:CD006583, 2008

Alessandri F, Lijoi D, Mistrangelo E, et al: Randomized study of laparoscopic versus minilaparotomic myomectomy for uterine myomas. J Minim Invasive Gynecol 13(2):92, 2006

American Association of Gynecologic Laparoscopists, Munro MG, Storz K, et al: AAGL practice report: practice guidelines for the management of hysteroscopic distending media. J Minim Invasive Gynecol 20(2):137, 2013

American College of Obstetricians and Gynecologists: Antibiotic prophylaxis for gynecologic procedures. Practice Bulletin No. 104, May 2009, Reaffirmed 2014

American College of Obstetricians and Gynecologists: Hysteroscopy. Technology Assessment No. 7, June 2011

American College of Obstetricians and Gynecologists: Prevention of deep vein thrombosis and pulmonary embolism. Practice Bulletin No. 84, August 2007, Reaffirmed 2013

American College of Obstetricians and Gynecologists: Robotic surgery in gynecology. Committee Opinion No. 628, March 2015

Audebert AJ, Gomel V: Role of microlaparoscopy in the diagnosis of peritoneal and visceral adhesions and in the prevention of bowel injury associated with blind trocar insertion. Fertil Steril 73(3):631, 2000

Baadsgaard SE, Bille S, Egeblad K: Major vascular injury during gynecologic laparoscopy: report of a case and review of published cases. Acta Obstet Gynaecol Scand 68:283, 1989

Barnett JC, Hurd WW, Rogers RM Jr, et al: Laparoscopic positioning and nerve injuries. J Minim Invasive Gynecol 14(5):664, 2007

Bergqvist D, Bergqvist A: Vascular injuries during gynecologic surgery. Acta Obstet Gynaecol Scand 66:19, 1987

Berguer R, Forkey DL, Smith WD: The effect of laparoscopic instrument working angle on surgeons' upper extremity workload. Surg Endosc 15(9):1027, 2001

Berman JM, Guido RS, Garza Leal JG, et al: Three-year outcome of the Halt trial: a prospective analysis of radiofrequency volumetric thermal ablation of myomas. J Minim Invasive Gynecol 21(5):767, 2014

Bhoyrul S, Vierra MA, Nezhat CR, et al: Trocar injuries in laparoscopic surgery. J Am Coll Surg 192(6):677, 2001

Bonjer HJ, Hazebroek EJ, Kazemier G, et al: Open versus closed establishment of pneumoperitoneum in laparoscopic surgery. Br J Surg 84:599, 1997

Boughey JC, Nottingham JM, Walls AC: Richter's hernia in the laparoscopic era: four case reports and review of the literature. Surg Laparosc Endosc Percutan Tech 13:55, 2003

Bradley LD, Falcone T: Hysteroscopy: Office Evaluation and Management of the Uterine Cavity. 1st ed. Philadelphia, Mosby Elsevier, 2009, p 4

Brandner P, Neis KJ, Ehmer C: The etiology, frequency, and prevention of gas embolism during CO_2 hysteroscopy. J Am Assoc Gynecol Laparosc 6:421, 1999

Brill A, Nezhat F, Nezhat C, et al: The incidence of adhesions after prior laparotomy (a laparoscopic appraisal). Obstet Gynecol 85:269, 1995

Bubenik LJ, Hosgood G, Vasanjee SC: Bursting tension of medium and large canine arteries sealed with ultrasonic energy or suture ligation. Vet Surg (3):289, 2005

Byron JW, Markenson G, Miyazawa K: A randomized comparison of Veress needle and direct trocar insertion for laparoscopy. Surg Gynecol Obstet 177:259, 1993

Camanni M, Bonino L, Delpiano EM, et al: Laparoscopy and body mass index: feasibility and outcome in obese patients treated for gynecologic diseases. J Minim Invasive Gynecol 17(5):576, 2010

Campbell ES, Xiao H, Smith MK: Types of hysterectomy: comparison of characteristics, hospital costs, utilization and outcomes. J Reprod Med 48:943, 2003

Caprini JA, Arcelus JI: Prevention of postoperative venous thromboembolism following laparoscopic cholecystectomy. Surg Endosc 8(7):741, 1994

Catarci M, Carlini M, Gentileschi P, et al: Major and minor injuries during the creation of pneumoperitoneum: a multicenter study on 12,919 cases. Surg Endosc 15:566, 2001

Chandler JG, Corson SL, Way LW: Three spectra of laparoscopic entry access injuries. J Am Coll Surg 192(4):478, 2001

Chapron C, Pierre F, Harchaoui Y, et al: Gastrointestinal injuries during gynaecological laparoscopy. Hum Reprod 14(2):333, 1999

Childers JM, Aqua KA, Surwit EA, et al: Abdominal-wall tumor implantation after laparoscopy for malignant conditions. Obstet Gynecol 84:765, 1994

Chopin N, Malaret JM, Lafay-Pillet MC, et al: Total laparoscopic hysterectomy for benign uterine pathologies: obesity does not increase the risk of complications. Hum Reprod (12):3057, 2009

Christianson MS, Barker MA, Lindheim SR: Overcoming the challenging cervix: techniques to access the uterine cavity. J Low Genit Tract Dis 12(1):24, 2008

Clayman RV: The safety and efficacy of direct trocar insertion with elevation of the rectus sheath instead of the skin for pneumoperitoneum. J Urol 174: 1847, 2005

Cohen SL, Einarsson JI, Wang KC, et al: Contained power morcellation within an insufflated isolation bag. Obstet Gynecol 124(3):491, 2014

Cooper JM, Brady RM: Intraoperative and early postoperative complications of operative hysteroscopy. Obstet Gynecol Clin North Am 27:347, 2000

Copeland C, Wing R, Hulka JF: Direct trocar insertion at laparoscopy: an evaluation. Obstet Gynecol 62:655, 1983

Corson SL, Batzer FR, Gocial B, et al: Measurement of the force necessary for laparoscopic trocar entry. J Reprod Med 34:282, 1989

Corson SL, Hoffman JJ, Jackowski J, et al: Cardiopulmonary effects of direct venous CO_2 insufflation in ewes: a model for CO_2 hysteroscopy. J Reprod Med 33:440, 1988

Cravello L, D'Ercole C, Roger V, et al: Laparoscopic surgery in gynecology: randomized, prospective study comparing pneumoperitoneum and abdominal wall suspension. Eur J Obstet Gynaecol Reprod Biol 83:9, 1999

Demyttenaere S, Feldman LS, Fried GM: Effect of pneumoperitoneum on renal perfusion and function: a systematic review. Surg Endosc 21(2):152, 2007

Dingfelder JR: Direct laparoscope trocar insertion without prior pneumoperitoneum. J Reprod Med 21:45, 1978

Einarsson JI, Cohen SL, Fuchs N, et al: In-bag morcellation. J Minim Invasive Gynecol 21(5):951, 2014

Einarsson JI, Sun J, Orav J, et al: Local analgesia in laparoscopy: a randomized trial. Obstet Gynecol 104(6):1335, 2004

Ellström M, Ferraz-Nunes J, Hahlin M, et al: A randomized trial with a cost-consequence analysis after laparoscopic and abdominal hysterectomy. Obstet Gynecol 91(1):30, 1998

Eltabbakh GH, Piver MS, Hempling RE, et al: Laparoscopic surgery in obese women. Obstet Gynecol 94(5 Pt 1):704, 1999

Eltabbakh GH, Shamonki MI, Moody JM, et al: Hysterectomy for obese women with endometrial cancer: laparoscopy or laparotomy? Gynecol Oncol 78(3 Pt 1):329, 2000

Epstein J, Arora A, Ellis H: Surface anatomy of the inferior epigastric artery in relation to laparoscopic injury. Clin Anat 17:400, 2004

Falcone T, Paraiso MF, Mascha E: Prospective, randomized clinical trial of laparoscopically assisted vaginal hysterectomy versus total abdominal hysterectomy. Am J Obstet Gynecol 180(4):955, 1999

Farley DR, Greenlee SM, Larson DR, et al: Double-blind, prospective, randomized study of warmed, humidified carbon dioxide insufflation vs standard carbon dioxide for patients undergoing laparoscopic cholecystectomy. Arch Surg 139(7):739, 2004

Fuller J, Scott W, Ashar B, et al: Laparoscopic trocar injuries: a report from a U.S. Food and Drug Administration (FDA) Center for Devices and Radiological Health (CDRH) Systematic Technology Assessment of Medical Products (STAMP) Committee. Finalized: November 7, 2003

Galen DI, Isaacson KB, Lee BB: Does menstrual bleeding decrease after ablation of intramural myomas? A retrospective study. J Minim Invasive Gynecol 20(6):830, 2013

Ghezzi F, Cromi A, Uccella S, et al: Transumbilical versus transvaginal retrieval of surgical specimens at laparoscopy: a randomized trial. Am J Obstet Gynecol 207(2):112.e1, 2012

Giannios NM, Gulani V, Rohlck K, et al: Left upper quadrant laparoscopic placement: effects of insertion angle and body mass index on distance to posterior peritoneum by magnetic resonance imaging. Am J Obstet Gynecol 201(5):522.e1, 2009

Goldberg JM, Maurer WG: A randomized comparison of gasless laparoscopy and CO_2 pneumoperitoneum. Obstet Gynecol 90:416, 1997

Greenberg JA, Einarsson JI: The use of bidirectional barbed suture in laparoscopic myomectomy and total laparoscopic hysterectomy. J Minim Invasive Gynecol 15(5):621, 2008

Groenman FA, Peters LW, Rademaker BM, et al: Embolism of air and gas in hysteroscopic procedures: pathophysiology and implication for daily practice. J Minim Invasive Gynecol 15(2):24, 2008

Gunenc MZ, Yesildaglar N, Bingol B, et al: The safety and efficacy of direct trocar insertion with elevation of the rectus sheath instead of the skin for pneumoperitoneum. Surg Laparosc Endosc Percutan Tech 15:80, 2005

Harkki-Siren P, Kurki T: A nationwide analysis of laparoscopic complications. Obstet Gynecol 89:108, 1997

Hasson HM: A modified instrument and method for laparoscopy. Am J Obstet Gynecol 110:886, 1971

Hasson HM: Open laparoscopy: a report of 150 cases. J Reprod Med 12:234, 1974

Hasson HM, Rotman C, Rana N, et al: Open laparoscopy: 29-year experience. Obstet Gynecol 96:763, 2000

Heinberg EM, Crawford BL III, Weitzen SH, et al: Total laparoscopic hysterectomy in obese versus nonobese patients. Obstet Gynecol 103(4):674, 2004

Ho HS, Saunders CJ, Gunther RA: Effector of hemodynamics during laparoscopy: CO_2 absorption or intra-abdominal pressure? J Surg Res 59(4):497, 1995

Horiuchi T, Tanishima H, Tamagawa K, et al: Randomized, controlled investigation of the anti-infective properties of the Alexis retractor/protector of incision sites. J Trauma 62(1)212, 2007

Howard FM, El-Minawi AM, DeLoach VE: Direct laparoscopic cannula insertion at the left upper quadrant. J Am Assoc Gynecol Laparosc (5):595, 1997

Hulka JF, Peterson HB, Phillips JM, et al: Operative hysteroscopy: American Association of Gynecologic Laparoscopists 1991 membership survey. J Reprod Med 38:572, 1993

Hurd WW, Amesse LS, Gruber JS, et al: Visualization of the epigastric vessels and bladder before laparoscopic trocar placement. Fertil Steril 80:209, 2003

Hurd WW, Bude RO, DeLancey JO, et al: The relationship of the umbilicus to the aortic bifurcation: implications for laparoscopic technique. Obstet Gynecol 80(1):48, 1992

Hurd WW, Wang L, Schemmel MT: A comparison of the relative risk of vessel injury with conical versus pyramidal laparoscopic trocars in a rabbit model. Am J Obstet Gynecol 173:1731, 1995

Ido K, Suzuki T, Kimura K, et al: Lower-extremity venous stasis during laparoscopic cholecystectomy as assessed using color Doppler ultrasound. Surg Endosc 9(3):310, 1995

Jansen FW, Vredevoogd CB, van Ulzen K, et al: Complications of hysteroscopy: a prospective multicenter study. Obstet Gynecol 96:266, 2000

Kho KA, Nezhat C: Parasitic myomas. Obstet Gynecol 114(3):611, 2009

Klauschie J, Wechter ME, Jacob K, et al: Use of anti-skid material and patient-positioning to prevent patient shifting during robotic-assisted gynecologic procedures. J Minim Invasive Gynecol 17(4):504, 2010

Lajer H, Widecrantz S, Heisterberg L: Hernias in trocar ports following abdominal laparoscopy: a review. Acta Obstet Gynaecol Scand 76:389, 1997

Lamberton GR, Hsi RS, Jin DH, et al: Prospective comparison of four laparoscopic vessel ligation devices. J Endourol 22(10):2307, 2008

Lamvu G, Zolnoun D, Boggess J, et al: Obesity: physiologic changes and challenges during laparoscopy. Am J Obstet Gynecol 191(2):669, 2004

Leibl BJ, Schmedt CG, Schwarz J, et al: Laparoscopic surgery complications associated with trocar tip design: review of literature and own results. J Laparoendosc Adv Surg Tech 9:135, 1999

Li TC, Saravelos H, Richmond M, et al: Complications of laparoscopic pelvic surgery: recognition, management and prevention. Hum Reprod Update 3: 505, 1997

Long JB, Giles DL, Cornella JL, et al: Open laparoscopic access technique: review of 2010 patients. JSLS 12(4):372, 2008

Lundorff P, Hahlin M, Källfelt B, et al: Adhesion formation after laparoscopic surgery in tubal pregnancy: a randomized trial versus laparotomy. Fertil Steril 55:911, 1991

Madeb R, Koniaris LG, Patel HR, et al: Complications of laparoscopic urologic surgery. J Laparoendosc Adv Surgical Tech A 14(5):287, 2004

Magrina JF: Complications of laparoscopic surgery. Clin Obstet Gynecol 45:469, 2002

Mais V, Ajossa S, Guerriero S, et al: Laparoscopic versus abdominal myomectomy: a prospective, randomized trial to evaluate benefits in early outcome. Am J Obstet Gynecol 174(2):654, 1996

Merlin TL, Hiller JE, Maddern GJ, et al: Systematic review of the safety and effectiveness of methods used to establish pneumoperitoneum in laparoscopic surgery. Br J Surg 90:668, 2003

Milad MP, Milad EA: Laparoscopic morcellator-related complications. J Minim Invasive Gynecol 21(3):486, 2014

Montz FJ, Holschneider CH, Munro MG: Incisional hernia following laparoscopy: a survey of the American Association of Gynecologic Laparoscopists. Obstet Gynecol 84:881, 1994

Morrison JE Jr, Jacobs VR: Replacement of expensive, disposable instruments with old-fashioned surgical techniques for improved cost-effectiveness in laparoscopic hysterectomy. J Soc Laparoendosc Surg 8:201, 2004

Munro MG: Laparoscopic access: Complications, technologies, and techniques. Curr Opin Obstet Gynecol 14:365, 2002

Nagler EV, Vanmassenhove J, van der Veer SN, et al: Diagnosis and treatment of hyponatremia: a systematic review of clinical practice guidelines and consensus statements. BMC Med 12:1, 2014

Negrin Perez MC, De La Torre FP, Ramirez A: Ureteral complications after gasless laparoscopic hysterectomy. Surg Laparosc Endosc Percutan Technol 9:300, 1999

Newcomb WL, Hope WW, Schmeltzer TM, et al: Comparison of blood vessel sealing among new electrosurgical and ultrasonic devices. Surg Endosc 23(1):90, 2009

Nezhat F, Brill AI, Nezhat CH, et al: Laparoscopic appraisal of the anatomic relationship of the umbilicus to the aortic bifurcation. J Am Assoc Gynecol Laparosc 5:135, 1998

Nieboer TE, Johnson N, Lethaby A, et al: Surgical approach to hysterectomy for benign gynaecological disease. Cochrane Database Syst Rev 3: CD003677, 2009

Nordestgaard AG, Bodily KC, Osborne RW Jr, et al: Major vascular injuries during laparoscopic procedures. Am J Surg 169:543, 1995

O'Hanlan KA, Lopez L, Dibble SL, et al: Total laparoscopic hysterectomy: body mass index and outcomes. Obstet Gynecol 102(6):1384, 2003

O'Rourke N, Kodali BS: Laparoscopic surgery during pregnancy. Curr Opin Anaesthesiol 19(3):254, 2006

Ott DE, Reich H, Love B, et al: Reduction of laparoscopic-induced hypothermia, postoperative pain and recovery room length of stay by pre-conditioning gas with the Insuflow device: a prospective randomized controlled multicenter study. JSLS 2(4):321, 1998

Palmer R: Safety in laparoscopy. J Reprod Med 13(1):1, 1974

Panici PB, Zullo MA, Angioli R, Muzii L. Minilaparotomy hysterectomy: a valid option for the treatment of benign uterine pathologies. Eur J Obstet Gynecol Reprod Biol 119(2):228, 2005

Park JY, Park SK, Kim DY, et al: The impact of tumor morcellation during surgery on the prognosis of patients with apparently early uterine leiomyosarcoma. Gynecol Oncol 122(2):255, 2011

Pearl J, Price R, Richardson W, et al: Guidelines for diagnosis, treatment, and use of laparoscopy for surgical problems during pregnancy. Surg Endosc 25(11): 3479, 2011

Peng Y, Zheng M, Ye Q, et al: Heated and humidified CO_2 prevents hypothermia, peritoneal injury, and intra-abdominal adhesions during prolonged laparoscopic insufflations. J Surg Res 151(1):40, 2009

Phillips DR, Nathanson HG, Milim SJ, et al: The effect of dilute vasopressin solution on the force needed for cervical dilatation: a randomized controlled trial. Obstet Gynecol 89(4):507, 1997

Pritts EA, Parker WH, Brown J, et al: Outcome of occult uterine leiomyosarcoma after surgery for presumed uterine fibroids: a systematic review. J Minim Invasive Gynecol 22(1):26, 2015

Propst AM, Liberman RF, Harlow BL, et al: Complications of hysteroscopic surgery: predicting patients at risk. Obstet Gynecol 96:517, 2000

Rahn DD, Phelan JN, Roshanravan SM, et al: Anterior abdominal wall nerve and vessel anatomy: clinical implications for gynecologic surgery. Am J Obstet Gynecol 202(3):234.e1, 2010

Ramirez PT, Frumovitz M, Wolf JK, et al: Laparoscopic port-site metastases in patients with gynecological malignancies. Int J Gynecol Cancer 14:1070, 2004

Reid K, Pockney P, Draganic B, et al: Barrier wound protection decreases surgical site infection in open elective colorectal surgery: a randomized clinical trial. Dis Colon Rectum 53(10):1374, 2010

Reynolds JD, Booth JV, de la Fuente S, et al: A review of laparoscopy for non-obstetric-related surgery during pregnancy. Curr Surg 60(2):164, 2003

Romanowski L, Reich H, McGlynn F, et al: Brachial plexus neuropathies after advanced laparoscopic surgery. Fertil Steril 60:729, 1993

Sammour T, Kahokehr A, Hill AG: Meta-analysis of the effect of warm humidified insufflation on pain after laparoscopy. Br J Surg 95(8):950, 2008

Scribner DR Jr, Walker JL, Johnson GA, et al: Laparoscopic pelvic and paraaortic lymph node dissection in the obese. Gynecol Oncol 84(3):426, 2002

Sepilian V, Della Badia C: Iatrogenic endometriosis caused by uterine morcellation during a supracervical hysterectomy. Obstet Gynecol 102(5 Pt 2): 1125, 2003

Sepilian V, Ku L, Wong H, et al: Prevalence of infraumbilical adhesions in women with previous laparoscopy. JSLS 11(1):41, 2007

Shah DK, Vitonis AF, Missmer SA: Association of body mass index and morbidity after abdominal, vaginal, and laparoscopic hysterectomy. Obstet Gynecol 125(3):589, 2015

Shamiyeh A, Glaser K, Kratochwill H, et al: Lifting of the umbilicus for the installation of pneumoperitoneum with the Veress needle increases the distance to the retroperitoneal and intraperitoneal structures. Surg Endosc 23(2): 313, 2009

Sharma KC, Brandstetter RD, Brensilver JM, et al: Cardiopulmonary physiology and pathophysiology as a consequence of laparoscopic surgery. Chest 110(3):810, 1996

Sharp HT, Dodson MK, Draper ML, et al: Complications associated with optical-access laparoscopic trocars. Obstet Gynecol 99:553, 2002

Sutton C: Hysteroscopic surgery. Best Pract Res Clin Obstet Gynaecol 20:105, 2006

Thomas D, Ikeda M, Deepika K, et al: Laparoscopic management of benign adnexal mass in obese women. J Minim Invasive Gynecol 13:311, 2006

Tulikangas PK, Nicklas A, Falcone T, et al: Anatomy of the left upper quadrant for cannula insertion. J Am Assoc Gynecol Laparosc 7(2):211, 2000

Unfried G, Wieser F, Albrecht A, et al: Flexible versus rigid endoscopes for outpatient hysteroscopy: a prospective randomized clinical trial. Hum Reprod 16:168, 2001

Uppal S, Frumovitz M, Escobar P, et al: Laparoendoscopic single-site surgery in gynecology: review of literature and available technology. J Minim Invasive Gynecol 18(1):12, 2011

van Det MJ, Meijerink WJ, Hoff C, et al: Optimal ergonomics for laparoscopic surgery in minimally invasive surgery suites: a review and guidelines. Surg Endosc 23(6):1279, 2009

Vellinga TT, De Alwis S, Suzuki Y, et al: Laparoscopic entry: the modified Alwis method and more. Rev Obstet Gynecol 2(3):193, 2009

Verbalis JG, Goldsmith SR, Greenberg A, et al: Diagnosis, evaluation, and treatment of hyponatremia: expert panel recommendations. Am J Med 126(10 Suppl 1):S1, 2013

Vilos GA, Ternamian A, Dempster J, et al: Laparoscopic entry: a review of techniques, technologies, and complications. J Obstet Gynaecol Can 29(5): 433, 2007

Wu MP, Ou CS, Chen SL, et al: Complications and recommended practices for electrosurgery in laparoscopy. Am J Surg 179:67, 2000

Zivanovic O, Sonoda Y, Diaz JP, et al: The rate of port-site metastases after 2251 laparoscopic procedures in women with underlying malignant disease. Gynecol Oncol 111(3):431, 2008

CHAPTER 42

Postoperative Considerations

Many problems following surgery can be avoided by the preoperative risk assessment and prevention strategies described in Chapter 39. However, despite ideal preparation, complications may still develop, and vigilance for these adverse events can help ensure successful convalescence for most patients.

POSTOPERATIVE ORDERS

These written instructions address support of each organ system, while normal function is gradually reestablished. Although orders are customized for each woman, goals are common among all surgical patients—resuscitation, pain control, and resumption of daily activities. Table 42-1 offers a template for both inpatient and outpatient postoperative orders.

■ Fluid and Electrolytes

Nearly half of the average female body's weight is water. Two thirds of this water is contained in the intracellular compartment, and the remainder is stored extracellularly. This extracellular compartment is divided into a vascular space filled with plasma and an interstitium, which is the collection of small spaces between cells. Of extracellular fluid volume, 25 percent makes up intravascular plasma, and 75 percent fills the interstitium. This 1 to 3 ratio is relevant during fluid resuscitation. Extracellular compartment osmolarity is controlled primarily by sodium and chloride, whereas potassium, magnesium, and phosphate are the major intracellular electrolytes. Osmotic balance is maintained by the free movement of water between the intra- and extracellular spaces.

To support these fluid volumes, the daily liquid requirement for an average adult approximates 30 mL/kg/day. Urine output and insensible losses offset these requirements (Marino, 2007). Thus, postoperatively, crystalloid fluids are primarily used for maintenance and in some cases for resuscitation. Sodium chloride is the main component of these fluids. Because sodium is most abundant in the extracellular space, the fluid is uniformly distributed between the interstitial areas. With crystalloid resuscitation, the primary effect is interstitial volume expansion rather than plasma volume growth. Two of the most commonly used crystalloid fluids for resuscitation and maintenance requirements are isotonic saline and lactated Ringer solution.

Compared with plasma, isotonic saline, also colloquially called normal saline, has a higher chloride concentration (154 mEq/L versus 103 mEq/L) and lower pH (5.7 versus 7.4). Thus, if isotonic saline is infused at large volumes, it can result in a hyperchloremic metabolic acidosis (Prough, 1999). The saline-induced acidosis usually has no adverse clinical consequences, but differentiating it from lactic acidosis (a marker of tissue necrosis) can be challenging in certain settings. Gastric secretions lost during vomiting or nasogastric tube suctioning are commonly replaced by a 5-percent dextrose in 0.45-percent normal saline solution with 20 mEq/L KCl added.

Also known as Hartmann solution, lactated Ringer solution contains potassium and calcium concentrations similar to plasma, but the sodium concentration (130 mEq) is comparatively reduced to that of isotonic saline to maintain cationic neutrality. The addition of 28 mEq/L of lactate necessitates a reduction in chloride concentrations to a level similar to plasma. In sum, the hyperchloremic metabolic acidosis risk observed with large-volume isotonic saline infusion is avoided. Disadvantageously, lactated Ringer solution leads to increased calcium binding of certain drugs that limits their efficacy (Griffith, 1986). Moreover, calcium can bind the citrated anticoagulant found in blood products and promote clot formation in donor blood. Advantageously, lactated Ringer solution does not significantly change serum lactate levels because only 25 percent of the infused volume remains intravascular. Therefore lactated Ringer solution is commonly employed in cases of isotonic dehydration, such as bowel sequestration in times of obstruction.

■ Pain Management

Postoperative pain management remains undervalued, and many patients continue to experience intense pain after surgery.

TABLE 42-1. Typical Postoperative Orders (Inpatient and Outpatient)

Postoperative Orders (Inpatient)	Postoperative Orders (Outpatient)
Admit to: recovery room/assigned hospital floor/ attending physician's name	Admit to: recovery room; transfer to DSU when cleared by anesthesia
Diagnosis: s/p what surgical procedure	Diagnosis: s/p what surgical procedure
Condition: stable	Condition: stable
Vital signs: q1h × 4, q2h × 2, then q4h	VS per routine
Activity: bed rest	Allergies: NKDA
Allergies: NKDA	Bed rest until A&A, then activity ad lib
Notify MD for: T >101°F; BP >160/110, < 90/60; P >130; RR >30, <10; UOP < 120 mL/4 hr; acute changes	NPO until A&A, then clear liquids IV fluids: LR at 125 mL/hr until tolerating PO, then D/C IV
Diet: NPO except ice chips IV fluids: LR at 125/hr	Notify MD for: T >101°F; BP >160/110, <90/60; P >130; RR >30, <10; acute changes
Special: Strict I/Os Turn, cough, deep breath q1h while awake IS to BS, q1h while awake Foley to gravity SCD hose to pump	D/C patient home when A&A, cleared by anesthesia, taking PO, ambulating, and able to void
Medications: 1. PCA orders: mix 30 mg MSO₄ in 30 mL NS; load 4–6 mg, then IV q6min on demand; lockout 20 mg in 4 hours 2. Phenergan 25 mg IV q6h prn N/V 3. ±Toradol 30 mg IM q6h × 24 h (only if Cr is okay)	F/U at _____ clinic in _____ weeks Write any necessary prescriptions
Labs: H & H in AM (or that afternoon if necessary)	

A&A = awake and alert; BS = bedside; Cr = creatinine; D/C = discontinue, discharge; DSU = day surgery unit; F/U = follow-up; H&H = hemoglobin and hematocrit; I/Os = input and output; IM = intramuscular; IS = incentive spirometry; IV = intravenous; LR = lactated Ringer; MSO₄= morphine sulfate; NKDA = no known drug allergies; NPO = nil per os; NS = normal saline; N/V = nausea and vomiting; P = pulse; PCA = patient-controlled analgesia; PO = per os; RR = respiratory rate; SCD = sequential compression device; s/p = status post; UOP = urine output; VS = vital signs.

A survey by Apfelbaum and colleagues (2003) revealed that more than 85 percent of respondents following surgery have moderate to severe pain. Poor pain control leads to decreased satisfaction with care, prolonged recovery time, increased use of health care resources, and increased costs (Joshi, 2005; McIntosh, 2009). Options for patient analgesia may be broadly classed as opiate-based or nonopioid.

Nonopioid Treatment Options

The two major classes of nonopioid therapies are acetaminophen and nonsteroidal antiinflammatory drugs (NSAIDs). Multimodal pain control postoperatively using intravenous (IV) NSAIDs and/or acetaminophen can reduce or enhance analgesia, lower narcotic needs, decrease the incidence of postoperative nausea and vomiting by as much as 30 percent, and reduce hospital length of stay (Akarsu, 2004; Chan, 1996; Khalili, 2013; Mixter, 1998; Santoso, 2014). In general, these drugs are well tolerated and carry a low risk of serious side effects. However, acetaminophen can be toxic to the liver in high doses. Thus, patients should avoid total doses exceed-

ing 4000 mg/day and use of alcohol while taking acetaminophen-containing products (Food and Drug Administration, 2011). A list of oral NSAIDs and their dosages are found in Table 10-1 (p. 239).

Opioid Treatment Options

Despite the common side effects that all opiates share—respiratory depression and nausea and vomiting—opiate therapy is the primary choice for managing moderate to severe pain. The three most common opiates prescribed after gynecologic surgeries are morphine, fentanyl, and hydromorphone. Meperidine, although commonly administered in many obstetric units, is avoided in part because of neurologic side effects associated with its active metabolite, normeperidine. Normeperidine is a cerebral irritant that can cause effects ranging from irritability and agitation to seizure.

Morphine is prescribed most frequently following gynecologic surgery and is a potent μ-opiate-receptor agonist. Action at this receptor accounts for the analgesia, euphoria, respiratory depression, and decreased gastrointestinal (GI) motility seen with morphine. Onset of action is rapid, and peak effects are seen within 20 minutes of IV administration. Its action typically lasts for 3 to 4 hours. Its active metabolite, morphine-6-glucuronide, is renally excreted and thus is well tolerated in low doses in those with liver disease.

Pruritus is common after administration, although its genesis is poorly understood. Some investigators theorize that central opiate receptors are stimulated, whereas others speculate a histamine release as evidenced by urticaria, wheals, and flushing. In these cases, changing to another pain medication is logical. For pruritus treatment, most evidence-based data derive from studies of regional analgesia. Success has been found with ondansetron, 4 mg IV (George, 2009). Antihistamines, such as diphenhydramine (Benadryl) 25 mg IV, are another option. Naloxone, an opioid antagonist, can be used but may reverse the analgesia provided by morphine.

Fentanyl, a potent synthetic opiate, is more lipophilic than morphine and displays a shorter duration of action and half-life. Peak analgesia is reached within minutes of IV administration and lasts for 30 to 60 minutes. Many conscious sedation protocols used during office gynecologic procedures combine fentanyl with a sedative such as midazolam (Versed).

Hydromorphone (Dilaudid), another semisynthetic analogue of morphine, is less lipophilic than fentanyl. It is available for delivery by multiple routes, including oral, intramuscular (IM), IV, rectal, and subcutaneous (SC). Hydromorphone achieves its peak analgesia 15 minutes after IV administration, and its effects last 3 to 4 hours. Although commonly used during epidural analgesia, hydromorphone is a suitable patient-controlled analgesia (PCA) alternative in patients with a morphine allergy. Table 42-2 provides a summary of various pain medications and dosage equivalents.

▪ Hormone Replacement Therapy

Some women will have significant menopausal symptoms after surgical removal of both ovaries. Symptoms can range from severe

TABLE 42-2. Opioid Equivalency Chart/Dosing Data for Opioids

Drugs	Approximate Opioid Equianalgesic Dose			Usual Starting Dose			
				Adults >50 kg Body Wt		Children and Adults <50 kg	
	Parenteral (mg)	Oral (mg)	Duration (h)	Parenteral	Oral	Parenteral	Oral
Morphine IR (Roxanol)	10	30	3–4	10 mg	30 mg	0.1 mg/kg	0.3 mg/kg
Morphine SR (Oramorph) (MS Contin)	—	30	8–12	—	30 mg	—	0.3 mg/kg
Meperidine (Demerol)	75	300	2–3	100 mg	NR	0.75 mg/kg	NR
Hydromorphone (Dilaudid)	1.5	7.5	3–4	1.5 mg	6 mg	0.015 mg/kg	0.06 mg/kg
Codeine	130	200	3–4	60 mg (IM/SC)	60 mg	NR	1 mg/kg
Oxycodone IR (Roxicet)[a] (Percocet)[a]	—	30	3–4	NA	10 mg	NA	0.2 mg/kg
Oxycodone SR (OxyContin)	—	30	8–12	NA	10 mg	NA	0.2 mg/kg
Hydrocodone (Lorcet)[a] (Lortab)[a] (Vicodin)	NA	30	6–8	NA	10 mg	NA	0.2 mg/kg
Methadone (Dolophine)	10	20	3–4	10 mg	20 mg	0.1 mg/kg	0.2 mg/kg
Fentanyl (Sublimaze) (Duragesic)	0.1	—	1	0.1 mg	—	—	—

[a]Narcotic/nonnarcotic combination product.
IM = intramuscular; IR = immediate release; NA = not available; NR = not recommended; SC = subcutaneous; SR = sustained release.

hot flashes to headaches or sudden mood swings. In these women, estrogen replacement therapy is considered for those without contraindications (Chap. 22, p. 494). For women completing surgery for endometriosis, a progestin may be added for those with residual disease, as discussed in Chapter 10 (p. 243).

PULMONARY COMPLICATIONS

Broad definitions hinder our ability to accurately assess the incidence of postoperative pulmonary complications, but reported estimates range from 9 to 69 percent (Calligaro, 1993; Hall, 1991). Postoperative pulmonary complications include atelectasis, pulmonary embolism (PE), and less commonly, pneumonia and acute respiratory distress syndrome (ARDS). All can potentially lead to acute respiratory failure.

Acute Respiratory Failure

In the general postsurgical population, acute respiratory failure (ARF) has an incidence ranging from 0.2 to 3.0 percent and an associated mortality rate that can exceed 25 percent (Arozullah, 2000; Johnson, 2007). ARF is classically divided into four subtypes defined by inadequate exchange of oxygen or carbon dioxide or both. Type 1 lesions exchange oxygen poorly, and examples include atelectasis, pneumonia, PE, and ARDS, all discussed subsequently.

Type 2 is typified by hypercapnia. It is seen in anesthesia overdose and muscle fatigue, in which ventilation suffers and carbon dioxide (CO_2) is retained. Also, increased metabolic processes such as fever, severe sepsis, overfeeding, and hyperthyroidism can generate excess CO_2. As a result, ventilatory work increases as the body attempts to maintain appropriate arterial pCO_2 levels. This can ultimately lead to respiratory failure.

Type 3 is similar to type 1 but merits a distinct category because of its common occurrence following anesthesia and surgery. Physiologically, general anesthesia reduces muscle tone to decrease lung volumes and airway diameters. The resulting atelectasis and airway closure can drive abnormal gas exchange and ventilation-perfusion mismatching, which creates a decrease in PaO_2. This hypoxemia is further aggravated by hypoventilation from central decreases in respiratory drive, residual effects of anesthetics, lung edema, or bronchospasm (Canet, 1989). To help circumvent type 3 ARF, important considerations include early treatment of hypoxemia, multimodal approaches to pain management, and chest physiotherapy.

Type 4 stems from shock and its associated cardiopulmonary hypoperfusion. For treatment, circulatory resuscitation, discussed in Chapter 40 (p. 864), accompanies oxygen therapy.

Atelectasis

This reversible closure or collapse of alveoli is seen in 90 percent of surgical patients (Lundquist, 1995). Development is associated with decreased lung compliance, gas exchange abnormalities, and increased pulmonary vascular resistance. Thus, characteristic signs are diminished breath sounds, dullness to percussion over affected lung fields, and decreased oxygenation. Pulse oximetry readings >92 percent represent adequate oxygenation, however, a PaO_2 measurement by arterial blood gas will most accurately assess a patient with hypoxic respiratory

failure. In addition to bedside findings, chest radiography typically shows linear densities in the lower lung fields. Classically, atelectasis is associated with low-grade fevers. However, Mavros and colleagues (2011) reviewed eight studies with a total of 998 patients and found no association between atelectasis and postoperative fever.

Prevention using lung expansion therapies is described in Chapter 39 (p. 827), and these can be used for treatment as well. Atelectasis is usually temporary (up to 2 days) and self-limited, and it rarely slows patient recovery or hospital discharge (Platell, 1997). Its importance mainly lies in its clinical similarity to PE and pneumonia. Thus, in women with risks for these more life-threatening complications, atelectasis may ultimately be a diagnosis of exclusion.

Hospital-acquired Pneumonia

This is the second most common nosocomial infection in the United States and carries high associated morbidity and mortality rates (Tablan, 2004). Its incidence in surgical patients varies and ranges from 1 to 19 percent depending on surgical procedure and hospital surveyed (Kozlow, 2003). With these infections, bacterial pathogens most typically include aerobic gram-negative bacilli, such as *Pseudomonas aeruginosa*, *Escherichia coli*, *Klebsiella pneumoniae*, and *Acinetobacter* species.

Clinically, pneumonia is diagnosed if chest radiography reveals a new or progressive radiographic infiltrate and if two of three clinical features (leukocytosis, fever >38°C, or purulent secretions) are present. Broad-spectrum antibiotic regimens are recommended for hospital-acquired pneumonia treatment (Table 42-3). If aspiration is highly suspected, specific treatment

TABLE 42-3. Empiric Antibiotic Therapy for Hospital-acquired Pneumonia[a]

Regimen Options	Dosage
Cefepime or ceftazidime	2 g every 8 hr
or	
Imipenem or meropenem	1 g every 8 hr
or	
Piperacillin–tazobactam	4.5 g every 6 hr
PLUS	
Aminoglycoside	
Gentamicin	7 mg/kg/d
Tobramycin	7 mg/kg/d
Amikacin	20 mg/kg/d
or	
Quinolone	
Levofloxacin	750 mg daily
Ciprofloxacin	400 mg every 8 hr

[a]In patients with late-onset disease or risk factors for multi-drug-resistant pathogens.
Adapted with permission from American Thoracic Society: Guidelines for the management of adults with hospital-acquired, ventilator-associated, and healthcare-associated pneumonia. Am J Respir Crit Care Med 2005 Feb 15; 171(4):388–416.

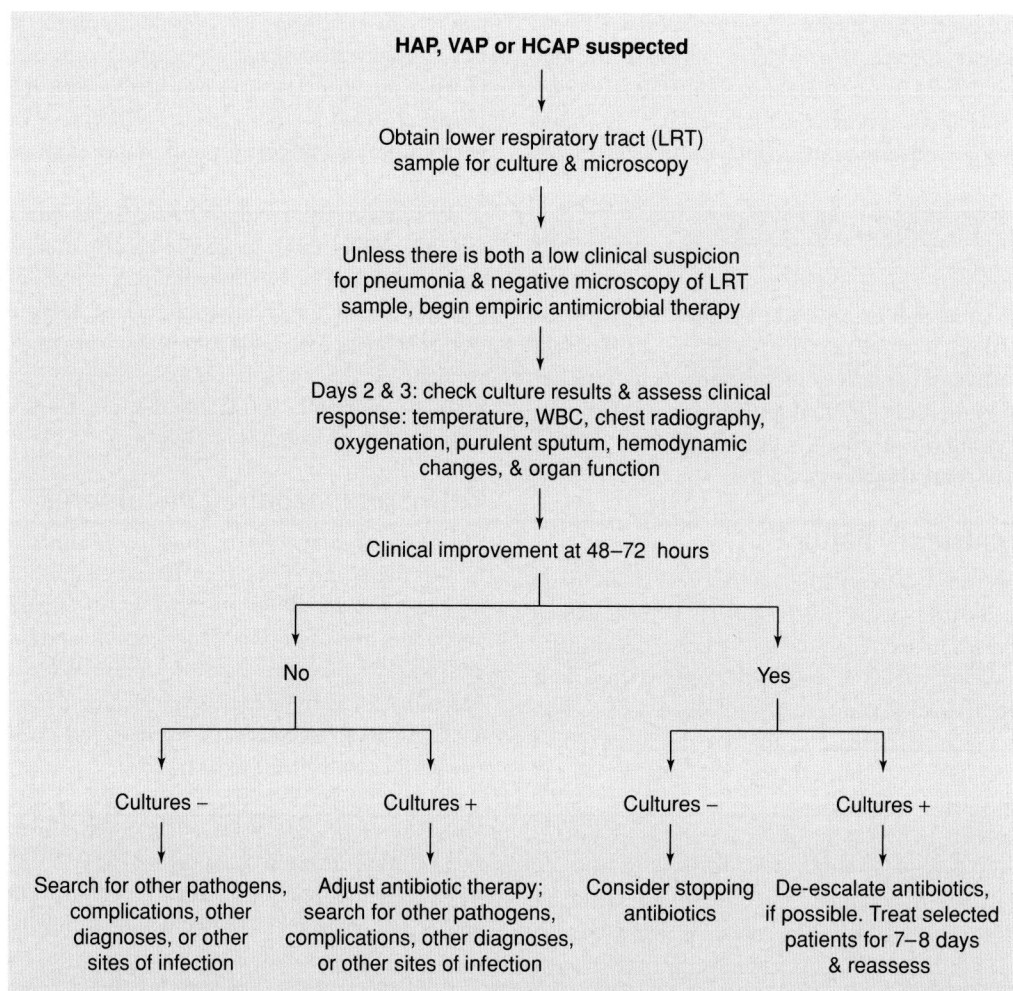

FIGURE 42-1 Algorithm describes management strategies for hospital-acquired pneumonia. HAP = hospital-acquired pneumonia; HCAP = health care-associated pneumonia; VAP = ventilator-associated pneumonia; WBC = white blood cells. (Reproduced with permission from American Thoracic Society: Guidelines for the management of adults with hospital-acquired, ventilator-associated, and healthcare-associated pneumonia. Am J Respir Crit Care Med 2005 Feb 15;171(4):388–416.)

for anaerobes with metronidazole or clindamycin is considered. An algorithm supported by the American Thoracic Society is shown in Figure 42-1. Preventive steps include substituting oral endotracheal and orogastric tubes in place of nasal tubes; elevating the head of the bed 30 to 45 degrees, particularly during feeding; and removing subglottic secretions in those unable to clear these (American Thoracic Society, 2005; Ferrer, 2010).

■ Pulmonary Embolism

If venous thromboembolism (VTE) is suspected, evaluation begins with clinical examination and risk estimation. Wells and colleagues (1995) described one of the most widely used pretest probability assessments for DVT (Table 42-4). When indicated, duplex sonography is highly sensitive for detecting proximal leg DVTs, with a false-negative rate of 0 to 6 percent (Gottlieb, 1999).

For PE, because symptoms may reflect other cardiopulmonary pathology, clinicians often initially elect chest radiography and electrocardiogram (ECG). The radiograph is typically abnormal but nonspecific, and findings can include atelectasis, elevated hemidiaphragm, cardiomegaly, and small pleu-

ral effusions (Worsley, 1993). ECG may display tachycardia or may reflect right heart strain by showing a large S wave in lead I, a Q wave in lead III, and inverted T wave in lead III (Stein, 1991). If suspicion for PE remains, then computed tomographic angiography (CTA) or less frequently, ventilation/perfusion (V/Q) scanning is ordered. These serve as alternatives to the invasive gold standards—pulmonary angiography or contrast venography.

Acute management of VTE involves anticoagulation with intravenous unfractionated heparin or subcutaneous low-molecular-weight heparin (Tables 42-5 and 42-6). After achieving adequate anticoagulation, oral vitamin K antagonists such as warfarin are initiated. To avoid paradoxical hypercoagulability, heparin is continued for at least 5 days after the initiation of warfarin (Houman Fekrazad, 2009). Once the international normalized ratio (INR) reaches a therapeutic range of 2 to 3, then heparin is stopped. Long term, anticoagulation therapy duration is dictated by clinical and patient circumstances. For those with a provoked first DVT or PE, anticoagulants are recommended for 3 months. Provocateurs include surgery, exogenous estrogen, or local trauma. Extended therapy is preferred for both those with unprovoked VTE or with second VTE,

TABLE 42-4. Pretest Probability for Deep-Vein Thrombosis

Major Points	Minor Points
Cancer	Recent trauma to
Immobilization	symptomatic leg
Recent major surgery	Unilateral edema
Thigh or calf tenderness	Erythema
Calf swelling	Dilated superficial veins
Family history of DVT	Hospitalized in last 6 months

Clinical Probability

High

>3 major points and no alternative diagnosis

>2 major points and >2 minor points + no alternative diagnosis

Low

1 major point + >2 minor points + has an alternative diagnosis

1 major point + >1 minor point + no alternative diagnosis

0 major points + >3 minor points + has an alternative diagnosis

0 major points + >2 minor points + no alternative diagnosis

Moderate

All other combinations

Adapted with permission from Wells PS, Hirsh J, Anderson DR, et al: Accuracy of clinical assessment of deepvein thrombosis. Lancet 1995 May 27;345(8961):1326–1330.

unless the risk of bleeding is high, in which case, treatment is halted at 3 months. For those with concurrent cancer, therapy is extended regardless of bleeding risk (Kearon, 2012).

■ Acute Respiratory Distress Syndrome

Acute lung injury that causes a form of severe permeability pulmonary edema and ARF is termed acute respiratory distress

TABLE 42-6. Characteristics of Some Low-Molecular-Weight Heparins

Name (Brand Name)	Dose
Enoxaparin (Lovenox)	1 mg/kg every 12 hr
	1.5 mg/kg daily
Tinzaparin (Innohep)	175 IU/kg daily
Dalteparin (Fragmin)	100 IU/kg every 12 hr
	200 IU/kg daily

IU = international units.

syndrome. This is a pathophysiologic continuum from mild pulmonary insufficiency to dependence on high inspired oxygen concentrations and mechanical ventilation. The theory that multiple insults lead to postoperative ARDS offers insight into modifiable intra- and postoperative alveolar damage prevention (Litell, 2011; Warner, 2000). Intraoperative strategies minimize lung trauma by keeping airway pressure and tidal volumes within set limits and by avoiding repeated alveolar opening and closing (Hemmes, 2013). Other measures strive to prevent infection, limit IV fluid volumes, and avoid blood product transfusion (Güldner, 2013).

CARDIAC COMPLICATIONS

■ Myocardial Infarction

Postoperative myocardial infarction (MI) is rare, and its generally reported incidence ranges from nearly 1 percent to as high as 37 percent among patients with surgery within 3 months following an MI (Mangano, 1990; Tinker, 1978). Declines in oxygen supply and increased demand classically underlie this coronary ischemia. Events that decrease oxygen supply include hypotension, lowered coronary perfusion, or poor carrying capacity caused by anemia. Increased afterload, tachycardia, and increased cardiac contractility can raise myocardial oxygen demands.

TABLE 42-5. Parkland Hospital Protocol for Continuous Heparin Infusion for Patients with Venous Thromboembolism

Initial Heparin Dose:
__ **units IV push (recommended 80 units/kg rounded to nearest 100, maximum 7500 units), then**
__ **units/hr by infusion (recommended 18 units/kg/hr rounded to nearest 50).**

Infusion Rate Adjustments—based on partial thromboplastin time (PTT):

PTT (sec)[a]	Intervention[b]	Baseline Infusion Rate Change[c]
<45	80 units/kg bolus	↑by 4 units/kg/hr
45–54	40 units/kg bolus	↑by 2 units/kg/hr
55–84	None	None
85–100	None	↓by 2 units/kg/hr
>100	Stop infusion 60 minutes	↓by 3 units/kg/hr

[a]PTT goal 55–84.
[b]Rounded to nearest 100.
[c]Rounded to nearest 50.

Most patients with postoperative MI do not have classic symptoms of chest pain or pressure. These are in part masked by postoperative analgesics (Muir, 1991). Dyspnea is the most common complaint and may be accompanied by acute cardiac failure or hemodynamic instability. ECG changes of postoperative MI tend to be less well defined, and most demonstrate a non-Q wave variant (Badner, 1998). CK isoenzyme (CK-MB) abnormalities are seen within 6 hours, and cardiac troponin I and T are highly specific later for diagnosis of MI (Zimmerman, 1999).

Postoperative MI treatment differs from that of nonsurgical patients, and its main tenets focus on shifting the oxygen delivery and utilization balance. Special attention is given to arrhythmia correction and hemodynamic status improvement. Ideally, these patients are cared for in a unit that provides intense monitoring, cardiopulmonary support, and cardiology consultation.

Hypertension

This is frequently encountered both preoperatively and postoperatively. As standard definitions are lacking, the reported incidence ranges from 3 to 90 percent, depending on the thresholds set and the type of surgery. Patients with poorly controlled hypertension preoperatively tend to have more blood pressure lability compared with normotensive patients or those with well-controlled hypertension. In general, a diastolic blood pressure greater than 110 mm Hg preoperatively best predicts those who will have postoperative hypertension issues.

Several possible triggers may raise blood pressures in the first 24 hours after surgery. First, abrupt withdrawal of β-blocker or of centrally acting sympatholytic agents such as clonidine can cause rebound hypertension. Pain and bladder distention may also contribute. Later in postoperative recovery, sympathetic hyperactivity may stem from inadequate pain management or from alcohol withdrawal. Last, return of excess interstitial fluid back into the vascular space may create fluid overload and hypertension.

Two approaches have been described for blood pressure treatment: fixed thresholds and relative changes from baseline. Charlson and colleagues (1990) demonstrated increased rates of postoperative cardiac and renal complications when the mean blood pressure rose 20 percent or more compared with preoperative levels. Given the paucity of good evidence, it is reasonable to initiate treatment if mean blood pressure readings rise by this percentage. With acute blood pressure management, the mean blood pressure should not be lowered by more than 20 percent or to a level less than 160/100 mm Hg.

GASTROINTESTINAL COMPLICATIONS

Postoperative Nausea and Vomiting

This is one of the most common complaints following surgery, and its incidence ranges from 30 to 70 percent in high-risk patients (Møller, 2002). Those at risk for postoperative nausea and vomiting (PONV) include females, nonsmokers, those with prior motion sickness or prior PONV, and those with extended surgeries (Apfelbaum, 2003).

A multimodal approach to prevention is recommended (Apfel, 2004). Currently, combinations of 4 to 8 mg of dexamethasone prior to anesthesia induction are followed, toward the end of surgery, by less than 1 mg of droperidol (Inapsine) and 4 mg of ondansetron (Zofran). This pretreatment significantly reduces symptoms by 25 percent. However, if symptoms develop within 6 hours of surgery, antiemetics from a different pharmacologic class than previously administered are considered (Habib, 2004). Persistent nausea may benefit from combining agents from different classes (Table 42-7).

Bowel Function and Diet Resumption

Normal GI function requires synchronized motility, mucosal transport of nutrients, and evacuation reflexes (Nunley, 2004).

TABLE 42-7. Commonly Used Medications for Nausea and Vomiting

Medication (Brand Name)	Usual Dosage	Route(s)
Antihistamines	**Every 6 hr**	
Diphenhydramine (Benadryl)	25–50 mg	IM, IV, PO
Hydroxyzine (Atarax, Vistaril)	25–100 mg	IM, PO
Meclizine (Antivert)	25–50 mg	PO
Benzamides	**Every 6 hr**	
Metoclopramide (Reglan)	5–15 mg	IM, IV, PO
Trimethobenzamide (Tigan)	250 mg	IM, PO, PR
Phenothiazines	**Every 6 hr**	
Prochlorperazine (Compazine)	5–10 (25 PR) mg	IM, IV, PO, PR
Promethazine (Phenergan)	12.5–25 mg	IM, IV, PO, PR
Serotonin Antagonists		
Ondansetron (Zofran)	8 mg every 8 hr	IV, PO
Granisetron (Kytril)	2 mg daily	IV, PO
Dolasetron (Anzemet)	100 mg daily	IV, PO

IM = intramuscular; IV = intravenous; PO = orally; PR = per rectum.

However, following intraabdominal surgery, dysfunction of enteric neural activity typically disrupts normal propulsion. Activity first returns in the stomach and is noted typically within 24 hours. The small intestine also exhibits contractile activity within 24 hours after surgery, but normal function may be delayed for 3 to 4 days (Condon, 1986; Dauchel, 1976). Rhythmic colonic motility resumes last, at approximately 4 days following intraabdominal surgery (Huge, 2000). Passage of flatus characteristically marks this return of function, and stool passage usually follows in 1 to 2 days.

Postoperative feeding is most effective when started early. It improves wound healing, promotes gut motility, decreases intestinal stasis, raises splanchnic blood flow, and stimulates reflexes that elicit GI hormone secretion to shorten postoperative ileus (Anderson, 2003; Braga, 2002; Correia, 2004; Lewis, 2001). The decision to initiate "early feeding" with liquids or with solid food has been studied prospectively (Jeffery, 1996). In patients who were given solid food as the first postoperative meal, the number of calories and amount of protein consumed on the first postoperative day were higher. In addition, the number of patients requiring diet changes to NPO (nil per os) was not statistically different (7.5 percent in regular diet and 8.1 percent in the clear diet groups). The improved tolerance and better palatability of solids makes this a reasonable option.

◼ Ileus

Postoperative ileus (POI) is a transient impairment of GI activity that leads to abdominal distention, hypoactive bowel sounds, nausea and vomiting related to GI gas and fluid accumulation, and delayed passage of flatus or stool (Livingston, 1990).

The genesis of POI is multifactorial. First, bowel manipulation during surgery leads to production of contributory factors. These include: (1) neurogenic factors related to sympathetic overactivity, (2) hormonal factors related to the release of hypothalamic corticotropin-releasing hormone (CRH), which plays a key role in the stress response, and (3) inflammatory factors (Tache, 2001). Second, perioperative opioid use also increases POI rates. Thus, in selecting opiates, clinicians balance the beneficial analgesia produced by central opioid receptor binding against the GI dysfunction that results from peripheral receptor binding effects (Holzer, 2004).

No single treatment defines POI management. Electrolyte repletion and IV fluids to reestablish euvolemia are traditional. In contrast, routine nasogastric tube (NGT) decompression to promote bowel rest has been challenged by multiple prospective randomized trials. A metaanalysis including nearly 5240 patients found routine NGT decompression unsuccessful and inferior to its selective use in symptomatic patients. Specifically, patients without NGTs had significantly earlier return of normal bowel function and decreased risks of wound infection and ventral hernia (Nelson, 2007). Additionally, tube-related discomfort, nausea, and hospital stays were reduced. For these reasons, postoperative NGTs are recommended only for symptomatic relief of abdominal bloating and recurrent vomiting (Nunley, 2004).

Gum chewing after laparotomy as a preventive modality for POI has been the focus of several small but randomized studies.

In these, sugarless gum is usually chewed 15 to 30 minutes at least three times daily. In evaluations, this practice is associated with earlier improvement in bowel motility markers (Ertas, 2013; Jernigan, 2014). However, compared with placebo, gum chewing achieves these goals on average only several hours earlier (Li, 2013).

◼ Bowel Obstruction

Obstruction of the small intestines may be partial or complete and can result from adhesions following intraabdominal surgery, infection, or malignancy. Of these, surgical adhesions are the most common cause (Krebs, 1987; Monk, 1994). Small bowel obstruction (SBO) develops following 1 to 2 percent of total abdominal hysterectomies, and nearly 75 percent of obstructions are complete (Al-Sunaidi, 2006). Obstruction may be remote from surgery, and the mean interval between primary intraabdominal procedure and SBO approximates 5 years (Al-Took, 1999).

Initial SBO management is similar to that for POI, but distinguishing between the two is important to prevent serious SBO sequelae. During SBO, the bowel lumen dilates proximal to the obstruction, and decompression may develop distally. Bacterial overgrowth in the proximal small bowel can promote bacterial fermentation and worsening dilation. The bowel wall also becomes edematous and dysfunctional (Wright, 1971). Progressive increases in bowel pressure compromise perfusion to the intestinal segment and can ultimately lead to ischemia or rupture (Megibow, 1991).

Clinical signs that may help distinguish SBO from POI include tachycardia, oliguria, and fever. Physical examination may reveal abdominal distention, high-pitched bowel sounds, and an empty rectal vault during digital examination. Last, leukocytosis with a neutrophil dominance should alert to possible coexistent bowel ischemia.

Computed tomography (CT) scanning is the primary imaging tool to identify SBO. Water-soluble contrast can safely help identify the cause and severity of an obstruction. Gastrografin, the most commonly used water-soluble dye, is a mixture of sodium amidotrizoate and meglumine amidotrizoate and may aid resolution of small bowel edema due to its high osmotic pressure. Gastrografin is also theorized to enhance smooth muscle contractility (Assalia, 1994). Although the use of oral Gastrografin does appear to reduce hospital length of stay, it has no therapeutic benefit in adhesion-related SBO (Abbas, 2007).

Treatment of SBO varies with the degree of obstruction. For partial obstruction, feedings are held, IV fluids and antiemetics are initiated, and an NGT is placed for significant nausea and vomiting. Continued surveillance monitors for signs of bowel ischemia. Symptoms in most cases of partial SBO improve within 48 hours. In contrast, for most of those with complete bowel obstruction, surgery to relieve the obstruction is indicated.

Colonic obstruction is rare following gynecologic surgery but carries a high mortality rate (Krstic, 2014). The colon can be obstructed by intrinsic lesions such as colon cancer or diverticulitis-related strictures or can be compressed by a pelvic mass or foreign body, such as a retained surgical sponge. An enlarged cecum found on an abdominal radiograph requires further evaluation by either a barium enema or colonoscopy. Immediate intervention is necessary when the cecal diameter exceeds 10 to 12 cm to minimize perforation risks.

▉ Diarrhea

Transient episodes of postoperative diarrhea are not uncommon after major gynecologic surgery as the GI tract returns to its baseline motility and function. Protracted episodes and excessive amounts of diarrhea almost always stem from infection and warrant further evaluation. Stool samples are examined for ova and parasites, cultured for bacteria, and assayed for *Clostridium difficile* toxin. Of potential etiologies, broad-spectrum antibiotics can impair normal GI flora growth and thereby promote *C difficile* toxin-associated pseudomembranous colitis. If toxin is identified, oral metronidazole or vancomycin is initiated and continued for 10 to 14 days after diarrhea resolution (Cohen, 2010). Regardless of the pathogen, aggressive fluid and electrolyte replacement is critical to prevent further aberrations that can delay recovery.

▉ Nutrition

The primary goals of postoperative nutrition are to improve immune function, promote wound healing, and minimize metabolic disturbances. Despite the additional stress in the immediate postoperative period, underfeeding is accepted for a brief period (Seidner, 2006). Table 42-8 offers a summary of basic immediate postoperative metabolic needs. However, extended protein calorie restriction in a surgical patient can lead to impaired wound healing, diminished cardiac and pulmonary function, bacterial overgrowth within the GI tract, and other complications that increase hospital stays and patient morbidity (Elwyn, 1975; Kinney, 1986; Seidner, 2006). If substantial oral caloric intake is delayed for 7 to 10 days, nutritional support is warranted.

In the absence of contraindications, enteral nutrition is preferred to a parenteral route, especially when infectious complications are compared (Kudsk, 1992; Moore, 1992). Other advantages of enteral nutrition include fewer metabolic disturbances and lower cost (Nehra, 2002).

URINARY COMPLICATIONS

▉ Oliguria
Prerenal Oliguria

Postoperative oliguria is defined as urine production less than 0.5 mL/kg/hr. Oliguria can be caused by a prerenal, intrarenal, or postrenal insult, and a systematic approach typically allows differentiation among these.

Prerenal oliguria is a physiologic response to hypovolemia, and coexistent tachycardia and orthostatic hypotension usually reflect this volume depletion. Causes of postoperative hypovolemia are varied and include acute hemorrhage, vomiting, severe diarrhea, and inadequate intraoperative volume replacement. In response to hypovolemia, the renin-angiotensin system is activated, and antidiuretic hormone (ADH) is released to prompt reabsorption of sodium and water by the renal tubules. Prerenal oliguria is the result of this sequence.

Treatment focuses on volume replacement. Thus, an accurate assessment of the patient's fluid deficit is critical. Tallying estimated surgical blood loss and data from the intraoperative fluid logs kept by the anesthesiologist will help begin the calculations. Insensible loss during laparotomy approximates 150 mL/hr.

Intrarenal Oliguria

Ischemic injury can lead to necrosis of the renal tubules and decreased filtration. This damage may be more common in a prerenal setting, in which the renal tubules are more vulnerable to insult from nephrotoxic agents such as NSAIDs, aminoglycosides, and contrast media. In many cases, intrarenal and prerenal oliguria can be differentiated by calculating the fractional excretion of sodium (FENa). Using sodium (Na^+) and creatinine (Cr) levels from both serum and urine, this is defined as:

$$(\text{Urine } Na^+/\text{plasma } Na^+) \div (\text{Urine Cr/plasma Cr}).$$

A ratio <1 suggests a prerenal source, whereas a ratio >3 indicates an intrarenal insult. Another difference is urine sodium levels. In prerenal oliguria, the level is typically <20 mEq/L, whereas in intrarenal states, it usually is >80 mEq/L.

Postrenal Oliguria

The most common cause of postrenal oliguria is urinary catheter obstruction. In those without a catheter, urinary retention is most

---

TABLE 42-8. Postoperative Nutritional Requirements

Nutritional Requirements	Recommendations
BEE in women	65.5 + 1.9 (height in cm) + 9.6 (weight in kg) − 4.7 (age in years)
Total calories	100% to 120% BEE
Glucose	50–70% total caloric intake. Maintain blood glucose level <200 mg/dL
Protein	1.5 g/kg/d of current weight (BMI <25) 2.0 g/kg/d of ideal weight (BMI >25)

BEE = Basal energy expenditure; BMI = body mass index.
Data from Nehra V: Fluid electrolyte and nutritional problems in the postoperative period. Clin Obstet Gynecol 2002 Jun;45(2):537–544.

likely. More seriously, ligation or laceration to the ureter or bladder may be sources. Importantly, partial or unilateral obstruction may exist despite adequate urine output. With this, associated findings may include hematuria, flank or abdominal pain, or ileus.

For diagnosis, renal sonography is highly sensitive and specific for confirming hydronephrosis. Additional diagnostic tools to identify ureteral obstruction include CT with IV contrast or retrograde pyelography. Importantly, IV contrast can be nephrotoxic, and thus CT with contrast may be a less than ideal choice for those with already elevated creatinine levels. As discussed in Chapter 40 (p. 868), the obstruction may be relieved with ureteral stenting alone or may require surgical repair.

■ Urinary Retention

Inability to void with a full bladder is common after gynecologic surgery, and incidences range from 7 to 80 percent depending on the definition used and surgical procedure (Stanton, 1979; Tammela, 1986). Overdistension can lead to prolonged difficulty with micturition and even permanent detrusor damage (Mayo, 1973). In addition to patient discomfort, recatheterization to treat retention increases the risk of urinary tract infection and may extend hospitalization.

Keita and colleagues (2005) prospectively evaluated risk factors potentially predictive of early postoperative urinary retention. Three major factors were independently associated with an increased risk—age greater than 50 years, intraoperative IV fluid administration greater than 750 mL, and bladder urine volume greater than 270 mL measured upon entry to the recovery room. Among gynecologic procedures, the risk is higher after laparotomy compared with laparoscopy (Bodker, 2003).

Despite identifiable risks, all women are advised on the need for immediate evaluation of absent or difficult voiding. Clinical markers that include pain, tachycardia, urge to void without success, and bladder enlargement by palpation or percussion are diagnostically equivalent to evaluation using bedside bladder sonography (Bodker, 2003).

Once retention is identified, catheterization and bladder drainage should follow. Lau and Lam (2004) sought to determine the best catheterization strategy for managing postoperative urinary retention. Compared with overnight bladder decompression with an indwelling catheter, episodic in-and-out catheterization is equally effective. Moreover, infectious morbidity rates do not significantly differ between the two.

Voiding Trials

Normal urination requires appropriate bladder contractility in the absence of significant urethral resistance (Abrams, 1999). Objective criteria that define normal function postoperatively vary and may be assessed using either active or passive voiding trials.

With an *active voiding trial*, the bladder is filled with a set volume, and following patient voiding, residual bladder urine volumes are calculated. To begin, the bladder is completely emptied by catheterization. It may be helpful for a woman to stand upright to clear the most dependent portions of her bladder. Next, sterile water infused under gravity is instilled into the bladder through the same catheter until approximately 300 mL is used or until a subjective maximum capacity is reached. A patient is then given up to 30 minutes to void spontaneously into a urine collection device. The difference between volume infused and volume retrieved is recorded as the *postvoid residual*.

The only published study evaluating the effectiveness of this strategy was reported by Kleeman and associates (2002). They evaluated women following surgery for incontinence and prolapse. In their study, a postvoid residual of less than 50 percent carried a recatheterization rate of 8 percent. If patients could spontaneously void greater than 70 percent of the instilled volume, there were no failures.

A *passive voiding trial* serves as an alternative, and residuals may be assessed following passive, physiologic filling of the bladder. To begin, the Foley catheter is removed, and a woman is encouraged to drink increased amounts of liquid. She is encouraged to void spontaneously at her first urge to urinate or after 4 hours, whichever is first. Urine volumes in a collection device are measured. An in-and-out catheterization or bladder sonogram is then performed to measure the postvoid residual (Fig. 23-12, p. 526).

An easy rule to remember for evaluating either active or passive voiding trials is the "75/75 rule," which is spontaneously voiding greater than 75 mL *and* voiding greater than 75 percent of the total volume. This constitutes a successful voiding trial and obviates the need for Foley catheter reinsertion. Alternatively, on the Urogynecology Service at Parkland Memorial Hospital, a postvoid residual of less than 100 mL constitutes a success.

PSYCHIATRIC COMPLICATIONS

Brief periods of confusion are not uncommon after general anesthesia. Delirium is estimated to complicate approximately 10 to 60 percent of all surgical cases (Ganai, 2007). Elderly patients have an elevated risk, which is associated with longer hospital stays, greater hospital costs, and even risk of death (Bilotta, 2013).

The clinical diagnosis of delirium is based on five criteria as outlined by the Diagnostic and Statistical Manual of Psychiatric Disorders (DSM-5): cognition changes, disturbance in attention and awareness, an acutely fluctuating time course, changes unrelated to a neurocognitive disorder, and a direct physiologic cause that underlies the delirium (American Psychiatric Association, 2013). There is no standard definition of postoperative delirium, but most studies note it between 24 and 72 hours after surgery. The Confusion Assessment Method (CAM) is a simple four-question tool, which has a sensitivity of 94 percent and specificity of 89 percent (Table 42-9) (Inouye, 2014).

Risk factors for postoperative delirium can be categorized as modifiable or nonmodifiable. Risks that can be altered include infection, pain, sodium and potassium electrolyte abnormalities, anemia, hypoxia, polypharmacy, sleep-wake cycle disruption, and certain medication classes (American Geriatric Society, 2015; Sanders, 2011). Notable groups are opiates, antihistamines, anticholinergics, benzodiazepines, and dihydropyridines, which include calcium-channel blocking agents. Nonmodifiable factors are increased age, preexisting cognitive deficits, poor preoperative functional status, and comorbid disease.

Treatment for postoperative delirium engages several strategies. First, oxygenation, electrolyte, and fluid imbalances are

TABLE 42-9. Confusion Assessment Method Short Form Questionnaire

Feature 1: Acute Onset and Fluctuating Course
Acute change in mental state from baseline?
Did this behavior fluctuate during interview?

Feature 2: Inattention
Did the patient have difficulty focusing attention?

Feature 3: Disorganized Thinking
Was the patient's thinking disorganized or incoherent?

Feature 4: Altered Level of Consciousness
Hyperalert, lethargic, stuporous, or unarousable?

Delirium is diagnosed if the following are present:
Feature 1 *and* feature 2 *PLUS* either feature 3 *or* 4.
Data from Inouye SK, van Dyck CH, Alessi CA, et al:
Clarifying confusion: the confusion assessment method.
A new method for detection of delirium. Ann Intern Med
1990 Dec 15;113(12):941–948.

corrected. Second, pain and potential infection are carefully assessed. In addition, all nonessential medications are halted to minimize confounding factors. Other strategies incorporate increased activity through physical therapy, establishment of distinct sleep-wake cycles, and even light therapy (de Jonghe, 2011; Ono, 2011).

FLUID AND ELECTROLYTE ABNORMALITIES

■ Hypovolemic Shock

Circulatory dysfunction decreases tissue oxygenation and results in multiorgan failure if not recognized and treated promptly. In gynecology, the most frequent cause of shock is hemorrhage-related hypovolemia, although cardiogenic, septic, and neurogenic shock are considered during patient evaluation. Hypovolemic shock may develop before, after, or during surgery, and a full discussion of the topic is found in Chapter 40 (p. 864).

■ Hyponatremia

This common imbalance is defined as a serum sodium level <135 mEq/L and may produce symptoms as levels drop below 125 mEq/L. Of causes, hypotonic fluid administration is often implicated. Aggressive IV crystalloid resuscitation with comparatively hypotonic fluids is one example. Another is venous absorption of large volumes of certain distending media during long operative hysteroscopy cases (Chap. 41, p. 904). Second, pain or drugs can induce water retention through a syndrome of inappropriate ADH (SIADH) (Steele, 1997). Alternatively, excessive renal excretion of sodium is seen with diuretic overuse and adrenal insufficiency. Last, extrarenal sodium losses may follow profuse diarrhea, vomiting, or nasogastric suctioning.

Severe hyponatremia can lead to metabolic encephalopathy with associated cerebral edema, seizures, increased intracranial pressure, and even respiratory arrest. Symptoms are not related to the specific serum sodium level as much as to the rate of change in these levels.

Treatment strategies incorporate the patient's extracellular volume status and the presence or absence of neurologic symptoms. The speed of correction ideally does not exceed 0.5 mEq/L/hr or a serum sodium goal of 130 mEq/L. Over aggressive correction can result in a specific demyelination disorder known as central pontine myelinolysis. In those without symptoms, careful replacement with isotonic fluids and treatment of underlying conditions will correct most cases. Frequent serum sodium levels are drawn to direct care. With associated hypervolemia, furosemide (Lasix) may be added. In those with acute neurologic symptoms, 3-percent saline can be given in a 100 mL infusion over 30 minutes and repeated an additional two times if needed (Nagler, 2014; Verbalis, 2013).

■ Hypernatremia

Hypernatremia is defined as a serum sodium concentration exceeding 145 mEq/L. Common causes are loss of hypotonic body fluids such as diarrhea, gastric secretions, and sweat. The resulting plasma hypertonicity draws water out of cells to maintain intravascular fluid compartment volume. Brain cell shrinkage can cause vascular bleeds and permanent neurologic damage. To restore brain cell volume, the brain metabolically generates compensatory compounds, termed idiogenic osmoles, which pull water back into its cells. Therefore, aggressive treatment with hypotonic fluids can overcorrect to create cerebral edema, seizure, coma, and even death (Adrogué, 2000). Volume replacement to correct hemodynamic instability is initiated with isotonic fluids or colloid fluids. Then, hypernatremia is corrected using hypotonic solutions.

Diabetes insipidus is a condition of renal water wasting, and an excessive amount of urine devoid of solutes is produced. Central diabetes insipidus is caused by a failure to release ADH whereas nephrogenic diabetes insipidus is caused by a deficit in the renal responsiveness to ADH. As treatment, the free water deficit is replaced over 2 to 3 days. In cases of central diabetes insipidus, the addition of ADH (vasopressin) prevents ongoing free water loss (Blevins, 1992).

■ Hypokalemia

This imbalance is defined as serum potassium below 3.5 mEq/L. Hypokalemia is usually caused by diarrhea or by abnormal renal loss secondary to metabolic alkalosis. Mild hypokalemia is often asymptomatic, but nonspecific symptoms seen with progression include generalized weakness and constipation. When the serum levels fall below 2.5 mEq/L, muscle necrosis can begin, and an ascending paralysis can develop with levels below 2.0 mEq/L. Hypokalemia in isolation does not produce cardiac arrhythmia, but it can promote dysfunction in combination with magnesium depletion, myocardial ischemia, and digitalis use (Schaefer, 2005).

The cornerstone of hypokalemia management is potassium replacement. Compared with IV replacement, oral potassium is safer, as it enters the circulation more slowly and reduces the risk of iatrogenic hyperkalemia. The maximum rate of IV potassium replacement is 20 mEq/hr, and the patient's cardiac rhythm is concurrently monitored (Kruse, 1990). Magnesium depletion can cause hypokalemia refractory to replacement efforts, and magnesium may need to be concomitantly replenished (Whang, 1985).

Hyperkalemia

This imbalance is defined as a serum potassium concentration exceeding 5.0 to 5.5 mEq/L. Pseudohyperkalemia can result from traumatic hemolysis, release from muscles distal to a tourniquet, or cellular release from a clotted specimen tube. Unsuspected findings in an asymptomatic patient should prompt a repeat measurement. Transcellular shifts in potassium are seen with digitalis and β-receptor antagonists. More importantly, medication-induced renal excretion impairment is one of the leading causes of hyperkalemia. The most commonly implicated medication classes are angiotensin-converting enzyme (ACE) inhibitors, potassium-sparing diuretics, and NSAIDs (Palmer, 2004; Perazella, 2000).

Hyperkalemia can slow electrical conduction in the heart. The earliest ECG findings of hypokalemia are narrowing and tenting of the T waves. As hyperkalemia progresses, the PR interval lengthens, P waves disappear, and QRS intervals ultimately widen.

Three principles govern hyperkalemia management: (1) protecting the myocardium, (2) shifting potassium intracellularly, and (3) enhancing potassium excretion. Intravenous calcium gluconate administered as 10 mL of a 10-percent solution over 2 to 3 minutes antagonizes the effect of potassium on myocardial repolarization and the conduction system. If there are no improvements in the ECG, calcium administration can be repeated 5 to 10 minutes later. Also, a combination of IV insulin (10 units) and 50 mL of 50-percent dextrose can temporarily shift potassium to the intracellular compartment. In addition, a β2 agonist, such as inhaled albuterol, can help by activating the Na$^+$/K$^+$-ATPase channel to also drive a potassium shift. Finally, potassium excretion can be cleared across the GI mucosa using sodium polystyrene sulfonate (Kayexelate), cleared renally using loop diuretics, or cleared with dialysis for those with impaired renal function.

POSTOPERATIVE FEVER

Pathophysiology

Fever is a response to inflammatory mediators, termed pyrogens, which originate either endogenously or exogenously. Circulating pyrogens lead to production of prostaglandins (primarily PGE$_2$), which elevate the thermoregulatory set point. The inflammatory cascade also produces several cytokines after various events, namely, surgery, cancer, trauma, and infection (Wortel, 1993). Thus, fever is common after surgery and is self-limited in most cases (Garibaldi, 1985). However, for those with persistent symptoms, a systematic approach to patient evaluation helps differentiate inflammatory from infectious etiologies.

Fevers that develop more than 2 days after surgery are more likely to be infectious. More broadly, causes may be categorized by the mnemonic, the "Five Ws," which represent wind, water, walking, wound, and "wonder" drug. First, pneumonia is considered, and women at greatest risk are those who have been mechanically ventilated for a prolonged period, have an NGT in place, or have preexisting chronic obstructive pulmonary disease (COPD). Second, catheterization places women at risk for urinary tract infection. Logically, catheterization duration correlates positively with this infection risk. Third, VTE may present with low-grade fever and other disease-specific symptoms. For example, women with DVT often complain of unilateral lower-extremity edema and erythema. Those with PE may note dyspnea, cough with blood-tinged sputum, chest pain, tachycardia, and symptoms of hypotension. Fourth, fever related to surgical site infections usually develops 5 to 7 days after surgery. These infections may involve the pelvis or abdominal wall layers. Last, medications commonly used postoperatively—such as heparin, β-lactam antibiotics, and sulfonamide antibiotics—may cause a rash, eosinophilia, or drug fever.

Clinical Evaluation

In multiple studies, fever evaluations that rotely include complete blood count (CBC), urinalysis, blood cultures, and chest radiographs are reported to be ineffective (Badillo, 2002; de la Torre, 2003; Schey, 2005). Thus, initial assessment of a woman with postoperative fever is individualized and begins with a focused history and physical examination. The simple diagnostic algorithm presented in Figure 42-2 can be used as one high-yield, cost-effective strategy. Treatment of wound infections is described in Chapter 3, whereas management of pulmonary complications and VTE were discussed earlier (p. 912).

POSTOPERATIVE WOUND

Acute Wound Healing

Wound healing has three phases—inflammatory reaction, proliferation, and remodeling (Li, 2007). Hemostasis by coagulation initiates the first step in the *inflammatory phase*. The infiltration of leukocytes and release of cytokines helps initiate the *proliferative phase* of wound repair. During this, two activities happen simultaneously—the growth of granulation tissue to fill the wound and the formation of epithelium to cover the wound. The final stage, *remodeling*, restores the structural integrity and functional aptitude of the new tissue.

Wound Dehiscence
Classification and Incidence

The depth to which a wound may open varies and may involve only the subcutaneous and skin layers. Such superficial separation can result solely from a hematoma or seroma, but more commonly is a consequence of wound infection. The reported incidence of superficial separations ranges from 3 to 15 percent (Owen, 1994; Taylor, 1998).

More seriously, separation can include the abdominal wall fascia. Fascial dehiscence occurs less frequently and is fatal in nearly 25 percent of cases (Carlson, 1997). Infection or sutures held under too much tension are notorious causes and lead to fascial necrosis. Sutures remain poorly anchored in necrotic fascia (Bartlett, 1985). These layers then separate with only minimal increases in intraabdominal pressure.

Prevention

Rates of wound dehiscence are affected by general patient health, surgical technique, and risks associated with wound infections. Of these, patient health factors may or may not be modifiable.

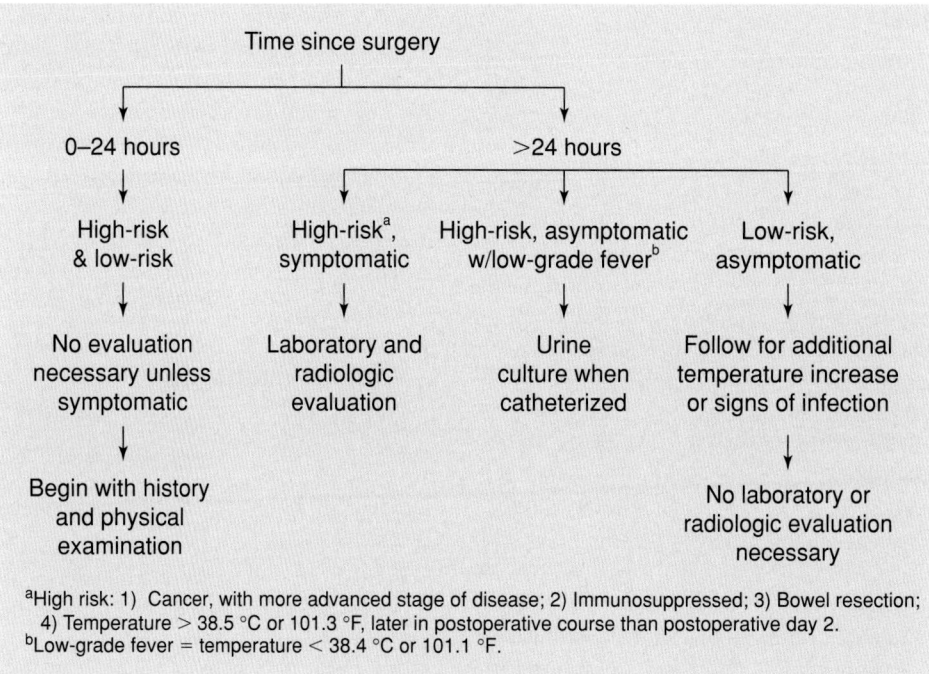

aHigh risk: 1) Cancer, with more advanced stage of disease; 2) Immunosuppressed; 3) Bowel resection; 4) Temperature > 38.5 °C or 101.3 °F, later in postoperative course than postoperative day 2.
bLow-grade fever = temperature < 38.4 °C or 101.1 °F.

FIGURE 42-2 Algorithm for evaluation of postoperative fever. (Reproduced with permission from de la Torre SH, Mandel L, Goff BA: Evaluation of postoperative fever: usefulness and cost-effectiveness of routine workup. Am J Obstet Gynecol 2003 Jun;188(6):1642–1647.)

Characteristics that confer an increased wound disruption risk include age greater than 65 years, pulmonary disease, malnutrition, obesity, malignancy, immunocompromised states, diabetes mellitus, and hypertension (Hodges, 2014; Riou, 1992).

Using proper surgical technique, a surgeon has multiple opportunities to lower wound disruption rates. Described in greater detail in Chapter 40 (p. 847), ideal technique advocates hemostasis, gentle tissue handling, removal of devitalized tissue, closure of dead space, use of monofilament suture in tissue at risk for infection, judicious use of closed-suction drains, and sustained normothermia (Mangram, 1999).

Last, infection is a common underlying cause of wound disruption. Risk factors for infection are numerous and are listed in Table 3-18 (p. 75). Of these, many conditions can be improved preoperatively (Table 42-10).

Diagnosis

Superficial wound separations usually present 3 to 5 days after surgery, with wound erythema and new drainage. A delay in evacuating inflammatory exudates from within subcutaneous-layer dead space can lead to fascial weakening and an increased risk of fascial dehiscence.

Fascial dehiscence generally presents within the first 10 days postoperatively. Superficial disruption of the subcutaneous layer and extensive leakage of peritoneal fluid or purulent drainage are indicative. Given the high mortality risk associated with fascial dehiscence and bowel evisceration, examination under anesthesia to estimate the extent of separation is often warranted.

Superficial Wound Dehiscence Treatment

Wet-to-dry Dressing Changes. With initial wound management, all hematomas, seromas, or pus are evacuated, and necrotic tissue is debrided. If needed, underlying infection is treated with antibiotics. As discussed in Chapter 3 (p. 80), most abdominal wound infections that follow clean cases originate from *Staphylococcus aureus*. In contrast, those after clean-contaminated cases have a greater chance of being polymicrobial. Thus, antibiotic regimens that cover gram-positive and gram-negative organisms are suitable (Table 3-20, p. 79). In these infections, anaerobes play a lesser role. Importantly, the number of infections caused by methicillin-resistant *Staphylococcus aureus* (MRSA) has increased dramatically, and coverage for this pathogen is considered.

After evacuation, wounds are typically gently filled with fluffed-out gauze to provide continued wound drainage and access for additional debridement. This dressing is usually removed daily and replaced with new moist gauze. Solutions used in this dressing remove surface bacteria without disrupting normal healing components. Thus, povidone iodine, iodophor gauze, dilute hydrogen peroxide, and Daiken solution, which are cytotoxic to white blood cells, should play a limited role in wound care (Bennett, 2001; O'Toole, 1996). In very necrotic wounds, allowing gauze to dry and pulling tissue adherent to the gauze with each change is acceptable. More frequent dressing changes are avoided as they lead to aggressive debridement of vital tissues and slow wound healing. Table 42-11 lists products used in modern wound care.

Negative-pressure Wound Therapy. This is primarily used for acute wounds to minimize scarring or for chronic wounds that have been resistant to other forms of wound care. The five mechanisms by which this technology aids wound healing are wound retraction, continuous wound cleaning, stimulation of granulation tissue formation, reduction of interstitial edema, and removal of exudates. The external forces create microdefects in individual cells that stimulate the cellular repair process and lead to cell proliferation within the wound. The negative pressure generated by such devices provides three wound care actions: (1) evacuates wound drainage to reduce bacterial

TABLE 42-10. Selected Interventions for Surgical Site Infection Prevention

Preoperative
Reduce hemoglobin A_{1c} levels to <7% before operation
Stop smoking 30 d before operation (Table 1-4, p. 11)
Administer specialized nutritional supplements or enteral nutrition for severe malnutrition for 7–14 d preoperatively
Adequately treat preoperative infections, such as UTI or cervicitis

Perioperative
Remove interfering hair immediately before surgery by clipping or depilatories; no perioperative shaving
Use an antiseptic surgical scrub or alcohol-based hand antiseptic for preoperative cleansing of the operative team members' hands and forearms
Prepare the skin around the operative site with an antiseptic agent based on chlorhexidine, alcohol, or iodine/iodophors
Administer prophylactic antibiotics for most clean-contaminated, contaminated, and dirty procedures (Table 39-6, p. 835).
Administer prophylactic antibiotics within 1 hr before incision (2 hr for vancomycin and fluoroquinolones)
Use higher dosages of prophylactic antibiotics for morbidly obese patients
Use vancomycin as a prophylactic agent only when there is a significant MRSA infection risk
Provide adequate ventilation, minimize operating room traffic, and clean instruments and surfaces with approved disinfectants
Avoid flash sterilization

Intraoperative
Carefully handle tissue, eradicate dead space, and adhere to standard principles of asepsis
Avoid use of surgical drains unless absolutely necessary
Leave contaminated or dirty-infected wounds open
Redose prophylactic antibiotics with short half-lives intraoperatively if operation is prolonged (for cefazolin if operation is >3 hr) or if there is extensive blood loss (>1500 mL)
Maintain intraoperative normothermia

Postoperative
Maintain serum glucose levels <200 mg/dL on postoperative days 1 and 2
Monitor wound infection

MRSA = methicillin-resistant *Staphylococcus aureus*; SSI = surgical site infection; UTI = urinary tract infection.
Adapted with pemission from Kirby JP, Mazuski JE: Prevention of surgical site infection. Surg Clin North Am 2009 Apr;89(2):365–389.

TABLE 42-11. Wound Care Products

Product	Description
Antifungal cream	Topical cream used as treatment for superficial fungal infections of the periwound skin; contains 2% miconazole nitrate.
Calcium alginate	Calcium alginate is a solid that exchanges calcium ions for sodium ions when it contacts any substance containing sodium such as wound fluid. The resulting sodium alginate is a gel that is nonadhesive, nonocclusive, and conformable to the wound bed. Indicated for moderately or highly draining wounds.
Enzymatic debrider	Topical solution that breaks down necrotic tissue by directly digesting the components of slough or by dissolving the collagen that holds necrotic tissue to the underlying wound bed.
Film	Thin, transparent polyurethane sheets coated on one side with acrylic, hypoallergenic adhesive. The adhesive will not stick to moist surfaces, and the film is impermeable to fluids and bacteria, but semipermeable to oxygen and water vapor. Indicated in superficial wounds with little or no exudate.
Foam	Polyurethane sheets containing open cells capable of holding fluids and pulling them away from the wound bed. Foams provide absorbency while keeping the wound moist. Indicated in moderately or highly draining wounds.
Gauze	Woven or nonwoven cotton or synthetic blends.
Hydrogel	Formulated in sheets or gels. Glycerin-, saline-, or water-based to hydrate the wound. Indicated in dry or minimally draining wounds.
Silver nitrate	Used to treat overgrown granulation tissue. Apply stick to hypergranulation tissue.

Reproduced with permission from Sarsam SE, Elliott JP, Lam GK: Management of wound complications from cesarean delivery. Obstet Gynecol Surv 2005 Jul;60(7):462–473.

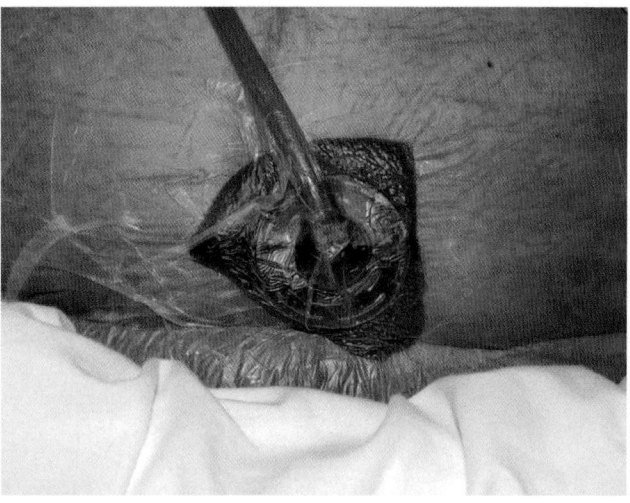

FIGURE 42-3 Wound vacuum in place. Porous synthetic sponge fills the wound. Negative pressure is created by one end of tubing placed within the sponge and the other attached to a suction-generating device. The sponge and wound are covered by an occlusive adhesive dressing, which helps to maintain the suction seal.

colonization, (2) promotes release of cytokines that are helpful in wound healing, and (3) increases blood flow and oxygenation to tissues to uniformly reduce wound size and improve angioneogenesis (Fabian, 2000; Morykwas, 1997; Sullivan, 2009).

The two most commonly used dressings are foam and moistened nonadherent cotton gauze. After the initial application, the dressing is typically changed within 48 hours and then two to three times a week thereafter. After the dressing is covered with an adhesive film dressing, a suction-generating evacuation tube runs through the dressing to help draw excessive exudates away from the wound and into a canister attached at the other end (Fig. 42-3). The vacuum pump offers either continuous or intermittent negative pressure.

Delayed Primary Closure. Approximately 4 days after wound disruption and resolution of subcutaneous infection, a superficial vertical mattress closure with delayed-absorbable suture may be used to reapproximate tissue edges (Wechter, 2005). Depending on wound depth and patient tolerances, this can be completed in the operating room or at the bedside using a local anesthetic complemented by systemic analgesia. Overall, this strategy reduces healing time by 5 to 8 weeks and significantly decreases the number of postoperative visits.

Fascial Dehiscence Treatment

Early recognition of abdominal wall separation is critical in reducing the serious morbidity and mortality rates. Fascial dehiscence is regarded as a surgical emergency, and a gynecologist must first determine if it is associated with evisceration of abdominal content. If abdominal contents are extruded, sterile towels soaked in saline and an outer abdominal binder can be used to cover and gently replace abdominal contents. Broadspectrum antibiotics are generally recommended to minimize ensuing peritonitis.

The final goal of treatment is fascial closure. For critically ill patients with significant edema, temporarily maintaining

anterior abdominal wall integrity with retention sutures until a patient is stable enough to tolerate a definitive operative closure is reasonable. After sufficient debridement of necrotic or infected tissue under general anesthesia, fascial closure may be performed. An interrupted mass closure using a no. 2 permanent suture is typically recommended. However, if primary fascial closure is under significant tension, a synthetic mesh bridge may be required. Typically considered a dirty wound, the subcutaneous layer is often left open. Wet-to-dry dressing changes are performed until the decision is made to proceed with delayed primary closure or allow secondary intention to compete the process (Cliby, 2002).

REFERENCES

Abbas S, Bissett IP, Parry BR: Oral water soluble contrast for the management of adhesive small bowel obstruction. Cochrane Database Syst Rev 3:CD004651, 2007

Abrams P: Bladder outlet obstruction index, bladder contractility index and bladder voiding efficiency: three simple indices to define bladder voiding function. Br J Urol Int 84:14, 1999

Adrogué HJ, Madias NE: Hypernatremia. N Engl J Med 342(20):1493, 2000

Akarsu T, Karaman S, Akercan F, et al: Preemptive meloxicam for postoperative pain relief after abdominal hysterectomy. Clin Exp Obstet Gynecol 31:133, 2004

Al-Sunaidi M, Tulandi T: Adhesion-related bowel obstruction after hysterectomy for benign conditions. Obstet Gynecol 108:1162, 2006

Al-Took S, Platt R, Tulandi T: Adhesion-related small-bowel obstruction after gynecologic operations. Am J Obstet Gynecol 180:313, 1999

American Geriatrics Society: Postoperative delirium in older adults: best practice statement from the American Geriatrics Society. J Am Coll Surg 220(2): 136, 2015

American Psychiatric Association: Diagnostic and Statistical Manual of Mental Disorders, Fifth Edition. Arlington, American Psychiatric Association, 2013

American Thoracic Society: Guidelines for the management of adults with hospital-acquired, ventilator-associated, and healthcare-associated pneumonia. Am J Respir Crit Care Med 171:388, 2005

Anderson AD, McNaught CE, MacFie J, et al: Randomized clinical trial of multimodal optimization and standard perioperative surgical care. Br J Surg 90:1497, 2003

Apfel CC, Korttila K, Abdalla M, et al: A factorial trial of six interventions for the prevention of postoperative nausea and vomiting. N Engl J Med 350:2441, 2004

Apfelbaum JL, Chen C, Mehta SS, et al: Postoperative pain experience: results from a national survey suggest postoperative pain continues to be undermanaged. Anesth Analg 97:534, 2003

Arozullah AM, Daley J, Henderson WG, et al: Multifactorial risk index for predicting postoperative respiratory failure in men after major noncardiac surgery. The National Veterans Administration Surgical Quality Improvement Program. Ann Surg 232:242, 2000

Assalia A, Schein M, Kopelman D, et al: Therapeutic effect of oral Gastrografin in adhesive, partial small-bowel obstruction: a prospective, randomized trial. Surgery 115:433, 1994

Badillo AT, Sarani B, Evans SR: Optimizing the use of blood cultures in the febrile postoperative patient. J Am Coll Surg 194:477, 2002

Badner NH, Knill RL, Brown JE, et al: Myocardial infarction after noncardiac surgery. Anesthesiology 88(3):572, 1998

Bartlett LC: Pressure necrosis is the primary cause of wound dehiscence. Can J Surg 28:27, 1985

Bennett LL, Rosenblum RS, Perlov C, et al: An in vivo comparison of topical agents on wound repair. Plast Reconstr Surg 108:675, 2001

Bilotta F, Lauretta MP, Borozdina A: Postoperative delirium: risk factors, diagnosis, and perioperative care. Minerva Anestesiol 79(9):1066, 2013

Blevins LS Jr, Wand GS: Diabetes insipidus. Crit Care Med 20(1):69, 1992

Bodker B, Lose G: Postoperative urinary retention in gynecologic patients. Int Urogynecol J 14:94, 2003

Braga M, Gianotti L, Gentilini O, et al: Feeding the gut early after digestive surgery: results of a nine-year experience. Clin Nutr 21:59, 2002

Calligaro KD, Azurin DJ, Dougherty MJ, et al: Pulmonary risk factors of elective abdominal aortic surgery. J Vasc Surg 18:914, 1993

Canet J, Ricos M, Vidal F: Early postoperative arterial oxygen desaturation. Determining factors and response to oxygen therapy. Anesth Analg 69(2):207, 1989

Carlson MA: Acute wound failure. Surg Clin North Am 77:607, 1997

Chan A, Dore CJ, Ramachandra V: Analgesia for day surgery: evaluation of the effect of diclofenac given before or after surgery with or without bupivacaine infiltration. Anaesthesia 51:592, 1996

Charlson ME, MacKenzie CR, Gold JP, et al: Intraoperative blood pressure. What patterns identify patients at risk for postoperative complications? Ann Surg 212(5):567, 1990

Cliby WA: Abdominal incision wound breakdown. Clin Obstet Gynecol 45:507, 2002

Cohen SH, Gerding DN, Johnson S, et al: Clinical practice guidelines for *Clostridium difficile* infection in adults: 2010 update by the Society for Healthcare Epidemiology of America (SHEA) and the Infectious Diseases Society of America (IDSA). Infect Control Hosp Epidemiol 31(5):431, 2010

Condon RE, Frantzides CT, Cowles VE, et al: Resolution of postoperative ileus in humans. Ann Surg 203:574, 1986

Correia MI, da Silva RG: The impact of early nutrition on metabolic response and postoperative ileus. Curr Opin Clin Nutr Metab Care 7:577, 2004

Dauchel J, Schang JC, Kachelhoffer J, et al: Gastrointestinal myoelectrical activity during the postoperative period in man. Digestion 14:293, 1976

de Jonghe A, van Munster BC, van Oosten HE, et al: The effects of melatonin versus placebo on delirium in hip fracture patients: study protocol of a randomised, placebo-controlled, double blind trial. BMC Geriatr 11:34, 2011

de la Torre SH, Mandel L, Goff BA: Evaluation of postoperative fever: usefulness and cost-effectiveness of routine workup. Am J Obstet Gynecol 188:1642, 2003

Elwyn DH, Bryan-Brown CW, Shoemaker WC: Nutritional aspects of body water dislocations in postoperative and depleted patients. Ann Surg 182:76, 1975

Ertas IE, Gungorduk K, Ozdemir A, et al: Influence of gum chewing on postoperative bowel activity after complete staging surgery for gynecological malignancies: a randomized controlled trial. Gynecol Oncol 131(1):118, 2013

Fabian TS, Kaufman HJ, Lett ED, et al: The evaluation of subatmospheric pressure and hyperbaric oxygen in ischemic full-thickness wound healing. Am J Surg 66:1136, 2000

Ferrer M, Liapikou A, Valencia M, et al: Validation of the American Thoracic Society—Infectious Diseases Society of America guidelines for hospital-acquired pneumonia in the intensive care unit. Clin Infect Dis 50(7):945, 2010

Food and Drug Administration: FDA drug safety communication: prescription acetaminophen products to be limited to 325 mg per dosage unit; boxed warning will highlight potential for severe liver failure. Silver Springs, U.S. Food and Drug Administration, 2011

Ganai S, Lee KF, Merrill A, et al: Adverse outcomes of geriatric patients undergoing abdominal surgery who are at high risk for delirium. Arch Surg 142(11):1072, 2007

Garibaldi RA, Brodine S, Matsumiya S, et al: Evidence for the non-infectious etiology of early postoperative fever. Infect Contr 6:273, 1985

George RB, Allen TK, Habib AS: Serotonin receptor antagonists for the prevention and treatment of pruritus, nausea, and vomiting in women undergoing cesarean delivery with intrathecal morphine: a systematic review and meta-analysis. Anesth Analg 109(1):174, 2009

Gottlieb RH, Widjaja J, Tian L, et al: Calf sonography for detecting deep venous thrombosis in symptomatic patients: experience and review of the literature. J Clin Ultrasound 27:415, 1999

Griffith CA: The family of Ringer's solutions. NITA 9(6):480, 1986

Güldner A, Pelosi P, de Abreu MG: Nonventilatory strategies to prevent postoperative pulmonary complications. Curr Opin Anaesthesiol 26(2):141, 2013

Habib AS, Gan TJ: Evidence-based management of postoperative nausea and vomiting: a review. Can J Anaesth 51:326, 2004

Hall JC, Tarala RA, Hall JL, et al: A multivariate analysis of the risk of pulmonary complications after laparotomy. Chest 99:923, 1991

Hemmes SN, Serpa Neto A, Schultz MJ: Intraoperative ventilatory strategies to prevent postoperative pulmonary complications: a meta-analysis. Curr Opin Anaesthesiol 26(2):126, 2013

Hodges KR, Davis BR, Swaim LS: Prevention and management of hysterectomy complications. Clin Obstet Gynecol 57(1):43, 2014

Holzer P: Opioids and opioid receptors in the enteric nervous system: from a problem in opioid analgesia to a possible new prokinetic therapy in humans. Neurosci Lett 361:192, 2004

Houman Fekrazad M, Lopes RD, Stashenko GJ, et al: Treatment of venous thromboembolism: guidelines translated for the clinician. J Thromb Thrombolysis 28(3):270, 2009

Huge A, Kreis ME, Zittel TT, et al: Postoperative colonic motility and tone in patients after colorectal surgery. Dis Colon Rectum 43:932, 2000

Inouye SK, Kosar CM, Tommet D, et al: The CAM-S: development and validation of a new scoring system for delirium severity in 2 cohorts. Ann Intern Med 160(8):526, 2014

Inouye SK, van Dyck CH, Alessi CA, et al: Clarifying confusion: the confusion assessment method. A new method for detection of delirium. Ann Intern Med 113(12):941, 1990

Jeffery KM, Harkins B, Cresci GA, et al: The clear liquid diet is no longer a necessity in the routine postoperative management of surgical patients. Am Surg 62:167, 1996

Jernigan AM, Chen CC, Sewell C: A randomized trial of chewing gum to prevent postoperative ileus after laparotomy for benign gynecologic surgery. Int J Gynaecol Obstet 127(3):279, 2014

Johnson RG, Arozullah AM, Neumayer L, et al: Multivariable predictors of postoperative respiratory failure after general and vascular surgery: results from the Patient Safety in Surgery study. J Am Coll Surg 204(6):1188, 2007

Joshi GP, Ogunnaike BO: Consequences of inadequate postoperative pain relief and chronic persistent postoperative pain. Anesthesiol Clin North Am 23:21, 2005

Kearon C, Akl EA, Comerota AJ, et al: Antithrombotic therapy and prevention of thrombosis, 9th ed: American College of Chest Physicians evidence based clinical practice guidelines. Chest 141:e419S, 2012

Keita H, Diouf E, Tubach F, et al: Predictive factors of early postoperative urinary retention in the postanesthesia care unit. Anesth Analg 101:592, 2005

Khalili G, Janghorbani M, Saryazdi H, et al: Effect of preemptive and preventive acetaminophen on postoperative pain score: a randomized, double-blind trial of patients undergoing lower extremity surgery. J Clin Anesth 25(3):188, 2013

Kinney JM, Weissman C: Forms of malnutrition in stressed and unstressed patients. Clin Chest Med 7:19, 1986

Kirby JP, Mazuski JE: Prevention of surgical site infection. Surg Clin North Am 89(2):365, 2009

Kleeman S, Goldwasser S, Vassallo B, et al: Predicting postoperative voiding efficiency after operation for incontinence and prolapse. Am J Obstet Gynecol 187:49, 2002

Kozlow JH, Berenholtz SM, Garrett E, et al: Epidemiology and impact of aspiration pneumonia in patients undergoing surgery in Maryland, 1999–2000. Crit Care Med 31:1930, 2003

Krebs HB, Goplerud DR: Mechanical intestinal obstruction in patients with gynecologic disease: a review of 368 patients. Am J Obstet Gynecol 157:577, 1987

Krstic S, Resanovic V, Alempijevic T, et al: Hartmann's procedure vs loop colostomy in the treatment of obstructive rectosigmoid cancer. World J Emerg Surg 9(1):52, 2014

Kruse JA, Carlson RW: Rapid correction of hypokalemia using concentrated intravenous potassium chloride infusions. Arch Intern Med 150(3):613, 1990

Kudsk KA, Croce MA, Fabian TC, et al: Enteral versus parenteral feeding: effects on septic morbidity after blunt and penetrating abdominal trauma. Ann Surg 215:503, 1992

Lau H, Lam B: Management of postoperative urinary retention: a randomized trial of in-out versus overnight catheterization. Aust N Z J Surg 74(8):658, 2004

Lewis SJ, Egger M, Sylvester PA, et al: Early enteral feeding versus "nil by mouth" after gastrointestinal surgery: systematic review and meta-analysis of controlled trials. BMJ 323:773, 2001

Li J, Chen J, Kirsner R: Pathophysiology of acute wound healing. Clin Dermatol 25(1):9, 2007

Li S, Liu Y, Peng Q, et al: Chewing gum reduces postoperative ileus following abdominal surgery: a meta-analysis of 17 randomized controlled trials. J Gastroenterol Hepatol 28(7):1122, 2013

Litell JM, Gong MN, Talmor D, et al: Acute lung injury: prevention may be the best medicine. Respir Care 56(10):1546, 2011

Livingston EH, Passaro EP Jr: Postoperative ileus. Dig Dis Sci 35:121, 1990

Lundquist H, Hedenstierna G, Strandberg A, et al: CT assessment of dependent lung densities in man during general anaesthesia. Acta Radiol 36:626, 1995

Mangano DT, Browner WS, Hollenberg M, et al: Association of perioperative myocardial ischemia with cardiac morbidity and mortality in men undergoing noncardiac surgery. The Study of Perioperative Ischemia Research Group. N Engl J Med 23(26):1781, 1990

Mangram AJ, Horan TC, Pearson ML, et al: Guideline for prevention of surgical site infection, 1999. Centers for Disease Control and Prevention (CDC) Hospital Infection Control Practices Advisory Committee. Am J Infect Control 27(2):97, 1999

Marino PL, Sutin KM (eds): The ICU Book. Philadelphia, Lippincott Williams & Wilkins, 2007, p 1065

Mavros MN, Velmahos GC, Falagas ME: Atelectasis as a cause of postoperative fever: where is the clinical evidence? Chest 140(2):418, 2011

Mayo ME, Lloyd-Davies RW, Shuttleworth KE, et al: The damaged human detrusor: functional and electron microscopic changes in disease. Br J Urol 45:116, 1973

McIntosh CA, Macario A: Managing quality in an anesthesia department. Curr Opin Anaesthesiol 22(2):223, 2009

Megibow AJ, Balthazar EJ, Cho KC, et al: Bowel obstruction: evaluation with CT. Radiology 180:313, 1991

Mixter CG III, Meeker LD, Gavin TJ: Preemptive pain control in patients having laparoscopic hernia repair: a comparison of ketorolac and ibuprofen. Arch Surg 133:432, 1998

Møller AM, Villebro N, Pedersen T, et al: Effect of preoperative smoking intervention on postoperative complications: a randomised clinical trial. Lancet 359:114, 2002

Monk BJ, Berman ML, Montz FJ: Adhesions after extensive gynecologic surgery: clinical significance, etiology, and prevention. Am J Obstet Gynecol 170:1396, 1994

Moore FA, Feliciano DV, Andrassy RJ, et al: Early enteral feeding, compared with parenteral, reduces postoperative septic complications: the results of a meta-analysis. Ann Surg 216:172, 1992

Morykwas MJ, Argenta LC, Shelton-Brown EI, et al: Vacuum-assisted closure: a new method for wound control and treatment: animal studies and basic foundation. Ann Plastic Surg 38:553, 1997

Muir AD, Reeder MK, Foëx P, et al: Preoperative silent myocardial ischaemia: incidence and predictors in a general surgical population. Br J Anaesth 67(4): 373, 1991

Nagler EV, Vanmassenhove J, van der Veer SN, et al: Diagnosis and treatment of hyponatremia: a systematic review of clinical practice guidelines and consensus statements. BMC Med 12:1, 2014

Nehra V: Fluid electrolyte and nutritional problems in the postoperative period. Clin Obstet Gynecol 45:537, 2002

Nelson R, Edwards S, Tse B: Prophylactic nasogastric decompression after abdominal surgery. Cochrane Database Syst Rev 3:CD004929, 2007

Nunley JC, FitzHarris GP: Postoperative ileus. Curr Surg 61:341, 2004

Ono H, Taguchi T, Kido Y, et al: The usefulness of bright light therapy for patients after oesophagectomy. Intensive Crit Care Nurs 27(3):158, 2011

O'Toole EA, Goel M, Woodley DT: Hydrogen peroxide inhibits human keratinocyte migration. Dermatol Surg 22:525, 1996

Owen J, Andrews WW: Wound complications after cesarean sections. Clin Obstet Gynecol 37:842, 1994

Palmer BF: Managing hyperkalemia caused by inhibitors of the renin-angiotensin-aldosterone system. N Engl J Med 351(6):585, 2004

Perazella MA: Drug-induced hyperkalemia: old culprits and new offenders. Am J Med 109(4):307, 2000

Platell C, Hall JC: Atelectasis after abdominal surgery. J Am Coll Surg 185: 584, 1997

Prough DS, Bidani A: Hyperchloremic metabolic acidosis is a predictable consequence of intraoperative infusion of 0.9% saline. Anesthesiology 90(5): 1247, 1999

Riou JP, Cohen JR, Johnson H Jr: Factors influencing wound dehiscence. Am J Surg 163:324, 1992

Sanders RD, Pandharipande PP, Davidson AJ, et al: Anticipating and managing postoperative delirium and cognitive decline in adults. BMJ 343:d4331, 2011

Santoso JT, Ulm MA, Jennings PW, et al: Multimodal pain control is associated with reduced hospital stay following open abdominal hysterectomy. Eur J Obstet Gynecol Reprod Biol 183: 48, 2014

Sarsam SE, Elliott JP, Lam GK: Management of wound complications from cesarean delivery. Obstet Gynecol Surv 60:462, 2005

Schaefer TJ, Wolford RW: Disorders of potassium. Emerg Med Clin North Am 23(3):723, 2005

Schey D, Salom EM, Papadia A, et al: Extensive fever workup produces low yield in determining infectious etiology. Am J Obstet Gynecol 192:1729, 2005

Seidner DL: Nutritional issues in the surgical patient. Cleve Clin J Med 73:S77, 2006

Stanton SL, Cardozo LD, Kerr-Wilson R: Treatment of delayed onset of spontaneous voiding after surgery for incontinence. Urology 13:494, 1979

Steele A, Gowrishankar M, Abrahamson S, et al: Postoperative hyponatremia despite near-isotonic saline infusion: a phenomenon of desalination. Ann Intern Med 126(1):20, 1997

Stein PD, Terrin ML, Hales CA, et al: Clinical, laboratory, roentgenographic, and electrocardiographic findings in patients with acute pulmonary embolism and no pre-existing cardiac or pulmonary disease. Chest 100(3):598, 1991

Sullivan N, Snyder DL, Tipton K, et al: Negative pressure wound therapy device. Technology assessment report. ECRI Institute. 2009. Available at: http://archive.ahrq.gov/research/findings/ta/negative-pressure-wound-therapy./ Accessed January 3, 2015

Tablan OC, Anderson LJ, Besser R, et al: Guidelines for preventing healthcare—associated pneumonia, 2003: Recommendations of CDC and the Healthcare Infection Control Practices Advisory Committee. MMWR 53:1, 2004

Tache Y, Martinez V, Million M, et al: Stress and the gastrointestinal tract: III. Stress-related alterations of gut motor function: role of brain corticotropin-releasing factor receptors. Am J Physiol Gastrointest Liver Physiol 280:G173, 2001

Tammela T, Kontturi M, Lukkarinen O: Postoperative urinary retention: I. Incidence and predisposing factors. Scand J Urol Nephrol 20:197, 1986

Taylor G, Herrick T, Mah M: Wound infections after hysterectomy: opportunities for practice improvement. Am J Infect Control 26:254, 1998

Tinker JH, Tarhan S: Discontinuing anticoagulant therapy in surgical patients with cardiac valve prostheses: observations in 180 operations. JAMA 239:738, 1978

Verbalis JG, Goldsmith SR, Greenberg A, et al: Diagnosis, evaluation, and treatment of hyponatremia: expert panel recommendations. Am J Med 126(10 Suppl 1):S1, 2013

Warner DO: Preventing postoperative pulmonary complications: the role of the anesthesiologist. Anesthesiology 92:1467, 2000

Wechter ME, Pearlman MD, Hartmann KE: Reclosure of the disrupted laparotomy wound: a systematic review. Obstet Gynecol 106:376, 2005

Wells PS, Hirsh J, Anderson DR, et al: Accuracy of clinical assessment of deep-vein thrombosis. Lancet 345:1326, 1995

Whang R, Flink EB, Dyckner T, et al: Magnesium depletion as a cause of refractory potassium repletion. Arch Intern Med 145(9):1686, 1985

Worsley DF, Alavi A, Aronchick JM, et al: Chest radiographic findings in patients with acute pulmonary embolism: observations from the PIOPED Study. Radiology 189(1):133, 1993

Wortel CH, van Deventer SJ, Aarden LA, et al: Interleukin-6 mediates host defense responses induced by abdominal surgery. Surgery 114:564, 1993

Wright HK, O'Brien JJ, Tilson MD: Water absorption in experimental closed segment obstruction of the ileum in man. Am J Surg 121:96, 1971

Zimmerman J, Fromm R, Meyer D, et al: Diagnostic marker cooperative study for the diagnosis of myocardial infarction. Circulation 99(13):1671, 1999

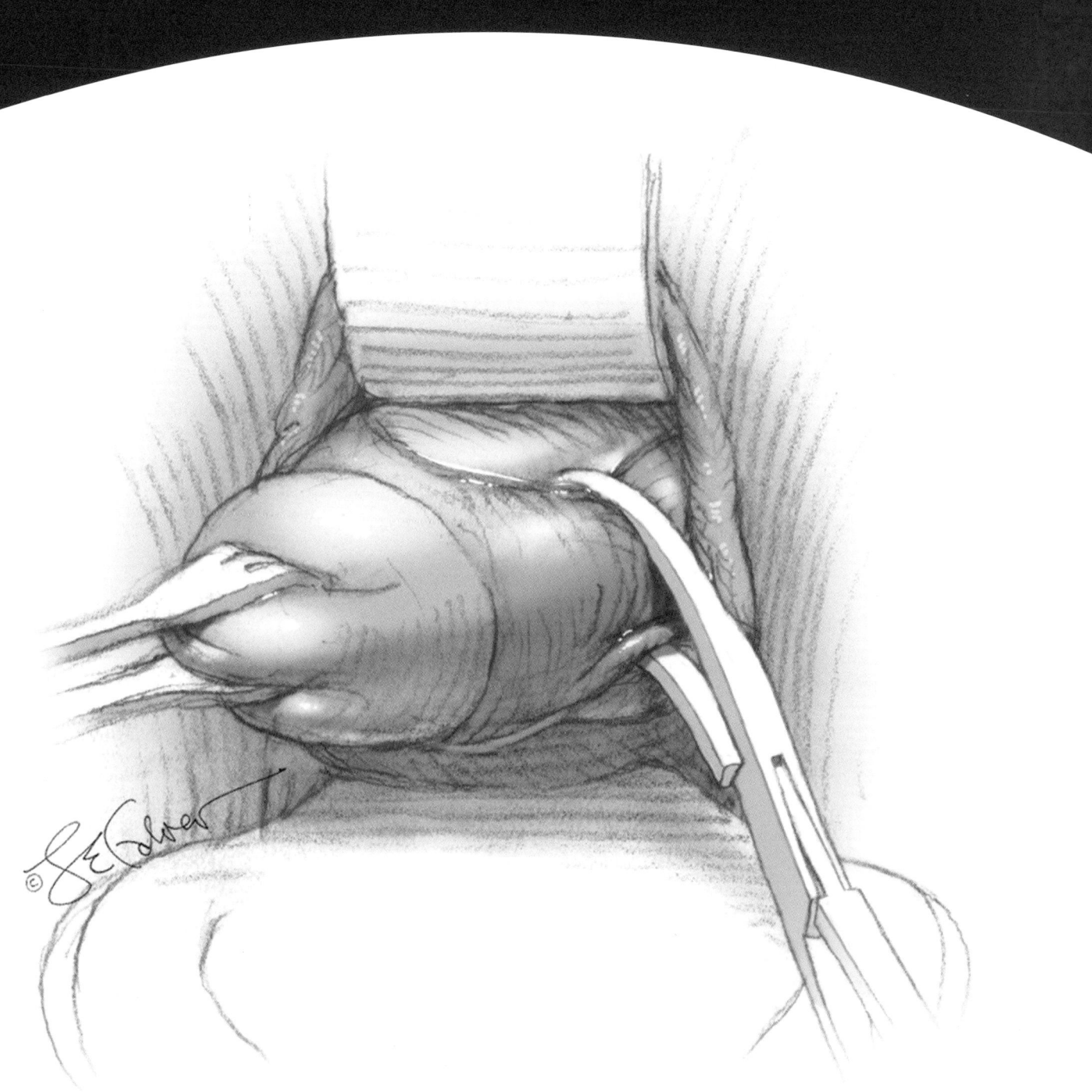

CHAPTER 43

Surgeries for Benign Gynecologic Disorders

43-1

Midline Vertical Incision

Abdominal entry is the first step for many gynecologic surgeries. Either vertical or transverse incisions may be used, and each offers particular advantages. Vertical incisions may be midline or paramedian, but of the two, the midline is chosen more often. This incision offers quick entry, minimal blood loss, superior access to the upper abdomen, generous operating room, and the flexibility for easy wound extension if greater space or access is needed. No important neurovascular structures traverse this incision. Thus, it may be favored for patients using anticoagulation agents. Despite advantages, midline incisions are more frequently associated with greater postoperative pain, poorer cosmetic results, and increased risks of wound dehiscence or incisional hernia compared with low transverse incisions. Last, for those with prior laparotomy, the incision type is typically repeated for subsequent surgeries.

PREOPERATIVE

▪ Consent

For abdominal entry, patients are informed of wound infection or dehiscence risks. Additionally, the chance of bowel or bladder injury is present with any abdominal entry, especially when extensive adhesions are encountered.

▪ Prophylaxis

Laparotomy per se does not require antibiotic prophylaxis or bowel preparation. These are dictated by the planned procedure. Prevention for venous thromboembolism is warranted, and options are described in Chapter 39 (p. 835).

INTRAOPERATIVE

Surgical Steps

❶ Anesthesia and Patient Positioning. After administration of adequate regional or general anesthesia, the patient is positioned supine. If needed, hair in the path of the planned incision is clipped; a Foley catheter is placed; and abdominal preparation is completed.

❷ Skin and Subcutaneous Layer. The skin is incised vertically in the midline beginning 2 to 3 cm above the symphysis pubis and extending cephalad to within 2 cm of the umbilicus. If less space is required, this incision may be shortened. For greater space or access, the incision may arch around the umbilicus and then continue cephalad in the upper abdominal midline. This extension passes to the left of the umbilicus to avert transection of the ligamentum teres. This remnant of the umbilical vein courses in the free border of the falciform ligament. The umbilicus itself contains attenuated fascia. Thus, the periumbilical incision should arch laterally enough to provide quality fascia on either side of the incision to allow an ultimately secure closure.

The subcutaneous layers of Camper and Scarpa are then incised either sharply with long even strokes or with electrosurgical blade to reach the linea alba fascia. Ideally, the number of blade strokes is minimized to avoid hatch marking the tissue, which increases tissue damage and wound infection risks.

❸ Fascia. Tendinous fibers from the anterior abdominal wall aponeuroses merge in the midline of the abdomen to form the linea alba. This fascia layer is sharply entered near the midpoint of the incision (Fig. 43-1.1). This incision is extended first cephalad and then caudally to mirror the length of the skin incision. To minimize injury to viscera during this extension, the linea alba is elevated by index fingers of the surgeon and assistant or by the open tips of a pean clamp (Fig. 43-1.2).

Once the fascia is incised, the right and left rectus abdominis muscle bellies are bluntly separated laterally. Inferiorly, sharp incision may be required to complete this. To avert injury to organs below, the rectus muscles are elevated during this division. Each half of the pyramidalis muscle lies atop its respective rectus belly, and this muscle is similarly divided sharply at the midline.

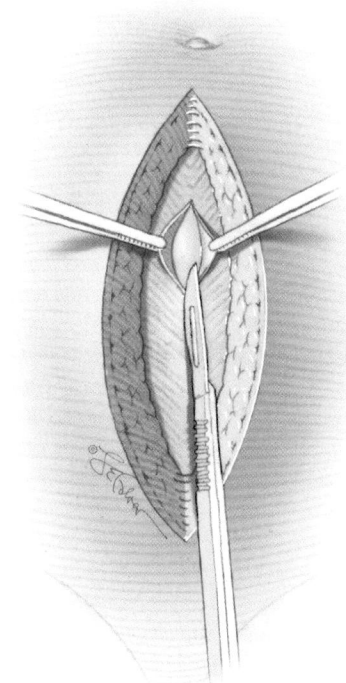

FIGURE 43-1.1 Fascial incision.

❹ Peritoneum. For entry, the peritoneum is identified between the rectus abdominis muscle bellies. It is grasped with two hemostats in the upper portion of the incision to avoid cystotomy. The interposed peritoneum should be palpated or visually examined to exclude intervening viscera. Only then is it sharply cut (Fig. 43-1.3). Next, an index finger sweeps directly beneath it to identify adhered bowel or omentum. If free, the peritoneum is elevated by fingers of the surgeon and assistant to protect viscera beneath. As the incision is extended cephalad above the arcuate line, the transverse fibers of the posterior rectus sheath are seen and are cut along with the peritoneum. As the incision is extended caudally, the transversalis fascia is found superficial to the peritoneum. To prevent bladder dome injury, this thin fascia layer is elevated by insinuating fingers beneath it and is cut, with the incision extending caudally. Next, the peritoneum beneath the transversalis fascia is similarly incised (Fig. 43-1.4). The bladder dome is identified by increasing tissue vascularity and thickness. Of note, the urachus, which is the remnant of the allantois, may be seen as a white cord extending from the bladder dome toward the umbilicus in the midline.

During abdominal entry, prior surgery may blur clear tissue planes. For example, the true midline may be deviated laterally, and after fascial incision, only rectus fibers may be seen. To find the midline after incising the fascia, fibers of the pyramidalis muscles can

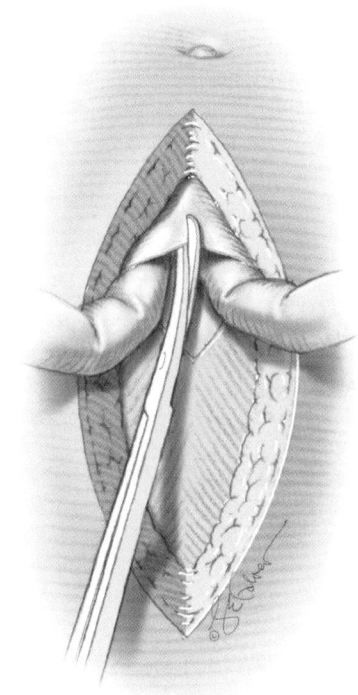

FIGURE 43-1.2 Fascial incision extended cephalad.

be followed as they angle toward the midline. Also, visually recreating a line between the symphysis and umbilicus can aid orientation. To reach the midline, the fascia closest to the presumed midline is grasped both

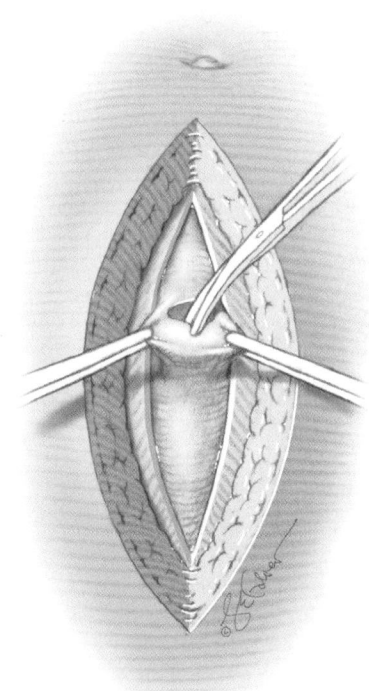

FIGURE 43-1.3 Peritoneal incision.

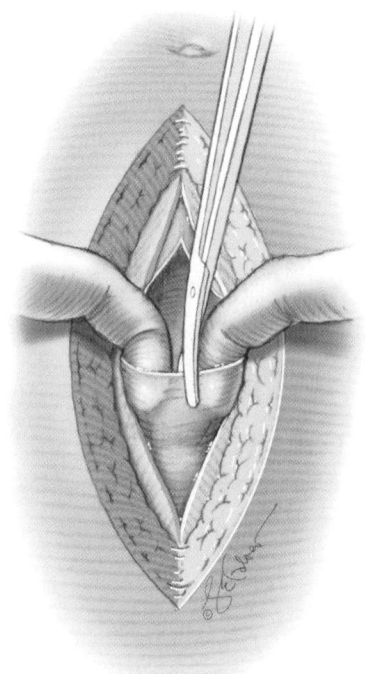

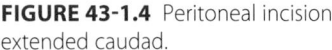

FIGURE 43-1.4 Peritoneal incision extended caudad.

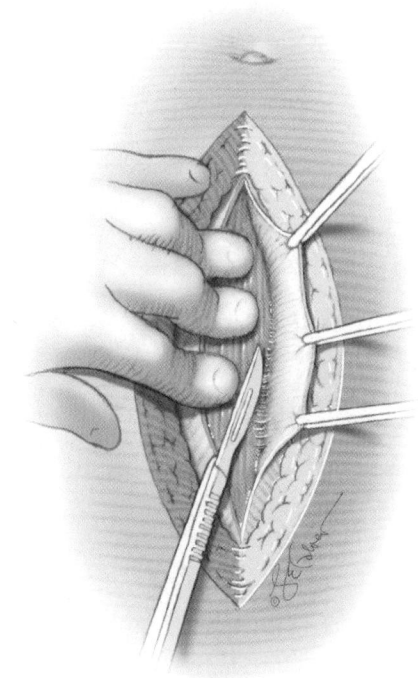

FIGURE 43-1.5 Lateral subfascial dissection.

cephalad and caudad along its length with Kocher clamps to create upward tension (Fig. 43-1.5). Simultaneously, downward manual pressure atop the ipsilateral rectus belly accentuates fibers between the fascia and underlying rectus belly. These fibers are then cut to permit lateral dissection of the fascia away from the rectus belly. This is continued laterally until the midline is identified. If the midline is not identified after some dissection on one side, the same steps can be repeated on opposite side.

Also with prior surgery, planes between the fascia, peritoneum, and viscera may be poorly defined. In these cases, a gradual layered entry is required to avoid organ injury. One technique uses Metzenbaum scissors. Scissor tips are insinuated between tissue layers such that the tips are seen each time prior to cutting. This minimizes the risk that the thicker bowel or bladder wall will be cut. If adhesions are found, they are divided. Dissection is maintained close to the fascial or peritoneal edge to minimize visceral injury.

❺ Operative Field. After abdominal entry, a self-retaining retractor is commonly placed to retract the bowel, omentum, and abdominal wall muscles. Moist laparotomy sponges are placed around the bulk of bowel and gently directed cephalad. Adhesiolysis may be required to adequately free intestines for this repositioning. Upper blades of the retractor assist in holding these loops up and away from the pelvis and operating field. The shortest blades possible are preferred for lateral

retraction. This reduces the risk of femoral or genitofemoral nerve compression by a blade resting atop the psoas major muscle. Once pelvic organs are adequately exposed, the planned abdominal surgery can proceed.

❻ Wound Closure. Closure of the visceral or parietal peritoneum is not required and is individualized (Chap. 40, p. 847). Starting from each end of the incision, the fascia is closed to its midpoint using a continuous running suture with a 0-gauge delayed-absorbable suture. These sutures are then tied together. If the subcutaneous layer measures less than 2 cm, then no closure is typically necessary. For deeper wounds, interrupted stitches of 2-0 to 4-0 gauge absorbable or delayed-absorbable suture are used to close this layer. The skin is closed with a subcuticular stitch using 4-0 gauge delayed-absorbable suture, staples, or other suitable method (Chap. 40, p. 847).

POSTOPERATIVE

For most gynecologic surgeries, recovery from the abdominal incision constitutes the greatest portion of postsurgical healing. Midline incisions lead to significant pain during ambulation, coughing, and deep breathing. As a result, women undergoing laparotomy are at greater risk of postoperative thrombotic and pulmonary complications. Prevention of these is warranted and described in Chapter 42 (p. 911). In addition, return of normal bowel function is commonly slowed, and signs of ileus should be monitored. Hospitalization typically varies from 1 to 3 days, and return of normal bowel function usually dictates this course. Postoperative activity in general can be individualized, although vigorous abdominal exercise is delayed for 6 weeks to allow for fascial healing. Driving can be resumed when pain does not limit the ability to brake quickly and when narcotic medications are not in use. Return to work is variable, although 6 weeks is commonly cited.

43-2

Pfannenstiel Incision

The Pfannenstiel, Cherney, and Maylard incisions are transverse abdominal incisions used for gynecologic procedures. Of these, the Pfannenstiel incision is the most commonly used incision for laparotomy in the United States. Because the transverse incision follows Langer lines of skin tension, excellent cosmetic results can be achieved. Additionally, decreased rates of postoperative pain, fascial wound dehiscence, and incisional hernia are noted. Use of the Pfannenstiel incision, however, is often discouraged for cases in which greater operating space or upper abdominal access is anticipated. Last, because of the layers created by incision of the internal and external oblique aponeuroses, purulent fluid can collect between these. Therefore, cases involving abscess or peritonitis favor use of a midline incision, which divides the fused linea alba.

PREOPERATIVE

Consent

General risks associated with transverse laparotomy incisions are similar to those for vertical incisions. Transverse incisions, however, carry risk of injury to the iliohypogastric and ilioinguinal nerves. These injuries frequently involve only transient sensory loss but rarely may lead to debilitating, chronic neuropathic pain.

INTRAOPERATIVE

Surgical Steps

❶ **Anesthesia and Patient Positioning.** After administration of adequate regional or general anesthesia, the patient is positioned supine. If needed, hair in the path of the planned incision is clipped; a Foley catheter is placed; and abdominal preparation is completed.

❷ **Skin and Subcutaneous Layer.** Two to 3 cm above the symphysis pubis, an 8- to 10-cm transverse incision is made with its lateral margins arching slightly cephalad. If less space is required, this length can be shortened. The incision is deepened sharply with scalpel or electrosurgical blade until the anterior rectus sheath is reached. The superficial epigastric vessels typically lie several centimeters from the midline and halfway between the skin and fascia. Coagulation of these vessels will limit incisional blood loss.

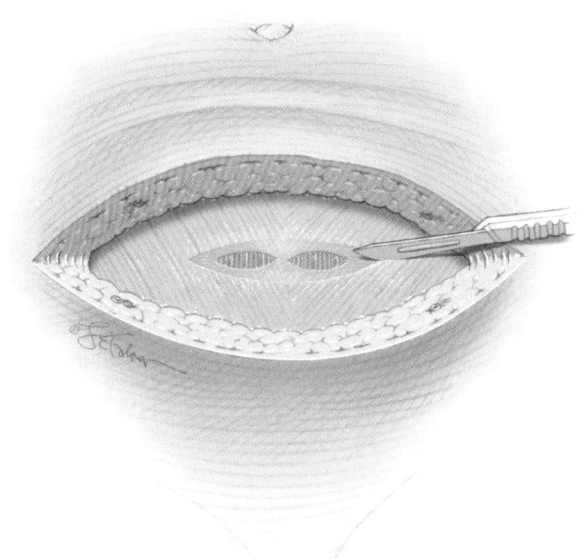

FIGURE 43-2.1 Fascial incision.

❸ **Fascia.** The anterior rectus sheath is sharply incised transversely in the midline (Fig. 43-2.1). At the level of the incision, the anterior rectus sheath is composed of two visible layers, the aponeuroses from the external oblique muscle and a fused layer containing aponeuroses of the internal oblique and transversus abdominis muscles. Lateral extension of the anterior rectus sheath incision requires cutting each layer individually (Fig. 43-2.2). This permits identification and ideally, avoidance of the iliohypogastric and ilioinguinal nerves as they run between these two fascial layers.

Of note, at the level of the incision, the inferior epigastric vessels typically lie outside the lateral border of the rectus abdominis muscle and beneath the fused aponeuroses of the internal oblique and transversus abdominis muscles. Thus, lengthening the incision farther laterally may cut these vessels. If significant lateral extension is required, these

vessels are identified, clamped, and ligated. This prevents bleeding and vessel retraction with later hemorrhage. In addition, risk of iliohypogastric and ilioinguinal nerve injury also increases as the incision is carried lateral to the rectus abdominis muscle borders (Rahn, 2010).

The superior edge of the fascial incision is grasped with a Kocher clamp on either side of the midline. Traction is directed cephalad and slightly outward. In the area superior to the initial incision, the anterior rectus sheath is then bluntly or sharply separated from the underlying rectus abdominis muscle (Fig. 43-2.3). With blunt dissection, upward facing fingers first push cephalad and then roll to direct pressure laterally. The fascia separates easily from the bellies of the rectus muscle, but it may be densely adhered along the midline and require sharp dissection (Fig. 43-2.4). Several small perforating nerves and vessels traverse the space between

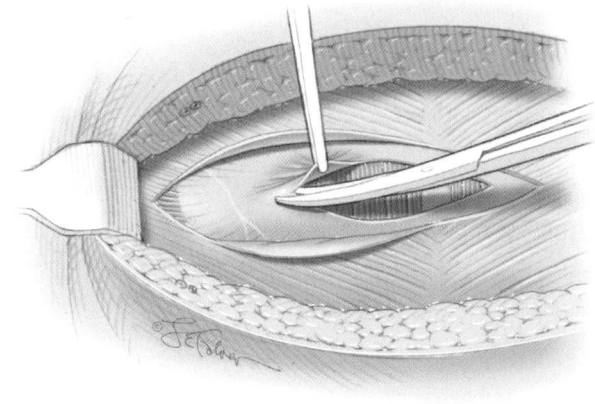

FIGURE 43-2.2 Incision extended laterally.

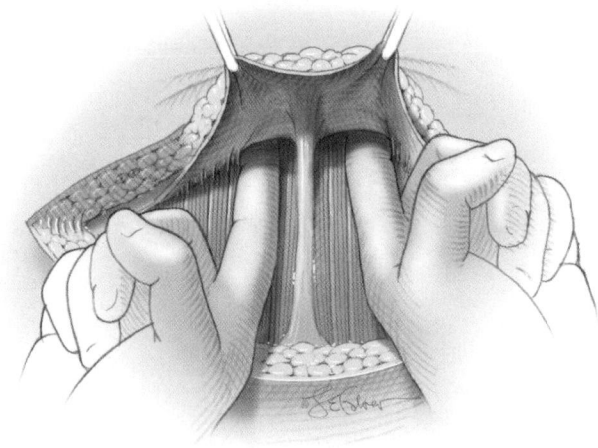

FIGURE 43-2.3 Blunt separation of anterior rectus sheath from underlying rectus abdominis muscle.

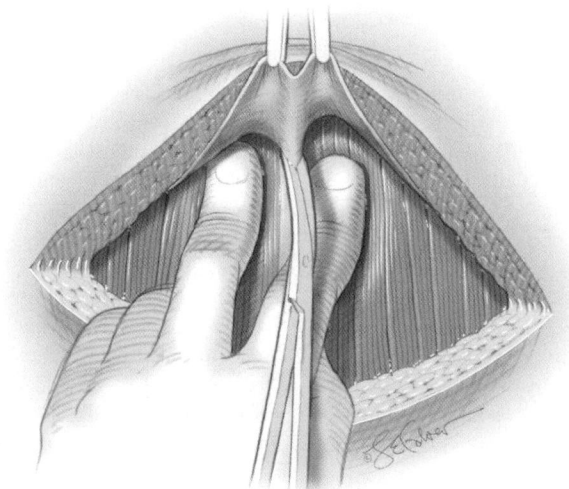

FIGURE 43-2.4 Sharp separation in the midline.

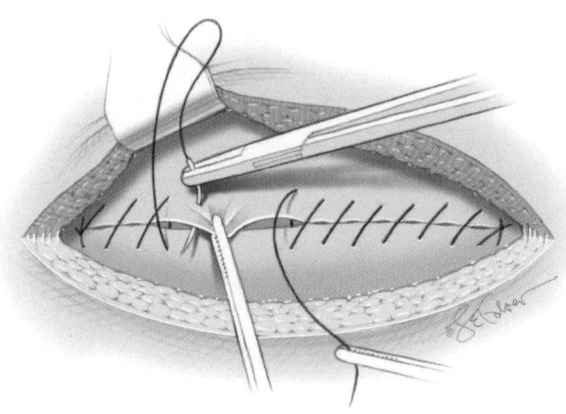

FIGURE 43-2.5 Fascial closure.

the anterior rectus sheath and rectus muscle. These vessels are coagulated to avoid laceration and bleeding. Upon completion of this dissection, a semicircular area with a radius of 6 to 8 cm has been created. A similar separation is performed in the area inferior to the initial fascial incision.

The rectus abdominis muscle bellies are then separated laterally from the midline either bluntly or sharply. The pyramidalis muscle, located superficial to the rectus muscle, usually requires sharp division at the midline.

❹ **Peritoneum.** Peritoneal entry is fully described and illustrated in Section 43-1, Steps 3 and 4 (p. 927). To summarize, upon separation of the rectus muscle bellies, the thin, filmy peritoneum is identified, grasped with two hemostats, and sharply incised. The peritoneal incision is then extended superiorly and inferiorly. Once the abdominal cavity has been entered and clear visualization established, the surgeon can proceed with the planned operation.

❺ **Wound Closure.** Closure of the visceral or parietal peritoneum is not required and is individualized. Starting from each end of the incision, the fascia is closed to its midpoint using a continuous running suture line with a 0-gauge delayed-absorbable suture (Fig. 43-2.5). These strands are then tied together. The subcutaneous layer and skin are closed similar to the midline vertical incision (Section 43-1, p. 928).

POSTOPERATIVE

The postoperative course for low transverse incisions follows that described for midline incisions (p. 928).

43-3
Cherney Incision

The Cherney incision is a transverse abdominal incision that is similar to the Pfannenstiel incision in its early steps. After the anterior rectus sheath is opened, however, the tendons of the rectus abdominis and pyramidalis muscles are transected 1 to 2 cm above their insertion into the symphysis pubis. These muscles are then lifted cephalad to provide access to the peritoneum. At this level, the inferior epigastric vessels run well lateral to the rectus bellies and typically are spared. However, if additional lateral extension is required, these vessels are ligated and transected.

This incision offers generous operating space and access to the space of Retzius. Thus, it may be a primary choice when these requirements are anticipated. Additionally, Pfannenstiel incisions may be converted to Cherney incisions when an unexpected need for additional space arises.

PREOPERATIVE

Preparation and consenting prior to Cherney incision are similar to that for Pfannenstiel incision (p. 929).

INTRAOPERATIVE

Surgical Steps

❶ **Initial Steps.** The initial steps mirror that of the Pfannenstiel incision (Steps 1-3, p. 929). Thus, the skin is incised transversely beginning 2 to 3 cm above the symphysis, the fascia is divided transversely, and the rectus sheath is dissected off the rectus abdominis muscle bellies. After these steps, however, the techniques diverge.

❷ **Fascia.** The fascial opening reveals the rectus abdominis and pyramidalis muscles. Cephalad to the symphysis pubis, fingers are insinuated beneath the rectus muscle tendons. This blunt dissection begins laterally and extends toward the midline. During insinuation, fingers exert pressure dorsally and against the bladder to protect it during tendon division. After this, fingers lift up the muscle tendons, which are then transected 1 to 2 cm above the symphysis pubis (Fig. 43-3.1). The muscles are flipped up and cephalad.

The peritoneum is grasped with two hemostats at a level above the bladder dome and is sharply incised. This incision is extended laterally. Once the abdominal cavity

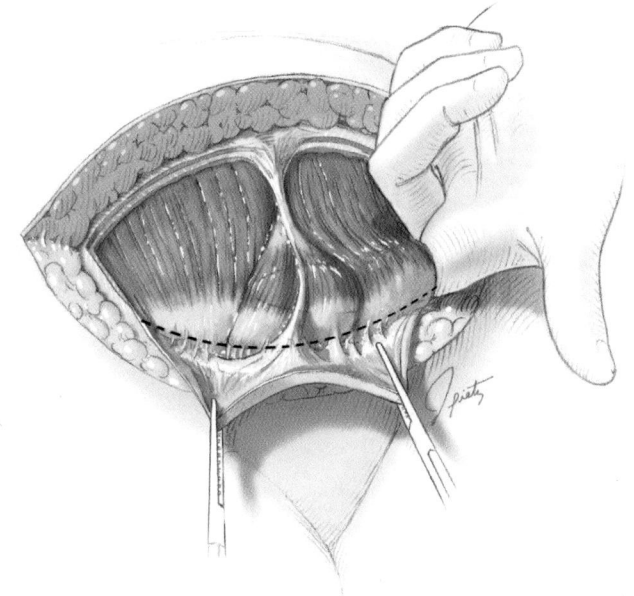

FIGURE 43-3.1 Tendon transection.

has been accessed, the planned surgery can proceed. Importantly, the risk of injury, particularly to the femoral and genitofemoral nerves, is increased when self-retaining retractors are used with this generally wider incision. This is also true for the Maylard incision. Thus, lateral retractor blades should fit just under the edges of the incision and not rest atop the psoas muscle.

❸ **Wound Closure.** During wound closure, the cut ends of the rectus muscle tendons are affixed with interrupted sutures of 0-gauge delayed-absorbable sutures to the undersurface of the inferior fascial edge (Fig. 43-3.2). To avoid osteitis pubis or

osteomyelitis, the tendons should not be affixed directly to the symphysis pubis.

Starting from each end of the incision, the fascia is closed to its midpoint using a continuous running suture with a 0-gauge delayed-absorbable suture. These strands are then tied together. The subcutaneous layer and skin are closed as with the midline vertical incision (p. 928).

POSTOPERATIVE

The postoperative course for low transverse incisions follows that described for midline incisions (p. 928).

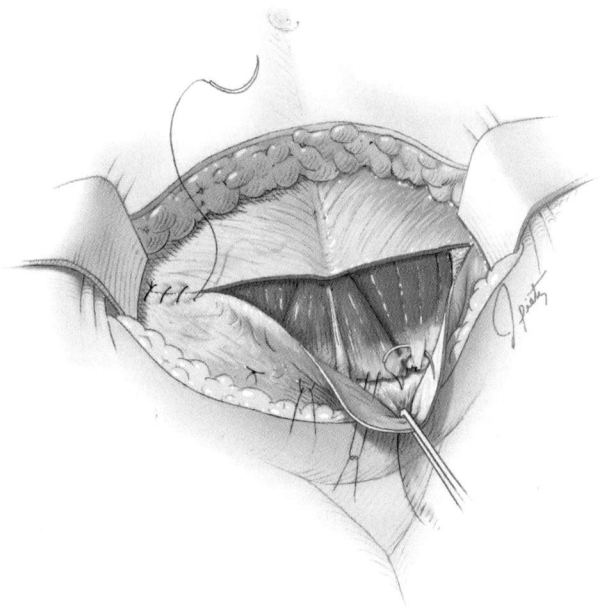

FIGURE 43-3.2 Wound closure.

43-4

Maylard Incision

The Maylard incision differs mainly from the Pfannenstiel incision in that the rectus sheath is not dissected away from the rectus abdominis muscle and that the bellies of the rectus abdominis muscle are transected. Transection affords extensive access to the pelvis. However, it is technically more difficult due to its required isolation and ligation of the inferior epigastric vessels. Moreover, the Maylard incision has been used infrequently because of concerns regarding greater postoperative pain, decreased abdominal wall strength, longer operating times, and increased febrile morbidity. Randomized studies, however, have not supported these concerns (Ghanbari, 2009; Mathai, 2013). The Maylard incision should be avoided in those patients in whom the superior epigastric vessels have been interrupted, as this leaves the rectus abdominis muscles with inadequate blood supply. Also, patients with significant peripheral vascular disease may rely on the inferior epigastric vessels for collateral blood supply to their lower extremities (Salom, 2007).

PREOPERATIVE

Preparation and consenting prior to Maylard incision are similar to that for Pfannenstiel incision (p. 929).

INTRAOPERATIVE

Surgical Steps

❶ **Initial Steps.** The initial steps mirror that of the Pfannenstiel incision (Steps 1 and 2, p. 929). Thus, the skin is incised transversely beginning 2 to 3 cm above the symphysis, and the fascia is divided transversely. After these steps, the techniques diverge, and in contrast to the Pfannenstiel incision, the anterior rectus sheath is not dissected away from the underlying rectus muscle.

The inferior epigastric vessels lie posterolateral to the rectus abdominis muscle bellies. Bilaterally, these vessels are identified, ligated, and transected. This step avoids their laceration and hemorrhage when the rectus abdominis muscle is transected.

❷ **Rectus Abdominis Muscle.** With fingers, the rectus abdominis muscle is bluntly dissected away from the underlying transversalis fascia and peritoneum. These latter are the encountered layers because the posterior

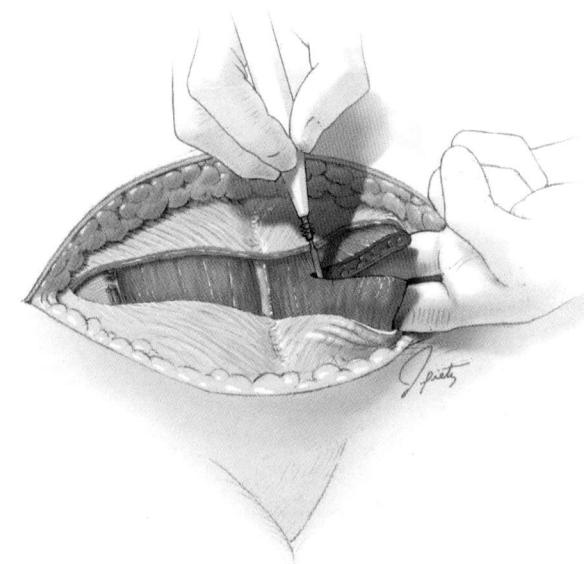

FIGURE 43-4.1 Rectus abdominis muscle transection.

rectus sheath ends at the arcuate line and is absent caudal to this line. The surgeon's fingers are slid behind the rectus muscle bellies, and this muscle is then transected using an electrosurgical blade (Fig. 43-4.1).

❸ **Peritoneum.** With two hemostats, the peritoneum is grasped, and it is sharply incised above the level of the bladder dome. This incision is then extended laterally (Fig. 43-4.2). After access is obtained to the abdominal cavity, planned surgery can proceed. As with Cherney incisions, careful self-retaining retractor placement is necessary to lessen the risk of femoral or genitofemoral nerve injury.

❹ **Wound Closure.** At incision closure, the fascia is closed with a running stitch using 0-gauge delayed-absorbable suture. Closing the fascia adequately reapproximates the transected muscle fibers, and therefore the divided muscle bellies are not directly sutured together. Starting from each end of the incision, the fascia is closed to its midpoint using a continuous running suture line with a 0-gauge delayed-absorbable suture. These strands are then tied together. The subcutaneous layer and skin are closed as with the midline vertical incision (p. 928).

POSTOPERATIVE

The postoperative course for low transverse incisions follows that described for midline incisions (p. 928).

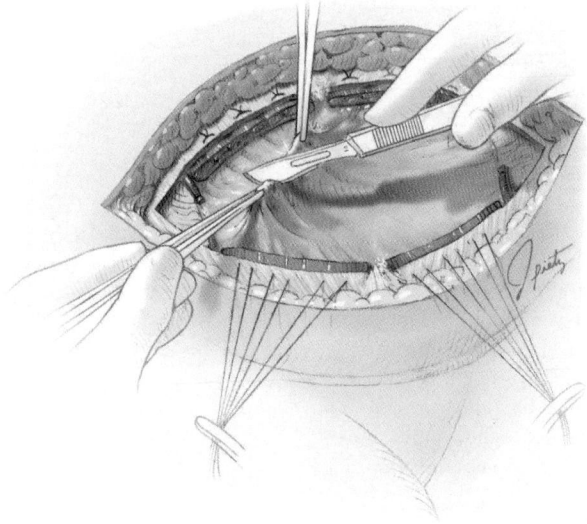

FIGURE 43-4.2 Suture placement through rectus abdominis muscle and fascia, and also peritoneal incision.

43-5

Ovarian Cystectomy

Ovarian cyst excision is typically prompted by patient symptoms or by ovarian qualities that suggest a lower concern for ovarian malignancy (Chap. 9, p. 215). Removal of the cyst alone can offer those with ovarian pathology an opportunity to preserve hormonal function and reproductive capacity. Accordingly, ovarian cystectomy goals include gentle tissue handling to limit postoperative adhesions and reconstruction of normal ovarian anatomy to aid the later transfer of ova to the fallopian tube.

In some women, a cystectomy may be performed laparoscopically rather than with laparotomy. Several studies support the safe and effective use of laparoscopy for this purpose (Chap. 9, p. 216). That said, there are settings in which its role is limited. In general, if a cyst is large, adhesive disease limits access and mobility, or the risk of malignancy is greater, then laparotomy is preferred.

PREOPERATIVE

Consent

In addition to general surgical risks of laparotomy, the major risk of cystectomy is extensive bleeding from or injury to the ovary that, in turn, necessitates removal of the entire ovary. Also, a variable degree of ovarian reserve may be lost with ovarian cystectomy. If ovarian cancer is suspected prior to surgery, patients should be educated regarding the possibility of surgical staging, including the need for hysterectomy and removal of both ovaries (Chap. 35, p. 748).

Many patients undergoing cystectomy for ovarian pathology have associated pain. Although in most cases cystectomy will be curative, in other instances, pain may persist despite cyst excision. This is especially true in those with coexistent endometriosis. Thus, patients are counseled that cystectomy may not relieve chronic pain in all cases.

Patient Preparation

Bowel preparation and antibiotics are typically not required preoperatively. If hysterectomy is required during ovarian staging, antibiotics may be given intraoperatively. Laparotomy dictates venous thromboembolism prophylaxis, and options are found in Table 39-8 (p. 836).

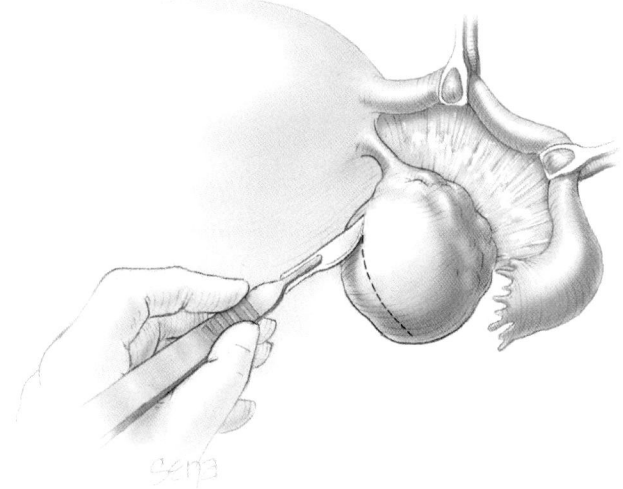

FIGURE 43-5.1 Ovarian incision.

INTRAOPERATIVE

Surgical Steps

❶ Anesthesia and Patient Positioning. Because of the potential for cancer staging in the upper abdomen if malignancy is found, general anesthesia is typically indicated for this inpatient procedure. The patient is supine. After anesthesia induction, hair in the planned incision path is clipped if needed; a Foley catheter is inserted; and abdominal preparation is completed. Because hysterectomy may be needed if malignancy is found, the vagina is also surgically prepared.

❷ Abdominal Entry. Most ovarian cysts can be removed through a Pfannenstiel incision. Extremely large cysts or those with a greater concern for malignancy usually require a vertical incision. This latter incision provides generous operating space and adequate upper abdomen access for cancer staging.

As described in Chapter 35 (p. 748), cell washings from the pelvis and upper abdomen are collected prior to ovarian manipulation and are saved if a cancer is found. The upper abdomen and pelvis are explored, and excrescences or suspicious areas are sampled and sent for intraoperative frozen-section analysis.

A self-retaining retractor is placed within the incision, and the bowel and omentum are packed from the operating field. The ovary is brought into view, and moist laparotomy sponges are placed in the cul-de-sac and beneath the ovary. This helps to minimize contamination of the pelvis if the cyst ruptures during excision.

❸ Ovarian Incision. The ovary is held between the surgeon's thumb and opposing fingers. The ovarian capsule that overlies the

dome of the cyst is then cut with either scalpel or electrosurgical needle tip. This incision is ideally placed on the antimesenteric surface of the ovary to minimize dissection into vessels at the ovarian hilum. The incision is ideally deepened to reach the cyst wall without entering and rupturing the cyst (Fig. 43-5.1). Allis clamps are then placed on the incised edges of the ovarian capsule to aid traction and countertraction during dissection.

❹ Cyst Dissection. Blunt dissection with fingertip or knife handle or sharp dissection with Metzenbaum scissor tips is used to develop the cleavage plane between the cyst wall and the remaining ovarian stroma (Fig. 43-5.2). If adhesions obliterate the cleavage plane, sharp dissection is preferred. As an assistant gently pulls the Allis clamps in a direction away from the cyst wall, the surgeon places fingers proximate to the advancing cleavage plane and pulls the cyst in the direction opposite the Allis clamps. Such traction and countertraction across the cleavage plane aid dissection. Because the surface of the cyst wall is often smooth and slippery, the surgeon may place an unfolded thin gauze sponge between fingers and the cyst wall to afford a better grip.

As dissection approaches completion, the highly vascular ovarian hilum is reached. If possible, a hemostat or pean clamp is placed across the small remaining tissue bridge between the cyst and normal ovary. The clamp is positioned closer to the ovary to allow space for scissors to cut the tissue pedicle and free the cyst without rupture. The pedicle is suture ligated with a fine absorbable suture. The ovarian bed is then examined, and bleeding points are coagulated or ligated.

❺ Cyst Excision. Once the cyst is removed, it may be sent to the pathology department for intraoperative frozen-section

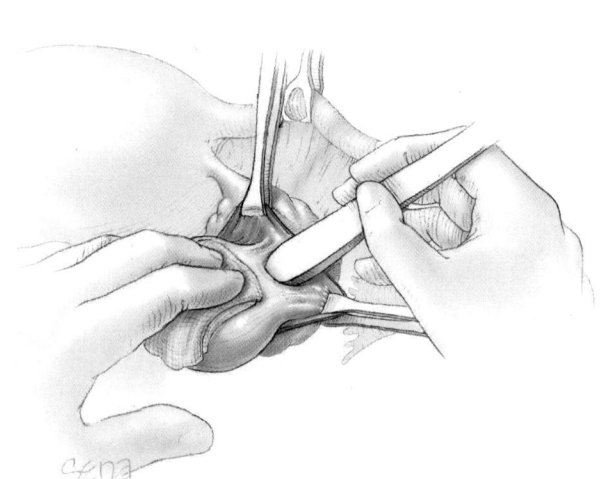

FIGURE 43-5.2 Cyst dissection.

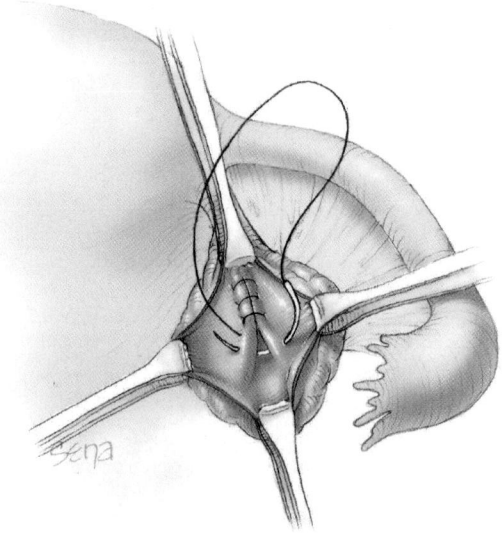

FIGURE 43-5.3 Ovarian closure.

analysis. In benign cases, excess capsule can be sharply trimmed from ovaries in which large cysts have stretched and thinned the ovarian surface. This excision is performed to help restore normal ovarian anatomy. But because ovarian follicles are contained within even extremely thinned capsules, this tissue is preserved whenever possible.

❻ Ovarian Closure. The ovarian bed is then closed in layers using 3-0 or 4-0 gauge delayed-absorbable suture. These sutures reapproximate the ovarian tissue that previously surrounded the cyst on both sides (Fig. 43-5.3). With a thinned ovarian cortex, the needle tip should not be driven through the capsule. Exposed suture on the ovarian surface may increase adhesion formation. The ovarian incision is closed with a running subcortical stitch (similar to subcuticular stitch) using 5-0 gauge delayed-absorbable suture.

❼ Incision Closure. Laparotomy sponges are removed from the cul-de-sac, and the pelvis is copiously irrigated with an isotonic solution such as lactated Ringer solution. Irrigation assumes an even greater importance with ovarian cyst rupture. For example, spill from a mature cystic teratoma (dermoid), if neglected, may induce a chemical peritonitis. Depending on the surgeon's preference and the patient's anatomy, an adhesion barrier may be placed around the ovary (Chap. 11, p. 261). The remaining packs and retractor are removed, and the abdominal incision is closed.

POSTOPERATIVE

After surgery, patient care in general follows that described for laparotomy (p. 928).

43-6

Salpingo-oophorectomy

Removal of the ovary and fallopian tube is more commonly performed by laparoscopy. However, laparotomy is typically indicated if the potential for malignancy is great, if the ovary is larger than 8 to 10 cm, or if extensive adhesions are anticipated. With either approach, the essential steps of salpingo-oophorectomy (SO) are: preventive identification of the ipsilateral ureter, infundibulopelvic (IP) ligament ligation, combined ligation of the proximal fallopian tube and uteroovarian ligament, and transection of the intervening mesovarium and mesosalpinx. Indications are varied and include suspicion for ovarian malignancy, ovarian cancer prevention for at-risk women, large symptomatic ovarian cysts in postreproductive females, and for reproductive-aged women, large, symptomatic ovarian cysts that are not suitable for cystectomy.

PREOPERATIVE

Patient Evaluation

This surgery is typically performed to remove ovarian pathology that has been evaluated sonographically. If anatomy is unclear, magnetic resonance (MR) imaging may add information. As listed in Chapters 35 and 36 (pp. 742 and 761), tumor markers are selectively drawn prior to surgery if malignancy is suspected.

Consent

In general, serious complications with SO are infrequent but include organ injury, especially to the ureter; hemorrhage; wound infection or dehiscence; and anesthesia complications. Ovarian pathology is the most common indication for SO. Thus, the possibility of cancer staging and a description of its steps are explained. Moreover, malignant cyst rupture and spillage are risks, and patients are informed that this will advance the cancer stage (Chap. 35, p. 748). Many women undergoing SO for ovarian pathology have associated pain. Although removal of the ovary in most cases will be curative, in other instances, pain may persist despite SO. Last, if performed bilaterally, SO dramatically curtails estrogen production. Thus, a preoperative discussion of consequences, as outlined on page 951, is recommended.

Patient Preparation

Bowel preparation and antibiotics are typically not required preoperatively. If hysterectomy is required during ovarian staging, antibiotics may be given intraoperatively. Laparotomy dictates venous thromboembolism prophylaxis, and options are found in Table 39-8 (p. 836).

INTRAOPERATIVE

Surgical Steps

❶ **Anesthesia and Patient Positioning.** Salpingo-oophorectomy performed via laparotomy typically requires general anesthesia to allow staging of the upper abdomen if malignancy is found. The patient is supine. After anesthesia induction, hair in the planned incision path is clipped if needed; a Foley catheter is inserted; and abdominal preparation is completed. Because of a possible need for hysterectomy if malignancy is found, the vagina is also surgically prepared.

❷ **Abdominal Entry.** Either a transverse or vertical incision may be used for SO. Clinical factors such as ovarian size and risk of malignancy influence this selection, as discussed on page 926.

Following abdominal entry, cell washings from the pelvis and upper abdomen are collected prior to ovarian manipulation. These are sent for pathologic evaluation if cancer is found. The upper abdomen and pelvis are explored. Peritoneal or omental implants are sampled and sent for intraoperative frozen-section analysis.

❸ **Exposure.** A self-retaining retractor such as an O'Connor O'Sullivan or Balfour retractor is placed, and the bowel is packed from the operating field. The affected adnexa is grasped and elevated from the pelvis. If extensive adhesions are found, normal anatomic relationships are restored.

❹ **Ureter Location.** Because of its close proximity to the IP ligament, the ureter is identified prior to clamp placement. In many instances, the ureter is seen beneath the posterior pelvic sidewall peritoneum. Here, it can often be identified as it enters the pelvis and crosses over the common iliac artery bifurcation just medial to the ovarian vessels. In other cases, retroperitoneal isolation of the ureter is required. For this, the peritoneum within the area bounded by the round and IP ligaments and the external iliac vessels is tented with tissue forceps and incised. This first peritoneal incision is extended cephalad toward the pelvic brim (Fig. 43-6.1). The incision also later assists in isolating the IP ligament for ligation. Once this peritoneal window is open, blunt dissection is directed deep, cephalad, and slightly medially through gauzy areolar connective tissue (see Step 6 of abdominal hysterectomy, p. 952). The ureter is typically found attached to the medial leaf of the incised peritoneum.

❺ **Infundibulopelvic Ligament.** The adnexa is lifted from the pelvis and inspected. To isolate the IP ligament, a second peritoneal opening is sharply created with Metzenbaum scissors or electrosurgical blade. It is made in the posterior leaf of the broad ligament below the IP ligament but above the ureter.

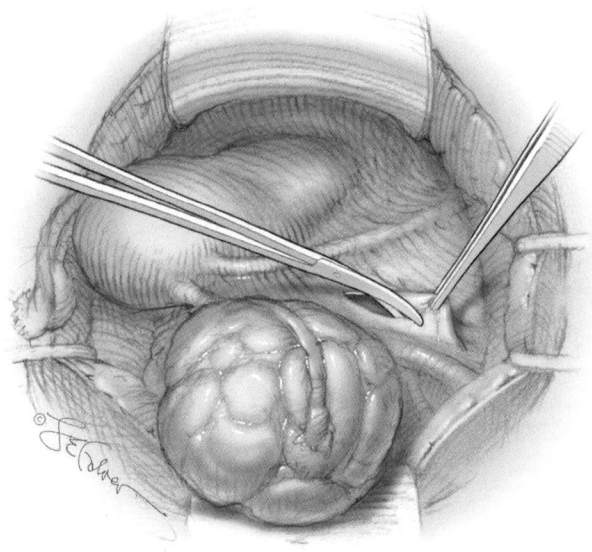

FIGURE 43-6.1 Retroperitoneal entry.

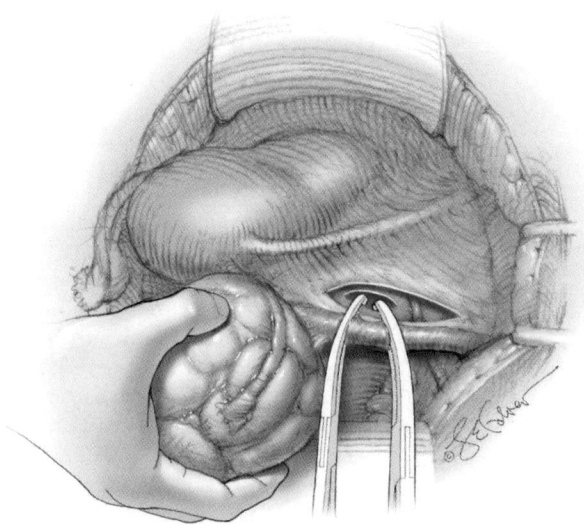

FIGURE 43-6.2 Infundibulopelvic ligament ligation.

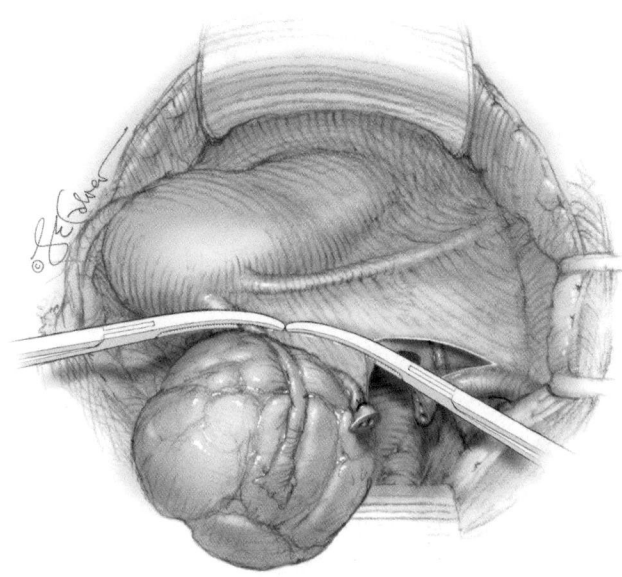

FIGURE 43-6.3 Ligation of uteroovarian ligament, fallopian tube ligation, and proximal adjacent mesovarium and mesosalpinx.

This incision is extended medially beneath the fallopian tube and uteroovarian ligament and toward the uterus. While remaining parallel to the IP ligament, it is also extended lateral and cephalad towards the pelvic brim. Ideally, the ureter is in view during this entire incision.

As a result of both peritoneal incisions, the IP ligament is isolated. This vascular ligament is then clamped with a Heaney or other sturdy clamp, and the clamp curve faces upward (Fig. 43-6.2). Of note, if SO is performed for cancer risk reduction, the clamp is brought across the IP close to the sidewall. A single Kelly (pean) clamp is placed across the IP at a distance medial to the Heaney clamp. During completion of adnexectomy, this medial clamp prevents "back-bleeding" and is removed with the specimen.

As shown, the ligament is transected between the Heaney and Kelly clamps. To ligate the IP pedicle, a free tie of 0-gauge delayed-absorbable suture is placed around the Heaney clamp. As the knot is secured,

this clamp is opened and closed quickly, that is, "flashed." Next, a transfixing suture is placed around the Heaney clamp (Fig. 40-22, p. 853). This suture is placed below the clamp yet distal to the first free tie to avoid hematoma formation by needle puncture of ovarian vessels. As this knot is cinched in place, the Heaney clamp is removed.

❻ **Fallopian Tube and Uteroovarian Ligament.** With the adnexa elevated, a Heaney or similar clamp is placed across both the proximal uteroovarian ligament and fallopian tube. It also incorporates some of the mesosalpinx and mesovarium. The clamp's curve faces the ovary. Next, another clamp enters laterally and is directed medially to close around the remaining mesosalpinx and mesovarium beneath the ovary (Fig. 43-6.3). Again, the clamp curve faces the ovary. Ideally, the tips of both clamps touch beneath the adnexa. Above both of these clamps are stacked second clamps, which lie a distance above their partners and closer to the ovary.

Tissue between the stacked clamps is cut with curved Mayo scissors to free the adnexa.

The freed adnexa is removed from the operative site and sent to pathology for evaluation. If malignancy is suspected, an intraoperative frozen section is requested. Tissue within each of the remaining two clamps is individually suture ligated with 0-gauge delayed-absorbable suture.

❼ **Wound Closure.** The retractor and packing sponges are removed from the abdomen. The abdominal incision is then closed as described for vertical or Pfannenstiel incisions (pp. 928 and 930).

POSTOPERATIVE

Patient recovery is similar to that described for laparotomy (p. 928). In reproductive-aged women, if only one ovary is removed, hormonal and reproductive function is preserved. However, if both are excised, then surgical menopause follows, and hormone replacement is considered (Chap. 22, p. 494).

Interval Partial Salpingectomy

Interval partial salpingectomy is similar to puerperal midsegment salpingectomy and differs mainly in procedure timing and in abdominal entry. In contrast to postpartum or postabortal sterilization, the term *interval* designates performance unrelated in time to pregnancy. Accordingly, for most women undergoing interval sterilization, the uterus is small and lies within the confines of the pelvis. Thus, fallopian tubes are reached either laparoscopically or through a low transverse incision.

In general with interval partial salpingectomy, a midtubal segment of fallopian tube is excised, and the severed ends seal by fibrosis and reperitonealization. Commonly used methods of interval sterilization include the Parkland and Pomeroy techniques.

Of tubal sterilization methods, interval partial salpingectomy is infrequently selected for U.S. women who elect sterilization (Peterson, 1996). More commonly, laparoscopic techniques are employed, mainly because of laparoscopy's postsurgical advantages (Chap. 41, p. 874). Accordingly, interval partial salpingectomy is typically selected for cases in which laparoscopy may not be indicated. Examples include cases complicated by extensive adhesions, those in which other concurrent pelvic pathology dictates laparotomy, or those in which laparoscopic equipment or surgical skills are lacking. Moreover, new recommendations advocate for risk reducing total salpingectomy when feasible as described on page 939. Thus, the opportunities for laparotomic interval salpingectomy may be few.

PREOPERATIVE

Patient Evaluation

As with any sterilization procedure, pregnancy should be excluded prior to the procedure by means of either urine or serum β-human chorionic gonadotropin (hCG) testing. Similarly, to limit the possibility of an early, undetected luteal-phase conceptus, sterilization is ideally performed during the follicular phase of the menstrual cycle, and an effective contraceptive method is used until surgery.

Consent

Partial salpingectomy is an effective method of sterilization. Pregnancy rates of less than 2 percent are typical. Failures may result from tubal recanalization or technical errors, such as ligation of the wrong structure.

Tubal sterilization is a safe surgical procedure, and complication rates are below 2 percent (Pati, 2000). Of these, anesthesia complications, organ injury, and wound infection are the most frequent. In addition, although pregnancy is uncommon following sterilization, when pregnancy does occur, the risk of ectopic pregnancy is high and approximates 30 percent (Peterson, 1996; Ryder, 1999). However, because tubal sterilization is highly effective contraception, the overall risk of pregnancy is low, and therefore also is the risk of ectopic pregnancy.

Aside from physical risks, some women experience regret following sterilization. Rates are highest in those 30 years or younger (Curtis, 2006; Hillis, 1999). Accordingly, prior to surgery women are counseled regarding the risk of regret, the permanence of the procedure, and alternative effective long-term contraceptive methods (American College of Obstetricians and Gynecologists, 2011).

INTRAOPERATIVE

Surgical Steps

❶ **Anesthesia and Patient Positioning.** Interval partial salpingectomy is usually an outpatient procedure, performed under general or regional anesthesia. Following administration of anesthesia, the patient is placed supine, the abdomen surgically prepared, and the bladder drained.

❷ **Minilaparotomy.** For most patients, a 4- to 6-cm transverse Pfannenstiel incision is sufficient. Small Richardson or army-navy retractors provide adequate intraabdominal visualization in most cases. A vaginally placed sponge stick or uterine manipulator can elevate the uterus to help bring fallopian tubes into view.

❸ **Tubal Identification.** A common reason for sterilization failure is ligation of the wrong structure, usually the round ligament. Identification and isolation of the fallopian tube prior to ligation and submission of tubal segments for pathologic confirmation is therefore required. In some cases, especially those with associated tubal adhesions, this step may be challenging. Lateral extension of the incision may be needed for improved exposure.

Initially, the uterine fundus is identified. At the cornu, insertion of the fallopian tube lies posterior to that of the round ligament, and this orientation can initially guide the surgeon to the correct structure. A primary Babcock clamp is used to elevate the fallopian tube proximally, while a second clamp grasps the tube more distally. The primary clamp is then moved again and is placed distal to the second. The second is then removed and again placed distal to the first. In this manner, the surgeon "marches" down the length of the tube to reach the ampulla and identify fimbria.

❹ **Parkland Method.** At the midpoint of the fallopian tube, an avascular space in the mesosalpinx is identified, and a hemostat is placed directly beneath the tube. The selected site should allow excision of a 2-cm tubal segment that does not incorporate the fimbria. Ligation of the fimbrial portion leads to a greater risk of tubal recanalization and higher failure rates.

The hemostat is bluntly advanced through the mesosalpinx as counterpressure is applied with the index finger. Once advanced through the defect, the hemostat tips are gently opened to expand the aperture (Fig. 43-7.1). The end of a 0-gauge chromic free tie is placed in the tip of the hemostat and pulled through the opening. This is repeated, bringing another tie through the rent. The midsegment is lifted, and the distal suture tied. The second tie is then secured around the proximal fallopian tube.

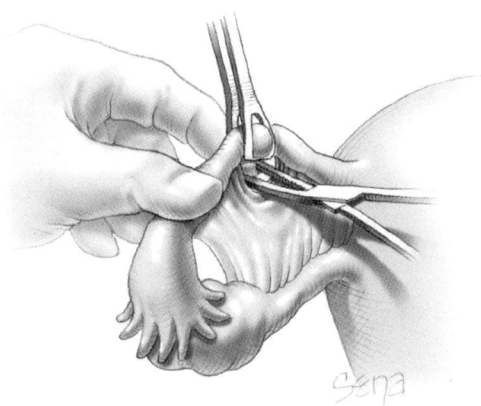

FIGURE 43-7.1 Parkland method: mesosalpinx opening created.

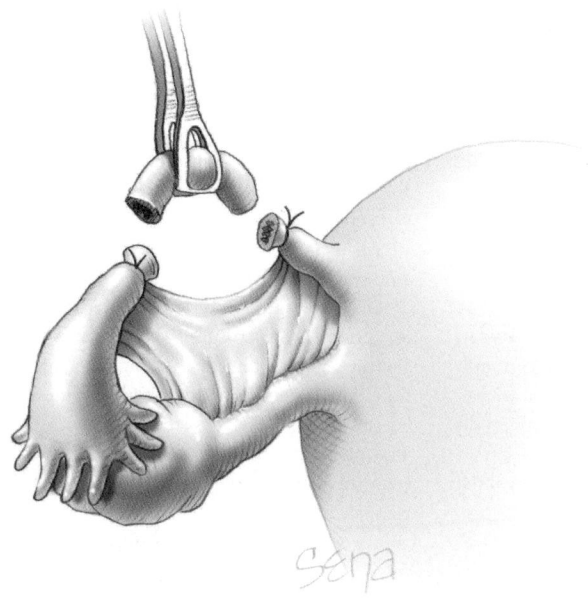

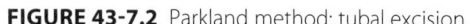

FIGURE 43-7.2 Parkland method: tubal excision.

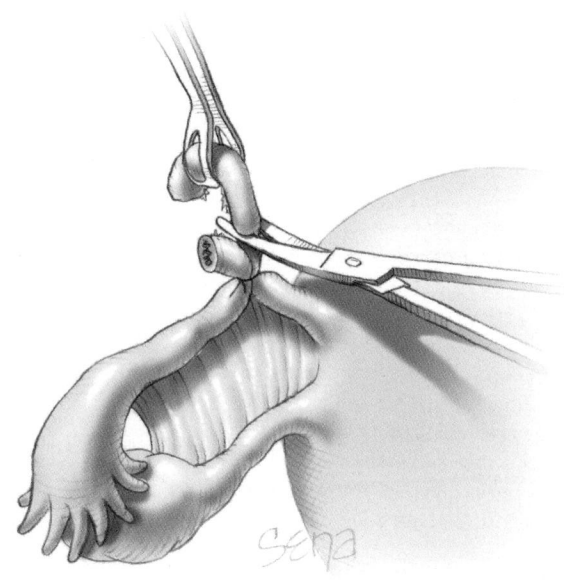

FIGURE 43-7.3 Pomeroy method.

❺ **Tubal Excision.** The Metzenbaum scissor tips are inserted through the mesosalpingeal defect, and the proximal portion of the fallopian tube is cut. A 0.5-cm pedicle is left to ensure that the tube will not slip through its ligature (Fig. 43-7.2). The tube is sharply dissected from the mesosalpinx toward the distal ligature, thereby freeing the tubal segment from the mesosalpinx. The distal part of the segment is excised to leave a 0.5-cm pedicle, and an adequate 2-cm tubal segment is obtained. The pedicles and mesosalpinx are inspected for hemostasis. The procedure is then repeated on the other side. Tubal segments are sent for histologic confirmation of complete transection.

❻ **Pomeroy Method.** This technique involves grasping and elevating a 2-cm midsegment of tube, ligating the tubal loop with a 2-0 plain catgut suture, and then excising the distal portion of the loop (Fig. 43-7.3). Prompt absorption of the suture following surgery causes the ligated ends to fall away, creating a resulting 2- to 3-cm gap that separates the ends.

❼ **Wound Closure.** The wound is closed as that for other transverse abdominal incisions (p. 930).

POSTOPERATIVE

The recovery following minilaparotomy is typically rapid and without complication, and women may resume regular diet and activities as tolerated. Sterilization is immediate following surgery, and intercourse may resume at the patient's discretion. Aside from regret, the risk of long-term physical or psychologic sequelae is low. Peterson and coworkers (2000) found that women who had undergone tubal sterilization were no more likely than those without this surgery to have menstrual abnormalities. Moreover, interval tubal ligation is unlikely to negatively affect sexual interest or pleasure (Costello, 2002).

43-8

Salpingectomy and Salpingostomy

Salpingostomy describes a lengthwise linear incision of the fallopian tube and is usually used to remove intraluminal ectopic pregnancy contents. In contrast, *salpingectomy* removes the fallopian tube with sparing of the ovary. Indications are varied, and this procedure may be selected for ectopic pregnancy removal, for sterilization, or for hydrosalpinx removal to improve in vitro fertilization success rates. Also, for ovarian cancer prevention, the Society of Gynecologic Oncology (2013) now recommends consideration of salpingectomy in lieu of tubal ligation or at the time of other pelvic surgery. The fallopian tube may be the origin of pelvic serous carcinomas (Chap. 35, p. 738).

Laparoscopic surgery offers patients the advantages of shorter hospitalizations, quicker recoveries, and less postoperative pain. Accordingly, laparoscopic treatment of ectopic pregnancy is generally preferred. As a result, laparotomic approaches for salpingectomy and salpingostomy are now reserved typically for patients with ruptured ectopic pregnancies who are hemodynamically unstable or in those with contraindications to laparoscopy. For hemoperitoneum, laparotomy offers fast entry into the abdomen for control of bleeding.

PREOPERATIVE

Consent

Most complications associated with salpingectomy and salpingostomy occur in conjunction with ectopic pregnancies, and the risk of bleeding is prominent. Injury to the ipsilateral ovary, however, is an attendant risk regardless of the indication. In certain cases, if severe, this damage can demand concurrent oophorectomy. Additionally, involvement of the ovary with tubal pathology may necessitate ovarian removal.

If salpingectomy is performed for sterilization, then consenting should mirror that for interval tubal sterilization found in Section 43-7.

Persistent Trophoblastic Tissue

Following any surgical treatment of ectopic pregnancy, trophoblastic tissue can persist. Remnant implants typically involve the fallopian tube, but extratubal trophoblastic implants have been found on the omentum and on pelvic and abdominal peritoneum. Peritoneal implants typically measure 0.3 to 2.0 cm and appear as red-black nodules. As expected, the risk of persistent trophoblast tissue is lower with salpingectomy compared with salpingostomy (Farquhar, 2005).

Preservation of Fertility

Most, but not all, studies show comparable subsequent fertility rates whether salpingectomy or salpingostomy is performed to treat ectopic pregnancy if the other tube is normal. This discussion is detailed in Chapter 7 (p. 172). Thus, with a healthy contralateral tube, neither salpingostomy nor salpingectomy offers a distinct fertility advantage. However, salpingostomy is considered a preferred option for tubal ectopic pregnancy if there is contralateral tubal disease and a desire for fertility. Unfortunately, in some cases of rupture, the extent of tubal damage or bleeding may limit tubal salvage, and salpingectomy may be required.

Patient Preparation

If performed for ectopic pregnancy, both salpingectomy and salpingostomy may be associated with substantial bleeding. Baseline complete blood count (CBC) and β-human chorionic gonadotropin (β-hCG) level are obtained. Patients undergo type and screen to establish blood type. Those with significant bleeding also require a type and crossmatch for packed red blood cells and other blood products as indicated. If performed for interval sterilization, then preparation follows that found in Section 43-7.

Salpingectomy and salpingostomy are associated with low infection rates. Accordingly, preoperative antibiotics are usually not required. Laparotomy dictates venous thromboembolism prophylaxis, and options are found in Table 39-8 (p. 836).

INTRAOPERATIVE

Surgical Steps

❶ **Anesthesia and Patient Positioning.** In most cases of ectopic pregnancy managed by laparotomy, surgery is an inpatient procedure and requires general anesthesia. For other indications, regional analgesia may be an option. The patient is supine. After anesthesia induction, hair in the planned incision path is clipped if needed; a Foley catheter is placed; and abdominal preparation is completed.

❷ **Abdominal Entry.** Most salpingectomy or salpingostomy procedures can be managed through a Pfannenstiel incision (p. 929). However, with a hemodynamically unstable patient and large hemoperitoneum, vertical incision may offer quicker entry.

❸ **Salpingectomy.** Once access to the pelvic organs has been achieved, the adnexa is elevated. Distal and proximal Babcock clamps are placed around the fallopian tube and direct the tube away from the uterus and ovary. This extends the mesosalpinx (Fig. 43-8.1).

Beginning at the distal, fimbriated end of the tube, one Kelly clamp or hemostat is placed across a 2-cm-long segment of the mesosalpinx, close to the fallopian tube. The clamp's curve faces the tube. Another clamp is similarly placed, but lies closer to the ovary. These clamps occlude vessels that traverse the mesosalpinx. Scissors then cut the interposed mesosalpinx.

The severed tissue pedicle that is closer to the ovary is tied with 2-0 or 3-0 gauge delayed-absorbable suture, and the clamp is removed. The clamp closer to the tube remains and leaves with the final specimen. Such clamping, cutting, and ligating are repeated serially,

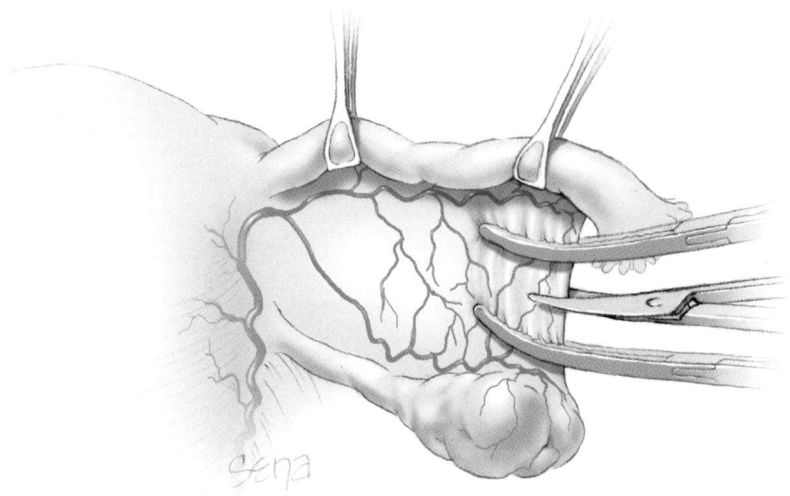

FIGURE 43-8.1 Salpingectomy.

with each clamp incorporating approximately 2 cm of mesosalpinx. Progression is directed from the ampullary end of the fallopian tube toward the uterus.

The last clamp is placed across the proximal mesosalpinx and fallopian tube. Scissors then cut the mesosalpinx and tube and free these from the uterus. This pedicle is similarly ligated.

❹ **Salpingostomy.** Surgical steps for salpingostomy mirror those used in laparoscopic salpingostomy and can be reviewed in Section 44-5 (p. 1013). To summarize, the affected fallopian tube is elevated with Babcock clamps. At the ectopic pregnancy site, the tube is sharply incised lengthwise on its antimesenteric border. The incision, usually 1 to 2 cm long, varies based on pregnancy

size. The products of conception are grasped and gently extracted or are delivered by hydrodissection. Bleeding sites are made hemostatic with electrosurgical coagulation, and the tubal incision is left to heal by secondary intention.

❺ **Wound Closure.** The pelvis is irrigated and rid of blood and tissue debris. The abdominal incision is closed as previously described for vertical or Pfannenstiel incision (pp. 928 and 930).

POSTOPERATIVE

In cases performed for ectopic pregnancy, salpingectomy or salpingostomy represents pregnancy termination. Accordingly, the Rh status of the patient should be evaluated.

Administration of 50 or 300 μg (1500 IU) of anti-D immune globulin intramuscularly within 72 hours after pregnancy termination in Rh negative women can dramatically lower the risk of alloimmunization in future pregnancies.

Because of the increased risk of persistent trophoblastic tissue in patients undergoing salpingostomy, serial weekly serum β-hCG levels should be measured until undetectable levels are reached. During this time, contraception should be used to avoid confusion between persistent trophoblastic tissue and a new pregnancy.

For elective sterilization, postoperative instructions follow those for interval tubal sterilization in Section 43-7. For all indications, resumption of activity and diet follow that for laparotomy (p. 928).

43-9

Cornuostomy and Cornual Wedge Resection

Interstitial pregnancy develops in a distensible portion of the tube surrounded by myometrium (Fig. 43-9.1). This location often permits pregnancies to attain greater size than ectopic pregnancy at other sites. Also, uterine rupture at the cornu, where uterine and ovarian arteries anastomose, can lead to brisk and significant hemorrhage. Fortunately, high-resolution sonography, β-hCG testing, and use of established diagnostic criteria have led to earlier diagnosis of interstitial pregnancy. This averts rupture in many circumstances.

In selected cases, this unusual type of ectopic pregnancy may be managed medically, but it is more frequently managed by various surgical techniques. *Cornuostomy* is analogous to linear salpingostomy for tubal ectopic pregnancy, whereas *cornual wedge resection* removes the interstitial pregnancy with its surrounding myometrium and fallopian tube (Moawad, 2010). Cornual wedge resection, often performed via laparotomy, has remained a cornerstone of therapy. However, many cases of interstitial pregnancy are now managed laparoscopically (Hwang, 2011). Factors to consider in selecting surgical route and specific procedure include gestational age, presence of rupture, hemodynamic stability, patient's desire for future fertility, and surgeon's preference and skill.

This discussion describes a laparotomic approach. However, the principles and surgical steps presented here are applicable to laparoscopic management with only minor modifications.

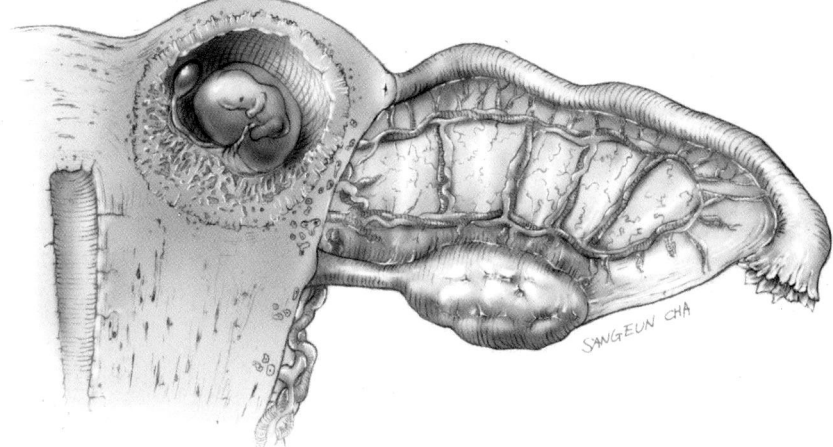

FIGURE 43-9.1 Interstitial pregnancy.

PREOPERATIVE

Patient Evaluation

In some cases, particularly those in which the cornu has ruptured and the woman is hemodynamically unstable, fluid resuscitation and blood transfusion are initiated preoperatively. Further, because there is risk for excessive intraoperative bleeding, a patient is typed and crossmatched for packed red blood cells and other blood products as indicated. A patient is counseled regarding the possible need for blood products, which includes anti-D immune globulin for those with Rh-negative blood. Baseline CBC and β-hCG levels are obtained.

Additional risks include removal of the ipsilateral ovary and the possibility of hysterectomy for uncontrollable bleeding. In the event that the patient has completed her childbearing, tubal ligation or bilateral salpingectomy or rarely even hysterectomy may be acceptable at the time of surgery.

Patient Preparation

Other than optimizing hemodynamic stability of the patient and ensuring blood availability, no special preparation is required. Prophylactic antibiotics or bowel preparation are generally not required. Laparotomy dictates venous thromboembolism prophylaxis, and options are found in Table 39-8 (p. 836).

INTRAOPERATIVE

Surgical Steps

❶ **Anesthesia and Patient Positioning.** Cornual wedge resection and cornuostomy are usually performed under general anesthesia, particularly if cornual rupture is suspected. The patient is supine. After anesthesia induction, hair in the planned incision path is clipped if needed; a Foley catheter is inserted; and abdominal preparation is completed.

❷ **Abdominal Entry.** Either a transverse or vertical incision may be used depending on the clinical situation as discussed in Section 43-1 (p. 926).

❸ **Exposure.** In the absence of cornual rupture and active bleeding, the bowel is packed away to provide adequate exposure of the pelvis. A self-retaining retractor may then be placed. If significant hemoperitoneum is encountered upon abdominal entry, the operator can attempt to remove obscuring blood with suction and laparotomy sponges. Failing this, the surgeon may consider manually elevating the uterus out of the pelvis where it may be inspected for rupture and hemorrhage. The uterus can be compressed between the operator's thumb and fingers to tamponade bleeding. Two heavy clamps can then be place across the base of the cornu. In rare cases, temporary compression of the aorta may be helpful if bleeding is torrential and poorly controlled.

❹ **Inspection of the Pelvis.** The location of the ectopic pregnancy is identified. Additional information including presence or absence of rupture, pregnancy size, amount of bleeding, and appearance of the contralateral (unaffected) adnexa is needed before deciding on the exact procedure to perform.

❺ **Vasopressin Injection.** For either cornuostomy or cornual wedge resection, dilute vasopressin (20 units in 30-100 mL of normal saline) may be injected into the myometrium surrounding the interstitial pregnancy to aid hemostasis. Needle aspiration prior to injection is imperative to avoid intravascular injection of this potent vasoconstrictor. The anesthesiologist is concurrently informed of vasopressin injection because a sudden increase in patient blood pressure may follow injection. Blanching at the injection site is expected.

❻ **Cornuostomy: Incision.** A linear incision is made through the uterine serosa and myometrium overlying the interstitial pregnancy (Fig. 43-9.2). As the incision is carried downward, some products of conception may extrude through the incision (Fig. 43-9.3). Products of conception may be removed by means of blunt, sharp, suction, or hydrodissection (Fig. 43-9.4). Despite vasopressin, bleeding from the myometrium is common and is best managed with electrosurgical coagulation or figure-of-eight stitches with 2-0 gauge absorbable or delayed-absorbable suture.

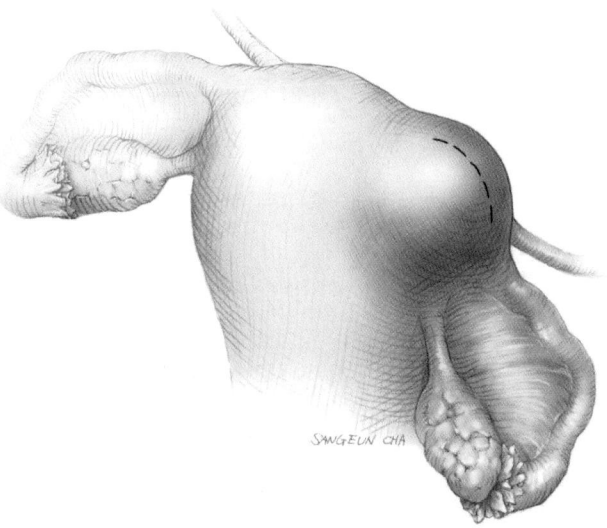

FIGURE 43-9.2 Incision line for cornuostomy.

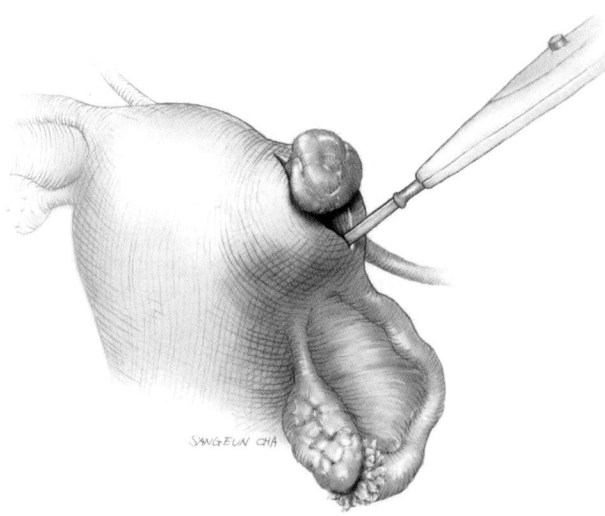

FIGURE 43-9.3 Cornuostomy with extrusion of products of conception.

❼ Cornuostomy: Incision Closure. The myometrial incision is usually closed with absorbable or delayed-absorbable suture in an interrupted or continuous running fashion (Fig. 43-9.5) A gauge of sufficient strength to prevent breakage during muscle approximation is selected, typically 2-0 or 0-gauge. For this, chromic suture may be preferred due to its slight elasticity that provides tensile strength and minimal tissue cutting. Closure may be completed with one layer of sutures or may require two to three layers to aid hemostasis, avert hematoma formation, and reapproximate myometrium. Additionally, some prefer a subserosal closure, similar to a subcuticular running stitch, as a final layer. This

theoretically minimizes the amount of exposed suture and thereby limits adhesion formation.

❽ Cornual Wedge Resection: Salpingectomy. With this approach, the pregnancy, surrounding myometrium, and ipsilateral fallopian tube are excised en bloc. The fallopian tube is removed to avoid future ectopic pregnancy in this tube. Such pregnancies form when the ipsilateral ovary's eggs are fertilized by sperm that travel out the contralateral tube and are transported by peritoneal fluid to the isolated and ligated tube.

Initially, salpingectomy is completed as described in Section 43-8.1 (p. 939). To summarize, the mesosalpinx is serially clamped

and ligated across its length (Fig. 43-9.6). This separates the tube from its mesosalpinx and ipsilateral ovary (Fig. 43-9.7).

❾ Cornual Wedge Resection: Myometrial Incision. Following vasopressin injection, the cornual serosa surrounding the pregnancy is incised with an electrosurgical blade (Fig. 43-9.8). The incision is angled inward as it is deepened. This creates a wedge into the myometrium (Fig. 43-9.9). Hemostasis can be achieved with electrosurgical blade coagulation or with sutures.

❿ Cornual Wedge Resection: Incision Closure. The myometrial incision is usually

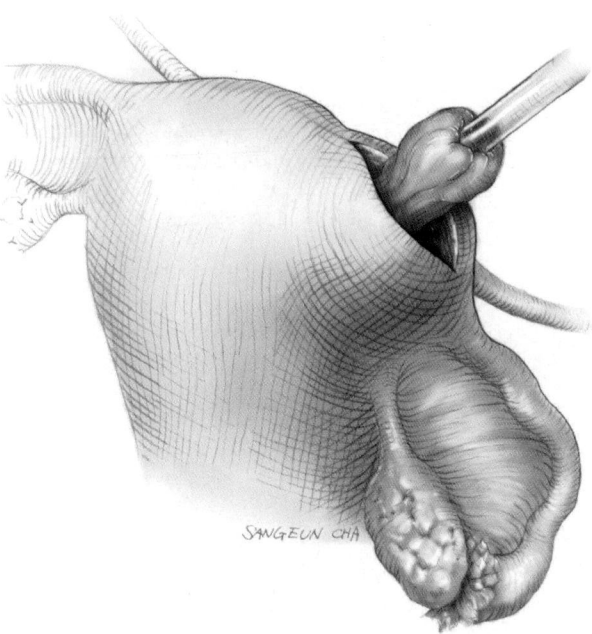

FIGURE 43-9.4 Suction removal of products of conception.

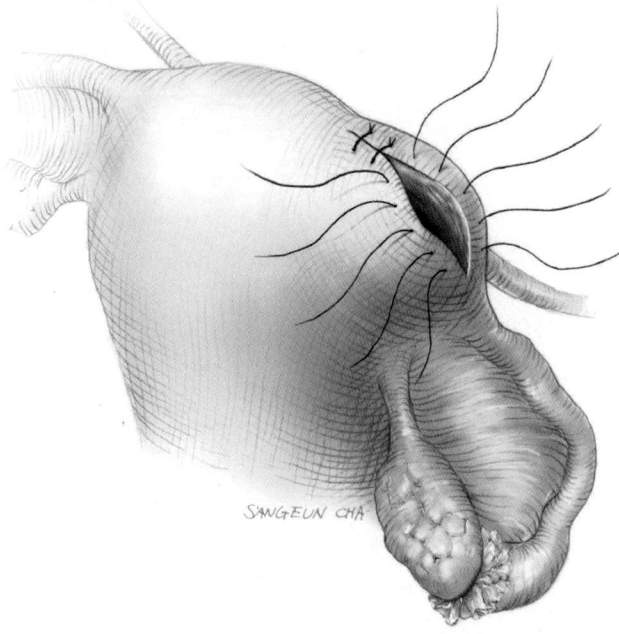

FIGURE 43-9.5 Myometrial incision closure.

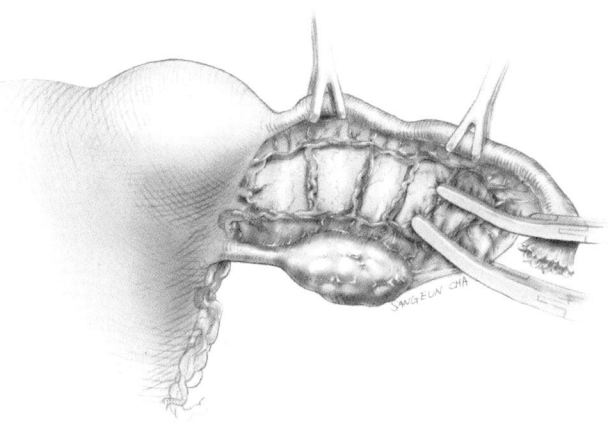

FIGURE 43-9.6 Mesosalpinx serially clamped and ligated.

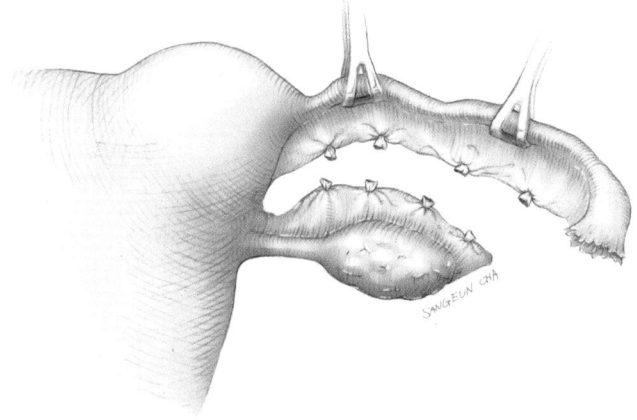

FIGURE 43-9.7 Salpingectomy completed.

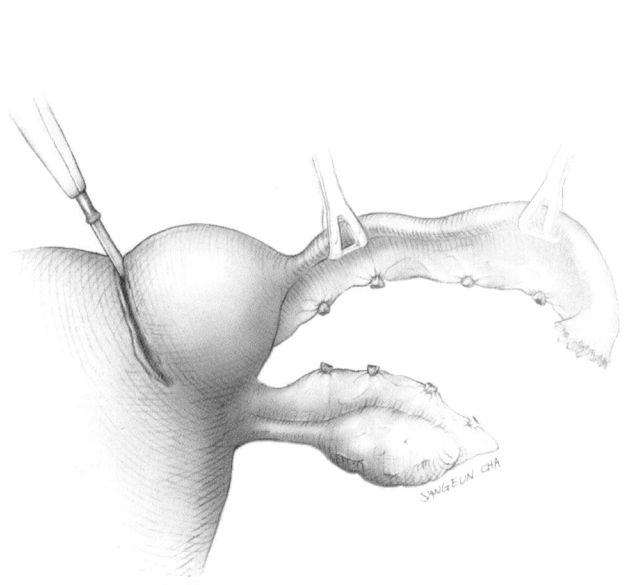

FIGURE 43-9.8 Myometrial incision.

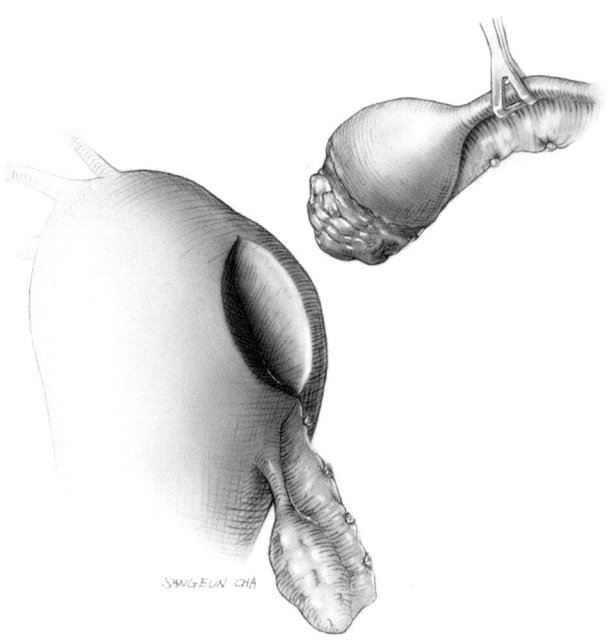

FIGURE 43-9.9 En bloc excision of interstitial pregnancy.

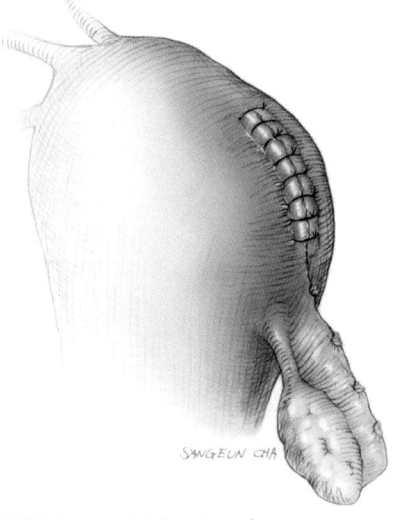

FIGURE 43-9.10 Incision closure.

closed in two to three layers with absorbable or delayed-absorbable suture in an interrupted or continuous running fashion. As with cornuostomy, some recommend a final subserosal layer closure. However, depending on the degree of wound tension created by the contracted myometrium, this suture may pull through the serosa, and a simple interrupted or running suture line may be required to approximate the serosa (Fig. 43-9.10).

As noted earlier, there can be cases with rupture and brisk bleeding, in which two clamps are quickly placed across the base of the cornu to halt hemorrhage. In these cases, salpingectomy is similarly completed.

Then, the cornual myometrium above these clamps is sharply removed. The myometrium within each clamp is then suture ligated with a transfixing stitch.

POSTOPERATIVE

After surgery, patient care in general follows that described for laparotomy (p. 928). As with salpingostomy for treatment of tubal pregnancy, there is increased risk of persistent trophoblastic tissue following cornuostomy. Therefore, serial β-hCG levels are followed postoperatively until a negative test result is obtained. For Rh-negative women, 50 or 300 μg (1500 IU) of anti-D immune globulin is given intramuscularly within 72 hours after pregnancy termination to lower the risk of alloimmunization in future pregnancies. Patients should also be counseled that there is also an increased risk of future ectopic pregnancy in the remaining tube following an interstitial pregnancy. Last, as is the case with other types of uterine surgery such as classical cesarean delivery or myomectomy, the uterine rupture rate in subsequent pregnancies and particularly during labor is increased. For this reason, delivery by cesarean at term before labor onset is generally recommended.

43-10

Abdominal Myomectomy

Myomectomy involves surgical removal of leiomyomas from their surrounding myometrium. Indications can include abnormal uterine bleeding, pelvic pain, infertility, and recurrent miscarriage. Hysterectomy is chosen to treat many of these indications. However, myomectomy is often selected by those desiring organ preservation for childbearing or those wishing to avoid hysterectomy.

Myomectomy often requires laparotomy. However, laparoscopic excision may be performed by those with skills in laparoscopic suturing and is described in Section 44-8 (p. 1022) (Seracchioli, 2000; Sizzi, 2007).

PREOPERATIVE

Patient Evaluation

Because of their influence on pre- and intraoperative planning, leiomyoma size, number, and location are evaluated prior to surgery with sonography, MR imaging, or hysteroscopy (Chap. 9, p. 206). For example, submucous tumors are more easily removed hysteroscopically (Section 44-14, p. 1040), whereas intramural and serosal types typically require laparotomy or laparoscopy. Leiomyomas may be small and buried within the myometrium. Thus, accurate information as to leiomyoma number and location aids complete excision. Last, multiple large tumors or those that are located in the broad ligament, encroach on the tubal ostia, or involve the cervix may increase the risk of conversion to hysterectomy. Patients are so counseled.

Consent

Myomectomy has several risks including significant bleeding and need for transfusion. Moreover, uncontrolled hemorrhage or extensive myometrial injury during tumor removal may force hysterectomy. Fortunately, rates of conversion to hysterectomy during myomectomy are low and range from 0 to 2 percent (Iverson, 1996; LaMorte, 1993; Sawin, 2000). Postoperatively, the risk of pelvic adhesion formation is significant. Also, leiomyomas can recur.

Patient Preparation

Hematologic Status. Abnormal uterine bleeding is a common indication for myomectomy. As a result, many women who elect to undergo this surgery are anemic. In addition, significant intraoperative blood loss during myomectomy is possible. Accordingly, attempts to resolve anemia and bleeding prior to surgery are pursued. Toward this goal, oral iron therapy, gonadotropin-releasing hormone (GnRH) agonists, and progesterone antagonists may have benefits (Chap. 9, p. 208).

GnRH Agonists. In addition to preoperative control of abnormal uterine bleeding, these agents have been shown to significantly decrease uterine volume after several months of use (Benagiano, 1996; Friedman, 1991). Decreased uterine size following treatment may allow a less invasive surgical procedure. For example, myomectomy may be completed through a smaller laparotomy incision or by laparoscopy or hysteroscopy (Lethaby, 2002; Mencaglia, 1993). These agents have also been found to diminish leiomyoma vascularity and uterine blood flow (Matta, 1988; Reinsch, 1994). For this surgery, there is conflicting evidence regarding a final benefit of adhesion prevention (Coddington, 2009; Imai, 2003).

The use of preoperative GnRH agonists, however, may also have disadvantages. Within leiomyomas, GnRH agonists can incite hyaline or hydropic degeneration, which may obliterate the pseudocapsule connective tissue interface between the tumor and the myometrium. Such obliterated cleavage planes may lead to tedious and lengthy tumor enucleation (Deligdisch, 1997). Moreover, studies have shown higher rates of leiomyoma recurrence in women treated with GnRH agonists prior to myomectomy (Fedele, 1990; Vercellini, 2003). Leiomyomas treated with these agents may shrink in volume and be missed during surgical removal.

For these reasons, GnRH agonists are not used routinely in all patients undergoing myomectomy. They can be recommended for preoperative use in women with greatly enlarged uteri or preoperative anemia or in cases in which a decrease in uterine volume would allow a less invasive approach to leiomyoma removal.

Similar to GnRH agonists, the oral progesterone agonists preoperatively shrink myoma volume and diminish menorrhagia (Donnez, 2012a,b). Currently available outside the United States, ulipristal acetate (Esmya) in dosages of 5 mg or 10 mg daily may be used during the 3 months prior to surgery.

Other Preoperative Methods. The risk of blood transfusion varies among studies and ranges from less than 5 percent to nearly 40 percent (Darwish, 2005; LaMorte, 1993; Sawin, 2000; Smith, 1990). Accordingly, in women with large uteri, especially those with multiple leiomyomas, cell-saver blood scavenger and reuse techniques may be selected (Son, 2014; Yamada, 1997). Indications, benefits, and limitations are discussed fully in Chapter 40 (p. 859).

Also with large leiomyomas, tourniquets or vasopressin may fail to adequately limit bleeding. For these, preoperative uterine artery embolization (UAE) on the morning of surgery may be an effective tool to limit blood loss. And unlike GnRH agonist use, UAE allows tissue planes to be preserved (Chua, 2005; Ngeh, 2004; Ravina, 1995).

Several disadvantages of UAE include risks for subsequent pregnancy complications, collateral ovarian infarction, and formation of uterine synechiae, among others discussed in Chapter 9 (p. 209). Thus, preoperative UAE may best be limited to patients with large uteri in whom excessive blood loss is expected and in those not seeking future pregnancy.

Prophylaxis. Few studies address the benefits of preoperative antibiotic use. Iverson and coworkers (1996), in their analysis of 101 myomectomy cases, found that although 54 percent of cases received prophylaxis, infectious morbidity was not lowered compared with cases in which antibiotics were not used. However, in cases performed for infertility, because of the potential for tubal adhesions associated with pelvic infection, antibiotic prophylaxis has been advocated (Milton, 2013). For those in whom prophylaxis is planned, selection can follow that for hysterectomy (Table 39-6, p. 835). For all cases, because the risk of conversion to hysterectomy is present, vaginal preparation immediately prior to surgical draping is warranted.

With myomectomy, the risk of bowel injury is low. Thus, bowel preparation is typically not required unless extensive adhesions are anticipated. Last, laparotomy dictates venous thromboembolism prophylaxis, and options are found in Table 39-8 (p. 836).

INTRAOPERATIVE

Surgical Steps

❶ **Anesthesia and Patient Positioning.** Myomectomy performed through a laparotomy incision is typically an inpatient procedure performed under general or regional anesthesia. The patient is supine. After anesthesia induction, hair in the planned incision path is clipped if needed; a Foley catheter is inserted; and abdominal preparation is completed.

❷ **Abdominal Entry.** The choice of Pfannenstiel incision is typically appropriate for uteri 14-weeks size or smaller (Section 43-2, p. 929). Larger uteri usually require a midline vertical abdominal incision.

❸ **Leiomyoma Identification.** Following abdominal entry, the surgeon inspects the serosal surface to identify leiomyomas to be removed. Additionally, squeezing palpation of the myometrium before and during the surgery will help identify firm buried intramural or submucous leiomyomas.

❹ **Use of Uterine Tourniquet.** Tourniquets have been used for years to temporarily occlude blood flow through the uterine arteries. Because the uterus receives collateral flow through the ovarian arteries, some tourniquet techniques include occlusion of both uterine and ovarian vessels. First, bilateral windows are created in the leaves of the broad ligament at the level of the internal cervical os. A Penrose drain or Foley catheter is threaded through the opening to encircle the uterine isthmus. Once in place, the Penrose drain is tied or the ends of the Foley catheter are clamped to compress the uterine vessels. Alternatively, the uterine arteries can be ligated bilaterally (Helal, 2010; Sapmaz, 2003). In combination with uterine artery compression, occlusion of the uteroovarian ligaments or infundibulopelvic ligaments to compress the ovarian arteries has been described (Al-Shabibi, 2009; Taylor, 2005). Large, isthmic, or broadligament leiomyomas, however, may limit the use of tourniquets in some.

❺ **Use of Vasopressin.** 8-Arginine vasopressin (Pitressin) is a sterile, aqueous solution of synthetic vasopressin. It is effective in limiting uterine blood loss during myomectomy because of its ability to cause vascular spasm and uterine muscle contraction. Compared with placebo, vasopressin injection significantly decreases blood loss during myomectomy (Frederick, 1994). Compared with tourniquet techniques, vasopressin injection has also been associated with either comparable or less intraoperative blood loss, with equally low patient morbidity, and lower myometrial hematoma formation rates (Darwish, 2005; Fletcher, 1996; Ginsburg, 1993).

Each vial of Pitressin is standardized to contain 20 pressor units/mL, and doses used for myomectomy are 20 U diluted in 30 to 100 mL of saline (Frishman, 2009). Vasopressin is typically injected along the planned serosal incision(s). The plasma half-life of this agent is 10 to 20 minutes. For this reason, injection of vasopressin is ideally discontinued 20 minutes prior to uterine repair to allow evaluation of bleeding from myometrial incisions (Hutchins, 1996).

The main risks associated with local vasopressin injection result from inadvertent intravascular infiltration and include transient increases in blood pressure, bradycardia, atrioventricular block, and pulmonary edema (Deschamps, 2005; Tulandi, 1996).

For these reasons, patients with a history of cardiovascular disease, cardiomyopathy, congestive heart failure, uncontrolled hypertension, migraine, asthma, and severe chronic obstructive pulmonary disease may not be candidates for vasopressin use. In addition to vasopressin, other less-researched agents for blood loss prevention have been reviewed by Kongnyuy and Wiysonge (2014).

❻ **Serosal Incision.** Because of postoperative adhesion formation risks, surgeons ideally minimize the number of serosal incisions and attempt to place incisions on the anterior uterine wall. Tulandi and colleagues (1993) found that posterior wall incisions result in a 94-percent adhesion formation rate compared with a 55-percent rate for anterior incisions.

For most patients, a midline vertical uterine incision allows removal of the greatest number of leiomyomas through the fewest incisions. The length should accommodate the approximate diameter of the largest tumor. The incision depth should afford access to all leiomyomas (Fig. 43-10.1). To reach lateral tumors, a surgeon may create lateral myometrial incisions within the initial central incision. However, at times, separate incision may be required to excise tumors. In these instances, a horizontal incision decreases the number of arcuate vessels transected.

❼ **Tumor Enucleation.** The first leiomyoma is grasped with a Lahey or single-tooth tenaculum (Fig. 43-10.2). Applying traction

on the leiomyoma outward and away from the myometrial incision aids in the development of a tissue plane between myometrium and leiomyoma. Sharp and blunt dissection of the pseudocapsule surrounding the leiomyoma frees the tumor from the adjacent myometrium.

❽ **Bleeding.** Hemorrhage during myomectomy primarily develops during tumor enucleation and is positively correlated with preoperative uterine size, total weight of leiomyomas removed, and operating time (Ginsburg, 1993). Approximately two to four main arteries feed each leiomyoma and enter the tumor at unpredictable sites. Accordingly, surgeons should watch for these vessels, ligate them prior to transection when possible, and be ready to immediately grasp them with hemostats for ligation or fulguration if lacerated during tumor excision (Fig. 43-10.3).

❾ **Myometrial Incision.** Smaller, internal incisions into the myometrium may be required to excise all leiomyomas. If the endometrial cavity is entered, it should be closed with a running suture of 4-0 or 5-0 gauge delayed-absorbable suture (Fig. 43-10.4).

❿ **Myometrial Closure.** After removal of all tumors, redundant serosa may be excised. Smaller internal myometrial incisions are closed first with delayed-absorbable suture (see Fig. 43-10.4). The myometrium is then closed in several layers to improve hemostasis

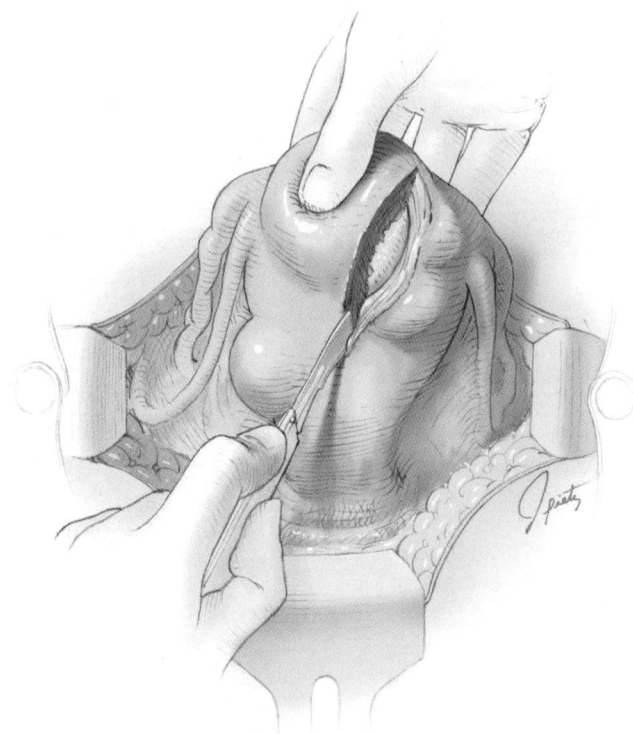

FIGURE 43-10.1 Uterine incision.

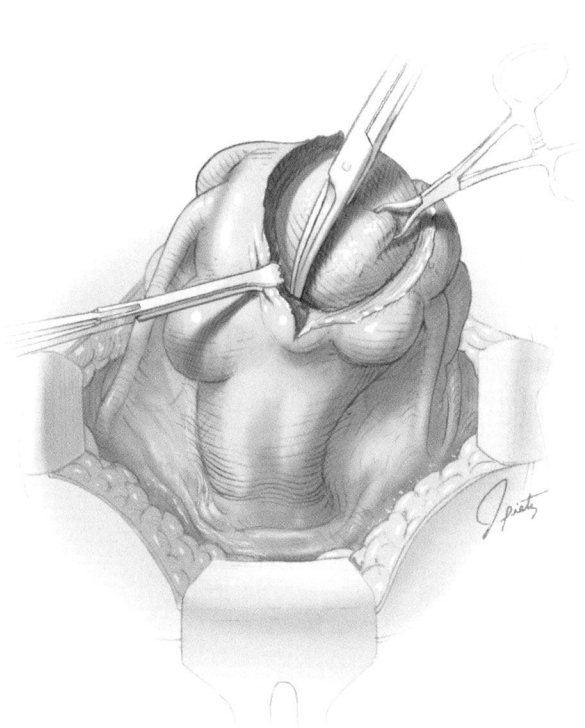

FIGURE 43-10.2 Tumor enucleation.

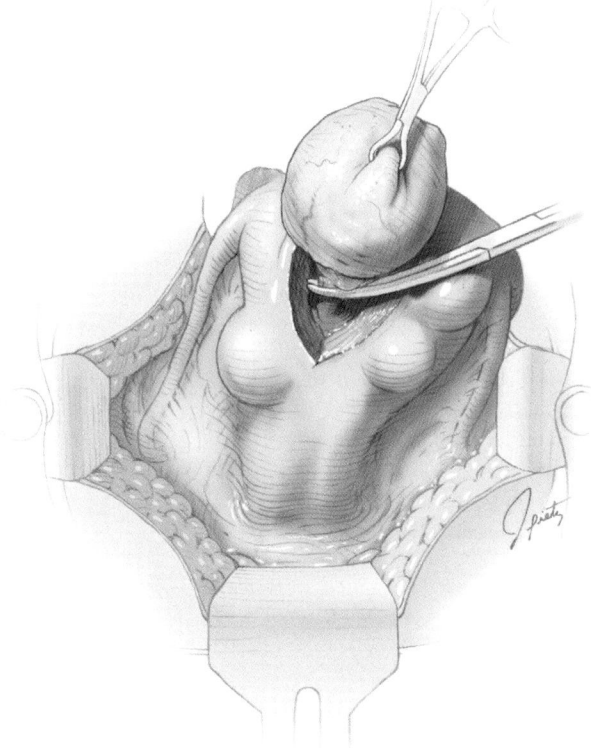

FIGURE 43-10.3 Vessel ligation.

and prevent hematoma formation. A gauge of sufficient strength to prevent breakage during muscle approximation is selected, typically 2-0 to 0-gauge.

⑪ **Serosal Closure.** Closure of the serosal incision using a running baseball stitch

or a subserosal running closure, similar to a running subcuticular closure, may help to limit adhesion formation. For this, 4-0 or 5-0 monofilament, delayed-absorbable suture may be selected. Moreover, absorbable adhesion barriers may help reduce the incidence of adhesion formation following

myomectomy (Ahmad, 2015; Canis, 2014; Tinelli, 2011).

POSTOPERATIVE

After surgery, care in general follows that described for laparotomy (p. 928). Febrile morbidity of greater than 38.0°C is a common event following myomectomy (Iverson, 1996; Rybak, 2008). Purported causes include atelectasis, myometrial incisional hematomas, and factors released with myometrial destruction. Although fever is common following myomectomy, pelvic infection is not. For example, LaMorte and colleagues (1993) noted only a 2-percent rate of pelvic infection in their analysis of 128 myomectomy cases.

Following myomectomy, there are no clear guidelines as to the timing of pregnancy attempts. Darwish and associates (2005) performed sonographic examinations on 169 patients after myomectomy. Following myometrial indicators, they concluded that wound healing is usually completed within 3 months. There are no clinical trials that address the issue of uterine rupture and therefore route of delivery of pregnancies occurring after myomectomy (American College of Obstetricians and Gynecologists, 2012). Management of these cases requires sound clinical judgment and individualization of care.

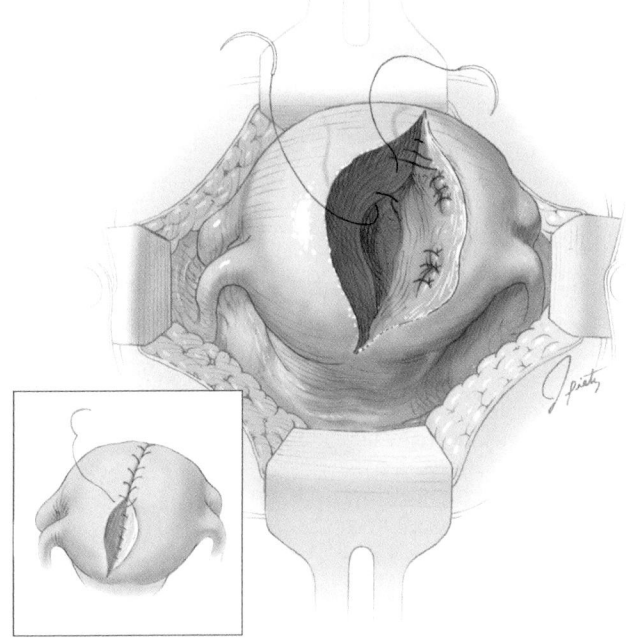

FIGURE 43-10.4 Uterine incision closure.

43-11

Vaginal Myomectomy for Prolapsed Leiomyoma

Prolapse of a pedunculated submucosal leiomyoma is an unusual occurrence but certainly not rare. Vaginal myomectomy is usually a relatively simple procedure and is frequently curative for the patient. Myoma and stalk size and patient discomfort are the most important variables for management. With a thin stalk, simply twisting the leiomyoma slowly off its stalk may be sufficient for removal. With larger stalk diameter or greater patient pain, removal in the operating room is typically preferred. Finally, for those with a large obstructive myoma on a thick, short stalk, hysterectomy may be necessary (Caglar, 2005; Golan, 2005).

PREOPERATIVE

Patient Evaluation

In many cases, diagnosis of a prolapsed pedunculated submucosal leiomyoma will be obvious, as will the size of the prolapsed myoma. However, as many of these patients present with abnormal uterine bleeding, evaluation for other less obvious causes of abnormal bleeding is appropriate. In other cases, only partial prolapse of a leiomyoma through the cervix may preclude assessment of total leiomyoma and stalk size, or the mass may be of unclear etiology. Accordingly, imaging studies, particularly transvaginal or transabdominal sonography or both, may yield additional information beyond pelvic examination. Specifically, uterine size, shape, and degree of involvement with additional leiomyomas or other pathology can be obtained. Moreover, biopsy of any mass of uncertain etiology is considered, and Tischler biopsy forceps may be selected (Fig. 29-16, p. 641). If required, Monsel solution can be applied to control bleeding from the biopsy site similar to that following colposcopic biopsy.

Consent

Risks with vaginal myomectomy are low. Uncontrollable bleeding and procedural failure are potential complications. Rarely, severing a stalk on great tension may concomitantly resect the attached uterine wall and injure intraabdominal organs. The possibility of hysterectomy and its consequences are also discussed with the patient beforehand. Leiomyoma prolapse recurrence is uncommon but may occur if additional submucosal leiomyomas are present or develop within the uterus.

Patient Preparation

In an otherwise healthy woman, little preparation is needed for vaginal myomectomy. However, uterine bleeding with leiomyoma prolapse is common, and hypovolemia and acute blood loss anemia are corrected as needed with crystalloid and blood products (Chap. 40, p. 864). If fever is present and infection of the prolapsed leiomyoma or lower genital tract is suspected, treatment with broad-spectrum antibiotics are initiated prior to vaginal myomectomy. Suitable options are found in Table 39-6 (p. 835). The need for thromboembolism prophylaxis will vary by patient age and anticipated length of surgery as outlined in Table 39-8 (p. 836).

INTRAOPERATIVE

Surgical Steps

❶ **Anesthesia and Patient Positioning.** The patient is placed in standard dorsal lithotomy position. Vaginal myomectomy may be performed under general or regional anesthesia, intracervical or paracervical blockade, conscious sedation, or intramuscular analgesia. For those women who are taken to the operating room at our institution, we usually prefer general anesthesia for several reasons. First, hysteroscopy is often done following vaginal myomectomy to further evaluate the uterine cavity and status of the stalk. Secondly, many leiomyomas are bulky and require at least a moderate amount of manipulation and vaginal retraction for removal.

An examination is done once the patient is relaxed to assess the size of the prolapsed leiomyoma; location, length, and thickness of the stalk; and general pelvic anatomy. The vagina is then surgically prepared, and the bladder is drained.

❷ **Leiomyoma Stalk Ligation.** To retract the posterior vaginal wall, an Auvard weighted vaginal speculum is positioned. Heaney retractors are used as needed for sidewall and anterior vaginal wall retraction. The prolapsed leiomyoma is grasped with a tenaculum. Traction is applied on the leiomyoma to allow access to the stalk (Fig. 43-11.1). Excessive traction on the leiomyoma is avoided. This can invert the uterine wall that is attached to the stalk and thereby risk resection of this wall rather than the proximal stalk. In addition, undue traction may avulse the tumor prior to stalk ligation.

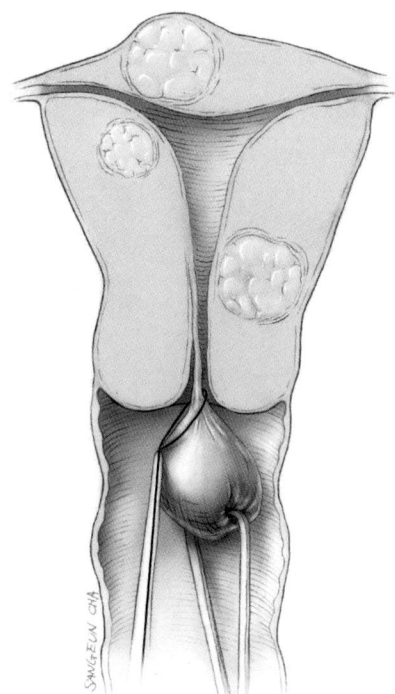

FIGURE 43-11.1 Suture loop surrounding leiomyoma stalk placed on tension.

The stalk is doubly ligated with delayed-absorbable suture. Preformed knotted loops with a knot pusher (as used in laparoscopy cases) work well in this setting (Fig. 41-35, p. 900). With this, the tenaculum is removed to place a loop and then reclamped. In

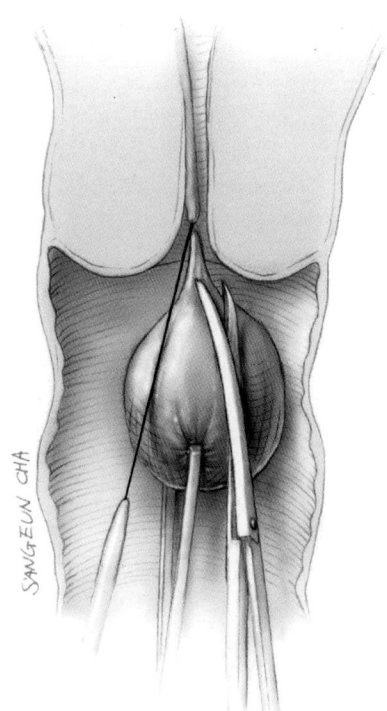

FIGURE 43-11.2 Suture loop cinched and tumor stalk transected.

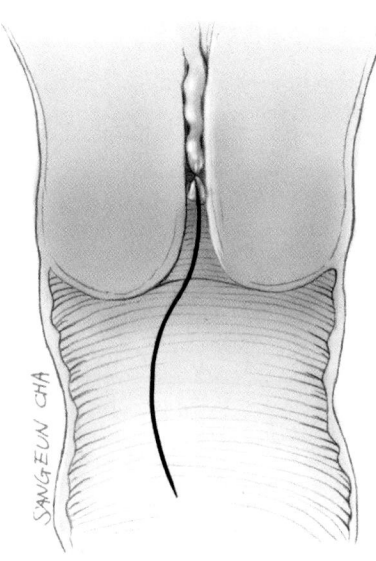

FIGURE 43-11.3 Leiomyoma excision completed.

contrast, manual knot tying may be technically difficult given the size of the obstructing leiomyoma, the stalk length (or lack thereof), and the cramped vaginal operating space. In such cases, tips of a Heaney right-angle clamp can be maneuvered past the myoma and then across the stalk.

❸ **Leiomyoma Removal.** The stalk is then sharply incised at an appropriate point distal to the ligature to prevent the ligature from slipping off (Fig. 43-11.2). With complete stalk transection, the prolapsed leiomyoma is freed for removal, and the ligated stalk retracts into the uterine cavity (Fig. 43-11.3). If a Heaney clamp has been placed, then the stalk is severed, the mass is removed, and a ligature is placed around the proximal stalk. As the suture is tied, the clamp is removed.

As alternatives, the stalk may be incised electrosurgically without ligature placement, or the leiomyoma can be twisted from its stalk if the stalk is not excessively thick. After leiomyoma removal, hysteroscopy may optionally be performed to assess hemostasis and the uterine cavity.

POSTOPERATIVE

No special care beyond routine postoperative surveillance is necessary following vaginal myomectomy for a pedunculated prolapsed leiomyoma. Regular diet and activities are resumed quickly and can be individualized.

43-12

Abdominal Hysterectomy

Hysterectomy is one of the most frequently performed gynecologic procedures, and more than 500,000 women undergo this procedure for benign disease annually in the United States (Jacoby, 2009). Of benign reasons, symptomatic leiomyomas and pelvic organ prolapse are the most frequent, although adenomyosis, endometriosis, chronic pain, and premalignant uterine or cervical disease are also relatively common.

PREOPERATIVE

Patient Evaluation

To reach the preoperative diagnosis, testing varies on clinical signs and symptoms and is discussed within the respective chapters covering specific etiologies. Prior to hysterectomy, all patients require cervical cancer screening. With abnormal findings, further evaluation is completed to exclude invasive cancer, which is treated instead with radical hysterectomy or chemoradiation. Similarly, women at risk for endometrial cancer and whose indication includes abnormal bleeding are also usually screened before surgery (Chap. 8, p. 184). Last, concurrent cervical infection or bacterial vaginosis is sought for preoperative eradication to lower postoperative infection risks.

Decision-making for Approach Selection

Hysterectomy may be completed using an abdominal, vaginal, laparoscopic, or robotic approach, and selection is influenced by many factors. For example, shape and size of the uterus and pelvis, surgical indications, presence or absence of adnexal pathology, extensive pelvic adhesive disease, surgical risks, hospitalization and recovery length, hospital resources, and surgeon expertise are all weighed once hysterectomy is planned. Each approach carries distinct advantages and disadvantages, discussed subsequently.

Vaginal Hysterectomy

Surgeons usually choose this approach if the uterus is relatively small, extensive adhesions are not anticipated, no significant adnexal pathology is expected, and some degree of pelvic organ descent is present. When this procedure is compared with abdominal hysterectomy, patients usually benefit from faster recovery and from reduced hospital stays, costs, and postoperative pain (Johnson, 2005; Nieboer, 2009).

Abdominal Hysterectomy

Despite the advantages of vaginal hysterectomy, most uteri in the United States are removed through an abdominal incision (Jacoby, 2009). Either a transverse or vertical incision may be selected depending on the clinical setting (p. 926).

Abdominal hysterectomy allows the greatest ability to manipulate pelvic organs. Thus, it may be preferred if large pelvic masses or extensive adhesions are anticipated. Additionally, an abdominal approach affords access to the ovaries if oophorectomy is desired, to the space of Retzius or presacral space if concurrent urogynecologic procedures are planned, or to the upper abdomen for cancer staging. However, for surgeons with advanced skills in minimally invasive surgery (MIS), most of these limitations are overcome, and their indications for abdominal hysterectomy may be few. That said, abdominal hysterectomy typically requires less operating time than laparoscopic or robotic hysterectomy and requires no advanced MIS expertise or instrumentation. Moreover, the Food and Drug Administration (FDA) (2014) has recently discouraged the use of laparoscopic power morcellators due to the potential dispersion of occult cancer cells. While data are being collected regarding this risk, many surgeons and patients may forego MIS hysterectomy for larger uteri, and thus rates of abdominal hysterectomy may increase.

Disadvantages of abdominal hysterectomy include longer patient recovery and hospital stays, increased incisional pain, and greater risk of postoperative fever and wound infection (Marana, 1999; Nieboer, 2009). Additionally, compared with a vaginal approach, abdominal hysterectomy is associated with greater risk for ureteral injury, but lower rates of bladder injury (Frankman, 2010; Gilmour, 2006).

Laparoscopic Hysterectomy

Selected more and more frequently, this hysterectomy group uses laparoscopic techniques to complete some or all steps of hysterectomy, and specific definitions are provided in Chapter 44 (p. 1026) (Turner, 2013). Although criteria vary depending on surgeon skill, this approach is often selected if the uterus is not excessively large, extensive adhesions are not expected, and some limitation deters vaginal hysterectomy alone. Patient recovery, hospital stays, and postoperative pain scores are comparable with those of vaginal hysterectomy, but a laparoscopic approach allows greater visualization and access to the abdomen and pelvis. This may be advantageous if oophorectomy is planned or if adhesive disease or bleeding is encountered. However, laparoscopy typically requires longer operating times, expensive equipment, and MIS expertise. In addition, in most studies, laparoscopic hysterectomy has been associated with greater rates of ureteral injury than either abdominal or vaginal hysterectomy (Frankman, 2010; Gilmour, 2006; Mamik, 2014).

Approach Selection

If all factors are equal, vaginal hysterectomy should be considered. However, with large pelvic masses or large uteri, with risk of gynecologic cancer, with extensive adhesions, or with poor uterine descent, either abdominal or laparoscopic hysterectomy may be required. Of note, surgical expertise is factored into the decision and strongly dictates the approach selected.

Total versus Supracervical Hysterectomy

Prior to hysterectomy, the decision to concurrently remove the cervix is discussed with the patient. Hysterectomy may include removal of the uterus and cervix, termed *total hysterectomy*, or may involve only the uterine corpus, called *supracervical hysterectomy (SCH)* (Fig. 43-12.1). The term *subtotal hysterectomy* is ambiguous and is not a preferred term.

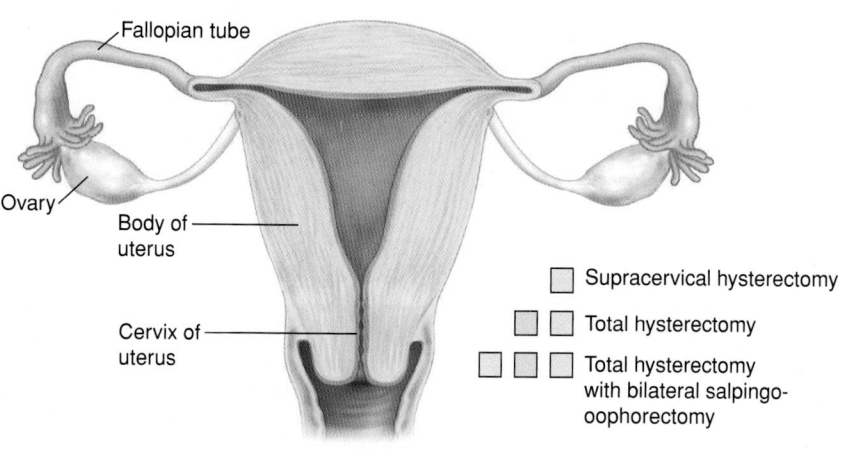

FIGURE 43-12.1 Hysterectomy classification.

Fallopian tube

Ovary

Body of uterus

Cervix of uterus

☐ Supracervical hysterectomy

☐ ☐ Total hysterectomy

☐ ☐ ☐ Total hysterectomy with bilateral salpingo-oophorectomy

Most hysterectomies performed are total, but SCH may be selected preoperatively. For example, SCH is purported to reduce the risk of mesh erosion at the cuff if concurrent hysterectomy and sacrocolpopexy are planned (Osmundsen, 2012; Tan-Kim, 2011). At one point, SCH was also suggested to improve urinary, bowel, or sexual function compared with total abdominal hysterectomy. But, several studies have shown no short- or long-term differences in these functions between total abdominal or supracervical hysterectomy (Learman, 2003; Lethaby, 2012; Thakar, 2002). Frequently, SCH may be an intraoperative decision during cases in which excision of the cervix risks increased bleeding, surrounding organ damage, or increased operating time.

As a disadvantage, 10 to 20 percent of women following SCH will still note cyclic vaginal bleeding, presumably from retained isthmic endometrium in the cervical stump. Procedures that ablate or core out the endocervical canal can help prevent this complication (Schmidt, 2011). Also, pelvic organ prolapse may develop (Hilger, 2005). For either complication, cervical stump excision, termed trachelectomy, may be required. Last, critics noted the persistent risk for cancer in the conserved stump. However, the risk for cervical cancer in these women is comparable to that in women without hysterectomy. Moreover, the prognosis for cervical stump cancer mirrors that in women with a complete uterus (Hannoun-Levi, 1997; Hellstrom, 2001).

In sum, SCH alone offers no distinct long-term advantages compared with total abdominal hysterectomy (American College of Obstetricians and Gynecologists, 2013b). The risk of persistent bleeding following surgery may deter many women and clinicians from its use. Moreover, although data are limited, trachelectomy following SCH may be surgically challenging due to scarring of bowel or bladder to the stump. Despite these disadvantages, if concurrent sacrocolpopexy is planned, SCH may lower mesh erosion rates. However, current data for this are limited and retrospective, and future research is needed.

Consent

For most women with indications, hysterectomy is a safe and effective treatment that typically leads to an improved postoperative quality of life and psychological outcome (Hartmann, 2004; Kuppermann, 2013). However, pelvic organs may be injured during surgery, and vascular, bladder, ureteral, and bowel injury are most commonly cited. Accordingly, these and the risks of wound infection, blood loss, and transfusion are discussed with the patient before surgery.

Infrequently, unintended adnexectomy may be required, and if bilateral, will create iatrogenic menopause. Importantly, patients should understand the sterilizing effects of hysterectomy.

Concurrent Adnexal Surgery

Hysterectomy is frequently performed with other operations. Pelvic reconstructive surgeries and bilateral salpingo-oophorectomy (BSO) or salpingectomy are among the most frequent.

Bilateral fallopian tubes and ovaries are prophylactically removed in approximately 40 percent of hysterectomy cases performed for benign indications in the United States (Asante, 2010). In a woman younger than 40 years, ovaries are typically conserved because continued estrogen production is expected until her late 40s. In those older than 50 years, BSO is common. However, for women in their 40s, the decision to prophylactically remove ovaries is controversial.

Proponents of prophylactic BSO between 40 and 50 argue that the procedure lowers future ovarian cancer risk and is estimated to prevent 1000 new cases of ovarian cancer each year (American College of Obstetricians and Gynecologists, 2014b). In addition, patients with retained ovaries may require future surgery for subsequent benign ovarian disease. This risk approximates 3 percent at 10 years posthysterectomy (Casiano, 2013). Specifically, women with endometriosis, pelvic inflammatory disease, and chronic pelvic pain are at greater risk for reoperation. And, if later oophorectomy is required, the risk of ureteral or bowel injury due to adhesions encasing the retained ovary is increased from that with primary BSO. Last, the duration of significant ovarian estrogen production for many will be shortened following hysterectomy. For example, Siddle and coworkers (1987) noted that the mean age of ovarian failure in a group undergoing hysterectomy was 45 years. This was significantly lower than the mean age of 49 years in a control group not receiving surgery.

However, arguments for ovarian conservation are convincing as well. If ovaries are retained during hysterectomy, ovarian cancer risk is still decreased 40 to 50 percent by the hysterectomy itself (Chiaffarino, 2005; Rice, 2013). Additionally, conservation delays the long-term effects of hypoestrogenism (Chap. 21, p. 474). Parker and colleagues (2013) noted higher ovarian and slightly elevated breast cancer rates but a lower all-cause mortality rate in women after hysterectomy with ovarian conservation compared with those electing BSO without estrogen replacement therapy (ERT). Although these rates became nearly equal in those electing BSO

and then receiving postoperative ERT, concerns regarding ERT compliance have been noted. Castelo-Branco and coworkers (1999) found that after 5 years following hysterectomy and BSO, only one third of patients still continued their ERT. Most stopped due to cancer concerns. In addition to loss of estrogen, ovarian androgen production is removed, and its importance in later life has not been entirely delineated (Olive, 2005). The American College of Obstetricians and Gynecologists (2014b) recommends strong consideration of ovarian retention in premenopausal women who are not at increased genetic risk for ovarian cancer. Trends in the United States show a significant decline in BSO rates for those younger than 55 (Novetsky, 2011; Perera, 2013).

Even if ovaries are conserved, the Society of Gynecologic Oncology (2013) encourages consideration of concurrent bilateral salpingectomy during hysterectomy. This practice is hoped to lower peritoneal serous carcinomas (Chap. 35, p. 738). That said, the degree of compromise of ovarian blood supply and long-term function by this resection is not fully known, and discussion of this point should be part of preoperative consenting.

Patient Preparation

Because of the risk of postoperative wound and urinary tract infection following hysterectomy, patients typically receive antibiotic prophylaxis with either a first- or second-generation cephalosporin (American College of Obstetricians and Gynecologists, 2014a). These and suitable alternatives are found in Table 39-6 (p. 835). As noted in Chapter 39 (p. 834), preoperative mechanical bowel preparation may be implemented depending on anticipated surgical circumstances. Fortunately, the risk of bowel injury with hysterectomy in general is low, and thus many forego evacuation measures for their patients. Laparotomy dictates venous thromboembolism prophylaxis, and options are found in Table 39-8 (p. 836).

INTRAOPERATIVE

Surgical Steps

❶ Anesthesia and Patient Positioning. Abdominal hysterectomy is typically performed under general or regional anesthesia. The patient is often supine. But if concomitant vaginal procedures are planned, the patient is placed in low lithotomy position in adjustable booted stirrups. After anesthesia induction, hair in the planned incision path is clipped if needed; a Foley catheter is inserted; and abdominal preparation is completed.

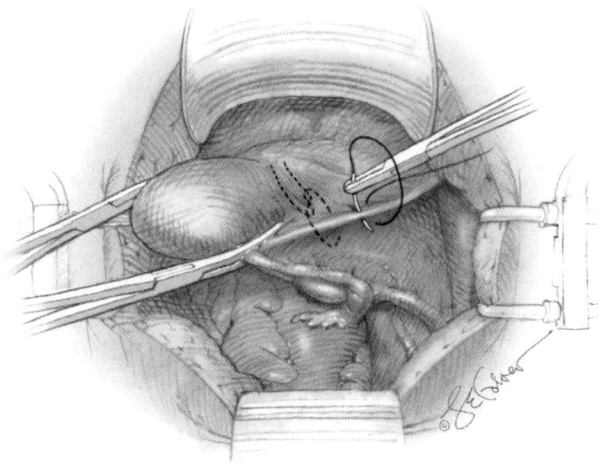

FIGURE 43-12.2 Round ligament ligation.

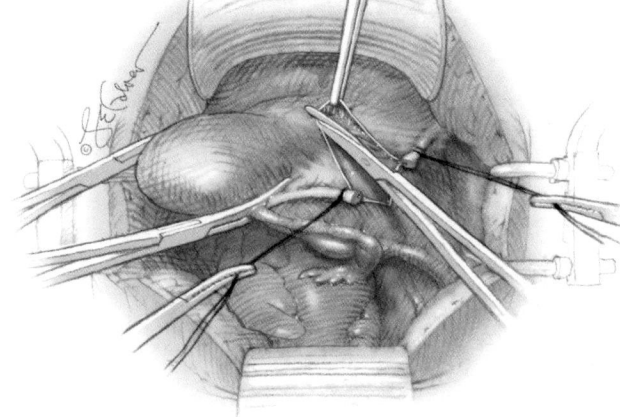

FIGURE 43-12.3 Opening of broad ligament anterior leaf.

❷ **Abdominal Entry.** Either a transverse or a vertical incision may be used for hysterectomy, and clinical factors influence selection (p. 926).

❸ **Exposure.** Following entry into the abdomen, a self-retaining retractor such as an O'Connor-O'Sullivan or a Balfour retractor is placed. The pelvis and abdomen are visually and manually explored, and the bowel is packed from the operating field. The uterus is grasped and elevated from the pelvis. If extensive adhesions are present, normal anatomic relationships are restored. Hysterectomy may be performed by one surgeon, but commonly two surgeons are present, with each typically operating on his or her side of the uterus.

❹ **Round Ligament Transection.** Curved Kelly (pean) clamps are placed immediately lateral to each uterine cornu to permit uterine manipulation. Hysterectomy begins with division of one round ligament at its midpoint (Fig. 43-12.2). This provides entry into the retroperitoneal space for ureter identification and access to the uterine artery and cardinal ligament for later transection. The round ligament is grasped with tissue forceps and elevated. A transfixing stitch using 0-gauge delayed-absorbable suture is placed approximately 1 cm lateral to the planned division site. The first bite of this stitch passes through an avascular site of the mesoteres beneath the round ligament, whereas the transfixing bite pierces the round ligament medial to first bite. This prevents hematoma formation between the transfixing stitch and pelvic sidewall. A second simple stitch of similar suture is placed 1 to 2 cm medial to the first and through an avascular site in the mesoteres and beneath the round ligament. These sutures prevent bleeding from Sampson artery and aid tissue manipulation. Once secured, sutures are held by hemostats and directed outward to create

tension along the interposed ligament. The round ligament is then divided, and the incision line is directed deeply into the first 1 to 2 cm of the broad ligament.

❺ **Anterior Broad Ligament Leaf.** With this action, the broad ligament separates to create anterior and posterior leaves. Between them, loose areolar connective tissue is seen. To incise the anterior leaf, the round ligament sutures are placed on tension. Metzenbaum scissors are introduced between the anterior leaf and underlying loose connective tissue. Both scissor tips are directed upward to be seen through the peritoneum as they advance. Gentle opening and closing of scissor blade tips during advancement separates the peritoneum from the underlying connective tissue. The tented anterior leaf is then incised sharply. The line of incision curves inferiorly and medially to the level of the vesicouterine

fold, which generally lies just below the uterine isthmus (Fig. 43-12.3).

Next, to further open the retroperitoneal space, the drape of peritoneum lying between the round ligament and infundibulopelvic (IP) ligament is grasped with smooth forceps and placed on tension. This peritoneum is incised with Metzenbaum scissors and with the same undermining technique used for the anterior leaf (Fig. 43-12.4). Lateral and parallel to the IP, the incision is extended cephalad toward the pelvic sidewall.

❻ **Ureter Identification.** This is accomplished by localized blunt dissection that is advanced downward with gentle cephalad and caudad strokes into gauzy retroperitoneal tissue above the presumed ureter path (Fig. 43-12.5). Dissection is directed downward, medially, and slightly cephalad toward the medial aspect of the posterior peritoneal

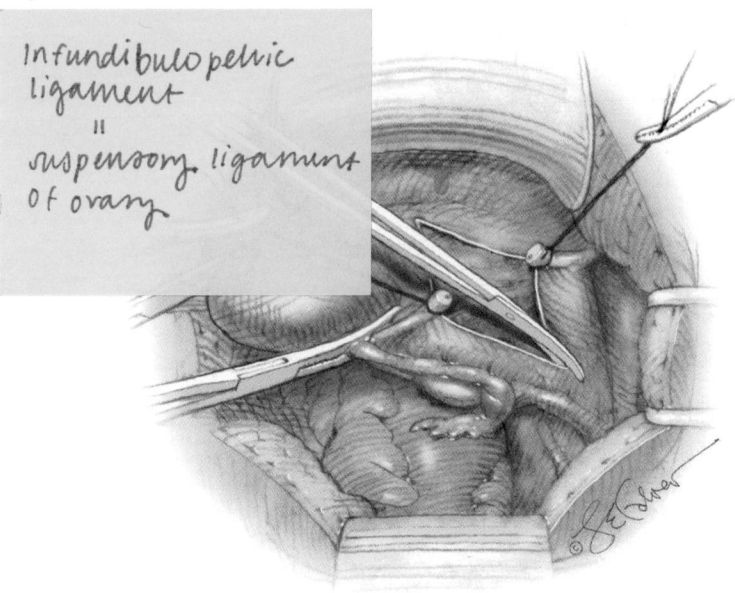

Infundibulopelvic ligament = suspensory ligament of ovary

FIGURE 43-12.4 Peritoneal incision extension.

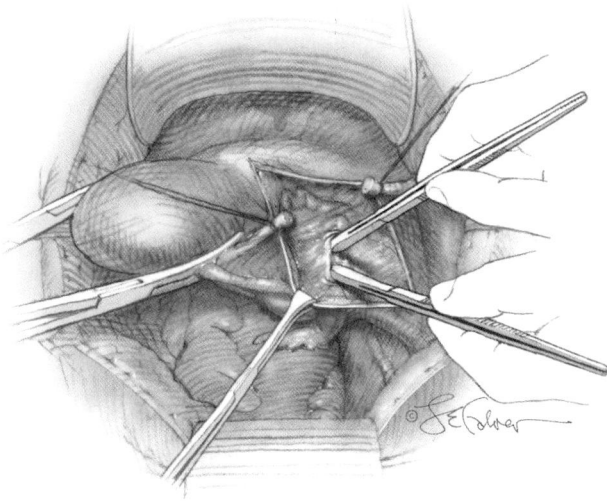

FIGURE 43-12.5 Ureter identification.

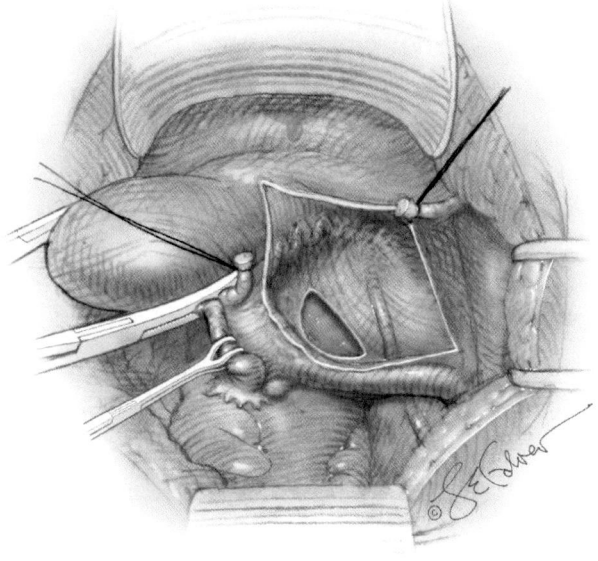

FIGURE 43-12.6 Posterior peritoneal window.

leaf, along which the ureter courses. Small vessels are coagulated as they are found.

❼ Posterior Broad Ligament Leaf. With the ureter directly visualized, the posterior peritoneal leaf is incised to create a window. If ovarian preservation is planned, this window is made beneath the uteroovarian ligament alone. If oophorectomy is planned, the posterior leaf of the broad ligament is incised parallel to the IP ligament. The incision is extended toward the pelvic brim and medially toward the uterus just below the uteroovarian ligament. This delineates the IP for ligation (Fig. 43-12.6).

❽ Adnexectomy. If the adnexa are to be removed, the fallopian tube and ovary are

grasped with a Babcock clamp and elevated medially to place the IP ligament on mild tension for improved delineation (Fig. 43-12.7). With the ureter visualized, a curved Heaney clamp can be placed around this ligament with its arc curving upward. The tips of the clamps are placed through the previously created peritoneal window. A Kelly clamp is placed medial to this and closer to the adnexa.

With clamps secured, the IP ligament is sharply transected above the Heaney clamp. A free tie of 0-gauge delayed-absorbable suture is placed around the Heaney clamp.

As the knot of this suture is secured, the Heaney clamp is quickly opened and closed, that is, "flashed." A transfixing stitch is then sutured below the clamp but above and distal to the first free tie. As the knot is cinched, the Heaney clamp is removed.

The adnexa is now freed from the pelvic sidewall, and its increased mobility may obstruct the surgeon's view. Accordingly, the adnexa can be tied to the Kelly clamp still located on the cornu. Alternatively, adnexa can be simply excised and removed.

❾ Ovarian Conservation. With the leaves of the broad ligament now open, if the ovary is to be preserved, then salpingectomy alone is now completed. This is fully described in Section 43-8 (p. 939). In summary, the mesosalpinx is serially clamped, cut, and ligated. Each clamp incorporates approximately 2 cm of mesosalpinx, and resection progresses from the fimbria to its union with the uterus.

To preserve the ovary, one Kelly clamp is already positioned at the cornu and across the uteroovarian ligament. A Heaney clamp is positioned lateral to this, and its arc faces the uterus (Fig. 43-12.8).

The intervening segment of uteroovarian ligament is incised between the Heaney and Kelly clamps. Ligation of the ligament is carried out as in Step 8. That is, a free tie of 0-gauge delayed-absorbable suture is placed around the Heaney clamp. As the knot is secured, the clamp is flashed. A transfixing stitch is then placed around the same clamp but distal to the first free tie. As the knot is cinched, the Heaney clamp is removed. The ovary is now freed from the uterus and can be placed laterally near the pelvic sidewall. The

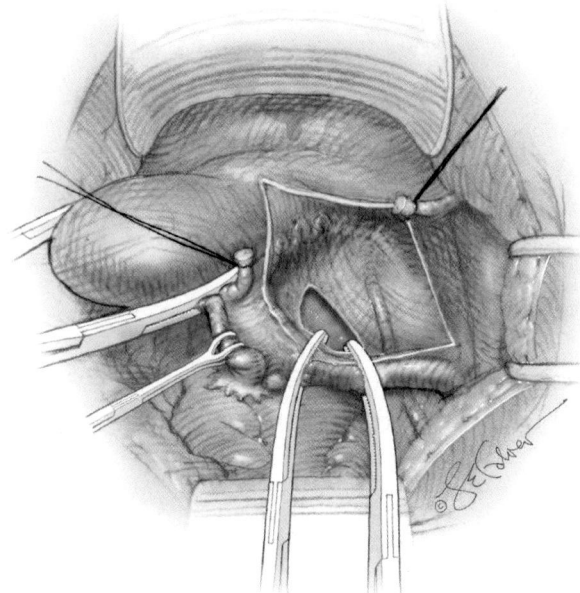

FIGURE 43-12.7 Infundibulopelvic ligament transection during oophorectomy.

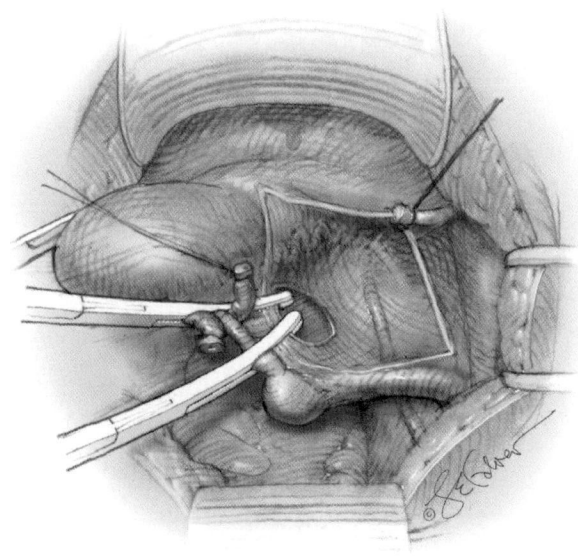

FIGURE 43-12.8 Uteroovarian ligament transection for ovarian conservation.

Kelly clamp is left in place at the cornu to prevent bleeding and allow uterine manipulation.

🔟 **Bladder Flap.** Steps 4 through 9 are completed bilaterally, and attention is next turned to the bladder. To avoid urinary tract injury, the bladder is moved caudad and away from the cervix. This is accomplished by first opening the vesicouterine space, the potential space between the bladder and cervix. Several techniques may be used, and at our institution, sharp dissection is preferred (Fig. 43-12.9). This method is particularly beneficial for patients with prior cesarean deliveries who may have scarring between the bladder and cervix. Alternatively, gentle blunt pressure from fingers or sponge stick can be used. Such pressure is directed beneath the bladder, against the cervix, and caudad. With either dissection method, taut uterine elevation creates helpful tension across the tissue planes to be separated. Tension is created by pulling upward on the Kelly clamps, previously placed at the cornua.

The peritoneum at the vesicouterine fold was previously incised bilaterally in Step 5. During dissection in the vesicouterine space, this peritoneum is grasped with atraumatic tissue forceps and elevated to create tension between it and the underlying cervix. Only loose connective tissue strands lie in this space, and they are easily cut with Metzenbaum scissors. Incision of these bands is kept close to the cervix to avoid cystotomy. Dissection in the midline minimizes laceration of vessels that course within the vesicocervical ligaments, colloquially termed *bladder pillars*. Once the correct plane is entered, the pearly white cervix and anterior vaginal wall are clearly differentiated from reddish bladder fibers.

The bladder is ideally dissected off the anterior vaginal wall at least 1 cm below the lower margin of the cervix. This averts incorporating bladder fibers within sutures or clamps placed during cuff closure. Thereby, bladder and distal ureteral injury, and later genitourinary fistulas, are prevented.

⓫ **Uterine Arteries.** The uterine artery and vein(s) are identified laterally along the uterus. At the level of the isthmus, some posterior peritoneum and loose areolar tissue still surrounds these vessels. Incising and removing such tissue from around any vessel is termed *skeletonizing*. This ultimately creates a smaller vascular pedicle and minimizes risks for vessel retraction during ligation.

To skeletonize, a surgeon individually grasps excess strips of perivascular connective tissue with fine smooth forceps and gently retracts them laterally and away from the uterine artery or vein. Metzenbaum scissors incise this tissue close to and parallel to the vessel, beginning superiorly and proceeding inferiorly. During this process, the remaining posterior broad ligament peritoneum is similarly incised parallel and close to the uterus (Fig. 43-12.10). Importantly, this step further "drops" the ureter away from the path of subsequent clamps.

Once skeletonized, the uterine vessels are clamped by a curved Heaney clamp at the uterine isthmus level. The clamp tips are placed horizontally across the vertical uterine vessels (Fig. 43-12.11). A Kelly clamp is placed medial and more vertical to the first

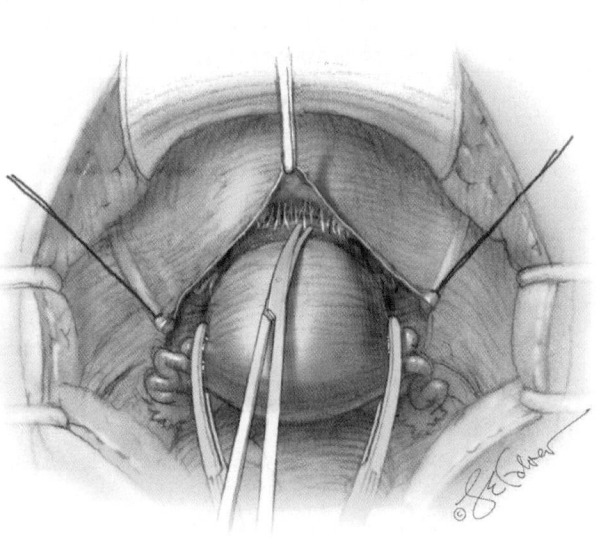

FIGURE 43-12.9 Dissection within vesicouterine space.

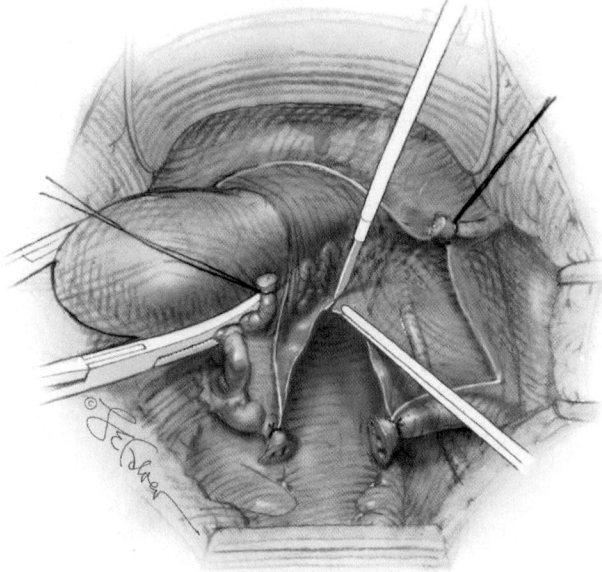

FIGURE 43-12.10 Uterine artery skeletonization.

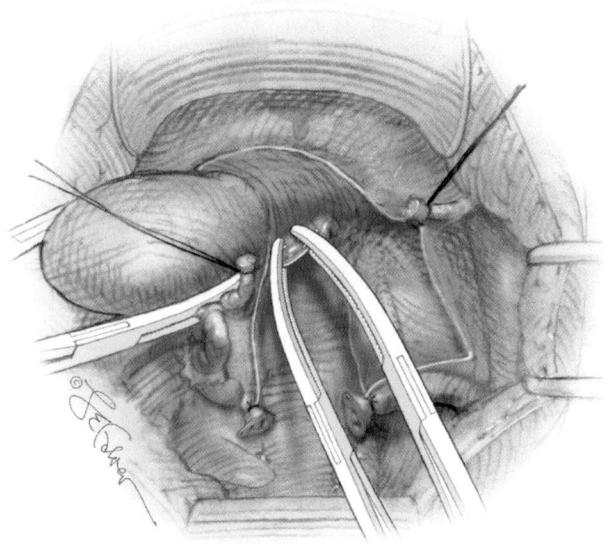

FIGURE 43-12.11 Clamps across uterine artery.

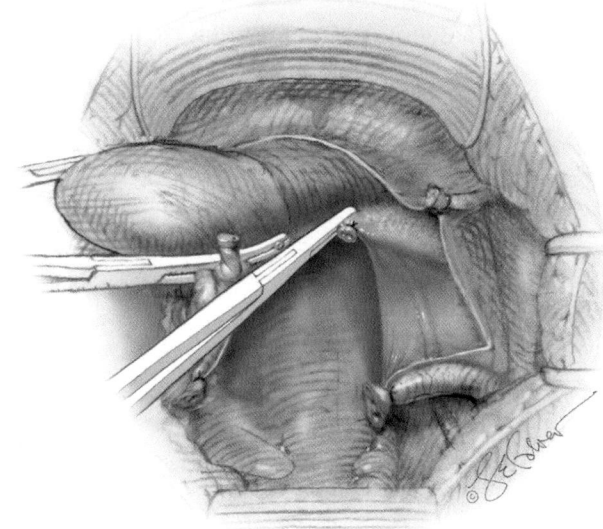

FIGURE 43-12.12 Clamp across cardinal ligament.

clamp and hugs the lateral uterus to prevent bleeding from severed vessels. Tissue between the clamps is then cut.

A simple stitch of 0-gauge delayed-absorbable suture is placed below the Heaney clamp's tip, and the suture ends are wrapped to the clamp's heel. As the knot is cinched, the Heaney clamp is slowly opened and removed. The Kelly clamp remains.

⑫ **Fundal Amputation.** After bilateral uterine artery ligation, if the uterus is large and bulky, the uterine fundus may be sharply severed from the cervix. After removal of the corpus, Kocher clamps are placed on the anterior and posterior walls of cervix for manipulation.

If supracervical hysterectomy is planned, no further transection is required. In premenopausal women, the upper endocervical canal is coagulated or removed by wedge resection to help avoid postoperative cyclic bleeding. The cervical stump is closed and rendered hemostatic with figure-of-eight stitches using 0-gauge delayed-absorbable suture. Each stitch passes through the posterior peritoneum, the posterior wall of the cervix, and then the anterior wall of the cervix before ligation. Conversely, if the cervical stroma is hemostatic, no suturing may be required.

⑬ **Cardinal and Uterosacral Ligament Transection.** These ligaments lie lateral to the uterus and inferior to the uterine vessels. A straight Heaney clamp is positioned across the cardinal ligament adjacent to the cervix and medial to the uterine artery pedicle (Fig. 43-12.12). As the Heaney clamp initially grasps the ligament, it is oriented parallel to the lateral side of the uterus. As the clamp is slowly closed, it is angled slightly away from the vertical axis of the cervix. A scalpel is

used to transect the portion of the cardinal ligament medial to the clamp. A transfixing stitch of 0-gauge delayed-absorbable suture is placed below the clamp, and the clamp is removed as the knot is cinched. For smaller bites through the cardinal ligament, a simple stitch without transfixion may suffice.

Depending on the ligament length, the above step may be repeated several times. In this manner, the cardinal ligament is transected and ligated from its superior to inferior extent down the lateral aspect of the cervix to the level of the upper vagina. When this is near completion, the uterosacral ligaments remain as final support structures attached to the cervix. These ligaments are more easily felt and seen by placing upward traction on the uterus. In most benign cases, these liga-

ments are incorporated within instruments used to clamp across the lower cardinal ligament and proximal vagina.

⑭ **Vagina Transection.** For this step, the surgeon's hand palpates through the anterior and posterior vaginal walls to identify the most inferior level of the cervix. Here, a curved Heaney clamp incorporates the uterosacral ligament and is placed across the anterior and posterior vaginal walls just below the cervix on one side. This is repeated on the other side, and the tips often meet in the midline (Fig. 43-12.13). Importantly, the bladder must be sufficiently mobilized away from this point to prevent injury.

The vaginal tissue above the level of these clamps is then transected. This procedure

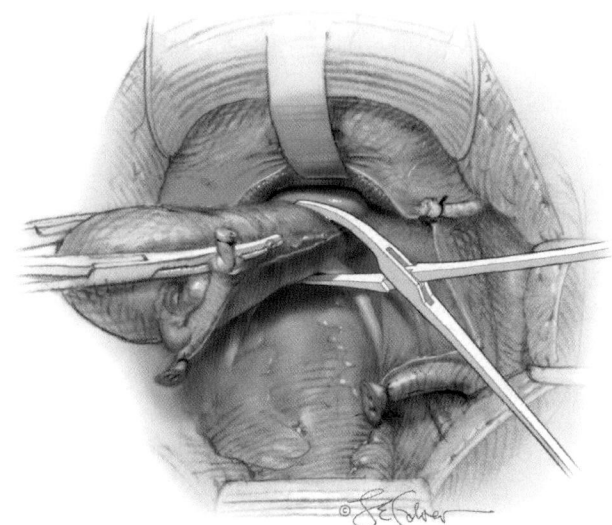

FIGURE 43-12.13 Clamp incorporating uterosacral ligament and proximal vagina.

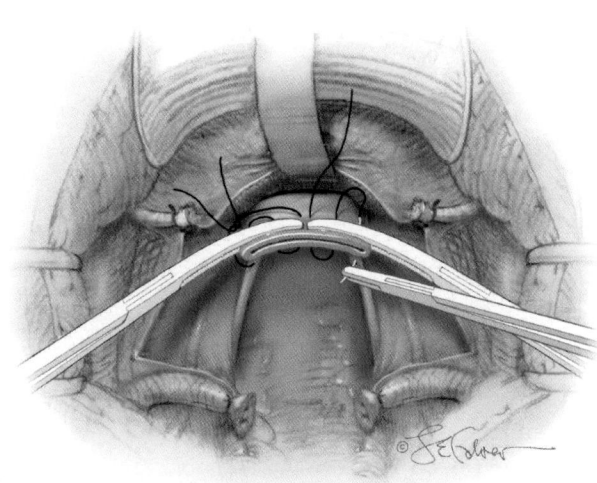

FIGURE 43-12.14 Clamps across proximal vagina. Two transfixing stitches for cuff closure.

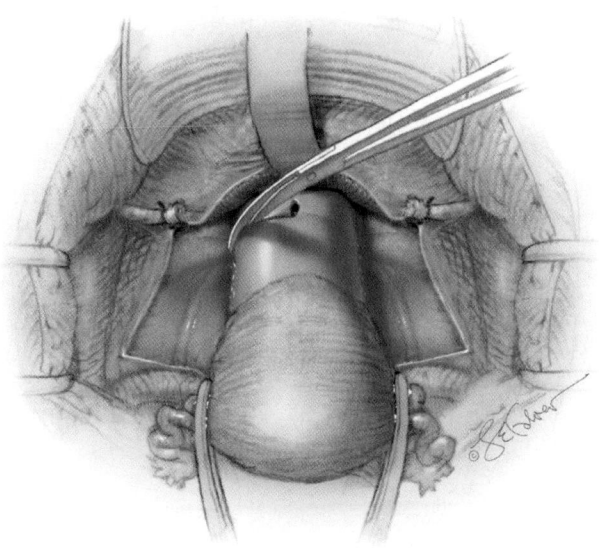

FIGURE 43-12.15 Circumferential vaginal incision.

frees the uterus from the pelvis. Transfixing sutures are placed below the Heaney clamps, and the clamps are removed (Fig. 43-12.14).

⓯ Vaginal Entry. During some cases, the cervix may be poorly appreciated between the vaginal walls. To avoid shortening the vagina or leaving cervix behind, the vagina can be entered to identify the cervix. For this, a small longitudinal incision is made in the midline of the upper anterior vaginal wall. A finger is inserted to palpate the cervical margin. Once this level is known, one blade of Jorgensen scissors is inserted into the vagina and positioned just below the cervix (Fig. 43-12.15). At this level, the vagina is then circumferentially cut. Kocher or Allis clamps are placed along the free cut vaginal edge as it forms.

⓰ Vaginal Cuff Closure. For support, a 0-gauge delayed-absorbable suture may be placed to suspend the vaginal apex to the uterosacral ligament pedicle on either side (Fig. 43-12.16). This stitch incorporates the anterior and posterior vaginal walls with the distal portion of the uterosacral ligament and helps prevent vaginal cuff prolapse following surgery.

These sutures are kept long and held by hemostats. Upward and lateral traction elevates the vaginal cuff. The full thicknesses of the incised anterior and posterior vaginal walls are then reapproximated with a running suture line using 0-gauge delayed-absorbable suture or with several figure-of-eight sutures. The peritoneum overlying the

posterior vaginal margin should be included in this closure to lessen the risk of postoperative oozing. Anteriorly, the bladder should be kept clear of the suture line. Once the vaginal cuff is hemostatic, the lateral suspending cuff sutures are cut.

⓱ Wound Closure. The abdominal incision is closed as described in Section 43-1 or 43-2 (p. 928).

POSTOPERATIVE

Postoperative care follows that for laparotomy, although sexual intercourse is usually delayed until 6 weeks after surgery to permit satisfactory vaginal cuff healing (p. 928).

Febrile morbidity is common following abdominal hysterectomy and exceeds that seen with vaginal or laparoscopic approaches (Peipert, 2004). Frequently, fever is unexplained. But, pelvic infections are common, and other sources of postoperative fever should be evaluated (Chap. 42, p. 919). Because of the high rate of unexplained fever, which resolves spontaneously, observation for 24 to 48 hours for mild temperature elevations is reasonable. Alternatively, antibiotic treatment may be initiated, and appropriate choices are found in Table 3-20 (p. 79). Additional testing, including transvaginal sonography or computed tomography (CT), may be indicated if a pelvic hematoma or abscess is suspected.

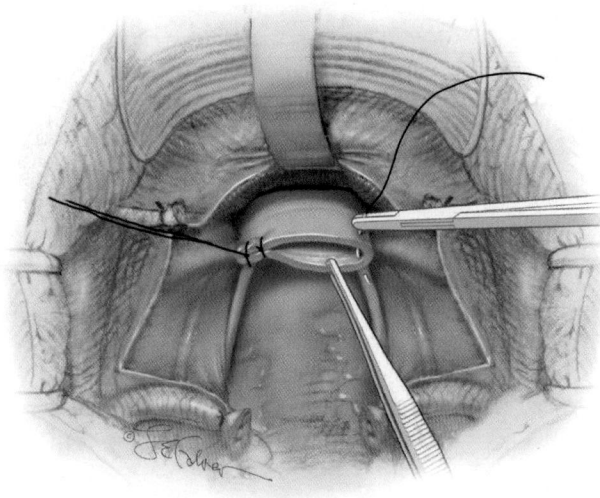

FIGURE 43-12.16 Vaginal cuff closure incorporating uterosacral ligament.

43-13

Vaginal Hysterectomy

In general, this approach is chosen by surgeons if the uterus is relatively small, extensive adhesions are not anticipated, no significant adnexal pathology is expected, and some degree of pelvic organ descent is present. Compared with abdominal hysterectomy, patients undergoing vaginal hysterectomy usually benefit from faster recovery and from reduced hospital stays, costs, and postoperative pain. During selection of hysterectomy approach described on page 950, if all factors are equal, then vaginal hysterectomy is preferred.

PREOPERATIVE

Patient evaluation, consenting, and patient preparation are similar to that for abdominal hysterectomy (p. 950).

INTRAOPERATIVE

Surgical Steps

❶ **Anesthesia and Patient Positioning.** After adequate general or regional anesthesia is administered, the patient is placed in standard dorsal lithotomy position (Fig. 40-4, p. 845). The vagina is surgically prepared, and the bladder is drained. Some surgeons may prefer to wait until the anterior peritoneum is entered before inserting a Foley catheter. This permits a gush of urine to signal inadvertent bladder laceration. Along the posterior vaginal wall, a short Auvard weighted vaginal speculum is placed, and a right-angle or other suitable retractor is placed anteriorly.

❷ **Vaginal Wall Incision.** To begin, one Lahey-thyroid clamp is used to grasp the anterior cervical lip, while a second one holds the posterior lip. For a smaller cervix, one clamp may easily grasp both lips together. The junction between the cervix and the anterior and posterior vaginal walls can be seen and palpated by in-and-out displacement of the cervix. Just proximal to this junction, a circumferential incision is made around the cervix and is guided by anatomy (Fig. 43-13.1). For example, if the cervix is flush with the vagina, then incision lies close to the remaining cervix to avoid rectal injury. In general, the incision is kept at a depth superficial to the cervical stroma to avert dissection into the cervix. To minimize blood loss during dissection, 10 to 15 mL of a dilute saline solution containing vasopressin (20 U diluted in 30–100 mL of saline) or 0.5-percent lidocaine and epinephrine (1:200,000 dilution) may be injected circumferentially along the incision path.

❸ **Posterior Entry.** Although described first here, the sequence of anterior and posterior entry is based on surgeon preference and intraoperative findings. The Lahey-thyroid clamp and cervix are lifted anteriorly to expose the posterior vaginal vault, and an Allis clamp is placed below the circumcised edge of the posterior vaginal wall. Downward traction on the Allis clamp creates tension across the incision. Curved Mayo scissors positioned across the incision line cut to enter the cul-de-sac of Douglas (Fig. 43-13.2). The posterior peritoneum may be affixed centrally to the posterior vaginal wall incision with a single stitch of delayed-absorbable suture. This approximation will assist with closure of the peritoneum at the procedure's end. The short Auvard speculum is replaced by one with a longer blade, which enters the cul-de-sac.

❹ **Anterior Peritoneal Entry.** This is generally considered the most challenging step of vaginal hysterectomy. First, the anterior vaginal wall is grasped near the circumferential incision in the midline and elevated with an Allis clamp. Tension is concurrently created by outward traction on the cervical Lahey-thyroid clamps. This traction reveals fibrous connective tissue bands connecting the bladder and cervix. These bands fill the vesicocervical space, which is typically 3 cm long (Balgobin, unpublished data). Although the proximal part of this space contains loose arcolar tissue, the distal portion contains

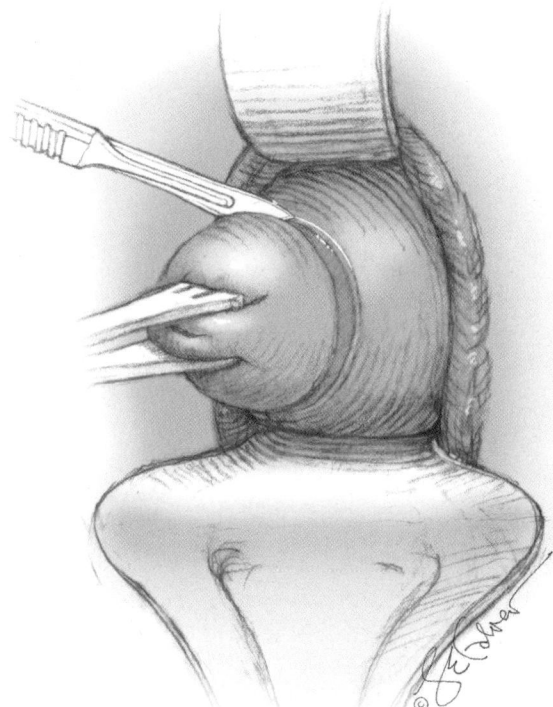

FIGURE 43-13.1 Circumferential cervical incision.

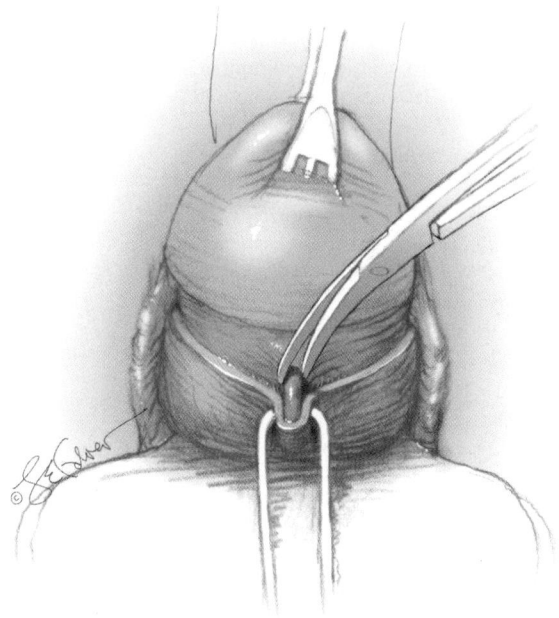

FIGURE 43-13.2 Entry into the cul-de-sac of Douglas.

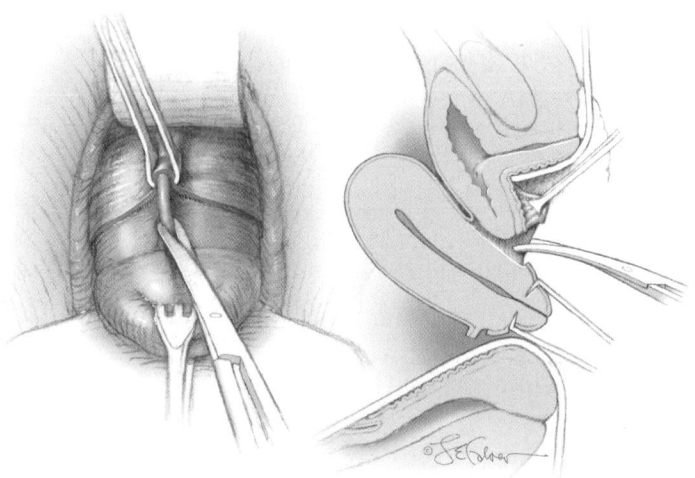

FIGURE 43-13.3 Sharp dissection of vesicouterine septum from two views.

thicker fibers. This knowledge permits calm, persistent dissection through this dense tissue rather than prematurely reorienting dissection, which risks "digging" into the cervix.

At our institution, sharp dissection is preferred (Fig. 43-13.3). This method is particularly beneficial for patients with prior cesarean deliveries, who may have scarring between the bladder and cervix. With traction established, the fibers are incised in the midline with Metzenbaum scissors. Tips are kept close and almost parallel to the cervix as dissection is extended cephalad. Bleeding vessels are frequently encountered during initial dissection and are coagulated. After the initial fibers are transected, gentle palpation with the index finger should indicate whether the upper part of the vesicocervical space has been reached. In the absence of scar tissue, these fibers are easily broken, and gentle blunt dissection is advanced cephalad until the vesicouterine fold is palpated. Alternatively, the entire vesicocervical space dissection can be completed with gentle blunt pressure from an index finger covered in surgical gauze. Such pressure is directed against the cervix and cephalad toward the vesicouterine fold.

This fold is a thin and transparent transverse peritoneal fold at the upper border of the cervix. With palpation, this smooth layer glides against the uterine serosa. This peritoneum is grasped with atraumatic tissue forceps, placed on tension, and incised (see Fig. 43-13.3). In cases with difficult anterior entry, the surgeon may enter the posterior cul-de-sac and wrap an index finger anteriorly to palpate and accentuate the vesicouterine fold for anterior entry.

Following vesicouterine fold incision, an index finger explores the opening to confirm peritoneal entry, exclude cystotomy, and identify unanticipated pelvic pathology. This finger then guides a curved Deaver retractor

into the opening to elevate the bladder and anterior vaginal wall.

❺ Transection of Uterosacral and Cardinal Ligaments. Outward traction on the Lahey-thyroid clamps pulls the supporting uterine ligaments into view. Such traction, along with upward bladder displacement, helps prevent ureteral injury. The uterosacral and cardinal ligaments are identified, clamped with a curved Heaney clamp, transected, and ligated with 0-gauge delayed-absorbable suture using a transfixing stitch (Fig. 43-13.4). Once the knot of this pedicle is tied, the suture ends are not cut but kept long for later identification. This step is then repeated on the opposite side.

Depending on the cardinal ligament length, similar clamping, cutting, and suturing may

need to be repeated. Advancement is cephalad, and along each side and parallel to the cervix. Each sequential clamp is placed medial to the prior pedicle to reduce ureteral injury risk.

❻ Uterine Arteries. The uterine artery is identified on one side and clamped with a curved Heaney clamp. The clamp is placed nearly perpendicular to the long axis of the uterus and medial to the prior cardinal ligament pedicle (Fig. 43-13.5). The tips should firmly abut the uterus to ensure enclosure of entire artery and vein(s) within the clamp. A more laterally placed clamp may not be completely enclose the artery. Following pedicle transection, a simple stitch is placed around the clamp and is secured at the clamp heel as the instrument is removed. Uterine arteries are ligated bilaterally.

❼ Cornua. Progressing cephalad, curved Heaney clamps are next placed across the round and uteroovarian ligaments and fallopian tube (Fig. 43-13.6). After transection, a simple stitch of 0-gauge delayed-absorbable suture is placed proximally around the clamp. As the knot is secured, the Heaney clamp is quickly flashed. A transfixing stitch is then sutured around the clamp and positioned distal to the first stitch. As this knot is cinched, the Heaney clamp is removed. This transection is repeated bilaterally. With ovarian preservation, these sutures are cut short after confirming pedicle hemostasis. However, for adnexectomy, the transfixing suture tails may be kept long to allow gentle traction to bring the adnexa toward the vagina.

For the above step, if the uterus is larger, the uteroovarian ligament and tube may be

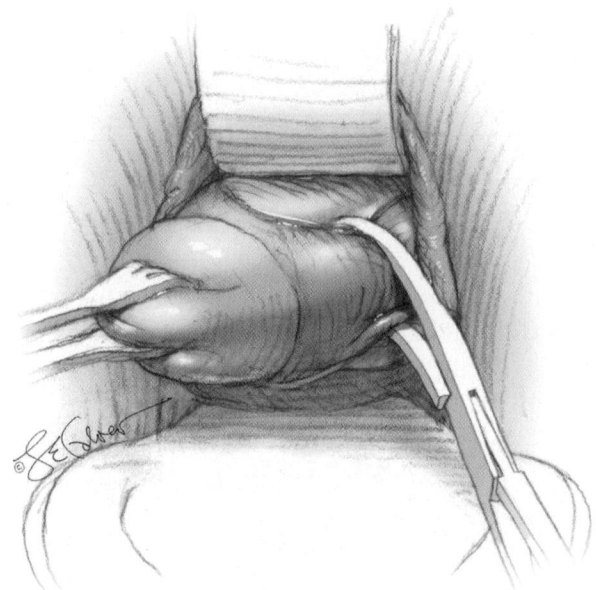

FIGURE 43-13.4 Clamp incorporating uterosacral and cardinal ligaments.

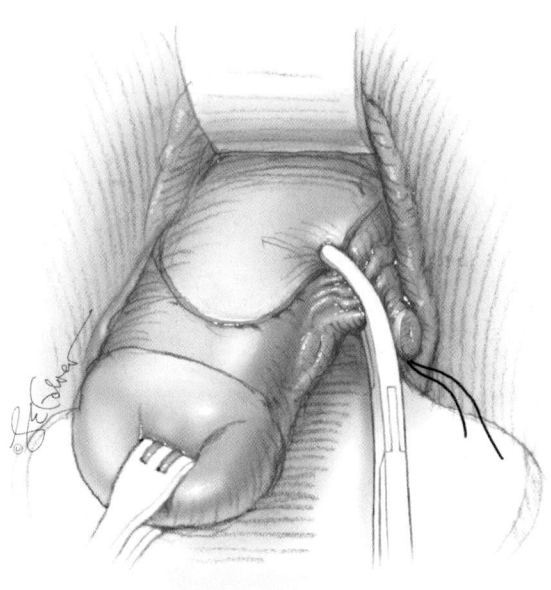

FIGURE 43-13.5 Clamp across uterine vessels.

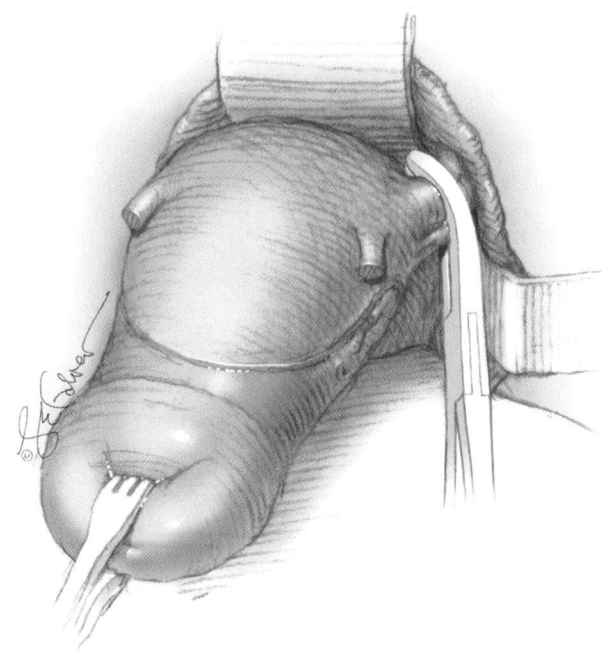

FIGURE 43-13.6 Clamp across uteroovarian ligament and fallopian tube.

difficult to reach and clamp. For this, the uterine corpus may be delivered through the posterior colpotomy incision to better expose these. To deliver the fundus, a tenaculum is placed on the upper posterior uterine wall, and it gently pulls the fundus into the vagina. Excessive traction may result in tissue avulsion and bleeding. Conversely, if the uterus is small and descent is adequate, the uteroovarian

and round ligaments and fallopian tube may be combined together in one curved Heaney clamp (Fig. 43-13.7). The pedicle is doubly ligated with a simple suture first placed proximally and then with a transfixing stitch placed distally.

With ovarian preservation, some recommend consideration of bilateral salpingectomy to lower high-grade peritoneal and

ovarian serous carcinoma rates. However, during vaginal hysterectomy, complete resection of the tube is typically more challenging than during abdominal approaches, and iatrogenic bleeding may lead to oophorectomy or conversion to laparotomy. If tube removal is desired, then adjunctive laparoscopic salpingectomy may be considered to ease safe removal of the entire tube.

❽ **Morcellation.** In some cases, the uterine fundus may be too large to deliver, and uterine debulking is required prior to ligation of the cornual attachments. This is performed only after both uterine artery pedicles have been secured.

One technique bisects the uterus using curved Mayo scissors, beginning at the cervix and moving toward the fundus. Near completion, fingers placed through the anterior colpotomy incision and behind the fundus help prevent scissor injury to adjacent organs (Fig. 43-13.8). Once completed, one half is elevated out of the operating field and into the pelvic cavity, whereas the other is brought into view for clamp placement across the uteroovarian and round ligaments and fallopian tube (Fig. 43-13.9). Other methods either enucleate individual large leiomyomas or involve cervix-to-fundus central coring to remove volume (Fig. 43-13.10). Once bulk is diminished, a Heaney clamp may be placed around the cornual structures as described in Step 7.

❾ **Adnexectomy.** For this, the adnexa is grasped with a Babcock clamp and gently pulled inferiorly and toward the contralateral side of the incision. This creates mild tension

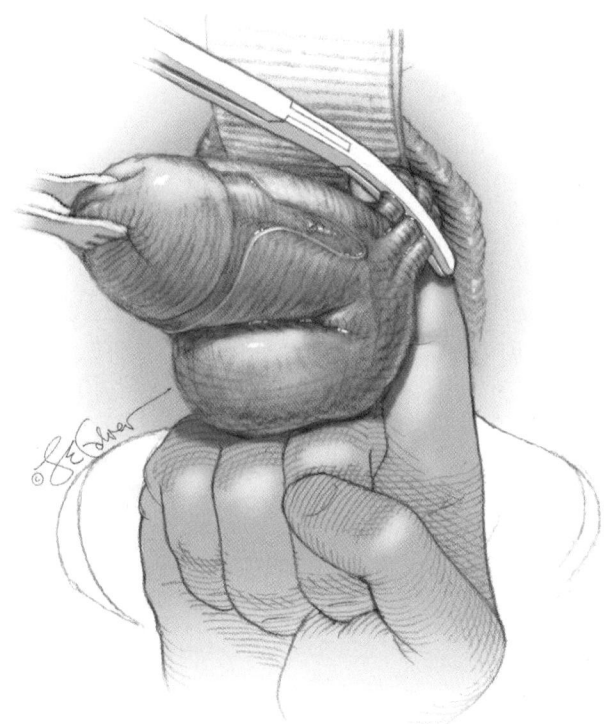

FIGURE 43-13.7 Fundal inversion to permit cornual structure clamping.

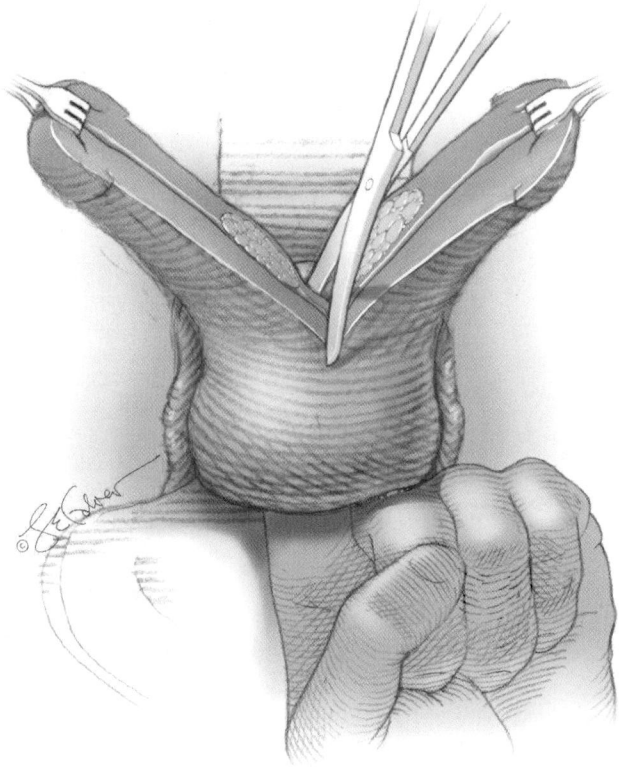

FIGURE 43-13.8 Uterus bisected.

FIGURE 43-13.9 Clamp across cornual structures.

on the infundibulopelvic (IP) ligament for improved delineation. To expand the operating field, a right-angle or similar retractor is positioned deep into the incision for vaginal sidewall retraction. This is coupled with upward traction from the originally placed anterior wall retractor.

A curved Heaney clamp is placed around the IP ligament, and its blades cover the entire pedicle width. For difficult angles, the surgeon's contralateral hand can push the ligament into correct position within the clamp. Prior to clamp closure, the surgeon confirms that no bowel or omentum is incor-

porated and that the entire ovary lies distal to the clamp. A moist sponge stick and slight Trendelenburg positioning can push the bowel away from the operative field.

The IP ligament is then clamped and transected (Fig. 43-13.11). First, a free tie of 0-gauge delayed-absorbable suture is placed

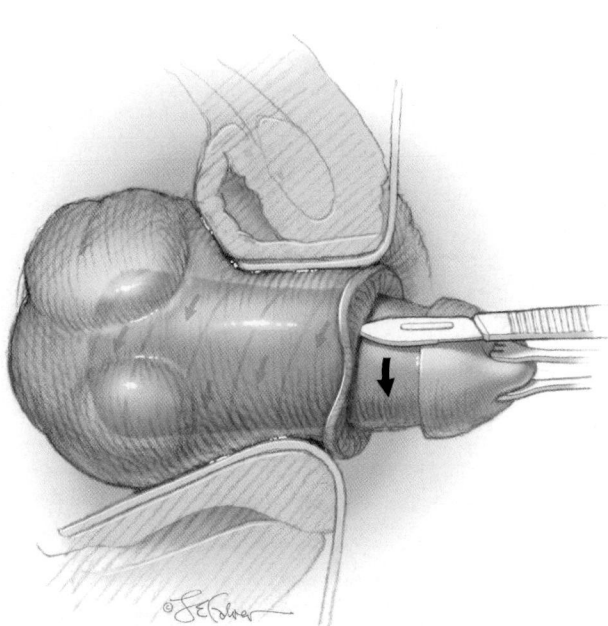

FIGURE 43-13.10 Coring of central uterine bulk.

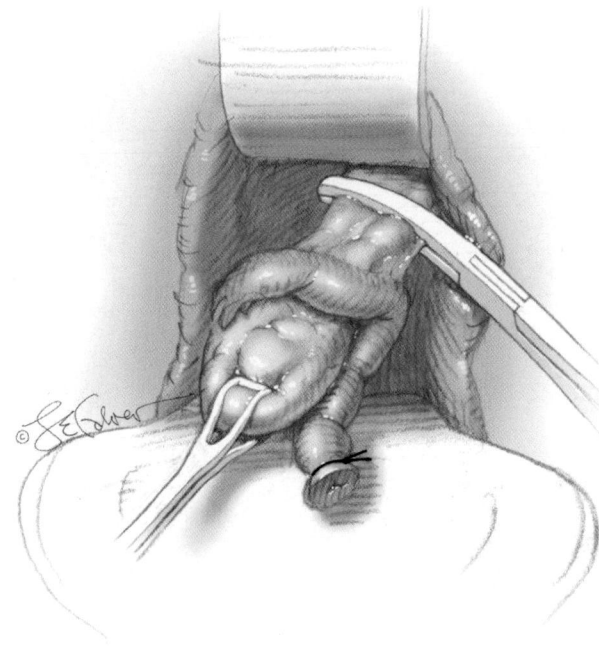

FIGURE 43-13.11 Clamp across infundibulopelvic ligament.

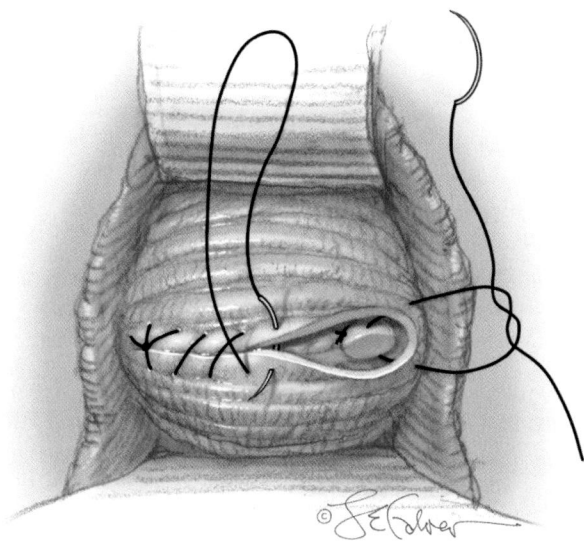

FIGURE 43-13.12 Vaginal cuff closure.

around the Heaney clamp. As the knot is secured, the clamp is flashed. A transfixing stitch is then placed around the same clamp but distal to the first free tie. As the knot is cinched, the Heaney clamp is removed. Excess traction on this pedicle is avoided to prevent avulsion or retraction of the ligament from the clamp. In such cases, resultant retroperitoneal bleeding may be difficult to control vaginally. Once hemostasis is ensured, the suture is cut. The opposite IP ligament is similarly clamped and transected.

⑩ Evaluation of Hemostasis. Following removal of the uterus, the surgical pedicles are inspected for bleeding. Electrosurgical coagulation or figure-of-eight sutures will typically control bleeding from discrete points. If indicated or preferred, a McCall culdoplasty may be performed (Section 45-22, p. 1116).

⑪ Vaginal Cuff Closure. The anterior and posterior vaginal walls are usually reapproximated by a horizontal suture line with interrupted or continuous running stitches of 0-gauge delayed-absorbable material. If short vaginal length is a concern, walls can be closed by a vertical suture line.

To help prevent later vaginal apex prolapse, the uterosacral ligament pedicles are incorporated within the cuff closure. For this, the interrupted or continuous running closure suture is initially passed through the anterior vaginal wall, through the ligament, through the posterior peritoneum, and finally through the posterior vaginal wall on one side (Fig. 43-13.12). This is repeated on the other side. Suturing then progresses from each side to the midline, or a single running suture may close the entire cuff line. During cuff closure, full thickness bites through the vaginal wall are taken. Also, the posterior peritoneum is incorporated with the closure to minimize risks of bleeding and cuff hematoma.

POSTOPERATIVE

In general, patients who undergo vaginal hysterectomy compared with abdominal hysterectomy, typically have faster return of normal bowel function, easier ambulation, and decreased analgesia requirements. Although diet and most activities are advanced quickly, intercourse is delayed for 6 weeks to permit vaginal cuff healing. Evaluation and treatment of postoperative complications mirrors that for abdominal hysterectomy.

43-14

Trachelectomy

For many women who have had supracervical hysterectomy, later surgical removal of the cervix, termed *trachelectomy*, is often indicated for complaints of vault prolapse, persistent cyclic bleeding, or preinvasive cervical lesions (Pasley, 1988). Hilger and associates (2005) reported on 335 women who underwent trachelectomy between 1974 and 2003. In half of them, trachelectomy was performed, on average, 26 years after supracervical hysterectomy. Of surgical indications, prolapse and pelvic mass are the most frequent. Bleeding accounts for nearly 10 percent of cases (Hilger, 2005; Kho, 2011).

The cervix may be removed either vaginally or abdominally, but for most women without concurrent pelvic pathology, vaginal trachelectomy is preferred (Pratt, 1976). With the resurgence of supracervical hysterectomy, now performed via laparoscopy, rates of trachelectomy for benign causes may rise.

Trachelectomy for benign indications is described here. Radical trachelectomy for invasive cervical cancer is gaining acceptance and is described in Chapter 30 (p. 670).

PREOPERATIVE

Patient Evaluation

As with hysterectomy, women require preoperative Pap test screening to exclude cervical cancer. Microscopic examination of cervicovaginal secretions will identify infections that merit treatment before surgery.

Consent

As with vaginal hysterectomy, patients are at risk for urinary tract and bowel injury. Similarly, postsurgical vaginal cuff complications may include hematoma, abscess, and cellulitis. Fortunately, complications are infrequent for most. Although Pratt and Jeffries (1976) noted complications in 91 of 262 patients, complication rates in several series range below 10 percent (Riva, 1961; Welch, 1959).

Patient Preparation

Entry into the peritoneal cavity is common during trachelectomy. Accordingly, as with vaginal hysterectomy, prophylaxis against postoperative infection and venous thromboembolism is warranted. Appropriate choices

are found in Tables 39-6 and 39-8 (p. 835). Enemas the evening prior to surgery aid in evacuation of the rectum.

INTRAOPERATIVE

Surgical Steps

❶ Anesthesia and Patient Positioning. Trachelectomy is performed as an inpatient procedure under general or regional anesthesia. The patient is placed in a standard dorsal lithotomy position, the vagina is surgically prepared, and a Foley catheter is placed.

❷ Incision and Extraperitoneal Dissection. The beginning steps of trachelectomy mirror those for vaginal hysterectomy (Step 2, p. 957). However, unlike vaginal hysterectomy, because the cervical stump lies outside the peritoneum, entry into the peritoneal cavity is not required for trachelectomy. Accordingly, once circumcision of the vaginal wall around the cervix is completed, dissection proceeds to the vesicouterine fold but without peritoneal entry.

In many cases, the bladder is more densely adhered to the anterior cervix, and the clear tissue planes often encountered during vaginal hysterectomy are absent. Moreover, if at completion of the original hysterectomy, the peritoneum was reapprox-

imated to cover the cervical stump, then the bladder may be draped over and scarred to the apex of the stump as well. For this reason, dissection of the vaginal wall, bladder, and rectum from the surface of the cervix typically requires sharp rather than blunt dissection (Fig. 43-14.1). As with vaginal hysterectomy, outward traction on the cervix in combination with counter traction of the vaginal wall aids dissection. To avoid cystotomy and proctotomy, scissor blades and dissecting pressure are directed against the cervix.

❸ Transection of Uterosacral and Cardinal Ligaments. Once dissected free from the vaginal wall, the uterosacral and cardinal ligaments are clamped and ligated as with vaginal hysterectomy (Fig. 43-14.2). The cervical branches of the uterine artery are typically clamped and ligated with the cardinal ligament. Depending on cervical length, serial transection and ligation of the cardinal ligament is continued cephalad until the stump apex is reached.

❹ Stump Excision and Cuff Closure. Once the apex is reached, sharp dissection across the top of the stump will free it from the vagina (Fig. 43-14.3). Next, incorporation of the uterosacral ligaments and reapproximation of the vaginal walls follows that for vaginal hysterectomy (Step 11, p. 961).

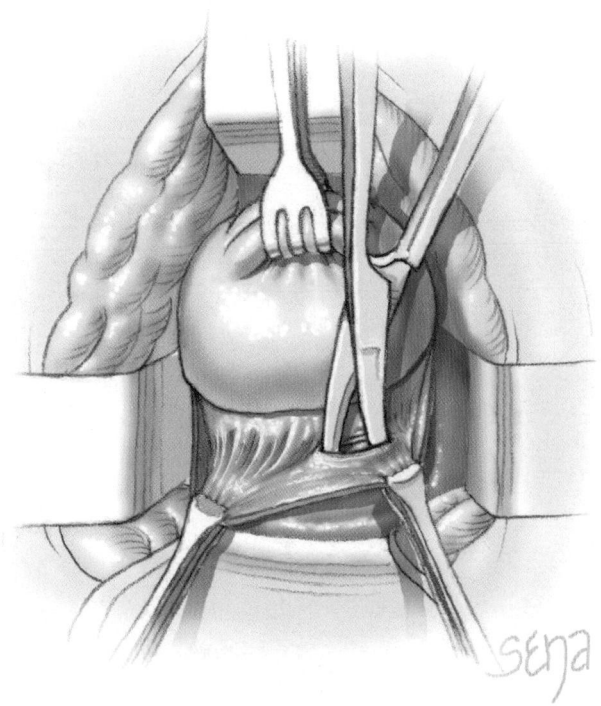

FIGURE 43-14.1 Extraperitoneal dissection.

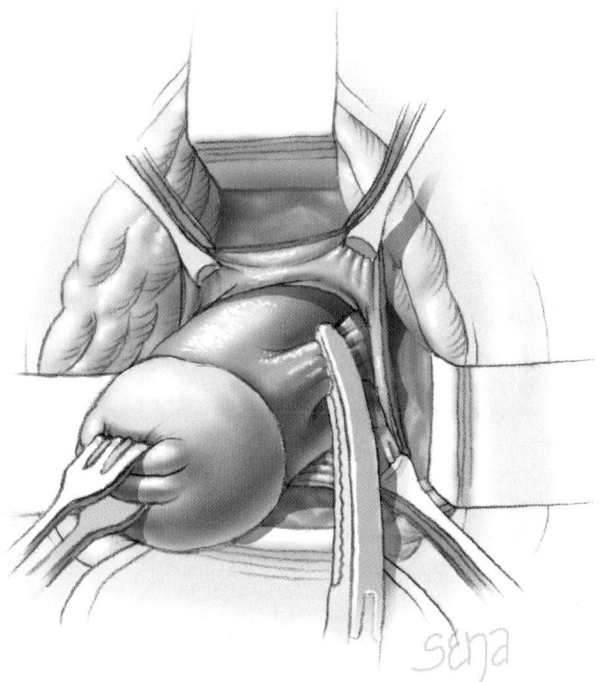

FIGURE 43-14.2 Uterosacral and cardinal ligament transection.

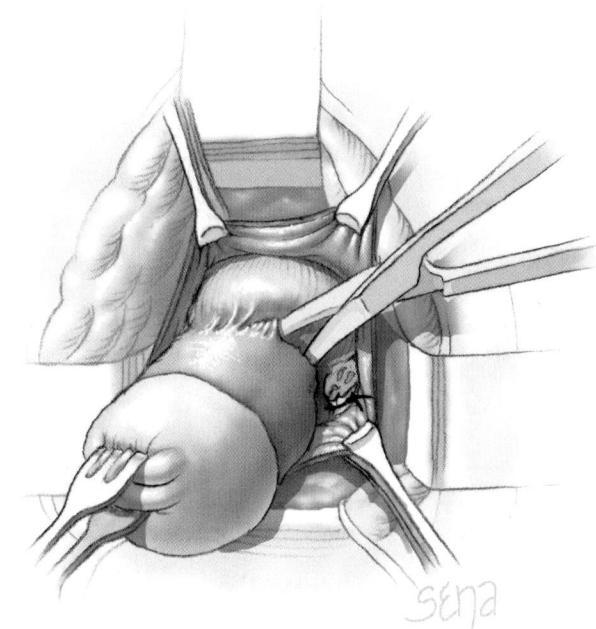

FIGURE 43-14.3 Stump excision.

POSTOPERATIVE

As with hysterectomy, a significant number of women will have unexplained febrile morbidity following trachelectomy. Pasley (1988) in his series of 55 cases noted a rate of 9 percent. Similar to hysterectomy, patients with persistent or high-degree fevers require evaluation and possible antibiotic treatment (Chap. 42, p. 919).

43-15

Sharp Dilatation and Curettage

This procedure is a primary tool for diagnostic evaluation and treatment of abnormal uterine bleeding. However, the indications for dilatation and sharp curettage (D & C) have decreased with the development of less invasive methods such as plastic endometrial samplers and transvaginal sonography (Chap. 8, p. 184).

For evaluation of abnormal uterine bleeding, sharp curettage may be used alone or more commonly in combination with hysteroscopy for those women with persistent bleeding despite normal findings with sonography and endometrial biopsy. In some, mechanical cervical dilatation followed by curettage may be required to gain access to the uterine cavity when a stenotic cervical os prohibits in-office endometrial sampling. Also, if uterine malignancy is suspected and initial biopsy is incomplete, D & C may permit a more thorough removal and interrogation of endometrial tissue.

In the treatment of severe acute menorrhagia, D & C may be used to remove hypertrophic endometrium if bleeding must be stopped promptly or if bleeding is refractory to medical management. Although suction curettage is used more commonly for removal of first-trimester pregnancy products (Chap. 6, p. 152), sharp D & C may also be an option. Finally, in women with suspected ectopic pregnancy, D & C sometimes is used to document the absence of intrauterine trophoblastic tissue (Chap. 7, p. 167).

PREOPERATIVE

Consent

For most women, sharp dilatation and curettage poses only a small risk of complication, and rates are typically below 1 percent (Radman, 1963; Tabata, 2001). Infection and uterine perforation are among the most frequent. With uterine perforation, concern for adjacent organ injury may require diagnostic laparoscopy or laparotomy and injury repair. Although rare, the possibility of hysterectomy is also discussed.

Patient Preparation

Because the indications for sharp D & C are diverse, diagnostic testing prior to evacuation will vary. Sonography is a frequent evaluation tool, and images are reviewed preoperatively to reorient the surgeon to uterine inclination and pathology.

Prophylactic antibiotic administration is typically not required when sharp D & C is performed for gynecologic indications. However, because pelvic infection may follow this procedure when performed in an obstetric setting, antibiotics are usually prescribed postoperatively. Doxycycline, 100 mg orally twice daily for 10 days, is a frequent choice (American College of Obstetricians and Gynecologists, 2014a). The risk of bowel injury or venous thromboembolism (VTE) with this procedure is rare. Thus, preoperative enema or VTE prophylaxis in those without additional risk factors is not mandatory.

INTRAOPERATIVE

Surgical Steps

❶ **Anesthesia and Patient Positioning.** Dilatation and curettage is typically performed as an outpatient procedure under general or regional anesthesia or with local nerve blockade combined with intravenous sedation. The patient is placed in standard dorsal lithotomy position, the vagina is surgically prepared, and the bladder drained.

A bimanual examination to determine uterine size and inclination is performed prior to introduction of vaginal instruments. Information obtained from this examination helps avoid uterine perforation. With insertion of instruments along the long axis of the uterus, there is less chance of injury.

❷ **Uterine Sounding.** Suitable vaginal exposure can be achieved with either a Graves speculum or individual vaginal retractors. The anterior lip of the cervix is grasped with a single-tooth tenaculum to stabilize the uterus during dilatation and curettage. A Sims uterine sound is then held like a pencil with the thumb and first two fingers (Fig. 43-15.1). The sound is slowly guided through the cervical os, into the uterine cavity, and to the fundus. To minimize perforation risks, instruments are not forced and are kept in the midline.

Once gentle resistance is met at the fundus, the distance from the fundus to the external os is measured by score marks along the length of the sound. Knowledge of the depth to which dilators and curettes can safely be inserted also decreases perforation risk.

At times, cervical stenosis may preclude easy access to the endocervical canal. In these cases, smaller caliber tools, such as a lacrimal duct probe, can be guided into the external cervical os to define the canal path. Sonography may be helpful when done simultaneously with D & C in these situations. Sonographic visualization of instruments as they are being passed may help assure proper placement (Christianson, 2008). In addition, pretreatment with the prostaglandin E_1 analogue misoprostol (Cytotec) may allow adequate cervical softening for instrument passage. Commonly used dosing options include 200 or 400 μg vaginally or 400 μg orally or sublingually once 12 to 24 hours prior to surgery. Song and coworkers (2014) noted equal efficacy but a patient preference for oral administration. Common side effects include cramping, uterine bleeding, or nausea.

❸ **Uterine Dilatation.** After the uterus is sounded, dilators of sequentially increasing caliber are inserted to open the endocervical canal and internal cervical os. A Hegar, Hank, or Pratt dilator, as shown on page 967, is held by the thumb and first two fingers, while the fourth and fifth fingers and heel of the hand rest on the perineum and buttock. Each dilator is gently and gradually advanced through the internal cervical os. Serial dilation continues until the cervix will admit the selected curette (Fig. 43-15.2).

During sounding or dilatation, uterine perforation may occur and is suspected when the instrument travels deeper than previously measured. Because of the blunt, narrow shape of these tools, risk of significant uterine or abdominal organ injury is low. In such cases, if significant bleeding is absent, reassessment of uterine inclination and completion of the D & C is reasonable. Alternatively, surgery may be terminated and repeated at a later date to allow myometrial healing. Importantly, lateral perforation may create a broad ligament hematoma, which if suspected merits

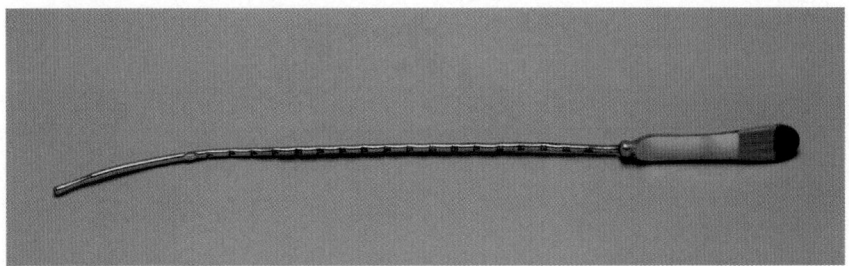

FIGURE 43-15.1 Sims uterine sound.

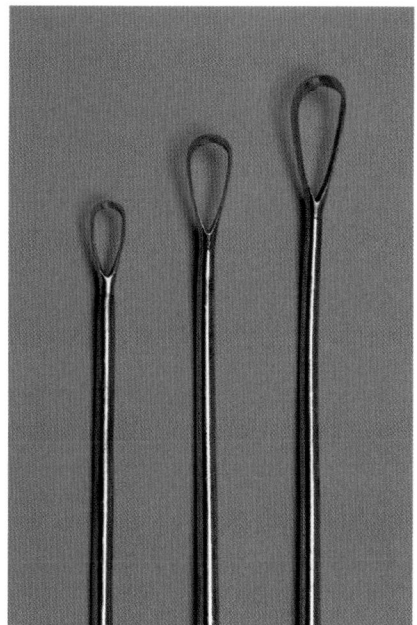

FIGURE 43-15.2 Uterine curettes.

laparoscopic evaluation or postoperative sur-veillance of hemodynamic status.

❹ **Uterine Curettage.** Prior to curettage, a sheet of nonadherent wound dressing mate-rial (Telfa pad) is spread out in the vagina beneath the cervix. The uterine curette is then inserted and advanced to the fundus, follow-ing the long axis of the corpus. The concave curve of the curette loop has a sharp edge, which allows curettage. On reaching the fun-dus, the sharp surface is positioned to contact the adjacent endometrium (Fig. 43-15.3). Pressure is exerted against the endometrium as the curette is pulled toward the internal cervical os.

After reaching the os, the curette is redi-rected to the fundus and positioned immedi-ately adjacent to the path of the first curettage pass. After several passes, tissue accumulated in the isthmic region is scraped out onto the Telfa pad. In this fashion, the entire uterine cavity is sequentially and circumferentially curetted. The collected specimen is sent for pathologic evaluation.

As with dilatation, the uterus may be per-forated during curettage. In contrast to the

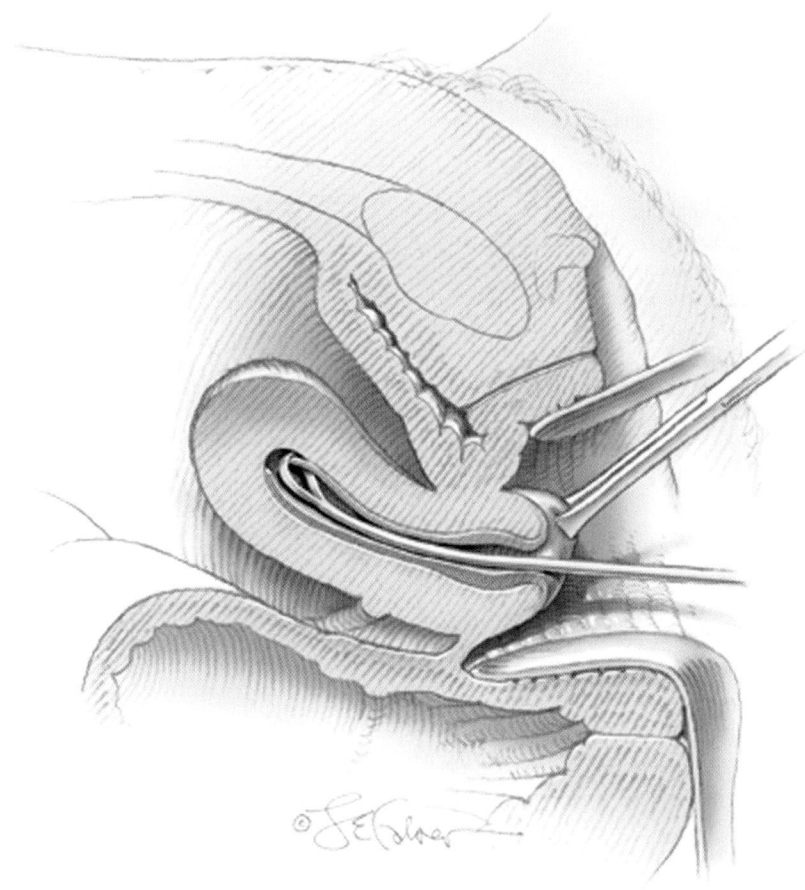

FIGURE 43-15.3 Uterine curettage.

metal sound or dilator, the sharp curette has the potential to lacerate bowel, vessels, and other abdominal organs. Accordingly, diag-nostic laparoscopy is considered to evaluate for such injuries.

❺ **Uterine Exploration.** Uterine polyps, both large and small, may be missed with sharp curettage. As described in Chapter 8 (p. 187), hysteroscopy is a more accurate means to diagnose and remove focal lesions and is often coupled with D & C. In areas without these resources or expertise, uter-ine exploration with Randall kidney stone forceps can be used to secure and remove polyps. For this, closed forceps are inserted into the endometrial cavity. Upon reaching

the fundus, forceps are opened against the uterine walls, closed, and then pulled away from the endometrium. With this technique, anterior, posterior, proximal, and distal cav-ity surfaces are explored. With capture of a polyp within the jaws, a tug against the closed forceps is felt as they are pulled away from the uterine wall. Firm traction typically frees the polyp. Removed tissue is sent for pathologic evaluation.

POSTOPERATIVE

Recovery from sharp D & C is typically fast and without complication. Light bleeding or spotting is expected, and patients may resume normal activities at their own pace.

43-16

Suction Dilatation and Curettage

Suction dilatation and curettage (D & C) is the most frequently used method to remove first-trimester products of conception. Vacuum aspiration, the most common form of suction curettage, requires a rigid plastic cannula attached to an electric-powered vacuum source. Alternatively, manual vacuum aspiration uses a similar cannula that attaches to a handheld syringe for its vacuum source (Lichtenburg, 2013).

PREOPERATIVE

Patient Evaluation

For most women, dilatation and curettage is preceded by transvaginal sonography. As discussed in Chapter 6 (p. 141), this imaging modality aids in documenting pregnancy nonviability, location, and size as well as uterine inclination. Images are reviewed preoperatively to reorient the surgeon to this information. In addition, complete blood count and blood typing results are reviewed. For women with significant preoperative bleeding, resuscitation as described in Chapter 40 (p. 864) is completed. Most molar pregnancies are treated with evacuation, and special preparation is described in Chapter 37 (p. 783). For Rh-negative women, administration of anti-D immune globulin intramuscularly within 72 hours of pregnancy termination can lower the risk of alloimmunization in future pregnancies. Doses of 300 μg (1500 IU) can be given for all gestational ages. Alternatively, dosing may be graduated, with 50 μg given IM for pregnancies ≤12 weeks and 300 μg given for those ≥13 weeks.

Consent

Suction D & C is a safe and effective method of uterine evacuation (Tunçalp, 2010). Short-term complication rates are low and have been cited at 1 to 5 percent (Hakim-Elahi, 1990; Zhou, 2002). Complications include uterine perforation, retained products, infection, and hemorrhage, and rates increase after the first trimester. Accordingly, sharp or suction curettage is ideally performed before 14 to 15 weeks' gestation.

The incidence of uterine perforation associated with uterine evacuation varies. Important determinants are surgeon skill, uterine position, and uterine size. Rates of perforation increase with a retroverted or large uterus and

with a less experienced surgeon. Accidental uterine perforation usually is recognized when the instrument passes without resistance deep into the pelvis. Observation may be sufficient if the uterine perforation is small, as when produced by a uterine sound or narrow blunt dilator. Considerable intraabdominal damage, however, can be caused by instruments—especially suction cannulas and sharp curettes—passed through a uterine defect into the peritoneal cavity. Because unrecognized bowel injury can cause severe peritonitis and sepsis, laparoscopy or laparotomy to examine the abdominal contents is often the safest course of action in these cases.

Rarely, women may develop cervical incompetence or intrauterine adhesions following D & C. Those undergoing this procedure should understand the potential for these rare but significant complications.

Patient Preparation

Suction D & C may be performed for cases of incomplete or inevitable abortion and require no cervical dilatation for procedure completion. However, other settings require physical dilatation of the cervical os with metal dilators, a procedural step closely associated with uterine perforation and patient discomfort. Therefore, to obviate this need, hygroscopic dilators may be placed in the endocervical canal to the level of the internal os. These dilators draw water from cervical proteoglycan complexes, which dissociate and thereby allow the cervix to soften and dilate.

Two dilator types are currently available in the United States. One type originates from the stems of *Laminaria digitata* or *Laminaria japonica,* a seaweed. The stems are cut, peeled, shaped, dried, sterilized, and packaged according to their hydrated size—small, 3 to 5 mm diameter; medium, 6 to 8 mm; and large, 8 to 10 mm (Fig. 43-16.1). Another type, Dilapan-S, is an acrylic-based hydrogel rod.

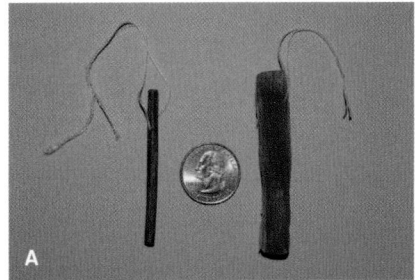

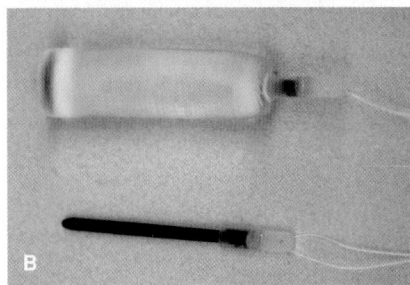

FIGURE 43-16.1 Hygroscopic dilators, dry and expanded. **A.** Laminaria. **B.** Dilapan-S.

For dilator placement, the cervix is cleansed with povidone-iodine or similar solution and grasped anteriorly with a tenaculum. A laminaria of appropriate size is then inserted using a uterine packing forceps so that the tip rests at the level of the internal os (Fig. 43-16.2). After 4 to 6 hours, the laminaria will have swollen to dilate the cervix sufficiently and allow easier D & C. Cramping frequently accompanies expansion of the device.

In addition to mechanical tools, various prostaglandin preparations have been investigated as cervical "ripening" agents. Misoprostol has been used effectively to induce uterine evacuation in properly selected patients. However, studies investigating its preoperative use to ease cervical dilatation prior to pregnancy evacuation show inconsistent results (Mittal, 2011; Sharma, 2005). Moreover, in comparison, laminaria prove more effective than misoprostol for ripening (Burnett, 2005; Firouzabadi, 2011).

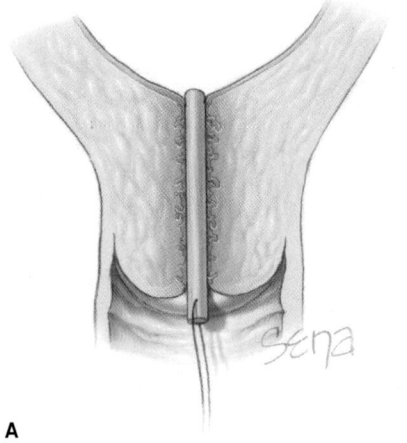

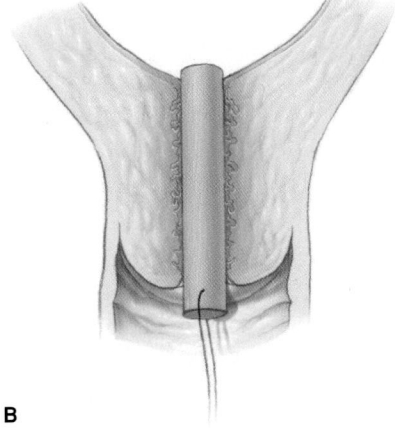

A   **B**

FIGURE 43-16.2 A. Correct laminaria placement. **B.** Expanded laminaria.

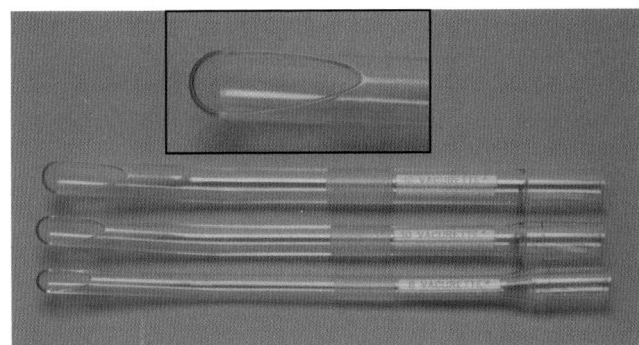

FIGURE 43-16.3 Karman cannulas (sizes 8 to 12 mm). Inset: Cannula tip.

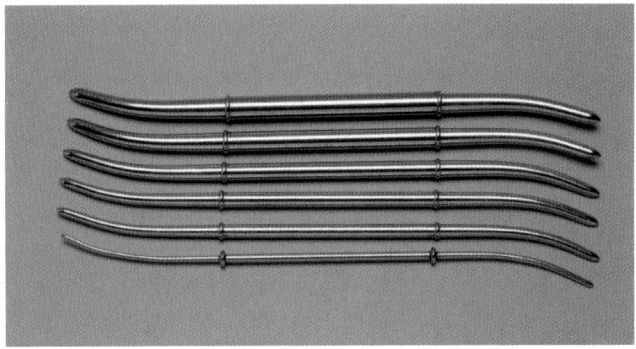

FIGURE 43-16.4 Hank dilators of serially increasing diameter.

Antibiotic prophylaxis is provided at the time of transcervical surgical pregnancy evacuation. Based on review of 11 randomized trials, Sawaya and associates (1996) concluded that perioperative antibiotics decreased the infection risk by 40 percent. Although no regimen appears superior, a convenient, inexpensive, and effective one is doxycycline, 100 mg orally twice daily for 10 days. Table 39-6 (p. 835) lists alternatives.

INTRAOPERATIVE

Instruments

Suction D & C requires an electric suction unit; stiff, translucent, large-bore sterile suction tubing; and sterile Karman suction cannulas (Fig. 43-16.3). Plastic suction cannulas are available in varying diameters. They also have a straight or slightly bent shaft, which can be select to conform to uterine cavity inclination. Choosing the most appropriately sized cannula balances competing factors. Small cannulas risk postoperative retention

of intrauterine tissue, whereas large cannulas risk cervical injury and greater discomfort. For most first-trimester evacuations, a no. 8 to 12 Karman cannula is sufficient.

Surgical Steps

❶ Anesthesia and Patient Positioning. In the absence of maternal systemic disease, abortion procedures do not require hospitalization. When abortion is performed outside a hospital setting, capabilities for cardiopulmonary resuscitation and for immediate transfer to a hospital must be available. Anesthesia or analgesia used varies and includes general anesthesia, paracervical block plus intravenous sedation, or intravenous sedation alone. After delivery of anesthesia or analgesia, the patient is placed in standard dorsal lithotomy position. Bimanual examination to determine uterine size and inclination is performed prior to introduction of vaginal instruments. Information obtained from this examination helps avoid uterine perforation. The vulva

and vagina are then surgically prepared, and the bladder is drained.

❷ Uterine Sounding and Cervical Dilatation. A Graves speculum or other suitable vaginal retractor(s) is positioned in the vagina to allow cervical access. A single-tooth tenaculum is placed on the cervical lip to provide gentle countertension during instrument passage. First, a Sims uterine sound (Fig. 43-15.1, p. 964) is placed through the cervical os and into the uterine cavity to measure the depth and inclination of the uterine cavity prior to dilatation.

If the cervix is closed or incompletely dilated, metal Pratt, Hegar, or Hank dilators (Fig. 43-16.4) of sequentially increasing diameter are placed through the external and internal os to gently open the cervix. The uterus is especially vulnerable to perforation during this step. Accordingly, the metal dilator is grasped as one would a pencil. The heel of the hand and fourth and fifth fingers rest

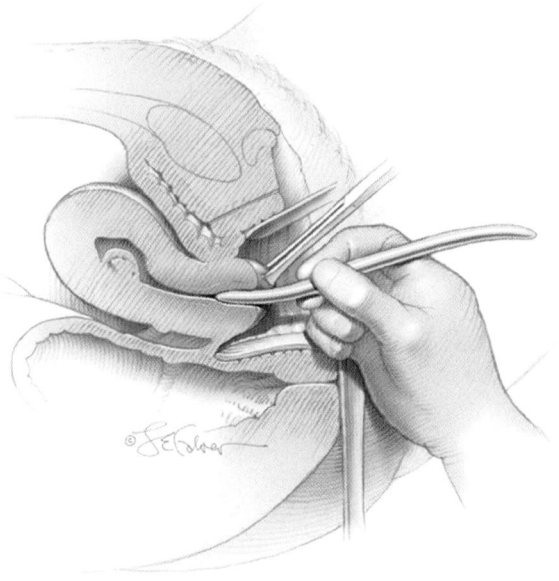

FIGURE 43-16.5 Uterine dilatation.

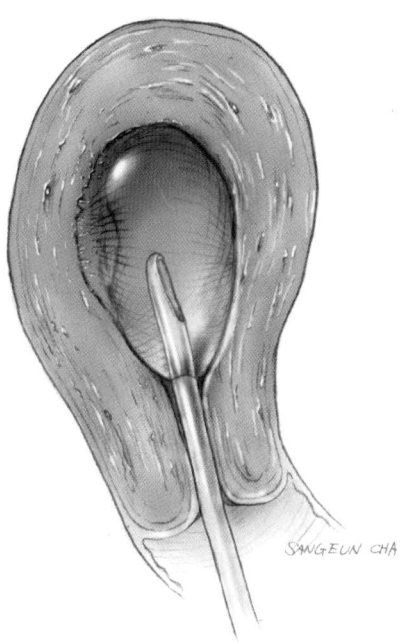

FIGURE 43-16.6 Suction cannula inserted into cavity and amnionic sac.

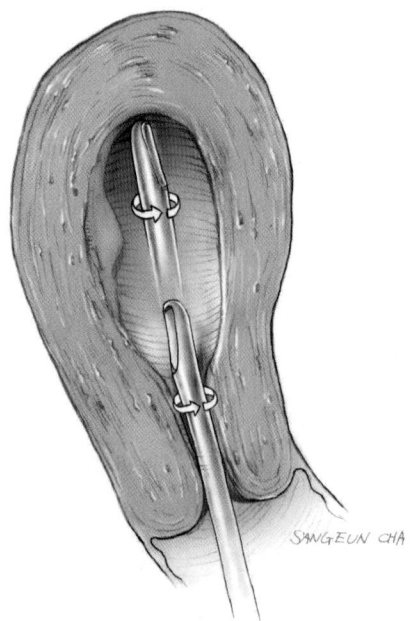

FIGURE 43-16.7 Suction cannula movement during curettage.

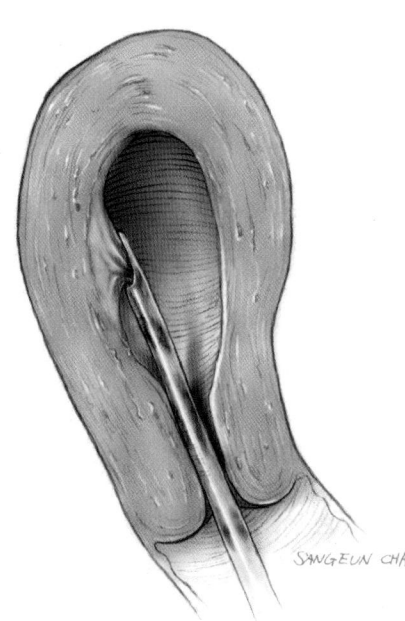

FIGURE 43-16.8 Removal of uterine contents.

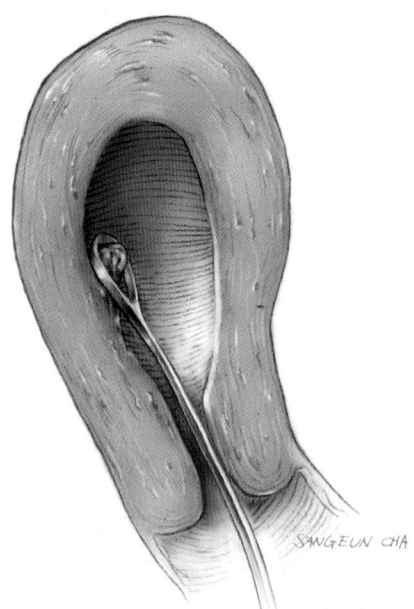

FIGURE 43-16.9 Sharp curettage.

on the perineum and buttock. Gentle pressure from only the thumb and first two fingers is used to push the dilator through the cervical os (Fig. 43-16.5).

❸ **Uterine Evacuation.** Through the now opened cervix, the Karman cannula is inserted into the endometrial cavity (Fig. 43-16.6). The suction unit is then turned on. The cannula is moved toward the fundus, then back toward the os, and is slowly turned circumferentially to cover the entire surface of the uterine cavity (Fig. 43-16.7). A gush of clear fluid into the tubing often heralds entry of the cannula into the gestational sac. This collapses the sac and

draws the placenta and membranes closer to the cannula for more expedient removal. Uterine contents are thereby removed (Fig. 43-16.8).

Tissue is collected in an attached container at the distal end of the tubing and is sent for pathologic evaluation. Occasionally, the Karman cannula may become obstructed with excess tissue. For this, the suction unit is turned off prior to cannula removal. Once the cannula opening is cleared of obstructing tissue, it may be reinserted, suction reestablished, and curettage completed.

❹ **Sharp Curettage.** Although no more tissue is aspirated, a gentle sharp curettage

is often completed to remove remaining placental or fetal fragments (Fig. 43-16.9). This is fully described in Section 43-15 (p. 964).

POSTOPERATIVE

Recovery from suction D & C is typically fast and without complication. Patients may resume normal activities as they desire, but abstinence from coitus is usually encouraged during the first week following surgery. Ovulation may resume as early as 2 weeks after an early pregnancy ends. Therefore, if contraception is desired, methods are initiated soon after abortion.

Hymenectomy

Imperforate hymen results from failure of the hymen to canalize during the perinatal period. Following menarche, menstrual blood accumulates behind this vaginal obstruction. Distention of the vagina and uterus with blood are *hematocolpos* and *hematometra*, respectively. For this reason, many cases are diagnosed after patients have become symptomatic, usually during adolescence. Accordingly, the indications for hymenectomy may include complaints of amenorrhea, pain, abdominal mass, and urinary and defecation dysfunction (Chap. 18, p. 415).

An asymptomatic imperforate hymen may also be found early, during childhood. If there is no associated mucocele, lesions can be managed expectantly. Elective hymenectomy can then be performed during puberty, when tissues are estrogenized, but prior to menarche to avoid hematometra or hematocolpos. The presence of estrogen aids surgical repair and healing.

PREOPERATIVE

Consent

Hymenectomy is a simple gynecologic procedure, and most patients recover with no short- or long-term complications. Uncommonly, the hymeneal edges may reepithelialize, and a repeat procedure may be required (Liang, 2003).

Patient Preparation

Bowel preparation and antibiotic or venous thromboembolism prophylaxis are not required for this brief surgery.

INTRAOPERATIVE

Surgical Steps

❶ **Anesthesia and Patient Positioning.** Hymenectomy is typically performed as a day surgery procedure using general anesthesia. The patient is placed in standard dorsal lithotomy position, the bladder is drained, and a sterile perineal prep is performed.

❷ **Hymen Incision.** To avert injury to the urethra anteriorly and to the rectum posteriorly, the surgeon avoids creating pure vertical and horizontal incisions. Instead, a cruciate incision is made anteroposteriorly from 10 to

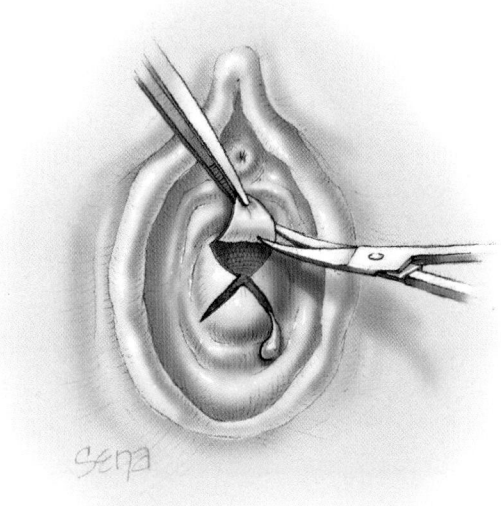

FIGURE 43-17.1 Hymenal leaflet trimming.

4 and from 2 to 8 o'clock into the hymeneal membrane (Fig. 43-17.1). Immediately, a stream of dark menstrual blood in the case of hematocolpos or mucoid fluid with mucocolpos will follow. The hymeneal leaflets are then sharply trimmed from the hymeneal ring. These are not excised too closely to the vaginal epithelium to avoid increased scarring at the hymeneal ring.

❸ **Irrigation.** The vagina is copiously irrigated using a sterile saline solution with either a red rubber catheter or bulb syringe. Intraoperative evaluation or manipulation of the upper vagina, cervix, and uterus is discouraged, as the walls of these organs may have been greatly thinned by hematocolpos or hematometra and are at risk for perforation.

❹ **Suturing.** The cut edges of the leaflet bases are then oversewn with interrupted stitches using 3-0 or 4-0 gauge delayed-absorbable suture, thus creating a ring of sutures (Fig. 43-17.2). A running interlocking suture line is avoided to minimize circumferential narrowing of the introitus.

Some use an alternative to sharp trimming and suturing of the leaflets. Instead,

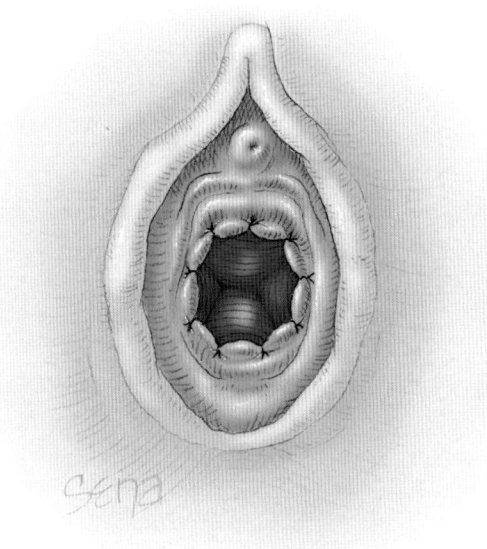

FIGURE 43-17.2 Suturing of leaflets' bases.

hemostats are placed across each leaflet base for approximately a minute to crush and seal fine vessels. After clamp removal, an incision with electrosurgical blade or scissors is carried through the crush line, excises distal leaflet tissue, and eliminates the need for suturing.

POSTOPERATIVE

Following surgery, the patient may use oral analgesics and topical anesthetics such as lidocaine ointment. Local wound care includes twice-daily sitz baths. The patient is counseled that retained fluid may continue to drain from the uterus and vagina for several days following the procedure. The patient is seen 1 to 2 weeks following surgery, at which time the introitus is inspected for patency and assessment of healing.

Bartholin Gland Duct Incision and Drainage

Bartholin gland duct cysts and abscesses are vulvar masses encountered routinely in office gynecology (Chap. 4, p. 97). Bartholin duct cysts typically measure 1 to 4 cm in diameter and are frequently asymptomatic. Patients with larger cysts, however, may complain of vaginal pressure or dyspareunia. In contrast, patients with gland duct abscesses typically complain of rapid unilateral vulvar enlargement and significant pain. Classically, a fluctuant mass is found on one side of the introitus, external to the hymenal ring, and at the lower aspects of the vulva.

Bartholin cysts or abscesses result from ductal opening obstruction followed by accumulation of mucus or pus within the gland duct. Bartholin gland abscesses are polymicrobial infections, and *Bacteroides* species, *Peptostreptococcus* species, *Escherichia coli,* and *Neisseria gonorrhoeae* are frequently found from culture of purulent drainage. Less typically, *Chlamydia trachomatis* may be involved (Bleker, 1990; Kessous, 2013).

Incision and drainage (I & D) alone may give immediate but sometimes only temporary relief. Often, unless a new duct ostium is created, the incised edges following I & D will seal and mucus or pus will reaccumulate. Therefore, I & D with subsequent steps to create a new ostium are surgical goals.

Permanent resolution of the cyst or abscess is the norm following either marsupialization or I & D with Word catheter placement. However, if obstruction recurs, repeating either of these procedures is preferable to gland excision for most cases. Bartholinectomy, described on page 975, carries significantly greater morbidity than either of these two less invasive procedures.

PREOPERATIVE

Consent

Repeated obstruction of the Bartholin gland duct following initial incision and drainage (I & D) is not uncommon during the weeks and months following drainage. Patients are informed of the possible need to repeat the procedure should the duct obstruct again. Dyspareunia is an infrequent long-term sequela, but patients are counseled regarding this potential. Rarely, deep tissue infection or rectovaginal fistula may develop postoperatively.

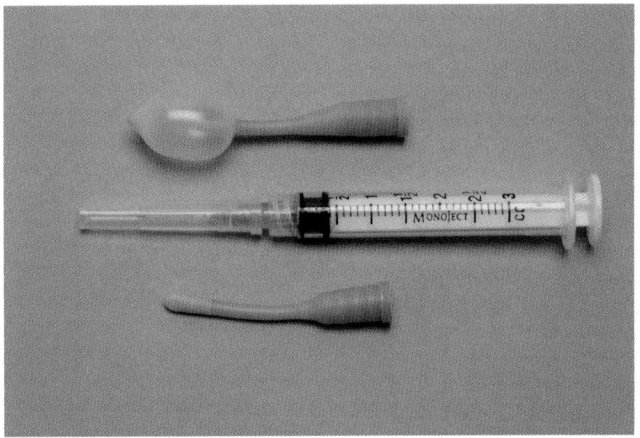

FIGURE 43-18.1 Word catheter. (Photograph contributed by Steven Willard.)

INTRAOPERATIVE

Instruments

The goal of Bartholin gland duct I & D is to empty the cystic cavity and create a new accessory epithelialized tract for gland drainage. For the latter, a Word catheter is used (Word, 1964). This is constructed of a 1-inch-long latex tube stem that has an inflatable balloon at one end and a saline-injection hub at the other (Fig. 43-18.1).

Surgical Steps

❶ Analgesia and Patient Positioning. Most procedures are performed as an outpatient procedure in the office or emergency room. Rarely, if the abscess is large or if adequate patient analgesia cannot be obtained, then I & D in the operative room may be required. The patient is placed in standard dorsal lithotomy position, and the ipsilateral labial skin is cleaned with a povidone-iodine solution or other suitable antiseptic agent.

Local analgesia is sufficient for most cases and can be obtained by infiltrating the skin overlying and adjacent to the planned incision with an aqueous 1-percent lidocaine solution. This may be augmented with mild intramuscular or intravenous analgesia.

❷ Drainage. A 1-cm incision is made using a scalpel with a no. 11 blade to pierce the skin and underlying cyst or abscess wall (Fig. 43-18.2). The incision is made atop the cyst, is placed just outside and parallel to the hymen at 5 or 7 o'clock (depending on the side involved), and is positioned medial to Hart line. This position mimics the normal anatomy of the gland duct opening and avoids creation of a fistulous tract to the outer labium majus (Hill, 1998). To minimize scalpel injury, some recommend use of a small Keyes punch biopsy to instead create a hole simultaneously through the skin and cyst wall.

General bacterial culture as well as samples specific for *Neisseria gonorrhoeae* and *Chlamydia trachomatis* identification can be obtained from spontaneously extruded pus.

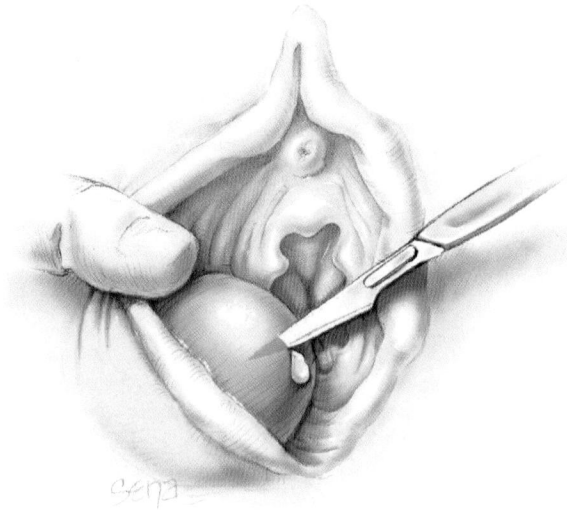

FIGURE 43-18.2 Abscess or cyst incision.

Mucus drained from a Bartholin cyst need not be cultured. Following drainage, the cavity is explored with a small cotton swab tip to open potential pus or mucus loculations. Probing is gentle to avoid perforation through the duct wall and into the nearby and highly vascular vestibular bulb (Fig. 38-26, p. 819). Cyst wall biopsy following cavity drainage to exclude rare Bartholin gland carcinoma is considered for women older than 40 years, for cysts with solid components, or for multiple cyst recurrences.

❸ **Word Catheter Placement.** A deflated Word catheter tip is placed into the empty cyst cavity. A syringe is used to inject 2 to 3 mL of sterile saline through the catheter hub to inflate the balloon. Inflation should reach a diameter sufficient to keep the catheter from falling out of the incision (Fig. 43-18.3). Alternatively, a nonlatex 14F Foley catheter is a suitable substitute for those with latex allergy or in settings without a Word catheter. In either case, insufflation with saline rather than air is preferred, as the latter is associated with premature balloon deflation. The hub end of the Word catheter can then be tucked inside the vagina to prevent it from being dislodged by traction from normal perineal movement.

POSTOPERATIVE

Bartholin gland duct cyst drainage does not require antibiotic treatment. In contrast,

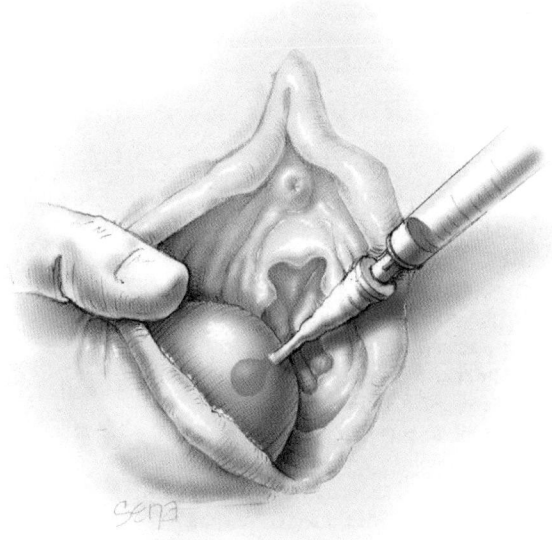

FIGURE 43-18.3 Word catheter in place.

abscesses are typically surrounded by significant cellulitis, and in such cases, antibiotics are warranted. Suitable choices include trimethoprim-sulfamethoxazole (Bactrim DS, Septra DS), doxycycline, or cephalexin (Keflex), prescribed for 7 to 10 days. At our institution, affected immunocompromised women are admitted for intravenous antibiotic therapy until fever or erythema improves.

Patients are encouraged to soak in warm tub baths twice daily. Coitus is avoided for patient comfort and to prevent Word catheter displacement. Ideally, the catheter is left in place for 4 to 6 weeks. Often, however, a catheter will be dislodged before this time. There is no need to try and replace the catheter if displaced, and attempts to reinsert it are typically not possible due to cavity closure.

43-19

Bartholin Gland Duct Marsupialization

As noted earlier (p. 971), a new duct ostium must be created following I & D of a Bartholin duct abscess to prevent the incised edges from adhering and allowing pus to reaccumulate. For this reason, marsupialization was developed as a means to create a new accessory tract for gland drainage.

With introduction of the Word catheter, however, use of marsupialization for cyst or abscess has declined. Word catheter placement offers several advantages over marsupialization, and recurrence rates are equal (Blakely, 1966; Jacobson, 1960). Marsupialization requires a greater degree of analgesia, a larger incision, placement of sutures, and longer procedure time. That said, this procedure may be selected for those with large abscesses or cysts, those with recurrences after Word catheter failures, or those with latex allergy.

PREOPERATIVE

Consent

The patient consenting discussion for marsupialization mirrors that for Bartholin gland duct I & D. Thus, patients are informed of possible abscess or cyst recurrence. Uncommon postoperative complications are dyspareunia, deep tissue infection, or rectovaginal fistula.

INTRAOPERATIVE

Surgical Steps

❶ **Anesthesia and Patient Positioning.** Marsupialization is an outpatient procedure typically performed in an operating suite using a unilateral pudendal nerve block or general anesthesia. Some authors, however, have described performance of the procedure in an emergency room setting (Downs, 1989). The patient is placed in standard dorsal lithotomy position, and the vulva and vagina are surgically prepared.

❷ **Skin Incision.** A vertical or elliptical incision measuring 2 cm is made across the skin overlying the cystic bulge using a scalpel with either a no. 10 or 15 blade. The incision is made atop the cyst, is placed just outside and parallel to the hymen at 5 or 7 o'clock (depending on the side involved), and is positioned medial to Hart line. This position mimics the normal gland duct opening anat-

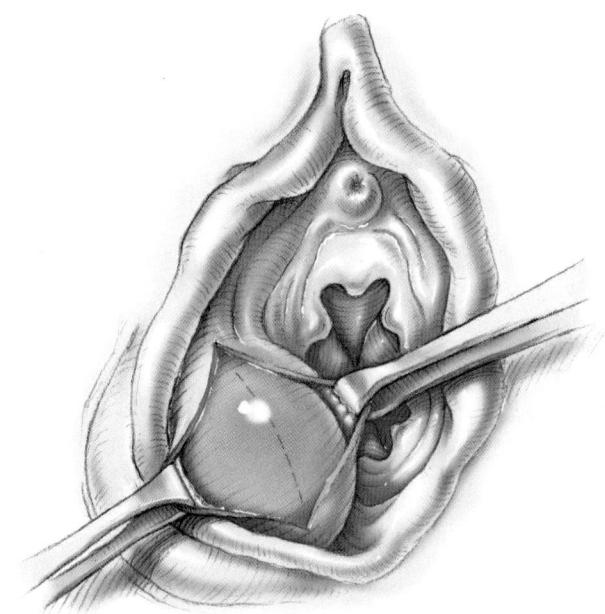

FIGURE 43-19.1 Skin incision.

omy and avoids creation of a fistulous tract to the outer labium majus (Fig. 43-19.1).

❸ **Cyst Incision.** A second vertical incision then opens the underlying cyst wall, and pus or mucus under pressure spills out. Pus may be cultured as described on page 971. Allis clamps are then placed on the superior, inferior, right, and left lateral cyst wall edges and fanned out.

Following drainage, the cavity is explored with a small cotton swab tip to open potential fluid loculations. Probing is gentle to avoid perforation through the duct wall and into the nearby and highly vascular vestibular bulb (Fig. 38-26, p. 819). In addition, cyst wall biopsy following cavity drainage to exclude rare Bartholin gland adenocarcinoma is considered if the patient is older than 40 years or if solid components accompany the cyst.

❹ **Wound Closure.** The edges of the cyst wall are sutured to adjacent skin edges with interrupted sutures using 2-0 or 3-0 gauge delayed-absorbable suture (Fig. 43-19.2).

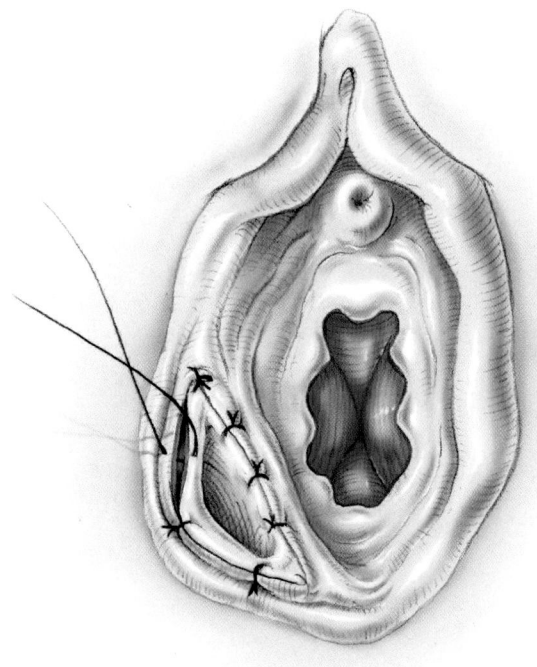

FIGURE 43-19.2 Cyst wall sutured open.

POSTOPERATIVE

Bartholin gland duct cyst drainage does not require antibiotic treatment. In contrast, abscesses are typically surrounded by significant cellulitis, and in such cases, antibiotics are warranted. Suitable choices include trimethoprim-sulfamethoxazole, doxycycline, or cephalexin, prescribed for 7 to 10 days.

At our institution, affected immunocompromised women are admitted for intravenous antibiotic therapy until fever or erythema improves.

Cool packs during the first 24 hours following surgery can minimize pain, swelling, and hematoma formation. After this time, warm sitz baths, one or two times daily, are suggested for pain relief and wound hygiene. Activities are resumed quickly, although intercourse is delayed until healing is complete.

Patients may be seen within the first week following surgery to ensure that ostium edges have not adhered to each other (Novak, 1978). Within 2 to 3 weeks, the wound shrinks to create a duct opening typically 5 mm or less. Recurrence rates following marsupialization are low. Jacobson (1960) noted only 4 recurrences in his series of 152 cases.

CHAPTER 43

43-20

Bartholin Gland Duct Cystectomy

Most Bartholin gland duct cysts can be managed with incision and drainage (I & D) and Word catheter placement or with marsupialization. Symptomatic cysts, however, which repeatedly recur and refill following I & D or marsupialization are typical candidates for excision. Others best managed with excision are cysts with solid components, which increases the concern for malignancy; massive cysts; or multilocular cysts, which may be incompletely drained by I & D. Bartholin gland duct abscesses are not suitable for excision and are instead incised and drained (p. 971).

Many had previously suggested excision of all Bartholin gland cysts in women older than 40 to exclude cancer. However, a study by Visco and Del Priore (1996) suggests that the morbidity of gland excision may not be justified for this rare cancer (Chap 4, p. 97). Instead, they recommend cyst I & D with cyst wall biopsy.

PREOPERATIVE

Consent

Complications are usually not encountered during bartholinectomy, but if the rich venous plexus of the nearby vestibular bulb is entered, bleeding can be significant (Fig. 38-26, p. 819). Additionally, gland excision can be associated with other morbidities such as postoperative wound cellulitis, hematoma formation, or pain from postoperative scarring. Rarely, recurrence from failure to remove the entire cyst wall, rectal injury, or rectovaginal fistula has been described.

Patient Preparation

No special antibiotic or venous thromboembolism prophylaxis is typically needed for this brief day surgery.

INTRAOPERATIVE

Surgical Steps

❶ **Analgesia and Patient Positioning.** Excision of most Bartholin gland duct cysts is performed as an outpatient procedure, in an operative suite, and under general anesthesia. The patient is placed in standard dorsal lithotomy position, and the vagina and perineum are surgically prepared.

❷ **Skin Incision.** A gauze sponge held by a ring forceps is placed inside the vagina by an assistant, and pressure is directed outward along the back wall of the cyst. This pushes the full extent of the cyst forward. The surgeon's fingers retract the labium minus laterally to expose the medial surface of the cyst.

A vertical incision that extends the length of the cyst is made on the medial surface of the labium minus. Care is taken to incise the skin but avoid puncture of the underlying cyst wall. Allis clamps are placed on the medial incision edge, which is fanned out medially and toward the contralateral labium.

❸ **Cyst Dissection.** To summarize the steps as an overview, dissection begins along the cyst's medial border, then along the lateral border, and finally deep vessels are ligated and transected to free the cyst. The greatest vascular supply to these cysts is located at their posterosuperior aspect. Accordingly, dissection of each border begins at the lower cyst pole and is directed superiorly.

To begin, medial traction on the Allis clamps and lateral fingertip traction against the cyst creates tension across connective tissue bands between the cyst wall and surrounding tissue. These bands are divided, and in this fashion, the inferomedial cyst wall is bluntly and sharply dissected free. Dissection planes are kept close to the cyst wall to avoid bleeding from the vestibular bulb and to avoid incision into the rectum (Fig. 43-20.1). Because the lowermost pole of a Bartholin gland cyst may extend to lie adjacent to the rectum, the rectum can be entered accidentally during dissection. Placing a finger at times into the rectum can help orient the surgeon to the spatial relationship between the two.

Following medial border dissection, Allis clamps are next placed on the lateral skin edges and fanned out laterally. Dissection then begins near the inferolateral cyst wall and moves superiorly.

During dissection, bleeding from the vestibular bulb can be troublesome. Most cases can be managed with ligation of individual vessels (if identified), placement of hemostatic sutures within the general bleeding area, closure of dead space, or a combination of these techniques.

❹ **Vessel Ligation.** As dissection is completed superiorly, the main deep vascular bundle to the cyst is identified and clamped with a hemostat (Fig. 43-20.2). The bundle is cut and ligated with 3-0 gauge delayed-absorbable or chromic suture.

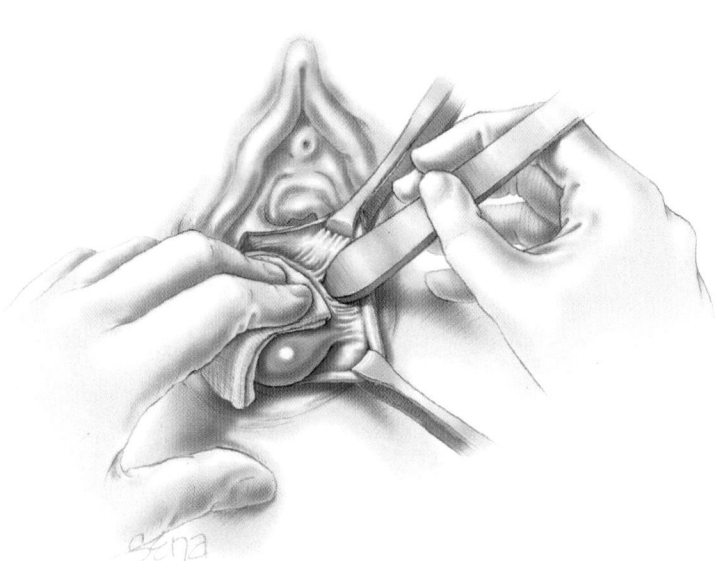

FIGURE 43-20.1 Cyst dissection.

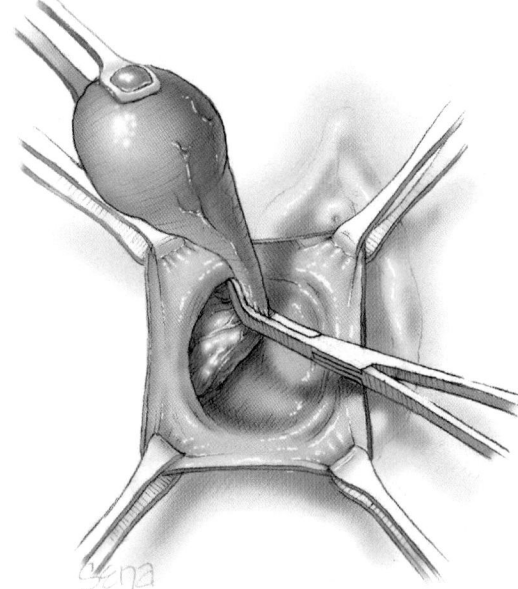

FIGURE 43-20.2 Vessel ligation.

❺ **Wound Closure.** The remaining cyst bed is closed in layers with running or interrupted suture line of 3-0 gauge delayed-absorbable suture. Typically, two layers are required prior to skin closure. However, with large or vascular cyst beds, additional layers may be required. The skin is approximated with a running subcuticular suture line of 4-0 gauge delayed-absorbable suture.

POSTOPERATIVE

Cool packs during the first 24 hours following surgery can minimize pain, swelling, and hematoma formation. After this time, warm sitz baths, one or two times each day, are suggested for pain relief and wound hygiene. Intercourse is delayed for several weeks to permit wound healing, and then resumption is typically dictated by patient comfort.

Vulvar Abscess Incision and Drainage

A patient with a vulvar abscess may typically present with pain, vulvar edema and erythema, and a fluctuant mass that should be differentiated from Bartholin gland duct abscess (Fig. 43-21.1). In some cases, the abscess may be draining spontaneously, and treatment consists of antibiotics to resolve surrounding cellulitis. In other cases, small abscesses measuring approximately 1 cm or less may be treated with local warm compresses or baths and oral antibiotics. Those with larger abscesses typically require incision and drainage (I & D) for infection resolution.

PREOPERATIVE

Patient Evaluation

In most cases, this is a visual diagnosis, and for those without comorbidities, no specific laboratory testing or imaging is needed. In obese patients, a serum glucose level is considered. Clear cases of necrotizing fasciitis require immediate debridement. However, in suspicious but not convincing cases, expeditious computed tomography can be useful (Chap. 3, p. 81).

Consent

Incomplete drainage and persistence of the abscess may follow initial incision and drainage, particularly if the abscess contains

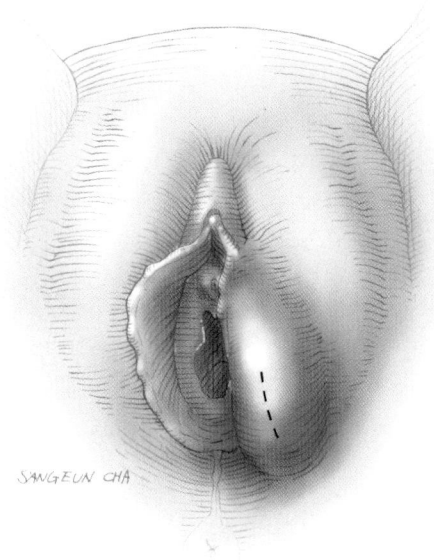

FIGURE 43-21.1 Vulvar abscess incision.

loculations. The abscess may also reform after drainage. Although uncommon, progression to or already coexisting necrotizing fasciitis may complicate the infection course.

Patient Preparation

For large abscesses or in the immunosuppressed, intravenous antibiotics are given preoperatively, and coverage for methicillin-resistant *Staphylococcus aureus* (MRSA) is considered. Thurman (2008) and Kilpatrick (2010) and their coworkers found MRSA to be a common pathogen in vulvar abscesses (43 and 64 percent, respectively).

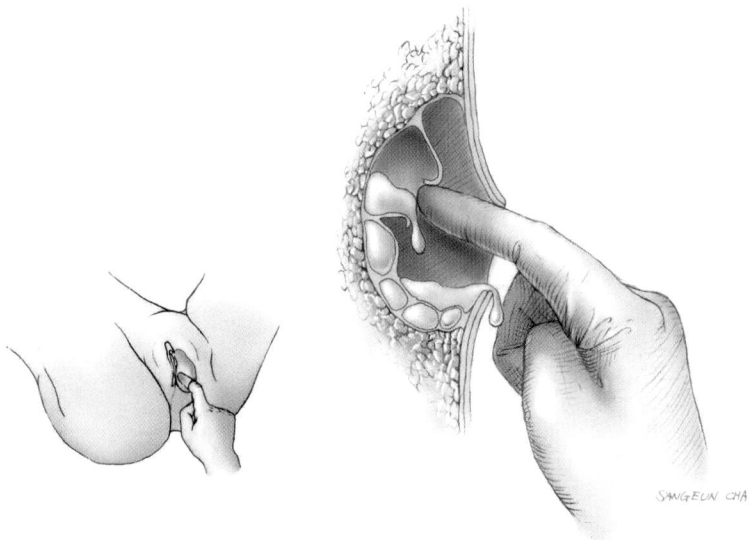

FIGURE 43-21.2 Digital exploration and disruption of abscess loculations.

INTRAOPERATIVE

Surgical Steps

❶ Anesthesia and Patient Positioning. Many patients with smaller abscesses can undergo incision and drainage in an ambulatory setting. In contrast, to attain adequate analgesia, larger abscesses often require drainage in the operating room under regional analgesia or general anesthesia.

The patient is placed in standard dorsal lithotomy position, and the involved area of the vulva is cleaned with povidone-iodine solution or other suitable antiseptic. If drainage is completed with local analgesia, the skin overlying the abscess is injected with a 1-percent lidocaine solution to achieve a field effect.

❷ Drainage. A 1- to 2-cm incision is made with a no. 11 scalpel blade into the site where the abscess wall is most thinned and is likely attempting to drain spontaneously. The incision penetrates into the abscess cavity with resultant extrusion of abundant pus. Aerobic and anaerobic cultures are obtained at this time. The abscess cavity is explored to bluntly dissect loculations within the cavity (Fig. 43-21.2). Digital or gentle cotton swab exploration is preferred to that with a pointed surgical instrument, which may tear vestibular bulb veins to create significant bleeding or hematoma.

❸ Procedure Completion. Depending on surgeon preference, a drain may be placed in the abscess cavity and brought out through a separate incision. The edges of the primary incision are then reapproximated with

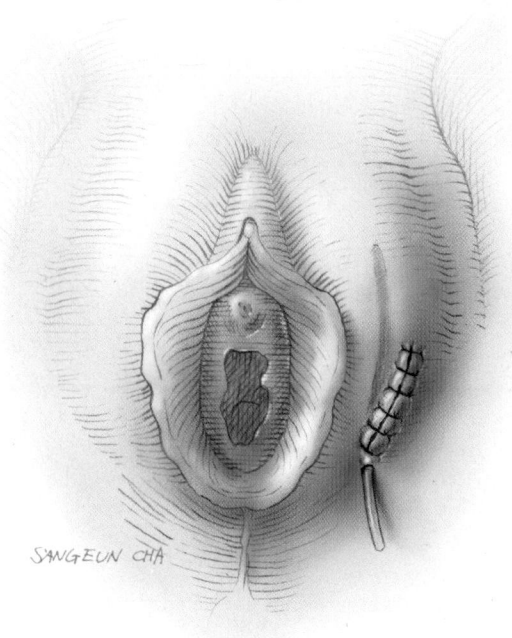

SANGEUN CHA

FIGURE 43-21.3 Drain placement and incision closure.

delayed-absorbable suture (Fig. 43-21.3). Alternatively, the wound may be packed with iodoform gauze. With a small abscess, the incision may simply be left open to allow for spontaneous healing.

POSTOPERATIVE

For small abscesses, the patient may be discharge following I & D, and reevaluation or wound repacking in 48 to 72 hours is reasonable. Appropriate antibiotic coverage are continued for several days, and trimethoprim-sulfamethoxazole (Bactrim, Septra) is a first-line oral agent against MRSA. Women with larger abscesses or greater surrounding cellulitis often warrant admission for pain control and intravenous antibiotic therapy. For MRSA, clindamycin or vancomycin is an effective intravenous choice. Most women with significant immunosuppression or diabetes also require hospital admission for antibiotic administration and comorbidity management. Specifically, Kilpatrick and colleagues (2010) noted that coexistent diabetes was significantly related to hospitalization for more than 7 days, reoperation, and progression to necrotizing fasciitis.

In those without gauze packing, warm sitz baths, one or two times each day, may aid pain relief and wound hygiene. With resolving fever and surrounding cellulitis, the drain is removed. For those with gauze packing, it may be changed once or twice daily until the cavity is nearly closed. In all cases, perineal hygiene and avoidance of labial shaving is emphasized.

43-22

Vestibulectomy

Anatomically, the vestibule extends along the inner labia minora, from the clitoris to the fourchette (Fig. 38-25, p. 818). Additional borders include the hymenal ring and Hart line, which lies along the inner labia minora and demarcates the boundary between keratinized and nonkeratinized epithelium. For some women, inflammation in this region can lead to vulvodynia and dyspareunia.

Most cases of vulvodynia are managed conservatively, but for refractory cases, three surgeries have been employed: vestibuloplasty, vestibulectomy, and perineoplasty (Edwards, 2003). Vestibuloplasty involves denervation of the vestibule by incising, undermining, and then closing the vulvar skin, but without excising the painful epithelium. It generally has been found to be ineffective (Bornstein, 1995).

Alternatively, vestibulectomy incorporates excision of vestibular tissue (Fig. 43-22.1). Incisions extend from the periurethral area down to the superior edge of the perineum and include the fourchette. The lateral incisions are carried along Hart line, and the medial incisions are placed so as to excise the hymen. In sum, mucous membrane, hymen, minor vestibular glands are removed, and Bartholin ducts are transected. Following excision, the vaginal mucosa is mobilized and pulled distally to cover the defect. In certain cases, a modified vestibulectomy is sufficient and extends only partially up the inner labia minora, well short of the periurethral area (Lavy, 2005).

Perineoplasty is the most extensive of the three procedures and extends from just below the urethra to the perineal body, usually terminating above the anal orifice (see Fig. 43-22.1). Similarly, following tissue resection, the vaginal epithelium is advanced to cover the defect. Although used to treat vulvodynia, perineoplasty may also treat fissuring and associated pain caused by lichen sclerosus (Kennedy, 2005; Rouzier, 2002).

PREOPERATIVE

Patient Evaluation

The most important factor for surgical success in treating vulvar pain is identifying the proper candidate (Chap. 4, p. 99). For example, vaginismus coexists in approximately half of patients with vulvodynia and is associated with lower rates of postsurgical pain relief (Goldstein, 2005).

Prior to anesthesia administration, the patient undergoes testing with a cotton swab to map areas of pain. These are marked with permanent marker prior to surgery to delineate the extent of excision (Haefner, 2005). Importantly, all sensitive areas are removed, even those adjacent to the urethra. If not, tender foci that should have been resected as part of the primary operation may remain (Bornstein, 1999).

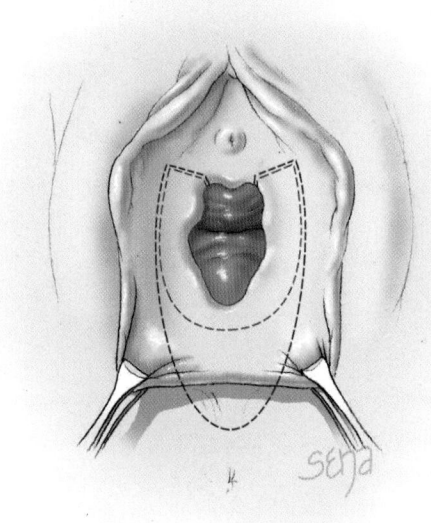

FIGURE 43-22.1 Incisions for vestibulectomy (*red line*) and for perineoplasty (*blue line*).

Consent

Operative treatments are effective in treating vulvodynia, and pain either resolves or significantly improves in nearly 65 and 80 percent of patients, respectively (Tommola, 2010). Complications are infrequent but may include bleeding, infection, wound separation, Bartholin duct cyst formation, anal sphincter weakness, vaginismus, vaginal stenosis, and failure to alleviate pain (Goetsch, 2009; Haefner, 2000).

Patient Preparation

Antibiotic prophylaxis is typically not required for this procedure. Venous thromboembolism prophylaxis may be required depending on anticipated surgical length and coexistent patient risk factors (Tables 39-7 and 39-8, p. 836). A preoperative enema may be employed to avoid immediate postoperative stool and thereby improve wound hygiene.

INTRAOPERATIVE

Surgical Steps

❶ **Anesthesia and Patient Positioning.** In most cases, vestibulectomy is an outpatient procedure, conducted using general or regional anesthesia. The patient is placed in standard dorsal lithotomy position, and the vulvovaginal area is surgically prepared.

❷ **Surgical Excision.** The primary incision, which is the lateral border, is made to a depth of 2 to 5 mm along Hart line. It is extended inferiorly to the fourchette. The medial incision is placed just proximal to the hymenal ring. The amount of tissue removed anteroposteriorly varies according to sensitivity mapping. Traditionally, it begins in the periurethral area and extends from the openings of the Skene ducts to the fourchette. Accordingly, care is taken to avoid urethral injury.

❸ **Vaginal Mucosal Advancement.** Following tissue excision, the incised edge of the vaginal mucosa is undermined 1 to 2 cm cephalad and then pulled distally to cover the defect (Fig. 43-22.2). To prevent hematoma and wound separation, hemostasis is achieved prior to final suturing.

❹ **Wound Closure.** A deep closure layer using interrupted 3-0 gauge delayed-absorbable sutures approximates the vaginal wall to its new site covering the vestibular defect. The superficial incision between the skin and vaginal epithelium is closed in an interrupted fashion with 4-0 gauge delayed-absorbable suture.

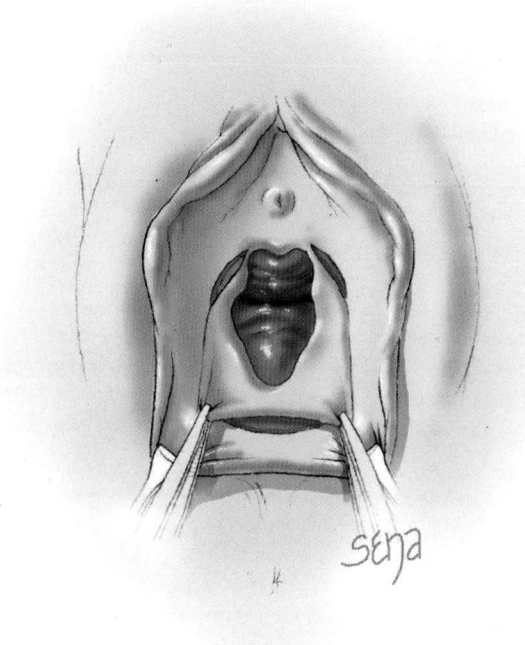

FIGURE 43-22.2 Vaginal mucosal advancement.

POSTOPERATIVE

Cool packs are used to relieve immediate discomfort, and sitz baths are initiated after the first 24 hours. Recovery is typically fast and without complications, and wound healing takes 4 to 8 weeks. Patients usually meet with their surgeon during this time and are instructed to gradually resume intercourse 6 to 8 weeks following surgery (Bergeron, 2001).

43-23

Labia Minora Reduction

When outstretched, most labia minora span 5 cm or less from their base to lateral edge. In some women, this span may be greater and may cause aesthetic dissatisfaction, discomfort with tight clothing, pain with exercise, and insertional dyspareunia. As a result, some elect to have their labia minora surgically reduced. Of note, many women seeking this surgery solely for aesthetic improvement have labial lengths well within normal standards (Crouch, 2011).

In appropriate candidates, goals of surgery include reduction in labial size and maintenance of normal vulvar anatomy. Early reductive procedures involved anteroposterior excision along the base of the labia and reapproximation of the surgical edges. Drawbacks to this approach include a marked color contrast at the suture line, where the labia minora's dark outer surface abuts the lighter inner surface. Moreover, the labial edge is often replaced by a stiff suture line. To reduce these effects, alternate techniques have incorporated labial V-, S-, Z- or W-plasty incisions, and surgeries are increasingly performed by plastic surgeons (Mirzabeigi, 2012).

PREOPERATIVE

Consent

Labia minora reductive surgery is a safe and effective means to remove excess labial tissues. As with any aesthetic procedure, women who are seeking cosmetic correction should have realistic expectations as to the final size, shape, and color of the labia. Wound complications such as hematoma, cellulitis, or incisional dehiscence are rare but should be discussed during counseling. Similarly, postoperative dyspareunia is uncommon but should be noted in the consenting process.

Patient Preparation

No specific radiologic imaging is needed for this condition or surgery. Antibiotic or venous thromboembolism prophylaxis is not required for this brief procedure in those without specific risks.

INTRAOPERATIVE

Surgical Steps

❶ **Anesthesia and Patient Positioning.** Labia minora reduction may be performed as an outpatient procedure using general or regional anesthesia. After anesthesia has been delivered, the patient is placed in standard dorsal lithotomy position, and the vulva is surgically prepared.

❷ **Labial Marking.** Excessive tissue removal is avoided because aggressive reduction may create anteroposterior narrowing and discomfort during subsequent intercourse. For this reason, during surgical marking, the surgeon may chose to place several fingers into the vagina to distend its caliber. The labia minora are then outstretched laterally.

The desired lateral span of each labium will vary between women, but most surgeons strive to create a final span of 1 to 2 cm. Asymmetry between labia is common, and surgical marking helps to even this difference. With a surgical marker, the surgeon draws a V-shaped wedge on the ventral and dorsal surfaces of the labia minora, demarcating the tissue for excision (Fig. 43-23.1, *left*). In other cases, a simple curved incision may suffice (*right*).

❸ **Wedge Excision.** The labia minora have a rich blood supply. To decrease bleeding, the incision may be infiltrated with a solution of 1-percent lidocaine and epinephrine in a 1:200,000 dilution. The tissue wedge or line is then sharply excised. Hemostasis may be achieved using electrosurgical coagulation and is important in avoiding hematoma formation.

❹ **Incision Closure.** For wedge incisions, the subcutaneous layers of the labia are reapproximated beginning proximally at the tip of the wedge (Fig. 43-23.2, *left*). Interrupted stitches of 4-0 gauge delayed-absorbable

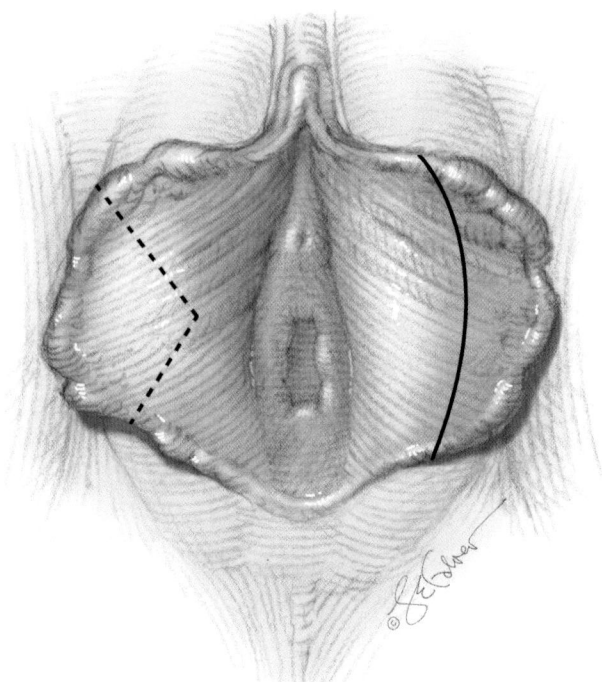

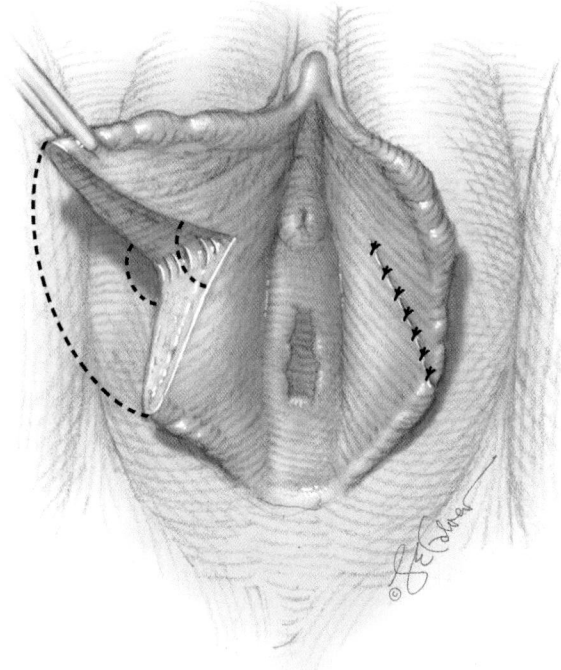

FIGURE 43-23.1 Incision lines. **A.** Wedge excision technique (*left*). **B.** Distal trimming technique (*right*).

FIGURE 43-23.2 Wedge incision closure (*left*) and final suture line (*right*).

suture are then added outward toward the lateral base to close the remainder of the wound. For linear incisions, dead space between skin edges is closed with interrupted stitches of similar suture. With either incision, the skin is reapproximated with 5-0 gauge delayed-absorbable suture in a running subcuticular or interrupted fashion (Fig. 43-23.2, *right*).

POSTOPERATIVE

Cool packs are used to relieve immediate discomfort, and sitz baths are initiated after the first 24 hours. Perineal hygiene is emphasized during the initial weeks following surgery. Exercise and intercourse may resume after wound healing.

43-24

Vaginal Septum Excision

As described in Chapter 18 (p. 404), incorrect embryologic development may lead to transverse or longitudinal septa at various levels of the vagina. Some septa have small fenestrations or are open ended to allow menstrual blood egress. Those without openings may lead to hematocolpos and hematometra.

Like the McIndoe procedure, vaginal septum excision is best performed in a mature adolescent or young adult rather than in a child. First, estrogen production following puberty can improve healing. Moreover, transverse vaginal septum excision requires some degree of postoperative vaginal dilatation to avoid stricture, and regimen compliance may be limited in young girls. Unfortunately, not all cases can be delayed. Patients may have persistent pain from hematocolpos and hematometra, and these are accompanied by an increased risk of endometriosis.

PREOPERATIVE

Patient Evaluation

Septa are frequently associated with other müllerian defects. Thus, anatomy and anomalies are usually preoperatively defined with sonography or more commonly with magnetic resonance imaging (Chap. 18, p. 416).

Consent

Risks of septum excision mirror those associated with the McIndoe procedure. However, skin grafting and its attendant risks are usually avoided except in cases with a thick vaginal septum. Vaginal stricture following excision is a significant risk. In their small series, Joki-Erkkilä and Heinonen (2003) found that two of three adolescents required reexcision of scar tissue following initial septum removal.

Patient Preparation

Antibiotic prophylaxis similar to that for hysterectomy is typically administered (Table 39-6, p. 835). Venous thromboembolism prophylaxis may be warranted for cases with greater anticipated length and complexity (Table 39-8, p. 836). Bowel preparation aids rectal decompression to permit greater vaginal distention for visualization. Also, digital rectal examination may be needed at times during surgery to direct septum excision and avoid

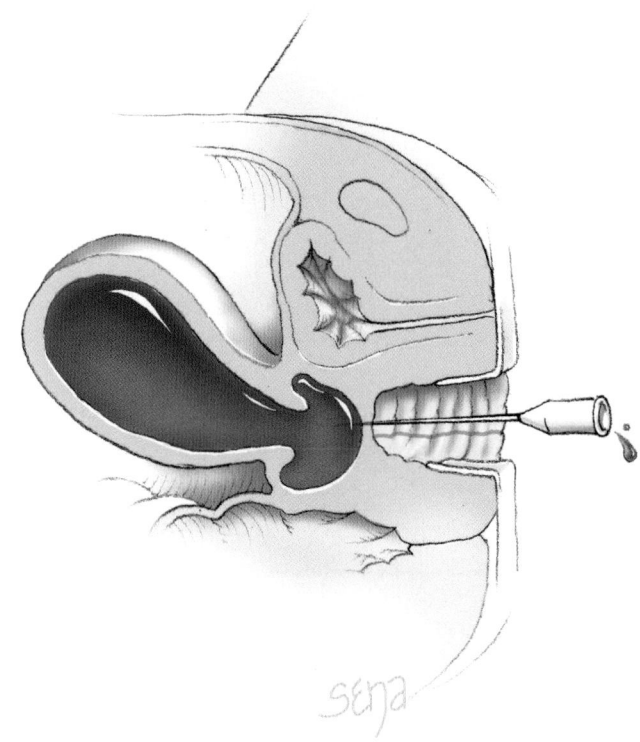

FIGURE 43-24.1 Diagnostic needle aspiration to direct dissection.

rectal laceration. Accordingly, an empty rectal vault may minimize wound contamination.

INTRAOPERATIVE

Surgical Steps

❶ **Anesthesia and Patient Positioning.** After administration of general anesthesia, the patient is placed in standard dorsal lithotomy position, and the perineum and vagina are surgically prepared. A Foley catheter serves as a guide to avoid urethral injury during septum excision.

❷ **Transverse Septum Incision.** First, retractors are placed to reveal the upper extent of the vagina. With higher-level septa, diagnostic needle aspiration of the suspected hematocolpos can help to locate the upper vagina to determine the direction of dissection (Fig. 43-24.1). The septum is then incised transversely at its center to avoid laceration of the urethra, bladder, or rectum.

A finger is placed through the transverse incision and is directed cephalad to delineate the upper vaginal walls and the circumferential margins of the septum. Similarly, the Foley catheter or a finger in the rectum may assist with orientation.

❸ **Excision.** Once the septal perimeter is defined, the initial transverse incision is

extended laterally to the vaginal wall margins. The septum is widely excised circumferentially along its base to minimize postoperative stricture (Fig. 43-24.2).

❹ **Wound Closure.** If the septum was thin, a simple circumferential ring of interrupted stitches is constructed using 2-0 gauge delayed-absorbable suture to reapproximate vaginal mucosal edges (Fig. 43-24.3). For thicker septa, the span between cephalad and caudad vaginal mucosal edges is greater. Accordingly, the mucosa may be undermined both cephalad and caudad to permit mucosal edge reapproximation without tension at the suture line. If the vaginal septum is thick and mucosal reapproximation is not possible, a skin graft can be taken and applied in a manner similar to the McIndoe procedure (p. 985). Finally, in all cases, a soft cylindrical stent is placed into the vagina to prevent stricture.

❺ **Unobstructed Longitudinal Septum.** With this septum, a soft tissue sheet attaches to and extends between the anterior and posterior vaginal walls. This divides the vaginal into right and left cylinders. To excise the anterior wall attachment, sharp or electrosurgical cutting is kept close to the union line of the septum and vaginal wall. This incision is extended cephalad until the attachment is freed or the cervix is reached. Incision stops short of the cervix to avoid its injury. The

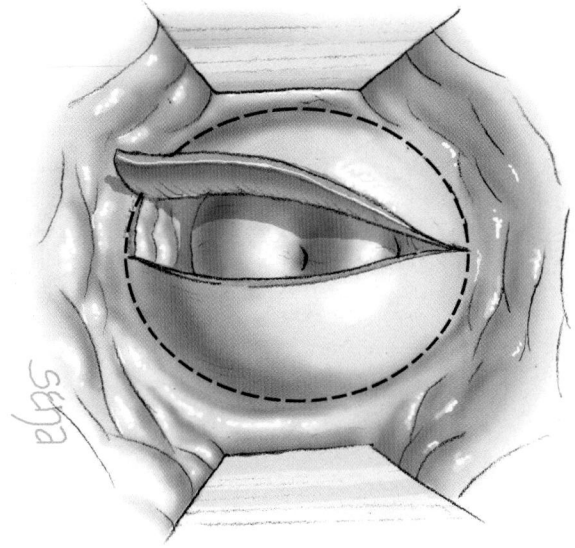

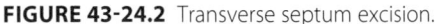

FIGURE 43-24.2 Transverse septum excision.

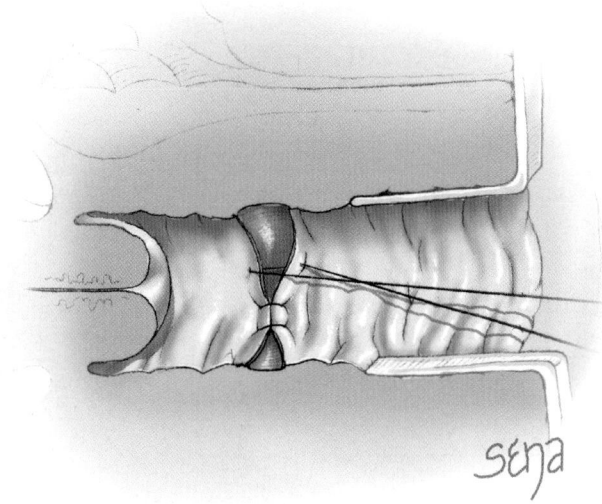

FIGURE 43-24.3 Vaginal mucosa reapproximation.

posterior wall attachment is similarly transected. For a lower partial septum, these two steps will free it. For high septa that extend between two cervices, a final anteroposterior incision across the septa and in front of the cervices will release it proximally.

❻ Obstructed Longitudinal Septum. With an oblique obstructive septum, its proximal end often originates between the two cervices of a uterine didelphys. The caudal end attaches to the lateral vaginal wall to

block outflow and distend the hemivagina. For this, a longitudinal incision is made centrally along the septum. Old blood is typically released with this. A finger is then placed through the incision to delineate the vaginal wall boundaries and identify the occult cervix. The Foley catheter tube in the urethra or a finger in the rectum may also assist with orientation. Once the septal perimeter is defined, the initial longitudinal incision is extended outward in an elliptical path to the vaginal wall margins.

❼ Wound Closure. With either longitudinal septum type, a simple line of interrupted stitches of 2-0 gauge delayed-absorbable suture is placed to reapproximate incised vaginal mucosal edges.

POSTOPERATIVE

The Foley catheter may be removed on the first postoperative day. The remaining postoperative care mirrors that for the McIndoe procedure, described next.

43-25

McIndoe Procedure

Creation of a functional vagina is the treatment goal for many women with congenital vagina agenesis. Although several surgical and nonsurgical approaches have been used, the McIndoe procedure is the most commonly employed in the United States (Chap. 18, p. 420). With this technique, a canal is formed between the urethra and urinary bladder anteriorly and the rectum posteriorly (McIndoe, 1938). A skin graft obtained from the patient's buttock or thigh is then wrapped around a soft mold and placed into the newly created vagina to allow epithelialization. Alternatively, other materials have been used to line the neovagina. These include buccal mucosa, cutaneous and myocutaneous flaps, amnionic membrane, and absorbable adhesion barrier (Creatsas, 2010; Fotopoulou, 2010; Li, 2014; Motoyama, 2003).

Vaginal stricture can be a significant complication following the McIndoe procedure. Thus, adherence to a postoperative regimen of vaginal dilatation is mandatory. For this reason, surgery may be postponed until the patient has reached the level of maturity needed to comply (American College of Obstetricians and Gynecologists, 2013a).

PREOPERATIVE

Patient Evaluation

Vaginal agenesis may be an isolated anomaly but is frequently associated with other müllerian defects. Thus, anatomy and anomalies are usually preoperatively defined with sonography or more commonly with magnetic resonance imaging (Chap. 18, p. 418).

Consent

Prior to surgery, patients are informed of overall success rates with this procedure. In a Mayo Clinic series of 225 patients, the McIndoe procedure provided a functional vagina to afford "satisfactory" intercourse in 85 percent of patients. In this review, the cumulative complication rate was 10 percent and included vaginal stricture, pelvic organ prolapse, graft failure, postcoital bleeding, and fistulas involving either the bladder or rectum (Klingele, 2003). Additionally, complications at the skin graft harvest site involved keloid formation, wound infection, and postoperative dysesthesias.

Patient Preparation

Antibiotic prophylaxis similar to that for hysterectomy is typically administered, and venous thromboembolism prophylaxis is planned (Tables 39-6 and 39-8, p. 835). Bowel preparation aids rectal decompression to permit greater room for blunt neovagina development. Also, digital rectal examination may be needed at times during surgery to direct dissection and avoid rectal laceration. An empty rectal vault may minimize wound contamination.

INTRAOPERATIVE

Instruments

Electrodermatome

The skin grafts used to line the neovagina are harvested from the donor site with the aid of an electrodermatome, which is able to shave grafts of varying size and depth. Both split-thickness and full-thickness skin grafts have been used in the McIndoe procedure, and the electrodermatome settings are adjusted to shave the desired depth.

Vaginal Mold

Following graft harvesting and neovagina formation, a stent is needed to apply the graft to the vaginal walls and hold it in place. Both soft and rigid forms have been used. Unfortunately, rigid or semirigid stents have led to graft loss, fibrosis, contracture, and pressure-related bladder or rectal fistulas.

Use of soft stents has decreased the number of these complications. Inflatable rubber stents or condoms filled with foam rubber or other soft compressible materials are examples (Adamson, 2004; Barutcu, 1998). The vagina graft produces abundant exudates, and poor drainage may lead to graft maceration, sloughing, and graft detachment. Accordingly, suction is attached to the soft

stents to aid drainage of the neovagina (Yu, 2004).

Surgical Steps

❶ **Anesthesia and Patient Positioning.** General anesthesia is administered, and the patient is initially positioned prone for skin graft harvesting from the buttock. Alternatively, skin may be obtained from the thigh or hip. Choosing a location that has minimal hair growth and is cosmetically discreet is desired. The assistance of a plastic surgeon may be enlisted for skin graft procurement.

❷ **Skin Graft.** The surgeon first marks the outline of the wound on the donor site skin, enlarging it by 3 to 5 percent to allow for skin shrinkage immediately after excision. The surgeon uses the electrodermatome to remove a single strip of skin that is typically 0.018 inch thick, 8 to 9 cm wide, and 18 to 20 cm long (Fig. 43-25.1). Alternatively, two smaller strips of 5 cm × 10 cm can be obtained from each buttock.

Following excision, the graft is placed in a pan of sterile saline. The harvest sites on the buttocks are sprayed with a topical hemostatic agent and dressed with a clear occlusive dressing (Tegaderm).

❸ **Perineal Incision.** The patient is then placed in standard dorsal lithotomy position, perineal cleansing is performed, and a Foley catheter inserted.

The lower edge of each labium minus is grasped with Allis clamps and extended laterally. A third Allis clamp is placed on the vestibular skin below the urethra and is lifted superiorly. A dimple in the vestibule is typically identified below the urethra, and a 2- to 3-cm transverse incision is made across the depression. Allis clamps are then placed on the superior and inferior edges of this incision and are retracted.

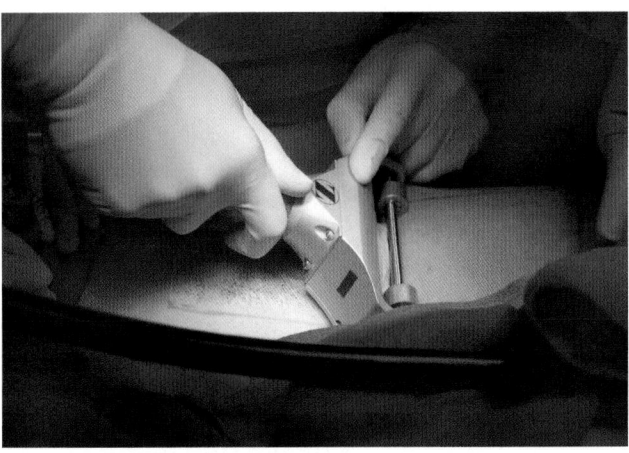

FIGURE 43-25.1 Skin graft harvest.

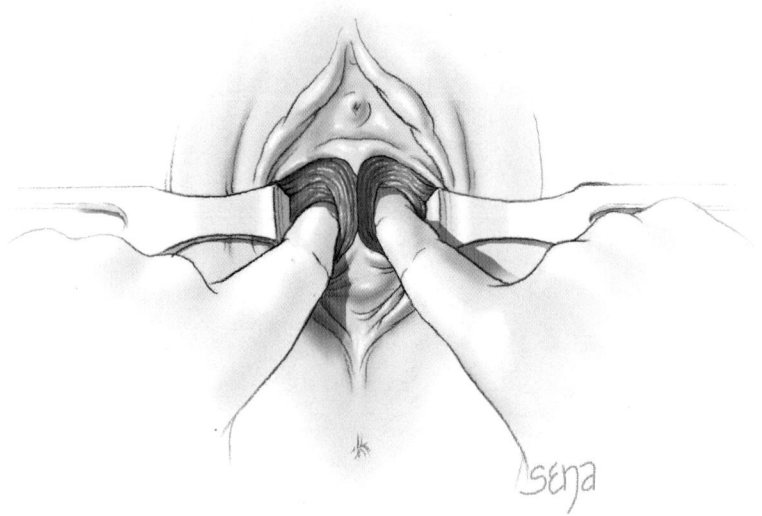

FIGURE 43-25.2 Neovaginal dissection.

❹ Neovaginal Dissection. With neovagina development, the goal is to create a canal that is bounded anteriorly by the pubovesical fascia that supports the urethra and bladder, posteriorly by the rectovaginal fascia and rectum, and laterally by the puborectalis muscles. Initially, two canals are created on either side of the median raphe, which is a midline collection of dense connective tissue bands that stretch between the urethra and bladder above and the rectum below (Fig. 43-25.2). The canals are initially formed using a spreading and gentle pushing motion with blunt-tipped scissors. Fingers are then insinuated into the forming tunnels, and pressure is exerted cephalad to extend the tunnel depth. To widen the canals, finger pads are rolled outward, and lateral pressure is applied. Posterior pressure should be avoided to prevent entering the rectum. Each canal is created to reach a depth of approximately 12 cm. Entering the cul-de-sac of Douglas is also avoided.

During dissection, several points are noteworthy. First, with initial caudal dissection,

the surgeon may meet greater resistance than with the more cephalad tissues. Second, remaining in the correct dissection plane can be difficult. Accordingly, the surgeon's finger may be placed into the rectum to identify its location and avert perforation. Similarly, the Foley catheter tubing may serve as an orienting tool anteriorly.

To expand the space, retractors can be placed along the lateral walls of the forming tunnels and stretched outward. Moreover, incising the medial fibers of the puborectalis muscles can add further width. These muscles are cut along the lateral aspect of each canal and at a level midway along the anteroposterior length of the canals.

Cephalad, the tunnel is extended to within 2 cm of the cul-de-sac of Douglas.

This leaves a layer of connective tissue affixed to the peritoneum. The skin graft will attach more effectively to this connective tissue than to a smooth peritoneal surface. Rates of subsequent enterocele formation are also lowered by this technique.

❺ Cutting the Median Raphe. Once the formation of the two tunnels is completed, the median raphe is cut. The final single canal measures approximately 10 to 12 cm deep and three fingerbreadths wide.

❻ Hemostasis. As collections of blood can separate the skin graft from the canal bed, hemostasis is required prior to mold insertion.

❼ Mold Preparation. The vaginal mold may now be covered with the harvested skin. The graft is removed from the saline bath. One end of the graft is placed at the base of one side of the mold with the skin's keratinized surface facing the mold. The long axis of the graft is laid parallel to the long axis of the mold. The graft is then draped up and over the mold tip (Fig. 43-25.3). Last, the lateral edges of the skin graft are approximated on either side of the mold using interrupted stitches of 3-0 catgut.

❽ Mold Customization. Adapting the mold to the size of the created neovaginal canal is essential. If the mold is too wide, pressure necrosis or inadequate drainage may result. Moreover, at the time of postoperative mold removal, a mold that is too

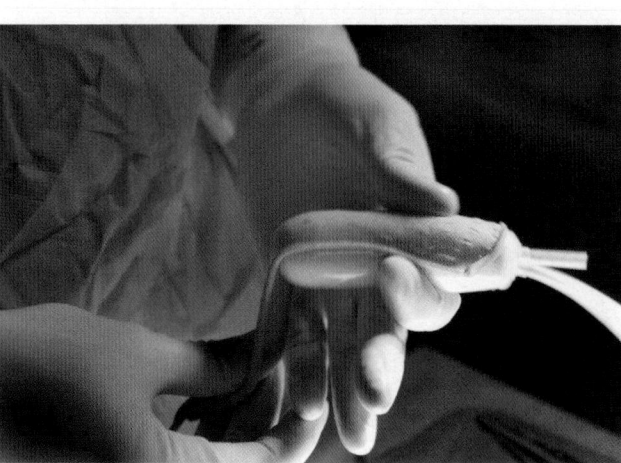

FIGURE 43-25.3 Mold creation.

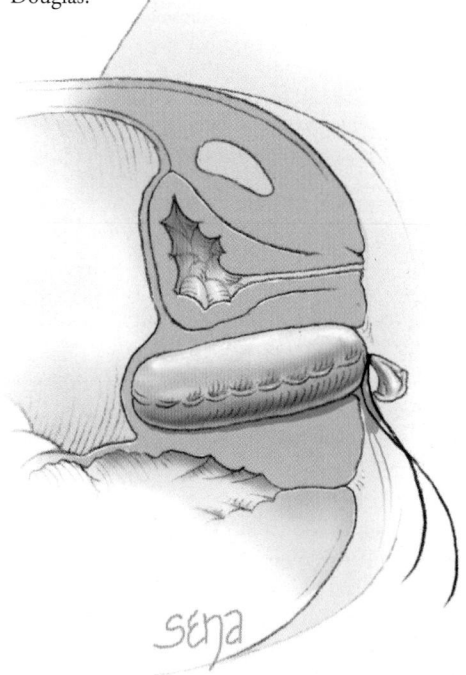

FIGURE 43-25.4 Skin graft and mold in place.

large and snuggly fitted into the neovagina may pull the graft loose. Once appropriately sized and constructed, the mold is then inserted (Fig. 43-25.4).

❾ Perineal Sutures. The edges of the skin graft at the distal end of the mold are then reapproximated to the distal circumferential opening of the neovagina using interrupted stitches of 4-0 or 5-0 gauge delayed-absorbable suture.

The labia minora, if sufficiently long, can be sutured together along the midline with 2-0 silk sutures to help hold the mold in place for the first 7 postoperative days. An elastic compression dressing is placed on the perineum.

POSTOPERATIVE

The soft stent and Foley catheter are left in place for 7 days following surgery. To minimize mold dislodgement and wound contamination, a low-residue diet and loperamide, 2 mg orally twice daily, is used to limit defecation.

At the time of mold removal, an operating room, general anesthesia, and standard dorsal lithotomy position are employed. Stitches in the labia minora are cut, and the mold is removed. To lessen the risk of graft avulsion, irrigation is used to reduce adherence between graft and mold.

Several schedules for postoperative dilatation have been described. Commonly, the size of the mold placed at surgery is too large for maintenance use. Therefore, a smaller dilator may initially be used and then gradually replaced with larger ones as the vagina stretches.

For the first 6 weeks following surgery, the dilator is worn continuously except during defecation. During the subsequent 6 weeks, it is used only at night. Following these initial 3 months, patients are then instructed to either wear the dilator at night or engage in intercourse at least twice each week.

43-26

Treatment of Preinvasive Ectocervical Lesions

LOOP ELECTROSURGICAL EXCISION PROCEDURE (LEEP)

In the United States, use of LEEP for cervical intraepithelial neoplasia (CIN) is popular and often preferred over cryotherapy or laser ablation. This procedure, also known as *large loop excision of the transformation zone (LLETZ)*, uses electric current through a monopolar wire electrode to either cut or coagulate cervical tissues. As such, these thin, semicircular electrodes allow clinicians to excise cervical lesions with minimal patient discomfort, cost, and complications. Moreover, unlike ablative procedures, LEEP permits submission of a surgical specimen for additional evaluation.

PREOPERATIVE

Patient Evaluation

In the United States, women typically receive colposcopic evaluation and histologic interpretation of cervical biopsies prior to LEEP. Less commonly, a "see and treat" approach is also acceptable for specific settings outlined in Chapter 29 (p. 637) (Numnum, 2005). With this, treatment is immediate and relies on initial diagnostic colposcopic findings rather than biopsy results.

For LEEP, part of patient evaluation includes her suitability for an in-office or an operating room procedure. Although office procedures offer lower cost and fewer anesthetic risks, several patient factors favor anesthesia in an operating room. First, markedly relaxed vaginal sidewalls may require significant and potentially uncomfortable retraction for adequate visualization. Second, a lesion or transformation zone that lies near the cervix periphery may risk vaginal or bladder injury during electrode-pass completion, especially if the patient moves unexpectedly. Last, patient comorbidities or anxiety and an inability to remain relatively motionless during an office procedure favor greater anesthesia and patient monitoring.

Consent

This procedure is associated with low morbidity, and overall complication rates approximate 10 percent (Dunn, 2004). Major complications are rare (0.5 percent) and may include bowel or bladder injury and hemorrhage (Dunn, 2003; Kurata, 2003). Short-term complications such as abdominal pain, heavier vaginal bleeding, and bladder spasm are treated symptomatically. Light vaginal bleeding or discharge is expected, and patients are so counseled.

Long-term complications include cervical stenosis and failure to completely treat the neoplasia. Persistent disease is typically noted in the initial surveillance Pap smear and in human papillomavirus (HPV) testing following LEEP. However, such treatment failure rates are low (approximately 5 percent) and are positively correlated with initial excised lesion size (Mitchell, 1998). Cervical stenosis is estimated to complicate less than 6 percent of cases. Risk factors include the presence of an endocervical lesion and excision of a large tissue volume (Baldauf, 1996; Suh-Burgmann, 2000).

The effects of LEEP with regard to obstetric outcomes are unclear. Several studies have shown that pregnancy does not appear to be adversely affected by LEEP, whereas others have noted increased risks of premature labor and premature rupture of membranes (Conner, 2014; Heinonen, 2013; Werner, 2010).

Patient Preparation

Ideally, LEEP is performed after completion of menses. This decreases the chance of a coexistent early pregnancy and allows cervical healing prior to the next menstrual cycle. With surgery prior to menses, abnormal postprocedural bleeding may be masked, and postsurgical swelling can block menstrual flow and intensify cramping. A normal bimanual examination is confirmed prior to surgery. If there is a possibility of pregnancy, β-hCG testing precedes treatment. Perioperatively, LEEP excision in general does not require antibiotic or venous thromboembolism prophylaxis. Similarly, bowel preparation is not needed.

INTRAOPERATIVE

Instruments

Tissue excision during LEEP requires an electrosurgical unit, wire loop electrodes, insulated speculum, and smoke evacuation system. Electrosurgical units used in LEEP procedures generate high-frequency (350–1200 kHz), low-voltage (200–500 V) electric current. Because of the risk for electric burns to the patient from stray current, grounding pads are placed on conductive tissue that is close to the operative site (Chap. 40, p. 858).

Similarly, an insulated speculum is used to limit the risk of stray current conductance to the patient. The insulated speculum has a port for smoke evacuation tubing, which assists in clearing smoke from the operating field to improve visualization and lower inhalation risks. Surgical smoke plumes can contain benzene, hydrogen cyanide, formaldehyde, and viruses, and thus local smoke evacuation systems are recommended (National Institute for Occupational Safety and Health, 1999). That said, transmission of infectious disease through surgical smoke has not been documented (Mowbray, 2013).

Electric current is directed to tissue via a 0.2-mm stainless steel or tungsten wire-loop electrode. These are available in various sizes to customize treatment according to lesion dimensions (Fig. 43-26.1). These instruments are disposable and discarded after each patient procedure.

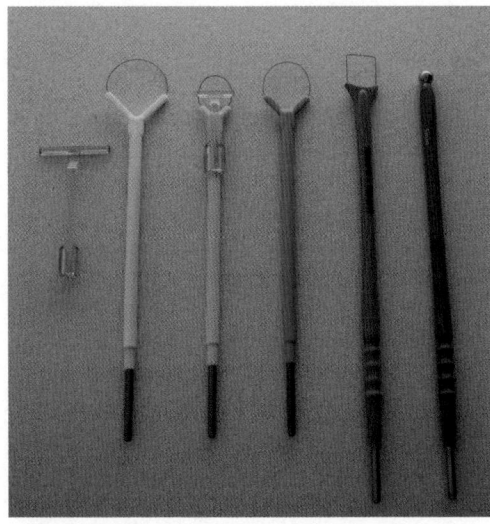

FIGURE 43-26.1 Various loop electrosurgical excision procedure (LEEP) electrodes.

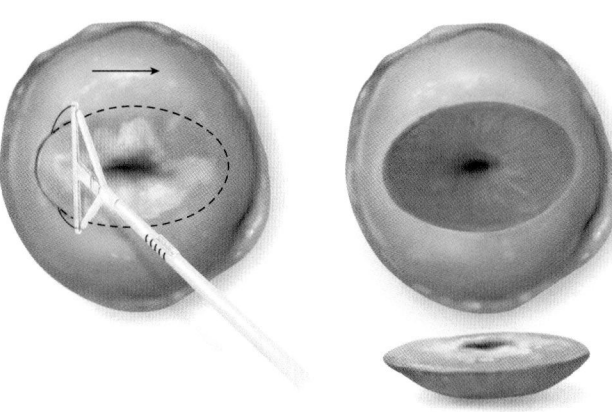

FIGURE 43-26.2 Single-pass loop electrosurgical excision.

Surgical Steps

❶ **Anesthesia and Patient Positioning.** The patient is placed in standard dorsal lithotomy position, and the electrosurgical grounding pad is placed on the upper thigh or buttock. The insulated speculum is inserted into the vagina, and smoke evacuation tubing is attached. The application of Lugol solution outlines lesion margins before starting the procedure (Chap. 29, p. 638).

For in office anesthesia, vasoconstricting solutions of either: (1) vasopressin in a 1-percent lidocaine solution (10 units Pitressin in 30 mL of lidocaine) or (2) 1-percent lidocaine with epinephrine (1:100,000 dilution) may be selected. A 25- to 27-gauge spinal needle is used to circumferentially inject 5 to 10 mL of either solution 1 to 2 cm deep into the cervix outside the area to be excised. Cervical blanching usually follows.

❷ **Single-pass Excision.** Ideally, the cervical transformation zone and CIN lesion is excised, and the appropriately sized loop is selected for this goal. If colposcopy is satisfactory, the correct loop diameter incorporates the transformation zone to a depth of 5 to 8 mm. The electrosurgical unit is set to cutting mode, and typically 30 to 50 W is used depending on the loop size. Larger loops require higher wattage.

To excise the transformation zone, a loop is positioned 3 to 5 mm outside the lateral perimeter of the area (Fig. 43-26.2). Current through the loop is activated prior to tissue contact, during which electric sparks at the loop tip may be seen. The loop is introduced to the cervix at a right angle to ectocervix. Once a 5 to 8-mm depth is reached, the loop is then drawn parallel to the surface until a point 3 to 5 mm outside the opposite border of the transformation zone and of the CIN lesion is reached. The loop is then withdrawn slowly, positioning it again at right angles to the surface. Current is stopped as soon as the loop exits the tissue. Following excision, the specimen is placed in formalin for pathologic evaluation.

❸ **Multiple-pass Excision.** Less commonly, bulky lesions may require multiple passes using a combination of loop electrode sizes (Fig. 43-26.3).

❹ **Control of Bleeding Sites.** Despite use of vasoconstrictors, bleeding following LEEP is common. Sites of active bleeding may be controlled using a 3- or 5-mm ball electrode, and the electrosurgical unit switched to coagulation mode. Alternatively, Monsel paste can be applied with direct pressure to bleeding sites.

POSTOPERATIVE

A watery vaginal discharge that develops after treatment usually requires light sanitary pad use, but tampons are discouraged. Vaginal spotting is expected and can persist for weeks. During the first few days following LEEP, patients may complain of diffuse mild lower abdominal pain or cramping for which nonsteroidal antiinflammatory drugs (NSAIDs) typically provide relief. Patients abstain from intercourse during the 4 weeks following surgery. Depending on patient symptoms, work and exercise may resume following treatment.

CERVICAL CRYOTHERAPY

For appropriate patients, cryotherapy has been used for decades to safely and effectively ablate the cervix transformation zone and CIN lesion. This method uses compressed gas to create extremely cold temperatures that necrose cervical epithelium. For this, the *cryoprobe*, an interfacing tip made of silver or copper, allows contact with and conduction of extreme cold across the cervix surface. When nitric oxide gas is used, probe temperatures can reach −65°C. Cell death occurs at −20°C (Gage, 1979).

As the cervical epithelium is cooled, an expanding layer of ice, called the *iceball*, forms beneath the center of the cryoprobe and grows circumferentially outward and past the probe margins. The expanding iceball grows in depth as well as circumference during treatment. The portion of the iceball in which temperatures fall below −20°C is termed the *lethal zone*. This zone spans from the center of the cryoprobe to a perimeter 2 mm *inside* the outer iceball edge. Past this perimeter, tissue temperatures are warmer, and necrosis may be incomplete. Thus,

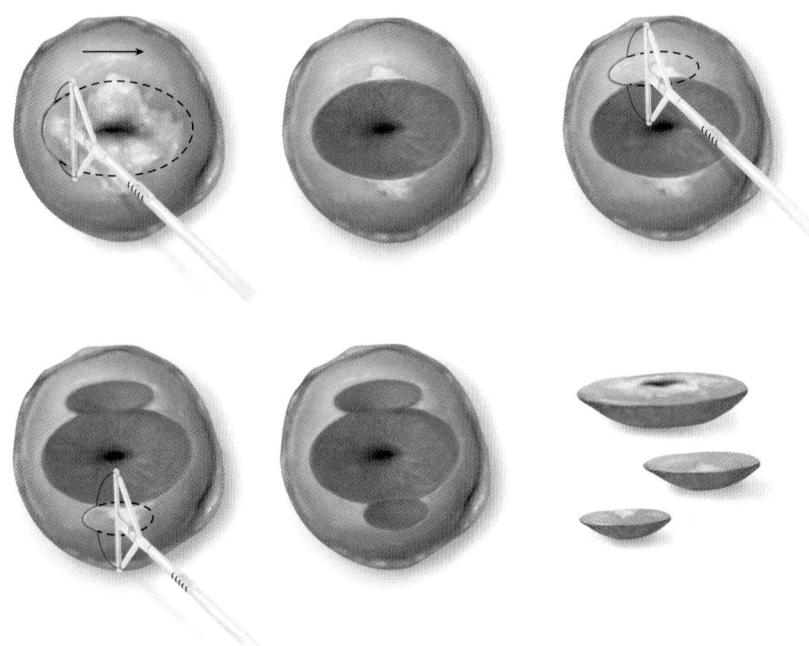

FIGURE 43-26.3 Multiple-pass excision.

when cryotherapy is performed, the iceball is allowed to enlarge until it reaches a mark 7 mm distal to the probe margin, that is, a 5-mm lethal zone and a 2-mm zone of indeterminate tissue death (Ferris, 1994).

Although some use these iceball dimensions to direct therapy, the World Health Organization (2014) recommends a double-freeze method for cryotherapy, described in the steps below. Importantly, a single-freeze method is not sufficient, and dysplasia recurs frequently in the first year following this treatment (Creasman, 1984; Schantz, 1984).

The specific indications and long-term rates of success for cryotherapy are discussed in Chapter 29 (p. 643). As reported in a national consensus guideline, randomized trials comparing different treatment modalities show similar efficacy (Massad, 2013). In general, cryotherapy is appropriate for squamous CIN that does not extend into the endocervical canal, does not span more than two quadrants of the ectocervix, is not associated with unsatisfactory colposcopic examination or abnormal glandular cytology, and is covered by the selected cryoprobe. Moreover, cryosurgery is generally not favored for treating CIN 3 due to higher rates of disease persistence following treatment and lack of a histologic specimen to exclude occult invasive cancer (Martin-Hirsch, 2013). Last, cryosurgery and other ablative techniques are not favored for women with CIN and human immunodeficiency virus (HIV) infection due to high failure rates (Spitzer, 1999).

PREOPERATIVE

Patient Evaluation

As with LEEP, women in the United States undergo colposcopy and histologic review of colposcopic biopsies prior to cryotherapy. Presurgical patient preparation mirrors that for LEEP (p. 988).

Consent

Intraoperative complications are uncommon, and hemorrhage is rare (Denny, 2005). Infrequently, women may experience a vasovagal reaction during treatment, and care is supportive. Perioperatively, patients are counseled that spotting, watery discharge, or cramping are typical, but infection is not. Long-term risks include cervical stenosis, squamocolumnar junction (SCJ) retraction into the endocervical canal, and treatment failure. Of these, treatment failures for CIN I and II have been cited at 6 to 10 percent (Benedet, 1981, 1987; Jacob, 2005; Ostergard, 1980). Last, infertility and pregnancy complications have not been associated with this treatment modality (Weed, 1978).

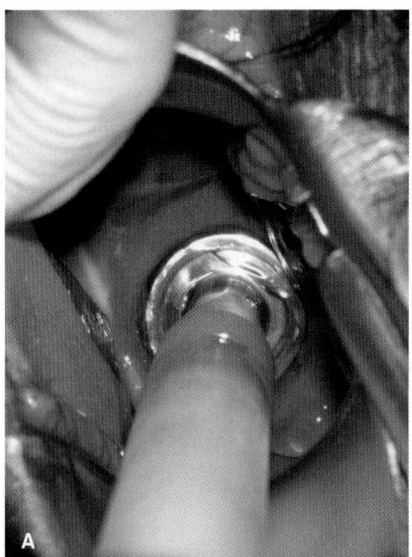
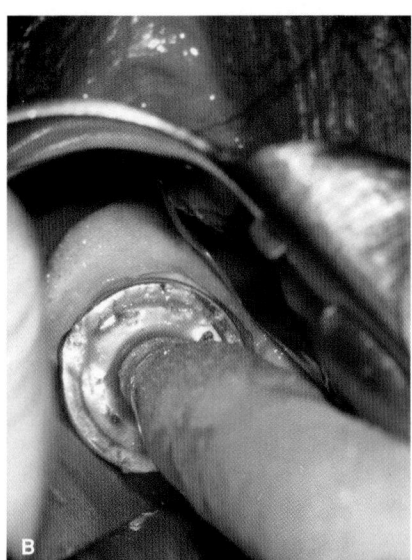

FIGURE 43-26.4 Cryotherapy. **A.** Cryotip applied to cervix. **B.** Creation of advancing iceball. (Used with permission from Dr. Claudia Werner.)

INTRAOPERATIVE

Instruments

Cryotherapy typically requires a tank of refrigerant gas plus a cryogun, connecting tubing, pressure gauge, and cryoprobe. Nitric oxide and carbon dioxide are frequently used refrigerant gases. Gas moves through connecting tubing, into the barrel of the cryogun, and then to the cryoprobe tip. Circumferential grooves at the cryoprobe base allow it to be screwed securely to the end of the cryogun.

Selection of an appropriate probe is individualized but should cover the transformation zone and lesion. Flat-faced probes are used for lesions located on the cervical portio. Advantageously, this shape has less of a tendency to push the resulting SCJ toward the endocervical canal, and it decreases the risk of unsatisfactory colposcopic examination following treatment.

❶ **Analgesia and Patient Positioning.** Cryotherapy may be performed in an office setting and requires no significant analgesia. However, to help attenuate associated uterine cramping, women are often given an NSAID prior to therapy.

The patient is positioned in standard dorsal lithotomy position, and a vaginal speculum is placed. No vaginal cleansing prep is required. The appropriate-sized cryoprobe is attached onto the end of the cryogun barrel. A water-based lubricant jelly is applied to the end of the cryoprobe to ensure even tissue contact.

❷ **Iceball Formation.** The probe is then pressed firmly against the cervix (Fig. 43-26.4). The cryogun trigger is squeezed, a light hissing

sound is typically heard, and frost begins to cover the probe. The trigger is held for 3 minutes as the iceball extends past the outer margin of the cryoprobe.

The cryoprobe should not contact the vaginal sidewalls. If this is identified, gas delivery is stopped to allow probe warming. The probe is then gently teased away from the wall, after which the procedure is continued.

❸ **First Thaw.** After the first freeze, the trigger is released. The probe quickly warms and can be removed from the cervix. Attempts to remove the probe prior to complete defrosting can cause patient discomfort and bleeding. The surface of the cervix is allowed to thaw during the following 5 minutes.

❹ **Second Cycle.** Subsequently, the freezing cycle is repeated for an additional 3 minutes. At completion of the second cycle, the cryoprobe and speculum are removed. Because vasovagal responses can be seen with this procedure, patients are assisted to a sitting position slowly.

POSTOPERATIVE

As noted, watery vaginal discharge that can persist for weeks, vaginal spotting, and cramping that responds to NSAIDs are expected. Infrequently, severe pain and cramping may result from necrotic tissue obstructing the endocervical canal. Removal of the obstructing tissue typically resolves symptoms.

Because a large area of the cervix is denuded after cryotherapy, the potential for infection is increased. Accordingly, patients abstain from intercourse during the 4 weeks following surgery. If abstinence is

CARBON DIOXIDE LASER CERVICAL ABLATION

The carbon dioxide (CO_2) laser produces a beam of infrared light that produces heat at its focal point sufficient to boil intracellular water and vaporize tissue. Indications and success rates are discussed more fully in Chapter 29 (p. 643). In general, laser ablation may be used for cases in which the entire transformation zone can be seen with satisfactory colposcopy. There should be no evidence of microinvasive, invasive, or glandular disease, and cytology and histology should positively correlate.

Although research has shown laser ablation to be an effective tool in treating CIN, its popularity has declined. Laser units are significantly more expensive than those used for cryotherapy and LEEP. Moreover, lesions are destroyed with ablation, and unlike LEEP, the opportunity for additional pathologic evaluation of surgical margins is lost. Last, physician and staff training and maintenance of certification are typically required for safe, effective use of laser equipment.

PREOPERATIVE

Consent

Laser ablation is considered a safe and effective means to treat CIN. As with any treatment of cervical dysplasia, patients should be counseled on the risks of disease persistence and recurrence following treatment. These risks and surgical complications are low and comparable with those for LEEP (Nuovo, 2000).

INTRAOPERATIVE

Instruments

Carbon dioxide lasers suitable for cervical ablation are mobile, self-contained units. Tissue effects vary depending on the interval at which energy bursts are released. As a result, continuous waves (cutting) or pulsed energy (coagulation) can be released. Laser guidance is accomplished through attachment to a colposcopic sled device.

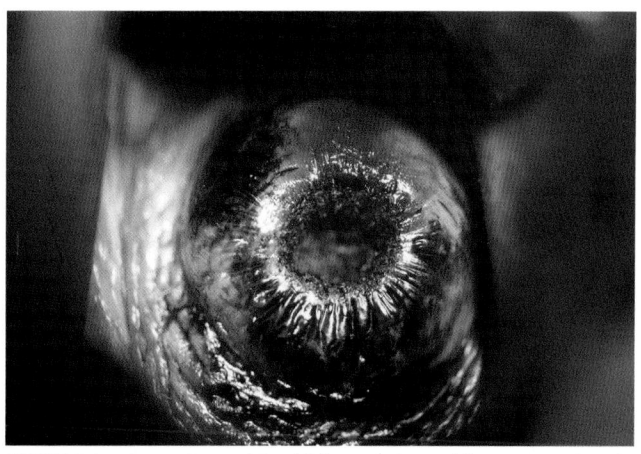

FIGURE 43-26.5 Cervical bed following laser ablation. (Used with permission from Dr. Eddie McCord.)

Because laser light is reflective, protective eyewear is required for the patient and all participants, and a sign is posted on the suite door warning that a laser procedure is in progress. For this same reason, a matte-surface speculum is necessary. As with LEEP, noxious smoke is generated, and a smoke evacuation system is required.

Surgical Steps

❶ Anesthesia and Patient Positioning. Laser ablation for many women is an outpatient procedure and performed in either an operating suite or an office, depending on laser equipment location and patient characteristics. In most cases, local analgesia combined with a vasoconstrictor is sufficient, and administration mirrors that used for LEEP (p. 989). The patient is placed in standard dorsal lithotomy position. A matte-surfaced speculum is inserted, and smoke evacuation tubing is attached to a port on the speculum. Misdirected laser energy can burn surrounding tissues and ignite paper drapes. Therefore, moistened cloth towels are draped outside the vulva to absorb misdirected energy. To delineate the area of excision, Lugol solution is applied.

❷ Laser Settings. The colposcope-laser assembly is brought into position and focused on the ectocervix. The laser is set to achieve a power density (PD) of 600 to 1200 W/cm^2 in a continuous wave mode. Average PD =

$100 \times W / D^2$. In this formula, D is the spot diameter in mm at 10 W at 0.1 sec pulse. Thus, a power of 10 W with a spot diameter of 1 mm will yield a PD of 1000 W/cm^2.

❸ Ablation. Initially, four dots are ablated at 12, 3, 6, and 9 o'clock positions on the perimeter of the cervix to surround the entire lesion. These dots serve as landmarks and are connected in an arching pattern to create a circle. Once encircled, the area is ablated to a depth of 5 to 7 mm (Fig. 43-26.5)

❹ Endocervical Eversion. To help prevent postoperative retraction of the SCJ cephalad into the endocervical canal, the tissue immediately surrounding the endocervix is ablated less deeply. This allows an apparent eversion of the endocervical lining and retention of the SCJ on the ectocervix.

❺ Hemostasis. Bleeding is common during CO_2 laser vaporization. A defocused laser beam and a lower power setting in a super pulse wave mode will coagulate vessels and aid hemostasis. Bleeding present at the end of surgery may also be controlled with an application of Monsel paste.

POSTOPERATIVE

Cramping is common following surgery, and light bleeding may persist for a week. Postoperative patient counseling is similar to that for LEEP (p. 989).

43-27

Cervical Conization

Cervical conization removes ectocervical lesions and a portion of the endocervical canal by means of a conical tissue biopsy (Fig. 43-27.1). It is a safe, effective means to treat CIN, carcinoma in situ (CIS), and adenocarcinoma in situ (AIS). Moreover, cervical conization is a standard treatment for women with unsatisfactory colposcopy and biopsies suggestive of high-grade CIN, those with positive endocervical curettage, or those with discordant cytologic and histologic findings. Excision may be completed via scalpel, termed *cold-knife conization.* Alternatively, laser or LEEP conization may be performed. Success rates for these excisional methods in the treatment of CIN are equivalent. However, LEEP conization has gained popularity because of its ease of use and cost effectiveness.

PREOPERATIVE

Patient Evaluation

Prior to conization, patients will have undergone colposcopic examination and histologic evaluation of biopsies. β-hCG testing is

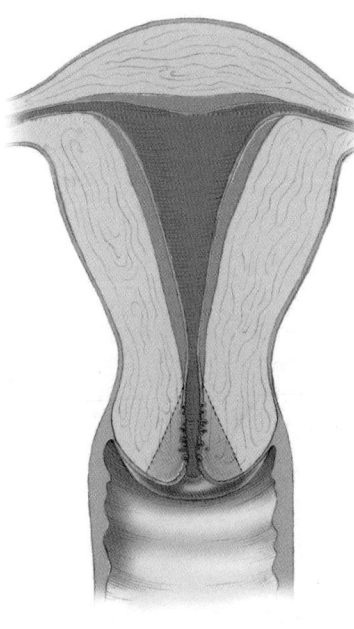

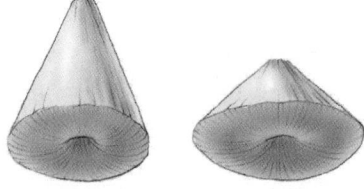

FIGURE 43-27.1 Cone-shaped tissue biopsies.

warranted prior to conization if pregnancy is suspected. If pregnancy is confirmed and invasion is not suspected colposcopically, postpartum patient management is reasonable. Conization during pregnancy has great morbidity because of increased vascularity and intraoperative bleeding.

Consent

Risks associated with conization mirror those for LEEP excision of ectocervical lesions. However, cold-knife conization has a greater risk of bleeding compared with that of laser and LEEP conization. Moreover, cold-knife and laser conizations carry higher risks of cervical stenosis compared with LEEP conization (Baldauf, 1996; Houlard, 2002). Increasing age and depth of endocervical excision are significant cervical stenosis risks. Penna and coworkers (2005) noted a lower risk of stenosis in postmenopausal women using estrogen replacement therapy compared with postmenopausal nonusers.

Cervical conization for CIN treatment has been associated with adverse outcomes in subsequent pregnancies that include preterm delivery, low-birthweight neonates, incompetent cervix, and cervical stenosis (Kristensen, 1993a,b; Raio, 1997; Samson, 2005). Although there is no major difference in obstetric outcome among the three techniques, increased cone biopsy size has been shown to positively correlate with rates of preterm delivery and premature membrane rupture (Mathevet, 2003; Sadler, 2004). Cold-knife conization generally removes more cervical stroma than other excisional methods.

COLD-KNIFE CONIZATION

Surgical Steps

❶ **Anesthesia and Patient Positioning.** For most women, cold-knife conization is a day-surgery procedure performed under general or regional anesthesia. Following administration of anesthesia, the patient is placed in the standard dorsal lithotomy position. The vagina is surgically prepared, the bladder drained, and vaginal sidewalls retracted to reveal the cervix. Areas of planned excision may be more easily identified following Lugol solution application.

❷ **Injection of Vasoconstrictors.** Associated bleeding during cold-knife conization can be brisk and obscure the operating field. Accordingly, preventative steps can be taken. First, vasoconstrictors as described for LEEP are injected circumferentially into the cervix (p. 989). Additionally, descending cervical branches of the uterine arteries, which supply

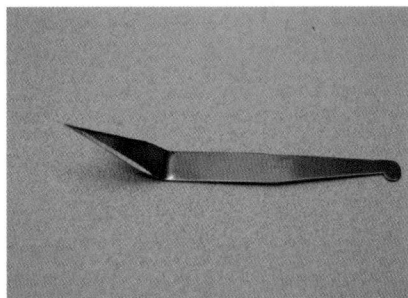

FIGURE 43-27.2 Beaver blade.

the cervix, can be ligated with figure-of-eight stitches using nonpermanent suture. These are placed along the lateral aspects of the cervix at 3 and 9 o'clock. After the knots are secured, the sutures are kept long and held by hemostats to manipulate the cervix.

❸ **Conization.** A uterine sound or small-caliber uterine dilator is placed into the endocervical canal to orient the surgeon as to the depth and direction of the canal. Using a no. 11 blade, the surgeon initiates the incision on the lower lip of the cervix. This limits blood from running downward and obscuring the planned incision path. Alternatively, a Beaver blade, which is a triangular-shaped knife blade with a 45-degree bend, may be used (Fig. 43-27.2). With either blade, a circumscribing incision creates a 2- to 3-mm border around the entire lesion (Fig. 43-27.3). The 45-degree angle of the blade is directed centrally and cephalad to excise a conical specimen. Toothed forceps or tissue hooks may be used to retract the ectocervix during cone creation. After incision of the ectocervix, a scalpel or Mayo scissors cuts the deep tip of the cone and releases the specimen. A suture is placed on the site of the specimen that corresponds to its 12 o'clock position in situ. The location of this suture is noted on the pathology requisition form and allows the pathologist to report positive and negative margin sites relative to their clock position.

❹ **Endocervical Curettage.** Following removal of the cone specimen, endocervical curettage is performed to evaluate for presence of residual disease proximal to the excised cone apex. This is sent as a separate specimen for evaluation.

❺ **Hemostasis.** With excision of the specimen, bleeding is common and can be controlled with individual suturing of isolated vessels, with electrosurgical coagulation, or with Sturmdorf sutures. In addition, a topical hemostatic agent such as absorbable methylcellulose mesh can be placed in the cone bed.

With placement of Sturmdorf sutures, a running locked suture line closes the cone

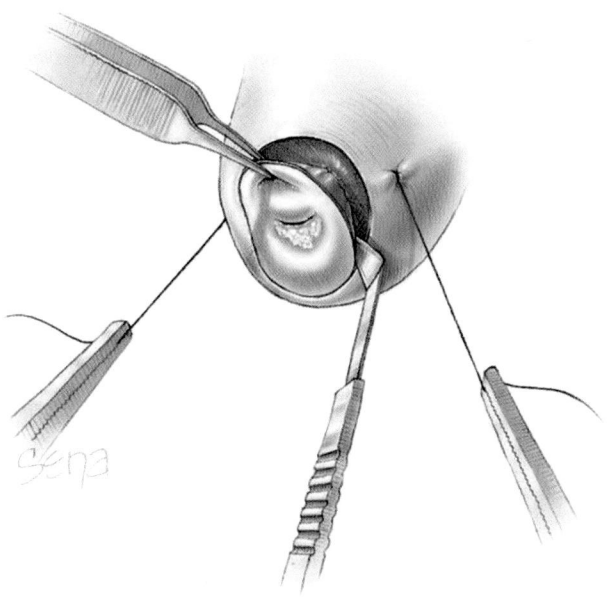

FIGURE 43-27.3 Conization incision.

bed by circumferentially folding the cut ectocervical edge inward toward the endocervix. This technique is less favored due to increased rates of postoperative dysmenorrhea, unsatisfactory postoperative surveillance Pap smears, and concerns that the flap might conceal residual disease (Kristensen, 1990; Trimbos, 1983).

LOOP ELECTROSURGICAL EXCISION PROCEDURE (LEEP) CONIZATION

Surgical Steps

The surgical steps for this more extensive LEEP mirror those used for excision of ectocervical lesions (p. 989). However, to remove a portion of the endocervical canal, a deeper pass must be made through the cervical stroma. This may be accomplished with a single deeper pass using a larger loop. Alternatively, in an effort to minimize the volume of tissue excised, a tiered or *top hat technique* can be selected. With this method, an initial pass is made to remove ectocervical lesions as previously described (see Fig. 43-26.2, p. 989). To remove endocervical canal tissue, a second smaller loop is passed more deeply into the cervical stroma (Fig. 43-27.4). As a result, the tissue is excised in two pieces, and both are sent for evaluation. Similar to cold-knife conization, the specimen is marked with suture to note its 12 o'clock position in situ.

LASER CONIZATION

Excision of a laser cone biopsy specimen uses techniques similar to those described for laser ablation (p. 991). However, rather than ablating the involved tissue, laser energy is directed to cut and remove the cone-biopsy specimen. A higher power density is used to create a cutting effect, for example, 25 W with a 1-mm spot size (PD = 2500 W/cm²). A cone-shaped specimen is then excised. During excision of the cone specimen, nonreflective tissue hooks may be needed to retract the ectocervical edge away from the

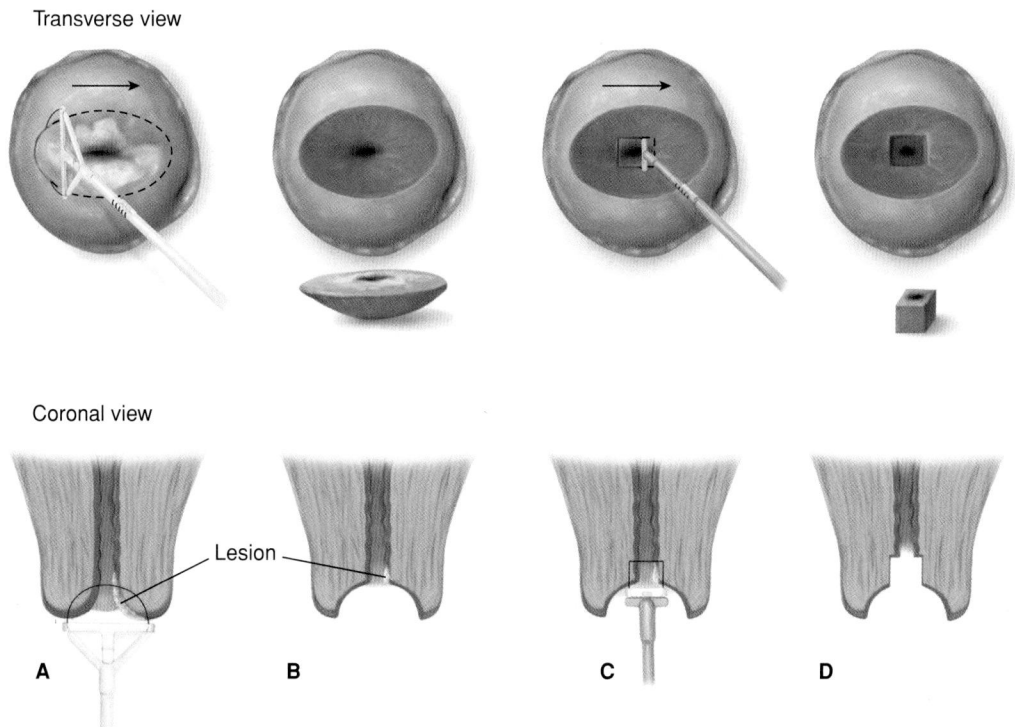

FIGURE 43-27.4 Loop electrosurgical excision procedure (LEEP) "top hat" cervical conization procedure transverse (*upper row*) and coronal (*lower row*) views. **A.** Excision of ectocervical portion of lesion. **B.** Appearance of cervix following ectocervical excision. **C.** Excision of endocervical portion of lesion. **D.** Appearance of cervix upon procedure completion.

laser beam path and to create tissue tension along the plane of incision.

POSTOPERATIVE

Recovery following all excisional methods is rapid and follows that for other surgeries of the cervix previously described (p. 989).

However, due to the greater incision, postoperative bleeding can develop more commonly and is treated with Monsel paste or other topical hemostat. Patients require postoperative surveillance for identification of disease persistence or recurrence, and this is described in detail in Chapter 29 (p. 644).

43-28

Treatment of Vulvar Intraepithelial Neoplasia

WIDE LOCAL EXCISION

With high-grade vulvar intraepithelial neoplasia (VIN), treatment goals include prevention of invasive vulvar cancer and when possible, the preservation of normal vulvar anatomy and function. For more widespread VIN, simple vulvectomy may be appropriate treatment and is described in Section 46-24 (p. 1208). However, less extensive methods such as wide local excision of lesions, ablative modalities, and medical treatments have also been evaluated as alternative options (Chap. 29, p. 649) (Hillemanns, 2006).

Of these, wide local excision of lesions is favored by many. It removes the preinvasive lesion, offers a tissue specimen for exclusion of invasive disease and evaluation of surgical margins, and compared with simple vulvectomy, lowers patient morbidity. In cases where excision involves the clitoris, urethra, or anus, a combined surgical excision and laser ablation approach is sometimes helpful. This combined technique uses CO_2 laser vaporization at sites where excision might lead to dysfunction or poor cosmesis (Cardosi, 2001).

PREOPERATIVE

Patient Evaluation

Prior to excision, full evaluation of the lower reproductive tract for evidence of invasive disease is completed as outlined in Chapter 29 (pp. 637 and 648). Importantly, vulvar biopsies are obtained during this evaluation and should exclude invasive disease, which would warrant more extensive excision (Chap. 31, p. 684).

Consent

Wide local excision of high-grade VIN successfully treats disease, and progression to invasive vulvar cancer is low (3 to 5 percent) (Jones, 2005; Rodolakis, 2003). However, VIN recurrence is common, and even in those patients with tissue margins negative for disease, recurrence ranges from 15 to 40 percent (Kuppers, 1997; Modesitt, 1998).

In the immunocompetent, surgical and postoperative risks are few and typically include wound infection or separation, chronic vulvodynia, dyspareunia, and scarring or altered

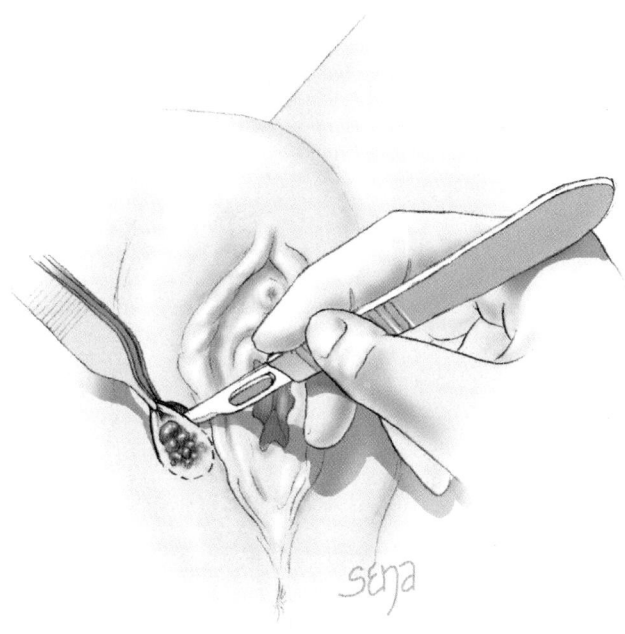

FIGURE 43-28.1 Vulvar incision.

vulvar appearance. Any vulvar operation requires thorough preoperative counseling regarding expectations for anatomic outcome and for sexual function.

INTRAOPERATIVE

Surgical Steps

❶ **Anesthesia and Patient Positioning.** The choice of anesthesia or analgesia will vary depending on the location and size of the treated lesion. Whereas smaller labial or perineal lesions may easily be excised using local analgesia in an office setting, larger lesions or those involving the urethra and/or clitoris may require general or regional anesthesia. The patient is placed in standard dorsal lithotomy position, pubic hair at the surgical site is clipped, and the vulva is surgically prepared.

❷ **Lesion Identification.** The area of excision should be well demarcated. For this, colposcopic examination following application of 3- to 5-percent acetic acid to the vulva will aid identification of lesion margins. Most recommend a 5-mm circumferential surgical margin surrounding the lesion (Joura, 2002). In the past, toluidine blue has been used to stain nuclear chromatin and enhance vulvar lesions. However, normal tissue can also absorb the stain and distort true disease margins, and use of toluidine blue is therefore not recommended.

❸ **Incision.** As shown here, a scalpel with a no. 15 surgical blade is used to incise smaller

lesions, whereas a no. 10 blade may be suitable for larger excisions (Fig. 43-28.1). An elliptical incision is preferred and aids wound reapproximation. Most VIN lesions fail to extend deeper than 1 mm on non-hair-bearing areas such as the labia minora. However, in hair-bearing areas of the vulva, VIN may extend to the deepest hair follicles. This is generally deeper than 2 mm, but not more than 4 mm. Thus, incision depth will vary depending on lesion location (Shatz, 1989). Once the incision is completed, Adson forceps or skin hooks can elevate and retract the skin margin away from the incision line. Dissection beneath the lesion begins at the incision periphery and progresses toward the center of the proposed excision area and then to the opposite incision margin.

Disease recurrence is related to the presence or absence of disease-free surgical margins. Thus, frozen sections of the specimen margins can be evaluated intraoperatively.

❹ **Margin Undermining.** Reapproximation of the wound edges without tension decreases the risk of postoperative superficial separation. Accordingly, a surgeon may need to sharply undermine the skin at the wound margins with fine scissors to mobilize the skin and immediate underlying subcutaneous tissue.

❺ **Wound Closure.** Prior to edge reapposition, the wound bed is rendered hemostatic to minimize hematoma formation and subsequent wound separation. The edges of the skin are then reapproximated with interrupted stitches using 3-0 or 4-0 gauge delayed-absorbable sutures.

POSTOPERATIVE

Without complication, recovery from wide local excision is typically rapid, and patients may resume normal activities as desired. Sitz baths and oral analgesics are usually recommended for the first week following surgery. Intercourse is delayed until wounds have fully healed, and this time will vary depending on wound site and size. Superficial wound separation is not uncommon, and sites of separation will heal by secondary intention.

Because of the significant risk for VIN recurrence, postprocedural surveillance is essential. Colposcopic vulvar examination is completed every 6 months for 2 years and then annually thereafter.

CAVITATIONAL ULTRASONIC SURGICAL ASPIRATION (CUSA)

Indications for use and mechanism of action of cavitational ultrasonic surgical aspiration are discussed more fully in Chapter 40 (p. 859). Briefly, cavitation causes fragmentation and disruption of tissue, which is then aspirated and collected. Thus, the tissue, although fragmented, can be sent for histologic or cytologic evaluation.

Treatment of high-grade VIN with CUSA usually produces excellent cosmetic results, and complications such as scarring and dyspareunia are rare. However, the recurrence rate is high, as it is with other treatment modalities for VIN, and especially in treated hair-bearing areas (Miller, 2002). Thus, it is generally reserved for vulvar skin without hair. Although the procedure allows for tissue evaluation, tissue disruption may preclude adequate examination of all parts of the specimen and their associated relationships. Cost is greater than for excisional therapy and is similar to the cost of laser therapy. Depending on lesion size, CUSA can be more time consuming compared with excision or laser ablation. However, compared with laser therapy, CUSA lacks a smoke plume and avoids the risks associated with radiant energy.

In addition to VIN treatment, CUSA works well for condyloma acuminata, particularly bulky or multifocal condyloma or condyloma that are refractory to topical treatment. Information regarding cavitational therapy for condyloma acuminata is included in this section due to the similarity of treatment for VIN.

PREOPERATIVE

Patient Evaluation

The same principles apply as for excisional treatment of VIN. Specifically, a full evaluation of the lower genital tract is indi-cated to exclude an invasive process. Although condyloma acuminata are often diagnosed and treated on the basis of clinical appearance, a complete evaluation of the lower genital tract should likewise be undertaken preoperatively.

Consent

Risks of cavitational therapy for VIN or condyloma are few and are similar to those of wide local excision. Postoperative healing is by secondary intention and may take several weeks.

INTRAOPERATIVE

Instruments

The CUSA unit consists of a console, an operative hand piece, and a foot pedal, by which the system is activated (Fig. 43-28.2). The console allows control of amplitude or intensity, irrigation, and aspiration. Amplitude determines the relative amount of tissue fragmentation. A setting at 1 will produce cellular fragmentation to a depth of 30 μm, whereas a setting at 10 will produce cellular fragmentation to a depth of 300 μm. Fragmentation of a specific tissue is dependent on its water content. Therefore, less power is required for tissues with high water content such as skin and condyloma. Irrigation is used to control the considerable heat generated by the vibrating titanium tip (23 kHz) of the hand piece and to suspend the fragmented tissue for suction removal. The tip has a hollow 2-mm diameter and will remove tissue within a 1- to 2-mm radius of the tip. Vaporized and fragmented tissue is aspirated through the hollow tip of

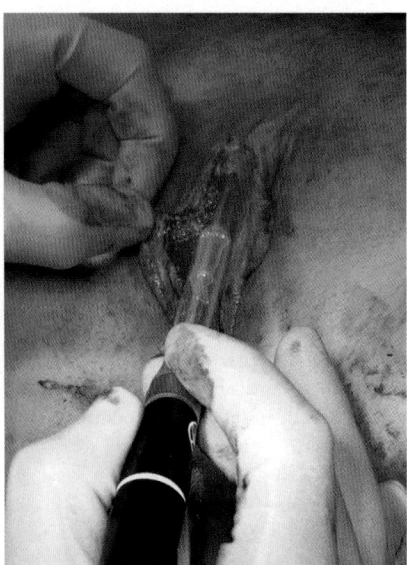

FIGURE 43-28.2 Operative handpiece of the cavitational ultrasonic surgical aspiration (CUSA) unit.

the hand piece and collected in a tissue trap. Each console setting may be varied depending on the needs of the operator.

Surgical Steps

❶ **Anesthesia and Patient Positioning.** CUSA is performed in the operating room under regional or general anesthesia. The patient is placed in standard dorsal lithotomy position. The vulva and the perianal region, if involved with disease, are surgically prepped.

❷ **Lesion Identification.** The same colposcopic identification techniques used prior to wide local excision apply for CUSA (p. 995). In Figure 43-28.3A, two areas of VIN are evident even prior to application 3- to 5-percent acetic acid. The larger of the two is located in the midportion of the right labium minus, and the smaller is more anterior and toward the clitoris.

❸ **Console Settings.** For treatment of VIN and condyloma acuminata, an amplitude setting of 5 to 6 produces cellular fragmentation to a tissue depth of 150 μm to 180 μm and should allow adequate removal of tissue without significant thermal injury. However, some studies have used amplitude settings at 6 to 8 for treatment of VIN (Miller, 2002). Irrigation and aspiration rates may be varied depending on the need of the operator. For example, if tissue fulguration is desired, a decrease in the irrigation rate will permit additional heat production at the hand-piece tip. Aerosolization can be minimized with proper balance of irrigation and aspiration rates.

❹ **Ablation.** As with wide local excision, the area of treatment should extend at least 5 mm beyond the identified lesion(s). The hand-piece tip is moved over the vulva in a back-and-forth motion. Only close contact with the skin of the vulva is required; no pressure is necessary. Repeat movements of the tip over the involved area dictate the depth of tissue removal. However, depth of destruction is often difficult to assess. Collagen bundles and elastic fibers become visible in the reticular dermis (Reid, 1985). Tissue destruction beyond this point increases the likelihood of scarring. For treatment of VIN, depth of treatment may vary between 1.5 and 2.5 mm (Miller, 2002; Rader, 1991). For condyloma acuminata, depth of treatment need not extend beyond the basement membrane (Ferenczy, 1983). Bleeding, if any, is usually minor and is controlled with pressure. Figure 43-28.3B shows the end result for the same patient shown in part A.

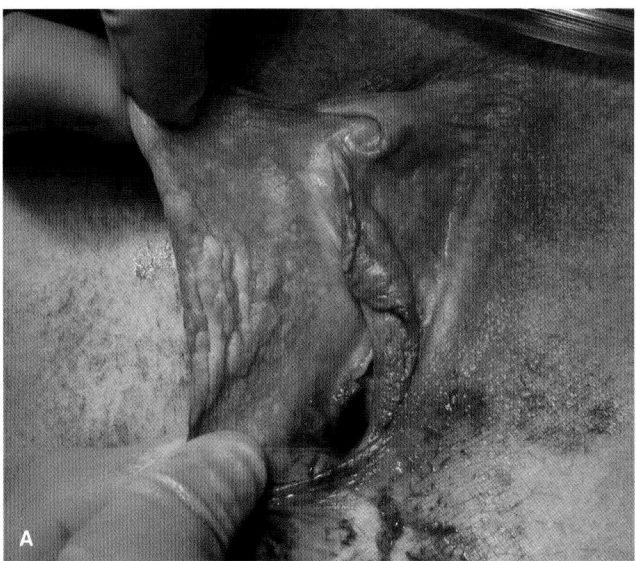 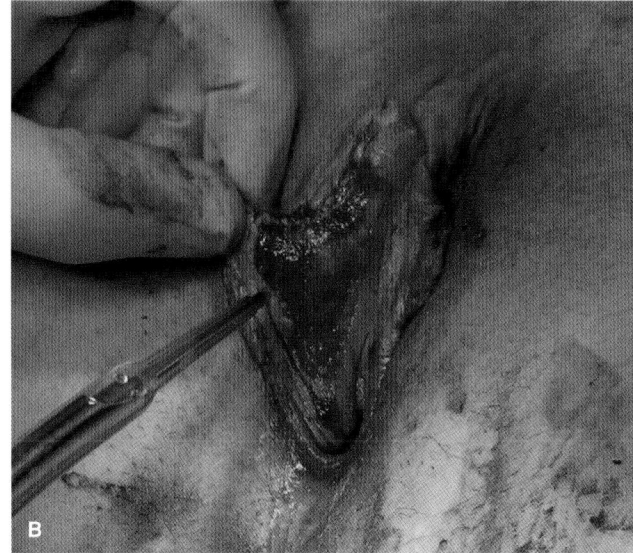

FIGURE 43-28.3 A. Vulvar intraepithelial neoplasia (VIN) involving the right labium minus. **B.** Cavitational ultrasonic surgical aspiration (CUSA) treatment of VIN completed.

POSTOPERATIVE

A 1-percent silver sulfadiazine cream may be applied to the vulva immediately following ablative therapy and continued once or twice daily for a short time. Oral analgesics and sitz baths are helpful in pain management following therapy. Patients may be seen for reevaluation 2 to 4 weeks postoperatively.

CARBON DIOXIDE LASER VAPORIZATION OF VIN

The CO_2 laser has been used for decades for treatment of VIN (Baggish, 1981). Success rates vary, however, and depend on factors such as length of patient surveillance, number of therapy courses, specific area of treatment, and total area of treated disease. In theory, the CO_2 laser is an ideal means to treat VIN. When used with the colposcope, the laser can accurately eradicate disease while preserving normal tissue structure and function. Associated bleeding is scant, healing is usually excellent, and scarring is minimal. Rates of significant complications are generally low. CO_2 laser vaporization may also be considered as an addition to an excisional procedure. One example is if there is multifocal disease involving both hair-bearing and non-hair-bearing areas, such as the clitoris, where excision may not be ideal. That said, Reid and colleagues (1985) recommend that only those surgeons experienced with CO_2 lasers attempt VIN vaporization by this method. Indeed, there is literally a thin margin between the depth of therapy needed to eradicate disease and a depth that may produce delayed healing, scarring, and a poor cosmetic result.

As with other destructive techniques, before laser vaporization is performed, invasive disease must be excluded. Since VIN is often multifocal, a thorough examination of the vulva and the lower genital tract with biopsy of any abnormal-appearing area is imperative. No tissue sample will be available for analysis following CO_2 laser vaporization.

PREOPERATIVE

Consent

As with other VIN treatment methods, recurrence or persistence following CO_2 laser vaporization is possible, and the patient is counseled on the need for postoperative surveillance. Pain, infection, fever, skin depigmentation, alopecia, scarring, and dyspareunia may result from treatment. Healing is generally complete in 4 to 6 weeks but may be delayed if treatment extends significantly into the dermis (Wright, 1987).

INTRAOPERATIVE

Instruments

A general description of the CO_2 laser is found on page 991. Recommendations regarding its use for cervical ablation of CIN are likewise appropriate for treatment of VIN.

Surgical Steps

❶ **Anesthesia and Patient Positioning.** Laser ablation of VIN is nearly always performed as an outpatient procedure either in an office setting or in an operative suite depending on laser availability. The procedure

may be performed under general, regional, or local anesthesia. Ferenczy and associates (1994) used disease greater than 6 cm^2 as a criterion for general anesthesia. The patient is placed in standard dorsal lithotomy position. To lessen the risk of injury from misdirected laser energy to tissues beyond those being treated, wet towels are positioned around the operative field. Paper drapes are avoided due to risk of fire. A moistened sponge is placed inside the rectum to prevent passage of flatus into the surgical field and possible gas ignition.

❷ **Laser Settings.** The laser is coupled to the colposcope, and the assembly is brought into focus on the vulva. A power density (PD) of 600 to 1200 W/cm^2 delivered in continuous mode is sufficient for therapy. However, Reid and associates (1985) caution that PD >600 W/cm^2 may be difficult to control on the vulva. Calculation of power density is described on page 991.

❸ **Examination of Treatment Area.** After a soaking application of 3- to 5-percent acetic acid solution is applied to the vulva, the area to be treated is examined colposcopically to delineate the zone of vaporization. This may be marked with the laser beam, incorporating a margin of 3 to 5 mm or upward to 1 cm of normal-appearing tissue (Helmerhorst, 1990; Hoffman, 1992).

❹ **Ablation.** The location of VIN will determine the needed depth of laser beam penetration for treatment. As hair root sheaths may harbor VIN up to a depth of 2.5 mm, involved hairy areas of the vulva will require laser penetration into the reticular dermis (Mene, 1985). Wright and Davies (1987) recommend a depth of 3 mm for hair-bearing areas and consider this depth to correspond well with destruction into the third surgical plane as described by Reid and coworkers (1985). Non-hair-bearing areas contain no adnexal structures and therefore, if laser is used, do not require deeper treatment. One millimeter or less of laser penetration is adequate for treatment of VIN in these areas, that is, no deeper than the basement membrane.

❺ **Reexamination.** After lasering, carbonized debris is removed, and 3- to 5-percent acetic acid solution is applied to the vulva, which is again examined colposcopically to confirm no remaining areas of disease.

POSTOPERATIVE

Care should be taken to avert adhesion formation (labial coaptation) of treated areas. Avoidance of restricting clothing and separation of the labia at least daily are recommended. Sitz bath two to three times per day is cleansing and frequently gives temporary relief of postoperative vulvar discomfort. Other measures that may be helpful include application of 1-percent silver sulfadiazine cream two to three times per day and oral analgesics. The patient should refrain from sexual activity until healing is complete.

The first postoperative visit may be scheduled at 4 to 6 weeks following the laser vaporization procedure. An acceptable schedule for surveillance of persistent or recurrent VIN is examination every 6 months for 2 years and then yearly thereafter. More frequent visits, particularly in the first year after treatment, may be warranted depending on individual patient characteristics.

REFERENCES

Adamson CD, Naik BJ, Lynch DJ: The vacuum expandable condom mold: a simple vaginal stent for McIndoe-style vaginoplasty. Plast Reconstr Surg 113:664, 2004

Ahmad G, O'Flynn H, Hindocha A, et al: Barrier agents for adhesion prevention after gynaecological surgery. Cochrane Database Syst Rev 4:CD00047, 2015

Al-Shabibi N, Chapman L, Madari S, et al: Prospective randomised trial comparing gonadotrophin-releasing hormone analogues with triple tourniquets at open myomectomy. BJOG 116(5):681, 2009

American College of Obstetricians and Gynecologists: Alternatives to hysterectomy in the management of leiomyomas. Practice Bulletin No. 96, August 2008, Reaffirmed 2012

American College of Obstetricians and Gynecologists: Antibiotic prophylaxis for gynecologic procedures. Practice Bulletin No. 104, May 2009, Reaffirmed 2014a

American College of Obstetricians and Gynecologists: Benefits and risks of sterilization. Practice Bulletin No. 46, September 2003, Reaffirmed 2011

American College of Obstetricians and Gynecologists: Elective and risk-reducing salpingo-oophorectomy. Practice Bulletin No. 89, January 2008, Reaffirmed 2014b

American College of Obstetricians and Gynecologists: Müllerian agenesis: diagnosis, management, and treatment. Committee Opinion No. 562, May 2013a

American College of Obstetricians and Gynecologists: Supracervical hysterectomy. Committee Opinion No. 388, November 2007, Reaffirmed 2013b

Asante A, Whiteman MK, Kulkarni A, et al: Elective oophorectomy in the United States: trends and in-hospital complications, 1998–2006. Obstet Gynecol 116(5):1088, 2010

Baggish MS, Dorsey JH: CO₂ laser for the treatment of vulvar carcinoma in situ. Obstet Gynecol 57:371, 1991

Baldauf JJ, Dreyfus M, Ritter J, et al: Risk of cervical stenosis after large loop excision or laser conization. Obstet Gynecol 88:933, 1996

Barutcu A, Akguner M: McIndoe vaginoplasty with the inflatable vaginal stent. Ann Plast Surg 41:568, 1998

Benagiano G, Kivinen ST, Fadini R, et al: Zoladex (goserelin acetate) and the anemic patient: results of a multicenter fibroid study. Fertil Steril 66:223, 1996

Benedet JL, Miller DM, Nickerson KG, et al: The results of cryosurgical treatment of cervical intraepithelial neoplasia at one, five, and ten years. Am J Obstet Gynecol 157:268, 1987

Benedet JL, Nickerson KG, Anderson GH: Cryotherapy in the treatment of cervical intraepithelial neoplasia. Obstet Gynecol 58:725, 1981

Bergeron S, Binik YM, Khalife S, et al: A randomized comparison of group cognitive-behavioral therapy, surface electromyographic biofeedback, and vestibulectomy in the treatment of dyspareunia resulting from vulvar vestibulitis. Pain 91:297, 2001

Blakely DH, Dewhurst CJ, Tipton RH: The long term results after marsupialization of Bartholin cysts and abscesses. J Obstet Gynaecol British Commonw 73:1008, 1966

Bleker OP, Smalbraak DJ, Schutte MF: Bartholin's abscess: the role of *Chlamydia trachomatis*. Genitourin Med 66:24, 1990

Bornstein J, Zarfati D, Goldik Z, et al: Perineoplasty compared with vestibuloplasty for severe vulvar vestibulitis. BJOG 102:652, 1995

Bornstein J, Zarfati D, Goldik Z, et al: Vulvar vestibulitis: physical or psychosexual problem? Obstet Gynecol 93:876, 1999

Burnett MA, Corbett CA, Gertenstein RJ: A randomized trial of laminaria tents versus vaginal misoprostol for cervical ripening in first trimester surgical abortion. J Obstet Gynaecol Can 27(1):38, 2005

Caglar GS1, Tasci Y, Kayikcioglu F: Management of prolapsed pedunculated myomas. Int J Gynaecol Obstet 89(2):146, 2005

Canis MJ, Triopon G, Daraï E, et al: Adhesion prevention after myomectomy by laparotomy: a prospective multicenter comparative randomized single-blind study with second-look laparoscopy to assess the effectiveness of PREVADH. Eur J Obstet Gynecol Reprod Biol 178:42, 2014

Cardosi RJ, Bomalaski JJ, Hoffman MS: Diagnosis and management of vulvar and vaginal intraepithelial neoplasia. Obstet Gynecol Clin North Am 28:685, 2001

Casiano ER, Trabuco EC, Bharucha AE, et al: Risk of oophorectomy after hysterectomy. Obstet Gynecol 121(5):1069, 2013

Castelo-Branco C, Figueras F, Sanjuan A, et al: Long-term compliance with estrogen replacement therapy in surgical postmenopausal women: benefits to bone and analysis of factors associated with discontinuation. Menopause 6:307, 1999

Chiaffarino F, Parazzini F, Decarli A, et al: Hysterectomy with or without unilateral oophorectomy and risk of ovarian cancer. Gynecol Oncol 97:318, 2005

Christianson MS, Barker MA, Lindheim SR: Overcoming the challenging cervix: techniques to access the uterine cavity. J Low Genit Tract Dis 12(1):24, 2008

Chua GC, Wilsher M, Young MPA, et al: Comparison of particle penetration with nonspherical polyvinyl alcohol versus trisacryl gelatin microspheres in women undergoing premyomectomy uterine artery embolization. Clin Radiol 60:116, 2005

Coddington CC, Grow DR, Ahmed MS, et al: Gonadotropin-releasing hormone agonist pretreatment did not decrease postoperative adhesion formation after abdominal myomectomy in a randomized control trial. Fertil Steril 91(5):1909, 2009

Conner SN, Frey HA, Cahill AG, et al: Loop electrosurgical excision procedure and risk of preterm birth: a systematic review and meta-analysis. Obstet Gynecol 123(4):752, 2014

Costello C, Hillis SD, Marchbanks PA, et al: The effect of interval tubal sterilization on sexual interest and pleasure. Obstet Gynecol 100:511, 2002

Creasman WT, Hinshaw WM, Clarke-Pearson DL: Cryosurgery in the management of cervical intraepithelial neoplasia. Obstet Gynecol 63:145, 1984

Creatsas G, Deligeoroglou E, Christopoulos P: Creation of a neovagina after Creatsas modification of Williams vaginoplasty for the treatment of 200 patients with Mayer-Rokitansky-Kuster-Hauser syndrome. Fertil Steril 94(5):1848, 2010

Crouch NS, Deans R, Michala L, et al: Clinical characteristics of well women seeking labial reduction surgery: a prospective study. BJOG 118(12):1507, 2011

Curtis KM1, Mohllajee AP, Peterson HB: Regret following female sterilization at a young age: a systematic review. Contraception 73(2):205, 2006

Darwish AM, Nasr AM, El Nashar DA: Evaluation of postmyomectomy uterine scar. J Clin Ultrasound 33:181, 2005

Deligdisch L, Hirschmann S, Altchek A: Pathologic changes in gonadotropin-releasing hormone agonist analogue treated uterine leiomyomata. Fertil Steril 67:837, 1997

Denny L, Kuhn L, De Souza M, et al: Screen-and-treat approaches for cervical cancer prevention in low-resource settings: a randomized, controlled trial. JAMA 294:2173, 2005

Deschamps A, Krishnamurthy S: Absence of pulse and blood pressure following vasopressin injection for myomectomy. Can J Anesth 52:552, 2005

Donnez J, Tatarchuk TF, Bouchard P, et al: Ulipristal acetate versus placebo for fibroid treatment before surgery. N Engl J Med 366(5):409, 2012a

Donnez J, Tomaszewski J, Vázquez F, et al: Ulipristal acetate versus leuprolide acetate for uterine fibroids. N Engl J Med 366(5):421, 2012b

Downs MC, Randall HW Jr: The ambulatory surgical management of Bartholin duct cysts. J Emerg Med 7:623, 1989

Dunn TS, Killoran K, Wolf D: Complications of outpatient LLETZ procedures. J Reprod Med 49:76, 2004

Dunn TS, Woods J, Burch J: Bowel injury occurring during an outpatient LLETZ procedure: a case report. J Reprod Med 48:49, 2003

Edwards L: New concepts in vulvodynia. Am J Obstet Gynecol 189:S24, 2003

Farquhar CM: Ectopic pregnancy. Lancet 366:583, 2005

Fedele L, Vercellini P, Bianchi S, et al: Treatment with GnRH agonists before myomectomy and the risk of short-term myoma recurrence. BJOG 97:393, 1990

Ferenczy A: Using the laser to treat condyloma acuminata and intradermal neoplasia. Can Med Assoc J 128:135, 1983

Ferenczy A, Wright JR, Richart RM: Comparison of CO₂ laser surgery and loop electrosurgical excision/fulguration for the treatment of vulvar intraepithelial neoplasia (VIN). Int J Gynecol Cancer 4:22, 1994

Ferris DG: Lethal tissue temperature during cervical cryotherapy with a small flat cryoprobe. J Fam Pract 38:153, 1994

Firouzabadi RD, Sekhavat L, Tabatabaii A, et al: Laminaria tent versus misoprostol for cervical ripening in missed abortion. Arch Gynecol Obstet 285(3):699, 2012

Fletcher H, Frederick J, Hardie M, et al: A randomized comparison of vasopressin and tourniquet as hemostatic agents during myomectomy. Obstet Gynecol 87:1014, 1996

Food and Drug Administration: FDA discourages use of laparoscopic power morcellation for removal of uterus or uterine fibroids. 2014. Available at: http://www.fda.gov/NewsEvents/Newsroom/PressAnnouncements/ucm393689.htm. Accessed April 27, 2014

Fotopoulou C, Sehouli J, Gehrmann N, et al: Functional and anatomic results of amnion vaginoplasty in young women with Mayer-Rokitansky-Küster-Hauser syndrome. Fertil Steril 94(1):317, 2010

Frankman EA, Wang L, Bunker CH, et al: Lower urinary tract injury in women in the United States, 1979–2006. Am J Obstet Gynecol 202(5):495.e1, 2010

Frederick J, Fletcher H, Simeon D, et al: Intramyometrial vasopressin as a haemostatic agent during myomectomy. BJOG 101:435, 1994

Friedman AJ, Hoffman DI, Comite F, et al: Treatment of leiomyomata uteri with leuprolide acetate depot: a double-blind, placebo-controlled, multicenter study. The Leuprolide Study Group. Obstet Gynecol 77:720, 1991

Frishman G: Vasopressin: if some is good, is more better? Obstet Gynecol 113(2 Pt 2):476, 2009

Gage AA: What temperature is lethal for cells? J Dermatol Surg Oncol 5:459, 1979

Ghanbari Z, Baratali BH, Foroughifar T, et al: Pfannenstiel versus Maylard incision for gynecologic surgery: a randomized, double-blind controlled trial. Taiwan J Obstet Gynecol 48(2):120, 2009

Gilmour DT, Das S, Flowerdew G: Rates of urinary tract injury from gynecologic surgery and the role of intraoperative cystoscopy. Obstet Gynecol 107(6):1366, 2006

Ginsburg ES, Benson CB, Garfield JM, et al: The effect of operative technique and uterine size on blood loss during myomectomy: a prospective, randomized study. Fertil Steril 60:956, 1993

Goetsch MF: Incidence of Bartholin's duct occlusion after superficial localized vestibulectomy. Am J Obstet Gynecol 200(6):688.e1, 2009

Golan A, Zachalka N, Lurie S, et al: Vaginal removal of prolapsed pedunculated submucous myoma: a short, simple, and definitive procedure with minimal morbidity. Arch Gynecol Obstet 271(1):11, 2005

Goldstein AT, Marinoff SC, Haefner HK: Vulvodynia: strategies for treatment. Clin Obstet Gynecol 48:769, 2005

Haefner HK: Critique of new gynecologic surgical procedures: surgery for vulvar vestibulitis. Clin Obstet Gynecol 43:689, 2000

Haefner HK, Collins ME, Davis GD, et al: The vulvodynia guideline. J Low Gen Tract Dis 9:40, 2005

Hakim-Elahi E, Tovell HM, Burnhill MS: Complications of first-trimester abortion: a report of 170,000 cases. Obstet Gynecol 76:129, 1990

Hannoun-Levi JM, Peiffert D, Hoffstetter S, et al: Carcinoma of the cervical stump: retrospective analysis of 77 cases. Radiother Oncol 43:147, 1997

Hartmann KE, Ma C, Lamvu GM, et al: Quality of life and sexual function after hysterectomy in women with preoperative pain and depression. Obstet Gynecol 104:701, 2004

Heinonen A, Gissler M, Riska A, et al: Loop electrosurgical excision procedure and the risk for preterm delivery. Obstet Gynecol 121(5):1063, 2013

Helal AS, Abdel-Hady el-S, Refaie E, et al: Preliminary uterine artery ligation versus pericervical mechanical tourniquet in reducing hemorrhage during abdominal myomectomy. Int J Gynaecol Obstet 108(3):233, 2010

Hellstrom AC, Sigurjonson T, Pettersson F: Carcinoma of the cervical stump: the radium-hemmet series 1959–1987. Treatment and prognosis. Acta Obstet Gynaecol Scand 80:152, 2001

Helmerhorst TJM, van der Vaart CH, Dijkhuizen GH, et al: CO_2-laser therapy in patients with vulvar intraepithelial neoplasia. Eur J Obstet Gynecol Repro Biol 34(1–2):149, 1990

Hilger WS, Pizarro AR, Magrina JF: Removal of the retained cervical stump. Am J Obstet Gynecol 193:2117, 2005

Hill DA, Lense JJ: Office management of Bartholin gland cysts and abscesses. Am Fam Physician 57:1611, 1998

Hillemanns P, Wang X, Staehle S, et al: Evaluation of different treatment modalities for vulvar intraepithelial neoplasia (VIN): CO_2 laser vaporization, photodynamic therapy, excision and vulvectomy. Gynecol Oncol 100:271, 2006

Hillis SD, Marchbanks PA, Tylor LR, et al: Poststerilization regret: findings from the United States Collaborative Review of Sterilization. Obstet Gynecol 93:889, 1999

Hoffman MS, Pinelli DM, Finan M, et al: Laser vaporization for vulvar intraepithelial neoplasia. J Reprod Med 37(2):135, 1992

Houlard S, Perrotin F, Fourquet F, et al: Risk factors for cervical stenosis after laser cone biopsy. Eur J Obstet Gynaecol Reprod Biol 104:144, 2002

Hutchins FL Jr: A randomized comparison of vasopressin and tourniquet as hemostatic agents during myomectomy. Obstet Gynecol 88:639, 1996

Hwang JH1, Lee JK, Lee NW, et al: Open cornual resection versus laparoscopic cornual resection in patients with interstitial ectopic pregnancies. Eur J Obstet Gynecol Reprod Biol 156(1):78, 2011

Imai A, Sugiyama M, Furui T, et al: Gonadotrophin-releasing hormones agonist therapy increases peritoneal fibrinolytic activity and prevents adhesion formation after myomectomy. J Obstet Gynaecol 23:660, 2003

Iverson RE Jr, Chelmow D, Strohbehn K, et al: Relative morbidity of abdominal hysterectomy and myomectomy for management of uterine leiomyomas. Obstet Gynecol 88:415, 1996

Jacob M, Broekhuizen FF, Castro W, et al: Experience using cryotherapy for treatment of cervical precancerous lesions in low-resource settings. Int J Gynaecol Obstet 89:S13, 2005

Jacobson P: Marsupialization of vulvovaginal (Bartholin) cysts. Am J Obstet Gynecol 79:73, 1960

Jacoby VL, Autry A, Jacobson G, et al: Nationwide use of laparoscopic hysterectomy compared with abdominal and vaginal approaches. Obstet Gynecol 114(5):1041, 2009

Johnson N, Barlow D, Lethaby A et al: Methods of hysterectomy: systematic review and meta-analysis of randomised controlled trials. BMJ 330(7506):1478, 2005

Joki-Erkkilä MM, Heinonen PK: Presenting and long-term clinical implications and fecundity in females with obstructing vaginal malformations. J Pediatr Adolesc Gynecol 16:307, 2003

Jones RW, Rowan DM, Stewart AW: Vulvar intraepithelial neoplasia: aspects of the natural history and outcome in 405 women. Obstet Gynecol 106:1319, 2005

Joura EA: Epidemiology, diagnosis and treatment of vulvar intraepithelial neoplasia. Curr Opin Obstet Gynecol 14:39, 2002

Kennedy CM, Dewdney S, Galask RP: Vulvar granuloma fissuratum: a description of fissuring of the posterior fourchette and the repair. Obstet Gynecol 105:1018, 2005

Kessous R, Aricha-Tamir B, Sheizaf B, et al: Clinical and microbiological characteristics of Bartholin gland abscesses. Obstet Gynecol 122(4):794, 2013

Kho RM, Magrina JF. Removal of the retained cervical stump after supracervical hysterectomy. Best Pract Res Clin Obstet Gynaecol 25(2):153, 2011

Kilpatrick CC, Alagkiozidis I, Orejuela FJ, et al: Factors complicating surgical management of the vulvar abscess. J Reprod Med 55:139, 2010

Klingele CJ, Gebhart JB, Croak AJ, et al: McIndoe procedure for vaginal agenesis: long-term outcome and effect on quality of life. Am J Obstet Gynecol 189:1569, 2003

Kongnyuy EJ, Wiysonge CS: Interventions to reduce haemorrhage during myomectomy for fibroids. Cochrane Database Syst Rev 11:CD005355, 2014

Kristensen GB, Jensen LK, Holund B: A randomized trial comparing two methods of cold knife conization with laser conization. Obstet Gynecol 76:1009, 1990

Kristensen J, Langhoff-Roos J, Kristensen FB: Increased risk of preterm birth in women with cervical conization. Obstet Gynecol 81:1005, 1993a

Kristensen J, Langhoff-Roos J, Wittrup M, et al: Cervical conization and preterm delivery/low birth weight: a systematic review of the literature. Acta Obstet Gynaecol Scand 72:640, 1993b

Kuppermann M, Learman LA, Schembri M, et al: Contributions of hysterectomy and uterus-preserving surgery to health-related quality of life. Obstet Gynecol 122(1):15, 2013

Kuppers V, Stiller M, Somville T, et al: Risk factors for recurrent VIN: role of multifocality and grade of disease. J Reprod Med 42:140, 1997

Kurata H, Aoki Y, Tanaka K: Delayed, massive bleeding as an unusual complication of laser conization: a case report. J Reprod Med 48:659, 2003

LaMorte AI, Lalwani S, Diamond MP: Morbidity associated with abdominal myomectomy. Obstet Gynecol 82:897, 1993

Lavy Y, Lev-Sagie A, Hamani Y, et al: Modified vulvar vestibulectomy: simple and effective surgery for the treatment of vulvar vestibulitis. Eur J Obstet Gynaecol Reprod Biol 120:91, 2005

Learman LA, Summitt RL Jr, Varner RE, et al: A randomized comparison of total or supracervical hysterectomy: surgical complications and clinical outcomes. Obstet Gynecol 102(3):453, 2003

Lethaby A, Mukhopadhyay A, Naik R. Total versus subtotal hysterectomy for benign gynaecological conditions. Cochrane Database Syst Rev 4:CD004993, 2012

Lethaby A, Vollenhoven B, Sowter M: Efficacy of pre-operative gonadotrophin hormone–releasing analogues for women with uterine fibroids undergoing hysterectomy or myomectomy: a systematic review. BJOG 109:1097, 2002

Li FY, Xu YS, Zhou CD, et al: Long-term outcomes of vaginoplasty with autologous buccal micromucosa. Obstet Gynecol 123(5):951, 2014

Liang CC, Chang SD, Soong YK: Long-term follow-up of women who underwent surgical correction for imperforate hymen. Arch Gynecol Obstet 269:5, 2003

Lichtenberg ES, Paul M, Society of Family Planning: Surgical abortion prior to 7 weeks of gestation. Contraception 88(1):7, 2013

Mamik MM, Antosh D, White DE, et al: Risk factors for lower urinary tract injury at the time of hysterectomy for benign reasons. Int Urogynecol J 25(8):1031, 2014

Marana R, Busacca M, Zupi E, et al: Laparoscopically assisted vaginal hysterectomy versus total abdominal hysterectomy: a prospective, randomized, multicenter study. Am J Obstet Gynecol 180:270, 1999

Martin-Hirsch PL, Paraskevaidis E, Bryant A: Surgery for cervical intraepithelial neoplasia. Cochrane Database Syst Rev 6:CD001318, 2013

Massad LS, Einstein MH, Huh WK, et al: 2012 updated consensus guidelines for the management of abnormal cervical cancer screening tests and cancer precursors. J Low Genit Tract Dis 17(5 Suppl 1):S1, 2013

Mathai M, Hofmeyr GJ, Mathai NE: Abdominal surgical incisions for caesarean section. Cochrane Database Syst Rev 5:CD004453, 2013

Mathevet P, Chemali E, Roy M, et al: Long-term outcome of a randomized study comparing three techniques of conization: cold knife, laser, and LEEP. Eur J Obstet Gynaecol Reprod Biol 106:214, 2003

Matta WH, Stabile I, Shaw RW, et al: Doppler assessment of uterine blood flow changes in patients with fibroids receiving the gonadotropin-releasing hormone agonist Buserelin. Fertil Steril 49:1083, 1988

McIndoe AH, Banister JB: An operation for the cure of congenital absence of the vagina. J Obstet Gynaecol Br Empire 45:490, 1938

Mencaglia L, Tantini C: GnRH agonist analogs and hysteroscopic resection of myomas. Int J Gynaecol Obstet 43:285, 1993

Mene A, Buckley CH: Involvement of the vulvar skin appendages by intraepithelial neoplasia. Br J Obstet Gynecol 92:634, 1985

Miller BE: Vulvar intraepithelial neoplasia treated with cavitational ultrasonic surgical aspiration. Gynecol Oncol 85:114, 2002

Milton SH: Gynecologic myomectomy. 2013. Available at: http://emedicine.medscape.com/article/267677-treatment#a1132. Accessed September 1, 2014

Mirzabeigi MN, Moore JH Jr, Mericli AF, et al: Current trends in vaginal labioplasty: a survey of plastic surgeons. Ann Plast Surg 68(2):125, 2012

Mitchell MF, Tortolero-Luna G, Cook E, et al: A randomized clinical trial of cryotherapy, laser vaporization, and loop electrosurgical excision for treatment of squamous intraepithelial lesions of the cervix. Obstet Gynecol 92:737, 1998

Mittal S, Sehgal R, Aggarwal S, et al: Cervical priming with misoprostol before manual vacuum aspiration versus electric vacuum aspiration for first-trimester surgical abortion. Int J Gynaecol Obstet 112(1):34, 2011

Moawad NS, Mahajan ST, Moniz MH, et al: Current diagnosis and treatment of interstitial pregnancy. Am J Obstet Gynecol 202:15, 2010

Modesitt SC, Waters AB, Walton L, et al: Vulvar intraepithelial neoplasia III: occult cancer and the impact of margin status on recurrence. Obstet Gynecol 92:962, 1998

Motoyama S, Laoag-Fernandez JB, Mochizuki S, et al: Vaginoplasty with Interceed absorbable adhesion barrier for complete squamous epithelialization in vaginal agenesis. Am J Obstet Gynecol 188:1260, 2003

Mowbray N, Ansell J, Warren N, et al: Is surgical smoke harmful to theater staff? A systematic review. Surg Endosc 27(9):3100, 2013

National Institute for Occupational Safety and Health: Control of smoke from laser/electric surgical procedures. Appl Occup Environ Hyg 14:71, 1999

Ngeh N, Belli AM, Morgan R, et al: Pre-myomectomy uterine artery embolisation minimises operative blood loss. BJOG 111:1139, 2004

Nieboer TE, Johnson N, Lethaby A, et al: Surgical approach to hysterectomy for benign gynaecological disease. Cochrane Database Syst Rev 3:CD003677, 2009

Novak F: Marsupialization of Bartholin cysts and abscesses. In Novak F (ed): Surgical Gynecologic Techniques. New York, Wiley, 1978, p 191

Novetsky AP, Boyd LR, Curtin JP: Trends in bilateral oophorectomy at the time of hysterectomy for benign disease. Obstet Gynecol 118(6):1280, 2011

Numnum TM, Kirby TO, Leath CA III, et al: A prospective evaluation of "see and treat" in women with HSIL Pap smear results: is this an appropriate strategy? J Low Gen Tract Dis 9:2, 2005

Nuovo J, Melnikow J, Willan AR, et al: Treatment outcomes for squamous intraepithelial lesions. Int J Gynaecol Obstet 68:25, 2000

Olive DL: Dogma, skepsis, and the analytic method: the role of prophylactic oophorectomy at the time of hysterectomy. Obstet Gynecol 106:214, 2005

Osmundsen BC1, Clark A, Goldsmith C, et al: Mesh erosion in robotic sacrocolpopexy. Female Pelvic Med Reconstr Surg 18(2):86, 2012

Ostergard DR: Cryosurgical treatment of cervical intraepithelial neoplasia. Obstet Gynecol 56:231, 1980

Parker WH, Feskanich D, Broder MS, et al: Long-term mortality associated with oophorectomy compared with ovarian conservation in the Nurses' Health Study. Obstet Gynecol 121(4):709, 2013

Pasley WW: Trachelectomy: a review of fifty-five cases. Am J Obstet Gynecol 159:728, 1988

Pati S, Cullins V: Female sterilization: evidence. Obstet Gynecol Clin North Am 27:859, 2000

Peipert JF, Weitzen S, Cruickshank C, et al: Risk factors for febrile morbidity after hysterectomy. Obstet Gynecol 103:86, 2004

Penna C, Fambrini M, Fallani MG, et al: Laser CO_2 conization in postmenopausal age: risk of cervical stenosis and unsatisfactory follow-up. Gynecol Oncol 96:771, 2005

Perera HK, Ananth CV, Richards CA, et al: Variation in ovarian conservation in women undergoing hysterectomy for benign indications. Obstet Gynecol 121:717, 2013

Peterson HB, Jeng G, Folger SG, et al: The risk of menstrual abnormalities after tubal sterilization. U.S. Collaborative Review of Sterilization Working Group. N Engl J Med 343:1681, 2000

Peterson HB, Xia Z, Hughes JM, et al: The risk of pregnancy after tubal sterilization: findings from the U.S. Collaborative Review of Sterilization. Am J Obstet Gynecol 174:1161, 1996

Pratt JH, Jefferies JA: The retained cervical stump: a 25-year experience. Obstet Gynecol 48:711, 1976

Rader JS, Leake JF, Dillon MB, et al: Ultrasonic surgical aspiration in the treatment of vulvar disease. Obstet Gynecol 77(4):573, 1991

Radman HM, Korman W: Uterine perforation during dilatation and curettage. Obstet Gynecol 21:210, 1963

Rahn DD, Phelan JN, Roshanravan SM, et al: Anterior abdominal wall nerve and vessel anatomy: clinical implications for gynecologic surgery. Am J Obstet Gynecol 202(3):234.e1, 2010

Raio L, Ghezzi F, Di Naro E, et al: Duration of pregnancy after carbon dioxide laser conization of the cervix: influence of cone height. Obstet Gynecol 90:978, 1997

Ravina JH, Bouret JM, Fried D, et al: Value of preoperative embolization of uterine fibroma: report of a multicenter series of 31 cases. Fertil Contracep Sex 23:45, 1995

Reid R, Elfont EA, Zirkin RM, et al: Superficial laser vulvectomy. II. The anatomic and biophysical principles permitting accurate control over the depth of dermal destruction with carbon dioxide laser. Am J Obstet Gynecol 152(3):261, 1985

Reinsch RC, Murphy AA, Morales AJ, et al: The effects of RU 486 and leuprolide acetate on uterine artery blood flow in the fibroid uterus: a prospective, randomized study. Am J Obstet Gynecol 170:1623, 1994.

Rice MS, Murphy MA, Vitonis AF, et al: Tubal ligation, hysterectomy and epithelial ovarian cancer in the New England Case-Control Study. Int J Cancer 133(10):2415, 2013

Riva HL, Hefner JD, Marchetti AA, et al: Prophylactic trachelectomy of cervical stump: two hundred and twelve cases. South Med J 54:1082, 1961

Rodolakis A, Diakomanolis E, Vlachos G, et al: Vulvar intraepithelial neoplasia (VIN): diagnostic and therapeutic challenges. Eur J Gynaecol Oncol 24:317, 2003

Rouzier R, Haddad B, Deyrolle C, et al: Perineoplasty for the treatment of introital stenosis related to vulvar lichen sclerosus. Am J Obstet Gynecol 186:49, 2002

Rybak EA, Polotsky AJ, Woreta T, et al: Explained compared with unexplained fever in postoperative myomectomy and hysterectomy patients. Obstet Gynecol 111(5):1137, 2008

Ryder RM, Vaughan MC: Laparoscopic tubal sterilization: methods, effectiveness, and sequelae. Obstet Gynecol Clin North Am 26:83, 1999

Sadler L, Saftlas A, Wang W, et al: Treatment for cervical intraepithelial neoplasia and risk of preterm delivery. JAMA 291:2100, 2004

Salom EM, Penalver M: Complications in gynecologic surgery. In Cohn SM, Barquist E, Byers PM, et al (eds): Complications in Surgery and Trauma. New York, Informa Healthcare USA, 2007, p 554

Samson SLA, Bentley JR, Fahey TJ, et al: The effect of loop electrosurgical excision procedure on future pregnancy outcome. Obstet Gynecol 105:325, 2005

Sapmaz E, Celik H. Comparison of the effects of the ligation of ascending branches of bilateral arteria uterina with tourniquet method on the intra-operative and post-operative hemorrhage in abdominal myomectomy cases. Eur J Obstet Gynecol Reprod Biol 111(1):74, 2003

Sawaya GF, Grady D, Kerlikowske K, et al: Antibiotics at the time of induced abortion: the case for universal prophylaxis based on a meta-analysis. Obstet Gynecol 87:884, 1996

Sawin SW, Pilevsky ND, Berlin JA, et al: Comparability of perioperative morbidity between abdominal myomectomy and hysterectomy for women with uterine leiomyomas. Am J Obstet Gynecol 183:1448, 2000

Schantz A, Thormann L: Cryosurgery for dysplasia of the uterine ectocervix: a randomized study of the efficacy of the single- and double-freeze techniques. Acta Obstet Gynaecol Scand 63:417, 1984

Schmidt T, Eren Y, Breidenbach M, et al: Modifications of laparoscopic supracervical hysterectomy technique significantly reduce postoperative spotting. J Minim Invasive Gynecol 18(1):81, 2011

Seracchioli R, Rossi S, Govoni F, et al: Fertility and obstetric outcome after laparoscopic myomectomy of large myomata: a randomized comparison with abdominal myomectomy. Hum Reprod 15(12):2663, 2000

Sharma S, Refaey H, Stafford M, et al: Oral versus vaginal misoprostol administered one hour before surgical termination of pregnancy: a randomised, controlled trial. BJOG 112:456, 2005

Shatz P, Bergeron C, Wilkinson EJ, et al: Vulvar intraepithelial neoplasia and skin appendage involvement. Obstet Gynecol 74(5):769, 1989

Siddle N, Sarrel P, Whitehead M: The effect of hysterectomy on the age at ovarian failure: identification of a subgroup of women with premature loss of ovarian function and literature review. Fertil Steril 47:94, 1987

Sizzi O, Rossetti A, Malzoni M, et al: Italian multicenter study on complications of laparoscopic myomectomy. J Minim Invasive Gynecol 14(4): 453, 2007

Smith DC, Uhlir JK: Myomectomy as a reproductive procedure. Am J Obstet Gynecol 162:1476, 1990

Society of Gynecologic Oncology: SGO Clinical Practice Statement: salpingectomy for ovarian cancer prevention. 2013. Available at: https://www.sgo.org/clinical-practice/guidelines/sgo-clinical-practice-statement-salpingectomy-for-ovarian-cancer-prevention./ Accessed April 25, 2014

Son M, Evanko JC, Mongero LB, et al: Utility of cell salvage in women undergoing abdominal myomectomy. Am J Obstet Gynecol 211(1):28.e1, 2014

Song T, Kim MK, Kim ML, et al: Effectiveness of different routes of misoprostol administration before operative hysteroscopy: a randomized, controlled trial. Fertil Steril 102(2):519, 2014

Spitzer M: Lower genital tract intraepithelial neoplasia in HIV-infected women: guidelines for evaluation and management. Obstet Gynecol Surv 54(2):131, 1999

Suh-Burgmann EJ, Whall-Strojwas D, Chang Y, et al: Risk factors for cervical stenosis after loop electrocautery excision procedure. Obstet Gynecol 96:657, 2000

Tabata T, Yamawaki T, Ida M, et al: Clinical value of dilatation and curettage for abnormal uterine bleeding. Arch Gynecol Obstet 264: 174, 2001

Tan-Kim J, Menefee SA, Luber KM, et al: Prevalence and risk factors for mesh erosion after laparoscopic-assisted sacrocolpopexy. Int Urogynecol J Pelvic Floor Dysfunct 22(2):205, 2011

Taylor A, Sharma M, Tsirkas P, et al: Reducing blood loss at open myomectomy using triple tourniquets: a randomised, controlled trial. BJOG 112:340, 2005

Thakar R, Ayers S, Clarkson P, et al: Outcomes after total versus subtotal abdominal hysterectomy. N Engl J Med 347:1318, 2002

Thurman AR, Satterfield TM, Soper DE: Methicillin-resistant *Staphylococcus aureus* as a common cause of vulvar abscesses. Obstet Gynecol 112:538, 2008

Tinelli A, Malvasi A, Guido M, et al: Adhesion formation after intracapsular myomectomy with or without adhesion barrier. Fertil Steril 95(5):1780, 2011

Tommola P, Unkila-Kallio L, Paavonen J: Surgical treatment of vulvar vestibulitis: a review. Acta Obstet Gynecol Scand 89(11):1385, 2010

Trimbos JB, Heintz AP, van Hall EV: Reliability of cytological follow-up after conization of the cervix: a comparison of three surgical techniques. BJOG 90:1141, 1983

Tulandi T, Beique F, Kimia M: Pulmonary edema: a complication of local injection of vasopressin at laparoscopy. Fertil Steril 66:478, 1996

Tulandi T, Murray C, Guralnick M: Adhesion formation and reproductive outcome after myomectomy and second-look laparoscopy. Obstet Gynecol 82:213, 1993

Tunçalp O, Gülmezoglu AM, Souza JP: Surgical procedures for evacuating incomplete miscarriage. Cochrane Database Syst Rev 9:CD001993, 2010

Turner LC, Shepherd JP, Wang L, et al: Hysterectomy surgical trends: a more accurate depiction of the last decade? Am J Obstet Gynecol 208(4):277.e1, 2013

Vercellini P, Trespidi L, Zaina B, et al: Gonadotropin-releasing hormone agonist treatment before

abdominal myomectomy: a controlled trial. Fertil Steril 79:1390, 2003

Visco AG, Del Priore G: Postmenopausal Bartholin gland enlargement: a hospital-based cancer risk assessment. Obstet Gynecol 87:286, 1996

Weed JC Jr, Curry SL, Duncan ID, et al: Fertility after cryosurgery of the cervix. Obstet Gynecol 52:245, 1978

Welch JS, Cousellor VS, Malkasian GD Jr: The vaginal removal of the cervical stump. Surg Clin North Am 39:1073, 1959

Werner CL, Lo JY, Heffernan T, et al: Loop electrosurgical excision procedure and risk of preterm birth. Obstet Gynecol 115(3):605, 2010

Word B: New instrument for office treatment of cysts and abscesses of Bartholin's gland. JAMA 190:777, 1964

World Health Organization: WHO Guidelines for Treatment of Cervical Intraepithelial Neoplasia 2–3 and Adenocarcinoma in situ: Cryotherapy, Large Loop Excision of the Transformation Zone, and Cold Knife Conization. Geneva, World Health Organization, 2014

Wright VC, Davies E: Laser surgery for vulvar intraepithelial neoplasia: principles and results. Am J Obstet Gynecol 156(2):374, 1987

Yamada T, Yamashita Y, Terai Y, et al: Intraoperative blood salvage in abdominal uterine myomectomy. Int J Gynaecol Obstet 56: 141, 1997

Yu KJ, Lin YS, Chao KC, et al: A detachable porous vaginal mold facilitates reconstruction of a modified McIndoe neovagina. Fertil Steril 81:435, 2004

Zhou W, Nielsen GL, Moller M, et al: Short-term complications after surgically induced abortions: a register-based study of 56,117 abortions. Acta Obstet Gynaecol Scand 81:331, 2002

CHAPTER 44

Minimally Invasive Surgery

44-1

Diagnostic Laparoscopy

Diagnostic laparoscopy provides a minimally invasive surgery (MIS) option for thorough evaluation of the peritoneal cavity and pelvic organs. It is often performed to evaluate pelvic pain or causes of infertility, to diagnose endometriosis, or to ascertain the extent of adhesive disease or qualities of a pelvic mass. Importantly, systematic evaluation of the peritoneal cavity is performed during every laparoscopy, either diagnostic or operative.

PREOPERATIVE

Consent

During the consenting process for diagnostic laparoscopy, a surgeon reviews procedure goals, including diagnosis and possible treatment of identified pathology. Among, others, this includes permission for lysis of adhesions, peritoneal biopsy, and excision or ablation of endometriosis. Importantly, a patient is counseled that diagnostic laparoscopy may not reveal any apparent pathology.

Laparoscopy is typically associated with few complications. Of these, organ injuries caused by puncture or by electrosurgery tools are the most common major complications and are summarized in Chapter 41 (p. 877). Patients are also counseled regarding possible need to complete the diagnostic evaluation via laparotomy. Reasons for conversion during diagnostic laparoscopy include failure to gain abdominal access, organ injury during entry, or extensive adhesions. Overall, the conversion risk to laparotomy is low and approximates 5 percent.

Patient Preparation

In general, laparoscopy is associated with lower rates of postoperative infection and venous thromboembolism (VTE) compared with laparotomy. For diagnostic laparoscopy, antibiotics are typically not required, and VTE prophylaxis is implemented for those with risk factors (Table 39-8, p. 836). In addition, for most patients, bowel preparation is not administered. However, if extensive adhesiolysis is anticipated and the risk of bowel injury is thereby increased, bowel preparation can be considered.

INTRAOPERATIVE

Instruments

Several instruments are especially helpful during diagnostic laparoscopy, and most are found in a standard laparoscopy instrument set. Of these, a blunt probe and atraumatic grasper are valuable to manipulate abdominal organs. A uterine manipulator that allows for chromopertubation is also considered if performing diagnostic laparoscopy for infertility evaluation. If this is planned, indigo carmine dye or methylene blue can be diluted and used. However, current indigo carmine shortages may favor methylene blue use. Either agent is diluted into 50 to 100 mL of sterile saline for injection through the cervical cannula.

Surgical Steps

❶ Anesthesia and Patient Positioning. Most laparoscopic surgery is performed in an operating room and requires general anesthesia. Much less commonly, in-office microlaparoscopy using 2- to 3-mm microlaparoscopes has been reported for second-look evaluation of cancer treatment, sterilization, and pelvic pain and infertility evaluation (Franchi, 2000; Mazdisnian, 2002; Mercorio, 2008; Palter, 1999).

In most cases, following anesthesia induction, the patient is placed in low dorsal lithotomy position in booted support stirrups to permit manipulation of the uterus. The patient's arms are tucked at her sides. Correct patient positioning is critical to avoid nerve injury and is discussed in Chapter 41 (p. 879). A bimanual examination is completed to determine uterine inclination. Inclination will direct positioning of the uterine manipulator, if used. The vagina and abdomen are surgically prepared, and the bladder is drained. If a longer procedure is anticipated, a Foley catheter may be required as a full bladder can obstruct the operating view or increase the risk of bladder injury.

❷ Uterine Manipulator Placement. Although not mandatory, a uterine manipulator may be placed to move the uterus during evaluation of the pelvis. Examples are shown in Chapter 41 (p. 881). For manipulator placement, a surgeon is gowned and doubly gloved. A Graves speculum or vaginal retractors are used to display the cervix. To stabilize the cervix, a single-tooth tenaculum is placed on the anterior cervical lip. A Cohen or other uterine manipulator is then inserted into the external os. Alternatively, after measurement of the uterine cavity with a uterine sound, the balloon end of an endometrial cavity manipulator may be threaded into the endometrial cavity, and the balloon inflated. The outer pair of surgical gloves is removed, and the surgeon moves to either side of the patient.

❸ Primary Trocar Entry. Abdominal access may be attained by any of the four basic techniques described in Chapter 41 (p. 889). These include Veress needle insertion, direct trocar insertion, optical-access insertion, or open entry methods. For diagnostic laparoscopy, no one method is superior to the others. The umbilicus is usually chosen as the site for abdominal entry. However, if a patient's history suggests periumbilical adhesions, then entry at Palmer point may be preferred. A 5-mm or 10-mm umbilical port will house a suitable laparoscope for diagnostic examination. Generally, starting with a 5-mm incision and laparoscope will allow for adequate visualization of the abdominopelvic cavity. Should improved optics be desired, this can be easily changed to a 10-mm size. Once safe initial entry is confirmed, the abdomen is insufflated to reach an intraabdominal pressure of 15 mm Hg or less.

❹ Additional Port Site Selection. Often during diagnostic laparoscopy, additional operative cannulas are needed. If minimal tissue manipulation is required, a suprapubic port may suffice. However, bilateral lower quadrant ports may be desired if lysis of adhesions or greater tissue manipulation is required. These are placed under direct laparoscopic visualization as described in Chapter 41 (p. 895).

❺ Upper Abdomen Evaluation. All laparoscopic procedures begin with a systematic and thorough diagnostic inspection of the entire peritoneal cavity, including the pelvis and upper abdomen. Once safe initial entry is confirmed, the area directly below the primary trocar entry site is evaluated for bleeding or other signs of entry trauma. Prior to Trendelenburg positioning, the upper abdomen is examined. Specifically, the liver surface, gallbladder, falciform ligament, stomach, omentum, and right and left hemidiaphragms are inspected. The ascending, transverse, and descending colon are also viewed. During inspection of the ascending portion, the appendix is identified. After Trendelenburg positioning, bowel and omentum fall toward the upper abdomen to expose the retroperitoneal structures. Now free of intestines, the area directly beneath the initial entry site is examined again. Previously unappreciated trauma to this area from initial abdominal entry might then be seen.

❻ Examination of Pelvis. After examination of the upper abdomen, attention is turned to the pelvis. First, the uterus is retroflexed with the aid of the uterine manipulator to provide clear viewing of the anterior cul-de-sac. Then, the manipulator tilts the uterus up and to the right to permit left pelvic sidewall inspection. The uterus is then anteflexed to provide access to the posterior cul-de-sac. Last, the uterus is tilted to the left, and the right pelvic sidewall is viewed. Peritoneal surfaces are thereby sequentially and methodically inspected. During this, endometriotic implants, peritoneal defects or windows, adhesions, fibrosis, or studding concerning for malignancy are sought.

Next, both ureters are visualized coursing from the pelvic brim, along the pelvic sidewall, and to the cervix. Both peristalsis and caliber are assessed. Uterine size, shape, and texture are also noted. To examine both fallopian tubes and ovaries, a surgeon may place a blunt probe into the cul-de-sac and sweep the probe forward and laterally. In doing so, the tubes and ovaries are lifted from the posterior cul-de-sac or ovarian fossa for inspection.

❼ Indicated Laparoscopic Procedures. After visual assessment of the pathology found, indicated procedures are then performed. If adhesions are encountered, they may be divided as described in Chapter 41 (p. 900).

❽ Abdomen Deflation and Port Removal. At laparoscopy completion, carbon dioxide (CO_2) insufflation is halted, and the gas tubing is disconnected from the primary cannula. The gas ports on all cannulas are opened to deflate the abdominal cavity. To prevent diaphragmatic irritation from retained CO_2, manual pressure is placed on the abdomen to help expel remaining gas. During this process, all secondary cannulas are removed using laparoscopic visualization. This allows exclusion of bleeding from punctured vessels that may have been tamponaded by these cannulas. Additionally, it prevents herniation of bowel or omentum up through the cannula track and into the anterior abdominal wall. Of note, pneumoperitoneum can also act as an intraoperative tamponade. Accordingly, potential bleeding sites are reinspected as the pneumoperitoneum is released. Next, the primary cannula is removed while leaving the laparoscope in the abdomen. Last, the laparoscope is slowly removed to visualize the abdomen and entry site for any evidence of bleeding and to prevent viscera from being pulled into the port site.

❾ **Incision Closure.** Depending on their size, incisions may require deep fascial stitches. To prevent incisional hernia formation, fascial closure is often recommended whenever trocars measuring ≥10 mm are employed (Lajer, 1997). Nonbladed trocars may decrease this risk (Liu, 2000). For closure, interrupted or running suture line using 0-gauge delayed absorbable suture is suitable.

If open entry was used, then sutures originally placed in the fascia are unthreaded from the trocar. Each of these sutures then is brought to the midline of the incision, and square knots are tied to close the fascial defect.

Skin incisions are closed with a subcuticular stitch of 4-0 gauge delayed-absorbable suture. Alternatively, the skin may be closed with cyanoacrylate tissue adhesive (Dermabond Topical Skin Adhesive) or skin tape (Steri-Strips) (Chap. 40, p. 847).

After incision closure, the uterine manipulator is removed.

POSTOPERATIVE

Depending on the procedure performed, most patients can be discharged home on the same day as surgery. For most, physical activities and diet can be resumed according to patient comfort.

44-2

Laparoscopic Sterilization

Approximately 650,000 tubal sterilization procedures are performed annually in the United States. Approximately half of these follow pregnancy delivery or termination, but the others are performed independent of pregnancy and are termed *interval sterilization* (Chan, 2010). Most interval procedures are performed laparoscopically, and most frequently they involve tubal occlusion by electrosurgical coagulation, by mechanical clips, by Silastic bands, or by suture ligation (Pati, 2000).

Current sterilization practices will likely change with recommendations now encouraging consideration of prophylactic salpingectomy at the time of sterilization, abdominal or pelvic surgery, or hysterectomy for women at average risk of ovarian cancer (American College of Obstetricians and Gynecologists, 2015). The rationale for this practice change to help decrease rates of certain epithelial ovarian cancers is described in Chapter 35 (p. 738).

PREOPERATIVE

Patient Evaluation

Several preventive steps can avoid sterilization procedures in women with early, undiagnosed pregnancies. Providing contraception well in advance of surgery, scheduling surgery in the follicular phase of the menstrual cycle, and preoperative serum β-human chorionic gonadotropin (β-hCG) level testing are effective methods to prevent or detect early pregnancy (American College of Obstetricians and Gynecologists, 2013a).

Patients who require treatment of advanced cervical epithelial abnormalities and who desire sterilization may choose hysterectomy rather than tubal occlusion as a means to serve both needs. For this reason, women ideally have cervical cancer screening results reviewed prior to surgery.

Consent

During the consenting process, patients are counseled regarding other reversible methods of contraception; other permanent methods, such as male sterilization; and the possibility of future regret (American College of Obstetricians and Gynecologists, 2009). Tubal sterilization is effective and should be considered a permanent procedure by the patient. Tubal sterilization is safe and associated complications are few. In general,

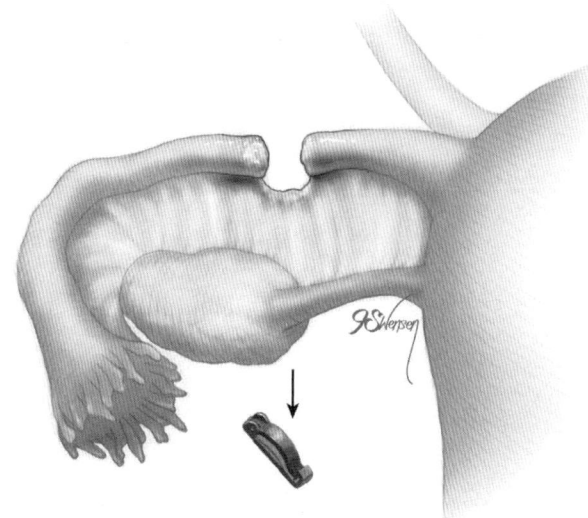

FIGURE 44-2.1 Filshie clip may fall away following fibrosis of fallopian tube ends.

the risks of laparoscopic sterilization mirror those of laparoscopy (Chap. 41, p. 877).

Sterilizing clips and bands routinely fall from around the tube once occluded ends necrose and fibrose (Fig. 44-2.1). Most ectopic clips are incidental findings without untoward patient effects, but less commonly they can incite local foreign body reactions. Rarely, cases of clip migration to sites such as the bladder, uterine cavity, and anterior abdominal wall have been reported (Gooden, 1993; Kesby, 1997; Tan, 2004).

Contraceptive failure and pregnancy rates related to each procedure are also discussed with the patient (Chap. 5, p. 116). Overall, these rates are low, and tubal sterilization is an effective method of contraception. If pregnancy does occur, however, there is a greater risk of ectopic pregnancy. Bipolar coagulation has the highest risk for this complication compared with that of clips or bands (Malacova, 2014; Peterson, 1996). Accordingly, amenorrhea following any sterilization procedure should prompt serum β-hCG testing to aid in identifying ectopic pregnancies.

Patient Preparation

For sterilization procedures, antibiotics and bowel preparation are typically not administered. VTE prophylaxis is implemented only for those at increased risk as listed in Table 39-8 (p. 836).

INTRAOPERATIVE

Surgical Steps

❶ **Anesthesia and Patient Positioning.** Most laparoscopic tubal sterilization procedures are performed using general anesthesia.

To reduce postoperative pain, investigators have evaluated the adjunctive use of bupivacaine solution injected or dripped onto the tubal serosa or delivered transcervically through balloon uterine manipulators into the fallopian tube lumen. Though results have varied, one metaanalysis suggests some benefit in diminishing immediate postoperative pain with these practices (Brennan, 2004; Harrison, 2014; Schytte, 2003; Wrigley, 2000).

To begin, the patient is placed in the low dorsal lithotomy position, and patient arms are tucked at the side. A bimanual examination is completed to determine uterine size and inclination. Uterine size will affect placement of the accessory trocar, and inclination will direct positioning of the uterine manipulator, if used. The vagina and abdomen are surgically prepared, and the bladder is drained. Most sterilization procedures are brief, and a Foley catheter is seldom required. Often, a uterine manipulator or sponge stick is then placed to provide uterine anteflexion or retroflexion during evaluation of the pelvis (p. (Chap. 41, p. 881).

❷ **Abdominal Entry and Accessory Ports.** For all of the sterilization procedures described, the initial steps of laparoscopic abdominal entry are performed as described in Chapter 41 (p. 889). In most instances, one accessory port is required and is placed suprapubically in the midline to provide an equal reach to both fallopian tubes. For a normal-sized uterus, this port is placed 2 to 3 cm above the symphysis pubis. However, for a larger uterus, this position is moved cephalad as needed to access both tubes. Once ports are in place, inspection of the abdomen and pelvis is completed prior to the planned procedure.

❸ **Filshie Clip.** The titanium Filshie clip is applied with the aid of a customized metal applicator that houses the clip within its single-action jaw. The applicator requires an 8-mm port for insertion into the abdominal cavity. As the jaw is closed, the shorter upper rim of the clip is forced beneath the longer lower clasp, and the clip is thereby locked into place around the fallopian tube.

❹ **Fallopian Tube Manipulation.** To begin, a blunt probe or atraumatic grasping forceps is placed through the accessory port. To aid clip positioning, the surgeon stretches the fallopian tube out horizontally and laterally. Concurrently, a uterine manipulator can be used to tilt the uterus laterally and in the opposite direction. The blunt probe is then removed from the single port for insertion of the clip applicator.

❺ **Applicator Insertion.** At the beginning of clip application, a Filshie clip is held within its applicator and inserted through the accessory cannula into the abdomen. A surgeon half closes the applicator's upper jaw to insert it and the clip through the cannula. The handle of the applicator is not gripped tightly, as this may prematurely close and lock the clip (Penfield, 2000).

Once the Filshie clip emerges through the cannula, the applicator is opened slowly. The jaw of the applicator has the potential to spring open more quickly than the clip can open. This can result in the clip falling off the applicator and into the abdomen. Fallen clips are preferably retrieved, but if an open clip becomes lost and hidden by loops of bowel, laparotomy is typically not required for retrieval.

❻ **Filshie Clip Placement.** After the clip is completely open, the clip and applicator are positioned with one jaw above and one below the fallopian tube at a site along the isthmic portion of the tube and 2 to 3 cm from the uterine cornu (Fig. 44-2.2). The entire width of the tube should lie across the base of the clip. The distal hooked end of the lower jaw should be visible through the mesosalpinx.

❼ **Filshie Clip Application.** Once satisfied that the clip is positioned correctly, a surgeon slowly squeezes the finger bar handle to its full limit, back toward the handle backstop. With this action, the upper ridge of the clip is slowly compressed and locked under the lower hooked end of the clip (Fig. 44-2.3). This flattens the entire tube within the clip (Fig. 44-2.4). As the applicator jaws are slowly opened, the clip releases automatically from the applicator as it has locked onto the tube. These steps are repeated on the opposite fallopian tube. If there is any doubt regarding proper clip placement, a second clip is applied correctly to the same tube.

Rarely, a fallopian tube may be transected by the clip. This is usually associated with a large fallopian tube, which has been clipped too quickly. For sterilization completion, a clip is applied to both ends of the transected tube.

❽ **Bipolar Electrosurgical Coagulation.** For this method, the fallopian tube is identified and grasped in the isthmic region at least 2 to 3 cm lateral to the cornu (Fig. 44-2.5). Placement here is important as pressure from retrograde menstrual flow against a coagulated stump that has been placed too close to the cornu can increase the risk of stump recanalization and fistula formation. Leaving a 2- to 3-cm segment allows ample space for absorption of intrauterine fluid without creating excess pressure against the stump.

❾ **Electrocoagulation.** The coagulating paddles of the bipolar forceps should span the tube. Overextending their grasp may lead to partial coagulation of the mesosalpinx and incomplete coagulation of the entire tube width. Before current is applied, the tube is slightly elevated and pulled away from other adjacent structures to prevent thermal injury to these. As current is applied, the tube swells and fluid often bubbles and pops from the tissue. Current is delivered until the tube is completely desiccated. Failure to reach this end point has been linked with higher contraceptive failure rates (Soderstrom, 1989). Because visual inspection of the tube is typically inadequate to assess complete desiccation, an ammeter is incorporated with most bipolar generators. Water conducts current through tissues. Thus, completely desiccated tissues are unable to conduct current. For this reason, current is maintained during coagulation until zero current flow across the tube is registered by the ammeter. The tube is then released.

A second site that is lateral but contiguous with the first coagulated segment is grasped and similarly coagulated. A total of three contiguous sites are serially coagulated. This occludes a total span of 3 cm along the tube's length (see Fig. 44-2.5). Coagulation of shorter distances along the tube can lead to recanalization and contraceptive failure (Peterson, 1999). These steps are then repeated on the opposite fallopian tube.

Occasionally following coagulation, the tube may stick to the bipolar paddles. To free the tube, the paddles are slowly opened and gently twisted to the right and then the left. Additionally, gentle fluid irrigation of the desiccated area may help release the tube.

❿ **Falope Ring (Silastic Band).** With this method, a Silastic Falope ring is applied with the aid of a custom metal applicator. To summarize the process, applicator tongs draw a portion of tube up into an inner sheath, and an outer sheath then pushes a Silastic band off the inner sheath and onto the fallopian tube loop.

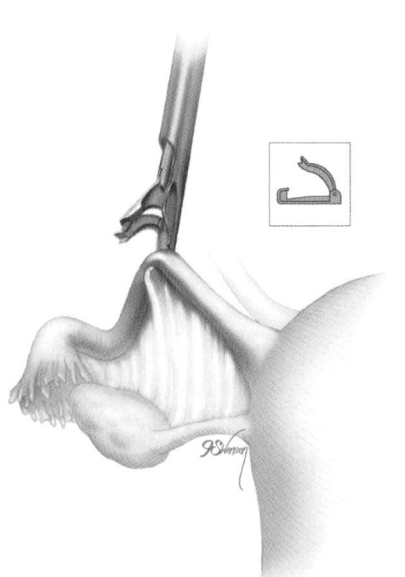

FIGURE 44-2.2 Open Filshie clip within applicator.

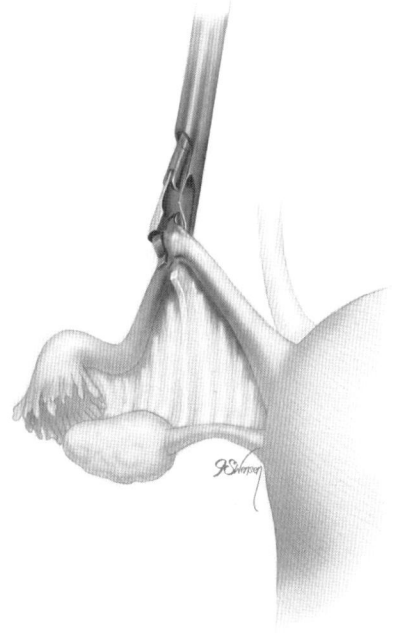

FIGURE 44-2.3 Clip application around fallopian tube.

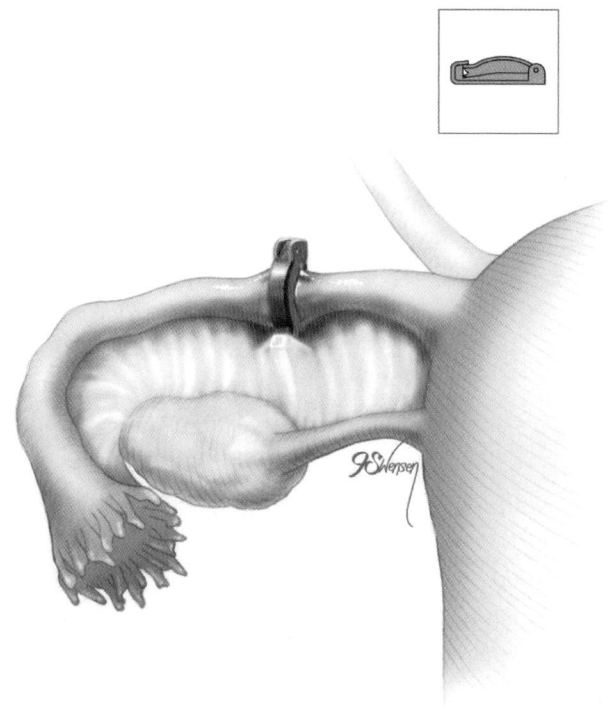

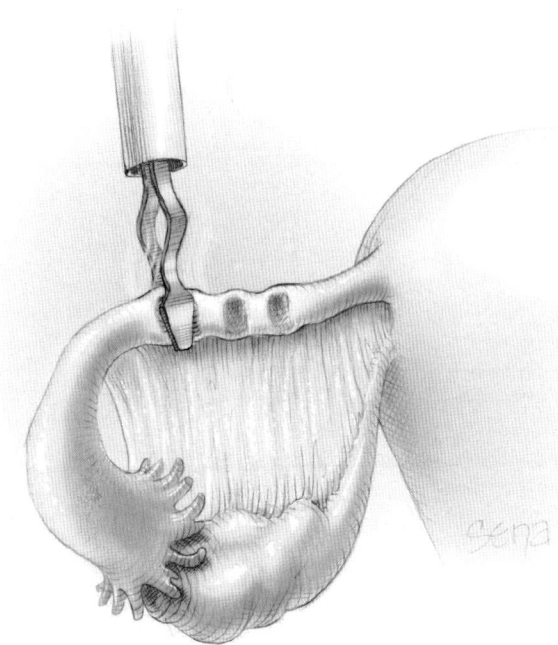

FIGURE 44-2.4 Closed clip around the tube.

FIGURE 44-2.5 Bipolar electrosurgical coagulation.

⓫ Ring Loading. Prior to its insertion into the abdomen, a Falope ring is stretched around the distal tip of the inner applicator sheath by means of a special ring loader and ring guide (Fig. 44-2.6).

⓬ Ring Placement. Once inserted through the accessory port, the applicator's tongs are opened and placed completely around the fallopian tube approximately 3 cm from the cornu. Tongs grasp the mesosalpinx directly at its attachment to the tube. This prevents excess mesosalpinx from being drawn into the inner sheath (Fig. 44-2.7).

⓭ Ring Application. A trigger on the applicator retracts the tongs and draws a loop of tube approximately 1.5 cm into the inner sheath. The total length of tube contained within the inner sheath is thus 3 cm (Fig. 44-2.8).

The outer sheath is then advanced toward the loop's base. This outer sheath pushes the Silastic band off the inner sheath and onto the loop base (Fig. 44-2.9). The loop base will blanch from ischemia following band placement (Fig. 44-2.10). These steps are repeated on the opposite fallopian tube.

⓮ Special Circumstances. Tubal transection is uncommon, and a Falope ring can be applied to each of the divided segments. Vessels of the mesosalpinx can occasionally tear and bleed as the tongs and tube are drawn into the inner sheath. The Silastic

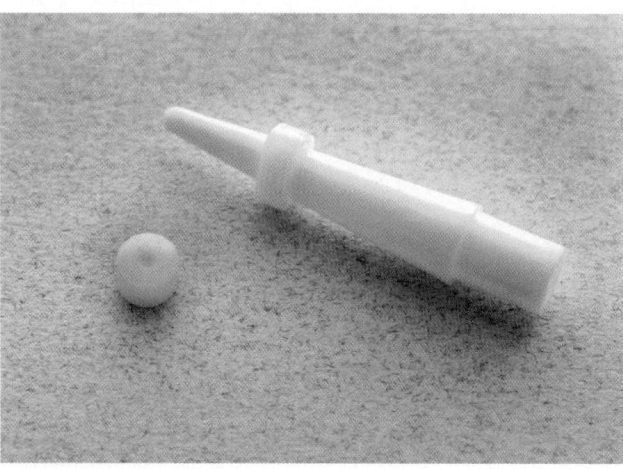

FIGURE 44-2.6 Falope ring (*left*) and ring stretched around applicator (*right*).

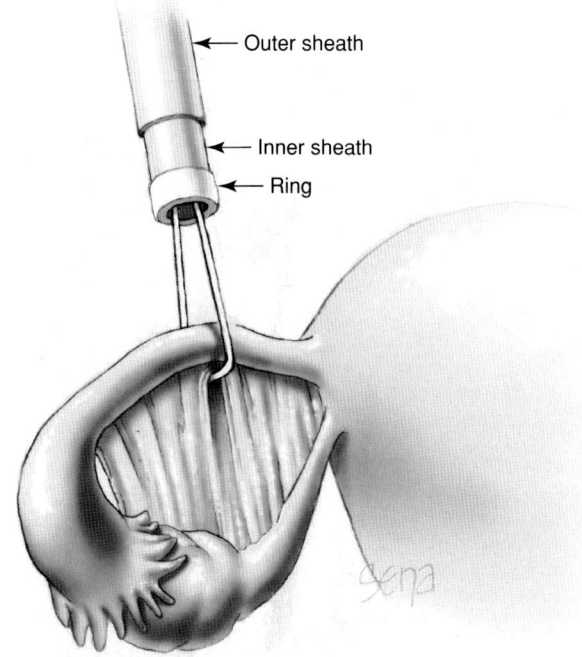

Outer sheath

Inner sheath

Ring

FIGURE 44-2.7 Falope ring applicator placement.

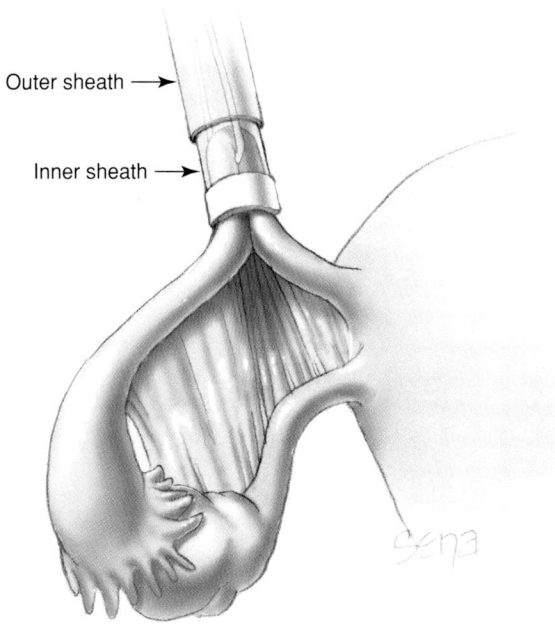

Outer sheath →

Inner sheath →

FIGURE 44-2.8 Tube drawn into inner sheath.

band, once applied to the loop base, will control bleeding in most instances. Thus, electrosurgical coagulation to achieve hemostasis is infrequently needed.

🄫 **Hulka Clip Application.** The plastic Hulka clip is also generically known as a spring clip because of the stiff outer metal spring that locks the clip into place. Required equipment includes the clips themselves and a custom metal applicator, which holds the clip during application.

🄬 **Fallopian Tube Manipulation.** To begin, a blunt probe or atraumatic grasping forceps is placed through the accessory port. The fallopian tube is outstretched horizontally and laterally to aid clip application. Concurrently, a uterine manipulator can be used to tilt the uterus laterally and in the opposite direction.

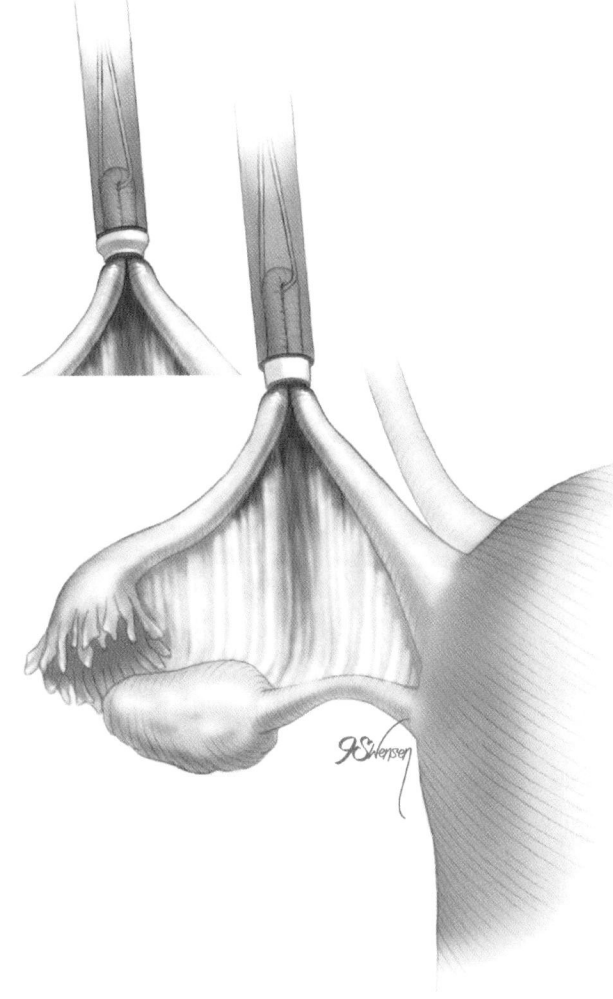

FIGURE 44-2.9 Outer sheath forces the Falope ring off the inner sheath (*inset*) and onto the fallopian tube.

🄭 **Clip Loading.** Before the applicator and its clip are inserted through the accessory trocar, the trigger of the applicator is gently squeezed by the surgeon's thumb. This action advances the outer rod of the applicator down and over the top of the clip. This closes the jaws of the clip to within 1 mm

of each of other. This is an unlocked position yet allows the clip and applicator to be threaded down the accessory cannula.

🄮 **Clip Application.** Once inside the abdomen, the applicator trigger is drawn backward, the outer rod retracts, and the upper jaw of the clip reopens. Held within the applicator jaws, the open clip is positioned across the narrow isthmic portion of the fallopian tube, 2 to 3 cm from the cornu, and perpendicular to the long axis of the tube (Fig. 44-2.11). The jaws are positioned around the tube in a manner that directs the tube deeply into the crux of the clip jaws. This aids in total occlusion of the tube as it is flattened across the base of the closing clip. Additionally, the applicator tip and clip are positioned such that when closed, the clip incorporates a small portion of adjacent mesosalpinx.

🄯 **Clip Closure.** Once the applicator jaws are appropriately positioned, the thumb-action trigger is slowly squeezed to push

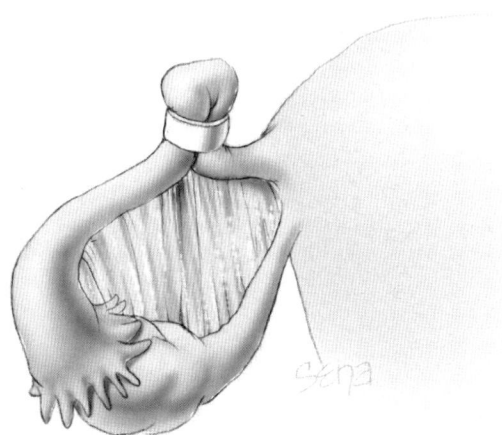

FIGURE 44-2.10 Falope ring in place.

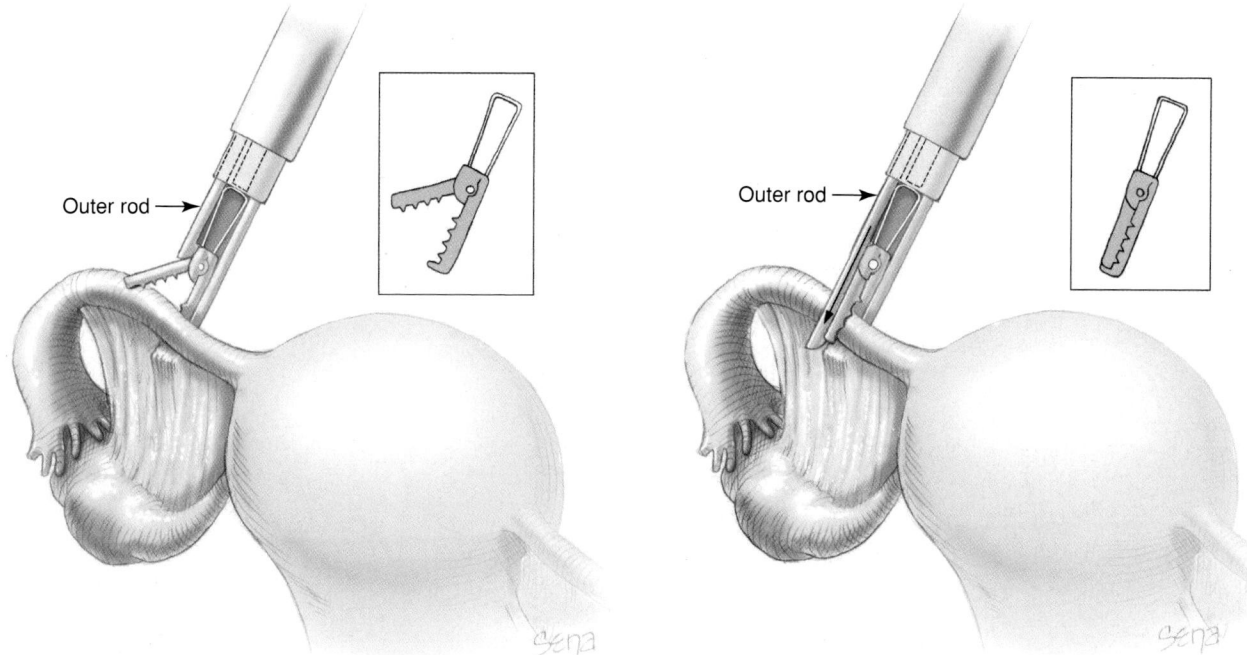

Outer rod →

FIGURE 44-2.11 Hulka clip application.

Outer rod →

FIGURE 44-2.12 Hulka clip closure.

forward the outer rod of the applicator and close the clip around the tube (Fig. 44-2.12). The clip application is inspected to ensure that it has completely encompassed the tube.

If placement is deemed correct, the trigger is fully depressed. This forces the center rod of the applicator forward against the butt of the clip's stiff metal spring (Fig. 44-2.13). The spring is pushed out and around the plastic frame of the clip to compress and lock the

upper and lower clip jaws in place. One clip is placed on each tube. If a clip is misapplied, a second clip can be placed lateral to the first.

㉑ **Pomeroy with Endoscopic Loop.** This procedure can be used as a sterilization technique but is more commonly used to excise fallopian tube ectopic pregnancies. A description and figures can be found in Section 44-3 (p. 1012).

㉑ **Wound Closure**
Subsequent surgery completion steps follow those of diagnostic laparoscopy (p. 1005).

POSTOPERATIVE

Postoperatively, patients are given instructions similar to those following diagnostic laparoscopy. Sterilization is immediate, and intercourse may resume at the patient's discretion.

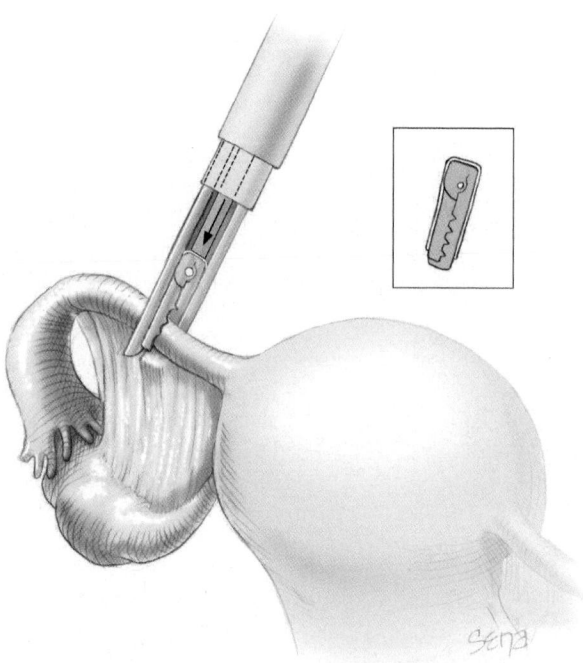

FIGURE 44-2.13 Inner rod forces the metal spring down and around the plastic clip to secure it.

Laparoscopic Salpingectomy

With surgical treatment of ectopic pregnancy, goals include hemodynamic support of the patient, removal of all trophoblastic tissue, repair or excision of the damaged tube, and preservation of fertility in those who desire it. For most women, the preferred surgical approach for ectopic pregnancy management is laparoscopic. It provides a safe and effective treatment of the affected fallopian tube while offering the advantages of laparoscopy. For some, laparoscopic salpingostomy is desired to treat and retain the affected tube. However, if fertility is not a consideration or if tubal damage or bleeding does not permit fallopian tube salvage, then laparoscopic salpingectomy may be selected due to its lower risk of persistent trophoblastic tissue.

Salpingectomy may also be used to remove hydrosalpinges in women undergoing in vitro fertilization. In this case, pregnancy rates are improved if such tubes are excised (Chap. 9, p. 224). Total salpingectomy can be used as a method of sterilization. This may be especially attractive if a primary sterilization technique has failed or if an ovarian cancer risk-reducing strategy is adopted (p. 1006). Last, in women with *BRCA* gene mutations, early bilateral salpingectomy followed by postmenopausal oophorectomy is one strategy to lower epithelial ovarian cancer risks yet provide extended estrogen benefits (Chap. 35, p. 738).

PREOPERATIVE

Consent

The general risks of laparoscopic surgery are discussed in Chapter 41 (p. 877). With salpingectomy, injury to the ipsilateral ovary is possible. Thus, the potential for oophorectomy and its effects on fertility and hormone function are discussed. Prior to cases for ectopic pregnancy, a patient's desire for future fertility is investigated. If she has completed her childbearing or has failed a prior sterilization procedure, then contralateral tubal ligation or bilateral salpingectomy may be acceptable at the time of surgery.

Following any surgical treatment of ectopic pregnancy, trophoblastic tissue can persist. The risk of this is lower with salpingectomy compared with salpingostomy and is discussed more fully on page 1013.

Patient Preparation

Baseline complete blood count (CBC), β-hCG level, and Rh status are routinely assessed. If salpingectomy is performed in the setting of an ectopic pregnancy, substantial bleeding may be encountered. Thus, the patient is typed and crossmatched for packed red blood cells and other blood products as indicated. Salpingectomy is associated with low rates of infection. Accordingly, preoperative antibiotics are usually not administered. For those undergoing laparoscopic salpingectomy for ectopic pregnancy, VTE prophylaxis is typically indicated due to the hypercoagulability associated with pregnancy (Table 39-8, p. 836). For prophylaxis in those with active bleeding, intermittent pneumatic compression devices are preferred.

INTRAOPERATIVE

Instruments

Most instruments required for salpingectomy are found in a standard laparoscopy instrument set. However, a suction irrigation system is commonly needed during salpingectomy to remove blood from a ruptured ectopic pregnancy. Depending on the size of the ectopic pregnancy or hydrosalpinges, an endoscopic retrieval bag may also be needed. For salpingectomy, the fallopian tube and mesosalpinx require ligation and excision. This may be accomplished using bipolar instruments, Harmonic scalpel, or laparoscopic suture loop (Endoloop). These may not be readily available in all operating suites, and desired tools are requested prior to surgery.

Surgical Steps

❶ **Anesthesia and Patient Positioning.** The patient is prepared and positioned for laparoscopic surgery (Chap. 41, p. 879).

❷ **Abdominal Entry.** The abdomen is entered with laparoscopic techniques, and typically two or three accessory trocar sites are added (Chap. 41, p. 889). Depending on the size of the ectopic pregnancy, at least one 10-mm or larger accessory port may be needed to allow specimen removal at surgery's end. Once ports are in place, inspection of the abdomen and pelvis is completed prior to the planned procedure.

❸ **Mesosalpingeal Incision.** The affected fallopian tube is lifted and held with an atraumatic grasping forceps. Kleppinger bipolar electrode forceps are placed across a proximal portion of the fallopian tube. A cutting current at 25 W should suffice (Fig. 44-3.1). When zero amperage of flow is noted, scissors can then cut the desiccated, blanched tube (Fig. 44-3.2).

The Kleppinger forceps are then advanced across the most proximal portion of mesosalpinx. Similarly, current is applied, and the desiccated tissue cut. This process serially moves from the proximal mesosalpinx to its distal extent under the tubal ampulla. As the distal mesosalpinx is cut, the tube is freed.

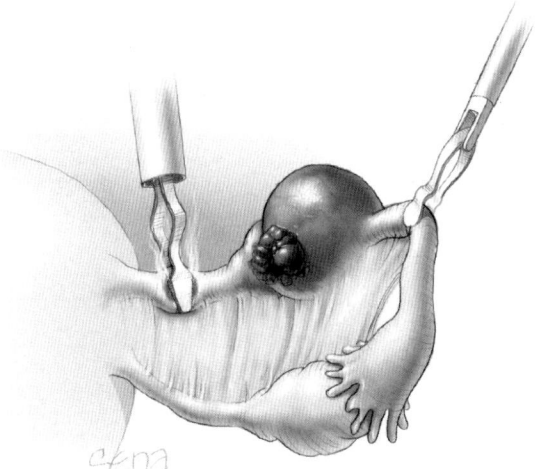

FIGURE 44-3.1 Fallopian tube desiccation.

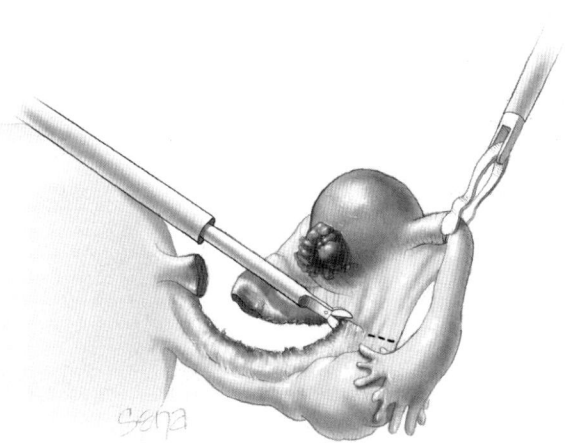

FIGURE 44-3.2 Mesosalpinx incision.

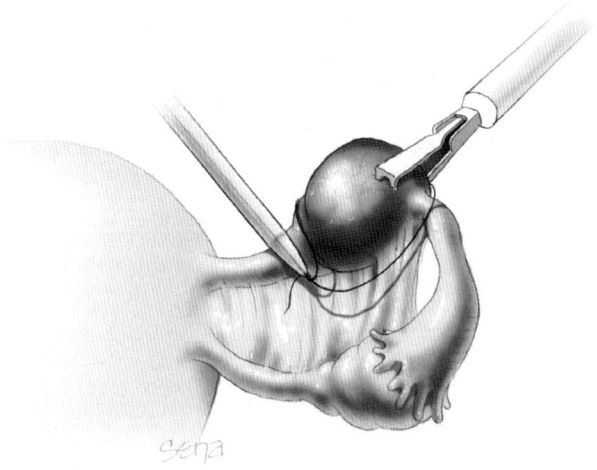

FIGURE 44-3.3 Endoscopic loop ligation.

Other energy sources also work well. Monopolar scissors themselves may be attached to current. In this technique, vessels within the mesosalpinx are first electrosurgically coagulated and then cut. Advanced bipolar technologies (LigaSure, ENSEAL), laser energy, and Harmonic scalpel are suitable options. A surgeon's expertise with a particular modality dictates selection. One or more of these may be preferred based on the surrounding pelvic pathology or adhesions. The major concern with any of these tools is the amount of thermal spread to surrounding tissues.

❹ **Endoscopic Loop Ligation.** Alternatively, the vascular supply to the fallopian tube within the mesosalpinx can be ligated. Figure 44-3.3 shows an endoscopic suture loop encircling a loop of fallopian tube that contains an ectopic pregnancy. Absorbable and delayed-absorbable suture loops are available, and either is suitable for ligation. Two or three suture loops are sequentially placed, and the tube distal to these ligatures is then cut free with scissors (Fig. 44-3.4).

❺ **Tissue Removal.** Most tubal ectopic pregnancies are small and pliant. Thus, they can be held firmly by grasping forceps and drawn up into one of the accessory site cannulas. The cannula, grasping forceps, and ectopic tissue can then be removed together. Larger tubal ectopic pregnancies may be placed in an endoscopic sac to prevent fragmentation as they are removed through the laparoscopic port site. Alternatively, larger ectopic pregnancies can be morcellated with scissors within an enclosed bag. Tissue removal techniques are presented on page 1019 and are also illustrated in Chapter 41 (p. 896).

❻ **Irrigation.** To remove all trophoblastic tissue, the pelvis and abdomen are irrigated and suctioned free of blood and tissue debris. Slow and systematic movement of the patient from Trendelenburg positioning to reverse Trendelenburg can also assist in dislodging stray tissue and fluid, which is then suctioned and removed from the peritoneal cavity.

❼ **Wound Closure.** Subsequent surgery completion steps follow those of diagnostic laparoscopy (p. 1005).

POSTOPERATIVE

As with most laparoscopic surgeries, patients can resume presurgical diet and activity levels according to their comfort, typically within days.

If salpingectomy is performed for ectopic pregnancy, Rh-negative patients are given a single 50- or 300-μg (1500 IU) $Rh_0(D)$ immune globulin dose intramuscularly within 72 hours. To identify patients in whom trophoblastic tissue may persist, serial serum β-hCG levels are monitored until undetectable (Seifer, 1997). Spandorfer and associates (1997) compared serum β-hCG levels 1 day postoperatively with those drawn prior to surgery. They found a significantly lower percentage of persistent trophoblastic tissue if the β-hCG level fell more than 50 percent and noted no cases if the level declined by greater than 77 percent. Until levels are undetectable, contraception is used to avoid confusion between persistent trophoblastic tissue and a new pregnancy. Ovulation may resume as early as 2 weeks after an early pregnancy ends. Therefore, if contraception is desired, methods are initiated soon after surgery. Last, patients are counseled regarding their increased risk of future ectopic pregnancy.

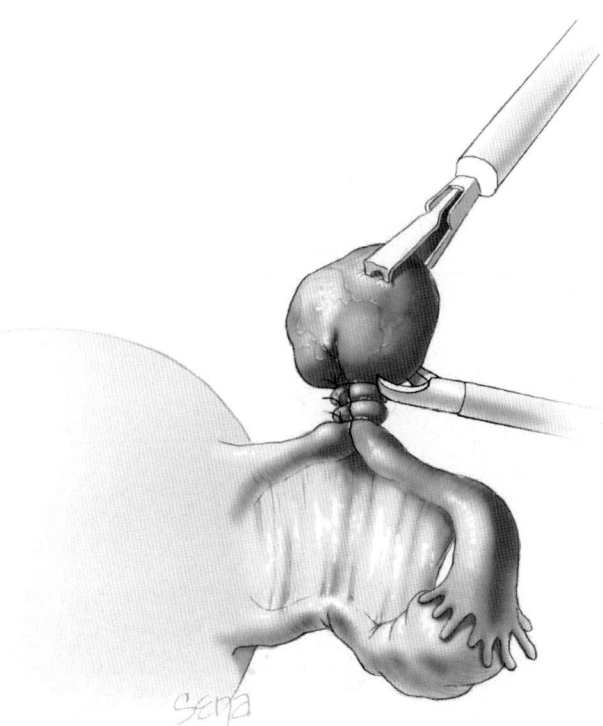

FIGURE 44-3.4 Looped portion of tube excised.

44-4

Laparoscopic Salpingostomy

For patients with ectopic pregnancy, laparoscopic linear salpingostomy offers the surgical advantages of laparoscopy and an opportunity to retain fertility by preserving the involved fallopian tube. Accordingly, suitable candidates are women with an unruptured isthmic or ampullary ectopic pregnancy and desiring future pregnancies. Success is mainly affected by the amount of bleeding, by the ability to control it, and by the degree of tubal damage.

PREOPERATIVE

Consent

Risks of laparoscopic salpingostomy mirror those for laparoscopic salpingectomy (p. 1011). Importantly, with salpingostomy, a patient is counseled regarding the possible need for salpingectomy if the tube is irreparably damaged or bleeding from the tube cannot be controlled. Also, rates of persistent trophoblastic disease are higher with salpingostomy compared with removal of the entire affected tubal segment.

Bleeding

Because trophoblastic tissue is vascular, disruption during ectopic pregnancy removal can lead to severe hemorrhage. The ability of tubal muscularis to contract is minimal, and thus, bleeding during salpingostomy must be controlled with external modalities such as electrosurgical coagulation. Many devices are appropriate, and the microbipolar device is effective for achieving hemostasis while creating minimal thermal spread. At times, bleeding may be extensive and persistent and necessitate salpingectomy.

To improve hemostasis, vasoconstrictive agents such as vasopressin have been evaluated. Dilutions of 20 U of vasopressin in 30 to 100 mL of saline are suitable. The mesosalpinx is then infiltrated with approximately 10 mL of solution. Because of the potential systemic vasoconstrictive effects of vasopressin, intravascular injection is avoided. Another approach is to inject the solution into the portion of the tube to be incised. This is dictated by surgeon preference. Additional complications and contraindications to vasopressin use are discussed on page 1023. Benefits to vasopressin include less frequent use of electrosurgery, shorter operating time, and lower conversion rates to laparotomy for surgery completion.

To avoid vasopressin's cardiovascular complications, Fedele and colleagues (1998) diluted 20 U of oxytocin in 20 mL of saline and similarly injected the mesosalpinx. Oxytocin is purported to contract the smooth muscle fibers of the tube and cause vasoconstriction of mesosalpinx vessels. These researchers noted easier pregnancy enucleation, less bleeding, and less frequent use of electrosurgery.

Persistent Trophoblastic Tissue

During treatment of ectopic pregnancy, trophoblastic tissue can persist in as many as 3 to 20 percent of cases. Remnant implants typically involve the fallopian tube, but extratubal trophoblastic implants have been found on the omentum and on pelvic and abdominal peritoneal surfaces. Peritoneal implants typically measure 0.3 to 2.0 cm and appear as red-black nodules (Doss, 1998). Severe postoperative bleeding is the most serious complication of this persistent tissue (Giuliani, 1998).

The risk of persistent trophoblast tissue is highest following laparoscopic salpingostomy, especially in women in whom small, early pregnancies are removed. In these pregnancies, the cleavage plane between the invading trophoblast and tubal implantation site is poor. This may lead to a more difficult dissection and failure to completely remove all products of conception. For all cases, preventive recommendations include irrigation and complete suctioning of the abdomen, limitation of Trendelenburg position to limit blood and tissue flow to the upper abdomen, and use of endoscopic bags for removal of larger ectopic pregnancies (Ben-Arie, 2001).

INTRAOPERATIVE

Instruments

Specific tools needed for salpingostomy mirror those for salpingectomy and should be available if salpingectomy is required (p. 1011).

Surgical Steps

❶ Anesthesia and Patient Positioning. The patient is prepared and positioned for laparoscopic surgery as described in Chapter 41 (p. 879).

❷ Abdominal Entry. The abdomen is accessed with laparoscopic techniques, and typically two or three accessory port sites are used. Depending on the ectopic pregnancy size, at least one 10-mm or larger accessory port may be necessary to allow specimen removal at surgery's end. Once cannulas are in place, systematic inspection of the abdomen and pelvis is completed prior to the planned procedure.

❸ Salpingostomy. The fallopian tube is lifted and held with atraumatic grasping forceps. By means of a 22-gauge needle through one of the accessory ports or through a separate abdominal wall needle puncture, a solution of vasopressin is injected into the mesosalpinx beneath the ectopic pregnancy. If the serosal layer overlying the ectopic tissue is injected instead, then a smaller 25-gauge needle may be used.

A monopolar needle tip electrode is set at a cutting voltage and used to create a 1- to 2-cm longitudinal incision (Fig. 44-4.1). The

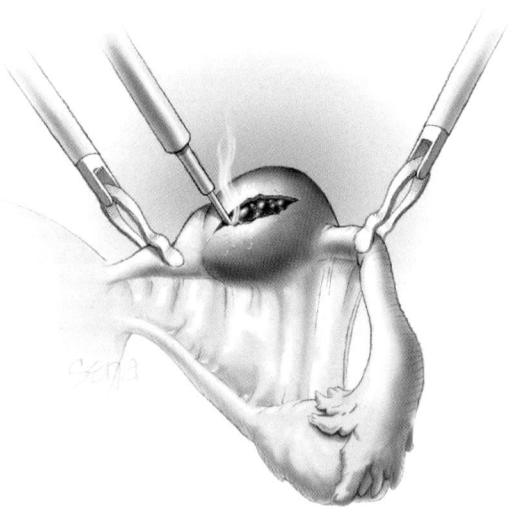

FIGURE 44-4.1 Salpingostomy.

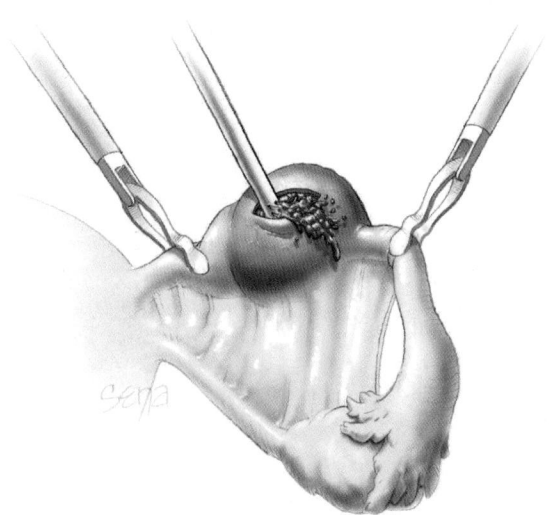

FIGURE 44-4.2 Hydrodissection.

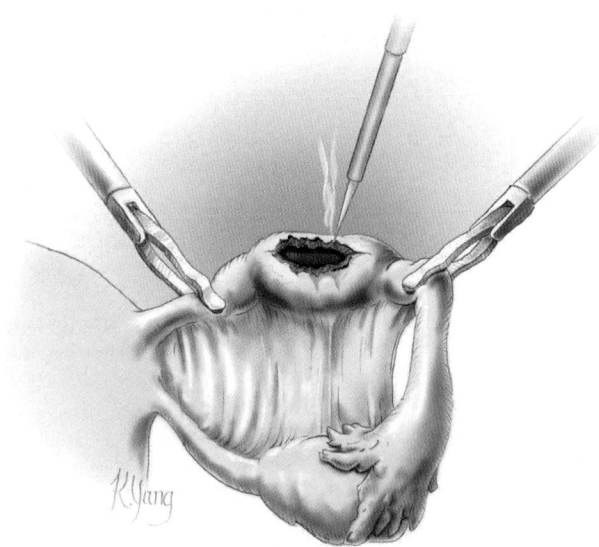

FIGURE 44-4.3 Coagulation of incision edges.

incision is positioned opposite the mesosalpinx and on the maximally distended portion of the tube that overlies the pregnancy. Laparoscopic scissors, CO_2 laser, bipolar needle, and Harmonic scalpel have also been used.

❹ **Pregnancy Removal.** For this step, atraumatic grasping forceps hold one edge of the incision while a suction-irrigation probe tip is insinuated into the tissue plane between the tubal wall and ectopic pregnancy (Fig. 44-4.2). Hydrodissection is performed on one side of the tube and then the other. A combination of high-pressure hydrodissection and gentle blunt dissection with the suction irrigator tip is used to remove the entire conceptus from the tube. Alternatively, the pregnancy or its fragments may require extraction by smooth grasping forceps.

❺ **Hemostasis.** Bleeding points can be controlled with monopolar or bipolar electrosurgical coagulation (Fig. 44-4.3). The tubal incision is left open to heal by secondary intention. Tulandi and Guralnick (1991) found no differences in subsequent fertility and adhesion formation between salpingotomy with or without tubal suturing. Use of topical fibrin products for hemostasis has been evaluated in limited studies and warrants further investigation with regard to adhesion prevention and future pregnancy effects (Mosesson, 1992).

❻ **Specimen Extraction.** Most ectopic pregnancies are small and pliant. Accordingly, they can be held firmly by grasping forceps and drawn up into one of the accessory cannulas. The cannula, grasping forceps, and ectopic tissue can then be removed together. Larger ectopic pregnancies may be placed in an endoscopic sac to prevent fragmentation as they are removed through the laparoscopic trocar site.

❼ **Irrigation.** To prevent persistent trophoblastic tissue postoperatively, the pelvis and abdomen are irrigated and suctioned free of blood and tissue debris.

❽ **Adhesion Prevention.** Adjuvants are available that can be used for the prevention of postoperative adhesion formation. However, although adhesion formation is lessened, no substantial evidence documents that their use improves fertility, decreases pain, or prevents bowel obstruction (American Society for Reproductive Medicine, 2013).

❾ **Wound Closure.** Subsequent surgery completion steps follow those of diagnostic laparoscopy (p. 1005).

POSTOPERATIVE

As with most laparoscopic surgeries, patients can resume presurgical diet and activity levels according to their comfort, typically within days. Postoperative topics specific to ectopic pregnancy include Rh_0 [D] immune globulin administration, surveillance for persistent trophoblastic disease, provision of contraception if desired, and counseling on future ectopic pregnancy risk as described on page 1012.

44-5

Laparoscopic Ovarian Cystectomy

Many studies have attested to the efficacy and safety of laparoscopic cystectomy for the management of ovarian cysts. Moreover, because of recovery-associated benefits, a laparoscopic technique is advocated by many as the preferred approach in women with ovarian cysts and a low risk of malignancy (Chap. 9, p. 216).

PREOPERATIVE

Patient Evaluation

Sonography is the primary tool used to diagnose ovarian pathology, and the sonographic characteristics of a cyst aid in determining preoperatively the malignant potential of a given lesion (Chap. 9, p. 217). In those patients with indeterminate ovarian cysts following sonography, magnetic resonance (MR) imaging may enhance discrimination.

The serum tumor marker cancer antigen 125 (CA125) is typically obtained preoperatively in postmenopausal patients and in any woman whose tumor displays other risk factors for ovarian epithelial cancer (Chap. 35, p. 742). Additionally, serum alpha-fetoprotein (AFP), lactate dehydrogenase (LDH), inhibin, and β-hCG levels may be measured to exclude germ cell or sex cord-stromal ovarian neoplasms, if these are suspected (Chap. 36, pp. 761 and 768).

Consent

Prior to surgery, patients are informed of the unique complications associated with laparoscopy itself (Chap. 41, p. 877). Specific to ovarian cystectomy, the risks of oophorectomy due to bleeding or extreme ovarian damage are discussed. Depending on the amount of oocyte-containing ovarian stroma that is stripped away with the cyst, diminished ovarian reserve is also a risk. Obviously, because many cysts are removed due to concerns of potential malignancy, patients should be familiar with the steps involved in the surgical staging of ovarian cancer.

Patient Preparation

Rates of pelvic and wound infection following ovarian cystectomy and laparoscopy are low, and antibiotic prophylaxis is typically not required. Bowel preparation is not usually required, but may be considered if extensive adhesions are suspected. VTE prophylaxis is typically not recommended for laparoscopic cystectomy. However, those with a greater risk of malignancy, with risks for VTE, or with an increased chance for conversion to laparotomy may benefit from these measures (Table 39-8, p. 836).

INTRAOPERATIVE

Instruments

Most instruments required for ovarian cystectomy are found in a standard laparoscopy instrument set. A suction irrigation system is commonly needed to remove cyst contents if rupture occurs. An endoscopic retrieval bag is also frequently used. Once contained in the sac, the cyst in some cases may be decompressed with a laparoscopic aspiration needle.

If oophorectomy is required, the infundibulopelvic ligament is ligated. This may be accomplished using bipolar instruments, Harmonic scalpel, laparoscopic suture loop, or stapler. These may not be readily available in all operating suites, and desired tools are requested prior to surgery.

Surgical Steps

❶ **Anesthesia and Patient Positioning.** The patient is prepared and positioned for laparoscopic surgery (Chap. 41, p. 879). A bimanual examination is completed to determine ovarian size and position and uterine inclination. Ovarian information will affect placement of the accessory ports, and uterine inclination will direct positioning of the uterine manipulator if used. A uterine manipulator may assist with moving the uterus and adnexa (p. 881). In anticipation of possible hysterectomy as a part of ovarian cancer staging, the vagina and abdomen are surgically prepared, and a Foley catheter is inserted. The patient is then draped to allow sterile access to the vagina and abdomen.

❷ **Abdominal Entry.** Primary and secondary trocars are placed as described in Chapter 41 (p. 889). For insertion of most endoscopic sacs, at least one 10-mm or larger accessory trocar may be necessary to allow specimen removal at surgery's end. Typically, two or three accessory trocars are required for cystectomy.

Once the abdomen is entered, a diagnostic laparoscopy is performed, inspecting the pelvis and upper abdomen for signs of malignancy such as ascites and peritoneal implants or for evidence of endometriosis. Suspicious areas are biopsied, and those concerning for cancer are sent for intraoperative analysis. Prior to ovarian cystectomy, adhesions are divided to restore proper anatomic relationships.

❸ **Ovarian Incision.** A blunt probe is placed under the uteroovarian ligament and posterior ovarian surface to elevate the ovary. An atraumatic grasping forceps then steadies the ovary, and the blunt probe is removed (Fig. 44-5.1). A monopolar needle tip electrode set at a cutting voltage is used to incise the ovarian capsule that overlies the cyst. Other suitable devices for incision include a monopolar scissor blade or Harmonic scalpel. This incision is ideally on the antimesenteric surface of the ovary to minimize dissection into extensive vascularity at the

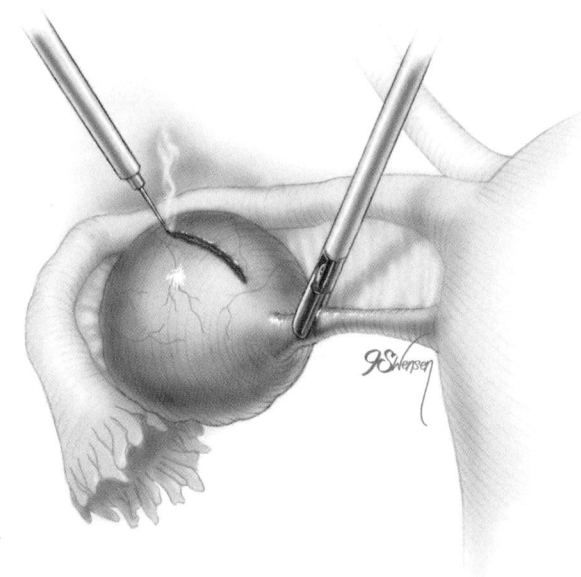

FIGURE 44-5.1 Ovarian incision.

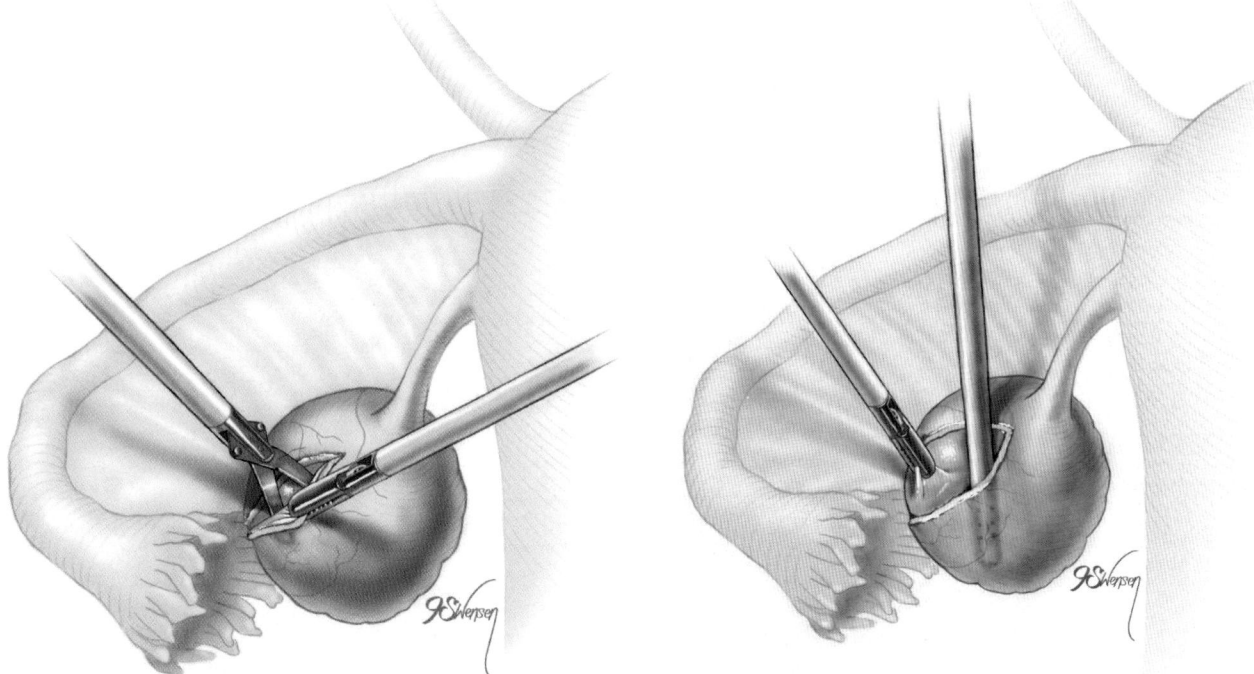

FIGURE 44-5.2 Dissection initiated.

FIGURE 44-5.3 Hydrodissection.

ovarian hilum. The incision is extended into the ovarian stroma to the level of the cyst wall but ideally does not rupture the cyst.

❹ **Cyst Dissection.** A space between the ovary and cyst wall is created using blunt forceps or dissecting scissors (Fig. 44-5.2). Atraumatic grasping forceps are used to hold one edge of the incision, while a blunt probe or suction-irrigation probe tip is insinuated in the tissue plane between the ovarian capsule and cyst wall (Fig. 44-5.3).

Blunt or hydrodissection is performed on one side of the cyst and then the other. Depending on the adherence of the cyst to its surrounding ovarian tissue, cystectomy may at times require sharp dissection with scissors. During dissection, points of bleeding may be coagulated, or isolated vessels may be grasped and coagulated (Fig. 44-5.4).

❺ **Cyst Removal.** Following enucleation from the ovary, the cyst is placed into an endoscopic bag (Fig. 44-5.5). The opening of the sac is closed and brought up to the anterior abdominal wall (Fig. 44-5.6). Depending on its size, the cyst and endoscopic bag may be removed in toto through one of the accessory cannulas. In this setting, the laparoscopic cannula is removed first, followed by the cyst contained within the sac.

Alternatively, with larger cysts, the cannula is removed, and the entire pursed opening of the bag is drawn up through the trocar incision and fanned out onto the skin surface. The open edges of the bag are pulled upward

to lift and press the cyst up against the incision. A needle tip is then directed into the incision and pierces the cyst contained within the endoscopic bag. An attached syringe is used to aspirate contents. Alternatively, the cyst may be ruptured by a toothed Kocher

clamp placed through the skin incision and into the sac (Fig. 44-5.7). Thereby, cyst fluid is retained within the endoscopic sac. The endoscopic sac and decompressed cyst wall are then removed together through the incision (Fig. 44-5.8). During removal, care is

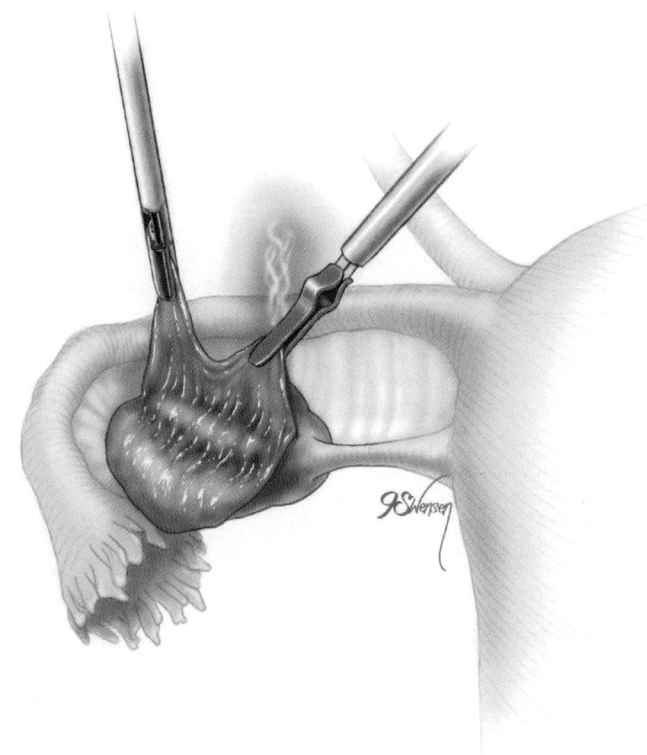

FIGURE 44-5.4 Following cyst enucleation, ovarian capsule edges are coagulated.

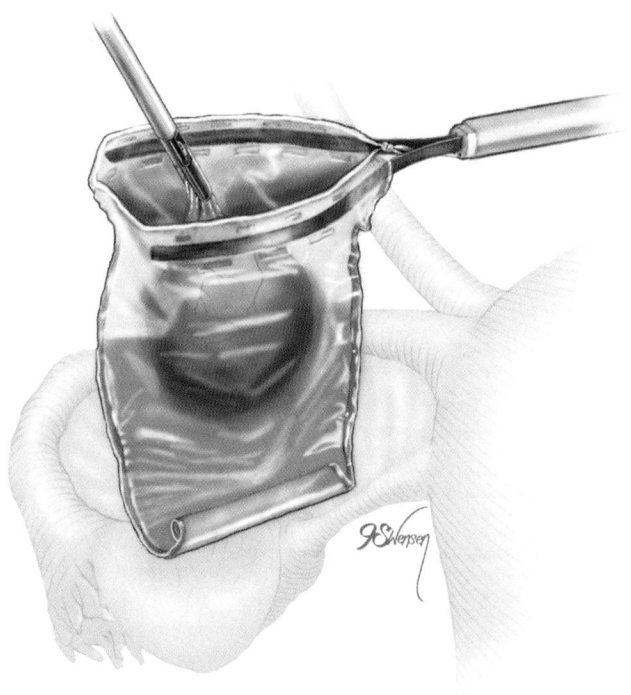

FIGURE 44-5.5 Cyst placed in endoscopic sac.

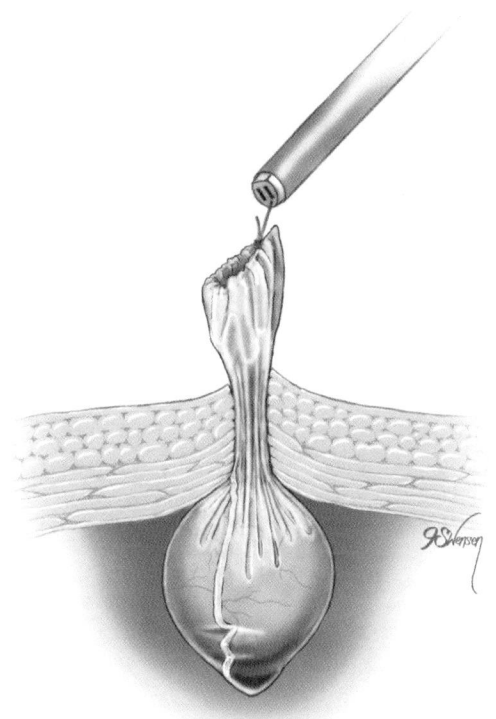

FIGURE 44-5.6 Endoscopic bag cinched and brought up to anterior abdominal wall.

taken to ensure that the endoscopic bag is not inadvertently punctured or torn, and all measures are used to prevent spillage of cyst contents into the abdomen or port site.

❻ Cyst Rupture. Not uncommonly during the dissection of the cyst away from the ovary, the cyst may rupture. The cyst wall is then removed using a "stripping" technique

(Fig. 44-5.9). With this, both the cyst wall and cyst capsule can be grasped near the dissection plane by atraumatic forceps. Traction and countertraction can separate filmy connective

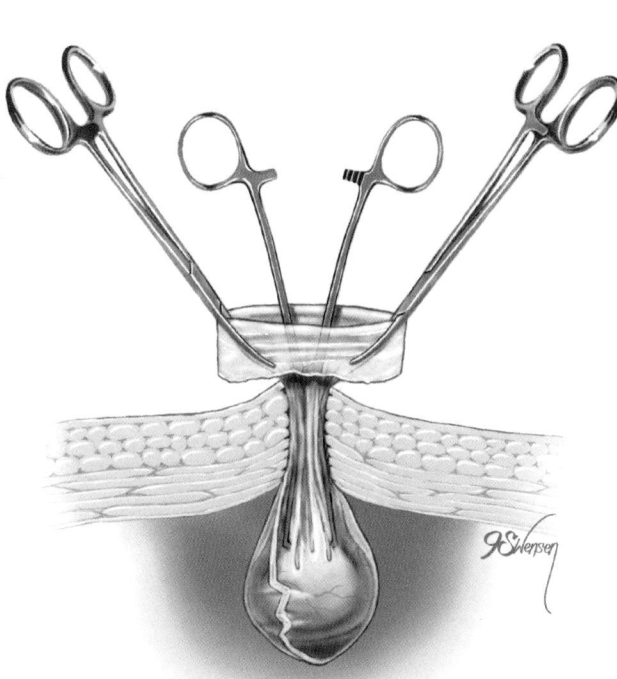

FIGURE 44-5.7 Cyst ruptured by toothed Kocher clamp within the endoscopic sac.

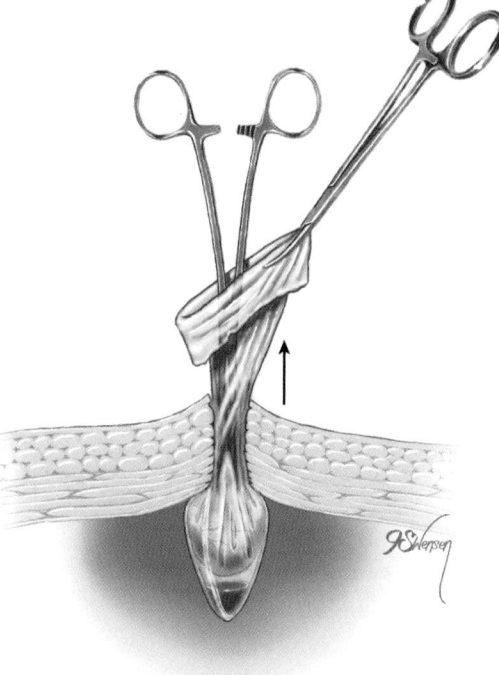

FIGURE 44-5.8 Sac and collapsed cyst are removed together.

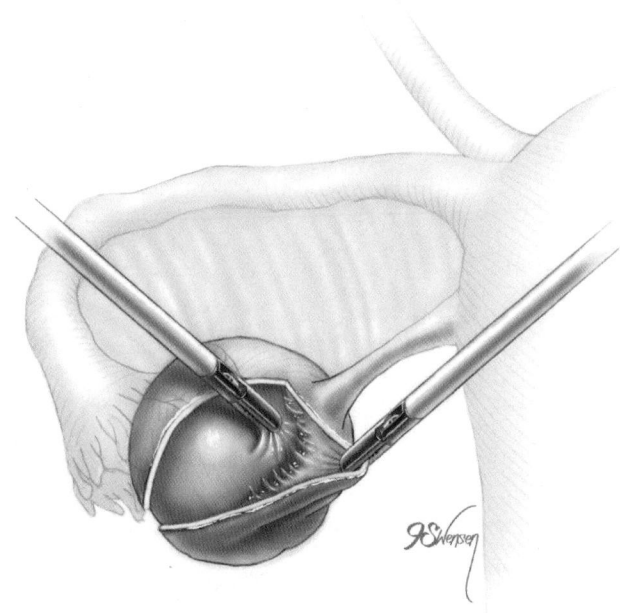

FIGURE 44-5.9 Stripping of collapsed cyst from ovarian capsule.

tissue between these to advance the dissection plane. As a result, the grasping forceps strip the cyst wall away from the underlying ovarian stroma. To prevent damage to the underlying healthy ovary, the dissection plane between the cyst and stroma should be clearly delineated by traction on each side to prevent tearing. Injection of dilute vasopressin into this space may also help delineate the dissection plane and minimize bleeding. Histologically, Muzii and colleagues (2002) showed that this technique in nonendometriotic lesions spared ovarian tissue and did not strip away normal ovarian tissue and follicles.

❼ Ovary Closure. Because of increased adhesion formation risk, technical difficulty, and time associated with laparoscopic suturing, in general the ovarian capsule is not sutured closed following cyst removal. Several studies show that leaving the capsule open does not lead to increased adhesion formation (Marana, 1991; Wiskind, 1990). Application of an adhesion barrier such as oxidized regenerated cellulose may be considered to prevent adhesion formation (Franklin, 1995; Wiseman, 1999). However, no substantial evidence documents that their use improves fertility, decreases pain, or prevents bowel obstruction (American Society for Reproductive Medicine, 2013).

❽ Wound Closure. If concerning for malignancy, the specimen is submitted in most cases for immediate frozen section analysis. If benign findings are noted, then steps toward surgical closure begin. If malignancy is found, then surgical staging should ensue. Of note, if a large mass was removed and the port site was likely extended during the removal, one should consider fascial closure to prevent port-site hernias. The finishing laparoscopic steps are similar to those for diagnostic laparoscopy (p. 1005).

POSTOPERATIVE

Following laparoscopic ovarian cystectomy, instructions similar to those for diagnostic laparoscopy are given (p. 1005).

44-6

Laparoscopic Salpingo-oophorectomy

Laparoscopy can be used to safely remove many adnexa and in most cases, offers a faster recovery and less postoperative pain compared with laparotomy. As discussed in Chapter 9 (p. 202), indications for adnexectomy vary but may include torsion, ovarian cyst rupture, suspicion of ovarian malignancy, and symptomatic ovarian remnant. In addition, prophylactic oophorectomy is often considered in women with or at genetic risk for cancers involving the breast, ovary, and colon (Chap. 35, p. 738).

Laparoscopy is a preferred approach when possible and can be safely performed in pregnancy, preferably in the early second trimester. However, for all patients, laparotomy may be preferred is certain clinical settings. These include a high suspicion of cancer, anticipation of extensive pelvic adhesions, and large ovarian size.

PREOPERATIVE

Patient Evaluation

Salpingo-oophorectomy is typically performed to remove ovarian pathology and sonography is the primary tool used for diagnosis. In cases in which anatomy may be unclear, MR imaging may add additional information. As discussed on page 1015, tumor markers may be drawn prior to surgery if malignancy is suspected.

Consent

Prior to surgery, patients are informed of the unique complications associated with laparoscopy (Chap. 41, p. 877). Specific to salpingo-oophorectomy, the risk of ureteral injury is discussed. Many adnexa are removed due to concerns of potential malignancy, and patients should be familiar with the steps involved in the surgical staging of ovarian cancer.

Patient Preparation

Unless an ovarian abscess is identified, laparoscopic salpingo-oophorectomy does not require antibiotic prophylaxis (American College of Obstetricians and Gynecologists, 2014b). If hysterectomy is required during ovarian staging, antibiotics may be given intraoperatively. Bowel preparation is not

usually required but may be considered if extensive adhesions are suspected. VTE prophylaxis is typically not recommended for laparoscopic cystectomy. However, those with a greater risk of malignancy, with underlying VTE risks, or with an increased chance for conversion to laparotomy may benefit from these measures (Table 39-8, p. 836).

INTRAOPERATIVE

Instruments

Most instruments required for ovarian cystectomy are found in a standard laparoscopy instrument set. However, a suction irrigation system is commonly needed to remove cyst contents if rupture occurs. An endoscopic retrieval bag is also frequently used. During oophorectomy, the infundibulopelvic ligament is ligated. This may be accomplished using bipolar instruments, Harmonic scalpel, laparoscopic suture loop, or stapler. These may not be readily available in all operating suites, and desired tools are requested prior to surgery.

Surgical Steps

❶ Anesthesia and Patient Positioning. The patient is prepared and positioned for laparoscopic surgery as described in Chapter 41 (p. 879). A bimanual examination is completed to determine ovarian size and position and uterine inclination. Ovarian information will affect placement of the accessory ports, and uterine inclination will direct positioning of the uterine manipulator if used. Because of possible hysterectomy as a part of ovarian cancer staging, the vagina and abdomen are surgically prepared, and a Foley catheter is inserted. A uterine manipulator may also be placed to assist with manipulation of the uterus and adnexa (p. 883).

❷ Abdominal Access. Primary and secondary trocars are placed as described in Chapter 41 (p. 889). Typically, two or three accessory ports are required. For insertion of most endoscopic sacs, at least one 10-mm or larger accessory port may be necessary to allow specimen removal at surgery's end.

❸ Pelvic Inspection and Washings. Once the abdomen is entered, a diagnostic laparoscopy is performed, inspecting the pelvis and upper abdomen for signs of malignancy such as ascites and peritoneal implants (p. 1004). Cellular washings from these areas are obtained and saved until frozen section analysis of the specimen has excluded malignancy. Similarly, identified peritoneal implants from these areas are biopsied and sent for intraoperative evaluation. Prior

to adnexectomy, adhesions are divided to restore proper anatomic relationships.

❹ Ureter Location. The ureter lies close to the infundibulopelvic (IP) ligament, and its course should be noted. If the location of the ureter is not clear, the peritoneum lateral to the ureter is incised, and retroperitoneal isolation of the ureter is completed (Fig. 44-6.1).

❺ Infundibulopelvic Ligament Coagulation. Ligation of the ovarian vessels within the IP ligament can be completed with endoscopic loop ligatures, electrosurgical coagulating devices, Harmonic scalpel, or stapler depending on surgeon preference (see Fig. 44-6.1). Once these vessels are occluded, the IP is severed distally.

❻ Opening of the Broad Ligament. After transection of the IP, the fallopian tube and ovary are gently elevated with atraumatic forceps. Incision of the broad ligament's posterior leaf is then extended to the round ligament (Fig. 44-6.2).

❼ Uteroovarian Ligament Coagulation. The uteroovarian ligament and proximal fallopian tube are identified posterior to the round ligament. Similarly to the IP, these may be coagulated, stapled, or ligated (Fig. 44-6.3). Distal to this occlusion, the uteroovarian ligament and fallopian tube are transected, and the adnexum is freed.

❽ Adnexum Removal. Various endoscopic bags are available for tissue removal (Chap. 41, p. 883). The specimen is dropped into the sac, which is closed and brought up to the anterior abdominal wall. Depending on its size, the adnexum and endoscopic bag may be removed in toto through one of the accessory port sites. In this setting, the laparoscopic cannula is removed first, followed by the specimen contained within the sac.

Alternatively, with larger cystic ovaries, the cannula is removed, and the entire pursed opening of the bag is drawn up through the incision and fanned out onto the skin surface. As illustrated in Section 44-5 (p. 1017), the open edges of the bag are pulled upward to lift and press the ovary against the incision. A needle tip is directed through the incision and into the sac. The ovary is pierced and aspiration drainage is completed by an attached syringe. Alternatively, the cyst may be ruptured by a toothed Kocher clamp placed through the skin incision and into the sac. Thereby, cyst fluid is retained in the endoscopic sac. The endoscopic sac and decompressed cyst wall are then removed together through the incision. During removal, care is taken to ensure that the endoscopic is

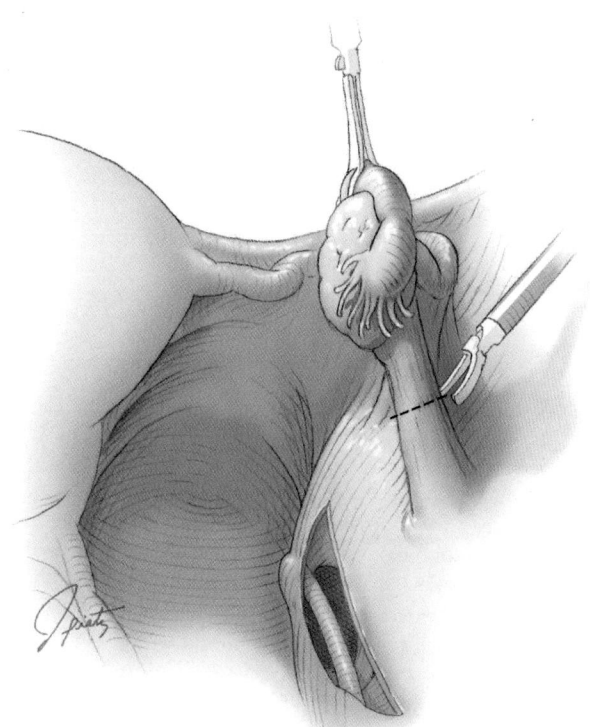

FIGURE 44-6.1 Infundibulopelvic ligament coagulation.

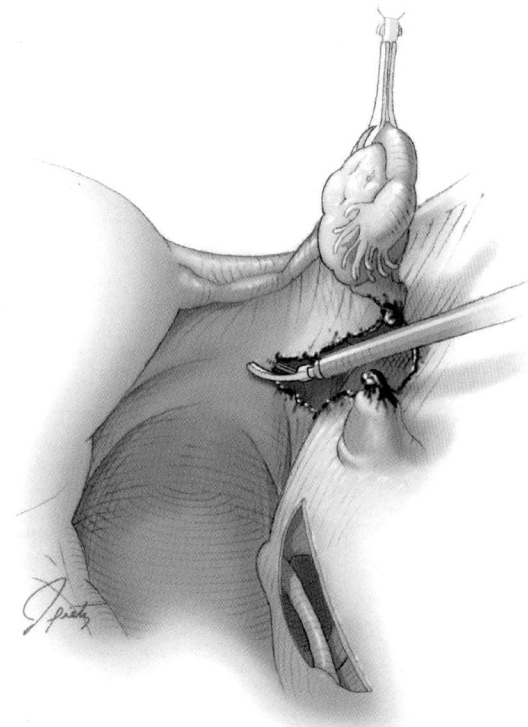

FIGURE 44-6.2 Opening of the broad ligament.

bag is not inadvertently punctured or torn, and all measures are used to prevent spill of cyst contents into the abdomen or port site. Additionally, to prevent spill or to remove a larger solid mass, one may remove the adnexa through a minilaparotomy incision or a col-

potomy incision as described on page 1031 and illustrated in Chapter 41 (p. 896).

❾ **Wound Closure.** If malignancy is suspected, the specimen is submitted for immediate frozen section analysis. If benign

findings are noted, then steps toward surgical closure begin (p. 1005). If malignancy is found, then surgical staging should ensue. Of note, if a large mass was removed and the port site was likely extended during the removal, one should consider fascial closure to prevent port-site herniation.

POSTOPERATIVE

Advantages to laparoscopy include a rapid return to normal diet and activities, and postoperative complication rates are low. If both adnexa are removed, then hormone replacement therapy is considered in appropriate candidates (Chap. 22, p. 494).

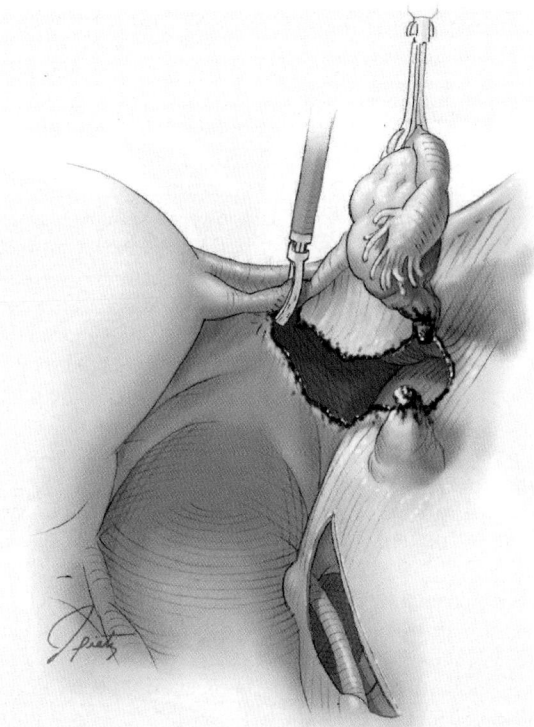

FIGURE 44-6.3 Fallopian tube and uteroovarian ligament coagulation to free the specimen.

44-7

Ovarian Drilling

Ovarian drilling is a technique of puncturing the ovarian capsule with a laser beam or an electrosurgical needle using a laparoscopic approach. Similar to ovarian wedge resection, this procedure's end goal is to reduce the amount of androgen-producing tissue in women with polycystic ovarian syndrome (PCOS). However, in wedge resection, a long cortical incision is required for this degree of resection. As a result, infertility secondary to adhesions complicates many postoperative courses (Buttram, 1975; Toaff, 1976). To minimize this risk and avoid the need for laparotomy, ovarian drilling techniques using laparoscopy were developed in the early 1980s.

Compared with gonadotropin stimulation to achieve pregnancy, ovarian drilling has lower rates of ovarian hyperstimulation syndrome (OHSS) and of multifetal gestation (Farquhar, 2012). Disadvantages include the surgical risks of laparoscopy, risks of pelvic adhesion formation, and concerns regarding long-term effects on ovarian function (Donesky, 1995; Farquhar, 2012). For these reasons, ovarian drilling is viewed as a second-line therapy. It can be useful in patients who fail to ovulate with clomiphene citrate, who are at risk for OHSS, or who desire to minimize their risk for multifetal gestation.

PREOPERATIVE

Consent

There appear to be relatively few complications that arise immediately after ovarian drilling. Hemorrhage, infection, and thermal bowel injury are infrequent. Similarly, ovarian atrophy following drilling is rare but has been reported (Dabirashrafi, 1989).

Adhesion formation following this procedure, however, is common. Most of these adhesions at second-look laparoscopy have typically been graded as minimal or mild (Gürgan, 1991). Moreover, researchers have described only a minimal, if any, decline in fertility from these adhesions (Gürgan, 1992; Naether, 1993). This risk, however, is discussed with the patient prior to surgery.

INTRAOPERATIVE

Instruments

Ovarian drilling has been described using monopolar or bipolar electrosurgical energy

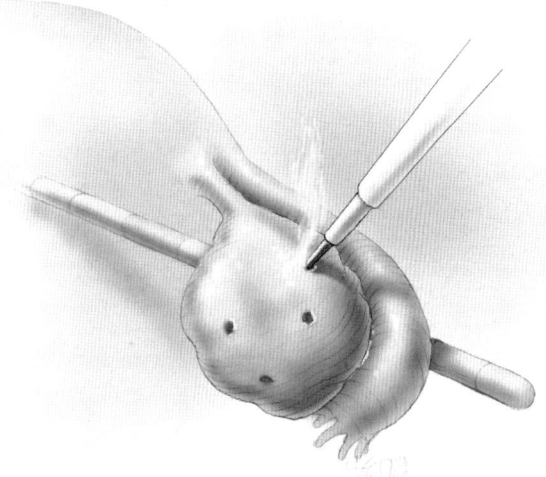

FIGURE 44-7.1 Ovarian drilling.

or using various lasers, all with the goal of causing focal damage to the ovarian stroma and cortex. Currently, no studies support the superiority of one modality (Strowitzki, 2005).

Number of Ovarian Punctures

Punctures into the ovarian capsule are typically 2 to 4 mm wide and 4 to 10 mm deep. Although techniques using as few as four or as many as 40 punctures per ovary have been described, few studies have investigated the optimum number of punctures (Farquhar, 2004). For example, Malkawi and Qublan (2005) showed that five punctures per ovary compared with 10 resulted in equally improved pregnancy rates and similarly low rates of postprocedural OHSS and multifetal gestation.

Surgical Steps

❶ **Anesthesia and Patient Positioning.** Patient positioning and anesthesia mirror those for other laparoscopic procedures (Chap. 41, p. 879).

❷ **Abdominal Entry.** Three incisions are used for this laparoscopic procedure. In addition to an umbilical incision, two bilateral lower abdominal incisions are made. These incisions serve as entry sites for the electrosurgical needle tip and grasping forceps.

❸ **Ovarian Drilling.** The ovary is elevated with a blunt grasper. The electrosurgical current is set at 30 to 60 W cutting mode. A monopolar electrosurgery needle tip is used to puncture the ovary perpendicular to the cortical surface and to pierce the follicular cysts that are characteristic of PCOS. Four to five punc-

tures are placed symmetrically on the antimesenteric surface of the ovary (Fig. 44-7.1). Drilling is avoided on the lateral surfaces of the ovaries to minimize adhesions to the pelvic sidewall and is avoided at the ovarian hilum to limit bleeding risks. The needle is inserted to a depth of 4 to 10 mm. Electrical current is applied for 3 to 4 seconds. The ovarian surface can be irrigated with saline or lactated Ringer solution to cool it (Strowitzki, 2005).

❹ **Adhesion Barriers.** Because of the risk for adhesion formation, some investigators use adhesion barrier products following ovarian drilling. Greenblatt and Casper (1993), however, showed no improvement in adhesion prevention following this procedure using Interceed adhesion barrier. No other studies have addressed the efficacy of other adhesion prevention products.

❺ **Wound Closure.** Subsequent surgery completion steps should follow those of diagnostic laparoscopy (p. 1005).

POSTOPERATIVE

Postoperatively, patients are given instructions similar to those following diagnostic laparoscopy (p. 1005).

44-8

Laparoscopic Myomectomy

Myomectomy involves surgical removal of leiomyomas from their surrounding myometrium, and accepted indications include selected cases of abnormal uterine bleeding, pelvic pain, infertility, and recurrent miscarriage. Historically, removal of serosal and intramural tumors required laparotomy. However, laparoscopic excision may be performed by those with advanced skills in operative laparoscopy and laparoscopic suturing. Robotic myomectomy has also increased in popularity for this indication (Visco, 2008).

In general, removal of subserosal and intramural leiomyomas are most appropriate for a laparoscopic approach. Submucous leiomyomas are best treated via hysteroscopic resection (p. 1040). The choice of abdominal or laparoscopic myomectomy is based on various factors that include tumor number, size, and location. Surgical experience and comfort with laparoscopic dissection, tissue extraction, and suturing are other requisites.

PREOPERATIVE

Patient Evaluation

Because of their impact on preoperative and intraoperative planning, leiomyoma size, number, and location are evaluated prior to surgery with sonography, MR imaging, and/or hysteroscopy, as described in Chapter 9 (p. 206). Specifically, leiomyomas may be small and buried within the myometrium. Therefore, accurate information as to tumor number and location ensures complete excision. Moreover, with a laparoscopic or robotic approach, the ability to palpate and appreciate smaller deep tumors may be compromised. In these cases, preoperative MR imaging may best assist with leiomyoma location and surgical planning. Last, multiple large masses or those that are located in the broad ligament, are near the cornua, or involve the cervix may increase the risk of conversion to hysterectomy, and patients are so counseled. Studies have also suggested that there is an increased risk of complications with the following: more than three leiomyomas, tumor size >5 cm, and intraligamental location (Sizzi, 2007). Accounting for these factors, a surgeon's expertise is the most important factor in determining approach to myomectomy.

Consent

Myomectomy can cause significant bleeding that requires transfusion. Moreover, uncontrolled hemorrhage or extensive myometrial injury during tumor removal may necessitate hysterectomy. Patients are also counseled regarding the risk of conversion to an open procedure, which ranges from 2 to 8 percent (American College of Obstetricians and Gynecologists, 2014a).

Postoperatively, serosal adhesions can form and leiomyomas can recur. In some series, the risk of leiomyoma recurrence after laparoscopic myomectomy appears to be higher than in conventional myomectomy (Dubuisson, 2000; Fauconnier, 2000). As one explanation, with laparoscopic myomectomy, small, deep intramural leiomyomas may be missed because a surgeon's tactile sensation is diminished.

The use of electrosurgical energy on the uterus and challenges of laparoscopic multilayer hysterotomy closure also heighten concerns regarding uterine rupture during a subsequent pregnancy (Hurst, 2005; Parker, 2010; Sizzi, 2007). Women undergoing myomectomy who do plan to have future pregnancies are counseled regarding the possible need for cesarean delivery based on the extent of myometrial disruption during the myomectomy.

Patient Preparation

Hematologic Status and Tumor Size. Many preparatory steps prior to myomectomy address associated patient anemia, anticipated intraoperative blood loss, and tumor size. First, many women who undergo this surgery are often anemic secondary to associated menorrhagia. Correction prior to surgery may include oral iron therapy, gonadotropin-releasing hormone (GnRH) agonist administration, or both. In anticipation of blood loss, a CBC and type and crossmatch for packed red blood cells is obtained. Autologous blood donation or cell saver devices may be considered if great blood loss is expected. In addition, uterine artery embolization may be performed the morning of surgery for large uteri to minimize blood loss. However, this is most often used prior to laparotomy for significantly sized uteri.

GnRH agonists may be considered to decrease leiomyoma size, lower intraoperative blood loss, and decreased adhesion rates. However, loss of pseudocapsule planes around the tumors and greater risk of recurrence due to missed smaller leiomyomas is the trade-off. A fuller evidence-based discussion of these same preoperative options is found in Section 43-10 (p. 945).

Prophylaxis

Few studies have addressed the benefits of preoperative antibiotic use. Iverson and coworkers (1996), in their analysis of 101 open myomectomy cases, found that although 54 percent of patients received prophylaxis, infectious morbidity was not lowered compared with patients in whom antibiotics were not used.

In cases of myomectomy performed for infertility, because of the potential for tubal adhesions associated with pelvic infection, antibiotic prophylaxis is commonly used. For those in whom prophylaxis is planned, 1 g of a first- or second-generation cephalosporin is appropriate (Iverson, 1996; Periti, 1988; Sawin, 2000).

The risk of bowel injury with this procedure is low, and bowel preparation is typically not required unless extensive adhesions are anticipated. Because the risk of conversion to hysterectomy is present, vaginal preparation immediately prior to surgical draping is performed. With laparoscopic gynecologic surgery, the decision to provide VTE prophylaxis factors patient- and procedure-related VTE risks (Gould, 2012). Thus, if longer operating times are anticipated or preexisting VTE risks are present, then prophylaxis as outlined in Table 39-8 (p. 836) is reasonable.

INTRAOPERATIVE

Instruments

Many instruments required for laparoscopic myomectomy are found in a standard laparoscopy instrument set. However, a laparoscopic injection needle may be required for vasopressin injection, and a suction irrigation system is frequently needed to remove blood following tumor enucleation. A myoma screw or tenaculum is helpful to create needed tissue tension and countertension for enucleation. After tumor excision, removal may be accomplished by several techniques described on page 1031. Thus, required endoscopic bags or morcellators are assembled preoperatively.

Surgical Steps

❶ **Anesthesia and Patient Positioning.** As with most laparoscopic procedures, the patient is placed in low dorsal lithotomy position in booted support stirrups after adequate general anesthesia has been delivered. A bimanual examination is completed to determine uterine size to aid port placement. Because of the risk of hysterectomy and because colpotomy may be used for tumor removal, both the vagina and abdomen are surgically prepared. A Foley catheter is inserted. A uterine manipulator may also be placed, including one that will allow chromotubation at the procedure's end (p. 881). If planned, indigo carmine or methylene blue dye is mixed with 50 to 100 mL of sterile saline for injection through the cervical cannula.

❷ Trocar and Laparoscope Insertion.
Primary and accessory trocars are placed as described in Chapter 41 (p. 889). Port placement is customized to assist uterine manipulation, leiomyoma excision, and hysterotomy repair. Depending on uterine height, the primary port may need to be placed supraumbilically. In general, a distance of at least 4 cm above the level of the fundus is helpful to provide a global view of the uterus. Typically, at least three accessory ports are required. If use of an electric morcellator is planned, one of the cannulas should be at least 12 mm to accommodate the morcellator. After the abdomen is safely entered, a diagnostic laparoscopy is performed, and the serosal uterine surface should be inspected to identify leiomyomas to be removed. Correlating with preoperative imaging, the surgeon selects the optimal uterine incision to minimize myometrial disruption and to remove the maximum number of tumors thorough one incision.

❸ Use of Vasopressin.
8-Arginine vasopressin (Pitressin) is a sterile, aqueous solution of synthetic vasopressin. It is effective in limiting uterine blood loss during myomectomy because of its ability to cause vascular spasm and uterine muscle contraction. Compared with placebo, vasopressin injection has been shown to significantly decrease blood loss during myomectomy (Frederick, 1994).

Each vial of vasopressin is standardized to contain 20 pressor units/mL. Suitable doses for myomectomy include 20 U diluted in a range from 30 to 100 mL of saline (Fletcher, 1996; Iverson, 1996). Vasopressin is typically injected along the planned serosal incision(s), between the myometrium and leiomyoma capsule (Fig. 44-8.1). A laparoscopic needle placed through one of the accessory ports or a 22-gauge spinal needle placed directly through the abdominal wall is suitable for injection. Needle aspiration prior to injection is imperative to avoid intravascular injection of this potent vasoconstrictor. The anesthesiologist is informed of vasopressin injection, as a sudden increase in patient blood pressure may potentially occur following injection. Blanching at the injection site is common. The plasma half-life of this agent is 10 to 20 minutes. For this reason, injection of vasopressin is discontinued 20 minutes prior to uterine repair to allow evaluation of bleeding from myometrial incisions (Hutchins, 1996).

The main risks associated with local vasopressin injection result from inadvertent intravascular infiltration and include transient increases in blood pressure, bradycardia, atrioventricular block, and pulmonary edema (Hobo, 2009; Tulandi, 1996). For these reasons, patients with a medical history of cardiac or pulmonary disease may be poor candidates for vasopressin use.

❹ Serosal Incision.
Because of postoperative adhesion formation risks, surgeons minimize the number of serosal incisions and attempt to place incisions on the anterior uterine wall. Tulandi and colleagues (1993) found for open myomectomy that posterior wall incisions result in a 94-percent adhesion formation rate compared with a 55-percent rate for anterior incisions.

After vasopressin injection, hysterotomy may be performed using a Harmonic scalpel, monopolar electrode, or laser. For most patients, an anterior midline vertical uterine incision allows removal of the greatest number of leiomyomas through the fewest incisions. The length should accommodate the approximate diameter of the largest tumor. The incision depth should afford access to all leiomyomas (Fig. 44-8.2).

❺ Tumor Enucleation.
Once the hysterotomy is created, the myometrium will generally retract, and the first leiomyoma may be grasped with a laparoscopic single-toothed tenaculum. Alternatively, a leiomyoma screw can also retract tissue to create tension between the myometrium and mass (Fig. 44-8.3). Using a blunt tool or suction-irrigator tip, blunt dissection of the pseudocapsule surrounding the leiomyoma frees the tumor from the

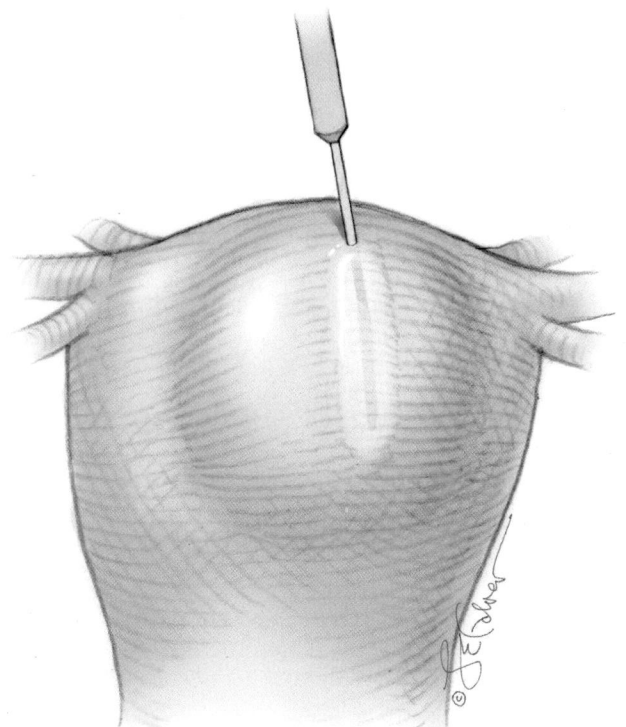

FIGURE 44-8.1 Vasopressin injection beneath serosa.

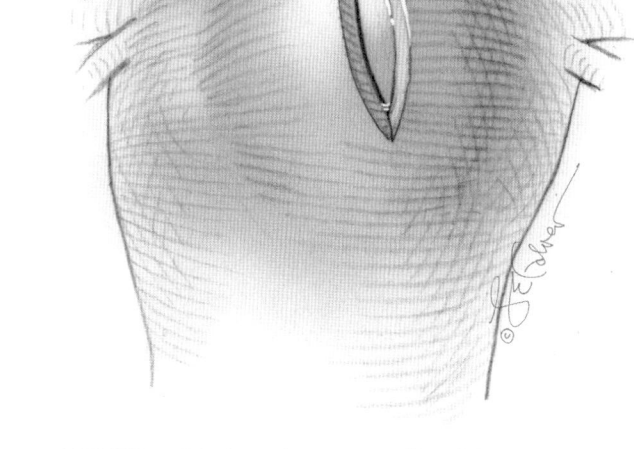

FIGURE 44-8.2 Serosal incision overlying leiomyoma.

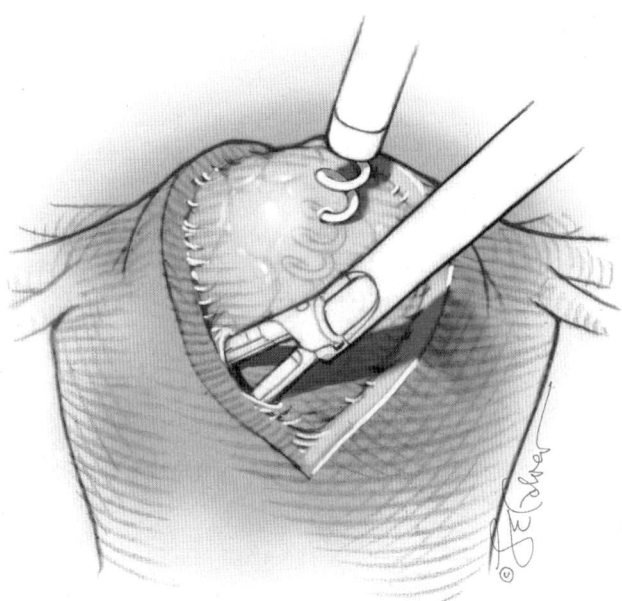

FIGURE 44-8.3 Tumor enucleation.

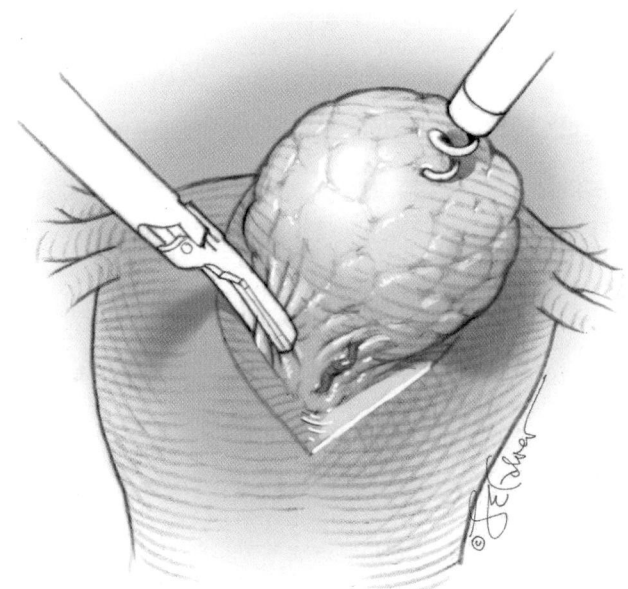

FIGURE 44-8.4 Coagulation of vascular attachments between the leiomyoma and the myometrium.

adjacent myometrium. Areas requiring sharp dissection from the myometrium may be freed with any of the electrosurgical instruments that were used for the uterine incision.

❻ **Bleeding.** Hemorrhage during myomectomy primarily develops during tumor enucleation and positively correlates with preoperative uterine size, total weight of leiomyomas removed, and operating time (Ginsburg, 1993). Approximately two to four main arteries feed each leiomyoma and enter the tumor at unpredictable sites. For this reason, surgeons must watch for these vessels, coagulate them prior to transection when possible, and be ready to immediately fulgurate remaining bleeding vessels (Fig. 44-8.4). To avoid myo-

metrial damage, the surgeon applies electrosurgical energy only when necessary.

❼ **Myometrial Closure.** Following removal of all tumors, redundant serosa may be excised. Laparoscopic suturing techniques described in Chapter 41 (p. 897) are used during incision reapproximation. The same general principles of myometrial closure for abdominal myomectomy are employed during laparoscopic myomectomy. In one method, for deep myometrial closure, a needle driver can be used with 0-gauge delayed-absorbable suture on a CT-2 needle in a continuous running fashion. Smaller internal myometrial incisions are closed first. The primary incision(s) is then closed in layers to

improve hemostasis and prevent hematoma formation (Fig. 44-8.5). A gauge of sufficient strength to prevent breakage during muscle approximation is selected, typically 0 to 2-0 gauge. Alternatively, barbed sutures can close myometrial defects during laparoscopic myomectomy. These obviate the need for knot tying and yield consistent wound opposition (Einarsson, 2010; Greenberg, 2008).

❽ **Serosal Closure.** Closure of the serosal incision using a running suture line with 4-0 or 5-0 gauge monofilament delayed-absorbable suture may help to limit adhesion formation (Fig. 44-8.6). Moreover, absorbable adhesion barriers have been shown to reduce the incidence of adhesion formation following myomectomy and may be introduced through laparoscopic ports (Ahmad, 2008). However, no substantial evidence documents that adhesion barrier use improves fertility, decreases pain, or prevents bowel obstruction (American Society for Reproductive Medicine, 2013).

❾ **Tissue Extraction.** Once amputated, the myomas must be removed, and options include minilaparotomy, colpotomy, and tissue morcellation. These are fully described in Section 44-10 (p. 1031) and illustrated in Chapter 41 (p. 896).

❿ **Laparoscopically Assisted Myomectomy (LAM).** Another MIS technique that may allow for safe and efficient myomectomy is LAM. The procedure is initiated as described above, and abdominal cavity assessment, uterine inspection, and incision of the serosa and myometrium are performed

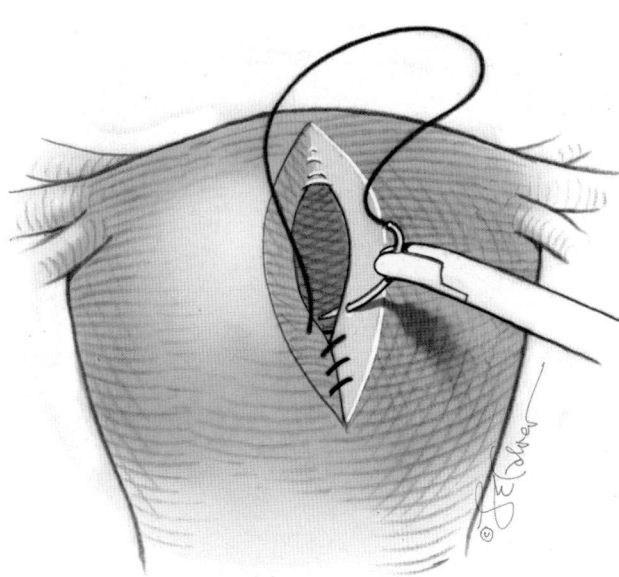

FIGURE 44-8.5 Myometrial closure.

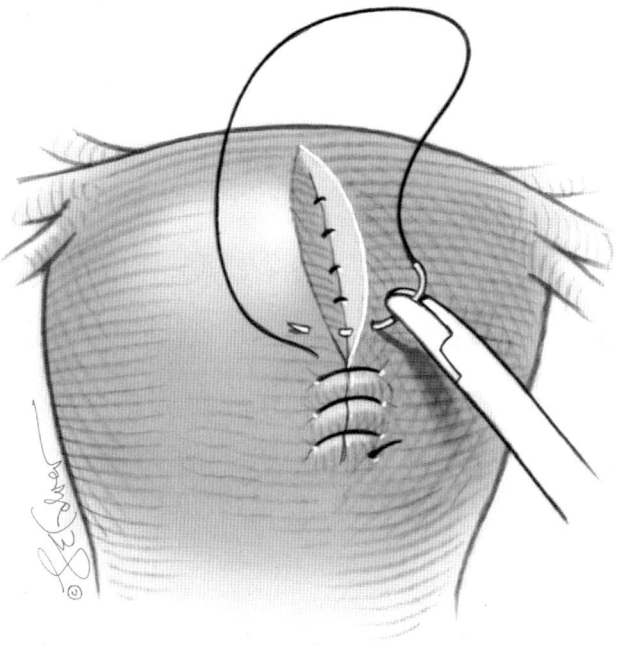

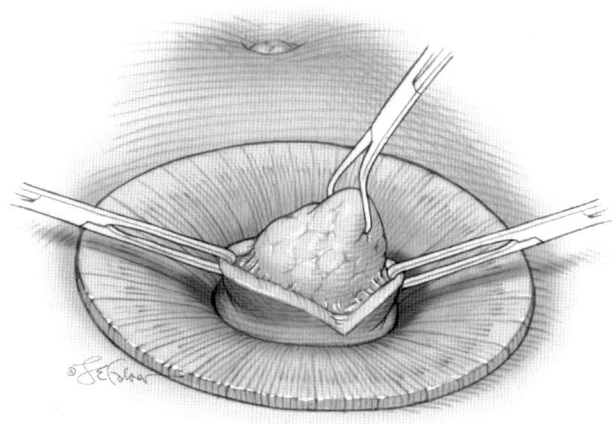

FIGURE 44-8.7 Tumor enucleation during laparoscopically assisted myomectomy.

FIGURE 44-8.6 Serosal closure.

laparoscopically. To aid in the laparoscopically challenging steps of myomectomy, LAM offers a hybrid approach. Specifically, tumor enucleation and uterine closure are completed through a 2- to 4-cm minilaparotomy incision placed suprapubically. With this, the pneumoperitoneum and visualization through the laparoscope are lost. Instead, application of a wound retraction system such as the Alexis or Mobius retractor provides visual access to the operative field. The uterus and leiomyoma are brought to the surface of the anterior abdominal wall and through the laparotomy incision. The tumors are then enucleated and divided through this incision (Fig. 44-8.7). This open incision also allows for conventional suturing techniques and aids suturing of large defects that require a multilayer closure (Fig. 44-8.8).

Advantages include decreased operative time, technical simplicity, improved tactile sensation to detect deep intramural leiomyomas, and easier removal of very large tumors (Prapas, 2009; Wen, 2010). Disadvantages stem mainly from the larger abdominal wall incision.

POSTOPERATIVE

Following abdominal myomectomy, postoperative care follows that for any major laparoscopic surgery. Hospitalization typically varies from 0 to 1 days, and febrile morbidity and return of normal bowel function usually dictate this course (Barakat, 2011). Postoperative activity in general can be individualized, although vigorous exercise is usually delayed until 4 weeks after surgery.

Fever

Febrile morbidity of greater than 38.0°C is common following myomectomy (Iverson, 1996; LaMorte, 1993; Rybak, 2008). Purported causes include atelectasis, myometrial incisional hematomas, and factors released with myometrial destruction. Although fever is common following myomectomy, pelvic infection is not. LaMorte and colleagues (1993) noted only a 2-percent rate of pelvic infection in their analysis of 128 open myomectomy cases.

Subsequent Pregnancy

There are no clear guidelines as to the timing of pregnancy attempts following myomectomy. Darwish and colleagues (2005) performed sonographic examinations on 169 patients following open myomectomy. Following myometrial indicators, they concluded that wound healing is usually completed within 3 months. There are no clinical trials that address the issue of uterine rupture and therefore route of delivery of pregnancies occurring after myomectomy (American College of Obstetricians and Gynecologists, 2014a). Management of these cases requires sound clinical judgment and individualization of care. In general, large incisions or those entering the endometrial cavity favor cesarean delivery.

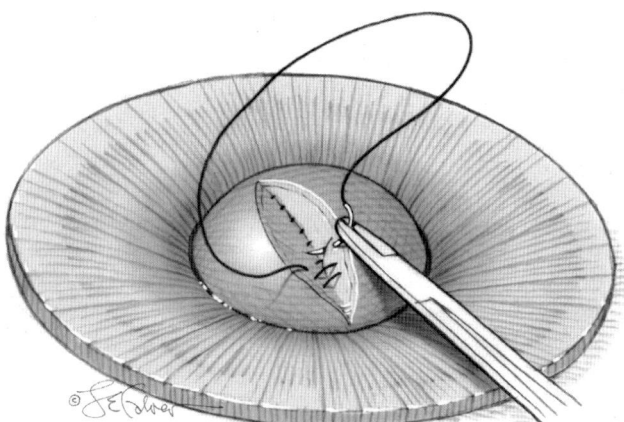

FIGURE 44-8.8 Myometrial closure during laparoscopically assisted myomectomy.

44-9

Laparoscopic Hysterectomy

Several laparoscopic techniques have been developed for hysterectomy and vary depending on the degree of laparoscopic dissection versus vaginal surgery required to remove the uterus (Garry, 1994). These include:

- Diagnostic laparoscopy prior to vaginal hysterectomy (VH)
- Vaginal hysterectomy assisted by laparoscopy, that is, lysis of adhesions and/or excision of endometriosis prior to VH
- Laparoscopically assisted vaginal hysterectomy (LAVH): laparoscopic dissection down to, but not including, uterine artery transection
- Laparoscopic hysterectomy (LH): laparoscopic dissection, including uterine artery transection, but completion of hysterectomy vaginally
- Total laparoscopic hysterectomy (TLH): complete laparoscopic excision of the uterus.

The laparoscopic approach offers advantages over traditional total abdominal hysterectomy (TAH). These include significant lower analgesia requirements, shorter hospital stays, rapid recovery, greater patient satisfaction, and lower rates of wound infection and hematoma formation (Kluivers, 2007; Schindlbeck, 2008). Disadvantageously, surgical time is lengthened, although the learning curve may be a factor. TLH offers fewer advantages compare with VH. Thus, in most cases, TLH should be an alternative to TAH (American College of Obstetricians and Gynecologists, 2011; Marana, 1999; Nieboer, 2009).

For all the hysterectomy types described in the following sections, plans for concurrent bilateral salpingo-oophorectomy (BSO) or for prophylactic salpingectomy are individualized. A detailed discussion of the surgical BSO is found in Chapter 43 (p. 951), whereas the advantages of risk-reducing salpingectomy are outlined in Chapter 35 (p. 738).

PREOPERATIVE

Patient Evaluation

A thorough pelvic examination and history reveal factors that help determine the optimal surgical route. Poor candidates for a vaginal approach include patients with minimal uterine descent, extensive abdominal or pelvic adhesions, a large uterus not amenable to tissue extraction methods, adnexal pathology, and a restricted vaginal vault or contracted pelvis. Patients with these findings are generally considered for TAH and also for TLH (Schindlbeck, 2008).

Of factors, uterine size and mobility are important. There is no agreed-upon size that precludes LH. However, a wide bulky uterus with minimal mobility may make it difficult to visualize vital structures, to manipulate the uterus during surgery, and to remove it vaginally. Once a patient has been deemed eligible for a laparoscopic approach, the same preoperative evaluation as for abdominal hysterectomy applies (Section 43-12, p. 950).

Consent

Similar to an open approach, possible risks of hysterectomy include increased blood loss and need for transfusion, unplanned adnexectomy, and injury to other pelvic organs, especially bladder, ureter, and bowel. The ureters are also at greater risk during LH compared with other hysterectomy approaches (Harkki-Siren, 1997, 1998). Kuno and colleagues (1998) evaluated ureteral catheterization to prevent such injury but found no benefit. Complications related specifically to laparoscopy include injury to the major vessels, bladder, and bowel during trocar placement (Chap. 41, p. 877).

The risk of conversion to an open procedure is also discussed. In general, conversion to laparotomy may be necessary if exposure and organ manipulation is limited or if bleeding is encountered that cannot be controlled laparoscopically.

Concurrent salpingectomy during hysterectomy may be considered to lower future rates of some epithelial ovarian cancers. For this, complete rather than partial salpingectomy is preferred. Operating time is minimally lengthened, but complication rates are not increased. Notably, the American College of Obstetricians and Gynecologists (2015) has emphasized that the planned route of hysterectomy should not be changed to complete prophylactic salpingectomy.

Patient Preparation

A blood sample is typed and crossmatched for potential transfusion. If considered, bowel preparation prior to laparoscopy may assist with colon manipulation and pelvic anatomy visualization by evacuating the rectosigmoid. Alternatively, enemas prior to surgery may be as effective for this goal. Antibiotic prophylaxis is administered within the hour prior to skin incision, and appropriate antibiotic options are listed in Table 39-6 (p. 835). Overall, the likelihood of VTE

during laparoscopic hysterectomy is significantly reduced when compared to abdominal hysterectomy (Barber, 2015). Thus, the decision to provide VTE prophylaxis should factor patient- and procedure-related VTE risks (Gould, 2012). If longer operating times are anticipated, conversion to laparotomy is a concern, or preexisting VTE risks are present, then prophylaxis as outlined in Table 39-8 (p. 836) is reasonable.

INTRAOPERATIVE

Instruments

Vessel occlusion is an important component of any hysterectomy. For this, suitable instruments include monopolar or bipolar instruments, Harmonic scalpel, stapling devices, traditional sutures, and suturing devices. Several of these can be used for dissection and hemostasis. The Harmonic scalpel is frequently used for its ability to cut with minimal smoke plume and little surrounding thermal tissue damage, although it should only be used to seal vessels up to 5 mm. Several advanced bipolar devices also offer improved vessel sealing. With various instruments, vessels measuring up to 5 mm (LigaSure, Gyrus Plasma Kinetic) and up to 7 mm (ENSEAL) can be coagulated with minimal thermal spread (Lamberton, 2008; Landman, 2003; Smaldone, 2008).

Surgical Steps

❶ Anesthesia and Patient Positioning. For most women, these procedures are performed in an inpatient setting under general anesthesia. The patient is placed in a low dorsal lithotomy position in booted support stirrups. A bimanual examination is completed to determine uterine size and shape to aid port placement. The abdomen and vagina are surgically prepared, a Foley catheter is inserted, and orogastric or nasogastric tube is placed. Uterine manipulators can assist with visualization. These are considered in cases in which anatomic distortion is anticipated or in those with large uteri.

❷ Initial Steps. The introductory steps for LH mirror that for other laparoscopic procedures (Chap. 41, p. 889). The number of ports and their caliber may vary, but in general, LH requires a 5- to 12-mm optical port placed at the level of the umbilicus or higher for larger uteri. Left upper quadrant entry is considered in cases of suspected periumbilical adhesions. For larger uteri, if the uterine fundus is close to or above the level of the umbilicus, the optical port is placed approximately 3 to 4 cm above the fundus for optimal viewing.

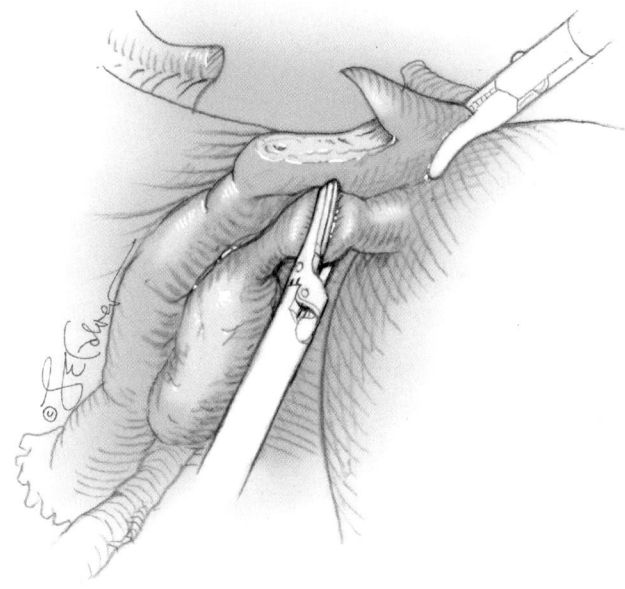

FIGURE 44-9.2 Uteroovarian ligament transection.

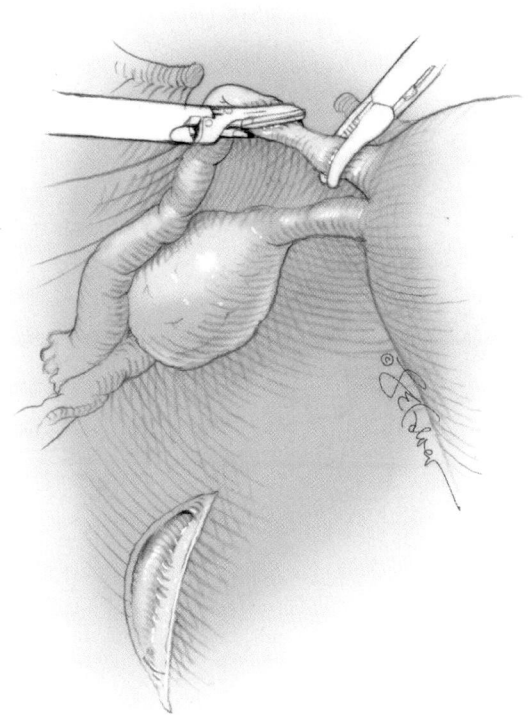

FIGURE 44-9.1 The ureter is first identified. With ovarian conservation, the round ligament is transected, and the fallopian tube is then grasped for transection.

Two or three accessory ports are also placed through the lower abdominal wall. Specifically, two ports are positioned beyond the lateral borders of the rectus abdominis muscle, whereas a third may be positioned centrally and cephalad to the uterine fundus.

❸ **Pelvic Evaluation.** With the ports and laparoscope inserted and the patient in Trendelenburg position, a blunt laparoscopic probe can aid organ manipulation. The pelvis and abdomen are visually explored. At this point, the decision is made whether to continue with LH or convert to laparotomy. If needed, adhesions are lysed to restore normal anatomy. The bowel is displaced from the pelvis into the abdomen to expand available operating space and viewing.

❹ **Ureter Identification.** Irrigating fluids and CO_2 used for insufflation can, with time, create edema of the peritoneum and hinder viewing of retroperitoneal structures. For this reason, the ureters are identified early. The ureters can often be seen easily beneath the pelvic peritoneum, or the peritoneum may be open to identify these. In such situations, the peritoneum medial to the infundibulopelvic (IP) ligament is grasped and tented using atraumatic forceps and incised with scissors. Hydrodissection techniques may be employed. The opening in the peritoneum

then is extended caudally and cephalad along the length of the ureter. Through this peritoneal window, the ureter is identified, and peristalsis should be noted (Fig. 44-9.1) (Parker, 2004).

❺ **Round Ligament Transection.** The proximal round ligament is grasped and divided.

❻ **Ovarian Conservation.** If ovarian preservation is planned, proximal portions of

the fallopian tube and uteroovarian ligament are also desiccated and transected (Figs. 44-9.1 and 44-9.2). With this, the tube and ovary are freed from the uterus and can be placed in the ovarian fossa.

❼ **Oophorectomy.** If removal of the ovaries is desired, the IP ligament is grasped and pulled up and away from retroperitoneal structures. The presence and path of the ureter is identified. The IP ligament is isolated and dissected away from the ureteral course. The pedicle is coagulated, desiccated, or stapled, and then divided (Fig. 44-9.3).

❽ **Broad Ligament Incision.** Following transection of the round ligament, the leaves of the broad ligament fall open and

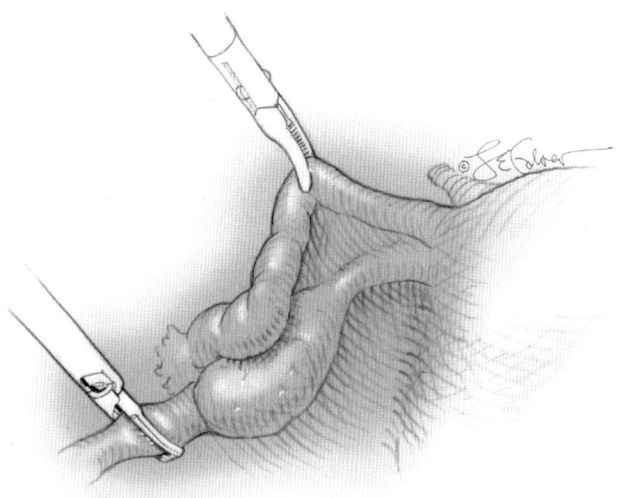

FIGURE 44-9.3 Infundibulopelvic ligament transection.

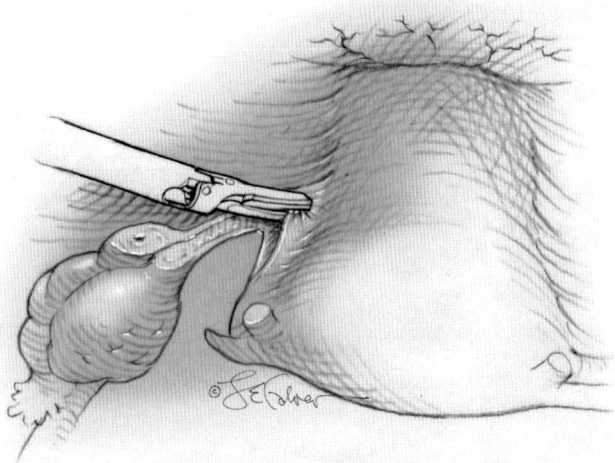

FIGURE 44-9.4 Anterior leaf of broad ligament incised caudally.

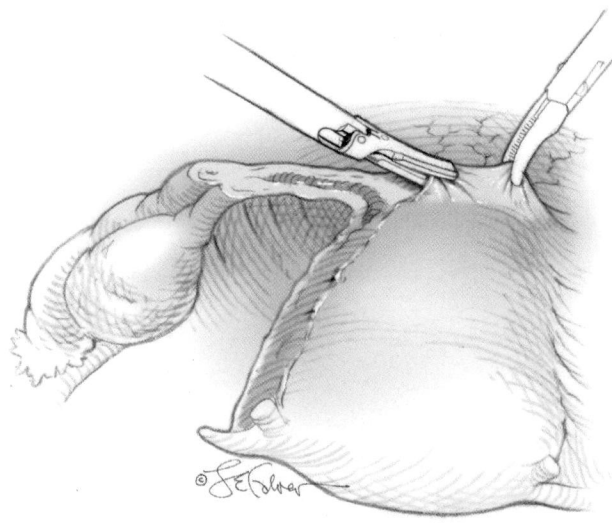

FIGURE 44-9.5 Vesicouterine fold incised.

loose gauzy connective tissue is found between these leaves. The anterior leaf is incised sharply (Fig. 44-9.4). This incision is directed caudally and centrally to the midline above the vesicouterine fold. The posterior leaf requires incision caudally to the level of the uterosacral ligament. The loose areolar tissue separating the anterior and posterior leaves is dissected as well. Ultimately, opening the broad ligament provides access to lateral uterine anatomy, which is important for subsequent uterine artery ligation.

❾ **Bladder Flap Development.** After broad ligament incision bilaterally, the vesicouterine fold is grasped with atraumatic forceps, elevated away from the underlying bladder, and incised (Fig. 44-9.5). This exposes connective tissue between the bladder and underlying uterus in the vesicouterine space. Loosely attached connections can be bluntly divided by gently pushing against the cervix and caudally to move the bladder caudad (Fig. 44-9.6). Denser tissue in the vesicouterine space is better divided sharply. With this, the tissue is elevated, and the

scissors are kept close to the surface of the cervix to minimize inadvertent cystotomy risk. As this tissue is dissected, the vesicouterine space is opened. Electrosurgery may be needed to coagulate small bleeding vessels. Creating cephalad traction on the uterus with the uterine manipulator may also help with this dissection. Development of this space allows the bladder to be moved caudally and off the lower uterus and upper vagina. This mobilization of the bladder is necessary for final colpotomy and uterus removal. Of the hysterectomy types, MIS approaches have the highest risk of bladder injury, and injury occurs most frequently to the dome during this sharp or blunt dissection (Harkki, 2001). This risk is increased if prior cesarean delivery or endometriosis has left scarring.

❿ **Uterine Artery Transection.** After the uterine arteries are identified, the areolar connective tissue surrounding them is grasped, placed on tension, and incised. This

skeletonizing of the vessels leads to superior occlusion of the uterine artery and vein. The arteries then are then coagulated and transected (Fig. 44-9.7). Alternatively, surgeons may elect to terminate the laparoscopic portion prior to uterine artery transection and complete artery ligation from a vaginal approach (LAVH).

⓫ **Vaginal Hysterectomy.** With LH, after the uterine arteries are transected, the surgical approach is converted to that for vaginal hysterectomy and is completed as outlined in Section 43-13 (p. 957). In this transition, the patient is repositioned from low dorsal lithotomy to standard lithotomy position.

⓬ **Abdominal Inspection.** After vaginal completion of the hysterectomy, attention is redirected to laparoscopic inspection of the pelvis for signs of bleeding. Before returning to the abdomen, surgeons will replace their

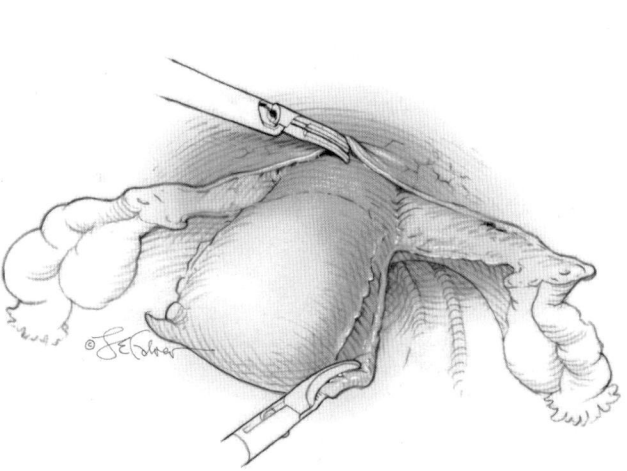

FIGURE 44-9.6 Bladder moved caudally.

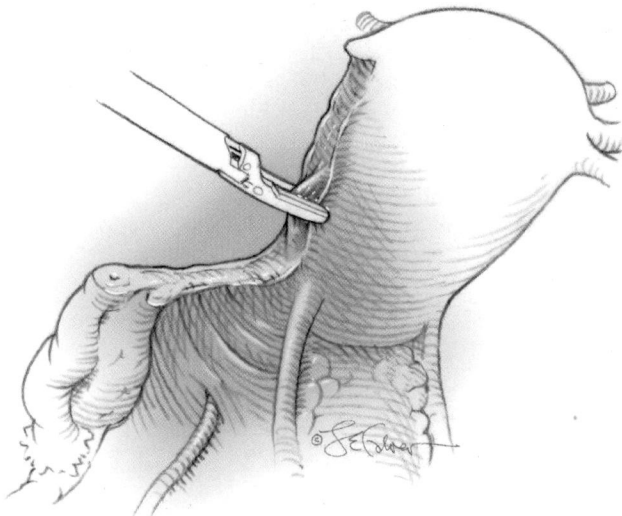

FIGURE 44-9.7 Uterine artery coagulation.

surgical gloves. Copious irrigation of the abdominopelvic cavity and confirmation of hemostasis is performed. During this inspection, intraabdominal pressures are lowered to better identify sources of bleeding. The laparoscopic procedure is terminated as outlined in Section 44-1 (p. 1005).

POSTOPERATIVE

Following LH, patient recovery mirrors that for vaginal hysterectomy. In general, compared with those undergoing abdominal hysterectomy, LH patients have faster return of normal bowel function, easier ambula-tion, and decreased analgesia requirements. A clear liquid diet can be initiated the day of surgery and advanced quickly as tolerated. Postoperative complications in general mirror those for abdominal hysterectomy with the exception that superficial surgical site infection rates are lower.

44-10

Laparoscopic Supracervical Hysterectomy

Laparoscopic supracervical hysterectomy (LSH) differs from total laparoscopic hysterectomy (TLH) in that the uterine corpus is amputated, but the cervix remains. Once freed, the corpus either is delivered through a posterior colpotomy or minilaparotomy incision or undergoes enclosed morcellation. Advantageously, the uterosacral and cardinal ligaments, which are important to pelvic support, are retained. It is also an excellent alternative for cases complicated by extensive scarring. Specifically, adhesions between the bladder and the lower uterine segment in the vesicouterine space or those in the cul-de-sac may make removal of the cervix difficult. Related to this, ureteral and bladder injury rates are decreased by avoiding difficult dissection.

Certain contraindications to preserving the cervix are excluded prior to selecting supracervical hysterectomy. Examples include Pap test findings of high-grade cervical dysplasia; endometrial hyperplasia with atypia or endometrial cancer; or a patient at risk for noncompliance with routine cervical cancer screening.

PREOPERATIVE

Patient Evaluation

A thorough pelvic examination and history reveal factors that help determine the optimal surgical route. Uterine size and mobility are important, although there is no agreed-upon size that precludes LSH. That said, a large bulky uterus with minimal mobility may be difficult to adequately manipulate, may limit exposure during surgery, and may be challenging to extract. Once a patient has been deemed eligible for a laparoscopic approach, the same preoperative evaluation as for an abdominal hysterectomy applies (Section 43-12, p. 950).

Consent

Similar to an open approach, possible risks of LSH include blood loss and need for transfusion, unplanned adnexectomy, and injury to other pelvic organs, especially bladder, ureter, and bowel. Complications related specifically to laparoscopy include injury to the major vessels, bladder, and bowel during trocar placement (Chap. 41, 877).

Postoperatively, endometrium within the lower uterine segment may be retained with LSH. As a result, the risk of cyclic long-term bleeding is a potential consequence. Rates quoted in early studies are as high as 24 percent but are lower in more recent investigations and range from 5 to 10 percent (Okaro, 2001; Sarmini, 2005; Schmidt, 2011; van der Stege, 1999). Techniques that resect more of the lower uterine and proximal endocervical tissue appear to decrease these long-term bleeding risks (Schmidt, 2011; Wenger, 2005).

In some case, secondary excision of the cervical stump may later be required. Termed trachelectomy, this excision may be indicated if refractory long-term bleeding or significant subsequent cervical neoplasia develops postoperatively. Trachelectomy has the additional indication for residual persistent infection, although this is more anecdotal and not quoted with a consistent incidence. Overall rates of trachelectomy appear to mimic the bleeding rates above and are on a downward trend.

The risk of conversion to an open procedure is also discussed. In general, conversion to laparotomy may be necessary if exposure and organ manipulation are limited or if bleeding is encountered that cannot be controlled with laparoscopic tools and techniques.

Patient Preparation

A blood sample is typed and crossmatched for potential transfusion. If considered, bowel preparation prior to laparoscopy may assist with colon manipulation and pelvic anatomy visualization by evacuating the rectosigmoid. Enemas prior to surgery may be as effective for this goal. Antibiotic prophylaxis is administered within the hour prior to skin incision, and appropriate antibiotic options are listed in Table 39-6 (p. 835). With laparoscopic gynecologic surgery, the decision to provide VTE prophylaxis factors patient- and procedure-related VTE risks (Gould, 2012). Thus, if longer operating times are anticipated, conversion to laparotomy is a concern, or preexisting VTE risks are present, then prophylaxis as outlined in Table 39-8 (p. 836) is reasonable.

INTRAOPERATIVE

Instruments

During cervical amputation, blunt scissors, Harmonic scalpel, laser, or monopolar needle or scissors may be used to excise the corpus. Vessel occlusion is an important component of any hysterectomy. For this, suitable instruments include monopolar or bipolar instruments, Harmonic scalpel, stapling devices, traditional sutures, and suturing devices. Many of these instruments may not be readily available in all operating suites, and desired tools should be requested prior to surgery. After tumor excision, removal may be accomplished by several techniques described in Steps 3, 4, and 5. Thus, required endoscopic bags or morcellators are assembled preoperatively.

Surgical Steps

❶ **Initial Steps.** The initial surgical steps for LSH mirror those for LH, including coagulation of the uterine vessels as described in Section 44-9, Steps 1 through 10 (p. 1026).

❷ **Uterine Amputation.** The corpus is amputated from the cervix at a point just below the internal cervical os and superior to the uterosacral ligaments (Fig. 44-10.1). To limit the possibility of residual endometrium, the incision is conical and extends

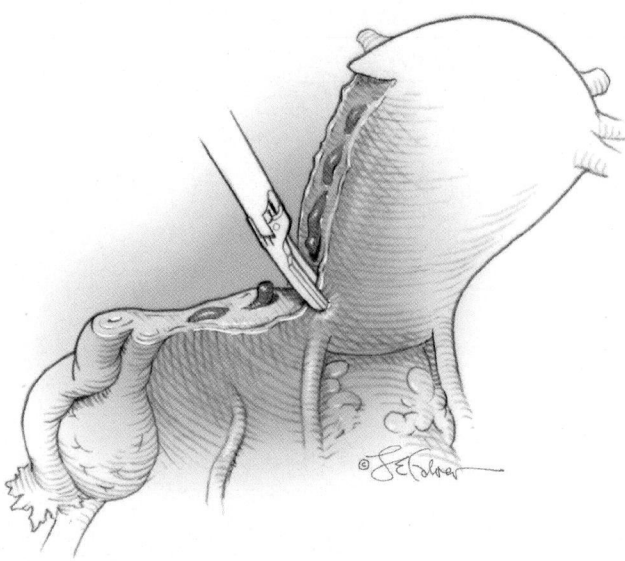

FIGURE 44-10.1 Incision initiated above uterosacral ligaments.

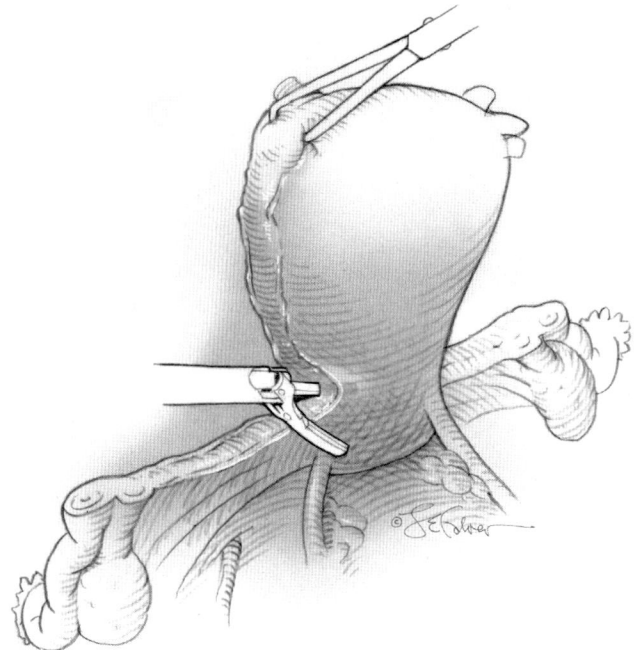

FIGURE 44-10.2 Incision extended posteriorly.

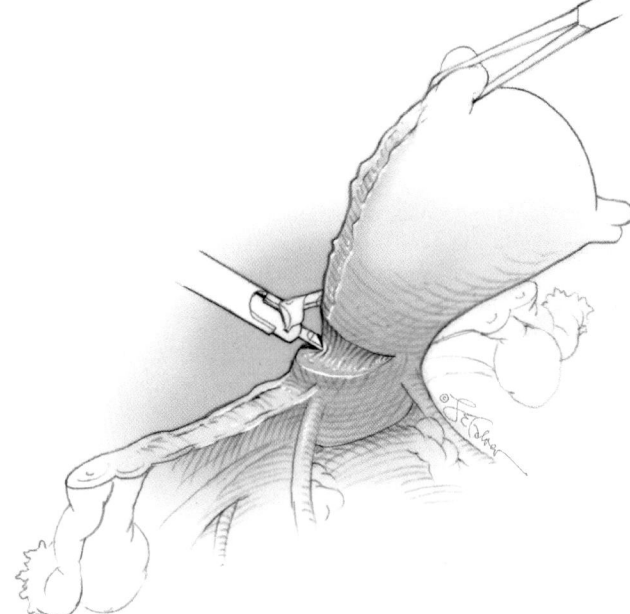

FIGURE 44-10.3 Cone-shape incision extended anteriorly.

down into the cervix (Figs. 44-10.2 through 44-10.4). Following amputation, adjunctive coring or ablation of the endocervical canal also may be performed to decrease the risk of postoperative cyclic bleeding (Fig. 44-10.5).

❸ **Tissue Extraction.** Once amputated, the uterine corpus must be removed, and options include minilaparotomy, colpotomy, and enclosed morcellation. Although

described here for the uterine corpus, these methods translate to surgical removal of other specimens.

First, for smaller specimens, a minilaparotomy incision ranging from 1 to 4 cm can be made to extract the corpus. Typically, a small Pfannenstiel incision is made, although a small midline vertical incision is also suitable. Both incisions are illustrated in Chapter 43 (p. 927).

For larger uteri, the addition of a tissue retrieval bag and self-retaining retractor can create a closed environment for manual morcellation. For this, a retrieval bag is initially placed into the abdomen. The bag containing the excised specimen is then brought to the surface and is fanned open outside and around the minilaparotomy incision. A self-retaining circular retractor is placed into the bag's interior and simultaneously opened within the incision (see Fig. 44-8.7). This creates a closed environment where the specimen can be sharply divided manually with scissors or knife. Long-term data on safety and efficacy are not currently available.

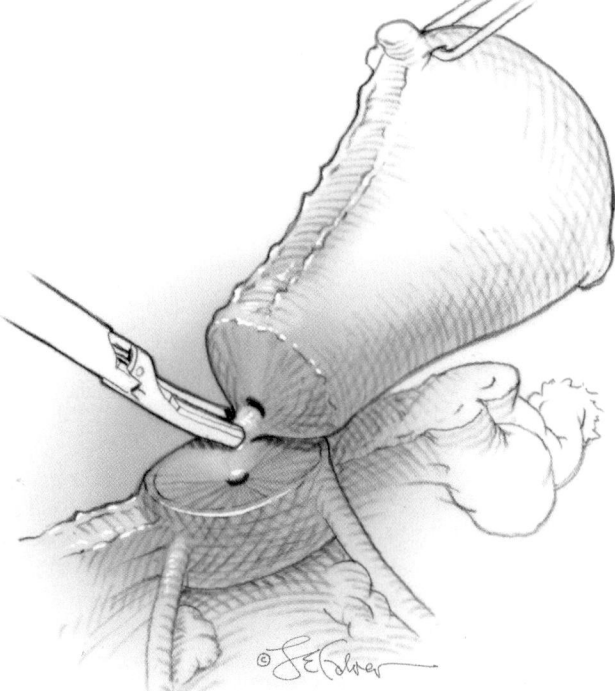

FIGURE 44-10.4 Excision completion.

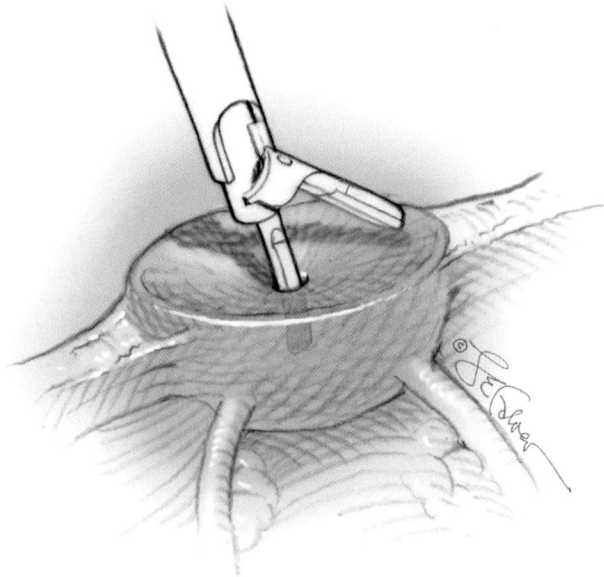

FIGURE 44-10.5 Endocervical canal coagulated.

❹ **Colpotomy.** As another option, a posterior colpotomy can be created similar to that for vaginal hysterectomy and shown in Figure 41-27 (p. 896). To enter the posterior cul-de-sac, attention is turned to the vagina, and handheld retractors are placed to expose the cervix and posterior fornix. The uterine manipulator is used to anteflex the uterus, and an Allis clamp is placed on the posterior vaginal wall 2 to 3 cm from the posterior cervicovaginal junction. The Allis clamp is pulled downward to create tension across the posterior vaginal wall. The posterior vaginal vault is then cut with curved Mayo scissors, and the cul-de-sac of Douglas is entered.

Alternatively, a colpotomy may be created laparoscopically by incising the posterior cul-de-sac with a monopolar instrument, a harmonic scalpel, or Endo Shears near the cervicovaginal junction. A uterine manipulator is used to reflect the uterus anteriorly to create space for the colpotomy, and a sponge stick may be used vaginally to help delineate the space. As Figure 41-28 illustrates, care is taken to avoid damage to the rectosigmoid and to the ureters, which lie lateral to the planned colpotomy.

With colpotomy, pneumoperitoneum is lost immediately. If a laparoscopic instrument is already holding the specimen, this can be passed through the colpotomy and removed vaginally.

For larger uteri, the addition of a tissue retrieval bag during tissue extraction can create a closed environment for scissor morcellation (Fig. 41-29). This reduces the risk of inadvertent tissue dissemination during fragmentation, although long-term safety data are needed (Cohen, 2014; Einarsson, 2014).

Following extraction, the vaginal incision is closed with interrupted stitches or a running suture line using 0-gauge delayed-absorbable suture. If colpotomy is used for specimen removal, a single prophylactic dose of antibiotics is administered. Suitable agents are listed in Table 39-6 (p. 835).

❺ **Morcellation.** A third method, enclosed power morcellation, is still being studied. For this, a large containment bag that can house the insufflation gas, can conform to the abdominal cavity, and can flatten against the intraperitoneal organs is introduced into the abdomen. Once in the abdomen, it is unfolded to allow the specimen and gas to be contained. Depending on the pathology, the bag may be

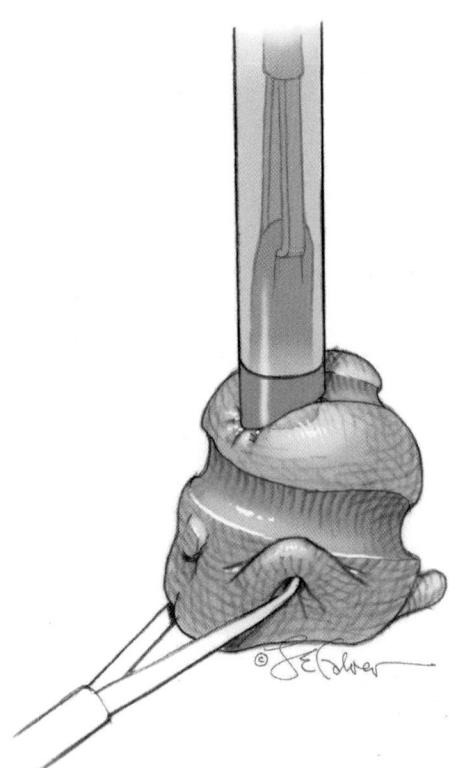

FIGURE 44-10.6 Uterine corpus morcellation.

exteriorized through one abdominal port or incision or may function simply as a liner that catches any disseminated tissue during power or manual morcellation (Einarsson, 2014).

During power morcellation, the corpus specimen is grasped securely with a toothed instrument such as a tenaculum and brought to the anterior abdominal wall. Because of the potential for surrounding organ injury, morcellators should not be moved toward the grasped tissue, but rather, those tissues should be brought to it (Fig. 44-10.6) (Milad, 2003). Importantly, the morcellator tip is always kept in laparoscopic view. A peeling rather than coring technique is used to pare down the mass. During this, the tenaculum holding the corpus is drawn up into the morcellator cylinder and well past the edge of the morcellating blade. This avoids metal-to-metal contact, which dulls the blade. In cases of prolonged morcellation, such as with large uteri, the blade may dull. For this, the generator allows a reverse in the blade's rotary direction. Improved cutting is usually restored with this step and generally offers enough blade life to complete the procedure.

Following morcellation, the gas is released, and bag and tissue fragments are removed.

Limitations of currently available retrieval bags involve pouch size, working aperture diameter, tensile strength of the bag, and bag permeability.

❻ **Hemostasis.** Points of bleeding are coagulated, and the surgeon may elect to reapproximate the anterior vesical and posterior cul-de-sac peritoneum to cover the cervical stump using 2-0 or 0-gauge delayed-absorbable suture. Alternatively, absorbable adhesion barriers (Interceed, Seprafilm) can be placed at the hemostatic surgical stump.

❼ **Laparoscopy Final Steps.** Completion of the procedure follows that for general laparoscopic procedures (p. 1005).

POSTOPERATIVE

Advantages of laparoscopy include a rapid return to normal diet and activities. With supracervical hysterectomy, there is no vaginal cuff that requires extended healing. Sexual intercourse, however, is delayed for 2 weeks following surgery to allow adequate internal healing.

44-11

Total Laparoscopic Hysterectomy

Total laparoscopic hysterectomy (TLH) is similar to LAVH, LSH, and LH with the exception that the procedure is completed entirely from a laparoscopic approach. After detachment, the specimen is removed vaginally or by tissue extraction techniques described on page 1031.

If all factors are equal, vaginal hysterectomy is considered for women undergoing hysterectomy. Ideal candidates for TLH are those not suitable for vaginal hysterectomy (American College of Obstetricians and Gynecologists, 2011). As such, TLH is viewed as a less invasive alternative to TAH. Compared with TAH, TLH benefits include rapid recovery, shorter hospitalizations, fewer minor complications of the wound or abdominal wall, and less blood loss (Nieboer, 2009; Walsh, 2009). These benefits are dependent on a learning curve and may not be readily apparent (Schindlbeck, 2008). Moreover, longer operative times and higher rates of urinary tract injuries are negative balancing factors.

PREOPERATIVE

Patient Evaluation

A thorough pelvic examination and history reveal factors that help determine the optimal surgical route. Uterine size and mobility are important, although there is no agreed-upon size that precludes TLH. That said, a wide bulky uterus with minimal mobility may be difficult to adequately manipulate, may limit exposure during surgery, and may be challenging to extract. Once a patient has been deemed eligible for a laparoscopic approach, the same preoperative evaluation as for an abdominal hysterectomy applies (Section 43-12, p. 950).

Consent

Similar to an open approach, possible risks of this procedure include increased blood loss and need for transfusion, unplanned adnexectomy, and injury to other pelvic organs, especially bladder, ureter, and bowel. Complications related to laparoscopy include entry injury to the major vessels, bladder, and bowel (Chap. 41, p. 877). The ureters are also at greater risk during laparoscopic hysterectomies compared with other hysterectomy approaches (Harkki-Siren, 1998). Kuno and colleagues (1998) evaluated the

use of ureteral catheterization to prevent such injury but found no benefit.

The risk of conversion to an open procedure is also discussed. In general, conversion to laparotomy may be necessary if exposure and organ manipulation is limited or if bleeding is encountered that cannot be controlled with laparoscopic tools and techniques.

Patient Preparation

A blood sample is typed and crossmatched for potential transfusion. If considered, bowel preparation prior to laparoscopy may assist with colon manipulation and pelvic anatomy visualization by evacuating the rectosigmoid. Alternatively, enemas prior to surgery may be as effective for this goal. Antibiotic prophylaxis is administered within the hour prior to skin incision, and appropriate antibiotic options are listed in Table 39-6 (p. 835). With laparoscopic gynecologic surgery, the decision to provide VTE prophylaxis factors patient and procedure-related VTE risks (Gould, 2012). Thus, if longer operating times are anticipated, conversion to laparotomy is a concern, or preexisting VTE risks are present, then prophylaxis as outlined in Table 39-8 (p. 836) is indicated.

PREOPERATIVE

Instruments

The same instruments that are used for the LH or LSH can be used for this procedure. In addition, a uterine manipulator that has a cupping device for delineating the cervicovaginal junction is helpful for colpotomy and also for final tissue extraction. If these are not available, a low-cost alternative is a right-angle retractor to delineate the anterior and posterior fornices for colpotomy.

Surgical Steps

❶ **Anesthesia and Patient Positioning.** For most women, TLH is performed as an inpatient procedure under general anesthesia. The patient is placed in low dorsal lithotomy position in booted support stirrups. A bimanual examination is completed to determine uterine size and shape to aid port placement. The abdomen and vagina are surgically prepared, a Foley catheter is inserted, and an orogastric or nasogastric tube is placed.

❷ **Uterine Manipulator.** A uterine manipulator with its attached cervical cup (VCare or KOH Cup with RUMI manipulator) is placed vaginally to assist uterine manipulation and delineate the cervicovaginal junction for colpotomy. To accomplish placement, the

cervical diameter and thickness are assessed. From this information, the manipulator-cup size, which is small, medium, or large, is selected. To permit manipulator insertion, the cervical os is dilated to accept a no. 8 cervical dilator. The uterus is also sounded to determine cavity depth for correct manipulator placement. The surgeon tests the balloon at the manipulator's end for patency by filling it with air via a port at the opposite end. Once again deflated, it is passed through the cervical os to the fundus and then reinflated to hold the manipulator in place (Fig. 44-11.1A). Two stay sutures of 0-gauge delayed-absorbable suture are placed at 6 and 12 o'clock or at 3 and 9 o'clock, depending on surgeon preference. To securely anchor the cup and cervix, stitches enter the ectocervix and exit just lateral to the endocervix. Each suture end is then passed through openings in the cup base (Fig. 44-11.1B). They are then tied firmly to the cervix on the outside face of the cup (Fig. 44-11.1C). Once in position, the proximal rim of the cup will delineate the cervicovaginal junction. With the VCare, the blue vaginal cup is then advanced to join the interior cup and is locked in place by a locking knob at the manipulator's distal end (Fig. 44-11.1D). If the KOH Cup is used, then a pneumo-occluding balloon is positioned behind the colpotomy cup.

❸ **Initial Laparoscopic Steps.** The introductory steps for LH mirror those for other laparoscopic procedures (Chap. 41, p. 889). The number of trocars and their caliber may vary, but in general, TLH requires a 5- to 12-mm optical port, usually at the umbilicus, and two or three accessory ports placed through the lower abdominal wall. Specifically, two trocars are placed beyond the lateral borders of the rectus abdominis muscle, whereas a third may be positioned centrally and cephalad to the uterine fundus. Left upper quadrant entry is considered for initial entry in cases with suspected periumbilical adhesions.

❹ **Pelvic Evaluation.** With the cannulas and laparoscope inserted and the patient in Trendelenburg position, a blunt laparoscopic probe aids bowel displacement. The pelvis and abdomen are thoroughly explored. At this point, the decision to continue with TLH or convert to laparotomy is made. If necessary, adhesions are lysed to restore normal anatomy.

❺ **Ureter Identification.** Irrigating fluids and CO_2 used for insufflation can with time create edema of the peritoneum and hinder visualization of structures beneath it. For this reason, the ureters are identified early. The ureters are often easily seen retroperitoneally, or the peritoneum may be opened to locate

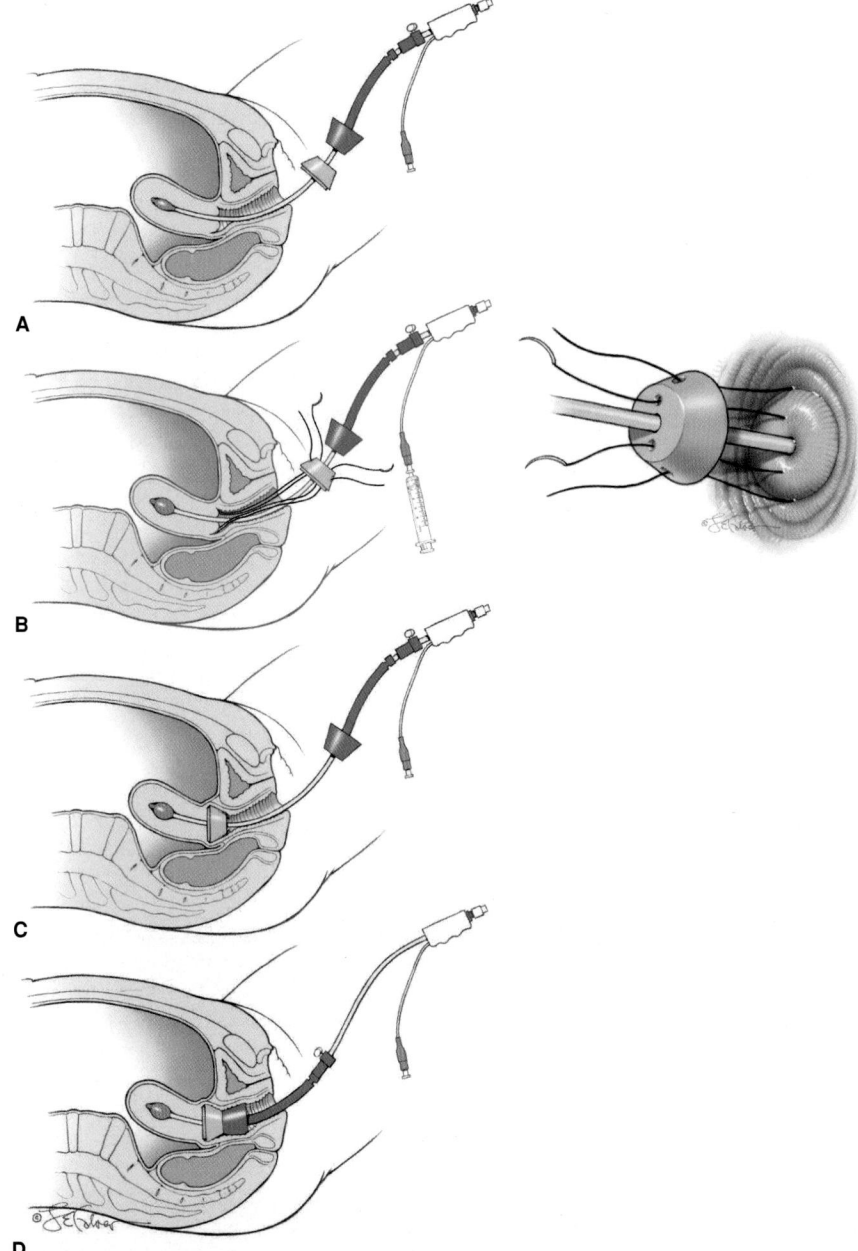

FIGURE 44-11.1 Uterine manipulator placement. **A.** Manipulator tip inserted into uterine cavity. **B.** Balloon tip inflated (*left*). Colpotomy cup sutured to cervix (*right*). **C.** Colpotomy cup sutured in place. **D.** Blue pneumo-occluding cup advanced and locked in place.

monopolar hook, or plasma kinetic needle point. Prior to incision, the uterine manipulator is pushed cephalad to allow the cervical cupping device to displace the ureters laterally and expose the optimal location for colpotomy. Additionally, dissection within the vesicouterine space should be sufficient to mobilize the bladder caudad and away from the planned colpotomy site.

With these preparatory steps completed, colpotomy is begun by placing the incising tool at the posterior cervicovaginal junction, which is delineated by the cervical cup. If a colpotomy cup is not used, a simple tool such as a right-angle retractor or sponge on a stick placed vaginally in the posterior fornix can also assist with delineating the cervicovaginal junction. The posterior vaginal wall is opened first (Fig. 44-11.3). By extending this incision, the uterosacral ligament is next transected (Fig. 44-11.4). The opposite uterosacral ligament is then divided close to the cervix. Last, the anterior colpotomy incision is created (Fig. 44-11.5). To minimize twisting and specimen disorientation, the lateral vaginal cuff points are transected last (Fig. 44-11.6). Hemostasis is generally maintained using this technique. To prevent vaginal tissue thermal damage and subsequent cuff dehiscence, surgeons use the minimum necessary amount of electrosurgery on the vaginal cuff.

❾ Removal of Uterus. The uterus is removed intact through the vaginal vault using the manipulator, unless uterine size limits this (Fig. 44-11.7). In the case of large uteri, the uterus is removed using tissue extraction techniques described on page 1031.

❿ Repair of the Vaginal Cuff. The cuff is closed laparoscopically with a running closure of absorbable suture, with interrupted figure-of-eight sutures, or with a suturing device. For this, delayed-absorbable material is preferred, and the uterosacral ligament is incorporated into the closure for vaginal cuff support (Fig. 44-11.8). If traditional suture is used, one must maintain tension to sufficiently close the cuff. If using barbed suture, the procedure is modified by manufacturer's recommendations to loosen stitch tension between the approximated cuff tissues. Moreover, if barbed suture is used, it is recommended to throw at least two bites in the opposite direction to the original direction of suture line closure to maintain tissue tension. For example, if closure is performed from right to left, the surgeon will reach the far left end and then will place two additional stitches in the left-to-right direction prior to final suture cutting. It is advisable to cut the suture flush with the tissue to decrease bowel damage risk from the barbed end. Confirmation of full-thickness closure is necessary to prevent

them. In such situations, the peritoneum medial to the infundibulopelvic (IP) ligament is grasped and tented using atraumatic forceps and incised with scissors. An irrigating probe is used to force water beneath and elevate the peritoneum for easier incision. The opening in the peritoneum then is extended a short distance caudally and cephalad over the suspected path of the ureter. Through this peritoneal window, the ureter is identified (see Fig. 44-9.1, p. 1027) (Parker, 2004).

❻ Round Ligament, Adnexa, and Uterine Artery. The initial steps for TLH mirror those for LH, described in Section

44-9, Steps 5 through 10 (p. 1027). These steps include transection of the round ligament, conservation or excision of the adnexa, caudad displacement of the bladder, and coagulation of the uterine vessels.

❼ Cardinal Ligament Transection. Following uterine artery coagulation, the cardinal ligaments are transected on each side to reach the level of the uterosacral attachments (Fig. 44-11.2).

❽ Colpotomy. Incision at the cervicovaginal junction may be performed with Harmonic scalpel, monopolar scissors,

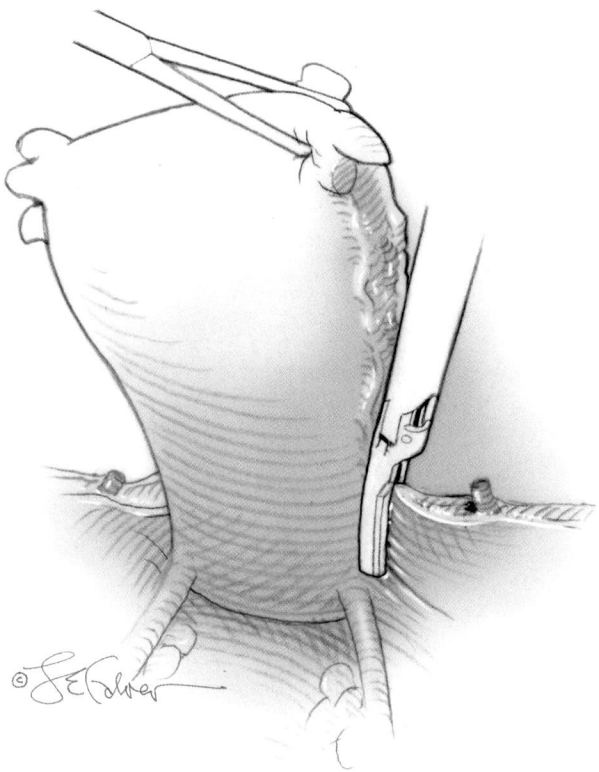

FIGURE 44-11.2 Cardinal ligament incised.

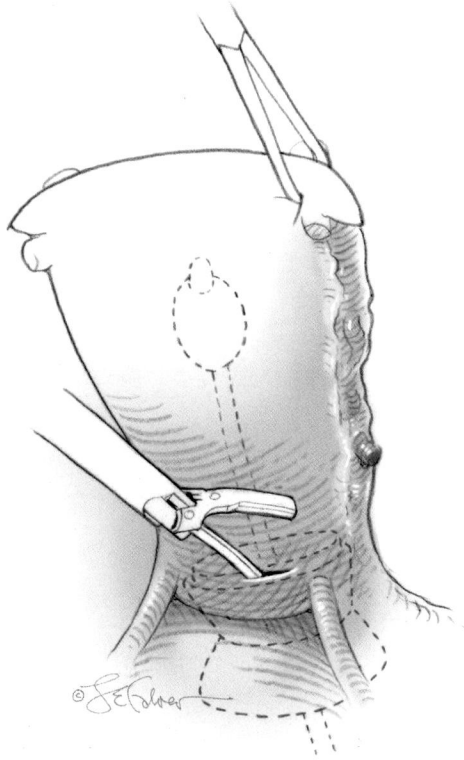

FIGURE 44-11.3 Posterior colpotomy.

later cuff dehiscence. Alternatively, for those less proficient with laparoscopic suturing, the cuff may be closed vaginally after removal of the uterus as described in Section 43-13 (p. 961).

After cuff closure, irrigation and confirmation of hemostasis is performed. Intra-abdominal pressures are lowered during this inspection to better identify sources of bleeding.

⓫ **Laparoscopy Final Steps.** Completion of this operation follows that for diagnostic laparoscopy (p. 1005).

POSTOPERATIVE

The advantages of a laparoscopic approach include a rapid return to normal diet and activities. Generally, the evening of the surgery, the Foley catheter is removed, diet is

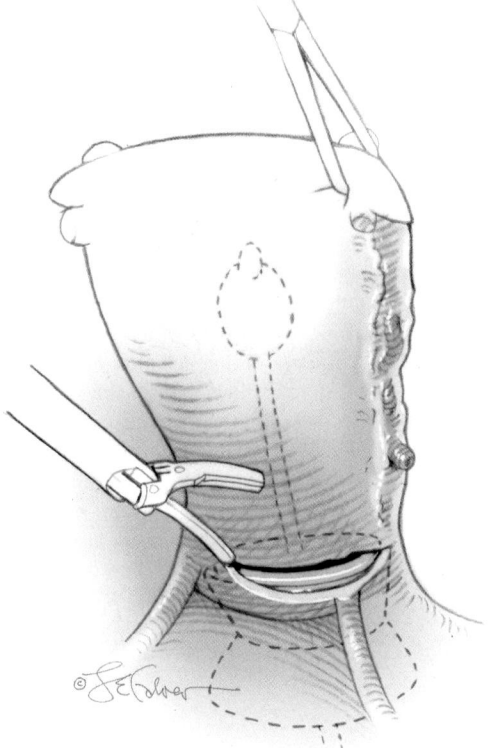

FIGURE 44-11.4 Right uterosacral ligament transected, and colpotomy extended toward the left.

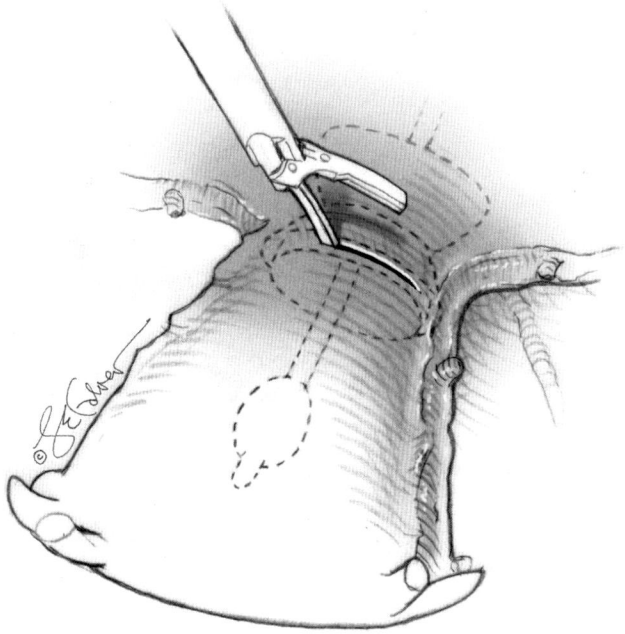

FIGURE 44-11.5 Anterior colpotomy.

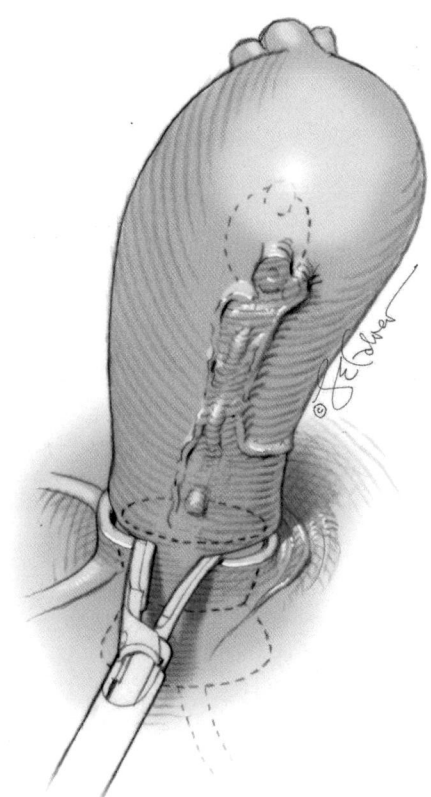

FIGURE 44-11.6 Joining anterior and posterior colpotomy incisions.

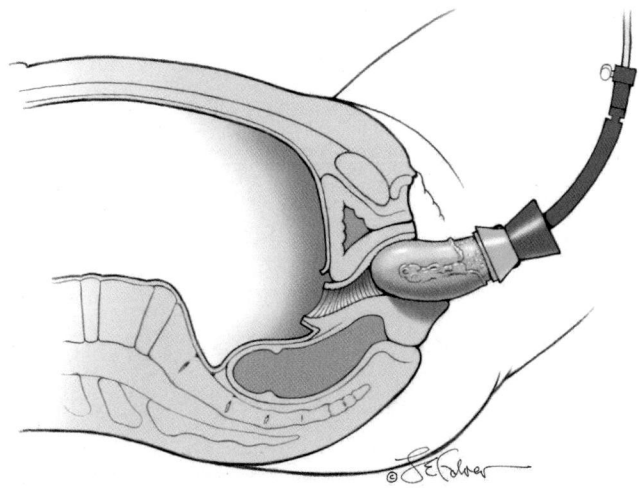

FIGURE 44-11.7 Uterus and manipulator removal.

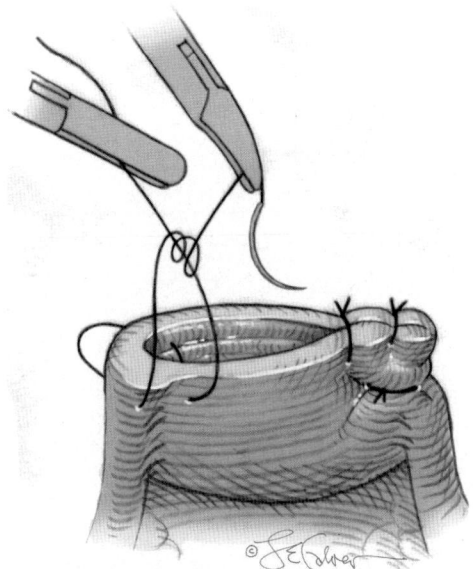

FIGURE 44-11.8 Vaginal cuff closure.

advanced, and the patient is allowed to ambulate. Oral analgesics are quickly adopted in place of parenteral options. The usual precautions for abdominal hysterectomy in regard to limitation of stress on the abdominal cavity by heavy lifting are followed. Delay of sexual activity mirrors that for abdominal hysterectomy, which is typically 6 weeks.

Vaginal cuff dehiscence is a serious postoperative complication that more frequently follows laparoscopic hysterectomy approaches compared with VH or TAH (Agdi, 2009; Walsh, 2007). In most cases, the precipitating event is sexual activity in premenopausal women and increased intraabdominal pressure coupled with a weak, atrophic vagina in postmenopausal women (Lee, 2009). Patients present with vaginal bleeding or evisceration. Typical treatment includes debridement of vaginal cuff edges, reapproximation with delayed-absorbable suture, and administration of antibiotic prophylaxis. However, compromised bowel may require more extensive surgeries to repair.

Preventatively, sound initial surgical technique strives to minimize electrosurgical damage during colpotomy creation and limit undue desiccation of the vaginal cuff. Approximation of all tissue planes, particularly full-thickness closure of the vaginal wall, should also be ensured. Reapproximation includes an adequate amount of viable tissue that is free of thermal effect. In addition, a two-layer closure may have an advantage over a single-layer figure-of-eight closure (Jeung, 2010).

Diagnostic Hysteroscopy

Hysteroscopy allows an endoscopic view of the endometrial cavity and tubal ostia. Indications are varied and include evaluation of abnormal uterine bleeding, infertility, or a sonographically identified uterine cavity mass. Contraindications to surgery include pregnancy and current reproductive tract infection.

PREOPERATIVE

Consent

Risks with diagnostic hysteroscopy are infrequent. Those described in Chapter 41 (p. 903) include uterine perforation and volume overload. Gas embolism is rare.

Patient Preparation

Infectious and VTE complications following hysteroscopic surgery are also rare. Accordingly, prophylaxis is typically not required (American College of Obstetricians and Gynecologists, 2013c, 2014b).

INTRAOPERATIVE

Surgical Steps

❶ **Anesthesia and Patient Positioning.** Diagnostic hysteroscopy can be performed in an outpatient setting under local anesthesia with or without intravenous sedation. Alternatively, a day-surgery setting and general anesthesia may be selected.

The patient is placed in standard lithotomy position, the vagina is surgically prepared, and the bladder is drained. Because diagnostic hysteroscopy is a short procedure with little if any blood loss, CO_2 or saline is typically selected for uterine distention. Trendelenburg positioning should be avoided to prevent the risk of gas embolism.

❷ **Hysteroscope Assembly.** For assembly, the hysteroscope is placed within its outer sheath and locked into place. The light source is then attached to the endoscope. By convention, during hysteroscope insertion, the light source is kept pointing toward the floor. The distention media tubing port is attached to a port that typically lies 180 degrees away from the light source connection.

❸ **Hysteroscope Introduction.** For most diagnostic hysteroscopic procedures, cervical

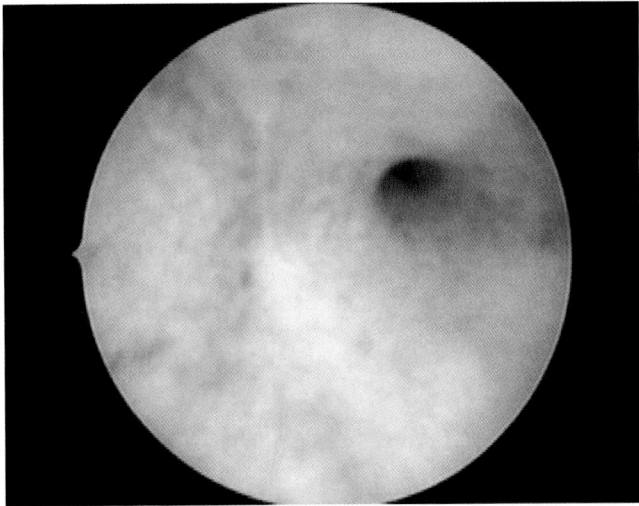

FIGURE 44-12.1 Hysteroscopic photograph of normal tubal ostia. (Used with permission from Dr. Kevin Doody.)

dilatation is not required to admit the 4- to 5-mm hysteroscope. Uterine sounding is not recommended by many because information regarding uterine depth and cavity inclination is provided by direct visualization during hysteroscope insertion. Moreover, the sound may disrupt the endometrium. This may alter endometrial anatomy prior to inspection and may cause obscuring bleeding.

For diagnostic purposes, a hysteroscope equipped with a 0-, 12-, or 30-degree forward oblique-view lens is suitable. A single-toothed tenaculum is placed on the anterior cervical lip, the flow of distention medium is begun, and the hysteroscope is introduced into the endocervical canal. Pressure exerted by the medium opens the endocervical canal and allows entry of the hysteroscope.

If using an angled lens, the surgeon should keep in mind that a panoramic image with a dark hole directly in the middle of the view is incorrect. The desired image would have the cervical canal at the bottom of the monitor if the light cord is directed downward, thus implying that the hysteroscope is in fact in the center of the cervical canal (Fig. 41-37, p. 902).

❹ **Hysteroscopic Evaluation.** As the hysteroscope is inserted, the endocervical canal is examined for abnormalities. Upon entering the cavity, the hysteroscope is held at the distal portion of the cavity to allow a panoramic evaluation. Systematically, the hysteroscope is moved to the fundus and then to the left and right to permit inspection of the tubal ostia (Fig. 44-12.1). If an angled lens is employed, the hysteroscope may remain just beyond the internal cervical os and the light cord moved in a 180-degree rotational arc to obtain a global assessment of the endometrial cavity. Some surgeons also advocate keeping the hysteroscope in the cav-

ity, evacuating it of distention medium, and evaluating the cavity in this decompressed stage. This helps identify lesions that may have been obliterated or flattened by the increased pressure of the distention medium.

❺ **Specific Procedures.** Following complete cavity inspection, if specific lesions are identified, they are typically biopsied under direct visualization with hysteroscopic forceps. If intrauterine device (IUD) removal is planned, most are grasped by the string or stem with hysteroscopic grasping forceps and are easily extracted as the entire hysteroscope is removed. However, embedded or fragmented devices may require removal in pieces. In these instances, a sturdy portion of the IUD is firmly grasped and traction on the forceps is exerted toward the vagina. For cases in which the IUD is deeply embedded, laparoscopy can assist in identifying uterine perforation and in determining whether the device is best removed hysteroscopically or laparoscopically.

❻ **Procedure Completion.** At the end of the procedure, the flow of distending medium is stopped, and the hysteroscope and then tenaculum are removed. A critical step at this point, and throughout the procedure, is to note the amount of distention fluid used and the amount retrieved. These values are used to calculate the fluid deficit, which is included in the operative report.

POSTOPERATIVE

Patient recovery is typically rapid and without complication and mirrors that following dilatation and curettage. Diet and activities may be resumed as desired by the patient. Spotting or light bleeding is not uncommon and typically stops within days.

44-13

Hysteroscopic Polypectomy

Indications for endometrial polyp removal include abnormal uterine bleeding, infertility, and risk of malignant transformation (Chap. 8, p. 188). Hysteroscopic excision of these growths may be completed by incision of the polyp base with hysteroscopic scissors or resectoscope loop, avulsion of the polyp with hysteroscopic forceps, or retrieval using suction and morcellation. Of these, the resectoscope and morcellator offer the most versatility in managing lesions, both large and small.

PREOPERATIVE

Patient Evaluation

In many women undergoing polypectomy, preoperative transvaginal sonography or saline infusion sonography examinations have been completed. Information regarding the size, number, and location of polyps is reviewed prior to surgery. Rarely, MR imaging may be indicated to fully distinguish a presumed polyp from a submucous leiomyoma. This often helps determine if myomectomy is instead required.

Consent

The complication rates for this procedure are low and mirror that for hysteroscopy in general (Chap. 41, p. 903). Thus, bleeding, infection, and uterine perforation, and rare fluid overload and gas embolism are described.

Patient Preparation

As with most hysteroscopic procedures, polypectomy is ideally performed during the follicular phase of the menstrual cycle, when the endometrial lining is thinnest and polyps would be most easily identified. Preoperative endometrial biopsy is optional but is generally considered part of abnormal uterine bleeding evaluation for those with endometrial cancer risks (Chap. 8, p. 184). Preoperative antibiotics or VTE prophylaxis is typically not required (American College of Obstetricians and Gynecologists, 2013c, 2014b).

INTRAOPERATIVE

Instruments

A resectoscope with a 90-degree loop electrode is ideal for polyp excision. Alternatively, an intrauterine morcellator has a hollow cannula that is attached to suction and can quickly excise small to large growths. For smaller polyps, polyp forceps may also be used through the 5F channel of the operative port.

Surgical Steps

❶ Anesthesia and Patient Positioning. Although simple polypectomy procedures under local analgesia in an office setting have been described, most cases are outpatient procedures performed under general or regional anesthesia. The complexity of fluid management, particularly with the use of hypotonic fluids, warrants a degree of safety that can be best provided in the operating suite. Following adequate anesthesia administration, the patient is placed in standard lithotomy position, the vagina is surgically prepared, and a Foley catheter is inserted.

❷ Media Selection. Hysteroscopic morcellation may be performed with a physiologic saline solution. However, if a monopolar resectoscope is used, then a nonelectrolyte solution is required. Because of the risks for hyponatremia with sorbitol and glycine, many prefer 5-percent mannitol. Alternatively, selection of a bipolar resecting system (Versapoint) allows performance within an isotonic electrolyte medium. The basics of medium selection are further described in Chapter 41 (p. 903). As with any hysteroscopic procedure, fluid volume deficits are calculated and noted regularly during surgery.

❸ Cervical Dilatation. The larger diameter of an 8- or 10-mm resectoscope or morcellator typically requires dilatation up to 9 mm with Pratt or similar dilators (Chap. 43, p. 967).

❹ Resection. Medium flow is begun, and the resectoscope is inserted into the endocervical canal under hysteroscopic visualization. Upon entering the cavity, a panoramic inspection is completed to identify the location and number of polyps. The resectoscope loop is then extended to reach behind the polyp. Electrosurgical current is applied as the loop is retracted toward the cervix to cut the polyp base. During resection, the loop should remain in view. The freed polyp is then grasped and delivered through the cervical os. This is similar to myoma excision, shown on page 1041.

In cases in which the polyp is large, several passes with the loop electrode may be required for complete excision. Passes begin at the polyp tip and progress until the base is reached. The uterus is not emptied after each pass. This practice maintains visualization of the polyp and minimizes the gas embolism and perforation risks associated with multiple introductions and reintroductions of instruments into the cavity. Instead, resected segments are allowed to float within the cavity as resection continues. Once the entire polyp is excised, then the fragments are collected on a Telfa sheet as they flow out of the cavity along with the distending medium. For larger polyps, the number of floating fragments will accrue. Thus, the cavity may need to be emptied prior to complete resection to permit an unobstructed view during resection.

❺ Morcellation. As with loop resection, distention medium flow is begun, and the morcellation unit is inserted. During morcellation,

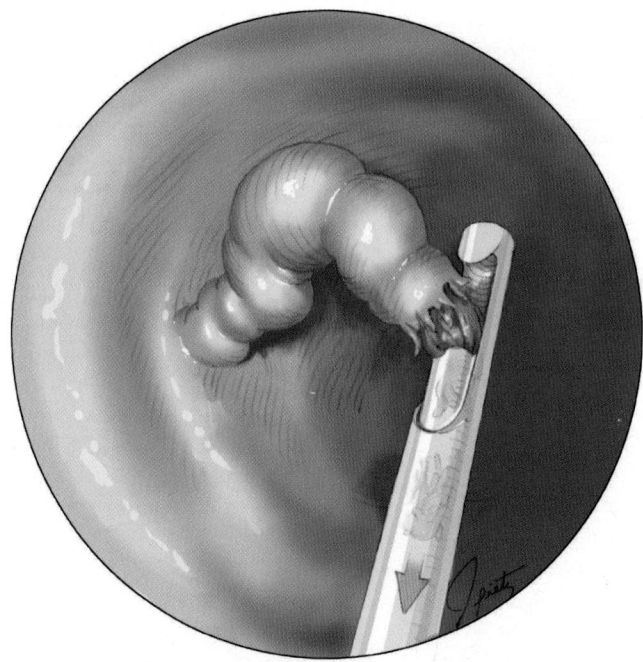

FIGURE 44-13.1 Hysteroscopic polypectomy.

it is important to work from the polyp tip toward the base (Fig. 44-13.1). Moreover, the mass is kept between the morcellator opening and the optics of the camera.

The morcellator also has suction action. This can be used to clear blood, tissue debris, and clots during resection of large growths. Better visual acuity and the continuous retrieval of the tissue are two of the advantages to this approach.

❻ **Control of Bleeding.** Bleeding sites may be coagulated with the same resection loop using a coagulating current. Alternatively, for heavy bleeding, a Foley catheter balloon may be inflated to tamponade vessels. This can be left in for several hours depending on bleeding severity. This is later removed, and vaginal bleeding is reassessed.

❼ **Instrument Removal.** The resectoscope or morcellator is removed, and the surgical specimen is sent for pathologic evaluation. At the end of the procedure, the flow of distending medium is stopped, and the hysteroscope and then tenaculum are removed. A critical step at this point, and throughout the procedure, is to note the amount of distention fluid used and retrieved to calculate the fluid deficit.

POSTOPERATIVE

Recovery following polypectomy is rapid, is typically without complication, and follows that for other hysteroscopic procedures (p. 1037).

44-14

Hysteroscopic Myomectomy

For symptomatic women with submucous leiomyomas, hysteroscopic resection of these tumors may provide relief of symptoms in most cases. Candidates may include those with abnormal uterine bleeding, with dysmenorrhea, or with infertility in which leiomyomas are suspected to be contributory. Tumors selected for resection should be either submucous or intramural with a prominent submucous component. During surgery, pedunculated submucous leiomyomas may be excised similarly to polyps (p. 1038). However, tumors with an intramural component require resection with a resectoscope, morcellator, or laser.

PREOPERATIVE

Patient Evaluation

Hysteroscopic myomectomy is a safe and effective option for most women. Contraindications to surgery, however, include pregnancy, potential endometrial cancer, current reproductive tract infection, and medical conditions sensitive to fluid volume overload.

Specific leiomyoma characteristics such as great size, large number, and greater degree of intramural penetration can increase the technical difficulty, complication rate, and clinical failure rate of this procedure (Di Spiezio Sardo, 2008). Thus, prior to resection, women typically undergo transvaginal sonography, saline infusion sonography (SIS), or hysteroscopy to evaluate leiomyoma characteristics. Alternatively, MR imaging can also accurately document uterine anatomy, but its expense and availability may limit its routine use.

During the evaluation by SIS or hysteroscopy, leiomyomas may be grouped according to criteria developed by Wamsteker and associates (1993) and adopted by the European Society for Gynaecological Endoscopy (ESGE).

Class 0: complete submucosal location
Class I: greater than 50-percent submucosal component
Class II: some submucosal involvement but greater than 50-percent myometrial component.

These criteria help predict which leiomyomas are suitable for hysteroscopic resection. A more recent classification has also been proposed by Lasmar and coworkers (2005, 2011). Similar to the ESGE system, their evaluation

grades the degree of tumor penetration into the myometrium. But, in addition, larger tumor size, wider tumor base, tumors in the upper portion of the cavity, or those found along the lateral wall receive higher scores. For higher scores, a nonhysteroscopic technique may be the safest and most successful.

Large or predominantly intramural tumors decrease clinical success rates, increase surgical risks, and increase the need for more than one surgical session to complete resection. For these reasons, many choose to resect only type 0 and I tumors and those measuring less than 3 cm (Vercellini, 1999; Wamsteker, 1993). More recent studies have reported resection of larger leiomyomas, although many need a two-step procedure and require a longer recovery (Camanni, 2010).

Consent

Complications of this procedure mirror that for hysteroscopy in general, and rates of 2 to 3 percent have been reported. Hysteroscopic myomectomy is associated with a greater risk of uterine perforation. This complication may follow cervical dilatation, but more frequently results during aggressive resection into the myometrium. Because of this risk, women are also consented for laparoscopy to assess and treat uterine or abdominal organ damage if perforation occurs.

Additionally, patients planning to seek pregnancy should be aware of possible intrauterine adhesion formation following resection and of rare uterine rupture during subsequent pregnancies (Batra, 2004; Howe, 1993).

During hysteroscopic myomectomy, distending medium is absorbed through venules that are opened during myometrial resection. Media is also absorbed across the peritoneum as the fluid flows in a retrograde direction through the fallopian tubes. Thus, resection of type I or II tumors or removal of large leiomyomas may be halted due to advancing fluid volume deficits. Patients are counseled that a second surgery may be required to finish resections in these cases. Fortunately, because of newer hysteroscopic morcellating tools, operating times and thus fluid deficits are decreased, even with large tumors.

Last, myomectomy is effective treatment, but 15 to 20 percent of patients will eventually require reoperation. This may be hysterectomy or repeat hysteroscopic resection at a later time for either persistent or recurrent symptoms (Derman, 1991; Hart, 1999).

Patient Preparation

GnRH agonists can preoperatively shrink leiomyomas to enable resection of large tumors or allow patients to rebuild their red

cell mass before surgery (Chap. 9, p. 208). However, disadvantages include preoperative hot flashes, difficulty in cervical dilatation, increased risk of laceration or perforations, and reduced intracavitary volume, which limits instrument mobility. Thus, GnRH agonist use is individualized.

To allow easier cervical dilatation and resectoscope insertion, misoprostol (Cytotec) can aid cervical softening. This practice is supported in some but not all studies, and postmenopausal women may benefit less from this pretreatment (Ngai, 1997, 2001; Oppegaard, 2008; Preutthipan, 2000). Commonly used dosing options include 200 or 400 μg vaginally or 400 μg orally once 12 to 24 hours prior to surgery. Common side effects include cramping, uterine bleeding, or nausea. Another alternative for cervical preparation prior to dilation is the use of dilute vasopressin (0.05 units/mL). Twenty milliliters of diluted vasopressin can be injected in divided doses intracervically at 4 and 8 o'clock. This method has the advantage of working rapidly at the time of surgery if the need for preoperative preparation was not anticipated (Phillips, 1997). Precautions with this potent vasocontrictor are outlined in Step 3 on page 1023.

Although the risk of postoperative infection is low, because pelvic infections can have devastating effect on future fertility, most recommend antibiotic prophylaxis prior to extensive hysteroscopic resections, as with myomectomy. Suitable agents are found in Table 39-6 (p. 835).

Concurrent Ablation

In those women with menorrhagia and with no desire for future fertility, endometrial ablation may be concurrently performed (p. 1043) (Loffer, 2005). However, because leiomyoma resection alone resolves abnormal bleeding in most women, we do not routinely perform concomitant endometrial ablation unless the patient desires hypomenorrhea.

INTRAOPERATIVE

Instruments

Hysteroscopic myomectomy can be performed using a resectoscope or hysteroscopic morcellator. Both procedures are described.

Surgical Steps

❶ **Anesthesia and Patient Positioning.** For most cases, hysteroscopic myomectomy is an outpatient procedure performed under general anesthesia. The patient is placed in standard lithotomy position, the vagina is surgically prepared, and a Foley catheter is inserted.

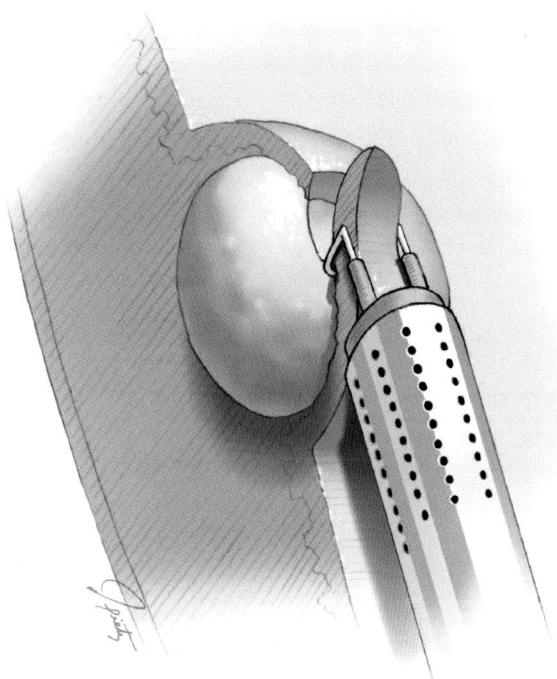

FIGURE 44-14.1 Hysteroscopic resection.

❷ **Medium Selection.** The choice of distending medium is dictated by the resecting tool used. Resection using a morcellator, bipolar electrosurgical loop, or laser can be performed in saline solution. Alternatively, cases using a monopolar electrosurgical loop require an electrolyte-free solution. Solution differences are discussed in Chapter 41 (p. 903).

❸ **Cervical Dilatation.** Using Pratt or other suitable dilators, the surgeon dilates the cervix as shown in Chapter 43 (p. 967).

❹ **Instrument Insertion.** The distending medium flow is begun, and the resectoscope or morcellator is inserted into the endocervical canal under direct visualization. Upon entering the endometrial cavity, a panoramic inspection is first performed to identify and assess leiomyomas.

❺ **Resection.** The electrosurgical unit is set to a continuous-wave mode (cutting). The resectoscope loop is advanced to lie behind the leiomyoma, and electric current is applied before the loop contacts the tissue. To minimize thermal injury and perforation, current is applied only as the loop is retracted and not when it is being extended. During resection, the loop should remain in view. Upon contact, the loop electrode is retracted toward the resectoscope (Fig. 44-14.1). To ensure a clean cut and complete excision of the shaved strip, current is not stopped until the entire loop is retracted. The shaved strip

of smooth muscle floats within the endometrial cavity.

This shaving process is repeated serially toward the myoma's base until the tumor is removed. Although strips can be removed from the cavity after each pass, this results in a repetitive loss of uterine distention. Repeated removal and reinsertion of a resectoscope increases the risk of perforation, gas embolism, and fluid intravasation. Thus in most cases, pushing removed strips to the fundus will help to adequately clear the operative field. However, if the view becomes obstructed, a pause in resection may be required to remove these strips.

❻ **Morcellation.** Morcellators currently available include Hologic's MyoSure, Smith & Nephew's TruClear system, and Boston Scientific's Symphion system. In general, sharp moving blades are contained within a hollow, rigid tube. By means of a vacuum source connected to the hollow tube, tissue is suctioned into the window opening at the device tip and is shaved off by the moving blade (Fig 44-14.2). Suction also removes morcellated tissue fragments through the device cylinder and allows collection for pathologic analysis.

In retrospective comparisons, hysteroscopic morcellation is faster than resectoscopy

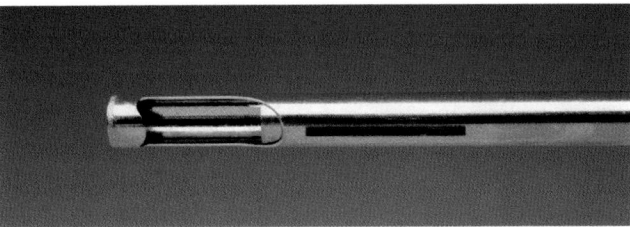

A

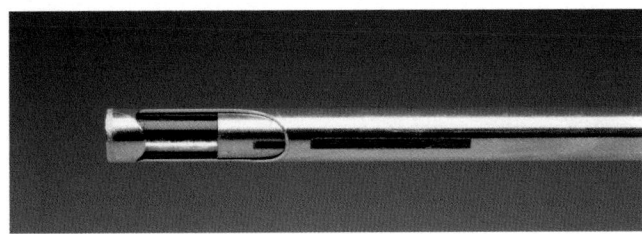

B

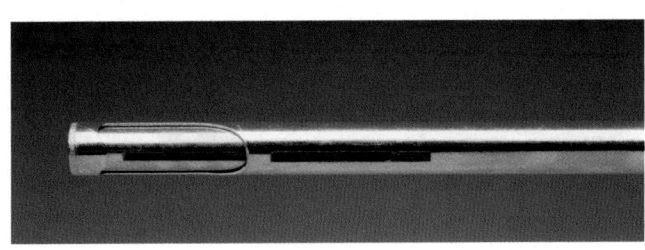

C

FIGURE 44-14.2 Hysteroscopic morcellator. **A.** Morcellator blade retracted. Suction draws tissue into the fluted opening. **B.** Blade partially advanced. The blade rapidly rotates as it is advanced and retracted. **C.** Blade is fully advanced and slices tissue drawn into the opening.

and appears easier to perform. It is associated with fewer fluid-related complications and has a shorter learning curve compared with conventional resectoscopy (Emanuel, 2005).

❼ **Intramural Leiomyomas.** During removal of leiomyomas with an intramural component, uterine perforation risks are increased if resection extends below the level of the normal myometrium. Therefore, when resection reaches this level, the surgeon should pause and wait for the surrounding myometrium to contract around the now smaller tumor. This delivers deeper portions of the leiomyoma into the uterine cavity. Diminishing the intrauterine pressure, by decreasing the fluid inflow pressure, can also help to deliver the myoma.

❽ **Fluid Volume Deficit.** Because of the hypervolemia risk during hysteroscopic myomectomy, fluid volume deficits are care-

fully monitored throughout the procedure. The final fluid deficit is noted in the operative report.

❾ **Hemostasis.** Bleeding is common during myomectomy and will often cease as the myometrium fibers contract due to the reduction in intracavitary volume. Vessels that are more actively bleeding may be coagulated with the edge of the resecting loop, and the electrosurgical unit set to a modulating (coagulating) current. At times, a ball electrode may be required to increase the surface area over which current is delivered. Global endometrial ablation offers a similar treatment in the case of multiple bleeding sites but is not suitable for patients desiring fertility. Rarely, bleeding may be poorly controlled with electrosurgical tools. In such cases, mechanical pressure applied to bleeding vessels by a Foley balloon inflated with 5 to 10 mL of saline may be required. This

can be left in for several hours depending on bleeding severity. The catheter is later removed, and vaginal bleeding is reassessed.

POSTOPERATIVE

Recovery following myomectomy is quick and typically without complication. Patients may resume diet and activities as tolerated. Spotting or light bleeding may follow surgery for 1 to 2 weeks.

For patients desiring pregnancy, conception may be attempted in the menstrual cycle after the resection, unless the leiomyoma was broadbased or had a significant intramural component. In these patients, barrier contraception is advised for three cycles. For women who fail to conceive or continue to have abnormal bleeding following resection, postoperative hysterosalpingography or hysteroscopy is recommended to evaluate for intrauterine synechiae.

44-15

Endometrial Ablation Procedures

Endometrial ablation broadly describes a group of hysteroscopic procedures that destroys or resects the endometrium and leads to eumenorrhea. For many women, ablation serves as a minimally invasive and effective treatment of abnormal uterine bleeding. Within the ablation group, techniques are defined as first- or second-generation depending on their temporal introduction into use and the need for hysteroscopic skills. First-generation tools require advanced hysteroscopic skills and longer operating times and can be associated with distention medium complications, such as volume overload. These techniques include endometrial vaporization with the neodymium:yttrium-aluminum-garnet (Nd-YAG) laser, rollerball electrosurgical desiccation, and endometrial resection by resectoscope.

Comparing first-generation methods, it appears that all three produce similar outcomes in terms of bleeding and patient satisfaction. However, resection methods have been associated with more surgical complications, and thus desiccation methods may be preferred for women without intracavitary lesions (Lethaby, 2002; Overton, 1997).

To reduce risks and required specialized training of these early ablative tools, second-generation nonresectoscopic methods have been introduced during the past 10 years. These tools use various modalities to destroy the endometrium but do not require direct hysteroscopic guidance. Modalities include thermal energy, cryosurgery, electrosurgery, and microwave energy.

PREOPERATIVE

Patient Evaluation

Prior to ablation, complete evaluation of abnormal uterine bleeding should be completed. Accordingly, the possibility of pregnancy, endometrial hyperplasia or endometrial cancer, and active pelvic infection is excluded. During evaluation of bleeding, transvaginal sonography (TVS), saline infusion sonography (SIS), and hysteroscopy may be used solely or in combination (Chap. 8, p. 188). However, many second-generation ablation techniques require a normal endometrial cavity, and endometrial pathology, if identified, can be treated concurrently by several of these ablative methods. Thus, SIS and hysteroscopy are more sensitive than TVS for focal lesions, and either is preferred

for preoperative evaluation. In addition, several second-generation techniques are not appropriate for large endometrial cavities. Thus, uterine depth is also assessed preoperatively by uterine sounding or sonography.

Myometrial thinning from prior uterine surgery may increase the risk of damage to surrounding viscera during ablation. Therefore, women with prior transmural uterine surgery are evaluated for type and location of uterine scar. A history of prior classical cesarean delivery or of abdominal or laparoscopic myomectomy may be considered a relative contraindication to ablation. Some experts advocate the sonographic evaluation of myometrial thickness to determine whether a patient is a candidate for ablation, although no specific thickness has been established (American College of Obstetricians and Gynecologists, 2013b).

Consent

Patients selecting ablation should be aware of success rates relative to other treatment options for abnormal bleeding (Chap. 8, p. 197). In general, rates of decreased menstrual flow range from 70 to 80 percent and of amenorrhea, from 15 to 35 percent (Sharp, 2006). Eumenorrhea, rather than amenorrhea, is considered the treatment goal. Therefore, a patient should not undergo ablation if guaranteed amenorrhea is desired. In addition, endometrial ablation effectively destroys the endometrium and is contraindicated in those who desire future fertility.

Endometrial tissue has tremendous regenerative capabilities. Therefore, premenopausal women are counseled before surgery regarding the need for adequate postoperative contraception. If pregnancy does occur, complications after ablation include prematurity, abnormal placentation, and perinatal morbidity. For this reason, many providers recommend concomitant tubal sterilization at the time of endometrial ablation (American College of Obstetricians and Gynecologists, 2013b).

However, in women with tubal sterilization, cornual hematometra or postablation tubal sterilization syndrome (PATSS) can develop from bleeding from regenerated or remnant endometrium. With cornual hematometra, blood is trapped between the postoperative cornual synechiae. With PATSS, blood collects between the occluded proximal tubal stump and synechiae to cause proximal hematosalpinx. Both conditions cause associated cyclic pain. Hysterectomy is commonly required for resolution (McCausland, 2002).

Following ablation, later evaluation of the endometrium for recurrent abnormal bleeding can be challenging. Namely, a Pipelle may not reach remnant endometrium, and endometrial stripe measurements may be less accurate. The American Society for Reproductive

Medicine (2008) advises against endometrial ablation in postmenopausal women because excluding malignancy in these women can be more difficult. Women with risks for endometrial cancer pose similar sampling challenges.

Complications associated with ablation mirror those with operative hysteroscopy, although the risk of fluid volume overload is avoided with second-generation tools.

Patient Preparation

During hysteroscopic surgeries, bacteria in the vagina may gain access to the upper reproductive tract and peritoneal cavity. However, postablation infection is rare, and preoperative prophylactic antibiotics are generally not indicated. Because the endometrium can thicken from only a few millimeters in the early proliferative phase to deeper than 10 mm in the secretory phase, all first-generation techniques and some of the second-generation ones are ideally performed in the early proliferative phase. Otherwise, drugs that induce endometrial atrophy such as GnRH agonists, combination oral contraceptives, or progestins may be used for 1 to 2 months prior to surgery. Alternatively, curettage may be performed immediately prior to ablation.

INTRAOPERATIVE

Surgical Steps

❶ **Anesthesia and Patient Positioning.** Endometrial ablation is typically a day-surgery procedure, performed under general anesthesia. Some studies state that second-generation techniques may be satisfactorily completed in an outpatient setting with intravenous sedation, local anesthetic blockade, or both (Sambrook, 2010; Varma, 2010). The patient is placed in dorsal lithotomy position, and the perineum and vagina are surgically prepared.

❷ **Selection of Distending Medium.** With first-generation procedures, distending medium is required and selected based on the destructive energy used as described in Chapter 41 (p. 903). In general, saline may be used for laser and bipolar electrical current, whereas monopolar tools require nonelectrolyte solutions.

❸ **Neodymium: Yttrium-Aluminum-Garnet Laser.** Introduced in the 1980s, the Nd-YAG laser was the first ablative tool. Under direct hysteroscopic observation and uterine distention with saline, a Nd-YAG laser fiber touches the endometrium and is dragged across the endometrial surface. This creates furrows of photocoagulated tissue that are 5 to 6 mm deep (Garry, 1995; Goldrath, 1981).

❹ Transcervical Resection of the Endometrium (TCRE). In addition to less expense, because of the larger loop diameter, TCRE can be completed more quickly than laser fiber ablation. The shorter procedure duration can reduce the risk of excess media absorption.

This method uses a resectoscope with monopolar or bipolar electrical current to excise strips of endometrium. The resection technique is similar to that described for hysteroscopic myomectomy (p. 1040). The excised tissue strips are sent for pathologic evaluation. In cases with concurrent intrauterine pathology such as endometrial polyps or submucous leiomyomas, TCRE can excise these lesions in addition to the endometrium.

However, TCRE has been associated with higher rates of perforation, especially at the cornua, where the myometrium is thinner. For this reason, many use a rollerball electrosurgical electrode in combination with TCRE, with the rollerball used in the cornua (Oehler, 2003).

❺ Rollerball. A 2- to 4-mm ball-shaped or barrel-shaped electrosurgical electrode can be rolled across the endometrium as an effective means of vaporizing the tissue (Vancaillie, 1989). Advantages to rollerball ablation compared with TCRE include shorter operating time, less fluid absorption, and lower perforation rates. Unfortunately, it is not effective in the treatment of intracavitary lesions, and pathology specimens are not obtained.

❻ Thermal Balloon Ablation. Several thermal balloon ablation systems are now currently used worldwide (Fig. 44-15.1). Of these, only the ThermaChoice III Uterine Balloon Therapy System is approved for use in the United States. Other balloon systems available in other countries include the Cavaterm Plus system or the Thermablate Endometrial Ablation System.

The ThermaChoice III Uterine Balloon Therapy System is a software-controlled device designed to destroy endometrial tissue using thermal energy. After cervical dilation to 5.5 mm, the Thermachoice device is inserted into the uterine cavity. Once inside the cavity, a 5-percent dextrose and water solution is instilled into a disposable silicone balloon at the tip and heated to coagulate the endometrium. During the treatment, the contained fluid within the balloon is circulated to maintain a temperature of 87°C (186°F) for 8 minutes. The balloon can be introduced without hysteroscopic assistance into the uterine cavity, and when inflated, it conforms to the cavity contour.

All hot-liquid balloon devices require no advanced hysteroscopic skills, and complication rates are low (Gurtcheff, 2003; Vilos, 2004). One disadvantage is the requirement for an anatomically normal uterine cavity.

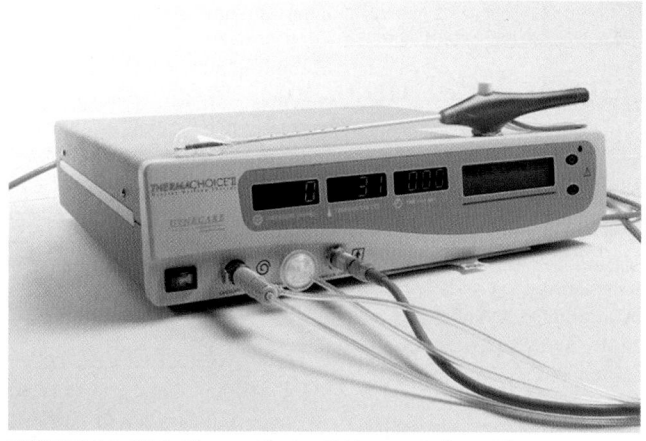

FIGURE 44-15.1 ThermaChoice III Uterine Balloon Therapy System. (©Ethicon, Inc. Reproduced with permission.)

Some studies, however, have demonstrated successful use in patients with submucosal leiomyomas (Soysal, 2001). Another limitation is the required pharmacologic thinning prior to thermal ablation. Alternatively, mechanical thinning can be accomplished with dilatation and curettage prior to ablation.

❼ Hysteroscopic Thermal Ablation. Several second-generation ablation procedures require a normal uterine cavity. However, the HydroThermAblator (HTA) system allows treatment of the endometrium concurrent with submucous leiomyomas, polyps, or abnormal uterine anatomy. Another advantage of this system is that it is performed under direct hysteroscopic visualization, allowing the surgeon to observe the endometrium being destroyed. However, the risk of external burns from circulating hot water appears to be higher using this method compared other second-generation methods (Della Badia, 2007).

This tool is designed to ablate the endometrial lining of the uterus by heating an uncontained saline solution to a temperature of 90°C and recirculating it through the uterus for 10 minutes (Fig. 44-15.2). Spill through the fallopian tubes is avoided because hydrostatic pressure during the procedure remains below 55 mm Hg, which is well below pressures needed to open the tubes to the peritoneal

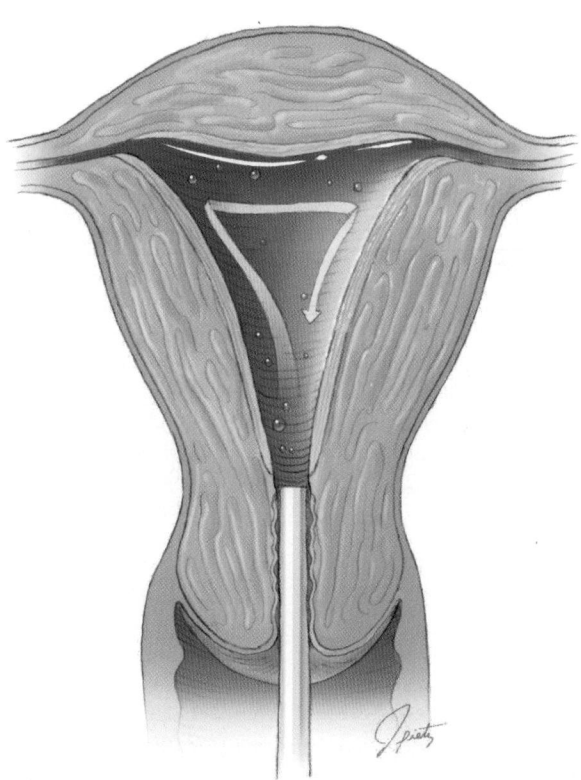

FIGURE 44-15.2 Hysteroscopic thermal ablation.

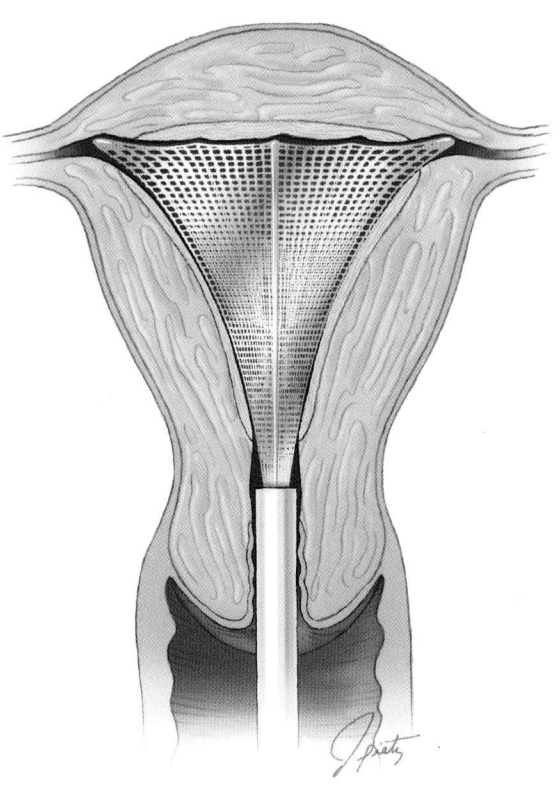

FIGURE 44-15.3 Impedance-controlled electrocoagulation.

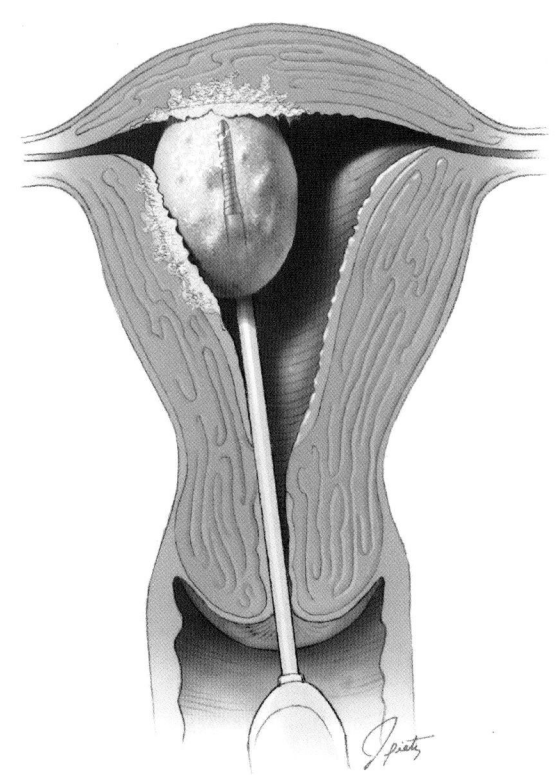

FIGURE 44-15.4 Cryoablation.

cavity. Similarly, the water seal created between the hysteroscope and internal cervical os prevents leakage of fluid into the vagina. For this reason, care is taken not to dilate the cervix to a diameter greater than 8 mm.

Initially, a hysteroscope is inserted into the 7.8-mm diameter disposable HTA sheath. This combination is introduced into the endometrial cavity to enable viewing while room-temperature saline is instilled into the uterine cavity. The fluid flow is then gradually heated and circulated to treat the endometrium. At the completion of the treatment phase, cool saline replaces the heated fluid, and the instrument is then removed (Glasser, 2003).

❽ **Impedance-controlled Electrocoagulation.** The NovaSure endometrial ablation system consists of a high-frequency (radiofrequency) bipolar electrosurgical generator and a single-use, fan-shaped device constructed of metal mesh. The mesh fan is designed to contour to the shape of the endometrial cavity. During treatment, an attachment provides suction to draw the endometrium and myometrium up against the mesh electrode for improved contact and to remove generated vapor (Fig. 44-15.3). The treatment time of 2 minutes results in desiccation of the endometrium. An advantage of this system is that it does not require preoperative endometrial preparation. Although Food and Drug Administration (FDA) approval studies evaluated the system in normal uterine

cavities, it has been used successfully in patients with small submucosal leiomyomas and polyps (Sabbah, 2006).

❾ **Cryoablation.** In addition to thermal damage, endometrial ablation can be achieved with extreme cold using the Her Option cryoablation system. Similar to the physics of cervical cryotherapy, gases compressed under pressure with this unit can generate temperatures of −100° to −120°C at the cryoprobe tip to produce an iceball. As an iceball grows, its leading edge advances through tissue, and cryonecrosis develops in those tissues reaching temperatures below −20°C (Chap. 43, p. 989).

The Her Option cryoablation system contains a metal probe, which is covered by a 5.5-mm disposable cryoprobe. After dilatation of the cervix, the cryoprobe's 1.4-inch cryotip is placed against one side of the endometrial cavity and advanced to one uterine cornu (Fig. 44-15.4). Concurrent transabdominal sonography is required to ensure accurate cryotip placement and surveillance of the increasing iceball diameter, which is seen as an enlarging hypoechoic area. The first freeze is terminated after 4 minutes or sooner, if the advancing iceball reaches to within 3 mm of the uterine serosa. The cryotip is allowed to warm, is moved from the cornu, and is redirected into the contralateral cornu. A second freeze is performed for 6 minutes or less based on iceball advancement.

❿ **Microwave Ablation.** The microwave endometrial ablation (MEA) technique uses microwave energy to destroy the endometrium. During the procedure, a microwave probe is inserted until the tip reaches the uterine fundus. Once placed, the probe tip is maintained at 75° to 80°C and moved slowly from side to side. Microwave energy is spread with a maximum penetration of 6 mm over the entire uterine cavity surface. Speed is an advantage, with the entire treatment completed in 2 to 3 minutes (Cooper, 1999). Due to complications of bowel burns in patients without evidence of uterine perforation, to obtain FDA approval, the manufacturers of the MEA system recommend preoperative myometrial thickness assessment to document at least a 10-mm thickness throughout the uterus (Glasser, 2009; Iliodromiti, 2011). MEA was FDA-approved in 2003, but Microsulis discontinued worldwide sales of the MEA device in 2011.

POSTOPERATIVE

Advantages to endometrial ablation include rapid patient recovery and low incidence of complications. Patients may resume normal diet and activities as tolerated. Patients may expect light bleeding or spotting during the first postoperative days as necrotic endometrial tissue is shed. A serosanguinous discharge follows for 1 week and is replaced by a profuse and watery discharge for another 1 to 2 weeks.

44-16

Transcervical Sterilization

Hysteroscopic sterilization is a minimally invasive, transcervical method to perform surgical sterilization. Currently, only two forms of transcervical sterilization are approved by the FDA. These are the *Essure Permanent Birth Control* system and *Adiana Permanent Contraception* system (Chap. 5, p. 117). However, the Adiana System is no longer manufactured, although not because of safety or efficacy concerns.

Essure employs a coil device, termed a *microinsert*, which is inserted into the proximal section of each fallopian tube. Once in place and released from its delivery catheter, the microinsert expands to anchor itself within the fallopian tube (Fig. 44-16.1). Over time, synthetic fibers within the microinsert incite a chronic inflammatory response and a local tissue ingrowth from the surrounding tube. This ingrowth leads to complete tubal lumen occlusion, which is documented by hysterosalpingography (HSG) at 3 months following surgery.

As with any permanent birth control method, candidates should be confident in their decision for sterilization. Contraindications include pregnancy or pregnancy termination within the prior 6 weeks, recent pelvic infection, known tubal occlusion, and for Essure, allergy to radiographic contrast medium or nickel.

PREOPERATIVE

Patient Evaluation

Pregnancy is excluded prior to sterilization using a serum or urine β-hCG test.

Consent

For many women, hysteroscopic sterilization is a safe and effective method of birth control. Efficacy rates are comparable with current laparoscopic sterilization rates, although long-term data are limited (Magos, 2004). With proper placement, Essure appears to have similar or superior contraceptive efficacy compared with other methods of sterilization (Levy, 2007).

Effective bilateral tubal occlusion or insert placement may not be possible in all patients due to tubal ostium stenosis or spasm or an inability to visualize the ostia (Cooper, 2003). Rates of successful placement average 88 to 95 percent (Kerin, 2003; Ubeda, 2004).

In general, complications of transcervical sterilization are similar to those of hysteroscopy. However, rates of fluid volume overload are low because in most cases procedure lengths are short (15 to 30 minutes) and opening of endometrial vascular channels is minimal. Uterine or tubal perforation has been noted. Rates approximate 1 to 2 percent, and in most cases, these are clinically insignificant (Cooper, 2003; Kerin, 2003). A perforated Essure insert may need to be removed from the peritoneal cavity to prevent complications. Chronic pelvic pain and insert erosion or migration can also occur.

Patient Preparation

Because menstrual bleeding and a thick endometrium can impair identification of tubal ostia, this procedure is typically performed during the early proliferative phase of the menstrual cycle. This also decreases the chance of an unidentified luteal-phase pregnancy. Preoperative analgesia may be considered and typically consists of a nonsteroidal antiinflammatory drug given 30 to 60 minutes before the procedure. Prophylactic antibiotics are not required.

INTRAOPERATIVE

Instruments

The Essure system is disposable and comes individually wrapped. It contains a handle, delivery catheter, release catheter, delivery wire, and microinserts. Each microinsert is attached to the end of a delivery wire, which is housed within a release catheter. In turn, the release catheter is surrounded by a delivery catheter.

Surgical Steps

❶ **Anesthesia and Patient Positioning.** Transcervical sterilization can be performed in an outpatient setting under local anesthesia with or without intravenous sedation. Alternatively, a day-surgery setting using general anesthesia may be selected. The patient is placed in the standard lithotomy position, and the vagina is surgically prepared.

❷ **Media Selection.** For the Essure system, electrosurgery is not required, and therefore, 0.9-percent saline is commonly used to avoid the increased expense and risk of hyponatremia associated with nonelectrolyte solutions. As with any hysteroscopic procedure, accurate calculation of fluid volume deficits during the procedure is essential. The final deficit is recorded within the operative note.

❸ **Hysteroscope Insertion.** Vaginal retractors or speculum provides access to the cervix, and a tenaculum may be used for adequate cervical traction to insert the hysteroscope. Depending on the diameter of the operative hysteroscope, standard cervical dilatation may or may not be required. A 12- to 30-degree hysteroscope is preferred to provide easy visualization of the cornua, and a 5F operating channel is needed.

❹ **Essure Microinsert Delivery.** Requisite for completion of the procedure, both tubal ostia must be visualized. To begin delivery, the outermost catheter of the system, the *delivery catheter*, is threaded through the operating channel of the hysteroscope. Its tip is inserted into one tubal ostium. This delivers the tightly coiled, collapsed insert into the ostium. The delivery catheter is then retracted into the Essure device handle, and an inner cannula, which is the *release catheter*, is now seen. As the release catheter is retracted, the microinsert begins to uncoil. Ideally, if correctly placed, three to eight coils of the microinsert trail into the endometrial cavity (Fig. 44-16.2). As a final step, a guide

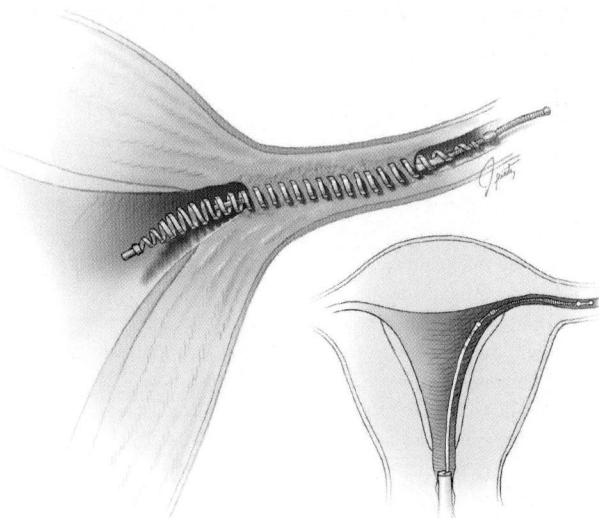

FIGURE 44-16.1 Microinsert placement and ingrowth of tissue.

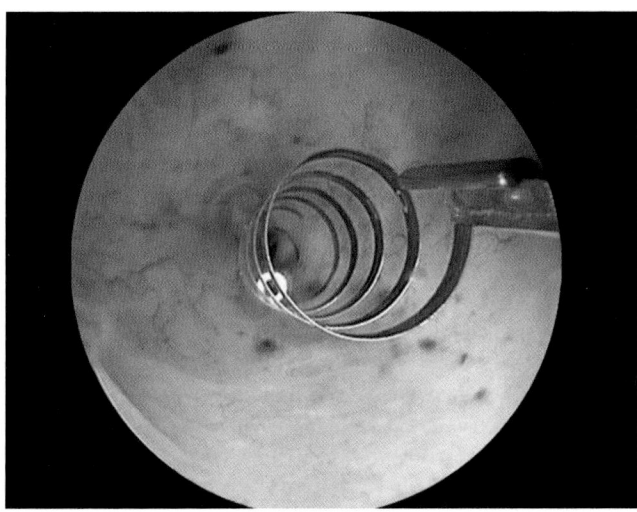

FIGURE 44-16.2 Hysteroscopic photograph of Essure microinsert coils within the tubal ostium. (Reproduced with permission from Bayer.)

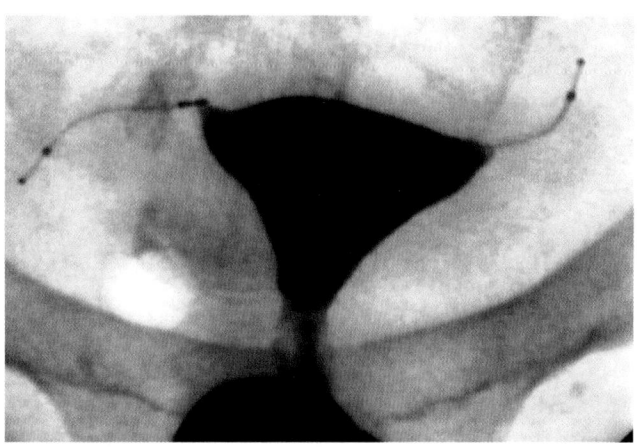

FIGURE 44-16.3 Hysterosalpingography displaying correct Essure microinsert placement. (Reproduced with permission from Bayer.)

wire that is attached to the distal end of the microinsert is detached and retracted. These steps are repeated at the opposite ostium.

POSTOPERATIVE

Patients typically resume normal diet and activity within the first 24 hours following surgery. Cramping is common within the first few days, and light spotting or bleeding may be noted during the week following surgery.

To document complete tubal occlusion, HSG is performed at 3 months following insertion (Fig. 44-16.3). Until this time, an alternative method of contraception should be used. Rarely, in those with correct placement, tubal occlusion may not be complete at 3 months, and a second HSG at 6 months may be required to document sterilization. Of note, although Essure microinserts are radiopaque with fluoroscopy, the Adiana silicone implant is not visible. Microinserts can be expelled. Thus, if no Essure device is identified during HSG or if 18 or more of its coils are seen trailing into the uterine cavity, then the microinsert should be replaced or an alternative method of contraception used (Magos, 2004).

Essure microinserts conduct thermal energy, and this is factored into future surgery across the proximal fallopian tube. Also, synechiae after endometrial ablation can obscure Essure HSG. Thus, ablation and Essure insertion are not performed concurrently. However, following HSG confirmation, Novasure, HTA, and Thermachoice III are thermal methods that can be performed with Essure inserts in place (Aldape, 2013). Last, MR imaging can safely be completed in those with Essure inserts.

44-17

Hysteroscopic Septoplasty

Most uterine septa form from incomplete regression of the medial portion of the müllerian ducts during their fusion (Fig. 44-17.1) (Chap. 18, p. 406). These septa rarely result in infertility. However, they have been associated with malpresentation and increased rates of first- and second-trimester spontaneous abortion. This serves as the main indication for septoplasty.

Before the popularity of operative hysteroscopy, septoplasty was performed abdominally and with a hysterotomy incision. Fortunately, hysteroscopic septoplasty affords MIS with decreased morbidity to the patient and uterus. *Septoplasty* refers to central division of the septum in a caudad-to-cephalad direction, generally with the use of hysteroscopic scissors. Bleeding is minimal due to the relative avascularity of the septum's fibroelastic tissue, which retracts upon incision. *Septum resection* is performed for broader, larger septa that have wider bases. A loop resectoscope or morcellator may be preferred for this.

PREOPERATIVE

Patient Evaluation

Diagnosis of a septate uterus follows guidelines outlined in Chapter 18 (p. 422) and includes HSG, SIS, and transvaginal sonography. Because of the frequent association between renal and müllerian anomalies, intravenous pyelography is also performed. Finally, although a septate uterus is associated with infertility and pregnancy loss, evaluation for other causes of these two conditions is completed prior to septum excision. Contraindications to septoplasty include

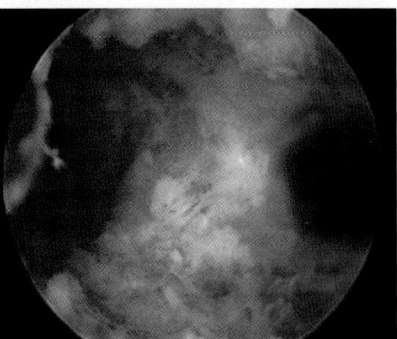

FIGURE 44-17.1 Hysteroscopic photograph of uterine septum. The dark uterine cavity is seen on either side.

pregnancy and active pelvic infection, and these should be excluded.

Consent

Hysteroscopic septoplasty is a safe and effective treatment for recurrent pregnancy loss, and postoperative live birth rates approximate 85 percent (Fayez, 1987). In general, complications mirror those for operative hysteroscopy, although the risk of uterine perforation appears increased. For this reason, concurrent laparoscopy in some cases is recommended to help inform a surgeon as to the proximity of the uterine serosa. As the hysteroscope nears the fundal serosa, transillumination of the hysteroscopic light indicates the potential for uterine perforation. Accordingly, a patient may also be consented for concurrent diagnostic laparoscopy as outlined on page 1003.

Patient Preparation

Infectious and VTE complications following hysteroscopic surgery are rare. Accordingly, preoperative antibiotics or VTE prophylaxis is typically not required (American College of Obstetricians and Gynecologists, 2013c, 2014b). Misoprostol may be used preoperatively to ease cervical dilatation (p. 901).

INTRAOPERATIVE

Instruments

Septum incision or resection can be completed using hysteroscopic scissors, resectoscope loop, Nd-YAG laser, or mechanical morcellators. Selection is according to septum dimensions and surgeon preference.

Surgical Steps

❶ Anesthesia and Patient Positioning. Hysteroscopic septoplasty is typically a day-surgery procedure performed under general anesthesia. A woman is placed in standard

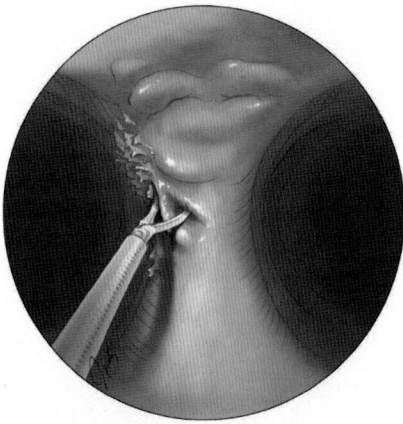

FIGURE 44-17.2 Septum incision.

lithotomy position, the vagina is surgically prepared, and a Foley catheter inserted. If surveillance laparoscopy is planned, then the abdomen is also prepared.

❷ Medium Selection. The choice of distending medium is dictated by the incising tool used. Sharp incision with scissors, Nd:YAG laser, or bipolar instrument is commonly selected and can be performed in any liquid medium. Monopolar technology will require a hypotonic nonconductive medium.

❸ Concurrent Laparoscopy. If planned concurrently, placement of the laparoscope follows the steps described in Chapter 41 (p. 889).

❹ Cervical Dilatation. A tenaculum is placed on the anterior cervical lip. Using a Pratt or other suitable dilator, the surgeon serially dilates the cervix.

❺ Instrument Insertion. The distending medium flow is begun, and the operative hysteroscope is inserted into the endocervical canal under direct visualization. Upon entering the endometrial cavity, a panoramic inspection is first performed to identify the septum.

❻ Septum Incision. If scissors are used, a surgeon attempts to keep the line of incision in the anteroposterior midline. Transection begins caudally, at the septum apex, and continues cephalad toward the fundus. Bites with the scissors are taken bilaterally and are directed toward the horizontal midline (Fig. 44-17.2). During incision of the septum, drifting from the vertical midline is common. Incisions typically drift posteriorly in an anteverted uterus and anteriorly in a retroverted one. Thus, a surgeon may pause and reorient periodically.

During septoplasty, incision rather than complete resection of the septum is sufficient. Septal stumps are retracted into the myometrium as the septum is transected. In most cases, the septum is relatively avascular, and cutting at its midpoint causes little bleeding. Signs that transection is complete include increasing tissue vascularity, serosal transillumination of the hysteroscope at the uterine fundus, and reaching a level in line with the tubal ostia.

❼ Septum Resection. In some cases, the septum is broad, wide, and difficult to simply incise. Thus, to achieve the desired uterine cavity, a surgeon must completely excise or resect the septum. In general, scissors may be used, but in some instances, vaporizing electrodes, loop electrodes, or morcellators are more useful. Instruments are selected according to surgeon skill and preference.

❽ Procedure Completion

After incision completion, the hysteroscope and tenaculum are removed. The final fluid deficit is noted in the operative report. Final steps of laparoscopy, if performed, follows those outlined in Chapter 41 (p. 1005).

POSTOPERATIVE

Recovery following septoplasty is rapid and typically without complication. Light bleeding or spotting may last 1 week or more. Patients may resume normal diet and activities as desired. Following resection, symptoms such as dysmenorrhea ultimately are greatly decreased.

To stimulate endometrial proliferation and prevent adhesion reformation, oral estrogen administration has proved effective. Although several regimens can be used, we prescribe 2 mg of estradiol, orally for 30 days.

Attempts at conception are delayed for 2 to 3 months following surgery. If septum resection appeared incomplete at the time of surgery or if recurrent miscarriage or amenorrhea develops, then postoperative HSG or a second hysteroscopy may be performed. Complete removal of the septum or adhesiolysis may be required (p. 1052). With subsequent pregnancy, if the myometrium was not entered, cesarean delivery is required only for obstetric indications.

44-18

Proximal Fallopian Tube Cannulation

Proximal fallopian obstruction may result from pelvic inflammatory disease, intratubal debris, congenital malformations, tubal spasm, endometriosis, tubal polyps, and salpingitis isthmica nodosa. It is generally diagnosed during evaluation of infertility when documentation of tubal patency is sought. Therapeutic options have the goal of a successful pregnancy. Therefore, approaches to occlusion in this portion of the tube include tubal cannulation, surgical tubocornual anastomosis, and in vitro fertilization (IVF) (Kodaman, 2004). During cannulation, attempts are made to flush debris from within the tubes and perform chromotubation.

Proximal fallopian tube cannulation may be used to treat up to 85 percent of proximal tubal obstructions, but the occlusion may recur following the surgery. It may be performed as an outpatient radiologic procedure using fluoroscopy (Papaioannou, 2003). Alternatively, cannula placement may be completed with hysteroscopic guidance (Confino, 2003). If a hysteroscopic approach is selected, laparoscopy is typically used concurrently. This allows evaluation and treatment of both proximal and distal tubal disease and provides identification of tubal perforation by the cannulating guide wire if this occurs.

PREOPERATIVE

Patient Evaluation

Proximal tubal occlusion is typically identified with HSG during evaluation of female infertility. To avoid disrupting an early pregnancy, preoperative β-hCG testing is warranted in most patients. Although this procedure may be performed at any time during the menstrual cycle, the early proliferative phase offers the advantage of a thinner endometrium to allow easy identification of tubal ostia and avoids disruption of an early luteal-phase pregnancy.

Consent

In addition to general complications associated with hysteroscopy and laparoscopy, patients undergoing proximal tubal cannulation are informed of the small risk of tubal perforation. Fortunately, because the guide wire measures only 0.5 mm in diameter, tubal damage is rarely significant and can be assessed by concurrent laparoscopic examination of the perforated tube.

In most cases, patients with combined proximal and distal tubal disease are best managed with IVF. As discussed in Chapter 9 (p. 224), hydrosalpinges, when present, can lower IVF success rates and are typically removed. Thus, consideration of and consent for salpingectomy should accompany plans for proximal tubal cannulation.

Patient Preparation

The risk of pelvic infection is low. However, because adhesions following such infection can have damaging effects on fallopian tube health, patients are given either a first- or second-generation cephalosporin prior to surgery. In addition, misoprostol may be used preoperatively to aid cervical softening and hysteroscope insertion.

INTRAOPERATIVE

Instruments

Fallopian tubes may be cannulated with a catheter system displayed in Figure 44-18.1. This system contains an outer cannula, inner cannula, and inner guide wire. The preset bend of the outer cannula aids placement of both the inner cannula and guide wire into the tubal ostium. Once the inner cannula has been threaded into the proximal fallopian tube, the guide wire is removed. The inner cannula, now emptied of the guide wire, can be used to flush debris from the fallopian tube and allow chromotubation, which is visualized laparoscopically (Fig. 19-9, p. 441).

Surgical Steps

❶ **Anesthesia and Patient Positioning.** Hysteroscopic tubal cannulation with concurrent laparoscopy is typically an outpatient procedure performed under general anesthesia. The patient is placed in standard lithotomy position, the abdomen and vagina are surgically prepared, and a Foley catheter is inserted.

❷ **Medium Selection.** No electrosurgery is required for tubal cannulation, thus saline is the preferred medium.

❸ **Laparoscopy.** The laparoscope is inserted as described in Chapter 41 (p. 889).

❹ **Cervical Dilatation.** Because a smaller diameter operative hysteroscope is required for tubal cannulation, cervical dilatation may not be required. If needed, it is performed as described in Chapter 43 (p. 967).

❺ **Hysteroscope Insertion.** The flow of saline is begun, and a 0- or 30-degree hysteroscope is inserted. A panoramic inspection of the entire cavity is performed, and the tubal ostia are identified.

❻ **Tubal Cannulation.** The catheter system is threaded through an operating port of the hysteroscope. Under direct visual guidance, the outer catheter is advanced and placed at one of the tubal ostia. The inner catheter is then threaded approximately 2 cm into the proximal fallopian tube (Fig. 44-18.2). The guide wire is removed.

❼ **Tubal Flushing.** The inner catheter is flushed with water-soluble dye. Indigo carmine dye or methylene blue can be diluted and used. However, current indigo carmine shortages may favor methylene blue use. Either agent is diluted into 50 to 100 mL of sterile saline for injection. The laparoscope is positioned to allow inspection of the distal tube to note the presence or absence of dye spill.

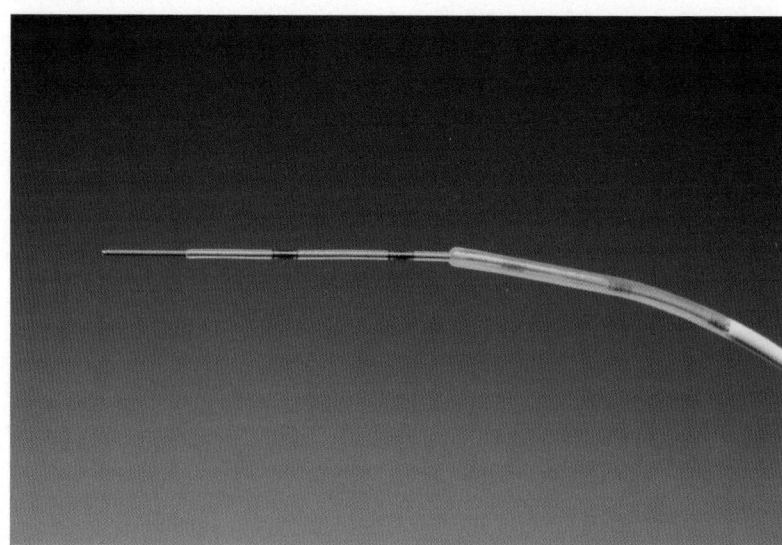

FIGURE 44-18.1 Hysteroscopic tubal cannulation catheter.

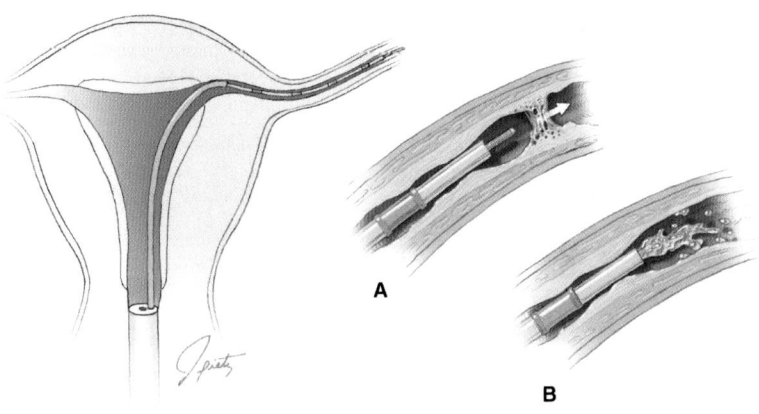

FIGURE 44-18.2 Tubal cannulation.

❽ Concurrent Procedures. If distal tubal adhesions are noted, laparoscopic lysis of adhesions may be concurrently performed.

❾ Procedure Completion. Following cannulation, the hysteroscope and cervical tenaculum are removed. Laparoscopy is completed as described in Chapter 41 (p. 1005).

POSTOPERATIVE

Recovery from hysteroscopic tubal cannulation and laparoscopy is typically quick and uncomplicated. Patients may resume diet, activity, and attempts at conception as desired.

CHAPTER 44

44-19

Lysis of Intrauterine Adhesions

Intrauterine adhesions, also called *synechiae,* may develop following uterine curettage (Fig. 44-19.1). Less commonly, they may result from pelvic radiation, tuberculous endometritis, or endometrial ablation. The presence of these adhesions, also termed *Asherman syndrome,* may lead to hypo- or amenorrhea, pelvic pain, and infertility or pregnancy loss.

Treatment goals include surgical re-creation of normal intrauterine anatomy and prevention of adhesion reformation. Surgery involves hysteroscopic transection rather than excision of adhesions. Thus, thin adhesions can usually be lysed using only gentle blunt force from the hysteroscopic sheath. However, dense adhesions usually require hysteroscopic division with scissors or laser.

Postsurgical pregnancy and live delivery rates are markers of surgical success, and these rates vary depending on the thickness of adhesions and degree of cavity oblitera-tion. For this reason, various adhesion clas-sification systems are useful to help predict the success of adhesiolysis for a given woman (Al-Inany, 2001).

PREOPERATIVE

Patient Evaluation

Although hysteroscopy and saline infusion sonography (SIS) can both accurately iden-tify adhesions, HSG is preferred initially,

because it allows concurrent assessment of tubal patency. However, after adhesions have been noted, diagnostic hysteroscopy is recom-mended to assess the thickness and density of these bands (Fayez, 1987). Additionally, completion of fertility assessment, including semen analysis and assessment of ovulation, is recommended prior to surgery to help predict chances of conception following the procedure.

Consent

In general, hysteroscopic adhesiolysis is an effective tool to correct menstrual disorders and improve fertility in women with uterine adhesions (Valle, 2003). Although overall cumulative delivery rates in those with no other fertility factors ranges from 60 to 70 percent, lower rates generally are associated with more severe disease (Pabuccu, 1997; Zikopoulos, 2004). In addition, pregnancies following surgery may be complicated by pla-cental implantation abnormalities or by pre-term labor (Dmowski, 1969; Pabuccu, 2008).

The complications mirror those for opera-tive hysteroscopy. However, the risk of uter-ine perforation may be increased. For this reason, patients should also be consented for diagnostic laparoscopy.

Patient Preparation

Infectious and VTE complications following hysteroscopic surgery are rare. Accordingly, preoperative antibiotics or VTE prophylaxis is typically not required (American College of Obstetricians and Gynecologists, 2013c, 2014b). Additionally, intraoperative intra-cervical dilute vasopressin or preoperative misoprostol may be used to soften the cervix and ease dilatation (Chap. 41, p. 901).

INTRAOPERATIVE

Surgical Steps

❶ **Anesthesia and Patient Positioning.** Hysteroscopic lysis of adhesions is typically a day-surgery procedure performed under general anesthesia. The patient is placed in standard lithotomy position, the vaginal is surgically prepared, and a Foley catheter inserted.

❷ **Medium Selection.** The choice of dis-tending medium is dictated by the tool used. Sharp transection with scissors, Nd:YAG laser, or bipolar instrument can be performed in any liquid medium. However, thick adhesions often require resection rather than division, and they are severed close to the myome-trium. Thus, the potential for creation of large denuded areas and fluid intravasation is great. Accordingly for many surgeons, 0.9-percent saline is preferred because hyponatremia less likely if fluid overload does develop.

❸ **Concurrent Laparoscopy.** There is an increased risk of uterine perforation in those with more severe obliteration of the cavity. Thus, adjunctive laparoscopy may guide sur-geons as to instrument proximity to the uter-ine serosa. The decision to use a laparoscope is individualized, and its placement follows the steps described in Chapter 41 (p. 889).

❹ **Cervical Dilatation.** Using Pratt or other suitable dilators, the surgeon serially dilates the cervix as described in Chapter 43 (p. 967).

❺ **Instrument Insertion.** The distend-ing medium flow is begun, and the operative hysteroscope is inserted into the endocervical canal under direct visualization. Upon entering the endometrial cavity, a panoramic inspection is first performed to identify adhesions.

❻ **Approach to Lysis.** In general, a system-atic approach to adhesiolysis begins with either blunt or sharp disruption of the most central adhesions and moves gradually to reach the most lateral. The size and qualities of adhesions may vary. Thin endometrial adhesions can usually be disrupted with gentle blunt force from the hysteroscopic sheath alone. More commonly, myofibrous and fibrous adhesions are denser and may require complete resection.

Adhesiolysis is continued until the endo-metrial cavity is restored to normal and the tubal ostia are seen. Importantly, procedures may require termination prior to this, if sig-nificant fluid volume deficits are reached.

❼ **Chromotubation.** At completion of adhesiolysis, transcervical chromotubation

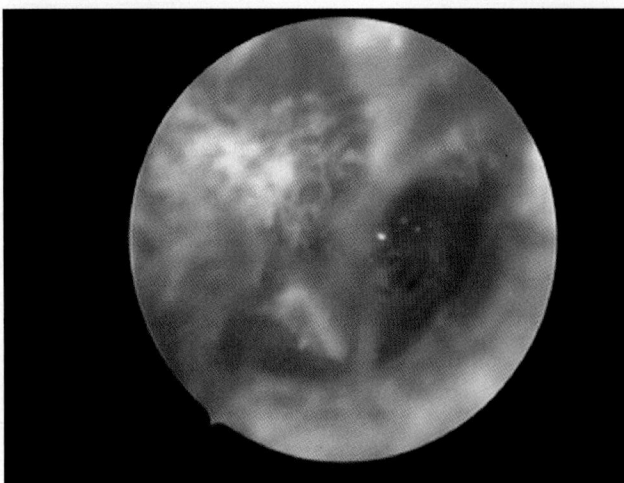

FIGURE 44-19.1 Hysteroscopic photograph of intrauterine adhe-sions. (Used with permission from Dr. Kevin Doody.)

is performed to document tubal patency. Chromotubation may be performed by injecting dye into the uterine cavity through a uterine manipulator during simultaneous laparoscopy. Alternatively, tubal cannulation as described previously may be performed to establish tubal patency (p. 1050).

❽ Mechanical Uterine Cavity Distention. This option has been used to prevent treated areas from adhering following surgery. Either a copper IUD, placed for 3 months, or an 8F pediatric Foley catheter balloon, used for 10 days, may be chosen. In a comparison of the two, Orhue and colleagues (2003) noted fewer new adhesions and greater pregnancy rates in women using the balloon. If a Foley balloon is placed, antibiotic prophylaxis with either doxycycline 100 mg orally twice daily or other appropriate antibiotic is recommended.

POSTOPERATIVE

Recovery from hysteroscopic resection is rapid and typically without complication. Patients may resume normal activities and diet as tolerated.

To stimulate endometrial proliferation and prevent reformation of adhesions, oral estrogen administration has proved effective. Although several regimens can be used, we prescribe 2 mg of estradiol, orally for 30 days following adhesiolysis. Conjugated equine estrogen (Premarin) 1.25 mg may also be used. Following IUD insertion, 6 to 8 weeks of oral estrogen supplementation is given.

New adhesions can form following adhesiolysis. In their early stages, these bands are thinner and thus more amenable to successful resection. For this reason, another hysteroscopy or HSG is typically performed at 3 months following the initial resection. If significant new adhesions are found, a second surgical lysis of adhesions is planned. To allow adequate uterine healing, attempts at pregnancy by the patient are delayed for 2 to 3 months.

REFERENCES

Agdi M, Al-Ghafri W, Antolin R, et al: Vaginal vault dehiscence after hysterectomy. J Minim Invasive Gynecol 16(3):313, 2009

Ahmad G, Duffy JMN, Farquhar C, et al: Barrier agents for adhesion prevention after gynaecological surgery. Cochrane Database Syst Rev 2: CD000475, 2008

Aldape D, Chudnoff SG, Levie MD: Global endometrial ablation in the presence of Essure microinserts. Rev Obstet Gynecol 6(2):80, 2013

Al-Inany H: Intrauterine adhesions: an update. Acta Obstet Gynaecol Scand 80:986, 2001

American College of Obstetricians and Gynecologists: Alternatives to hysterectomy in the management of leiomyomas. Practice Bulletin No. 96, August 2008, Reaffirmed 2014a

American College of Obstetricians and Gynecologists: Antibiotic prophylaxis for gynecologic procedures. Practice Bulletin No. 104, May 2009, Reaffirmed 2014b

American College of Obstetricians and Gynecologists: Benefits and risks of sterilization. Practice Bulletin No. 133, February 2013a

American College of Obstetricians and Gynecologists: Choosing the route of hysterectomy for benign disease. Committee Opinion No. 444, November 2009, Reaffirmed 2011

American College of Obstetricians and Gynecologists: Endometrial ablation. Practice Bulletin No. 81. May 2007, Reaffirmed 2013b

American College of Obstetricians and Gynecologists: Prevention of deep vein thrombosis and pulmonary embolism. Practice Bulletin No. 84, August 2007, Reaffirmed 2013c

American College of Obstetricians and Gynecologists: Salpingectomy for ovarian cancer prevention. Committee Opinion No. 620, January 2015

American College of Obstetricians and Gynecologists: Sterilization of women, including those with mental disabilities. Committee Opinion No. 371, July 2007, Reaffirmed 2009

American Society for Reproductive Medicine: Indications and options for endometrial ablation. Fertil Steril 90(5 Suppl):S236, 2008

American Society for Reproductive Medicine: Pathogenesis, consequences, and control of peritoneal adhesions in gynecologic surgery: a committee opinion. Fertil Steril 99(6):1550, 2013

Barakat EE, Bedaiwy MA, Zimberg S, et al: Robotic-assisted, laparoscopic, and abdominal myomectomy: a comparison of surgical outcomes. Obstet Gynecol 117(2 Pt 1):256, 2011

Barber EL, Neubauer NL, Gossett DR: Risk of venous thromboembolism in abdominal versus minimally invasive hysterectomy for benign conditions. Am J Obstet Gynecol 212(5):609, 2015

Batra N, Khunda A, O'Donovan PJ: Hysteroscopic myomectomy. Obstet Gynecol Clin North Am 31:669, 2004

Ben-Arie A, Goldchmit R, Dgani R, et al: Trophoblastic peritoneal implants after laparoscopic treatment of ectopic pregnancy. Eur J Obstet Gynecol Reprod Biol 96(1):113, 2001

Brennan MC, Ogburn T, Hernandez CJ, et al: Effect of topical bupivacaine on postoperative pain after laparoscopic tubal sterilization with Filshie clips. Am J Obstet Gynecol 190:1411, 2004

Buttram VC Jr, Vaquero C: Post-ovarian wedge resection adhesive disease. Fertil Steril 26:874, 1975

Camanni M, Bonino L, Delpiano EM, et al: Hysteroscopic management of large symptomatic submucous uterine myomas. J Minim Invasive Gynecol 17(1):59, 2010

Chan LM, Westhoff CL: Tubal sterilization trends in the United States. Fertil Steril 94(1):1, 2010

Cohen SL, Einarsson JI, Wang KC, et al: Contained power morcellation within an insufflated isolation bag. Obstet Gynecol 124(3):491, 2014

Confino E: Tubal Catheterization and falloposcopy. In Bieber EJ, Loffer FD (eds): Hysteroscopy, Resectoscopy, and Endometrial Ablation. Boca Raton, Parthenon Publishing Group, 2003, p 113

Cooper JM, Carignan CS, Cher D, et al: Microinsert noninciscional hysteroscopic sterilization. Obstet Gynecol 102:59, 2003

Cooper KG, Bain C, Parkin DE: Comparison of microwave endometrial ablation and transcervical resection of the endometrium for treatment of heavy menstrual loss: a randomised trial. Lancet 354:1859, 1999

Dabirashrafi H: Complications of laparoscopic ovarian cauterization. Fertil Steril 52:878, 1989

Darwish AM, Nasr AM, El Nashar DA: Evaluation of postmyomectomy uterine scar. J Clin Ultrasound 33:181, 2005

Della Badia C, Nyirjesy P, Atogho A: Endometrial ablation devices: review of a manufacturer and user facility device experience database. J Minim Invasive Gynecol 14:436, 2007

Derman SG, Rehnstrom J, Neuwirth RS: The long-term effectiveness of hysteroscopic treatment of menorrhagia and leiomyomas. Obstet Gynecol 77:591, 1991

Di Spiezio Sardo A, Mazzon I, Bramante S, et al: Hysteroscopic myomectomy: a comprehensive review of surgical techniques. Hum Reprod Update 14(2):101, 2008

Dmowski WP, Greenblatt RB: Asherman's syndrome and risk of placenta accreta. Obstet Gynecol 34:288, 1969

Donesky BW, Adashi EY: Surgically induced ovulation in the polycystic ovary syndrome: wedge resection revisited in the age of laparoscopy. Fertil Steril 63:439, 1995

Doss BJ, Jacques SM, Qureshi F, et al: Extratubal secondary trophoblastic implants: clinicopathologic correlation and review of the literature. Hum Pathol 29:184, 1998

Dubuisson JB, Fauconnier A, Babaki-Fard K, et al: Laparoscopic myomectomy: a current view. Hum Reprod Update 6:588, 2000

Einarsson JI, Cohen SL, Fuchs N, et al: In-bag morcellation. J Minim Invasive Gynecol 21(5): 951, 2014

Einarsson JI, Vellinga TT, Twijnstra AR, et al: Bidirectional barbed suture: an evaluation of safety and clinical outcomes. JSLS 14(3):381, 2010

Emanuel MH, Wamsteker K: The Intra Uterine Morcellator: a new hysteroscopic operating technique to remove intrauterine polyps and myomas. J Minim Invasive Gynecol 12:62, 2005

Farquhar C, Brown J, Marjoribanks J, et al: Laparoscopic drilling by diathermy or laser for ovulation induction in anovulatory polycystic ovary syndrome. Cochrane Database Syst Rev 6:CD001122, 2012

Farquhar CM: The role of ovarian surgery in polycystic ovary syndrome. Best Pract Res Clin Obstet Gynaecol 18:789, 2004

Fauconnier A, Chapron C, Babaki-Fard K, et al: Recurrence of leiomyomata after myomectomy. Hum Reprod Update 6:595, 2000

Fayez JA, Mutie G, Schneider PJ: The diagnostic value of hysterosalpingography and hysteroscopy in infertility investigation. Am J Obstet Gynecol 156:558, 1987

Fedele L, Bianchi S, Tozzi L, et al: Intramesosalpingeal injection of oxytocin in conservative laparoscopic treatment for tubal pregnancy: preliminary results. Hum Reprod 13:3042, 1998

Fletcher H, Frederick J, Hardie M, et al: A randomized comparison of vasopressin and tourniquet as hemostatic agents during myomectomy. Obstet Gynecol 87:1014, 1996

Franchi M, Ghezzi F, Beretta P, et al: Microlaparoscopy: a new approach to the reassessment of ovarian cancer patients. Acta Obstet Gynaecol Scand 79:427, 2000

Franklin RR: Reduction of ovarian adhesions by the use of Interceed. Ovarian Adhesion Study Group. Obstet Gynecol (3):335, 1995

Frederick J, Fletcher H, Simeon D, et al: Intramyometrial vasopressin as a haemostatic agent during myomectomy. BJOG 101:435, 1994

Garry R, Reich H, Liu CY: Laparoscopic hysterectomy: definitions and indications. Gynaecol Endosc 3:1, 1994

Garry R, Shelley-Jones D, Mooney P, et al: Six hundred endometrial laser ablations. Obstet Gynecol 85:24, 1995

Ginsburg ES, Benson CB, Garfield JM, et al: The effect of operative technique and uterine size on blood loss during myomectomy: a prospective, randomized study. Fertil Steril 60:956, 1993

Giuliani A, Panzitt T, Schoell W, et al: Severe bleeding from peritoneal implants of trophoblastic tissue after laparoscopic salpingostomy for ectopic pregnancy. Fertil Steril 70:369, 1998

Glasser MH: Practical tips for office hysteroscopy and second-generation "global" endometrial ablation. J Minim Invasive Gynecol 16(4):384, 2009

Glasser MH, Zimmerman JD: The Hydro ThermAblator system for management of menorrhagia in women with submucous myomas: 12- to 20-month follow-up. J Am Assoc Gynecol Laparosc 10:521, 2003

Goldrath MH, Fuller TA, Segal S: Laser photovaporization of endometrium for the treatment of menorrhagia. Am J Obstet Gynecol 140:14, 1981

Gooden MD, Hulka JF, Christman GM: Spontaneous vaginal expulsion of Hulka clips. Obstet Gynecol 81:884, 1993

Gould MK, Garcia DA, Wren SM, et al: Prevention of VTE in nonorthopedic surgical patients: Antithrombotic Therapy and Prevention of Thrombosis, 9th ed: American College of Chest Physicians Evidence-Based Clinical Practice Guidelines. Chest 141(2 Suppl):e227S, 2012

Greenberg JA, Einarsson JI: The use of bidirectional barbed suture in laparoscopic myomectomy and total laparoscopic hysterectomy. J Minim Invasive Gynecol 15(5):621, 2008

Greenblatt EM, Casper RF: Adhesion formation after laparoscopic ovarian cautery for polycystic ovary syndrome: lack of correlation with pregnancy rate. Fertil Steril 60:766, 1993

Gürgan T, Kisnisci H, Yarali H, et al: Evaluation of adhesion formation after laparoscopic treatment of polycystic ovarian disease. Fertil Steril 56(6):1176, 1991

Gürgan T, Urman B, Aksu T, et al: The effect of short-interval laparoscopic lysis of adhesions on pregnancy rates following Nd:YAG laser photo-coagulation of polycystic ovaries. Obstet Gynecol 80(1):45, 1992

Gurtcheff SE, Sharp HT: Complications associated with global endometrial ablation: the utility of the MAUDE database. Obstet Gynecol 102:1278, 2003

Harkki P, Kurki T, Sjoberg J, et al: Safety aspects of laparoscopic hysterectomy. Acta Obstet Gynaecol Scand 80:383, 2001

Harkki-Siren P, Sjoberg J, Makinen J, et al: Finnish national register of laparoscopic hysterectomies:

a review and complications of 1165 operations. Am J Obstet Gynecol 176:118, 1997

Harkki-Siren P, Sjoberg J, Tiitinen A: Urinary tract injuries after hysterectomy. Obstet Gynecol 92:113, 1998

Harrison MS, DiNapoli MN, Westhoff CL: Reducing postoperative pain after tubal ligation with rings or clips: a systematic review and meta-analysis. Obstet Gynecol 124(1):68, 2014

Hart R, Molnar BG, Magos A: Long-term follow-up of hysteroscopic myomectomy assessed by survival analysis. BJOG 106:700, 1999

Hobo R, Netsu S, Koyasu Y, et al: Bradycardia and cardiac arrest caused by intramyometrial injection of vasopressin during a laparoscopically assisted myomectomy. Obstet Gynecol 113(2 Pt 2):484, 2009

Howe RS: Third-trimester uterine rupture following hysteroscopic uterine perforation. Obstet Gynecol 81:827, 1993

Hurst BS, Matthews ML, Marshburn PB: Laparoscopic myomectomy for symptomatic uterine myomas. Fertil Steril 83:1, 2005

Hutchins FL Jr: A randomized comparison of vasopressin and tourniquet as hemostatic agents during myomectomy. Obstet Gynecol 88:639, 1996

Iliodromiti S, Murage A: Multiple bowel perforations requiring extensive bowel resection and hysterectomy after microwave endometrial ablation. J Minim Invasive Gynecol 18(1):118, 2011

Iverson RE Jr, Chelmow D, Strohbehn K, et al: Relative morbidity of abdominal hysterectomy and myomectomy for management of uterine leiomyomas. Obstet Gynecol 88:415, 1996

Jeung IC, Baek JM, Park EK, et al: A prospective comparison of vaginal stump suturing techniques during total laparoscopic hysterectomy. Arch Gynecol Obstet 282(6):631, 2010

Kerin JF, Cooper JM, Price T, et al: Hysteroscopic sterilization using a micro-insert device: results of a multicentre phase II study. Hum Reprod 18:1223, 2003

Kesby GJ, Korda AR: Migration of a Filshie clip into the urinary bladder seven years after laparoscopic sterilisation. BJOG 104:379, 1997

Kluivers KB, Hendriks JC, Mol BW, et al: Quality of life and surgical outcome after total laparoscopic hysterectomy versus total abdominal hysterectomy for benign disease: a randomized, controlled trial. J Minim Invasive Gynecol 14(2):145, 2007

Kodaman PH, Arici A, Seli E: Evidence-based diagnosis and management of tubal factor infertility. Curr Opin Obstet Gynecol 16:221, 2004

Kuno K, Menzin A, Kauder HH, et al: Prophylactic ureteral catheterization in gynecologic surgery. Urology 52:1004, 1998

Lajer H, Widecrantz S, Heisterberg L: Hernias in trocar ports following abdominal laparoscopy: a review. Acta Obstet Gynaecol Scand 76:389, 1997

Lamberton GR, Hsi RS, Jin DH, et al: Prospective comparison of four laparoscopic vessel ligation devices. J Endourol 22(10):2307, 2008

LaMorte AI, Lalwani S, Diamond MP: Morbidity associated with abdominal myomectomy. Obstet Gynecol 82:897, 1993

Landman J, Kerbl K, Rehman J, et al: Evaluation of a vessel sealing system, bipolar electrosurgery, harmonic scalpel, titanium clips, endoscopic gastrointestinal anastomosis vascular staples and sutures for arterial and venous ligation in a porcine model. J Urol 169(2):697, 2003

Lasmar RB, Barrozo PR, Dias R, et al: Submucous myomas: a new presurgical classification to evaluate the viability of hysteroscopic surgical treatment—preliminary report. J Minim Invasive Gynecol 12(4):308, 2005

Lasmar RB, Xinmei Z, Indman PD, et al: Feasibility of a new system of classification of submucous myomas: a multicenter study. Fertil Steril 95(6):2073, 2011

Lee CK, Hansen SL: Management of acute wounds. Surg Clin North Am 89(3):659, 2009

Lethaby A, Hickey M: Endometrial destruction techniques for heavy menstrual bleeding: a Cochrane review. Hum Reprod 17:2795, 2002

Levy B, Levie MD, Childers ME: A summary of reported pregnancies after hysteroscopic sterilization. J Minim Invasive Gynecol 14(3):271, 2007

Liu CD, McFadden DW: Laparoscopic port sites do not require fascial closure when nonbladed trocars are used. Am Surg 66(9):853, 2000

Loffer FD: Improving results of hysteroscopic submucosal myomectomy for menorrhagia by concomitant endometrial ablation. J Minim Invasive Gynecol 12(3):254, 2005

Magos A, Chapman L: Hysteroscopic tubal sterilization. Obstet Gynecol Clin North Am 31:705, 2004

Malacova E, Kemp A, Hart R, et al: Long-term risk of ectopic pregnancy varies by method of tubal sterilization: a whole-population study. Fertil Steril 101(3):728, 2014

Malkawi HY, Qublan HS: Laparoscopic ovarian drilling in the treatment of polycystic ovary syndrome: how many punctures per ovary are needed to improve the reproductive outcome? J Obstet Gynaecol Res 31:115, 2005

Marana R, Busacca M, Zupi E, et al: Laparoscopically assisted vaginal hysterectomy versus total abdominal hysterectomy: a prospective, randomized, multicenter study. Am J Obstet Gynecol 180:270, 1999

Marana R, Luciano AA, Muzii L, et al: Reproductive outcome after ovarian surgery: suturing versus nonsuturing of the ovarian cortex. J Gynecol Surg 7:155, 1991

Mazdisnian F, Palmieri A, Hakakha B, et al: Office microlaparoscopy for female sterilization under local anesthesia: a cost and clinical analysis. J Reprod Med 47:97, 2002

McCausland AM, McCausland VM: Frequency of symptomatic cornual hematometra and postablation tubal sterilization syndrome after total rollerball endometrial ablation: a 10-year follow-up. Am J Obstet Gynecol 186(6):1274, 2002

Mercorio F, Mercorio A, Di Spiezio Sardo A, et al: Evaluation of ovarian adhesion formation after laparoscopic ovarian drilling by second-look minilaparoscopy. Fertil Steril 89(5):1229, 2008

Milad MP, Sokol E: Laparoscopic morcellator-related injuries. J Am Assoc Gynecol Laparosc 10:383, 2003

Mosesson MW: The roles of fibrinogen and fibrin in hemostasis and thrombosis. Semin Hematol 29(3):177, 1992

Muzii L, Bianchi A, Croce C, et al: Laparoscopic excision of ovarian cysts: is the stripping technique a tissue-sparing procedure? Fertil Steril 77:609, 2002

Naether OG, Fischer R, Weise HC, et al: Laparoscopic electrocoagulation of the ovarian surface in infertile patients with polycystic ovarian disease. Fertil Steril 60:88, 1993

Ngai SW, Chan YM, Ho PC: The use of misoprostol prior to hysteroscopy in postmenopausal women. Hum Reprod 16:1486, 2001

Ngai SW, Chan YM, Liu KL, et al: Oral misoprostol for cervical priming in non-pregnant women. Hum Reprod 12(11):2373, 1997

Nieboer TE, Johnson N, Lethaby A, et al: Surgical approach to hysterectomy for benign gynaecological disease. Cochrane Database Syst Rev 3:CD003677, 2009

Oehler MK, Rees MC: Menorrhagia: an update. Acta Obstet Gynaecol Scand 82:405, 2003

Okaro EO, Jones KD, Sutton C: Long term outcome following laparoscopic supracervical hysterectomy. BJOG 108:1017, 2001

Oppegaard KS, Nesheim BI, Istre O, et al: Comparison of self-administered vaginal misoprostol versus placebo for cervical ripening prior to operative hysteroscopy using a sequential trial design. BJOG 115(5):663, 2008

Orhue AA, Aziken ME, Igbefoh JO: A comparison of two adjunctive treatments for intrauterine adhesions following lysis. Int J Gynaecol Obstet 82:49, 2003

Overton C, Hargreaves J, Maresh M: A national survey of the complications of endometrial destruction for menstrual disorders: the MISTLETOE study (Minimally invasive surgical techniques—Laser, endothermal or endoresection). BJOG 104:1351, 1997

Pabuccu R, Atay V, Orhon E, et al: Hysteroscopic treatment of intrauterine adhesions is safe and effective in the restoration of normal menstruation and fertility. Fertil Steril 68:1141, 1997

Pabuccu R, Onalan G, Kaya C, et al: Efficiency and pregnancy outcome of serial intrauterine device-guided hysteroscopic adhesiolysis of intrauterine synechiae. Fertil Steril 90(5):1973, 2008

Palter SF: Microlaparoscopy under local anesthesia and conscious pain mapping for the diagnosis and management of pelvic pain. Curr Opin Obstet Gynecol 11:387, 1999

Papaioannou S, Afnan M, Girling AJ, et al: Diagnostic and therapeutic value of selective salpingography and tubal catheterization in an unselected infertile population. Fertil Steril 79:613, 2003

Parker WH: Total laparoscopic hysterectomy and laparoscopic supracervical hysterectomy. Obstet Gynecol Clin North Am 31:523, 2004

Parker WH, Einarsson J, Istre O, et al: Risk factors for uterine rupture after laparoscopic myomectomy. J Minim Invasive Gynecol 17(5):551, 2010

Pati S, Cullins V: Female sterilization: evidence. Obstet Gynecol Clin North Am 27:859, 2000

Penfield AJ: The Filshie clip for female sterilization: a review of world experience. Am J Obstet Gynecol 182:485, 2000

Periti P, Mazzei T, Orlandini F, et al: Comparison of the antimicrobial prophylactic efficacy of cefotaxime and cephazolin in obstetric and gynaecological surgery: a randomised multi-centre study. Drugs 35:133, 1988

Peterson HB, Xia Z, Hughes JM, et al: The risk of pregnancy after tubal sterilization: findings from the U.S. Collaborative Review of Sterilization. Am J Obstet Gynecol 174:1161, 1996

Peterson HB, Xia Z, Wilcox LS, et al: Pregnancy after tubal sterilization with bipolar electrocoagulation. U.S. Collaborative Review of Sterilization Working Group. Obstet Gynecol 94:163, 1999

Phillips DR, Nathanson HG, Milim SJ, et al: The effect of dilute vasopressin solution on the force needed for cervical dilatation: a randomized controlled trial. Obstet Gynecol 89(4):507, 1997

Prapas Y, Kalogiannidis I, Prapas N: Laparoscopy vs laparoscopically assisted myomectomy in the management of uterine myomas: a prospective study. Am J Obstet Gynecol 200(2):144.e1, 2009

Preutthipan S, Herabutya Y: Vaginal misoprostol for cervical priming before operative hysteroscopy: a randomized, controlled trial. Obstet Gynecol 96:890, 2000

Rybak EA, Polotsky AJ, Woreta T, et al: Explained compared with unexplained fever in postoperative myomectomy and hysterectomy patients. Obstet Gynecol 111(5):1137, 2008

Sabbah R, Desaulniers G: Use of the NovaSure Impedance Controlled Endometrial Ablation System in patients with intracavitary disease: 12-month follow-up results of a prospective, single-arm clinical study. J Minim Invasive Gynecol 13:467, 2006

Sambrook AM, Jack SA, Cooper KG: Outpatient microwave endometrial ablation: 5-year follow-up of a randomised controlled trial without endometrial preparation versus standard day surgery with endometrial preparation. BJOG 117(4):493, 2010

Sarmini OR, Lefholz K, Froeschke HP: A comparison of laparoscopic supracervical hysterectomy and total abdominal hysterectomy outcomes. J Minim Invasive Gynecol 12(2):121, 2005

Sawin SW, Pilevsky ND, Berlin JA, et al: Comparability of perioperative morbidity between abdominal myomectomy and hysterectomy for women with uterine leiomyomas. Am J Obstet Gynecol 183:1448, 2000

Schindlbeck C, Klauser K, Dian D, et al: Comparison of total laparoscopic, vaginal and abdominal hysterectomy. Arch Gynecol Obstet 277(4):331, 2008

Schmidt T, Eren Y, Breidenbach M: Modifications of laparoscopic supracervical hysterectomy technique significantly reduce postoperative spotting. J Minim Invasive Gynecol 18, 81, 2011

Schytte T, Soerensen JA, Hauge B, et al: Preoperative transcervical analgesia for laparoscopic sterilization with Filshie clips: a double-blind, randomized trial. Acta Obstet Gynaecol Scand 82:57, 2003

Seifer DB: Persistent ectopic pregnancy: an argument for heightened vigilance and patient compliance. Fertil Steril 68:402, 1997

Sharp HT: Assessment of new technology in the treatment of idiopathic menorrhagia and uterine leiomyomata. Obstet Gynecol 108(4):990, 2006

Sizzi O, Rossetti A, Malzoni M, et al: Italian multicenter study on complications of laparoscopic myomectomy. J Minim Invasive Gynecol (4): 453, 2007

Smaldone MC, Gibbons EP, Jackman SV: Laparoscopic nephrectomy using the EnSeal Tissue Sealing and Hemostasis System: successful therapeutic application of nanotechnology. JSLS 12(2):213, 2008

Soderstrom RM, Levy BS, Engel T: Reducing bipolar sterilization failures. Obstet Gynecol 74:60, 1989

Soysal ME, Soysal SK, Vicdan K: Thermal balloon ablation in myoma-induced menorrhagia under local anesthesia. Gynecol Obstet Invest 51:128, 2001

Spandorfer SD, Sawin SW, Benjamin I, et al: Postoperative day 1 serum human chorionic gonadotropin level as a predictor of persistent ectopic pregnancy after conservative surgical management. Fertil Steril 68:430, 1997

Strowitzki T, von Wolff M: Laparoscopic ovarian drilling (LOD) in patients with polycystic ovary syndrome (PCOS): an alternative approach to medical treatment? Gynecol Surg 2:71, 2005

Tan BL, Chong HC, Tay EH: Migrating Filshie clip. Aust N Z J Obstet Gynaecol 44:583, 2004

Toaff R, Toaff ME, Peyser MR: Infertility following wedge resection of the ovaries. Am J Obstet Gynecol 124:92, 1976

Tulandi T, Beique F, Kimia M: Pulmonary edema: a complication of local injection of vasopressin at laparoscopy. Fertil Steril 66:478, 1996

Tulandi T, Guralnick M: Treatment of tubal ectopic pregnancy by salpingotomy with or without tubal suturing and salpingectomy. Fertil Steril 55:53, 1991

Tulandi T, Murray C, Guralnick M: Adhesion formation and reproductive outcome after myomectomy and second-look laparoscopy. Obstet Gynecol 82:213, 1993

Ubeda A, Labastida R, Dexeus S: Essure: a new device for hysteroscopic tubal sterilization in an outpatient setting. Fertil Steril 82:196, 2004

Valle RF: Intrauterine adhesion. In Bieber EJ, Loffer FD (eds): Hysteroscopy, Resectoscopy, and Endometrial Ablation. Boca Raton, Parthenon Publishing Group, 2003, p 93

Vancaillie TG: Electrocoagulation of the endometrium with the ball-end resectoscope. Obstet Gynecol 74:425, 1989

van der Stege JG, van Beek JJ: Problems related to the cervical stump at follow-up in laparoscopic supracervical hysterectomy. JSLS 3(1):5, 1999

Varma R, Soneja H, Samuel N, et al: Outpatient Thermachoice endometrial balloon ablation:

long-term, prognostic and quality-of-life measures. Gynecol Obstet Invest 70(3):145, 2010

Vercellini P, Zaina B, Yaylayan L, et al: Hysteroscopic myomectomy: long-term effects on menstrual pattern and fertility. Obstet Gynecol 94:341, 1999

Vilos GA: Hysteroscopic and nonhysteroscopic endometrial ablation. Obstet Gynecol Clin North Am 31:687, 2004

Visco AG, Advincula AP: Robotic gynecologic surgery. Obstet Gynecol 112(6):1369, 2008

Walsh CA, Sherwin JR, Slack M: Vaginal evisceration following total laparoscopic hysterectomy: case report and review of the literature. Aust N Z J Obstet Gynaecol 47(6):516, 2007

Walsh CA, Walsh SR, Tang TY, et al: Total abdominal hysterectomy versus total laparoscopic hysterectomy for benign disease: a meta-analysis. Eur J Obstet Gynecol Reprod Biol 144(1):3, 2009

Wamsteker K, Emanuel MH, de Kruif JH: Transcervical hysteroscopic resection of submucous fibroids for abnormal uterine bleeding: results regarding the degree of intramural extension. Obstet Gynecol 82:736, 1993

Wen KC, Chen YJ, Sung PL, et al: Comparing uterine fibroids treated by myomectomy through traditional laparotomy and 2 modified approaches: ultraminilaparotomy and laparoscopically assisted ultraminilaparotomy. Am J Obstet Gynecol 202(2):144.e1, 2010

Wenger JM, Spinosa JP, Roche B, et al: An efficient and safe procedure for laparoscopic supracervical hysterectomy. J Gynecol Surg 21(4): 155, 2005

Wiseman DM, Trout JR, Franklin RR, et al: Metaanalysis of the safety and efficacy of an adhesion barrier (Interceed TC7) in laparotomy. J Reprod Med 44(4):325, 1999

Wiskind AK, Toledo AA, Dudley AG, et al: Adhesion formation after ovarian wound repair in New Zealand White rabbits: a comparison of ovarian microsurgical closure with ovarian nonclosure. Am J Obstet Gynecol 163:1674, 1990

Wrigley LC, Howard FM, Gabel D: Transcervical or intraperitoneal analgesia for laparoscopic tubal sterilization: a randomized, controlled trial. Obstet Gynecol 96:895, 2000

Zikopoulos KA, Kolibianakis EM, Platteau P, et al: Live delivery rates in subfertile women with Asherman's syndrome after hysteroscopic adhesiolysis using the resectoscope or the VersaPoint system. Reprod Biomed Online 8:720, 2004

Diagnostic and Operative Cystoscopy and Urethroscopy

During gynecologic surgery, the lower urinary tract may be injured. Thus, diagnostic cystoscopic evaluation is often warranted following procedures in which the bladder and ureters have been placed at risk. Additionally, operative cystoscopy is within the scope of many gynecologists for the passage of ureteral stents, lesion biopsy, and foreign-body removal. Of these, ureteral stenting may be indicated to delineate the ureter's course during cases with abnormal pelvic anatomy or to assess ureteral patency following gynecologic surgery.

Rigid and flexible cystoscopes are available, although in gynecology, a rigid scope is typically used. A cystoscope is composed of an outer sheath, bridge, endoscope, and obturator. The sheath contains one port for fluid infusion and a second port for fluid egress. For office cystoscopy, a sheath measuring 17F affords greater comfort. However, for operative cases, a 21F or wider-diameter cystoscope is preferred to allow rapid fluid infusion and easier instrument and stent passage. The sheath's end tapers, and in women- with a narrow urethral meatus, an obturator can be placed inside the sheath to create a rounded tip for smooth introduction. In selected instances, gentle dilation of the external urethral opening using narrow cervical dilators is needed prior to sheath introduction. The next piece,

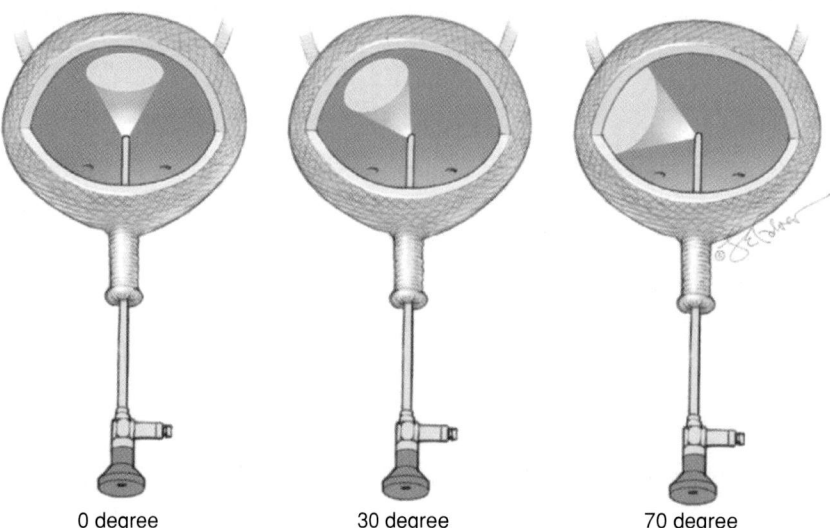

0 degree   30 degree   70 degree

FIGURE 45-1.1 Cystoscopic optical views.

the bridge, attaches to the proximal portion of the sheath and allows coupling between the endoscope and sheath. Additional ports are present on the bridge and are generally used to introduce stents or instruments.

Several endoscope viewing angles are available and include 0-, 30-, and 70-degree optical views (Fig. 45-1.1). Zero-degree endoscopes are used for urethroscopy. For cystoscopy, a 70-degree endoscope is superior for providing the most comprehensive view of the lateral, anterior, and posterior walls; trigone; and ureteral orifices. To achieve a comparable view, a 30-degree endoscope requires additional manipulation. However, a 30-degree endoscope does offer advantages and allows surgeons greater flexibility as it can be used for either urethroscopy or cystoscopy during a given examination. For operative cystoscopic cases in which instruments are passed down the sheath, a 30-degree endoscope should be used because with 0- and 70-degree endoscopes, operative instruments generally lie outside the field of view.

PREOPERATIVE

Prior to office cystoscopy, urinary tract infection (UTI) is excluded to avoid upper tract infection. If diagnostic cystoscopy is performed properly, complications are rare. Of these, infection is the most common and results from the significant incidence of bacteriuria following cystoscopy.

INTRAOPERATIVE

Surgical Steps

❶ **Anesthesia and Patient Positioning.** Cystoscopy may be performed in low or standard lithotomy position with the legs positioned in stirrups. For office cystoscopy, 2-percent lidocaine jelly is instilled into the urethra 5 to 10 minutes prior to cystoscope insertion. For operative procedures, an additional 50 mL of 4-percent lidocaine solution may be instilled via catheter into the bladder. The perineum and urethral meatus are surgically prepared prior to urethral manipulation.

❷ **Distention Media.** The bladder must be adequately distended to fully visualize all surfaces, and for diagnostic purposes, saline or sterile water is suitable. To ensure adequate medium flow, an infusion bag is elevated significantly above the level of the symphysis. The volume needed may vary but is reached when bladder walls are not collapsing inward. Overdistending the bladder is also avoided as it may result in temporary urinary retention. If the bladder is distended beyond its capacity, excess fluid will leak out the urethral meatus and around the cystoscope rather than rupturing the bladder, which is rare.

❸ **Indigo Carmine.** If intraoperative cystoscopy is performed to document ureteral patency, ½ to 1 ampule of indigo carmine is administered intravenously prior to the procedure to aid visualization of urine jets. Less commonly, methylene blue may be used instead but carries the risk of methemoglobinemia in patients with glucose-6-phosphate dehydrogenase deficiency. However, its use may increase given current shortages of indigo carmine (American Urogynecologic Society, 2014a).

❹ **Cystoscopy.** The anterior urethral wall is sensitive, and discomfort may result if the sheath's tapered edge is directed anteriorly. Thus, the sheath is inserted into the urethral meatus with the bevel directed posteriorly. Immediately following insertion into the external urethral opening, medium flow is begun.

The cystoscope is advanced toward the bladder under direct visualization. Often, in women with anterior wall prolapse, the urethra slopes downward, and the scope tip is similarly directed. During the procedure, the cystoscope can be steadied with one hand holding the sheath near the urethral meatus (Fig. 45-1.2).

❺ **Bladder Inspection.** Upon entry into the bladder, the cystoscope is slowly withdrawn until the bladder neck is identified. The cystoscope is then advanced and rotated 180 degrees so that the light-source cable is pointing down. In this position, an air bubble is noted at the dome, which provides orientation for the remainder of the cystoscopic examination. When a 70- or 30-degree scope is used, the cystoscope is angled upward to view this bubble. To maintain orientation during rotation, the camera is held static while the light cord and cystoscope are rotated (Fig. 45-1.3).

As the distended bladder assumes a spherical shape, it is systematically inspected on each side from apex to internal urethral opening. First, to view the entire left side of the bladder, the cystoscope and light cable are rotated

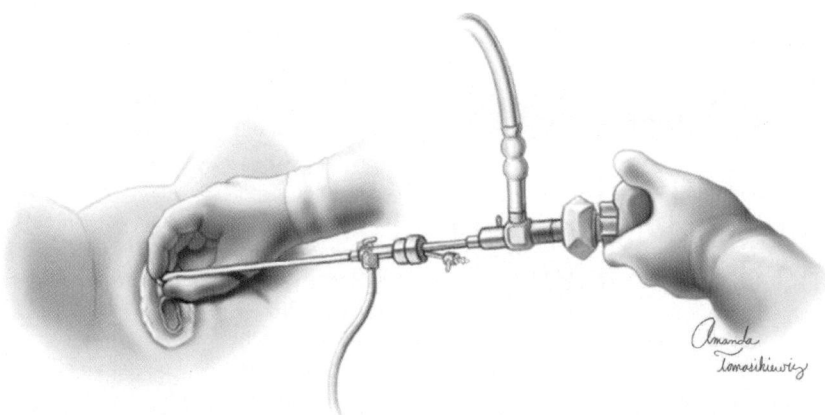

FIGURE 45-1.2 Cystoscope steadied during procedure.

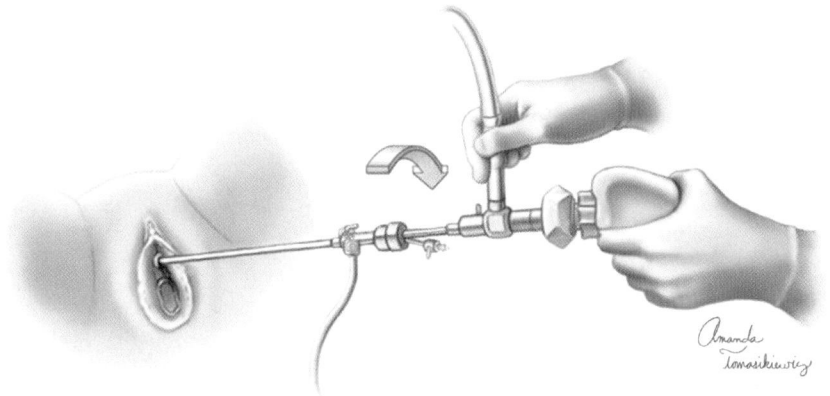

FIGURE 45-1.3 Orientation during cystoscopy is maintained by holding the camera steady while the light cord and cystoscope are rotated.

approximately 90 degrees in a clockwise fashion. The surgeon's left hand is used to prevent awkward hand crossing. To examine the bladder wall from 12 to 3 o'clock positions, the cystoscope is initially angled upward and then pans down to the 3 o'clock position, at which point the scope is parallel to the floor. Next, inspection from 3 to 6 o'clock requires gradual downward angling of the cystoscope. The left ureteral orifice is generally found at the 5 o'clock position, approximately 3 to 4 cm proximal to the internal urethral opening. During bladder inspection, especially the base or posterior wall, digital elevation of the anterior vaginal wall to lift the bladder floor and orifices to a more anatomically correct position is beneficial if pelvic organ prolapse is present. Moreover, accentuated angling may be needed. Once the left orifice is noted, further subtle clockwise rotation of the cystoscope along the interureteric ridge permits isolation of the right ureteral orifice.

The cystoscope is again rotated so that the light-source cable is again pointing downward and the bubble at the dome is again identified. For the right side, counterclockwise movement of the cystoscope and light cord with the surgeon's right hand averts awkward hand crossing. The right wall of the bladder is then similarly examined.

While horizontal to the floor, the cystoscope is withdrawn to the bladder neck and then angled downward to provide a second view of the trigone and both ureteral orifices and to document ureteral patency. Brisk urine flow, with or without indigo carmine, should be seen from each orifice. Peristalsis of the ureteral orifice alone, without flow, is insufficient to document patency. Moreover, scant flow may indicate partial ureteral obstruction and merits further evaluation.

The average time to efflux approximates 10 minutes but can be longer. After 20 minutes, absent jets bilaterally more often reflect hypovolemia and resolve with fluid bolus.

Following this bolus, 10 to 20 mg of furosemide (Lasix) can be added as needed to promote diuresis. Underlying renal disease may also delay efflux. During inspection, a unilateral jet is more concerning for ureteral injury. To evaluate, the surgeon can attempt to thread a stent through the ureteral orifice and into the ureter, as described in Step 8. Repair of ureteral injury is described in Chapter 40 (p. 868).

❻ **Operative Cystoscopy.** For this procedure, the operative instrument (biopsy or grasping forceps or scissors) is introduced through the operating port, until viewed at the end of the cystoscope. Prior to instrument insertion, a rubber adapter cap is positioned over the operating port to create a watertight seal with the operative instrument. Once in view, the instrument and cystoscope are moved together as a unit toward the area of interest.

❼ **Ureteral Stenting.** Ureteral stents may be placed at several junctures during surgery. They may be inserted at the beginning of surgery and left through its duration to define anatomy in cases in which the ureter is at high surgical risk of injury. Alternatively, they may be threaded intraoperatively to document ureteral patency and exclude injury. Finally, ureteral stents may be positioned and left in place at the conclusion of surgery if ureteral injury is suspected or identified. Duration of postoperative stenting is variable and based on indications.

Ureteral stents are available in various sizes, and those ranging from 4 to 7 F are commonly used. Stents vary in length from 20 to 30 cm, and a 24-cm length is appropriate for most adults. Generally, open-ended or whistle-tip stents are used to delineate anatomy or to exclude obstruction. Double- or single-pigtail stents are used in situations that require prolonged ureteral drainage.

❽ **To Exclude Ureteral Obstruction.** A 4F to 6F open-ended or whistle-tip stent is threaded through the operating channel of a 30-degree cystoscope and into the field of view. By advancing both the stent and cystoscope toward the orifice, the stent is passed into the ureteral orifice. After the stent has entered the opening, it is manually threaded and advanced. Alternatively, an Albarrán bridge may be used. This specialized bridging sheath allows deflection and guidance of a stent into an orifice.

Once inserted, a stent is advanced past the level of suspected obstruction. If a stent threads easily, obstruction is excluded. In most gynecologic surgery, this would not be higher than the pelvic brim, which should be 12 to 15 cm from the ureteral orifice in adults. When passing a stent, undue pressure is avoided during advancement to avoid ureteral perforation. Efflux should be documented after stent removal.

If ureteral transection or stricture is suspected from the above steps, a cone-tip ureteral catheter is inserted, and dye is injected into the distal ureter to locate extravasation or point of narrowing. This is done intraoperatively with fluoroscopic guidance. If dye flows to the renal pelvis easily and no extravasation noted, ureteral injury is unlikely.

If gross blood issues from an orifice prior to ureteral manipulation, the ureter may be partially transected. Even if good efflux is noted, many insert and maintain a double-J stent for approximately 4 weeks. In such cases, a computed tomography (CT) urogram or renal sonogram is completed 4 to 12 weeks after stent removal to exclude stricture.

After the above interrogations, absent efflux from one orifice may uncommonly reflect a long-standing unilateral nonfunctioning kidney. For this, postoperative CT and nuclear scan can be selected.

❾ **To Delineate Anatomy.** For this purpose, the stent is advanced until resistance is met, which indicates that the renal pelvis has been reached. The stent is tied securely to the transurethral catheter and drains into the cystoscopy drape. At the conclusion of surgery, the stent is removed.

❿ **Ureteral Stenting.** In cases in which a ureteral stent is required postoperatively, a double-pigtail stent is used. The proximal coil of the stent prevents renal pelvis injury, and the distal coil secures placement in the bladder.

For placement, a guide wire is first threaded into the ureteral orifice and passed to the renal pelvis. The pigtail stent is then placed over the guide wire and advanced by a pusher device until the distal end enters the bladder. The guide wire is removed, allowing the ends to coil in the renal pelvis and bladder, respectively. Correct upper coil positioning is confirmed intraoperatively using fluoroscopy or plain film radiograph. Stents are usually kept for 2 to 8 weeks depending on the injury identified or suspected. They are generally removed in the office with cystoscopic guidance.

⓫ Biopsy and Foreign Body Removal.
Mucosal lesions can be biopsied with minimal risk or discomfort to the patient. A biopsy instrument is introduced into the cystoscope's operating port and brought into the operative field. With the instrument in view, the cystoscope is moved directly to the lesion. Biopsy is performed, and the cystoscope and instrument are withdrawn through the urethra together. In this way, a biopsy specimen is not pulled through the sheath and possibly lost. Bleeding is usually minor and will stop by itself. For brisk bleeding, electrosurgical coagulation can be used if a nonconducting solution was selected as the distention medium. As described in Chapter 41 (p. 903), electrolyte solutions such as saline cannot be used with monopolar electrosurgery. These solutions conduct current, thus dissipating the energy and thereby rendering the instrument useless.

Foreign bodies, such as stones, are removed using the same technique as biopsy. The instrument is used to grasp the foreign body and then removed together with the cystoscope.

⓬ Suprapubic Teloscopy.
This is a technique used to visualize the bladder through an abdominal approach. We have found suprapubic teloscopy to be valuable when the ureters must be assessed during a difficult cesarean delivery or during a laparotomy in which a woman has not been positioned to allow easy cystoscopic access to the urethra.

The bladder is distended using the transurethral Foley catheter until the bladder wall is tense. A wide purse-string using 2-0 gauge absorbable suture is then placed

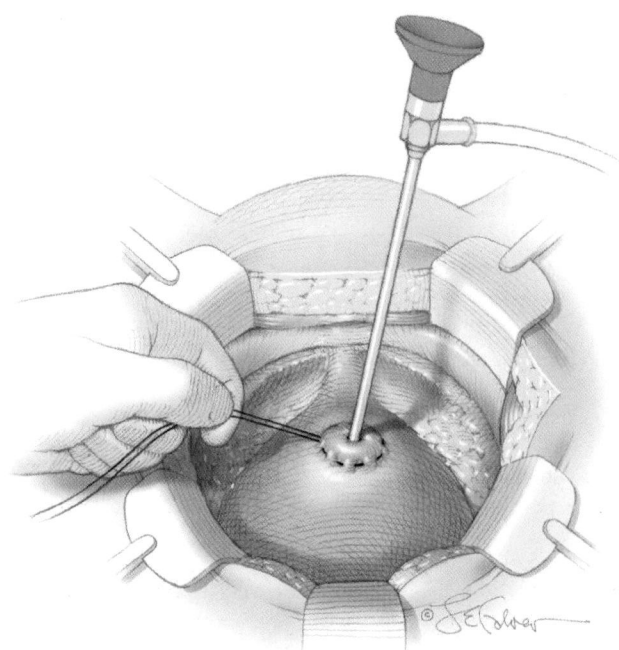

FIGURE 45-1.4 Suprapubic teloscopy.

at the bladder dome, taking deep bites into the bladder muscularis (Fig. 45-1.4). The two suture ends are elevated but held loosely. A small stab incision is then made in the purse-string's center, and a cystoscope is introduced into the bladder. This incision is preferably made in the retropubic or extraperitoneal portion of the bladder dome to minimize risk of fistula formation. For suprapubic teloscopy, a 30-degree cystoscope is most effective. The two suture ends are then pulled up and held tightly to prevent the escape of distending fluid. To allow visualization of the trigone and ureteral orifices, the Foley bulb is deflated but left in place. Indigo carmine or methylene blue is given if necessary to document ureteral efflux. If the ureteral orifices still cannot be visualized, the bladder incision is extended inferiorly into the retropubic portion to allow direct visualization. At the conclusion

of teloscopy, the cystoscope is removed, and the purse-string suture is tied, closing the cystotomy.

POSTOPERATIVE

Office cystoscopy does not require specific postoperative management except for prophylactic antibiotics to cover common urinary tract pathogens. At our institution, we prescribe a single perioperative dose. With operative cystoscopy, hematuria may develop, but it generally clears within a few days and is considered significant only if associated with symptomatic anemia.

With long-term ureteral stenting, additional complications may include ureteral spasm, which typically presents as back pain. Stone formation and stent fragmentation are less common but can occur if length of catheterization exceeds 8 weeks.

Burch Colposuspension

Abdominal antiincontinence procedures attempt to correct stress urinary incontinence (SUI) by stabilizing the anterior vaginal wall and urethrovesical junction in a retropubic location. Specifically, the Burch procedure, also known as *retropubic urethropexy*, uses the strength of the iliopectineal ligament (Cooper ligament) to stabilize the anterior vaginal wall and anchor the wall to the musculoskeletal framework of the pelvis (Fig. 38-24, p. 817).

The Burch colposuspension is usually performed through a Pfannenstiel or Cherney incision. In the past 20 years, some have introduced laparoscopic approaches that use suture or mesh to affix the paravaginal tissues to Cooper ligament (Ankardal, 2004; Zullo, 2004). Compared with open Burch colposuspension, laparoscopic approaches offer similar postoperative rates of subjective cure, despite some evidence for poorer objective outcomes (Carey, 2006; Dean, 2006). Longer-term results will also define its role.

PREOPERATIVE

Patient Evaluation

Prior to surgery, patients undergo complete urogynecologic evaluation. Although not required for uncomplicated demonstrable SUI, urodynamic testing can help differentiate stress and urgency incontinence and assess bladder capacity and voiding patterns (Chap. 23, p. 526).

Many women with SUI may also have associated pelvic organ prolapse. For this reason, other indicated pelvic reconstructive surgeries commonly accompany Burch colposuspension. A required hysterectomy does not appear to improve or worsen Burch procedure success rates (Bai, 2004; Meltomaa, 2001).

Consent

For most women with SUI, Burch colposuspension offers a safe, effective long-term treatment for incontinence. In one systematic review, overall continence rates ranged from 85 to 90 percent at 1 year and declined to 70 percent by 5 years (Lapitan, 2012). Surgical risks compare similarly with other surgeries for SUI (Green, 2005; Lapitan, 2003). Intraoperative complications are rare and may include ureteral injury, bladder or urethral

perforation, and hemorrhage (Galloway, 1987; Ladwig, 2004).

Complications following surgery, however, are not uncommon and may include urinary tract or wound infection, voiding dysfunction, de novo urinary urgency, and pelvic organ prolapse—primarily enterocele formation (Alcalay, 1995; Demirci, 2000, 2001; Norton, 2006). Overcorrection of the urethrovesical angle has been suggested as a cause of these long-term urinary and prolapse complications.

Patient Preparation

The American College of Obstetricians and Gynecologists (2014) recommends antibiotic prophylaxis prior to urogynecologic surgery, and appropriate choices mirror those for hysterectomy (Table 39-6, p. 835). For all patients undergoing major gynecologic surgery, thromboprophylaxis is also recommended (Table 39-8, p. 836). Bowel preparation is based on surgeon preference and on concurrent surgeries planned.

INTRAOPERATIVE

Surgical Steps

❶ Anesthesia and Patient Positioning. Burch colposuspension may be performed under general or regional anesthesia as an

inpatient procedure. The patient is placed supine with legs in booted support stirrups in low lithotomy position. The abdomen and vagina are surgically prepared, and a Foley catheter is inserted.

❷ Abdominal Incision. A low Pfannenstiel or Cherney incision is performed (Section 43-2, p. 929). Surgery in the space of Retzius (retropubic space) is easier to accomplish if the incision is placed low on the abdomen, approximately 1 cm above the upper border of the pubic symphysis. If hysterectomy, culdoplasty, or other intraperitoneal procedure is planned, the peritoneum is entered and concurrent surgery completed prior to colposuspension. If the procedure is done in isolation, fascia of the anterior abdominal wall muscles and then transversalis fascia are incised, but entry into the peritoneal cavity is not required to reach the retropubic space.

❸ Entry into the Space of Retzius. Between the lower anterior abdominal wall peritoneum and pubic bone lies an avascular plane, that is, the space of Retzius. To enter this retropubic space, the fingers of one hand gently dissect along the cephalad surface of the pubic bone. Alternatively, gentle sponge dissection can be used to open this space (Fig. 45-2.1). Loose areolar tissue is found behind the symphysis within this space and easily separates from the bone. However,

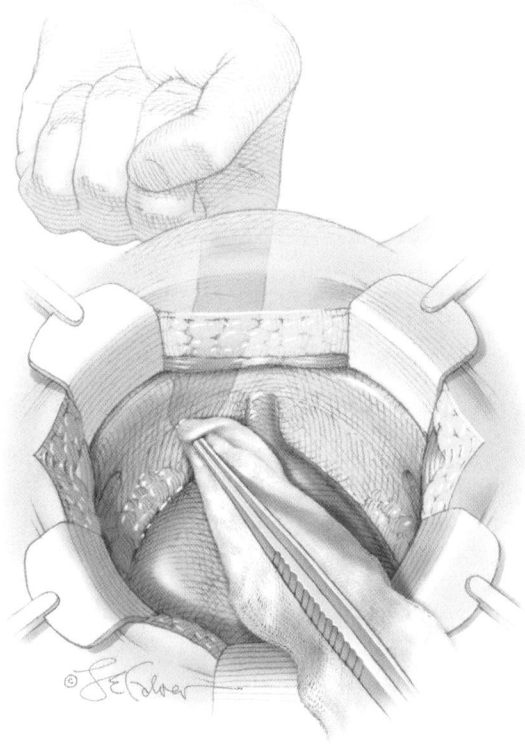

FIGURE 45-2.1 Entry into the space of Retzius.

entry into the wrong tissue plane risks bleeding and bladder injury. Direct exposure of the back of the pubic bone ensures that the correct space has been entered. The bladder and urethra are gently pulled downward and away from the pubic bone, and the space of Retzius opens.

In those with prior surgery, sharp dissection is generally required. Dissection begins with the curved tips of Metzenbaum scissors placed directly on the pubic bone and progresses dorsally until the space is exposed. Sutures can be used to control bleeding from torn paravaginal vessels.

During space of Retzius dissection, the obturator canal is identified early to avoid neurovascular injury to the obturator vessels and nerves. The canal is typically found 1.5 to 2.5 cm below the upper border of the iliopectineal ligament and approximately 5 to 7 cm from the midline of the upper border of the symphysis pubis (Drewes, 2005). Accessory obturator vessels that commonly pass over Cooper ligament to enter the obturator canal are also identified. These can be lacerated during pronounced retraction to expose Cooper ligament.

❹ Exposing the Anterior Vaginal Wall.

After opening this space, fingers of the surgeon's nondominant hand are placed intravaginally at the vagina's midlength and just behind the pubic bone. With one on each side, the finger pads straddle the urethra and push the vagina ventrally. Working within the retropubic space and beginning at the lateral borders of the urethra, gentle downward and lateral pressure against the finger pad bluntly dissects away fat. This exposes the pearly white periurethral tissue between the arcus tendineus fascia pelvis (ATFP), which lies laterally, and urethra, which is medial. If necessary, a surgeon can use a Kittner (peanut) sponge or gauze sponge stick. Importantly, to protect the delicate urethral musculature, this dissection remains lateral to the urethra.

Aggressive dissection or Burch sutures may lacerate vessels within the Santorini plexus of paravaginal veins and risk significant bleeding (Fig. 38-24, p. 817). This is easily controlled with upward pressure from the vaginal fingers. Identified vessels can then be ligated.

❺ Urethrovesical Junction.

Identifying this site aids correct suture placement. To isolate the urethrovesical junction, the surgeon's vaginal hand positions the Foley catheter balloon at the bladder neck. Undue

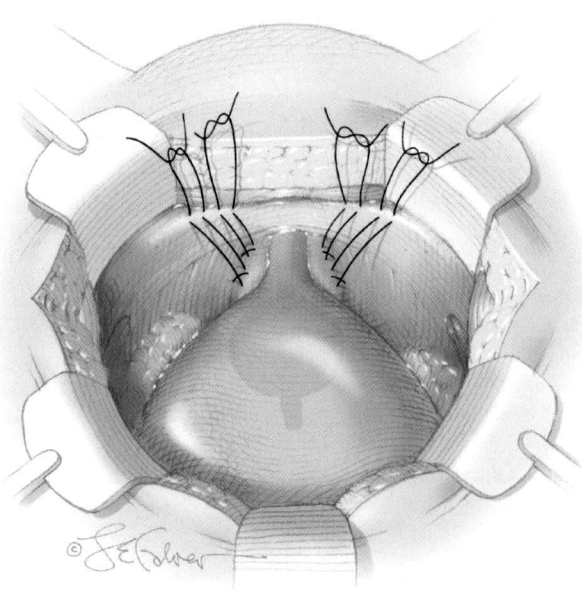

FIGURE 45-2.2 Suture placement.

tension on the Foley catheter is avoided as this can drag the bladder into the operative field and increase the risk of sutures entering the bladder.

❻ Suture Placement.

For exposure, the surgeon's vaginal finger presses upward, and the bladder neck is gently displaced by an assistant to the contralateral side by a narrow retractor. To suspend tissue, a double-armed suture of 2-0 gauge nonabsorbable material is placed laterally on each side of the urethra. A first suture is placed 1.5 to 2 cm lateral to the proximal third of the urethra. The needle point is directed toward the vaginal finger, and a thimble may be used to avoid needle-stick injury. For this suturing, a figure-of-eight stitch is used and incorporates vaginal wall while excluding epithelium. A second suture is then placed 1.5 to 2 cm lateral to the urethrovesical junction. Identical sutures are placed on the opposite side of the urethra (Fig. 45-2.2).

Both ends of each suture are then placed through the nearest point of the ipsilateral iliopectineal ligament. Slack is removed from each suture, and knots are tied above the ligament. With knot securing, suture bridges are expected, and these should stabilize but not elevate the anterior vaginal wall and urethrovesical junction. The vaginal wall is stabilized approximately at the level of the distal portion of the ATFP and not significantly higher. Greater elevation of the bladder neck risks postoperative voiding dysfunction.

❼ Cystoscopy.

Following suture ligation, cystoscopy is performed. This allows identification and removal of any errant sutures that may traverse the bladder or urethral mucosa. Moreover, it enables a surgeon to inspect the ureteral orifices and document efflux.

❽ Catheterization.

After colposuspension, the Foley catheter may remain to drain the bladder. Alternatively, a suprapubic catheter may be placed. Investigators comparing the two have found no differences in antiincontinence procedure success rates, length of hospitalization, or rates of infection. Urethral catheterization, however, was linked with a shorter duration of catheterization but also greater patient discomfort (Dunn, 2005; Theofrastous, 2002).

❾ Incision Closure.

The anterior abdominal wall peritoneum is generally closed to prevent displacement of small bowel into the retropubic space. The remaining abdominal wall incision is closed as described in Section 43-2 (p. 930).

POSTOPERATIVE

In general, recovery follows that associated with laparotomy and varies depending on concurrent surgeries and incision size. A voiding trial as described in Chapter 42 (p. 917) is performed prior to hospital discharge.

Tension-Free Vaginal Tape

The tension-free vaginal tape procedure (TVT) is the most commonly performed operation worldwide for stress urinary incontinence. The procedure is one of the most widely studied incontinence operations, and cure rates up to 17 years approximate 80 percent (Holmgren, 2005; Nilsson, 2013; Song, 2009). The TVT procedure has also become the prototype for a host of other incontinence operations, which include the TOT (transobturator tape), TVT-O (tension-free vaginal tape obturator), and single-incision midurethral slings ("minislings"). These are all considered midurethral slings (MUS) and are based on the concept that midurethral support is vital to continence.

Tension-free vaginal tape placement is indicated for SUI that is secondary to urethral hypermobility or intrinsic sphincteric deficiency (Chap. 23, p. 522). It is used for primary cases and for women who have had prior antiincontinence procedures.

During TVT, a permanent sling material is placed underneath the midurethra, traverses the periurethral tissue, passes behind the pubic bone through the space of Retzius, and exits through the anterior abdominal wall. Once positioned, tissue ingrowth ultimately holds the mesh in place. During placement, the TVT needle is directed blindly through the space of Retzius and can lacerate vessels there to create significant bleeding. A modification of the TVT, the TOT was developed to avoid hemorrhage in this space and to decrease bladder and bowel perforation risks (p. 1063). However, the TVT remains the primary standard operation for SUI.

The TVT device consists of a permanent polypropylene mesh covered with a plastic sheath that is removed after the mesh is positioned. The plastic sheath is believed to prevent bacterial contamination of the mesh as it passes through the vagina and to protect the mesh from being damaged during passage. Once these plastic sheaths are removed, the mesh remains fixed in position. The mesh is attached to two metal disposable needles that are connected to a reusable metal introducer during placement. A metal catheter guide is used to displace the urethra away from the needle during the procedure.

PREOPERATIVE

Patient Evaluation

Prior to TVT procedures, a diagnosis of SUI must be made as described in Chapter 23 (p. 523). Importantly, in some women, SUI can be occult and masked by pelvic organ prolapse that kinks and partially obstructs the urethra. Accordingly, prolapse replacement to reestablish more normal anatomy during urodynamic testing may help unmask this potential SUI. Also of note, caution is exercised in patients who are Valsalva voiders. These women void with abdominal straining rather than with detrusor contraction and urethral relaxation. Most incontinence procedures prevent leakage by closing the urethra during cough or Valsalva maneuver. Therefore, these surgeries, when performed in women who rely on the Valsalva maneuver to urinate, will often result in voiding dysfunction. This tenet applies to all midurethral sling procedures.

Consent

The consenting process for TVT should include an honest discussion of outcomes. At best, the 5-year cure rate is 85 percent, with another 10 percent significantly improved. However, some patients will develop postoperative urgency incontinence, and others will develop bothersome voiding dysfunction. Additionally, with time and aging, incontinence may recur secondary to factors not related to urethral support.

As for all antiincontinence procedures, prior to surgery, the patient is provided surgical success rates from the literature and those of the individual surgeon. Moreover, the definition of "outcome success" varies from woman to woman. For example, in a patient with severe incontinence and 20 leakage episodes per day, improvement to one leakage episode every other day would be considered successful. However, in a woman with rare leakage, it may be more difficult to achieve an outcome considered satisfactory. Therefore, patient's expectations are discussed prior to surgery.

The short-term complications of the TVT procedure include incomplete bladder emptying requiring drainage with Foley catheter or intermittent self-catheterization for several days. A small percentage of patients will develop long-term urinary retention requiring reoperation for tape division or excision (p. 1072). In these women, continence rates decrease. The TVT procedure is associated with a learning curve, and urinary retention rates decline as the number of cases a physician performs accrues. Postoperatively, vaginal mesh erosion may develop as an early or late complication. This is managed by simple excision of the piece of eroding tape and vaginal wall revision. Of note, the American Urogynecologic Society (2014b) considers the mesh used for this sling to be safe and effective.

Intraoperative complications include hemorrhage, bladder perforation, and rarely, bowel injury. Major vessels are injured in less than 1 percent of cases.

Patient Preparation

The American College of Obstetricians and Gynecologists (2014) recommends antibiotic prophylaxis prior to urogynecologic procedures, and appropriate choices mirror those for hysterectomy (Table 39-6, p. 835). For all patients undergoing major gynecologic surgery, thromboprophylaxis is recommended (Table 39-8, p. 836). Bowel preparation is based on surgeon preference and mainly on concurrent surgeries planned.

INTRAOPERATIVE

Surgical Steps

❶ **Anesthesia and Patient Positioning.** The procedure was initially described as an ambulatory surgical procedure performed under local anesthesia. However, it can also be performed with regional or general anesthesia. If performed solely, TVT in most cases is a day-surgery operation. The procedure is performed in standard lithotomy position. The vagina is surgically prepared, and an 18F Foley catheter, which allows passage of a rigid catheter guide, is inserted to assist in deflection of the urethra during needle passage.

❷ **Abdominal Incisions.** To begin, two ½-cm skin incisions are made at the level of the upper border of the symphysis, and each lies no further than 2 cm from the midline. More lateral placement risks ilioinguinal nerve injury (Geis, 2002).

❸ **Vaginal Incisions.** A midline incision is made sharply in the vaginal epithelium and superficial vaginal muscularis beginning 1 cm proximal to the external urethral opening and is extended 1.5 to 2 cm cephalad. Allis clamps are placed on the edges of the vaginal incision for traction. Using Metzenbaum scissors, bilateral periurethral tunnels are created beneath the vaginal epithelium on either side of the urethra. These tunnels extend several centimeters toward the inferior pubic rami to allow placement of the TVT needle just behind the pubic bone.

❹ **Catheter-guide Placement.** A rigid guide is placed through the 18F Foley catheter. During passage of TVT needles, a surgical assistant uses the catheter guide to deflect the urethra to the contralateral side to lower urethral injury risks.

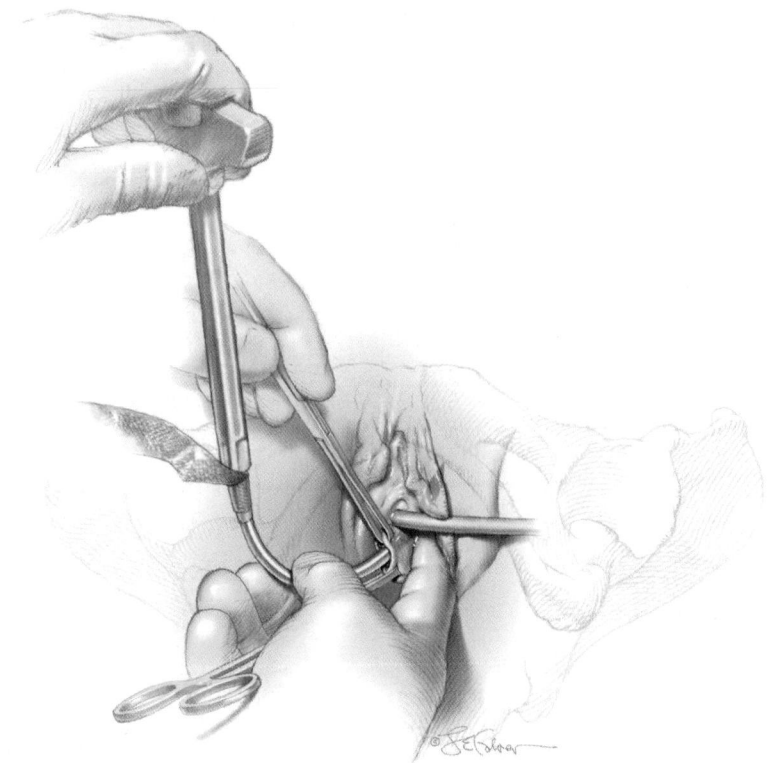

FIGURE 45-3.1 Needle placed through periurethral tunnel.

❺ Mesh Placement. The TVT needle and mesh are attached to the introducer. The needle is placed through one of the periurethral tunnels so that its point touches the front surface of the ipsilateral pubic ramus (Fig. 45-3.1). A hand placed in the vagina then carefully guides the needle around the back of the ramus. The needle is then curved upward toward the ipsilateral abdominal incision, perforates the periurethral tissue just behind the pubic bone, and enters the

retropubic space (Rahn, 2006). During this, the needle is always directly behind the pubic bone. Pressure is applied to the introducer handle with the other hand, but the vaginal hand controls the needle's direction. The handle of the introducer always remains parallel to the ground to avoid lateral excursion into major vessels and obturator nerve (Fig. 45-3.2). Additionally, after the needle passes around the pubic ramus and behind the symphysis, its tip is always directed

toward the abdominal wall incisions. The bladder may be perforated if excessive pressure is applied and if the needle is aimed cephalad rather than toward the abdominal wall (Fig. 45-3.3). Small changes in the position of the hand applying handle pressure can lead to bladder perforation.

❻ Cystourethroscopy. After the needle perforates the abdominal wall, the Foley and catheter guide are removed, and cystourethroscopy is performed with a 70-degree cystoscope. The bladder is distended with 200 to 300 mL of fluid, and inspection for cystotomy is completed. Generally, perforation will be obvious, and the TVT needle will be seen entering and exiting the bladder. In this situation, the needle is removed and redirected, and correct placement is confirmed by cystoscopy. Inspection of the urethra is also essential and can be performed with the same 70-degree angle scope. Alternatively, a 0-degree or 30-degree endoscope may be used. Iatrogenic trocar bladder injury, if identified intraoperatively does not appear to influence continence outcomes or increase postoperative voiding dysfunction or infection rates (Zyczynski, 2014).

In contrast to bladder perforation, urethral perforation theoretically carries a risk of urethrovaginal fistula. Thus, if urethral perforation is noted, most surgeons abort the procedure and postpone until several months later.

After cystoscopy, the introducer is unscrewed from the needle. The needle is brought through the abdominal wall. The needle is then cut from the mesh, and the mesh is held with a hemostat. Next, the other TVT needle is attached to the introducer and is placed on the other side of the urethra in a similar fashion. Cystourethroscopy is then repeated.

❼ Setting Mesh Position. A hemostat or similar instrument is placed between the suburethral tissue and the tape to act as a spacer and create distance between the mesh and urethra (Fig. 45-3.4). This spacing avoids excessive mesh tension and lowers the risk for postoperative urinary retention and voiding dysfunction.

Prior to sheath removal, the vaginal sulci are inspected to exclude perforation of the vaginal epithelium occurring during needle guidance. If perforated mesh is seen, the tape is removed, and the TVT needle is again passed through a newly created periurethral tunnel that lies slightly medial to the original. The vaginal perforation defect is repaired with one or two simple interrupted delayed-absorbable sutures.

❽ Sheath Removal. Once the tape is satisfactorily positioned, an assistant then removes the plastic covering around the

A   **B**

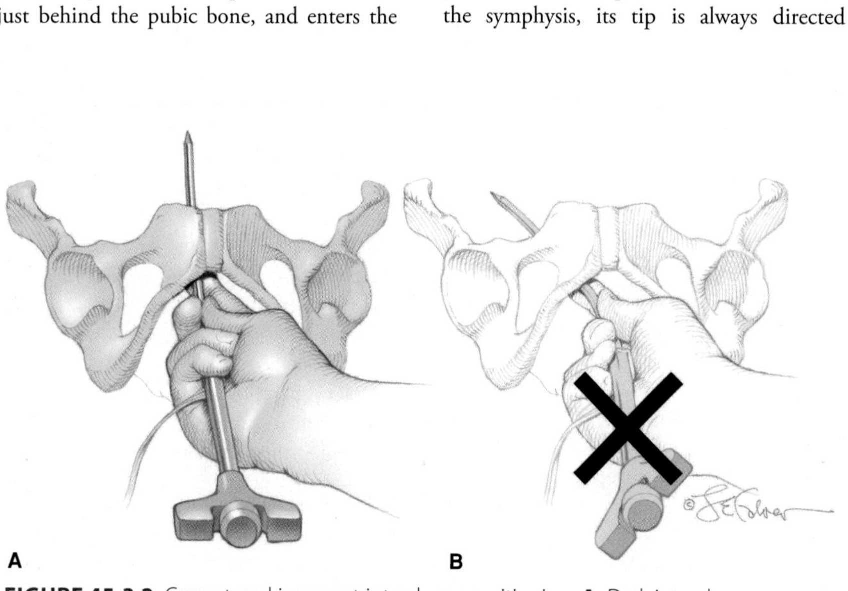

FIGURE 45-3.2 Correct and incorrect introducer positioning. **A.** Dark introducer, correct position. The tip is directed in the midline to a position behind the pubic bone. The handle is parallel to the ground. **B.** White introducer, incorrect position. The tip is directed laterally.

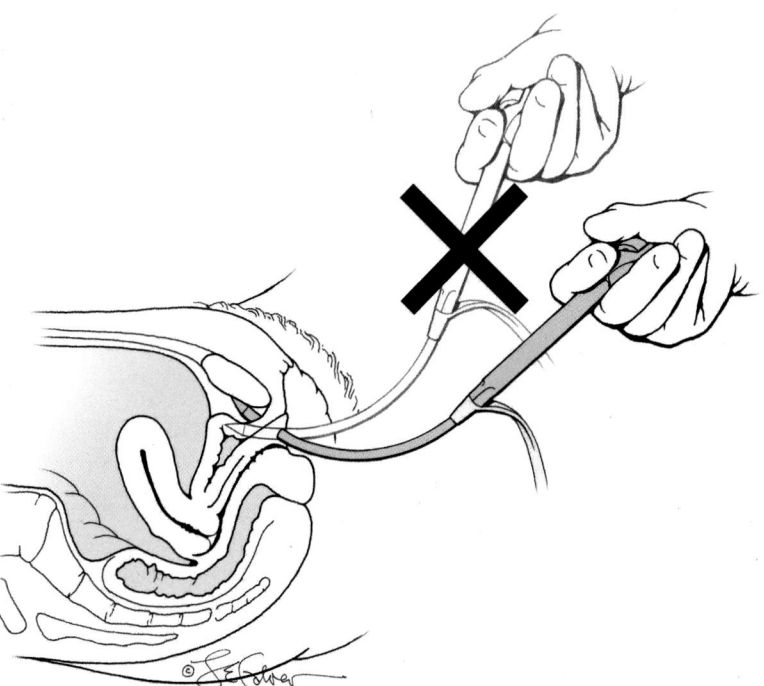

FIGURE 45-3.3 Correct (*dark introducer*) and incorrect (*light introducer*) hand and introducer positioning.

mesh, while the surgeon holds the mesh at the desired distance from the urethra using the spacer instrument. The plastic covering is lifted away from both sides with minimal tension to avoid mesh stretching or undue urethral elevation. With ideal positioning, a few millimeters of free space separate the suburethral tissue and mesh. The mesh is trimmed just below the skin at the abdominal incisions (Fig. 45-3.5).

❾ **Wound Closure.** The vaginal incision is closed in a running fashion with 2-0 gauge delayed-absorbable suture. The abdominal incisions may be closed with Dermabond or with a single interrupted 4-0 gauge delayed-absorbable skin suture.

POSTOPERATIVE

Prior to discharge from a day-surgery unit, an active voiding trial is performed (Chap. 42, p. 917). If the patient fails this trial, a Foley catheter is replaced and kept for 1 to 3 days prior to a second voiding trial. Alternatively, a patient can be taught self-catheterization. This is continued until postvoid residual volumes fall below about 100 mL.

Normal diet and activity can resume during the first postoperative days. Intercourse, however, is postponed until the vaginal incision is healed, usually at 6 weeks. The time to resumption of exercise and strenuous physical activity is controversial. A standard recommendation has been to delay these at least 2 months, although there are no data supporting this. However, logic would suggest that this is reasonable for adequate healing.

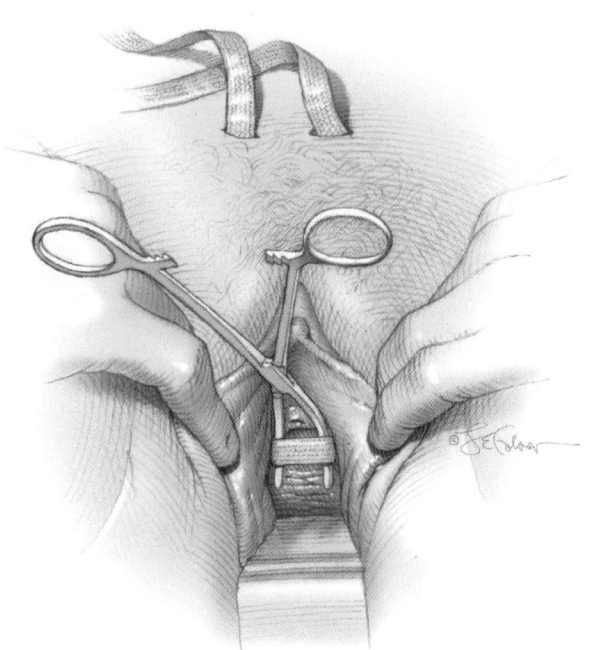

FIGURE 45-3.4 Setting mesh position.

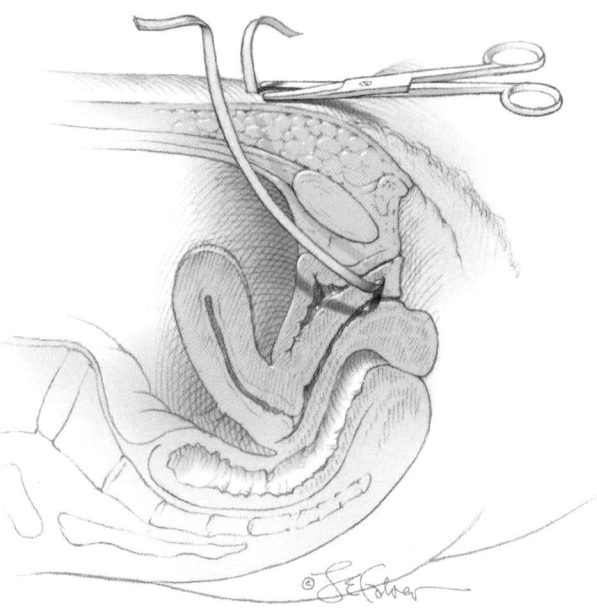

FIGURE 45-3.5 Sheath removal and tape trimming.

45-4

Transobturator Tape Sling

The transobturator tape (TOT) sling procedure is a variation of the midurethral sling procedures, which began with tension-free vaginal tape (TVT) (p. 1063). With the TOT procedure, a permanent sling material is inserted bilaterally through the obturator foramen and extends underneath the midurethra. As a result, the space of Retzius is avoided and thereby minimizes the potential for associated bladder and bowel injuries. Bleeding in the space of Retzius is a primary TVT complication, and avoiding this space is an attractive TOT feature. Additionally, in patients who have had prior incontinence procedures and have scarring in the space of Retzius, bladder perforation may be averted by avoiding dissection in this space.

The procedure has several important differences from TVT, and there are also several modifications of the TOT procedure itself. Several companies produce kits containing required mesh and placement needles for TOT. The two major types of TOT procedures are defined by whether needle placement begins inside the vagina and is directed outward, termed an *in-to-out approach,* or starts outside the vagina and is directed inward, called an *out-to-in approach.* Limited data do not show superiority of one over the other (Debodinance, 2007). Currently, the out-to-in technique is more commonly performed and is described here.

Generally, TOT is indicated for primary SUI secondary to urethral hypermobility (Chap. 23, p. 525). In patients with SUI secondary to intrinsic sphincteric deficiency, the value of TOT is unclear, as results are conflicting and data are limited (Rechberger, 2009; Richter, 2010).

PREOPERATIVE

Patient Evaluation

Evaluation and preparation prior to TOT mirrors that for TVT (p. 1063).

Consent

As with other surgeries for incontinence, the major risks of this procedure are voiding dysfunction, urinary retention, development of urgency incontinence, and failure to correct SUI. Groin and thigh pain appear to be another potential postoperative problem. Long-term complications may be associated

with the supporting mesh and include mesh erosion (Schimpf, 2014).

Intraoperatively, there is some risk of bladder or urethral perforation, although this is believed to be significantly less than that with TVT. Inappropriate TOT trocar placement rarely can lead to significant hemorrhage or neurologic deficits if obturator nerve and vessel branches are damaged in the thigh compartment.

INTRAOPERATIVE

Instruments

A TOT kit will contain two TOT needles and synthetic mesh tape. The TOT needle is designed to navigate the path from the entry point around the pubic rami to the midurethral vaginal wall incision. A plastic sheath surrounds the mesh tape and allows the mesh to be pulled into position smoothly. However, once these plastic sheaths are removed, the mesh remains fixed in position.

Surgical Steps

❶ **Anesthesia and Patient Positioning.** If performed solely, a TOT procedure in most cases is a day-surgery procedure. It is performed in standard lithotomy position under general, regional, or local anesthesia. The vagina is surgically prepared, and a Foley catheter is placed to assist in determination of urethral location.

❷ **Vaginal Incisions.** A midline incision is made sharply in the vaginal epithelium and superficial muscular layer beginning 1 cm proximal to the external urethral opening

and is extended 2 to 3 cm cephalad. Allis clamps are placed on the edges of the vaginal incision for traction. Using Metzenbaum scissors and blunt finger dissection, bilateral periurethral tunnels are created beneath the vaginal epithelium on either side of the urethra. These tunnels extend up to and behind the ischiopubic rami.

❸ **Thigh Incisions.** A 0.5- to 1-cm entry incision is made bilaterally in the thigh-crease skin (genitocrural fold), 4 to 6 cm lateral to the clitoris, and at the point where the adductor longus insertion can be palpated. This muscle arises from the superior ramus of the pubis and inserts medially at the midlength of the femur.

To summarize the needle's path, insertion starts along the lateral edge of the ischiopubic ramus just below the insertion of the adductor longus tendon and arches around the ramus. During this arc, the needle sequentially penetrates the gracilis, adductor brevis, and obturator externus muscles, obturator membrane, obturator internus muscle, and periurethral endopelvic fascia and exits through the vaginal incision.

❹ **Mesh Placement.** The TOT needle is grasped, and the tip is placed in one of the thigh incisions (Fig. 45-4.1). The tip is directed cephalad until the obturator membrane is perforated, and a "popping" sensation is felt. A vaginal finger is placed in the ipsilateral vaginal tunnel and is positioned up to and behind the ischiopubic ramus. Using the curve of the TOT needle, the surgeon then directs the needle tip to the end of his finger and passes the needle into the vagina (Fig. 45-4.2). At this time, the vaginal sulcus is inspected to exclude perforation.

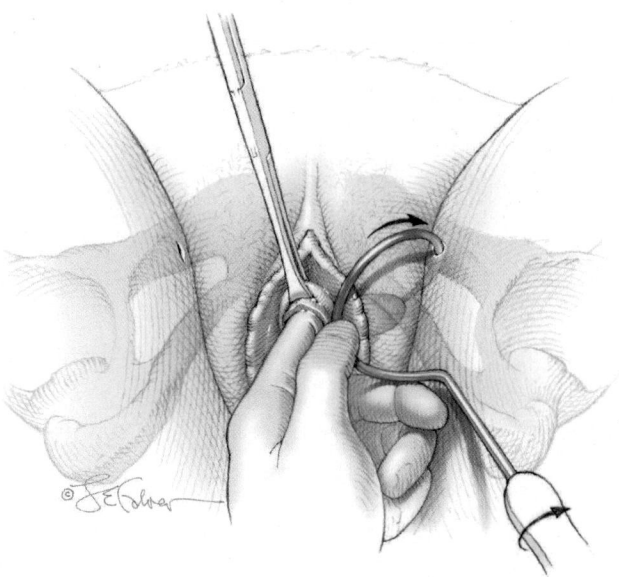

FIGURE 45-4.1 Needle introduction.

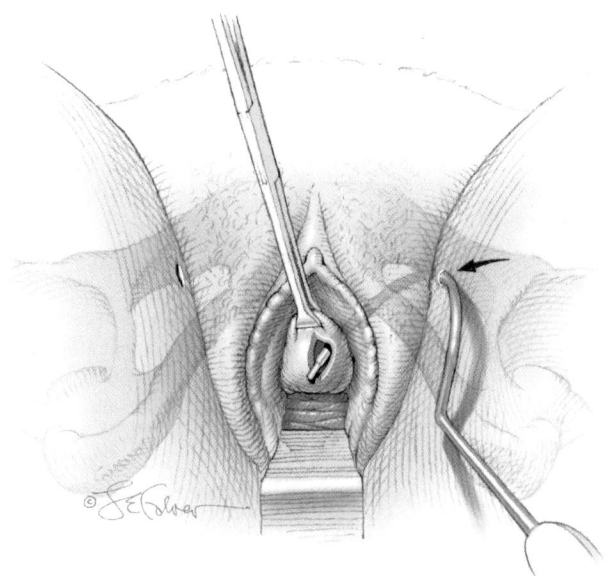

FIGURE 45-4.2 Needle passage.

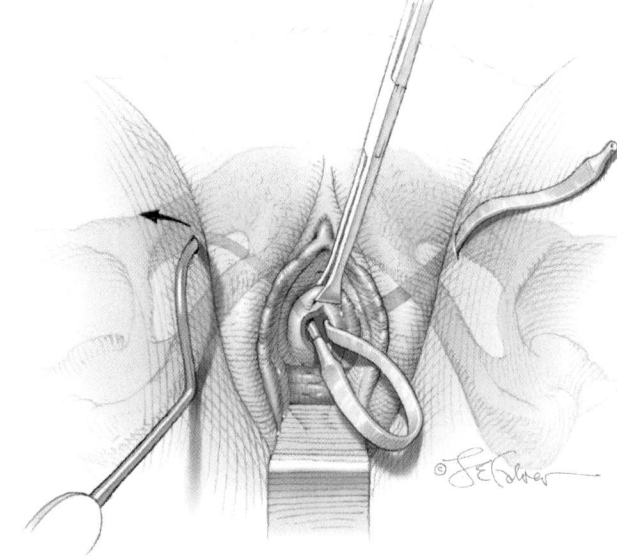

FIGURE 45-4.3 Tape placement.

If the needle has perforated the sulcus epithelium, it is removed and reinserted correctly. Next, the TOT covered mesh is attached to the needle end, and the needle retraces its original path as it is withdrawn back through the thigh incision. With this, the covered mesh is threaded into position. The mesh is then removed from the needle. The procedure is repeated on the other side (Fig. 45-4.3).

❺ **Setting Mesh Position.** A hemostat or similar instrument is placed and opened between the urethra and mesh to act as a spacer and create distance between the mesh and the urethra (Fig. 45-4.4). This spacing avoids excessive urethral elevation and lowers postoperative urinary retention risks. Prior to sheath removal, the vaginal sulci are again

inspected to exclude perforation. If mesh is seen in a sulcus, the tape is removed and reinserted on the affected side.

❻ **Sheath Removal.** An assistant surgeon then removes the plastic covering of the mesh from each of the thigh incisions. Concurrently, the surgeon holds the mesh at the desired distance from the urethra using the spacer instrument. The plastic covering is removed with minimal tension to avoid mesh stretching. The mesh is trimmed just inside thigh incisions.

❼ **Wound Closure.** The vaginal incision is closed in a running fashion with 2-0 gauge delayed-absorbable suture. The thigh incisions may be closed with a single interrupted subcuticular suture with 4-0 gauge delayed-

absorbable suture or with other suitable skin closure methods (Chap. 40, p. 847).

❽ **Cystourethroscopy.** The procedure is marketed as one in which cystoscopy is not necessary. However, because the bladder and urethra can be injured, we recommend postprocedural cystoscopy.

POSTOPERATIVE

Prior to discharge from a day-surgery unit, an active voiding trial is performed (Chap. 42, p. 917). If significant residuals persist, a Foley catheter remains. A second voiding trial can be repeated in a few days or at the surgeon's discretion. Alternatively, a patient can be taught self-catheterization. This is continued until postvoid residuals fall below approximately 100 mL.

Normal diet and activity can resume during the first postoperative days. Intercourse, however, is delayed until the vaginal incision is healed. The time to resumption of exercise and strenuous physical activity is controversial. A standard recommendation delays these at least 2 months. Data to support this are lacking, however, logic would suggest that this is reasonable to allow adequate healing.

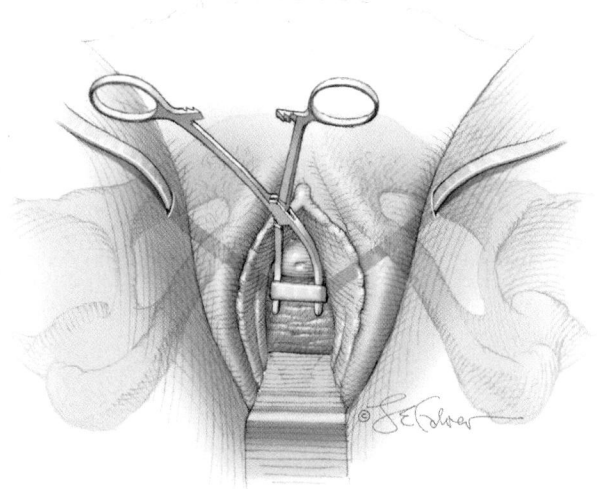

FIGURE 45-4.4 Setting mesh position.

45-5

Pubovaginal Sling

Pubovaginal sling is a standard procedure for SUI. It has traditionally been used for SUI stemming from intrinsic sphincteric deficiency (Chap. 23, p. 522). In addition, this procedure may also aid patients with prior failed antiincontinence operations. It is generally not employed in a woman having her first surgery for incontinence.

In the past, different materials had been used for the sling, however, autologous fascia is currently preferred. Generally, this fascia is obtained from the patient's rectus sheath, although fascia lata from the thigh may alternatively be harvested. With this surgery, a strip of fascia is placed at the proximal urethra through the space of Retzius, and ends are secured either to each other or to the rectus fascia above the rectus abdominis muscle.

In contrast to midurethral slings, which generally employ premade kits and standardized procedural steps, the technical aspects of autologous fascia pubovaginal slings have greater variability. These include size and location of harvested tissue, anchoring method of the sling to the rectus fascia, and technique for determining mesh tension across the proximal urethra. Steps for the rectus fascial sling are described here.

PREOPERATIVE

■ Patient Evaluation

As with other antiincontinence procedures, patients require urogynecologic evaluation, including urodynamic testing to confirm SUI and intrinsic sphincteric deficiency. Additionally, SUI often accompanies pelvic organ prolapse. Thus, the need for concurrent repair of associated prolapse is assessed prior to surgery (Chap. 24, p. 545).

■ Consent

In addition to general surgical risks, patients are counseled regarding the risk of recurrent incontinence, urinary retention, and voiding dysfunction following surgery (Albo, 2007). Overall, traditional slings seem to be as effective as minimally invasive slings but have higher rates of adverse effects (Rehman, 2011).

■ Patient Preparation

Antibiotics and thromboprophylaxis are given as outlined in Tables 39-6 and 39-8 (p. 835). Bowel preparation is based on surgeon preference and mainly on concurrent surgeries planned.

INTRAOPERATIVE

■ Surgical Steps

❶ **Anesthesia and Patient Positioning.** Pubovaginal sling may be performed under general or regional anesthesia as an inpatient procedure. The patient is placed in standard lithotomy position, with lower extremities positioned in candy-cane or booted support stirrups. The abdomen and vagina are surgically prepared, and a Foley catheter is inserted.

❷ **Graft Harvest.** A transverse skin incision is made 2 to 4 cm above the symphysis and is large enough to allow removal of a transverse fascial strip that measures, at minimum, 1.5 cm wide × 6 cm long. The incision is carried down through subcutaneous tissue to the fascia.

The fascia to be harvested is outlined and then incised, sharply dissected away from the underlying rectus muscle bellies, and removed. Following removal, the strip is cleaned of fat and adventitial tissue. A helical stitch using 0-gauge polypropylene suture is then placed through the fascia at each end of the strip. This stitch is repeated at the other end. These sutures are not tied. The fascial incision is then closed in a running fashion with 0-gauge delayed-absorbable suture.

❸ **Vaginal Incision.** At a point 2 cm proximal to the external urethral orifice, a 3- to 5-cm midline vertical incision is made sharply in the anterior vaginal wall and extended cephalad. Alternatively, a U-shaped incision is made at the level of the bladder neck. Sharp and blunt dissection is used to separate the vaginal epithelium from the underlying fibromuscular layer. The space of Retzius is then entered with a combination of sharp and blunt dissection bilaterally by penetrating the periurethral connective tissue (Fig. 45-5.1). Entry into this space is confirmed by the surgeon's finger palpating the dorsal surface of the pubic bone (Fig. 45-5.2). During entry, Santorini's venous plexus can be lacerated, and bleeding is controlled with compression or stitches of 2-0 gauge absorbable suture.

❹ **Fascia Placement.** A 0.5- to 1-cm long fascial incision is made no further than 2 cm from the midline on each side. These are placed caudal to the prior harvest incision and just above the pubic bones. A long

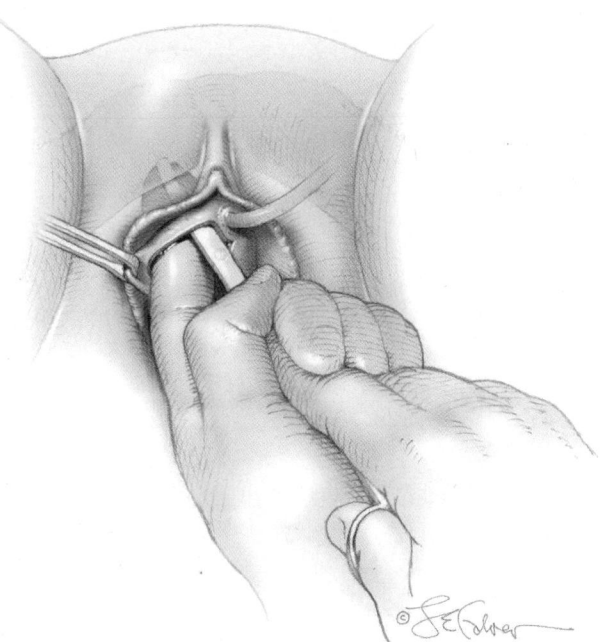

FIGURE 45-5.1 Entry into the space of Retzius.

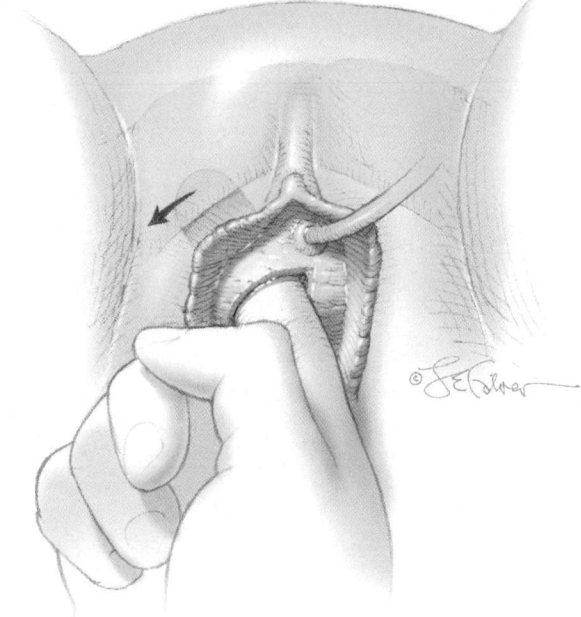

FIGURE 45-5.2 Palpation of pubic bone.

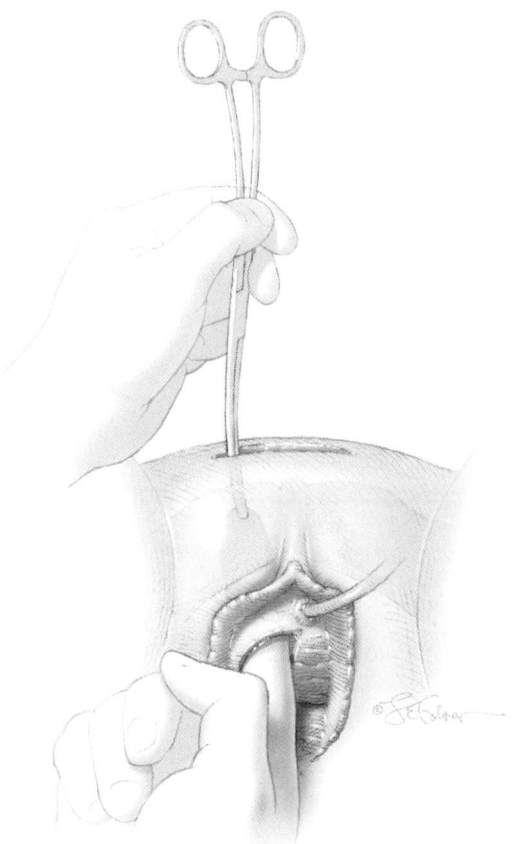

FIGURE 45-5.3 Passing of dressing forceps.

dressing or packing forceps or needle ligature carrier is placed into one of these incisions and from above, perforates the rectus tendon. The instrument is placed against the back of the pubic bone and advanced toward the vagina. Concurrently, the surgeon guides the instrument to his finger within the space of Retzius and advances it into and through the vaginal incision (Fig. 45-5.3). At this time, cystourethroscopy is performed to exclude bladder or urethral perforation.

The suture ties at one end of the fascial strip are grasped with the perforating forceps and threaded up through the abdominal incision on one side of the urethra. With the other end of the sling, this step is repeated on the other side of the urethra. As a result, the fascial sling lies positioned below the bladder neck (Fig. 45-5.4). Usually four 2-0 gauge delayed-absorbable sutures may be used to fix the proximal and distal edges of the sling beneath the bladder neck to prevent displacement during sling positioning. Stitches are placed lateral to the urethra.

❺ **Setting Sling Position.** Within the laparotomy incision, sutures attached to the sling ends from each side meet and are tied together above the rectus sheath. During knot tying, a space of two to three fingerbreadths is left between the knot and fascia to pre-

vent bladder neck obstruction and urinary retention. In addition, a hemostat is placed between the suburethral tissue and the fascial sling to create distance between the sling and urethra (see Fig. 45-4.4). After the knot

is secured, there should be no upward angulation of the urethra or bladder neck, and a few millimeters of free space should be noted between the fascial sling and the bladder neck.

❻ **Cystourethroscopy.** Cystoscopy is again performed to exclude bladder or urethral perforation. In addition, excessive resistance noted during passage of the cystoscope into the bladder may suggest undue sling tension, which can lead to postoperative obstructive symptoms. If such resistance is noted, the sling is loosened.

❼ **Vaginal Incision.** The vaginal incision is closed with 2-0 gauge delayed-absorbable suture in a running fashion. A Foley catheter is left in place. In the past, suprapubic tube insertion was common practice. However, with a trend toward tying the fascial sling with less tension, the risk of prolonged urinary retention is lowered, and suprapubic drainage is therefore not typically required.

❽ **Abdominal Incision.** The two prior 1-cm fascial incisions are closed with an interrupted stitch of delayed-absorbable suture. The remaining abdominal incision is closed as described in Section 43-2 (p. 930).

POSTOPERATIVE

In general, recovery follows that associated with laparotomy and is heavily dependent on incision size. A voiding trial as described in Chapter 42 (p. 917) is performed prior to hospital discharge.

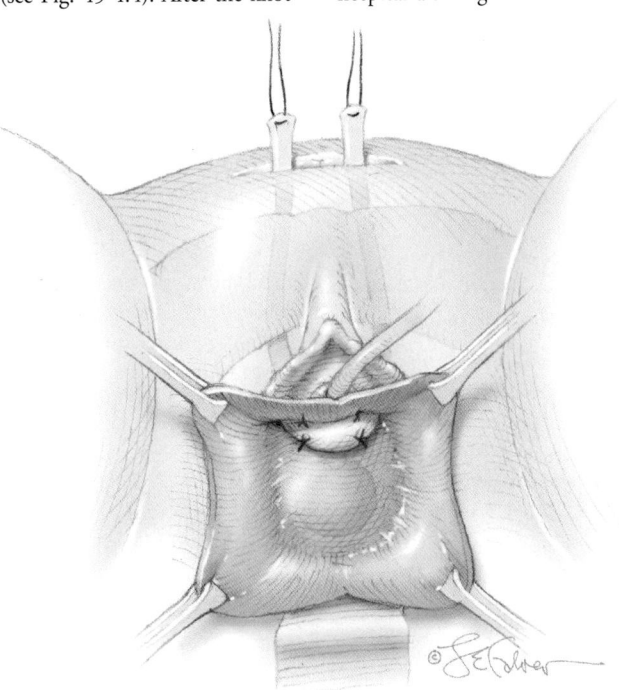

FIGURE 45-5.4 Fascial sling placed and sutured in place on vaginal side.

45-6

Urethral Bulking Injections

Injection of bulking agents into the urethral submucosa is one method available to treat SUI that results from intrinsic sphincter deficiency (ISD) (Chap. 23, p. 522). Although mechanisms are not completely clear, effectiveness may result from expansion of the urethral walls, which allows them to better approximate or *coapt*. As a result, intraluminal resistance to flow is increased and continence is restored. Alternatively, injections elongate the functional urethra, and this may allow more even distribution of abdominal pressures across the proximal urethra to resist opening during stress (Monga, 1997).

Although traditionally recommended for treatment of SUI solely due to ISD, some evidence suggests it can be used to treat SUI resulting from combined ISD and urethral hypermobility (Bent, 2001; Herschorn, 1997; Steele, 2000).

Urethral injection offers a cystoscopically assisted, minimally invasive treatment of SUI. It can be performed in an office under local anesthesia and is associated with a low risk of complications. For these reasons, it is often chosen for women who wish to avoid surgery or who are not surgical candidates due to other comorbidities. Urethral injections can be performed both peri- and transurethrally. The transurethral approach is more often used and allows for more accurate placement of the bulking agent (Faerber, 1998; Schulz, 2004). Currently available agents in the United States approved for use include autologous fat and several synthetic agents described later.

PREOPERATIVE

Patient Evaluation

Complex urodynamic testing with assessment of urethral structure and function is completed. To assess for ISD, maximum urethral closure pressure or leak point pressure are specifically evaluated (Chap. 23, p. 527). Additionally, urethral mobility is assessed.

Consent

Procedure efficacy is discussed, and success rates in general are lower than those for surgery. Specifically, 1-year rates of curing or improving SUI range from 60 to 80 percent (Bent, 2001; Corcos, 2005; Lightner, 2002, 2009; Monga, 1995). Continence

rates diminish with time, as would be intuitive, with the breakdown of collagen and fat. However, Chrouser (2004) found similar rates of decline with time even when synthetic material was compared with collagen. Accordingly, these injections are viewed as a nonpermanent treatment of SUI, and sustained continence is found in only 25 percent of patients at 5 years following injection (Gorton, 1999).

One major advantage to urethral injection is its low associated risk of complications. Side effects of injection are generally transient and may include vaginitis, acute cystitis, and voiding symptoms. Of these, urinary retention for a few days postprocedure is the most frequent. Long-term retention, however, is not a significant risk. A more serious complication is persistent de novo urgency, which may develop in as many as 10 percent of women following injection (Corcos, 1999, 2005).

Patient Preparation

Prior to urethral injection, UTI and anatomic pathology such as urethral diverticula are excluded. Anecdotally, we have seen bulking agent migration into such diverticula. As noted, UTI can commonly follow urethral injection. Therefore, a single dose of an antibiotic to cover uropathogens is administered orally after procedure completion. Thromboprophylaxis is not typically required for this brief office procedure.

INTRAOPERATIVE

Choice of Bulking Agent

In the United States, currently used agents for urethral injection are carbon-coated synthetic microspheres (Durasphere), calcium hydroxylapatite particles (Coaptite), and polydimethylsiloxane (Macroplastique). These synthetic agents are effective. However, no randomized trials compare results among these three, and long-term data are lacking (Shah, 2012; Zoorob, 2012).

Of agents no longer used, autologous fat provided limited success for SUI due to rapid degradation and reabsorption (Haab, 1997; Lee, 2001). A bovine collagen product (Contigen) was commonly selected, but manufacturing ceased due to an inadequate supply of medical-grade collagen. Ethylene vinyl alcohol copolymer (Uryx/Tegress) was withdrawn due to urethral erosion complications.

Surgical Steps

❶ **Anesthesia and Patient Positioning.** Urethral injection for most patients can be

performed in an office setting with cystoscopic capability. The patient is placed in the dorsal lithotomy position, the vulva is prepared and draped, and the bladder drained. Two-percent lidocaine jelly is instilled into the urethra 10 minutes prior to the procedure. If necessary, topical 20-percent benzocaine can be used as an analgesic on the vulva, and 4 mL of 1-percent lidocaine can be injected in divided doses at the 3 and 9 o'clock positions of the external urethral orifice.

❷ **Transurethral Approach to Needle Placement.** A cystoscope is positioned within the distal urethra, so that the midurethra, proximal urethra, and bladder neck are viewed simultaneously. A 22-gauge spinal needle attached to a syringe carrying the bulking agent is introduced through the cystoscopic sheath. With the bevel pointing toward the urethral lumen, the needle is directed at a 45-degree angle to the lumen and inserted through the urethral wall at the 9 o'clock position and at the level of the midurethra. After the needle tip penetrates the urethral wall, the bevel is no longer seen. The needle is then advanced parallel to the urethral lumen for 1 to 2 cm. This positions the needle at the level of the proximal urethra.

❸ **Injection.** The bulking agent is injected under constant pressure, and the submucosal lining begins to rise (Fig. 45-6.1). The needle is withdrawn slowly to bulk the proximal and midurethra. Bulking agent is administered until coaptation of the mucosa has developed (Fig. 45-6.2). In general, 1 to 2 syringes (2.5 to 5 mL) of agent are used per procedure. These steps are then repeated at the 3 o'clock position.

Ideally, the number of needle holes made into the urethral wall is minimized to avoid leakage of bulking agent through these punctures. Thus, if a second syringe of agent is required to achieve coaptation, the originally positioned needle remains in place, and a second syringe of agent is attached.

❹ **Cystoscope Removal.** Once coaptation of the mucosa is achieved, the cystoscope is removed, taking care not to advance proximal to the injection site. This avoids forceful compression of the deposited agent by the cystoscope tip and loss of coaptation.

POSTOPERATIVE

Women are discharged home following their first postinjection void, and single-dose oral antibiotic prophylaxis is prescribed. Women abstain from intercourse for 10 days following injection but may otherwise resume usual activities.

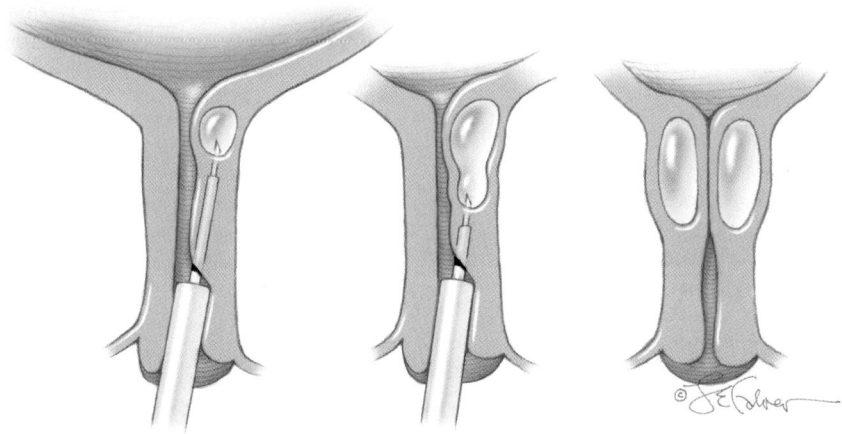

FIGURE 45-6.1 Injection of bulking agent.

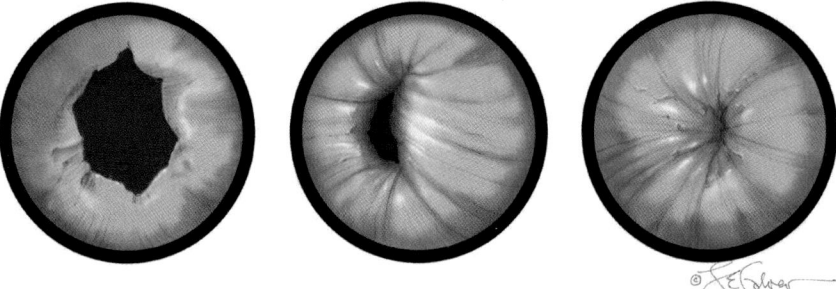

FIGURE 45-6.2 Corresponding cystoscopic views of urethral coaptation as bulking agent is injected, as shown in Figure 45-6.1.

If urinary retention develops, then intermittent self-catheterization is begun and continued until retention resolves. For those unable to self-catheterize, a temporary Foley catheter is placed. However, catheter placement can potentially compress deposited bulking agent and diminish urethral coaptation.

Two weeks following injection, we assess treatment success. If a patient fails to achieve desired degrees of continence, additional injections are planned to improve urethral coaptation.

45-7

Urethrolysis

Urethrolysis is the loosening or release of a prior urethral suspension repair. This release is used in women with urethral obstruction symptoms including urinary retention and voiding dysfunction following suspension. It can be performed either vaginally or abdominally. A vaginal approach is predominantly used. An abdominal approach, however, may afford a better opportunity to mobilize the bladder from the pubic symphysis and may also be selected in instances in which the initial surgery was performed via laparotomy.

Debate exists as to the need of a concurrent antiincontinence procedure to compensate for urethral support lost with urethrolysis. However, in many cases, residual scarring prevents SUI, and our belief is to avoid repeating a second potentially obstructing procedure. Accordingly, this decision is individualized.

PREOPERATIVE

Patient Evaluation

In women with bladder neck obstruction, symptoms usually begin soon after initial surgery. Objective assessment with urodynamic testing is performed to determine the cause of voiding dysfunction and differentiate between a hypotonic bladder and obstruction. Obstruction may result from bladder neck obstruction or

pelvic organ prolapse. Thus, a thorough examination for prolapse is completed.

Consent

In addition to usual surgical risks, bleeding may be a significant complication due to vascularity in the space of Retzius. Additionally, dissection of dense scarring around the urethra and bladder may place these structures at risk of laceration.

Due to scar tissue reformation, initial obstruction improvement can worsen over time, as scar tissue may variably reform. In contrast, postoperative incontinence may follow deconstruction of prior antiincontinence support or from denervation injury during extensive periurethral dissection.

Patient Preparation

As with all genitourinary procedures, UTI is excluded prior to surgery. Antibiotic prophylaxis is administered prior to surgery to decrease risks of postoperative wound and urinary tract infection (Table 39-6, p. 835). Thromboprophylaxis is provided as outlined in Table 39-8 (p. 836).

INTRAOPERATIVE

Surgical Steps—Vaginal Approach

❶ **Anesthesia and Patient Positioning.** Urethrolysis may be performed under general or regional anesthesia. The patient is placed

in standard lithotomy position with lower extremities in candy-cane or booted support stirrups. The vagina is surgically prepared, and a Foley catheter is inserted into the bladder.

❷ **Vaginal Incision.** Traction is placed on the Foley catheter to identify the bladder neck and assess the degree of scarring. A 2- to 3-cm long incision, either vertical midline or U-shaped, is made in the anterior vaginal wall. The incision site will vary along the vaginal length depending on the location of the original sling or sutures (Fig. 45-7.1). Sharp dissection is used to separate the vaginal epithelium from underlying fibromuscular tissue and is extended bilaterally toward the inferior edge of each pubic rami.

Dissection frees the urethra by dividing scar tissue or prior sling material or sutures that lie between the urethra and pubic rami (Fig. 45-7.2). If prior supporting material is identified, it may be incised or if necessary, excised. Bleeding is frequently encountered and can be controlled with direct pressure or vessel ligation.

After this lateral dissection, the periurethral tissue is perforated, and the space of Retzius is entered. Careful blunt dissection within this space and at the back of the pubic symphysis will additionally mobilize the proximal urethra. Dissection is kept close to the dorsal surface of the pubic bone to avoid cystotomy in a bladder that is generally densely adhered to the pubic bone.

❸ **Incision Closure.** Following adequate mobilization of the urethra, the vaginal incision

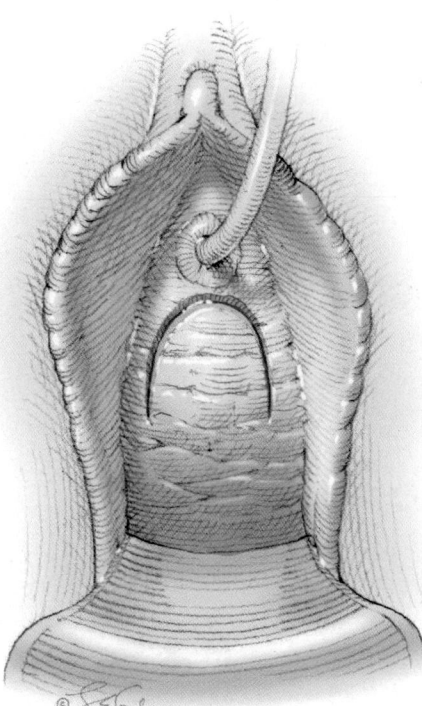

FIGURE 45-7.1 Vaginal incision.

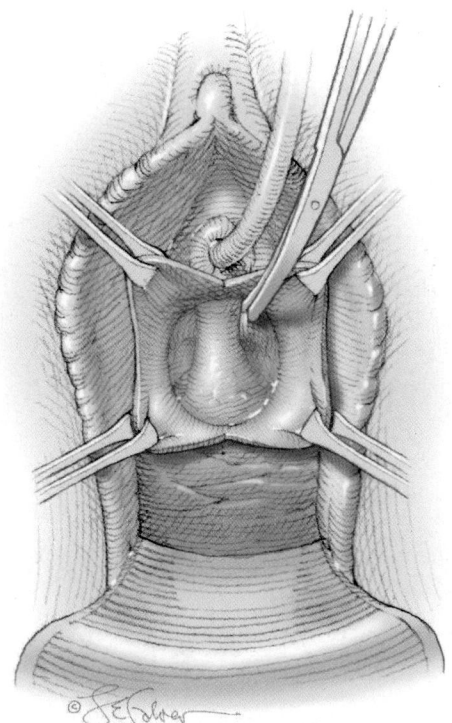

FIGURE 45-7.2 Periurethral dissection.

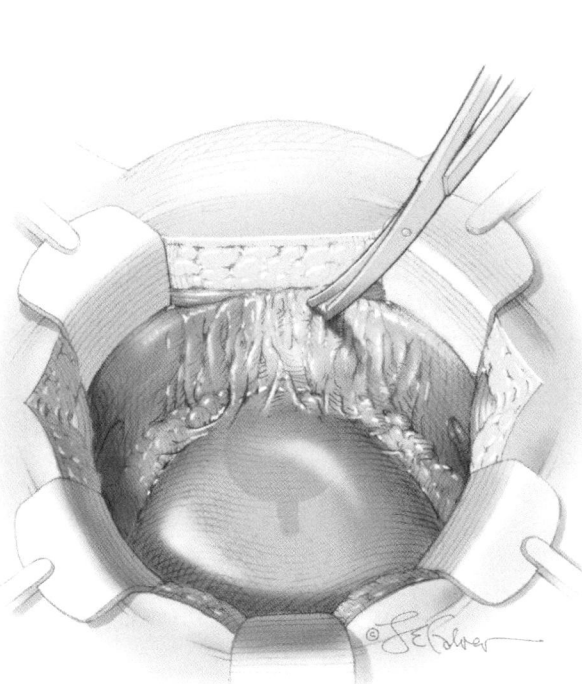

FIGURE 45-7.3 Dissection in the space of Retzius.

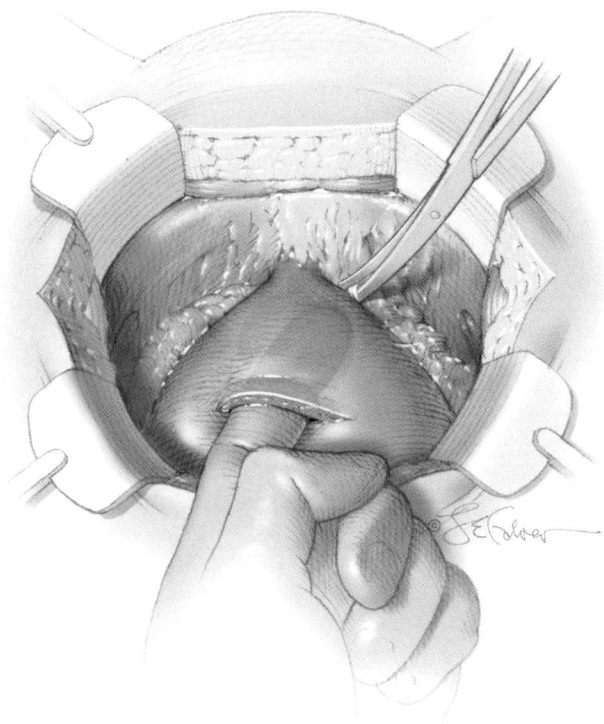

FIGURE 45-7.4 Intentional cystotomy to aid bladder and urethral dissection.

is reapproximated with a running closure using 2-0 gauge delayed-absorbable suture.

Surgical Steps— Abdominal Approach

❶ **Anesthesia and Patient Positioning.** As with a vaginal approach, urethrolysis may be completed under general or regional anesthesia. For an abdominal approach, booted support stirrups and low lithotomy positioning are preferred. This positioning allows vaginal access for the surgeon's hand during dissection and for cystoscopy. The abdomen and vagina are surgically prepared, and a Foley catheter is inserted into the bladder.

❷ **Abdominal Incision.** A low transverse incision is typically preferred for this procedure to permit easy access to the space of Retzius. Either Pfannenstiel or Cherney incisions are usually selected (Sections 43-2 and 43-3, p. 929). If the procedure is done in isolation, fascia of the anterior abdominal wall muscles and then transversalis fascia are incised, but entry into the peritoneal cavity is not necessary to reach the space of Retzius.

❸ **Entry into the Space of Retzius.** The correct plane of dissection to enter the space of Retzius lies directly behind the pubic bone. Loose areolar tissue is gently dissected downward in a mediolateral fashion with fingers or sponge, beginning immediately behind the pubic bone. If the correct plane is entered, this potential space opens easily. However, women requiring urethrolysis have typically had prior surgery within this space. As a result, tissue can be densely adhered and sharp downward dissection along the dorsal surface of the symphysis may be preferred to enter this space (Fig. 45-7.3).

❹ **Bladder Dissection and Urethrolysis.** The bladder is also typically densely adhered to the back of the symphysis. Sharp dissection with the curved surface of scissors facing the symphysis is directed against the symphysis to minimize cystotomy risk. At times, however, an intentional cystotomy may be required so that a finger can be placed inside the bladder to aid dissection (Fig. 45-7.4).

Sharp dissection is continued inferiorly and laterally down the inner surface of the symphysis and pubic bones to free the bladder and eventually also the proximal urethra.

Bleeding is common during dissection and may be controlled with absorbable sutures.

❺ **Abdominal Closure.** The abdomen is closed in a standard fashion (Sections 43-2 or 43-3, p. 930).

POSTOPERATIVE

An active bladder test is performed following catheter removal. If large residual volumes are found, intermittent self-catheterization or Foley catheter replacement is required. If cystotomy was performed, the duration of catheterization is dependent on cystotomy size and location. For example, small cystotomies in the bladder dome typically require drainage for 7 days or less. For larger cystotomies at the bladder base, however, drainage for several weeks may be needed. Antibiotic suppression is not required with this catheter use.

Normal diet and activity can resume during the first postoperative days. With a vaginal approach, however, intercourse is postponed until the vaginal incision is well healed. Recovery from an abdominal approach follows that for laparotomy (Section 43-1, p. 928).

45-8

Midurethral Sling Release

Symptoms of voiding obstruction may develop following urethral sling procedures, specifically TVT and TOT procedures. For most patients, postoperative urinary retention resolves in days or 1 to 2 weeks. However, voiding dysfunction requiring surgery develops in up to 3 percent and generally is identified days to weeks after surgery (Jonsson Funk, 2013; Nguyen, 2012; Richter, 2010). If obstruction is diagnosed soon after the index procedure, surgical release is performed and involves simple cutting of the sling material.

PREOPERATIVE

Patient Evaluation and Preparation

Inability to fully empty the bladder may stem from urethral obstruction or a hypotonic bladder. New-onset urinary retention after a midurethral sling procedure (TVT or TOT) is usually due to sling tightness. However, other factors can be involved, such as preexisting or de novo bladder hypotonia. Thus, prior to TVT urethrolysis, urodynamic testing is often performed to prove that symptoms are due to obstruction rather than to bladder hypotonicity. Additionally, tape may erode into the bladder or urethra in cases of obstruction, and cystoscopy allows exclusion of this complication.

Perioperatively, no specific patient preparation is required, as midurethral sling release is a minor surgical procedure.

Consent

Associated with midurethral sling release, the risks of incontinence recurrence, failure to adequately relieve retention, fistula formation, and intraoperative bladder or urethral injury are discussed during consenting.

INTRAOPERATIVE

Surgical Steps

❶ **Anesthesia and Patient Positioning.** This surgery can be performed with local,

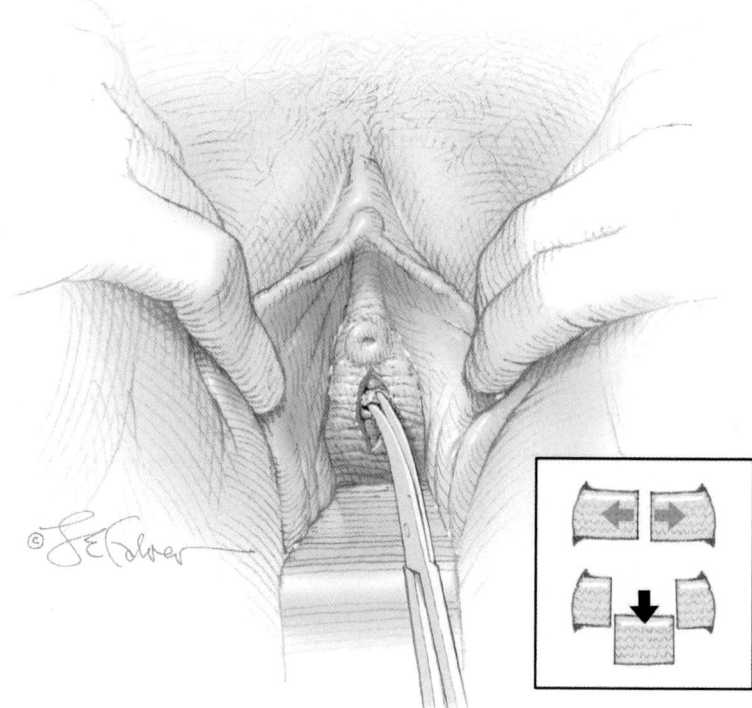

FIGURE 45-8.1 Mesh transection through vaginal incision. Inset top: Mesh incision and retraction. Inset bottom: Partial mesh excision.

regional, or general anesthesia as an outpatient procedure. A patient is placed in standard lithotomy position within candy-cane or booted support stirrups. The vagina is surgically prepared, and a Foley catheter is inserted.

❷ **Vaginal Incision and Tape Identification.** A midline suburethral incision that follows the prior primary surgical incision is made sharply. Careful dissection is used to expose the sling material and to define the urethral borders. Alternatively, with prior TOT, tight tissue bands may be palpated in the sulci. In this case, the vagina can be incised at one sulcus, and the tape transected or partially excised here.

Often because of increased sling tension, sling material is stretched and measures only half its expected width. Additionally, there is usually extensive tissue ingrowth into the sling material, and identification and mobilization can be difficult. Occasionally, a sling may migrate to the proximal urethra. In these instances, the vaginal incision may require cephalad extension.

❸ **Incision of Sling Material.** Following mobilization of the material, a hemostat is opened between the sling and urethra.

Metzenbaum scissors are used to cut the sling material. In general, incision leads to immediate retraction of sling ends (Fig. 45-8.1, top inset). If retraction does not follow, a 1-cm segment of material is then excised (see Fig. 45-8.1, bottom inset). If the sling is deeply embedded and near the urethral lumen, one to two imbricating layers are placed through the vaginal muscularis following sling excision using 2-0 or 3-0 gauge delayed-absorbable suture.

❹ **Incision Closure.** After vigorous irrigation, the vaginal epithelium is closed in a continuous running fashion using 2-0 gauge delayed-absorbable suture.

POSTOPERATIVE

Prior to discharge, an active voiding trial is performed (Chap. 42, p. 917). If a Foley catheter remains, a second voiding trial can be repeated in a few days or at the surgeon's discretion. If a woman is performing self-catheterization, this is continued until postvoid residuals fall below approximately 100 mL. Normal diet and activity can resume during the first postoperative days. Intercourse, however, should be postponed until the vaginal incision is healed.

45-9

Urethral Diverticulum Repair

The approach to urethral diverticulum repair varies and depends on diverticular sac location, size, and configuration. For those near the bladder neck, partial ablation is often chosen to avoid damage to the bladder neck and continence mechanism. For midurethral diverticula, simple diverticulectomy is typically performed. For those located at the external urethral orifice, again, simple diverticulectomy is preferred to the Spence procedure. The latter is rarely performed and can alter final urethral orifice anatomy. Last, for those with a complex diverticulum that may surround the urethra, a combination of techniques may be necessary. Of these options, complete vaginal excision of the urethral diverticulum is preferred (Antosh, 2011).

PREOPERATIVE

Patient Evaluation

As described in Chapter 26 (p. 585), urethral diverticula can be difficult to diagnose due to their often varied and nonspecific presentations. Once identified, accurate information regarding diverticular anatomy is essential to surgical planning and patient counseling. Compared with transvaginal sonography or voiding cystourethrography, magnetic resonance (MR) imaging is a superior radiographic study to delineate diverticular configuration, especially with complex diverticula (Ockrim, 2009).

Additionally, cystoscopy is valuable in locating sac openings along the urethral length and demonstrates high specificity, as transurethral visualization of an ostium is unlikely to be associated with other diagnoses. That said, our frequency of urethral diverticulum detection (sensitivity) was only 39 percent (Pathi, 2013).

Women with diverticulum can present with urinary incontinence. In such cases, we typically perform baseline urodynamic testing but generally defer antiincontinence procedures until after postoperative reevaluation.

Consent

With diverticular repair, damage to urethral continence mechanism may lead to postoperative incontinence. Alternatively, urethral stricture or stenosis or urinary retention may develop depending on the extent and location of surgery. Additionally, urethrovaginal

fistula and bladder injury can result. Recurrence rates of 10 to 25 percent have been reported, especially with a horseshoe or circumferential configuration or previous surgical intervention (Antosh, 2011; Ingber, 2011). Failures are believed secondary to incomplete diverticulum excision. Moreover, urethral pain can persist or arise after diverticulectomy (Ockrim, 2009). Recurrent UTI can also persist. Last, with the Spence marsupialization technique, a distal diverticulum and urethral orifice are sharply opened together to form a large single meatus. Thus, external urethral orifice anatomy is usually altered, and a spraying pattern with urination may result.

Patient Preparation

Any acute diverticular infection or cystitis is treated prior to surgery. Preventatively, antibiotic and venous thromboprophylaxis are given as outlined in Tables 39-6 and 39-8 (p. 835).

INTRAOPERATIVE

Surgical Steps— Diverticulectomy

❶ **Anesthesia and Patient Positioning.** Diverticulum excision is typically performed as an inpatient procedure under general or regional anesthesia. A patient is placed in standard lithotomy position within candy-cane or booted support stirrups. The vagina is surgically prepared, and a Foley catheter containing a 10-mL balloon is placed in the bladder to assist in identifying the bladder neck.

❷ **Cystourethroscopy.** This procedure is performed at the procedure's onset to attempt diverticular opening identification and exclude other abnormalities.

❸ **Vaginal Incision.** To begin, a midline or U-shaped incision is made on the anterior vaginal wall over the diverticulum, and the vaginal epithelium is dissected sharply off the fibromuscular layer of the vaginal wall (Fig. 45-9.1). Ample epithelium is freed to allow adequate exposure and to permit final tissue approximation without suture-line tension.

❹ **Diverticulum Exposure.** Next, the fibromuscular layer of the vagina and urethra is incised with a longitudinal or transverse incision to reach the diverticular sac. Anatomically, the distal vaginal and urethral walls are fused, and it may be difficult or impossible to separate tissue planes. Thus, sharp dissection is needed to completely mobilize the diverticular sac away from the vaginal and urethral fibromuscular layer and to the level of the diverticular sac neck (Fig. 45-9.2). During dissection, the sac may be inadvertently or intentionally entered. With this, the diverticular walls can be grasped with Allis clamps to create tension across the connective tissue fibers between the diverticular

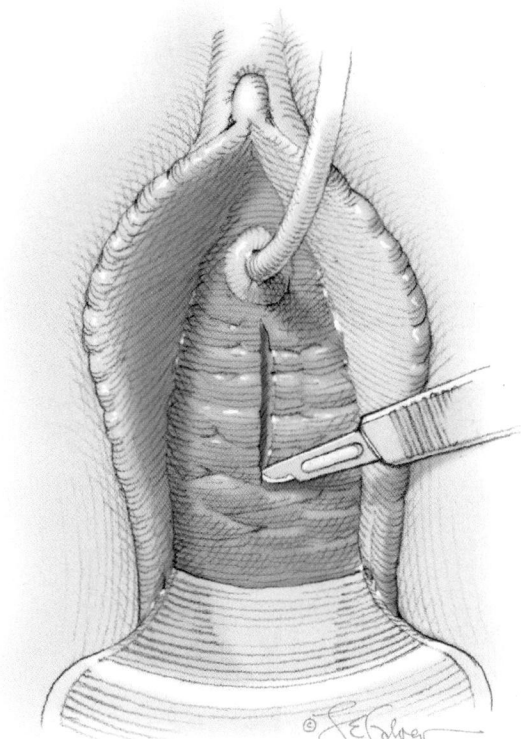

FIGURE 45-9.1 Vaginal incision.

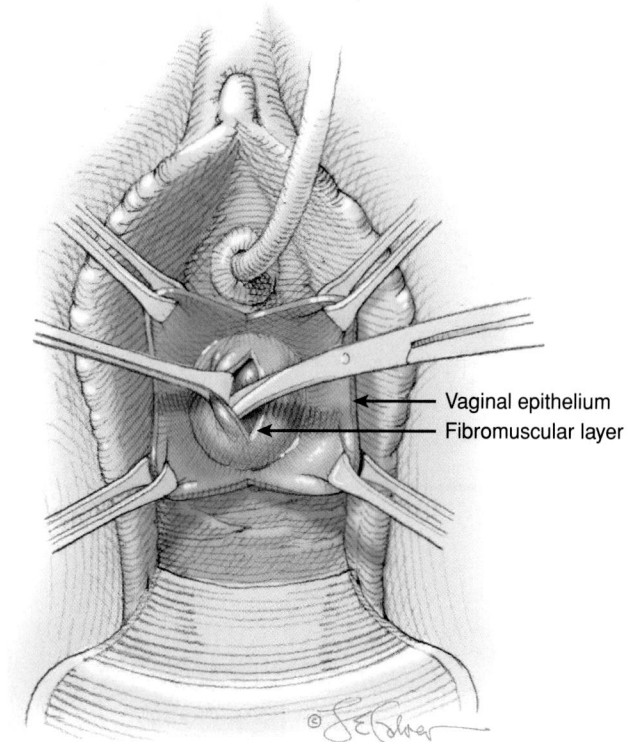

FIGURE 45-9.2 Diverticular sac dissection.

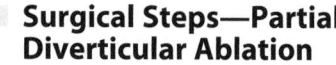

FIGURE 45-9.3 Diverticulum excision.

walls and the vaginal fibromuscular layer to aid dissection. Similarly, an index finger placed within the sac can recreate sac fullness to stretch these same connective tissue fibers. Dissection is then continued until the diverticulum's communication with the urethra is isolated. Caution and awareness of urethral location are essential to avoid damage.

❺ **Diverticulum Excision.** At its neck, the diverticulum is excised from the urethra (Fig. 45-9.3).

❻ **Urethral Closure.** The urethral defect is closed with interrupted 4-0 gauge delayed-absorbable sutures over the Foley catheter (Fig. 45-9.4). Fibromuscular layers of the

urethra and vagina are then reapproximated off tension in two or more layers. For this closure, a vest-over-pants method with 2-0 gauge delayed-absorbable suture is preferred when possible to avoid overlapping suture lines (Fig. 45-9.5). Redundant vaginal epithelium is trimmed, and the epithelium is closed in a running fashion with 2-0 gauge delayed-absorbable suture.

Surgical Steps—Partial Diverticular Ablation

If extensive dissection is required around the trigone, consideration is given to leaving the proximal portion of the sac in place to avoid direct injury or denervation injury. In addition, ureteral stents may be beneficial during the dissection.

❶ **Vaginal Incision.** Again, a midline or U-shaped incision is made on the anterior vaginal wall over the diverticulum, and the vaginal epithelium is dissected sharply off the fibromuscular layer of the vaginal wall. Ample epithelium is freed to allow adequate exposure and later defect closure off tension. The Foley catheter and balloon can be placed on gentle tension to aid in identifying the bladder and bladder neck to avoid injury.

❷ **Diverticulum Exposure.** A longitudinal incision is made through the fibromuscular layer to the diverticular sac, and sharp dissection is used to completely mobilize and expose the sac. The diverticulum is opened,

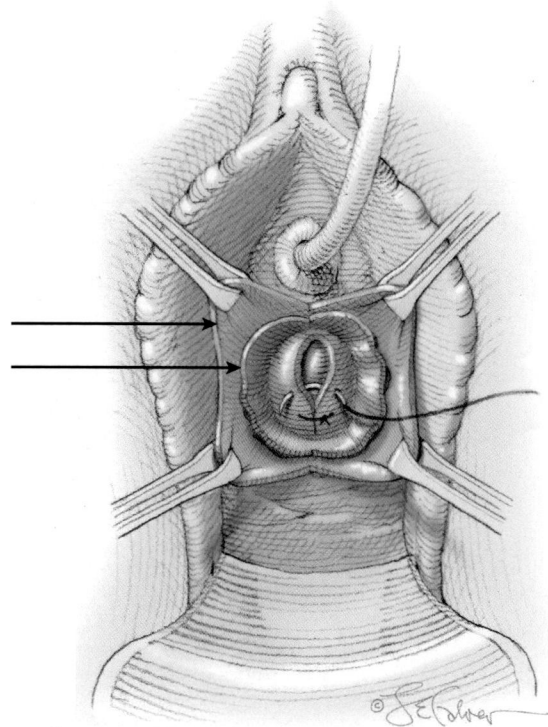

FIGURE 45-9.4 Urethral defect closure.

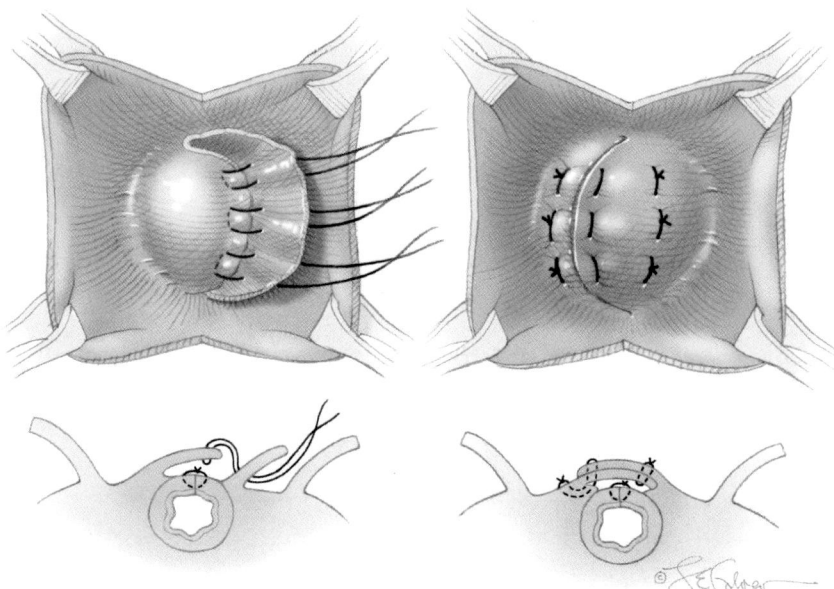

FIGURE 45-9.5 Fibromuscular layer reapproximation.

and the communication with the urethra is identified. To avoid injury to the proximal urethra and bladder neck, the diverticular sac, but not the neck of the diverticulum, is sharply excised. As much of the sac as can be accessed is removed.

❸ **Sac Closure.** The base of the sac is then sutured side to side with 3-0 gauge delayed-absorbable suture to cover the urethral defect. A second, and possibly a third, imbricating layer using the vaginal muscularis is

created with similar suture. Excess vaginal epithelium that had previously covered the diverticulum is excised. The vaginal epithelium is closed in a running fashion with a 2-0 gauge delayed-absorbable suture.

Surgical Steps—Spence Marsupialization

❶ **External Urethral Orifice Incision.** Tips of Metzenbaum scissors are inserted

into the urethral orifice and vagina. An incision is made that incorporates and simultaneously incises the posterior urethral wall, entire thickness of the diverticulum, and distal anterior vaginal wall. By this incision, the external urethral orifice ring is opened and its communication into the diverticular sac is enlarged.

❷ **Marsupialization.** For marsupialization, cut edges of the diverticular sac are reapproximated to the vaginal epithelium in a running pattern using 4-0 gauge delayed-absorbable suture. Ultimately, the urethral orifice is widened by this incorporation of the diverticular sac diameter.

POSTOPERATIVE

Catheter management is an important aspect of postoperative care. Although no consensus guidelines exist, most experts recommend catheter placement for 5 to 7 days. Surgeries of increasing complexity may require longer duration. Antibiotic suppression is not required with this catheter use. Normal diet and activity can resume during the first postoperative days. Intercourse, however, is postponed until the vaginal incision is well healed.

45-10

Vesicovaginal Fistula Repair

Vesicovaginal fistulas may be repaired either vaginally or abdominally. A vaginal approach is preferred for most fistulas seen in the United States, which are posthysterectomy, apical fistulas. This approach offers comparable success rates, lower morbidity, and faster patient recovery. Of vaginal methods, the one most commonly performed by gynecologists is the Latzko technique. With this, surrounding vaginal epithelium is reflected away from the fistulous tract. The tract is then resected, but the portion into the bladder is not excised. This avoids a large bladder defect, which can develop with resection of even relatively small fistulas. Following excision, layered closure of the vaginal incision seals the leak. If performed for fistulas at the vaginal apex, then both anterior and posterior vaginal wall epithelia are reflected for tract access. In this location, the final layered closure simulates the steps of colpocleisis, and thus the Latzko technique for apical fistulas is often likened to a proximal partial colpocleisis (p. 1120).

Alternatively, in some cases, the fistulous tract can be completely excised vaginally, and a layered repair of the bladder and then vaginal wall follows. This is preferred by many if the fistulous opening is less than 5 mm in diameter and distant from ureteral orifices.

At times, an abdominal approach may be necessary for women in whom fistula location prohibits effective surgical access or in whom prior vaginal repairs have been unsuccessful. The most commonly described abdominal approach, termed the O'Conor technique, is outlined here and involves bisecting the bladder wall to enter the fistulous tract. Modifications to this as well as an extravesical approach have been described, especially during laparoscopic or robotic routes to fistula repair (Miklos, 2015). With any abdominal approach, omentum or peritoneum can be mobilized and interposed between the bladder and vagina in an attempt to prevent recurrence.

One principle of fistula repair dictates that a repair be performed in noninfected and noninflamed tissues. A second states that tissue must be approximated without excess tension. Last, a multilayer, watertight closure aids reestablishment of bladder integrity. If these guidelines are followed, success rates are typically good and approximate 95 percent (Rovner, 2012). In the United States, most fistulas follow hysterectomy for benign causes, and repair of these fistulas is associated with high cure rates. In contrast, fistulas associated with gynecologic cancer and radiation therapy may require adjunctive surgical procedures such as vascular or myocutaneous flaps. These flaps provide supportive blood supply to defects that develop in poorly vascularized or fibrotic tissue. Even with these measures, success rates are lower.

PREOPERATIVE

Patient Evaluation

Prior to repair, a fistula should be well characterized, and complex fistulas with multiple tracts or a primary or concomitant ureterovaginal fistula should be identified. Proper evaluation typically includes cystoscopy and imaging that displays the upper and lower urinary tract such as CT urography (pyelography) or intravenous pyelography (IVP) (Fig. 26-2, p. 580). Ureterovaginal fistulas are usually associated with upper tract abnormalities such as hydroureter and hydronephrosis. Therefore, normal IVP or CT findings are reassuring that ureteral involvement is absent. Additionally, this imaging complements cystoscopy in ascertaining the proximity of ureters relative to a fistula for surgical planning. In general, routine posthysterectomy vesicovaginal fistulas develop midline at the vaginal apex and usually away from the ureters, which enter the bladder at the midlength of the vagina. However, lateral fistulas raise concern for ureteral involvement or proximity.

Whether or not surgery can be performed vaginally largely depends on the ability to adequately expose the fistula. Thus, during physical examination, a surgeon assesses if a fistula can be brought down into the surgical field and if a patient's pelvis affords adequate space. Some degree of prolapse of the vaginal apex is helpful for fistula repair. However, a final decision on the repair route is sometimes made intraoperatively, when muscle relaxation from anesthesia allows better assessment of access.

Additionally, tissue infection or inflammation is sought, and if it is identified, fistula repair is delayed until resolution. Fistulas recognized within a few days following hysterectomy may be repaired immediately, prior to the brisk inflammatory response. However, if surgical repair is not undertaken within a few days following the initial surgery, a delay of approximately 6 weeks is recommended to permit tissue inflammation abatement.

Consent

Fistulas may redevelop following repair, and patients are counseled that initial surgery may not be curative. With the Latzko procedure, the vagina is moderately shortened in most cases. Thus, the risk of postoperative dyspareunia is included during surgical consenting. However, a recent study showed that fistula repair improves sexual function and quality of life, with no attributed difference between vaginal and abdominal routes (Mohr, 2014).

Patient Preparation

Immediately prior to surgery, intravenous antibiotics and thromboprophylaxis are commonly administered (Tables 39-6 and 39-8, p. 835). The necessity of bowel preparation for this procedure is unclear, and administration is individualized.

INTRAOPERATIVE

Surgical Steps—Vaginal Repair

❶ **Anesthesia and Patient Positioning.** In most cases, repair is performed with general or regional anesthesia, and postoperative hospitalization is individualized. The patient is placed in standard dorsal lithotomy position, and the vagina is surgically prepared. If ureters lie close to a fistula, ureteral stents are placed (p. 1059). Cystoscopy is required during the procedure to document ureteral patency and assess bladder integrity.

❷ **Delineating a Fistulous Tract.** Initially, the course of a fistulous tract is identified. If a tract is wide enough to accept a pediatric catheter, the tube is threaded through the fistulous tract, and the balloon is inflated within the bladder. If a tract cannot be delineated in this manner, then lacrimal duct probes, ureteral stents, or other suitable narrow dilators are used to trace the tract course and direction. Subsequently, attempts are made to dilate the tract and place a pediatric catheter.

❸ **Exposure.** For repair, the fistula is brought into the operative field. If catheterization of the tract is possible, tension on the catheter will allow this. Alternatively, four sutures can be placed in the vaginal wall surrounding the fistula and used to pull the fistula into the operative field (Fig. 45-10.1). Some advocate performing a mediolateral episiotomy to gain exposure, although this is not our practice.

❹ **Vaginal Incision.** A vaginal incision is made circumferentially approximately 1 to 2 cm around the fistulous tract (Fig. 45-10.2). Vaginal epithelium surrounding the tract is sharply mobilized laterally and away from vaginal fibromuscular wall and then excised with Metzenbaum scissors.

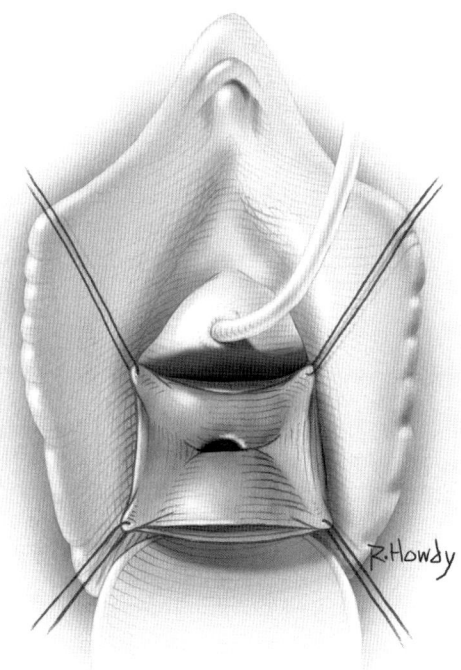

FIGURE 45-10.1 Stay sutures in the vaginal wall improve fistula access.

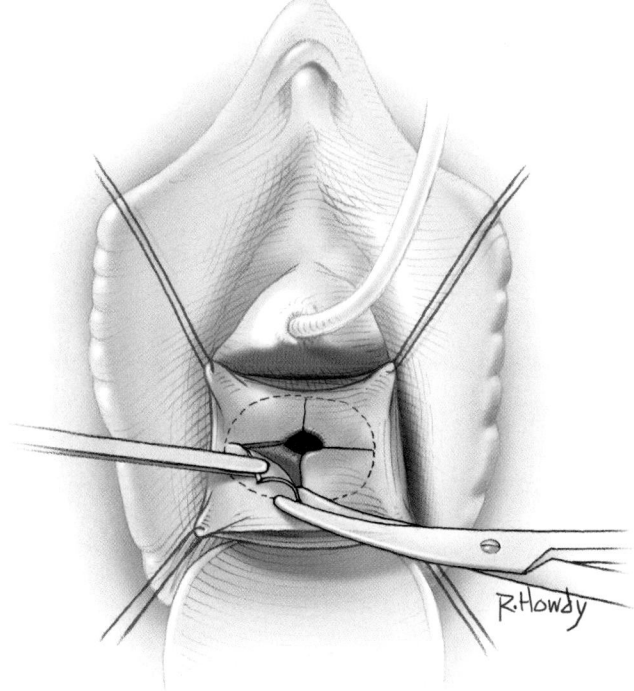

FIGURE 45-10.2 Vaginal epithelium incision.

❺ Tract Excision. The fistula tract may or may not be totally excised to the level of the bladder. As noted earlier, complete tract excision creates a larger bladder defect for repair. Also, we prefer not to excise a fistulous tract lying near a ureteral orifice to avert potential ureteral injury and need for reimplantation (Blaivas, 1995).

❻ Fistula Closure. If a tract is totally excised, the bladder mucosa is reapproximated with 3-0 gauge delayed-absorbable suture in an interrupted or running fashion. Following this closure, the bladder is retrograde filled with at least 200 mL of fluid to exclude leaks. If a defect is found, additional reinforcing sutures are placed until a watertight repair is achieved.

Regardless of whether the tract is completely or partially excised, anterior and posterior bladder and vaginal muscular layers are then approximated over the fistula site. For this, an interrupted or running suture line of 3-0 or 2-0 gauge delayed-absorbable sutures is created (Fig. 45-10.3). Beginning proximally and adding distally, sequential suture lines are layered (Fig. 45-10.4).

After muscular layers of the bladder and vaginal walls are closed, the vaginal epithelium is closed in a continuous running fashion using 3-0 or 2-0 gauge delayed-absorbable suture.

❼ Cystoscopy. Cystoscopy is again performed to document ureteral patency and to inspect the incision site.

Surgical Steps— Abdominal Repair

❶ Anesthesia and Patient Positioning. In most cases, abdominal repair is performed under general anesthesia. The patient is placed in low lithotomy position within booted support stirrups. With the patient's thighs parallel to the ground and the legs separated, access to the vagina is maximized. The abdomen and vagina are surgically prepared, and a Foley catheter is inserted.

❷ Abdominal Incision and Bladder Entry. A low transverse or midline abdominal

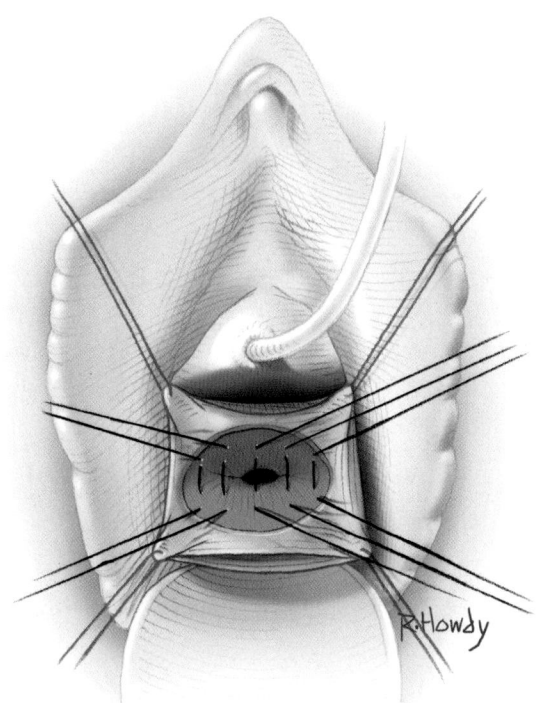

FIGURE 45-10.3 First-layer closure over fistula.

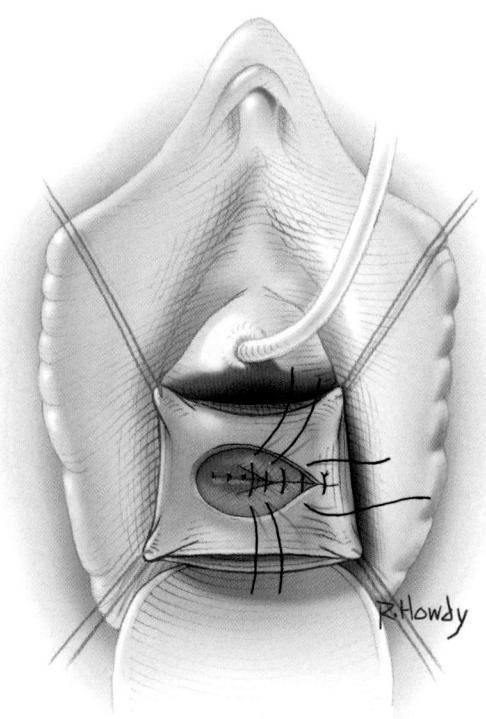

FIGURE 45-10.4 Second fibromuscular layer closure over fistula and vaginal epithelium reapproximation.

entry incision can be used. If mobilization of the omentum is anticipated, a vertical midline incision can provide greater access to the upper abdomen. A Maylard or Cherney incision may alternatively be selected (Section 43-3, p. 931). After the peritoneum is entered, the abdomen is explored, bowel is packed from the operating field, and a self-retaining abdominal wall retractor is placed. The space of Retzius is opened using the technique described on page 1061. Next, a vertical midline extraperitoneal incision is made into the bladder dome. Prior to this incision, pushing the Foley balloon up or filling the bladder helps avoid grasping and then cutting the posterior bladder wall.

❸ **Fistulous Tract Delineation and Excision.** After cystotomy, the fistula and ureteral orifices are seen from within the bladder. If the fistulous tract is near the orifices, ureteral stents are placed. From the dome, the cystotomy incision is extended over the top and then back of the bladder to reach the circular fistulous opening (Fig. 45-10.5). A lacrimal probe or catheter may be placed into the fistulous tract to delineate its course. The tract is then excised.

In contrast and less commonly, if a fistula tract lies close to the trigone, extension of the bladder incision to the fistulous tract may not be desired, as the resulting bladder defect would be extensive. In these cases, the entire fistulous tract is directly excised using only the bladder dome incision. However, vascular flap interposition with this approach is limited as the bladder wall is not significantly dissected off the vaginal wall.

❹ **Separation of the Bladder and Vagina.** In cases with bladder bisection, sharp dissection is used to separate the vagina away from the bladder in the area of the fistula (Fig. 45-10.6). Scarring may be extensive, and sharp rather than blunt dissection is preferred. To assist, the rounded tip of an end-to-end anastomosis (EEA) sizer can be placed in the vagina to manipulate and accentuate the dissection plane (Fig. 46-21.4, p. 1202). The vagina is widely separated from the bladder to allow omentum or peritoneal flap placement between the two.

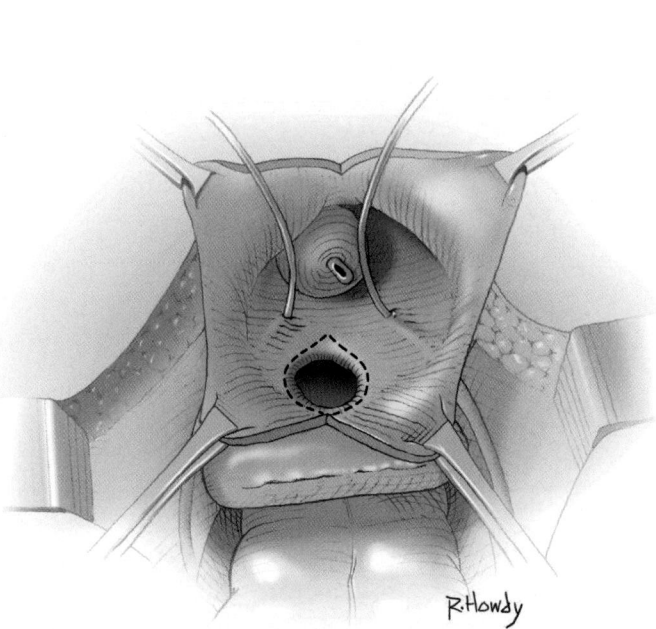

FIGURE 45-10.5 Bladder incision.

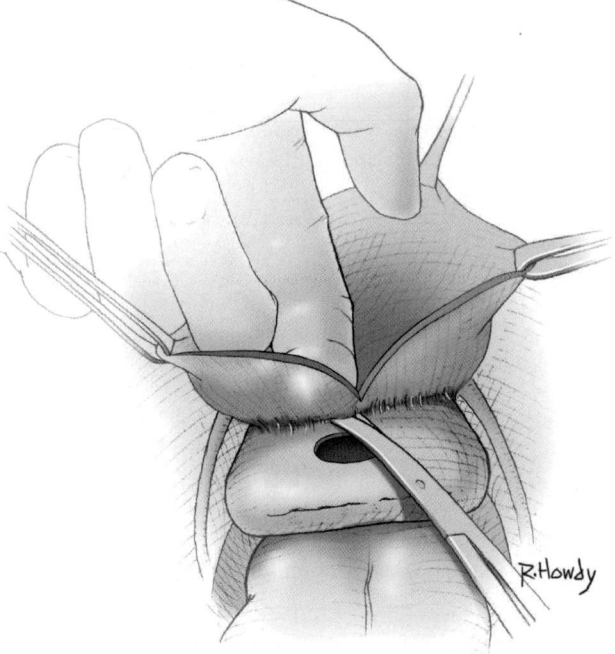

FIGURE 45-10.6 Separation of the bladder and vagina.

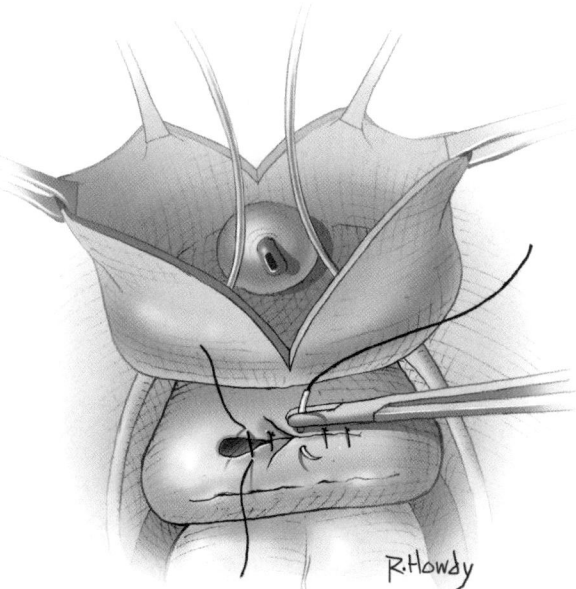

FIGURE 45-10.7 Vaginal closure.

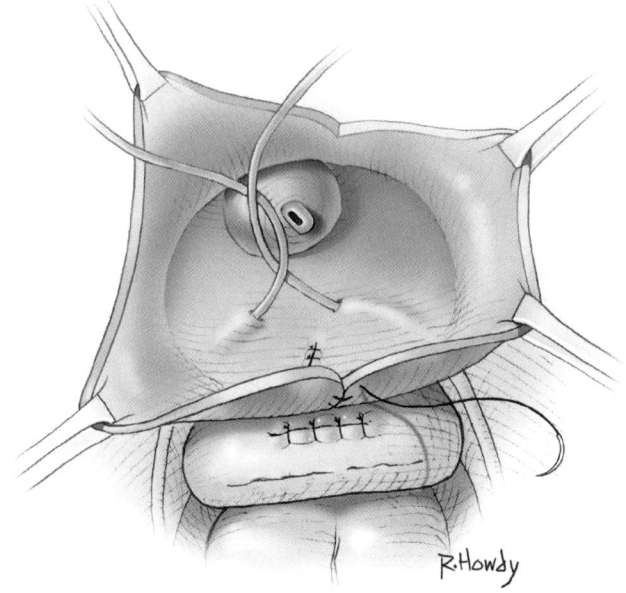

FIGURE 45-10.8 First-layer bladder closure.

❺ **Vaginal Closure.** The vagina is closed in one or two layers with 2-0 gauge delayed-absorbable suture and running or interrupted stitches (Fig. 45-10.7). The EEA sizer or fingers within the vagina can accentuate the vaginotomy margins to aid closure.

❻ **Bladder Closure.** The entire bisecting bladder incision is closed in two or three layers using running sutures of 3-0 gauge absorbable suture (Fig. 45-10.8). As with the vaginal approach, after the first layer, the bladder is retrograde filled with at least

200 mL, and incision-line leaks are sought. If defects are noted, additional reinforcing sutures are placed to achieve a watertight repair. During bladder closure, each subsequent layer is imbricated such that the preceding suture line is covered and tension is released (Fig. 45-10.9).

If the bladder is not bisected and the fistulous tract is directly excised solely through the bladder dome cystotomy, then the muscular wall of vagina is first repaired in one or two layers as in Step 5. Second, the bladder wall at the fistula excision site is closed in one or two

layers using a running stitch of 3-0 absorbable suture. Next, the bladder mucosa is reapproximated with a single-layer running stitch of 3-0 absorbable suture. Last, the entry bladder dome incision is closed similarly, except the bladder mucosa is reapproximated first and followed by bladder wall closure in layers.

❼ **Omental or Peritoneal Interposition.** As described in Section 46-14 (p. 1186), the omentum can be mobilized to create a J-flap. The omentum is then sutured to the anterior wall of the vagina to cover the incision

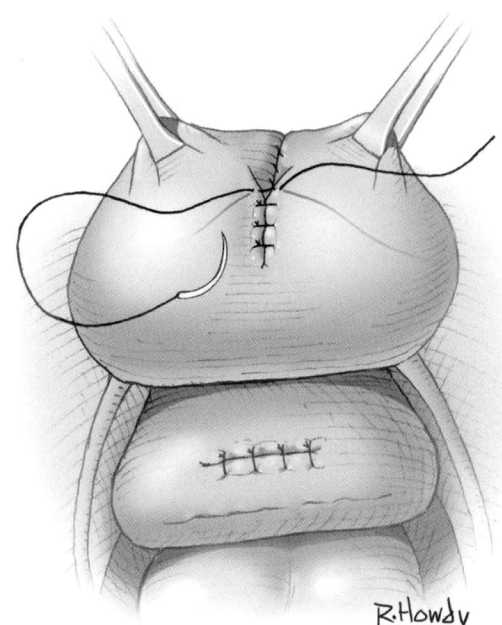

FIGURE 45-10.9 Second-layer bladder closure.

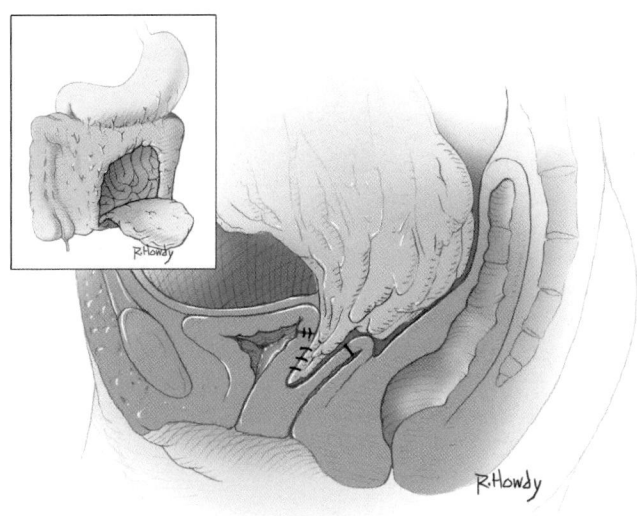

FIGURE 45-10.10 Omentum interposition.

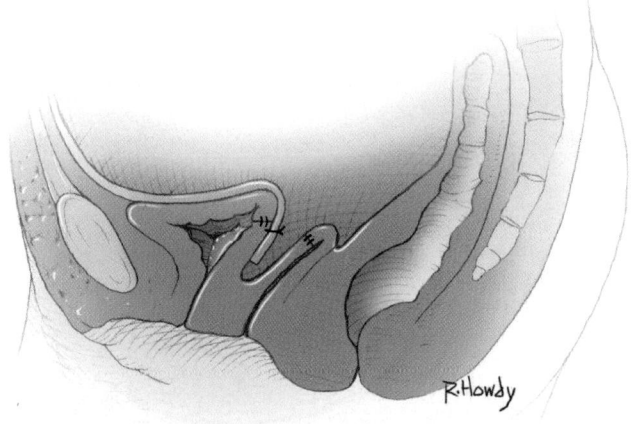

FIGURE 45-10.11 Peritoneum interposition.

line (Fig. 45-10.10). This provides a tissue layer between vagina and bladder, increases vascular flow to the area, and may improve tissue healing. Alternatively, if the omentum cannot be mobilized, peritoneum, although less vascular, can be interposed and creates another barrier layer between the bladder and vagina (Fig. 45-10.11).

❽ **Cystoscopy.** Cystoscopy is performed to document ureteral patency and inspect the incision site.

❾ **Incision Closure.** The abdominal incision is closed as described in Chapter 43 (p. 931).

POSTOPERATIVE

The bladder is drained postoperatively to prevent overdistention and suture disruption. Either transurethral or suprapubic catheter placement will ensure adequate drainage in the immediate postoperative period. At our institution, we generally continue catheterization for at least 2 weeks following vesicovaginal fistula repair. Antibiotic suppression is not required with this catheter use.

45-11

Martius Bulbocavernosus Fat Pad Flap

This vascular graft contains the fat pad overlying the bulbospongiosus (formerly called bulbcocavernosus) muscle and brings a supportive blood supply to repairs involving avascular or fibrotic tissue. As such, this graft is commonly used in complex urethral diverticulum excisions or in complex rectovaginal or vesicovaginal fistula repairs. However, of these indications, there is some evidence supporting successful repair of certain recurrent fistulas without vascular graft interposition (Miklos, 2015; Pshak, 2013).

During graft placement, one end of the bulbocavernosus fat pad is dissected free and subsequently brought to the repair site through the primary vaginal incision. Thus, due to its anatomic origin and limited length, this fat pad, when indicated, is selected for defects involving the low to mid-vagina.

PREOPERATIVE

Patient Evaluation

In most instances, graft placement is anticipated for those with prior radiation or with fistula recurrence. Thus, preoperative planning includes assessment of tissue vascularity, connective tissue strength, and ability to adequately mobilize vaginal tissues to create a multilayered repair closure. For this procedure, a woman must have adequate labial fat, which is also assessed prior to surgery.

Consent

During consenting, women are informed of the potential for postoperative vulvar numbness, pain, paresthesias, or hematoma. Because one of the labia majora is repositioned as the graft, patients are counseled regarding the cosmetic consequences.

Patient Preparation

Because of the risk of poor wound healing in these complicated repairs, antibiotic prophylaxis listed in Table 39-6 (p. 835) is warranted. Thromboprophylaxis is given as outlined in Table 39-8 (p. 836. The necessity of bowel preparation for this procedure is unclear, and administration is individualized based on concomitant procedures.

INTRAOPERATIVE

Surgical Steps

❶ **Anesthesia and Patient Positioning**
In most cases, a Martius flap graft and fistula repair can be performed with general or regional anesthesia, and the need for postoperative hospitalization is individualized. The patient is positioned in standard lithotomy position, the vagina is surgically prepared, and a Foley catheter is inserted.

❷ **Fistula or Diverticulum Repair.** The specific defect is repaired as outlined in its respective section of this chapter.

❸ **Labial Incision.** After repair completion, the lateral margin of one labium majus is incised (Fig. 45-11.1). The length of the incision is tailored to specific labial anatomy and graft size needed. In many cases, a 6- to 8-cm incision is made beginning below the level of the clitoris and is extended inferiorly.

❹ **Mobilization of the Fat Pad.** The vulvar incision edges are retracted laterally, and sharp dissection is used to free the labial fat pad (Fig. 45-11.2). This tissue is vascular, and vessels ideally are ligated or coagulated prior to transection. For rectovaginal fistulas, a broad base is left inferiorly, and the fat pad is detached superiorly. For vesicovaginal and urethrovaginal fistulas or urethral diverticula, the broad base of the pad is maintained superiorly, while the fat pad is detached inferiorly. In each instance, releasing the pad with this specific polarity anatomically permits the largest possible graft to cover the repair site. Occasionally, bilateral fat pads are needed.

❺ **Graft Placement.** After the pad is freed, a tunnel is created by bluntly dissecting with a hemostat that travels from the vulvar incision, underneath the vaginal epithelium, and to the vaginal incision at the repair site. The tunnel must be sufficiently broad to avoid vascular compression and graft necrosis. A suture is placed at the graft tip and used to pass the graft through the tunnel and into the vagina (Fig. 45-11.3).

❻ **Graft Fixation.** The graft is secured to the vaginal muscularis overlying the repair site with several interrupted stitches using 3-0 gauge delayed-absorbable suture (Fig. 45-11.4).

❼ **Incision Closure.** With hemostasis established, the vulvar incision is closed along its length using continuous or interrupted stitches of 3-0 gauge delayed-absorbable

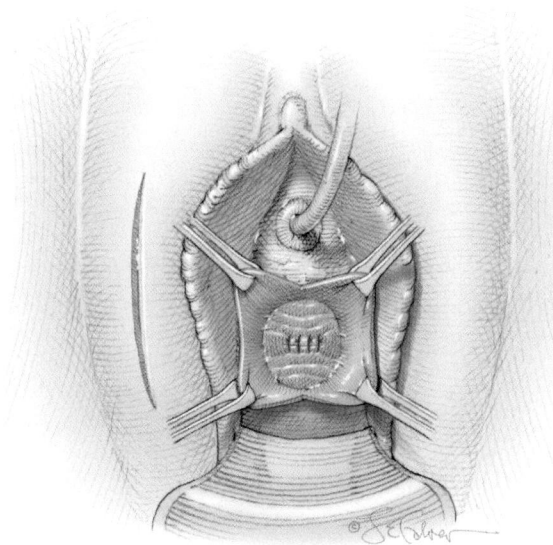

FIGURE 45-11.1 Labial incision.

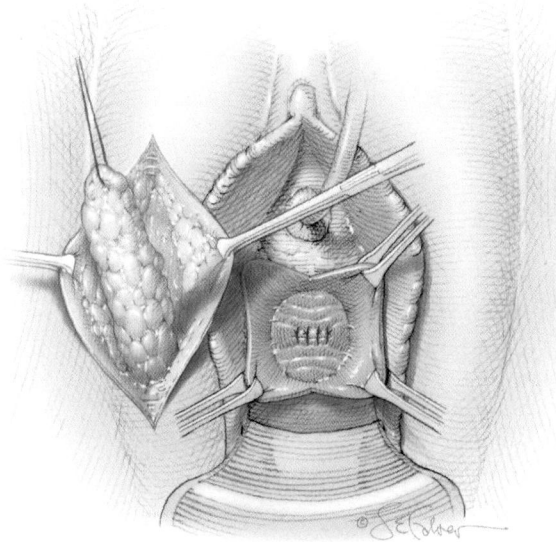

FIGURE 45-11.2 Mobilization of the fat pad.

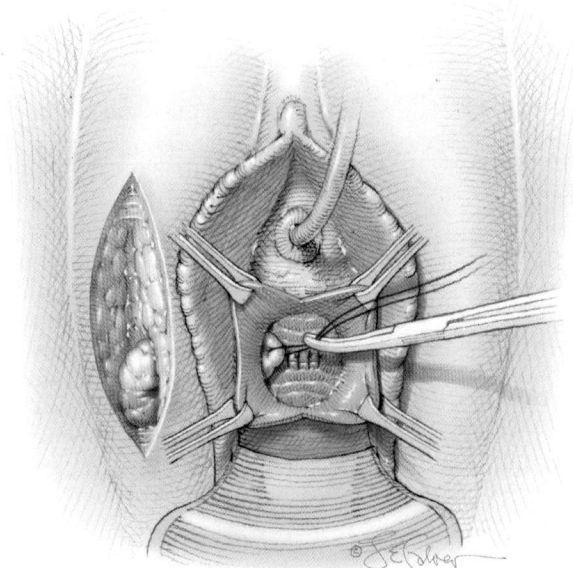

FIGURE 45-11.3 Graft placement.

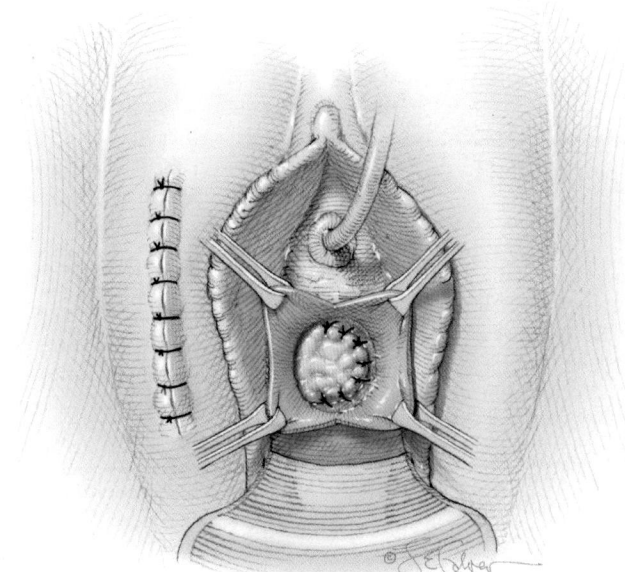

FIGURE 45-11.4 Graft fixation.

sutures. For a deep cavity at the harvest site, fatty tissue may be reapproximated in layers to close this space with several interrupted 2-0 or 3-0 gauge delayed-absorbable sutures. Alternatively, a drain may be placed in the cavity. The vaginal epithelium overlying the defect repair is closed in a continuous running fashion using 3-0 gauge delayed-absorbable suture.

POSTOPERATIVE

Care after surgery is predominantly dictated by the associated defect repair. Ideally, the vaginal and perineal sites are kept dry rather than wet, and baths are avoided during the first 6 weeks. After each void or stool, patients rinse with a water-filled squirt bottle and gently pat dry.

45-12

Sacral Neuromodulation

Sacral neuromodulation or sacral nerve stimulation (SNS) electrically stimulates the sacral nerves to modulate reflexes that influence the bladder, sphincters, and pelvic floor (Noblett, 2014). Currently, the InterStim System is the only implantable SNS device that is Food and Drug Administration (FDA)-approved for the following primary indications: urgency-frequency, urgency urinary incontinence, nonobstructive urinary retention, and fecal incontinence. Although not FDA-approved for chronic pelvic pain, interstitial cystitis/painful bladder syndrome, or chronic idiopathic constipation, it may sometimes be used if these symptoms coexist with the previously listed primary indications. This surgery is typically offered to women who have failed to adequately improve with multiple other conservative therapies. The mechanism of action is unclear, but one explanation describes modulation of reflex neural pathways involved with bladder storage and emptying and with innervation of the pelvic floor. Of these, pudendal afferent somatic fibers are thought to play an important role (deGroat, 1981; Gourcerol, 2011).

SNS is generally completed in two phases. First, during a test phase, a slender, 30-cm long permanent lead that conducts electrical impulses to its tip is placed into one posterior sacral foramen and adjacent to a sacral nerve root, most commonly S3. This lead is connected to a temporary external pulse generator to permit an efficacy trial lasting 1 to 2 weeks. If symptoms are decreased by at least 50 percent, then the patient is deemed a suitable candidate for permanent generator implantation. During the second or implantation phase, the lead is connected a permanent implantable pulse generator (IPG), and the IPG is tucked within a subcutaneous pocket created in the buttock. This staged approach is illustrated in these atlas pages.

A variation of these classic steps, termed percutaneous nerve evaluation (PNE), inserts a *temporary* lead through the S3 foramen in the office, under local anesthesia, and generally without fluoroscopic guidance. However, despite these advantages, the trial period with PNE is brief (3 to 7 days), and the less securely anchored temporary lead more easily migrates away from the target nerve.

PREOPERATIVE

Patient Evaluation

Preoperative testing will vary depending on the indication. For urinary symptoms, women undergo full evaluation including urodynamic testing, voiding diary, cystoscopy, and other selected tests described in Chapter 23 (p. 523). For fecal incontinence, colonoscopy, endoanal sonography, manometry, and possibly pudendal nerve testing, described in Chapter 25 (p. 564), are completed during evaluation.

Consent

Failure to significantly improve symptoms may follow either SNS phase. However, approximately 70 percent of those who undergo permanent IPG implantation achieve a greater than 50-percent symptom improvement (Van Kerrebroeck, 2012). Pain at the IPG site and superficial wound infection may also complicate either phase. Long-term adverse changes include altered bowel or bladder function, undesirable sensations, neurostimulator site numbness, lead migration, and surgical device revision, replacement, or required removal. The IPG device is a relative contraindication for MR imaging, although certain IPG models permit head imaging.

Patient Preparation

A single prophylactic antibiotic dose may or may not be administered according to surgeon preference. Although not rigorously studied, prophylaxis is recommended by some due to needle passage from skin

to perineural tissue in the presacral space. Thromboprophylaxis is typically not required given the procedure's short duration.

INTRAOPERATIVE

Surgical Steps

❶ **Anesthesia and Patient Positioning.** Although the procedure can be performed using local anesthesia and intravenous sedation, we prefer general anesthesia for the test phase. Importantly, neuromuscular blockade prohibits adequate motor response evaluation and is contraindicated. The patient is positioned prone on a Wilson frame or with a pillow under the lower abdomen to flex the hip 30 degrees for easier access to the sacrum. Pillows are also placed under the shins to allow the toes to move freely during test stimulation. The drape is positioned to permit inspection of the pelvic floor and soles for muscle responses. The area from the lower back to the perineum is surgically prepared. A Foley catheter is typically not required due to the surgery's brevity.

❷ **Identification of S3 Foramina.** These landmarks for lead placement are located approximately 9 cm above the coccyx and 1 to 2 cm lateral to the midline (Fig. 45-12.1). Fluoroscopy is currently the most common method of identifying the necessary bony landmarks intraoperatively. The fluoroscopic C-arm is draped and moved into the anteroposterior (AP) position to allow mapping of the sacral region including foramina. With this, the skin overlying the S3 foramina is outlined with a surgical marker.

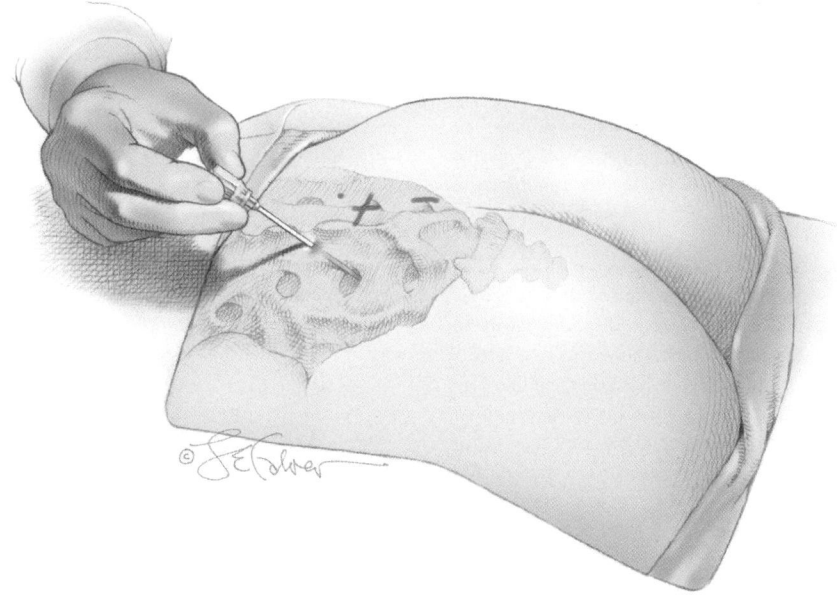

FIGURE 45-12.1 Foramen needle insertion.

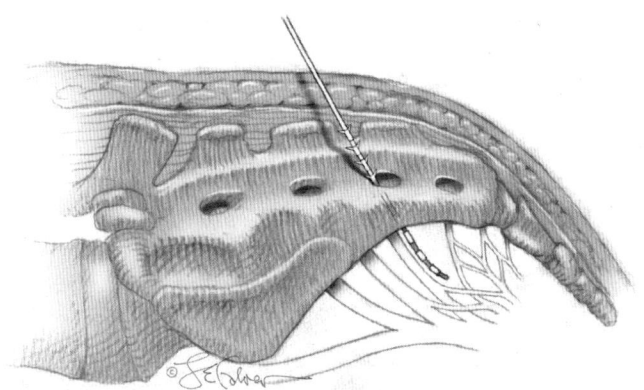

FIGURE 45-12.2 Correct lead positioning.

❸ **Foramina Needle Insertion.** An insulated foramen needle is inserted through the skin at a site approximately 2 cm lateral to the midline, 2 cm superior to the sciatic notch, and cephalad to the inked outline of the foramen. The needle is guided at a 60-degree angle caudally until the S3 foramen is penetrated. Optimally, the needle is placed into the medial and superior aspect of the S3 foramen. The needle penetrance depth, which is usually 2.5 to 4.0 cm, is confirmed and adjusted with fluoroscopic guidance by a laterally positioned C-arm.

Once in place, the needle is used to conduct electrical test impulses to the S3 nerve. This nerve contracts the levator ani muscles to create an inward retraction or "bellows" movement. S3 stimulation also causes the great toe to flex downward, that is, plantar flexion. In anesthetized patients, a sensory response cannot be elicited, but evidence suggests that motor responses may be more or at least as predictive of success (Cohen, 2006; Govaert, 2009; Peters, 2011). The typical patient sensation with S3 stimulation is a tapping or vibration in the vagina, rectum, or perineum. Once the desired S3 motor reflexes are obtained ("bellows and toe"), lead placement is initiated. If these are absent, needle depth or angle is adjusted to achieve the desired responses. Also, a needle in the contralateral foramen or in a foramen up or down one vertebral space may be tried.

❹ **Lead Placement.** Once positioned, the stylet present within the foramen needle is removed and replaced with a guide wire to the appropriate depth. The foramen needle is then removed while holding the guide wire in place. A small incision is made on either side of the guide wire, and a combined introducer sheath/hollow dilator tool is then slid over the guide wire to occupy the foramen needle's former position. The hollow dilator is unscrewed from the introducer sheath, and the dilator and guide wire are removed together. This leaves only the introducer sheath in place.

Next, using fluoroscopy, the long, flexible lead is passed down the introducer sheath into the S3 foramen. To aid threading, the lead contains a temporary stiff inner stylet. A recently introduced curved stylet better follows anatomic contours to position the lead close to the nerve root (Jacobs, 2014). The lead also contains four circumferential electrode bands arranged in series at its tip, and proximal to these lie four plastic barbs or tines to ultimately anchor the lead within soft tissues (Fig. 45-12.2).

With correct lead positioning as shown, the most proximal of the four electrode bands are fluoroscopically visible just anterior to the sacrum. All four electrodes on the lead should conduct pulses and elicit S3 motor responses. If necessary, the lead can be repositioned within the foramen. Once correctly positioned, the introducer sheath and then the curved lead stylet are removed. As the introducer sheath is removed, the four tines or barbs lock into place. Thus, the lead cannot be retracted after this point. All four electrodes are again tested to confirm the previously observed responses.

If lead advancement is needed, its stylet is replaced and the lead advanced. Retraction is more problematic. The lead is removed using gentle traction, and Steps 3 and 4 are repeated. The desired range of stimulation amplitude to achieve desired motor responses is 1 to 2 milliamps. Responses at lower amplitudes may indicate that the lead lies too close to the nerve, whereas requisite higher amplitudes can decrease battery longevity.

❺ **Pulse Generator Incision and Lead Passage.** Several centimeters below the iliac crest, a 4-cm transverse incision is made over the lateral portion of the buttock that is ipsilateral to the selected foramen. Sharp and blunt dissection is used to create a deep pocket that can house the extension device for the temporary external pulse generator and eventually, the permanent IPG. The pocket should remain above the gluteal muscle fascia but is made sufficiently deep to accommodate the final IPG.

After the pocket is created, a pointed passing device is used to create a narrow tunnel between the lead and the pocket (Fig. 45-12.3). The core of the passing device is removed, leaving a hollow straw within the tunnel (inset). The lead is then manually threaded laterally

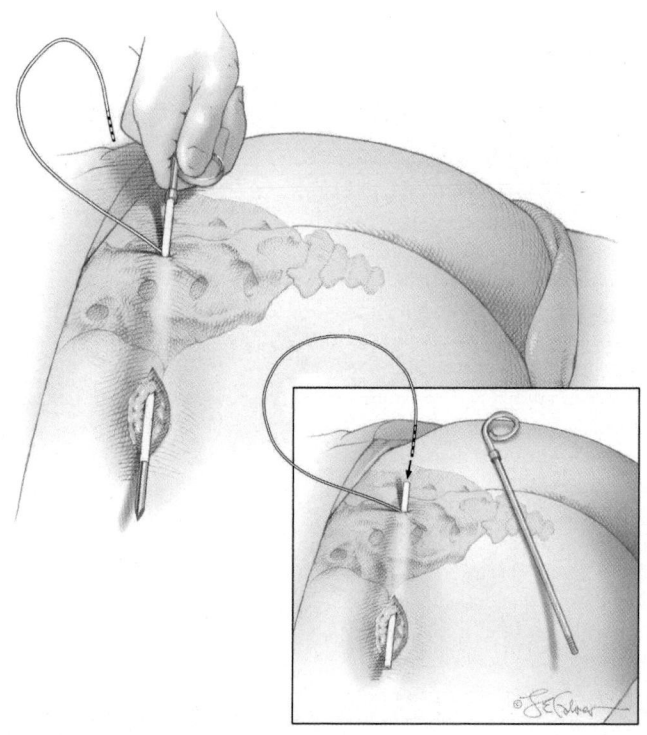

FIGURE 45-12.3 Pulse generator incision and lead passage.

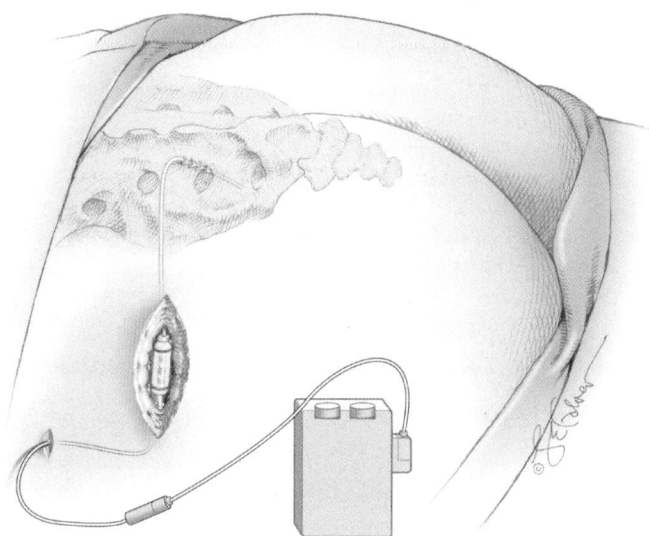

FIGURE 45-12.4 Within pocket, lead joins extension wire that extends to temporary pulse generator.

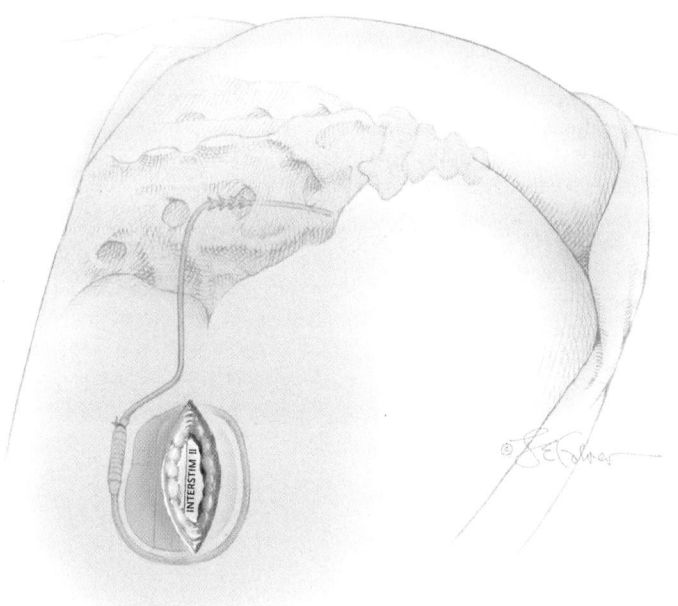

FIGURE 45-12.5 Final implanted pulse generator.

through this straw and into the pocket. The straw is then removed laterally.

❻ Placement of the Extension Device (First Phase). Within the subcutaneous pocket, the lead is next connected to an extension wire that serves to join the lead to the temporary pulse generator (Fig. 45-12.4). A stab incision is then created lateral to the pocket. The passing device is again used and, this time, guides the extension wire through a second tunnel between the pocket and stab incision. The subcutaneous tissue is then closed over the connector in the pocket with 2-0 gauge delayed-absorbable suture in an interrupted or running fashion. The skin is closed with a subcuticular stitch using 4-0 gauge delayed-absorbable suture or with other suitable skin closure methods. Similarly, the stab incision is closed. Last, the extender wire is joined to a temporary external pulse generator, which is used for 1 to 2 weeks (see Fig. 45-12.4).

❼ Implantable Pulse Generator Placement (Second Phase). If significant symptom relief is obtained, the permanent IPG is placed 1 to 2 weeks after initial surgery. The procedure is performed with the patient prone and usually with general anesthesia for airway control. The buttock incision is opened down to the connector. The connector and extension wire are removed. The permanent IPG is connected to the lead, and then placed into the subcutaneous pocket (Fig. 45-12.5). The incision is closed again as in Step 6.

POSTOPERATIVE

Pain or erythema at the incision site suggests cellulitis, abscess, or seroma. These symptoms are evaluated as soon as possible, and antibiotics are instituted if needed. Unusual pain is also evaluated immediately as this could suggest lead malfunction. A woman can turn the device off by herself if necessary. Primary symptoms are continually assessed postoperatively, and the IPG is reprogrammed as needed. Reprogramming the device or changing leads will often lead to symptom improvement.

SECTION 6

45-13

Anterior Colporrhaphy

The anterior vaginal wall is the most frequent site of clinically recognized prolapse (Brincat, 2010). One method to correct this is anterior colporrhaphy, which reapproximates attenuated fibromuscular tissue between the vagina and bladder to elevate the bladder to a more anterior and anatomically normal position. Anatomic success rates following this surgery are modest at 1 year (Altman, 2011; Weber, 2001). Thus, strategies to improve these colporrhaphy rates include: (1) concurrent vaginal paravaginal defect repair (PVDR), (2) concurrent apical support surgeries, or (3) synthetic or biologic mesh placement instead of or in addition to colporrhaphy.

Of these, PVDR attempts to provide lateral support to the anterior vaginal wall. However, the vaginal PVDR is less favored as its required dissection creates a large defect within tissue that carries significant nerves and vessels. Also, efficacy data are lacking.

Synthetic mesh placement is associated with improved anterior prolapse anatomic outcomes (61 versus 35 percent) (Altman, 2011). But this disparity in anatomic success does not always reflect symptom success rates (Chmielewski, 2011). Symptom improvement rates for mesh range from 75 to 96 percent compared with ranges of 62 to 100 percent for native tissue (Lee, 2012). Moreover, mesh use significantly increases risks of mesh erosion, vaginal lumen narrowing, and pelvic abscess (Maher, 2013). These may be associated with dyspareunia, urinary complaints, and chronic pelvic pain (Food and Drug Administration, 2011). Currently, few data guide patient selection for mesh placement, which may be best reserved for those with recurrent prolapse or those with medical comorbidities that preclude alternative procedures (American College of Obstetricians and Gynecologists, 2011). Moreover, surgeons using mesh need adequate training and experience, and patients are educated regarding risks and benefits. Alternatively, cadaveric fascia has been similarly used, but surgical success using this tissue is not significantly improved compared with colporrhaphy alone (Gandhi, 2005).

Last, increasing data suggest that vaginal apex support plays a critical role in anterior vaginal wall suspension (Lowder, 2008; Summers, 2006). Thus, anterior colporrhaphy is now often complemented by apical support procedures.

PREOPERATIVE

Patient Evaluation

As stated, women with anterior wall prolapse often have other compartment defects, and a complete POP-Q examination, described in Chapter 24 (p. 540), aids surgical planning. In addition, anterior vaginal wall prolapse is frequently associated with stress urinary incontinence (SUI) (Borstad, 1989). Even those who are continent, however, may have occult SUI unmasked following prolapse correction. Thus, preoperative urodynamic evaluation is often recommended. During this evaluation, the prolapse is reduced to its anticipated postoperative position to mimic pelvic floor anatomy and dynamics following surgery (Chaikin, 2000; Yamada, 2001). The decision to perform a concurrent prophylactic antiincontinence procedure is then dictated by individual urodynamic findings and adequate patient counseling.

Consent

For most women, anterior colporrhaphy has low complication rates. Of these, recurrence of the anterior vaginal wall defect is one of the most frequent. De novo SUI described earlier, prolonged catheter use for urinary retention, and voiding dysfunction are also discussion points. Although infrequent, postoperative dyspareunia is another cited complication. However, preoperative symptoms related to sexual function in general improve with anterior colporrhaphy (Weber, 2001). Uncommonly, serious hemorrhage, cystotomy, or ureteral injury may occur intraoperatively.

If mesh is used, these latter risks may be increased, and bowel or ureteral injury is possible. Accordingly, intraoperative cystoscopy is recommended. Less common short-term postoperative mesh complications include wound infection or hematoma. Long-term data from randomized trials show mesh erosion rates that range from 5 to 19 percent; chronic pain, up to 10 percent; and dyspareunia, 8 to 28 percent (American College of Obstetricians and Gynecologists, 2011).

Patient Preparation

Bowel preparation is generally not indicated for isolated anterior colporrhaphy but may be recommended at the surgeon's discretion if other compartmental repairs are planned. Antibiotic prophylaxis with a first- or second-generation cephalosporin is recommended immediately prior to surgery as cystoscopy is also performed. Thromboprophylaxis is given as outlined in Table 39-8 (p. 836).

INTRAOPERATIVE

Surgical Steps

❶ **Anesthesia and Patient Positioning.** After adequate general or regional anesthesia is administered, a patient is placed in standard lithotomy position, the vagina is surgically prepared, and a Foley catheter inserted. A short Auvard weighted speculum may be positioned to retract the posterior vaginal wall.

❷ **Concurrent Surgery.** Anterior colporrhaphy can be performed with the uterus in situ or alternatively, following hysterectomy. If other reconstructive surgeries are required, they may precede or follow anterior colporrhaphy.

❸ **Vaginal Incision.** In those with prior hysterectomy and adequate apical support, two Allis clamps are placed on each side of the midline, 1 to 2 cm distal to the vaginal apex or at the upper extent of the anterior vaginal wall prolapse (Fig. 45-13.1) Clamps are gently pulled laterally to create tension, and the vaginal wall between them is incised transversely. If hysterectomy precedes the repair, the two Allis clamps are placed at the opened cuff edge on either side of midline.

A third clamp is placed in the midline vaginal wall, 3 to 4 cm distal to the apical transverse incision. All three clamps are held, creating gentle outward tension. Metzenbaum scissors tips are insinuated beneath the epithelium in the midline of the previously made transverse incision and directed away from the vaginal apex. Scissor blades are opened and closed, while the surgeon exerts gentle

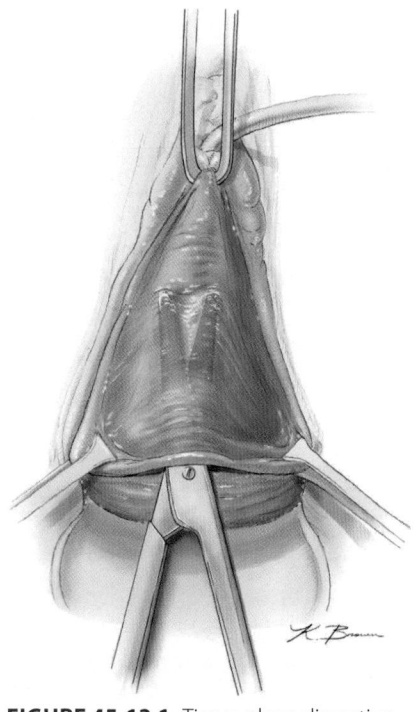

FIGURE 45-13.1 Tissue plane dissection.

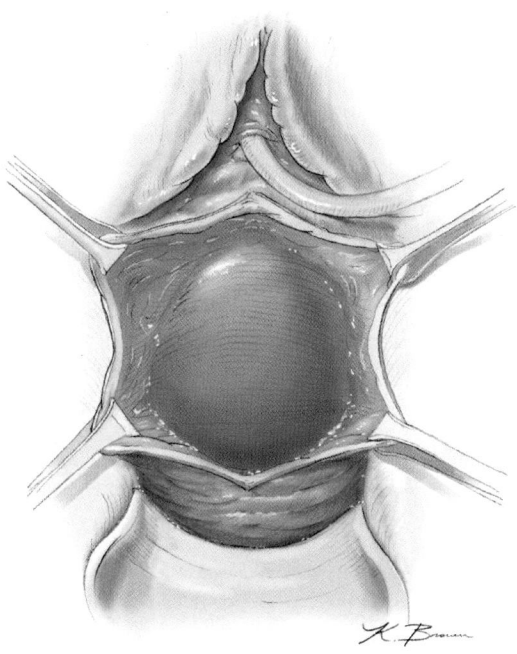

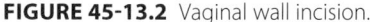

FIGURE 45-13.2 Vaginal wall incision.

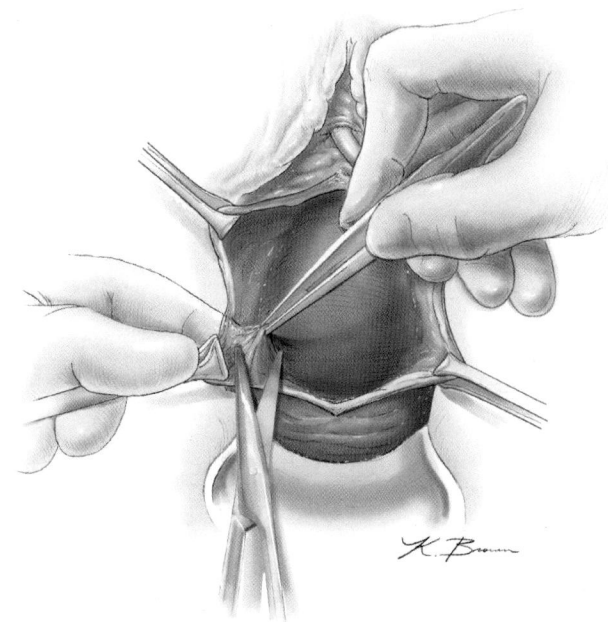

FIGURE 45-13.3 Separation of epithelium from fibromuscular layer.

forward pressure that is parallel to and within the plane beneath the vaginal epithelium. This technique allows separation of the epithelium from the fibromuscular layer. This dissection continues caudad to reach the distal, midline Allis clamp. The undermined vaginal wall is then incised in the midline longitudinally. The midline Allis clamp is then replaced more distally, and the process continues until the vaginal epithelium has been divided to within 2 to 3 cm of the external urethral opening (Fig. 45-13.2). This ending spot corresponds to a midpoint along the length of the urethra. If the anterior wall prolapse does not extend distally beyond the bladder neck, then the distal epithelial incision terminates at the neck. In addition, if a concurrent midurethral sling is planned, the colporrhaphy incision terminates just proximal to the bladder neck to allow a separate incision for sling placement.

❹ **Lateral Dissection.** Along the freed epithelial edges, additional Allis or Allis-Adair clamps are placed to create gentle outward tension, while the vaginal epithelium is dissected laterally off the vagina's fibromuscular wall (Fig. 45-13.3). This is accomplished with one finger placed behind the epithelium to accentuate the dissection plane, while scissors are held parallel to the vagina and cut connective tissue fibers between the epithelium and fibromuscular layer. Once the desired tissue plane is entered, a combination of sharp and blunt dissection readily separates the layers. Simultaneous countertraction on the fibromuscular layer by an assistant using tissue forceps or a gauze-covered finger can aid dissection. This separation is extended laterally toward the pelvic walls until substantial fibromuscular tissue is exposed to permit mid-

line plication. The steps are then repeated on the contralateral side.

❺ **Traditional Anterior Colporrhaphy.** Plication of the fibromuscular layer to the midline is then begun. For this, an interrupted stitch of 2-0 gauge delayed-absorbable suture is placed on one side of the midline beginning nearest the apex. This same needle and suture are carried to the other side of the midline, and a mirror stitch is placed the same distance from the apex. To plicate tissue, the bites of each stitch are generously spaced to bring together the wide lateral

span of attenuated tissue. However, excessive tension is avoided to prevent sutures from pulling through the fibromuscular tissue or from significantly narrowing the vagina. As sutures are tied, the midline bladder bulge is elevated by the surgeon gently upward and away from the incision line. Such plication creates a firm fibromuscular wall layer to support the bladder and if indicated, the urethra (Fig. 45-13.4).

❻ **Vaginal Paravaginal Defect Repair.** If vaginal PVDR is to be performed, the vaginal dissection described above is extended

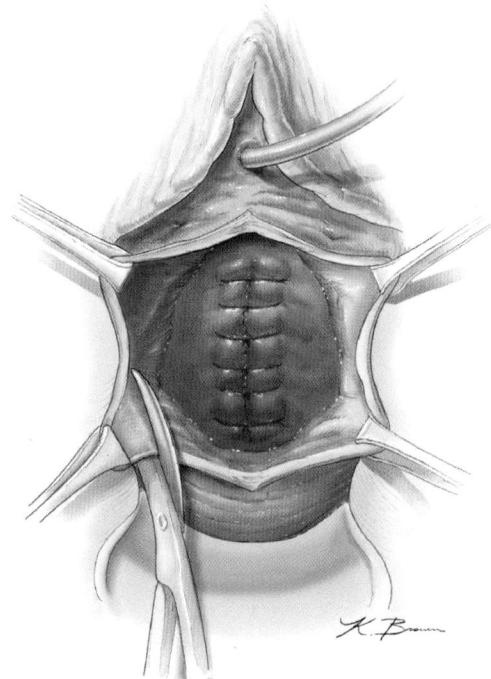

FIGURE 45-13.4 Midline plication completed.

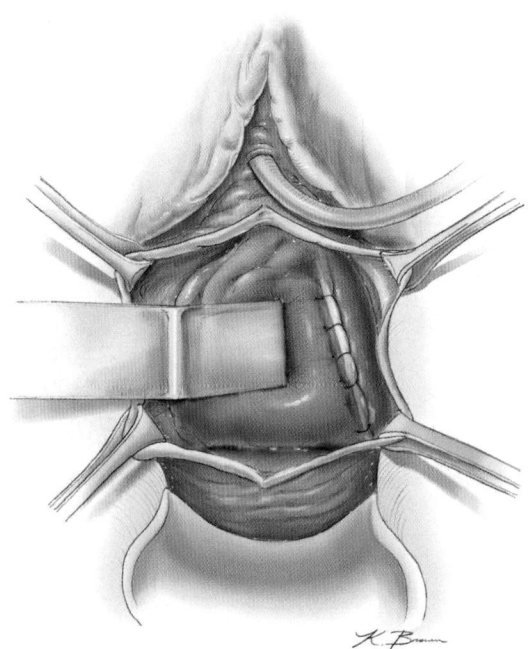

FIGURE 45-13.5 Vaginal paravaginal defect repair.

❽ Mesh Placement. Various marketed mesh kits are available, and full descriptions for placement are provided by individual manufacturers. In general, a broad mesh sling supports the proximal anterior vaginal wall and has mesh arms that extend and anchor to the sacrospinous ligaments (SSLs) to provide apical support. Concurrently, the distal extent of the mesh ends at the level of the bladder neck.

For placement of anterior and apical mesh repair kits, the paravesical space is entered by lateral dissection similar to the steps for vaginal PVDR (Step 6). The ATFP and the ischial spines are palpated. A finger also slides medially over the SSL. The recommended fixation point on this ligament is 2 to 3 cm medial to the ischial spine, which is similar to the fixation point for the traditional SSL fixation procedure (p. 1112).

❾ Cystoscopy. Kwon and coworkers (2002) performed cystoscopy following 346 anterior colporrhaphy procedures and found unexpected injury in 2 percent of cases. These each required suture removal and replacement. Accordingly, cystoscopy is warranted to document integrity of the ureteral orifices, bladder, and urethral lumen.

POSTOPERATIVE

For most women, recovery following anterior colporrhaphy is rapid and associated with few complications. Urinary retention or UTI, however, is common. Prior to discharge, an active voiding trial is performed. If a Foley catheter remains, a second voiding trial can be repeated in a few days or at the surgeon's discretion.

As with other vaginal surgery, diet and activity can be advanced as tolerated. Women, however, abstain from intercourse until wound healing is complete, typically at 6 to 8 weeks following repair.

laterally to the pelvic side walls at the level of the arcus tendineus fascia pelvis (ATFP) (Chap. 38, p. 808). Dissection also generally extends from the dorsal surface of the pubic bones to the ischial spines. Blunt dissection is typically used to enter the space of Retzius. If a paravaginal defect is present, the space is easily entered. Visualization of the pelvic sidewall is aided by Breisky-Navratil and lighted retractors. If present, the ATFP appears as a white line running from pubic bone's dorsal surface to the ischial spine. In some cases, the ATFP is attenuated and indistinct, and stitches are instead anchored to the obturator internus muscle's investing fascia. For repair, a series of four to six 2-0 gauge permanent sutures are placed in the ATFP or obturator fascia and attached to the paravaginal connective tissue (Fig. 45-13.5).

❼ Incision Closure. Depending on the size of the original anterior wall defect, some redundant vaginal wall will likely be present and require trimming (see Fig. 45-13.4). Liberal trimming, however, can place the vaginal wall incision on excessive tension, affect wound healing, and narrow the vagina. The vaginal epithelium is reapproximated in a running fashion with a 2-0 gauge delayed-absorbable suture.

Abdominal Paravaginal Defect Repair

Paravaginal defect repair (PVDR) is a prolapse procedure that aims to correct lateral defects in the anterior vaginal wall. The procedure involves attachment of the lateral vaginal wall to the arcus tendineus fascia pelvis (ATFP) (Fig. 38-24, p. 817). This procedure is rarely performed alone and is more often combined with other prolapse procedures, especially abdominal sacrocolpopexy. PVDR is ineffective treatment for stress urinary incontinence (SUI). That said, abdominal PVDR may be performed in conjunction with the antiincontinence Burch colposuspension if a lateral anterior wall defect and prolapse complaints coexist with SUI. PVDR can also be performed laparoscopically or robotically by those with advanced skills. If sutures can be placed the same as in the abdominal approach, the results are expected to be equivalent, but data are limited.

PREOPERATIVE

Patient Evaluation

Demonstration of lateral vaginal wall defects on physical examination is required prior to surgery. If significant anterior wall prolapse is identified, evaluation for SUI or occult SUI is pursued. In women who have a paravaginal defect, other pelvic support defects such as apical or posterior vaginal prolapse commonly coexist. Thus, attempts to identify these defects precede surgery.

Consent

Paravaginal defect repair provides support to the lateral vaginal walls, but as with other prolapse procedures, long-term success rates may diminish with time. The procedure involves surgery in the space of Retzius, which has the potential for significant blood loss. In particular, risks of bleeding and bladder injury are generally greater in patients with prior space of Retzius surgery as dense adhesions between bladder and pubic bone are common. Inaccurate suture placement can result in injury to the bladder and/or ureters, although this is infrequent.

Patient Preparation

As with most abdominal urogynecologic surgeries, antibiotic prophylaxis is given to pre-

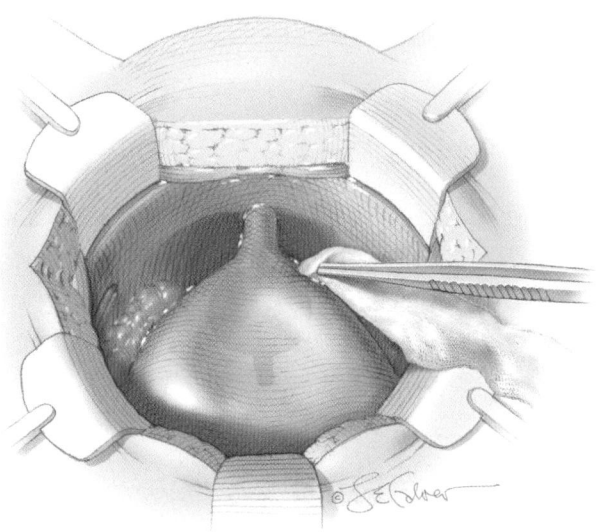

FIGURE 45-14.1 Dissection in the space of Retzius.

vent wound infection (Table 39-6, p. 835). Bowel preparation may be implemented at the surgeon's discretion if additional procedures are planned. Thromboprophylaxis is given as outlined in Table 39-8 (p. 836).

INTRAOPERATIVE

Surgical Steps

❶ **Anesthesia and Patient Positioning.** When performed in conjunction with apical or other repairs, this surgery is typically performed as an inpatient procedure under general anesthesia. Following administration of anesthesia, the patient is placed in low lithotomy position in booted support stirrups. Adequate exposure to the vagina is vital because a vaginal hand is used to elevate and dissect the paravaginal/paravesical space. The abdomen and vagina are surgically prepared, and a Foley catheter with a 10-mL balloon is inserted.

❷ **Abdominal Incision.** A low transverse incision placed 1 to 2 cm cephalad to the symphysis pubis affords the best exposure to the space of Retzius. This procedure is typically done in conjunction with abdominal sacrocolpopexy, and the abdominal cavity is entered (Section 43-2, p. 929). If performed in isolation or with a Burch colposuspension, entry into the peritoneal cavity is not necessary to open the space of Retzius.

❸ **Entering the Space of Retzius.** After incision of the fascia, the rectus muscles are separated in the midline and retractors are used to hold them apart. To open the space of Retzius, the correct dissection plane lies directly behind the pubic bone, deep to the transversalis fascia but superficial to the perito-

neum. Loose areolar tissue is gently dissected in a lateral-to-medial fashion with atraumatic forceps or scissors beginning immediately behind the pubic bone (Fig. 45-14.1). If the correct plane is entered, this avascular potential space opens easily and without significant hemorrhage. Small bleeding vessels within the loose areolar tissue are coagulated as encountered. If significant bleeding does occur, the wrong tissue plane has likely been entered. From prior surgery in this space, the bladder often adheres to the pubic bone and anterior abdominal wall and thus sharp dissection is indicated.

After the medial portion of the space of Retzius is opened, the obturator canal is identified bilaterally so that its associated vessels and nerve can be avoided. The canal is generally found 5 to 6 cm lateral from the pubic symphysis midline and 1 to 2 cm below the iliopectineal line. The ischial spine is then palpated 4 to 6 cm below and posterior to the obturator canal. The remainder of the paravaginal space is opened with gentle blunt dissection using a gauze sponge. This dissection is generally directed lateromedially, that is, from obturator fascia to lateral bladder border, to expose the ATFP and paravaginal tissue. To assist, a vaginal hand pushing up into the space creates a firm surface to dissect against. In addition, a malleable retractor gently displaces the bladder to the contralateral side.

Large paravaginal blood vessels are often noted along the lateral vaginal wall. Bleeding from these vessels can be controlled by upward pressure of the vaginal hand while hemostatic sutures are placed.

❹ **Identification of the Arcus Tendineus Fascia Pelvis.** The ATFP runs along the pelvic sidewall between the pubic bone and

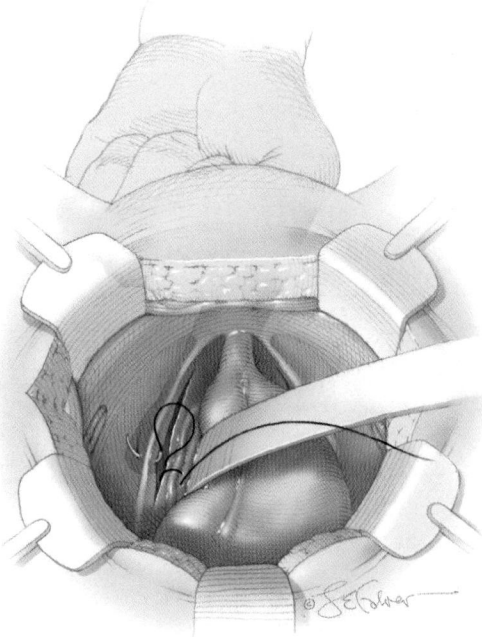

FIGURE 45-14.2 Placement of paravaginal sutures.

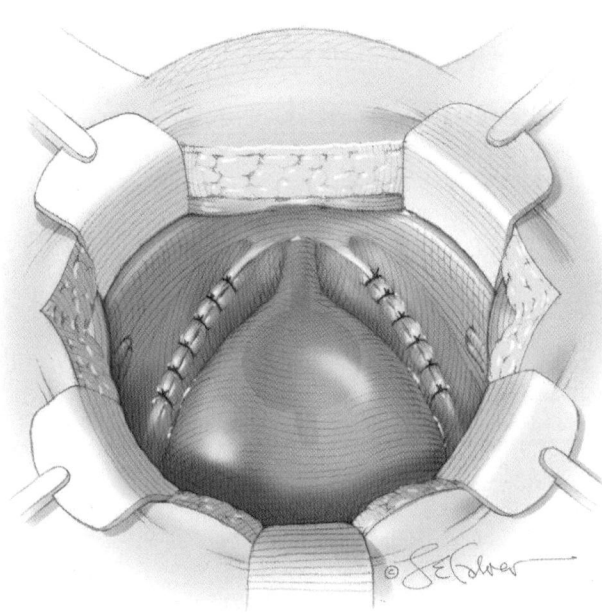

FIGURE 45-14.3 Final suture placement.

the ischial spine as a white connective tissue condensation. In those with defects, it may be attenuated, torn in the middle, or completely avulsed from the sidewall. Even in these cases, the distal third of the ATFP is generally preserved and easily identified.

❺ Placement of Paravaginal Sutures. One or two fingers of the surgeon's nondominant hand are placed in the vagina to elevate the lateral vaginal wall on the planned side of defect repair. At the same time, a medium-sized malleable retractor is used to reflect the bladder medially and protect it and the ureter from inadvertent suture placement or entrapment.

Usually four to six interrupted 2-0 gauge permanent sutures placed approximately 1 cm apart are needed to obliterate the paravaginal defect. The ultimate suture line extends from the level of the ischial spine to the level of the bladder neck or proximal

urethra (Fig. 45-14.2). Each suture passes through the paravaginal tissue just lateral to the bladder wall and through the ATFP or obturator internus fascia and tied. A vaginal finger covered by a thimble for protection presses upward against the lateral vaginal wall to help isolate the paravaginal tissue and assess suture penetration. If a suture punctures the vaginal lumen, it is removed, discarded, and replaced by a more superficial stitch. If bleeding follows, the suture may be tied to constrict involved vessels. Prior to suture placement, the obturator canal and neurovascular bundle are identified and avoided. After all sutures are placed, the procedure is repeated on the other side of the vagina (Fig. 45-14.3).

❻ Cystoscopy. This is performed to note efflux from both ureteral orifices and to exclude bladder-perforating sutures. A

misplaced suture might be seen as a dimple in the bladder wall. If found, sutures entering the bladder are removed abdominally and properly placed.

❼ Incision Closure. After vigorous irrigation of the space of Retzius, the abdomen is closed in a standard fashion (Section 43-2, p. 930). If the peritoneum was opened, closure is recommended to prevent small bowel adhesions in the space of Retzius.

POSTOPERATIVE

In general, recovery follows that associated with laparotomy or endoscopy and varies depending on concurrent surgeries and incision size. A voiding trial as described in Chapter 42 (p. 917 is performed prior to hospital discharge.

45-15

Posterior Colporrhaphy

Posterior colporrhaphy, also colloquially termed posterior repair, is traditionally used to repair prolapse of the posterior vaginal compartment. Specifically, posterior colporrhaphy techniques attempt to reinforce the fibromuscular tissue layer between the vagina and rectum to prevent prolapse of the rectum into the vaginal lumen. The tissue plicated in the midline is often reapproximated distally to the level of the hymen and here includes reapproximation of the perineal body tissue. This is especially important for women who display "perineal descent" during preoperative evaluation. Women with such poor perineal strength may often reinforce (or splint) the perineal body to aid defecation. For these women, perineorrhaphy is often carried out concurrently. Often, the posterior vaginal wall apex must also be suspended to obtain successful repair and prevent recurrence. The apex may be suspended vaginally to the uterosacral or sacrospinous ligament or abdominally to the anterior longitudinal ligament of the sacrum. Thus, a careful preoperative evaluation is essential to restore anatomy.

There are three current transvaginal repairs of posterior wall prolapse. First, traditional midline plication of levator ani muscles, also known as levator myorrhaphy or levatorplasty, plicates the puborectalis muscle in the midline (Francis, 1961). Second, midline vaginal wall plication without levator myorrhaphy brings together the vaginal wall muscularis and adventitial layers in the midline. Tissue previously referred to as "rectovaginal fascia" is in fact these muscularis and adventitial layers, as histologic studies of normal anatomy illustrate a lack of true fascia between the vagina and rectum. Last, defect-directed, also called site-specific, repair reapproximates attenuated vaginal wall at specific bulge sites rather than rotely in the midline. Among these, evidence suggests that midline plication without levator myorrhaphy has superior objective outcomes compared with site-specific repair and has lower dyspareunia rates than levator myorrhaphy (Karram, 2013). For these reasons, midline plication without levator myorrhaphy is the procedure of choice for posterior compartment prolapse except perhaps in select cases, such as women with large genital hiatus undergoing colpocleisis.

Importantly, compared with these methods, a biologic or synthetic graft in the posterior compartment does not improve anatomic or functional outcomes (Maher, 2013; Paraiso, 2006; Sung, 2012). Well-designed studies that demonstrate efficacy and safety of newly developed grafts are needed before surgeons incorporate these materials into their practices.

PREOPERATIVE

Patient Evaluation

A detailed discussion of symptoms begins every patient evaluation prior to colporrhaphy. Often, patients may associate all of their bowel symptoms to a posterior wall bulge, but the two may not be related. Specifically, if constipation is a major complaint, further evaluation and trial of nonsurgical treatment is typically indicated (Chap. 25, p. 569). Symptoms most likely to be cured or improved by posterior repair include the sensation of vaginal bulge and the need to digitally compress the rectal vault for defecation. Also termed vaginal splinting, compression involves placing fingers in the vagina and pushing downward over the defect or sweeping forward to help empty bowel. As another compensatory action, a digit may be inserted in the rectum to scoop out stool.

Posterior wall prolapse commonly accompanies other support defects, and patients undergo a complete pelvic organ prolapse examination. If concurrent anterior vaginal wall or vaginal apex prolapse is present, these are also repaired.

Consent

In addition to standard surgical risks, this procedure may be associated with failure to correct symptoms or anatomy. Accordingly, a patient and surgeon identify treatment goals and clarify expectations. In the few completed randomized studies, current techniques give a less than optimal anatomic repair, and success rates approximate 70 percent. Another frequent postoperative risk is dyspareunia, which is more common following the levator ani muscle plication discussed earlier. Accordingly, levator plication is not recommended in women who desire to preserve coital function. Injury to the rectum or rectovaginal fistula is another rare but potential complication.

Patient Preparation

Depending on surgeon preference, patients may be instructed to take in only clear liquids the day prior to surgery and complete one or two enemas that night or the morning of surgery. Ballard and associates (2014), however, noted no distinct advantage to this. Antibiotics and thromboprophylaxis are given as outlined in Tables 39-6 and 39-8 (p. 835).

INTRAOPERATIVE

Surgical Steps

❶ **Anesthesia and Patient Positioning.** If done in isolation, posterior colporrhaphy is typically a day-surgery procedure for healthy women and performed under general or regional anesthesia. A patient is placed in standard lithotomy position in candy-cane or booted support stirrups. The vagina is surgically prepared, and a Foley catheter inserted.

❷ **Concurrent Surgery.** Posterior colporrhaphy can be performed with the uterus in situ or alternatively, following hysterectomy. If other reconstructive surgeries are required, they may precede or follow posterior colporrhaphy. Notably, completion of the posterior repair prior to vaginal apex suspension permits the plicated and thus more substantial tissue to be anchored to selected ligaments during apical suspension.

❸ **Vaginal Incision and Dissection.** Two Allis clamps are placed on the posterolateral wall of the distal vagina on either side of the midline. Clamps are gently pulled laterally to create tension, and the vaginal wall between them is incised transversely at or just proximal to the level of the hymen and superficial to the perineal body. A third Allis clamp is placed in midline and 3 to 4 cm proximal to the introitus. All three clamps are held, creating gentle outward tension. Metzenbaum scissors tips are insinuated beneath the epithelium in the midline of the previously made transverse incision and directed cephalad (Fig. 45-15.1). Scissor blades are opened and closed, while the surgeon exerts gentle forward pressure that is parallel to and within the plane beneath the vaginal epithelium. This technique allows separation of the epithelium from the fibromuscular layer. This dissection continues cephalad to reach the proximal midline Allis clamp. The undermined vaginal epithelium is then incised in the midline longitudinally.

The midline Allis clamp is then replaced further cephalad, and the process continues until the vaginal epithelium has been divided to the level of the vaginal apex. If a concurrent hysterectomy has been performed, the colporrhaphy incision generally extends to the cuff incision. In either case, if only a simple discrete distal to mid-vagina defect is present, then the midline colporrhaphy incision stops just cephalad to that defect's proximal border.

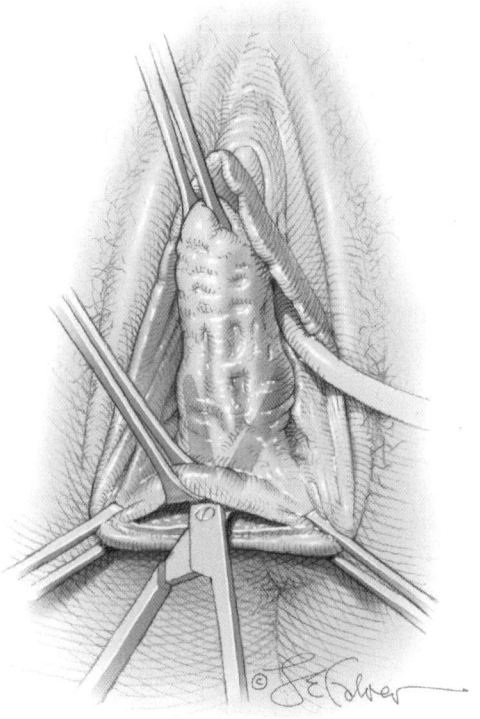

FIGURE 45-15.1 Vaginal incision and dissection.

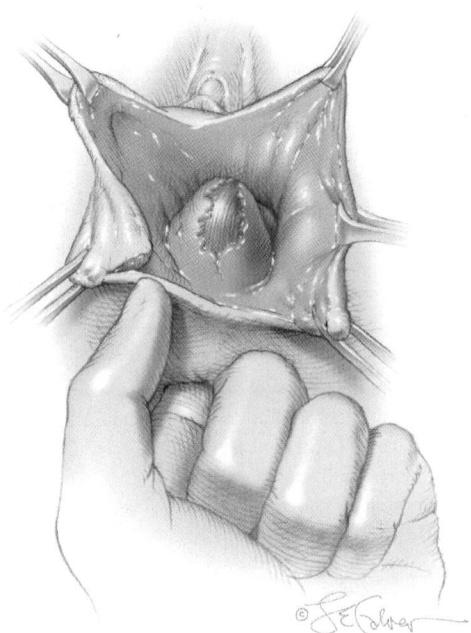

FIGURE 45-15.2 Rectal examination.

❹ **Lateral Dissection.** Along the freed epithelial edges, additional Allis or Allis-Adair clamps are placed to create gentle outward tension, while the vaginal epithelium is dissected laterally off the vagina's fibromuscular wall. This is accomplished with one finger placed behind the epithelium to accentuate the dissection plane. Scissors are held parallel to the vagina and cut connective tissue fibers between the epithelium and fibromuscular layer.

During this early lateral dissection, the perineal body is fused with the vaginal wall fibromuscular layer, and scarring may be present from prior episiotomy. Thus, clear tissue planes are not typically present, and sharp dissection is required. Cephalad to the perineal body, once the desired tissue plane is entered, a combination of sharp and blunt dissection readily separates the layers. Simultaneous countertraction on the fibro-

muscular tissue by an assistant using tissue forceps or a gauze-covered finger can aid dissection. Separation in the correct tissue plane is essential. Deep dissection can enter rectum, whereas superficial dissection can create holes in the vaginal epithelium, often called "button holes."

This tissue separation is extended laterally toward the pelvic walls until substantial fibromuscular tissue is exposed to permit

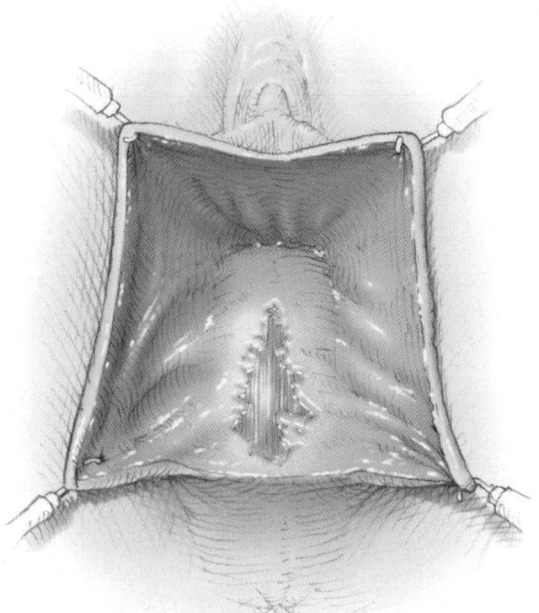

FIGURE 45-15.3 Midline defect.

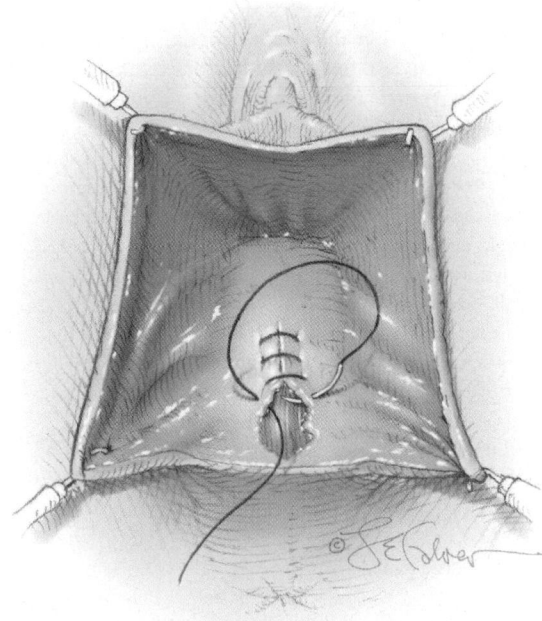

FIGURE 45-15.4 Midline plication.

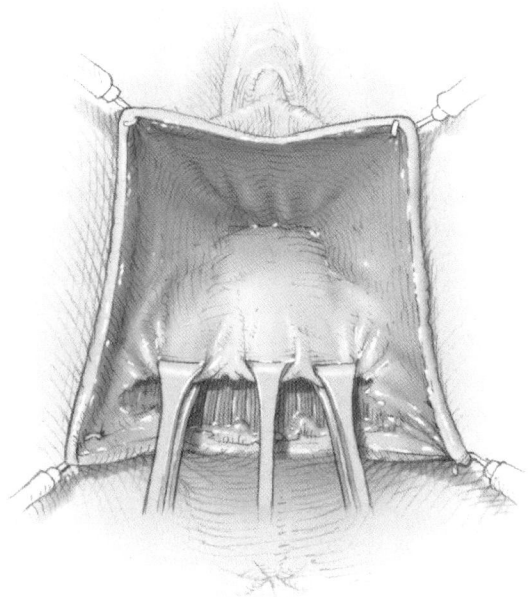

FIGURE 45-15.5 Distal defect.

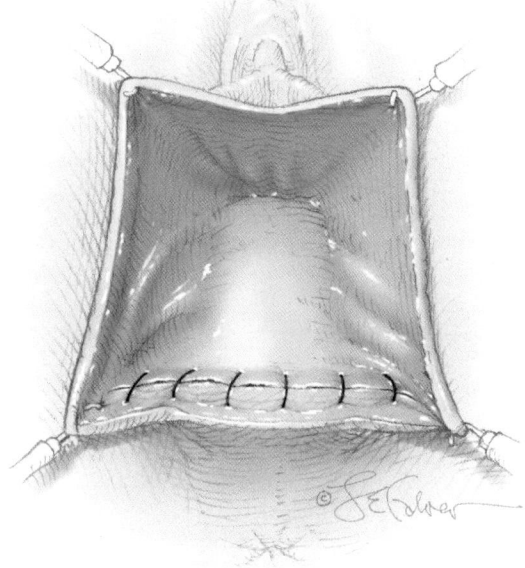

FIGURE 45-15.6 Defect-directed repair.

midline plication. The steps are then repeated on the contralateral side.

❺ Rectal Examination. Rectal examination is performed to exclude rectal injury and to help identify the edges of the fibromuscular wall to be plicated (Fig. 45-15.2).

❻ Midline Plication. A series of interrupted 2-0 gauge delayed-absorbable sutures are used to plicate the vaginal muscularis and perineal body tissue along the length of the posterior vaginal wall (Figs. 45-15.3 and 45-15.4). As noted, levator plication is avoided in patients who desire to preserve coital function as the risks of vaginal lumen narrowing and dyspareunia may be higher. To plicate tissue, an interrupted stitch of 2-0 gauge delayed-absorbable suture is placed on one side of the midline beginning nearest the apex. This same needle and suture are carried to the other side of the midline, and a mirror stitch is placed the same distance from the apex. The the bites of each stitch are generously spaced to bring together the wide lateral span of attenuated tissue. Such plication creates a firm fibromuscular wall layer to support the rectum and if indicated, the perineal body. However, excessive tension is avoided to prevent sutures from pulling through the

fibromuscular tissue or from significantly narrowing the vagina. As sutures are tied, the midline rectal bulge is gently pushed downward by the surgeon and away from the incision line.

Rectal examination is again performed after all sutures are placed to exclude inadvertent suture placement into the rectum. If identified, these are removed and correct suture placement completed.

❼ Defect Assessment. In some instances, a discrete defect is identified in the posterior fibromuscular layer after the initial dissection. Defects may be lateral, midline, apical, or perineal (Figs. 45-15.5 and 45-15.6). Repair focuses solely on the defect, which is closed by interrupted stitches of 2-0 gauge delayed-absorbable sutures. This is generally a one-layer closure. This repair may be complemented by a midline plication if significant tissue attenuation is still noted.

❽ Indicated Apical Suspension. If indicated, apical suspension is performed after vaginal wall plication. The proximal posterior vagina is affixed to either the uterosacral or sacrospinous ligament, as described on page 1107. If perineorrhaphy is planned, it is also completed prior to incision closure.

❾ Incision Closure. Following plication, redundant vaginal wall often remains and requires trimming. Liberal trimming, however, can narrow the vagina and can place the vaginal wall incision on excessive tension that impairs wound healing. The vaginal mucosa is reapproximated in a running fashion using a 2-0 gauge delayed-absorbable suture. Widely positioned sutures are avoided as they can create accordion-type bunching of the vaginal epithelium and subsequent vaginal shortening when the final suture is tied.

POSTOPERATIVE

Patients are instructed on perineal hygiene. Constipation and straining are avoided, and stool softeners are usually prescribed. As with other vaginal surgery, diet and activity can be advanced as tolerated. Women, however, abstain from intercourse until wound healing is complete, typically at 6 to 8 weeks following repair. Some women have urinary retention after posterior repairs, even without an antiincontinence procedure. If unable to void spontaneously by the time of discharge, a patient can go home with a catheter and be seen again within a week for removal.

45-16

Perineorrhaphy

The perineal body serves as core support of the distal vagina, rectum, and pelvic floor. Therefore, a damaged or weakened perineal body may contribute to distal prolapse. Reinforcement of this structure, that is, *perineorrhaphy*, is often performed in conjunction with other reconstructive procedures, such as posterior colporrhaphy. To reestablish distal support, perineorrhaphy lengthens the anteroposterior dimension of a shortened perineal body, while the genital hiatus is concurrently narrowed.

PREOPERATIVE

Patient Evaluation

During assessment, the length of the genital hiatus is measured in centimeters both at rest and with Valsalva maneuver from the external urethral opening at 12 o'clock to the posterior aspect of the hymeneal ring at 6 o'clock. The perineal body is measured from the hymeneal ring at 6 o'clock to the mid-anus.

With perineorrhaphy planning, the degree to which the perineal body is lengthened can be tailored according patient symptoms, surgical goals, and clinical findings. With typical perineorrhaphy, the degree of perineal body lengthening is minimized to create or maintain a genital hiatus wide enough to preserve comfortable intercourse. Moreover, in sexually active postmenopausal women whose partners have decreased erectile tone, entry into the vagina may be difficult if the introitus is too narrow. Thus, following perineorrhaphy, 2 to 3 fingers ideally comfortably pass through the introitus.

For women with "perineal descent" who have to splint to defecate or in those with distal defects and attenuated perineal body tissue, perineorrhaphy may be coupled with posterior colporrhaphy. As described on page 1093, the distal extent of the plicated rectovaginal wall can be reattached to the perineal body. This reestablishes continuity of connective tissue support in the posterior vaginal compartment.

In some women, pelvic support takes precedence, and coital function is also not desired. With "high" perineorrhaphy, the superior-to-inferior extent of the perineal body is lengthened and generally accompanied by plication of the levator ani muscle fascia at the superior aspect of the perineal body. The result of this extensive perineorrhaphy is a shorter genital hiatus length and narrower introitus and vaginal lumen. This may be an advanta-geous adjunct to colpocleisis. However, data showing improved colpocleisis outcomes by adding levator myorrhaphy are limited (Gutman, 2009).

Consent

A patient preparing for perineorrhaphy is counseled regarding risks of postoperative dyspareunia, prolapse recurrence, or wound complications, such as a stitch abscess. Bleeding from perineal skin tearing during intercourse may also result and require minor surgical revision.

Patient Preparation

Because of the surgical site's close proximity to the anus and also because bowel injury is possible, antibiotic prophylaxis is administered prior to surgery to minimize wound infection risks (Table 39-6, p. 835). Bowel preparation, which may employ clear liquid diet and enemas, mirrors that for posterior repair (p. 1093). Thromboprophylaxis is given as outlined in Table 39-8 (p. 836).

INTRAOPERATIVE

Surgical Steps

❶ **Anesthesia and Patient Positioning** Perineorrhaphy is typically performed under general or regional anesthesia, and this choice is often dictated by concurrent surgeries planned. The patient is placed in standard lithotomy position in candy-cane or booted support stirrups. A vaginal and rectal examination under anesthesia is again performed to assess the size of the perineal body and defects of the posterior vaginal wall, which may also require repair. The vagina is surgically prepared, and a Foley catheter inserted.

❷ **Concurrent Surgery.** If concurrent surgeries have been included, perineorrhaphy is the final procedure in most cases.

❸ **Incision.** To determine the approximate appearance of the final repair, Allis clamps are placed on the posterolateral walls of the vagina at or just proximal to the hymen. These are brought together in the midline and 2 or 3 fingers should easily pass through the intended genital hiatus. If the resulting opening is too narrow, both Allis clamps are moved closer to the midline, and the above steps are repeated. With this technique, a surgeon can judge the final size of the introitus and perineal body. Because scarring and retraction can develop, it is prudent to err on the side of leaving the genital hiatus larger rather than smaller. To begin, a diamond-shape incision is made with its cephalad tip extending 2 to 3 cm into the vagina and the caudal tip extending to a point approximately 2 cm above the anus.

❹ **Removal of Skin and Mucosa.** For traction, Allis clamps are placed at each corner of the diamond. Metzenbaum scissors are used to excise the perineal skin and vaginal epithelium within the diamond away from the underlying tissue. During dissection, the scissor tips are held parallel to the perineal and vaginal tissues, respectively.

Sharp dissection must be performed over the perineal body. This area contains a normal condensation of tissue, and scarring may also be present. As a result, development of good tissue planes is often not possible. A dilute vasopressin solution may be injected to decrease bleeding from extensive venous sinuses that are typically encountered in this region from obstetric or vaginal delivery scars. Frequent rectal examination during dissection may be required to assess the amount of tissue present between the anal and vaginal epithelium to prevent entry into the rectum.

❺ **Suture Placement.** One centimeter caudal to the hymeneal ring, a 0-gauge delayed-absorbable suture on a CT-1 needle is used to approximate the connective tissue surrounding the perineal muscles (bulbospongiosus and superficial transverse perineal muscles) in the midline. In suturing this tissue, a wide lateral bite is taken, and suture is directed first in an inward-to-outward and then outward-to-inward sequence (Fig. 45-16.1). This suture technique ultimately buries knots below the plicated muscles. However, initially, the first suture is held and not tied.

Downward traction is placed, and a second suture is placed approximately 1 cm cephalad. This suture ideally reapproximates the separated ends of the perineal membrane. As with the first, this suture is not tied. A third suture can be placed 1 cm further cephalad to this, if necessary. In a similar fashion, one to two stitches are placed 1 cm apart and caudad to the primary suture. These lower stitches plicate the connective tissue surrounding the superficial transverse perineal muscles and upper extent of the external anal sphincter muscle in the midline. The sutures are then progressively tied beginning with the lowermost. In some cases, a second, more superficial layer is placed in the perineal body for additional support.

❻ **Vaginal and Perineal Closure.** Starting at the vaginal apex, the vaginal epithelium is closed in a running fashion using 2-0 gauge delayed-absorbable suture (Fig. 45-16.2). When creating a running suture line in the

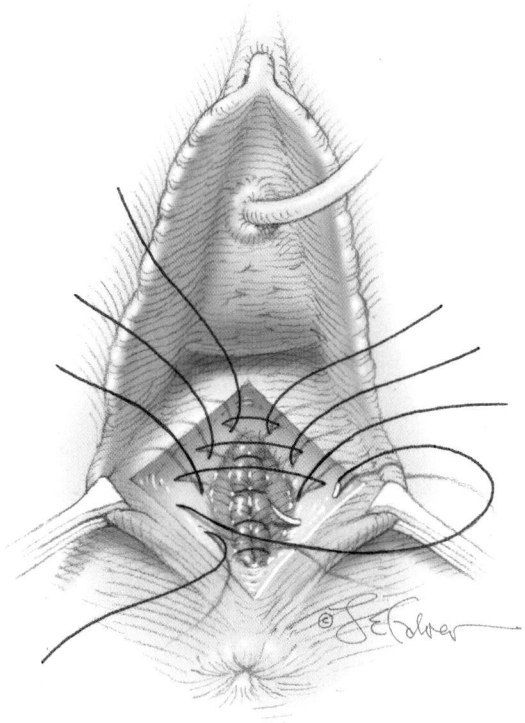

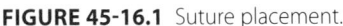

FIGURE 45-16.1 Suture placement.

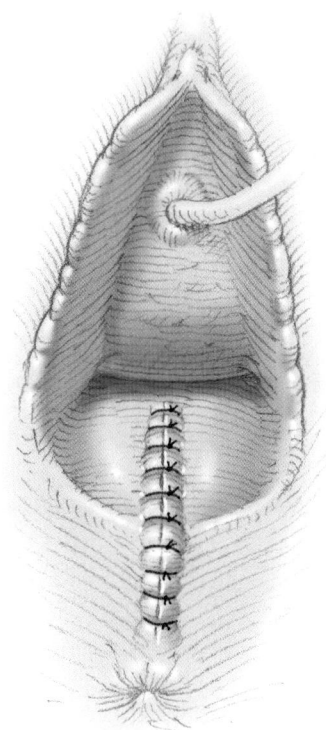

FIGURE 45-16.2 Wound closure.

vagina, stitches are placed close together. If suture bites are placed far apart during epithelial closure, the vagina can be shortened.

The running suture reapproximates the hymeneal ring and then is brought into the perineal area. The same suture may be used in a running mattress method to reapproximate the subcutaneous tissue to the end of the incision, near the anus. The skin is then reapproximated in an interrupted or running fashion using 3-0 gauge delayed-absorbable suture.

POSTOPERATIVE

Patients are instructed on perineal hygiene. Constipation is avoided and stool softeners are usually prescribed. As with other vaginal surgery, diet and activity can be advanced as tolerated. Women, however, abstain from intercourse until wound healing is complete, typically at 6 to 8 weeks following repair. Some women have urinary retention after perineorrhaphy, even without an antiincontinence procedure. If unable to void spontaneously by the time of discharge, a patient can go home with a catheter and be seen again within a week for removal.

45-17

Abdominal Sacrocolpopexy

Abdominal sacrocolpopexy (ASC) using graft material is a widely accepted transabdominal prolapse operation, and many consider it the preferred procedure to correct advanced apical prolapse. Grafts of autologous, cadaveric, or synthetic materials may be used, but permanent (synthetic) mesh has the best success rate and is selected unless otherwise contraindicated (Culligan, 2005). The graft augments native tissue and suspends the upper third of the vagina to the anterior longitudinal ligament of the sacrum. In addition to correcting apical prolapse, the graft also covers proximal portions of the anterior and posterior vaginal walls. As such, ASC also corrects apical segment prolapse of the anterior vagina wall ("apical" or "transverse" cystoceles) and of the posterior vaginal wall (enteroceles and "high" rectoceles). A modification of the procedure, sacrocolpoperineopexy, is used if concomitant perineal descent is present and believed to contribute to patient symptoms (Cundiff, 1997).

One advantage to ASC is its durability, and long-term success rates for apical suspension approximate 90 percent. It may be used as a primary procedure or alternatively as a repeat surgery for patients with recurrences after other prolapse repair failures. In addition, ASC is often chosen for women believed to be at high risk for recurrence and for whom mesh would augment their own tissue. Examples include those with connective tissue disease, history of recurrent hernia, obesity, or chronically increased intraabdominal pressure such as chronic obstructive pulmonary disease or chronic constipation. Abdominal synthetic mesh aids durability, but its use is balanced against the potential for complications, as discussed later.

Although the vaginal apex can also be successfully suspended with vaginal approach procedures such as sacrospinous ligament fixation (p. 1112) and uterosacral ligament suspension (p. 1107), ASC offers distinct advantages. First, ASC maintains or lengthens the vagina, in contrast to vaginal approaches, which may shorten it. Second, the use of synthetic "permanent" mesh with multiple attachment sites to the vagina has a very low risk of apical failure. Finally, unlike vaginal approaches, in which the vaginal apex is directly affixed to a structure such as the uterosacral or sacrospinous ligament, ASC repositions the vaginal apex to its nearly normal anatomic position using intervening graft material. Thus, the apex typically remains mobile, which possibly lowers dyspareunia rates.

Sacrocolpopexy can be performed by laparotomy, by conventional laparoscopy, and with robotic assistance. If minimally invasive surgery (MIS) is performed in the same manner as the open operation, similar results can be expected (p. 1103). However, only limited data are currently available on long-term success rates with these MIS approaches (Freeman, 2013; Maher, 2013; Paraiso, 2011).

PREOPERATIVE

Patient Evaluation

Prolapse of the vaginal apex often coexists with other prolapse sites along the vagina. Accordingly, a careful preoperative search is performed for other prolapse sites. If necessary, ASC can be completed concurrently with paravaginal defect repair, posterior repair, or other prolapse surgeries. Beer and Kuhn (2005) found that approximately 70 percent of ASC procedures were performed with other pelvic reconstructive operations. With the technique we describe, a concurrent enterocele will be repaired by the colpopexy, and other enterocele repairs are thus unnecessary.

Prior to ASC, patients with symptoms of urinary incontinence undergo simple or complex urodynamic testing to clarify the type of incontinence and determine if an antiincontinence procedure will be beneficial. For those with SUI, a concurrent antiincontinence operation is generally performed. Because prolapse correction can unmask occult SUI in some women, clinicians also test those without incontinence while manually reducing the prolapse. Last, apical suspension can predispose to later development of anterior vaginal wall prolapse and SUI. Thus, stress-continent women undergoing ASC may elect a prophylactic SUI procedure. To evaluate this practice, the CARE (Colpopexy After Reduction Efforts) trial found that continent women undergoing ASC *plus* a prophylactic urethropexy had a 2-year postoperative SUI incidence of 32 percent. Without preventive urethropexy, SUI rates following ASC were 45 percent (Brubaker, 2006, 2008). Importantly, adding an antiincontinence procedure decreases, but does not eliminate, the risk of later de novo SUI. At this time, it is unclear how best to extrapolate these findings to women who elect to have sacrocolpopexy and midurethral sling procedures.

Consent

Recurrent prolapse is common following any corrective surgery. Thus, a surgeon should be aware of recurrence rates quoted in the literature and his or her own personal rates. Although apical prolapse recurrence is infrequent, later prolapse of the anterior and posterior vaginal walls is more common. An extension of the CARE trial used a clinically based definition of anatomic failure. It showed that by 5 years, nearly one third of women met the composite definition of failure (Nygaard, 2013). However, 95 percent had no retreatment for their prolapse.

Mesh erosion develops in 2 to 10 percent of cases. It is generally found at the apex and occurs more often if hysterectomy is performed concurrent with ASC. Erosion may arise soon after surgery or years later (Beer, 2005; Nygaard, 2004, 2013). Many technical points described in the following steps aim to prevent this complication.

Patient Preparation

Bowel preparation will vary depending on surgeon preference. Patients can be instructed to take only clear liquids the day prior to surgery and complete one or two enemas that night or the morning of surgery. Alternatively, a mechanical bowel preparation using agents listed in Chapter 39 (p. 835) may be preferred. Ballard and associates (2014), however, noted no distinct advantage to this for urogynecologic operations. Antibiotics and thromboprophylaxis are given as outlined in Tables 39-6 and 39-8 (p. 835).

For postmenopausal women, vaginal estrogen cream use during the 6 to 8 weeks prior to surgery has been routinely recommended. Estrogen treatment is thought to enhance vascularity and thereby increase tissue strength and promote healing. Although this is logical and commonly practiced, no data suggest that preoperative vaginal estrogen cream decreases mesh erosion or prolapse recurrence rates.

INTRAOPERATIVE

Instruments and Materials

The upper vagina must be elevated and distended by a vaginal manipulator to allow adequate dissection and delineation of the vaginal wall fibromuscular layers for mesh placement. The manipulator may be a cylindrical Lucite rod or a large EEA (end-to-end anastomosis) sizer, which is present in most operating rooms and shown in Figure 46-21.4 (p. 1202).

The ideal bridging material for this procedure is permanent, nonantigenic, easily cut or customized, and readily available. The ideal mesh has a large pore size to allow host tissue ingrowth, is monofilament to decrease bacterial adherence, and is flexible. Currently, polypropylene mesh is the most common synthetic graft used (American Urogynecologic Society, 2013, 2014b).

Surgical Steps

❶ Anesthesia and Patient Positioning. Following administration of general anesthesia, the patient is positioned in a modified supine position with thighs parallel to the ground and legs in booted support stirrups. Correct positioning prevents nerve injury and allows access to the vagina for manipulation and examination, to the bladder for cystoscopy, and to the abdomen for proper self-retaining retractor placement. The buttocks are positioned at the table edge or slightly distal to allow full range of vaginal manipulator motion. The vagina and abdomen are surgically prepared, and a Foley catheter is inserted.

❷ Incision. A vertical or transverse abdominal incision may be used, and selection is directed by a woman's body habitus and by planned concurrent procedures. A Pfannenstiel incision generally provides adequate access to the sacrum and deep pelvis. If a Burch colposuspension, paravaginal defect repair, or other surgery in the space of Retzius is planned, then a low transverse incision that is positioned closer to the symphysis may be preferred.

❸ Bowel Packing. A self-retaining retractor, preferably a Balfour type, is placed, and the bowel is packed up and out of the pelvis with moist laparotomy sponges. Bowel packing attempts to shift the sigmoid colon farther to the patient's left, thereby permitting access to the midline and right aspects of the sacrum.

❹ Concomitant Hysterectomy. Some data suggest that hysterectomy at the time of ASC leads to higher mesh erosion rates (Culligan, 2002; Griffis, 2006). To reduce erosion risks at the cuff, some surgeons advocate supracervical hysterectomy, theorizing that the cervical stump may act as a barrier to prevent ascending infection and erosion (McDermott, 2009). If a total abdominal hysterectomy is performed, the vaginal apex is closed with absorbable suture such as 0-gauge polyglactin 910 (Vicryl) in a running or interrupted fashion. A second imbricating layer using the same suture may be placed to reduce potential mesh erosion. Another preventive measure is avoiding mesh fixation near the cuff suture line. Specifically, a 1-cm margin from this suture line may avert early mesh erosion during the cuff's healing phase.

❺ Identification of Pelvic Anatomy. Important boundaries during presacral space dissection are identified beneath the peritoneum prior to the posterior peritoneal incision. These include the aortic bifurcation, iliac vessels, right ureter, right uterosacral ligament, medial border of the rectosigmoid colon, and sacral promontory, which is the upper anterior surface of the S1 vertebra. An understanding that the right ureter, right common iliac artery, and left common iliac vein all lie within 3 cm of the sacral promontory's midline may lower rates of their injury during surgery in the presacral space (Good, 2013b; Wieslander, 2006). Moreover, both ureters are threatened during dissection of the bladder off the anterior vaginal wall and during suturing of the anterior mesh strip.

❻ Peritoneal Incision. The rectosigmoid colon is gently retracted to the left with a malleable ribbon or similar retractor. The peritoneum overlying the sacral promontory, between the rectosigmoid colon's medial border and the right ureter, is elevated with tissue forceps and incised sharply. The incision is extended caudally into the posterior cul-de-sac of Douglas. As the incision approaches the deeper portion of the cul-de-sac, it is kept between the medial border of the rectum and the right uterosacral ligament. A vaginal manipulator directed ventrally to create tension aids dissection. The incision may then be continued to the posterior vaginal wall and toward the vaginal apex.

Maintaining proper orientation is critical during this step as inadvertent deviation can cause ureteral or iliac vessel injury on the right, or colon injury on the left. Similarly, if the initial peritoneal incision is extended above the sacral promontory, the left common iliac vein should be identified and avoided. This vessel can lie less than 1 cm from the promontory and is generally difficult to visualize or palpate due to its absent pulsatility and decreased tone. Final closure of this peritoneal incision allows the mesh to lie retroperitoneally. This may lower the risk of bowel-to-mesh adhesions and of bowel obstruction from small-bowel loops entrapped below the bridging mesh strip.

❼ Identification of Anterior Longitudinal Ligament. Following peritoneal incision, the loose connective tissue between the peritoneum and the sacrum is sharply and bluntly dissected to expose the anterior longitudinal ligament lying along the sacrum's vertical midsection. Generally, this presacral space dissection is started at the promontory and continued 3 to 4 cm inferiorly to the upper extent of the S2 vertebra. Within the connective tissue of the presacral space, fibers of the superior hypogastric nerve plexus, right and left hypogastric nerves, and the inferior mesenteric and superior rectal artery and vein are embedded (Fig. 38-23, p. 816). Of these, the right hypogastric nerve is the most common structure identified during dissection. Below the aortic bifurcation, this midline cordlike nerve courses laterally and at the lower sacral levels, reaches the right pelvic sidewall. Transection of this nerve is ideally avoided.

Also of seminal importance, the middle sacral vessels typically adhere to the anterior surface of the ligament. Once found in the area exposed for mesh attachment, middle sacral vessels can be avoided, ligated, or coagulated depending on surgeon's preference and operative findings. The middle sacral vein also forms anastomoses with the lateral sacral veins that contribute to the sacral venous plexus. Vessels of this plexus can be extensive, especially in the lower part of the sacrum.

❽ Presacral Space Hemorrhage. Careful exposure of the anterior longitudinal ligament and overlying vessels helps prevent bleeding during suture placement. Despite these efforts, laceration of the sacral venous plexus can lead to rapid and substantial blood loss, and several steps are critical to its control. First, pressure is applied immediately and held for several minutes. This may be particularly effective for venous bleeding. Sutures and clips may be useful, but tearing of small veins frequently worsens with suturing. Additionally, as vessels retract into the bone, isolation and ligation becomes difficult. Sterile thumbtacks directed through lacerated vessels and pushed into the sacrum can effectively compress such vessels. Unfortunately, these tacks are not routinely found in many operating rooms.

Alternatively, various topical hemostatic agents have been used to control bleeding refractory to these initial steps (Table 40-5, p. 861). Of these, the fibrin sealant family allows conformation to irregular wounds, which is a distinct advantage for presacral space hemorrhage. In refractory cases, vascular surgery consultation may be prudent. Also, injury to the iliac vessels or aorta necessitates immediate consultation.

❾ Sacral Suture Site Selection. To anchor the suspending mesh strips proximally, a surgeon must decide whether to place sutures through the anterior longitudinal ligament at higher or lower sacral levels. Suture placement at the S3 or S4 vertebral bodies increases the risk of sacral venous plexus laceration, and this practice has largely been abandoned. Suture placement above the sacral promontory risks left common iliac vein injury and penetration of the L5-S1 disc, which may lead to painful discitis or osteomyelitis (Good, 2013a; Wieslander, 2006). However, this disc is the most protuberant structure in the presacral space, and mesh is commonly affixed here, especially during the learning phase of ASC (Abernathy, 2012).

For correct sacral promontory identification, the steep angle of descent between L5 and S1 can be used. That said, even correct suture placement at S1 and the sacral

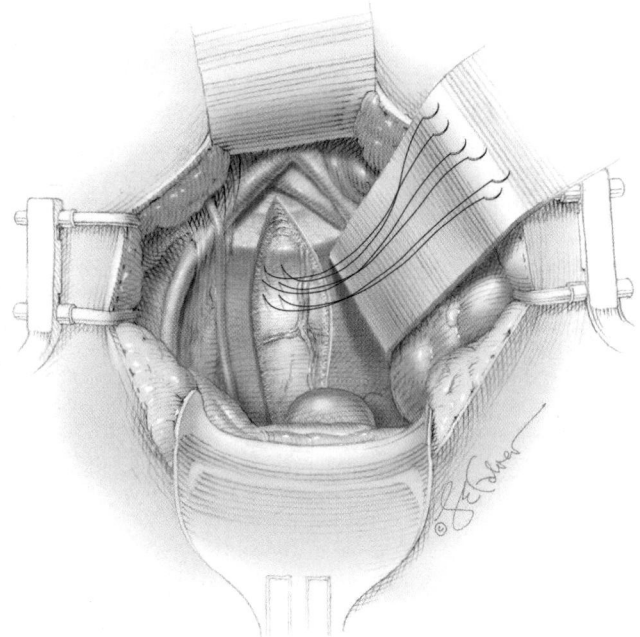

FIGURE 45-17.1 Placement of sacral sutures.

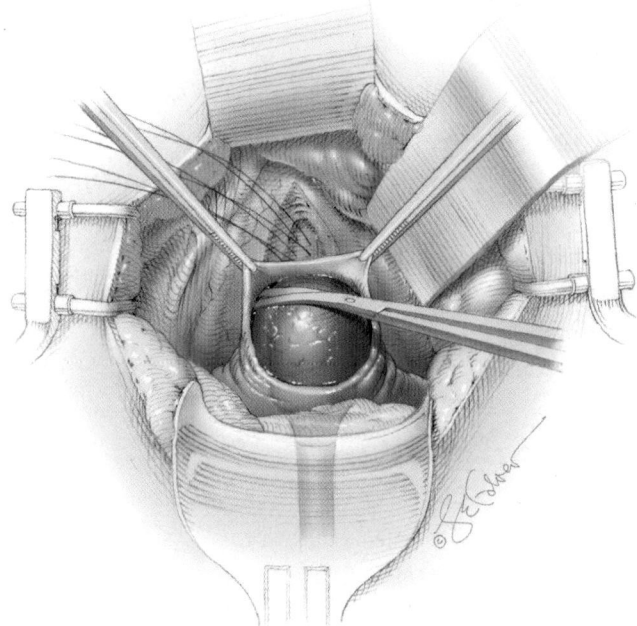

FIGURE 45-17.2 Dissection of the anterior vaginal wall.

promontory still risks middle sacral vessel laceration. However, at S1, the middle sacral vessels are visible and can be easily isolated and avoided or when necessary, clipped or coagulated. Additionally at S1, the anterior longitudinal ligament is thicker and stronger than at lower sacral levels (White, 2009). Affixing sutures here minimizes suture avulsion risks. Finally, attachment of the mesh at S1 may result in a more anatomic suspension of the vaginal apex (Balgobin, 2013).

For these reasons, we prefer to affix mesh to the anterior surface of S1, with the most cephalad suture placed at or just below the sacral promontory. If safe suture placement over the S1 vertebra is prohibited, then the level of the L5-S1 disc is an alternative. Shallow tissue "bites" are needed here to avoid the disc as the anterior longitudinal ligament is only 1 to 2 mm thick.

⑩ **Sacral Suture Placement.** Typically, three or four serial permanent sutures are used to affix the sacral portion of mesh to the anterior longitudinal ligament. These stitches can be placed first, as described here, or later after vaginal mesh attachment. Needle passage moves from right to left with each stitch, and sutures are aligned vertically. Starting with the lowest suture, they are spaced approximately 0.5 to 1 cm apart. With suturing, 2-0 gauge permanent material, each double-armed with SH needles, is passed through the full thickness of the anterior longitudinal ligament (Fig. 45-17.1). During this, based on findings, suture "bites" either encompass or avoid vessels. Once completed, sutures are held by a hemostat

and not tied. Their needles are covered with a surgical towel to avoid stick injuries.

⑪ **Anterior Vaginal Wall Dissection.** Prior to mesh attachment, the peritoneum and bladder must be dissected off the proximal vagina. Dissection of the bladder from the upper third of the anterior vaginal wall is aided by the vaginal manipulator. The cervical stump or vaginal apex is displaced cephalad and dorsally, and its covering peritoneum is incised transversely and proximal to the bladder's cephalad margin. With prior hysterectomy, careful identification of the vaginal apex and superior extent of bladder is critical to avoid cystotomy. This is especially important in women with short vaginal lengths or vesicovaginal adhesions. In these cases, retrograde bladder filling and Foley bulb identification may help delineate the upper bladder margin. With cystotomy, several options are possible. If the cystotomy is small and close to the bladder dome, then a two- to three-layered bladder closure, followed by an interposition flap (omental or peritoneal), may be considered. However, if the cystotomy is large or nears the trigone, an alternative approach to vault suspension using native tissue may be considered to minimize mesh erosion into the bladder or fistula formation. Alternatively, the cystotomy can be repaired, and ASC deferred for a later time.

Once the correct vesicovaginal space is entered, the bladder is sharply dissected from the anterior vaginal wall for a distance of approximately 4 to 6 cm caudad to create an extensive surface for mesh fixation. However, the extent of this dissection varies depending

on intraoperative anatomy. Sharp rather than blunt dissection is preferred in the vesicovaginal space (Fig. 45-17.2). Electrosurgical energy use is minimized to reduce risks of delayed thermal bladder injury. Dissection progresses at a depth above the fibromuscular layer of the vaginal wall. Entry into this proper plane lowers the rate of incidental entry into the vagina, which may increase future mesh erosion risks. If the vaginal lumen is entered, the opening is irrigated copiously and closed in two imbricated layers using 2-0 or 3-0 gauge delayed-absorbable suture.

⑫ **Posterior Vaginal Wall Dissection.** To expose an area of adequate size for mesh fixation, the rectovaginal space is entered, and the rectum is separated from the posterior vagina. For this, the vaginal manipulator now displaces the vaginal apex ventrally. The reflection of the rectum against the posterior vaginal wall is identified, and the peritoneum is incised transversely 2 to 3 cm proximal to this reflection line. The right and left uterosacral ligaments are used as lateral dissection boundaries. With gentle outward traction on the peritoneum, the rectovaginal space is developed with a combination of sharp and blunt dissection. In the absence of adhesions or fibrosis, the rectovaginal space easily opens inferiorly to the superior margin of the perineal body, which lies 3 to 4 cm above the hymen. Identification of loose gauzy connective tissue fibers usually indicates dissection in the correct plane. Also, the white, glistening posterior vaginal wall provides another visual clue, and dissection is kept close to this tissue to avoid inadvertent rectal entry.

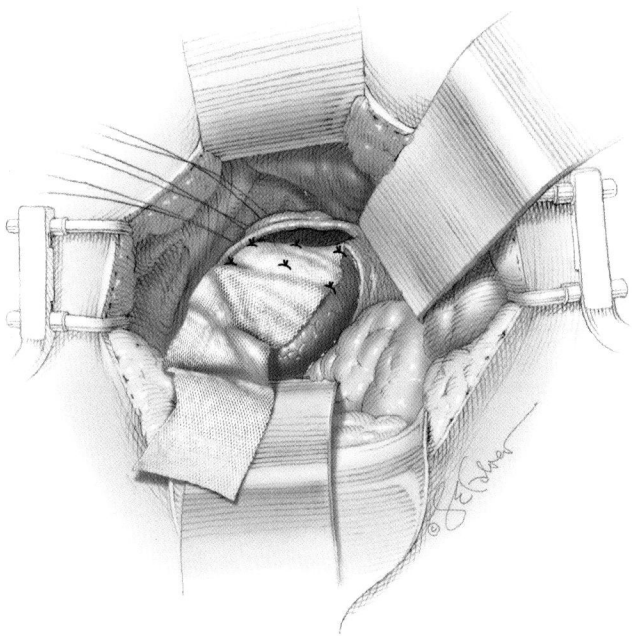

FIGURE 45-17.3 Posterior mesh secured and draped forward. Initially placed sacral sutures are seen in the background.

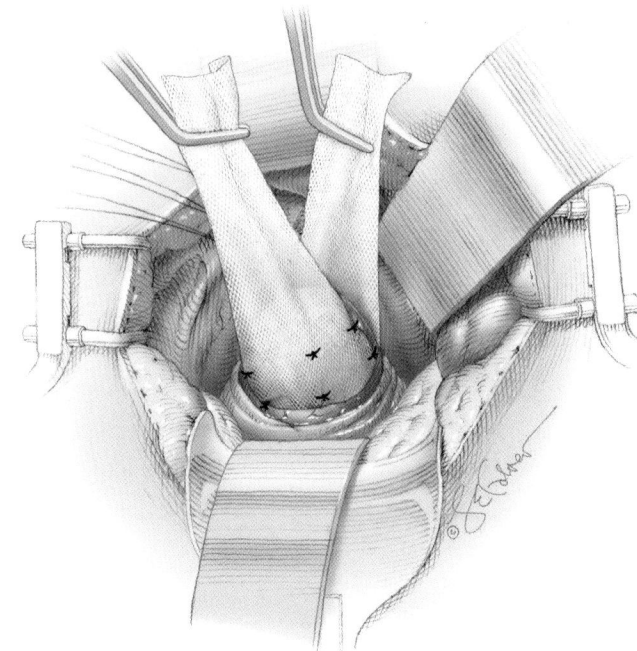

FIGURE 45-17.4 Anterior and posterior mesh in place.

In contrast, fatty tissue or excessive bleeding generally indicates incorrect plane dissection and potential proximity to the rectum.

⓭ Graft Principles. Whether two separate strips of self-cut mesh or a commercially preformed Y-shaped mesh is used, several surgical principles are generally followed. First, depending on the extent of dissections, six to 12 sutures on the anterior and a similar number on the posterior vaginal wall are placed through the mesh and the vaginal wall muscularis. Sutures ideally do not enter the vaginal lumen because epithelial healing over the stitches may be incomplete, especially with braided suture. However, if the fibromuscular layer is thin, this may not be possible. In this setting, many select monofilament, delayed-absorbable suture, which has a greater propensity for epithelialization postoperatively.

Second, sutures are tied down loosely to avoid tissue strangulation and vaginal wall necrosis, which may lead to mesh or suture erosion. Third, the lower extent of the mesh does not abut the bladder or rectal reflections to minimize potential risks of pelvic organ dysfunction or mesh erosion of into these organs. Last, mesh is positioned symmetrically across the width of both the anterior and posterior vaginal walls.

At our institution, we fashion the two mesh strips only after vaginal dissection is completed. The broader area of each strip will cover the dissected anterior vaginal surface and posterior vaginal surface, respectively. Each strip also has a narrowed portion that will extend to the sacrum and be affixed to the anterior longitudinal ligament. This narrowed portion reduces mesh bulk, especially near the rectum on the left and the iliac vessels and ureter on the right, to lower mesh erosion rates. However, excessive narrowing may compromise overall repair strength (Balgobin, 2011). Generally, the narrow portion of mesh measures approximately 2 cm. Lengthwise, the proximal end of mesh is initially left long to allow correct positioning to the sacrum and later is trimmed.

⓮ Mesh Placement. To begin, the vaginal manipulator is pushed cephalad and ventrally to fully expose the dissected posterior vaginal wall and stabilize the vagina for suturing. The mesh is commonly attached to the posterior vaginal wall with two to four rows of 2-0 gauge permanent or delayed-absorbable sutures, and rows are placed approximately 1.5 cm apart (Fig. 45-17.3). Depending on the vaginal width and the lateral extent of dissection, each row consists of two to three sutures spaced 1 to 1.5 cm apart. The inferior and lateral extents of the dissected vagina are adequately exposed prior to suture placement to avoid incorporation of rectum into a stitch.

For the anterior vaginal wall, mesh is sutured in exactly the same fashion as was performed on the posterior wall (Fig. 45-17.4).

⓯ Mesh Sizing and Sacral Attachment. For this step, the prior sacral dissection is again exposed, and the two proximal portions of each mesh strip are held together by a right-angle clamp for maneuvering. The vaginal manipulator is removed and replaced by surgeon fingers. Then, by digital pressure directed cephalad, the cuff is gently elevated, and the proximal portions of mesh are extended to the earlier placed sacral sutures. Alternatively, the cuff can be gently elevated by the vaginal manipulator. With correct positioning, apical suspension reduces prolapse of the apex and the apical segments of the anterior and posterior vaginal walls. Moreover, the mesh segment between the vagina and sacrum should be tension free. Once the desired mesh position and length are determined, the excess mesh above the most cephalad sacral suture is trimmed off. This avoids mesh contact with the right ureter, iliac vein, and other vascular structures that all lie within 1 to 2 cm of the fixation site (Kohli, 1998; Nygaard, 2004).

The six needles of the three double-armed sacral sutures are then passed through the proximal portions of both mesh strips (Fig. 45-17.5). Each of the three sutures is then tied to secure the proximal mesh to the anterior longitudinal ligament (Fig. 45-17.6). To prevent air knots while the lowest sacral suture is secured, the surgeon gently pushes the vaginal apex against the lower part of the sacrum with the vaginal manipulator.

⓰ Peritoneal Closure. Reapproximation of the peritoneum over the mesh can be accomplished in a running or interrupted fashion using 3-0 or 2-0 gauge absorbable suture (Fig. 45-17.7). Placing this mesh retroperitoneally theoretically may lower the risk of bowel obstruction, but this complication has been reported despite peritoneal reapproximation (Pilsgaard, 1999). During closure, the right ureter is kept in constant view to avoid kinking or direct injury.

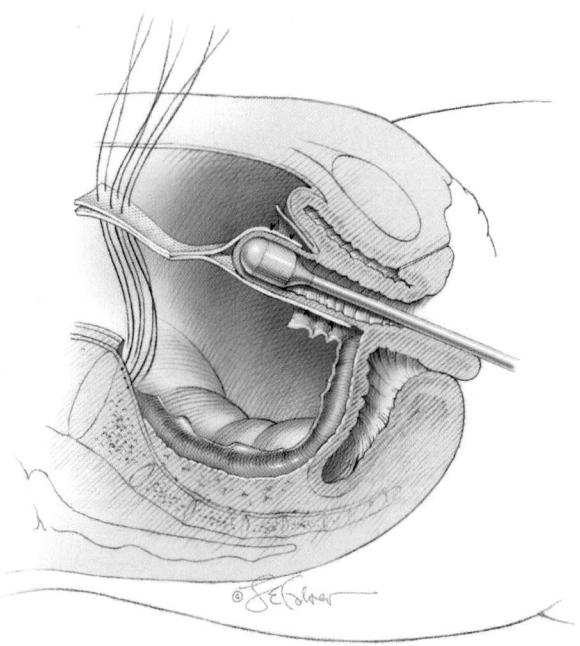

FIGURE 45-17.5 Mesh attachment to the sacrum.

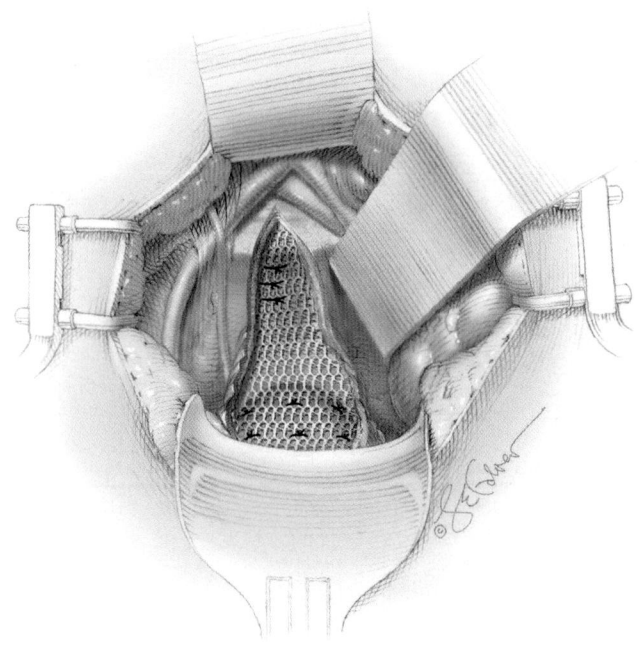

FIGURE 45-17.6 Final mesh placement.

⑰ Cystoscopy. Cystoscopy is routinely performed prior to laparotomy closure to document ureteral integrity and absence of bladder sutures or injury. Urethral examination is important if an antiincontinence procedure is also performed.

⑱ Abdominal Closure. The abdomen is closed in a standard fashion (Section 43-1 or 43-2, p. 928).

POSTOPERATIVE

Patient Care

Postoperative in-hospital management is similar to that for other intraabdominal surgeries.

Specific to ASC, a passive or active voiding trial can be performed on postoperative day 1 or 2, depending on the patient's condition and extent of dissection. Some women have urinary retention after apical suspension, even without an antiincontinence procedure. If unable to void spontaneously by the time of discharge, a patient can go home with a catheter and be seen again within a week for removal. A stool softener is prescribed when regular diet is tolerated, and constipation and straining are ideally avoided.

At routine postoperative visits, the patient is evaluated for prolapse recurrence and mesh or suture erosion. Symptoms of pelvic floor dysfunction are also elicited. Anatomic suc-

cess does not always correlate with functional success, and vice versa. Thus, continual evaluation of surgical results is based on anatomy and on symptoms such as urinary incontinence, defecatory dysfunction, pelvic pain, and sexual dysfunction.

Complications

Following ASC, the graft material or its attaching sutures can erode through the vaginal epithelium. On average, symptoms develop 14 months following surgery, and vaginal bleeding and discharge are classic symptoms (Kohli, 1998). The diagnosis is generally straightforward, as mesh or sutures can be seen directly during speculum examination.

Mesh erosion through the vaginal mucosa may initially be treated with a 6-week or longer course of intravaginal estrogen cream. For those with exposed mesh and symptoms, surgical removal in an operating suite may be performed vaginally. Epithelium around the erosion site is sharply dissected from the mesh and undermined. The mesh is grasped, placed on gentle tension, dissected off the overlying tissue, and as much mesh as can be identified is resected. The vaginal epithelial edges are then trimmed to freshen edges and reapproximated in a running or interrupted fashion using 2-0 gauge delayed-absorbable suture. Failure of these wounds to heal is interpreted as a sign of graft or tissue infection, and more extensive or complete removal of the graft is considered. Sutures that are eroding into the vagina may be cut and removed in the office. Fortunately, removal of sutures or portions of eroding mesh does not generally compromise prolapse correction.

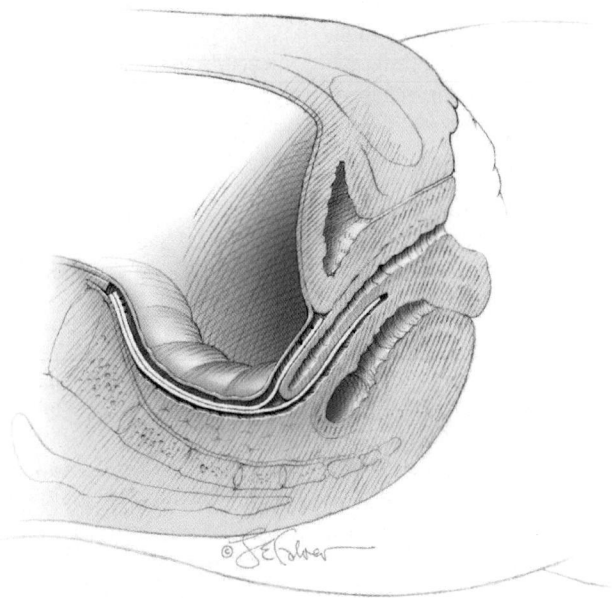

FIGURE 45-17.7 Peritoneal closure.

45-18

Minimally Invasive Sacrocolpopexy

Sacrocolpopexy (SC) is increasingly being performed with a minimally invasive approach using conventional laparoscopy or robot-assisted laparoscopy. The basic procedural steps are the same as for laparotomic ASC and differ mainly by abdominal entry method and instruments used. Steps are outlined here, but a fuller discussion is found in Section 45-17.

Although not as extensively studied as abdominal sacrocolpopexy (ASC), limited data suggest that minimally invasive SC has similar short-term functional and anatomic results, shorter hospitalization, but longer operating times and greater cost (Judd, 2010; Siddiqui, 2012). Several randomized trials have compared outcomes and costs of laparoscopic sacrocolpopexy (LSC) with robotic sacrocolpopexy (RSC) (Anger, 2014; Paraiso, 2011). Compared with LSC, RSC carries increased cost, operative time, and higher pain scores, but short-term anatomic and functional outcomes and complications are similar. Data also show a longer robotic learning curve to achieve proficiency. That said, as robotic technology and training continues to develop, operative time, costs, and complications will likely decline.

PREOPERATIVE

Patient Evaluation

Candidates for minimally invasive SC undergo the same prolapse and incontinence evaluation as for ASC (p. 1098). As discussed in Chapter 41 (p. 874), factors influencing approach include patient overall health, restrictions to prolonged anesthesia, body habitus, intraabdominal adhesions, and surgeon skill.

Consent

Consent considerations mirror those for ASC. Additionally, with the minimally invasive approach, patients are counseled and consented for laparotomy if surgery cannot be completed by MIS. In addition, complications more common to laparoscopy are discussed (Chap. 41, p. 877). These include puncture injury to organs and vessels during abdominal entry, positioning neuropathies, and delayed thermal injury to intraabdominal organs from electrosurgical tools.

Patient Preparation

This mirrors preparation for ASC and covers antibiotics and thromboembolism prophylaxis and bowel preparation options (p. 1098).

INTRAOPERATIVE

Surgical Steps

❶ **Anesthesia and Patient Positioning.** Following administration of general anesthesia, the patient is positioned for laparoscopy in booted support stirrups as fully described in Chapter 41 (p. 879). The buttocks are positioned slightly distal to the table edge to compensate for mild upward patient migration that often occurs in the steep Trendelenburg position needed for laparoscopy. Correct positioning decreases nerve injury rates, provides access to the vagina, and allows full rotation of vaginal manipulator and laparoscopic instruments. The vagina and abdomen are surgically prepared, and a Foley catheter is inserted.

❷ **Incision and Trocar Placement.** A full description of minimally invasive entry is found in Chapter 41 (p. 889). For LSC, four ports are generally used (Fig. 45-18.1). A 10-mm umbilical port houses the laparoscope; one 5-mm port is placed subcostally and lateral to the rectus abdominis muscle on either side for tissue manipulation; and two 10-mm ports, one in each lower quadrant, allow needle-bearing sutures to be threaded into the abdomen. Knots are tied using an extracorporeal technique, illustrated in Chapter 41 (p. 899).

For RSC, five ports are placed in a shallow "W" formation. One 12-mm umbilical port houses the laparoscope; one 8- or 10-mm assistant port is placed subcostally lateral to the rectus abdominis muscle on the right; and three 8-mm robotic ports are positioned in bilateral lower quadrants, with two on the left and one on the right. We dock the robotic cart on the patient's left to permit manipulation of the vagina. Knots are tied using intracorporeal knot-tying techniques.

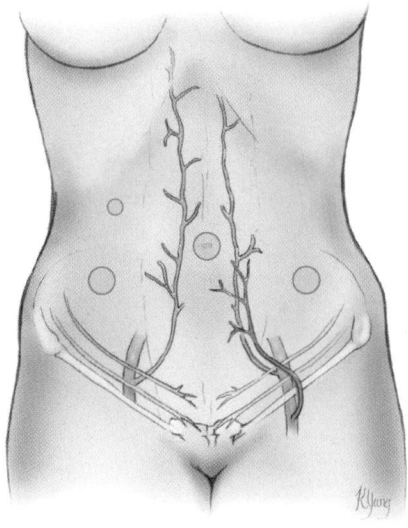

FIGURE 45-18.1 Port placement.

❸ **Concomitant Hysterectomy.** The same considerations described for ASC apply to minimally invasive SC. An additional concern with minimally invasive total hysterectomy is the use of electrosurgery to amputate the uterus and its potential for greater cuff dehiscence and mesh erosion rates (Chap. 44, p. 1036). Moreover, limited data currently suggest that total hysterectomy at the time of minimally invasive sacrocolpopexy significantly increases the mesh erosion risk (Tan-Kim, 2011). Accordingly, in appropriately selected patients, supracervical hysterectomy (SCH) is preferred. During the final steps of SCH, to prepare for subsequent sacrocolpopexy, the serosal edges of the cervix may be reapproximated over the exposed endocervical canal using three to five interrupted 2-0 or 0-gauge polyglactin 910 (Vicryl) sutures.

❹ **Pelvic Anatomy Delineation.** To begin sacrocolpopexy, the bowel is gently swept out of the pelvis and above the pelvic brim. With LSC, the rectosigmoid epiploicae may be sutured to the left pelvic sidewall to aid presacral space visualization. With RSC, to accomplish the same goal, an atraumatic grasper used through the third robotic port gently displaces the rectosigmoid laterally. Next, the aortic bifurcation and iliac vessels are identified, and the sacral promontory is visualized and probed in the midline. With RSC, promontory palpation using conventional laparoscopic instruments prior to robot docking is important. This provides tactile anatomic information that is not obtainable robotically. Last, other structures and boundaries are identified as described for ASC.

❺ **Peritoneal Incision.** The peritoneum overlying the sacral promontory in the midline is elevated with tissue forceps and incised sharply with endoscopic scissors (Fig. 45-18.2). The incision is extended caudally into the posterior cul-de-sac of Douglas and then to the vaginal apex (Fig. 45-18.3). Upward and outward traction on the right and left peritoneal edges aids with dissection. Monopolar energy delivered through the scissors is intermittently used for peritoneal dissection and to control small-vessel bleeding.

❻ **Anterior Longitudinal Ligament Identification.** Following peritoneal incision, the loose connective tissue between the peritoneum and the sacrum is sharply and bluntly dissected to expose presacral space anatomy similar to that for ASC. Gentle dissection with scissors or atraumatic tissue forceps removes fat and areolar tissue from the sacrum. Beneath these tissues, the shiny white anterior longitudinal ligament is seen overlying the bone in the midline. A gauze sponge introduced through the assistant port

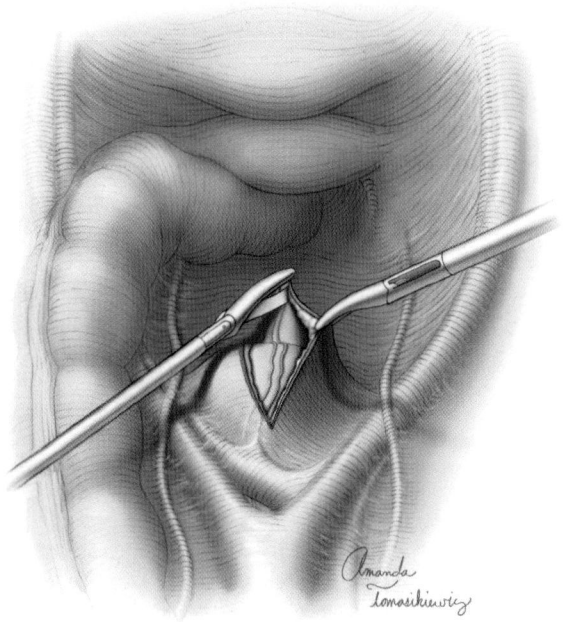

FIGURE 45-18.2 Peritoneal incision overlying the sacrum.

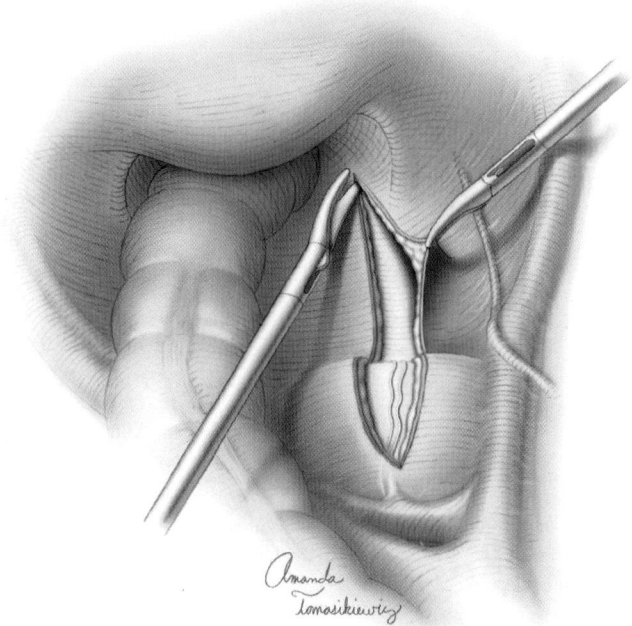

FIGURE 45-18.3 Peritoneal incision extended caudad.

or a laparoscopic Kittner can assist this dissection.

During dissection, significant hemorrhage can occur. To apply bleeding site pressure, a gauze sponge and atraumatic forceps can be introduced through an assistant port. Bleeding management otherwise follows that during ASC (Step 8, p. 1099).

❼ **Sacral Suture Site Selection.** This is completed in a similar manner to that described for ASC. The anterior surface of S1 may be poorly seen with a 0-degree laparoscope due to this vertebral surface's steep angle of descent. In these cases, switching from a 0-degree to a 30-degree scope and directing it downward improves viewing.

❽ **Anterior Vaginal Wall Dissection.** A vaginal manipulator is placed to elevate the vaginal apex, and the peritoneum covering it is incised transversely. Sharp and blunt dissection is used to separate the peritoneum and bladder from the anterior vaginal wall (Fig. 45-18.4). The use of electrosurgery during dissection is limited in an effort to minimize delayed thermal injury to the bladder or ureters.

❾ **Posterior Vaginal Wall Dissection.** The cervical stump or vaginal apex is next directed cephalad and ventrally. The peritoneum covering the posterior vaginal wall is incised transversely at a level proximal to the reflection of the rectum against the posterior vaginal wall (Fig. 45-18.5). The right and left uterosacral ligaments are used as lateral dissection boundaries. With gentle outward

traction on the peritoneum, the rectovaginal space is entered and developed with a combination of sharp and blunt dissection similar to that with ASC.

During minimally invasive procedures, with patients positioned in steep Trendelenburg, angling a straight vaginal manipulator may be difficult and thus may limit posterior wall exposure. Access can be

improved by instead using a medium-sized Deaver retractor in the vagina with its tip directed anteriorly.

❿ **Mesh Placement.** Affixing mesh to the posterior proximal vagina mirrors that in ASC. One strip of mesh is threaded into the peritoneal cavity through one of the 8- or 10-mm assistant cannulas. With graspers

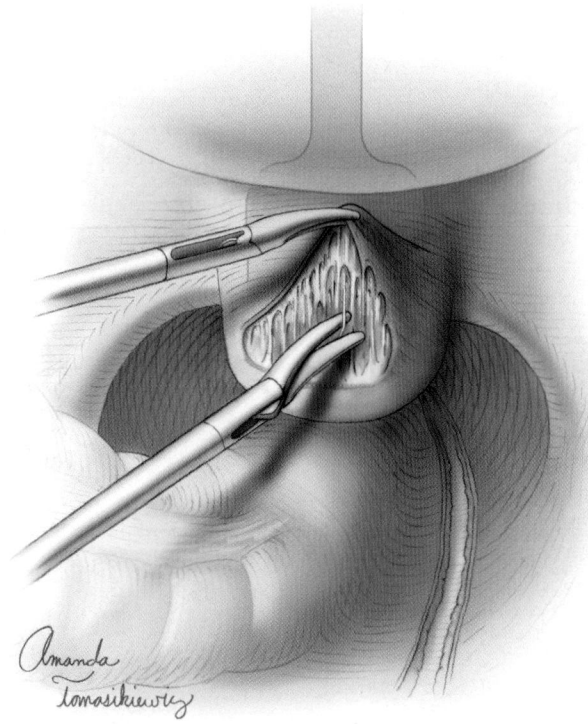

FIGURE 45-18.4 Dissection of the anterior vaginal wall.

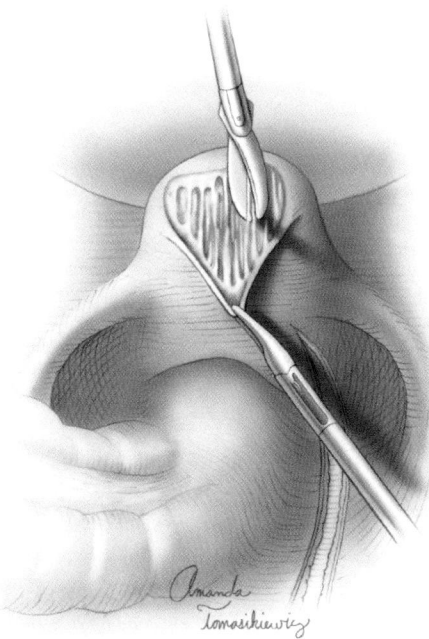

FIGURE 45-18.5 Dissection of the posterior vaginal wall.

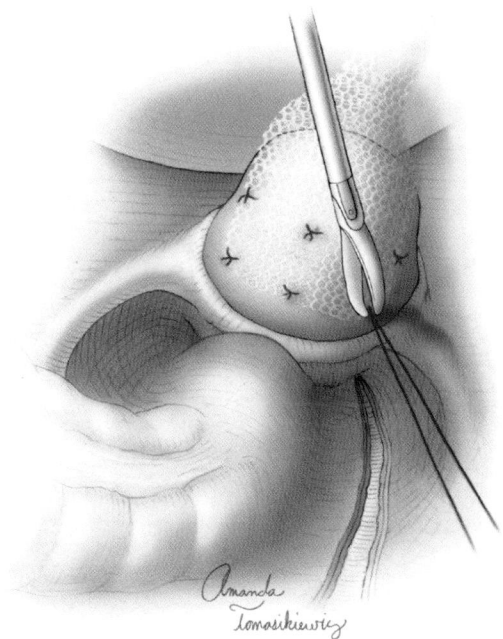

FIGURE 45-18.6 Posterior mesh placement.

placed through a contralateral operating port, the mesh is guided into place and held against the dissected portion of posterior vaginal wall. The same sutures and suturing principles used for ASC are used for minimally invasive sacrocolpopexy (Fig. 45-18.6). Sutures are placed through the mesh and the vaginal wall using laparoscopic or robotic needle drivers. However, with LSC, the knots are secured using the extracorporeal knot tying technique, but with RSC, the intracorporeal technique is used. Accordingly, long sutures, usually 30 to 36 inches, are used for LSC,

but short sutures, approximately 6 inches, are used for RSC.

With the vaginal manipulator serving as a support, a second strip of mesh is sutured to the anterior vaginal wall in the same manner as on the posterior vaginal wall (Figs. 45-18.7 and 45-18.8).

⓫ Mesh Sizing and Sacral Attachment. For this step, the prior sacral dissection is again exposed, and the two proximal portions of mesh are held together by an atraumatic tissue forceps for maneuvering.

Using the vaginal manipulator, the cuff is gently elevated, and the proximal portions of mesh are extended to the earlier exposed ligament over the S1 vertebra. With correct positioning, apical suspension reduces prolapse of the apex and the apical segments of the anterior and posterior vaginal walls. Moreover, the mesh segment between the vagina and sacrum should be tension free.

⓬ Sacral Suture Placement. Once desired mesh position and length are determined,

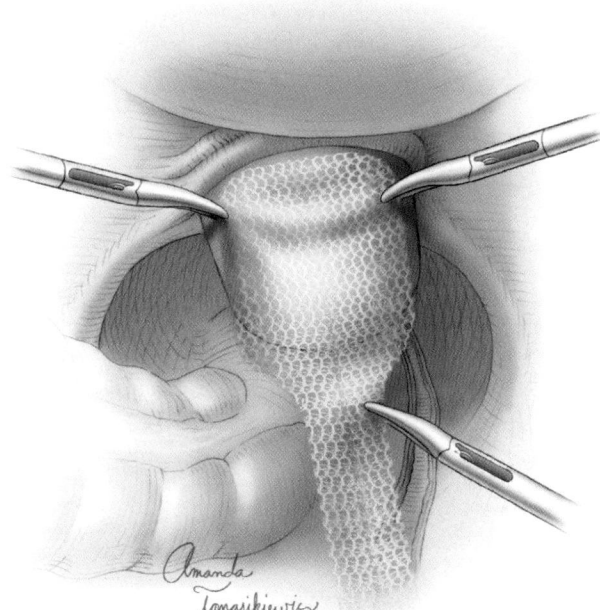

FIGURE 45-18.7 Anterior mesh placement.

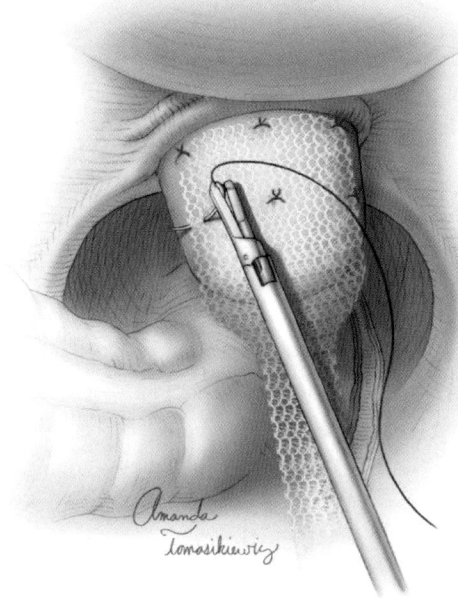

FIGURE 45-18.8 Anterior mesh sutured.

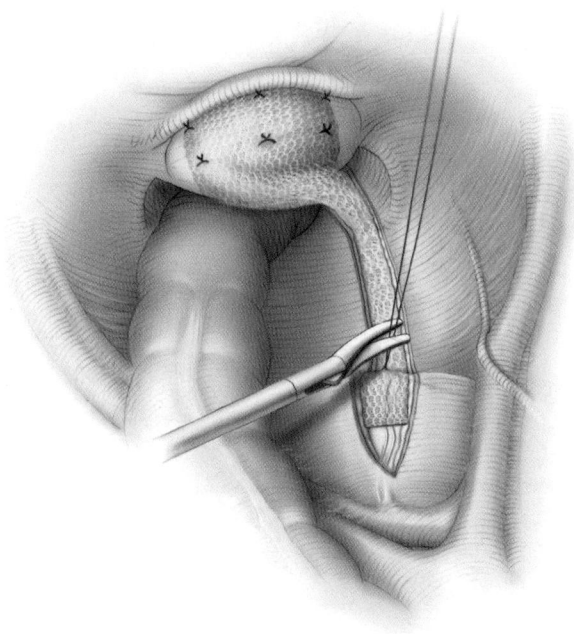

FIGURE 45-18.9 Mesh attachment to the sacrum.

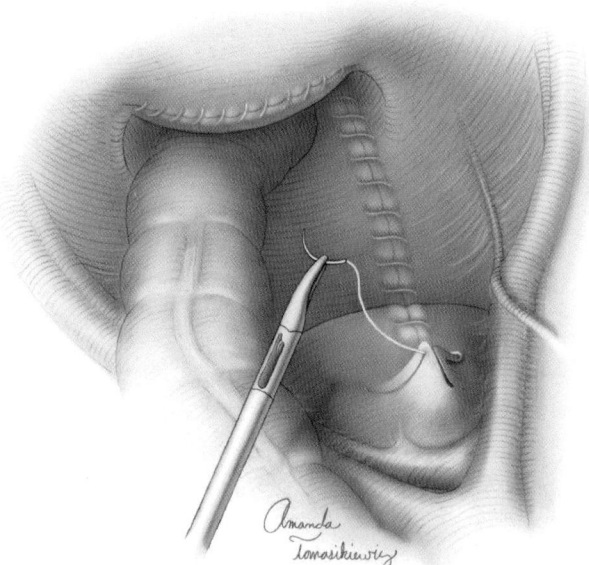

FIGURE 45-18.10 Peritoneal closure.

excess fabric above the planned most cephalad sacral suture is trimmed off. The sacral portion of the mesh is then secured to the anterior longitudinal ligament with three to four stitches that ultimately are aligned vertically along the S1 vertebra. For this, the proximal portions of both mesh strips are held against the ligament, and each stitch travels from right to left. The lowest stitch is placed first, and the needle enters the right side of the mesh, drives through the longitudinal ligament under direct visualization, and exits on the mesh's left side. To prevent air knots as the lowest sacral suture is secured, the surgeon elevates the vaginal manipulator to gently push the vaginal apex closer to and against the lower part of the sacrum.

Two or three additional sutures are next placed in the same fashion, each at a more cephalad level. Ideally, each suture lies approximately ½ cm from the previous one, and the most cephalad suture is at or just below the level of the promontory (Fig. 45-18.9).

⓭ **Peritoneal Closure.** The peritoneum is closed over the intervening and sacral portions of the mesh with 2-0 delayed-absorbable suture in a running fashion (Fig. 45-18.10). If desired, the peritoneum over the vaginal apex is closed over the exposed mesh in a similar fashion.

⓮ **Return to Supine Position.** With RSC, the robot is undocked at this point. With both RSC and LSC, the patient is returned to a supine position, and the abdomen deflated prior to cystoscopy.

⓯ **Cystoscopy.** This is routinely performed prior to port closure to document ureteral integrity and exclude bladder sutures or injury. Urethral examination is important if an anti-incontinence procedure is also performed.

⓰ **Wound Closure.** Subsequent surgery completion steps follow those of laparoscopy (Chap. 41, p. 897).

POSTOPERATIVE

Patients are usually discharged from the hospital on postoperative day 1. As with other minimally invasive surgery, diet is advanced as tolerated and early ambulation is encouraged. Other postoperative management specific to sacrocolpopexy mirrors that for ASC.

45-19

Vaginal Uterosacral Ligament Suspension

The vaginal apex can be effectively suspended with various vaginal or abdominal surgeries. Of these, suturing the apex to the high (proximal) portion of each uterosacral ligaments (USL), that is, uterosacral ligament suspension (USLS), is more commonly performed vaginally, although abdominal and laparoscopic approaches are suitable. Although often modified, the ultimate USLS goal is vaginal apex support restoration by affixing the anterior and posterior vaginal walls to the uterosacral ligaments at and above the level of the ischial spines. The steps described here outline our preferred approach, which is a modification of the USLS procedure described by Shull and associates (2000).

Another vaginal apical suspension procedure, sacrospinous ligament fixation (SSLF), also strives to correct apical prolapse. However, if USLS and SSLF are compared, USLS maintains the normal vaginal axis orientation and was thought to lower rates of dyspareunia and anterior vaginal wall prolapse. However, authors of the Operations and Pelvic Muscle Training in the Management of Apical Support Loss (OPTIMAL) trial compared outcomes of these two and found that after 2 years, both showed equal composite success scores nearing 60 percent (Barber, 2014). These rates are lower than the 70- to 90-percent success rates generally reported for these apical suspension procedures, but retreatment rates remained low at 5 percent (Margulies, 2010). Of complications in the OPTIMAL trial, neurologic pain persisted in 4 percent of SSLF cases, but ureteral obstruction was more frequent after USLS and approximated 3 percent.

In addition to apical prolapse correction, vaginal USLS effectively repairs apical enteroceles, and thus other enterocele repairs are unnecessary. However, apical prolapse commonly develops in conjunction with anterior and posterior compartment prolapse. Thus, vaginal USLS is often performed with other surgeries such as colporrhaphy and perineorrhaphy to correct these defects.

PREOPERATIVE

Patient Evaluation

As just noted, apical prolapse often coexists with other sites of prolapse, and a careful preoperative assessment is performed.

Also prior to vaginal USLS, patients with urinary incontinence symptoms undergo simple or complex urodynamic testing to clarify the type of incontinence. For those with SUI, a concurrent antiincontinence operation is generally performed. Because prolapse correction can unmask occult incontinence, clinicians also test continent women while manually reducing the prolapse with a moderately full bladder. Women with such occult SUI are carefully counseled and may also elect to also undergo antiincontinence surgery. Last, fully continent women undergoing vaginal prolapse surgery are also at risk for later development of postoperative SUI.

To evaluate whether a prophylactic midurethral sling (MUS) placed during apical and anterior vaginal prolapse surgery reduces this risk in stress-continent women, the OPUS (Outcomes Following Vaginal Prolapse Repair and Midurethral Sling) trial was conducted. Investigators concluded that prophylactic MUS in these asymptomatic women leads to a 27-percent postoperative SUI incidence at 1 year compared with a 43-percent rate without concomitant prophylactic MUS (Wei, 2012). These results support earlier findings of the CARE trial (p. 1098). Importantly, adding an antiincontinence procedure decreases, but does not eliminate, the risk of de novo SUI.

As another preoperative step, some suggest that estrogen may increase the vaginal wall thickness for easier dissection and suture placement. However, randomized controlled trials analyzing this treatment for reducing suture erosion or prolapse recurrence risks are lacking.

Consent

Recurrent prolapse is common following any corrective surgery. Thus, a surgeon should be aware of recurrence rates quoted in the literature and his or her own personal rates. As noted in the prior section, urinary incontinence or voiding or defecatory dysfunction may follow USLS. Also, USLS fixes the upper vagina to the USL and has a potential to shorten the vaginal canal. Accordingly, dyspareunia is another postoperative risk. Moreover, sacral plexus nerve injury with subsequent neuropathy ensues in up to 7 percent of women following vaginal USLS (Barber, 2014; Montoya, 2012). Thus, women are counseled regarding the possible need for suture release if severe buttock pain that radiates to the posterior thigh develops postoperatively. Mild buttock pain without associated radiation and without motor deficits generally resolves during several weeks of expectant management that incorporates analgesics. Last, apical suspension suture erosion and vaginal granulation tissue are frequently reported complications (Barber, 2014).

Patient Preparation

Bowel preparation will vary depending on surgeon preference. Patients can be instructed to take only clear liquids the day prior to surgery and complete one or two enemas the night prior to or the morning of surgery. Alternatively, a mechanical bowel preparation, listed in Chapter 39 (p. 835), may be preferred. Ballard and associates (2014), however, noted no distinct advantage to this for urogynecologic operations. Antibiotics and thromboprophylaxis are given as outlined in Tables 39-6 and 39-8 (p. 835).

❶ **Anesthesia and Patient Positioning.** Vaginal USLS is typically performed under general anesthesia. The patient is placed in standard lithotomy position using candycane or booted support stirrups. Examination under anesthesia assesses the degree of prolapse and confirms the need for planned surgeries. The vagina and abdomen are surgically prepared, and a Foley catheter is inserted.

❷ **Vaginal Apex Incision.** The initial incision can be made in various ways. If complementing vaginal hysterectomy, the vaginal cuff is already open, and each USL transfixing suture is already held by a hemostat. However, if the patient has previously undergone hysterectomy, the vaginal apex is grasped with Allis clamps, and the overlying epithelium is incised vertically or horizontally depending on circumstances. For example, for concurrent colporrhaphy, a midline vertical apical incision that extends distally along the anterior and/or posterior vaginal wall is preferred.

Alternatively, in patients with large apical enteroceles and redundant apical tissue, a diamond-shaped portion of epithelium can be excised and a new apex created. However, excessive tissue excision that may result in vaginal shortening is avoided. Stitches may then be placed at the lateral boundaries of the intended new apex for later identification. With enterocele, epithelial dissection at the apex typically reveals a peritoneal sac, which is incised to allow peritoneal cavity entry. Last, if a clear dissection plane is not identified, USLS can be performed by an extraperitoneal approach, or SSLF may be performed instead.

❸ **Packing, Retraction, and Identification.** Bowel must be adequately packed away for proper USL visualization to avoid bowel injury when high uterosacral sutures are placed. First, a Deaver retractor displaces the bladder upward. Then, a right-angle retractor or two fingers in the posterior cul-de-sac gently displace the posterior peritoneum and underlying rectum downward to avoid

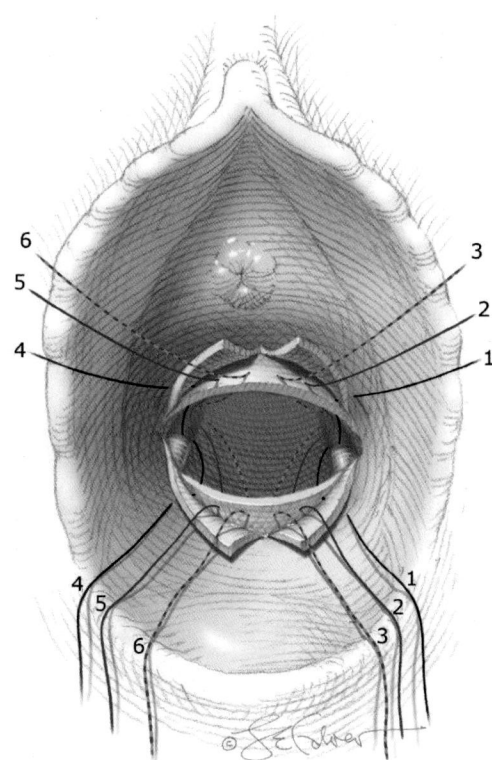

FIGURE 45-19.1 Vaginal view of sutures placed into uterosacral ligaments and vaginal walls.

peritoneum tearing, which creates bleeding and difficult USL identification. Two moist laparotomy sponges tied together are then gently threaded into the posterior cul-de-sac to pack bowel into the upper pelvis. The Deaver retractor is then repositioned to cover the laparotomy sponges. Gentle upward retractor traction exposes the mid and proximal USL portions and the deep posterior cul-de-sac close to the sacrum.

Two Allis clamps are next placed at approximately 5 and 7 o'clock positions on the posterior vaginal wall and incorporate the posterior peritoneum. Gentle downward Allis clamp traction tenses the USLs, which are then traced with the contralateral index finger. The strong ligament fibers can be traced from their distal attachments in the vagina to their proximal sacral attachment. Concurrently, the ischial spines, which protrude from the lateral pelvic walls and lie anterolateral to the USLs, are palpated. Ureters are usually indistinct to touch, but they course anterolateral to the USLs. A lighted Breisky-Navratil retractor is useful for retracting the rectum medially to further expose the USLs. A second similar retractor is often positioned on the opposite side for improved visualization of the proximal USL.

❹ **Suture Placement into the Uterosacral Ligament.** Following adequate exposure, two to three sutures are placed through one USL. Sutures are equally spaced along the mid to proximal length of each ligament. Long, straight needle drivers are useful for this. The sutures are individually tagged as they are placed, preferably with labeled clamps numbered 1 through 3 for one side and 4 through 6 for the other. Sutures are then loosely secured to the ipsilateral surgical drape. For the most distal stitch, we use a 2-0 gauge delayed-absorbable suture (*black*) with a swaged on SH needle. For the more proximal stitch(es), a similar gauge permanent material (*blue*) is selected instead (Fig. 45-19.1).

To begin, the distal absorbable suture perforates the USL at its midlength, which lies at approximately the level of the ischial spine. The subsequent, more proximal sutures are placed approximately 0.5 cm to 1 cm cephalad from each prior suture. Two or three sutures are placed on each side, and this number is guided by surgeon preference, the extent of USL exposed, and vaginal cuff width.

With each stitch placement, the needle tip ideally passes through the most medial portion of the ligament in a lateral-to-medial direction. These specifics attempt to minimize ureteral entrapment or kinking risks. Moreover, to lower rectal injury rates, an assistant retracts the rectum to the contralateral side, and suture purchases do not extend too medial, that is, beyond the ligament width. Similarly, suture bites that are too deep risk injury to internal iliac vessels or sacral nerves (Wieslander, 2007). At comple-

tion, gentle traction on each suture should confirm correct placement and incorporation of adequate USL tissue. Excess laxity during such USL traction usually indicates insufficient tissue to provide adequate apical support, and the suture is replaced.

Hematomas form occasionally following inadvertent laceration of pelvic sidewall veins. Application of pressure with a sponge stick will typically control bleeding.

❺ **Other Procedures.** Once all the suspensory sutures are placed through each USL, colporrhaphy is completed if indicated. If a perineorrhaphy or midurethral sling procedure is planned, we defer these until the USLS operation is completed.

❻ **Vaginal Wall Suture Placement.** Vaginal packing is first removed, and ultimately, four to six sutures (two or three from each USL) are placed along the vaginal cuff width. If one begins on the patient's left side, the free end of the left distal absorbable USLS suture (suture 1) is threaded into a Mayo needle. The needle and suture then pierce the left lateral anterior vaginal wall at the apex. The other needle-bearing suture end similarly penetrates the posterior wall (see Fig. 45-19.1). Each suture strand traverses the full vaginal wall thickness, including the epithelium.

Next, the proximal (permanent) USLS suture(s) are similarly passed through the anterior and posterior vaginal walls, each medial to the previous suture. To lower suture erosion rates, permanent sutures traverse the full thickness of the fibromuscular layer but not the epithelium. However, a substantial thickness of fibromuscular wall is incorporated to prevent tissue tearing, which can create suture bridges that are bowel obstruction risks. The same steps are then repeated on the right.

Ultimately, on each side, the most cephalad USLS sutures (sutures 3 and 6) are placed most medially on the vaginal cuff. The most distal USLS sutures (sutures 1 and 4) are placed most laterally on the vaginal cuff. For organization, all completed sutures are held within numbered clamps on their respective sides.

At this point, indigo carmine or methylene blue dye is given intravenously in preparation for cystoscopy that follows knot tying. Knots are secured starting with most medial cuff sutures (sutures 3 and 6) and ending with the most lateral (sutures 1 and 4) (Fig. 45-19.2). The vaginal wall is confirmed to approximate the ULSs. Both this approximation and the order in which sutures are tied may prevent suture bridges. All sutures are held with their corresponding numbered clamps after tying until cystoscopy is completed.

❼ **Cystoscopy.** This is performed to document ureteral patency and exclude bladder

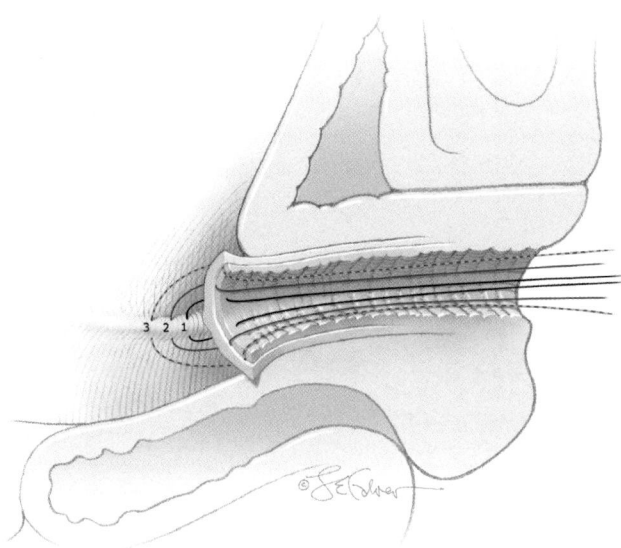

FIGURE 45-19.2 Lateral view of sutures placed into the left utero-sacral ligament.

sutures or cystotomy. The ureter lies closest to the lower portion of the USL. Thus, if ureteral obstruction is suspected, the most distal USLS suture on the ipsilateral side is released first, and cystoscopy is repeated. If no flow is noted, the next most proximal suture is released, and this is continued cephalad in a stepwise fashion until efflux is seen.

❽ **Rectal Examination.** The rectum is digitally explored to confirm approximation of the cuff against the USLs and exclude sutures entering the rectum.

❾ **Closure of the Vaginal Cuff.** The suspension suture ends are now cut, and the vaginal cuff is reapproximated in a running fashion with 2-0 gauge delayed-absorbable suture. Alternatively, four interrupted 2-0 absorbable sutures are placed through the full thickness of the anterior and posterior vaginal cuff prior to tying of the USL sutures and held for later cuff closure. This practice aids cuff closure with high suspensions, in which vaginal edges may be inaccessible without pulling that in turn disrupts the repair.

POSTOPERATIVE

Following vaginal USLS, postoperative care mirrors that for vaginal surgery. Postoperative activity in general can be individualized, although intercourse is usually delayed until after 6 weeks following surgery. A voiding trial can be completed on postoperative day 1, depending on the patient's condition and general progress. Some patients have urinary retention after apical suspension, even without an antiincontinence procedure. If unable to void spontaneously by the time of discharge, the patient can be discharged with a catheter and followed up within a week for removal. Patients are screened for lower extremity neuropathy prior to discharge. Suture erosion with granulation tissue can be a short- or long-term complication and is managed as described on page 1102.

45-20

Abdominal Uterosacral Ligament Suspension

Uterosacral ligament suspension (USLS) is more commonly performed vaginally (p. 1107). But for some situations, an abdominal approach, either via laparotomy or laparoscopy, offers advantages. For example, with advanced apical prolapse, many consider abdominal sacrocolpopexy (ASC) the preferred procedure. However, limited data suggest that total hysterectomy concurrent with ASC leads to higher mesh erosion rates. Thus, with total abdominal hysterectomy, abdominal USLS represents an ASC alternative to reduce graft erosion. A second possible indication is the setting of iatrogenic cystotomy during ASC. In this case, to minimize mesh erosion into the bladder or fistula formation, ASC can be aborted and USLS performed instead (p. 1102). Last, although not evidence-based, for women with concurrent pelvic cancer, mesh placement may not be ideal, and thus, USLS may be preferred.

During abdominal USLS, the mid to proximal span of both USLs is sutured to the anterior and posterior vaginal walls at the vaginal apex. Because of this suspension, enteroceles are effectively closed. Abdominal USLS is effective, and limited data show that success rates for the apical suspension approximate 90 percent (Lowenstein, 2009; Rardin, 2009). However, as with other apical procedures, subsequent anterior or posterior compartment defects are later risks.

PREOPERATIVE

Before surgery, patients are examined to identify other prolapsed sites, which could be concurrently repaired. Similarly, overt or occult SUI is excluded. In addition, consenting includes a discussion regarding prophylactic antiincontinence surgery. As with other apical suspension procedures, and as described fully on page 1098, even stress-continent women may benefit in many cases from a prophylactic antiincontinence procedure performed concurrently. However, for abdominal USLS, data on this prophylactic practice are lacking and must be extrapolated from ASC and vaginal USLS studies. Last, as another preoperative step, some suggest that estrogen aids dissection and suture placement, as the vaginal wall thickness is increased (Rahn, 2014, 2015). However, no randomized controlled trials have analyzed

this treatment's ability to improve dissection or reduce suture erosion or prolapse recurrence risks.

Consenting mirrors that for vaginal USLS (p. 1107). Antibiotics and thromboprophylaxis are given as outlined in Tables 39-6 and 39-8 (p. 835). Bowel preparation is selected according to surgeon preference as for vaginal USLS.

INTRAOPERATIVE

Surgical Steps

❶ **Anesthesia and Patient Positioning.** Following administration of general anesthesia, the patient is positioned in a low lithotomy position with thighs parallel to the ground and legs in booted support stirrups. The vagina and abdomen are surgically prepared, and a Foley catheter is inserted.

❷ **Incision.** A midline vertical or low transverse abdominal incision is suitable, and a self-retaining retractor and bowel packing clears the operative field. With a laparoscopic approach, port placement is similar to that described for laparoscopic sacrocolpopexy (p. 1103).

❸ **Ureter Identification.** The ureters are identified early, as these can be trapped during suture placement through the USL and can be kinked with suture tying. Thus, frequent confirmation of ureter location and cystoscopy after the suspension sutures are tied are essential steps.

❹ **Identification of Uterosacral Ligaments.** Prior to hysterectomy, a surgeon identifies each USL by applying contralateral and upward uterine traction. With this technique, the USLs are stretched and more easily seen or palpated. In women with prior hysterectomy, the vaginal cuff is similarly elevated and deviated by a vaginal manipulator. The USLs run medial and posterior to the ureters, and their proximity explains the significant ureteral injury rate, which can reach 11 percent with vaginal USLS (Barber, 2000). The USL midpoint generally lies at the level of the ischial spines, which are located anterolateral to the USLs. In women with normal support, the cervix and upper vagina are located roughly at the level of these spines. Thus, this bony landmark is generally chosen as the site for the most distal USL suture. However, this site may be modified according to vaginal length and intraoperative findings.

❺ **Uterosacral Ligament Suture Placement.** Following adequate exposure, two to three sutures are placed through one USL. Sutures are equally spaced along the mid to proximal length of each ligament. During suture placement, the vaginal cuff is elevated to accentuate the USLs. For the most distal stitch, we use a 2-0 gauge delayed-absorbable suture (*black*) with a swaged-on SH needle. For the more proximal stitch(es), a similar gauge permanent material (*blue*) is selected instead (Fig. 45-20.1).

To begin, the distal absorbable suture perforates the USL at its midlength, which lies approximately at the level of the ischial spine.

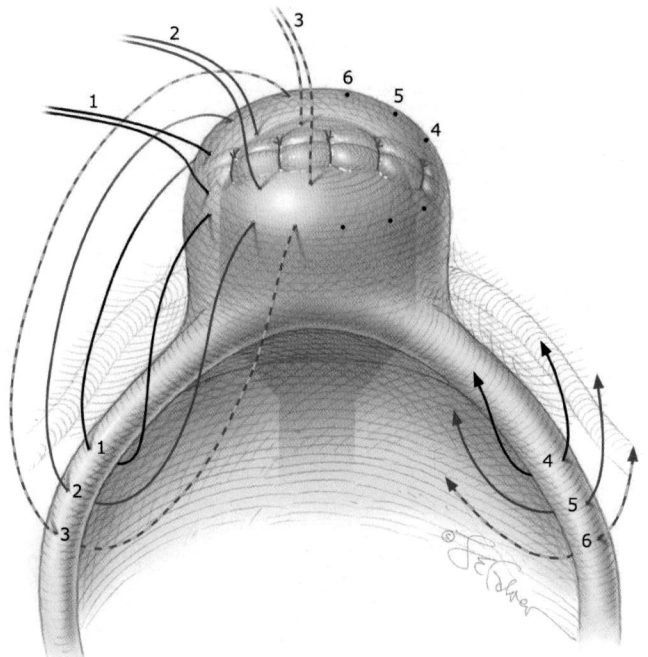

FIGURE 45-20.1 Uterosacral ligament suture placement.

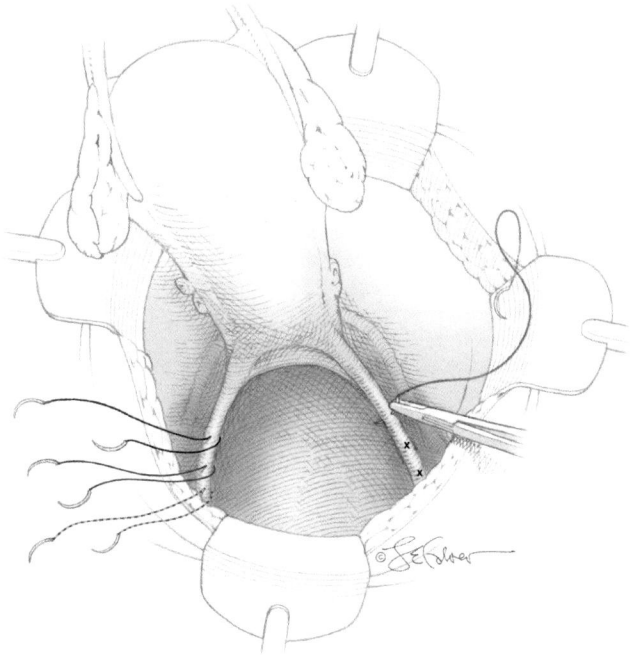

FIGURE 45-20.2 Vaginal cuff suture placement.

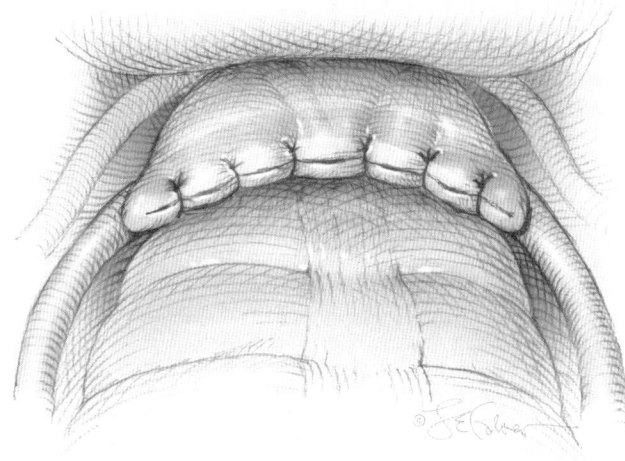

FIGURE 45-20.3 All sutures secured.

The subsequent, more proximal sutures are placed approximately 0.5 to 1 cm cephalad from each prior suture. Two or three sutures may be placed on each side, and this number is guided by surgeon preference, the extent of USL exposed, and vaginal cuff width.

With stitch placement, each needle tip ideally passes through the most medial portion of the ligament in a lateral-to-medial direction. Moreover, the assistant retracts the rectum to the contralateral side, and suture purchases do not extend too medial, that is, beyond the ligament width. Similarly, suture bites that are too deep risk injury to internal iliac vessels or sacral nerves (Wieslander, 2007). At completion, gentle traction on each suture should confirm correct placement and incorporation of adequate USL tissue. If not, the suture is replaced.

Following each placement, sutures with needles still attached are then individually tagged, preferably with labeled clamps, and are loosely secured to the ipsilateral drape. This series is repeated on the other side.

❻ Hysterectomy. These suspensory sutures may be placed through the USL before or after hysterectomy based on surgeon preference and intraoperative findings (Fig. 45-20.2). If sutures are placed prior to hysterectomy, they are held by numbered hemostats and not tied. Their needles are covered with a surgical towel to avoid stick injuries. Hysterectomy is then completed, and the cuff is closed.

❼ Vaginal Wall Suture Placement. Ultimately, four to six sutures (two or three

from each USL) are placed along the vaginal cuff width. An EEA sizer or similar blunt manipulator is placed in the vagina for cuff movement. If one begins on the patient's left side, the free end of the left distal absorbable USLS suture (suture 1) is threaded into a Mayo needle. The needle and suture then pierce the left lateral anterior vaginal wall at the apex. The other needle-bearing suture end similarly penetrates the posterior wall (see Fig. 45-20.1). Each suture strand may traverse the full vaginal wall thickness, including the epithelium.

Next, the proximal (permanent) USLS sutures are passed through the anterior and posterior vaginal walls, each medial to the previous suture on the cuff. To lower suture erosion rates, permanent sutures traverse the full thickness of the fibromuscular walls but not the epithelium. However, a substantial thickness of fibromuscular wall should be incorporated to prevent tissue tearing, which can create suture bridges that are bowel obstruction risks. The same steps are repeated on the right side of the cuff.

Ultimately on each side, the most cephalad USLS suture (suture 3 or 6) is placed most medially along the vaginal cuff width. The most distal USLS suture (suture 1 or 4) is placed most laterally on the vaginal cuff. For organization, all completed sutures are held within numbered clamps on their respective sides.

At this point, knots are secured starting with the most medial sutures (sutures 3 and 6) and ending with the most lateral (sutures 1 and 4). The vaginal wall is confirmed to

approximate the ULSs (Fig. 45-20.3). Both this approximation and the order in which sutures are tied may prevent suture bridges. All sutures are held with their corresponding numbered clamps after tying until cystoscopy is completed.

❽ Cystoscopy. To document ureteral patency and exclude bladder sutures or cystotomy, cystoscopy is performed after all suspension sutures are tied. The ureter lies closest to the lower portion of the USL. Thus, if ureteral obstruction is suspected, the most distal USLS suture on the ipsilateral side is released first, and cystoscopy is repeated. If no flow is noted, the next most proximal suture is released, and this is continued cephalad in a stepwise fashion until efflux is seen.

❾ Rectal Examination. This is performed to confirm approximation of the cuff to the USLs and exclude sutures entering the rectum.

❿ Incision Closure. The abdomen is closed in a standard fashion (Chap. 43, p. 928).

⓫ Concurrent Procedures. If necessary, a paravaginal defect repair or other abdominal antiincontinence procedure may be performed prior to incision closure. If posterior repair or vaginal antiincontinence surgery is required, these will follow incision closure.

POSTOPERATIVE

Following abdominal USLS, postoperative care mirrors that for abdominal sacrocolpopexy (p. 1102).

45-21

Sacrospinous Ligament Fixation

Extending between the ischial spine and lower sacrum, the sacrospinous ligament (SSL) lies deep to the coccygeus muscle and adds significant stability to the bony pelvis. Fixation of the vaginal apex to this coccygeus-sacrospinous ligament (C-SSL) complex—namely, sacrospinous ligament fixation (SSLF)—is often selected for apical prolapse repair. Although there are many SSLF modifications, apex fixation to the right ligament is most often described, likely due to the left-sided location of the rectosigmoid (Goldberg, 2001; Kearney, 2003).

Gaining access to the SSL also varies. In a more traditional approach, the pararectal space and SSL are accessed through a posterior colporrhaphy incision, and only the right aspect of the apical posterior vaginal wall is attached to the ligament. Alternatively, in the *Michigan four-wall modification,* the SSL is accessed through an apical incision, dissection to the SSL remains extraperitoneal, and both anterior and posterior vaginal walls are directly affixed to the SSL by four points that span the vaginal apex width. Advantageously, this technique may avoid anterior enterocele, contralateral vaginal wall descent, and the need for bilateral suspension (Larson, 2013). A modification of the original Michigan approach is described here (Morley, 1988).

Success rates are comparable to those for other vaginal approaches for vault suspension (Barber, 2014; Maher, 2013). However, SSLF compares less favorably with abdominal sacrocolpopexy. But, SSLF averts abdominal surgery and is associated with shorter operating times and quicker recovery. For these reasons, it is often preferred for women with comorbidities. Additionally, this approach allows other concurrent support defects to be repaired vaginally as well.

PREOPERATIVE

Patient Evaluation

Before surgery, patients are examined to identify other prolapsed sites, which could be concurrently repaired. Similarly, overt or occult SUI is excluded. In addition, consenting includes a discussion regarding prophylactic antiincontinence surgery. As with other apical suspension procedures, and as described fully on page 1098, even stress-continent women may benefit in many cases from a prophylactic antiincontinence procedure performed concurrently. Last, as another preoperative step, some suggest that estrogen aids dissection and suture placement, as the vaginal wall thickness is increased (Rahn, 2014, 2015). However, no randomized controlled trials have analyzed this treatment's ability to improve dissection or reduce suture erosion or prolapse recurrence risks.

Consent

Because the vagina is fixed and laterally deviated with SSLF, dyspareunia is one postoperative risk. Also, recurrent prolapse is common following any corrective surgery. Although the apical prolapse rate following SSLF is below 10 percent, anterior vaginal wall prolapse rates can approach 30 percent (Barber, 2009). This anterior prolapse is attributed to the exaggerated posterior deflection of the vaginal axis, which exposes the anterior vaginal wall to greater intraabdominal stresses than other apical suspensions (Weber, 2005). Despite this theoretical vulnerability, the OPTIMAL trial cited earlier (p. 1107) compared SSLF and vaginal USLS 2-year outcomes and found equal composite success scores nearing 60 percent (Barber, 2014). These percentages are lower than the 70- to 90-percent success rates generally reported for these procedures. That said, actual retreatment rates remained low at 5 percent (Margulies, 2010).

For most women, SSLF has low associated risks for serious complications, but neurovascular injury can occur. First, low-pressure vessel bleeding encountered during dissection and exposure of the pararectal space is generally attributed to retractor or needle injury of the extensive venous plexus that drains the rectum and vagina. This bleeding can usually be controlled with sustained pressure from pararectal space packing. Second, arterial bleeding may follow aggressive retraction and subsequent middle rectal artery avulsion or laceration. The internal pudendal and inferior gluteal arteries are also at risk if a needle inadvertently extends past the proximal SSL border. Arterial bleeding is best controlled by vessel ligation or clipping. An internal iliac ligation for such bleeding is ineffective due to extensive collateral circulation in the pelvis.

The pudendal nerve and lower sacral nerves such as S3 and S4 can also be damaged if the needle exits or enters past the ligament's proximal (upper) margin. Sutures that are placed too close to the sacrum risk injury to S4 or the nerve to the levator ani muscles (Roshanravan, 2007). Even sutures that are placed in the recommended mid and lower aspect of the SSL can entrap or lacerate the nerve to the levator ani muscles. Pelvic floor muscle spasms, buttock pain, and dyspareunia may be manifestations.

Moreover, sacral plexus nerve injury with subsequent neuropathy has followed vaginal SSLF. As described on page 1107, persistent neurologic pain was noted in 4 percent of SSLF cases in the OPTIMAL trial. Accordingly, women are counseled that additional surgery for suture release may be needed if severe buttock pain that radiates to the posterior thigh persists postoperatively. Mild buttock pain without associated radiation or without motor deficits is common and generally resolves within several weeks and with expectant management that incorporates analgesics. This buttock pain is generally attributed to entrapment of the nerve to the levator ani muscle.

Of other complications, ureteral and rectal injuries and ileus are rare, mainly because this procedure is extraperitoneal. In addition, as with any apical suspension procedure, voiding and defecatory dysfunction can develop.

Patient Preparation

Bowel preparation will vary depending on surgeon preference. Patients can be instructed to take only clear liquids the day prior to surgery and complete one or two enemas that night or the morning of surgery. Alternatively, a mechanical bowel preparation using agents listed in Chapter 39 (p. 835) may be preferred. Ballard and associates (2014), however, noted no distinct advantage to this for urogynecologic operations. As with most vaginal surgery, because of the risk posed by the normal vaginal flora for postoperative wound cellulitis and abscess, preoperative antibiotics are warranted. Typical agents are found in Table 39-6 (p. 835). Additionally, thromboprophylaxis is provided as outlined in Table 39-8 (p. 836).

INTRAOPERATIVE

Surgical Instruments

Suture placement into the SSL can be performed with various ligature carriers and include the Deschamps ligature carrier, Miya hook, Capio ligature carrier, and Endo Stitch. Alternatively, a Mayo needle and long, straight needle driver can be used. Using the Deschamps ligature carrier, a surgeon threads the suture through an eye at the needle-shaped carrier tip. Arcs and curves constructed into the instrument aid ease of suture placement. Once the tip of the Deschamps carrier passes through the ligament, the suture is retrieved with a nerve hook, as shown in atlas Step 4. Disadvantages to this device, however, include the relative thickness of the needle tip, which may be difficult to drive through the ligament. Alternatively, disposable devices have become popular, in particular the Capio ligature carrier. This device is easier to manipulate

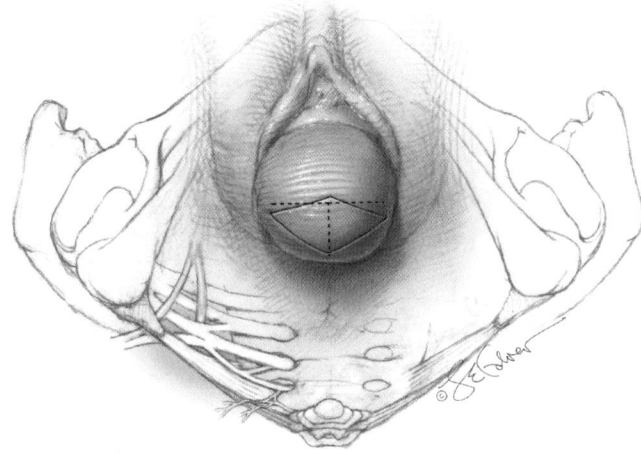

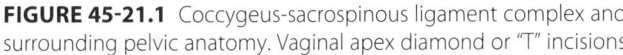

FIGURE 45-21.1 Coccygeus-sacrospinous ligament complex and surrounding pelvic anatomy. Vaginal apex diamond or "T" incisions.

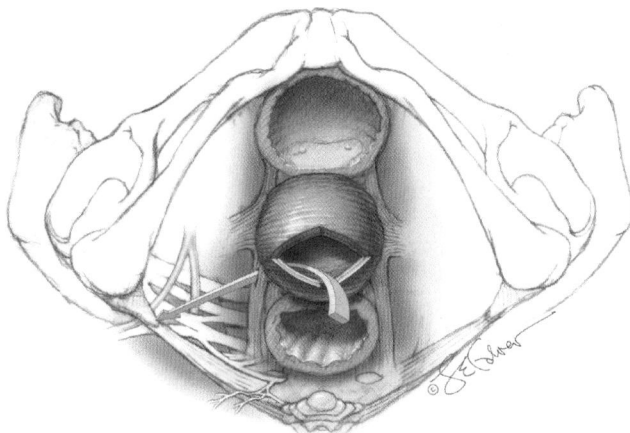

FIGURE 45-21.2 Entry into right pararectal space through rectal pillar.

than the Miya hook. Also, its design aids placement of sutures using ligament palpation and thus obviates the need for extensive dissection. To expose the ligament, Deaver and Breisky-Navratil retractors are commonly used.

Surgical Steps

❶ **Anesthesia and Patient Positioning.** After general anesthesia has been administered, a woman is placed in standard lithotomy position. The vagina is surgically prepared, and a Foley catheter is inserted. Initially, vaginal vault prolapse is reduced to place the vagina in a normal anatomic position.

❷ **Vaginal Wall Incision.** *In the setting of vaginal cuff prolapse,* the apex is grasped and brought to the level of the ligament to confirm adequate vaginal length or need for redundant tissue excision. With advanced prolapse, a new apex site is required and most often lies posterior to the former hysterectomy scar (Kearney, 2003). When indicated, excess vaginal tissue will be excised. At the planned apex, four points in a diamond configuration are grasped with Allis clamps, are directed inward, and individually brought to lie against the SSL. This ensures fixation off tension and correction of any anterior and posterior vaginal wall redundancy. These points include one midline anterior, one midline posterior, and two lateral ones. Once determined, the diamond-shaped redundant vaginal wall within these four Allis clamps is incised to a depth reaching the underlying loose preperitoneal connective tissue (Fig 45-21.1). If this diamond lies posterior to the prior cuff scar, the peritoneum is generally easily identified and the enterocele sac may be entered intentionally or inadvertently. If this diamond lies anterior to the prior cuff, then

dissection proceeds more superficially to avoid bladder entry.

If vaginal shortening is a concern, then a transverse incision is made at the new apex site and no tissue is excised. Next, a vertical incision that extends several centimeters posteriorly from this transverse incision's midpoint creates a "T" incision that aids access into the pararectal space (Fig. 43-21.1, dotted line). With either incision configuration, the intended apex site is marked with sutures or clamps to maintain proper orientation during fixation.

In the setting of concomitant vaginal hysterectomy, after hysterectomy completion, the lateral edges of the anterior and posterior vaginal walls are grasped with Allis clamps and brought into direct contact with the SSL to similarly assess for excess tension or redundancy. A vertical incision is then made through the midline posterior vaginal wall at the open cuff and extended 2 to 3 cm distally. The extraperitoneal space between the vaginal wall and the peritoneum is entered. Then, the pararectal space is entered as described next.

❸ **Access to the Right Sacrospinous Ligament.** Whether the SSL is accessed through the apex (Michigan modification) or through the posterior vaginal wall (traditional approach), the same retroperitoneal spaces are entered. Namely, the rectovaginal space and then the pararectal space are entered sequentially to reach the SSL (Fig. 45-21.2). Following entry into the rectovaginal space, traction on the vaginal epithelium with an Allis clamp and countertraction on peritoneum with tissue forceps are applied, while sharp or blunt dissection is directed toward the right ischial spine. Important anatomic structures during entry into the right pararectal space include the rectum, which lies medially and is retracted leftward to avoid injury; blood vessels and peritoneum, which lie ventrally and superiorly; and the levator ani muscles, which

are found dorsal and laterally. To enter the pararectal space, the rectal pillars, also known as deep uterosacral ligament fibers, are perforated as shown by the *arrow* in Figure 45-21.2. This tissue is typically attenuated in women with advanced prolapse and thus easier to perforate. In some cases, perforation with a hemostat or similar instrument is needed. Once in the pararectal space, the ischial spine tip is palpated, and the index finger moves gently medially toward the lower, lateral border of the sacrum to delineate the C-SSL complex (Fig. 45-21.3). This step also allows blunt digital dissection of loose connective tissue from the ligament's midportion.

❹ **Retractor Positioning.** Two to three retractors are positioned to adequately expose the C-SSL complex (Fig. 45-21.4). We prefer a small Deaver to displace the peritoneum and blood vessels superiorly, a Breisky-Navratil retractor to displace the rectum medially, and a second Breisky-Navratil retractor to displace the levator muscles inferiorly and further expose the ligament's lower portion. Retraction is gentle to avoid vessel or rectal injury. A rectal examination at this point aims to exclude rectal laceration. During dissection and retractor positioning, vessels in the area may be lacerated, and hemostasis is obtained with direct pressure, electrosurgical coagulation, or ligatures.

❺ **SSL Suture Placement.** Once the C-SSL complex is delineated, sutures are placed approximately two fingerbreadths or 2 to 3 cm medial to the ischial spine, which roughly corresponds to the SSL midportion (Roshanravan, 2007; Walters, 2007). Sutures placed too close to the spine risk injury to the pudendal nerves or vessels. Needle entry or exit points ideally remain within the mid to lower portion of the ligament. This lowers injury risk to the inferior gluteal vessels and pudendal

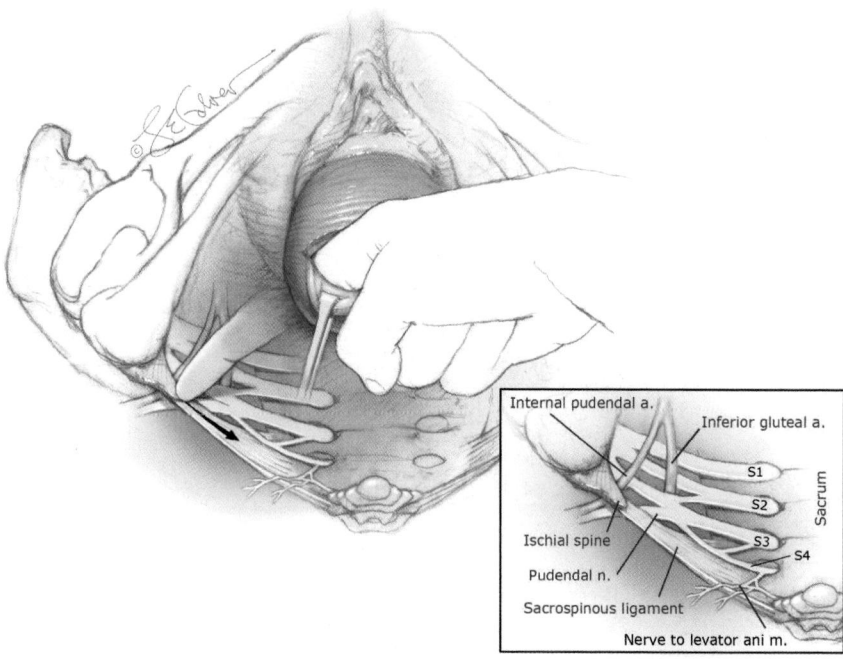

FIGURE 45-21.3 Anatomy delineated.

or sacral nerves, which course in close proximity to the upper SSL margin.

We use the Deschamps ligature carrier or a tapered Mayo needle with a half-circle radius to ultimately pass four sutures (two absorbable and two permanent) through the ligament (see Fig. 45-21.4). To begin, two long sutures, one delayed-absorbable (*black*) and one permanent (*blue*) are threaded through the carrier eye. For the absorbable sutures, we select either 2-0 or 0-gauge polydioxanone (PDS II), and for the permanent sutures, we use similar-gauge polypropylene (Prolene). Thus, with a single ligament penetration, four sutures ends are available Alternatively, four delayed-absorbable sutures using 0-gauge polydioxanone can be used.

When the Deschamps ligature carrier is used, sutures are retrieved using a nerve hook, as shown. Once the suture ends are retrieved, suture traction is applied to test their anchorage. Firm resistance during traction confirms proper placement. Laxity indicates superficial placement through the coccygeus muscle or overlying fascia, and the sutures are replaced deeper into C-SSL. At this point, the four suture ends are paired by color, tagged by individually numbered hemostats, and loosely secured to the surgical drape.

The second carrier pass is then completed approximately 1 cm medial to the first. Based on intraoperative findings, the order of the carrier passes may be reversed, that is, the lateral suture is placed second. Adequate anchorage

is similarly confirmed, and these sutures are then paired and tagged. Ultimately, these two carrier passes result in four suture pairs that will later be sutured to the anterior, posterior, and lateral vaginal walls.

Adequate suture labeling (1 through 4) avoids suture tangling and later suture bridging at the fixation site. The delayed-absorbable suture (*black*), which is placed most laterally on the ligament is labeled "1" and will be placed through the right lateral aspect of the vaginal cuff. The delayed-absorbable suture (*black*) placed most medial on the ligament is labeled "4" and will be placed through the left lateral aspect of the vaginal cuff. Sutures 3 and 4 correspond to the permanent sutures (*blue*). These ultimately will be placed through the medial portion of the cuff.

If indicated, anterior colporrhaphy is performed at this time. If performed, the anterior vaginal wall is reapproximated with 2-0 or 3-0 gauge absorbable suture to the level of the cuff. Rectoceles are often corrected with SSLF, and posterior colporrhaphy is not frequently required. If a posterior midline plication, perineorrhaphy, or midurethral sling is planned, we prefer to complete this after apical suspension.

❻ Vaginal Apex Suturing. The SSL sutures are then sequentially anchored to the anterior and posterior fibromuscular walls of the vagina apex along the vaginal cuff width. To begin, the two ends of suture 1 are grasped. The end that is most cephalad on the ligament is threaded through the Mayo needle eye. This is then driven through the full thickness of the lateral right anterior vaginal wall including the epithelium, at the site of the initial intended-apex marking suture. The other end of suture 1 is then driven through the lateral right posterior wall. Similar steps are subsequently repeated on the cuff's left side with delayed-absorbable suture 4 (Fig. 45-21.5). Suture ends are not tied but instead held on their respective sides by a hemostat.

Attention is then directed to the permanent sutures (2 and 3). First and medial to those of suture 1, the ends of suture 2 are driven through the anterior and posterior fibromuscular vaginal walls at a point right of the cuff midline. To lower suture erosion rates, permanent sutures traverse the full thickness of the fibromuscular walls but not the epithelium. However, a substantial fibromuscular wall thickness is incorporated to prevent tissue tearing, which can create suture bridges and incomplete healing of the vaginal wall to the ligament. Second and medial to those of suture 4, the ends of suture 3 are driven through the anterior and posterior fibromuscular vaginal walls at a point left of the cuff midline.

❼ Suspension of the Vaginal Vault. At this point, knots are secured starting with suture 4 and ending with suture 1. A pulley

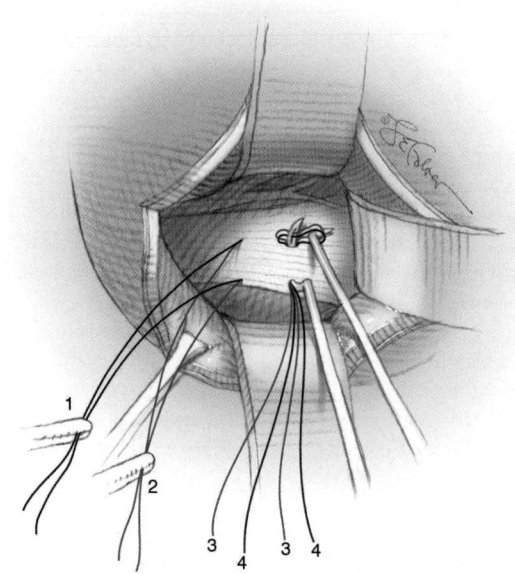

FIGURE 45-21.4 Retractor exposure and ligature placement.

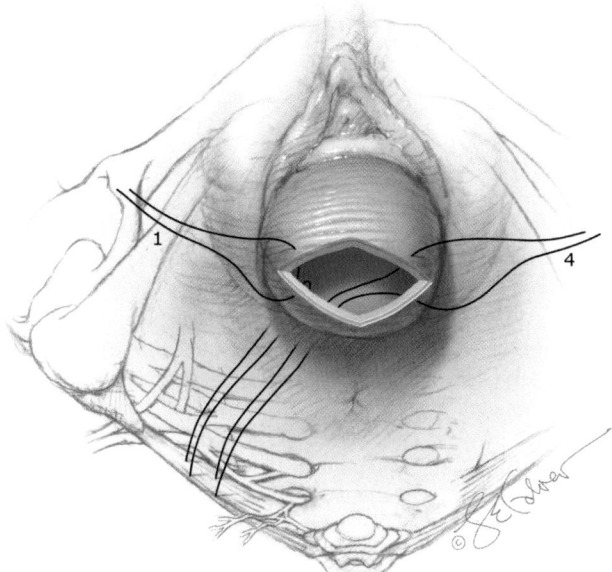

FIGURE 45-21.5 Lateral apex suturing.

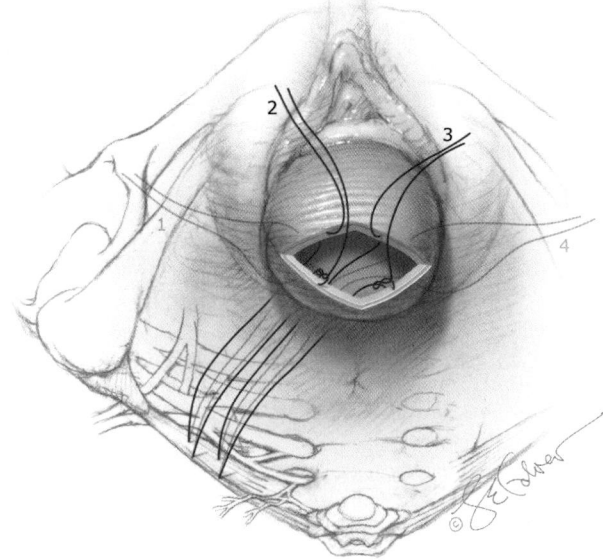

FIGURE 45-21.6 Permanent suture placement (*blue strands*).

stitch may be used for the permanent sutures. With this stitch, a knot is secured on the vaginal wall (posterior wall in this case) (Fig. 45-21.6). As shown in Figure 45-21.7, traction on the other suture end (anterior dashed strand) pulls the tied wall (posterior) to the SSL. However, with the four-wall modification, this type of stitch is not necessary. Each suture is tied down to ensure direct apposition of the vaginal walls to the SSL (Fig. 45-21.8). Both this snug approximation and the order in which sutures are tied may prevent suture bridges. All sutures are held with their corresponding numbered clamps after tying until cystoscopy is completed. Rectal examination confirms apposition of the vaginal cuff to the SSL and excludes rectal injury.

❽ **Cuff closure.** If needed, the remainder of the vaginal cuff may be closed in a running fashion using 2-0 gauge delayed-absorbable suture.

POSTOPERATIVE

Following SSLF, postoperative care mirrors that for vaginal surgery. Postoperative activity in general can be individualized, although intercourse is usually delayed until after 6 weeks following surgery. A voiding trial can be completed on postoperative day 1, depending on the patient's condition and general progress. Some patients have urinary retention after apical suspension, even without an antiincontinence procedure. If unable to void spontaneously by the time of discharge, the

patient can be discharged with a catheter and followed up within a week for removal.

Patients are screened for lower extremity neuropathy prior to discharge. Mild gluteal pain is common and typically resolves within several weeks. Severe gluteal pain that radiates down the posterior thigh and leg is a sign of sacral nerve entrapment and is generally treated by prompt suture release. Dyspareunia is commonly attributed to the posterolateral deflection of the vaginal axis. However, given the anatomic position of the nerves to the coccygeus and levator ani muscles, entrapment of these nerves may possibly lead to transient or sustained muscle spasm and dysfunction (Roshanravan, 2007). If levator muscle tenderness is identified, physical therapy may be helpful.

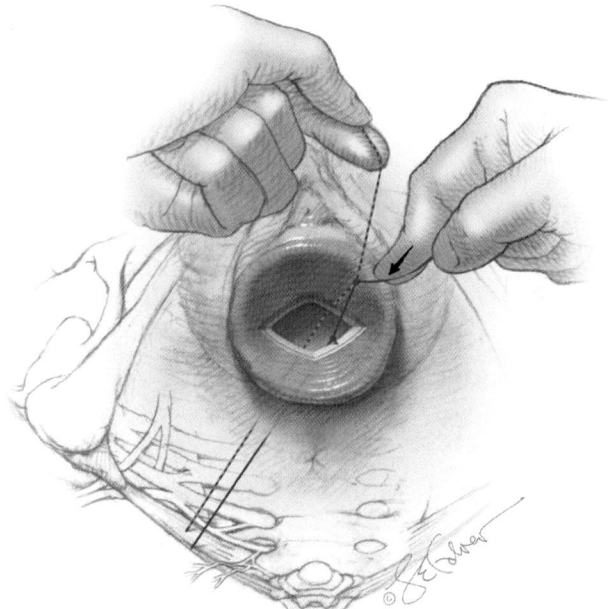

FIGURE 45-21.7 Pulley stitch.

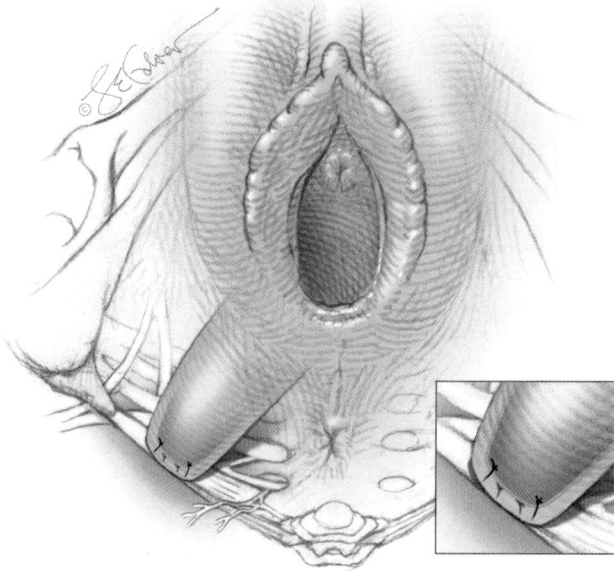

FIGURE 45-21.8 Vaginal apex approximated to ligament.

45-22

McCall Culdoplasty

Culdoplasty techniques are used to obliterate the posterior cul-de-sac of Douglas and prevent herniation of small bowel into the vaginal wall, that is, enterocele. Thus, culdoplasty usually complements procedures that further expose the posterior cul-de-sac to enterocele, such as retropubic urethropexy procedures. However, evidence-based studies have not borne out these benefits, and current concepts of specific pelvic-support defect repair have decreased the popularity of culdoplasty. Nevertheless, this procedure is still performed and may have value when completed in conjunction with other prolapse procedures.

Of these, McCall culdoplasty is most commonly performed during vaginal hysterectomy to close the cul-de-sac, add support to the posterior vaginal apex, and possibly prevent enterocele formation. With traditional McCall culdoplasty, two to three horizontal *internal* rows using permanent sutures are placed from one uterosacral ligament (USL) to the other to obliterate the posterior cul-de-sac (McCall, 1957). The term *internal* denotes that these sutures remain totally intraabdominal and do not penetrate into the vaginal lumen. In addition, one to two rows of absorbable *external* sutures are similarly placed through the USLs, but these pass through the posterior vaginal cuff.

Several modifications aim to provide better vaginal apex support. These include the Mayo/McCall culdoplasty and the modified McCall culdoplasty. The steps described next outline our approach. Importantly, if significant vaginal apex prolapse or enterocele is already present, then we prefer an apical suspension procedure such as sacrocolpopexy, sacrospinous ligament fixation, or vaginal uterosacral ligament suspension, as more data support their efficacy.

PREOPERATIVE

Patient Evaluation

McCall culdoplasty is generally performed following vaginal hysterectomy in patients with enterocele or preventively in those without. Because the degree of pelvic organ prolapse will dictate reconstructive surgeries planned, a thorough prolapse evaluation is performed.

Consent

As with any pelvic reconstructive surgery to correct prolapse, the risk of enterocele formation or recurrence is discussed. In addition, because this procedure involves placement of sutures through the uterosacral ligaments, risks similar to uterosacral ligament suspension procedures are addressed and include dyspareunia, ureteral or bowel injury, and sacral plexus nerve damage (p. 1107). Suture erosion risks are low.

Patient Preparation

Bowel preparation will vary depending on surgeon preference and is typically dictated by concurrent surgery planned. Antibiotics and thromboprophylaxis are given as outlined in Tables 39-6 and 39-8 (p. 835).

INTRAOPERATIVE

Surgical Steps

❶ **Anesthesia and Patient Positioning.** McCall culdoplasty is typically performed under general anesthesia, although epidural or spinal regional methods may also be appropriate in select cases. The patient is placed in standard lithotomy position using candy-cane or booted support stirrups. The vagina is surgically prepared, and a Foley catheter is inserted. Vaginal hysterectomy is completed as described in Section 43-13 (p. 957), but the vaginal cuff is left open for culdoplasty completion. Excess peritoneum or vaginal wall may be excised at this time if indicated.

❷ **Packing.** After vaginal hysterectomy, a moist pack is placed into the posterior cul-de-sac to prevent descent of bowel or omentum.

❸ **Identification of Uterosacral Ligaments and Ureters.** This mirrors that described for the vaginal uterosacral ligament suspension procedure (p. 1107). Briefly, a Deaver retractor displaces the bladder upward, and gentle upward retractor traction exposes the distal to mid-USL portions. Two Allis clamps are next placed at approximately 5 and 7 o'clock positions on the posterior vaginal wall and incorporate the posterior peritoneum. Gentle downward Allis clamp traction tenses the USLs, which are then traced with the contralateral index finger from their distal attachments in the vagina toward the sacrum. Ureters are typically indistinct to touch, but they course anterolateral to the USLs. Lighted Breisky-Navratil retractors are useful on either side to further expose the USLs.

❹ **Suture Placement.** For the internal McCall sutures, we use 2-0 gauge permanent suture with a swaged-on SH needle. For the external McCall sutures, a similar-gauge delayed-absorbable material is selected. The number of suture rows placed is guided by cul-de-sac depth, vaginal cuff width, and surgeon preference. Generally, two to three internal and one to two external rows are placed.

Of the internal sutures, the first suture row is the most distal of these, and each subsequent row is placed progressively cephalad across the posterior cul-de-sac. Each row begins with a stitch into one USL. The needle tip pierces the most medial portion of the left USL and travels in a lateral-to-medial direction. As with other USL suspension procedures, these specifics attempt to minimize ureteral entrapment risks. Moreover, to reduce rectal injury rates, the rectum is retracted to the contralateral side, and suture purchases do not extend too medial, that is, beyond the ligament width. The needle then travels through the cul-de-sac peritoneum or rectal serosa with intervening suture bites and exits through the opposite USL. Each row is spaced approximately 0.5 cm to 1 cm cephalad from the previous one. The internal McCall sutures are tagged, held, and tied only after placement of the external McCall sutures.

Following these internal rows, the first external suture is placed through the full thickness of the posterior vaginal wall and incorporates the posterior peritoneum and USL (Fig. 45-22.1). Progressive left-to-right bites are then taken serially through the rectal serosa to reach the opposite uterosacral ligament (Fig. 45-22.2). Finally, the suture enters the opposite uterosacral ligament, passed through the posterior peritoneum, and exits through the full vaginal wall thickness to reenter the vagina.

❺ **Suture Tying.** The internal sutures are tied first. These sutures are sequentially tied beginning with the most proximal sutures and progressing caudad. The external sutures are then tied, and again the most cephalad of these is tied first.

❻ **Rectal Examination.** The rectum is digitally explored to exclude sutures entering the rectum.

❼ **Cystoscopy.** This is performed after all McCall culdoplasty sutures are tied to document ureteral patency and exclude bladder sutures or cystotomy.

❽ **Vaginal Cuff Closure.** Upon completion of McCall culdoplasty, the remaining steps of vaginal hysterectomy will follow as described in Section 43-13 (p. 961).

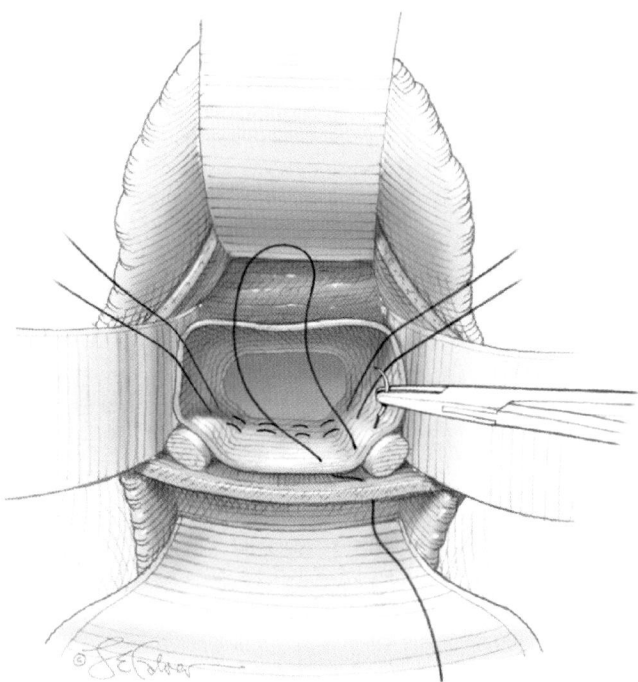

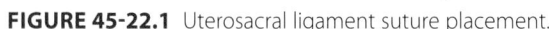

FIGURE 45-22.1 Uterosacral ligament suture placement.

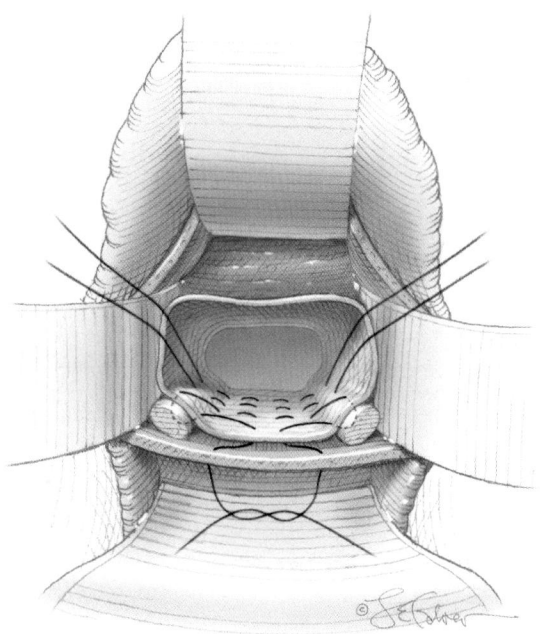

FIGURE 45-22.2 Suture reenters the vagina prior to securing.

POSTOPERATIVE

Following vaginal hysterectomy and McCall culdoplasty, postoperative care mirrors that for vaginal surgery. Activity in general is individualized, although intercourse is usually delayed until 6 weeks. As with other uterosacral ligament suspension procedures, patients are screened for lower extremity neuropathy prior to discharge. Suture erosion with granulation tissue can be a short- or long-term complication and is managed as described on page 1102.

45-23

Abdominal Culdoplasty Procedures

Included in this group are the Moschcowitz and Halban operations. As with other culdoplasty techniques, the goal is posterior cul-de-sac obliteration to prevent enterocele. However, evidence-based studies have not borne out these benefits, and the popularity of culdoplasty has declined. Nevertheless, this procedure is still performed and may have value when completed with other prolapse procedures.

Selection of either the Halban or Moschcowitz procedure is based on surgeon preference and concurrent abdominal or vaginal pathology. Permanent sutures are generally used to close the cul-de-sac, and procedures differ by the orientation of suture placement. No trials have compared these techniques' efficacy head-to-head.

PREOPERATIVE

Patient Evaluation

Culdoplasty is typically performed with other prolapse surgeries. Thus, thorough pelvic organ prolapse evaluation is performed, and all prolapse sites are considered when planning surgical correction. As with other prolapse procedures, patients are evaluated for existing or occult urinary incontinence.

Consent

As with any pelvic reconstructive surgery to correct prolapse, the risk of enterocele recurrence following abdominal culdoplasty is discussed. Additionally, risks of ureteral and bowel injury are included in the consenting process. During Halban and Moschcowitz culdoplasty, the rectosigmoid is plicated to the posterior vaginal wall. Accordingly, defecatory dysfunction and technical difficulty in performing subsequent colonoscopy have been reported following these culdoplasty procedures. Adhesion formation and difficulty with dissection in this space during subsequent operation may also be encountered.

Patient Preparation

Bowel preparation will vary by surgeon preference. Patients can drink only clear liquids the day before surgery and complete one or two enemas the night prior to or the morning of surgery. Alternatively, mechanical bowel preparation, listed in Chapter 39 (p. 835), may be selected. Antibiotics and thromboprophylaxis are given as outlined in Tables 39-6 and 39-8 (p. 835)

INTRAOPERATIVE

Surgical Steps

❶ Anesthesia and Patient Positioning. Abdominal culdoplasty is typically performed under general anesthesia. Patient positioning mirrors that described more fully for ASC on page 1099. Thus, following administration of general anesthesia, the patient is positioned in a low lithotomy position with thighs parallel to the ground and legs in booted support stirrups. The vagina and abdomen are surgically prepared, and a Foley catheter is inserted.

❷ Surgical Incision. Either transverse or vertical incision may be used for culdoplasty. Incision choice is dependent on concurrent surgeries planned. A self-retaining abdominal retractor is placed and concurrent surgeries such as hysterectomy and vault suspension are performed.

❸ Special Considerations. Following completion of initial procedures, the cul-de-sac is exposed and evaluated for suture placement. Additionally, an end-to-end anastomosis (EEA) sizer may be placed within the vagina or rectum to identify borders of the posterior cul-de-sac and allow correct suture placement. Prior to culdoplasty, both ureters are identified again.

In the past, these procedures have focused on suturing peritoneal and serosal surfaces. However, it is currently believed that a more effective approach incorporates deep bites into the muscularis of the vagina and rectosigmoid but avoiding entry into bowel and vaginal lumens. Also, adjacent rectosigmoid veins are protected to avert hematomas from needle sticks. If bleeding develops, direct vascular compression provides effective control in most instances.

❹ Halban Culdoplasty. Several rows of 2-0 gauge permanent sutures are placed longitudinally through the serosa and muscularis of the rectosigmoid (Fig. 45-23.1). Rows are placed approximately 1 cm apart. The same sutures are then advanced through the peritoneum of the deep cul-de-sac and up toward the apex of the posterior vaginal wall. As much of the cul-de-sac as possible is obliterated, but to avoid ureteral injury, sutures are not placed lateral to the uterosacral ligaments.

❺ Moschcowitz Culdoplasty. Concentric 2-0 gauge permanent sutures are placed in the cul-de-sac beginning at the base and are directed upward almost to the level of the vaginal apex (Fig. 45-23.2). During placement, sutures are placed through the posterior vaginal wall and then advanced through the right uterosacral ligament, the rectosigmoid colon muscularis, and finally the left uterosacral

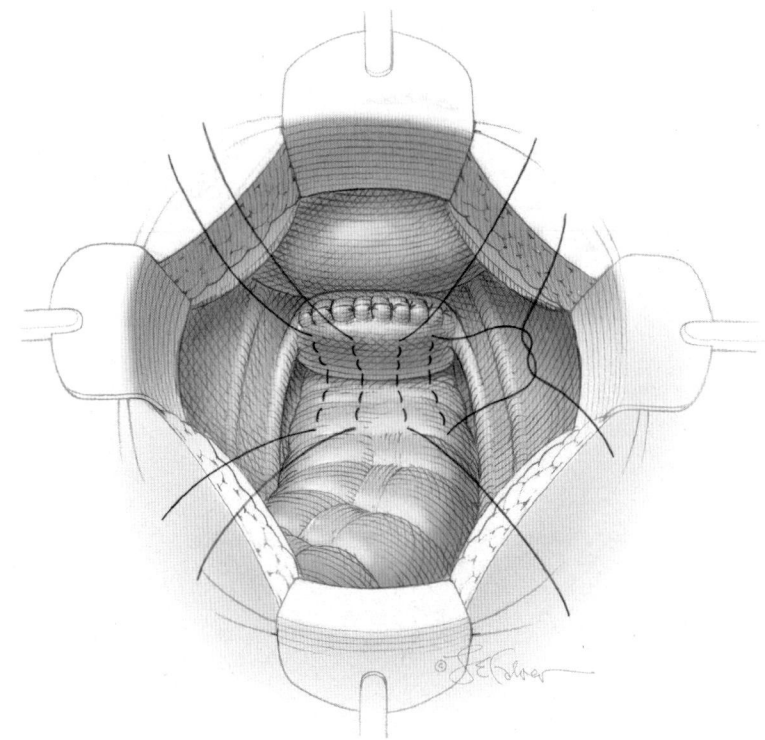

FIGURE 45-23.1 Halban culdoplasty.

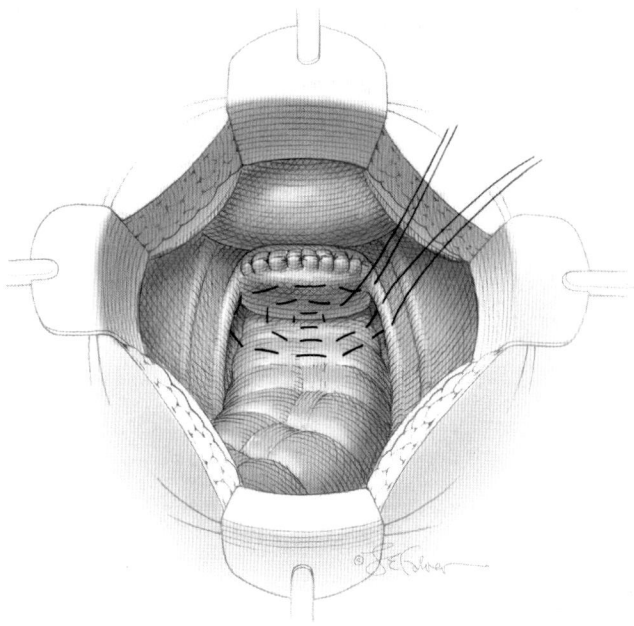

FIGURE 45-23.2 Moschcowitz culdoplasty.

ligament. The number of concentric rings required depends on the cul-de-sac depth, and usually three to four rings are sufficient. Rings are positioned 1 to 2 cm apart. As with the Halban procedure, to reduce ureteral kinking, the lateral extent of the each suture ring should incorporate only the medial width of the uterosacral ligament.

❻ Rectal Examination. This is performed to exclude sutures entering the rectum.

❼ Cystoscopy. Cystoscopy is performed after all culdoplasty sutures are tied to document ureteral patency.

❽ Incision Closure. The abdominal incision is closed as described in Chapter 43 (p. 928).

POSTOPERATIVE

Following culdoplasty, postoperative care follows that for any major abdominal surgery. Hospitalization typically varies from 1 to 3 days, and return of normal bowel function usually dictates this course. Postoperative activity in general can be individualized, although intercourse is usually delayed until 6 weeks.

45-24

Colpocleisis

Pelvic organ prolapse surgery can broadly be grouped as reconstructive or obliterative. Colpocleisis, also known as colpectomy, vaginal extirpation, and vaginectomy, is an obliterative surgery for advanced vaginal or uterovaginal eversion. To correct prolapse, all obliterative procedures close the vaginal canal and thus are only indicated in symptomatic women who do not desire to preserve vaginal anatomy or coital function or who are medically unsuitable for reconstructive surgery. Specifically, this operation may be performed quickly with general, regional, or local anesthesia.

The two main obliterating surgeries are partial colpocleisis and complete colpocleisis. With the partial procedure, also called LeFort colpocleisis, central rectangular sections of vaginal epithelium are dissected from the anterior and posterior vaginal walls, and the denuded fibromuscular layers are apposed and sewn together. This elevates the prolapse back into the pelvic cavity effectively and closes the vagina. The remaining lateral epithelial strips are fashioned into drainage tracts on either side for genital tract fluid egress. Thus, this surgery is appropriate for women with or without a uterus (Fig. 45-24.1).

In contrast, with total or complete colpocleisis, the entire circumference of vaginal epithelium is resected before vaginal walls are approximated. Drainage tracts are lacking, thus, it is typically used for posthysterectomy vault prolapse. If the uterus is present, concurrent total vaginal hysterectomy and closure of the peritoneum and vaginal cuff are performed prior to complete colpocleisis.

Obliterative procedures are effective, and success rates range from 91 to 100 percent (Abassy, 2010; Fitzgerald, 2006; Weber, 2005). However, these rates are interpreted in the context of patients' shorter life expectancies, limited activity levels, and variable outcome definitions. Anatomic success following colpocleisis is likely due to the amount of vaginal tissue sutured together to create a shelf of support. Several studies evaluating symptom improvement have also found high rates of patient satisfaction and functional improvement yet low rates of regret for sexual function loss (Barber, 2007; Fitzgerald, 2008; Gutman, 2009; Hullfish, 2007).

SUI following colpocleisis is common, thus prophylactic antiincontinence surgery is considered. Additionally, high perineorrhaphy (p. 1096) or levator myorrhaphy (p. 1093) is recommended to narrow the genital hiatus and potentially decrease the recurrent prolapse risk. Last, concurrent hysterectomy eliminates the risk of uterine or cervical cancer and of postoperative hemato- or pyometra.

However, patient morbidity, including greater blood loss, increased transfusion risk, and longer procedure time, is increased with hysterectomy. Also, support success rates following colpocleisis are similar whether or not the uterus is removed (Abassy, 2010; Fitzgerald, 2006; Weber, 2005). Thus, hysterectomy is selected based on a woman's general health, surgical goals, and comorbid genital tract disease risks.

PREOPERATIVE

Patient Evaluation

Because access to the cervix and endometrial cavity is not possible following this procedure, preinvasive lesions should be excluded. Specifically, a normal cervical cancer screening result is documented prior to surgery, and evaluation of the endometrium with either endometrial biopsy or sonography is recommended.

The full extent of prolapse should be defined prior to surgery. Importantly, colpocleisis is difficult in women with good distal support of either the anterior or posterior vaginal walls.

Women with advanced prolapse often do not display SUI because the urethra is kinked by prolapsing organs. However, with replacement of the prolapse, many with occult SUI do manifest symptoms. Thus, cough stress test or urodynamic testing has traditionally been performed with the prolapse elevated and replaced to search for occult SUI. Urinalysis and a postvoid residual measurement are also evaluated. For those who demonstrate SUI or occult SUI, antiincontinence surgery is recommended. However, even without SUI, a prophylactic antiincontinence procedure is considered to prevent later de novo SUI. Still, benefits of an additional procedure are weighed against the potential risk of urinary retention. For SUI, midurethral slings or urethral bulking agents are suitable options.

Last, women with global prolapse frequently have some degree of ureteral kinking and obstruction. Thus, preoperative pyelography, CT urography, or renal sonography may be elected to identify or exclude ureteral obstruction. Alternatively, preoperative or intraoperative cystoscopy prior to the colpocleisis can be used to document ureteral patency. Known preexisting obstruction will assist with interpretation of cystoscopy findings performed at the procedure's end. Also, with known ureteral obstruction, preoperative stent placement is considered to potentially assist with ureter identification during surgery. Colpocleisis ideally will unkink the ureter, and this can be documented during intraoperative cystoscopy after prolapse correction.

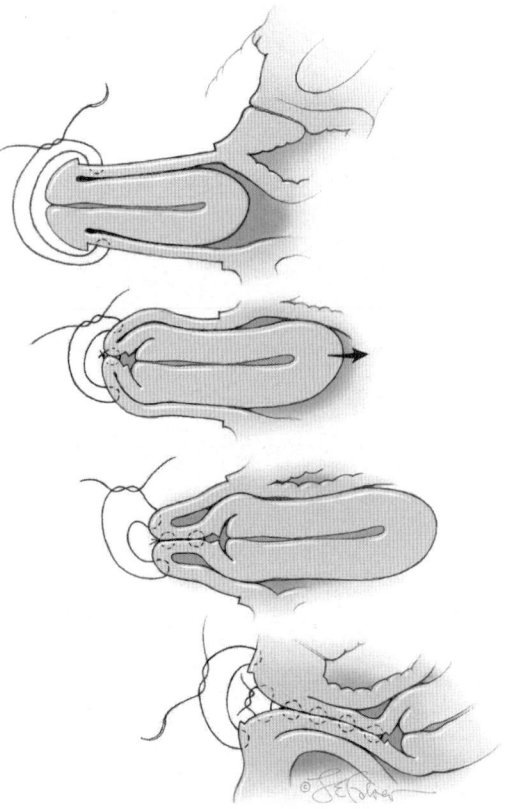

FIGURE 45-24.1 Prolapse correction following placement of serial sutures.

Consent

Women considering this procedure must be fully aware that future vaginal intercourse is not possible. Thus, a patient's partner is ideally included in the decision and consenting process. Patients expressing hesitation or doubt are excluded as candidates.

First, as with any prolapse surgery, prolapse recurrence risk is discussed, although this risk is low with colpocleisis. Of note, later de novo rectal prolapse is disproportionately prevalent, and this unique complication was reported in 4 percent of women in one study (Collins, 2007). Second, as discussed, urinary incontinence may develop postoperatively. In addition, ureteral injury has been described. Third, in the unlikely situation that cervical or uterine malignancy develops after LeFort partial colpocleisis, the diagnosis may be potentially delayed. Finally, postoperative morbidity and mortality are especially pertinent in the elderly, and risks for cardiac, thromboembolic, pulmonary, or cerebrovascular events approximate 5 percent (Fitzgerald, 2006).

Patient Preparation

Bowel preparation, if any, will vary depending on surgeon preference. Patients can be instructed to take only clear liquids the day before surgery and complete one or two enemas the night prior to or the morning of surgery. Alternatively, a mechanical bowel preparation, listed in Chapter 39 (p. 835), may be elected. Antibiotic and thromboprophylaxis are given as outlined in Tables 39-6 and 39-8 (p. 835).

INTRAOPERATIVE

Anesthesia and Patient Positioning

General or regional anesthesia is preferred, although colpocleisis can be performed under local anesthesia. A patient is placed in standard lithotomy position using candy-cane or booted support stirrups, the vagina is surgically prepared, and a Foley catheter is inserted.

Surgical Steps—LeFort Partial Colpocleisis

As noted, LeFort partial colpocleisis may be performed in women with or without a uterus, but the following description outlines steps in women without prior hysterectomy.

❶ Vaginal Marking. Throughout the descriptions of both colpocleisis procedures, *proximal* and *distal* will describe prolapsed anatomy rather than final prolapse-corrected anatomy. To begin, the rectangular areas of vaginal mucosa on the anterior and poste-

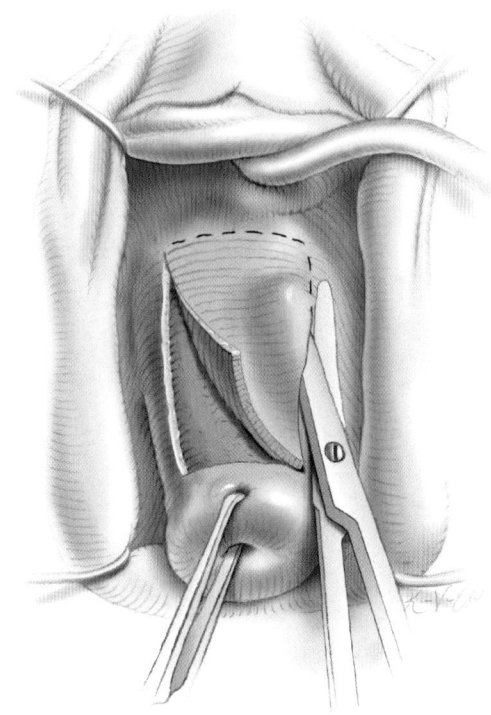

FIGURE 45-24.2 Anterior vaginal wall incision.

rior vaginal walls are outlined with a surgical marker or electrosurgical blade. The size of these areas to be removed is determined by the length and width of vaginal walls. On the anterior wall, the proximal edge of the rectangle extends to within 1 to 2 cm of the bladder neck . On the posterior wall, the proximal rectangle edge extends to within 1 to 3 cm of the posterior hymenal ring. The distal rectangle edges reach to within 1 to 2 cm of the cervicovaginal junction both anteriorly and posteriorly. The lateral edges of each rectangle are drawn to leave approximately 2-cm wide lateral epithelial borders on either side. These will be fashioned into lateral channels of adequate caliber to conduct drainage.

❷ Vaginal Infiltration. The rectangular areas of the vaginal wall to be removed may be thoroughly infiltrated with 50 mL of a dilute hemostatic solution. One example is 20 units of synthetic vasopressin (Pitressin) in 60 mL of saline. This infiltration extends beyond the anticipated incision boundaries. Without infiltration, bleeding can be significant during epithelial excision.

Needle aspiration prior to injection is imperative to avoid intravascular injection of this potent vasoconstrictor. The anesthesiologist is also informed of vasopressin administration, as patient blood pressure may suddenly rise following injection. Blanching at the injection site is common.

Due to the vasoactive effects of vasoconstrictors, patients with certain comorbidities may not be suitable candidates for their

use. These can include a history of angina, myocardial infarction, cardiomyopathy, congestive heart failure, uncontrolled hypertension, migraine, asthma, and severe chronic obstructive pulmonary disease.

❸ Vaginal Dissection. Previously outlined areas are sharply incised down to the fibromuscular layer. If the anterior dissection is performed first, the vaginal wall epithelium within the previously marked anterior rectangle is dissected off the underlying vaginal wall fibromuscular layer using both sharp and blunt dissection (Fig. 45-24.2). Dissection in the correct plane will prevent inadvertent bladder or bowel entry. One effective technique places a finger behind the vaginal wall, while cephalad dissection with Metzenbaum scissors advances parallel to the vaginal wall epithelium. Bleeding during dissection can generally be controlled with pressure and electrosurgical coagulation. Occasionally, figure-of-eight stitches of 2-0 gauge absorbable suture are needed if large venous sinuses are cut. Next, the vaginal wall epithelium within the previously marked posterior rectangle is similarly dissected off the fibromuscular layer on the posterior vaginal wall (Fig. 45-24.3). Of note, some prefer to dissect posteriorly first to avoid obscuring blood from the anterior wall that may ooze into the surgical field.

❹ Apical and Lateral Channels. After these rectangles are removed, a row of interrupted stitches using 2-0 gauge delayed-absorbable suture are placed through the

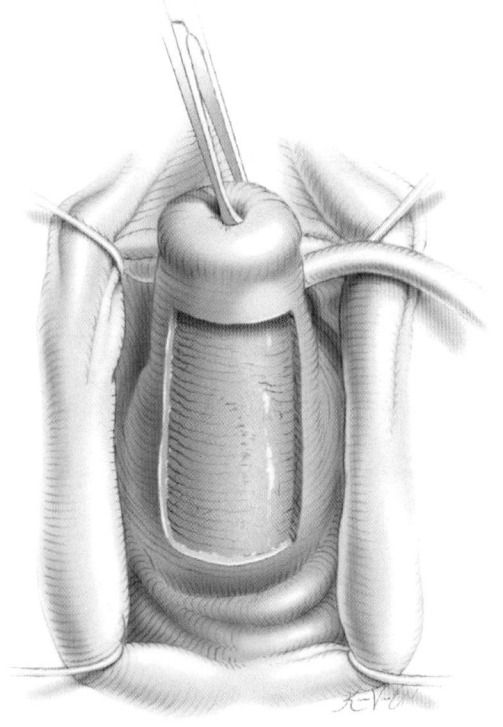

FIGURE 45-24.3 Posterior vaginal wall incision.

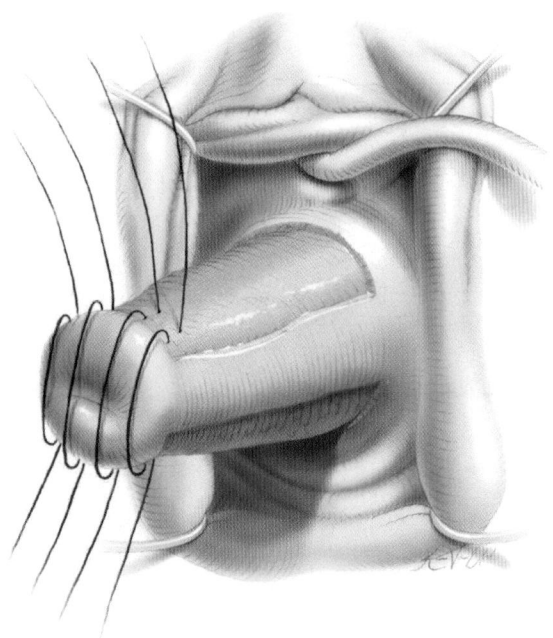

FIGURE 45-24.4 Initial suture placement.

anterior and posterior distal transverse epithelial edges (Fig. 45-24.4). These will effectively close the fibromuscular layer over the cervix and create the apical channel. Next, lateral channels on each side are formed and connect with this apical channel. For this, the lateral anterior and posterior epithelial edges are approximated along their full length (Fig. 45-24.5). This lateral row of

sutures begins distally and progresses proximally to the original proximal transverse incision near the bladder neck. The lateral channels can be created in a stepwise fashion, alternating from one side to the other.

❺ **Anterior-to-Posterior Vaginal Wall Approximation.** With the lateral canals now fashioned, the uterus can be sequentially

elevated into the pelvic cavity. For this, a surgeon places progressive rows of interrupted 2-0 gauge permanent or delayed-absorbable sutures that approximate the anterior and posterior fibromuscular layers along the distal prolapsed-tube width (Fig. 45-24.6). Successive transverse tiers of sutures are placed approximately 1 cm apart until the proximal transverse incision is reached (Fig. 45-24.7). These rows create a tissue septum that elevates and supports the uterus (see Fig. 45-24.1).

❻ **Cystoscopy.** With either colpocleisis procedure, cystoscopy is performed to exclude urinary tract injury and document ureteral patency.

❼ **Closure of the Vaginal Epithelium.** This layer is then reapproximated in a running fashion with 2-0 or 3-0 gauge delayed-absorbable suture (Fig. 45-24.8). Importantly, the ostia of the bilateral drainage tracts remain patent.

❽ **Concurrent Surgery.** At this point, an antiincontinence procedure may be completed as needed. Perineorrhaphy may be performed before or after vaginal wall closure (p. 1096).

Surgical Steps—Complete Colpocleisis

❶ **Vaginal Infiltration.** The vaginal cuff is placed on traction, and a vasoconstrictive agent may be injected in a similar fashion

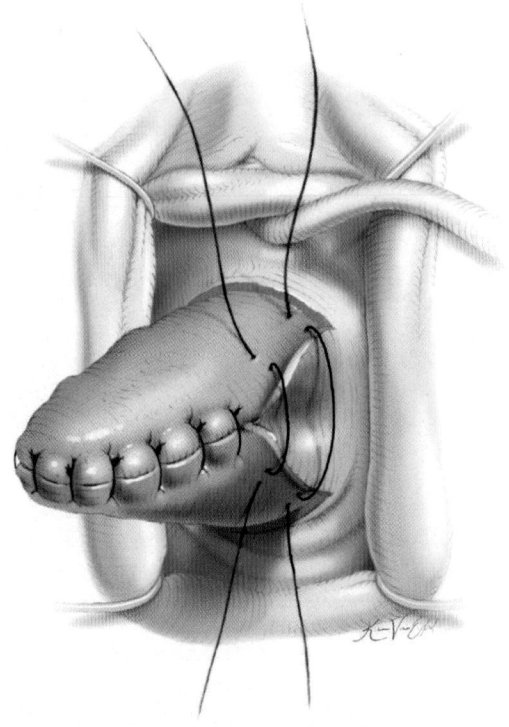

FIGURE 45-24.5 Creation of lateral drainage canals.

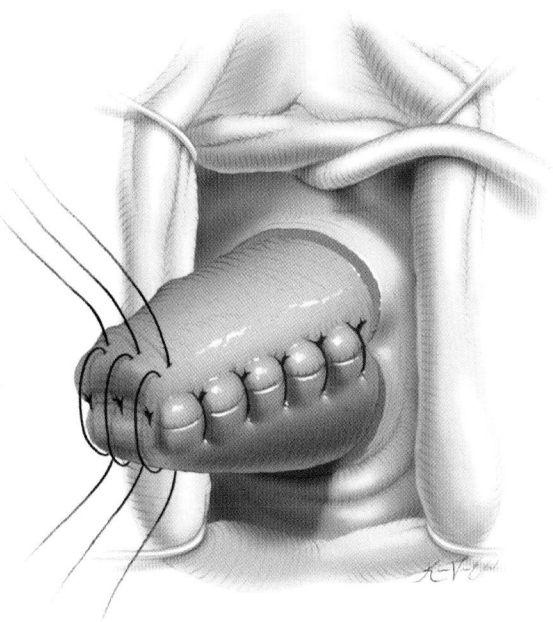

FIGURE 45-24.6 Second row of sutures.

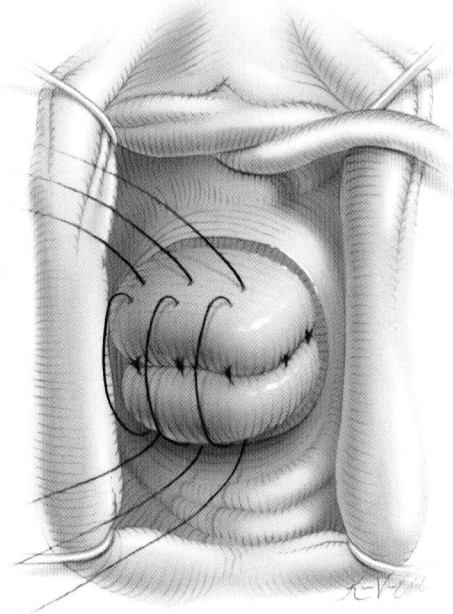

FIGURE 45-24.7 Subsequent row of sutures.

to that described for the LeFort partial colpocleisis.

❷ **Vaginal Incision and Dissection.** To begin, the borders of planned dissection are marked circumferentially with a pen or electrosurgical blade. When redundant tissue is present, marking three to four smaller rectangles over the entire prolapsed vaginal tube helps maintain orientation during dissection.

First, the vaginal epithelium is incised anteriorly at a point 1 to 2 cm distal to the bladder neck. Ultimately, this will be a point that lies approximately 1 cm proximal to the neck. Incision placement here will prevent

downward displacement of the bladder neck and the proximal urethra during apposition of the anterior and posterior vaginal walls. Additionally, it will allow room for the midurethral sling if one is planned. As the incision is swept circumferentially around the prolapse tube, a 1- to 2-cm distance is maintained distal to the hymeneal ring.

The vaginal epithelium is sharply and bluntly dissected off the underlying

fibromuscular layer (Figs. 45-24.9 and 45-24.10). Dissection is kept close to the epithelium to avoid inadvertent bladder or rectal entry. Once the desired plane is identified, sharp and blunt dissection can proceed quickly until the entire vaginal epithelium is removed. One technique for sharp dissection involves positioning a finger behind the vaginal wall and dissecting with Metzenbaum scissors parallel to the vaginal wall and close

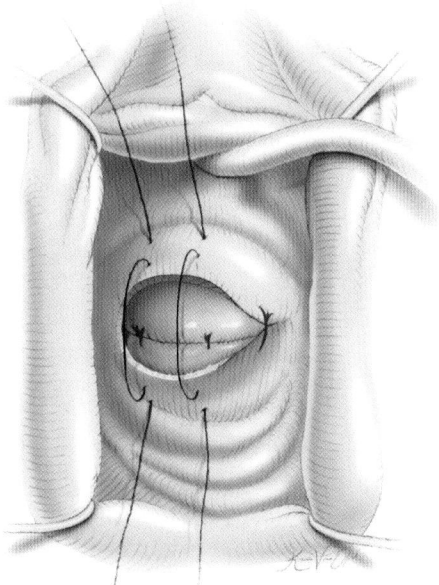

FIGURE 45-24.8 Vaginal mucosa closure.

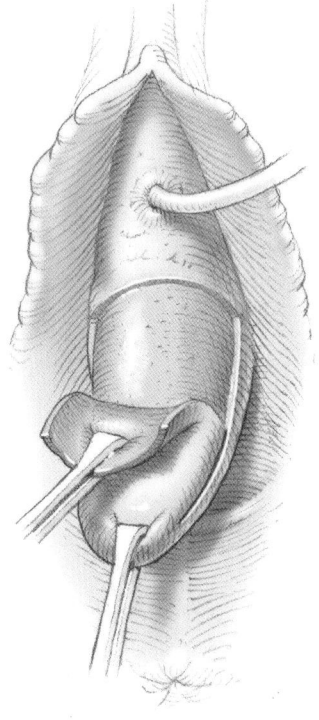

FIGURE 45-24.9 Anterior vaginal wall incision.

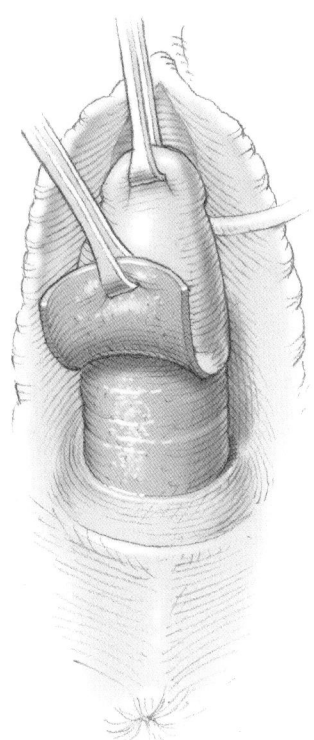

FIGURE 45-24.10 Posterior vaginal wall incision.

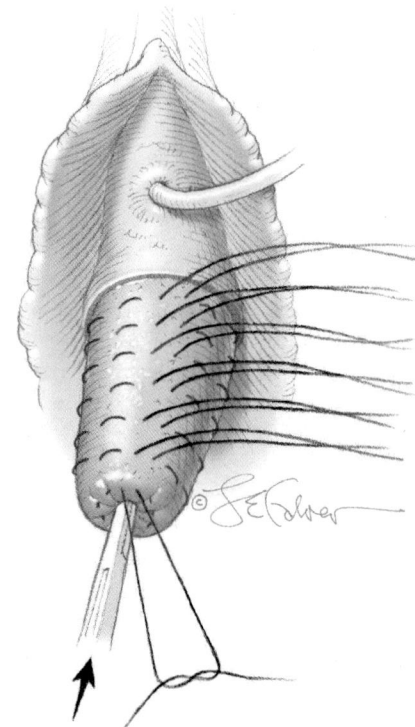

FIGURE 45-24.11 Circumferential suturing.

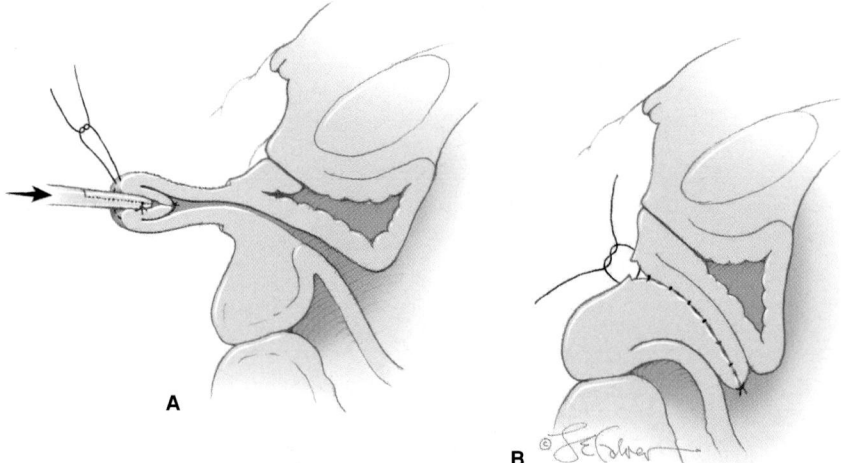

FIGURE 45-24.12 A. Cephalad pressure against telescoping vaginal tube as serial sutures are secured. **B.** Completely inverted vaginal tube.

to the epithelium. After entry into the correct plane, blunt dissection with a gauze-covered index finger may allow rapid and wide development of this avascular space. There are areas where dissection may be difficult. For example, upon reaching the prolapsed vaginal apex and uterosacral ligament remnants, extensive scarring may be present that requires sharp dissection. The entire vaginal epithelium is removed from the prolapsed vaginal tube.

❸ **Suture Placement.** To plicate the vaginal walls together and elevate the everted vagina, a surgeon places a series of circumferential purse-string sutures around the vaginal tube. With 2-0 gauge permanent or delayed-absorbable suture, stitches incorporate the

fibromuscular layer but avoid deep penetration into the bladder, ureter, or rectum (Fig. 45-24.11).

The first purse-string suture is placed approximately 1 cm from the cuff, and tied while the cuff is inverted with atraumatic forceps or a hemostat (Fig. 45-24.12). The cut suture tails are held with a clamp and the second suture is placed 1 cm proximally. The hemostat tip inverts the vagina while the second suture is tied, and used again to tag the second suture. Progressive purse-string sutures are placed similarly 1 cm apart until the proximal edge of cut vaginal epithelium is reached. These serial steps telescope the prolapsed vaginal tube cephalad and toward the pelvic cavity. Depending on the size of the prolapse, approximately six to eight suture rings are needed to completely invert the prolapsed vaginal tube.

❹ **Finishing Steps.** Final steps are similar with both colpocleisis procedures. First, cystoscopy is performed to exclude urinary tract injury and document ureteral patency. The vaginal epithelium is then reapproximated in a running fashion with 2-0 or 3-0 gauge

delayed-absorbable suture. At this point, an antiincontinence procedure may be performed. Perineorrhaphy may be performed before or after vaginal wall closure (p. 1096).

POSTOPERATIVE

Hospital admission is often prudent given the usual older age and comorbidities of these patients. A normal diet can be given immediately. Oral analgesics are usually sufficient. A voiding trial is performed prior to discharge as all patients can experience urinary retention from a levator myorrhaphy or perineorrhaphy. Patients with urinary retention can return within a week for a subsequent voiding trial and catheter removal.

In general, recovery with colpocleisis is quick and typically without complication. Postoperative bleeding is not anticipated, save for spotting from the surgical site. As with any prolapse procedure, constipation is avoided to protect repair strength during healing. Thus, stool softeners are recommended. Resumption of normal activities is encouraged with the exception of heavy lifting for several months.

45-25

Anal Sphincteroplasty

External anal sphincter (EAS) and/or internal anal sphincter (IAS) repair is most commonly performed in patients with acquired fecal incontinence (FI) and an anterior sphincter defect. One of two methods may be selected for sphincter repair and include an end-to-end technique or an overlapping method. The end-to-end technique is most often used by obstetricians at delivery to reapproximate torn anal sphincter ends. However, in women remote from delivery, the overlapping technique is often selected, and with this, disrupted ends are overlapped and then sutured.

In cases remote from delivery, the overlapping method is preferred. However, the optimal technique or suture material for repair and the effects of pudendal neuropathy on treatment outcome are not well known (Madoff, 2004). With the overlapping method, short-term continence rates up to 85 percent were previously reported (Fleshman, 1991; Sitzler, 1996). However, newer reports show significant deterioration of FI during long-term postoperative surveillance (Bravo Gutierrez, 2004; Zutshi, 2009).

In cases at delivery, no evidence shows that either method yields superior results (Fitzpatrick, 2000; Garcia, 2005). Moreover, overlapping repair requires increased technical skills and carries the potential for increased blood loss, operating time, and pudendal neuropathy. Accordingly, the end-to-end technique is likely to remain the standard method for sphincter reapproximation at delivery until further data from randomized controlled trials are available.

PREOPERATIVE

Patient Evaluation

Because the etiology of FI in patients with documented sphincter defects may be multifactorial, careful preoperative evaluation attempts to distinguish underlying sources. Evaluation for structural gastrointestinal (GI) tract pathology typically involves colonoscopy and/or barium enema. Additionally, radiographic bowel transit studies can be used to diagnose slow transit time, which may be related to defecatory dysfunction.

Specific to the anorectum, endoanal sonography can accurately define structural disruption of the EAS and IAS (Fig. 25-7, p. 568) and is generally performed prior to sphincter repair. Exceptions are cloacal-like defects or chronic fourth-degree lacerations.

In these, the absent anterior portion of the sphincter(s) is easily identified clinically.

Anal manometry and pudendal nerve conduction studies may identify physiologic dysfunction such as neuropathy. Although these tests provide additional information and can be used during counseling, they are not necessary in patients with FI and a documented sphincter defect. In fact, the relationship of pudendal nerve function, typically assessed by determining pudendal nerve terminal motor latency, to sphincteroplasty outcome remains controversial (Madoff, 2004). One study found no association between pudendal nerve status and long-term anal continence (Malouf, 2000).

Clinicians have attempted to improve success rates by selecting only those women who may benefit most from surgery. Patient age, preoperative anal manometry readings, and pudendal nerve motor function have been evaluated as possible outcome predictors. However, research findings are conflicting, and none of these consistently predicts outcome (Bravo Gutierrez, 2004; Buie, 2001; El-Gazzaz, 2012; Gearhart, 2005).

Consent

Although many women may have improved FI immediately following anal sphincteroplasty, repair durability is poor. For example, 3 to 5 years following correction, only approximately 10 percent of women are fully continent of solid and liquid stool (Halverson, 2002; Malouf, 2000). Retrospective data show that no patients are continent 10 years following sphincteroplasty (Zutshi, 2009). However, despite FI based on validated questionnaires, the quality of life in these patients notably did not decline.

Reasons for worsening continence following initial improvement remain unknown but may include aging, scarring, and progressive pudendal neuropathy either from initial injury or from the sphincter repair (Madoff, 2004). In addition, skeletal muscle repair is thought to have poor success because resting muscle tone places incision lines on constant tension. Thus, preoperative counseling informs that most individuals will improve after the procedure, but continence is rarely perfect and deteriorates over time.

In addition to persistent FI, sphincteroplasty is associated with other surgical risks. More common serious complications are wound dehiscence and fistula formation. Ha and coworkers (2001) noted a wound complication in 12 percent and fistula formation in 4 percent. Dyspareunia is a risk, especially if levator myorrhaphy (p. 1093) is concomitantly performed in sexually active women. Moreover, we believe levator myorrhaphy is

a nonanatomic repair and do not perform it with sphincteroplasty.

Patient Preparation

Because of the high associated risk of wound complications, antibiotic prophylaxis is warranted to minimize wound infection following surgical contamination from vaginal and rectal flora. We use a combination of ciprofloxacin and metronidazole to obtain broad bacterial coverage. Additionally, we often continue this same antibiotic coverage orally for approximately 7 days postoperatively to help reduce wound complications (Maldonado, 2014). Although benefits from mechanical bowel preparation have not been demonstrated, some form of bowel preparation is typically administered the day or night before surgery. Options are listed in Chapter 39 (p. 835). Thromboprophylaxis is also provided as outlined in Table 39-8 (p. 835).

INTRAOPERATIVE

Surgical Steps

❶ **Anesthesia and Patient Positioning.** After administration of either general or regional anesthesia, a woman is placed in standard lithotomy position using candy-cane or booted support stirrups. The vagina and perineum are surgically prepared and draped, and a Foley catheter is inserted.

❷ **Incision and Dissection.** A downward-arching curvilinear incision is placed between the fourchette and anus, and this connects with a midline posterior vaginal wall incision (Fig. 45-25.1). The vaginal incision edges are placed on tension with Allis clamps. Along the distal 3 to 4 cm of the posterior vaginal wall, the vaginal epithelium is then sharply dissected off its underlying fibromuscular layer and off the perineal body.

On the perineum, dissection continues distally and laterally with Metzenbaum scissors. Advancement is kept just deep to the perianal skin and progresses until the scarred and usually retracted edges of the EAS are identified within the ischioanal fossa. Dissection proceeds until the EAS muscle is sufficiently mobile to ensure a tension-free overlapping repair.

As the inner arch of the EAS is sharply separated from the anal submucosa, care is taken to avoid anal lumen entry. To assist, a surgeon's index finger within the anus can guide dissection depth, and concomitant upward traction by an assistant on the sphincter's scarred ends helps accentuate the best dissection plane. Internal pudendal vessel branches

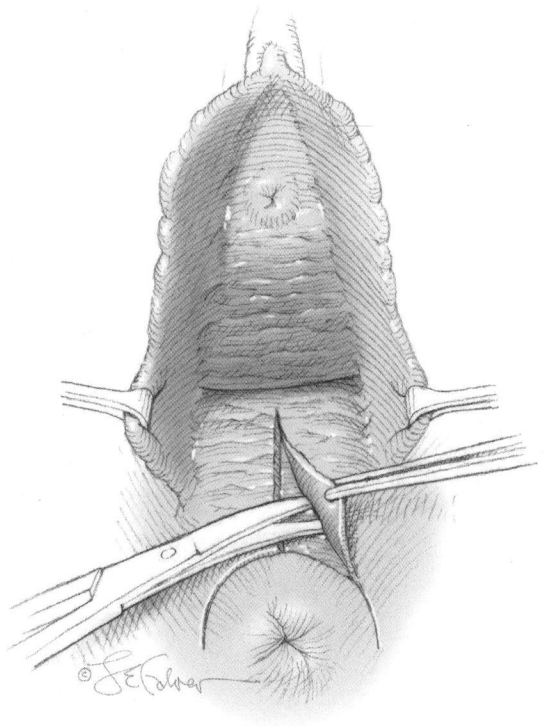

FIGURE 45-25.1 Vaginal dissection.

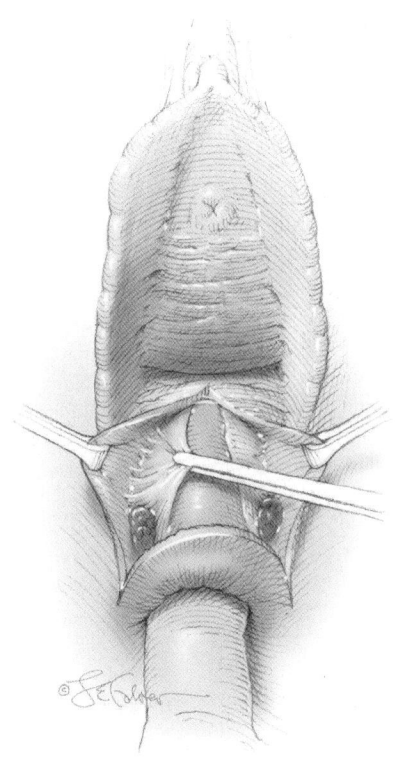

FIGURE 45-25.2 Internal anal sphincter identification.

can be lacerated or inferior rectal nerve injured, especially if lateral dissection extends beyond the 3 and 9 o'clock positions. Thus, if extensive lateral dissection is anticipated, the end-to-end method of repair is preferred.

Scarring in the midline may be cut but is not excised. This fibrous tissue adds strength to the sphincter muscle approximation. However, with extensive scarring, sphincter muscle fibers may be difficult to isolate. A nerve stimulator or a needle tip electrosurgical blade can assist in delineating these fibers. Current will often contract them.

❸ **Suture Placement within the Internal Anal Sphincter.** The IAS contributes significantly to the anal canal resting tone, and its reapproximation is included in the repair. Grasped in Figure 45-25.2, the IAS is a smooth, rubbery, thickened white sheet lying deep to the EAS and superficial to the anal mucosa and submucosal layers. This muscle usually retracts laterally when severed.

For suturing, we prefer monofilament, delayed-absorbable suture. First, because both the IAS and EAS muscles are under constant contraction, direct tissue reapproximation by these longer-acting sutures in theory allows adequate scar formation during the critical first 3 months of postoperative healing. Second, use of permanent suture for sphincteroplasty has been associated with high rates of suture erosion and wound dehiscence (Luck, 2005).

With suturing, the disrupted IAS edges are approximated in a continuous or interrupted fashion using 3-0 or 2-0 gauge monofilament, delayed-absorbable sutures such as polydioxanone PDS II (Fig. 45-25.3). Sutures are spaced approximately 0.5 cm apart. As the distal extent of the IAS is generally several millimeters cephalad to the distal extent of the EAS, reapproximation of the IAS ends above the anal verge. Suture placement and

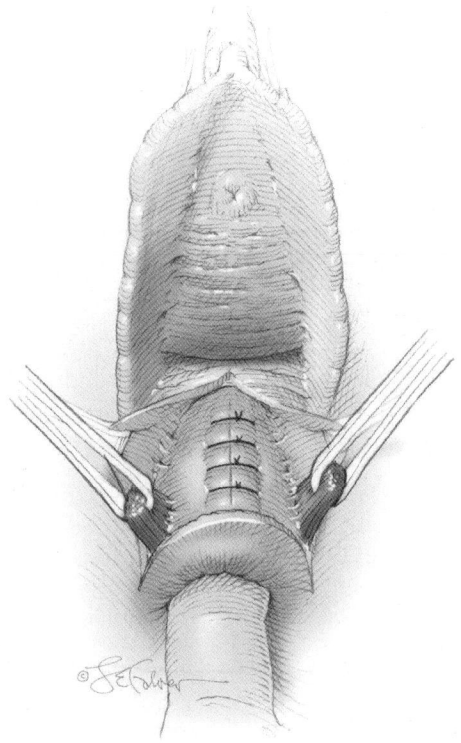

FIGURE 45-25.3 Following internal anal sphincter reapproximation, the external anal sphincter is identified and grasped.

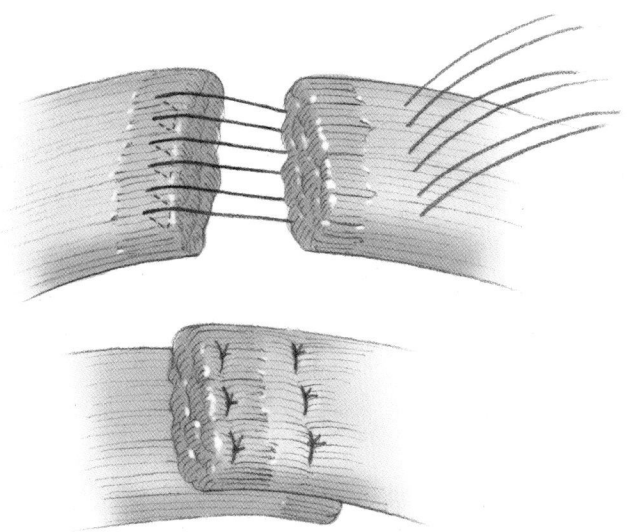

FIGURE 45-25.4 Overlapping sphincteroplasty.

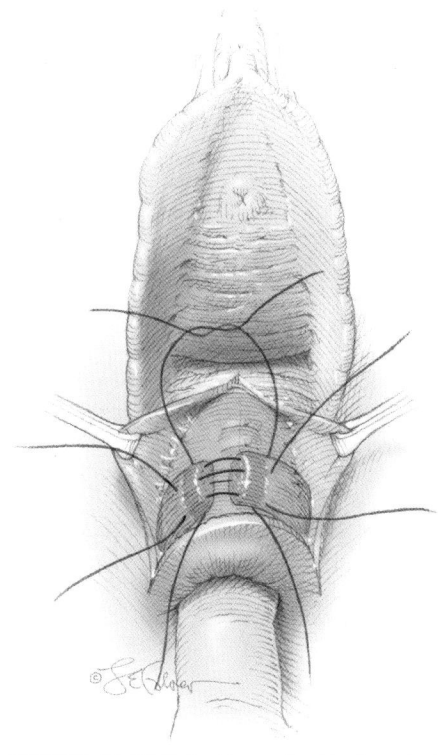

FIGURE 45-25.5 End-to-end sphincteroplasty.

exposure of the IAS is aided by a finger in the rectum.

In many cases when an IAS defect is diagnosed remote from delivery, both the IAS and the EAS are usually identified as a unit. This unit is repaired en-bloc as described next.

❹ **Overlapping External Anal Sphincteroplasty.** The overlapping repair of the EAS or EAS/IAS muscle unit is accomplished by placing two rows of mattress stitches using 2-0 or 3-0 gauge monofilament, delayed-absorbable suture. Within each row, the first stitch is the most cephalad, and more caudal stitches are added sequentially. The first row of mattress sutures begins at a distance (1 to 1.5 cm) from the severed edge of the overlying muscle. These then travel through the distal end of the underlying muscle (Fig. 45-25.4). A final upward pass again through the overlying muscle completes the stitch. To aid viewing, the suture ends in this row are held until the second suture row is placed. The second row of stitches then traverses through and through to secure the free end of the overlying muscle to the underlying muscle.

With the overlapping method, either the right or left dissected end of the muscle can be used as the overlying muscle based on intraoperative findings. If significant mobilization cannot be achieved due to scarring or missing sphincter, then an end-to-end repair is performed.

❺ **End-to-End External Anal Sphincteroplasty.** When performed for FI remote from delivery, each end of the disrupted EAS and surrounding scar tissue is identified and grasped with an Allis clamp (see Fig. 45-25.3). The ends of the EAS and its surrounding fibrous tissue are brought to the midline and reapproximated using three to four interrupted stitches of delayed-absorbable, monofilament suture (Fig. 45-25.5).

❻ **Perineal Body Reconstruction.** Patients with anal sphincter defects often have a deficient perineal body. In these cases, perineal body reconstruction is performed following reapproximation of the IAS and EAS muscles. This mirrors Step 4 of perineorrhaphy in Section 45-16 (p. 1096). For this, the connective tissue surrounding the separated ends of the bulbospongiosus and superficial transverse perineal muscles are identified and reapproximated. A combination of 2-0 and 0-gauge absorbable sutures is used for this repair. Deep suture bites at the level of the hymen also reunite the perineal membrane, which attaches to both the vaginal walls and the perineal body at the level of the hymen.

❼ **Incision Closure.** Excision of excess perineal skin and/or vaginal epithelium may be required prior to closing the incision. Vaginal epithelium and then perineal skin is reapproximated in a running or interrupted fashion using 2-0 or 3-0 gauge absorbable suture, again similar to perineorrhaphy.

POSTOPERATIVE

Pain varies postoperatively, and some women can be discharged home on postoperative day 2, whereas others require longer hospitalization. The Foley catheter is removed on postoperative day 1 or 2. An active voiding trial is performed, and some women may have difficulty voiding due to pain, inflammation, and levator ani muscle spasm. To limit trauma to the healing repair, we try to delay defecation for several days. Although data are lacking, we encourage patients to forego food and drink on day 1. They are subsequently advanced to clear liquids for 3 or 4 days. Stool softeners are given when a solid diet is begun and are continued for at least 6 weeks. Diet or agents that add bulk to the stool are discouraged as this may increase the repair breakdown risk. Local wound care involves perineal cleansing with a plastic water bottle following urination or defecation. Ambulation is encouraged, but physical exercise and sexual intercourse are delayed for 8 weeks. The first postoperative visit is typically 4 weeks following surgery.

45-26

Rectovaginal Fistula Repair

In general, rectovaginal fistulas (RVFs) encountered by gynecologists are those complicating obstetric events and develop in the distal third of the vagina just above the hymen. Surgical management of these "low" RVFs varies by the condition of the external anal sphincter (EAS) but is usually achieved by a transvaginal or transanal approach. Midlevel RVFs are found in the middle third of the vagina and are also usually due to obstetric trauma. These can often be repaired transvaginally or transanally by a tension-free layered closure. High RVFs may follow hysterectomy or radiation therapy and lie close to the cervix or the vaginal cuff, and these are most commonly repaired abdominally.

Fistulas identified during or shortly after delivery are suitable for immediate repair. However, fistulas are not repaired in the setting of inflammation, induration, or infection. Moreover, fistulas that are associated with radiation therapy and recurrent fistula, due to poor tissue vascularity, often require interposition of a vascular flap.

Outcomes vary depending on the underlying cause and repair method. Success rates following obstetric injury repair range from 78 to 100 percent (Khanduja, 1999; Tsang, 1998). However, in cases with episioproctotomy, the reported success rate is 74 percent, and in those repaired by rectal advancement flap, rates reach only 40 to 50 percent (Mizrahi, 2002; Sonoda, 2002). Fistulas from radiation, cancer, or active inflammatory bowel disease are more difficult to treat successfully. In general, success rates are highest with the first surgical attempt at repair (Lowry, 1988).

PREOPERATIVE

Patient Evaluation

As outlined in Chapter 25 (p. 574), a thorough evaluation is necessary to assess the etiology and delineate the full extent of a fistula. Unless RVFs are obviously from a prior obstetric event, fistulous tract biopsy is indicated to exclude malignancy or inflammatory conditions. Proctoscopy or colonoscopy is warranted if inflammatory bowel disease, malignancy, or gastrointestinal infection is suspected. If there are questions regarding the etiology, complexity, or number of fistulas, then imaging may be needed. At times, pinpoint fistulas are difficult to identify and may require examination under anesthesia with lacrimal duct probing. Coexisting anal incontinence is assessed, as this may be related to sphincter damage or other etiologies and is likely to persist after fistula repair.

Consent

Specific risks following rectovaginal fistula repair include fistula recurrence, dyspareunia, and vaginal narrowing or shortening. Fecal incontinence can follow some repairs if the anal sphincter is disrupted during surgery, as with episioproctotomy, or if coexistent sphincter defects are not recognized and repaired.

Patient Preparation

A rigorous bowel preparation is preferred to clear all stool from the rectal vault. Accordingly, a mechanical bowel preparation is advised the day prior to surgery, and options are listed in Chapter 39 (p. 835). If stool is still present in the rectum at the beginning of surgery, then a povidone-iodine (Betadine) flush with a Malecot drain may be needed. Antibiotic prophylaxis is given concurrent with surgery, however, additional doses during the days before surgery are not indicated. We use a combination of ciprofloxacin and metronidazole to obtain broad bacterial coverage. Additionally, thromboprophylaxis is provided as outlined in Table 39-8 (p. 836).

INTRAOPERATIVE

Surgical Steps

❶ **Anesthesia and Patient Position.** Rectovaginal fistula repair is typically an inpatient procedure, performed under general or regional anesthesia. A patient is placed in standard lithotomy position in candy-cane or booted support stirrups. The vagina is surgically prepared, and a Foley catheter is inserted.

❷ **Fistula Identification.** The fistula is identified and its course is traced with a probe or dilator. Small fistulas may be dilated to improve identification of the tract.

❸ **Vaginal Incision.** For a midlevel or low RVF not involving the external anal sphincter, a circular incision is made in the vaginal epithelium surrounding the fistula (Fig. 45-26.1). The incision is made sufficiently wide to permit tract excision and generous mobilization of surrounding tissues for closure without excess suture-line tension (Fig. 45-26.2). Remember that tenets of proper fistula repair emphasize tension-free, multilayered closure, and excellent hemostasis. The entire fistula tract is then excised (Fig. 45-26.3). This creates an anal or rectal opening that is often significantly larger than that found preoperatively.

❹ **Closure of the Rectal Wall.** Using 3-0 gauge delayed-absorbable suture, the edges of the anal mucosal defect are reapproximated

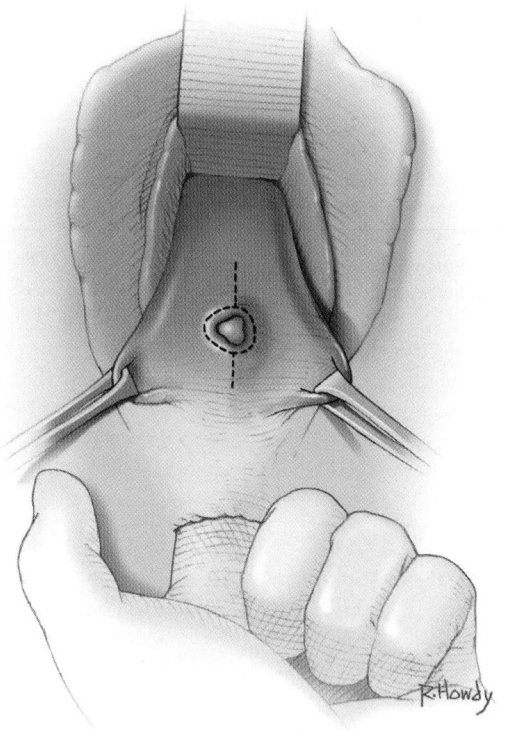

FIGURE 45-26.1 Vaginal incision.

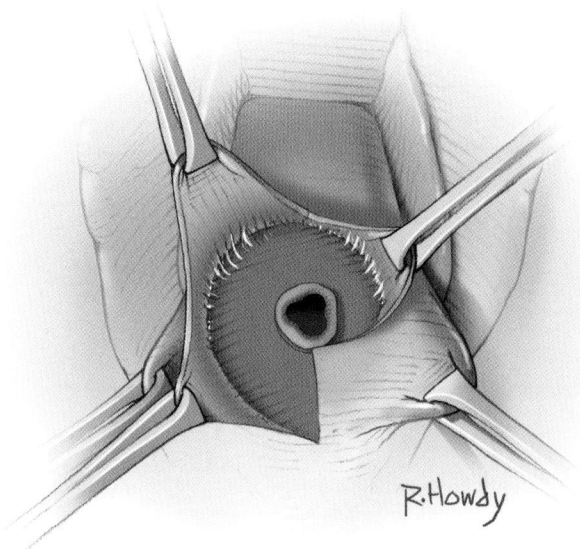

FIGURE 45-26.2 Mobilization of surrounding vaginal mucosa.

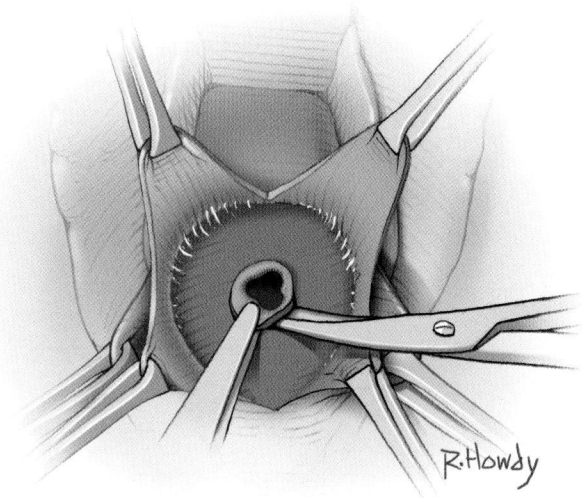

FIGURE 45-26.3 Fistulous tract excision.

in a running or interrupted fashion. Each bite or suture is spaced no more than 5 mm apart (Fig. 45-26.4). Although absorbable sutures can be placed into the rectal lumen, we prefer to reapproximate the submucosal tissue without needle or suture entering the rectum. One or two additional layers of the same gauge suture are placed in the anal or rectal wall muscularis to reinforce the submucosal closure. If the internal anal sphincter (IAS) but not the EAS is involved, the above additional layers incorporate the torn IAS edges.

This step ideally reduces the postoperative anal incontinence risk.

Alternatively, with very small RVFs, a purse-string suture can be placed to encircle the anal defect, and its perimeter lies a few millimeters from the resected fistulous tract rim. This suture is tied and inverts the defect's edges into the bowel lumen. Additional reinforcing layers are then placed as described above.

❺ **Closure of the Vaginal Fibromuscular Layer.** The fibromuscular layer of the vagina

is next reapproximated with 2-0 gauge delayed-absorbable sutures in a running or interrupted fashion (Fig. 45-26.5). If possible, two layers are completed to minimize incision tension and reinforce the repair. With anovaginal fistulas, these additional layers also reapproximate perineal body tissue.

If the fistula involves the EAS, an episioproctotomy—that is, conversion of the defect into a fourth-degree laceration—can be elected. Following excision of the fistulous tract and mobilization of surrounding tissue, repair of the episioproctotomy is similar to the layered repair of an obstetric fourth-degree laceration. Briefly, the anal submucosa is reapproximated with 3-0 gauge

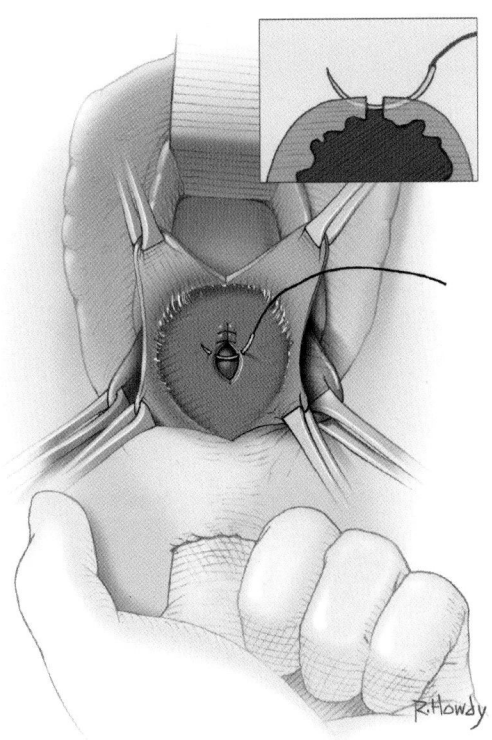

FIGURE 45-26.4 Closure of the rectal wall.

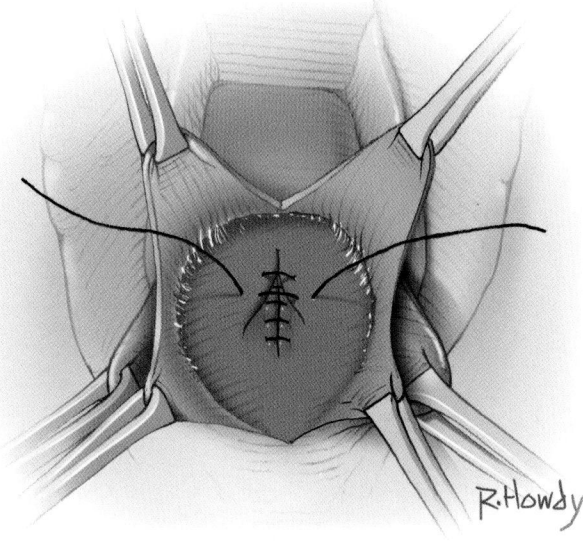

FIGURE 45-26.5 Closure of the fibromuscular layer.

absorbable suture in a running or interrupted fashion. Repair of the IAS, EAS, and perineal body reconstruction mirror that for anal sphincteroplasty (p. 1125).

⑥ Martius Bulbocavernosus Fat Pad Graft. In cases in which avascular or fibrotic tissue is extensive, a Martius graft may be placed between the fibromuscular layer and vaginal epithelium (p. 1083).

⑦ Vaginal Wall Closure. Excess vaginal mucosa is trimmed, and the vaginal mucosa is closed in a continuous running fashion using 3-0 gauge absorbable or delayed-absorbable suture.

POSTOPERATIVE

Normal activity can resume during the first postoperative days. Intercourse, however, is delayed at least 6 weeks or until the vaginal incision is healed. To limit trauma to the healing repair, dietary modifications are instituted similar to those for sphincteroplasty (p. 1127).

REFERENCES

Abassy S, Kenton K: Obliterative procedures for pelvic organ prolapse. Clin Obstet Gynecol 53: 86, 2010

Abernathy M, Vasquez E, Kenton K, et al: Where do we place the sacrocolpopexy stitch: an MRI investigation. Female Pelvic Med Reconstr Surg 18:s74, 2012

Albo ME, Richter HE, Brubaker L, et al: Burch colposuspension versus fascial sling to reduce urinary stress incontinence. N Engl J Med 356:2143, 2007

Alcalay M, Monga A, Stanton SL: Burch colposuspension: a 10–20 year follow up. BJOG 102: 740, 1995

Altman D, Väyrynen T, Engh ME, et al: Anterior colporrhaphy versus transvaginal mesh for pelvic-organ prolapse. N Engl J Med 364(19): 1826, 2011

American College of Obstetricians and Gynecologists: Antibiotic prophylaxis for gynecologic procedures. Practice Bulletin No. 104, May 2009, Reaffirmed 2014

American College of Obstetricians and Gynecologists: Vaginal placement of synthetic mesh for pelvic organ prolapse. Committee Opinion No. 513, December 2011

American Urogynecologic Society: Indigo carmine shortage. AUGS Guidelines Development Committee, Washington, 2014a

American Urogynecologic Society: Position Statement on Restriction of Surgical Options for Pelvic Floor Disorders. Washington, 2013

American Urogynecologic Society; Society of Urodynamics, Female Pelvic Medicine and Urogenital Reconstruction: Position statement on mesh midurethral slings for stress urinary incontinence. Washington, 2014b

Anger JT, Mueller ER, Tarnay C, et al: Robotic compared with laparoscopic sacrocolpopexy: a randomized controlled trial. Obstet Gynecol 123(1):5, 2014

Ankardal M, Ekerydh A, Crafoord K, et al: A randomised trial comparing open Burch colposuspension using sutures with laparoscopic colposuspension using mesh and staples in women with stress urinary incontinence. BJOG 111:974, 2004

Antosh DD, Gutman RE: Diagnosis and management of female urethral diverticulum. Female Pelvic Med Reconstr Surg 17(6):264, 2011

Bai SW, Kim BJ, Kim SK, et al: Comparison of outcomes between Burch colposuspension with and without concomitant abdominal hysterectomy. Yonsei Med J 45:665, 2004

Balgobin S, Fitzwater JL, White AB, et al: Effect of mesh width on vaginal apical support after abdominal sacrocolpopexy. Female Pelvic Med Reconstr Surg 17:S9, 2011

Balgobin S, Good MM, Dillon SJ, et al: Lowest colpopexy sacral fixation point alters vaginal axis and cul-de-sac depth. Am J Obstet Gynecol 208(6):488.e1, 2013

Ballard AC, Parker-Autry CY, Markland AD, et al: Bowel preparation before vaginal prolapse surgery: a randomized controlled trial. Obstet Gynecol 123(2 Pt 1):232, 2014

Barber MD, Amundsen CL, Paraiso MF, et al: Quality of life after surgery for genital prolapse in elderly women: obliterative and reconstructive surgery. Int Urogynecol J Pelvic Floor Dysfunct 18(7):799, 2007

Barber MD, Brubaker L, Burgio KL, et al: Comparison of 2 transvaginal surgical approaches and perioperative behavioral therapy for apical vaginal prolapse: the OPTIMAL randomized trial. JAMA 311(10):1023, 2014

Barber MD, Brubaker L, Menefee S, et al: Operations and pelvic muscle training in the management of apical support loss (OPTIMAL) trial: design and methods. Contemp Clin Trials 30: 178, 2009

Barber MD, Visco AG, Weidner AC, et al: Bilateral uterosacral ligament vaginal vault suspension with site-specific endopelvic fascia defect repair for treatment of pelvic organ prolapse. Am J Obstet Gynecol 183:1402, 2000

Beer M, Kuhn A: Surgical techniques for vault prolapse: a review of the literature. Eur J Obstet Gynecol Reprod Biol 119:144, 2005

Bent AE, Foote J, Siegel S, et al: Collagen implant for treating stress urinary incontinence in women with urethral hypermobility. J Urol 166:1354, 2001

Blaivas JG, Heritz DM, Romanzi LJ: Early versus late repair of vesicovaginal fistulas: vaginal and abdominal approaches. J Urol 153(4):1110, 1995

Borstad E, Rud T: The risk of developing urinary stress-incontinence after vaginal repair in continent women: a clinical and urodynamic follow-up study. Acta Obstet Gynaecol Scand 68:545, 1989

Bravo Gutierrez A, Madoff RD, Lowry AC, et al: Long-term results of anterior sphincteroplasty. Dis Colon Rectum 47:727, 2004

Brincat CA, Larson KA, Fenner DE: Anterior vaginal wall prolapse: assessment and treatment. Clin Obstet Gynecol 53(1):51, 2010

Brubaker L, Cundiff GW, Fine P, et al: Abdominal sacrocolpopexy with Burch colposuspension to reduce urinary stress incontinence. N Engl J Med 354:1557, 2006

Brubaker L, Nygaard I, Richter HE, et al: Two-year outcomes after sacrocolpopexy with and without Burch to prevent stress urinary incontinence. Obstet Gynecol 112(1):49, 2008

Buie WD, Lowry AC, Rothenberger DA, et al: Clinical rather than laboratory assessment predicts continence after anterior sphincteroplasty. Dis Colon Rectum 44:1255, 2001

Carey M, Goh J, Rosamilia A, et al: Laparoscopic versus open Burch colposuspension: a randomised controlled trial. BJOG 113:999, 2006

Chaikin DC, Groutz A, Blaivas JG: Predicting the need for anti-incontinence surgery in continent women undergoing repair of severe urogenital prolapse. J Urol 163:531, 2000

Chmielewski L, Walters MD, Weber AM, et al. Reanalysis of a randomized trial of 3 techniques of anterior colporrhaphy using clinically relevant definitions of success. Am J Obstet Gynecol 205:69.e1, 2011

Chrouser KL, Fick F, Goel A, et al: Carbon coated zirconium beads in β-glucan gel and bovine glutaraldehyde cross-linked collagen injections for intrinsic sphincter deficiency: continence and satisfaction after extended follow-up. J Urol 171:1152, 2004

Cohen BL, Tunuguntla HS, Gousse A: Predictors of success for first stage neuromodulation: motor versus sensory response. J Urol 175:2178, 2006

Collins SA, Jelovsek JE, Chen CC, et al: De novo rectal prolapse after obliterative and reconstructive vaginal surgery for urogenital prolapse. Am J Obstet Gynecol 197(1):84e1, 2007

Corcos J, Collet JP, Shapiro S, et al: Multicenter randomized clinical trial comparing surgery and collagen injections for treatment of female stress urinary incontinence. Urology 65:898, 2005

Corcos J, Fournier C: Periurethral collagen injection for the treatment of female stress urinary incontinence: 4-year follow-up results. Urology 54:815, 1999

Culligan PJ, Blackwell L, Goldsmith LJ, et al: A randomized controlled trial comparing fascia lata and synthetic mesh for sacral colpopexy. Obstet Gynecol 106:29, 2005

Culligan PJ, Murphy M, Blackwell L, et al: Long-term success of abdominal sacral colpopexy using synthetic mesh. Am J Obstet Gynecol 187:1473, 2002

Cundiff GW, Harris RL, Coates K, et al: Abdominal sacral colpoperineopexy: a new approach for correction of posterior compartment defects and perineal descent associated with vaginal vault prolapse. Am J Obstet Gynecol 177(6):1345, 1997

Dean NM, Ellis G, Wilson PD, et al: Laparoscopic colposuspension for urinary incontinence in women. Cochrane Database Syst Rev 3:CD002239, 2006

Debodinance P: Trans-obturator urethral sling for the surgical correction of female stress urinary incontinence: outside-in (Monarc) versus inside-out (TVT-O). Are the two ways reassuring? Eur J Obstet Gynecol Reprod Biol 133(2):232, 2007

deGroat WC: Changes in the organization of the micturition reflex pathway of the cat after transection of the spinal cord. Exp Neurol 71:22, 1981

Demirci F, Petri E: Perioperative complications of Burch colposuspension. Int Urogynecol J 11:170, 2000

Demirci F, Yucel O, Eren S, et al: Long-term results of Burch colposuspension. Gynecol Obstet Invest 51:243, 2001

Drewes PG, Marinis SI, Schaffer JI, et al: Vascular anatomy over the superior pubic rami in female cadavers. Am J Obstet Gynecol 193(6):2165, 2005

Dunn TS, Figge J, Wolf D: A comparison of outcomes of transurethral versus suprapubic catheterization after Burch cystourethropexy. Int Urogynecol J 16:60, 2005

El-Gazzaz G, Zutshi M, Hannaway C, et al: Overlapping sphincter repair: does age matter? Dis Colon Rectum 55:256, 2012

Faerber GJ, Belville WD, Ohl DA, et al: Comparison of transurethral versus periurethral collagen injection in women with intrinsic sphincter deficiency. Tech Urol 4:124, 1998

Fitzgerald MP, Richter HE, Bradley CS, et al: Pelvic support, pelvic symptoms, and patient satisfaction after colpocleisis. Int Urogynecol J Pelvic Floor Dysfunct 19(12):1603, 2008

Fitzgerald MP, Richter HE, Siddique S, et al: Colpocleisis: a review. Int Urogynecol J 17:261, 2006

Fitzpatrick M, Behan M, O'Connell PR, et al: A randomized clinical trial comparing primary overlap with approximation repair of third-degree obstetric tears. Am J Obstet Gynecol 183(5): 1220, 2000

Fleshman JW, Peters WR, Shemesh EI, et al: Anal sphincter reconstruction: anterior overlapping muscle repair. Dis Colon Rectum 34(9):739, 1991

Food and Drug Administration: UPDATE on serious complications associated with transvaginal placement of surgical mesh for pelvic organ prolapse: FDA safety communication. 2011. Available at: http://www.fda.gov/MedicalDevices/Safety/AlertsandNotices/ucm262435.htm. Accessed October 18, 2014

Francis WJ, Jeffcoate TN: Dyspareunia following vaginal operations. J Obstet Gynaecol Br Commonw 68:1, 1961

Freeman RM, Pantazis K, Thomson A, et al: A randomised controlled trial of abdominal versus laparoscopic sacrocolpopexy for the treatment of post-hysterectomy vaginal vault prolapse: LAS study. Int Urogynecol J 24(3):377, 2013

Galloway NT, Davies N, Stephenson TP: The complications of colposuspension. Br J Urol 60:122, 1987

Gandhi S, Goldberg RP, Kwon C, et al: A prospective, randomized trial using solvent dehydrated fascia lata for the prevention of recurrent anterior vaginal wall prolapse. Am J Obstet Gynecol 192:1649, 2005

Garcia V, Rogers RG, Kim SS, et al: Primary repair of obstetric anal sphincter laceration: a randomized trial of two surgical techniques. Am J Obstet Gynecol 192(5):1697, 2005

Gearhart S, Hull T, Floruta C, et al: Anal manometric parameters: predictors of outcome following anal sphincter repair? J Gastrointest Surg 9:115, 2005

Geis K, Dietl J: Ilioinguinal nerve entrapment after tension-free vaginal tape (TVT) procedure. Int Urogynecol J Pelvic Floor Dysfunct 13(2):136, 2002

Goldberg RP, Tomezsko JE, Winkler HA, et al: Anterior or posterior sacrospinous vaginal vault suspension: long-term anatomic and functional evaluation. Obstet Gynecol 98(2):199, 2001

Good MM, Abele TA, Balgobin S, et al: L5-S1 discitis—can it be prevented? Obstet Gynecol 121(2 Pt 1):285, 2013a

Good MM, Abele TA, Balgobin S, et al: Vascular and ureteral anatomy relative to the midsacral promontory. Am J Obstet Gynecol 208(6):486.e1, 2013b

Gorton E, Stanton S, Monga A, et al: Periurethral collagen injection: a long-term follow-up study. Br J Urol Int 84:966, 1999

Gourcerol G, Vitton V, Leroi AM, et al: How sacral nerve stimulation works in patients with faecal incontinence. Colorectal Dis 13(8):e203, 2011

Govaert B, Melenhorst J, van Gemert WG, et al: Can sensory and/or motor reactions during percutaneous nerve evaluation predict outcome of sacral nerve modulation? Dis Colon Rectum 52:1423, 2009

Green J, Herschorn S: The contemporary role of Burch colposuspension. Curr Opin Urol 15:250, 2005

Griffis K, Evers MD, Terry CL, et al: Mesh erosion and abdominal sacrocolpopexy: a comparison of prior, total, and supracervical hysterectomy. J Pelvic Med Surg 12(1):25, 2006

Gutman RE, Bradley CS, Ye W, et al: Effects of colpocleisis on bowel symptoms among women with severe pelvic organ prolapse. Int Urogynecol J 21(4):461, 2009

Ha HT, Fleshman JW, Smith M, et al: Manometric squeeze pressure difference parallels functional outcome after overlapping sphincter reconstruction. Dis Colon Rectum 44:655, 2001

Haab F, Zimmern PE, Leach GE: Urinary stress incontinence due to intrinsic sphincteric deficiency: experience with fat and collagen periurethral injections. J Urol 157:1283, 1997

Halverson AL, Hull TL: Long-term outcome of overlapping anal sphincter repair. Dis Colon Rectum 45:345, 2002

Herschorn S, Radomski SB: Collagen injections for genuine stress urinary incontinence: patient selection and durability. Int Urogynecol J 8:18, 1997

Holmgren C, Nilsson S, Lanner L, et al: Long-term results with tension-free vaginal tape on mixed and stress urinary incontinence. Obstet Gynecol 106(1):38, 2005

Hullfish KL, Bovbjerg VE, Steers WD: Colpocleisis for pelvic organ prolapse: patient goals, quality of life, and satisfaction. Obstet Gynecol 110 (2 Pt 1):341, 2007

Ingber MS, Firoozi F, Vasavada SP, et al: Surgically corrected urethral diverticula: long-term voiding dysfunction and reoperation rates. Urology 77(1):65, 2011

Jacobs SA, Lane FL, Osann KE, et al: Randomized prospective crossover study of interstim lead wire placement with curved versus straight stylet. Neurourol Urodyn 33(5):488, 2014

Jonsson Funk M, Siddiqui NY, Pate V, et al: Sling revision/removal for mesh erosion and urinary retention: long-term risk and predictors. Am J Obstet Gynecol 208:73.e1, 2013

Judd JP, Siddiqui NY, Barnett JC, et al: Cost-minimization analysis of robotic-assisted, laparoscopic, and abdominal sacrocolpopexy. J Minim Invasive Gynecol 17(4):493, 2010

Karram M, Maher C: Surgery for posterior vaginal wall prolapse. Int Urogynecol J 24:1835, 2013

Kearney R, DeLancey JO: Selecting suspension points and excising the vagina during Michigan four-wall sacrospinous suspension. Obstet Gynecol 101(2):325, 2003

Khanduja KS, Padmanabhan A, Kerner BA, et al: Reconstruction of rectovaginal fistula with sphincter disruption by combining rectal mucosal advancement flap and anal sphincteroplasty. Dis Colon Rectum 42(11):1432, 1999

Kohli N, Walsh PM, Roat TW, et al: Mesh erosion after abdominal sacrocolpopexy. Obstet Gynecol 92:999, 1998

Kwon CH, Goldberg RP, Koduri S, et al: The use of intraoperative cystoscopy in major vaginal and urogynecologic surgeries. Am J Obstet Gynecol 187:1466, 2002

Ladwig D, Miljkovic-Petkovic L, Hewson AD: Simplified colposuspension: a 15-year follow-up. Aust N Z J Obstet Gynaecol 44:39, 2004

Lapitan MC, Cody JD: Open retropubic colposuspension for urinary incontinence in women. Cochrane Database Syst Rev 6:CD002912, 2012

Lapitan MC, Cody DJ, Grant AM: Open retropubic colposuspension for urinary incontinence in women. Cochrane Database Syst Rev 1:CD002912, 2003

Larson KA, Smith T, Berger MB, et al: Long-term patient satisfaction with Michigan four-wall sacrospinous ligament suspension for prolapse. Obstet Gynecol 122(5):967, 2013

Lee PE, Kung RC, Drutz HP: Periurethral autologous fat injection as treatment for female stress urinary incontinence: a randomized, double-blind controlled trial. J Urol 165:153, 2001

Lee U, Wolff EM, Kobashi KC: Native tissue repairs in anterior vaginal prolapse surgery: examining definitions of surgical success in the mesh era. Curr Opin Urol 22(4):265, 2012

Lightner D, Rovner E, Corcos J, et al: Randomized controlled multisite trial of injected bulking agents for women with intrinsic sphincter deficiency: mid-urethral injection of Zuidex via the Implacer versus proximal urethral injection of Contigen cystoscopically. Urology 74(4):771, 2009

Lightner DJ, Itano NB, Sweat SD, et al: Injectable agents: present and future. Curr Urol Rep 3:408, 2002

Lowder JL, Park AJ, Ellison R, et al: The role of apical vaginal support in the appearance of anterior and posterior vaginal prolapse. Obstet Gynecol 111: 152, 2008

Lowenstein L, Fitz A, Kenton K, et al: Transabdominal uterosacral suspension: outcomes and complications. Am J Obstet Gynecol 200(6):656e1, 2009

Lowry AC, Thorson AG, Rothenberger DA, et al: Repair of simple rectovaginal fistulas. Influence of previous repairs. Dis Colon Rectum 31(9):676, 1988

Luck AM, Galvin SL, Theofrastous JP: Suture erosion and wound dehiscence with permanent versus absorbable suture in reconstructive posterior vaginal surgery. Am J Obstet Gynecol 192:1626, 2005

Madoff RD: Surgical treatment options for fecal incontinence. Gastroenterology 126:S48, 2004

Maher C, Feiner B, Baessler K, et al: Surgical management of pelvic organ prolapse in women. Cochrane Database Syst Rev 4:CD004014, 2013

Maldonado PA, Good MM, McIntire DD, et al: Overlapping sphincteroplasty for cloacal defect following obstetrical injury: presenting characteristics and subjective long-term outcomes. Female Pelvic Med Reconstr Surg 20(4);Suppl:S111, 2014

Malouf AJ, Norton CS, Engel AF, et al: Long-term results of overlapping anterior anal-sphincter repair for obstetric trauma. Lancet 355:260, 2000

Margulies RU, Rogers MA, Morgan DM: Outcomes of transvaginal uterosacral ligament suspension: systematic review and metaanalysis. Am J Obstet Gynecol 202(2):124, 2010

McCall ML: Posterior culdeplasty; surgical correction of enterocele during vaginal hysterectomy; a preliminary report. Obstet Gynecol 10(6):595, 1957

McDermott CD, Hale DS: Abdominal, laparoscopic, and robotic surgery for pelvic organ prolapse. Obstet Gynecol Clin North Am 36: 585, 2009

Meltomaa SS, Haarala MA, Taalikka MO, et al: Outcome of Burch retropubic urethropexy and the effect of concomitant abdominal hysterectomy: a prospective long-term follow-up study. Int Urogynecol J 12:3, 2001

Miklos JR, Moore RD: Laparoscopic extravesical vesicovaginal fistula repair: our technique and 15-year experience. Int Urogynecol J 26(3): 441, 2015

Mizrahi N, Wexner SD, Zmora O, et al: Endorectal advancement flap: are there predictors of failure? Dis Colon Rectum 45(12):1616, 2002

Mohr S, Brandner S, Mueller MD, et al: Sexual function after vaginal and abdominal fistula repair. Am J Obstet Gynecol 211:74.e1, 2014

Monga AK, Robinson D, Stanton SL: Periurethral collagen injections for genuine stress incontinence: a 2-year follow-up. Br J Urol 76:156, 1995

Monga AK, Stanton SL: Urodynamics: prediction, outcome and analysis of mechanism for cure of stress incontinence by periurethral collagen. BJOG 104:158, 1997

Montoya TI, Luebbehusen HI, Schaffer JI, et al: Sensory neuropathy following suspension of the vaginal apex to the proximal uterosacral ligaments. Int Urogynecol J 23(12):1735, 2012

Morley GW, DeLancey JO: Sacrospinous ligament fixation for eversion of the vagina. Am J Obstet Gynecol 158:872, 1988

Nguyen JN, Jakus-Waldman SM, Walter AJ, et al: Perioperative complications and reoperations after incontinence and prolapse surgeries using prosthetic implants. Obstet Gynecol 119(3):539, 2012

Nilsson CG, Palva K, Aarnio R, et al: Seventeen years' follow-up of the tension-free vaginal tape procedure for female stress urinary incontinence. Int Urogynecol J 24(8):1265, 2013

Noblett KL, Cadish LA: Sacral nerve stimulation for the treatment of refractory voiding and bowel dysfunction. Am J Obstet Gynecol 210(2):99, 2014

Norton P, Brubaker L: Urinary incontinence in women. Lancet 367:57, 2006

Nygaard I, Brubaker L, Zyczynski HM, et al: Long-term outcomes following abdominal sacrocolpopexy for pelvic organ prolapse. JAMA 309(19):2016, 2013

Nygaard IE, McCreery R, Brubaker L, et al: Abdominal sacrocolpopexy: a comprehensive review. Obstet Gynecol 104:805, 2004

Ockrim JL, Allen DJ, Shah PJ, et al: A tertiary experience of urethral diverticulectomy: diagnosis, imaging and surgical outcomes. BJU Int 103(11):1550, 2009

Paraiso M, Barber M, Muir T, et al: Rectocele repair: a randomized trial of three surgical techniques including graft augmentation. Am J Obstet Gynecol 195:1762, 2006

Paraiso MF, Jelovsek JE, Frick A, et al: Laparoscopic compared with robotic sacral colpopexy for vaginal prolapse. A randomised controlled trial. Obstet Gynecol 118(5):1005, 2011

Pathi SD, Rahn DD, Sailors JL, et al: Utility of clinical parameters, cystourethroscopy, and magnetic resonance imaging in the preoperative diagnosis of urethral diverticula. Int Urogynecol J 24(2):319, 2013

Peters KM, Killinger KA, Boura JA: Is sensory testing during lead placement crucial for achieving positive outcomes after sacral neuromodulation? Neurourol Urodynam 30:1489, 2011

Pilsgaard K, Mouritsen L: Follow up after repair of vaginal vault prolapse with abdominal colposacropexy. Acta Obstet Gynecol Scand 78:66, 1999

Pshak T, Nikolavsky D, Terlecki R, et al: Is tissue interposition always necessary in transvaginal repair of benign, recurrent vesicovaginal fistulae? Urology 82(3):707, 2013

Rahn DD, Good MM, Roshanravan SM, et al: Effects of preoperative local estrogen in postmenopausal women with prolapse: a randomized trial. J Clin Endocrinol Metab 99(10):3728, 2014

Rahn DD, Marinis SI, Schaffer JI: Anatomical path of the tension-free vaginal tape: reassessing current teachings. Am J Obstet Gynecol 195(6):1809, 2006

Rahn DD, Ward RM, Sanses TV, et al: Vaginal estrogen use in postmenopausal women with pelvic floor disorders: systematic review and practice guidelines. Int Urogynecol J 26(1):3, 2015

Rardin CR, Erekson EA, Sung VW, et al: Uterosacral colpopexy at the time of vaginal hysterectomy: comparison of laparoscopic and vaginal approaches. J Reprod Med 54(5):273, 2009

Rechberger T, Futyma K, Jankiewicz K, et al: The clinical effectiveness of retropubic (IVS-02) and transobturator (IVS-04) midurethral slings: randomized trial. Eur Urol 56:24, 2009

Rehman H, Bezerra CCB, Bruschini H, et al: Traditional suburethral sling operations for urinary incontinence in women. Cochrane Database Syst Rev 1:CD001754, 2011

Richter HE, Albo ME, Zyczynski HM, et al: Retropubic versus transobturator midurethral slings for stress incontinence. N Engl J Med 362(22):2066, 2010

Roshanravan SM, Wieslander CK, Schaffer JI, et al: Neurovascular anatomy of the greater sciatic foramen and sacrospinous ligament region in female cadavers: implications in sacrospinous ligament and iliococcygeal fascia vaginal vault suspension. Am J Obstet Gynecol 197(6):660.e1, 2007

Rovner ES: Urinary tract fistulae. In Kavoussi LR, Novick AC, Partin AW, et al (eds): Wein: Campbell-Walsh Urology, 10th ed. Philadelphia, Saunders, 2012

Schimpf MO, Rahn DD, Wheeler TL, et al: Sling surgery for stress urinary incontinence in women: a systematic review and metaanalysis. Am J Obstet Gynecol 211(1):71.e1, 2014

Schulz JA, Stanton SL, Baessler K, et al: Bulking agents for stress urinary incontinence: short-term results and complications in a randomized comparison of periurethral and transurethral injections. Int Urogynecol J Pelvic Floor Dysfunct 15:261, 2004

Shah SM, Gaunay GS: Treatment options for intrinsic sphincter deficiency. Nat Rev Urol 9(11):638, 2012

Shull BL, Bachofen C, Coates KW, et al: A transvaginal approach to repair of apical and other associated sites of pelvic organ prolapse with uterosacral ligaments. Am J Obstet Gynecol 183(6):1365, 2000

Siddiqui NY, Geller EJ, Visco AG: Symptomatic and anatomic 1-year outcomes after robotic and abdominal sacrocolpopexy. Am J Obstet Gynecol 206:435.e1, 2012

Sitzler PJ, Thomson JP: Overlap repair of damaged anal sphincter. A single surgeon's series. Dis Colon Rectum 39(12):1356, 1996

Song PH, Kim YD, Kim HT, et al: The 7-year outcome of the tension-free vaginal tape procedure for treating female stress urinary incontinence. BJU Int 104(8):1113, 2009

Sonoda T, Hull T, Piedmonte MR, et al: Outcomes of primary repair of anorectal and rectovaginal fistulas using the endorectal advancement flap. Dis Colon Rectum 45(12):1622, 2002

Steele AC, Kohli N, Karram MM: Periurethral collagen injection for stress incontinence with and without urethral hypermobility. Obstet Gynecol 95:327, 2000

Summers A, Winkel LA, Hussain HK, et al: The relationship between anterior and apical compartment support. Am J Obstet Gynecol 194:1438, 2006

Sung VW, Rardin CR, Raker CA, et al: Porcine subintestinal submucosal graft augmentation for rectocele repair: a randomized controlled trial. Obstet Gynecol 119(1):125, 2012

Tan-Kim J, Menefee SA, Luber KM, et al: Prevalence and risk factors for mesh erosion after laparoscopic-assisted sacrocolpopexy. Int Urogynecol J 22(2):205, 2011

Theofrastous, Cobb DL, Van Dyke AH, et al: A randomized trial of suprapubic versus transurethral bladder drainage after open Burch urethropexy. J Pelvic Surg 872, 2002

Tsang CB, Madoff RD, Wong WD, et al: Anal sphincter integrity and function influences outcome in rectovaginal fistula repair. Dis Colon Rectum 41(9):1141, 1998

Van Kerrebroeck PE, Marcelissen TA: Sacral neuromodulation for lower urinary tract dysfunction. World J Urol 30(4):445, 2012

Walters MD, Karram MM (eds): Surgical treatment of vaginal vault prolapse and enterocele. In Urogynecology and Reconstructive Pelvic Surgery, 3rd ed. Philadelphia, Mosby, 2007, p 262

Weber AM, Richter HE: Pelvic organ prolapse. Obstet Gynecol 106: 615, 2005

Weber AM, Walters MD, Piedmonte MR, et al: Anterior colporrhaphy: a randomized trial of three surgical techniques. Am J Obstet Gynecol 185:1299, 2001

Wei JT, Nygaard I, Richter HE, et al: A midurethral sling to reduce incontinence after vaginal prolapse repair. N Engl J Med 366:2358, 2012

White AB, Carrick KS, Corton MM, et al: Optimal location and orientation of suture placement in abdominal sacrocolpopexy. Obstet Gynecol 113(5):1098, 2009

Wieslander CK, Rahn DD, McIntire DD, et al: Vascular anatomy of the presacral space in unembalmed female cadavers. Am J Obstet Gynecol 195:1736, 2006

Wieslander CK, Roshanravan SM, Schaffer JI, et al: Uterosacral ligament suspension sutures: anatomic relationships in unembalmed female cadavers. Am J Obstet Gynecol 197(6):672.e1, 2007

Yamada T, Ichiyanagi N, Kamata S, et al: Need for sling surgery in patients with large cystoceles and masked stress urinary incontinence. Int J Urol 8:599, 2001

Zoorob D, Karram M: Bulking agents: a urogynecology perspective. Urol Clin North Am 39(3):273, 2012

Zullo F, Palomba S, Russo T, et al: Laparoscopic colposuspension using sutures or Prolene meshes: a 3-year follow-up. Eur J Obstet Gynaecol Reprod Biol 117:201, 2004

Zutshi M, Hull T, Bast J, et al: Ten-year outcome after anal sphincter repair for fecal incontinence. Dis Colon Rectum 52:6, 2009

Zyczynski HM, Sirls LT, Greer WJ, et al: Findings of universal cystoscopy at incontinence surgery and their sequelae. Am J Obstet Gynecol 210(5):480.e1, 2014

Surgeries for Gynecologic Malignancies

Radical Abdominal Hysterectomy (Type III)

The five "types" of hysterectomy are defined in Chapter 30 (p. 669). Of these, radical hysterectomy differs from simple hysterectomy in that the parametrium, paravaginal tissue, and their lymphatics are widely resected to achieve negative tumor margins. Described in this section, type III (radical) hysterectomy is chiefly indicated for stage IB1 to IIA cervical cancer or small central recurrences following radiation therapy, or for clinical stage II endometrial cancer when tumor has extended to the cervix (Koh, 2015).

Type III radical hysterectomy is increasingly being performed by minimally invasive approaches (p. 1142). With these techniques, the principles of the abdominal operation are still applied. Namely, radical hysterectomy is a dynamic operation that requires a focused, consistent surgical approach but also significant intraoperative decision making. Familiarity with its concepts continues to be critically important in developing expertise in complex pelvic surgery.

PREOPERATIVE

Patient Evaluation

Radical hysterectomy is not appropriate for women with higher-stage cancers. Thus, accurate clinical staging is critical prior to selection of this surgery. Pelvic examination under anesthesia with cystoscopy and proctoscopy is not mandatory for smaller cervical cancer lesions, but the clinical staging described in Chapter 30 (p. 663) should be completed before proceeding surgically. To refine patient selection, for most patients with grossly visible cervical tumors, abdominopelvic computed-tomography (CT) or magnetic resonance (MR) imaging is also performed to identify nodal metastases or undetected local tumor extension. That said, there are limitations on what can be reliably detected preoperatively (Chou, 2006).

Consent

Women undergoing hysterectomy are specifically counseled regarding the loss of fertility. In those considering bilateral salpingo-oophorectomy (BSO), a discussion of menopause and hormone replacement is included and detailed in Chapter 43 (p. 951). The tone of the consenting process should reflect the extent of the operation required to hopefully cure or at least begin treatment of the malignancy. Moreover, a patient must be advised that the procedure may be aborted if metastatic disease or pelvic tumor extension is found (Leath, 2004).

Radical abdominal hysterectomy can result in significant morbidity from short- and long-term complications. These complications may develop more frequently in women with obesity, prior pelvic infections, and previous abdominal surgery, in whom surgery may be more difficult (Cohn, 2000). Of potential intraoperative complications, the most common is acute hemorrhage. Blood loss may reach 500 to 1000 mL, and transfusion rates are variable, but high (Estape, 2009; Naik, 2010). Subacute postoperative complications may include significant postoperative bladder or bowel dysfunction from surgical denervation (20 percent), symptomatic lymphocyst formation (3 to 5 percent), and uretero-vaginal or vesicovaginal fistula (1 to 2 percent) (Franchi, 2007; Hazewinkel, 2010; Likic, 2008). With any cancer surgery, risk for venous thromboembolism (VTE) is also increased. Additionally, long-term effects on sexual function and other body functions are candidly reviewed and are detailed on page 1139 (Jensen, 2004; Serati, 2009).

Patient Preparation

For this, a blood sample is typed and cross-matched for potential transfusion. Pneumatic compression devices or subcutaneous heparin or both is planned because of the typically longer surgery and postoperative recovery times and the increased VTE risk associated with cancer (Table 39-8, p. 836) (Martino, 2006).

Bowel preparation with a polyethylene glycol-electrolyte solution (GoLYTELY) is no longer commonly used. Inadvertent bowel injury is rare unless extenuating circumstances are identified. However, it may be helpful to empty the colon to limit fecal spill if extensive pelvic adhesions are anticipated due to prior infection, endometriosis, or radiation therapy.

Suitable perioperative antibiotic prophylaxis to prevent most surgical site infection is found in Table 39-6 (p. 835). Typically, a third-generation cephalosporin is given intravenously at spaced intervals. Compared with simple hysterectomy, the high-volume blood loss during radical hysterectomy clears antibiotics more rapidly from the operative site, and longer surgery may extend past the antibiotic half-life. Both necessitate the additional doses (Bouma, 1993; Sevin, 1991).

Concurrent Surgery

Early-stage cervical cancer most frequently spreads via the lymphatics. Thus, adjunctive lymph node removal seeks to identify occult metastases. Pelvic lymphadenectomy is typically completed just before or immediately after radical hysterectomy, and paraaortic lymphadenectomy may also be indicated in some circumstances (p. 1169) (Angioli, 1999).

Spread to the adnexa is much less common than via the lymphatics. Thus, the decision for BSO depends on a woman's age and potential for metastases (Shimada, 2006). If ovaries are preserved, then salpingectomy alone is recommended to reduce future risk of some epithelial ovarian cancers (Society of Gynecologic Oncology, 2013). In candidates for ovarian preservation, transposition of ovaries out of the pelvis may be considered in young women if postoperative radiation is anticipated. However, ovarian function may be short-lived. Also, in transposed ovaries, symptomatic periadnexal cysts are commonplace (Buekers, 2001). Oocyte and ovarian cryopreservation techniques have advanced and may soon be a more widespread option (Chap. 20, p. 466).

INTRAOPERATIVE

Surgical Steps

❶ Anesthesia and Patient Positioning. General anesthesia is mandatory, but epidural

placement may be considered for postoperative pain control (Leon-Casasola, 1996). Bimanual examination is performed in the operating room before scrubbing to reorient a surgeon to the patient's individual anatomy. The patient is positioned supine. After anesthesia administration, hair in the path of the planned incision is clipped if needed; a Foley catheter is placed; and abdominal preparation is completed.

❷ Abdominal Entry. A midline vertical abdominal incision provides excellent exposure, but typically prolongs hospital stays and increases postoperative pain. Alternatively, Cherney or Maylard incisions offer postoperative advantages found with transverse incisions and allow access to the lateral pelvis (Chap. 43, p. 931). However, upper paraaortic nodes are not readily accessible through these transverse incisions. A Pfannenstiel incision offers limited exposure and is reserved only for selected patients (Orr, 1995).

❸ Exploration. After abdominal entry, a surgeon first thoroughly explores the abdomen for obvious metastatic disease. Firm, enlarged lymph nodes and any other suspect lesions are removed or biopsied. Confirmation of metastases or pelvic tumor extension leads to a decision on whether to proceed or abort an operation based on overall intraoperative findings and clinical situation (Leath, 2004).

❹ Entering the Retroperitoneal Space. The uterus is placed on traction with curved Kelly clamps at the cornua. The round ligament is sutured with 0-gauge delayed-absorbable suture as laterally as possible, and the tie is held on tension to aid entry into the retroperitoneal space. Lateral round ligament transection later aids excision of the parametrium out to the pelvic sidewall. Once the round ligament is divided, the broad ligament beneath separates into thin anterior and posterior leaves that contain loose areolar connective tissue between.

Similar to simple hysterectomy, the anterior leaf of the broad ligament is placed on traction and is sharply dissected to the vesicouterine fold. The posterior leaf of the broad ligament is then placed on traction and sharply dissected along the pelvic sidewall parallel to the infundibulopelvic (IP) ligament.

❺ Ureter Isolation. Loose areolar connective tissue of the retroperitoneal space is bluntly dissected in the area lateral to the IP until the external iliac artery is palpated just medial to the psoas major muscle. The index and middle fingers are placed on either side of the artery, and the areolar connective tissue is bluntly finger dissected toward the patient's head using a backward "walking" motion (Fig. 46-1.1).

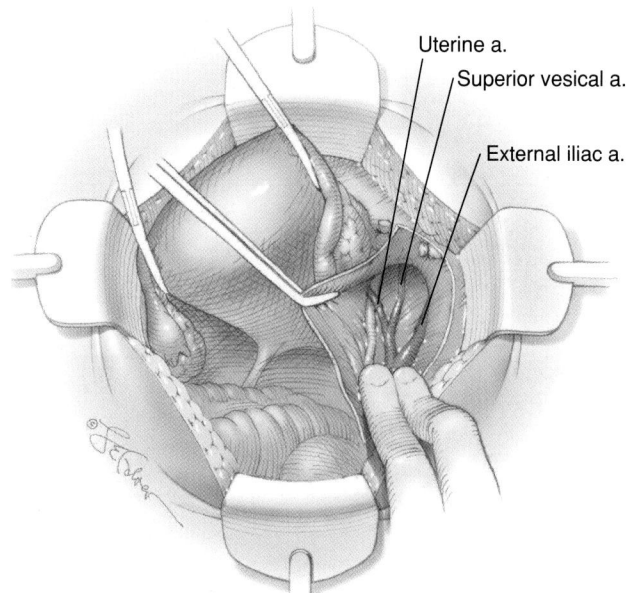

Uterine a.
Superior vesical a.
External iliac a.

FIGURE 46-1.1 Finding the ureter.

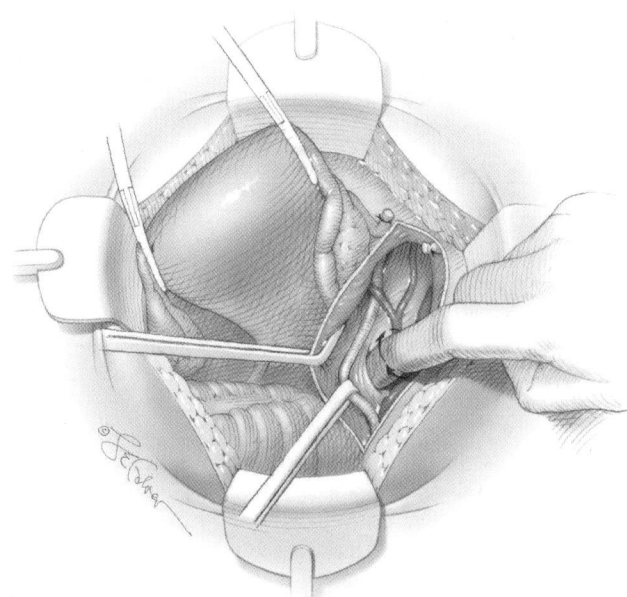

FIGURE 46-1.2 Opening the pararectal space.

To permit further cephalad inspection, the medial portion of the broad ligament's posterior leaf is elevated. This permits direct identification of the common iliac artery bifurcation and origins of the external and internal iliac arteries. Here, the ureter crosses over the bifurcation. To isolate the ureter at this site, the surgeon bluntly dissects with a finger or suction tip in a sweeping motion from top to bottom along the medial peritoneal leaf to identify and sufficiently mobilize the lateral surface of the ureter.

To free the medial surface, a Babcock clamp grasps the ureter, and Mixter right-angle clamp tips are opened and closed parallel to the ureter to develop an avascular space between it and its medial peritoneal attachment. Through this space, clamp tips are then passed beneath the ureter to grasp a quarter-inch-wide Penrose drain. The drain is then pulled through this space to surround and isolate the ureter. This assists in identifying its location throughout the remainder of surgery.

❻ Creating Spaces. The parametrium that will be removed with the hysterectomy specimen lies between the paravesical and pararectal spaces. Thus, creation of these spaces is needed to isolate the parametrium for transection. The pararectal space is developed by gently placing the right index finger lateral to the IP and between the internal iliac artery and ureter. The finger tracks in a gentle swirling motion at a 45-degree angle downward toward the midline and aiming for the coccyx (Fig. 46-1.2). Once formed, this space is bordered by the rectum and ureter medially, internal iliac artery laterally, cardinal ligament anteriorly, and the sacrum posteriorly.

In contrast, the paravesical space is formed by holding the lateral tie of the round ligament and bluntly following the external iliac artery caudally to the pubic ramus. The index and middle finger of the right hand then sweep intervening avascular areolar tissue deeply and medially toward the midline. The developed paravesical space is bounded by the bladder and superior vesical artery medially, the external iliac vessels laterally, the pubic symphysis anteriorly, and the cardinal ligament posteriorly. Once paravesical and pararectal spaces are created, the parametrium is now isolated between these two openings.

❼ Adnexa. With hysterectomy, ovaries may be retained or removed. If uninvolved with cancer, indications are similar to those for benign hysterectomy (Chap. 43, p. 951). If ovarian preservation is planned, the surgeon performs salpingectomy by serially clamping, cutting, and ligating the mesosalpinx (Section 43-6, p. 939). The uteroovarian ligament is then clamped, cut, and ligated close to uterus. The ovary is tucked laterally during hysterectomy completion. Alternatively, if BSO is planned, the IP ligament is doubly clamped, cut, and ligated. The uteroovarian ligament is left intact and the adnexa are ultimately removed with the uterine specimen.

❽ Uterine Artery Ligation. For this step, lateral reflection of the broad ligament's lateral leaf just distal to the round ligament will reveal the superior vesical artery. This vessel is bluntly dissected to better define its location and is grasped with a Babcock clamp and placed on lateral traction. A right-angle clamp is used to develop an avascular space beneath the vessel that should accommodate a

narrow curved Deaver retractor. Lateral traction on the superior vesical artery prevents its inadvertent ligation and aids in identification of the uterine artery (Fig. 46-1.3).

Next, a surgeon's left hand is inserted into the pelvis with the middle finger placed in the paravesical space, the index finger in the pararectal space, and the uterus with attached Kelly clamps cupped in the palm. The uterus is held on firm medial traction to expose the lateral pelvic sidewall. To visualize the uterine artery, a surgeon sharply dissects parametrial attachments and intervening areolar connective tissue beginning at the internal iliac artery and continuing caudad to the superior vesical artery. The origin of the uterine artery is found during this caudal dissection.

Tissues surrounding the uterine artery are bluntly dissected, and a right-angle clamp is placed beneath this artery to retrieve a 2-0 gauge silk suture. The uterine artery tie is placed as close as possible to its origin from the internal iliac artery. The process is repeated to place a separate silk suture far enough medial to enable vessel transection. Black silk ties help identify the proximal and distal portions of the uterine artery throughout the remainder of the operation. A small vascular clip (Hemoclip) can also be placed lateral to the silk tie on the proximal uterine artery for additional security of hemostasis. The uterine artery is then cut. The underlying uterine vein may also then be isolated, clipped or tied, and cut.

❾ Uniting Paravesical and Pararectal Spaces. The parametrial tissues have been pressed together by development of the paravesical and pararectal spaces. Parametrial resection to unite the upper (ventral) portion

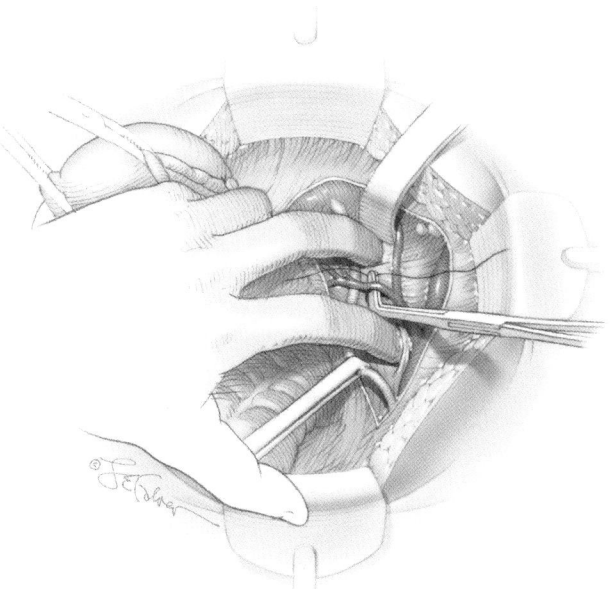

FIGURE 46-1.3 Ligating the uterine artery.

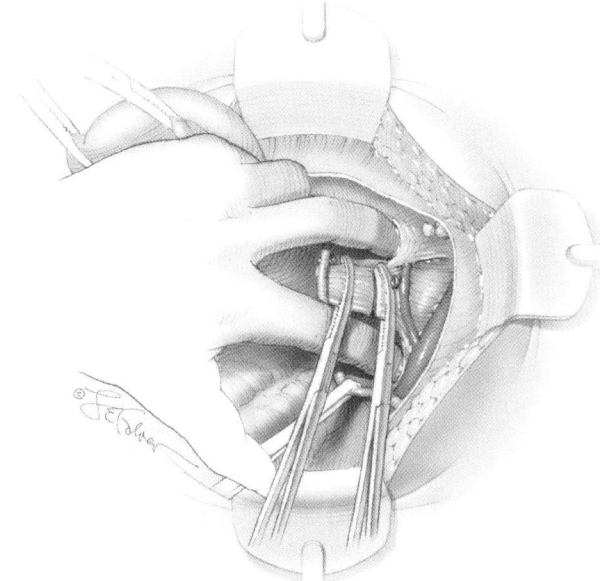

FIGURE 46-1.4 Uniting the spaces by parametrial resection.

of these spaces begins near the sidewall, moves medially, and can be performed by several methods. These include: (1) clamping, cutting, and suturing, (2) stapling with gastrointestinal anastomosis (GIA) stapler, (3) electrosurgical blade dissection in which a right-angle clamp elevates and isolates parametrial tissue, or (4) use of an electrothermal bipolar coagulator (LigaSure) (Fig. 46-1.4). Dissection is continued until the parametrium overlying the ureter is mobile.

⑩ Ureter Mobilization. In this same area of the pelvis, tips of a right-angle clamp are positioned between the ureter and peritoneal leaf. As previously described, opening and closing the tips downward and parallel to the ureter develops an avascular plane to

bluntly dissect the ureter from the medial peritoneal leaf. The ureter is placed on gentle lateral traction by grasping the previously placed Penrose drain with the left hand. The right index finger carefully sweeps the ureter downward and laterally until a "tunnel" through the paracervical tissue can be palpated ventromedially as the ureter enters this tissue (Fig. 46-1.5). Additional parametrial dissection is often required to ensure that the uterine artery and surrounding soft tissue has been lifted medially and off the ureter.

⑪ Bladder Dissection. Electrosurgical dissection is performed to free the bladder distally from the cervix and onto the upper vagina. This may need to be repeated several times as the tunnel is progressively unroofed and the

ureter is more directly visible. To allow adequate vaginal margins, the bladder will eventually need to be dissected so that it lies several centimeters distal to the cervical portio and onto the upper vagina.

⑫ Unroofing the Ureteral Tunnel. The uterus is placed on lateral traction, and the proximal ureter is held on traction to straighten it by gently pulling on the Penrose drain. The previously created tunnel opening is palpated. Concurrently, a right-angle clamp is inserted with its tips directed upward, while direct visualization of the underlying ureter is confirmed. The tips are then directed medially toward the cervix, "pop" through the paracervical tissue, and create a new distal opening (Fig. 46-1.6). One tip of a second

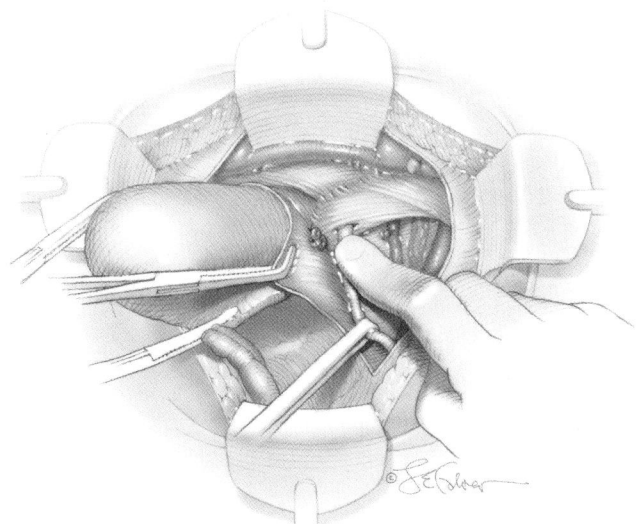

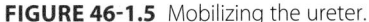

FIGURE 46-1.5 Mobilizing the ureter.

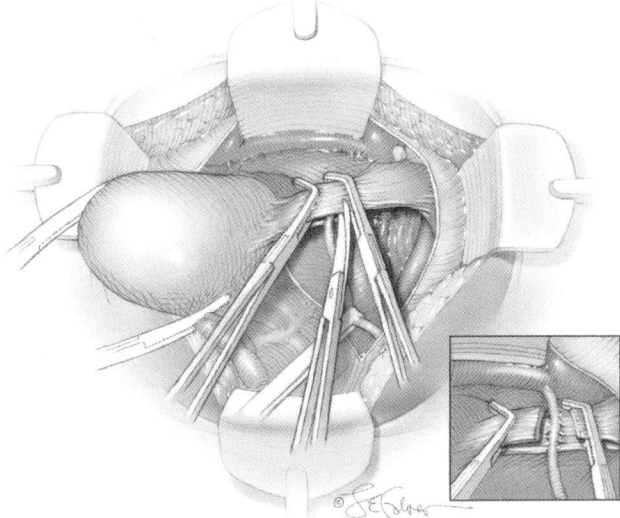

FIGURE 46-1.6 Unroofing the ureteral tunnel.

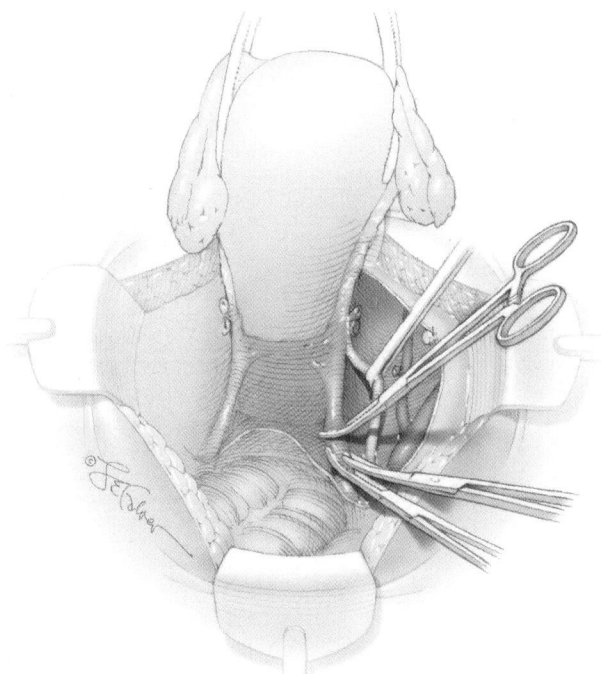

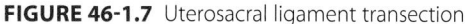

FIGURE 46-1.7 Uterosacral ligament transection.

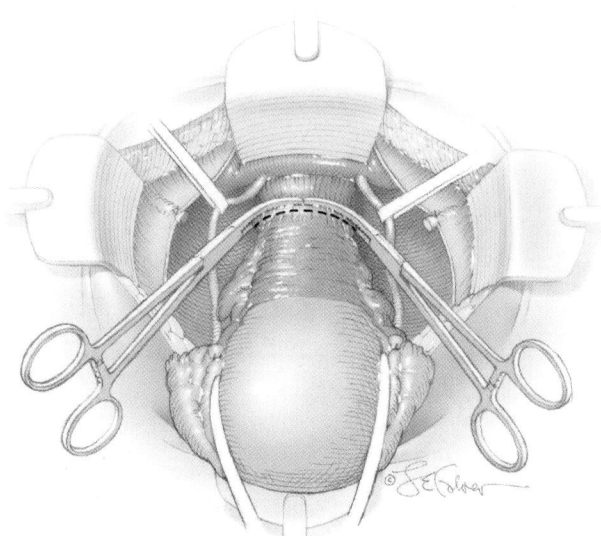

FIGURE 46-1.8 Vaginal transection.

clamp is placed through the tunnel and then through the new distal opening. The clamp then closes around the paracervical tissue that lies above and lateral to the ureter.

Within the tunnel, the ureter is bluntly dissected and pushed posteriorly toward the tunnel floor. It should be visible below before cutting the overlying paracervical tissue. Delayed-absorbable 3–0 suture ties are used to secure the paracervical tissue pedicles that are held by the right-angle clamps, but significant bleeding is commonplace during these steps. The same procedure may be repeated several times caudally to completely unroof the tunnel and expose the ureter. The dissection proceeds in a proximal to distal fashion with direct visualization of the ureter at all times to prevent injury. After being unroofed, the ureter is retracted upward, and filmy attachments between the it and tunnel bed are sharply divided.

⓭ **Uterosacral Resection.** Posterior radical dissection is often best performed near the operation's end because exposed retroperitoneal tissues typically ooze until the vaginal cuff is closed. The cervical external os is palpated, and at this level, the electrosurgical blade is used to superficially incise or "score" the peritoneum between the uterosacral ligaments. This score line joins the incision line of the previously cut posterior broad ligament peritoneum.

Between the uterosacral ligaments, a plane is developed by gently pressing a finger toward the vaginal wall without poking through and into the vaginal vault. This rectovaginal plane is developed by gentle pressure toward the sacrum and enlarged laterally until three fingers can be comfortably inserted. This maneuver frees the rectosigmoid from the uterosacral ligaments and prevents inadvertent bowel injury. Remaining peritoneal attachments are sharply dissected to fully expose the rectovaginal space. The exposed uterosacral ligaments can be visualized, palpated, clamped at the pelvic sidewall, then cut, and ligated with 0-gauge delayed-absorbable suture (Fig. 46-1.7). This procedure may need to be repeated to complete transection of the uterosacral ligament and adjacent supportive tissues.

⓮ **Vaginal Resection.** At this point in the operation, the radical hysterectomy specimen is held in place only by the paracolpium and vagina. The bladder and ureters are further bluntly and sharply dissected free until at least 3 cm of upper vagina will be included with the resected specimen. Curved clamps are placed on the lateral paracolpium. The ureter should be lateral and directly visible. Tissue is then cut and suture ligated with 0-gauge delayed-absorbable suture.

The upper vagina can then be: (1) clamped, cut, and suture ligated, (2) stapled, or (3) sharply transected with electrosurgical blade and suture ligated (Fig. 46-1.8). The specimen is carefully examined to ensure an adequate upper vaginal segment and grossly negative margins.

⓯ **Suprapubic Catheter Placement.** This catheter may aid postoperative voiding trials in carefully selected, motivated patients (Pikaart, 2007).

⓰ **Ovarian Transposition.** For those in whom ovarian function preservation is desired, transposing adnexa out of the anticipated pelvic radiation field is an option. A distal portion of the ovary is grasped with a Babcock clamp. Using traction, dissection is performed to mobilize the IP ligament so that the ovary can be lifted into the upper abdomen. For future radiography or CT interpretation, a large vascular clip is placed on the residual uteroovarian ligament stump to serve as an ovarian location marker. For transposition, a 0-gauge silk suture is placed at this stump site and tied. Its needle is covered but remains attached to the suture.

A handheld abdominal retractor is then used to expose an area of the lateral posterior peritoneum as high as possible in the abdomen. The silk suture needle is then uncovered and placed through the peritoneum, and the ovary is elevated by this "pulley-stitch" and tied. The lateral pelvic defect is closed with a continuous running stitch using 0-gauge delayed-absorbable suture to prevent internal herniation, that is, entrapment of bowel within the peritoneal defect. Ovaries are inspected before abdominal closure to exclude vascular compromise by transposition.

⓱ **Final Steps.** Active bleeding should be immediately controlled when the radical hysterectomy specimen has been removed. A dry laparotomy sponge may be held firmly deep in the pelvis for several minutes to tamponade raw surfaces. Topical hemostatic agents may be employed (Table 40-5, p. 861). With bleeding controlled, a surgeon then assesses the vascular support to the ureter and other sidewall structures. To structures that appear particularly devascularized, an omental J-flap may provide additional blood supply (Section 46-14, p. 1186) (Fujiwara, 2003; Patsner, 1997). Routine pelvic suction drainage and closure of the peritoneum are not necessary (Charoenkwan, 2014; Franchi, 2007).

POSTOPERATIVE

Immediate postoperative care following radical hysterectomy in general follows that for laparotomy. Early ambulation after radical hysterectomy is especially important to prevent thromboembolic complications (Stentella, 1997). Moreover, following laparotomy for cancer, anticoagulants are continued for 2 to 4 weeks postoperatively (American College of Obstetricians and Gynecologists, 2013). Early feeding, including rapid initiation of a clear liquid diet, may also shorten the hospital stay (Kraus, 2000).

Bladder tone returns slowly, and a major cause is thought to be partial sympathetic and parasympathetic denervation during radical dissection (Chen, 2002). Thus, Foley catheter drainage is commonly continued until a patient is passing flatus because improving bowel function typically accompanies resolving bladder hypotonia. Removal of the catheter or clamping of the suprapubic tube should be followed by a successful voiding trial (Chap. 42, p. 917). A voiding trial may be attempted prior to hospital discharge or at the first postoperative visit. Patients with adequate function are instructed to press gently on the suprapubic area for several days afterward to help completely empty the bladder during voiding and prevent retention. Successful voiding may take several weeks to achieve. In addition to urinary retention, tenesmus and constipation are frequent immediate symptoms that should improve significantly over months or years (Butler-Manuel, 1999; Sood, 2002). Postoperative stool softeners are often prescribed.

Nerve-sparing radical hysterectomy is a method demonstrating improved postoperative bladder function (Raspagliesi, 2006). However, many patients have preexisting abnormal urodynamic findings that are simply exacerbated by radical hysterectomy (Lin, 1998, 2004). In the 3 percent of women who develop long-term bladder hypotonia or atony, intermittent self-catheterization is preferred to indwelling urinary catheterization (Chamberlain, 1991; Naik, 2005).

For cervical cancer patients undergoing BSO, estrogen replacement therapy is not contraindicated and may be initiated in the hospital at the discretion of the treating oncologist. Cervical cancer survivors treated with radical hysterectomy have much better sexual functioning than those who receive radiation therapy. Despite this, more than half of surgical patients postoperatively report a worse sex life (Butler-Manuel, 1999). Severe orgasmic problems, uncomfortable intercourse due to reduced vaginal length, and severe dyspareunia may develop but often resolve within 6 to 12 months. However, persistent lack of sexual interest and poor lubrication may be long-term or permanent changes (Jensen, 2004). Disturbed vaginal blood flow response during sexual arousal may account for much of the reported constellation of symptoms (Maas, 2004). Eventually, patients treated by surgery alone can expect a quality of life and overall sexual function similar to peers without a history of cancer (Frumovitz, 2005).

46-2

Modified Radical Abdominal Hysterectomy (Type II)

Four procedural differences distinguish a modified radical hysterectomy (type II) hysterectomy from the more radical type III procedure (Section 46-1, p. 1134). First, the uterine artery is transected where it crosses the ureter (rather than at its origin from the internal iliac artery). Second, only the medial half of the cardinal ligament is resected (instead of division at the sidewall). Additionally, the uterosacral ligament is divided halfway between the uterus and sacrum (rather than at the sacrum). And last, a smaller margin of upper vagina is removed. These modifications serve to reduce surgical time and associated morbidity, while still enabling complete resection of smaller cervical tumors (Cai, 2009; Landoni, 2001).

Clear indications for modified radical hysterectomy are few and controversial (Rose, 2001). Stage IA1 (with lymphovascular space invasion) or IA2 cervical cancer are the most common diagnoses (Koh, 2015). Type II hysterectomy is also performed on occasion for: (1) preinvasive or microinvasive disease when a more invasive lesion cannot be excluded, (2) selected stage IB1 disease with <2 cm lesions, and (3) small central postirradiation recurrences (Cai, 2009; Coleman, 1994; Eisenkop, 2005). In addition, a variation of this operation may be performed if

more extensive dissection is required for known benign disease. Anatomic landmarks that distinguish a type II hysterectomy are somewhat vague, and thereby allow a surgeon to sculpt the procedure to a patient's specific situation (Fedele, 2005). Similar to the type III radical procedure, modified radical hysterectomy is increasingly being performed using a minimally invasive approach.

PREOPERATIVE

Preparation for surgery should proceed with the same care and discretion that is essential for the success of radical (type III) abdominal hysterectomy (Section 46-1, p. 1135).

INTRAOPERATIVE

Surgical Steps

❶ Anesthesia and Patient Positioning. Modified radical hysterectomy is performed under general anesthesia with the patient supine. Bimanual examination is performed in the operating room before scrubbing to reorient a surgeon to a patient's individual anatomy. The abdomen is surgically prepared, and a Foley catheter is placed.

❷ Abdominal Entry. Modified radical hysterectomy may be safely performed through a midline vertical or low transverse incision (Fagotti, 2004).

❸ Retroperitoneal Dissection. The initial steps of modified radical (type II) hysterectomy mirror those of the type III procedure.

The retroperitoneum is opened to identify structures, the ureter is mobilized, and the paravesical and pararectal spaces are developed to exclude the possibility of parametrial tumor extension before proceeding with this less radical operation (Scambia, 2001). As with radical hysterectomy, adnexa may be spared or removed (p. 1135).

❹ Uterine Artery Ligation. At this point, type II hysterectomy begins to differ from the radical type III procedure. The superior vesical artery does not have to be identified, nor does the entire extent of the internal iliac artery need to be dissected free of adventitial tissue. The ureteral tunnel opening is palpated, and the uterine vessels divided at that location (Fig. 46-2.1). Ligation of the uterine artery as it crosses the ureter allows preservation of distal ureteral blood supply.

❺ Cardinal Ligament Resection. The bladder is mobilized distally off the cervix and onto the upper vagina. Parametrial tissue at the sidewall does not require mobilization over and off the ureter (as in a type III hysterectomy). Posterolateral attachments of the ureter remain intact, and only the medial halves of the cardinal ligaments are resected by successive clamping, cutting, and suture ligation of the paracervical tissue that lies medial to the ureter (Fig. 46-2.2). In contrast to the type III hysterectomy, the ureter is not dissected out of the tunnel bed, but is rolled laterally to expose the medial cardinal ligament.

❻ Uterosacral Resection. Posterior dissection is also modified. Uterosacral ligaments are only clamped halfway to the pelvic sidewall (instead of "at" the pelvic sidewall)

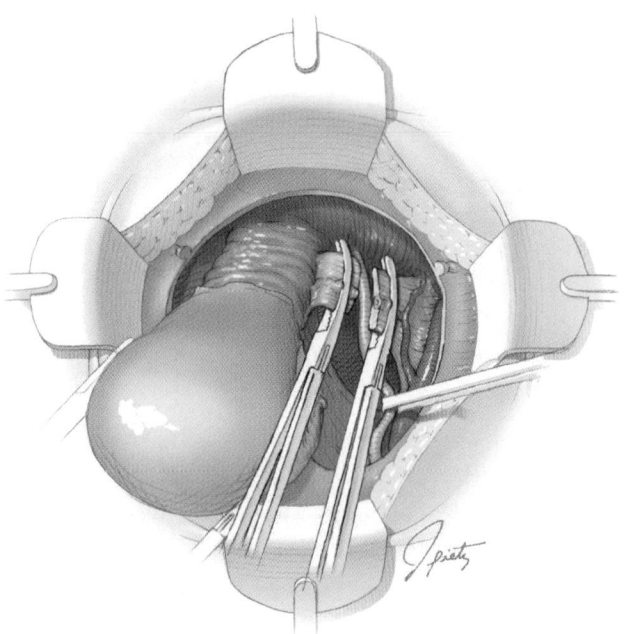

FIGURE 46-2.1 Uterine artery ligation.

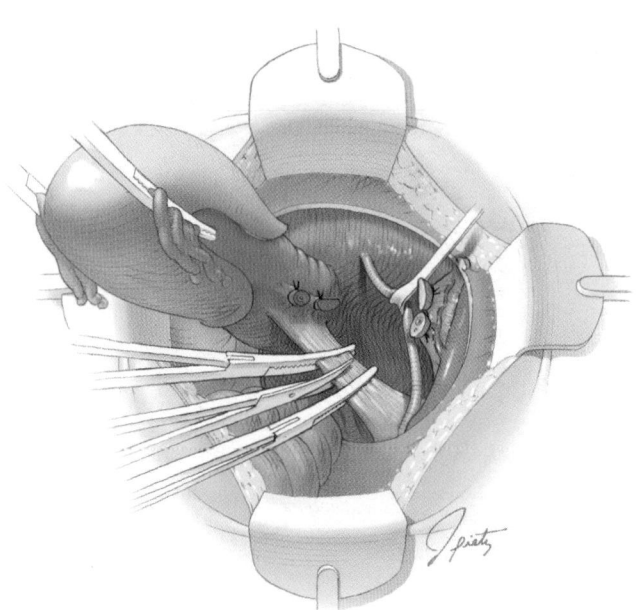

FIGURE 46-2.2 Cardinal ligament transection.

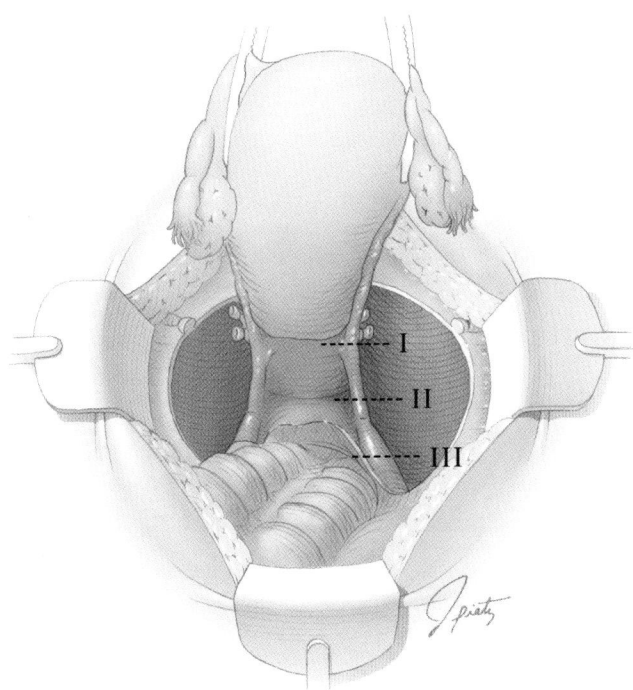

FIGURE 46-2.3 Uterosacral ligament transection.

and transected (Fig. 46-2.3). The uterus and adjacent parametrium can then be lifted well out of the pelvis and any additional tissues also clamped, cut, and ligated.

❼ **Vaginal Resection.** At this point, the modified radical hysterectomy specimen is held in place only by the paracolpium and vagina. The bladder and ureters are further bluntly and sharply dissected free until at least 2 cm of upper vagina will be included in the specimen (instead of 3 to 4 cm). Curved clamps are placed on the lateral paracolpium, cut, and suture ligated.

The upper vagina can then be: (1) clamped, cut, and suture ligated, (2) stapled, or (3) sharply transected with electrosurgical blade and suture ligated. The specimen is carefully examined to ensure an adequate upper vaginal segment and grossly negative margins.

POSTOPERATIVE

In general, postoperative care follows that for radical hysterectomy, but the incidence of complications is lower (Cai, 2009). Partial sympathetic and parasympathetic denervation should be much less extensive with a modified radical hysterectomy. Thus, bladder dysfunction is much less likely than following a type III radical hysterectomy, and successful voiding begins much earlier (Landoni, 2001; Yang, 1999). Foley catheter drainage may be discontinued on the second postoperative day and is followed by a voiding trial (Chap. 42, p. 917). In addition, bowel and sexual dysfunction should also be less pronounced.

46-3

Minimally Invasive Radical Hysterectomy

Since the 1990s, experience with this procedure has accrued, and rates of both laparoscopic and robotic radical hysterectomy have increased (Wright, 2012). Compared with laparotomy, a minimally invasive surgery (MIS) approach appears to offer comparable cancer survival rates and has similar rates of most surgical complications (Lee, 2010; Yan, 2011). With MIS, less intraoperative blood loss and shorter hospital stays are noted, but operative times can be longer depending on surgeon proficiency (Soliman, 2011).

Whether radical hysterectomy with pelvic lymphadenectomy is completed via laparotomy or with MIS, the cancer indications and surgical steps are the same. Thus, compared with simple hysterectomy (type I), greater resection of parametrial and paracolpium tissue and their lymphatics is essential to help ensure tumor-free surgical margins. This degree of resection requires significantly more retroperitoneal dissection, during which the ureter and major vessels must be identified to aid resection and avoid injury.

PREOPERATIVE

Patient Evaluation

Thorough preoperative pelvic examination reveals factors that help determine the optimal surgical approach for a given patient. For example, a large broad or bulky uterus may be difficult to manipulate during MIS, may block views, and may be too large for vaginal removal. Importantly, morcellation is avoided with any gynecologic malignancy.

General challenges to MIS, such as obesity, are described in Chapter 41 (p. 874). That said, laparoscopy can be a successful option for many obese patients and offers lower rates of postoperative wound infection, which is often a major complication after laparotomy in these patients (Park, 2012). Once a patient is deemed eligible for an MIS approach, the same preoperative evaluation as for an open procedure applies (p. 1135).

Consent

Risks of MIS radical hysterectomy mirror those listed for radical abdominal hysterectomy (p. 1135). Patient factors that contribute include older age, previous abdominal surgery, and prior radiotherapy (Chi, 2004).

General complications related to MIS are discussed in Chapter 41 (p. 877). With minimally invasive radical hysterectomy specifically, there is also increased concern for nerve injury from a longer operation in lithotomy and steep Trendelenburg position. Additionally, the risk of conversion to an open procedure is discussed. This risk may be increased if exposure and organ manipulation are limited.

Patient Preparation

Preoperative preparation is the same as for an open procedure (p. 1135). Thus, antibiotics and VTE prophylaxis are warranted (Tables 39-6 and 39-8, p. 835). Benefits of mechanical bowel preparation can be debated and are individualized. If considered, an evacuated rectosigmoid may improve colon manipulation and pelvic anatomy visualization. Options are found in Chapter 39 (p. 835).

Concurrent Surgery

Pelvic lymphadenectomy is typically completed just before or immediately after radical hysterectomy, and paraaortic lymphadenectomy may also be indicated in some circumstances. An MIS approach to lymph node removal in these areas is described in Section 46-12 (p. 1176).

Planned oophorectomy should depend on a woman's age and potential for metastases (Hu, 2013). Ovarian metastasis is rare with early-stage cervical cancer, and particularly with squamous cell carcinoma. Thus, if preservation is chosen, the ovary can be transposed with MIS techniques to the upper abdomen. This is done to help extend ovarian function if later radiotherapy is required. However, ovarian longevity may be shortened postoperatively, and symptomatic ovarian cysts are common. Moreover, advancements in oocyte and ovarian cryopreservation may soon provide suitable alternatives.

Regardless of ovarian preservation, salpingectomy is now encouraged for all women undergoing hysterectomy (Society of Gynecologic Oncology, 2013). As explained in Chapter 35 (p. 738), this practice is hoped to lower rates of high-grade ovarian and peritoneal serous carcinomas.

INTRAOPERATIVE

Instruments

Basic MIS tools for laparoscopic or robotic surgery are required. Important instruments for radical hysterectomy include 5- and 12-mm trocars, combined irrigation/suction device, vaginal probe, and energy devices for cutting and vessel sealing. For the

latter, several electrosurgical and ultrasonic energy-based devices are adapted for either laparoscopic or robotic cases. These include Harmonic scalpel, electrosurgical monopolar instruments, and electrothermal bipolar coagulator devices (LigaSure, ENSEAL, PK Dissecting Forceps). For laparoscopy, the argon-beam coagulator is another option. While operating in the pelvis, a 0-degree laparoscope can be used, although a laparoscope with a 30-degree lens system may also be advantageous in certain circumstances to provide superior lateral views.

Surgical Steps

❶ **Anesthesia and Patient Positioning.** The patient is initially supine for general endotracheal anesthesia induction. For VTE prophylaxis, lower extremity compression devices are placed. Legs are then positioned in adjustable booted support stirrups in low lithotomy to permit adequate perineal access. Positioning should permit a transvaginal uterine manipulator to move easily in all directions. As described in Chapter 41 (p. 879), appropriate positioning of legs within the stirrups and arms at the side is crucial to reduce nerve injury risks.

Bimanual examination is performed in the operating room before scrubbing to reorient a surgeon to the patient's individual anatomy. The abdomen, perineum, and vagina are then surgically prepared, and a Foley catheter is inserted. To avoid stomach puncture by a trocar during primary abdominal entry, an orogastric or nasogastric tube is placed to decompress the stomach.

During MIS radical hysterectomy, a manipulator is frequently placed to aid uterine repositioning and help acquire adequate vaginal surgical margins. Several uterine manipulators are described and illustrated in Chapter 44 (p. 1033). Popular options include a RUMI manipulator/KOH ring combination or a V-Care device. However, in cervical cancer cases, if a bulky cervical lesion is present, a blunt vaginal probe in the vaginal fornix may be all that can be inserted.

❷ **Port Placement.** An illustrated description of MIS entry into the abdominal cavity is found in Chapter 41 (p. 889). Suitable entry methods include the open technique, direct trocar insertion, or transumbilical insertion of a Veress needle. For gynecologic oncology cases, the open technique is often used to minimize vascular or bowel puncture risk. With primary entry, an umbilical or supraumbilical site is preferred. Following entry, a 10- or 12-mm Hassan trocar with a blunt obturator is placed into the abdominal cavity and is secured to the fascia.

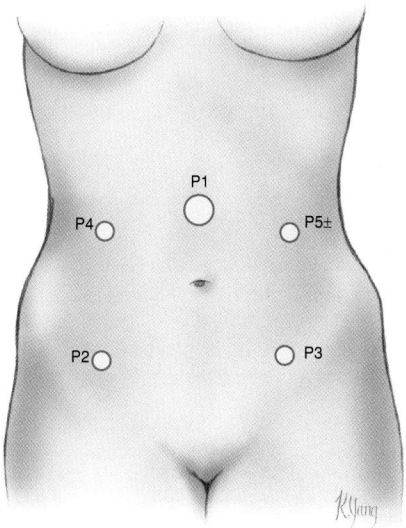

FIGURE 46-3.1 Port placement for minimally invasive radical hysterectomy.

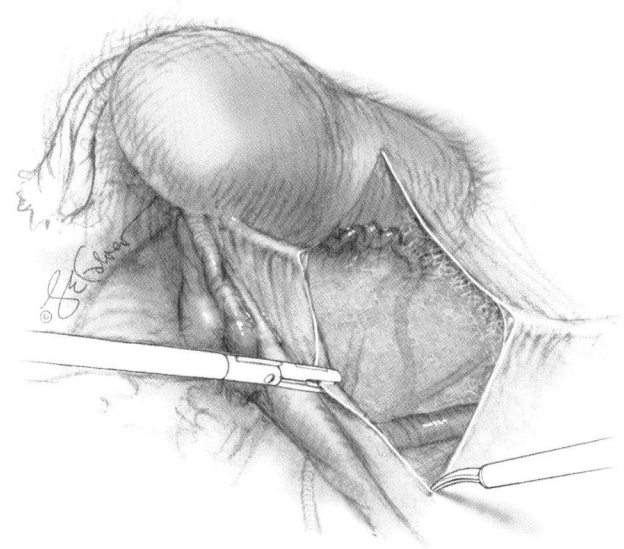

FIGURE 46-3.2 Opening the broad ligament leaf.

Through the trocar, the obturator is removed and replaced by a 10-mm laparoscope.

After abdominal insufflation, the abdomen and pelvis are thoroughly inspected to assess the extent of disease and adhesions. At this point, confirmation of metastatic disease or pelvic tumor extension should prompt a surgeon to decide whether to proceed or abort the operation based on intraoperative findings and clinical situation. Moreover, the decision is made to proceed laparoscopically or convert to laparotomy.

For laparoscopy, the surgeon stands on one side of the patient, whereas one assistant occupies the opposite side and another stands between the patient's legs. To proceed, other ports are placed under direct laparoscopic visualization. Anatomic landmarks are identified to guide port placement and avert vascular puncture injuries. For complex MIS gynecologic procedures, four port sites are preferred (Fig. 46-3.1). Additional ports are placed according to surgeon preference. These ideally have a minimum of 8 cm between them to allow ample range of motion and for robotic cases, to avoid arm collision.

❸ **Opening the Retroperitoneum.** This is the initial step to opening the paravesical and pararectal spaces bilaterally and identifying the ureter. Development of these spaces allows the parametrial tissue to be isolated and later resected.

First, the assistant angles the uterus to the contralateral side of dissection using a uterine manipulator and/or a grasper holding one cornu. This creates tension across the round ligament, which is divided at its midpoint. Transection may be accomplished using any of the energy-based devices previously listed.

Once the round ligament is transected, the broad ligament beneath it separates into thin anterior and posterior leaves, with loose areolar connective tissue between them. The anterior leaf is tented upward by graspers and sharply incised with monopolar scissors or other energy-based device. Incision extends caudally and medially toward the vesicouterine fold and halts near the midline.

To further expand the retroperitoneal opening, the drape of peritoneum lying between the divided round ligament and infundibulopelvic (IP) ligament is elevated with smooth graspers. Incision of this tented peritoneum is extended cephalad toward the pelvic brim but remains lateral and parallel to the IP (Fig. 46-3.2). This exposes the external iliac vessels and provides access to the ureter.

❹ **Ureteral Identification.** This is accomplished by precise sharp and blunt dissection just lateral to the medial leaf of the opened peritoneum. For this, a blunt probe or the closed tips of a grasper may be selected. Dissection is advanced downward, medially, and slightly cephalad with gentle back-and-forth cephalad-caudad strokes into the gauzy retroperitoneal tissue and over the presumed ureter path (Fig. 46-3.3). The ureter is identified and traced along the medial leaf of the peritoneum.

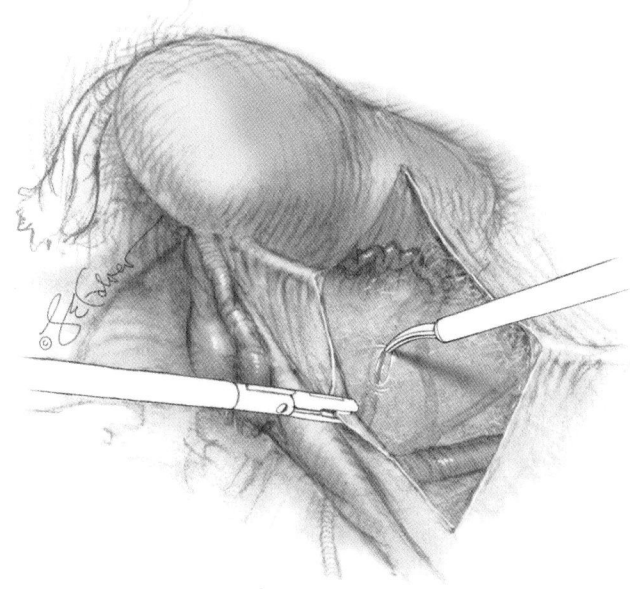

FIGURE 46-3.3 Locating the ureter.

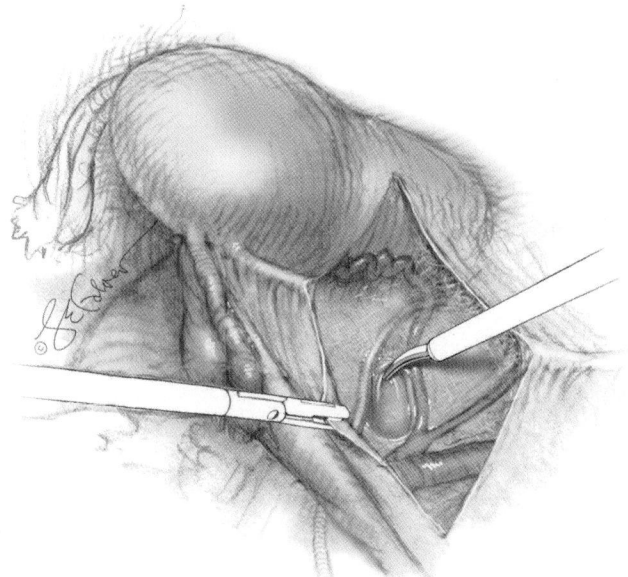

FIGURE 46-3.4 Opening the pararectal space.

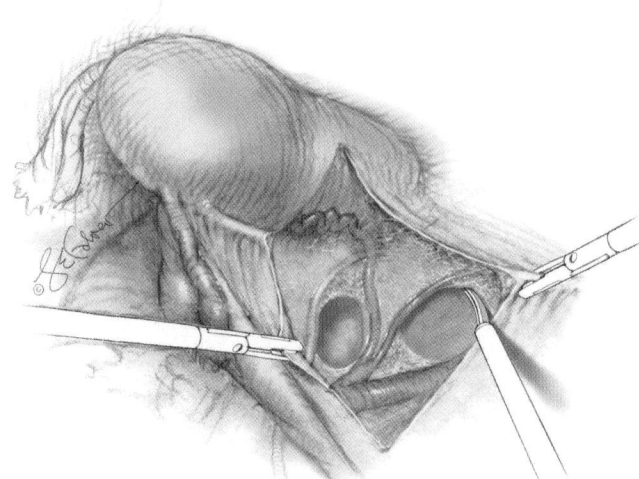

FIGURE 46-3.5 Opening the paravesical space.

❺ Creating Spaces. The uterus remains deviated to the contralateral side to develop the pararectal space. This avascular space is bounded by the rectum and ureter medially, the internal iliac artery laterally, the cardinal ligament and uterine artery caudally, and sacrum cephalad. Within these borders, the tips of closed scissors or other blunt tip push downward and medially through loose connective tissue (Fig. 46-3.4). The surgeon directs dissection downward toward the midline, aims for the pelvic floor, and stops once the levator ani muscles are reached.

For the paravesical space, boundaries are the external iliac vessels laterally, the bladder and obliterated umbilical ligament medially, the pubic symphysis caudally, and the cardinal ligament cephalad. To open this space, the previously incised edge of the broad ligament's anterior leaf is lifted at a point between the bladder and pelvic sidewall. Superficial loose connective tissue lies medial to the external iliac vessels and is bluntly dissected with closed scissors or grasper (Fig. 46-3.5). Staying medial to the external iliac vein and lateral to the superior vesicle/obliterated umbilical artery, dissection is directed caudally until the curve of the pubic ramus is reached.

Once the paravesical and pararectal spaces are opened, the parametria is now isolated between these two spaces for later resection. This dissection also helps to mobilize the bladder, discussed next, and to expose the external iliac vessels, which will aid later pelvic lymphadenectomy.

❻ Bladder Mobilization. During radical hysterectomy, the bladder is dissected free from the cervix and upper vagina. The mobile

bladder is moved caudad and protected during final vaginal transection. To mobilize the bladder, the peritoneum at the vesicouterine fold is grasped with atraumatic graspers and elevated to create tension between it and the underlying cervix (Fig. 46-3.6). The vesicouterine space, the potential space between the bladder and cervix, is opened using sharp and blunt dissection. Only loose connective tissue fibers lie in this space and are easily cut. Incision of these bands is kept close to the cervix to avoid cystotomy. Dissection in the midline minimizes laceration of vessels that course within the vesicocervical ligaments, colloquially termed bladder pillars. Once the

correct plane is entered, the pearly white cervix and anterior vaginal wall below are clearly differentiated from the more opaque bladder.

Ultimately, the bladder is moved sufficiently caudad to permit excision of up to 3 cm of proximal vagina at the procedure's end. This aids acquisition of tumor-free surgical margins. Generous dissection also avoids incorporating bladder fibers into the cuff closure, which could lead to bladder injury or to later genitourinary fistula.

❼ Uterine Artery Ligation. For this step, the pelvic sidewall vessels are exposed. By visually moving from the common iliac artery

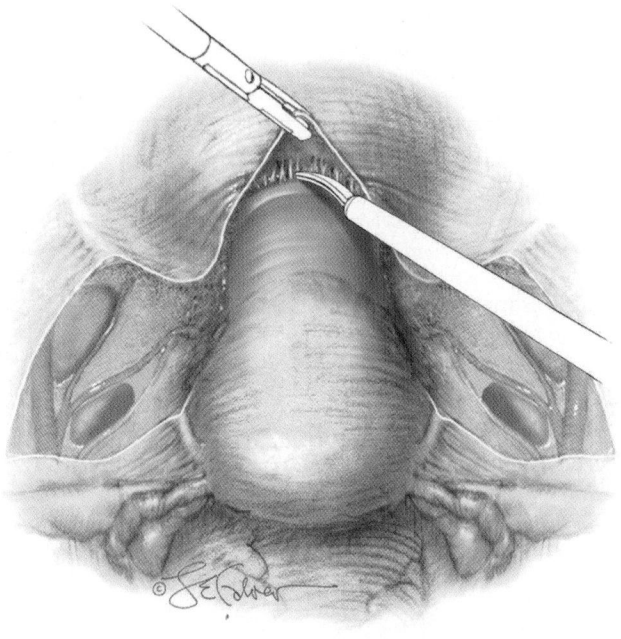

FIGURE 46-3.6 Dissection in the vesicovaginal space.

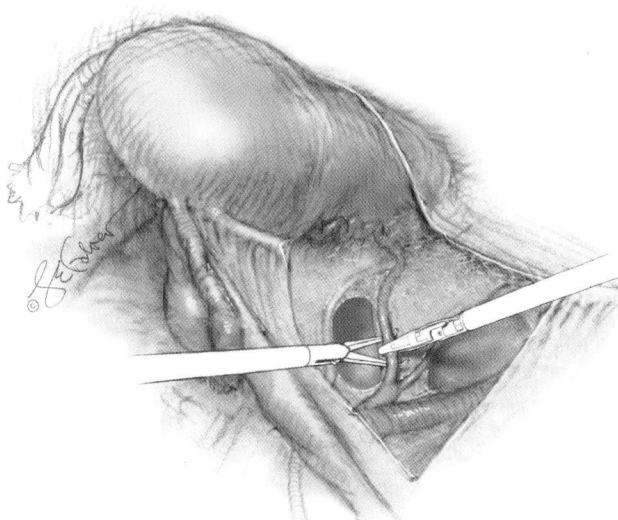

FIGURE 46-3.7 Uterine artery ligation.

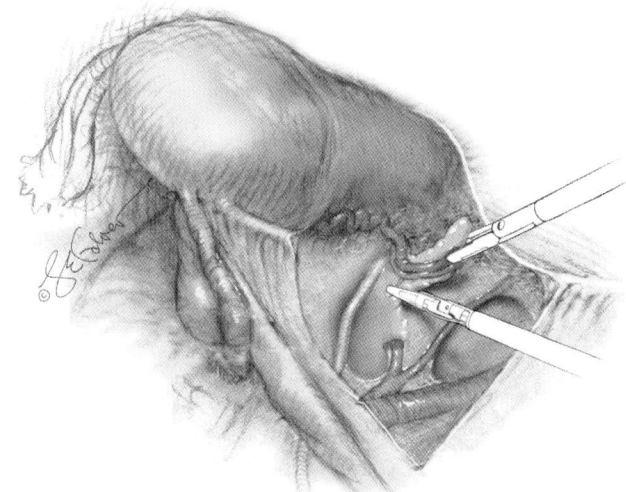

FIGURE 46-3.8 Lifting the parametrium off the ureter.

toward its bifurcation, a surgeon can identify the internal iliac artery. The first anterior branch of the internal iliac artery is the umbilical artery. The uterine artery is the second branch and courses medially and over the ureter.

Alternatively, to isolate the uterine artery, the superior vesical artery is identified by blunt dissection on the medial border of the paravesical space. The vessel is followed cephalad to identify the uterine artery origin. In most instances, the uterine artery originates from the internal iliac artery and is identified by its medial course toward and over the ureter.

To isolate the uterine artery for ligation at its origin from the internal iliac artery, tips of a grasper are positioned beneath the vessel. Opening and closing the grasper tips, while directing dissection downward, develops an avascular plane around the artery. Importantly, the uterine vein lies just beneath the artery, and its injury can compromise visibility from brisk bleeding. Once isolated, the uterine artery is coagulated using a vessel-sealing device and divided (Fig. 46-3.7). The artery ends are then elevated to identify the uterine vein, which is similarly isolated, coagulated, and divided.

❽ Ureteral Mobilization and Parametrial Dissection. Ultimately, during a radical procedure, the ureter is freed in stages from surrounding tissue until its insertion into the bladder is reached. This dissection allows the ureter to be reflected laterally and protected during the wide parametrial excision required for radical hysterectomy.

During early dissection, atraumatic graspers tent up the medial posterior peritoneal leaf to which the ureter is attached. The tips of a right-angle grasper are then positioned between the ureter and peritoneum. Opening and closing the tips downward and parallel to the ureter develops an avascular plane to dissect the ureter free.

Such dissection continues caudally until parametrial tissue surrounding the ureter is met. This tissue is confined between the paravesical and pararectal spaces, contains the divided uterine vessels, and will be dissected medially and up and off the ureter. For this, connective tissue around the medial coagulated end of the uterine artery is grasped laterally and then lifted up and medially (Fig. 46-3.8). Loose connective tissue bands holding the artery and vein and surrounding parametria to the pelvic floor are coagulated and sharply transected. Dissection is continued medially until the lateral border of the ureter is reached.

For ureterolysis, caudally directed tips of a Maryland grasper are insinuated and opened within the avascular space overlying the ureter. This exposes tissue pedicles on the ureter's lateral aspect, which are then coagulated and cut. The uterine vessels and parametrium are then pulled medially and reflected off the ureter. They will be removed with the final specimen.

During continued caudal ureterolysis, the ureter is seen to enter a "tunnel" within the pubocervical ligament (Fig. 46-3.9). To open this tunnel and free the ureter, the ureter is retracted downward and laterally. Within the tunnel, caudally directed grasper

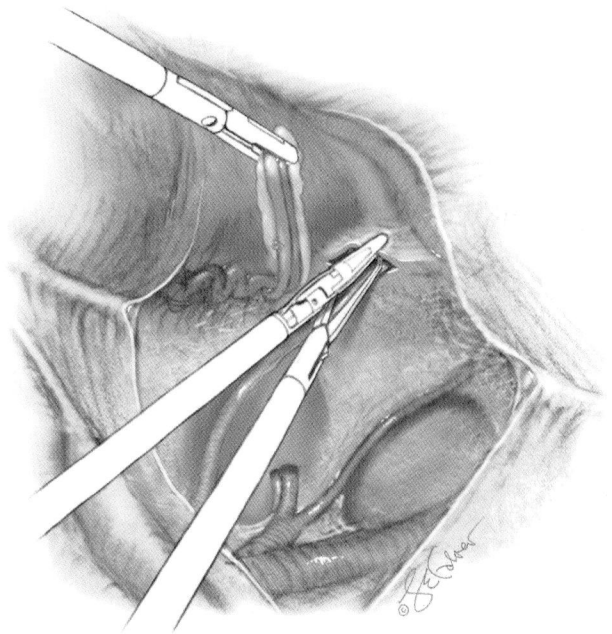

FIGURE 46-3.9 Unroofing the ureter.

tips are insinuated and opened within the space overlying the ureter. Tips of an energy-based tool then elevate the tunnel roof above and away from the ureter. This pubocervical ligament roof and the veins within it are then transected. The roof is divided in small increments caudally until completely opened. At this point, the ureteral insertion into the bladder can be identified. The ureter can then be bluntly rolled off the tunnel "floor" and moved laterally with an atraumatic tool to allow later cardinal ligament transection without ureteral injury.

❾ **Adnexectomy or Ovarian Preservation.** The IP ligament or the uteroovarian ligament will be transected depending on whether the ovary is removed or retained, respectively. Steps for both mirror those with benign hysterectomy and are fully illustrated in Section 43-12 (p. 953). For these steps, a window is made in the posterior broad ligament below the IP ligament. The window can be made bluntly or with an energy-based tool, and the window is then enlarged. The incision is opened parallel to the IP ligament and is extended cephalad toward the pelvic brim and medially toward the uterosacral ligament. The ureter should be clearly identified to avoid its injury.

For adnexectomy, the IP ligament is divided with a vessel-sealing device followed by cutting. In contrast, if the ovary is to be preserved, then salpingectomy alone is first completed. For this, the mesosalpinx is divided with a vessel-sealing and cutting device, and resection progresses from the fimbria to its union with the uterus. Next, the uteroovarian ligament is transected with the same device, and the ovary is tucked over to the sidewall until hysterectomy completion.

If ovarian preservation is chosen, the ovary can be transposed laparoscopically. With this, the IP ligament is further dissected cephalad by extending the peritoneal incision on both the medial and lateral sides of the IP ligament. This mobilizes the ovary, whose uteroovarian ligament stump is then sutured to the lateral peritoneum in the upper abdomen as described on page 1138. Importantly, following transposition, the ovary is inspected to confirm adequate blood supply. A clip can be placed at the uteroovarian stump so that it can be delineated on future imaging studies.

At this point, steps 3 through 9 are completed on the contralateral side.

❿ **Rectovaginal Space.** Developing this potential space moves the rectum downward to isolate the uterosacral ligaments for wide resection. It also permits adequate excision of the proximal vagina for tumor-free margins without rectal injury. First, the uterus

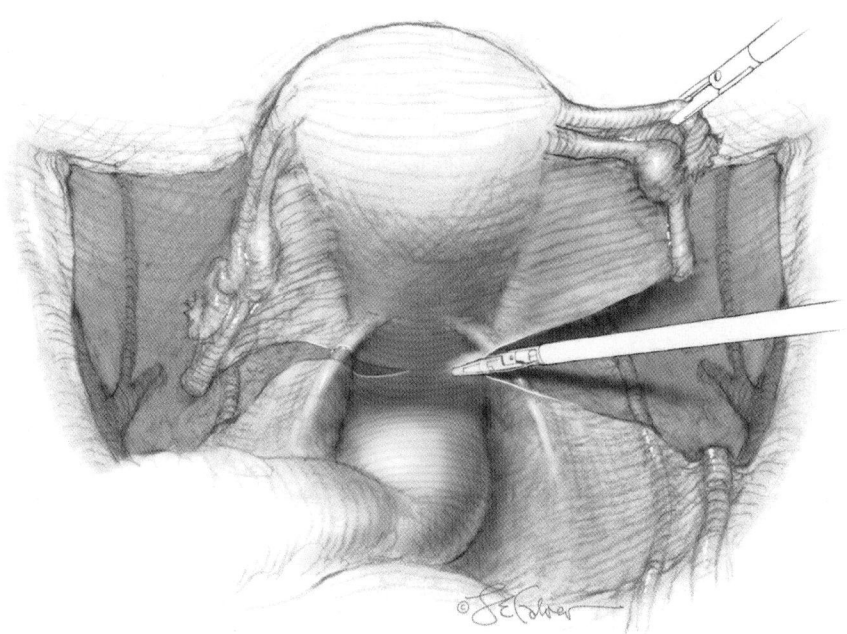

FIGURE 46-3.10 Incising the posterior peritoneum.

is retracted upward in the midline, and the peritoneum between the uterosacral ligaments is incised at the level of the external cervical os (Fig. 46-3.10). The peritoneal edge closer to the rectum is then grasped and tented outward with atraumatic graspers, and the rectovaginal space is open with a blunt dissector moved side to side. This exposes connective tissue bands and small vessels between the rectum and vagina. These bands are cauterized and transected close to the vagina with an energy-based device (Fig. 46-3.11). Dissection continues 4 cm caudally to ultimately allow a 3-cm vaginal resection.

⓫ **Uterosacral Ligament Transection.** The uterosacral ligaments, which are now isolated, can then be ligated as close to the sacrum as possible with an energy-based tool (Fig. 46-3.12). Before division of the ligament, the ureter is retracted laterally for protection.

⓬ **Cardinal Ligament Division.** Next, the lateral attachments of the cervix to the pelvic sidewalls are coagulated and transected with an energy-based device in a caudal direction (Fig. 46-3.13). During this step, the deep uterine vein is usually encountered and should be sufficiently sealed and divided. Also, the

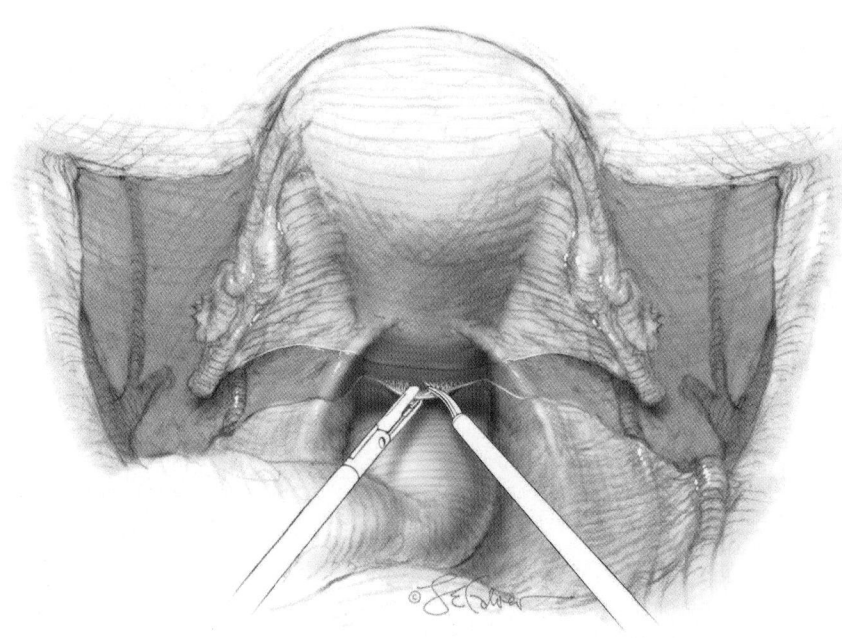

FIGURE 46-3.11 Opening the rectovaginal space.

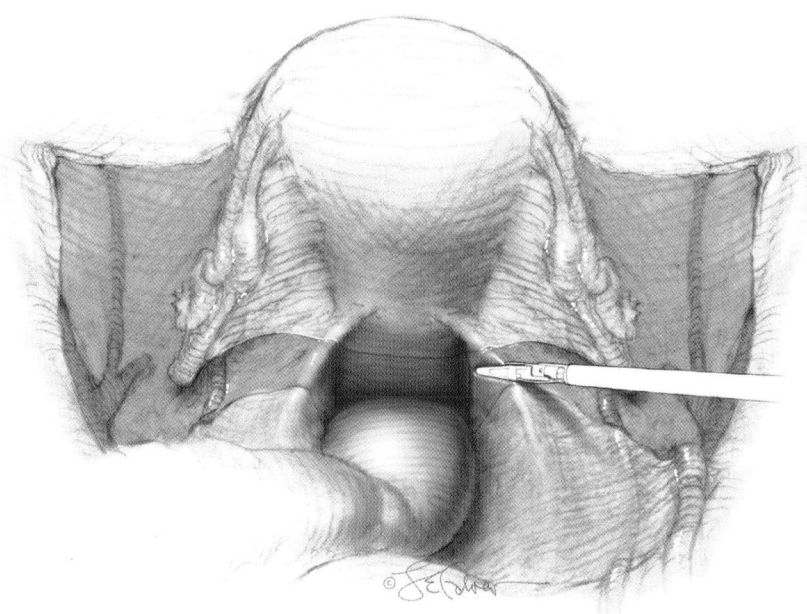

FIGURE 46-3.12 Uterosacral ligament transection.

plane of transection stays at or slightly below the level of the ureter. This avoids extensive autonomic pelvic plexus damage, which exacerbates bladder and possibly bowel and sexual dysfunction.

⑬ Vaginal Resection. With complete mobilization of the bladder and rectum, the anterior and posterior vagina should be easily identified. The radical hysterectomy specimen is now held in place only by the paracolpium and vagina. The goal of radical hysterectomy

resection is to remove approximately 3 cm of the upper vagina. For this, transverse anterior and posterior colpotomy incisions are made and extended circumferentially around the cervix (Fig. 46-3.14). Delineating marks on the uterine manipulator can help direct colpotomy.

The uterus, cervix, vaginal margin, and parametrial tissue are then freed. The specimen is removed intact through the vagina. The final specimen is labeled "radical hysterectomy specimen" and includes cervix,

uterus, vaginal margin, and parametrial tissue (Fig. 46-3.15).

⑭ Vaginal Cuff Closure. Closure of the vaginal cuff can be performed by multiple methods. As noted earlier, one option is cuff closure from a vaginal approach as done during simple vaginal hysterectomy (Section 43-13, p. 961). Alternatively, suitable endoscopic closure techniques are described and detailed in Section 44-11 (p. 1034). Following cuff closure, lymphadenectomy is begun and is described in Section 46-12 (p. 1176).

Both the ureters and bladder can be injured during these procedures. If injury is suspected, cystoscopy at the end of the procedure can aid injury recognition (Section 45-1, p. 1057).

⑮ Port Removal and Fascial Closure. Once procedures have been completed, an inspection for hemostasis is performed. Ports are then removed under direct visualization. All fascial defects larger than 10 mm are closed with 0-gauge delayed-absorbable suture to avoid hernia development at the site. Various methods of skin closure are described in Chapter 40 (p. 847).

POSTOPERATIVE

Immediate postoperative care following minimally invasive radical hysterectomy in general mirrors that for other minimally invasive procedures. Diet is advanced more quickly than with open procedures, and

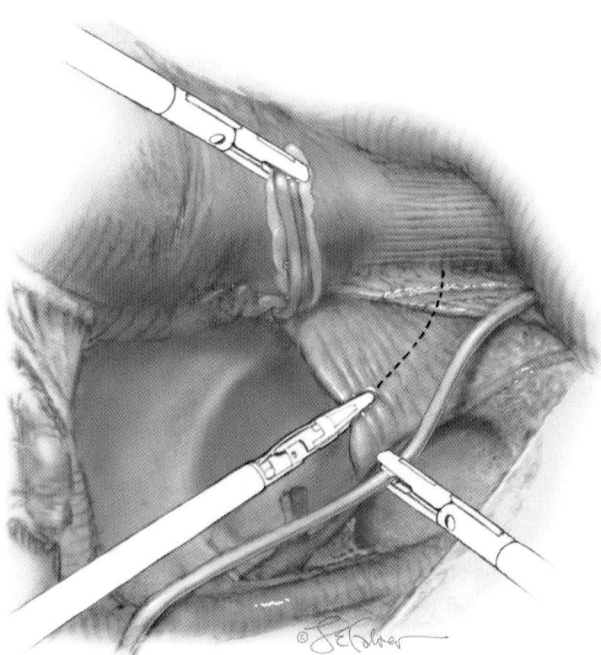

FIGURE 46-3.13 Paracolpium transected.

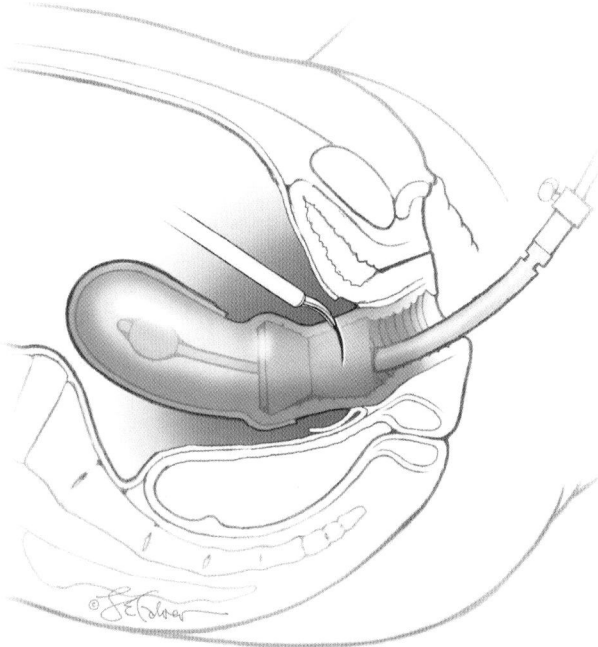

FIGURE 46-3.14 Colpotomy created.

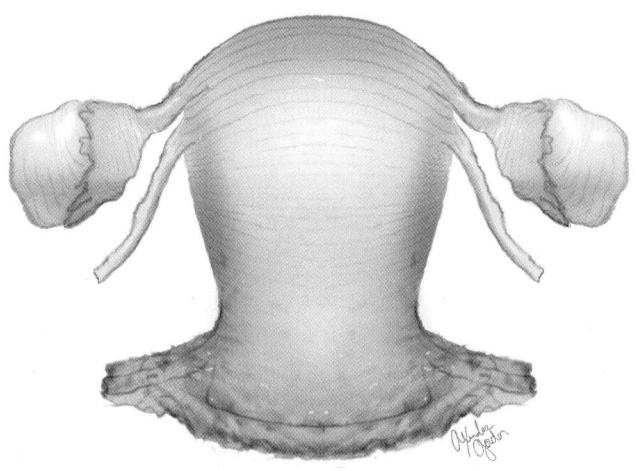

FIGURE 46-3.15 Anterior view of a radical hysterectomy specimen including uterus, cervix, portion of vagina, and parametria.

most patients will tolerate a regular diet early on postoperative day 1. Patients are often discharged home on postoperative day 1 or 2 since their pain is well controlled. As with open radical procedures, the same principles for retaining a Foley catheter do apply. Therefore, many patients will be sent home with the Foley catheter and return to clinic for a voiding trial (Chap. 42, p. 917).

Following minimally invasive radical hysterectomy, patients may be at increased risk for vaginal cuff dehiscence compared with an open approach. In one series, the rate was 1.7 percent and was similar whether surgery was completed laparoscopically or robotically (Nick, 2011). The closure technique of the vaginal cuff is the suggested cause. Thus, many advocate vaginal rather than endoscopic cuff closure to decrease this risk (Fanning, 2013; Uccella, 2011).

Total Pelvic Exenteration

Total pelvic exenteration removes the bladder, rectum, uterus (if present), and surrounding tissues. It is generally indicated for curative situations when less radical surgery, chemotherapy, or radiation options have been exhausted. The most common indication is centrally persistent or recurrent cervical cancer after radiation therapy. Less frequent indications include some instances of recurrent endometrial adenocarcinoma, uterine sarcoma, or vulvar cancer; locally advanced carcinoma of the cervix, vagina, or endometrium when radiation is contraindicated such as prior radiotherapy or malignant fistula; and melanoma of the vagina or urethra (Berek, 2005; Goldberg, 2006; Maggioni, 2009). Palliative exenterations may be of benefit on rare occasions when selected patients have severe, unrelenting symptoms (Guimarães, 2011).

Because exenteration commonly follows radiation therapy, the uterus and cervix usually have lost their distinct tissue architecture and boundaries. As a result, traditional hysterectomy steps and anatomic landmark identification are typically not possible. Minimally invasive exenterative procedures have been reported and may rarely be indicated in highly selected patients (Martinez, 2011; Puntambekar, 2006).

Total pelvic exenterations are subclassified based on the extent of pelvic floor muscle and vulvar resection (Table 46-4.1) (Magrina, 1997). Supralevator (type I) exenteration may be indicated when a lesion is relatively small and does not involve the lower half of the vagina. Most total pelvic exenterations will be infralevator (type II). This type is selected if vaginal contracture, prior hysterectomy, or the inability to otherwise achieve adequate margins is present. Rarely, tumor extension warrants an infralevator exenteration with vulvectomy (type III).

PREOPERATIVE

Patient Evaluation

Initially, biopsy confirmation of recurrent invasive disease is performed. With confirmation, the single most important preoperative challenge is to search for metastatic disease that would abort plans for surgery. Chest radiography is mandatory. Abdominopelvic CT is also routinely indicated, but a positron emission tomography (PET) scan may be particularly helpful (Chung, 2006; Husain, 2007). Hydroureter and hydronephrosis are not absolute contraindications unless they are due to obvious pelvic sidewall disease.

Patients often initially reject the entire concept of this operation even when faced with the knowledge that it represents their only chance for cure. Counseling is essential, and overcoming denial may take several visits. Regardless, not all eligible women will wish to proceed.

Consent

The consenting process is the ideal time to finalize plans for the type and location of urinary conduit, plans for colostomy or low rectal anastomoses, and need for vaginal reconstruction or other ancillary procedures. A patient is also advised that the procedure may need to be aborted based on intraoperative findings.

For those who undergo exenteration, the perioperative mortality rate approaches 5 percent (Marnitz, 2006; Sharma, 2005). However, the mortality rate from progressive cancer would otherwise be 100 percent. Patients should be prepared for admission to an intensive care unit (ICU) postoperatively. Infection, wound breakdown, bowel obstruction, and venous thromboembolic events are common short-term complications. Additionally, intestinal fistulas or anastomotic leaks or strictures may develop. Reoperation may be required. Most women will experience significant morbidity and unforeseen complications (Berek, 2005; Goldberg, 2006; Maggioni, 2009). Preexisting medical problems, morbid obesity, and malnutrition increase these risks.

Long-term effects on sexual function and other body functions are candidly reviewed. Patients with two ostomies have a lower quality of life and poorer body image. However, in those who retain vaginal capacity, quality of life and sexual function is reportedly improved compared with those without reconstruction. Thus, counseling regarding vaginal reconstruction is part of the preoperative dialogue (Section 46-9, p. 1165). In general, a woman returns to baseline functioning within a year postoperatively, but quality of life is often affected by worries regarding tumor progression (Hawighorst-Knapstein, 1997; Rezk, 2013). Patients should be aware that more than half will develop recurrent disease despite exenterative surgery (Benn, 2011; Westin, 2014).

Patient Preparation

Prior to surgery, stoma sites are marked, the consent form is reviewed, and final questions are answered. To minimize fecal contamination during bowel excision, aggressive bowel preparation such as with a polyethylene glycol with electrolyte solution (GoLYTELY) is mandatory. Ileus is common following exenteration and nutritional demands are increased. Thus, total parenteral nutrition (TPN) is often initiated as early as possible when needed. In addition, routine antibiotic prophylaxis has been shown to decrease infectious complications (Goldberg, 1998). Pneumatic compression devices or subcutaneous heparin is particularly important due to the anticipated long operation and extended postoperative recovery. Patients are typed and crossmatched for potential blood product replacement. Critical care team consultation may be indicated, and an ICU bed is requested.

INTRAOPERATIVE

Instruments

To prepare for complicated resections, a surgeon should have access to all types and sizes of bowel staplers. These include end-to-end anastomosis (EEA), gastrointestinal anastomosis (GIA), and transverse anastomosis (TA) staplers. Additionally, an electrothermal bipolar coagulator (LigaSure) may speed pedicle ligation while decreasing blood loss (Slomovitz, 2006).

Surgical Steps

❶ **Anesthesia and Patient Positioning.** General anesthesia with or without epidural placement for postoperative pain management is mandatory. An arterial line for monitoring is typically added as a necessary precaution. Bimanual examination is performed to

TABLE 46-4.1. Differences among Type I (Supralevator), Type II (Infralevator), and Type III (with Vulvectomy) Pelvic Exenterations

Pelvic Structure	Degree of Resection		
	Type I	**Type II**	**Type III**
Viscera	Above levator	Below levator	Below levator
Levator ani muscles	None	Limited	Complete
Perineal membrane	None	Limited	Complete
Vulvoperineal tissues	None	None	Complete

reorient a surgeon to a patient's individual anatomy. The abdomen, perineum, and vagina are surgically prepared, and a Foley catheter is inserted. Legs should be positioned in low lithotomy in booted support stirrups to permit adequate perineal access.

❷ Abdominal Entry. The type of abdominal entry may be dictated by an intended rectus abdominis flap, which requires a low transverse incision. Otherwise, a midline vertical incision is ideal. A less commonly employed option is to initially assess by laparoscopy a patient's suitability for exenteration. This minimally invasive approach may avoid unnecessary laparotomy in up to half of candidate patients (Kohler, 2002; Plante, 1998).

❸ Exploration. The most common reason that exenterations are aborted is the presence of metastatic peritoneal disease (Miller, 1993). Thus, following positioning of an abdominal self-retaining retractor, a surgeon thoroughly explores for disseminated disease that may not have been suspected preoperatively. Typically, numerous adhesions must also be lysed to inspect and palpate abdominal contents. Suspicious lesions are removed or biopsied.

❹ Lymph Node Dissection. A significant number of exenterations will be aborted intraoperatively due to identification of lymph node metastases (Miller, 1993). For this reason, pelvic and paraaortic node sampling and frozen section analysis is performed to exclude metastatic disease before proceeding. Additionally, retroperitoneal dissection provides a surgeon with a sense of the degree of pelvic sidewall fibrosis, which may render the vessels, ureters, and other important structures virtually indistinguishable from the surrounding soft tissue.

❺ Pelvic Sidewall Exploration. As described in Section 46-1 (p. 1135), the retroperitoneum is entered and the external iliac and internal iliac artery bifurcation is bluntly dissected free of overlying areolar connective tissue. The ureter is placed on a Penrose drain for identification. The paravesical and pararectal spaces are developed.

Parametrial tumor extension is the third most common reason for aborting exenteration (Miller, 1993). Thus, the pelvic sidewall should be verified to be clinically free of disease by inserting one finger into the paravesical space, another into the pararectal space, and palpating the intervening tissue down to the levator plate. There must be a grossly negative margin at the pelvic sidewall to proceed. Tissues may be biopsied and frozen section analysis performed to confirm this impression. Often, it is difficult to know with absolute certainty whether the margins are clear due to the varying extent of retroperitoneal fibrosis encountered.

❻ Bladder Mobilization. The bladder blade is removed from the self-retaining retractor to permit entry into the space of Retzius and blunt reflection of the bladder from the back of the pubic symphysis. To achieve this, downward traction on the bladder and urethra will expose filmy attachments that may be electrosurgically incised (Fig. 46-4.1). Laterally positioned false ligaments of the bladder are divided between clamps or transected with an electrothermal bipolar coagulator. This joins the retropubic and paravesical spaces. The bladder should be floppy in the pelvis from loss of its supporting pelvic attachments and is completely freed ventrally. However, the urethra is still attached to the bladder.

❼ Rectal Mobilization. Following mobilization of the bladder, the ureters are held laterally, and the overlying peritoneum at the pelvic brim is divided on each side in a medial direction up to the sigmoid colon mesentery. By inserting a finger into each pararectal space and sweeping medially, it should be possible to develop the avascular plane between the rectosigmoid and the sacrum (retrorectal space).

Surgeons should be confident that there is no sacral tumor invasion and that they will be able to lift the rectosigmoid out of the pelvis to achieve a posterior margin that is tumor free. This is the last decision to be made before dividing the bowel and beginning steps of the operation that are irreversible.

Once all the tumor boundaries have been assessed, exenteration proceeds by dividing the sigmoid colon with a GIA stapler and dividing the intervening mesenteric tissue (Section 46-21, p. 1201). The proximal sigmoid colon is then packed into the upper abdomen. The distal rectosigmoid is held ventrally and cephalad while a hand is inserted posteriorly to bluntly dissect the adventitial tissue between the rectum and sacrum in the midline (Fig. 46-4.2). This maneuver is continued distally to the coccyx

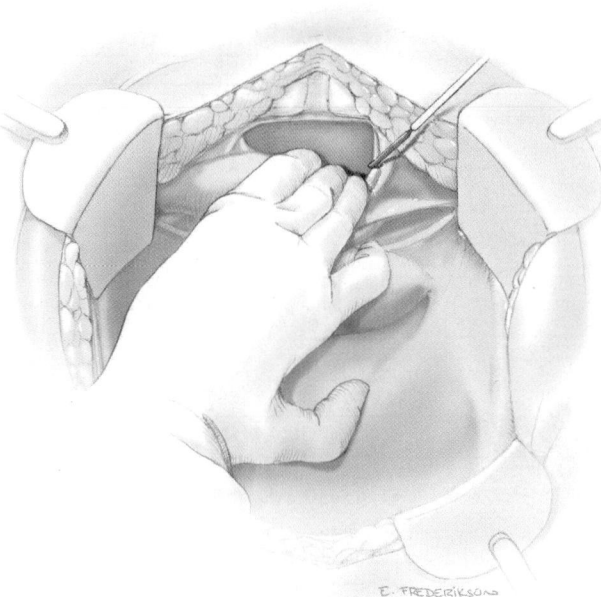

FIGURE 46-4.1 Mobilizing the bladder.

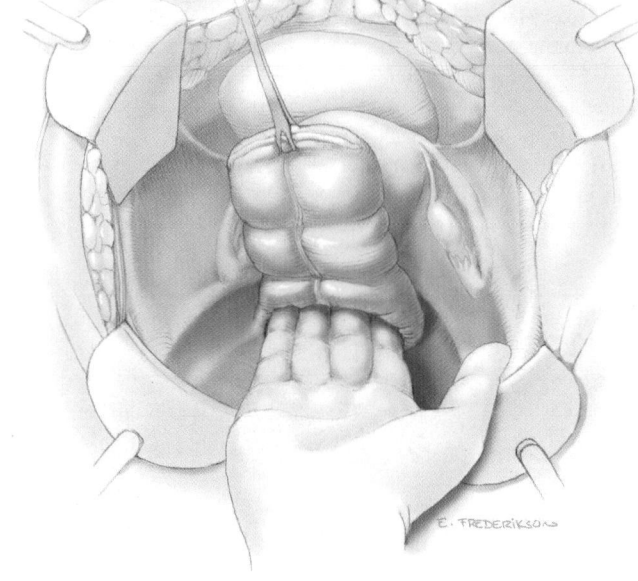

FIGURE 46-4.2 Mobilizing the rectum.

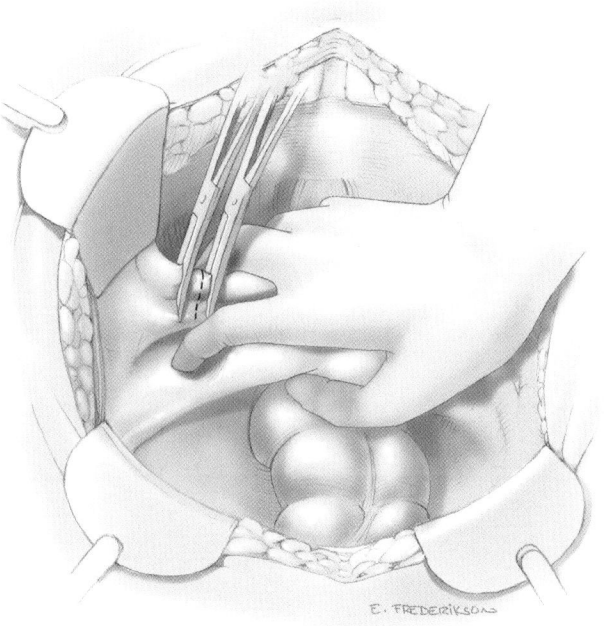

FIGURE 46-4.3 Dividing the cardinal ligaments.

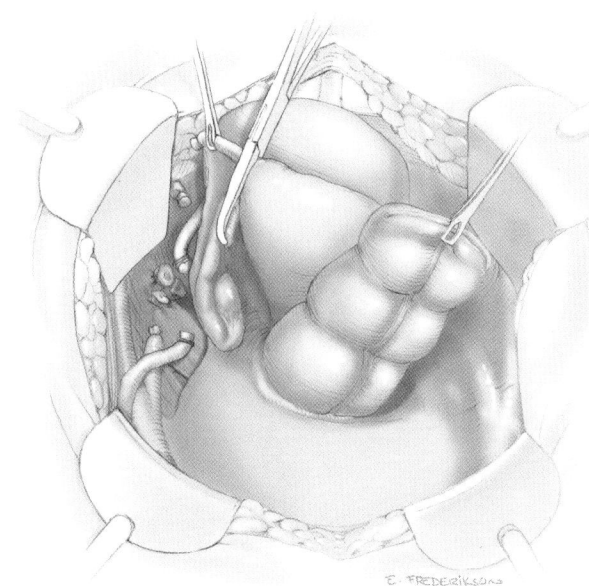

FIGURE 46-4.4 Dividing the hypogastric vessels and ureter.

to develop the retrorectal space and isolate the laterally located rectal pillars.

❽ Cardinal Ligament Division. The mobilized bladder and distal rectum with uterus (if present) are held together on contralateral traction, while a hand is placed with one finger in the paravesical space and the other in the pararectal space to isolate the lateral pelvic attachments. The cardinal ligaments, internal iliac vessels, and ureter are often not distinguishable in a typically radiated field, but lie within this tissue.

Beginning anteriorly, these fibrous attachments are serially divided at the pelvic sidewall (Fig. 46-4.3). Vascular clips should be available in case of tissue slippage or inadvertent bleeding.

❾ Internal Iliac Vessels and Ureter Division. As the pelvic sidewall dissection continues dorsally, the anterior branches of the internal iliac artery, venous channels, and distal ureter ideally are individually located and ligated to optimize hemostasis (Fig. 46-4.4). However, blood vessels and

ureters frequently will lie within fibrous tissue and may be relatively indistinguishable. Thus, clamps or the electrothermal bipolar coagulator are placed around smaller pedicles to minimize the possibility of inadvertent blood loss. At minimum, the ureter is located, isolated, and divided as distally as possible to provide extra length for reaching the urinary conduit. Later, any damage at the distal tip can be trimmed as needed to ensure healthy tissue for urinary conduit creation. A large vascular clip is placed on the proximal end of the ureter to distend the lumen

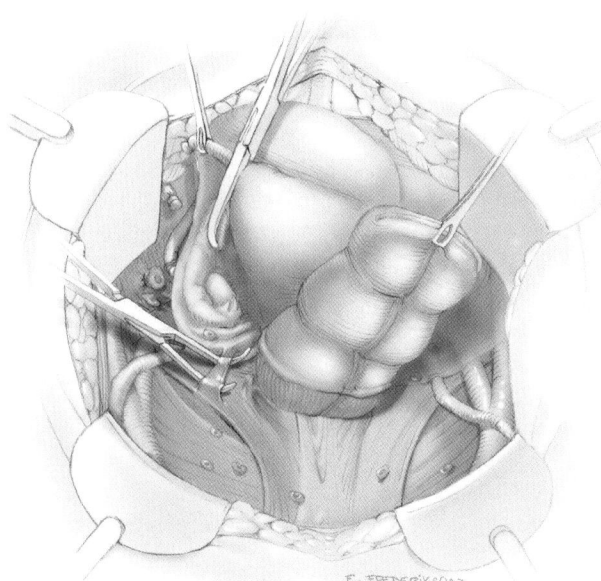

FIGURE 46-4.5 Dividing the rectal pillars.

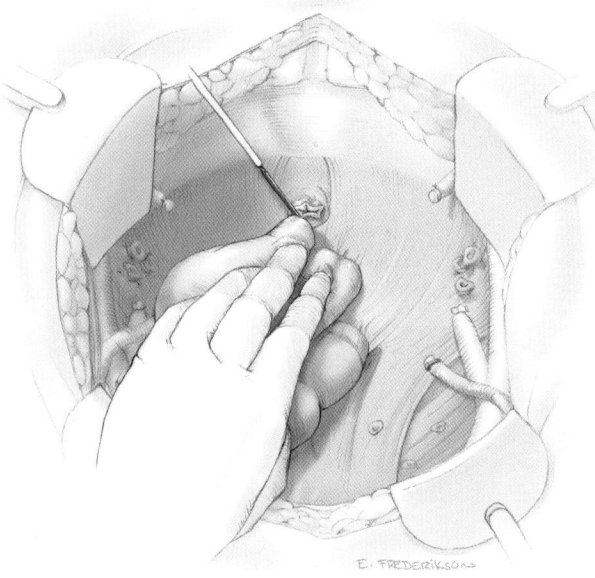

FIGURE 46-4.6 Supralevator exenteration: dividing the urethra.

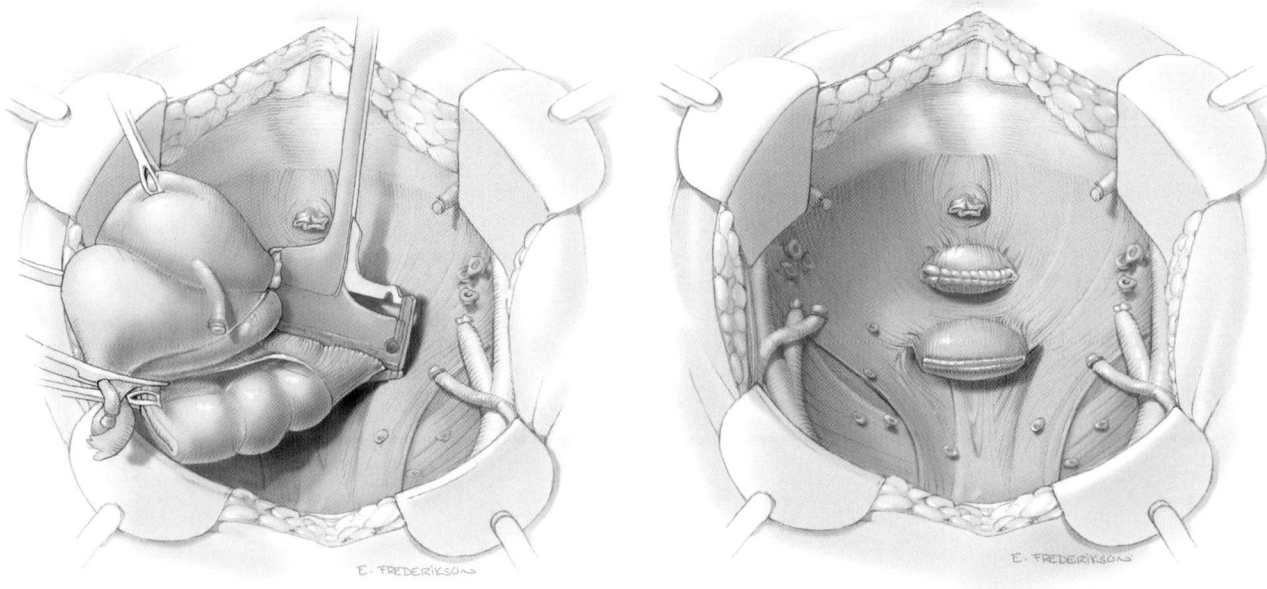

FIGURE 46-4.7 Supralevator exenteration: dividing the rectum.   **FIGURE 46-4.8** Supralevator exenteration: appearance of the pelvic floor.

and aid later anastomosis into the planned conduit. Dissection is then repeated on the contralateral side, and any remaining lateral attachments along the levator ani muscles are divided as the pelvic floor curves toward the perineum.

❿ Rectal Pillar Division. The exenteration specimen is now chiefly tethered by the rectal stalks and distal mesenteric attachments posteriorly. These can be skeletonized with a right-angle clamp and divided along the pelvic floor (Fig. 46-4.5). This maneuver is continued distally to expose the entire posterior pelvic floor. The exenteration specimen is then circumferentially inspected and additional dissection is performed to completely release it from all attachments leading through the levator ani muscles. At this point, steps diverge depending on whether supralevator or infralevator exenteration is planned.

⓫ Supralevator Exenteration: Final Steps. Removal of the specimen above the levator muscles begins by posterior traction on the bladder. The Foley catheter should be palpable within the urethra, and all surrounding tissue should already be dissected away. An electrosurgical blade is used to transect the distal urethra (Fig. 46-4.6). The distal opening does not require closure and may function as a natural orifice drain postoperatively. Next, the vagina is transected and then closed with 0-gauge delayed-absorbable suture in a running fashion. The transverse anastomosis (TA) or curved cutter stapler

(Contour) is placed across the distal rectum and fired (Fig. 46-4.7). This completes detachment of the specimen, which includes bladder, uterus, rectum, and surrounding tissue. The pelvic floor is then carefully assessed to identify bleeding points (Fig. 46-4.8). A laparotomy pad is packed firmly into the pelvis to tamponade any surface oozing, while the exenteration specimen is inspected to confirm grossly negative margins.

⓬ Infralevator Exenteration: Perineal Phase. With infralevator exenteration, once abdominal dissection reaches the levator muscles, a second surgical team begins the perineal phase. The use of two teams typically shortens operative time and reduces bleeding. The planned perineal resection is outlined to encompass the tumor. As shown in Figure 46-4.9, resection may require infralevator exenteration with or without vulvectomy.

The perineal incision ideally begins concomitantly with division of the levator muscles

by the abdominal team. At the perineum, a skin incision is first performed, followed by use of an electrosurgical blade to dissect through the subcutaneous tissues surrounding the urethra, vaginal opening, and anus.

⓭ Infralevator Exenteration: Partial Resection of the Levator Muscles. Within the abdomen, the primary surgical team places the specimen on traction. Electrosurgical blade dissection is used to circumferentially incise the levator muscles lateral to the area of tumor extension (Fig. 46-4.10). The dissection proceeds distally toward the perineum.

⓮ Infralevator Exenteration: Connecting the Perineal and Abdominal Spaces. After the perineal incision has reached the fascial plane, four spaces are developed: subpubic space, left and right vaginal spaces, and retrorectal space. It is helpful to have the abdominal surgeon place a hand deep into

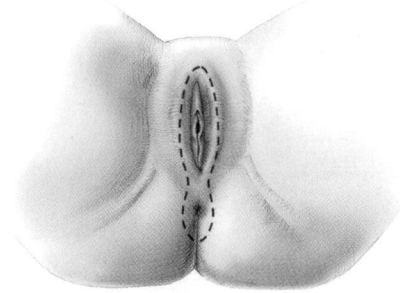
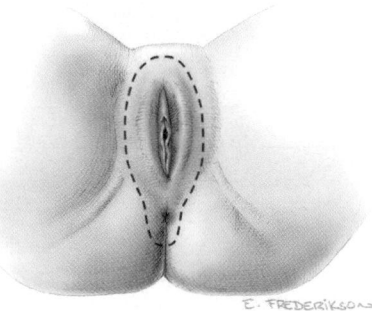

FIGURE 46-4.9 Infralevator exenteration: perineal phase incisions.

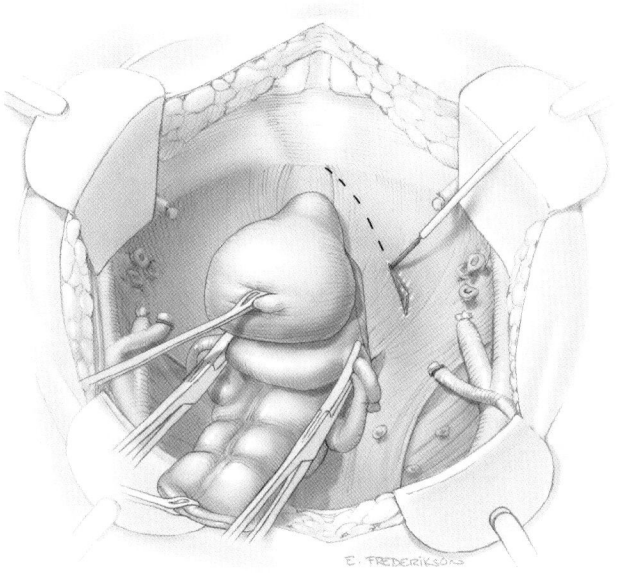

FIGURE 46-4.10 Infralevator exenteration: partial resection of the levator muscles.

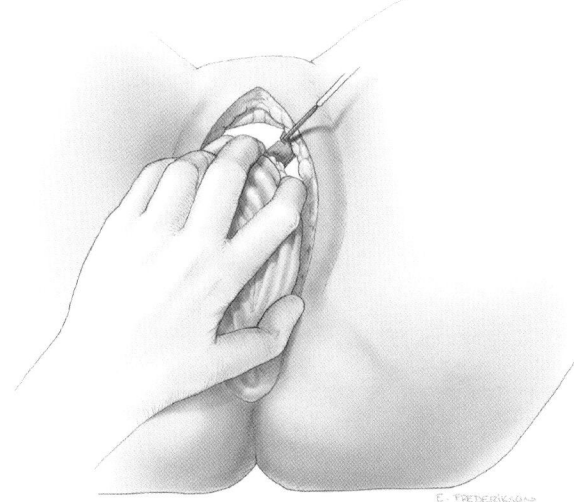

FIGURE 46-4.11 Infralevator exenteration: connecting the perineal and abdominal spaces.

the pelvis and guide the electrosurgical dissection by the perineal team (Fig. 46-4.11). Five pedicles are identified that separate these avascular spaces: two pubourethral pedicles, two rectal pillar pedicles, and the midline posterior anococcygeal pedicle. Electrosurgical dissection that is directed by the abdominal surgeon's finger is performed to open the intervening spaces. From below, the five vascular pedicles are divided and ligated using the electrothermal bipolar coagulator.

⑮ Infralevator Exenteration: Removal of the Specimen. Circumferential dissection will result in complete detachment of the specimen that can be removed either vaginally or abdominally (Fig. 46-4.12). Hemostasis is

then achieved with a series of sutures, vascular clips, or clamps and ties. Finally, the pelvic floor and pedicle sites are carefully reinspected (Fig. 46-4.13).

⑯ Infralevator Exenteration: Simple Closure. If vaginal reconstruction in not planned, the most straightforward and quickest way to close the perineum is for the second team to perform a layered closure of the deep tissues with 0-gauge delayed-absorbable suture (Fig. 46-4.14). The perineal skin is

closed with the same type of delayed-absorbable suture in a running fashion.

⑰ Final Steps. A dry laparotomy pad may be held firmly deep in the pelvis to tamponade surface oozing, while the conduit, colostomy or bowel anastomosis, other surgical procedures, or vaginal reconstruction are performed. In some instances, intraoperative radiation therapy may be a useful adjunct for an obviously positive or clinically suspicious resection margin (Backes, 2014; Foley, 2014; Koh,

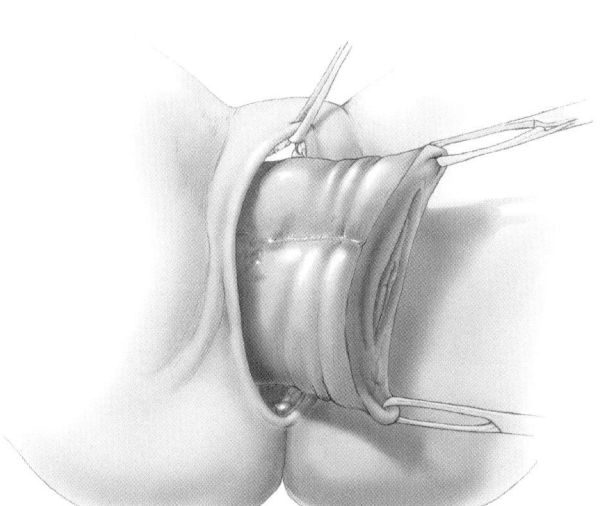

FIGURE 46-4.12 Infralevator exenteration: removal of the specimen.

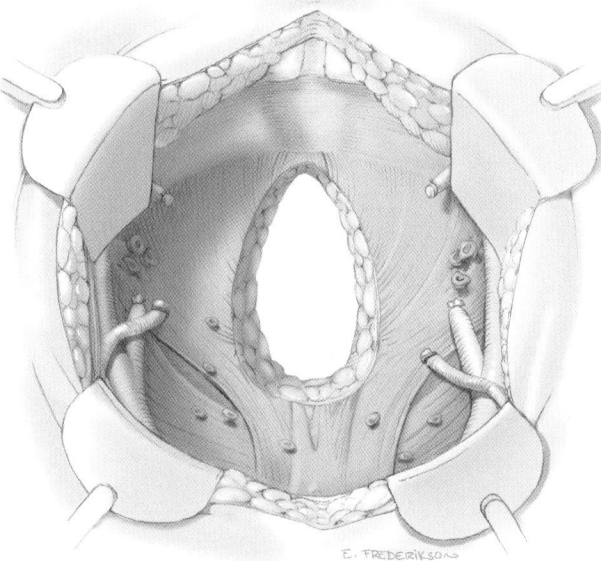

FIGURE 46-4.13 Infralevator exenteration: pelvic floor.

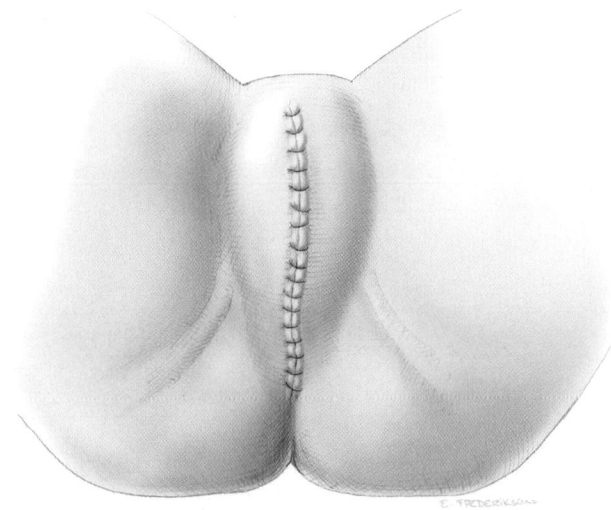

FIGURE 46-4.14 Infralevator exenteration: simple perineal closure.

2015). An omental J-flap may provide additional blood supply to the irradiated, denuded pelvic floor (Section 46-14, p. 1186). The type of postoperative suction drainage may be dictated by these ancillary procedures but should be used judiciously (Goldberg, 2006).

POSTOPERATIVE

The morbidity of total pelvic exenteration depends on various factors, which include preoperative health of the patient, intraoperative events, extent of the procedure, ancillary procedures, and postoperative vigilance. Hospitals that treat a relatively high volume of such patients report lower surgical in-hospital mortality rates (Maggioni, 2009). However, unlike a few decades ago, few institutions perform this operation on a regular basis.

The immediate life-threatening concerns are massive bleeding, acute respiratory distress syndrome, pulmonary embolism, and myocardial infarction (Fotopoulou, 2010). Every effort is made to encourage early ambulation as soon as the patient is stable. A prolonged ileus or partial small bowel obstruction will typically respond to expectant management but may require TPN for weeks. Intestinal fistulas and leaks are more common when using mesh to cover the pelvic floor or when performing low rectal anastomoses. Omental pedicle grafts and rectus abdominis or gracilis myocutaneous flaps may prevent such complications. Pelvic abscess and septicemia are additional subacute complications that develop commonly (Berek, 2005; Goldberg, 2006; Maggioni, 2009).

Anterior Pelvic Exenteration

Removal of the uterus, vagina, bladder, urethra, distal ureters, and parametrial tissues with preservation of the rectum is meant to be a less morbid operation than total pelvic exenteration (Section 46-4, p. 1149). Patients are carefully selected for this more limited procedure to still achieve negative surgical margins. Women who have previously had a hysterectomy are not usually good candidates, because a complete resection of a central recurrence involving the vaginal cuff would typically require removal of both bladder and rectosigmoid colon. The most common indications include small recurrences confined to the cervix or anterior vagina after pelvic radiation. In gynecologic oncology, up to half of all exenterations performed are anterior (Berek, 2005; Maggioni, 2009).

PREOPERATIVE

The preoperative evaluation is similar to that described for total pelvic exenteration (Section 46-4, p. 1149). Although preservation of the rectum is planned, patients are advised that potentially unforeseen clinical circumstances may dictate bowel resection and colostomy or low rectal anastomosis. Accordingly, a complete bowel preparation is still mandatory.

INTRAOPERATIVE

Surgical Steps

❶ **Initial Steps.** Anterior exenteration is technically similar to total pelvic exenteration, described earlier. Patients are positioned in low lithotomy in booted support stirrups, the appropriate skin incision is made, the abdomen is explored, lymph nodes are removed, and spaces are developed to exclude metastatic or unresectable disease. The procedure begins to differ after the bladder has been mobilized. A surgeon then makes the final decision to leave the rectum intact and proceed with anterior pelvic exenteration.

❷ **Developing the Rectovaginal Space.** Instead of mobilizing the rectum and dividing the sigmoid colon, the rectovaginal space is developed much as in a type III radical hysterectomy. The uterosacral ligament and the entire length of the rectal pillars are divided to free the exenteration specimen posteriorly.

❸ **Lateral Pelvic Attachments.** The mobilized bladder and uterus are held medially to

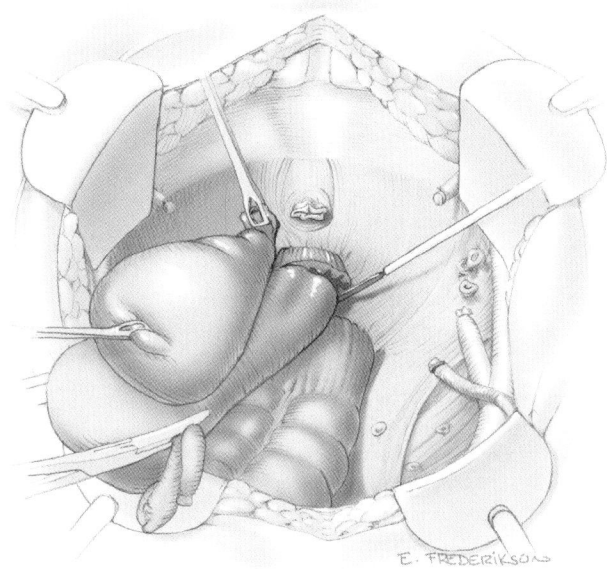

FIGURE 46-5.1 Removal of the specimen.

aid in isolation of the cardinal ligaments, internal iliac vessels, and ureter. These structures are successively divided with an electrothermal bipolar coagulator (LigaSure) or clamped, cut, and individually ligated.

❹ **Removal of the Specimen.** After the anterior pelvic exenteration specimen has been completely mobilized, the urethra and vagina are divided (Figs. 46-5.1 and 46-5.2). The urethra is left open, and the vaginal cuff is closed with 0-gauge delayed-absorbable suture in a running fashion.

❺ **Final Steps.** Typically, the lesion is small and lies above the levator ani muscles, thus a perineal phase is not required. For

this reason, placement of a myocutaneous flap for vaginal reconstruction may be more problematic in these patients due to limited space in the pelvis.

POSTOPERATIVE

Morbidity of anterior pelvic exenteration is comparable with that of total pelvic exenteration (Section 46-4, p. 1149) (Sharma, 2005). Ideally, the operation is shorter and restoration of bowel function is more rapid. Some patients will experience tenesmus or long-term rectal symptoms that likely stem from interruption of the autonomic nervous system in surrounding tissue.

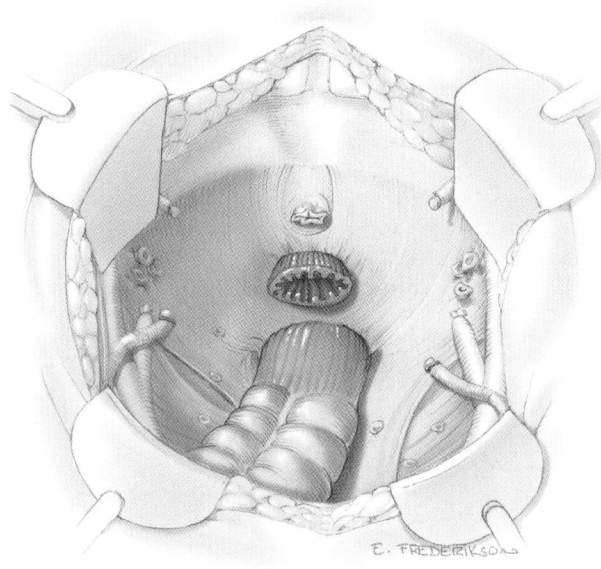

FIGURE 46-5.2 Appearance of the pelvic floor.

46-6

Posterior Pelvic Exenteration

Removal of the uterus, vagina, rectum, and parametrial tissues with preservation of the ureters and bladder is meant to be a less morbid operation than total pelvic exenteration (Section 46-4, p. 1149). Patients are carefully selected for this more limited procedure to still achieve negative surgical margins. For this reason, women who have previously had a hysterectomy are not usually good candidates. The most common indications include small postirradiation recurrences primarily involving the posterior vaginal wall or coexisting with a rectovaginal fistula. In gynecologic oncology, fewer than 10 percent of exenterations are posterior (Berek, 2005; Maggioni, 2009).

PREOPERATIVE

Preoperative evaluation is largely identical to that described for total pelvic exenteration (Section 46-4, p. 1149). A surgeon's judgment and experience are critical in deciding to proceed with a more limited operation. However, patients are advised that potentially unforeseen clinical circumstances may dictate resection of the ureters and bladder with formation of a urinary conduit.

INTRAOPERATIVE

Surgical Steps

❶ **Initial Steps.** Posterior pelvic exenteration is technically similar to a type III radical hysterectomy but with the addition of rectosigmoid resection and a more extended vaginectomy (Section 46-1, p. 1134). The operation begins as a total pelvic exenteration. Patients are positioned in low lithotomy in booted support stirrups, the appropriate skin incision is made, the abdomen is explored, lymph nodes are removed, and spaces are developed to exclude metastatic or unresectable disease (Section 46-4, p. 1150).

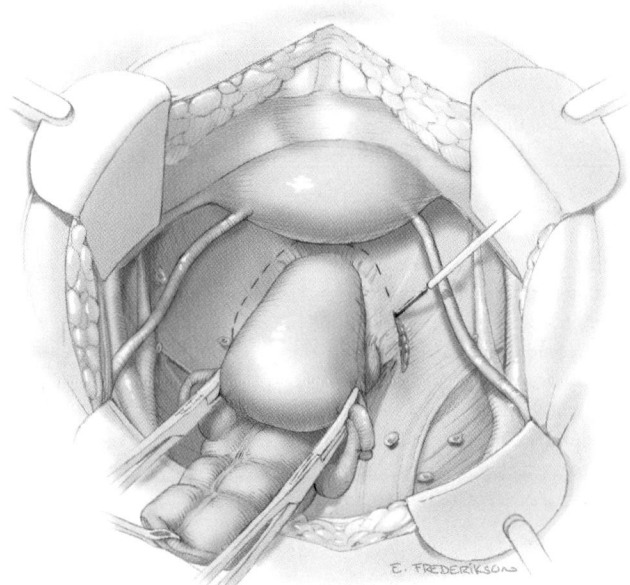

FIGURE 46-6.1 Incising the levator muscles.

A surgeon then makes the final decision to leave the bladder intact and proceed with posterior exenteration.

❷ **Ureteral Dissection.** As with type III radical hysterectomy, the retroperitoneum is entered, ureters are mobilized, uterine arteries are ligated at their internal iliac artery origin, and parametrial tissue is divided at the pelvic sidewall. The bladder is then mobilized away from the cervix and vagina, and ureters are unroofed from the paracervical tunnels. The lateral attachments are then divided all the way to the levator ani muscles. However, typically these steps are much more tedious in a previously irradiated field because of tissue fibrosis and scarring.

❸ **Mobilizing the Rectum.** The sigmoid colon is divided with the mesentery and peritoneal attachments, as described for low anterior resection (p. 1201). The retrorectal space is bluntly dissected to mobilize the rectum and enable transection of the rectal pillars and uterosacral ligaments.

❹ **Removal of the Specimen.** The entire specimen may then be placed on traction to aid placement of the transverse anastomosis (TA) or curved cutter stapler (Contour) and

division of the rectum. The rectum is divided below the tumor to leave grossly negative margins.

To encompass the tumor for removal, dissection is continued circumferentially to (or through) the levator ani muscles (Fig. 46-6.1). The distal vagina is transected and sewn closed in a running fashion with 0-gauge delayed-absorbable suture. The specimen is removed.

❺ **Final Steps.** Typically, the lesion is small and lies above the levator ani muscles, and thus a perineal phase is usually not required. As a result, placement of a myocutaneous flap for vaginal reconstruction may be more problematic in such patients due to limited space in the pelvis.

POSTOPERATIVE

Morbidity of posterior pelvic exenteration is comparable with that of total pelvic exenteration (Section 46-4, p. 1149) (Sharma, 2005). Ideally, the operation is shorter and urinary complications are less frequent. However, posterior exenteration in a previously irradiated patient frequently results in a contracted bladder and intractable urinary incontinence.

Incontinent Urinary Conduit

Removal of the bladder during total or anterior exenteration is the main indication for an incontinent urinary conduit. Less commonly, an otherwise irreparable postirradiation vesicovaginal fistula may warrant urinary diversion. Following cystectomy, an isolated resected segment of bowel that maintains its mesenteric connection and vascular supply is used as the new urine reservoir. A stoma is crafted using one end of the bowel segment and an opening in the anterior abdominal wall. Ureters are reimplanted into the opposite end of this isolated bowel segment.

Various techniques are available to create such urinary conduits, and these are categorized as *incontinent diversions* or *continent diversions*. An incontinent diversion is the simplest to create, but postoperatively a patient must continuously wear an ostomy bag. These conduits are often preferable for medically compromised patients, the elderly, and anyone with a short life expectancy. Alternatively, a continent urinary reservoir can be created that is emptied by intermittent patient self-catheterization of the bowel stoma.

Of incontinent diversions, an *ileal conduit* has historically been the most common urinary diversion used in gynecologic oncology (Goldberg, 2006). However, this bowel segment and distal ureters invariably lie within a previously irradiated field. Conduit construction with radiation-damaged bowel may lead to higher rates of stenosis or leakage at the ureteral anastomotic sites (Pycha, 2008). More recently, the *transverse colon conduit* has proven to be a very successful alternative for previously irradiated patients (Segreti, 1996b; Soper, 1989). *Sigmoid* conduits are generally less desirable due to preexisting radiation damage and proximity to a concurrent colostomy site. The *jejunal conduit* is another rarely used option that typically lies outside the radiation field.

The basic principles of constructing an incontinent urinary conduit are the same, regardless of the intestinal segment used. First, healthy-appearing bowel with a good blood supply is selected. Second, wide-caliber ureterointestinal anastomoses and stenting are essential to minimize the risk of anastomosis stenosis. Third, sufficient mobility of the ureters and bowel segment is important to prevent tension that might lead to anastomotic leaks. Fourth, creation of a straight tunnel through the abdominal wall helps prevent bowel kinking and obstruction.

PREOPERATIVE

Patient Evaluation

The preoperative evaluation is usually dictated by the preceding exenterative procedure. The specific decision is whether to plan for an incontinent or continent urinary conduit. Patients are extensively counseled regarding the differences. The type of conduit selected should be considered permanent, although later conversions are possible (Benezra, 2004).

Consent

Patients are advised that intraoperative findings may dictate revision of an original surgical plan. Postoperatively, urinary infections with or without pyelonephritis are very common with any type of conduit. Anastomotic leaks are less frequent with routine ureteral stent placement but can contribute to a prolonged ileus, the need for CT-guided drainage, or potentially, surgical reexploration with revision. Episodes of small bowel obstruction are possible and often develop at the site where the bowel segment was harvested and the remaining bowel ends were reanastomosed. In the long term, ureteral strictures or stenosis may compromise renal function. Infrequently, reoperation is necessary for complications that do not respond to conservative management (Houvenaeghel, 2004).

Patient Preparation

Bowel preparation is mandatory, but preparation is typically dictated by the preceding exenterative surgery (Section 46-4, p. 1149). Ideally, an enterostomal therapist is available to mark a conduit stoma site, typically on the patient's right side, that is unobstructed in the supine, sitting, and standing positions.

INTRAOPERATIVE

Surgical Steps

❶ **Initial Steps.** To avoid unnecessary traction on its anastomoses, the incontinent urinary conduit is constructed as the last major intraabdominal step during exenterative surgery. Hemostasis is achieved before beginning the conduit. Anesthesia, patient positioning, and skin incisions are typically dictated by the preceding operation.

❷ **Exploration.** The bowel segment for the planned conduit is carefully inspected. It must be healthy appearing, not tethered, and lie close to the distal ureters. The final decision is now made regarding which type of incontinent conduit is best for the circumstances. If the distal ileum has the typical leathery, pale, mottled appearance of radiation injury, a conduit should be prepared from the transverse colon. Overlooking the importance of this decision can lead to various otherwise preventable complications intraoperatively and postoperatively.

❸ **Ileal Conduit: Preparing the Bowel Segment.** The ileocecal junction is located, and the ileum is elevated to identify a bowel segment with the most mobility to reach the right side of the anterior abdominal wall where the stoma will be located. Ideally, the proximal end of the segment lies 25 to 30 cm from the ileocecal valve. At the selected site, the mesentery is scored on each side with an electrosurgical blade to aid insertion of a hemostat directly beneath the bowel loop. A Penrose drain is pulled through to mark this proximal end along the ileum that will eventually become the distal part of the conduit and will form the abdominal wall stoma.

The conduit length depends on subcutaneous tissue depth and ileum mobility but should measure approximately 15 cm. The conduit's butt end will house the ureteral anastomoses and is selected by measuring the ileum that lies distal to the Penrose drain, and again the mesentery is scored. The gastrointestinal anastomosis (GIA) stapler is then inserted to divide the distal bowel segment (Fig. 46-7.1). The point of division should ideally be at least 12 cm from the ileocecal valve. The conduit is remeasured prior to dividing the proximal ileum, to account for possible shrinkage of the intervening segment and to again ensure sufficient length.

Once the bowel is stapled and divided, the conduit mesentery is also carefully divided on each end of the segment. This tissue division is angled inward and toward the base of the mesentery near its insertion to the posterior abdominal wall. This provides adequate mobility. The vasculature may be compromised if too much mesentery is divided, whereas too little will result in tension on the conduit. A perfect balance is required.

When convenient, intestinal continuity, minus the excised segment, is reestablished anterior to the conduit. This is completed by end-to-end small-bowel reanastomosis using the GIA and TA staplers as described in Section 46-20 (p. 1198).

❹ **Ileal Conduit: Preparing the Ureters.** The staple line is excised from the stomal end of the conduit, and the conduit is irrigated into a basin. The ureters should now be engorged from the vascular clips placed earlier during exenteration. The distal end of the ureters should have a stay suture placed for traction. To prevent focal necrosis that may impede successful anastomosis, ureters are never directly grasped with forceps

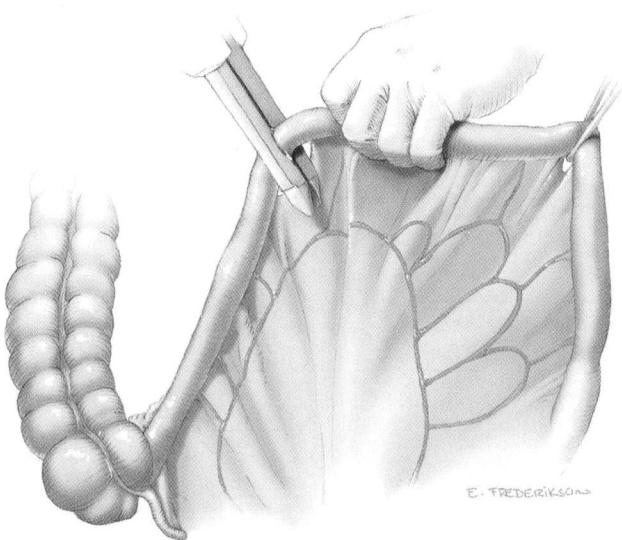

FIGURE 46-7.1 Ileal conduit: preparing the bowel segment.

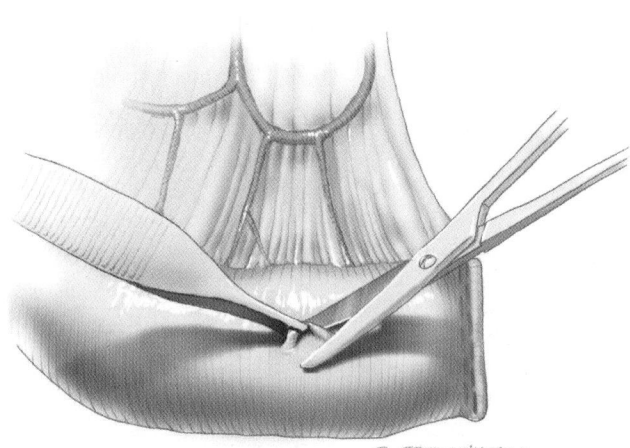

FIGURE 46-7.2 Ileal conduit: ileal incision.

or roughly handled. They are sharply freed from their retroperitoneal attachments so that they easily reach past the point of their planned anastomosis into the conduit. The left ureter is brought *under* the inferior mesenteric artery (IMA) to prevent acute angulation and kinking. This ureter ultimately exits from beneath the base of the sigmoid colon mesentery to reach the conduit.

❺ Ileal Conduit: Ureteral Anastomoses.
Adson forceps are used to grasp a small

section of the ileal serosa to which the left ureter will reach. This site is ideally approximately 2 cm from the butt end of the conduit on the anterior side of the antimesenteric surface. Metzenbaum scissors remove a small, full-thickness section of bowel wall (Fig. 46-7.2). The ileal mucosa should be easily visible.

The distal tip of the left ureter is cut at a 45-degree angle just behind the vascular clip placed during exenteration. If the distal ends of the ureters exhibit fibrosis, they are trimmed to reach healthy-appearing tissue. The prior distal stay-suture is removed with this trimming. Urine will drain into the abdomen while a 4–0 delayed-absorbable stay suture is placed outside-to-in through

the ureter's distal tip. The needle is left on this traction stitch since it will be the final suture in the anastomosis. Fine tip scissors are used to spatulate the ureter for approximately 1 cm, but the length is customized depending on the caliber of the ureteral lumen (Fig. 46-7.3). This maneuver helps to reduce the possibility of future ureteral stenosis.

The first suture is placed at the apex of the spatulation with a full-thickness bite through the ureteral wall and bowel mucosa (Fig. 46-7.4). Two or three adjoining mucosa-to-mucosa sutures are placed. A 7F ureteral stent is then placed through the stomal end of the conduit and advanced through the anastomosis into the left renal pelvis. The stent is held against the wall of the midsection of

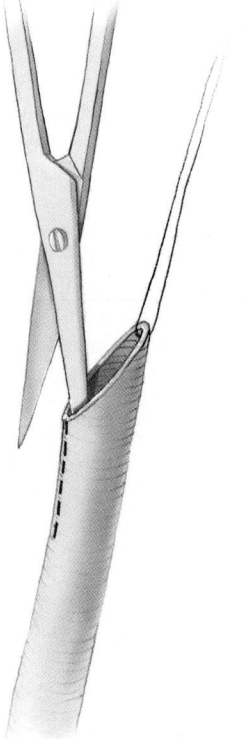

FIGURE 46-7.3 Ileal conduit: spatulating the ureter.

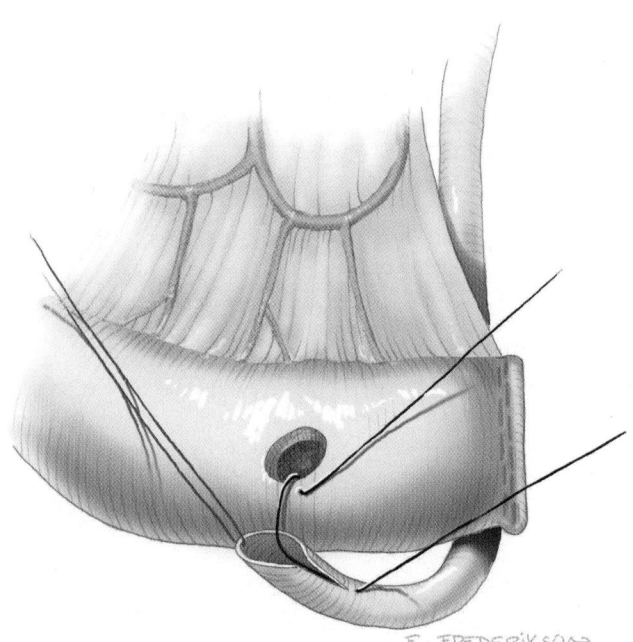

FIGURE 46-7.4 Ileal conduit: suturing ureter and ileal segment.

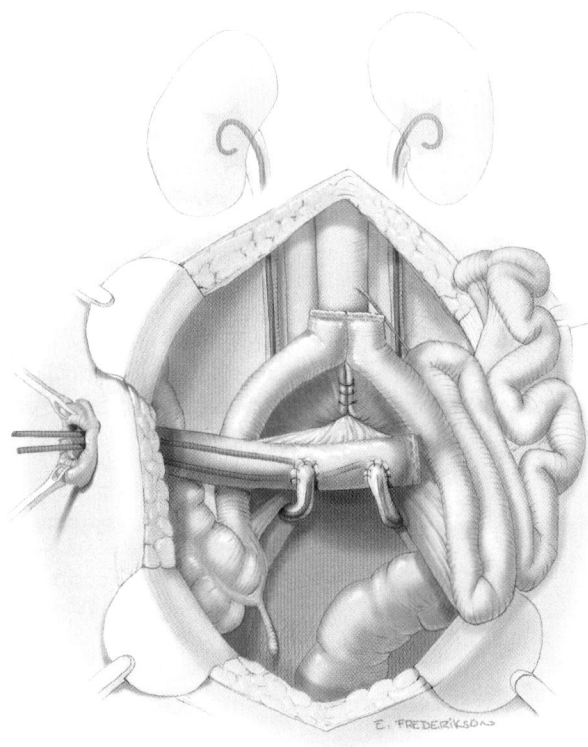

FIGURE 46-7.5 Ileal conduit: stoma with stents carefully pulled through abdominal incision.

the conduit with one hand and secured with a 3–0 or 4–0 gauge chromic catgut suture through the entire bowel wall and around the stent to hold it in place. The left ureteral anastomosis is completed with additional circumferential sutures to achieve a watertight closure (Fig. 46-7.5).

The anastomotic site for the right ureter is selected at least 2 to 3 cm distal to that of the left along the length of the conduit. The entire procedure is then repeated. Saline with methylene blue dye is used to fill the conduit and observe for watertight integrity. Any anastomotic leaks must be reinforced

with additional sutures and retested. If leakage persists or if there is concern about the mucosa-to-mucosa apposition, then the entire anastomosis should be redone.

This butt end of the conduit is next secured to the sacral promontory, iliopsoas muscle, or posterior peritoneum with two or three delayed-absorbable sutures through the seromuscular layer of the conduit. Stabilizing the conduit in this way will prevent undue tension on the ureteral anastomoses when the patient is upright and gravity allows the intestines to slide into the pelvis.

❻ Ileal Conduit: Stoma Creation. The skin at the proposed stoma site is elevated with a Kocher clamp. An electrosurgical blade, set on cutting mode, is used to excise a small circle of skin. The subcutaneous fat is separated by blunt dissection until the fascia is visible. A cruciate incision is made with an electrosurgical blade (Fig. 46-7.6). The rectus abdominis muscle is split longitudinally and another cruciate incision is created in the peritoneum. The opening is bluntly expanded until it easily accommodates two fingers.

The stoma and stents are carefully pulled through the incision until at least 2 cm of ileum protrudes through the skin. The mesentery may need to be trimmed or the abdominal wall opening further dissected to accommodate the conduit. The mucosal edge of the bowel is everted. The stoma is completed with 3–0 gauge delayed-absorbable "rosebud" stitches that include the ileal mucosa, intervening bowel serosa, and skin dermis (Fig. 46-7.7). Circumferential sutures

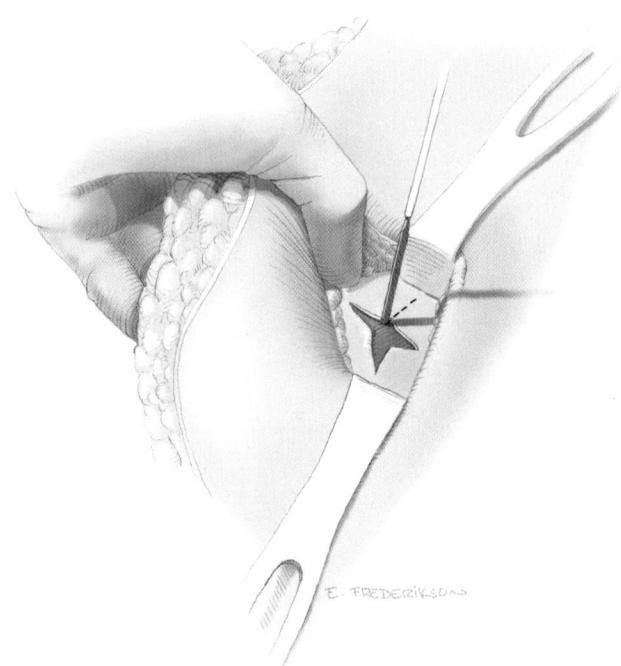

FIGURE 46-7.6 Ileal conduit: making the stoma.

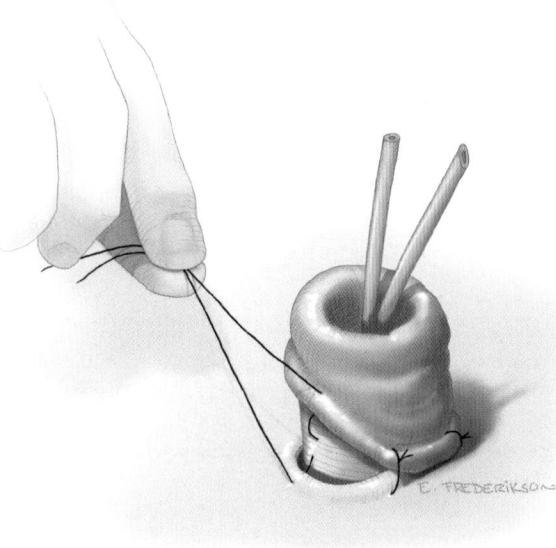

FIGURE 46-7.7 Ileal conduit: suturing the stoma.

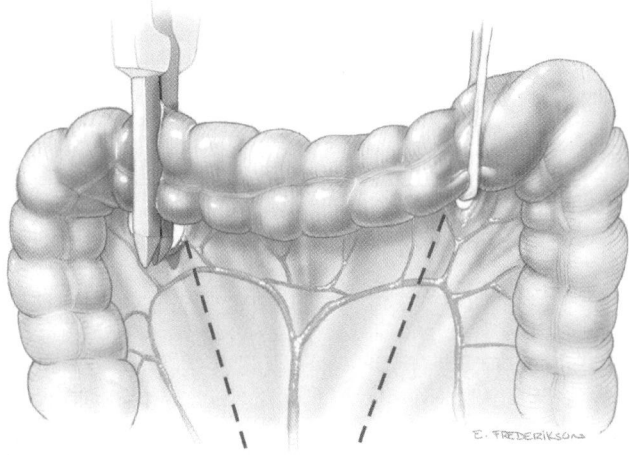

FIGURE 46-7.8 Transverse colon conduit: preparing the bowel segment.

are placed. Both stents are trimmed to fit in the stoma bag. To enable correct identification postoperatively, the right ureteral stent is cut at a "right" angle. Individual silk sutures placed through each stent may be secured at the skin to prevent stent dislodgment over the first few postoperative days.

❼ **Transverse Colon Conduit.** For this type of conduit, the hepatic and splenic flexures of the transverse colon are fully mobilized. In addition, the omentum is detached. Division points are marked with Penrose drains and transected (Fig. 46-7.8). The transverse mesocolon is then divided, as shown by the dotted lines, to provide sufficient mobility while preserving the middle colic artery. When performed in the usual setting of an exenteration with left lower quadrant colostomy, the bowel segment must measure approximately 20 cm to reach the right lower quadrant. Often, this requires incorporation of the hepatic flexure into the conduit and yields an antiperistaltic orientation, that is, urine ultimately flows through the conduit in the opposite direction that fecal waste would normally be propelled. Thus, the proximal bowel segment (nearest the cecum) will be the end of the conduit that eventually is brought through the abdominal wall.

Ureters are sufficiently mobilized in the retroperitoneal space, and both are brought out through a commodious peritoneal opening to reach the conduit. The left ureter will need to be brought across the aorta *proximal* to the IMA (unlike the ileal conduit). The ureteral anastomoses are then completed, ideally at the teniae coli, over stents. To prevent postoperative sliding and tension on the anastomoses, the conduit's butt end is secured to the sacrum, iliopsoas muscle, or posterior peritoneum with interrupted

delayed-absorbable suture. Intestinal continuity is reestablished anterior to the conduit by a functional end-to-end anastomosis using EEA and TA staplers, as described in Section 46-18 (p. 1195). The stoma can be made at the preselected site, but it can be repositioned almost anywhere that the conduit will comfortably reach. The stomal end of the conduit is brought through the anterior abdominal wall and secured (Fig. 46-7.9).

❽ **Final Steps.** Mesenteric defects require closure to prevent internal hernias but not so tightly as to compromise blood supply. A suction drain may be placed if integrity of the anastomoses and leakage is a concern. If the stoma appears dusky, the abdominal wall tunnel may be too tight, the mesentery may be twisted or placed on too much tension, or the blood supply may not be

sufficient. The last circumstance is the worst, and it generally requires trimming of the distal end of the bowel or occasionally redoing the entire conduit. Either is preferable to avoid problematic retraction, stricture, or necrosis.

POSTOPERATIVE

The stoma is regularly checked for viability during the immediate postoperative recovery period. Both stents should be functioning. A dry stent that does not respond to irrigation should prompt an imaging study to exclude ureteral obstruction. Urinary fistulas and ureteral obstruction are uncommon but are potentially life-threatening if not addressed with percutaneous drainage or reoperation. Prolonged bowel dysfunction may indicate an anastomotic urine leak or small-bowel obstruction.

Patients often are readmitted within a few weeks of surgery due to partial small bowel obstruction, urinary infection, wound separation, or other relatively minor complications of exenteration. These typically resolve with targeted supportive care. Long-term complications include ureteral stenosis and renal loss. Renal function may deteriorate due to chronic infection and reflux. When patients cannot be otherwise managed, they may require long-term percutaneous nephrostomy tubes, indwelling stents, or reoperation and conduit or stoma revision.

Predictably, the overall morbidity of creating an incontinent conduit is much higher in previously irradiated patients (Houvenaeghel, 2004). Tissue quality and mobility are especially important in these patients.

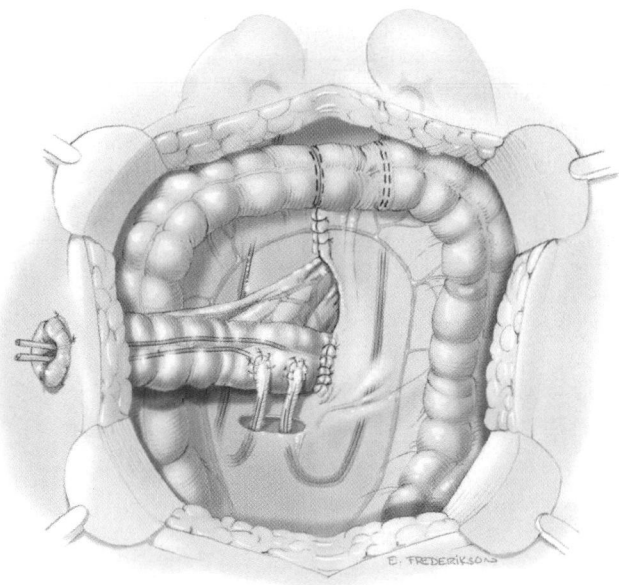

FIGURE 46-7.9 Transverse colon conduit: final appearance.

46-8

Continent Urinary Conduit

Removal of the bladder during total or anterior exenteration is the main indication for a continent urinary conduit. Vesicovaginal fistulas and disabling incontinence following radiation therapy are other less common reasons. Following cystectomy, urine is diverted into a reservoir created from a resected bowel segment. Depending on their construction, these diversions may render a woman continent or incontinent. An incontinent conduit reservoir chronically drains into an ostomy bag, whereas that of a continent conduit does not leak urine. Patients empty the reservoir by intermittent self-catheterization.

Continent conduits, however, may not be appropriate for all patients. The operation is more complex than an incontinent diversion procedure and may lead to more postoperative complications (Karsenty, 2005). It also requires a highly motivated patient who is capable of long-term self-catheterization. An ideal candidate for a continent conduit is a young, otherwise healthy woman without a colostomy.

There are several continent diversion methods. In gynecologic oncology, the continent ileocolonic urinary reservoir (Miami pouch) has become the most popular choice (Salom, 2004). This pouch is technically straightforward to construct and uses tissues that characteristically lie in nonirradiated areas (Penalver, 1998).

A Miami pouch includes a distal ileum segment, the ascending colon, and a portion of transverse colon. The basic steps involve opening the colon segment along the length of the tenia and folding it onto itself. The walls of the ascending and transverse colon are then sewn together to achieve a reservoir with low intraluminal pressure. The ileal segment is tapered and purse-string sutures are placed at the level of the ileocecal valve to achieve continence. The free ileal segment end is then exteriorized as a stoma to allow catheterization (Penalver, 1989).

PREOPERATIVE

Patient Evaluation

Preoperative evaluation is usually dictated by the preceding exenterative procedure. The specific decision is whether to plan for an incontinent or continent urinary conduit. Patients are extensively counseled regarding the differences. The presence of a permanent colostomy removes the apparent advantage of a continent conduit and an abdominal wall without draining stomas. Catheterization may be more problematic in very obese women. In addition, some patients with prior high-dose radiation or chronic bowel disease may also not be good candidates due to poor tissue quality and increased associated risks of anastomotic leaks, ureteral stricture, or fistula.

Consent

Patients are advised that intraoperative findings such as poor bowel appearance and dense adhesions may dictate a change in surgical plans. In addition, complications are common and should be reviewed. Even in experienced centers, half of patients will have one or more early pouch-related complications: ureteral stricture with obstruction, anastomotic leak, fistula, difficulty in catheterization, pyelonephritis, or sepsis. One third will develop late complications beyond 6 weeks. Ten percent of patients will ultimately require reoperation to revise the Miami pouch (Penalver, 1998). As a result, many patients would not choose the continent urinary conduit again (Goldberg, 2006).

Patient Preparation

Bowel preparation is mandatory but generally is dictated by the preceding exenterative surgery. Ideally, an enterostomal therapist is available to mark a conduit stoma site in the right lower abdomen that is unobstructed in the supine, sitting, and standing positions.

INTRAOPERATIVE

Surgical Steps

❶ **Initial Steps.** To avoid unnecessary traction on anastomoses, the continent urinary conduit is constructed as the last major intraabdominal procedure during exenterative surgery. Before beginning the conduit, hemostasis should be achieved. Anesthesia, patient positioning, and skin incisions are typically dictated by the preceding operation.

❷ **Exploration.** The conduit bowel segment is carefully inspected. It must be healthy appearing and lack severe radiation injury. At this point, the final decision to proceed with creation of a Miami pouch is made.

❸ **Preparing the Bowel Segment.** The right colon is freed along the white line of Toldt from the cecum, around the hepatic flexure, to the proximal transverse colon. The white line of Toldt marks the lateral attachment of ascending and descending colon's peritoneum to the posterior abdomen's parietal peritoneum. The conduit will require approximately 25 to 30 cm of colon and at least 10 cm of ileum. With these

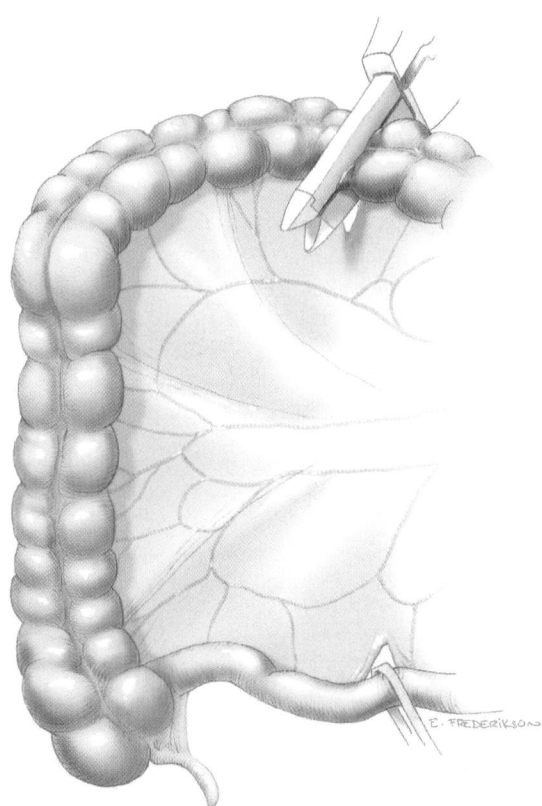

FIGURE 46-8.1 Preparing the bowel segment.

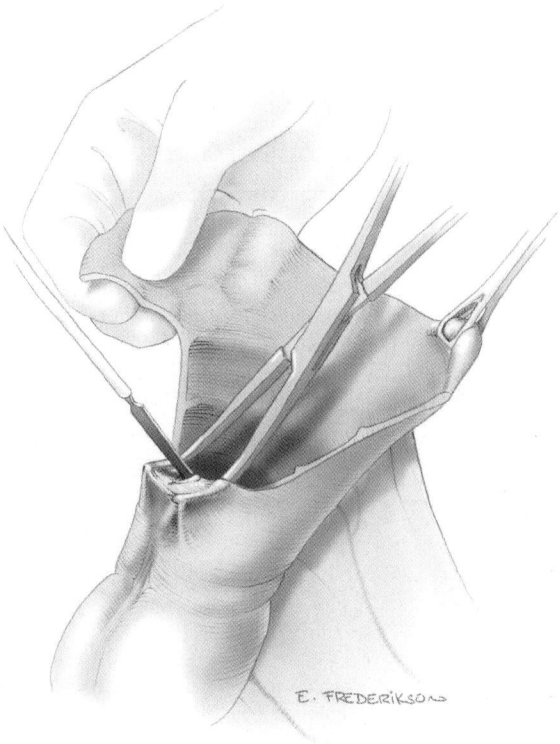

FIGURE 46-8.2 Detubularizing the bowel.

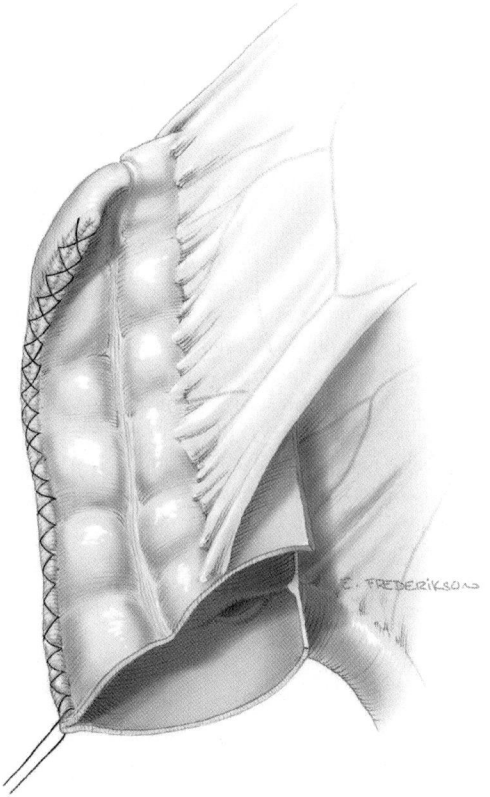

FIGURE 46-8.3 Creating the reservoir.

measurements in mind, a surgeon selects sites to divide the bowel.

The mesentery is scored with an electrosurgical blade, and a Penrose drain is placed around the sections to be divided. Within the mesentery, the underlying vasculature is reviewed to ensure sufficient conduit blood supply. A gastrointestinal anastomosis (GIA) stapler is used to divide the bowel at both sites marked with the Penrose drains (Fig. 46-8.1).

The mesenteries are incised down through the avascular areas to the posterior peritoneum. At this point, intestinal continuity is reestablished by a functional end-to-end stapled ileotransverse enterocolostomy using the GIA and transverse anastomosis (TA) staplers. The mesenteric defect is closed with 0-gauge delayed-absorbable suture in a running fashion to prevent internal herniation.

❹ Detubularizing the Bowel. The conduit staple lines on both ends of the bowel segment are removed with Metzenbaum scissors, and the bowel is irrigated into a basin. Of this bowel segment, the entire colonic portion is opened with an electrosurgical blade along the tenia of the antimesenteric border to "detubularize" the bowel (Fig. 46-8.2). This is extended to remove the appendix.

❺ Creating the Pouch. The colon segment is folded in half and four delayed-absorbable stay sutures are placed at the

corners to begin creation of the pouch. The lateral edge is closed in two layers with 2–0 and 3–0 gauge delayed-absorbable suture in a running fashion (Fig. 46-8.3).

❻ Tapering the Ileum. A 14F red rubber catheter is inserted through the terminal ileum segment into the pouch. Two pursestring, 0-gauge delayed-absorbable sutures are placed 1 cm apart at the ileocecal junction. The ileum is elevated with Babcock clamps, and a GIA stapler is used to taper the terminal ileum on its antimesenteric border over the

catheter (Fig. 46-8.4). An anterior abdominal wall opening is made in the right lower quadrant so that the ileal segment of the conduit can be pulled through to approximate its final position.

❼ Ureteral Anastomoses. Both ureters are further mobilized from their retroperitoneal attachments and brought into position under the ascending mesocolon using a 4–0 gauge delayed-absorbable stay suture at the tip. Manipulation with this suture avoids crush injury by forceps and subsequent

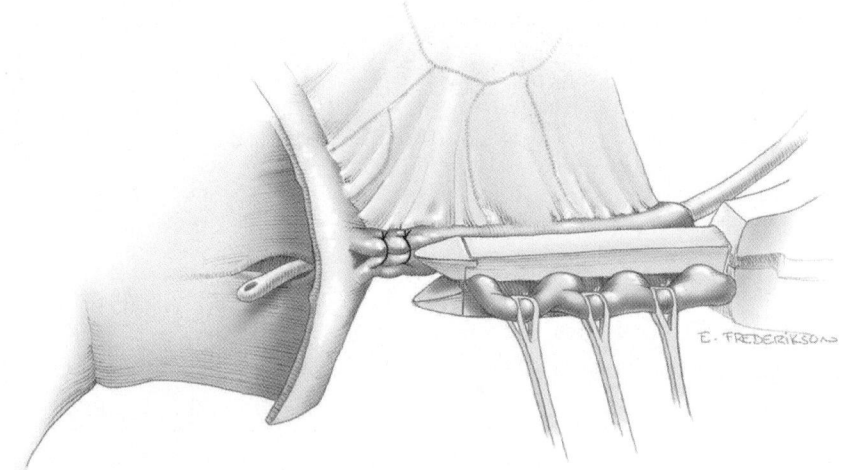

FIGURE 46-8.4 Tapering the ileum.

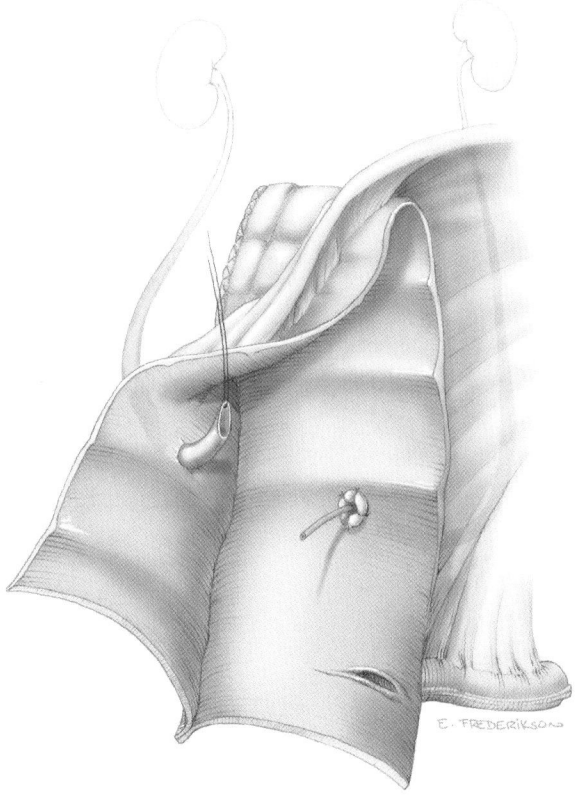

FIGURE 46-8.5 Ureteral anastomoses.

necrosis. As in the transverse colon conduit, the left ureter is brought over the aorta and *above* the origin of the inferior mesenteric artery (IMA).

The ureteral anastomotic sites to the pouch are selected based on ureter length and their ability to have a straight course to the pouch. One ureter is usually brought through on either side of the pouch suture line. The ureters are trimmed and spatulated (see Fig. 46-7.3, p. 1158). In creating the openings for the ureters, the bowel mucosa is incised at sites away from the suture line. A hemostat is poked through the bowel wall, grasps the ureteral stay suture, and thereby pulls 2 cm of each ureter into the pouch.

Each ureter is secured to the bowel mucosa with interrupted stitches of 4–0 gauge delayed-absorbable suture (Fig. 46-8.5). Single-J ureteral stents (7F) are inserted and sutured to the bowel wall with 3–0 gauge chromic to stabilize their placement. To enable correct identification postoperatively, the right ureteral stent is cut at a "right" angle.

❽ **Closing the Pouch.** A large Malecot catheter is brought into the pouch through an incision made away from the ileocecal valve. The ureteral stents are brought out through the pouch next to the Malecot (Fig. 46-8.6). Here, where the catheters exit the pouch, a watertight purse string using 3–0 plain catgut suture is placed. Absorbable

suture is used for this purse string, as the Malecot catheter will be removed only 2 to 3 weeks postoperatively.

The remaining edges of the pouch are closed with two layers of 2–0 and 3–0 gauge

delayed-absorbable suture in a running fashion. Continence may be tested by inserting a red rubber catheter through the plicated ileum, filling the pouch with 250 to 300 mL of saline, removing the red rubber catheter, and gently squeezing the pouch. Additional purse-string sutures may be placed at the ileocecal valve if incontinence is demonstrated. The completed pouch (Fig. 46-8.7) is now ready to be brought to the abdominal wall.

❾ **Final Steps.** The two stents and Malecot drain are brought out through a separate stab wound on the abdominal wall away from the stoma site. The Malecot drain is individually fixed to the skin with nylon sutures. The ileal segment is pulled through the abdominal wall and may require trimming to sit flush. The pouch is stabilized by suturing it to the undersurface of the abdominal wall, and the stoma is created by placing interrupted stitches of 3–0 gauge delayed-absorbable suture between the dermis and ileal mucosa as described in Section 46-7, Step 6 (p. 1159). A red rubber catheter is inserted and withdrawn to make sure that the pouch can be easily accessed. A Jackson-Pratt (JP) drain is then placed near the pouch to monitor for urine leakage and is brought out through a separate stab wound away from the stoma.

POSTOPERATIVE

The Miami pouch initially requires more care than an incontinent urinary conduit. Mucus will be produced by the colonic bowel

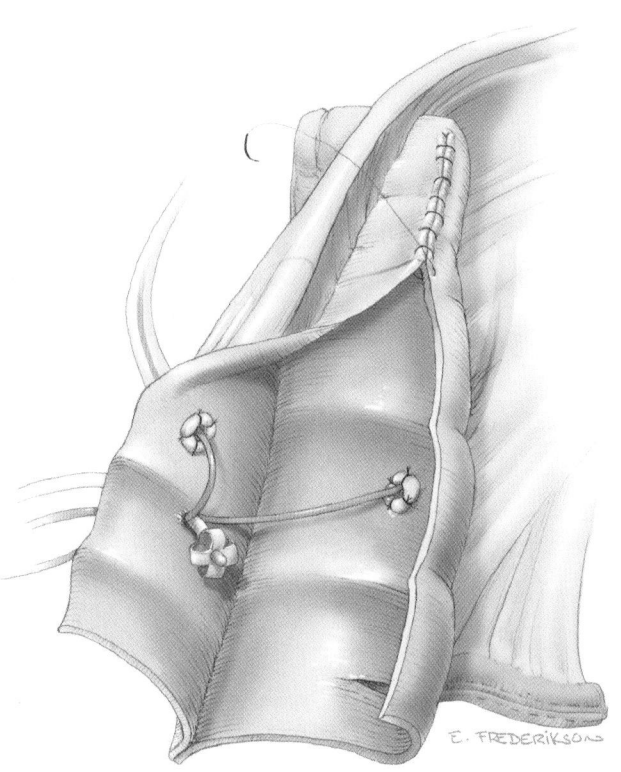

FIGURE 46-8.6 Closing the reservoir.

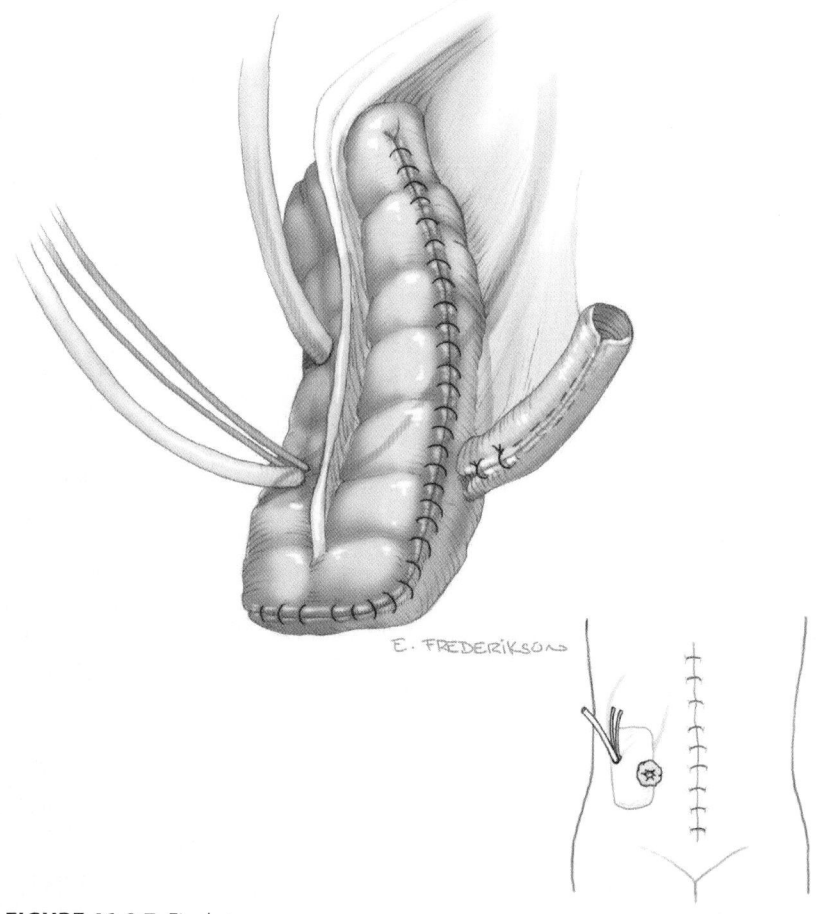

E. FREDERIKSON

FIGURE 46-8.7 Final steps.

segment. Therefore, the Malecot catheter is irrigated every few hours to permit urine drainage. In contrast, the ureteral stents are irrigated only if one of the catheters becomes obstructed. Two to 3 weeks postoperatively, an intravenous pyelogram (IVP) and gravity pouchogram are performed. The IVP excludes anastomotic leaks, ureteral stricture, and fistulas. The pouchogram involves retrograde filling of the conduit to search for leaks. If these tests are normal, the ureteral stents, Malecot catheter, and JP suction drainage tube may all be removed. The hole in the conduit that housed these tubes will heal secondarily.

A patient is taught self-catheterization using an 18F to 22F red rubber catheter and antiseptic technique. The interval between catheterizations is progressively increased over weeks to reach 6 hours during the day and span sleep hours at night. In addition, the pouch requires periodic irrigation to remove mucus. An IVP, pouchogram, and serum electrolyte and creatinine level measurement are performed at 3 months postoperatively and then every 6 months to evaluate the pouch, renal function, and upper urinary tracts.

More than half of patients will have a conduit-related complication postoperatively. Fortunately, most may be successfully managed conservatively without the need for reoperation (Ramirez, 2002). The most common urinary complications are ureteral stricture or obstruction, difficult catheterization, and pyelonephritis (Angioli, 1998; Goldberg, 2006). The gastrointestinal complication rate attributed to Miami pouch is less than 10 percent and includes fistulas (Mirhashemi, 2004).

46-9

Vaginal Reconstruction

Patients undergoing exenterative surgery are typical candidates for creation of a new vagina. Other less common indications include congenital absence of the vagina, postirradiation stenosis, and total vaginectomy. There are innumerable ways to perform the procedure, and the type of reconstruction is typically determined by both the surgeon's personal experience and the patient's clinical circumstances.

Vaginal reconstruction at the time of exenteration is a very personal choice. Not every woman will desire a new vagina, and others will be unhappy with the functional result (Gleeson, 1994a). Moreover, reconstruction may significantly prolong an already lengthy operation and lead to additional perioperative morbidity (Mirhashemi, 2002). However, proponents suggest that filling the large pelvic defect and bringing in a new source of blood supply may actually prevent postoperative fistula or abscess formation (Goldberg, 2006; Jurado, 2000).

To create a functional neovagina, one of the following is performed: (1) surrounding skin and subcutaneous tissue is mobilized and positioned into the defect (skin flap), (2) skin from another part of the body is harvested and transferred to replace the vaginal mucosa (split-thickness skin graft), or (3) skin and underlying tissue outside the radiated field are mobilized on an attached section of muscle with its dominant blood supply (myocutaneous flap). Of the three choices for vaginal reconstruction, skin flaps, such as *rhomboid flaps*, *pudendal thigh fasciocutaneous flaps*, and *advancement* or *rotational flaps*, are technically the easiest to perform (Burke, 1994; Gleeson, 1994b; Lee, 2006). *Split-thickness skin grafts (STSG)* provide the ability to cover large surfaces if primary closure is not possible. However, these require that most of the native subcutaneous tissue has been retained at the neovagina site and require months of stenting with a vaginal mold to prevent stricture (Kusiak, 1996). *Rectus abdominis myocutaneous (RAM) flaps* and *gracilis myocutaneous flaps* are technically more challenging and take longer to perform, but they demonstrate the most satisfying functional results (Lacey, 1988; Smith, 1998). Importantly, RAM flaps may be inappropriate in those with a prior Maylard incision or any other procedure that resulted in ligation of the inferior epigastric artery, which is the dominant blood supply to this type of flap.

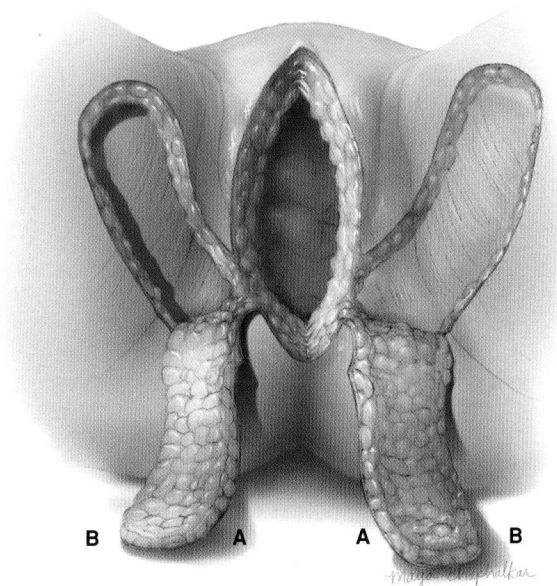

FIGURE 46-9.1 Raising the perineal flaps.

Regardless of reconstruction technique, sexual function is often significantly impaired in women after pelvic exenteration (Hockel, 2008; Ratliff, 1996). Other techniques are used less commonly and are not covered in this section.

PREOPERATIVE

Patient Evaluation

The surgeon should have an open discussion with the patient regarding the risks and benefits of vaginal reconstruction. Some women may have unrealistic expectations that are important to address preoperatively. Others may not wish to incur additional morbidity. The patient should also be aware that intraoperative complications may dictate a change of plans and the need to abort reconstruction.

Consent

The potential morbidity of the neovagina depends on the type of reconstruction. Flap necrosis, prolapse, wound separation, or other complications may require reoperation and/or lead to an unsatisfying end result. Postoperative patient concerns are expected and include self-consciousness about being seen in the nude by their partner and vaginal dryness or discharge (Ratliff, 1996).

Patient Preparation

The preceding exenterative surgery typically dictates preoperative preparation. Modifications may be required, depending on the type of neovaginal reconstruction. For example, the legs may need to be surgically prepped beyond the knees for a gracilis flap or a suitable donor site identified for STSG.

INTRAOPERATIVE

Surgical Steps

❶ Anesthesia and Patient Positioning. General anesthesia is required for vaginal reconstruction. The abdomen, perineum, and vagina have been surgically prepared, and a Foley catheter inserted. Legs are positioned in standard lithotomy in booted support stirrups to permit adequate perineal access.

❷ Pudendal Thigh Fasciocutaneous Flap. From a perineal approach, the planned incisions are marked along the skin from the non-hair-bearing areas just lateral to the labia majora. Flaps are roughly 15 × 6 cm. The most inferior skin margin should be level with the lower part of the gaping perineal defect. The skin incision is begun at the superior flap margin and dissected to include the underlying subcutaneous tissue and fascia lata (Fig. 46-9.1). The posterior labial artery, a branch of the internal pudendal artery, provides blood supply (Fig. 38-28, p. 822).

The flap's edges are approximated in a running, subcuticular suture line with 4–0 gauge delayed-absorbable suture. The edges both marked "A" in the figure are joined, as are both edges marked "B." The tubular neovagina is inserted into the perineal defect such that the end labeled with letters becomes the new vaginal apex. The incision sites are closed with interrupted stitches of 3–0 gauge delayed-absorbable suture, and bilateral JP drains are placed beneath these suture lines. The perineal defect requires sculpting of

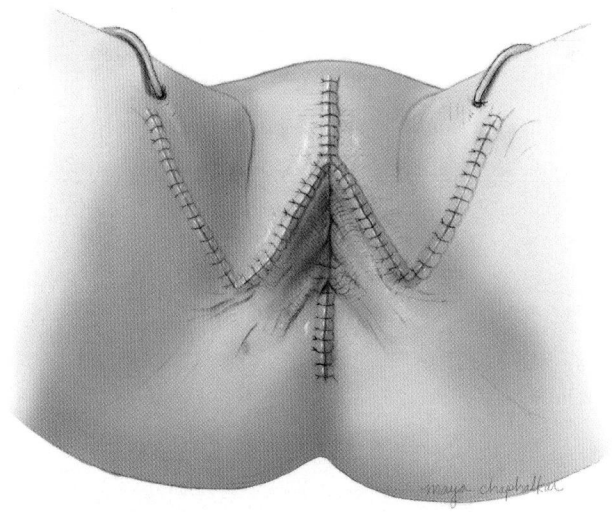

FIGURE 46-9.2 Perineal flap closure.

tissue folds and suturing to form a functional end result (Fig. 46-9.2). The apex of the neovagina may then be abdominally sutured to the hollow of the sacrum as in a traditional sacrocolpopexy (Section 45-17, p. 1098). Intraabdominally, the neovagina is then covered with an omental J-flap to provide additional neovascularization.

❸ **Split-Thickness Skin Graft with Omental J-Flap.** Modification of the omental flap, which is normally used to close off

the pelvic inlet after exenteration, can create a cylinder for a new vagina. Notably, in thin patients, a thin, poorly vascularized, attenuated omentum may be inadequate to form a substantial cylinder and cover the mold.

From an abdominal approach, the omentum is detached from the stomach with a ligate-divide-staple (LDS) device or electrothermal bipolar coagulator (LigaSure). Resection is usually from right to left, until it will comfortably reach the pelvis as a J-flap (Section 46-14, p. 1186). Only three quarters of the omentum

is divided, so as to preserve the left gastro-epiploic artery for blood supply. The distal omentum is rolled into a cylinder and sutured together with interrupted stitches of 3–0 gauge delayed-absorbable suture (Fig. 46-9.3).

The proximal end can be closed abdominally with similar interrupted sutures or the transverse anastomosis (TA) stapler without dividing it entirely. From the perineal side, the omental cylinder is then sutured to the vaginal introitus.

Next, the STSG is harvested from the donor site and sutured over a vaginal mold with 4–0 gauge delayed-absorbable suture in a manner similar to the McIndoe procedure described in Section 43-25 (p. 985). The mold is placed into the neovaginal space and sutured into place at the introitus (Fig. 46-9.4). Each of the remaining smaller perineal defects, now above and below the neovagina, is closed in the midline with interrupted stitches of 3–0 gauge delayed-absorbable suture.

❹ **Gracilis Myocutaneous Flap.** From a perineal approach, a reference line is drawn on the medial thigh from the pubic tubercle to the medial tibial plateau following the adductor longus muscle. Inferior to this line, an island of skin, its associated subcutaneous tissue, and the gracilis muscle will serve as the flap. The planned elliptic incision is marked, and a full-thickness skin incision through the

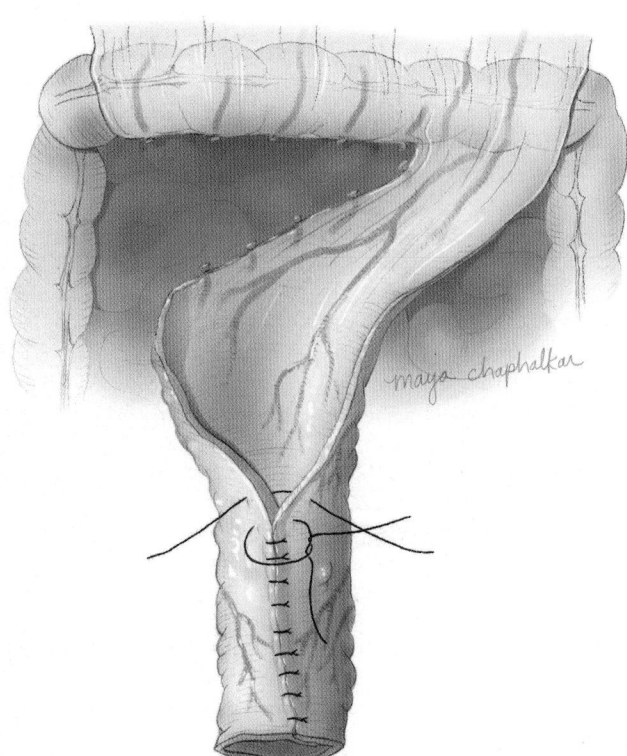

FIGURE 46-9.3 Raising the omental J-flap.

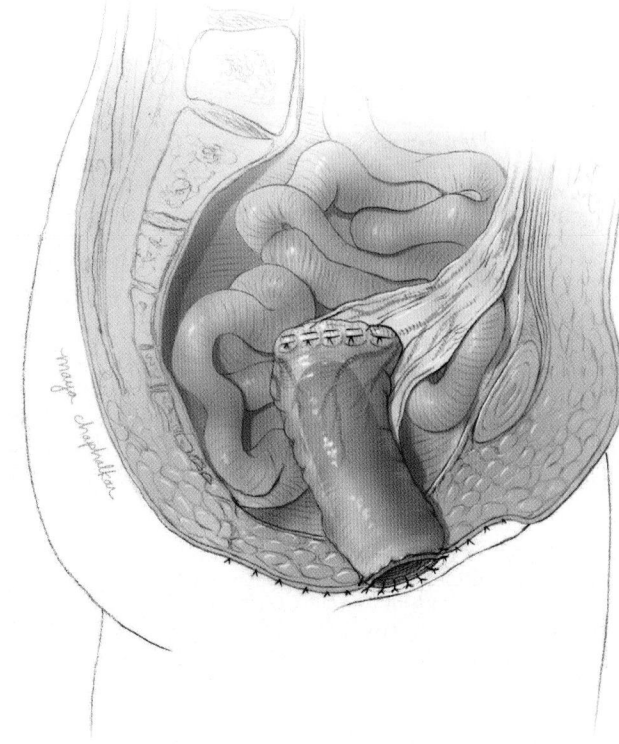

FIGURE 46-9.4 Insertion of the split-thickness skin graft.

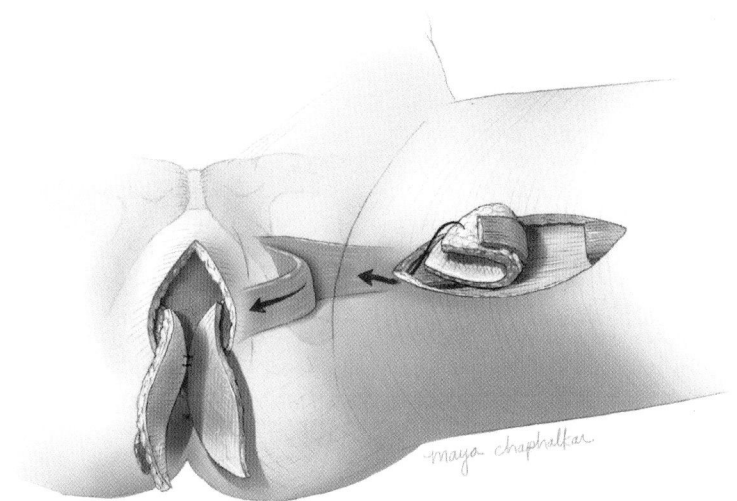

FIGURE 46-9.5 Gracilis myocutaneous flap.

reference line is continued through the subcutaneous fat and the fascia lata. The belly of the gracilis muscle is isolated at its distal margin and divided. The remainder of the incision is completed around the marked skin island margin. The gracilis muscle is fully mobilized with blunt and sharp dissection from distal to proximal. This preserves the dominant vascular pedicle—a branch of the medial femoral circumflex artery—as it enters the deep anterior belly of the muscle 6 to 8 cm from the pubic tubercle.

Through the operative site on the thigh, a subfascial tunnel is bluntly developed medially to the open perineal defect. The left gracilis muscle flap is rotated *clockwise* against the thigh, that is, rotated first posteriorly and then medially. It is placed through the tunnels and allowed to hang freely between the patient's legs. The right flap is rotated *counterclockwise* and similarly positioned (Fig. 46-9.5).

Beginning at the distal tip, the tubular gracilis neovagina is constructed by suturing the skin edges of the right and left skin islands together with interrupted stitches using 4–0 gauge delayed-absorbable suture. The proximal opening should accommodate two or three fingers. The neovagina is rotated cephalad into the pelvis and posteriorly anchored to the levator plate abdominally with interrupted stitches of 0-gauge delayed-absorbable suture to prevent vaginal prolapse. Redundant flap skin is trimmed, and the proximal skin is sutured to the introitus with interrupted stitches of 3–0 gauge delayed-absorbable suture.

Each of the remaining smaller perineal defects, now above and below the neovagina, is closed in the midline with interrupted stitches of 3–0 gauge delayed-absorbable suture. Each thigh incision is similarly closed.

❺ **Rectus Abdominis Myocutaneous (RAM) Flap.** A skin and muscle island can be harvested from any location on the abdominal wall as long as the base of its shape is at the umbilicus. Typically, a 10 × 15 cm skin island is marked. At the superior border of the island, which will ultimately form the vaginal opening, the skin, subcutaneous tissue, and anterior rectus sheath are incised. One belly of the rectus abdominis muscle is freed with blunt dissection from the posterior sheath. The belly is divided proximally, and its anastomotic vessels connecting to the superior epigastric system are ligated.

The remaining borders of the skin island are incised through the anterior rectus sheath to the arcuate line. The subcutaneous fat is mobilized along the lateral and medial margins of the rectus muscle belly. The rectus muscle is then bluntly dissected from the posterior sheath until reaching the arcuate line, which is the caudal margin of this sheath. Next, the posterior peritoneum is cut inferiorly along the full length of the midline incision well beyond the flap. The RAM flap is now fully detached, but it needs to be further mobilized on its vascular pedicle to be able to swing into the pelvis. At the distal portion of the skin island, the rectus muscle is then bluntly dissected inferiorly from the anterior sheath to its insertion onto the pubic bone.

The flap, consisting of skin, subcutaneous tissue, anterior sheath, and rectus belly, is coiled around a syringe to form a tube (Fig. 46-9.6). The skin edges are approximated with 4–0 gauge delayed-absorbable suture. The syringe is removed, and the tube is placed into the pelvis. The pelvic end of the tube is closed. The RAM flap must be put into the pelvis without tension to prevent occlusion of its dominant vascular supply from the inferior epigastric artery.

The open end of the neovagina is brought out under the pubic symphysis to the perineum where it is attached to the vulvar defect using interrupted vertical mattress stitches using 0-gauge delayed-absorbable

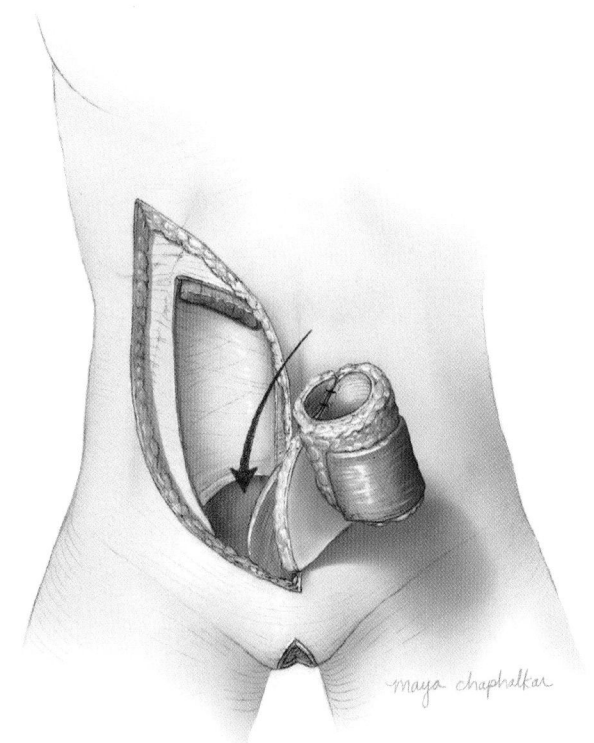

FIGURE 46-9.6 Rectus abdominis myocutaneous flap.

suture. An omental J-flap may also be prepared to provide additional blood supply.

Each of the remaining smaller perineal defects, now above and below the neovagina, is closed in the midline with interrupted stitches of 3–0 gauge delayed-absorbable suture. Abdominal wall posterior rectus fascia is reapproximated with no. 1 polydioxanone monofilament (PDS). Skin is closed with staples.

POSTOPERATIVE

The presence of a vagina significantly improves quality of life for many women, as well as reducing sexual problems after exenteration (Hawighorst-Knapstein, 1997). Reconstruction may be beneficial to a woman's self-image, and the knowledge that intercourse is possible may be reassuring even if she chooses not to be sexually active postoperatively. Morbidity from the procedure largely depends on the type of neovagina.

Pudendal thigh flaps are reliable and easy to harvest, but perhaps are the most likely to be nonfunctional. Long-term sequelae may include vulvar pain, chronic vaginal discharge, hair growth, and protrusion of the flaps. These symptoms may discourage patients and their partners from attempting sexual activity (Gleeson, 1994b).

STSG neovaginas may become infected at the donor or recipient site. Graft sloughing due to vascular compromise or development of a seroma is another common complication. Postoperatively, patients must initially be immobilized to aid healing, and stenting with a vaginal mold is required for months to prevent vaginal stenosis or contracture (Fowler, 2009).

Gracilis myocutaneous flaps may be difficult to pass into the pelvis during the procedure and have the potential for partial or complete tissue loss due to necrosis from an inherently tenuous blood supply (Cain, 1989). Flap loss is significantly more common if rectosigmoid anastomosis is performed concurrently during exenteration (Soper, 1995). Long-term prolapse is another relatively common problem. Residual scarring on the legs is a frequent, albeit relatively minor, complaint postoperatively.

Rectus abdominis muscle flaps are perhaps the best choice for vaginal reconstruction at the time of pelvic exenteration (Jurado, 2009). Ideally, they fill pelvic dead space, reduce the risk of fistulas, and provide fulfilling sexual activity (Goldberg, 2006). However, the donor site may be difficult to close primarily or may lead to a postoperative hernia or dehiscence. The operating time is also increased because, unlike a gracilis flap where the abdominal team can be proceeding with exenteration while the perineal team is beginning the reconstruction, two surgical teams are not possible when performing a RAM flap. Flap necrosis, enterocutaneous fistula, and vaginal stenosis are other frequent complications (Soper, 2005).

46-10

Pelvic Lymphadenectomy

Pelvic lymph node removal and evaluation is a fundamental tool in accurate cancer staging. As such, it is commonly indicated in women undergoing surgery for uterine, ovarian, or cervical cancer. Also, in those with grossly involved nodes, pelvic lymphadenectomy may serve to optimally debulk tumor burden.

The aim of lymphadenectomy is bilateral *complete* removal of all fatty lymphatic tissue from the areas predicted to carry nodal metastases (Cibula, 2010). These nodes lie within well-defined anatomic boundaries that include: the midportion of the common iliac artery (cephalad), deep circumflex iliac vein (caudad), psoas muscle (laterally), ureter (medially), and obturator nerve (dorsally) (Whitney, 2010). Ideally, the procedure yields numerous pelvic nodes from multiple sites within these boundaries (Huang, 2010). Groups specifically sampled are the external iliac artery, internal iliac artery, obturator, and common iliac artery nodal groups. Removal of at least four lymph nodes from each side (right and left) is a minimum requirement to validate that an "adequate" lymphadenectomy has been performed (Whitney, 2010). In general, the extent of pelvic lymphadenectomy will depend on the clinical circumstances, such as degree of associated scarring and patient habitus.

Additional definitions are commonly used in association with lymphadenectomy. For example, pelvic lymph node "sampling" is a more limited procedure within the same anatomic boundaries and is particularly intended to remove any enlarged or suspicious nodes (Whitney, 2010). Sampling is limited to easily accessible pelvic regions and does not address all nodal groups (Cibula, 2010). Pelvic lymph node "dissection" is a vague term that may range from sampling to lymphadenectomy.

Pelvic lymphadenectomy can be performed via laparotomy or a minimally invasive abdominal approach (p. 1176). In contrast, although the pelvic lymph nodes lie retroperitoneally, a lateral abdominal wall approach to reach these without entering the peritoneal cavity, that is, *extraperitoneal pelvic lymphadenectomy*, is not commonly performed (Larciprete, 2006). Last, emerging advancements in lymphatic mapping and sentinel node techniques are designed to limit the short- and long-term complications associated with extensive lymphatic resection.

PREOPERATIVE

Patient Evaluation

Imaging studies such as CT, MR, or PET imaging may suggest pelvic lymphadenopathy and help guide a surgeon to suspicious areas. However, the ability to preoperatively detect microscopic metastases is limited.

Consent

With proper technique, pelvic lymphadenectomy is a straightforward procedure with relatively few complications. These include postoperative lymphocele, nerve and vascular injury, acute hemorrhage, infection, and chronic lymphedema.

Patient Preparation

Bleeding is a common problem with pelvic lymphadenectomy and may be exacerbated with obese patients, grossly enlarged or densely adhered lymph nodes, and pelvic vessel anatomic variants. Accordingly, units of packed red blood cells are typed and cross-matched. Topical hemostatic agents may also prove valuable.

Routine bowel preparation and antibiotic prophylaxis are not required for lymphadenectomy but may be indicated for other concurrent surgeries. Prevention of VTE is warranted, and options are listed in Table 39-8 (p. 836).

INTRAOPERATIVE

Surgical Steps

❶ Anesthesia and Patient Positioning. This surgery may be performed under general or regional anesthesia with a patient supine. A Foley catheter is placed, and the abdomen is surgically prepared.

❷ Abdominal Entry. A midline vertical or low transverse abdominal incision that allows access to the previously noted anatomic boundaries is appropriate for this procedure. A Pfannenstiel incision offers limited exposure and is reserved for only selected patients.

❸ Abdominal Exploration. Pelvic and paraaortic lymph nodes are routinely inspected during initial abdominal exploration. Unexpected grossly positive nodes may indicate that a proposed operative plan should be abandoned (for example, radical hysterectomy for cervical cancer) or revised (Whitney, 2000).

❹ Retroperitoneal Exploration. The retroperitoneal space has typically already

been entered through the round ligament during preceding surgical procedures. However, to extend retroperitoneal access, a surgeon may further incise the anterior and posterior leaves of the broad ligament.

Palpation of the external iliac artery pulsation just medial to the psoas major muscle is the starting point. Its identification permits a surgeon to locate relevant anatomy, as vascular anomalies are regularly encountered. Blunt dissection is then performed cephalad to see the common iliac artery bifurcate into the external and internal iliac arteries. The ureter is isolated as previously described (p. 1135). The remaining pelvic sidewall structures are covered with fatty-lymphoid tissue and are not yet easily visible.

To summarize the planned en bloc specimen excision, dissection begins proximally along the psoas major muscle and external iliac artery and proceeds distally to reach the inguinal ring where the nodal specimen is reflected medially and off the external iliac vein. Next, dissection along the internal iliac artery begins cephalad and moves caudad, and last enters the obturator space for nodal dissection here. The entire nodal bundle is lifted and removed. Separately, nodes excised from along the distal common iliac artery can be included in the final specimen.

❺ External Iliac Nodes. For this nodal group, an index finger is placed atop the psoas major muscle and lateral to the external iliac artery at a point distal to the common iliac artery bifurcation. The finger bluntly dissects caudally and parallel to the external iliac artery to separate the lateral preperitoneal fat from the fatty-lymphoid tissue covering the external iliac vessels (Fig. 46-10.1). The general absence of lateral branches from these vessels enables more aggressive blunt separation to be performed unless there is significant fibrosis. The genitofemoral nerve, which is visible parallel to the external iliac artery, can often be spared with careful dissection. Injury to this nerve results in ipsilateral labium majus and proximal thigh numbness.

Next, forceps traction is typically required to lift all adventitial tissue up and above the external iliac artery beginning at the common iliac artery bifurcation. This countertraction helps maintain the correct dissection plane moving distally as bands between nodal tissue and the artery are divided using electrosurgical cutting (Fig. 46-10.2).

As dissection continues caudally, the distal self-retaining retractor blade may be temporarily removed to allow resection of all pelvic nodes heading toward the inguinal canal. For this, the fatty nodal tissue overlying the caudal portions of the psoas major muscle and external iliac artery is grasped with forceps. With an incision made parallel and superficial

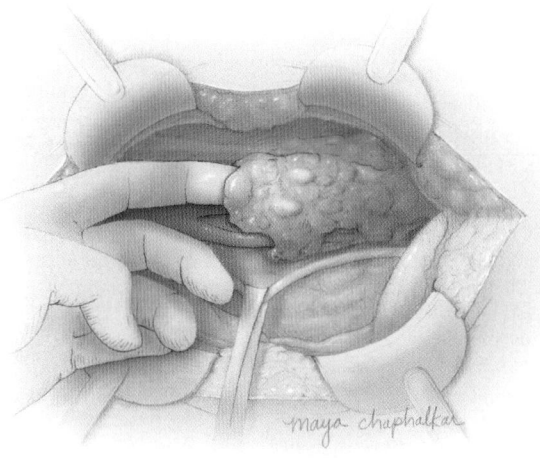

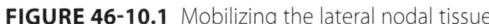

FIGURE 46-10.1 Mobilizing the lateral nodal tissue.

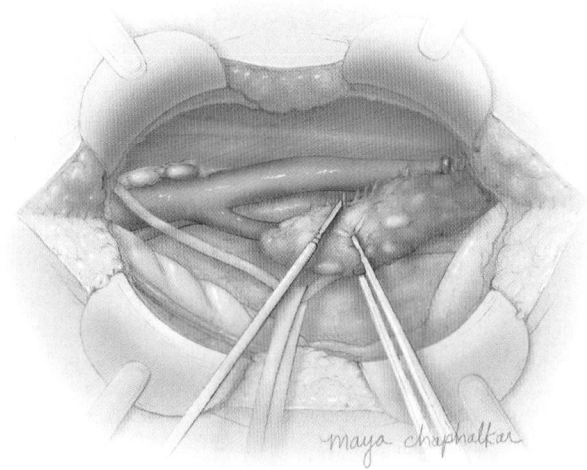

FIGURE 46-10.2 Medial dissection over the vein.

to the artery, distal nodal tissue is freed. Mobilization of this tissue exposes the deep circumflex iliac vein, which crosses laterally over the distal external iliac artery. The deep circumflex iliac vein originates from the distal part of the external iliac vein and serves as the caudal boundary for this nodal group.

The mobilized nodal tissue is next reflected medially to reveal the entire external iliac artery. Medial traction is applied with forceps, and fine adventitial bands that connect the nodes to the underlying external iliac vein are transected using electrocautery cutting or Metzenbaum scissors. Once completed, this external iliac nodal group dissection later permits safe entry into the obturator space, outlined in Step 7.

❻ Internal Iliac Nodes. Next, ureterolysis, if not previously performed, is completed (Section 46-1, Step 5, p. 1135). The ureter is moved and held medially by a Penrose drain or narrow retractor for protection and improved pelvic sidewall visualization. Spatially, nodes that have been dissected off the external iliac vessels and the fatty nodal tissue bridging the external iliac vein and the internal iliac artery lie in the same plane. Beginning at the common iliac artery bifurcation, the free nodal bundle is elevated and placed on tension. Initial sharp dissection of the internal iliac nodal group continues caudally along the internal iliac vessels and then along the superior vesical artery. As dissection approaches the distal aspect of the superior vesical artery, the nodal attachments are fine and enable electrocautery dissection without the need for clips or ligatures. At this point, both the external iliac and internal iliac nodes are completely dissected and can be submitted as one specimen or combined with obturator fossa lymph nodes, depending on surgeon preference.

❼ Obturator Fossa Node Group. To reach this nodal group, an index finger is gently inserted between the psoas major muscle and external iliac artery, and blunt dissection progresses downward to the obturator fossa. Lateral arterial or venous branches may need vascular clip application and transection. During this dissection, nodal tissue may be identified behind the external iliac vessels and added to the specimen.

As a result, the external iliac vein is mobilized and can be retracted upward and laterally by a vessel retractor to expose the obturator fossa (Fig. 46-10.3). If present, nodal tissue along the inferomedial wall of the external iliac vein is transected with blunt and electrosurgical blade dissection. Also, accessory venous branches may be identified and clipped.

With the vein retractor in place, the obturator nodal tissue is grasped with forceps. This nodal bundle lies deep to the external iliac vein but superficial to the obturator

nerve. With upward traction applied, blunt forceps or a suction tip moved gently side-to-side disrupts nodal tissue attachments to the obturator nerve. The blunt dissection is performed in the center of the fossa to minimize injury to surrounding deep pelvic vasculature. This also clears off tissue to permit obturator nerve identification.

Once this nerve is localized, dissection should purposely remain superficial to it. Firm fibrotic attachments may be electrosurgically transected under direct visualization. As the caudal end of the bundle is reached, it is usually tethered to the sidewall. To free it, a vascular clip is placed distal to the bundle, and the tethered attachment is divided proximal to the clip. At the cephalad end of the bundle, nodes are carefully separated sharply from the inferior aspect of the external iliac vein while avoiding obturator nerve injury.

Nodal tissue deep to the obturator nerve is not routinely removed since the obturator artery and vein traverse this area. Laceration of

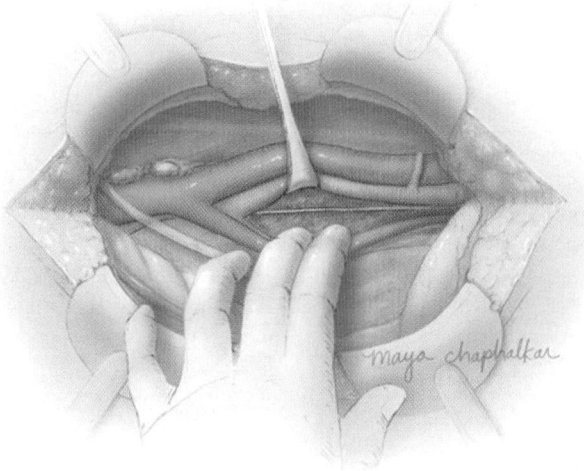

FIGURE 46-10.3 Obturator fossa dissection.

CHAPTER 46

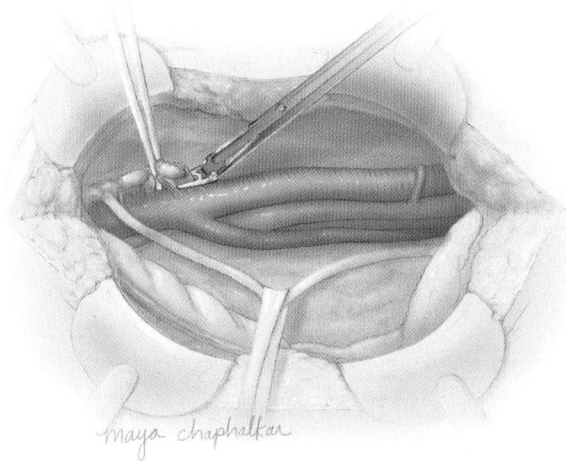

FIGURE 46-10.4 Distal common iliac dissection.

either vessel can result in retraction and catastrophic hemorrhage that is difficult to control.

❽ Distal Common Iliac Lymph Nodes. To remove this group, the upper retractor blade is readjusted to expose the distal half of the common iliac artery. The colon may require mobilization using electrosurgical dissection along the white line of Toldt. Once this line is incised, bowel can then be retracted sufficiently to allow access to the common iliac nodes. The ureter is further mobilized medially before beginning node dissection.

Lateral fatty-lymphoid tissue may be removed by first grasping and elevating with forceps and using electrosurgical dissection to establish a plane. Blunt dissection to further separate the nodal tissue from the artery is continued cephalad. Electrosurgical coagulation or clips plus sharp incision are used to detach these nodes (Fig. 46-10.4). Laterally, the nodes are dissected off the psoas major muscle. Importantly, on the patient's right side, the common iliac vein and inferior vena cava (IVC) lie beneath the lateral margin of the common iliac artery, and thus, careful dissection is warranted. Further dissection is performed atop the distal common iliac artery, which serves as the medial border of dissection for this nodal group.

❾ Final Steps. Gauze sponges may be opened and tightly placed into the obturator fossa and medial to the external iliac vein to tamponade any surface oozing while additional procedures are performed. Topical hemostatic agents are employed as needed (Table 40-5, p. 861). Closing the retroperitoneal space and using suction drainage does not minimize hematoma or lymphocele development (Charoenkwan, 2014).

POSTOPERATIVE

Neurologic injuries involving the obturator, ilioinguinal, iliohypogastric, genitofemoral, or femoral nerves may result from direct surgical trauma, stretch injury, suture entrapment, or retractor placement (Cardosi, 2002). Their specific neurologic deficits and management are described in Chapter 40 (p. 843). Notably, transection of the obturator nerve is ideally immediately noted intraoperatively and an epineural repair performed (Vasilev, 1994).

Surgical blunt dissection techniques decrease the risk of inadvertent vessel or nerve injury, but these may increase the chance of postoperative lymphocele formation. Also known as lymphocyst, these usually asymptomatic and transient lymph collections may form a thick fibrotic wall. Postoperative pelvic hematomas are also not uncommon.

46-11

Paraaortic Lymphadenectomy

Removal of paraaortic lymph nodes typically follows pelvic lymphadenectomy to surgically stage women with uterine and ovarian cancer because of these cancers' unpredictable lymphatic dissemination patterns (Burke, 1996; Negishi, 2004). Moreover, removal of enlarged paraaortic nodes may provide optimal debulking of ovarian cancer and may also confer a survival benefit in selected endometrial and cervical cancer patients (Cosin, 1998; Havrilesky, 2005).

Paraaortic lymphadenectomy implies bilateral complete removal of all nodal tissue from within an area with well-defined anatomic boundaries: inferior mesenteric artery (cephalad), midlength of common iliac artery (caudad), ureter (lateral), and aorta (medial). The completeness of the procedure will vary by clinical setting, but an adequate dissection requires that lymphatic tissue at least be demonstrated pathologically from both the right and left sides (Whitney, 2010).

Paraaortic lymphadenectomy can be performed via laparotomy or minimally invasive approach (p. 1176). The proximal dissection is usually only extended to the inferior mesenteric artery (IMA), unless a "high" lymphadenectomy is indicated (Whitney, 2010). With this modification, a surgeon extends dissection to reach the renal veins. Most often, this is performed during ovarian cancer staging or in high-risk endometrial cancer cases to debulk tumor and more accurately stage these cancers (Mariani, 2008; Morice, 2003).

PREOPERATIVE

Patient Evaluation

As described earlier (p. 1169), imaging studies may help guide a surgeon to the most suspicious lymph nodes but are not entirely reliable in identifying small nodal metastases.

Consent

Paraaortic lymphadenectomy is not routinely performed worldwide due to the procedure's technical difficulty and potential for complications (Fujita, 2005). Of these, acute hemorrhage and postoperative ileus occur most often. Other complications should be infrequent. In obese women, operative visibility is hindered, and thus, procedure complexity and operative times are considerably greater.

Patient Preparation

Bleeding is a common problem with this lymphadenectomy. Accordingly, units of packed red blood cells are typed and cross-matched. Topical hemostatic agents may also prove valuable. Routine bowel preparation and antibiotic prophylaxis are not typically required. However, other concurrent surgeries may dictate their use. Prevention of VTE is warranted, and options are listed in Table 39-8 (p. 836).

INTRAOPERATIVE

Surgical Steps

❶ **Anesthesia and Patient Positioning.** Lymphadenectomy may be performed under general or regional anesthesia with a patient supine. A Foley catheter is placed, and the abdomen is surgically prepared.

❷ **Abdominal Entry.** A midline vertical abdominal incision that allows access to the previously noted anatomic boundaries is appropriate for this procedure. Low transverse incisions offer limited exposure and are reserved for only selected patients.

❸ **Abdominal Exploration.** Paraaortic lymph nodes are routinely palpated during initial abdominal exploration. A hand is placed beneath the small bowel mesentery to palpate the aorta. The index and middle fingers are then used to straddle the aorta and palpate for lymphadenopathy. Suspicious or grossly positive paraaortic nodes are typically removed as an initial step. Unexpected positive nodes may indicate that the proposed operative plan should be abandoned or revised (Whitney, 2000). For most instances, in which no adenopathy is present, the dissection is usually performed last due to the possibility of triggering catastrophic bleeding that might otherwise limit further surgery.

❹ **Visualization.** Exposure and proper retractor positioning is perhaps the most important part of this procedure. Thus, a self-retaining retractor is positioned to allow access to the aorta. The sigmoid colon and descending colon are gently retracted in a lower left direction, whereas small bowel and transverse colon are packed into the upper abdomen by laparotomy sponges. Modified Trendelenburg patient positioning is also helpful to shift bowel from the operative field. Additional sharp dissection along the right paracolic gutter peritoneum (white line of Toldt) may be necessary to sufficiently mobilize and move the cecum from the dissection field. Once bowel has been cleared, the peritoneum overlying the aorta and right

common iliac artery should be visible. Both vessels are palpated before proceeding. Also, as described on page 1135, the ureter is isolated and held laterally on a Penrose drain to avoid its injury.

❺ **Opening the Retroperitoneal Space.** Beginning atop the midportion of the right common iliac artery, a right-angle clamp is used to guide electrosurgical blade incision of the posterior parietal peritoneum. Following each vessel's course, the incision moves cephalad and medially over the right common iliac artery and then cephalad atop the aorta (Fig. 46-11.1). Staying directly above these arteries is recommended to avoid inadvertent laceration of the right common iliac vein or IVC. Continuing cephalad in the midline, sharp incision of the peritoneum is extended through the caudal and then left lateral aspect of the duodenal peritoneal reflection to mobilize the duodenum cephalad. An upper midline self-retaining retractor blade is repositioned to retract this bowel.

❻ **Right Paraaortic Nodes.** With the ureter still held laterally, the surgeon first establishes the medial border of the right paraaortic nodal group. Atop the midportion of the right common iliac artery, the lymph node bundle is elevated with forceps to reveal fibrous bands connecting it to the artery. A right-angle clamp is placed beneath these bands, which are then sharply divided to free the distal bundle from the artery. Using electrosurgical cutting atop the right common iliac artery, cephalad and slightly medial dissection continues following the vessel course. Once the aortic bifurcation is reached, cephalad dissection progresses atop the right lateral border of the aorta to reach the level of the IMA. Small perforating vessels may be encountered and are coagulated.

To establish the lateral border of this nodal group, the ureter is again held laterally. Blunt cephalad dissection with a suction tip atop the iliopsoas muscle separates the retroperitoneal fat from the right border of the IVC. The upper right abdominal retractor blade may need to be repositioned to improve visibility.

At this point, the right paraaortic node bundle has been largely detached medially, distally, and laterally. Next, the bundle is again grasped distally with forceps and elevated as gentle sharp dissection beneath this bundle in the midline is directed cephalad. Delicate perforating veins along the IVC warrant meticulous dissection to reduce bleeding. One of these, the "fellow's vein," is routinely encountered near the level of the aortic bifurcation and is occluded with a vascular clip for hemostasis (Fig. 46-11.2). Upon reaching the level of the IMA, the

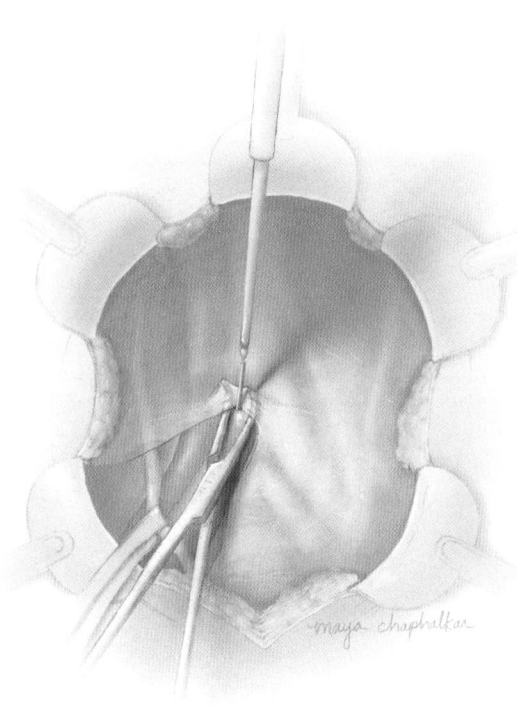

FIGURE 46-11.1 Opening the retroperitoneal spaces.

nodal bundle can be removed by placing large vascular clips across the cephalad end and transecting it before the clip. Once excised, this right nodal bundle is sent as a separate specimen.

❼ Repair of Venous Bleeding. A surgeon should prepare for small lacerations in the wall of the IVC or common iliac veins caused by inadvertent avulsion of perforating venous tributaries. Hemorrhage may be copious and immediate. Initially, pressure is applied with a sponge-stick or finger, and anesthesia staff is informed of the potential for increased blood loss. Second, exposure is assessed. Blood is suctioned from the abdominal cavity, retractors are repositioned, and incisions are extended if necessary. Last, proper vascular instruments are obtained. Lacerated veins can usually be simply repaired with vascular clips (Fig. 46-11.3).

❽ Left Paraaortic Nodes. The medial border of this nodal group is developed using electrosurgical dissection that begins at the IMA. To advance, the medial side of the bundle is elevated with forceps to create tension across fibrous bands connecting it to the aorta. These fibers are sharply divided and free the proximal bundle. Moving caudally, continued similar dissection progresses atop the left border of the aorta toward its bifurcation. Upon reaching the bifurcation, dissection then advances caudally and slightly lateral to follow atop the left common iliac artery's course. This artery's midlength marks the caudad border.

Once this medial dissection is completed, fibrovascular attachments between the sigmoid colon mesentery and left side of the distal aorta are sharply transected. This aids access to laterally located paraaortic nodes.

To develop the lateral border of this nodal group, fingers or suction tip carefully separate the lateral fatty lymphoid tissue from the overlying sigmoid colon mesentery and from the underlying ovarian vessels and

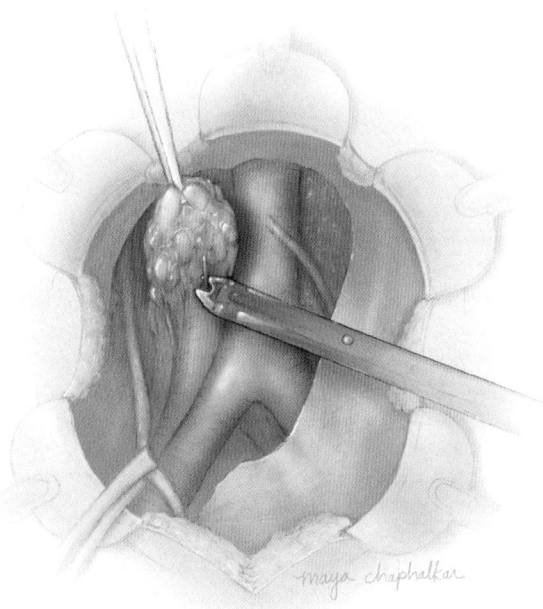

FIGURE 46-11.2 Removal of right paraaortic nodes.

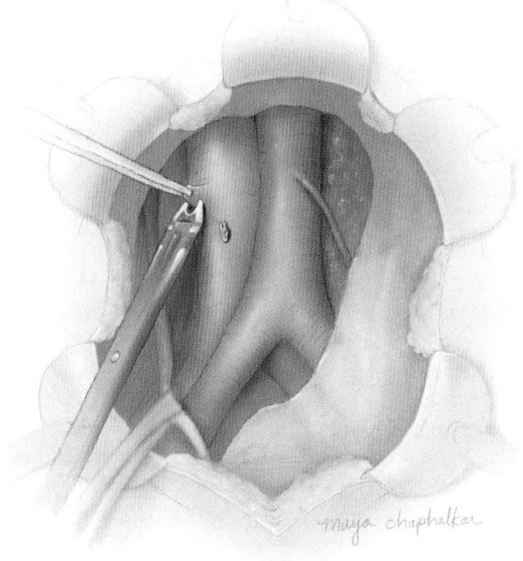

FIGURE 46-11.3 Repair of venous bleeding.

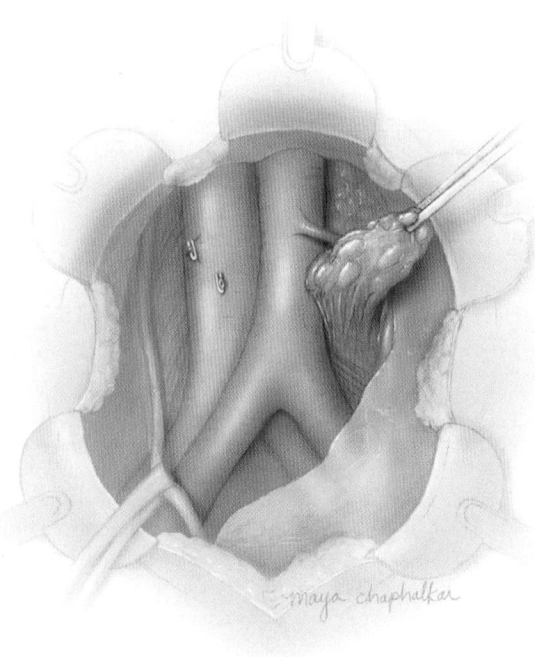

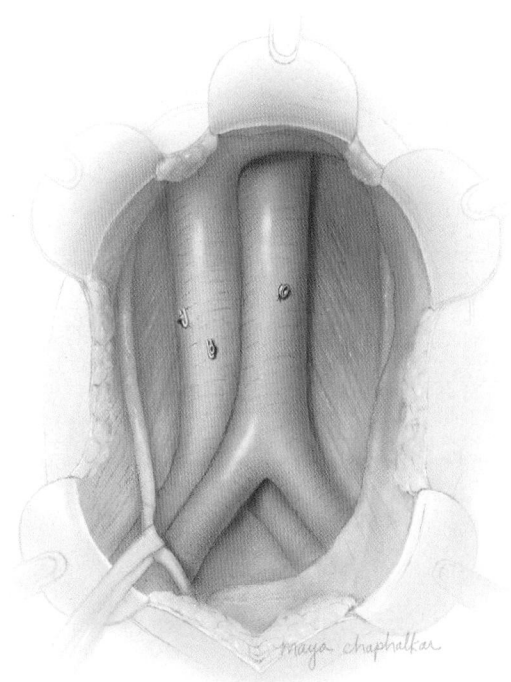

FIGURE 46-11.4 Removal of left paraaortic nodes.

FIGURE 46-11.5 Completed high paraaortic lymphadenectomy.

ureter. Opening this potential space allows clear identification of the ureter and the ovarian vessels, which lie medial to the ureter. A handheld vein retractor is positioned to gently lift up the sigmoid colon mesentery, its adjoining vessels, and ureter.

Establishing these medial and lateral borders delineates the left paraaortic lymph node bundle for removal. To free this bundle caudally, nodal tissue over the common iliac artery is elevated on traction with forceps. A vascular clip is placed across the bundle's caudal end, which is transected before the clip and freed. The distal nodal bundle is next elevated and lifted cephalad (Fig. 46-11.4). Fibrovascular attachments between the bundle and the medial aorta and lateral iliopsoas muscle are transected with electrosurgical blade or with vascular clips and Metzenbaum scissors as dissection moves progressively cephalad to the level of the IMA. Importantly, dissection into the lumbar vessels, which originate from the aorta's posteromedial aspect, is avoided. At the level of the IMA, the cephalad end of the left paraaortic lymph node bundle is clipped and transected. The entire nodal group is removed in toto and submitted as an individual specimen.

❾ **Interiliac Nodes.** Optionally, additional lymph nodes may be removed by excising the fatty tissue between the common iliac vessels. For this, the posterior peritoneum at the aortic bifurcation is grasped, and electrosurgical incision is extended caudally atop

the inner side of both common iliac arteries. The crossing left common iliac vein is visible directly beneath.

The peritoneum is reflected caudally, and the fatty tissue beneath is grasped and placed on tension. Sharp dissection is performed along the surface of both common iliac veins, which have very few small perforating vessels. Once mobilized between the common iliac vessels, the triangle-shaped area of fatty-lymphoid tissue is freed by electrosurgical division of bands connecting it to the sacrum.

❿ **High Paraaortic Lymphadenectomy.** For this extended lymph node removal, anatomic boundaries begin caudally at the level of the IMA and reach cephalad to the entry level of the right ovarian vein and left renal vein (Whitney, 2010). To begin, the former midline peritoneal incision atop the aorta is incised further cephalad, and the duodenal loop is bluntly dissected off the aorta. Repositioning of the retractor blade to move this loop cephalad aids exposure.

On the aorta's right side, the caudal end of the high paraaortic nodal bundle is grasped with blunt forceps, and dissection atop the right lateral border of the aorta is continued cephalad until the right ovarian vein, before its insertion into the IVC. Here, the nodal bundle can be clipped, divided, and incorporated within the specimen.

On the left side, high paraaortic node dissection begins with identification, clipping, and

cutting of the IMA between ties, which allows access to upper nodal tissue. The mesenteric circulation has an extensive collateral network that permits IMA ligation without subsequent bowel ischemia. Alternatively, the IMA may be preserved if adequate exposure is available. This avoids potential bowel ischemia in those with poorly developed collateral vessels.

Dissection continues cephalad atop the left border of the aorta and reaches the left renal vein, which was exposed by prior cephalad displacement of the duodenum. Removal of the left paraaortic nodes includes elevation of the distal nodal bundle and sharp dissection to isolate and electrosurgically divide lymphatic attachments. At the left renal vein, the bundle is clipped and transected (Fig. 46-11.5).

⓫ **Retroaortic Lymphadenectomy.** This more extended dissection is optional and begins after left-sided paraaortic lymphadenectomy has been completed. The left-sided lumbar arteries can be seen branching directly from the aorta. These vessels may be clipped and cut to allow manual rolling of the aorta from left to right, which provides access to the retroaortic nodal chain. Typically, this procedure is performed when imaging studies have demonstrated suspicious nodes in the region.

⓬ **Final Steps.** Gauze sponges may be opened and gently placed in areas of nodal dissection to tamponade any surface oozing. Closing the retroperitoneal space or routinely using suction drainage does not minimize hematoma or lymphocele development (Morice, 2001).

POSTOPERATIVE

The postoperative course following paraaortic lymphadenectomy in general follows that after laparotomy. However, the incidence of postoperative ileus is increased due to longer operative time, increased bowel manipulation, incision extension, and additional blood loss. As with pelvic lymphadenectomy, lymphoceles and hematomas may develop.

46-12

Minimally Invasive Staging for Gynecologic Malignancies

Minimally invasive surgery (MIS) can often be used for surgical staging that includes pelvic and paraaortic lymph node excision and sometimes omentectomy and peritoneal biopsy. Also, for those without comprehensive staging at their primary surgery, MIS may allow a less morbid completion of cancer staging. Specific MIS qualities that are suited to lymphadenectomy include expanded magnified views within deep or narrow spaces and the ability to achieve fine dissection. In terms of landmarks and fields of dissection, MIS lymphadenectomy procedural steps are the same as those with the open abdominal approach described on pages 1169 and 1172. However, with an MIS approach to cancer staging, paraaortic lymphadenectomy is typically completed first. The needed pneumoperitoneum gradually distends bowel, and thus surgery higher in the abdomen is performed early to permit adequate bowel manipulation and displacement.

PREOPERATIVE

Patient Evaluation

A thorough pelvic examination and history reveal factors that help determine the optimal surgical route for an individual patient. As described in Chapter 41 (p. 874), when considering MIS, patients with suspected extensive adhesive disease, morbid obesity, or significant cardiopulmonary disease may be poor candidates. Regardless of approach, preoperative imaging studies prior to lymphadenectomy may help guide the surgeon to suspicious lymph nodes.

Consent

General complications related to MIS are discussed in Chapter 41 (p. 877) and include entry injury to the major vessels, bladder, ureters, and bowel. More specific to MIS staging, acute hemorrhage is the most commonly associated complication. Additionally, ureteral damage, postoperative lymphocele, and nerve injuries can occur, particularly to the obturator and genitofemoral nerve. In addition, the risk of conversion to an open procedure is discussed. Conversion to laparotomy may be necessary if exposure and

organ manipulation are limited or if acute hemorrhage cannot be controlled with MIS techniques. Finally, port-site metastasis is a rare but possible complication.

Patient Preparation

As mentioned, bleeding is a frequent problem with pelvic lymphadenectomy and may be exacerbated by retroperitoneal fibrosis. Accordingly, units of packed red blood cells are typed and crossmatched. Topical hemostatic agents may also prove valuable. Routine bowel preparation and antibiotic prophylaxis are not required for lymphadenectomy but may be indicated for other concurrent surgeries. Thromboembolism prophylaxis is warranted because of the VTE risk associated with cancer. Options are listed in Table 39-8 (p. 836).

INTRAOPERATIVE

Instruments

Important basic MIS tools for laparoscopy include blunt graspers and scissors, whereas the EndoWrist monopolar scissors and the EndoWrist bipolar Maryland grasper are used with the robot. Additional instruments needed for lymphadenectomy include a combined irrigation/suction device, which clears fluid and bluntly dissects; endoscopic bag for node removal; two to three 5-mm instrument ports; 10-mm laparoscope port; 12-mm endoscopic-bag port; and energy devices for cutting and vessel sealing. For the last, several electrosurgical and ultrasonic energy-based devices are adapted for either laparoscopic or robotic cases. These include Harmonic scalpel, electrosurgical monopolar instruments, and electrothermal bipolar coagulator devices (LigaSure, ENSEAL, PK Dissecting Forceps). For laparoscopy, the argon-beam coagulator is another option. Laparoscope selection varies by surgeon, and a 0-degree scope is frequently used. For others, a 30-degree scope permits greater visibility in tight or angulated spaces.

Surgical Steps

❶ **Anesthesia and Patient Positioning.** Laparoscopic lymphadenectomy is performed under general anesthesia. For VTE prophylaxis, lower extremity compression devices are placed, and legs are then positioned in adjustable booted support stirrups. Typically, low lithotomy position is selected due to concurrent hysterectomy, although supine may be appropriate for restaging procedures. As described in Chapter 41 (p. 879), appropriate positioning of legs within the stirrups and

arms at the side is crucial to reduce nerve injury risks. Also, the patient is secured to the bed by means of a gel pad or bean bag with appropriate protective padding. This keeps the patient from sliding when placed in steep Trendelenburg position, which is needed to reflect bowel for retroperitoneal access.

To avoid stomach puncture by a trocar during primary abdominal entry, an orogastric or nasogastric tube is placed to decompress the stomach. To avert similar bladder injury, a Foley catheter is inserted. The abdomen is then surgically prepared. If hysterectomy is planned, then vaginal preparation is also done.

❷ **Port Placement.** As described in Section 46-3 (p. 1142), a 10-mm primary trocar for the laparoscope is placed either at or approximately 1 to 2 cm above the umbilicus using an open abdominal entry method. For paraaortic dissection, this port is placed far enough cephalad to permit visualization of the lower aorta. Accessory ports include a right and left lateral abdominal trocar and one above one of the anterior superior iliac spines, as shown in Figure 46-3.1 (p. 1143).

Additional ports are placed according to surgeon preference or clinical circumstances. All ports ideally have a minimum of 8 cm between them to allow ample range of motion and for robotic procedures, to avoid arm collision.

❸ **Visual Inspection.** Following insertion of the laparoscope, lymph nodes are grossly inspected during initial abdominal exploration. Unexpected positive nodes may alter a proposed operative plan in certain cases, particularly with cervical cancer. In addition, a decision is made to proceed with the MIS approach or convert to laparotomy.

❹ **Paraaortic Lymphadenectomy: Opening the Retroperitoneal Space.** With the patient in steep Trendelenburg position, the small bowel is gently moved into the right and left upper quadrants. The first landmarks identified are the aortic bifurcation and right common iliac artery. The peritoneum over the midlength of the right common iliac artery is grasped, elevated, and sharply incised. This peritoneal incision is extended superiorly atop the right common iliac artery and then atop the aorta. Following each vessel's course, the incision progresses to the curve of duodenum overlying the aorta (Fig. 46-12.1). Once the peritoneum is opened at this level, it is held anteriorly and cephalad by an assistant surgeon using graspers. Blunt and sharp dissection is performed by the surgeon to lift and displace the duodenum cephalad to expose the aorta. This small bowel is progressively lifted until the level of the inferior mesenteric artery

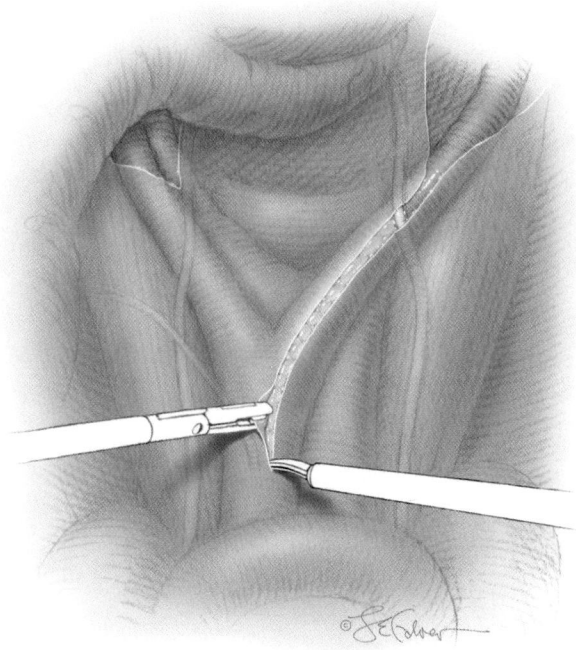

FIGURE 46-12.1 Opening peritoneum over common iliac artery and aorta.

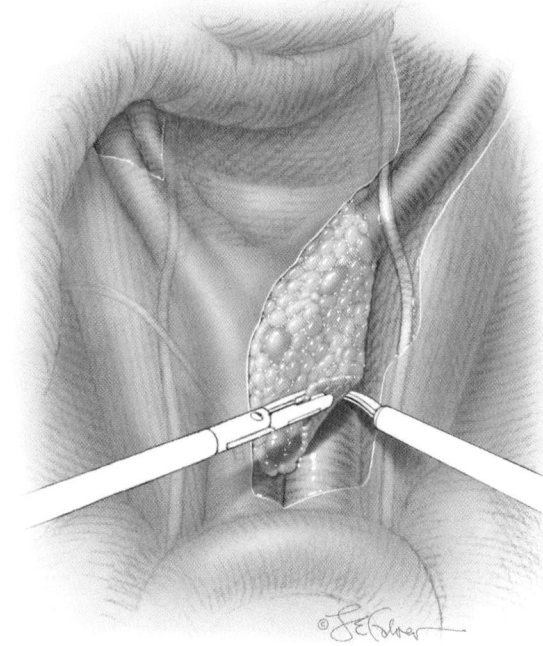

FIGURE 46-12.2 Dissection over the inferior vena cava.

(IMA) is reached as it exits from the aorta on the left.

❺ **Ureter Identification.** For this, the lateral peritoneal cut edge atop the right common iliac artery is grasped and elevated. Blunt dissection beneath this peritoneum progresses laterally until the right ureter is located as it crosses the common iliac artery. Once identified, the ureter is directed laterally with gentle blunt traction. This lowers ureteral injury risks during the remaining nodal dissection.

❻ **Right Paraaortic Lymph Nodes.** To summarize lymphadenectomy within this anatomic area, the caudal end of the fatty, lymph node-containing tissue bundle is freed first. The surgeon then develops medial, lateral, and deep bundle margins and last frees the cephalad tip to permit bundle removal.

To begin, with the ureter held laterally and the inferolateral peritoneal edge elevated, the surgeon first develops the caudal border of this nodal group. Dissection begins at the midlength of the right common iliac artery and atop this artery's lateral border. Within the overlying fatty tissue, small spaces are bluntly developed to create fibrous pedicles that can be lysed or coagulated and divided. In doing so, the distal end of the nodal bundle is progressively freed from the artery and can be elevated and brought cephalad.

Dissection then follows the artery's course and moves medially atop its lateral border. During this dissection, small fibrous bands

between the nodal bundle and the right common iliac artery are sequentially transected. Crossing the IVC and reaching the lower aorta, dissection continues atop the right lateral margin of the aorta until reaching the level of the IMA.

To establish the lateral border of this nodal group, the surgeon revisits the dissection's starting point at the right common iliac artery's midlength. Here, a plane is bluntly developed between the lateral border of the IVC and psoas major muscle. Blunt dissection in this plane frees the retroperitoneal fat and is extended cephalad to the level of the IMA.

At this point, the right paraaortic node bundle has been largely detached medially, distally, and laterally, and division of the deep bundle attachments can be performed. The nodal tissue is elevated and separated from the underlying IVC with gentle blunt dissection progressing cephalad. This dissection moves proximally atop the IVC to reach the level of the IMA (Fig. 46-12.2). During this progression, small pedicles that often contain minor vessels are developed. These pedicles and their multiple perforating vessels are sequentially isolated, clipped or coagulated, and divided. Typically, this is the most difficult part of the dissection because inadvertently avulsed vessels may bleed profusely. For control, hemostatic clips or coagulation can be used. Moreover, a small gauze sponge can be prophylactically placed into the abdomen to provide quick tamponade if required.

At the level of the IMA, the nodal bundle can be excised by placing large vascular clips across the cephalad end and transecting it before the clip. Lymph nodes are extracted intact using an endoscopic bag through a 12-mm port. Once removed, this right nodal bundle is sent as an individual specimen.

❼ **Left Paraaortic Lymph Nodes.** Acquisition of the left paraaortic lymph nodes begins atop the aorta at the level of the IMA. As on the right side, after the initial bundle tip is freed, the medial, lateral, and deep margins are developed. However, dissection moves caudally rather than cephalad and ends at the left common iliac artery's midlength.

The cephalad end of this nodal group is first developed using sharp or electrosurgical dissection that begins just below the IMA (Fig. 46-12.3). Small spaces within the fatty tissue are bluntly opened to create fibrous pedicles that can be lysed or coagulated and divided. This frees the proximal end of the nodal bundle.

To advance, the lateral peritoneal edge and colon mesentery are elevated to the left on tension, and fibrovascular attachments to left side of the distal aorta are sharply transected. This permits lateral retraction of the colon mesentery for exposure. The medial side of the bundle is next elevated with forceps to create tension across fibrous bands connecting the nodal bundle and aorta. These fibers are sharply divided. Similar dissection continues caudally atop the left border of the

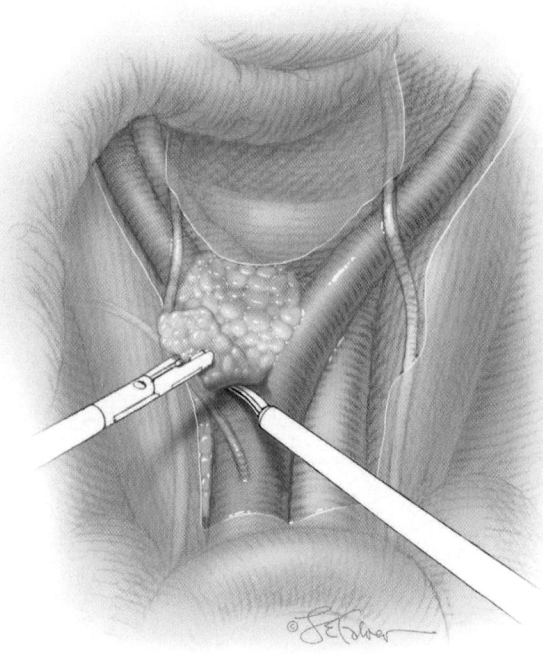

FIGURE 46-12.3 Dissection over the aorta.

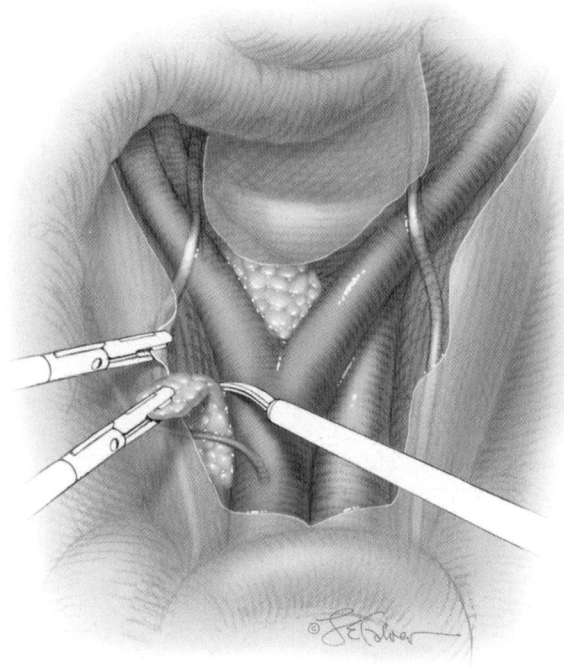

FIGURE 46-12.4 Dissection to the level of the inferior mesenteric artery.

aorta toward its bifurcation. Upon reaching the bifurcation, dissection then moves caudally and slightly laterally atop the left common iliac artery's lateral border to finish at this artery's midlength.

To access the lateral border of this nodal group, a blunt tip carefully sweeps laterally to separate the lateral fatty lymphoid tissue from the overlying sigmoid colon mesentery and from the underlying ureter. The ureter serves as the lateral boundary of this nodal group. Opening this potential space allows the ureter and the ovarian vessels, which lie medial to the ureter, to be clearly identified. A blunt probe is then repositioned to gently lift the colon mesentery, its adjoining vessels, and ureter. With this lateral border now developed, dissection of nodal attachments continues caudad, staying medial to the ureter and reaching the midlength of the left common iliac artery.

After establishing the medial and lateral boundaries of the left paraaortic nodal group, the caudad tip of the nodal bundle is again grasped and elevated. From the midlength of the left common iliac artery, dissection beneath the bundle moves cephalad while transecting deep attachments between it and the lateral aorta and between it and the psoas major muscle (Fig. 46-12.4). Upon reaching the level of the IMA, the cephalad end of the fatty tissue is clipped and transected. The entire nodal group bundle is removed in toto within an endoscopic bag through the 12-mm port. It is submitted as an individual specimen.

❽ High Paraaortic Lymphadenectomy. In some instances, a surgeon may elect an extended laparoscopic dissection. The anatomic boundaries of a high paraaortic lymphadenectomy begin distally at the IMA and reach proximally to the entry level of the right ovarian vein and left renal vein into the IVC, respectively (Whitney, 2010). Typically, this extension is possible only in selected patients with favorable anatomy, such as thin body habitus. Otherwise, upper abdominal exposure is problematic. Other helpful maneuvers include having a second surgical assistant and placing additional right and left upper quadrant trocars. In contrast, robotic paraaortic lymphadenectomy stops at the level of the IMA. High paraaortic dissection to the level of the renal vein is technically difficult and infrequently performed. Reasons include poor visualization, limitations in spanning the distance with the robotic arms, and inability to turn the patient around without undocking and placing additional ports.

To begin laparoscopically, the peritoneum overlying the aorta at the level of the IMA is grasped and elevated cephalad to displace small intestine into the upper abdomen and provide exposure to the aorta. The surgeon dissects retroperitoneally atop the aorta to further mobilize the duodenum and displace it cephalad. Often a laparoscopic fan retractor positioned in the retroperitoneal space aids exposure of the upper aorta.

To develop the medial border of the right high paraaortic nodal group, the nodal bundle overlying the IVC is regrasped and held on traction to dissect and divide the fibrous attachments from the aorta's anterior surface and right border. This begins caudally at the level of the IMA and ends cephalad at the right ovarian vein.

For the lateral border of this nodal group, the right ureter is identified and again retracted to the right. The lateral portion of the nodal bundle is then bluntly separated from the psoas muscle in a proximal direction. The ovarian vein will be encountered and may be individually sealed and divided depending on its proximity to lymph nodes slated for removal.

With both lateral and medial borders defined, the deep middle attachments of this nodal bundle are freed by gentle cephalad dissection over the IVC until the level of the right ovarian vein is reached. Last, the proximal border of the nodal bundle is detached and removed as described earlier.

Dissection of the high left paraaortic nodal group begins by placing laparoscopic clips on the IMA and dividing between using a vessel-sealing device. Alternatively, the IMA may be preserved if adequate exposure is available. This avoids potential bowel ischemia in those with poorly developed collateral vessels. The left ureter is again identified as the lateral border of this high nodal group and is held laterally by an assistant.

The surgeon performs blunt dissection with intermittent coagulation and division of fibrous or vascular pedicles to detach the nodal bundle in a cephalad direction. Dissection continues until it reaches the left renal vein, where the bundle is detached and removed.

❾ Pelvic Lymphadenectomy: Retroperitoneal Entry.

For this nodal resection, lymphoid tissue is removed within the area bounded by the psoas major muscle (lateral), the superior vesical artery (medial), the midlength of the common iliac artery (cephalad), and the deep circumflex iliac vein (caudad). To begin, the round ligament is transected, and the peritoneal leaf between the round and infundibulopelvic (IP) ligament is grasped, elevated, and incised parallel to the IP. Gentle traction is again applied to the round ligament, and the broad ligament's anterior peritoneal leaf is opened to reach the vesicouterine fold in the midline. If radical hysterectomy is planned after pelvic lymphadenectomy, then pararectal and paravesical spaces are completely developed as described on page 1144 prior to pelvic lymph node removal.

❿ Pelvic Lymphadenectomy: Distal Common Iliac Nodes.

Bowel is first retracted sufficiently to allow access to the distal half of the common iliac artery. To remove this nodal group, the prior peritoneal incision atop the common iliac artery is extended from its midlength caudally to expose the artery. Ureterolysis, if not previously performed, is completed as described in Section 46-3, Step 4 (p. 1143). The ureter is then bluntly retracted medially before beginning node dissection.

Lateral fatty lymphoid tissue may be removed by first elevating it with a blunt grasper and using electrosurgical dissection atop the common iliac artery's lateral margin to establish a plane between the nodal bundle and artery. Blunt dissection to further separate the nodal tissue from the artery is continued caudad. Electrosurgical coagulation plus sharp incision is used to detach these nodes. Importantly, on the patient's right side, the common iliac vein and inferior vena cava lie beneath the common iliac artery's lateral margin, and thus careful node excision is prudent. Further dissection is performed atop the distal common iliac artery, which serves as the medial border for this nodal group. Upon reaching the common iliac artery bifurcation, lymphatic tissue excision continues caudally to incorporate the external iliac nodal group.

⓫ External Iliac Nodes.

Removal of this lymph node group starts by freeing its lateral border. Tissue previously resected along the common iliac artery is elevated and placed on tension. Dissection then extends caudally along the lateral side of the external iliac artery until reaching the deep circumflex iliac vein. This vein crosses the distal external iliac artery and serves as the caudal boundary of this nodal group. Along this path, dissection bluntly develops a plane between medially located lymphoid tissue and lateral preperitoneal fat found above the psoas major muscle (Fig. 46-12.5). During dissection, the genitofemoral nerve running atop the psoas major muscle is ideally identified and protected.

Next, grasper traction is typically required to lift the nodal bundle above the external iliac artery beginning at the common iliac artery bifurcation. During caudal dissection, a blunt tool gently pushes into the fibrofatty tissue to create distinct pedicles that attach the nodal bundle to the artery. These pedicle attachments can then be coagulated and divided. Electrosurgery can be also used to obtain hemostasis as the lymph node bundle is progressively excised caudally.

The mobilized nodal bundle is next reflected medially to reveal the entire external iliac artery (Fig. 46-12.6). Medial traction is applied with forceps, and fine adventitial bands that connect nodes to the underlying external iliac vein are transected using electrosurgical cutting. In contrast to open surgery, the pneumoperitoneum and Trendelenburg position used during laparoscopy result in vein collapse. As a result, the external iliac vein is harder to distinguish and can be easily injured. Once completed, this external iliac nodal group dissection later permits safe entry into the obturator space, outlined in Step 13.

⓬ Internal Iliac Nodes.

The ureter is moved and held medially by a blunt instrument for protection and improved pelvic sidewall visualization. Beginning at the distal aspect of the superior vesical artery, the free

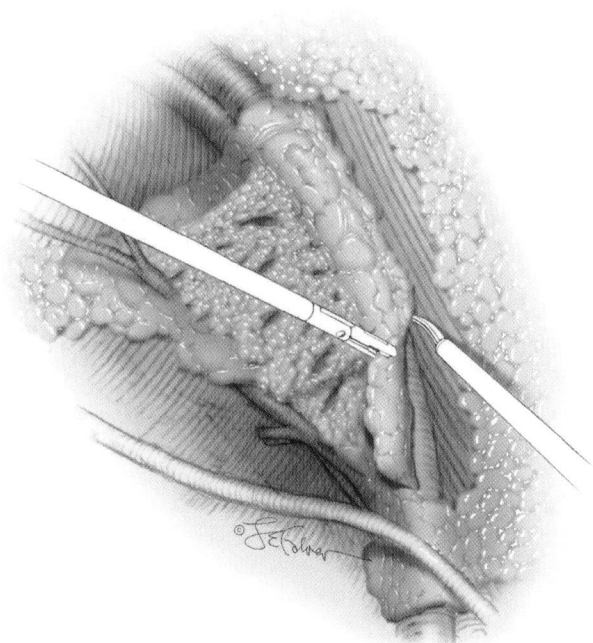

FIGURE 46-12.5 Dissection between the external iliac artery and psoas major muscle.

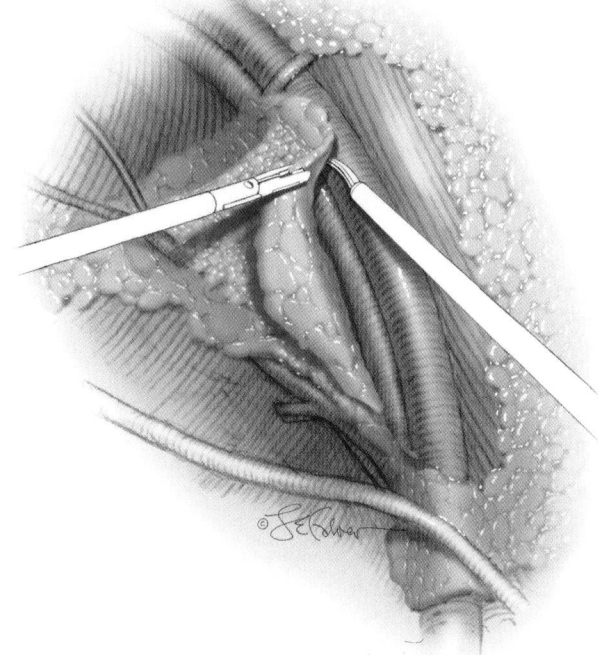

FIGURE 46-12.6 Dissection off the external iliac vessels.

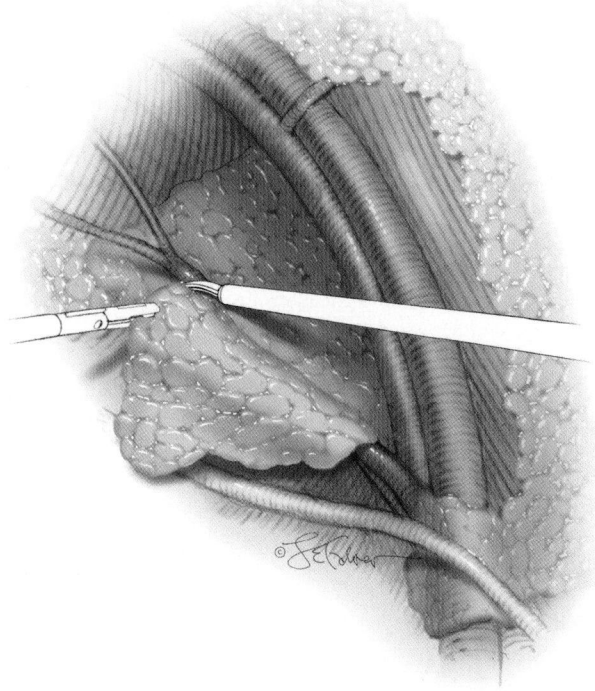

FIGURE 46-12.7 Dissection off the internal iliac artery.

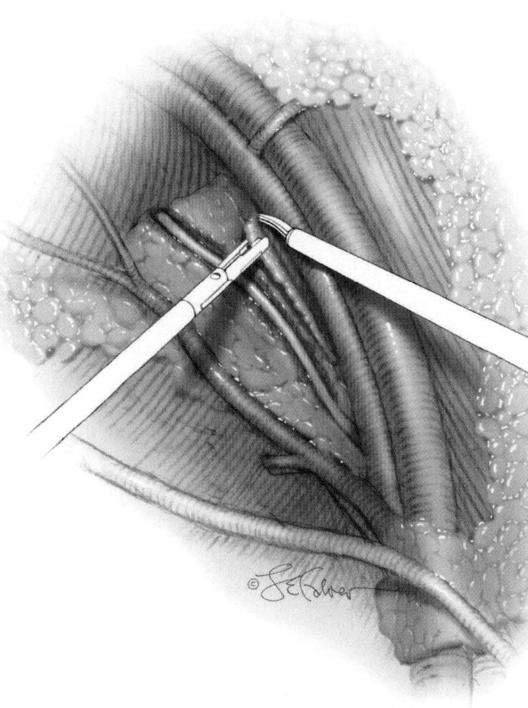

FIGURE 46-12.8 Dissection above the obturator artery.

nodal bundle is again elevated and placed on tension. Initial sharp excision of the internal iliac nodal group continues cephalad along the superior vesical artery and then along the internal iliac vessels (Fig. 46-12.7). As dissection approaches the common iliac artery bifurcation, the nodal attachments are fine and allow blunt disruption. At this point, both the external iliac and internal iliac nodes are completely dissected and can be submitted as one specimen or combined with obturator fossa lymph nodes, depending on surgeon preference.

⓭ **Obturator Fossa Nodes.** With the assistant surgeon holding medial traction on the superior vesical artery, the obturator fossa can be exposed. This fossa may be entered medially, between the external iliac artery and the psoas major muscle. Thereafter, the external iliac vessels are retracted medially so that the obturator space can be accessed from a lateral approach. Or, the obturator space can suitably be entered medially.

If present, nodal tissue along the inferomedial wall of the external iliac vein is transected with blunt and electrosurgical dissection. Also, accessory venous branches may be identified and coagulated.

Within the exposed fossa, obturator nodal tissue is grasped with forceps. This nodal bundle lies deep to the external iliac vein but superficial to the obturator nerve. With upward traction applied, blunt forceps or a suction/irrigation device tip moved gently side-to-side disrupts nodal tissue attachments to the obturator nerve (Fig. 46-12.8). This blunt dissection is performed in the center of the fossa to minimize injury to surrounding deep pelvic vasculature. This also clears off tissue to permit obturator nerve identification.

Once this nerve is localized, dissection should purposely remain superficial to it. Firm fibrotic attachments may be electrosurgically transected under direct visualization. As the caudal end of the bundle is reached, it is usually tethered to the sidewall and freed sharply. At the cephalad end of the bundle, nodes are carefully separated sharply from the inferior aspect of the external iliac vein while avoiding obturator nerve injury. Nodal tissue deep to the obturator nerve is not routinely removed since the obturator artery and vein traverse this area. Laceration of either vessel can result in retraction and catastrophic hemorrhage that is difficult to control.

Pelvic lymph nodes are then removed in toto via endoscopic bag. The identical procedure is performed on the contralateral side.

⓮ **Completion of Laparoscopic Staging and Omentectomy.** The staging procedure for ovarian cancer includes obtaining multiple peritoneal biopsies from the cul-de-sac, pelvic sidewalls, and pelvic gutters, and from the diaphragm bilaterally. This can be performed with a blunt grasper and laparoscopic scissors, with or without electrosurgical coagulation. The surgical staging for ovarian cancer and for certain histologic subtypes of endometrial cancer (papillary serous and clear cell carcinoma) also includes omentum removal.

A laparoscopic omentectomy is performed by identifying and elevating the omentum away from the transverse colon. Avascular windows are created within the proximal omentum. The intervening vascular attachments are then ligated with a vessel-sealing energy tool or endoscopic stapler. Once completely dissected, the omentum is placed in an endoscopic bag and removed through a transabdominal 12-mm port. In many women, the omentum is large and therefore is brought through the vagina if a laparoscopic hysterectomy is performed. All specimens undergo minimal manipulation and are removed through an endoscopic bag to help decrease the risk of port-site or intraabdominal tumor implantation.

⓯ **Port Removal and Fascial Closure.** Once procedures are completed, areas are inspected for bleeding. Topical hemostatic agents may be used and are listed in Table 40-5 (p. 861). If hemostasis is achieved, trocars are removed and port sites closed. Fascial defects larger than 10 mm are sutured to decrease the risk of herniation at those sites. Interrupted stitches of 0-gauge delayed-absorbable suture are placed to reapproximate this fascia. Alternatively, a dedicated trocar-site closure device, described in Chapter 41 (p. 897), can be used. Regardless of technique, the defect is palpated to confirm adequate closure.

POSTOPERATIVE

The postoperative course following MIS staging lymphadenectomy generally follows that after other major laparoscopic surgery. Patients usually are able to tolerate clear liquids quickly, followed by a regular diet and discharge on postoperative day 1. With their pain typically controlled with oral pain medication, patients ambulate early.

Postoperative complications may include pelvic lymphocele formation, neurologic injuries, or trocar-site herniation. One long-term potential complication of pelvic lymphadenectomy is lymphedema. The exact incidence is unknown, but estimates range from 1 to 27 percent after surgical staging for endometrial cancer (Todo, 2010). The risk increases if more lymph nodes are removed or if pelvic radiation is administered after surgery. Treatments, which may or may not be successful, often include compression stockings, lower extremity wrapping, and massage therapy to manipulate lymph channels. Although generally not associated with an adverse outcome, this complication can significantly lower a patient's quality of life postoperatively.

46-13

En Bloc Pelvic Resection

Ovarian cancer with contiguous encasement of the reproductive organs, pelvic peritoneum, cul-de-sac, and sigmoid colon is the main indication for en bloc pelvic resection. Also known as radical oophorectomy, this effective technique aids a maximal cytoreductive surgical effort. As a result of removing all microscopic and infiltrative peritoneal tumor in the pelvis, improved survival rates can be expected in patients with advanced epithelial ovarian cancer (Aletti, 2006b). Moreover, pelvic recurrence rates are low and reflect the completeness of pelvic tumor eradication (Hertel, 2001). Many of the principles of en bloc pelvic resection mirror those of other procedures in gynecologic oncology.

PREOPERATIVE

Patient Evaluation

Pelvic examination may reveal a relatively immobile mass, and abdominopelvic CT images typically demonstrate a pelvic mass and ascites. With the presumed diagnosis of advanced ovarian cancer, patients are prepared for anticipated cytoreductive surgery. However, the need for en bloc resection is usually dictated by intraoperative findings rather than preoperative testing.

Consent

In general, women with advanced ovarian cancer undergoing cytoreductive surgery are at significant risk for complications. Minor postoperative problems such as incisional cellulitis, superficial wound dehiscence, urinary tract infection, or ileus are common. Major postoperative complications of en bloc resection include anastomotic leaks and various fistulas (Bristow, 2003; Park, 2006).

Patient Preparation

Primary anastomosis without colostomy is typical for most patients. Thus, bowel preparation is commonplace for any type of cytoreductive ovarian cancer surgery, but particularly if en bloc pelvic resection is a possibility. One or more bowel resections may be required to achieve optimal debulking, and often, preoperative determination of the exact location of tumor infiltration is not entirely accurate. The combination of pneumatic compression devices and subcutaneous

heparin is particularly important due to the anticipated longer operation length, coagulability risk associated with malignancy, and possibility of extended postoperative recovery. Moreover, patients are routinely typed and crossmatched for packed red blood cell replacement, as transfusions are frequently indicated (Bristow, 2003).

INTRAOPERATIVE

Instruments

En bloc pelvic resection requires access to multiple sizes of bowel staplers, including gastrointestinal anastomosis (GIA), transverse anastomosis (TA), and end-to-end anastomosis (EEA) staplers. Additionally, a ligate-divide-staple (LDS) device or electrothermal bipolar coagulator (LigaSure) may be used to divide vascular tissue pedicles.

Surgical Steps

❶ **Anesthesia and Patient Positioning.** Bimanual examination under general anesthesia is especially important to confirm the need for low lithotomy leg positioning in booted support stirrups. Access to the perineum is crucial any time the EEA device may need to be placed in the rectum. Sterile preparation of the abdomen, perineum, and vagina is performed, and a Foley catheter is placed.

❷ **Abdominal Entry.** Typically, a vertical incision is selected for ovarian cancer debulking surgery since the extent of disease cannot

be precisely known beforehand and upper abdominal disease requires excision. At first, the incision extends up to the umbilicus. After exploration and determination of tumor resectability, it can be lengthened as needed.

❸ **Exploration.** The abdomen is thoroughly explored to first determine whether all gross disease can be safely removed. For example, unresectable upper abdominal tumor makes the prospect of a radical pelvic operation less attractive.

Frequently during exploration, it is difficult to distinguish uterus, adnexa, and adjacent tumor. As shown in Figure 46-13.1, both ovaries may be grossly enlarged with tumor and densely fixed into the posterior cul-de-sac with contiguous involvement of the uterus, rectosigmoid, and lateral sidewalls. Moreover, superficial implants often coat the fallopian tubes, the vesicouterine fold, and much of the surrounding pelvic peritoneum. En bloc pelvic resection will allow removal of all this gross disease.

❹ **Lateral Pelvic Dissection.** For cases in which the round ligaments cannot be located with certainty, the lateral peritoneum is grasped with an Allis clamp, and an electrosurgical blade is used to enter the retroperitoneum (Fig. 46-13.2). The loose areolar connective tissue of this space is bluntly dissected and the overlying peritoneum is sharply incised to create an opening in which the external iliac artery can be palpated. This artery is bluntly followed to the bifurcation with the internal iliac artery. The medial peritoneal leaf of the

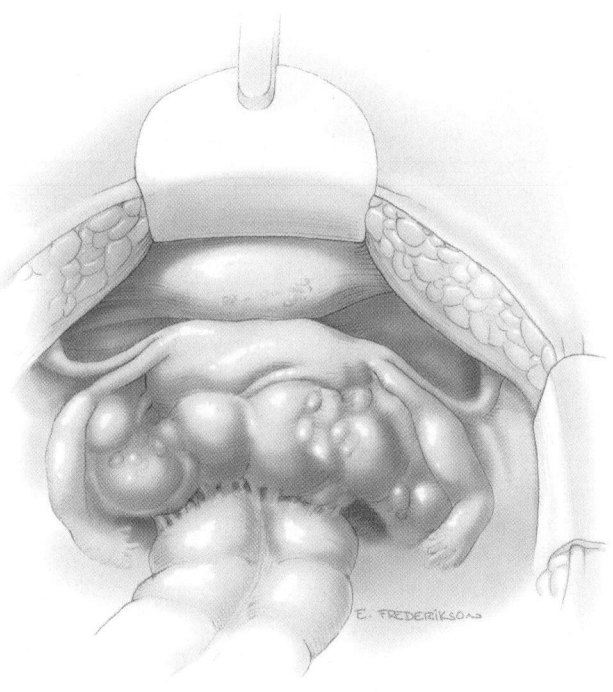

FIGURE 46-13.1 Extensive ovarian cancer.

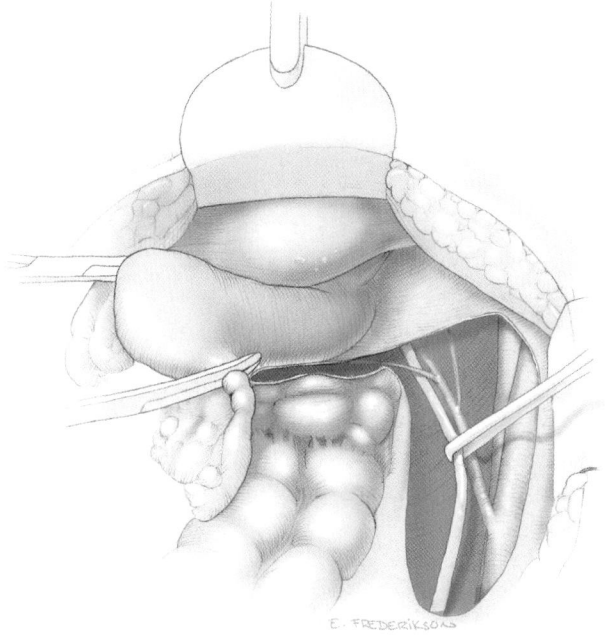

FIGURE 46-13.2 Lateral pelvic dissection.

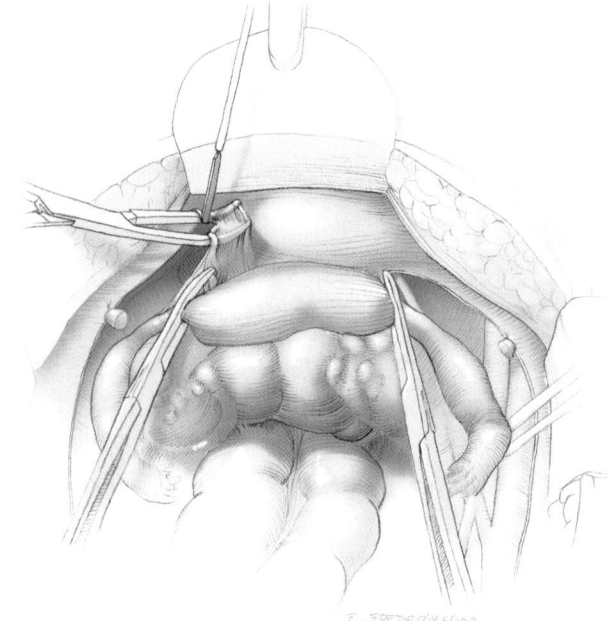

FIGURE 46-13.3 Vesicouterine dissection.

broad ligament is elevated to identify the ureter, around which a one-quarter inch Penrose drain is looped.

The infundibulopelvic (IP) ligament will typically not be entirely distinguishable due to induration and anatomic distortion by tumor. A window is bluntly opened just superior to the ureter as it crosses above the pelvic brim to isolate a tissue pedicle that will include the IP ligament. The ligament is isolated, clamped, cut, and tied with 0-gauge delayed-absorbable suture. The entire sequence is repeated on the contralateral side. The ureter may then be mobilized distally, and the anterior portion of the broad ligament is incised toward the vesicouterine fold using an electrosurgical blade. The round ligament will be identified during this dissection and separately divided.

❺ **Vesicouterine Dissection.** The anterior broad ligament dissection is continued with a right-angle clamp guiding the electrosurgical blade (Fig. 46-13.3). The peritoneum is typically edematous and thick. En bloc removal of tumor implants within the vesicouterine fold will require a wide excision of the peritoneum over the bladder dome. Thus, the proximal end of the vesicouterine fold may be held on traction, and an electrosurgical blade used to sharply dissect in a caudal direction toward the cervix while encompassing the tumor. The bladder mucosa is typically not entered, but it may be simply repaired if an inadvertent cystotomy occurs (Chap. 40, p. 867). After removal of this peritoneum, the bladder may then be advanced distally in the usual manner as for simple hysterectomy. The whitish cervix will be visualized

through the anterior vaginal wall. The ureters are held laterally while the uterine vessels are freed of surrounding connective tissue (skeletonized), clamped, cut, and ligated.

❻ **Dividing the Sigmoid Colon.** This step mirrors those in Steps 5 and 6 of low anterior resection, illustrated on page 1201. First, the ureters are held laterally, while a right-angle clamp guides an electrosurgical blade during posterior peritoneum incision. This incision moves medially on each side to reach the midline sigmoid colon mesentery. The sigmoid colon segment that lies proximal to the tumor is selected, and the underlying mesentery is superficially incised on each side with the electrosurgical blade. A GIA stapler is then inserted to divide the bowel.

After colon division, the remaining mesentery is scored superficially with the electrosurgical blade and divided with the electrothermal bipolar coagulator. Larger pedicles, such as those including the inferior mesenteric vessels, will need to be clamped, cut, and ligated separately. As during total pelvic exenteration, the avascular retrorectal space between the rectum and the sacrum may then be bluntly dissected to completely mobilize the rectosigmoid down to the cervix (Fig. 46-13.4).

❼ **Retrograde Hysterectomy.** The bladder is separated from the upper vagina with sharp electrosurgical blade dissection. The anterior vaginal wall distal to the tumor margin is grasped with a Kocher clamp. The anterior vaginal wall is then incised at 12 o'clock with the electrosurgical blade, and the incision is extended laterally to the right

and left. The cervix is grasped with a Kocher clamp and retracted to expose the posterior vaginal wall. An electrosurgical blade is used to incise this wall transversely and enter the rectovaginal space. Two Allis clamps grasp the upper vagina to apply caudad traction and aid further dissection. A retrorectal hand is placed to assess whether the tumor extends into the rectovaginal septum beyond the cervix. With large masses, distal dissection may be required into the rectovaginal septum to reach a point distal to the tumor's leading edge. If so, further distal vaginal wall excision may be needed to reach tumor-free margins. Alternatively, smaller tumors may allow proximal dissection in the rectovaginal septum. This gains additional rectal length distal to the tumor and allows for creation of a higher colon reanastomosis. Finally, the remaining uterosacral and cardinal ligaments are clamped, analogous to that during radical hysterectomy, but in a retrograde fashion. With this, distal portions of the cardinal ligament are transected first, and then more cephalad portions are clamped, cut, and ligated. For protection, ureters are held laterally (Fig. 46-13.5).

❽ **Distal Rectal Division.** The mucosa of the rectal segment distal to the tumor is circumferentially dissected free of mesenteric attachments and rectal pillars by constant traction on the en bloc specimen. The TA or contour cutting (Contour) stapler is inserted into the pelvis and fired to transect the rectum (Fig. 46-13.6, dotted line). The specimen, which contains the uterus, adnexa, rectosigmoid, and surrounding peritoneum,

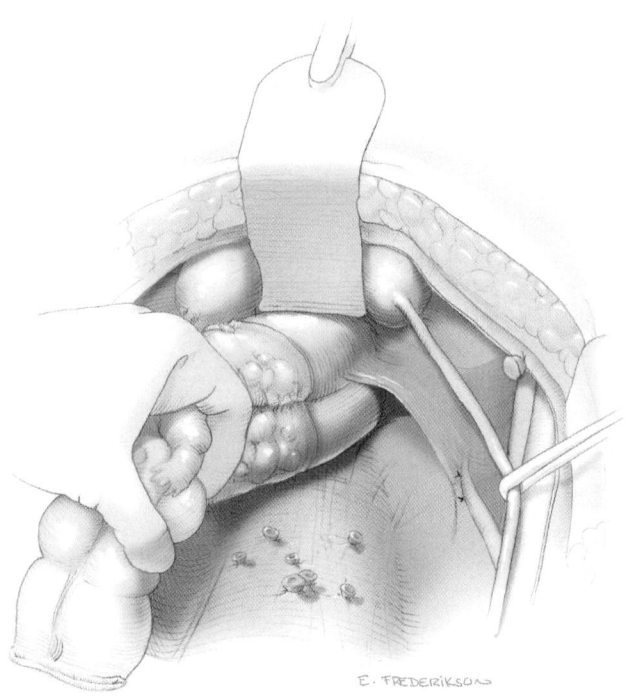

FIGURE 46-13.4 Dividing the rectosigmoid.

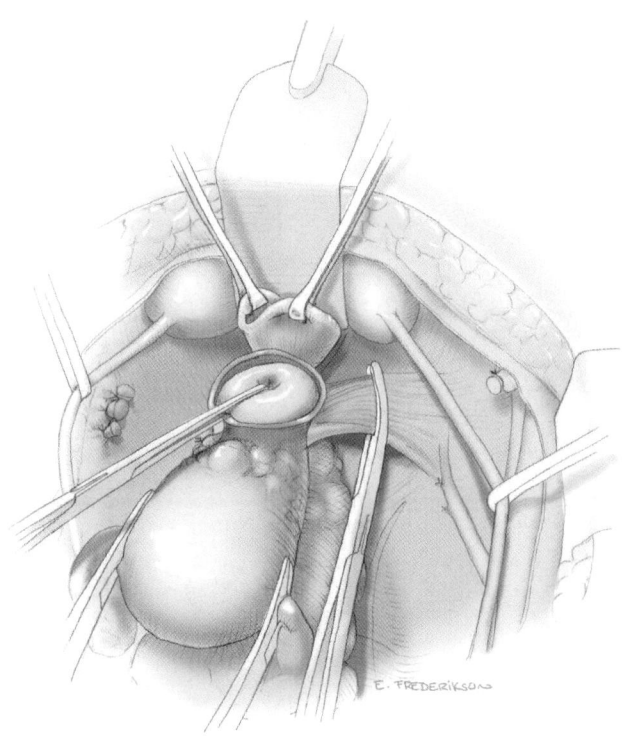

FIGURE 46-13.5 Retrograde hysterectomy.

is then lifted out of the pelvis. The vaginal opening is closed in a running fashion with 0-gauge delayed-absorbable suture. The final appearance Fig. 46-13.7 is shown with completed rectosigmoid anastomosis, which is described in Section 46-21 (p. 1200).

❾ **Final Steps.** A surgeon then proceeds with additional procedures if necessary to complete the ovarian cancer debulking surgery. A colostomy or rectosigmoid anastomosis may require mobilization of the splenic flexure and is performed near the end of

surgery. Postoperative drains may be placed at the surgeon's discretion. Occasionally, the bladder may also be retrograde filled to exclude cystotomy during vesicouterine dissection. All pedicles sites are reexamined for hemostasis.

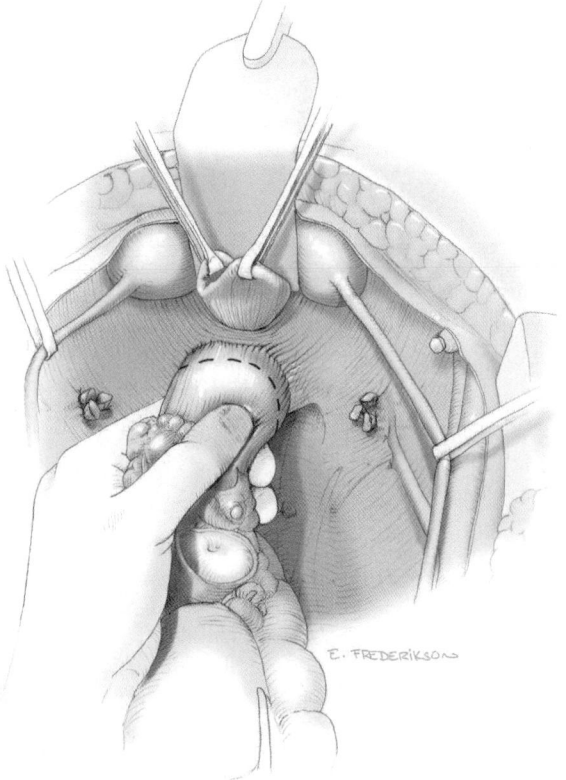

FIGURE 46-13.6 Rectosigmoid resection.

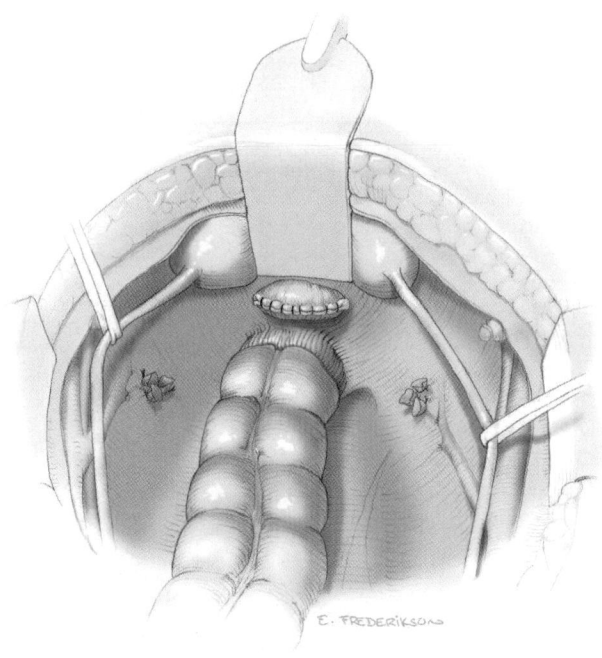

FIGURE 46-13.7 Final appearance.

POSTOPERATIVE

En bloc pelvic resection of primary and recurrent ovarian cancer permits a high rate of complete debulking with acceptable morbidity and mortality rates (Park, 2006). Urinary tract infection, pneumonia, deep-vein thrombosis, wound cellulitis, and postoperative ileus are relatively common events following major abdominal surgery for ovarian cancer. Reoperation for anastomotic breakdown or postoperative hemorrhage specific to en bloc pelvic resection is uncommon (Bristow, 2003; Clayton, 2002).

46-14

Omentectomy

The omentum is typically removed for two reasons: (1) tumor debulking or (2) cancer staging. First, patients who present with advanced ovarian cancer almost invariably have metastases to the omentum. The extent of this "omental cake" may be massive and involve the upper gastrocolic ligament, anterior abdominal wall, splenic hilum, and transverse colon (Fig. 35-14, p. 748). Thus, a surgeon is prepared to encompass the entire tumor with an adequate resection. Second, omentectomy is routinely indicated for staging patients with ovarian cancer or with uterine papillary serous carcinoma who do not have obvious metastatic disease (Boruta, 2009; Koh, 2014; Whitney, 2010).

As a reminder, the proximal omentum has two leaves. Its anterior leaf attaches to the greater curvature of the stomach via the gastrocolic ligament. Its posterior leaf attaches to the caudal margin of the transverse colon. The lesser omental sac lies between these two proximal leaves. *Infracolic omentectomy* describes transection of the anterior leaf (gastrocolic ligament) at a level below the transverse colon. This is sufficient for most clinical circumstances. Supracolic (total) omentectomy describes transection of the anterior leaf (gastrocolic ligament) at a level above the transverse colon and close to the stomach's greater curvature. It may be indicated for a large omental cake.

Omentectomy may be completed by laparotomy, as described here. It is also amenable to a MIS approach, as described in Section 46-12, Step 14 (1180).

PREOPERATIVE

Patient Evaluation

Imaging studies may suggest an omental cake, but its extent is difficult to ascertain until exploration in the operating room.

Consent

Although bleeding may follow inadequate vessel ligation, complications from omentectomy are rare. Obesity and intraabdominal adhesive disease, however, may increase these risks. Obesity results in a much thicker omentum that has thicker vascular pedicles, which may slip from clamps or ligatures. Additionally, prior upper abdominal surgery—particularly gastric bypass—may cause adhesions and a more difficult resection. In addition to these risks, women with an omental cake are informed of a possible need for bowel resection, splenectomy, or other radical debulking procedures to remove the entire tumor.

Patient Preparation

The risk of infection following omentectomy is low, however, this surgery is typically performed with other gynecologic procedures that warrant antibiotics and VTE prophylaxis, as listed in Tables 39-6 and 39-8 (p. 835). The decision to administer a bowel preparation regimen is individualized by surgeon preference and clinical setting. Suitable options are found in Chapter 39 (p. 835).

INTRAOPERATIVE

Surgical Steps

❶ **Anesthesia and Patient Positioning.** Omentectomy is typically performed as an inpatient procedure under general anesthesia. A patient is positioned supine, a Foley catheter is placed, and the abdomen is surgically prepared.

❷ **Abdominal Entry.** Infracolic omentectomy may be performed through any type of incision. However, because of the uncertain extent of disease that accompanies these cases, a midline vertical incision is most commonly selected. If only a portion of the omentum needs to be removed for staging purposes, the incision does not necessarily need to be extended above the umbilicus since the omentum is often accessible. In all other situations, the incision is extended cephalad to provide sufficient exposure.

❸ **Exploration.** Palpation of the omentum is often the first step in exploring the abdomen. This organ is directly beneath a midline vertical incision and should be readily visible. Omentectomy is typically the first procedure performed in women with an omental cake and presumed ovarian cancer. The omentum can usually be quickly removed and sent for frozen section analysis while a surgeon places a self-retaining retractor and proceeds with the remainder of a planned operation.

❹ **Visualization.** A surgeon gently grasps the infracolic omentum and pulls it out of the abdomen through the incision. The borders of any omental cake can be seen directly or palpated. The extent of resection can then be determined, and the abdominal wall incision extended if necessary.

❺ **Entrance into the Lesser Sac.** The posterior leaf of the omentum is best accessed by flipping the omental drape cephalad. Filmy adventitial tissue with some traversing small vessel tributaries joins this leaf and colon, and these attachments are electrosurgically cut and vessels divided by a ligate-divide-staple (LDS) device or an electrothermal bipolar coagulator (LigaSure). Dissection generally begins as far to the right as possible and continues as far to the left as possible. A right-angle clamp is opened beneath the omentum to guide the direction of the electrosurgical blade (Fig. 46-14.1). Once the posterior leaf is transected, the lesser sac is entered.

Entrance into the lesser sac mobilizes the colon and provides access to the tumor-free proximal gastrocolic ligament.

❻ **Gastrocolic Ligament Division.** Next, attention turns to the anterior omental leaf, and the omental drape is now flipped caudad. For an infracolic omentectomy, dissection of the omentum is performed inferior to the level of the transverse colon. Dissection again generally begins on the far right and moves to the left. Numerous vertically coursing vessels can be seen, but others are covered by fatty tissue and difficult to appreciate. A right-angle clamp is used by the surgeon to "pop" through an avascular portion of the gastrocolic ligament that is near, but safely distal to, the colon. The clamp is then opened in a vertical direction (parallel to the vessels) and held in place to guide the LDS or electrothermal bipolar coagulator in safely and quickly dividing the tissue (Fig. 46-14.2).

This procedure is continued across the entire gastrocolic ligament, and the omental specimen is handed off. However, if a J-flap is planned instead of an omentectomy, then only three quarters of the omentum is divided from right to left. This preserves the left gastroepiploic artery for blood supply. The distal tip of the flap is brought into the pelvis and tacked to adjoining peritoneum with 2–0 or 3–0 gauge delayed-absorbable suture to provide additional blood supply wherever desired. Regardless of whether removing the infracolic omentum or fashioning a J-flap, the drape will need to be rotated back and forth intermittently to make certain that dissection remains away from the colon.

❼ **Supracolic Omentectomy.** In cases in which an omental cake has extended proximally, a supracolic (total) omentectomy is indicated. This procedure requires a midline vertical incision to provide better exposure to the upper abdomen. Resection may simply involve transecting the omentum at a higher level in the gastrocolic ligament. Alternatively, anatomic boundaries of resection may need to be extended to the hepatic flexure, the stomach, and the splenic flexure to encompass the entire tumor.

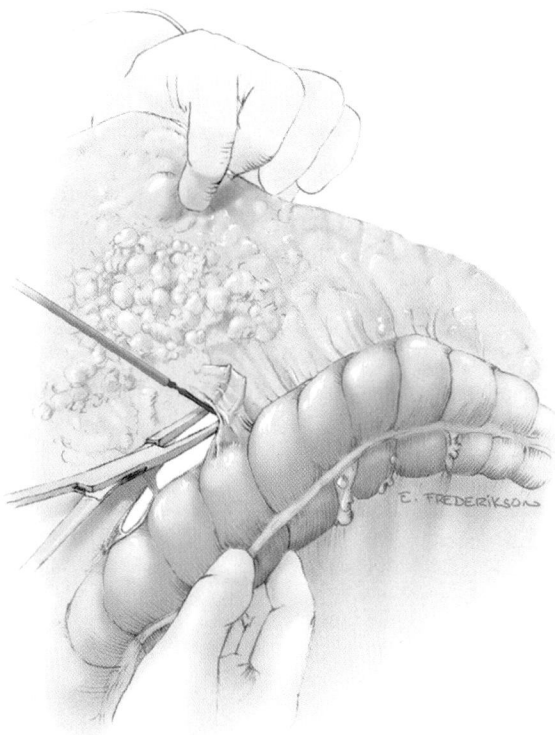

FIGURE 46-14.1 Posterior omental leaf transection to enter the lesser sac.

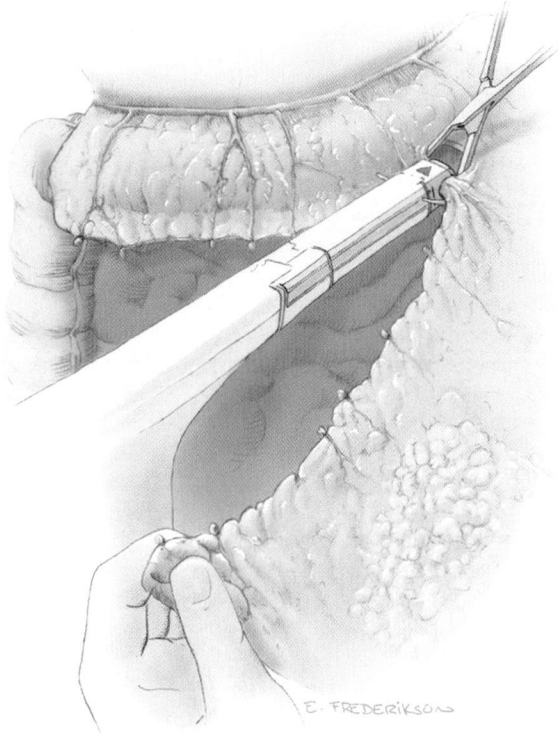

FIGURE 46-14.2 Anterior ligation of gastrocolic ligament.

Dissection again proceeds from right to left, detaching the posterior leaf of the omentum from its attachment to the transverse colon. Mobilization of the ascending colon around the hepatic flexure may be necessary to perform a gastrocolic omentectomy. The right gastroepiploic artery is ligated, and the dissection is continued to the left by dividing the short gastric vessels until the lateral-most portion of the tumor is reached. Mobilization of the descending colon and takedown of the splenic flexure may be required if tumor extends that far laterally.

❽ **Incision Closure.** The remaining omentum should be reexamined at the completion of surgery before closing the abdomen. Occasionally, small bleeding vessels or a hematoma will need to be addressed with additional ligation. The abdominal entry incision is then closed as described in Section 43-1 (p. 928).

POSTOPERATIVE

Nasogastric tube placement is required only if a total omentectomy has been performed. Decompression of the stomach for 48 hours protects the ligated gastric vessels from postoperative dislodgement due to gastric dilation. The remaining postoperative course follows that for laparotomy or for other specific concurrent surgeries performed.

46-15

Splenectomy

In gynecologic oncology, removal of the spleen is occasionally required to achieve optimal surgical cytoreduction of metastatic ovarian cancer. Most commonly, tumor is found directly extending from the omentum into the splenic hilum during primary debulking surgery. Splenectomy and other extensive upper abdominal resection techniques have been shown to improve survival with acceptable morbidity (Chi, 2010; Eisenhauer, 2006). However, the number of patients who will actually have their spleen removed during their initial operation ranges from 1 to 14 percent (Eisenkop, 2006; Goff, 2006). Splenectomy is also indicated for selected patients with isolated parenchymal recurrences to assist optimal secondary surgical cytoreduction of ovarian cancer (Manci, 2006). In some instances, a laparoscopic or hand-assisted approach may be possible (Chi, 2006). Last, intraoperative splenic trauma is the least common indication and usually is unanticipated (Magtibay, 2006).

PREOPERATIVE

Patient Evaluation

Preoperative diagnosis of splenic involvement is often difficult to predict with certainty prior to primary cytoreduction. Typically, in such cases, an omental cake is seen on CT images, but its proximity to the spleen is difficult to ascertain. Splenic involvement is more commonly distinguishable at the time of secondary cytoreduction. Ideally, relapsed patients have isolated disease and have had an extended progression-free survival of at least 12 months before they are considered for splenectomy.

Consent

Patients with presumed advanced ovarian cancer are consented for possible splenectomy, but the decision to perform the procedure will only be finalized intraoperatively. Although removal of the spleen results in a longer operative time, greater blood loss, and longer hospital stay, it may ultimately determine whether tumor is optimally debulked or not (Eisenkop, 2006). Possible serious complications include hemorrhage, infection, and pancreatitis.

INTRAOPERATIVE

Surgical Steps

❶ **Anesthesia and Patient Positioning.** Splenectomy is performed under general anesthesia and with the patient supine. The abdomen is surgically prepared, and a Foley catheter is inserted.

❷ **Abdominal Entry and Exploration.** During laparotomy, splenectomy requires a vertical incision for adequate exposure. Following entry, a surgeon carefully assesses the entire abdomen and pelvis to confirm the ability to resect all gross disease. Ideally, splenectomy is performed only if optimal tumor debulking can thereby be achieved. The spleen is grasped to assess its mobility, degree of tumor involvement, and potential difficulty in removal. As a brief review, the spleen has ligamentous attachments to its surrounding organs. These include the gastrosplenic, splenocolic, and splenophrenic ligaments. All are transected during splenectomy.

❸ **Entrance into the Lesser Sac.** The gastrocolic ligament, which lies between the stomach's greater curvature and the transverse colon, is opened to the left of midline by dividing vascular pedicles as described in Section 46-14, Step 6 (p. 1186). Dissection is continued in two directions (Fig. 46-15.1). For one, dissection moves along the superior transverse colon with mobilization of the

entire splenic flexure of the colon to reach the splenocolic ligament. For the other, dissection progresses upward to the greater curvature of the stomach toward the gastrosplenic ligament. The intervening portion of omentum is often involved with tumor and is removed.

❹ **Mobilization of the Spleen.** The spleen is grasped, elevated, and pulled medially to expose the splenophrenic ligament. A surgeon uses alternating electrosurgical blade and blunt finger dissection to further mobilize the spleen. Additional blunt and sharp dissection is then performed circumferentially to free the spleen from the gastrosplenic and splenocolic ligaments. Notably, the gastrosplenic is the most vascular and contains the short gastric arteries. These are carefully ligated and divided. To avoid pancreatic injury, it is important to continually review the anatomy.

❺ **Ligating the Splenic Vessels.** The spleen is elevated into the incision, and the peritoneum overlying the splenic hilum is carefully incised. To aid this approach, a left index finger is held against the spleen, and the pancreatic tail, which lies close to the splenic hilum (often within 1 cm), is displaced medially with the left thumb.

Blunt dissection parallel to the expected course of the splenic artery and vein aids identification of these vessels. The artery, vein, and vascular tributaries are individually ligated. The artery is first isolated to prevent splenic engorgement (Fig. 46-15.2). A

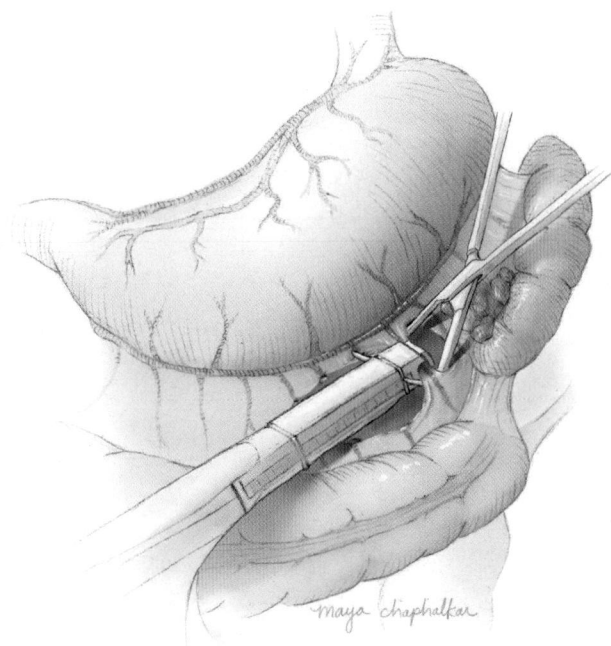

FIGURE 46-15.1 Mobilizing the spleen.

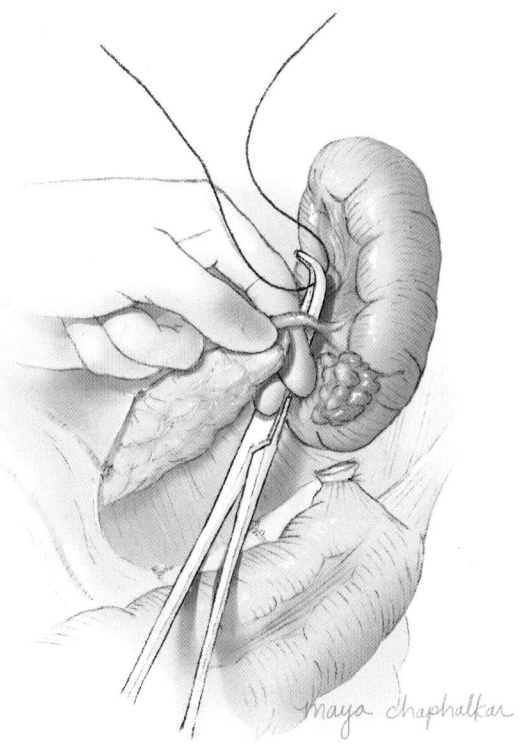

FIGURE 46-15.2 Vessel ligation.

right-angle clamp is placed beneath the artery, and a 2–0 silk suture is pulled through and tied. A second silk tie is placed more distally, directly at the hilum. The proximal end of the artery is again tied or occluded with a vascular clip. The artery is then divided, and the procedure is repeated for the splenic vein. Vascular tributaries are similarly divided. The remaining peritoneal attachments are incised with an electrosurgical blade to remove the spleen.

❻ **Final Steps.** The distal pancreas is carefully inspected to exclude injury. The splenic vessels are also reexamined prior to abdominal closure. Suspicion of pancreatic trauma or bleeding usually prompts placement of a suction drain in the splenic bed. Otherwise, drainage is not routinely required. A nasogastric tube is placed to decompress the stomach and prevent displacement of gastric vessel staples.

POSTOPERATIVE

Hemorrhage is the most serious immediate complication and typically, originates from the short gastric or splenic vessels. Bleeding can be profuse, and thus the initial 12 to 24 postoperative hours require particular vigilance (Magtibay, 2006).

The most common postoperative "complication" is left lower lobe lung atelectasis. This will typically resolve with ambulation, pulmonary therapy, and time. Development of a postoperative intraabdominal abscess usually results from inadvertent injury to the stomach, splenic flexure, or distal pancreas.

Excessive pancreatic manipulation or laceration may lead to pancreatitis or leaking. When a distal pancreatectomy is required due to tumor adherence or injury, approximately one quarter of patients will develop a pancreatic leak. According to one set of criteria, this leak is defined by a left upper quadrant collection of fluid seen on imaging after postoperative day 3, and this fluid contains an amylase level >3 times that of serum amylase. If a drain has been placed, fluid may be sent to the laboratory if this complication is suspected. Pancreatic leak usually presents early in the postoperative period and can be managed conservatively with percutaneous drainage (Kehoe, 2009).

Patients undergoing splenectomy will be at lifelong risk for episodes of overwhelming sepsis. Accordingly, the pneumococcal and meningococcal vaccines are recommended and the *Haemophilus influenzae* type b is considered postoperatively (Kim, 2015). Importantly, these vaccines may be given together but are not administered earlier than 14 days following splenectomy. In addition, patients are instructed to seek immediate medical attention for fevers, which may rapidly progress to serious illness.

46-16

Diaphragmatic Surgery

Patients with advanced ovarian cancer will often have tumor implants or confluent plaques involving the diaphragm. The right hemidiaphragm is most frequently affected. Implants are typically superficial, but invasive disease can extend through the peritoneum to the underlying muscle. Accordingly, gynecologic oncologists are prepared to perform diaphragmatic ablation, stripping (peritonectomy), or full-thickness resection. These surgical procedures increase the rate of optimal tumor debulking and correlate with improved survival (Aletti, 2006a; Tsolakidis, 2010).

PREOPERATIVE

Patient Evaluation

Imaging studies may suggest diaphragmatic nodularity, but the extent is difficult to ascertain until exploration in the operating room.

Consent

Patients with presumed advanced ovarian cancer are informed of the possible need for extensive upper abdominal surgery to achieve optimal cytoreduction. Pulmonary complications after diaphragmatic surgical techniques most commonly include atelectasis and/or pleural effusion. However, empyema, subphrenic abscess, and pneumothorax are also possible (Chereau, 2011; Cliby, 2004).

INTRAOPERATIVE

Instruments

It is generally advisable to have a cavitational ultrasonic surgical aspiration (CUSA) system and/or argon beam coagulator (ABC) available for ovarian cancer debulking procedures, since one or both can be useful in eradicating diaphragmatic disease. These tools are discussed further in Chapter 40 (p. 859).

Surgical Steps

❶ **Anesthesia and Patient Positioning.** As with other major intraabdominal surgeries, diaphragmatic surgery requires general anesthesia. The patient is positioned supine, the abdomen is surgically prepared to accommodate an incision to the sternum, and a Foley catheter is inserted.

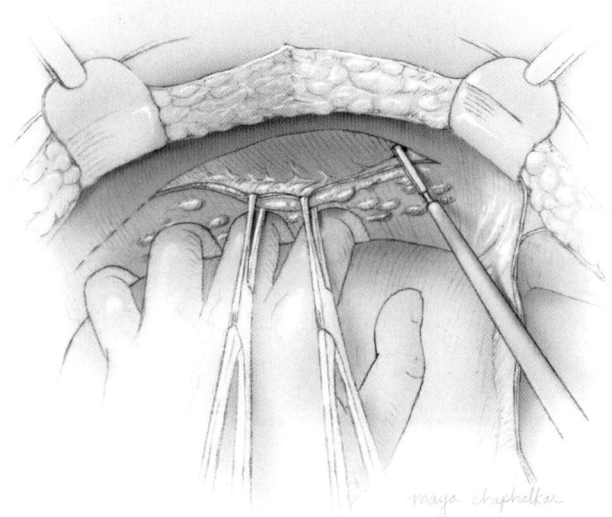

FIGURE 46-16.1 Diaphragm stripping.

❷ **Abdominal Entry.** Diaphragmatic surgery requires a vertical midline incision that has been extended to the sternum, passing to the right side of xiphoid process, for maximum exposure. Following abdominal entry, a surgeon carefully assesses the entire abdomen and pelvis to confirm the ability to resect all gross disease. Ideally, diaphragmatic surgery is performed only if optimal tumor debulking can thereby be achieved.

❸ **Diaphragmatic Ablation.** A few scattered, small tumor implants on the surface of the right or left hemidiaphragm can usually be easily ablated with the CUSA or ABC. This simple technique may be all that is required.

❹ **Diaphragmatic Stripping.** Confluent plaques of tumor or extensive implants indicate the need for resection of the peritoneum. For this, the right side of the anterior rib cage is retracted sharply upward. The liver is manually retracted downward and medially to aid division of the falciform ligament, right coronary ligament, and right triangular ligament of the liver with sharp dissection using an electrosurgical blade. This maneuver significantly mobilizes the liver and allows it to be held medially away from the diaphragm.

Dissection begins on the right side of the diaphragm, where the diaphragmatic peritoneum meets the anterior abdominal wall. Allis clamps are used to grasp the peritoneum above the tumor plaque and place it on tension. The peritoneal incision is created transversely above the tumor with an electrosurgical blade, and a plane is developed with blunt dissection to separate the peritoneum from the underlying muscle fibers of the

diaphragm. The free peritoneal edge is placed on tension with Allis clamps to maintain traction. The incision is then extended medially and laterally to encompass the implants (Fig. 46-16.1). The specimen eventually becomes large enough to grasp with a left hand to aid in "stripping" the peritoneum off the diaphragm. Electrosurgical blade dissection proceeds dorsally until all implants are contained within the peritoneal specimen. At this point, it can be detached.

❺ **Diaphragmatic Resection.** Occasionally, tumor has penetrated through the peritoneum, and a plane cannot be developed to strip the diaphragm. In these circumstances, fullthickness diaphragmatic resection is required. A self-retaining retractor is placed, and the liver mobilized. A transverse peritoneal incision is made above the tumor plaque, and at this point, the inadequacy of stripping is determined.

The ventilator is temporarily turned off to avoid lung parenchymal injury, and an electrosurgical blade is used to cut through the diaphragmatic muscle into the pleural cavity above the tumor. Ventilation may then be resumed while Allis clamps are placed to retract the specimen into the peritoneal cavity. Both pleural and peritoneal surfaces should be visible to aid in complete resection of the disease. After resection, primary mass closure of the diaphragmatic defect is then performed with a running stitch using 0-gauge polydioxanone monofilament (PDS) suture or interrupted stitches of silk suture.

To evacuate the pneumothorax, a red rubber catheter is placed through the defect into the pleural space prior to securing the final knot. The ventilator is turned off at the end of inspiration to maximally inflate the lungs while the catheter is placed on suction. The catheter is removed concomitantly with tying the knot, and mechanical ventilation is resumed (Bashir, 2010). Grafts are not typically needed, even for large defects (Silver, 2004).

❻ **Final Steps.** The patient is placed in Trendelenburg position at the completion of stripping or resection to check the integrity of the diaphragmatic closure. The upper abdomen is filled with saline and observed for air leaks as the patient is ventilated. The presence of air bubbles indicates the need to reintroduce the red rubber catheter through the hole, resuture the defect, and retest the closure. Chest tubes are not routinely required.

POSTOPERATIVE

Atelectasis is common with any diaphragmatic surgery, and routine postoperative respiratory expansion techniques are appropriate (Chap. 39, p. 827). Diaphragmatic stripping is associated with an increased incidence of pleural effusion, especially when the pleural space is entered. Fortunately, most will self-resolve, and only a few will require postoperative thoracentesis (Dowdy, 2008). Patients having full-thickness diaphragmatic resection are carefully monitored with chest radiographs for evidence of a pneumo- or hemothorax. Those few who do not resolve with supportive care measures may require chest tube drainage to aid lung reexpansion (Bashir, 2010).

46-17

Colostomy

A colostomy is a surgical anastomosis between created openings in the colon and anterior abdominal wall to divert bowel contents into an external collection bag. Colostomies serve several purposes and may be used: (1) to protect distal bowel repair from disruption or contamination by feces, (2) to decompress an obstructed colon, and (3) to evacuate feces if the distal colon or rectum is excised. In gynecologic oncology, specific indications for performing a colostomy are innumerable. Some of the more common ones include rectovaginal fistula, severe radiation proctosigmoiditis, bowel perforation, and rectosigmoid resection in which reanastomosis is not feasible.

A colostomy may be temporary or permanent, and its duration is dictated by clinical circumstances. For instance, recurrent end-stage cervical cancer with obstruction may warrant a permanent colostomy. In contrast, only temporary diversion is needed to allow healing of an intraoperative bowel injury that occurred during benign gynecologic surgery.

In addition, the location of the stoma and the decision to perform an end or loop colostomy are also clinically based. A loop colostomy is constructed by creating an opening in a loop of colon and bringing both ends through the stoma. Alternatively, an end colostomy stoma contains only the proximal end of the transected colon. The distal end is stapled and left intraabdominally.

Regardless of the clinical circumstances, the same surgical principles apply during colostomy: adequate bowel mobilization, sufficient blood supply, and a tension-free tunnel through the abdominal wall without bowel constriction. Strict attention to these seemingly straightforward steps ensures the best possible outcome. In some circumstances, a laparoscopic colostomy may be possible (Jandial, 2008).

PREOPERATIVE

Patient Evaluation

The colostomy site, typically on the patient's left, is ideally marked preoperatively by an enterostomal therapist to ensure that the postoperative stoma will be located in an easily accessible area when sitting and standing.

Consent

Concerns regarding postoperative quality of life changes are common with this procedure.

Accordingly, a surgeon carefully describes a colostomy's medical purpose and its expected temporary or permanent duration. Much of the fear regarding "wearing a bag" can be assuaged with compassionate preoperative counseling and education. Many times, postoperative results are actually superior to a patient's current symptoms and quality of life.

Perioperative complications may include fecal leakage into the abdomen or retraction of the stoma. Long-term complications involve parastomal hernia, stricture, and the potential need for surgical revision.

Patient Preparation

To minimize fecal contamination during bowel incision, aggressive bowel preparation such as with a polyethylene glycol with electrolyte solution (GoLYTELY) may be considered the day prior to surgery unless contraindicated, such as with bowel obstruction or perforation. Additionally, broad-spectrum antibiotics are given preoperatively due to the possibility of stool contamination of the operative site. With stool spill, postoperative antibiotic doses for 24 to 48 hours and a drain near the anastomosis are reasonable.

INTRAOPERATIVE

Surgical Steps

❶ **Anesthesia and Patient Positioning.** Colostomy is performed under general anesthesia with the patient positioned supine. Prior to surgery, the abdomen is surgically prepared, and a Foley catheter is inserted.

❷ **Abdominal Entry and Exploration.** Although concurrent surgery may dictate the approach, a midline vertical incision, due to its superior exposure, is generally preferred when colostomy is a possibility. The bowel segment is selected as distally as possible to preserve normal bowel. Dissection and adhesiolysis are performed as necessary to mobilize the bowel to obtain sufficient length before creating the abdominal wall stoma opening. The colon is elevated to ensure that it will reach the selected stoma site without tension. If the bowel fails to reach the selected site without tension despite maximal mobilization, then the proposed stoma site is moved to accommodate the available bowel length.

❸ **End Colostomy.** This type of diversion is commonly used for rectovaginal fistulas and severe proctosigmoiditis after radiation. Ideally, a more distal colon site is used since bowel content becomes progressively more solid and less voluminous as it moves from

the cecum to the rectum. As a result, the ostomy bag does not need to be changed as often, and the risk of dehydration or electrolyte abnormalities is reduced. If performing an end sigmoid colostomy, the distal bowel may simply be stapled closed and left in the pelvis (Hartmann pouch). In contrast, a more proximal end colostomy performed for a distal colonic obstruction will require that the distal bowel also be brought to the abdominal wall and opened, either at the same site or as a second ostomy. This distal-bowel-loop ostomy serves as a "mucus fistula" to prevent a closed loop obstruction and subsequent colonic perforation from mucus or gas accumulation.

The stoma site for a sigmoid colostomy is selected based on an imaginary line drawn from the umbilicus to the left-sided anterior superior iliac spine. The site is sufficiently lateral from the midline to allow application of the ostomy appliance. But, it is located sufficiently medial because stoma support from the rectus muscle lowers stoma-site hernia risks.

To begin, a Kocher clamp is used to elevate the skin and an electrosurgical blade, set to a cutting mode, is used to remove a 3-cm circle of skin. The fascia is exposed by blunt dissection. In obese patients, a cone through the subcutaneous fat with its tip at the fascia may need to be removed to prevent bowel constriction. A cruciate incision is made on the anterior sheath. The fibers of the rectus abdominis muscle are bluntly separated, and another cruciate incision is cut on the posterior sheath. The opening is bluntly expanded to accommodate two or three fingers.

After the colon is divided as described in Section 46-21, Step 5 (p. 1201), the proximal bowel is mobilized by incising the peritoneum toward the splenic flexure along the white line of Toldt, which is the reflection of posterior abdominal parietal peritoneum over the mesentery of the descending colon. A Babcock clamp is then placed through the skin opening to grasp the stapled end of bowel and lift it through the abdominal opening (Fig. 46-17.1). The bowel should appear pink, and its mesentery must not be twisted. The primary vertical abdominal incision is then closed.

The stoma is not ordinarily "matured" until the abdominal wall and skin are closed, with a dressing in place. First, the table is tilted to the left to minimize bowel spillage and fecal contamination of the incision site, and then the intestinal staple line is excised. Circumferential interrupted 3–0 and 4–0 gauge delayed-absorbable sutures are placed through the bowel mucosa and skin dermis (Fig. 46-17.2). The ostomy bag appliance may then be attached.

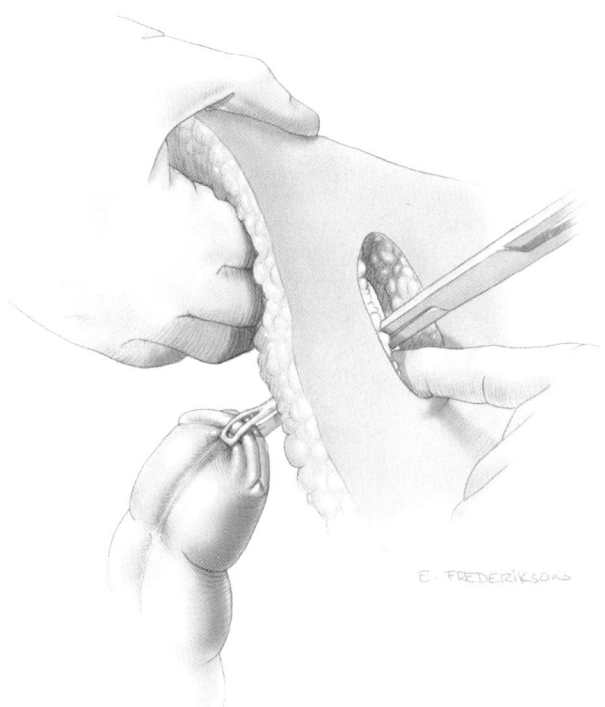

FIGURE 46-17.1 End-sigmoid colostomy: bowel pulled through abdominal wall incision.

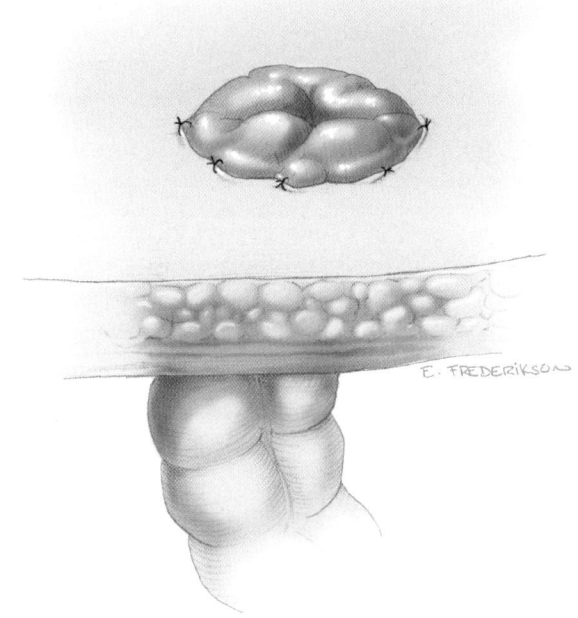

FIGURE 46-17.2 End-sigmoid colostomy: bowel mucosa sutured to skin.

❹ **Loop Colostomy Principles.** The typical indications for this type of procedure include protection of a distal anastomosis, relief of colonic obstruction, and colonic perforation. Accordingly, loop colostomy can be performed at any site along the colon where indicated. A loop colostomy in general is intended to be a temporary or palliative procedure. It is easier to take down, often simpler to perform, and does not necessarily require designation of loops as distal or proximal. However, fecal matter will eventually pass through to the distal segment. As a result, this type of colostomy is not a permanent solution to a fistula or proctosigmoiditis.

❺ **Transverse Loop Colostomy.** As a stand-alone procedure, a transverse loop colostomy is most often performed to relieve a distal obstruction and can be used in an emergent or palliative setting. This colostomy is performed in the left upper quadrant by creating a 5-cm transverse incision over the rectus abdominis muscle midway between the costal margin and the umbilicus. The anterior and posterior fascia, rectus abdominis muscle, and peritoneum are opened longitudinally by sharp and blunt dissection. The omentum is separated from the underlying transverse colon along enough length to allow the bowel segment to be pulled up through the incision without it. Next, a one-quarter inch Penrose drain is placed through the mesocolon for traction, and the bowel loop is brought through the incision (Fig. 46-17.3). A Hollister

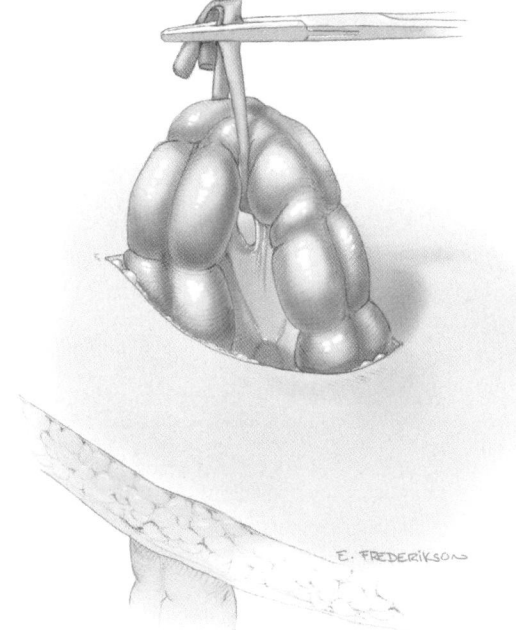

FIGURE 46-17.3 Transverse loop colostomy: bowel segment elevated.

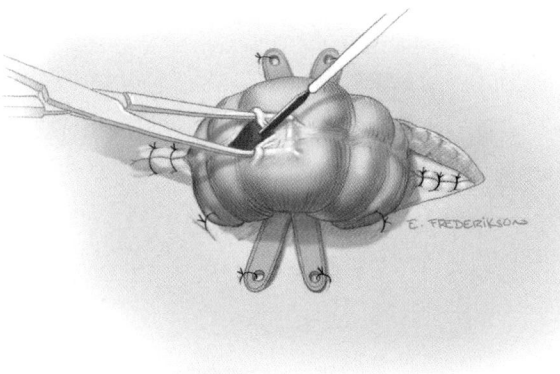

FIGURE 46-17.4 Transverse loop colostomy: bowel opened.

bridge or similar device is passed through the mesenterotomy in place of the Penrose drain. The skin incision is then closed around the bowel loop without constricting it.

The bowel is then "matured" by opening the antimesenteric half of the bowel along the tenia with an electrosurgical blade and leaving a 1-cm margin on each end (Fig. 46-17.4). The colostomy edges are sutured to the skin with interrupted stitches of 3–0 gauge delayed-absorbable suture.

❻ **Final Steps.** The stoma is carefully inspected and ideally is pink and comfortably positioned. A dusky color may indicate bowel ischemia, which can lead to sloughing, necrosis, and retraction. Tension on the bowel may be improved with additional colon mobilization. Constriction of a loop colostomy within the abdominal wall opening can be improved by broadening the fascial incision or removing additional subcutaneous fat. With end colostomy, on occasion, the tip may need to be transected further distally to reach a viable bowel segment. All of these steps are cumbersome but are much easier to perform during the operation rather than postoperatively after complications become obvious.

POSTOPERATIVE

Morbidity is comparable for end and loop colostomies (Segreti, 1996a). Complications may be immediate or not evident for several months. Common complications specific to a colostomy may include wound infection, necrosis, bowel obstruction, hematoma, retraction, fistula, fecal leakage, sepsis, stricture, and parastomal herniation (Hoffman, 1992). Many of these complications are manageable with supportive care and local measures. Dramatic symptoms are infrequent but may require operative revision. Careful attention during initial surgery will prevent most of these morbidities.

46-18

Large Bowel Resection

Partial colectomy is most often performed as part of cytoreductive surgery for ovarian cancer, although other indications include radiation injury and colonic fistula. Surgical principles are similar, whether a bowel segment to be removed is from the ascending, transverse, or descending colon. Rectosigmoid (low anterior) resection is somewhat more complex and is reviewed in Section 46-21 (p. 1200).

Ideally during colectomy, a surgeon will achieve meticulous hemostasis, remove the smallest required length of colon, avoid fecal spill, and confirm bowel continuity by excluding possible sites of proximal or distal intestinal obstruction. In addition, bowel must be sufficiently mobilized to create a tension-free anastomosis that is watertight, large caliber, and supported by adequate blood supply. During surgery planning, insufficient bowel length for reanastomosis, a malnourished patient, questionable vascular supply, or undue anastomosis tension may instead require a permanent or temporary diverting colostomy.

A general familiarity with colonic blood supply is important for partial colectomy. The ascending and transverse colon are supplied by the superior mesenteric artery via the ileocolic, right colic, and middle colic branches. The descending and sigmoid colon are supplied by the left colic and sigmoid branches of the inferior mesenteric artery. As a result, these vessels form an effective anastomotic vascular network that allows large bowel resection at virtually any segment of the colon.

PREOPERATIVE

Patient Evaluation

The need for partial colectomy during ovarian cancer cytoreductive surgery is usually decided intraoperatively and is based on clinical circumstances. For example, although preoperative CT images may suggest tumor at multiple sites near the colon, these lesions are often superficial and may be removed without colectomy. Typically, the need for colectomy is more obvious preoperatively for those with radiation damage or fistula. However, the extent of resection will still generally be unclear until the operation is underway.

Consent

Patients are fully informed of the potential for colostomy, anastomotic leak, and abscess formation. A postoperative ileus should also be anticipated.

Patient Preparation

To minimize fecal contamination during bowel incision, most surgeons still recommend aggressive bowel preparation. One choice, a polyethylene glycol with electrolyte solution (GoLYTELY), may be considered the day prior to surgery unless contraindicated, such as with bowel obstruction or perforation. However, there is no evidence that patients benefit from this practice, and bowel preparation may not lower the risk of postoperative complications (Guenaga, 2009; Zhu, 2010). If a bowel obstruction is present, then cleansing only the distal colon with enemas is a secondary option. The patient is also marked for a colostomy if that is a possibility. Moreover, if a complicated resection or prolonged recovery is anticipated, postoperative TPN administration is considered. Preoperative antibiotics and perioperative VTE prophylaxis are warranted, and options are listed in Tables 39-6 and 39-8 (p. 835).

INTRAOPERATIVE

Instruments

To prepare for complicated resections, a surgeon should have access to all types and sizes of bowel staplers. These include end-to-end anastomosis (EEA), gastrointestinal anastomosis (GIA), and transverse anastomosis (TA) staplers. Additionally, a ligate-divide-staple (LDS) device or electrothermal bipolar coagulator (LigaSure) may aid in vessel ligation.

Surgical Steps

❶ **Anesthesia and Patient Positioning.** Rectovaginal examination under anesthesia is mandatory before positioning any patient for abdominal gynecologic cancer surgery. A palpable mass with compression of the rectum or rectovaginal septum indicates the need for low lithotomy with legs comfortably positioned in booted support stirrups to prepare for possible low anterior resection and anastomosis. Supine positioning is otherwise appropriate. Sterile preparation of the abdomen, perineum, and vagina is completed, and a Foley catheter is inserted.

❷ **Abdominal Entry.** A midline vertical incision is preferable if partial colectomy is anticipated as this incision provides access to the entire abdomen. Required dissection, adhesiolysis, or other unanticipated findings may render exposure from a transverse incision inadequate.

❸ **Exploration.** A surgeon first explores the entire abdomen to lyse adhesions, to "run" the bowel and evaluate its appearance from duodenum to rectum, to exclude other potential sites of obstruction proximally or distally, and to determine the extent of the bowel resection. Colonic blood supply at the splenic flexure, hepatic flexure, and ileocecal valve can be tenuous. As a result, resection boundaries ideally lie beyond these areas if possible. For example, in Figure 46-18.1, because of the known tenuous blood supply at the hepatic flexure, the proximal line of transection includes several centimeters of transverse colon. Similarly, the distal line of transection includes 8 to 10 cm of the terminal ileum because the ileocecal artery is sacrificed. Leaving this terminal ileum would render it vulnerable to necrosis from insufficient remaining vascular support.

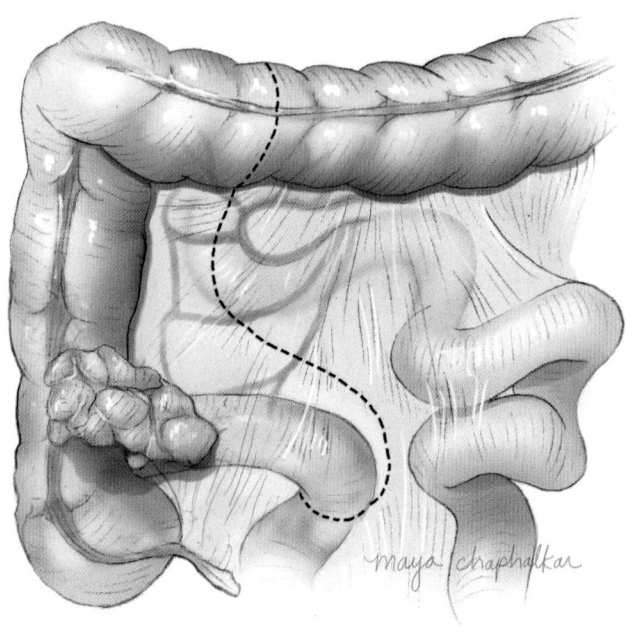

FIGURE 46-18.1 Area of resection encompasses tumor.

Once the segment is selected, a window is made in the mesocolon proximal and distal to the lesion. A one-quarter inch Penrose drain is pulled through each location's opening to provide traction.

❹ Mobilization of the Colon. The bowel is next mobilized by incising peritoneum along the white line of Toldt and/or along the hepatic or splenic flexures—depending on the resection site. For the case shown in Figure 46-18.1, the right retroperitoneal space is entered at the mid-ascending colon, continued along the white line of Toldt, and extended toward and around the cecum to a site beyond the distal Penrose drain. The entry opening is created with an electrosurgical blade just lateral to the colon. This space is bluntly expanded, and electrosurgical dissection is next guided cephalad past the proximal Penrose drain while providing countertraction on the colon. The bowel segment may be bluntly mobilized medially as necessary. Partial infracolic omentectomy may be required for resections involving the transverse colon.

❺ Resection. A GIA stapler is inserted to replace one Penrose drain, is positioned around the entire colon diameter, and is fired. This stapler lays two rows of staples and transects interposed bowel. A second stapling and transection is then repeated at the other Penrose drain site. Staying close to the bowel segment's wall, the bowel segment may then be detached from its underlying mesentery, using an LDS device, electrothermal bipolar coagulator, or individual clamps and 0-gauge delayed-absorbable suture ligation. During this process, as much of the mesentery as possible is preserved to provide adequate blood supply to the anastomosis. The specimen is then removed.

❻ Side-to-Side Anastomosis. The proximal and distal bowel ends are held parallel against each other to estimate their position following anastomosis. Typically, additional mobilization of the bowel by incising adhesions and peritoneum is required using a combination of electrosurgical blade and blunt dissection. The two segments must comfortably approximate antimesenteric borders without tension. For larger resections, the mesentery of each segment may also need to be dissected to achieve sufficient mobility. The proximal and distal stapled bowel ends are skeletonized of fatty tissue to create an anastomosis with maximal mucosa-to-mucosa contact. To accomplish this, the proximal staple line is elevated with two Allis clamps at its lateral edges. DeBakey forceps grasp surrounding fatty tissue and place it on traction, while an electrosurgical blade is used to dissect this tissue away from the bowel serosa. The dissection is then performed on the distal rectal segment in similar fashion.

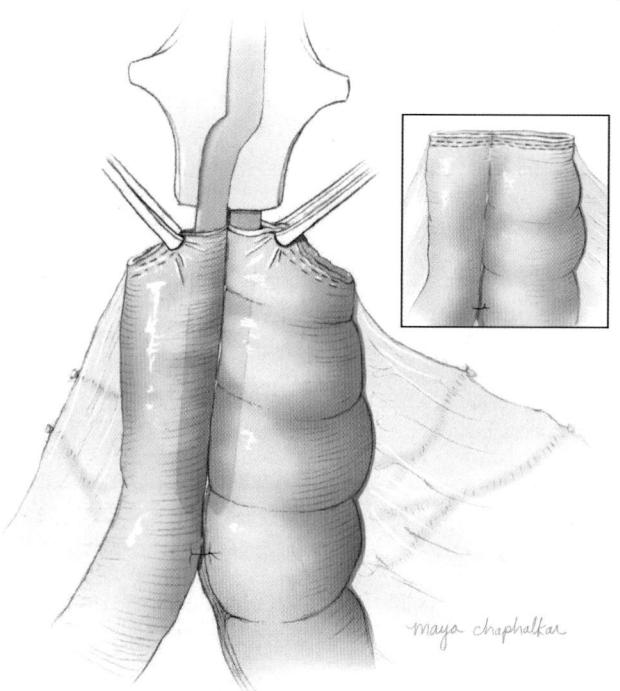

FIGURE 46-18.2 GIA stapler creates a side-to-side anastomosis of the ileum (*left*) and transverse colon (*right*). Inset: TA stapler line closes the distal end of the anastomosis.

The antimesenteric tip of each staple line is excised with scissors, and the bowel is held vertically by Allis clamps to prevent fecal spill. One or two seromuscular silk stay sutures may be placed distally on each bowel end to help align the correct position and prevent slippage. One fork of the GIA stapler is then inserted as deeply as possible into each of the bowel lumens (Fig. 46-18.2). The bowel segments are evenly positioned, and the device is then fired along the antimesenteric surfaces and removed. This stapler places two staggered rows of titanium staples and simultaneously transects tissue between these rows.

The bowel interior should be examined for bleeding sites, which may be electrosurgically coagulated. The remaining opening may then be stapled across with a TA stapler, and residual bowel tissue above the TA staple line is excised. The mesenteric defect is reapproximated with interrupted or running 0-gauge delayed-absorbable suture to prevent an internal hernia.

❼ Final Steps. The abdomen is irrigated with copious warmed saline at the conclusion of any bowel resection, especially if feces have spilled during the procedure. Drains are not routinely required and may impair healing.

POSTOPERATIVE

Morbidity after large bowel resection is significantly increased by various factors, but especially by preexisting obstruction, malignancy, obesity, radiation damage, or sepsis. Moreover, patients undergoing multiple bowel resections have greater blood loss and longer hospital stay (Salani, 2007). Anastomotic leaks are the most specific complication and typically present as an abscess or fistula, or as peritonitis within days or weeks of surgery. Some localized leaks can be managed with initiation of TPN, CT-guided drainage, antibiotic administration, and bowel rest for a couple of weeks. However, urgent reoperation is indicated for nonlocalized intraperitoneal perforation and its resulting peritonitis. This will usually require temporary colostomy (Kingham, 2009).

Pelvic abscesses may also result from intraoperative fecal spillage or hematoma superinfection. Usually these will resolve with CT-guided drainage and antibiotics. Gastrointestinal hemorrhage should be rare with stapled procedures. In addition, symptomatic anastomotic strictures are infrequent and often present as colonic obstruction. Some strictures can be managed with endoscopic stents, but often they require reoperation. Small or large bowel may also become obstructed by postoperative adhesions or tumor progression. Last, a prolonged ileus can develop and be slow to resolve. Most of these complications will depend primarily on the patient's underlying nutrition and the clinical circumstances prompting the primary surgery.

46-19

Ileostomy

Relatively few patients will require ileostomy for management of a gynecologic malignancy. For those who do, loop ileostomy is usually a temporary procedure that is performed to protect a distal anastomosis (Nunoo-Mensah, 2004). Palliation of a large-bowel obstruction or diversion of a colonic fistula may be other indications (Tsai, 2006). On occasion, ovarian cancer will involve the entire colon, requiring colectomy with a permanent end ileostomy and formation of a Hartmann pouch (Song, 2009).

PREOPERATIVE

Patient Evaluation

Stoma placement is particularly important for an ileostomy since the effluent will be more corrosive than that of a colostomy. Ideally, the site is marked preoperatively by an enterostomal therapist.

Consent

In general, many of the complications from this procedure mirror those of colostomy: retraction, stricture, obstruction, and herniation. Patients are informed that temporary loop ileostomies can be taken down later without a laparotomy.

Patient Preparation

Bowel preparation is preferred whenever there is a potential for more extensive bowel resection. However, ileostomy can safely be performed in virtually all circumstances without cleansing. Antibiotics and VTE prophylaxis are warranted, and options are listed in Tables 39-6 and 39-8 (p. 835).

INTRAOPERATIVE

Surgical Steps

❶ Anesthesia and Patient Positioning. Ileostomy is performed under general anesthesia. Patients are generally supine, but low lithotomy is acceptable.

❷ Abdominal Entry. A midline vertical incision is preferable for most situations in which an ileostomy is considered.

❸ Exploration. After abdominal entry, a surgeon first explores the abdomen, lyses

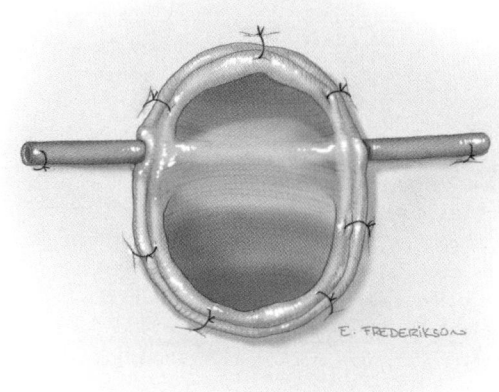

FIGURE 46-19.1 Ileal loop opened with cautery.

adhesions, "runs" the bowel length to identify obstructive sites, and determines the need for ileostomy. An ileum loop is selected that will reach several centimeters above the skin. Additionally, to reduce the effluent volume, the selected loop is located as distally along the bowel length as possible. On occasion, tethering of small bowel by carcinomatosis or radiation injury will significantly reduce mobility and will require a more proximal diversion.

❹ Loop Ileostomy. A one-quarter inch Penrose drain is placed through a mesenterotomy at the selected loop's apex. The loop can then be approximated to the stoma site, which is created to accommodate two fingers as described for an ileal conduit (Section 46-7, p. 1159). The loop is pulled through the abdominal wall opening so that several centimeters protrude above the skin surface. The Penrose drain is removed and replaced with either the cut end of a red rubber catheter or another device that can be sewn to the skin to elevate the loop. The loop should be tension-free and patent. The proximal end of the loop is placed in the lower position to reduce fecal flow into the distal bowel. The skin of the abdominal wall is then closed around the stoma.

The ileostomy is "matured" by longitudinally incising the bowel loop and everting its walls with Allis clamps. Circumferential interrupted stitches of 3–0 and 4–0 gauge delayed-absorbable sutures are placed through the dermis and bowel mucosa (Fig. 46-19.1). An ostomy bag may then be applied.

❺ End Ileostomy. If a total colectomy is performed or if the bowel is too tethered or the patient too obese for a loop to reach the abdominal wall, the distal ileum may need to be divided instead of brought out as a loop.

The segment is selected, a mesenterotomy is made, and the GIA stapler is fired. An appropriate stoma site is identified, and with a few modifications, the end ileostomy is matured as in colostomy (Section 46-17, p. 1192). Typically, the abdominal wall opening will be smaller in diameter. Unless there is a distal colon obstruction necessitating creation of a mucus fistula, the distal bowel segment can be left in the peritoneal cavity.

An attempt is made to evert the single stoma by turning the bowel wall over on itself using Allis clamps. In each quadrant of the stoma, stitches of 3–0 gauge delayed absorbable suture are placed through the dermis, the seromuscular layer of the bowel at the skin level, and a full-thickness bite at the cut edge of the everted bowel.

POSTOPERATIVE

The stoma is carefully examined postoperatively for its appearance and function. The loop supporting rod may be removed in 1 to 2 weeks, but potentially earlier if the stoma becomes dusky or the loops seem constricted or are obstructed.

Ileostomy may be associated with significant postoperative complications. High-output effluent may result in electrolyte abnormalities that are difficult to correct. In addition, approximately 10 percent of patients will require early reoperation for small-bowel obstruction or intraabdominal abscess (Hallbook, 2002). Specifically, if loop ileostomy is indicated to protect a low anterior anastomosis, it is more commonly associated with bowel obstruction and ileus than is loop colostomy (Law, 2002). Long-term complications such as a peristomal hernia or retraction are also possible.

46-20

Small Bowel Resection

Indications for small bowel resection in gynecologic oncology are numerous and include obstruction, tumor invasion, perforation, intraoperative injury, fistulas, or radiation damage. Unlike the large bowel, where greater attention is required to ensure an adequate blood supply to the anastomotic site, the small intestine has a consistent cascade of vessels that all arise from the superior mesenteric artery. However, unique situations such as radiation damage, obstructive dilatation, and edema can compromise this vasculature dramatically. In these situations, meticulous dissection is especially crucial to prevent inadvertent removal of the bowel serosa, enterotomy, and bowel damage that will impair anastomotic healing. In general, surgical principles with this procedure are much the same as those for large bowel resection (Section 46-18, p. 1195).

PREOPERATIVE

Patient Evaluation

Small bowel obstructions (SBOs) that do not resolve with nasogastric suction decompression and bowel rest may result from postoperative adhesions or tumor progression. Patients with recurrent gynecologic malignancy, particularly those with ovarian cancer, are preoperatively imaged by abdominopelvic CT with oral contrast. Numerous sites of obstruction may be suspected that would indicate a woman with end-stage disease who might be better served by placement of a palliative percutaneous draining gastrostomy tube. Patients with an SBO following pelvic radiation often have stenosis at the terminal ileum. This vulnerability stems from its proximity to the radiation field of many gynecologic cancers and its limited mobility compared with other small-bowel segments.

Consent

Depending on circumstances, patients are counseled regarding the intraoperative decision-making process to decide on anastomosis, bypass, or ileostomy. Leaking, obstruction, and/or fistula formation are possible complications. Less common outcomes include short-bowel syndrome and vitamin B_{12} deficiency, both described later.

Patient Preparation

Aggressive bowel preparation is often contraindicated, particularly in patients with obstruction. Antibiotics and VTE prophylaxis are provided (Chap. 39, p. 835). If a complex fistula is present or an extensive resection for radiation damage is anticipated, then postoperative TPN may be advisable.

INTRAOPERATIVE

Instruments

The surgeon should have access to all types and sizes of bowel staplers, such as end-to-end anastomotic (EEA), gastrointestinal anastomotic (GIA), and transverse anastomotic (TA) staplers, to prepare for complicated resections.

Surgical Steps

❶ **Anesthesia and Patient Positioning.** Small bowel resection is performed under general anesthesia. Patients are generally supine, but low lithotomy or other positioning with access to the anterior abdominal wall is acceptable.

❷ **Abdominal Entry.** A midline vertical incision is preferable for most situations in which a small-bowel resection is considered.

❸ **Exploration.** The surgeon explores the entire abdomen first to identify the obstruction. Infrequently, an adhesion may be located and lysed to quickly relieve an obstruction, thereby avoiding small bowel resection. More often, an area is discovered that warrants removal. Importantly, the remainder of the bowel must be examined to exclude other obstructive sites.

Peritoneum and adhesions attached to the involved portion of small bowel are dissected to mobilize the bowel. The small intestine can be damaged easily by rough handling and extensive blunt dissection—particularly if the bowel is edematous, densely adhered, or previously irradiated. Trauma is minimized to reduce spillage of intestinal contents by inadvertent enterotomy. Ideally, healthy-appearing serosa for anastomosis is identified at sites both proximal and distal to the lesion while preserving a maximum amount of intestine.

❹ **Dividing Small Bowel.** The involved bowel is brought through the abdominal incision. A one-quarter inch Penrose drain is pulled through a mesenterotomy at the proximal and distal sites to be approximated. A GIA stapler is inserted to replace the Penrose drain and is fired. This is repeated at the other bowel site (Fig. 46-20.1). These staple lines minimize contamination of the abdomen with bowel contents.

A wedge of mesentery then is "scored" by superficially creating a V shape with an electrosurgical blade. The mesentery is divided by a ligate-divide-staple (LDS) device, electrothermal bipolar coagulator (LigaSure), or clamps and 0-gauge delayed-absorbable suture ligatures. Achieving hemostasis will be more difficult with edematous or inflamed tissue, and thus smaller mesentery pedicles should be sequentially divided. The bowel specimen is then removed.

❺ **Performing Side-to-Side Anastomosis.** The proximal and distal bowel segments are elevated with Allis clamps and matched parallel along their antimesenteric borders.

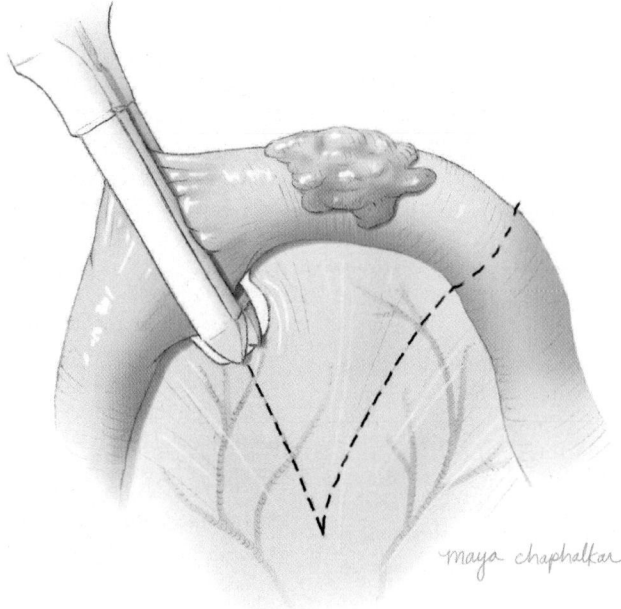

FIGURE 46-20.1 Identifying proximal and distal sites.

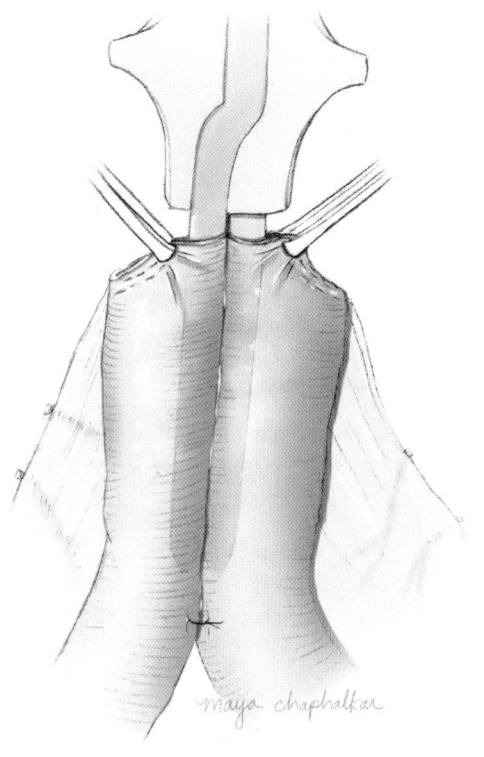

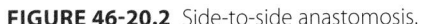

FIGURE 46-20.2 Side-to-side anastomosis.

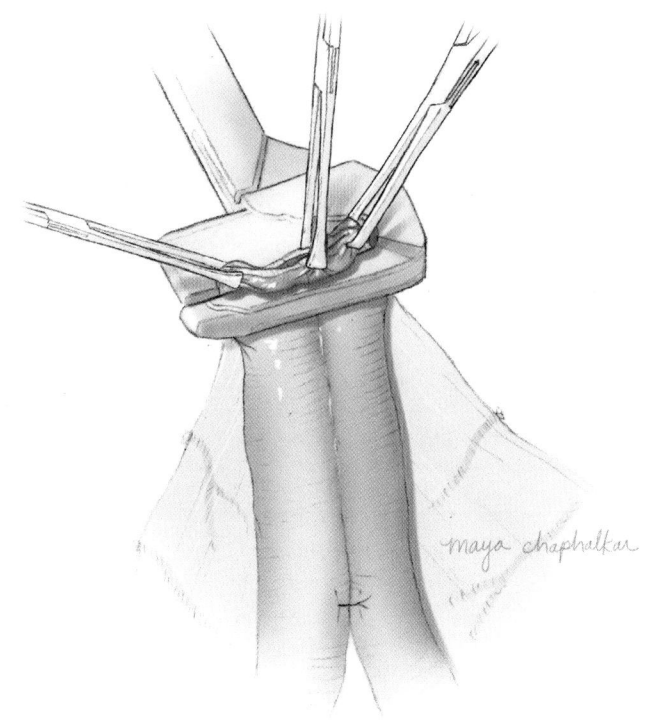

FIGURE 46-20.3 Closing the enterotomy.

To help alignment, one or two silk stay sutures are placed through the antimesenteric border of each segment beyond the tip of where the GIA stapler fork will reach. The antimesenteric corner of each segment is excised at the staple line just deeply enough to enter the lumen and sufficiently widely to permit passage of one GIA stapler fork. Massively distended bowel from an obstruction may be decompressed by inserting a pool suction tip into the proximal bowel end.

Allis clamps are replaced on the bowel at the edge of each opening. These clamps and silk stay sutures assist insertion of one fork of the GIA stapler into each segment and aid in bowel positioning (Fig. 46-20.2). The bowel is rotated to bring the antimesenteric borders together, Allis clamps are removed, and the GIA stapler is closed and fired.

The remaining enterotomy is regrasped with three Allis clamps to approximate for closure. The TA stapler is placed around the bowel beneath the Allis clamps and is closed (Fig. 46-20.3). The Allis clamps elevate the enterotomy and assist with correct positioning of the TA stapler. The stapler is fired, excess tissue above the stapler is trimmed sharply, and the stapler is opened and removed. The mesenteric defect may be closed next with running 0-gauge delayed-absorbable suture to prevent internal herniation—that is, herniation of bowel or omentum through the mesenteric defect.

❻ Final Steps. The abdomen is copiously irrigated with warmed saline. This is performed at the conclusion of any bowel resection, but particularly if bowel contents spill during the procedure. Drains are not required routinely and may impair healing. In general, it is prudent to place a nasogastric tube to decompress the stomach postoperatively until bowel function has resumed. Palpation of the stomach will confirm correct placement, or else the anesthesiologist can be directed to advance or pull back the tube as needed. If this is overlooked, correct location can only be reliably confirmed postoperatively by chest radiography.

POSTOPERATIVE

The underlying health of the patient, diagnosis, and indications for small bowel resection will dictate much of the potential postoperative morbidity. Ileus is common. Fistula formation, anastomotic leakage, and obstruction are more serious problems that may require reoperation. Two specific complications are unique to extensive small bowel surgery.

First, short-bowel syndrome may develop. More than half the small intestine can be removed without impairing nutritional absorption as long as the remaining bowel is functional. Accordingly, this syndrome is more likely to develop from extensive radiation damage than from surgical resection. Symptoms include diarrhea and dehydration. Maldigestion, malabsorption, nutritional deficiencies, and electrolyte imbalance are often noted. As a result, home TPN may be required in some patients (King, 1993).

A second complication, vitamin B_{12} deficiency, results from inadequate absorption and depletion of available stores. The ileum measures on average 300 cm in length, and vitamin B_{12} and bile salts are only absorbed in the ileum's distal 100 cm. Malabsorption in this segment may result from radiotherapy or extensive intestinal resection (Bandy, 1984). If vitamin B_{12} deficiency is suspected, a complete blood count (CBC), peripheral blood smear, and serum cobalamin (B_{12}) level are collected as part of an initial laboratory assessment. Accepted lower limits of serum vitamin B_{12} levels in adults range between 170 and 250 ng/L. One option for replacement is 1 mg intramuscularly weekly for 8 weeks, followed by long-term monthly injections (Centers for Disease Control and Prevention, 2011).

46-21

Low Anterior Resection

Rectosigmoid resection, also known as low anterior resection, is mainly used in gynecologic oncology to achieve optimal cytoreduction of primary or recurrent ovarian cancer (Mourton, 2005). This procedure is distinguished from other types of large bowel resection in that it requires mobilization and transection of the rectum distally, below the peritoneal reflection. Following resection of the involved rectosigmoid segment, proximal and distal bowel ends are usually anastomosed.

Low anterior resection is the most common bowel operation for primary tumor debulking (Hoffman, 2005). For example, en bloc pelvic resection combines low anterior resection with hysterectomy, bilateral salpingo-oophorectomy, and removal of surrounding peritoneum (Section 46-13, p. 1182) (Aletti, 2006b). In addition, total and posterior pelvic exenterations incorporate many of the same principles of tissue dissection to remove centrally recurrent cervical cancer and achieve widely negative soft tissue margins. Other less common indications for low anterior resection are radiation proctosigmoiditis and intestinal endometriosis (Urbach, 1998). Occasionally, additional large or small bowel resections will be performed concomitantly with low anterior resection (Salani, 2007).

PREOPERATIVE

Patient Evaluation

Bowel symptoms may or may not be present in women with rectosigmoid involvement of ovarian cancer. However, a surgeon should have greater suspicion if patients describe rectal bleeding or progressive constipation. A rectovaginal examination may help predict a need for low anterior resection. Additionally, CT images may suggest rectosigmoid invasion of tumor. However, prediction prior to surgery is difficult. Many ovarian cancers intraoperatively may be easily lifted away from the bowel, or surface tumors may be removed without resection.

Consent

Patients should be prepared for the possibility of low anterior resection any time ovarian cytoreductive surgery is discussed. The survival benefit of achieving minimal residual disease warrants the risks of this procedure. However, low anterior resection significantly extends operative time, and hemorrhage may contribute to a need for blood transfusion (Tebes, 2006).

In general, progressively higher complication rates and poorer long-term bowel function follow anastomoses that are more distal and approach the anal verge. However, the operation is designed to encompass the tumor. Thus, an end sigmoid colostomy with Hartmann pouch is another, albeit less attractive, option for very low resections. In general, a protective loop colostomy or ileostomy is not required, but patients are counseled for that possibility in the event of poor nutrition, tenuous bowel blood supply, or anastomosis tension. Anastomotic leaks develop in fewer than 5 percent of procedures (Mourton, 2005).

Patient Preparation

To minimize fecal contamination during resection, bowel preparation such as with a polyethylene glycol with electrolyte solution (GoLYTELY) is generally considered prior to surgery. Antibiotics and VTE prophylaxis are warranted, and suitable options are found in Tables 39-6 and 39-8 (p. 835).

INTRAOPERATIVE

Instruments

All types and sizes of bowel staplers such as end-to-end anastomosis (EEA), gastrointestinal anastomosis (GIA), and transverse anastomosis (TA) staplers should be available. Additionally, a ligate-divide-staple (LDS) device or electrothermal bipolar coagulator (LigaSure) may be used for vessel ligation.

Surgical Steps

❶ **Anesthesia and Patient Positioning.** Low anterior resection via laparotomy requires general anesthesia. Rectovaginal examination under anesthesia is performed before positioning any patient for abdominal gynecologic cancer surgery. A palpable mass with compression of the rectum or rectovaginal septum prompts patient positioning in low lithotomy with legs safely placed in boot support stirrups. This allows access to the rectum in cases requiring EEA stapler insertion for anastomosis. Alternatively, supine positioning may be appropriate if no mass is palpable by rectovaginal examination. In such cases, if a mass is more proximally located, low rectal anastomosis can be performed entirely within the pelvis.

❷ **Abdominal Entry.** A midline vertical incision provides generous operating space and upper abdominal access. This is preferable if low rectal anastomosis is anticipated because the descending colon may need to be mobilized around and beyond the splenic flexure of the colon. Transverse incisions often fail to provide sufficient exposure.

❸ **Exploration.** A surgeon first explores the entire abdomen to determine if disease is resectable. If not, then the procedure's benefit is reevaluated. On occasion, imminent bowel obstruction, infection, or other clinical circumstances may dictate resection regardless of residual tumor. The pelvis and rectosigmoid are palpated to mentally plan for the resection and determine whether en bloc pelvic resection or an exenterative procedure is indicated.

❹ **Visualization.** The bowel is packed into the upper abdomen, and retractor blades are positioned to allow access to the deep pelvis and the entire rectosigmoid colon. Ureters are identified at the pelvic brim and are held laterally on Penrose drains to expose the peritoneum and mesentery that can next be safely dissected.

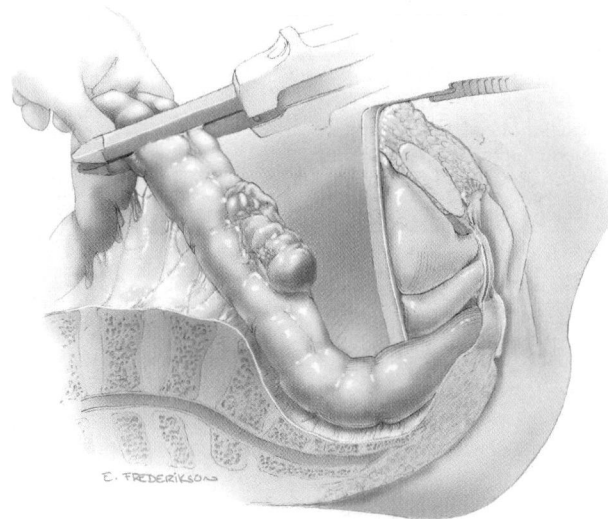

FIGURE 46-21.1 Dividing the proximal end.

❺ Dividing the Proximal Sigmoid Colon.
The sigmoid colon is held on traction proximal to the tumor and in the approximate area where it will be divided. The ureter is located, and a right-angle clamp is used to guide superficial electrosurgical blade dissection of the peritoneum and mesentery up to the bowel serosa. A similar dissection is repeated on the other side. Blunt dissection may then be performed to define the entire circumference of the sigmoid colon. Epiploica and adjacent fatty tissue are held with DeBakey forceps and dissected away with an electrosurgical blade from the proposed area of transection. The GIA stapler is placed across the sigmoid colon, fired, and removed (Fig. 46-21.1).

❻ Dividing the Mesentery. Occasionally, the tumor is small and superficially located, requiring only a wedge resection of underlying mesentery to remove it with the bowel segment. More frequently, the entire mesentery needs to be divided to provide access to the avascular plane between the rectosigmoid and the sacrum (retrorectal space). For this, a right-angle clamp is placed through sections of the mesentery, and an LDS device or electrothermal bipolar coagulator divides this tissue. Dissection is continued caudally to divide the mesentery (Fig. 46-21.2). Typically, one or more pedicles will have a blood vessel that slips out and requires clamping with a right-angle clamp and ligation with 0-gauge delayed-absorbable suture.

Blunt dissection is performed in the pelvic midline to identify the large superior rectal vessels, which are branches of the inferior mesenteric artery. This artery and vein are large and are separately doubly clamped, cut, and ligated with 0-gauge delayed-absorbable suture. From this midline, dissection then progresses laterally on both sides until no tissue is visible between the ureters. The common iliac artery bifurcation and sacrum are entirely visible.

❼ Dividing the Rectum. The proximal sigmoid colon and attached mesentery are repacked into the upper abdomen to improve pelvic exposure. The rectosigmoid is held superiorly, and blunt dissection is performed caudally in the retrorectal space to mobilize the distal bowel beyond the tumor to define the location of planned resection. The ureters are traced along the pelvic sidewall. Lateral blunt dissection is performed to further mobilize the rectosigmoid. Lateral mesenteric attachments are isolated and divided with an LDS device or electrothermal bipolar coagulator or are grasped between Pean clamps, cut, and ligated. Self-retaining retractor blades may require repositioning as dissection proceeds more distally.

The anterior bowel serosa is generally visible throughout its course beyond the peritoneal

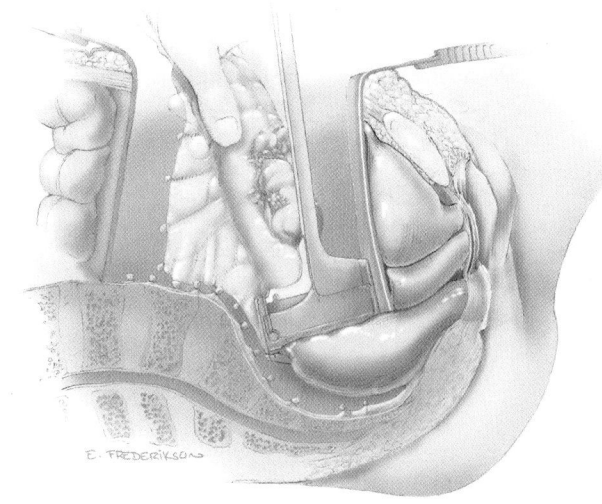

FIGURE 46-21.2 Dividing the distal end.

reflection and into the levator muscles. Lateral and posterior bowel margins are surrounded by fatty tissue, mesentery, and rectal pillars. The distal rectum beyond the tumor is grasped and rotated to aid exposure of these attachments. Attachments are divided using alternating electrosurgical blade dissection and vascular pedicle division and/or right-angle clamping and transection. Division continues circumferentially until the rectal serosa is entirely visible.

The curved cutter stapler (Contour) is a good choice for the limited space of the deep pelvis. The rectosigmoid is held on traction, while the stapler is gently inserted into the pelvis around the rectal segment. The ureters and any lateral tissue are pushed safely away, the stapler is fired, and the low anterior resection specimen is removed (see Fig. 46-21.2). The pelvis is irrigated, and a laparotomy sponge is left in place to tamponade any surface oozing.

❽ Mobilization. The final decision is now made to perform an anastomosis instead of an end sigmoid colostomy. The upper abdominal retractors are removed, and the proximal sigmoid colon is mobilized by incising peritoneum along the white line of Toldt toward and/or around the splenic flexure (Fig. 46-21.3). A combination of electrosurgical

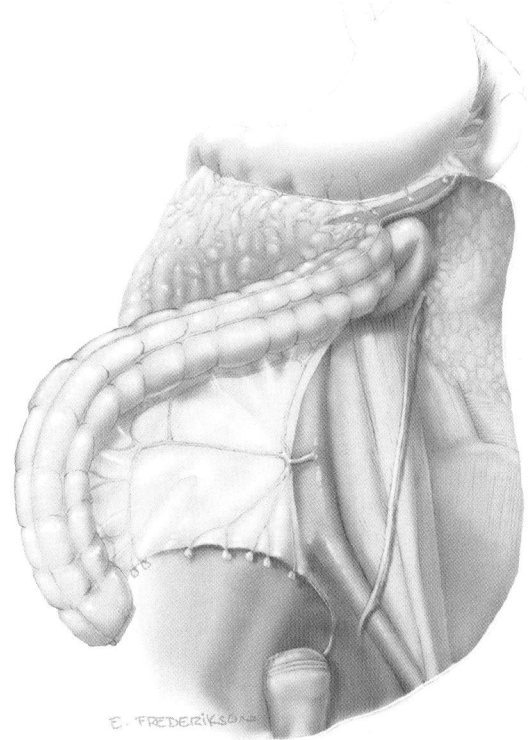

FIGURE 46-21.3 Mobilizing the descending colon.

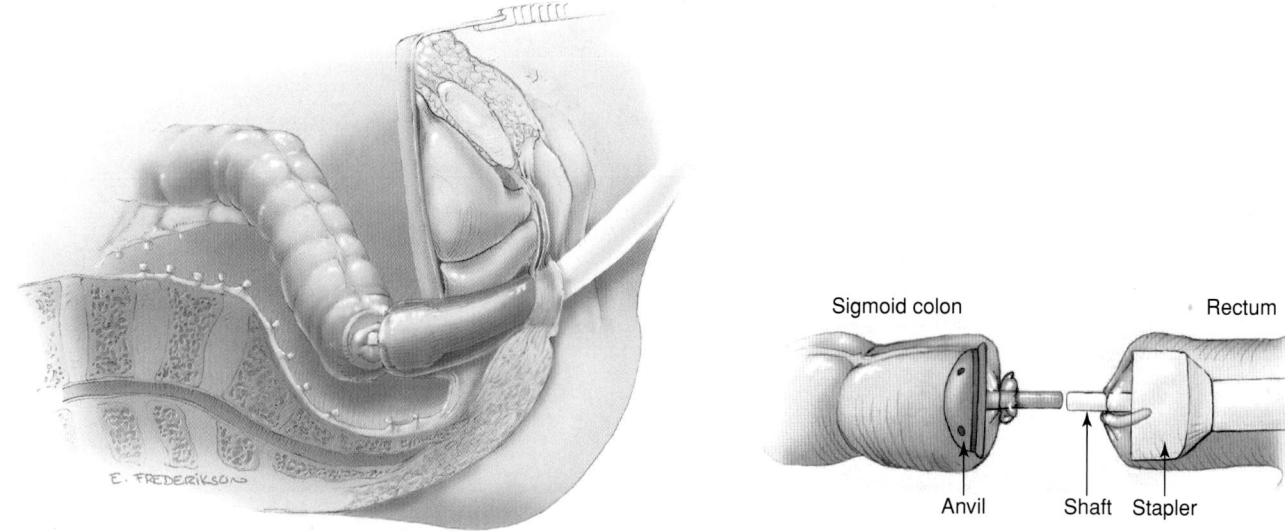

Sigmoid colon　　　　　Rectum

Anvil　　　Shaft　Stapler

E. FREDERIKSON

FIGURE 46-21.4 Performing end-to-end anastomosis. Inset: The EEA stapler device head.

blade and blunt dissection is typically used. The proximal sigmoid colon is intermittently placed into the deep pelvis to assess the extent of further dissection needed to achieve a tension-free anastomosis. Ideally, the proximal sigmoid colon sits comfortably on top of the distal rectum. To achieve this, mobilization may encompass the entire splenic flexure of the colon. Occasionally, the hepatic flexure may also need to be mobilized. Sufficient mobility is critical to ensure a tension-free anastomosis.

❾ **Preparing the Anastomotic Sites.** The proximal and distal stapled bowel ends now must be cleared of fatty tissue or epiploica to allow sufficient mucosa-to-mucosa contact during anastomosis. The staple line of the proximal sigmoid colon is grasped with two Allis clamps at the lateral edges and elevated. Adson forceps are used to delicately place any surrounding fatty tissue on traction, and an electrosurgical blade is used to dissect these away from the bowel serosa. This can be particularly difficult in patients with prominent diverticulosis. A similar dissection may also be required on the distal rectal segment.

❿ **Placing the Anvil.** The largest possible EEA circular stapler that will fit the bowel segments, typically the 31-mm size, is used. This provides a commodious anastomosis that will lessen the chances of symptomatic rectal stenosis. The proximal sigmoid colon is again held with Allis clamps, and scissors are used to remove the entire staple line. The Allis clamps are replaced to grasp the mucosa/serosa and hold open the proximal sigmoid colon. Sizing instruments may be used if necessary to decide which EEA instrument is best. The EEA device contains

an anvil that will be placed in the proximal bowel and a stapler that is placed in the distal bowel. Articulation of the anvil and stapler head allows firing of a staple ring at this articulation site to form the anastomosis.

First, the anvil is detached from the stapler, lubricated, and gently inserted by rotating it into the proximal sigmoid colon. Its concave surface faces proximally, away from the anticipated anastomotic site (Fig. 46-21.4 inset). Sequential stitches that pierce through bowel serosa, muscularis, and mucosa create a purse string around the anvil. These "through-and-through" stitches using 2–0 Prolene suture are placed 5 to 7 mm from the mucosal edge. The purse string begins and ends on the outside of the bowel serosa around the anvil spike and is then tied securely. Allis clamps are removed. A quicker alternative is to use a stapler purse-string suture device. Irrigation may be performed if bowel contents have spilled.

⓫ **Placing the Stapler.** The distal rectal stump is reexamined to ensure that all surrounding fatty tissue has been dissected free. The surgical team then reviews the details of using an EEA instrument. A phantom application is helpful. After this, the shaft of the stapler is extended and its spike is attached. The shaft and spike are then retracted into the instrument. The EEA is lubricated and gently inserted into the anus until the circular outline is visible and seen to be gently pressing on the rectal staple line. A wing nut located on the device handle is gently rotated, and this extends the shaft and its spike. This is guided by the abdominal surgeon so that the spike is brought out just posterior to the staple midline. In the abdomen, gentle countertraction against the rectum may be helpful as the sharp

spike tip pops through the entire bowel wall thickness. The shaft subsequently becomes visible and the spike is removed.

⓬ **Stapling.** The abdominal surgeon lowers the proximal sigmoid colon to the distal rectum and connects the hollow tip of the anvil into the metal shaft of the EEA. An audible "click" should be heard to confirm articulation. The tip of the EEA is held perfectly still, while the wing nut is again rotated to retract the shaft back into the EEA until the handle indicator is in the correct position. This draws the anvil into apposition with the stapler head. The safety is released, and the instrument is fired by squeezing and depressing the handles completely. Incomplete squeezing can result in partial stapling. The wing nut is then turned to the specified position to release the staple line. The EEA with its attached anvil is then gently rotated and slowly removed from the rectum. The anastomosis is visualized by the abdominal surgeon throughout the process. Distal retraction of the anastomosis or inability to remove the EEA suggests that the stapler was not completely fired. This situation may be salvaged by gently pulling the EEA through the anus and cutting inside the staple line to release the anastomosis. The anvil is removed from the EEA instrument and inspected to confirm that two completely intact circular "donuts" of rectal tissue are present.

⓭ **Rectal Insufflation.** Warmed saline is irrigated into the pelvis. The integrity of the anastomosis may now be checked by gently inserting a proctoscope or red rubber catheter into the anus, but distal to the anastomosis. Air is then insufflated into the bowel. The abdominal surgeon gently palpates the sigmoid colon to make certain that air is

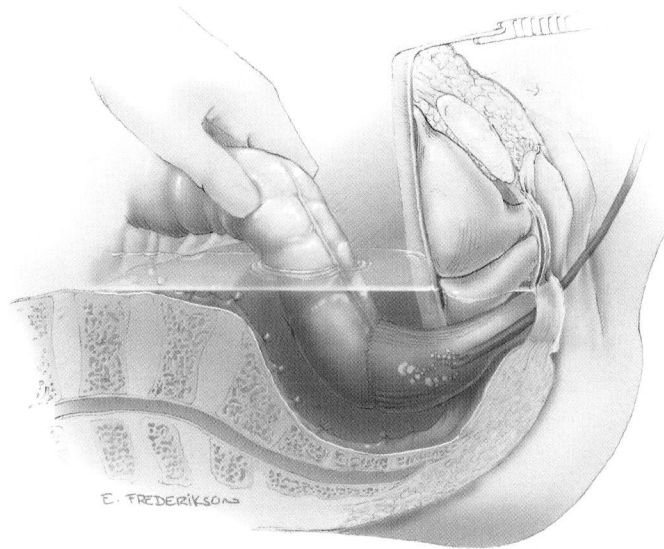

FIGURE 46-21.5 Testing the anastomosis.

entering the sigmoid colon proximal to the anastomotic site. No air bubbles are visible if the connection is watertight (Fig. 46-21.5). The appearance of bubbles suggests a leak, but this should be double-checked for authenticity. Occasionally, air is being erroneously pumped into the vagina rather than the rectum due to incorrect placement of the red rubber catheter. If there is any valid suspicion for a leak, the distal rectum should be divided again and the anastomosis redone. Reinforcing interrupted suture to close the

air leak may be attempted in select situations, but this is riskier. Diverting colostomy may also be considered if the problem cannot otherwise be managed.

⓮ **Final Steps.** All pedicles sites are rechecked for hemostasis, and the pelvis is irrigated. Nasogastric suction is not routinely required. In addition, prophylactic suction drainage of the pelvis does not improve outcome or influence the severity of complications (Merad, 1999).

POSTOPERATIVE

The most common early postoperative complications are similar to those for other major abdominal operations and include fever, self-limiting ileus, wound separation, and anemia requiring transfusion. Serious events such as bowel obstruction and fistula develop infrequently (Gillette-Cloven, 2001). Long-term, some patients will have a poor functional result, including fecal incontinence or chronic constipation (Rasmussen, 2003).

Low rectal anastomoses have much higher intraperitoneal leakage rates than large bowel anastomoses. Leakage of stool leads to fever, leukocytosis, lower abdominal pain, and ileus. These should prompt abdominopelvic CT imaging with oral contrast. If a leak is present, it may appear as a pelvic abscess, or at times, contrast extravasation can be demonstrated into the fluid collection. Occasionally, this complication can be successfully managed with percutaneous drainage of the abscess, bowel rest, and broad-spectrum antibiotics. Otherwise, a temporary diverting loop ileostomy or colostomy may be required (Mourton, 2005). Risk factors for postoperative leakage include previous pelvic irradiation, diabetes mellitus, low preoperative serum albumin, long surgical duration, and a low anastomosis (≤6 cm from the anal verge) (Matthiessen, 2004; Mirhashemi, 2000; Richardson, 2006).

46-22

Intestinal Bypass

This bowel anastomotic procedure typically connects a section of the ileum to the ascending or transverse colon and thereby "bypasses" a portion of diseased bowel. Following anastomosis, the closed, bypassed small-bowel segment remains.

There are relatively few indications for intestinal bypass in gynecologic oncology, and this procedure accounts for less than 5 percent of all bowel operations performed for these cancers (Barnhill, 1991; Winter, 2003). In all circumstances, removal of diseased bowel and end-to-end anastomosis is preferable. However, some patients will have unresectable tumor, dense adhesions, extensive radiation injury, or other prohibitive factors. In these cases, a poor decision to proceed with an aggressive dissection can result in numerous enterotomies, hemorrhage, or other intraoperative catastrophes with major postoperative sequelae. Instead, an intestinal bypass can often quickly be performed with minimal morbidity. Many times a bypass is selected because it is the easiest palliative maneuver for a terminally ill patient. The main purpose is to relieve an obstruction, reestablish an adequate bowel communication, and restore the patient's ability to take oral nourishment.

PREOPERATIVE

Patient Evaluation

The intestinal tract is evaluated by CT scanning. Invariably, pelvic radiation injuries are located at the terminal ileum, but there may be complex fistulas or multiple sites of obstruction to be addressed. In most circumstances in which a bypass is considered, a surgeon should anticipate limitations in adequately exploring the abdomen intraoperatively. Careful analysis of preoperative findings will help ensure that bypass encompasses the entire lesion and does not leave a distal obstruction.

Consent

Patients usually have a miserable quality of life when bypass is considered, and the operation's goal is mainly to improve patient symptoms. The counseling process should emphasize that intraoperative judgment will dictate whether a small bowel resection, ileostomy, large bowel resection, colostomy, or bypass is indicated. Many risks are similar to those of other intestinal surgical procedures and include anastomotic leaks, obstruction, abscess formation, and fistula. Blind loop syndrome, discussed

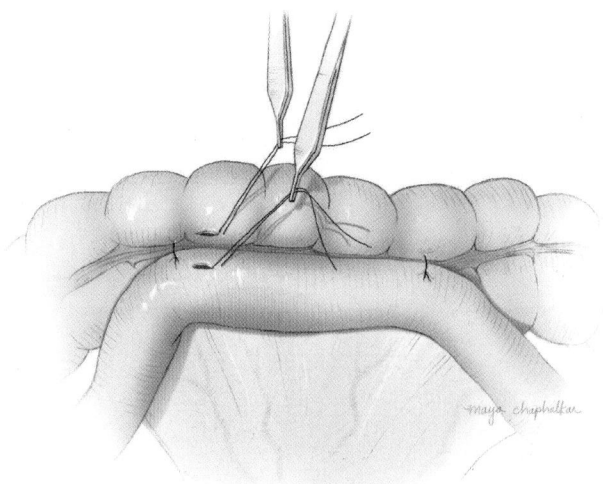

FIGURE 46-22.1 Aligning the bowel.

later, is one long-term complication that is specific to the bypass procedure.

Patient Preparation

Aggressive bowel preparation with oral agents is usually contraindicated due to bowel obstruction or other dire circumstances. Broad-spectrum antibiotics are given perioperatively due to the possibility of stool contamination, and VTE prophylaxis is provided. If a prolonged recovery is anticipated, postoperative TPN is considered.

INTRAOPERATIVE

Instruments

To prepare for complicated resections, bowel staplers such as an end-to-end anastomosis (EEA), gastrointestinal anastomosis (GIA), and transverse anastomosis (TA) staplers should be available.

Surgical Steps

❶ Anesthesia and Patient Positioning. Bypass is performed under general anesthesia with the patient positioned supine. Prior to surgery, the abdomen is surgically prepared, and a Foley catheter is inserted.

❷ Abdominal Entry and Exploration. Colostomy generally requires a midline vertical incision for adequate exposure. A surgeon first explores the entire abdomen to identify bowel lesions. In addition, the remaining bowel is examined to exclude other obstructive sites. Healthy-appearing bowel proximal and distal to the lesion is selected with the intent of preserving the maximal amount of intestine. Typically, the bypass will entail

connecting a section of the ileum to the ascending or transverse colon.

❸ Aligning the Bowel. The two bowel segments selected for the anastomosis are aligned side-to-side without tension or twisting. The hepatic or splenic flexure of the transverse colon may require mobilization from its peritoneal attachments to achieve a tension-free connection. The antimesenteric borders of the bowel segments are held in position by 2–0 silk stay sutures that are placed approximately 6 cm apart along the length of the aligned bowel segments. Two Adson forceps are used to hold up the small-bowel serosa laterally and transversely on traction. An electrosurgical blade is used to enter the small bowel lumen on its antimesenteric surface (Fig. 46-22.1). The same maneuver is performed on the teniae coli to enter the colon.

❹ Performing the Side-to-Side Anastomosis. One fork of the GIA stapler is inserted into each bowel segment lumen. The bowel is adjusted, if necessary, to position the antimesenteric surfaces between the stapler forks. The stapler is then closed and fired (Fig. 46-22.2). With stapling, the initial small bowel openings that were cut to admit the stapler forks are fused into one open defect. This opening can be closed with the TA stapler and the excess bowel trimmed. As a result this TA staple line, the diseased bowel loop is also simultaneously sealed.

❺ Final Steps. Occasionally, small bleeding sites on the staple line will need spot electrosurgical coagulation. The anastomosis is also palpated to verify an adequate lumen. The bowel is reexamined to make certain that the connection is watertight and that there is no tension on the anastomosis.

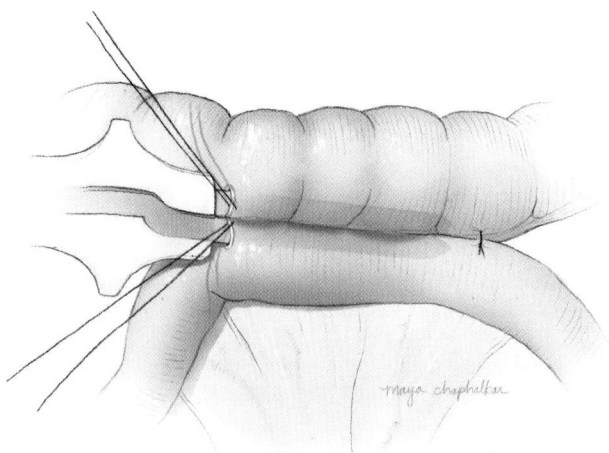

FIGURE 46-22.2 Performing side-to-side anastomosis.

POSTOPERATIVE

Recovery after bypass surgery should be rapid compared with that following a large resection with anastomosis. In general, postoperative ileus will resolve in several days, and patients may begin oral alimentation. The underlying clinical situation prompting the need for bypass surgery will dictate most of the clinical course. Relatively minor complications such as febrile morbidity and wound infection or wound separation occur commonly. Fistulas, obstruction, anastomotic leaks, abscesses, peritonitis, and perforation are more difficult to manage and often lead to a prolonged postoperative course or death.

Blind loop syndrome is a condition of vitamin B_{12} malabsorption, steatorrhea, and bacterial overgrowth of the small intestine. The usual scenario is a bypass procedure that leaves a segment of nonfunctional, severely irradiated bowel behind. Stasis of the intestinal contents leads to dilatation and mucosal inflammation. Symptoms resemble a partial small bowel obstruction and include nausea, vomiting, diarrhea, abdominal distention, and pain. Bowel perforation is possible. Antibiotics will often alleviate the condition, but recolonization and resumption of the blind loop syndrome is common (Swan, 1974). The only definitive therapy for recurrent episodes is exploration with resection of the bypassed segment. To avoid this syndrome, a surgeon may still perform the side-to-side anastomosis. But, the closed loop can be relieved by creation of a mucus fistula at the abdominal wall.

46-23

Appendectomy

Removal of the appendix may be indicated during gynecologic surgery for various reasons. The need, however, is commonly not recognized until an operation is already underway, as signs and symptoms of benign gynecologic conditions can mimic appendicitis (Bowling, 2006; Fayez, 1995; Stefanidis, 1999).

In addition, malignancies may involve the appendix. Ovarian cancer frequently metastasizes to the appendix, which thereby often warrants removal (Ayhan, 2005). Primary tumors of the appendix are rare but commonly metastasize to the ovaries. Thus, the initial surgical intervention is often performed by a gynecologic oncologist (Dietrich, 2007). Pseudomyxoma peritonei is the classic type of mucinous tumor of appendiceal origin that spreads to the ovaries and may implant throughout the abdomen (Prayson, 1994).

Elective coincidental appendectomy is defined as the removal of an appendix at the time of another surgical procedure unrelated to appreciable appendiceal pathology. Possible benefits include preventing a future emergency appendectomy and excluding appendicitis in patients with chronic pelvic pain or endometriosis. Other groups that may benefit include women in whom pelvic or abdominal radiation or chemotherapy is anticipated, women undergoing extensive pelvic or abdominal surgery in which major adhesions are anticipated postoperatively, and patients such as the developmentally disabled in whom making the diagnosis of appendicitis may be difficult because of diminished ability to perceive or communicate symptoms (American College of Obstetricians and Gynecologists, 2014).

PREOPERATIVE

Specific preoperative tests or preparations are not required prior to appendectomy. In general, the consenting process for gynecologic surgery includes a discussion of possible "other indicated procedures" such as appendectomy when anticipated intraoperative findings and the potential for performing an appendectomy are uncertain.

Most studies suggest that there is, at most, a small increased risk of nonfatal complications associated with elective coincidental appendectomy at the time of gynecologic surgery, whether performed during laparotomy or during laparoscopy (Salom, 2003). Hematoma formation at the mesoappendix may cause an ileus or partial small bowel obstruction. Perforation of the stump is rare and typically follows insecure suture placement.

INTRAOPERATIVE

Surgical Steps

❶ **Anesthesia and Patient Positioning.** Appendectomy is performed under general anesthesia in a supine position. Postoperative hospitalization is individualized and is dependent on concurrent surgeries and associated clinical symptoms.

❷ **Abdominal Entry.** Appendectomy can be performed through almost any incision. A laparoscopic approach or an oblique McBurney incision in the right lower quadrant of the abdomen is traditionally selected for appendectomy. However, in gynecologic cases, the needs of planned concurrent procedures will commonly dictate incision choice.

❸ **Locating the Appendix.** The appendix is located by first grasping the cecum and gently elevating it upward into the incision. Insertion of the terminal ileum should be visible, and the appendix is typically obvious at this point. Infrequently, an appendix is retrocecal or otherwise difficult to identify. In this situation, the convergence of the three teniae coli can be followed to locate the appendiceal base.

❹ **Mesoappendix Division.** The appendix tip is elevated with a Babcock clamp, and the cecum is held laterally to place the mesoappendix on gentle traction. The appendiceal artery is usually very difficult to distinguish reliably due to abundant surrounding fatty tissue. Thus, curved hemostats are used to successively clamp the mesoappendix and its vessels to reach the appendiceal base (Fig. 46-23.1).

The first hemostat is placed horizontally—aiming directly toward the base of the appendix. The second hemostat is placed at a 30-degree angle so that the tips meet, but Metzenbaum scissors have room to cut between the two clamps. The mesoappendix pedicle is ligated with 3–0 gauge delayed-absorbable suture. This step is typically repeated once or twice to comfortably reach the base of the appendix. An alternative is to use an electrothermal bipolar coagulator (LigaSure) to divide the mesoappendix.

❺ **Appendix Ligation.** At this point, the appendix has been completely isolated from the mesoappendix and is still held vertically by a Babcock clamp. A first hemostat is placed at the appendiceal base, and a second is positioned directly above (Fig. 46-23.2). A third hemostat is closed with a few millimeters of intervening tissue to allow for passage of a knife blade. The knife then cuts between

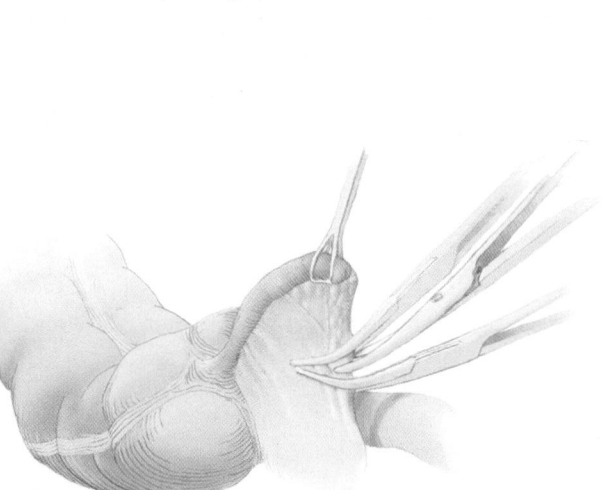

FIGURE 46-23.1 Clamping the mesoappendix.

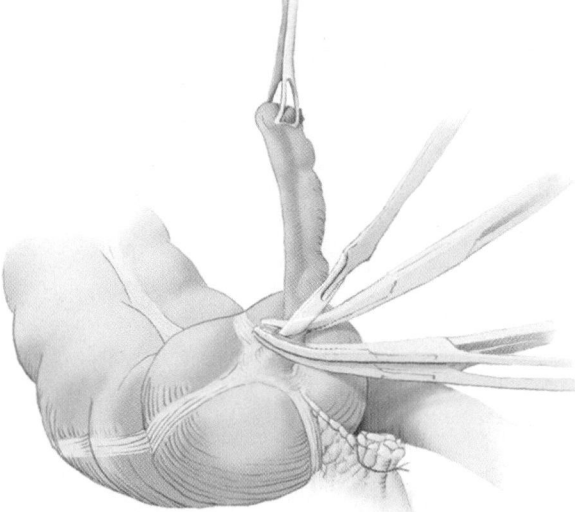

FIGURE 46-23.2 Ligation of the appendix.

the second and third clamps, and the appendix is removed. The contaminated knife and appendix are then handed off the field.

A 2–0 silk suture is tied beneath the first hemostat as that clamp is slowly removed. A separate suture is then tied underneath the second hemostat for added security of the appendiceal stump. Gentle electrosurgical coagulation at the stump surface may also be performed.

❻ **Final Steps.** There is no need to invert the stump or to place a purse-string suture around it. The cecum may be returned to the abdomen, and remaining concurrent surgeries completed.

POSTOPERATIVE

Patient care postoperatively is dictated by other surgeries performed. Delayed initiation of oral intake or administration of additional antibiotics is not required for appendectomy alone.

46-24

Skinning Vulvectomy

The term *skinning vulvectomy* implies a wide, superficial resection that encompasses both sides of the vulva, that is, a complete simple vulvectomy. The surgical procedure is straightforward and removes the entire lesion. It is distinguished from a *radical complete vulvectomy* in that skinning vulvectomy removes only the squamous epithelium and dermis and preserves the subcutaneous fat and deeper tissues. A less extensive, unilateral procedure is better referred to as a *wide local excision* or *partial simple vulvectomy* (Section 43-28, p. 995).

The usual indication for skinning vulvectomy is a woman with confluent, bilateral vulvar intraepithelial neoplasia (VIN) 2 to 3 who is not a candidate for directed ablation with carbon dioxide (CO_2) laser or cavitational ultrasonic surgical aspirator (CUSA) (Section 43-28, p. 996). Fortunately, individuals with such extensive VIN are infrequently encountered. Paget disease without underlying adenocarcinoma and vulvar dystrophies refractory to standard therapy are other rare indications (Ayhan, 1998; Curtin, 1990; Rettenmaier, 1985).

Despite its less radical resection, skinning vulvectomy can still be disfiguring and psychologically devastating. In addition, the defect is often large and cannot be closed primarily without a split-thickness skin graft (STSG) or other type of flap (Section 46-28, p. 1219).

PREOPERATIVE

Patient Evaluation

Colposcopy with directed diagnostic biopsy is required to exclude a squamous lesion with invasion, which would warrant a more radical procedure. Familiarity with an array of possible STSGs or flaps is crucial to planning the operation in the event primary closure is not possible.

Consent

Patients are informed that other more limited treatment options either have been exhausted or are inappropriate. The surgery may result in significant sexual changes, which may be permanent. Accordingly, surgeons emphasize that all efforts will be made to restore a functional, normal-appearing vulva. Fortunately, most physical complications are minor and include cellulitis or partial wound dehiscence.

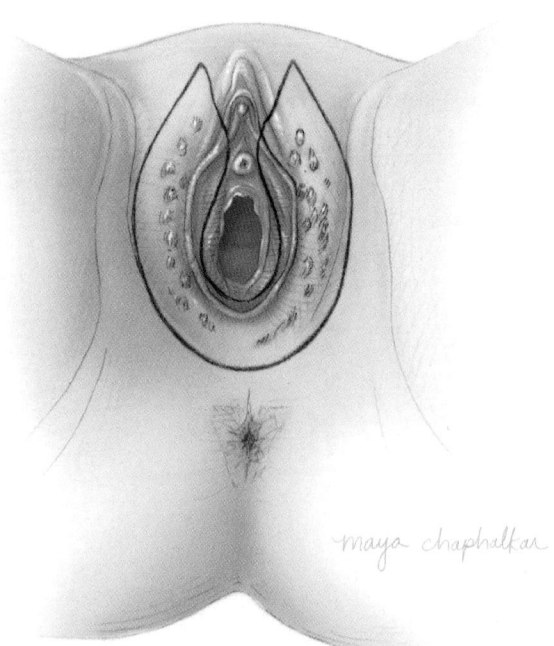

FIGURE 46-24.1 Marking the incisions.

Patient Preparation

Complete bowel preparation is influenced by surgeon preference and only indicated if perianal skin is to be excised. In these cases, bowel preparation may minimize fecal soiling and permit initial wound healing prior to the first stool. Otherwise, enemas are sufficient. Antibiotics and VTE prophylaxis are typically given. Grafts are typically taken from the upper thigh, and donor site selection for STSG is described in Section 46-28 (p. 1219).

INTRAOPERATIVE

Surgical Steps

❶ **Anesthesia and Patient Positioning.** Regional or general anesthesia is generally required. The patient is placed in standard lithotomy position, and adjustments provide access to the entire lesion. Vulvar hair should be clipped. Intraoperative colposcopy may be needed to better delineate VIN lesion margins.

❷ **Skin Incision.** The inner and outer incision lines are drawn to encompass the disease with margins of at least a few millimeters (Fig. 46-24.1). As an overview, once final markings are placed, the skin is dissected off one side of the vulva. The skin on the opposite side of the vulva is then removed, and the bridging skin overlying the perineal body is excised last. In performing this, the clitoris may be spared in many cases by making a horseshoe-shaped incision (as shown).

To begin, if preserving the clitoris, the outer incision is started on one side of the

vulva at the anterolateral margin of the clitoris and is continued inferiorly along the length of the labium majus at least halfway to the perineal body. The inner incision on that same side of the vulva is then also taken through the full skin thickness to the same inferior halfway point. Incising the skin in stages reduces blood loss.

❸ **Beginning the Dissection.** The specimen edge may then be reflected with an Allis clamp to provide traction as the avascular plane underneath the skin is dissected from the subcutaneous fatty tissue (Fig. 46-24.2). When the anterior skin edge is large enough, a hand is placed underneath to reflect the specimen more firmly and guide dissection inferiorly. The outer and inner skin incision is then extended on that same side downward toward the perineal body. Electrosurgical coagulation is used to achieve hemostasis before repeating the process on the contralateral side.

❹ **Removal of the Specimen.** The left and right outer skin incisions are joined in the midline superficial to the perineal body. The posterior vulvar tissue is held with an Allis clamp to provide traction for upward dissection toward the inner incision. The inner incision is made sufficiently proximal to encompass disease. This portion of the skinning vulvectomy is typically performed last because an avascular tissue plane superficial to the subcutaneous tissue is absent, and bleeding can be brisk. The specimen can be removed following detachment from the inner incision.

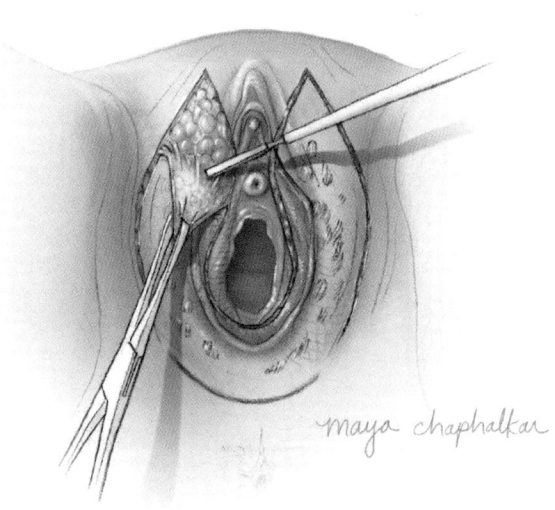

FIGURE 46-24.2 Performing the dissection.

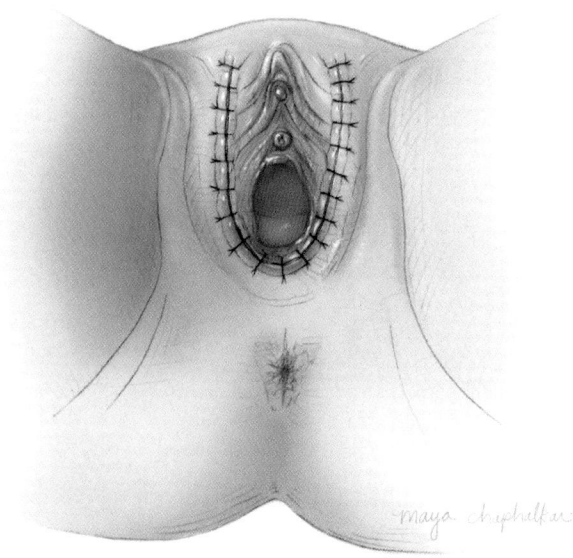

FIGURE 46-24.3 Primary closure.

The skinning vulvectomy specimen is carefully examined to grossly determine margins. A frozen section may be warranted if close VIN margins are suspected, to determine if more tissue requires excision. However, the margins of vulvar Paget disease cannot reliably be judged visually or by frozen-section analysis (Fishman, 1995). A stitch is placed on the specimen and noted on the pathology requisition form to orient the pathologist.

❺ Closure of the Defect. A dry laparotomy pad is held against the vulvar defect and slowly rolled downward to halt surface bleeding and aid meticulous electrosurgical coagulation of vessels. The operative site is irrigated and assessed.

If the width of the defect is sufficiently narrow to permit primary closure, the surrounding tissue is mobilized. Lateral undermining may be particularly useful for a tension-free closure. Typically, 0 or 2–0 gauge delayed-absorbable vertical mattress sutures are then placed circumferentially with the knots laterally positioned (Fig. 46-24.3). However, if a split-thickness skin graft is required, the graft is now harvested and placed as described on page 1219.

❻ Final Steps. A CO_2 laser may be used to vaporize multifocal lesions outside the operative field. This is described in Section 43-28 (p. 997).

POSTOPERATIVE

If a primary closure is performed, postoperative care is essentially the same as described for patients undergoing radical partial vulvectomy (p. 1212). Long-term surveillance is mandatory regardless of margin status to identify recurrent or de novo sites of preinvasive disease. The Foley catheter can be removed without regard to urine spill unless a graft is placed or the patient is otherwise immobile.

46-25

Radical Partial Vulvectomy

For vulvar cancer, to reduce the high morbidity associated with radical complete vulvectomy yet avoid sacrificing a cure, a less extensive resection may be used. Patients with well-localized, unifocal, clinical stage I invasive lesions are ideal candidates (Stehman, 1992). *Radical partial vulvectomy* is a somewhat ambiguously defined operation that generally refers to complete removal of the tumor-containing portion of the vulva, wherever it is located, with 1- to 2-cm skin margins and excision to the perineal membrane (Whitney, 2010). *Radical hemivulvectomy* refers to a larger resection that may be anterior, posterior, right, or left. Vulvectomy is typically performed concurrently with inguinofemoral lymphadenectomy to add prognostic information. However, in those with microinvasive disease undergoing wide local excision or skinning vulvectomy, lymphadenectomy is not required.

The chief concern in performing a less extensive operation for vulvar cancer is the possibility of an increased risk of local recurrence due to multifocal disease. However, survival after partial or complete radical vulvectomy is comparable if negative margins are obtained (Chan, 2007; Landrum, 2007; Scheistroen, 2002; Tantipalakorn, 2009). Following radical partial vulvectomy, 10 percent of patients will develop a recurrence on the ipsilateral vulva, and this may be treated by reexcision (Desimone, 2007).

PREOPERATIVE

Patient Evaluation

Biopsy confirmation of invasive cancer is mandatory. An isolated squamous lesion with less than 1 mm of invasion, that is, microinvasion, may be adequately managed with only wide local excision (Section 43-28, p. 995). Multiple microinvasive lesions may require skinning vulvectomy (p. 1208). In general, patients undergoing radical partial vulvectomy do not require reconstructive grafts or flaps to cover operative defects.

Consent

Morbidity after radical vulvar surgery is common. Wound separation or cellulitis develops frequently. Long-term changes may include displacement of the urine stream, dyspareunia, vulvar pain, and sexual dysfunction. Surgeons should be sensitive to these possible sequelae and counsel patients appropriately, emphasizing the curative intent and limited scope of the operation.

Patient Preparation

Bowel preparation is influenced by surgeon preference and may be indicated with posteriorly located resections. In such instances, bowel preparation may minimize fecal soiling and permit initial wound healing prior to the first stool. Antibiotics and VTE prophylaxis are typically given prior to incision (Tables 39-6 and 39-8, p. 835).

INTRAOPERATIVE

Surgical Steps

❶ **Anesthesia and Patient Positioning.** Radical partial vulvectomy has been performed under local anesthesia combined with sedation in medically compromised patients (Manahan, 1997). However, regional or general anesthesia is typically required.

Inguinal lymphadenectomy (p. 1216) is typically performed before vulvar resection. Patients may then be repositioned to standard lithotomy position to provide full exposure to the vulva. The vulva is surgically prepared, and a Foley catheter is inserted.

❷ **Radical Partial Vulvectomy: Variations.** The area of tissue to be removed when radically excising a small cancer depends on the size and location of the tumor. In Figure 46-25.1, the dotted line indicates a planned skin incision for: (A) a 1-cm right labium majus tumor with 2-cm margins, (B) a 2.5-cm periclitoral tumor necessitating anterior hemivulvectomy, and (C) a 2.5-cm midline posterior fourchette tumor requiring posterior hemivulvectomy.

❸ **Right Hemivulvectomy: Making the Lateral Incision.** The planned excision is drawn on the vulva with a surgical marking pen to provide 2-cm margins (Fig. 46-25.2). Tapering the incision anteriorly and posteriorly will aid in a tension-free closure. The lateral skin incision is made with a knife (no. 15 blade) into the subcutaneous fat. Forceps are used to place the skin edges on traction and aid electrosurgical dissection downward until reaching the perineal membrane (Fig. 46-25.3). An index finger can then be used to develop the plane between the fat pad of the labium majus and the subcutaneous tissue of the lateral thigh.

❹ **Right Hemivulvectomy: Completing the Resection.** Tissue medial to this lateral resection border is next mobilized medially by blunt and electrosurgical dissection along the perineal membrane. The skin edge of the specimen is then placed on lateral traction, and the medial (vaginal mucosa) incision is incised from anterior to posterior. The labial fat pad is transected anteriorly, and the entire radical right hemivulvectomy specimen is placed on downward traction to aid final dissection along the mucosal incision in an anterior-to-posterior direction (Fig. 46-25.4). Notably, the vascular vestibular bulb is

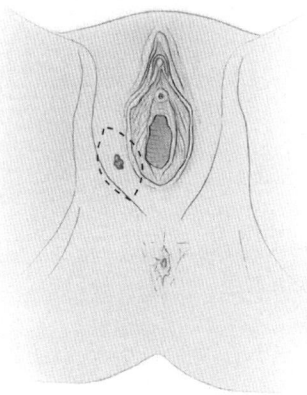

A

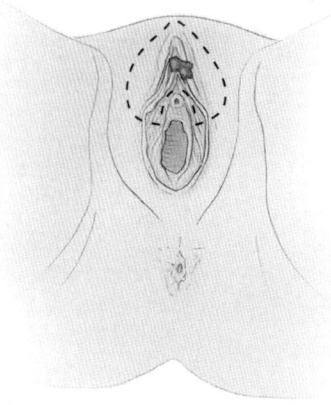

B

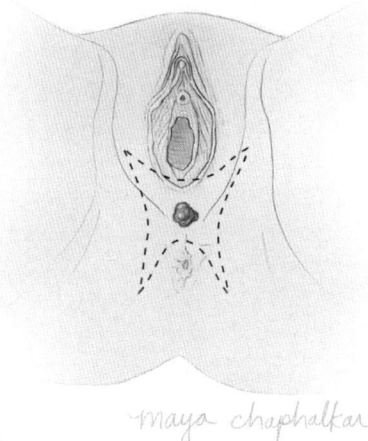

C

maya chaphalkar

FIGURE 46-25.1 Radical partial vulvectomy: variations.

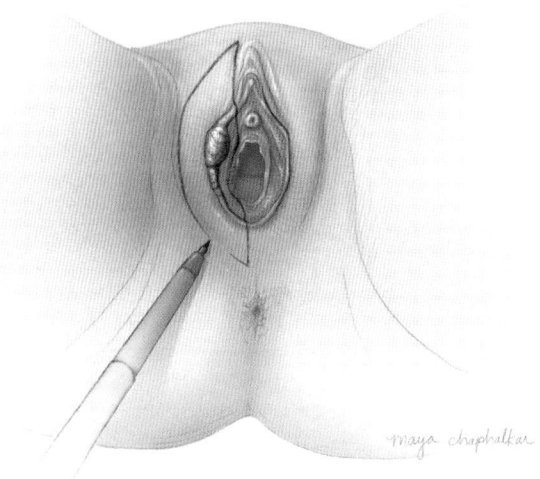

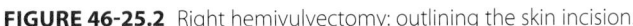

FIGURE 46-25.2 Right hemivulvectomy: outlining the skin incision.

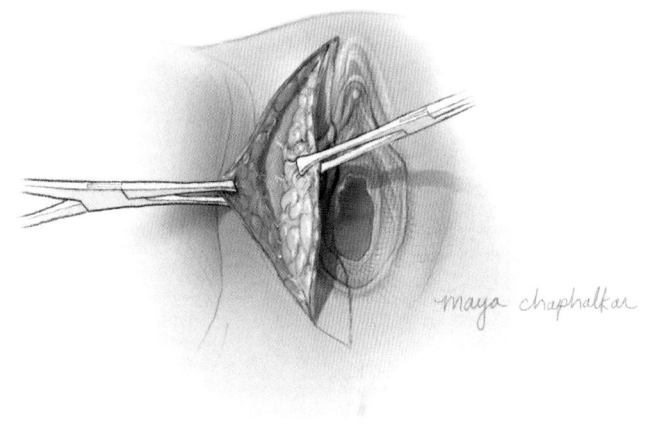

FIGURE 46-25.3 Right hemivulvectomy: lateral dissection to the fascia lata.

typically encountered as the posterior resection is completed. Suture ligation of bleeding sites is often required.

After completed resection, the specimen is examined to ensure adequate margins. It is marked at 12 o'clock with an orienting stitch, and this is noted on the pathology requisition form.

❺ **Right Hemivulvectomy: Defect Closure.** A gauze sponge may be held firmly in the cavity and rolled downward to guide the electrosurgical blade in achieving hemostasis. The defect can then be irrigated and evaluated to determine requirement for a tension-free closure while minimizing anatomic distortion (Fig. 46-25.5). Several pedicles are visible, particularly at the

vaginal margin, where vessels were clamped and tied.

In general, lateral undermining of the subcutaneous tissue will provide sufficient mobility to allow primary closure. Interrupted 0-gauge delayed-absorbable suture is used to create a layered reapproximation of deeper tissues. Interrupted vertical mattress sutures, often alternating 0 and 2–0 gauge suture, with knots placed laterally are used to close the skin (Fig. 46-25.6).

❻ **Anterior Hemivulvectomy.** This variation requires removal of the clitoris and partial resection of the labia minora, labia majora, and mons pubis. The most anterior portion of the incision is first created on the mons and carried down to the pubic symphysis. The

specimen is reflected posteriorly to guide dissection. In the midline, the clitoral vessels are separately clamped, divided, and ligated with 0-gauge delayed-absorbable suture.

The posterior incision is made above the urethral meatus, and careful attention to Foley catheter location helps avoid urethral injury. Layers of interrupted 0-gauge delayed-absorbable sutures are used to reapproximate deep tissue. Then, 3–0 gauge absorbable suture is used to close the defect in a direction that places the least tension on the suture line. Usually, the area surrounding the urethral meatus is left to granulate secondarily.

❼ **Partial Urethral Resection (Optional).** If an anterior lesion encroaches on the urethral meatus, then a distal urethrectomy may be required to achieve a negative margin. Prior to this, the radical partial vulvectomy should otherwise be almost entirely completed. The

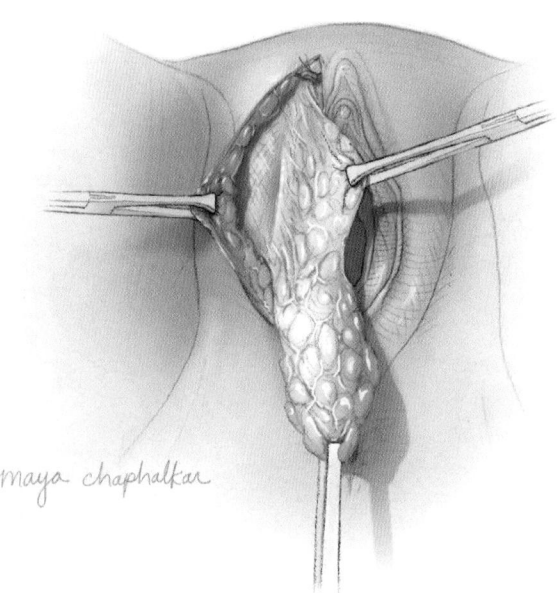

FIGURE 46-25.4 Right hemivulvectomy: removal of the specimen.

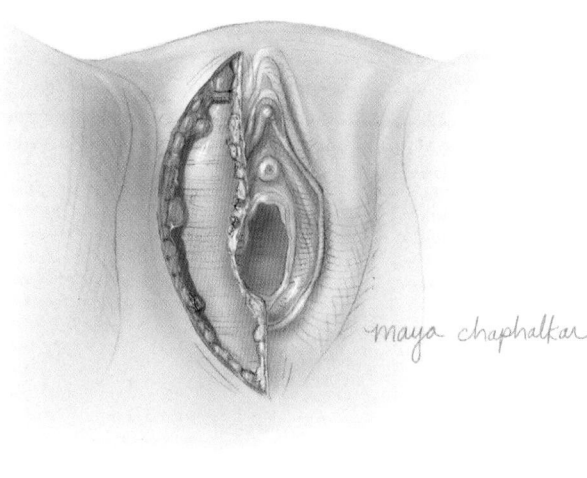

FIGURE 46-25.5 Right hemivulvectomy: evaluation of the surgical defect.

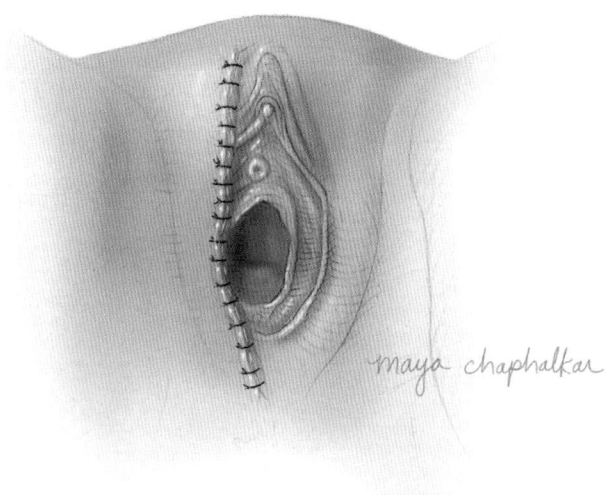

FIGURE 46-25.6 Right hemivulvectomy: closure of the surgical defect.

urethra may be transected anywhere distal to the pubic arch. For this, the meatus is held with an Allis clamp, and the specimen placed on traction. The posterior urethra is incised with a knife, and the underlying uroepithelium and mucosa are sewn jointly to the adjacent vestibule skin at the 6 o'clock position with 4–0 gauge delayed-absorbable suture. The urethral incision is extended laterally, followed by additional sutures at 3 and 9 o'clock. The Foley balloon is deflated and removed from the bladder. Transection is completed, and a final stitch is placed at 12 o'clock. The Foley catheter is then replaced. Alternatively, the surgeon may forgo stitch placement altogether and allow the meatus to heal by secondary intent. Although urethral plication may be indicated in selected cases, resection of 1 to 1.5 cm of the distal urethra does not ordinarily result in a significant increase in urinary incontinence (de Mooij, 2007).

❽ Posterior Hemivulvectomy. This variation entails removal of a portion of the labia majora, Bartholin glands, and upper perineal body. It is generally necessary to compromise the deep margin in this resection because of proximity to the anal sphincter and rectum.

The skin is first incised posteriorly, and a finger is placed into the rectum to guide proximal dissection. The specimen is gradually retracted upward off the sphincter. From the midline, dissection then proceeds laterally on each side until the anterior margin at the introitus can be incised to complete the resection. The perineal body is reinforced with interrupted sutures of 0-gauge delayed-absorbable material to provide bulk and to allow reapproximation of skin edges for a tension-free closure. Rectal examination is performed at the end of surgery to confirm the absence of palpable stitches or stenosis. Incontinence of flatus or stool may develop postoperatively despite efforts to preserve the sphincter.

❾ Final Steps. Suction drains are not typically required but are at least considered in some circumstances. Copious irrigation is indicated at various times during closure of the defect to minimize postoperative infection. No formal dressing is applied. However, fluffed-out gauze may be placed at the perineum and held in place with mesh underwear to tamponade any subcutaneous bleeding and to promote a clean and dry operative site in the immediate postoperative period.

POSTOPERATIVE

Meticulous care of the vulvar wound is mandatory to prevent morbidity. The vulva is kept dry by use of a blow dryer or fan. Within a few days, brief sitz baths or bedside irrigation followed by air drying will help keep the incision clean. Patients are instructed not to wear tight-fitting underwear upon discharge from the hospital. Moreover, instructions encourage loose-fitting gowns to aid healing and efforts to minimize wound tension. For posteriorly located defects near the anus, a low-residue diet and stool softeners will prevent straining and potential perineal incision disruption.

Typically, the Foley catheter is removed postprocedure or at least on postoperative day 1. If a distal urethrectomy was performed or extensive periurethral dissection was required, then the catheter is removed within a few days. This permits tissue swelling and obstructive urinary retention concerns to abate. Early removal prevents ascending urinary infection. If immobility is encouraged to aid reconstructive graft or flap healing, then the timing of catheter removal is individualized. Notably, urine that comes in contact with the vulvar incision during normal voiding is of little clinical concern.

Incision separation is the most common postoperative complication and often will involve only a portion of the incision (Burke, 1995). Stitches are removed as needed and affected portions of the wound are debrided. Efforts to keep the site clean and dry are continued. Granulation tissue will eventually allow healing by secondary intention, but recovery time will be significantly extended. Although negative-pressure wound therapy (wound vacuum-assisted closure) may be practical in rare instances, the location of most defects precludes effective device placement.

Sexual dysfunction may stem from a sense of disfigurement. Scarring may also result in discomfort or altered sensation that lowers a woman's sexual satisfaction. Clinician sensitivity to these concerns enables a dialogue to develop that can lead to possible management options (Janda, 2004).

46-26

Radical Complete Vulvectomy

If cancers are so extensive that no meaningful portion of the vulva can be preserved, radical complete vulvectomy is indicated rather than the more limited radical partial vulvectomy (p. 1210). The operation is typically performed concurrently with bilateral inguino-femoral lymphadenectomy (p. 1216). With the radical complete vulvectomy technique currently used, intact skin bridges remain between the three incisions (vulvectomy incision and two lymphadenectomy incisions) to aid wound healing. Traditionally, the en bloc incision, colloquially termed the *butterfly* or *longhorn* incision, removed these skin bridges and the underlying lymphatic channels that potentially harbored tumor emboli "in transit" between the vulvar tumor and nodes (Gleeson, 1994c). However, such recurrences are rare, and the en bloc technique has been largely abandoned (Rose, 1999). Thus, the three-incision procedure is preferred because survival rates are equivalent and major morbidity is dramatically reduced (Helm, 1992).

Removal of an extensive vulvar lesion with an adequate margin and with resection down to the perineal membrane usually creates a large surgical defect. In some cases, wound margins may be primarily closed without tension by undermining and mobilizing adjacent tissues. On other occasions, a split-thickness skin graft, lateral skin transposition, rhomboid flap, or other reconstructive procedure, described on page 1219, will be indicated to reduce the chances of wound separation.

PREOPERATIVE

Patient Evaluation

Biopsy confirmation of invasive cancer should precede surgery. Depending on the location of the tumor, the clitoris-sparing modification of radical complete vulvectomy is an option (Chan, 2004). Frequently, patients are elderly, obese, or have significant coexisting medical problems that must be considered.

Consent

Major morbidity is common soon after radical complete vulvectomy, and partial wound separation or cellulitis occurs frequently. Complete wound breakdown is more problematic, and weeks of aggressive hospital care may be required to promote secondary healing. Premature hospital discharge may result in

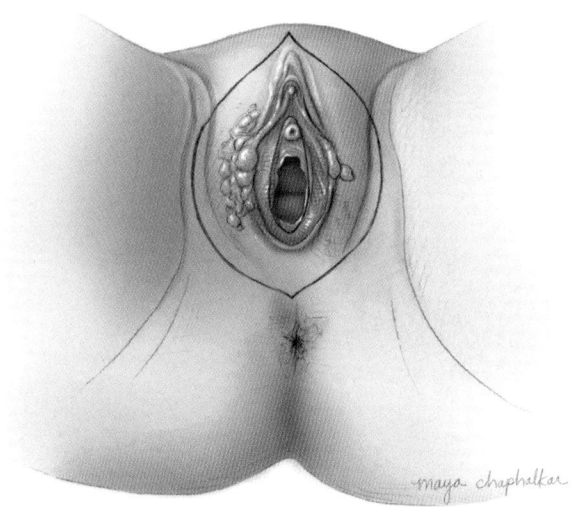

FIGURE 46-26.1 Incisions.

poor home wound care, and subsequent tissue necrosis often requires readmission and surgical debridement. Thus, meticulous attention to the wound is critical during patient admission and frequent office visits thereafter.

Long-term changes may include displacement of the urine stream, dyspareunia, vulvodynia, and sexual dysfunction. Accordingly, surgeons counsel on these possible sequelae yet emphasize the curative intent of the operation and the need for adequate tumor-free margins to lessen local recurrence risks.

Patient Preparation

Bowel preparation is guided by surgeon preference and may be indicated with posteriorly located lesions. In addition, evaluation of potential graft donor sites is completed. Antibiotics and VTE prophylaxis are typically given prior to initial incision (Tables 39-6 and 39-8, p. 835).

INTRAOPERATIVE

Surgical Steps

❶ Anesthesia and Patient Positioning. Regional or general anesthesia is required, and inguinofemoral lymphadenectomy is performed first. The patient is then placed in standard lithotomy position. Exposure and surgical preparation of the operative field is planned to accommodate resection and reconstruction. Sites of potential donor graft harvest are also prepared as described on page 1219.

❷ Planning the Skin Incision. The medial and lateral incisions are drawn to encompass the tumor and provide a 1- to 2-cm margin around the tumor. The clitoris is included if necessary. Tapering the incision

anteriorly and posteriorly will also aid in a tension-free closure (Fig. 46-26.1).

❸ Anterior Dissection. The skin incision begins anteriorly with the knife (no. 15 blade) cutting into the subcutaneous fat. The incision is extended downward approximately three quarters of its length. The remainder of the posterior skin incision is completed later to decrease blood loss. Much of the anterior dissection is described in the preceding section on radical partial vulvectomy (Section 46-25, step 6, p. 1211). However, use of the Harmonic scalpel or bipolar electrocoagulation device (LigaSure) in this more extensive resection may decrease operative time and blood loss compared with use of a conventional electrosurgical blade (Pellegrino, 2008).

Briefly, the incision is carried down to the pubic symphysis. The specimen is reflected downward on traction to guide dissection. The vascular base of the clitoris is clamped in the midline, transected, and suture ligated with 0-gauge delayed-absorbable suture (Fig. 46-26.2). Electrosurgical or Harmonic scalpel dissection then proceeds dorsally off the pubic bone until the inner incision line is reached anteriorly. This inner anterior incision is made above the urethral meatus to avoid injury to the urethra unless a distal urethrectomy is required (46-25, step 8, p. 1212).

❹ Lateral Dissection. Blunt finger dissection is performed to establish a plane lateral to the labial fat pads and at a depth to reach the perineal membrane. The vulvectomy specimen is placed on traction to guide dissection medially to reach the vaginal walls. Along the lower lateral sides of the vagina, the vascular vestibular bulb is encountered. Vessels are divided with the Harmonic scalpel or clamped, cut, and ligated with 0-gauge

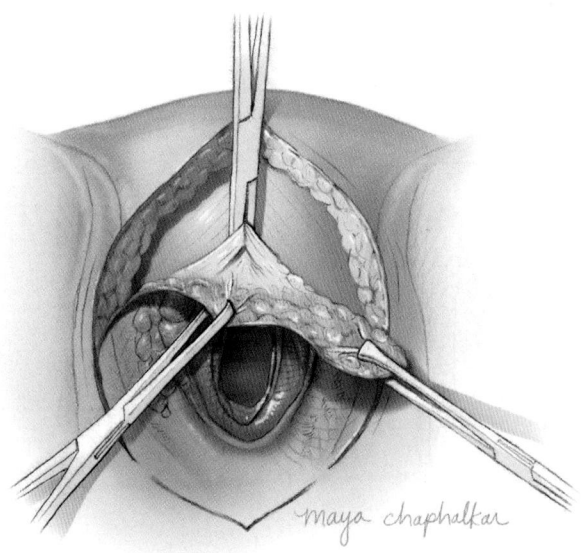

FIGURE 46-26.2 Anterior dissection.

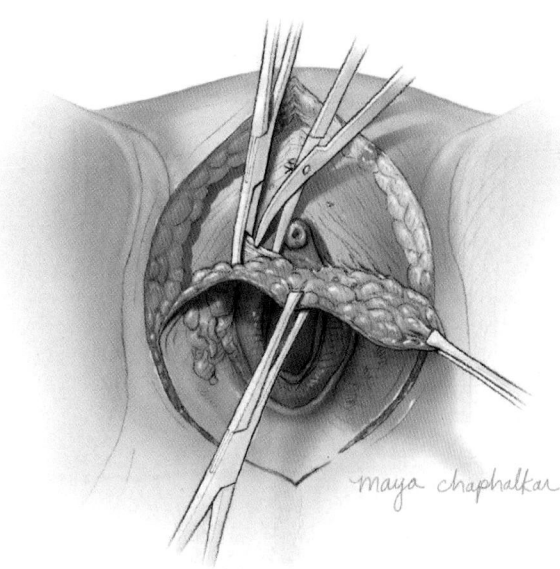

FIGURE 46-26.3 Medial dissection.

delayed-absorbable suture to reduce bleeding (Fig. 46-26.3).

❺ **Posterior Dissection.** An outer skin incision is completed inferiorly with a knife as the vulvectomy proceeds posteriorly toward the perineal body. A finger is then placed into the rectum to prevent inadvertent injury, and the specimen is now held upward on traction (Fig. 46-26.4). Electrosurgical dissection along the deep fascia plane extends the outer incisions toward the midline. The dissection continues anteriorly away from the

anus until the inner incision can be made. With this, the entire complete radical vulvectomy specimen is detached.

❻ **Evaluating the Specimen.** A stitch is placed at 12 o'clock on the specimen and noted on the laboratory requisition form to orient the pathologist. Skin retraction of the specimen will make it appear narrower and smaller than the defect. However, it is carefully inspected to assess its margins. Additional lateral or medial tissue margins can be separately sent if necessary.

Alternatively, a frozen section analysis can be requested to evaluate an equivocal margin.

❼ **Closing the Defect.** The wound is copiously irrigated, and hemostasis is achieved with a combination of electrosurgical coagulation and clamping with suturing. The defect is then evaluated to determine the best method of closure (Fig. 46-26.5). Undermining lateral tissues will aid a tension-free primary closure. Deeper tissues are first reapproximated with 0-gauge delayed-absorbable suture and interrupted stitches. The vulvar skin is then

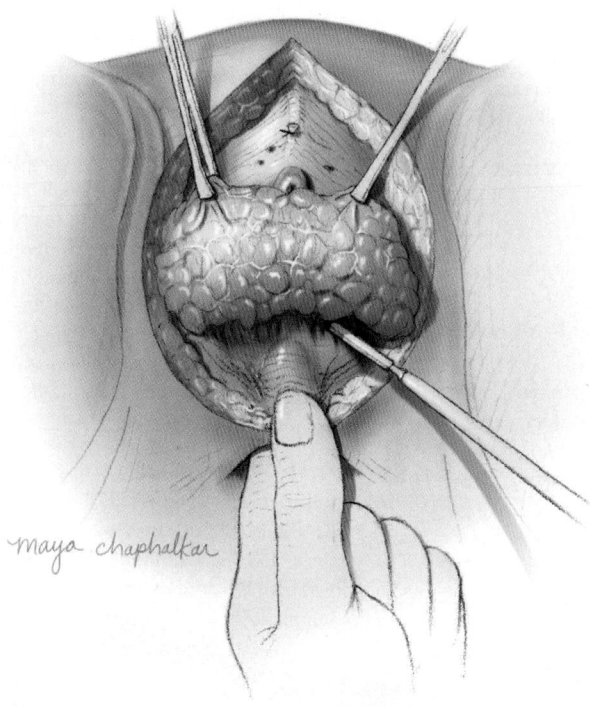

FIGURE 46-26.4 Posterior dissection.

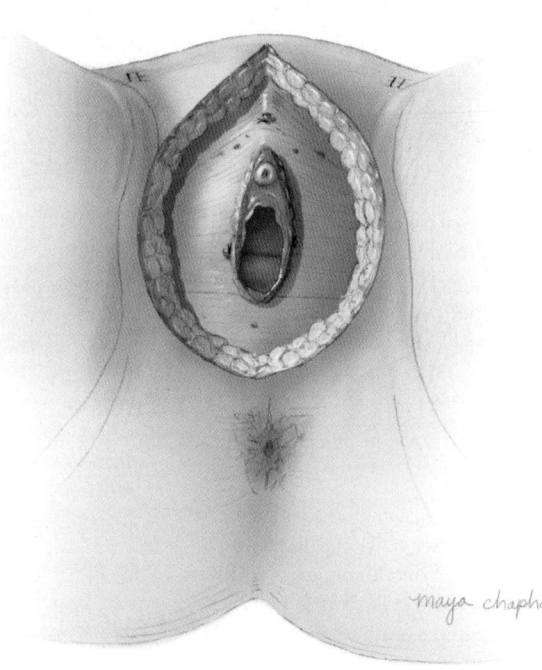

FIGURE 46-26.5 Surgical defect.

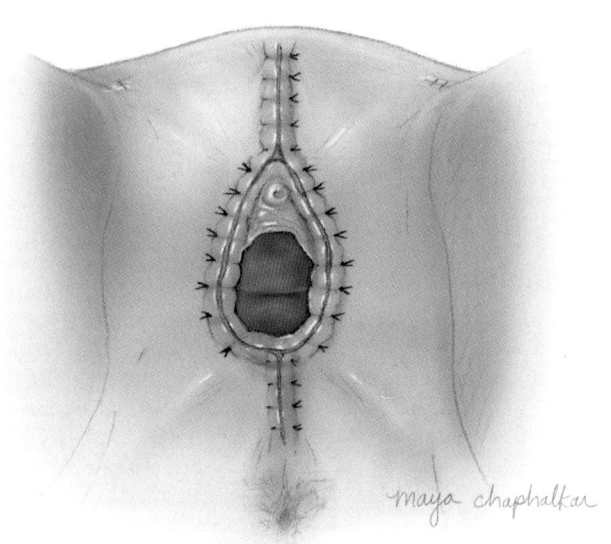

FIGURE 46-26.6 Simple closure.

closed with 0-gauge, or alternating with 2–0 gauge, delayed-absorbable vertical mattress sutures (Fig. 46-26.6). No stitches are placed between the skin and urethra if this displaces the urethra or creates tension on it. Instead, this area can be allowed to heal secondarily by granulation. If a split-thickness skin graft or flap is required to close the incision, the graft is now harvested and placed as described on page 1219.

❽ **Final Steps.** Suction drains do not prevent wound infection or breakdown but may be considered in some cases if the defect is large (Hopkins, 1993). If primary closure is performed, then fluffed-out gauze may be placed at the perineum and held in place with mesh underwear to keep the operative site clean and dry in the immediate postoperative period.

POSTOPERATIVE

If a primary closure is performed, postoperative care is essentially the same as described for patients undergoing radical partial vulvectomy (p. 1212). Because of a larger operative defect, the likelihood of morbidity is correspondingly increased. Management of reconstructive grafts and flaps is reviewed on page 1220.

46-27

Inguinofemoral Lymphadenectomy

Vulvar cancer staging is the primary indication for removal of groin nodes. Inguinal metastases are the most significant prognostic factor in vulvar squamous cancer, and their detection will necessitate additional therapy (Chap. 31, p. 682) (Homesley, 1991). Occasionally, in patients with ovarian or uterine cancer, suspicion of inguinal metastases will prompt removal.

In general, lymphatic drainage from the vulva rarely bypasses the superficial nodes. Thus, a superficial node dissection is integral. These lymph nodes lie within the fatty tissue along the saphenous, superficial external pudendal, superficial circumflex iliac, and superficial epigastric veins. After superficial nodes are addressed, deep nodes may be removed. These nodes are consistently located just medial and parallel to the femoral vein within the fossa ovalis. To reach these, cribriform fascia preservation is recommended to avoid major morbidity (Bell, 2000).

Generally, for patients with unilateral lesions distant from the midline, ipsilateral lymphadenectomy is usually sufficient (Gonzalez Bosquet, 2007). For bilateral lesions or those that encroach on the midline, bilateral lymphadenectomy is indicated.

Sentinel lymph node mapping is a promising modality that has demonstrated great potential in reducing the radicality of detecting inguinal metastases (Van der Zee, 2008). This minimally invasive strategy is emerging as the future standard for vulvar cancer staging and is described in Chapter 31 (p. 686).

PREOPERATIVE

Patient Evaluation

Clinical palpation is not an accurate means of evaluating the groin nodes (Homesley, 1993). MR imaging and PET scanning are also relatively insensitive (Bipat, 2006; Cohn, 2002; Gaarenstroom, 2003). Fixed, large, clinically obvious groin metastases that appear unresectable are treated preoperatively with radiation before attempting removal.

Consent

Patients should understand the need for unilateral or bilateral groin dissection and its relationship to their cancer treatment. They should be prepared for a potentially several-week recovery in which postoperative complications are common and may include cellulitis, wound breakdown, chronic lymphedema, and lymphocyst formation. These events may develop within a few days, several months, or even years later. In contrast, intraoperative complications are less common, and hemorrhage from the femoral vessels is rarely encountered.

Patient Preparation

When both groins are dissected, a two-team approach is ideal to reduce operative time. Prophylactic antibiotics may be administered, but they have not been shown to prevent complications (Gould, 2001). VTE prophylaxis is also provided.

INTRAOPERATIVE

Surgical Steps

❶ **Anesthesia and Patient Positioning.** General or regional anesthesia may be used. Inguinal lymphadenectomy is performed prior to partial or complete radical vulvectomy. Legs are placed in booted support stirrups in low lithotomy position, are abducted approximately 30 degrees, and are flexed minimally at the hip to flatten the groin. Rotation of the thigh a few degrees outward will open the femoral triangle.

❷ **Skin Incision.** The groin is incised 2 cm below and parallel to the inguinal ligament starting 3 cm caudal and medial to the anterior superior iliac spine—aiming toward the adductor longus tendon (Fig. 46-27.1). The incision is 8 to 10 cm long and is taken through full skin thickness and 3 to 4 mm into the fat.

❸ **Developing the Upper Flap.** Adson forceps elevate and provide traction to the upper skin edge while a hemostat is opened underneath to begin cephalad dissection down through the subcutaneous fat and Scarpa fascia—aiming for a position in the midline of the incision and 3 cm above the inguinal ligament. Dissection proceeds downward until the glistening white aponeurosis of the external oblique muscle is identified. Adson forceps are then replaced with skin hooks to provide better traction.

A semicircle of fatty tissue is rolled inferiorly and laterally along the aponeurosis using electrosurgical dissection and intermittent blunt dissection. During dissection, the superficial circumflex iliac vessels are divided with a Harmonic scalpel or clamped and ligated. Additionally, superficial epigastric and superficial external pudendal vessels are divided as they are encountered (Fig. 38-29, p. 823). Dissection proceeds until the lower margin of the inguinal ligament is exposed (Fig. 46-27.2).

❹ **Developing the Lower Flap.** The posterior skin flap is now raised in a similar manner to the upper flap. Dissection progresses through the subcutaneous fat to the deep fascia of the thigh—aiming approximately 6 cm from the inguinal ligament toward the apex of the femoral triangle. As shown in Figure 46-27.1, the femoral triangle is bordered by the inguinal ligament superiorly, by the sartorius muscle laterally, and by the adductor longus muscle medially. Blunt finger dissection along the inner portion of the sartorius and adductor longus muscles aids development of the lower flap boundaries. The dissection progressively becomes deeper into the subcutaneous tissue of the thigh, but remains superficial to the fascia lata. The tissue exiting at the apex of the femoral triangle is divided. Dissection progresses toward the fossa ovalis in circumferential path (Fig. 38-29, p. 823). Node-bearing tissue is held on traction to aid its dissection. Venous tributaries are ligated as they are encountered.

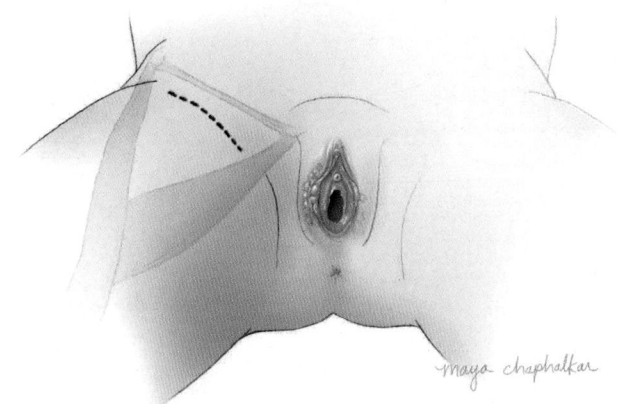

FIGURE 46-27.1 Incisions.

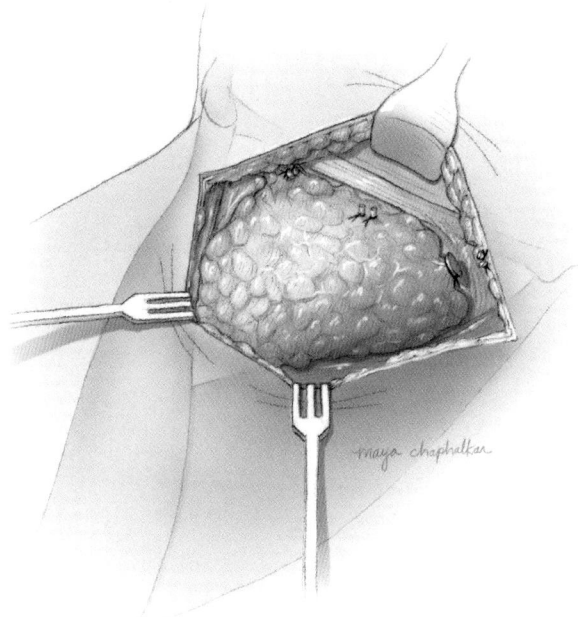

FIGURE 46-27.2 Dissection of the upper flap.

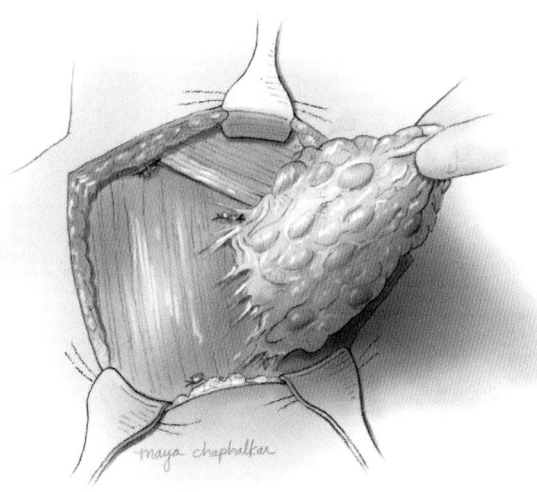

FIGURE 46-27.3 Dissection of the lower flap and removal of superficial nodes.

❺ **Removal of the Superficial Nodes.** The superficial lymph nodes lie within the fatty tissue just mobilized. The saphenous vein is encountered during the dissection of the medial side of the fat pad. The distal end this vein is individually transected and ligated with permanent suture for identification. If desired, saphenous vein transection can be avoided, and the vein can be salvaged by dissecting it from the fat pad. Circumferential dissection is next performed to isolate and remove the nodal bundle as it overlies the fossa ovalis (Fig. 46-27.3). The proximal end of the saphenous vein is separately ligated, unless the vessel has been preserved and can be dissected away from the nodal bundle. Remaining attachments are dissected from the cribriform fascia or clamped and cut to remove the specimen.

❻ **Removal of the Deep Nodes.** The femoral vein should be visible within the fossa ovalis. The deep groin nodes lie just medial and parallel to this vessel. Of these, Cloquet node is the uppermost. The residual deep femoral nodal tissue is excised by removing any fatty tissue along the anterior and medial surfaces of the femoral vein above the deep limit of the fossa ovalis. The femoral sheath and cribriform fascia remain intact if possible.

If a clinically positive deep node cannot otherwise be reached, the cribriform fascia may be unroofed by making a longitudinal incision distally along the overlying femoral sheath (Fig. 46-27.4). Seven or eight underlying deep inguinal nodes are revealed, and these deep nodes are typically located in

a more orderly fashion than the superficial nodes. Fatty-lymphoid tissue is then dissected from the anterior and medial surfaces of the femoral vein. Following node removal, the femoral sheath edges may then be reapproximated using 3–0 gauge delayed-absorbable suture and/or covered with the sartorius muscle.

❼ **Sartorius Muscle Transposition (Optional).** The fascia lata is incised to allow blunt dissection of the sartorius muscle (Fig. 46-27.5). The proximal sartorius muscle is then transected at its insertion to the anterior

superior iliac spine. A finger is wrapped around the upper part of the muscle to aid electrosurgical blade transection directly off the spine. Transection is as high as possible, with care taken to avoid the lateral femoral cutaneous nerve. The muscle is then further mobilized to cover the femoral vessels and sutured to the inguinal ligament with 2 0 gauge delayed-absorbable suture.

❽ **Wound Closure.** The surgical defect is carefully examined, made hemostatic, and irrigated. The groin is closed with layers of delayed-absorbable suture, and a

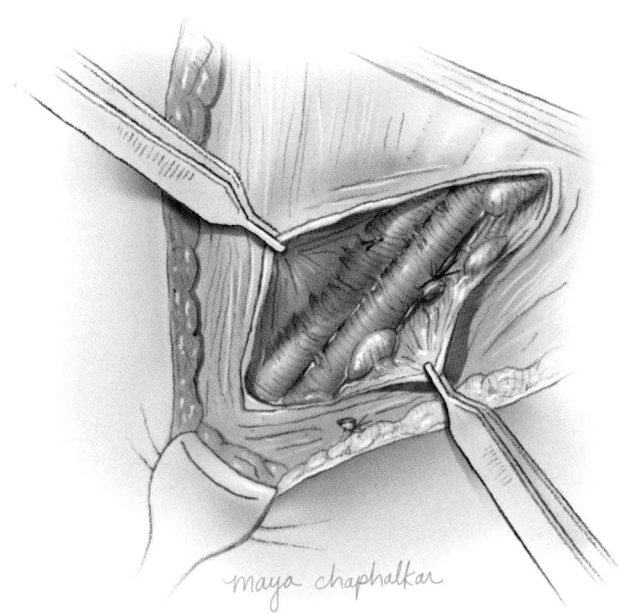

FIGURE 46-27.4 Unroofing the cribriform fascia to remove deep nodes.

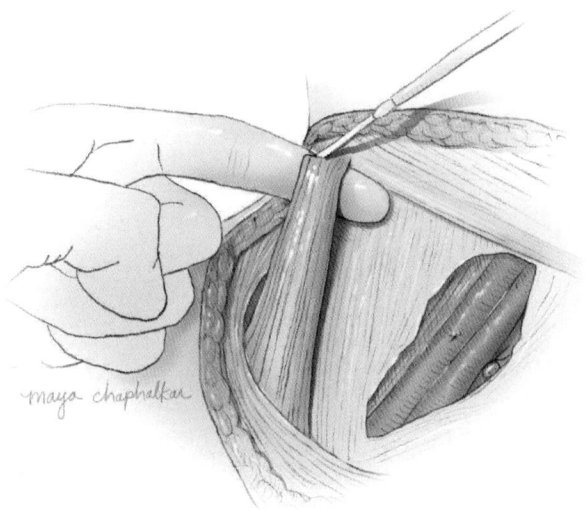
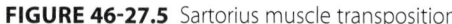

FIGURE 46-27.5 Sartorius muscle transposition.

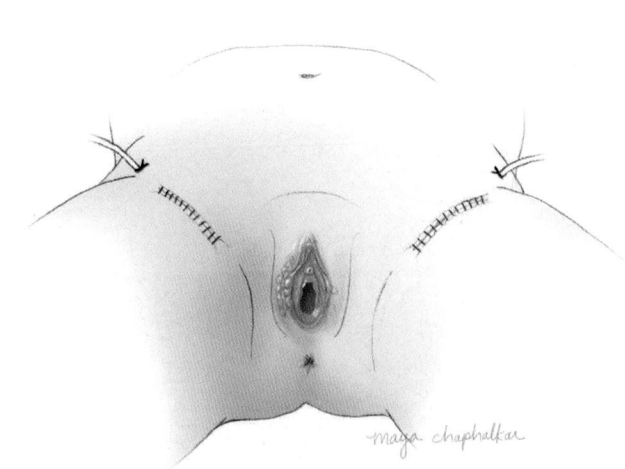

FIGURE 46-27.6 Wound closure.

Blake or Jackson-Pratt drain is brought out superolaterally and tied in place with permanent suture (Fig. 46-27.6). Staples are placed to reapproximate skin edges.

POSTOPERATIVE

Suction drainage enables the incision to heal and the underlying space to be obliterated. Drain tubing is manually milked or stripped three times daily with index finger and thumb toward the suction device to prevent blockage. Drains may be removed when output declines to 20 to 25 mL per day. Typically,

this requires approximately 2 weeks (Gould, 2001). Premature removal may result in a symptomatic lymphocyst that requires drain reinsertion or outpatient needle aspiration.

The groin incision remains uncovered and is regularly examined. Postoperative complications are common, particularly wound cellulitis and breakdown. Preoperative radiation and removal of bulky, fixed nodes increase the risk of these. Unroofing the deep fascia can also unnecessarily expose the femoral vessels to erosion or sudden hemorrhage. A protective sartorius muscle transposition may be especially indicated in these selected

situations to prevent morbidity (Judson, 2004; Paley, 1997).

Chronic lymphedema is another frequent complication of inguinal lymphadenectomy. In most reports, preservation of the saphenous vein has been shown to reduce the incidence (Dardarian, 2006; Gaarenstroom, 2003). Regardless, this condition is typically much more problematic with the addition of groin radiation. Supportive management is meant to minimize the edema and prevent symptomatic progression. Foot elevation, compression stockings, and, on occasion, diuretic therapy may be helpful.

Reconstructive Grafts and Flaps

Primary closure of a vulvar wound is typically not advised if closure of a large defect would create excessive incision tension or if other untoward factors are present. In these cases, a reconstructive skin graft or flap is preferable to a defect healing by secondary intent. In general, the simplest procedure that will achieve the best functional result should be selected.

The decision to perform a split-thickness skin graft (STSG), lateral skin transposition, or rhomboid skin flap depends on clinical circumstances and surgeon experience. Variations of these techniques are occasionally used in gynecologic oncology (Burke, 1994; Dainty, 2005; Saito, 2009). Typical candidates for a skin graft or flap have undergone a large wide local excision, skinning vulvectomy, or partial or complete radical vulvectomy. Myocutaneous flaps, most commonly using the rectus abdominis and gracilis muscles, are used primarily in patients with prior radiation, very large defects, or a need for vaginal reconstruction (Section 46-9, p. 1167). However, a full description of the innumerable types of local flaps is beyond the scope of this section.

PREOPERATIVE

Patient Evaluation

Fortunately, a broad range of operative procedures are available—each with their advantages and disadvantages (Weikel, 2005). The size of the lesion and the anticipated postsurgical defect will largely dictate reconstructive options. In some complicated cases, plastic surgery consultation may be indicated.

Consent

A woman's body image may be significantly altered following extensive vulvar surgery, and sexual dysfunction may be a problem (Green, 2000). When discussing these effects, patient responses vary widely. Some express minimal concern, whereas others are devastated by the thought of a disfiguring result. Accordingly, counseling is individualized, specifically addressing patient concerns.

In addition, wound separation, infection, and wound healing by secondary intention are common. Moreover, patients are advised that recurrences of their underlying disease may recur within the graft or flap (DiSaia, 1995).

Patient Preparation

Prophylactic antibiotics are typically given, and bowel preparation is generally influenced by surgeon preference. Early ambulation may be detrimental to graft or flap healing. Therefore, to prevent VTE, use of pneumatic compression devices or subcutaneous heparin is especially warranted (Table 39-8, p. 836).

For patients undergoing STSG, the hip, buttock, and inner thigh are carefully examined. The selected donor sites should contain healthy skin, should be hidden by a patient's clothing postoperatively, and must be accessible in the operating room. Typically, a graft is taken from the upper thigh.

INTRAOPERATIVE

Surgical Steps

❶ **Anesthesia and Patient Positioning.** General or regional anesthesia is required. The patient will need to be positioned in low lithotomy with complete access to the vulva, upper thighs, and mons pubis. Sterile preparation of the lower abdomen, perineum, thighs, and vagina is performed, and a Foley catheter is placed. Infrequently, the buttock or hip will be selected as the STSG donor site—this will require additional repositioning.

❷ **Evaluating the Surgical Defect.** After the vulvar resection has been completed and hemostasis is achieved, the wound is examined to confirm that primary closure is impossible (Fig. 46-28.1). The best graft or flap that will adequately cover a defect is determined.

❸ **Split-thickness Skin Graft (STSG).** A dermatome device is required to harvest the graft from the donor site when performing a STSG. At a setting of 18/1000ths to 22/1000ths, normal epithelium is harvested from the donor site (Fig. 43-25, p. 985). The STSG is placed in a basin and moistened with saline. The donor site is then sprayed with thrombin, covered with a transparent film dressing (Tegaderm), and wrapped firmly with gauze.

The recipient site is irrigated with antibiotic solution, and hemostasis must be absolute. The graft is then held over the defect and cut to fit so that there is some overlap. Meticulous care is required to smooth graft wrinkles and avoid graft tension. Edges are then sutured to the skin with interrupted 3–0 gauge nylon suture (Fig. 46-28.2). Moistened gauze or cotton balls are placed over the graft and covered with opened and fluffed gauze squares to provide light pressure. To create a stable dressing, a few ties are usually placed through the covering dressing and lateral to the graft site. Alternatively, fibrin tissue adhesives and/or vacuum-assisted closure devices

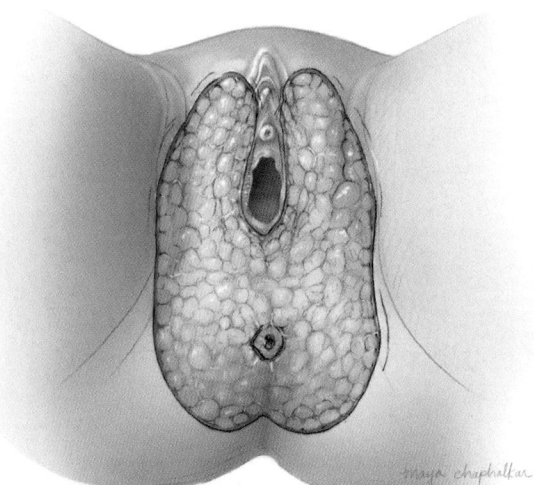

FIGURE 46-28.1 Large vulvar surgical defect.

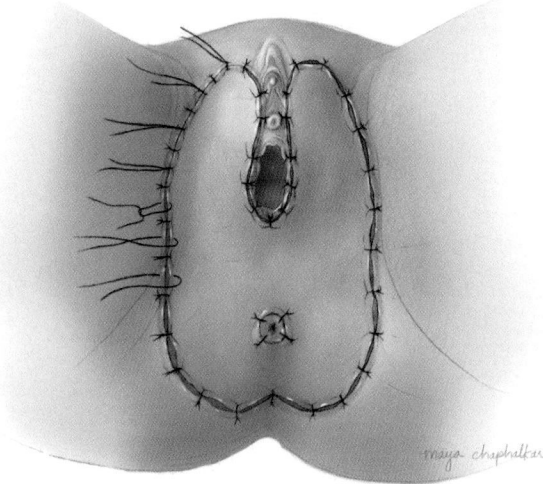

FIGURE 46-28.2 Split-thickness skin graft.

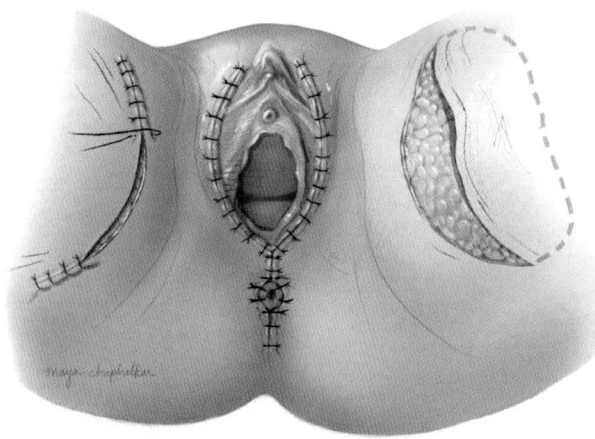

FIGURE 46-28.3 Lateral skin transposition.

may further augment graft adherence and viability (Dainty, 2005).

❹ **Lateral Skin Transposition.** In some cases, the skin lateral to the surgical defect is extensively undermined but still may not be able to cover a large defect and reach the medial skin margin. To perform a lateral skin transposition, a surgeon makes separate curvilinear relaxing upper thigh skin incisions bilaterally. As shown in Figure 46-28.3, the relaxing incisions are each undermined to the dotted line, which represents to lateral boarder of this dissection. The resulting mobility of the intervening vulvar skin bridge should allow for a tension-free primary closure using interrupted vertical mattress sutures. Last, the relaxing incisions are closed with interrupted 0-gauge delayed-absorbable suture.

❺ **Rhomboid Flaps.** A rhomboid is a four-sided parallelogram with unequal angles

at its corners. When creating a rhomboid flap from adjacent tissue, a marking pen is used to draw all sides the same length as the short axis of the defect (A-C; Fig. 46-28.4). This minimizes wound tension and prevents necrosis. The diagonal A-C is continued in a straight line onto the adjacent vulvar skin lateral to the defect, and marked so that the length of AC = CE. The remaining rhomboid sides are drawn in parallel.

Incisions are made through the skin and into the subcutaneous fat. A flap is developed to include underlying fatty tissue and is mobilized medially to cover the surgical defect. In repositioning the flap, (as shown by the arrow), line CE swings medially to appose line AB and is secured with stay sutures at the corners CA and EB. Flap edges are reapproximated with vertical mattress stitches using 0-gauge delayed-absorbable suture (Fig. 46-28.5). Typically, excess tissue folding at the corners requires significant trimming or

undermining to provide a reasonably smooth contour and is needed to aid closure of the remaining defects above and below the flap. Finally, a suction drain is placed at the donor site to prevent seromas caused by extensive tissue dissection and that could otherwise result in wound dehiscence.

POSTOPERATIVE

Patients are kept relatively immobile for the first 5 to 7 postoperative days to prevent tension on the reconstruction. Foley catheter drainage is also continued during these initial postoperative days. A low-residue diet, diphenoxylate hydrochloride (Lomotil), or loperamide hydrochloride (Imodium) tablets will aid healing by delaying defecation and preventing straining (Table 25-6, p. 570). Thromboembolic prophylaxis is continued until the patient is ambulatory.

During the first few days postoperatively, the wound is examined frequently to identify signs of hematoma or infection. For STSGs, the transparent dressing may be removed from the donor site after approximately 7 days, and an antibiotic ointment applied. For skin flaps, positioning changes or release of some sutures may be helpful if ischemia is noted at the margins. Suction drains are discontinued when output is less than 30 mL per 24 hours.

Women experience significant sexual dysfunction after vulvectomy. However, the extent of the surgery and need for reconstruction is less important than preexisting depression and hypoactive sexual dysfunction. Accordingly, postoperative psychologic counseling and treatment of depression may be particularly helpful (Green, 2000; Weijmar Schultz, 1990).

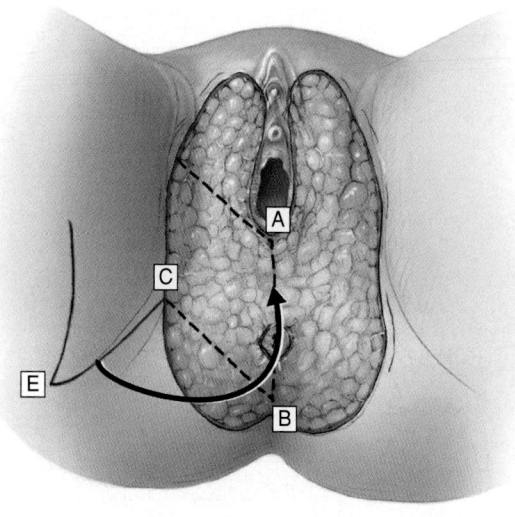

FIGURE 46-28.4 Rhomboid flap: flap positioning.

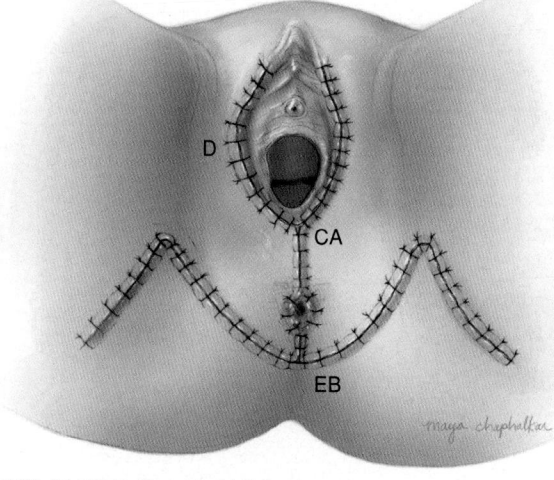

FIGURE 46-28.5 Rhomboid flap: closure.

REFERENCES

Aletti GD, Dowdy SC, Podratz KC, et al: Surgical treatment of diaphragm disease correlates with improved survival in optimally debulked advanced stage ovarian cancer. Gynecol Oncol 100:283, 2006a

Aletti GD, Podratz KC, Jones MB, et al: Role of rectosigmoidectomy and stripping of pelvic peritoneum in outcomes of patients with advanced ovarian cancer. J Am Coll Surg 203:521, 2006b

American College of Obstetricians and Gynecologists: Elective coincidental appendectomy. Committee Opinion No. 323, November 2005, Reaffirmed 2014

American College of Obstetricians and Gynecologists: Prevention of deep vein thrombosis and pulmonary embolism. Practice Bulletin No. 84, August 2007, Reaffirmed 2013

Angioli R, Estape R, Cantuaria G, et al: Urinary complications of Miami pouch: trend of conservative management. Am J Obstet Gynecol 179:343, 1998

Angioli R, Estape R, Salom E, et al: Radical hysterectomy for cervical cancer: hysterectomy before pelvic lymphadenectomy or vice versa? Int J Gynecol Cancer 9:307, 1999

Ayhan A, Gultekin M, Taskiran C, et al: Routine appendectomy in epithelial ovarian carcinoma: is it necessary? Obstet Gynecol 105:719, 2005

Ayhan A, Tuncer ZS, Dogan L, et al: Skinning vulvectomy for the treatment of vulvar intraepithelial neoplasia 2–3: a study of 21 cases. Eur J Gynecol Oncol 19:508, 1998

Backes FJ, Billingsley CC, Martin DD, et al: Does intra-operative radiation at the time of pelvic exenteration improve survival for patients with recurrent, previously irradiated cervical, vaginal, or vulvar cancer? Gynecol Oncol 135(1):95, 2014

Bandy LC, Clarke-Pearson DL, Creasman WT: Vitamin-B$_{12}$ deficiency following therapy in gynecologic oncology. Gynecol Oncol 17:370, 1984

Barnhill D, Doering D, Remmenga S, et al: Intestinal surgery performed on gynecologic cancer patients. Gynecol Oncol 40:38, 1991

Bashir S, Gerardi MA, Giuntoli RL 2nd, et al: Surgical technique of diaphragm full-thickness resection and trans-diaphragmatic decompression of pneumothorax during cytoreductive surgery for ovarian cancer. Gynecol Oncol 119:255, 2010

Bell JG, Lea JS, Reid GC: Complete groin lymphadenectomy with preservation of the fascia lata in the treatment of vulvar carcinoma. Gynecol Oncol 77:314, 2000

Benezra V, Lambrou NC, Salom EM, et al: Conversion of an incontinent urinary conduit to a continent urinary reservoir (Miami pouch). Gynecol Oncol 94:814, 2004

Benn T, Brooks RA, Zhang Q, et al: Pelvic exenteration in gynecologic oncology: a single institution study over 20 years. Gynecol Oncol 122(1):14, 2011

Berek JS, Howe C, Lagasse LD, et al: Pelvic exenteration for recurrent gynecologic malignancy: survival and morbidity analysis of the 45-year experience at UCLA. Gynecol Oncol 99:153, 2005

Bipat S, Fransen GA, Spijkerboer AM, et al: Is there a role for magnetic resonance imaging in the evaluation of inguinal lymph node metastases in patients with vulva carcinoma? Gynecol Oncol 103(3):1001, 2006

Boruta DM 2nd, Gehrig PA, Fader AN, et al: Management of women with uterine papillary serous cancer: a Society of Gynecologic Oncology (SGO) review. Gynecol Oncol 115:142, 2009

Bouma J, Dankert J: Infection after radical abdominal hysterectomy and pelvic lymphadenectomy: prevention of infection with a two-dose peri-operative antibiotic prophylaxis. Int J Gynaecol Cancer 3:94, 1993

Bowling CB, Lipscomb GH: Torsion of the appendix mimicking ovarian torsion. Obstet Gynecol 107:466, 2006

Bristow RE, del Carmen MG, Kaufman HS, et al: Radical oophorectomy with primary stapled colorectal anastomosis for resection of locally advanced epithelial ovarian cancer. J Am Coll Surg 197:565, 2003

Buekers TE, Anderson B, Sorosky JI, et al: Ovarian function after surgical treatment for cervical cancer. Gynecol Oncol 80:85, 2001

Burke TW, Levenback C, Coleman RL, et al: Surgical therapy of T1 and T2 vulvar carcinoma: further experience with radical wide excision and selective inguinal lymphadenectomy. Gynecol Oncol 57:215, 1995

Burke TW, Levenback C, Tornos C, et al: Intraabdominal lymphatic mapping to direct selective pelvic and paraaortic lymphadenectomy in women with high-risk endometrial cancer: results of a pilot study. Gynecol Oncol 62:169, 1996

Burke TW, Morris M, Levenback C, et al: Closure of complex vulvar defects using local rhomboid flaps. Obstet Gynecol 84:1043, 1994

Butler-Manuel SA, Summerville K, Ford A, et al: Self-assessment of morbidity following radical hysterectomy for cervical cancer. J Obstet Gynaecol 19:180, 1999

Cai HB, Chen HZ, Zhou YF, et al: Class II radical hysterectomy in low-risk IB squamous cell carcinoma of cervix: a safe and effective option. Int J Gynecol Cancer 19:46, 2009

Cain JM, Diamond A, Tamimi HK, et al: The morbidity and benefits of concurrent gracilis myocutaneous graft with pelvic exenteration. Obstet Gynecol 74:185, 1989

Cardosi RJ, Cox CS, Hoffman MS: Postoperative neuropathies after major pelvic surgery. Obstet Gynecol 100:240, 2002

Centers for Disease Control and Prevention: Vitamin B$_{12}$: dietary supplement fact sheet. 2011. Available at: http://ods.od.nih.gov/factsheets/VitaminB12-HealthProfessional/#h5. Accessed March 7, 2015

Chamberlain DH, Hopkins MP, Roberts JA, et al: The effects of early removal of indwelling urinary catheter after radical hysterectomy. Gynecol Oncol 43:98, 1991

Chan JK, Sugiyama V, Pham H, et al: Margin distance and other clinico-pathologic prognostic factors in vulvar carcinoma: a multivariate analysis. Gynecol Oncol 104:636, 2007

Chan JK, Sugiyama V, Tajalli TR, et al: Conservative clitoral preservation surgery in the treatment of vulvar squamous cell carcinoma. Gynecol Oncol 95:152, 2004

Charoenkwan K, Kietpeerakool C: Retroperitoneal drainage versus no drainage after pelvic lymphadenectomy for the prevention of lymphocyst formation in patients with gynaecological malignancies. Cochrane Database Syst Rev 1:CD007387, 2014

Chen GD, Lin LY, Wang PH, et al: Urinary tract dysfunction after radical hysterectomy for cervical cancer. Gynecol Oncol 85:292, 2002

Chereau E, Rouzier R, Gouy S, et al: Morbidity of diaphragmatic surgery for advanced ovarian cancer: retrospective study of 148 cases. Eur J Surg Oncol 37(2):175, 2011

Chi DS, Abu-Rustum NR, Sonoda Y, et al: Laparoscopic and hand-assisted laparoscopic splenectomy for recurrent and persistent ovarian cancer. Gynecol Oncol 101:224, 2006

Chi DS, Abu-Rustum NR, Sonoda Y, et al: Ten-year experience with laparoscopy on a gynecologic oncology service: analysis of risk factors for complications and conversion to laparotomy. Am J Obstet Gynecol 191:1138, 2004

Chi DS, Zivanovic O, Levinson KL, et al: The incidence of major complications after the performance of extensive upper abdominal surgical procedures during primary cytoreduction of advanced ovarian, tubal, and peritoneal carcinomas. Gynecol Oncol 119:38, 2010

Chou HH, Chang TC, Yen TC, et al: Low value of [^{18}F]-fluoro-2-deoxy-D-glucose positron emission tomography in primary staging of early-stage cervical cancer before radical hysterectomy. J Clin Oncol 24:123, 2006

Chung HH, Kim SK, Kim TH, et al: Clinical impact of FDG-PET imaging in post-therapy surveillance of uterine cervical cancer: from diagnosis to prognosis. Gynecol Oncol 103(1):165, 2006

Cibula D, Abu-Rustum NR: Pelvic lymphadenectomy in cervical cancer—surgical anatomy and proposal for a new classification system. Gynecol Oncol 116:33, 2010

Clayton RD, Obermair A, Hammond IG, et al: The Western Australian experience of the use of en bloc resection of ovarian cancer with concomitant rectosigmoid colectomy. Gynecol Oncol 84:53, 2002

Cliby W, Dowdy S, Feitoza SS, et al: Diaphragm resection for ovarian cancer: technique and short-term complications. Gynecol Oncol 94:655, 2004

Cohn DE, Dehdashti F, Gibb RK, et al: Prospective evaluation of positron emission tomography for the detection of groin node metastases from vulvar cancer. Gynecol Oncol 85:179, 2002

Cohn DE, Swisher EM, Herzog TJ, et al: Radical hysterectomy for cervical cancer in obese women. Obstet Gynecol 96:727, 2000

Coleman RL, Keeney ED, Freedman RS, et al: Radical hysterectomy for recurrent carcinoma of the uterine cervix after radiotherapy. Gynecol Oncol 55:29, 1994

Cosin JA, Fowler JM, Chen MD, et al: Pretreatment surgical staging of patients with cervical carcinoma: the case for lymph node debulking. Cancer 82:2241, 1998

Curtin JP, Rubin SC, Jones WB, et al: Paget's disease of the vulva. Gynecol Oncol 39:374, 1990

Dainty LA, Bosco JJ, McBroom JW, et al: Novel techniques to improve split-thickness skin graft viability during vulvo-vaginal reconstruction. Gynecol Oncol 97:949, 2005

Dardarian TS, Gray HJ, Morgan MA, et al: Saphenous vein sparing during inguinal lymphadenectomy to reduce morbidity in patients with vulvar carcinoma. Gynecol Oncol 101:140, 2006

de Mooij Y, Burger MP, Schilthuis MS, et al: Partial urethral resection in the surgical treatment of vulvar cancer does not have a significant impact on urinary incontinence. A confirmation of an authority-based opinion. Int J Gynecol Cancer 17:294, 2007

Desimone CP, Van Ness JS, Cooper AL, et al: The treatment of lateral T1 and T2 squamous cell carcinomas of the vulva confined to the labium majus or minus. Gynecol Oncol 104(2):390, 2007

Dietrich CS III, Desimone CP, Modesitt SC, et al: Primary appendiceal cancer: gynecologic manifestations and treatment options. Gynecol Oncol 104:602, 2007

DiSaia PJ, Dorion GE, Cappuccini F, et al: A report of two cases of recurrent Paget's disease of the vulva in a split-thickness graft and its possible pathogenesis-labeled "retrodissemination." Gynecol Oncol 57:109, 1995

Dowdy SC, Loewen RT, Aletti G, et al: Assessment of outcomes and morbidity following diaphragmatic peritonectomy for women with ovarian carcinoma. Gynecol Oncol 109:303, 2008

Eisenhauer EL, Abu-Rustum NR, Sonoda Y, et al: The addition of extensive upper abdominal surgery to achieve optimal cytoreduction improves survival in patients with stages III-IV epithelial ovarian cancer. Gynecol Oncol 103(3):1083, 2006

Eisenkop SM, Spirtos NM, Lin WC: Splenectomy in the context of primary cytoreductive operations for advanced epithelial ovarian cancer. Gynecol Oncol 100:344, 2006

Eisenkop SM, Spirtos NM, Lin WM, et al: Laparoscopic modified radical hysterectomy: a strategy for a clinical dilemma. Gynecol Oncol 96:484, 2005

Estape R, Lambrou N, Diaz R, et al: A case matched analysis of robotic radical hysterectomy with lymphadenectomy compared with laparoscopy and laparotomy. Gynecol Oncol 113:357, 2009

Fagotti A, Fanfani F, Ercoli A, et al: Minilaparotomy for type II and III radical hysterectomy: technique, feasibility, and complications. Int J Gynaecol Cancer 14:852, 2004

Fanning J, Kesterson J, Davies M, et al: Effects of electrosurgery and vaginal closure technique on postoperative vaginal cuff dehiscence. JSLS 17(3):414, 2013

Fayez JA, Toy NJ, Flanagan TM: The appendix as the cause of chronic lower abdominal pain. Am J Obstet Gynecol 172:122, 1995

Fedele L, Bianchi S, Zanconato G, et al: Tailoring radicality in demolitive surgery for deeply infiltrating endometriosis. Am J Obstet Gynecol 193:114, 2005

Fishman DA, Chambers SK, Schwartz PE, et al: Extramammary Paget's disease of the vulva. Gynecol Oncol 56:266, 1995

Foley OW, Rauh-Hain JA, Clark RM, et al: Intraoperative radiation therapy in the management of gynecologic malignancies. Am J Clin Oncol March 28, 2014 [Epub ahead of print] [KL1]

Fotopoulou C, Neumann U, Kraetschell R, et al: Long-term clinical outcome of pelvic exenteration in patients with advanced gynecological malignancies. J Surg Oncol 101:507, 2010

Fowler JM: Incorporating pelvic/vaginal reconstruction into radical pelvic surgery. Gynecol Oncol 115:154, 2009

Franchi M, Trimbos JB, Zanaboni F, et al: Randomised trial of drains versus no drains following radical hysterectomy and pelvic lymph node dissection: a European Organisation for Research and Treatment of Cancer–Gynaecological Cancer Group (EORTC-GCG) study of 234 patients. Eur J Cancer 43:1265, 2007

Frumovitz M, Sun CC, Schover LR, et al: Quality of life and sexual functioning in cervical cancer survivors. J Clin Oncol 23:7428, 2005

Fujita K, Nagano T, Suzuki A, et al: Incidence of postoperative ileus after paraaortic lymph node dissection in patients with malignant gynecologic tumors. Int J Clin Oncol 10:187, 2005

Fujiwara K, Kigawa J, Hasegawa K, et al: Effect of simple omentoplasty and omentopexy in the prevention of complications after pelvic lymphadenectomy. Int J Gynaecol Cancer 13:61, 2003

Gaarenstroom KN, Kenter GG, Trimbos JB, et al: Postoperative complications after vulvectomy and inguinofemoral lymphadenectomy using separate groin incisions. Int J Gynaecol Cancer 13:522, 2003

Gillette-Cloven N, Burger RA, Monk BJ, et al: Bowel resection at the time of primary cytoreduction for epithelial ovarian cancer. J Am Coll Surg 193:626, 2001

Gleeson N, Baile W, Roberts WS, et al: Surgical and psychosexual outcome following vaginal reconstruction with pelvic exenteration. Eur J Gynaecol Oncol 15:89, 1994a

Gleeson NC, Baile W, Roberts WS, et al: Pudendal thigh fasciocutaneous flaps for vaginal reconstruction in gynecologic oncology. Gynecol Oncol 54:269, 1994b

Gleeson NC, Hoffman MS, Cavanagh D: Isolated skin bridge metastasis following modified radical vulvectomy and bilateral inguinofemoral lymphadenectomy. Int J Gynaecol Cancer 4(5):356, 1994c

Goff BA, Matthews BJ, Wynn M, et al: Ovarian cancer: patterns of surgical care across the United States. Gynecol Oncol 103(2):383, 2006

Goldberg GL, Sukumvanich P, Einstein MH, et al: Total pelvic exenteration: the Albert Einstein College of Medicine/Montefiore Medical Center experience (1987–2003). Gynecol Oncol 101: 261, 2006

Goldberg JM, Piver MS, Hempling RE, et al: Improvements in pelvic exenteration: factors responsible for reducing morbidity and mortality. Ann Surg Oncol 5:399, 1998

Gonzalez Bosquet J, Magrina JF, Magtibay PM, et al: Patterns of inguinal groin metastases in squamous cell carcinoma of the vulva. Gynecol Oncol 105(3):742, 2007

Gould N, Kamelle S, Tillmanns T, et al: Predictors of complications after inguinal lymphadenectomy. Gynecol Oncol 82:329, 2001

Green MS, Naumann RW, Elliot M, et al: Sexual dysfunction following vulvectomy. Gynecol Oncol 77:73, 2000

Guenaga KK, Matos D, Wille-Jorgensen P: Mechanical bowel preparation for elective colorectal surgery. Cochrane Database Syst Rev 1:CD001544, 2009

Guimarães GC, Baiocchi G, Ferreira FO, et al: Palliative pelvic exenteration for patients with gynecological malignancies. Arch Gynecol Obstet 283(5):1107, 2011

Hallbook O, Matthiessen P, Leinskold T, et al: Safety of the temporary loop ileostomy. Colorectal Dis 4:361, 2002

Havrilesky LJ, Cragun JM, Calingaert B, et al: Resection of lymph node metastases influences survival in stage IIIC endometrial cancer. Gynecol Oncol 99:689, 2005

Hawighorst-Knapstein S, Schonefussrs G, Hoffmann SO, et al: Pelvic exenteration: effects of surgery on quality of life and body image—a prospective longitudinal study. Gynecol Oncol 66:495, 1997

Hazewinkel MH, Sprangers MA, van der Velden J, et al: Long-term cervical cancer survivors suffer from pelvic floor symptoms: a cross-sectional matched cohort study. Gynecol Oncol 117:281, 2010

Helm CW, Hatch K, Austin JM, et al: A matched comparison of single and triple incision techniques for the surgical treatment of carcinoma of the vulva. Gynecol Oncol 46:150, 1992

Hertel H, Diebolder H, Herrmann J, et al: Is the decision for colorectal resection justified by histopathologic findings: a prospective study of 100 patients with advanced ovarian cancer. Gynecol Oncol 83:481, 2001

Hockel M, Dornhofer N: Vulvovaginal reconstruction for neoplastic disease. Lancet Oncol 9:559, 2008

Hoffman MS, Barton DP, Gates J, et al: Complications of colostomy performed on gynecologic cancer patients. Gynecol Oncol 44:231, 1992

Hoffman MS, Griffin D, Tebes S, et al: Sites of bowel resected to achieve optimal ovarian cancer cytoreduction: implications regarding surgical management. Am J Obstet Gynecol 193:582, 2005

Homesley HD, Bundy BN, Sedlis A, et al: Assessment of current International Federation of Gynecology and Obstetrics staging of vulvar carcinoma relative to prognostic factors for survival (a Gynecologic Oncology Group study). Am J Obstet Gynecol 164:997, 1991

Homesley HD, Bundy BN, Sedlis A, et al: Prognostic factors for groin node metastasis in squamous cell carcinoma of the vulva (a Gynecologic Oncology Group study). Gynecol Oncol 49:279, 1993

Hopkins MP, Reid GC, Morley GW: Radical vulvectomy: the decision for the incision. Cancer 72:799, 1993

Houvenaeghel G, Moutardier V, Karsenty G, et al: Major complications of urinary diversion after pelvic exenteration for gynecologic malignancies: a 23-year mono-institutional experience in 124 patients. Gynecol Oncol 92:680, 2004

Hu T, Wu L, Xing H, et al: Development of criteria for ovarian preservation in cervical cancer patients treated with radical surgery with or without neoadjuvant chemotherapy: a multicenter retrospective study and meta-analysis. Ann Surg Oncol 20(3):881, 2013

Huang M, Chadha M, Musa F, et al: Lymph nodes: is total number or station number a better predictor of lymph node metastasis in endometrial cancer? Gynecol Oncol 119:295, 2010

Husain A, Akhurst T, Larson S, et al: A prospective study of the accuracy of ^{18}Fluorodeoxyglucose positron emission tomography (^{18}FDG PET) in identifying sites of metastasis prior to pelvic exenteration. Gynecol Oncol 106:177, 2007

Janda M, Obermair A, Cella D, et al: Vulvar cancer patients' quality of life: a qualitative assessment. Int J Gynecol Cancer 14:875, 2004

Jandial DD, Soliman PT, Slomovitz BM, et al: Laparoscopic colostomy in gynecologic cancer. J Minim Invasive Gynecol 15:723, 2008

Jensen PT, Groenvold M, Klee MC, et al: Early-stage cervical carcinoma, radical hysterectomy, and sexual function: a longitudinal study. Cancer 100:97, 2004

Judson PL, Jonson AL, Paley PJ, et al: A prospective, randomized study analyzing sartorius transposition following inguinal-femoral lymphadenectomy. Gynecol Oncol 95:226, 2004

Jurado M, Bazan A, Alcazar JL, et al: Primary vaginal reconstruction at the time of pelvic exenteration for gynecologic cancer: morbidity revisited. Ann Surg Oncol 16:121, 2009

Jurado M, Bazan A, Elejabeitia J, et al: Primary vaginal and pelvic floor reconstruction at the time of pelvic exenteration: a study of morbidity. Gynecol Oncol 77:293, 2000

Karsenty G, Moutardier V, Lelong B, et al: Long-term follow-up of continent urinary diversion after pelvic exenteration for gynecologic malignancies. Gynecol Oncol 97:524, 2005

Kehoe SM, Eisenhauer EL, Abu-Rustum NR, et al: Incidence and management of pancreatic leaks after splenectomy with distal pancreatectomy performed during primary cytoreductive surgery for advanced ovarian, peritoneal and fallopian tube cancer. Gynecol Oncol 112:496, 2009

Kim DK, Bridges CB, Harriman HK, et al: Advisory Committee on Immunization Practices recommended immunization schedule for adults aged 19 years or older: United States, 2015. Ann Intern Med 162:214, 2015

King LA, Carson LF, Konstantinides N, et al: Outcome assessment of home parenteral nutrition in patients with gynecologic malignancies: what have we learned in a decade of experience? Gynecol Oncol 51:377, 1993

Kingham TP, Pachter HL: Colonic anastomotic leak: risk factors, diagnosis, and treatment. J Am Coll Surg 208:269, 2009

Koh WJ, Greer BE, Abu-Rustum NR, et al: Cervical cancer, version 2.2015. J Natl Compr Canc Netw 13(4):395, 2015

Koh WJ, Greer BE, Abu-Rustum NR, et al: Uterine neoplasms, version 1.2014. J Natl Compr Canc Netw 12(2):248, 2014

Kohler C, Tozzi R, Possover M, et al: Explorative laparoscopy prior to exenterative surgery. Gynecol Oncol 86:311, 2002

Kraus K, Fanning J: Prospective trial of early feeding and bowel stimulation after radical hysterectomy. Am J Obstet Gynecol 182:996, 2000

Kusiak JF, Rosenblum NG: Neovaginal reconstruction after exenteration using an omental flap and split-thickness skin graft. Plast Reconstr Surg 97:775, 1996

Lacey CG, Stern JL, Feigenbaum S, et al: Vaginal reconstruction after exenteration with use of gracilis myocutaneous flaps: the University of California, San Francisco, experience. Am J Obstet Gynecol 158:1278, 1988

Landoni F, Maneo A, Cormio G, et al: Class II versus class III radical hysterectomy in stage IBIIA cervical cancer: a prospective, randomized study. Gynecol Oncol 80:3, 2001

Landrum LM, Lanneau GS, Skaggs VJ, et al: Gynecologic Oncology Group risk groups for vulvar carcinoma: improvement in survival in the modern era. Gynecol Oncol 106:521, 2007

Larciprete G, Casalino B, Segatore MF, et al: Pelvic lymphadenectomy for cervical cancer: extraperitoneal versus laparoscopic approach. Eur J Obstet Gynaecol Reprod Biol 126:259, 2006

Law WL, Chu KW, Choi HK: Randomized clinical trial comparing loop ileostomy and loop transverse colostomy for faecal diversion following total mesorectal excision. Br J Surg 89:704, 2002

Leath CA III, Straughn JM Jr, Estes JM, et al: The impact of aborted radical hysterectomy in patients with cervical carcinoma. Gynecol Oncol 95:204, 2004

Lee CL, Wu KY, Huang KG, et al: Long-term survival outcomes of laparoscopically assisted radical hysterectomy in treating early-stage cervical cancer. Am J Obstet Gynecol 203(2):165.e1, 2010

Lee PK, Choi MS, Ahn ST, et al: Gluteal fold V-Y advancement flap for vulvar and vaginal reconstruction: a new flap. Plast Reconstr Surg 118:401, 2006

Leon-Casasola OA, Karabella D, Lema MJ: Bowel function recovery after radical hysterectomies: thoracic epidural bupivacaine-morphine versus intravenous patient-controlled analgesia with morphine: a pilot study. J Clin Anesth 8:87, 1996

Likic IS, Kadija S, Ladjevic NG, et al: Analysis of urologic complications after radical hysterectomy. Am J Obstet Gynecol 199:644.e1, 2008

Lin HH, Sheu BC, Lo MC, et al: Abnormal urodynamic findings after radical hysterectomy or pelvic irradiation for cervical cancer. Int J Gynaecol Obstet 63:169, 1998

Lin LY, Wu JH, Yang CW, et al: Impact of radical hysterectomy for cervical cancer on urody-

namic findings. Int Urogynaecol J Pelvic Floor Dysfunct 15:418, 2004

Maas CP, ter Kuile MM, Laan E, et al: Objective assessment of sexual arousal in women with a history of hysterectomy. BJOG 111:456, 2004

Maggioni A, Roviglione G, Landoni F, et al: Pelvic exenteration: ten-year experience at the European Institute of Oncology in Milan. Gynecol Oncol 114:64, 2009

Magrina JF, Stanhope CR, Weaver AL: Pelvic exenterations: supralevator, infralevator, and with vulvectomy. Gynecol Oncol 64:130, 1997

Magtibay PM, Adams PB, Silverman MB, et al: Splenectomy as part of cytoreductive surgery in ovarian cancer. Gynecol Oncol 102:369, 2006

Manahan KJ, Hudec J, Fanning J: Modified radical vulvectomy without lymphadenectomy under local anesthesia in medically compromised patients. Gynecol Oncol 67:166, 1997

Manci N, Bellati F, Muzii L, et al: Splenectomy during secondary cytoreduction for ovarian cancer disease recurrence: surgical and survival data. Ann Surg Oncol 13:1717, 2006

Mariani A, Dowdy SC, Cliby WA, et al: Prospective assessment of lymphatic dissemination in endometrial cancer: a paradigm shift in surgical staging. Gynecol Oncol 109:11, 2008

Marnitz S, Kohler C, Muller M, et al: Indications for primary and secondary exenterations in patients with cervical cancer. Gynecol Oncol 103:1023, 2006

Martinez A, Filleron T, Vitse L, et al: Laparoscopic pelvic exenteration for gynaecological malignancy: is there any advantage? Gynecol Oncol 120(3):374, 2011

Martino MA, Borges E, Williamson E, et al: Pulmonary embolism after major abdominal surgery in gynecologic oncology. Obstet Gynecol 107:666, 2006

Matthiessen P, Hallbook O, Andersson M, et al: Risk factors for anastomotic leakage after anterior resection of the rectum. Colorectal Dis 6:462, 2004

Merad F, Hay JM, Fingerhut A, et al: Is prophylactic pelvic drainage useful after elective rectal or anal anastomosis? A multicenter controlled randomized trial. Surgery 125:529, 1999

Miller B, Morris M, Rutledge F, et al: Aborted exenterative procedures in recurrent cervical cancer. Gynecol Oncol 50:94, 1993

Mirhashemi R, Averette HE, Estape R, et al: Low colorectal anastomosis after radical pelvic surgery: a risk factor analysis. Am J Obstet Gynecol 183:1375, 2000

Mirhashemi R, Averette HE, Lambrou N, et al: Vaginal reconstruction at the time of pelvic exenteration: a surgical and psychosexual analysis of techniques. Gynecol Oncol 87:39, 2002

Mirhashemi R, Lambrou N, Hus N, et al: The gastrointestinal complications of the Miami pouch: a review of 77 cases. Gynecol Oncol 92:220, 2004

Morice P, Joulie F, Camatte S, et al: Lymph node involvement in epithelial ovarian cancer: analysis of 276 pelvic and paraaortic lymphadenectomies and surgical implications. J Am Coll Surg 197:198, 2003

Morice P, Lassau N, Pautier P, et al: Retroperitoneal drainage after complete para-aortic lymphadenectomy for gynecologic cancer: a randomized trial. Obstet Gynecol 97:243, 2001

Mourton SM, Temple LK, Abu-Rustum NR, et al: Morbidity of rectosigmoid resection and primary anastomosis in patients undergoing primary cytoreductive surgery for advanced epithelial ovarian cancer. Gynecol Oncol 99:608, 2005

Naik R, Jackson KS, Lopes A, et al: Laparoscopic assisted radical vaginal hysterectomy versus radical abdominal hysterectomy—a randomized phase II trial: perioperative outcomes and surgicopathological measurements. BJOG 117:746, 2010

Naik R, Maughan K, Nordin A, et al: A prospective, randomised, controlled trial of intermittent self-catheterisation vs supra-pubic catheterisation for post-operative bladder care following radical hysterectomy. Gynecol Oncol 99:437, 2005

Negishi H, Takeda M, Fujimoto T, et al: Lymphatic mapping and sentinel node identification as related to the primary sites of lymph node metastasis in early stage ovarian cancer. Gynecol Oncol 94:161, 2004

Nick AM, Lange J, Frumovitz M, et al: Rate of vaginal cuff separation following laparoscopic or robotic hysterectomy. Gynecol Oncol 120(1):47, 2011

Nunoo-Mensah JW, Chatterjee A, Khanwalkar D, et al: Loop ileostomy: modification of technique. Surgeon 2:287, 2004

Orr JW Jr, Orr PJ, Bolen DD, et al: Radical hysterectomy: does the type of incision matter? Am J Obstet Gynecol 173:399, 1995

Paley PJ, Johnson PR, Adcock LL, et al: The effect of sartorius transposition on wound morbidity following inguinal-femoral lymphadenectomy. Gynecol Oncol 64:237, 1997

Park JY, Kim DY, Kim JH, et al: Laparoscopic compared with open radical hysterectomy in obese women with early-stage cervical cancer. Obstet Gynecol 119(6):1201, 2012

Park JY, Seo SS, Kang S, et al: The benefits of low anterior en bloc resection as part of cytoreductive surgery for advanced primary and recurrent epithelial ovarian cancer patients outweigh morbidity concerns. Gynecol Oncol 103(3):977, 2006

Patsner B, Hackett TE: Use of the omental J-flap for prevention of postoperative complications following radical abdominal hysterectomy: report of 140 cases and literature review. Gynecol Oncol 65:405, 1997

Pellegrino A, Fruscio R, Maneo A, et al: Harmonic scalpel versus conventional electrosurgery in the treatment of vulvar cancer. Int J Gynaecol Obstet 103:185, 2008

Penalver MA, Angioli R, Mirhashemi R, et al: Management of early and late complications of ileocolonic continent urinary reservoir (Miami pouch). Gynecol Oncol 69:185, 1998

Penalver MA, Bejany DE, Averette HE, et al: Continent urinary diversion in gynecologic oncology. Gynecol Oncol 34:274, 1989

Pikaart DP, Holloway RW, Ahmad S, et al: Clinical-pathologic and morbidity analyses of Types 2 and 3 abdominal radical hysterectomy for cervical cancer. Gynecol Oncol 107:205, 2007

Plante M, Roy M: Operative laparoscopy prior to a pelvic exenteration in patients with recurrent cervical cancer. Gynecol Oncol 69:94, 1998

Prayson RA, Hart WR, Petras RE: Pseudomyxoma peritonei: a clinicopathologic study of 19 cases with emphasis on site of origin and nature of associated ovarian tumors. Am J Surg Pathol 18:591, 1994

Puntambekar S, Kudchadkar RJ, Gurjar AM, et al: Laparoscopic pelvic exenteration for advanced pelvic cancers: a review of 16 cases. Gynecol Oncol 102(3):513, 2006

Pycha A, Comploj E, Martini T, et al: Comparison of complications in three incontinent urinary diversions. Eur Urol 54:825, 2008

Ramirez PT, Modesitt SC, Morris M, et al: Functional outcomes and complications of continent urinary diversions in patients with gynecologic malignancies. Gynecol Oncol 85:285, 2002

Rasmussen OO, Petersen IK, Christiansen J: Anorectal function following low anterior resection. Colorectal Dis 5:258, 2003

Raspagliesi F, Ditto A, Fontanelli R, et al: Type II versus type III nerve-sparing radical hysterectomy: comparison of lower urinary tract dysfunctions. Gynecol Oncol 102(2):256, 2006

Ratliff CR, Gershenson DM, Morris M, et al: Sexual adjustment of patients undergoing gracilis myocutaneous flap vaginal reconstruction in conjunction with pelvic exenteration. Cancer 78:2229, 1996

Rettenmaier MA, Braly PS, Roberts WS, et al: Treatment of cutaneous vulvar lesions with skinning vulvectomy. J Reprod Med 30:478, 1985

Rezk YA, Hurley KE, Carter J, et al: A prospective study of quality of life in patients undergoing pelvic exenteration: interim results. Gynecol Oncol 128(2):191, 2013

Richardson DL, Mariani A, Cliby WA: Risk factors for anastomotic leak after recto-sigmoid resection for ovarian cancer. Gynecol Oncol 103(2):667, 2006

Rose PG: Skin bridge recurrences in vulvar cancer: frequency and management. Int J Gynaecol Cancer 9:508, 1999

Rose PG: Type II radical hysterectomy: evaluating its role in cervical cancer. Gynecol Oncol 80:1, 2001

Saito A, Sawaizumi M, Matsumoto S, et al: Stepladder V-Y advancement medial thigh flap for the reconstruction of vulvoperineal region. J Plast Reconstr Aesthet Surg 62:e196, 2009

Salani R, Zahurak ML, Santillan A, et al: Survival impact of multiple bowel resections in patients undergoing primary cytoreductive surgery for advanced ovarian cancer: a case-control study. Gynecol Oncol 107:495, 2007

Salom EM, Mendez LE, Schey D, et al: Continent ileocolonic urinary reservoir (Miami pouch): the University of Miami experience over 15 years. Am J Obstet Gynecol 190:994, 2004

Salom EM, Schey D, Penalver M, et al: The safety of incidental appendectomy at the time of abdominal hysterectomy. Am J Obstet Gynecol 189:1563, 2003

Scambia G, Ferrandina G, Distefano M, et al: Is there a place for a less extensive radical surgery in locally advanced cervical cancer patients? Gynecol Oncol 83:319, 2001

Scheistroen M, Nesland JM, Trope C: Have patients with early squamous carcinoma of the vulva been overtreated in the past? The Norwegian experience 1977–1991. Eur J Gynaecol Oncol 23:93, 2002

Segreti EM, Levenback C, Morris M, et al: A comparison of end and loop colostomy for fecal diversion in gynecologic patients with colonic fistulas. Gynecol Oncol 60:49, 1996a

Segreti EM, Morris M, Levenback C, et al: Transverse colon urinary diversion in gynecologic oncology. Gynecol Oncol 63:66, 1996b

Serati M, Salvatore S, Uccella S, et al: Sexual function after radical hysterectomy for early-stage cervical cancer: is there a difference between laparoscopy and laparotomy? J Sex Med 6:2516, 2009

Sevin BU, Ramos R, Gerhardt RT, et al: Comparative efficacy of short-term versus long-term cefoxitin prophylaxis against postoperative infection after radical hysterectomy: a prospective study. Obstet Gynecol 77:729, 1991

Sharma S, Odunsi K, Driscoll D, et al: Pelvic exenterations for gynecological malignancies: twenty-year experience at Roswell Park Cancer Institute. Int J Gynaecol Cancer 15:475, 2005

Shimada M, Kigawa J, Nishimura R, et al: Ovarian metastasis in carcinoma of the uterine cervix. Gynecol Oncol 101(6):234, 2006

Silver DF: Full-thickness diaphragmatic resection with simple and secure closure to accomplish complete cytoreductive surgery for patients with ovarian cancer. Gynecol Oncol 95:384, 2004

Slomovitz BM, Ramirez PT, Frumovitz M, et al: Electrothermal bipolar coagulation for pelvic exenterations. Gynecol Oncol 102:534, 2006

Smith HO, Genesen MC, Runowicz CD, et al: The rectus abdominis myocutaneous flap: modifications, complications, and sexual function. Cancer 83:510, 1998

Society of Gynecologic Oncology: SGO clinical practice statement: salpingectomy for ovarian cancer prevention. November 2013. Available at: https://www.sgo.org/clinical-practice/guidelines/sgo-clinical-practice-statement-salpingectomy-for-ovarian-cancer-prevention/. Accessed January 11, 2015

Soliman PT, Frumovitz M, Sun CC, et al: Radical hysterectomy: a comparison of surgical approaches after adoption of robotic surgery in gynecologic oncology. Gynecol Oncol 123(2):333, 2011

Song YJ, Lim MC, Kang S, et al: Total colectomy as part of primary cytoreductive surgery in advanced Mullerian cancer. Gynecol Oncol 114:183, 2009

Sood AK, Nygaard I, Shahin MS, et al: Anorectal dysfunction after surgical treatment for cervical cancer. J Am Coll Surg 195:513, 2002

Soper JT, Berchuck A, Creasman WT, et al: Pelvic exenteration: factors associated with major surgical morbidity. Gynecol Oncol 35:93, 1989

Soper JT, Havrilesky LJ, Secord AA, et al: Rectus abdominis myocutaneous flaps for neovaginal reconstruction after radical pelvic surgery. Int J Gynaecol Cancer 15:542, 2005

Soper JT, Rodriguez G, Berchuck A, et al: Long and short gracilis myocutaneous flaps for vulvovaginal reconstruction after radical pelvic surgery: comparison of flap-specific complications. Gynecol Oncol 56:271, 1995

Stefanidis K, Kontostolis S, Pappa L, et al: Endometriosis of the appendix with symptoms of acute appendicitis in pregnancy. Obstet Gynecol 93:850, 1999

Stehman FB, Bundy BN, Dvoretsky PM, et al: Early stage I carcinoma of the vulva treated with ipsilateral superficial inguinal lymphadenectomy and modified radical hemivulvectomy: a prospective study of the Gynecologic Oncology Group. Obstet Gynecol 79:490, 1992

Stentella P, Frega A, Cipriano L, et al: Prevention of thromboembolic complications in women undergoing gynecologic surgery. Clin Exp Obstet Gynecol 24:58, 1997

Swan RW: Stagnant loop syndrome resulting from small-bowel irradiation injury and intestinal bypass. Gynecol Oncol 2:441, 1974

Tantipalakorn C, Robertson G, Marsden DE, et al: Outcome and patterns of recurrence for

International Federation of Gynecology and Obstetrics (FIGO) stages I and II squamous cell vulvar cancer. Obstet Gynecol 113:895, 2009

Tebes SJ, Cardosi R, Hoffman MS: Colorectal resection in patients with ovarian and primary peritoneal carcinoma. Am J Obstet Gynecol 195:585, 2006

Todo Y, Yamamoto R, Minobe S, et al: Risk factors for postoperative lower-extremity lymphedema in endometrial cancer survivors who had treatment including lymphadenectomy. Gynecol Oncol 119:60, 2010

Tsai MS, Liang JT: Surgery is justified in patients with bowel obstruction due to radiation therapy. J Gastrointest Surg 10:575, 2006

Tsolakidis D, Amant F, Van Gorp T, et al: Diaphragmatic surgery during primary debulking in 89 patients with stage IIIB-IV epithelial ovarian cancer. Gynecol Oncol 116:489, 2010

Uccella S, Ghezzi F, Mariani A, et al: Vaginal cuff closure after minimally invasive hysterectomy: our experience and systematic review of the literature. Am J Obstet Gynecol 205(2):119.e1, 2011

Urbach DR, Reedijk M, Richard CS, et al: Bowel resection for intestinal endometriosis. Dis Colon Rectum 41:1158, 1998

Van der Zee AG, Oonk MH, De Hullu JA, et al: Sentinel node dissection is safe in the treatment of early-stage vulvar cancer. J Clin Oncol 26:884, 2008

Vasilev SA: Obturator nerve injury: a review of management options. Gynecol Oncol 53:152, 1994

Weijmar Schultz WC, van de Wiel HB, Bouma J, et al: Psychosexual functioning after the treatment of cancer of the vulva: a longitudinal study. Cancer 66:402, 1990

Weikel W, Hofmann M, Steiner E, et al: Reconstructive surgery following resection of primary vulvar cancers. Gynecol Oncol 99:92, 2005

Westin SN, Rallapalli V, Fellman B, et al: Overall survival after pelvic exenteration for gynecologic malignancy. Gynecol Oncol 134(3):546, 2014

Whitney CW: GOG Surgical Procedures Manual. Gynecologic Oncology Group, 2010. Available at: https://gogmember.gog.org/manuals/pdf/surgman.pdf. Accessed March 7, 2015

Whitney CW, Stehman FB: The abandoned radical hysterectomy: a Gynecologic Oncology Group study. Gynecol Oncol 79:350, 2000

Winter WE, McBroom JW, Carlson JW, et al: The utility of gastrojejunostomy in secondary cytoreduction and palliation of proximal intestinal obstruction in recurrent ovarian cancer. Gynecol Oncol 91:261, 2003

Wright JD, Herzog TJ, Neugut AI, et al: Comparative effectiveness of minimally invasive and abdominal radical hysterectomy for cervical cancer. Gynecol Oncol 127(1):11, 2012

Yan X, Li G, Shang H, et al: Twelve-year experience with laparoscopic radical hysterectomy and pelvic lymphadenectomy in cervical cancer. Gynecol Oncol 120(3):362, 2011

Yang YC, Chang CL: Modified radical hysterectomy for early Ib cervical cancer. Gynecol Oncol 74:241, 1999

Zhu QD, Zhang QY, Zeng QQ, et al: Efficacy of mechanical bowel preparation with polyethylene glycol in prevention of postoperative complications in elective colorectal surgery: a meta-analysis. Int J Colorectal Dis 25:267, 2010

INDEX